NORMAL HEART RATES FOR INFANTS AND CHILDREN

AGE	RATE (beats/minute) RESTING (AWAKE)	RESTING (SLEEPING)	EXERCISE (FEVER)
Newborn	100-180	80-160	Up to 220
1 week to 3 months	100-220	80-200	Up to 220
3 months to 2 years	80-150	70-120	Up to 200
2 years to 10 years	70-110	60-90	Up to 200
10 years to adult	55-90	50-90	Up to 200

From Gillette, P.C.: Dysrhythmias. In Adams, F.H., and Emmanouilides, G.C., editors: Moss' heart disease in infants, children, and adolescents, ed. 3, Baltimore, 1983, Williams & Wilkins.

NORMAL RESPIR

AGE	RATE (breaths/minute)
Newborn	35
1 to 11 months	30
2 years	25
4 years	23
6 years	21
8 years	20
10 years	19
12 years	19
14 years	18
16 years	17
18 years	16-18

NORMAL BLOOD PRESSURE READINGS FOR CHILDREN

BOYS

SYSTOLIC BLOOD PRESSURE PERCENTILE

AGE	5th	10th	50th	90th	95th
1 day	54	58	73	87	92
3 days	55	59	74	89	93
7 days	57	62	76	91	95
1 mo	67	71	86	101	105
2 mo	72	76	91	106	110
3 mo	72	76	91	106	110
4 mo	72	76	91	106	110
5 mo	72	76	91	105	110
6 mo	72	76	90	105	109
7 mo	71	76	90	105	109
8 mo	71	75	90	105	109
9 mo	71	75	90	105	109
10 mo	71	75	90	105	109
11 mo	71	76	90	105	109
1 yr	71	76	90	105	109
2 yr	72	76	91	106	110
3 yr	73	77	92	107	111
4 yr	74	79	93	108	112
5 yr	76	80	95	109	113
6 yr	77	81	96	111	115
7 yr	78	83	97	112	116
8 yr	80	84	99	114	118
9 yr	82	86	101	115	120
10 yr	84	88	102	117	121
11 yr	86	90	105	119	123
12 yr	88	92	107	121	126
13 yr	90	94	109	124	128
14 yr	93	97	112	126	131
15 yr	95	99	114	129	133
16 yr	98	102	117	131	136
17 yr	100	104	119	134	138
18 yr	102	106	121	136	140

DIASTOLIC BLOOD PRESSURE* PERCENTILE

AGE	5th	10th	50th	90th	95th
1 day	38	42	55	68	72
3 days	38	42	55	68	71
7 days	37	41	54	67	71
1 mo	35	39	52	64	68
2 mo	33	37	50	63	66
3 mo	33	37	50	63	66
4 mo	34	37	50	63	67
5 mo	35	39	52	65	68
6 mo	36	40	53	66	70
7 mo	37	41	54	67	71
8 mo	38	42	55	68	72
9 mo	39	43	55	68	72
10 mo	39	43	56	69	73
11 mo	39	43	56	69	73
1 yr	39	43	56	69	73
2 yr	39	43	56	68	72
3 yr	39	42	55	68	72
4 yr	39	43	56	69	72
5 yr	40	43	56	69	73
6 yr	41	44	57	70	74
7 yr	42	45	58	71	75
8 yr	43	47	60	73	76
9 yr	44	48	61	74	78
10 yr	45	49	62	75	79
11 yr	47	50	63	76	80
12 yr	48	51	64	77	81
13 yr	45	49	63	77	81
14 yr	46	50	64	78	82
15 yr	47	51	65	79	83
16 yr	49	53	67	81	85
17 yr	51	55	69	83	87
18 yr	52	56	70	84	88

Reprinted with permission from the Second Task Force on Blood Pressure Control in Children, National Heart, Lung and Blood Institute, Bethesda, MD. Tabular data prepared by Dr. B. Rosner, 1987.

*K4 was used for ages less than 13; K5 was used for ages 13 and over.

Nursing Care of Infants and Children

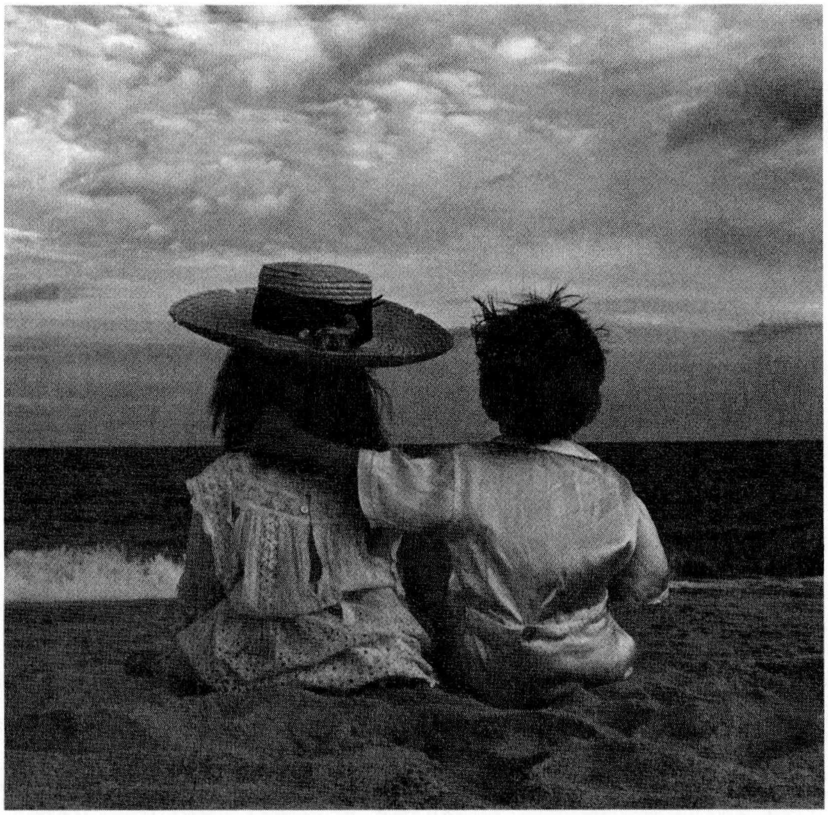

Nursing Care of Infants and Children

LUCILLE F. WHALEY, R.N., Ed.D.

Specialist, Parent-Child Nursing;
Professor Emeritus,
San Jose State University,
San Jose, California

DONNA L. WONG, R.N., Ph.D., P.N.P., C.P.N., F.A.A.N.

Nurse Consultant,
Saint Francis Hospital Children's Center,
Tulsa, Oklahoma;
Children's Medical Center of Dallas,
Dallas, Texas;
Adjunct Associate Professor,
Department of Pediatrics,
University of Oklahoma
College of Medicine—Tulsa,
Tulsa, Oklahoma

FOURTH EDITION

With 738 illustrations and 24 color plates

Mosby
Year Book

St. Louis Baltimore Boston Chicago London Philadelphia Sydney Toronto

Mosby Year Book

Dedicated to Publishing Excellence

SPONSORING EDITOR Linda L. Duncan
SENIOR DEVELOPMENTAL EDITOR Sally Adkisson
PROJECT MANAGER Patricia Gayle May
PRODUCTION EDITOR Judith Bange
MANUSCRIPT EDITORS Mary Cusick Drone and Roger McWilliams
LAYOUT ARTIST Kathleen L. Teal
DESIGNER Diane Beasley

COVER ART William Hunt: *Playing Field Hospital.* Courtesy of Coe Kerr Gallery, New York, N.Y. Private Collection.

FRONTISPIECE PHOTOGRAPH *Two Children.* Copyright 1987 by Betsy Cameron.

FOURTH EDITION

Printed in the United States of America

Mosby–Year Book, Inc.
11830 Westline Industrial Drive
St. Louis, Missouri 63146

Library of Congress Cataloging-in-Publication Data

Whaley, Lucille F.
Nursing care of infants and children / Lucille F. Whaley, Donna L. Wong.—4th ed.
p. cm.
Includes bibliographical references.
Includes index.
ISBN 0-8016-5378-9
1. Pediatric nursing. I. Wong, Donna L. II. Title.
[DNLM: 1. Pediatric Nursing. WY 159 W552n]
RJ245.W47 1991
610.73′62—dc20
DNLM/DLC 90-13695
for Library of Congress CIP

93 94 95 CL/VH 9 8 7 6 5 4 3

To Bert, Kathy, and Reen

LUCILLE F. WHALEY

To my husband, Ting,
for the love and support
that make it all possible

To my daughter, Nina,
whose commitment to her goals
is an inspiration to me

And to my father, Rudy,
for always being there
to help, no matter what the request

DONNA L. WONG

CONTRIBUTORS

Annette L. Baker, R.N., M.S.N.
Kawasaki Nurse Coordinator,
Cardiology Department,
The Children's Hospital,
Boston, Massachusetts

Dorothy C. Blome, R.N.,C., M.N.
Clinical Education Specialist,
Children's Medical Center of Dallas,
Dallas, Texas

Jeanne T. Boisvert, R.N., B.S.N.
Staff Nurse III,
The Children's Hospital,
Boston, Massachusetts

Marilyn Cox Borgersen, R.N., M.S.N., C.D.E.
Endocrine Clinical Nurse Specialist,
Children's Medical Center of Dallas,
Dallas, Texas

†Frederick W. Bozett, R.N., D.N.S.
Professor,
College of Nursing,
University of Oklahoma Health Sciences Center,
Oklahoma City, Oklahoma

Jeanette M. Broering, R.N., M.S., C.P.N.P.
Assistant Clinical Professor,
Departments of Family Health Care Nursing and Pediatrics,
Division of Adolescent Medicine,
University of California—San Francisco,
San Francisco, California

Marion E. Broome, R.N., Ph.D.
Associate Professor and Assistant Chairperson,
College of Nursing,
Maternal-Child Nursing,
Rush–Presbyterian–St. Luke's Medical Center,
Chicago, Illinois

Lydia DeSantis, R.N., Ph.D.
Associate Professor,
University of Miami,
School of Nursing,
Miami, Florida

Jeanne O'Connor Egan, R.N., M.S.N.
Pediatric Neurosurgery Clinical Specialist,
Children's Hospital National Medical Center,
Washington, D.C.

Joann Gephart, R.N., M.S.N.
Nurse Consultant,
Maternal and Child Health Bureau,
Department of Health and Human Services,
Rockville, Maryland

Ann Burns Gerraughty, R.N., M.S.
Critical Care Clinical Nurse Specialist,
Cardiac Intensive Care Unit,
The Children's Hospital,
Boston, Massachusetts

Caryn Stoermer Hess, R.N., M.S.
Nursing Consultant,
Englewood, Colorado

Elizabeth J. Heywood, R.N., M.S.N., P.N.P.
Nephrology Pediatric Nurse Practitioner,
Children's Hospital National Medical Center,
Washington, D.C.

Marilyn Hockenberry-Eaton, R.N., M.S.N., C.P.N.P.
Assistant Professor,
Graduate Pediatric Oncology Program,
Emory University School of Nursing,
Atlanta, Georgia

Elizabeth E. Hogue, J.D.
Elizabeth E. Hogue, Chartered,
Baltimore, Maryland

Christina Algiere Kasprisin, R.N., M.S.
Quality Attainment Coordinator,
Saint Francis Hospital;
Assistant Clinical Professor,
University of Oklahoma College of Nursing,
Tulsa, Oklahoma

Charmaine Kleiber, R.N., M.S., C.P.N.P.
Clinical Nurse Specialist,
Pediatric Nursing Division,
University of Iowa Hospital and Clinics,
Iowa City, Iowa

Lindyce A. Kulik, R.N., B.S.N.
Staff Nurse III,
Education Coordinator,
Cardiac Intensive Care Unit,
The Children's Hospital,
Boston, Massachusetts

Marilyn McCubbin, R.N., Ph.D.
Assistant Professor,
University of Wisconsin—Madison,
School of Nursing,
Madison, Wisconsin

Paula Moynihan, R.N., B.S.N.
Staff Nurse III,
Quality Assurance Coordinator,
Cardiovascular Intensive Care Unit,
The Children's Hospital,
Boston, Massachusetts

†Deceased.

Patricia O'Brien, R.N.,C., M.S.N., P.N.P.
Cardiovascular Clinical Nurse Specialist,
Departments of Cardiology and Cardiac Surgery,
The Children's Hospital,
Boston, Massachusetts

Patricia A. O'Hara, R.N., B.S.N.
Nurse Manager,
Cardiac Medical/Surgical Unit,
The Children's Hospital,
Boston, Massachusetts

Suzanne J. Reidy, R.N., B.S.N.
Staff Nurse III,
The Children's Hospital,
Boston, Massachusetts

Carole T. Roberts, R.N., M.S., P.N.P.
Cardiology Nurse Practitioner,
The Children's Hospital,
Boston, Massachusetts

Judy Holt Rollins, R.N., M.S.
Child Health Care Consultant,
National Consultant for Very Special Arts,
Washington, D.C.

Kathleen Rossman, R.R.T.
Special Projects Coordinator,
Eastern Oklahoma Perinatal Center,
Saint Francis Hospital,
Tulsa, Oklahoma

Patricia Rotondi, R.N., M.S.
Nurse Manager,
Cardiac Intensive Care Unit,
The Children's Hospital,
Boston, Massachusetts

Cindy Hylton Rushton, R.N.,C., M.S.N., F.A.A.N.
Clinical Educator III, Neonatal/Infant Specialist,
Children's National Medical Center;
Doctoral Student,
The Catholic University of America,
School of Nursing,
Washington, D.C.

Mercedes Sandaval, Ph.D.
Chairperson, Arts and Sciences Department,
Inter-American Center,
Miami-Dade Community College,
Miami, Florida

Donna Phillips Smith, R.N., M.S.
Pediatric Nurse Consultant,
Clinical Nurse I, Pediatrics,
Saint Francis Hospital;
Clinical Assistant Professor,
University of Oklahoma,
College of Nursing,
Tulsa, Oklahoma

Allison T. Weber, R.N., B.S.N.
Electrophysiology Nurse,
Cardiac Dysrhythmia Service,
The Children's Hospital,
Boston, Massachusetts

REVIEWERS

Jeanette Adams, R.N., M.S.N., Dr.P.H.
Assistant Professor,
The University of Texas Health Science Center,
School of Nursing,
Houston, Texas

Stephanie Allen, R.N., B.S.N.
Program Coordinator, Nursing Education,
Children's Medical Center of Dallas,
Dallas, Texas

Elizabeth Alseth, R.N., M.S.
Diabetes Clinical Nurse Specialist,
Children's Hospital of Wisconsin,
Milwaukee, Wisconsin

Catherine C. Ayoub, R.N., M.N., Ed.M.
Clinical Fellow in Psychology,
Clinical Nurse Consultant,
Judge Baker Children's Center,
Boston Children's Hospital,
Boston, Massachusetts

Connie Morain Baker, M.S.
Child Life Coordinator,
Children's Hospital of Oklahoma,
Oklahoma City, Oklahoma

Jane W. Ball, R.N., Dr.P.H.
EMS Education Coordinator,
Children's Hospital National Medical Center,
Washington, D.C.

Dorothy C. Blome, R.N.,C., M.N.
Clinical Education Specialist,
Children's Medical Center of Dallas,
Dallas, Texas

Marilyn Cox Borgersen, R.N., M.S.N., C.D.E.
Endocrine Clinical Nurse Specialist,
Children's Medical Center of Dallas,
Dallas, Texas

Cheryl Boyd, R.N., M.S.
Diabetes Nurse Educator,
Children's Medical Center,
Tulsa, Oklahoma

†Frederick W. Bozett, R.N., D.N.S.
Professor,
College of Nursing,
University of Oklahoma Health Sciences Center,
Oklahoma City, Oklahoma

Regina D. Bridwell, M.P.H.
Programs and Projects Specialist,
Arizona Department of Health Services,
Phoenix, Arizona

Wendy Royce Brittain, R.N.P., B.S.N.
Apnea and Sleep Disorders Specialty Nurse,
Arkansas Children's Hospital,
Little Rock, Arkansas

Jeanette M. Broering, R.N., M.S., C.P.N.P.
Assistant Clinical Professor,
Departments of Family Health Care Nursing and Pediatrics,
Division of Adolescent Medicine,
University of California—San Francisco,
San Francisco, California

Marion E. Broome, R.N., Ph.D.
Associate Professor and Assistant Chairperson,
College of Nursing,
Maternal-Child Nursing,
Rush–Presbyterian–St. Luke's Medical Center,
Chicago, Illinois

Jack A. Campbell
Certified Orthopedic Technician,
Eastern Oklahoma Orthopedic Center,
Tulsa, Oklahoma

Van G. Chauvin, R.N.,C., M.S., M.H.S.
Family Nurse Practitioner,
School Nurse Practitioner Program,
Dallas Independent School District,
Dallas, Texas

Lynn Clutter, R.N., M.S.N.
Child Health and Parenting Consultant,
Tulsa, Oklahoma

Kellie L. Cyrus, R.N., B.S.N.
Pediatric Endocrinology Clinical and Research Nurse,
Children's Medical Center,
Tulsa, Oklahoma

Juanita Conkin Dale, R.N., Ph.D., C.P.N.P.
Pediatric Nurse Practitioner/Research Liaison,
Department of Nursing Education and Research,
Children's Medical Center of Dallas,
Dallas, Texas

Mary Ann Davis, M.Ed.
Program Director,
Oklahoma Society to Prevent Blindness,
Oklahoma City, Oklahoma

†Deceased.

Patricia Dean, R.N., B.S.N.
Department of Nursing,
Miami Children's Hospital,
Miami, Florida

Judith P. Doll, M.S.
Associate Coordinator,
Automotive Safety for Children Program,
James Whitcomb Riley Hospital for Children,
Indianapolis, Indiana

Bonnie Uthoff Dolson, R.N., M.S.
Former Assistant Professor,
Houston Baptist University,
BSN Department of Nursing,
Houston, Texas

Candace C. Colombo Dye, R.N., M.S., N.N.P.
Clinical Nurse Specialist,
Assistant Clinical Professor, Pediatrics,
University of California—Irvine Medical Center,
Orange, California;
Assistant Clinical Professor,
School of Nursing,
University of California—Los Angeles,
Los Angeles, California

Martha E. Eddy, R.N., M.A., C.P.N.P.
Nurse Clinician,
Adjunct Clinical Instructor,
University of Iowa College of Nursing,
Iowa City, Iowa

Jeanne O'Connor Egan, R.N., M.S.N.
Pediatric Neurosurgery Clinical Specialist,
Children's Hospital National Medical Center,
Washington, D.C.

Suzanne L. Feetham, R.N., Ph.D., F.A.A.N.
Special Expert,
Office of Planning, Analysis, and Evaluation,
National Center for Nursing Research,
Bethesda, Maryland;
Senior Fellow Distinguished Scholar,
School of Nursing,
University of Pennsylvania,
Philadelphia, Pennsylvania

David Fournier, Ph.D.
Associate Professor,
Department of Family Relations and Child Development,
Oklahoma State University,
Stillwater, Oklahoma

William K. Frankenburg, M.D., M.S.P.H.
Pediatrics and Preventive Medicine Professor,
University of Colorado Health Sciences Center,
Denver, Colorado

Sandra L. Gardner, R.N., M.S., P.N.P.
Neonatal/Perinatal/Pediatric Consultant;
Director, Professional Outreach Consultation,
Denver, Colorado

Debra A. Gayer, R.N., M.S., C.P.N.P.
Pediatric Pulmonary Clinical Nurse Specialist,
University of Missouri Hospital and Clinics,
Columbia, Missouri

Barbara A. Hannah, R.N., M.S.
Director of Nursing,
Cleveland Area Hospital,
Cleveland, Oklahoma;
Chairman, BLS Affiliate Faculty Task Force,
American Heart Association—Oklahoma Affiliate,
BLS National Faculty,
American Heart Association

Janice S. Hayes, R.N., Ph.D.
Associate Dean for Academic Programs,
University of Miami School of Nursing;
Research Consultant,
Miami Children's Hospital,
Miami, Florida

Mary Henley, R.N.
Research Nurse and Clinical Coordinator,
Tulsa Cystic Fibrosis Center,
Oklahoma University College of Medicine,
Tulsa, Oklahoma

Caryn Stoermer Hess, R.N., M.S.
Nursing Consultant,
Englewood, Colorado

Elizabeth J. Heywood, R.N., M.S.N., P.N.P.
Nephrology Pediatric Nurse Practitioner,
Children's Hospital National Medical Center,
Washington, D.C.

Marilyn Hockenberry-Eaton, R.N., M.S.N., C.P.N.P.
Assistant Professor,
Graduate Pediatric Oncology Program,
Emory University School of Nursing,
Atlanta, Georgia

Elizabeth E. Hogue, J.D.
Elizabeth E. Hogue, Chartered,
Baltimore, Maryland

Joan L. Holihan, R.N., M.S.N., P.N.P.
Clinical Educator for the Critical Care Unit,
The Children's Hospital National Medical Center,
Washington, D.C.

Debra P. Hymovich, R.N., Ph.D., F.A.A.N.
Postdoctoral Fellow,
University of Pennsylvania,
School of Nursing,
Philadelphia, Pennsylvania

Marguerite M. Jackson, R.N., M.S., C.I.C.
Director, Epidemiology Unit,
University of San Diego Medical Center,
San Diego, California

Sandra L. Jacobs, R.N., C.P.N.
Apnea Nurse Clinician,
Children's Hospital, Inc.,
Columbus, Ohio

Judy Johnson-Russell, R.N., M.S.
Assistant Professor,
Texas Woman's University,
College of Nursing,
Dallas, Texas

Jacqueline C. Jones
Education Assistant,
Automotive Safety for Children Program,
James Whitcomb Riley Hospital for Children,
Indianapolis, Indiana

Christina Algiere Kasprisin, R.N., M.S.
Quality Attainment Coordinator,
Saint Francis Hospital;
Assistant Clinical Professor,
University of Oklahoma College of Nursing,
Tulsa, Oklahoma

Sylvia Kerr, R.N., M.S.
Associate Professor,
College of Nursing and Applied Health Sciences,
University of Tulsa,
Tulsa, Oklahoma

Charmaine Kleiber, R.N., M.S., C.P.N.P.
Clinical Nurse Specialist,
Pediatric Nursing Division,
University of Iowa Hospitals and Clinics,
Iowa City, Iowa

Bernice Kopel, Ed.D., R.D., L.D.
Associate Professor,
Food, Nutrition, and Institution Administration Department,
Oklahoma State University,
Stillwater, Oklahoma

Jean M. Koviach, R.N., B.S.N., C.P.N.P.
Clinic Coordinator/Nurse Clinician,
Pediatric Allergy/Pulmonary Clinic,
University of Iowa Hospitals and Clinics,
Iowa City, Iowa

John Kramer, M.D.
Tulsa Cystic Fibrosis Center,
Utica Square Medical Center,
Tulsa, Oklahoma

Edgar O. Ledbetter, M.D.
Director, Department of Maternal, Child, and Adolescent Medicine,
American Academy of Pediatrics,
Elk Grove Village, Illinois

Rosemary Liguori, R.N., M.S.N., C.P.N.A./P.
Assistant Professor,
Division of Nursing,
Northeastern State University,
Tahlequah, Oklahoma

Bobbie Mackay, R.N., M.S.N., M.S.W.
Pulmonary Clinical Specialist,
Cystic Fibrosis Program Coordinator,
St. Louis, Missouri

Ida Martinson, R.N., Ph.D., F.A.A.N.
Professor and Chair,
Department of Family Health Care Nursing,
School of Nursing,
University of California—San Francisco,
San Francisco, California

Margo McCaffery, R.N., M.S., F.A.A.N.
Consultant in the Nursing Care of Patients with Pain,
Santa Monica, California

Marilyn A. McCubbin, R.N., Ph.D.
Assistant Professor,
University of Wisconsin—Madison,
School of Nursing,
Madison, Wisconsin

John C. McCullers, Ph.D.
Professor Emeritus,
Department of Family Relations and Child Development,
Oklahoma State University,
Stillwater, Oklahoma

Frances Lynn McCullough, R.N.P., M.N.Sc.
Orthopaedic Clinical Nurse Specialist,
Arkansas Spine Center, P.A.,
Little Rock, Arkansas

Shirley W. Menard, R.N., M.S.N., C.P.N.P.
Assistant Professor,
University of Texas Health Science Center,
School of Nursing,
San Antonio, Texas

Angela Ciolfi Murphy, R.N., Ph.D.
Department of Nursing,
Rhode Island College,
Providence, Rhode Island

Bobbie Crew Nelms, R.N., Ph.D., C.P.N.P.
Professor,
Department of Nursing,
California State University—Long Beach,
Long Beach, California

Kristie Nix, R.N., Ed.D.
Associate Professor,
College of Nursing and Applied Health Sciences,
University of Tulsa,
Tulsa, Oklahoma

Myung K. Park, M.D.
Department of Pediatrics,
University of Texas Health Science Center,
San Antonio, Texas

David P. Parks, M.D.
Fellow Associate,
Pulmonary Allergy—Pulmonary Division,
University of Iowa Hospitals and Clinics,
Iowa City, Iowa

Kaaren Pederschmidt, R.N., M.S.
Educator, Pediatrics and Pediatric Critical Care,
Stanford University Hospital,
Stanford, California

Judy Holt Rollins, R.N., M.S.
Child Health Care Consultant,
National Consultant for Very Special Arts,
Washington, D.C.

Kathleen Rossman, R.R.T.
Special Projects Coordinator,
Eastern Oklahoma Perinatal Center,
Saint Francis Hospital,
Tulsa, Oklahoma

Cindy Hylton Rushton, R.N.,C., M.S.N., F.A.A.N.
Clinical Educator III, Neonatal/Infant Specialist,
Children's National Medical Center;
Doctoral Student,
The Catholic University of America,
School of Nursing,
Washington, D.C.

Cheryl Seifert, Ph.D.
The Chicago Counseling and Psychotherapy Center,
Chicago, Illinois

Janice Selekman, R.N., D.N.Sc.
Associate Professor,
Generic Baccalaureate Program Director,
Thomas Jefferson University,
Philadelphia, Pennsylvania

Cecilia E. Shaw, R.N.,C., B.S.N., O.C.N.
Clinical Supervisor/Research Coordinator,
Cancer Care Associates,
Tulsa, Oklahoma

Donna Phillips Smith, R.N., M.S.
Pediatric Nurse Consultant,
Clinical Nurse I, Pediatrics,
Saint Francis Hospital;
Clinical Assistant Professor,
University of Oklahoma,
College of Nursing,
Tulsa, Oklahoma

Rosemarie E. Steffen, R.N., M.S.N.
Professor of Nursing,
El Centro College,
Dallas, Texas

Karen Bruner Stroup, Ph.D.
Research Associate,
Automotive Safety for Children Program,
James Whitcomb Riley Hospital for Children,
Indianapolis, Indiana

Ralph C. Underwager, Ph.D.
Institute for Psychological Therapies,
Northfield, Minnesota

Dwight A. Vance, R.Ph.
Drug Information Pharmacist,
Saint Francis Hospital,
Tulsa, Oklahoma

Hollida Wakefield, M.A.
Institute for Psychological Therapies,
Northfield, Minnesota

Barbara J. Walker
Director, Traffic Safety;
Program Coordinator,
Indiana Department of Transportation,
Indianapolis, Indiana

Holly Webster, R.N., M.S.
Director, Nursing Education,
Primary Children's Medical Center,
Salt Lake City, Utah

Janet K. Williams, R.N., M.A.
Genetic Associate of Pediatrics,
Division of Medical Genetics,
University of Iowa Hospitals and Clinics,
Iowa City, Iowa

Ding-Djung Yang, Ph.D.
Research Associate,
Department of Chemistry,
University of Chicago,
Chicago, Illinois

Heidi Zwick, R.N., B.S.N.
Trauma Coordinator,
Children's Hospital National Medical Center,
Washington, D.C.

PREFACE

In offering this fourth edition of *Nursing Care of Infants and Children,* we find ourselves grateful for the support given to the book over the years. The book you are holding has been the leading book in pediatric nursing since it was first published in 1979. Today, it is the most widely used book in nursing education throughout the world. This kind of support places a special responsibility on us to earn your future support again and again, with each new edition. So, with your encouragement and comments, we offer the most extensive revision this book has ever undergone.

While carefully preserving aspects of the book that have met with such universal acceptance—its logical organization, its writing style, and its emphasis on nursing research—we have also made some dramatic departures from past editions.

For the first time, we have enlisted the assistance of 31 nurse experts to revise content in increasingly complex specialty areas. While we have always sought the advice, reviews, and expertise of specialists, we also always organized and revised each chapter ourselves. But the rapid development of knowledge in pediatric nursing has continued to amaze us, so we decided to invite some highly expert nurse specialists to revise portions of the text on areas undergoing rapid and complex change.

Yet, in making this specialized expertise available to our readers, we were determined to do so in a way that would not compromise the strengths of a text that has been used happily by hundreds of thousands of nurses. Consequently, we carefully supervised each of the revisions and in many cases reorganized and revised the material ourselves, to maintain the consistent organization and writing style that, over the years, have proved so effective in the teaching of pediatric nursing. We remain acutely aware that, in the end, the purpose of the book is to teach.

ORGANIZATION OF THE BOOK

The same general approach to the presentation of content has been preserved from the first edition, although much content has been added, deleted, condensed, and rearranged within this framework to improve the flow and minimize duplication. The book is divided into two broad parts. Part I, sometimes called the "age and stage" approach, considers infancy and childhood in a developmental context. It emphasizes the nurse's role in health promotion and maintenance and in making the family the focus of care. In this developmental context, the care of common health problems is presented, giving readers a sense of the normal problems expected in otherwise healthy children and showing them when in the course of childhood these problems are most likely to be manifested. The remainder of the book, Part II, presents the more serious health problems of infancy and childhood that are not peculiar to any particular age-group and that frequently require hospitalization or major medical and nursing intervention.

Unit I provides a longitudinal view of the child as an individual on a continuum of developmental changes from birth through adolescence and as a member of a family unit maturing within a culture and a community. Chapter 1 includes a discussion of morbidity and mortality in infancy and childhood and child health care from a historical perspective. Because of the importance of injuries as the leading cause of death in children, an overview of this topic is included. The nursing process, with emphasis on nursing diagnosis, and the role of the nurse in caring for infants and children are discussed. Besides extensive updating of vital statistics, including Canadian child mortality, the section on evaluation of health care has been revised to reflect current legislative changes, and a new section on ethical decision making has been included under Role of the Pediatric Nurse.

The child in the context of family, culture, and community has been elaborated and broadened to emphasize this important influence on development. Chapter 2 provides the opportunity to expand the discussion of social, cultural, and religious influences on child development and health promotion, including socioeconomic factors, customs and folkways, and health beliefs and practices. Additional cultural groups, Haitians and Cubans, are addressed, as well as the homeless—an increasingly prevalent minority group. Chapter 3, devoted to the family, further emphasizes the importance of this social group on the health and welfare of children. Family theories establish the tone of the chapter, which has been expanded to include a variety of parenting situations that reflect contemporary society. An important example is a new section on gay/lesbian families. Family strengths are addressed, and current findings on adoption, divorce, single-parenting, stepfamilies, and dual-earner families have been incorporated.

The basic overview of child development in Chapter 4 maintains the same general organization and expands on the theoretic approach to personality development and learning. Biologic systems development is deemphasized in this chapter and discussed more fully in relation to major systems dysfunction later in the book. Chapter 5 now focuses on hereditary influences in health promotion. The content on prenatal influences has either been deleted or placed elsewhere, such as under Multiple Births in Chapter 3.

Unit II is concerned with the principles and skills of nursing assessment, including communication and interviewing, observation, physical and behavioral assessment, and health guidance. Chapter 6 contains guidelines for communicating with both children and their families and a detailed description of a health assessment, including an extensive discussion of family assessment and nutritional assessment. Other areas that have been expanded include sleep assessment, psychosocial history, and cultural assessment. Chapter 7 continues to provide a comprehensive approach to physical examination and developmental assessment, with new material added on temperature and blood pressure measurement and the Denver II, a major revision and restandardization of the Denver Developmental Screening Test.

Unit III stresses the importance of the neonatal period, a time of greatest risk to survival, and includes the addition of several health concerns encountered in the vulnerable first month of life. Some of the additions to this unit include increased emphasis on the family during the birth process and in those instances when a newborn is critically ill or dies, as well as home care for phototherapy.

In Chapter 8 several areas have been updated to reflect current issues and developments, such as reusable vs disposable diapers, benefits vs hazards of neonatal circumcision, and formula feeding vs breast-feeding. The strong emphasis on the family remains, with additional attention given to fathers, siblings, and multiple births.

Chapter 10 stresses the nurse's role in care of the high-risk newborn and the importance of acute observations to the survival of this vulnerable group of infants. Rapid advances in the field of neonatal care require extensive revision of content. New to this edition is a discussion of feeding resistance, a problem encountered frequently in infants on long-term parenteral and intragastric (nasogastric, gastrostomy) feeding. Infant stress, including its recognition and management, and developmental intervention have been elaborated. The section also includes a separate discussion of cocaine exposure in the neonate.

The basic content of congenital defects in Chapter 11 remains essentially similar to that in previous editions with updated management and nursing care. New to this chapter is a section on the neonatal surgical patient, including the pain experience.

Units IV through VII present the major developmental stages outlined in Unit I, which are expanded to provide a broader concept of these stages and the health problems most often associated with them. Special emphasis is placed on the preventive aspects of care. The chapters on health promotion follow a standard approach that is used consistently for each age-group. New areas and those receiving expanded coverage are development of body image, development of sexuality, sleep problems, alternate child care arrangements, spoiled-child syndrome, and dental health. Topics that have been greatly revised to reflect the numerous and ongoing changes in these areas are immunizations and car seat safety. As the book goes to press, major changes in the schedule for *Haemophilus influenzae* type b vaccine are occurring, which could not be included in Chapter 12 but are presented in Appendix G.

The chapters on health problems in these units primarily reflect more typical and age-related concerns. The information on many disorders has been rewritten to reflect recent changes. Examples include food sensitivity, failure to thrive, sudden infant death syndrome, apnea of infancy, infantile autism, sexual abuse, Lyme disease, attention deficit–hyperactivity disorder, homosexuality, and teenage pregnancy, especially in relation to abortion and confidentiality. Additional conditions that are now addressed are stomatitis, wound healing, drug reactions, erythema multiforme (including Stevens-Johnson syndrome), toxic epidermal necrolysis, tic disorders, Tourette syndrome, posttraumatic stress disorder, testicular cancer, human papillomavirus, and human immunodeficiency virus. Discussions of some disorders have been moved to other chapters.

Unit VIII deals with children who have the same developmental needs as growing children but who, because of congenital or acquired physical, cognitive, or sensory impairment, require alternative interventions to facilitate development. Chapter 22 reflects current trends in the care of families and children with chronic illness or disability such as home care, normalizing children's lives, focusing on developmental needs, enabling and empowering families, and providing early intervention. A detailed Nursing Care Plan has been added to summarize the nursing needs of the child and of the family. The developmental aspects pertaining to the child with special needs are summarized in an extensive table.

The focus in Chapter 23 is primarily on the impact of life-threatening illness and death on the child and family. The sections on hospice and home care, tissue donation, the child's right to die, and the impact of the death on siblings have been expanded. A Nursing Care Plan for the dying child has been added. The content in Chapters 24 and 25 on cognitive and sensory impairments has been reduced, since much of this care is highly specialized. The one exception is the discussion on fragile X syndrome, which is completely rewritten to include current findings on this disorder.

Unit IX is concerned with the impact of hospitalization on the child and the family and continues to present a comprehensive overview of the stressors imposed by hospitalization and nursing interventions to prevent or eliminate them. Chapter 26 has greatly expanded discussions of pain assessment and management. The section on discharge planning and home care provides the basic concepts for implementing home care for children with complex health needs. Chapter 27 continues to present information on the safe implementation of procedures with children. We have tried to include as much available research as possible to base the nursing intervention on scientific findings, not traditional practice. Examples include parental presence during procedures (including induction of anesthesia), controlling elevated temperature, controlling infection, collecting urine specimens, administering intramuscular injections, and measuring the length of nasogastric tubes for feeding. Additional sections have been included on gastric routes for administration of medications, and the section on intravenous administration of medication has been expanded.

Units X through XIV consider serious health problems of infants and children primarily from biologic systems orientation, which has the practical organizational value of permitting health problems and nursing considerations to relate to specific pathophysiologic disturbances. Some important changes are evident in these chapters, including those that reflect such advancements in pediatric care as improved survival in childhood cancer and earlier, more successful correction of congenital heart defects. All of the chapters in these units have been updated, and several discussions have been greatly expanded, such as respiratory procedures and common respiratory problems, asthma, diabetes, cancer treatment, and nursing care related to such topics. Some important content added or revised includes a discussion of venous access devices, hypoplastic left heart syndrome, hypercholesterolemia, hypoxia, acquired immune deficiency syndrome, and tissue transplantations, in particular bone marrow and heart.

The content in some chapters has been extensively reorganized to present a more logical presentation of information and newer concepts. In Chapter 34 the heart defects are classified according to physiologic changes related to pulmonary blood flow, obstruction to blood flow, or both, rather than the traditional system of cyanotic or noncyanotic defects. Physiologic consequences of congenital heart disease—congestive heart failure and hypoxia—are discussed before the defects are presented, since the major effects of the anatomic alterations result in one or both of these conditions. In Chapter 36, a general discussion of nursing care related to childhood cancer is presented as a unit, with the specific types of cancer and unique nursing considerations following this review.

The content in Chapters 39 and 40 has been reorganized and retitled to reflect a more logical aggregation of disorders that affect mobility. Health problems related to skeletal and articular dysfunction are found in Chapter 39. This chapter now includes sports injuries and heat injury. Chapter 40 is devoted to neuromuscular dysfunction.

UNIFYING PRINCIPLES

Several unifying principles have guided the organizational structure of this book since its inception. These principles have been strengthened in the revision to produce a text that is consistent in approach throughout each chapter.

An Integrated Approach to Development

Children are whole people. No book on pediatric nursing is complete without extensive coverage of communication, nutrition, play, safety, dental care, sexuality, sleep, self-esteem, and, or course, parenting. Nurses promote the healthy expression of all these dimensions of personhood. To function effectively in this role, nurses need to understand how these functions are expressed by different children at different developmental ages and stages. Even effective parenting depends on the parent's knowledge of development, and it is often the nurse's responsibility to provide parents with a developmental awareness of their children's needs. For these reasons, we have elected to integrate coverage of the many dimensions of childhood. Safety concerns, for instance, are much different for a toddler than for an adolescent. Sleep needs change with age, and so do nutritional needs. As a result, the units on each age of childhood contain complete information on all these functions as they relate to the specific age. In the unit on the school-age child, for instance, information is presented on nutritional needs; age-appropriate play and its significance; safety concerns characteristic of the age-group; appropriate dental care; sleep characteristics; and means of promoting self-esteem, a particularly significant concern for school-age children. The challenges of being the parent of a school-age child are presented, and interventions are suggested that nurses can use to promote more healthy parenting. It is our belief that the various functions of personhood ought not be artificially separated and presented in isolation of the human beings from which they derive their meaning. Using the integrated approach, students gain an appreciation for the unique characteristics and needs of children at every age and stage.

The Family as the Unit of Care

The child is an integral member of the family unit. Nursing care is most effective when it is rendered with the belief that the family is the unit of care. This belief permeates our book. When a child is healthy, the child's health is enhanced when the family is a fully functioning, health-promoting system. The family unit can be manifested in a myriad of structures; each has the potential to provide a caring, supportive environment in which the child can grow, mature, and maximize his or her human potential.

In addition to family-centered care being integrated into every chapter, an entire chapter is devoted to understanding the family as the basic unit in children's lives. Another chapter discusses the social, cultural, and religious influences that impact family beliefs. Separate sections in another chapter deal in depth with family communication and family assessment. The impact of illness, hospitalization, and death of a child are covered extensively in two additional chapters. The needs of the family are emphasized throughout the text under Nursing Considerations in a separate section called Family Support. Numerous Parent Guidelines are included to assist nurses in providing helpful information to families.

The Critical Role of Research

The information presented in this book is supported insofar as humanly possible with research performed and published by nurses, as well as that of other professionals engaged in the care of children and their families. This revision is in fact the product of an exhaustive review of the literature published since the book was last revised. In the field of pediatric nursing, much research remains to be done, and in some cases we have performed our own research to clarify ambiguous aspects of the nursing care of infants and children. Wherever possible, we indicate areas in need of further research, and we often summarize the state of the research when controversial issues are encountered through a device called Questions and Controversies. Many readers and researchers have come to rely on our copious bibliographies, in which the majority of entries are less than 5 years old, reflecting the most recent social, behavioral, medical, and nursing applications to pediatric research and health care.

Nursing Care

While the information in this text incorporates information from numerous disciplines (medicine, pathophysiology, pharmacology, nutrition, psychology, sociology), its primary purpose is to provide information on the nursing care of children and families. Discussions of all disorders conclude with a section on Nursing Considerations. In addition, 49 care plans have been included in this fourth edition. Taken together, they provide coverage of the nursing care for virtually every disease, disorder, condition, and crisis of childhood. In a sense, by emphasizing specific health problems through the vehicle of care plans, students gain an intuitive sense of the major health problems of childhood.

The purpose of the care plans, like every other feature of the book, is to teach, to convey information. They include all the current nursing diagnoses approved by NANDA through its Ninth Conference that have a potential bearing on the health problem. Although the care plans can be individualized for use with a specific patient in a clinical setting, that is not their main purpose. For every diagnosis, appropriate goals, extensive possible interventions, and sample evaluation outcomes are presented. Thus a complete range of nursing care is presented within the context of a care plan and the nursing process.

For almost every health problem for which a care plan is included, the surrounding narrative text is presented according to the nursing process. In these instances, specific headings for assessment, nursing diagnoses, planning, implementation, and evaluation, with identifying logos for each step, present appropriate information that is then amplified in the care plan, presented in a standard nursing practice context. In keeping with our general purpose of providing practical as well as conceptual information on every page of this book, the care plans provide excellent prototypes for high-quality nursing practice.

NURSING LEARNING TOOLS

Much of our effort as authors is directed toward making this book easy to teach from and, more important, easy to learn from. Therefore we continue to offer numerous pedagogic devices that enhance student learning:

- CHAPTER OUTLINES with page numbers have been provided at the beginning of each chapter to allow readers to quickly locate topics of interest.
- PARENT GUIDELINES boxes have been included to help nurses and students teach parents about the special needs of their infants and children.
- Other GUIDELINES boxes summarize important interventions for a variety of situations and conditions.
- EMERGENCY TREATMENT boxes and other emergency management are flagged by means of red thumb tabs and are listed on the endpapers, enabling the reader to quickly locate interventions for crisis situations.
- QUESTIONS AND CONTROVERSIES highlight important areas of research regarding controversial or sensitive issues in the care of children and their families.
- KEY POINTS, located at the end of each chapter, help the reader summarize major points, make connections, and synthesize information.
- PRINTED ENDPAPERS, located on the inside front and back covers of the book, provide essential information the nurse needs to refer to often, such as vital signs, blood pressure, and conversion tables.
- Hundreds of numbered TABLES and BOXES highlight key concepts and nursing interventions.
- A functional TWO-COLOR DESIGN visually segments the organization of each chapter and draws the reader's attention to material of special interest.
- A highly detailed, cross-referenced INDEX allows readers to quickly access discussions.

Building on this group of valuable learning tools, we are pleased to present some additional aids that we hope will benefit both educators and students:

- RELATED TOPICS, which appear at the beginning of every chapter, allow readers to turn to any chapter where they think a given topic will be discussed. At the beginning of the chapter, they will see the topic listed in the chapter outline with a page number or in the RELATED TOPICS section, indicating the chapter or chapters where the appropriate discussion(s) can be found. When turning to the cross-referenced chapter(s), readers will then find the topic listed in the chapter outline with a page number.
- GLOSSARIES have been provided at the beginning of the chapters so that new terms and abbreviations can be found, referred to, and mastered quickly, allowing the student to put the language of pediatric nursing to work.
- NURSING ALERTS call the reader's attention to some consideration that, if ignored, could lead to a deteriorating or emergency situation. Key assessment data, risk factors, and danger signs are among the kinds of information we alert readers to.
- NURSING TIPS present handy information of a nonemergency nature that makes patients more comfortable and the nurse's job a little easier.
- THERAPEUTIC DIALOGUES describe realistic nurse-child-family interactions, a vital aspect of nursing care.
- A DETAILED TABLE OF CONTENTS has been provided, in addition to a BRIEF TABLE OF CONTENTS, to enable readers to locate specific topics and discussions.

CANADIAN CONTENT

In this edition we have made reference to Canadian statistics regarding infant and child health in Chapter 1 and to Canadian immunization schedules in Chapter 12. In addition, we have included numerous Canadian service organizations throughout the text. We appreciate the wide usage of our book in Canada and hope that these supplements are of value to the Canadian reader.

TEACHING/LEARNING PACKAGE

For the fourth edition of our text we are pleased to offer an extensive number of ancillary products for instructors and students to use in class and clinical settings:

Instructor's Resource Manual. This valuable resource manual, prepared by Angela Murphy and Caryn Hess, follows the textbook chapter by chapter and includes chapter outlines, chapter overviews, learning objectives/resources, potential student problem areas, audiovisual and supplementary materials, recommendations for guest lecturers, student learning activities, and topics for research papers. Many chapters also include experiential exercises and case studies. A ***Test Bank*** containing 600 test items has also been provided. An answer key with page number rationales is included at the back of the manual. A special section featuring student study activities has also been provided. Instructors may photocopy these activities for classroom use.

Overhead Transparencies. One hundred two-color transparency acetates that focus on key material in the text assist instructors in increasing student understanding.

Pediatric Quick Reference. New to this edition is our *Pediatric Quick Reference,* a handy pocket-sized resource that accompanies every copy of the text. The guide features commonly referred-to information such as assessment data, pain management strategies, fluid requirements, emergency information, and laboratory values.

MicroTest III. Available in IBM and Apple versions, *MicroTest III* is the computerized version of the *Test Bank* from the *Instructor's Resource Manual.* Complete with user's guide, *MicroTest III* allows instructors to edit, add, delete, or select questions on the computer.

▪ ▪ ▪

Just as children and their families bring with them a vast and unique background that affects their role within the health care system, so it is that each nurse brings to each child and family an individual set of characteristics and values that will affect their relationship. Although we have attempted to present a total picture of the child in each age-group both in wellness and in illness, no one child, family, or nurse will be found in this book. We hope that each page, chapter, and unit builds a foundation on which the nurse can begin to construct the ideal of comprehensive, individualized nursing care for infants and children.

Lucille F. Whaley
Donna L. Wong

ACKNOWLEDGMENTS

With each edition of *Nursing Care of Infants and Children* more and more of our colleagues have become involved in the revision of the book. We are grateful to the many nursing faculty, practitioners, and students who have offered their comments, recommendations, and suggestions. We are especially indebted to the contributors who revised selected chapters of this edition and the reviewers for their constructive criticism and suggestions.

Our primary goal in revising this edition has been to present the most current and accurate data available at the time of publication. In reviewing the literature, we have not always been able to locate published updates on certain topics or to use the published data in its existing form. To obtain current and usable data, we contacted several individuals and organizations who generously provided us with what we needed. We are especially grateful to the following people and organizations:

Bernard Rosner, Ph.D., Associate Professor of Preventive Medicine and Clinical Epidemiology (Biostatistics), Harvard Medical School, compiled the blood pressure percentiles from the Second Task Force on Blood Pressure Control in Children into tabular form for our use on the inside front cover. We thank the National Heart, Lung, and Blood Institute for granting us permission to use these data.

William Frankenburg, M.D., shared with us the latest information on the Denver II and granted permission for duplication of the testing form in Appendix B. The Canadian Center for Health Information provided statistics on childhood mortality for Chapter 1, and the American Cancer Society provided statistics on cancer incidence in children for Chapter 36. Ross Laboratories compiled data on infant feeding habits, which appear in Chapter 12. The American Academy of Pediatrics kept us informed of the latest developments in several areas of pediatrics, especially immunizations.

We again extend thanks to those institutions that have welcomed us to the units providing care to infants and children: Saint Francis Hospital, Tulsa, Oklahoma; Children's Medical Center of Dallas, Dallas, Texas; Children's Hospital of Wisconsin, Milwaukee, Wisconsin; Miami Children's Hospital, Miami, Florida; Children's Hospital National Medical Center, Washington, D.C.; James Whitcomb Riley Hospital for Children, Indianapolis, Indiana; Arkansas Children's Hospital, Little Rock, Arkansas; Santa Clara Valley Medical Center, San Jose, California; Stanford University

Medical Center, Palo Alto, California; El Camino Hospital, Mountain View, California; Prince of Wales Children's Hospital, Sydney, Australia; Royal Children's Hospital, Melbourne, Australia; and Adelaide Children's Hospital, Adelaide, Australia.

We appreciate the efforts of the library staffs of many of these institutions for assisting in the extensive research needed to update the book, and Barbara Brown, Milton J. Chatton Medical Library, for her generosity with library facilities. We especially thank Peggy Cook, librarian at Hillcrest Medical Center, Tulsa, Oklahoma, for the scores of computer searches and hundreds of articles she provided, as well as the many citations she checked for accuracy, that made it possible to update the content through 1990. We also thank Dwight Vance, R.Ph., Drug Information Pharmacist at Saint Francis Hospital, for his efforts in checking the accuracy of pharmaceutical agents.

We are especially indebted to the many families who allowed us to take photographs and those individuals, especially Caryn Hess, Peggy Cook, and Earl Fillmore, who shared with us photographs of family members. Special thanks are extended to Patti Muller, R.N., Ed.D., Director of Educational Resources; John Roy, medical photographer; Vicky Nongard, graphics coordinator, and Rob Riley, graphics illustrator, for the generous use of their facilities at Saint Francis Hospital. We also thank David Wilson, R.N., M.S., and Kathleen Rossman, R.R.T., for coordinating some of the new photography with John Roy.

We are especially grateful to our own "resident" photographer, Ting Kin Wong, for the many long hours spent in his darkroom. We again wish to thank George Wassilchenko, Oral Roberts University, for the additional illustrations he has contributed to this edition and Kathleen Whaley for the new illustrations she has prepared.

No book is ever a reality without the dedication and perseverance of the editorial staff, and although it is impossible to list every individual at Mosby–Year Book who has made exceptional efforts to produce this text, we are especially grateful to William Brottmiller, Sally Adkisson, Judi Bange, and Gayle May for their patience and commitment to excellence. In addition, we wish to thank our typists, Maureen Whaley and Lynne Murtha, for the superb job they did and for their efforts in meeting very stringent deadlines.

As always, we wish to thank the members of our families, Bert, Maureen, and Kathy Whaley, Ting and Nina Wong, and Rudy Mitchko, whose devotion, patience, and forbearance are a constant source of support and encouragement. Truly, without their willingness to assume many of the tasks necessary to produce a text of this size and their sacrifices, which allowed us the time needed to revise it, this book would never have been completed. And last, we thank each other for the shared excitement of exploration and the stimulation and mutual esteem associated with this collaboration.

Lucille F. Whaley
Donna L. Wong

BRIEF CONTENTS

NURSING CARE PLANS

COLOR PLATES*

Color plates follow p. xxxii

*Plates 1, 3 to 12, 14, 15, and 18 from Habif, T.P.: Clinical dermatology: a color guide to diagnosis and therapy, ed. 2, St. Louis, 1990, Mosby–Year Book, Inc. Plates 2, 13, 16, and 17 from Seidel, H.M., and others: Mosby's guide to physical examination, ed. 2, St. Louis, 1991, Mosby-Year Book, Inc. Plates 19 and 20 from Thompson, J.M., and others: Clinical nursing, ed. 1, St. Louis, 1986, Mosby–Year Book, Inc. Plates 21 to 24 courtesy Hillcrest Medical Center, Tulsa, OK.

DETAILED CONTENTS

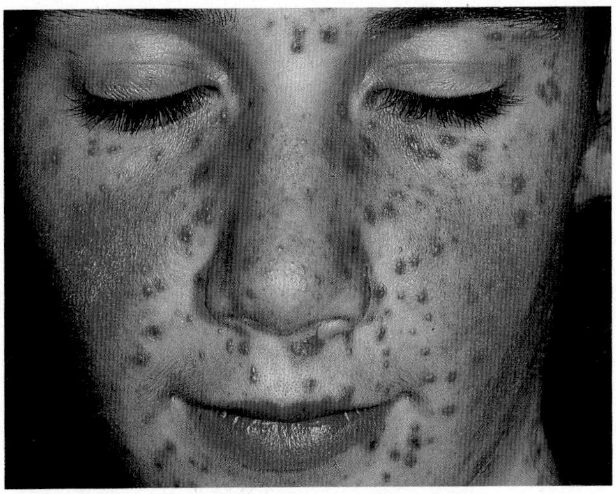

Plate 1. Varicella (chickenpox).

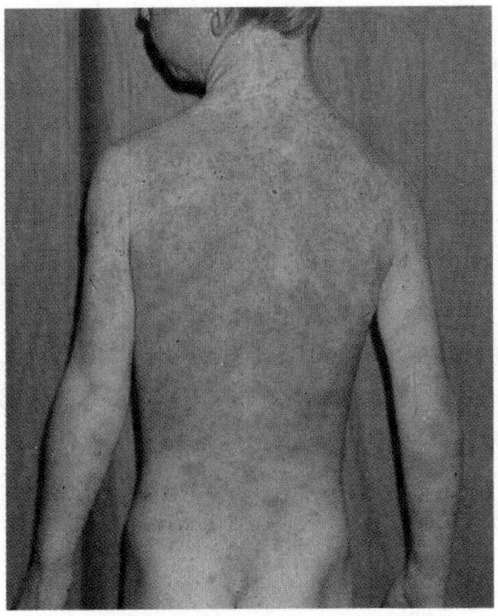

Plate 2. Rubeola (measles).

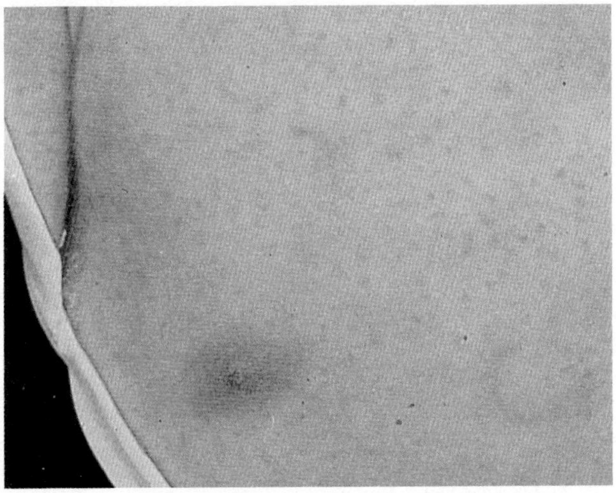

Plate 3. Rubella (German measles).

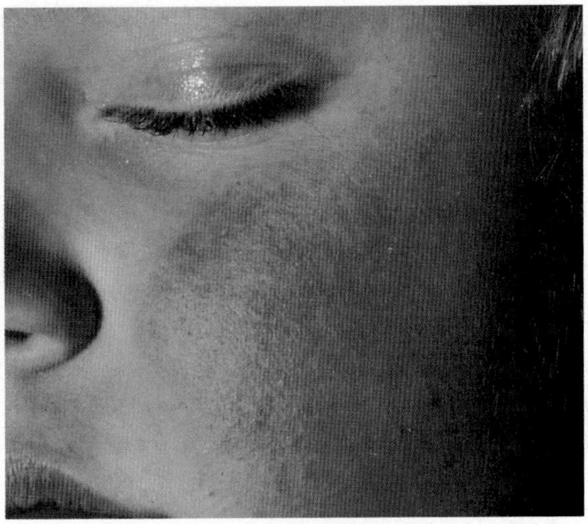

Plate 4. Erythema infectiosum.

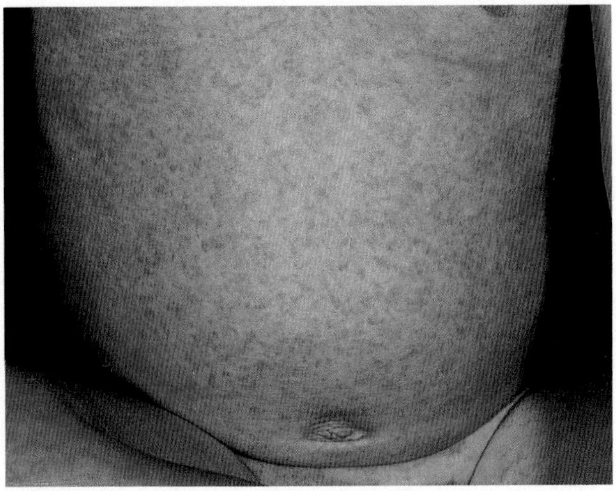

Plate 5. Roseola infantum.

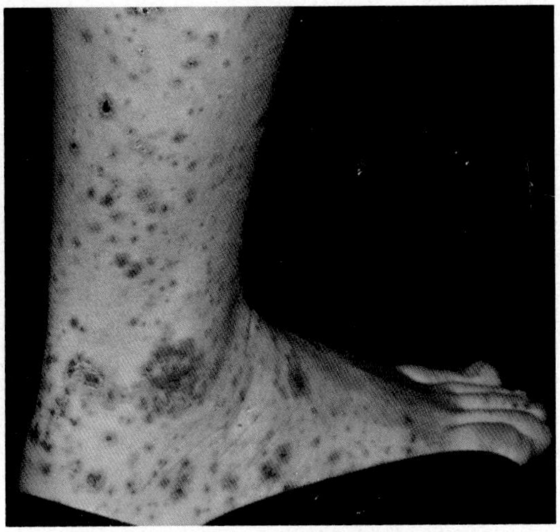

Plate 6. Henoch-Schönlein purpura.

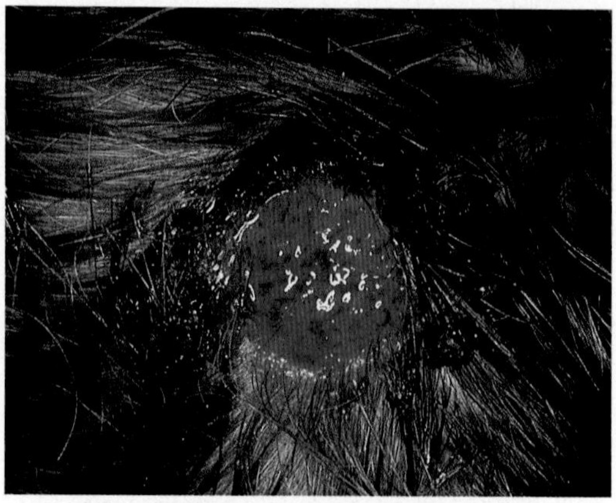

Plate 7. Tinea capitis.

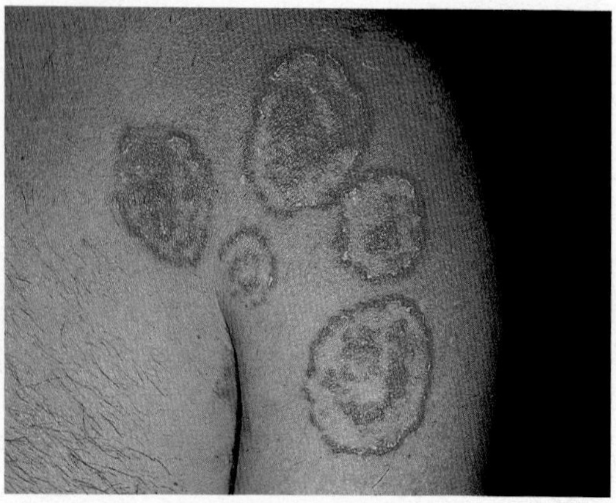

Plate 8. Tinea corporis.

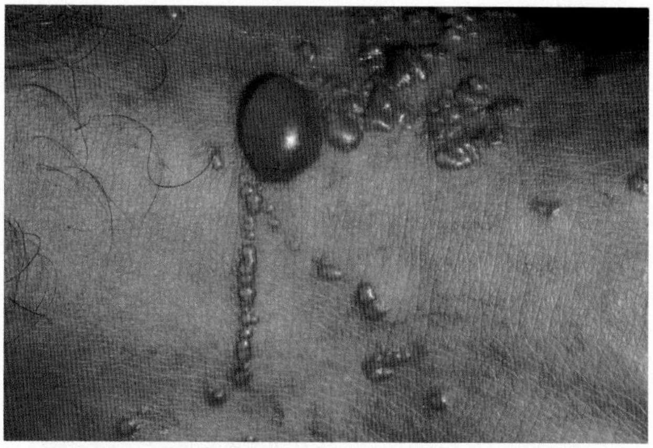

Plate 9. Poison ivy.

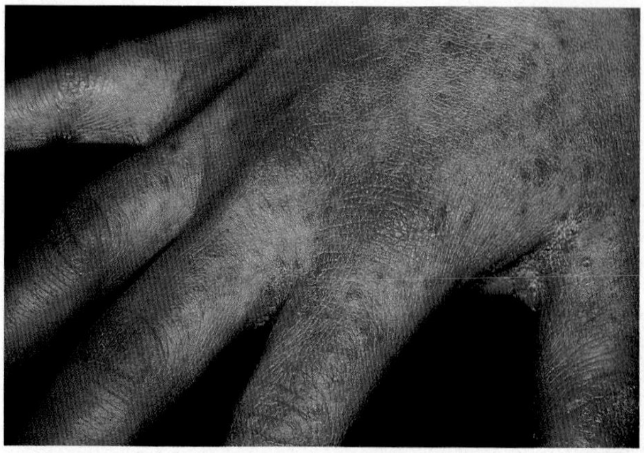

Plate 10. Scabies.

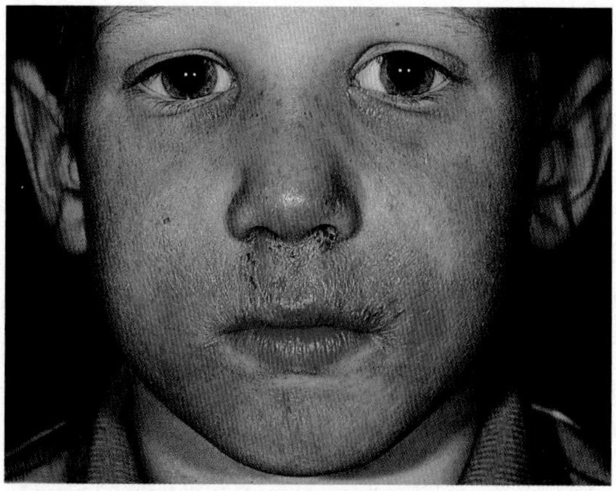

Plate 11. Atopic dermatitis.

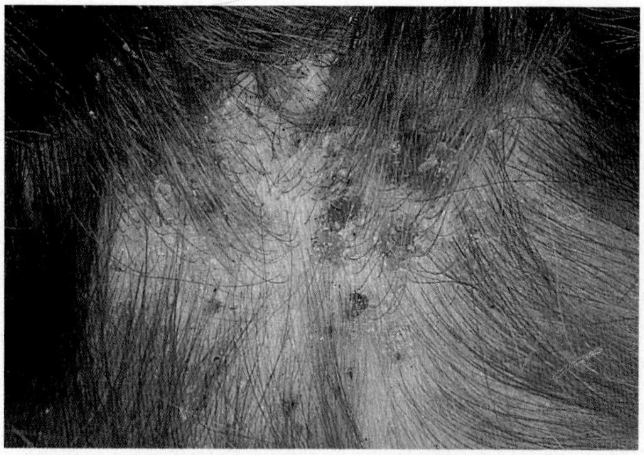

Plate 12. Pediculosis capitis.

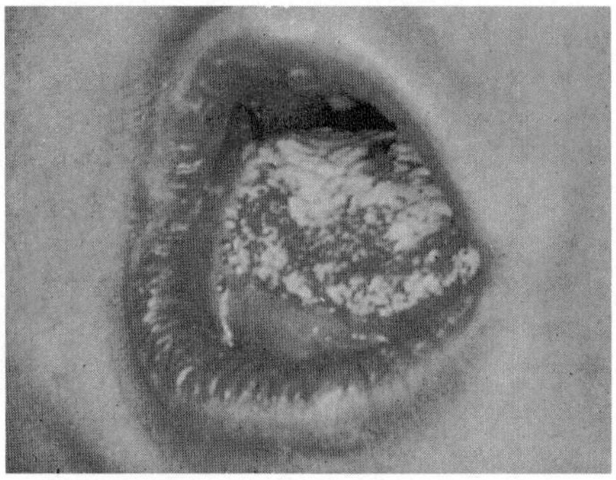

Plate 13. Candidiasis (thrush).

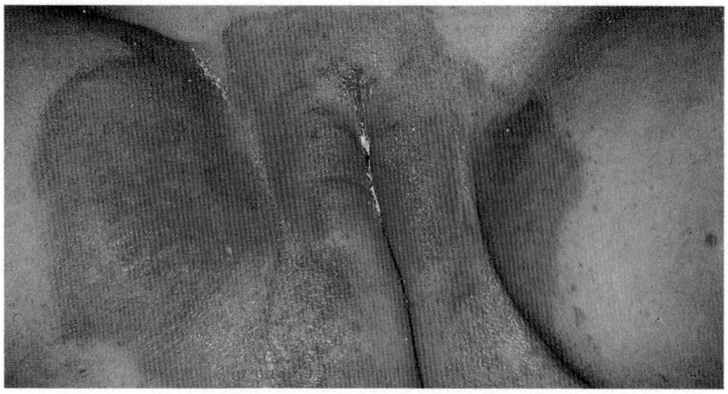

Plate 14. Irritant dermatitis.

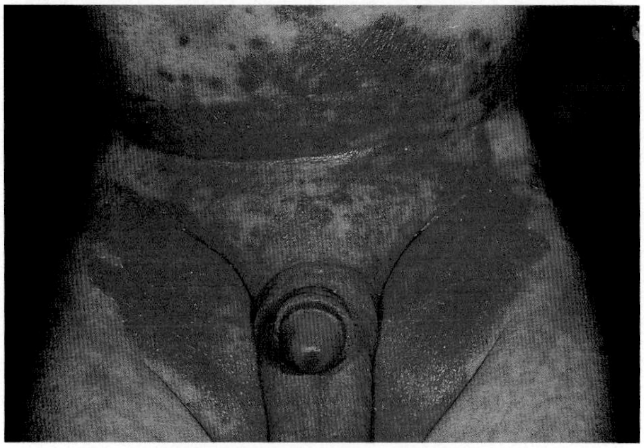

Plate 15. Candida dermatitis.

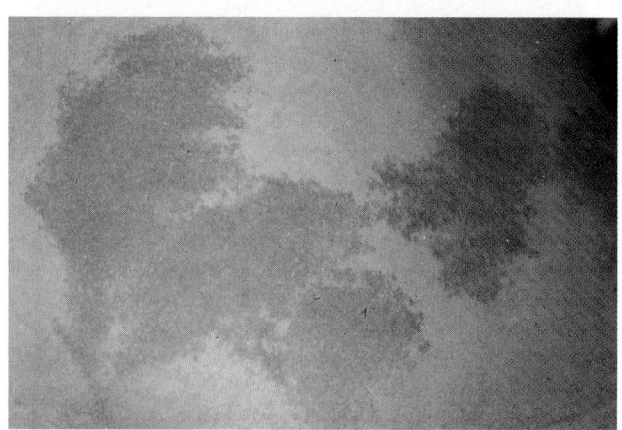

Plate 16. Café-au-lait patches.

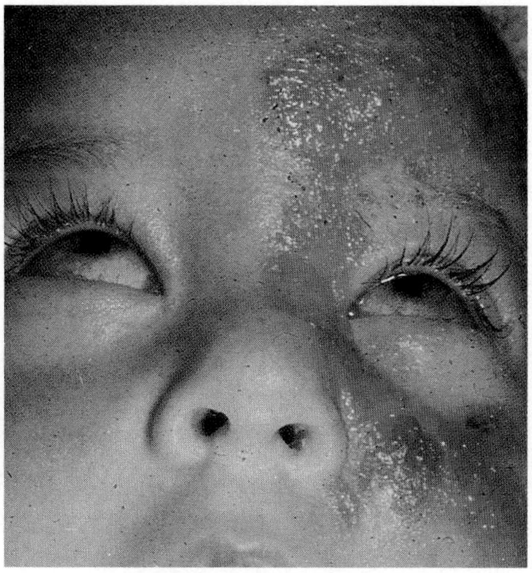

Plate 17. Impetigo.

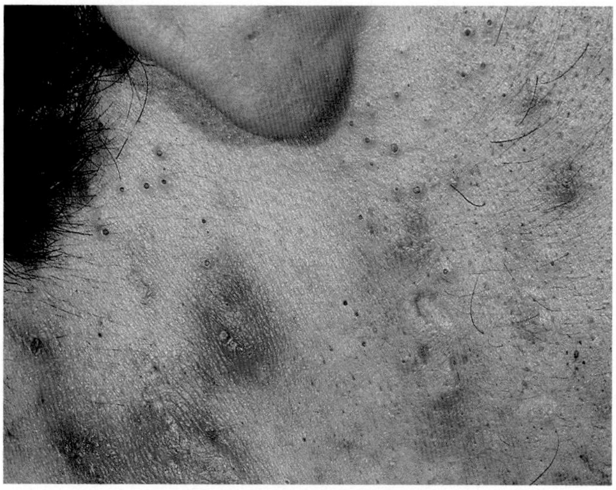

Plate 18. Localized cystic acne.

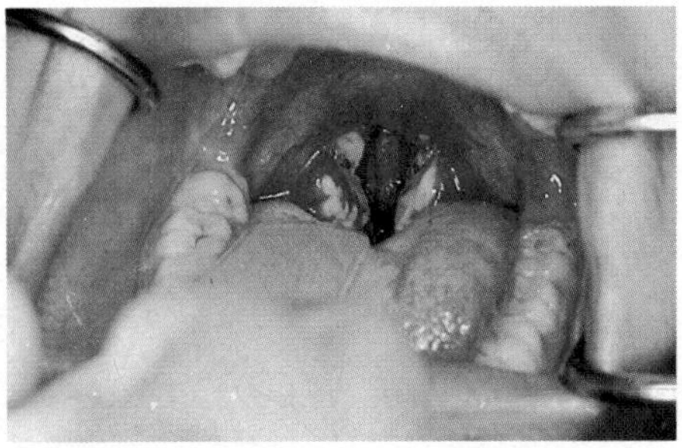

Plate 19. Tonsillitis and pharyngitis.

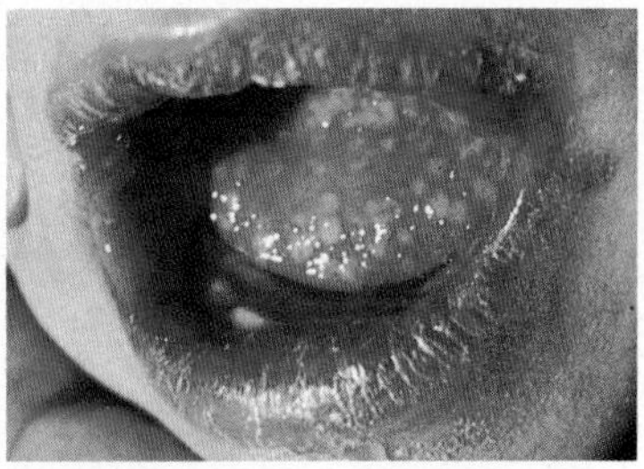

Plate 20. Primary gingivostomatitis.

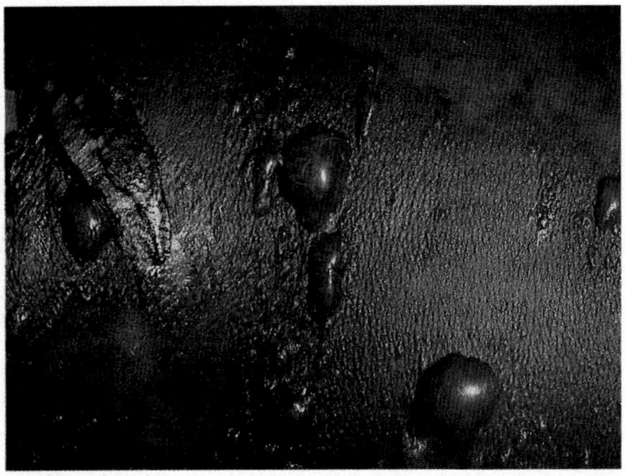

Plate 21. Superficial partial-thickness burns (blisters intact).

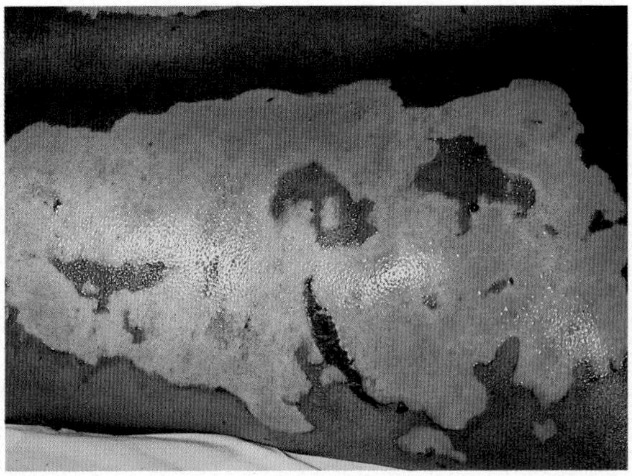

Plate 22. Superficial partial-thickness burns (blisters removed).

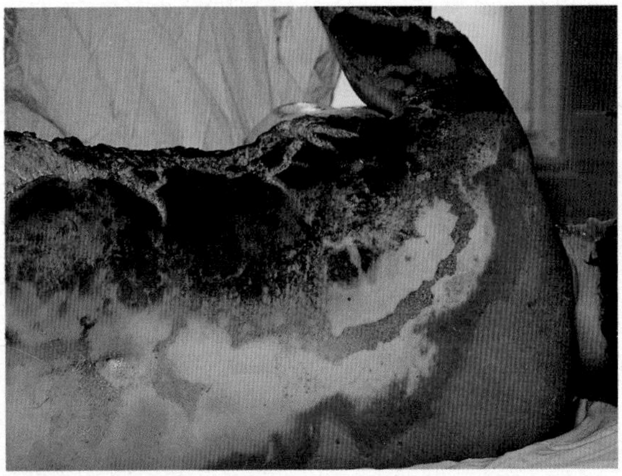

Plate 23. *From bottom to top,* Deep superficial burn (red area); full-thickness burn (white area); full-thickness burn with eschar (brown area).

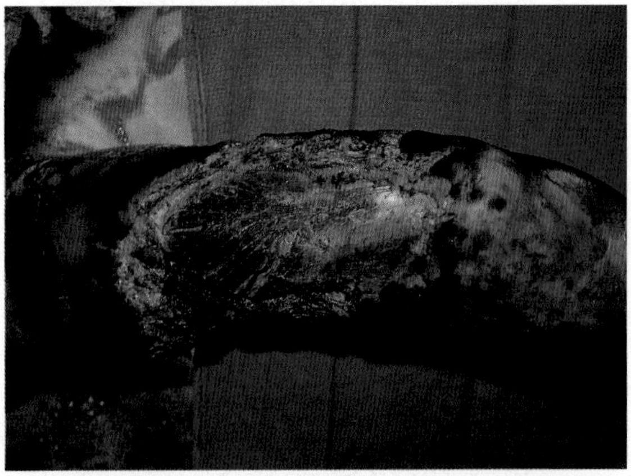

Plate 24. Full-thickness burn (muscle and fascia involved).

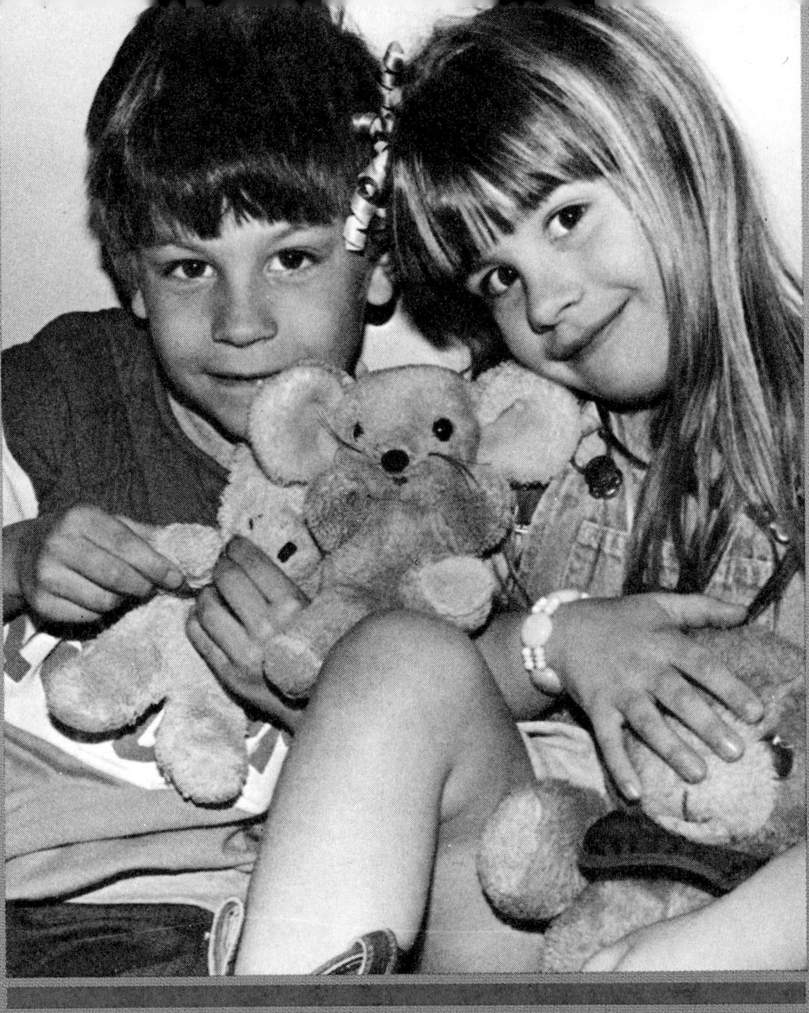

CHILD HEALTH PROMOTION AND MAINTENANCE

PART

I

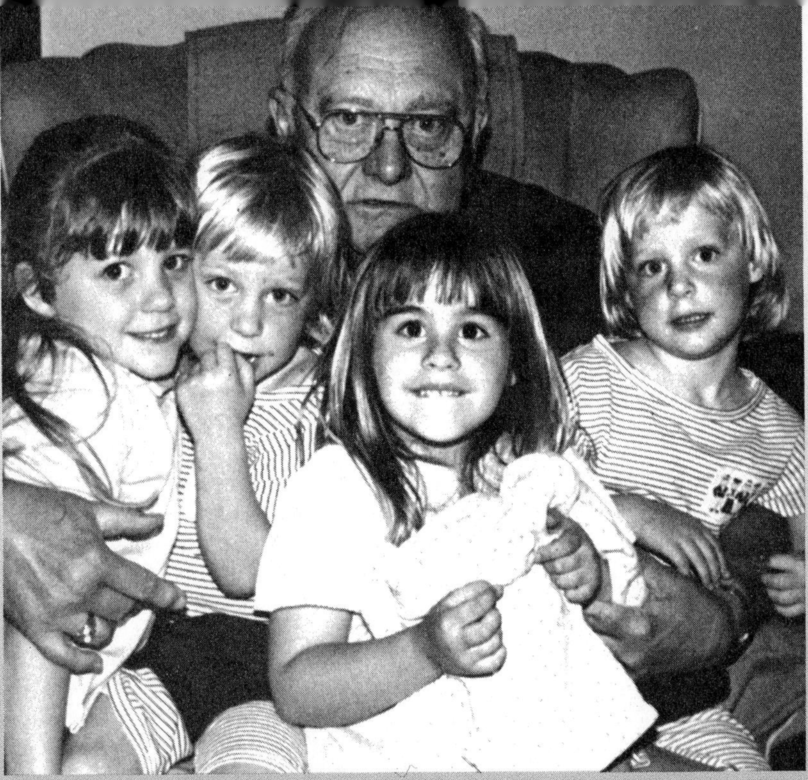

Children, Their Families, and the Nurse

UNIT I

Chapter 1, *Perspectives of Pediatric Nursing,* emphasizes a child-family–centered rather than a disease-centered approach to nursing of infants and children. Childhood health is viewed from the perspective of mortality and morbidity trends at various ages, with special attention to injuries, the leading cause of death. A historical overview of child health care in the United States serves as a basis for understanding changes that have occurred in pediatrics. Nursing is viewed as a process and the nurse as a person who can work effectively with infants and children and help create conditions in which others, particularly parents, can function more effectively in child care.

Chapter 2, *Social, Cultural, and Religious Influences on Child Health Promotion,* considers the way in which the societal and cultural-religious background of the family affects children, their health, and their relationships. The emphasis is on differences in health practices, environmental influences, and perspectives on health and health care providers.

Chapter 3, *Family Influences on Child Health Promotion,* is concerned with children in their family setting. It includes selected family theories, family constellations, and family influences on development. The child's place within the family is examined with emphasis on family members' roles in shaping the child's attitudes and behavior.

Chapter 4, *Growth and Development of Children,* provides a vertical or longitudinal view of the alterations that take place during growth and development and serves as a preface to the horizontal age-specific discussions in the chapter on health promotion. Children are presented as unique individuals on a lifelong developmental continuum; they differ physiologically, morphologically, and emotionally from adults, from other children, and from the children they were and will become.

Chapter 5, *Hereditary Influences on Health Promotion of the Child and Family,* discusses genetic factors affecting the growth and health of children. It includes cytogenetic disorders, major inheritance patterns, and effects of heredity on common diseases and conditions. The major emphasis is on the nurse's role in dealing with families coping with genetic disease or disability.

CHAPTER 1

Perspectives of Pediatric Nursing

RELATED TOPICS

Cancer in children, Ch. 36
The child and trauma, Ch. 39
Chronic illness/disability: scope of the problem, Ch. 22
Classification of high-risk newborns, Ch. 10
Cultural/religious influences on health care, Ch. 2
Injury prevention: infant, Ch. 12; toddler, Ch. 14; preschooler, Ch. 15; school-age child, Ch. 17; and adolescent, Ch. 19
Interpersonal relationships, Ch. 4
Preschool or daycare experience, Ch. 15
Suicide, Ch. 21
Temperament, Ch. 4

GLOSSARY

AFDC Aid to Families of Dependent Children
ATV All-terrain vehicle
CCS Crippled Children's Services
CNS Clinical nurse specialist
CSHN Children with Special Health Needs
DHHS Department of Health and Human Services
DRG Diagnosis related group
HIV Human immunodeficiency virus
ICD International Classification of Diseases
JCAHO Joint Commission on Accreditation of Healthcare Organizations
LBW Low birth weight
infant mortality rate The number of deaths per 1000 live births during the first year of life
MCH Maternal-child health
morbidity Illness
morbidity statistics Prevalence of a specific illness in the population at a particular time
mortality Death
mortality statistics The incidence or number of individuals who have died over a specific period of time
MV Motor vehicle
NANDA North American Nursing Diagnosis Association
NCHS National Center for Health Statistics
neonatal mortality rate The number of deaths per 1000 live births before 28 days of life
perinatal mortality rate The number of infant deaths under 7 days of life per 1000 live births and fetal deaths (fetus $\geq$ 28 weeks of gestation)
PHS Public Health Service
PNP Pediatric nurse practitioner
postneonatal mortality rate The number of deaths per 1000 live births from 28 days to 1 year of life
SSA Social Security Act
vital statistics Numerical figures describing rates of occurrence for events, such as mortality or morbidity
WIC Women, Infants, and Children (special supplemental food program)

Health care of children has changed dramatically in the past century. It has paralleled society's changing view of children from "miniature adults," whose value to the community was measured in productivity, to a recognition and appreciation of children as unique individuals with special needs and qualities. There has been a shifting focus in child care from treatment of disease to prevention of illness and promotion of health. Nurses are no longer solely involved in the episodic care of children during an acute illness. They are increasingly responsible for providing comprehensive, distributive care that attempts to meet the needs of children and their families.

This chapter presents an overview of child health through discussion of past and present trends in childhood mortality and morbidity, with special attention to injuries, the leading cause of death in children. It offers a brief history of the evolution of child health care in the United States. The role of the pediatric nurse in both traditional and extended-role situations is also discussed. The process of nursing children and families is briefly reviewed because it is the basis of all nursing action.

HEALTH DURING CHILDHOOD

Health is a complex phenomenon. As defined by the World Health Organization (WHO), it is "a state of complete physical, mental, and social well-being and not merely the absence of disease." Despite this broad definition, health is traditionally assessed by observing *mortality* (death) and *morbidity* (illness) rates over a period of time. Therefore the *presence* of disease becomes a prime indicator of health.

Based on these parameters, the health of children in the United States is better than ever before. As is discussed in the following sections, mortality rates for all ages of children have dropped dramatically since the beginning of the of the 1900s. However, there remains cause for concern. In 1979, the Surgeon General of the United States established a set of 1990 Health Objectives for the Nation in the area of infant and child health (Promoting health, 1980):

1. To reduce infant mortality to fewer than 9 deaths per 1000 live births
2. To reduce deaths among children 1 through 14 years of age to fewer than 34 per 100,000 children
3. To reduce deaths among persons 15 through 24 years of age to fewer than 93 per 100,000 children
4. To reduce motor vehicle accident deaths among children less than 15 years of age to no more than 5.5 per 100,000 children
5. To reduce home accident deaths among children less than 15 years of age to no more than 5 per 100,000 children
6. To reduce deaths from homicide among black males 15 through 24 years of age to fewer than 60 per 100,000 children
7. To reduce deaths from suicide among persons 15 through 24 years of age to fewer than 11 per 100,000

During the past decade, five of the seven objectives have been met. However, most discouraging is the slow progress that has been made toward reducing the infant mortality rate to fewer than 9 deaths per 1000 live births. In addition, the achievement of reduced deaths from suicide seems highly unlikely. In fact, the suicide death rate among young persons has increased rather than decreased during this time (Hoekelman and Pless, 1988; The 1990 Health Objectives, 1986). Objectives for the year 2000 continue to address these two areas. For example, one objective is to reduce infant mortality to no more than 7 deaths per 1000 live births (Healthy people, 1990).

Other areas of concern regarding children's health in the United States include the following (Eisenberg, 1987; Hughes and others, 1987; Wise and Meyers, 1988):

1. The infant and child death rate is still high in the United States when compared with rates in most other well-developed countries, and progress has slowed during the 1980s.
2. Depending on race, nonwhite children, particularly black children, have up to a 50% higher mortality rate than white children.
3. The United States rate for teenage pregnancy, abortion, and childbearing is the highest among industrialized countries; pregnancy rates among 15- to 17-year-old girls in Canada are half the rate in the United States; pregnancies of mothers less than 19 years of age result in almost twice as many low-birth-weight (LBW) neonates as pregnancies of mothers 20 and older.
4. The poverty rate for children has increased in recent years; 20% of all children live in poverty (defined in 1989 as annual income of $10,060 or less for a family of three); almost 50% of black children and more than one third of Hispanic children live in poverty (AAP special report, 1989).
5. Other areas of concern are low immunization levels among preschool children, malnutrition, increasing incidence of tuberculosis in Asian and Hispanic populations, increasing incidence of sexually transmitted disease, dental problems, injuries, homelessness, substance abuse, especially "cocaine babies," and suicide.

Information concerning mortality and morbidity is important to nurses. Such data yield significant information about (1) the causes of death and illness, (2) high-risk age-groups for certain disorders or hazards, (3) advances in treatment and prevention, and (4) specific areas of health counseling. By being aware of such information nurses can better guide their planning and delivery of care.

MORTALITY

Figures describing rates of occurrence for events such as death in children are often referred to as *vital statistics. Mortality statistics* describe the incidence or number of individuals who have died over a specific period of time. They are usually presented as rates per 100,000 population because of their lower frequency of occurrence than statistics such as infant mortality. Mortality rates are calculated from a sample of death certificates.

In the United States the National Center for Health Statistics (NCHS), under the Department of Health and Human Services (DHHS), Public Health Service (PHS), has the responsibility for collection, analysis, and dissemination of data on the health of the American people. Because of the complexity of compiling such data, statistics may vary in different reports and should be interpreted cautiously. For example, figures may be *estimated* (from previously collected data), *provisional* (from temporary current data), or *final* (from complete provisional data). It is not unusual for final statistics to be published 2 or more years after original collection of the data.

Causes of death are categorized according to the International Classification of Diseases (ICD). The ICD is revised approximately every 10 years. As of 1975 the Ninth Revision has been used. This has produced many changes in the classification system, making comparisons between causes of death before and after 1976 difficult. This should be kept in mind when reviewing mortality statistics from different sources and for various time intervals. For example, the causes of infant death are markedly different in the Eighth and Ninth Revisions. In the Ninth Revision there is the addition of respiratory distress syndrome and sudden infant death syndrome in the list of 10 leading causes of death. However, deaths due to human immunodeficiency virus (HIV) infections are not in the Ninth Revision and are classified separately (Wegman, 1989).

Infant Mortality

Infant mortality rate is defined as the number of deaths per 1000 live births during the first year of life. It may be further divided into *neonatal* (<28 days of life) and *postneonatal* (28 days to 1 year) mortality. Rates of infant mortality are sensitive indicators of a wide range of factors affecting children's health. Only a minority of infants with specific problems die; many more survive with health conditions that affect childhood mortality and morbidity (American Academy of Pediatrics, 1986).

In the United States there has been a dramatic decrease in the infant mortality rate. At the beginning of the twentieth century the mortality rate was about 1 in 6 live births; in 1987 the infant mortality rate dropped to 1 in 100 live births, the lowest rate ever recorded in the United States. This decrease has primarily been a result of infectious disease control and nutritional advances during the early 1900s and the advent of antibiotic and antibacterial agents in the late 1930s.

However, when viewed from a worldwide perspective, the United States lags significantly behind other well-developed countries. In 1987 it ranked twenty-first among the 25 countries with the lowest infant mortality rates, Japan having the lowest rate (Wegman, 1989) (Table 1-1). This is far behind neighboring countries such as Canada, which ranked fifth. Reasons for the decline in improvement of infant mortality rates include a diminishing return from the previous advances, proportionately less funding of maternal-infant services in relation to existing need, and poor utilization of existing prenatal care especially among pregnant teenagers, who tend to have LBW infants.

Birth weight is considered the major determinant of neonatal death in the developed countries of the world. There is an inverse relationship between birth weight and mortality; that is, the lower the birth weight, the higher the mortality. The relatively high incidence of LBW (<2500 g) in the United States is considered a key factor in its higher neonatal mortality rates when compared with other countries. Other factors that increase the risk of infant mortality include black race, male sex, short or long gestation, birth order (all but second), maternal age (younger or older), lower level of maternal education, and lack of prenatal care during the first trimester (Centers for Disease Control, 1989).

While there has been a steady and significant decline in infant mortality, the number of deaths occurring in the first year of life is still proportionately high when compared with mortality rates at other ages. This is true of other countries, such as Canada (Table 1-2). As Table 1-3 shows, the infant death rate in the United States is almost as great as the cumulative rates for ages 1 through 54 years. It is not until age 55 and over that the death rate per age interval begins to exceed the infant death rate.

During the first half of this century neonatal mortality rates had not shown the remarkable reduction observed in postnatal infant mortality. In the early 1960s attention focused on perinatal health care in an effort to decrease the number of neonatal deaths. The *perinatal mortality rate* is commonly defined as the number of infant deaths under 7

Table 1-1 Infant mortality for 25 countries with population over 2.5 million, 1987 (rate per 1000 live births)

COUNTRY	RATE
Japan	5.0
Sweden	5.7*
Finland	6.1
Switzerland	6.8
Canada	7.3
Hong Kong	7.4
Ireland	7.4
Singapore	7.4*
France	7.6*
Netherlands	7.6
Denmark	8.3
German Federal Republic	8.3
Norway	8.4
German Democratic Republic	8.5*
Spain	8.5* (1985)
Australia	8.7
United Kingdom	9.1*
Belgium	9.7*
Austria	9.8
New Zealand	10.0
Italy	10.1
United States of America	10.1
Israel	11.5
Greece	12.6*
Czechoslovakia	13.1*

From Wegman, M.E.: Annual summary of vital statistics—1988, Pediatrics 84(6):943-956, 1989.
*Provisional data.

Table 1-2 Death rates for children, Canada, 1988 (rates per 100,000 population)

AGE (YEARS)	RATE TOTAL	MALE	FEMALE
Under 1	717.9	801.6	630.0
1-4	41.4	45.9	36.2
5-9	21.7	26.8	16.4
10-14	24.6	31.0	17.8
15-19	70.8	103.4	36.3
20-24	90.5	138.8	41.1

Data from Canadian Center for Health Information, Statistics Canada, 1988.

Table 1-3 Death rates by age, United States, 1987 (estimated rates per 100,000 in specified group)

AGE (YEARS)	RATE
Under 1	1018.5
1-4	51.6
5-14	26.5
15-24	99.4
25-34	133.2
35-44	214.1
45-54	498.0
55-64	1241.3
65-74	2751.3
75-84	6282.5
85 and over	15,320.8

From National Center for Health Statistics: Advance report of final mortality statistics, 1987, Monthly vital statistics report 38(suppl. 5):15, DHHS Pub. No. (PHS) 89-1120, 1989.

days per 1000 live births and fetal deaths (fetuses of 28 weeks or more gestation), although other definitions exist that affect the reported data. As a result of the efforts in perinatal care, the perinatal mortality rate declined from 33 per 1000 live births/fetal deaths in 1950 to a rate of 10.8 in 1985. In contrast to the trend of minimal improvement in infant mortality rates in the past decade, perinatal mortality rates have continued to decline significantly (National Center, 1989b). This drop has been largely the result of better treatment of perinatal illnesses, particularly asphyxia, immaturity, respiratory disorders, and gastrointestinal problems.

The leading causes of infant mortality are listed in Table 1-4. Among the 10 leading causes of infant death, the first 4—congenital anomalies, sudden infant death syndrome, disorders relating to short gestation and unspecified LBW, and respiratory distress syndrome—accounted for just over half of all deaths of infants under 1 year of age in 1987. The next 6 causes accounted for only 14% of all infant deaths. Because of an increase in the number of deaths assigned to the category accidents and adverse effects, the rank of this cause changed from the eighth leading cause in 1986 to the sixth in 1987 (National Center, 1989a).

Table 1-4 Leading causes of death in infants under 1 year of age, United States, 1987 (estimated rates per 100,000 live births)

RANK	CAUSE OF DEATH	RATE
. . .	All causes	1,008.2
1	Congenital anomalies	207.0
2	Sudden infant death syndrome	137.3
3	Disorders relating to short gestation and unspecified low birth weight	88.0
4	Respiratory distress syndrome	86.2
5	Newborn affected by maternal complications of pregnancy	36.7
6	Accidents and adverse effects	24.9
7	Infections specific to the perinatal period	22.6
8	Newborn affected by complications of placenta, cord, and membranes	22.0
9	Intrauterine hypoxia and birth asphyxia	20.8
10	Pneumonia and influenza	17.7
. . .	All other causes	345.0

From National Center for Health Statistics: Advance report of final mortality statistics, 1987, Monthly vital statistics report 38 (suppl. 5):31, DHHS Pub. No. (PHS) 89-1120, 1989.

Although a number of perinatal problems have benefited from improved treatment, congenital anomalies continue to be the leading cause of infant mortality, accounting for about 20% of those deaths. The most frequent type of birth defect is cardiovascular, followed by central nervous system defects and then respiratory system defects (Contribution of birth defects, 1989). However, the frequency and the types of congenital malformations vary greatly among minority groups in the United States. Certain racial/ethnic groups have a higher incidence of some malformations than others. In an analysis of the 18 major birth defects by racial/ethnic groups, the American Indian had the highest total rate followed by whites, blacks, Asians, and Hispanics (Chavez, Cordero, and Becerra, 1988). The incidence of most birth defects has neither substantially decreased nor increased. Some notable exceptions are a slight decline in spina bifida and anencephaly and an increase in heart defects. The increased incidence of patent ductus arteriosus is probably due to improved survival of LBW infants and better diagnosis, but the increase in ventricular septal defect is likely to reflect a true increase. The relative stability of the incidence of congenital anomalies suggests the need for discovering and implementing improved prevention strategies (Kalter and Warkany, 1983).

When infant mortality rates are categorized according to race, a disturbing difference is seen. The infant mortality rates for whites are considerably lower than for all other races in the United States, with blacks having almost twice the rate for whites. Although the infant mortality rate of both groups has declined, the gap has remained fairly constant.

One encouraging note is that the gap in mortality rates between nonwhite races has been narrowing. Since the Indian Health Service assumed responsibility for the health of American Indians and Alaska Natives in 1955, infant mortality has declined by 75% (Indian Health Service, 1984). This improvement, however, is primarily due to declines in the neonatal mortality rate. The postneonatal death rates for Native Americans remain twice as high as those for the white race. This suggests that Native Americans leave the hospital healthy but go to unsafe environments, which decrease their chances of survival past the first year. This phenomenon is not unique to the United States, because postneonatal mortality rates for northwest Ontario Indians are reported to be four times the Canadian all-race rate (Honigfeld and Kaplan, 1987).

Childhood Mortality

For children older than 1 year of age, death rates have always been less than those for infants, as Table 1-5 shows. Death rates are 20 times less for 1- to 4-year-old children and 40 times less for 5- to 14-year-old children as compared with death rates for infants. The school-age years have the lowest rate of death, especially for males. However, a sharp rise occurs during later adolescence primarily from injuries, homicide, and suicide—all potentially preventable conditions. A general trend in racial differences that occurs in infant mortality is also apparent in childhood deaths for all ages and for both sexes. Whites have fewer deaths for all ages, and for both racial groups male deaths outnumber female deaths. Of particular note is the trend toward an unchanged rate or an increasing rate in the 15- to 19-year-old age-group for four of the five leading causes of deaths.

After 1 year of age there is a dramatic change in the causes of death, with injuries (accidents) being the leading cause until people reach their early forties. Injuries account for about 45% of all childhood deaths from ages 1 to 14 years (Table 1-6). In young adults ages 15 to 24, injuries, homicide, and suicide are responsible for about 75% of all deaths. Because of their critical importance in child health, injuries are discussed separately on p. 11 and suicide is discussed in Chapter 21.

Violent deaths have been steadily increasing among children. Fortunately, there has been a leveling off and decline in the homicide rate among children, although homicide remains the second leading cause of death in the 15- to 19-year age-group. Suicide, on the other hand, has been increasing and is currently the third leading cause of death in the 15- to 19-year age-group. Children 4 years of age and younger are most likely to be killed by a parent, at home, and by a blunt instrument. Children 12 years and older tend to be killed by non–family members and most frequently by firearms or knives. Homicides that occur in children between 3 and 12 years of age appear to be a mixture of the latter two types (Paulson and Rushforth, 1986).

Fatalities from violence represent only the tip of the iceberg. Nonfatal intentional injuries occur as much as 100 times more frequently. A common misconception about violence is that it is interracial. While blacks are overrepresented in the homicide statistics, little violence is actually racially instigated. Eighty percent of homicides occur between members of the same race. The overrepresentation of blacks in violence statistics reflects their increased incidence of living in poverty. When poverty is controlled as an influencing factor, the difference in incidence of violent deaths among blacks and whites disappears (Spivak, Prothrow-Stith, and Hausman, 1988).

Table 1-5 Death rates of children at selected age intervals according to sex and race, United States, 1987 (rates per 100,000 population in specified group)*

AGE INTERVAL (YEARS)	WHITE		ALL OTHER	
	MALE	FEMALE	MALE	FEMALE
Under 1	942.1	742.9	1,938.0	1,571.5
1-4	52.0	40.5	81.1	65.8
5-9	27.4	17.9	36.6	25.0
10-14	32.8	17.9	43.3	21.9
15-19	116.3	48.7	133.9	46.0

From National Center for Health Statistics: Annual report of final mortality statistics, 1987, Monthly vital statistics report 38(suppl. 5):13, DHHS Pub. No. (PHS) 89-1120, 1989.

*Infant death rates may differ from infant mortality rates, which are based on live births.

The causes of increased violence against children are not fully understood. In young children, the increase may represent more accurate identification of child abuse. In all cases, the problem of child homicides is an extremely complex one, involving numerous social, economic, and other influences. Prevention lies in a better understanding of the social and psychologic factors that lead to the high rates of homicide and suicide. Nurses need to be especially aware of young people who are depressed, repeatedly in trouble with the criminal justice system, or associated with groups known to be violent. Prevention requires identification of these youngsters as well as therapeutic intervention by qualified professionals.

The major declines in death rates during childhood have been due to gastrointestinal diseases, infectious diseases, perinatal conditions, neoplasms, and injuries. The absence of infectious diseases as a leading cause of death is testimony to the role antibacterial agents and immunizations have played in the declining mortality rates and the specific causes of death. More effective treatment of severe infections has resulted in other disorders becoming more prominent in the list of leading killers. Most notable among these are the neoplasms. (The incidence of cancer in children is discussed in Chapter 36.)

However, infectious disease may again play a prominent role in childhood mortality. Of particular concern is the increasing incidence of HIV infection in children. Among children younger than 15 years of age, 360 deaths were reported in 1988, an increase of more than 70% from the 1987 estimate (Wegman, 1989). HIV infection is already the ninth

Table 1-6 Five leading causes of death in children at selected age intervals, United States, 1987 (rates per 100,000)

RANK	AGES 1-4	RATE	AGES 5-14	RATE	AGES 15-24	RATE
	All causes	51.6	All causes	25.6	All causes	99.4*
1	Accidents	20.2	Accidents	12.3	Accidents	48.9*
2	Congenital anomalies	6.4	Cancer	3.3	Homicide	14.0*
3	Cancer	3.8	Congenital anomalies	1.3	Suicide	12.9*
4	Homicide	2.3*	Homicide	1.2*	Cancer	5.1
5	Heart disease	2.2	Heart disease	.9*	Heart disease	2.8*
	HIV infection† (9)	0.7			HIV infection (7)	1.3

National Center for Health Statistics: Advance report of final mortality statistics, 1987, Monthly vital statistics report 38(suppl. 5):19, DHHS Pub No. (PHS) 89-1120., 1989.
*Rates remained unchanged or increased since 1983.
†Human immunodeficiency virus: rank for each age-group in parentheses if HIV in 10 leading causes of death.

leading cause of death among children 1 to 4 years of age and the seventh in young people between the ages of 15 and 24 years. If the current trends continue, acquired immunodeficiency syndrome (AIDS) can be expected to move into the top five leading causes of death in the 1- to 4-year age-group by 1992 (Novello and others, 1989).

MORBIDITY

Morbidity statistics describe the prevalence of a specific illness in the population at a particular time. These are generally presented as rates per 1000 population because of their greater frequency of occurrence. Unlike mortality statistics, morbidity is very difficult to define and may denote acute illness, chronic disease, or disability. The source of data also greatly influences the resulting statistics. Common sources include reasons for visits to physicians, diagnosis for hospital admission, or household interviews, such as the National Health Interview Survey (NHIS), Child Health Supplement. Unlike death rates, which are updated annually, morbidity statistics are revised much less frequently and do not necessarily represent the general population. The following discussion is intended to present an overview of illness in children from a variety of perspectives.

Childhood Morbidity

Acute illness may be defined as symptoms severe enough to limit activity or require medical attention. According to the National Health Interview Survey, children under 5 years of age have about 3.5 acute illnesses per year with 8.8 days of restricted activity. Children 5 to 14 years of age have 2.9 episodes and 9.4 days of disability. As a general rule acute illness is less common in children under 6 months of age, increases thereafter until 3 or 4 years of age, and then gradually decreases throughout middle and older childhood. There is a slight peak again during the first year or two of school, probably as a result of increased exposure to new contagions (Green and Haggerty, 1984).

Infections account for nearly 80% of all childhood illnesses, and respiratory infections lead the list, occurring two to three times as often as all other illnesses combined. The chief illness of childhood is the common cold. The types of diseases that children contract during childhood vary according to age. For example, upper respiratory tract infection and enuresis tend to decrease with age, whereas other disorders, such as acne and headaches, tend to increase with age. Also, children who have any type of problem are more likely to have that problem again than are children in the general population. Morbidity is not distributed randomly in children. Certain children have more than their share of illnesses, even those of the common childhood variety (Starfield and others, 1984). Children from poor families tend to have more health problems than children from nonpoor families, despite the fact that poor families seek medical care less frequently. This finding suggests the need for heightened efforts to improve access to health care for low-income children (Newacheck and Starfield, 1988).

Recent concern has focused on groups of children who have increased morbitity—homeless children, children living in poverty, children of LBW, children with chronic illnesses, foreign-born adopted children, and children in daycare centers. A number of different factors account for these at-risk groups. A major cause is barriers to health care, especially for the homeless, the poverty stricken, and those with chronic health problems (see p. 17). Even in regard to LBW, the physical, social, and psychologic environment after birth probably has the largest impact on the health status of these children (Overpeck and others, 1989). Other reasons include improved survival of children with chronic health problems, particularly infants of very LBW. Children residing in certain at-risk environments, such as country of origin (for adopted children) and daycare centers, are more likely to have a variety of medical conditions, especially infections (Bell and others, 1989; Jenista and Chapman, 1987).

Injury-related morbidity is also significant. Almost 16 million children are seen in emergency rooms for their injuries—600,000 children are hospitalized, and about 30,000 youngsters suffer permanent disability from injuries each year (Division of Injury Control, 1990).

Probably the most important aspect of morbidity is the degree of disability it produces. Disability can be measured in days off from school or days confined to bed. It can be the result of an acute or chronic disorder. On an average, a child loses 5.3 days per year because of injury or illness. Girls miss somewhat more school than boys; however, boys are more likely to miss school because of injuries. Of all children under 17 years of age, over 95% are not disabled in any way. About 2% have mild disability, another 2% have moderate disability, and 0.2% are severely disabled (Pless, 1987). (The incidence of chronic conditions is discussed in Chapter 22.)

Although childhood is a time of relative health, it is the rare child who never becomes ill. Most children experience one or more episodes of acute illness annually and may be disabled for a short time. The rapidity with which children become ill often causes great anxiety for parents, who fear that the illness is serious. Part of nurses' intervention is education of parents regarding the usual types of childhood illness and recognition of those symptoms that require treatment, such as signs of respiratory distress or dehydration. Nurses should also be aware of signs of potentially fatal illnesses. However, the future progress in decreasing childhood morbidity, as in childhood mortality, rests more on parent education than on scientific discoveries such as the antibiotic. Nurses play a vital role in advancing child care through health promotion.

The New Morbidity

In addition to disease and injury, children face other problems that can significantly alter their health. These include behavioral, social (family), and educational problems that are sometimes referred to as the "new morbidity" or "pediatric social illness." Examples of such conditions include child abuse and neglect, nonorganic failure to thrive, injuries, childhood adjustment disorders, learning disorders, and attention deficit-hyperactivity disorder. Estimates on the incidence of these problems vary, but they probably represent at least 5% and as much as 25% to 30% in specific age-groups, social classes, and medical facilities (Starfield, 1980).

One of the dilemmas of the new morbidity is its identification in children. For example, the proportion of children with these problems is *greater* than the number of visits children make to health care facilities with a "new morbidity" diagnosis. Consequently many children seen at a health center have another primary disorder, usually somatic, and are only then diagnosed with a psychosocial or psychosomatic problem. There is greater emphasis from health professionals on organic deviations than on mental or social ones, and since insurance companies generally do not reimburse for counseling required in the care of psychosocial

Table 1-7 Mortality from leading types of injuries, United States, 1986 (rates per 100,000 population in each age-group)

TYPE OF ACCIDENT	AGE (YEARS)			
	UNDER 1	1-4	5-14	15-24
▪ Males				
All causes	1152.7	57.9	31.7	151.4
Accidents (all types)	25.5	23.7	16.8	78.5
Motor vehicle	4.9 (3)*	7.8 (1)	8.9 (1)	58.2 (1)
Drowning†	2.4 (5)	6.0 (2)	2.9 (2)	6.3 (2)
Fires and burns	2.8 (4)	5.0 (3)	1.5 (3)	1.3 (5)
Firearms	—	—	1.0 (4)	2.0 (3)
Ingestion of food/object	5.0 (2)	1.0 (4)	—	—
Mechanical suffocation	5.7 (1)	—	—	—
Falls	—	0.7 (5)	0.3 (5)	—
Poisoning	—	—	—	1.7 (4)
Accidents as a percent of all deaths	2.2%	41%	53%	52%
▪ Females				
All causes	905.8	45.8	19.9	52.3
Accidents (all types)	22.7	16.9	7.9	23.3
Motor vehicle	4.8 (1)	6.2 (1)	4.9 (1)	19.5 (1)
Drowning†	2.6 (5)	3.1 (3)	0.9 (3)	0.5 (4)
Fires and burns	3.6 (3)	4.0 (2)	1.1 (2)	0.8 (2)
Firearms	—	—	0.2 (4)	0.3 (5)
Ingestion of food/object	3.3 (4)	0.7 (4)	—	—
Mechanical suffocation	4.3 (2)	—	—	—
Falls	—	0.4 (5)	<0.05 (5)	—
Poisoning	—	—	—	0.7 (3)
Accidents as a percent of all deaths	2.5%	37%	40%	45%

Modified from National Center for Health Statistics, Public Health Service, U.S. Department of Health and Human Services, as cited in Accident facts, Chicago, 1989, National Safety Council.
*Indicates rank among the leading types of accidents.
†Exclusive of deaths in water transportation.

problems, there is a distinct disincentive to diagnose them. However, children do have such problems, and those working with children, especially nurses in primary care facilities, need to be aware of their potential existence and to deliberately investigate them.

Although no conclusive characteristics have been identified for children with new morbidity problems, some findings are significant in terms of defining a high-risk group. These include children (1) from the lowest socioeconomic strata, (2) ages 7 to 14 years, (3) of male gender, (4) from one-parent families, (5) with a presenting complaint of a chronic physical disorder, (6) with reading skills below grade level, and (7) with higher rates of school absenteeism (Goldberg and others, 1984; Gortmaker and others, 1990; Nader and others, 1981).

INJURIES—THE LEADING KILLER

Injuries, the leading cause of death in children over age 1 year, cause more deaths and disabilities in children than do all causes of disease combined. As children grow older, the percentage of deaths from injuries increases (Table 1-7). Injuries have not shown the dramatic declines seen in other areas of childhood mortality. Some of the reasons include (Committee on Trauma Research, 1985):

1. Injury has traditionally been regarded as an unavoidable accident or a behavioral problem, rather than a health problem. The term *accident* suggests a chaotic, random event that is "luck" or "chance"; the term *injury* is preferred because it connotes a sense of responsibility and control.
2. Injury control, including research, has not received high priority or sufficient financial support. No central agency coordinates or is responsible for reducing the incidence of injuries.
3. Research on injuries has not been based on a theoretical framework, as has been done with diseases. There is a need to view injuries in terms of *host,* the affected person, *environment,* the time and place, and *agent,* the object that is the direct cause.

Host and Agent

The type of injury and the circumstances surrounding it are closely related to normal growth and developmental behavior (Box 1-1). As children develop, their innate curiosity impels them to investigate activities and to mimic the behavior of others. This is essential in order to acquire competency as an adult, but it predisposes them to numerous hazards during childhood.

The developmental stage of the child partially determines the types of injuries that are most likely to occur at a specific age and thus helps provide clues to preventive measures. For example, small infants are helpless in any environment, and when they begin to roll over or otherwise propel themselves, they can fall from unprotected surfaces. The crawling infant with a natural tendency to place objects in the mouth is at risk of aspiration or poisoning. The mobile toddler with the instinct to explore and investigate and the ability to run and climb is subject to a variety of injuries, including falls, burns, and collision with objects. As children grow older, their absorption with play often makes them oblivious to environmental hazards such as street traffic or water, and the need to conform and gain acceptance compels older children and adolescents to accept challenges and dares. Although the highest incidence of injury is in children less than 9 years of age, most fatal injuries occur in later childhood and adolescence.

Children's personalities can be a factor in their susceptibility to injuries, although the evidence for "accident proneness" is contradictory. The temperament characteristics most consistently identified with an increased risk of injury are aggression and overactivity (Bijur, Golding, and Haslum, 1988; Bijur, Stewart-Brown, and Butler, 1986; Bijur

Box 1-1 CHILDHOOD INJURIES: RISK FACTORS

Sex—preponderance of males; difference mainly due to behavioral characteristics, especially aggression
Temperament—children with difficult temperament profile (see Chapter 4), especially persistence, high activity, and negative reactions to new situations (Hyman, 1987)
Stress—predisposes to increased risk taking and self-destructive behavior; general lack of self-protection
Alcohol and drug use—associated with higher incidence of motor vehicle injuries, drownings, homicide, and suicide
Previous history of injury—associated with increased likelihood of another injury, especially if initial injury required hospitalization
Developmental characteristics
- —mismatch between child's developmental level and skill required for activity, for example, all-terrain vehicles
- —natural curiosity to explore environment
- —desire to assert self and challenge rules
- —older child—desire for peer approval and acceptance

Cognitive characteristics (age specific)
- *Infancy*—sensorimotor: explores environment through taste and touch
- *Young child*
  - —object permanence: actively searches for attractive object
  - —cause and effect: unaware of consequential dangers
  - —transductive reasoning: may fail to learn from experiences; for example, falling from step is not perceived as same type of danger as climbing a tree
  - —magical and egocentric thinking: cannot comprehend danger to self or others; cannot take place of others to realize danger; if thinking something is safe, believes it to be so
- *School-age child*—transitional cognitive processes: unable to fully comprehend causal relationships; attempts dangerous acts without detailed planning regarding consequences
- *Adolescent*—formal operations: preoccupied with abstract thinking and loses sight of reality; may lead to feeling of vulnerability

Anatomic characteristics (especially in young children)
- *Large head*—predisposes to cranial injury
- *Large spleen and liver with wide costal arch*—predisposes to direct trauma to these organs
- *Small and light body*—may be thrown easily, especially inside a moving vehicle

Other factors—poverty, family stress (i.e., maternal illness, recent environmental change), substandard alternative child care, young maternal age, low maternal education, multiple siblings (Scheidt, 1988)

and others, 1988). These two traits may explain why boys at all ages have more injuries than girls, a trend that increases as children grow older.

The pattern of deaths caused by injuries, especially from motor vehicles, drowning, and burns, is remarkably consistent in most Western societies, such as Canada. Table 1-7 compares the leading causes of deaths from injuries for each age-group according to sex. The overwhelming cause of death in children over 1 year of age is motor vehicle (MV)–related fatalities, including passenger, pedestrian, bicycle, and motorcycle deaths (Fig. 1-1) (Paulson, 1989). Even though the *percentage* of infants dying from MV injuries is small compared with the total number of deaths in that age-group, children under 1 year of age have a high death rate from MV passenger deaths (primarily from failure to be properly restrained).

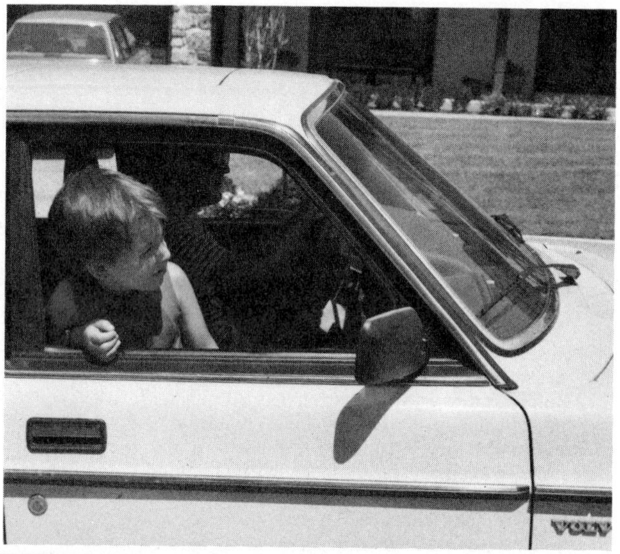

Fig. 1-1. Motor vehicle injuries are the leading cause of death in children over age 1 year.

Although MV injuries accounted for 57% of accidental deaths among the young in 1975 and 65% in 1984, the death rate from MV injuries actually decreased from 22 to 19.6 per 100,000 young persons during that period (Hoekelman and Pless, 1988). The incidence of vehicular injuries, especially among young children, has been declining, probably as a result of child passenger restraint laws (see Questions and Controversies, p. 14). Currently, all states in the United States have enacted legislation requiring young children to be properly restrained in motor vehicles. However, seat belt laws vary from state to state in terms of the ages of children covered, types of vehicles affected, penalties for noncompliance, and other special provisions (Faber, 1986). Therefore, the effect of mandatory seat belt laws on mortality varies according to different reports.

With the decline in deaths from automobile accidents, recent attention has turned to injuries to riders on bicycles, all-terrain vehicles (ATVs), buses, and airplanes, and to pedestrians. Approximately 400 to 500 children die each year in the United States from bicycling injuries, and the majority of these deaths are due to head injury (Weiss, 1986). Despite the banning of three-wheel ATVs in 1988, four-wheel ATVs are sold and present a danger to young riders, especially those under 16 years of age (Dolan, Knapp, and Andres, 1989) (see also Motor Vehicle Injury, Chapter 17). Buses are exempt from mandatory seat belt laws, and there is evidence that such protection would save lives (Spital,

A

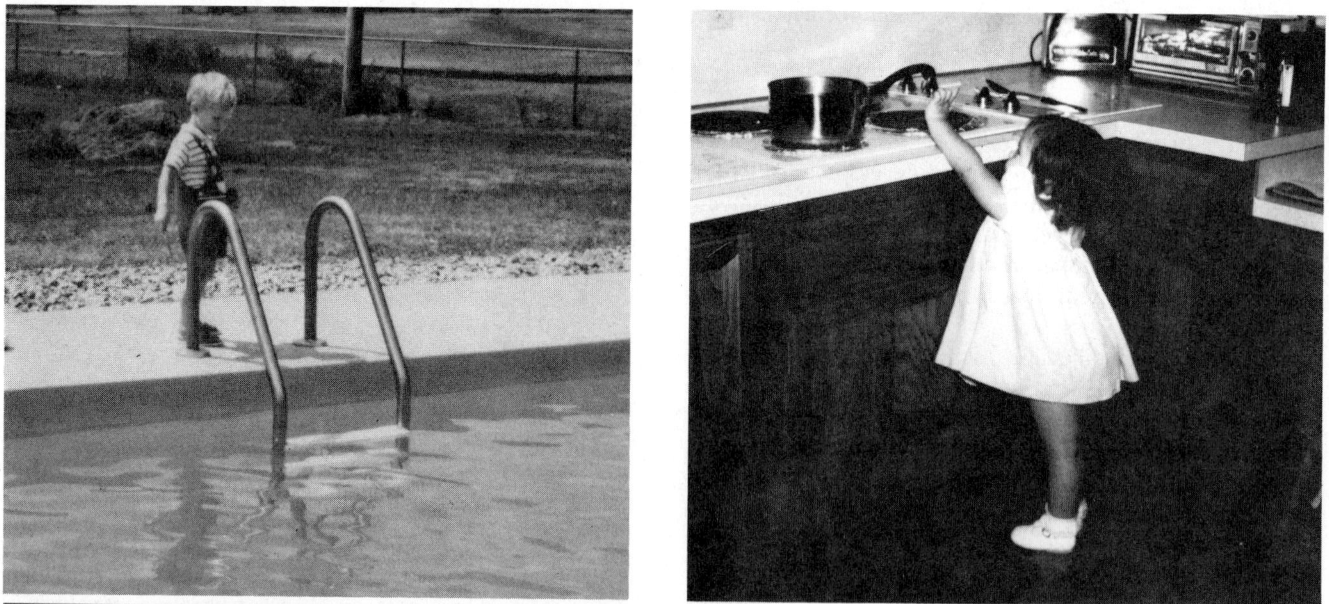

B

Fig. 1-2. A, Drowning is the second leading cause of death in boys and the third in girls ages 1 to 14 years. **B,** Burns are the second leading cause of death from injury in girls and the third in boys ages 1 to 14 years.

Spital, and Spital, 1986). Airlines are also considering seat requirements for children under 2 years, an age-group that has been allowed to travel free on an adult's lap (Nelms, 1990). About 44% of children under age 15 who die from automobile-related injuries are pedestrians (Committee on Accident, 1987). Sadly, parents may not be as aware of the dangers of this activity as they should be, thus exposing children to this risk (Rivara, Bergman, and Drake, 1989).

When accidental deaths are compared according to sex and age, the causes of death differ. Drowning and burns are the second and third leading causes of death in boys ages 1 to 14, but the order is reversed in girls (Fig. 1-2). In addition, firearms are a major cause of death in males but not in females (Fig. 1-3). During infancy, more males succumb to death from aspiration than do females (Fig. 1-4). More than half of all poisonings occur in children under 2 years of age (Fig. 1-5). By age 4 to 5 years, nonintentional poisonings are uncommon. Another increase occurs in the 15- to 24-year age-group, where it is the fourth leading cause of death from injury. Poisoning in this age-group is typically intentional and usually represents death from suicide (especially females) or drug abuse.

Analyzing deaths from specific types of injuries by age

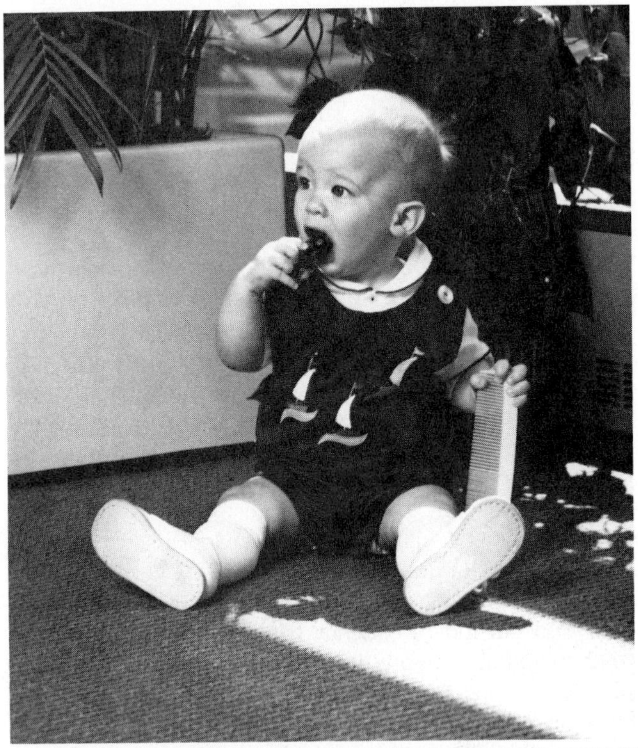

Fig. 1-4. Aspiration/suffocation is the leading cause of death from injury in infants, especially in males.

Fig. 1-3. Firearms are the fourth leading cause of death in boys and girls ages 5 to 14 years and the third cause in boys ages 15 to 24.

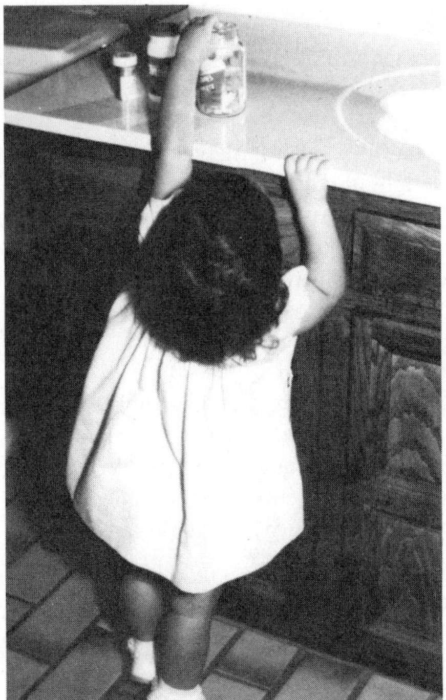

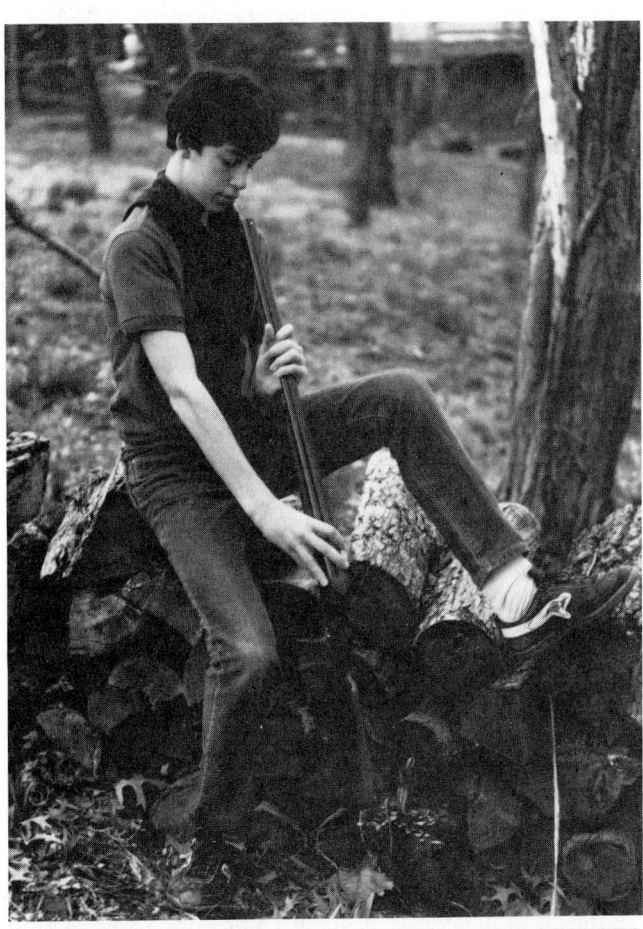

Fig. 1-5. Poisoning causes a considerable number of injuries in children under 4 years of age, but is the third and fourth leading causes of death from injury in females and males, respectively, ages 15 to 24.

and sex is useful in identifying high-risk groups. When comparing accidental deaths with other causes of childhood mortality, it is clear that preventing injuries offers the greatest promise for improving survival. Nurses certainly play a major role in providing anticipatory guidance to parents and older children regarding hazards during each age period.

Environment

A number of environmental factors, such as place, time, and equipment, contribute to injuries. The highest number of injuries occurs in the home, especially in children younger than 6 years of age. Older children have almost as many injuries outside the home, especially at school and recreational sites. Among recreational and sports activities, football is one of the most hazardous athletic activities, accounting for 20 injuries per 100,000 participants per year. Serious, potentially fatal injuries result from spinal cord trauma. Among females, gymnastics appears to pose the greatest risks (Runyan and Gerken, 1989).

Injuries from bicycling, a common recreational activity, tend to occur most frequently between 4 and 8 PM and on road conditions that are described as hazardous, for example, bumps, potholes, and gravel. In addition, the child's bicycle is often in need of repair (Selbst and Alexander, 1987). For drowning, the second leading cause of death, the risk factors include living in a warm climate, swimming in undesignated areas, inability to swim, not using or misusing a personal flotation device, and using open boats (Gulaid and others, 1988).

Recent attention has focused on the incidence of injuries on farms, where many children reside and work. Injuries occur most frequently among males ages 10 to 19 years and result primarily from farm machinery (tractors, wagons, and trucks) (American Academy of Pediatrics, 1988; Salmi and others, 1989).

Identification of environmental hazards has in some instances had tremendous influence on reducing the incidence of fatal injuries; for example, placing fences around swimming pools and guards on windows has decreased the incidence of fatal drownings and falls (see Questions and Controversies).

Injury Prevention

Theoretically all injuries are preventable, and one of the chief nursing responsibilities is to anticipate and recognize where safety measures are applicable. Injury prevention necessitates protection, education, and legislation. The two major strategies for injury prevention are:

1. **Passive strategies,** which provide automatic protection by product and environmental design, for example, the use of automatic seat belts or airbags. Such devices require no active participation by the individual and have the greatest success rate.
2. **Active strategies,** which *persuade* individuals to change their behavior for increased self-protection, such as using seat belts voluntarily, or *require* compliance with safety regulations, such as laws that mandate use of safety restraints in young children. Persuasion through education has been much less effective than legislated change, although it remains a key strategy.

QUESTIONS AND CONTROVERSIES

How effective are injury prevention programs in reducing the incidence of injuries in children?

The success of injury prevention programs has been variable. The most effective interventions for injury prevention have been passive strategies and legislation, including the following:

Mandatory seat belt laws—have reduced motor vehicle deaths and nonfatal injuries in all age-groups, especially young children but less so among adolescents (Chorba, Reinfurt, and Hulka, 1988; Orsay and others, 1988; Sewell and others, 1986; Wagenaar and Webster, 1986). However, the eventual decline in seat belt use after initiation of the legislation and the high misuse of child restraint systems continue to be major problems (Faber, 1986; Margolis, Wagenaar, and Molnar, 1988).

Increasing minimum drinking age—has reduced fatal motor vehicle crashes among youth; one program demonstrated a 33% decline in alcohol-related motor vehicle deaths among persons ages 15 through 18 years and a 38% decline among persons 19 through 20 years (Decker, Graitcer, and Shaffner, 1988).

Federal Hazardous Substances Labeling Act and the Poison Prevention Packaging Act—have significantly reduced the number of poisonings by limiting the number of tablets in a container, using child-resistant closures, and limiting exposure to the toxin (Walton, 1982).

Flammable Fabrics Act and the use of smoke detectors—have reduced deaths from burns (Miller and others, 1982).

Use of window guards—has reduced falls from windows in one city by 50% (Spiegel and Lindaman, 1977).

Unfortunately, educational programs to reduce childhood injuries have been less successful. For example, less than 5% of children wear bicycle safety helmets, despite evidence that they can reduce risk of death and serious head injury. One study showed an 85% reduction in the risk of head injury in persons involved in bicycle injuries (Thompson, Rivara, and Thompson, 1989). Initial results of a community-wide helmet campaign to increase the use of safety helmets has been promising, but long-term compliance is unknown (DiGuiseppi and others, 1989). Although driver education is thought to promote safe driving skills, increasing the availability of driver education increases the involvement of teenagers in motor vehicle crashes. Thus, such programs may have a negative impact (Runyan and Gerken, 1989). Obviously, injury prevention is a complex process and one that requires controlled studies to document its short- and long-term success in reducing fatal and nonfatal injury.

The preventive aspects of child care are an ongoing part of health promotion throughout childhood. To protect the child from injury, persons who are responsible for children need to be aware of the normal behavior characteristics that render children vulnerable to injuries and to be alert to factors in the environment that create a hazard to their safety. Parents and others are often surprisingly unaware of their child's developmental progress and capabilities. Anticipatory guidance regarding developmental expectations serves to alert the parents to the type of injuries that are most likely to occur at any given age and to environmental circumstances that might precipitate an injury. For example, infants must not be left where they can fall or roll over and toddlers must not be given objects or toys with small removable parts or sharp edges or given unsupervised access to places where they can fall, drown, or be burned.

Very early in the parent-child relationship the parents need to learn how to provide a safe environment for their child, what kinds of behaviors they can expect of the child at various stages in the child's development, and their responsibility for the safety of their child. This is particularly important for first-time parents. Safety responsibility in such areas as purchase of infant equipment, especially a car restraint, should begin *before* the child is born.

It cannot be assumed that parents of one or more children are familiar with all areas of child safety. Moreover, the addition of a new child brings up the issue of sibling rivalry and the unwelcome but realistic possibility that the new child may be at risk from a jealous older sibling. For example, the parents should be cautioned against leaving the infant alone with the older child who feels threatened by the newcomer.

Providing a safe environment for the child involves the combined efforts of family, nurses, and community. At each age level there are environmental attractions that are hazardous to the safety of the child. The specific hazards vary according to season (drowning, injuries related to winter heating devices), geographic area (water injuries in areas with swimming pools, rivers, lakes; heater burns in cold climates), and socioeconomic level (lead poisoning and street injuries in slum areas, bicycle injuries in middle-class areas).

Cultural factors also need to be considered when instituting safety instruction, since noncompliance is one of the major deterrents to injury prevention. For example, cultural characteristics, such as the lack of future orientation and resistance to changing long-standing habits, can interfere with a cultural group's acceptance of injury prevention practices (Foss, 1987). One study found that efforts regarding the use of seat belts among Mexican-American parents were more effective when the dominant decision-making male in the family and the influential older woman, often a grandmother, were included in the educational efforts (Faber, 1986).

Safety should be an intrinsic element of nursing practice. Nurses who themselves practice safety, who are alert to safety needs in the environment, and who recognize the need for safety education contribute to injury reduction. The special problems and preventive measures are discussed as appropriate throughout the book and are related to the various age levels and conditions that predispose to specific hazards.

EVOLUTION OF CHILD HEALTH CARE IN THE UNITED STATES*

Children in colonial America were born into a world with many hazards to their health and survival. Epidemics were common, and no control or treatment was known. Physicians were few, and only a small number had any formal training. Midwives also were untrained, basing their practice on past experiences. Books providing information on child care and feeding were scarce and, when available, were useful only to a minority of literate parents.

Medical care by physicians was limited to wealthy European families who lived in or could travel to more developed cities. Children who lived on farms were mainly cared for by another family member or by a competent neighbor. Traveling medicine men, with their various forms of quackery, were common. Black children who were bought as slaves or born to slaves had only as much care as their owner was able or willing to provide (Scott and Winston, 1976). American Indian children were treated for disease according to the tradition of each tribe, which was often a mixture of medicine, magic, and religion (Sayre and Sayre, 1976). With the colonization of America the Indians were exposed to many new diseases, which were fatal to large numbers of them.

Statistics on childhood mortality during the colonial period are largely unavailable. Epidemic diseases were prevalent, however, and included smallpox, measles, mumps, chickenpox, influenza, diphtheria, yellow fever, cholera, and whooping cough, but the disease that surpassed all others as a cause of childhood death was dysentery. Sometimes entire families succumbed to this illness. Other diseases that were major contributors to childhood illness were the "slow epidemic" of tuberculosis, nutritional diseases, and injuries (Schmidt, 1976).

Although scientific knowledge was accumulating, especially from work done in Europe, there were no organized efforts in the United States to apply that knowledge to the care of the sick. It was not until the Industrial Revolution was well under way in the nineteenth century that the consequences of childhood illness and injury and the effects of child labor, poverty, and neglect became more widely recognized. The end of the nineteenth century is often regarded as the dark ages of pediatrics, and the first half of the twentieth century as the dawn of improved health care for children (Cone, 1976).

The study of pediatrics began in the last half of the 1800s, particularly under the influence of a Prussian-born physician, Abraham Jacobi (1830-1919), who is referred to as the Father of Pediatrics (Leopold, 1957). He was awarded the first professorship in pediatrics in America in 1870, started pediatric departments in several New York hospitals, and was one of the founders of the American Pediatric Society in 1888. With several other physicians he pioneered in the scientific and clinical investigation of childhood diseases. One outstanding achievement was the es-

*JoAnn Gephart, R.N., M.S.N., assisted in the revision of this section.

tablishment of "milk stations," where mothers could bring sick children for treatment and learn the importance of pure milk and its proper preparation.

The crusade for pure milk helped bring the dairy industry under legal control and led to the establishment of infant welfare stations. The remarkable decline in infant mortality since 1900 has been achieved through prevention and health-promoting measures such as improved sanitation and pasteurization of milk. Before these regulations existed, the unsanitary milk supply was a chief source of infantile diarrhea and bovine tuberculosis. Cows were often kept in filthy stables and fed garbage and distillery wastes. Milk from cows fed distillery wastes was reported to make infants "tipsy." Some of the cows were so diseased with tuberculosis that they had to be raised on cranes to be milked (Cone, 1976).

At about the same time increasing concern developed for the social welfare of children, especially those who were homeless or employed as factory laborers. The work of one such reformer, Lillian Wald (1867-1940), had far-reaching effects on child health and nursing. She founded the Henry Street Settlement in New York City, which eventually provided nursing service, social work, and an organized program of social, cultural, and educational activities. Wald is regarded as the founder of public health or community nursing. She was instrumental in establishing the role of the first full-time school nurse, Lina Rogers. Soon other nurses were employed to teach parents and children about the prevention or need for treatment of minor skin conditions, malnutrition, and other impairments or illnesses identified in the school. An outgrowth of nursing involvement in school health was the development of pediatric courses and specialized clinical experience in schools of nursing.

As more causes of disease were identified, there was an emphasis on isolation and asepsis. In the early 1900s children with contagious diseases were isolated from adult patients. Parents were prohibited from visiting because they might transmit disease to and from the home. Even toys and personal articles of clothing were kept from the child. It was not until the 1940s and the famous work of Spitz and Robertson on institutionalized children that the effects of isolation and maternal deprivation were recognized. This brought forth a surge of interest in the psychologic health of children and resulted in changes for hospitalized children, such as rooming-in, sibling visitations, child life (play) programs, prehospitalization preparation, parent education, and hospital schooling.

Influenced by social reformers such as Lillian Wald, national leaders began to take action to improve children's living conditions. In 1909 President Theodore Roosevelt called the first White House Conference on Children. It focused on care of dependent children and attempted to address the deplorable working conditions of youngsters. As a result of this conference, the U.S. Children's Bureau was established under the jurisdiction of the Department of Labor, since at that time laws to regulate child labor were seen as the greatest need. Later, the Bureau was placed under the Department of Health, Education and Welfare (now the Department of Health and Human Services). White House conferences were held approximately every 10 years until 1980 to address the welfare, health, education, social, economic, and psychologic needs of children.

The establishment of the Children's Bureau in 1912 marked the beginning of a period of studies of economic and social factors related to infant mortality, maternal deaths, and maternal and infant care in rural areas, all of which created the basis for stimulating better standards of care for mothers and children. This helped lead to the first Maternity and Infancy Act (Sheppard-Towner Act) in 1921, which provided grants to states to develop a Division of Maternal and Child Health (MCH) as a unit of the health department. However, this bill eventually lapsed because of opposition from those who viewed it as a socialist movement.

With the passage of Title V of the Social Security Act (SSA) in 1935, a federal-state partnership was established under the administration of the Children's Bureau. Title V included federal grants-in-aid to states, matched by state funds, for three types of work: maternal and child health (MCH), Crippled Children's Services (CCS), and child welfare services. The first programs provided by Title V were prenatal, postnatal, and child health clinics and training of personnel; the early programs also emphasized casefinding, multidisciplinary teams, demonstrations, and special projects. The early emphasis of the CCS Program was on orthopedic care. With the recognition that a child's ability to function could also be limited by a chronic illness, state CCS programs became involved with children with developmental, behavioral, and educational problems and more recently with home care of children with complex medical conditions. This broadened concept was officially reflected in the 1985 passage of legislation that changed the name of the CCS to the Program for Children with Special Health Needs (CSHN). Most of the states have replaced the words "crippled children" in their official designations with more current terms such as "special children's services" or "handicapped children's program."

The passage of the Omnibus Budget Reconciliation Act of 1981 (P.L. 97-35) (OBRA) created the MCH Services Block Grant and provided for continuation of Title V of the SSA as a state-federal partnership. The MCH Services Block Grant consolidated seven existing categorical programs (Maternal and Child Health/Crippled Children's Services — Title V; Social Security Income [SSI]; Hemophilia; Sudden Infant Death Syndrome; Lead-Based Paint Poisoning Prevention; Genetic Diseases; and Adolescent Health Services) into one block, allowing each state to develop its own programs and set its own priorities.

The MCH Block Grant, administered under the MCH Bureau of the DHHS, is a principal source of support to states, assisting them in their efforts to maintain and strengthen the planning, promoting, and coordinating of health care of mothers and children. Of the total MCH block grant appropriation, 85% provides funds to state health agencies and 15% is set aside for use as Special Projects of Regional and National Significance (SPRANS) and to support overall MCH efforts. Examples of these efforts are infant mortality reviews, breast-feeding promotion, child health systems development, reduction and prevention of violence and injury, family-centered comprehensive community-based coordinated care models for children with special health care needs, and integrated adolescent health program models.

Other federal programs have had a major impact on maternal and child health. In 1965 Medicaid was created under Title XIX of the SSA to reduce financial barriers to health care for the poor. Under Medicaid, the Early and Periodic Screening Diagnosis and Treatment Program (EPSDT) provides preventive and curative services to children younger than 21 years of age. However, not all poor children are eligible for Medicaid. Financial eligibility varies considerably from state to state. For example, some states set payment standards at or above 75% of the federal poverty level, whereas a few states set their standards at 25% of the poverty level or lower (Report to Congress, 1988).

In 1966 the Special Supplemental Food Program for Women, Infants, and Children (WIC) was passed. It provides nutritious food and nutrition education to low-income, pregnant, postpartum, and lactating women and to infants and children up to age 5. Other nutrition programs include Food Stamps, National School Lunch Program, School Breakfast Program, and Child Care Food Program, which provides financial assistance for nutritious meals to children in daycare centers, family and group daycare homes, and Head Start centers.

The last two decades have witnessed significant legislation regarding individuals with chronic conditions. In 1975 the Education for All Handicapped Children Act (P.L. 94-142) was passed to provide a free appropriate public education to all handicapped children from ages 3 to 21 and to provide for those supportive services (speech, counseling, and so on) that ensure the benefit of special education.

In 1986 the Education of the Handicapped Amendments Act (P.L. 99-457) was enacted to broaden the scope of the earlier law by expanding services for infants and toddlers and their families. A significant aspect of this new law calls for the development of an Individualized Family Service Plan (IFSP), which requires that each infant or toddler and family served receive a multidisciplinary assessment of their particular strengths and needs in order to receive appropriate services.

One of the most drastic changes in health care delivery has been the establishment of a prospective payment system based on diagnosis related groups (DRGs). The DRG categories allow pretreatment (prospective) billing for almost all United States hospitals reimbursed by Medicare. With hospitals now financially responsible when Medicare patients exceed the allotted admission stay, more patients are being discharged early. This has created an immense need for home care and other sources of community-based services. The exact impact DRGs will have on pediatric care is uncertain, but with containment of health care cost a national priority, it is inevitable that some form of prospective payment will affect children. Nurses need to be aware of the changing economics and prepared to meet the challenges.

Despite the number of federal and state programs available to assist children and families, there are serious barriers to health care in the United States. For example, 16 million children under the age of 21 years are uninsured, and 1 out of every 5 children lives in poverty. These barriers to care include *financial barriers*, such as not having insurance or having insurance that does not cover certain services; *system barriers*, such as having to travel great distances for health care or state-to-state variations in Medicaid benefits; or *knowledge barriers*, such as not knowing about the need or value of prenatal or child health supervision or being unaware of the services that are available (AAP Special Report, 1989). The current thrust in health care initiative is to improve children's and families' access to health care.

PEDIATRIC NURSING

Nursing of infants and children is consistent with the definition of nursing as "the diagnosis and treatment of human responses to actual or potential health problems" (Nursing, 1980). Its purpose is to promote the highest possible state of health in each child. Pediatric nursing consists of preventing disease or injury; assisting children, including those with a permanent disability or health problem, to achieve and maintain an optimum level of health and development; and treating or rehabilitating children who have health deviations. At all times nursing of children incorporates the family in the scope of care.

ROLE OF THE PEDIATRIC NURSE

Pediatric nurses are involved in every aspect of a child's growth and development. Nursing functions vary according to regional job structures, individual education and experience, and personal career goals. Just as clients (children and their families) present a vast and unique background, so it is that each nurse will bring to the clients an individual set of variables that will affect their relationship. No matter where pediatric nurses practice, their primary concern is the welfare of the child and family.

Family Advocacy

Although the nurse is responsible to self, the profession, and the institution of employment, primary responsibility is to the recipient of nursing services, the child and family. The nurse must work with members of the family, identifying their goals and needs, and plan interventions that best meet the defined problems. As a consumer advocate the nurse has the goal of ensuring that families are aware of all available health services, informed adequately of treatments and procedures, involved in the child's care when possible, and encouraged to change or support existing health care practices. The pediatric nurse is aware of the United Nations Declaration of the Rights of the Child (Box 1-2) and practices within these guidelines to ensure that every child receives optimum care.

Box 1-2 UNITED NATIONS DECLARATION OF THE RIGHTS OF THE CHILD

Preamble

Whereas the peoples of the United Nations have, in the Charter, reaffirmed their faith in fundamental human rights, and in the dignity and worth of the human person, and have determined to promote social progress and better standards of life in larger freedom,

Whereas the United Nations has, in the Universal Declaration of Human Rights, proclaimed that everyone is entitled to all the rights and freedoms set forth therein, without distinction of any kind, such as race, color, sex, language, religion, political or other opinion, national or social origin, property, birth or other status,

Whereas the child, by reason of his physical and mental immaturity, needs special safeguards and care, including appropriate legal protection, before as well as after birth,

Whereas the need for such special safeguards has been stated in the Geneva Declaration of the Rights of the Child of 1924, and recognized in the Universal Declaration of Human Rights and in the statutes of specialized agencies and international organizations concerned with welfare of children,

Whereas mankind owes to the child the best it has to give

Now Therefore the General Assembly Proclaims

This Declaration of the Rights of the Child to the end that he may have a happy childhood and enjoy for his own good and for the good of society the rights and freedoms herein set forth, and calls upon parents, upon men and women as individuals and upon voluntary organizations, local authorities and national governments to recognize these rights and strive for their observance by legislative and other measures progressively taken in accordance with the following principles:

Principle 1

The child shall enjoy all the rights set forth in this Declaration. All children, without any exception whatsoever, shall be entitled to these rights, without distinction or discrimination on account of race, color, sex, language, religion, political or other opinion, national or social origin, property, birth or other status, whether of himself or his family.

Principle 2

The child shall enjoy special protection, and shall be given opportunities and facilities, by law and by other means, to enable him to develop physically, mentally, morally, spiritually and socially in a healthy and normal manner and in conditions of freedom and dignity. In the enactment of laws for this purpose the best interests of the child shall be the paramount consideration.

Principle 3

The child shall be entitled from his birth to a name and a nationality.

Principle 4

The child shall enjoy the benefits of social security. He shall be entitled to grow and develop in health; to this end special care and protection shall be provided both to him and to his mother, including adequate pre-natal and post-natal care. The child shall have the right to adequate nutrition, housing, recreation and medical services.

Principle 5

The child who is physically, mentally or socially handicapped shall be given the special treatment, education and care required by his particular condition.

Principle 6

The child, for the full and harmonious development of his personality, needs love and understanding. He shall, wherever possible, grow up in the care and under the responsibility of his parents, and in any case in an atmosphere of affection and of moral and maternal security; a child of tender years shall not, save in exceptional circumstances, be separated from his mother. Society and the public authorities shall have the duty to extend particular care to children without a family and to those without adequate means of support. Payment of state and other assistance toward the maintenance of children of large families is desirable.

Principle 7

The child is entitled to receive education, which shall be free and compulsory, at least in the elementary stages. He shall be given an education which will promote his general culture, and enable him on a basis of equal opportunity to develop his abilities, his individual judgment, and his sense of moral and social responsibility, and to become a useful member of society.

The best interests of the child shall be the building principle of those responsible for his education and guidance; that responsibility lies in the first place with his parents.

The child shall have full opportunity for play and recreation, which shall be directed to the same purposes as education; society and the public authorities shall endeavor to promote the enjoyment of this right.

Principle 8

The child shall in all circumstances be among the first to receive protection and relief.

Principle 9

The child shall be protected against all forms of neglect, cruelty and exploitation. He shall not be the subject of traffic, in any form.

The child shall not be admitted to employment before an appropriate minimum age; he shall in no case be caused or permitted to engage in any occupation or employment which would prejudice his health or education, or interfere with his physical, mental or moral development.

Principle 10

The child shall be protected from practices which may foster racial, religious and any other form of discrimination. He shall be brought up in a spirit of understanding, tolerance, friendship among peoples, peace and universal brotherhood and in full consciousness that his energy and talents should be devoted to the service of his fellow men.

Box 1-3 PEDIATRIC BILL OF RIGHTS—A CHILD'S VIEW

Any person regardless of age has the right to refuse pedeatric care.
Any person regardless of age has the right to pick there own pedeatrision, if there a girl they can pick a girl, if there a boy they can pick a boy.
Any person regardless of age has the right to not take there medicen if they dont want to.
Any person regardless of age has the right not to wear those paperthings at the doctors office.
Any person regardless of age has the right not to get weighed at the doctors office.

Andreasen, S.: Pediatrics 55(3):370, 1975. Copyright American Academy of Pediatrics 1975.

Of special significance is the nurse's role as child advocate. The Pediatric Bill of Rights, composed by a 10-year-old child, clearly states the child's views regarding the desired "rights" (Box 1-3). Unfortunately, most of these "rights" are not in the child's best interest when health care is needed. However, they emphasize the need for nurses to consider the child's feelings and to individualize care to allow for personal preferences, fears, and dislikes. The concept of atraumatic care is particularly important to the pediatric nurse. *Atraumatic care* is the provision of therapeutic care in settings, by personnel, and through the use of interventions that eliminates or minimizes the psychologic and physical distress experienced by children and their families in the health care system (Wong, 1989). The overriding principle in providing atraumatic care is first do no harm. A concern for the child's total welfare is the priority.

Throughout the text there are numerous examples relating to special needs of children in various age-groups. As child advocate the nurse uses this knowledge to adapt care for the child's optimum physical and emotional well-being. Examples of this may be fostering the parent-child relationship during hospitalization, preparing the child before any unfamiliar treatment or procedure, allowing the child privacy, providing play activities for expression of fear, aggression, or loss of control, and respecting cultural differences relating to childrearing practices.

The nurse is aware of the needs of children and works with all caregivers to ensure that these fundamental requirements are met. This often necessitates that the nurse expand the boundaries of practice to less traditional settings. The nurse may be involved in education, political/legislative change, rehabilitation, screening, administration, and even engineering and architecture. Regardless of how removed from direct patient care individual nurses become, they continue to foster health care practices that promote the well-being of children by incorporating knowledge of child growth and development into particular roles of practice. For example, as educator the nurse has the primary responsibility of helping others learn about and care for children. The audience for this information may be other nurses, parents, schoolteachers, other members of the health team, or the general public. In some states nurses are involved in mass media programs for immunization of all children.

Illness Prevention/Health Promotion

The emerging trend toward health care has been prevention of illness and maintenance of health, rather than treatment of disease or disability. Nursing has kept pace with this change, especially in the area of child care. In 1965 specialized *pediatric nurse practitioner (PNP)* programs began to develop that have led to several specialized ambulatory or primary care roles for nurses. The thrust of these programs has been to educate nurses beyond the basic preparational stage in areas of child health maintenance so that all children can receive high-quality care. The practitioner programs have expanded to prepare school nurse practitioners, hospital nurse practitioners, and other specialists, such as the developmental pediatric nurse practitioner. Although the curriculum varies from program to program, the course content generally includes history taking, physical diagnosis, growth and development, health education, counseling, common childhood problems, and planning care for individuals and groups.

The *clinical nurse specialist (CNS)* role has been developed in an attempt to provide expert nursing care. The term *nurse clinician* is based on a primary philosophy of clinical competence in direct patient care. The clinical specialist is competent in providing nursing care during all stages of illness or wellness and functions in any of the settings where patients may be found—the hospital, home, community, clinic, or long-term facility. The CNS role has developed within each of the traditional specialty areas, as well as in other areas. The educational preparation includes a graduate degree in nursing that may incorporate the practitioner skills. In some settings the roles of the PNP and CNS are merging to create a new professional—advanced practice nurse (Gleeson and others, 1990).

The pediatric CNS plays an important role in the care of children, performing all the functions of the pediatric nurse. In addition, however, the CNS should serve as a role model to the staff for clinical practice, a researcher to validate nursing observations and interventions, a change agent within the health care system, and a consultant/teacher to the health care team.

Every nurse involved with child care must practice preventive health. Regardless of the identified problem, the role of the nurse is to plan care that fosters every aspect of growth and development. Based on a thorough assessment process, problems related to nutrition, immunizations, safety, dental care, development, socialization, discipline, or schooling frequently become obvious. Once the problem is identified, the nurse acts to intervene directly or to refer the family to other health persons or agencies.

The best approach to prevention is education and anticipatory guidance. In this book each chapter on health promotion includes sections on anticipatory guidance. An appreciation of the hazards or conflicts of each developmental period enables the nurse to guide parents regarding childrearing practices aimed at preventing potential problems. One of the most significant examples is safety. Since each age-group is at risk for special types of injuries, preventive teaching can help prevent most injuries, thus significantly lowering permanent disability and mortality from injuries in children.

Prevention also involves less obvious aspects of child care. Besides preventing physical disease or injury, the nurse's role is also to promote mental health. For example, it is not sufficient to administer immunizations without regard for the psychologic trauma associated with the procedure. Optimum health involves the practice of good medicine with a humane approach to health care; the nurse is often the one professional capable of ensuring "humanity." Because of the current educational emphasis on holistic care, the extended and less formal interaction with the family, and the nursing role within the health team, the nurse's role is often one of *facilitator* of care rather than direct intervenor.

Health Teaching

Health teaching is inseparable from family advocacy and prevention. Health teaching may be a direct goal of the nurse, such as during parenting classes, or may be indirect, such as informing parents and children of a diagnosis or medical treatment, encouraging children to ask questions about their bodies, referring families to health-related professional or lay groups, and supplying patients with appropriate literature. Anticipatory guidance is one of the most important types of health teaching.

Health teaching is often one area in which nurses feel competent because it involves translating information rather than receiving messages, translating them, and planning intervention. In other words, it is a concrete, structured type of communication as opposed to other emotionally laden, nondirected types of interaction. However, the nurse focuses on giving appropriate health teaching with generous feedback and evaluation to promote learning.

Support/Counseling

Attention to emotional needs requires support and sometimes counseling. Frequently, the role of child advocate or health teacher is supportive by the very nature of the individualized approach. Support can be offered in many ways, the most common of which include listening, touching, and physical presence. The last two are most helpful with children because they facilitate nonverbal communication.

Counseling involves a mutual exchange of ideas and opinions that provides the basis for mutual problem solving. Although it is similar to health teaching, its focus is broader and more intense because it frequently implies some crisis or upsetting event that needs intervention. It involves support as well as teaching, techniques to foster expression of feelings or thoughts, and approaches to help the family cope with stress. Optimally counseling not only results in a resolved problem but also helps the family attain a higher level of functioning, greater self-esteem, and closer relationships. Although counseling is often the role of nurses in more specialized areas, counseling techniques are discussed in various sections of the text to help students and nurses cope with immediate crises and refer families for additional professional assistance.

Therapeutic Role

The most basic of all nursing roles is the restoration of health through caregiving activities. Nurses are intimately involved with meeting the physical and emotional needs of children, including feeding, bathing, toileting, dressing, security, and socialization. Although they are responsible for instituting physicians' orders, they are also held singularly accountable for their own actions and judgments regardless of written orders.

A significant aspect of restoration of health is continual assessment and evaluation of physical status. Indeed, the concentrated focus throughout the text on physical assessment, pathophysiology, and scientific rationale for therapy is to assist the nurse in decision making regarding health status. Only when aware of normal findings can the nurse intelligently identify and document deviations. In addition, the pediatric nurse never loses sight of the emotional and developmental needs of the individual child, which can significantly influence the course of the disease process.

Coordination/Collaboration

The nurse, as a member of the health team, collaborates and coordinates nursing services with the activities of other professionals. Working in isolation does not serve the child's best interest. First, the concept of "holistic care" can only be realized through a unified interdisciplinary approach. Second, aware of individual contributions and limitations to the child's care, the nurse must collaborate with other specialists to provide for high-quality health services. Failure to recognize limitations can be nontherapeutic at best and destructive at worst. For example, the nurse who feels competent in counseling but who is really inadequate in this area may not only prevent the child from dealing with a crisis but may also impede future success with a qualified professional.

Even nurses who practice in isolated geographic areas widely separated from other health professionals cannot be considered independent. Every nurse works interdependently with the child and family, collaborating on needs and interventions so that the final care plan is one that truly meets the child's needs. Unfortunately, this is one aspect of collaboration and coordination that is lacking in health care planning. Often numerous disciplines work together to formulate a comprehensive approach without consulting with clients regarding their ideas or preferences. The nurse is in a vital position to include consumers in their care, either directly or indirectly, by communicating their thoughts to the health team.

Ethical decision making*

Ethical dilemmas arise when competing moral considerations underlie various alternatives. Parents, nurses, physi-

*This section was written by Cindy Hylton Rushton, R.N.C., M.S.N.

cians, and other health care team members may reach different but morally defensible decisions by assigning different weight to the competing moral values. Thus, nurses are forced to determine the most beneficial or least harmful action within the framework of societal mores, professional practice standards, the law, institutional rules, religious traditions, the family's value system, and the nurse's personal values.

When ethical conflicts occur, nurses may experience conflicting loyalties to their profession, colleagues, patients and families, institutions, and society. Moreover, the nurse's role in ethical decision making can be ambiguous. A nurse may be obliged to carry out procedures based on physician orders or hospital policy that are inconsistent with the patient's best interest. At times, members of the health care team do not seek the nurse's input or involvement, leaving the nurse with incomplete information about the clinical situation or without a voice in decision making.

The role of nurses as members of the health care team justifies their participation in collaborative ethical decision making. Nurses routinely use systematic problem-solving skills to resolve clinical problems. Each decision requires the nurse to collect pertinent physiologic and psychosocial data, assess relevant values held by the patient and family, and incorporate those data into a plan of care. Each of these activities is a crucial component of ethical decision making.

Furthermore, since nurses spend the most time directly caring for the child, they are in a unique position to provide insight about the patient's condition and response to therapy. In addition, they assist families in dealing with their grief and stress and often interpret information regarding the child's condition, prognosis, and treatment options to help families make informed decisions. Because of their relationship to families, nurses are often able to represent the child's and parents' values, beliefs, and preferences, thus serving as an important liaison for communication between the family and other health team members.

Participation in ethical decision making requires knowledge of ethical theory and principles, and skills in moral reasoning, communication, and group process. Nurses have an individual responsibility to clarify their personal values and beliefs and to be informed about contemporary ethical thinking and legal, institutional, public policy, as well as professional guidelines such as the Code for Nurses. Therefore, nurses must prepare themselves systematically for collaborative ethical decision making. This can be accomplished through formal coursework, continuing education, contemporary literature, and working to establish an environment conducive to ethical discourse.

The nurse can also use the professional code of ethics for guidance. A code of ethics provides one means for professional self-regulation. The Code for Nurses by the American Nurses' Association focuses on the nurse's accountability and responsibility to the client and emphasizes the nursing role as an independent professional role that upholds its own legal liability (Box 1-4).

Nurses may face ethical issues regarding patient care, such as the use of lifesaving measures for severely impaired newborns or the terminally ill child's right to refuse treatment. Throughout the text such dilemmas are addressed under a section titled "Questions and Controversies." The conflicting ethical arguments are presented to help nurses clarify their value judgments when confronted with similar sensitive issues.

Box 1-4 CODE FOR NURSES

1. The nurse provides services with respect for human dignity and the uniqueness of the client unrestricted by considerations of social or economic status, personal attributes, or the nature of health problems.
2. The nurse safeguards the client's right to privacy by judiciously protecting information of a confidential nature.
3. The nurse acts to safeguard the client and the public when health care and safety are affected by the incompetent, unethical, or illegal practice of any person.
4. The nurse assumes responsibility and accountability for individual nursing judgments and actions.
5. The nurse maintains competence in nursing.
6. The nurse exercises informed judgment and uses individual competence and qualifications as criteria in seeking consultation, accepting responsibilities, and delegating nursing activities to others.
7. The nurse participates in activities that contribute to the ongoing development of the profession's body of knowledge.
8. The nurse participates in the profession's efforts to implement and improve standards of nursing.
9. The nurse participates in the profession's efforts to establish and maintain conditions of employment conducive to high-quality nursing care.
10. The nurse participates in the profession's effort to protect the public from misinformation and misrepresentation and to maintain the integrity of nursing.
11. The nurse collaborates with members of the health professions and other citizens in promoting community and national efforts to meet the health needs of the public.

American Nurses' Association, 1976, 1985. Reproduced with permission of the American Nurses' Association.

Research

Practicing nurses rarely consider themselves researchers, yet they are the individuals most likely to observe human responses to health and illness. Unfortunately, few nurses systematically record or analyze such observations. For example, pediatric nurses devise innovative methods to encourage children to comply with treatments. Only if these interventions are shared with other nurses, especially through publications, can a body of knowledge on nursing practice develop.

Research also implies a questioning of *why* something is effective and *if* there is a better approach. Evaluation is essential to the nursing process, and research is one of the best evaluators. Therefore nurses need to be more involved in research and in applying research findings to their practice. Throughout the text research relevant to nursing of children and families is incorporated as appropriate and is also highlighted in the Questions and Controversies section. Research findings are presented to encourage nurses to base their practice on theoretical foundations, not tradition, and additional questions may be proposed in the hope of stimulating research in a particular area.

Health Care Planning

Up to this point the nurse's role has been viewed through the nucleus of a family. However, the nursing role is far more extensive and includes the community or society as a whole. Traditionally nurses have been involved in public health care, on either a continuous or an episodic basis. Rarely, however, have nurses been involved in health care planning, especially on a political or legislative level. Their role must also involve the decision-making body of government. Nursing, as the largest health profession, needs to have a voice, especially as family/consumer advocate. This does not mean that the nurse must hold public office. Rather it suggests knowledge and awareness of community needs, interest in government formulation of bills, support of politicians to ensure passage (or rejection) of significant legislation, and active involvement in groups dedicated to the welfare of children, such as professional nursing societies, Parent-Teacher Organizations, parent support groups, religious organizations, and voluntary organizations.

Health care planning involves not only providing new services but also promoting the highest quality of existing ones. Nursing needs to ensure the excellence of its own profession through each individual member, who practices according to the Code of Nurses and standards of practice. A *standard of practice* is the level of performance that is expected of a professional. Pediatric nurses are obligated to follow the Standards of Maternal-Child Health Nursing (Box 1-5) and specific standards for their specialty, such as pediatric oncology nursing or school nursing.* They should also be involved in making certain their colleagues implement the standards, through education, role modeling, and supervision.

Throughout the text the highest standards of nursing practice are continually reflected in the emphasis on thorough assessment, focus on scientific rationale as the basis for care, summary of nursing care goals and responsibilities, and comprehensive discussion of growth and development. Family-centered principles are continually evident in the consideration of dynamics affecting the child, parents, siblings, and extended members. The nurse is viewed as a vital component of the health care delivery system. Although nursing functions are clearly outlined, nursing responsibilities must be equally emphasized. It is hoped that the roles briefly described here will be studied, practiced, and implemented to the ultimate benefit of all children.

Future Trends

The present shift in focus from treatment of disease to promotion of health is likely to further expand nurses' roles in ambulatory care, with prevention and health teaching receiving a major emphasis. As prospective payment becomes a certainty in pediatric care, the need for home care and community health services will necessitate that nurses become more independent and highly skilled beyond the traditional care settings. Both of these trends are illustrated throughout the book with increased emphasis on prevention through anticipatory guidance, child health and family assessment, and discharge planning and home care.

Technologic advances will also influence pediatric nurses' roles. Increasing technical skills related to patient care, as well as the demand for computer knowledge in the work setting, are inevitable future trends. As more positions are created in the health care system that do not require a nursing background, such as "patient care educator," nurses

Box 1-5 AMERICAN NURSE'S ASSOCIATION STANDARDS OF MATERNAL AND CHILD HEALTH NURSING PRACTICE

Standard I
The nurse helps children and parents attain and maintain optimum health.

Standard II
The nurse assists families to achieve and maintain a balance between the personal growth needs of individual family members and optimum family functioning.

Standard III
The nurse intervenes with vulnerable clients and families at risk to prevent potential developmental and health problems.

Standard IV
The nurse promotes an environment free of hazards to reproduction, growth and development, wellness, and recovery from illness.

Standard V
The nurse detects changes in health status and deviations from optimum development.

Standard VI
The nurse carries out appropriate interventions and treatment to facilitate survival and recovery from illness.

Standard VII
The nurse assists clients and families to understand and cope with developmental and traumatic situations during illness, childbearing, childrearing, and childhood.

Standard VIII
The nurse actively pursues strategies to enhance access to and utilization of adequate health care services.

Standard IX
The nurse improves maternal and child health nursing practice through evaluation of practice, education, and research.

From American Nurse's Association: Standards of Maternal and Child Health Nursing Practice, American Nurses' Association, Kansas City, 1983.

*Available from the Association of Pediatric Oncology Nurses, 11512 Allecingie Parkway, Richmond, VA 23235, (804) 379-9150; and the National Association of School Nurses, Lamplighter Lane, P.O. Box 1300, Scarborough, ME 04074, (207) 883-2117.

will be required to continually update their knowledge and prove their unique contribution.

Changing demographics will also impact on pediatric nursing. While the actual number of children under age 18 years will increase from 64.3 million in 1990 to an estimated 67.4 million in 2000, their relative importance in terms of proportion of the total population will decrease from 26% to 25%. In other words, the adult population is growing faster than the pediatric population. With this trend is a decrease in younger children and an increase in older children, as well as a decrease in the white population with an increase in nonwhite groups (Evans, 1989). Such changes will impact delivery of health care, with problems of adolescents and minority groups taking on more significance. As the elderly comprise a larger percentage of the population, health care dollars will be split between the youngest and the oldest groups, with shrinking resources having to meet the needs of both. Nurses will need to keep abreast of developments in adolescent medicine and continually adapt their care to the cultural milieu in which they practice. An ever-present challenge will be cost containment without sacrificing quality care. Such demands may be overwhelming, but they also provide challenge and creativity.

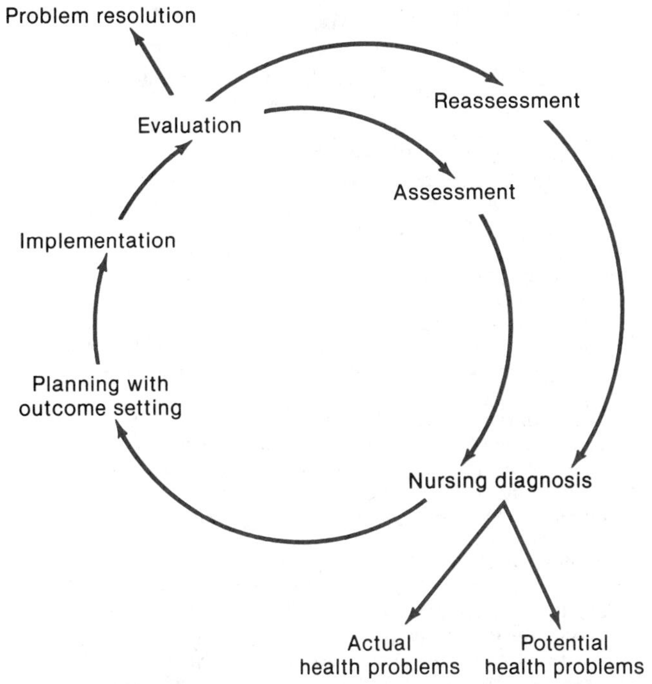

Fig. 1-6. Stages of the nursing process.

PROCESS OF NURSING CHILDREN AND FAMILIES

A systematic thought process is essential to a profession, as it assists the professional in meeting the needs of a client. The nursing process is the framework for the practice of professional nursing. It is a method of problem identification and problem solving that describes what the nurse actually does. The five-step model accepted as the nursing process includes assessment, diagnosis (problem identification), planning (with outcome development), implementation, and evaluation. The nursing process can be envisioned as a continuous cycle. The nurse assesses the child and family and compares the gathered information with expected information. Based on the assessment, the nurse identifies actual health problems and anticipates potential health problems. These are formulated into nursing diagnoses. A plan of care is devised and then implemented. When evaluation is performed, patient status is reassessed and a new cycle begins with modifications instituted as needed to achieve the desired outcomes (Fig. 1-6).

Assessment

Assessment is a continuous process that is operative at all phases of problem solving and is the foundation for decision making. Derived through multiple nursing skills, it consists of the purposeful collection, classification, and analysis of data from a variety of sources. To ensure an accurate and comprehensive assessment, the nurse must consider information about the patient's biophysical, psychologic, sociocultural, and spiritual background.

Nursing Diagnosis

Analysis and synthesis of the collected data result in problem identification. In order to solve a problem it is essential to acknowledge that it exists and to describe its nature. The problem may involve an unmet need, an unrealized expectation, an interrupted process, or a community crisis. In some instances no actual problem is identified, but present health practices or coping mechanisms may need to be maintained. Potential problems, such as infection, may be recognized because of the identified risk, such as altered defense mechanisms. *Nursing diagnoses* are used to describe these problems or concerns.

The North American Nursing Diagnosis Association's (NANDA's) currently accepted definition states that a nursing diagnosis is "a clinical judgment about individual, family, or community responses to actual and potential health problems/life processes. Nursing diagnoses provided the basis for selection of nursing interventions to achieve outcomes for which the nurse is accountable."* Currently accepted nursing diagnoses are listed in Appendix F. NANDA is responsible for the clinical testing and approval of proposed nursing diagnoses.

Currently, work is under way to develop a classification system or taxonomy for nursing diagnoses. Both NANDA and Marjory Gordon have developed frameworks; NANDA bases its framework on 9 human response patterns, and Gordon bases hers on 11 functional health patterns (Box 1-6). In clinical practice, the classification systems, especially Gordon's patterns, serve as a framework for organizing a nursing assessment and standardizing data collection. Additional research is needed to broaden the list of nursing diagnoses, especially for specialty areas such as pediatrics, and refine a universally accepted taxonomy. However, the

*From NANDA, Ninth Conference, 1990.

Box 1-6 CLASSIFICATION SYSTEMS FOR NURSING DIAGNOSES

Human Response Patterns*

Exchanging—involves mutual giving and receiving
Communicating—involves sending messages
Relating—involves establishing bonds
Valuing—involves the assigning of relative worth
Choosing—involves the selection of alternatives
Moving—involves activity
Perceiving—involves the reception of information
Knowing—involves the meaning associated with information
Feeling—involves the subjective awareness of information

Functional Health Patterns†

Health perception–health management pattern—perceptions related to general health management and preventive practices
Nutritional-metabolic pattern—intake of food and fluids related to metabolic requirements
Elimination pattern—regularity and control of excretory functions, bowel, bladder, skin, and wastes
Activity-exercise pattern—activity patterns that require energy expenditure and provide for rest
Sleep-rest pattern—effectiveness of the sleep and rest periods
Cognitive-perceptual pattern—adequacy of language, cognitive skills, and perception related to required or desired activities; includes pain perception
Self-perception–self-concept pattern—beliefs and evaluation of self-worth
Role-relationship pattern—family and social roles, especially parent-child relationships
Sexuality-reproductive pattern—problems or potential problems with sexuality or reproduction
Coping–stress tolerance pattern—stress tolerance level and coping patterns, including support systems
Value-belief pattern—values, goals, or beliefs that influence health-related decisions and actions

*Modified from the North American Nursing Diagnosis Association, St. Louis, 1986.
†From Gordon, M.: Nursing diagnosis: process and application, ed. 2, New York, 1987, McGraw-Hill Book Co.

development of nursing diagnoses is the beginning of a scientific basis for nursing practice.

(Throughout the text the nursing care plans incorporate nursing diagnoses that relate to the specific condition or disorder. Since nursing diagnoses should only prescribe interventions that nurses can perform independently, nursing interventions related to medical management are identified by an asterisk.)

Planning

Once the nursing diagnoses have been identified, a plan of care is developed and outcomes or goals are established. The *outcome* is the projected change in a patient's health status, clinical condition, or behavior that occurs after nursing interventions are instituted. The ultimate goal of nursing care is to convert the nursing diagnoses into a desired health state. The plan must be formulated before the interventions are developed and implemented.

The end point of the planning phase is the development of the nursing plan of care. The standard nursing care plans in this text provide guidelines for the care of children and families with a particular problem and differ from individualized care plans (Table 1-8). *Standard care plans* are plans that are sufficiently broad to account for situations that may develop in patients with particular problems. For this reason the care plans often have numerous nursing diagnoses, both expected and potential. These possible nursing diagnoses guide patient observation and data collection in monitoring the development of adverse reactions.

Individualized care plans are plans that are concerned with only those diagnoses that apply to the particular patient situation. Consequently, in actual practice all the problems presented in a standard care plan may not be relevant. In clinical practice, nursing care plans include an average of three nursing diagnoses (McLane, 1987). When a standard nursing care plan is used as a guide in developing an individualized plan of care, the problems not pertinent to the situation are eliminated and the outcomes individualized to the specific situation. To help the reader develop an

Table 1-8 Characteristics of standard and individualized nursing care plans

	STANDARD CARE PLAN*	INDIVIDUALIZED CARE PLAN
1. Assessment	Information is specific only to problem	Information specific to both identified problem and the child and family
2. Nursing diagnosis	All probable nursing diagnoses with general etiologic factors are considered	Only nursing diagnoses specific to the child and family are considered; the cause of the disease directs actual plan of care
3. Planning	Goals are broad and represent nursing goals	Goals are specific and reflect patient outcomes
4. Implementation	Nursing interventions are broad and applicable to most patients with problem	Nursing interventions are specific and provide direction for nursing care of individual patient
5. Evaluation	Progress the patient is *expected* to make is identified	Progress the patient has actually made toward the outcome is identified

*Describes format used in nursing care plans in the text that may differ from other types of standardized nursing care plans.

individualized care plan, the nursing diagnoses in the text are listed in order of priority. In general, potential problems are discussed toward the end of the plan, except in instances where nursing interventions are essential in preventing a potential problem from becoming an actual problem. An example is the nursing diagnosis of potential for suffocation in the care of a child with epiglottitis, where the intervention of avoiding examination of the throat is essential to prevent complete airway obstruction.

Implementation

The phase of implementation begins when the nurse puts the selected intervention into action and accumulates feedback regarding its effects. The feedback returns in the form of observation and communication and provides a data base on which to evaluate the outcome of the nursing intervention. Throughout the implementation stage, the patient's physical safety and psychologic comfort are the main concerns.

Evaluation

Evaluation is the last step in the decision-making process. The nurse gathers, sorts, and analyzes data to determine if (1) the goal has been met, (2) the plan requires modification, or (3) another alternative should be considered. Observations guidelines are included in the standard care plans to help the reader identify methods of evaluating whether the goals or outcomes are achieved. The evaluation stage either completes the nursing process or serves as the basis for selection of other alternatives for intervention in solving the specific problem.

Documentation

Although not a step in the nursing process, documentation is an essential part of nursing practice. The initial assessment is recorded, followed by evidence of the diagnostic process. Then the written plan of care is made available. All nursing interventions are recorded as they are performed, along with the patient response to these interventions. Finally, the evaluation is documented in order to compare current patient status against expected patient outcomes.

The nursing process has become an integral part of professional practice. The Joint Commission on Accreditation of Healthcare Organizations (JCAHO) has incorporated the nursing process into the accreditation requirements for health care agencies desiring this method of voluntary recognition for meeting recognized standards of care. Although accreditation is optional, agencies receiving federal/state government reimbursement (i.e., Medicaid or Medicare) must be approved by JCAHO.

Primary Nursing

Inherent in the decision-making process is accountability. Nurses are responsible for their actions, in both the legal and the ethical senses. Part of the trend in nursing practice is a stronger commitment to accountability. One of the outgrowths of this has been the movement toward *primary nursing.* Primary nursing involves 24-hour responsibility and accountability by one nurse for the care of a small group of patients. The primary nurse becomes the bedside nurse, with few if any duties delegated to other staff. If responsibilities are shared, it is usually with an associate primary nurse who maintains continuity of care when the primary nurse is not on duty.

One of the traditional problems with primary nursing is providing consistency in scheduling the same nurse and associate. An approach that minimizes this difficulty is to designate one primary nurse and as many associates as are needed to ensure that the same group of nurses care for the child. This *primary core group* requires that at least one nurse be assigned to the patient for each shift and that additional nurses be assigned for these individuals' days off. By identifying the core group in advance for a specific period, all the nurses working with the child can plan care jointly, with the primary nurse maintaining overall responsibility.

The philosophy of primary care is supported throughout the discussion of nursing of children and families. In some instances the one-to-one relationship between child and nurse is emphasized because of its therapeutic benefit, such as in nonorganic failure to thrive. However, primary nursing is universally a supportive intervention in pediatric nursing because it provides a consistent caregiver for the child and focuses on the family unit as an integral component in the planning and implementation of care.

KEY POINTS

- Health as defined by WHO, is "a state of complete physical, mental and social well-being and not merely the absence of disease."
- Although the infant mortality rate in the United States is at an all-time low, the United States lags significantly behind other well-developed countries, such as Finland, Japan, Canada.
- Low birth weight is the leading cause of neonatal death in developed countries.
- Injuries are the leading cause of death in children over age 1 year, with the majority of injuries being due to motor vehicle mishaps.
- Childhood morbidity, although difficult to define, encompasses acute illness, chronic disease, and disability.
- Eighty percent of childhood illnesses are attributable to infections, with respiratory infections occurring two to three times as often as all other illnesses combined.
- The "new morbidity," or "pediatric social illness," refers to behavioral, social, and educational problems that can significantly alter a child's health.
- Children's developmental stage and their environment are important determinants in the prevalence of injuries at a given age and thus help to direct preventive measures.

- Two strategies for injury prevention in children are (1) *passive,* which provides automatic protection by product and environmental design; and (2) *active,* which persuades people to change their behaviors for increased self-protection.
- During the first half of the 1900s, public health initiatives, such as environmental strategies to control infection and the development of antibiotics, were the major advances leading to decreased childhood deaths.
- During the latter half of the 1900s, the advancement and application of medical knowledge and technology, specifically in care of high-risk and low-birth-weight newborns, lowered the number of deaths in children, especially the neonatal mortality rate.
- The pediatric nurse's roles include family advocacy, illness prevention/health promotion, health teaching, support-counseling, therapeutic role, coordination/collaboration, ethical decision making, research, and health care planning.
- With the shift in focus from treatment of disease to promotion of health, nurses' roles may expand in ambulatory care, with emphasis on prevention and health teaching.
- The process of nursing children and families includes accurate and comprehensive *assessment,* analysis and synthesis of assessment data to arrive at a *nursing diagnosis, planning* of care, *implementation* of the plan, and *evaluation* of interventions.
- Primary nursing involves care and accountability by one nurse for a small patient population.

REFERENCES

AAP special report: barriers to care, Elk Grove Village, IL, 1989, American Academy of Pediatrics.

American Academy of Pediatrics, Committee on Accident and Poison Prevention: Rural injuries, Pediatrics 81(6):902-903, 1988.

American Academy of Pediatrics, Task Force on Infant Mortality: Statement on infant mortality, Pediatrics 78(6):1155-1160, 1986.

Bell, D., and others: Illness associated with child day care: a study of incidence and cost, Am. J. Public Health 79(4):479-484, 1989.

Bijur, P., Golding J., and Haslum, M.: Persistence of occurrence of injury: can injuries of preschool children predict injuries of school-aged children? Pediatrics 82(5):707-712, 1988.

Bijur, P., Stewart-Brown, S., and Butler, N.: Child behavior and accidental injury in 11,966 preschool children, Am. J. Dis. Child. 140(5):487-492, 1986.

Bijur, P., and others: Behavioral predictors of injury in school-age children, Am. J. Dis. Child. 142(12):1307-1312, 1988.

Centers for Disease Control: National infant mortality surveillance (NIMS), 1980, MMWR 38(No. SS-3):1-46, 1989.

Chavez, G., Cordero, J., and Becerra, J.: Leading major congenital malformations among minority groups in the United States, 1981-1986, MMWR 37(No. SS-3):17-24, 1988.

Chorba, T., Reinfurt, D., and Hulka, B.: Efficacy of mandatory seat-belt use legislation, the North Carolina experience from 1983 through 1987, JAMA 260(24):3593-3597, 1988.

Committee on Accident and Poison Prevention: Injury control for children and youth, Elk Grove Village, IL, 1987, American Academy of Pediatrics.

Committee on Trauma Research, Commission on Life Sciences, National Research Council and the Institute of Medicine: Injury in America: a continuing public health problem, Washington, DC, 1985, National Academy Press.

Cone, T.E., Jr.: Highlights of two centuries of American pediatrics, 1776-1976, Am. J. Dis. Child. 130:762-775, 1976.

Contribution of birth defects to infant mortality—United States, 1986, MMWR 38(37):633-635, 1989.

Decker, M., Graitcer, P., and Schaffner, W.: Reduction in motor vehicle fatalities associated with an increase in the minimum drinking age, JAMA 2060(24):3604-3610, 1988.

DiGuiseppi, C., and others: Bicycle helmet use by children: evaluation of a community-wide helmet campaign, JAMA 262(16):2256-2261, 1989.

Division of Injury Control, Center for Environmental Health and Injury Control, Centers for Disease Control: Childhood injuries in the United States, Am. J. Dis. Child. 144(6):627-646, 1990.

Dolan, M., Knapp, J., and Andres, J.: Three-wheel and four-wheel all-terrain vehicle injuries in children, Pediatrics 84(4):694-698, 1989.

Eisenberg, L.: Preventive pediatrics: the promise and the peril, Pediatrics 80(3):415-422, 1987.

Evans, V.: Sociodemographic trends toward the 21st century. In Feeg, V., editor: Pediatric nursing: forum on the future: looking toward the 21st century, Pitman, NJ, 1989, Anthony J. Jannetti, Inc.

Faber, M.: A review of efforts to protect children from injury in car crashes, Fam. Community Health 9(3):25-41, 1986.

Foss, R.: Sociocultural perspective on child occupant protection, Pediatrics 80(6):886-893, 1987.

Gleeson, R., and others: Advanced practice nursing: a model of collaborative care, MCN 15(1):9-12, 1990.

Goldberg, I.R., and others: Mental health problems among children seen in pediatric practice: prevalence and management, Pediatrics 73(3):278-292, 1984.

Gortmaker, S., and others: Chronic conditions, socioeconomic risks, and behavioral problems in children and adolescents, Pediatrics 85(3):267-276, 1990.

Green, M., and Haggerty, R.: Episodic problems. In Green, M., and Haggerty, R., editors: Ambulatory pediatrics III, Philadelphia, 1984, W.B. Saunders Co.

Gulaid, J., and others: Differences in death rates due to injury among blacks and whites, 1984, MMWR 37(SS-3):25-33, 1988.

Healthy people, 2000—national health promotion and disease prevention objectives, Washington, DC, 1990, U.S. Public Health Service.

Hoekelman, R., and Pless, B.: Decline in mortality among young Americans during the 20th century: prospects for reaching national mortality reduction goals for 1990, Pediatrics 82(4):582-595, 1988.

Honigfeld, L., and Kaplan, D.: Native American postneonatal mortality, Pediatrics 80(4):575-578, 1987.

Hughes, D., and others: The health of America's children, Washington, DC, 1987, Children's Defense Fund.

Indian Health Service Chart Book Series, June 1984, U.S. Department of Health and Human Services, Public Health Service, Health Resources and Services Administrations.

Jenista, J., and Chapman, D.: Medical problems of foreign-born adopted children, Am. J. Dis. Child. 141(3):298-302, 1987.

Kalter, H., and Warkany, J.: Congenital malformations: etiologic factors and their role in prevention, part I, N. Engl. J. Med. 308:424-431, Feb. 1983; part II, 308:491-497, March 1983.

Leopold, J.: Abraham Jacobi. In Veeder, B.S., editor: Pediatric profiles, St. Louis, 1957, Mosby–Year Book, Inc.

Margolis, L., Wagenaar, A., and Molnar, L.: Recognizing the common problem of child automobile restraint misuse, Pediatrics 81(5):717-729, 1988.

McCarthy, E., and Kozak, L.J.: Hospital use by children: United States, 1983, DHHS Pub. No. (PHS) 85-1250, 1985.

McLane, A.M., editor: Classification of nursing diagnosis: proceedings of the Seventh Conference, North American Nursing Diagnosis Association (NANDA), St. Louis, 1987, Mosby–Year Book, Inc.

Miller, R., and others: Pediatric counseling and subsequent use of smoke detectors, Am. J. Public Health 72:392-393, 1982.

Nader, P., and others: The new morbidity: use of school and community health care resources for behavioral, educational and social-family problems, Pediatrics 67(1):53-60, 1981.

National Center for Health Statistics: Advance report of final mortality statistics, 1987, Monthly vital statistics report, 38(suppl. 5), DHHS Pub. No. (PHS) 89-1120, 1989a.

National Center for Health Statistics: Perinatal mortality in the United States: 1981-85, Monthly vital statistics report 37(suppl. 10) DHHS Pub. No. (PHS) 89-1120, 1989b.

Nelms, B.: Travel may be dangerous, J. Pediatr. Health Care 4(3):115-116, 1990.

Newacheck, P., and Starfield, B.: Morbidity and use of ambulatory care services among poor and nonpoor children, Am. J. Public Health 78:927-933, 1988.

The 1990 Health Objectives for the Nation: a midcourse review, 1986, U.S. Department of Health and Human Services, Public Health Service.

Novello, A., and others: Final report of the United States Department of Health and Human Services Secretary's Work Group on pediatric human immunodeficiency virus infection and disease: content and implications, Pediatrics 84(3):547,1989.

Nursing: a social policy statement, Kansas City, MO, 1980, American Nurses' Association.

Nyman, G.: Infant temperament, childhood accidents, and hospitalization, Clin. Pediatr. 26(8):398-404, 1987.

Orsay, E., and others: Prospective study of the effect of safety belts on morbidity and health care costs in motor-vehicle accidents, JAMA 23(30):3598-3603, 1988.

Overpeck, M., and others: A comparison of the childhood health status of normal birth weight and low birth weight infants, Public Health Rep. 104(1):58-70, 1989.

Paulson, J.: Injuries: the leading cause of death in children, Curr. Opin. Pediatr. 1(1):192-202, 1989.

Paulson, J., and Rushforth, N.: Violent death in children in a metropolitan county: changing patterns of homicide, 1958-1982, Pediatrics 78(6):1013-1020, 1986.

Pless, I.: Morbidity and mortality among the young. In Hoekelman, R.A., and others, editors: Primary pediatric care, St. Louis, 1987, Mosby–Year Book, Inc.

Promoting health/preventing disease: objectives for the nation, Washington, DC, U.S. Department of Health and Human Services, Public Health Service, 1980.

Report to Congress and the Secretary by the Task Force on Technology-Dependent Children: Fostering home and community-based care for technology-dependent children, April 7, 1988.

Rivara, F., Bergman, A., and Drake, C.: Parental attitudes and practices toward children as pedestrians, Pediatrics 84(6):1017-1021, 1989.

Runyan, C., and Gerken, E.: Epidemiology and prevention of adolescent injury: a review and research agenda, JAMA 262(16):2273-2279, 1989.

Salmi, L., and others: Fatal farm injuries among young children, Pediatrics 83(2):267-271, 1989.

Sayre, J.W., and Sayre, R.F.: American children and the "children of nature," Am. J. Dis. Child. 130:716-723, 1976.

Scheidt, P.: Behavioral research toward prevention of childhood injury, Am. J. Dis. Child. 142(6):612-617, 1988.

Schmidt, W.M.: Health and welfare of colonial American children, Am. J. Dis. Child. 130:694-701, 1976.

Scott, R., and Winston, M.: The health and welfare of the black family in the United States, Am. J. Dis. Child 130:704-707, 1976.

Selbst, S., and Alexander, O.: Bicycle injuries: a description of the problem, Am. J. Dis. Child. 141(2):140-144, 1987.

Sewell, C., and others: Child restraint law effects on motor vehicle accident fatalities and injuries: the New Mexico experience, Pediatrics 78(6):1079-1084, 1986.

Spiegel, C., and Lindaman, F.: Children can't fly: a program to prevent childhood morbidity and mortality from window falls, Am. J. Public Health 67(12):1143-1147, 1977.

Spital, M., Spital, A., and Spital, R.: The compelling case for seat belts on school buses, Pediatrics 78(5):928-932, 1986.

Spivak, H., Prothrow-Smith, D., and Hausman, A.: Dying is no accident, Pediatr. Clin. North Am. 35(6):1339-1347, 1988.

Starfield, B.: Psychosocial and psychosomatic diagnoses in primary care of children, Pediatrics 66 (2):159-163, 1980.

Starfield, B., and others: Morbidity in childhood—a longitudinal view, N. Engl. J. Med. 310(13):824-829, 1984.

Thompson, R., Rivera, F., and Thompson, D.: A case-control study of the effectiveness of bicycle safety helmets, N. Engl. J. Med. 320(21):1361-1367, 1989.

Wagenaar, A., and Webster, D.: Preventing injuries to children through compulsory automobile safety seat use, Pediatrics 78(4):662-672, 1986.

Walton, W.: An evaluation of The Poison Prevention Packaging Act, Pediatrics 69(3):363-370, 1982.

Wegman, M.: Annual summary of vital statistics—1988, Pediatrics 84(6):943-956, 1989.

Weiss, B.: Bicycle helmet use by children, Pediatrics 77(5):677-679, 1986.

Wise, P., and Meyers, A.: Poverty and child health, Pediatr. Clin. North Am. 35(6):1169-1186, 1988.

Wong, D.: Principles of atraumatic care. In Feeg, V., editor: Pediatric nursing: forum on the future: looking toward the 21st century, Pitman, NJ, 1989, Anthony J. Jannetti, Inc.

BIBLIOGRAPHY

Mortality and Morbidity

American Academy of Pediatrics, Committee on Adolescence: Suicide and suicide attempts in adolescents and young adults, Pediatrics 81(2):322-324, 1988.

Diaz, C., and others: Ill health and use of medical care: community-based assessment of morbidity in children, Med. Care 24(9):848-856, 1986.

Feeg, V.: New legislative efforts to improve child health and decrease infant mortality, Pediatr. Nurs. 15(2):145-148, 1989.

Gould, J., Davey, B., and LeRoy, S.: Socioeconomic differentials and neonatal mortality: racial comparison of California singletons, Pediatrics 83(2):181-186, 1989.

Jason, J., and Jarvis, W.: Infectious diseases: preventable causes of infant mortality, Pediatrics 80(3):335-341, 1987.

Kitchen, W., and others: Children of birth weight $<$1000 g: changing outcome between ages 2 and 5 years, J. Pediatr. 110(2):283-288, 1987.

Mutch, L., and others: Secular changes in rehospitalization of very low birth weight infants, J. Pediatr. 78(1):164-171, 1986.

National Center for Health Statistics: Annual summary of births, marriages, divorces, and deaths, United States, 1988, 37(13), Hyattsville, MD, 1989.

Report of the National Commission to Prevent Infant Mortality: Death before life: the tragedy of infant mortality, Washington, DC, 1988, The Commission.

Urtis, J., Clayton, D., and Jay, S.: Infant morbidity: a measurement of severity and occurrence of illness in preterm and term infants, J. Pediatr. Nurs. 3(2):110-117, 1988.

U.S. Congress, Offices of Technology Assessment: Healthy children: investing in the future, OTA-H-345, Washington, DC, Feb. 1988, U.S. Government Printing Office.

Victora, C., and others: Influence of birth weight on mortality from infectious diseases: a case-control study, Pediatrics 81(6):807-811, 1988.

Wegman, M.: Low birth weight, vital records, and infant mortality, Pediatrics 78(6):1143-1145, 1986.

Wise, P., and others: Infant mortality increase despite high access to tertiary care: an evolving relationship among infant mortality, health care, and socioeconomic change, Pediatrics 81(4):542-548, 1988.

Injuries

Baker, S.: Injury science comes of age, JAMA 262(16):2284-2285, 1989.
Bourguet, C., and McArtor, R.: Unintentional injuries: risk factors in preschool children, Am. J. Dis. Child. 143(5):556-559, 1989.
Bowman, M., Sanson-Fisher, R., and Webb, G.: Interventions in preschools to increase the use of safety restraints by preschool children, Pediatrics 79(1):103-109, 1987.
Christophersen, E.: Accident prevention in primary care, Pediatr. Clin. North Am. 33(4):925-933, 1986.
Fingerhut, L., and Kleinman, J.: Firearm mortality among children and youth. Advance data from vital and health statistics: No 178. Hyattsville, MD, 1989, National Center for Health Statistics.
Katcher, M., Landry, G., and Shapiro, M.: Liquid-crystal thermometer use in pediatric office counseling about tap water burn prevention, Pediatrics 83(5):766-771, 1989.
Kelly, B., Sein, C., and McCarthy, P.: Safety education in a pediatric primary care setting, Pediatrics 79(5):818-824, 1987.
Lee, E., Jacobson, J., and Levanas, V.: Stressful life events and accidents at school, Pediatr. Nurs. 15(2):140-142, 1989.
Meller, J., and Shermeta, D.: Falls in urban children, Am. J. Dis. Child. 141(12):1271-1275, 1987.
Moore, E., and others: Protecting our children through Kid Safe, Pediatr. Nurs. 14(1):32-36, 1988.
Ridenour, M.: Elementary school playgrounds: safe play areas or inherent dangers? Percept. Mot. Skills 64:447-451, 1987.
Schor, E.: Unintentional injuries: patterns within families, Am. J. Dis. Child. 141(12):1280-1284, 1987.
Wilson, M.: Injury prevention: protecting the under-6 set, Contemp. Pediatr. 5(5):19-34, 1988.
Zuckerman, B.S., and Duby, J.C.: Development approach to injury prevention, Pediatr. Clin. North Am. 32(1):17-29, 1985.

Evolution of Child Health Care

Arnold, L., and others: Lessons from the past, MCN 14(2):75-82, 1989.
Cherry, B., and Carty, R.: Changing concepts of childhood in society, Pediatr. Nurs. 12(6):421-424, 1986.
Cone, T.E., Jr.: History of American pediatrics, Boston, 1980, Little, Brown & Co., Inc.
DeGraw, C., and others: Public law 99-457: new opportunities to serve young children with special needs, J. Pediatr. 113(6):971-974, 1988.
Donahue, M.P.: Nursing: the finest art, an illustrated history, St. Louis, 1985, Mosby–Year Book, Inc.
Farel, A.: Public health in early intervention: historic foundations for contemporary training, Inf. Young Child. 1(1):63-70, 1988.
Gale, C.: Inadequacy of health care for the nation's chronically ill children, J. Pediatr. Health Care 3(1):20-27, 1989.
Kilmon, C., and Poteet, G.: Child care needs of nursing personnel: the challenge for the future, Pediatr. Nurs. 6(3):369-374, 1988.
Meisels, S., and Margolis, L.: Is the early and periodic screening, diagnosis, and treatment program effective with developmentally disabled children? Pediatrics 81(2):262-271, 1988.
Murphy, M.: What price success: can we afford "saved" babies? J. Pediatr. Health Care 3(6):285-286, 1989.
Oberg, C.: Medically uninsured children in the United States: a challenge to public policy, Pediatrics 85(5):824-833, 1990.
Report to Congress and the Secretary by the Task Force on Technology-Dependent Children: fostering home and community-based care for technology-dependent children, vols. 1 and 2, U.S. Department of Health and Human Services, Health Care Financing Administration, HCFA Pub. No. 88-02171, 1988.
Velsor-Friedrich, B.: The federal government and child health, J. Pediatr. Nurs. 5(1):56-58, 1990.

Pediatric Nursing

Bru, G.: Using the revised APON standards of practice, J. Pediatr. Oncol. Nurs. 7(1):17-21, 1990.
Doxiadis, S.: Ethical issues in preventive pediatrics, Pediatrics 83(2): 309-310, 1989.
Ethics in Nursing: position statements and guidelines, Kansas City, MO, 1988, American Nurses' Association.
Fost, N.: Ethical issues in pediatrics, Curr. Opin. Pediatr. 1(1):176-178, 1989.
Fowler, M.: Ethical decision making in clinical practice, Nurs. Clin. North Am. 24(4):955-965, 1989.
Fry, S.: Ethical decision making. I. Selecting a framework, Nurs. Outlook 37(5):248, 1989.
Fry, S.: Ethics. I. Issues in nursing, Nurs. Clin. North Am. 24(2):461-577, 1989.
Graham, S.: Research and treatment: ethical distinctions related to the care of children, J. Pediatr. Nurs. 2(1):23-29, 1987.
Gurile, P., and Harter, I.: Getting standards off the shelf and into practice, J. Pediatr. Nurs. 2(5):295-301, 1987.
Gurile, P., and Harter, I.: Testing child health standards in a clinical setting, J. Pediatr. Nurs. 2(5):302-307, 1987.
Guzzetta. C., and others: Clinical assessment tools for use with nursing diagnoses, St. Louis, 1989, Mosby–Year Book, Inc.
Hanna, D., and Wyman, N.: Assessment + diagnosis = care planning: a tool for coordination, Nurs. Manage. 18(11):106-109, 1987.
Johnson, P., and Gaines, S.: Helping families to help themselves, MCN 13(5):336-339, 1988.
Keefe, M., and Kotzer, A.: Integrating clinical practice and research: a challenge for the pediatric nurse practitioner, J. Pediatr. Health Care 2(6):275-280, 1988.
Lane, K., and Peppe, K.: Where are the standards? J. Pediatr. Nurs. 2(5):291-294, 1987.
Levin, R., and others: Diagnostic content validity of nursing diagnoses, IMAGE J. Nurs. Sch. 21(1):40-44, 1989.
Lynn, M.: Children have rights too, J. Pediatr. Nurs. 1(5):345-348, 1986.
Lyons, J., and Hester, N.: Research-generated nursing diagnoses for healthy school-age children, Issues Compr. Pediatr. Nurs. 10(3):149-159, 1987.
Lyons, N., and others: Too busy for research? Collaboration: an answer, MCN 15(2):67-72, 1990.
McFarland, G., and McFarland, E.: Nursing diagnosis & intervention: planning for patient care, St. Louis, 1989, Mosby–Year Book, Inc.
McLane, A.: Measurement and validation of diagnostic concepts: a decade of progress . . . review of nursing diagnosis research, Heart Lung 16(6):616-624, 1987.
McVety, D.: Old-fashioned care still makes the difference, MCN 14(2):126-127, 1989.
Montana, J.: Computers and nursing care, J. Pediatr. Nurs. 3(1):48-53, 1988.
Nelms, B.: Child advocacy: the need is great, J. Pediatr. Health Care 3(1):1-2, 1989.
Olson, R., Heater, B., and Becker, A.: A meta-analysis of the effects of nursing interventions on children and parents, MCN 15(2):104-108, 1990.
Rushton, C.: Ethical decision-making in critical care. I. The role of the pediatric nurse, Pediatr. Nurs. 14(5):411-412, 1988.
Rushton, C.: Ethical decision-making in critical care. II. Strategies for nurse preparation, Pediatr. Nurs. 14(6):497-502, 1988.
Rushton, C.: Ethical unrest: implications for the future. In Feeg, V., editor: Pediatric nursing: forum on the future: looking toward the 21st century, Pitman, NJ, 1989, Anthony J. Jannetti, Inc.
Starn, J., and Niederhausen, V.: An MCN model for nursing diagnosis to focus intervention, MCN 15(3):180-183, 1990.
Thompson, J., and Thompson, H.: Living with ethical decisions with which you disagree, MCN 13(4):245-250, 1988.

CHAPTER 2

Social, Cultural, and Religious Influences on Child Health Promotion

RELATED TOPICS

Communicating with families through an interpreter, Ch. 6
Family assessment: cultural and religious traditions, Ch. 6
Family influences on child health promotion, Ch. 3
Lactose intolerance, Ch. 13
Nutritional assessment, Ch. 6
Sickle cell anemia, Ch. 35
Skin, Ch. 7
Spiritual development: general, Ch. 4; toddler, Ch. 14; preschooler, Ch. 15; school-age child, Ch. 17; and adolescent, Ch. 19
Vegetarian diets, Ch. 13

GLOSSARY

acculturation Gradual changes produced in a culture by the influence of another culture that cause one or both cultures to be more similar to the other

cultural shock Feelings of helplessness and discomfort in a state of disorientation experienced by an outsider attempting to adapt to a different cultural group

culture Way of life developed by a group of people in adaptation to the physical and social circumstances in which they find themselves

ethnicity Shared racial, cultural, social, and linguistic heritage

ethnocentrism Emotional attitude that one's own ethnic group is superior to other ethnic groups

race Group of people with similar physical characteristics, such as color, that are transmitted through generations and are sufficient to characterize the group as a distinct human race

role Expected behavior of individuals in a particular culture

socialization The process by which individuals learn the ways of a given society in order to function within that group

stereotyping Labeling and a lack of recognition of differences among individuals within a particular cultural, ethnic, or religious group

subculture Smaller gorup within a culture that possesses many characteristics of the larger culture while contributing its own unique values

transcultural nursing Nursing that focuses on the comparative study and analysis of different cultures to provide culture-specific and sensitive care practices

The future of any society depends on its children. If it is to survive, the society must make provision for their care, nurture, and socialization. Cultural survival depends on whether the customs and values of the culture are transmitted from one generation to the next through the medium of the family. The culture into which children are born outlines the roles of their parents, structures their relationships with other people, and determines much of the behavior they acquire. A holistic view of any child requires that nurses develop some understanding of the ways that culture contributes to the development of social and emotional relationships and influences childrearing practices and attitudes toward health. This orientation to transcultural nursing includes an awareness of the nurse's own cultural frame of reference and a concerted effort to recognize and appreciate the views and beliefs of the health care recipients to deliver culture-specific and sensitive care.

■ CULTURE

Culture is the "way of life developed by a group of people in adaptation to the physical and social circumstances in which they find themselves" (Elkin and Handel, 1989). Culture differs from both race and ethnicity. *Race* generally refers to a group of people with similar physical characteristics such as skin color that are transmissible by descent and sufficient to characterize it as a distinct human type. One system of classification includes three recognized types: caucasoid (white), negroid (black), and mongoloid (yellow). *Ethnicity* refers to a shared racial, cultural, social, and linguistic heritage (Martinson, 1989). *Socialization* is the process by which individuals learn the ways (beliefs, values, and behaviors) of a given society in order to function within that group (Elkin and Handel, 1989).

A culture is composed of individuals who share a set of values, beliefs, practices, and information that is learned, integrative, social, and satisfying. Culture is not a surface veneer that covers a basic outlook shared by all human beings but an ingrained orientation to life that serves as a frame of reference for individual perception and judgment. People from one culture differ from those in other cultures in the ways they think, solve problems, perceive, and structure the world. Culture is, essentially, the way of life of a group of people that incorporates experience s of the past, influences thought and action in the present, and transmits these traditions to future group members. Adaptation is necessary, however, for the culture to survive in an ever-changing world. Consciously and unconsciously, the members abandon, modify, or assume new patterns to meet the needs of the group.

The observable components of a culture, such as material objects (dress, art, utensils, and other artifacts) and actions, are sometimes termed the *material, overt,* or *manifest culture; nonmaterial covert culture* refers to those aspects that cannot be observed directly, such as the ideas, beliefs, customs, and feelings of the culture. Related to the large culture are many *subcultures,* each with an identity of its own. Children are socialized into a particular subculture rather than into the culture as a whole. Subcultural influences, such as ethnicity and social class, are discussed in more detail later in this chapter.

The culture in which children are reared determines the type of food they will eat, the language they will speak, the ideals of behavior they will follow, and the way they will conduct themselves in social roles. To be acceptable members of the culture, children must learn how the culture expects them to behave toward others in the group. In turn, they learn how they can expect others to behave toward them.

Cultures and subcultures contribute to the uniqueness of child members in such a subtle way and at such an early age that children grow up to feel that their beliefs, attitudes, values, and practices are the "correct" or "normal" ones; those of other cultures may be viewed as "deviant" or "wrong." A set of values learned in childhood is apt to characterize children's attitudes and behavior for life, guiding their long-range strivings and monitoring their short-range, impulsive inclinations. Thus every ongoing society socializes each succeeding generation to its cultural heritage.

The manner and sequence of the growth and development phenomenon are universal and fundamental features of all children; however, the variations in behavioral responses that children display to similar events are believed to be determined by cultures. Inborn temperament and modes of behavior that prompt children to behave in their own preferred and highly individual manner may be in harmony or in conflict with the culture. Such forces as heredity and maturation impose limits on the influence that parents and other social groups may bring to bear.

The culture fosters and reinforces those behaviors deemed desirable and appropriate; it attempts to depress or extinguish those at conflict with cultural norms. Some cultures encourage aggressive behaviors in their children; others favor amiability and compliance. Some foster individual resourcefulness and competition; others emphasize cooperation and submission to group interest. The child from a culture that values cooperation will not respond to a challenge such as, "I'll bet you can eat your breakfast faster than Johnny can," whereas a child from a culture that emphasizes individual achievement will be stimulated by the challenge.

Cultures may also differ in whether status in the group is based on age or on skill. Even children's play and their types of games are culturally determined. In some cultures children play in groups composed of members of the same sex; in others they play in mixed-sex groups. In some cultures team games predominate; in others most play is limited to individual games.

Standards and norms vary from culture to culture and location to location; a practice that is accepted in one area may meet with disapproval or create tension in another. The extent to which cultures tolerate divergence from the established norm varies among cultures and subcultural groups. Although conformity provides a degree of security, it is a decided deterrent to change.

SOCIAL ROLES

Much of children's self-concept is derived from their ideas about their social roles. Roles are cultural creations; therefore, the culture prescribes patterns of behavior for persons in a variety of social positions. All persons who hold similar social positions have the obligation to behave in a particular manner. A role prohibits some behaviors and allows for others. Because it delineates and clarifies roles, the culture is a significant influence on the development of children's self-concept, that is, the attitudes and beliefs they have about themselves.

A social group consists of a system of roles carried out in both primary and secondary groups. A *primary group* is characterized by intimate, continued face-to-face contact, mutual support of the members, and the ability to order or constrain a considerable proportion of individual members' behavior. Two such groups are the family and the peer group, both of which exert a great deal of influence on the child. *Secondary groups* are groups that have limited, intermittent contact and in which there is generally less concern for members' behavior. These groups offer little in terms of support or pressure toward conformity except in rigidly limited areas. Examples of secondary groups are professional associations and church organizations (also considered in relation to subgroups).

A concept of social role also depends largely on whether a child is reared in a primary- or secondary-group community. Children are subjected to perceptively different forms of parental training in these two types of environments.

Primary Group Influence

In a primary-group community (e.g., some contemporary rural, religious, or ethnic communities), all members know each other, most belong to the same subgroups, and all are concerned about each member's behavior. There is a high degree of material and psychologic support among the community members, and since there is one traditional set of values that the entire group agrees on and supports, there is little conflict of values. In a stable community where the members remain within comparatively defined limits and relatives are likely to live close together, young members have ample opportunity to observe and absorb the practices and customs of the culture. Any member of the community feels justified in evaluating and censuring the conduct of another member.

Children reared in a primary-group community learn that there is only one acceptable way to respond to any given situation. The entire group agrees, and any tendency to deviate is met with collective disapproval. It is the parents' duty to see that the children learn and adhere to social roles and modes of behavior defined and strengthened by the views of the community.

Secondary Group Influence

The childrearing orientation in a secondary-group environment, such as urban communities, differs considerably from that of a primary-group community. An urban community is dynamic and rapidly changing. Many of the traditional behaviors and values do not meet the needs of the changing society. Consequently parents are often uncertain about what to teach their children. They may wish to rear their children with values consistent with their own, but the differences in experience between the generations are too great. As a result, they often grant their children autonomy in some areas of decision making early in the developmental process, and other secondary groups assume a greater influence. The children are exposed to an assortment of social groups with diverse sets of values and expectations. None of the groups is highly dominant in its influence; therefore the children are exposed to an eclectic set of values, some in agreement and some at conflict with the others. From these they must ultimately select those that they determine to be best for them and adopt them to form a consistent set of roles and behaviors to be incorporated into the self-concept.

Guilt and Shame Orientation

Conditioning children to feel either guilt or shame for misdeeds is a technique used by a culture to control social behavior—to internalize the norms and expectations of others. Some cultural groups value a well-developed conscience (superego) and condition their children to feel guilt following wrongdoing. Offenders want to purge themselves and get an uncomfortable physical feeling. Since guilt is based within the individual, successful conditioning produces self-regulated persons who punish themselves without their being caught in the act of wrongdoing.

In many cultural groups guilt is lacking and social controls are based on the use of shame. Offenders do not want anyone to see them when they have been guilty of wrongful deeds. Sometimes children in these groups learn that anything is acceptable as long as one is not caught; the shame results when the forbidden act is found out by others.

Although both techniques are used by members of both primary- and secondary-group communities, shame is apt to be more successful in a primary-group community because most behaviors are quite public. In secondary-group communities it is less effective; persons are not as apt to be caught and, if caught, can withdraw and join a group that is unaware of the misdeed. Guilt probably has a greater influence on behavior in urban communities and, although it is characteristic of most American cultures, many authorities believe that the trend in urban America is shifting away from a guilt orientation. Rapid changes in the American culture leave parents unsure of their own values; therefore much of their function is abandoned to the school and peers. Peers are notorious for the use of shame as a disciplinary technique.

SUBCULTURAL INFLUENCES

Except in rare situations, children grow and develop in a blend of cultures and subcultures, those smaller groups within a culture that possess many characteristics of the larger culture while contributing their own particular values. In a large, complex society such as the United States, different groups have their own set of standards, values, and expectations within the collective ways of the large culture.

Most were formed when groups of people clustered together by preference, by external pressures from the majority culture, or by geographic isolation. Although many cultural differences are related to geographic boundaries, subcultures are not always restricted by location.

There are even subcultures related to the age stages of development that have traditions, games, loyalties, and rules. Age-related subcultures are easily identified in the behavior of school-age children and adolescents. The culture is handed down by word of mouth from one "generation" to the next, and its rituals and behavior standards are highly resistant to outside influence.

Children's membership in a cultural subgroup is, for the most part, involuntary. They are born into a family with a specific ethnic and/or racial heritage, socioeconomic level, and religious beliefs. Although in the complex American society there are countless subcultures and considerable variation in the way of life, those subcultures that seem to exert the greatest influence on childrearing are ethnicity, social class, and occupational role. Additionally, schools and peer-group subcultures are strong influences in the socialization of the child.

Ethnicity

Ethnicity is the classification of or affiliation with any of the basic groups or divisions of mankind or any heterogeneous population differentiated by customs, characteristics, language, or similar distinguishing factors. Ethnic differences extend to many areas and include such manifestations as family structure, language, food preferences, moral codes, and expression of emotion. Some standards of behavior result from the cultural heritage of the specific ethnic group as, for example, the traditional role of the father. Others reflect the interaction between subcultures, most notably between members of the majority culture and a minority subculture.

To establish their place in the group, children learn how to adhere to a mode of behavior that is in accordance with standards distinctive to the group and learn how they can expect others to behave toward them. They take their cues from observing and imitating those to whom they are exposed. For example, children of a racial minority form a perception of their role as a group member by observing the manner in which role models within the subgroup respond to treatment by people outside the subgroup. When they see group members display an attitude of inferiority, they assume this to be the appropriate behavior. These perceptions are then incorporated into their own self-concept.

In the United States the cross-cultural lines are becoming blurred as subcultures are assimilated and blended into the larger culture (Fig. 2-1). Although ethnic differences in childrearing are probably diminishing, they remain important. It is particularly difficult for persons to attempt to maintain an identity with a subculture while living and conforming to the requirements of the larger culture. Universal customs and language of the dominant culture used in commercial and educational systems are different from those of the minority culture. Often the values are in conflict. Consequently children reared in this environment are

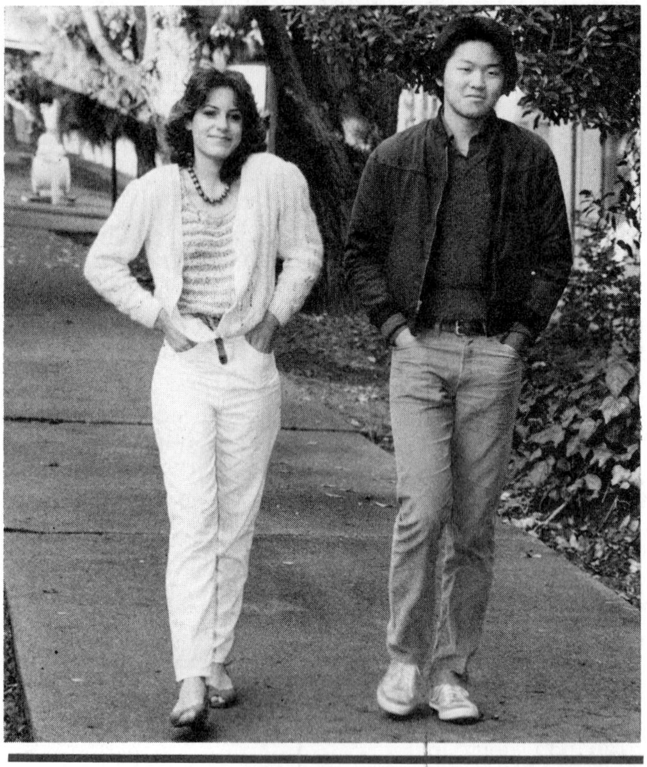

Fig. 2-1. Youngsters from different cultural backgrounds interact within the larger culture.

confused about roles and values, and they usually adopt those of the more influential or higher-status culture. Youth, in particular, are influenced by the locally dominant group.

Ethnocentrism. Ethnocentrism is the emotional attitude that one's own ethnic group is superior to others, that one's values, beliefs, and perceptions are the correct ones, and that the group's ways of living and behaving are the best way. Ethnic *stereotyping* or labeling stems from ethnocentric views of people (Friedman, 1990). Ethnocentrism implies that all other groups are inferior and that their ways are not in the best interests of the group. This attitude strongly influences the ability of one person to evaluate the beliefs and behaviors of others objectively. This inherent viewpoint of individuals tends to bias their interpretation and understanding of the behavior of others.

Social Class/Occupation

Although there are exceptions, probably the greatest influence on childrearing practices and their consequences is the social class of the family into which a child is born. Differences in childrearing goals and practices as well as attitudes toward health, have been found to be greater between social classes than between races or ethnic groups. In North America social class and socioeconomic level are essentially synonymous and are most easily determined by occupation; for example, the upper middle class consists primarily of professional and business people, almost all with a college education. The working class includes employees in manufacturing, trades, and service occupations (such as barbers or hairdressers) who have a high school education. In the lower class, the breadwinners are typically unskilled laborers or unemployed families who may or may not be on public assistance (Elkin and Handel, 1989). Since children are reared differently by parents who vary in respect to education, occupation, and income, social class can be expected to produce substantial variation in their upbringing.

Upper- and middle-class children live in an enriched environment that provides material comforts and broader opportunities. The parents are usually educated, and other authority figures such as teachers with whom the children are routinely in contact are usually from a middle-class background and have activities and expectations for the children that are similar to those of the parents. Parents have occupations that require judgment, creativity, and resourcefulness, and these attributes are fostered in their children.

Because members of the upper classes, or the power elite, do not participate in studies, information on childrearing practices in these groups is limited. Attitudes toward children appear to be generally permissive; however, much of the actual child care in upper-class families is delegated to surrogates, such as housekeepers, governesses, or private schools. In middle-class families child care is more likely to consist of daycare, babysitters, and nursery school rather than these more expensive alternatives.

Although differences in parental behavior in different social classes are less marked than they have been in the past, one of the distinctions that is observed in middle classes but not in lower classes is the willingness to delay gratification. The uncertainty of their life leads members of the lower classes to take advantage of gratifications when they are available. This characteristic has caused lower classes to be labeled as present oriented, whereas middle classes seem to be future oriented. With better job security through unionization, unemployment compensation, and other welfare features, some segments of the lower classes are finding life more predictable. They are less apt to seize gratifications lest the opportunity vanish and are beginning to develop long-range goals, including an increased interest in education for their children. Middle-class parents have higher educational and occupational aspirations for their children and use long-range planning to meet these goals (Shaffer, 1985).

Intellectual skills. There appear to be differences in intellectual skills and scholastic achievement between children in the upper and middle classes and those in the lower classes. The more apparent differences lie in the areas of abstract thinking and manipulation. Although the relative merits of testing techniques and standards are a matter of question, there is a higher incidence of academic failure in children from the lower class with its attendant dropout rate. It has been found that lower-class parents value the concrete and tangible rather than the abstract and are therefore less inclined to encourage these qualities in their children. Their own educational level discourages these parents from reading to their children and providing other means for learning in the home. There are no role models in the family to support the value of education, and numerous provisions for intellectual growth are restricted by cost. To compound this, lower-class neighborhoods have the poorest schools, and the children are often hampered in their learning by poor health and inadequate nutrition. In addition children from the lower classes are often penalized within the school because they do not possess the symbols, attitudes, and behaviors characteristically valued by the dominant class group. There is a social class bias in educative influence. Most teachers come from the middle classes, and school board members are from middle and upper classes.

Communication skills. Any concept that occurs to a person can be expressed in language. However, ease of communication and use of language codes vary among the social classes. Language is much more restricted in the lower classes, and the classes are more easily differentiated by grammar than by pronunciation. Persons in the middle classes use different grammar from those from the lower classes and are able to express more complicated ideas; persons in the lower classes use very simple grammar and are less likely to offer explanations. For example, a middle-class parent may tell a child, "I'd rather you made less noise because I am trying to read a book." A lower class parent may say, "Shut up" (Elkin and Handel, 1989).

These communication differences are highly significant in relation to school achievement. School is constructed around the elaborate language codes of the middle class; therefore children from the lower classes must learn these language skills, which places them at a decided disadvantage. This is particularly true for bilingual children and children from ethnic groups who have developed a dialect unique to their own group. For example, black English, essentially another language and treated as such, is not spoken by other groups, including middle-class blacks. Many regional dialects and variations in language usage must be taken into consideration when communicating with persons from these groups. English words that sound like another word in a foreign language can cause considerable misunderstanding. For example, when a nurse tried to explain to Spanish parents that their infant died of SIDS (sudden infant death syndrome), the parents thought the nurse said SIDA, the Spanish abbreviation for AIDS (acquired immune deficiency syndrome) (Lawson, 1990).

Aspirations. Middle-class parents are positively oriented toward change, whereas working-class parents remain tradition oriented. Consequently the working class emphasizes conformity to parental values and external regulations, whereas middle-class parents are more concerned with producing self-directed children. This attitude difference reflects the occupation orientation of the different classes. Middle-class occupations tend to involve more self-direction and getting ahead; lower-class occupations tend to be standardized with direct supervision. Middle-class parents encourage their children in activities that foster achievement and that they believe will make them well-rounded, self-directed adults. They involve their children in such activities as dancing lessons, athletics, and scouting. Working-class parents tend to be more concerned that their children grow up to be moral, upright, and religious. Lower-class parents are less interested in the direction of their children's activities than with their conduct; they are more concerned that their children stay out of trouble.

With few exceptions, parents in all classes love their children and in a broad sense have similar goals regarding childrearing. Differences lie in the parental behavior toward the children in attempting to help them to reach these goals. Lower-class parents are more restrictive and rely on coercive techniques in child training. They stress obedience and conformity, and the most frequently used form of discipline for undesirable behavior is physical punishment. Middle-class parents are more apt to make use of manipulative techniques such as reasoning and drawing on the child's sense of guilt. They tend to scold and use isolation rather than physical punishment. There is more concern regarding the *intent* of the act than the *consequence* of the act. Upper middle–class parents are more permissive and foster desirable behavior through more lenient disciplinary methods, such as natural consequences and positive reinforcement. Lower-class parents tend to use more restrictive disciplinary methods, such as assertion of authority, deprivation, and punishment. However, these more punitive strategies can be modified with early intervention (Portes, Dunhan, and Williams, 1986).

The very poor in the society who consistently exist on or below the poverty level live in a perpetual state of despair. Their limited skills give them no bargaining power in the job market, and the education needed to improve their status is beyond them. The poor desire better things for their children but are trapped in a circular pattern that perpetuates their life condition. Their powerlessness to control their fate or condition is a source of fatalism and resignation that is characteristic of the group in general. Optimism, when it is manifest, is more likely to be expressed in terms of luck or chance. This fatalistic attitude is a significant impediment to occupational and educational aspirations and to seeking health care. It also inhibits them from seeking health care or practicing preventive health care measures. For example, if someone is injured or killed in an automobile injury, it is bad luck, not something that could have been prevented by wearing a seat belt.

Poverty

A subcultural influence closely related to but different from social class is the condition known as poverty. It is a relative concept and is usually associated with the general standards of a population. An *absolute standard* of poverty attempts to delimit some basic set of resources needed for adequate existence; a *relative standard* reflects the median standard of living in a society and is the term used in referring to childhood poverty in the United States (Bauwens and Anderson, 1984). That is, what appears to be deprivation in one area may be a standard or norm in another.

In the United States, rates of poverty have changed dramatically—to the detriment of children. Presently it is estimated that 20% of all children live in poverty (defined in 1989 as annual income of $10,060 or less for a family of three). Almost 50% of black children and more than one third of Hispanic children live in families with incomes below the poverty level. What is even more alarming is the fact that over the past three decades, rates for childhood poverty have increased by 37%, whereas rates for the elderly have fallen by 49%. These trends have left childhood in a precarious position—the concentration of poverty rates in children has never been as great as it currently is (Wise and Meyers, 1988).

For the majority of children who experience poverty, it is not necessarily a persistent state of living. Rather, evidence indicates that families go in and out of financial scarcity. Nearly half of the children in the United States are in a vulnerable economic position at least once during their childhood. Persistent poverty is a way of life for 2½ million children under age 15, and intermittent poverty affects the lives of an additional 3½ million children.

The factor most related to the child's probability of experiencing poverty is race, with black children more likely than any other racial or ethnic group to experience poverty. The reasons for this increased prevalence of poverty among black children is not entirely clear. For example, the expected prevalence of poverty for black children living in intact two-parent families is about the same as for white children who live in one-parent families. In transitory childhood poverty, the single most important event for both black and white children is loss of one or more wage earners (Duncan and Rodgers, 1988).

Approximately half of all poor children live in households headed by females; however, the presence of a working father is no guarantee that the family will not live in poverty. More than 70% of the increase in the number of poor children that occurred in the early 1980s was due to rising poverty in families with a man present. In addition, approximately one fourth of children in families with married parents would be poor if they depended on the father's income alone. Although these trends have complex origins, they illustrate the growing inability of the American family to provide economic essentials that all children need (Wise and Meyers, 1988). Two groups of children who live in poverty include the homeless and migrant workers.

Homeless. One of the most pressing problems in the United States is the growing number of homeless families. Homeless individuals are those persons who lack resources and community ties necessary to provide for their own adequate shelter. In the past the homeless population traditionally included single adults, mostly males. Currently, the fastest growing segment of the homeless consists of families, most commonly single mothers with two or three children, who comprise more than 33% of the homeless population, with estimates in some cities exceeding 50%. More than half of homeless children are less than 5 years of age and are predominantly from minority groups (American Academy of Pediatrics, 1988; Alperstein and Arnstein, 1988).

Another group of homeless children are the "runaway" and "throwaway" adolescents. Nationwide it has been estimated that this group numbers between 250,000 and 500,000. Over 90% tend to come from minority ethnic groups and usually from troubled families, including mentally and physically abusive parents (Alperstein and Arnstein, 1988).

Many families are becoming homeless because of financial and housing problems, such as loss of job and income, loss of welfare benefits, being victims of robbery, and eviction (Wood, 1989). A recent trend that has displaced some poor families from their residences is the renovation of lower-class, urban neighborhoods by middle- or upper middle–class groups, a phenomenon known as *gentrification* (Skolnick, 1987). Lack of a permanent dwelling deprives children of the most basic necessities for proper growth and development. Children who are homeless suffer from physical and mental disorders that exceed those found in poor families who have a permanent residence (Bassuk and Rosenberg, 1990).

Migrant families. One of the most disadvantaged groups is migrant farm workers and their children. Estimates indicate that in the United States there are between 3 and 5 million migrant and seasonal workers and their dependents, whose average yearly income is well below the poverty level. In addition, most of the families have no health care insurance (American Academy of Pediatrics, 1989).

The low position of these families on the economic scale and their rootless, mobile existence subjects them to inadequate sanitation, substandard housing, social isolation, and lack of educational and medical facilities. This life-style is especially deleterious to the children. Schooling and health care are inadequate. Children are apt to live in a number of localities and attend a variety of schools in the course of a year with no continuity in either education or health care. Because both parents work in the fields, children receive little adult supervision; therefore, injury rates are high and meals are erratic. Except where prohibited by law, children are even recruited to work in the fields along with the adults.

Some migrants have a home base to which they return at the end of a growing season; others travel continuously, migrating north in summer and south in winter. With most there is little if any integration into the dominant culture; therefore migrant groups suffer social isolation. Groups who travel together, especially those with the same ethnic background, develop a cohesiveness and form their own set of values and customs. Sometimes a migrant family will leave the migration stream and become a part of a permanent community. However, this involves adaptation to a new environment and life-style that can be stress provoking to these families.

Affluence

On the opposite end of the socioeconomic spectrum are the children of affluent members of society. Although they can live within the warmth of a positive family relationship, many of them appear to be just as deprived as the poverty stricken (Grinker, 1978). Wealth does not provide protection against many of life's problems and disappointments, especially in the area of parent-child relationships. Like their counterparts in the poverty groups, children of the affluent suffer from social discrimination (too rich or not rich enough to meet different standards), inadequate parenting, or unsatisfactory role models.

Children of the wealthy suffer most from lack of parental contact. There may be long separations from loving, caring parents because of social or business interests. Some have a cold, sometimes hostile parent, who is rarely available to the children. Even their places of residence contribute to their isolation and loneliness. Purchased parent surrogates such as servants, sports professionals (such as tennis or swimming instructors), and private school personnel provide their adult companionship and authority. The children of the wealthy are especially subject to psychologic problems and antisocial behavior. The difference between behavior in the rich and the poor is that self-indulgent behavior in the rich is often viewed as acceptable (Grinker, 1978).

Many children from wealthy families, just like those from poor families, seem to thrive and flourish, making positive contributions to their families and society. However, a large number grow up to display a lack of motivation or self-discipline and boredom. They also may fail to acquire the necessary skills to handle responsibility and money, especially third-generation rich who are born into wealth and have developed less of the work ethic of earlier generations (Conatser, 1986).

Religion

Probably the most influential factor in shaping the culture of the United States is the Judeo-Christian faith. Many immigrants came to the country for religious freedom and established a religious and moral atmosphere that persists today. However, there are individual differences that are part of the general culture.

The religious orientation of the family dictates a code of morality as well as influencing the family's attitudes toward education, male and female role identity, and attitudes regarding their ultimate destiny (Fig. 2-2). It may also determine the school that the children attend, the companions with whom they associate, and often their mate selection. In many cultures the religious beliefs are such an integral part of the culture that it is difficult to distinguish one from the other. In a few instances, such as the Mennonites and Amish communities, religion is the basis of a common way of life that determines where the children are reared and a totally individualistic life-style. (See also Religious Beliefs, p. 49)

Schools

When children enter school, their radius of relationships extends to include a wider variety of peers and a new focus of authority. Although parents continue to exert the major influence on the children, in the school environment teachers have the most significant psychologic impact on their development and socialization. The function of teachers is primarily limited to teaching, but, like parents, they are concerned about the emotional welfare of the children. Both parents and teachers must constrain behavior, and both are in a position to enforce standards of conduct.

Socialization. Next to the family the schools exert the major force in providing continuity between generations by conveying a vast amount of culture from the older members

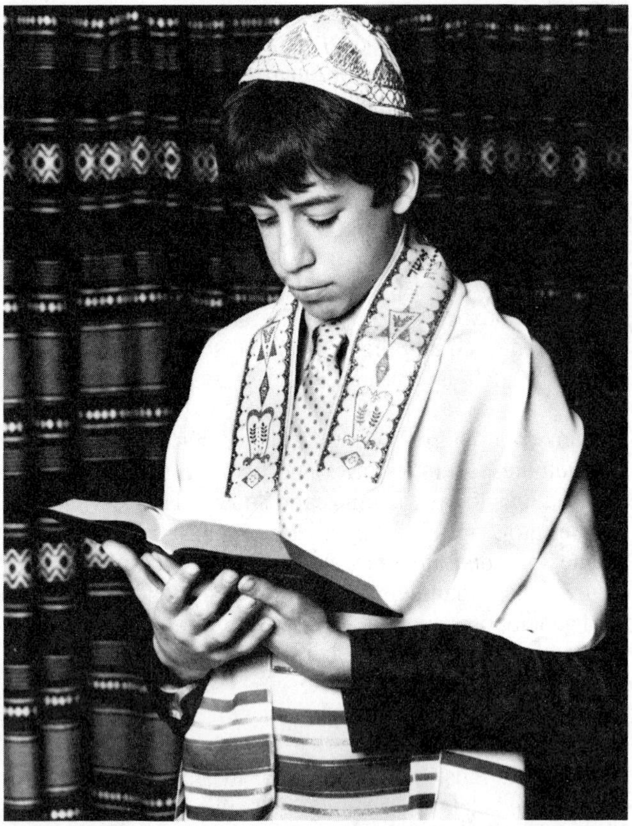

Fig. 2-2. A boy during his bar mitzvah ceremony.

to the young. In this way children are prepared to carry out the traditional social roles they are expected to assume as adults in society. School is the center of "cultural diffusion" wherein the cultural standards of the larger group are mediated to the local community. It governs what is taught and, to a large extent, how it is taught. School rules and regulations regarding attendance, authority relationships, and the system of sanctions and rewards based on achievement transmit to the child the behavioral expectations of the adult world of employment and relationships. School is often the only institution in which children systematically learn about the negative consequences of behaviors that deviate from social expectations. In addition, the school provides an opportunity for some children to participate in the larger society in rewarding ways and often provides avenues for social mobility for both students and teachers. Through education individuals in the lower classes are offered the opportunity for further education and the capacity to move up in the social strata.

Teachers have the responsibility for transmitting the knowledge and values of the dominant culture, that is, those values on which there is broad consensus. They are expected to stimulate and guide the intellectual development of children and their sense of esthetics and to foster their capacity for creative problem solving.

Traditionally the socialization process of school began when the child entered kindergarten or the first grade. With over 60% of mothers working outside the home, this socialization process begins much earlier for a significant number of children in a variety of daycare settings (Ziegler and Hall, 1988). Considering that the majority of mothers work because of economic necessity, this trend toward out-of-home care for children will probably continue.

Peer Cultures

Peer groups also have an impact on the socialization of children (Fig. 2-3). Peer relationships become increasingly important and influential as children proceed through school. In school children have what can be regarded as a culture of their own. It is most apparent in the school and in the unsupervised play group. The play group presents this culture in a much purer form than does the school, which is partly produced by adults.

During their lives children are exposed to value systems such as those of the family, ethnic group, and social class. In peer-group interaction they are confronted with a variety of these sets of values. The values imposed by the peer group are especially compelling because children must accept and conform to them in order to be accepted as members of the group. When the peer values are not too different from those of family and teachers, the mild conflict created by these small differences serves to separate children from the adults in their lives and to strengthen the feeling of belonging to the peer group.

The kind of socialization provided by the peer group depends on the special subculture that develops from the background, interests, and capabilities of its members. Some groups support school achievement, others focus on athletic prowess, and still others are decidedly antithetic to educative goals. Scholastic achievement is strongly related to the value system of the peer groups. Many conflicts between teachers and students and between parents and students can be attributed to fear of rejection by peers. There is always a conflict between what is expected from parents regarding academic achievement and what is expected from the peer culture. This is especially pronounced in high school and is discussed further in Chapter 19.

Although it has neither the traditional authority of the parents nor the legal authority of the schools for teaching information, the peer group manages to convey a substantial amount of information to its members, especially about taboo subjects such as sex and drugs. Children's need for the friendship of their peers brings them into an increasingly complex social system. The world of the peer group is different from the adult world and, through peer relationships, children learn ways in which to deal with dominance and hostility and to relate with persons in positions of leadership and authority. Another function of the peer subculture is to relieve boredom and to provide recognition that individual members do not receive from teachers and other authority figures.

The peer-group culture has secrets, mores, and codes of ethics with which they promote feelings of group solidarity and detachment from adults. They have traditions and folkways that are transferred from "generation to generation" of

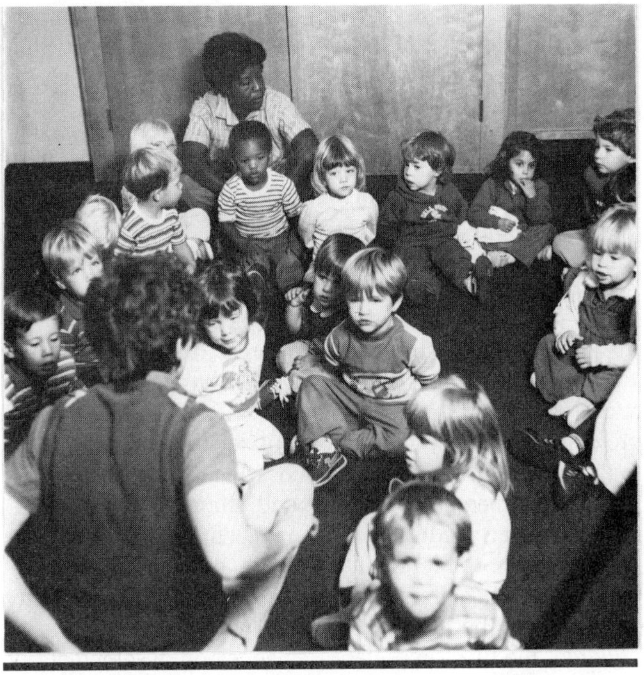

Fig. 2-3. Children from a variety of cultural and ethnic backgrounds begin to socialize in the daycare setting.

school children and that have a great influence over the behavior of all members of the group. There are age-related games and other activities and, as children move from one level to the next, folkways of the younger group are discarded as those of the new are adopted. For example, a school-age child rides a bicycle to school; the high-school student prefers a car. As they advance, children are forward oriented only—they look forward with anticipation but look backward with contempt.

Biculture

Some children are exposed to the values, role relationships, and life-styles of two cultures—a virtual "straddling" of two cultures. This is sometimes observed in the play group but usually is not a significant factor until children enter school. Children of two cultures must unlearn some of the established practices of one culture in order to become socialized in the other, especially in role relationships. For example, children from Hispanic and Oriental cultures are taught to look away when scolded; in United States schools the teacher expects direct eye contact—"Look at me when I speak to you" (Sloat and Matsuura, 1990). Children learn new roles and social behavior more rapidly than their adult counterparts.

This biculture is particularly marked in language differences. The bilingual child is said to be at a disadvantage in school situations of the dominant culture, in which there is controversy over bilingual education. On the one hand those supporting bilingual education adhere to the principle that children will understand more readily and perform more realistically (especially in testing situations) if learning is directed in their own language; others contend that children living in a dominant culture should adopt the ways of that culture, including language.

Another aspect of biculture occurs when children meld the elements of the dominant culture and the minority culture with the characteristics of a subculture that is uniquely their own.

THE CHILD AND FAMILY IN NORTH AMERICA

America is an aggregate of numerous Old and New World cultures that are blended with the unique heritage of pioneering frontiersmen. Models of childrearing appear to reflect the history of the country. The early philosophic standards of the Protestant ethic, which resulted in a pleasureless, hard-driven, independent individual, is gradually being replaced in contemporary American society by the social ethic, which emphasizes a group-oriented and other-directed philosophy.

The frontier background of the American culture has also contributed to the overall orientation to life and childrearing. There has always been a basic optimistic view of the world, a belief that things can be better and that the children can and will be better off than the parents. This hopeful outlook and a general future orientation together with the possibility of upward social mobility have created a pervasive overall attitude of optimism. Increasing development of self-confidence and autonomy in children is fostered and encouraged. Children are generally permitted a greater degree of freedom than in more tradition-oriented cultures, where individuals remain in one social class for life.

Family life in America is characterized by increasing geographic and economic mobility. Here there is less reliance on tradition, families are fragmented, and there is limited opportunity to transmit and acquire the traditional and accepted customs of a culture. Consequently young adults rely to a greater extent on the professed experts, peers, and the mass media for acquisition of acceptable patterns of behavior, including childrearing practices. Each generation, as it adapts to the new, discards the inadequacies of previous generations. This often constitutes a source of confusion and frustration as parents attempt to adjust to rapid changes; tradition and precedent no longer meet needs and challenges of rapid change that require new approaches and innovation for problem solving. Competent parents attempt to determine the comparatively stable, essential components of the culture and transmit these to their children. Awareness of an attention to changing cultural norms during childrearing helps the parent to adapt to the new demands of the culture that are different from those they learned as children.

Minority-Group Membership

The United States has more racial, ethnic, and religious minority groups than any other country (McGoldrick, 1987). Ethnic minority groups are becoming increasingly important because each group is expected to produce children at a faster rate than the majority white population (Table 2-1).

Table 2-1 Number of children by race and Spanish origin

	NUMBER IN MILLIONS		
	1980	1990	2000
Race/Spanish origin			
White	52.2	51.9	53.5
Nonwhite*	11.2	12.4	13.9
Black	9.5	10.3	11.4
Spanish origin	NA	7.1	8.7

Modified from U.S. children and their families: current conditions and recent trends, Select Committee on Children, Youth, and Families, Washington, DC, 1987, U.S. Government Printing Office. Cited in Evans (1989), p. 37.
**Nonwhite* refers to all races other than white and includes blacks, Indians, Japanese, Chinese, and any other race except white. Blacks comprise the great majority of nonwhites. People of Spanish origin can be of any race.

The increases are due to higher fertility rates in many of the minority groups and the immigration of minority adults of childbearing age. Blacks are the largest minority group, followed closely by Hispanics (Evans, 1989).

The definition of various minority groups is not universal. In the 1990 United States census form, *blacks* included persons identified, for example, as African- or Afro-American, Haitian, Jamaican, West Indian, or Nigerian. Persons of *Spanish/Hispanic origin* included Mexican, Mexican-American, Chicano, Puerto Rican, Cuban, Argentinean, Columbian, Costa Rican, Dominican, Ecuadoran, Guatemalan, Honduran, Nicaraguan, Peruvian, and Salvadoran persons, as well as persons from other Spanish-speaking countries or the Caribbean or Central or South America. *Mexican-American* referred only to persons of Mexican origin or ancestry. In some writings, the term *Latino* refers to individuals from Mexico and Central America (Friedman, 1990).

One of the difficulties with including diverse groups of people under ethnic labels, such as black or Hispanic, is that the groups can differ tremendously in their own cultural heritage. Just as the majority white population differs according to various subcultures, such as socioeconomic status and occupation, so do the minority groups. For example, black families may be upper class (10%), middle class (about 40%), or lower class (about 50%), with subdivisions within these categories (Skolnick, 1987). The reader should be aware that any of the generalizations made in this chapter to an ethnic group may not apply to certain groups and individuals.

When minority groups immigrate to another country, a certain degree of cultural/ethnic blending occurs through the process of *acculturation,* those gradual changes produced in a culture by the influence of another culture that cause one or both cultures to be more similar to the other. However, the changes occur to various degrees in different families and groups. At one time is was believed that the great diversity among the ethnic groups in the United States would result in a great "melting pot" where the differences among different cultures would eventually diminish to produce a homogeneous society. However, this does not appear to be the case. Many groups continue to identify with their traditional heritage while adapting to the ill-defined concept of the "American way."

Studies in the past indicate that early in life children become aware of their racial or ethnic status and of the discriminatory attitudes of the majority culture toward their group. The direct effects of discrimination are anger and low self-esteem, which become manifest in a variety of behaviors. Inner conflicts and suppressed hostility that focus children's attention inward may be factors in the failure of many children to achieve in other areas.

Evidence indicates that changes in attitudes are slowly taking place in some groups and in some places. With growing awareness, interest, and understanding by increasing numbers of the majority group, which has accompanied the recent emergence of racial and ethnic pride, minority-group children are becoming more secure and confident in their racial or ethnic identity. Individuals vary in their reactions to membership in a minority group, and much of this variation can be attributed to familial factors. As with all children, the most important influences on development of the positive self-image are warm, understanding parents who take an active interest in fostering their children's growth. Parents who accept their children and react positively and constructively rather than in a negative and self-defeating manner will help their children develop feelings of self-worth, self-esteem, and self-acceptance. The more adequate children feel, the more positive will be their attitudes toward both majority and minority children, the greater will be their ability to withstand prejudice and intolerance, and the less will be their need for counteraggressive behavior.

CULTURAL SHOCK

The term *cultural shock* describes the "feelings of helplessness and discomfort and a state of disorientation experienced by an outsider attempting to comprehend or effectively adapt to a different cultural group because of differences in cultural practices, values, and beliefs" (Leininger , 1978). This state occurs with both clients and health care providers who move from one culture to another culture or setting. It can happen to persons who immigrate to a new country (such as the Asian refugees) or persons from a subcultural group who must adjust to the ways of an unfamiliar subgroup (such as children entering the school subculture or clients who enter the hospital subculture). Cultural shock is characterized by the inability to respond to or function in a new or strange situation.

Numerous factors influence the reactions to a new environment. Language barriers, including dialects and jargon (such as medical language) specific to a subcultural group, inhibit effective communication. Habits and customs (such as different role behaviors or etiquette) and differences in attitudes and beliefs are puzzling to the stranger in the new environment. The outsider experiences an intense sense of isolation and feelings of loneliness and nonrelatedness.

Nurses entering an unfamiliar cultural situation can reduce the cultural shock by becoming familiar with the cultural groups with which they work and by learning tolerance of the values, beliefs, and customs of these groups.

Immigrants and refugees from cultures in which children are taught to respect and obey their elders and in which females are considered inferior to males, such as most Asian cultures, may find difficulty dealing with the consequences of Western egalitarianism. When children enter the school system, they learn to question authority and are confronted with the movement for equality of the sexes in all aspects of life. This often creates conflict within the family, especially in families such as the Vietnamese, who consider education highly valuable for their children.

CULTURAL/RELIGIOUS INFLUENCES ON HEALTH CARE

Cultural beliefs and practices are an important part of data gathering in the nursing assessment. Nurses continually encounter beliefs and practices that may facilitate or impede nursing interventions, including attitudes toward family planning, food habits, and folkways that are firmly entrenched in the culture. The language of the client may be different from that of the larger culture, or there may be regional or ethnic peculiarities in the use of basic English. Subcultural influences, such as some religious beliefs and practices, may be in conflict with standard health practices and therapeutic interventions.

SUSCEPTIBILITY TO HEALTH PROBLEMS

Some groups of people are more susceptible and others more resistant to certain illnesses than are persons from other groups. An innate susceptibility is acquired through generations of evolutionary changes that take place within constrained or segregated populations. The proximity to disease, environmental factors, and the general physical status are significant factors associated with health problems.

Hereditary Factors

The genetic constitution of individuals as groups influences the degree to which they are susceptible to a specific disorder. It may be the result of an inherent lack of resistance to a disease organism, a trait that is an advantage in one environment but which places the possessor at a disadvantage in another, or it may be the consequence of intermarriage within a relatively narrow range of geographic, ethnic, or religious restrictions.

A geographic constraint is illustrated by the classic example of the common communicable disease rubeola. The rubeola virus, or the populations that were continually exposed to it, became altered in such a way that the disease was considered to be a universal disease of childhood from which the majority of children suffered without ill effects. When other populations (e.g., the inhabitants of the Hawaiian Islands) were exposed to the virus by explorers and missionaries, they experienced a violent response that resulted in high mortality.

Another communicable disease, tuberculosis, appears to be more prevalent in certain ethnic groups such as the Native Americans of the Southwest, Vietnamese immigrants, and Mexican-Americans (Orque, 1983b). In many populations it is difficult to determine how much the increased incidence can be attributed to ethnic factors and how much is related to the life-styles in the lower social strata.

A number of diseases show ethnic or racial differences. For example, Tay-Sachs disease, characterized by early neurologic deterioration and mental retardation, affects primarily Ashkenasi Jewish families, particularly those of Northeastern European origin, while Sephardic Jewish families appear to be no more at risk for the disease than other populations. The incidence of cystic fibrosis is highest in whites, it is almost nonexistent in Orientals, and the rare affected blacks are usually in areas where there is apt to be mixed ancestry. Some selected genetic disorders that are more prevalent in certain populations are listed in Table 2-2. Racial and ethnic differences are further considered in relation to diseases and defects as they are discussed throughout the book.

Other groups appear to have a predisposition for certain diseases. Although sickle cell disease is a classic disorder of blacks, especially Africans, cardiovascular disease, pneumonia, and diabetes are also high among blacks. Hispanics are more likely to suffer from diabetes and infectious/parasitic diseases than their Anglo counterparts, and Native Americans have particularly high rates of tuberculosis, diarrhea, alcoholism, and suicide (Bullough and Bullough, 1982; Markides and Coreil, 1986).

Common food items and drugs may cause health problems in certain racial groups. For example, persons with glucose-6-phosphate dehydrogenase (G-6-PD) deficiency develop acute hemolytic anemia after they ingest fava (horse or broad) beans or certain drugs such as aspirin preparations, sulfonamides, or primaquine. The deficiency is the most common enzyme abnormality and is found in a large percentage of people around the world, especially those of Mediterranean, African, Near Eastern, and Asian origin (Cohen, 1984).

The sensitivity to foods containing lactose is a common hereditary characteristic of several cultural groups, especially southern Europeans, Jews, Arabs, blacks, Asians, and Native Americans. Lactose intolerance usually does not become a problem until the child reaches 3 to 5 years of age. However, lactose-intolerant children become uncomfortable with distention, flatus, and diarrhea after ingesting milk or milk products. Unknowing but well-meaning health workers may be responsible for these symptoms in their clients when they prescribe foods containing lactose as sources of nutrients.

An example of resistance to disease, or selective advantage, of a population is found in persons who possess the sickle cell trait. Persons with sickle cell trait are highly resistant to a form of malaria, and in the parts of the world

Table 2-2 Distribution of selected genetic traits and disorders by population or ethnic group

ETHNIC OR POPULATION GROUP	GENETIC OR MULTIFACTORIAL DISORDER PRESENT IN RELATIVELY HIGH FREQUENCY
Åland Islanders	Ocular albinism (Forsius-Erikkson type)
Amish	Limb-girdle muscular dystrophy (IN—Adams, Allen counties) Ellis-van Creveld (PA—Lancaster county) Pyruvate kinase deficiency (OH—Mifflin county) Hemophilia B (PA—Holmes county)
Armenians	Familial Mediterranean fever Familial paroxysmal polyserositis
Blacks (African)	Sickle cell disease Hemoglobin C disease Hereditary persistence of hemoglobin F G-6-PD deficiency, African type Lactase deficiency, adult β-Thalassemia
Burmese	Hemoglobin E disease
Chinese	Alpha thalassemia G-6-PD deficiency, Chinese type Lactase deficiency, adult
Costa Rican	Malignant osteopetrosis
Druze	Alkaptonuria
English	Cystic fibrosis Hereditary amyloidosis, type III
Eskimos	Congenital adrenal hyperplasia Pseudocholinesterase deficiency Methemoglobinemia
Finns	Congenital nephrosis Generalized amyloidosis syndrome, V Polycystic liver disease Retinoschisis Aspartylglycosaminuria Diastrophic dwarfism
French Canadians (Quebec)	Tyrosinemia Morquio syndrome
Gypsies (Czech)	Congenital glaucoma
Hopi Indians	Tyrosinase positive albinism
Iceland	Phenylketonuria
Irish	Phenylketonuria Neural tube defects
Japanese	Acatalasemia Cleft lip/palate Oguchi disease
Jews	
Ashkenazi	Tay-Sachs disease (infantile) Niemann-Pick disease (infantile) Gaucher disease (adult type) Familial dysautonomia (Riley-Day syndrome) Bloom syndrome Torsion dystonia Factor XI (PTA) deficiency
Sephardi	Familial Mediterranean fever Ataxia-telangiectasia (Morocco) Cystinuria (Libya) Glycogen storage disease III (Morocco)
Lapps	Congenital dislocation of hip
Lebanese	Dyggve-Melchoir-Clausen syndrome
Mediterranean people (Italians, Greeks)	G-6-PD deficiency, Mediterranean type β-Thalassemia Familial Mediterranean fever
Navaho Indians	Ear anomalies
Nova Scotia Acadians	Niemann-Pick disease, type D
Oriental	Dubin-Johnson syndrome (Iran) Ichthyosis vulgaris (Iraq, India) Werdnig-Hoffman disease (Karaite Jews) G-6-PD deficiency, Mediterranean type Phenylketonuria (Yemen) Metachromatic leukodystrophy (Habbanite Jews, Saudi Arabia)
Polish	Phenylketonuria
Polynesians	Clubfoot
Portugese	Joseph disease
Scandinavians (Norwegians, Swedes, Danes)	Cholestasis-lymphedema (Norwegians) Sjögren-Larsson syndrome (Swedes) Krabbe disease Phenylketonuria
Scots	Phenylketonuria Cystic fibrosis Hereditary amyloidosis, type III
Thai	Lactase deficiency, adult Hemoglobin E disease
Zuni Indians	Tyrosinase positive albinism

Data from Cohen, F.L.: Clinical genetics in nursing practice, Philadelphia, 1984, J.B. Lippincott Co., pp. 23-24; Damon, A.: Race, ethnic group and disease, Soc. Biol. 16:69, 1969; Der Kaloustian, V.M., Maffah, J., and Loiselet, J.: Genetic diseases in Lenanon, Am. J. Med. Genet. 7:187, 1980; Goodman, R.M.: Genetic disorders among the Jewish people, Baltimore, 1979, Johns Hopkins University Press; McKusick, V.: Mendelian inheritance in man, ed. 8, Baltimore, 1988, Johns Hopkins University Press; Tamot, B.: Genetic polymorphisms and diseases in man, New York, 1974, Academic Press, Inc.; Stanbury, J.B.: The metabolic basis of inherited disease, New York, 1983, McGraw-Hill, Inc.; Ferak, V., Genčík, A., and Genčíkova, A.: Population genetical aspects of primary congenital glaucoma, Hum. Genet. 61:193, 1982.

where the organisms are prevalent, there is a high frequency of the trait. However, in an environment where malaria is not a threat, possession of the trait has no advantage and only the negative aspects of the condition remain (risk of sickle cell anemia in offspring).

Physical characteristics. Among racial groups there are observable differences in physical appearance. The most obvious are skin and hair coloring and texture. Skin color is determined by the amount of melanin pigment present in the skin. Persons from countries located near the equator have darkly pigmented skin, which serves to protect the skin from the year-round exposure to the sun's rays; persons from the northern countries have very light skin, which provides for maximum exposure to the sun's rays (necessary for vitamin D metabolism) during the short daylight hours. There can be wide variations in skin color between these two extremes in terms of geographic origin or from intermixing of dark and light skin color.

As a consequence of the dark pigmentation, the detection of skin color changes can be difficult and requires modification of assessment techniques. For example, vasomotor alterations, cyanosis, and jaundice observable in the skin are not easily recognized in very dark or black skin. Variations in the skin color can alter the appearance of the skin in a given circumstance (see Table 7-8).

Variations in the newborn are often related to racial or ethnic origin. For example, newborn infants of Asian and black parents are smaller than infants of white parentage (David, 1990). Bluish pigmented areas (mongolian spots) on the sacral region are a common observation on Oriental, black, Native American, and Mexican-American infants.

Evaluation of stature and body build reveals some racial tendencies. Oriental children are usually smaller at all ages and black children are taller and heavier between ages 5 and 14 than white children of the same age (see growth measurements, Appendix C). This difference in stature can lead to misinterpretation of health status and capabilities. Black children who appear normal for their age may, in fact, be underdeveloped when compared with other black children (Bloch, 1983). In communication and education a child who is smaller than the average may appear precocious and one who is larger might appear to be slow. Expectations determined on this basis can be detrimental to the child.

Socioeconomic Factors

The most overwhelming adverse influence on health is socioeconomic status. A higher percentage of lower-class individuals are suffering from some health problem at any one time than are those in any other group. The sum of all aspects of their situation contributes to and compounds health problems; this includes crowded living conditions and poor sanitation, which facilitate transfer of disease. There is a higher incidence of lead poisoning in children from lower-class families, where there is more ready access to lead in the environment, such as paint and other lead-containing compounds or utensils, pottery with lead-containing glazes, and burning of lead-containing batteries for heat in winter.

In the lower classes, children are less likely to be immunized against preventable diseases than are children in the upper and middle classes. Lack of funds or inaccessibility to health services inhibits treatment for any but severe illness or injury. Sometimes health care is inadequate because of ignorance. In some areas a disorder is so commonplace that it is looked on as unavoidable; it is not recognized as something that requires (or is amenable to) treatment. The parents may not have information regarding causes, treatment, outcome of the illness, or preventive measures.

Poverty. A high correlation between poverty and the prevalence of illness has long been observed. Impoverished families suffer from poor nutrition; they have little if any preventive health care, inadequate health maintenance, and very limited access to health services. One of the most significant health problems related to poverty is a high infant mortality rate (Wise and Myers, 1988). Health care often ranks low on their list of priorities. Day-to-day needs of food, clothing, and lodging take precedence as long as the ailing person feels able to perform activities of daily living.

Poor families are denied access to many health institutions for emergency or other hospital care. Frequently they must travel long distances to service centers that are willing to assume their care. In an emergency they must find money for taxi fare, borrow an automobile, or seek other means of transportation. They must find care for dependents, such as other infants and small children, or have them accompany them when taking the ill child for care. Families tend to delay preventive care indefinitely unless health services are relatively accessible. They are more likely to consult folk practitioners or other persons within their community.

Poor nutrition accounts for many health problems in the lower classes. Lack of funds and ignorance result in a diet that may be seriously lacking in essential food substances, especially protein, vitamins, and iron. This inadequate diet often leads to nutritional deficiency disorders and growth retardation in children. In many the total intake is insufficient to support normal growth. Unstructured eating patterns and irregularly scheduled mealtimes can also contribute to erratic food intake and a proportionately larger consumption of nonnourishing snacks, which can result in excessive weight gain.

Because of deficient preventive care, dental problems are more prevalent. Lack of standard immunizations together with reduced resistance from poor nutrition renders the exposed children in poor segments of the population vulnerable to communicable diseases. Poor sanitation and crowded living conditions also contribute to the higher incidence and perpetuation of illness. In general poor people become ill more frequently and remain ill for longer periods of time than persons in the general population.

Homeless. Homeless children experience all of the health problems associated with poverty, as well as other types of disorders. Preventive health care, especially immunization and dental care, is seriously lacking. Both delayed growth and overweight problems are common (Miller and Lin, 1988). Developmental delays, severe depression, anxiety, and learning difficulties have been reported (Bass and others, 1990; Bassuk and Rosenberg, 1990). The erratic chaotic life-style of these children increases their vulnerability to any number of physical and psychosocial problems, including child abuse, illicit drug use, and prostitution (Alperstein and Arnstein, 1988).

Migrant families. Migrants generally suffer more illness, both acute and chronic, than does the general population. They are subject to unhealthy environments, poverty, and insufficient medical care; their health-seeking behavior in general is an illness- or injury-oriented recourse to medical care. Affected persons will postpone seeking care for themselves or their children until physical pain or suffering is almost unbearable (O'Brien, 1982).

When medical care is provided to a migrant family, follow-up care is usually impossible because of their transient life-style. Compliance to medical therapies is primarily related to accessiblity and availability. For example, medications provided by health workers are more likely to be taken than those that must be obtained at a pharmacy. In addition, medications are often discontinued following self-perceived recovery. Treatment regimens that do not interfere with work or family responsibilities are most likely to be adhered to. Their entire approach to health care is described by O'Brien (1982) as "pragmatic survivalism," a concept "symbolizing a pattern of health-illness attitudes and behaviors that focus on the achievement and maintenance of low-level wellness in the most practical manner possible for the continuance of productive life."

The health problems of migrant children appear to be dental caries, upper respiratory tract infections, otitis media, scabies and lice, intestinal parasites, pesticide exposure, injuries, teenage pregnancy, and growth and development delay (American Academy of Pediatrics, 1989).

CUSTOMS AND FOLKWAYS

Nurses are becoming increasingly aware of the need to consider cultural differences in clients when providing health care. An understanding of the various beliefs regarding the causation of illness and disease as well as traditional health practices is essential to successful intervention. The more nurses know about the values, beliefs, and customs of other ethnic groups, the better able they are to meet the needs of these families and to gain their cooperation and compliance.

Relationships with Health Care Providers

The manner of relating with health care providers differs considerably among cultural groups. One area of conflict to some nurses is the attitude toward time and waiting that is part of some cultures. The time orientation of Hispanic and black ethnic groups is in the present. For example, blacks are very flexible in their time orientation; a black family may be late for or miss appointments because other issues take precedence over the appointment and they may not communicate this to the health agency (Bloch, 1983). Hispanics, too, have a very relaxed view of time. Whereas the dominant culture in the United States says that "time flies," the Hispanic says, "time walks." The Japanese, on the other hand, consider time to be valuable and to be used wisely. They tend to be punctual for medical appointments and persistent in following prescribed regimens (Hashizume and Takano, 1983). A Vietnamese family will subordinate time to values considered to be more significant, such as propriety. They may be late for an appointment because of an overextended visit by a friend in their home. The Vietnamese do not hurry personal visits in order to maintain social harmony (Orque, 1983b).

In many cultural groups the mother assumes the responsibility for health care; in others both parents are involved equally in relationships with health workers. A somewhat different approach is apparent in some of the Oriental cultures. For example, the father in Vietnamese families, as unquestioned head of the family, is traditionally the family member who interacts with persons, including health care providers, outside the family unit. Therefore, he is the one who represents the family in health matters. In the Hispanic family the father, as head of the house, makes decisions regarding illness and treatment of family members, but the grandmother in the extended family is consulted regarding child care. Usually the family confers with other members before reaching a decision regarding treatment or hospitalization of a child. The Arab family also relies on others to give advice and guidance in a time of crisis (Meleis, 1981). A Japanese father may appear to be passive and uninvolved but actually is involved according to his own cultural standards (Tseng and others, 1982). In working with families, it is essential for nurses to identify key members—failure to include these significant individuals in teaching can seriously hinder adherence to the plan of care (Faber, 1986; Foss, 1987).

Nurses should make themselves aware of any specific attitudes regarding the manner of approach to a child in a given culture. Navajo Indians do not like a stranger near their infants. It is feared that the stranger may "witch" the child and cause the child harm. On the other hand, if a stranger, particularly a woman, lavishes attention on a Hispanic infant but fails to touch the child, the infant will develop symptoms of the "evil eye" (see p. 46). Vietnamese and Korean families may become upset if a newborn is admired at length for fear the evil spirits will overhear and desire the infant (Hollingsworth, Brown, and Brooten, 1980).

Some ethnic groups consider a child's admission to the hospital a family affair, with all members gathering to support and console the child and the parents. In others, such as the Samoan family, the family is willing to relinquish the care of the child to the hospital authority without interference. Their visits with the child are short, although intense, but this behavior may be misinterpreted by the hospital staff as disinterest or abandonment.

All ethnic groups are proud people who are entitled to be treated with dignity and respect. Family members are addressed by their last names: many groups consider it an affront to be called by their first names. Stereotyping is to be condemned. Persons are individuals who are evaluated in relation to their cultural standards, needs, and preferences (Fig. 2-4).

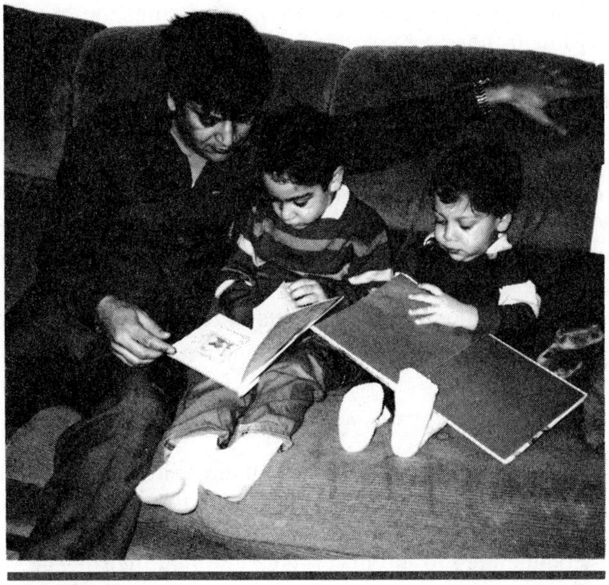

Fig. 2-4. Fathers from many cultures assume an active parenting role.

Nurses who are members of a majority culture may encounter tension and distrust in a child from a minority culture as a result of the child's learned conception or relationships with other persons in the majority group. Based on these perceptions, minority children often suspect that nurses may have hostile feelings toward them and fear ill treatment. When such children are hospitalized, this feeling compounds the feelings of loneliness, helplessness, and retribution that accompany fearful happenings and separation from families. The reverse situation may be encountered by a nurse from a minority culture attempting to meet the needs of a child who has been conditioned to view the nurse's cultural or ethnic group as inferior.

Communication. Communication is basic to all human relationships, but it may be a source of distress and misunderstanding between persons from different ethnic groups, especially if the languages are different. Ideally, conversations with families who are unable to speak the dominant language are best conducted by a health care worker who speaks the language of the family. If this is not possible, it may be necessary to engage the services of an interpreter. However, use of an interpreter can be a source of misunderstanding if the interpreter is unfamiliar with the medical terminology or if there are no corresponding words in the second language to express the ideas and concepts under discussion (see Communicating with Families Through an Interpreter, Chapter 6).

Some persons with poor or limited language comprehension may simply smile and nod in agreement if they do not understand the questions or directives. It is vital that the family fully understand all implications of a child's care and management before they sign permits for special procedures or assume responsibility for the child's care. It is not uncommon for an Oriental family to indicate "yes" when in fact they mean "no" in order to avoid social disharmony. They tend to use indirectness rather than confrontation and may become evasive when direct questioning makes them feel uncomfortable (Chen-Louie, 1983; Orque, 1983b).

Nonverbal communication is a practiced art in many American Indian tribes, and the members are highly sensitive to body language. They emphasize periods of silence to formulate thoughts in preparation for speech and often remain silent after listening to statements by others in order to properly assimilate what has been said. Interruption, interjection, or haste to arrive at abrupt conclusions is perceived as immature behavior.

Eye contact is viewed differently in cultures. It is not uncommon for persons in some ethnic groups to avoid eye contact and become uncomfortable when conversing with health workers. In non-Western cultures, a patient may not look directly into the nurse's eyes, as a sign of respect. Some Native Americans will make eye contact during the initial greeting, but continued, unwavering eye contact is considered insulting and disrespectful (Wilson, 1983).

There may be reluctance on the part of families to question or otherwise initiate contact with health professionals. In the Asian cultures, for example, it is considered a sign of disrespect to question those who are viewed as persons of authority (Orque, 1983b). A Japanese family may wait silently rather than ask or question. They believe that the health professionals know best and will meet their needs without being asked (Hashizume and Takano, 1983). It is also important to avoid criticism. Criticism can cause the Japanese-American to "lose face," to feel ashamed, which is highly undesirable.

It is necessary to speak slowly and carefully, not loudly, when conversing with families who have poor language comprehension. Many persons are able to read and write English better than they can speak or understand it. Also, the dominant language usually takes over in anxiety-provoking situations, even in persons who are able to communicate satisfactorily under ordinary circumstances.

Terms of address and use of first and last names vary among cultures and can create confusion in institutions. For example, in Asian cultures, the family name is given first in respect for the family and the given names follow. Therefore all siblings in a family have the same first name (in some families it may be the middle names that are the same). Ethiopians use no last names but have a very complex system whereby women retain their last names after marriage and the paternal grandfather's name becomes a child's last name. The Mennonites refer to children as sons and daughters of a particular parent, such as "Josiah's son," rather than by the son's name (Elkin and Handel, 1989).

Although all people share the basic emotions, there are decided ethnic variations in the way emotions are expressed. In some cultures (e.g., persons of Latin or Jewish background) emotions are expressed openly and members are accustomed to share their sorrows and joys with family and friends. Conversely, Nordic and Asian groups are more restrained in expressing emotion.

Nurses caring for persons of another culture will be better able to communicate if they understand the common names used to describe symptoms and diseases: for example, *miseries* (pain) and *locked bowels* (constipation) in black people and *caida de la mollera* (fallen fontanel from dehydration), *susto* (fright), and *la diarrhea* (diarrhea) in Latinos.

Food Customs

Food customs and symbolism of various cultural, ethnic, and religious groups have become an integral part of their lives. Although in a large country such as the United States most persons have adopted the eclectic food habits that have evolved over countless generations, many ethnic and geographic food traditions and preferences are retained. Special holidays, ceremonies, and life experiences such as births, birthdays, weddings, and death are often marked by special food items or feasts. In many cultures specific food practices are followed during pregnancy in the belief that certain foods damage the developing fetus.

The distinctive food customs of ethnic groups are a product of their native environment, determined by availability. Fish is a staple food of persons living near the ocean, such as people from Japan, Polynesia, and Scandinavia. Fruit and vegetable preferences are also directly related to the climate in which these grow naturally or can be cultivated. The types of grain that are ethnically associated are also those that grow best in their native lands. For example, rice is the staple grain of the Orient and Pacific islands, wheat of the temperate climates of Europe, rye in Scandinavia, and corn of the North American Indians. The diet of the Eskimo is predominantly fish and meat, depending on which is the most easily procured in the area. Even in the continental United States there are regional favorites, such as rice, hominy grits, and okra in the southern states. In some cultures food is highly spiced; in others foods tend to be bland. Table 2-3 lists the food items common to all cultures, and Table 2-4 outlines some of the foods associated with some specific ethnic groups.

There are a number of restrictions related to food items. Some have a physiologic origin, such as lack of dairy foods in the diets of some persons of African or Asian ancestry with lactose intolerance. Others have religious restrictions, such as kosher foods and food preparation of the Orthodox Jewish faith and the vegetarian diet of Seventh Day Adventists (see Vegetarian Diets, Chapter 13).

Children in a strange environment, such as the hospital, feel much more comfortable when they are served foods to which they are accustomed (Fig. 2-5). The hospital food often tastes strange and bland, especially to children who enjoy the highly seasoned foods of their culture. The family may be concerned that the child is receiving foods appropriate to their culture and beliefs (see Health Beliefs, p. 46). Where possible, it is advisable to provide children's ethnic foods or allow families to bring favorite foods that are not available on the hospital menu. Concern for differences in food habits and patterns projects an attitude of respect of the family's ethnic or religious heritage.

HEALTH BELIEFS AND PRACTICES

The nurse encounters people of many different racial and ethnic origins in the process of meeting the health needs of children and families. Some of these families have become so enculturated to the majority culture that their health beliefs and practices are consistent with those of the health care system. There are still numerous families, however, whose traditional practices and beliefs are an integral part

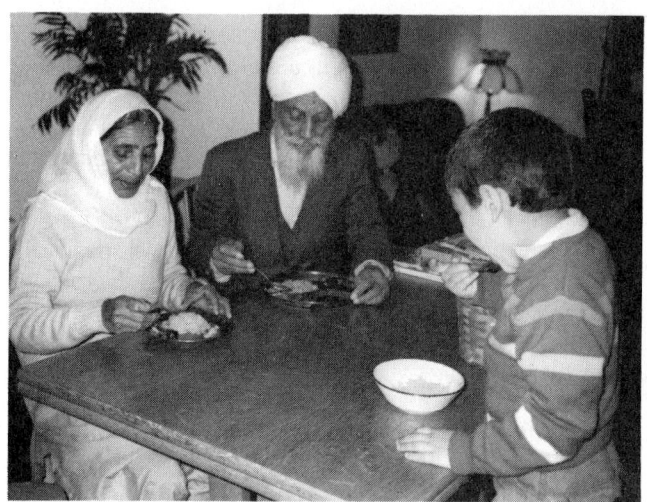

Fig. 2-5. Food customs outside the home can differ significantly from traditional cultural practices.

Table 2-3 Foods common to most ethnic food patterns

MEAT AND ALTERNATES	MILK AND MILK PRODUCTS	GRAIN PRODUCTS	VEGETABLES	FRUITS	OTHERS
Pork*	Milk, fluid	Rice	Carrots	Apples	Fruit juices
Beef	Ice cream	White bread	Cabbage	Bananas	
Chicken		Noodles, macaroni, spaghetti	Green beans	Oranges	
Eggs		Dry cereal	Greens (especially spinach)	Peaches	
			Sweet potatoes or yams	Pears	
			Tomatoes	Tangerines	

From Endres, J.B., and Rockwell, R.E.: Food, nutrition, and the young child, St. Louis, 1980, Mosby–Year Book, Inc., p. 180.
*May be restricted due to religious custom.

Table 2-4 Characteristic food choices for six groups

VEGETABLES	FRUITS	MEATS AND ALTERNATIVES	GRAIN PRODUCTS	OTHERS
Black				
Broccoli, corn, greens (mustard, collard, kale, turnips, beet, etc.), lima beans, okra, peas, pumpkin	Grapefruit, grapes, nectarine, plums, watermelon	Sausage, pig's feet, ears, etc., bacon, luncheon meat, organ meats, turkey, catfish, perch, red snapper, tuna, salmon, sardines, shrimp, kidney beans, red beans, black-eyed peas, peanuts, and peanut butter	Corn bread, hominy grits, biscuits, muffins, cooked cereal, crackers	Chitterlings, salt pork, gravies, buttermilk
Hispanic-American				
Avocado, chilies, corn, lettuce, onion, peas, potato, prickly pear (cactus leaf called *nopales*), zucchini	Guava, lemon, mango, melons, prickly pear (cactus fruit called *tuna*), zapote (or sapote)	Lamb, tripe, sausage *(chorizo)*, bologna, bacon, pinto beans, pink beans, garbanzo beans, lentils, peanuts, and peanut butter	Tortillas, corn flour, oatmeal, sweet bread *(pan dulce)*	Salsa (tomato-pepper, onion relish), chili sauce, guacamole, lard *(manteca)*, pork cracklings
Japanese				
Bamboo shoots, broccoli, burdock root, cauliflower, celery, cucumbers, eggplant, gourd *(Kampyo)*, mushrooms, napa cabbage, peas, peppers, radishes (daikon or pickles called *takuwan*), snow peas, squash, sweet potatoe, turnips, water chestnuts, yamaimo	Apricot, cherries, grapefruit, grapes, lemon, lime, melons, persimmon, pineapple, pomegranate, plums (dried pickled *umeboshi*), strawberries	Turkey, raw tuna or sea bass *(sashimi)*, mackerel, sardines *(mezashi)*, shrimp, abalone, squid, octopus, soybean curd *(tofu)*, soybean paste *(miso)*, soybeans, red beans *(azuki)*, lima beans, peanuts, almonds, cashews	Rice crackers, noodles (whole-wheat noodle called *soba* or *udon*), oatmeal	Soy sauce, Nori paste (used to season rice), bean thread *(konyaku)*, ginger (*shoga;* dried form called *denishoga*)
Chinese				
Bamboo shoots, bean sprouts, bok choy, broccoli, celery, Chinese cabbage, corn, cucumbers, eggplant, greens (collard, Chinese, broccoli, mustard, kale), leeks, lettuce, mushrooms, peppers, scallions, snow peas, taro, water chestnuts, white turnips, white radishes, winter melon	Figs, grapes, kumquats, loquats, mango, melons, persimmon, pineapple, plums, pomegranate	Organ meats, duck, white fish, shrimp, lobster, oyster, sardines, soybeans, soybean curd *(tofu)*, black beans, chestnuts *(kuri)*	Barley, millet	Soy sauce, sweet and sour sauce, mustard sauce, ginger root, plum sauce, red bean paste
Vietnamese*				
Bamboo shoots, bean sprouts, cabbage, carrots, cucumbers, greens, lettuce, mushrooms, onions, peas, spinach, yams	Apple, banana, eggfruit *(o-ma)*, grapefruit, jackfruit, lychee, mandarin, mango, orange, papaya, pineapple, tangerine, watermelon	Beef, blood, brain, chicken, duck, eggs, fish, goat, kidney, lamb, liver, pork, shellfish, soybeans	French bread, rice, rice noodles, wheat noodles	Fish sauce, fresh herbs, garlic, ginger, lard, MSG, peanut oil, sesame seeds, sesame seed oil, vegetable oil

From Endres, J.B., and Rockwell, R.E.: Food, nutrition, and the young child, St. Louis, 1980, Mosby–Year Book, Inc., pp. 182-183. Modified from Nutrition during pregnancy and lactation, California Department of Public Health, revised 1975.

NOTE: Foods common to all ethnic groups have been omitted.

*Information supplied by Hanh-Trang Tran-Viet, Carbondale, Ill.

Continued.

Table 2-4 Characteristic food choices for six groups—cont'd

VEGETABLES	FRUITS	MEATS AND ALTERNATIVES	GRAIN PRODUCTS	OTHERS
▪ **Indian *(East)***				
Cauliflower, carrots, cucumber, corn-gourds, leeks, eggplant, beets, radishes, hot pepper, bell pepper, peas, French beans, okra, pumpkin, red and white cabbage, mung sprouts, bean sprouts, potatoes, tapioca root, sweet potatoes	Oranges, limes, grapes, watermelon, mango, guava, honeydew, chiku, cantaloupe, pineapple, green, yellow, and red bananas, berries, custard apples	Lamb, beef, duck, chicken, shrimp, catfish, buffalo, sunfish, sardines, fresh crab, lobster, peanuts, cashews, almonds, chick-peas, split peas, black-eyed peas, dry mung beans	Rice pancakes wheat chapati, puri, mixed grain flour bread	Fresh coconut juice, curries, tomato sauce, tamarind sauce, dried grain curries *(pulses)*, yogurt-curry garnished with coriander (fresh leaves)

of their daily lives. It is important for health care workers to be aware that "other people may live by different rules and priorities from those of the health care provider, and these rules and priorities decisively influence health-related behavior" (Bauwens and Anderson, 1984).

Health Beliefs

The beliefs related to the cause of illness and the maintenance of health are an integral part of the cultural heritage of families. Often inseparable from religious beliefs, they influence the way that families cope with health problems and the way that they respond to health care providers. Predominant among most cultures are beliefs related to natural forces, supernatural forces, and imbalance between forces.

Natural forces. The most common natural forces held responsible for ill health if the body is not adequately protected include cold air entering the body, impurities in the air, or other natural sources. For example, the Chinese parent will overdress the infant in an effort to keep cold wind from entering the child's body. The Chinese believe that cold weather, rain, or wind is responsible for "cold" conditions (Chen-Louie, 1983). They also believe that an innate energy called *chi* enters and leaves the body through the mouth, nose, and ears and flows through the body in definite pathways, or meridians, at specific times and locations. Lack of *chi* and blood is believed to be a cause of fatigue, low energy, and a variety of ailments.

In the black culture natural phenomena such as phases of the moon, seasons of the year, and planet positions are believed to affect the body and its processes; therefore health maintenance is strongly associated with the ability to read "the signs" (Bloch, 1983). Some cultures consider such behavior as overeating, overwork, anxiety, and inadequate food and sleep as natural causes of illness. Most Native Americans consider health to be a state of harmony with nature and the universe (Wilson, 1983).

Supernatural forces. High on the list of causes of illness are forces beyond comprehension and logical explanation. Evil influences such as voodoo, witchcraft, or evil spirits are viewed in some cultures as causes of adverse health, especially those illnesses that cannot be explained by other means.

A health belief that is common among people from Latin America, Mediterranean, Near East, some Asian, and some African societies is the concept of the "evil eye" (*mal ojo* is the Hispanic term). It is part of the concept of health as a state of balance; illness is a state of imbalance (see below). Strength and power are associated with the evil eye; therefore, as long as an individual's strength and weakness remain in balance, he or she is unlikely to become a victim of the evil eye. Weaknesses are not necessarily physical. For example, an excess of some emotion, such as envy, can create a weakness. Infants and small children, because of immature development of their internal strength-weakness states, are especially vulnerable to the gaze of the evil eye (Pasquale, 1984). Consequently, the evil eye serves to rationalize an inexplicable onset of illness in children who display such symptoms as restlessness, crying, diarrhea, vomiting, and fever.

Although seldom expressed to health care providers, the belief that a witch can cast a spell or curse over another person at the request of someone who wishes the person ill or dead is found in Hispanic, African, and Australian aboriginal cultures. The victim is often tortured in effigy by pins driven into a doll at the location where the intended victim is to be hurt. "Voodoo deaths" have occurred from the victim's belief in the curse and may result from dehydration as the victim gives up the will to live and refuses to drink (Chidester, 1990).

Imbalance of forces. The concept of balance or equilibrium is widespread throughout the world. One of the most common imbalances supported by the Hispanic, Filipino, Chinese, and Arab cultures is that which exists between "hot" and "cold." This belief is reputedly derived from Hippocratic theory of humoral pathology, which states that illness is caused by an imbalance of the four humors: phlegm, blood, black bile, and yellow bile. Hot and cold describe certain properties and conditions completely unrelated to temperature. Diseases, areas of the body, foods, and illnesses are classified as either "hot" or "cold." In Chinese health belief the forces are termed *yin* (cold) and *yang* (hot) (Chen-Louie, 1983). In order to maintain health and prevent illness these hot and cold forces must be kept in balance.

Illness is treated by restoring normal balance through the application of appropriate "hot" or "cold" remedies. A "cold" condition such as a respiratory disease is believed to be caused by exposure to cold weather, rain, or cold wind entering the body; it is treated by administration of "hot" foods, herbs, or drugs. Menstruation is considered to be a "hot" condition; therefore, women are cautioned against ingesting "hot" foods that might increase menstrual flow or produce cramping. Ingesting too much of either "hot" or "cold" foods can also be interpreted as a cause of illness.

Health care workers who are aware of this belief are better able to understand why some persons refuse to eat certain foods. It is often useful to discuss the diet with the family to determine their feelings and beliefs regarding food choices. It is possible to help families devise a diet that contains the necessary balance of basic food groups prescribed by the medical subculture while conforming to the beliefs of the ethnic subculture.

The hot-cold food classification may have adverse effects. For example, newborn infants are often started on evaporated milk formulas. Evaporated milk is considered to be a hot food, while whole milk is viewed as a cool food. Infants tend to develop rashes, which are believed to be caused by "hot" foods; in such cases parents may decide to switch to whole milk. However, parents fear that it is dangerous to change too rapidly, so they often feed the child some type of neutralizing substance, which may create additional health problems (Murillo-Rohde, 1980). Such a problem might be averted if the family's preference is determined before discharge from the hospital and a formula prescribed that is agreeable to both the family and the practitioner.

Health Practices

There are numerous similarities among cultures regarding prevention and treatment of illness. All cultures have some types of home remedies that they apply before seeking help from other persons. Within the ethnic community folk healers who are endowed with the ability to "cure" maladies are sought for special situations and when home remedies are unsuccessful. There is the *curandero* (male) or *curandera* (female) of the Mexican-American community whose healing powers are believed to be a gift from God. The Asian consults a herbalist, knowledgeable in medicines, and/or an ethnic practitioner practiced in Asian therapies, including acupuncture (insertion of needles), acupressure (application of pressure), and moxibustion (application of heat). Native Americans consult a variety of healers with specific skills and knowledge. Specialized medicine persons diagnose illness, provide nonsacred treatments (usually by way of massage and herbs), and care for souls. Other specialists perform services or affect cures through spiritual means.

The folk healers are very powerful persons in their community and have the ability to acquire information about an illness without resorting to probing questions. They "speak the language" of the family who seeks help and often combine their rituals and potions with prayer and entreaties to God. They also are able to create an atmosphere conducive to successful management. Furthermore, they exhibit a sincere interest in the family and their problem.

Often it will be found that the folk remedies are compatible with the medical regimen and can be used as a means to reinforce the treatment plan. For example, most of the foods contraindicated for a person with peptic ulcer are "hot" foods and would be avoided by the person's belief system. Also, aspirin (a "hot" medication) is an appropriate therapy for "cold" diseases such as the common cold and arthritis (Murillo-Rohde, 1980). It is not uncommon to discover that a folk prescription has a scientific basis. However, numerous health remedies or preventive practices have no scientific basis, such as the use of *asafetida,* a piece of rotten flesh that looks like a dried sponge and is worn around the neck to prevent contagious diseases, or the wearing of copper or silver bracelets to protect the wearer. Since they do no harm, these practices should be respected.

To overcome the effect of the evil eye usually requires specialized rituals conducted by the appropriate practitioner. For example, the Chicano curandera ascertains that the condition is truly the result of the evil eye by performing an assessment ritual and, upon a confirmed diagnosis, performs a curative ritual. There are prescribed rituals for other maladies such as the *moller caida.* Sometimes the faith in the folk practitioner delays obtaining needed medical treatment, although the practitioner will usually suggest medical care if his or her ministrations are unsuccessful.

Health practices of different cultures may also present problems of assessment and interpretation. For example, the Vietnamese practice of "coining" may produce weltlike lesions on the child's back when a coin, held on edge, is repeatedly rubbed lengthwise on the oiled skin to rid the body of the disease (Feldman, 1984). Another such custom is the Old World practice of cupping (also practiced by the Vietnamese). A container, such as a tumbler, bottle, or jar, containing steam is placed against the skin surface to "draw out the poison" or other evil. When the heated air within the container cools, a vacuum is created that produces a bruiselike blemish on the skin directly beneath the mouth of the container (Asnes and Wisotsky, 1981; Holland and Sweeney, 1985). Both of these remedies can be misdiagnosed as evidence of "child abuse" by uninformed professionals.

Other cultural health remedies that are detrimental to health include eating clay or excessive amounts of salt. A mercury compound, *azogue* (the Spanish name for quicksilver), is commonly used in Mexico and sometimes sold illegally to low-income Hispanic families in the United States as a "remedy" for diarrhea. Alert health care workers know that the drug can cause permanent central nervous system damage. A careful history can reveal these practices, but it may require the collaboration of a folk healer to convince a user to stop the practice.

Faith healing and religious rituals are closely allied with many folk-healing practices. Wearing of amulets, medals, and other religious relics believed by the culture to protect the individual and facilitate healing is a common practice. It is important for health workers to recognize the value of this practice and keep the items where the family has placed them or nearby. It offers comfort and support and rarely impedes medical and nursing care. If an item must be removed during a procedure, it should be replaced, if possible, when the procedure is completed. The reason for its temporary removal is explained to the family, and they are reassured that their wishes will be respected.

Although most subcultures in the large developed countries have become acculturated to the Western medical system, many still maintain faith in traditional healing practices and practitioners. When the folk practices do not interfere with the welfare of the patient, they need not be discouraged. Often a compromise can be reached that accomplishes the goal of the nurse while it maintains the dignity and self-esteem of the client.

Folklore Related to Prenatal Influences

Since ancient times the striking appearance of abnormal human development has been of concern, as evidenced by descriptions in primitive drawings and on clay tablets, and has served as the origin of numerous legendary and mythologic creatures. Consequently the processes of pregnancy and birth have been surrounded with strongly held beliefs and superstitions that involve taboos and prescriptions for behavior directed toward assuring the well-being of the unborn child. Even in the face of scientific advances, these superstitions and folkways have survived for generations and may still persist in various forms as part of a cultural heritage. The degree to which these beliefs are expressed depends on the strength of the cultural influence, the attitudes of the individual families, and the confidence and credibility engendered by the health care providers.

One of the most universal explanations of defective development has been maternal impressions. It has been a widespread belief that the appearance of the unborn child will be improved if the pregnant woman looks at beautiful people or things. The same concept in reverse has been used to explain birth defects. For example, if a pregnant woman was frightened by a rabbit, it was believed that her child would be born with a cleft ("hare") lip; a microcephalic infant was attributed to the mother's seeing a monkey during pregnancy; and the mother's viewing a person with missing limbs would cause the unborn child to be similarly affected. Activities such as a mother reaching her arms above her head, walking in circles, or tying knots were believed to cause the umbilical cord to be knotted or twisted around the neck of the fetus. Even the shape of birthmarks and other skin defects is sometimes believed to reflect maternal impressions. For example, eating strawberries by the mother is associated with nevi. Articles of apparel or adornment, food cravings, emotions such as fright and anger, undesirable thoughts, and the time and manner of announcing the pregnancy are all believed to influence the well-being of the unborn child.

Expectant mothers who are able to rationalize the illogical nature of the beliefs will, through a normal fear of hav-

TABLE 2-5 Religious beliefs that affect nursing care

RELIGION	BELIEFS ABOUT BIRTH AND DEATH	BELIEFS ABOUT DIET AND FOOD PRACTICES
Adventist (Seventh Day Adventist; Church of God)	*Birth:* Opposed to infant baptism Baptism in adulthood	Meat prohibited in some groups No alcohol, coffee, or tea
Baptist (27 groups)	*Birth:* Opposed to infant baptism Believers baptize by immersion as adults *Death:* Counsel and prayer with clergy, family, patient	Some groups discourage coffee, tea, and alcohol
Black Muslim	*Birth:* No baptism *Death:* Carefully prescribed procedure for washing and shrouding dead	Prohibit alcohol, pork and meat of dead animals, or foods traditional among American blacks, e.g., corn bread, collard greens
Buddhist Churches of America	*Birth:* No infant baptism Infant presentation *Death:* Last rite chanting often practiced at bedside soon after death Priest should be contacted	No requirements or restrictions Some sects are strictly vegetarian Discourage use of alcohol and drugs

Data from Recognizing your patients' spiritual needs, Nursing 77 7(12):64-68, 1977; Beliefs that can affect therapy, Pediatr. Nurs. 5(3):40-43, 1979; Carpenito, L.J.: Nurs-1987, Addison-Wesley Publishing Co.; Spector, R.E.: Cultural diversity in health and illness, ed. 2, New York, 1985, Appleto' ˜entury-Crofts; personal communications.

ing an abnormal infant, conform to the superstitions. In most instances these customs are relatively harmless and are not in conflict with sound health practices. However, there are situations when conformity to cultural or subcultural beliefs may compromise the health and well-being of either mother or fetus, for example, the practice of eating clay, cornstarch, chalk, or other substances. Understanding and judicious management on the part of nurses and other health care workers are required to explore with the mother all the ramifications of the practice without creating undue stress and guilt in the mother.

Not all of these beliefs are unfounded. There is evidence that maternal emotions may indeed affect the fetus. Prolonged stimulation of the autonomic nervous system caused by extreme stress or long-term anxiety produces physiologic changes in the maternal system, such as increased heart rate, vasoconstriction, and decreased gastric motility. In addition to the indirect effect produced by constriction of uterine blood flow, the stress hormones cross the placental membrane to affect the fetus directly. Assisting the expectant mother in dealing with her stresses or securing counseling services for her is part of the nursing considerations.

RELIGIOUS BELIEFS

Religion influences the life-styles of most cultures. Among many groups illness, injury, or death is believed to be sent by God as a punishment for sin. Some may believe that health workers will be unable to help a person whom God is punishing and may express a fatalistic attitude toward treatment, stating that it is "the will of God." Others view it as a test of strength, as the testing of Job in the Bible, and strive to remain faithful and overcome the conflicts.

Religious affiliation has implications for many health-related functions and procedures. It is comforting to the family of an ill child to have this need recognized and respected. Nurses need to determine if there are any special considerations related to spiritual practices that are important to the family. Dietary restrictions are clarified, especially in denominations in which there may be a number of variations. Where specific religious practices do not interfere with the health of the child or the therapy (such as fasting), the wishes of the family are respected. Family members are asked whether they want a clergy member present and whether they prefer hospital staff to call or to do this on their own.

It is important to determine the wishes of the family regarding baptism, rites or practices related to death, and other religious rituals (such as circumcision, communion, or use of amulets or icons). An important role of the nurse is to be aware of spiritual needs of families and convey an attitude of concern for this important element of the child's care. Religion, which offers families understanding and spiritual support, is a valuable asset to health care. Characteristics of selected religions with beliefs that affect health care are outlined in Table 2-5.

BELIEFS REGARDING MEDICAL CARE	COMMENTS
Some believe in divine healing and practice annointing with oil and use of prayer May desire communion or baptism when ill Believe in man's choice and God's sovereignty Some oppose hypnosis as therapy	Sabbath: Saturday for many Accept Bible literally
"Laying on of hands" (some) May encounter some resistance to some therapies, such as abortion Believe God functions through physician Some believe in predestination; may respond passively to care	Fundamentalist and conservative groups accept Bible as inspired word of God
Faith healing unacceptable Always maintain personal habits of cleanliness	General adherence to Moslem tenets overlaid, in many instances, by antagonism to whites especially Christians and Jews Do not indulge in activities (such as sleeping) more than is necessary to health
Illness believed to be a trial to aid development of soul; illness due to Karmic causes May be reluctant to have surgery or certain treatments on holy days Cleanliness believed to be of great importance Family may request Buddhist priest for counseling	Optimistic outlook; teach ways to overcome fears, anxieties, apprehension

ing diagnosis: application to clinical practice, ed 3, Philadelphia, 1989, J.B. Lippincott Co.; Kozier, B., and Erb, G.: Fundamentals of nursing, ed. 3, Menlo Park, CA,

Continued.

TABLE 2-5 Religious beliefs that affect nursing care—cont'd

RELIGION	BELIEFS ABOUT BIRTH AND DEATH	BELIEFS ABOUT DIET AND FOOD PRACTICES
Church of Christ Scientist (Christian Science)	*Birth:* No baptism *Death:* No last rites	No requirements or restrictions
Church of Jesus Christ of Latter Day Saints (Mormon)	*Birth:* No baptism at birth Infant is "blessed" by church official at first opportunity after birth (in church) Baptism by immersion at 8 years *Death:* No special rites	Prohibit tea, coffee, alcohol Encourage sparing use of meats Fasting for 24 hours on first Sunday each month (from after evening meal Saturday until evening meal Sunday)
Eastern Orthodox (Turkey, Egypt, Syria, Rumania, Bulgaria, Cyprus, Albania, etc.)	*Birth:* Most believe in infant baptism by immersion 8 to 40 days after birth *Death:* Last rites obligatory for impending death	Restrictions depend on specific sect
Episcopal (Anglican)	*Birth:* Infant baptism mandatory; urgent if poor prognosis* *Death:* Last rites available but not mandatory	Abstain from meat on fast days May fast on Wednesday, Friday, during Lent, and before Christmas Some fast for 6 hours before receiving Holy Communion
Friends (Quakers)	*Birth:* No baptism Infant's name recorded in official book	No requirements or restrictions Most practice moderation Avoid alcohol and illicit drugs
Greek Orthodox	*Birth:* Baptism considered important Performed 40 days after birth If not possible to baptize by sprinkling or immersion, Church allows child baptism "in the air" by moving the child in the form of a cross* as appropriate words are said *Death:* Last rites, administration of Sacrament of Holy Communion Should be performed while dying person is still conscious	Church prescribed fast periods—usually occur on Wednesday, Friday, and during Lent; consist of avoiding meat and (in some cases) dairy products If health compromised, priest may be contacted to convince family to forego fasting
Hindu	*Birth:* No ritual *Death:* Special prescribed rites Priest pours water into the mouth of dead child, ties a thread around neck or wrist to signify blessing (should not be removed) Family washes body and is particular about who touches body	Many dietary restrictions Beef and veal not eaten Some strict vegetarians
Islam (Muslim/Moslem)	*Birth:* No baptism *Death:* Patient must confess sins and beg forgiveness before death; family should be present Family washes and prepares body, then turns it to face Mecca Only relatives and friends may touch body	Prohibit all pork products Daylight fasting practiced during ninth month of Muhammadan year (Ramadan) Strict Muslims do not use alcohol

*See Baptism, Chapter 10.

BELIEFS REGARDING MEDICAL CARE	COMMENTS
Deny the existence of health crisis; see sickness and sin as errors of mind that can be altered by prayer Oppose human intervention with drugs or other therapies; however, accept legally required immunizations Many adhere to belief that disease is a human mental concept that can be dispelled by "spiritual truth" to extent that they refuse all medical treatment	Many desire services of Practitioner or Reader; will sometimes refuse even emergency treatment until they have consulted a Reader Unlikely to donate organs for transplant
Devout adherents believe in divine healing through annointment with oil and "laying on of hands" by church officials (elders) Medical therapy not prohibited	Married adults wear special undergarments May request Sacrament on Sunday while in hospital Financial support for sick available through well-funded welfare system Discourage cremation Discourage use of tobacco
Annointment of the sick No conflict with medical science	Discourage cremation
Some believe in spiritual healing Rite for annointing sick available but not mandatory	Religious icons very important Communion four times yearly: Christmas, Easter, June 30, and August 15; may be mandatory for some
No special rites or restrictions	Believe in plain speech and dress Pacifists
Each health crisis handled by ordained priest; deacon may also serve in some cases Holy Communion administered in hospital Some may desire Sacrament of the Holy Unction performed by priest	Oppose euthanasia Believe every reasonable effort should be made to preserve life until termination by God Discourage autopsies that may cause dismemberment Prefer burial to cremation
Illness or injury believed to represent sins committed in previous life Accept most modern medical practices	Cremation preferred
Faith healing not acceptable unless psychologic condition of patient is deteriorating; performed for morale Ritual washing after prayer; prayer takes place five times daily (upon rising, midday, afternoon, early evening, and before bed); during prayer, face Mecca and kneel on prayer rug	Older Muslims often have a fatalistic view that may interfere with compliance to therapy May oppose autopsy

Continued.

TABLE 2-5 Religious beliefs that affect nursing care—cont'd

RELIGION	BELIEFS ABOUT BIRTH AND DEATH	BELIEFS ABOUT DIET AND FOOD PRACTICES
Jehovah's Witness	*Birth:* No baptism *Death:* No last rites	Eat nothing to which blood has been added; can eat animal flesh that has been drained
Judaism (Orthodox and Conservative)	*Birth:* No baptism Ritual circumcision of male infants on eighth day; performed by Mohel (ritual circumciser familiar with Jewish law and aseptic technique) Reform Jews favor ritual circumcision, but not as a religious imperative *Death:* Remains are ritually washed by members of the Ritual Burial Society Burial should take place as soon as possible	Numerous dietary kosher laws exist that may be influenced by local practices and family and cultural tradition Allowed only meat from animals that are vegetable eaters, are cloven hoofed, chew their cud, and are ritually slaughtered; fish that have scales and fins Prohibit any combination of meat and milk; milk products served first can be followed by meat in a few minutes but milk may not be consumed for several hours after eating meat. Fasting for 24 hours is part of Yom Kippur observance Matzo replaces leavened bread during Passover week
Lutheran	*Birth:* Baptize only living infants shortly after birth *Death:* Last rites optional	No requirements or restrictions
Mennonite (similar to Amish)	*Birth:* No baptism in infancy Baptism during early or middle teens	No requirements or restrictions
Methodist	*Birth:* No baptism at birth; performed on children or adults *Death:* No ritual	No requirements or restrictions
Nazarene	*Birth:* Baptism optional *Death:* No last rites	No requirements or restrictions Alcohol prohibited
Pentecostal (Assembly of God, Four-square)	*Birth:* No baptism at birth Baptism by complete immersion after age of accountability *Death:* No last rites	Abstain from alcohol, eating blood, strangled animals, or anything to which blood has been added Some individuals may resist pork
Orthodox Presbyterian	*Birth:* Infant baptism by sprinkling* *Death:* Last rites not a sacramental procedure; scripture reading and prayer	No requirements or restrictions
Roman Catholic	*Birth:* Infant baptism mandatory; especially urgent in poor prognosis, when it may be performed by anyone* *Death:* Rite for Annointing of the sick is mandatory Family or patient may request annointing if prognosis is grave	Fasting and abstaining from meat mandatory on Ash Wednesday and Good Friday; fasting optional during Lent; no meat on Fridays during Lent as general rule Most hospital patients exempt from fasting Some older Catholics may adhere to older rule of no meat on Friday
Russian Orthodox	*Birth:* Baptism by priest only *Death:* Traditionally after death arms are crossed, fingers set in a cross	No meat or dairy products on Wednesday, Friday, and during Lent
Unitarian Universalist	*Birth:* Some practice infant baptism; most consider it unnecessary *Death:* No ritual	No requirements or restrictions

*See Baptism, Chapter 10.

BELIEFS REGARDING MEDICAL CARE	COMMENTS
Adherents are generally absolutely opposed to blood transfusions, including banking of own blood; individuals can sometimes be persuaded in emergencies May be opposed to use of albumin, globulin, factor replacement (hemophilia), vaccines	Often possible to obtain a court order appointing a hospital official as temporary guardian to consent to a child's transfusion when parents refuse consent Autopsy approved only as required by law
May resist surgical procedures during Sabbath, which extends from sundown Friday until sundown Saturday Seriously ill and pregnant women are exempt from fasting Illness is grounds for violating dietary laws, e.g., patient with congestive heart failure does not have to use kosher meats, which are high in sodium	Oppose all forms of mutilation, including autopsy; body parts not donated or removed; amputated limbs, organs, or surgically removed tissues should be made available to family for burial Donation or transplantation of organs requires rabbinical consent May oppose prolongation of life after irreversible brain damage
If grave prognosis, family may request annointing and blessing of sick or visit by church official	Accept scientific developments
No illness rituals Deep concern for dignity and self-determination of individual that would conflict with shock treatment or medical treatment affecting personality or will	
Communion may be requested before surgery or similar crisis	Encourage donation of body or body parts to medical science
Church official administers communion and laying on of hands Adherents believe in divine healing but not exclusive of medical treatment	Cremation permitted
No restrictions regarding medical care Deliverance from sickness is provided for in atonement; may pray for divine intervention in health matters and seek God in prayer for themselves and others when ill	Some insist illness is divine punishment; most consider it an intrusion of Satan Practice glossolalia (speaking in tongues)
Communion administered when appropriate and convenient Blood transfusion accepted when advisable Pastor or elder should be called for ill person Believe science should be used for relief of suffering	Full forgiveness granted for any illness connected with a sin
Encourage anointing of sick, although this may be interpreted by older members of church as equivalent to the old terminology "extreme unction" or "last rites"; they may require careful explanation if reluctance associated with fear of imminent death Traditional church teaching does not approve of contraceptives or abortion	Family may request that major amputated limb be buried in consecrated ground Transplant accepted as long as loss of organ does not deprive donor of life or functional integrity of body Autopsy acceptable Religious articles important
Cross necklace is important and should be removed only when necessary and replaced as soon as possible Adherents believe in divine healing, but not exclusive of medical treatment	Opposed to autopsy, embalming, or cremation
Believe God helps those who help themselves Some may prefer not to have clergy visit them in hospital	Cremation preferred to burial

IMPORTANCE OF CULTURE AND RELIGION TO NURSES

To begin to understand and to deal effectively with families in a multicultural community or in a unicultural community that is different from one's own, it is most important that nurses be aware of their own attitudes and values regarding a way of life, including health practices. Nurses, too, are a product of their own cultural background and education. Frequently, nurses and other health care workers are not aware of their own cultural values and how those values influence their thoughts and actions. Those who are aware of their own culturally founded behavior are more sensitive to cultural behavior in others. To recognize that a behavior may be characteristic of a culture rather than an "abnormal" behavior places nurses at an advantage in their relationships with families. When nurses respect cultural differences of a family, they are better able to determine whether the behavior is distinctive to the individual or a characteristic of the culture. What appears to be puzzling behavior may simply be the customary response in the culture (e.g., expression of emotion).

Cultural standards and values, the family structure and function, and past experiences with health care influence a family's feelings and attitudes toward health, their children, and health care delivery systems. It is often difficult for nurses to be nonjudgmental and objective in working with families whose behaviors and attitudes differ from or conflict with their own. To be aware of one's own feelings and attitudes, as well as to respect those of the family, is essential to a helping relationship and achievement of nursing goals. To rely on one's own values and experiences for guidance can result only in frustration and disappointment.

Table 2-6 Cultural characteristics related to health care of children

CULTURAL GROUP	HEALTH BELIEFS	HEALTH AND DIET PRACTICES
Asian Americans		
Chinese	A healthy body viewed as gift from parents and ancestors and must be cared for Health is one of the results of balance between the forces of *yin* (cold) and *yang* (hot), energy forces that rule the world Illness caused by imbalance Believe blood is source of life and is not regenerated *Chi* is innate energy Lack of *chi* and blood results in deficiency that produces fatigue, poor constitution, and long illness	Goal of therapy is to restore balance of *yin* and *yang* Acupuncturist applies needles to appropriate meridians identified in terms of *yin* and *yang* Acupressure and *tai chi* replacing acupuncture in some areas Moxibustion is application of heat to skin over specific meridians Wide use of medicinal herbs procured and applied in prescribed ways Folk healers are herbalist, spiritual healer, temple healer, fortune healer Meals may or may not be planned to balance hot and cold Milk intolerance relatively common Use of condiments, e.g., monosodium glutamate and soy sauce, may create difficulty with some diet regimens, e.g., low-salt diets
Japanese	Three major belief systems: *Shinto* religious influence Humans inherently good Evil caused by outside spirits Illness caused by contact with polluting agents, e.g., blood, corpses, skin diseases Chinese and Korean influence Health achieved through harmony and balance between self and society Disease caused by disharmony with society and not caring for body Portuguese influence Upholds germ theory of disease	Believe evil removed by purification Energy restored by means of acupuncture, acupressure, massage, and moxibustion along affected meridians *Kampō* medicine—use of natural herbs Believe in removal of diseased parts Trend is to use both Western and Oriental healing methods Care for disabled viewed as family's responsibility Take pride in child's good health Seek preventive care, medical care for illness Older persons avoid some food combinations (e.g., milk and cherries, watermelon and crab) and believe pickled plums to have special properties

Sources: Bloch, 1983; Chen-Louie, 1983; Chow, 1976; Char, 1981; Ehling, 1981; Greathouse and Miller, 1981; Hashizume and Takano, 1983; Holland and Sweeney, 1985; Hollingsworth, Brown, and Brooten, 1980; Jacques, 1976; Lacay, 1981; Monrroy, 1983; Orque, 1983a, 1983b; Sodetaini-Shebata, 1981.

It is one thing to know what is needed to deal with a health problem; it is often quite another to implement a fruitful course of action unless nurses work within the cultural and socioeconomic framework of the family.

It is beneficial to make an effort to adapt ethnic practices to the health needs of the family rather than attempt to change long-standing beliefs. To aid their efforts to understand and respect the cultural beliefs of families, nurses should have a readily available resource file containing pertinent information about the cultural and subcultural characteristics of the community in which they practice (e.g., traditional practices related to infant feeding practices and the time and manner of weaning and toilet training). Bridging cultural gaps in delivery of health care to children requires the establishment of a close relationship with families and other influential persons in the community (such as the local folk healer) and periodic assessment of one's own attitudes and behaviors and those of other health workers toward people of other racial or ethnic origins.

Some characteristics of selected cultures are outlined in Table 2-6. These generalizations are presented to assist nurses in learning the unique beliefs and practices of various groups and are not meant to be stereotypes of any group. Learning about culture must begin somewhere; Tables 2-5 and 2-6 are presented as beginning frameworks for practicing transcultural nursing. Each nurse must assess individuals and families to identify in what ways they are similar to and different from their cultural and religious backgrounds (see Box 6-18).

FAMILY RELATIONSHIPS	COMMUNICATION	COMMENTS
Extended family pattern common Strong concept of loyalty of young to old Respect for elders taught at early age—acceptance without questioning or talking back Children's behavior a reflection on family Family and individual honor and "face" important Self-reliance and self-restraint highly valued; self-expression repressed Males valued more highly than females; women submissive to men in family	Open expression of emotions unacceptable Often smile when do not comprehend	Do not react well to painful diagnostic workup; are especially upset by drawing of blood Deep respect for their bodies and believe it best to die with bodies intact; therefore may refuse surgery Believe in reincarnation Older members fear hospitals; often believe hospital is a place to go to die Children sometimes breast-fed for up to 4 or 5 years*
Close intergenerational relationships Family provides anchor Family tends to keep problems to self Value self-control and self-sufficiency Concept of *haji* (shame) imposes strong control; unacceptable behavior of children reflects on family Many adopt practices of contemporary middle class Concern for child's missing school may result in sending to school before fully recovered from illness	*Issei*—born in Japan; usually speak Japanese only *Nisei, Sansei,* and *Yonsei* have few language difficulties New immigrants able to read and write English better than to speak or understand it Make significant use of nonverbal communication with subtle gestures and facial expression Tend to suppress emotions Will often wait silently	Generational categories: *Issei*—1st generation to live in U.S. *Nisei*—2nd generation *Sansei*—3rd generation *Yonsei*—4th generation *Issei* and *Nisei*—tolerant and permissive childrearing until 5 or 6, then emphasis on emotional reserve and control Cleanliness highly valued Time considered valuable and used wisely Tendency to practice emotional control may make assessment of pain more difficult

*Most Asian cultures consider the child 1 year old at the time of birth. Traditional Chinese custom adds 1 year on January 1 regardless of the birthday—a child born in December is 2 years old the next January.

Continued.

Table 2-6 Cultural characteristics related to health care of children—cont'd

CULTURAL GROUP	HEALTH BELIEFS	HEALTH AND DIET PRACTICES
Vietnamese	Good health considered to be balance between *yin* (cold) and *yang* (hot) Believe person's life has been predisposed toward certain phenomena by cosmic forces Health believed to be result of harmony with existing universal order, harmony attained by pleasing good spirits and avoiding evil ones Belief in *am duc,* the amount of good deeds accumulated by ancestors Many use rituals to prevent illness Practice some restrictions to prevent incurring wrath of evil spirits	Family uses all means possible before using outside agencies for health care Fortune-tellers determine event that caused disturbance May visit temple to procure divine instruction Use astrologer to calculate cyclical changes and forces Regard health as family responsibility; outside aid sought when resources run out Certain illnesses considered only temporary (such as pustules, open wounds) and ignored Seek generalist health healers May use special diets to prevent illness and promote health Lactose intolerance prevalent
Filipino	Believe God's will and supernatural forces govern universe Illness, accidents, and other misfortunes are God's punishment for violations of His will Widely accept "hot" and "cold" balance and imbalance as cause of health and illness	Some use amulets as a shield from witchcraft or as good luck pieces Catholics substitute religious medals and other items
American black	Illness classified as: Natural—affected by forces of nature without adequate protection, e.g., cold air, pollution, food and water Unnatural—evil influences, e.g., witchcraft, voodoo, hoodoo, hex, fix, rootwork; symptoms often associated with eating Believe serious illness sent by God as punishment, e.g., parents punished by illness or death of child Believe serious illness can be avoided May resist health care because illness is "will of God"	Self-care and folk medicine very prevalent Folk therapies usually religious in origin Attempt home remedies first; poorer people do not seek help until illness serious Usually seek help from: "Old lady"—woman in community with a common knowledge of herbs; consults regarding pediatric care Spiritualist—has received gift from God for healing incurable diseases or solving personal problems; strongly based in Christianity Priest (voodoo priest/priestess)—most powerful healer Root doctor—meets need for herbs, oils, candles, and ointments Prayer is common means for prevention and treatment
Haitian*	Illnesses have a supernatural or natural origin Supernatural illness are caused by angry voodoo spirits, enemies, or the dead, especially deceased ancestors Natural illnesses are based on conceptions of natural causation: Irregularities of blood volume, flow, purity, viscosity, color and/or temperature (hot/cold) Gas *(gaz)* Movement and consistency of mother's milk Hot/cold imbalance in the body Bone displacement Movement of diseases Health is maintained by good dietary and hygienic habits	Health is a personal responsibility Foods have properties of "hot"/"cold" and "light"/"heavy" and must be in harmony with one's life cycle and bodily states Natural illnesses are treated by home remedies first Supernatural illness treated by healers: voodoo priest *(houngan)* or priestess *(mambo),* midwife *(fam saj),* and herbalist or leaf doctor *(dokte fey)* Amulets and prayer used to protect against illness due to curses or willed by evil people

*This section was written by Lydia DeSantis, Ph.D., R.N.

FAMILY RELATIONSHIPS	COMMUNICATION	COMMENTS
Family is revered institution Multigenerational families Family is chief social network Children highly valued Individual needs and interests are subordinate to those of family group Father is main decision maker Women taught submission to men Parents expect respect and obedience from children	Many immigrants are not proficient in speaking and understanding English May hesitate to ask questions Questioning authority is sign of disrespect; asking questions considered impolite Use indirectness rather than forthrightness in expressing disagreement May avoid eye contact with health professionals as a sign of respect	Consider status more important than money Children taught emotional control Time concept more relaxed—consider punctuality less significant than other values, i.e., propriety Place high value on social harmony
Family is highly valued with strong family ties Multigenerational family structure common, often with collateral members as well Personal interests are subordinated to family interests and needs Members avoid any behavior that would bring shame on the family	Immigrants and older persons may not be able to speak or understand English	Tend to have a fatalistic outlook on life Believe time and providence will solve all
Strong kinship bonds in extended family; members come to aid of others in crisis Less likely to view illness as a burden Augmented families common (unrelated persons living in same household) Place strong emphasis on work and ambition Sex-role sharing among parents	Alert to any evidence of discrimination Place importance on nonverbal behavior May use nonstandard English or "black English" Use "testing" behaviors to assess personnel in health care situations before seeking active care Best to use simple, direct, but caring approach	High level of caution and distrust of majority group Social anxiety related to tradition of humiliation, oppression, and loss of dignity Will elect to retain dignity rather than seek care if values are compromised Strong sense of peoplehood High incidence of poverty Black minister a strong influence in black community Visits by family minister are sought, expected, and valued in helping to cope with illness and suffering
Maintenance of family reputation is paramount Lineal authority supreme; children in a subordinate position in family hierarchy Children valued for parental social security in old age and expected to contribute to family welfare at an early age Children viewed as "gifts from god" and treated with indulgence and affection	Recent immigrants and older persons may speak only Haitian creole May prefer family/friends to act as translators and confidants Often smile and nod in agreement when do not understand Quiet and gentle communication style and lack of assertiveness lead health care providers to falsely believe they comprehend health teaching and are compliant Will not ask questions if health care provider is busy or rushed	Will use biomedical and ethnomedical (folk) systems simultaneously, Resistant to dietary and work restrictions Adherence to prescribed treatments directly related to perceived severity of illness

Continued.

Table 2-6 Cultural characteristics related to health care of children—cont'd

CULTURAL GROUP	HEALTH BELIEFS	HEALTH AND DIET PRACTICES
Hispanic American		
Mexican-American (Latino, Chicano, Raza-Latino)	Health beliefs have strong religious association Believe in body imbalance as a cause of illness, especially imbalance between *caliente* (hot) and *frio* (cold) or "wet" and "dry" Some maintain good health is a result of "good luck"—a reward for good behavior Illness prevented by performing properly, eating proper foods, and working proper amount of time; accomplished through prayer, wearing religious medals or amulets, and sleeping with relics at home Illness is a punishment from God for wrongdoing, forces of nature, and the supernatural	Seek help from *curandero* or *curandera,* especially in rural areas Curandero(a) receives his/her position by birth, apprenticeship, or a "calling" via dream or vision Treatments involve use of herbs, rituals, and religious artifacts Practice for severe illness—make promises, visit shrines, offer medals and candles, offer prayers Adhere to "hot" and "cold" food prescriptions and prohibitions for prevention and treatment of illness
Puerto Rican	Subscribe to the "hot-cold" theory of causation of illness Believe some illness caused by evil spirits and forces	Infrequent use of health care systems Seek folk healers—use of herbs, rituals Consult spiritualist medium for mental disorders *Santeria* is system and practitioners are called *santeros* Treatments classified as "hot" or "cold"
Cuban-American†	Prevention and good nutrition are related to good health	Diligent users of the medical model, in part because of aggressive public health practices on the island prior to and after the revolution Eclectic health-seeking practices, including preventive measures, extensive use of the medical model, and, in some instances, folk medicine of both religious and nonreligious origins; home remedies; in many instances seek assistance of *santeros* (Afro-Cuban healers) and spiritualists to complement medical treatment Nutrition is important; parents show overconcern with eating habits of their children and spend a considerable part of the budget on food; traditional cuban diet is rich in meat and starch; consumption of fresh vegetables added in U.S.
Native American (numerous tribes)	Believe health is state of harmony with nature and universe Respect of bodies through proper management All disorders believed to have aspects of supernatural Violation of a restriction or prohibition thought to cause illness Fear of witchcraft May carry objects believed to guard against witchcraft Theology and medicine strongly interwoven	Medicine persons: Altruistic persons who must use powers in purely positive ways Persons capable of both good and evil—perform negative acts against enemies Diviner-diagnosticians—diagnose but do not have powers or skill to implement medical treatment Specialists—use herbs and curative but nonsacred medical procedures Medicine persons—use herbs and ritual Singers—cure by the power of their song obtained from supernatural beings, effect cures by laying on of hands

†This section was written by Mercedes Sandaval, Ph.D.

FAMILY RELATIONSHIPS	COMMUNICATION	COMMENTS
Traditionally men considered breadwinners, women homemakers Males are considered big and strong *(macho)* Strong kinship; extended families include *compadres* (godparents) established by ritual kinship Children valued highly and desired, taken everywhere with family Many homes contain shrines with statues and pictures of saints	May use nonstandard English Most bilingual; many only speak Spanish May have a strong preference for native language and revert to it in times of stress	High degree of modesty—often a deterrent to seeking medical care Youngsters often reluctant to share communal showers in schools Relaxed concept of time—may be late for appointments Magicoreligious practices common May view hospital as place to go to die
Family usually large and home-centered—the core of existence Father has complete authority in family—family provider and decision-maker Wife and children subordinate to father Children valued—seen as a gift from God Children taught to obey and respect parents; corporal punishment to ensure obedience	May use nonstandard English Spanish speaking or bilingual Strong sense of family privacy—may view questions regarding family as impudent	Relaxed sense of time Pay little attention to *exact* time of day Suspicious and fearful of hospitals
Strong family ties with mother and father kinships Children supported and assisted by parents long after becoming adults Elderly cared for at home	Most are bilingual (English/Spanish) except for segments of the senior population	In less than 30 years Cubans have been able to obtain a higher standard of living than other Hispanic groups in U.S. Have been able to retain many of their former social institutions: bilingual and private schools, clinics, social clubs, the family as an extended network of support, etc. Many do not feel discriminated against nor harbor feelings of inferiority with respect to Anglo-Americans or "mainstream" population
Extended family structure—usually includes relatives from both sides of family Elder members assume leadership roles	Most continue to speak their Indian language as well as English Nonverbal communication	Time orientation—present Respect for age Going to hospital associated with illness or disease; therefore may not seek prenatal care since pregnancy viewed as natural process

KEY POINTS

- Nurses have a responsibility to understand the influence of culture, race, and ethnicity on the development of social and emotional relationships, childrearing practices, and attitudes toward health.
- A culture is composed of individuals with a set of values, beliefs, practices, and information that is learned, integrative, social, and satisfying.
- A child's self-concept evolves from ideas about his or her social roles.
- Primary groups are characterized by intimate contact, mutual support, and behavior constraint among members.
- Secondary groups have limited intermittent contact, little mutual support, and no pressure for conformity.
- Guilt and shame are two behaviors commonly conditioned in children to control social behavior.
- Important subcultural influences on children include ethnicity, social class, occupation, poverty, affluence, religion, schools, peers, and biculture.
- A trend that has significantly influenced the American family is increasing geographic and economic mobility.
- Membership in a minority group presents special challenges for children, although changes in societal attitudes are slowly taking place.
- A child's physical characteristics and susceptibility to health problems are strongly related to ethnic and cultural variations of hereditary and socioeconomic forces.
- Hereditary and socioeconomic forces play an important role in a child's susceptibility to health problems.
- Groups of children suffering from greater physical and mental health problems are those living in poverty who are homeless or have migrant families.
- Drug response, food sensitivity, disease resistance, physical characteristics, and disease states may demonstrate ethnic or cultural variations.
- Because verbal and nonverbal communication is an important culture consideration, nurses need to acknowledge and respect their patient's practices in order for productive interaction to occur.
- Cultural beliefs related to cause of illness and maintenance of health may focus on natural forces, supernatural forces, or imbalance of forces.
- In planning and implementing patient care, nurses need to strive to adapt ethnic practices to the family's health needs rather than attempt to change long-standing beliefs.

REFERENCES

Alperstein, G., and Arnstein, E.: Homeless children—a challenge for pediatricians, Pediatr. Clin. North Am. 35(6):1413-1425, 1988.

American Academy of Pediatrics: Health needs of homeless children, Pediatrics 82(6):938-940, 1988.

American Academy of Pediatrics: Health care for children of migrant families, Pediatrics 84(4):739-740, 1989.

Asnes, R.S., and Wisotsky, D.H.: Cupping lesions simulating child abuse, J. Pediatr. 99:267-268, 1981.

Bass, J.L., and others: Pediatric problems in a suburban shelter for homeless families, Pediatrics 85(1):33-38, 1990.

Bassuk, E.L., and Rosenberg, L.: Psychosocial characteristics of homeless children and children with homes, Pediatrics 85(3):257-261, 1990.

Bauwens, E., and Anderson, S.: Social and cultural influences on health care. In Stanhope, M., and Lancaster, J.: Community health nursing, St. Louis, 1984, Mosby–Year Book, Inc.

Beliefs that can affect therapy, Pediatr. Nurs. 5(3):40-43, 1979.

Bloch, B.: Nursing care of black patients. In Orque, M.S., Bloch, B., and Monrroy, L.S.A.: Ethnic nursing care, St. Louis, 1983, Mosby–Year Book, Inc.

Bullough, V.L., and Bullough, B.: Health care for the other Americans, New York, 1982, Appleton-Century-Crofts.

Carpenito, L.J.: Nursing diagnosis: application to clinical practice, ed. 3, Philadelphia, 1989, J.B. Lippincott Co.

Char, E.L.: The Chinese American. In Clark, A.L., editor: Culture and childrearing, Philadelphia, 1981, F.A. Davis Co.

Chen-Louie, T.: Nursing care of Chinese American patients. In Orque, M.S., Bloch, B., and Monrroy, L.S.A.: Ethnic nursing care, St. Louis, 1983, Mosby–Year Book, Inc.

Chidester, D.: Patterns of transcendence: religion, death, and dying, Belmont, CA, 1990, Wadsworth Publishing Co.

Chow, E.: Cultural health traditions: Asian perspectives. In Branch, M.F., and Paxon, P.P., editors: Providing safe nursing care for ethnic people of color, New York, 1976, Appleton-Century-Crofts.

Clark, A.L., editor: Culture and childrearing, Philadelphia, 1981, F.A. Davis Co.

Cohen, F.L.: Clinical genetics in nursing practice, Philadelphia, 1984, J.B. Lippincott Co.

Conatser, C.: Effect of wealth on approach to patient care, J. Assoc. Pediatr. Oncol. Nurses 3(2):14-19, 1986.

David, R.: Race, birthweight, and mortality rates, J. Pediatr. 116(1):101-102, 1990.

Duncan, G.J., and Rodgers, W.L.: Longitudinal aspects of childhood poverty, J. Marriage Fam. 50(4):1007-1021, 1988.

Ehling, M.B.: The Mexican American (El Chicano). In Clark, A.L., editor: Culture and childrearing, Philadelphia, 1981, F.A. Davis Co.

Elkin, F., and Handel, G.: The child and society: the process of socialization, New York, 1989, Random House, Inc.

Evans, V.: Sociodemographic trends toward the 21st century. In Feeg, V., editor: Pediatric nursing: forum on the future: looking toward the 21st century, Pitman, NJ, 1989, Anthony J. Jannetti, Inc.

Faber, M.: A review of efforts to protect children from injury in car crashes, Fam. Community Health 9(3):25-41, 1986.

Feldman, K.W.: Pseudoabusive burns in Asian refugees, Am. J. Dis. Child. 138:768-769, 1984.

Flynn, B.C., and Miller, M.H.: Current perspectives in nursing: social issues and trends, St. Louis, 1980, Mosby–Year Book, Inc.

Foss, R.: Sociocultural perspective on child occupant protection, Pediatrics 80(6):886-893, 1987.

Friedman, M.: Transcultural family nursing: application to Latino and black families, Pediatr. Nurs. 5(3):214-222, 1990.

Greathouse, B., and Miller, V.G.: The black American. In Clark, A.L., editor: Culture and childrearing, Philadelphia, 1981, F.A. Davis Co.

Grinker, R.R.: The poor rich: the children of the super-rich, Am. J. Psychiatry 135:913-916, 1978.

Hashizume, S., and Takano, J.: Nursing care of Japanese patients. In Orque, M.S., Bloch, B., and Monrroy, L.S.A.: Ethnic nursing care, St. Louis, 1983, Mosby–Year Book, Inc.

Henderson, G., and Premeaux, M., editors: Transcultural health care, Menlo Park, CA, 1981, Addison-Wesley Publishing Co., Inc.

Holland, S., and Sweeney, E.: Vietnamese children and families: the impact of culture, Washington, DC, 1985, Association for Care of Children's Health.

Hollingsworth, A.O., Brown, L.P., and Brooten, D.A.: The refugees and childbearing: what to expect, RN 43(11):45-48, 1980.

Jacques, G.: Cultural traditions: a black perspective In Branch, M.F., and Paxton, P.P.: Providing safe nursing care for ethnic people of color, New York, 1976, Appleton-Century-Crofts.

Lacay, G.: The Puerto Rican in mainland America. In Clark, A.L., editor: Culture and childrearing, Philadelphia, 1981, F.A. Davis Co.

Lawson, L.V.: Culturally sensitive support for grieving parents, MCN 15(2):76-79, 1990.

Leininger, M.: Transcultural nursing, New York, 1978, John Wiley & Sons, Inc.

Leslie, G.R.: The family in social context, ed. 5, New York, 1982, Oxford University Press, Inc.

Markides, K.S., and Coreil, J.: The health of Hispanics in the southwestern United States: an epidemiologic paradox (review), Public Health Rep. 101(3):253-265, 1986.

Martinson, I.M.: The challenge of culturally diverse pediatric clients. In Feeg, V, editor: Pediatric nursing: forum on the future: looking toward the 21st century, Pitman, NJ, 1989, Anthony J. Jannetti, Inc.

McGoldrick, M.: Ethnicity, families, and psychosocial problems. In Leahey, M., and Wright, L.: Families and psychosocial problems, Springhouse, PA, 1987, Springhouse Corp.

Meleis, A.I.: The Arab American in the health care system, Am. J. Nurs. 81:1180-1183, 1981.

Miller, D.S., and Lin, E.H.B.: Children in sheltered homeless families: reported health status and use of health services, Pediatrics 81(5):668-673, 1988.

Monrroy, L.S.A.: Nursing care of Raza/ Latina patients. In Orque, M.S., Bloch, B., and Monrroy, L.S.A.: Ethnic nursing care, St. Louis, 1983, Mosby–Year Book, Inc.

Murillo-Rohde, I.: Health care for the Hispanic patient, Crit. Care Update 7(5):29-36, 1980.

O'Brien, M.E.: Pragmatic survivalism: behavior patterns affecting low-level wellness among minority group members, Adv. Nurs. Sci. 4(3):13-26, 1982.

Orque, M.S.: Nursing care of Filipino American patients. In Orque, M.S., Bloch, B., and Monrroy, L.S.A.: Ethnic nursing care, St. Louis, 1983a, Mosby–Year Book, Inc.

Orque, M.S.: Nursing care of South Vietnamese patients. In Orque, M.S., Bloch, B., and Monrroy, L.S.A.: Ethnic nursing care, St. Louis, 1983b, Mosby–Year Book, Inc.

Pasquale, E.A.: The evil eye phenomenon, Home Healthcare Nurse 2(3):32-35, 1984.

Portes, P., Dunham, R., and Williams, S.: Assessing child-rearing style in ecological settings: its relation to culture, social class, early age intervention and scholastic achievement, Adolescence 21(83):723-735, 1986.

Salzer, J.L., and Nelson, N.A.: Health care of Ethiopian refugees, Pediatr. Nurs. 9:449-452, 1983.

Schwartz, A.J.: The schools and socialization, New York, 1975, Harper & Row, Publishers, Inc.

Shaffer, D.C.: Developmental psychology: theory, research and application, Monterey, CA, 1985, Brooks/Cole Publishing Co.

Skolnick, A.: The intimate environment: exploring marriage and the family, ed. 4, Boston, 1987, Little, Brown & Co, Inc.

Sloat, A., and Matsuura, W.: Intercultural communication. In Craft, M., and Denehy, J., editors: Nursing interventions for infants and children, Philadelphia, 1990, W.B. Saunders Co.

Sodetani-Shibata, A.E.: The Japanese American. In Clark, A.L., editor: Culture and childrearing, Philadelphia, 1981, F.A. Davis Co.

Spradley, B.W.: Community health nursing, Boston, 1981, Little, Brown & Co, Inc.

Tseng, W., and others: Cross-cultural differences in parent-child assessment: U.S.A and Japan, Int. J. Soc. Psychiatry 28:305-317, 1982.

Valentine, C.A.: Culture and poverty, Chicago, 1968, University of Chicago Press.

Wilson, U.M.: Nursing care of American Indian patients. In Orque, M.S., Bloch, B., and Monrroy, L.S.A.: Ethnic nursing care, St. Louis, 1983, Mosby–Year Book, Inc.

Wise, P.H., and Meyers, A.: Poverty and child health, Pediatr. Clin. North Am. 35(6):1169-1186, 1988.

Wood, D.: Homeless children: their evaluation and treatment, J. Pediatr. Health Care 3(4):194-199, 1989.

Zigler, E., and Hall, N.: Day care and its effect on children: an overview for pediatric health professionals, J. Dev. Behav. Pediatr. 9(1):38-46, 1990.

BIBLIOGRAPHY

General

Ablon, J., and Ames, G.M.: Culture and family. In Gilliss, C.L., and others, editors: Toward a science of family nursing, Menlo Park, CA, 1989, Addison-Wesley Publishing Co., Inc.

Anderson, A.B., and Frideres, J.S.: Ethnicity in Canada: theoretical perspectives, Toronto, 1981, Butterworths.

Bauwens, E.E., and Anderson, S.: Social and cultural influences on health care. In Stanhope, M., and Lancaster, J.: Community health nursing, St. Louis, 1984, Mosby–Year Book, Inc.

Brink, P.J.: Value orientations as an assessment tool in cultural diversity, Nurs. Res. 33:198-203, 1984.

Carpio, B.: The adolescent immigrant, Can. Nurse 7(3):27-29, 1981.

Chen-Louie, T.T.: Bicultural experiences, social interactions, and health care implications. In Reinhardt, A.M., and Quinn, M.D., editors: Family-centered community nursing, vol. 2, St. Louis, 1980, Mosby–Year Book, Inc.

Choi, E.S., and Hamilton, R.K.: The effects of culture on mother-infant interaction, JOGNN 15:256-261, 1986.

DeFriese, G.H., and Hetherington, J.S.: Child health and the problem of access to care, Fam. Community Health 4(3):71-83, 1982.

Dobson, S.: Bringing culture into care, Nurs. Times 78:2106-2109, 1982.

Fitzgerald, F.T.: Patients from other cultures: how they view you, themselves, and disease, Consultant 28(3):65-67, 1988.

Flynn, B.C., and Miller, M.H.: Current perspectives in nursing: societal issues and trends, St. Louis, 1980, Mosby–Year Book, Inc.

Fong, C.M: Ethnicity and nursing practice, Top. Clin. Nurs. 7(3):1-10, 1985.

Frenkel, S.I., and others: Does patient contact change racial perceptions? Am. J. Nurs. 80:1340-1342, 1980.

Germain, C.P.: Cultural concepts in critical care, Crit. Care. Q. 5(3):61-78, 1982.

Handelman, L., Menahem, S., and Eisenbruch, I.M.: Transcultural understanding of a hereditary disorder: mucopolysaccharidosis VI in a Vietnamese family, Clin. Pediatr. 28(10):470-473, 1989.

Harwood, A., editor: Ethnicity and medical care, Cambridge, MA, 1981, Harvard University Press.

Hautman, M.A., and Harrison, J.K.: Health beliefs and practices in a middle-income Anglo-American neighborhood, Adv. Nurs. Sci. 4(3):49-63, 1982.

Henry, B.M., and DiGiacomo-Geffers, E.: The hospitalized rich and famous, Am. J. Nurs. 80:1426-1429, 1980.

Johnston, M.: Cultural variations in professional and parenting practices, J. Obstet. Gynecol. Nurs. 9:9-13, 1980.

Kleinman, A.: Patients and healers in the context of culture, Berkeley, 1980, University of California Press.

Kubricht, D.W., and Clark, J.A.: Foreign patients: a system for providing care, Nurs. Outlook 30:55-57, 1982.

LaFargue, J.P.: Mediating between two views of illness, Top. Clin. Nurs. 7(3):70-77, 1985.

Lanara, V.A.: Cultural value—influence on the delivery of care, Intensive Care Nurs. 4(1):3-8, 1988.

Lash, M.E.: Community health nursing in a minority setting, Nurs. Clin. North Am. 15(2):339-348, 1980.
Linley, J.F.: Mothers' attitudes regarding health care for their children, MCN 9:37-39, 1984.
Lipson, J.G., and Meleis, A.I.: Culturally appropriate care: the case of immigrants, Top. Clin. Nurs. 7(3):48-56, 1985.
Louie, K.B.: Transcending cultural bias: the literature speaks, Top. Clin. Nurs. 7(3):78-84, 1985.
Low, S.M.: The cultural basis of health, illness and disease, Soc. Work Health Care 9(3):13-23, 1984.
Maheady, D.C.: Cultural assessment of children, MCN 11(2):128, 1986.
Mandelbaum, J.K.: The food square: helping people of different cultures understand balanced diets, Pediatr. Nurs. 9:20-21, 1985.
Marchant, R.: Caring for hospitalized inner-city children, Pediatr. Nurs. 11:129-131, 1985.
Morse, J.M.: Transcultural nursing: its substance and issues in research and knowledge, Recent Adv. Nurs. 18:129-141, 1987.
O'Brien, M.E.: Transcultural nursing research—alien in an alien land, Image 13:37-39, 1981.
Orque, M.S., Bloch, B., and Monrroy, L.S.A.: Ethnic nursing care, St. Louis, 1983, Mosby–Year Book, Inc.
Queen, S.A., Haberstein, R.W., and Quadagno, J.S.: The family in various cultures, New York, 1985, Harper & Row, Publishers, Inc.
Reichenback, M.B.: A framework for the nature and development of health beliefs in children, Matern. Child Nurs. J. 15(3):119-128, 1986.
Ruiz, M.C.J.: Open-mindedness, intolerance of ambiguity and nursing faculty attitudes toward culturally different patients, Nurs. Res. 30:177-181, 1981.
Spector, R.E.: Cultural diversity in health and illness, ed. 2, New York, 1985, Appleton-Century-Crofts.
Spinetta, J.J.: Measurement of family function, communication, and cultural effects, Cancer 53(suppl. 10):2330-2337, 1984.
Stern, P.N.: Solving problems of cross-cultural health teaching, Image 13:47-50, 1981.
Thiederman, S.B.: Ethnocentrism: a barrier to effective health care, Nurs. Pract. 11(8):52-59, 1986.
Tripp-Reimer, T.: Research in cultural diversity, West. J. Nurs. Res. 6:353-355, 1984.
Tripp-Reimer, T., and Afifi, L.A.: Cross-cultural perspectives on patient teaching, Nurs. Clin. North Am. 24(3):613-619, 1989.
Tripp-Reimer, T., Brink, P.J., and Saunders, J.M.: Cultural assessment: content and process, Nurs. Outlook 32:78-82, 1984.
Tripp-Reimer, T., and Lauer, G.: Ethnicity and families with chronic illness. In Wright, L., and Leahey, M: Families and chronic illness, Springhouse, PA, 1987, Springhouse Corp.

Poverty, Homeless

Berne, A.S., and others: A nursing model for addressing the health needs of homeless families, Image 22(1):8-13, 1990.
Oberg, C.N.: Pediatrics and poverty, Pediatrics 79(4):567-568, 1987.
Parker, S., Greer, S., and Zuckerman, B.: Double jeopardy: the impact of poverty on early child development, Pediatr. Clin. North Am. 35(6):1227-1240, 1988.
Rafferty, M.: Standing up for America's homeless, Am. J. Nurs. 89(12):1614-1617, 1989.

Religion

Abbott, D.A., Berry, M., and Meredith, W.H.: Religious beliefs and practice: a potential asset in helping families, Fam. Relations 39(4):443-448, 1990.
Adams, C.E., and others: The effects of religious beliefs on the health care practices of the Amish, Nurs. Pract. 11(3):58-67, 1986.
D'Antonio, W.V.: The American Catholic family: signs of cohesion and polarization, J. Marriage Fam. 47:395-402, 1985.
Ellis, D.: What happened to the spiritual dimension? Can. Nurs. 76(9):42-43, 1980.
Gershan, J.A.: Judaic ethical beliefs and customs regarding death and dying, Crit. Care Nurse 5(1):32-34, 1985.
Lutwak, R.A., Ney, A.M., and White, J.E.: Maternity nursing and Jewish law, MCN 13(1):44-46, 1988.
Masulis, K.: When parents refuse treatment for their children . . . Jehovah's Witnesses, J. Christ. Nurs. 4(2):10-12, 1987.
Nelson, M., and Joranoric, L.: Pregnancy, diabetes, and Jewish dietary law, J. Am. Diet. Assoc. 87(8):1054-1057, 1987.
Shelly, J.A.: Spiritual care: Planting seeds of hope, Crit. Care Update 9(2):7-15, 1982.
Sodestrom, K.E., and Martinson, I.M.: Patients' spiritual coping strategies: a study of nurse and patient perspectives, Oncol. Nurs. Forum 14(2):41-46, 1987.
Stoll, R.T.: Guidelines for spiritual assessment, Am. J. Nurs. 79:1574-1577, 1979.
Swan, R.: The law should protect all children . . . children in faith-healing sects, J. Christ. Nurs. 4(2):40, 1987.
Thornton, A.: Reciprocal influences of family and religion in a changing world, J. Marriage Fam. 47:381-394, 1985.
Thurkauf, G.E.: Understanding the beliefs of Jehovah's Witnesses, Focus Crit. Care 16(3):199-204, 1989.

Ethnic Groups: Asian American

Aquino, C.J.: The Filipino in America. In Clark, A.L., editor: Culture and childrearing, Philadelphia, 1981, F.A. Davis Co.
Aslam, M., and others: Asian medicine: in the best tradition? Nurs. Mirror 153(4):34-36, 1981.
Brown, B.S.: Growing up healthy: the Chinese experience, Pediatr. Nurs. 9:255-257, 1983.
Choi, E.: Unique aspects of Korean-American mothers, JOGNN 15(5):394-400, 1986.
Dung, T.N.: Understanding Asian families: a Vietnamese perspective, Child. Today 13(2):1012, 1984.
Egan, M.G.: A family assessment challenge: refugee youth and foster family adaptation, Top. Clin. Nurs. 7(3):64-69, 1985.
Floriani, C.M.: Southeast Asian refugees: life in a camp. Am. J. Nurs. 80:2028-2030, 1980.
Gordon, V.C., Matousek, I.M., and Lang, T.A.: Southeast Asian refugees: life in America, Am. J. Nurs. 80:2031-2036, 1980.
Grosso, C., and others: The Vietnamese American family . . . and grandma makes three, MCN. 6:177-180, 1981.
Joe, V.: A new lifestyle in a new land, Can. Nurse 7(3):6-10, 1981.
Kwok, A.W.H.: Culture conflict: a study of the problems of Chinese immigrant adolescents in Canada, Can. Nurs. 78(3):32-34, 1982.
Leyn, R.B.: The challenge of caring for child refugees from Southeast Asia, MCN 3:178-182, 1978.
Marrio, E.B., and Hall, R.R.: Asian family traditions and their influence in transcultural health care delivery, Child. Health Care 15(3):172-177, 1987.
Martinson, I.M.: Impact of childhood cancer on family care in Taiwan, Pediatr. Nurs. 15(6):636-637, 1989.
Muecke, M.A.: Caring for Southeast Asian refugee patients in the USA, Am. J. Public Health 73:431-438, 1983.
Pickwell, S.M.: Primary health care for Indochinese refugee children, Pediatr. Nurs. 8:104-107, 1982.
Rocereto, L.V.: Selected health beliefs of Vietnamese refugees, J. School Health 51:63-64, 1981
Rorabaugh, M.L.: The pediatric nurse practitioner in Southeast Asia: a personal account, Pediatr. Nurs. 9:263-266, 1983.
Rosenburg, J.A.: Health care for Cambodian children: integrating treatment plans, Pediatr. Nurs. 12:118-125, 1986.
Schultz, S.L.: How Southeast-Asian refugees in California adapt to unfamiliar health care practices, Health Soc. Work 7:148-156, 1982.
Stern, P.N.: Solving problems of cross-cultural health teaching: the Filipino childbearing family, Image 13:47-50, 1981.
Yeatman, W., and Dang, V.: Coa Gia (coin rubbing), JAMA 244:2748-2749, 1980.

Ethnic Groups: Black American

Capers, C.F.: Nursing and the Afro-American client, Top. Clin. Nurs. 7(3):11-17, 1985.

Levy, D.R.: White doctors and black patients: influence of race on the doctor-patient relationship, Pediatrics 75(4):639-643, 1985.

Pass, C.M.: Psychological factors, childbearing, and black female adolescents, J. Pediatr. Nurs. 1:247-259, 1986.

Powers, B.A.: The use of orthodox and black American folk medicine, Adv. Nurs. Sci. 4(3):35-47, 1982.

Roberson, M.H.B.: The influence of religious beliefs on health choices of Afro-Americans, Top. Clin. Nurs. 7(3):57-63, 1985.

Ethnic Groups: Hispanic American

Charles, C.: Mental health services for Haitians. In Lefley, H.P., and Pederson, P.B., editors: Cross-cultural training for mental health professionals, Springfield, IL, 1986, Charles C Thomas, Publisher.

Chesney, A.P., and others: Mexican American folk medicine: implications for the family physician, J. Fam. Pract. 11:567-574, 1980.

daSilva, G.C.: Awareness of Hispanic cultural issues in the health care setting, Assoc. Care Child. Health 13(1):4-10, 1984.

DeSantis, L.: Childrearing beliefs and practices of Cuban and Haitian parents: implications for nurses. In Carter, M.A., editor: Proceedings of the tenth annual conference of the Transcultural Nursing Society, Salt Lake City, 1985, Transcultural Nursing Society.

DeSantis, L.: Infant feeding practices of Haitian mothers in South Florida: cultural beliefs and acculturation, Matern. Child Nurs. J. 15:77-89, 1986.

DeSantis, L.: Cuban and Haitian perspectives on child health: a transcultural view. In Wang, J.F., Simoni, P.S., and Nath, C.L., editors: Proceedings of the West Virginia Nurses' Association research symposium, Charleston, WV, 1988, West Virginia Nurses' Research Conference Group.

Foreman, J.T.: *Susto* and the health needs of the Cuban refugee population, Top. Clin. Nurs. 7(3):40-47, 1985.

Gonzales-Swafford, M.J.: Ethno-medical beliefs and practices of Mexican-Americano, Nurs. Pract. 8(10):29-30, 32, 34, 1983.

Guendelman, S.: Developing responsiveness to the health needs of Hispanic children and families, Soc. Work Health Care 8(4):1-15, 1983.

Guendelman, S.: At risk: health needs of Hispanic children, Health Soc. Work 10:183-190, 1985.

Laguerre, M.S.: Haitian Americans. In Harwood, A., editor: Ethnicity and medical care, Cambridge, MA, 1984, Harvard University Press.

Mardiros, M.: A view toward hospitalization: the Mexican American experience, J. Adv. Nurs. 9:469-478, 1984.

Ramirez, A.G.: A media-based acculturation scale for Mexican-Americans: application to public health education programs, Fam. Community Health 9(3):63-71, 1986.

Richardson, L.: Breakthrough to nursing. 2. Folk medicine in a Hispanic population, Imprint 29:72-77, 1982.

Tamez, E.G.: Familism, machismo, and child rearing practices among Mexican Americans, J. Psychosoc. Nurs. 19(9):21-25, 1981.

Zepeda, M.: Selected maternal-infant care practices of Spanish-speaking women, J. Obstet. Gynecol. Nurs. 11:371-374, 1982.

Ethnic Groups: Other Cultures

Backup, R.W.: Health care of the American Indian patient, Crit. Care Update 7(2):16-22, 1980.

Drakulic, L., and Tanaka, W.: The East Indian family in Canada, Can. Nurse 7(3):24-26, 1981.

Gershan, J.A.: Judaic ethical beliefs and customs regarding death and dying, Crit. Care Nurs. 5:32-34, 1985.

Macdonald, A.C.: Folk health practices among north costal Peruvians: implications for nursing, Image 13:51-55, 1981.

Meleis, A.I., and Sorrell, L.: Arab American women and their birth experiences, MCN. 6:171-176, 1981.

Niederhauser, V.P.: Health care of immigrant children: incorporating culture into practice, Pediatr. Nurs. 15(6):569-574, 1989.

Rozendal, N.: Understanding Italian American cultural norms, J. Psychosoc. Nurs. Ment. Health Serv. 25(2):29-35, 1987.

Satz, K.J.: Integrating Navajo tradition into maternal-child nursing, Image 14:89-91, 1982.

Tripp-Reimer, T.: Barriers to health care: variations in interpretation of Appalachian client behavior by Appalachian and non-Appalachian health professionals, West. J. Nurs. Res. 4:179-191, 1982.

Tripp-Reimer, T.: Retention of a folk-healing practice (matiasma) among four generations of urban Greek immigrants, Nurs. Res. 32:97-101, 1983.

van Breda, A.: Health issues facing Native American children, Pediatr. Nurs. 15(6):575-577, 1989.

Wiggins, L.R.: Health and illness beliefs and practices among the Old Order Amish, Health Values 7(6):24-29, 1983.

CHAPTER 3

Family Influences on Child Health Promotion

RELATED TOPICS

Adolescent pregnancy, Ch. 20
Alternate child care arrangements, Ch. 12
Communicating with families, Ch. 6
Family assessment, Ch. 6
Growth and development of children, Ch. 4
Impact of chronic illness or disability on the child and family, Ch. 22
Limit-setting and discipline, Ch. 14
Multiple births and subsequent children, Ch. 8
Preschool or daycare experience, Ch. 15
Promotion of parent-infant bonding (attachment), Ch. 8
Sibling rivalry, Ch. 14
Social, cultural, and religious influences on child health promotion, Ch. 2

GLOSSARY

adoption Legal process that establishes a legal relationship of parent and child between persons not related by birth, with the same rights and obligations of parents and biologic children

authoritarian Parental style of control in which parents make strict rules and rigidly enforce behavior, without involving the child in the decision-making process

authoritative Parental style of control in which parents establish rules, provide rationales for the rules, discuss these with their children, emphasize behavior rather than the child as a person, and help the child develop inner-directed self-control

blended or **combined family** Both married adults have children from a previous marriage residing in the household

consanguineous Blood relationships
dual-earner family Both parents have job responsibilities, usually outside the home
DZ Dizygotic or fraternal twins; arise from two separately fertilized eggs; have separate genetic characteristics just as any other pair of siblings
extended or **consanguineous family** Nuclear unit with other relatives living in the same household
family Two or more people who are emotionally involved with each other and usually live in close geographic proximity
function Family interaction; duties performed by family members
household Persons sharing a common dwelling; often used synonymously with *family*
MZ Monozygotic or identical twins; result from a single egg that, once fertilized, divides into two eggs, resulting in children sharing the exact same genetic characteristics
nuclear or **conjugal family** Husband, wife, and children (natural or adopted) who live in a common household
permissive Parental style of control that allows children to regulate their own behavior without much parental guidance or intervention
single-parent family Mother or father has children residing in the household
stepfamily or **reconstituted family** One or both married adults have children from a previous marriage residing in the household
structure Composition of the family; arrangement of roles within family system

Societies, to maintain and perpetuate themselves, have established institutions designed to rear and to educate their children. The primary institution for this responsibility is the family, and, as the basic interpersonal group, it is a universal characteristic of all human societies. The family provides each newborn member of society with legitimacy, that is, a family connection (usually symbolized by a family name) and an ascribed position in the societal strata. It serves as the link between individual members and the larger society (Johnson, 1984). Socialization patterns and the organization of roles and relationships within the community are largely determined in the context of the family.

Although the structure and subordinate goals of the family vary among and within cultures and change at different times and in different places, the overall purpose of the family is to provide for the future of a society and the stability of its culture. During the long time required for human infants to reach a level of independence, individual families assume the responsibility for their rearing, although such families differ considerably in form, complexity, and goals of socialization.

The term *family* has many meanings, has provided a fertile field for study, and has been defined in a number of ways and for a number of purposes according to the individual's own frame of reference, value judgment, or the discipline (Johnson, 1984). For example, biology describes the family as fulfilling the biologic function of perpetuation of the species. Psychology emphasizes the interpersonal aspects of the family and its responsibility for personality development. Economics views the family as a productive unit providing for material needs, while sociology depicts it as the social unit that reacts with the larger society. Others define family in relation to the persons who comprise the family unit: *consanguinal* (blood relationships), *affinal* (marriage relationships), and *fictive* (invented relationships, such as godparents or groups who call themselves a family). Still others attempt to describe the family as a combination of these elements or in terms of what a family ought to be.

No consensus on a definition of family has been reached. Earlier definitions emphasized that family members were related by legal ties or genetic relationships and lived in the same household with specific roles (Burgess, Locke, and Thomas, 1963). Later definitions have been broadened to reflect both structural and functional changes. Friedman (1986) defines family as "composed of [two or more] people who are emotionally involved with each other and live in close geographical proximity." According to Friedman (1986), emotional involvement is "a perception of reciprocal obligations, a sense of commonness, and a sharing of certain obligations, coupled with a caring commitment to each other." Geographic proximity may no longer be a necessary component of a definition of family, since it is increasingly common for family members, such as the breadwinner, to live apart from the household for variable intervals. This all-encompassing definition can include communal, cohabitative, heterosexual, and homosexual relationships; single-parent families; childless couples; and dual-earner families.

Traditionally a family has been conceptualized as a group with the belief that both a mother and father are needed to rear a child. Nearly all societies grant a very high rank to the married status, although this concept has undergone considerable modification. Some of the newer forms of family—such as communal families and homosexual families—have been controversial. To maintain the viability of the family, each culture has devised standards of familial behavior, systems that reward those who support or conform to these standards, and systems that punish those who do not.

In an effort to include persons and situations that might be excluded in definitions of family, the term *household* is used to describe a variety of family styles and other combi-

This chapter was coauthored by Marilyn McCubbin, R.N., Ph.D.

nations of persons sharing a common dwelling. A household includes such nontraditional groups as (1) persons who have never married and who have no family or other form of union but who are members of a household, (2) the one-parent family consisting of a single parent and child(ren), (3) two homosexuals living together in a stable union, and (4) stable consensual unions, with or without children (World Health Organization, 1978). A household can also consist of a single, never-married person or married persons who choose not to have children. Although the concept of household is recognized and appreciated, the term *family* is used consistently throughout this book to indicate the relationships between dependent children and one or more protective adults. It also implies relationships among siblings. Family members share a sense of belonging to their own family that deeply affects their lives.

FAMILY THEORIES

A family theory can be viewed as a "set of lenses" (Hill and Hansen, 1960) used to describe families and how the family unit responds to events both within and outside the family. Each family theory makes certain assumptions about the family and has inherent strengths and limitations (Table 3-1). Although no single "grand" theory encompasses all the complexities of contemporary family life, three theories in widespread use for many years are developmental, structural-functional, and interactional. Other useful theories are family systems theory, family stress theory, exchange theory, and conflict theory. Most nurses use a combination of these theories in their work with children and families. Examples of applications of these theories to specific family situations are included in Table 3-1.

DEVELOPMENTAL THEORY

Developmental theory is an outgrowth of several theories of development. Foremost among the developers are Duvall (1977), who described eight developmental tasks of the family throughout its life span (Box 3-1), derived from Erikson's eight stages of man (see Chapter 4), and Rogers (1962), who incorporated role theory into the developmental concept. The family is described as a small group, a semiclosed system of personalities that interacts with the larger cultural social system. As an interrelated system, changes do not occur in one part without a series of changes in other parts.

Developmental theory addresses family change over time by using Duvall's family life-cycle stages, based on the predictable changes in the structure, function, and roles of the family, with the age of the oldest child as the marker for stage transition. Thus, the arrival of the first child marks the transition from stage I to stage II. As the first child grows and develops, the family enters subsequent stages. In every stage, the family is faced with certain developmental tasks. At the same time, each member of the family must achieve individual developmental tasks as part of each family life-cycle stage.

Developmental theory can be applied to nursing practice in a number of ways, such as assessing how well new parents are accomplishing the individual and family developmental tasks associated with transition to parenthood. One drawback of the developmental theory as presently constructed, however, is the difficulty in applying it to nonnuclear families, such as single-parent families and stepfamilies, which may omit some stages, pass through others not included here, or approach developmental stages and tasks in different sequences.

Box 3-1 DUVALL'S DEVELOPMENT STAGES OF THE FAMILY

Stage I: Marriage and an Independent Home: The Joining of Families
Reestablish couple identity
Realign relationships with extended family
Make decisions regarding parenthood

Stage II: Families with Infants
Integrate infants into the family unit
Accommodate to new parenting and grandparenting roles
Maintain the marital bond

Stage III: Families with Preschoolers
Socialize children
Parents and children adjust to separation

Stage IV: Families with School Children
Children develop peer relations
Parents adjust to their children's peer and school influences

Stage V: Families with Teenagers
Adolescents develop increasing autonomy
Parents refocus on midlife marital and career issues
Parents begin a shift toward concern for the older generation

Stage VI: Families as Launching Centers
Parents and young adults establish independent identities
Renegotiate marital relationship

Stage VII: Middle-Aged Families
Reinvest in couple identity with concurrent development of independent interests
Realign relationships to include in-laws and grandchildren
Deal with disabilities and death of older generation

Stage VIII: Aging Families
Shift from work role to leisure and semiretirement or full retirement
Maintain couple and individual functioning while adapting to the aging process
Prepare for own death and dealing with the loss of spouse and/or siblings and other peers

Modified from Wright, L.M., and Leahey, M.: Nurses and families: a guide to family assessment and intervention, Philadelphia, 1984, F.A. Davis Co.

Table 3-1 Summary of family theories and applications

FAMILY THEORY	ASSUMPTIONS	STRENGTHS	LIMITATIONS	APPLICATIONS
Developmental theory	Families develop and change over time in similar and consistent ways Family and its members must perform certain time-specific tasks set by themselves and by persons in the broader society Family role performance at one stage of the family life cycle influences family's behavioral options at next stage Family tends to be in stage of disequilibrium entering a new life-cycle stage and strives toward homeostasis within stages	Provides a dynamic, rather than static, view of family Addresses both changes within family and changes in family as a social system over its life history Anticipates potential stressors that normally accompany transitions to various stages and when problems may peak because of lack of resources	More easily applied to two-parent families with children Use of age of oldest child and marital duration as marker of stage transition may be problematic (e.g., in stepfamilies, single-parent families)	Anticipatory guidance, educational strategies, and developing/strengthening family resources for management of: transition to parenthood; family adjustment to children entering school, becoming adolescents, leaving home; management of "empty nest" years and retirement
Structural-functional theory	Family performs at least one societal function (e.g., reproduction, socializing children, producing/consuming goods and services) while also meeting family needs Family, as a social system, tends toward stability Family behaviors are largely determined by norms	Considers interplay within family, as well as between family and the larger social system (school, workplace) Views family as both open to outside influence and transactions and as a system that tends to maintain boundaries	Strong emphasis on family stability and maintaining status quo	Dual-career or dual-worker families and management of combined work and family roles and responsibilities Relationships of family unit with schools, other societal institutions
Symbolic interactional theory	Family is a unit of interacting persons, with each occupying a position within the family to which a number of roles are assigned. Family relationships are continually in flux The definition family members make of situations partially determines the effects situations have for them Family members communicate through symbols that have both meaning and value attached to them	More culture and value free, less normative and prescriptive Views family as a living social unit and examines both behavior and perceptions	Looks more at family at one point in time Focuses on internal family interactions and processes; less emphasis on family-community/society interactions and relationships Complex framework with many concepts, assumptions	Family communications, decision making, problem solving
Exchange theory	Overall assumption is that humans, families, groups, associations, and even nations seek rewarding statuses, relationships, interactions, and feeling states so that their rewards are maximized and/or their costs are minimized	Breadth and versatility Applicable to various family forms, to families of other cultures and countries Can be applied to individuals, families, groups, organizations, societies	What constitutes a reward or cost is not clear Does not directly address how individuals or families acquire meaning and value in determining what is a reward and/or cost	Rewards and costs associated with paid employment of mothers, decision to have children or be child free, parenting responsibilities, kin and intergenerational relationships, marital dissolution

Continued.

Table 3-1 Summary of family theories and applications—cont'd

FAMILY THEORY	ASSUMPTIONS	STRENGTHS	LIMITATIONS	APPLICATIONS
Family systems theory	A change in any one part of a family system affects all other parts of the family system (circular causality) Family systems are characterized by periods of rapid growth and change and periods of relative stability Both too little change and too much change are dysfunctional for the family system; therefore, a balance between morphogenesis (change) and morphostasis (no change) is necessary Family system can initiate change as well as react to it	Applicable for family in normal everyday life, as well as for family dysfunction and pathology Useful for families of varying structure and various stages of life cycle	More difficult to determine cause-and-effect relationships because of circular causality	Mate selection, courtship processes, family communication, boundary maintenance, power and control within family, parent-child relationships, adolescent pregnancy and parenthood
Conflict theory	Families are viewed as ongoing competitive social systems The conflict inherent in family relationships can be managed by negotiation and problem solving Complete suppression of conflict in a family system is likely to have negative consequences for the family unit and/or its members	Applicable to all family forms and structures Appropriate for examining many situations families are facing in today's society Can see how family conflict changes over time	Can be perceived as having a "negative" focus Can view all conflict as power struggle, which severely limits its use of this theory Needs further use and testing	Divorce, remarriage, stepfamily relationships, conflict over any aspect of family life—relationships with children, in-laws, work-family issues, caretaking of dependent members (children, elders), family violence
Family stress theory	Stress is an inevitable part of family life, and any event, even if positive, can be stressful for family Family encounters both normative expected stressors and unexpected situational stressors over life cycle Stress has a cumulative effect on family Families cope and respond to stressors with a wide range of responses and effectiveness	Potential to explain and predict family behavior in response to stressors and to develop effective interventions to promote family adaptation Focuses on positive contribution of resources, coping, and social support to adaptive outcomes Can be used by many disciplines in health field	Relationships between all variables in framework not yet adequately described Do not yet know if certain combinations of resources, coping strategies are applicable to all stressful events	Transition to parenthood and other normative transitions, single-parent families, families experiencing work-related stressors (dual-earner, unemployment), acute or chronic childhood illness or disability, infertility, death of a child, divorce, teenage pregnancy and parenthood

STRUCTURAL-FUNCTIONAL THEORY

Structural-functional theory, one of the dominant orientations in modern sociology, has been most systematically applied by Parsons (Rodman, 1965). In analyzing families, this theory focuses less on family change and more on the interrelatedness, interdependence, and integration between family members and all aspects of society and its subcultures, particularly the occupational subsystem. *Structure* refers to the arrangement of roles that comprise a social system; *function* is the contribution made by an activity or role to the whole and the consequences of the activity for the system. The family is described as a social system with members who have specific roles and functions. The family process is directed toward maintaining an equilibrium between the complementary roles within the family—for example, husband-wife, father-daughter, mother-son, or wife–mother-in-law.

Internal relationships involve the division of labor between family members and the functions of these divisions for family maintenance. "Expressive" roles are seen in integrative or solidifying activities, such as hugging, that bring emotional satisfaction to the family members. "Instrumental" roles are activities, such as earning an income, that occur external to the family but that also include satisfactory goal attainment of the family. Traditionally, expressive roles have been assigned to the wife-mother, while the husband-father has assumed the instrumental roles. However, the classic breadwinner husband, homemaker wife, and two children now comprise only a small proportion of families in developed countries. Both expressive and instrumental roles are becoming less gender-specific.

From a structural-functional viewpoint, the major goal of the family is socialization of its members into society. Families perform certain functions ultimately directed toward this goal. Functions of the family as outlined by Friedman (1986) are:

1. **Reproductive** to ensure family continuity
2. **Affective** to meet the psychologic needs of family members
3. **Socialization** and **social placement** to help children become productive members of society
4. **Economic** to provide and allocate sufficient resources for the family
5. **Health care** for the provision of physical necessities, such as food, shelter, and a high level of wellness

This framework can be applied in nursing practice to assess how well the family is accomplishing these five functions in relation to its overall goal.

Structural-functional theory focuses heavily on the integration of the family within the occupational system. In many instances occupational roles are segregated from family roles. However, with increasing numbers of women in the work force and greater emphasis on careers, negotiating work-family conflicts in dual-earner families has become a significant facet of family life.

SYMBOLIC INTERACTIONAL THEORY

Interactional theory, which views the family as a unit of interacting personalities, was first advanced by Burgess (1926). The focus is on family interactions only, not on broader social systems. The family is described as a unit of interacting personalities that exists as long as the interaction takes place. Individuals have a position, or a status, in the family structure because they possess attitudes and behaviors that are consistent with the norms and expectations of culturally and socially defined roles. They play these roles in interactions within the group, and the responses of others in the family serve to reinforce or to challenge the individual's role behaviors. A role cannot exist without some other role toward which it is oriented. Basic to the interactional approach is communication, since actions of the family result from the communication process.

Family members communicate by the use of symbols. Words, ideas, gestures, and inflections are all symbols with learned meanings, and the family is the source of these meanings (Burr and others, 1979). The important developmental concepts of self and role continually evolve as a result of interactions with other family members. Rather than approaching families with predefined views, the nurse using this theory needs to determine how family members perceive themselves and their roles. For example, the nurse might ask new mothers and fathers how they see their roles as parents and, after learning what these perceptions are, observe how they are translated into actual behavior (Knafl, 1986).

EXCHANGE THEORY

Exchange theory provides a rationale to explain human interactions and predict behavior. It is based on the assumption that individuals interact through the give-and-take of a broad range of commodities, resources, or skills. It asserts that all individuals have needs whose fulfillment constitutes a reward. Also, individuals attempt to maximize rewards and minimize costs in their exchanges in order to obtain the most profitable outcomes. Behavior is positively reinforced when it is associated with reward and negatively reinforced when it is associated with punishment (Singelmann, 1972). Therefore knowledge of a person's needs, anticipations, and expectations is important if the appropriate reinforcement is to be employed.

Applied to the family, exchange theory can help explain patterns of behavior among family members and determine why these relationships are either positive or negative. Fundamental to the theory is the concept of *reciprocity*. In the complex set of interactions that characterize family life, it is assumed that family members act in a manner designed to obtain what they think they deserve, or at least attain the best possible outcome under the circumstances.

A disadvantage of the theory is the frequent failure to define what constitutes a reward. In some cases a conflict over what two family members regard as a reward makes behavior difficult to analyze. For instance, one parent may try to preserve a failing marriage, while the other seeks a divorce. In other cases, rewards may not be apparent because of the complexity of human motivation. For example, parents may feel rewarded by the day-to-day social and psychologic joys of seeing their children develop. Others may feel more motivated by the delayed gratification of seeing their children grow into responsible, productive adults or may even look forward to the day when they can depend on their children for their own care, in exchange for the care they provided for their children when they were young. Exchange theory may not adequately account for the habitual or emotional responses family members have for each other, and rewards that are altruistic or moral in nature may be difficult to quantify and analyze.

Nevertheless, the theory offers the nurse a useful tool in helping family members understand many aspects of their behavior. For example, the theory can be applied to help new parents understand their reasons for choosing parenthood and evaluate and anticipate the costs and rewards of being parents.

FAMILY SYSTEMS THEORY

Family systems theory is derived from general systems theory, a science of "wholeness" that is characterized by interaction among the components of the system and between the system and the environment. General systems theory expanded scientific thought from a simplistic view of direct cause and effect (*A* causes *B*) to a more complex and interrelated theory (*A* influences *B*, but *B* also affects *A*). In family systems theory the family is viewed as a system that continually interacts with its members and the environment. The emphasis is on the *interaction* between the members, such that a change in one family member creates a change in other members, which in turn results in a new change in the original member. Consequently, a problem or dysfunction does not lie in any one member but rather in the type of interactions used by the family. Since it is the interactions, rather than individual members, that are viewed as the source of the problem, the family becomes the patient and the focus of care. Examples of the application of family systems theory to clinical problems are nonorganic failure to thrive and child abuse. According to family systems theory, the problem does not rest solely with the parent or child but in the type of interactions between the parent and child, as well as in a host of other factors that affect their relationship.

Understanding family systems theory requires knowledge of numerous basic definitions and concepts that are beyond the focus of this discussion. However, some general concepts that are unique to this theory and have significance to understanding family dynamics are presented.

The family is viewed as a whole that is different from the sum of the individual members. For example, in a household of parents and one child there are not only three individuals, but also three relationships (or subsystems) that characterize the family system. These include the marital relationship, the mother-child relationship, and the father-child relationship. This concept of *nonsummativity*—"the whole is greater than the sum of its parts"—implies that when working with a family, the nurse must be aware of the relationships between family members. To effect positive change in a family, it is necessary to work with and through the several subsystems of the family.

Another important concept, *adaptability*, views the family as a highly adaptable unit. When problems exist within the family, change can be effected by altering the interaction or feedback messages that perpetuate disruptive behavior. *Feedback* refers to processes within the family that help identify strengths and needs and determine how well goals are being accomplished. Positive feedback initiates change, while negative feedback resists change.

When the family system is disrupted, change can occur at any point in the system. Consequently, it is not necessary to go back into the family history or an individual's life to find out the "cause" of the problem, as recommended by other theories, such as psychoanalytic theory. In family systems theory the emphasis is on what is occurring now in the family and on intervening to change that pattern. This focus allows for sometimes rapid and dramatic changes.

A major factor that influences a family's adaptability is its boundary, an imaginary but very real line that exists between the family and its environment. This boundary, or line, may be open or closed. If open, the family welcomes input into its system by accepting new ideas, information, resources, and opportunities. This type of family reaches out for help and uses the available support systems. In contrast, a closed family resists input by viewing change as threatening. The family is suspicious of any available support and strives to maintain the family system by avoiding outside influences. Having knowledge of boundaries is critical when teaching or counseling families. Although open families are receptive to intervention, closed families typically resist assistance and more effort is required to gain their trust and acceptance.

CONFLICT THEORY

Grounded in the Marxist philosophy of class conflict, conflict theory is based on the assumption that conflict is natural and inevitable in all human interaction and should not be viewed as bad or disruptive (Eshleman, 1981). When family members are in conflict, the goal is how to manage and resolve the conflict, not how to avoid it. Family situations involve perpetual give-and-take, and harmony can be satisfactorily maintained only through negotiation (Sprey, 1979).

Conflict arises from a variety of sources, but the most frequent is a perceived unequal exchange between marriage partners. The outcome can be continued conflict, dissolution of the relationship, or resolution of the conflict. Resolution of the conflict requires three ingredients (Beckman, 1978): (1) open communication, (2) accurate perceptions regarding the degree and nature of conflict, and (3) constructive efforts to resolve conflict. Efforts include a willingness on the part of each member to consider the point of view of the other, to consider alternative solutions, and to compromise if necessary.

Conflict theory can be applied to dual-earner parents who have difficulty sharing various responsibilities for child care. Using this theory, the nurse would assist the parents with problem solving, negotiating, and compromising in an effort to redefine and restructure the situation. The goal is often to reach a compromise, since with many family issues reaching a consensus, wherein both parties see each other's side the same way, is not possible.

FAMILY STRESS THEORY

Family stress theory explains how families react to stressful events and suggests factors that promote adaptation to these events. Families encounter stressors, including those that are predictable (e.g., parenthood) and those that are unpredictable (e.g., illness or unemployment), as an inevitable part of life. These stressors are cumulative, involving simultaneous demands from work, family, and community life. Too many stressful events occurring within a relatively short period of time—usually 1 year—can overwhelm the family's ability to cope, thus placing the family system at risk for breakdown or its members at risk for physical and emotional health problems. When the family experiences too many stressors for it to cope adequately, a state of crisis ensues. For adaptation to occur under these circumstances, a change in family structure and/or interaction is necessary.

Family stress theory also encompasses certain capabilities the family can use to manage a crisis brought on by too many stressors. The Typology Model of Adjustment and Adaptation (McCubbin and McCubbin, 1989), a comprehensive family stress model, summarizes these capabilities through four components: (1) basic attributes of the family—the family type—that explain how the family typically operates and behaves; (2) resources of individual family members, the family unit, and the community, including social support from extended family, friends, neighbors, and health professionals; (3) the way the family defines the situation, its impact, and their ability to manage; and (4) coping behaviors or strategies that family members or the family unit can use to keep the family functioning as a unit, decrease an individual member's tension, anxiety, and distress, and increase understanding of the particular situation or problem. For example, expectant parents seek to learn more about parenthood through parenting classes, books about childrearing, or other parents. In these ways they are coping with this anticipated transition by increasing their knowledge.

Applying the Typology Model to the desired outcome of family adaptation, the concept of "fit" is defined at two levels: the individual family members within the family and the family within the community (McCubbin and McCubbin, 1989; McCubbin and Patterson, 1982). Adaptation occurs over time and is not always a smooth process; Hill (1949) called the process a "roller coaster of family adaptation."

FAMILY STRUCTURE AND FUNCTION

Structure is a manner of organization or the arrangement of a number of parts that are interrelated in specified, recurring ways. Function refers to a special duty or performance required in the course of work or activity; it may also refer to the interactions of family members, specifically the quality of the relationships. The structure of a family may vary according to the composition of its component parts and according to its life cycle. Both structure and function are altered and modified as the needs of the family change.

FUNCTIONS OF THE FAMILY

Authorities agree families serve society in many ways. They play a vital role in the economy, since they produce and consume goods and services. They also are the basic unit for replacing dying members of the society. Furthermore, society, to maintain its continuity, must transmit its knowledge, customs, values, and beliefs to the young. However, where children are not an economic necessity, their primary function is to receive and to give love. Not only do they appear to be loved more, but they are loved as children for a longer period. Children depend on their families to meet the primary requirements for growth and development and to establish for them an atmosphere of security. Although goals for socialization and childrearing practices differ from one culture to another, in most societies the family appears to have three major objectives in relation to children: caregiving, nurturing, and training.

FAMILY STRUCTURE

The family structure, or family composition, consists of individuals, each with a socially recognized status and position, who interact with one another on a regular, recurring basis in socially sanctioned ways. When members are gained or lost through events (e.g., marriage, divorce, birth, death, abandonment, incarceration), the family composition is altered and roles must be redefined or redistributed.

Traditionally the family structure refers to either *nuclear* or *extended families.* However, family composition has assumed new configurations in recent years, with the single-parent family and stepfamilies becoming prominent forms. In any case, the predominant structural pattern in any society depends to a large extent on the mobility of families as they pursue economic goals and as relationships change. It is not uncommon for children to belong to several different family groups during their lifetime. In general, extended families are associated with agricultural societies, whereas small conjugal units are characteristic of more advanced, industrialized societies.

Nuclear Family

The nuclear, or conjugal, family consists of a husband, wife, and their children (natural or adopted) who live in a common household. This is the reproductive unit in which the marital tie (legally or otherwise sanctioned) is the chief binding force. A strongly functional nuclear family is the prototype of human relationships and the basic unit from which more complex familial forms are composed. In some instances one or more additional persons (e.g., a relative, friend, foster child, or others) may reside in the same household. Nuclear families can be combined into larger units in one of two ways: through plural marriage (polygamous families) or through extension of the parent-child relationship (extended family). Some authorities classify childless couples as a nuclear family because the alliance is conjugal with the theoretic potential for reproduction.

The nuclear family is more characteristic of an urban, mobile society. It is highly adaptable, with the ability to adjust and reshape its structure when needed. It is free to move where there is opportunity for higher income with concomitant improvement in other areas, such as social class and prestige. It is not economically bound to a geographic area nor dependent on the cooperative efforts of other members. The family members are employed on an individual basis, and economic resources are in the form of money. The present-day family must purchase the services of specialized individuals and groups, whereas previously these needs and services were met on a cooperative basis by the extended family members.

Although extended families residing in the same household are rapidly disappearing in American society, the isolated nuclear family without relatives within easy visiting distance is uncommon. This is most often seen where there has been extreme mobility of separate generations, such as wide geographic separations or marriages into different social strata, religious backgrounds, or roles. Most consanguineous family members maintain contact through visits, telephone calls, letters, and gift exchanges. Having no relatives readily available for advice and assistance with child care, as is common in extended families, parents in some nuclear families are more likely to turn to "experts" for childrearing guidance.

The majority of nuclear families in America are associated with an extended kinship network of nuclear families living in separate households but in close geographic proximity. This concept, sometimes referred to as a modified extended family, describes a meaningful aspect of daily existence that is reflected in frequent visiting and the exchange of services and financial aid. This family association meets the members' psychologic needs to a greater extent than do experts, friends, or organizations. It is not uncommon for families to reject the opportunity for social or economic advancement rather than leave such kinship associations.

Affiliative relationships. Although the nuclear family is predominantly a legally sanctioned institution, there are a number of families in which the attachment is only affiliative, that is, nonmarital cohabitation. These families consist primarily of two adults, the "couple households" (Macklin, 1980), but may include children. The mother and father live together, often with children from previous matings, and share family responsibilities. However, the family unit is less stable and relationships are subject to change. Instability of the social environment in the home has been associated with juvenile delinquency, which appears to be related to the number of family constellations (changes in the adult members of the household) experienced during childhood. This is probably a reflection of repeated adjustment to a variety of authority figures (Mednick and Baker, 1980).

Single-Parent Family

The single-parent family, a result of recent social phenomena, is now recognized as a family and has emerged partially as a consequence of women's rights movements wherein more women (and men) have established separate households because of divorce, death, desertion, or illegitimacy. In addition, a more liberal attitude in the courts has made it possible for single persons, both male and female, to adopt children, whereas, previously, rigid prerequisites specified that both a father and a mother must be present in the home. Although single-parent families are usually headed by the mother, it is becoming increasingly common for fathers to be awarded custody of dependent children in divorce settlements. A significant number of single-parent families result from a single mother who wishes to have a child but does not choose to have a husband. Also, unmarried mothers often choose to keep and raise their children rather than place them for adoption or marry, and are frequently absorbed into the extended family. With the increased psychologic independence of women as a whole and the increased acceptability of illegitimacy in society, more unmarried women are deliberately choosing mother-child families. The challenges of these single-parent families are discussed on p. 96.

Binuclear Family

Binuclear family is a term used to describe the situation that allows parents to continue the parenting role while terminating the spousal unit (Ahrons, 1979). The degree of cooperation between households and the time the child spends with each can vary. In *joint custody* the court assigns divorcing parents equal rights and responsibilities to the minor child or children. These alternate family forms are efforts on the part of those concerned to view divorce as a process of reorganization and redefinition of a family rather than as a family dissolution. Joint custody and coparenting are discussed further on p. 95 in relation to special parenting situations.

Stepfamily

Stepfamilies, also referred to as *reconstituted families,* are those in which one or both of the married adults have children from a previous marriage residing in the household. The term *blended families* or *combined families* more often refers to families composed of parents and the children each of them brings from a previous marriage. Stepfamilies are discussed further on p. 97.

Extended Family

The extended, or consanguineous, family is one mode of combining nuclear families into larger units through the parent-child relationship. It consists of the nuclear family plus lineal or collateral relatives. More often it is composed of two or more residential units of three or more generations affiliated through extension of the parent-child relationship, that is, grandparents, parents, and grandchildren. An extended family can be compounded by either monogamous or polygamous relationships. Broader views recognize the affiliation of collateral relatives as an extended family—not necessarily organized into nuclear families.

Extended family structure is more functional in areas where land is the basis of wealth and sustenance. Today the best examples of extended family units can be found among successful farmers, Native Americans, and certain recent immigrants. Here the family serves as the basic social, educational, and productive unit, providing services and sharing resources. Extended families may form under conditions of either extreme poverty in order to pool resources or extreme wealth in order to consolidate resources. Extended families direct cooperative efforts for common goals; the needs of the individual are sublimated to the welfare of the family enterprise and survival. The children learn early in life to respect their elders, and this value is reinforced through observation of their parents' behavior toward older family members (Fig. 3-1).

In the extended family childrearing is often a shared responsibility. Relatives are always present and available to help young mothers with household chores and child care activities. Daily lives of the children are organized around the needs and requirements of the family with assigned tasks and obligations. Family ties between the nuclear unit and the main extended family are strong, although there is a high degree of competition between individual nuclear units for acquisition of power and resources.

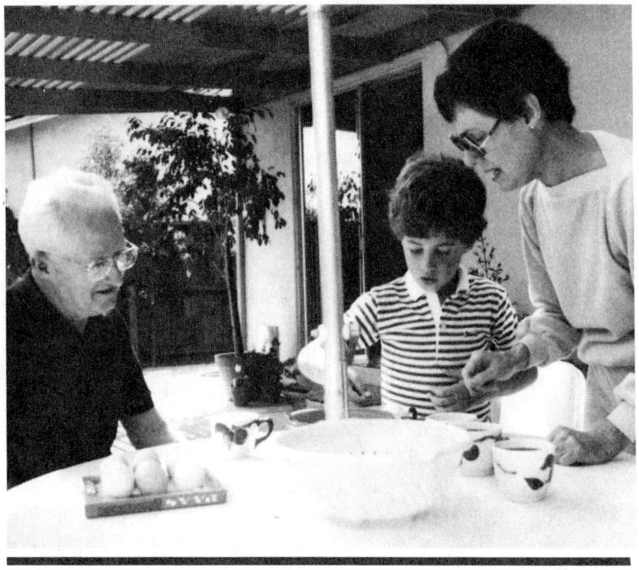

Fig. 3-1. Children benefit from interaction with grandparents even when they do not share the same household.

Polygamous Family

Although it is not legally sanctioned in the United States, sometimes the conjugal unit can be extended by the addition of spouses in polygamous matings. Polygamy generally refers to either wives *(polygyny)* or, very rarely, husbands *(polyandry)*. Many societies practice polygyny that is further designated as *sororal,* in which the wives are sisters, or *nonsororal,* in which the wives can be unrelated. Sororal polygyny is widespread throughout the world, and although plural marriages produce problems of adjustment for the members, co-wives who are sisters are more likely to get along with each other and display less jealousy than co-wives who are not. Most often mothers and their children share a husband and father, usually with each mother and her children maintaining a separate household, particularly when the wives are unrelated.

A special form of sororal polygyny is the *sororate,* in which a cultural rule specifies that the preferred mate for a widower is the sister of his deceased wife. In a sororate the marriages are successive rather than concurrent.

Where it exists, polygamy is usually accorded a higher status than monogamy. It may be limited to ruling families or to high-status persons and tends to be practiced by a small segment of the population. This is probably a result of economic factors and the unequal sex ratio in some areas at the time of biologic maturity.

Communal Family

The communal family emerged, as have all previous experimental communities, from a disenchantment with most contemporary life choices. Although communal families may have divergent beliefs, practices, and organization, the basic impetus for formation has been dissatisfaction with social systems and life goals of the larger communities and with the nuclear family structure, in particular, as it exists from either an ideologic or a practical perspective. Relatively uncommon today, communal groups share common ownership of property and goods; in cooperatives there is private ownership of property, but certain goods and services are shared and exchanged cooperatively without monetary consideration. There is strong reliance on group members and material interdependence. Both provide collective security for nonproductive members, share homemaking and childrearing functions, and help overcome the problem of interpersonal isolation or loneliness.

Unlike the traditional extended family, nuclear units in a commune may come and go at will. There is no consanguineous tie between the units. The mother-child tie is strong during infancy and early childhood, but many parents are happy to relinquish older children to the care of others. Although the parents maintain primary responsibility for the health and well-being of the children, the children are free to form close relationships with a number of adults in the commune and are encouraged to do so.

Gay/Lesbian Family*

The most common means by which homosexuals acquire children is through legal marriage. Gay men and lesbians marry partners of the opposite sex for a variety of reasons, including love for the spouse, desire for children, family and peer pressure, desire for companionship, and fear of loneliness (Bozett, 1987b, 1988a; Ross, 1983). Some homosexuals may not be aware of their homosexuality at the time of marriage, while others may marry hoping that a heterosexual relationship will abolish their homosexual desires.

While most children in gay/lesbian households are biologic from a former, legal marriage, there are other means by which homosexuals acquire children. For example, they may be foster or adoptive parents (Ricketts and Achtenberg, 1987), lesbian mothers may conceive through artificial fertilization (this is becoming increasingly common) (Pies, 1987), or a gay male couple may become parents through use of a surrogate mother.

There are a number of research studies on children reared in lesbian mother households (Green, 1978; Green and others, 1986; Hoeffer, 1981; Huggins, 1989; Steckel, 1987). In none of the studies was the mother's sexual orientation found to be detrimental to the children. According to Green (1978), "Children being raised by transsexual or homosexual parents do not differ appreciably from children raised in more conventional family settings on macroscopic measures of sexual identity." In the only reported study of children of gay fathers, Bozett (1987a, 1988b) found that if the children, who ranged in age from 14 to 35, had mutual interests and feelings in common with their father and if they believed the father's homosexuality was not outwardly discernible, then the children were more accepting of their father as gay. If there was little mutuality and they thought their father's homosexuality was externally evident, then the children exerted greater control in relation to when, where, and with whom they would be seen in public with their father. Younger children who lived with their father were also more selective in whom they would invite home. However,

*This section was written by Frederick Bozett, R.N., D.N.S.

in no instance did any of "the children express any difficulty with their father in the parental role. . . . even though several of the children thought that homosexuality was immoral, many of them considered their father a friend, confidante, and adviser" (Bozett, 1988b).

In child custody disputes when parental homosexuality is an issue, the courts have expressed concern that the children may become gay, that they may be molested, that the home environment is immoral, and that the children will be harassed by their peers (Rivera, 1987). However, according to reported research, children in gay/lesbian households are no more likely to be gay than are children reared in heterosexual households (Bell, Weinberg, and Hammersmith, 1981; Green, 1978); 85% to 90% of child molestation is perpetrated by heterosexual men (Geiser, 1979); and the quality of parenting and home life of gay men and lesbians, whether they are single or in a partner relationship, is equivalent to that of nongay parents (Bozett, 1984; Harris and Turner, 1986; Turner, Scadden, and Harris, 1985). It is true that children may be taunted if their peers know their mother or father is homosexual. However, this kind of harassment is similar to that experienced by children in other minority groups, and like other minority parents, gays and lesbians tend to help their children manage these situations constructively as they arise.

Disclosure of parental homosexuality ("coming out") to children may also be a concern. It has been found that generally it is best for children to be told. However, there are a number of factors to consider before telling children: parents should be fairly comfortable with their own gayness before disclosing it to children; it should be discussed with them before they know or suspect; the disclosure should be planned and should take place in a quiet setting where interruptions are unlikely; and children should be assured that the parent's relationship with them will not change as a result of disclosure (Bigner & Bozett, in press; Miller, 1987; Schulenburg, 1985).

Parents should also be prepared for questions from their children such as "What does being gay mean?" "What makes a person gay?" "Will I be gay, too?" and, "What should I tell my friends about it?" Also, the earlier children are informed, the easier it is for them to deal with the information. Moreover, after disclosure the parent-child relationship may become closer (Bozett, 1980; Moses and Hawkins, 1982; Schulenburg, 1985; Turner, Scadden, and Harris, 1985). However, even though most children are accepting, during their own sexual awakening in adolescence they may have difficulty dealing with the fact of their parent's homosexuality. In addition, if the parent develops a partner relationship in which the couple live together in a spouselike relationship (in no state is marriage legal between two persons of the same sex), the children may develop a resentment toward the partner or have other problems similar to those seen in heterosexual stepparent families (Baptiste, 1987).

Because this family form is more common than most persons may realize, it is important for the nurse to understand that homosexual families are simply different from the heterosexual family form, not better or worse. The gay/lesbian family environment can be just as healthy as any other. Nurses need to be nonjudgmental and to learn how to accept differences rather than demonstrate a homophobic prejudice that can have a detrimental effect on the nurse–child/family relationship. Moreover, the more knowledge of the child's family constellation and life-style the nurse has, the greater benefit he or she can be to the gay or lesbian parent and the child.

Box 3-2 TRAITS OF A HEALTHY FAMILY

1. Communicates and listens
2. Affirms and supports one another
3. Teaches respect for others
4. Develops a sense of trust
5. Has a sense of play and humor
6. Exhibits a sense of shared responsibility
7. Teaches a sense of right and wrong
8. Has a strong sense of family in which rituals and traditions abound
9. Has a balance of interaction among members
10. Has a shared religious core
11. Respects the privacy of one another
12. Values service to others
13. Fosters family table time and conversation
14. Shares leisure time
15. Admits and seeks help with problems

From Curran, D.: Traits of a healthy family, New York, 1983, Ballantine Books.

Family Strengths

Increasing interest has been shown in the characteristics that make families strong, especially since the family has undergone many structural changes over the last few decades (Dubowitz and others, 1988). The family strengths approach can be applied to all families, whatever their structure, because it focuses on what makes the family endure and survive when faced with demanding events and changes.

Stinnet and associates (1977, 1981, 1985) have identified the following family strengths: ability to deal with crisis in a positive manner, spending time together, love, appreciation and commitment, respect for individuality, good communication patterns, and high degree of religious orientation. Curran (1983) has also identified traits of the healthy family (Box 3-2). Not every trait is found in every healthy family, and dysfunctional families may have one or more of these traits. Awareness of family strengths can assist health professionals in identifying healthy families and those in need of developing more healthy characteristics.

FAMILY ROLES AND RELATIONSHIPS

Each individual has a position, or status, in the family structure, and each occupant of a position plays culturally and socially defined roles in interactions within the group. Within prescribed guidelines for behavior set by the culture, subcultures (including the family group) establish variations in role definition and may specify different requirements for playing the same role. Each family has its own traditions and values and sets its own standards for interaction within and outside the family group. Each determines the experiences the children should have, those they are to be shielded from, and how each of these experiences meets the needs of family members. Conformity to group norms is directly related to the strength and nature of group ties. Where family ties are strong, social control is highly effective, and most members play their roles willingly and with commitment.

PARENTAL ROLES

In all family groups the socially recognized status of father and mother exists with socially sanctioned roles that prescribe appropriate sexual behavior and childrearing responsibilities. The guides for behavior in these roles serve to control sexual conflict in society and provide for prolonged care of children. The degree to which parents are committed and the way they play their respective roles are influenced by a number of variables. Each individual is affected by a unique socialization experience.

Role definitions are changing as a result of the changing economy and the women's liberation movement. Women are achieving equality with men in education, more of them are entering the labor force, and the number of women who choose to have fewer children or none at all is increasing. During childhood, particularly in the upper and middle classes, the trend is toward deemphasizing the basic male-female characteristics of aggression, dependence, and achievement. As the role of the woman changes, there must necessarily be a change in the complementary role of the male. Fathers are taking a more active role in childrearing and household activities, which is most evident in middle-class families. Marital roles, on the other hand, are most segregated in the lower classes. Redefinition of sex roles in the American family is taking place, but a cultural lag of the persisting traditional role definitions creates role conflicts in many of these families.

ROLE LEARNING

Roles are learned through the socialization process. During all stages of development children learn and practice, through interaction with others and in their play, a set of social roles and something of the characteristics of other roles. They behave in patterned and more or less predictable ways because they learn roles that define mutual expectations in typical and recurring social relationships. Role conceptions are transmitted by socializing agents (parents, peers, authority figures) who use positive and negative sanctions to ensure conformity to their norms. Role behaviors positively reinforced by rewards such as love, affection, friendship, and honors are strengthened. Negative reinforcement takes the form of ridicule, withdrawal of love, expressions of disapproval, or banishment. Types of roles are described in Box 3-3.

Box 3-3 TYPES OF ROLES

Ascribed roles are those that are strictly defined by the culture, and very little deviation is allowed in modifying them. Ascribed roles apply to general traits such as sex, age, kinship, social class, and ethnic origin. There are culturally determined behaviors that must be adhered to regarding these roles, and they are expected to be learned in the home. For example, a child who attempts to change an ascribed role (such as sex) will be confronted with serious problems.

Achieved roles are those acquired through effort, and children must do something to attain them. Achieved roles include educational, occupational, religious, and recreational roles. These are based on performance and are acquired through satisfaction of specified requirements. The direction of these role achievements is strongly influenced by values conveyed to the children by their parents. For example, some parents believe that a college education is essential; others encourage children to seek occupational gratification.

Adopted roles are those that are sometimes transient, such as the role of patient or traveler. More often, adopted behavior patterns become fixed into what are known as character roles and apply to the unique behaviors that the child displays in a given situation. Such roles as the leader, the follower, the clown, or the show-off are examples of adopted roles. They are frequently adopted when playing the role meets a need or is the response to a complementary role in another.

Assumed roles are those related to fantasy and are especially important in childhood. This is one of the dominant means for children's adjustment and socialization. Children continually assume roles of persons they observe in their environment. The environment is a primary resource for learning the conduct that befits their position or status. Assumed roles only become a problem if they persist into the world of reality. For example, a child who persistently plays an infantile role is severely hampered in relationships with peers.

Continuity and Discontinuity

Anthropologists who make a study of societies throughout the world have determined that there are decided differences from culture to culture in the continuity with which young children are prepared for adult roles. In some cultures children begin to learn adult roles and behaviors at a very early age and continue to do so throughout childhood. For example, cultures that value courage and aggressiveness continuously encourage these behaviors in their children. In other cultures children are taught roles and behaviors that are in direct opposition to those they are expected to assume as adults. For example, in the United States, children are expected to be submissive in childhood, but individuals are expected to be dominant as adults. Continuity in the rearing of females in Western cultures has generally been more consistent in terms of role identification than that experienced by males. With expanding female roles, however, this continuity is becoming less apparent.

Role Structuring in Children

One responsibility of the family is to develop in the children culturally appropriate role behavior. Children learn to perform in expected ways consistent with their position in the family and culture at a very early age. The observed behavior of each child is a single manifestation—a combination of social influences as well as individual psychologic processes. In this way the uniting of the child's intrapersonal system (the self) with the interpersonal system (the family) is comprehended simultaneously as the conduct of the child.

Role structuring initially takes place within the family unit, where the children fulfill a set of roles and respond to the complementary roles of their parents and other family members. The roles of the children are shaped primarily by the parents, who apply direct or indirect pressures in an attempt to induce or force children into the desired patterns of behavior or direct their efforts toward modification of the role responses of the child on a mutually acceptable basis. Each set of parents has their own techniques, and each will determine the course that the process of socialization is to follow (see Discipline: Shaping Behavior, p. 86).

Children respond to life situations according to behaviors learned in reciprocal transactions. As they acquire important role-taking skills, their relationships with others change. They become proficient at understanding others as they acquire the ability to discriminate their own perspectives from those of others. The children who get along well with others and attain status in the peer group have well-developed role-taking skills (see Role Learning in Children, Chapter 4).

FAMILY SIZE AND CONFIGURATION

The size and composition of the family directly influence child development. No two children grow in exactly the same environment, although identical twins more nearly approximate this. For example, in a nuclear family with two children—even of the same sex—one will live in a family with an older sibling, whereas the other will be reared in a family with a younger sibling. In a family where there is a 10-year age span between the children, one may be born to a 20-year-old mother, the other to a 30-year-old mother. For the child in each situation the environment is different.

Family Size

Parenting practices differ between small and large families. In small families more emphasis is placed on the individual development of the children. Parenting is intensive rather than extensive, and there is constant pressure to measure up to family expectations. Children's development and achievement are measured against that of other children in the neighborhood and social class. In small families there is more democratic participation by the children than in larger families. Adolescents in small families identify more strongly with their parents and rely more on their parents for advice. They have well-developed, autonomous inner controls as contrasted with adolescents from larger families who rely more on adult authority.

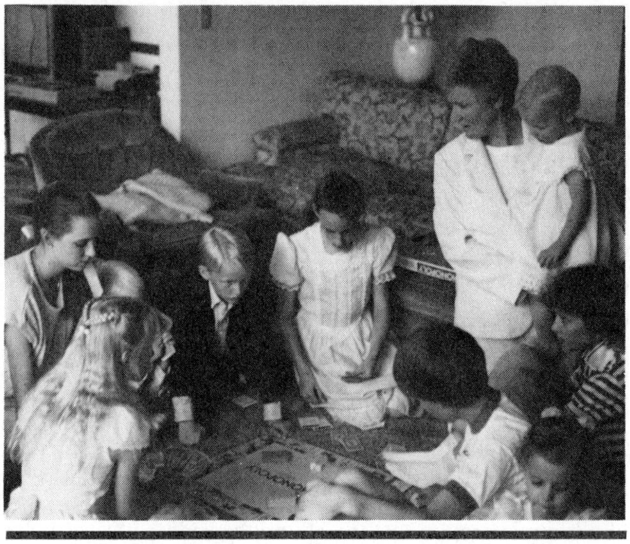

Fig. 3-2. Innumerable relationships and activities are possible in a large family.

Children in a large family are able to adjust to a variety of changes and crises. There is more emphasis on the group and less on the individual (Fig. 3-2). Cooperation is essential, often because of economic necessity. The large number of persons sharing a limited amount of space requires a greater degree of organization, administration, and authoritarian control. The control is wielded by a dominant family member—a parent or an older child. The number of children reduces the intimate, one-to-one contact between the parent and any individual child. Consequently, children turn to each other for what they cannot get from their parents. The reduced parent-child contact encourages individual children to adopt specialized roles in an attempt to gain recognition in the family.

Discipline is often administered by older siblings in large families. Siblings are usually better attuned to what constitutes misbehavior, and sibling disapproval or ostracism is frequently a more meaningful disciplinary measure than parental interventions. In situations such as death or illness of a parent, an older sibling assumes responsibility for the family at considerable personal sacrifice. Large families seem to generate a sense of security in the children fostered by sibling support and cooperation. However, adolescents from a large family are more peer oriented than family oriented.

Spacing of Children

Age differences between siblings affect the childhood environment, but to a lesser extent than does the sex of the siblings. The arrival of a sibling has the greatest impact on the older child, and a 2- to 4-year difference in age appears to be most threatening. When the older child is very young, the self-image is too immature to be threatened. At an older age the child is better able to understand the situation and therefore is less likely to see the newcomer as a threat, although the child does feel the loss of the only-child status.

In general, the narrower the spacing between siblings,

the more the children influence one another, especially in emotional characteristics; the wider the spacing, the greater the influence of the parents. Also, younger children tend to identify with older siblings. Consequently they assume some of the personality characteristics of the older child. Girls with brothers frequently have more "traditionally" masculine characteristics than girls raised with sisters. They are, on the whole, more aggressive and ambitious and perform better on tests of intellectual ability, which is probably related to the more stimulating environment created by competitive, aggressive boys. Boys with older sisters, especially if the age difference is slight, are generally less aggressive and daring than boys raised with older boys, which is probably a reflection of the identification process and the greater power exerted by the older sibling (Maccoby, 1980).

Sibling Interaction

Relationships between siblings in the family group duplicate, to some extent, many of the social interaction experiences of later years. Through relationships with siblings, children learn patterns of loyalty, competition, dominance, and other interactional skills. Such factors as whether a child is the firstborn, a middle child, or the youngest child or whether there is an age span of 1 or 6 years separating the child from the closest sibling affect the child's view of the world and relationships with others inside and outside the family. None of these characteristics is absolute, however; nor do they apply to all children and all parents. The potential effects depend on all other intrafamilial factors operating, such as parenting practices, the number of children in the family, and age, sex, and birth order difference between older and younger siblings (Fig. 3-3).

Sibling rivalry begins at an early age (see Chapter 14). It has been observed that the character of interactions between children and their parents is much more positive than between siblings (Baskett and Johnson, 1982). Children often talk to, laugh with, and display affection toward

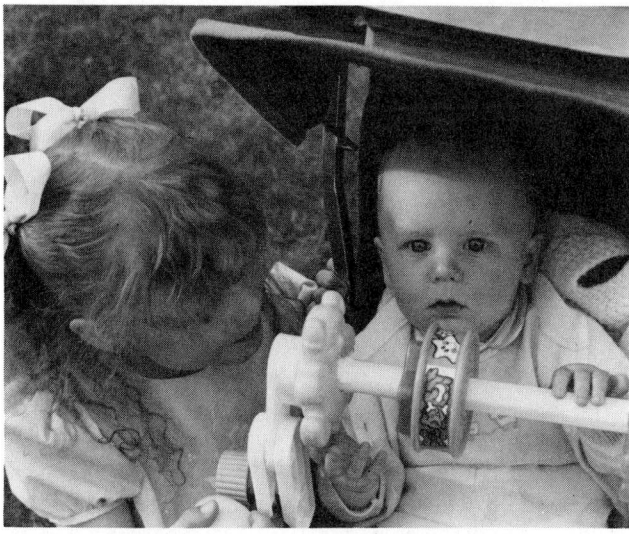

Fig. 3-3. Older children may have some doubts about a younger sibling.

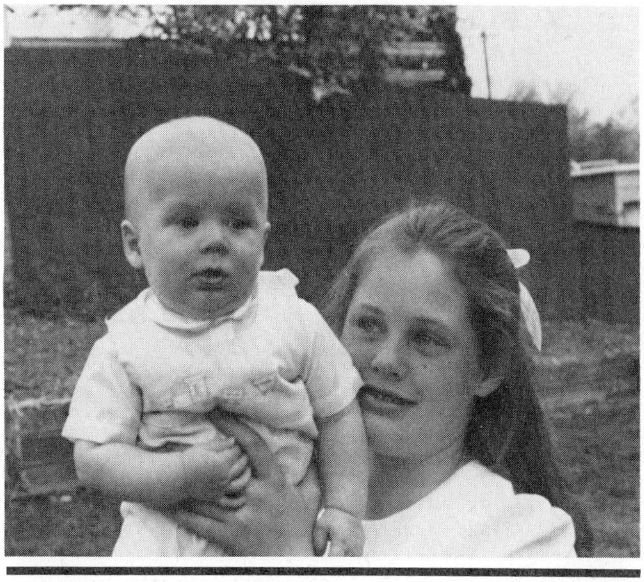

Fig. 3-4. Older school-age children can take responsibility for the care of younger children.

their parents, but direct behaviors such as hitting, yelling, and various annoying physical antics toward their siblings. Brothers and sisters are more coercive than parents and tend to respond less positively to a sibling's social overtures. Quarrels are most often initiated by the older sibling and become more frequent and intense as the younger child becomes more mature and is better able to retaliate. Same-sex siblings engage in more positive interaction than cross-sex siblings. Much of this behavior can be attributed to maternal behaviors. Mothers have been observed to direct more attention to the younger sibling who differs in gender from the older one (Dunn and Kendrick, 1981).

Although competition is commonplace among siblings, especially those who are nearly the same age, there are positive aspects of sibling interactions. Positive social responses outnumber negative ones in total interactions between siblings and acts of kindness are typically more common than hateful or rivalrous conduct. In many societies older children are the principal caregivers of infants and toddlers, and school-age children often assume some care of younger children in other cultures. Even older preschool children become sources of emotional support to younger ones in situations when parents are not around. Older siblings become role models for younger ones who imitate their behavior and often take over toys abandoned by them. Older children also serve as teachers, which is of benefit to both the younger and the older children (Fig. 3-4).

Ordinal Position

It has been observed for some time that the birth position of children affects their personalities. Parents treat children differently, and sibling interactions are different depending on the children's position within the family. Also, power is unequally distributed among siblings. Older siblings attempt to dominate younger ones; therefore, younger siblings develop interpersonal skills, the ability to negotiate,

Box 3-4 INFLUENCE OF ORDINAL POSITION ON CHILDREN

Firstborn Children

Are more achievement oriented
Receive more physical punishment
Are allowed to show more aggression to siblings
Have stronger consciences, are more self-disciplined and inner directed
Are prone to feelings of guilt
Identify more with parents than with peers
Are subject to greater parental expectations
Are more likely to attend college
Demonstrate higher intellectual achievement
Plan better and experience fewer frustrations
Are likely to be most wanted

Middle Children

Have more demands made on them for household help
Are praised less often
Receive less of the parents' time
Learn to compromise and be adaptable
Are less stimulated toward achievement
Are more difficult to characterize because of a variety of positions in the family

Youngest Children

Are less dependent than firstborn children
Are less tense, more affectionate, and more good-natured
Tend to identify more with peer group than with parents
Are popular with classmates
Have fewer demands placed on them for household help

and an ability to accept unfavorable outcomes to a greater extent than older siblings. Later-born children are obliged to interact with other siblings from birth and seem to be more outgoing and make friends more easily than firstborns (Steelman and Powell, 1985). However, children vary tremendously; these generalizations represent averages and do not apply in all situations. For general characteristics of children in the various ordinal positions, see Box 3-4.

The only child. Being the only child in a family has traditionally been considered to be a disadvantage. Only children have been described as selfish, spoiled, dependent, and lonely. However, a review of 141 research studies indicates that there are no essential personality differences between a child reared alone and one who is reared with one or more siblings (Polit and Falbo, 1987). They display no more evidence of maladjustment or self-centeredness than any other children and tend to strongly resemble firstborn children in such respects as higher educational goals. Only children perform better on cognitive tests, are more mature and cultivated, are more socially sensitive, and demonstrate superiority in language facility.

Only children also enjoy the advantage of having parents who, without the distraction of other children, are able to devote more time to them, talk to them, and stimulate them in intellectual activities. However, parents also exert greater pressure for mature behavior at an early age and for achievement. Relative isolation from peers contributes to intellectual pursuits and encourages a rich fantasy life, independence, and originality.

The effects of onliness on personality are questionable. Only children do not have the stereotyped concept of sex-appropriate behavior and often exhibit some characteristics associated with both sexes, but the significant influence is the quality of the parent-child relationship. Because of the wide differences among parents, a typical personality cannot be assigned to the only child. An unusually large number of only children live with a single parent, primarily as a result of divorce, and parents of only children tend to be somewhat older (Pines, 1981).

Multiple Births

A deviation in early development that occurs with variable frequency is multiple births. Twins are not uncommon in the population, but triplets are rare and quadruplets or quintuplets are extremely unusual. In any of these situations the offspring can be of the like or unlike sex, that is, derived from a single ovum, from multiple ova, or a combination of the two, which can involve one or more cell divisions. The cause of twinning is unknown, but the increase in the number of larger multiples (quintuplets, sextuplets) during recent years has been associated with the administration of fertility drugs to the mother.

Twins are of two distinct types: *identical,* or *monozygotic (MZ);* and *fraternal,* or *dizygotic (DZ).* These two types are separate and apparently unrelated phenomena. DZ twins are derived from the fertilization of two ova that are released nearly simultaneously from the ovary. They may be of like sex or opposite sexes, and they differ both physically and in genetic constitution. They are merely siblings who happen to be born at the same time. MZ twins are the result of one fertilized ovum that becomes separated at a very early stage of development, with each part developing into a complete individual. MZ twins are always alike in both gene complement and physical characteristics, including sex (Fig. 3-5). The term "identical," used to describe MZ twins, is not entirely accurate, because no two individuals are ever exactly alike in every detail.

The frequency of twin births varies according to ethnic origin, maternal age, and heredity, and these differences are related almost exclusively to the incidence of DZ twins. MZ twins occur with relatively uniform frequency in all populations (approximately 1:200 to 285 births) and appear to be random events. DZ twinning, on the other hand, shows variable frequency among racial populations, the highest being in the black races and the lowest in the Asian races, with the white races in the intermediate range. In the United States the overall twinning rate is approximately 1:80 pregnancies and consists of one third MZ and two thirds DZ twins.

DZ twinning becomes increasingly common with advancing maternal age, rising to a maximum between ages 35 and 39 years and then decreasing rapidly. Maternal age has little if any effect on the MZ twinning rate. MZ twinning is unaffected by heredity, but DZ twins show a marked familial tendency. The tendency toward DZ twinning is a he-

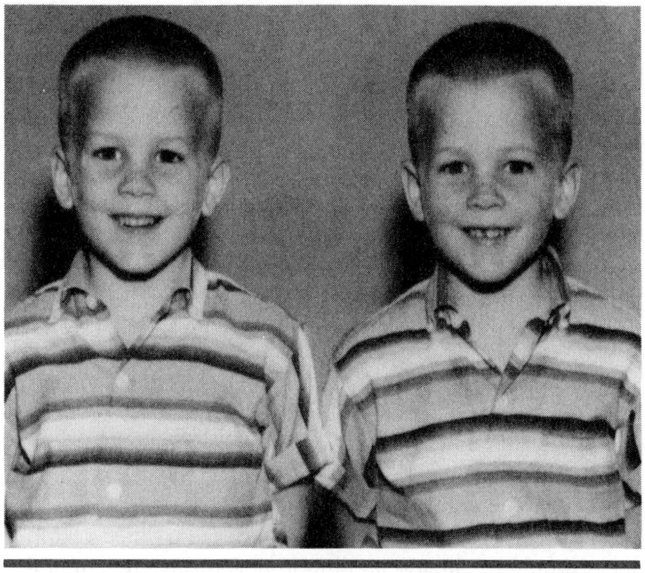

Fig. 3-5. Monozygotic, or identical, twins.

reditary trait expressed only in the female. There is an increase in twins among relatives of mothers of twins (e.g., female siblings and offspring of DZ twins) but not among relatives of the fathers (e.g., brothers of DZ twins and offspring of a DZ twin). Fathers, however, do appear to transmit the disposition toward double ovulation to their daughters.

Twins have always been a source of interest and have provided an appealing theme for dramatists and novelists. The distinctive characteristics of the two types of twins have also been of special interest to both geneticists and environmentalists in their efforts to obtain information regarding the "nature-nurture" controversy. Regardless of whether they are identical or fraternal, twins share a common environment.

A special kind of sibling relationship is observed in twins, although getting along with each other and quarreling are not too different from any other two siblings, especially if they are different-sex fraternal twins. Twins generally tend to work out a relationship that is reasonably satisfactory to both and demonstrate early independence from parental attention. They develop a remarkable capacity for cooperative play and considerable loyalty and generosity toward each other. It is not uncommon for them to evolve a private language between themselves that may interfere with development of the family language.

In a twinship, one member of the pair, to a greater or lesser extent, is more dominant, outgoing, and aggressive than the other, often to the consternation of their parents. However, the seemingly more passive twin is able to accomplish as much and get his or her way as frequently as the more aggressive twin.

It has also been observed that there is a difference in behavior between identical and fraternal twins. Whereas there is near unison in the actions of identical twins (although they alternate in assuming the leadership), fraternal twins, even of the same sex, do not display this quality. Sibling rivalry can be quite pronounced in fraternal twins, especially in mixed-sex twins. A demanding, rapidly developing girl can be particularly troublesome to her twin brother.

Identical twins also differ in their response to the tendency of some parents to treat twins exactly alike. The present philosophy is to determine the degree to which the children demonstrate an inclination toward togetherness. Some twins thrive best when they are constantly in each other's company; others prefer more individuality and separateness. The conservative approach is to allow the children to follow their natural inclinations. Early years of togetherness are often the basis of the children's security. To separate them too early may produce unnecessary stresses. The tendency is to foster individual differences as they are evidenced in order to ease the process of separation when it becomes advisable.

Any multiple birth attracts the interest of others, and parents should be prepared for the added attention the twins will attract, including the interest of researchers who will ask the parents' permission to include their children in studies of twins. Friends and relatives will lavish attention on them, and people on the street will stop to admire them.

Parental adjustment. The entrance of any new member into a household creates a number of stresses, but with multiple births two or more new members must be incorporated into the family at the same time. The problems are obvious. Two infants must be provided with physical care, including feeding, diapering, and all the purchasing and preparation that accompany the care of any infant. Scheduling becomes crucial, and each advancement in development brings new problems and adjustments (e.g., space and sleeping arrangements, selecting a stroller and other equipment). Care must be observed in selecting toys. As play becomes a serious business, some toys that would be safe and appropriate for a single child become weapons when two infants share a playpen. It is a good idea to select different toys for the children as they grow older and encourage sharing.

It is especially important for parents to maintain relationships with each other and other family members. It is doubly important for parents to arrange time together as often as possible. The **National Organization of Mothers of Twins Clubs, Inc.*** has local chapters throughout the United States to offer information and support to parents of twins and is highly recommended as a resource for all new parents of twins. The **Twins Foundation†**—an organization founded by a group of twins and designed to aid twins and other multiples—is recommended for older children.

Another problem faced by parents of twins occurs at the time of birth. Not only are the parents faced with double the work and care of the newborns, but the process of attachment may also be impeded. The mother first forms an attachment to the twins as a unit before she is able to form an attachment to each child individually (see Multiple Births

---

*12404 Princess Jeanne, N.E., Albuquerque, NM 87112-4640; (505) 275-0955.

†P.O. Box 9487, Providence, RI 02940-9487; (401) 274-8946.

and Subsequent Children, Chapter 8). As they develop, the children, who are facing the task of differentiating themselves from their environment, must learn to differentiate themselves not only from the mother but from one another as well.

Forming separate attachments is especially difficult if one of the twins must remain in the hospital. Therefore it is recommended that, if possible, both infants should stay in the hospital until they can be discharged together (Jimenez and Jungman, 1980). However, this would be impractical when one is a seriously ill infant who requires lengthy care.

It has been found that there is an increased risk for child abuse and neglect among families with twins (Groothuis and others, 1982). The increased stress related to the care of two young children is probably a factor, but it has been demonstrated that large families and inadequate spacing of children predispose to child abuse. Families with a multiple birth incorporate both of these factors.

Promoting individuation. All children proceed through a separation-individuation process as they grow and develop. For twins the process is complicated in a number of ways. Unlike singletons, twins lack a perception of separateness, and the close physical and emotional attachment between them inhibits development of individuality. In addition, twin children are frequently thought of and treated as a unit, and efforts they make in the direction of individuality are often impeded by others (Sater, 1979). There are a number of ways in which parents and others can aid twins in achieving individuation. Box 3-5 outlines suggestions for behaviors that promote individuation.

Box 3-5 PROMOTING INDIVIDUATION OF TWINS

Select different-sounding names.
Take separate photographs of the children (beginning at birth) so each child will have a picture of "me." Be certain to label each picture.
Avoid dressing children alike.
Use their given names. Avoid referring to them as "the twins."
Take each child on separate short outings occasionally while the other is at home with another family member or a sitter.
Build a one-to-one relationship with each child.
Hold and cuddle each child. Provide frequent body contact with each one.
Play and participate in learning with each child and to the same extent as with a singly born child.
Provide toys according to individual preferences, needs, and interests.
Entertain each as much as feasible. Avoid leaving them to entertain each other for long periods of time.
Provide separate rooms, if possible.
Praise each child individually and, preferably, at different times.
Discipline twins individually.
Provide separate feeding and care schedules according to the needs of the individual child.
Arrange for frequent opportunities for individual contact with other adults.
Encourage play with other children the same age.

Modified from Sater, J.: Appraising and promoting a sense of self in twins, MCN 4:218-226, 1979.

PARENTING

The biologic route to parenthood is the same regardless of cultural background, age, or the motivation of the couple. Although the impulse for sexual union is spontaneous and not seasonally limited, the union for purposes of procreation can be timed according to needs and desires of the family and based on rational attachment to and the care and welfare of another individual, a great deal of which involves total dependency. It is a developmental stage in the life cycle, one that may be viewed by the parents as an endurance contest, a dismal failure, or the most rewarding and pleasurable experience of their lives.

There are ties that bind the parents to their children throughout a lifetime. Parenthood never truly ends until the death of the parent. As in all developmental processes, parenthood is influenced by past experiences, and current events affect the future of the parents. Many events and feelings regarding the past are brought out as parents care for their own children. In addition, the child is a reflection of the parent. If parents like what they see in the child, their own self-esteem is increased. A successful relationship with a child builds the parents' self-image and contributes to a better acceptance of themselves.

PARENTHOOD

A characteristic in all societies is that adults are expected to become parents and to be gratified by the experience. Pressures of tradition, sentiment regarding the state of motherhood, and religious exhortations to fulfill divine commands of fertility profoundly influence decision making, since conformity to social-role expectations is a strong influence in family planning.

Motivation for Parenthood

Conscious and unconscious motivation may enter into the decision to initiate a pregnancy. For a number of parents the motivation is based on the simple assumption that all normal people get married and have children. For many it provides proof of their biologic adequacy or demonstrates their adulthood. Some may wish to fulfill a parent's wish for grandchildren or to perpetuate the family name and fortune. To have a child in an attempt to cement a tenuous marriage is a hazardous motive. A corollary to this is the woman who desires a child to compensate for the lack of a meaningful relationship with her husband and to combat a feeling of inner loneliness and boredom. A child may be the only means for some persons to fulfill the urge to create something of value. Some persons have children in order to experience the full potential of their sexuality. In a few societies individuals are not considered to have reached full maturity until they have children. Other motivating factors include the need to seek stimulation and novelty, to have power, to influence a life, or to compete with others. However, in most instances the couple sincerely wish to become parents.

The decisions for second and subsequent children may be as varied as the initial motivation for parenthood. Parents may reason that a single child will benefit from interaction with a sibling to provide companionship, sharing, and experience with conflict in human relationships. Occasionally disappointment with a first child may prompt parents to try again in the hope for a more gratifying experience. Many find parenthood a satisfying experience and enjoy the presence of children. In other families the advent of a child is an unplanned event that is met with mixed emotions.

The number of children that a couple choose to have is an individual matter. Whether this choice is fulfilled may depend on how effectively the couple practice contraception as well as on their changing values and attitudes toward more or fewer children. Family-size preferences do not remain the same throughout marriage. Factors that are likely to influence family size are social class, religion, economic resources, race, type of conjugal-role relationships, and the social-psychologic aspects of sexual relations. If a time comes when all parenthood becomes a matter of choice without religious, societal, or family pressures, it might be interesting to speculate on what types of people will choose to become parents.

Preparation for Parenthood

There is little or no evidence to support the existence of a "parental instinct" or a "maternal instinct." There appear to be no internal mechanisms to guide parental behavior; therefore parental behaviors must be learned through the socialization process. Adults in North America as a whole are ill-prepared for the monumental task of parenthood. Education in North American schools is notably deficient in courses that are relevant to most aspects of family life, such as sex, child care, home management, and interpersonal relationships. There are programs designed to prepare for childbirth during pregnancy, but few that prepare young adults for the life process. Some new parents have had limited experience caring for younger siblings or for the children of siblings, while the experience of others has been confined to occasional baby-sitting for neighbors during adolescence.

New parents approach parenthood with meager experience and scant knowledge, although no other task can compare, in overall consequences, with that of rearing a human being. Parents learn by trial and error, committing the same mistakes that have been committed by countless other parents, but they somehow manage to accomplish the task, becoming more skilled with each additional child. Tradition rather than rational planning furnishes the chief norms for childrearing.

The empiric preparation for parenthood is begun in the parent's own childhood. It has been established that the amount and quality of parenting that individuals have experienced in their own childhood significantly influence their later relationships with others and their ability to assume the role of parents in adulthood. By observation and imitation of their own parents and other role models—such as acquaintances, married siblings, and persons in the mass media—individuals learn culturally defined, sex-appropriate roles. Their own parents are probably the only persons that parents observe intimately in the parental role; this results in a *generational continuity*—parents rear their own children in much the same way as they themselves were reared—which is evident in the way that individuals fulfill their parental role.

Goals of Parenting

The family, in order to fulfill one of its primary functions, provides for the caregiving, nurturing, and training of children. In the process of childrearing, parents have at least three basic goals for their children:

1. **Survival**—to promote the physical survival and health of their children, thereby ensuring that the children live long enough to produce children of their own
2. **Economic**—to foster the skills and behavioral capacities that the children will need for economic self-maintenance as adults
3. **Self-actualization**—to foster behavioral capabilities for maximizing cultural values and beliefs

Parental Development

Parents proceed through parental developmental stages as a function of individual adult developmental tasks. In the process of parent-child development, the behavior of each influences the behavior of the other. The ways in which the child and the parents influence one another are discussed in subsequent chapters at greater length in relation to each major stage of child development. Briefly, development of a parental sense can be divided into four phases (Friedman, 1957):

1. **Anticipation.** Looking forward to parenthood, a young couple think about and discuss becoming parents and the way in which they will rear their children. They wonder what changes will develop in their relationship and what kind of parents they will be.
2. **Honeymoon.** This is the early interpersonal adjustment to the infant in which an attachment is formed between the parents and the child and new role learning takes place. The transition in self-image from a nonparent to a parent is made.
3. **Plateau.** The long middle period of parental development parallels child development:
   The child as infant—parents learn to interpret the child's needs.
   The child as toddler—parents learn to accept growth and development.
   The child as preschooler—parents and child learn to separate.
   The child as grade-schooler—parents learn to accept rejection and still be supportive.
   The child as teenager—parents begin to rebuild their lives.
4. **Disengagement.** This phase ends the active parental role, usually at the time of the child's marriage.

TRANSITION TO PARENTHOOD

The transition to parenthood is abrupt. Although the parents have anticipated the child's arrival, birth means the sudden imposition of totally dependent care 24 hours a day for the new member of the family. Some have described the birth of an infant as a crisis, and it may very well be a crisis if the event is perceived as disturbing old habits and relationships and eliciting new responses. It requires role changes, destroys or significantly modifies former relationships, and means adjusting to new role realignments. Whereas previously the roles of a couple were husband and wife, they now become, in addition, father and mother. It is difficult to adjust to being parents, but it is a normal human experience and a tool for personal growth.

The advent of a new family member requires that the family cope with greater financial responsibilities, a possible loss of income, changes in sleeping habits, and less time for husband and wife to spend with each other (especially if it is a firstborn) and/or with other children. If the events are perceived as aversive, it could well disrupt the husband-wife bond. Some investigators find that the birth of a first child results in a reduction of spousal intimacy and affection, while others report that the adjustment to parenthood is only mildly stressful. It appears that the impact of a new baby on the marital relationship is less severe or disruptive when the parents are older, conceive after the marriage ceremony, and have been married longer before conceiving (Belsky, 1981). In other words, mature, well-adjusted couples who have chosen to be parents are more likely to experience fewer difficulties as they make the transition to parenthood. However, numerous other factors can affect this adjustment.

Parental Factors Affecting Transition to Parenthood

The birth of an infant is a highly significant event that alters the behavior of both mothers and fathers. No amount of preparation can truly and fully prepare prospective parents for the constant and immediate needs of an infant. The importance of early parent-infant interactions is addressed in the discussion of the neonate, especially early mother-infant bonding and the attachment process (see Chapter 8). Some of the predominant factors affecting parenting are the age of the parents, the quality of the parental relationship, the amount of previous experience with childrearing, parental support systems, and the effects of stress on parental behavior.

Parental age. The most satisfactory age for childbearing has been established as the years between 18 and 35. During this time parents are considered to be in optimum health and with a predicted life span that allows sufficient time and vigor to raise a family. Increased life span, the trend toward dual careers, and the desire for financial security before childbearing, however, have altered childbearing behaviors.

Statistics indicate that the age at which parents begin their families has increased recently. There has been a substantial increase in the birth rate for women 30 to 44 years of age and a decline for women 20 to 29 years of age in the United States (National Center for Health Statistics, 1990b, 1990c). One of the obvious outgrowths of the increased rate of first births for older parents is a decrease in the numbers of subsequent children born to a family.

Research has determined that the age of parents has an effect on mother-child interactions. Older mothers are quite responsive to their children and appear to derive more pleasure from interactions with their children (Ragozin and others, 1982). Younger mothers express less favorable attitudes about childrearing and are likely to be less responsive to their infants. The issue of teenage parents is discussed under Adolescent Pregnancy in Chapter 20. See also Questions and Controversies.

Previous experience. Parents appear to be more relaxed and experience less conflict in disciplinary relationships with later-born than with firstborn children. They have had experience with and are more cognizant of normal growth and development expectations. However, much is contingent on the spacing of subsequent children. Frustrations can increase when parents are faced with two or more children who do not vary significantly in age. However, children are able to entertain one another, and older children assume some responsibility for the care of younger children, thereby allowing parents more freedom for some activities. (See also Family Size, p. 76.)

Marital relationship. The birth of an infant is highly significant and usually alters the behavior of both mothers and fathers and may even affect the quality of their relationship. For example, sex typing of new parents is affected. New mothers feel more "feminine" and exhibit more femi-

QUESTIONS AND CONTROVERSIES

How is childrearing affected when the parents have delayed having a first child until their thirties or even early forties?

Current trends indicate that more women are delaying having children. The rate of first-time births for women between the ages of 30 and 45 has increased since 1970. In prior decades the birth of the *last* child was occurring at this time in the lives of women. Reasons for postponing childbearing are related to more women entering career paths; individual and couple needs to achieve educational and occupational goals and attain more financial security; and a sense of commitment in a relationship (Soloway and Smith, 1987). Some women who initially decide not to have children change their mind as the "biologic time clock" begins to run out. Although there has been considerable research on the transition to parenthood, the impact of delayed childbearing on the couple, the child, and the family unit has not been fully explored (Koo, Suchindran, and Griffith, 1987). Questions posed by this trend also include: How does delayed childbearing affect not only the infant but the child, who in later years may have "relatively old" parents in comparison with peers? What is the impact on the child who experiences the death of grandparents at a relatively young age? Is support from relatives and friends altered when childbearing occurs later in life? Do improved socioeconomic factors, often associated with older first-time parents, help in the transition to parenthood for these families? Will families undergo new stresses as some older parents are faced with caring for their children and their own aging parents at the same time?

nine behaviors and engage in fewer masculine activities, thus behaving in the more traditionally sex-typed manner. On the other hand, new fathers become less traditionally sex typed. Although they maintain the frequency of masculine role behaviors, fathers display an increase in feminine activities and their self-concept becomes less "masculine" (Feldman and Aschenbrenner, 1983).

Marital relationships can affect infants indirectly when the behavior of one parent influences the behavior of the other. For example, marital tension or strife can alter a mother's caregiving routines and interfere with her enjoyment of her infant (Belsky, 1981), or both parents may be unresponsive to their infant. As indicated in the discussion of family theories, every family member influences the behavior of every other member—even very early in the transition to parenthood.

More positive indirect effects occur in situations where parents serve as sources of mutual support and encouragement (Crnic and others, 1983). For example, fathers are more involved with their infants in families where the parents frequently discuss their infants. Even infants who may be at risk for later emotional problems will establish satisfying relationships with their parents unless the parents are unhappily married (Belsky, 1981).

Father involvement. Until recently the bulk of research and concern has been related to mother-infant interactions, partly because mothers attend more to their infants than fathers do and partly because of the stereotypic view of motherhood. However, current practices that encourage early father-infant interaction have indicated that fathers appear to be just as intrigued with their newborns as mothers are (see Paternal Engrossment, Chapter 8). Even fathers who have little initial contact with their neonates will become involved with them over the next few months (Easterbrooks and Goldberg, 1984), although the type of interaction will be different from that of the mother (Fig. 3-6). For example, whereas mothers are likely to hold, soothe, care for, or play quietly with their infants, fathers are more boisterous, engaging in more physically stimulating activities that infants seem to enjoy. However, fathers are more than simply playmates. They are often successful at soothing a distressed infant. Furthermore, a secure attachment to the father can help offset the consequences of an insecure attachment to the mother (Main and Weston, 1981).

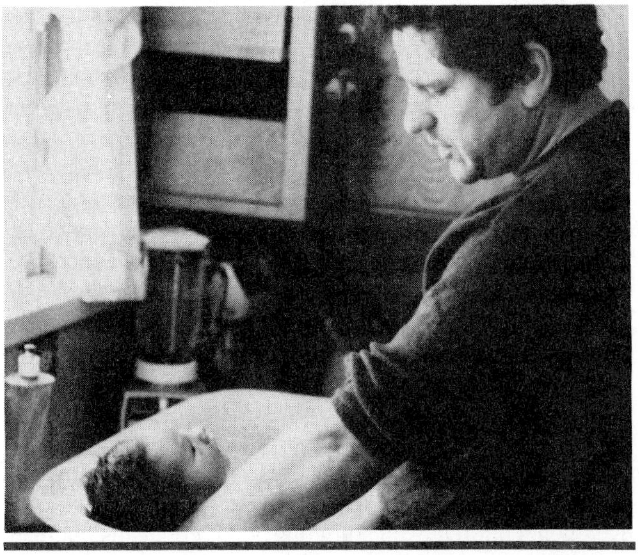

Fig. 3-6. Fathers assume care of their children soon after birth.

Effects of stress. The effect of stress on parental behavior cannot be denied. Parents who are tired, worried, ill, or feeling unable to control the events that affect their lives may not exhibit the patience or understanding or take the time to reason with or otherwise cope with their children's behavior that they would at other times. They often find it difficult to set aside their own immediate needs in order to respond to their children. Under stressful conditions parents are less responsive to their children and are less likely to play with them, talk with them, or help them.

One of the areas in which parents, especially the mother, are subject to stress is in balancing parenthood and a career. The change from more or less equal roles to that of more stereotyped roles is a source of stress to some families. The challenges of dual-earner families are discussed further on p. 98.

Infant characteristics. The behavior of the infant and child can also influence initial adjustment and subsequent childrearing. Parents of temperamentally difficult infants find more disruption of activities than parents with more quiet infants. Parents of children who require special care often encounter problems not only with their children but with the quality of their relationships with each other as well. Both of these issues are discussed in association with each stage of child development and in Chapter 22 in relation to the child with a chronic illness or disability.

Support Systems

Successful adaptation to the stress of transition to parenthood involves at least two types of family resources (McCubbin and Patterson, 1982). First are the internal resources of the family, such as *adaptability* and *integration.* Changing from an orderly, predictable life to a relatively disordered, unpredictable one is a universal adaptation families must make. Rigid schedules are impossible to maintain, and former activities must be curtailed or abandoned. Adaptation is reflected in learning to be patient, becoming better organized, and becoming more flexible.

Integration involves an attempt of the couple to continue some activities in which they were engaged before the advent of parenthood. In this way couples are able to maintain a sense of continuity and appreciate the importance of the husband-wife relationship. In some families the birth of an infant brings the couple closer together, increases their interdependence, and expands their feelings of unity and cohesion. The adjustment to parenthood can be facilitated when parents discuss their own role expectations and the role expectations of the spouse. This is especially important for first-time fathers.

The second kind of resource for coping with stress is the use of coping strategies that strengthen the organization

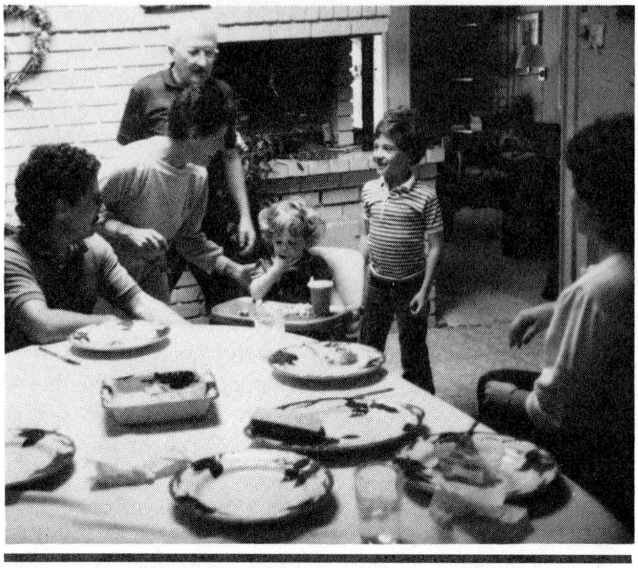

Fig. 3-7. Maintaining relationships with the extended family is important.

and functioning of the family. These include the use of community resources, the use of social support, and the adoption of a future orientation. Interpersonal supports that provide information, advice, and caretaking are derived from friends, relatives, and neighbors. Relationships with family, friends, and community are essential (Fig. 3-7). Arranging for time away from the infant (child or children) is beneficial. Fathers can assume care of the family to allow the mother some time to herself at home or away from the home, even for an afternoon or evening. Adoption of a future orientation provides reassurance to parents that things will get better, that they will cope, and that it is realistic to plan for the time when they are able to engage in self-fulfilling activities.

It is also reassuring to know that others experience ambivalent feelings toward parenthood and share the same difficulties and frustrations. Exchanging ideas and experiences with other parents provides an opportunity to voice concerns and to learn new ways of coping with the multiple problems of childrearing. Whether it is family, friends, or community resources, parents need persons to whom they can turn for advice, comfort, and assistance—persons with whom they can share the joys and difficulties of childrearing.

ESSENTIALS OF PARENTING

There are some essential types of knowledge and skills parents need in order for them to feel more comfortable in the parenting role. Experience in having been nurtured as a child is an essential component of successful parenting. Parents tend to rear their children in much the same manner as they themselves were reared, although this influence can be modified and improved parenting skills can be learned.

Skills that parents must learn include a basic understanding of childhood growth and development and the way in which it affects behavior. The behavior of infants and children is less bewildering and mysterious when parents are able to anticipate and prepare for it. Parents also need to know some of the basic skills needed to feel comfortable (e.g., physical care skills, such as bathing, feeding) and how to use play to facilitate child development and interpersonal interactions.

Probably the most important skills used by parents are interpersonal skills. Infants communicate their needs to others by crying, and parents must learn to interpret and respond to this basic communication. As children grow and develop, their interpersonal skills change and become more complex. Both parents and children expand their ability to communicate their needs, to respond to the needs of others, and to become sensitive to the feelings of others.

PARENTING BEHAVIORS

Parents' overall acceptance of a child and their disciplinary orientation have a profound impact on the way in which children view themselves and relate with others. Adults' attitudes as parents are influenced by their conception of their roles in relation to children. Childrearing may be viewed as restricting and controlling child behavior, as taming the child's innate rebellious and uncivilized nature, or as guidance to provide a suitable role model for the child to emulate. Much depends on the parents' own background, their mental health, their attitudes toward childrearing in general, and their attitudes toward any individual child.

Attitudes Toward Childrearing

There are infinite variations in the way parents rear their children. Some are related to cultural influences; others to social class and economic resources. The results of numerous studies suggest that parents differ from one another in two major attitudinal continuums.

Permissiveness-restrictiveness. Permissiveness and restrictiveness refer to the degree of autonomy that parents allow their children. Some parents exercise close, restrictive control over much of their children's behavior. They limit their children's freedom of expression by imposing many demands and actively surveying their children's behavior to ensure that they comply with rules and regulations. Permissive parents make few demands and allow their children considerable freedom in exploring their environment, expressing their opinions and emotions, and making decisions about their activities. Many find a balance between the two extremes. It is not uncommon to find that many parents become less restrictive as both they and their children mature.

Warmth-hostility. Although almost all parents feel affection for their children, how openly or frequently this affection is expressed and the degree to which affection is mixed with feelings of rejection or hostility vary considerably from parent to parent. Parents described as warm and nurturant are those who often smile at, praise, and encourage their children while limiting their criticisms, punishments, and signs of disapproval.

Within the wide range of families the amount of affection

that parents show their children may vary considerably and be influenced by cultural factors and individual differences in the personality and temperament of both the parents and the children. Children who come from homes in which they are loved and accepted display socially acceptable behavior and are generally good-natured, cheerful, friendly, cooperative, and emotionally stable. Because they are loved and accepted themselves, they are able to form satisfactory relationships with others.

Cool, hostile, or rejecting parents are quick to criticize, belittle, punish, or ignore their children while limiting their expressions of affection or approval. It is important to be aware that these measures of parental warmth or coldness reflect parental behavior in a large number of situations. For example, a parent may be cool and rejecting when a child misbehaves but warm and affectionate in other contexts. Such a parent would be considered high in parental warmth. On the other hand a parent who demonstrates warmth when the child praises him or her but who is critical, punitive, or indifferent in most other situations would be classified as aloof and rejecting.

Rejection. A small minority of parents display a rejecting attitude toward their children that appears in a number of forms and occurs for a number of reasons. Rejection may be subtle or blatant, and manifestations may be extensive, ranging from neglect and belittling to emotional and physical abuse. Rejecting parents overtly or covertly express feelings of dislike for the child, indicate that the child is unwanted, or state that caring for the child is burdensome. Children who are rejected develop feelings of insecurity and inferiority; they believe that if they are unworthy of parental love, they must be of no value. Many develop an avoidant relationship with the rejecting parent(s). Others attempt to win parental affection through attention-getting behaviors that frequently serve only to compound the rejecting behavior of the parents. When these tactics fail, the child may become either hostile and aggressive or withdrawn and submissive.

Sometimes rejected children find social acceptance and adjustment through identification with peers, but more often they develop feelings of isolation, inadequacy, and generally lowered self-esteem. A persistent pattern of rejection can have pervasive and long-range effects on a child's personality. The problems of disturbed parent-child relationships that are severely damaging to children are discussed in relation to failure-to-thrive syndrome, the abused child, and some of the emotional problems of childhood.

Parental Styles of Control

The extent to which parents restrict children's behavior or allow them autonomy and freedom significantly affects the psychologic atmosphere in the home. Although there are variations and degrees in parenting styles, they can generally be described as either authoritarian, permissive, or authoritative.

Authoritarian. Authoritarian, or dictatorial, parents try to control their children's behavior and attitudes through unquestioned mandates. They establish rules and regulations or a standard of conduct that they expect to be followed rigidly and unquestioningly. They value and reward absolute obedience, mute acceptance of their word, and unfailing respect for the family's principles and beliefs. They forcefully punish any behavior that is contrary to parental standards. Parental authority is exercised with little explanation and little involvement of the child in decision making. The message is: "Do it because I say so."

Punishment need not be corporal but may be stern withdrawal of love and approval. The familiar saying—"Children are to be seen, not heard"—typifies this type of childrearing. Careful training often results in rigidly conforming behavior in the children, who tend to be sensitive, shy, self-conscious, retiring, and submissive. They are more apt to be courteous, loyal, honest, and dependable but docile. These behaviors are more typically observed when parental arbitrary power assertion is accompanied by close supervision and a reasonable level of affection. If not, arbitrary power assertion is more likely to be associated with both defiant and antisocial behavior (Maccoby, 1980).

Permissive. At the other extreme are permissive, or laissez-faire, parents who exert little or no control over their children's actions. These well-meaning parents sometimes confuse permissiveness with license. They avoid imposing their own standards of conduct and allow their children to regulate their own activity as much as possible. These parents consider themselves to be resources for the children, not role models. If rules do exist, the parents explain the underlying reason, encourage the children's opinions, and consult them in decision-making processes. They employ lax, inconsistent discipline, do not set sensible limits, and do not prevent the children from upsetting the home routine. The parents rarely punish the children, since most behavior is considered acceptable. Consequently, the children, in effect, control the parents. Children of submissive parents are often disobedient, disrespectful, irresponsible, aggressive, and generally defiant of authority.

Authoritative. Authoritative, or democratic, parents combine some childrearing practices from both the foregoing extremes. They direct their children's behavior and attitudes by emphasizing the reason for rules and negatively reinforcing deviations. They respect the individuality of each of their children and allow them to voice their objections to family standards or regulations. Parental control is firm and consistent but tempered with encouragement, understanding, and security. Control is focused on the issue, not on withdrawal of love or the fear of punishment. These parents foster "inner-directedness," a conscience that regulates behavior based on feelings of guilt or shame for wrongdoing, not on fear of being caught or punished. Parents' realistic standards and reasonable expectations produce children with high self-esteem who are self-reliant, assertive, inquisitive, content, and highly interactive with other children.

The most successful type of childrearing seems to be the authoritative method. Parents do not set rigid, arbitrary limits but maintain firm control, particularly in areas of parent-child disagreement. Permissiveness, necessary for children to develop their full potential, is tempered with reasonable and consistent setting of limits. Parental power is shared, and both parents provide leadership but listen to what the children have to contribute. There is more flexibility in decision making and demands on the children, and discipline is more apt to be based on reasoning with encouragement of verbal give-and-take. However, it is very clear that parents are the final authority in areas of dispute. This approach to childrearing is more likely to facilitate the development of competence in children, which is evidenced by independent and responsible behavior on the part of the children.

Discipline: Shaping Behavior

Discipline is not punishment. Rather it is the teaching of desirable behavior. Children need to learn the rules governing behavior in the home, the neighborhood, the school, and the community at large. To learn acceptable behavior that permits them to live enjoyably with themselves and others, children need the steady, firm guidance of loving parents and others in authority roles. Good discipline provides children with protection from dangers (from within and without) and relieves them of the burden of decisions that they are not prepared to make, yet allows them to develop independence of thought and action within a secure framework.

Children who learn to live within reasonable rules are happier and more secure children. Without the stabilizing influence of controls, children feel uncertain and insecure. Too often, inexperienced and insecure parents fear the loss of a child's love, suffer feelings of guilt over disciplinary action, or may even relinquish their authority to the child. To discipline is to teach reality. Sensible, mature parents establish fair rules and regulations in the home and then see that they are carried out. Parents should never exploit children's love for them as a means to control their children. Children's anxiety lest they lose that love is already great. Discipline based on love of the child and carried out with conviction, confidence, and consistency will produce a self-reliant, buoyant, and self-controlled child.

Disciplinary strategies are discussed in chapters related to health promotion of children; a general discussion is presented in Chapter 14 under Limit-Setting and Discipline.

INFLUENCE OF THE "EXPERTS"

Evidence indicates that there have been decided shifts in the overall philosophy of childrearing during the twentieth century. Directions on childrearing, with parental roles and practices defined by the experts, have been transmitted as advice to parents through a steady flow of pamphlets, books, and articles. Recent changes in the opinions of these experts are the result of alterations in the concept of child development and behavior and of research into the effects of parent-child interaction.

The earlier view of child care that advocated rigid scheduling, early weaning and toilet training, and prohibition of devices that provided the child with passive pleasures (such as pacifiers) has been replaced by an easier, warmer, and more relaxed approach toward coping with child behavior that emphasizes "tender loving care" as the basis for satisfactory physical and emotional well-being. Some believe, however, that this approach generates too much permissiveness and produces some undesirable long-term consequences. The current trend in parenting manuals is to reassure parents that they will not be "perfect" parents, that mistakes are allowed, and that while they should keep trying to do a good job of rearing their children, at the same time they should try to be relaxed and spontaneous, and enjoy their children. These manuals attempt to convey the idea that parents are more capable than they think they are.

Parents turn to guidebooks because of an optimistic belief in progress, a faith in the future, and a typical desire to do better—better than they have been doing, better than their own parents, and better than their relatives and neighbors. Through these popular how-to parent books, parents can gain some of the accumulated knowledge of significant researchers in child development that they would be unable to acquire by attempting to read and synthesize the original texts. These guidebooks do not attempt to provide all the answers and are less authoritarian than those of the past. Most are written on the assumption that parents want to raise successful children and need support to view themselves as competent adults whose decisions are valid. Parents must deal with parenting problems on the spot at the same time that they are assimilating helpful advice and new information. They must be made to feel confident in their values and judgment during this process.

Since popular parenting manuals vary in their approaches, it is probably best to suggest that parents review some of those that are available and select at least two for use rather than relying on the advice of a single resource. In addition to the three most widely sold authors of childrearing books—Haim G. Ginott *(Between Parent and Child* and *Between Parent and Teenager),* Fitzhugh Dodson *(How to Parent),* and Benjamin Spock *(Baby and Child Care)*—there are at least 300 other books by experts such as Lee Salk, Thomas Gordon, Bruno Bettelheim, and T. Berry Brazelton.

In the past, one of the primary deficiencies in how-to books was a disregard for alternate life-styles, cultural variations, or class differences in the population. With few exceptions the standard manuals concentrated on early childhood growth and development and on the family as an isolated entity, and portrayed the mother as the primary caregiver. The working mother was ignored or discouraged, and daycare was seldom mentioned. Fortunately, recent manuals tend to reflect the realities of our more complex society. Some books have also appeared that offer guidelines for single parents, adoptive parents, parents with a child who is disabled, stepparents, and families in the process of divorce. These are primarily authored by individuals who offer help based on their own experiences or by authorities who have made a study of a special problem. Parents can receive some assistance from these supplemental publications to help them cope with the additional stresses imposed by their special circumstances.

■ SPECIAL PARENTING SITUATIONS

Parenting is a demanding task under the most ideal circumstances, but when parents and children are faced with situations that deviate from what is considered to be the norm, the potential for family disruption is increased. Some of the issues that are encountered frequently are divorce and the accompanying challenges of single parenthood and/or reconstituted families. Adoption and dual-career families, too, face unique challenges. The problems associated with children of alcoholic parents, parents with physical disabilities, homeless parents, or incarcerated parents are ones that are not addressed in the following discussions but may be topics that the reader may wish to investigate.

PARENTING THE ADOPTED CHILD

"Adoption is the method provided by law to establish the legal relationship of parent and child between persons who are not so related by birth, with the same rights and obligations that exist between children and their natural parents" (Child Welfare League of America, 1968). Adoptive parents are those who, whatever the motivation, assume the sociologic and ethical responsibility of biologic parents, and the ties of affection between them and their children are just as strong as biologic ties.

Motivation

Persons are motivated to adopt a child for different reasons. Most instances involve an adopting couple who find it impossible to have children of their own, and agencies in the past regarded this as the major criterion for placement of adoptable children. However, today many people consider adoption for other reasons. Some feel a responsibility to provide a home for a child who needs one; others are able to have more children of their own but are seriously concerned about overpopulation and elect to increase their family through adoption; many families are finding "room for one more" with whom to share their love. In addition, single, divorced, and widowed persons who believe that they have love and security to offer a child are seeking to adopt.

The demand for white infants with no physical or mental problems far exceeds the supply. However, there has been an increase in the number of children with special needs, formerly considered to be unadoptable, who are finding homes through the adoptive process. These include children with disabilities, older children, children who are of minority or mixed racial ancestry, and children from foreign countries. However, the attitude that adoptive parents want only a "perfect" child has been so ingrained that health care workers are often unaware that there are families who have enough love and nurturing capacity to accept a child with an "imperfection."

The decision to adopt should be a joint one, and various attitudes and feelings must be examined before the couple can assume the responsibility for an adopted child. Most adults assume that they will be able to have children of their own. To discover that they are unable to do so is often accompanied by feelings of inferiority, doubts about masculinity or femininity, and feelings of guilt or blame in relation to the spouse. These feelings and frustrations, superimposed on the anxious waiting for pregnancy, feelings of loss, and the endless medical procedures to establish the cause of infertility, provide an adoptive couple with their own unique preparation for parenthood.

Whatever motivates a couple to seek adoption as an alternative means to acquire a family, the decision should be based on emotionally healthy needs. The welfare of the child should be the primary consideration in placement, and such motives as the need to strengthen an unstable marriage, to treat emotional problems (including grief over the death of a child), or to treat psychogenic sterility should be carefully explored. Also, when adoption satisfies the needs of only one of the two parents, the outcome is questionable.

Sources of Adoptive Children

In the past the major source of adoptable infants was socially unsanctioned pregnancies, primarily of unwed mothers, since society accords a very high rating to the married status. Although adoption as a means of creating a family is openly acceptable, having children outside the marriage state is generally met with societal disapproval. However, with the widespread use of contraception, more liberalized abortion laws, and more liberal attitudes toward single parents, the number of these children available for adoption has decreased significantly.

Almost half the adoptable children in the United States are adopted by relatives, either extended family members or stepparents. Nonrelative adoptions are primarily arranged through licensed social agencies. A small proportion are arranged independently by individuals such as physicians, lawyers, nurses, and members of the clergy. It is well recognized that the safest and most satisfactory adoptions are those conducted through a licensed social agency, either public or voluntary. Although adoption through an authorized agency can be time-consuming, with sometimes frustrating and disappointing delays, the decision to pursue an independent adoption should be made with caution. While independent adoptions are frequently faster than agency adoptions, independent adoptions sometimes result in serious problems. They are generally more costly, and some are arranged by persons seeking a profit. The child's anonymity may not be guaranteed, and the child's health or legal status may be unclear. Also, since independent contractors frequently do not investigate the adoptive family, unlike adoption agencies, an independent adoption may not always be in the child's best interests.

Risks related to agency adoptions are usually less than those encountered in family life. Careful screening of infants can detect all but the more obscure defects, and subsequent development of defects or illnesses is no less predictable than in natural families. However, inherent emotional difficulties may be intensified in the case of adoption. Common reactions to adoption include anxiety associated with the waiting period until the adoption is legally final, uncertainty regarding whether adoption is the right choice, parents' concerns about their ability to love and parent the child, and coping with the reactions and questions of relatives, other children (if any) in the family, and friends. However bonding can be as strong and immediate for adoptive parents and children as it is for natural parents—sometimes even stronger.

Preparation for Adoption

Unlike natural parents who prepare for their child's birth with prenatal classes and the support of friends and relatives, adoptive parents have few sources of support and preparation for the new addition to their family. Nurses who offer services to adoptive parents can provide the information, support, and reassurance needed to reduce parental anxiety regarding the adoptive process and refer them to state parental support groups that provide guidance for adoptive parents. Such sources can be contacted through a state or county welfare office. Prospective parents seeking information on international adoptions can contact **Families Adopting Children Anywhere.***

Preadoption counseling should include measures to help parents overcome feelings of inadequacy and make preparations for receiving the child, such as instruction in infant care. Adoptive parents need to prepare for the possibility that the confidentiality or the identity of the biologic parents may not be guaranteed. Some agencies even advise the adoptive parents to maintain an ongoing information store about the natural parents so that they can answer the child's questions and thereby reduce the excessive fantasizing that children may engage in later during identity formation.

Parenting Adopted Children

Most problems faced by adoptive parents are no different from those encountered by natural parents. All parents want to be good parents, but this desire is often intensified in adoptive parents. Adoptive parents have been portrayed as more apprehensive and insecure than biologic parents, and in need of more assistance. According to a recent study, however, adoptive parents feel the need for less assistance than biologic parents. This feeling is probably due to the adoptive parents' completely voluntary decision to become parents, the relatively long time they had to prepare for parenting, and the maturity associated with adopting (Edwards, 1987).

The sooner infants enter their adoptive home, the better for purposes of parent-infant attachment; the more caregivers the infant has had before adoption, the more problems are likely to be encountered in attachment. The infant must break the bond with the previous caregiver and form a new bond with the adoptive parents. The difficulties in forming an attachment will depend on the amount of time the infant has spent with earlier caregivers, such as the birth mother, nurse, or adoption agency personnel (Clore and Newberry, 1981).

Siblings, adopted or natural, who are old enough to understand should be included in decisions regarding the commitment to adopt, with reassurance that they are not being replaced. Ways that the siblings can interact with the adopted child should be stressed (Fig. 3-8).

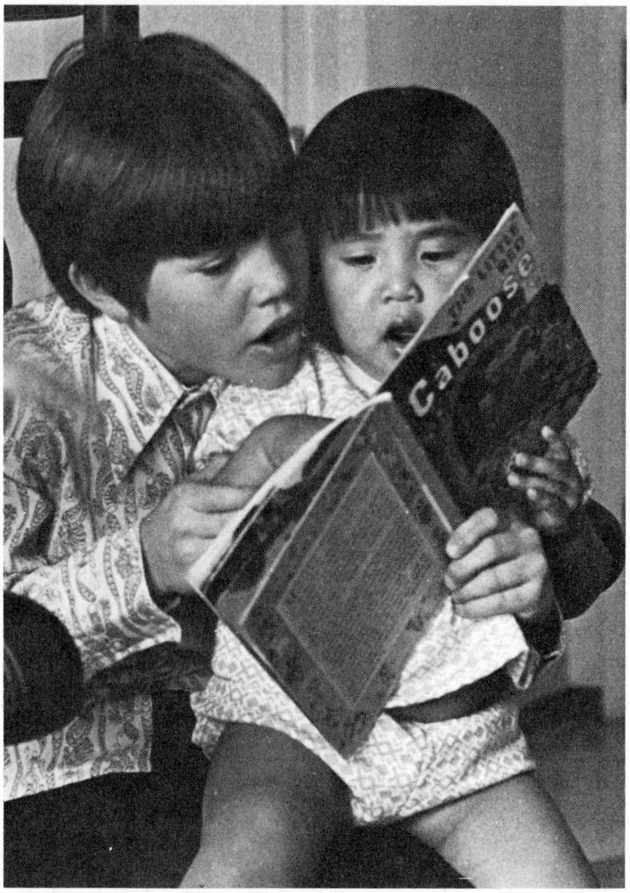

Fig. 3-8. A big brother reads a story to his adopted sister.

Acceptance by extended family members and friends may create additional stresses for the family. Parents are encouraged to discuss the issue of adoption with other members of the family, especially the grandparents, whose feelings and attitudes about adoption may not be compatible. This may be a particularly difficult problem when the adopted children are members of different ethnic groups. It should be made clear to everyone that the child is the parents' child, not their "adopted" child.

Issues of origin. The task of telling children that they are adopted is a cause of deep concern and anxiety. There are no clear-cut guidelines for parents to follow in determining precisely when and at what age children are ready for the information, and parents are naturally reluctant to present the children with such unsettling news. However, it is an important aspect of their parental responsibilities, and although they may be tempted to withhold the fact from the child, it is an essential component of the child's identity.

The timing seems to arise naturally as parents become aware of the child's readiness. Most authorities believe that children should be informed at an age young enough so that, as they grow older, they do not remember a time when they did not know that they were adopted. The time must be

*P.O. Box 28058, Northwood Station, Baltimore, MD 21239; (301) 488-2656.

right for both the parents and the child and is highly individual; it may be when children ask where babies come from, at which time children can also be told the facts of their adoption. If they are told in such a way as to convey the idea that they were active participants in the selection process, they will be less apt to feel that they were abandoned victims in a helpless situation. For example, parents can tell children that their personal qualities drew the parents to them. It is wise for parents who have not previously discussed adoption to tell children that they are adopted before the children enter school to avoid third parties inadvertently telling the children before the parents have the opportunity. Complete honesty between parents and children usually strengthens the relationship.

Earlier advice to adoptive parents stressed the need to treat adopted children exactly the same as any biologic siblings and to make them feel no different. This approach, however, denies the differences that adopted children actually feel. At age 5 or 6, children begin to realize that someone had to give them up for them to be "chosen" by the adoptive family. To deny these feelings may actually hurt the child (Brodzinsky, 1988). For both the child and the adoptive parents, it is important to acknowledge the differences in the adoptive situation.

Acknowledging and encouraging discussion of the child's feelings help the child develop a positive self-image. Once the child has been told about the adoption, the child's feelings about it do not end; rather, adjusting to one's own adoption is a continuous process often characterized by a sense of loss and a search for identity throughout childhood and adolescence and even continuing when adopted children become adults and have their own children (Sherry, 1986). Adopted children, however, seem to adapt more easily if the family is comfortable with the adoption, talks about the birth circumstances openly, and has acceptance and support from the extended family, friends, and neighbors. When they are emotionally and developmentally ready, adopted children may benefit from learning about their birth parents and may even decide to contact them, although this is usually recommended only after adolescence in closed adoptions, because of the identity crises and turmoil surrounding the event.

Children should be encouraged to ask questions. Parents can anticipate many of the questions, although children may hesitate to ask about the birth parents, hoping that the adoptive parents will initiate the discussion. This is probably one of the most difficult tasks facing adoptive parents. However, it is not so much what is said to the children but the attitudes and feelings that are communicated. Children should be told about their illegitimacy, if this is an actuality, and the most complete picture possible of the birth parents should be provided (Clore and Newberry, 1981).

Parents can anticipate some behavior changes following the disclosure—especially in children who are older. Children may use the fact of their adoption as a weapon to manipulate and threaten parents. There is the inevitable "My real mother would not treat me like this," or "You don't love me as much because I'm adopted." Statements such as these hurt parents and increase their feelings of insecurity, so that as parents they may become overpermissive. Adopted children need the same undemanding love, combined with firm discipline and limit-setting, as any other child.

Adoptive parents may experience unwelcomed curiosity and even cruel remarks from others about the child's adoption and appearance. Questions about the child's "real" birth parents, jokes that an infertile mother will now get pregnant, or misguided attempts to match physical characteristics of the child with the adoptive parents can be distressing. Nurses in contact with adoptive parents can help counter the effects of these thoughtless remarks by affirming the parental role, asking the parents about the child's arrival, and listening to their reports about the child's development and accomplishments.

Adolescence. Adolescence may be an especially trying time for parents of adopted children. The normal confrontations of adolescents and parents may assume more painful aspects in adoptive families. Adolescents may use their adoption as a tool in defying parental authority or as a justification for aberrant behavior. As they attempt to master the task of identity formation, the feeling of abandonment by their natural parents may come to awareness or may be intensified. Sex differences in reacting to adoption may surface. It has been shown that girls have more difficulty accepting their sexuality, since they may not be able to identify with a nonfertile female parent.

The children fantasize about their parents, and they may feel the need to discover the identity of their natural parents in order to define themselves and their identity—one of the major tasks of adolescent development. It is important for parents to keep lines of communication open and to reassure the youngsters that they understand the feelings of needing to search for their identities. In some states birth certificates are made legally available to adopted children when they come of age. It is important for parents to be honest with questioning adolescents and to tell them of this possibility (the parents themselves are unable to obtain the birth certificate; it is the children's responsibility if they desire it).

A candid approach that may or may not be suitable for the adoptive situation is the "open adoption" program. The mother who gives her child for adoption is invited to write an explanatory letter to the child and the adoptive parents, who usually respond with a letter and pictures. It is a voluntary exchange handled through the agency, which keeps all names and addresses confidential. When these exchanges are eventually read by the adopted children, it helps them realize the circumstances of their adoption.

Special Adoptive Situations

The difficulty in finding infants to adopt has created an increased opportunity for adoptive parents to provide homes for children with special needs. The additional burdens of care for children with physical or emotional disabilities are no different from those of naturally born children with similar problems, with the possible exception that adoptive parents are aware of the nature of the disabilities before they receive the children. However adoption of older children and/or those of a different racial or ethnic origin poses some special considerations for both parents and children.

Older children. Adopting older children constitutes an emotional experience for everyone concerned—children, parents, siblings (if any), and, often, extended family members. It involves a commitment on the part of both the adopting family and the adopted child. Adoptive families should learn as much as possible about the child before they make a final commitment.

Children awaiting adoption are usually from foster homes, group homes, or institutions. Visits between the potential adoptive family and the child can take place in the child's present home or on some type of outing during which the individuals involved are able to interact, such as on a picnic or a trip to the zoo or a playground. Visits by the child to the home of the adoptive family begin with short excursions such as an afternoon, then a day, followed by a weekend or a week. The number and frequency of visits depend on the needs of the child and the family. During the visits the child and the family determine whether or not they will be able to make a commitment (Brockhaus and Brockhaus, 1982).

One of the difficulties of rearing adopted older children is helping them to deal with having had another set of parents. The children may have lost, in addition to their biologic parents, siblings, grandparents, friends, and personal possessions. Often they have lived in several foster homes in which they formed attachments. They need time and assistance in working through the grief process that is an integral part of any loss. At the same time, they must adjust to a new household and relationships. Children who have experienced many losses and disappointments find adjustment more difficult and take a longer period of time to overcome fear of rejection and to develop affectionate ties to the new family. They grieve for those they left behind and may be afraid to love in case they must again move on.

Children who are adopted after age 2 maintain an image of the previous parenting persons that may cause the adopting parents some insecurity. The parents may not feel as close to these children as they would to children adopted in infancy. It is necessary that children who can remember them maintain an image of the natural parents. As they grow, children are able to clearly distinguish between the parents who loved and cared for them and those who were merely responsible for their birth. Some of the early difficulties of adaptation are related to the change in surroundings, a change that is difficult for all children.

Early in the process of forming lasting relationships the families alter routines and activities to accommodate the children and avoid conflicts. The children are excited but somewhat frightened that they will be unable to behave in such a way that will ensure acceptance and prevent their being sent away. Eventually the parents and the children are unable to maintain the host-houseguest roles and behaviors and begin a stormy period of adjustment. Children continually test families, who must repeatedly reassure the children that they are wanted. Children may withdraw or act angry for months. Many conflicts can arise, particularly in the area of parental expectations and discipline. Children's past experiences, good and bad, are brought to the fore, especially during holidays. Although the children are relieved and happy to be in a new home, they often miss the familiar times and relationships. During this time the families may require considerable support and encouragement from sources outside the immediate family unit.

Eventually expectations become more realistic, and family members learn to cope more effectively. The children are increasingly able to integrate past with present. They develop trust and confidence in the parents, and all the members develop into a family unit with autonomy, stability, and identification (Brockhaus and Brockhaus, 1982).

Cross-racial and international adoption. Adoption of children of racial backgrounds different from that of the family is relatively commonplace. In addition to the problems faced by adopted children of any age, children of a cross-racial adoption must deal with their differentness. It is advised that parents who adopt such children do everything to preserve the adopted children's racial heritage.

Adoptive parents are urged to investigate the culture of their children's country, maintain their children's family name as a middle name (in some cultures this is a link to the village of their ancestors), and teach children the history and heroes of their native country. Persons from the children's country can provide information about eating and sleeping patterns that will help the family make the adopted children's adaptation easier. Even music, a few words of the native language, and foods from their native country will appeal to the children's senses.

Although the children are full-fledged members of an adopting family and citizens of the adopted country, if they have a foreign appearance or other decided racial characteristics, problems may be encountered outside the family. Bigotry exists that may appear among relatives and friends. Strangers may make thoughtless comments and talk about the children as though they were not members of the family. It is vital that the family make it clear to others that this is their child and a cherished member of the family.

In international adoptions the medical information the parents receive may be quite complete or very sketchy (Hostetter and Johnson, 1989). Many internationally adopted children were born prematurely, and common health problems such as infant diarrhea may delay growth and development. Some children may have serious or multiple health problems, and this can be very stressful for the parents. Cultural practices, such as constant holding rather than letting the child explore, may further affect the child's progress. On arrival, regardless of age, some internationally adopted children may experience temporary adjustment problems. Sleep disturbances, malaise without fever, abdominal pain, avoidance of school, and preoccupation with food have all been reported (Hostetter and Johnson, 1989). In addition to giving advice on medical management, nurses should provide these parents with opportunities to discuss their feelings and situations.

PARENTING AND DIVORCE

From the mid-1960s to the early 1980s the divorce rate rose significantly, peaking at a rate of 5.3 divorces per 1000 population in 1979 and 1981. Between 1982 and 1986 the rates stabilized at 4.9 divorces per 1000 population in 1986. The 1989 rate of 4.7 divorces per 1000 population was the lowest rate since 1974 (National Center for Health Statistics, 1990a). More than 1 million children under the age of 18 have been involved in a divorce, however, in every year since 1972. In 1987 there were 1,038,000 of these children, 2% fewer than in 1986 and fewer than in any year since 1973 (National Center for Health Statistics, 1990a). Many of these children are very young, since half of the couples who divorce were married for less than 7 years.

Authorities agree that marital factors within the home significantly influence the development of children. Children from a happy, relaxed atmosphere in the home are less likely to have a negative outlook than are those from stressed homes. The effect of the parents' inability to adapt influences the adjustment and personality growth of young children. The interpersonal tension created by parental insecurity and anxiety is communicated to children, who often do not have the ego resources to cope with these feelings of tension and the vague threat of a change in their world. Even in the best divorces there will be fear, pain, uncertainty, and other emotional effects.

The process of divorce begins with a period of marital conflict of varying length and intensity, a separation, the actual legal divorce, and the reestablishment of different living arrangements (Box 3-6). Since a function of parenthood is to provide for the security and emotional welfare of children, disruption of the family structure often engenders strong feelings of guilt in the parents. Some may feel resentment toward their children—who are making the situation more difficult—and may attempt to compensate with overprotective behavior and excessive concern for their children's welfare. Some even blame the children for their problems. Children become scapegoats and find themselves dragged into their parent's problems. Some children take advantage of this opportunity to play one parent against the other.

During a divorce, parental capacity may be compromised. The parents may be much too preoccupied with their own feelings, needs, and life changes to be available and supportive to their children. Newly employed parents, usually mothers, are likely to leave children with new sitters, in strange settings, or alone after school. Searching for and establishing new relationships impinge on time that could be spent at home, including weekends that may have formerly been spent with the children. Moreover, divorcing parents need to know what to do, and there are few acceptable models on which they can rely.

When adults find themselves alone for the first time in years, they may become frightened and begin to depend on their children. Such children may be forced to grow up too quickly and assume the responsibility of an absent parent or become a substitute for the absent parent. Assumption of adultlike roles places an enormous burden on children. Role reversal frequently takes place wherein the child supports the adult and is burdened not only with his or her own problems but with many of the parents' problems as well.

Box 3-6 STAGES OF THE DIVORCE PROCESS

Acute Phase

The decisive separation of the married couple with legal steps of filing for dissolution of the marriage and, usually, the departure of the father from the home. The duration of this phase lasts from several months to over a year and is accompanied by familial stress and a chaotic atmosphere.

Transitional Phase

Adults and children assume unfamiliar roles and relationships within a new family structure. This phase is often accompanied by a change of residence, a reduced standard of living and altered life-style, a larger share of the economic responsibility shouldered by the mother, and radically altered parent-child relationships.

Stabilizing Phase

Postdivorce family reestablishes a stable, functioning family unit. Remarriage frequently occurs, with concomitant changes in all areas of family life.

Modified from Wallerstein, J.S.: Children of divorce: stress and developmental tasks. In Garmezy, N., and Rutter, M., editors: Stress, coping, and development in children, New York, 1983, McGraw-Hill, Inc.

Disorder is characteristic in the custodial household following separation and divorce; coercive types of control, inflammable tempers in both parents and children, reduced parental competence, and a greater sense of parental helplessness are common, as well as greater disorder, poorly enforced discipline, and diminished regularity in enforcing household routines. Noncustodial parents also are seldom prepared for the role of visitor and may not have a residence suitable for children's visits. They may be concerned about maintaining the visiting arrangement over the years to follow (Wallerstein, 1983).

Impact of Divorce on Children

The conventional belief has been that unhappily married couples should stay together for the good of the children; however, research indicates that the eventual escape from parental conflict may be the most positive outcome of divorce for many children (Hetherington, 1981). Children who are under the continual stress of intact but unhappy homes often feel more secure and happy after the marital relationship is dissolved, if one of the parents is able to form a family of better quality. In fact, a couple might well *divorce* for the good of the children (Wallerstein and Kelly, 1980). However, in a number of situations the children continue to experience open parental discord for a considerable time following marriage dissolution (Wallerstein, 1983). In many ways divorce is similar to a surgical procedure—a cure for a problem when "medical" methods fail—with trauma, convalescence, and the aftermath of permanent scars.

The impact of divorce on children continues to be a major concern of researchers, but it is incorrect to view divorce as having uniform consequences for all children

(Demo and Acock, 1988). Factors related to the child's adjustment to divorce include age and gender, number of siblings, predivorce adjustment and well-being, available supports, level of family conflict at various times in the divorce process, emotional stability of the parents (especially the custodial parent), amount of contact with both the custodial and the noncustodial parent, quality of the parent-child relationship, and socioeconomic status of the family (Green, 1988).

Most children go through two phases when adjusting to a divorce: a *crisis phase,* which often lasts for a year or longer and is accompanied by an emotional upheaval that affects the relationship with the custodial parent, and an *adjustment phase,* in which children settle down and begin to adapt to life in a single-parent home (Hetherington, 1981).

Complications sometimes associated with divorce include efforts on the part of one parent to subvert the child's loyalties to the other, abandonment to other caregivers, and adjustment to a stepparent. In the majority of divorce cases the mother receives custody of the child; this has an effect on the male child's identification with a father figure in addition to all the other ramifications of living in a family without a father or in a single-parent family. Many divorced mothers with small children move in with parents, other relatives, or friends in some kind of dependent or sharing arrangement.

Children may feel a sense of shame and embarrassment concerning the family situation. Such feelings cause children to see themselves as different, inferior, or unworthy of love, especially if they feel any responsibility for the family dissolution. Although the social stigma attached to divorce no longer produces the emotions it has in the past, it may still exist in some small towns and can reinforce children's negative self-image. The lasting effects of divorce depend on the children's and the parents' adjustment to the transition from an intact family to a single-parent family and, often, to a reconstituted family.

Telling the children. Many parents do not tell their children about the divorce, either because they do not know what to tell the children or because they believe that the children will not understand. Although news of a pending divorce is an unhappy shock, most children are remarkably resilient and are more capable of accepting painful realities and stresses than parents expect. What is difficult for children to handle is the anxiety, uncertainty, and confusion of not knowing what is happening to their family. Children need to be told what is taking place early in the process. Frank disclosure, even when painful, helps to build trust and provides children with the security of knowing what is going on.

If possible, the initial disclosure should include both parents and all siblings, followed by later discussions with children individually. Ample time should be set aside for the discussions, and they should take place during a period of calm, not after an argument. Parents who physically hold or touch their children provide them with a feeling of warmth that is reassuring. The discussions should include the reason for the divorce—minimizing blame—and reassurance that the divorce is not the fault of the children. Children may feel guilty, as though they have somehow failed or are being punished for misbehavior. They wonder what role they played in the divorce, or failure to keep the family together. Children assume that they have a tremendous power over parents (some actually do).

Parents need not fear open expression of their emotions. Tears express love, and if parents cry, it offers permission for children to cry, also. Children need to ventilate their feelings. They normally feel anger and resentment and should be allowed to communicate these feelings without punishment. Parents need to listen to what the children are saying in order to gain an understanding of what they are experiencing.

The primary concern of children involved in family dissolution is to know what will happen to them. They have feelings of terror and abandonment, see themselves apart from the family, feel alone and isolated, and long for consistency and order in their lives. They fear the uncertain future and need to know where they will live, who will take care of them, if they will be with their siblings, and if there will be enough money to live on. They worry that they might be left alone—if parents can divorce one another, can they not divorce the children? They need help in deciding what to tell their friends and teachers. They wonder if the parents will marry someone else. They need to be taught that relationships change, how to deal with new relationships, and that they will still retain the love and affection of the parents.

Age-related responses to divorce. The feelings and behaviors of children may differ according to age (Box 3-7), but all suffer stress second only to the stress produced by the death of a parent. Some research has indicated that the adverse effects of divorce are more common in younger children (Hetherington, Cox, and Cox, 1979; Kurdek, Blisk, and Siesky, 1981; Wallerstein and Kelly, 1975). Older children have some obvious advantages over their younger counterparts. They can talk about their experience with their friends, many of whom are also children of divorce. They can understand that they are not personally responsible and recognize the finality of the situation. They can appreciate both parents for their personal qualities, and they can recognize that one of the benefits of reduced conflict between their parents is an improved relationship between themselves and each parent (Kurdek and Siesky, 1980). Other research, however, paints a darker view of the effect of divorce on older children. Adolescents certainly feel a sense of emotional and physical abandonment (Wallerstein and Blakeslee, 1989), and this can have a delayed effect in young adulthood that is characterized by anxiety and an inability to establish a loving, intimate relationship with a potential partner. Many are fearful they will repeat the mistakes of their parents.

Egocentric preschoolers, who see and understand things only in relation to themselves, assume themselves to be the cause of parental distress and interpret the separation as punishment. They feel sadness and strong feelings of responsibility for the loss of the absent parent. Moreover, they consciously fear that they may be abandoned by the remaining parent. Consequently, it is essential to establish

Box 3-7 FEELINGS AND BEHAVIORS OF CHILDREN RELATED TO DIVORCE

Infancy
Effects of reduced mothering or lack of mothering
Increased irritability
Disturbance in eating, sleeping, and elimination
Interference with attachment process

Early Preschool Children (Ages 2-3 Years)
Frightened and confused
Blame themselves for the divorce
Fear of abandonment
Increased irritability, whining, tantrums
Regressive behaviors (e.g., thumbsucking, loss of elimination control)
Separation anxiety

Later Preschool Children (Ages 3-5 Years)
Fear of abandonment
Blame themselves for the divorce; decreased self-esteem
Bewilderment regarding all human relationships
Become more aggressive in relationships with others (e.g., siblings, peers)
Engage in fantasy to seek understanding of the divorce

Early School-Age Children (Ages 5-6 Years)
Depression and immature behavior
Loss of appetite and sleep disorders
May be able to verbalize some feelings and understand some divorce-related changes
Increased anxiety and aggression
Feel abandoned by departing parent

Middle School-Age Children (Ages 6-8 Years)
Panic reactions
Feelings of deprivation—loss of parent, attention, money, and secure future
Profound sadness, depression, fear, and insecurity
Feelings of abandonment and rejection
Fear regarding the future
Difficulty expressing anger at parents
Intense desire for reconciliation of parents
Impaired capacity to play and enjoy outside activities
Decline in school performance
Altered peer relationships—become bossy, irritable, demanding, and manipulative
Frequent crying, loss of appetite, sleep disorders
Disturbed routine, forgetfulness

Later School-Age Children (Ages 9-12 Years)
More realistic understanding of divorce
Intense anger directed at one or both parents
Divided loyalties
Able to express feelings of anger
Ashamed of parental behavior
Feel the need for revenge; may wish to punish the parent they hold responsible
Feel lonely, rejected, and abandoned
Altered peer relationships
Decline in school performance
May develop somatic complaints
May engage in aberrant behavior such as lying, stealing

Adolescents (Ages 12-18 Years)
Able to disengage themselves from parental conflict
Feel a profound sense of loss—of family, childhood
Feelings of anxiety
Worry about themselves, parents, siblings
Express anger, sadness, shame, embarrassment
May withdraw from family and friends
Disturbed concept of sexuality
May engage in acting-out behaviors

some kind of stability for these children; otherwise, they will convert their energies to restabilization efforts rather than to growth and development. They need frequent, repeated, and concrete explanations of what is going to happen to them and how they will be cared for, and assurance that something new will take the place of the old and that they will not be deserted. In order that they do not imagine things, explanations, such as where they will live, who will prepare their meals when the parent is at work, and when they will see the absent parent again, should be specific. They need to focus on reality.

School-age children are able to deal with parental separation better than younger children, even though they feel intense pain, loneliness, and deprivation. Younger children are preoccupied with the departure of one parent, usually the father, and grieve openly and long for his return, fearing replacement. Older children are more likely to perceive one parent as responsible, become angry with both parents, and express this anger with behavior distressing to one parent. School performance may be affected because they are unable to focus on learning; therefore teachers and school counselors should be informed so that they have a better understanding of alterations in the children's behavior and performance. Somatic complaints may be observed, such as gastrointestinal complaints, headaches, asthma, a low energy level, fatigability, clumsiness, and susceptibility to injury. Often children must move to an unfamiliar environment or new neighborhood and form new relationships in addition to coping with the alteration in their family structure. They almost invariably wish for the parents to reunite.

Adolescents may be highly resentful, since their lives are already sufficiently difficult and stressful. Although they are able to comprehend the divorce and are less likely to feel responsibility, adolescents find the divorce of their parents extraordinarily painful. Adolescents' sexual identity is affected by disturbed parental relationships, a precipitous deidealization of both parents, and concern about their own future as a marital partner. They are anxious about the availability of money for future needs. However, the separation of the parents may provide some space in which the older adolescent can develop an emotional detachment from the family and individualization—normal developmental tasks of adolescence.

Sex differences. Some observers have noted sex differences in the way children respond to the stress of divorce and living in a single-parent family. The primary effect of absence of either parent from the home is that children experience difficulty adjusting to and developing a sexual identity. This is more marked when the parental absence occurs early in the child's life and when it is the same-sex parent. Girls from homes where fathers are absent depend more on their mothers and show some anxiety about relationships with males during adolescence. Boys from homes without fathers tend to be less aggressive, are more apt to have emotional and social problems, and demonstrate cognitive patterning more similar to that of girls. Overprotectiveness, extreme indulgence, and often prolonged physical contact with the mother over many years may contribute to serious sex-identity problems in male children.

Children from homes in which one or both parents are frequently absent are highly susceptible to peer-group influence; this appears to be related to lack of attention and concern at home rather than to a positive attraction of the peer group. In addition, the peer group frequently serves a role identification function for young males from homes where the father is absent or ineffectual.

Some research indicates that in the younger age-groups boys are more affected by divorce than girls (Hetherington, Cox, and Cox, 1985; Peterson and Zill, 1986). However, these findings could not be confirmed in a recent analysis of national survey data (Baydar, 1989). Girls tend to have more difficulty when they are adolescents or young adults (Wallerstein and Blakeslee, 1989). Perhaps boys who show a poor adjustment to divorce are those who were very close to their fathers (Shaffer, 1985). Boys who are raised in homes where the father has custody seem to be better adjusted than those living with their mothers; girls living with their fathers are less well adjusted than those living with their mothers (Santrock and Warshak, 1979). Regular visits by the father appear to help children, especially boys, to make a positive adjustment to life in a single-parent family (Hess and Camara, 1979). One factor that seems to predict children's postdivorce relations with their parents is the quality of their relationship with each parent in the year *preceding* the divorce (Fine, Moreland, and Schwebel, 1983).

Family differences. Family characteristics may be more critical to children's well-being than specific child characteristics, such as age or sex. High levels of ongoing family conflict are related to problems of social development, emotional stability, and cognitive skills for the child. Greater marital conflict before divorce has been found to be predictive of a more problematic parent-child relationship after separation, which is associated with poorer adjustment in the child (Tschann and others, 1990). Conflict, whether in divorced or intact families, leads to lower self-esteem, increased anxiety, and loss of self-control (Slater and Haber, 1984) and reduces the child's attraction to the parents (White, Brinkerhoff, and Booth, 1985). In contrast, children's adjustment is facilitated when there is less parental conflict both before and after the divorce (Guidubaldi and others, 1986; Porter and O'Leary, 1980).

Support from extended family and friends can help buffer the effects of divorce; grandparents may extend considerable assistance to both their adult child and their grandchildren (Johnson, 1988). On the other hand, relationships with former in-laws tend to deteriorate immediately after separation (Ambert, 1988). Family finances are almost always negatively affected by divorce (Christensen, Dahl, and Retlig, 1990; Weitzman and Adair, 1988). Changes in life-style, financial instability, and loss of status may contribute indirectly to altered childrearing practices and fewer opportunities for children to participate in outside enrichment activities (Demo and Acock, 1988).

■ ■ ■

Research on the adverse effects of divorce on children must be viewed with some caution and scrutiny. Many of the samples are small, drawn from one area of the country, or selected from clinical rather than general populations. The lack of a control group in many studies also limits the conclusions.

Some positive outcomes of divorce have been reported, including more androgynous behavior—not following strict gender roles, thus allowing both boys and girls to assume both instrumental and expressive roles by following the more androgynous model of the single custodial parent. Greater maturity, feelings of self-efficacy, and an internal locus of control are also positive outcomes. However, emotional adjustment is closely associated with the child's personal adjustment before the divorce (Demo and Acock, 1988).

Developmental Tasks

Wallerstein and Blakeslee (1989) describe seven developmental tasks in an attempt to conceptualize the responses of children to divorce over a period of time (Box 3-8). The first two must be dealt with immediately, others within the first few months. Successful mastery of the early tasks is linked with maintenance of developmental pace and resumption of school following an expected diminished learning effectiveness and academic performance. Later tasks are associated with a more leisurely pace and extend over the remainder of the growth period.

Custody and Parenting Partnerships

Traditionally when parents separated, the mother was given custody of the children. Now both parents and the courts are seeking alternatives. The present belief is that neither fathers nor mothers should be awarded custody automatically. Rather, custody should be awarded to the parent who is best able to provide for the children's welfare.

In most divorce cases the mother still receives custody of the child with visitation agreements for the father. However, more courts are now awarding custody to fathers. Men usually make more money and can offer more material benefits than many women are able to provide. The incidence of delinquent support payments to custodial mothers is a matter of universal knowledge and concern. The single-parent family is commonplace, but many divorced mothers with small children move in with parents, other relatives, or friends in some kind of dependent or sharing arrangement. No matter what type of custody arrangement is awarded, the primary consideration is the welfare of the children.

Characteristics of the various types of postseparation parenting arrangements are outlined in Box 3-9. This typology, derived from studies by Durst, Wedemeyer, and Zurcher (1985), includes joint custody (discussed later) but does not address the issue of divided custody in which the

Box 3-8 PSYCHOLOGIC TASKS FOR CHILDREN AFTER DIVORCE

Task I: Understanding the Divorce
Young children: Understand the immediate changes and differentiate fantasy from reality; manage concerns regarding abandonment, placement in foster care, not seeing departed parent again.
Adolescents/young adults: Understand what led to marital failure; evaluate parents' actions; draw useful conclusions for their own lives.

Task II: Strategic Withdrawal
Acknowledge concern and provide appropriate help to parents and siblings; remove divorce from being their total focus and get back to their own interests, pleasures, activities, peer relationships, etc.
Parents must help children to remain children to complete this task.

Task III: Dealing with Loss
Deal with loss of intact family and loss of presence of one parent, usually the father.
May be most difficult task.
Deal with feelings of rejection and blame for making one parent leave.
Task is easier if child has good relationship with both parents.

Task IV: Dealing with Anger
Manage anger at parents for deciding to divorce, yet be aware of parents' needs, anxiety, and loneliness.
Diminished anger and forgiveness come about together.

Task V: Working Out Guilt
Guilt for causing marital difficulties and driving wedge between parents
Need to separate guilty ties and get on with their lives.

Task VI: Accepting Permanence of Divorce
Early denial and fantasies of parents getting back together.
May not be overcome until parent remarries or child separates from parents and leaves.

Task VII: Taking a Chance on Love
Most important task for growing children—adolescents and young adults.
Remain open to love, commitment, marriage, fidelity.
Be able to turn away from parents' model.

Data from Wallerstein, J., and Blakeslee, S.: Second chances: men, women, and children a decade after divorce, New York, 1989, Ticknor & Fields.

Box 3-9 PARENTING PARTNERSHIPS

Type I: Mother and Nonparent Father
Father never enters fathering role
Mother assumes sole responsibility for child from birth
Father's contact with children infrequent and unpredictable
Father does not engage in guidance or caretaking of children
Father functions as entertainer only
Spousal boundaries highly variable—communication usually written

Type II: Mother and Father as Friends
Father had participated in child care before divorce
Mother has responsibility for children
Father maintains predictable schedule of visits for some time, often 2 to 3 days per month; overnight stays frequent
Father-child interaction is primarily "father as friend"
Close relationship between parents based on common interests, past history, and mutual affection

Type III: Mother and Restricted Father
Court-ordered inflexible visiting schedule for father
Father feels restricted; mother satisfied with visiting arrangement
Father's parenting role ambiguous
Father participates little in children's development
Considerable hostility between spouses
Low level of communication between spouses
Parents often need intermediary for communication

Type IV: Time-Sharing Parents
Equal sharing of children in terms of time
Lack of shared decision making
Low level of communication between parents
Each parent functions as "sole custodian"—each functions independently, not cooperatively
Burden of smooth-running arrangement primarily children's responsibility

Type V: Co-parents
Parents are full partners in parenting
Joint decision making
Clear, flexible boundaries between spousal and parental subsystems
Time-sharing variable

From Durst, P.L., Wedemeyer, N.V., and Zurcher, L.A.: Parenting partnerships after divorce: implications for practice, Soc. Work 30:423-428, 1985.

custody of the children is divided between the parents. The problems of custodianship when the mother or the father is awarded custody of the children are discussed in relation to single-parenthood (see next section).

Joint custody. When both parents believe that they are equally capable of raising the children and both want custody, joint custody is a viable alternative that is becoming more common. Co-parenting offers substantial benefits for the family: children can be close to both parents, and life with each parent can be more normal as opposed to a disciplinarian mother and a recreational father. However, the long-term effects of joint custody are still unknown.

Parents consider themselves full partners in parenting and do not base this definition on the amount of time spent with the children. The advantage of this arrangement is that neither parent feels more powerful or dominant than the other, and each is more likely to get dependable, mature adult help with problems of childrearing. The relationship between the parents is one of cooperation but limited to matters related to parental functioning.

The joint custody plan can be almost anything that both parents agree on, but both parents must be truly dedicated to making it work. It usually assumes one of two forms (Charnas, 1983). In one form the children reside with one parent with the other having liberal visitation, but unlike the sole custody situation, both parents are the children's legal guardians and both participate in childrearing. This type of arrangement is especially advantageous for participants whose job or geographic location prevents easy access to the children or for those who have difficulty cooperating.

In the second form of joint custody the parents alternate having physical care and control of the children on a reasonably equitable basis while maintaining shared parenting responsibilities legally. This type of custody arrangement works well for families who live in closer proximity and whose occupations allow an active role in the care and rearing of the children. The arrangement is more effective when each parent maintains some personal regard and civility toward the other.

Variations of joint custody are endless. However, to be successful, the parents must place a high value on the commitment to provide as normal parenting as possible and be able to separate their marital conflicts from the parenting roles. The parents can expect some differing views on childrearing, just as with parents in intact families. Another requisite is that the children should have access to both parents unless the physical or psychologic welfare of the children is in jeopardy. In some cases of joint custody the children live with neither parent. For example, the child lives at a school and alternates vacations and holidays between the father and the mother.

Divided custody. Another parenting option is divided, or split, custody. For example, sons might live with the father and the daughters with the mother. The arrangements vary according to the needs and desires of the families. Children visit with the other parent and children. Most such families maintain an open-house policy whereby children are free to visit with little or no interference with their outside activities. The cooperation between parents is as variable as in other forms of custody. This arrangement usually requires flexibility and the ability of both families to work together to make it a success.

▪ ▪ ▪

The two-parent family has long been considered to be the most desirable for childrearing. Any departure from this may present risks to the child's overall development and well-being. Children reared in two-parent households, research shows, have a more stable environment for personality development, as well as appropriate role models for learning sex-role behavior (Demo and Acock, 1988).

SINGLE-PARENTING

Single-parent status is acquired by means of divorce, separation, or death, or through birth or adoption of a child by a single person. Although divorce rates have stabilized, the number of single-parent households continues to rise, with the majority of single parents being women (Burden, 1986). It is estimated that at least half the children born during the 1970s and 1980s will spend part of their time in a family headed by a divorced, separated, widowed, or never-married mother (Norton and Glick, 1986). Although some women are single parents by choice, most of these women never planned on being single parents, and many feel pressure to marry or remarry.

Managing shortages of money, time, and energy are major concerns of single parents (Quinn and Allen, 1989; Weitzman, 1985) (Box 3-10). Studies repeatedly confirm the financial difficulties of single-parent families. In fact, the stigma of poverty may be more keenly felt than the discrimination associated with being a single parent (Richards, 1989). In addition, these families are often forced by their financial status to live in communities where inadequate housing and personal safety are concerns. Moreover, single parents may feel guilty about the time spent away from their children. Divorced mothers from marriages where the father assumed the breadwinning role and the mother the householding and parenting roles have been found to have the most difficulty in adjusting to becoming the breadwinner for the family (Fassinger, 1989). Many single parents have trouble arranging for adequate child care, and care for sick children is especially difficult to obtain. Single mothers trying to balance work, chores, and child care may frequently give up personal activities, recreation, and even rest (Burden, 1986; Sanik and Mauldin, 1986).

Box 3-10 TOP TEN EVERYDAY STRESSES OF SINGLE MOTHERS

1. Economics/finances/budgeting
2. Guilt for not accomplishing more
3. Insufficient "me" time
4. Self-image/self-esteem/feelings of unattractiveness
5. Children's behavior/discipline/sibling fighting
6. Unhappiness with work situation
7. Housekeeping standards
8. Communicating with children
9. Insufficient family playtime
10. Lack of shared responsibility in the family

From Curran, D.: Stress and the healthy family, Minneapolis, 1985, Winston Press.

Although the life of single mothers is often portrayed bleakly, many single mothers do remarkably well and feel contentment in their lives (Fig. 3-9). Many feel they are excellent parents and are proud of their ability to manage their multiple roles effectively (Quinn and Allen, 1989; Richards, 1989). These women have a positive attitude and an acceptance of their work status (in and out of the home), and can often count on someone else, such as a boyfriend, relative, or an older child, to help out (Quinn and Allen, 1989).

Supports and resources for single-parent families include health care services that are open evenings and weekends, high-quality child care, respite child care to relieve parental exhaustion and burnout, and parent enhancement centers for advancing education and job skills, providing recreational activities, and offering parenting education. Groups for single-parent fathers and grandparents who are primary caregivers are also important (Strett, 1989). There is a need on the part of the parent for social contacts and a life separate from the children for the emotional growth of both parent and child. The single parent can find support and en-

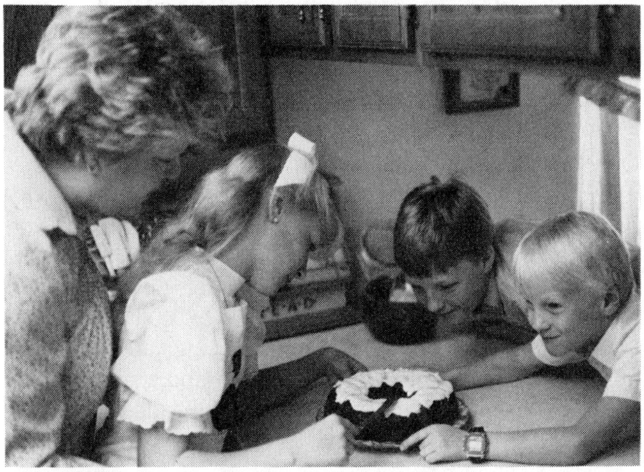

Fig. 3-9. Single parents take every opportunity to engage in activities with their children.

couragement from **Parents Without Partners,*** an organization designed to meet the needs of this increasingly important group.

Single Fathers

Fathers who have custody of their children have many of the same problems as divorced mothers. They feel overburdened by the responsibility, depressed, and concerned about their ability to cope with the emotional needs of the children, especially the needs of the girls (Hetherington, 1981). The lack of homemaking skills is characteristic of most fathers. They find it difficult at first to coordinate household tasks, school visits, and other activities associated with managing a household alone. Fathers often demand more assistance with household tasks and more independence from their children than custodial mothers do, and they are likely to make use of alternative caregiving and support systems.

STEPFAMILIES

Since 1980 the number of stepfamilies has stabilized. Approximately 10 million children live in stepfamilies. While 17.4% of married-couple families with young children were stepfamilies in 1987, up to 40% of all families will become stepfamilies before the children reach the age of 18 (Glick, 1989). Most of these families experience major change in their lives within 3 years of a divorce—a return to a nuclear family and the sudden acquisition of a stepparent when the custodial parent remarries. Most stepfamilies involve a mother, her children, and a stepfather; less often it is a father with children and a stepmother. Sometimes two single-parent families join to form a single household.

*International Headquarters, 7910 Woodmont Ave., Washington, DC 20014; or P.O. Box 8506, Silver Spring, MD 20907; (202) 638-1320.

Box 3-11 TIPS FOR "LIVING IN STEP"

1. Let relationships develop slowly and naturally. Don't expect too much too soon, from the children, from your spouse, or from yourself.
2. Don't criticize or belittle lost (or new) parents, or try to erase or replace them. Stepparents are additional parents.
3. Expect confused feelings, anxieties, competition for attention, bids for loyalty. Decide on standards of discipline and behavior and stick to them.
4. Communicate. Don't pretend everything is fine if it isn't. Look at problems squarely and deal with them openly.
5. If you need help, admit it and get it. Read a book, get counseling, join a support group, call a family meeting.

From Stein, B.: Yours, mine, and ours: a look at stepfamilies, Growing Parent 12(9):1-5, 1984.

Stepparenting

The term "parenting coalition" has been suggested to describe the situation where there are more than two parents for a child, as in stepfamilies (Visher and Visher, 1989). This term implies the need for cooperation rather than competition between the biologic parents and the stepparents. Cooperative parenting relationships can allow more time for each set of parents to be alone to establish their own relationship. Under ideal circumstances, power conflicts between the two households can be reduced, and tension and anxiety can be lessened for all family members. In addition, the children's self-esteem can be increased, and there is a greater likelihood of continued contact with grandparents (Visher and Visher, 1989). The development of a parenting coalition requires time and corresponds to the stages of stepfamily development described by Papernow (1984): (1) bonding between the couple; (2) recognition that all parenting adults are important to the children's well-being; (3) definition and clarification of acceptable stepparent roles; and (4) ability to share among adults in both households in terms of childrearing decisions and responsibilities. Flexibility, mutual support, and open communication are critical in successful relationships in stepfamilies and stepparenting situations (Rosen, 1987).

Unfortunately, stepfamilies usually do not seek help to prevent problems from arising. Typically, information and counseling are sought only when problems have surfaced and can no longer be ignored. A preventive rather than remedial approach to stepfamilies and stepparenting is needed (Ganong and Coleman, 1989) (Box 3-11).

Effects on Children

Although there has been a great deal of research on the impact of divorce on children, there are relatively little data on the outcomes for children in stepfamilies (Hobart, 1988). Becoming a stepchild is often a stressful transition (Crosbie-Burnett and Skyles, 1989; Hetherington, Cox, and Cox, 1985; Wallerstein and Blakeslee, 1989). Several transitional factors have been demonstrated to have an effect on children. The relationship with the noncustodial parent usually decreases. Divided loyalties between the two sets of parents may be exacerbated. As time goes on, the entry of new children from the remarriage can cause a stepchild from a previous marriage to have less favored status. In stepfamilies the possibility of a second divorce situation is very critical, since the children have already experienced significant losses in both relationships and environmental and circumstantial changes. Despite these risks and stresses, studies to date have not demonstrated long-term negative effects on children in remarried families (Amato, 1987).

PARENTING IN DUAL-EARNER FAMILIES

No change in family life-style has had more impact than the large numbers of women entering the workplace. As women moved away from the traditional homemaker pattern, the numbers of dual-earner families increased dramatically; now 60% of women with children 5 years of age or younger are in the labor force (Dawson and Cain, 1990). This trend is unlikely to diminish. As a result, the family is subjected to considerable stress as members attempt to meet the challenge of the often competing demands of occupational needs and those regarded as necessary for a rich family life.

Role definitions are frequently altered to arrange an equitable division of time and labor, as well as to resolve conflicts between earlier and later norms, especially those related to the traditional norms of the culture (Fig. 3-10). Overload is a common source of stress in a dual-earner family, and social activities are significantly curtailed. Time demands and scheduling are major problems, and when there are children, the demands can be even more intense; dual-earner couples may increase the strain on themselves in order to avoid creating stress for their children, although there is no evidence to indicate that the dual-earner life-style, as such, is stressful to children. However, the stress experienced by the parents may affect the children indirectly.

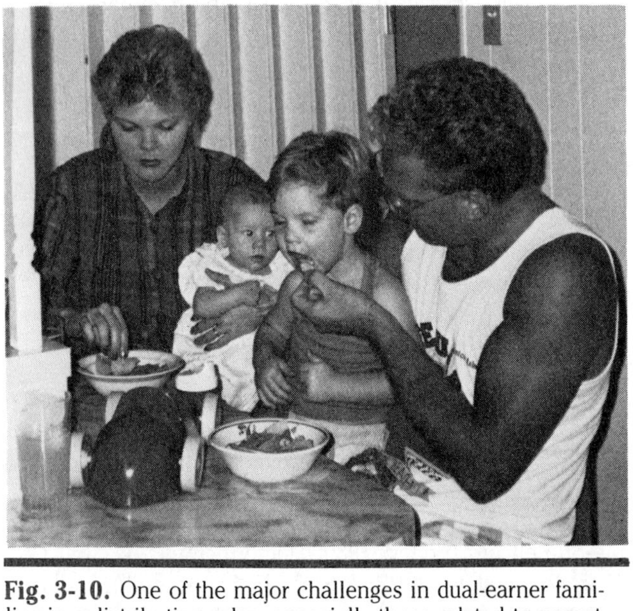

Fig. 3-10. One of the major challenges in dual-earner families is redistributing roles, especially those related to parenting.

Working Mothers

Only 7% of all American families reflect the traditional stereotype of two-parent families with the father as breadwinner and the mother staying at home (Otto, 1988). Even though working mothers have become the norm, disapproving attitudes from some health care workers and some child care books, lack of a national policy on child care, and "scripts" from their own childhood of being cared for by an at-home mother contribute to the torn and guilty feelings many working mothers experience (Balk and Christoffel, 1988).

QUESTIONS AND CONTROVERSIES

How does daycare influence the cognitive, social, and emotional development of the child?

Although children in daycare settings experience daily separation from their parent(s) and spend a good portion of their day in nonparental child care, the parents and family remain the primary influence on the child's development (Phillips and Howes, 1987). Child care, however, is a collaborative arrangement between the daycare provider and the family. In a review of the research on daycare since 1980, King and MacKinnon (1988) note that the quality of interactions between both the child and parent and the child and caregiver are very important for the child's development, but the latter are very difficult to regulate through licensing requirements. It was found that frequent individual contact with adult caregivers that was nonrestrictive and positive with less controlling, demanding, or punishing overtones promoted more positive cognitive development (Clarke-Stewart, 1987). Across many socioeconomic levels and from toddlerhood to early school-age, children with daycare experience exceeded home-reared children in social interaction with peers, confidence in social situations, friendliness, and more socially mature behaviors (Ramey, Dorval, and Baker-Ward, 1981; Schindler, Moley, and Frank, 1987). Some research has found daycare children to be more aggressive (Haskins, 1985), with different reasoning about rules and transgressions (i.e., not as apt to perceive social misbehavior as needing punishment) (Siegal and Storey, 1985). Emotional development is usually measured by attachment; insecure attachment is usually not a problem in daycare children 2 years of age and older (Rutter, 1982). The effects of daycare on infants under 1 year, however, remain unclear. This is due to controversy on how to measure attachment in infants and whether the avoidant behavior seen in daycare infants is really an adaptive behavior of children who routinely separate from the parent (Clarke-Stewart, 1987) or an indication of greater insecurity that will lead to the possibility of social maladjustment in the preschool and school-age years (Belsky, 1988). Longitudinal research involving infants cared for in a variety of daycare settings is particularly needed to more fully answer: what are the long-term effects of daycare on the child's development when out-of-home care is started in the first year of life?

The mother's status as a working woman has not been found consistently to have either positive or negative effects on children's development and educational outcomes (Balk and Christoffel, 1988; Bianchi and Spain, 1986; Hayes and Kamerman, 1983). Working women who scored high on measures of emotional well-being, sensitivity to and acceptance of their children, satisfaction with nonwork time, and positive feelings about their marriage were more likely to have securely attached infants, regardless of child care arrangements (Belsky, 1988). One consistent finding is that the "consequences of maternal employment" (mental health, marital satisfaction, children's well-being) are favorable when the woman's employment status is consistent with her and her husband's preferences about it (Spitzke, 1988).

The source and quality of child care are persistent concerns for all working parents. Child care can be provided by the employer, the other parent on an alternate work schedule, a formal group (e.g., daycare center), relatives (the most frequent source), or baby-sitters, either in the child's or the babysitter's home (Spitzke, 1988). Five characteristics of daycare that are important to the child's development are (1) the timing of entry into care, (2) the amount of time in daycare, (3) the stability of the care, (4) the setting, and (5) the quality of the care (King and MacKinnon, 1988). Any research on the effects of daycare must be examined carefully; the characteristics of the daycare setting and the measures used for child outcomes, such as attachment, must be taken into consideration (see Questions and Controversies).

KEY POINTS

- Although there is no agreement about the definition of *family,* families typically consist of two or more individuals who are emotionally involved with each other and reside in proximity.
- Theories that have been used to describe families include developmental theory, structural-functional theory, symbolic interactional theory, exchange theory, family systems theory, conflict theory, and family stress theory.
- Family composition refers to individuals with socially recognized statuses and positions who interact on a recurring basis in socially sanctioned ways.
- Although the traditional family structure has been nuclear or extended, in recent years other forms, such as the single-parent family, have emerged.
- Family size and positioning within the family structure have a strong impact on a child's development.
- Interpersonal skills and a basic understanding of childhood growth and development are two essential areas of focus for parents.
- Parents tend to demonstrate differences in one of two dimensions of childrearing: permissiveness-restrictiveness or warmth-hostility.
- The three styles of parental control, which influence approaches to discipline, are authoritarian, permissive, and authoritative.
- Marital factors within the home significantly influence a child's development. The impact of divorce on a child depends on age and sex, outcome, and quality of parental care following the divorce.

REFERENCES

Ahrons, C.R.: The binuclear family: two households, one family, Altern. Lifestyles 2:499-515, 1979.

Amato, P.R.: Family processes in one-parent, stepparent, and intact families: the child's point of view, J. Marriage Fam. 49:327-337, 1987.

Ambert, A.: Relationships with former in-laws after divorce: a research note, J. Marriage Fam. 50:679-686, 1988.

Balk, S., and Christoffel, K.: Advising the working mother, Contemp. Pediatr. 5(9):56-85, 1988.

Baptiste, D.A.: The gay and lesbian stepparent family. In Bozett, F.W., editor: Gay and lesbian parents, New York, 1987, Praeger Publishers.

Baskett, L.M., and Johnson, S.M.: The young child's interaction with parents versus siblings: a behavioral analysis, Child Dev. 53:643-650, 1982.

Beckman, L.J.: Couples' decision-making processes regarding fertility. In Tauber, K.E., Burgess, L.L., and Sweet, J.A., editors: Social demography, New York, 1978, Academic Press, Inc.

Bell, A.P., Weinberg, M.S., and Hammersmith, S.K.: Sexual preference, Bloomington, IN, 1981, Indiana University Press.

Belsky, J.: Early human experience: a family perspective, Dev. Psychol. 17:3-23, 1981.

Belsky, J.: The "effects" of infant day care reconsidered, Early Childhood Res. Q. 3(3):235-272, 1988.

Bianchi, S., and Spain, D.: American women in transition, New York, 1986, Russell Sage Foundation.

Bigner, J.J., and Bozett, F.W.: Parenting by gay fathers, Marriage Fam. Rev. (in press).

Bozett, F.W.: How and why gay fathers disclose their homosexuality to their children, Fam. Relations 29:173-179, 1980.

Bozett, F.W.: Parenting concerns of gay fathers, Top. Clin. Nurs. 6:60-71, 1984.

Bozett, F.W.: Children of gay fathers. In Bozett, F.W., editor: Gay and lesbian parents, New York, 1987a, Praeger Publishers.

Bozett, F.W.: Gay fathers. In Bozett, F.W., editor: Gay and lesbian parents, New York, 1987b, Praeger Publishers.

Bozett, F.W.: Gay fatherhood. In Bronstein, P., and Cowan, C.P., editors: Fatherhood today: men's changing role in the family, New York, 1988a, John Wiley & Sons, Inc.

Bozett, F.W.: Social control of identity by children of gay fathers, West. J. Nurs. Res. 10:550-565, 1988b.

Brockhaus, J.P.D., and Brockhaus, R.H.: Adopting an older child—the emotional process, Am. J. Nurs. 82:288-291, 1982.

Brodzinsky, D.: As cited in Hering, R.: Chosen and given, N.Y. Times Magazine, Sept. 11, 1988.

Burden, D.: Single parents and the work setting: the impact of multiple job and homelife responsibilities, Fam. Relations 35:37-43, 1986.

Burgess, E.W.: The family as a unit of interacting personalities, Family 7:3-9, 1926.

Burgess, E., Locke, H., and Thomas, M.: The family, ed. 3, New York, 1963, American Book.

Burr, W., and others: Symbolic interaction and the family. In Burr, W., and others, editors: Contemporary theories about the family, vol. 2, New York, 1979, Free Press.

Charnas, J.F.: Joint child-custody counseling—divorce 1980s style, Soc. Casework 64:546-554, 1983.

Child Welfare League of America: Standard for adoption services, New York, 1968, The League.

Christensen, D.H., Dahl, C.M., and Rettig, K.D.: Noncustodial mothers and child support: examining the larger context, Fam. Relations 39(4):388-394, 1990.

Clarke-Stewart, L.: Predicting child development from day care forms and features: the Chicago study. In Phillips, D.A., editor: Quality in child care: what does the research tell us? Washington, DC, 1987, National Association for the Education of Young Children.

Clore, E.R., and Newberry, Y.S.G.: Nurse practitioner guidance for the adoptive family from birth to adolescence, Pediatr. Nurs. 7(6):16-25, 1981.

Crnic, K.A., and others: Effects of stress and social support on mothers and premature and full-term infants, Child Dev. 54:209-217, 1983.

Crosbie-Burnett, M., and Skyles, A.: Stepchildren in school and colleges: recommendations for educational policy changes, Fam. Relations 38:59-64, 1989.

Curran, D.: Traits of a healthy family, New York, 1983, Ballantine Books.

Curran D.: Stress and the healthy family, Minneapolis, 1985, Winston Press.

Dawson, D.A., and Cain, V.S.: Child care arrangements: health of our nation's children, United States; 1988, Advance data from vital and health statistics; No. 187, Hyattsville, MD, 1990, National Center for Health Statistics.

Demo, D., and Acock, A.: The impact of divorce on children, J. Marriage Fam. 50:619-648, 1988.

Dubowitz, H., and others: The changing American family, Pediatr. Clin. North Am. 35:1291-1311, 1988.

Dunn, J., and Kendrick, C.: Social behavior of young siblings in the family context: differences between same-sex and different-sex dyads, Child Dev. 52:1265-1273, 1981.

Durst, P.L., Wedemeyer, N.V., and Zurcher, L.A.: Parenting partnerships after divorce: implications for practice, Soc. Work 10:423-428, 1985.

Duvall, E.R.: Family development, ed. 5, Philadelphia, 1977, J.B. Lippincott Co.

Easterbrooks, M.A., and Goldberg, W.A.: Toddler development in the family: impact of father involvement and parenting characteristics, Child Dev. 55:740-752, 1984.

Edwards, J.: Perceived needs of adoptive and biologic parents, Issues Compr. Pediatr. Nurs. 10:223-234, 1987.

Eshleman, J.R.: The family: an introduction, ed. 3, Boston, 1981, Allyn & Bacon, Inc.

Fassinger, P.: Becoming the breadwinner: single mothers' reactions to changes in their paid work lives, Fam. Relations 38:404-411, 1989.

Feldman, S.S., and Aschenbrenner, B.: Impact of parenthood on various aspects of masculinity and femininity: a short-term longitudinal study, Dev. Psychol. 19:278-289, 1983.

Fine, M.A., Moreland, J.R., and Schwebel, A.I.: Long-term effects of divorce on parent-child relationships, Dev. Psychol. 19:703-713, 1983.

Freidman, D.: Parent development, Calif. Med. 86:25-28, 1957.

Friedman, M.: Family nursing: theory and assessment, ed. 2, Norwalk, CT, 1986, Appleton-Century-Crofts.

Ganong, L., and Coleman, M.: Preparing for remarriage: anticipating the issues, seeking solutions, Fam. Relations 38:28-33, 1989.

Geiser, R.L.: Hidden victims: the sexual abuse of children, Boston, 1979, Beacon Press.

Glick, P.: Remarried families, stepfamilies, and stepchildren: a brief demographic profile, Fam. Relations 38:24-27, 1989.

Green, M.: Reaching out to children of divorce, Contemp. Pediatr. 5:22-42, 1988.

Green, R.: Sexual identity of 37 children raised by homosexual or transsexual parents, Am. J. Psychiatry 135:692-697, 1978.

Green, R., and others: Lesbian mothers and their children: a comparison with solo parent heterosexual mothers and their children, Arch. Sex. Behav. 15:167-184, 1986.

Groothuis, J.R., and others: Increased child abuse in families with twins, Pediatrics 70(5):769-773, 1982.

Guidubaldi, E.M., and others: The role of selected family environment factors in children's post-divorce adjustment, Fam. Relations 35:141-151, 1986.

Harris, M.B., and Turner, P.H.: Gay and lesbian parents, J. Homosex. 12:103-113, 1986.

Haskins, R.: Public school aggression among children with varying day care experience, Child Dev. 56:689-703, 1985.

Hayes, C., and Kamerman, S., editors: Children of working parents: experiences and outcomes, Washington, DC, 1983, National Academy Press.

Hess, R.D., and Camara, K.A.: Post divorce family relationships as mediating factors in the consequences of divorce for children, J. Soc. Issues 35:79-96, 1979.

Hetherington, E.M.: Children and divorce. In Henderson, R.W., editor: Parent-child interaction: theory, research, and prospects, New York, 1981, Academic Press, Inc.

Hetherington, E.M., Cox, M., and Cox, R.: Play and social interaction in children following divorce, J. Soc. Issues 35:26-49, 1979.

Hetherington, E.M., Cox, M., and Cox, R.: The aftermath of divorce. In Contemporary readings in child psychology, ed. 2, New York, 1981, McGraw-Hill, Inc.

Hetherington, E.M., Cox, M., and Cox, R.: Long-term effects of divorce and remarriage on the adjustment of children, J. Am. Acad. Child Psychiatry 24:518-530, 1985.

Hill, R.: Families under stress, New York, 1949, Harper & Row, Publishers, Inc.

Hill, R., and Hansen, D.: The identification of conceptual frameworks utilized in family study, Marriage Fam. Liv. 22:299-311, 1960.

Hobart, C.: The family system in remarriage: an exploratory study, J. Marriage Fam. 50(3):649-661, 1988.

Hoeffer, B.: Children's acquisition of sex-role behavior in lesbian-mother families, Am. J. Orthopsychiatry 51:536-544, 1981.

Hostetter, M., and Johnson, D.: International adoption: an introduction for physicians, Am. J. Dis. Child. 143:325-332, 1989.

Huggins, S.: A comparative study of self-esteem of adolescent children of divorced lesbian mothers and divorced heterosexual mothers, J. Homosex. 18(1/2):123-135, 1989.

Jimenez, S.L., and Jungman, R.G.: Supplemental information for the family with a multiple pregnancy, MCN 5:320-325, 1980.

Johnson, C.: Postdivorce reorganization of relationships between divorcing children and their parents, J. Marriage Fam. 50:221-231, 1988.

Johnson, R.: Promoting the health of families in the community. In Stanhope, M., and Lancaster, J.: Community health nursing, St. Louis, 1984, Mosby–Year Book, Inc.

King, D., and MacKinnon, C.: Making difficult choices easier: a review of research on day care and children's development, Fam. Relations 37:392-398, 1988.

Knafl, K.: The concept of family. In Logan, B., and Dawkins, C., editors: Family-centered nursing in the community, Menlo Park, CA, 1986, Addison-Wesley Publishing Co., Inc.

Koo, H., Suchindran, C., and Griffith, J.: The completion of childrearing: change and variation in timing, J. Marriage Fam. 49:281-293, 1987.

Kurdek, L., Blisk, D., and Siesky, A.: Correlates of children's long-term adjustment to their parents' divorce, Dev. Psychol. 17:565-579, 1981.

Kurdek, L., and Siesky, A.: Children's perceptions of their parents' divorce, J. Divorce 3:339-378, 1980.

Maccoby, E.E.: Social development: psychological growth and the parent-child relationship, New York, 1980, Harcourt Brace Jovanovich, Inc.

Macklin, E.D.: Nontraditional family forms: a decade of research, J. Marriage Fam. 42:175-192, 1980.

Main, M., and Weston, D.R.: The quality of the toddler's relationship to mother and to father: related to conflict and the readiness to establish new relationships, Child Dev. 52:932-940, 1981.

McCubbin, H.I., and Patterson, J.M.: Family adaptation to crisis. In McCubbin, H.I., Cauble, E., and Patterson, J.M., editors: Family stress, coping, and social support, Springfield, IL, 1982, Charles C Thomas, Publisher.

McCubbin, M., and McCubbin, H.: Theoretical orientation to family stress and coping. In Figley, C., editor: Treating families under stress, New York, 1989, Brunner/Mazel, Inc.

Mednick, B., and Baker, R.: Consequences of family structure and maternal state for child and mother's development, Final report, NICHD (contract N 01-HD-82807), 1980.

Miller, B.: Counseling gay husbands and fathers. In Bozett, F.W., editor: Gay and lesbian parents, New York, 1987, Praeger Publishers.

Moses, A.E., and Hawkins, R.O.: Counseling lesbian women and gay men: a life issues approach, St. Louis, 1982, Mosby–Year Book, Inc.

National Center for Health Statistics: Advance report of final divorce statistics, 1987, Monthly Vital Statistics Rep. 38(12, suppl. 2):2, 1990a.

National Center for Health Statistics: Annual summary of births, marriages, divorces, and deaths: United States, 1989, Monthly Vital Statistics Rep. 38(13):5, 1990b.

National Center for Health Statistics: Births, marriages, divorces, and deaths for 1989, Monthly Vital Statistics Rep. 38(12):1, 1990c.

Norton, A., and Glick, P.: One-parent families: a social and economic profile, Fam. Relations 35:8-17, 1986.

Otto, L.: America's youth: a changing profile, Fam. Relations 37:385-391, 1988.

Papernow, P.: The stepfamily cycle: an experiential model of stepfamily development, Fam. Relations 33:355-363, 1984.

Peterson, J., and Zill, N.: Marital disruption, parent-child relationships, and behavior problems in children, J. Marriage Fam. 48:295-307, 1986.

Phillips, D., and Howes, C.: Indicators of quality child care: review of research. In Phillips, D.A., editor: Quality in child care: what does the research tell us? Washington, DC, 1987, National Association for the Education of Young Children.

Pies, C.: Considering parenthood: psychosocial issues for gay men and lesbians choosing alternative fertilization. In Bozett, F.W., editor: Gay and lesbian parents, New York, 1987, Praeger Publishers.

Pines, M.: Only isn't lonely (or spoiled or selfish), Psychol. Today 15(3):15-19, 1981.

Polit, D., and Falbo, T.: Only children and personality development, J. Marriage Fam. 49:309-325, 1987.

Porter, B., and O'Leary, D.: Marital discord and childhood behavior problems, J. Abnorm. Child Psychol. 8:287-295, 1980.

Quinn, P., and Allen, K.: Facing challenges and making compromises: how single mothers endure, Fam. Relations 38:390-395, 1989.

Ragozin, A.S., and others: Effects of maternal age on parenting role, Dev. Psychol. 18:627-634, 1982.

Ramey, C., Dorval, B., and Baker-Ward, L.: Day care and the socially disadvantaged. In Kilmer, S., editor: Advances in early education and day care, Greenwich, CT, 1981, JAI.

Richards, L.: The precarious survival and hard-won satisfaction of white single-parent families, Fam. Relations 38:396-403, 1989.

Ricketts, W., and Achtenberg, R.: The adoptive and foster gay and lesbian parent. In Bozett, F.W., editor: Gay and lesbian parents, New York, 1987, Praeger Publishers.

Rivera, R.R.: Legal issues in gay and lesbian parenting. In Bozett, F.W., editor: Gay and lesbian parents, New York, 1987, Praeger Publishers.

Rodman, H.: Talcott Parsons' view of the changing American family. In Rodman, H., editor: Marriage, family, and society, New York, 1965, Random House, Inc.

Rogers, R.H.: Improvement in the construction and analysis of family life cycle categories, Kalamazoo, MI, 1962, Western Michigan University.

Rosen, M.: Stepfathering, New York, 1987, Ballantine Books.

Ross, M.W.: The married homosexual man: a psychological study, London, 1983, Routledge & Kegan Paul, Inc.

Rutter, M.: Socioemotional consequences of day care for preschool children. In Zigler, E., and Gordon, E., editors: Day care: scientific and social policy issues, Boston, 1982, Auburn.

Sanik, M., and Mauldin, T.: Single vs. two-parent families: a comparison of mothers' time, Fam. Relations 35:53-56, 1986.

Santrock, J.W., and Warshak, R.A.: Father custody and social development in boys and girls, J. Soc. Issues 35:112-125, 1979.

Sater, J.: Appraising and promoting a sense of self in twins, MCN 4:218-226, 1979.

Schindler, P., Moley, B., and Frank, A.: Time in day care and social participation of young children, Dev. Psychol. 23:255-261, 1987.

Schulenburg, J.: Gay parenting, New York, 1985, Doubleday & Co.

Shaffer, D.R.: Developmental psychology: theory, research, and applications, Monterey, CA, 1985, Brooks/Cole Publishing Co.

Sherry, S.: Helping families adapt to adoption, Contemp. Pediatr. 3:96-111, 1986.

Siegal, M., and Storey, R.: Day care and children's conceptions of moral and social rules, Child Dev. 56:1001-1008, 1985.

Singelmann, R.B.: Exchange as symbolic interaction: convergences between two theoretical perspectives, Am. Soc. Rev. 37:414-424, 1972.

Slater, E., and Haber, J.: Adolescent adjustment following divorce as a function of familial conflict, J. Consult. Clin. Psychol. 52:920-921, 1984.

Soloway, N., and Smith, R.: Antecedents of late birth-timing decisions of men and women in dual-career marriages, Fam. Relations, 36:258-262, 1987.

Spitzke, G.: Women's employment and family relations: a review, J. Marriage Fam. 50(3):595-618, 1988.

Sprey, J.: Conflict theory and the study of marriage and the family. In Burr, W.R., and others, editors: Contemporary theories about the family, vol. 2, New York, 1979, Free Press.

Steckel, A.: Psychosocial development of children of lesbian mothers. In Bozett, F.W., editor: Gay and lesbian parents, New York, 1987, Praeger Publishers.

Steelman, L.C., and Powell, B.: The social and academic consequences of birth order: real, artifactual, or both? J. Marriage Fam. 47:117-124, 1985.

Stinnet, N.: In search of strong families, In Stinnet, N., Chesser, B., and DeFrain, J., editors: Building family strengths: blueprints for addiction, Lincoln, 1981, University of Nebraska Press.

Stinnet, N.: Secrets of strong families, Boston, 1985, Little, Brown & Co., Inc.

Stinnet, N., and Sauer, K.: Relationship characteristics of strong families, Fam. Perspect. 11:3-11, 1977.

Strett, R.: Support services for single parents, Early Childhood Update 5:6, winter 1989.

Tschann, J., and others: Family process and children's functioning during divorce, J. Marriage Fam. 51:431-444, 1990.

Turner, P.H., Scadden, L., and Harris, M.B.: Parenting in gay and lesbian families. Paper presented at the First Future of Parenting Symposium, Chicago, March 1985.

Visher, E., and Visher, J.: Parenting coalitions after remarriage: dynamics and therapeutic guidelines, Fam. Relations 38:65-70, 1989.

Wallerstein, J.S.: Children of divorce: stress and developmental tasks. In Garmezy, N., and Rutter, M., editors: Stress, coping, and development in children, New York, 1983, McGraw-Hill, Inc.

Wallerstein, J.S., and Blakeslee, S.: Second chances: men, women, and children a decade after divorce, New York, 1989, Ticknor & Fields.
Wallerstein, J.S., and Kelly, J.B.: The effects of parental divorce: the experiences of the preschool child, J. Am. Acad. Child Psychiatry 14:600-616, 1975.
Wallerstein, J.S., and Kelly, J.B.: California's children of divorce, Psychol. Today, pp. 67-76, Jan. 1980.
Weitzman, L.: The divorce revolution, New York, 1985, Free Press.
Weitzman, M., and Adair, R.: Divorce and children, Pediatr. Clin. North Am. 35(6):1313-1323, 1988.
White, L., Brinkerhoff, D.B., and Booth, A.: The effect of marital disruption on child's attachment to parents, J. Fam. Issues 6:5-22, 1985.
World Health Organization: Health and the family: studies in the demography of family life cycles and their health implication, Geneva, Switzerland, 1978, The Organization.

BIBLIOGRAPHY

General

Abidin, R.A., and Wilfong, E.: Parenting stress and its relationship to child health care, Child. Health Care 18(2):114-116, 1989.
Aldous, J., Osmond, M.W., and Hicks, M.W.: Men's work and men's families. In Burr, W.R., and others, editors: Contemporary theories about the family, vol. 1, New York, 1979, Free Press.
Atkinson, A.M.: Providers' evaluations of the effect of family day care on own family relationships, Fam. Relations 37(4):399-404, 1988.
Barranti, C.C.R.: The grandparent/grandchild relationship: family resource in an era of voluntary bonds, Fam. Relations 34:343-352, 1985.
Brandt, M.A.: Consider the patient part of the family, Nurs. Forum 11:19-23, 1984.
Brody, C.J., and Steelman, L.C.: Sibling structure and parental sex-typing of children's household tasks, J. Marriage Fam. 47:265-273, 1985.
Callan, V.J.: Comparisons of mothers of one child by choice with mothers wanting a second birth, J. Marriage Fam. 47:155-164, 1985.
Clemen-Stone, S., Eigsti, D., and McGuire, S.: Comprehensive family and community health nursing, ed. 3, St. Louis, 1991, Mosby–Year Book, Inc.
Clements, I.W., and Roberts, F.B., editors: Family health: a theoretical approach to nursing care, New York, 1983, John Wiley & Sons, Inc.
Felson, R.B., and Zielinski, M.A.: Children's self-esteem and parental support, J. Marriage Fam. 51(3):727-736, 1989.
Fsife, B.L.: A model for predicting the adaptation of families to a medical crisis: an analysis of role integration, Image 17:108-112, 1985.
Gilliss, C.L., and others, editors: Toward a science of family nursing, Menlo Park, CA, 1989, Addison-Wesley Publishing Co., Inc.
Glick, P.C.: Fifty years of family demography: a record of social change, J. Marriage Fam. 50(4):861-873, 1988.
Kaufman, D.H.: An interview guide for helping children make health-care decisions, Pediatr. Nurs. 11:365-367, 1985.
Klaus, M.H., and Kennell, J.H.: Parent-infant bonding, ed. 2, St. Louis, 1982, Mosby–Year Book, Inc.
Lamb, M.E.: Mothers, fathers, and children in a changing world. In Tyson, R.L., Call, J., and Galenson, E., editors: Infancy in a changing world, New York, 1985, Basic Books, Inc., Publishers.
LaRossa, R.: Fatherhood and social change, Fam. Relations 37(4):451-457, 1988.
Leahey, M., and Wright, L., editors: Families and life-threatening illness, Springhouse, PA, 1987, Springhouse Corp.
Lewis, J.M.: How's your family? New York, 1979, Brunner/Mazel, Inc.
Mancini, J.A., and Orthner, D.K.: The context and consequences of family change, Fam. Relations 37(4):363-366, 1988.
McCubbin, H.I., and Figley, C.R., editors: Stress and the family: coping with normative transitions, New York, 1983, Brunner/Mazel, Inc.
McCubbin, H.I., and others: Family types and strengths, Edina, MN, 1988, Burgess International Group, Inc.
Moriarty, H.J.: Key issues in the family research process: strategies for nurse researchers, Adv. Nurs. Sci. 12(3):1-14, 1990.
Neal, A.G., Groat, H.T., and Wicks, J.W.: Attitudes about having children: a study of 600 couples in the early years of marriage, J. Marriage Fam. 51(2):313-328, 1989.
Newman, B.M., and Newman, P.R.: Development through life: a psychosocial approach, ed 3, Homewood, IL, 1984, The Dorsey Press.
Wright, L.M., and Leahey, M., editors: Nurses and families: a guide to family assessment and intervention, Philadelphia, 1984, F.A. Davis Co.
Wright, L., and Leahey, M., editors: Families and chronic illness, Springhouse, PA, 1987, Springhouse Corp.
Wright, L., and Leahey, M., editors: Families and psychosocial problems, Springhouse, PA, 1987, Springhouse Corp.

Family Theories

Beutler, I.F., and others: The family realm: theoretical contributions for understanding its uniqueness, J. Marriage Fam. 51(3):805-815, 1989.
Hurley, P.M.: Family assessment: systems theory and the genogram, Child. Health Care 10:76-82, 1982.
Nye, F.I.: Choice, exchange, and the family. In Burr, W., and others, editors: Contemporary theories about the family, vol. 2, New York, 1979, Free Press.
Simon, F.B., Stierlin, H., and Wynne, L.C.: The language of family therapy, New York, 1985, Family Process Press.
Sprey, J.: Current theorizing on the family: an appraisal, J. Marriage Fam. 50(4):875-890, 1988.

Gay/Lesbian Family

Baptiste, D.A.: Psychotherapy with gay/lesbian couples and their children in "stepfamilies": a challenge for marriage and family therapists, J. Homosex. 14:223-238, 1987.
Bigner, J.J., and Jacobsen, R.B.: Parenting behaviors of homosexual and heterosexual fathers, J. Homosex. 18(1/2):173-186, 1989.
Bozett, F.W.: Gay fathers: evolution of the gay-father identity, Am. J. Orthopsychiatry 51(3):552-559, 1981.
Bozett, F.W.: Heterogeneous couples in heterosexual marriages: gay men and straight women, J. Marital Fam. Ther. 8(1):81-89, 1982.
Bozett, F.W.: Gay men as fathers. In Hanson, S.M.H., and Bozett, F.W., editors: Dimensions of fatherhood, Beverly Hills, CA, 1985, Sage Publications, Inc.
Bozett, F.W., editor: Gay and lesbian parents, New York, 1987, Praeger Publishers.
Bozett, F.W.: Intervening with gay families with an overweight adolescent. In Leahey, M., and Wright, L.M., editors: Families and chronic illness, Springhouse, PA, 1987, Springhouse Corp.
Bozett, F.W.: Gay fathers: a review of the literature, J. Homosex. 18(1/2):137-162, 1989.
Cramer, D.: Gay parents and their children: a review of research and practical implications, J. Counsel. Dev. 64(8):504-507, 1986.
Fishel, A.H.: Gay parents, Issues Health Care Women 4:139-164, 1983.
Golombok, S., Spencer, A., and Rutter, M.: Children in lesbian and single-parent households: psychosexual and psychiatric appraisal, J. Child Psychol. 24:551-572, 1983.
Green, G.D.: Lesbian mothers: mental health considerations. In Bozett, F.W., editor: Gay and lesbian parents, New York, 1987, Praeger Publishers.
Hall, M.: Lesbian families: cultural and clinical issues, Soc. Work 23:380-385, 1987.
Hitchens, D.: Social attitudes, legal standards, and personal trauma in child custody cases, J. Homosex. 5:89-95, 1980.
Hitchens, D., and Kirkpatrick, M.: Lesbian mothers/gay fathers. In Benedek, E., editor: Child psychiatry and the law, vol. 2, New York, 1985, Brunner/Mazel, Inc.

Hotvedt, M.E., and Mandel, J.B.: Children of lesbian mothers. In Paul, W., and others, editors: Homosexuality: social, psychological, and biological issues, Beverly Hills, CA, 1982, Sage Publications, Inc.

Jay, K., and Young, A.: The gay report, New York, 1987, Summit Books.

Lewin, E., and Lyons, T.: Everything in its place: the coexistence of lesbianism and motherhood. In Paul, W., and others, editors: Homosexuality: social, psychological, and biological issues, Beverly Hills, CA, 1982, Sage Publications, Inc.

Lewis, K.G.: Children of lesbians: their point of view, Soc. Work 25:198-203, 1980.

Maddox, B.: Married and gay, New York, 1982, Harcourt Brace Jovanovich, Inc.

Matteson, D.R.: The heterosexually married gay and lesbian parent. In Bozett, F.W., editor: Gay and lesbian parents, New York, 1987, Praeger Publishers.

McCandlish, B.M.: Against all odds: lesbian mother family dynamics. In Bozett, F.W., editor: Gay and lesbian parents, New York, 1987, Praeger Publishers.

Miller, B.: Identity resocialization in moral careers of gay husbands and fathers. In Davis, A., editor: Papers in honor of Gordon Hirabayashi, Edmonton, Canada, 1986, University of Alberta Press.

Nungesser, L.G.: Theoretical bases for research on the acquisition of social sex-roles by children of lesbian mothers, J. Homosex. 5:177-187, 1980.

Pagelow, M.: Heterosexual and lesbian single mothers: a comparison of problems, coping, and solutions, J. Homosex. 5:189-204, 1980.

Paul, J.P.: Growing up with a gay, lesbian, or bisexual parent: an exploratory study of experiences and perceptions, doctoral dissertation, Berkeley, 1986, University of California—Berkeley.

Pennington, S.B.: Children of lesbian mothers. In Bozett, F.W., editor: Gay and lesbian parents, New York, 1987, Praeger Publishers.

Richardson, D.: Lesbian mothers. In Hart, J., and Richardson, D., editors: The theory and practice of homosexuality, Boston, 1981, Routledge & Kegan Paul, Inc.

Robinson, B.E.: Gay fathers. In Robinson, B.E., and Barret, R.L.: Fatherhood, New York, 1986, Guilford.

Skeen, P., Walters, L., and Robinson, B.: How parents of gays react to their children's homosexuality and to the threat of AIDS, J. Psychosoc. Nurs. 26(12):7-10, 1988.

Wismont, J.M., and Reame, N.E.: The lesbian childbearing experience: assessing developmental tasks, Image 21(3):137-141, 1989.

Family Configuration/Parenting

Abramovitch, R., Corter, C., and Pepler, D.J.: Observations of mixed-sex sibling dyads, Child Dev. 51:1268-1271, 1980.

Brazelton, T.: "Middle child" label is unfair. In Families today, Wis. State J., March 7, 1990.

Brazelton, T.: Middle child patterns reflect all kids' needs. In You and your child, Milwaukee J., March 11, 1990.

Falbo, T., and Polit-O'Hara, D.F.: Only children: what do we know about them? Pediatr. Nurs. 11:356-360, 1985.

Goshen-Gottstein, E.R.: The mothering of twins, triplets, and quadruplets, Psychiatry 70:769-773, 1982.

Lewis, M., and Feiring, C.: Some American families at dinner. In Laosa, L.M., and Sigel, I.E., editors: Families as learning environments for children, New York, 1982, Plenum Publishing Corp.

Mulhern, R.K., and Passman, R.H.: Parental discipline as affected by sex of parent, sex of child, and the child's apparent responsiveness to discipline, Dev. Psychol. 17:604-613, 1981.

Riley, D., and Cochran, M.M.: Naturally occurring childrearing advice for fathers: utilization of the personal social network, J. Marriage Fam. 47:275-286, 1985.

Slevin, K.F.: Motherhood, culture, and change, Pediatr. Nurs. 8:405-408, 1982.

Steffensmeier, R.H.: A role model of the transition to parenthood, J. Marriage Fam. 44:319-323, 1982.

Stewart, R.B.: Sibling attachment relationships: child-infant interactions in the strange situation, Dev. Psychol. 19:192-199, 1983.

Ventura, J.N.: Parent coping behaviors, parent functioning, and infant temperament characteristics, Nurs. Res. 31:269-273, 1982.

Webster-Stratton, C., and Kogan, K.: Helping parents parent, Am. J. Nurs. 80:240-241, 1980.

Adoption

American Academy of Pediatrics, Committee on Early Childhood, Adoption, and Dependent Care: Health care of foster children, Pediatrics 79(4):644-646, 1987.

American Academy of Pediatrics, Task Force on Pediatric AIDS: Infants and children with acquired immunodeficiency syndrome: placement in adoption and foster care, Pediatrics 83(4):609-612, 1989.

Bachrach, C.A., and others: Adoption in the 1980s. Advance data from vital and health statistics, No. 181, Hyattsville, MD, 1989, National Center for Health Statistics.

Brockhaus, J.P.D., and Brockhaus, R.H.: Adopting an older child—the legal process, Am. J. Nurs. 82:292-294, 1982.

Hill, M., and Peltzer, J.: A report of thirteen groups for white parents of Black children, Fam. Relations 31:557-565, 1982.

Hostetter, M.K., and others: Unsuspected infectious diseases and other medical diagnoses in evaluation of internationally adopted children, Pediatrics 83(4):559-564, 1989.

Messer, M.M., and Rasmussen, N.H.: Southeast Asian children in America: the impact of change, Pediatrics 78(2):323-329, 1986.

Ritchie, C.W.: Adoption: an option often overlooked, Am. J. Nurs. 89:1156-1157, 1989.

Schor, E.L.: Foster care, Pediatr. Clin. North Am. 35(6):1241-1252, 1988.

Sherwen, L.N., Smith, D.W., and Cueman, M.A.: Common concerns of adoptive mothers, Pediatr. Nurs. 10:127-130, 1984.

Smith, D.W., and Sherwen, L.N.: Mothers and their adopted children: the bonding process, New York, 1983, Tiresias Press.

Smith, D.W., and Sherwen, L.N.: The bonding process of mothers and adopted children, Top. Clin. Nurs. 6(3):38-48, 1984.

Divorce

Arditti, J.A.: Noncustodial fathers: an overview of policy and resources, Fam. Relations 39(4):460-465, 1990.

Booth, A., and Edwards, J.N.: Age at marriage and marital instability, J. Marriage Fam. 47:67-75, 1985.

Bray, J.H., and Berger, S.H.: Noncustodial father and paternal grandparent relationship in stepfamilies, Fam. Relations 39(4):414-419, 1990.

Coucouvanis, J.A., and Solomons, H.C.: Handling complicated visitation problems of hospitalized children, MCN 8:131-134, 1983.

Depner, C.E., and Bray, J.H.: Modes of participation for noncustodial parents: the challenge for research, policy, practice and education, Fam. Relations 39(4):378-381, 1990.

Ferreiro, B.W.: Presumption of joint custody: a family policy dilemma, Fam. Relations 39(4):420-426, 1990.

Furstenberg, F., and others: The life course of children of divorce: marital disruption and parental contact, Am. Soc. Rev. 48:656-668, 1983.

Jackson, P.L.: Caring for children from divorced families, MCN 8:126-130, 1983.

Johnston, J.R.: Role diffusion and role reversal: structural variation in divorced families and children's functioning, Fam. Relations 39(4):405-413, 1990.

Kimard, E., and Reinherz, H.: Effects of marital disruption on children's school aptitude and achievement, J. Marriage Fam. 48:285-293, 1986.

Lebowitz, M.L.: Divorce and the American teenager, Pediatrics 76:695-698, 1985.

Lowery, C.R.: Child custody in divorce: parents' decisions and perceptions, Fam. Relations 34:241-249, 1985.

Lowery, C.R., and Settles, S.A.: Effects of divorce on children: differential impact of custody and visitation patterns, Fam. Relations 34:455-463, 1985.

Mitchell, A.K.: Adolescents' experiences of parental separation and divorce, J. Adolesc. 6:175-187, 1983.

Parish, G.D.: Perceptions of personal and familial adjustment by children from intact, single-parent, and reconstituted families, Psychol. Schools 21:166-174, 1983.

Rankin, R.P., and Maneker, J.S.: The duration of marriage in a divorcing population: the impact on children, J. Marriage Fam. 47:43-52, 1985.

Rhyne, M.C.: Understanding and supporting families in the process of divorce, Nurse Practitioner 11(12):37-51, 1986.

Schilling, L.S.: The effects of divorce on children: a perspective for the pediatric health care provider, J. Assoc. Care Child. Health 11:92-96, 1983.

Wallerstein, J.: Children of divorce: preliminary report of a ten-year follow-up of young children, Am. J. Orthopsychiatry 54:444-458, 1984.

Webster-Stratton, C.: The relationship of marital support, conflict, and divorce to parent perceptions, behaviors, and childhood conduct problems, J. Marriage Fam. 51(2):417-430, 1989.

Single Parenting

Burns, C.E.: The hospitalization experience and single-parent families: a time of special vulnerability, Nurs. Clin. North Am. 19:285-293, 1984.

Grief, G.L.: Children and housework in the single father family, Fam. Relations 34:353-357, 1985.

Grief, G.L.: Single fathers rearing children, J. Marriage Fam. 47:185-191, 1985.

Hanson, S.: Single custodial fathers and the parent-child relationship, Nurs. Res. 30:202-204, 1981.

Hughes, C.B., and Scoloveno, M.: The single father, Top. Clin. Nurs. 6(3):1-9, 1984.

McLanahan, S., and Booth, K.: Mother-only families: problems, prospects, and politics, J. Marriage Fam. 51(3):557-580, 1989.

Risman, B.J., and Park, K.: Just the two of us: parent-child relationships in single-parent homes, J. Marriage Fam. 50(4):1049-1062, 1988.

Weinberg, T.S.: Single fatherhood: How is it different? Pediatr. Nurs. 11:173-175, 1985.

Stepfamilies

Cherlin, A., and McCarthy, J.: Remarried couple households: data from the June 1980 current population survey, J. Marriage Fam. 47(4):23-30, 1985.

Clawson, J.F., and Sears, J.: A stepmother in the family, Pediatr. Nurs. 15(3):249-251, 1989.

Clingempeel, W., Ievoli, G., and Brand, E.: Structural complexity and the quality of stepfather-stepchild relationships, Fam. Process 23:547-560, 1984.

Coleman, M., and Ganong, L.: Stepfamily self-help books: brief annotations and ratings, Fam. Relations 38(1):90-96, 1989.

Crosbie-Burnett, M.: Application of family stress theory to remarriage: a model for assessing and helping stepfamilies, Fam. Relations 38(3):323-331, 1989.

Ganong, L.H., and Coleman, M.: The effects of remarriage on children: a review of the empirical literature, Fam. Relations 33:389-406, 1984.

Ganong, L.H., and Coleman, M.: Do mutual children cement bonds in stepfamilies? J. Marriage Fam. 50(3):687-698, 1988.

Peek, C.W., and others: Patterns of functioning in families of remarried and first-married couples, J. Marriage Fam. 50(3):699-708, 1988.

Pill, C.J.: Stepfamilies: redefining the family, Fam. Relations 39(2):186-193, 1990.

Pink, J.E.T., and Wampler K.S.: Problem areas in stepfamilies: cohesion, adaptability, and the stepfather-adolescent relationship, Fam. Relations 34:327-335, 1985.

Poppen, W.A., and White, P.N.: Transition to the blended family. Elem. Sch. Guid. Coun. 19:50-61, 1984.

Reuter, L., and Strang, V.: Yours, mine, and ours: stepparents and their children, MCN 11:264-266, 1986.

Romanczuk, A.N.: Helping the stepparent parent, MCN 12:106-110, 1987.

Dual-Earner Family

American Academy of Pediatrics, Committee on Psychosocial Aspects of Child and Family Health: The mother working outside the home, Pediatrics 73:874-875, 1984.

Atkinson, A.: Providers' evaluation of the effect of family day care on own family relationships, Fam. Relations 37:399-404, 1988.

Brazelton, T.: Working and caring, Reading, MA, 1987, Addison-Wesley Publishing Co., Inc.

Floge, L.: The dynamics of child-care use and some implications for women's employment, J. Marriage Fam. 47:143-154, 1985.

Heins, M., and others: Attitudes of pediatricians toward maternal employment, Pediatrics 72:283-290, 1983.

Kutzner, S.K., and Toussie-Weingarten, C.: Working parents: the dilemma of child rearing and career, Top. Clin. Nurs. 6(3):30-37, 1984.

Sinal, S.H., and Herndon, A.: Attitude of pediatricians toward maternal employment and substitute child care, South. Med. J. 77:726-729, 1984.

Thomas, V.G.: Determinant of global life happiness and marital happiness in dual-career black couples, Fam. Relations 39(2):174-178, 1990.

Tiedje, L.B., and Collins, C.: Combining employment and motherhood, MCN 14:9-14, 1989.

CHAPTER 4

Growth and Development of Children

RELATED TOPICS

Activity: infant, Ch. 12; toddler, Ch. 14; preschooler, Ch. 15; school-age child, Ch. 17; and adolescent, Ch. 19
Biologic development: infant, Ch. 12; toddler, Ch. 14; preschooler, Ch. 15; school-age child, Ch. 17; and adolescent, Ch. 19
Cognitive development: infant, Ch. 12; toddler, Ch. 14; preschooler, Ch. 15; school-age child, Ch. 17; and adolescent, Ch. 19
Dental health: infant, Ch. 12; toddler, Ch. 14; preschooler, Ch. 15; school-age child, Ch. 17; and adolescent, Ch. 19
Development of body image: infant, Ch. 12; toddler, Ch. 14; preschooler, Ch. 15; school-age child, Ch. 17; and adolescent, Ch. 19
Development of sexuality: infant, Ch. 12; toddler, Ch. 14; preschooler, Ch. 15; school-age child, Ch. 17; and adolescent, Ch. 19
Fears: infant, Ch. 12; toddler, Ch. 14; preschooler, Ch. 15; school-age child, Ch. 17; and adolescent, Ch. 19
Language development: infant, Ch. 12; toddler, Ch. 14; preschooler, Ch. 15; school-age child, Ch. 17; and adolescent, Ch. 19
Moral development: toddler, Ch. 14; preschooler, Ch. 15; school-age child, Ch. 17; and adolescent, Ch. 19
Nutrition: infant, Ch. 12; toddler, Ch. 14; preschooler, Ch. 15; school-age child, Ch. 17; and adolescent, Ch. 19
Play: infant, Ch. 12; toddler, Ch. 14; preschooler, Ch. 15; school-age child, Ch. 17; and adolescent, Ch. 19
Psychosocial development: infant, Ch. 12; toddler, Ch. 14; preschooler, Ch. 15; school-age child, Ch. 17; and adolescent, Ch. 19
Sleep: infant, Ch. 12; toddler, Ch. 14; preschooler, Ch. 15; school-age child, Ch. 17; and adolescent, 19
Social development: infant, Ch. 12; toddler, Ch. 14; preschooler, Ch. 15; school-age child, Ch. 17; and adolescent, Ch. 19
Spiritual development: toddler, Ch. 14; preschooler, Ch. 15; school-age child, Ch. 17; and adolescent, Ch. 19
Stress: toddler, Ch. 14; preschooler, Ch. 15; school-age child, Ch. 17; and adolescent, Ch. 19
Temperament: infant, Ch. 12; toddler, Ch. 14; preschooler, Ch. 15; school-age child, Ch. 17; and adolescent, Ch. 19

GLOSSARY

cephalocaudal Head-to-tail direction of growth
cross-sectional Method of child study that measures a group of children at the same point in time
development A gradual change and expansion; advancement from lower to more advanced stages of complexity; the emerging and expanding of the individual's capacities through growth, maturation, and learning
developmental task A set of skills and competencies peculiar to each developmental stage that children must accomplish or master in order to deal effectively with their environment
differentiation Processes by which early cells and structures are systematically modified and altered to achieve specific and characteristic physical and chemical properties; sometimes used to describe the trend of mass to specific; development from simple to more complex activities and functions
growth An increase in number and size of cells as they divide and synthesize new proteins; results in increased size and weight of the whole or any of its parts
longitudinal A method of child study that compares the same child at different points in time
maturation An increase in competence and adaptability; aging; usually used to describe a qualitative change; a change in the complexity of a structure that makes it possible for that structure to begin functioning; to function at a higher level
proximodistal near-to-far direction of growth

Growth and development are complex processes involving numerous components that are subject to a wide variety of influences. All facets of the child's body, mind, and personality develop simultaneously, although not independently, and emerge at varying rates and sequences. Infants, except for limited reflex responses, depend totally on adults for satisfaction of even the most basic needs. As development proceeds, children begin to communicate their needs verbally and nonverbally and to assume increasing responsibility for their basic need gratification.

Those who care for children come to understand the physical changes that take place during the process of development and the special needs generated by these changes, for example, the nature and quantity of the food intake, the method and frequency of feeding, and the amount of sleep and activity that change during childhood. Health and safety hazards associated with every phase of development require provisions for the child's physical safety, including prevention of injuries and disease and education of children, families, and communities regarding these potential threats to health and well-being.

This chapter is devoted to some of the ongoing maturational changes in children from a longitudinal perspective. The reader is introduced to the general progression and flow of developmental changes that take place throughout childhood. Also included are preliminary discussions of some of the major concepts and needs that accompany, are precipitated by, or in some way influence normal development. In subsequent chapters the topics introduced here are elaborated in discussions of major developmental stages to provide a holistic view of a child at a specific stage in development.

GROWTH AND DEVELOPMENT

All children are basically alike. They follow the same pattern of development and maturation, while at the same time, their hereditary, cultural, and experiential backgrounds make each child distinct from every other child. They differ in their rate of growth, their ultimate size and capabilities, and the way in which they respond to their environment.

Because they do not have the resources for coping with the world, children need to be surrounded by caring people who are willing to share their pleasures and help them through troubling times. Although the emphasis and classification may vary according to the interpreter, the essential needs of children during all stages of development are physical, biologic, and emotional, including love, emotional security, discipline, appropriate independence, and self-esteem. However, regardless of the stage of development, the state of health, or the situation, *the child is first of all a child.*

FOUNDATIONS OF GROWTH AND DEVELOPMENT

Growth and development, usually referred to as a unit, expresses the sum of the numerous changes that take place during the lifetime of an individual. The entire course is a dynamic process that encompasses several interrelated dimensions: growth, development, maturation, and differentiation (see Glossary).

All of these processes are interrelated. Although they are simultaneous, ongoing processes, none occurs apart from the others. The child's body becomes larger and more complex; the personality simultaneously expands in scope and complexity. Very simply, growth can be viewed as a *quantitative* change, and development as a *qualitative* change. Children "grow" by maintaining a positive balance of increase over loss in size; they "grow up" by maturing in structure and function.

Stages of Growth and Development

Most authorities in the field of child development conveniently categorize child growth and behavior into approximate age stages or in terms that describe the features of an age-group. The age ranges of these stages are admittedly arbitrary, and since they do not take into account individual differences, they cannot be applied to all children with any degree of precision. However, this categorization affords a convenient means to describe the characteristics associated with the majority of children at periods when distinctive developmental changes appear and specific developmental tasks must be accomplished. It is also significant for nurses to know that there are characteristic health problems peculiar to each major phase of development. The sequence of descriptive age periods and subperiods that is used here and elaborated on in subsequent chapters is listed in Box 4-1.

Methods of Studying Growth and Development

The early growth period in the human being extends over a longer time than that of any other mammalian species. The long period of childhood allows for more elaborate brain development, body growth, and the development of those characteristics of personality that distinguish man from lower animals. During these early years children prepare for adulthood in several dimensions: they increase in size and acquire increasingly intricate motor capacities, their personality emerges, and they assimilate their culture.

To determine whether or not growth and development have taken place, the child can be compared with a representative group of children at the same point in time (*cross-sectional* method), or the same child can be measured and compared at different points in time (*longitudinal* method). Standards or norms for the study of developmental progress have been established by these two contrasting methods.

Cross-sectional. The cross-sectional method, which tests or measures the characteristics of a number of children representing the various ages or stages of development, is the more common. The observations of children are made at the same point in time. For example, a group of schoolchildren, ages 6 to 12 years, are measured for specific characteristics such as height, weight, mental ability, motor ability, or vocabulary. The data collected and averaged on a group of 6-year-old children, for instance, provide information on the expected achievement of a child in that age-group. If large groups are used, the results are expressed as averages, but the meaning of these results is directly related to the similarities within the groups, such as race, sex, and socioeconomic level. Most norms or averages are determined in this way and are helpful when comparing groups. For instance, the average height of 8-year-old children in Chicago can be compared with the average height of 8-year-old Mexican children. This method is espe-

Box 4-1 DEVELOPMENTAL AGE PERIODS

Prenatal period: Conception to birth
GERMINAL: conception to approximately 2 weeks
EMBRYONIC: 2 to 8 weeks
FETAL: 8 to 40 weeks (birth)
A rapid growth rate and total dependency make this one of the most crucial periods in the developmental process. The relationship between maternal health and certain manifestations in the newborn emphasizes the importance of adequate prenatal care to the health and well-being of the infant.

Infancy period: Birth to 12 or 18 months
NEONATAL: Birth to 28 days
INFANCY: 1 to approximately 12 months
The infancy period is one of rapid motor, cognitive, and social development. Through mutuality with the caregiver (parent), the infant establishes a basic trust in the world and the foundation for future interpersonal relationships. The critical first month of life, although part of the infancy period, is often differentiated from the remainder because of the major physical adjustments to extrauterine existence and the psychologic adjustment of the parent.

Early childhood: 1 to 6 years
TODDLER: 1 to 3 years
PRESCHOOL: 3 to 6 years
This period, which extends from the time the children attain upright locomotion until they enter school, is characterized by intense activity and discovery. It is a time of marked physical and personality development. Motor development advances steadily. Children at this age acquire language and wider social relationships, learn role standards, gain self-control and mastery, develop increasing awareness of dependence and independence, and begin to develop a self-concept.

Middle childhood: 6 to 11 or 12 years
Frequently referred to as the "school age," this period of development is one in which the child is directed away from the family group and is centered around the wider world of peer relationships. There is steady advancement in physical, mental, and social development with emphasis on developing skill competencies. Social cooperation and early moral development take on more importance with relevance for later life stages. This is a critical period in the development of a self-concept.

Later childhood: 11 to 19 years
PREPUBERTAL: 10 to 13 years
ADOLESCENCE: 13 to approximately 18 years
The tumultuous period of rapid maturation and change known as adolescence is considered to be a transitional period that begins at the onset of puberty and extends to the point of entry into the adult world—usually high school graduation. Biologic and personality maturation are accompanied by physical and emotional turmoil, and there is redefining of the self-concept. In the late adolescent period the child begins to internalize all previously learned values and to focus on an individual, rather than a group, identity.

cially useful to establish norms for a given age-group with or without other factors.

Longitudinal. The longitudinal method is often used to determine growth trends and rates. Each child in a group of children is observed and measured periodically over a number of years and through successive stages of growth and development. This approach is also useful in assessing the long-term or delayed effects of an early experience, such as a prolonged illness, malnutrition, or maternal rejection. Although the longitudinal method is more difficult to carry out, the growth and development of a child can be compared at any moment with a representative group of children and can be followed through successive stages to determine the speed and direction of that child's distinctive growth.

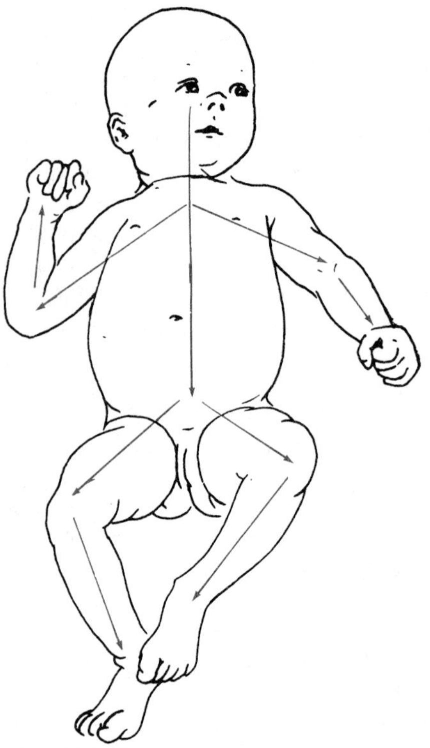

Fig. 4-1. Directional trends in growth.

Patterns of Growth and Development

There are definite and predictable patterns in growth and development that are continuous, orderly, and progressive. These patterns, sometimes referred to as trends or principles, are universal and basic to all human beings. Although they are more apparent with respect to physical growth, most of these patterns apply to psychologic and social growth as well and follow predetermined trends in direction, sequence, and pace. However, each human being accomplishes these in a manner and time unique to that individual.

Directional trends. Growth and development proceed in regular, related directions or gradients and reflect the physical development and maturation of neuromuscular functions (Fig. 4-1). The first pattern is the *cephalocaudal*, or head-to-tail, direction. The head end of the organism develops first and is very large and complex, whereas the lower end is small and simple and takes shape at a later period. The physical evidence of this trend is most apparent during the period before birth, but it also applies to postnatal behavioral development. Infants achieve structural control of the head before the trunk and extremities, hold their back erect before they stand, use their eyes before their hands, and gain control of their hands before they have control of their feet.

Second, the *proximodistal,* or near-to-far, trend applies to the midline-to-peripheral concept. A conspicuous illustration is the early embryonic development of limb buds, followed by rudimentary fingers and toes. In the infant, shoulder control precedes mastery of hands, the whole hand is used as a unit before the fingers can be manipulated, and the central nervous system develops more rapidly than the peripheral nervous system.

These trends or patterns are bilateral and appear to be symmetric; each side develops in the same direction and at the same rate as the other. For some of the neurologic functions, this symmetry is only external because of unilateral differentiation of function at an early stage of postnatal development. For example, by the age of approximately 5 years children demonstrate a decided preference for the use of one hand over the other, although previously they used either one.

The third trend in directional growth, *mass to specific* (sometimes referred to as differentiation), describes development from simple operations to more complex activities and functions. From very broad, global patterns of behavior, more specific, refined patterns emerge. All areas of development (physical, mental, social, emotional) proceed in this direction. Through the processes of development and differentiation, early embryonal cells with vague, undifferentiated functions progress to an immensely complex organism composed of highly specialized and diversified cells, tissues, and organs. Generalized development will precede specific or specialized development; gross, random muscle movements take place before fine muscle control. The child will at first run and jump for the sake of motion, but eventually these activities take the more complex form of a race or hopscotch. Infants will respond to people in general before they recognize and prefer their parents.

Sequential trends. In all dimensions of growth and development there is a definite, predictable sequence. It is orderly and continuous, with each child normally passing through every stage. Each stage is affected by those preceding it and affects those that follow. Sequential patterns have been described for motor skills such as locomotion and use of hands, and types of behavior such as language and social skills. Children crawl before they creep, creep before they stand, and stand before they walk. Children first play alone, then with others in increasing numbers and increasingly complex activities.

New biologic parts and behaviors arise out of and build on those already established. This continuity with the past, or *epigenesis,* serves as a foundation for the future and requires interaction with a suitable environment at the proper time. In very early physical development, fingers arise from webbed appendages on limb buds, the nervous system develops from a neural plate derived from an area of embryonic ectoderm, and sexual organs differentiate from a morphologically neutral primitive gonad. Later, facets of the personality are built on the early foundation of trust. The child babbles, then forms words and, finally, sentences; writing emerges from scribbling.

Developmental pace. Although there is a fixed, precise order to development, it does not progress at the same rate or pace in all children. There are periods of accelerated growth and periods of decelerated growth in both total body growth and growth of subsystems. The very rapid growth rate before and after birth gradually levels off throughout early childhood. Relatively slow during middle childhood, the rate increases markedly at the beginning of adolescence and levels off in early adulthood.

The focus of development and growth shifts at successive stages in development. For instance, the head grows most rapidly before birth, while other body parts grow more slowly; after birth other structures grow faster than the head. This growth pattern accounts for shifts in body proportion, facial characteristics, and voice. Similarly, one type of development seems to take precedence over another during various periods of growth. At times of rapid growth, other development may reach a plateau. For example, when children begin to walk, the thrills of upright locomotion take precedence over other activity such as speech, and they may not learn any new words for 3 to 4 months. Schoolwork may suffer during the early adolescent growth spurt.

Sensitive periods. There are limited times during the process of growth when children interact with a particular environment in a specific manner. The terms *critical periods, sensitive periods,* and *vulnerable periods* have been applied to those times in an organism's lifetime when it is more susceptible to positive or negative influences. Colombo (1982) describes a "critical" period as one when the developing organism is more sensitive to beneficial stimulation or more susceptible to detrimental influence. Touwen (1989) suggests that "critical" period implies the need for specific stimulation, while "sensitive" and "vulnerable" periods of maturation are those during which external conditions may be particularly harmful to specific tissues, organs, or systems.

The quality of interactions during these sensitive periods determines whether the effects on the children will be beneficial or harmful. The character and extent of the interaction's consequences depend on the nature of the environmental influences and the stage of development. For example, physiologic maturation of the central nervous system is influenced by adequacy and timing of contributions from the environment, such as stimulation and nutrition. The first 3 months of prenatal life is a sensitive period for physical growth. During this period of accelerated growth and differentiation, specific organs and systems are most vulnerable to environmental influences; the earlier the impact, the more far-reaching are the effects.

The terms *critical, sensitive,* and *optimal periods* apply to all aspects of growth and development. During fetal development there are times during the period of tissue differentiation when interference by a detrimental influence can alter the normal course of events. Such alterations can produce a physical or mental defect that can have either minor or far-reaching effects.

Psychologic development also appears to have sensitive periods when an environmental event has maximum influence on the developing personality. Observers have identified periods in development when behavior patterns are most readily acquired. For example, primary socialization occurs during the first year, when infants make their initial social attachments and establish a basic trust in the world. At this time a warm relationship with the caregiver is fundamental to a healthy parent-child relationship (Mitchell and Mills, 1983) (see Promotion of Parent-Infant Bonding [Attachment], Chapter 8).

The sensitive period concept might also be applied to readiness for learning skills such as toilet training or reading. In these instances there appears to be an opportune time when the skill is best learned. However, if the skill is not learned at this time, acquisition at a later time is still possible. The optimum time for school entry has been based on the readiness to acquire the specific types of skills learned in the school setting.

Individual Differences

Each child grows in his or her own unique and personal way. Great individual variation exists in the age at which developmental milestones are reached. The sequence is predictable; the exact timing is not. Rates of growth vary from one individual to another, and measurements are defined in terms of ranges to allow for individual differences among children. Some children are fast growers, others are moderate, and some are slower to reach maturity. For example, periods of fast growth, such as the pubescent growth spurt, may begin earlier or later in some children than in others. Children may grow fast or slow during the spurt and may finish sooner or later than other children. The sex of the child is an influential factor because girls seem to be more advanced in physiologic growth at all ages.

Terminal points and optimum tendency. The terminal points in growth vary immensely from one child to another. For example, some individuals will grow until reaching a height of over 180 cm (6 feet), others will cease growing at 150 cm (5 feet); the majority will achieve varying heights between the two. Females as a group reach both height and weight terminal points before males, with average terminal height in males exceeding that for females.

There appears to be a tendency for organisms to strive for optimum developmental potential in both structure and function. When environmental factors interfere with normal development for a time (e.g., during periods of inadequate food supply or illness), children's bodies will usually make up for the interrupted period and return to their characteristic pattern of growth. For instance, children born prematurely will demonstrate delayed development during the early months but will usually "catch up" to others of the same age by the time they enter school. However, if the deprivation is severe or occurs throughout a critical period, development may be permanently impaired.

Interrelatedness. Children develop as whole beings, not in pieces and parts. They are a product of the past environment in which they have grown and their current stresses and satisfactions. Factors affecting one part will influence others. For example, children deprived of love and affection will be delayed in physical and mental development. Although there are exceptions, children who deviate from the average with respect to one aspect of growth will probably deviate in others.

Secular Trend in Growth and Development

Measurements and observations recorded over the past century indicate a significant worldwide trend in the rate and age of maturation. Children from widely different populations are maturing earlier and becoming larger at each age. There appears to be a slight but not so marked increase in average adult height because, although children are growing faster, they also stop growing sooner. On the average young men reach their full height at approximately age 20, whereas in 1900 they did not reach their final height until about 25. The average size increase since 1900 is nearly 1 cm (3/8 inch) per decade in height, 1 kg (2½ pounds) in weight in preschool children, and 2.5 cm (1 inch) and 2.5 kg (5½ pounds) per decade during puberty. In girls the age of menarche has advanced progressively.

Many theories have been advanced to explain this phenomenon. Improved environmental factors, such as nutrition and socioeconomic conditions, are important factors, as well as the sharp decrease in infant mortality during this century. Since body size is an inherited trait, the tendency toward the selection of mates from wider geographic areas is an important factor. The trend appears to reach a plateau in populations with optimum environments, which suggests there is a maximum end point.

BIOLOGIC GROWTH AND DEVELOPMENT

As children grow, their external dimensions change. These changes are accompanied by corresponding alterations in structure and function of internal organs and tissues, reflecting the gradual acquisition of physiologic competence. These alterations, although progressive and interdependent, are not a uniform process but are characterized by cycles of accelerated and slow development that vary from organ to organ and system to system. Each part has its own rate of growth, and many growth rates are directly related to alterations in the size of the child (e.g., heart rate). Skeletal muscle growth approximates whole body growth; brain, lymphoid, adrenal, and reproductive tissues follow distinct and individual patterns (Fig. 4-2).

External Proportions

Variations in the growth rate of different tissues and organ systems produce significant changes in body proportions during childhood. The cephalocaudal trend of development is most evident in total body growth as indicated by these changes (Fig. 4-3). During fetal development the head is the fastest growing part, and at 2 months of gestation the head comprises 50% of total body length. During infancy growth of the trunk predominates; the legs are the most rapidly growing part during childhood; then, in adolescence, the trunk once again elongates. In the newborn the lower limbs are one third of the total body length but only 15% of the total body weight; in the adult the lower limbs comprise one half of the total body height and 30% of total body weight. As growth proceeds, the midpoint in head-to-toe measurements gradually descends from a level even with the umbilicus at birth to the level of the symphysis pubis at maturity.

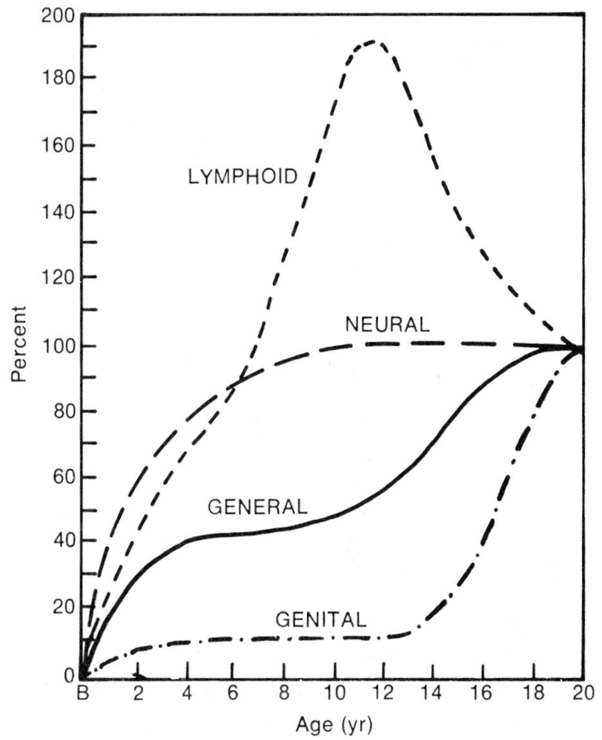

Fig. 4-2. Growth rates for body as a whole and three types of tissues. *Lymphoid type:* thymus, lymph nodes, and intestinal lymph masses; *neural type:* brain, dura, spinal cord, optic apparatus, and head dimensions; *general type:* body as a whole, external dimensions, and respiratory, digestive, renal, circulatory, and musculoskeletal systems.

Modified from Harris, J.A., and others: The measurement of man, Minneapolis, 1930, University of Minnesota Press.

The first year is a period of rapid growth dominated by lengthening of the trunk and accumulation of subcutaneous fat. When infants begin to walk, their large head, heavy trunk, and protuberant abdomen atop short, bowed legs force them to walk with a wide stance, outward rotation of the hips, and everted feet. The high center of gravity created by this disproportionate bulk causes infants to walk unsteadily and contributes to frequent falls.

After the first year and extending to puberty, the legs grow more rapidly than any other part. The bowlegged appearance disappears with locomotion, the abdomen is held in, and the body becomes slender and elongated. Until puberty this slender, long-legged build is characteristic of both sexes; in similar clothes and hairstyle the two sexes are indistinguishable. With the onset of puberty there is a marked alteration in body proportion when all structures show the effects of the pubertal growth spurt. The feet and hands are first to increase in rate of growth; therefore during this transient period they appear large and ungainly in relation to the rest of the body, often a source of embarrassment to the adolescent. The trunk again grows faster than the legs, so that a large portion of the increase in height at adolescence is a result of trunk growth.

Since the legs continue to grow until puberty, early-maturing children have shorter than average legs, and the legs of later-maturing children are longer. Inasmuch as the onset of puberty is approximately 2½ years earlier in girls, for a while girls are larger than boys, and girls' legs are shorter than boys' legs. Laterality of growth follows rapid linear growth; both boys and girls proceed to "fill out" during the later stages of adolescent growth.

One of the more outstanding features of changing body proportion is shoulder and hip breadth as a result of hormone secretion from the maturing gonads. Shoulder and hip growth increases in both sexes, but the shoulder width in boys is considerably greater than in girls. The anteroposterior hip diameter increases in girls, and the female pelvis becomes wider, shallower, and roomier than the male pelvis. The differences in deposition of fat produce the distinctive feminine contours in girls, whereas boys lose subcutaneous fat.

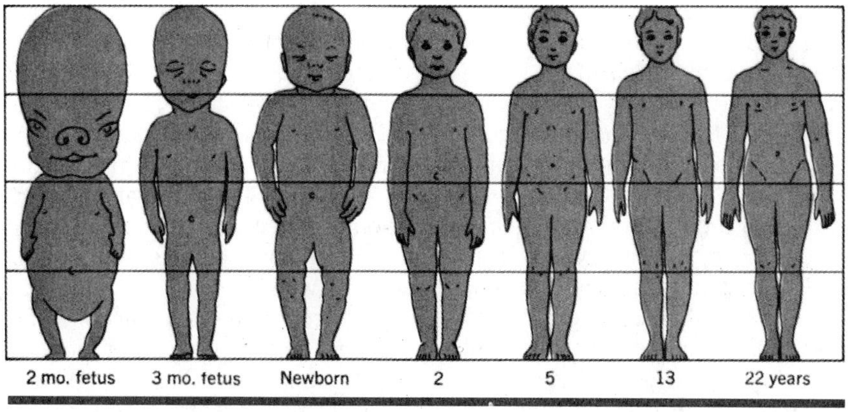

Fig. 4-3. Changes in body proportions from before birth to adulthood.

From Crouch, J.E., and McClintic, J.R.: Human anatomy and physiology, ed. 2, New York, 1976, John Wiley & Sons, Inc.

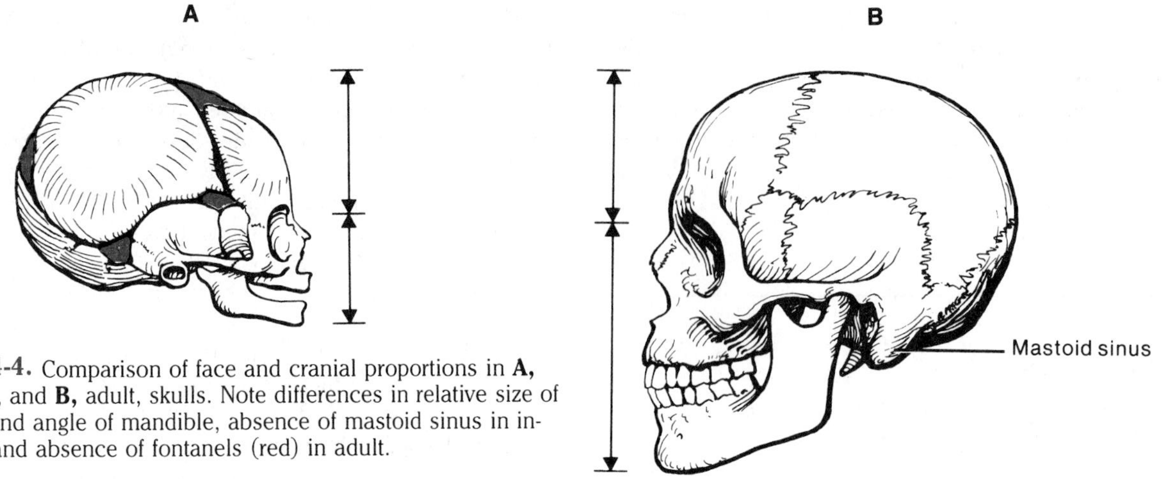

Fig. 4-4. Comparison of face and cranial proportions in **A,** infant, and **B,** adult, skulls. Note differences in relative size of face and angle of mandible, absence of mastoid sinus in infant, and absence of fontanels (red) in adult.

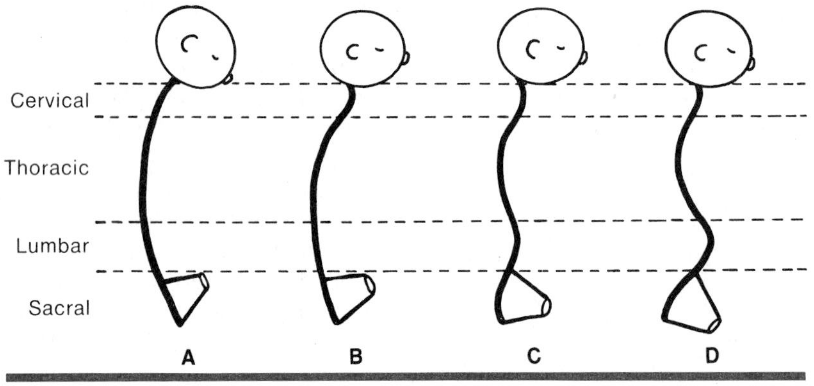

Fig. 4-5. Development of spinal curvatures. **A,** Newborn infant. **B,** Cervical secondary curvature. **C,** Lumbar secondary curvature. **D,** Lordosis.

Physique. Physique refers to the body form, build, or shape of an individual. A number of classification systems have been advanced that attempt to describe specific body types. The most important was developed by Sheldon (1940), who described three general body types: *endomorphic,* "soft and round" persons with short, fat builds; *mesomorphic,* well-muscled, thick-chested, and broad-shouldered persons; and *ectomorphic,* tall and thin persons. Children seldom exhibit these three body builds in pure form, but every body contains all three components in varying degrees. Consequently, current classification systems expand on these forms with rating scales that incorporate all components. Body build is primarily of interest in determining exercise and sports participation.

Facial proportions. Facial proportions show characteristic changes during childhood. In infancy and early childhood the face is small in relation to the skull (Fig. 4-4). The size of the cranial vault reflects the advanced development of the brain. The brain has achieved 25% of its adult size at birth and 50% at the end of 1 year. Over 90% of the growth of the brain cavity has been reached by the end of the fifth year, and 98% has been achieved at age 15 years.

After the first year the facial skeleton grows more rapidly than the brain case. The principal growth occurs in the jaws as they enlarge to accommodate the teeth and in the muscles of mastication as they develop. The face grows first in width and then in length, so that the child's face appears to emerge from underneath the skull, particularly during adolescence.

The size of the face relative to the skull has implications for health in the infant and young child. The large, heavy cranium is the primary site of injury in falls. The changing dimensions of the face alter the diameter and angle of ear structures, particularly the external auditory meatus and the eustachian tube. The latter contributes significantly to the incidence of middle ear infection.

Posture. Posture is also altered by growth and maturation of various structures. Within the narrow confines of the uterus the prenatal posture is one of total flexion. The spine curves with the head and extremities bent upon the child. The bones in the vertebral column of the newborn form two primary curvatures, one in the thoracic region and one in the sacral region (Fig. 4-5, *A*). Both are forward, concave curvatures that rely largely on the shape of their component bones. The thoracic curve is relatively stable, and movement is limited in scope and amount by thin, intervertebral discs and oblique spinous processes. The sacral curve eventually becomes fused and permanently fixed.

As the infant gains head control, at approximately 3 months of age, a secondary curvature appears in the cervical region (Fig. 4-5, *B*). This curve, unlike the primary curvatures, is convex forward, and its mobility is maintained by thick intervertebral discs and the tension of muscles stretched across its convexity.

To maintain a sitting posture, another secondary curvature develops in the lumbar region (Fig. 4-5, *C*). Like the cervical curve, the lumbar curve is convex, mobile, depends largely on intervertebral discs, and is controlled by the large postural muscles of the spine. When children assume an upright posture in their initial efforts to walk, they compensate for a high center of gravity and the weight of a large liver by an exaggerated lumbar curvature, or *lordosis* (Fig. 4-5, *D*). With advancing skill in locomotion there is a gradual progression toward normal upright posture. When situations cause a delay in holding up the head or sitting, the secondary curvatures may fail to develop at the expected time.

Biologic Determinants of Growth and Development

A prominent feature of childhood and adolescence is physical growth. In some tissues growth is continuous (e.g., bone growth and dentition); in others significant alterations occur at specific stages (e.g., appearance of secondary sex characteristics). Satisfactory growth achievement is most commonly judged in terms of increase in body weight, height, and skeletal growth. Serial measurements taken over time and compared with standardized norms can assess a child's developmental progress with a high degree of confidence. Table 4-1 and Fig. 4-6 indicate the general trends in height and weight gain during childhood.

Height. Linear growth, or height, occurs almost entirely as a result of skeletal growth and is considered to be a stable measure of general growth. It is not uniform throughout life, but when maturation of the skeleton is complete, linear growth ceases. The maximum growth in length occurs before birth, but the newborn continues to grow at a rapid, though slower, rate. As the months pass, the growth rate rapidly decelerates. By 2 years of age children normally have achieved 50% of their adult height. By age 4 birth length has usually doubled.

At approximately 3 years of age the child begins a relatively stable and steady growth rate of 5 to 6 cm (2 to 2½ inches) per year that continues for the next 9 years. (Occasionally a child will exhibit a transitory midgrowth height increase at age 6 or 7.) This long midgrowth period is ended by a sudden and marked acceleration, the adolescent growth spurt. Although there is wide variation, this increase, which begins about ages 10½ to 11 in girls and 12½ to 13 in boys, lasts approximately 2 to 2½ years. During this

TABLE 4-1 General trends in height and weight gain during childhood

AGE	WEIGHT*	HEIGHT*
Infants		
Birth–6 months	Weekly gain: 140-200 g (5-7 oz) Birth weight doubles by end of first 4-7 months†	Monthly gain: 2.5 cm (1 inch)
6-12 months	Weight gain: 85-140 g (3-5 oz) Birth weight triples by end of first year	Monthly gain: 1.25 cm (½ inch) Birth length increases by approximately 50% by end of first year
Toddlers	Birth weight triples by 14-17 months† Birth weight quadruples by age 2½ Yearly gain: 2-3 kg (4½-6½ lb)	Height at age 2 is approximately 50% of eventual adult height Gain during second year: about 12 cm (4¾ inches) Gain during third year: about 6-8 cm (2⅜-3¼ inches)
Preschoolers	Yearly gain: 2-3 kg (4½-6½ lb)	Birth length doubles by age 4 Yearly gain: 5-7.5 cm (2-3 inches)
School-Age Children	Yearly gain: 2-3 kg (4½-6½ lb)	Yearly gain after age 7: 5 cm (2 inches) Birth length triples by about age 13
Pubertal Growth Spurt		
Females—10-14 years	Weight gain: 7-25 kg (15-55 lb) Mean: 17.5 kg (38⅛ lb)	Height gain: 5-25 cm (2-10 inches); approximately 95% of mature height achieved by onset of menarche or skeletal age of 13 Mean: 20.5 cm (8¼ inches)
Males—11-16 years	Weight gain: 7-30 kg (15-65 lb) Mean: 23.7 kg (52⅛ lb)	Height gain: 10-30 cm (4-12 inches); approximately 95% of mature height achieved by skeletal age of 15 years Mean: 27.5 cm (11 inches)

*Yearly height and weight gains for each age-group represent averaged estimates from a variety of sources.
†Jung and Czajka-Narins, 1985.

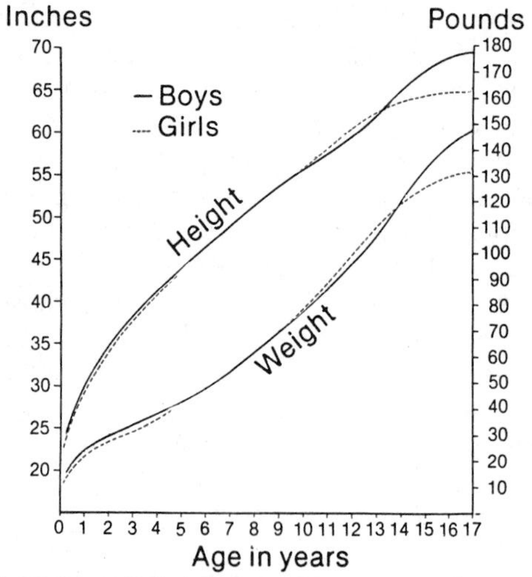

Fig. 4-6. Average height and weight curves for boys and girls. The earlier increase for girls at adolescence is clearly shown. Most girls are larger than boys between ages 11 and 13, probably a result of earlier influence of sex hormones on physical growth.

From Lowrey, G.H.: Growth and development of children, ed. 8, St. Louis, 1986, Mosby–Year Book, Inc.

Table 4-2 Percentage of mature height attained at different ages

CHRONOLOGIC AGE (YEARS)	PERCENT OF EVENTUAL HEIGHT	
	BOYS	GIRLS
1	42.2	44.7
2	49.5	52.8
3	53.8	57.0
4	58.0	61.8
5	61.8	66.2
6	65.2	70.3
7	69.0	74.0
8	72.0	77.5
9	75.0	80.7
10	78.0	84.4
11	81.1	88.4
12	84.2	92.9
13	87.3	96.5
14	91.5	98.3
15	96.1	99.1
16	98.3	99.6
17	99.3	100.0
18	99.8	100.0

From Bayley, N.: Growth curves of height and weight for boys and girls, scaled according to physical maturity, J. Pediatr. 48:187-194, 1956.

time a boy may add 20 cm (8 inches) to his height and a girl 16 cm (6½ inches). Usually, 98% of the terminal height is reached by age 16½ in girls but not until age 17¾ in boys (Table 4-2).

From analysis of data derived from longitudinal studies, it is possible to state the percentage of terminal height that has been achieved at any given age and to predict the future height of an individual from measurements taken in childhood. Predictions are of little value until the second year of life. By this time the child has frequently compensated for any deviations related to prematurity or other prenatal influences. However, children with lower birth weights are likely to remain shorter and lighter throughout childhood (Binkin and others, 1988). Variability in the onset of puberty may also alter the predictive value in this age-group.

Such predictions are valuable tools to help parents and their slow-maturing children accept the child's unique pattern of growth and to help these puzzled children understand why they are different from their taller age-mates. Predictions are sometimes useful in preventing possible disappointment in the preparation for occupations or careers that have height restrictions and require early beginning physical preparation (e.g., ballet dancing). More important, if parents are satisfied that a child's apparently small size merely reflects the normal expectations based on their own adult size, they will be less likely to force-feed the child, which can result in obesity or food refusal and poor appetite. For the young girl whose predicted adult height is excessively tall, this early indication provides time to initiate therapy, if advisable, and to help the child develop the capacity to deal with the potential problems associated with this trait.

Weight. At birth, weight is more variable than height and to a greater extent is a reflection of the intrauterine environment. The rate of weight gain increases rapidly for a short time after birth but soon decreases markedly. After the second year the "normal" rate of weight gain, just like the growth rate in height, assumes a steady annual increase—approximately 2 to 2.75 kg (4½ to 6 pounds) per year— until the adolescent growth spurt. The weight gain usually lags behind the gain in height by about 3 months.

Lifetime weight gain is subject to numerous intrinsic and extrinsic factors that are discussed as they apply to specific situations or conditions. Growth responses become apparent by changes in weight before they appear in other aspects of growth. Weight gain is usually considered to be an indication of satisfactory growth progress in a child and is probably the best index of nutrition and growth. However, it may be difficult to determine if this increase in weight is caused by healthy tissue development or by an unhealthy deposition of fat or accumulation of fluid.

Bone age and dentition. Both bone age determinations and state of dentition are used as indicators of growth. Since both are discussed elsewhere (for bone age, see below; see p. 117, Chapter 12, and Chapter 17 for dentition), neither is elaborated here.

Skeletal Growth and Maturation

Growth of the skeleton follows a genetically programmed developmental plan that not only furnishes the best indicator of general growth progress but also provides the best estimate of biologic age. Some degree of assessment can be achieved by observation of facial bone development (i.e., nasal bridge height, prominence of malar eminences, and

A 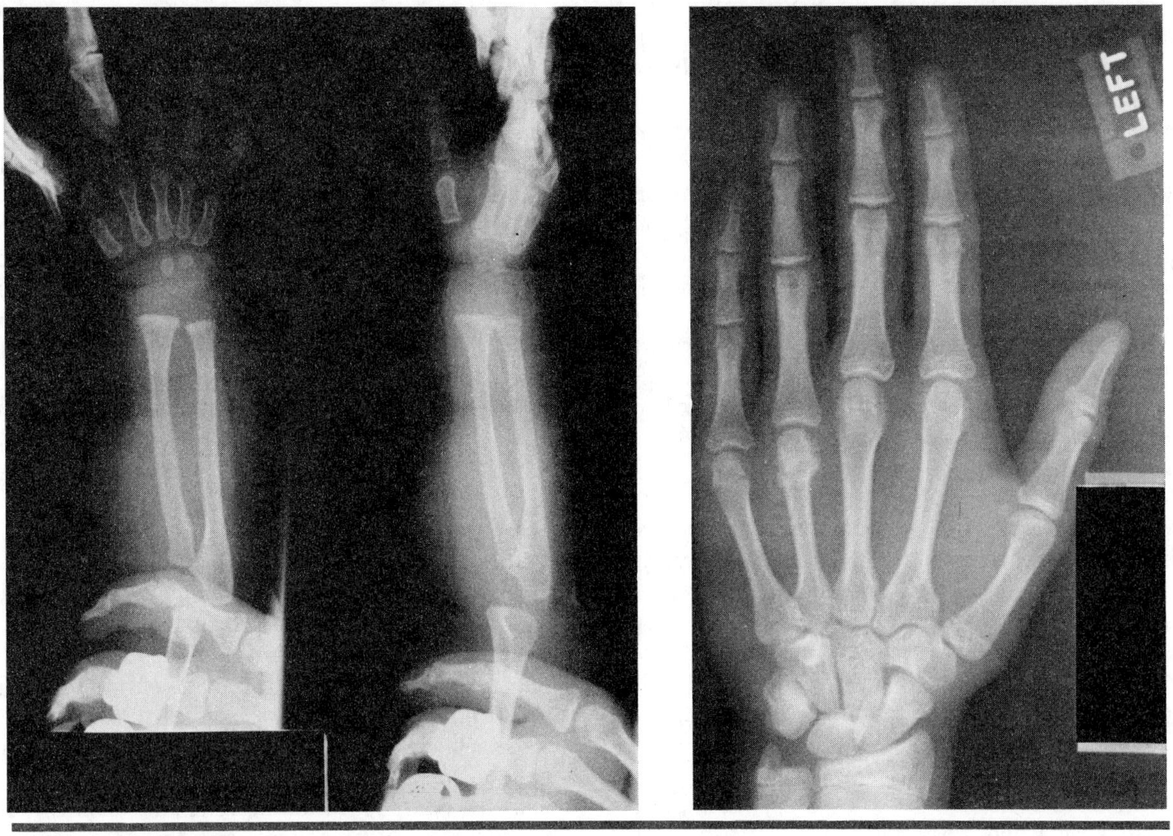 B

Fig. 4-7. Radiographs illustrating bone age in children. **A,** Eight-month-old (note complete ossification in adult fingers holding the child's arm). **B,** Fourteen-year-old, epiphyses visible.

mandibular size), but the most accurate measure of general development is the determination of osseous maturation by radiography. Skeletal age appears to correlate more closely with other measures of physiologic maturity (e.g., onset of menarche) than with chronologic age or height. This "bone age" is determined by comparing the mineralization of ossification centers and advancing bony form to age-related standards. Skeletal maturation begins with the appearance of centers of ossification in the embryo and ends when the last epiphysis is firmly fused to the shaft of its bone.

In the healthy child skeletal growth and development consist of two concurrent processes: (1) the creation of new cells and tissues (growth), and (2) the consolidation of these tissues into a permanent form (maturation). Early in fetal life closely packed connective tissue forms cartilage, which enlarges within the forming structures and builds successive layers on the surface of the mass. Bone formation begins during the second month of fetal life, when calcium salts are deposited in the intercellular substance (matrix) to form calcified cartilage first and then true bone. There are some differences in this bone formation. In small bones the bone continues to form in the center and cartilage continues to be laid down on the surfaces. Bones of the face and cranium are laid out in a tough membrane and directly ossified into bone during fetal life.

In long bones ossification takes place in two centers. It begins in the *diaphysis* (the long central portion of the bone) from a "primary" center and continues in the *epiphysis* (the end portions of the bone) at "secondary" centers of ossification. Situated between the diaphysis and the epiphysis, an epiphyseal cartilage plate unites with the diaphysis by columns of spongy tissue, the *metaphysis.* At this site the active growth in length takes place, and interference with this growth site by trauma or infection can result in deformity. Under the influence of hormones, principally pituitary growth hormone and thyroid hormone, bones increase in circumference by the formation of new bone tissue beneath the membrane surrounding the bone (periosteum) and in length by proliferation of cartilage.

Over the growth period of approximately 19 to 20 years, this development can be divided into three distinct but overlapping phases: (1) ossification of the diaphysis, (2) ossification of the epiphysis, and (3) invasion and subsequent replacement of growth cartilage plates with bony fusion of epiphysis and diaphysis. These changes do not take place in all bones simultaneously but appear in a specific order and at a specific time. Although the speed of bone growth and amount of maturity at specific ages vary from one child to another, the order of ossification is constant.

The first centers of ossification appear in the 2-month-old embryo, and at birth the number is approximately 400, about half the number at maturity. New centers appear at regular intervals during the growth period and provide the basis for assessment of bone age. Postnatally, at 5 to 6 months of age, the earliest centers to appear are those of the capitate and hamate bones in the wrist. Therefore radiographs of the hand and wrist provide the most useful areas for screening to determine skeletal age, especially before age 6 years (Fig. 4-7). These centers appear earlier in girls than in boys.

Skeletal development advances until maturity through growth of ossification centers and lengthening of long bones at the metaphysis and cartilage plates. Linear growth can continue as long as the epiphysis is separated from the diaphysis by the cartilage plate; when the cartilage disappears, the epiphysis unites with the diaphysis and growth ceases. Epiphyseal fusion also follows an orderly sequence; thus the timing of epiphyseal closure furnishes another medium for measuring skeletal age.

Neurologic Maturation

In contrast to other body tissues, which grow rapidly after birth, the nervous system grows proportionately more rapidly before birth. Two periods of rapid brain cell growth occur during fetal life: a dramatic increase in the number of neurons between 15 and 20 weeks of gestation, and another increase at 30 weeks, which extends to 1 year of age. The rapid growth of infancy continues during early childhood, then slows to a more gradual rate during later childhood and adolescence.

It is believed that no new nerve cells appear after the sixth month of fetal life. Postnatal growth consists of increasing the amount of cytoplasm around the nuclei of existing cells, increasing the number and intricacy of communications with other cells, and advancing their peripheral axions to keep pace with expanding body dimensions. This allows for increasingly complex movement and behavior. Neurophysiologic changes also provide the foundation for language, learning, and behavior development. Neurologic and electroencephalographic development are sometimes used as indicators of maturational age in the early weeks of life.

Brain. Brain volume is reflected in head circumference, which increases six times as much during the first year as it does in the second year of life (see Appendix C). One half of the postnatal brain growth is achieved by 1 year of age, 75% by age 3, and 90% by age 6. The brain comprises 12% of the body weight at birth, doubles in weight in the first year, and has tripled by age 5 or 6 years. Thereafter growth slows until the brain is only about 2% of total body weight in adulthood.

Surface configuration also changes with development. The early embryonic brain surface is smooth, but sulci deepen with advancing development throughout childhood. At birth the cortex is only about one half its adult thickness, resulting in very little cortical control over body movements at birth. Movements are guided principally by primitive reflexes (see Chapter 8). With advancing development and maturation the brain, through association pathways, exercises increasing control over much of reflex activity. This allows the growing child to perform progressively complex tasks requiring coordinated movements. Persistence of primitive reflexes may suggest defective cortical development.

Cortical control is closely associated with the acquisition of a myelin coating on the nerves. Although nerve fibers are able to conduct impulses without this myelin sheath, the impulses travel at a slower rate and with more likelihood of diffusion. Myelinization of the various nerve tracts in the central nervous system accelerates rapidly after birth and follows the cephalocaudal and proximodistal sequence, which allows progressively complex neuromotor function. Myelinization begins with spinal cord and cranial nerve fibers, followed by the brainstem and corticospinal tracts. Myelinization accelerates rapidly after birth and follows the cephalocaudal and proximodistal directional sequence, beginning with the spinal and cranial nerve fibers, followed by the brainstem and corticospinal tracts. In general the pathways concerned with sensation are myelinated before the motor pathways.

The acquisition of motor skills depends on this myelinization and maturation, and no amount of special training or practice will hasten the process. Most of the advancing performance of an infant is a direct result of brain development and depends only indirectly on environmental stimuli.

Spinal cord. The spinal cord also demonstrates alterations relative to the vertebral column during prenatal and early postnatal growth. In the embryo the spinal cord extends the entire length of the vertebral canal. However, because the vertebral column and the cord have different growth rates, the cord in the newborn ends at the level of the third and fourth lumbar vertebrae. As growth continues, the cord becomes higher in relation to the vertebrae until it ends at the level of the first lumbar vertebra in the adult (Fig. 4-8).

The disparity in growth rates also involves the spinal nerves attached to the cord. In the early developing embryo the spinal nerves are directed nearly horizontal to the intervertebral foramina, through which they emerge from the spinal column. At full growth the upper cervical nerves are still directed on a horizontal plane, but lower nerves become directed more and more obliquely downward toward their intervertebral foramina. The sacral and coccygeal nerves are so arranged in relation to one another and in a vertical direction that they resemble the arrangement of hairs on a horse's tail, hence the term "cauda equina."

Lymphoid Tissues

Lymphoid tissues contained in the lymph nodes, thymus, spleen, tonsils, adenoids, and blood lymphocytes follow a distinctive growth pattern unlike that of other body tissues. These tissues are small in relation to total body size, but they are well developed at birth. They increase rapidly to reach adult dimensions by 6 years of age and continue to grow. At about age 10 to 12 years the tissues reach a maximum development approximately twice their adult size, followed by a rapid decline to stable adult dimensions by the end of adolescence.

Lymph nodes are large, and the superficially located nodes are often palpable. The tonsils, massive during early

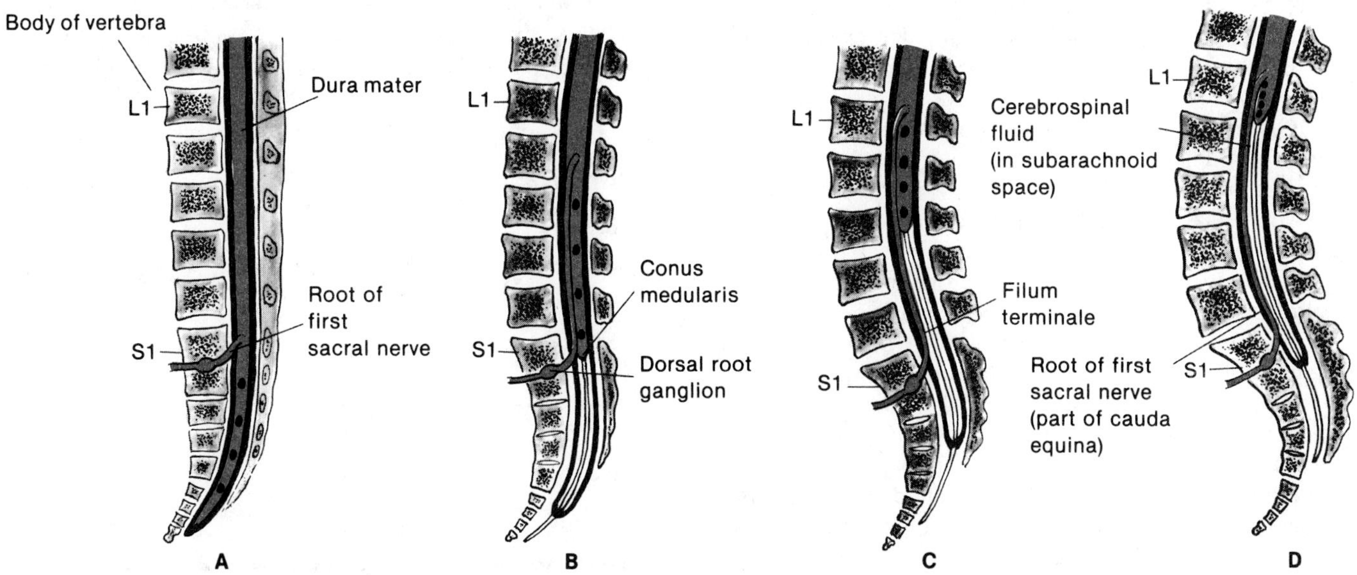

Fig. 4-8. Diagrams showing position of caudal end of spinal cord in relation to vertebral column and meninges at various stages of development. Increasing inclination of root of first sacral nerve is also illustrated. **A,** Eight weeks. **B,** Twenty-four weeks. **C,** Newborn. **D,** Adult. *L1,* First lumbar vertebra; *S1,* first sacral vertebra.

childhood, become inconspicuous in the adult. The thymus gland beneath the sternum, a prominent feature in infancy, may be impossible to detect in an adult. The growth pattern of lymphatic tissues parallels the development of immunity and probably reflects the repeated exposure to new infectious agents.

Dentition

The course of dentition is sometimes divided into four major stages: (1) growth, (2) calcification, (3) eruption, and (4) attrition. The primary teeth arise as outgrowths of the oral epithelium during the sixth week of embryonic life and begin to calcify during the fourth to sixth months. Tooth buds form at 10 different points in each arch and eventually become the enamel organs for the 20 primary (deciduous) teeth. All the buds are present at birth, but the amount of enamel laid down varies with each set of teeth.

Teeth are divided into quadrants of the mandible and maxilla and are named for their location in each quadrant of the dental arch, such as central incisor, lateral incisor, and first and second molars. Teeth are also named after their specific function in the mastication of food. The knifelike or scissorslike, central and lateral incisors cut the food. The single-pointed cuspids, also called *canines,* tear the food. The two premolars, called *bicuspids* because of their two-pointed crown, crush the food. The permanent molars, which have four or five cusps, grind the food.

The teeth and their care are discussed further in relation to time of eruption (see Chapters 12 and 17). Because of its relative regularity, the eruption of teeth is sometimes used as a criterion for developmental assessment, especially the 6-year molar, which seems to be the most universally consistent in timing. However, dental maturation does not correlate well with bone age and is less reliable as an index of biologic age. Retarded eruption is more common than accelerated eruption and may be caused by heredity or may indicate health problems such as endocrine disturbance, nutritional factors, or malposition of teeth.

Development of Organ Systems

All tissues and organ systems undergo changes during development. Some are striking; others are more subtle. Many have implications for assessment and care. Since the major importance of these changes relates to their dysfunction, the developmental characteristics of various systems and organs are discussed throughout the book as they relate to these areas. Physical characteristics and function of the body systems are described in relation to assessment (Chapter 7). Physical characteristics and physiologic changes that vary with age are included in age-group descriptions. For example, the relationship of surface area to body mass is of primary importance during very early development; physical characteristics related to hormonal changes are most significant during adolescence and are discussed as they apply to problems associated with this phase.

Catch-Up Growth

When there has been a secondary cause of growth deficiency, such as severe illness or acute malnutrition, recovery from the illness or the establishment of an adequate diet will produce a dramatic acceleration of the growth rate that usually continues until the child's individual growth pattern is resumed. Although the phenomenon has not been satisfactorily explained, during this period the biologic timing mechanism is apparently unaffected. When the problem is corrected, children tend to catch up to the developmental stage at which they would be normally. For example, newborns exhibit a transitory weight loss shortly after birth and then rapidly regain the weight. In addition, during the early months of life the developmental achievements of prematurely born infants lag behind those of full-term infants of the same chronologic age. The deficit in the attainment of developmental landmarks closely corresponds to the degree of prematurity; however, the differences become less conspicuous as the infant matures. Children usually catch up to age-mates during the preschool years.

Catch-up growth involves growth in both length and weight, but the extent of inadequacy depends on the timing, severity, duration, and character of the source of the secondary deficiency. In general, any serious interruption in progress will have an impact, although small, on the ultimate size of the individual. Growth retardation that is prolonged or that occurs during a sensitive period may not be compensated. Catch-up growth applies to those tissues that can increase in size and to those that still retain the capacity to increase cell numbers. Growth deficiency in tissues such as the brain results in a permanent deficit when the problem occurs during a sensitive period in its development.

PHYSIOLOGIC CHANGES

Physiologic changes that take place in all organs and systems are discussed as they relate to dysfunction. Others, such as pulse and respiratory rates and blood pressure, are an integral part of physical assessment (see Chapter 7). In addition, there are changes in basic functions including metabolism, temperature, and patterns of sleep and rest.

Metabolism

Metabolism—all chemical and energy transformations in the body—is affected by an assortment of intrinsic and extrinsic factors (e.g., body size, age, sex, emotions, exercise, climate, hormones, environmental temperature). Therefore metabolic needs vary among individuals and within each individual. The rate of metabolism when the body is at rest (basal metabolic rate, or BMR) demonstrates a distinctive change throughout childhood. Highest in the newborn infant, BMR closely relates to the proportion of surface area to body mass, which changes as the body increases in size. Most authorities consider surface area to be the best estimate of the amount of functioning protoplasm present in the organism (see Fig. 27-19 for computation of surface area). In both sexes the proportion decreases progressively to maturity. The BMR is slightly higher in boys at all ages and further increases during pubescence over that in girls.

The rate of metabolism determines the caloric requirements of the child. The basal energy requirement of infants is about 108 kcal/kg of body weight and decreases to 40 to 45 kcal/kg at maturity (Table 4-3). The daily water requirements show a similar modification. Children's energy needs vary considerably at different ages and with changing circumstances. The greatest proportion of calories in infancy is used for basal metabolic needs and growth.

Table 4-3 Recommended daily requirements for calories and protein through adolescence*

AGE (YEARS)	ENERGY ALLOWANCE (kcal/kg)	PROTEIN (g)
Infants		
0-½	108	13
½-1	98	14
Children		
1-3	102	16
4-6	90	24
7-10	70	28
Males		
11-14	55	45
15-18	45	49
Females		
11-14	47	46
15-18	40	44

*Data from Food and Nutrition Board: Recommended daily allowances, ed. 10, Washington, DC, 1989, National Academy Press.

The energy requirement to build tissue steadily decreases with age, following the general growth curve; however, exercise needs vary with the individual child and may be considerably more. For short periods (e.g., during strenuous exercise) and more prolonged periods (e.g., illness), the needs can be very high. For example, each degree of fever increases the basal metabolism 10% with a corresponding fluid requirement. The *specific dynamic action* (SDA) refers to the energy required to ingest and assimilate food. A very small portion of ingested calories is lost in stools during normal metabolism, but much more may be lost in this way when the child suffers from conditions that impair digestion or absorption.

Temperature

Body temperature, reflecting metabolism, displays the same decrement from infancy to maturity (see inside front cover). Following the unstable regulatory ability in the neonatal period, heat production steadily declines as the infant grows into childhood. Individual differences of 0.5° to 1° F are normal, and occasionally a child normally displays an unusually high or low temperature. Beginning at approximately 12 years of age, girls display a temperature that remains relatively stable, while the temperature in boys continues to fall for a few years longer. Females maintain a temperature slightly above that of males throughout life.

Even with improved temperature regulation, infants and young children are highly susceptible to temperature fluctuations. Body temperature responds to changes in environmental temperature and is increased with active exercise, crying, and emotional upset. Infections can cause a higher and more rapid temperature increase in infants and young children than in older children. In relation to body weight, an infant produces more heat per unit than children near maturity. Consequently, during active play or when heavily clothed, an infant or small child is likely to become overheated.

Motor Development

Closely allied to biologic development and maturation is the development of basic motor responses. Children's ability to perform motor functions depends on the state of maturation of bones, muscles, and the nervous system and follows the patterns of development described earlier in the chapter. As in all maturation processes motor behavior follows a developmental sequence (Box 4-2).

SLEEP AND REST

Sleep, a protective function in all organisms, allows for repair and recovery of tissues following activity. As in most aspects of development, a wide variation exists among individual children and ages of children in the amount and distribution of sleep. As the child matures, not only does a change occur in the quantity of time spent in sleep but also in the quality of that sleep. Also, family influences, social expectations, and cultural variations in sleep patterns must be considered when analyzing sleep problems.

Time and Quality of Sleep

The length of time spent in sleep decreases throughout childhood. Newborns sleep much of the time not occupied with feeding and other aspects of their care. Larger newborns sleep for longer periods than smaller ones because of their larger stomach capacity. As infants mature total time spent in sleep gradually decreases, and they remain awake for longer periods and sleep longer at night. During the later part of the first year, most children sleep through the night and take one or two naps during the day. By the time they are 1½ years old, most children have eliminated the second nap. After age 3 years children have usually given up daytime naps, except in those cultures in which an afternoon nap or siesta is customary. From ages 4 to 10 sleep time declines slightly, then increases somewhat during the pubertal growth spurt. The changes in length of sleep in relation to age are illustrated in Fig. 4-9.

Alterations take place in the percentage of sleep time spent in each of the two different identified sleep cycles: (1) active sleep characterized by irregular pulse and expirations, many body movements, and short, rapid eye movements (paradoxic, or REM, sleep); and (2) quiet sleep in which breathing and heartbeat are regular and body and eye movements are absent (slow-wave, or non-REM, sleep).

REM sleep is characterized by activity. More oxygen is used, blood flow to the brain is increased, the temperature rises, and brain waves show increased activity. Sensory paths transmit inpulses in much the same manner as during waking hours. Later these visual, auditory, and vestibular stimuli are believed to be incorporated by the brain into dream imagery.

During non-REM sleep the heart rate and breathing pattern are regular, and this cycle is believed to provide most of the restorative functions attributed to sleep. Four stages of non-REM sleep are described. Stage 1 consists of drowsiness with decreasing awareness of the external world. Sleep progresses from drowsiness through stage 2, from which a sleeping person can be easily wakened and, if wakened, may not admit to having been asleep. Sleep in stage 3 becomes increasingly deep, breathing and heart rate are very stable, muscles are relaxed, and brain waves are very slow. Stage 4 is the deepest sleep, from which it is difficult to be roused except by important stimuli. A child can be moved from one place to another without waking. Making the difficult transition to wakefulness from stage 4 non-REM sleep is significant in some sleep disorders of children.

The sleep of newborns consists of approximately 50% REM sleep, in contrast to approximately 20% in older children. The large amount of active REM sleep in early infancy is believed to serve as an endogenous source of stimulation to the higher brain centers and is important for normal development at a time when exogenous sources are minimal because of the short periods of arousal. REM sleep is probably more important in early months and may be necessary for development of higher brain centers. The decrease in REM sleep as development progresses may indicate that with longer periods of wakefulness, the more mature brain has less need for this endogenous stimulation. The deep, restful non-REM sleep increases proportionately with age; children who have recently given up napping take a longer time to get into REM sleep during the initial sleep cycle than do either older or younger children, which suggests they are more fatigued.

Sleep Cycles

Once non-REM sleep has developed, a single nighttime sleep period contains all four stages of sleep and is arranged in cycles, which remain constant throughout life. However, the length of the sleep cycles and the amounts of REM and non-REM sleep vary among individuals and developmental ages. The length of a sleep cycle (time between

Box 4-2 DEVELOPMENT OF MOTOR BEHAVIORS

Reflexive or rudimentary movements are acquired during infancy and form the foundation of all other movements, including sitting, crawling, creeping, reaching, standing, and walking.

General fundamental skills are common to all children and develop during early childhood. The order in which both rudimentary and fundamental skills normally develop is the same for all children, but there is wide variation in children's abilities to perform skills. Fundamental skills include such activities as running, jumping, balancing, catching, and throwing.

Specific skills develop during later childhood as general fundamental skills become more refined, fluid, and automatic. There is greater emphasis on form, accuracy, and adaptability and children begin to apply these skills to sports and other activities that require body movement.

Specialized skills evolve slowly from late childhood through adolescence and depend on the amount of repetition and concentrated application.

Data from Zaichkowsky, L.D., Zaichkowsky, L.B., and Martinek, T.J.: Growth and development: the child and physical activity, St. Louis, 1980, Mosby–Year Book, Inc.

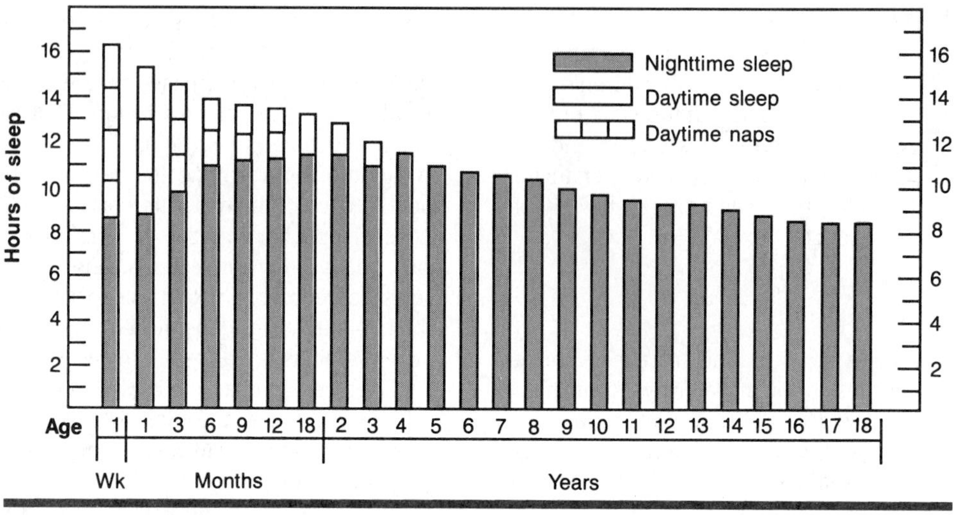

Fig. 4-9. Changes in number of hours of sleep with increasing age.
Modified from Ferber, R.: Solve your child's sleep problems, New York, 1985, Simon & Schuster.

two consecutive appearances of the same sleep state) increases with age. For example, the length of a sleep cycle in the newborn infant increases from about 50 minutes to about 90 in adolescence. The amount of stage 4 non-REM sleep also decreases but accounts for about 25% of a child's total sleep at all ages.

Partial waking is also characteristic of normal sleep. After about 1 hour of stage 4 sleep the child will arouse for a brief period, which will last a few seconds or up to several minutes. During this waking period the child may exhibit a variety of behaviors. Mild behaviors include rubbing the face, turning over, brief crying, adjusting covers, looking around, and/or unintelligible speech. The child may open the eyes or sit up briefly before returning to sleep. More conspicuous behaviors include sleepwalking, confused threshing, or bedwetting. Periodic wakenings are normally followed by rapid return to sleep and take place several times during the sleep period. They should not be mistaken for sleeplessness. (See Chapters 12, 15, and 17 for a discussion of sleep disturbances.)

TEMPERAMENT

Temperament is defined as "the manner of thinking, behaving, or reacting characteristic of an individual" (Chess and Thomas, 1985) and refers to the way a person deals with life. From the time of birth, children exhibit marked individual differences in the way they respond to their environment. These differences significantly influence the way others, particularly parents, respond to them and their needs. Temperament is a categoric term with no implications of good or bad, and without etiologic connections, and as with other characteristics, it is influenced by the environment as development progresses.

A genetic basis has been suggested for some differences in temperament. It has been found from studies of young children that identical twins are more alike than fraternal twins in temperamental attributes (Goldsmith and Gottesman, 1981; Matheny, 1980). Since temperament is identified primarily by parental perceptions, a child described as difficult at one time may be reported as easy at a later time. Parental relationships with a child can strongly affect behavior. As parental competency increases, the child's behavior may be less difficult or may appear easier to the parent.

Box 4-3 ATTRIBUTES OF TEMPERAMENT

Activity—level of physical motion during activity, such as sleep, eating, play, dressing, and bathing.
Rhythmicity—regularity in the timing of physiologic functions, such as hunger, sleep, and elimination.
Approach-withdrawal—nature of initial responses to a new stimulus, such as people, situations, places, foods, toys, and procedures. *Approach* responses are positive, displayed by activity or expression; *withdrawal* responses are negative expressions or behaviors.
Adaptability—ease or difficulty with which the child adapts or adjusts to new or altered situations.
Threshold of responsiveness (sensory threshold)—amount of stimulation, such as sounds or light, required to evoke a response in the child.
Intensity of reaction—energy level of the child's reactions, regardless of quality or direction.
Mood—amount of pleasant, happy, friendly behavior compared with unpleasant, unhappy, crying, unfriendly behavior exhibited by the child in various situations.
Distractibility—ease with which a child's attention or direction of behavior can be diverted by external stimuli.
Attention span and persistence—length of time a child pursues a given activity *(attention)* and the continuation of an activity in spite of obstacles *(persistence)*.

Characteristics of Temperament

The characteristics of behavioral individuality, derived from parental interviews, were identified, categorized, and rated in the New York Longitudinal Study (NYLS) of child behavior. The temperamental attributes established from analysis of the information are outlined in Box 4-3 (Chess and Thomas, 1983).

Categories of Temperament

Further analysis of the NYLS data revealed that most of the behavior characteristics cluster in constellations or combinations. For example, highly active children are frequently irritable and irregular in behaviors such as sleeping, feeding, and elimination, whereas passive children are more likely to be good natured and regular in their habits. These temperamental patterns appear to persist over time and can affect children's adjustment to a variety of settings and situations throughout childhood.

From these observations, most children can be placed in one of three common categories based on their overall pattern of temperamental attributes. However, there are wide ranges in degree of manifestations, and varying combinations can be observed within normal limits. Approximately 30% of children do not appear in any of the following three groups (Chess and Thomas, 1983):

1. **The easy child.** Easygoing children are even-tempered, regular, and predictable in their habits, and have a positive approach to new stimuli. They are open and adaptable to change, and display a mild to moderately intense mood that is typically positive. Approximately 40% of NYLS children fall into this category.
2. **The difficult child.** Difficult children are highly active, irritable, and irregular in their habits. Negative withdrawal responses are typical, and they require a more structured environment. These children adapt slowly to new routines, people, or situations. Mood expressions are usually intense and primarily negative. They exhibit frequent periods of crying, and frustration often produces violent tantrums. This group comprises about 10% of the NYLS children.
3. **The slow-to-warm-up child.** Slow-to-warm-up children typically react negatively and with mild intensity to new stimuli and, unless pressured, adapt slowly with repeated contact. They respond with only mild but passive resistance to novelty or changes in routine. They are quite inactive and moody but show only moderate irregularity in functions. Fifteen percent of children in the NYLS studies demonstrate this temperament pattern.

Significance of Temperament

Observations indicate that children who display the difficult or slow-to-warm-up patterns of behavior are more vulnerable to the development of behavior problems in early and middle childhood. Any child can develop behavior problems if there is dissonance between the child's temperament and the environment. Demands for change and adaptation that are in conflict with children's capacities can become excessively stressful. However, authorities emphasize that it is not children's temperament patterns that place them at risk but the degree of *fit* between children and their environment, specifically their parents, that determines the degree of vulnerability. The greater the dissonance between the child's temperament and the ability of the parents to accept and deal with the behavior, the greater the likelihood of subsequent behavior problems (Chess and Thomas, 1983). (See Failure to Thrive, Chapter 13.)

Early identification of temperament provides a useful tool for caregivers in anticipating probable areas of difficulty or risk associated with development. For example, "difficult" children may be prone to colic in infancy, active children require more vigilance to prevent injury, and school entry will require different approaches for children with different temperaments.

Several parental questionnaires have been devised to facilitate assessment of temperament. Nurses who employ these assessment tools are better able to help parents interpret their children's behavior and to provide anticipatory guidance regarding numerous aspects of childrearing. The concept of temperament is also discussed in relation to child development at various ages and coping with the experiences of hospitalization. The most commonly used questionnaires for assessing infant and child temperament are those developed by Carey and McDevitt (Carey and McDevitt, 1978; Fullard, McDevitt, and Carey, 1984; Hegvik, McDevitt, and Carey, 1982).

DEVELOPMENT OF MENTAL FUNCTION AND PERSONALITY

Personality and cognitive skills develop in much the same manner as biologic growth—new accomplishments build on previously mastered skills. Many aspects depend on physical growth and maturation. This is not a comprehensive account of the multiple facets of personality and behavior development. Many aspects are integrated with the child's emotional and social development in later discussion of various age-groups. Table 4-4 summarizes some of the developmental theories.

THEORETIC FOUNDATIONS OF PERSONALITY DEVELOPMENT

According to Freud, all human behavior is energized by psychodynamic forces, and this psychic energy is divided among three components of personality: the id, the ego, and the superego. The *id* is the inborn component that is driven by instincts. The id obeys the pleasure principle of immediate gratification of needs regardless of whether the object or action can actually do so. The *ego* serves the reality principle. It functions as the conscious or controlling self that is able to find realistic means for gratifying the instincts while blocking the irrational thinking of the id. The *superego* functions as the moral arbitrator and represents the ideal. It is the mechanism that prevents individuals from expressing undesirable instincts that might threaten the social order.

TABLE 4-4 Summary of personality, moral, and cognitive development theories

STAGE/age	RADIUS OF SIGNIFICANT RELATIONSHIPS (SULLIVAN)	PSYCHOSEXUAL STAGES (FREUD)	PSYCHOSOCIAL STAGES (ERIKSON)	COGNITIVE STAGES (PIAGET)	MORAL JUDGMENT STAGES (KOHLBERG)
I Infancy Birth to 1 year	Maternal person (unipolar-bipolar)	Oral sensory	Trust vs mistrust	Sensorimotor (birth to 18 months)	
II Toddlerhood 1-3 years	Parental persons (tripolar)	Anal-urethral	Autonomy vs shame and doubt	Preoperational thought, preconceptual phase (transductive reasoning) (e.g., specific to specific) (2-4 years)	Preconventional (premoral) level Punishment and obedience orientation
III Early childhood 3-6 years	Basic family	Phallic-locomotion	Initiative vs guilt	Preoperational thought, intuitive phase (transductive reasoning) (4-7 years)	Preconventional (premoral) level Naive instrumental orientation
IV Middle childhood 6-12 years	Neighborhood, school	Latency	Industry vs inferiority	Concrete operations (inductive reasoning and beginning logic)	Conventional level Good-boy, nice-girl orientation Law-and-order orientation
V Adolescence 13-19 years	Peer groups and outgroups Models of leadership Partners in friendship, sex, competition, cooperation	Genitality	Identity and repudiation vs identity confusion	Formal operations (deductive and abstract reasoning)	Postconventional or principled level Social-contract orientation Universal ethical principle orientation (no longer included in revised theory)
VI Early adulthood	Divided labor and shared household		Intimacy and solidarity vs isolation		
VII Young and middle adulthood	Mankind "My kind"		Generativity vs self-absorption		
VIII Later adulthood			Ego integrity vs despair		

Psychosexual Development (Freud)

Freud also considered the sexual instincts to be significant in the development of the personality. However, he used the term *psychosexual* to describe any *sensual pleasure.* Many simple body functions, considered asexual in the usual sense, were viewed as "erotic" activities by Freud and these activities were thought to be motivated by the general life force he called the *sex instinct.* Personality development was viewed as the growth or unfolding of these instincts.

According to Freud's theory, during childhood certain regions of the body assume a prominent psychologic significance as the source of new pleasures, and new conflicts gradually shift from one part of the body to another at particular stages of development. Each stage builds on the previous one, and the maturation of the sex instinct leaves distinct imprints on the developing psyche. Freud believed that children who encounter severe conflicts at any stage may be reluctant to move to the next phase, causing further development to be arrested or impaired. In addition, they may retreat to earlier stages of development if they experience too much anxiety or too many conflicts at a subsequent stage of development.

Although Freud was the first to provide a systematic explanation for human behavior, the theory focuses on a single motive governing behavior—the desire to satisfy biologic needs (dominated by sexual instincts), thereby releasing tensions. The theory, derived from retrospective studies of adults and not from direct observation, is difficult to verify or disconfirm and is of little value in predicting future behaviors.

Oral stage (birth to 1 year). During infancy the major source of pleasure seeking centers on oral activities such as sucking, biting, chewing, and vocalizing. Children may prefer one of these practices over the others, and the preferred method of oral gratification can provide some indication of the personality they develop. Examples of oral personality traits are pessimism or optimism, determination or submission, gullibility or suspiciousness, admiration or envy, and cockiness or self-belittlement (DiCaprio, 1983).

Anal stage (1 to 3 years). Interest during the second year of life centers on the anal region as sphincter muscles develop and children are able to withhold or expel fecal material at will. At this stage the climate surrounding toilet training can have lasting effects on children's personalities. Examples of anal personality traits are stinginess or overgenerosity, constrictedness or expansiveness, rigid punctuality or tardiness, stubbornness or acquiescence, and orderliness or messiness.

Phallic stage (3 to 6 years). During the phallic stage the genitals become an interesting and sensitive area of the body. Children recognize differences between the sexes and become curious about the dissimilarities. This is the period associated with the controversial issues of the Oedipus and Electra complexes, penis envy, and castration anxiety. Examples of phallic personality traits are brashness or bashfulness, stylishness or plainness, gaiety or sadness, blind courage or timidity, and gregariousness or isolationism.

Latency period (6 to 12 years). During the latency period children elaborate on previously acquired traits and skills. Physical and psychic energy are channeled into acquisition of knowledge and vigorous play.

Genital stage (age 12 and over). The last significant stage begins at puberty with maturation of the reproductive system and production of sex hormones. The genital organs become the major source of sexual tensions and pleasures, but energies are also invested in forming friendships and preparation for marriage.

Psychosocial Development (Erikson)

The theory of personality development advanced by Erikson (1963) is the most widely accepted and used. Although built on Freudian theory, it emphasizes a healthy personality as opposed to a pathologic approach. It involves predictable age-related stages during which specific changes are assumed to take place. Erikson also uses the biologic concepts of critical periods and epigenesis, describing key conflicts or core problems the individual strives to master during critical periods in personality development. Successful completion or mastery of each of these core conflicts is built on the satisfactory completion or mastery of the previous core conflict.

At each stage of psychosocial development, children are confronted with a unique problem requiring the integration of personal needs and skills with social demands and cultural expectations. Erikson refers to the individual's efforts to adjust as a *crisis.* Crisis in this context implies the normal stresses as opposed to an extraordinary set of events. The tension produced by societal demands must be reduced in order that the favorable outcome can be achieved.

Each psychosocial stage has two components, the favorable and unfavorable aspects of the core conflict, and progress to the next stage depends on resolution of this conflict. No core conflict is ever mastered completely but remains a recurrent problem throughout life. No life situation is ever secure. Each new situation presents the conflict in a new form. For example, when children who have satisfactorily achieved a sense of trust encounter a new experience (e.g., hospitalization), they must again develop a sense of trust in those responsible for their care in order to master the situation.

Erikson's eight stages or "psychosocial crises" are outlined in the following segments. The lasting outcome, or ego quality (Erikson, 1978), of each stage, achieved through a central process (Newman and Newman, 1984), provides the resources for coping. Specific persons in the environment become the key socializing agents in the process (Shaffer, 1984). All eight stages are included, since the later age stages are important to family functions and have an impact on the development of children.

Although Erikson's theory stresses the rational and adaptive nature of persons, it does not clearly indicate the kinds of experiences needed to cope with and resolve the various crises. There is no concern for individual differences. Regardless of its shortcomings, Erikson's theory provides an excellent framework for explaining children's behaviors in mastering developmental tasks.

Trust vs mistrust (birth to 1 year). The first and most important attribute of a healthy personality to develop is a basic trust. Establishment of basic trust dominates the first year of life and describes all the child's satisfying experiences at this age. Corresponding to Freud's oral stage, it is a time of "getting" and "taking in" through all the senses. It exists only in relation to something or someone; therefore consistent, loving care by a mothering person is essential to development of trust. *Mistrust* develops when trust-promoting experiences are deficient or lacking or when basic needs are inconsistently or inadequately met. Shreds of mistrust are sprinkled throughout the personality, but through the process of mutuality with the primary caregiver the individual develops the ego quality *hope*, an enduring belief that one can attain one's deep and essential wishes. The result is faith and optimism.

Autonomy vs shame and doubt (1 to 3 years). Corresponding to Freud's anal stage, the problem of autonomy can be symbolized by the holding on and letting go of the sphincter muscles. The development of autonomy during the toddler period is centered around children's increasing ability to control their bodies, themselves, and their environment. They want to use their powers to do things for themselves, using their newly acquired motor skills of walking, climbing, and manipulating and mental powers of selection and decision making. They also learn to conform to social rules. Negative feelings of *doubt* and *shame* arise when children are made to feel small and self-conscious, when their choices are disastrous, when others shame them, or when they are forced to be dependent in areas in which they are capable of assuming control. They come to doubt their abilities. The central process for achieving autonomy is imitation, and the key socializing agents are the parents. The favorable outcomes are *self-control* and *willpower.*

Initiative vs guilt (3 to 6 years). The stage of industry corresponds to Freud's phallic stage and is characterized by vigorous, intrusive behavior, enterprise, and a strong imagination. Children explore the physical world with all their senses and powers. They develop a conscience. No longer guided only by outsiders, children respond to an inner voice that warns and threatens. Children sometimes undertake goals or activities that are in conflict with those of parents or others, and being made to feel that their activities or imaginings are bad produces a sense of *guilt.* Excessive guilt inhibits initiative, but children must learn to retain a sense of initiative without impinging on the rights and privileges of others. The central process is identification, and the key socializing agent is the family. The lasting outcomes are *direction* and *purpose;* the courage to imagine and pursue is a valued goal.

Industry vs inferiority (6 to 12 years). This stage correlates with the latency period of Freud. Having achieved the more crucial stages in personality development, children are now ready to be workers and producers. They want to engage in tasks and activities they can carry through to completion; they need and want real achievement. Children learn to compete and to cooperate with others, and they learn the rules. When children succeed in their efforts they develop a sense of mastery and self-assurance. It is a decisive period in their social relationships with others. Feelings of inadequacy and *inferiority* may develop if too much is expected of them or if they believe that they cannot measure up to the standards set for them by others. Without experiencing mastery children will shun new activities. The key socializing agents are teachers and peers, and the central process is education. The ego quality developed from a sense of industry is *competence,* the free exercise of skill and intelligence in the completion of tasks.

Identity vs role confusion (12 to 18 years). Corresponding to Freud's genital stage, the development of identity is characterized by rapid and marked physical changes. Previous trust in their bodies shaken, children become overly preoccupied with the way they appear in the eyes of others as compared with their own self-concept. Adolescents struggle to fit the roles they have played and those they hope to play with the current roles and fashions adopted by their peers, to integrate their concepts and values with those of society, and to come to a decision regarding an occupation. Inability to solve the core conflict results in *role confusion.* The central processes are peer pressure and role experimentation; the key socializing agent is the society of peers. The outcome of successful mastery is devotion and *fidelity,* the ability to sustain loyalties freely committed in early adolescence to others and loyalties freely pledged in later adolescence to values and ideologies.

Intimacy vs isolation (early adulthood). A sense of intimacy is established on a sense of identity. *Intimacy* is the capacity to develop an intimate love relationship with another and intimate interpersonal relationships with friends, partners, and other significant persons. Without intimacy the individual feels *isolated* and alone. The central process is mutuality among peers, and the key socializing agents are lovers, spouses, and close friends. The favorable outcome is affiliation and *love,* the capacity for mutuality that transcends childhood dependency.

Generativity vs stagnation (young and middle adulthood). Central to this stage of development is the creation and care of the next generation. The essential element is to nourish and nurture. It may be directed toward one's own children, children of others, or other products of creativity. The individual who fails in this component of personality development becomes self-absorbed and *stagnant.* The key socializing agents are the spouse, children, and cultural norms, and the central process is person-environment fit and creativity. The favorable outcome is production and *care,* the commitment to be concerned for what has been generated.

Ego integrity vs despair (old age). A sense of integrity results from satisfaction with life and acceptance of what has been; *despair* arises from remorse for what might have been. The central process is introspection, and the favorable outcome is renunciation and *wisdom,* the detached yet active concern with life in the face of death.

Interpersonal Development (Sullivan)

Also built on Freudian theory, the interpersonal development theory by Sullivan (1953) emphasizes the interpersonal relationships in which children engage and the importance of social approval and disapproval in developing a self-concept. What children interpret as unfavorable interactions result in tension and anxiety; the outcome of favorable relationships is a sense of comfort and security. Through repeated interactions children acquire a repertoire of actions and behaviors that produce a feeling of security and avoid anxiety.

The first interactions are those between infants and their "mothering" figure, usually the mother, who gratifies and comforts. This bipolar relationship gradually extends to include others in the family group. Between the ages of 2 and 5, children not only become more outgoing but also direct their social gestures to a wider audience outside but near the home and family, such as relatives and neighborhood children. They engage in peer play, family events, and other aspects of social learning. Observational studies suggest that 2- to 3-year-olds are more likely than older children to remain near an adult and to seek physical affection, while the sociable behaviors of 4- to 5-year-olds normally consist of playful bids for attention or approval that are directed at peers rather than adults.

During the school years children enter into a wider range of relationships with other persons and authority figures at school and in the community. They develop "chumships," the special relationship between two peers—the shared intimacy and common interests of genuine friendships that are lacking in earlier relationships. Personal identity in adolescence is an outgrowth of intimate relationships, first with friends of the same sex, then with friends of the opposite sex.

Although Sullivan's theory recognizes the importance of environment in development and has some predictive value, it does not recognize the biologic maturation process.

THEORETIC FOUNDATIONS OF MENTAL DEVELOPMENT

The term *cognition* refers to the process by which developing individuals become acquainted with the world and the objects it contains. Children are born with inherited potentialities for intellectual growth, but they must develop into that potential through interaction with the environment. By assimilating information through the senses, processing it, and acting on it, they come to understand relationships between objects and between themselves and their world. With cognitive development, children acquire the ability to reason abstractly, to think in a logical manner, and to organize intellectual functions or performances into higher-order structures.

Cognitive Development (Piaget)

Cognitive development consists of age-related changes that occur in mental activities. The best-known theory regarding children's thinking, and a more comprehensive developmental theory than those already described, has been developed by the Swiss psychologist Jean Piaget (1969). He believes intelligence enables individuals to make adaptations to the environment that increase the probability of survival and that through their behavior individuals establish and maintain equilibrium with the environment.

Piaget proposes three stages of reasoning: (1) *intuitive,* (2) *concrete operational,* and (3) *formal operational.* When they enter the stage of concrete logical thought at about age 7 years, children are able to make logical inferences, classify, and deal with quantitative relationships about concrete things. Not until adolescence are they able to reason abstractly with any degree of competence.

According to Piaget, children proceed through the stages of mental activity in an orderly and sequential manner. The mechanisms that enable them to adapt to new situations and to move from one stage to the next are assimilation and accommodation. By *assimilation* children incorporate new knowledge, skills, ideas, and insights into cognitive schemes (Piaget uses the term *schema**) already familiar to them. To new situations that do not fit into an established schema, children *accommodate.* They change and organize existing schemas to solve more difficult tasks and form new schemas. Children's understanding of a new experience is based on all relevant previous experiences. They achieve equilibrium over and over again by applying schemas already available to them. Thus children achieve an accurate understanding of reality and come to deal with increasingly complex problems in an increasingly effective manner.

One of the most prominent criticisms of Piaget's theory is that it ignores the important concept of unconscious motivation and its impact on behavior. Nor does it account for individual differences and unevenness in cognitive development—some children demonstrate more advanced behavior in one area than in another. Although it emphasizes biologic factors in human development, Piaget's theory provides one of the dominant frameworks for understanding children's thinking. Piaget was very conservative in his descriptions of children's abilities. Recent studies indicate that children, especially preschool children, are capable of more advanced thought than Piaget acknowledged.

Development of logical thinking. Piaget believes there are four major stages in the development of logical thinking. Each is derived from and builds on the accomplishments of the previous stage in a continuous, orderly process. The course of intellectual development is both maturational and invariant and is divided into the following periods, subperiods, and stages (ages are approximate).

Sensorimotor (birth to 2 years). The sensorimotor stage of intellectual development consists of six substages (see Chapter 12) that are governed by sensations through which simple learning takes place. Children progress from reflex activity through simple repetitive behaviors to imitative behavior. They develop a sense of "cause and effect" as they direct behavior toward objects and solve problems primarily through trial and error. They display a high level of curiosity, experimentation, and enjoyment of novelty. As a result of interactions with their environment, children begin to develop a sense of self as they are able to differentiate themselves from their environment.

Children become aware that an object has *permanence*, that it exists even though it is no longer visible. The awareness of object permanence is extremely important because it is a prerequisite for all other mental activity. All concepts begin with or involve objects in one way or another. Toward the end of the sensorimotor period children begin to use language, and representational thought appears as they imitate the behavior of others, even in the absence of these other persons.

Preoperational (2 to 7 years). The predominant characteristic of this period of intellectual development is *egocentricity.* Egocentricity in this sense does not mean selfishness or self-centeredness, but rather the inability to put oneself in the place of another. Children interpret objects and events not in terms of general properties, but in terms of their relationships or their use to them. They are unable to see things from any perspective other than their own; they cannot see another's point of view, nor can they see any reason to do so.

Preoperational thinking is concrete and tangible. Children cannot reason beyond the observable, and they lack the ability to make deductions or generalizations. Thought

*A schema is a pattern of action and/or thought.

is dominated by what they see, hear, or otherwise experience. However, they are increasingly able to use language and symbols to represent objects in their environment. Through imaginative play, questioning, and interacting, they begin to elaborate concepts and make simple associations between ideas. One of the most salient features of preoperational thought is lack of conservation or reversibility; children at this stage cannot understand that for every action or operation there is an action or operation that cancels it. For example, children in this age-group are unable to grasp the idea that a ball of clay can be changed and brought back to the original shape. In the latter stage of this period their reasoning is *intuitive* (e.g., the stars have to go to bed just as they do), and they are only beginning to deal with problems of weight, length, size, and time.

Concrete operational (7 to 11 years). During this period thought becomes increasingly logical and coherent. Children are able to classify, sort, order, and otherwise organize facts about the world to use in problem solving. They develop a new concept of permanence—conservation (see Developing Concrete Operations [Piaget], Chapter 17). They realize that volume, weight, and number remain the same even though outward appearances are changed. They are able to deal with a number of different aspects of a situation simultaneously. They do not have the capacity to deal in abstraction; they solve problems in a concrete, systematic fashion based on what they can perceive. Reasoning is inductive. Through progressive changes in thought processes and relationships with others, thought becomes less self-centered. Children can consider points of view other than their own. Thinking has become socialized.

Formal operational (12 to 15 years). Formal operational thought is characterized by adaptability and flexibility. Adolescents can think in abstract terms, use abstract symbols, and draw logical conclusions from a set of observations. They can make hypotheses and test them; they can consider abstract, theoretic, and philosophic matters. Although they may confuse the ideal with the practical, they can deal with and resolve most contradictions in the world.

Moral Development (Kohlberg)

It is theorized that children develop moral reasoning in an invariant developmental sequence. To understand the stages in the development of moral judgment, it is important to be aware of the stages of logical thought and the relationship to cognitive development as well as to moral behavior. Moral development is based on cognitive developmental theory and consists of three major levels, each with two stages (Kohlberg, 1968).

Kohlberg's theory allows for prediction of behavior but pays little attention to individual differences. Questions arise relative to observed sex differences in attainment of the various sequences of moral development (Holstein, 1976). It is argued that the theory was derived from interviews with male adults and may not reflect the feminine moral reasoning (Gilligan, 1977).

Preconventional level. The preconventional level of morality parallels the preconceptual level of cognitive development and intuitive thought. At this level morality is external, since children conform to rules imposed by authority figures. Culturally oriented to the labels of good/bad and right/wrong, children integrate these labels in terms of the physical or pleasurable consequences of their actions. The two stages of this level are:

Stage 1: *The punishment-and-obedience orientation.* Children determine the goodness or badness of an action in terms of its consequences. They avoid punishment and obey unquestioningly those who have the power to determine and enforce the rules and labels. They have no concept of the underlying moral order that supports these consequences.

Stage 2: *The instrumental-relativist orientation.* The right behavior consists of that which satisfies the child's own needs (and sometimes the needs of others). Although elements of fairness, reciprocity, and equal sharing are evident, they are interpreted in a very practical, concrete manner without the elements of loyalty, gratitude, or justice.

Conventional level. At this stage children are concerned with conformity and loyalty, actively maintaining, supporting, and justifying the social order, as well as personal expectations of those significant in their lives. They value the maintenance of family, group, or national expectations regardless of consequences. This level correlates with the concrete operational stage in cognitive development and consists of two stages:

Stage 3: *The interpersonal concordance* or *"good boy–nice girl" orientation.* Behavior that meets with approval and pleases or helps others is viewed as good. Conformity to the norm is the "natural" behavior, and one earns approval by being "nice."

Stage 4: *The "law and order" orientation.* Obeying the rules, doing one's duty, showing respect for authority, and maintaining the social order is the correct behavior. The rules and authority can be social or religious, depending on which is most valued.

Postconventional, autonomous, or principled level. At the postconventional level children have reached the cognitive formal operational stage and endeavor to define moral values and principles that are valid and applicable beyond the authority of the groups and persons holding these principles. This level is not associated with the individual's identification with these groups. Level 3 also has two stages, but Stage 6 has been eliminated because Kohlberg determined that it is so rarely attained that is serves no useful purpose in a discussion such as this:

Stage 5: *The social-contract, legalistic orientation.* Correct behavior tends to be defined in terms of general individual rights and standards that have been examined and agreed on by the entire society. Although procedural rules for reaching consensus become important with emphasis on the legal point of view, there is also emphasis on the possibility of changing law in terms of societal needs and rational considerations. Agreement and contract outside the legal realm are binding elements of obligation.

Spiritual Development

Spiritual beliefs are closely related to the moral and ethical portion of children's self-concepts and as such must be considered as part of children's basic needs assessment. Children need to have meaning, purpose, and hope in their lives, and the need for confession and forgiveness is present even in very young children. The research in spiritual development is both limited and subject to criticism, particularly in relation to age-stage theories. However, the stage theories provide a useful means for the reader to assess the approximate level of development for any given child.

Fowler (1974) has identified four stages in the development of faith that parallel and are closely associated with cognitive and psychosocial development:

Stage 0: *Undifferentiated.* This stage of development encompasses the period of infancy when children have no concept of right or wrong, no beliefs, and no convictions to guide their behavior. However, the beginnings of a faith are established with the development of basic trust through their relationships with the primary caregiver.

Stage 1: *Intuitive-projective.* Toddlerhood is primarily a time of imitating the behavior of others. Children imitate the religious gestures and behaviors of others without comprehending any meaning or significance to the activities. During the preschool years children assimilate some of the values and beliefs of their parents. Parental attitudes toward moral codes and religious beliefs convey to children what they consider good and bad. Children follow parental beliefs as part of their daily lives rather than through an understanding of their basic concepts.

Stage 2: *Mythical-literal.* Through the school-age years spiritual development parallels cognitive development and is closely related to children's experiences and social interaction. Most children have a strong interest in religion during the school-age years. The existence of a deity is accepted, and petitions to an omnipotent being are important and expected to be answered; good behavior is rewarded and bad behavior is punished. Children's developing conscience bothers them when they disobey. They have a reverence for many thoughts and matters and are able to articulate their faith. They may even begin to question its validity.

Stage 3: *Synthetic-convention.* As children approach adolescence they become increasingly aware of spiritual disappointments. They recognize that prayers are not always answered (at least on their own terms). They begin to reason, to question some of the established parental religious standards, and to drop or modify some religious practices.

Stage 4: *Individuating-reflexive.* Adolescents become more skeptical and begin to compare the religious standards of their parents with others. They attempt to determine which to adopt and incorporate into their own set of values. They also begin to compare religious standards with the scientific viewpoint. It is a time of searching rather than reaching. Adolescents are uncertain about many religious ideas but will not achieve profound insights until late adolescence or early adulthood.

THEORETIC FOUNDATIONS OF LANGUAGE DEVELOPMENT

Children learn the complex symbol system of language with astonishing speed. Infants use abstract signifiers (words) to refer to objects and activities before they can walk. They can express hundreds of different messages by age 2 years, and know and use most of the syntactic structures of their native tongue by age 5 years. However, at all stages of language development, children's comprehension vocabulary is greater than their expressed vocabulary, and the acquisition of vocabulary and language keeps pace with cognitive advancement.

Children are born with the mechanism and capacity to develop speech and language skills: intact physiologic function of (1) the respiratory system, (2) speech control centers in the cerebral cortex, and (3) articulation and resonance structures of the mouth and nasal cavities. In addition, acquisition of language requires (1) an intact and discriminating auditory apparatus, (2) intelligence, (3) a need to communicate, and (4) stimulation.

Components of Language

Children first achieve a knowledge of *phenology,* referring to the basic units of sound, which are combined to produce words. Each language uses only a portion of all the sounds that humans are capable of generating, and children must learn to hear and to pronounce the speechlike sounds peculiar to their language. Then they learn how to combine these basic sounds into words.

Next children learn the *semantics* of language, that is, that words and sentences convey an expressed meaning. Use of semantics progresses to knowledge of *syntax,* the form or structure of their language—the rules that specify how words are combined to form meaningful sentences. The rules of syntax vary considerably from one language to another, but the basic principle is true of all; that is, individual words in a sentence interact with sentence structure to give the entire sentence a meaning.

Children must also acquire the important component of language, *pragmatics,* the principles specifying how language is to be used in different social contexts and situations. Pragmatic abilities and social editing skills evolve gradually over the course of childhood. All children in all cultures go through the same stages of language acquisition regardless of the structure of the language they are learning.

Stages of Language Development

Children proceed through several stages in the development of language. Infants can discriminate speech from other sound patterns and pay particularly close attention to speech from the beginning. By the time they enter school, children have mastered most of the syntactic rules of their native language and can produce a variety of sophisticated, adultlike messages (Box 4-4).

Theories of Language Development

There are three major theories of language acquisition: learning theory, nativism, and the interactional approach. *Learning theorists* believe that language is acquired as children hear and respond to the speech of their companions. However, some disagreement exists among them regarding how children learn to speak. One faction believes that language is learned through operant conditioning as adults reinforce children for their attempts to produce grammatical speech. Others argue that children acquire language by lis-

Box 4-4 STAGES IN DEVELOPMENT OF LANGUAGE

Prelinguistic stage—the period before children utter their first meaningful words; develops in steplike fashion over first 10 to 12 months from crying through cooing to babbling.
Holophrastic stage—the period when children's speech consists of one-word utterances, some of which are thought to be holophrases (single-word utterances that represent the meaning of an entire sentence); begins at about 1 year of age.
Telegraphic stage—the period when children's speech consists solely of content words, omitting the less meaningful parts of speech (such as articles, prepositions, and auxiliary verbs); begins at about 18 to 24 months of age.
Preschool period—the period when children begin to produce some very lengthy sentences and speech increases in complexity; ages 30 months to 5 years.
Middle childhood period—the period when children refine their language skills and increase linguistic competence; ages 6 to 14 years. They use bigger words, produce longer and more complex utterances, and learn subtle exceptions to grammatical rules. They begin to understand even the most complex syntactic structures of their native language.

tening to and imitating the speech of their older companions.

Nativists propose that human beings have an inborn linguistic processor, or language acquisition mechanism, that is specialized for language learning. They also believe that there is a critical period for language development and that humans are most proficient at language learning between 2 years of age and puberty.

The *interactional* proponents acknowledge that children are biologically prepared to acquire language but suggest that what may be innate is the development and maturation of the nervous system rather than a special linguistic processor. They also recognize the crucial role of environment in language learning, because children must hear simplified versions of adult speech in order to acquire the needed linguistic concepts.

Factors Affecting Language Acquisition

Girls are more advanced in language development than boys. Firstborn children develop language earlier than do later-born children, and children of multiple births (twins, triplets) develop language later than children of single births. Delayed, lack of, or impaired speech can result from a variety of sources, including congenital structural defects of the mouth and nasopharynx, a hearing deficit, neurologic dysfunction (including mental retardation), maternal deprivation, and emotional factors. Some of these factors are discussed in relation to health problems in which impaired speech is a symptom or a consequence. It is also important to note that some of the organ systems and organs on which speech depends, such as the respiratory system for gas exchange and the tongue for eating, are responsible for higher priority functions that take precedence over the lesser important function of communication. During illness or trauma children may direct their limited energy to the more vital functions of these systems: breathing and eating.

THEORETIC FOUNDATIONS OF SOCIAL LEARNING

Learning occurs when behavior changes as a result of experience, and learning theories attempt to explain the ways in which controlled changes in the environment produce predictable changes in behavior. Basically children acquire new behaviors and produce alterations in existing behaviors through (1) forming associations through conditioning and (2) observing models.

Conditioning (Skinner)

Conditioning is learning by association, that is, establishing a connection between a stimulus and a response. In *classical*, or Pavlovian, conditioning two events that occur simultaneously or close together in time come to have similar meanings to the child and thus evoke the same response. For example, infants learn very early to associate the sight of the mother's face and the sound of her voice with feeding and other pleasant sensations. Consequently an infant will cease crying or somehow indicate pleasure when she speaks or enters the infant's visual field. This type of learning appears to be the predominant form that takes place during infancy, particularly in the first 6 months, before the development of motor control.

Operant, or *instrumental*, conditioning involves the use of rewards or reinforcements to encourage the performance of specific behaviors. Reinforcing desired responses whenever they occur increases the likelihood that they will be repeated. These reinforcements can be inner satisfactions or externally applied reward systems. Behavior that is not in some way reinforced or rewarded will be extinguished. The principles of instrumental conditioning are especially applicable to learning that takes place naturally in toddlers and preschool children. These children can appreciate the significance of rewards and punishments even though they may not be able to conceptualize the context or framework in which they are operating. A substantial proportion of early childhood learning, such as acquisition of motor skills, consists of simple operant conditioning.

Avoidance conditioning discourages undesired behaviors through the use of punishment and fear of punishment. The effectiveness of rewards and punishments depends on the child's subjective assessment of the reward or punishment. Some rewards are not reinforcing, and punishments do not generate fear if they are inappropriate to the developmental level, emotional stage, or value system of the individual child. Punishment is effective in controlling behavior, but it must be correctly timed, brief, appropriate to the child and the undesired behavior, and tempered with love.

Operant conditioning is the basis of behavior-modification procedures that have achieved varying degrees of success in speech therapy and in modifying behavior in overly aggressive and mentally retarded children. Behavior is shaped by reinforcing closer and closer approximations to the behavior being taught.

Modeling or Observational Learning (Bandura)

Much of childhood learning takes place because of children's innate tendency to observe and imitate the behavior of those who are significant in their lives. Children learn many new behaviors from observing parents, siblings, and peers. Learning is immediate, and children can often correctly imitate a behavior on the first attempt. They are more apt to imitate those whom they believe to be prestigious and those whom they see being rewarded for their behavior.

As children gain more complex cognitive skills and the use of language, learning assumes broader dimensions, involving creativity, problem solving, and abstract conceptualization. Modeling requires no reinforcement, although in most situations children imitate a behavior because they are in some way reinforced for doing so. A child may proudly proclaim to be doing something "just like mommy and daddy." Apparently modeling is its own reward (Fig. 4-10).

Role Learning in Children

A *role* is a set of duties, rights, obligations, and expected behaviors that accompanies a given position in a social structure. Children are expected to play a variety of roles such as son or daughter, sister or brother, student, classmate, and playmate. They learn and practice these roles and learn something of the characteristics of other roles through interaction with others and in their play. Children will behave in patterned and more or less predictable ways because they learn roles that define mutual expectations in typical and recurring social relationships (see Chapter 3).

Individuals bring their own unique temperaments, skills, and values to the interpretation and enactment of the roles they play. Because most roles exist independently of the individuals who play them, the functions and norms associated with any given role influence the way persons play the roles and the responses of the people associated with those persons. For example, expectations about the role of teacher affect the behavior of persons playing that role, and those expectations serve as a guide to others in the evaluation of persons in that role.

As their relationships expand, children also become increasingly proficient in understanding other people. They develop the ability to distinguish their own perspectives from those of their companions through role taking. This ability is acquired in a progressive developmental sequence that parallels the invariant cognitive stages of Piaget (see p. 125). Selman's stages of social role taking are outlined in Box 4-5.

The ability to interact successfully with other people is closely related to role-taking skills. Relationships change as children recognize that others have different motives and intentions. For example, in Selman's stage 1 a friend is someone who not only lives nearby but also does nice things

Box 4-5 STAGES OF ROLE TAKING

0. **Egocentric or undifferentiated perspective** (approximately 3 to 6 years). Children are unaware of any perspective other than their own—whatever is right for them is agreeable to others.
1. **Social-informational role taking** (approximately 6 to 8 years). Children recognize that people can have perspectives that differ from their own but only because these persons have received different information. Children are unable to think about the thinking of others and imagine how others will react to an event.
2. **Self-reflective role taking** (approximately 8 to 10 years). Children know that their own and others' viewpoints may conflict even when they receive the same information. They are able to consider another's point of view and recognize that others can place themselves in their shoes. Consequently, children are able to anticipate another's reactions to their behavior but are unable to consider their own and another's perspective at the same time.
3. **Mutual role taking** (approximately 10 to 12 years). Children can consider their own and another's point of view simultaneously and realize that others are able to do the same. They can also assume the perspective of a disinterested child and anticipate the way the active participants (self and other) will react to the viewpoint of either participant.
4. **Social and conventional system role taking** (approximately 12 to 15 years). Young persons now attempt to understand the perspective of another by comparing it with that of the social system in which they operate. They expect others to consider and assume perspectives on events congruent with most persons in their social group.

From Selman, R.L.: The growth of interpersonal understanding, New York, 1980, Academic Press, Inc.

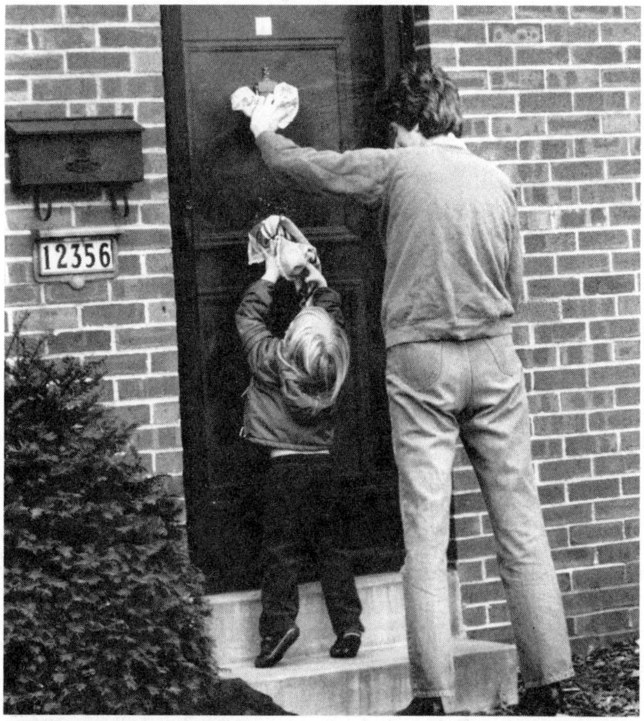

Fig. 4-10. Children learn by imitating the behavior of others.

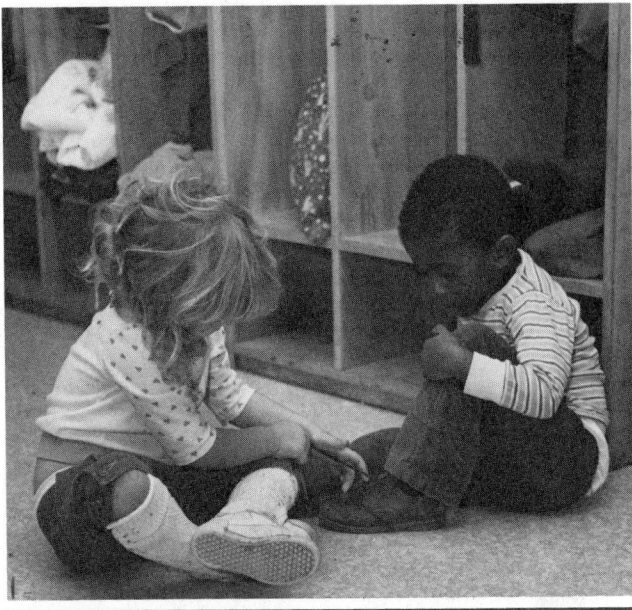

Fig. 4-11. A friend is someone who does nice things.

(Fig. 4-11); at stage 2 the term *friend* implies a reciprocal relationship with mutual respect, kindness, and affection (Furman and Bierman, 1983). In adolescence friendship becomes a relationship of common interests and values with a reasonably well-coordinated outlook on life, and a "friend" becomes someone with whom intimate information can be shared (Berndt, 1982). It has also been found that children who are adept in role-taking abilities are better able to establish intimate friendships (McGuire and Weisz, 1982) and are more popular with classmates (Kurdek and Krile, 1982).

DEVELOPMENT OF SELF-CONCEPT

Self-concept is all the notions, beliefs, and convictions that constitute children's knowledge of themselves and that influence their relationships with others. It is not present at birth but develops gradually as a result of each child's unique experiences within the self, with significant others, and with the realities of the world (Stuart and Sundeen, 1987). However, the self-concept is subjective and therefore may or may not reflect reality.

The content of the self-concept differs at various stages of development and results from the cognitive capacities and the dominant motives of individuals coming in contact with stage-related cultural expectations. In infancy self-concept is primarily an awareness of one's independent existence learned in part as a result of social contacts and experiences with other people. The process becomes more active during toddlerhood as children explore the limits of their capacities and the nature of their impact on others (Newman and Newman, 1984).

School-age children are more aware of differences in perspectives among people, social norms, and moral imperatives. They are sensitive to social pressures and become preoccupied with issues of self-criticism and self-evaluation. Because school-age children depend on adults for material and emotional resources, the self-concept is likely to be most vulnerable during this time. Little change in self-concept occurs during early adolescence when children anxiously focus on their physical and emotional changes and peer acceptance. Self-concept crystallizes during later adolescence as young people review and evaluate their childhood experiences and organize their self-concept around a set of values, goals, and competencies (Newman and Newman, 1984).

Body Image

Body image, a vital component of the self-concept, is the subjective concepts and attitudes that individuals have toward their own bodies as objects in space. Central to the concept of self, body image is the picture of the body formed in the mind, including feelings about size, function, appearance, and potential. The picture appears to be a learned phenomenon that may be conscious or unconscious and may be cognitive and/or emotional. Body image has physical, psychologic, and social components and includes present and past perceptions. It changes with advancing development and is continually modified by new perceptions and experiences.

The significant others in their lives exert the most important and meaningful impact on children's body image. Labels that are attached to them (such as "skinny," "pretty," or "fat") or body parts (such as "ugly mole," "bug eyes," or "yucky skin") are incorporated into the body image. Because they lack the understanding of deviations from the physical standard or norm, children notice prominent differences in others and unwittingly make "rude" and often cruel remarks about such minor deviations as large or widely spaced front teeth, large or small eyes, moles, or extreme variations in height.

Development during growth. Infants receive input about their bodies through self-exploration and sensory stimulation from others. As they begin to manipulate their environment, they become aware of their bodies as separate from others. Toddlers learn to identify the various parts of their bodies and are able to use symbols to represent objects. Preschoolers become aware of the wholeness of their bodies and discover the genitals. Exploration of the genitals and the discovery of differences between the sexes become important. There is only a vague concept of internal organs and function (Selekman, 1983; Stuart and Sundeen, 1987).

School-age children begin to learn about internal body structure and function and become aware of differences in the body size and configurations of others. They are highly influenced by the cultural norms of society and the fads of the times. Children whose bodies deviate from the norm are often subject to criticism and ridicule.

Adolescence is the age when children become most concerned about the physical self. The familiar body changes and the new physical self must be integrated into the self-concept. Adolescents face conflicts over what they see and what they visualize as the ideal body structure. Body image formation during adolescence is a crucial element in the shaping of an identity, the psychosocial crisis of adolescence.

Self-Esteem

Self-esteem is described as the affective component of the self, and the self-concept is the cognitive component; however, the two are almost indistinguishable, and the terms are often used interchangeably (Stanwyck, 1983). Self-esteem is a personal, subjective judgment of one's worthiness derived from and influenced by the social groups in the immediate environment and the individual's perceptions of how he or she is valued by others. Self-esteem is primarily a function of being loved and of gaining the respect of others.

Self-esteem is a product of both competence and social acceptance that changes with development. Throughout childhood children experience an increased ability to differentiate components of competence, an increased concern with a variety of significant others who may give or withhold approval, and an increased capacity to experience guilt when internal norms for either competence or social acceptance are violated (Newman and Newman, 1984). *High self-esteem* is described as a feeling based on unconditional acceptance of oneself as a worthy and important being (Stuart and Sundeen, 1987).

Highly egocentric toddlers are unaware of any difference between competence and social approval. They are the center of their world, and to them all positive experiences are evidence of their importance and value. Preschool and early school-age children, on the other hand, are increasingly aware of the discrepancy between their competencies and the abilities of more advanced children. They are expected to evaluate a situation and anticipate the consequences of their behavior before they act. The acceptance of adults and peers outside the family group becomes more important to them. Since these valued persons may not be as proud of their achievements or as understanding of their limitations as their families are, their recently acquired capacity for guilt may lead to anxiety over failure, and they will be more vulnerable to feelings of worthlessness and depression. As their competencies increase and they develop meaningful relationships, their self-esteem rises. Their self-esteem is again at risk during early adolescence when they are defining an identity and sense of self in the context of their peer group.

Unless children are continually made to feel incompetent and of little worth, a decrease in self-esteem during vulnerable periods is only temporary. Transitory periods of lowered self-esteem at the stages of development are expected when they must set new goals or when there are very obvious discrepancies in competence. A constant source of anxiety arises from the endless number of separations that occur in the process of acquiring autonomy, independence, and individuality. As an expression of their own urgencies, parents often set overambitious goals for their children and expect them to perform beyond the limits of their capacity. Also, children's attempts at autonomy and achievement are often thwarted by parental overprotection, because either the parents fear the children will be hurt or the parents find it more convenient to do things for them.

In order to develop and preserve self-esteem, children need to feel that they are worthwhile individuals who are in some way different from, superior to, and more lovable than any other individual in the world. They need recognition for their achievements and the approval of parents and peers. Parents and other authority figures can foster a positive self-concept by providing appropriate encouragement and recognition for achievement and by discouraging inappropriate behaviors. However, when authority figures express disapproval, they must convey to a child that the *behavior* is unacceptable, not the child. Constructive communication, such as the use of "I" messages, conveys feeling and needs without destroying the child's self-esteem.

Children who experience warm, affectionate relationships with their family and who are aware of their parents' acceptance and positive attitudes toward them are more accepting of themselves. Children who have a strong sense of their own worth are confident, able to initiate activities, explore their environment, and take risks in their behavior when confronted with new or novel situations. They approach tasks and relationships with the expectation that they will be well received and successful. Such is the focus of nursing—to allow children and their families to grow and to prosper from their experiences in times of both health and illness.

DEVELOPMENT OF SEXUALITY

From the moment of birth children are treated differently by their families based on their biologic sex. Almost immediately infants are placed in male or female categories with given names that clearly indicate a sex, dressed in pink if girls or blue if boys, and referred to as either "he" or "she." Thus information regarding a sexual identity is conveyed to children and to the world, and along with these overt messages a set of sex-related attitudes toward them emerges. The outcome of the identification process depends on the characteristics of the parents and other role models, the innate capacities and preferences of the child, and the cultural and familiar value placed on the child's sex.

Families recognize the importance of sex differences and even in infancy treat boys differently from girls. Parental attitudes and expectations regarding sex-appropriate behaviors, acquired from the parents' own upbringing, influence how they react to their children from infancy. These attitudes and expectations are transmitted to infants first in subtle, then in more obvious, ways. For example, family members relate to infants differently: little girls are handled more tenderly; little boys are stimulated with boisterous activity and vigorous motor play. Families provide sex-appropriate toys and encourage play consistent with the sex-role expectations of the children.

Four dimensions appear to be involved in the development of sex-role identification. Children (1) learn to apply appropriate gender labels to themselves, (2) acquire sex-appropriate standards of behavior, (3) develop a preference for being the sex that they are, and (4) identify with their parent of the same sex.

Gender Label

The gender label is achieved early and subtly through imitation of the parents' expressions as they refer to children's gender, for example, "That's a good girl" or "That's a good boy." Since it is such an important and basic component of children's total identity, the appropriate gender must be assigned as soon as possible in rare cases where the sex of the infant is in doubt (see Aberrant Sexual Development, Chapter 11). The gender orientation has more effect on development than does chromosomal determination of sex.

However, with the increasing number of nontraditional gender roles portrayed on prime time television, children's stereotypical perceptions of men and women may be changing. Children who are familiar with shows that depict men performing traditionally feminine tasks such as cooking, cleaning, and caring for children and women employed outside the home have a more flexible view of sex-related roles (Rosenwasser, Lingenfelter, and Harrington, 1989).

Sex-Role Standards

Beginning when children are toddlers, sex-role standards are differentiated and continuously developed throughout childhood. By the time children are 3 years old, they know whether they are boys or girls, and they have acquired considerable knowledge of and a preference for sex-appropriate behaviors. They can differentiate one sex from the other even before they learn anatomic differences; 2-year-old children can identify others as girls or boys based on external appearances.

Preschool children have definite impressions of masculinity and femininity, and they are reflected in overt play. Most children in this age-group engage in stereotyped sex-appropriate play activities. Little girls are more likely to play at housekeeping, taking care of dolls, dressing up, and cooking; boys choose trucks, blocks, and more physically active play. Boys are generally more aggressive in their play, and in disagreements with peers they are more apt to react with shouting or fighting. Girls tend to be more dependent and introverted in their play (Maccoby and Jacklin, 1974).

With the strong women's movement, more liberal views regarding sex-role typing, and the unisex trend in all areas of interaction, these sex-associated characteristics are less apparent than they have been in the past. For example, although boys and younger girls were observed to pay more attention and learn more about objects labeled for their sex, older girls were much more flexible regarding what they consider correct for their sex (Bradbard and others, 1986). However, the United States, like most cultures, still has a strong masculine orientation, with males generally accorded more privileges than females.

Families expect children to learn appropriate sex-role behavior early and to deviate little from it. Each family has its own concept of what constitutes male or female attributes and the types of sex-linked behavior they wish to cultivate in their children. These beliefs are conveyed to the children by a variety of means, and parents exert special efforts to gain compliance with their expectations. Experiences the children are exposed to, toys selected for them, and activities they are encouraged to participate in all reflect some aspect of the family's sex-role conformity to standards of achievement, competition, self-assertiveness, and independence with control of feelings and repression of emotions. With girls the family usually places more emphasis on passive activities and development of interpersonal sensitivity, docility, interrelatedness with others, and nurturance.

Observing siblings' interaction at play can provide insight into sex-role relationships. Sibling relationships mirror parent relationships within a given family—divorced or intact. For example, older boys from discordant families have been observed to bully their younger sisters (MacKinnon, 1989).

In the case of boys the prohibition against effeminate behavior is very strong. Boys are rewarded less often for displaying behavior considered appropriate for their sex, but they are discouraged from exhibiting undesirable behavior by negative reinforcement. Parents emphasize the things that boys should *not* do or be, that is, those things that might label them as "sissies." Avoidance of the opposite sex-role behavior is a major means of sex-role learning in the American culture, especially for boys. This emphasis seems to be stronger in lower-class families, where sex roles are more clearly defined and segregated. In middle-class homes sex-role differentiation is less clear-cut. Mothers often work outside the home, and male role models are more apt to help with behaviors traditionally assigned to the female, such as housework and baby-sitting.

The family situation may be more influential for sex-role development of girls than of boys, since boys are more apt to learn much of their masculine behaviors from role models outside the home. For example, in lower-class black families in which the father is frequently absent, a male child often associates with gangs to learn a masculine role, whereas a Hispanic youth who has a male model in the home may join such gangs to escape the paternal dominance and be free to express his masculine role.

Girls, on the other hand, are dealt with more leniently in America. Their role is less rigidly defined than that of boys. Girls are permitted to engage in masculine games and activities, to wear pants, and to be a tomboy without strong cultural disapproval. This greater variance may create some confusion in establishing a sex-role identity. A girl's acceptance of a parental role model depends a great deal on whether the role model of her mother is congruent with the girl's concept of a sex role.

Gender Preference

Gender preference for the sex children are born is acquired over a long time and depends on several things. Children will prefer to be a member of their own sex when their behaviors and competence closely approximate the sex-role standards, when they like their parent of the same sex, and when they believe their sex is valued. The sexes are not always valued equally in all cultures nor in all families. In cultures where males are more highly valued and are given higher status, boys are likely to develop a firm preference for their sex. However, girls in these cultures may be less certain regarding their gender assignment, even to the point of rejecting their sex group. A deterrent to sex-role preference by children can exist in families where the parents, at a specific birth, had hoped strongly for a child of the opposite sex. The environmental cues within the family will convey to these children that the opposite sex is a preferred one.

Gender Identity

The process by which children style themselves after their parent of the same sex and internalize that parent's values and outlook is *identification*. Most children wish to be like their parent of the same sex, and although the motivation for identification is still unsettled, children are more willing to share these parental attributes when they are able to see a degree of similarity between themselves and their parents. Children become aware of the similarity when they perceive actual physical and psychologic similarities, adopt parental behaviors, and are told of similarities by others. Once this identification is formed, it can be strengthened by the continued positive conception of the role model or weakened if the child does not perceive the model as desirable. Identification is not a total, all-or-nothing happening. To some extent children identify with both parents, and as their sphere of social contacts widens, they identify with peers and other adults outside the family.

■ ROLE OF PLAY IN DEVELOPMENT

Through the universal medium of play children learn what no one can teach them. They learn about their world and how to deal with this environment of objects, time, space, structure, and people. They learn about themselves operating within that environment—what they can do, how to relate to things and situations, and how to adapt themselves to the demands society makes on them. It has been said that play is the *work* of the child. In play children continually practice the complicated, stressful processes of living, communicating, and achieving satisfactory relationships with other people. In addition, while promoting and advancing development and relationships, play is an intrinsically motivated, often purposeless, and satisfying activity—something children do for the sheer fun of it.

CLASSIFICATION OF PLAY

From a developmental point of view, patterns of children's play can be categorized according to *content* and *social character*. In both there is an additive effect; each builds on past accomplishments, and some element of each is maintained throughout life. At each stage in development the new predominates.

Content of Play

The content of play involves primarily the physical aspects of play, although social relationships cannot be ignored. The content of play follows the directional trend of the simple to the complex.

Social-affective play. Play begins with social-affective play, wherein infants take pleasure in relationships with people. As adults talk, fondle, nuzzle, and in various ways elicit a response from an infant, the infant soon learns to provoke parental emotions and responses with such behaviors as smiling, cooing, or initiating games and activities. The type and intensity of the adult behavior with children vary among cultures.

Sense-pleasure play. Sense-pleasure play is a nonsocial stimulating experience that originates from without. Objects in the environment—light and color, tastes and odors, textures and consistencies—attract children's attention, stimulate their senses, and give pleasure. Pleasurable experiences are derived from handling raw materials (water, sand, food), from body motion (swinging, bouncing, rocking), and from other uses of senses and abilities (smelling, humming) (Fig. 4-12).

Skill play. Once infants have developed the ability to grasp and manipulate, they persistently demonstrate and exercise their newly acquired abilities through skill play, repeating an action over and over again. The element of sense-pleasure play is often evident in the practicing of a new ability, but all too frequently the determination to conquer the elusive skill produces pain and frustration (e.g., learning to ride a bicycle).

Unoccupied behavior. In unoccupied behavior children are not playful but focus their attention momentarily on anything that strikes their interest. Children daydream, fiddle with clothes or other objects, or walk aimlessly. This role differs from that of onlookers, who actively observe the activity of others.

Dramatic, or pretend, play. One of the vital elements in children's process of identification is dramatic play, also known as *symbolic* or *pretend play*. It begins in late infancy (11 to 13 months) as children engage in

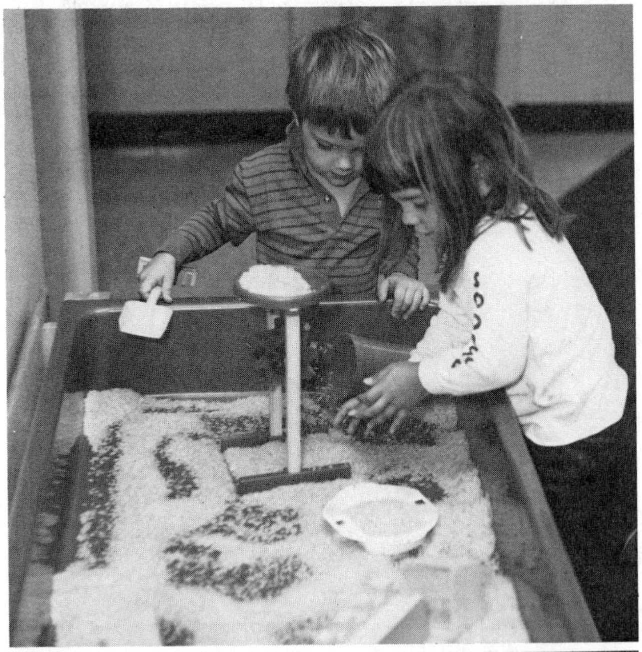

Fig. 4-12. Children derive pleasure from handling raw materials.

simple pretending with familiar activities, such as eating, sleeping, or drinking from a cup. In toddlerhood the activities are still primarily those that are familiar. As children enter the preschool stage their play becomes further removed from everyday activities and much more complex. Dramatic play is the predominant form of play in the preschool child.

Once children begin to invest situations and people with meanings and to attribute affective significance to the world, they can pretend and fantasize almost anything. By acting out events of daily life, children learn and practice the roles and identities modeled by the members of their family and society. Pretend play provides a framework within which mature behaviors are tested and assimilated (Connolly, Doyle, and Reznick, 1988).

Children's toys, replicas of the tools of society, provide a medium for learning about adult roles and activities that may be puzzling and frustrating to them. Interacting with the world is one way children get to know it. The simple, imitative, dramatic play of the toddler, such as using the telephone, driving a car, or rocking a doll, evolves into more complex, sustained dramas of the preschooler, which extend beyond common domestic matters to the wider aspects of the world and the society, such as playing policeman, storekeeper, teacher, or nurse (Fig. 4-13). Older children work out elaborate themes, act out stories, and compose plays.

Games. Children in all cultures engage in games alone and with others. Solitary activity involving games begins as very small children participate in repetitive activities and progress to more complicated games that challenge their independent skills, such as solving puzzles, solitaire, and computer or video games. When children interact with others, games assume the same developmental trends. Very young children participate in simple, *imitative games* such as pat-a-cake and peekaboo.

Preschool children learn and enjoy *formal games* that begin with ritualistic, self-sustaining games, such as ring-around-a-rosy and London Bridge. With the exception of some simple board games, preschool children do not engage in *competitive games*. They do play competitively but find it difficult not to take competition seriously. Preschoolers hate to lose and will try to cheat, want to change rules, or demand exceptions and opportunities to change their moves. Competitive games are the province of school-age children and adolescents who enjoy a variety of games including cards, checkers, chess, and physically active games such as baseball.

Social Character of Play

The play interactions of infancy are between a child and an adult. Children continue to enjoy the company of an adult but are increasingly able to play alone. As age advances, interaction with age-mates increases in importance and becomes an essential part of the socialization process (Fig. 4-14). Through interaction, highly egocentric infants, unable to tolerate delay or interference, ultimately acquire concern for others and the ability to delay gratification or even to re-

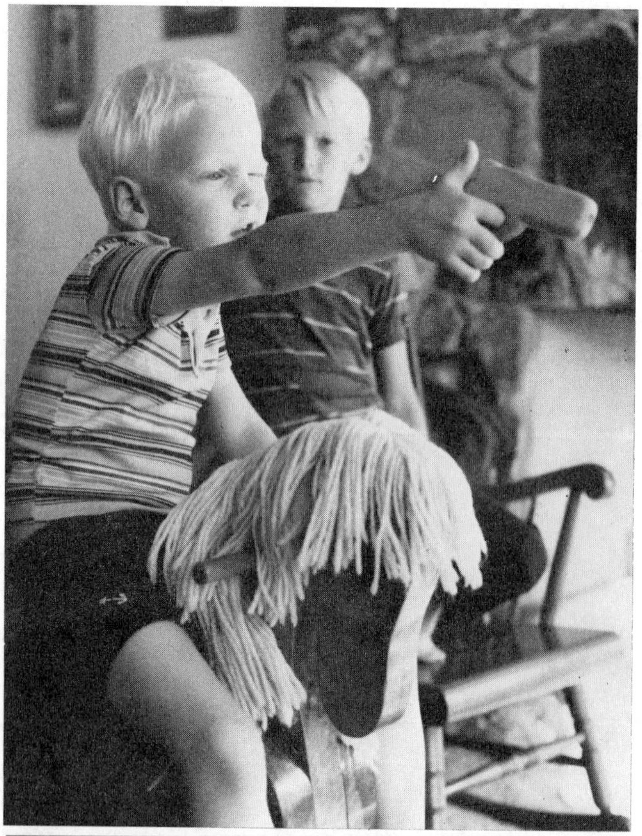

Fig. 4-13. Preschoolers spend considerable time in pretend play.

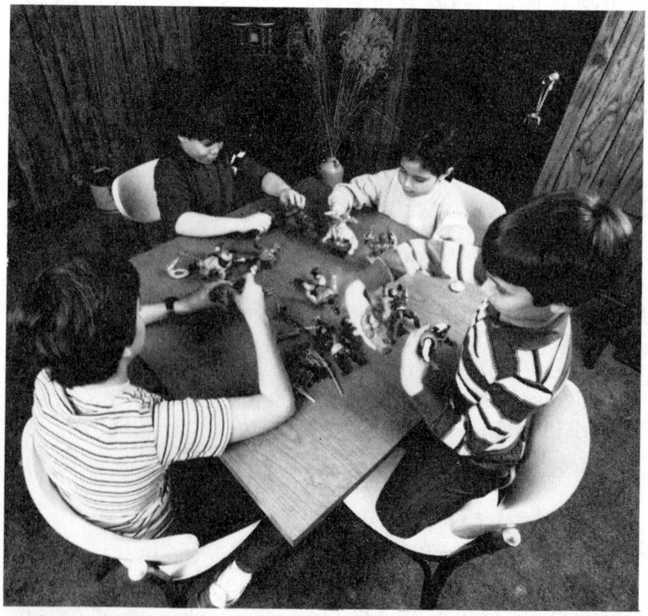

Fig. 4-14. Children show interest and pleasure in the company of others.

ject gratification at the expense of another. A pair of toddlers engage in considerable combat because their personal needs cannot tolerate delay or compromise. By the time they reach age 5 or 6 years, children are able to arrive at a compromise or make use of arbitration, usually after individual children have attempted but failed to gain their own way. Through continued interaction with peers and the growth of conceptual abilities and social skills, children are able to increase participation with others.

Onlooker play. During onlooker play children watch what other children are doing but make no attempt to enter into the play activity. There is an active interest in observing the interaction of others but no movement toward participating. Watching television is a common example of the onlooker role.

Solitary play. Children who independently play alone with toys different from those used by other children in the same area are engaging in *solitary play.* They enjoy the presence of other children but make no effort to get close or speak to them. Their interest is centered on their own activity, which they pursue with no reference to the activities of the others.

Parallel play. During parallel activities children play independently but among other children. They play with toys like those the children around them are using, but as each child sees fit, neither influencing nor being influenced by the other children. Each plays beside, but not with, other children (Fig. 4-15). There is no group association. Parallel play is the characteristic play of toddlers, but it may also occur in other groups of any age. Individuals who are involved in a creative craft with each person separately working on an individual project are engaged in parallel play.

Associative play. When children play together and are engaged in a similar or even identical activity, but there is no organization, division of labor, leadership assignment, or mutual goal, the play is *associative.* Children borrow and

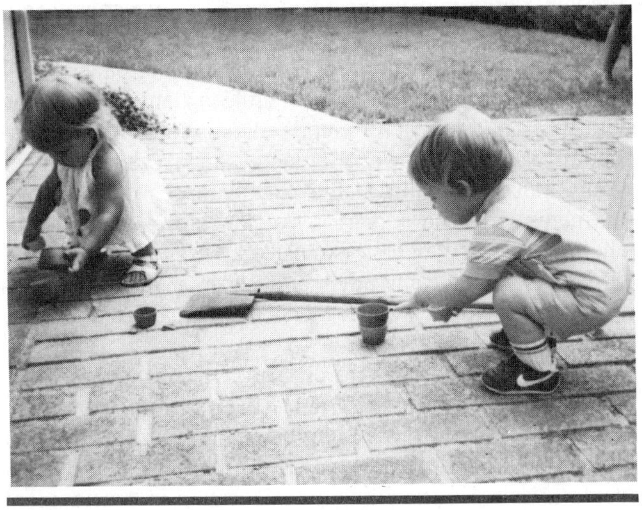

Fig. 4-15. Parallel play.

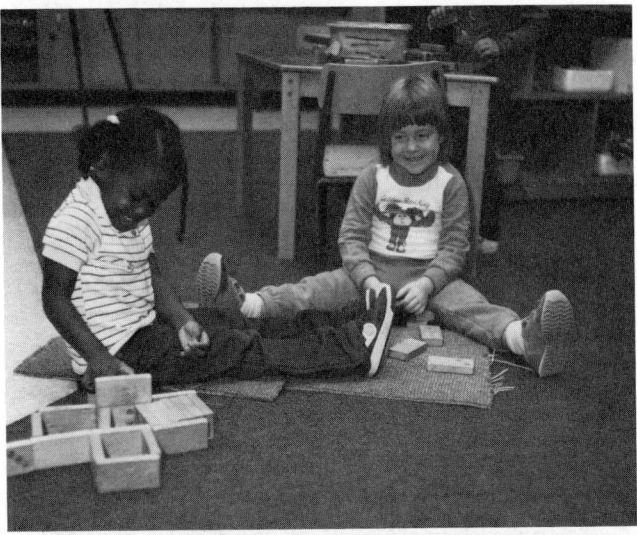

Fig. 4-16. Associative play.

lend play materials, follow each other with wagons and tricycles, and sometimes attempt to control who may or may not play in the group. Each child acts according to his own wishes; there is no group goal (Fig. 4-16). For example, two children play with dolls, borrowing articles of clothing from each other and engaging in similar conversation, but neither directs the other's actions nor establishes rules regarding the limits of the play session. There is a great deal of behavioral contagion: when one child initiates an activity, the entire group follows the example.

Cooperative play. Cooperative play is organized, and the children play in a group *with* other children. The children discuss and plan activities for the purposes of accomplishing an end—to make something, to attain a competitive goal, to dramatize situations of adult or group life, or to play formal games. The group is loosely formed, but there is a marked sense of belonging or not belonging. The goal and its attainment require organization of activities, division of labor, and playing roles. The leader-follower relationship is definitely established, and the activity is controlled by one or two members who assign roles and direct the activity of the others. The activity is organized to allow one child to supplement another's function in order to complete the goal.

FUNCTIONS OF PLAY

The specific values of play or the functions that it serves throughout childhood include sensorimotor development, intellectual development, socialization, creativity, self-awareness, and therapeutic and moral value.

Sensorimotor Development

Sensorimotor activity is a major component of play at all ages and is the predominant form of play in infancy. Active play is essential for muscle development and serves a useful purpose as a release for surplus energy. Through sen-

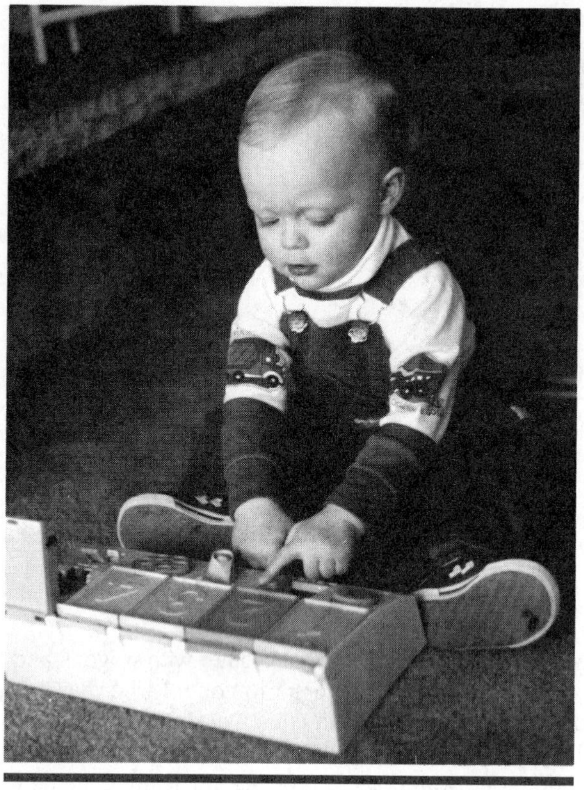

Fig. 4-17. Children learn through exploration with shapes and textures.

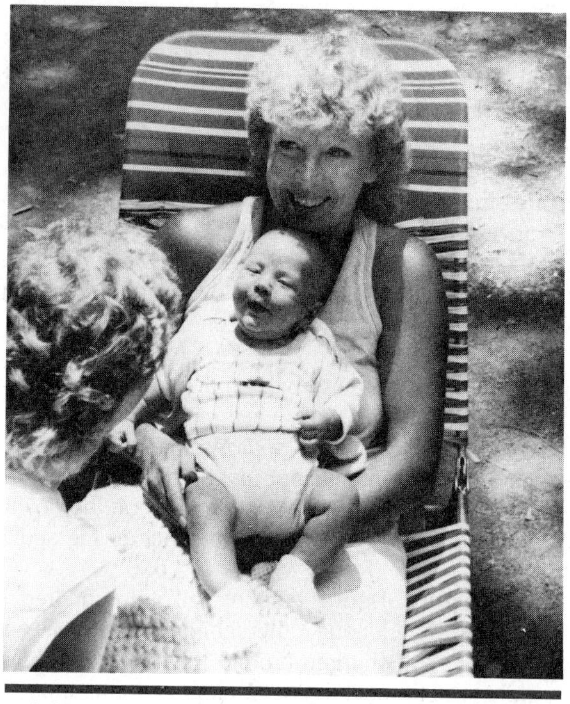

Fig. 4-18. The socialization process begins in early infancy.

sorimotor play, children explore the nature of the physical world. Infants gain impressions of themselves and their world through tactile, auditory, visual, and kinesthetic stimulation. Toddlers and preschoolers revel in body movement and exploration of things in space. Children continue to engage in sensorimotor play, although with increasing maturity, the play becomes more differentiated and involved. Whereas very young children run for the sheer joy of body movement, older children incorporate or modify the motions into increasingly complex and coordinated activities such as races, games, roller skating, and bicycle riding.

Intellectual Development

Through exploration and manipulation, children learn colors, shapes, sizes, textures, and the significance of objects (Fig. 4-17). They learn the significance of numbers and how to use them, they learn to associate words with objects, and they develop an understanding of abstract concepts and spatial relationships, such as up, down, under, and over. Activities such as puzzles and games help them develop problem-solving skills. Books, stories, films, and collections expand knowledge and provide enjoyment as well. Play provides a means to practice and expand language skills. Through play children continually rehearse past experiences to assimilate them into new perceptions and relationships. Play helps children comprehend the world in which they live and distinguish between fantasy and reality.

Socialization

From very early infancy children show interest and pleasure in the company of others (Fig. 4-18). Their initial social contact is with the mothering person, but through play with other children, they learn to establish social relationships and solve the problems associated with these relationships.

Children pass through four distinct phases in developing social competence in play during their first 5 years. Infants under a year of age investigate other infants in much the same manner as they investigate other objects in their environment. Children between ages 2 and 3 years generally engage in considerable pretend play with mutually dependent roles such as mother and baby, physician and patient, grocer and customer. Their social circle expands to include both short- and long-term friends. When they reach the preschool years children become increasingly aware of a peer group and can identify stable characteristics of individual playmates. They have one or two favorite playmates with whom they play almost exclusively. They can verbalize judgments about each other and sense a distinction between good friends and mere acquaintances (Howes, 1987).

In play children learn to give and take, which is more readily learned from critical peers than from more tolerant adults. They learn the sex role that society expects them to fulfill, as well as approved patterns of behavior and deportment. Closely associated with socialization is development of moral values and ethics. Children learn right from wrong, the standards of the society, and to assume responsibility for their actions.

Creativity

In no other situation is there more opportunity to be creative than in play. Children can experiment and try out their ideas in play through every medium at their disposal, including raw materials, fantasy, and exploration. Creativity is stifled by pressure toward conformity; therefore striving for peer approval may inhibit creative endeavors in the school-age or adolescent child. Creativity is primarily a product of solitary, as opposed to group, activity. Once children feel the satisfaction of creating something new and different, they transfer this creative interest to situations outside the world of play.

Self-Awareness

Beginning with active explorations of their bodies and awareness of themselves as separate from the caregiver. the process of self-identity is facilitated through play activities. Children learn who they are and what their place is in the world. They become increasingly able to regulate their own behavior, to learn what their abilities are, and to compare their abilities with those of others. Through play children are able to test their abilities, assume and try out various roles, and learn the effect their behavior has on others.

Therapeutic Value

There is no doubt that play is therapeutic at any age. It provides a means for release from the tension and stress encountered through the environment. In play children can express emotions and release unacceptable impulses in a socially acceptable fashion. Children are able to experiment and test fearful situations and can assume and vicariously master the roles and positions they are unable to perform in the world of reality. Children reveal much about themselves in play. Children are able to communicate to the alert observer through play the needs, fears, and desires they are unable to express with their limited language skills. Throughout their play children need the presence and acceptance of adults to help them control aggression and channel their destructive tendencies.

Moral Value

Although children learn at home and at school those behaviors considered right and wrong in the culture, the interaction with peers during play contributes significantly to their moral training. Nowhere is the enforcement of moral standards so rigid as in the play situation. If they are to be acceptable members of the group, children must adhere to the culturally accepted codes of behavior—fairness, honesty, self-control, and consideration for others. Children soon learn that their peers are less tolerant of violations than are adults, and to maintain a place in the play group they must conform to the standards of the group.

CHARACTERISTICS OF PLAY

There are several aspects of play that display developmental changes and that differentiate children's play from adult play.

Tradition

In general the play of small children varies little from generation to generation within a culture. Each generation of children imitates the play of the preceding generation; in this way the more satisfying forms of play are perpetuated. Many types of play are characteristic of all cultures, for example, playing with balls, some form of doll, or some type of walking toy to help children just beginning to walk to maintain balance.

Seasonal changes are accompanied by traditional forms of toys and play activities. Sledding and ice skating are popular in winter; jump rope, bicycling, and roller skating are played in spring and summer.

Time and Age

The amount of time that children spend in play decreases with age. Older children have less time available for play because of an increase in schoolwork and other responsibilities. With advancing age and development, the number and variety of play activities diminish and play becomes less physically active, but the time spent in specific activities increases as interests narrow and the attention span lengthens. The number of playmates decreases with age as children progress from play with anyone available to play with a few selected and special age-mates.

Children's play can be divided into the following four categories: (1) imitative, (2) exploratory, (3) testing, and (4) model building. At all ages each of these types is evident in children's play, but one type will predominate over the others at specific ages. For example, imitative play can be seen in the infant who mimics the actions of another (pat-a-cake), but it reaches its peak in the dramatic play of preschoolers who play "house," "astronaut," or "school." It can also be observed in circular group singing and rhythmic games such as ring-around-a-rosy.

As children grow older, play activities become less spontaneous, more formal and structured, and increasingly sex appropriate. Whereas infants and small children of both sexes play in much the same way, by the time they enter school, children engage in activities deemed appropriate for their sex. Little boys in particular are clearly aware they do not play with certain toys, and they avoid their girl playmates.

Patterns of Development

Throughout childhood certain play activities are popular at one age and not at another (Box 4-6). These activities are so consistent and predictable that childhood is sometimes divided into age stages according to the types of play characteristic of each particular phase of development.

As they grow older, children also use materials in more meaningful ways. For example, an infant or small child first

Box 4-6 AGE CHARACTERISTICS OF PLAY

Exploratory Stage
Age: Approximately 3 to 12 months
Activities: Grasping, holding, and examining articles
Exploration via creeping or crawling

Toy Stage
Age: 1 to 7 or 8 years
Activities: Imitating adult behavior with replicas of adult tools

Play Stage
Age: 8 to 12 years
Activities: Interest in toys diminishes
Interest in games, sports, and hobbies increases

Daydreaming Stage
Age: Characteristic of older children and pubescents
Activities: Playing the martyr misunderstood and mistreated by everyone or the hero or beauty admired by everyone (Fig. 4-19)

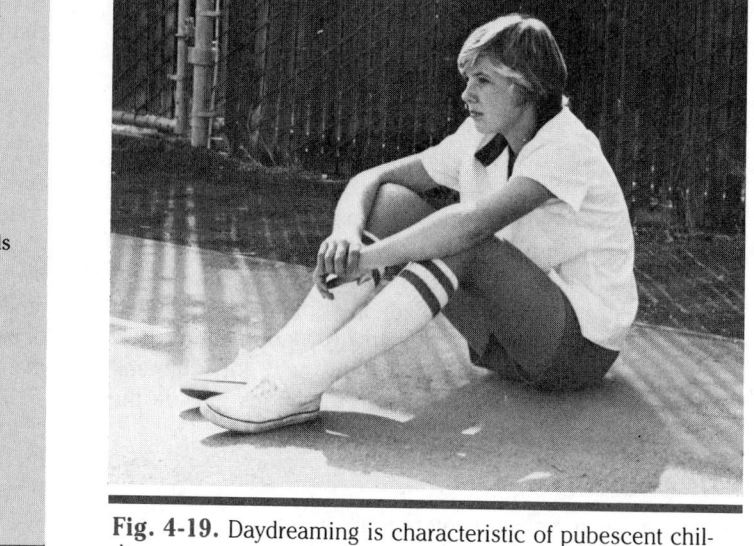

Fig. 4-19. Daydreaming is characteristic of pubescent children.

uses a block as something to handle or throw, then as something to represent another object, such as an airplane or car. To older children a block is a building material with which they can construct increasingly complex structures. Instead of representative objects, they require replicas of cars and airplanes. Eventually these materials are discarded altogether.

TOYS

Toys are the inanimate objects with which children interact, and cognitive development appears to be related to the variety and accessibility of objects for children to explore, experiment with, and come to know. Access to playthings, particularly during the earlier years, correlates with the accessibility of caregivers who make objects available, react to children's response to the objects, encourage further exploration, and talk about what is happening. Consequently, although they can be significant in themselves, playthings assume an especially important aspect as a medium of social interchange.

Selecting Toys

The type of toys chosen by and/or provided for children can facilitate learning and development in the areas just described. Toys that are small replicas of the culture and its tools help children assimilate their culture and learn sex and occupational roles. Toys that require pushing, pulling, rolling, and manipulating teach them about physical properties of the items and help to develop muscles and coordination. Rules and the basic elements of cooperation and organization are learned through board games.

Because they can be employed in a variety of ways, raw materials or multidimensional toys are best for enhancing skills and stimulating the imagination. Through manipulation, playthings such as boxes, clay, and blocks can assume a multitude of symbolic objects and inspire creative impulses. For example, building blocks can be used to construct a variety of things, to count, and to learn shapes and sizes. "Educational" toys are less flexible. There are several ways in which families can encourage children's toy play (see Parent Guidelines).

PARENT GUIDELINES
Encouraging Play

Realize that play teaches skills and abilities that are the center of intelligence.
Play with your child, enroll the child in a play group that meets several times a week, or hire a baby-sitter who can act as a playmate.
Do not turn every play activity into an educational lesson.
Respect your child's likes and dislikes; remember that learning is best acquired in an enjoyable situation.
Observe your child at play so that you come to know favorite types of toys and activities.

From Lewis, M., and Block, J.R.: Toy play: IQ building, Mother's Manual, Sept./Oct. 1982, pp. 31-32.

Play materials need not be expensive or elaborate. Infants and small children derive enjoyment from simple kitchen utensils such as wooden spoons and small plastic plates to bang, pot lids to clang together, and a nest of measuring spoons to rattle. Empty cartons, especially oversized ones used to pack furniture for shipping, can assume the function of clubrooms, hideaways, and other private places. A large mound of dirt (3 to 4 feet high) can become a place for small children to roll toy cars and balls and dig holes

PARENT GUIDELINES
Toy Safety

Select toys that suit the skills, abilities, and interests of the child.
Select toys that are safe for the specific child; look for a label that indicates the intended age-group. Toys that are safe at one age may not be safe for another.
Make certain all parts are present and directions for use are clear and appropriate to the child.
Check for safety labels such as "flame retardant" or "flame resistant."
Select toys durable enough to survive rough play.
Select toys light enough that they will not cause harm if one falls on a child.
Look for toys with smooth, rounded edges. Avoid toys with sharp edges that can cut or sharp points. Points on the inside of the toy can puncture if the toy is broken.
Avoid toys with any small parts that can be swallowed or aspirated, especially for children under 3 years of age.
Avoid toys with any shooting or throwing objects that can injure eyes. This includes toys into which other missiles, such as sticks or pebbles, might be used as substitutes for the intended projectiles. Arrows and darts used by children should have blunt tips and be manufactured from resilient materials; make certain tips are securely attached.
Make certain that materials in toys are nontoxic.
Avoid toys that make loud noises that might be damaging to a child's hearing. Even some squeaking toys are too loud when held close to the ear.
Remove and discard plastic wrapping from toys that could suffocate a child.
Playthings meant for older children should be safely stowed away on high shelves, in locked closets, or in other areas unavailable to younger children.
Make certain an older child understands that a toy inappropriate for smaller children should be kept out of the hands of younger brothers and sisters.
Teach the child the proper way to unplug an electric toy—pull on the plug, not the cord.
Teach the child the safe use of utensils that under certain circumstances can cause injury—scissors, knives, needles, heating elements, or loops, long string, or cord (a potential for strangulation in very young children).
Teach children to beware of electrical appliances and even electrically operated playthings. Children are unfamiliar with the hazards of electricity in association with water.
Provide a safe place for the child to store toys.
Select a toy chest or toy box that is ventilated, is free of self-locking devices that could trap a child inside, and has a lid designed not to pinch a child's fingers or fall on a child's head.
Teach the child to store toys safely in order to prevent accidental injury from stepping or falling on a toy.
Remove large toys, bumper pads, and boxes from playpens; an adventuresome child can use such items as a means of climbing or falling out.
Check all toys periodically for breakage, loose parts, and other potential hazards.
Check movable parts to make certain they are attached securely to the toy. Sometimes pieces that are safe when attached to the toy become a danger when detached.
Repair or discard broken toys.
Make certain that toys are constructed with nontoxic materials, and use only paint labeled "nontoxic" to repaint toys, toy boxes, or children's furniture.
Sand sharp wooden toys or splintered surfaces smooth.
Examine all outdoor toys regularly for rust and weak or sharp parts that could become a danger to a child.
Maintain toys in good repair, without signs of possible hazards such as sharp edges, splinters, weak seams, rust; keep electrical cords and plugs in good condition.

during summer and a place for sliding in winter. Paper is a fascinating and versatile raw material for children of any age, and most books on toy materials include recipes for play dough and finger paint.

Toy Safety

Selection of toys and play equipment is a joint effort between parents and children, but evaluation of their safety is the responsibility of the adult. Government agencies do not inspect and police all toys on the market. Therefore adults who purchase, supervise purchases, or allow children to use play equipment need to evaluate such equipment for its safety, including toys that are gifts or those purchased by the children themselves. Children need toys and activities that increase their sense of competence but that do not create a threat to their health and safety (see Parent Guidelines).

FACTORS THAT INFLUENCE DEVELOPMENT

Children are engaged in a continuous, dynamic, and reciprocal relationship with their environment in order to achieve and maintain an equilibrium. This equilibrium, or balance, is continually upset and regained through numerous and varied complex interactions. It is impossible to include a discussion of all the complex and interrelated factors that influence the development of children as unique individuals. However, some of the major areas of importance are presented.

PHYSIOLOGIC FACTORS

Children are affected by physical factors such as the climate, physiologic influences such as their innate characteristics and susceptibilities, the value system of their families and culture, and psychologic influences such as the quality of parenting and the number, sex, and personalities of the significant persons in their lives. Some factors that may be facilitated, modified, or otherwise influenced by nursing interventions are mentioned in this section, although specific activities and elaboration are discussed elsewhere when appropriate.

Children's basic needs for food, water, air, warmth, elimination, and shelter must be met. Infants, except for limited reflex responses, are totally dependent on adults for satisfaction of even the most basic needs. As development proceeds, children begin to communicate their needs verbally and nonverbally and to assume increasing responsibility for their basic needs gratification.

Those who care for children come to understand the physical changes that take place during the process of development and the special needs generated by these changes, for example, the nature and quantity of food intake, the method and frequency of feeding, and the amount of sleep and activity, which change during childhood. Health and safety hazards associated with every phase of development require provisions for children's physical safety, including prevention of injuries and disease and education of children, families, and communities regarding these potential threats to health and well-being.

Heredity

Inherited characteristics have a profound influence on development. A high correlation exists between parent and child with regard to traits such as height, weight, and rate of growth. The sex of a child, determined by random selection at the time of conception, directs both the pattern of growth and the behavior of others toward the child. In all cultures attitudes and expectations are different with respect to the sex of the child. Sex plus other hereditary determinants strongly affects growth rate and the end result of that growth.

Most physical characteristics, including shape and form of features, body build, and physical peculiarities, are inherited and can influence the way children grow and interact with their environment. Children's heritage may cause a deviation from established overall physical standards for growth and development. For example, Japanese children are smaller than average at all ages. Some children are taller and heavier than the average from early childhood and usually achieve their linear growth sooner. Black girls begin the pubertal growth spurt at a slightly earlier age than white girls and for a brief period are slightly taller (Lowrey, 1986).

The relative importance of heredity and environment in molding development has been deliberated by scientists, educators, and health professionals. It is now commonly accepted that the end product is not a result of the *action* of one or the other of these processes but the *interaction* of one with the other. For example, children who receive genes for above-average height can only achieve full potential with an optimum environment, including good diet, love, and freedom from disease. On the other hand, children who inherit genes for less-than-average height will never attain a height greater than their programmed stature even in a superior environment. Children with limited intellectual capability can never excel in a field that requires highly intellectual skills, no matter to what extent they are pushed. But children with superior mentality will be wasted without an environment that stimulates and encourages their innate capacity.

The area that has provoked the greatest controversy is the contribution of heredity and environment to behavior characteristics and intelligence. Intellectual diversity of individuals is undisputed, but the extent to which large human groups differ in intelligence on a genetic basis is continually challenged. Infant and early childhood stimulation programs and innovative educational techniques at all levels of intellectual endowment have substantiated the positive influence of appropriate environmental stimulation on achievement. On the other hand, early childhood deprivation and the alarming effects of inadequate nutrition during critical periods of development are areas of concern to health professionals.

The influences on behavior traits are more difficult to assess. The culture dictates that some hereditary characteristics (e.g., sex) imply conformity to specific behavioral expectations. Many dimensions of personality that appear to be hereditary (e.g., the degree of responsiveness or unresponsiveness, activity level, extroversion or introversion, the degree of deliberateness or impulsiveness) and various constitutional traits (e.g., beauty, ugliness, physical deformity, sensory handicaps, learning impairment) affect the way others react to children and the interpersonal behavior children display in response. A display of undesirable behavior requires careful evaluation to determine the degree to which the behavior can be attributed to the interpersonal environment or to hereditary influences. This determination can be a significant factor in assessing whether or not such children would profit from therapy or if they should be removed from that environment.

Differences in health and vigor of children may be attributed to hereditary traits. An inherited physical or mental defect or disorder will alter or modify children's physical and/or emotional growth and interactions. The extent to which handicapping conditions interfere with children's growth and well-being are considered in relation to numerous disabilities throughout the remainder of the book.

Neuroendocrine

It has been suggested there may be a growth center in the hypothalamic region responsible for maintaining genetically determined growth patterns. It is believed that some functional relationship exists between the hypothalamus and the endocrine system that influences growth. There is also evidence, based on observations of denervated skeletal muscles, that the peripheral nervous system may influence growth, because muscles deprived of nerve supply degenerate. Many of these effects are not sufficiently explained by disuse or diminished blood supply. For example, nail growth on an extremity with a severed nerve will lag behind the nail growth on the corresponding extremity, but the growth returns to normal with regeneration of the nerve. There is no satisfactory explanation for this revived growth rate; the process may involve a chemical substance secreted by nerve cells that modifies the growth and repair processes.

Hormones. Probably all hormones affect growth in some fashion. Three hormones—growth hormone, thyroid hormone, and androgens—when given to persons deficient in these hormones, stimulate protein anabolism and thereby produce retention of elements essential for building protoplasm and bony tissue. It appears that each of the hormones that has a significant influence on growth manifests its major effect at a different period of growth (see Table 38-1).

Upright Posture

Evidence indicates that the amount of time infants spend in the vertical position influences the age they reach important motor milestones. For example, infants who are placed in the upright posture develop accelerated muscular growth and strength in the legs, neck, and trunk that promotes development of motor skills (Thelen and Fisher, 1982). This is partially supported by observations that infants from Third World countries who are carried vertically in slings walk at an earlier age than children in Western countries who spend more time in the horizontal position. Also, very young infants (2 to 8 weeks old) who are held upright and allowed to practice the "stepping" reflex walk at an earlier age than infants who do not receive this early experience (Zelazo, Zelazo, and Kolb, 1972). Thus experience may be as important as maturation in determining motor development.

Sex

The sex of the child has some influence on growth and development, although it is not always apparent which differences are related to cultural expectations as opposed to innate characteristics. Extensive research (Maccoby and Jacklin, 1974) indicates there are few actual differences but many myths regarding differences between girls and boys. There is no substantial evidence to indicate that girls are more social and suggestible, lack motivation to achieve, have a lower self-esteem, or are better at learning by rote than boys. Nor is there validity to the myth that boys are more analytic and better at high-level tasks than girls. In most studies boys and girls are equally dependent on caregivers, equally susceptible to persuasive communications, and equally motivated to achieve.

There are sex differences that influence behavior in childhood. In general, boys are more aggressive physically; girls verbally (Archer, Pearson, and Westeman, 1988). Boys also more frequently engage in rough and tumble play and aggressive fantasies. This behavior persists through the college years, although aggression diminishes with age in both sexes. Competitive behavior has been observed more often in boys than in girls in some studies, but there is some question as to the validity of this; other studies find the sexes to be similar in this aspect. Both sexes are alike in their willingness to explore a novel environment.

Studies differ in regard to differences between the activity levels of boys and girls, which may reflect the situations in which the measurements were conducted. The play of both boys and girls is equally organized and planned. Some studies find that boys seem to have more difficulty sitting still, engage in more exploratory behavior, and are stimulated to bursts of high activity in the presence of other boys. Boys exhibit greater impulsiveness and have difficulty resisting distractions, as reflected by the greater incidence of injuries in boys at all ages. However, boys tend to be outside more than girls, and many activities are influenced by motivational factors such as fear, anger, and curiosity.

Both sexes are highly responsive to social situations, although there are some sex differences in social relationships. Boys and girls show interest in confronting social stimuli (e.g., human faces and voices), in imitating models, and in understanding the emotional reactions and needs of others. However, boys have a more extensive sphere of relationships, are highly oriented toward a peer group, and congregate in large groups, whereas girls are more likely to associate in pairs or small groups and become involved in a more intense relationship with a few close friends. Girls appear to be more concerned with the welfare of the group and therefore are more apt to compromise in situations involving conflict.

The sexes are similar in overall self-confidence and self-satisfaction but differ in the areas in which they seem to feel the greatest self-confidence. Boys are apt to view themselves as more powerful and with more control over events. They respond to a challenge, especially when it appeals to their ego or competitive feelings, in order to attain a higher level of achievement. Little difference exists between the sexes regarding motivation to achieve, although some studies find girls to be superior in this respect.

During childhood girls are more likely to comply with adult commands and directions. However, this ready compliance does not extend to relationships with peers. Boys, on the other hand, appear to be more concerned about maintaining status in the peer group, which may render them more vulnerable to pressures and challenges from the group.

Girls have always been considered to demonstrate more nurturant or helping behavior than boys, but this is not established to the satisfaction of child psychologists. Girls between the ages of 6 and 10 are more often seen behaving in nurturing ways than boys, but many studies of nursery school children have not observed this difference. Much of this type of behavior is the result of imitation and modeling; as with other popular beliefs about differences between girls and boys, there is little basis in fact. It may be a result of selective attention of casual observers whose ideas are confirmed or strengthened by behaviors that are consistent with their prior beliefs. Behavior inconsistent with expectations is more likely to go unnoticed, and consequently entrenched ideas are perpetuated.

Disease

Altered growth and development is one of the clinical manifestations in a number of hereditary disorders. Growth impairment is particularly marked in skeletal disorders, such as the various forms of dwarfism and at least one of the chromosomal anomalies (Turner syndrome). Many of the disorders of metabolism, such as vitamin D–resistant rickets, mucopolysaccharidoses, and the numerous endocrine disorders, interfere with the normal growth pattern. In other disorders the tendency is toward the upper percentile of height, for example, Klinefelter syndrome and Marfan syndrome.

Many chronic illnesses associated with varying degrees of growth failure are related to congenital cardiac anomalies and respiratory disorders such as cystic fibrosis. Any disorder characterized by the inability to digest and absorb body nutrients will have an adverse effect on growth and development. These include the malabsorption syndromes and defects in digestive enzyme systems. Almost any disease state that persists over an extended period, particularly during a critical period of development, may have a permanent effect on growth. For example, children on long-term corticosteroid therapy exhibit growth retardation.

Children in a prolonged state of disequilibrium caused by illness, such as chronic infections, are under a constant inner stress that inhibits their response to adult demands and contributes to their difficulty in managing stimulating environmental experiences. Behaviors that these children display as they cope with outside stimuli, as well as inner irritations, can be misinterpreted as distractibility and lack of persistence toward a goal. A prolonged illness that occurs in the second year during the phase of rapid acquisition of motor control and autonomy may cause a child to lose the natural impetus peculiar to this stage of development. Such a child may remain passive and require special stimulation to develop the independence that would have developed spontaneously under normal circumstances.

PHYSICAL ENVIRONMENT

Some physical conditions have been shown to have some effect on growth, although their influence is less evident than factors such as heredity, nutrition, or hormonal excesses or deficiencies.

Season, Climate, and Oxygen Concentration

There is some evidence that season and climate may have an influence on growth. Growth in height appears to be faster in the spring and summer months, whereas growth in weight proceeds more rapidly during the autumn and winter. These observations have not been satisfactorily explained. This phenomenon may have a hormonal basis, or it may be related to seasonal differences in activity levels.

It was formerly believed that persons living in a warm climate were smaller than those from a cold climate. However, it is much too difficult to separate the effects of climate from other factors such as race, nutrition, or disease. There does seem to be more evidence regarding the effects of hypoxia on growth. Children with disorders that produce a chronic hypoxia are characteristically small when compared with children of the same chronologic age. In addition, children native to high altitudes are smaller than those living at lower altitudes (Yip, Binkin, and Trowbridge, 1988).

Environmental Hazards

Hazards in the environment are a source of concern to health care providers and others interested in health and safety. No aspect of the potential dangers of daily living has escaped investigation by some group or individual, and more types and sources of environmental pollution are detected as populations and technology expand. Physical injuries are the most prevalent consequences of environmental dangers, and these are discussed extensively throughout the book as they apply in relation to age, specific hazards, and selected physical disabilities. The harmful agents most often associated with health risks are chemicals and radiation.

The sources and routes of exposure to chemical hazards are surprisingly extensive. Water, air, and food contamination from a variety of origins are well documented and discussed. Newer, recognized sources of exposure are substances carried home (usually from the workplace) on clothes or other objects, chemicals secreted in breast milk (especially prescribed drugs and nicotine), and contamination within well-insulated homes (especially from disinfectants or burning of substances that produce toxic fumes) (Rogan, 1980). Passive inhalation of tobacco smoke by infants and children has been found to be a hazard at all stages of development.

The harmful effects of large doses of radiation are unquestioned although the long-term consequences are still under investigation. The effects of low-dose or short-term radiation are still debatable, as are the safe vs harmful dosage levels. However, the ubiquitous gas radon (and especially its isotopes) has been determined to be an ever-present danger (American Academy of Pediatrics, 1989).

Socioeconomic Level

Evidence indicates that the socioeconomic level of children's families has a significant impact on children's body size. At all ages children from upper- and middle-class families are taller than comparative children of families in the lower socioeconomic strata. Girls from upper- and middle-class families also reach menarche up to 3 months earlier than girls from the lower socioeconomic levels.

The cause of these differences is less definite although the general health and nutrition of lower socioeconomic levels are probably significant factors. Nutritious food sources (especially proteins) are scarce, and other factors (e.g., larger family size and regularity in eating, sleeping, and exercise) may play a role.

NUTRITION

Probably the single most important influence on growth is nutrition. Dietary factors regulate growth at *all* stages of development, and their effects are exerted in numerous and complex ways. Adequate nutrition provides the essential nutrients in the amount and balance necessary to sustain physiologic needs. These needs vary widely according to age, level of activity, and environmental conditions. Inadequacies in any or all of these essential nutrients will be reflected in altered growth.

The nutritional requirements of childhood are directly related to the rate and direction of growth. During the rapid prenatal growth period, faulty nutrition may negatively influence development from the time of implantation of the ovum until birth. The nutritional needs are met entirely through the maternal system; as a result, maternal deficiencies or abnormalities in the supplementary intrauterine structures will be manifest in fetal development.

During infancy and childhood the demand for calories is relatively great, as evidenced by the rapid increase in both height and weight. Protein and caloric requirements are higher at this time than at almost any period of postnatal development. As the growth rate slows with its concomitant decrease in metabolism, a corresponding reduction in caloric and protein requirement occurs (see Table 4-3). Growth is uneven during the periods of childhood between infancy and adolescence, when there are plateaus and small growth spurts. The child's appetite fluctuates in response to these variations until the turbulent growth spurt of adolescence, when adequate nutrition is extremely important but may be subject to numerous emotional influences. Children's caloric intake must equal their energy output plus that needed for growth. It is estimated that the average child (e.g., the 6- to 10-year-old child) expends 55% of the energy for metabolic maintenance, 25% for physical activity, 8% in fecal loss, and 12% for growth. See Table 4-5 for servings per day of the basic food groups during childhood. Sample menus for various age-groups are included in discussions on nutrition in the chapters on health promotion of children in specific age-groups.

Adequate nutrition is closely related to good health throughout life, and an overall improvement in nourishment is evidenced by the gradual increase in size and early maturation of children in this century. In the growing child, inadequate nutrition is dangerous, particularly during those periods critical for growth. Inadequate nutrition has the greatest impact during the critical periods of rapid cell division. For example, normal development of the central nervous system depends on adequate nutrition during fetal life and throughout the first 2 years of postnatal life.

Malnutrition

The term *malnutrition* in its strictest sense is usually used to describe undernutrition, primarily that resulting from insufficient caloric intake. However, malnutrition may result from the following: (1) a dietary intake that is quantitatively or qualitatively inadequate, or both, including overnutrition; (2) disease that interferes with appetite, digestion, or absorption while increasing nutritional requirements; (3) excessive physical activity or inadequate rest; or (4) disturbed interpersonal relationships and other environmental or psychologic factors. Severe malnutrition during the critical periods of development, particularly the first 6 months of life, is positively correlated with diminished height, weight, and intelligence scores. The importance of nutrition as a vital aspect of health promotion during all phases of the illness-

Table 4-5 Servings per day for children based on basic four food groups

FOOD GROUP	SERVINGS PER DAY
Milk or equivalent (for calcium) ½ cup whole milk equals: ¾ ounce cheese ½ cup yogurt, milk pudding 1 cup cottage cheese	2-3 cups for child 4 cups for adolescent Usual serving size: Toddler and preschooler—½ to ¾ cup School-age and older—1 cup
Meat, fish, poultry, or equivalent 1 ounce meat equals: 1 egg 1 ounce cheese 2 tablespoons peanut butter ½ cup cooked legumes	2 for child and adolescent Usual serving size: Toddler and preschooler—1 egg, 1 to 2 ounces meat School-age and older—1 egg, 3 ounces meat
Vegetables and fruits Citrus equivalents: 1 orange or tomato ½ cup orange or grapefruit juice ¾ cup strawberries	4 for child and adolescent 1 citrus daily; 1 yellow or dark green vegetable 3 to 4 times weekly Usual serving size: Toddler and preschooler—2 to 4 tablespoons to ¼ to ½ cup School-age and older—½ cup
Breads and cereals 1 slice enriched bread equals: ¾ cup dry cereal ½ cup cooked pasta, rice, or cereal ½ hamburger bun 1 small muffin or biscuit	4 for child and adolescent Usual serving size: Toddler and preschooler—½ slice bread, ¼ cup School-age and older—1 slice bread, ½ cup

*Fats and carbohydrates should be served sparingly to meet caloric needs.

wellness continuum is included as it relates to developmental phases and specific health problems.

INTERPERSONAL RELATIONSHIPS

Solid interpersonal relationships are essential to psychologic well-being. Relationships with significant others play an important role in development, particularly in emotional, intellectual, and personality development. Not only do the quality and quantity of contacts with other persons exert an influence on growing children, but the widening range of contacts is essential to learning and the development of a healthy personality (Fig. 4-20). During the formative years, culturally determined, age-appropriate behaviors are reinforced and consequently repeated. Thus patterns of reward, punishment, and modeling continually modify children's individuality of character and temperament. Children behave in a manner that elicits rewards from the persons most significant in their lives.

Significant Others

Normal children routinely turn to parents, teachers, and friends for comfort, protection, education, acceptance, and material needs. Parents and caregiving persons are unquestionably the most influential persons during early infancy. They meet the infants' basic needs of food, warmth, comfort, and love, provide stimulation for their senses, and facilitate their expanding capacities. Through these individuals children learn to trust the world and feel secure to venture in increasingly wide relationships. Through constant reinforcement children learn the behaviors that bring satisfaction to the nurturing persons and incorporate them. Eventually these behaviors become self-motivating. For example, children learn that evacuating the bowel in a proper receptacle produces a positive response from the parents, resulting in a lifetime behavioral pattern.

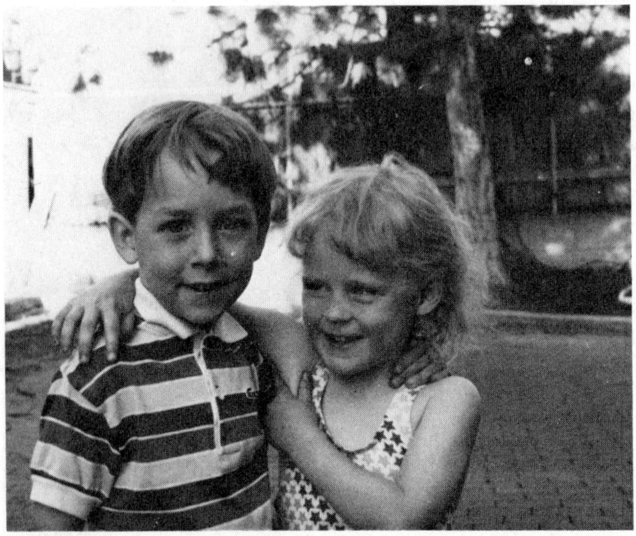

Fig. 4-20. Preschool children develop friendships outside the family group.

As they get older, children seek approval from a widening sphere of persons, including other members of their family, their peers, and to a lesser degree other authority figures (e.g., teachers). The increasing importance of the peer group in determining the behavior of school-age children and adolescents is well documented. However, it is the quality of the parent-child relationship that determines to a large extent the impact of peer influence on a child.

Generally the parents are most influential in helping children to assume sex-role identification. Parents define and reinforce acceptable sex-role behavior and provide sex-appropriate role models for the children. In the absence of a suitable sex-role model in the family setting, children may adopt some characteristics of the opposite-sex parent or sibling. Frequently children identify with a teacher or other significant person of the same sex.

Siblings are children's first peers, and the way they learn to relate to each other can affect later interactions with peers outside the family group. For example, firstborn children who are accustomed to a position of leadership with siblings tend to assume the same position with peers; younger children are more often followers. Ease in relationships with peers of the same or opposite sex is frequently associated with similar associations in the home.

Pets can also serve as an object for love and affection (Ross, 1981), and play an important role in the lives of many young children. They provide close, nonjudgmental companionship, are on call 24 hours a day, and can be an excellent tool for helping build children's self-esteem. By assuming responsibility for helping care for a pet, children can develop confidence in their abilities and gain respect for a job well done (Pets are Wonderful Council, 1985). They can also be a first step in developing a concern for other people.

Love and Affection

The single most important emotional need of children is to be loved and to feel secure in that love. Children strive above all else to gain the love and acceptance of those who are significant in their lives. When they feel secure in this love, they are able to withstand the normal crises associated with growing up and those unexpected crises (e.g., illness or loss) that are superimposed on the anticipated course of development.

Children cannot receive too much love. However, this love must be communicated to them through words and actions that tell them they are loved, not for their actions or achievement, but for what they are or simply *because they are*. Although love is closely associated with discipline, independence, and other factors that influence the child's self-concept, it should be an undemanding, accepting love that is indispensable to the development of a healthy personality. Unconditional love, freely bestowed, helps establish a sense of security and a positive sense of self within children that will persist throughout their lifetime (Fig. 4-21). Children must know they are loved and that whatever happens they can depend on this love. For many children spiritual love is a very significant source of complete, undemanding love. Without the security of loving relationships,

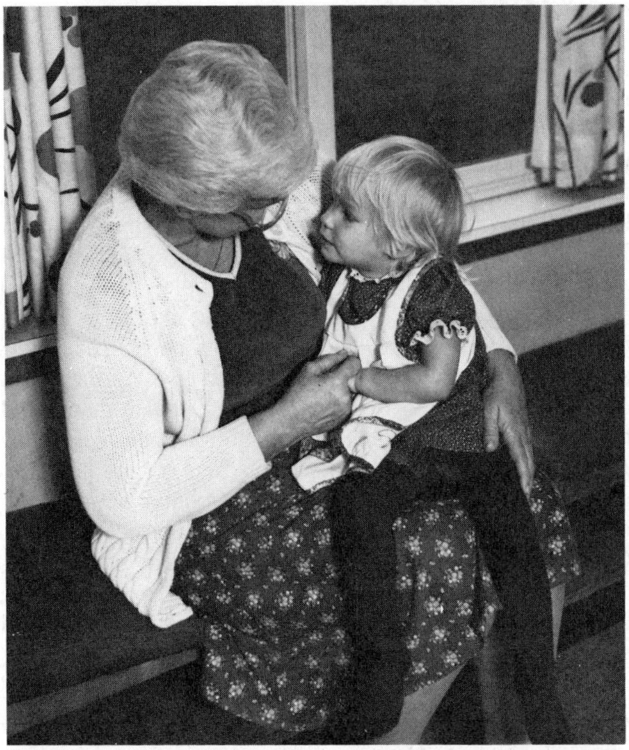

Fig. 4-21. A grandmother is a primary source of unconditional love and comfort.

children may become tense and insecure and develop undesirable behavior patterns as they attempt to obtain that love or try to compensate for its loss.

The primary source of love, particularly during infancy, is the parent, usually the mother or mothering person. The establishment of this early love attachment (or bonding) profoundly influences subsequent interpersonal relationships. With ever-widening relationships, children need the love and acceptance of others. They need to feel they are wanted, accepted, and belong in whatever relationships are important to them at each stage of development.

Parents may truly love their children but be unable to communicate this love to them. Parents who are insecure in their parenting skills frequently seek advice and reassurance from health professionals. Nurses aware of indications of parental insecurity will be able to provide assistance and reassurance that can preserve and enhance the parent-child relationship and build a sense of confidence in the parent.

Security

Closely allied to the need for love is the need for a sense of security. As they grow and develop in a complex world, children encounter many threats to their sense of security. Indeed, most childhood behavior problems are associated with an element of insecurity. Every change in themselves or their environment creates a feeling of uncertainty. Faced with confusing, conflicting adjustments, young children need the security provided by relatively stable situations and dependable human relationships. The degree to which they can cope with these stresses depends on the patience and support they receive from those most closely involved in their care.

A multitude of factors exists that can generate a feeling of insecurity in children. Ordinarily the parents, who are sources of comfort, guidance, and encouragement, provide a measure of security in an insecure world. To achieve this security, children need the warm acceptance of loving parents, a stable family unit, and judicious handling of stress-provoking situations such as sibling rivalry, relocation to a new neighborhood, and illness in themselves or other members of the family. A disturbed home environment caused by such factors as marital discord, illness of a parent or family member, or death of a family member can shatter their equilibrium.

Infants are disturbed by physical threats, such as hunger, cold, or discomfort. Small children are physiologically disturbed by emotions such as anger, fear, and grief, which they can release only in overt behavior. They can obtain a measure of relief from these feelings by the reassurance that their physical needs will be met, restraints will be placed on their behavior, and expectations that keep pace with their inner controls will be held. Rejection by significant persons, social ineptitude, and physical handicaps often produce insecurity in a child. The number and variety of stressful factors originating within or outside the child are often difficult to determine; therefore those responsible for the child's care must be alert for cues that reveal threats to this sense of security.

Discipline and Authority

Because children live in an organized society, they must be prepared to accept restrictions on their behavior. Discipline is not punishment. Rather it is the teaching of desirable behavior. Children need to learn the rules governing behavior in the home, the neighborhood, the school, and the community at large. To learn acceptable behavior that permits them to live enjoyably with themselves and others, children need the steady, firm guidance of loving parents and others in authority roles. Good discipline provides children with protection from dangers within and without and relieves them of the burden of decisions they are not prepared to make, yet allows them to develop independence of thought and action within a secure framework.

Children who learn to live within reasonable rules are happier and more secure children. Without the stabilizing influence of controls, children feel uncertain and insecure. Too often, inexperienced and insecure parents fear the loss of a child's love, suffer feelings of guilt over disciplinary action, or even relinquish their authority to the child. To discipline is to teach reality. Sensible, mature parents establish fair rules and regulations in the home and then see that they are carried out. Parents should never exploit children's love for them as a means to control their children. Children's anxiety lest they lose that love is already great. Discipline based on love of the child and carried out with conviction, confidence, and consistency will produce a self-reliant, buoyant, and self-controlled child.

Dependence and Independence

As children grow and mature, they are increasingly able to direct their own activities and to make more independent decisions. However, there are great fluctuations in their ability to function independently. Even with a compelling inner drive to master and achieve, they are not always able to cope with difficult and frustrating problems or conflicts. All children feel the urge to grow up and move toward maturity, but they have at their disposal only those energies not being used to maintain mastery over old conflicts. Independence should be permitted to grow at its own rate.

Periods of regression and dependence not only are normal but are often necessary and helpful. If children feel sufficiently comfortable and content in a situation or relationship and reasonably certain that they can return to this safety and security, they will venture into the untried and untested on their own. If they feel doubtful concerning their abilities to cope, regression to a more comfortable level of competence allows them to replenish their inner resources and prepare to move ahead once again. Independence grows out of dependence; one cannot be considered as distinct from the other.

Children will learn independence of thought and decision making provided the opportunity is not withheld from them. If they are pushed into acting independently before they feel themselves ready, they may withdraw from independence. When they choose not to relinquish the joys of independence and autonomy or to move ahead to new worlds of independence, they will dawdle. Parents, teachers, nurses, and others responsible for the child's care must be able to adjust their expectations and support to meet the child's needs of the moment. It is important to recognize when to help and when not to help children experiment with their immature and imperfect self-control, when to make demands requiring children's utmost ability, and when to allow them to function temporarily on a more immature level. They need these freedoms and controls in the process of becoming mature, self-reliant adults.

Emotional Deprivation

The most prominent feature of emotional deprivation, particularly during the first year, is developmental retardation. Much of the information regarding the adverse effects of interpersonal influences on development has been acquired through retrospective studies of gross deprivation and trauma. The most notable instances involved homeless infants who were placed in institutions for care. These infants, who did not receive consistent caregiving, failed to gain weight even with an adequate diet; they were pale, listless, and immobile, and unresponsive to stimuli that usually elicit a response (such as a smile or cooing) in the normal infant. If the emotional deprivation continues for a sufficient length of time, the child does not survive.

Harlow's classic experiments with infant monkeys illustrate the far-reaching effects of emotional and social deprivation in infancy (Harlow and Harlow, 1962). In these experiments the monkeys were raised by substitute, inanimate "mothers" made of cloth-covered wire from whom they derived nourishment and a measure of comfort but no mothering. These monkeys developed abnormal play and sex behavior. The few who bore offspring were unable to "mother" them. However, those who were allowed peer associations developed normal play and social-sex behavior. By correlating these findings with retrospective studies of human infants in comparable age-groups, attempts have been made to explain some of the behaviors observed in these children in later interpersonal relationships.

Although the most remarkable examples of emotional deprivation were first recognized among infants in institutions, the term *masked deprivation* has been used to describe children who are reared in homes where there is a distorted parent-child relationship or otherwise disordered home environment. Infants do not thrive if the caregiving person is hostile, fearful of handling them, or indifferent to them and their needs. Such children exhibit poor growth even though they are apparently free of physical disease. Children past the age of infancy who evidence physical underdevelopment are also retarded in bone age. These same infants and children display "catch-up" growth in a changed environment.

STRESS IN CHILDHOOD

Stress has been defined and described by numerous authorities from both a physiologic and an emotional point of view. Most discussions are centered on adult responses, but children are frequently among the most affected victims of a wide range of threatening events. Essentially it is "an imbalance between environmental demands and a person's coping resources that . . . disrupts the equilibrium of the person" (Masten and others, 1988).

Most research related to children has been restricted to specific stressors and stress-provoking experiences such as hospitalization, separation and loss, and pain. A description of all the stressors to which children are exposed is beyond the scope of this segment; however, the more common manifestations and stressful events are discussed briefly. Since stress is a normal aspect of life, stressors and some coping strategies are discussed in relation to specific situations throughout the book. For children's response to a intensely stressful event (such as a natural disaster, bombing, or schoolyard shooting) see Posttraumatic Stress Disorder, Chapter 18.

Although children are not strangers to stress, some children appear to be more vulnerable than others. Children's age, temperament, life situation, and state of health affect their vulnerability, reactions, and ability to handle stress. Also, the responses to a stressor can be behavioral, psychologic, or physiologic. It is impossible, unrealistic, and undesirable to protect children from stress, but providing them with interpersonal security helps them develop coping strategies for dealing with stress. The concept of an emotional bank can help parents and caregivers maintain a proper perspective regarding the effects of stress and coping. According to Usdin (1988), children have an emotional bank in which deposits, as well as withdrawals, can be

Box 4-7 WARNING SIGNS: CHILDHOOD STRESS

Bed-wetting
Boasts of superiority
Complaints of feeling afraid or upset without being able to identify the source
Complaints of neck or back pains
Complaints of pounding heart
Complaints of stomach upset, queasiness, or vomiting
Compulsive cleanliness
Compulsive ear tugging, hair pulling, or eyebrow plucking
Cruel behavior toward people or pets
Decline in school achievement
Defiance
Demand for constant perfection
Depression
Dirtying pants
Dislike of school
Downgrading of self
Easily startled by unexpected sounds
Explosive crying
Extreme nervousness
Frequent daydreaming and retreats from reality
Frequent urination or diarrhea
Headaches
Hyperactivity, or excessive tension or alertness
Increased number of minor spills, falls, and other accidents
Irritability
Listlessness or lack of enthusiasm
Loss of interest in activities usually approached with vigor
Lying
Nightmares or night terror
Nervous laughter
Nervous tics, twitches, or muscle spasms
Obvious attention-seeking
Overeating
Poor concentration
Poor eating
Poor sleep
Psychosomatic illnesses
Stealing
Stuttering
Teeth grinding (sometimes during sleep)
Thumb-sucking
Uncontrollable urge to run and hide
Unusual difficulty in getting along with friends
Unusual jealousy of close friends and siblings
Unusual sexual behavior, such as spying or exhibitionism
Unusual shyness
Use of alcohol, drugs, or cigarettes
Withdrawal from usual social activities

From Kuczen, B.: Childhood stress: don't let your child be a victim, New York, 1982, Delacorte Press.

made. "If the child has a good positive balance in the account, he or she can tolerate significant withdrawal experiences. If the child has a low balance, then even a minor withdrawal may bankrupt the account, causing it to be overdrawn."

Parents and other caregivers can try to recognize signs of stress (Box 4-7) in order to help children deal with stresses before they become overwhelming. If a number of stresses are imposed on children at the same time, the children are more vulnerable. When a succession of stresses produces an excessive stress load, children may experience a serious change in health and/or behavior. An adaptation of the Holmes and Rahe stress scale for adults appears in Box 4-8, which provides a tool to alert parents or caregivers to situations children experience that are not always viewed by adults as stressful.

It is most important that parents and persons working with children understand the nature of childhood stress and ways it can be recognized or anticipated. Caregivers must *listen* to children so they are aware of children's fears and concerns and must let them know that they are important and what they say matters. Physical contact is comforting and reassuring to children. Simply holding, touching, or hugging children is both relaxing and comforting and facilitates communication. Spending unhurried time with children, family outings, vacations, and exposing children to positive influences help build children's strength and security. Solid interpersonal relationships are essential to the psychologic well-being of children.

Coping

Coping is defined as "flexible strategies for dealing with environmental challenges" (Murphy and Moriarity, 1976). It refers to a special class of individual reactions to stressors—specifically, a reaction to a stressor that resolves, reduces, or replaces the affect state classified as stressful. Children, like adults, respond to everyday stress by trying to change the circumstances (primary control coping) or trying to adjust to circumstances the way they are (secondary control coping) (Band and Weisz, 1988). An example of primary control is via tantrums or aggressive behavior; with-drawal and submission are examples of secondary control.

Any strategy that provides relaxation is effective in reducing stress, and most children have their own natural methods, for example, withdrawal, physical activity, reading, listening to music, working on a project, or taking a nap. The list is endless. Some turn to parents to solve their problems, or they may develop socially unacceptable strategies such as cheating, stealing, or lying (Kuczen, 1982).

Children can be taught stress-reduction techniques to use in coping. First, they must be helped to recognize signs of tension in themselves and then taught any of a variety of appropriate strategies—special exercises, relaxation and breathing, mental imagery, and numerous other simple activities. Also, parents and other caregivers can anticipate possible stress-provoking events and prepare children for coping by role playing a scenario or "talking it through" beforehand. Most of the stress-reducing strategies discussed

Box 4-8 STRESS SCALE FOR CHILDREN

Life Event	Value
1. Death of a parent	100
2. Divorce of parents	73
3. Separation of parents	65
4. Parent's jail term	63
5. Death of a close family member (e.g., grandparent)	63
6. Personal injury or illness	53
7. Parent's remarriage	50
8. Suspension or expulsion from school	47
9. Parent's reconciliation	45
10. Long vacation (summer, etc.)	45
11. Parent or sibling illness	44
12. Mother's pregnancy	40
13. Anxiety over sex	39
14. Birth or adoption of a new baby	39
15. New school or classroom or new teacher	39
16. Money problems at home	38
17. Death or moving away of close friend	37
18. Changes in studies	36
19. More quarrels with parents (or parents quarreling more)	35
20. Change in school responsibilities	29
21. Sibling going away to school	29
22. Family arguments with grandparents	29
23. Winning school or community awards	28
24. Mother or father going to work or stopping work	26
25. School beginning or ending	26
26. Family's living standard changing	25
27. Change in personal habits (e.g., bedtime, homework, etc.)	24
28. Trouble with parents (e.g., lack of communication, hostility, etc.)	23
29. Change in school hours, schedule of courses	23
30. Family's moving	20
31. New sports, hobbies, family recreation activities	20
32. Change in church activities (more involvement or less)	19
33. Change in social activities (e.g., new friends, loss of old ones, peer pressures)	18
34. Change in sleeping habits, giving up naps, etc.	16
35. Change in number of family get-togethers	15
36. Change in eating habits (e.g., going on or off diet, new way of family cooking)	13
37. Vacation	13
38. Christmas	12
39. Breaking home, school, or community rules	11

Add up the points for items that have touched the child's life in the last 12 months.

Score below 150, the child is carrying an average stress load.

Score between 150 and 300, the child has a better-than-average chance of showing some symptoms of stress.

Score over 300, the child's stress load is heavy and there is a strong likelihood for experiencing a serious change in health and/or behavior.

From Saunders, A., and Remsberg, B.: The stress-proof child: a loving parent's guide, New York, 1984, Holt, Rinehart & Winston, pp. 72-73.

in Chapter 26 in relation to managing pain are effective for any stress situation.

Probably the most useful tool that children can learn is how to solve problems. When children can view any new situation as a problem to be solved and an opportunity to learn, they are not vulnerable to the control of others. It provides them with a sense of mastery over their own lives and reinforces the fact that they have within themselves the ability and information to handle whatever comes their way. Problem-solving skill gives them the confidence to know where and how to seek help when they need it.

Childhood Fears

Fear is a normal function, a self-preservation signal that mobilizes the physiologic resources of the organism. *Fear* and *anxiety* are often used interchangeably, and the physical reactions to both are almost identical. *Fear* is an emotional reaction to a specific real or unreal threat or danger; *anxiety* refers to a general uneasiness, apprehension, or feeling of impending doom. Fear is a momentary reaction to danger based on a low estimate of one's own power. Fearful children perceive a threat (person, animal, or situation) as being stronger than themselves and thus capable of harming them. When the balance of power is altered, the fear disappears. For example, children's fears can be alleviated by the presence of an adult whom they perceive as a source of protection; or fear can be overcome by familiarity with the source of the threat, such as a dog or a dark room. Anxiety is general, lasting, internally generated, and reflects overall feelings of weakness, ineptitude, and helplessness (Wolman, 1978).

In childhood the distinction between fear and anxiety is important because childhood fears are specific, and except for the specific fear (or fears), children are happy and active. Childhood fears are limited problems, and most are alleviated with growth and children's increased self-confidence and faith in themselves. Unrealistic fears are abandoned with maturation and learning, to be replaced by realistic fears. As with other stresses, there are individual differences in susceptibility to fear, and certain fears are age related (Table 4-6). Fears that are likely to persist into adulthood are fear of physical danger, death, sickness, body injury, physical assault, car accidents, airplane crashes, and war.

Children often come to fear things they did not fear at a younger age because of their lack of awareness (e.g., a busy street), or they may become fearful of familiar things. With the development of imaginative ability, imaginary creatures and situations may become a source of fear. Also, children with superior intelligence are likely to be more aware of real dangers, are less likely to succumb to imaginary fears, and have fewer fears than other children. These

Table 4-6 Typical childhood fears

AGE	FEARS
0-6 months	Loss of support, loud noises, bright lights; sudden movement
7-12 months	Strangers, sudden appearance of unexpected and looming objects (including people), animals, heights
Toddler 1-3 years	Separation from parent, the dark, loud or sudden noises, injury, strangers (including strange peers), certain persons (e.g., the doctor), certain situations (e.g., trip to the dentist), animals, large objects or machines, change in environment
Preschool 3-5 years	Separation from parent, supernatural beings such as monsters or ghosts, animals, the dark, noises, "bad" people, injury, death
School-age 6-12 years	Supernatural beings, injury, storms, the dark, staying alone, separation from parent, things seen on television or in movies, injury, tests and failure in school, consequences related to unattractive physical appearance, death
Adolescence	Inept social performance, social isolation, sexuality, drugs, war, divorce, crowds, gossip, public speaking, plane and car crashes, death

From Feiner, J., and Schachter, R.: When your child is afraid. In Schachter, R., and McCauley, C.S.: Why your child is afraid, New York, 1988, Simon & Schuster.

observations are probably related to cognitive capacities (Wolman, 1978).

Coping with fears is the same as coping with other stresses. To help children overcome their fears, parents and others should not shame or show disapproval for their fears, encourage their unreasonable fears, overprotect them, or force them into a situation they fear. For example, throwing a fearful child into deep water will probably increase a fear of water to the point of a lasting phobia. Parents can serve as models by demonstrating strength, decisiveness, and self-confidence. For instance, the parents can take their children by the hand and gently guide them into shallow water or around a dark room. Desensitization by gradually facing the fearsome object or situation is effective with most children. Parents can allow their children to express their fears and encourage them to cope with certain dangers. Most of all, parents need to make their children feel that they will always be loved and will be protected whenever necessary. (See also Posttraumatic Stress Disorder, Chapter 18.)

RESILIENCY

Some children manage to achieve stable personalities and a sense of competence despite adverse conditions and a series of stressful events in their childhood, such as biologic insults, a pathologic family environment, or the negative effects of poverty. This ego-resiliency has been observed in a number of studies (Anthony and Cohler, 1987; Garmezy and Rutter, 1983; Sroufe, 1983; Werner and Smith, 1982). The findings of these observations have determined that resilient children share a number of characteristics in common. They were active, alert, responsive, and sociable as infants, with the ability to elicit positive responses from other people, and acquired a strong sense of autonomy. As children they enjoy school, often using it as a refuge from a disordered home, and are well liked by peers.

Ego-resilient children use a wide variety of coping strategies, have hobbies and interests that give them a sense of mastery and pride, and have problem-solving and communication skills that they use effectively (Werner, 1987). Central in the histories of all these children, regardless of the type and extent of their adversity, is that they had the opportunity to establish a secure relationship with at least one stable person who accepted them uncritically.

Persons other than the significant other in children's lives can play an enabling role when the person who provides support is unavailable. Other significant persons can promote the competencies of these and other children by assuming a nurturing role and encouraging their independence, teaching them self-help skills, and boosting their self-confidence (see Questions and Controversies, p. 549).

INFLUENCE OF THE MASS MEDIA

There is no doubt that the communications media provide children with a means for extending their knowledge about the world in which they live and have contributed to narrowing the differences between classes.

Reading Materials

The oldest form of mass media—books, newspapers, and magazines—contributes to children's competence in almost every direction, as well as providing enjoyment. Recognition of the impact of reading matter used in the schools on the value system and socialization processes prompted reevaluation of textbook content in terms of the biased presentation of male and female role models, the sugar-coated view of life situations, and the unrealistic, biased history of minority groups.

Fairy tales, for generations the mainstay of young children's literature, for a time suffered condemnation as being sexist, overly violent in content, and riddled with unfavorable stereotypes, such as the wicked stepmother, dwarfs, and physical unattractiveness associated with evil. They are now believed to provide an excellent medium for explaining puzzling and important topics such as death, stepparents, and inner feelings and turmoils. To a young child the world is peopled by giants, adults who control their lives and threaten their autonomy, who want children to do something against their will. Children can see these giants overcome. The split view of parents is also portrayed in fairy tales: the "good" parents who give children whatever they want and the "mean" parents who deprive their children of things. Although they do not provide solutions, fairy tales confront children with emotional predicaments and offer suggestions for dealing with them.

Comic books and other pulp reading material have been popular in every generation, usually at the expense of literature provided by schools, libraries, and parents. Many children have nothing else to read. The easy reading, quick action, and adventure in brief episodes seem to fulfill a need for children who are striving to understand both aggression in others and their own impulses. Reading ability, intelligence, and school adjustment apparently have no relationship to the number and type of comic books read. Most comic books appear to be relatively harmless to the majority of children and are in some ways even beneficial. Comic books seem to have only a minor influence on acquisition of beliefs, values, and behaviors. The popularity of this medium has prompted some educators to encourage translations of literature into comic book form in order to stimulate the interest of students in the classics.

Movies

Movies, not closely bound to reality and often portraying an assortment of socially approved behaviors, perhaps make a contribution to children's value systems, but they do provide opportunities for desirable social learning. On the other hand, children, especially adolescents, flock to the "macho" movies and those whose heroes resort to violent resolution of problems, such as the use of karate techniques and wild automobile chases. The carryover of these influences into daily life and relationships may account in part for the increase in violent behavior of young persons.

A recent concern is the plethora of "slasher" and R-rated movies available to children and teenagers, in theaters, cable television, and video cassettes. The content of movies has changed markedly during the past few years with mutilation as the major theme. To children who are unable to distinguish between reality and fantasy these films play on their deepest fears, resulting in bedtime fears, nightmares, and a fearful view of the world (Schmitt, 1989).

Young children can be frightened by some of the movies considered to be safe for family viewing. For example, Bambi can be frightening to young children, and the villainous witches in *Snow White* and the *Wizard of Oz* are terrifying figures. Also, some of the classic Disney movies such as *Snow White* and *Cinderella,* which depict stepmothers as evil, destructive persons, can have a deleterious effect on children-stepmother relationships or can be confusing to children who have developed a positive relationship with a stepmother.

Television

The medium that has the most impact on children in America today is television, which has become one of the most significant socializing agents in the life of young children. The content of programs and commercials provides multiple sources for acquiring information, modeling behaviors, and observing value orientations. Besides producing a leveling effect on class differences in general information and vocabulary, TV exposes children to a wider variety of topics and events than they encounter in day-to-day life. Television always has time to talk to children and is a form of access to the adult world.

Ninety-eight percent of households in the United States have a TV set, usually situated prominently in the most used room. Children between the ages of 3 and 11 watch an average of 3 to 4 hours of TV a day, and by the time they reach age 18 they will have spent more time watching television than in any other single activity except sleeping (Liebert, Sprafkin, and Davidson, 1982). Similar findings have been reported on TV usage in Australia, Canada, and some European countries (Murray, 1980).

Considerable controversy has been generated and continues regarding the favorable vs deleterious influence of television on child development and behavior. Some indict the content of television; others accuse the medium itself (see Questions and Controversies). Several factors encourage the learning or performing of TV-influenced behaviors (Box 4-9).

Interventions. It is clear that parents need to supervise the amount and type of TV programs their children watch and to teach their children how to watch TV (see Parent Guidelines, p. 152). Since children see television as pieces of reality, parents can point out to them that what they see on the screen is not reality, that it is people who make the programs. Parents should restrict viewing violent programs and encourage watching programs with characters who cooperate, help, and care for each other (Murray, 1989). Older children can be encouraged to make short films to illustrate the point.

Parents can help children evaluate TV violence by pointing out the subtleties children miss, such as the aggressor's motives and intentions and the unpleasant consequences the perpetrators suffer as a result of their aggressive acts. Often the consequence is separated from the act by a commercial and children cannot make the correlation. Parents need to point out that conflicts can be resolved without resorting to violent behavior. They can also stress the purpose of the programs—primarily entertainment—and explain why they like or dislike something on TV, for example, "This show is trying to tell you that crime does not pay and, if one does wrong, one will go to jail." Explanations and discussions can take place between shows (with the volume turned down), and young children can learn from older children as well as from adults. These discussions can be very effective when begun early and carried out consistently.

It is especially important to identify at-risk children and control their viewing. House rules that specify the type and amount of television help children understand limits, and video-recorded selections of appropriate programs can be substituted for less desirable offerings. Parents need to carefully monitor cable and other pay TV programming, since these popular options present more uncensored programming. Locked boxes are available for cable receivers that allow families to prevent children from viewing R-rated or other programs when unsupervised. The effects of Music

QUESTIONS AND CONTROVERSIES

Does television viewing have a positive, negative, or neutral effect on child development and behavior?

Television has been accused of "shortening attention span, reducing school achievement, displacing reading, creating a passive intellect, inducing obesity, fostering sexual and racial stereotyping, and causing violent behavior" (Anderson, 1989). However, the findings are inconclusive.

Influence of the medium

Much of the adverse influence of TV depends on the susceptibility of the individual child. Also, one study (Argenta, Stoneman, and Brody, 1986) found that different television programs have different effects on children 3 to 5 years of age. For example, girls imitate program content more than boys and interacted with their peers more during viewing; boys were more involved with toys in the room. Younger children showed more attention to Sesame Street; older children conversed more and played with toys during the show and appreciated the humor in situation comedies. Observing cartoons engaged the attention of both sexes at all ages.

Television is a solitary activity and as such may increase passivity and decrease physical activity and social interaction. Insecure children with strong feelings of rejection may become addicted to the medium in order to meet a need they are unable to satisfy in other ways. It encourages low energy and apathy and may contribute to development of obesity in susceptible children (Dietz and Gortmaker, 1985). Too often TV can become a substitute for play and other activities.

Probably the most serious impact of television on children is the preempting of valuable time that could be devoted to other pursuits and stifling of imaginative play. It is the leading leisure activity of children. The American Academy of Pediatrics has issued statements (1984, 1986, 1988) on the behavior of children and adolescents. Children have been found to use their imagination more when listening to stories on the radio than when they view stories on television (Greenfield, Farrar, and Beagles-Roose, 1986).

Research indicates that children who do not have TV available read comic books, go to movies, listen to the radio, or engage in roughly equivalent forms of entertainment (Huston and Wright, 1982). Also, popular children who engage in sports and extracurricular activities tend to read often as well as watch a lot of TV. Before television children spent time at the movies, reading comic books, and listening to the radio. Without television would children spend their time in other activities, such as reading, doing homework, and engaging in intellectual and social activities, or would they spend their time principally with other media?

There is evidence to indicate that television can have a positive influence on cognitive development and school achievement of children, especially disadvantaged children (Strasburger, 1986). However, TV is a one-way medium in which the viewer is a passive recipient as opposed to an active processor of information. There is a significant negative correlation between the number of hours children spend watching TV and their reading grades (Ridley-Johnson, Cooper, and Chance, 1983) and reading comprehension scores (Morgan and Gross, 1980). However, recent research indicates that effects on reading do not affect all children equally (Beentjes and Van der Voort, 1988). Three hours of television per day is likely to slow academic progress of children with high IQs and socioeconomic status; children with few resources occasionally benefit from the added stimulation of television.

Influence of the message

Television is indicted for teaching violence, simplistic social judgments, and unhealthful attitudes toward sexuality, nutrition, and drugs. It has been lauded for teaching tolerance, conflict resolution, social problem solving, and providing important health information (Anderson, 1989).

Most programming stresses the triumph of good over evil, but with an unrealistically rapid resolution of problems, including moral dilemmas, often accompanied by pain or violence. Programs fail to portray the complex internal dynamics that are generally part of children's moral dilemmas. Physical solutions to problems are common, with violence as the first alternative for problem solving.

On the positive side, television has been shown to be a positive influence on children's abilities to deal with a variety of social issues, such as divorce, the arrival of a new baby, discrimination, honesty, and helpfulness. Children who view educational programming (e.g., *Mister Rogers' Neighborhood* and *Sesame Street*) for a long period of time become more affectionate, considerate, cooperative, and helpful toward their playmates.

An increasing concern is the effect of television on adolescent behavior, especially regarding drinking and casual sexual activity. Adults are portrayed drinking beer, wine, and liquor more often than any other beverages. Television represents adults involved in casual sexual relationships, and a 1988 Harris poll counted over 14,000 sexual references and inneundos on regular programming (exclusive of commercials) (Zylke, 1988).

The average child in the United States is exposed to nearly 20,000 TV commercials each year. Many of these extol the virtues of various toys, fast-food items, high-sugar treats, and other articles that the parents may not wish to purchase. Although young children do not actually purchase products, they continually ask for products they have seen advertised. When parents deny requests, conflicts often ensue. In addition to the resentment and anger toward adults, peer relationships may be affected when children evaluate peers on the basis of whether or not they possess a valued object popularized in commercials.

The effect of TV advertising on health and safety behaviors is also a concern. Children see vitamins and medications in commercial messages and are convinced of their value, even asking for specific products when they do not feel well (Rossiter and Robertson, 1980). Although few television characters smoke on prime-time television, many consume alcohol; and seat belts and bicycle helmets are not used routinely by many television characters.

A late innovation that has been imposed on television-viewing children and their families, toy-based television programs, requires that children must buy a toy to interact with the television set. Not only is the content of these programs objectionable (violent themes), but using the toys interferes with the creative aspects of play that require children to use their imagination. The American Academy of Pediatrics (1988) opposes these toys and the growing commercialization of children's television.

Continued.

QUESTIONS AND CONTROVERSIES—cont'd

Does viewing violence on television increase violent behavior in children?

Children learn from watching television, and there is ample recent documentation to support earlier studies that implicated television as a source for learned antisocial behavior (Huesmann and Eron, 1986; Lefkowitz and others, 1988; Singer, Singer, and Rapaczniski, 1984). For example, it has been shown that viewing violence on television adds aggressive strategies to the children's repertoire of responses. The aggression may even be enhanced if the target of the aggression shares some characteristic with the victim observed on television (Green and Tomas, 1986). However, at least one review of the literature states that the findings offer little support for the media aggression hypothesis (Gadow and Sprafkin, 1989).

Evidence also indicates that children may become sensitized to violence and therefore are likely to tolerate aggressive behaviors they witness in real-life altercations. Incidences have also been reported in which parents' inappropriate behavior toward their children was attributed to television models (Wharton and Mandell, 1985). However, viewing violence may provide children with the means for vicarious release of aggressive impulses. An additional question arises: Does the violence viewed on television influence children's aggressive behavior or are children predisposed to violence attracted to this type of programming?

Box 4-9 FACTORS THAT ENCOURAGE LEARNING OR PERFORMING TV-INFLUENCED BEHAVIORS

Age. Younger children focus on behaviors rather than on motives or consequences. They view alternatives in a concrete manner, and they are unable to differentiate between central and peripheral plot information. Small children remember various assorted items in the program, for example, they remember the *act,* not the motive or consequences.

Identification with characters or situations. Children will more often imitate behaviors of persons and situations similar to those in their own lives.

Reward and punishment syndrome. Children will imitate behaviors they see rewarded or *not* punished when it is expected. They are less likely to repeat an act they see punished; their attention is immediately attracted when they see an act committed that they know should be punished but is not.

Opportunity to reproduce behaviors. Children will imitate behaviors when given the right environment or when violence seems an accepted solution. When children see a situation on television, they will use this information when they encounter a similar situation that requires a solution.

Motivation to reproduce behaviors. Children will imitate behavior when given the appropriate incentives: expectation of reward or lack of punishment. Some children have self-control; others do not.

Television (MTV) on young viewers has yet to be fully evaluated.

It is permissible to use the TV as a "baby-sitter" under certain circumstances; for example, it can keep the children quiet while the parent gets organized after a difficult day and thus can prevent an explosive situation.

Nurses and parents can be powerful forces in influencing the media. They can watch closely for an increase in violence and other undesirable programming and complain to sponsors and TV stations if they believe it is not appropriate. Good programming can be both educational and entertaining.

PARENT GUIDELINES
Television Viewing

Construct a time chart of the child's activities (homework, TV viewing, scheduled outside activities, playing with friends).

Discuss with the child what both believe to be a balanced set of activities.

At the beginning of each week select appropriate programs from television schedules.

Allow the child to select programs from this approved list.

Rule out TV at specific times, e.g., before breakfast or on school nights).

Make a list of alternative activities, e.g., riding a bicycle, reading a book, or working on a hobby.

Require that the child choose to do something from this list before watching TV.

Watch the programs with the child.

Turn the TV off after the selected program is over.

Provide a positive role model for the child—if parents watch a lot of TV, the child probably will also.

Data from Murry, J.P.: Using TV sensibly, Child Behav. Dev. Lett. 5 (9):1, 4-5, 1989.

KEY POINTS

- Growth and development of children are strongly influenced by both genetic and environmental factors.
- The major development phases are the prenatal, infancy, early childhood, middle childhood, and later childhood, or adolescent, phases.
- Information about normal growth and development is derived from both cross-sectional and longitudinal studies.
- Growth and development follow predictable patterns in direction, sequence, and pace.
- Biologic growth is determined by height, weight, bone age, and dentition.

- External proportions and organ systems change with advancing age.
- Critical periods in development are those times when the child is more sensitive to beneficial stimulation or more susceptible to detrimental influences.
- Temperament is a way of thinking, behaving, and reacting to people and situations.
- Temperamental attributes of children can be described as easy, difficult, or slow-to-warm-up.
- According to Freud's psychosexual theory, during childhood certain regions of the body assume a prominent psychologic significance as the source of new pleasures.
- Erikson's psychosocial theory emphasizes the concept of critical periods in personality development when children strive to master core conflicts; each successive stage is built on successful completion of early stages.
- Piaget's theory of cognitive development describes children's progress through stages of mental activity in an orderly, sequential manner that enables them to make adaptations to the environment.
- Moral and spiritual development are accomplished in conjunction with cognitive development.
- Children are born with the capacity for speech and language and master rules of language by the time they enter school.
- According to social learning theory, children learn appropriate behavior through conditioning and observation of role models.
- In the context of the family children learn to apply appropriate sex labels to themselves, acquire sex-appropriate behaviors, develop a preference for their biologic sex, and identify with the parent of the same sex.
- To develop a positive self-concept children need recognition for their achievements and the approval of others.
- Through play children learn about their world and how to relate to things, people, and situations.
- Play provides a means of development in the areas of sensorimotor and intellectual progress, socialization, creativity, self-awareness, and moral behavior; it serves as a means for release of tension and expression of emotions.
- Growth and development are affected by a variety of conditions and circumstances, including heredity, physiologic function, sex of the child, disease, physical environment, nutrition, and interpersonal relationships.
- Children's vulnerability and reaction to stress depend to a large extent on their age, coping behaviors, and support systems.
- The mass media can be influential in children's learning and behavior.

REFERENCES

American Academy of Pediatrics, Committee on Adolescence: Sexuality, contraception, and the media, Pediatrics 78:535-536, 1986.

American Academy of Pediatrics, Committee on Communications: Commercialization of children's television and its effect on imaginative play, Pediatrics 81:900-901, 1988.

American Academy of Pediatrics, Committee on Environmental Hazards: Radon exposure: a hazard to children, Pediatrics 83:799-802, 1989.

American Academy of Pediatrics, Task Force on Children and Television: Children, adolescence, and television, Elk Grove Village, IL, 1984, American Academy of Pediatrics.

Anderson, D.R.: Television and children: not necessarily bad news, Child Behav. Dev. Lett., 5(9):1-3, 1989.

Anthony, E.J., and Cohler, B., editors: The invulnerable child, New York, 1987, Guilford Press.

Archer, J.A., Pearson, N.A., and Westeman, K.E.: Aggressive behavior of children aged 6-11: gender differences and their magnitude, Br. J. Soc. Psychol. 27:371-384, 1988.

Argenta, D.M., Stoneman, Z., and Brody, G.H.: The effects of three different television programs on young children's peer interactions and toy play, J. Appl. Dev. Psychol. 7:355-371, 1986.

Band, E.B., and Weisz, J.R.: How to feel better when it feels bad: children's perspectives on coping with everyday stress, Dev. Psychol. 24:247-253, 1988.

Beentjes, J.W.J., and Van der Voort, T.H.A.: Television's impact on children's reading skills: a review of research, Read. Res. Q. 23:389-413, 1988.

Berndt, T.J.: The features and effects of friendship in early adolescence, Child Dev. 53:1447-1460, 1982.

Binkin, N.J., and others: Birth weight and childhood growth, Pediatrics 82:828-834, 1988.

Bradbard, M.R., and others: Influence of sex stereotypes on children's exploration and memory: a competence versus performance distinction, Dev. Psychol. 22:481-486, 1986.

Carey, W., and McDevitt, S.: Revision of the Infant Temperament Questionnaire, Pediatrics 61:735-739, 1978.

Chess, S., and Thomas, A.: Individuality: dynamics of individual behavioral development. In Levine, M.D., and others, editors: Developmental-behavioral pediatrics, Philadelphia, 1983, W.B. Saunders Co.

Chess, S., and Thomas, A.: Temperamental differences: a critical concept in child health care, Pediatr. Nurs. 11:167-171, 1985.

Colombo, J.: The critical period concept: research, methodology and theoretical issues, Psychol. Bull. 81:260-275, 1982.

Connolly, J.A., Doyle, A.B., and Reznick, E.: Social pretend play and social interaction in preschoolers, J. Appl. Dev. Psychol. 9:301-313, 1988.

DiCaprio, N.S.: Personality theories: a guide to human nature, ed. 2, New York, 1983, Holt, Rinehart & Winston General Book.

Dietz, W.H., and Gortmaker, S.L.: Do we fatten our children at the television set? Obesity and television viewing in children and adolescents, Pediatrics 75:807-812, 1985.

Erikson, E.H.: Childhood and society, ed. 2, New York, 1963, W.W. Norton & Co., Inc.

Erikson, E.H.: Reflections on Dr. Borg's life cycle. In Erikson, E.H., editor: Adulthood, New York, 1978, W.W. Norton & Co., Inc.

Fowler, J.W.: Toward a developmental perspective on faith, Religious Educ. 69:207-219, 1974.

Fullard, W., McDevitt, S., and Carey, W.: Assessing temperament in one to three year old children, J. Pediatr. Psychol. 9:205-217, 1984.

Furman, W., and Bierman, K.L.: Developmental changes in young children's conception of friendship, Child Dev. 54:549-556, 1983.
Gadow, K.D., and Sprafkin, J.: Field experiments of television violence with children: evidence for an environmental hazard? Pediatrics 83:399-405, 1989.
Garmezy, N., and Rutter, M., editors: Stress, coping, and development in children, New York, 1983, McGraw-Hill Book Co.
Gilligan, C.: In a different voice: women's conceptions of self and morality, Harvard Educ. Rev. 47:481-517, 1977.
Goldsmith, H.H., and Gottesman, I.I.: Origins of variation in behavioral style: a longitudinal study of temperament in young twins, Child Dev. 52:91-103, 1981.
Green, R.G., and Thomas, S.L.: The immediate effects of media violence on behavior, J Soc. Issues 42:7-27, 1986.
Greenfield, P., Farrar, D., and Beagles-Roose, J.: Is the medium the message? An experimental comparison of the effects of radio and television on imagination, J. Appl. Dev. Psychol. 7:201-218, 1986.
Harlow, H.F., and Harlow, M.K.: Social deprivation in monkeys, Sci. Am. 203:136-146, Nov. 1962.
Hegvik, R., McDevitt, S., and Carey, W.: The Middle Childhood Temperament Questionnaire, J. Dev. Behav. Pediatr. 3:197-200, 1982.
Holstein, C.: Irreversible, stepwise sequence in the development of moral judgment: a longitudinal study of males and females, Child Dev. 47:51-61, 1976.
Howes, C.: Social competence with peers in young children: developmental sequences, Dev. Rev. 7:252-272, 1987.
Huesmann, L.R., and Eron, L.D., editors: Television and the aggressive child: a cross-national comparison, Hillsdale, NJ, 1986, Lawrence Erlbaum Associates, Inc.
Huston, A., and Wright, J.C.: Effects of communications media on children. In Kopp, C.B., and Krakow, J.B., editors: The child: development in a social context, Reading, MA, 1982, Addison-Wesley Publishing Co., Inc.
Jung, F.E., and Czajka-Narins, D.M.: Birth weight doubling and tripling times: an updated look at the effects of birth weight, sex, race and type of feeding, Am. J. Clin. Nutr. 42:182-189, 1985.
Kohlberg, L.: Moral development. In Sills, D.L., editor: International encyclopedia of the social sciences, New York, 1968, Macmillan, Inc.
Kuczen, B.: Childhood stress, New York, 1982, Delacorte Press.
Kurdek, L.A., and Krile, D.: A developmental analysis of the relation between peer acceptance and both interpersonal understanding and perceived social self-competence, Child Dev. 53:1485-1491, 1982.
Lefkowitz, M.M. et al: Growing up to be violent: a longitudinal study of the development of aggression, New York, 1988, Pergamon Press, Inc.
Liebert, R.M., Sprafkin, J.N., and Davidson, E.S.: The early window: effects of television on children and youth, New York, 1982, Pergamon Press, Inc.
Lowrey, G.H.: Growth and development of children, ed. 8, St. Louis, 1986, Mosby–Year Book, Inc.
Maccoby, E.E., and Jacklin, C.N.: The psychology of sex differences, Stanford, CA, 1974, Stanford University Press.
MacKinnon, C.E.: An observational investigation of sibling interactions in married and divorced families, Dev. Psychol. 25:36-44, 1989.
Masten, A., and others: Competence and stress in school children: moderating effects of individual and family qualities, J. Child Psychol. Psychiatry 29:747-764, 1988.
Matheny, A.P.: Bayley's Infant Behavior Record: behavioral components and twin analysis, Child Dev. 51:1157-1167, 1980.
McDevitt, S., and Carey, W.: The measurement of temperament in 3 to 7 year old children, J. Child Psychol. Psychiatry 19:245-253, 1978.
McGuire, K.D., and Weisz, J.R.: Social cognition and behavioral correlates of preadolescent chumship, Child Dev. 53:1478-1484, 1982.
Mitchell, K., and Mills, N.M.: Is the sensitive period in parent-infant bonding overrated? Pediatr. Nurs. 9(2):91-94, 1983.
Morgan, M., and Gross, L.: Television viewing, IQ, and academic achievement, J. Broadcasting 24:117-133, 1980.
Murphy, L.B., and Moriarity, A.E.: Vulnerability, coping and growth, New Haven, CT, 1976, Yale University Press.
Murray, J.P.: Television and youth: 25 years of research and controversy, Boys Town, NE, 1980, Boys Town Center for the Study of Youth Development.
Murray, J.P.: Using TV sensibly, Child Behav. Dev. Lett. 5(9):1, 4-5, 1989.
Newman, B.M., and Newman, P.R.: Development through life: a psychosocial approach, ed. 3, Homewood, IL, 1984, The Dorsey Press.
Pets Are Wonderful Council in consultation with Dr. Lee Salk: Raising better children: how a pet can help, Chicago, 1985, Pets Are Wonderful Council.
Piaget, J.: The theory of stages in cognitive development, New York, 1969, McGraw-Hill Book Co.
Ridley-Johnson, R., Cooper, H., and Chance, J.: The relation of children's television viewing to school achievement and IQ, J. Educ. Res. 20:294-297, 1983.
Rogan, W.J.: The sources and routes of childhood chemical exposures, J. Pediatr. 97(5):861-865, 1980.
Rosenwasser, S.M., Lingenfelter, A.F., and Harrington, A.F.: Nontraditional gender role portrayals on television and children's gender role perceptions, J. Appl. Dev. Psychol. 10:97-105, 1989.
Ross, S.B., Jr.: Children and companion animals, Feelings Med. Signif. July-Aug. 1981, pp. 13-16.
Rossiter, J.R., and Robertson, T.S.: Children's dispositions toward proprietary drugs and the role of television drug advertising, Public Opinion Q. 44:316-329, 1980.
Schmitt, B.D.: Nightmares on main street (editorial), Am. J. Dis. Child. 143:649, 1989.
Selekman, J.: The development of body image in the child: a learned response, Top. Clin. Nurs. 5(1):13-21, 1983.
Shaffer, D.R.: Developmental psychology: theory, research, and applications, Monterey, CA, 1984, Brooks/Cole Publishing Co.
Sheldon, W.H.: The varieties of human physique, New York, 1940, Harper & Row, Publishers, Inc.
Singer, J.L., Singer, D.G., and Rapaczynski, W.S.: Family patterns and television viewing as predictors of children's beliefs and aggressions, J. Commun. 34:73-89, 1984.
Sroufe, L.A.: Infant-caregiving attachment and patterns of adaptation and competence. In Perlmutter, M., editor: Minnesota symposia in child psychology, vol. 16, Hillsdale, NJ, 1983, Lawrence Erlbaum Associates, Inc.
Stanwyck, D.J.: Self-esteem through the life span, Top. Clin. Nurs. 6(2):11-28, 1983.
Strasburger, V.C.: Does television affect learning and school performance? Pediatrician 13:141-147, 1986.
Stuart, G.W., and Sundeen, S.J.: Principles and practice of psychiatric nursing, ed. 3, St. Louis, 1987, Mosby–Year Book, Inc.
Sullivan, H.S.: The interpersonal theory of psychiatry, New York, 1953, W.W. Norton & Co., Inc.
Thelen, E., and Fisher, D.M.: Newborn stepping: an explanation for a disappearing reflex, Dev. Psychol. 18:760-775, 1982.
Touwen, B.C.L.: Perspective: critical periods of early brain development, Inf. Young Child. 1:vii-x, 1989.
Usdin, G.: Investing in the "emotional bank" concept, Child. Teens Today 8(6):7, 1988.
Werner, E.E.: The roots of resiliency, Early Childhood Update 3(4):1-2, 5, 1987.
Werner, E.E., and Smith, R.S.: Vulnerable but invincible: a longitudinal study of children and youth, New York, 1982, McGraw-Hill Book Co.
Wharton, R., and Mandell, F.: Violence on television and imitative behavior: impact on parenting practices, Pediatrics 75:1120-1123, 1985.
Wolman, B.B.: Children's fears, New York, 1978, Grosset & Dunlap, Inc.
Yip, R., Binkin, N.J., and Trowbridge, F.L.: Altitude and childhood growth, J. Pediatr. 113:486-489, 1988.
Zelazo, P.R., Zelazo, N.A., and Kolb, S.: "Walking" in the newborn, Science 176:314-315, 1972.

Zylke, J.W.: More voices join medicine in expressing concern over amount, content of what children see on TV (letter), JAMA 260: 1831, 1835, 1988.

BIBLIOGRAPHY

General

American Academy of Pediatrics, Committee on Genetics and Environmental Hazards: Special susceptibility of children to radiation effects, Pediatrics 72:890, 1983.
Aquilino, M.L.: Healthy sexual development in childhood, Child. Nurse 4(5):1-4, 1986.
Bradley, R.H., and others: Home environment and cognitive development in the first 3 years of life: a collaborative study involving six sites and three ethnic groups in North America, Dev. Psychol. 25:217-235, 1989.
Brazelton, T.B.: Forces for development in infants and parents, Early Childhood Update 2:1-2, 1986.
Brown, M.S., and others: Type A behavior in children: what a pediatric nurse practitioner needs to know, J. Pediatr. Health Care 3:131-136, 1989.
Castiglia, P.T.: Growth and development, J. Pediatr. Health Care1:48-49, 1986.
Clark, M.K.: Exercise and physical fitness for good health in children, Child. Nurse 4(1):1-3, 1986.
Ferber, R.: Solve your child's sleep problems, New York, 1985, Simon & Schuster.
Ferber, R.: The sleepless child. In Guilleminault, C., editor: Sleep and its disorders in children, New York, 1987, Raven Press.
Guilleminault, C., editor: Sleep and its disorders in children, New York, 1987, Raven Press.
Harlow, H.F., and Harlow, M.K.: Learning to love, Am. Sci. 54:244-272, 1966.
Havighurst, R.J.: Developmental tasks and education, ed. 3, New York, 1972, David McKay Co., Inc.
Honig, A.S.: Development of academically competent children, Early Childhood Update (3)1:2, 1987.
Howes, C.: Pressuring children to learn versus developmentally appropriate education, J. Pediatr. Health Care 3:181-186, 1989.
Lewis, C.E., Siegel, J.M., and Lewis, M.A.: Feeling bad: exploring sources of distress among pre-adolescent children, Am. J. Public Health 74:117-122, 1984.
Messer, D.J, and others: Relation between mastery behavior in infancy and competence in early childhood, Dev. Psychol. 22:366-372, 1986.
Miller, S.A.: Promoting self-esteem in the hospitalized adolescent: clinical interventions, Issues Compr. Pediatr. Nurs. 10:187-194, 1987.
Mussen, P.H., editor: Handbook of child psychology, New York, 1983, John Wiley & Sons, Inc.
Parker, S., Greer, S., and Zuckerman, B.: Double jeopardy: the impact of poverty on early child development, Pediatr. Clin. North Am. 35:1227-1240, 1988.
Phillips, J.L.: The origins of intellect: Piaget's theory, San Francisco, 1969, W.H. Freeman & Co., Publishers.
Post, E.M., and Richman, R.A.: A condensed table for predicting adult stature, J. Pediatr. 98:440-442, 1981.
Power, T.G., and Parke, R.D.: Patterns of early socialization: mother- and father-infant interaction in the home, Int. J. Behav. Dev. 9:331-341, 1986.
Rankin, W.W.: Listening with the heart, J. Pediatr. Nurs. 3(2):127-129, 1988.
Raymond, C.L., and Benbow, C.P.: Gender differences in mathematics: a function of parental support and student sex typing? Dev. Psychol. 6:808-819, 1986.
Seidner, B., Stipek, D.J., and Feshbach, N.D.: A developmental analysis of elementary school-aged children's concepts of pride and embarrassment, Child Dev. 59:367-377, 1988.
Shaffer, D.R.: Developmental psychology: theory, research, and applications, Monterey, CA, 1985, Brooks/Cole Publishing Co.
Sherwen, L.N: Separation: the forgotten phenomenon of child development, Top. Clin. Nurs. 5:1-11, 1983.
Sigman, M., and others: Infant attention in relation to intellectual abilites in childhood, Dev. Psychol. 6:788-792, 1986.
Snow, M.E., Jacklin, C.N., and Maccoby, E.E.: Sex-of-child differences in father-child interaction at one year of age, Child Dev. 54:227-232, 1983.
Stone, L.J., and Church, J.: Childhood and adolescence, ed. 5, New York, 1984, Random House, Inc.
Tanner, J.M., and Davies, P.S.W.: Clinical longitudinal standards for height and height velocity of North American children, J. Pediatr. 107:317-329, 1985.
Thomas, R.M.: Comparing theories of child development, ed. 2, Belmont, CA, 1985, Wadsworth, Inc.
Withrow, C., and Fleming, J.W.: Pediatric social illness: a challenge to nurses, Issues Compr. Pediatr. Nurs. 6:261-275, 1983.

Temperament

Carey, W.B.: Temperament: a tool for coping with problem behavior, Contemp. Pediatr. 6(1):139-153, 1989.
Chess, S., and Thomas, A.: Temperament in clinical practice, New York, 1986, Guilford Press.
Koniak-Griffin, D., and Rummell, M.: Temperament in infancy: stability, change, and correlates, Matern. Child Nurs. J. 17(1):25-40, 1988.
Little, D.L.: Written explanation of temperament scores, Pediatrics 75:275-277, 1985.
Ruddy-Walace, M.: Temperaments: assessing individual differences in hospitalized children, J. Pediatr. Nurs. 2:30-36, 1987.
Turecki, S.: Temperamentally difficult children, Feelings Med. Signif. 32(1):1-4, 1990.
Wallace, M.R.: Temperament: a variable in children's pain management, Pediatr. Nurs. 15:118-121, 1989.
Washington, J., and Goldberg, S.: Temperament in preterm infants: style and stability, J. Am. Acad. Child Psychiatry 25:493-502, 1986.
Worobey, J., and Blajda, V.M.: Temperament ratings at 2 weeks, 2 months, and 1 year: differential stability of activity and emotionality, Dev. Psychol. 25:257-263, 1989.

Moral and Spiritual Development

Betz, C.L.: Faith development in children, Pediatr. Nurs. 7(2):22-25, 1981.
Colby, A., and others: A longitudinal study of moral judgment, Chicago, 1983, Society for Research in Child Development.
Dettmore, D.: Spiritual care: remembering your patients' forgotten needs, Nursing '84 14(10):46, 1984.
Ferszt, G.G., and Taylor, P.B.: When your patient needs spiritual comfort, Nursing '88, pp. 48-49, April 1988.
Johnson, D.F., and Goldman, S.: Children's recognition and use of rules of moral conduct in stories, Am. J. Psychol. 100:205-224, 1987.
McCown, D.E.: Moral development in children, Pediatr. Nurs. 10:42-44, 1984.
Rankin, W.W.: Children and morality, J. Pediatr. Nurs. 3:412-413, 1988.
Ryan, J.: The neglected crisis, Am. J. Nurs. 84:1257-1258, 1984.
Shelly, J.A.: Spiritual care: planting seeds of hope, Crit. Care Update 9(12):7-15, 1982.

Language

Bonvillian, J.D., Orlansky, M.D., and Novack, L.L.: Developmental milestones: sign language acquisition and motor development, Child Dev. 54:1435-1445, 1983.
Castiglia, P.T.: Speech-language development, J. Pediatr. Health Care 1:165-167, 1987.

Dunn, J., and Shatz, M.: Becoming a conversationalist despite (or because of) having an older sibling, Child Dev. 60:399-410, 1989.
LeNormand, M.T.: A developmental exploration of language used to accompany symbolic play in young, normal children, Child Care, Health and Dev. 12:121-134, 1986.
Leonard, L.V., and others: Three hypotheses concerning young children's imitations of lexical items, Dev. Psychol. 17:591-601, 1983.
McCabe, A.E.: Differential language learning styles in young children: the importance of context, Dev. Rev. 9:1-20, 1989.
Menyuk, P.: Language development in a social context, J. Pediatr. 109:217-224, 1986.
Rosenthal, M.K.: Vocal dialogues in the neonatal period, Dev. Psychol. 18:17-21, 1982.
Sande, D.R., and Billingsley, C.S.: Language development in infants and toddlers, Nurse Pract. 10(9):39-47, 1985.

Play

Axelsson, A., and Jerson, T.: Noisy toys: a possible source of sensorineural hearing loss, Pediatrics 76:574-578, 1985.
Bellack, J.P., and Fleming, J.W.: Theoretical practical aspects of play: a universal need. In Fore, C., and Poster, E.C., editors: Meeting psychosocial needs of children and families in health care, Washington, DC, 1985, Association of Care of Children's Health.
Betz, C.L., and Poster, E.C.: Incorporating play into the care of the hospitalized child, Issues Compr. Pediatr. Nurs. 7:343-355, 1984.
Brown, C.C., and Gottried, A.W., editors: Play interactions: the role of toys and parental involvement in children's development, Skillman, NJ, 1985, Johnson & Johnson Baby Products Co.
Cohen, D.: The development of play, New York, 1987, New York University Press.
Lee, J., and Fowler, M.D.: Merely child's play? Developmental work and playthings, J. Pediatr. Nurs. 1:260-270, 1986.
Marino, B.L.: Assessments of infant play: applications to research and practice, Issues Compr. Pediatr. Nurs. 11:227-240, 1988.
Oppenheim, J.F.: Buy me! Buy me! The Bank Street guide to choosing toys for children, New York, 1987, Pantheon Books, Inc.

Nutrition

American Academy of Pediatrics, Committee on Nutrition: Toward a prudent diet of children, Pediatrics 71:78-80, 1983.
American Academy of Pediatrics, Committee on Nutrition: Prudent lifestyle for children: dietary fat and cholesterol, Pediatrics 78:521-525, 1986.
Barness, L.A., and others: Straight talk about feeding young children, Contemp. Pediatr. 5(6):22-55, 1988.
Dwyer, J.: Promoting good nutrition for today and the year 2000, Pediatr. Clin. North Am. 33:799-822, 1986.
Endres, J.B., and Rockwell, R.E.: Food, nutrition, and the young child, ed. 2, St. Louis, 1985, Mosby–Year Book, Inc.
Georgieff, M.K., and others: Effect of neonatal caloric deprivation on head growth and 1-year developmental status in preterm infants, J. Pediatr. 107:581-582, 1985.
Pipes, P.L.: Nutrition in infancy and childhood, ed. 4, St. Louis, 1989, Mosby–Year Book, Inc.
Walker, W.A., and Hendricks, K.M.: Manual of pediatric nutrition, Philadelphia, 1985, W.B. Saunders Co.
Williams, S.R.: Nutrition and diet therapy, ed. 5, St. Louis, 1985, Mosby–Year Book, Inc.

Stress and Fear

Berman, B.D., and Boyce, W.T.: Environmental stresses and protective factors in child health and development, Curr. Opin. Pediatr. 1:172-175, 1989.
Busen, N.H.: Societal values: a cause of stress in children, J. Pediatr. Health Care 2:300-306, 1988.
Colton, J.A.: Childhood stress: perceptions of children and professionals, J. Psychopathol. Behav. Assess. 7(2):155-173, 1985.
Compas, B.E.: Coping with stress during childhood and adolescence, Psychol. Bull. 101:393-403, 1987.
Garmezy, N.: Stressors of childhood. In Garmezy, N., and Rutter, M. editors: Stress, coping, and development in children, New York, 1983, McGraw-Hill Book Co.
Grey, M., and Hayman, L.L.: Assessing stress in children: research and clinical implications, J. Pediatr. Nurs. 2:316-327, 1987.
Hobbie, C.: Relaxation techniques for children and young people, J. Pediatr. Health Care 3:83-87, 1989.
Honig, A.S.: Research in review: stress and coping in children, part 1, Young Child. 41(4):50-63, 1986.
Honig, A.S.: Research in review: stress and coping in children, part 2, Young Child. 41(5):47-59, 1986.
Kagan, J.: Stress and coping in early development. In Garmezy, N., and Rutter, M., editors: Stress, coping, and development in children, New York, 1983, McGraw-Hill Book Co.
Langbaum, T.: What are children worrying about? Clin. Pediatr. 3(12):79, 82, 1986.
Lee, M.A.: Helping children cope with a national disaster, MCN 12:87-88, 90, 1987.
Lewis, C.E., Siegel, J.M., and Lewis, M.A.: Feeling bad: exploring sources of distress among pre-adolescent children, Am. J. Public Health 74:117-122, 1984.
Rankin, W.W.: Fear and courage, J. Pediatr. Nurs. 3(1):46-47, 1988.
Rutter, M.: Stress, coping, and development: some issues and some questions. In Garmezy, N., and Rutter, M., editors: Stress, coping, and development in children, New York, 1983, McGraw-Hill Book Co.
Schor, E.L.: Use of health care services by children and diagnoses received during presumably stressful life transitions, Pediatrics 77:834-841, 1986.
Witmer, D., and Crouthamel, C.S.: Overcoming the common fears of childhood, Contemp. Pediatr. 3(9):76-90, 1986.

Mass Media

Comstock, G.A.: Influences of mass media on child health behavior, Health Educ. Q. 8(1):32-38, 1981.
Dail, P.W., and Way, W.L.: What do parents observe about parenting from prime time television, Fam. Rel. 34:491-499, 1985.
Eron, L.D., and others: Age trends in the development of aggression, sex-typing, and related television habits, Dev. Psychol. 19:71-77, 1983.
Lorch, E.P., Bellack, D.R., and Augsbach, L.H.: Young children's memory for televised stories: effects of importance, Child Dev. 58:453-463, 1987.
Pearl, D., Bouthilet, L., and Lazar, J.: Television and behavior: ten years of scientific progress and implications for the eighties, vols. 1 and 2, Washington, DC, 1982, U.S. Department of Health and Human Services.
Rothenberg, M.B.: In my opinion . . . role of television in shaping the attitudes of children, Child. Health Care 13:148-150, 1985.
Silverman, W.K., Jaccard, J., and Burke, A.E.: Children's attitudes toward products and recall of product information over time, J. Exp. Child Psychol. 45:365-381, 1988.
Singer, D.G.: Does violent television produce aggressive children? Pediatr. Ann. 14:804-810, 1985.
Strasburger, V.C.: When parents ask about . . . the influence of TV on their kids, Contemp. Pediatr. 2:18-27, 1985.
Zuckerman, D.M., and Zuckerman, B.S.: Television's impact on children, Pediatrics 75:233-240, 1985.

CHAPTER 5

Hereditary Influences on Health Promotion of the Child and Family

RELATED TOPICS

Aberrant sexual development, Ch. 11
Birth of a child with a physical defect, Ch. 11
Cleft lip and/or palate, Ch. 11
Cranial deformities, Ch. 11
Cystic fibrosis, Ch. 32
Defects in physical development, Ch. 11
Down syndrome, Ch. 24
Fragile X syndrome, Ch. 24
Hypertrophic pyloric stenosis, Ch. 33
Impact of chronic illness or disability on the child and family, Ch. 22
Klinefelter syndrome, Ch. 20
Malformations of the central nervous system, Ch. 11
Multiple births, Ch. 3
Muscular dystrophies, Ch. 40
Phenylketonuria, Ch. 9
Retinoblastoma, Ch. 36
Skeletal defects, Ch. 11
Turner syndrome, Ch. 20

GLOSSARY

autosome A chromosome other than a sex (X or Y) chromosome

carrier An individual who possesses and can transmit the gene for a given trait but does not exhibit the trait

chromosomal aberration The addition, loss, or structural alteration of a chromosome

congenital A condition present at birth; causes may be genetic, nongenetic, or both

dominant Refers to a gene that produces an effect (is expressed) whenever it is present

eugenics The science concerned with the improvement of the genetic potential of the human population by control of heredity through voluntary social action

euthenics The science concerned with improvement of the human race through control of environmental factors

familial A disorder that "runs in families" or is present in more members of a family than would be expected by chance

genetic Caused by a single gene, several genes, or a deviation in chromosome number or structure; may or may not be apparent at birth

genotype The genetic constitution that determines the physical and chemical characteristics of an individual

heterozygous Having dissimilar genes at a given position (locus) on a pair of chromosomes

homozygous Having the same genes at a given position (locus) on a pair of chromosomes

inherited (heritable, hereditary) Synonymous with genetic, used in the past to describe a disorder appearing in parent and offspring over several generations

malformation Morphogenic defect of an organ, part of an organ, or larger region of the body resulting from an intrinsically abnormal developmental process. Monogenetic—caused by a single gene

mosaic Presence of two or more genotypically different cell lines in the same individual

multifactorial A complex interaction of both genetic and environmental factors

mutation A hereditary change in genetic material; can be either a change in a single gene or a change in chromosome characteristics

nondisjunction Failure of two chromatids or two homologous chromosomes to separate during division so that both members of a pair pass to the new cell

pedigree Family tree

phenocopy A condition or trait produced by environmental factors that is indistinguishable from one due to genetic factors

phenotype The physical or chemical characteristics of an individual; produced by interaction of the environment on the genotype

PKU Phenylketonuria

polygenic Inheritance involving many genes at separate loci whose combined, additive effects produce a given phenotype

proband (index case) An affected individual (regardless of sex) through whom a family comes to the attention of an investigator

recessive Refers to a gene that produces its effect (is expressed) only when it is present in the homozygous state

syndrome A recognized pattern of malformations with a single, specific etiology

translocation The transfer of all or part of a chromosome to another location on the same chromosome or to a different chromosome following chromosome breakage

X-linked Refers to a gene located on the X chromosome

Child development begins before birth and is directed by the action of many genetic mechanisms controlled by a strict chronology. But no less significant are the influences of environment, particularly during the time of critical differentiation. The physical, biochemical, and mental characteristics of the child include not only those traits that create the individuality of each child but also those characteristics that produce unpleasant symptoms or undesirable physical abnormalities that are interpreted as disease.

Numerous defects and diseases seen frequently in the population show an increased incidence in some families or under certain environmental conditions. Parents and health workers alike are concerned with the probability that a specific disease or disorder will recur in a family. To better counsel families and to anticipate probable problems, the nurse needs a fundamental understanding of the principles of genetics and the importance of heredity as an etiologic factor in diseases and disorders of childhood. This chapter is concerned with some genetic factors that play a role in growth and development and with counseling the family regarding problems related to hereditary disorders.

GENETIC INFLUENCES ON HEALTH

Hereditary influences on health and disease are assuming increasing importance to persons in the health professions. Medical science has made rapid advances in the control of infectious diseases and nutritional disorders that formerly accounted for the major share of deaths in infancy. At the same time, contributions from the fields of biochemistry and cytology have established a genetic basis and the means for identification of an increasing number of diseases and defects. Consequently there has been a corresponding increase in the proportion of conditions in which genetic factors are prominent, especially in the pediatric population.

HEREDITY IN HEALTH PROBLEMS

There is probably a genetic component in all disease processes. In some disorders the genetic defect is known; in others the precise nature of the genetic component is more obscure. In some the disorder is apparent at birth; in others the manifestations do not appear for weeks, months, or years (Table 5-1). Some diseases and disorders are determined by the genetic constitution of the individual, such as muscular dystrophy, Marfan syndrome, and Down syndrome. Other diseases, although genetically determined, do not become clinically apparent until environmental factors precipitate the onset of symptoms. For instance, an infant with phenylketonuria, a disorder caused by lack of an enzyme essential for the metabolism of the protein phenylalanine, does not display any symptoms until a sufficient amount of milk containing the protein is ingested. Also, the serious effects of sickle cell anemia develop under conditions of lowered oxygen tension.

Other disorders result primarily from environmental factors. These include most infectious diseases and trauma. Development of the disease depends on environmental con-

Table 5-1 Characteristic age of onset for manifestations of some genetic diseases

AGE OF ONSET	CONDITION
Lethal during prenatal life	Some chromosomal aberrations Some gross malformations
Birth	Congenital malformations Chromosomal aberrations, e.g., Down syndrome Some forms of adrenogenital syndrome Some forms of deafness
Soon after birth	Phenylketonuria Galactosemia Cystic fibrosis (sometimes)
Infancy	Tay-Sachs disease Werdnig-Hoffman disease Maple syrup urine disease
Early childhood	Cystic fibrosis Duchenne muscular dystrophy Sickle cell anemia
Near puberty	Limb-girdle muscular dystrophy Some forms of adrenogenital syndrome
Young adulthood	Acute intermittent porphyria Hereditary juvenile glaucoma
Variable onset age	Diabetes mellitus (0 to 80 years) Facioscapulohumeral muscular dystrophy (2 to 45 years) Huntington chorea (15 to 65 years) Myotonic dystrophy (birth to old age)

tact with the etiologic agent, but there is strong evidence to indicate a decided genetic element in the susceptibility to most diseases (e.g., tuberculosis, poliomyelitis, and measles in some populations). However, the bulk of common diseases and disorders have varying degrees of genetic influence. This category contains most of the birth defects, the allergic disorders, many neurologic defects, and some metabolic diseases.

Genetic diseases can usually be classified into one of the following three broad categories according to the hereditary factors that produce the observed effect: cytogenetic, monogenetic, and multifactorial.

CYTOGENETIC DISORDERS

An aberration is defined as a deviation from that which is normal or typical. Chromosomal aberrations, or cytogenetic disorders, are deviations in either structure or number of a chromosome, and the consequences in either situation can be readily observed in the affected individual. Although the types of cytogenic disorders are not as varied as those caused by a single gene, the incidence for many of the specific abnormalities is significantly higher than that for any of the single-gene (monogenic) disorders.

A structural aberration involves loss, addition, rearrangement, or exchange of some of the genes of a chromosome. If there is sufficient remaining genetic material to render the organism viable, structural alterations can produce an endless variety of clinical manifestations. Also fragile, or weak, sites have been identified on both autosomes and on the X chromosome and have been associated with physical and mental abnormalities, such as the "fragile X" syndrome.

Deviations in chromosome number involve the gain or loss of a chromosome and are designated with the suffix *-somy.* A cell that contains one less than the total number of chromosomes is called a *monosomy* because of the loss of one member of a chromosome pair; a cell that contains one more than the total number of chromosomes resulting from the addition of an extra member to a normal pair is called a *trisomy.* A number of deviations that are compatible with life occur in humans, especially those involving the sex chromosomes, but the more serious outcomes are related to abnormalities of the autosomes. Trisomies are the chromosomal aberrations encountered most commonly by health workers.

The clinical consequences that attend variations in chromosome number frequently consist of discrete, identifiable syndromes, particularly in regard to the trisomies (see Tables 5-2 and 5-3). The chromosomal structural anomalies form a more diverse group of reported physical deviations with few recognized syndromes. Some of the chromosomal disorders, such as Down syndrome, can be identified on the basis of physical characteristics; all require chromosomal analysis to establish a chromosomal abnormality as a causative factor.

Causes of Chromosome Defects

There is considerable speculation regarding the precise cause of chromosome errors. Ionizing radiation has been found to be a cause of chromosome breaks, rearrangements, and nondisjunction—especially the large doses from radiographic tests and studies (mother) and from occupational exposure (father). The duration of unstable, or fragile, abnormalities may disappear in 3 to 5 years; stable, or permanent, alterations probably persist for more than 20 years. It is difficult to determine the effect on germ cells, however.

Autoimmune diseases appear to have a role in the pathogenesis of nondisjunction during cell division. Viruses have also been implicated, especially in relation to chromosome breakage.

Most of the information regarding factors that cause chromosome errors is related to parental age. The incidence of trisomic births corresponds strongly with increasing maternal age, regardless of the number of pregnancies. For example, the risk for trisomy 21, or Down syndrome, increases dramatically for mothers more than 35 years of age (see Down Syndrome, Chapter 24, for further discussion). There is no positive explanation for this observation. However, throughout a lifetime the germ cells are vulnerable to a variety of exogenous influences and to the normal effects of the aging process. Recent evidence indicates that increasing paternal age is also a factor, although the coinci-

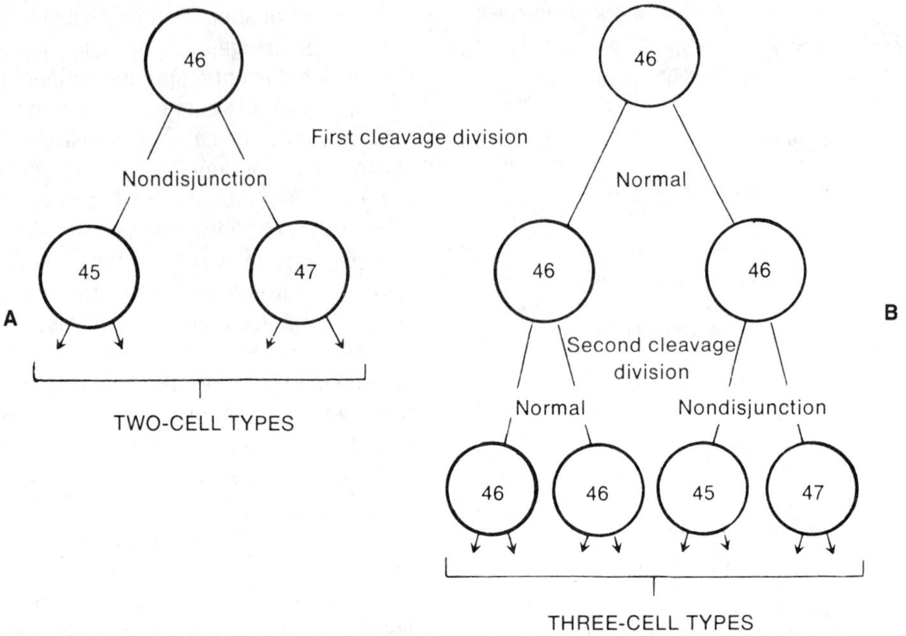

Fig. 5-1. Nondisjunction in early mitotic division of zygote, which produces mosaic genotype. **A,** Nondisjunction at first mitotic division. **B,** Nondisjunction during second mitotic division.

dence of increasing maternal age and increasing paternal age hampers such investigation. Currently the risk appears to be significant only in men older than 55 years of age.

Maldistribution of Chromosomes

The complex nature of cell division makes it highly susceptible to mechanical error, which can occur during the critical processes of germ cell (gamete) formation and in the early divisions of the zygote following fertilization *(nondisjunction)*. In a few cases the unequal distribution of genetic material results from fusion of two nonhomologous chromosomes to form one large chromosome *(translocation)*.

Nondisjunction. The mechanism that is considered to be responsible for maldistribution of chromosomes in the majority of cases is nondisjunction during meiosis. Nondisjunction is failure of the separation and migration of chromosomes during cell division. The consequence of this prolonged attachment during division is an unequal distribution of chromosomes between the two resulting cells. Nondisjunction can take place during ova formation or sperm formation and can involve autosomes or sex chromosomes. The ratio of trisomic gametes that are produced depends on whether nondisjunction occurs during the first or second meiotic division (Fig. 5-1).

Nondisjunction that occurs during early cell division following fertilization will result in an individual with mixed cell lines. The types of cells and their ratio depend on whether nondisjunction occurs at the first or later divisions. Nondisjunction during the first division produces two cell types: half will contain 45 chromosomes, and half will contain 47 chromosomes (Fig. 5-1, *A*). Nondisjunction that occurs in one of the normal cells during the second division will produce cells with both normal and abnormal chromosome constitutions (Fig. 5-1, *B*). An individual whose cells display mixed chromosome counts is called a *mosaic*. Because monosomic cells are nonviable (with the exception of the X monosomy, which is discussed later), most mosaic individuals have an intermixture of normal and trisomic cells. The extent of clinical manifestations is determined by the type of tissues that contain cells with abnormal chromosome numbers and may vary from near normal to a fully manifested syndrome. If a germ cell contains a trisomy, it will be transferred to half the gametes, with a 50% risk that it will be transmitted to the offspring.

Translocation. *Translocation* is a defect in chromosome structure that occurs when one chromosome becomes attached to another to create one large chromosome. Translocations can occur between any two chromosomes, although those encountered most commonly are those between wishbone-shaped chromosomes, the best known being the fusion of a D group chromosome (13, 14, 15) and a G group chromosome (21, 22) or between two G group chromosomes. Because the cells of a person with a translocated chromosome have the normal amount of genetic material, no physical abnormalities are associated with its possession even though the total chromosome count is only 45. The attached chromosomes behave as a single chromosome during cell division and can be transmitted from parent to offspring. During the first meiotic division of gamete formation in such cases, there may be a balanced or an unbalanced distribution of genetic material. Fig. 5-2 shows the possible distribution of genetic material during germ cell formation and the results of the combination of these various cells with gametes of normal chromo-

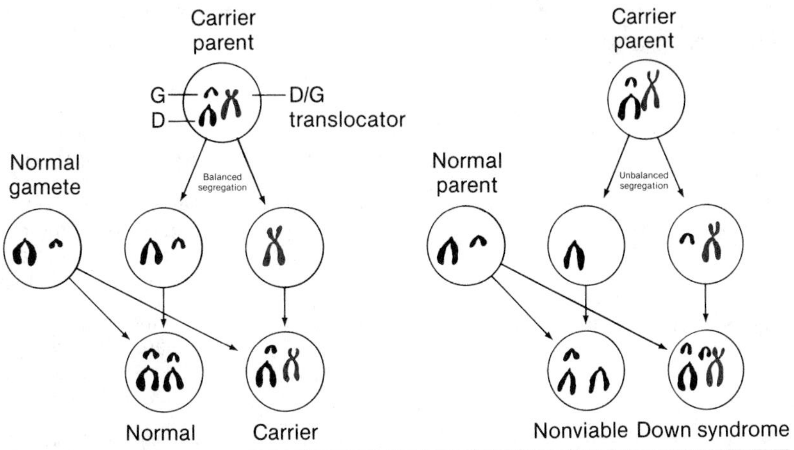

Fig. 5-2. Possible offspring from mating of somatically normal carrier of D/G translocation with genetically and somatically normal individual. D/G = Translocated chromosomes D and G.

some constitution. Persons who are clinically affected because of a translocation have extra chromosome material, although their chromosome count is 46.

Unlike nondisjunction, translocation is not related to increasing parental age. A child affected as a result of a translocated chromosome often has parents in the younger age-groups. There is frequently a history of spontaneous abortion in previous pregnancies, or there may be a family history of abortions. Usually one parent is found to be a carrier of the translocated chromosome, displaying normal characteristics but a chromosomal complement of 45 chromosomes.

In a situation where a parent has a translocation involving a group D or G chromosome, the chances for an affected offspring are estimated to be 1:5 when the mother is the carrier and less than 1:20 when the father carries the translocation.

An uncommon translocation occurs when the two members of chromosome 21 are fused together in a somatically normal individual. Such a person can produce nothing but affected offspring because the gametes that are formed will contain either (1) no chromosome 21 and be nonviable or (2) only the translocated chromosome and produce Down syndrome.

Abnormalities of Autosomes

Both numeric and structural abnormalities of autosomes account for a variety of disorders of infancy and childhood. A few are associated with a group of characteristics that clearly indicate the precise chromosomal anomaly. The first and the most common disorder in which an associated chromosomal abnormality was demonstrated is Down syndrome (see Chapter 24).

Recognizing autosomal anomalies. The best known viable trisomies (21, 18, 13) are easily identified, and the diagnosis can nearly always be made early on physical characteristics alone—usually in the delivery room or newborn nursery (Table 5-2). Often nurses in the newborn nursery see infants who have a facial appearance that sets them apart from other infants. The infant may have no obvious congenital malformation, but on closer inspection may evidence other variations, the sum of which disclose the specific features of known syndromes.

It need not be appearance only that suggests more careful scrutiny of such infants. They may exhibit hypotonia and other neurologic manifestations such as an unusual cry, poor feeding behavior, or abnormal reflex responses. These observations in appearance have been shown to be clinically significant in the diagnosis of most of the identified chromosomal abnormalities and are also useful in recognizing many syndromes associated with other disorders having a genetic basis. Less is known about the features of the deletion syndromes.

Abnormalities of Sex Chromosomes

The possible mechanisms by which sex chromosome abnormalities may occur are the same as those previously described, that is, prefertilization nondisjunction during one of the meiotic divisions of gametogenesis in either parent or in the early postfertilization divisions of the zygote. Most are a result of an increase in sex chromosome number as a result of nondisjunction during meiosis. An increase in the number of sex chromosomes does not produce the profound effects that are associated with the autosomal trisomies, although some degree of mental deficiency accompanies a number of them.

This reduced disability in children with multiple sex chromosomes, compared with the severe effects in children with additional autosomes, is attributed to an unusual characteristic of sex chromosomes—*X inactivation.* In all body cells only one X chromosome is biologically active; the other (or others) is in some way "switched off," or *inactivated,* during the very early divisions of the zygote and remains so throughout life.

Table 5-2 Common autosomal aberrations

SYNDROME	CHROMOSOMAL ABNORMALITY AND NOMENCLATURE	AVERAGE INCIDENCE (LIVE BIRTH)*	MAJOR CLINICAL MANIFESTATIONS
Cri du chat	Deletion of short arm of No. 5 chromosome—46,XY,5p−	1:50,000	Distinctive weak, high-pitched, mewlike cry resembling the cry of a cat; small head; hypertelorism; failure to thrive; severe mental retardation—profound with age
Trisomy 13 (Patau)	Trisomy of No. 13 chromosome—47,XY,13+	1:4000-15,000	Multiple anomalies, including cleft lip and palate (frequency bilateral); ear malformations; microphthalmia; polydactyly; eye defects; mental retardation; early death
Trisomy 18 (Edwards)	Trisomy of No. 18 chromosome—47,XY,18+	1:3500-8000	Deformed and low-set ears; micrognathia; rocker-bottom feet; overlapping (index over third) fingers; prominent occiput; hypertelorism; failure to thrive and early death; mental retardation
Trisomy 21 (Down)	Trisomy of No. 21 chromosome—47,XY,21+ (trisomy); 46,XY (translocation); 46,XY/47,XY,21+ (mosaic)	1:700†	Brachycephaly with flat occiput; inner epicanthal folds; small ears, nose, and mouth with protruding tongue; muscular hypotonia; broad, short hands with stubby fingers and transverse palmar crease; broad, stubby feet with wide space between big and second toes; mental retardation; variable life expectancy

*Data from Nora, J.J., and Fraser, F.C.: Medical genetics: principles and practice, ed. 3, Philadelphia, 1989, Lea & Febiger.
†Risk related to maternal age: age 30 years = 1:1500; age 35 years = 1:300; age 40 years = 1:100; age 45 years = 1:25. Previously 50% were born to mothers over 35 years of age; now only 20% are born to women in that age-group, in large part because of the availability of prenatal diagnosis.

Table 5-3 Common sex chromosome abnormalities

SYNDROME	CHROMOSOMAL NOMENCLATURE	PHENOTYPE	OCCURRENCE	CLINICAL MANIFESTATIONS
Turner	45,X	Female	1:2500 female births*	Short stature; webbed neck; low posterior hairline; shield-shaped chest with widely spaced nipples; sterile
Triple X	47,XXX (can also be 48,XXXX or 49,XXXXX)	Female	1:850-1250 female births	Normal female characteristics; usually tall; variable mental capacity and behavior; at risk for language, neuromotor, learning skills, and psychosocial adaptation; fertile
XYY male	47,XYY (can also be 48,XYYY or mosaic)	Male	1:900 male births*	Usually normal sex development; tendency to be tall with long head; poor coordination; may demonstrate aberrant behavior; at risk for learning disabilities
Klinefelter	47,XXY (48,XXYY, 48,XXXY, 49,XXXXY, and so on, mosaics)	Male	1:850 male births*	Tall with long legs; hypogenitalism; sterile; male secondary sex characteristics may be deficient; may demonstrate aberrant behavior
Fragile X	46,XY, 46,XX	Predominantly male	1:2000 male births*	Normocephaly or macrocephaly; prominent mandible; large ears; macroorchidism; mental retardation

*Data from Nora, J.J., and Fraser, F.C.: Medical genetics: principles and practice, ed. 3, Philadelphia, 1989, Lea & Febiger.

A number of sex chromosome abnormalities have been described, and some are listed in Table 5-3. The more common of these, Klinefelter and Turner syndromes, are discussed further in Chapter 20 in relation to developmental problems of later childhood. Some general characteristics of chromosomal abnormalities of sex chromosome numbers are listed in Box 5-1.

The fragile X syndrome (see Chapter 24) is attributed to a fragile (unstable) site, or specific point, on the X chromosome. It appears at the same point in a given family and demonstrates some of the characteristics of an X-linked inheritance pattern.

MONOGENIC (SINGLE-GENE) DISORDERS

Disorders for which a simple, definite inheritance pattern can be identified are rare individually, but collectively they constitute a significant portion of health problems seen in infants and children. They can involve any system in the body. They can be of such minor importance that they have little effect on the child, or so severe as to cause serious disability or to be incompatible with life.

Conditions that can be directly attributed to a single gene are distributed in families in characteristic patterns according to the basic Mendelian principles. Genes are either dominant or recessive in their effect, and most disorders caused by a single gene can be recognized readily by the simple family patterns that they display.

Some generalizations can be made regarding diseases and malformations caused by a single gene on either the autosomes or sex chromosomes. Disorders resulting from structural defects seem to be primarily the result of dominant genes; most metabolic defects appear to be caused by recessive genes. Dominant traits are seen more frequently and are usually less severe than are recessive traits. This is probably because of the "double-dose" effect. Whereas recessive traits are only manifest when both genes are present, a dominant disorder usually involves a single gene from a heterozygous parent. The presence of a normal gene appears to overcome the effect of a recessive gene.

Codominance occurs when both genes of a heterozygous pair are expressed equally; neither is recessive to the other. This is characteristic of the major blood groups, such as the ABO blood groups in which both the A and the B antigens are dominant. The O trait, without antigens, behaves as a recessive gene. Codominance is clearly illustrated by type AB blood.

Some examples of single gene disorders are outlined in Table 5-4, including the inheritance pattern, basic defect, and manifestations.

Box 5-1 CHARACTERISTICS OF SEX CHROMOSOME ABNORMALITIES

There is a direct relationship between the male or female phenotype and the presence or absence of a Y chromosome. It appears that the Y chromosome is essential for development of male characteristics.

The severity of defects is not related to the number of extra X chromosomes, except for mental retardation, which increases proportionately with each X chromosome.

The presence of more than one Y chromosome appears to have variable but as yet not well-defined effects on the phenotype.

Table 5-4 Partial list of single-gene disorders

DISEASE	INHERITANCE	BASIC DEFECT	MANIFESTATIONS	THERAPY
Achondroplasia	Autosomal dominant	Defect in ossification at epiphyseal plate (growth portion of bones)	Very short limbs; large head; lordosis	Supportive
Adrenogenital syndrome (Ch. 38)				
Albinism (ocular)	Autosomal recessive	Deficiency of tyrosinase; failure to convert tyrosine to dopa, and, hence, lack of melanin synthesis	Lack of pigment in skin, hair, and eyes; eye defects	Symptomatic Avoid exposure to sunlight Ophthalmologic care
Cystic fibrosis (Ch. 32)				
Galactosemia (Ch. 9)				
Hemophilia A (Ch. 35)				
Hemophilia B (Ch. 35)				
Hypothyroidism (familial)	Autosomal recessive	Deficiency of iodotyrosine deiodinase	Lethargy; stunted growth; mental retardation	Early administration of thyroid hormone

Continued.

Table 5-4 Partial list of single-gene disorders—cont'd

DISEASE	INHERITANCE	BASIC DEFECT	MANIFESTATIONS	THERAPY
Maple syrup urine disease	Autosomal recessive	Defective metabolism of branched-chain amino acids	Onset in early infancy; neurologic disorders; odor of urine similar to that of maple syrup	Diet low in branched-chain amino acids
Marfan syndrome (arachnodactyly	Autosomal dominant	Defect in elastic fibers of connective tissues	Tall and thin, with long tapering fingers; poorly developed musculature; associated defects include aortic aneurysm, dislocation of optic lens, winged scapula	Supportive Surgical correction of deformities
Muscular dystrophy (Ch. 40)				
Nephrogenic diabetes insipidus (Ch. 30)				
Neurofibromatosis (von Recklinghausen disease) (Ch. 18)				
Noonan syndrome	Autosomal dominant	Unknown	Small stature, shield-shaped chest, webbed neck, low posterior hairline, narrow maxilla, low-set ears, ptosis, hypertelorism, cardiac anomalies (pulmonic stenosis)	Correct cardiac anomalies Supportive
Osteogenesis imperfecta (Ch. 39)				
Phenylketonuria (Ch. 9)				
Retinoblastoma (Ch. 36)				
Severe combined immune deficiency (Ch. 35)				
Tay-Sachs disease (amaurotic familial idiocy)	Autosomal recessive	Deficiency of hexosaminidase; defect in synthesis of gangliosides	Predominantly in Ashkenazi Jews; progressive neurologic deterioration; blindness, cherry-red spot in macula; early death	Supportive
Thalassemias (Ch. 35)				
Werdnig-Hoffmann disease (Ch. 40)				
Wiskott-Aldrich syndrome (Ch. 35)				
von Willebrand disease (Ch. 35)				

Variation in Gene Action

Several factors influence the way in which genes behave or are manifest. The most notable of these is *mutation*. Mutations usually occur naturally *(spontaneous)*, or can be *induced* by a variety of external agents, or *mutagens*, including temperature, certain chemicals, and radiation. Other factors may influence gene mutation. For example, the incidence of mutation increases with parental age, especially that of the father. This phenomenon is most apparent in the autosomal dominant disorders.

A number of other variables are observed in many disorders that modify the basic inheritance patterns. The degree to which a gene exerts its effect or the differences in effects that a given gene may produce sometimes appear to contradict the established concepts of inheritance and, again, are more apparent in dominant disorders (Box 5-2).

Autosomal Inheritance Patterns

The characteristic major inheritance patterns are described and accompanied by sample pedigree charts. Because there are 44 autosomes and only 2 sex chromosomes, the majority of hereditary disorders are a result of defective genes on an autosome.

Autosomal dominant inheritance. Usually the first case in a family appears suddenly as the result of a fresh mutation and, depending on the degree of disability the condition imposes on the individual, will either die out or continue to be passed on through several generations (Fig. 5-3). Incomplete penetrance is common, and there is wide variability in expression. The basic defect, probably a structural protein, is unknown in most autosomal dominant disorders; therefore, screening of undetected persons, including prenatal diagnosis, is usually not possible. Later onset is common. Examples of an autosomal-dominant disorder include achondroplasia, polydactyly, and Marfan syndrome.

Box 5-2 VARIATIONS IN GENE ACTION

Penetrance—regularity with which an inherited trait is manifest in the phenotype
- *Full penetrance:* The gene produces its effect each time it is present in the genotype.
- Example: achondroplastic dwarfism
- *Nonpenetrance:* The gene recognized is not manifest in a person who carries the responsible gene; expressed as percentage.
- Example: retinoblastoma with 80% penetrance

Variable expressivity—degree of severity of, or variability in, manifestations seen in persons of a particular genotype; ranges from being almost undetectable (mild) to incapacitating (severe)
- Example: polydactyly; location and number of digits vary

Pleiotropy—multiple, different, and seemingly unrelated phenotypic effects associated with a particular genotype—the varied clinical features that constitute a syndrome
- Example: Marfan syndrome

Heterogeneity—same or similar manifestations that result from:
- Different genes at the same locus on a chromosome
- Genes at different loci on a chromosome
- Examples: the hemophilias and the muscular dystrophies that exhibit different inheritance patterns

Autosomal recessive inheritance. Children who display an autosomal recessive disorder will always be homozygous for that trait. The heterozygous person, with only one gene for a rare recessive disorder, remains undetected in the population (Fig. 5-4). It is estimated that each person carries from three to eight genes for such a severe genetic disease. However the probability of mating between two persons who carry the same gene is highly unlikely. If they are blood relatives, the likelihood is increased. The chances are also increased if the mating occurs between persons who select a mate because of geographic, ethnic, or religious restrictions. For example, there is a higher risk that Ashkenazi Jews will be carriers of the gene for Tay-Sachs disease. The age of onset for autosomal recessive disorders is early, and, because they are usually biochemical defects, heterozygote detection and prenatal diagnosis are often possible. Examples of an autosomal recessive disorder include cystic fibrosis, phenylketonuria (PKU), and galactosemia.

X-Linked Inheritance Patterns

Genes on the X chromosome differ from those on the Y chromosome; therefore, the transmission of traits caused by these genes will vary according to the sex of the individual who carries the gene. The two X chromosomes in the female are alike in gene constitution, with two genes for each trait. Genes on the X chromosome have no counterpart on the Y chromosome; therefore a characteristic determined by a gene on the X chromosome is *always* expressed in the male. One of the most significant aspects of X-linked inheritance is the absence of father-to-son transmission. Although it is essential for development of the male phenotype, the Y chromosome carries no known medically significant characteristics.

X-linked dominant inheritance. Superficially this pattern resembles an autosomal dominant inheritance pattern (Fig. 5-5). This type of inheritance is relatively uncommon, and because the effects in the male are severe and usually fatal, transmission of the gene takes place primarily in the female. An example of an X-linked dominant disorder is hypophosphatemic vitamin D–resistant rickets.

		Affected parent	
	Gametes	A	a
Normal parent	a	A a Affected	a a Normal
	a	A a Affected	a a Normal

Characteristics of autosomal dominant inheritance

Males and females are affected with equal frequency.
Affected individuals will have an affected parent (unless the condition is caused by a fresh mutation).
Half the children of a heterozygous affected parent will have the probability of possessing the defective gene, although it may be nonpenetrant.
Unaffected children of affected parents will have unaffected children (unless the gene is nonpenetrant).
Traits can be traced vertically through previous generations—a positive family history.

Fig. 5-3. Possible offspring of mating between normal parent and one with autosomal dominant trait.

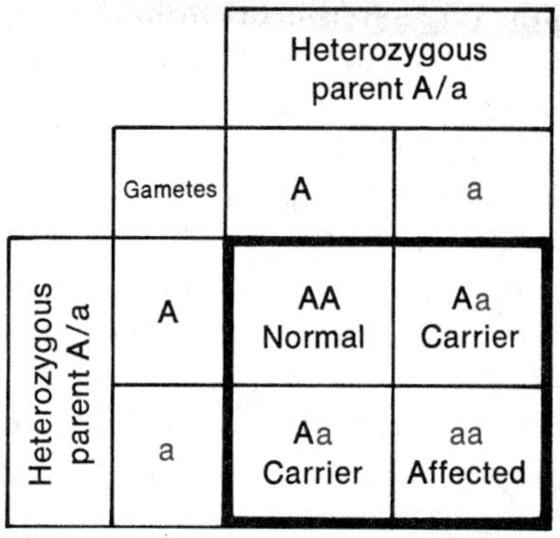

Heterozygous parent A/a
Gametes
A
a
Heterozygous parent A/a
A
a
AA Normal
Aa Carrier
Aa Carrier
aa Affected

Characteristics of autosomal recessive inheritance

Males and females are affected with equal frequency.
Affected individuals will have unaffected parents who are heterozygous for the trait.
There is a 1 in 4 chance that any child of two unaffected heterozygous parents will be affected.
Two affected parents will have affected children exclusively.
Affected individuals mated to unaffected individuals will have normal children, all of whom will be carriers.
There is usually no evidence of the trait in previous generations—a negative family history.

Fig. 5-4. Possible offspring of mating between two parents with recessive gene on an autosome.

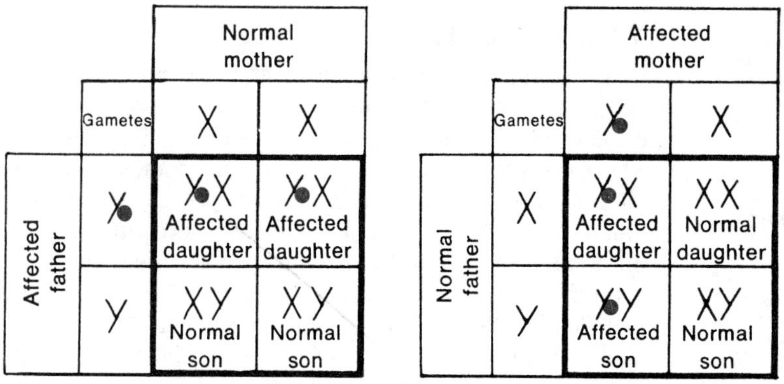

Characteristics of X-linked dominant inheritance

Affected individuals will have an affected parent.
All the daughters but none of the sons of an affected male have the probability of being affected.
Half the sons and half the daughters of an affected female will be affected.
Normal children of an affected parent will have normal offspring.
There are no carriers.
The inheritance pattern shows a positive family history.

Fig. 5-5. Sex differences in offspring ratios in X-linked dominant inheritance. ● = Dominant allele on X chromosome.

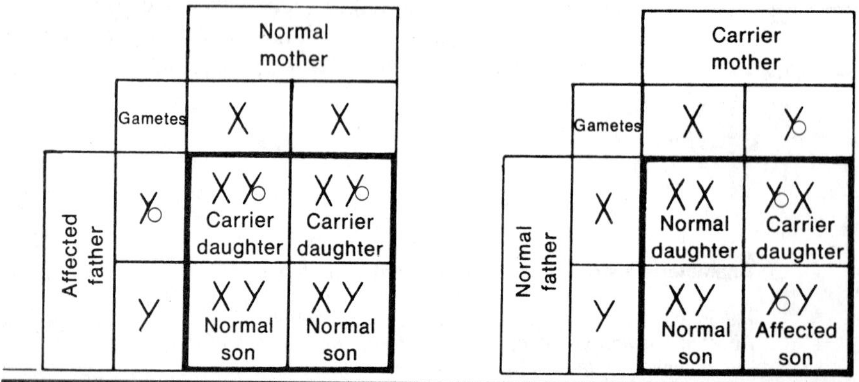

Characteristics of X-linked recessive inheritance

Affected individuals are principally males.
Affected individuals will have unaffected parents (except in the rare possibility that the father is affected and the mother is a carrier).
Half the female siblings of an affected male have the probability of being carriers of the trait.
Unaffected male siblings of an affected male cannot transmit the disorder.
Sons of an affected male are unaffected.
Daughters of an affected male are carriers.
The unaffected male children of a carrier female do not transmit the disorder.

Fig. 5-6. Sex differences in offspring ratios in X-linked recessive inheritance. ○ = Recessive allele on X chromosome.

X-linked recessive inheritance. The abnormal gene behaves as any recessive gene; that is, its effect will be hidden by a normal dominant gene. Therefore two recessive genes are usually present for manifestations in the female (Fig. 5-6). However, unequal X inactivation can produce manifestations in a carrier female. Fresh mutations are not rare. Examples of an X-linked recessive disorder include hemophilia and Duchenne muscular dystrophy.

MULTIFACTORIAL DISORDERS

A number of diseases and defects that are encountered frequently in the population show an increased incidence in some families, but show no clear-cut affected-unaffected classification. Although the incidence is higher than would be expected by chance, no specific mode of inheritance can be identified. In some, environmental factors appear to play an important role. These are the conditions classified as *multifactorial*—disorders in which a genetic susceptibility combined with the appropriate environmental agents interact to produce a disease state. Disorders that are considered to be multifactorial include most congenital defects and many common diseases.

A term used in relation to, and sometimes interchangeably with, multifactorial is *polygenic* (literally meaning many genes), which is usually used to describe the genetic component of multifactorial inheritance. Polygenes are quantitative and additive; that is, a number of minor genes in the right combination produce a given characteristic—each making a small contribution to the total effect.

When the laws of inheritance are applied to polygenic characteristics, it is expected that relatives will have more genes in common and that these genes will be expressed more often when united with a similar combination of genes. Table 5-5 indicates the proportion of genes that relatives can have in common. The more distant the relationship, the fewer the shared genes. In families where there is an increased incidence of a disorder, the frequency in first-degree relatives may be 3 to 15 times that in the population as a whole. The appearance of more than one affected family member indicates a greater number of polygenes in common. However, socioeconomic differences or seasonal distribution might suggest environmental influences.

Table 5-5 Proportion of genes in common in various relationships

RELATIONSHIP	PROPORTION OF GENES IN COMMON
First-degree relatives	
Parent, child, sibling	½
Second-degree relatives	
Grandparent, grandchild, uncle, aunt, nephew, niece, half-sibling	¼
Third-degree relatives	
First cousins	⅛
Second cousins	1/32

Common Diseases

The appearance of clinical manifestations in multifactorial disorders requires a strong genetic predisposition that places susceptible individuals at a point of risk where environmental influences determine whether (and in some cases to what extent) they will be affected. Examples in this category include such infectious diseases as tuberculosis, rubeola, and paralytic poliomyelitis. In some diseases a genetic trait can be identified. For example, the development of peptic ulcer occurs more frequently in persons with type O blood; however, environmental stresses are also important etiologic factors. Other diseases with multifactorial causes include diabetes mellitus, psoriasis, and schizophrenia.

HLA system. The inherited histocompatibility (tissue) antigens, similar to the blood group antigens, have been implicated in the development of many diseases. These antigens, termed the *human leukocyte antigen* (HLA) system and also known as the *major histocompatibility complex* (MHC), are present on the cell membrane of almost all body cells. They occur in linked pairs and are inherited in the same manner as the blood group antigens. A number of these antigens have been identified and have been classified as follows: class 1—the HLA-A, HLA-B, and HLA-C antigens; class 2—the HLA-D and HLA-DR (D-related) antigens; and class 3—certain complement factors with genes in the HLA region.

A relationship between the HLA system has been shown for several disorders, for example, insulin-dependent diabetes mellitus, hemochromatosis, psoriasis vulgaris, celiac disease, myasthenia gravis, and several forms of arthritis. Most notable is the striking association between HLA-B27 and idiopathic ankylosing spondylitis in 90% to 95% of affected persons. Although significant associations have been identified in only a few disorders, risk estimates can be determined regarding the frequency with which one of these diseases develops in an individual carrying a specific HLA antigen compared with the frequency of the disease in persons who do not carry the HLA antigen.

Drug sensitivity. Pharmacogenetics is that branch of genetics concerned with drug responses and their genetic modification. In many drug-sensitive persons a mode of inheritance can be identified, but the disease is not manifest unless the individual is exposed to the drug in question. Examples of disorders precipitated by contact with a drug are malignant hyperthermia, which occurs in some anesthetized patients; the porphyrias, in which symptoms are produced by exposure to alcohol or certain drugs; and glucose-6-phosphate dehydrogenase (G-6-PD) deficiency, in which affected persons develop a hemolytic crisis when they take certain drugs, are exposed to naphthalene mothballs, or ingest fava beans.

A number of persons show a resistance or sensitivity to certain drugs. For example, there is a genetically related ability of some persons to resist the anticoagulant coumadin and for some individuals to metabolize the antituberculin drug isoniazid more slowly than others. Persons with some disorders display altered responses to therapeutic agents, for example PKU and catecholamines, Down syndrome and atropine, and familial dysautonomia and norepinephrine.

Congenital Anomalies

The development of an organism, especially during embryogenesis, is an intricate process in which all parts must be properly integrated to ensure a coordinated whole. The rate must be such that one part is ready when needed by another part; otherwise, either part may cease to grow or may deviate from its normal path. Congenital anomalies, or birth defects, can arise at any stage of development and show wide variability in determining factors as well as in type, extent, and frequency of defects. Some defects result when a state, present in one phase of development as a normal condition, persists into another phase as abnormal. For example, a cleft lip is normal in a young embryo, and a patent ductus arteriosus is essential during fetal life. Any agent that interferes with these complex processes will produce a defect in development ranging in severity from an insignificant local anomaly to complete degeneration.

A few congenital defects are clearly caused by a single gene, some are associated with chromosomal abnormalities, and others are produced by known intrauterine environmental factors. However many of the more common and severe defects (e.g., pyloric stenosis, central nervous system malformations, cataracts, and congenital heart disease) appear to be consistent with polygenic inheritance.

Nongenetic factors can produce a congenital anomaly that imitates, or is indistinguishable from, one genetically determined. Such a condition is termed a *phenocopy.* For example, deafness, hypothyroidism, and cataracts can each be caused by a mutant gene, but they may also be caused by exogenous agents. Deafness can be a result of a number of different agents, rubella virus can cause congenital cataracts, and lack of iodine in a child can produce hypothyroidism. In addition, many single-gene and chromosomal abnormalities manifest one or more physical or mental defects. Some such defects include cleft lip and palate, clubfoot, congenital dislocated hip, congenital heart defects, and mental retardation. Assigning a cause of mental retardation presents a particularly difficult problem.

Mental retardation is a manifestation of a variety of syndromes, both single-gene and chromosomal, and numerous environmental agents are known to be damaging to brain tissue, for example, lack of oxygen as a result of anesthesia or drugs during labor and delivery. For these reasons it is extremely important that such exogenous factors be ruled out before any given congenital defect is labeled hereditary.

Because of the steady decline in infant mortality from other causes, congenital anomalies are responsible for an ever-increasing proportion of all deaths in infancy and constitute an increasing proportion of infants requiring intensive newborn care. Some defects are of such minor significance that they have little or no effect on survival or the quality of life; others are so severe as to be incompatible with life or are a serious threat to survival. There is also a high correlation between the incidence of congenital anomalies and the infant who is small for gestational age. The more severe the growth retardation, the more likely the chance for abnormal development. Multiple anomalies are not uncommon and tend to appear together in patterns or relationships.

THERAPEUTIC MANAGEMENT OF GENETIC DISEASE

There is no cure for genetic disease at present, although preventive and corrective therapy is helping to reduce the harmful effects in an increasing number of conditions. Genetic research is making progress in the art of altering the genetic material directly. Meanwhile the major goal of therapy is modification of the internal or external environment to correct or minimize the effects of the genetic defect.

Therapeutic Modalities

The therapeutic modalities available for genetic disorders are few when compared with the infinite variety of conditions afflicting the population, but with increased understanding of the basic defects and the technical advances being made, an increasing number are becoming amenable to treatment.

Surgical repair. Surgical repair of structural defects has made it possible to prolong life in a number of multifactorial disorders, such as congenital heart disease and pyloric stenosis. Numerous facial and limb deformities can be altered by plastic and reconstructive techniques. In cases of familial polyposis coli, surgical removal of the colon eliminates the countless polyps that invariably become cancerous. Splenectomy prevents the trapping of abnormal blood cells in that organ in several hereditary disorders of red blood cells. Early diagnosis and enucleation in retinoblastoma have reduced the mortality from this dreaded eye tumor.

In the last few years there has been some interest in fetal surgery for some life-threatening anomalies, particularly urinary tract abnormalities. Although some procedures are possible, such as decompression of the hydronephrotic kidney or hydrocephalic ventricles, the Council on Scientific Affairs of the American Medical Association has issued a resolution that emphasizes the need for further animal experimentation before the practice can be considered safe and beneficial.

Diet modification. For disorders in which an enzyme deficiency causes a toxic accumulation of a substance or its by-products, restricting the intake of foods containing the offending substance often prevents irreversible damage from the improper metabolism of these compounds. Examples include the low-phenylalanine diet prescribed for children with PKU, elimination of dairy products containing lactose for infants and children with hereditary lactase deficiency, avoidance of foods containing or producing galactose for children with galactosemia, and a diet low in branched-chain amino acids for infants and children with maple syrup urine disease.

Product replacement. In some deficiency diseases, supplying the missing product that cannot be synthesized prevents undesirable effects. For example, thyroid extract is prescribed to prevent the damaging effects of hypothyroidism, and providing the missing blood factors prevents life-threatening and debilitating hemorrhages in the hemophilias. Other examples are insulin for diabetes mellitus, growth hormone for pituitary dwarfism, and corticosteroids for adrenogenital syndrome.

Avoidance of drugs or other substances. In drug-induced disease, such as glucose-6-phosphate dehydrogenase (G-6-PD) deficiency and the porphyrias, avoidance of the drugs that precipitate a reaction provides a simple preventive measure.

Removal of toxic substances. Removal of toxic substances that accumulate in vital tissues as a result of a hereditary disease can prevent disabling complications. Some of the deleterious effects of hemochromatosis, a hereditary disorder characterized by an excess accumulation of iron in the liver, heart, and pancreas, can be reduced with the removal of iron by administration of chelating agents.

Immunologic prevention. The administration of immunoglobulin to Rh-negative mothers following birth of an Rh-positive infant is effective in preventing Rh-antibody formation that causes hemolytic disease of the newborn in subsequent births.

Transplantation. Replacement of nonfunctioning organs with normal organs is increasing the survival of children with defective organs because the problems of tissue incompatibility are better controlled. Examples of organ transplants include kidneys in hereditary polycystic kidneys, heart in severe cardiac myopathy, liver in hepatic atresia, pancreas in diabetes mellitus, and bone marrow in hereditary diseases affecting the blood-forming organs, such as thalassemia.

Cofactor administration. Diet supplements can be given when the body is unable to synthesize or effectively use some substances needed as cofactors in metabolism, such as vitamin B_{12} in pernicious anemia, in which absorption of this vitamin is absent.

Recombinant DNA. The transfer of modified genetic material from one organism (a virus) to another causes the viral DNA to become integrated into the cellular DNA of the recipient cell. This recombinant DNA multiplies, producing the missing substance (such as insulin) in the cells of the recipient.

Gene transfer. Fragments of DNA from a normal gene can be introduced directly into a recipient cell lacking such a gene. This approach has been attempted in humans with the transfer of normal gene copies of beta hemoglobin into bone marrow cells in an effort to treat a form of beta thalassemia. It may also hold promise in sickle cell anemia.

Other therapies. Other methods such as enzyme repression and competitive inhibition are providing effective treatment in some metabolic disorders. Future therapies include the possibility of replacement or stabilization by injection or oral administration of a substance that the patient lacks.

Environmental Manipulation

Inherited diseases or defects for which there is no therapeutic modality can be modified to enhance the quality of life for the affected individual. Some examples of environmental manipulation include hearing aids for deaf children, glasses or vision enhancers such as enlarged print and books in braille for the visually impaired, mobilizing devices such as braces and wheelchairs for persons with muscle and bone impairment, prosthetic devices for limb deficiencies, and infant stimulation programs to maximize the potential of mentally retarded children.

GENETICS AND SOCIETY

There is no doubt that diseases constitute a significant portion of world health problems, and the advantages of improving the human race are seldom questioned. Controversy exists, however, between those who advocate improvement in the species by selective breeding and those who recommend providing a better environment. Improvement of the race through altering the genetic makeup of the individual is termed *eugenics;* improvement of the human race by modifying the environment is called *euthenics.*

Eugenics

Eugenics is essentially planned breeding designed to alter future generations. Such practice has been successfully used for many years by animal and plant breeders in developing superior food products. For many persons any discussion of controlling heredity creates visions of Hitler's interpretation and misuse of directed evolution; some racial groups view it as the code word for genocide; and religious groups protest that it is tampering with God's creation. Eugenics can be further segregated into *positive eugenics* and *negative eugenics.*

Positive eugenics. Positive eugenics is the attempt to encourage reproduction among individuals who are considered to possess superior or beneficial characteristics. Suggested means for accomplishing this purpose include selected mating of individuals who are considered to possess superior traits. Other methods are the establishment of sperm banks, with sperm from a small, select number of donors to be frozen and used to impregnate a large number of suitable women, and the production, asexually, of replicas of desirable persons by cloning (replacing the cell nucleus of a fertilized ovum with the nucleus of a cell from the desired individual; asexual reproduction). Some of the qualifications considered superior might be physical characteristics, socially desirable behavior, and superior intellect, as well as absence of genetically determined defects or disease.

Negative eugenics. Negative eugenics is the discouragement or prohibition of reproduction among individuals who are considered to be physically or mentally handicapped. Voluntary or legal prohibition of reproduction by persons with these characteristics might be accomplished with marriage laws, sterilization, and abortion. The arguments for and against the relative merits and objections of eugenics will continue for years to come.

Euthenics

An opposite point of view is taken by those who support euthenics, which advocates the modification of the environment to allow an individual with a genetic defect to live a relatively normal life. Examples of euthenic measures are prescription glasses for nearsighted persons and special schools for the deaf. Medical treatments such as special diets for children with inborn errors of metabolism, hormone replacement such as insulin for diabetic persons and thyroid for persons with cretinism, and special orthopedic appliances and prosthetic devices can be considered environmental manipulation. Providing better nutrition and home environment for children during the growing stages and educational and social stimulation are prime examples of euthenics.

IMPACT OF HEREDITARY DISORDERS ON THE FAMILY

The presence of a genetically or prenatally derived disorder presents multiple problems and concerns to the family and to health workers. The disorder may have been present in a family for generations, or it may appear suddenly in a family. In either situation the family is faced with decisions regarding their reproductive future.

GENETIC SCREENING

Tests to detect the presence of a defective gene are rapidly assuming greater importance in management of genetic disorders as more defects are identified and techniques are developed for easy application. It is probable that with improved technology, mass screening for numerous defects may eventually be a routine procedure. However, to be truly effective, screening programs depend on education of both health professionals and the public regarding these programs. The religious, moral, and ethical issues revolving around screening and prenatal diagnosis are extensive and beyond the scope of this discussion; therefore only a few are mentioned, and the reader is encouraged to investigate these issues further in other resources.

> **QUESTIONS AND CONTROVERSIES**
>
> **Should society allow a couple to have children when one or both have a severely disabling condition known to be hereditary that inhibits or impairs their ability to function?**
>
> In order to solve such a dilemma a number of issues need to be addressed. How is the competence or incompetence of the involved family to be determined (Kilpack, 1986)? Do persons with a disability have the same right to procreate as persons without a physical or mental disability? If society is to have a voice in such decisions, society will need to determine what constitutes a "disabling condition." Who will determine whether a condition is disabling (physicians, lawyers, politicians)? How will such a decision be enforced (Kilpack, 1985)?
>
> Also, should insurance companies be expected to pay for the care of a child with a disease such as cystic fibrosis, born to parents who were fully aware that they had the causative gene?

Purposes of Screening

Genetic screening is presumptive identification of an unrecognized genotype in individuals or populations. There are several purposes for this screening: (1) to detect the presence of disease, incipient or overt, (2) to provide reproductive information, and (3) to gain information concerning the incidence of a disorder in the population.

Screening for disease. The rationale for screening for disease is to discover persons who (1) have the disease, either manifest or incipient, or (2) may, in time or under special circumstances, develop the disease. The purpose of this knowledge is to anticipate serious consequences and provide the individual with treatment and management that will prevent, reverse, or diminish the adverse effects of the disorder. An example is the generalized, systematic screening of newborn infants for PKU, hypothyroidism, and galactosemia. The mass screening programs have indicated that many of these disorders are more prevalent than formerly believed. Others that are included in some screening programs are congenital adrenal hyperplasia, homocystinuria, maple syrup urine disease, sickle cell disease and other hemoglobinopathies, tyrosinemia, histidinemia, Hartnup disease, adenosine deaminase deficiency, and various other aminoacidurias and urea cycle disorders.

A number of technologies are available for detecting disease—biochemical assays, protein iontophoresis, chromosome analysis, and the newer testing with DNA molecular probes. It has even been suggested that the DNA of an affected child be banked and used to identify markers in other family members at a later date, such as a subsequent pregnancy.

Screening for reproductive information. Screening for heterozygotes (carriers) can detect unaffected persons with certain genes who, when they mate with an individual who carries a similar gene, are at high risk of producing an affected offspring. These individuals are thus provided with the knowledge they need for use in decisions about family planning. Carriers of a number of diseases can be detected by laboratory tests, but because of the rarity of these diseases, mass screening is not feasible except in persons or populations known to be at risk. Persons at risk include close relatives of persons with an inborn error of metabolism or other detectable disorder, or certain ethnic populations known to have a high incidence of a specific disease, such as sickle cell anemia in blacks, Tay-Sachs disease in Ashkenazi Jews, and thalassemia in persons of Mediterranean ancestry.

Screening for epidemiologic information. Public health officials may use screening as a method of monitoring the incidence of diseases or malformations in a population in order to detect environmental or other causes that might significantly influence incidence of the disorder. For example, the observation that the incidence of a syndrome was significantly increased in a population 8 to 10 months after a rubella epidemic led to the discovery that this disease has a significant damaging impact on the unborn child during the first trimester of pregnancy.

Prenatal Diagnosis

A variety of techniques are available for diagnosing a number of diseases and defects in the fetus. As more and more diseases can be diagnosed prenatally and parents at risk are recognized early, these procedures provide the means to detect defects that are best corrected soon after delivery, conditions that may require preterm delivery for early correction, conditions that may require cesarean delivery, conditions that may require medical or surgical treatment before birth, and conditions on which a decision may be based to terminate a pregnancy.

Prenatal diagnosis by amniocentesis has become relatively commonplace. Although it carries a certain amount of risk, this technique has been employed to detect a variety of inborn errors of metabolism, chromosomal abnormalities, and sex of the fetus in sex-related disorders. Fetuses at risk for some central nervous system abnormalities can be identified by examination of maternal serum alpha-fetoprotein (MSAFP). Other techniques available in selected medical facilities include DNA testing, ultrasonography, fetoscopy, chorionic villi sampling, and fetal blood sampling. Amniography, fetography, and radiography are used less often.

A number of genetic diseases can now be detected prenatally, and with advancing technology more are being added to the list. Identification of chromosomal aberrations and some diseases prominent in some races has been available for some time. More recent additions, using DNA molecular probes, include prenatal detection of cystic fibrosis, sickle cell anemia, and Duchenne muscular dystrophy. Nurses interested in current information about a particular disorder should contact the nearest genetic counseling center. A national directory of these centers is available from the U.S. Department of Health and Human Services.*

The primary dilemma faced by families when a disorder is diagnosed prenatally is the option for terminating the pregnancy. When the disorder is one that produces a major disability, the problem involves the care and management of the affected infant. Parents may choose to terminate a pregnancy in which the child will require special care that the parents are unable or unwilling to provide. A more difficult decision involves a relatively minor defect, such as cleft lip, for which there is definitive therapy but such therapy is beyond the family's physical, emotional, or financial resources.

*National Center for Education in Maternal and Child Health, 38th and R Streets N.W., Washington, DC, 20057, (301) 443-4513.

QUESTIONS AND CONTROVERSIES

Should parents of an unborn child known to have a disorder involving a serious mental defect be allowed to continue the pregnancy when they will be unable or unwilling to care for the child after birth? Can society deny services to the child after birth because of the family's decision, or, if the society must assume responsibility for care of the child, should society have a voice in the decision?

The physical, emotional, and monetary burdens of lifetime care for a child with a physical or mental defect can drain the resources of many families and institutions. Some families are incapable of providing adequate care for a child with physical or mental defects. Institutions are continually faced with diminished funding for the care of these children.

It is important that families with increased risk of having a child with an abnormality are made aware of this risk and are informed of any tests that could detect the presence of a defect. Health professionals can be held liable if such information is not conveyed to the clients so that they can use the knowledge in making decisions about reproduction (Rhodes, 1989). For example, pregnant women over the age of 35 years should be informed of the increased risk for Down syndrome in that age-group and the availability of amniocentesis.

Significance of Screening to Families

Mass screening programs have not been enthusiastically endorsed and carried out by all members of the health professions or wholeheartedly accepted by the public—especially compulsory screening. The reasons for this resistance are justified in many instances. Many practitioners are unfamiliar with the techniques required for genetic screening, and some of the tests are not completely accurate. The cost of screening for a variety of genetic defects is beyond the means of most childbearing families, and the stigma attached to the carriers of a disease is a prohibiting factor. However, with the success of several well-organized or legislated programs and their significance in the prevention of disease or of the damaging effects of disease, an increasing number of programs are gaining acceptance and support.

In the majority of situations families support screening for genetic disease. They express a sense of relief to know their status: it is comforting to be assured that they do not carry the defective gene, or to have the information on which to make decisions when they are found to be carriers. Families have a strong desire to know what is being done to their infants, and knowledge of the procedure can lessen anxiety and help them prepare for possible consequences, such as repeat tests.

Much of family concern regarding screening centers around the issues of informed consent and the use to be made of the information from the screening. Some states re-

QUESTIONS AND CONTROVERSIES

Should parents have the right to refuse permission for routine screening of their newborn to detect the presence of a disease for which therapy is now available? Should screening be required to detect the presence of a disease for which no therapy is presently available?

Screening for some biochemical defects (phenylketonuria, hypothyroidism, galactosemia) is mandatory or common practice (American Academy of Pediatrics, 1982). Initiation of treatment before irreversible damage occurs has improved the quality of life for persons with these disorders, and the cost of the screening has been less than the cost to society for institutional care of untreated victims. It has also eliminated much of the financial and other less tangible burdens to the family; that is, the cost and burden of special diets or medication are less burdensome than the care and management of a disabled child.

However, some parents strenuously object to screening procedures on the basis of religious and personal biases. Should they be given the option of refusal, inasmuch as these diseases are not a threat to other infants or children? On the other hand, if the screening is mandatory, are the parents in fact asking health professionals to break the law in submitting to their wishes?

Technology is available for detection of many more diseases for which there is no available remedy. Should the child and family be subjected to the procedures when no help can be offered? On the other hand, persons with a disorder for which there is at present no remedy can be contacted if one should become available. However, screening for these diseases is expensive.

QUESTIONS AND CONTROVERSIES

Should routine genetic screening be performed for a disease with no known adverse clinical consequences? Also, should incidental but unexpected findings of genetic screening be disclosed? To whom?

Some argue that screening for a disease with no known clinical repercussions is desirable because it allows follow-up that may reveal subtle consequences unrecognized before (Cohen, 1984). However, there is no reason to subject children and families to the stress of screening procedures if there is no visible evidence of disease and no untoward symptoms.

Sometimes screening information alters family relationships. Disruption of parent-child bonding can occur in the newborn period. The common consequences of detecting a genetic disease in a child are blaming, overprotectiveness of the child resulting in impaired psychologic development, and guilt feelings in the family. Knowledge that they have a disease can seriously alter identity information in adolescents. It makes them "different" from their peers, and persons who are carriers of a genetic disease often exhibit an altered self-concept.

Unexpected information that might seriously alter family relationships includes nonpaternity and discovery of a disorder other than the one for which the individual was screened (Korsch, 1984).

quire written consent, some specify the tests to be performed, and some describe the risks, benefits, and the right to be informed of uncertain results, including the process in the event of an abnormal finding. Institutions may provide classes for families to explain the screening program, provide verbal explanation, or distribute written materials. In some areas exemptions from mandated screening are allowed in certain situations, such as objections on religious grounds if there is a conflict with religious practices and beliefs of an established church. Others impose penalties for noncompliance (Cohen, 1984).

The nature and purposes of the procedure should be clearly explained to clients in language that they can understand. The issue of divulging unexpected findings is subject to debate. It is not unusual to detect one disorder while screening for another. Also, if a genetic trait is detected in a child but not in a parent (such as the sickle cell trait), the question of paternity can become an issue. It is also important to help families understand the meaning of false positive and false negative results of testing.

Release of information to persons other than the family is also subject to debate. At present the reporting of genetic findings is not mandatory, as it is for certain contagious diseases, and it is questionable whether this would be desirable. A family may not wish for other family members or even the family practitioner to receive the results of screening. Third parties who might make use of such information are insurance companies and employers. All of these possibilities should be made clear to families in order to provide them with some selective control.

The social stigma attached to the carrier of a defective gene may be a side effect of screening. In some families such knowledge is a source of embarrassment and damaging to the self-esteem of its members. Teenagers are especially vulnerable to the effects of knowing they carry a specific defective gene at a time when identity formation and peer approval are extremely important. Cultural views regarding this knowledge can have profound effects on the members of some ethnic groups. In some cases, social status within the cultural group can be impaired.

Probably the most important area for nursing practice is teaching. Families need an understanding of why the screening is proposed, what the results mean, and how the family can interpret false positive and false negative results. Parents are concerned, and their anxiety is greater when they have not received sufficient information about the screening or testing process and its significance for the health of their infant (Sorenson and Mangione, 1984). The need for retesting, no matter what the reason, can be extremely stressful to families, and they also have a right to know who assumes the cost of the screening—the family or the state. The nurse is a valuable resource person in making families aware of alternatives and in helping them select the one that best suits their particular situation.

Prenatal diagnosis of fetal sex is becoming more popular with expectant parents. When the pregnancy is at risk for an X-linked recessive disorder, such as Duchenne muscular dystrophy, there is a 50% chance that a male offspring will be affected, and many families choose to terminate a pregnancy involving a male fetus. However, there is also a 50% chance that the infant will be unaffected. More controversial is the issue of determining sex to satisfy parental curiosity or as a means of sex selection.

GENETIC COUNSELING

In recent years the significance of heredity as an etiologic agent in disease and disability has assumed a more prominent place in the nursing care of infants and children. With the expanded recognition of genetic diseases and defects, an increasingly well-informed public, assuming more responsibility for the quality of future populations, is creating a justified demand for accurate information regarding risks to present and future generations. The actual number of persons who need advice is relatively small compared with those who have many other health problems, but their need is great. When expert counseling is not accessible, these persons may become victims of well-meaning but uninformed quasi-professionals or misguided relatives and acquaintances.

It is estimated that only a small proportion of persons who need counseling are seen by professional counselors. Many families who might benefit from counseling do not recognize the need, or this special need is not apparent to those who supervise their care. Unfortunately, families who need counseling are rarely referred to counselors unless they themselves request the service. Nurses in the field of infant and child care continually encounter genetic diseases and families in which there is a risk that a disorder may be transmitted to an offspring. It is a responsibility of nurses to be alert to situations in which families could benefit from genetic counseling, to become familiar with facilities in their areas where genetic counseling is available, and to learn the basic principles of heredity. In this way they will be able to direct individuals and families to take advantage of needed counseling services and to be active participants in the counseling process. They should be knowledgeable regarding special services that are available to help in management and support of affected children.

A comprehensive definition of genetic counseling prepared by a group of eminent medical geneticists states that genetic counseling is a communication process that deals with the human problems associated with the occurrence, or risk of occurrence, of a genetic disorder in a family. This process involves an attempt by one or more appropriately trained persons to help the individual or family (Fraser, 1974):

- Comprehend the medical facts, including the diagnosis, the probable course of the disorder, and the available management
- Appreciate the way heredity contributes to the disorder, and the risk of recurrence in specified relatives
- Understand the options for dealing with the risk of recurrence
- Choose the course of action that seems appropriate to them in view of their risk and their family goals and act in accordance with that decision
- Make the best possible adjustment to the disorder in an affected family member and/or to the risk of recurrence of that disorder

Clients

The clients, or persons who seek advice, must first be aware that there is a genetic problem or potential problem. They may be referred to counseling by a family practitioner, a specialist, a nurse, a friend, or a relative, or they may seek counseling as a result of information in the media. Some simply view genetic counseling as a new service of which they should take advantage.

Clients may or may not be affected themselves, but request genetic counseling about the heritability of a trait that may be deleterious, beneficial, or merely troublesome. Clients might be a young couple contemplating marriage or childbearing who are concerned about a disorder in one of their families, no matter how remote the relationship, or may seek advice because they are related. A couple who are both members of a population at risk for certain diseases may wish to determine whether they carry the harmful gene (e.g., blacks and sickle cell anemia, Ashkenazi Jews and Tay-Sachs disease, or persons of Mediterranean ancestry and thalassemia). A couple planning adoption might seek counseling regarding a prospective child.

More often persons who inquire about the possibility of recurrence of a disease or disorder are parents of a child with a specific disease or defect that significantly impairs fitness who are concerned that they might produce another similarly affected child. This advice may be sought before the couple initiates another pregnancy, after the mother is already pregnant, or after the birth of another child. There is often concern regarding the risk to unaffected siblings of the affected child or to the affected child's future children.

More than ever before, parents plan and feel responsible

QUESTIONS AND CONTROVERSIES

Should parents be permitted prenatal diagnosis for sex determination unrelated to X-linked disease?

Prenatal ultrasonography and chromosome analysis from amniotic fluid allow determination of sex before birth. It has long been employed for detecting sex in carrier mothers at risk of passing a sex-linked disorder to a male offspring. Parents are also informed of the sex of the fetus when amniocentesis is performed to rule out a chromosomal anomaly or some other undesirable disorder. The technique could easily be employed for sex determination alone. To date, the long-term effects on society if parents are allowed to selectively terminate a pregnancy with a fetus of the "wrong sex" are unknown. However, it is well-known that a male is the preferred firstborn (Fletcher, 1979).

for their children. They need to know the risk in *their particular situation* and how it relates to the random risk for *any* prospective parents. It has been found that when families understand the risks involved, they normally make sensible decisions regarding family planning.

Some families may need counseling regarding the advisability of sterilization, artificial insemination, prenatal diagnosis, or termination of a pregnancy. Infertility or recurrent abortion in a family may indicate a need for counseling. Occasionally a counselor becomes involved in cases of disputed paternity, questioned maternity (when it is suspected that infants have been substituted for one another at birth), rape, or incestuous matings. Delayed or abnormal sexual development may also be a reason to seek genetic advice.

Special risk situations. When health personnel are alerted to the possibility of an inherited disease in a family, this knowledge makes possible the early detection and subsequent treatment of the disorder. This is increasingly important as treatments are becoming available for more genetically determined diseases and is especially true in situations where treatment is effective only when initiated early. The history of a condition in an older sibling, such as PKU or galactosemia, provides a clue for specific and thorough testing for the condition in a newborn. In this way early therapy can be initiated when indicated, thus minimizing or eliminating the effects of the disease or defect.

Information Essential for Genetic Counseling

Unlike a medical prognosis that predicts the outcome of a disease, a genetic prognosis directly involves other persons: the affected child, members of the immediate family, relatives, and future offspring. Effective genetic counseling requires a thorough evaluation of each situation. Information from which the counselor derives risks of recurrence is acquired from several sources: an accurate diagnosis, a thorough family history, and an extensive knowledge of genetics.

Accurate diagnosis. The first and most important component in the counseling process is an accurate diagnosis. The disorder in question may be diagnosed by the attending practitioner who refers the family for counseling, or the practitioner can call on the services of a counseling unit for a definitive diagnosis by special biochemical or cytogenetic tests, particularly in cases of very rare and unusual syndromes. There are over 3000 known inherited disorders, many of which have similar clinical manifestations but totally different modes of inheritance. For example, symptoms in the early stages of severe X-linked muscular dystrophy appear much like those of the milder autosomal recessive and autosomal dominant varieties, autosomal recessive neurogenic muscular atrophies, and nongenetic poliomyelitis. The significance of the risks related to each type of disorder is readily apparent. It is especially difficult to assign a cause to deafness and mental retardation.

Family history. A careful, detailed family history is necessary to the counseling process. Not only does it provide a picture of the *proband* (the affected person, or *index case*) in relation to other family members, but it may also serve to identify other persons who are similarly affected or who might be at risk to produce affected children. Analyzing the pattern of affected members of the family can assist in confirming a tentative diagnosis or in determining the level of risk in multifactorial inheritance.

Knowledge of genetics. In order to counsel families regarding their particular problem, a counselor must have a thorough understanding of genetic principles, a knowledge of the risks related to multifactorial inheritance, and up-to-date information on genetic diseases.

Estimation of Risks

The mode of inheritance determines the degree of risk in the major categories of genetic disorders (Box 5-3). In general, the more definite and clear-cut the genetics, the greater the risks; as the causative factors become more obscure, the outlook is more hopeful.

Interpretation of Risks

When explaining risk estimates, the counselor does not attempt to make recommendations or decisions for consultants. The counselor provides appropriate and accurate information about the nature of the disorder, the extent of the risk involved, the probable consequences, and alternative solutions but remains nondirective, leaving the final decision to the persons concerned. In some instances genetic information will increase the family's distress; in others their anxiety will be reduced, depending on their makeup and the meaning that the disorder has for that particular family.

It is helpful to explain risks in different ways and to use examples from games of chance to aid in understanding the meaning of probabilities. Most persons do not have an adequate knowledge of genetics and human biology to fully

Box 5-3 ESTIMATION OF GENETIC RISK

High-Risk Situations

Conditions caused by a factor that segregates during cell division
Recurrence risk: 1:10 or greater
  Can be predicted with high degree of accuracy
  Based on mendelian ratios
Examples: single-gene disorders, translocated chromosome disorder

Moderate-Risk Situations

Conditions that are multifactorial
Recurrence risk: less than 1:10; usually less than 1:20
  Based on prior experience and observation of the disorder under similar circumstances (empiric)
Examples: pyloric stenosis, spina bifida, congenital heart defects

Random-Risk Situations

Conditions caused by environmental agents and not likely to recur in another pregnancy under normal circumstances unless the agent is still operative
Recurrence risk: approximately 1:30
Examples: rubella syndrome, fresh mutation, most chromosomal aberrations

comprehend these complex concepts. However, there are few people who have not had experience with flipping coins, baseball pools, lotteries, horse racing, and other games based on probabilities. Flipping coins can be used effectively to illustrate the probabilities in single-gene disorders, and weather reports and horse racing are well-known examples of empiric risk estimates.

✦ **NURSING ALERT** Families may misunderstand probabilities, even when they are fully explained. It is important to impress on them that *each pregnancy is an independent event.* It is not uncommon for parents who are told that a recessive disorder carries a 1:4 risk of recurrence to feel secure with one affected child. They incorrectly reason that because they already have one affected child the next three will be unaffected. Chance has no memory; the risk is 1:4 for each and every pregnancy.

NURSES AND GENETIC COUNSELING

Nurses skilled in counseling techniques are in a unique position to help meet the counseling needs of families in which there is a genetic disease or disorder. Public health nurses work with a family in a close, sustained relationship and earn the family's confidence and trust; genetics nurse specialists, with advanced preparation in genetic theory, are assuming a prominent position on counseling teams; and practitioners in the specialty areas of maternity and pediatric nursing are constantly involved with families in which there is a genetic defect. Nurses are frequently the persons who recognize clues that indicate a genetics-related problem, who assist the family in obtaining the needed services for diagnosis and treatment, and who provide follow-up care.

Counseling Services

The most efficient counseling service consists of a group of specialists that may include physicians, geneticists, psychologists, biochemists, cytologists, nurses, social workers, and other auxiliary personnel. The services are most often under the leadership of a physician trained in medical genetics, who assumes responsibility for the medical aspects of the problem. The counseling service may serve only as a referral group, or it may conduct a regular clinic service. Most often it is associated with a large medical center, many of which have extensive outreach programs with satellite clinics throughout adjacent areas. There are also numerous specialty clinics that deal with specific genetic disorders (such as cystic fibrosis, muscular dystrophy, hemophilia, diabetes) and provide their own genetic counseling services. Unfortunately, these units are concentrated in and around large metropolitan areas. As a result, counseling is not always accessible to the large number of persons who would benefit from the service.

Role of the Nurse in Genetic Counseling

It is a nurse who is frequently the family's initial contact with a counseling service. An intake interview is conducted before the primary counseling session or diagnostic workup to assess the needs of the family and attempt to reduce their anxiety; therefore, ample time should be allotted. Ideally, both spouses should attend, but small children should be excluded. If possible, childcare facilities should be made available as part of the counseling service. If this is impossible, some distraction in the form of toys and play equipment can be provided. In the interview the nurse takes a family history for pertinent information and explains the clinic procedures carefully. Many families are concerned about such things as whether they will be required to undress, if blood is to be drawn, if they can accompany the child during the visit, or if they will be told what to do about reproduction. Families who have a relaxed and nonstressful initial discussion are able to gain more from a counseling session.

Taking a family history. The person taking a family history must allow a liberal amount of time. When possible, it is best to include both parents in the interview in order to elicit information about relatives on both sides of the family. Medical records, birth and death records, family Bibles, and photograph albums are helpful resources, and persons being interviewed should be instructed to bring such items if they are available. It may be necessary to consult other members of the family. The level of education and the degree of understanding vary widely among informants and influence the reliability of the information. There may be reticence on the part of informants, particularly if they view the disorder as something to be ashamed of or in some way threatening. Sometimes true relationships may be concealed, such as illegitimacy.

The family history is recorded in the form of a pedigree chart or family tree (in some disciplines the pedigree chart is termed a *genogram*) using standard symbols to indicate persons, relationships, and significant details related to them (Fig. 5-7). Construction of a pedigree (Box 5-4) begins with the affected child (proband, index case, original patient) and *all* the mother's pregnancies (Fig. 5-8, *A*). Next the maternal family history is explored in a similar manner (Fig. 5-8, *B*); then information about relatives on the father's side is gathered in the same manner (Fig. 5-8, *C*). It is important at this point to determine whether the couple might be related in any way.

It is important to include information about births—live births, stillbirths, and abortions; matings—legally sanctioned, consanguineous, multiple, unwed, and other complex relationships; and health of family members, including any diseases or disorders, and death and causes of death. Sometimes the place of birth and ethnic background are significant. For example, the incidence of Tay-Sachs disease is higher in Ashkenazi Jews from eastern Europe than in Jews from other geographic origins. Also, when a pedigree chart is being evaluated, the fact that a sister died in infancy as a "blue baby" might be genetically significant, whereas a healthy sibling who drowned at age 1 year would not. Information concerning first-degree relatives is most important and should be complete.

Follow-up care. The success of counseling is measured by the way in which the family uses the information presented to them. Maintaining contact with the family or

Box 5-4 GUIDELINES FOR PEDIGREE CONSTRUCTION

1. Begin diagram in the center of a large sheet of paper.
2. Represent males in a family with a square and females with a circle.
3. Indicate the proband with an arrow (if the counselee is not the proband, indicate the relationship of the counselee with a "C" under that person's symbol).
4. Use a horizontal bar to designate a marriage; place the male on the left and the female on the right (use a broken line to indicate an unwed mating and a double bar for a consanguineous mating).
5. Suspend symbols for outcome of all pregnancies (including offspring, abortions, and stillbirths) vertically from the mating line in order of birth from left to right, regardless of sex and outcome.
6. Designate offspring with Arabic numerals.
7. Include significant information about all the mother's pregnancies (e.g., bleeding, anemia, radiographs, infectious disease, drugs taken).
8. Place maternal and paternal relatives in proper relationship to the proband.
9. Designate generations by Roman numerals with the earliest generation at the top.
10. Include at least three generations: parents, siblings, grandparents, aunts, uncles, first cousins, and offspring of proband (if appropriate).
11. Include name of each person (including maiden names for married women), their date of birth, health problems, and date and cause of death.
12. Date the pedigree.

referral to an agency that can provide a sustained relationship—usually the public health agency in their locality— is one of the most important aspects of the counseling process. Some families do not choose to have follow-up visits, but in most instances these visits make the family feel that they have not been abandoned and facilitate the process of adjustment to the problem.

Follow-up visits to the counseling service or in the home provide the family with the opportunity to ask questions that they did not ask on previous visits. Often the family members have not really "heard" the information presented to them or have misinterpreted what they have heard, so that it may be necessary to repeat and reinforce counseling. In some disorders a diagnosis in one family member places relatives at risk and is an indication for further screening.

One very important aspect of follow-up care is support and assistance in management of the affected child. For example, a disorder such as PKU requires conscientious diet management; therefore, it is important to make certain that the family understands and follows instructions. Children born subsequently must be carefully observed for early detection of symptoms. Genetic and specialty clinics devote a great deal of their time and efforts in helping families cope with the consequences of genetic disease.

Nurses should be prepared to help families arrive at tentative decisions regarding the future, including family planning, education or institutionalization of a handicapped child, plans for adoption, and many other problems related to their specific problems. Initial and ongoing assessments

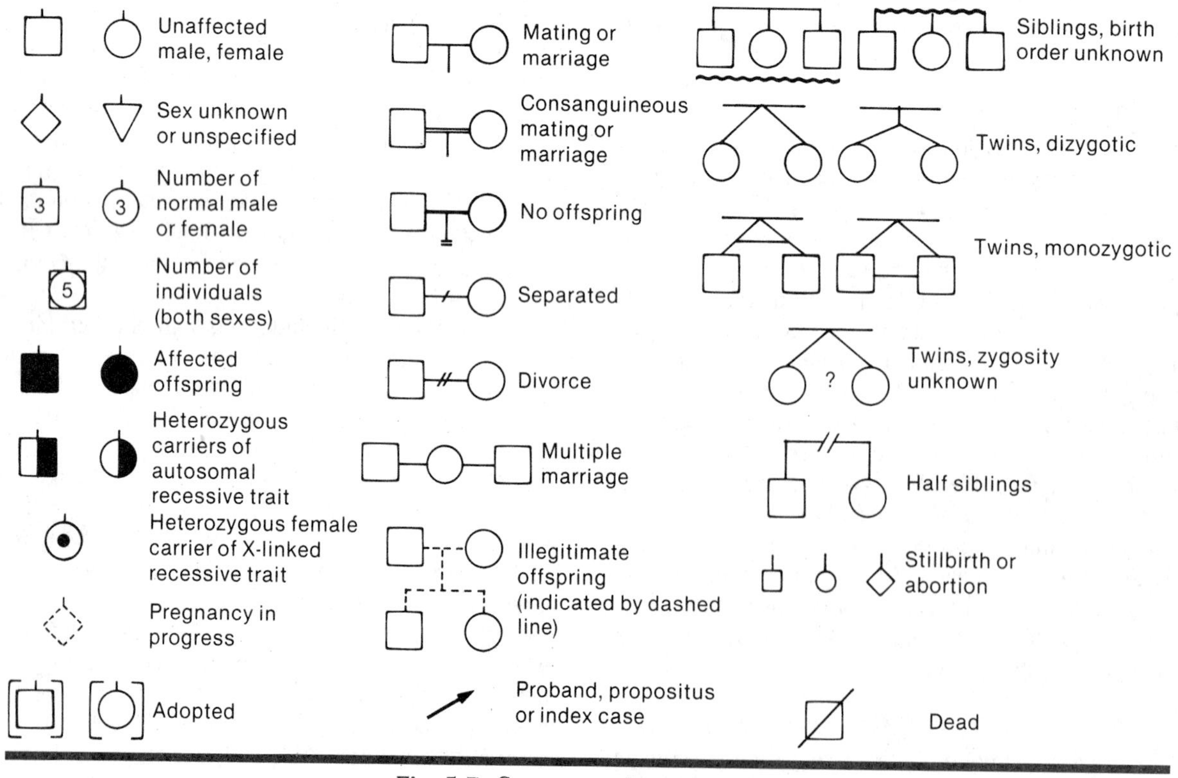

Fig. 5-7. Common pedigree symbols.

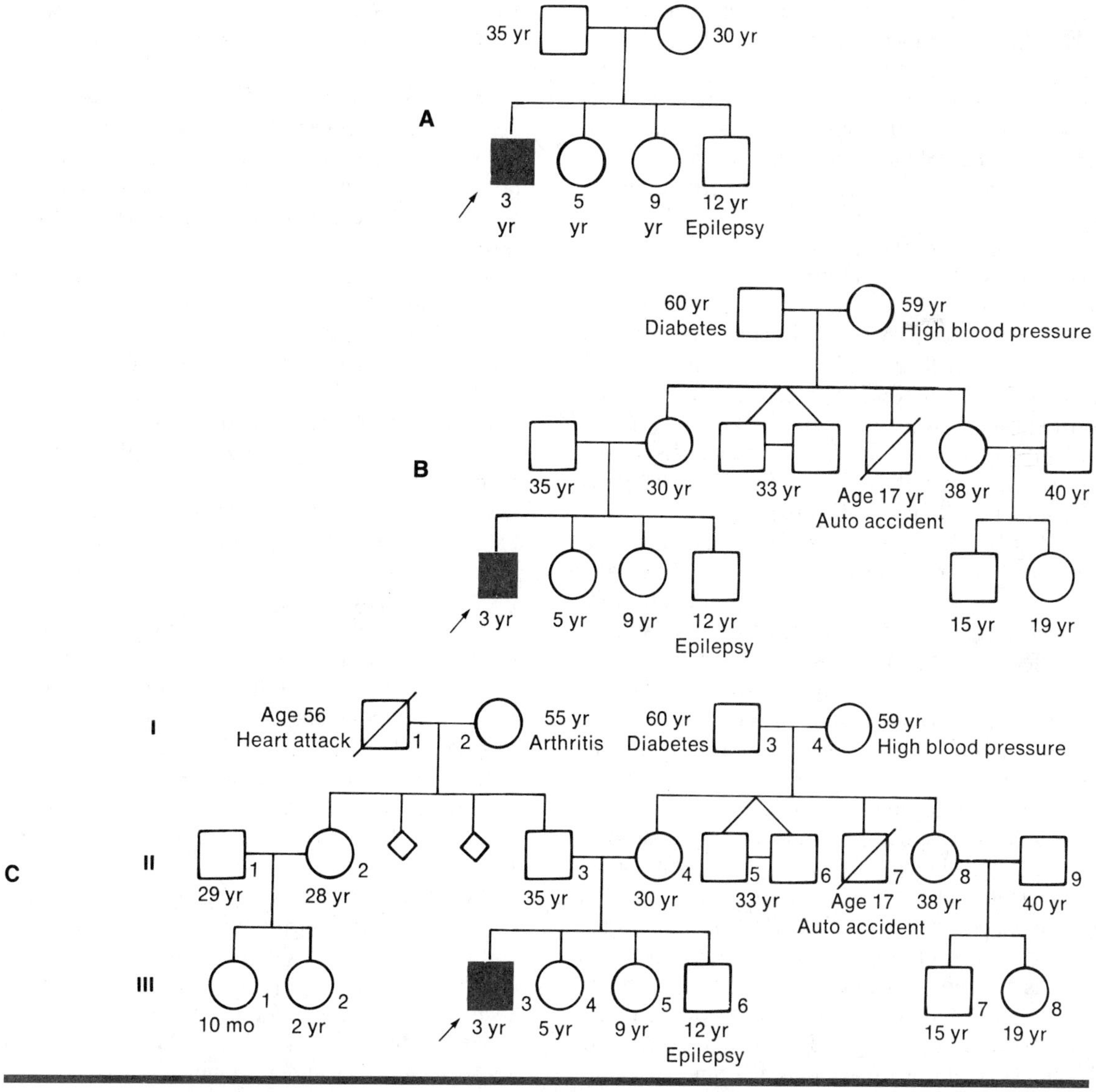

Fig. 5-8. Construction of a pedigree. **A,** Proband, siblings, and parents. **B,** Maternal relatives. **C,** Paternal relatives added.

of the family's coping abilities, resources, and support systems are vital in order to determine their need for additional assistance and support. Also, nurses should be alert for evidence of risk factors that indicate poor adjustment (e.g., child abuse, divorce, or other maladaptive behaviors). Locating agencies and clinics specializing in a specific disorder or its consequences that can provide services (e.g., equipment, medication, and rehabilitation), educational programs, and parent groups is part of the nurse's resources.

Supportive Counseling

It requires time and understanding to deal with the emotional tension and anxiety generated in families who are faced with the prospect of a genetic disorder. Knowledge of and the ability to deal with the range of psychologic responses and all their ramifications (e.g., the grief reaction, guilt, anger, and coping mechanisms) are essential components of the nursing role in genetic counseling. Many of these factors determine the degree to which a counselor's message is understood and influence the family's attitudes and the use they make of counseling information. Awareness and understanding of these feelings make the difference between a genetic informant and a genetic counselor.

Timing of the counseling requires careful evaluation. Some families may not be ready to listen immediately after a diagnosis is made; many do not listen effectively the first time information is presented to them. Families who seek genetic counseling, spontaneously or by referral, are apprehensive and know that decisions made on the basis of the information that they receive may alter their lives significantly and may even alter their view of themselves. There may be numerous blocks to getting information across to families. Often they are so angry or frightened that they do not hear what is being said to them; they may feel guilty, embarrassed, or somehow inferior or inadequate. It is sometimes necessary to wait a week or more to allow the family sufficient time to absorb the initial impact of the situation before they are ready to assimilate any new information.

It is important early in counseling to get a clear understanding of the family's initial concerns, their state of knowledge about the disease, their attitudes and beliefs concerning the condition, and to determine the kind and amount of information they need or want. Some are not sure they should be at a counseling service. Whether the persons needing help are parents who have given birth to an affected child, relatives of an affected individual, or persons who have been identified as carriers of a deleterious gene, their feelings, attitudes, and fears must be dealt with.

It is almost certain that the counselor will be misunderstood. Most clients do not understand what they hear, and because misunderstandings are so prevalent, the follow-up interviews are especially important. Some clients say they want to know all about the disease and its implications, but this may not be true. Information often seems to go "in one ear and out the other." Others really do want to know and will ask questions until they understand. Careful interviewing and assessment will determine the extent and type of information needed and desired by the clients.

Guilt and self-blame are very natural and universal reactions. Nurses must deal with parents' feelings of guilt about carrying "bad genes" or having "made my child sick." For example, the young father of a child with Down syndrome refused to submit to chromosome analysis for fear he might be identified as a carrier of a translocated chromosome and thought he could not endure the guilt this knowledge would generate. Often the counseling person is in a position to absolve the parents of guilt by explaining the random nature of segregation during both gamete formation and fertilization. Sometimes there is comfort in knowing that everyone carries defective genes and that it is mere chance that a particular couple happen to carry the same abnormal gene. Reactions may be different in situations where one member can pinpoint the "blame" (dominant or X-linked disorders), whereas there is some reassurance in recessive disorders for the couple to know that it is not just one of them who carries the defective gene. Anxieties generated by old wives' tales, superstitions, and misconceptions can be dispelled.

It is important to stress that there is nothing shameful about an inherited or congenital defect and to emphasize any appropriate remedy. Families have a tendency to be more ashamed of a hereditary disorder than of one caused by self-indulgence, such as alcoholism. The threat of a hereditary "taint" often creates intrafamilial strife, hostility, and marital disharmony, sometimes to the point of family disintegration. Relatives frequently cease reproduction after the diagnosis of a hereditary defect, or the decision to marry may be deferred on the basis of a disorder, even a remote one, in a partner's family. While people may understand the situation intellectually, this does not help them emotionally. A large and vital part of the nurse's role in genetic counseling is that of sympathetic and supportive listener.

Burden of genetic defect. The way in which members of a family respond to the probability of a genetic disorder will depend a great deal on the nature of the condition and the burden, actual or perceived, that it may place on them. A burden is considered to be the total amount of distress, economic and emotional, that is placed on persons, their families, and society by the birth of an affected child—the anticipated burden as well as the threat of disability. Various factors that are associated with disorders produce a burden in different ways to determine the total impact on a family. These include severity, chronicity, age of onset, mortality, morbidity, presence or absence of chronic pain, mental retardation, and cosmetic disfigurement.

There is a great deal of variability in the ability of individuals and families to withstand stress, and persons respond differently to probabilities. A degree of risk that is reassuring to one may be threatening or intolerable to another. Also, two individuals will respond differently to a hazard that both perceive as threatening. Some parents will choose to have children even in the face of high risk; others believe that even a moderate risk is too much to take. Some may risk having a child with a disorder that produces a minor defect or even one that causes early death but elect not to risk having a child with a lifelong disability. The longer the duration of the disability, the greater the financial and emotional burden.

In some disorders, such as Down syndrome, the burden of the disease rests primarily on the family rather than on the affected child. In diseases with severe crippling effects, such as muscular dystrophy, the impact of the disease affects both the child and the family.

All of these matters confront a family when they must make a decision about whether to risk a pregnancy that might result in a child with a disability, and nurses should be prepared to explore these probabilities with them. Decisions are often irrevocable; therefore the choice must be mutually achieved. Parents who elect to have children in spite of a fairly high risk of recurrence can be helped by education. By learning about the disorder, they will be alert to signs of the disease so that early treatment can be initiated to minimize the ill effects of the disorder.

Barriers to effective counseling. Obstacles to the use of genetic counseling involve the attitudes of both the family and the counselor. Frequent obstacles to an objective use of information are religious attitudes toward conception and opposition to sterilization and to abortion in situations where there is a high risk of recurrence or where prenatal diagnosis has indicated a defective fetus. Many persons fatalistically accept "the will of God." Another obstacle is the right of the individual—the right of the fetus to come to full term and the right of parents to conceive. A person with a high risk of producing a disabling condition in an offspring may believe that he or she is entitled to the same rights as anyone else, including the right of procreation.

Differences in the ability to comprehend what is said probably interfere most with effective use of counseling information. Clients vary in experiences, education, and intellectual level, and even with careful explanation many are still unable to understand the basic fundamentals of inheritance. They may be able to repeat information but fail to grasp its significance.

Sometimes nurses themselves create barriers with their own biases. There are some diseases that have a special impact on individual nurses, and in such cases it is difficult to be nonjudgmental. Families may become defensive if they believe that the nurse is bringing undue pressure to bear on their decision. Others may pressure the nurse to make the decision for them. "What would you do if you were in this situation?" is a common question. In some instances nurses (intentionally or unintentionally) do influence families. They are often tempted to direct the decisions of the clients, especially less intelligent persons who may be judged to be less responsible for their actions. In genetic counseling families should be given all the facts and possible consequences, then assisted, without coercion, in their problem solving. However, the decision concerning a course of action should be left to them.

KEY POINTS

- There is a probably a genetic component in all disease processes.
- Genetic diseases are usually classified as those produced by chromosomal aberrations, those caused by a single mutant gene, or those resulting from interaction of genetic and environmental factors (multifactorial).
- Chromosomal aberrations are caused by deviations in either chromosome structure or number.
- Alterations in chromosome number occur as a result of unequal distribution of genetic material during gamete formation or early cell division of the zygote.
- Disorders caused by a single gene are distributed in families according to predictable Mendelian principles of inheritance.
- Mutant genes can be dominant or recessive and can be located on an autosome or an X chromosome.
- Variations in gene action include the regularity with which it is manifest (penetrance), the severity or variability of its expression (expressivity), and the different and seemingly unrelated effects associated with the basic defect (pleiotropy).
- Congenital defects, errors or morphogenic development, may arise at any stage of development and demonstrate wide variability in causative factors.
- Although no cure for genetic disease is presently available, various therapeutic measures are used to modify or correct the basic defect.
- Eugenics refers to measures aimed at controlling heredity in order to alter future generations.
- Euthenics involves modifying the environment to allow a genetically abnormal individual to live a relatively normal life.
- The objectives of genetic screening are to detect the presence of disease in individuals, detect unaffected carriers of a disease, and monitor the incidence of disease and/or malformations in a population.
- Genetic counseling is directed toward providing individuals and families with information needed to make decisions about a course of action appropriate to them.
- Nurse's roles in genetic counseling include identifying cases, interviewing families, educating families about their disease and its therapy, and providing follow-up care and support.

REFERENCES

American Academy of Pediatrics, Committee on Genetics: New issues in newborn screening for phenylketonuria and congenital hypothyroidism, Pediatrics 69:104-106, 1982.

Cohen, F.L.: Clinical genetics in nursing practice, Philadelphia, 1984, J.B. Lippincott Co.

Fletcher, J.C.: Ethics and amniocentesis for fetal sex identification, N. Engl. J. Med. 301:550-552, 1979.

Fraser, F.C.: Genetic counseling, Am. J. Hum. Genet. 26:636-659, 1974.

Kilpack, V.: Ethical issues in procedural dilemmas in measuring patient competence. In Chinn, P.L., editor: Ethical issues in nursing, Rockville, MD, 1986, Aspen Systems.

Korsch, B.M.: What do patients and parents want to know? What do they need to know? Pediatrics (suppl.), pp. 917-919, 1984.

Rhodes, A.M.: Cases on the tort of "wrongful life," MCN 14:279, 1989.

Sorenson, J.R., and Mangione, T.W.: Parental response to repeat testing of infants with "false-positive" results in a newborn screening program, Pediatrics 73(2):183-187, 1984.

BIBLIOGRAPHY

General

Buyse, M.L., editor: Encyclopedia of birth defects, New York, 1988, Alan R. Liss, Inc.

Cohen, F.L.: Clinical genetics in nursing practice, Philadelphia, 1984, J.B. Lippincott Co.

Cooper, D.N., and Schmidtke, J.: Diagnosis of genetic disease using recombinant DNA, Hum. Genet. 73:1-14, 1986.

Darras, B.R., Harper, J.F., and Francke, U.: Prenatal diagnosis and detection of carriers with DNA probes in Duchenne's muscular dystrophy, N. Engl. J. Med. 316:985-992, 1987.

Forsman, I.: Education of nurses in genetics, Am. J. Hum. Genet. 43:552-558, 1988.

Gilbert-Barness, E., Opitz, J.M., and Barness, L.A.: The pathologist's perspective of genetic disease, Pediatr. Clin. North Am. 36:163-187, 1989.

McKusick, V.A.: Mapping and sequencing the human genome, N. Engl. J. Med. 320:910-915, 1989.

Naeye, R.L., and Peters, E.C.: Working during pregnancy: effects on the fetus, Pediatrics 69:724-727, 1982.

Preus, M.: Numerical classification of syndromes, Hosp. Pract. 20(6):111-117, 1985.

Pritchard, D.J.: Foundations of developmental genetics, London, 1986, Taylor & Frances.

Shaw, M.W.: Genetic services: necessity or luxury? Am. J. Med. Genet. 15:373-378, 1983.

Smith, D.W.: Recognizable patterns of human malformation, ed. 3, Philadelphia, 1982, W.B. Saunders Co.

Stainton, M.C.: The fetus: a growing member of the family, Fam. Rel. 34:321-326, 1985.

Tinley, S.T.: Nurses' and geneticists' role expectations for the genetics nurse clinician, J. Pediatr. Nurs. 2:259-264, 1987.

Weiss, J.O., and others: Genetic disorders and birth defects in families and society, Birth Defects 20(4):1-8, 1984.

Williams, J.K.: Pediatric nurse practitioners' knowledge of genetic disease, Pediatr. Nurs. 9:119-121, 1983.

Williams, R.R.: Nature, nurture, and family predisposition, N. Engl. J. Med. 318:769-770, 1988.

Winter, R.M.: A combined method for grouping cases with multiple malformations, J. Med. Genet. 25:119-126, 1988.

Genetic Disorders

Linden, M.G., and others: 47,XXX: what is the prognosis? Pediatrics 82:619-630, 1988.

Marion, R.W., and others: Trisomy 18 score: a rapid, reliable diagnostic test for trisomy 18, J. Pediatr. 113:45-48, 1988.

McKusick, V.A.: Mendelian inheritance in man, ed. 8, Baltimore, 1988, Williams & Wilkins.

Nyhan, W.L.: Cytogenetic diseases, Clin. Symp. 35(1) entire issue, 1983.

Rovet, J., and Netly, C.: The triple X chromosome syndrome in childhood: recent empirical findings, Child Dev. 54:831-845, 1983.

Salbenblat, J.A., and others: Gross and fine motor development in 47,XXY and 47,XYY males, Pediatrics 80:240-244, 1987.

Schinzel, A.: Catalogue of unbalanced chromosome aberrations in man, New York, 1984, Walter de Gruyter, Inc.

Schwartz, S., and Palmer, C.G.: Chromosomal findings in 164 couples with repeated spontaneous abortions: with special consideration to prior reproductive history, Hum. Genet. 63:28-34, 1983.

Sinclair, L.: Metabolic disease in childhood, Oxford, 1982, Blackwell Scientific Publications, Ltd.

Stene, J., and others: Paternal age and Down's syndrome: data from prenatal diagnosis, Hum. Genet. 59:119, 1981.

Wilkins, L.E., and others: Clinical heterogeneity in 80 home-reared children with cri du chat syndrome, J. Pediatr. 102:528-529, 1983.

Multifactorial Disorders

Cohen, M.M., Jr.: The child with multiple birth defects, New York, 1982, Raven Press.

Gilbert-Barness, E., Opitz, J.M., and Barness, L.A.: The pathologist's perspective of genetic disease: malformations and dysmorphology, Pediatr. Clin. North Am. 36:163-187, 1989.

Golub, H.L.: Infant cry: a clue to diagnosis, Pediatrics 69:197-201, 1982.

McDevitt, H.O.: The HLA system and its relation to disease, Hosp. Pract., July 15, 1985, pp. 57-72.

Osband, B.A.: Multifactorial inheritance: implications for perinatal and neonatal nurses, J. Perinat. Neonatal Nurs. 2(4):43-52, 1989.

Peter, D.: HLA antigens and disease, Diagn. Med. 4:54-81, 1981.

Schaller, J.G., and Hansen, J.A.: HLA relationships to disease, Hosp. Pract., May 1981, pp. 41-49.

Wilson, G.N.: Recurrence risks of malformations, J. Reprod. Med. 27:607-612, 1982.

Therapeutic Management

Cederbaum, S.D.: Introduction to recombinant DNA, Pediatrics 74:408-410, 1984.

Dunn, P.: Surgery for the unborn, Nurs. Life 4(5):19-21, 1984.

Gaffney, S.E.: Intrauterine fetal surgery: the ramifications for nurses, MCN 10:250-254, 1985.

Hirschhorn, R.: Therapy of genetic disorders (editorial), N. Engl. J. Med. 316:623-624, 1987.

Ledley, F.D.: Somatic gene therapy for human disease: background and prospects, part 1, J. Pediatr. 110:1-8, 1987.

Ledley, F.D.: Somatic gene therapy for human disease: background and prospects, part 2, J. Pediatr. 110:167-174, 1987.

Merz, B.: Gene therapy: correcting the errors in life's blueprint, Med. World News 25(19):46-50, 1984.

Scarpa, M., Jones, S.N., and Caskey, C.T.: Advances toward gene therapy, Curr. Opin. Pediatr. 1:453-464, 1989.

Thomson, E.J.: A genetics primer for early service providers, Inf. Young Child. 2(2):37-48, 1989.

Genetic Screening

American Academy of Pediatrics Committee on Genetics: New issues in newborn screening for phenylketonuria and congenital hypothyroidism, Pediatrics 69:104, 1982.

American Academy of Pediatrics Committee on Genetics: Alpha-fetoprotein screening, Pediatrics 80:444-445, 1987.

American Academy of Pediatrics Committee on Genetics: Newborn screening fact sheets, Pediatrics 83:449-464, 1989.

Berry, H.K.: Neonatal screening: the spectrum of metabolic disorders, part 3, Diagn. Med. 7(3):39-41, 44, 46, 1984.

Black, R.B.: Prenatal diagnosis: the experience in families who have children, Am. J. Hum. Genet. 19:729-739, 1984.

Black, R.B., and Furlong, R.: Impact of prenatal diagnosis in families, Soc. Work Health Care 9(3):37-50, 1984.

DiMaio, M.S., and others: Screening for fetal Down's syndrome in pregnancy by measuring maternal serum alpha-fetoprotein levels, N. Engl. J. Med. 317:342-345, 1987.

Faden, R.R., and others: Parental rights, child welfare, and public health: the case of PKU screening, Am. J. Publ. Health 72:396-400, 1982.

Faden, R.R., and others: A survey to evaluate parental consent as public policy for neonatal screening, Am. J. Publ. Health 72:1347, 1982.

Fisher, D.A.: Second International Conference on Neonatal Thyroid Screening: progress report, J. Pediatr. 103:653-654, 1983.

Fleischer, A.C., Kirchner, S.G., and Thieme, G.A.: Prenatal detection of fetal anomalies with sonography, Pediatr. Clin. North Am. 32:1523-1536, 1985.

Fletcher, J.C., and Evans, M.I.: Maternal bonding in early fetal ultrasound examinations, N. Engl. J. Med. 308:392-393, 1983.

Furlong, R.M., and Berkowitz, R.L.: Intrauterine treatment: meeting the psychosocial needs of the family, Health Soc. Work 10:55-62a, 1985.

Grace, J.T.: Does a mother's knowledge of fetal gender affect attachment? MCN 9:42-45, 1984.

Green, D, and Malin, J.: When reality shatters parents' dreams, Nursing '88 18(2):61-64, 1988.

Hammer, R.M., and Tufts, M.A.: Chorionic villi sampling for detecting fetal disorders, MCN 11:29-31, 1986.

Harvey, E.B., and others: Prenatal x-ray exposure and childhood cancer in twins, N. Engl. J. Med. 312:541-545, 1985.

Hogge, J.S., Hogge, W.A., and Golbus, M.S.: Chorionic villus sampling, JOGNN 15(1):24-28, 1986.

Holtzman, N.A.: Ethical issues in the prenatal diagnosis of phenylketonuria, Pediatrics 74:424-427, 1984.

Jones, S.L.: Decision making in clinical genetics: ethical implications for perinatal practice, J. Perinat. Neonatal Nurs. 1:11-23, 1988.

Lopez, E.I.: Prenatal diagnosis by ultrasound, J. Perinat. Neonatal Nurs. 2(4):34-42, 1989.

Morgan, C.D., and Elias, S.: Prenatal diagnosis of genetic disorders, J. Perinat. Neonatal Nurs. 2(4):1-12, 1989.

National Institutes of Health Consensus Development Conference Statement: Newborn screening for sickle cell disease and other hemoglobinopathies, Bethesda, MD, 1987, National Institutes of Health.

Nussbaum, R.L., and others: Newborn screening for sickling hemoglobinopathies, Am. J. Dis. Child. 138:44-48, 1984.

Ornoy, A., and others: Pathological confirmation of cystic fibrosis in the fetus following prenatal diagnosis, Am. J. Med. Genet. 28:935-948, 1987.

Ostrer, H.: Prenatal diagnosis of genetic disorders by DNA analysis, Pediatr. Ann. 18:701-713, 1989.

Ostrer, H., and Hejtmancik, J.F.: Prenatal diagnosis and carrier detection of genetic disease by analysis of deoxyribonucleic acid, J. Pediatr. 112:679-687, 1988.

President's Commission for the Study of Ethical Problems in Medicine and Biomedical and Behavioral Research: Screening and counseling for genetic conditions, 1983, Washington, DC, U.S. Government Printing Office.

Rowley, P.T.: Genetic screening: marvel or menace? Science 225:138-144, 1984.

Scriver, C.R.: Genetic screening: implications for preventive medicine, Am. J. Publ. Health 73:243, 245, 1983.

Sorensen, J.R., and others: Parental response to repeat testing of infants with "false-positive" results in a newborn screening program, Pediatrics 73:183-187, 1984.

Stringer, M.R.: Chorionic villi sampling: a nursing perspective, JOGNN 17(1):19-22, 1988.

Wertz, D.C., and Fletcher, J.C.: Ethical issues in prenatal diagnosis, Pediatr. Ann. 18:739-749, 1989.

Williams, J.K.: Screening for genetic disorders, J. Pediatr. Health Care 3:115-121, 1989.

Williamson, R., and Murray, J.C.: Molecular analysis of genetic disorders. In Pitkin, R.M., and Scott, J., editors: Clinical obstetrics and gynecology, Philadelphia, 1988, J.B. Lippincott Co.

Worthington, S: Genetic screening, J. Obstet. Gynecol. Nurs. (suppl.) 13(2):32s-37s, 1984.

Genetic Counseling

Baird, P.A., and Sadovnick, A.D.: Maternal age-specific rates for Down syndrome: changes over time, Am. J. Med. Genet. 29:917-928, 1988.

Buri, C.E., and Hecht, F.: Tort liability in genetic diagnosis and genetic counseling, Am. J. Hum. Genet. 34:353-355, 1982.

Clark, M.H.: A pedigree primer, J. Pediatr. Nurs. 4:112-118, 1989.

Coplan, J.: Wrongful life and wrongful birth: new concepts for the pediatrician, Pediatrics 75:65-72, 1985.

dYdewalle, G., and others, editors: Experiments on genetic risk perception and decision-making: explorative studies, Birth Defects 23(2):209-225, 1987.

Ekwo, E.E., Kim, J., and Gosselink, C.A.: Parental perceptions of the burden of genetic diseases, Am. J. Med Genet. 28:955-964, 1987.

Farrell, C.D.: Genetic counseling: the emerging reality, J. Perinat. Neonatal Nurs. 2(4):21-33, 1989.

Fibison, W.J.: The nursing role in the delivery of genetic services, Health Care Women 4:1-15, 1983.

Fleisher, L.D.: Wrongful births: when is there liability for prenatal injury? Am. J. Dis. Child. 141:1260-1265, 1987.

Hamilton, A.K., and Noble, D.N.: Assisting families through genetic counseling, Soc. Casework 64:14-19, 1983.

Kenen, R.H.: Genetic counseling: the development of a new interdisciplinary occupational field, Soc. Sci. Med. 18:541-549, 1984.

Korsch, B.M.: What do patients and parents want to know? What do they need to know? Symposium of Pediatric Patient Educations: Challenge for the 80s, 1983.

LaRochelle, D.: Prenatal genetic counseling: ethical and legal interfaces with the nurse's role, Health Care Women 4:77-92.

Lin, A.E., and Garver, K.L.: Genetic counseling for congenital heart defects, J. Pediatr. 113:1105-1109, 1988.

Nora, J.J., and Nora, A.H.: Update on counseling the family with a first-degree relative with a congenital heart defect, Am. J. Med. Genet. 29:137-142, 1988.

Reilly, P.R.: Ethical, legal, and social issues in genetics, Curr. Opin. Pediatr. 1:448-452, 1989.

Rhodes, A.M.: Minimizing the liability risks of genetic counseling, MCN 14:313, 1989.

Rhodes, A.M.: Wrongful birth and wrongful life, MCN 14:171, 1989.

Sankaranalayanan, K.: Prevalence of genetic and partially genetic diseases in man and the estimation of genetic risks of exposure to ionizing radiation, Am. J. Hum. Genet. 42:651-660, 1988.

Somer, M., Mustonen, H., and Norio, R.: Evaluation of genetic counselling: recall of information, post-counselling reproduction, and attitude of the counsellees, Clin. Genet. 34:352-365, 1988.

Thurman, T.F.: Genetic counseling: practical concepts about risks and risk management, Consultant 25(6):50-52, 56, 1985.

VanRegemorter, N., and others: Congenital malformations in 10,000 consecutive births in a university hospital: need for genetic counseling and prenatal diagnosis, J. Pediatr. 104:386-390, 1984.

Wilson, G.N.: Counseling parents of children with genetic disorders, Feelings Med. Signif. 25:(4)13-16, 1983.

Williams, J.K.: Counseling adolescents about environmental teratogens, Pediatr. Nurs. 12:292-295, 1986.

Williams, J.K.: Genetic counseling in pediatric nursing care, Pediatr. Nurs. 12:287-290, 1986.

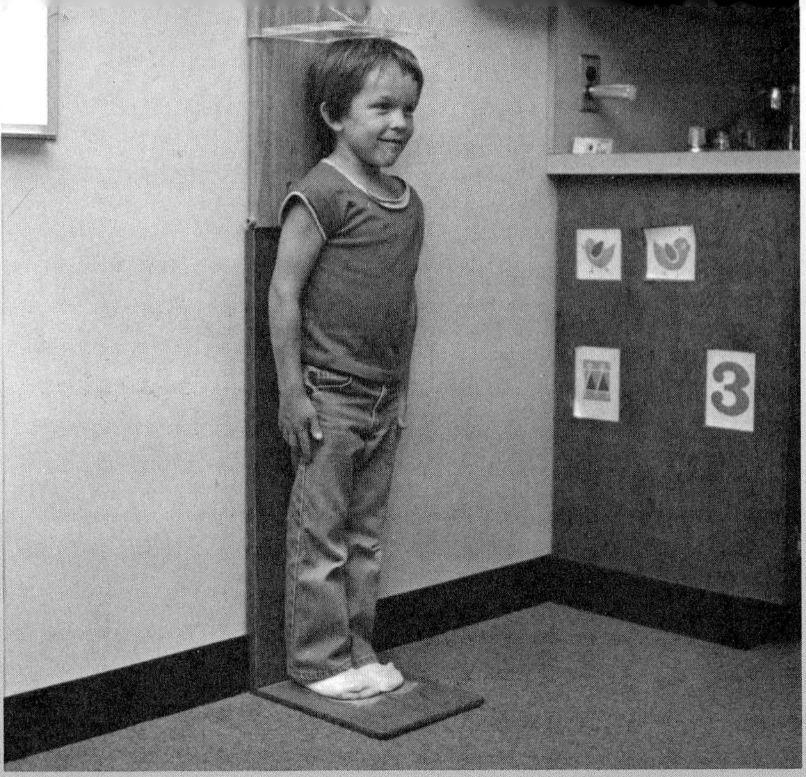

Assessment of the Child and Family

UNIT II

Assessment is fundamental to the nursing process. Establishing a data base on which to formulate a nursing diagnosis, plan interventions, and evaluate outcomes of care is essential, whether the nurse is caring for a child who is well or ill. Assessment facilitates identification of present problems and prevention of future ones. Although the assessment process primarily focuses on the child, it permits an exploration into family dynamics and often is the first clue to cultural, environmental, socioeconomic, or religious traditions that influence the child's total well-being.

Assessment primarily involves some form of communication. Chapter 6, *Communication and Health Assessment of the Child and Family,* is concerned with general aspects of communication as they relate to the nurse, family, and child. It also discusses the interview process specifically in terms of history-taking, with special emphasis on assessment of the family and nutrition.

Chapter 7, *Physical and Developmental Assessment of the Child,* deals with the procedures and skills required to perform a complete pediatric physical assessment, including sensory and developmental testing. Findings primarily related to normal structure and function are emphasized, with notation of those deviations that require referral and further evaluation.

CHAPTER 6

Communication and Health Assessment of the Child and Family

RELATED TOPICS

Assessment of family strengths and level of adjustment (chronic health conditions), Ch. 22
Development of self-concept, Ch. 4
Developmental assessment, Ch. 7
Family structure and function, Ch. 3
Family theories, Ch. 3
Growth measurements, Ch. 7
Immunizations, Ch. 12
Nutritional disturbances, Ch. 13
Pain assessment, Ch. 26
Preparation for procedures, Ch. 27
Role of play in development, Ch. 4
Sex education, Chs. 15 and 17
Sexually transmitted diseases, Ch. 20
Sleep disturbances, Chs. 12 and 15
Social, cultural, and religious influences on child health promotion, Ch. 2
Use of play in procedures, Ch. 27
Use of play to minimize stress, Ch. 26
Taking a family history, p. 175
Traits of a healthy family, p. 74

GLOSSARY

CC Chief complaint
FAPGAR Family AGPAR (Adaptability, Partnership, Growth, Affection, and Resolve)
HOME Home Observation and Measurement of the Environment
HSQ Home screening questionnaire
KFD Kinetic family drawing
NLP Neurolinguistic programming
PH Past history
PI Present illness
ROS Review of systems

Communication is essential to the nursing of children. It is the most important skill used in assessment of children and their families and the most important feature in forming trusting relationships with them. Communication consists of all those behaviors by which one person, consciously or unconsciously, affects another. All behavior transmits a message; even the attempt not to communicate creates a particular impression. Inherent in communication are the power of observation, the use of all the senses, and the intangible reaction of intuition.

This chapter is concerned with the communication process as it relates to health assessment. In the first section, strategies for communication and interviewing are reviewed, and specific suggestions for communicating with parents and children are presented. The second section deals with a particular type of interview—the health history. It is presented in some detail to give nurses the opportunity to learn to take a history, as well as to facilitate understanding those histories recorded by other members of the health team. Because of the importance of the family and nutrition in ensuring optimal emotional and physical health, special sections on family and nutritional assessment are included.

COMMUNICATION

Communication may be verbal, nonverbal, or abstract. *Verbal* communication may involve language and its expression, such as vocalizations in the form of laughs, moans, and squalls, or the implications of what is not said in light of what has been said. *Nonverbal* communication is often called body language and includes gestures, movements, facial expressions, postures, and reactions. *Abstract* communication takes such forms as play, artistic expression, symbols, photographs, and choice of clothing. Because it is possible to exert greater conscious control over verbal communication, it is a less reliable indicator of true feelings, especially in relationships with children.

Many factors influence the communication process. To be successful (gratifying), communication must be appropriate to the situation, properly timed, and clearly delivered. This implies that nurses understand and use techniques of effective communication. Verbal and nonverbal messages must be congruous; that is, two or more messages sent via different levels must not be contradictory.

Nurses need to recognize their own feelings and attempt to recognize those of the persons with whom the communicative interchange takes place. Biases and judgments interfere with all aspects of the process. The tendency to approve or disapprove of another's statements inhibits positive reactions. In addition, the transmission and reception of messages may be altered by influences of intimacy or distance, trust and mistrust, security and insecurity, or caring and not caring on the part of the participants. The value of effective communication is increased understanding between the nurse, child, and family. Since nursing of infants and children always involves the inclusion of a caregiver, nurses must be able to communicate not only with children of all ages but with the adults in their lives as well.

VERBAL COMMUNICATION—THE POWER OF WORDS

Words shape reality, and thus they hold tremendous power. One can change another's perception of reality by the choice of words each uses (Cassell, Coulehan, and Putnam, 1989). For example, if the diagnosis of cancer is always referred to as a tumor, cyst, malignancy, or carcinoma, patients may never really know that they have cancer. Consequently they may assume less responsibility for their care than if they were aware of the seriousness of the condition. By learning to recognize how patients and health professionals use language to manipulate reality, one can also learn how to change perceptions and communicate more effectively.

Avoidance Language

Probably the most common way people try to alter reality is by avoiding words that truly describe it. For example, euphemisms such as "passed on" are used instead of the word "death." Avoidance language usually indicates that a person wants to hide something, especially feelings. As a rule, accepting a person's use of euphemisms only serves to perpetuate the fears and never helps the person deal with them. In contrast, use of straightforward, precise, descriptive language lends perspective to the situation and allows the person to discuss the fears. Most often, imagined fears are far greater than the actual reality. (For a discussion of explaining death to children, see Chapter 23.)

Distancing Language

Sometimes people use impersonal words to shield themselves from the painful reality of a situation. For example, parents may state that they know *someone* with a child who is slow and actually be talking about personal fears regarding *their* child. By realizing that parents need to talk about this difficult subject, the nurse can provide sensitive statements that ease them into discussing their situation.

One of the dangers in supporting distancing language is that the parent may effectively deny that a problem exists. To return to the previous example, if the issue of retardation is never approached directly but is allowed to be "someone else's problem," the parents may not be able to make decisions for special schools or individualized training.

Sometimes distancing is desirable because the topic may be too painful to discuss directly. The use of third-person technique (p. 194) may be very therapeutic by allowing an individual the opportunity to indirectly approach a subject and receive feedback but still remain in control.

NONVERBAL COMMUNICATION—PARALANGUAGE

In addition to the spoken word, messages are relayed through nonverbal means, or paralanguage, which involves pitch, pause, intonation, rate, volume, and stress in speech (Cassell, Coulehan, and Putnam, 1989). Young children become very adept at understanding paralanguage; long before they know the meaning of words, they sense anxiety or fear by the rise in pitch or the accelerated rate of the parent's voice. By careful attention to the spoken word, nurses can better understand the meaning of another's verbal message and more accurately control their own paralanguage.

Because most people do not exert conscious control over paralanguage, it is a valuable clue to such things as feelings and concerns. For example, *pausing* may signify a need to formulate thoughts, recall information, or sometimes fabricate a story. Frequent pauses, however, often make the speaker sound insecure. Long pauses may mean that the individual needs more information.

Rate also sends unspoken messages. Talking too fast usually makes the speaker sound glib and insensitive. Talking slowly with a firm tone and appropriate pauses conveys authority. Therefore, a person is much more likely to "hear" instructions if the latter approach is used. Children, in particular, respond attentively to a slow, even, steady voice.

Confirming and Disconfirming Behaviors

People respond to each other through *confirming behaviors*, such as nodding the head, using direct eye contact, repeating or requesting clarification, and making appropriate comments, or *disconfirming behaviors*, such as tapping fingers or a foot, turning away from the speaker, avoiding eye contact, and interrupting (Heineken and Roberts, 1983). Since there is a reciprocal relationship between such behaviors, nurses need to use confirming behaviors to receive confirmation in return. This "mirroring" effect is particularly evident in children because of their sensitivity to nonverbal cues.

GUIDELINES FOR COMMUNICATION AND INTERVIEWING

The most widely used method of communicating with parents on a professional basis is the interview process. Interviewing, unlike social conversation, is a specific form of goal-directed communication. As nurses converse with children and adults, they endeavor to focus on the individuals to determine the kind of persons they are, their usual mode of handling problems, whether help is needed, and the way in which they react to counseling. Developing interviewing skills requires time and patience, but adherence to some guiding principles and avoiding some obstacles facilitate this process.

ESTABLISHING A SETTING FOR COMMUNICATION

Part of the success in interviewing depends on the type of physical and psychologic setting the interviewer constructs. Appropriate introduction, role clarification, explanation of the reason for the interview, preliminary acquaintance with the family, and assurance of privacy and confidentiality are prerequisites for establishing a setting conducive to communication.

Appropriate Introduction

Nurses should introduce themselves to, and ask the name of, each family member who is present. During the interview, each person is addressed by name, after asking them their preference regarding form of address. Using the person's preferred name conveys respect and communicates a personal interest in each family member. The preferred name should be recorded on the medical record and communicated to other staff members (Elizabeth, 1989).

At the beginning of the visit, children are included in the interaction by asking them their name, age, and other information. Nurses often direct all questions to adults, even when children are old enough to speak for themselves. This serves to terminate one extremely valuable source of information, the patient. If the child is included, the general rules for communicating with children are followed (p. 192).

Role Clarification and Explanation of the Interview

During the introduction it is also necessary to clarify the nurse's particular role in the health setting. For example, nurses performing interviews may be pediatric nurse practitioners, inpatient staff nurses, clinic nurses, office nurses, visiting nurses, or school nurses. A parent is much more likely to reveal personal information about the child and family if the relevance and importance of the interview are stressed. If this is not done, parents may refuse to elaborate on certain areas because they feel it has no bearing on the "problem." In addition, since more than one member of the health team may take a history during the course of a hospital admission, it is important to clarify the reason for each interview.

Another reason for role clarification is education of the health consumer. With expanded roles in nursing, it is not unusual for families to think that the examiner is a physician, not a nurse. Role clarification is especially important because some parents may feel deceived if they later are made aware of the nurse's identity. Since the general consumer acceptance of pediatric nurse practitioners has been very favorable, it is also important to acknowledge the expertise of the nurse by emphasizing the nurse's role.

Preliminary Acquaintance

Because of the personal and private nature of an in-depth interview, the person being interviewed must trust the interviewer in order to reveal such extensive information. Therefore, it is best to begin with some general conversation. Comments such as, "How have things been since your last visit?" "Tell me about Johnny," or (to the child) "What do you think is going to happen today?" allow the parent or child to express the main concern in a casual, relaxed atmosphere.

The preliminary acquaintance conversation also reveals how responsive the informant may be to questions. For example, using open-ended statements may lead the person into a lengthy detailed discussion. In this case it is more beneficial to direct questions toward specific answers to avoid tangential remarks. At other times a person may respond to open-ended questions with only minimal information, in which case the continued use of open-ended questions probably will reveal more data than "yes" or "no" type questions.

Assurance of Privacy and Confidentiality

The place where the interview is conducted is almost as important as the interview itself. The physical environment should allow for as much privacy as possible with distractions, such as interruptions, ambient noise, or other visible activity, kept to a minimum. At times it is necessary to turn off a television or radio. The environment should also have some play provision for young children to keep them occupied during the parent-nurse interview (Fig. 6-1). Parents who are constantly interrupted by their children are unable to concentrate fully and tend to give short, brief answers to terminate the interview as quickly as possible.

Confidentiality is also an essential component of the initial phase of the interview. Since the interview is usually shared with other members of the health team or the teacher (as in the case of students), it is the interviewer's responsibility and obligation to inform the family of the confidential limits of the conversation. If there is concern regarding confidentiality in a situation, such as talking to a parent suspected of child abuse or a teenager contemplating suicide, the nurse must deal with this directly and inform the person that in such instances confidentiality cannot be ensured.

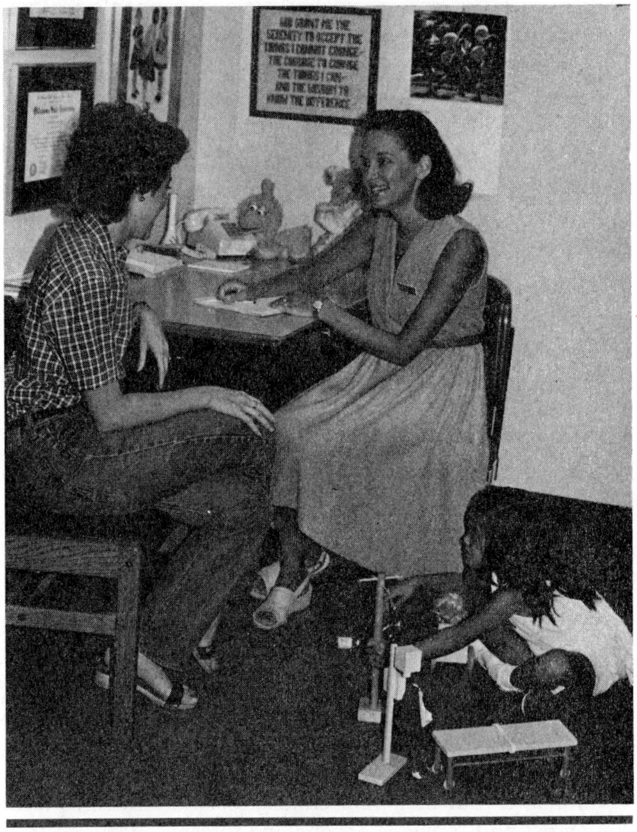

Fig. 6-1. Child plays while nurse interviews parent.

COMMUNICATING WITH FAMILIES

Communicating with the family is a triangular process involving the nurse, parents, and child. Although the following discussion focuses primarily on this triad, in many circumstances significant others, for example, siblings, relatives, or other caregivers, may be part of the communication process.

COMMUNICATING WITH PARENTS

Although the parent and child are separate and distinct entities, relationships with the child are frequently mediated via the parent, particularly in the case of younger children. For the most part, information about the child is acquired by direct observation or communicated to the nurse by the parents. Usually it can be assumed that, because of the close contact with the child, the information imparted by the parent is reliable. Making an assessment of the child requires input from the child (verbal and nonverbal), information from the parent, and the nurse's own observations of the child and interpretation of the relationship between the child and the parent. Counseling and guidance must be directed to the caregiver of infants and small children; when children are old enough to be active participants in their own health maintenance, the parent becomes a collaborator in health care.

Encouraging the Parent to Talk

Interviewing parents not only offers the nurse an opportunity to determine the health and developmental status of the child but also offers information about all factors that influence the child's life. Whatever the parent sees as a problem should be a concern of the nurse. These problems are not always easy to identify. Nurses need to be alert for clues and signals by which a parent communicates worries and anxieties. Careful phrasing with broad open-ended questions such as "What is Jimmy eating now?" provides more information than several single-answer questions such as "Is Jimmy eating what the rest of the family eats?" that can be answered with "yes" or "no."

Sometimes the parent will take the lead without stimulation. Other times it may be necessary for the nurse to direct another question on the basis of an observation such as "Connie seems unhappy today," or "How do you feel when David cries?" If the parent appears to be tired or distraught, the nurse might ask, "What do you do to relax?" or "What help do you have with the children?" A comment such as "You handle the baby very well. What kinds of experience have you had with babies?" to new mothers who appear comfortable with their first child gives them positive reinforcement and provides an opening for any questions they might have regarding the care of the infant. Often all that is required to keep the parent talking is a nod and saying "yes," or "un-huh."

When attempting to elicit feelings and covert problem areas, it is best to avoid closed-ended questions that begin with "Does . . .," "Did . . .," or "Is . . .," which usually require only a single response. In addition, asking questions such as, "Does your son have any problems at school?" subtly implies a lack of parental skills and evokes defensiveness. Instead, it is helpful to say "What . . .," "How . . .," "Tell me about . . .," and encourage elaboration with "You were saying . . .," "You say that . . .," or reflecting back key words or phrases, such as "He was depressed?" Open-ended questions are nonthreatening and encourage description.

Another useful approach is to elicit information about a topic and compare the answer to the person's perception of what "things" should be. For example, after the parent describes what the child is eating, it is helpful to ask, "What do you think your child should be eating?" If there is a discrepancy between the two answers, it is important to ask the parent to comment on how important the difference is. This approach allows the parent to discuss areas of concern that may not be disclosed otherwise.

Directing the Focus

Ability to direct the focus of the interview while allowing for maximum freedom of expression is one of the most difficult goals in effective communication. One approach is the use of open-ended or broad questions, followed by guiding statements. For example, if the parent proceeds to list the other children by name, the nurse can also say, "Tell me their ages, too." If the parent continues to describe each child in depth, which is not the purpose of the interview, the nurse can redirect the focus by stating, "Let's talk about the other children later. You were beginning to tell me about Paul's activities at school." This approach conveys interest in the other children but focuses the data collection on the patient.

In the event that the parent has suggested that a problem exists with one of the other children, the nurse should reintroduce this subject at the end of the interview to assess the need for further family follow-up. Saying to the parent, "Before you were mentioning that your older son is having trouble in school. Tell me what you see as the problem," reintroduces this subject but only in terms of the possible problem.

Listening

Listening is the most important component for effective communication. When listening is truly aimed at understanding the client, it is an active process that requires concentration and attention to all aspects of the conversation—verbal, nonverbal, and abstract. One of the greatest blocks to listening is environmental distraction and premature judgment.

The attitudes and feelings of the nurse are easily injected into an interview. Often nurses' perceptions of a parent's behavior are influenced by their own perceptions, prejudices, and assumptions, which may include racial, religious, and cultural stereotypes. What may be interpreted as passive hostility or disinterest in a parent may be shyness or an expression of anxiety. For example, in Western cultures eye contact and directness are signs of paying attention. However, in many non-Western cultures, including Native Americans, directness, such as looking someone in the eye, is considered rude. Children are taught to avert their gaze and to look down when being addressed by an adult, especially one with authority (Sloat and Matsuura, 1990). Therefore, judgments about "listening" need to be made with an appreciation of cultural differences.

Although it is necessary to make some preliminary judgments, the nurse must attempt to listen with as much objectivity as possible by clarifying meanings and attempting to see the situation from the parent's point of view. Effective interviewers use conscious control over their reactions, responses, and the techniques they use.

Use of minimal verbal activity with active listening facilitates parent involvement. It is tempting to spend time explaining, describing, and interpreting health information when the opportunity presents itself. However, it is possible to provide effective health education by properly timing the information and presenting only as much as is necessary at the moment.

Careful listening facilitates the use of clues, verbal leads, or signals from the interviewer to move the interview along. Frequent references to an area of concern, repetition of certain key words, or a special emphasis on something or someone serve as cues to the interviewer for the direction of inquiry. Concerns and anxieties are usually mentioned in a casual, offhand manner. Even though they are casual, they are important and deserve more careful scrutiny to identify problem areas. For example, a parent who is concerned about a child's habit of bed-wetting may casually mention that the child's bed was "wet this morning."

Because the interview is almost always triangular—nurse, child, and parent—the parent may wish to convey information in such a way as to prevent the child from hearing it. This requires active listening on the part of the nurse to hear the unspoken message. The following example illustrates this point:

> During a routine health visit the nurse performed a complete history and physical examination on a 4-year-old girl. The child was accompanied by her mother, who appeared to be a reliable, well-informed, and talkative informant. During the child's birth history, the mother gave all the information asked. However, during the family history, the mother stated to the nurse, "I had a hysterectomy 6 years ago." Because the nurse gave no indication of acknowledging the significance of this statement, the mother repeated it, only this time she stressed the "6 years." The nurse, who had not been listening as attentively as she should have, realized that the mother was telling her something very important. The mother raised her eyebrows and gently shook her head "no," warning the nurse not to explore this area too openly. The nurse correctly read the cues and stated, "Let's return to your health history later."
>
> At the completion of the physical examination, the nurse brought the child to the Health Center's playroom and took the opportunity to investigate this contradictory information of a "4-year-old child born to a woman with a hysterectomy 6 years ago." The mother revealed that this child was adopted. The mother was greatly concerned about the fact that the child was unaware of this and requested the nurse's advice.
>
> Fortunately the nurse had "listened" carefully enough to realize the significance of this woman's concern and allowed her the opportunity to discuss it in private.

Listening is also helpful in assessing reliability. For example, the answers elicited at the beginning of the interview may differ from those at the end, when the parent feels more confident in revealing problems. It is important to identify any discrepancies and reintroduce those topics for further investigation.

Using Silence

Silence as a response is often one of the most difficult interviewing techniques to learn. It requires a sense of confidence and comfort on the part of the interviewer to allow the interviewee space in which to think uninterrupted. Silence permits the interviewee to sort out thoughts and feelings and search for responses to questions, and allows for sharing of feelings in which two or more people absorb the emotion to its depth.

Sometimes it is necessary to break silence and reopen communication. This should be done in such a way that the person is given a choice to continue talking about what is considered important. Breaking a silence by introducing a new topic or by prolonged talking essentially terminates the interviewee's opportunity to use the silence. Suggestions for breaking the silence include statements such as, "Is there anything else you wish to say?" "I see you find it difficult to continue; how may I help?" or "I don't know what this silence means. Perhaps there is something you would like to put into words but find difficult to say."

Being Empathic

Empathy means feeling and participating in the inner feelings of another while remaining objective. The empathic interviewer attempts to see the world from the interviewee's perspective with as much understanding as possible. Empathy differs from sympathy, which is subjectively thinking or feeling like the other person. Although important and necessary at times, sympathy is not always therapeutic in the helping relationship. Empathy, however, is a very beneficial supportive technique (see Questions and Controversies).

QUESTIONS AND CONTROVERSIES

What are parents' concerns, and what kinds of support are beneficial?

Two studies demonstrate that a minority of parents' concerns (about 30%) are related to medical problems. Over half are child/family concerns, such as eating, sleeping, crying, parenting skills, language development, socializing the child, discipline, safety, and adjustment to divorce; about 15% are nutritional concerns, such as breast-feeding, weaning, and eating habits (Hickson and others, 1983; Ryberg and Merrifield, 1984). The use of structured forms significantly increases the identification of parental concerns and appropriate professional counseling regarding these issues (Ertel and Ertel, 1986; Triggs and Perrin, 1986).

Many parental concerns warrant supportive intervention. Wasserman and others (1984) report on the effectiveness of three supportive behaviors: (1) *encouragement,* the expression of positive reinforcement or good feelings in regard to a parent's actions; (2) *reassurance,* assuagement of a parent's concern or worry; and (3) *empathy,* the expression of intellectual appreciation of a parent's situation. Reassurance was used most frequently, followed by encouragement and empathy. In this study nurse practitioners provided significantly more reassurance and total support than physicians. However, in another study of nurse practitioners' interactions with parents, the process of assessing and intervening was dominated by questions, commands, and opinions. Rarely did the nurse practitioners encourage parents to ask questions, problem solve, or share their knowledge on an issue (Webster-Stratton, Glascock, and McCarthy, 1986).

To evaluate the impact of providing different kinds of support, Wasserman and others (1984) compared visit outcomes as measured by various methods with mothers who received high or low levels of support. Mothers exposed to high levels of encouragement had significant improvement in their opinions of clinicians and higher satisfaction. Mothers exposed to high levels of empathy had higher satisfaction and greater reduction in concerns. No significant differences in outcome were found for high levels of reassurance. From this study it appears that empathy, the least used form of support, is the most beneficial and reassurance, the most used type of support, is least beneficial.

Some individuals are naturally empathic and easily "feel" with another person. However, empathy can be learned by attending to the verbal and nonverbal language of the interviewee. Neurolinguistic programming (NLP), which is concerned with the manner of accessing and understanding information, is an excellent method of increasing empathic communication and will be discussed later (p. 194).

Defining the Problem

To arrive at a solution to a problem or concern, the nurse and the parent must agree that one exists. If neither believes that there is a problem, there is certainly no need to create one. Sometimes the parent may believe that there is a problem that the nurse is unable to see. For example, a mother was overly concerned about every small sniffle, sneeze, or cough in her infant who had been carefully examined and found to be healthy with no evidence of a respiratory problem. On careful questioning, the nurse discovered that a previous child had died of pneumonia in infancy. Consequently, the nurse was able to better understand the mother's concern. Once the nurse acknowledges the mother's fear, she can help the mother deal with her special anxieties about her infant and teach her how to recognize when there is need for concern.

Occasionally the nurse identifies a problem that the parent denies exists. In this case the nurse should pursue the situation and either find a way to deal with it or enlist the aid of other health team members. For example, the parents of a child with Down syndrome may refuse to believe that their child is different from any other child of the same age. They may say, "He is just a little slow," and "All the child needs to do is to try harder." A child with an obvious behavior problem may be described by the parents as "just stubborn" or "just behaving that way to spite us." Such statements may be clues that the parents have not progressed past the stage of denial in adjusting to the disability.

Solving the Problem

Once the problem is identified and agreed on by parent and nurse, they can begin to arrive at a solution. A parent who is included in the problem-solving process is more apt to follow through with a course of action. Such questions as "What have you tried so far?" or "What have you thought about doing?" provide leads for exploration and give the parents the feeling that their ideas and solutions are worthwhile. These can be followed by "What prevents you from trying that?" "That sounds like a good plan," and "You seem to be stumped. Have you considered trying this?" Such approaches encourage participation and reinforce rather than belittle parents' efforts to solve problems.

Sometimes a parent arrives at a solution that the nurse does not consider to be the best alternative. If it can be ascertained that it will do no harm and the parents are convinced of its merits, it is usually best to allow them to continue with the plan. A course of action is more likely to be carried out when parents can reach their own conclusions. However, when parental decisions may be hazardous, nurses are obligated to discuss the risks with the family and try to reach a more beneficial solution. Whenever possible, decisions should be theirs, with the nurse serving as a *facilitator* in problem solving.

Providing Anticipatory Guidance

The ideal way to handle a situation is to deal with it *before* it becomes a problem. The best preventive measure is anticipatory guidance. One of the most significant areas in pediatrics is injury prevention through appropriate anticipatory guidance. Beginning prenatally, parents need specific instructions on home safety. Because of the child's maturing developmental skills, home safety changes must be implemented early to minimize risks to the child.

Many normal developmental changes can disturb unprepared parents, such as a toddler's diminished appetite, negativism, altered sleeping patterns, and anxiety toward strangers. Such topics are discussed in the chapters on health promotion to provide the nurse with knowledge to counsel parents.

Avoiding Blocks to Communication

A number of blocks to communication can adversely affect the quality of the helping relationship. Many of these blocks are initiated by the interviewer, such as giving unrestricted advice or forming prejudged conclusions. Another type of block occurs primarily with the interviewees and deals with information overload. When individuals are presented with too much information or information that is overwhelming, they will often demonstrate signals of increasing anxiety or decreasing attention. Such signals should alert the interviewer to give less information or to clarify what has been said. Some of the more common blocks to communication and signs of information overload are listed in Boxes 6-1 and 6-2.

Communication blocks can be corrected by careful analysis of the interview process. One of the best methods for improving interviewing skills is audiotape and/or videotape feedback. With supervision and guidance, the interviewer can recognize the blocks and consciously avoid them.

Box 6-1 BLOCKS TO COMMUNICATION

- Socializing
- Giving unrestricted and sometimes unasked-for advice
- Offering premature or inappropriate reassurance
- Giving overready encouragement
- Defending a situation or opinion
- Using stereotyped comments or cliches
- Limiting expression of emotion by asking directed, closed-ended questions
- Interrupting and finishing the person's sentence
- Talking more than the interviewee
- Forming prejudged conclusions
- Deliberately changing the focus

Box 6-2 SIGNS OF INFORMATION OVERLOAD

Long periods of silence
Wide eyes and fixed facial expression
Constant fidgeting or attempting to move away
Nervous habits, e.g., tapping, playing with hair
Sudden disruptions, e.g., asking to go to the bathroom
Looking around
Yawning
Frequently looking at a watch or clock
Attempting to change topic of discussion

Box 6-3 GUIDELINES FOR USING AN INTERPRETER

Explain to interpreter reason for interview and type of questions that will be asked.
Clarify whether a detailed or brief answer is required and whether the translated response can be general or literal.
Introduce interpreter to family and allow some time before actual interview so that they can become acquainted.
Communicate directly with family members when asking questions to reinforce interest in them and to observe nonverbal expressions.
Refrain from interrupting family member and interpreter while they are conversing.
Avoid commenting to interpreter about family members since they may understand some English.
Respect cultural differences; it is often best to pose questions about sex, marriage, or pregnancy indirectly—ask about child's "father" rather than mother's "husband."
Allow time following interview for interpreter to share something that he or she felt could not be said earlier; ask about interpreter's impression of nonverbal clues to communication and family members' reliability or ease in revealing information.
Arrange for family to speak with same interpreter on subsequent visits whenever possible.

Communicating with Families Through an Interpreter

Sometimes communication is impossible because two people speak different languages. In this case it is necessary to obtain information through a third party, the interpreter. When an interpreter is used, the same guidelines for interviewing are used. Specific guidelines for using an adult interpreter are presented in Box 6-3.

Communicating with the families through an interpreter requires sensitivity to cultural, legal, and ethical considerations. For example, in some cultures using a child as an interpreter is considered an insult to an adult, because children are expected to show respect by not questioning their elders. In some cultures, class differences between the interpreter and the family may cause the family to feel intimidated and less inclined to offer information. Therefore, care should be exercised in choosing someone to translate, and time should be provided for the interpreter and family to establish rapport (Sloat and Matsuura, 1990).

Issues of legal and ethical concerns may also arise. For example, in obtaining informed consent through an interpreter, it is important that the family be fully informed of all the aspects of the particular procedure that they are consenting to. Issues of confidentiality may arise when family members related to another patient are asked to interpret for the family, thus revealing sensitive information that may be shared with other families on the unit.

When no one is available to translate, children within the family are often asked to assume this role. In this situation it is important to stress *literal* translation of parent responses. To maximize correct translations, it may be necessary to interrupt the parent and ask the child to translate every few sentences. When children are used as interpreters, the nurse needs to ask questions directed at specific answers and must assess the interpreted translation in terms of nonverbal expressions of communication.

COMMUNICATING WITH CHILDREN

Although the greatest amount of verbal communication may usually be carried out with the parent, the child should not be excluded during the interview. Periodic attention to infants and younger children through play or by occasionally directing questions or remarks to them makes children participants in the interview. Older children can be actively included as informants.

In communication with children of all ages, the nonverbal components of the communication process convey the most significant messages. It is difficult to disguise feelings, attitudes, and anxiety when relating to children. They are very alert to surroundings and attach meaning to every gesture and move that is made. This is particularly true with very young children.

Active attempts to make friends with children before they have had an opportunity to evaluate an unfamiliar person tend to increase their anxiety. A helpful tactic is to continue to talk to the child and parent but go about activities that do not involve the child directly, thus allowing him to carry out his observations from a safe position. If the child has a special toy or doll, it is helpful to "talk" to the doll first (Fig. 6-2). Asking simple questions such as, "Does your teddy bear have a special name?" may ease the child into conversation. Other guidelines for communicating with children are presented in Box 6-4. Specific guidelines for preparing children for procedures, a common nursing function, are discussed in Chapter 27.

Communication Related to Development of Thought Processes

The normal development of language and thought offers a frame of reference in knowing how to communicate with children. Thought processes progress from concrete to

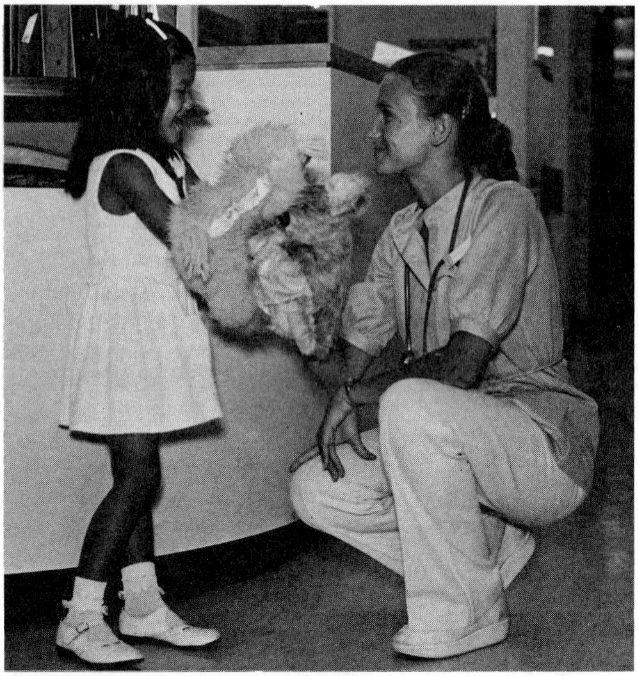

Fig. 6-2. Nurse talks to child using puppets and assumes position at child's level.

Box 6-4 GUIDELINES FOR COMMUNICATING WITH CHILDREN

Allow children time to feel comfortable with the nurse.
Avoid sudden or rapid advances, broad smiles, extended eye contact, or other gestures that may be seen as threatening.
Talk to the parent if child is initially shy.
Communicate through transition objects such as dolls, puppets, or stuffed animals before questioning a young child directly.
Give older children the opportunity to talk without the parents present.
Assume a position that is at eye level with the child.
Speak in a quiet, unhurried, and confident voice.
Speak clearly, be specific, use simple words, and short sentences.
State directions and suggestions *positively.*
Offer choices only when one exists.
Be honest with children.
Allow them to express their concerns and fears.
Use a variety of communication techniques.

functional and finally to abstract, formal operations.

Infancy. Because they are unable to use words, infants primarily use and understand nonverbal communication. Infants communicate their needs and feelings through nonverbal behaviors and vocalizations that can be interpreted by someone who is around them for a sufficient amount of time. Infants smile and coo when content and cry when distressed. Crying is provoked by unpleasant stimuli from inside or outside, such as hunger, pain, body restraint, or loneliness. Adults interpret this to mean that an infant needs something and consequently try to alleviate the discomfort and reduce tension. Crying (or the desire to cry) persists as a part of everyone's communication repertoire.

Infants respond to adults' nonverbal behaviors. They become quiet when they are cuddled, patted, or receive other forms of gentle, physical contact. They derive comfort from the sound of a voice, even though they do not understand the words that are spoken. Until infants reach the age at which they experience stranger anxiety, they readily respond to any firm, gentle handling and quiet, calm speech. Loud, harsh sounds and sudden movements are frightening.

Older infants' attentions are centered on themselves and their parents; therefore, any stranger is a potential threat until proved otherwise. Holding out the hands and asking the child to "come" is seldom successful, especially if the infant is with the parent. If infants must be handled, the best approach is simply to pick them up firmly without gestures. It is helpful to observe the position in which the parent holds the infant. Most infants have learned to prefer a particular position and manner of handling. In general, infants are more at ease upright than horizontal. It is also best to hold infants in such a way that they can keep their parents in view. Until they have developed the understanding that an object (in this case the parent) removed from sight can still be present, they have no way of knowing that the object is still there.

Early childhood. Children under 5 years of age are almost completely egocentric. They see things only in relation to themselves and from their point of view. Therefore, any communication to them should be focused on *them.* They need to be told what they can do or how they will feel. Experiences of others are of no interest to them. It is futile to use another child's experience as an attempt to gain the cooperation of very small children. They should be allowed to touch, examine, and familiarize themselves with articles that will come in contact with them. A stethoscope bell will feel cold; palpating a neck might tickle. Although they have not yet acquired sufficient language skills to express their feelings and wants, toddlers are able to communicate effectively with their hands to transmit ideas without words. They push an unwanted object away, pull another person to show them something, point, and cover the mouth that is saying something they do not wish to hear.

Everything is direct and concrete to small children. They are unable to work with abstractions and base all deductions on literal formulations. Analogies escape them because they are unable to separate fact from fantasy. For example, they attach literal meaning to such common phrases as "two-faced," "sticky fingers," or "coughing your head off." Children who are told they will get "a little stick in the arm" may not be able to envision an injection (Fig. 6-3). Nurses must be aware of inadvertently using a phrase that might be misinterpreted by a small child.

Language should be used that is consistent with the child's developmental level. For example, in talking with a toddler, it is best to use simple, *short* sentences, repeat

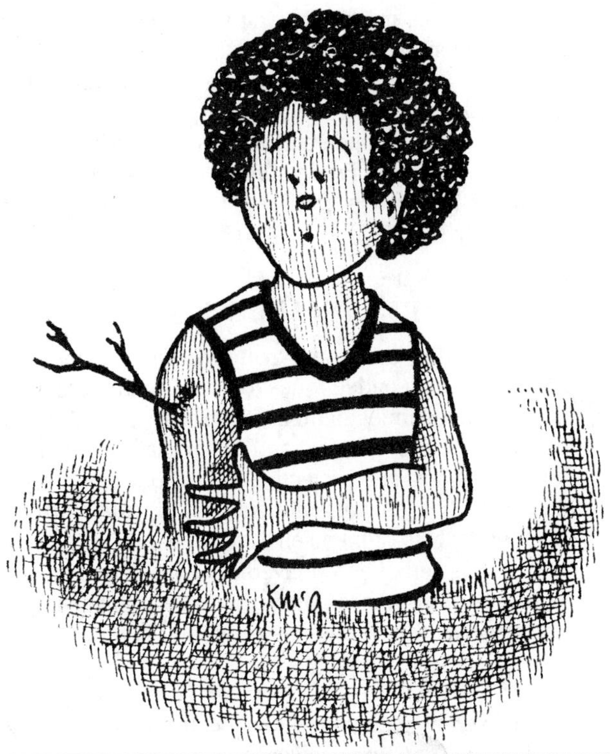

Fig. 6-3. To a young child the expression "a little stick in the arm" is taken literally.

words that are *familiar* to the child, and limit descriptions to *concrete* explanations.

Children in this age category assign human attributes to inanimate objects. They endow mechanical devices and instruments with living characteristics. Consequently they fear that these objects may jump, bite, cut, or pinch all by themselves. Children do not know that these devices are unable to perform without human direction. Unfamiliar equipment is kept out of view until needed. When equipment is used, explanations are kept simple.

School-age years. Children ages 5 to 8 years rely less on what they see and more on what they know when faced with new problems. They want explanations and reasons for everything but require no verification beyond that. They are interested in the functional aspect of all procedures, objects, and activities. They want to know why an object exists, why it is used, how it works, and the intent and purpose of its user. They need to know what is going to take place and why it is being done to *them* specifically. For example, to explain a procedure such as taking a blood pressure, the nurse might show the child how squeezing the bulb pushes air into the cuff and makes the "silver" in the tube go up. The child should be permitted to operate the bulb. An explanation for the reason might be as simple as, "I want to see how far the silver goes up when the cuff squeezes your arm." Consequently the child becomes an enthusiastic participant. Allowing children to ask questions about what is happening to them and maintaining a permissive atmosphere are conducive to questioning.

Children at this age have a heightened concern about body integrity. Because of the special importance and value they place on their body, they are overly sensitive to anything that constitutes a threat or suggestion of injury to it. This concern extends to their possessions also, so that they may appear to overreact to loss or threatened loss of treasured objects. Helping children to voice their concerns enables the nurse to provide reassurance and to implement activities that reduce their anxiety. For example, if a reticent child fears being the single object of probing inquiry, the nurse can ignore that particular child by talking and relating to other children in the family or group. When children no longer feel like single targets, they will usually interject personal ideas, feelings, and interpretations of events.

Older children have an adequate and satisfactory use of language. They still require relatively simple explanations, but their ability to think concretely can facilitate communication and explanation. Commonly they have sufficient experience with health and health workers to understand what is transpiring and generally what is expected of them.

Adolescence. As children move into adolescence, they fluctuate between child and adult thinking and behavior. They are riding a current that is moving them rapidly toward a maturity that may be beyond their coping ability. Therefore, when tensions rise, they may seek the security of the more familiar and comfortable expectations of childhood. Anticipating these shifts in identity allows the nurse to adjust the course of interaction to meet the needs of the moment. No single approach can be relied on consistently, and one can expect to encounter cooperation, hostility, anger, bravado, and a variety of other behaviors and attitudes. It is as much a mistake to regard the adolescent as an adult with an adult's wisdom and control as it is to confine to the teenager the concerns and expectations of a child.

Frequently adolescents are more willing to discuss their concerns with an adult outside the family, and they often welcome the opportunity to interact with a nurse. They are extremely susceptible to the advances of anyone who displays a genuine interest in them. However, adolescents are quick to reject persons who attempt to impose their values on them, whose interest is feigned, or who appear to have little respect for who they are and what they think or say.

As with all children, adolescents need to express their feelings. Generally they talk quite freely when given an opportunity. However, what adolescents say cannot always be taken at face value. When emotional factors are involved, the feelings that are interjected into words are as significant as the words that are used. The best way to give support is to be attentive, try not to interrupt, and avoid comments or expressions that convey disapproval or surprise. Prying and asking embarrassing questions should be avoided, and any impulse to give advice should be resisted. Frequently adolescents reveal their feelings or a source of concern or ask a question when they are involved in routine matters such as a physical assessment.

Teenagers characteristically have a language and culture all their own that further sets them apart from others. To avoid misinterpretation, frequent clarification of terms is ad-

Box 6-5 GUIDELINES FOR COMMUNICATING WITH ADOLESCENTS

Build a Foundation
Spend time together.
Encourage expression of ideas and feelings.
Respect their views.
Tolerate differences.
Praise good points.
Respect their privacy.
Set a good example.

Communicate Effectively
Give undivided attention.
Listen, listen, listen.
Be courteous, calm, and open-minded.
Try not to overreact. If you do, take a break.
Avoiding judging or criticizing.
Avoid the "third degree."
Choose important issues when taking a stand.
After taking a stand:
  Think through all options.
  Make expectations clear.

visable. Occasionally adolescents are reticent and answer only in monosyllables. Usually this happens when they are opposed to the contact with the nurse or do not yet feel safe enough to reveal themselves. In this instance the best approach is to confine discussions to irrelevant topics to reduce the element of threat until such time as they feel more secure. The nurse must be alert for signals that indicate they are ready to talk. The major sources of concern for adolescents are attitudes and feelings toward sex, relationships with parents, peer group acceptance, and developing a sense of identity.

Interviewing the adolescent presents some special situations to the interviewer. The first may be whether to talk to the adolescent alone, with the parents, or to each individually. Of course, if the adolescent is alone, there is no question, except that the nurse might want to suggest to the teenager that she may talk with the parents at another time. If parents and teenager are together, talking with the adolescent first has the advantage of immediately identifying with the young person, thus fostering the interpersonal relationship. However, talking with the parents initially may provide insight into the family relationship. Whichever decision is made, both parties need an opportunity to be included in the interview. If time constraints are important, such as during history-taking, these need to be clarified at the onset to avoid appearing to "take sides" by talking more with one person than the other.

Confidentiality is of great importance when interviewing adolescents. Parents and teenagers need to know the limits of confidentiality, specifically that young persons' disclosures will be kept between them and the nurse. However, exceptions also must be clarified, such as breaking confidence if it is necessary for the welfare of adolescents, as in the case of suicidal behavior.

Another dilemma in interviewing adolescents is that two views of a problem frequently exist—the teenager's and the parents'. Clarification of the problem is a major task. However, providing both parties with an opportunity to discuss their perceptions in an open and unbiased atmosphere can, by itself, be therapeutic. By demonstrating positive communication skills, the nurse can help families communicate more effectively (Box 6-5).

COMMUNICATION TECHNIQUES

In addition to such conventional interviewing methods as reflection and open-ended questions, a number of techniques encourage family members to express their thoughts and feelings in a less directive and confrontational manner. Several approaches are projective—they present nonspecific material that enables individuals to externalize or project inner aspects of themselves to others (Krahn, 1985).

The following verbal and nonverbal approaches are helpful in a variety of instances. Throughout the book examples are given that use the techniques described here.

Verbal Techniques

A variety of verbal techniques can be used to encourage communication. The interviewer can use some of these techniques to pose questions or explore concerns in a less threatening manner. Others can be presented as "word games" that are often well received by children.

Third-person technique. The third-person technique involves expressing a feeling in terms of a third person (he, she, they). This technique is less threatening than directly asking individuals how they feel, because it gives them the opportunity to agree or disagree without being defensive. For example, the nurse may comment, "Sometimes when people are sick a lot they feel angry and sad because they cannot do what others can," and either wait silently for a response or encourage a reply with a statement such as, "Did you ever feel that way?" This approach allows three choices: (1) to agree and, hopefully, express how they feel (2) to disagree, or (3) to remain silent, in which case they may have such feelings but are unable to express them at that time. Demonstrating to parents how useful such techniques are also helps them learn new ways of communicating with the child.

Another variation of the third-person technique is to ask about friends, for example, "Do any of your friends smoke or drink alcohol?" Since peer group activity often reflects the children's activity, this may introduce the topic in such a way that young persons are able to talk about their habits or concerns.

Neurolinguistic programming. Neurolinguistic programming (NLP) deals with the *manner* in which individuals access and understand information. Although people may use all of the following sensory modalities to communicate, usually one modality predominates: visual, auditory, or kinesthetic. The specific sensory mode is identified by observing the type of verbs, adjectives, and adverbs the person uses. By using the same sensory mode, the nurse can enhance rapport and communicate information more effectively (Box 6-6). Visual people also benefit from visual aids, such as diagrams and illustrations. The auditory person uses words or sounds. Children tend to use the kinesthetic mode and learn from manipulating objects (Brockopp, 1983; Knowles, 1983).

One technique used in NLP is *anchoring*, the process of associating an internal response with some external trigger. Anchors may be visual, auditory, or kinesthetic in nature or a combination of these sensory modes. For example, stroking a person's face may be associated with a loving response. Therefore, when the nurse strokes the person's face, that initial association with affection is triggered (Molsberry and Shogan, 1990). (See also the discussion of touch on p. 197.)

Facilitative responding. Facilitative responding is the careful listening and reflecting back to patients the feelings and content of their statements. Such responses are empathetic and nonjudgmental and legitimize the person's feelings. The formula for facilitative responses is, "You feel because ____________" (Henrich and Bernheim, 1981). For example, if a child states, "I hate coming to the hospital and getting shots," a facilitative response is, "You feel unhappy because of all the things that are done to you."

Storytelling. Storytelling uses the language of children to probe into areas of their thinking while bypassing conscious inhibitions or fears. Children respond to a variety of storytelling techniques. The simplest is asking them to relate a story about an event, such as "being in the hospital." Another approach involves showing children a picture of a particular event, such as a child in a hospital with other people in the room, and asking them to describe the scene. Comic strips cut from a newspaper with the words removed or originally drawn to depict a particular scenario are excellent vehicles when children ascribe their own statements to each comic scene (Epstein, 1975; Walker, 1988) (Fig. 6-4). Cartoon storytelling can also involve children's serial drawings of some event with short verbal communications added as appropriate.

Mutual storytelling involves a more therapeutic approach. It not only serves to uncover children's thinking but also attempts to change their perceptions or fears by retelling a somewhat different story. It is a powerful tool and must be used wisely. It begins by asking the child to tell a story about something, followed by another story told by the nurse that is similar to the child's tale but that has differences that help the child in problem areas. A typical example is the child's story of going to the hospital and never seeing the parents again. The nurse's story is also of a child (using different names but similar circumstances) in a hospital whose parents visit every day, but in the evening after coming home from work. In this way the child's fears of abandonment and separation are handled.

Sometimes children need help in beginning a story with encouragements, such as "Once upon a time . . ." or the use of a tape recorder. For less verbal children, having them draw pictures or write about an event may help them relate stories.

Another approach to mutual storytelling is the *squiggle-drawing game*. The game begins with the interviewer drawing a squiggle (any straight, curved, wavy, or zigzag line) and asking the child to make a drawing out of the squiggle and to tell a story about the drawing. Then the interviewer asks questions about the drawing and story. This process is

Box 6-6 NEUROLINGUISTIC PROGRAMMING

Sensory Mode Communication	Appropriate Response
Visual mode: I can *see* that I do not *look* well.	Tell me what you *see*.
Auditory mode: From what I *hear* the doctor *saying*, my child won't get better.	What have you *heard* that makes you see things this way?
Kinesthetic mode: I *feel* that my child's prognosis is *weak*.	Tell me more about *feeling* that her prognosis is weak.

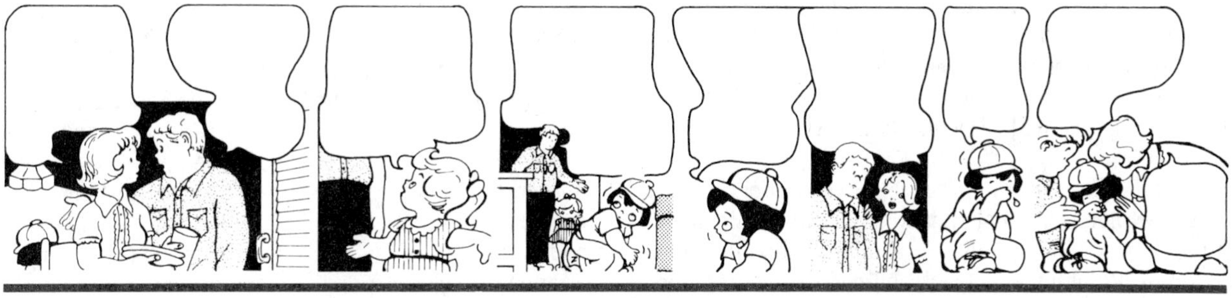

Fig. 6-4. Filling in the blanks on a comic strip is an effective communication technique with older children.

reversed with the child making a squiggle and the interviewer then making a drawing out of it. It is preferable for the child to develop the first story so that the interviewer can decide what theme to use when it is his or her turn to draw and tell a story (Claman, 1980).

Bibliotherapy. Bibliotherapy involves the use of books in a therapeutic and supportive process. Its goal is to help children express feelings and concerns through the familiar activity of being read to or reading to themselves. Although it incorporates an educational component, it involves more than using a book for its preparatory value, such as familiarizing a child with hospitalization or a procedure. Bibliography provides children with an opportunity to explore an event that is similar to their own but sufficiently different to allow them to distance themselves from it and remain in control. Since children tend to trust the characters in a book, they are able to feel familiar with the content even if they are suspicious of the person who reads the story. A book is essentially nonthreatening because the child can close it or stop reading it at any time. General guidelines for using bibliotherapy are presented in Box 6-7.

Fantasy. A special type of bibliotherapy uses fantasy or fairy tales, such as *Hansel and Gretel*, *Cinderella*, or *Jack and the Beanstalk*. The figures and events of fairy tales personify and illustrate universal inner conflicts, such as the need to be loved, the fear that one is worthless, the love of life, and the fear of death. They subtly suggest how these conflicts may be solved, and the endings give reassurance and hope for the future (Bettelheim, 1976). Without explanation, children find meaning in the stories to meet their needs.

Dreams. Dreams often reveal unconscious and repressed thoughts and feelings. Although interpretation of dreams is a specialized area of psychotherapy, asking a child or parent to talk about a dream may uncover areas that were previously unknown to the nurse. For example, a mother whose child had been diagnosed with a life-threatening illness described dreams about her son's dying. As she relayed the dream, she also commented that she feared her dream would "cause" his death. Subsequently the nurse and mother were able to explore guilt feelings that were very disturbing to the parent.

Another approach toward using dreams is *guided imagery*. For example, a critically ill child dreamed that "the black angel" was in the room. When talking to the child about the nightmare, the nurse tried to have him imagine that he could tell the angel anything he wanted. He stated, "I would tell her to go away." They then talked about fears of being left alone or taken away. The nurse stressed that the child was safe and that no one would let anything happen to him. This calmed the child, and the nightmare did not recur.

"What if" questions. "What if" questions encourage children to explore potential situations and to consider different problem-solving options. For example, the nurse can ask children, "What if you got sick and had to go to the hospital?" Their responses reveal what they know already and what makes them curious. Their thoughts concerning a new experience are elicited in a nonthreatening manner. This type of communication is excellent for helping children learn coping skills, especially in potentially dangerous situations. For example, parents might ask, "What if a stranger comes to school to pick you up and tells you your mommy is sick?" to prepare a child for appropriate responses.

Three wishes. A strategy for engaging children in conversation is the "three wishes" technique. One simply asks, "If you could have any three things in the world, what would they be?" One child's answer to this was most revealing. He responded, "I don't want to be sick anymore." When asked about the other two wishes, he replied, "If that one came true, so would every other wish, so I don't have any more." Following this dialogue, the nurse and boy were able to talk about what being sick meant to him. Although the nurse could not make him better, she was able to make some of the other "wishes" come true. One of them was to arrange for school friends to visit the child during his hospitalization and convalescence at home. Before this conversation the youngster's desire for peer companionship had never been revealed.

Box 6-7 GUIDELINES FOR USING BIBLIOTHERAPY

Assess the child's emotional and cognitive development in terms of readiness to understand the book's message.
Be familiar with the book's content (intended message or purpose) and the appropriate age for which it is written.
Read the book to the child, if the child if unable to read.
Explore the meaning of the book with the child by having the child:
- Retell the story
- Read a special section together
- Draw a picture related to the story and discuss the drawing
- Talk about the characters
- Summarize the moral or meaning of the story

Resources for Books

Association for the Care of Children's Health: Books for children and teenagers about hospitalization, illness, and disabling conditions, Washington, DC, 1987, The Association.
Berg, P.J., Devlin, M.K., and Gedaly-Duff, V.: Bibliotherapy with children experiencing loss, Issues Compr. Pediatr. Nurs. 4:37-50, 1980.
Dreyer, S.: The Bookfinder 4: when kids need books, Circle Pines, MN, 1989, American Guidance Service.
Fassler, J.: Helping children cope: mastering stress through books and stories, London, 1978, The Free Press.
Fosson, A., and Husband, E.: Bibliotherapy for hospitalized children, South. Med. J. 77(3):342-346, 1984.
Griffin, B.: Special needs bibliography: current books for/about children and young adults regarding social concerns, emotional concerns, the exceptional child, Dewitt, NY, 1986, The Griffin.
Oppenheim, J., Brenner, B., and Boegehold, B.: Choosing books for kids, New York, 1986, Ballantine Books.
Rubin, R.: Bibliotherapy sourcebook, Phoenix, AZ, 1978, Oryx Press.
Wallace, N.E.: Special books for special children, Child. Health Care 12(1):34-36, 1983.

Rating game. The rating game is particularly helpful in encouraging older children to talk. Instead of asking youngsters how they feel, the nurse asks how their day has been "on a scale from 1 to 10, with 10 being the best." With a reply of "today is a 2," one can begin exploring why this day rates so poorly. An extension of this is to have children keep a log of each day's rating and expand it into a diary. For children who are too young to understand the concept of numbers, a series of happy and sad faces can be used to rate feelings (see Faces Scale, Table 26-3).

Word association game. Another approach is the word association game. One can begin by having a list of key words and asking children to say the first word that they think of when they hear the word. It is best to start with neutral words and then introduce more anxiety-producing words, such as illness, needles, hospitals, and operation. The key words should be chosen to relate to some event in the child's life that is relevant.

Sentence completion. Without directly asking about feelings, one can probe into areas of concern by presenting a statement and having the child complete it. This is particularly useful with older school-age children and adolescents. Some sample statements are:

The thing I like best (least) about school is ____________.
The best (worst) age to be is ____________.
The most (least) fun thing I ever did was ____________.
The thing I like most (least) about my parents is ____________.
If I could change one thing about my family, it would be ____________.
If I could be anything I wanted, I would be ____________.
The thing I like most (least) about myself is ____________.

The beginning statements are more neutral than the last ones, which center on feelings about oneself.

Pros and cons. A somewhat different approach to encouraging exploration of feelings is to select a topic, such as "being in the hospital," and have the child list "five good things and five bad things" about it. This is an exceptionally valuable technique when applied to relationships. For example, family members are asked to write down five things they like and dislike about each other. In reviewing the lists, each member has the opportunity to discuss his or her feelings in a nonjudgmental atmosphere. However, when this technique is used, the nurse must be prepared to handle feelings and issues that can surface unexpectedly.

Nonverbal Techniques

Many children and adults find talking about their feelings difficult. For them verbal communication may be more stressful than supportive. Several nonverbal techniques can be used to encourage communication.

Touch. Touch is one of the most meaningful forms of communication, particularly when communicating feelings and attitudes. Children are particularly sensitive to messages conveyed by touch, and the nurse can use touch in a most therapeutic manner. Numerous types of touch can be used, such as massaging, stroking, and swaddling. A more structured form is *therapeutic touch*, which refers to the art of interpersonal energy transfer for the purpose of healing. A number of different strategies are used in therapeutic touch, which involves placing the hands above the person's body to direct the transfer of energy (Krieger, 1986; Thayer, 1990).

Regardless of the particular method of touch that is used to communicate to the child or adult, nurses must assess what is considered positive touch. For example, a child may be frightened by premature touching that may be perceived as an aggressive attack, whereas another child might be comforted by light stroking or rubbing. When using touch, the duration, location, intensity, and sensation must be altered to find the correct balance for the child, especially the neonate. (See Developmental Intervention, Chapter 10.)

Writing. Writing is an alternative communication approach for older children and adults. Specific suggestions include (1) keeping a journal or diary, (2) writing feelings or thoughts that are difficult to express, (3) writing "letters" that are never mailed (a variation is making up a "pen pal" to write to), or (4) keeping an account of the child's progress from both a physical and an emotional viewpoint.

To encourage writing about feelings, it is helpful to give some instruction while keeping the format as open-ended as possible. For example, rather than asking children to write about things that worry them, it is better to request them to complete the specific statement, "These are the things that upset me today: . . ." Therefore, the format for diaries or journals might include these types of specific questions, sentences with blanks for completion, check lists, or lists for rankings (Sorensen, 1989). Any form of writing can also be supplemented with drawings.

To initiate a conversation, the nurse can inquire about the writing, possibly even asking to read some of it. Frequently, as one writes down ideas, thoughts, or feelings, there is also an urge to discuss them. Once they are written, they are more real and tangible but often less frightening than when kept locked inside one's mind.

Writing can also have a long-term benefit. After the experience there can be growth in rereading about it. One mother used her journal to help her teenage daughter understand a serious childhood illness that had threatened the youngster's life. The adolescent had become resentful of comments about "when she was ill," but after reading the journal with the mother, she realized what a stressful time those earlier years had been and gained a deeper appreciation of her parents' continuing concern for her health.

Drawing. Drawing is one of the most valuable forms of communication—both nonverbal, from looking at the drawing, and verbal, from the child's story of the picture. Children's drawings tell a great deal about them because they are projections of their personality. Children's drawings are usually of themselves, their experiences, or those who are significant to them. Besides communicating about themselves, art also provides children with a natural activity that helps them deal with both conscious and unconscious feelings.

Drawing can be spontaneous or directed. *Spontaneous drawings* involve giving children a variety of art supplies (older children like felt-tipped pens) and providing the op-

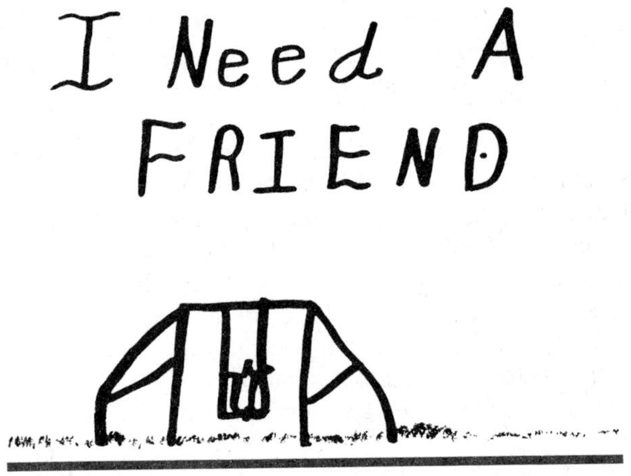

Fig. 6-5. Using the three themes approach, this child chose the theme, "the first day of school." The drawing and title reveal the child's loneliness and insecurity in a new setting.

Box 6-8 GUIDELINES FOR EVALUATING DRAWINGS

Use spontaneous drawings and evaluate more than one drawing whenever possible.
Interpret drawings in light of other available information about the child and family.
Interpret drawings as a whole rather than on specific details of the drawings.
Consider individual elements of the drawing that may be significant:
- **Sex of figure drawn first**—usually relates to the child's perception of own sex role.
- **Size of individual figures**—expresses importance, power, authority.
- **Order in which figures are drawn**—expresses priority in terms of importance.
- **Child's position to other family members**—expresses feelings of status or alliance.
- **Exclusion of a member**—may denote feeling of not belonging or desire to eliminate.
- **Accentuated parts**—usually express concern for areas of special importance; for example, large hands may be sign of aggression.
- **Absence of or rudimentary arms and hands**—suggests timidity, passivity, or intellectual immaturity; tiny, unstable feet may be expressions of insecurity, and hidden hands may signify guilt feelings.
- **Placement of drawing on the page and type of stroke**—free use of paper and firm continuous strokes express security, whereas drawings restricted to a small area and lightly drawn in broken or wavering lines may be a sign of insecurity.
- **Erasures, shadings, or cross-hatching**—expresses ambivalence, concern, or anxiety with particular area.
- **Dominant color**—may indicate a number of various emotions:
  - **Red**—hostility and aggression
  - **Blue**—stability, self-confidence, and self-sufficiency
  - **Yellow**—outgoing and emotionally expressive but possibly dependent on adults for approval
  - **Green**—maturity and self-reliance
  - **Dark colors, such as purple or black**—cry for help or indication of unhappiness or depression

portunity to draw. The only encouragement may be the statement, "Draw something for me." *Directed drawing* involves a more specific direction, such as "draw a person." In isolated figure drawings the children's responses tend to be predominantly intellectual, in that they will produce a more complete picture with more parts than those they draw in a group picture. Figure drawings are the basis for certain intellectual tests (see Goodenough Draw-a-Person Test, Chapter 7).

If the child needs encouragement to draw, the "three themes" approach is helpful. This technique involves writing three statements about the child at the bottom of the paper and asking the child to choose one and draw a picture (Fig. 6-5).

The basic assumption in interpreting drawings is that children are revealing something about themselves. However, interpretation must be undertaken with an understanding of normal development in art expression (see Gross and Fine Motor Behavior, Chapter 15). For example, it is normal for a 4-year-old to draw arms attached to a head but highly questionable in a 6-year-old. Understanding how to interpret and use drawings takes considerable time, experience, and study. It is just as dangerous to "read" too much into drawing and mislabel a person as it is to disregard a drawing as meaningless. When studying a drawing, every detail must be evaluated, as well as relationships of one part to another. It is helpful to label the characters (mother, father, and so on) and to denote the order in which each was drawn. When evaluating drawings, the guidelines presented in Box 6-8 should be followed. Although not a complete inventory for analyzing drawings, they provide initial guidelines that can offer much information about the child. One caution is that interpretation must be viewed in light of the child's particular circumstances. For example, while cross-hatching is generally a sign of anxiety, it can also be an attempt to reproduce a design in a particular artistic effect, in which case it may have no significance.

Kinetic family drawing. Group drawings are highly influenced by the child's feelings, and the response is predominantly emotional. Consequently, group drawings are valuable in disclosing what children think about themselves and others. The most valuable group drawing is of the family. A special type is the *kinetic family drawing (KFD)* (Burns, 1982; Burns and Kaufman, 1972), in which the child is asked to "Draw your family doing something." In giving directions, only a general statement of encouragement is offered to avoid suggesting themes. Drawing the family is appropriate for children over 4 years of age.

The focus of the KFD is not only the family unit but also the activity and interaction of each family member. The drawing describes the child's perspective of family dynamics and his or her place in the family matrix. In evaluating a KFD, either subjective impressions or an objective scoring system may be used (Burns, 1982; Spinetta and others, 1981). Suggestions for evaluating a KFD are listed in Box 6-9.

Sociogram. Drawing need not be limited to children. Adults can be asked to draw, although they are much less

Box 6-9 GUIDELINES FOR EVALUATING KINETIC FAMILY DRAWINGS

Note omission of family members; if someone is missing, ask the child if everyone in the family has been included in the drawing.
Ask child to explain what each family member is doing.
Encourage child to tell as much as possible about the drawing.
Note signs of physical intimacy or distance, such as people close to each other or touching.
Note placement of people in the drawing, such as top or bottom of drawing and proximity to each other.
Note facial expressions, such as happy, sad, blank, or bored.
Note which members are facing each other or turned away from each other and how they are grouped together.

Modified from Burns, R.: Self growth in families: kinetic family drawings (KFD)—research and application, New York, 1982, Brunner/Mazel, Inc.

likely to comply and may deliberately try to hide disclosures by drawing a very simple sketch. One type of drawing that is useful with adults and children as young as 5 years is the *sociogram (life-space drawing)* or *family circle.* For the sociogram or life-space drawing, the person is given blank paper and a pencil with the instructions: "Draw a circle to represent you. Around the circle draw circles to represent the most significant persons in your life and label each. Draw the circles in proximity to your circle to represent closeness. For example, the person who is most significant is the circle closest to you."

In the family circle the directions differ slightly (Thrower, Bruce, and Walton, 1982): "Draw a circle to represent your family. Draw in smaller circles to represent you and the most significant persons in your life. People can be inside or outside the family circle. Draw the circles large or small, depending on their significance or influence to you." Family members can label the relationships as supportive with a plus sign or negative with a minus sign.

The sociogram or family circle is an immediate portrait of significant persons in the individual's life. Drawing it is also a task that can uncover hidden or repressed relationships. For example, one mother drew a circle inside her circle to represent a severely retarded child who had been institutionalized for several years. She remarked that she had not realized how unresolved her feelings of attachment to this child were until she had to graphically place him in her life (Fig. 6-6).

After completing the sociogram or family circle, the family can be encouraged to explore their feelings further with questions such as the following:

How would you change the circles to improve relationships?
How do you think you could accomplish these changes?
If one person in the circle were to change, what effect do you think that would have on others in the circle?

Conjoint family drawing. Another useful technique with children and adults is the *conjoint family drawing.* The family is given a large sheet of white paper and a box of colored pencils, pens, or crayons. Each member is asked to select a different color pen and not to exchange colors. They are instructed to work together on a drawing but without talking to each other. After the drawing is completed, each member is asked to discuss it. Emphasis is placed on the process or "how" the drawing took place, rather than on the symbolic meaning of each part. Suggestions for assessing the process are presented in Box 6-10.

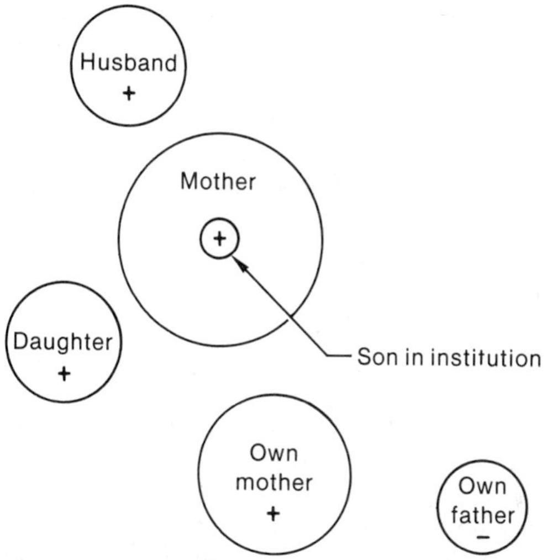

Fig. 6-6. Sociogram of mother with strong, but unresolved feelings toward son placed in an institution.

Box 6-10 GUIDELINES FOR ASSESSING THE CONJOINT FAMILY DRAWING

Who initiates the drawing?
Who uses the most or least space?
Does anyone infringe on another's "space"?
Do "subsystems" appear, or is anyone deleted?
Does someone take the lead in organizing the drawing?
Who copies another's theme, or who draws something completely different?

The conjoint family drawing is a valuable tool in uncovering family dynamics and relationships. It can be used as a learning experience to help "well" families learn more about themselves. In a hospital setting it can be used with groups of children to discover their patterns of leadership and cooperation. When it is used with dysfunctional families, nurses must have sufficient skill in handling issues and feelings that may arise.

Play. Play is a universal language of children. It is one of the most important forms of communication and can be an effective technique in relating to them. Clues about physical, intellectual, and social developmental progress can often be gleaned from the form and complexity of a child's play behaviors. Play requires a minimum of equipment or none at all. Therapeutic play is often used to reduce the trauma of illness and hospitalization (Chapter 26) and to prepare children for therapeutic procedures (Chapter 27).

Because their ability to perceive precedes their ability to transmit, small infants respond to activities that register on their senses. Patting, stroking, and other skin play convey messages. Repetitive actions, such as stretching infants' arms out to the side while they are lying on the back and then folding them across the chest or raising and revolving the legs in a bicycling motion, will elicit pleasurable sounds. Colorful items to catch the eye or interesting sounds such as a ticking clock, chimes, bells, or singing can be used to attract children's attention.

Older infants respond to simple games. The old game of peekaboo is an excellent means of initiating communication with infants while maintaining a "safe," nonthreatening distance. After this intermittent eye-to-eye contact, the nurse is no longer viewed as a stranger but as someone who is a friend. This can be followed by touch games. Clapping an infant's hands together for pat-a-cake or wiggling the toes for "this little piggy" delights an infant or small child. Much of the nursing assessment can be carried out with the use of games and simple play equipment while the infant remains in the safety of the parent's arms or lap. Talking to a foot or other part of the child's body is an effective tactic.

The nurse can capitalize on the natural curiosity of small children by playing games such as "Which hand do you take?" and "Guess what I have in my hand" or by manipulating items such as a flashlight or stethoscope. Finger games are very useful. More elaborate materials, such as puppets and replicas of familiar or unfamiliar items, serve as excellent means to communicate with small children (see Fig. 6-2). The variety and extent are limited only by the nurse's imagination.

Through play children reveal their perceptions of interpersonal relationships with their family, friends, or hospital personnel. Children may also reveal the wide scope of knowledge they have acquired from listening to others around them. For example, through needle play, children may disclose how carefully they have watched each procedure by precisely duplicating the technical skills. They may also reveal how well they remember those who performed procedures. One child who painstakingly reenacted every detail of a tedious medical procedure also played the role of the physician who had repeatedly shouted at her to be still for the long ordeal. Her anger at him was most evident during the play session and revealed the cause for her abrupt withdrawal and passive hostility toward the medical and nursing staff following the test.

Play sessions serve not only as assessment tools for determining children's awareness and perception of their illness but also as methods of intervention and evaluation. In the previous example, when the child revealed anger toward the physician, the nurse acted the part of the patient, but this time did not accept the physician's harsh commands to stay still. Instead the nurse said to the physician all the things the child had wished she could say.

Subsequent play sessions can also be used for evaluation of the child's progress. A change in the type of drawing or the theme of the play may indicate progression toward or away from ability to deal with anxiety.

■ HISTORY-TAKING

This section deals with interviewing as it relates to the health history. The precise depth and extent of a nursing history vary with its intended purpose. The nurse uses judgment in deciding what data are necessary and relevant for the identification of problems or concerns.

The format used resembles a medical history, but the objective of each assessment area is the identification of nursing diagnoses. The value in following the well-established medical approach is that it is systematic and familiar to members of the health team. The categories listed in Box 6-11 encompass the children's current and past health status and information about their psychosocial environment.

PERFORMING A HEALTH HISTORY

The methods used to perform a health history are innumerable. Each examiner will devise a unique approach. However, one important component of every history is organized and systematic data collection.

A systematic approach has several important functions:

1. Ensures consistency and completeness
2. Allows for individualized nursing care based on a comprehensive data base
3. Maximizes the amount and quality of data for future evaluation of health status and efficacy of care
4. Provides an immediate basis for decision-making regarding the planning of nursing care.

The format used for history-taking may be (1) *direct*—the nurse asks for information via direct interview with the informant—or (2) *indirect*—the informant supplies the information by completing some type of questionnaire. The direct method is superior to the indirect approach or a combination of both. However, in view of time constraints, the direct approach is not always practical. If the direct approach cannot be used, it is important to review parents' written responses and question them regarding any unusual answers.

The direct method loses its value if the nurse asks questions directly from a form. In essence the parent is completing the form by listening to it rather than reading it. Using a systematic approach does not imply rote memory of a specific outline. Rather, it means using categories to define what areas of information are required. If nurses use as a model the basic categories outlined in the box and understand the objective of each, they can then obtain the required information as it arises during the course of the interview. However, the history is recorded using the established format.

Identifying Information

Much of the identifying information may already be available from other recorded sources. However, if the parent

Box 6-11 OUTLINE OF A PEDIATRIC HEALTH HISTORY

Identifying information
1. Name
2. Address
3. Telephone
4. Birthdate and place
5. Race
6. Sex
7. Religion
8. Nationality
9. Date of interview
10. Informant

Chief complaint (CC): to establish the major *specific* reason for the child's and parents' seeking professional health attention

Present illness (PI): to obtain *all* details related to the chief complaint

Past history (PH): to elicit a profile of the child's previous illnesses, injuries, or operations
1. Birth history (pregnancy, labor, and delivery, perinatal history)
2. Previous illnesses, injuries, or operations
3. Allergies
4. Current medications
5. Immunizations
6. Growth and development
7. Habits

Review of systems (ROS): to elicit information concerning any potential health problem
1. General
2. Integument
3. Head
4. Eyes
5. Ears
6. Nose
7. Mouth
8. Throat
9. Neck
10. Chest
11. Respiratory
12. Cardiovascular
13. Gastrointestinal
14. Genitourinary
15. Gynecologic
16. Musculoskeletal
17. Neurologic
18. Endocrine

Family medical history: to identify the presence of genetic traits or diseases that have familial tendencies and to assess exposure to a communicable disease in a family member and family habits that may affect the child's health, such as smoking and other chemical use

Psychosocial history: to elicit information about the child's self-concept

Sexual history: to elicit information concerning the child's sexual concerns and/or activities and any pertinent data regarding adults' sexual activity that influence the child

Family history: to develop an understanding of the child as an individual and as a member of a family and a community
1. Family composition
2. Home and community environment
3. Occupation and education of family members
4. Cultural and religious traditions
5. Family function and relationships

Nutritional assessment: to elicit information on the adequacy of the child's nutritional intake and need
1. Dietary intake
2. Clinical examination

seems anxious, the nurse may use this opportunity to ask about such information to help the parent feel more comfortable.

Informant. One of the important areas under identifying information concerns the informant, the person(s) who furnished the information. The nurse should record certain data about the informant, such as (1) who the person is (child, parent, and so on), (2) an impression of reliability and willingness to communicate, and (3) any special circumstances, such as the use of an interpreter or conflicting answers by more than one person.

Assessing reliability is one of the more important judgments to make. A totally reliable informant will always give the same answers to questions. Several generalizations can be made in considering the parent's reliability (Hoekelman, Kelly, and Zimmer, 1976):

1. Concrete facts, such as birth weight, length, and date, are recalled most accurately.
2. Minor illnesses are forgotten more easily than major ones.
3. Mothers, particularly those of firstborns, tend to exaggerate the child's achievement of developmental skills.
4. Mothers of several children tend to be less accurate in their recall of most items than mothers of single children.
5. The mother's educational level is directly related to the accuracy of recall for some items, such as immunizations.
6. More specific and detailed questioning considerably increases the accuracy of recall.

The last generalization is particularly significant. Nurses who use these suggestions for approaches to history-taking are more likely to positively influence reliable parent recall than are those who fail to consider such factors.

An example of a statement that gives identifying information about an informant is: "Mother, reliability questionable, answers items with hesitation, speaks primarily Spanish, interpreter (Mrs. ____________) present for history."

Chief Complaint

The chief complaint is the specific reason for the child's visit to the clinic, office, or hospital. Six guidelines determine appropriate recording of the chief complaint: it should (1) consist of a brief statement, (2) be restricted to one or two symptoms, (3) refer to a concrete complaint, (4) be recorded in the child's or parent's own words, (5) avoid the use of diagnostic terms or translations, and (6) state the duration of the symptoms.

The nurse elicits the chief complaint by asking open-ended, neutral questions such as, "Tell me what seems to be the matter," "How may I help you?" or "Why did you come here today?" Labeling-type questions such as, "How are you sick?" or "What is the problem?" are avoided, since the reason for the visit may not be an illness or a problem. For example, the visit may be for a routine health assessment, or the chief complaint may be of a nonphysical nature.

Examples of properly recorded chief complaints for a variety of situations may be: (1) ambulatory clinic—"My child has had a runny nose and sore throat for 4 days, but today it is worse"; (2) hospital admission—child states: "I need to have my tonsils fixed"; has had sore throat and repeated earaches for 5 years; and (3) health center—"We are here for a routine checkup"; last visit 1 year ago.

If the visit is for a well-child examination, one can ask, "Before we begin, is there anything of particular concern that you would like to discuss?" This type of statement encourages the parent (or child) to bring up an issue that may not surface during routine interviewing.

Occasionally it is difficult to isolate one symptom or problem as the chief complaint because the parent may identify many. In this situation it is important to be as specific as possible when asking questions. For example, asking informants to state which *one* problem or symptom caused them to seek help *now* may help them focus on the most immediate concern.

Present Illness

The history of the present illness* is a narrative of the chief complaint from its earliest onset through its progression to the present. The four major components are (1) details of *onset,* (2) complete *interval* history (from onset to present), (3) *present* status, and (4) reason for seeking help *now.* The focus of the present illness is on all factors that are relevant to the main problem, even if they have disappeared or changed during the onset, interval, and present status of the complaint.

Analyzing a symptom. Since pain is often the most characteristic symptom denoting onset of a physical problem, it is used as a prototype for analysis of a symptom. Assessment includes (1) type, (2) location, (3) severity, (4) duration, and (5) influencing factors.

The *type* or character of pain should be as specific as possible. However, for young children with limited verbal skills, describing the pain is difficult. Asking the parents how they know the child is in pain may help describe its type, location, and severity. For example, a mother stated, "My child must have a severe earache because she pulls at her ears, rolls her head on the floor, and screams. Nothing seems to help."

The nurse can help older children describe the pain or "hurt" by asking them if, for example, it is sharp, throbbing, dull, aching, or stabbing. Whatever words they use should be recorded in quotes (see also Pain Assessment, Chapter 26).

The *location* of the pain also must be specific. "Stomach pains" is too general a description. Older children can better localize the pain if the nurse asks them to "point with one finger to where it hurts." The nurse can also determine if the pain radiates by asking, "Does the pain stay there or move? Show me where it goes with your finger."

The *severity* of pain is best determined by finding out how it affects the child's usual behavior. Pain that prevents a child from playing, interacting with others, sleeping, and eating is most often severe.

Duration of pain includes the duration, onset, and frequency of attacks. It may be necessary to describe this in terms of activity and behavior, such as "pain lasted all night because child refused to sleep and cried intermittently."

Influencing factors are anything that causes a change in the type, location, severity, or duration of the pain. These include (1) precipitating events (those that cause or increase the pain), (2) relieving events (those that lessen the pain, such as medications), (3) temporal events (times when the pain is relieved or increased), (4) positional events (e.g., standing, sitting, and lying down), and (5) associated events (e.g., meals, stress, and coughing).

A standard method of analyzing a symptom is listed in Box 6-12. The three categories—onset, characteristics, and course since onset—comprise the essential data for the present illness. Although the analysis of a symptom has concentrated on discussion of physical complaints, the same process of description and investigation can be used for emotional or psychosocial problems.

Determining the reason for seeking help. The preceding discussion deals primarily with a description of the problem. However, since most chief complaints have a "duration," it follows that something significant must have occurred to motivate the person to seek help at this time. Such factors may be a change in physical status, a change in behavioral reaction, or a result of social pressure. Elicit-

Box 6-12 GUIDELINES FOR ANALYZING A SYMPTOM

Onset
Date of onset
Manner of onset (gradual or sudden)
Precipitating and predisposing factors related to onset (e.g., emotional disturbance, physical exertion, fatigue, bodily function, pregnancy, environment, injury, infection, toxins and allergens, therapeutic agents)

Characteristics
Character (quality, quantity, consistency, or other)
Location and radiation (of pain)
Intensity or severity
Timing (continuous or intermittent, duration of each, temporal relationship to other events)
Aggravating and relieving factors
Associated symptoms

Course Since Onset
Incidence (single acute attack, recurrent acute attacks, daily occurrences, periodic occurrences, continuous chronic episode)
Progress (better, worse, unchanged)
Effect of therapy

*NOTE: The term *illness* is used in its broadest sense to denote any problem or concern of a physical, emotional, or psychosocial nature. It is actually a history of the chief complaint.

ing such information may alter the possible nursing diagnosis and plan of care. The following example illustrates the potential significance of determining why a person seeks help at a particular time:

> ***Chief complaint:*** "I can't control my son. It's been a problem, but for the past year and a half it has become worse."
>
> ***Present history:*** Child has had temper tantrums since infancy. He "throws things, hits and kicks people, yells and screams." It occurs whenever he "doesn't get his way." They usually last "a minute or two" and occur at least weekly. Mother has responded to them in a variety of ways: hits him, ignores him, takes a special object or privilege away, insults him. Nothing seems to work. Mother admits that ignoring the behavior is the most difficult approach, and she rarely can do so without eventually hitting or scolding him. Mother is not able to identify why she sought help now.

Further physical history revealed nothing unusual. However, family history disclosed several significant facts, especially that (1) the father had died 2 months earlier, and (2) he had been ill for 1½ years before his death. The nurse focused the history on events that had occurred since the beginning of the father's illness, which coincided with the son's increased behavior problems. The mother revealed that during her husband's illness she had had too little time to concern herself with her son's behavior, other than realizing that it was a problem. However, after her husband's death, she could no longer ignore the severity of her son's behavior or its disruptive effect on the family. As she verbalized these thoughts, she began to identify the specific reason for seeking help now. She stated, "I used to wait for my husband to come home to take the children off my hands. When he was sick, I was too busy worrying about him. But now I am home all alone. When dinnertime comes, there is no one to relieve me."

Although the interventions included several approaches to managing the problem, one of them focused on providing the mother with some freedom from the responsibility of total parenting. Had the nurse not concentrated on uncovering the mother's reason for seeking help at this particular time, a very important clue in planning care might have been missed.

Past History

The past history contains information relating to all previous aspects of the child's health status and concentrates on several areas that are ordinarily deleted in the history of an adult, such as birth history, detailed feeding history, immunizations, and growth and development. Since a large amount of data is included in this section, it is more efficient for nurses to use a combination of open-ended and fact-finding questions. For example, the nurse may begin interviewing for each section with an open-ended statement, such as "Tell me about your child's birth," to provide informants with the opportunity to relate what they think is most important. Fact-finding questions related to specific details are asked whenever necessary to focus the interview on certain topics.

Birth history. Birth history includes all data concerning (1) the mother's health during pregnancy, (2) the labor and delivery, and (3) the infant's condition immediately after birth. Since prenatal influences have significant effects on a child's physical and emotional development, a thorough investigation of birth history is important. However, the extent of the history depends on the child's age—the younger the child, the more detailed the birth history. With older children, parents may question the relevance of inquiry regarding pregnancy and birth. To address this concern, the nurse may state: "I will be asking you some questions about your pregnancy and ________'s (refer to child by name) birth. Your answers will give me a more complete picture of his overall health."

Pregnancy, labor, and delivery. An obstetric history begins with an overview of the pregnancy, preferably by an open-ended question, such as, "How was your pregnancy?" This allows the mother to state what she considered most significant. Most important, the nurse should ask about the use of medications or other remedies that the mother used to relieve physical symptoms.

Basic information in an obstetric history includes maternal age, number of pregnancies (gravida), outcome of pregnancies (parity), length of gestation, and any complications. (For a more detailed obstetric history refer to maternity texts.) Because emotional factors also affect the outcome of pregnancy and the subsequent parent-child relationship, it is important to investigate (1) concurrent crises during pregnancy and (2) prenatal attitudes toward the fetus.

The topic of parental acceptance of pregnancy is best approached through indirect questioning. Asking parents if the pregnancy was planned is a leading statement because they may respond affirmatively for fear of criticism if the pregnancy was unexpected. The nurse can encourage parents to disclose their true reactions by referring to specific facts relating to the pregnancy, such as the spacing between offspring, an extended or short interval between marriage and conception, or the concurrent experience of pregnancy and adolescence. The parent can choose to explore such statements with further explanations or, for the moment, may not be able to reveal such feelings. Silence should alert the nurse to the importance of refocusing on this topic later in the interview.

Perinatal history. The perinatal period is the time from birth to 27 days of life, but the primary focus is on the immediate period after birth and during hospitalization. Specific data include (1) weight and length at birth; (2) loss of weight following delivery; (3) time of regaining birth weight; (4) condition of health immediately after birth, such as quality of cry, level of activity (feeble or vigorous), and color of skin; (5) Apgar score (some parents may be aware of this); and (6) possible problems, such as fever, convulsions, hemorrhage, snuffles, skin eruptions, desquamation, paralysis, birth injuries, deformities, or congenital anomalies.

Dietary history. Because parental concerns related to eating are so common and nursing interventions to ensure optimal nutrition so important, the dietary history is discussed separately toward the end of this chapter under Nutritional Assessment.

Previous illnesses, injuries, and surgeries. When inquiring about past illnesses, the nurse can begin with a general statement, such as, "What other illness has your child had?" Since parents are most likely to recall serious health problems, it is important to specifically ask about colds, earaches, and common childhood diseases, such as measles, rubella (German measles), chickenpox, mumps, pertussis (whooping cough), diphtheria, scarlet fever, strep throat, tonsillitis, or allergic manifestations. It is best not to accept simple statements from the parents regarding the nature of the disease. Rather, encourage them to give onset, symptoms, course, and termination. For example, it is not uncommon for parents to confuse measles with rubella or strep throat with tonsillitis. Other important information concerning previous illnesses includes occurrence of similar symptoms in other children at the same time, course of convalescence with or without complications or sequelae, and geographic incidence of the disease.

In addition to illnesses, questions about injuries that required medical intervention, operations, and any other reason for hospitalization, including dates of each incident, are asked. It is important to focus on injuries such as falls, poisonings, choking, or burns, since these may be potential areas for parental guidance. While obtaining a history of the injury, the nurse should ascertain what happened before the injury (who was the child with, where were the parents, had this ever happened before) as well as what immediate action the parent took.

Inquiries about the child's emotional reactions to each experience are important. For example, one mother stated that her 4-year-old daughter had recently been admitted to the hospital for respiratory distress and had become very afraid of medical personnel, procedures, and equipment. The nurse realized from this information that the child needed special preparation for the physical examination.

Allergies. The nurse should ask about commonly known allergic disorders, such as hay fever and asthma, as well as unusual reactions to drugs, food, or contact agents, such as poisonous plants, animals, household products, or fabrics. Information about allergic reactions to drugs is essential. Failure to document a serious reaction places the child at risk if the drug is given; misdiagnosing a reaction as a serious allergy may deprive the child of effective treatment. If asked appropriate questions, most people can give reliable information about drug reactions (Box 6-13).

NURSING ALERT Penicillin allergy is associated with an immediate onset (within an hour of administration) or accelerated onset (1 to 72 hours after administration) skin eruption, especially an urticarial rash, or more serious symptoms such as laryngeal edema or anaphylactic shock.*

Box 6-13 GUIDELINES FOR TAKING A DRUG ALLERGY HISTORY

Are you allergic to any medication? If yes, what is (are) the medication(s) you are allergic to?
What dosage form did you take?
What type of reaction did you have?
How soon after the therapy was started did this occur?
How long ago did the reaction occur?
Who told you that it was an allergic reaction?
Have you taken this drug or other drugs of similar class after this reaction occurred? If yes, did you experience similar problems?

From Pau, A., Morgan, J., and Terlingo, A.: Drug allergy documentation by physicians, nurses and medical students, Am. J. Hosp. Pharm. 46(3):570-573, 1989.

Current medications. In addition to any allergies to drugs, questions about current drug regimens, including vitamins, aspirin, antibiotics, antihistamines, decongestants, or antitussives, are asked. All medications should be listed, including name, dose, schedule, duration, and reason for administration. Not infrequently parents are unaware of the actual name of the drug. Whenever possible, it is advisable to ask parents to bring the containers with them during the next visit. It is also possible to ask them for the name of the pharmacy and to call directly for a list of all the child's recent prescription medications. However, this approach does not reveal over-the-counter medications.

Immunizations. A record of all immunizations or "baby shots" is essential. Since many parents are unaware of the exact name and date of each immunization, the most reliable source of information is a hospital, clinic, or private physician's record. All immunizations and "boosters" should be listed, stating (1) name of the specific disease, (2) number of injections, (3) dosage, if known (sometimes lesser amounts are given if a reaction is anticipated), (4) ages when administered, and (5) the occurrence of any reaction following the immunization.

Growth and development. Questions about growth and development are an essential part of the child's history. The American Academy of Pediatrics recommends developmental appraisal at each health visit (see Recommendations for Health Supervision, Chapter 7). Asking parents about their perception of the child's development is important, since their concerns are good indicators that a problem exists (Glascoe, Altemeier, and MacLean, 1989). Whenever possible, parental responses are compared to existing health records or to current evaluation of actual growth (height, weight, dentition) and developmental performance (screening tests, grades in school, scholastic achievement, play activities, social relationships) (see Development Assessment, Chapter 7).

The most important previous growth patterns to record are (1) approximate weight at 6 months, 1 year, 2 years, and 5 years of age; (2) approximate length at 1 and 4 years; and (3) dentition, including age of onset, number of teeth, and symptoms during teething. Developmental milestones include (1) age of holding up head steadily, (2) age of sitting

*From Penicillin allergy in childhood, Lancet 1(8635):420, 1989.

alone without support, (3) age of walking without assistance, and (4) age of saying first words with meaning.

Specific and detailed questions are essential when inquiring about developmental milestones. For example, "sitting up" can mean many different activities, such as sitting propped up, sitting in one's lap, sitting with support, sitting up alone but in a hyperflexed position for assisted balance, or sitting up unsupported with the back slightly rounded. The clue to misunderstanding of the requested activity is an unusually early age of achievement.

Probing the area of developmental or intellectual performance can be a delicate one for parents, especially if there is concern for the child's progress. Therefore, it is best to approach such questioning with broad questions, such as, "How is Jimmy doing in school?" rather than with qualifying statements, such as, "Does Jimmy do well in school?" If the parents' response is vague and general, follow with questions such as, "How does he do in spelling, reading, or math?" Since these questions are appropriate for older children, they should be addressed directly to the child, as well as to the parent, for comparison of responses and increased reliability.

A school history is taken because it provides a general index of the child's functioning outside of the home. General questions, such as, "How's school?", are followed by specific questions about present grade in school and scholastic achievement in various subjects. At this point the child may feel at ease in giving opinions about such areas as the best and worst things at school, favorite teachers or subjects, or groups of friends. The nurse should also ask about after-school activities, such as hobbies and sports. (A school history may also be taken during the personal/social history.)

Habits. Habits are an important area to explore because, despite the normalcy of practices such as ritualistic behaviors, numerous parental concerns (Box 6-14) may be uncovered. One of the most common concerns among parents, especially those of young children, relates to sleep. Many children develop a normal sleep pattern, and all that is required during the assessment is a general overview of nighttime sleep and nap schedules. However, a number of children also develop sleep problems (see Sleep Disturbances, Chapters 12 and 15). When sleep problems occur, a more detailed sleep history is required (Box 6-15). Since sleep problems have multiple causes, a thorough history is essential in order to guide appropriate interventions.*

Habits related to use of chemicals apply primarily to older children and adolescents. If a youngster admits to smoking, drinking, or drug use, the quantity and frequency are recorded. Asking questions such as "Have you ever had a drinking or drug problem?" or "When was the last time you had a drink or took drugs?" was found to yield more reliable data than questions such as "How much do you drink?" or "How often do you drink or take drugs?" (Cyr and Wartman, 1988). If older children deny use of chemical substances, it is advisable to inquire about past experimentation. Asking, "You mean you never tried to smoke or drink?" implies that the nurse expects some such activity and consequently is likely to be nonjudgmental of an affirmative answer. One should also be aware of the confidential nature of such questioning, the adverse effect that the parents' presence may have on the adolescent's willingness to answer, and that self-report may not be an accurate account of chemical abuse (Zuckerman, Amaro, and Cabral, 1989).

*A sleep chart for the family to record the child's daily sleep and wake activities is available in Wong, D. and Whaley, L.: Clinical manual of pediatric nursing, ed. 3, St. Louis, 1990, Mosby–Year Book, Inc.

Box 6-14 HABITS TO EXPLORE DURING HEALTH INTERVIEW

Behavior patterns, such as nail biting, thumbsucking, pica (habitual ingestion of nonfood substances), rituals ("security" blanket or toy), and unusual movements (head-banging, rocking, overt masturbation, and walking on toes)
Activities of daily living, such as hour of sleep and arising, duration of nighttime sleep and naps, type and duration of exercise, regularity of stools and urination, age of toilet training, and occurrences of daytime or nighttime bedwetting
Unusual disposition, as well as response to frustration
Use or abuse of alcohol, drugs, coffee, and cigarettes

Review of Systems

Review of systems is exactly what the title implies—a specific review of each body system, similar to the order of the physical examination. Often the history of the present illness provides a complete review of the system involved in the chief complaint. Since asking questions about other body systems may appear unrelated and irrelevant to the parents or child, it is important to precede the questioning with an explanation of why the data are needed (similar to the explanation concerning relevance of birth history) and reassurance that the child's main problem has not been forgotten.

The review of a specific system is begun with a broad statement, such as, "How has your child's general health been?" or "Has your child had any problems with his eyes?" If the parent states that there have been past problems with some body function, this is pursued with an encouraging statement, such as, "Tell me more about that." If the parent denies any problems, it is best to query for specific symptoms, such as, "No headaches, bumping into objects, or squinting?" If the parent reconfirms the absence of such symptoms, positive statements to this effect are recorded in the history, such as, "Mother denies child is having headaches, bumping into objects, or squinting." In this way, anyone who reviews the health history is aware of exactly what symptoms were investigated.

An outline of suggested areas for review of each body system is presented in Box 6-16. Although medical terminology may be used to record a symptom, only terms understood by the family are used during the interview.

Box 6-15 GUIDELINES FOR ASSESSING SLEEP PROBLEMS IN CHILDREN*

General History of Chief Complaint

Ask parents/child to describe sleep problems; record in their words.
Inquire about onset, duration, character, frequency, and consistency of sleep problems:
- Circumstances surrounding onset (birth of sibling, start of toilet training, death of significant other, move from crib to bed)
- Circumstances that aggravate problem, i.e., overtiredness, family conflict, or disrupted routine (visitors)
- Remedies used to correct problem and results of interventions

24-Hour Sleep History

Time and regularity of meals†
- Family members present
  - Activities afterward, especially evening meal

Time of night and day sleep periods
- Hours of sleep and waking
- Hours of being put to bed and taken out of bed
  - How bedtime is decided (when child looks tired or at a time decided by parent; do both parents agree on bedtime?)

Prebedtime or nap rituals (bath, bottle or breast-feeding, snack, television, active or quiet playing, story)
- Mood before nap or bedtime (wide awake, sleepy, happy, cranky)
- Which parent(s) participates in nap or bedtime rituals?

Nap and bedtime rituals
- Where is child allowed to fall asleep? (own bed or crib, couch, parent's bed, someone's lap, other)
- Is child helped to fall asleep? (rocked, walked, patted, given pacifier or bottle, placed in room with light, television, radio, or tape recorder on, other)
- Are patterns consistent each time or do they vary?
- Does child awake if sleep aids are changed or taken away? (placed in own bed, television turned off, other)
- Does child verbally insist that parents stay in room?

Child's behaviors if refuses to go to sleep or stay in room
- If child complains of fears, how convincing are the fears?

Sleep environment
- Number of bedrooms
- Location of bedrooms, especially in relation to parent(s)' room
- Sensory features (light on, door open or closed, noise level, temperature)

Nightwakings
- Time, frequency, and duration
- Child's behavior (call out, cry, come out of room, appear frightened, confused, or upset)
- Parent(s)' responses (let child cry, go in immediately, take to own bed, feed, pick up, rock, give pacifier, talk, scold, threaten, other)
- Conditions that reestablish sleep
  - Do they always work?
  - How long do the interventions take to work?
  - Which parents intervene?
  - Do both parents use same or different approach?

Daytime sleepiness
- Occurrence of falling asleep at inappropriate times (circumstances, suddenness and irresistibility of onset, length of sleep, mood on awakening)
- Signs of fatigue (yawning, lying down, as well as overactivity, impulsivity, distractibility, irritability, temper tantrums)

Past Sleep History

Sleep patterns since infancy, especially age when slept during the night, stopped daytime naps, later bedtime
Response to changes in sleep arrangements (crib to bed, different room or house, other)
Sleep behaviors (restlessness, snoring, sleepwalking, nightmares, partial wakings [young child may wake confused, crying, and thrashing, but does not respond to parent; falls asleep with intervention if not excessively disturbed])
Parent(s)' perception of child's sleep habits (good or poor sleeper, light or deep sleeper, needs little sleep)
Family history of sleep problems (sibling behavior imitated by child; some sleep disorders, e.g., narcolepsy and enuresis, tend to recur in families)

Modified from Ferber, R.: Assessment procedures for diagnosis of sleep disorders in children. In Noshpitz, J., editor: Sleep disorders for the clinician, London, 1987, Butterworths, pp. 185-193.
*Not all of these areas need to be assessed with every family. For example, if nightwakings are not a problem, this section of the interview can be eliminated.
†A convenient point to start the 24-hour history is the evening meal.

Family Medical History

The family medical history is used primarily for the purpose of discovering the potential existence of hereditary or familial diseases in the parents and child and family habits that may affect the child's health, such as smoking and other chemical use. In general it is confined to first-degree relatives (parents, siblings, and grandparents and their children) and is mose easily recorded using a pedigree chart or genogram (see p. 176). Information for each family member includes age, marital status, state of health if living, cause of death if deceased, and any evidence of the following conditions: heart disease, hypertension, cancer, diabetes mellitus, obesity, congenital anomalies, allergy, asthma, tuberculosis, sickle cell disease, mental retardation, convulsions, insanity or other emotional problems, syphilis, or rheumatic fever. In the case of genetic diseases, a more in-depth inquiry into family transmission of the disorder is performed (see Role of the Nurse in Genetic Counseling, Chapter 5). The accuracy of the reported disorders is confirmed by inquiring about the symptoms, course, treatment, and sequelae of each diagnosis.

Geographic location. One of the important areas to explore when assessing the family health history is geographic location, including birthplace and travel to different areas in or outside of the country for identification of possible exposure to endemic diseases. Although the primary in-

Box 6-16 GUIDELINES FOR REVIEW OF SYSTEMS

General: Overall state of health, fatigue, recent and/or unexplained weight gain or loss (period of time for either), contributing factors (change of diet, illness, altered appetite), exercise tolerance, fevers (time of day), chills, night sweats (unrelated to climatic conditions), frequent infections, general ability to carry out activities of daily living

Integument: Pruritus, pigment or other color changes, acne, eruptions, rashes (location), tendency to bruising, petechiae, excessive dryness, general texture, disorders or deformities of nails, hair growth or loss, hair color change (for adolescent, use of hair dyes or other potentially toxic substances, such as hair straighteners)

Head: Headaches, dizziness, injury (specific details)

Eyes: Visual problems (ask about behaviors indicative of blurred vision, such as bumping into objects, clumsiness, sitting very close to the television, holding a book close to the face, writing with head near desk, squinting, rubbing the eyes, bending the head in an awkward position), cross-eye (strabismus), eye infections, edema of lids, excessive tearing, use of glasses or contact lenses, date of last optic examination

Nose: Nosebleeds (epistaxis), constant or frequent running or stuffy nose, nasal obstruction (difficulty in breathing), alteration or loss of sense of smell

Ears: Earaches, discharge, evidence of hearing loss (ask about behaviors, such as need to repeat requests, loud speech, inattentive behavior), results of any previous auditory testing

Mouth: Mouth-breathing, gum bleeding, toothaches, toothbrushing, use of fluoride, difficulty with teething (symptoms), last visit to dentist (especially if temporary dentition is complete), response to dentist

Throat: Sore throats, difficulty in swallowing, choking (especially when chewing food—may be from poor chewing habits), hoarseness, or other voice irregularities

Neck: Pain, limitation of movement, stiffness, difficulty in holding head straight (torticollis), thyroid enlargement, enlarged nodes or other masses

Chest: Breast enlargement, discharge, masses, enlarged axillary nodes (for adolescent female, ask about breast self-examination)

Respiratory: Chronic cough, frequent colds (number per year), wheezing, shortness of breath at rest or on exertion, difficulty in breathing, sputum production, infections (pneumonia, tuberculosis), date of last chest x-ray examination, and skin reaction from tuberculin testing

Cardiovascular: Cyanosis or fatigue on exertion, history of heart murmur or rheumatic fever, anemia, date of last blood count, blood type, recent transfusion

Gastrointestinal: (Much of this in regard to appetite, food tolerance, and elimination habits has been asked elsewhere), nausea, vomiting (not associated with eating, may be indicative of brain tumor or increased intracranial pressure), jaundice or yellowing skin or sclera, belching, flatulence, recent change in bowel habits (blood in stools, change of color, diarrhea, and constipation)

Genitourinary: Pain on urination, frequency, hesitancy, urgency, hematuria, nocturia, polyuria, unpleasant odor to urine, force of stream, discharge, change in size of scrotum, date of last urinalysis (for adolescent, sexually transmitted disease, type of treatment; for male adolescent, ask about testicular self-examination)

Gynecologic: Menarche, date of last menstrual period, regularity or problems with menstruation, vaginal discharge, pruritus, date and result of last Pap smear (include obstetric history as discussed under birth history when applicable); if sexually active, type of contraception

Musculoskeletal: Weakness, clumsiness, lack of coordination, unusual movements, back or joint stiffness, muscle pains or cramps, abnormal gait, deformity, fractures, serious sprains, activity level

Neurologic: Seizures, tremors, dizziness, loss of memory, general affect, fears, nightmares, speech problems, any unusual habits

Endocrine: Intolerance to weather changes, excessive thirst and/urination, excessive sweating, salty taste to skin, signs of early puberty

terest focuses on the child's temporary residence in various localities, the nurse should also inquire about close family members' travel, especially during tours of military service or business trips. Children are especially susceptible to parasitic infestation in areas of poor sanitary conditions and to vector-borne diseases, such as those from mosquitoes or ticks in warm and humid or heavily wooded regions.

Psychosocial History

In the traditional medical history a personal and social section is included that concentrates on children's personal status, such as school adjustment and any unusual habits, and on the family and home environment. Since several personal aspects are covered under development and habits, and the social aspects are discussed in detail under Family Assessment, only those issues related to children's general view of themselves in terms of self-concept are presented here (see Development of Self-concept, Chapter 4).

Through observation the nurse can obtain a general idea of how children handle themselves in terms of confidence in dealing with others and ability to answer questions. Observing the parent-child relationship can indicate the types of messages sent to children about their self-worth. Do the parents treat the children with respect, focusing on their strengths, or is the interaction one of constant reprimands, with emphasis on the children's weaknesses and faults?

Messages about body image are also conveyed through the parent-child interaction. Do the parents label the children and body parts, such as bad boy, skinny legs, or ugly scar? The type of touch can also be revealing. Are children handled gently, using soothing touch to calm an anxious child, or they are treated roughly, using slaps or restraint to force compliance? When children touch certain parts of the body, such as the genitals, do parents make comments that suggest a negative connotation?

With older children, many of the communication strategies discussed earlier in the chapter are useful in eliciting more definitive information about their self-concept. Children can write down five things they like and dislike about themselves. Sentence completion with statements such as "The thing I like best (or worst) about myself is ____________" or "If I could change one thing about myself it would be ____________," can be used. Drawing offers numerous possibilites for offering insight. Children can draw a picture of an "ideal person" and then discuss how their characteristics are the same as or different from this portrait. Another activity is to have children make a collage using cutouts from magazines to represent themselves (Winkelstein, 1989). Through play with puppets, dolls, or stuffed animals, children can reveal how they relate to others, often reflecting their own self-image.

Sexual History

Sexual history is an essential component of adolescents' health assessment. The history uncovers areas of concern related to sexual activity, alerts the nurse to circumstances that may indicate screening for sexually transmitted diseases, and provides information related to the need for sexual counseling, such as safe sex practices (Andrist, 1988).

One approach toward initiating a conversation about sexual concerns is to begin with a history of peer interactions. Open-ended statements such as "Tell me about your social life," or "Who are your closest friends?" generally lead into a discussion of dating and sexual issues. To probe further, questions about the adolescent's attitudes on such topics as sex education, "going steady," "living together," and premarital sex can be included. Questions are phrased to reflect concern and not judgment or criticism of sexual practices.

In any conversation regarding sexual history, the nurse must be aware of the language that is used in either eliciting or conveying sexual information. Phrases such as "sexually active" have many meanings. For example, one adolescent denied being sexually active despite a positive pregnancy test. When asked again about whether or not she was sexually active, she denied the activity stating that "I lie perfectly still during intercourse." "Are you having sex with anyone?" is suggested as the most direct and best understood question (Strasburger, 1986).

Other questions to ask adolescents include "Are you using any type of contraception? Why not? Have you discussed this relationship with your parents? If you did, what would their reaction be?" If teenagers deny sexual activity, it is just as important to discuss with them their concerns about not being sexually active as it is to discuss concerns with teenagers who are sexually active. Most teenagers tend to feel "Everyone is doing it but me," and this becomes a major issue for them (Strasburger, 1986).

Since homosexual experimentation may occur, all sexual contacts should be referred to in nongender terms, such as "anyone" or "partners," rather than "girlfriends" or "boyfriends." A detailed account of sexual partners is needed if the patient has a history of, displays any of the symptoms of, or asks for treatment of a sexually transmitted disease. A difficult but necessary part of the interview is to determine the sites of possible infection. Since sexual diseases can be contracted at any of the body orifices, the adolescent should be informed that a sexually transmitted disease can be acquired without visible signs of disease at nongenital sites, such as the mouth.

The degree of inquiry into the parents' sexual activity depends on many factors. For example, it may be limited to a brief discussion of their plans regarding future children or contraception. In instances in which overt adult sexual activity may be having an adverse effect on the children, a more detailed exploration of this area is warranted. The nurse must make this decision based on facts learned during the interview since this line of questioning should never be wanton prying. If parents ask the relevance of revealing such matters, the nurse must be prepared to offer a sound and logical explanation. It is every person's right to refuse to disclose personal information, especially if not informed of its significance or value.

FAMILY ASSESSMENT

Assessment of the family, both its structure and function, is an essential component of the history-taking process. Numerous studies demonstrate that the quality of the functional relationship between the patient and family members is a major factor in emotional and physical health. Because of its significance in nursing of children, family assessment is discussed separately and in greater detail apart from the more traditional health history.

Family assessment is the collection of data about the composition of the family and the relationships among its members. In its broadest sense the family refers to all those individuals who are significant to the nuclear unit, including relatives, friends, and other social groups, such as the school and church (see also Chapter 3).

Family assessment differs from family therapy in several ways. First, the primary goal of family assessment is to collect information for planning care, intervention, evaluation, or referral. In family therapy, data collection is only the initial stage in the process of family counseling. Second, the skills required for family therapy exceed those needed for assessment. Third, family assessment is a process often used with healthy families who may or may not be coping with stressful events. Family therapy is used primarily with families needing additional support to cope successfully with stress. Despite these differences, family assessment can and frequently is therapeutic. The process of involving family members in discussing family characteristics and activities often stimulates productive discussion and insight into family dynamics and relationships.

Because of the time involved in performing an in-depth family assessment as presented here, the nurse should be selective in deciding when knowledge of family function may facilitate nursing care. Indications for initiating a comprehensive family assessment are presented in Box 6-17.

In addition to the discussion of family assessment presented here, assessment issues specific to the family of a child with a chronic illness or disability are included in Chapter 22.

Box 6-17 GUIDELINES FOR INITIATING A COMPREHENSIVE FAMILY ASSESSMENT

Children receiving comprehensive well child care
Children experiencing major stressful life events, e.g., chronic illness, disability, parental divorce, or death of a family member
Children requiring extensive home care
Children with developmental delays
Children with repeated accidental injuries and those with suspected child abuse
Children with behavioral or physical problems that suggest family dysfunction as the etiology

ASSESSMENT OF FAMILY STRUCTURE

Family structure refers to the composition of the family—who lives in the home and those social, cultural, religious, and economic characteristics that influence the child's and family's overall psychobiologic health (see also Chapter 2). Since the information elicited in this part of the history is often the most personal and confidential, it is left to the end of the interview, when the nurse-parent-child rapport is well established.

Structural Assessment Interview

The most common method of eliciting information on family structure is interviewing family members. The principal areas of concern are (1) family composition, (2) home and community environment, (3) occupation and education of family members, and (4) cultural and religious traditions.

Family composition. Family composition is primarily concerned with the immediate members of the household, but should also include a review of the family's extended support system. For example, in a single-parent family, the household members may consist of the mother and two children, but the mother's parents may be very significant sources of childcare and financial support. Although the interview method can be used to collect information about household members—their relationship, ages, and roles within the family, as well as significant individuals outside the family unit—other efficient methods include those discussed under Structural Assessment Tools.

In assessing family composition it is sometimes difficult to ascertain the status of the adult relationships. For example, the parent may fail to mention the other parent. In this case the nurse can then ask, "Where is the child's father (or mother)?" It is best to avoid the term *husband* or *wife* because that precludes the existence of nonmarital relationships. If the parent states that the child's father (or mother) is not part of the household, the nurse can explore this by inquiring about his or her continued relationship with the child and the presence of any other significant male (or female) within the home. The nurse should also inquire about previous marriages, separations, death of spouses, or divorces. It is important to ask about the children's reaction to any of these events, which usually have a tremendous effect on their general physical and emotional health.

Home and community environment. Information about the home environment includes:

1. Type of dwelling (private home, apartment, multiple dwelling, or trailer)
2. Number of rooms, including sleeping arrangements, floors, and occupants
3. Accessibility of stairs or elevators
4. Adequacy of utilities
5. Safety features (fire escape, guard rails on high-rise windows, smoke detectors, and use of car restraints)
6. Housing problems (insects, poor sanitation, or flaking paint)

Recent stresses or changes in the home should be explored, such as relocation, change in employment status, marital discord or divorce, and addition of a new sibling. If any are identified, the nurse should inquire about the child's adjustment to the change.

Information regarding the community environment may vary according to geographic location, such as an urban or rural setting. It is the nurse's responsibility to have at least a general knowledge of the locality in order to focus questions on specific areas of significance. However, some general topics for investigation include:

1. Type of neighborhood (residential or industrial, relative age of neighboring families, willingness of neighbors to help one another, interracial or ethnic problems)
2. Location of and distance to school
3. Usual transportation to school
4. Availability of age-mates for the child
5. Available play areas
6. Potential dangers in the community environment (e.g., proximity to industrial centers; i.e., an asbestos or chemical factory); incidence of crime; and potential sources of injury (i.e., swimming pool, drainage ditch, or other adjacent body of water, steep hill or cliff, or heavy street traffic)

Occupation and education of family members. The occupational history of the parents consists of more than a listing of their career and place of employment. It should focus on (1) type of activity (manual or sedentary, individually paced or highly pressured), (2) number of hours away from the home, (3) exposure to environmental hazards (chemicals, coal, radiation, lead, carbon monoxide, or fire), and (4) satisfaction associated with the employment.

The occupational history should also lead into a discussion of the family's financial status. Since some parents may resist disclosing their annual income, the nurse can assess the adequacy of financial resources by inquiring about source of income when unemployed, usual housing expenses, and expenditures for food, shelter, clothing, and recreation. A general statement, such as, "The cost of living is certainly high today. How do you make ends meet?" may encourage parents to discuss any financial hardships without fear of criticism. Assessment of the family's medical insurance is very important, since availability of financial assistance is directly related to use of health care (U.S. Congress, 1988).

Ascertaining the parents' educational preparation usually follows a discussion of occupation. By the end of the inter-

Box 6-18 GUIDELINES FOR ASSESSING CULTURE

Does the family identify with a particular religious/ethnic group? Are both parents from that group?
How is religious/ethnic background a part of the family's life?
What special religious/cultural traditions are practiced in the home (e.g., food choices and preparation)?
Where were family members born, and how long have they lived in this country?
What language does the family speak most frequently?
Do they speak/understand English?
What do they believe causes health or illness?
What religious/ethnic beliefs influence the family's perception of illness and its treatment?
What methods are used to prevent illness or treat an illness?
How does the family know when a health problem needs medical attention?
Who is the first person the family contacts when a member is ill?
Does the family rely on cultural/religious healers or remedies? If so, ask them to describe the type of healer or remedy.
Who does the family go to for support (clergy, medical healer, relatives)?
Does the family experience discrimination because of their race, beliefs, or practices? If so, ask them to describe instances of discrimination.

view, the nurse has probably made some personal judgment regarding the parent's level of formal and/or informal education. However, since many people are embarrassed to admit failure to complete the usual academic learning, it is best to approach the area of years in school indirectly whenever possible. For example, the nurse can ask about the type of training, education, or acquisition of special skills that may be required for the parents' vocation. This information is highly valuable in planning implementation of care (e.g., counseling, guidance, or teaching) and is another reason to refrain from actual intervention until the history (and physical examination whenever warranted) is completed.

Cultural and religious traditions. Knowledge of the family's cultural traditions and religious practices is essential in planning care. The influence of culture and religion on the family is discussed in Chapter 2. Cultural traditions and religious practices that should be assessed in the family history include childrearing beliefs, attitudes toward health care, and personal faith in a deity. Cultural practice in relation to nutrition is discussed in Chapter 2. Guidelines for assessing culture are presented in Box 6-18.

Structural Assessment Tools

Several structural assessment tools are valuable in collecting and recording data about family composition and environment. Like the interview method these tools also provide information about relationships, although several additional methods should be used to assess family function.

Tools that involve drawing have several advantages. They:

1. Provide an immediate visual presentation of the family tree and extended support systems
2. Yield extensive information in a short period of time
3. Are easily updated
4. May stimulate productive and meaningful communication among family members

Two tools involving drawing are presented below; the sociogram and kinetic family drawing are discussed on p. 198.

Genogram. The genogram (family tree, family diagram) uses symbols to diagrammatically record data about family structure. It is a modification of the pedigree chart used in genetics to record the family medical history. Symbols often used in the genogram are presented in Fig. 5-7. Because there is no universal list of symbols, those used by other health professionals may differ. If in doubt regarding which symbol to use, or if one does not exist, it is best to write in the word describing the relationship, such as *foster child.* Since the genogram is also concerned with the *strength* of family relationships, attachment symbols are often added as additional information on family functioning is obtained (see Fig. 6-8). Because a genogram can become complex, it is helpful to circle the nuclear family on the diagram. Instructions for beginning a genogram are similar to those for a pedigree (see p. 176).

Ecomap. The ecomap is a visual presentation of the family's support system outside the home. It begins with the genogram of the immediate family inside one circle and uses other smaller circles to represent each member's relationship with other significant people, agencies, or institutions (Hartman, 1979). A blank ecomap is shown is Fig. 6-7. The size of the circles is not important; rather, symbols of attachment (Fig. 6-8) are used to signify the type of relationship, and arrows may be drawn along the connecting lines to denote flow of energy or resources.

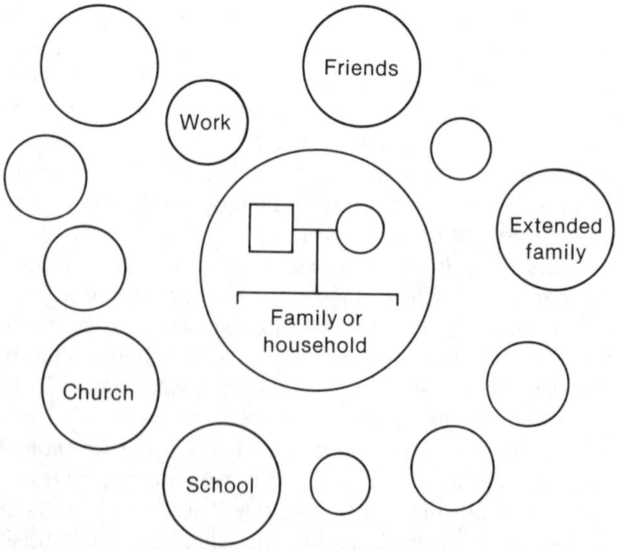

Fig. 6-7. Ecomap. Genogram is completed for immediate family members and circles are labeled as appropriate.
Modified from Hartman, A.: Finding families: an ecological approach to family assessment in adoption, Beverly Hills, CA, 1979, Sage Publications.

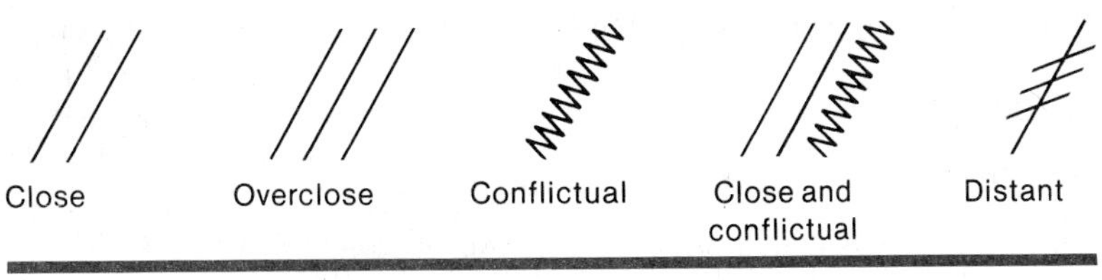

Fig. 6-8. Symbols of attachment or intensity of relationship.

ASSESSMENT OF FAMILY FUNCTION

Family function is concerned with how the family behaves toward one another and the quality of the relationships (see also Chapter 3). It is considered the most important component in determining "family health." Assessment of function requires more skill on the part of the interviewer than does assessment of structure and is best approached after structure is assessed.

Family Function Interview

As in assessment of family structure, the more traditional method of eliciting information on family function is interviewing family members. The principal areas of concern are the following characteristics, which are generally cited as significant variables in determining family health (see also Chapter 3).

Family interaction and roles. Family interaction refers to the ways family members relate to each other. The chief concern is the amount of intimacy and closeness among the members, especially the spouses. *Roles* refer to the behaviors of people as they assume different statuses or positions. The more flexibility and sharing of roles, the better family members are able to meet each other's needs. In assessing interactions and roles, general observations are made about the family's response to one another (e.g., cordial, hostile, cool, loving, patient, or short-tempered), obvious roles of leadership versus submission, and support and attention shown to various members.

Asking questions concerning with whom the child shares a room, the child's household chores, and activities the family performs together gives some idea of how the family interacts. It is best to avoid direct questions such as, "How does your family get along with each other?" because the usual response is "OK." An effective way of approaching this topic, especially with adolescents, is use of the third-person technique (see p. 194). For example, the nurse may say, "Teenagers and parents have a way of seeing things differently, especially when it comes to money, dating, clothes, using the car, and curfew. Have you and your parents ever disagreed about such things?" (For a more detailed discussion of family communication strategies, see pp. 187-200.)

Other assessment questions include:

Whom do you talk to when something is bothering you?
Who usually oversees what is happening with the children, such as at school or concerning their health?
What activities does your family do together?
What are the different family members' household chores?
How easy or difficult is it for your family to change or accept new responsibilities for household tasks?

Power, decision making, and problem solving. Power and control in the family is a critical issue. Several family therapists conclude that clear boundaries of power, that is, shared power by the parents in rearing the children, is essential for family health. Knowledge of who has power and how decisions are made usually offers clues to how problems are solved. One of the best methods of collecting data is to offer a hypothetic conflict or problem, such as a child with failing school grades, and ask the family how they would handle this situation. By observing the group dynamics, conclusions can be drawn about how the family typically deals with conflicts or problems.

Assessment questions include:

Who usually makes the decisions in your family
(Directed to the child) If one parent makes a decision, can you appeal to the other parent to change it?
(Directed to the parents) What input do the children have in making decisions or discussing rules?
Who makes and enforces the rules?
What happens when a rule is broken?

Communication. In interviewing the family, the nurse is concerned with the clarity and directness of communication patterns. Clear communication relays messages that are understood by all members. Direct communication is sent to the intended receiver. Assessments are made by observing who speaks to whom, if one person speaks for another or interrupts, if members appear disinterested when certain individuals speak, and if there is agreement between verbal and nonverbal messages. To further assess communication, the nurse can periodically ask family members if they understood what was just said and to repeat the message.

Assessment questions include:

How often do family members wait until others are finished talking before "having their say"?
(Directed to the child) Do your parents encourage you to share your opinion with them?
(Directed to the parents) Do your children tend to listen to you, such as when you ask them to do things?
(Directed to the parents) Do your children tend to come to you with their problems and discuss their feelings?

Expression of feelings and individuality. Healthy families allow expression of feelings and promote the development of individuality while encouraging family closeness. There is the space and freedom to grow with the limits and structure needed for guidance. Observing patterns of communication offers clues to how freely feelings are expressed.

Assessment questions include:

Is it OK to get angry or sad in your house?
Who gets angry most of the time? What do they do?
If you are upset, how do other family members try to comfort you?
Who comforts you?
When you want to do something new, such as try out for a new sport or get a job, what is the family's response (offer assistance, discourage you, or leave it to you to work out)?

Family Function Assessment Tools

In addition to observing and interviewing the family to assess family function, several other methods are available and should be used as needed to obtain a comprehensive assessment. The following section discusses selected instruments that are appropriate for the nurse to use. They are reliable and valid but require little formal training and minimal time to administer. The reader is referred to the discussion on the conjoint family drawing on p. 199 and to reviews of other instruments for further information (Dunst, Trivette, and Deal, 1988; Humenick, 1982; McCubbin and Thompson, 1987; Smilkstein, 1984; Speer and Sachs, 1985).

Family APGAR. The Family APGAR (FAPGAR) is a brief screening questionnaire designed to reflect a family member's satisfaction with the functional state of the family (Smilkstein, 1978) (see Appendix A). The acronym APGAR is for Adaptability, Partnership, Growth, Affection, and Resolve (commitment) (Box 6-19). The acronym was chosen because it is familiar to health professionals, but it bears no relationship to the Apgar scoring system for newborns. It can be completed in about 5 minutes and can be used by nuclear families, as well as families with alternative lifestyles.

The responses to the five questions are scored as follows: "Almost always"—2; "Some of the time"—1; and "Hardly ever"—0. Each score is totaled. Scores of 7 to 10 suggest a highly functional family; 4 to 6, a moderately dysfunctional family; and 0 to 3 a severely dysfunctional family. The questions in the box can be used in the interview without the APGAR ratings to elicit similar types of information.

Feetham Family Functioning Survey. The Feetham Family Functioning Survey provides information about family members' *perception* of relationships that contribute to or are affected by family functioning (Feetham and Humenick, 1982).* Although recommended primarily as a research instrument, it can be used clinically without scoring the items to identify areas that may be of concern to the family.

*The survey is available for a fee from Suzanne Feetham, Ph.D., R.N., F.A.A.N., Nursing Research and Development, Children's Hospital National Medical Center, 111 Michigan Ave., N.W., Washington, DC 20010; (202) 939-4980.

Box 6-19 FAMILY APGAR

Definition	Function Measured by the Family APGAR	Relevant Open-Ended Questions
Adaptation is the use of intrafamilial and extrafamilial resources for problem-solving when family equilibrium is stressed during a crisis.	How resources are shared, or the degree to which a member is satisfied with the assistance received when family resources are needed.	How have family members aided each other in time of need? In what way have family members received help or assistance from friends and community agencies?
Partnership is the sharing of decision-making and nurturing responsibilities by family members.	How decisions are shared, or the member's satisfaction with mutuality in family communication and problem-solving.	How do family members communicate with each other about such matters as vacations, finances, medical care, large purchases, and personal problems?
Growth is the physical and emotional maturation and self-fulfillment that is achieved by family members through mutual support and guidance.	How nurturing is shared, or the member's satisfaction with the freedom available within the family to change roles and attain physical and emotional growth or maturation.	How have family members changed during the past years? How has this change been accepted by family members? In what ways have family members aided each other in growing or developing independent life-styles? How have family members reacted to your desires for change?
Affection is the caring or loving relationship that exists among family members.	How emotional experiences are shared, or the member's satisfaction with the intimacy and emotional interaction that exists in the family.	How have members of your family responded to emotional expressions such as affection, love, sorrow, or anger?
Resolve is the commitment to devote time to other members of the family for physical and emotional nurturing. It also usually involves a decision to share wealth and space.	How time (and space and money) is shared, or the member's satisfaction with the time commitment that has been made to the family by its members.	How do members of your family share time, space, and money?

Modified from Smilkstein, G.: The Family APGAR: a proposal for a family function test and its use by physicians, J. Fam. Pract. 6(6):1231-1239, 1978.

Box 6-20 SAMPLE QUESTION FROM THE FEETHAM FAMILY FUNCTIONING SURVEY

The amount of time you spend with your *spouse*.

a. How much is there now?

LITTLE						MUCH
1	2	3	4	5	6	7

b. How much should there be?

LITTLE						MUCH
1	2	3	4	5	6	7

c. How important is this to me?

LITTLE						MUCH
1	2	3	4	5	6	7

Reproduced with the permission of Suzanne L. Feetham, Ph.D., R.N., F.A.A.N., Children's Hospital National Medical Center, Washington, DC, Developed from research funded by Division of Nursing, H.R.A., H.H.S., NU00632, Wayne State University, Detroit, MI, 1977-1980.

The survey consists of 27 questions in the following areas of family functioning (Box 6-20): household tasks; child care; sexual and marital relationships; interaction with family, children, and friends; community involvement; and sources of emotional support. Questions are answered on a seven-point scale that rates "what is," "what should be," and "how important it is." Discrepancy between the first two ratings, together with degree of importance, contributes to clinical assessment of the members' perceptions of family functioning. The survey takes less than 10 minutes to complete, but persons with less than a high school education have some difficulty with the format.

Home Observation and Measurement of the Environment and Home Screening Questionnaire. Ideally a thorough assessment includes observing the child and family in a variety of settings. Undoubtedly the richest environment for observing a child's development and interactions with family members is the home. Two tools that can be used to assess the child's home environment are the Home Observation for Management of the Environment (HOME)* (Caldwell and Bradley, 1984) and the Home Screening Questionnaire (HSQ) (Frankenburg and Coons, 1986).† Both are divided into two age-groups—birth to 3 years of age and 3 to 6 years of age (see Appendix A). HOME has an additional inventory for children 6 to 10 years; forms are also available for children with moderate to severe disabilities in each of the three age-groups for visual, auditory, orthopedic, and cognitive impairments.

Some of the HOME items require direct observation, whereas others necessitate questioning of the parents. Each item receives a "yes" or "no" response. The number of "yes" scores correlates with the amount of appropriate environmental stimulation. Any "no" scores indicate possible areas for intervention and counseling. Use of HOME requires about a 1-hour home visit with both the child and major caregiver.

The HSQ was developed using HOME as a guide. The 0- to 3-year form consists of 30 items plus a checklist of toys available to the child in the home. The 3- to 6-year form has 34 items and a similar toy checklist. The questions are written at approximately a third to sixth grade reading level and, unlike the HOME, can be completed by the parents in any setting in about 15 to 20 minutes. Scoring directions are detailed in the manual and are based on credits for different answers. For each age-group there is a minimum score for determining suspect or nonsuspect results.

In making a home or school visit, specific objectives for assessing the environment are listed in Box 22-8.

*The forms and an administration manual are available for a fee from the Center for Research on Teaching and Learning, College of Education, University of Arkansas at Little Rock, 2801 S. University Ave., Little Rock, AK 72204; (501) 569-3422.

†The forms and manual are available for a fee from Denver Developmental Materials, Inc., P.O. Box 6919, Denver, CO 80206-0919; (303) 355-4729.

NUTRITIONAL ASSESSMENT

A nutritional assessment is an essential part of a complete health appraisal. Its purpose is to evaluate the child's nutritional status, the state of balance between nutrient intake and nutrient expenditure or need (Krause and Mahan, 1984). A thorough nutritional status assessment includes: (1) dietary intake, (2) clinical examination, and (3) biochemical analysis.

DIETARY INTAKE

Knowledge of the child's dietary intake is a useful and practical component of a nutritional assessment. However, it is also one of the most difficult factors to assess. Individuals' recall of food consumption, especially amounts eaten, is frequently unreliable. In addition, people may be hesitant to reveal their eating patterns if they sense criticism from the nurse. People from different cultures may have difficulty adequately describing the types of food they eat. Despite these obstacles, however, a food intake record is essential. Several methods are available.

Dietary History

Regardless of the format used in recording food intake, every nutritional assessment should begin with a dietary history. The exact questions used to elicit a dietary history vary with the child's age. In general, the younger the child, the more specific and detailed the history should be. Box 6-21 provides a sample dietary history for children with additional questions regarding infant feeding.

The broad overview elicited from the dietary history can be helpful in evaluating food intake records (Box 6-22). It also is concerned with financial and cultural factors that influence food selection and preparation. Because cultural practices are very prevalent in food preparation, it is important to consider carefully the kind of questions that are asked and the judgment made in regard to counseling. For example, some cultures (e.g., Hispanic, black, and Native American) include many vegetables, legumes, and starches

Box 6-21 DIETARY HISTORY

What are the family's usual mealtimes?
Do family members eat together or at separate times?
Who does the family grocery shopping and meal preparation?
How much money is spent to buy food each week?
How are most foods prepared—baked, broiled, fried, other?
How often does the family or your child eat out?
- What kinds of restaurants do you go to?
- What kinds of food does your child typically eat at restaurants?

Does your child eat breakfast regularly?
Where does he eat lunch?
What are your child's favorite foods, beverages, and snacks?
- What are the average amounts eaten per day?
- What foods are artificially sweetened?
- What are your child's snacking habits?
- When are sweet foods usually eaten?
- What are your child's toothbrushing habits?

What special cultural practices are followed?
- What ethnic foods are eaten?

What foods and beverages does your child dislike?
How would you describe his usual appetite (hearty eater, picky eater)?
What are his feeding habits (breast, bottle, cup, spoon, eats by self, needs assistance, any special devices)?
Does he take vitamins or other supplements; do they contain iron or fluoride?
Are there any known or suspected food allergies; is your child on a special diet?
Has your child lost or gained weight recently?
Are there any feeding problems (excessive fussiness, spitting up, colic, difficulty sucking or swallowing); any dental problems or appliances, such as braces, that affect eating?
What types of exercise does your child do regularly?
Is there a family history of cancer, diabetes, heart disease, high blood pressure, or obesity?

Additional Questions for Infants
What was the infant's birth weight; when did it double, triple?
Was the infant premature?
Are you breast-feeding or have you breast-fed your infant? For how long?
If you use a formula, what is the brand?
- How long has the infant been taking it?
- How many ounces does he drink a day?

Are you giving the infant cow's milk (whole, low-fat, skimmed)?
- When did you start?
- How many ounces does he drink a day?

Do you give your infant extra fluids (water, juice)?
If he takes a bottle to bed at nap or nighttime, what is in the bottle?
At what age did you start cereal, vegetables, meat or other protein sources, fruit/juice, finger food, table food?
Do you make your own baby food or use commercial foods, such as infant cereal?
Does the infant take a vitamin/mineral supplement? If so, what type?
Has the infant shown an allergic reaction to any food(s)? If so, list the foods and describe the reaction.
Does the infant spit up frequently, have unusually loose stools, or have hard, dry stools? If so, how often?
How often do you feed your infant?
How would you describe your infant's appetite?

in their diet that together provide sufficient essential amino acids, even though the actual amount of meat or dairy protein is low. (See Chapter 2 for cultural food practices.)

Twenty-four-hour recall. The most common and probably easiest method of assessing daily intake is the 24-hour recall. The child or parent recalls every item eaten in the past 24 hours and the approximate amounts. The 24-hour recall is most beneficial when it is representative of a typical day's intake. Some of the difficulties with a daily recall are the family's inability to remember exactly what was eaten and inaccurate estimation of portion size. To increase accuracy of reporting portion sizes, the use of food models and additional questioning are recommended. In general, this method is most useful in providing *qualitative* information about the child's diet.

Food diary. To improve the reliability of the daily recall, the family can complete a food diary by recording every food and liquid consumed for a certain number of days. A 3-day record consisting of 2 weekdays and 1 weekend day represents most people's eating patterns. Providing specific charts to record intake can improve compliance. The family should record items immediately after eating.

Food frequency record. A food frequency questionnaire or record provides information about the number of times in a day, week, or month a child consumes items from the four food groups (Box 6-22). In general, it provides more of a qualitative overview but has the advantage of avoiding recall based on a "typical" day. It is especially useful when verifying a food history or diary.

CLINICAL EXAMINATION

A significant amount of information regarding nutritional adequacy is elicited from a clinical examination, especially from assessing the skin, hair, teeth, gums, lips, tongue, and eyes. Hair, skin, and mouth are vulnerable to nutritional deficiency or excess because of the rapid turnover of epithelial and mucosal tissue. Table 6-1 summarizes clinical signs of possible nutritional deficiency or excess. Few are diagnostic for a specific nutrient, and if suspicious signs are found, they must be confirmed with dietary and biochemical data. Generally the clinical examination does not reveal children at risk for a deficiency or excess.

Anthropometry

An essential parameter of nutritional status is anthropometry, the measurement of height, weight, head circumference in young children, proportions, skinfold thickness, and arm

Box 6-22 FOOD FREQUENCY RECORD*

Food Group	Number of Servings (Day, Week)	Serving Size (in Cup, Tablespoon, or Ounce Portions)	Food Group	Number of Servings (Day, Week)	Serving Size (in Cup, Tablespoon, or Ounce Portions)
Milk/cheese Milk Cheese Yogurt Pudding Ice cream Other			*Fruits/juice* Citrus (orange, grapefruit, tangerine) Noncitrus Other		
Protein foods Meat Fish Poultry Egg Peanut butter Legumes (dried beans, peas) Nuts Other			*Fats* Butter, oil, margarine, mayonnaise, salad dressing		
Breads/cereals Bread, tortilla Cooked, pasta, rice, hot cereal Dry cereal (not presweetened) Crackers Muffins Other			*Sweets* Soda, punch Cake/cookie, etc. Candy Presweetened cereal		
Vegetables Yellow or orange Green/leafy Other					

*For comparison of actual intake with recommended intake, see Table 4-5.

circumference. Height and head circumference reflect past nutrition, whereas weight, skinfold thickness, and arm circumference reflect present nutritional status, especially of protein and fat reserves. Skinfold thickness is a measurement of the body's fat content since approximately one half of the body's total fat stores are directly beneath the skin. The upper arm muscle circumference is correlated with measurements of total muscle mass. Since muscle serves as the body's major protein reserve, this measurement is considered an index of the body's protein stores (Gray and Gray, 1980). Ideally growth measurements are recorded over a period of time, and comparisons are made regarding the *velocity* of growth based on previous and present values. Techniques for anthropomorphic measurement are discussed in Chapter 7 under Growth Measurements.

Biochemical Analysis

Numerous biochemical tests are available for assessing nutritional status and include analysis of plasma, blood cells, urine, or tissues from liver, bone, hair, and fingernails. Many of these tests are complicated and are not performed routinely. Common laboratory procedures for nutritional status include measurement of hemoglobin, hematocrit, albumin, creatinine, and nitrogen. Laboratory values for these tests and more specific nutrient measurements are given in Appendix D.

EVALUATION OF NUTRITIONAL ASSESSMENT

After collecting the data needed for a thorough nutritional assessment, the nurse should evaluate the findings to plan

Table 6-1 Clinical Assessment of Nutritional Status

EVIDENCE OF ADEQUATE NUTRITION	EVIDENCE OF DEFICIENT OR EXCESS NUTRITION	DEFICIENCY/EXCESS*
▪ General Growth		
Within 5th and 95th percentiles for height, weight, and head circumference	Below 5th or above 95th percentiles for growth	Protein, calories, fats, and other essential nutrients, especially A, pyridoxine, niacin, calcium, iodine, manganese, zinc
Steady gain with expected growth spurts during infancy and adolescence	Absence of or delayed growth spurts; poor weight gain	
Sexual development appropriate for age	Delayed sexual development	Excess vitamin A, D
▪ Skin		
Smooth, slightly dry to touch	Hardening and scaling	Vitamin A
Elastic and firm	Seborrheic dermatitis	Excess niacin
Absence of lesions	Dry, rough, petechiae	Riboflavin
Color appropriate to genetic background	Delayed wound healing	Vitamin C
	Scaly dermatitis on exposed surfaces	Riboflavin, vitamin C, zinc
	Wrinkled, flabby	Niacin
	Crusted lesions around orifices, especially nares	Protein and calories Zinc
	Pruritus	Excess vitamin A, riboflavin, niacin
	Poor turgor	Water, sodium
	Edema	Protein, thiamin Excess sodium
	Yellow tinge (jaundice)	Vitamin B_{12} Excess vitamin A, niacin
	Depigmentation	Protein, calories
	Pallor (anemia)	Pyridoxine, folic acid, vitamin B_{12}, C, E (in premature infants), iron Excess vitamin C, zinc
	Paresthesia	Excess riboflavin
▪ Hair		
Lustrous, silky, strong, elastic	Stringy, friable, dull, dry, thin	Protein, calories
	Alopecia	Protein, calories, zinc
	Depigmentation	Protein, calories, copper
	Raised areas around hair follicles	Vitamin C
▪ Head		
Even molding, occipital prominence, symmetric facial features	Softening of cranial bones, prominence of frontal bones, skull flat and depressed toward middle	Vitamin D
Fused sutures after 18 months	Delayed fusion of sutures	Vitamin D
	Hard tender lumps in occiput	Excess vitamin A
	Headache	Excess thiamin
▪ Neck		
Thyroid not visible, palpable in midline	Thyroid enlarged; may be grossly visible	Iodine
▪ Eyes		
Clear, bright	Hardening and scaling of cornea and conjunctiva	Vitamin A
Conjunctiva—Pink, glossy	Burning, itching, photophobia, cataracts, corneal vascularization	Riboflavin
Good night vision	Night blindness	
▪ Ears		
Tympanic membrane—Pliable	Calcified (hearing loss)	Excess vitamin D
▪ Nose		
Smooth, intact nasal angle	Irritation and cracks at nasal angle	Riboflavin Excess vitamin A

Table 6-1 Clinical assessment of nutritional status—cont'd

EVIDENCE OF ADEQUATE NUTRITION	EVIDENCE OF DEFICIENT OR EXCESS NUTRITION	DEFICIENCY/EXCESS*
▪ Mouth		
Lips—Smooth, moist, darker color than skin	Fissures and inflammation at corners	Riboflavin Excess vitamin A
Gums—Firm, coral pink color, stippled	Spongy, friable, swollen, bluish-red or black color, bleed easily	Vitamin C
Mucous membranes—Bright pink, smooth, moist	Stomatitis	Niacin
Tongue—Rough texture, no lesions, taste sensation	Glossitis	Niacin, riboflavin, folic acid
	Diminished taste sensation	Zinc
Teeth—Uniform white color, smooth intact	Brown mottling, pits, fissures	Excess fluoride
	Defective enamel	Vitamin A, C, D, calcium, phosphorus
	Caries	Excess carbohydrates
▪ Chest		
In infants, shape is almost circular	Depressed lower portion of rib cage	Vitamin D
In children, lateral diameter increases in proportion to anteroposterior diameter	Sharp protrusion of sternum	
Smooth costochondral junctions	Enlarged costochondral junctions	Vitamin C, D
Breast development—Normal for age	Delayed development	See General Growth, above, especially zinc
▪ Cardiovascular system		
Pulse and blood pressure (BP) within normal limits	Palpitations	Thiamin
	Rapid pulse	Potassium Excess thiamin
	Arrhythmias	Magnesium, potassium Excess niacin, potassium
	Increased BP	Excess sodium
	Decreased BP	Thiamin Excess niacin
▪ Abdomen		
In young children, cylindric and prominent	Distended, flabby, poor musculature	Protein, calories
Older children, flat	Prominent, large	Excess calories
Normal bowel habits	Potbelly, constipation	Vitamin D
	Diarrhea	Niacin Excess vitamin C
	Constipation	Excess calcium, potassium
▪ Musculoskeletal system		
Muscles—Firm, well-developed, equal strength bilaterally	Flabby, weak, generalized wasting	Protein, calories
	Weakness, pain, cramps	Thiamin, sodium, chloride, potassium, phosphorus, magnesium Excess thiamin
	Muscle twitching, tremors	Magnesium
	Muscular paralysis	Excess potassium
Spine—Cervical and lumbar curves (double S curve)	Kyphosis, lordosis, scoliosis	Vitamin D
Extremities—Symmetric; legs straight with minimum bowing	Bowing of extremities, knock-knees	Vitamin D, calcium, phosphorus
	Epiphyseal enlargement	Vitamin A, D
	Bleeding into joints and muscles, joint swelling, pain	Vitamin C
Joints—Flexible, full range of motion, no pain or stiffness	Thickening of cortex of long bones with pain and fragility, hard tender lumps in extremities	Excess vitamin A
	Osteoporosis of long bones	Calcium Excess vitamin D

Continued.

Table 6-1 Clinical assessment of nutritional status—cont'd

EVIDENCE OF ADEQUATE NUTRITION	EVIDENCE OF DEFICIENT OR EXCESS NUTRITION	DEFICIENCY/EXCESS*
▪ Neurologic system		
Behavior—Alert, responsive, emotionally stable	Listless, irritable, lethargic, apathetic (sometimes apprehensive, anxious, drowsy, mentally slow, confused)	Thiamin, niacin, pyridoxine, vitamin C, potassium, magnesium, iron, protein, calories Excess vitamin A, D, thiamin, folic acid, calcium
	Masklike facial expression, blurred speech, involuntary laughing	Excess manganese
Absence of tetany, convulsions	Convulsions	Thiamin, pyridoxine, vitamin D, calcium, magnesium Excess phosphorus (in relation to calcium)
Intact peripheral nervous system	Peripheral nervous system toxicity (unsteady gait, numb feet and hands, fine motor clumsiness)	Excess pyridoxine
Intact reflexes	Diminished or absent tendon reflexes	Thiamin, vitamin E

*Nutrients listed are deficient unless specified as excess.

appropriate counseling. From the data, the child can be assessed as (1) malnourished, (2) at risk for becoming malnourished, or (3) well nourished with adequate reserves.

Often the majority of the findings are from dietary intake, anthropometry, and clinical examination. Singly no one of these measures nutritional status. For example, dietary intake is important in assessing the quality of nutrient consumption, in managing the child at risk of malnutrition, and in determining if the prescribed intake goals are being met.

The daily food diary is analyzed for inclusion of selections in each of four basic food groups. For example, if the list includes no vegetables, the nurse should ask the reason for this rather than assume that the child dislikes vegetables because it may be that the parent did not serve any. Also the information obtained needs to be evaluated in terms of the family's ethnic practices and financial resources. To encourage increased protein intake with additional meat may be in conflict with food practices that use meat sparingly, such as in Asian meal preparation, or unfeasible for families on a limited budget. Based on the specific details of the nutrition history, appropriate counseling can be planned. More elaborate analysis can be done by calculating either by hand or with a computer the amounts of every nutrient in each food consumed.

Findings from clinical examination and anthropometry are evaluated with the data obtained from the dietary intake. For example, findings suggestive of anemia and a dietary record of iron-poor foods necessitate laboratory analysis of hemoglobin. Any suspicious findings are referred to the practitioner for further evaluation.

KEY POINTS

- Communication, the most important skill nurses must possess in the care of children, has verbal, nonverbal, and abstract components.
- To effectively establish a setting for communication, nurses must make an appropriate introduction, clarify their role and the purpose of the interview, and ensure privacy and confidentiality.
- When communicating with parents, nurses need to encourage parental involvement, listen carefully, use silence, and be empathic.
- Communication with children must reflect their development stage.
- Verbal communication techniques that have proved effective include the third-person technique, neurolinguistic programming, facilitative responding, storytelling, bibliotherapy, the use of "what if" questions, and other word games.
- Nonverbal communication with children may take the form of touch, writing, drawing, and play.
- The objectives of performing a health history are to identify pertinent information, determine the chief complaint, analyze the present illness, secure the past history, and record a family and sexual history.
- Family assessment is the collection of data about family composition and relationships among members; it focuses on home and community environment, occupation and education, and cultural and religious traditions.
- The family function interview examines interaction and roles, power, decision-making, problem-solving, communication, and expression of feelings and individuality.
- Nutritional assessment is performed by determination of dietary intake, clinical examination, and biochemical analysis.

REFERENCES

Andrist, L.: Taking a sexual history and educating clients about safe sex, Nurs. Clin. North Am. 23(4):959-973, 1988.

Bettelheim, B.: The uses of enchantment: the meaning and importance of fairy tales, New York, 1976, Alfred A. Knopf, Inc.

Brockopp, D.Y.: What is NLP? Am. J. Nurs. 83(7):1012-1014, 1983.

Burns, R.: Self growth in families: kinetic family drawings (KFD)—Research and application, NY, 1982, Brunner/Mazel, Inc.

Burns, R.C., and Kaufman, S.H.: Actions, styles, and symbols in kinetic family drawings, (KFD): research and application, New York, 1972, Brunner/Mazel, Inc.

Caldwell, B., and Bradley, R.: Home observation for measurement of the environment, rev. ed., Little Rock, AR, 1984, University of Arkansas.

Cassell, E., Coulehan, J., and Putnam, S.: Making good interview skills better, Patient Care 23(6):145-148, 1989.

Claman, L.: The squiggle-drawing game in child psychotherapy, Am. J. Psychother. 34(3):414-425, 1980.

Cyr, M., and Wartman, S.: The effectiveness of routine screening questions in the detection of alcoholism, JAMA 1259:51-54, 1988.

Dunst, C., Trivette, C., and Deal, A.: Enabling and empowering families: principles and guidelines for practice, Cambridge, MA, 1988, Brookline Books.

Elizabath, J.: Form of address: an addition to history taking?, Br. Med. J. 298(6668):257, 1989.

Epstein, C.: Nursing the dying patient, Reston, VA, 1975, Reston Publishing Co., Inc.

Ertel, I., and Ertel, P.: The role of a structured encounter form in improving the quality of child health supervision, Am J. Dis. Child. 140(4):313, 1986.

Feetham, S., and Humenick, S.: Feetham Family Functioning Survey. In Humenick, S., editor: Analysis of current assessment strategies in the health care of young children and childbearing families, Norwalk, CT, 1982, Appleton-Century-Crofts.

Frankenburg, W., and Coons, C.: Home Screening Questionnaire: its validity in assessing home environment, J. Pediatr. 108(4):624-626, 1986.

Glascoe, F., Altemeier, W., and MacLean, W.: The importance of parents' concerns about their child's development, Am. J. Dis. Child. 43:955-958, 1989.

Gray, G.E., and Gray, L.K.: Anthropometric measurements and their interpretation: principles, practices, and problems, J. Am. Diet. Assoc. 77(11):534-539, 1980.

Hartman, A.: Finding families: an ecological approach to family assessment in adoption, Beverly Hills, CA, 1979, Sage Publications, Inc.

Heineken, J., and Roberts, F.B.: Confirming, not disconfirming: communicating in a more positive manner, MCN 8(1):78-80, 1983.

Henrich, A.P., and Bernheim, K.F.: Responding to patients' concerns, Nurs. Outlook 29(7):428-433, 1981.

Hickson, G., and others: Concerns of mothers seeking care in private pediatric offices: opportunities for expanding services, Pediatrics 72(5):619-624, 1983.

Hoekelman, R.A., Kelly, J., and Zimmer, A.W.: The reliability of maternal recall, Clin. Pediatr. 15(3):261-265, 1976.

Humenick, S., editor: Analysis of current assessment strategies in the health care of young children and childbearing families, Norwalk, CT, 1982, Appleton-Century-Crofts.

Knowles, R.D.: Building rapport through neuro-linguistic programming, Am. J. Nurs. 83(7):1010-1014, 1983.

Krahn, G.: The use of projective assessment techniques in pediatric settings, J. Pediatr. Psychol. 10:179-193, 1985.

Krause, M.V., and Mahan, L.K.: Food, nutrition, and diet therapy, Philadelphia, 1984, W.B. Saunders Co.

Krieger, D.: The therapeutic touch, New York, 1986, Prentice Hall Press.

McCubbin, H., and Thompson, A., editors: Family assessment inventories for research and practice, Madison, WI, 1987, The University of Wisconsin–Madison.

Molsberry, D., and Shogan, M.: Communicating through touch. In Craft, M., and Denehy, J., editors: Nursing interventions for infants and children, Philadelphia, 1990, W.B. Saunders Co.

Ryberg, J., and Merrifield, E.: Tuning in to parents' concerns, Child. Nurse 2(2):1-4, 1984.

Sloat, A., and Matsuura, W.: Intercultural communication. In Craft, M., and Denehy, J., editors: Nursing interventions for infants and children, Philadelphia, 1990, W.B. Saunders Co.

Smilkstein, G.: The family APGAR: a proposal for a family function test and its use by physicians, J. Fam. Pract. 6(6):1231-1239, 1978.

Smilkstein, G.: The physician and family function assessment, Fam. Systems Med. 2(3):263-279, 1984.

Sorensen, E.: Using children's diaries as a research instrument, J. Pediatr. Nurs. 4(6):427-431, 1989.

Speer, J., and Sachs, B.: Selecting the appropriate family assessment tool, Pediatr. Nurs. 11(5):349-355, 1985.

Spinetta, J., and others: The kinetic family drawing in childhood cancer. In Spinetta, J., and Deasy-Spinetta, P.: Living with childhood cancer, St. Louis, 1981, Mosby–Year Book, Inc.

Strasburger, V.: The challenge of adolescent medicine in the 1980s, Child Care Newsletter 5(1):1-3, 1986.

Thayer, M.: Touching with intent: using therapeutic touch, Pediatr. Nurs. 16(1):70-72, 1990.

Thrower, S., Bruce, W., and Walton, R.: The Family Circle Method for integrating family systems concepts in family medicine, J. Fam. Pract. 15(3):451-457, 1982.

Triggs, B., and Perrin, E.: Improving communication about behavior and development by using a checklist, Am. J. Dis. Child. 140(4):313, 1986.

U.S. Congress, Offices of Technology Assessment, Healthy children: investing in the future, OTA-H-345, Washington, DC, U.S. Government Printing Office, February 1988.

Walker, C.: Stress and coping in siblings of childhood cancer patients, Nurs. Res. 37(4):208-212, 1988.

Wasserman, R., and others: Pediatric clinicians' support for parents makes a difference: an outcome-based analysis of clinician-parent interaction, Pediatrics 74(6):1047-1053, 1984.

Webster-Stratton, C., Glascock, J., and McCarthy, A.: Nurse practitioner-patient interactional analyses during well-child visits, Nurs. Res. 35(4):247-249, 1986.

Winkelstein, M.: Fostering positive self-concept in the school-age child, Pediatr. Nurs. 15(3):229-233, 1989.

Zuckerman, B., Amaro, H., and Cabral, H.: Validity of self-reporting of marijuana and cocaine use among pregnant adolescents, J. Pediatr. 115(5,Part 1):812-815, 1989.

BIBLIOGRAPHY

Communication Strategies/Health Interview

Able-Boone, H., Dokecki, P., and Smith, M.: Parent and health care provider communication and decision making in the intensive care nursery, Child. Health Care 18(3):113-141, 1989.

Baretich, D., Stephenson, P., and Igoe, J.: Using art to understand children's perceptions of roles in physician's office visits, Pediatr. Nurs. 15(4):356-360, 1989.

Bossert, E., and Martinson, I.: Kinetic family drawings—revised: a method of determining the impact of cancer on the family as perceived by the child with cancer, J. Pediatr. Nurs. 5(3):204-213, 1990.

Cameron, C.O., Juszczak, L., and Wallace, N.: Using creative arts to help children cope with altered body image, Child. Health Care 12(3):108-112, 1984.

Clutter, L. and others: Communicating effectively with young children, Child. Nurse 5(4):1-4, 1987.

Clutter, L. and others: Communicating effectively with older children, Child. Nurse 6(1):1-4, 1988.

Denehy, J.: Communicating with children through drawings. In Craft, M., and Denehy, J., editors: Nursing interventions for infants and children, Philadelphia, 1990, W.B. Saunders Co.

DiLeo, J.H.: Interpreting children's drawings, New York, 1983, Brunner/Mazel, Inc.

DiLeo, J.H.: Children's drawings as diagnostic aids, New York, 1980, Brunner/Mazel, Inc.

Faber, A., and Mazlish, E.: How to talk so kids will listen and listen so kids will talk, New York, 1980, Avon Books.

Ferber, R.: Assessment procedures for diagnosis of sleep disorders in children. In Noshpitz, J., editor: Sleep disorders for the clinician, London, 1987, Butterworths.

Fosson, A., and deQuan, M.M.: Reassuring and talking with hospitalized children, Child. Health Care 13(1):37-44, 1984.

Furth, G.M.: The use of drawings made at significant times in one's life. In Kubler-Ross, E.: Living with death and dying, New York, 1981, Macmillan Publishing Co., Inc.

Garbarino, J., and others: What children can tell us: eliciting, interpreting, and evaluating information from children, San Francisco, 1989, Jossey-Bass Inc., Publishers.

Hahn, K.: Therapeutic storytelling: helping children learn and cope, Pediatr. Nurs. 13(3):175-178, 1987.

Hudson, C., and others: Storytelling: a measure of anxiety in hospitalized children, Child. Health Care 16(2):118-122, 1987.

Johnson, B.: Children's drawings as a projective technique, Pediatr. Nurs. 16(1):11-16, 1990.

Kaufman, D.H.: An interview guide for helping children make healthcare decisions, Pediatr. Nurs. 11(5):365-367, 1985.

Kennedy, C., and Garvin, B.: Nurse-physician communication, Appl. Nurs. Res. 1(3):122-127, 1988.

Koppitz, E.M.: Psychological evaluation of children's human figure drawings, New York, 1968, Grune & Stratton, Inc.

Lynn, M.: Projective technique: a way of getting "hidden" information, part I, J. Pediatr. Nurs. 1(6):58-60, 1986.

Monsen, R.: Phases in the caring relationship: from adversary to ally to coordinator, MCN 11(5):316-318, 1986.

Moss, M., and Schleutermann, J.: Assessment of the pediatric client. In Malasanos, L., and others, editors: Health assessment, ed. 3, St. Louis, 1986, Mosby–Year Book, Inc.

Pau, A., Morgan, J., and Terlingo, A.: Drug allergy documentation by physicians, nurses, and medical students, Am. J. Hosp. Pharm. 46(3):570-573, 1989.

Pazola, K., and Gerberg, A.: Privileged communication-talking with a dying adolescent, MCN 15(1):16-23, 1990.

Pederson, C.J., and Anderson, J.M.: Factors that impact data collection from children, Cancer Nurs. 3(6):439-444, 1980.

Perlman, N., and Abramovitch, R.: Visit to the pediatrician: children's concerns, J. Pediatr. 110(6):988-990, 1987.

Pontious, S.L.: Practical Piaget: helping children understand, Am. J. Nurs. 82(1):114-117, 1982.

Rollins, J.: Childhood cancer: siblings draw and tell, Pediatr. Nurs. 16(1):21-27, 1990.

Sabbeth, B.: Trial balloons: when families of ill children express needs in veiled ways, Child. Health Care 17(2):87-92, 1988.

Smith, J., and Felice, M.: Interviewing adolescent patients: some guidelines for the clinician, Pediatr. Ann. 9:238-243, 1980.

Stickler, G.: Clinical guidelines for the pediatrician, Pediatrics 80(1):118-120, 1987.

Tiedman, M., Simon, K., and Clatworthy, S.: Communicating through therapeutic play. In Craft, M., and Denehy, J., editors: Nursing interventions for infants and children, Philadelphia, 1990, W.B. Saunders Co.

Walker, C.: Use of art and play therapy in pediatric oncology, J. Pediatr. Oncol. Nurs. 6(4):121-126, 1989.

Younger, J.: Literary works as a mode of knowing, Image 22(1):39-43, 1990.

Family Assessment

Allmond, B., Buckman, W., and Gofman, H.: The family is the patient: an approach to behavioral pediatrics for the clinician, St. Louis, 1979, Mosby–Year Book, Inc.

Beavers, W., Hampson, R., and Hulgus, Y.: Commentary: the Beavers systems approach to family assessment, Fam. Process 24:398, 1985.

Bradley, R., and Caldwell, B.: Using the home inventory to assess the family environment, Pediatr. Nurs. 14(2):97-103, 1988.

Calloway, S.: Home Observation for Measurement of the Environment. In Humenick, S., editor: Analysis of current assessment strategies in the health care of young children and childbearing families, Norwalk, CT, 1982, Appleton-Century-Crofts.

Clark, M., Frankel, M., and Trowbridge, D.: A pedigree primer, J. Pediatr. Nurs. 4(2):112-118, 1989.

Gilliss, C., and others: Toward a science of family nursing, Menlo Park, CA, 1989, Addison-Wesley Publishing Co., Inc.

Jolly, W., Froom, J., and Rosen, M.G.: The genogram, J. Fam. Pract. 10:251-255, 1980.

Lapp, C., Diemert, C., and Enestvedt, R.: Family-based practice: discussion of a tool merging assessment with intervention, Fam. Community Health 12(4):21-28, 1990.

Lewis, J.M.: How's your family? New York, 1979, Brunner/Mazel, Inc.

Lipman, T.: Assessing family strengths to guide plan of care using Hymovich's framework, J. Pediatr. Nurs. 4(3):186-196, 1989.

Martinson, I.: The challenge of culturally diverse pediatric clients, Pediatric Nursing: Forum on the future: looking toward the 21st century. Pitman, NJ, 1989, Anthony J. Jannetti, Inc.

McCubbin, H., and McCubbin, M.: Family system assessment in health care. In McCubbin, H., and Thompson, A., editors: Family assessment inventories for research and practice, Madison, WI, 1987, The University of Wisconsin–Madison.

Roberts, C., and Feetham, S.: Assessing family functioning across three areas of relationships, Nurs. Res. 31(4):321-325, 1982.

Rogers, J., and Durkin, M.: The semi-structured genogram interview. I. Protocol, II. Evaluation. Fam. Systems Med. 2(2):176-187, 1984.

Whall, A.L.: Nursing theory and the assessment of families, J. Psychiatr. Nurs. 19(1):30-36, 1981.

Wright, L., and Leahey, M.: Nurses and families: a guide to family assessment and intervention, Philadelphia, 1984, F.A. Davis Co.

Nutritional Assessment

American Academy of Pediatrics, Committee on Nutrition: Assessment of nutritional status. In Pediatric nutrition handbook, ed. 2, Elk Grove Village, IL, 1985, The Academy.

Benjamin, D.: Laboratory tests and nutritional assessment: protein-energy status, Pediatr. Clin. North Am. 36(1):139-161, 1989.

Hinson, L.: Nutritional assessment and management of the hospitalized patient, Crit. Care Nurs. 5:53-60, 1985.

Mahan, L.K., and Rees, J.M.: Nutrition in adolescence, St. Louis, 1984, Mosby–Year Book, Inc.

Pipes, P.L.: Nutrition in infancy and childhood, ed. 4, St. Louis, 1989, Mosby–Year Book, Inc.

Simko, M., Cowell, C., and Hreha, M.: Practical nutrition: a quick reference for the health care practitioner, Rockville, MD, 1989, Aspen Publishers, Inc.

Solomons, N.W.: Assessment of nutritional status: functional indicators of pediatric nutriture, Pediatr. Clin. North Am. 32(2):319-334, 1985.

Stuff, J.E., and others: A comparison of dietary methods in nutritional studies, Am. J. Clin. Nutr. 37:300-306, 1983.

Todd, K.S., Hudes, M., and Calloway, D.H.: Food intake measurement: problems and approaches, Am. J. Clin. Nutr. 37:139-146, 1983.

CHAPTER 7

Physical and Developmental Assessment of the Child

RELATED TOPICS

Anthropometry, Ch. 6
Assessment of cardiac function, Ch. 34
Biologic development: adolescent, Ch. 19
Dental disorders, Ch. 18
Disorders affecting the skin, Ch. 18
Growth and development, Ch. 4
The gynecologic examination, Ch. 20
History-taking, Ch. 6
Hearing impairment; vision impairment, Ch. 25
Physical assessment: newborn, Ch. 8
Preparation for procedures, Ch. 27
Sexually transmitted diseases, Ch. 20
Systemic hypertension, Ch. 34

GLOSSARY

AI Apical impulse; most lateral cardiac impulse
anterior or ventral Nearer the front of the body
auricle Pertaining to the ear
auscultation Listening for sounds produced by the body
DD Disc diameter
DDST-R Denver Developmental Screening Test (Revised)
fundus Back of the eyeball
ICS Intercostal space
lateral Toward the side of the body
MCL Midclavicular line
medial Nearer the middle of the body
NCHS National Center for Health Statistics
ophthalmoscope Instrument used to view the interior of the eye
optic or ophthalmic Pertaining to the eye
otic Pertaining to the ear
otoscope Instrument used to view the interior of the ear
palpation Use of touch to detect superficial and deeper structures of the skin
percussion Striking or tapping the body surface to produce sounds
PERRLA Pupils equal, round, react to light, and accommodation
PMI Point of maximum intensity
posterior or dorsal Nearer the back of the body
recumbent length Refers to length measured supine
R-PDQ Revised Denver Prescreening Developmental Questionnaire
sphygmomanometer Instrument used for measuring blood pressure
stature Refers to standing height
transverse Crosswise
tympanic membrane Eardrum

Physical and developmental assessment is a continuous process that begins during the interview, primarily through inspection or observation, and continues to some degree throughout the professional relationship. Although the assessment resembles that of a medical physical examination, the objective of each assessment area is to formulate nursing diagnoses and evaluate the effectiveness of interventions.

This chapter discusses the influence of age on the preparation of children for physical examination, the tools used for assessment of health status, the performance of the examination, and methods of developmental assessment.

GENERAL CONCEPTS OF PEDIATRIC PHYSICAL ASSESSMENT

The physical examination is more than a series of technical maneuvers. It demands the same sensitivity to the child's physical and psychologic needs as any other strange and unfamiliar experience. This discussion is concerned with the recommended schedule for health supervision, the sequence of the assessment process, and the preparation of the child for the examination.

RECOMMENDATIONS FOR HEALTH SUPERVISION

The objectives of pediatric health supervision are maintenance of optimum wellness and prevention of illness. The concept of prevention necessitates an orderly and routine schedule of activities—of which physical examination plays an essential role—that are aimed at meeting these two objectives. The American Academy of Pediatrics recommends the schedule shown in Box 7-1 for the care of well children who receive competent parenting and who have no serious health problems. Circumstances that may indicate the need for additional visits or procedures include families of diverse socioeconomic and cultural backgrounds, especially those with foreign-born adopted children (Jenista and Chapman, 1987) or foster children (American Academy of Pediatrics, 1987); one-parent families; or those with children who have chronic illnesses or disabilities.

Box 7-1 RECOMMENDATIONS FOR HEALTH SUPERVISION

	INFANCY						EARLY CHILDHOOD					LATE CHILDHOOD					ADOLESCENCE[1]			
AGE[2]	By 1 mo.	2 mos.	4 mos.	6 mos.	9 mos.	12 mos.	15 mos.	18 mos.	24 mos.	3 yrs.	4 yrs.	5 yrs.	6 yrs.	8 yrs.	10 yrs.	12 yrs.	14 yrs.	16 yrs.	18 yrs.	20+ yrs.
HISTORY Initial/Interval	●	●	●	●	●	●	●	●	●	●	●	●	●	●	●	●	●	●	●	●
MEASUREMENTS Height and Weight	●	●	●	●	●	●	●	●	●	●	●	●	●	●	●	●	●	●	●	●
Head Circumference	●	●	●	●	●	●														
Blood Pressure										●	●	●	●	●	●	●	●	●	●	●
SENSORY SCREENING Vision	S	S	S	S	S	S	S	S	S	S	○	○	○	○	S	○	○	S	○	○
Hearing	S	S	S	S	S	S	S	S	S	S	○	○	S[3]	S[3]	S[3]	○	S	S	○	S
DEVEL./BEHAV.[4] ASSESSMENT	●	●	●	●	●	●	●	●	●	●	●	●	●	●	●	●	●	●	●	●
PHYSICAL EXAMINATION[5]	●	●	●	●	●	●	●	●	●	●	●	●	●	●	●	●	●	●	●	●
PROCEDURES[6] Hered./Metabolic[7] Screening	●																			
Immunization[8]		●	●	●			●	●	●			●					●			
Tuberculin Test[9]	←					●→	←		●		→						←		●	→
Hematocrit or Hemoglobin[10]	←				●	→	←		●		→	←		●		→	←		●	→
Urinalysis[11]	←			●		→	←		●		→	←		●		→	←		●	→
ANTICIPATORY[12] GUIDANCE	●	●	●	●	●	●	●	●	●	●	●	●	●	●	●	●	●	●	●	●
INITIAL DENTAL[13] REFERRAL										●										

1. Adolescent-related issues (e.g., psychosocial emotional, substance usage, and reproductive health) may necessitate more frequent health supervision.
2. If a child comes under care for the first time at any point on the schedule, or if any items are not accomplished at the suggested age, the schedule should be brought up to date at the earliest time.
3. At these points, history may suffice: if problem suggested, a standard testing method should be employed.
4. By history and appropriate physical examination: if suspicious, by specific objective development testing.
5. At each visit, a complete physical examination is essential, with infant totally unclothed, older child undressed and suitably draped.
6. These may be modified, depending upon entry point into schedule and individual need.
7. Metabolic screening (e.g., thyroid, phenylketonuria, galactosemia) should be done according to state law.
8. Schedule(s) per Report of Committee on Infectious Disease, *1986 Red Book.**
9. For low-risk groups, the Committee on Infectious Diseases recommends the following options: (1) no routine testing or (2) testing at three times—infancy, preschool, and adolescence. For high-risk groups, annual TB skin testing is recommended.
10. Present medical evidence suggests the need for reevaluation of the frequency and timing of hemoglobin or hematocrit tests. One determination is therefore suggested during each time period. Performance of additional tests is left to the individual practice experience.
11. Present medical evidence suggests the need for reevaluation of the frequency and timing of urinalyses. One determination is therefore suggested during each time period. Performance of additional tests is left to the individual practice experience.
12. Appropriate discussion and counseling should be an integral part of each visit for care.
13. Subsequent examinations as prescribed by dentist.

From Committee on Psychosocial Aspects of Child and Family Health, 1985-1988: Guidelines for health supervision II, 1987, Elk Grove Village, IL, American Academy of Pediatrics.

Note: Special chemical, immunologic, and endocrine testing are usually carried out upon specific indications. Testing other than newborn (e.g., inborn errors of metabolism, sickle disease, lead) are discretionary with the physician.

***Author's note:** For more current recommendations see Immunizations, Chapter 12.

The services required by each child must be individualized by the practitioner. Nurses should look for opportunities to review children's previous schedules of health care and institute specific measures or referrals to update the health record. For example, during hospitalization children's overall record should be reviewed to ensure that they have had sensory screening, appropriate immunizations, and a yearly dental examination.

SEQUENCE OF THE EXAMINATION

Ordinarily the examining sequence follows a head-to-toe direction to provide a general guideline for assessment of each body area in order to minimize omitting segments of the examination. The typical organization of a physical examination is listed in the chapter outline.

In examining children, this orderly sequence is frequently altered to accommodate the child's developmental needs, although written recording follows the traditional model. Using developmental and chronologic age as the main criteria for assessing each body system accomplishes several goals:

1. Minimizes stress and anxiety associated with assessment of various body parts
2. Fosters a trusting nurse-child-parent relationship
3. Allows for maximum preparation of the child
4. Preserves the essential security of the parent-child relationship, especially with young children
5. Maximizes the accuracy and reliability of assessment findings.

PREPARATION OF THE CHILD

While the physical examination consists of painless procedures, to a child the use of a tight arm cuff, probes in ears and mouth, pressing on the abdomen, and listening to the

Box 7-2 GENERAL GUIDELINES FOR PERFORMING PEDIATRIC PHYSICAL EXAMINATION

- Perform examination in appropriate, nonthreatening area.
  - Have room well lit and decorated with neutral colors.
  - Have room temperature comfortably warm.
  - Place all strange and potentially frightening equipment out of sight.
  - Have some toys, dolls, stuffed animals, and games available for the child.
  - If possible, have rooms decorated and equipped for different-age children.
  - Provide privacy, especially for school-age children and adolescents.
- Provide time for play and becoming acquainted.
- Observe behaviors that signal child's readiness to cooperate:
  - Talking to the nurse
  - Making eye contact
  - Accepting the offered equipment
  - Allowing physical touching
  - Choosing to sit on examining table rather than parent's lap
- If signs of readiness are not observed, use the following techniques:
  - Talk to parent while essentially "ignoring" child; gradually focus on child or a favorite object, such as a doll.
  - Make complimentary remarks about the child, such as appearance, dress, or a favorite object.
  - Tell a funny story or play a simple magic trick.
  - Have a nonthreatening "friend" available, such as a hand puppet to "talk" to child for the nurse (see Fig. 7-33, *A*)
- If child refuses to cooperate, use the following techniques:
  - Assess reason for uncooperative behavior; consider that a child who is unduly afraid may have had a previous traumatic experience.
  - Try to involve child and parent in process.
  - Avoid prolonged explanations about examining procedure.
  - Use a firm, direct approach regarding expected behavior.
  - Perform examination as quickly as possible.
  - Have attendant gently restrain child.
  - Minimize any disruptions or stimulation.
    - Limit number of people in room.
    - Use isolated room.
    - Use quiet, calm, confident voice.
- Begin the examination in a nonthreatening manner for young children or children who are fearful:
  - Use those activities that can be presented as games, such as test for cranial nerves (see Table 7-18) or parts of developmental screening tests (p. 288).
  - Use approaches such as "Simon says" to encourage child to make a face, squeeze a hand, stand on one foot, and so on.
  - Use the "paper-doll" technique.
    - Lay child supine on an examining table or floor that is covered with a large sheet of paper.
    - Trace around child's body outline.
    - Use the body outline to demonstrate what will be examined, such as drawing a heart and listening with the stethoscope before performing the activity on the child.
- If several children in the family will be examined, begin with the most cooperative child to provide modeling of desired behavior.
- Involve child in the examination process:
  - Provide choices, such as sitting on the table or in the parent's lap.
  - Allow child to handle or hold equipment.
  - Encourage child to use equipment on a doll, family member, or examiner.
  - Explain each step of the procedure in simple language.
- Examine child in a comfortable and secure position:
  - Sitting in parent's lap
  - Sitting upright if in respiratory distress
- Proceed to examine the body in an organized sequence (usually head to toe) with the following exceptions:
  - Alter sequence to accommodate needs of different-age children (see Table 7-1).
  - Examine painful areas last.
  - In emergency situation, examine vital functions (airway, breathing, and circulation) and injured area first.
- Reassure child throughout examination, especially about bodily concerns that arise during puberty.
- Discuss the findings with the family at the end of the examination.
- Praise child for cooperation during examination; give reward such as small toy or sticker.

chest with a cold piece of metal can be considerably stressful. Therefore, the same considerations discussed in Chapter 27 for preparing children for procedures are followed here. In addition to that discussion, general guidelines related to the examining process are presented in Box 7-2. The physical examination should be as pleasant as possible, as well as educational. For example, with preschool and older children, the nurse can use a detailed drawing or anatomically correct doll* to help them learn about their bodies (Vessey, Braithwaite, and Weidmann, 1990). The "paper-doll" technique is a useful approach to teaching children about the part of the body that is being examined (Fig. 7-1). At the conclusion of the visit, the child can bring home the paper doll as a memento of the experience.

In most instances, children cooperate best when their parents remain with them. There are occasions, however, when older children, particularly adolescents, prefer to be examined alone, such as during the genital examination. Frequently, the child being examined is also accompanied by a sibling. The sibling can be disruptive because of boredom. A helpful tactic is to involve the sibling in the examination by allowing the child to hold the stethoscope or a tongue blade and praising the "help" during the assessment.

*Information about an anatomically correct doll (Jamie doll) is available from Judith A. Vessey, Ph.D., R.N.,C., University of California, San Francisco, Department of Family Health Care Nursing, N411Y, San Francisco, CA 94143-0605; (415) 476-4632.

Table 7-1 summarizes guidelines for positioning, preparing, and examining children at various ages. Since no child fits precisely into one age category, it may be necessary to vary the approach after a preliminary assessment of the child's developmental achievements and needs. Even when the best approach is used, many toddlers are uncooperative

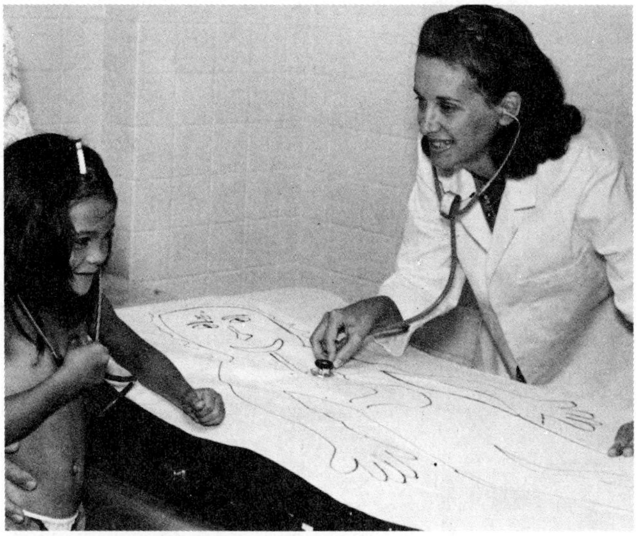

Fig. 7-1. Using paper-doll technique to prepare child for physical examination.

Table 7-1 Age-specific approaches to physical examination during childhood

AGE	POSITION	SEQUENCE	PREPARATION
Infant	Before sits alone: supine or prone, preferably in parent's lap; before 4 to 6 months: can place on examining table After sits alone: use sitting in parent's lap whenever possible If on table, place with parent in full view	If quiet, auscultate heart, lungs, abdomen Record heart and respiratory rates Palpate and percuss same areas Proceed in usual head-toe direction Perform traumatic procedures last (eyes, ears, mouth [while crying], rectal temperature [if taken]) Elicit reflexes as body part examined Elicit Moro reflex last	Completely undress if room temperature permits Leave diaper on male Gain cooperation with distraction, bright objects, rattles, talking Smile at infant; use soft, gentle voice Pacify with bottle of sugar water or feeding Enlist parent's aid for restraining to examine ears, mouth Avoid abrupt, jerky movements
Toddler	Sitting or standing on/by parent Prone or supine in parent's lap	Inspect body area through play: "count fingers," "tickle toes" Use minimal physical contact initially Introduce equipment slowly Auscultate, percuss, palpate whenever quiet Perform traumatic procedures last (same as for infant)	Have parent remove outer clothing Remove underwear as body part examined Allow to inspect equipment; demonstrating use of equipment usually ineffective If uncooperative, perform procedures quickly Use restraint when appropriate; request parent's assistance Talk about examination if cooperative; use short phrases Praise for cooperative behavior
Preschool child	Prefers standing or sitting Usually cooperative prone/supine Prefers parent's closeness	If cooperative, proceed in head-toe direction If uncooperative, proceed as with toddler	Request self-undressing Allow to wear underpants if shy Offer equipment for inspection; briefly demonstrate use (may demonstrate on parent)

Continued.

Table 7-1 Age-specific approaches to physical examination during childhood—cont'd

AGE	POSITION	SEQUENCE	PREPARATION
Preschool child—cont'd			Make up "story" about procedure: "I'm seeing how strong your muscles are" or "I am going to give your arm a hug with this special cloth" (blood pressure) Use paper-doll technique Give choices when possible Expect cooperation; use positive statements: "Open your mouth"
School-age child	Prefers sitting Cooperative in most positions Younger child prefers parent's presence Older child may prefer privacy	Proceed in head-toe direction May examine genitalia last in older child Respect need for privacy	Request self-undressing Allow to wear underpants Give gown to wear Explain purpose of equipment and significance of procedure, such as otoscope to see eardrum, which is necessary for hearing Teach about body functioning and care
Adolescent	Same as for school-age child Offer option of parent's presence	Same as older school-age child	Allow to undress in private Give gown Expose only area to be examined Respect need for privacy Explain findings during examination: "Your muscles are firm and strong" Matter-of-factly comment about sexual development: "Your breasts are developing as they should be" Emphasize normalcy of development Examine genitalia as any other body part; may leave to end May use mirror during examination of genitalia to allow youngster to view area examined about personal anatomy

and unable to be consoled for much of the physical examination. However, some seem intrigued by the new surroundings and unusual equipment and respond more like preschoolers than toddlers. Likewise, some early preschoolers may require more of the "security measures" employed with younger children, such as continued parent-child contact, and less of the preparatory measures used with preschoolers, such as playing with the equipment before and during the actual examination (Fig. 7-2).

Although the variations in the general approaches are numerous, some of them are elaborated here because they are more common. For example, the suggested sequence may change considerably when the child is in pain or when obvious physical defects are present. In either situation it is preferable to examine the affected area last to minimize distress early in the examination and to focus on normal, healthy, or functioning body parts.

Positioning may also be altered because of physical distress. For example, the child who is having difficulty breathing may not be able to lie down; thus as much of the physical examination as possible should be performed in a sitting or slightly reclining position, or the examination should be completed at another time.

ASSESSMENT SKILLS

The traditional four categories of assessment skills include inspection, palpation, percussion, and auscultation. Each involves a set of tools to facilitate its performance, usefulness, and accuracy. Although the trend has been to incorporate more specialized and technical equipment into nursing assessment, the nurse is equipped with all of the tools necessary for a fairly comprehensive and detailed physical examination. The use of sight, smell, hearing, and sometimes taste are necessary for inspection. The hands and fingers are the main tools of palpation and percussion, and the ear can be used for auscultation. Although several specific instruments refine the examination, few of them can replace the human tools of skill, knowledge, and interpretation.

Inspection

Inspection is the most valuable, least mechanical, and most difficult skill to learn. It involves the use of the senses, primarily vision, to make judgments, comparisons, and decisions. Because inspection is a highly subjective process, it requires skill, repetition, and practice to establish reliable findings for distinguishing among ranges of normal, borderline, and abnormal.

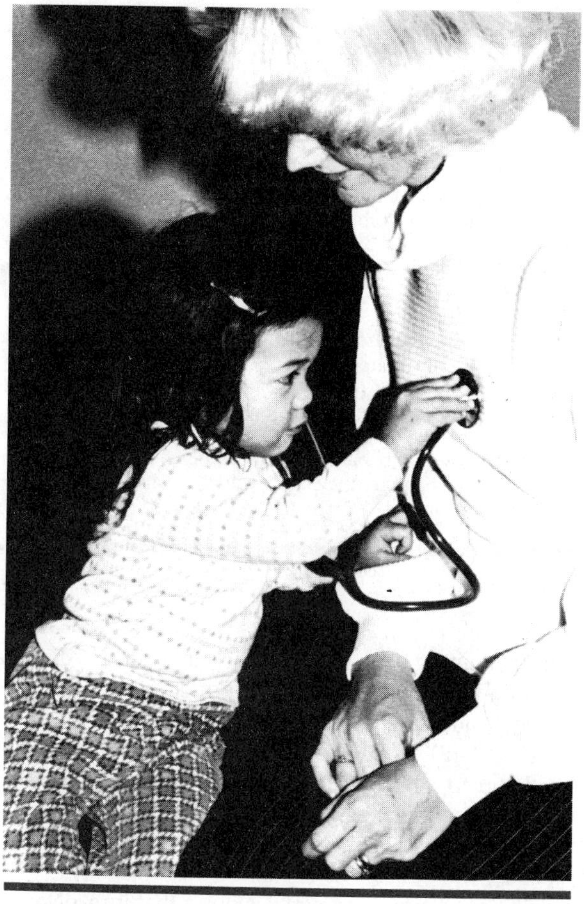

Fig. 7-2. Preparing child for physical examination.

Methods of inspection. One of the keys to competent inspection is the conscious, systematic, and active use of the senses. As each body part is examined, the visible areas are deliberately inspected for color, texture, firmness, hygiene, masses, hair distribution, tone, movement, behavior, tension, flaccidity, symmetry, location, position, and temperature. As each of these aspects is observed, it is compared with normal anatomy and physiology. Although the objective is not to "diagnose" an abnormality by labeling it as a specific disorder, defect, or disease, it is the nurse's responsibility to recognize and record any deviation from expected findings.

Inspection may be combined with specific instruments for better visualization, such as the otoscope for the ear (p. 256), and with measurements to validate subjective impressions. For example, the nurse may observe that the child appears thin; this impression is substantiated by recording height and weight on a growth chart, comparing the values, and judging those measurements in terms of genetic background, previous growth trends, physical status, and nutritional intake. After establishing a thorough data base, the nurse then proceeds to draw conclusions and formulate nursing diagnoses.

Frequently competent inspection involves intangible skills for which no yardstick exists. The most common example relates to measuring the emotional state or behavior. An experienced nurse may look at a child and suspect a health problem without any further assessment. Often, however, the nurse is unable to state specifically what behaviors have led to that conclusion. One way of developing assessment skills is to consciously analyze behaviors, such as appearance, movement, relationships, activity, verbal interaction, mood, and orientation, and to record what is observed, not what is interpreted. For example, a *factual* statement is, "An 11-year-old Oriental male, color is pale, moves slowly, holds right lower quadrant of abdomen, occasional facial grimaces, answers questions slowly and briefly." An *interpretative* statement is, "An 11-year-old Oriental male in distress, pain in lower right abdomen, and refuses to talk." Interpretative statements are much more liable to erroneous or altered interpretations by others than factual statements, which describe what is observed.

Palpation

Palpation is primarily the use of touch or the tactile sense to detect both superficial and deeper characteristics of the body. It is combined with inspection, since in many instances it validates a visual impression, such as texture of the skin. Palpation uses touch to assess temperature, position, form, size, consistency, moisture, and movement, such as vibration or pulsation. It is used to examine all accessible parts of the body, such as organs, glands, blood vessels, bones, muscles, hair, skin, and mucosa. A thorough knowledge of anatomy is essential in differentiating palpation of normal body structures from abnormal ones, such as masses.

Methods of palpation. Palpation involves the use of the fingers and hands for superficial and deep examination of body parts (Box 7-3). When deeper organs are palpated, particularly those in the abdomen, a *bimanual maneuver* may be used. One hand is placed on the abdomen, and the other hand applies pressure to the first hand. Palpation is done with the cushions and palmar surfaces of the contact hand, not with the fingernails (which should be kept short and trimmed). In small children the distal palmar surfaces of the fingers are directly applied to the skin, and the other hand may or may not be used to apply pressure to the contact hand. Frequently the nonpalpating hand is placed against the child's back directly underneath the area to be

Box 7-3 METHODS OF PALPATION

Fingertips—for small areas, such as the neck for lymph glands or the infant's skull for fontanels, or when fine tactile discriminations are made, such as texture of the skin

Fingertips and dorsa (backs) of the hands—for temperature differences

Palmar surfaces of the fingers and hand—for detecting vibration, such as heart thrills or the point of maximum impulse of the heart on the chest wall

Grasping action of the fingers—to evaluate consistency, position, and size of organs or masses

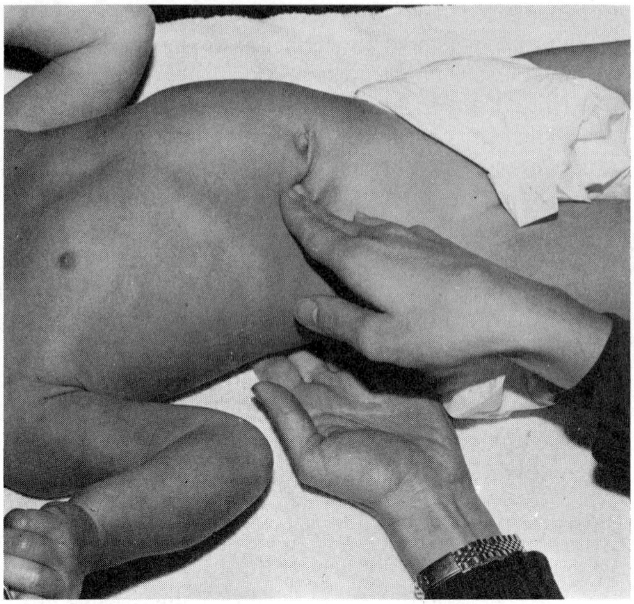

Fig. 7-3. Bimanual palpation.

Box 7-4 GUIDELINES FOR PROMOTING RELAXATION

Position the child comfortably, such as in a semireclining position in the parent's lap, with the knees flexed.
Warm the hands before touching the skin.
Use distraction, such as telling stories or talking to the child.
Teach the child to use deep breathing and to concentrate on an object.
Give the infant a bottle or pacifier.
Begin with light, superficial palpation and gradually progress to deeper palpation.
Palpate any tender or painful areas last.
Have the child hold the parent's hand and squeeze it if the palpation is uncomfortable.
Use the nonpalpating hand to comfort the child, such as placing the free hand on the child's shoulder while palpating the abdomen.

palpated. In this way the organ is "caught" or felt between both hands (Fig. 7-3). Bilateral and symmetric palpation is performed to compare the findings on one side of the body with those on the other side.

For any type of palpation to be effective, but especially for deep palpation of internal organs, the child must be relaxed; otherwise the tense muscles act like a wall between the hand and the organ. Guidelines for helping the child relax are presented in Box 7-4.

Percussion

Percussion is the striking or tapping of the body surface to produce sounds that correlate with the type of underlying tissue density. The principles of percussion are the same as those used to produce sounds in a musical instrument, such as the drum. For example, hollow, air-filled spaces, such as the lungs, create a low-pitched, well-sustained note called *resonance.* Dense, solid objects, such as organs or masses, create a high-pitched, short, thudding sound called *dullness.* Percussion sounds are described in terms of *tones* and *notes* (Table 7-2). Because sounds are difficult to describe in words, practice in percussing different areas of the body and comparing the emitted sounds is fundamental to developing skill and competence.

Methods of percussion. Techniques for percussion may be direct or indirect. *Direct* percussion is striking or tapping the body surface directly with the finger (Fig. 7-4, *A*). It is useful for percussing well-defined areas, such as a bone or the borders of an organ. It is also advantageous for greater accuracy when examining infants or small children, where body organs are in proximity.

In the *indirect* method the tapping is performed by striking a stationary finger positioned on the body. Some practitioners prefer this method because there is less perception by the patient of being hit or struck than in the direct approach. Indirect percussion is performed by (1) placing the index or middle finger against the body area to be percussed and (2) using the tip of the middle finger of the other hand to strike the base of the distal phalanx of the nonpercussing finger (Fig. 7-4, *B*).

Auscultation

Auscultation is similar to percussion in that it involves evaluation of body sounds. It differs in that it concerns those sounds produced by the body, such as sounds arising from the heart, lungs, and abdomen. The characteristics of auscultatory sounds are the same as those used to describe percussion tones, that is, intensity, pitch, duration, and quality (see Table 7-2).

Methods of auscultation and types of stethoscopes. As with percussion, the direct or indirect method of listening for sounds can be used. In the *direct* method the examiner's ear is applied directly to the body surface. In some instances loud sounds, such as grade VI murmurs or expiratory wheezes, can be heard by placing the ear close to the child, but not directly against the skin. The direct approach has disadvantages in terms of patient modesty, aversion to skin-to-skin contact, or possible infection to the examiner from skin lesions.

Indirect auscultation involves the use of a stethoscope to transmit internal body sounds to the ear. The main types of stethoscopes are the open bell and the closed diaphragm. The *open-bell,* or *Ford, chestpiece* consists of a short cone or funnel-shaped horn joined to a binaural headset and eartips with flexible tubing. It has the advantage of conducting sounds with virtually no distortion of pitch and is better for the perception of certain low-pitched sounds, such as diastolic murmurs. However, it must be placed firmly against the body surface for an airtight seal. Normally the diameter of the bell does not exceed 2.5 cm (1 inch). A larger-width bell would not permit a tight seal on bony or small sur-

Table 7-2 Definition of percussion sounds

PERCUSSION SOURCE	EXAMPLES
▪ Tones*	
Intensity—amplitude or loudness of tone	Loud tones—produced by more hollow, air-filled spaces, such as the lungs Soft tones—produced by more dense or solid masses, such as the heart
Pitch—frequency or number of vibrations per second; the greater the number of vibrations, the higher the pitch; the fewer the number, the lower the pitch	Low-pitched—air-filled lungs High-pitched—consolidated lung
Duration—time period of vibrations and length of time the sound lasts	Long duration—normal lungs Short duration—high-density organ, such as the heart
Quality of timbre—subjective evaluation that depends on the source of the sound	The same musical note from two different instruments produces a different quality or timbre of sound; for example, sounds of equal loudness and pitch from different organs, such as the lungs and heart, produce sounds of varying quality
▪ Notes	
Resonance—clear hollow note, low pitch, long duration, relatively loud (heard with ease)	Normal lungs
Tympany—clear hollow note, higher pitched than resonance, musical with rich overtones (quality), long duration	Tympanic sound can be produced by lightly tapping an air-filled cheek with the finger; similar sound when percussing an air-filled stomach
Hyperresonance—cross between resonance and tympany; lower pitch than normal resonance, high intensity, and long duration	Usually indicates less density, such as increased amount of air or decreased amount of tissue; usually pathologic, such as pneumothorax or asthma
Dullness—high-pitched, short duration, soft (low intensity), and thudding	Related to increased density and solidity, such as the heart
Flatness—absolute dullness, high-pitched, very short, nonmusical in quality	Solid tissue, such as the thigh

*These same terms are used to describe any sound and are used in physical assessment to record auscultatory sounds.

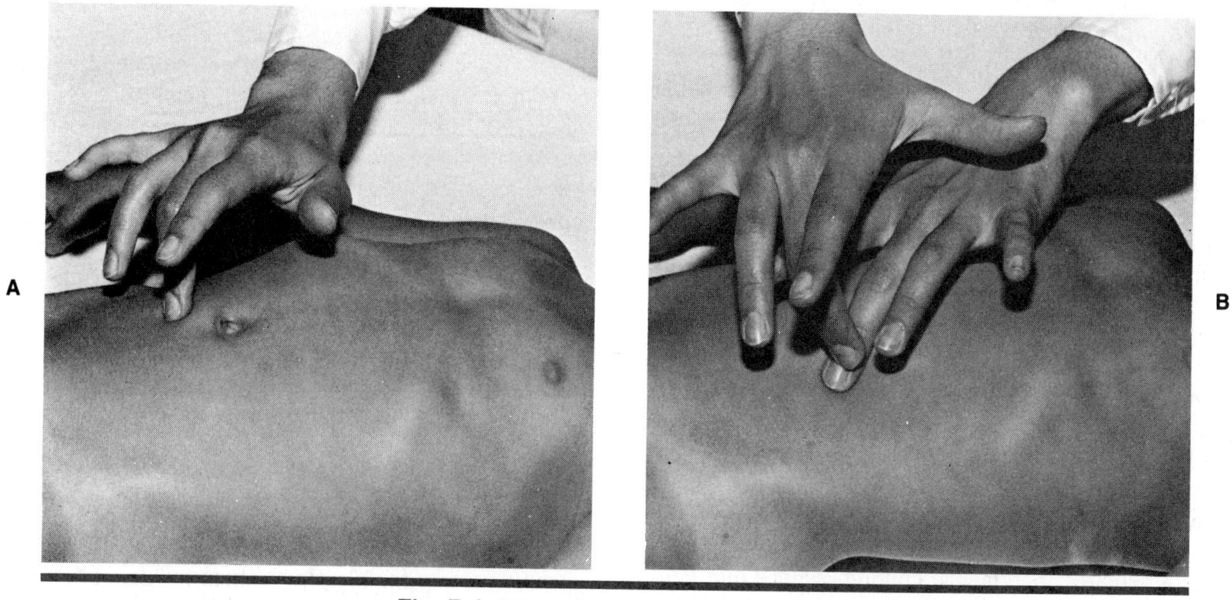

Fig. 7-4. Percussion. **A,** Direct. **B,** Indirect.

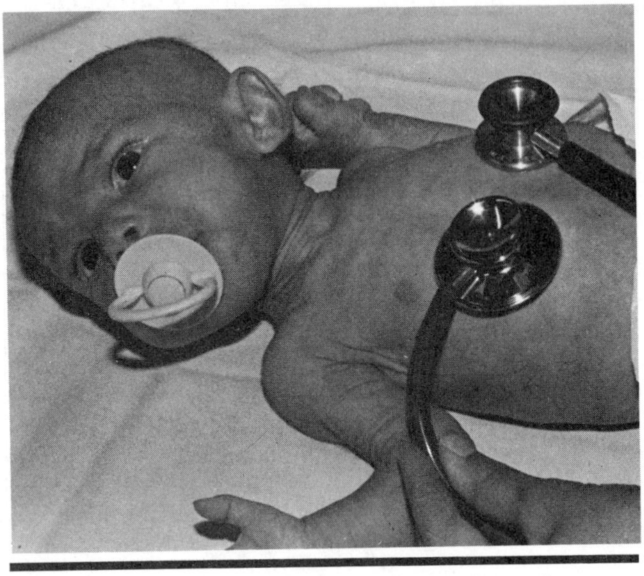

Fig. 7-5. Comparison of pediatric and adult-size stethoscopes on infant's chest. Closed-diaphragm chestpiece is against skin and open-bell chestpiece is facing upward.

faces, thus resulting in admittance of ambient sounds. This restriction in size limits the volume of sound it can accumulate.

The larger, flatter, and less bulky *closed-diaphragm*, or *Bowles, chestpiece* is sealed by its own diaphragm. These features afford it several advantages. Its larger diaphragm admits a greater quantity of sound and is more sensitive to high-pitched sounds. The diaphragm filters out low-frequency vibrations, so that sounds appear to be of higher pitch than when heard through the bell. The self-sealing diaphragm obviates the need for an airtight skin seal, so that a larger diaphragm is still accurate when placed on a bony or small chest. However, a close-fitting seal is still recommended in order to decrease the admittance of environmental sounds. In infants and small children, especially premature infants, the use of a specially sized pediatric diaphragm is recommended both to achieve sufficient skin contact and to localize sounds in segmented areas of the chest (Fig. 7-5).

Using the stethoscope properly involves knowledge of how it works and factors that interfere with its performance. As with percussion, skill requires considerable practice, particularly in listening to normal body sounds. Although descriptions of auscultatory sounds are discussed in examination of the specific body system, general guidelines for effective auscultation are described in Box 7-5.

Auscultation, like inspection, requires the mental discipline of concentrating on one aspect of many simultaneous stimuli. The nurse must consciously listen for one sound, such as breathing, while deliberately disregarding other sounds, such as the heartbeat or environmental noises. This is particularly important in children, whose thin chest wall effectively transmits sounds throughout the thoracic cavity. Because accurate auscultation requires additional time for the beginning practitioner, it is always thoughtful to explain to parents or older children why one is listening for so long, in order to allay their fears that some abnormality is suspected.

Box 7-5 GUIDELINES FOR EFFECTIVE AUSCULTATION

Make sure the child is relaxed and not crying, talking, or laughing.
Check that the room is a comfortable temperature and is quiet as possible.
Warm the stethoscope before placing it against the skin.
Apply firm pressure on the chestpiece but not enough to prevent vibrations and transmission of sound.
Avoid placing the stethoscope over hair or clothing, moving it against the skin, breathing on the tubing, or sliding fingers over the chestpiece, which may cause sounds that falsely resemble pathologic findings.
Use a symmetric and orderly approach to compare sounds.

PHYSICAL EXAMINATION

Although the approach to and sequence of the physical examination differ according to the child's age, the following discussion outlines the traditional model for physical assessment. It emphasizes normal findings, variations from the norm that may cause parents or children concern but that require little or no intervention, and abnormalities that necessitate appropriate referral. Although the focus includes all pediatric age-groups, the reader is referred to Chapter 8 for a detailed discussion of a newborn assessment for procedures and findings unique to the neonate.

GROWTH MEASUREMENTS

Measurement of physical growth in children is a key element in evaluation of the health status of children. Physical growth parameters include weight, height (length), skinfold thickness, arm circumference, and head circumference. Values for these growth parameters are plotted on percentile charts, and the child's measurements in percentiles are compared with those of the general population.

The most commonly used growth charts in the United States are from the National Center for Health Statistics (NCHS) and are available for boys and girls ages (see Appendix C):

1. **Birth to 36 months**—records weight by age, recumbent length by age, weight for length, and head circumference by age
2. **Two to 18 years**—records weight by age, stature by age
3. **Prepubescence**—records weight for stature

✦NURSING ALERT The prepubescent charts are only appropriate for plotting values for prepubescent boys and girls, regardless of chronologic age, and not for any child showing signs of pubescence, such as breast budding, testicular enlargement, or growth of axillary or pubic hair.

Two sets of charts include data for children 2 to 3 years; the major difference between the two charts is that one set (birth to 36 months) is based on recumbent length, and the other set (2 to 18 years) uses stature (standing height). These two methods of measuring length are not equivalent. Measurements using recumbent length are greater by as much as 2 cm, or nearly 1 inch, in this age-group than measurements obtained using stature. This amount of difference between measurements can lead to an erroneous conclusion of delayed growth if length is plotted during one visit and stature during the next visit on the birth to 36-month chart.

NURSING ALERT Plot only recumbent length on the birth to 36-month NCHS growth charts and stature on the 2- to 18-year growth charts.

The NCHS growth charts use the 5th and 95th percentiles as criteria for determining which children are outside the normal limits for growth. In general, those whose height or weight falls below the 5th percentile are considered underweight or small in stature; those whose measurements are above the 95th percentile are considered overweight or large in stature. The use of the NCHS growth charts for children from different ethnic groups is discussed in Questions and Controversies.

Percentile charts for skinfold thickness and arm circumference are also available and may be used as reference data. However, they should not be considered standards or norms, because values between the 5th and 95th percentile are not ranges of normal.

Overall evaluation of growth requires judgment in interpretation of growth percentiles. Generally, children whose height or weight falls below the 5th percentile or above the 95th percentile should be followed closely. However, small or large size may be genetic (Fig. 7-6). Comparing children's growth trends with those of their parents is essential in evaluating adequate growth. Special charts are available for parent-specific adjustments for evaluation of the child's height (Himes and others, 1985). Breast-fed infants grow

QUESTIONS AND CONTROVERSIES

How accurate are the United States growth charts for evaluating the growth of children from different ethnic and socioeconomic backgrounds?

A study by Habicht and others (1974) showed that differences in height and weight among well-nourished preschool children of different ethnic backgrounds were relatively small (3% for height and about 6% for weight), but the differences between these children and those of a poorer socioeconomic level, regardless of ethnic background, were high (about 12% for height and 30% for weight). A more recent study found that 72% of elementary-age Indochinese refugee children fell below the 10th percentile for weight for age and height for age on the United States (NCHS) growth charts. However, when weight for stature was compared, the results were within the normal range (Pickwell, 1982). Growth of Mexican-American children has also been found to be less than that of the reference population used for the NCHS growth charts. Mexican-American adolescents are short in stature according to the chart (Martorell, Mendoza, and Castillo, 1989). However, whether the differences for these groups are the result of nutritional factors or genetic background is still unclear.

Such findings indicate that the present United States growth charts can serve as a *reference guide* for all racial or ethnic groups if used from the perspective that different groups of children have varying normal distributions on the growth curves. For example, the average weight and height for Chinese children based on standards from China (see Appendix C) fall on the 10th percentile, not the 50th percentile, on the NCHS growth charts. The NCHS charts can be used for United States black children because this group was included in the sample population (Moore and Roche, 1982).

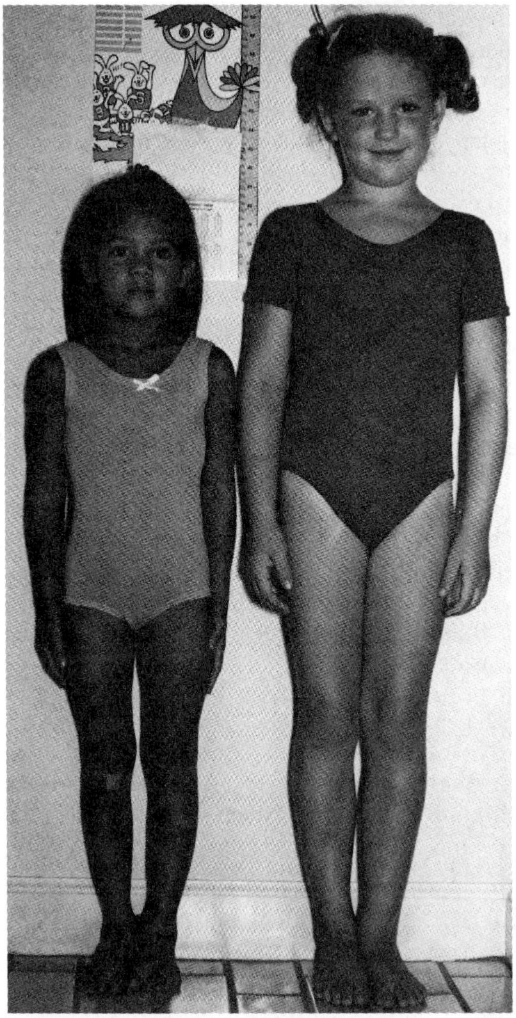

Fig. 7-6. These children of identical age (5¾ years) are markedly different in size. Child on left, of part Oriental descent, is at 5th percentile for height and weight. Child on right is above 95th percentile for height and weight. However, both children demonstrate normal growth patterns. (For growth measurements of Chinese children, see Appendix C.)

slower than bottle-fed infants, especially during the second half of the first year. This slower growth is normal although it may be at or below the 5th percentile (Dewey and Others, 1989).

Other children whose growth may be questionable include:

1. Children whose height and weight percentiles are widely disparate, for example, height in the 10th percentile and weight in the 90th percentile, especially with above-average skinfold thickness
2. Children who fail to show the expected growth rates in height and weight, especially during the rapid growth periods of infancy and adolescence (Table 7-3)
3. Children who show a sudden increase, except during puberty, or decrease in a previously steady growth pattern
4. Since growth is a continuous but uneven process, the most reliable evaluation lies in comparison of growth measurements over a prolonged time.

Length

Length refers to measurements taken when children are lying down supine (also referred to as recumbent length). Until children are 24 months old (36 months if the birth to 36-month chart is used), recumbent length is measured. Because of the normally flexed position during infancy, measuring length requires full extension of the body by (1) holding the head in midline, (2) grasping the knees together gently, and (3) pushing down on the knees until the legs are fully extended and flat against the table. If a measuring board is used, the head is placed firmly at the top of the board and the heels of the feet are placed firmly against the footboard.

If such a measuring device is not available, length is measured by placing the child on a paper-covered surface, marking the end points of the top of the head and heel of the feet, and measuring between these two points (Fig. 7-7). For accurate measurement the writing utensil is held at a right angle to the table when the cephalic point is marked, and the feet are positioned with the toes pointing directly to the ceiling when the heel point is marked. Regardless of the method used, assistance in holding the child's head in midline is enlisted while the nurse extends the legs and takes the measurements.

Table 7-3 Expected growth rates at various ages

AGE	EXPECTED GROWTH RATE (IN CM/YEAR)
1 to 6 months	18-22
6 to 12 months	14-18
2nd year	11
3rd year	8
4th year	7
5th to 10th years	5-6

From Human growth and growth disorders: an update, South San Francisco, 1989, Genentech, Inc.

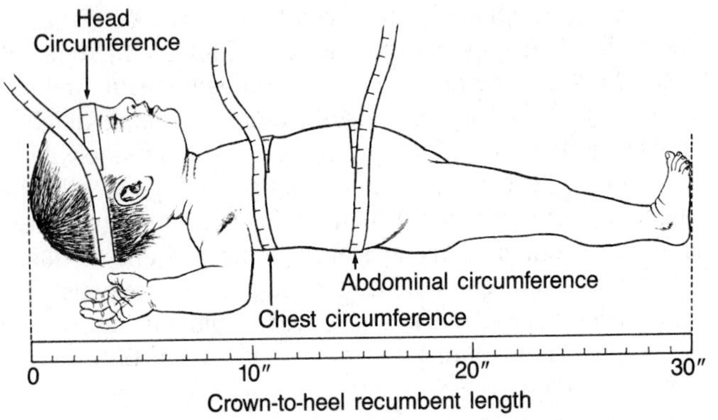

Fig. 7-7. Measurement of head, chest, and abdominal circumference and crown-to-heel (recumbent) length.

Height

Height refers to the measurement taken when children are standing upright (also referred to as stature). Height is measured by having the child, with shoes removed, stand as tall and straight as possible, with the head in midline and the line of vision parallel to the ceiling or floor. The child's back is to the wall or other vertical flat surface, with the heels, buttocks, and back of the shoulders touching the wall and the medial malleoli touching if possible (Fig. 7-8). Any flexion of the knees, slumping of the shoulders, or raising of the heels of the feet is checked and corrected (see Nursing Tip).

The vertical distance is measured by placing a firm, flat surface against the vertex or crown of the head. For the most accurate measurement, a wall-mounted unit (stadiometer) should be used. The movable measuring rod of platform scales is accurate only if it maintains a parallel position to the floor and rests securely on the topmost part of the crown. One way of improvising a flat surface for measuring length is to attach a paper or metal tape or yardstick to the wall, position the child adjacent to the tape, and place a three-dimensional object, such as a thick book or box, on top of the head. The side of the object must rest firmly against the wall to form a right angle. Length or stature is measured to the nearest 1 mm or ⅛ inch.

Occasionally special length measurements are taken, such as *sitting height* or *crown-to-rump length* (see General Measurements, Chapter 8, for the newborn). In older infants and children, sitting height is most easily determined by having the child sit against the wall and measuring between the vertex of the head and the sitting surface. Although not a usual measurement, this method is used for children sus-

NURSING TIP: MEASURING HEIGHT

Normally height is less if measured in the afternoon than in the morning. To minimize this variation, apply modest upward pressure under the jaw or the mastoid processes.

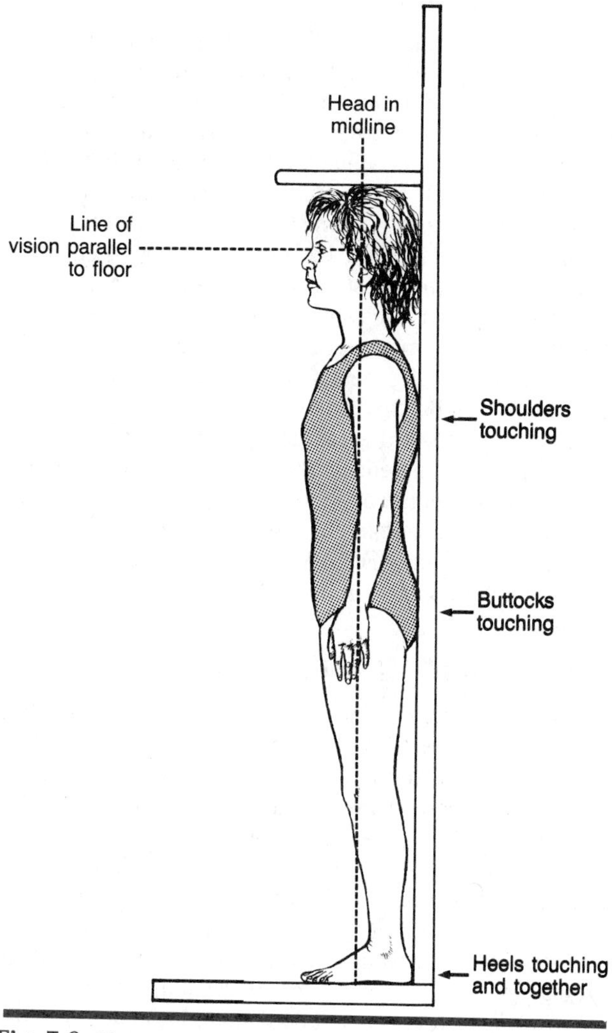

Fig. 7-8. Measurement of height.
Redrawn from Human growth and growth disorders: an update, South San Francisco, 1989, Genentech, Inc.

pected of being dwarfs to help distinguish true dwarfism from small stature. Normally sitting height accounts for 70% of total body length at birth, 60% at 2 years, and about 52% at age 10 years.

Weight

Weight is measured with an appropriately sized beam balance scale, which measures weights to the nearest 10 g or ½ ounce for infants and 100 g or ¼ pound for children. Before the child is weighed, the scale is balanced by setting it at zero and noting if the balance registers exactly in the middle of the mark. If the end of the balance beam rises to the top or bottom of the mark, more or less weight, respectively, is added. Some scales are designed to allow for self-correction, but others need to be recalibrated by the manufacturer. Scales vary in their accuracy; infant scales tend to be more accurate than adult platform scales, and newer scales more accurate than older ones, especially at the upper levels of weight measurement. When precise measurements are needed, two nurses should take the weight independently, and if there is a discrepancy, a third reading should be taken (Burke, Roberts, and Maloney, 1988).

A

B

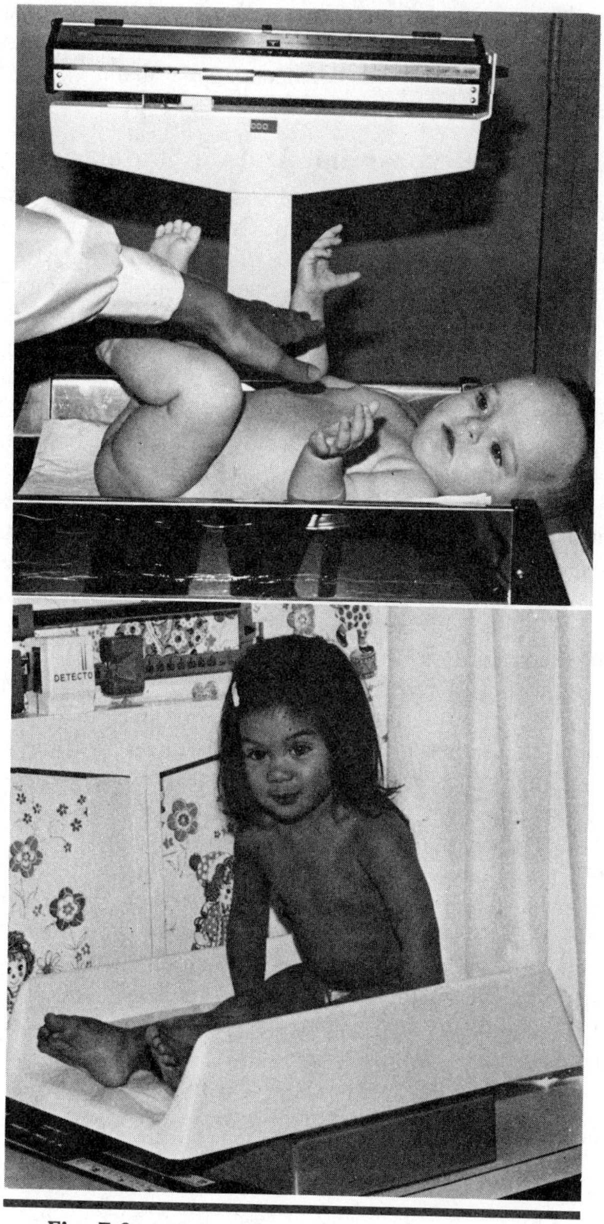

Fig. 7-9. A, Infant on scale. **B,** Toddler on scale.

Measurements are made in a comfortably warm room. When the birth to 36-months growth charts are used, children should be weighed nude. Older children are usually weighed while wearing their underpants or a light gown. However, with all children, the need for privacy is always respected. If the child must be weighed wearing some article of clothing or some type of special device, such as a prosthesis, this is noted when the weight is recorded. Children who are measured for recumbent length are usually weighed on a large platform type of infant scale and placed in a lying-down or sitting position. When weighing infants, the nurse places the hand lightly above the body to prevent them from accidentally falling off the scale (Fig. 7-9, *A*).

Once stature is taken, weight can also be measured on an upright platform scale. For maximum asepsis, either type of scale is covered with a clean sheet of paper that is changed between each child's measurement.

Skinfold Thickness and Arm Circumference

Measures of relative weight and stature cannot distinguish between adiposity or muscularity. One convenient measure of body fat is skinfold thickness, which is increasingly recommended as a routine measurement (see also Anthropometry, Chapter 6). Skinfold thickness is measured with special calipers, such as the Lange calipers. However, such instruments are costly and often are not available for general use. Plastic calipers, such as the Ross Adipometer,* have been shown to be an accurate substitute for the standard instruments (Jung and others, 1984; Ryan, 1985). The most common sites for measuring skinfold thickness are the triceps (most practical for routine clinical use), subscapula, suprailiac, abdomen, and upper thigh. For greatest reliability the exact procedure for measurement must be followed and the average of at least two measurements of one site recorded (Box 7-6).

Arm circumference is an indirect measure of muscle mass and is also recommended in the evaluation of nutritional status. Measurement of arm circumference follows the same procedure for skinfold thickness except the midpoint is measured with a paper or steel tape. For ease in locating the midpoint, a special tape is available (Inser-tape*) that has a midpoint mark of 0 and a centimeter scale beginning with 1 on either side of the 0. The tape is placed vertically along the posterior aspect of the upper arm until the same measurement appears at the acromial process and olecranon process; 0 is the midpoint. Percentiles for triceps skinfold and arm circumference in children are listed in Appendix C.

*Available from Ross Laboratories' local representative.

Box 7-6 GUIDELINES FOR MEASURING TRICEPS SKINFOLD THICKNESS

With child's right arm flexed 90 degrees at elbow, mark midpoint between acromion and olecranon on posterior aspect of arm.
With arm hanging freely, grasp a fold of skin between thumb and forefinger 1 cm above midpoint.
Gently pull fold away from underlying muscle and continue to hold until measurement is completed.
Place caliper jaws over skinfold at midpoint mark; if a plastic caliper (e.g., Ross Adipometer) is used, apply pressure with thumb to align lines on caliper; follow directions for using other calipers.
Estimate reading to nearest 1.0 mm, 2 to 3 seconds after applying pressure.
Take measurements until duplicates agree within 1 mm.

Head Circumference

Head circumference is usually measured in children up to 36 months of age and in any child whose head size is questionable. The head is measured at its greatest circumference, usually slightly above the eyebrows and pinna of the ears and around the occipital prominence at the back of the skull (see Fig. 7-7). Since head shape can affect the location of the maximum circumference, more than one measurement at points above the eyebrows may need to be taken to obtain the most accurate measure. A paper or metal tape is used because a cloth tape can stretch and give a falsely small measurement. For greatest accuracy, devices with tenths of a centimeter are used and recorded, since the percentile charts have only 0.5 cm increments.

The head size is plotted on the appropriate growth chart under head circumference. Generally, head and chest circumferences are equal at about 1 to 2 years of age. During childhood chest circumference exceeds head size by about 5 to 7 cm (2 to 3 in). (For newborns see General Measurements, Chapter 8.)

PHYSIOLOGIC MEASUREMENTS

Physiologic measurements, key elements in evaluating physical status of vital functions, include temperature, pulse, respiration, and blood pressure. Each physiologic recording is compared with normal values for that age-group (see inside front cover). In addition, the nurse compares the values taken on preceding health visits with present recordings. For example, a falsely elevated blood pressure reading may not indicate hypertension if previous recent readings have been within normal limits. The isolated recording may indicate some stressful event in the child's life.

As in most procedures carried out with children, older children and adolescents are treated much the same as are adults. Special consideration must be given to preschool children, whose fear of body mutilation is intensified with any intrusive procedure (see Development of Body Image, Chapter 15). Rectal temperatures are particularly threatening and should be avoided whenever possible.

For best results in taking vital signs of infants, the usual order of approach is reversed. Respirations are counted first, before the infant is disturbed, the pulse next, and temperature last. If vital signs cannot be taken without disturbing the child, the child's behavior (e.g., crying) is recorded with the measurement.

Temperature

Temperature can be measured at several sites in the body. Temperature measurement using a mercury thermometer is taken by the oral, rectal, or axillary route. The only difference in selection of thermometers is that the rectal type has a more rounded blunt bulb as compared with the oral type, which has a more slender, elongated tip.

Recent substitutes for the mercury thermometer are the electronic thermometer, the tympanic membrane sensor, the plastic strip, and the digital thermometer. These devices offer several advantages to children, since they measure temperature rapidly and/or avoid oral or rectal intrusion.

The *electronic thermometer* is ideally suited to pediatric use because the plastic sheath is unbreakable, the child's mouth can remain open when an oral temperature is taken, and the temperature registers within 60 seconds. Reports regarding the accuracy of the electronic thermometer measurement for all three routes is conflicting, with some research supporting the accuracy (Barrus, 1983) and other research casting doubt on the accuracy, particularly for the axillary route (Heidenreich and Giuffre, 1990; Ogren, 1990).

The *tympanic membrane sensor* gathers the infrared energy emitted from the tympanic membrane, which serves as an excellent site because both the eardrum and the hypothalamus (temperature-regulating center) are perfused by the same circulation. The covered probe tip is placed gently at the external opening of the auditory canal, and a temperature reading is given in only 1 second. The sensor is unaffected by cerumen, and the presence of suppurative or nonsuppurative otitis media does not significantly affect the measurement (Kenney and others, 1990; Weir and Weir, 1989). Research on the validity of the device demonstrates that it correlates well with oral, rectal, and axillary measurement of core body temperature (Hancock, 1987). In addition, the procedure is well accepted by infants and children (Barber and Kilmon, 1989). Unfortunately, both the electronic thermometer and the tympanic membrane sensor are expensive devices.

The *plastic strip thermometer* changes color in response to sensed temperature changes. The strip is placed on the forehead until a color change occurs, which usually takes less than 15 seconds. Research findings on the accuracy of the strips have been variable. In one study the strip correlated more closely with rectal measurements than with axillary measurements taken with mercury thermometers. The readings were frequently higher than mercury readings, giving a false impression of fever (Martyn and others, 1988). The strip's advantages for home use include simple instructions and minimal cost.

The *digital thermometer* consists of a probe that connects to a microprocessor chip. The chip translates the signals into degrees and sends the figure to a digital display. The digital thermometer is more accurate and easier to read, but somewhat more expensive than the mercury or plastic strip thermometer.

Measurement using mercury thermometers. *Oral temperatures* are taken in children who can be trusted to keep the thermometer under their tongue with their mouth closed without biting on the glass. Some institutions have a specific age for permitting oral temperatures, such as after 5 or 6 years. In some instances even younger children can cooperate.

When an oral temperature is being taken, the thermometer is placed under the tongue in the right or left posterior sublingual pocket, not in the front of the tongue. Contrary to traditional belief, the sublingual site indicates rapid changes in core body temperature *better* than the rectum. The sublingual area has a rich blood supply derived from the carotid arteries, which are close to the temperature-regulating center in the brain and the central circulation at the heart (Erickson, 1980). However, several factors can affect temporarily the temperature of the mouth, such as hot or cold beverages, smoking, and open-mouth breathing (Neff and others, 1989; Terndrup, Allegra, and Kealy, 1989). While there is some evidence that oxygen by mask lowers oral temperature, the clinical significance of the difference is questionable (Dressler, Smejkal, and Ruffolo, 1983).

Axillary temperatures are often recommended for children who object strongly to a rectal temperature but for whom an oral temperature is not feasible. Axillary temperatures have the advantage of avoiding an intrusive procedure and eliminating the risk of rectal perforation and possible peritonitis, especially in newborn and premature infants. To take an axillary temperature, the thermometer is placed in the axilla with the arm kept close to the child's side (Fig. 7-10, *A*). Axillary temperatures may be affected by poor peripheral perfusion (lower value) or the use of radiant warmers (higher value) (Haddock, Merrow, and Vincent, 1988).

Rectal temperatures should be taken only when no other route or device can be used. This may include children whose mental age or temperament precludes cooperation and understanding instructions, agitated children, and those who have had oral and axillary injuries or surgery. They are contraindicated in newborns (because of the risk of rectal perforation), in anyone who has had rectal surgery, and in children receiving chemotherapy that affects the mucosa. One factor affecting the accuracy of rectal measurements is the presence of stool in the rectum.

For measurement of rectal temperature, children are placed in a side-lying, supine, or prone position. A convenient position for infants is supine with the knees flexed toward the abdomen. This position is maintained with one hand while the other hand is used to insert the lubricated bulb of the thermometer a maximum of 2.5 cm (1 inch). Further insertion increases the risk of perforation, because the colon curves at a depth of about 3 cm (1¼ inches) (Figure 7-10, *B*). It is advisable to cover the penis, because this procedure often stimulates urination.

There is no universal agreement regarding the length of time mercury thermometers should be kept in place. Recommendations based on research using children are 7 minutes for an oral reading, 4 minutes for a rectal reading (Nichols and others, 1972), and 5 minutes for an axillary temperature (Eoff and Joyce, 1981) (see also General Measurements, Chapter 8, for research on neonates). However, these times may not represent *clinically significant* differences in temperature readings taken for shorter intervals (see Nursing Tip, p. 236).

Normal body temperature registers 37.0° C (98.6° F) via the oral route. Traditionally it has been assumed that rectal temperatures are 1° F higher and axillary temperatures 1° F lower than oral temperatures. However, it has been demonstrated that this difference may be considerably less, with axillary and rectal readings differing by an average of 0.49° C (0.9° F) or less (Eoff and Joyce, 1981; Haddock, Vincent, and Merrow, 1986). Because of these variations, the route is charted along with the recorded temperature reading.

A

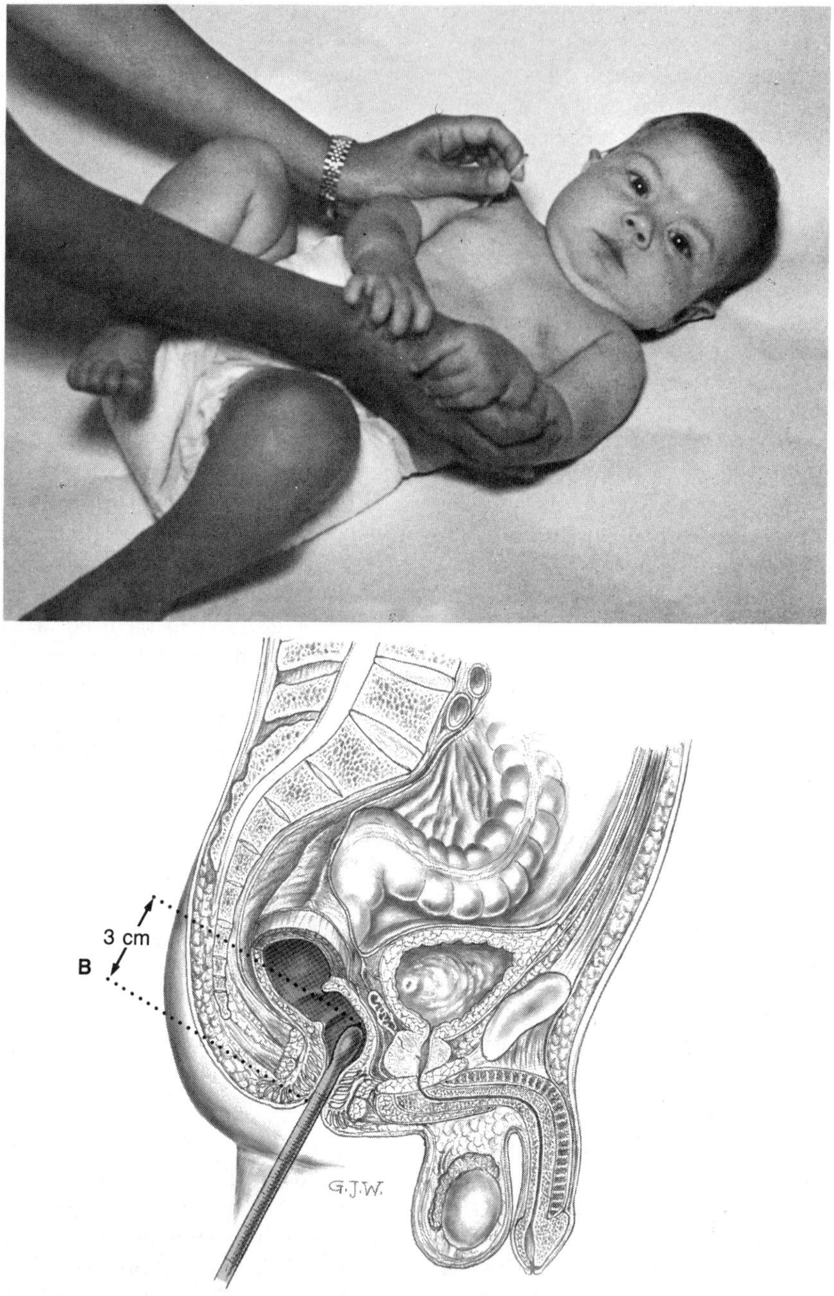

Fig. 7-10. A, Position for taking axillary temperature. **B,** Cross-section of rectum illustrates curve at approximately 3 cm from anus, where risk of perforation from thermometer is greatest.

A characteristic of some small children is the tendency toward a rapid temperature elevation with the associated risk of precipitating seizures. Whenever a child feels extra warm to the touch, the temperature should be taken, even if it was found to be normal only a short time before. Children under 3 years of age are especially vulnerable to febrile seizures.

NURSING TIP: THERMOMETER INSERTION TIME

If in doubt about the optimum length of insertion time, reinsert the mercury thermometer after the first reading for a short time and recheck the scale for a rise. If the value is increased, reinsert the thermometer until the next reading is the same as the previous reading.

Pulse

A satisfactory pulse can be taken radially in children over 2 years of age. However, in infants and young children the

Table 7-4 Grading of pulses

GRADE	DESCRIPTION
0	Not palpable
+1	Difficult to palpate, thready, weak, easily obliterated with pressure
+2	Difficult to palpate, may be obliterated with pressure
+3	Easy to palpate, not easily obliterated with pressure (normal)
+4	Strong, bounding, not obliterated with pressure

apical impulse (heard through a stethoscope held to the chest at the apex of the heart) is more reliable. (See Fig. 7-41 for location of pulses.) The pulse is counted for 1 full minute in infants and young children because of possible irregularities in rhythm. Pulses may be graded according to the criteria in Table 7-4. A comparison of radial and femoral pulses should be done at least once during early childhood to detect the presence of circulatory impairment, such as coarctation of the aorta. Because of the marked variability in heart rate with activity, the child's behavior is also recorded. (See inside front cover for normal rates for pediatric age-groups.)

Respiration

The respiratory rate is counted in the same manner as for the adult patient, except that in infants the movements are primarily diaphragmatic and therefore observed by abdominal movement. Since the movements are irregular, they should be counted for 1 full minute for accuracy (see also p. 268). (See inside front cover for normal respiratory rates in children.)

Blood Pressure

Blood pressure measurement by noninvasive methods is part of a routine vital sign determination. Blood pressure should be measured annually in children 3 years of age through adolescence, and in children with symptoms of hypertension, children in emergency rooms and intensive care units, and high-risk infants (Report of the Second Task Force, 1987). Several authorities also recommend routine measurements in low-risk neonates (American Academy of Pediatrics and American Academy of Obstetricians and Gynecologists, 1988).

Measurement devices. A number of devices are available for measuring blood pressure. The most commonly used instrument is the *mercury-gravity* or *aneroid sphygmomanometer*. Both types are reliable and accurate, but the mercury-gravity manometer does not require recalibration as does the aneroid type.

Blood pressure can also be measured using electronic devices that employ oscillometric or Doppler techniques. In *oscillometry*, pressure changes are transmitted through the arterial wall to the pressure cuff, and the oscillations are detected by a pressure sensitive indicator. Oscillometers have digital readouts for systolic, diastolic, and mean arterial pressures (MAP), and pulse. The MAP is not the same as the mean blood pressure (arithmetic average of systolic and diastolic pressures). Rather, it is a weighted average of the two pressures and generally falls about one third of the way between the diastolic low and the systolic peak—a value somewhat lower than the arithmetic mean of systolic and diastolic blood pressures (Looney, 1978). Blood pressure readings using oscillometry, such as Dinamap, are generally higher and correlate better with direct radial artery values than measurements using auscultation (see Table 7-7) (Park and Menard, 1987).

The *Doppler ultrasound* translates changes in ultrasound frequency caused by blood movement within the artery to audible sound by means of a transducer in the cuff. The Doppler is useful for systolic pressure measurement but is unreliable for diastolic pressure measurement. Oscillometric and Doppler instruments are very useful in measuring blood pressure in infants and have largely replaced the flush method, which reflects only the mean blood pressure.

Selection of cuff. No matter what type of noninvasive technique is used, the most important factor in accurately measuring blood pressure is the use of an appropriately sized cuff (cuff size refers only to the inner inflatable bladder, not the cloth covering). Unfortunately, authorities disagree on the correct method for determining cuff size. The Report of the Second Task Force (1987) recommends a method based on *limb length* (Table 7-5):

Width sufficient to cover approximately 75% of upper arm between top of shoulder and olecranon
Length sufficient to completely encircle circumference of limb with or without overlapping
Enough room at antecubital fossa to place bell of stethoscope
Enough room at upper edge of cuff to prevent obstruction of axilla

The American Heart Association (Frohlich, 1988) recommends a method based on *limb circumference* (Table 7-6):

Width 40% to 50% of limb circumference; measured at upper arm midway between top of shoulder and olecranon
Length sufficient to completely or nearly completely encircle circumference of limb without overlapping

Table 7-5 Commonly available blood pressure cuffs

CUFF NAME*	BLADDER WIDTH (CM)	BLADDER LENGTH (CM)
Newborn	2.5-4.0	5.0-9.0
Infant	4.0-6.0	11.5-18.0
Child	7.5-9.0	17.0-19.0
Adult	11.5-13.0	22.0-26.0
Large arm	14.0-15.0	30.5-33.0
Thigh	18.0-19.0	36.0-38.0

From Report of the Second Task Force on Blood Pressure Control in Children—1987, Pediatrics 79(1):1-25, 1987.
*Cuff name does not guarantee that the cuff will be appropriate size for a child within that age range.

Table 7-6 Recommended bladder dimensions for blood pressure cuffs

ARM CIRCUMFERENCE AT MIDPOINT (CM)	CUFF NAME*	BLADDER WIDTH (CM)	BLADDER LENGTH (CM)
5-7.5	Newborn	3	5
7.5-13	Infant	5	8
13-20	Child	8	13
24-32	Adult	13	24
32-42	Wide adult	17	34
42-50	Thigh	20	42

From Frohlich, E.D., and others: Recommendations for human blood pressure determination by sphygmomanometers: report of a special task force appointed by the Steering Committee, American Health Association, Circulation 77:501A, 1988.
*Cuff name does not guarantee that the cuff will be appropriate size for a child within that age range.

The guidelines using limb length for selecting cuff width may produce satisfactory blood pressure readings in children with average weight for height, but inaccurate readings in children with thick arms. Using limb circumference for selecting cuff width more accurately reflects direct arterial blood pressure than using limb length because this method takes into account the varying thickness of the arm and the amount of pressure required to compress the artery (Park and Guntheroth, 1989). For measurement sites other than the upper arms, the limb circumference guidelines can be used although the shape of the limb (i.e., conical shape of the thigh) may prevent appropriate placement of the cuff) and result in inaccurate reflection of intraarterial blood pressure.

Cuffs that are either too narrow or too wide affect the accuracy of blood pressure measurements, although wide cuffs tend to affect blood pressure readings less. When the correctly sized cuff is used, the inflated cuff transmits the same pressure on the underlying arterial wall as the pressure registered on the manometer. If the cuff is too small, the pressure around the artery may be less than that registered on the manometer, so that the reading on the device is falsely high. If the cuff is too large, the excessive cuff width reduces the kinetic energy of blood flow, resulting in a perceived lower pressure; this effect is probably more marked with the auscultatory method than with the oscillometric method (Fig. 7-11) (Park and Guntheroth, 1989).

✦ **NURSING ALERT** In choosing cuff sizes, use an appropriately sized cuff. When the correct size is not available, use an oversized cuff rather than an undersized one or use another site that more appropriately fits the cuff size. Do not choose a cuff based on the name of the cuff (i.e., an "infant" cuff may be too small for some infants).

When another site is used, blood pressure measurements using noninvasive techniques may differ. Generally, pressure in the lower sites is greater than pressure in the upper sites because of a phenomenon known as "amplification of systolic pressure." For example, systolic pressure in the thigh may be 10 to 20 mm Hg higher than in the arm. This difference may also occur because of the lack of a well-designed cuff for the thigh. The systolic pressure in the thigh using noninvasive techniques should be at least equal to that in the arm (Park, 1988).

✦ **NURSING ALERT** Compare blood pressure in the upper and lower extremities at least once to detect abnormalities, such as coarctation of the aorta, in which the lower extremity pressure is less than the upper extremity pressure.

Measurement and interpretation. Measuring and interpreting blood pressure in infants and children requires additional attention to correct procedure because (1) limb sizes vary and cuff selection must accommodate the circumference, (2) excessive pressure on the antecubital fossa affects the Korotkoff sounds, (3) children easily become anxious, which can elevate the blood pressure, and (4) blood pressure values change with age and growth. Larger children, especially in terms of height, have higher normal blood pressures than smaller children of the same age (de Swiet and others, 1989).

Although the technique of blood pressure measurement in children is generally the same as that used for adults (Box 7-7), some aspects of the procedure require special attention. Because children are easily upset by unfamiliar procedures, every effort is made to prepare them for blood pressure measurement. For children of preschool age and above, each step of the procedure is explained and they are told how the cuff will feel, such as a tight feeling or an arm hug. Explanations such as "I want to see how strong your muscle is" or "Let's watch the silver rise in the tube" are especially appealing to young children.

Since the child should be quiet and relaxed during the procedure, blood pressure is measured before any anxiety-producing procedures are performed. Infants and small children may be more quiet if the reading is taken while they are sitting in the parent's lap.

A pediatric stethoscope using the bell is helpful for hearing blood pressure sounds in small children and infants. If ausculation is not possible, a systolic reading alone can be obtained by palpation and is measured as the point at which the pulse at the radial or brachial artery reappears as the cuff is deflated.

The average blood pressure readings at various ages throughout childhood using sphygmomanometry are listed on the inside front cover and readings using oscillometry are listed in Table 7-7 (see Nursing Tip, p. 240). Blood pressure values are defined as follows (see also discussion of hypertension in Chapter 34):

Normal blood pressure—systolic and diastolic blood pressure less than the 90th percentile for age and sex

High normal blood pressure—systolic and diastolic blood pressure between the 90th and 95th percentiles for age and sex

High blood pressure—systolic and diastolic blood pressure at or above the 95th percentile for age and sex

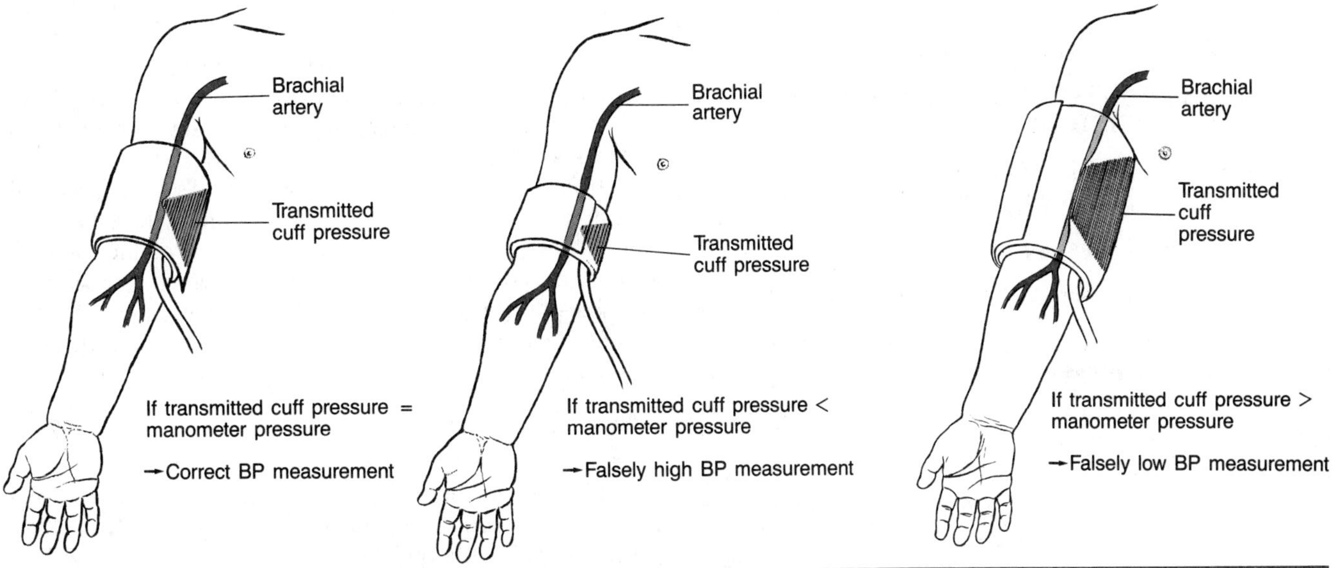

Fig. 7-11. Effect of cuff size on blood pressure measurement.

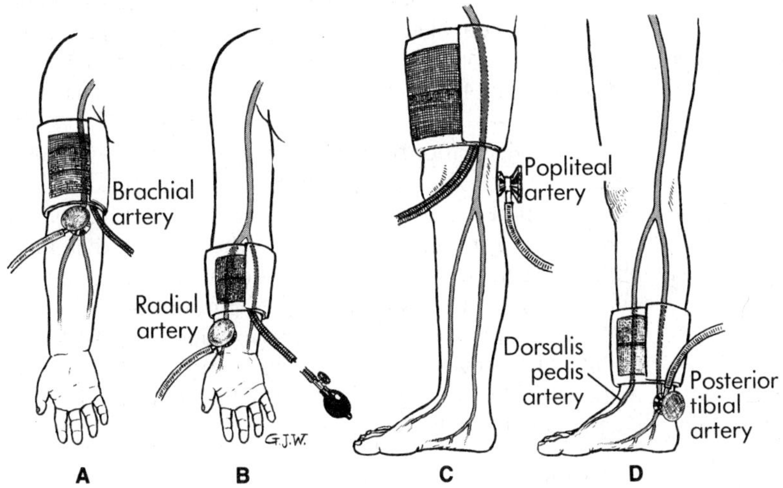

Fig. 7-12. Sites for measuring blood pressure. **A,** Upper arm. **B,** Lower arm or forearm. **C,** Thigh. **D,** Calf or ankle.

Box 7-7 GUIDELINES FOR DETERMINING BLOOD PRESSURE

Use an appropriately sized cuff.
Use same position, preferably sitting, and right arm for brachial artery site (Fig. 7-12, *A*).
Use alternate site as needed to accommodate available cuff sizes:
- Use smaller size on forearm: place cuff above wrist and auscultate radial artery (Fig. 7-12, *B*).
- Use larger size on thigh: place cuff above knee and auscultate popliteal artery (Fig. 7-12, *C*).
- Use larger size on calf: place cuff above malleoli or at midcalf and auscultate posterior tibial or dorsal pedal artery (Fig. 7-12, *D*).

Position limb at level of heart.
Rapidly inflate cuff to about 20 mm Hg above point at which radial pulse disappears.
Release cuff pressure at a rate of about 2 to 3 mm Hg per second during auscultation of artery.
Read mercury-gravity manometer at eye level.
Record systolic value as onset of a clear tapping sound (first Korotkoff sound).
Record diastolic pressure as:
- Fourth Korotkoff sound (K4) (low-pitched, muffled sound) for children up to age 12 years
- Fifth Korotkoff sound (K5) (disappearance of all sound) for children 13 to 18 years

Record also limb, position, cuff size, and method of measurement.
If using electronic monitor, follow manufacturer's instructions and guidelines for correct cuff size.
- With oscillometric device (i.e., Dinamap), all four limb sites can be used, but reserve the thigh for last, since it is the most uncomfortable.
- Stabilize the limb during cuff deflation, since movement interferes with the device's ability to measure blood pressure accurately.

NURSING TIP: QUICK GUIDE TO NORMAL SYSTOLIC BP VALUES

Use the following formula to approximate the average **systolic blood pressure** for children:

1 to 7 years: age in years + 90

8 to 18 years: (2 × age in years) + 83

Use the following formula to approximate the average **diastolic blood pressure** for children:

1 to 5 years: 56

6 to 18 years: age in years + 52

Table 7-7 Normative Dinamap BP values (systolic/diastolic, mean arterial pressure in parentheses)

AGE-GROUP	MEAN	90TH PERCENTILE	95TH PERCENTILE
Newborn (1-3 days)	65/41(50)	75/49(59)	78/52(62)
1 month to 2 years	95/58(72)	106/68(83)	110/71(86)
2-5 years	101/57(74)	112/66(82)	115/68(85)

From Park, M., and Menard, S.: Normative oscillometric blood pressure values in the first 5 years in an office setting, Am. J. Dis. Child. 143(7):860-864, 1989.

GENERAL APPEARANCE

The general appearance of the child is a cumulative, subjective impression of the child's physical appearance, state of nutrition, behavior, personality, interactions with parents and nurse (also siblings if present), posture, development, and speech. Although general appearance is recorded in the beginning of the physical examination, it encompasses all the observations of the child during the interview and physical assessment.

Physical Appearance

The description of physical appearance notes the *facies,* the facial expression and appearance of the child. For example, the facies may give clues to children who are in pain, have difficulty in breathing, feel frightened, discontent, or happy, are mentally deficient, or are acutely ill.

Posture, position, and types of *body movement* also are important in the overall assessment of physical appearance. The child with hearing or vision loss may characteristically tilt the head in an awkward position to facilitate perception of sound or sight. The child in pain may favor a body part. The child with low self-esteem or a feeling of rejection may assume a slumped, careless, and apathetic pose or posture. Likewise, a child with confidence, a feeling of self-worth, and a sense of security usually demonstrates a tall, straight, well-balanced posture. Although the nurse observes such "body language," it must not be interpreted too freely but rather recorded objectively.

Hygiene is noted in terms of the child's state of cleanliness, unusual body odor, the condition of the hair, neck, nails, teeth, and feet, and the condition of the clothing. Such observations give excellent clues to possible instances of neglect, inadequate financial resources, housing difficulties (e.g., no running water), or lack of knowledge of children's needs.

Nutrition

General appearance includes an overall impression of the child's state of nutrition. This impression is more than a statement describing body weight or stature, such as "slender and tall." It is an estimation of the quality, as well as quantity, of nutritional intake. For example, two children can be of the same height and weight, yet one can appear overweight because of flabby, loose skin, while the other child appears strong, robust, and well built because of firm, well-defined musculature. Likewise, a small, slender child may be well nourished with no signs of chronic undernutrition, such as bony prominences, protuberant abdomen, flat buttocks, gaunt facies, and poor muscle tone with evidence of wasting.

The impression of nutritional state is compared with the parents' history of feeding practices. Discrepancies between the two "impressions" may be a valuable area for nutritional counseling. For example, parents who believe that their child is too thin and eats too little, despite evidence of adequate growth and physical signs of proper nutrition, may find it helpful to keep a daily diary in order to calculate the child's cumulative food intake. Many parents are surprised at the quantity of food ingested, even though the amounts at each meal or snack are small.

Behavior

Behavior includes the child's personality; level of activity; reaction to stress, requests, or frustration; interactions with others, primarily the parent and nurse; degree of alertness; and response to stimuli. It is one of the most important observations that the nurse makes during a child's health assessment (Box 7-8; see also Box 7-12).

Development

Although gross developmental achievement can usually be assessed from careful and detailed observation of the child, the impressions should be documented with screening tests, such as the Denver Developmental Screening Test (DDST). Various tests for assessing development, speech, vision, and hearing are discussed later in this chapter and in Chapter 25.

An overall estimate of the child's speech development, motor skills, degree of coordination, and recent area of achievement is recorded under general appearance. For example, the following statement may apply to an 18-month-old child: "Motor development advanced for age; climbs, runs, jumps (most recent motor skill), manipulates small

Box 7-8 GUIDELINES FOR OBSERVING BEHAVIOR

What is the child's overall personality—calm, anxious, tense, content, outgoing, shy, talkative, aggressive, introverted, stable, or moody?
Is the child active, sedentary, fidgety, or restless?
Does the child have a long attention span, or is the child easily distracted?
Does the child sit quietly on the examining table or parent's lap, or does the child climb, run, open doors, and otherwise explore the environment?
How does the child react to commands—with fear or willingness to obey?
How advanced is the child's ability to follow requests? Can the child follow two or three commands in succession without the need for repetition? Is the child attentive to requests, or must they be repeated several times?
Is the child cooperative, belligerent, or argumentative?
What is the child's response to delayed gratification or frustration? Is the child able to withstand momentary discomfort and wait for the requests to be met?
In what tone of voice does the child make requests or talk to the parents?
Does the child seek approval and gain satisfaction from it?
Does the child use eye-to-eye contact during conversation?
Does the child agree with the parent's answers or find reasons to disagree, interrupt, or argue? What is the child's reaction to the nurse—respectful, friendly, reserved, apprehensive, or uninterested?
Is the child interested in the surroundings? Does the child look around the room, ask questions about unfamiliar objects, seem to enjoy exploring them, or attempt to break or destroy them?
Can the child follow directions for using the instruments or imitate their use? Is the child quick or slow to grasp explanations?

objects with ease; excellent coordination and balance; beginning to name many objects; uses two-word phrases; and enjoys 'talking' to self and others."

SKIN

Skin is assessed for color, texture, temperature, moisture, and turgor. Hair is also inspected for color, texture, quality, distribution, and elasticity. Examination of the skin and its accessory structures primarily involves inspection and palpation.

Physical Factors Influencing Assessment

Examination of the child is conducted in a well-illuminated room with nonglare lighting. Ideally the room should be neutral in color. Colors such as pink, blue, yellow, or orange cast deceiving glows on the skin. The room should also be comfortably warm, since air-conditioning can cause a cold-induced cyanosis and excessive heat can produce flushing. Poor hygiene and artificial paint on nails or lips also mask true determination of color. Sometimes it is necessary to clean the skin with soap and water and to remove cosmetics before beginning inspection. Although not a common situation in pediatrics, the nurse should remember that such factors can hide signs of ecchymoses, petechiae, pallor, or cyanosis.

Texture, temperature, moisture, and turgor can be subjectively inspected, but palpation must be done for greater accuracy. Clothing always interferes with palpation; thus the nurse needs to examine each area of the body nude, either as part of the general overall examination or combined with assessment of each body system. Since texture is affected by climatic exposure, such as cold, sun, and wind, the texture of protected areas of the body is compared with that of exposed areas.

Genetic Factors Influencing Assessment of Color

The normal color in light-skinned children varies from a milky-white and rosy color to a more deeply hued pink color. In general, cyanosis or bluish discolorations are not normal, except in the newborn (see Table 8-3). Dark-skinned children, such as those of American Indian, Hispanic, black, Latin, Mediterranean, or Oriental descent, have inherited various brown, red, yellow, olive-green, and bluish tones in their skin, which can falsely alter assessment. For example, some children of Mediterranean origin normally have bluish-tinged lips, suggestive of cyanosis. Oriental persons, whose skin is normally of a yellow tone, may appear to be jaundiced. Full-blooded black individuals often have normal bluish pigmentation of the gums, buccal cavity, borders of the tongue, and nail beds. The visible portion of their sclera may contain speckled deposits of brown melanin that resemble petechiae.

Physiologic Factors Influencing Assessment of Color

Edema of the skin affects color in all individuals because it increases the amount of interstitial fluid, thereby increasing the distance between the outermost layers of the epidermis and the pigmented and vascular layers. Edema decreases the intensity of skin color, sometimes producing a false pallor.

Exposure to sunlight, on the other hand, stimulates the melanocytes to produce more melanin, thereby increasing the color of the skin. Individuals who are deeply suntanned require as careful observation as those who are genetically dark skinned.

In general, the amount of adipose tissue does not markedly affect skin color, because deposition of fat cells is below the pigmented layers of the skin. Overnutrition may not mean adequate nutrition, and pallor that may indicate nutritional iron deficiency is carefully assessed.

Reliable Areas for Assessment of Color

Color changes are most reliably assessed in those areas of the body where melanin production is least: sclera, conjunctiva, nail beds, lips, tongue, buccal mucosa, palms, and soles. These areas are rarely affected by edema or amount of adipose tissue but are sensitive to changes from physical factors, such as use of cosmetics, ingestion of colored food substances, or poor hygiene.

Table 7-8 Differences in color changes of racial groups

COLOR CHANGE	LIGHT SKIN	DARK SKIN
Cyanosis	Bluish tinge, especially in palpebral conjunctiva (lower eyelid), nail beds, earlobes, lips, oral membranes, soles, and palms	Ashen-gray lips and tongue
Pallor	Loss of rosy glow in skin, especially face	Ashen-gray appearance in black skin More yellowish-brown color in brown skin
Erythema	Redness easily seen anywhere on body	Much more difficult to assess; rely on palpation for warmth or edema
Ecchymosis	Purplish to yellow-green areas; may be seen anywhere on skin	Very difficult to see unless in mouth or conjunctiva
Petechiae	Purplish pinpoints most easily seen on buttocks, abdomen, and inner surfaces of the arms or legs	Usually invisible except in oral mucosa, conjunctiva of eyelids, and conjunctiva covering eyeball
Jaundice	Yellow staining seen in sclera of eyes, skin, fingernails, soles, palms, and oral mucosa	Most reliably assessed in sclera, hard palate, palms, and soles

Variations in Skin Color

Many of the specific color changes peculiar to the newborn are described in Table 8-3. Differences in assessment of color changes in ethnic groups are presented in Table 7-8.

Pallor and cyanosis. The skin receives its pigmented color of yellow, brown, and black from melanin and its shades of red or blue from the color of hemoglobin. Oxygenated hemoglobin in the superficial capillaries of the dermis gives a rosy, pink glow. Reduced (deoxygenated) hemoglobin reflects a bluish tone through the skin, called *cyanosis,* which is evident when reduced hemoglobin levels reach 5 mg/dl of blood or more, regardless of the total hemoglobin. In general, the darker the skin pigmentation, the greater the amount of deoxygenated hemoglobin must be for cyanosis to be evident.

Pallor, or paleness, may be a sign of anemia, chronic disease, edema, or shock. However, it may be a normal complexion characteristic or an indication of indoor living.

Pallor or cyanosis can be compared to the color change normally produced by blanching. For example, in nonpigmented nails, pressing down on the free edge of the nail on the index or middle finger of a child with good skin color produces marked blanching or whitening as compared with the return blood flow. In a child with pallor the difference in color change will be slight. The blanching color change can be observed in dark-skinned individuals by gently applying pressure to their lips or gums.

Erythema. Erythema, or redness of the skin, may be the result of increased temperature from climatic conditions, local inflammation, or infection. It may also appear as a sign of skin irritation, allergy, or other dermatoses. The degree of redness reflects the amount of increased blood flow to the area. The nurse notes any reddening and describes its location, size, presence of warmth, itching, type of distribution (e.g., diffuse, clearly circumscribed, parallel to a vein), and the presence of characteristic lesions, such as macules, papules, or vesicles (see Chapter 18 for a description of skin lesions).

Plethora. Plethora is also redness of the skin but is caused by increased numbers of red blood cells as a compensatory response to chronic hypoxia. Intense redness of the lips or cheeks occurs.

Ecchymosis and petechiae. Ecchymosis and petechiae are caused by extravasation or hemorrhage of blood into the skin; the only difference between the two is size. Ecchymoses are large, diffuse areas, usually black and blue in color, and are typically the result of accidental injuries in healthy, active children. Since ecchymotic areas may indicate systemic disorders or child maltreatment, the nurse should always investigate the reported cause of the bruises, especially when they are located in suspicious areas, such as the back or buttocks, rather than on the knees, shins, elbows, or forearms.

Petechiae are small, distinct pinpoint hemorrhages 2 mm or less in size, which can denote some type of blood disorder, such as decreased platelets in leukemia. Because of their size, ecchymoses are more readily observed than are petechiae, which may be visible only in areas of very light-colored skin. Areas of erythema can be distinguished from ecchymosis or petechiae by blanching the skin. Since erythema is a result of increased blood flow *to* the area, exerting pressure will momentarily empty the engorged vessels and produce blanching. Because the other discolorations are produced by blood leaking *into* tissue spaces, blanching will not occur.

Jaundice. Jaundice, a yellow staining of the skin usually caused by bile pigments, is always a significant finding. If a yellow-orange cast is noted in an otherwise healthy child, the nurse should inquire about the quantity of ingested yellow vegetables, such as carrots, which in excess produce a yellow-orange color from deposits of carotene in the skin, a condition called carotenemia.

Texture

The nurse palpates the skin for texture, noting moisture and temperature. Any marks or scars that are suggestive of healed injuries are noted, and inquiries are made about their origin. Normally the skin of young children is smooth, soft, and slightly dry to the touch, not oily or clammy. Any variations from these findings are noted, because they may indicate common problems of childhood such as cradle cap, eczema, diaper rash, or excessive dryness (xeroderma) all over the body from too frequent bathing, exposure to the weather, or vitamin A deficiency. Excessively moist, clammy skin may indicate serious health problems, particularly heart disease.

Temperature

Temperature is evaluated by symmetrically feeling each part of the body and comparing upper areas with lower ones. Any distinct difference in temperature is noted. Although not a common anomaly, one of the key signs for coarctation of the aorta is warm upper extremities and cool lower ones. The nurse also observes the skin temperature of the dressed child. Young children produce heat rapidly, and they quickly become overheated if dressed too warmly. Many parents do not realize this and fail to change the amount of clothing to accommodate climatic variations.

Turgor

Tissue turgor refers to the amount of elasticity in the skin. It is best determined by grasping the skin on the abdomen between the thumb and index finger, pulling it taut, and quickly releasing it. Elastic tissue immediately assumes its normal position without residual marks or creases. In children with poor skin turgor the skin remains suspended or tented for a few seconds before slowly falling back on the abdomen. Skin turgor is one of the best estimates of adequate hydration and nutrition.

While evaluating turgor, the nurse also inspects for signs of *edema,* normally evident as swelling or puffiness. Periorbital edema is a sign of several systemic disorders, such as kidney diseases, but may normally be evident in children who have been crying or sleeping or who have allergies. Edema is evaluated for change according to position, its specific location, and response to pressure. For example, in pitting edema, pressing a finger into the edematous area will cause a temporary indentation.

Accessory Structures

Inspection of the accessory structures of the skin, namely the hair, nails, and dermatoglyphics, may be performed while the skin is being examined or when the scalp and extremities are being assessed.

Hair. The hair is inspected for color, texture, quality, distribution, and elasticity. Children's scalp hair is usually lustrous, silky, strong, and elastic. Genetic factors affect the appearance of hair. For example, the hair of black children is usually curlier and coarser than that of white children. Hair that is stringy, dull, brittle, dry, friable, and depigmented may suggest poor nutrition. Any bald or thinning spots are recorded. Although alopecia can be a sign of various skin disorders, such as tinea capitis, loss of hair in infants is often the result of lying in the same position and may be a clue for counseling parents concerning the child's stimulation needs.

General cleanliness of the hair and scalp is noted. Various ethnic groups condition their hair with oils or lubricants, which, if not thoroughly washed from the scalp, clog the sebaceous glands, causing scalp infections. The nurse also inspects hair shafts for lice, whose ova appear as grayish translucent flakes. Ova or nits are distinguished from dandruff because the eggs adhere to the hair. If pediculosis capitis is suspected, the nurse should be careful to guard against self-infestation of the lice by wearing gloves and handwashing.

The scalp is also inspected for ticks, which appear as grayish or brown oval bodies. Although they can be found anywhere on the body, the most common sites are exposed parts, such as the head. Although not all dog or wood ticks transmit serious disease, a notation of removal is made on the child's chart in case symptoms appear.

Unusual hairiness anywhere on the body, such as arms, legs, trunk, or face, is noted. Tufts of hair anywhere along the spine, especially over the sacrum, are significant because they can mark the site of spina bifida occulta.

In older children who are approaching puberty, the nurse looks for growth of secondary hair as a sign of normally progressing pubertal changes (see Figs. 19-7 and 19-8). Precocious or delayed appearance of hair growth is noted because, although not always suggestive of hormonal dysfunction, it may be of great concern to the early- or late-maturing adolescent.

Nails. The nails are inspected for color, shape, texture, and quality. Normally the nails are pink, convex in shape, smooth, and hard but flexible, not brittle. The edges, which are usually white, should extend over the fingers. Dark-skinned individuals may have more deeply pigmented nail beds. Variation in color, such as blueness, suggests cyanosis, and a yellow tint may indicate jaundice. Bluish-black discoloration usually indicates hemorrhage under the nail from trauma. Fungal infections cause the entire nail to become whitish with a pitting surface. Short, ragged nails are typical of habitual biting. Uncut nails with dirt accumulated under the edge sometimes indicate poor hygiene.

Changes in the shape of nails are also significant. For example, concave curves or "spoon nails," called *koilonychia,* are sometimes seen in iron-deficiency anemia, a common nutritional problem of children. Clubbing of the nails is always a significant finding and usually is associated with chronic cyanosis. In clubbing, the base of the nail becomes visibly swollen and feels springy when palpated, rather than firm as in the normal nail (see Fig. 31-8).

Dermatoglyphics. Each individual has a distinct set of

handprints and footprints. The patterns, or *dermatoglyphics,* are unique to the individual and vary a great deal in detail and complexity of patterns. Flexion creases also appear on the palm of the hand and the sole of the foot. The palm normally shows three flexion creases (Fig. 7-13, *A*). In some situations, such as Down syndrome, the two distal horizontal creases are fused to form a single horizontal crease called a *single palmar crease,* or *simian crease* (Fig. 7-13, *B*). If grossly abnormal lines or folds are observed, the nurse should sketch a picture to describe them and refer the finding to a specialist for further investigation.

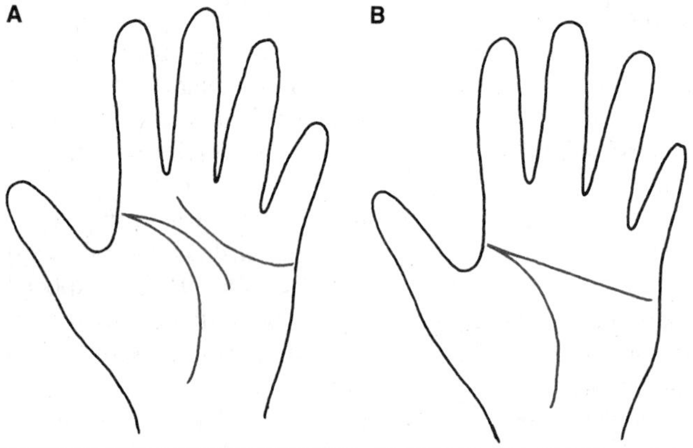

Fig. 7-13. Examples of flexion creases on palm. **A,** Normal. **B,** Simian crease.

LYMPH NODES

The body's extensive lymph system is usually assessed when examining the part of the body in which the glands are located. The usual sites for palpating accessible lymph nodes are shown in Fig. 7-14. Since the major function of lymph nodes is to collect and filter the lymph of bacteria and other foreign matter as it returns to the circulatory system, the nurse must have knowledge of the lymph's directional flow. Tender, enlarged warm lymph nodes are generally indicative of infection or inflammation *proximal* to their location. For example, occipital or postauricular adenopathy is often seen in local scalp infection, such as pediculosis, tick bite, or external otitis. Cervical adenopathy usually accompanies acute infections in or around the mouth or throat. In children, however, small, nontender, movable nodes are frequently normal.

Nodes are palpated with the distal portion of the fingers by gently but firmly pressing in a circular motion along the regions where nodes are normally present. During assessment of the nodes in the head and neck, the child's head is tilted upward slightly but without tensing the sternocleidomastoid or trapezius muscle. This position facilitates palpation of the *submental, submaxillary, tonsillar,* and *cervical nodes.* The *axillary nodes* are palpated with the arms relaxed at the side but slightly abducted. The *inguinal nodes* are best assessed with the child in the supine position. Size, mobility, temperature, and tenderness are noted, in addition to reports by the parents regarding any visible change of enlarged nodes.

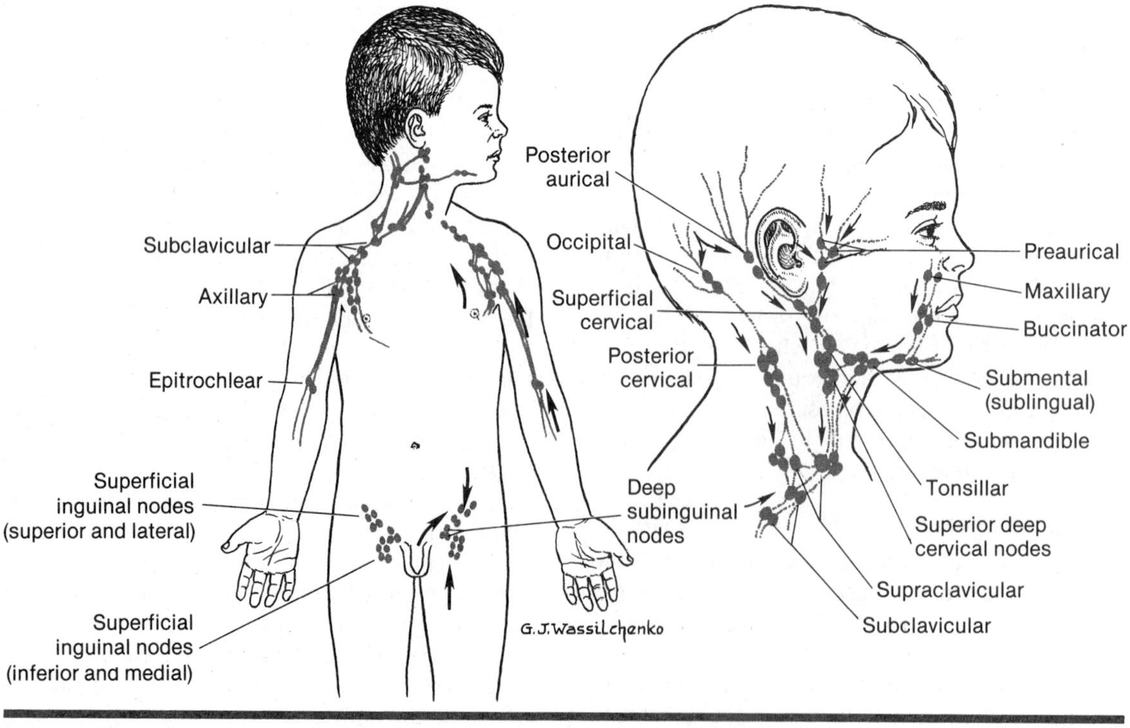

Fig. 7-14. Location of superficial lymph nodes. Arrows indicate directional flow of lymph.

HEAD

The head is inspected for general *shape* and *symmetry*. A flattening of one part of the head, such as the occiput, may indicate that the child continually lies in this position. Marked asymmetry is usually abnormal and may indicate premature closure of the sutures (craniosynostosis).

Head control in infants and head posture in older children are noted. Most infants by 4 months of age should be able to hold the head erect and in midline when in a vertical position.

✦ **NURSING ALERT** Significant head lag after 6 months of age strongly indicates cerebral injury and is referred for further evaluation.

Range of motion is evaluated by asking the older child to look in each direction (to either side, up, and down) or manually putting the younger child through each position. Limited range of motion may indicate wryneck, or *torticollis,* a result of injury to the sternocleidomastoid muscle, in which the child holds the head to one side with the chin pointing toward the opposite side. Hyperextension of the head (opisthotonos) with pain on flexion is a serious indication of meningeal irritation (see also Fig. 7-60 on Brudzinski sign).

The *skull* is palpated for patent sutures, fontanels, fractures, and swellings. Normally the posterior fontanel closes by the second month of life and the anterior fontanel fuses between 12 and 18 months of age. Early or late closure is noted, since either may be a sign of a pathologic condition. For a more detailed discussion of the cranial bones, see Chapter 8.

While the head is being examined, the *face* is inspected for symmetry, movement, and general appearance. Asking the child to "make a face" assesses symmetric movement and discloses any degree of paralysis. Any unusual facial proportion is noted, such as unusually high or low forehead, wide- or close-set eyes, or small, receding chin.

The nurse also notes any unusual swellings or sites of edema that may be associated with specific disorders, such as nephrosis, Cushing syndrome, or steroid therapy. Visible and palpable swelling anterior to the earlobe and above the angle of the jaw is characteristic of parotid gland enlargement in mumps. It gives the child a characteristic "chipmunk" appearance.

Generally the head and face are not auscultated or percussed, with the exception of the sinuses. The *sinuses* are air cavities within certain bones adjacent to the nasal cavity (Fig. 7-15). The sinuses develop as outpouchings of the nasal airway as the skull bones enlarge throughout infancy and childhood. The maxillary and ethmoid sinuses are present soon after birth (Glasier, Mallory, and Steele, 1989). The frontal and sphenoid sinuses develop later in childhood. Normally the sinuses are not percussed unless there are signs of an infection, such as headache and congestion.

NECK

Besides assessing motility of the head and neck, the nurse also inspects the neck as to size and palpates it for associated structures. The neck is short with skin folds between the head and shoulders during infancy; however, it lengthens during the next 3 to 4 years. A short or webbed neck is associated with various anomalies, such as Turner syndrome. Marked edema of the neck may indicate mumps, local throat or mouth infections, or diphtheria. Distended neck veins often indicate difficulty on expiration, such as in asthma or cystic fibrosis.

The *trachea* is palpated by placing the thumb and index finger on each side and sliding them back and forth to note any masses. Normally the trachea is in the midline or slightly to the right of the midline. Any shift is noted, since

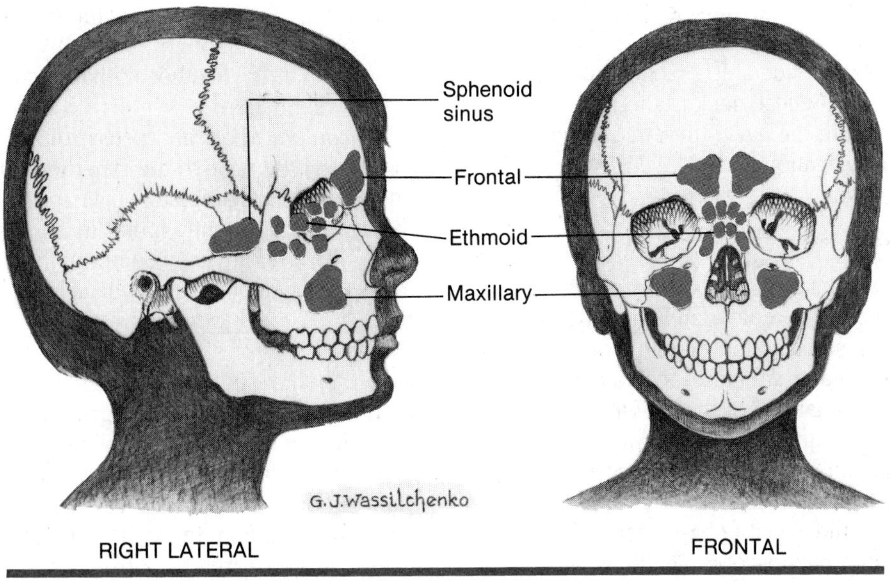

Fig. 7-15. Location of sinuses.

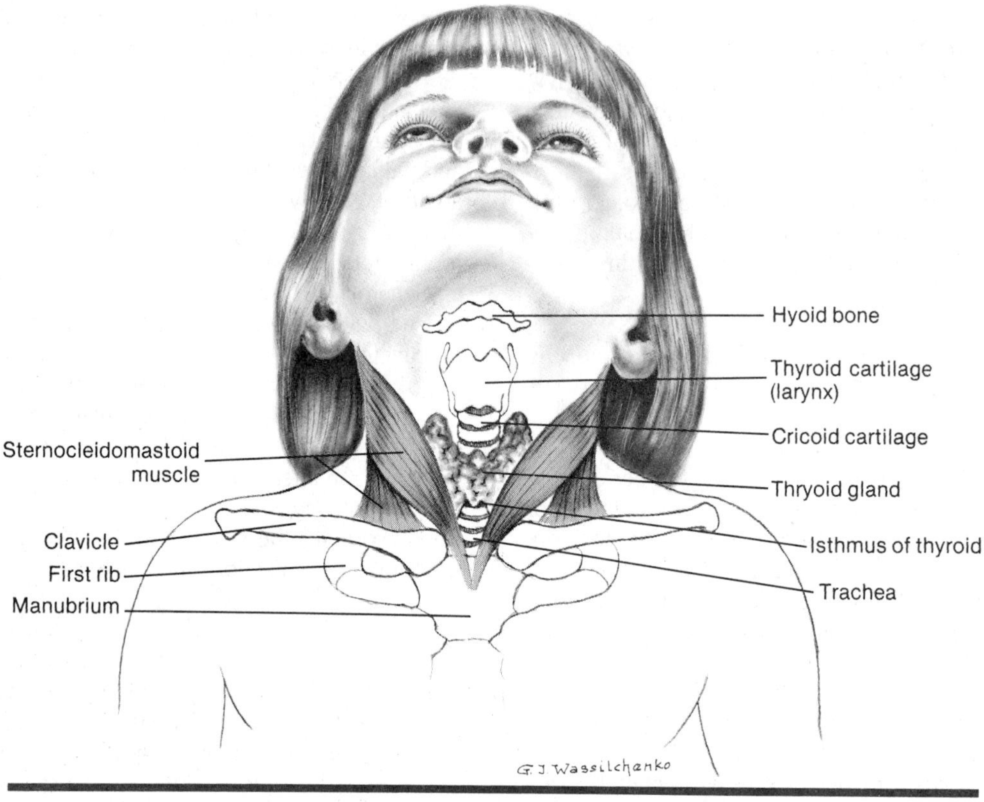

Fig. 7-16. Anterior view of structures in neck.

it can signify serious lung problems, such as a tumor or foreign body in the lung.

The *thyroid gland,* which is located at the base of the neck, is palpated. This butterfly-shaped gland straddles the trachea and has two lateral lobes connected by an isthmus or band of glandular tissue. The isthmus is the only portion of the thyroid that is usually palpable, because the lobes that curve posteriorly around the trachea are partially covered by the sternocleidomastoid muscle (Fig. 7-16). Normally the thyroid rises as the child swallows. However, palpating the thyroid takes considerable practice and is especially difficult in an infant, whose neck is short and thick. If any masses are detected in the neck, they are recorded and reported for further investigation.

EYES

Examination of the eyes involves inspection of all exterior structures for size, symmetry, color, and motility, and inspection of the interior surfaces for examination of retinal structures. To examine each structure accurately requires an understanding of the anatomy of the eyeball (Fig. 7-17). The retinal examination requires the use of an ophthalmoscope and is a highly skilled procedure. Discussion of the funduscopic examination includes the basic normal findings that the nurse should be able to discern with some practice in using the ophthalmoscope. The third part of the examination involves vision testing.

Placement and Alignment

The eyes are judged for relative placement on the face, symmetry of location, and general slant of the palpebral fissures or lids (Fig. 7-18). If any possible abnormality of placement is observed, these findings can be substantiated by measuring the interpupillary distance, which is approximately 4.5 to 5.5 cm (1¾ to 2¼ inches) or the inner canthal distance, which averages about 2.5 cm (1 inch) (Laestadius, Aase, and Smith, 1969). Large spacing between the eyes is called *hypertelorism.* Although a normal variant in some children, hypertelorism with other midfacial anomalies may suggest mental retardation.

Epicanthal folds, an excess fold of skin extending from the roof of the nose to the inner termination of the eyebrow and partially or completely overlapping the inner canthus of the eye, are frequently found in children of Asiatic descent (Fig. 7-18, *B*). They may be normally present in non-Oriental infants, but they usually disappear as the child grows older.

The *palpebral slant* is inspected. The degree of slant is judged by drawing an imaginary line through the two points of the medial canthus and across the outer orbit of the eyes and aligning each eye on the line. Usually the palpebral fissures lie horizontally. However, in Oriental persons the slant is normally upward (Fig. 7-18, *C*). Since eye abnormalities are common in many chromosomal disorders, the nurse must be careful to observe and record any deviations from the expected. For example, children with Down syn-

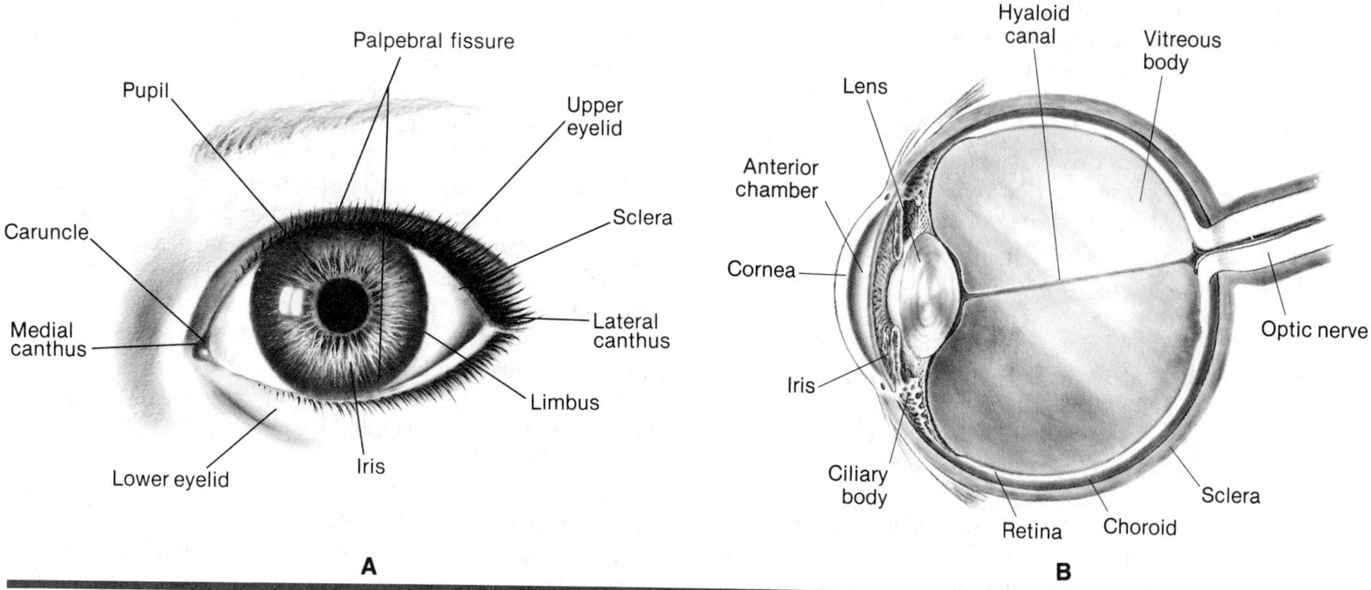

Fig. 7-17. Normal structure of eye. **A,** Anterior view. **B,** Cross-sectional view.

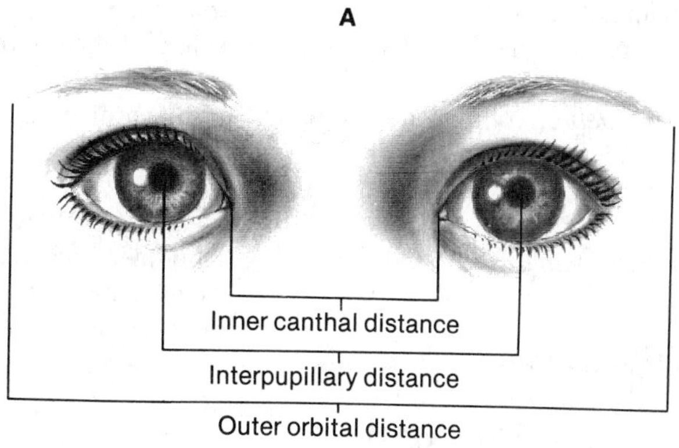

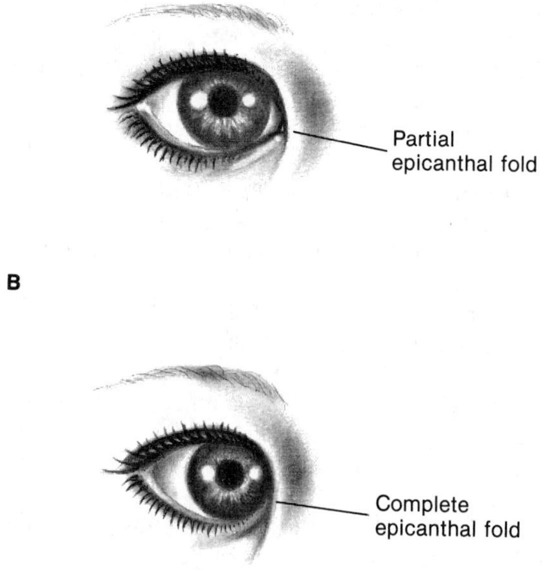

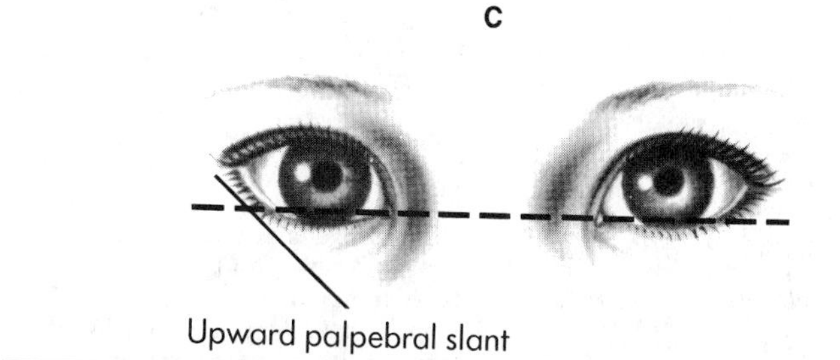

Fig. 7-18. A, Anatomic landmarks of eye. **B,** Epicanthal folds. **C,** Upward palpebral slant. (Note imaginary line to determine slant.)

drome characteristically demonstrate hypertelorism, epicanthal folds, and upward palpebral slant.

The *lids* are inspected for proper placement on the eye. When the eye is open, the upper lid should fall somewhere between the upper iris and upper rim of the pupil. *Ptosis* refers to a lid that covers part of the pupil or the lower part of the iris. The term *sunset eyes* or the *setting-sun sign* refers to an upper lid that covers no part of the iris, allowing some of the sclera or "white-of-the-eye" to show. Although either can be a normal variant of lid placement, it can also be a sign of several disorders.

When the eyes are closed, the lids should completely cover the cornea and sclera. Failure to do so can result in chronic eye irritation and infection. When the lids are opened or closed, no palpebral conjunctiva should be visible. Malposition of the eyelids includes *ectropion*, a rolling-out of the lids with exposed conjunctiva, and *entropion*, a turning-in of the lid. The latter is normally found in some Oriental children. The nurse should check to see if the inturned lid causes irritation of the cornea.

Inspection of External Structures

The lids are also observed for color (any sign of hemorrhage), size (any evidence of edema), and mobility. Normally the lids contain the same amount of pigmentation as does the rest of the skin. Inflammation or erythema along the lid is noted. Some of the more common lid disorders are listed in Box 7-9.

The lining of the lids, the *palpebral conjunctiva*, is inspected. Inspecting the lower conjunctival sac is easily accomplished by pulling the lid down while the child looks up. To evert the upper lid, the upper lashes are held and gently pulled *down* and *forward* while the child looks down. If this is not successful, a tongue blade or stem of a cotton-tipped applicator can be placed 1 cm above the edge of the lid margin. With this in place, the nurse gently pushes down on the lid with the stick and rolls the lid upward. As soon as the lid is everted, the fingers holding the lashes are used to keep the lid everted.

Normally the conjunctiva appears pink and glossy. Vertical yellow striations along the edge are the *meibomian* or *sebaceous glands* near the hair follicle. Located in the inner or medial canthus and situated on the inner edge of the upper and lower lids is a tiny opening called the *lacrimal punctum*. Any excessive tearing or inflammation of the lacrimal apparatus is noted.

The lids are observed for blinking movement. Excessive blinking can indicate eyestrain or a nervous habit. Asymmetric or infrequent blinking can be a sign of paralysis or muscle weakness. The blink reflex is tested by making a quick movement toward the eye.

The *eyelashes* are inspected for distribution, direction of growth, and pigmentation. Normally the upper lashes curl upward and the lower lashes curve downward. Lashes that turn inward toward the eyeball can cause conjunctival irritation.

The *bulbar conjunctiva*, which covers the eye up to the limbus or junction of the cornea and sclera, should be transparent, revealing the white color of the underlying sclera. Dilation of the blood vessels in the conjunctiva makes it appear red. Although this redness is characteristic of many disorders, it can also indicate eyestrain, irritation, or fatigue.

The *sclera*, or white covering of the eyeball, should be clear. Any yellow staining is noted, since this may indicate jaundice. Tiny black marks in the sclera of heavily pigmented individuals are normal and do not indicate petechiae or the presence of a foreign body. A bluish tone may indicate disorders such as osteogenesis imperfecta or glaucoma.

The *cornea*, or covering of the iris and pupil, should be clear and transparent. Any opacities are recorded since they can be signs of scarring or ulceration, which can interfere with vision. The best way to test for opacities is to illuminate the eyeball by shining a light at an angle (obliquely) toward the cornea.

The *pupils* are compared for size, shape, and movement. They should be round, clear, and equal. Their *reaction to light* is tested by quickly shining a source of light toward the eye and removing it. As the light approaches, the pupils constrict; as the light fades, the pupils dilate. *Accommodation*, or the focusing ability of the eyes to produce clear vision at different distances, is tested by having the child look at a bright, shiny object at a distance and quickly moving the object toward his face. The pupils constrict as the object is brought near the eye. The normal findings when examining the pupil may be recorded as PERRLA, which means "pupil equal, round, reacts to light and accommodation."

The *iris* is inspected for size, color, and clarity. The iris should be perfectly round; a cleft or notch at its outer edge

Box 7-9 INFLAMMATIONS OF THE EYELID

Hordeolum or stye	Inflammation of sebaceous glands near lashes, usually on lower lid; painful, red, swollen areas
Internal stye	Acute inflammation of meibomian glands of upper lid; if upper lid is everted, stye appears as a yellow line across the tarsus (edge of eyelid)
Chalazion	Granulomas or cysts of internal sebaceous glands (meibomian glands); localized, nontender, firm, discrete swellings covered with freely movable skin
Marginal blepharitis	Inflammation of edge of lid; red, scaly, crusted lid edges; may include pustules around base of lashes and pus from meibomian glands
Dacryocystitis	Inflammation and blockage of lacrimal sac or duct; swelling, redness, and pain, below and to nasal side of inner canthus, with purulent discharge

is called a *coloboma.* Since a visual field defect coincides with the coloboma, this finding warrants further ophthalmologic evaluation. Permanent eye color is usually established by 6 to 12 months of age. Lack of usual eye color and a pink glow to the iris are characteristic of albinism. The pink color is a reflection of the red reflex of the retina. Black-and-white speckling of the iris, known as *Brushfield spots,* is seen in Down syndrome.

As the iris and pupil are inspected, the *lens* is also examined. Normally the lens is not visible while looking into the pupil. White or gray spots usually indicate opacities or cataracts in the lens. Complete opacities prevent funduscopic examination of internal retinal structures.

Inspection of Internal Structures

Inspection of internal structures necessitates the use of a special instrument, the ophthalmoscope. The following discussion describes this instrument, outlines preparation of the child for the examination, and presents the major funduscopic findings.

Use of the ophthalmoscope. The ophthalmoscope permits visualization of the interior of the eyeball with a system of lenses and a high-intensity light. The "ophthalmic head" contains plus lenses (magnifiers), which are usually indicated by black numbers, and minus lenses (minifiers), which are indicated by red numbers. The lenses are changed by rotating a disk on the outside of the head. These lenses permit clear visualization of eye structures at different distances from the nurse's eye and correct visual acuity differences in the examiner and child.

If the nurse wears corrective lenses or glasses, they should be worn when the ophthalmoscope is being used. If the child wears glasses, these should be removed unless they are worn to correct severe astigmatism, which can cause distortion of the images. The lens of the ophthalmoscope can grossly detect visual acuity problems in the child if the nurse who has 20/20 vision is forced to use plus or minus lenses to see the retinal structures clearly. With hyperopia, or farsightedness, higher plus or convex lenses are needed; with myopia, or nearsightedness, more minus or concave lenses are used. Use of the ophthalmoscope requires practice to know which lens setting produces the clearest image.

The interior of the eye is illuminated by a light source within the ophthalmic head, which shines through the lens from a small window. There is also a light dial that changes the type of light emitted through the window. For general purposes the small, white circular light is used for the undilated pupil and the larger white circular light is used for the dilated pupil.

Manipulating the ophthalmoscope. The ophthalmoscope is held by its body in the examiner's dominant hand, and the instrument is placed lightly against the examiner's cheek so that the lens remains directly in front of the eye and the light shines toward the child's eye. With the instrument in position the nurse moves toward the child, approaching from the side at a 15-degree angle, not directly toward the eye. When examining the left eye, the nurse uses the left eye, and vice versa. This is to prevent eyestrain and to approach the child in the best juxtaposition. The nurse's free hand may be used to attract the child's attention away from the instrument's light source and toward a point directly in front of the child to help in guidance while moving as close as possible to the child. The examination should be done in a dimly lit, but not necessarily dark, room.

From a distance of about 1 foot, the examination of the cornea, iris, and lens begins with a lens setting of +8 to +2. Once near the child's face, the lens is changed to 0 or −2. Since the light source falls on only part of the retina at a time, the ophthalmoscope is systematically moved up and down and from side to side to visualize each structure within the fundus (Fig. 7-19).

Preparing the child. The nurse can prepare the child for the ophthalmic examination by showing the child the instrument, demonstrating the light source and how it shines in the eye, and explaining the reason for darkening the room. For infants and young children who do not respond to such explanations, it is best to try to use distraction to encourage them to keep their eyes open. Forcibly parting the lids results in an uncooperative, watery-eyed child and a frustrated nurse. Usually, with some practice, the nurse can elicit a red reflex almost instantly while approaching the child and may also gain a momentary inspection of the blood vessels, macula, or optic disc.

Funduscopic examination. Fig. 7-20 shows the structures of the back of the eyeball, or the *fundus.* The fundus is immediately apparent as the *red reflex.* The intensity of the color increases in darkly pigmented individuals.

✦ **NURSING ALERT** A brilliant, uniform red reflex is an important sign because it virtually rules out almost all serious defects of the cornea, aqueous chamber, lens, and vitreous chamber. Any dark shadows or opacities are recorded because they indicate some abnormality in any of these structures.

As the ophthalmoscope is brought closer to the eye, the most conspicuous feature of the fundus is the *optic disc,* the area where the blood vessels and optic nerve fibers enter and exit from the eye. The round or vertically oval disc is creamy pink but lighter than the surrounding fundus and derives its color from the rich capillary network. Its size is important because other structures of the fundus are measured in relationship to the disc diameter (DD). Most discs have a small, pale depression in their center, called the *physiologic cup* or *depression,* which represents the blind spot of the retina. It is not always visible but, when large enough to be seen, should not extend to the disc margin. Blurring of the disc margins, loss of the depression, and a bulging disc are important signs of papilledema or swelling of the optic nerve, which clinically indicates increased intracranial pressure.

After the optic disc is located, the area is inspected for *blood vessels.* The central retinal artery and vein appear in the depths of the disc and emanate outward with visible branching. The veins are darker in color and about one fourth larger in size than the arteries. A narrow band of

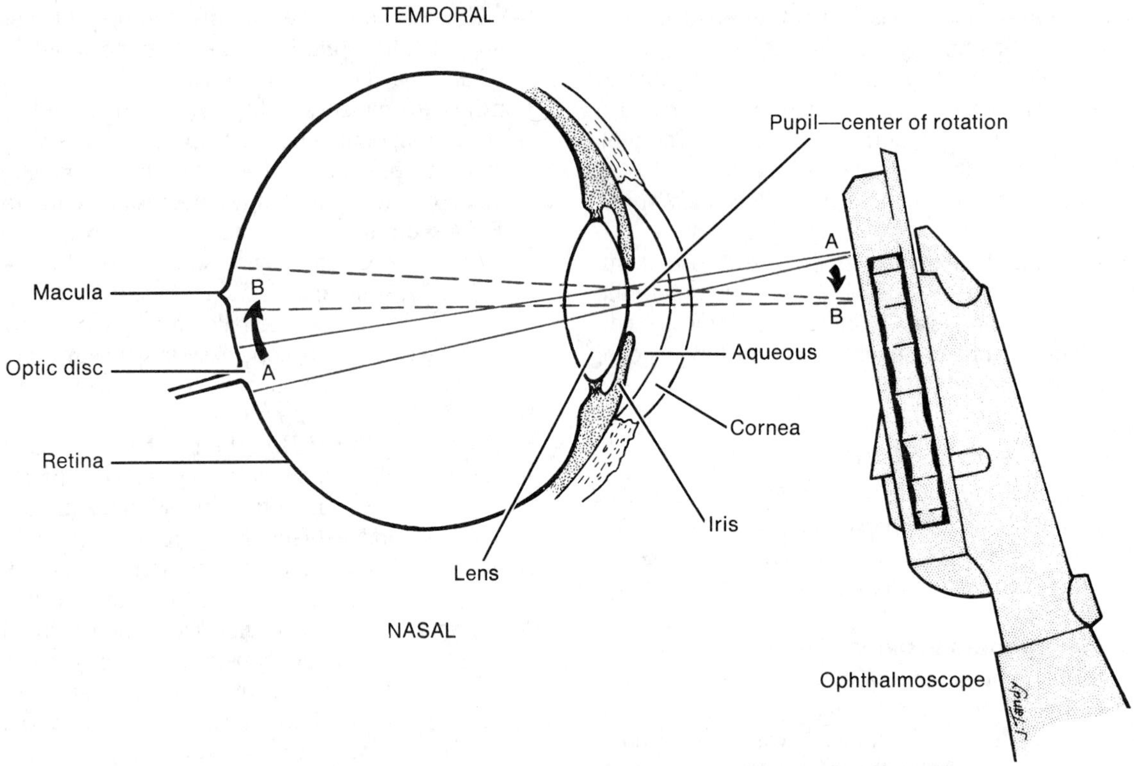

Fig. 7-19. Visual axis through ophthalmoscope. Beam of light **(A)** and its corresponding visual field is usual view when approaching child from side at 15-degree angle. **B** represents a direct visualization with child staring at light.

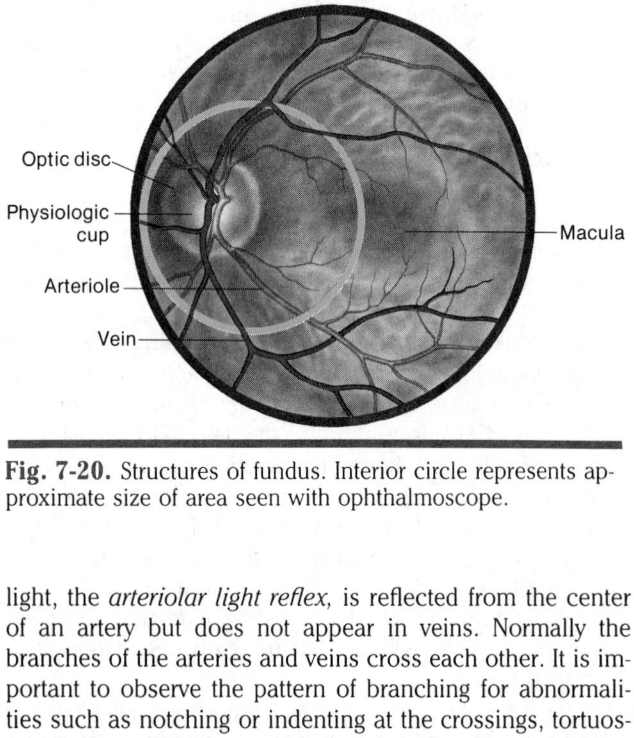

Fig. 7-20. Structures of fundus. Interior circle represents approximate size of area seen with ophthalmoscope.

light, the *arteriolar light reflex,* is reflected from the center of an artery but does not appear in veins. Normally the branches of the arteries and veins cross each other. It is important to observe the pattern of branching for abnormalities such as notching or indenting at the crossings, tortuosity or dilation of the vessels, or small hemorrhages (dark areas) along the branches. Any of these findings are reported for further investigation.

About 2 DD temporal to the disc is the *macula,* the area of the fundus with the greatest concentration of visual receptors. It is about 1 DD in size and darker in color than the fundus (red reflex) or optic disc. The intensity of the color directly correlates with the individual's skin pigmentation; that is, the darker the skin, the darker the color of the macula. In the center of the macula is a minute glistening spot of reflected light called the *fovea centralis,* the area of most perfect vision.

Although abnormalities of the macula are usually not apparent unless the eye is dilated, permitting more detailed inspection, the nurse should at least note its presence. If locating the macula is difficult, the child is asked to look directly at the light. As Fig. 7-19 shows, a light shone directly into the eye falls on the fovea. However, since this is the most light-sensitive area of the retina, the nurse must be careful to focus on the macula only momentarily. If direct visualization does *not* cause the light to fall on the center of the fovea, strabismus may exist because fixation is occurring at a point other than the center of the macula. Recognition of this deviation is of great importance in determining the type of treatment for strabismus, because in this situation the usual regimen of occlusive therapy (covering the stronger eye to force the weaker or deviating eye to focus) will not benefit the child (Havener, 1984).

Vision Testing

Several tests are available for assessing vision. This discussion focuses on four areas: (1) binocularity, (2) visual acu-

A

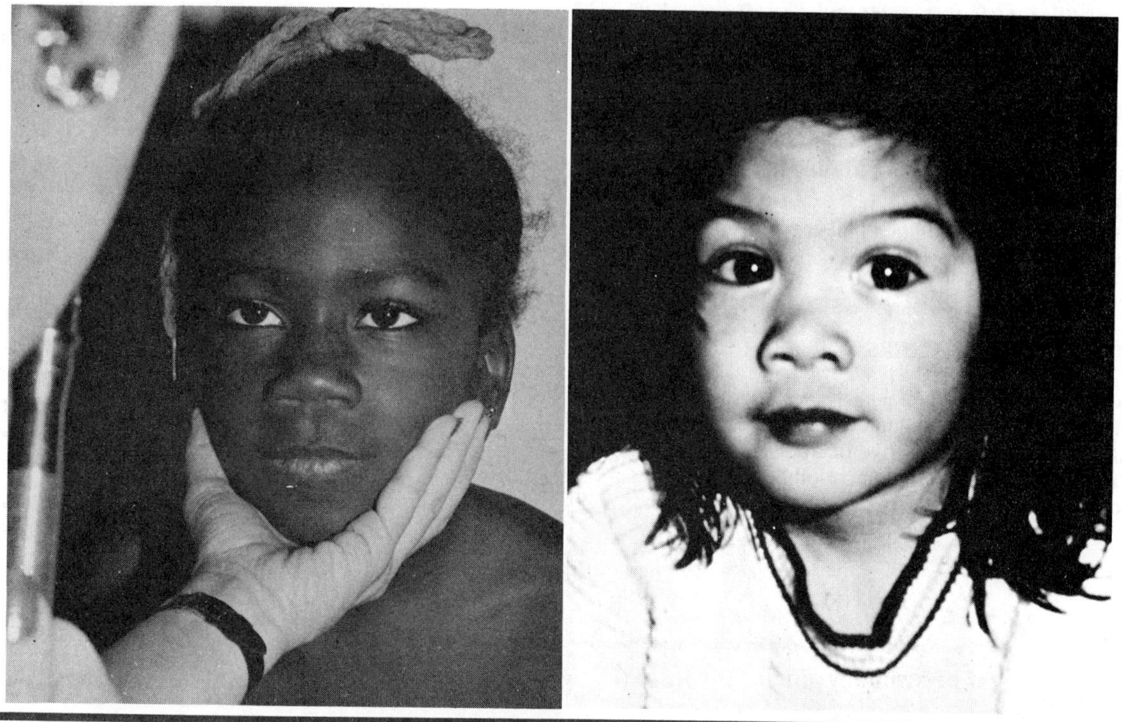

B

Fig. 7-21. A, Corneal light reflex test demonstrating orthophoric eyes. B, Pseudostrabimus. Inner epicanthal folds cause eyes to appear malaligned; however, corneal light reflexes fall perfectly symmetrically.

ity, (3) peripheral vision, and (4) color vision. The reader is also referred to Chapter 25 for behavioral and physical signs that indicate visual impairment.

Binocularity. Normally, by the age of 3 to 4 months, children achieve the ability to fixate on one visual field with both eyes simultaneously (binocularity). One of the most important tests for binocularity is alignment of the eyes to detect nonbinocular vision or strabismus. In strabismus, or "cross-eye," one eye deviates from the point of fixation. If the malalignment is constant, the weak eye becomes "lazy" and eventually the brain suppresses the image produced by that eye. If strabismus is not detected and corrected by age 4 to 6 years, a type of blindness, called *amblyopia*, may result.

Two tests commonly used to detect malalignment are the corneal light reflex and the cover tests. In the *corneal light reflex test* (also called *red reflex gemini test* or *Hirschberg test*), a flashlight or the light of the ophthalmoscope is shined directly into the eyes from a distance of about 40.5 cm (16 inches). If the eyes are orthophoric or normal, the light falls symmetrically within each pupil (Fig. 7-21, *A*) or twin red reflexes are observed. If the light falls off center in one eye, the eyes are malaligned. Epicanthal folds may give a false impression of malalignment of the eyes (pseudostrabismus) (Fig. 7-21, *B*).

Terms for describing the types of strabismus are:

Esotropia or **esophoria**—inward deviation of the eye (see Fig. 25-3)
Exotropia or **exophoria**—outward deviation of the eye
Phoria—malalignment that is not obvious until fusion is disrupted
Tropia—constant or intermittent malalignment of the eyes; more severe and more likely to result in amblyopia than phoria

In the *cover test*, one eye is covered and the movement of the *uncovered* eye is observed while the child gazes on a near (33 cm, or 13 inches) or distant (50 cm, or 20 inches) object. If the uncovered eye does not move, it is aligned. If the uncovered eye moves, a malalignment is present because when the stronger eye is temporarily covered, the weaker eye attempts to fixate on the object.

In the *uncover test*, occlusion is shifted back and forth from one eye to the other eye and movement of the *covered* eye is observed while the child is fixating at a point in front of him. If normal alignment is present, shifting the cover from one eye to the other eye will not cause movement of the covered eye. If malalignment is present, the covered eye will move from its position when covered to a straight position when uncovered. This test takes more practice than the other cover test because the occluder must be moved back and forth quickly and accurately in order to see the eye move (see Nursing Tip, p. 252). Since deviations can occur at different ranges, particularly in the case of phorias, it is important to perform the cover tests at both near and far distances.

Visual acuity testing in young and school-age children. Visual acuity refers to the ability to see near and far objects clearly. The most commonly used test for measuring acuity is the *Snellen Letter Chart* (see Appendix B). It consists of lines of letters in decreasing size. Each line is given a value, for example, line 7 is "20."

During testing children stand 20 feet from the chart (with heels at the 20-foot line) and read each line. If they can read line 7, they have 20/20 vision, the accepted standard for normal acuity. If they can read only line 2, they have 20/100 vision—they are able to see at a distance of 20 feet what people with 20/20 or normal eyesight can see at 100 feet.

NURSING TIP: OCCLUDERS FOR THE COVER TEST

The cover test is usually easier to perform if the examiner uses his or her own hand rather than a card-type occluder (Fig. 7-22). Attractive occluders fashioned like an ice cream cone or happy face lollipop cut from cardboard are also well received by young children.

Other letter or symbol screening tests are described in Table 7-9. Many of the tests that are suitable for preschoolers can also be used for difficult-to-test children, such as those with developmental delays. The Snellen symbol chart is frequently used to screen preschool children (see Appendix B). However, many young children have difficulty because of confusion in identifying the direction of the E, rather than inability to see the symbol clearly. To avoid this problem, the Blackbird Preschool Vision Screening System was developed by a nurse (Fig. 7-23). The screening system uses a modified E that resembles a bird and a story about the Blackbird to help engage children's attention. Testing is done with flash cards or a wall-mounted chart, and the children are instructed to indicate the direction of the bird's flight. Some have reported a higher percentage of children successfully tested with the Blackbird System than with the Snellen E (Sato-Viacrucis, 1986). The Blackbird System also contains guidelines for vision screening the noncommuni-

Table 7-9 Letter or symbol vision acuity tests

TEST	DESCRIPTION	COMMENTS*
Snellen Letter†	Uses letters of the English alphabet for testing at 20 feet	Suitable for most children above the second grade who are familiar with reading the alphabet
Snellen E†	Uses the capital letter E pointing in four directions; children "read" the chart by showing the direction of the letter E or using a large duplicate E to match the chart E at 20 feet	For illiterate or non-English-speaking people and preschool children and grade 1 Preschool children often have difficulty with direction despite adequate vision
Home Eye Test for Preschoolers‡	Uses a large letter E for demonstration and an E chart for testing at 10 feet	Designed for use by parents for children 3 to 6 years
Blackbird Preschool Vision Screening System§	Uses a modified E to resemble a flying bird; children identify which way the bird is flying Uses flash cards, story-telling, and disposable cardboard eyeglass occluders	Designed for children as young as 3 years
Blackbird Storybook Home Eye Test§	Similar to above	Designed for use by parents for children as young as 2½ years
HOTV or Matching Symbol†	Uses the four letters H, O, T, and V on a chart for testing at 10 or 20 feet Child names the letters on the chart or matches them to a demonstration card	Suitable for children as young as 3 years Avoids the problem with image reversal and eye-hand coordination that can occur with the letter E
Faye Symbol Chart†	Use pictures of a house, apple, and umbrella on a chart for testing at 10 feet	Suitable for children as young as 27 to 30 months
Denver Eye Screening Test (DEST)‖	Uses single cards for the letter E, one for demonstration and one for testing at 15 feet Also uses Allen Picture Cards (a tree, birthday cake, horse and rider, telephone, car, house, and teddy bear) for testing at 15 feet	Suitable for children 2½ years and older May be reliably used with cooperative children from the age of 24 months
Dot Test†	Uses a series of different-sized dots; child points to one of the nine dots randomly positioned on a disk	Suitable for children as young as 24 months

*Ages for testing are based on published reports. Proper instruction of young children is essential for successful screening.
†Available from Good-Lite Company, 1540 Hannah Ave., Forest Park, IL 60130; (312) 366-3860.
‡Available from the National Society to Prevent Blindness, 500 E. Remington Rd., Schaumburg, IL 60173; (800) 331-2020.
§Available from Blackbird Vision Screening System, PO Box 277424, Sacramento, CA 95827; (916) 363-6884.
‖Available from Denver Developmental Materials, Inc., PO Box 6919, Denver, CO 80206-0919; (303) 355-4729.

A

B

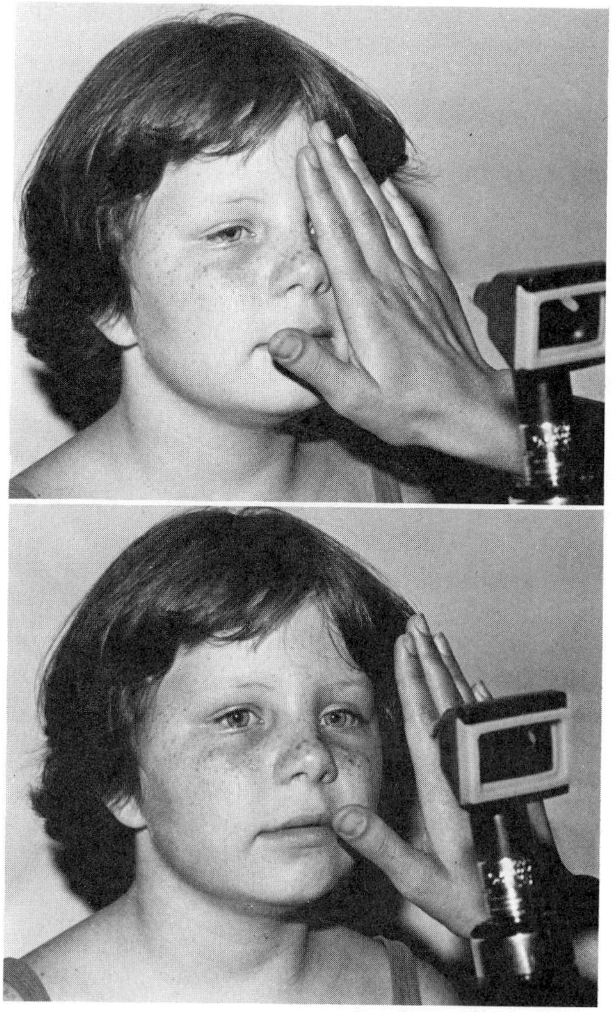

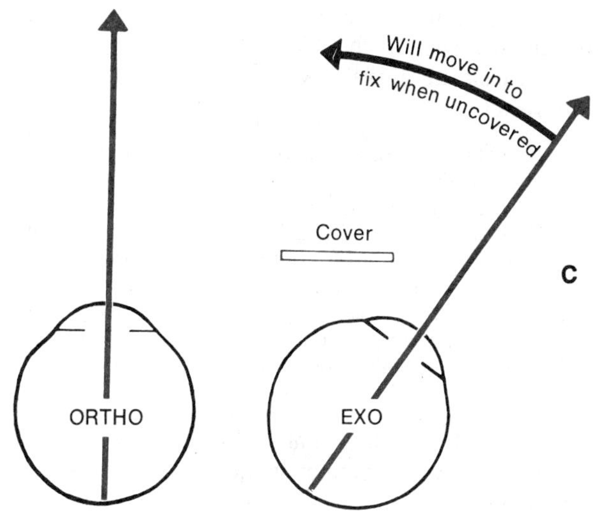

Fig. 7-22. Uncover test for strabismus. **A,** Eye is occluded, child is fixating on light source. **B,** If eye does not move when uncovered, eyes are aligned. **C,** Exophoria. As eye is uncovered, it shifts to fixate on object.

C from Prior, J.A., Silberstein, J.S., and Stang, J.M.: Physical diagnosis: the history and examination of the patient, ed. 6, St. Louis, 1981, Mosby–Year Book, Inc.

cative, nonreaders, or non-English-speaking children to assist screeners with more difficult-to-test populations, and the Blackbird Storybook Home Eye Test is designed for parents to prescreen young children at home.

Although most chart tests are designed for testing at 20 feet, modifications can be made for testing at closer ranges because it is easier to engage children's attention at a closer range, and the charts require less space for the screening lane. Measurements at closer range are converted to the standard 20-foot scale by multiplying the two numbers by the number that converts the first one to 20. For example, 10/25 is equivalent to 20/50. When closer ranges are used, proper positioning of the child (e.g., with heels on the 10-foot mark) is essential. Because young children are active, their tendency to move or lean forward can affect the testing more at close distances than at farther ones. Both the Snellen Letter and Snellen Symbol charts for use at 10 feet are available from the National Society to Prevent Blindness and from the Good-Lite Company (for addresses, see Table 7-9).

The Snellen charts are usually used for testing far visual acuity to detect myopia (nearsightedness). However, in school-age children they can also be used to test for hyperopia (farsightedness). The *plus lens test for hyperopia* involves having the child wear a pair of convex or plus lenses. With these lenses the child should be *unable* to read the 20/20 or 20/30 line. Ability to see these lines clearly indicates excessive farsightedness and represents a need for referral.

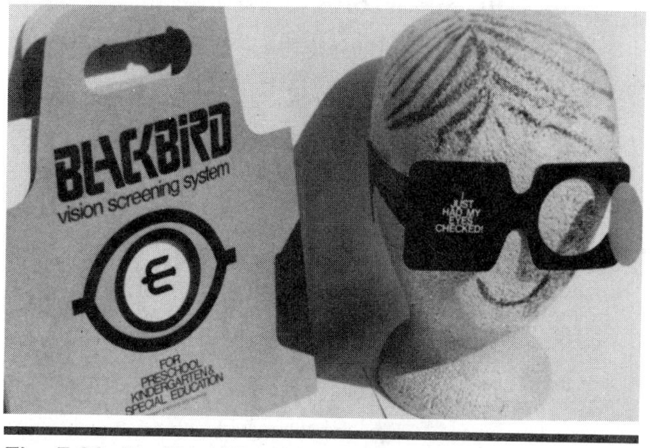

Fig. 7-23. Blackbird Vision Screening System. Note Blackbird symbol and special "eyeglass" occluder.

Vision performance can also be measured using optical instruments, such as the *Titmus Vision Tester.** Three sections of tests are available with the Professional Model Titmus Tester:

1. The Michigan Pre-School Test, which tests visual acuity and binocularity using the letter E in children from 3½ years of age through grade 1
2. The Massachusetts Vision Test, which tests visual acuity, hyperopia (plus lens test), and binocularity (both near and far) using the letter E in elementary school children
3. The Adult Series, which tests near and far visual acuity using the standard Snellen letters, binocularity, and color perception in secondary school children and adults

There are no universal criteria for referring children when using the Snellen charts. The American Academy of Pediatrics (1986) recommends the following criteria for vision referral:

1. Children before their fifth birthday who are unable to read the 20/40 line or less
2. Children 5 years and older who are unable to read at the 20/30 line or less
3. A 2-line difference of visual acuity between the eyes, even within the passing range

The National Society to Prevent Blindness (1988) recommends the following criteria for referral of children for a complete eye examination:

1. Three-year-old children with vision in either eye of 20/50 or less (inability to correctly identify one more than half the symbols on the 40-foot line) or a two-line difference in visual acuity between the eyes in the passing range, for example, 20/20 in one eye and 20/40 in the other eye
2. All other ages and grades with vision in either eye of 20/40 or less (inability to correctly identify one more than half the symbols on the 30-foot line)
3. All children who consistently show any signs of possible visual disturbances, regardless of visual acuity (see Chapter 25)

*Manufactured by Titmus Optical, Inc., Petersburg, VA 23804.

Visual acuity testing in infants and difficult-to-test children. In newborns, vision is tested mainly by checking for *light perception* by shining a light into the eyes and noting responses such as pupillary constriction, blinking, following the light to midline, increased alertness, or refusal to open the eyes after exposure to the light. Although the simple maneuver of checking light perception and eliciting the pupillary light reflex indicates that the anterior half of the visual apparatus is intact, it does not confirm that the infant can see. In other words, this test does not assess whether the brain receives the visual message and interprets the signals.

Another test of visual acuity is the infant's ability to fix on and follow a target. Although any brightly colored or patterned object can be used, the human face is excellent. The infant is held upright while the nurse's face moves slowly from side to side. If visual fixation and following are not present by 3 to 4 months of age, further ophthalmologic evaluation is needed (Nelson and others, 1984).

Other signs that may indicate visual loss include fixed pupils, marked strabismus, constant nystagmus, setting-sun sign, and slow lateral movements. Unfortunately it is very difficult to test each eye separately; the presence of such signs in one eye could indicate unilateral blindness.

Special tests are available for testing infants and other

Table 7-10 Special tests of visual acuity and estimated visual acuity at different ages

TEST	DESCRIPTION	BIRTH	4 MONTHS	1 YEAR	AGE OF 20/20 VISION
Optokinetic nystagmus	A striped drum is rotated or a striped tape is moved in front of infant's eyes. Presence of nystagmus indicates vision. Acuity is assessed by using progressively smaller stripes.	20/400	20/200	20/60	20-30 months
Forced choice preferential looking*	Either a homogeneous field or a striped field is presented to infant; an observer monitors the direction of the eyes during presentation of pattern. Acuity is assessed by using progressively smaller striped fields.	20/400	20/200	20/50	18-24 months
Visually evoked potentials	Eyes are stimulated with bright light or pattern, and electrical activity to visual cortex is recorded through scalp electrodes. Acuity is assessed by using progressively smaller patterns.	20/100 to 20/200	20/80	20/40	6-12 months

Data from Hoyt, C., Nickel, B., and Billson, F.: Ophthalmological examination of the infant: development aspects, Surv. Ophthalmol. 26:177-189, 1982.
*One type of preferential looking test is the *Teller Acuity Card Test,* in which a set of rectangular cards containing different black and white patterns or grading is presented to the child as an observer looks through a central peephole in the card. The observer, who is hidden from view, observes the variety of visual cues, such as fixation, eye movements, head movements, or pointing. The finest grading the child is judged to be able to see is taken as the acuity estimate. The test is appropriate for children from birth to 24 to 36 months of age. (Teller, D., and others: Assessment of visual acuity in infants and children: the acuity card procedure, Dev. Med. Child Neurol. 28:779-789, 1986.)

difficult-to-test children to assess acuity and/or confirm blindness. These tests are presented in Table 7-10 with the estimated visual acuity at different ages. The discrepancy between the acuities obtained by the various techniques probably reflects the testing of different responses of the developing infant's brain (Hoyt, Nickel, and Billson, 1982).

Peripheral vision. In children who are old enough to cooperate, peripheral vision, or the visual field of each eye, is estimated. The test is performed by having children fixate on a specific point directly in front of them as an object, such as a finger or a pencil, is moved from beyond the field of vision into the range of peripheral vision. Each eye is checked separately and for each quadrant of vision. As soon as children see the object, they tell the nurse to stop moving it. At that point the angle from the anteroposterior axis of the eye (straight line of vision) to the peripheral axis (point at which the object is first seen) is measured. Normally children see about 50 degrees upward, 70 degrees downward, 60 degrees nasalward, and 90 degrees temporally. Limitations in peripheral vision may indicate blindness from damage to structures within the eye or to any of the visual pathways.

Color vision. Another important test is for color vision. It is estimated that from 8% to 10% of white males and less than half that percentage of black males have inherited the X-linked disorder known as *color vision deficit* (less acceptable term, *color blindness*). From 0.5% to 1% of white females are affected. Although the severity of impaired perception of color varies considerably, the two most common types are *protanomaly,* in which the child confuses gray with pink or pale blue with green, and *deuteranomaly,* in which the child confuses gray with pale purple or green. In most of these individuals, the color vision deficit causes no major problems. However, some of the difficulties encountered by individuals with more severe deficits may be inability to distinguish amber or red traffic lights, failure to see a red brake light on the rear of a car, difficulty in distinguishing green traffic lights from certain types of incandescent street lamps, and a poor sense of color coordination of clothing. For school-age children the greatest difficulty lies in performance of academic skills that use color as a visual aid. Adolescents may be ineligible for certain vocational opportunities, such as electronics, photography, printing, interior decorating, pharmaceuticals, textiles, police work, and for several types of military service (Kovalesky, 1985).

The tests available for color vision include the *Ishihara test* and the *Hardy-Rand-Rittler* (HRR) *test*. Each consists of a series of cards (pseudoisochromatic) on which is printed a color field composed of spots of a certain "confusion" color. Against the field is a number or symbol similarly printed in dots but of a color likely to be confused with the field color by the person with a color vision deficit. As a result the figure or letter is invisible to an affected individual but is clearly seen by a person with normal vision. By using the HRR test, which uses symbols rather than numbers, reliable testing can be done on children as young as 3 years of age (Kovalesky, 1985). Nurses administering the test must be familiar with the testing materials and should be able to inform the parents of the disorder's effects on practical areas of living, its genetic transmission, and its irreversibility.

EARS

Like the eyes, examination of the ears involves inspection of the external auditory structures, visualization of the internal landmarks using the otoscope, and screening for hearing ability.

Placement and Alignment

The entire external earlobe is called the *pinna,* or *auricle,* and is located on each side of the head. The height alignment of the pinna is measured by drawing an imaginary line from the outer orbit of the eye to the occiput or most prominent protuberance of the skull. The top of the pinna should meet or cross this line (Fig. 7-24, *A*). Low-set ears (Fig. 7-24, *B*) are commonly associated with renal anomalies or mental retardation. The angle of the pinna is measured by draw-

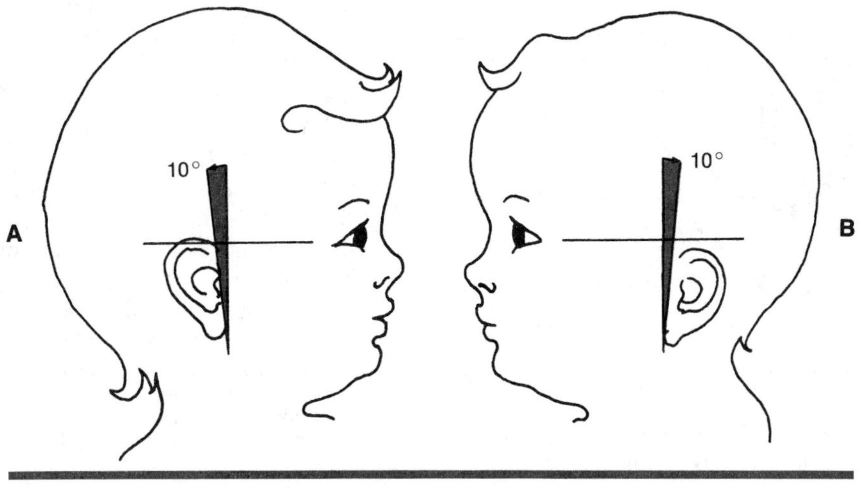

Fig. 7-24. Ear alignment. **A,** Normal. **B,** Abnormal.

ing a perpendicular line from the imaginary horizontal line and aligning the pinna next to this mark. Normally the pinna lies within a 10-degree angle of the vertical line (Fig. 7-24, *A*). If it falls outside this area (Fig. 7-24, *B*), the nurse records the deviation and looks closely for other anomalies.

Normally the pinna extends slightly outward from the skull. Except in newborn infants, ears that are flat against the head or protruding away from the scalp may indicate problems. For example, masses or swelling make the pinna stand forward and may indicate mastoiditis, mumps, or postauricular abscesses. Flattened ears in infants may suggest a frequent side-lying position and may offer a clue to the parents' lack of understanding of the child's stimulation needs.

Inspection of External Structures

The pinna, or auricle, can be considered an "oracle" because deviations in structure can be a sign of possible middle ear anomalies and congenital conductive hearing loss (Jaffe, 1976). Fig. 7-25 shows the usual landmarks of the pinna. The *helix* is the prominent outer rim of the pinna. The *antihelix* is a second curved rim that is adjacent and almost parallel to the helix. The *concha* is a deep cavity, within and partly surrounded by the antihelix, that leads into the external auditory canal. Lying anterior to the concha is a prominent protuberance called the *tragus*, and opposite to this is the *antitragus*, below which is the *lobule*. In some children the lobule is adherent with the helix in an upward and backward slant. An adherent lobule is considered a normal variation. Each of the major projections of the pinna forms corresponding depressions. There is remarkable similarity among external pinnas; the nurse should be familiar with eminences and depressions in order to note deviations.

The skin surface around the ear is inspected for small openings, extra tags of skin, or sinuses. If a sinus is found, a special notation of this is made, since it may represent a fistula that drains into some area of the neck or ear. Cutaneous tags represent no pathologic process but may cause parents concern in terms of the child's appearance.

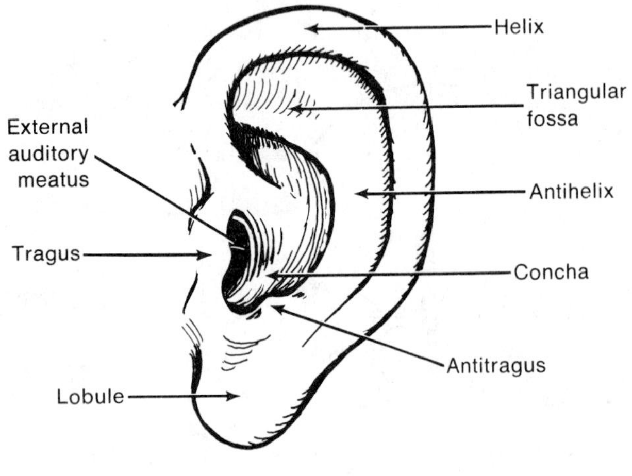

Fig. 7-25. Usual landmarks of pinna.

The ear is also inspected for general hygiene. An otoscope is not necessary to look into the external canal to note the presence of *cerumen*, a waxy substance produced by the ceruminous glands in the outer portion of the canal. If the ear canal appears totally free of cerumen, the nurse should inquire as to how the ears are cleaned. Occasionally parents insert cotton-tipped swabs or thin objects, such as bobby pins, into the canal to remove wax. Deep insertion of such objects can damage the drum or walls of the canal, as well as push the wax against the tympanic membrane to form a plug. It is best to question parents about ear cleaning by remarking how clean the ears are and casually asking how they remove the wax. This approach is more likely to yield an honest answer than is direct questioning about the use of specific instruments.

In general, it is best to advise parents or children to clean the ears with a washcloth and, if they use a swab, to gently wipe only the outermost portion of the canal. They should always avoid using any sharp, hard object in the ear. If the cerumen is hard and dry (appears dark and crusted, rather than yellow-brown and soft), it can be softened and removed by instilling 2 or 3 drops of mineral oil into the ear for a few days and then rinsing the canal with an ear syringe. Commercial products (Cerumenex, Murine, Debrox) are also available without prescription to aid in removing desiccated cerumen.* Cerumen must be removed to adequately examine an ear if otitis media is suspected. Removal is most easily accomplished with irrigation, using room temperature tap water or normal saline and a Water-Pik or rubber ball syringe (Watkins, Moore, and Phillips, 1984).

The presence, color, and odor of any discharge from the aural canal are noted. If discharge is present in one canal, care is taken to prevent transmitting potentially infectious material to the other ear or to another child through handwashing, using disposable specula, or sterilizing reusable specula between each examination (Lowrey and others, 1988).

Inspection of Internal Structures

Inspection of internal structures necessitates the use of the otoscope. The following discussion describes the instrument and its use, outlines positioning and preparation of the child for the examination, and presents the major otoscopic findings.

Use of the otoscope. The otic head permits visualization of the tympanic membrane by use of a bright light, a magnifying glass, and a speculum. Some otoscopes have an attachment for a pneumatic device to insert air into the canal when a determination of membrane compliance (movement) is needed. The speculum comes in a variety of sizes (2, 3, 4, and 5 mm) to accommodate different canal widths. The largest speculum that fits comfortably into the ear should be used to achieve the greatest area of visualization.

*A booklet for families regarding ear care is *Caring for Your Ears*, available from Ross Laboratories, Customer Relations, 625 Cleveland Ave., Columbus, OH 43216; (614) 229-7921.

The lens or magnifying glass is movable, allowing the examiner to insert an object, such as a curette, into the ear canal through the speculum while still viewing the structures through the lens. The handle is the same as for the ophthalmic head and operates similarly. The nurse should become familiar with the instrument and practice attaching the otic head to the handle.

Positioning the child. Before beginning the otoscopic examination, the child is positioned properly and restrained if necessary. Older children usually are cooperative and do not need restraint. However, the nurse should prepare them for the procedure by allowing them to play with the instrument, demonstrating how it works, and stressing the importance of remaining still. A helpful suggestion is letting them observe the nurse examining the parent's ear. Older children can view the inside of the ear. With younger children one can explain that he or she is looking for a "big elephant" in the ear. This kind of "fairy tale" is an absorbing distraction and usually elicits cooperation. After the ear has been examined, it is important to clarify that "looking for elephants" was only pretending.

As the speculum is inserted into the meatus, it is moved around the outer rim to accustom the child to the feel of something entering the ear. If examining a painful ear, it is helpful to touch some nonpainful part of the affected ear, then examine the unaffected ear, and finally return to the painful ear. By this time the child is usually less fearful of anything causing discomfort to the ear and will be more cooperative.

For their protection and safety infants and toddlers must be restrained for the otoscopic examination. There are two general positions of restraint. In one the child is seated sideways in the parent's lap with one arm "hugging" the parent and the other arm at the side. The ear to be examined is toward the nurse. With one arm the parent holds the child's head firmly against his or her chest, and with the other arm "hugs" the child, thereby securing the child's free arm. The ear is examined using the same procedure for holding the otoscope as described later (Fig. 7-26, *A*).

The other position involves placing the child on the side or abdomen with the arms at the side and the head turned so that the ear to be examined points toward the ceiling. The nurse leans over the child and uses the upper part of the body to restrain the arms and upper trunk movements and the examining hand to stabilize the head. This position is practical for young infants or for older children who need minimum restraining, but it may not be feasible for other children who protest vigorously. For safety the nurse should enlist the parent's help in immobilizing the head by firmly placing one hand above the ear and the other on the child's back or side (Fig. 7-26, *B*).

With cooperative children the ear can be examined with the child in a side-lying, sitting, or standing position. One disadvantage to standing is that the child may "walk away" as the otoscope enters the canal. If the child is standing or sitting, proper positioning of the head is essential to achieve a full view of the membrane. The head is tilted slightly away from the nurse or toward the child's opposite shoulder to bring the drum to a 90-degree angle (Fig. 7-27).

Manipulating the otoscope. With the thumb and forefinger of the free (usually nondominant) hand, the nurse grasps the auricle. For the two positions of restraint, the otoscope is held upside down at the junction of its head and handle with the thumb and index finger. The other fingers are placed against the skull to allow the otoscope to move with the child in case of sudden movement. In examining a cooperative child, the handle can be held with the otic head upright or upside down. The dominant hand can be used to examine both ears, as shown in Figs. 7-26 and 7-27, or reversed for each ear, whichever is more comfortable.

A

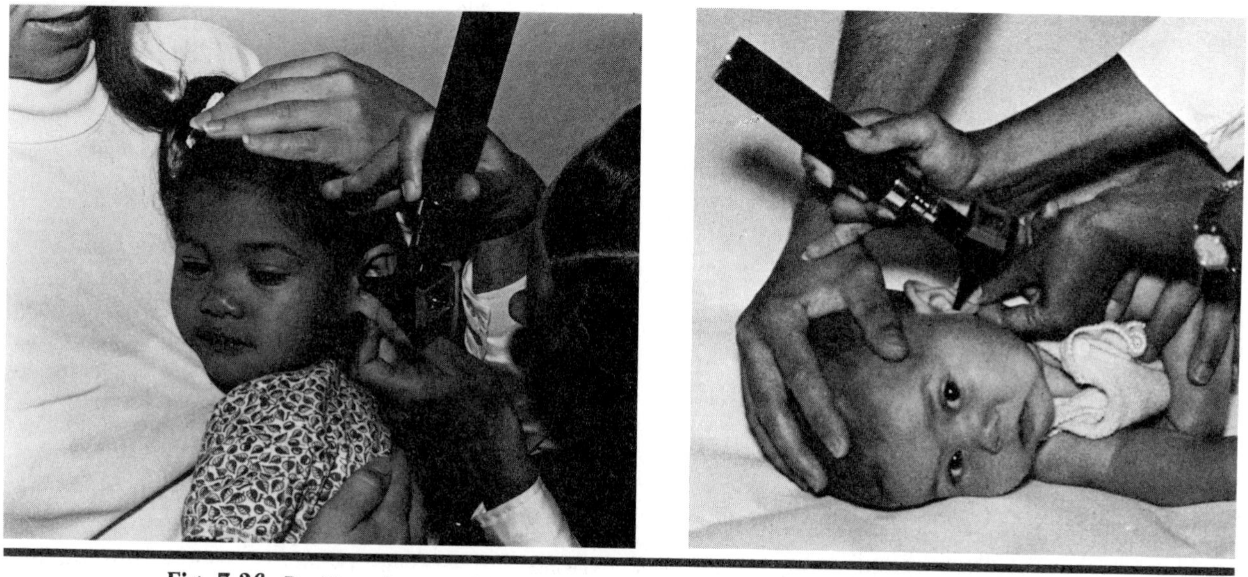

B

Fig. 7-26. Positions for restraining child, **A,** and infant, **B,** during otoscopic examination.

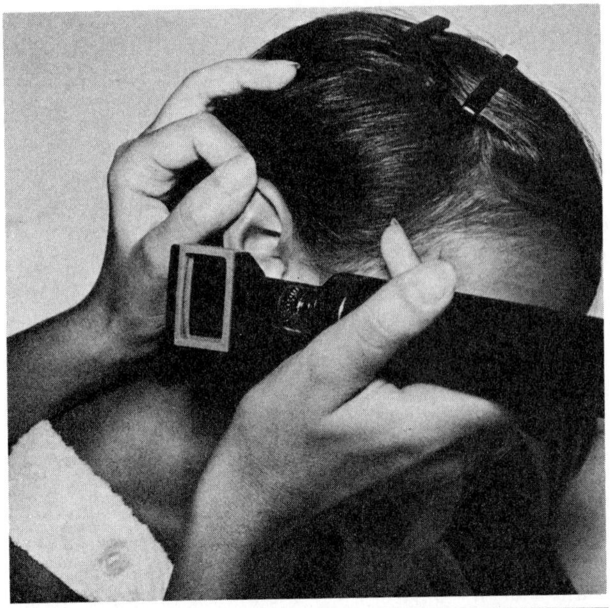

Fig. 7-27. Positioning head by tilting it toward opposite shoulder for full view of tympanic membrane.

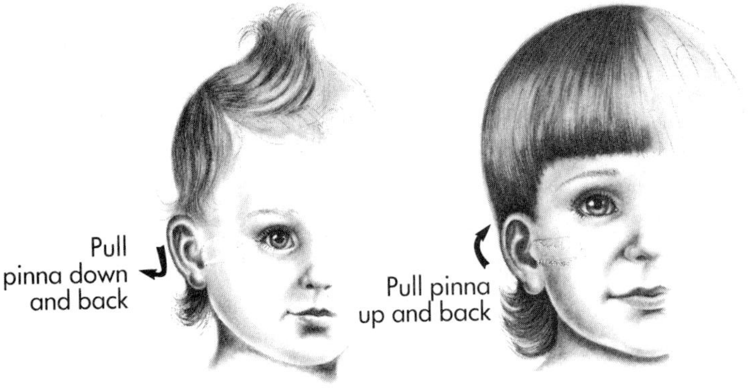

Fig. 7-28. Straightening the canal to view the eardrum in infant, **A,** and child over 3 years of age, **B.**

Entering the canal. Before the otoscope is introduced into the canal, the nurse visualizes the external ear and the tympanic membrane as superimposed on a clock (see Fig. 7-30). The numbers become important geographic landmarks. The speculum is introduced into the meatus between the 3 and 9 o'clock positions in a *downward* and *forward* position. Because the canal is curved, the speculum does not permit a panoramic view of the tympanic membrane unless the canal is straightened. In infants the canal curves upward and the tympanic membrane lies almost horizontally along the upper wall of the canal. The pinna must be pulled *downward* and *backward* to the 6 to 9 o'clock range to straighten the canal (Fig. 7-28, *A*).

With older children, usually those over 3 years of age, the canal curves downward and forward, and the drum, although more vertical, slopes inward and forward. Therefore the pinna is pulled *upward* and *back* toward a 10 o'clock position (Fig. 7-28, *B*). If there is difficulty in visualizing the membrane, it can be brought into view by repositioning the head, introducing the speculum at a different angle, and pulling the pinna in a slightly different direction.

In neonates and young infants the walls of the canal are pliable and floppy because of the underdeveloped cartilaginous and bony structures. Therefore the very small 2 mm speculum usually needs to be inserted deeper into the canal than in older children. Great care must be exercised not to damage the walls or drum. Because the small opening of the speculum permits a limited view, each quadrant of the membrane must be systematically inspected. In older children the speculum need not be inserted past the cartilaginous (outermost) portion of the canal, usually a distance of 0.60 to 1.25 cm (¼ to ½ inch). The entire canal is about 2.5

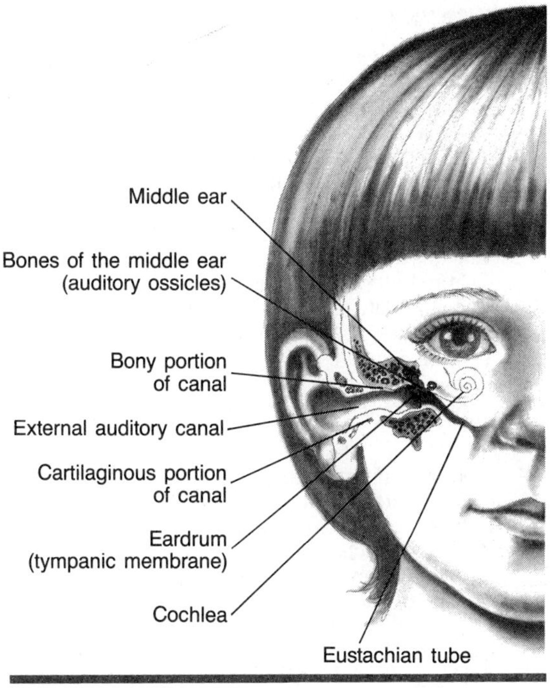

Fig. 7-29. Cross-section of external, middle, and parts of inner ear.

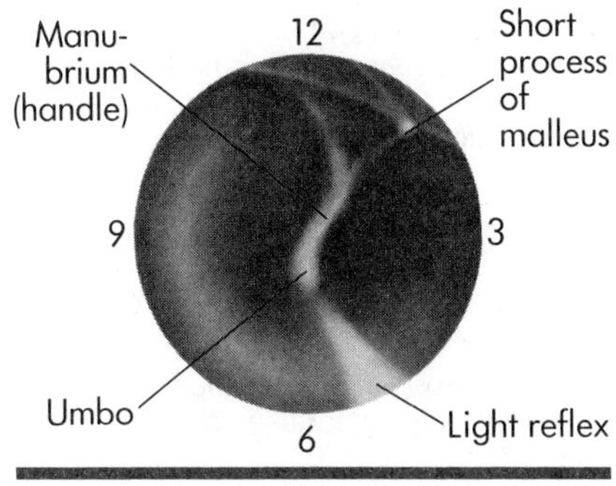

Fig. 7-30. Landmarks of tympanic membrane with "clock" superimposed.

cm (1 inch) long. Insertion of the speculum into the posterior or bony portion of the canal causes pain (Fig. 7-29).

Otoscopic examination. As the speculum is introduced into the external canal, the walls of the canal, the color of the tympanic membrane, the light reflex, and the usual landmarks of the bony prominences of the middle ear are inspected (Fig. 7-30).

The *walls* of the external auditory canal are pink, although they are more pigmented in dark-skinned children. Minute hairs are evident in the outermost portion, where cerumen is produced. Signs of irritation, foreign bodies, or infection are noted.

Foreign bodies in the ear are not uncommon in children and range from erasers to beans. Symptoms may include pain, discharge, and affected hearing. Soft objects, such as paper or insects, can be removed with forceps. Small, hard objects, such as pebbles, can be removed with a suction tip, a hook, or irrigation. However, irrigation is contraindicated if the object is vegetative matter, such as beans or pasta, which swells when in contact with fluid.

✦ **NURSING ALERT** If there is any doubt about the type of object in the ear and the appropriate method to remove it, refer the child to the appropriate practitioner.

The *color* of the *tympanic membrane* is a translucent, light pearly pink or gray. Marked erythema (which may indicate suppurative otitis media), a dull nontransparent grayish color (sometimes suggestive of serous otitis media), or ashen-gray areas (signs of scarring from a previous perforation) are noted. A black area usually suggests a perforation of the membrane that has not healed; perforations are commonly located at the periphery of the drum. Slight redness is normal in the newborn because of increased vascularity and is often evident in older infants and young children as a result of crying.

The characteristic tenseness and slope of the tympanic membrane cause the light of the otoscope to reflect at about the 5 or 7 o'clock position. The *light reflex* is a fairly well-defined cone-shaped reflection, which normally points away from the face. Absence of the light reflex is always recorded, since it signifies bulging of the membrane and loss of its usual contours.

The *bony landmarks* of the drum are formed by the following structures. The *umbo,* or tip of the malleus bone, appears as a small, round, opaque concave spot near the center of the drum. The *manubrium* (long process or handle) of the malleus appears to be a whitish line extending from the umbo upward to the margin of the membrane. At the upper end of the long process near the 1 o'clock position (in the right ear) is a sharp knoblike protuberance, representing the *short process* of the malleus. Sometimes a shadow is seen at about the 10 or 11 o'clock position. This is the junction of the *incus* and the *stapes* bones.

Loss of any of these landmarks is noted, since it is probably caused by the bulging of the membrane as a result of fluid accumulation in the middle ear. Retraction of the drum with abnormal prominence of the bony landmarks suggests serous otitis media.

Auditory Testing

Several types of hearing tests are available. Some of them, such as audiometric testing, involve specialized equipment that measures the degree of hearing loss. Others, such as tests for the startle reflex in neonates, are rough estimations of perception of sound. The nurse must operate under a high index of suspicion for those children who may have conditions associated with hearing loss and who may have developed behaviors that indicate auditory impairment. Types of hearing loss, causes, clinical manifestations, and appropriate treatment are discussed in Chapter 25.

One of the most frequently used tests is *audiometry,* which measures the threshold of hearing for pure-tone fre-

Table 7-11 Selected hearing tests

TEST	DESCRIPTION	COMMENTS
Clinical hearing tests	In newborns, elicit the startle reflex and observe other neonatal responses to loud noises, such as facial grimaces, blinking, gross motor movement, quiet if crying or crying if quiet, opening the eyes, or ceasing sucking activity. During infancy note child's reaction to a noise. Stand about 18 inches away from infant, to the side, and out of child's peripheral field of vision. With the room silent and infant sitting in parent's lap, distracted by some object, make a voice sound such as PS or PHTH (high-pitched), or OO (low-pitched), ring a bell or a rattle, or rustle tissue paper.	An objective sign of alerting to sound may be an increase in heart rate or respiratory rate. Absence of alerting behaviors suggests hearing loss. Eliciting the startle reflex is used only in infants from birth to 4 months. Test is usually inadequate for children beyond infancy because of their tendency to ignore sounds or be distracted. Compare response of localizing sound to expected age response (see Box 12-3).
Crib-o-gram	Neonatal screening tool that analyzes hearing responses by comparing the infant's motor activity before, during, and after a sound is introduced. A motion-sensitive transducer is placed beneath the crib or Isolette mattress, and a microprocessor "reads" the infant's movements.	Both administration of the test and its scoring are totally automated. The test is repeated several times to increase reliability. A consistent change in activity that coincides with the test sound is scored as a pass. Neonates who are premature or ill may not respond to sound despite adequate hearing.
Tympanometry	Measures tympanic membrane compliance (or mobility) and estimates middle ear air pressure. A soft rubber cuff is pressed over the external canal to produce an airtight seal; an automatic reading of air pressure registers on the machine.	Detects middle ear disease and abnormalities but does not indicate the degree of hearing loss or the interpretation of sound. Difficult to perform in young children because of inability to maintain an adequate seal or excessive movement by the child.
Conduction tests	**Rinne test**—Stem of tuning fork is placed against the mastoid bone until the sound ceases to be audible. Tuning fork is then moved so that the prongs are held near, but not touching, the auditory meatus. Child should again hear the sound *(Rinne positive)*. If sound is not again audible *(Rinne negative)*, some abnormality is interfering with the conduction of air through the external and middle chambers.	Requires the cooperation and ability of the child to signal when the sound is no longer audible and when it is again heard. Not useful for most children before preschool age.
	Weber test—Stem of tuning fork is held in the midline of the head. Child should hear the sound equally in both ears *(Weber positive)*. With air conductive loss child will hear the sound better in the affected ear *(Weber negative)*.	Frequently not suitable for young children because of their difficulty in discriminating between "better, more, or less."
Audiometry	Electrical audiometer measures the threshold of hearing for pure-tone frequencies and loudness. A sound is transmitted to the child's ear and reduced until child indicates the sound is no longer heard; this procedure is repeated for several sounds covering the range found in conversation. In an air conduction audiogram the sounds are transmitted through earphones. In a bone conduction audiogram the sounds are passed through a plaque placed over the mastoid bone.	Provides valuable information regarding the severity of the hearing loss, the sound cycles involved, and the possible location of the defect. Requires specialized training of personnel, expensive equipment, and cooperation from the child in terms of confirming the perception of sound. For children 24 months to about 5 years play audiometry can be used; it is based on behavior modification and involves reinforcement for correct response.
Brainstem-evoked auditory response (BEAR)	Through electrode wires attached to the infant's or child's scalp, electrical or brain wave potentials generated within the auditory system are transmitted to a computer for analysis. Following repetitive acoustic stimulation, the waveforms from a normal sleeping or quiet infant consist of several peaks and valleys that reflect activations of neural structures of the brain.	Requires specialized training of personnel and expensive equipment.

Any child who is suspected of a hearing loss because of poor performance using any of the first four screening tests is referred for special audiometric or BEAR testing.

quencies (measured in Hertz [Hz]) at various levels of loudness (measured in decibels [dB]). An audiogram is a record of the audiometric testing.

In a *threshold acuity test* a sound is transmitted to the child's ear at a level the child can easily hear, and then the loudness is reduced until the child indicates the sound (usually by holding up a hand or pushing a button) is no longer heard. This procedure is repeated for frequencies between 500 and 8000 Hz. The sounds are usually delivered through headphones that can be compared to a "space helmet." Since the child is listening to very soft sounds, audiometry is best performed in a soundproof room.

Audiometry can also be used as a screening test or "sweep check" by presenting several different frequencies at either 20 or 25 dB. Another screening device is the Audioscope,* which incorporates audiometric hearing screening and otoscopy in a single instrument. The Audioscope produces pure tones at 500, 1000, 2000, and 4000 Hz at a fixed hearing level of 25 dB. Failure to respond to any frequency is considered a failure. The instrument is reliable for children 5 years of age and older. Children as young as 3 years of age may be able to respond to the screening if adequately prepared by having a practice session in which they can become acquainted with the directions (Orlando and Frank, 1987). Other hearing tests that may be used in infants and children are described in Table 7-11.

Another test that indirectly provides clues to a potential hearing loss is measurement of tympanic membrane compliance (mobility). Normally the pressure on both sides of the membrane is equal, allowing the drum to move easily when negative or positive pressure is applied. Decreased or low compliance usually indicates middle ear effusion (otitis media), a potential cause of conductive hearing loss.

Membrane compliance can be measured by *pneumatic otoscopy (pneumootoscopy)*. Pressure to the tympanic membrane is applied by means of a bulb attached to the head of the otoscope, and the movement of the drum is observed. A limitation of the test is that the pressures needed to properly assess tympanic membrane mobility and accurately screen for middle ear abnormalities are not known (Cavanaugh, 1989).

Another test is *tympanometry*, a simple, reliable, and easily performed procedure that measures the compliance of the tympanic membrane and middle ear pressure. A disadvantage of tympanometry is that it is difficult to perform in young children, because a tight seal must be achieved between the instrument and the external auditory canal and excessive movement by the child interferes with the reading. Unlike tympanometry, another device, the Acoustic Otoscope, does not require a seal at the eardrum and is effective even if the child is crying (Schwartz and Schwartz, 1987.)

Vestibular Testing

Vestibular testing for inner ear function concerning equilibrium is evaluated in young children by holding them at a 30-degree angle and rotating them in a complete circle in each direction. The normal response is nystagmus (movement of the eyes) in the direction of the rotation while being swung and in the opposite direction when the movement stops. This same procedure can be done by using a swivel chair for older children or by having them pivot quickly to one side, then the other.

*Manufactured by Welch Allyn, Skaneateles Falls, NY 13153.

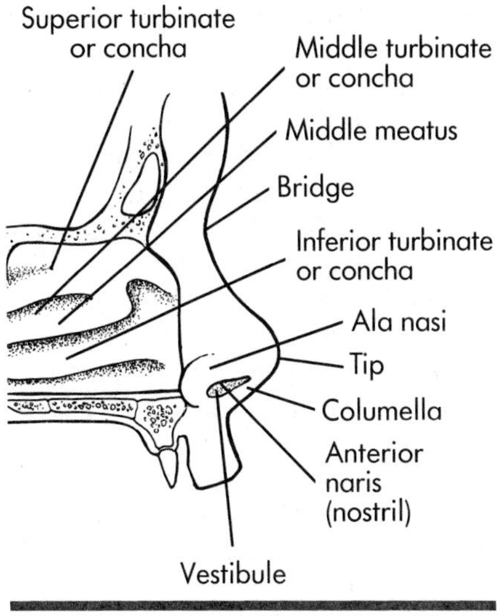

Fig. 7-31. External landmarks and internal structures of nose.

NOSE

The nose marks the beginning of the passageway through the respiratory tract. It is an important organ for filtration, temperature control, and humidification of inspired air, and a sensory organ for olfaction (smell). Each of these functions depends on the patency of the passageways and the mucosal lining of the nasal cavity. Inspection is primarily used for assessing the external and internal structures.

Inspection of External Structures

The nose is located in the middle of the face just below the eyes and above the lips. Its placement and alignment can be compared by drawing an imaginary vertical line from the center point between the eyes down to the notch of the upper lip. The nose should lie exactly vertical to this line, with each side exactly symmetric. Its location, any deviation to one side, and asymmetry in overall size and in diameter of the nares (nostrils) are noted. The bridge of the nose is sometimes flat in Oriental and black children. The alae nasi are noted for any sign of flaring, which indicates respiratory difficulty. Fig. 7-31 illustrates the usual landmarks used in describing the external structures of the nose.

Inspection of Internal Structures

The anterior vestibule of the nose is inspected by pushing the tip upward, tilting the head backward, and illuminating the cavity with a flashlight or otoscope without the attached ear speculum. For a deeper view of the inferior and middle turbinates and the middle meatus, a nasal speculum is used, such as a 9 mm speculum with a very short barrel that attaches to the otoscope head. Forceps specula are not routinely used in children. The short, wide speculum is inserted into the nares, slightly away from the septum, and the otoscope is tilted upward to straighten the passageway toward the posterior wall of the cavity. Pushing against the septum is avoided because it causes pain. Generally inspection is adequate without the speculum, unless one decides that a closer examination of the nasal membranes is warranted. If the nasal speculum is used, the process is explained to the child, similar to the type of preparation for using the otoscope.

The *color* of the *mucosal lining,* which is normally redder than the oral membranes, is noted, as well as any swelling, discharge, dryness, or bleeding. Nasal membranes that are abnormally pale, grayish pink, and swollen suggest nasal allergies. Red, swollen membranes are usually characteristic of the common cold. These differences in appearance are important diagnostic clues to distinguishing between allergy and cold symptoms.

Normally, there should be no discharge from the nose. However, if the child has been crying, a watery discharge is normal. At other times a thin, clear exudate may indicate allergies, chronic rhinitis, or sinusitis. Purulent discharge is caused by infection and can indicate upper respiratory tract infections resulting from either a viral or a bacterial agent. Discharge from one nostril may be caused by a foreign body. If possible, it is removed with forceps (tweezers). If it is deep in the cavity, the child is referred to a more experienced practitioner.

Looking deeper into the nose, the nurse inspects the *turbinates,* or *concha,* plates of bone enveloped by mucous membrane that jut into the nasal cavity. The turbinates greatly increase the surface area of the nasal cavity as air is inhaled. The spaces or channels between the turbinates are called the *meatus* and correspond to each of the three turbinates. Normally the front end of the inferior and middle turbinate and the middle meatus can be seen. They should be the same color as the lining of the vestibule. Enlarged, boggy, pale, grayish mucosa should be noted. Swollen turbinates greatly occlude the passageways for entry of air.

Inside the nose, the *septum,* which should equally divide the vestibules, is inspected. Any deviation is noted, especially if it causes an occlusion of one side of the nose. A perforation may be evident within the septum. If this is suspected, the nurse can shine the light of the otoscope into one naris and look for admittance of light through the perforation to the other nostril.

Since olfaction is an important function of the nose, testing for smell may be done at this point or as part of cranial nerve assessment (see Table 7-18).

MOUTH AND THROAT

The mouth is the beginning of the passageway to the digestive tract, but it also functions in the entry or exit of air. The major structure of the exterior of the mouth is the *lips.* Inspection of the lips for color has been discussed in the section on skin (p. 241). Any deviations are noted, such as *cheilitis,* the presence of painful, inflamed, and dried cracks or fissures of the lips. Cheilitis may be caused by exposure to harsh climatic conditions, habitual licking or biting of the lips, mouth breathing from respiratory distress, or dehydration, particularly with fever in systemic disease. *Cheilosis,* or angular stomatitis, is fissuring at the angles or corners of the lips and may indicate deficiencies of riboflavin or niacin.

Any lesions on the lips are noted. The herpes simplex virus produces singular or clusters of vesicular eruptions on the lip, which are often called "cold sores." The lip may also be the site of a primary syphilitic chancre, which appears as a firm nodule that ulcerates and crusts. Whenever potentially infectious lesions are examined, gloves are worn.

Inspection of Internal Structures

The mouth and throat are divided into three areas: (1) the *oral cavity,* which extends from the lips to the palatopharyngeal arches, (2) the *oropharynx,* which extends from the epiglottis to the lower edge of the adenoids, and (3) the *nasopharynx,* which extends from above the lower edge of the adenoids to the nasal cavity. The major structures that are visible on examination within the oral cavity and oropharynx are the mucosal lining of the lips and cheeks, gums or gingiva, teeth, tongue, palate, uvula, tonsils, and posterior oropharynx (Fig. 7-32). Other pharyngeal structures that are not visible on examination are the epiglottis, lingual tonsils, and pharyngeal tonsils or adenoids.

With a cooperative child almost the entire examination can be done without the use of a tongue blade. The nurse asks the child to open the mouth wide, to move the tongue in different directions for full visualization, and to say "ahh," which depresses the tongue for full view of the back of the mouth (tonsils, uvula, oropharynx). For a closer look at the buccal mucosa or lining of the cheeks, the nurse can ask children to use their fingers to move the outer lip and cheek to one side (see also Nursing Tips).

Infants and toddlers, however, usually resist attempts to keep the mouth open. Because inspecting the mouth is an upsetting part of the examination, it is reserved until last (with examination of the ears) or performed during episodes of crying. However, the use of a tongue blade to de-

NURSING TIPS: EXAMINATION OF MOUTH

To encourage the child to open the mouth for examination:

- Perform the examination in front of a mirror.
- Let the child first examine someone else's mouth, such as the parent, the nurse, or a puppet (Fig. 7-33, *A*) and then examine the child's mouth.

If the child resists opening the mouth, pinch the nostrils closed; this forces the child to open the mouth to breathe.

press the tongue is necessary. The tongue blade is placed along the *side* of the tongue, not the center back area where the gag reflex is elicited. Fig. 7-33, *B*, illustrates proper positioning of the child for oral examination.

All areas lined with *mucous membranes* (inside the lips and cheeks, gingiva, underside of tongue, palate, back of pharynx) are inspected. The membranes should be bright pink, smooth, glistening, uniform, and moist. Any deviations are noted, such as color, white patches or ulceration, bleeding, and sensitivity. For example, reddened areas with white ulcerated centers may be canker sores (aphthae), which may be caused by trauma to the gums during toothbrushing or chewing. White curdy plaques or patches anywhere on the oral mucosa, but particularly on the surface of the tongue and hard palate, that bleed when scraped are signs of moniliasis (candidiasis).

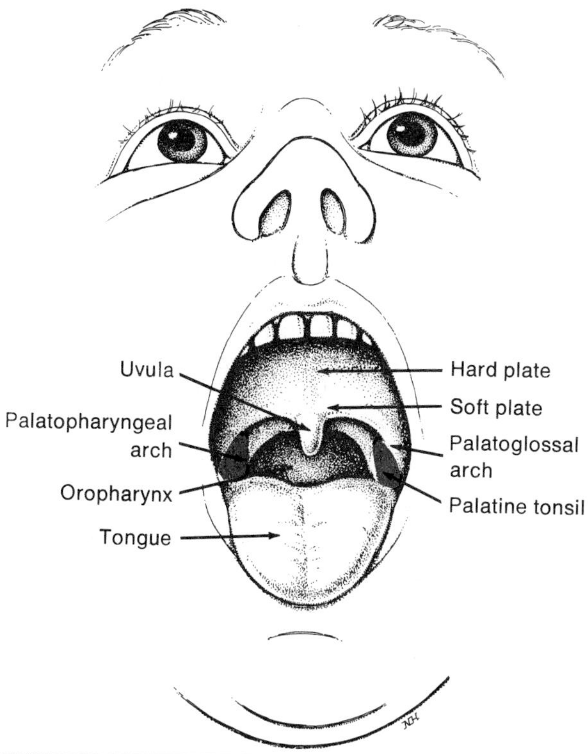

Fig. 7-32. Interior structures of mouth.

As the nurse observes the lining of the mouth, any odor (halitosis) is noted. Mouth odors are characteristic of a number of important health problems, such as poor dental hygiene, gingival disease, chronic constipation, dehydration, malnutrition, or systemic illness. A sudden, foul odor in the mouth may indicate a foreign body in the nose, particularly a bean or pea.

The *teeth* are inspected for number in each dental arch, hygiene, and occlusion or bite. The general rule for estimating the number of temporary teeth in children who are 2 years of age or younger is: *the child's age in months minus 6 months equals the number of teeth.* Discoloration of tooth enamel with obvious plaque (whitish coating on the surface of the teeth) is a sign of poor dental hygiene and indicates a need for dental counseling. Brown spots in the crevices of the crown of the tooth or between the teeth may be caries. Teeth that appear greenish black may be stained from oral ingestion of supplemental iron. Although unsightly, this disappears after the iron is no longer given.

Malocclusion or poor biting relationship of the teeth is evaluated in terms of (1) how the jaws relate to each other in vertical, transverse, and anteroposterior directions (e.g., the "bucktoothed" appearance that results when the maxilla is forward in relation to the mandible), (2) how the teeth are aligned, and (3) how the teeth interdigitate when in occlusion. Although parents frequently express concern regarding thumb-sucking and the development of orthodontic

A

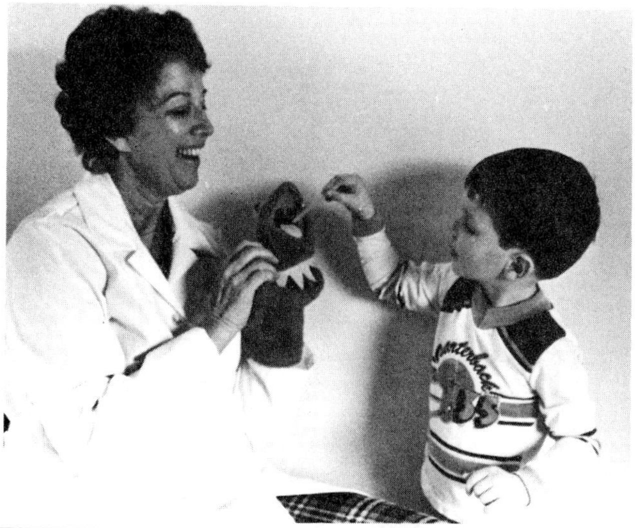

B

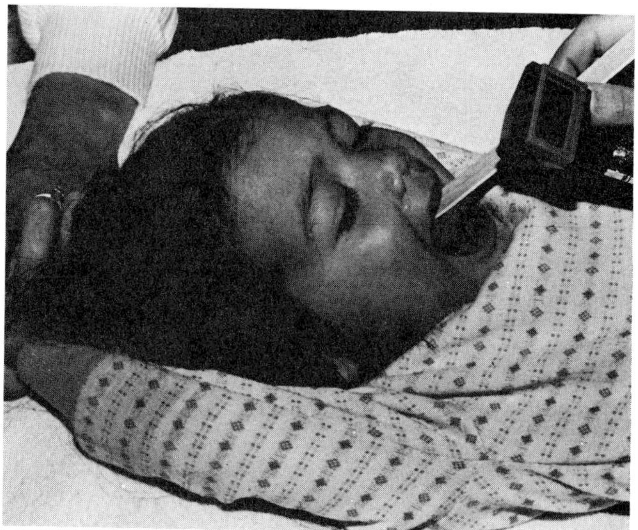

Fig. 7-33. A, Encouraging child to cooperate. **B,** Positioning child for examination of mouth.

problems, thumb-sucking that ceases before the permanent teeth erupt does little harm.

The *gums* surrounding the teeth are examined. The color is normally coral pink, and the surface texture is stippled, similar to the appearance of orange peel. In dark-skinned children the gums are more deeply colored and a brownish area is often observed along the gum line.

The *tongue* is inspected for the presence of papillae, small projections that contain several taste buds each and give the tongue its characteristic rough appearance. Changes in the surface texture are noted, such as (1) "geographic tongue," unusual patterns of papillae formation and denuded areas, (2) coated tongue, such as in candidiasis, or (3) an exceptionally beefy red and swollen tongue, which is a sign of various systemic diseases.

The size and mobility of the tongue are noted, especially protrusion, which is frequently seen in children with mental retardation. Normally the tip of the tongue extends to the lips. If the child is unable to move the tongue forward to this point, the frenulum, or central band of mucous membrane, which attaches the tongue to the floor of the mouth, may be too short. "Tongue-tie" can result in speech problems.

The roof of the mouth consists of the *hard palate,* near the front of the cavity, and the *soft palate,* toward the back of the pharynx, which has a small midline protrusion called the *uvula.* Both are carefully inspected to be sure that they are intact. Sometimes there is a pinpoint cleft in the soft palate that may go undetected unless carefully inspected. Such a cleft is especially important if the uvula is bifid, or separated into two appendages. A submucosal cleft may result in speech problems later on, since air cannot be effectively trapped for vocalization. The arch of the palate should be dome shaped. A narrow-flat roof or high-arched palate affects the placement of the tongue and can cause feeding and speech problems. Movement of the uvula is tested by eliciting a gag reflex, which moves the uvula upward to close off the nasopharynx from the oropharynx.

As the recesses of the oropharynx are inspected, the size and color of the *palatine tonsils* are also noted. They are normally the same color as the surrounding mucosa, glandular rather than smooth in appearance, and barely visible over the edge of the palatoglossal arches. Enlargement, redness, and white patches on the tonsils and surrounding area are recorded. Such signs indicate suppurative tonsillitis or pharyngitis.

CHEST

Although the thoracic cavity (part of the body between the neck and the respiratory diaphragm encased by ribs) houses two vital organs, the heart and lungs, the anatomic structures of the chest wall are important sources of information concerning cardiac and pulmonary function, skeletal formation, and secondary sexual development. The chest is inspected for size, shape, symmetry, movement, breast development, and the presence of the bony landmarks formed by the ribs and sternum.

The *rib cage* consists of 12 ribs and the sternum, or breast bone, located in the midline of the trunk (Fig. 7-34).

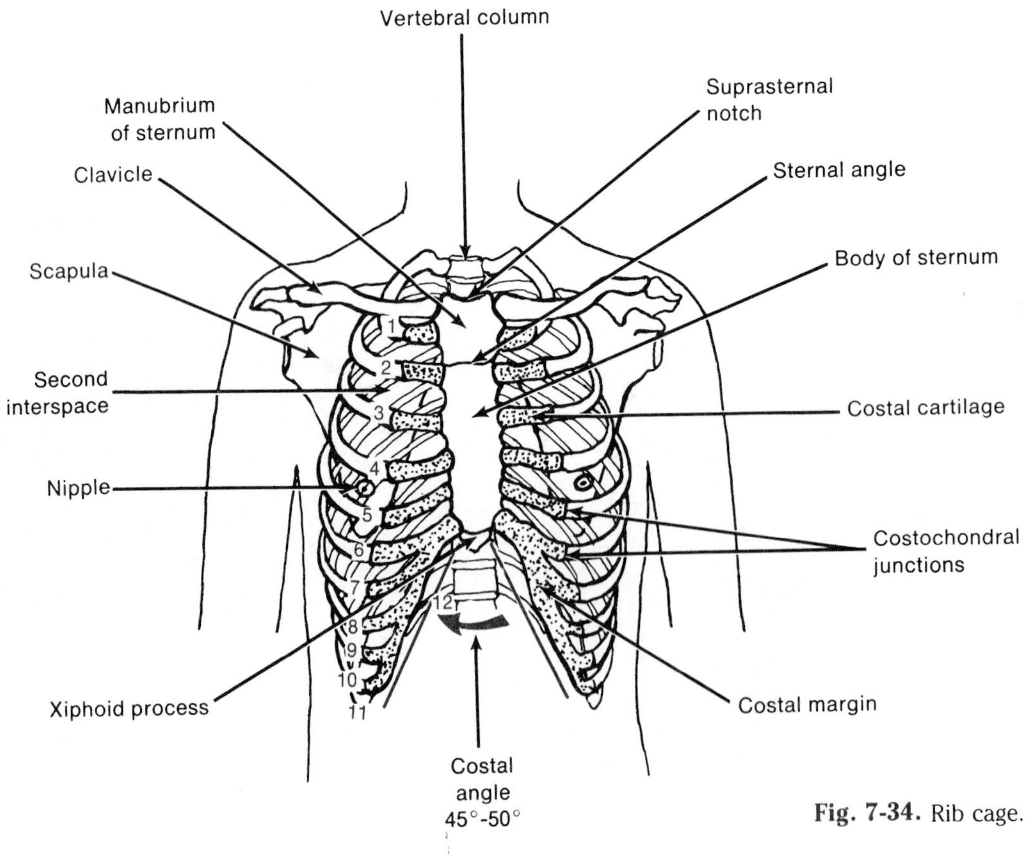

Fig. 7-34. Rib cage.

The first seven ribs, often called *true ribs,* attach directly to the costal cartilages of the sternum at the costochondral junction. The next five ribs are called *false ribs* because they do not attach directly to the costal cartilages of the sternum. The eighth, ninth, and tenth ribs attach to the costal cartilages below the seventh rib, and the last two ribs, often called *floaters,* have no direct attachment to the sternum or anterior ribs, other than their posterior attachment to the vertebral column.

The *sternum* is composed of three main parts. The *manubrium,* the uppermost portion, can be felt at the base of the neck at the *suprasternal notch.* The largest segment of the sternum is the *body,* which forms the *sternal angle (angle of Louis)* as it articulates with the manubrium. At the end of the body is a small, movable process called the *xiphoid.* The angle of the costal margin as it attaches to the sternum is called the *costal angle* and is normally about 45 to 50 degrees. These bony structures are important landmarks in the location of ribs and intercostal spaces. The first rib attaches directly to the manubrium. The second rib attaches directly to the body of the sternum below the sternal angle. The sternal angle is felt as a ridge a few centimeters below the suprasternal notch. The space immediately below a rib is its corresponding *intercostal space (ICS).*

The nurse must become familiar with locating and properly numbering each rib, because ribs are geographic landmarks for palpating, percussing, and auscultating underlying organs. Normally all the ribs can be counted by palpating inferiorly from the second rib. The tip of the eleventh rib can be felt laterally, and the tip of the twelfth rib can be felt posteriorly. Other helpful landmarks include the nipples, which are usually located between the fourth and fifth ribs or at the fourth interspace and, posteriorly, the tip of the scapula, which is located at the level of the eighth rib or interspace. In children with thin chest walls, correctly locating the ribs presents little difficulty.

The *thoracic cavity* is also divided into segments by drawing imaginary lines on the chest and back. Fig. 7-35 illustrates the anterior, lateral, and posterior divisions.

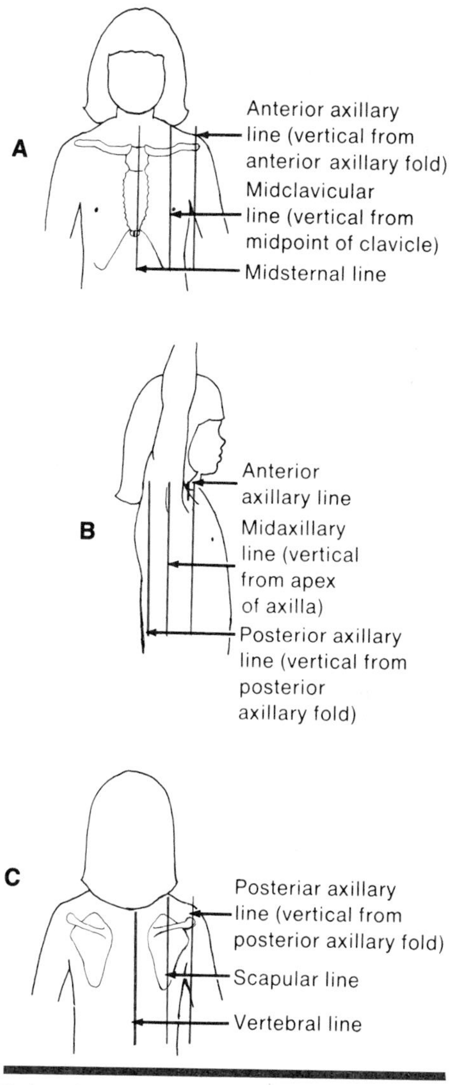

Fig. 7-35. Imaginary landmarks of chest. **A,** Anterior. **B,** Right lateral. **C,** Posterior.

The *size* of the chest is measured by placing the tape around the rib cage at the nipple line (see Fig. 7-7). For greatest accuracy at least two measurements are taken, one during inspiration and the other during expiration, and the average recorded. Chest size is important mainly in comparison with its relationship with head circumference, which is discussed on p. 234. Marked disproportions are always recorded, because most are caused by abnormal head growth, although some may be the result of altered chest shape, such as barrel chest or pigeon chest.

During infancy the *shape* of the chest is almost circular, with the anteroposterior diameter equaling the transverse or lateral diameter. As the child grows, the chest normally increases in the transverse direction, causing the anteroposterior diameter to be less than the lateral diameter. In an older child the characteristic barrel shape of an infant's chest is a significant sign of chronic obstructive lung disease, such as asthma or cystic fibrosis. Other variations in shape that are usually variants of the normal configuration are *pigeon breast,* or *pectus carinatum,* in which the sternum protrudes outward, increasing the anteroposterior diameter, and *funnel chest,* or *pectus excavatum,* in which the lower portion of the sternum is depressed. A severe depression may impair cardiorespiratory function and may indicate the presence of an underlying heritable connective tissue disorder, such as the Marfan syndrome (Arn and others, 1989). However, in general, neither condition causes pathologic dysfunction, although they often cause parents and children concern regarding acceptable physical appearance.

The *angle* made by the lower costal margin and the sternum ordinarily is about 45 degrees. A larger angle is characteristic of lung diseases that also cause a barrel shape of the chest. A smaller angle may be a sign of malnutrition. As the rib cage is inspected, the junction of the ribs to the costal cartilage (costochondral junction) and sternum is noted. Normally the points of attachment are fairly smooth. Swellings or blunt knobs along either side of the sternum are known as the *rachitic rosary* and may indicate vitamin D deficiency. Another variation in shape that may either be nor-

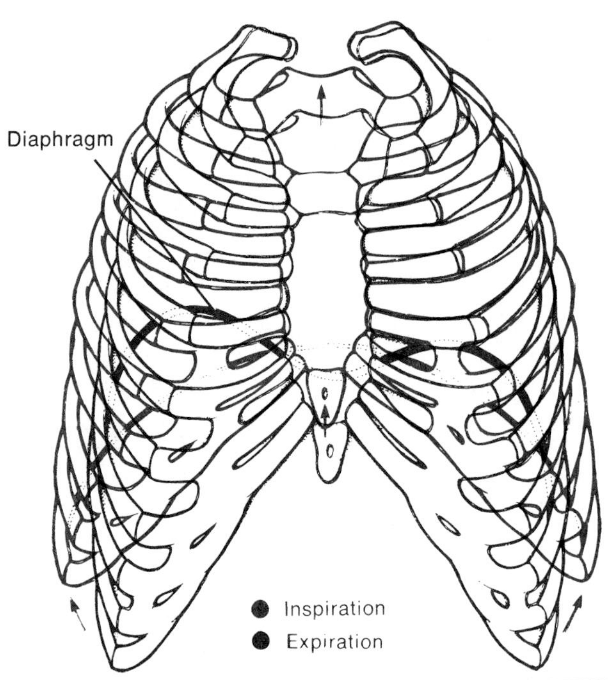

Fig. 7-36. Movement of chest during respiration.

mal or may suggest rickets (vitamin D deficiency) is *Harrison groove,* which appears as a depression or horizontal groove where the diaphragm leaves the chest wall. Usually marked flaring of the rib cage below the groove is an abnormal finding.

Body *symmetry* is always an important notation during inspection. Asymmetry in the chest may indicate serious underlying problems, such as cardiac enlargement (bulging on the left side of rib cage) or pulmonary dysfunction. However, asymmetry is most often a sign of scoliosis, lateral curvature of the spine. Asymmetry warrants further medical investigation.

Movement of the chest wall should be symmetric bilaterally and coordinated with breathing. During inspiration the chest rises and expands, the diaphragm descends, and the costal angle increases. During expiration the chest falls and decreases in size, the diaphragm rises, and the costal angle narrows (Fig. 7-36). In children under 6 or 7 years of age, respiratory movement is principally abdominal or diaphragmatic. In older children, particularly females, respirations are chiefly thoracic. In either type the chest and abdomen should rise and fall together.

Any asymmetry of movement is an important pathologic sign and must be reported. Decreased movement on one side of the chest may indicate pneumonia, pneumothorax, atelectasis, or an obstructive foreign body. Marked *retraction* of muscles either between the ribs (intercostal), above the sternum (suprasternal), or above the clavicles (supraclavicular) is always noted, because it is a sign of respiratory difficulty (see Fig. 31-7).

As the skin surface of the chest is inspected, the position of the *nipples* is observed, as well as any evidence of *breast* development. Normally the nipples are located slightly lateral to the midclavicular line between the fourth and fifth ribs. Symmetry of nipple placement and normal configuration of a darker pigmented areola surrounding a flat nipple in the prepubertal child are noted.

Pubertal breast development usually begins in girls between 10 and 14 years of age (see Fig. 19-6). Precocious or delayed breast development is recorded, as well as evidence of any other secondary sexual characteristics. In males gynecomastia may be caused by hormonal or systemic disorders, but more commonly it is the result of adipose tissue from obesity or a transitory body change during early puberty. In either situation the nurse should investigate the child's feelings regarding breast enlargement.

In adolescent females who have achieved sexual maturity, the breasts are palpated for evidence of any masses or hard nodules. This opportunity should also be taken to discuss the importance of routine self-breast examination. Although carcinoma of the breast is rare in women under 20 years of age, it is advisable to stress the value of routine self-breast examination so that it becomes a practiced habit during later years. The vast majority of palpable masses are benign (Marks and Fisher, 1987). This fact is emphasized to decrease any fear or concern that results when a mass is felt.

LUNGS

The lungs are situated inside the thoracic cavity, with one lung on each side of the sternum. Each lung is divided into an *apex,* which is slightly pointed and rises above the first rib; a *base,* which is wide and concave and rides on the dome-shaped diaphragm; and a body, which is divided into *lobes.* The right lung has three lobes: the upper, middle, and lower. The left lobe has only two lobes, the upper and lower, because of the space occupied by the heart. The two surfaces of the lung are the *costal surface,* which faces the chest wall and backs up to the vertebral column, and the *mediastinal surface,* which faces the space lying between the lungs, the mediastinum. The center of the mediastinal surface is called the *hilus,* where the bronchus and blood vessels enter the lung (Fig. 7-37, *A*).

Examination of the lungs requires knowledge of their location and their relationship to the rib cage. The trachea bifurcates slightly below the level of the sternal angle. The apex of each lung rises about 2 to 4 cm above the inner third of the clavicles. The lower costal margin crosses the sixth rib at the midclavicular line and the eighth rib at the midaxillary line. The posterior base of the lungs crosses the eleventh rib at the vertebral line. The upper border of the right middle lobe parallels the inferior surface of the fourth rib. Fig. 7-37 illustrates the position of the lobes within the thoracic cavity during relaxation. Respiration causes displacement of the lobes upward (expiration) or downward (inspiration).

Inspection

Inspection of the lungs involves primarily observation of respiratory movements, which are discussed on p. 237. Respirations are evaluated for (1) rate (number per minute), (2) rhythm (regular, irregular, or periodic), (3) depth (deep or

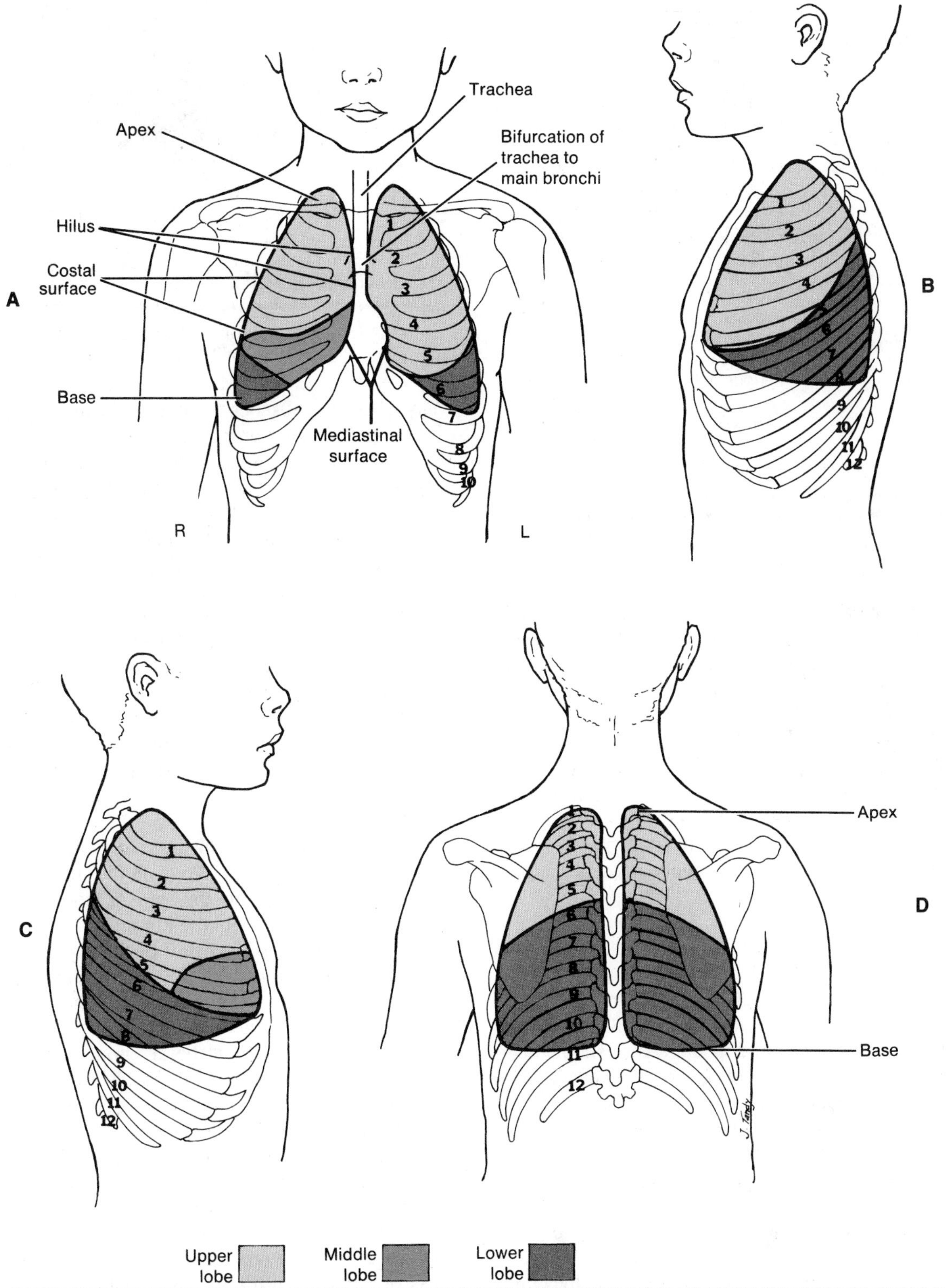

Fig. 7-37. Location of lobes of lungs within thoracic cavity. **A,** Anterior view. **B,** Left lateral view. **C,** Right lateral view. **D,** Posterior view.

Table 7-12 Various patterns of respiration

TERM	DESCRIPTION
Tachypnea	Increased rate
Bradypnea	Decreased rate
Dyspnea	Distress during breathing
Apnea	Cessation of breathing
Hyperpnea	Increased depth
Hypoventilation	Decreased depth (shallow) and irregular rhythm
Hyperventilation	Increased rate and depth
Kussmaul breathing	Hyperventilation, gasping and labored respiration, usually seen in diabetic coma or other states of respiratory acidosis
Cheyne-Stokes respirations	Gradually increasing rate and depth with periods of apnea
Biot breathing	Periods of hyperpnea alternating with apnea (similar to Cheyne-Stokes except that the depth remains constant)
Seesaw (paradoxic) respirations	Chest falls on inspiration and rises on expiration

shallow), and (4) quality (effortless, automatic, difficult, or labored). The nurse also notes the character of breath sounds based on inspection without the aid of auscultation, such as noisy, grunting, snoring, or heavy. Usual terms for describing various patterns of respiration are listed in Table 7-12.

Respiratory rate is always evaluated in relation to general physical status. For example, tachypnea is expected with fever, because for every degree Fahrenheit elevation in temperature, the respiratory rate increases four breaths per minute. The usual ratio of breaths to heartbeats is 1:4 (see inside front cover for normal respiratory rates at various ages).

Palpation

Respiratory movements are felt by placing each hand flat against the back or chest with the thumbs in midline along the lower costal margin of the lungs. The child should be sitting during this procedure and if cooperative should take several deep breaths. During respiration the hands will move with the chest wall. The amount of respiratory excursion is evaluated and any asymmetry of movement is noted. Normally in older children the posterior base of the lungs descends 5 to 6 cm (about 2 inches) during a deep inspiration.

The nurse also palpates for *vocal fremitus,* the conduction of voice sounds through the respiratory tract. With the palmar surfaces of the nurse's hands on the chest, the child repeats words, such as "ninety-nine," "one, two, three," or "eee-eee." Vibrations are felt as the hands move symmetrically on either side of the sternum and vertebral column. In general, vocal fremitus is most intense in the apex and least prominent at the base of the lungs. Decreased vocal fremitus in the upper airway may indicate several gross pulmonary changes. Absence of fremitus usually indicates obstruction of a major bronchus, which may occur as a result of aspiration of a foreign body. Decreased or absent fremitus is always recorded and reported for further investigation.

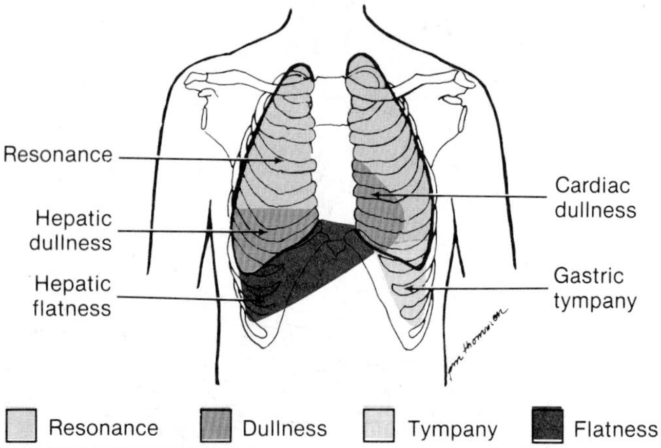

Fig. 7-38. Percussion sounds found in normal thorax.

During palpation other vibrations that indicate pathologic conditions are noted. One is a *pleural friction rub,* which has a grating sensation. It is synchronous with respiratory movements and is the result of opposing surfaces of the inflamed pleural lining rubbing against one another.

Crepitation is felt as a coarse, cracking sensation as the hand presses over the affected area. It is the result of the escape of air from the lungs into the subcutaneous tissues caused by injury or surgical intervention. Both pleural friction rubs and crepitation can usually be both heard and felt.

Percussion

The lungs are percussed in order to evaluate the densities of the underlying organs. Fig. 7-38 illustrates the expected percussion sounds within the anterior thorax. *Resonance* is heard over all the lobes of the lungs that are not adjacent to other organs. *Dullness* is heard beginning at the fifth interspace in the right midclavicular line. Percussing downward to the end of the liver, a *flat* sound is heard because the liver no longer overlies the air-filled lung. *Cardiac dullness* is felt over the left sternal border from the second to the fifth interspace medially to the midclavicular line. Below the fifth interspace on the left side, *tympany* results from the air-filled stomach. Deviations from these expected sounds are always recorded and reported.

In percussing the chest, the anterior lung is percussed from apex to base, usually with the child in the supine or sitting position. Each side of the chest is percussed in sequence in order to compare the sounds, such as the dullness of the liver on the right side with the tympany of the stomach on the left side. When the posterior lung is percussed, the procedure and sequence are the same, although the child should be sitting. Normally only resonance is heard when percussing the posterior thorax from the shoulder to the eighth or tenth rib. At the base of the lungs dullness is heard as the diaphragm is percussed.

NURSING TIPS: ENCOURAGING DEEP BREATHS

To encourage a young child to take deep breaths while the lungs are being auscultated:

- Ask the child to "blow out" the light on an otoscope; discreetly turn off the light on the last try so that the child feels successful (Fig. 7-39).
- Place a cotton ball in the child's palm; ask the child to blow the ball into the air and have the parent catch it.
- Place a small tissue on the top of a pencil and ask the child to blow the tissue off.
- Purchase an inexpensive pinwheel and have the child blow to make it turn.

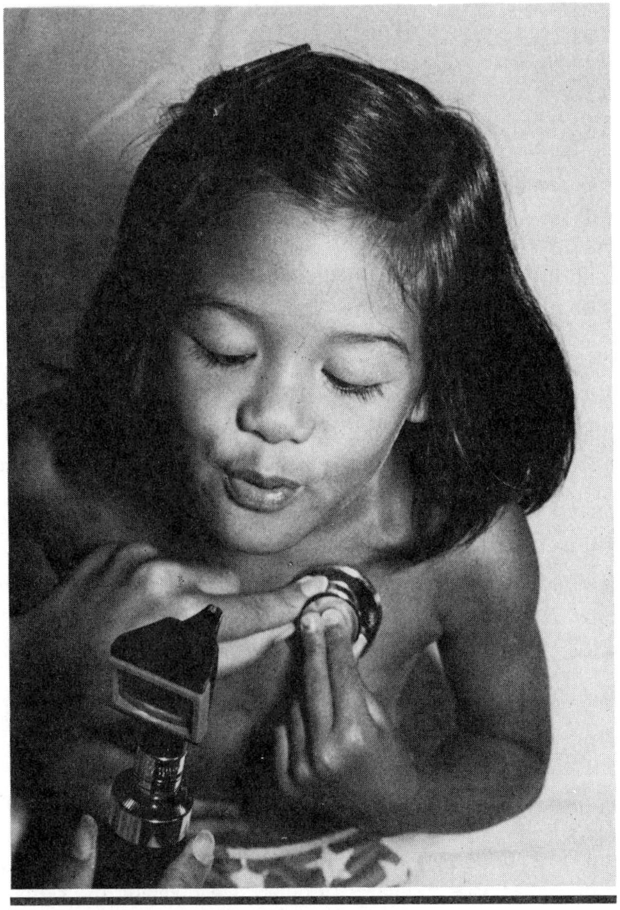

Fig. 7-39. Auscultating lungs while child "blows out" otoscope light.

Auscultation

Auscultation involves using the stethoscope to evaluate breath and voice sounds. Breath sounds are best heard if the child inspires deeply (see Nursing Tips). In the lungs, breath sounds are classified as vesicular, bronchovesicular, or bronchial (Box 7-10).

Absent or *diminished breath sounds* are always an abnormal finding warranting investigation. Fluid, air, or solid masses in the pleural space all interfere with the conduction of breath sounds, although in young children breath sounds are easily transmitted through the thin chest wall, so that unilateral breath sounds may not be heard. Diminished breath sounds in certain segments of the lung suggest pulmonary areas that may benefit from postural drainage and percussion. Increased breath sounds following pulmonary therapy indicate improved passage of air through the respiratory tract.

Voice sounds are also part of auscultation of the lung. Normally vocal resonance or voice sounds are heard, but the syllables are indistinct. They are elicited in the same manner as vocal fremitus, except that the nurse listens with the stethoscope. Consolidation of lung tissue produces three types of abnormal voice sounds:

1. **Whispered pectoriloquy.** Words are whispered, and syllables are heard.
2. **Bronchophony.** Spoken words are not distinguishable, but the vocal resonance is increased in intensity and clarity.
3. **Egophony.** "Ee" is heard as the nasal sound "ay" through the stethoscope.

Decreased or absent vocal resonance is caused by the same conditions that affect vocal fremitus.

Various pulmonary abnormalities produce *adventitious sounds* that are not normally heard over the chest. They are not alterations of normal breath sounds but additional abnormal sounds (Table 7-13). Considerable practice with an experienced tutor is necessary to differentiate the various types of adventitious sounds.* Often it is best to describe the type of sound heard in the lungs rather than trying to label it correctly.

The other adventitious sound of importance is the *pleural friction rub,* discussed on p. 268. Its sound can be simulated by cupping one hand to the ear and rubbing a finger

Box 7-10 CLASSIFICATION OF NORMAL BREATH SOUNDS

Vesicular Breath Sounds

Heard over entire surface of lungs, with exception of upper intrascapular area and area beneath manubrium.
Inspiration is louder, longer, and higher pitched than expiration.
Sound is soft, swishing noise.

Bronchovesicular Breath Sounds

Heard over manubrium and in upper intrascapular regions where trachea and bronchi bifurcate.
Inspiration is louder and higher in pitch than in vesicular breathing.

Bronchial Breath Sounds

Heard only over trachea near suprasternal notch.
Inspiratory phase is short, and expiratory phase is long.

*A suggested resource for becoming familiar with normal and abnormal lung sounds is Wilkins, R., Hodgkin, J., and Lopez, B.: Lung sounds: a practical guide (book and audio tape), St. Louis, 1988, Mosby–Year Book, Inc.

Table 7-13 Description of abnormal lung sounds

TERM	CHARACTERISTICS	SIMILAR SOUND	CAUSE
Coarse crackle	Discontinuous, interrupted explosive sounds Loud, low in pitch	Agitating a container of moderately heated salt	Air passing through larger airways containing fluid
Fine crackle	Discontinuous, interrupted explosive sounds Less loud than above and of shorter duration; higher in pitch than coarse crackles	Strands of hair rolled between fingers; separating Velcro	Air passing through smaller airways containing fluid
Wheeze	Continuous sounds High-pitched; a hissing sound	Two marble plates coated with oil are suddenly separated	Airway narrowed by asthma or partially obstructed by tumor or foreign body
Rhonchus	Continuous sounds Low-pitched; a snoring sound	Cooing of a wood pigeon, croaking of a frog, or snoring	Large upper airway partially obstructed by thick secretions

Data from Ward, J.: Lung sounds: easy to hear, hard to describe, Respir. Care 34(1):763-770, 1989; Murphy, R., and Holford, S.: Lung sounds, Respir. Care 25(7):763-770, 1980.

of the other hand across the cupped hand. The most common site for a friction rub to be heard is the lower anterolateral chest wall (between the midaxillary and midclavicular lines), the area of greatest thoracic mobility.

HEART

Knowledge of the anatomy and physiology of the normal heart is essential in order to properly evaluate the findings. In addition to the discussion below, the normal circulation of the blood through the heart chambers, major blood vessels, and valves is discussed in Chapter 34.

The heart is situated in the thoracic cavity between the lungs in the mediastinum and above the diaphragm (Fig. 7-40). About two thirds of the heart lies within the left side of the rib cage, with the other third on the right side as it crosses the sternum. Most of the anterior cardiac surface is occupied by the right ventricle. Part of the right atrium and left ventricle also faces anteriorly, whereas the left atrium lies primarily in a posterior position.

The heart is positioned in the thorax like a trapezoid:

Vertically along the right sternal border (RSB) from the second to the fifth rib
Horizontally (long side) from the lower right sternum to the fifth rib at the left midclavicular line (LMCL)
Diagonally from the left sternal border (LSB) at the second rib to the LMCL at the fifth rib
Horizontally (short side) from the RSB and LSB at the second intercostal space (ICS)—base of the heart

The most important skill in examining the heart is auscultation, which is performed when the child is quiet. Inspection and palpation also yield important information. However, percussion is of little value in assessing cardiac size or function.

Inspection

When the chest is examined, any obvious bulging is noted, especially on the left side, which may indicate cardiac enlargement. This is best done by observing the child sitting in a semi-Fowler position and looking at the anterior chest wall from an angle, comparing both sides of the rib cage with each other. Normally they should be symmetric. In children with thin chest walls, the PMI is sometimes apparent as a pulsation.

Since comprehensive evaluation of cardiac function is not limited to the heart, other findings are also considered, such as the presence of all pulses (especially the femoral pulses) (Fig. 7-41), distended neck veins, clubbing of the fingers, peripheral cyanosis, edema, blood pressure, and respiratory status.

Palpation

Palpation is used to determine the location of the *apical impulse (AI)*, the most lateral cardiac impulse that may correspond to the apex. The AI is found:

- Just lateral to the left MCL and fourth ICS in children < 7 years of age
- At the left MCL and fifth ICS in children > 7 years of age

Although the AI gives a general idea of the size of the heart (with enlargement, the apex is lower and more lateral), its normal location is quite variable, making it a rather unreliable indicator of heart size (O'Neill and others, 1989).

The *point of maximum intensity (PMI)*, as the name implies, is the area of most intense pulsation. Usually, the PMI is located at the same site as the AI, but it can occur elsewhere. For this reason, the two terms should not be used synonymously. For example, in newborns the PMI is found *medial* to the left MCL at the fourth to fifth ICS because of greater right ventricular activity.

Thrills are palpable vibrations most commonly produced by the flow of blood from one chamber of the heart to another through a narrowed or abnormal opening, such as a stenotic valve or a septal defect. They are best felt with the ball of the hand (palmar surface at the base of the fingers)

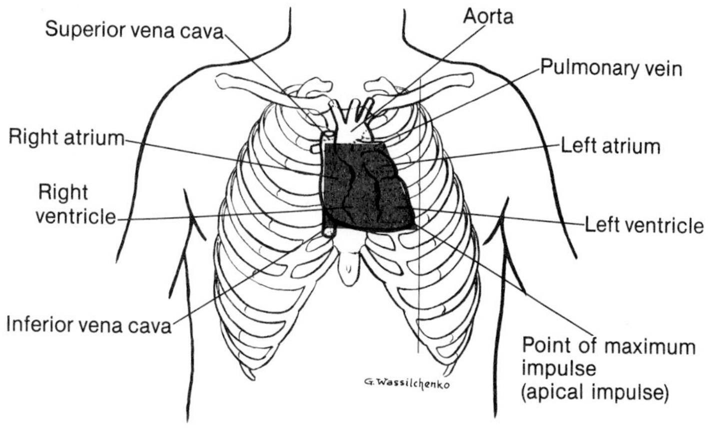

Fig. 7-40. Position of heart within thorax.

and during expiration. Thrills feel similar to the placing of one's hand on a purring cat.

Pericardial friction rubs are scratchy, high-pitched grating sounds, similar to pleural friction rubs, except that they are not affected by changes in respiration. This is a useful clue in differentiating the two rubs, because the pleural rub will cease if the child holds the breath, but the pericardial rub will not. Both thrills and rubs are abnormal and must be reported for further evaluation.

Palpation is also used to assess *capillary filling time*—an important test for peripheral circulation. The skin is pressed lightly on a central site, such as the forehead, or a peripheral site, such as the top of the hand, to produce a slight blanching. The time it takes for the blanched area to return to its original color is the capillary refill time.

✦ **NURSING ALERT** Capillary refill should be brisk—in 1 to 2 seconds; prolonged refill may be associated with poor systemic perfusion.

Auscultation

Auscultation involves listening for heart sounds with the stethoscope, similar to the procedure used in assessing breath sounds.

Origin of heart sounds. The heart sounds are produced by the opening and closing of the valves and the vibration of blood against the walls of the heart and vessels. Normally two sounds—S_1 and S_2—are heard, which correspond respectively to the familiar "lub dub" often used to describe the sounds. S_1 is caused by the closure of the *tricuspid* and *mitral* valves (sometimes called the *atrioventricular* valves). Right ventricular contraction follows tricuspid valve closure, and left ventricular contraction follows mitral valve closure. The contractions (systole) occur almost simultaneously, although the mitral valve (left side) closes slightly before the tricuspid valve (right side). Normally this split of the sounds is so close that it is not audible, except occasionally at the apex of the heart.

S_2 is the result of the closure of the *pulmonic* and *aortic* valves (sometimes called *semilunar* valves). Aortic valve

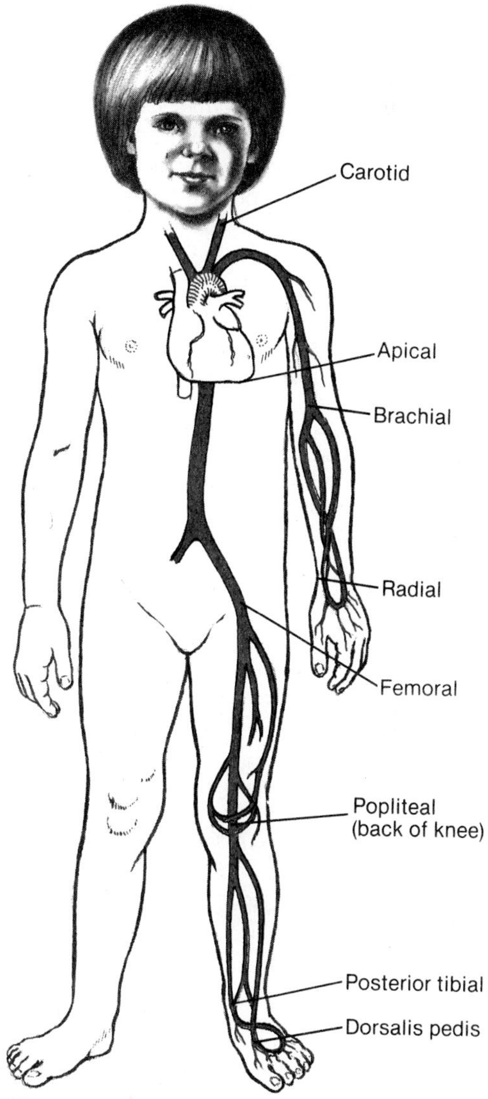

Fig. 7-41. Location of pulses.

closing (left side) occurs slightly before pulmonic valve closing (right side). The flow of blood into the aorta and pulmonary artery occurs following closure of their respective valves. The interval between S_2 and S_1 is diastole, or relaxation, of the heart. Normally the split of the two sounds in S_2 is distinguishable and widens during inspiration, since inspiration prolongs right ventricular filling and delays pulmonic valve closure. *Physiologic splitting* is a significant normal finding that should be elicited.

✦ **NURSING ALERT** "Fixed splitting," in which the split in S_2 does not change during inspiration, is an important diagnostic sign of atrial septal defect.

The approximate anatomic position of the valves within the heart chambers and the auscultatory sites are shown in Fig. 7-42. The auscultatory sites, located in the direction of the blood flow through the valves, correspond to the area where the sounds are heard best.

Two other heart sounds—S_3 and S_4—may be produced. *S_3* is the result of vibrations produced during ventricular filling. It is normally heard only in some children and young adults, but it is considered abnormal in older individuals. *S_4* is caused by the recoil of vibrations between the atria and ventricles following atrial contraction at the end of diastole. It is rarely heard as a normal heart sound and indicates the need for further cardiac evaluation.

Another important category of heart sounds is *murmurs,* which are produced by vibrations within the heart chambers or in the major arteries from the back and forth flow of blood (see Assessment of Cardiac Function, Chapter 34, for a more detailed discussion). Murmurs are classified as:

1. **Innocent.** No anatomic or physiologic abnormality exists.
2. **Functional.** No anatomic cardiac defect exists but a physiologic abnormality such as anemia is present.
3. **Organic.** A cardiac defect with or without a physiologic abnormality exists.

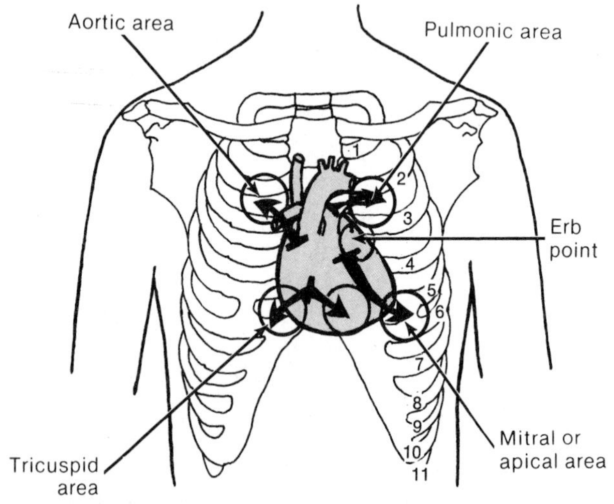

Fig. 7-42. Direction of heart sounds from anatomic valve sites.

The description and classification of murmurs are skills that require considerable practice and training. In general, the nurse should be able to recognize murmurs as distinct swishing sounds that occur in addition to the normal heart sounds and should record the following:

1. **Location** of the area of the heart where the murmur is heard best
2. **Time** of the occurrence of the murmur within the S_1S_2 cycle
3. **Intensity**—evaluation in relationship to the child's position
4. **Loudness**—estimation

The usual subjective method of grading the loudness or intensity of a murmur is listed in Table 7-14. Characteristics of innocent murmurs as opposed to organic murmurs are described in Box 7-11.

There are a number of other abnormal sounds, such as ejection clicks, snaps, gallops, and hums. It is beyond the scope of this discussion to elaborate on such adventitious heart sounds. The best approach is to become familiar with normal heart sounds and to refer any questionable heart sound for further evaluation.

Table 7-14 Grading of the intensity of heart murmurs

GRADE	DESCRIPTION
I	Very faint, frequently not heard if child sits up
II	Usually readily heard, slightly louder than grade I, audible in all positions
III	Loud, but not accompanied by a thrill
IV	Loud, accompanied by a thrill
V	Loud enough to be heard with the stethoscope barely on the chest, accompanied by a thrill
VI	Loud enough to be heard with the stethoscope not touching the chest; often heard with the human ear close to the chest, accompanied by a thrill

Box 7-11 CHARACTERISTICS OF INNOCENT MURMURS

Systolic (occur with or after S_1)
Short duration and have no transmission to other areas of the heart
Grade III or less in intensity and do not increase over time
Loudest in the pulmonic area (second or third intercostal space along the left sternal border)
Variable in relationship to position, respiration, and activity (e.g., audible in the supine position but absent in the sitting position; may be louder with exercise, fever, anxiety, or anemia)
Not associated with any physical signs of cardiac disease
Low-pitched, musical, or groaning quality

Differentiating normal heart sounds. In referring to Fig. 7-42, it is apparent that normally S_1 is louder at the apex of the heart in the mitral and tricuspid area and that S_2 is louder near the base of the heart in the pulmonic and aortic area. Each sound is auscultated by inching down the chest in the sequence outlined in Table 7-15 (see Nursing Tip). In addition to the areas listed in Table 7-15, the following areas should be auscultated for sounds, such as murmurs, which may radiate to these regions: the sternoclavicular area above the clavicles and manubrium, along the sternal border, along the left midaxillary line, and below the scapulae.

The heart is auscultated with the child in at least two positions, sitting and reclining (Fig. 7-43). If adventitious sounds are detected, they are further evaluated with the child standing, sitting and leaning forward, and lying on the left side. For example, atrial sounds such as S_4 are heard best with the person in a recumbent position and usually fade if the person sits or stands.

Heart sounds are evaluated for:

1. **Quality,** which should be clear and distinct, not muffled, diffuse, or distant
2. **Intensity,** especially in relation to location or auscultatory site, not weak or pounding
3. **Rate,** which should be the same as the radial pulse
4. **Rhythm,** which should be regular and even

A particular arrhythmia that occurs normally in many children is *sinus arrhythmia,* in which the heart rate increases with inspiration and decreases with expiration. This can be differentiated from a truly abnormal arrhythmia by having

NURSING TIP: HEART SOUNDS

To distinguish between S_1 or S_2 heart sounds, simultaneously palpate the carotid pulse with the index and middle fingers and listen to the heart sounds; S_1 is synchronous with the carotid pulse.

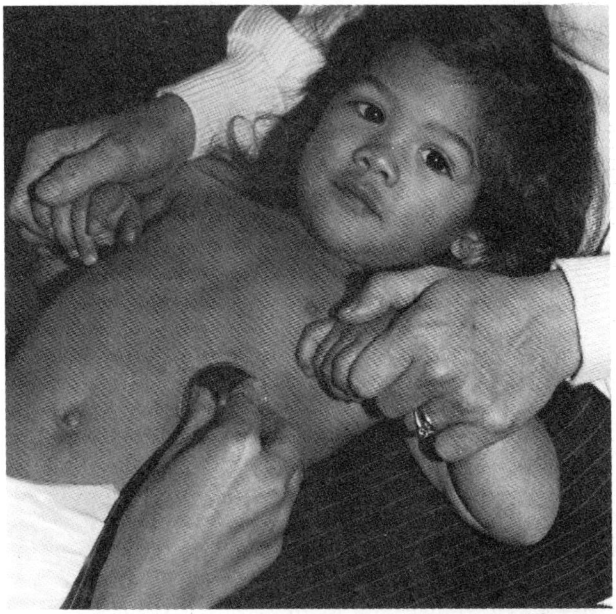

Fig. 7-43. Reclining position in parent's lap for auscultation of heart.

Table 7-15 Sequence of auscultating heart sounds*

AUSCULTATORY SITE	CHEST LOCATION	CHARACTERISTICS OF HEART SOUNDS
Aortic area	Second right intercostal space close to sternum	S_2 heard louder than S_1; aortic closure heard loudest
Pulmonic area	Second left intercostal space close to sternum	Splitting of S_2 heard best, normally widens on inspiration; pulmonic closure heard best
Erb point	Second and third left intercostal space close to sternum	Frequent site of innocent murmurs and those of aortic or pulmonic origin
Tricuspid area	Fifth right and left intercostal space close to sternum	S_1 heard as louder sound preceding S_2 (S_1 synchronous with carotid pulse)
Mitral or apical area	Fifth intercostal space, left midclavicular line (third to fourth intercostal space and lateral to left midclavicular line in infants)	S_1 heard loudest; splitting of S_1 may be audible because mitral closure is louder than tricuspid closure S_3 heard best at beginning of expiration with child in recumbent or left side-lying position, occurs immediately after S_2, sounds like word "Ken-tuc-ky" S_1 S_2 S_3 S_4 heard best during expiration with child in recumbent position (left side-lying position decreases sound), occurs immediately before S_1, sounds like word "Ten-nes-see" S_4 S_1 S_2

*Use both diaphragm and bell chestpieces when auscultating heart sounds. Bell chestpiece is necessary for low-pitched sounds of murmurs, S_3, and S_4.

Table 7-16 Various patterns of heart rate or pulse

TERM	DESCRIPTION
Tachycardia	Increased rate
Bradycardia	Decreased rate
Pulsus alternans	Strong beat followed by weak beat
Pulsus bigeminus	Coupled rhythm in which beat is felt in pairs because of premature beat
Pulsus paradoxus	Intensity or force of pulse decreases with inspiration
Sinus arrhythmia	Rate increases with inspiration, decreases with expiration
Water-hammer or Corrigan pulse	Especially forceful beat caused by a very wide pulse pressure (systolic blood pressure minus diastolic blood pressure)
Dicrotic pulse	Double radial pulse for every apical beat
Thready pulse	Rapid, weak pulse that seems to appear and disappear

children hold their breath. In sinus arrhythmia, cessation of breathing causes the heart rate to remain steady. Table 7-16 lists variations in patterns of heart rate or pulse. Like respiratory rate, heart rate is always evaluated in relation to the child's general physical status. For example, the pulse rate is usually increased by 8 to 10 beats per minute for each degree Fahrenheit elevation in temperature. Athletic children occasionally have lowered heart rates that may even reach rates suggestive of bradycardia (below 60 beats per minute) but that represent a highly developed and efficient heart muscle (see inside front cover for normal heart rates at various ages).

ABDOMEN

Examination of the abdomen involves the usual four skills, except that the order is altered. Inspection is followed by auscultation, percussion, and palpation last because it may distort the normal abdominal sounds. The sequence of examination changes according to the age and cooperativeness of the child. Frequently all four types of assessment are performed at different times. For example, the nurse may auscultate for bowel sounds following evaluation of heart and lung sounds at the beginning of the examination when the child is quiet. Inspection may occur at any time during the examination. Percussion usually follows lung percussion, and palpation may be done toward the end of the examination when the child is relaxed and more trusting.

Knowledge of the anatomic placement of the abdominal organs is essential to differentiate normal, expected findings from abnormal ones (Fig. 7-44). The *abdominal cavity* is the portion of the trunk from directly beneath the diaphragm and thoracic cavity to the region of the pelvic cavity. For descriptive purposes the abdominal cavity is divided into four quadrants by drawing a vertical line midway from the sternum to the pubic symphysis and a horizontal line across the abdomen through the umbilicus (Fig. 7-44). This method of division actually includes the pelvic cavity. Each section is designated as follows:

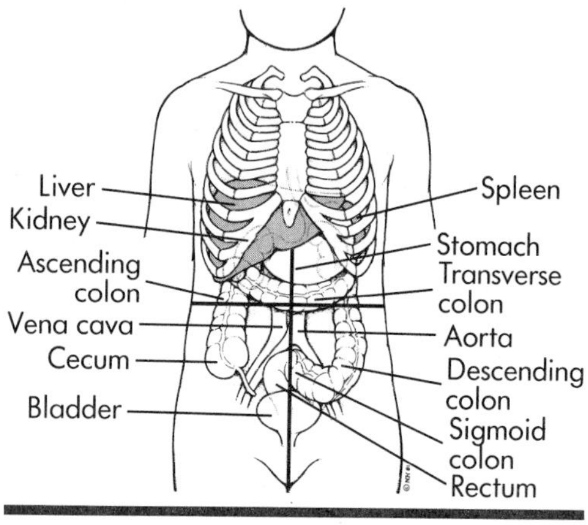

Fig. 7-44. Location of structures in abdomen.

Right upper quadrant (RUQ)
Right lower quadrant (RLQ)
Left upper quadrant (LUQ)
Left lower quadrant (LLQ)

The abdominal cavity contains the major organs of digestion, and the pelvic cavity houses the internal reproductive organs, the lower parts of the digestive tract, and the urinary bladder. However, in infancy the bladder is an abdominal organ.

Inspection

The *contour* of the abdomen is inspected while the child is erect and supine. Normally the abdomen of infants and young children is quite cylindric and, in the erect position, fairly prominent because of the physiologic lordosis of the spine. In the supine position the abdomen appears flat. During adolescence the usual male and female contours of the pelvic cavity change the shape of the abdomen to form characteristic adult curves, especially in the female.

The *size* and *tone* of the abdomen also give some indication of general nutritional status and muscular development. A large, prominent, flabby abdomen is often seen in obese children, whereas a concave abdomen suggests undernutrition. However, careful note is made of a protruding abdomen, which may indicate pathologic states such as abdominal distention, ascites, tumors, or organomegaly. A protuberant abdomen with spindly extremities and flat, wasted buttocks suggests severe malnutrition that may occur from inadequate nutritional intake such as kwashiorkor or from diseases such as cystic fibrosis. A midline protrusion from the xiphoid to the umbilicus or pubic symphysis is usually *diastasis recti,* or failure of the rectus abdominis muscles to join in utero. In a healthy child a midline protrusion is usually a variation of normal muscular development.

✦ **NURSING ALERT** A tense, boardlike abdomen is a serious sign of paralytic ileus and intestinal obstruction.

The *skin* covering the abdomen should be uniformly taut, without wrinkles or creases. Sometimes silvery, whitish striae are seen, especially if the skin has been stretched as in obesity or with distention resulting from ascites. Any scars, ecchymotic areas, excessive hair distribution, or distended veins are noted. Superficial veins may be visible in thin, light-skinned children, but distended veins are an abnormal finding, suggesting vascular or abdominal obstruction or abdominal distention.

Movement of the abdomen is observed. In infants and thin children *peristaltic waves* may be visible through the abdominal wall, and they always warrant careful evaluation. They are best observed by standing at eye level to and across from the abdomen. Visible peristaltic waves most often indicate pathologic states, particularly intestinal obstruction such as pyloric stenosis. Abdominal movement in relation to respiration is discussed on p. 237.

The *umbilicus* is inspected for herniation, discharge, hygiene, and fistulas, such as a patent urachus (an abnormal connection between the umbilicus and bladder). If a herniation is present, the sac is palpated for abdominal contents and the approximate size of the opening is estimated. *Umbilical hernias* are common in infants, especially in black children. Since "home remedies" for treatment such as taping coins over the umbilicus or using "belly binders" may be harmful to the skin and actually delay natural closure, the nurse should ask parents whether such procedures have been used. Umbilical hernias normally protrude and expand when the child coughs, cries, or strains.

Hernias may exist elsewhere on the abdominal wall, such as in the inguinal or femoral region (Fig. 7-45). An *inguinal hernia* is a protrusion of peritoneum through the abdominal wall in the inguinal canal. It occurs mostly in males, is frequently bilateral, and may be visible as a mass in the scrotum. It is palpated by sliding the little finger into the external inguinal ring at the base of the scrotum and asking the child to cough. If a hernia is present, it will hit the tip of the finger (see Nursing Tip below and Inguinal Hernia, Chapter 11).

A *femoral hernia,* which occurs more frequently in girls, is felt or seen as a small mass on the anterior surface of the thigh just below the inguinal ligament in the femoral canal (a potential space medial to the femoral artery). Its location is estimated by placing the index finger of the right hand on the child's right femoral pulse (left hand for left pulse) and the middle ring finger flat against the skin toward the midline. The ring finger lies over the femoral canal, where the herniation occurs. Palpation of hernias in the pelvic region, particularly inguinal ones, is often part of the examination of genitalia.

NURSING TIP: TESTING FOR INGUINAL HERNIA

If the child is too young to cough, have the child blow up a balloon or laugh to raise the intraabdominal pressure sufficiently to demonstrate the presence of an inguinal hernia.

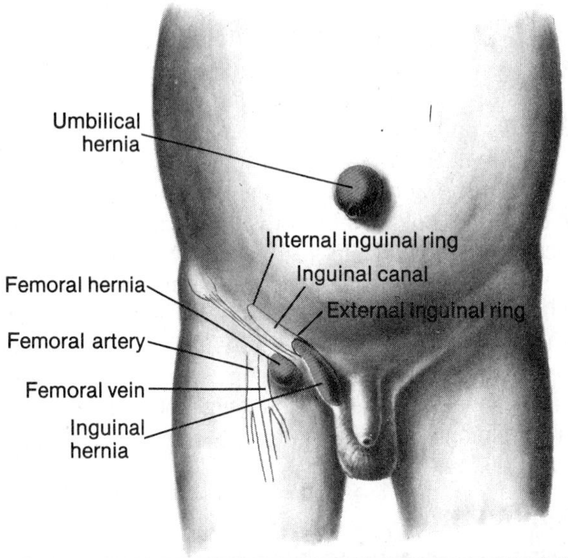

Fig. 7-45. Location of hernias.

Auscultation

Each of the four quadrants should be auscultated using the diaphragm and bell chestpieces. Unlike listening to the heart or lungs, in which the stethoscope rests gently on the skin, to hear bowel sounds the stethoscope must be pressed firmly against the abdominal surface. With the diaphragm chestpiece this usually presents no difficulty, but with the bell chestpiece, especially one with a short cone, the skin may occlude the opening and prevent transmission of sound.

The most important sound to listen for is *peristalsis,* or *bowel sounds,* which sound like short metallic clicks and gurgles. Loud grumbling noises, known as *borborygmi,* are the familiar "stomach growls," usually denoting hunger. Depending on when the child last ate, a sound may be heard every 10 to 30 seconds, and its frequency per minute is recorded. Bowel sounds may be stimulated by stroking the abdominal surface with a fingernail. Absence of bowel sounds or hyperperistalsis is recorded and reported, since either usually denotes abdominal disorder.

Various other sounds may be heard in the abdominal cavity. Normally the pulsation of the aorta is heard in the epigastrium. Sounds that resemble murmurs (called *bruits*), hums, or rubs are always referred for further evaluation.

Percussion

Percussion of the abdomen is performed in the same manner as percussion of the lungs (see Fig. 7-38). Normally dullness or flatness is heard on the right side at the lower costal margin because of the location of the liver. Tympany is typically heard over the stomach on the left side and in the rest of the abdomen. An unusually tympanitic sound, like the beating of a tight drum, denotes air in the stomach, which is commonly caused by mouth breathing. However, it can also denote a pathologic condition such as low intestinal obstruction or paralytic ileus. Lack of tympany may occur normally when the stomach is full after a meal, but in other situations it may denote the presence of fluid or solid masses. Variation in percussion tones not explained by normal physiologic processes warrants referral for further investigation.

Palpation

Two types of palpation are performed, superficial and deep. In *superficial palpation* the hand is placed lightly against the skin and each quadrant is felt, noting any areas of tenderness, muscle tone, and superficial lesions, such as cysts. Skin turgor, discussed on p. 243, is also tested.

Since superficial palpation is often perceived as tickling, several techniques can be used to minimize this sensation (see Nursing Tips). Admonishing the child to stop laughing only draws attention to the sensation and decreases cooperation. Positioning the child supine with the legs flexed at the hips and knees helps relax the abdominal muscles (see Box 7-4).

Tenderness or pain anywhere in the abdomen during superficial palpation is always noted. There are two types of abdominal pain:

Visceral, which arises from the viscera or internal organs, such as the intestines, and is usually dull, poorly localized, and difficult for the patient to describe

Somatic, which arises from the walls or linings of the abdominal cavity such as the peritoneum, and is generally sharp, well localized, and more easily described

When assessing abdominal pain, it is important to remember that children often respond with an "all-or-none" reaction—either there is no pain or great pain. At times it is difficult to distinguish pain from fear. One approach is to ask children "how thin" and "how fat" they can make them-

NURSING TIPS: AVOIDING TICKLING SENSATION

To minimize the sensation of tickling during palpation:

- Have children "help" with the palpation by placing their hand over the palpating hand.
- Have them place their hand on the abdomen with the fingers spread wide apart and palpate between their fingers.
- Distract them with statements such as "I am trying to feel what you ate today."
- Maintain conversation about their eating habits to distract them from the palpation.

NURSING TIP: ASSESSING ABDOMINAL PAIN

When a child complains of abdominal pain, observe whether the child's eyes are opened or closed during palpation of the abdomen. The natural reaction of patients with genuine abdominal tenderness is to watch the palpating hand carefully to avoid unnecessary pain—the opened eyes sign (Gray, Dixon, and Collin, 1988).

selves. If this produces discomfort, then some degree of peritoneal irritation is probably present (see also Nursing Tip).

A special phenomenon called *rebound tenderness,* or *Blumberg sign,* may be performed if the child complains of abdominal pain. It is produced by pressing firmly over part of the abdomen distal to the area of tenderness. When the pressure is suddenly released, the child feels pain in the original area of tenderness. This response is found only when the peritoneum overlying a diseased organ is inflamed, such as in appendicitis.

Deep palpation is used for palpating organs and large blood vessels and for detecting masses and tenderness not discovered during superficial palpation. If the child complains of abdominal pain, that area of the abdomen is palpated *last.* Normally palpation of the midepigastrium causes pain as pressure is exerted over the aorta, but this should not be confused with visceral or somatic tenderness.

The abdominal organs are palpated by pressing them against the free hand, which is placed on the child's back (see Fig. 7-3). Palpation begins in the lower quadrants and proceeds upward. In this way the edge of an enlarged liver or spleen is not missed. Except for palpating the liver, successful identification of other organs, such as the spleen, kidney, and part of the colon, requires considerable practice with tutored supervision.

The lower edge of the *liver* is sometimes palpable in infants and young children as a superficial mass 1 to 2 cm (3/8 to 3/4 inch) below the right costal margin (the distance is sometimes measured in fingerbreadths). Normally the liver descends during inspiration as the diaphragm moves downward. This downward displacement should not be mistaken for a sign of hepatomegaly. In older children the liver frequently is not palpable.

The *spleen* is palpated by feeling it between the hand placed against the back and the one palpating the left upper quadrant. The spleen is much smaller than the liver and positioned behind the fundus of the stomach. The tip of the spleen may be felt during inspiration as it descends within the abdominal cavity. It is sometimes palpable 1 to 2 cm below the left costal margin in infants and young children.

NURSING ALERT If the liver is palpable 3 cm below the right costal margin or the spleen is palpable more than 2 cm below the left costal margin, these organs are enlarged—a finding that is always reported for further medical investigation.

Other anatomic structures that are sometimes palpable in children include the kidney, bladder, cecum, and sigmoid colon. Palpation of the *kidney,* which is discussed in Chapter 8 under assessment of the neonate, is quite difficult because of its deep position within the abdominal cavity. Normally only the tip of the right kidney is palpable because of its lower placement within the cavity and is best felt during inspiration. The *bladder* may be palpated slightly above the pubic symphysis in infants and young children. It descends deeper into the pelvic cavity during adolescence, when it is not palpable except if distended. Occasionally parts of the colon are palpable. The *cecum* is a soft, gas-filled mass in the right lower quadrant. The *sigmoid colon* is felt as a sausage-shaped mass that is freely movable over the pelvic brim in the left lower quadrant and is normally tender.

Although most of these structures are not routinely felt, awareness of their relative location and characteristics is necessary to avoid mistaking them for abnormal masses that require additional investigation. The most common palpable mass in children is feces, which may be associated with pain in the right lower quadrant from a distended cecum. In sexually active pubescent females a palpable mass in the lower abdomen may be a pregnant uterus.

During palpation of the abdomen the *femoral pulses* are felt by placing the tips of two or three fingers (index, middle, and/or ring) along the inguinal ligament about midway between the iliac crest and pubic symphysis. Both pulses are felt simultaneously to make certain that they are equal and strong (Fig. 7-46).

NURSING ALERT Absence of femoral pulses is a significant sign of coarctation of the aorta and is referred for medical evaluation.

When the abdomen is examined, *abdominal reflexes* are tested by scratching the skin toward the umbilicus. The normal response is for the umbilicus to move toward the stimulus or quadrant that was stroked. Normally the response may be absent in children under 1 year of age. Asymmetry or absence of response is noted and reported, although there is great variability in correctly eliciting a response.

GENITALIA

Examination of genitalia conveniently follows assessment of the abdomen while the child is still supine. In adolescents, inspection of the genitalia may be left to the end of the examination. This part of the physical appraisal is usually uneventful for infants or toddlers but begins to be anxiety-producing for older preschoolers, school-age children, and adolescents, mainly because of their concern for modesty and privacy. The best approach is to examine the genitalia matter-of-factly, placing no more emphasis on this part of the assessment than on any other segment. It helps to relieve children's and parents' anxiety by stating the results of the findings, for example, "Everything looks fine here." If it is necessary to ask questions about deviations, such as about discharge or difficulty in urinating, consideration for the child's privacy is observed by covering the lower abdomen with the gown or underpants.

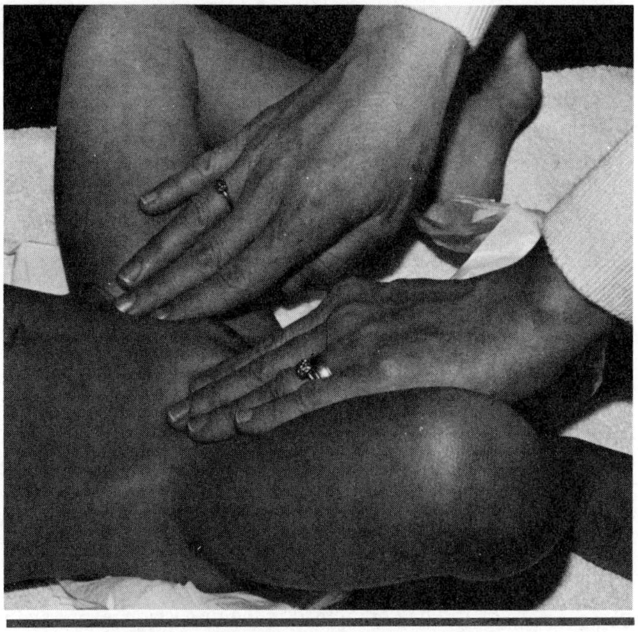

Fig. 7-46. Palpating for femoral pulses.

In examining the genitalia, gloves are worn whenever body substances are contacted. It might be helpful for the adolescent to know that wearing gloves also prevents skin-to-skin contact. Each step of the examination is explained before it is performed, such as checking the scrotum for an inguinal hernia (discussed on p. 275) and the reason for asking the boy to cough. If male adolescents have an erection during the examination, they are reassured that this is a normal involuntary reflex to touch, not a sexual response, and the rest of the examination is then completed (Church and Baer, 1987).

The examination of female genitalia is limited to inspection and palpation of external structures. If a vaginal examination is required, an appropriate referral is made unless the nurse is qualified to perform the procedure. Guidelines for performing a pelvic examination are available in a number of sources (Gemberling, 1987; Marks and Fisher, 1987; Talbot, 1986). Both sexes need preparation, reassurance, and privacy for and during the examination. Older children and adolescents should be given the choice of whether or not they wish to be accompanied by a family member (Phillips, Bohannon, and Heald, 1986). Whenever possible, the sex of the examiner should also be an option for the teenager. Studies show that some young people feel more comfortable with an examiner of the same sex, although males and females report feeling comfortable with a female examiner (Neinstein and others, 1989; Seymore and others, 1986). For females, the semisitting position has been found to be less stressful that the supine position for the pelvic examination (Seymore and others, 1986).

The genital examination is an excellent time for eliciting questions of concern about body functioning or sexual activity (see Therapeutic Dialogue, p. 278). The nurse can

THERAPEUTIC DIALOGUE

Sexual Concerns During Adolescence

Following examination of the genitalia, the nurse comments to a 13-year-old girl, "Everything looks fine here. You are becoming a young woman. Are there any questions you would like to ask about how you are developing?"

ADOLESCENT: No. (Eyes are downcast; face has a sad expression.)

NURSE: During this time many young people have a lot of questions, but they are embarrassed to ask them. Have you ever felt that way? (Nurse uses third-person technique; see p. 194)

ADOLESCENT: Yes. (Eyes look teary.)

NURSE: I think that this is very difficult for you to talk about. The tears are hard to hold back, aren't they?

(Adolescent begins to cry, nurse moves closer to her, and hands her a tissue.)

NURSE: Sometimes talking helps. I am here to listen.

ADOLESCENT: Most of my friends have their period and have boyfriends. I don't have either.

SUMMARY

With the adolescent's admission of her concerns, the nurse and teenager were able to discuss different rates of growth, both physically and emotionally. The nurse also suggested that the youngster talk with her mother about her worries. The mother, who had been in the room but had not joined in the discussion, expressed that she too had menstruated late and had felt left out among her peers. She encouraged her daughter to talk with her more because she did understand some of the pains of growing up.

also use this opportunity to increase or reinforce the child's knowledge of reproductive anatomy by naming each body part and explaining its function. For example, many females are unaware of the existence of two openings within the vulva. They assume that the passage of urine occurs from the vagina. For males, this part of the health assessment is an opportune time to teach self-testicular examination.

One of the most important factors in successfully performing the examination is that the nurse recognize any personal fears or anxieties and deal with them. Transfer of anxiety, especially in the beginning practitioner, can be the greatest deterrent to lessening the child's concern or fear.

Male Genitalia

The external appearance of the glans and shaft of the penis, the prepuce, the urethral meatus, and the scrotum is noted (Fig. 7-47). The size of the *penis* is generally small in infants and young boys until puberty, when it begins to increase in both length and width. A very small penis may actually be an enlarged clitoris in a genetically female child. In an obese child the penis often looks abnormally small because of the folds of skin partially covering it at the base. An enlarged penis in a young child may denote precocious puberty. One should be familiar with normal pubertal growth of the external male genitalia in order to compare the findings with the expected sequence of maturation (see Fig. 19-8).

The *glans* (head of the penis) and *shaft* (portion between the perineum and prepuce) are examined for signs of swelling, skin lesions, inflammation, or other irregularities. Any of these signs may denote underlying disorders, especially sexually transmitted diseases. Confirmation of a sexu-

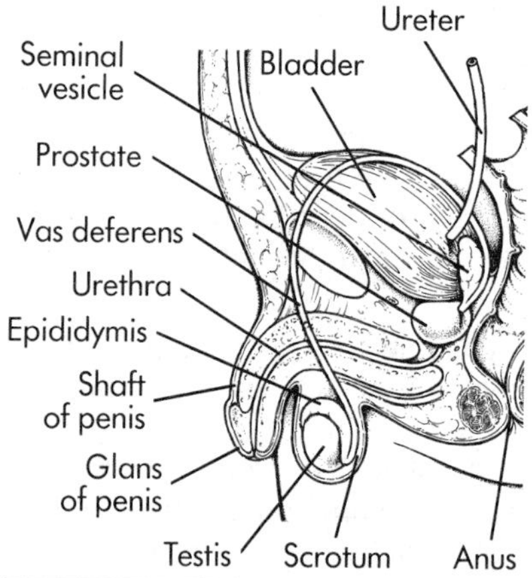

Fig. 7-47. Major structures of genitalia in circumcised prepubertal male.

ally transmitted disease should alert the nurse to the possibility of sexual abuse, especially in young children.

If the child is uncircumcised, the *prepuce* or foreskin covering the glans of the penis is inspected. In infants the prepuce is normally tight and is not retracted for examination, since accidental tearing of the thin membrane may cause scarring and adhesion formation later on. In children the foreskin is gently retracted for examination of the glans and the meatus and then replaced. A tight foreskin that cannot be retracted is called *phimosis.*

The *urethral meatus* is carefully inspected for location and evidence of discharge. Normally it is centered at the tip of the shaft. If it opens on the ventral or underneath side of the glans or shaft, it is called *hypospadias.* An opening on the dorsal or top part of the penis is termed *epispadias.* If the urethral meatus opens into the perineum at the junction of the scrotum, the nurse carefully inspects for signs suggestive of ambiguous genitalia. If feasible during inspection, the strength and direction of the urinary stream during micturition are noted.

The size of the *scrotum* is noted. In infants the scrota appear large in relation to the rest of the genitalia. Normally, the left scrotum hangs lower than the right and both hang freely from the perineum behind the penis. Scrota that are small, close to the perineum, or with evidence of any midline separation, which could be enlarged labia, are noted. An abnormally large scrotal sac may indicate an inguinal hernia, a hydrocele, or inflammation of the internal reproductive structures, particularly the epididymis.

The skin of the scrotum is usually loose and highly rugated (wrinkled). During early adolescence the skin normally becomes redder and coarser. In dark-skinned children the scrota are more deeply pigmented. A smooth, shiny surface with pigmentation that varies markedly from the surrounding skin should be reported.

Hair distribution is also noted. Normally before puberty no pubic hair is present. Soft downy hair at the base of the penis is an early sign of pubertal maturation. In older adolescents the typical male pattern of hair distribution is diamond shaped from the anus to the umbilicus.

Palpation of the scrotum includes identification of the testes, epididymis, spermatic cords, and, if present, inguinal hernias. The two *testes* are felt as small ovoid bodies, about 1.5 to 2 cm (½ to ¾ inch) long—one in each scrotal sac. They do not enlarge until puberty, when they approximately double in size. Normally the testes descend during the last trimester of uterine development, usually by the eighth month of gestation. Therefore undescended testes *(cryptorchidism)* is a common finding in premature infants.

Palpating for the presence of the testes requires an understanding of the normal anatomy and physiology of the coverings of the testes and scrotal sac. The scrotum and testes are surrounded by cremasteric fascia, which extends to the cremaster muscle. The muscle attaches to a point in the abdomen and extends downward along the inner surface of the thigh. The muscle or *cremasteric reflex* is stimulated by cold, touch, emotional excitement, or exercise. When contracted, the muscle causes the skin of the scrotum to shrink and pulls the testes higher into the pelvic cavity.

Several measures are useful in preventing the cremasteric reflex during palpation of the scrotum. First, the hands should be warm, not cold. Second, if old enough, the child is examined while sitting in a tailor or "Indian" position, which stretches the muscle, preventing its contraction (Fig. 7-48, *A*). Third, the normal pathway of ascent of the testes can be blocked by placing the thumb and index finger over the upper part of the scrotal sac along the inguinal canal (Fig. 7-48, *B*). If there is any question concerning the existence of two testes, the index and middle fingers are placed in a scissors fashion to separate the right and left scrota. If after using these techniques the testes have not been palpated, the inguinal canal and perineum are felt to locate masses that may be undescended testes (see Nursing Tips: Testicular Examination, p. 511). Although undescended testes may descend at any time during childhood and are checked at each visit, failure to palpate testes is reported.

The *epididymis* is palpated as a vertical ridge of soft nodular tissue behind the testes. The *spermatic cord* consists of the blood vessels, nerves, lymphatic glands, and the ductus deferens of the testes. Any masses, swelling, or tenderness is noted and reported.

Female Genitalia

A convenient position for examination of the genitalia involves placing the young child supine on the examining table or in a semireclining position on the parent's lap with the feet supported on the nurse's knees as the nurse sits facing the child. The child's attention is diverted from the examination by instructing her to try to keep the soles of her feet pressed against each other. The labia majora (see below) are separated with the thumb and index finger and retracted outward in order to expose the labia minora, urethral meatus, and vaginal orifice. The child can use her hands "to help" (Fig. 7-49).

The genitalia are inspected for size and location of the structures of the *vulva* or *pudendum* (area of the external genital organs) (Fig. 7-50). The *mons pubis* is a pad of adipose tissue over the symphysis pubis. At puberty the mons is covered with hair, which extends along the labia. The usual pattern of female *hair distribution* is an inverted triangle. Any extension of hair along the linea alba to the umbilicus is noted. The appearance of soft downy hair along the labia majora is an early sign of sexual maturation.

The *clitoris* is an erectile organ located at the anterior end of the labia minora. It is covered by a small flap of skin, the *prepuce.* Its size is noted because, although variable, a large protruding clitoris may represent an underdeveloped phallus.

The *labia majora* are two thick folds of skin running posteriorly from the mons to the posterior commissure of the vagina. Internal to the labia majora are two folds of skin called the *labia minora.* Although the labia minora are prominent in the newborn, they gradually atrophy and are almost invisible until their enlargement during puberty.

The inner surface of the labia should be pink and moist. Any skin lesions such as chancres, blisters, or warts (condylomata acuminata) are noted and investigated since they may be sexually transmitted. The size of the labia and any evidence of fusion, which may suggest male scrota, are noted. Normally no masses are palpable within the labia. However, in genitalia of an ambiguous nature, palpable masses may represent descended testes.

The urethral meatus and vaginal orifice are located in the space between the labia, the *vestibule.* The *urethral meatus* is located posterior to the clitoris and is surrounded by Skene glands and ducts. Although not a prominent structure, the meatus can be more readily identified by wiping downward along the vestibule toward the perineum. It will appear as a small V-shaped slit. Its location is noted, especially if it opens from the clitoris or inside the vagina. The

A

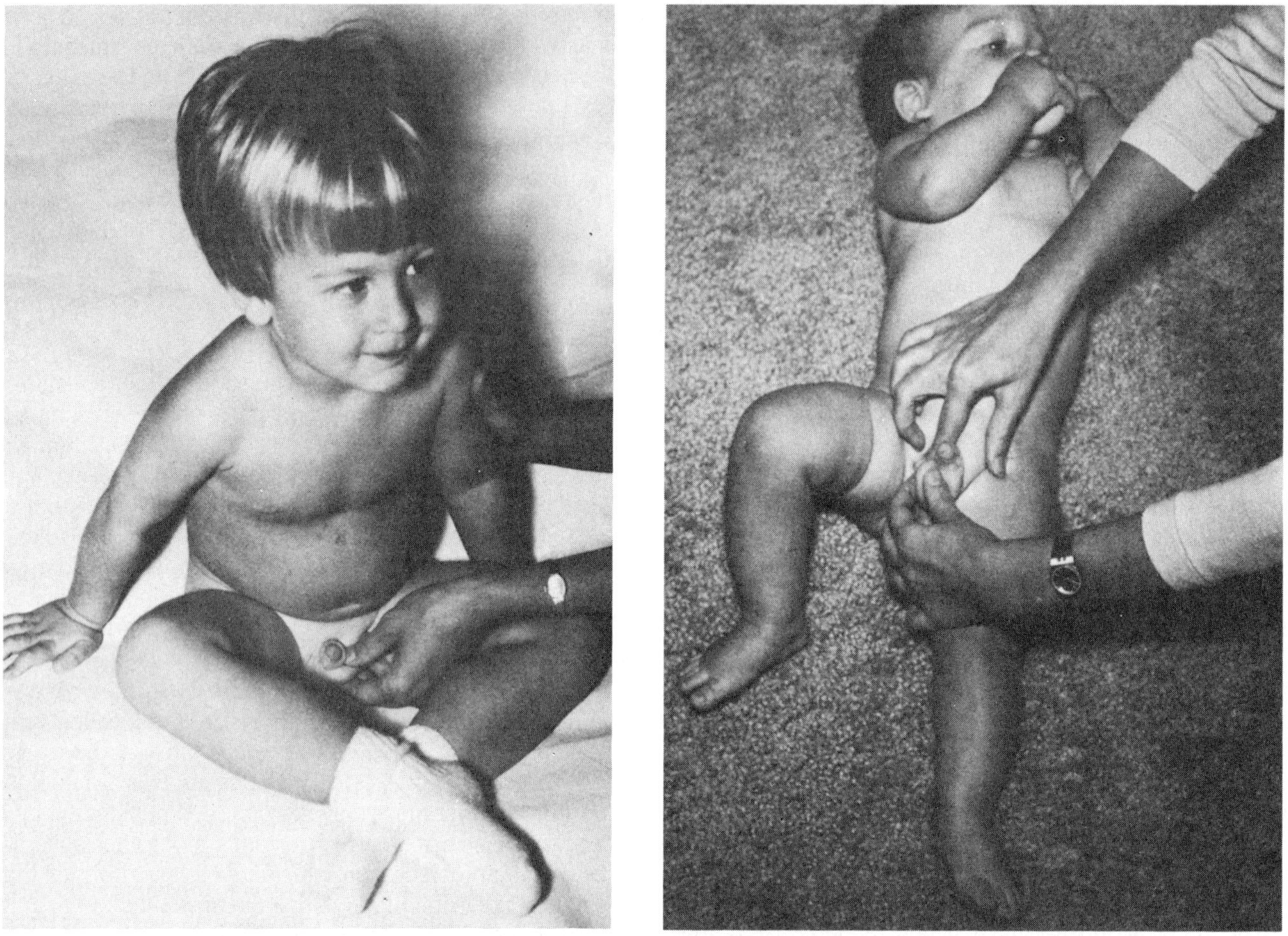

B

Fig. 7-48. A, Preventing cremasteric reflex by having child sit in "tailor" position. **B,** Blocking inguinal canal during palpation of scrotum for descended testes.

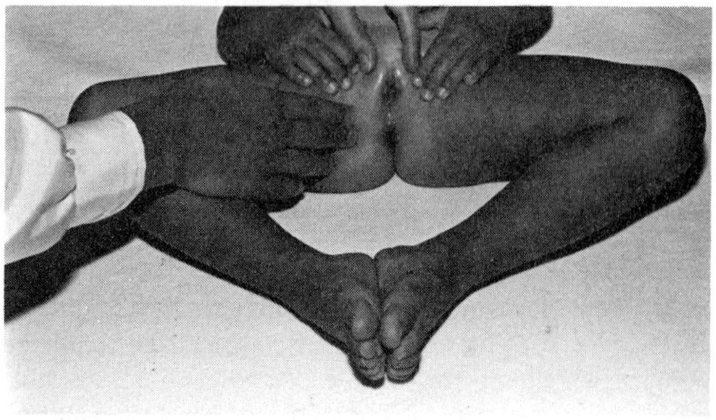

Fig. 7-49. Position for examining genitalia in female child.

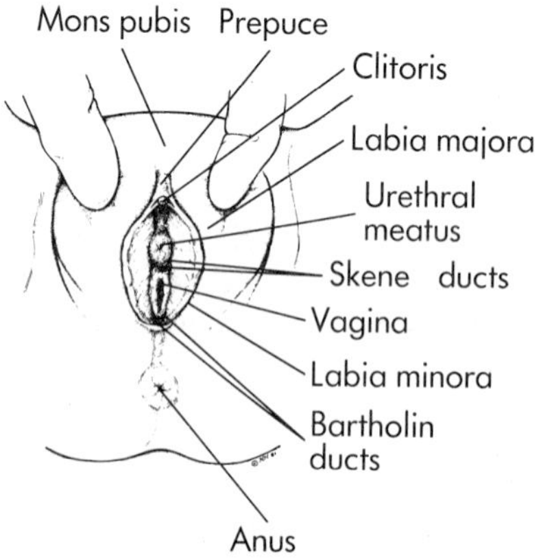

Fig. 7-50. External structures of genitalia in prepubertal female. Labia are spread to reveal deeper structures.

glands, which are common sites of cysts and sexually transmitted disease, are gently palpated.

The *vaginal orifice* is located posterior to the urethral meatus. Its appearance is variable depending on individual anatomy and sexual activity. Ordinarily examination of the vagina is limited to inspection. However, in the presence of signs suggesting ambiguous genitalia, the nurse may decide to refer or perform a manual examination to determine if a vaginal vault exists.

In virgins a thin crescent-shaped or circular membrane, called the *hymen,* may cover part of the vaginal opening. In some instances, it completely occludes the orifice. After rupture, small rounded pieces of tissue called *caruncles* remain. Although an imperforate hymen denotes lack of penile intercourse, a perforate one does not necessarily indicate sexual activity (see also Sexual Abuse, Chapter 16).

Surrounding the vaginal opening are *Bartholin glands,* which secrete a clear, mucoid fluid into the vagina for lubrication during intercourse. The ducts are palpated for cysts. The discharge from the vagina is also noted, which is usually clear or whitish. Variations in the appearance, such as white and cheesy or yellow-greenish, and odor may indicate infection. Sudden, foul-smelling, and profuse discharge may suggest a foreign body inside the vaginal vault. The presence of feces or urine from the vagina usually suggests a fistula from the rectum or urethra. Any swelling, inflammation, or prolapsed area around the vagina is noted. Any such findings are referred for further gynecologic evaluation.

ANUS

Following examination of the genitalia, one can easily observe the anal area, although the child should be placed on the abdomen. The general firmness of the buttocks and symmetry of the gluteal folds are noted. The tone of the anal sphincter is assessed by eliciting the *anal reflex.* Scratching or gently pricking the anal area results in an obvious quick contraction of the external anal sphincter.

The sphincter area is inspected for *fissures,* small cuts or tears in the mucosa that are painful and often lead to constipation as the child refrains from defecating; *prolapse* of the rectum, which is evident as a tubelike protrusion that can be retracted manually; *polyps,* cherry-red protrusions that often cause bleeding; and *hemorrhoids,* dark protrusions of blood vessels. Each of these, although not common, is reported for further medical investigation. Benign protrusions are small *mucosal tabs* of skin attached to the anal sphincter.

The skin around the anal area is inspected for lesions, the most common of which are caused by diaper rash. If the child complains of perianal itching, testing for pinworms is recommended.

BACK AND EXTREMITIES

While the child is prone, the spine, extremities, joints, and muscles are inspected. However, they are also observed with the child sitting and standing.

Spine

The general *curvature* of the spine is noted. Normally the back of a newborn is rounded or C-shaped from the thoracic and pelvic curves. The development of the cervical and lumbar curves approximates development of various motor skills, such as cervical curvature with head control, and gives the older child the typical double-S curve (see Fig. 4-5).

Marked curvatures in posture are abnormal (see Fig. 39-30). *Scoliosis,* lateral curvature of the spine, is an important childhood problem, especially in females. Although scoliosis may be palpated by feeling along the spine and noting a sideways displacement, more objective tests include:

1. With the child standing erect, clothed only in underpants (and bra if older girl), observe from behind, noting asymmetry of the shoulders and hips.
2. With the child bending forward so that the back is parallel to the floor, observe from the side, noting asymmetry or prominence of the rib cage.

A slight limp, a crooked hemline, or complaints of a sore back are other signs and symptoms of scoliosis.

The *back,* especially along the spine, is inspected for any tufts of hair, dimples, or discoloration. A small dimple (usually with a tuft of hair), called a *pilonidal cyst,* may indicate an underlying spina bifida occulta. The spine is palpated to identify each spiny process of the vertebrae or lack of them.

Mobility of the vertebral column is easily assessed in most children because of their propensity for constant motion during the examination. However, mobility can be specifically tested for by asking the child to sit up from a prone position or to do a modified sit-up exercise. Maintaining a rigid straightness when performing these maneuvers is considered abnormal and may indicate central nervous system infection or irritation. However, some individuals who are unable to relax, despite normal skeletal function, may also retain a rigid posture.

Movement of the cervical spine is an important diagnostic sign for neurologic problems, such as meningitis. Normally movement of the head in all directions is effortless.

NURSING ALERT Hyperextension of the neck and spine, called *opisthotonos,* which is accompanied by pain when the head is flexed, is always referred for immediate medical evaluation.

Extremities

Each extremity is inspected for symmetry of length and size; any deviation is referred for orthopedic evaluation. The fingers and toes are counted to be certain of the normal number. This normalcy is so often taken for granted that an extra digit *(polydactyly)* or fusion of digits *(syndactyly)* may go unnoticed. The fingers and toes are also inspected for any evidence of clubbing, cyanosis, disorders of the nails (including habitual nail biting), and general hygiene. These have been discussed in more detail under assessment of the skin (p. 241). If there is any doubt regarding symmetry of leg length, the legs are measured from the anterior iliac spine (felt as the point of the pelvis) to the medial malleolus (ankle bone).

The arms and legs are inspected for *temperature, color, tenderness,* and *masses.* Temperature in each extremity should be equal, although the feet may normally be colder than the hands. Coolness denotes decreased blood circulation, such as from occlusion of a blood vessel, whereas heat denotes increased blood flow, such as an infection or inflammation. Enlargement of bone, such as from swelling, with redness, heat, and tenderness needs further evaluation. It may signify trauma, infection, or an underlying disease process (e.g., sickle cell disease). A solid mass palpable along a bone with or without pain may be a tumor. Although not all masses are malignant, they must be evaluated further.

Since accidental fractures are common in children, the nurse should be familiar with assessing orthopedic injuries. The five main criteria are (1) pain, (2) pulse, (3) paresthesia (abnormal sensation, such as numbness), (4) pallor, and (5) paralysis. Palpation over a possible fractured bone may elicit crepitation, a grating sound produced by movement of the broken ends of the bone.

The *shape* of bones is assessed. Several variations of bone shape may be observed in children. Although many of them cause parents concern, most are benign and require no treatment. *Bowleg,* or *genu varum,* is lateral bowing of the tibia. It is clinically present when the child stands with the medial malleoli (rounded prominence on either side of the ankle) in apposition and the space between the knees is greater than approximately 5 cm (2 inches) (Fig. 7-51). Toddlers are usually bowlegged after beginning to walk until all their lower back and leg muscles are well developed. Unilateral or asymmetric bowlegs that are present beyond the age of 2 to 3 years, particularly in black children, may represent pathologic conditions requiring further investigation.

Knock-knee, or *genu valgum,* appears as the opposite of bowleg, in that the knees are close together but the feet are spread apart. It is determined clinically by using the same method as for genu varum but by measuring the distance between the malleoli, which normally should be less than 7.5 cm (3 inches) (Fig. 7-52). Knock-knee is normally present in children from about 2 to 7 years of age. Knock-knee that is excessive (as measured roentgenographically by the tibiofemoral angle), asymmetric, accompanied by shortened stature, or evident in a child nearing puberty requires further evaluation.

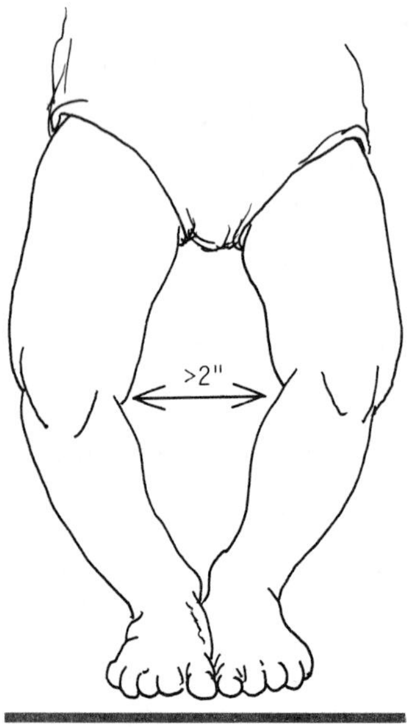

Fig. 7-51. Bowleg.

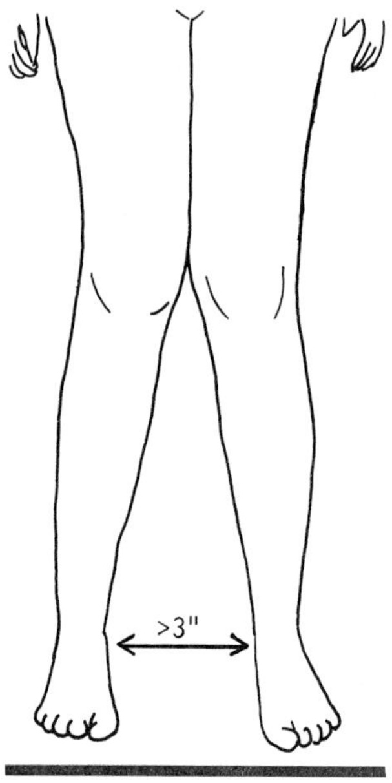

Fig. 7-52. Knock-knee.

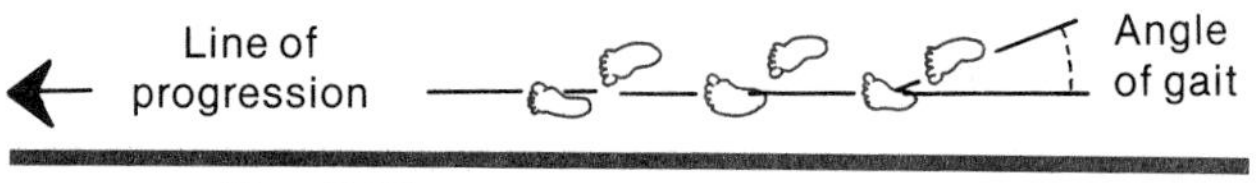

Fig. 7-53. Measurement of angle of gait.

The *feet* are observed for arch development and correct gait. Infants' and toddlers' feet appear flat because the foot is normally wide and the arch is covered by a fat pad. Development of the arch occurs naturally from the action of walking. Normally at birth the feet are held in a valgus (outward) or varus (inward) position. To determine whether a foot deformity at birth is the result of intrauterine position or development, the outer, then inner, side of the sole is scratched. If the foot position is self-correctable, it will assume a right angle to the leg.

Gait is assessed by having the child walk and estimating the angle of gait, which is the angle between the axis of the foot (imaginary line drawn through center of foot) and the line of progression (Fig. 7-53). Normally the feet turn outward less than 30 degrees and inward less than 10 degrees. Variations in foot positions are described in Table 11-3.

Toddlers have a "toddling" or broad-based gait, which facilitates walking by lowering the center of gravity. As the child reaches preschool age, the legs are brought closer together. By school age the walking posture is much more graceful and balanced.

The most common gait problem in young children is pigeon toe or toeing in, which usually results from torsional deformities, such as internal tibial torsion (abnormal rotation or bowing of the tibia). Tests for tibial torsion include measuring the thigh-foot angle, which requires considerable practice for accuracy.

The *plantar* or *grasp reflex* is tested while examining the feet. It is elicited by exerting firm but gentle pressure with the tip of the thumb against the lateral sole of the foot from the heel upward to the little toe and then across to the big toe. The normal response in children who are walking is flexion of the toes. *Babinski sign,* dorsiflexion of the big toe and fanning of the other toes, is normal during infancy but abnormal after about 1 year or when locomotion begins (see Fig. 8-10, *B*). A positive Babinski sign after age 1 year is an indication of spinal cord lesions and requires further neurologic examination.

Joints

The joints are evaluated for *range of motion.* Normally this requires no specific testing if the nurse has been observant of the child's movements during the examination. However, the hips should be routinely investigated in infants for congenital dislocation. Signs of congenital hip dislocation are discussed in Chapter 11. Any evidence of joint immobility or hyperflexibility is reported.

The joints are routinely palpated for *heat, tenderness,* and *swelling.* These signs, as well as redness over the joint, may indicate infection or any of the collagen diseases. Such findings warrant further investigation.

Muscles

Much of the examination of the spine, extremities, and joints indicates muscular development, the shape and contour of the body in both a relaxed and tensed state. If there is asymmetry of development, the circumference of the muscle mass is measured with a tape measure and compared with the measurement of the contralateral muscle. Marked disparity between the two sizes is reported.

Development is closely associated with *tone* or the balance between the muscle mass and nervous stimulation. Tone is estimated by grasping the muscle and feeling its firmness when it is relaxed and contracted. A common site for testing tone is the biceps muscle of the arm. Children usually willingly "make a muscle" by clenching their fist.

Strength is estimated by having the child use an extremity to push or pull against resistance, as in the following example:

1. **Arm strength:** Child holds the arms outstretched in front of the body and tries to raise the arms while downward pressure is applied.
2. **Hand strength:** Child squeezes one or two fingers of the nurse's hand.
3. **Leg strength:** Child sits on a table or chair with the legs dangling and tries to raise the legs while downward pressure is applied.

Symmetry of strength is estimated in the extremities, hands, and fingers. Evidence of paresis or weakness is reported.

NEUROLOGIC ASSESSMENT

The assessment of the nervous system is the broadest and most diverse, since every human function, both physical and emotional, is controlled by neurologic impulses. This discussion focuses primarily on a general appraisal of behavior, cognitive-perceptual development, sensory and cerebellar functioning, deep tendon reflexes, the cranial nerves, and "soft" signs.

Assessment of neurologic function requires the use of a few additional tools. A reflex hammer, which has a small rounded rubber head, is used to test deep tendon reflexes. A pin and cotton are useful when testing sensory function. For the assessment of the cranial nerves, some flavors to taste and some odors to smell are necessary, although nothing elaborate is required (see Table 7-18). Motor development is best evaluated with screening tests, such as the Denver Developmental Screening Test (DDST).

Behavior

There is no special testing for behavior. Rather, it is an overall impression of the child's personality, affect, level of activity, social interaction, and attention span. Some aspects of assessing behavior are discussed elsewhere (see p. 240). Difficulties at home, at school, and in social situations suggest the need for additional psychologic assessment.

Another approach toward assessing behavior is the use of a behavioral checklist (Box 7-12). It is completed by parents of children 6 to 12 years old and focuses on five major areas: mood, play, school, friends, and family relations. Scoring is based on a point system of 0 for "never," 1 for "sometimes," and 2 for "often." The scores are summed; a total score equal to or higher than 28 suggests the need for further evaluation of the child (Jellinek and others, 1988).

State of consciousness is a specific area for behavior under neurologic assessment. Hyperirritability, hyporeactivity, lethargy, delirium, stupor, or coma requires immediate referral. Levels of consciousness are described in Chapter 37. The nurse should always question parents' perceptions of change in behavior, which usually precedes an altered level of consciousness.

Cognitive-Perceptual Development

Cognitive-perceptual development is best assessed using a formal screening test such as the DDST. Adaptive and speech-comprehension development are significant indicators of intellectual functioning. If intellectual or perceptual impairment is suspected or learning difficulties exist, the child should be referred to an appropriate developmental study team for further evaluation. "Soft" signs that should suggest minimum or borderline brain dysfunction are dis-

Box 7-12 PEDIATRIC SYMPTOM CHECKLIST

1. Complains of aches or pains
2. Spends more time alone
3. Tires easily, little energy
4. Fidgety, unable to sit still
5. Has trouble with a teacher
6. Less interested in school
7. Acts as if driven by a motor
8. Daydreams too much
9. Distracted easily
10. Is afraid of new situations
11. Feels sad, unhappy
12. Is irritable, angry
13. Feels hopeless
14. Has trouble concentrating
15. Less interest in friends
16. Fights with other children
17. Absent from school
18. School grades dropping
19. Is down on himself or herself
20. Visits physician, but physician finds nothing wrong
21. Has trouble with sleeping
22. Worries a lot
23. Wants to be with you more than before
24. Feels he or she is bad
25. Takes unnecessary risks
26. Gets hurt frequently
27. Seems to be having less fun
28. Acts younger than children his or her age
29. Does not listen to rules
30. Does not show feelings
31. Does not understand other people's feelings
32. Teases others
33. Blames others for his or her troubles
34. Takes things that do not belong to him or her
35. Refuses to share

From Jellinek, M.S., and others: Pediatric symptom checklist: screening school-age children for psychosocial dysfunction, J. Pediatr. 112(2):201-209, 1988.

cussed at the conclusion of assessment of the neurologic system (p. 288).

Motor Functioning

Motor ability primarily involves assessment of voluntary muscle contraction and acquisition of age-specific developmental milestones for gross and fine motor skills (see Denver Developmental Screening Test, p. 290). One of the most important milestones in motor development is head control. Since development proceeds in the cephalocaudal direction, head lag suggests early brain damage. Head control is usually acquired by 4 months of age, although, as discussed in Chapter 8, even the newborn demonstrates some head control.

Handedness is also observed. Infants and toddlers may show preference for one hand, but they usually do not display marked preference until the preschool years. Sole use of one hand may indicate paresis on the opposite side. Failure to demonstrate handedness by a school-age child suggests failure of the brain to develop dominance, but its diagnostic significance is controversial.

Box 7-13 TESTS FOR SENSORY DISCRIMINATION

Touch the skin with a pin or piece of cotton and ask the child to describe the different sensations.
Place a cold or warm object on the skin (the rubber and metal heads of the reflex hammer work well) and have the child differentiate between them.
Touch different parts of the body simultaneously and see if the child can localize both points.

Box 7-14 TESTS FOR CEREBELLAR FUNCTION

Finger-to-nose test. With the child's arm extended, ask the child to touch the nose with the index finger with the eyes open and then closed.
Heel-to-shin test. While standing, have the child run the heel of one foot down the shin or anterior aspect of the tibia of the other leg, both with the eyes opened and then closed.
Romberg test. With the eyes closed, have the child stand with the heels together; falling or leaning to one side is abnormal and is called *Romberg sign.*

Sensory Functioning

Sensory functioning is mainly assessed in terms of the sensory cranial nerves, in particular, vision and hearing and peripheral sensation. This discussion is devoted to testing of peripheral sensation. Testing of the cranial nerves is discussed on p. 288, and vision and auditory testing are discussed on pp. 250 and 259, respectively.

Peripheral sensation. With children old enough to cooperate, *sensory discrimination* is assessed by performing the following with the child's eyes closed (Box 7-13). Because these tests are similar to playing a game, they may be performed at the beginning of the examination in order to decrease the child's anxiety and foster trust.

✦ **NURSING ALERT** Decreased sensation or hyperesthesia (excessive sensation) are abnormal and must be referred for further neurologic evaluation.

Cerebellar Functioning

The cerebellum mainly controls balance and coordination. Much of the assessment of cerebellar functioning involves observing the child's posture, body movements, gait, and development of fine and gross motor skills. Tests such as balancing on one foot and the heel-to-toe walk in the DDST also assess balance. Coordination is tested by asking the child to reach for a toy, button clothes, tie shoes, or draw a straight line on a piece of paper, provided the child is old enough to accomplish these activities.

Several tests for cerebellar function are described in Box 7-14 and can be performed as games. When the Romberg test is done, the nurse should sit beside the child if there is a possibility that the child may fall.

School-age children should be able to perform these tests, although preschoolers normally can bring the finger only within 5 to 7.5 cm (2 to 3 inches) of their nose. Difficulty in performing these exercises indicates a poor sense of position (especially with the eyes closed) and incoordination (especially with the eyes opened). Coordination can also be tested by any sequence of rapid successive movements, such as quickly touching each finger with the thumb of the same hand. Cerebellar testing is particularly significant in children with symptoms of hyperactivity or learning difficulty.

Reflexes

Testing reflexes is an important part of the neurologic examination. Persistence of primitive reflexes, loss of reflexes, or hyperactivity of deep tendon reflexes is usually the result of a cerebral insult. This discussion is primarily concerned with reflexes found in children past infancy. The primitive reflexes of the newborn are discussed in Chapter 8.

In eliciting reflexes, it is important to have some understanding of their basic physiology. A *reflex* is an involuntary response to a stimulus. However, three characteristics are unique: (1) the individual is aware of the movement, (2) the person may be able to inhibit it, such as by tensing the muscle, but (3) when the activity occurs, it does so without the person's conscious assistance. Although reflexes are under the control of higher brain centers, they may continue to function even though the influence of the brain has been lost. This commonly occurs in spinal cord injury, when the child is unable to walk but still demonstrates the patellar reflex.

Reflexes can be elicited by using the rubber head of the reflex hammer, flat of the finger, or side of the hand. If the child is easily frightened by equipment, it is best to use one's hand or finger. Although testing reflexes is a simple procedure to perform, the child may inhibit the reflex by unconsciously tensing the muscle. The nurse should try to distract younger children with toys or by talking to them. Older children can concentrate on the exercise of grasping their two hands in front of them and trying to pull them apart to divert their attention from the testing and cause involuntary relaxation of the muscles.

Several *superficial reflexes* are present, such as the abdominal, cremasteric, anal, and plantar. These have already been discussed throughout the chapter. *Deep tendon reflexes* are stretch reflexes of a muscle. The most common deep tendon reflex is the *knee jerk,* or *patellar reflex* (sometimes called *quadriceps reflex*). The reflexes normally elicited are described in Figs. 7-54 through 7-58. Reflexes are evaluated by using the grading system in Table 7-17. Absent or hyperactive reflexes are reported for further evaluation.

Several other reflexes are normally present or absent but are not elicited unless specific indications exist. For example, in the presence of symptoms suggestive of meningeal irritation, the Kernig sign and the Brudzinski signs are elicited. To test for Kernig sign the child lies supine and the leg is flexed at the hip and knee. Resistance or pain on extending the leg at the knee is abnormal and is called a positive *Kernig sign* (Fig. 7-59). The test for Brudzinski sign is performed by flexing the child's head while supine. If this causes pain or the knees and hips to flex involuntarily, *Brudzinski sign* is positive (Fig. 7-60).

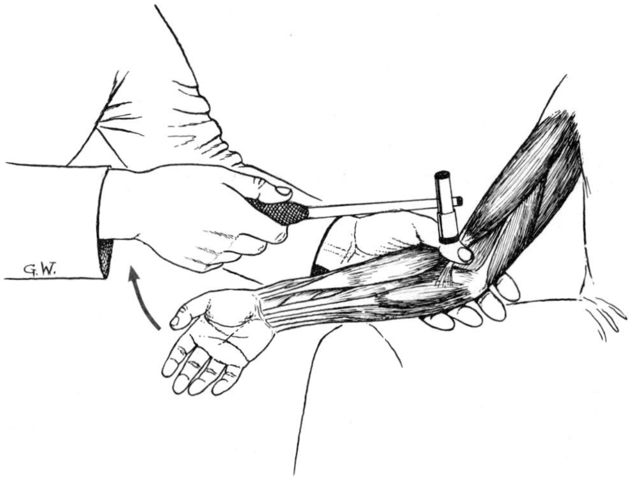

Fig. 7-54. Testing for biceps reflex. Child's arm is held by placing partially flexed elbow in examiner's hand with thumb over antecubital space. Examiner's thumbnail is struck with hammer. Normal response is partial flexion of forearm.

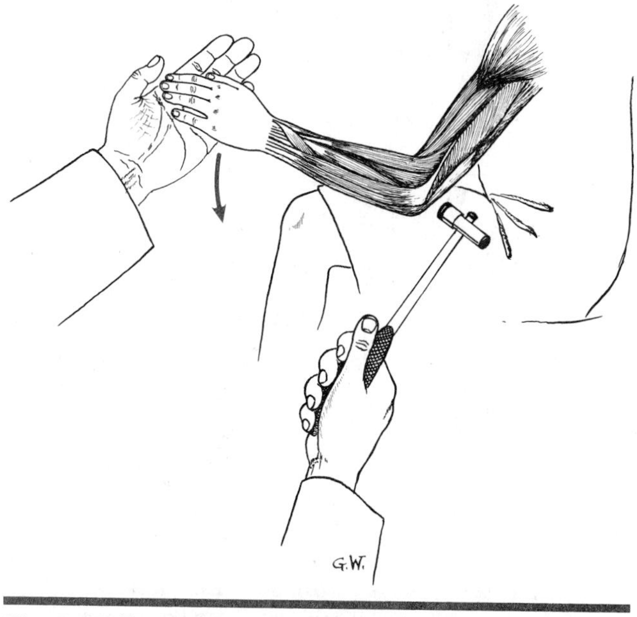

Fig. 7-55. Testing for triceps reflex. Child's arm is flexed at the elbow and child's hand is placed in examiner's palm. Triceps tendon is struck. Alternate position: child is placed supine, with his forearm resting over the chest. Child's arm is abducted, with upper arm supported and forearm allowed to hang freely. Normal response is partial extension of forearm.

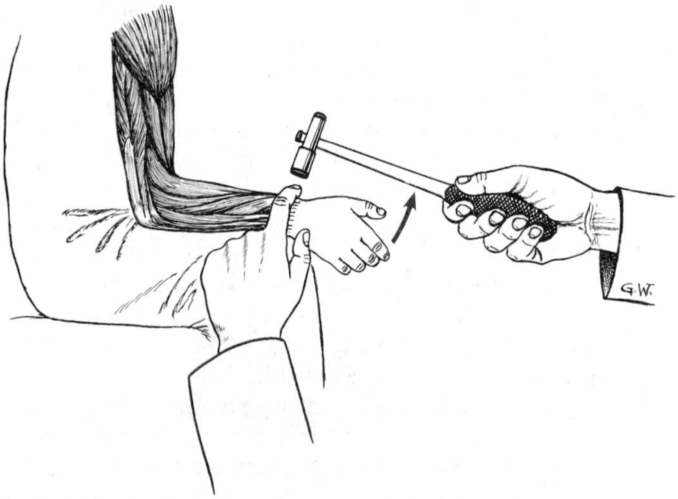

Fig. 7-56. Testing for brachioradialis reflex. Child's forearm is placed on his lap or abdomen, with arm flexed at elbow and the palm down. Radius is struck about 1 inch (depending on child's size) above wrist. Normal response is flexion of forearm and supination (turning upward) of palm.

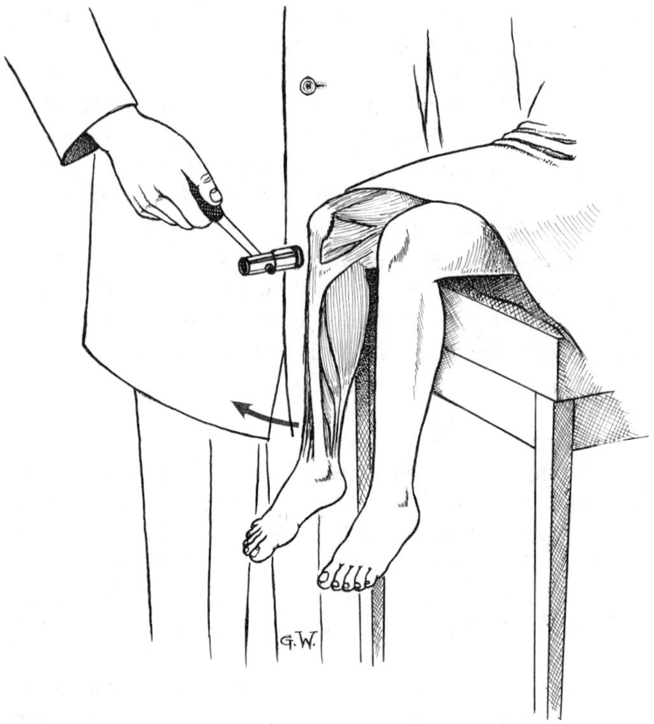

Fig. 7-57. Testing for patellar, or knee jerk, reflex. Child sits on edge of examining table (or on parent's lap) with lower legs flexed at knee and dangling freely. Patellar tendon is tapped just below kneecap. Normal response is partial extension of lower leg.

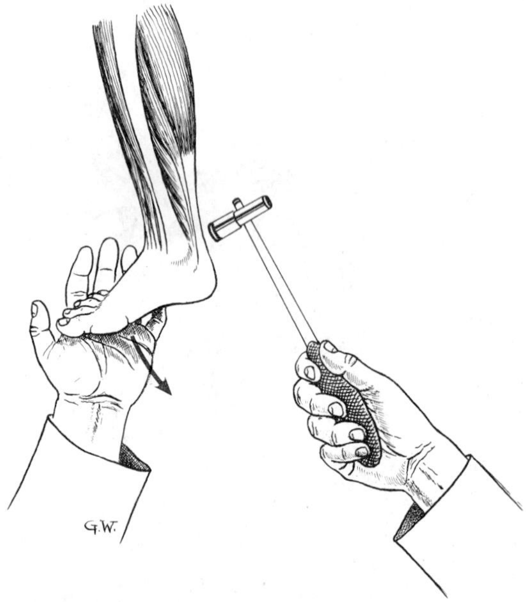

Fig. 7-58. Testing for Achilles reflex. Same position employed in eliciting knee jerk reflex is used. Foot is supported lightly in examiner's hand, and Achilles tendon is struck. Normal response is plantar flexion of foot (foot pointing downward).

Table 7-17 Grading of reflexes

GRADE	DESCRIPTION
4+	Extremely brisk, hyperactive
3+	Brisker than normal
2+	Average, normal
1+	Diminished
0+	Absent

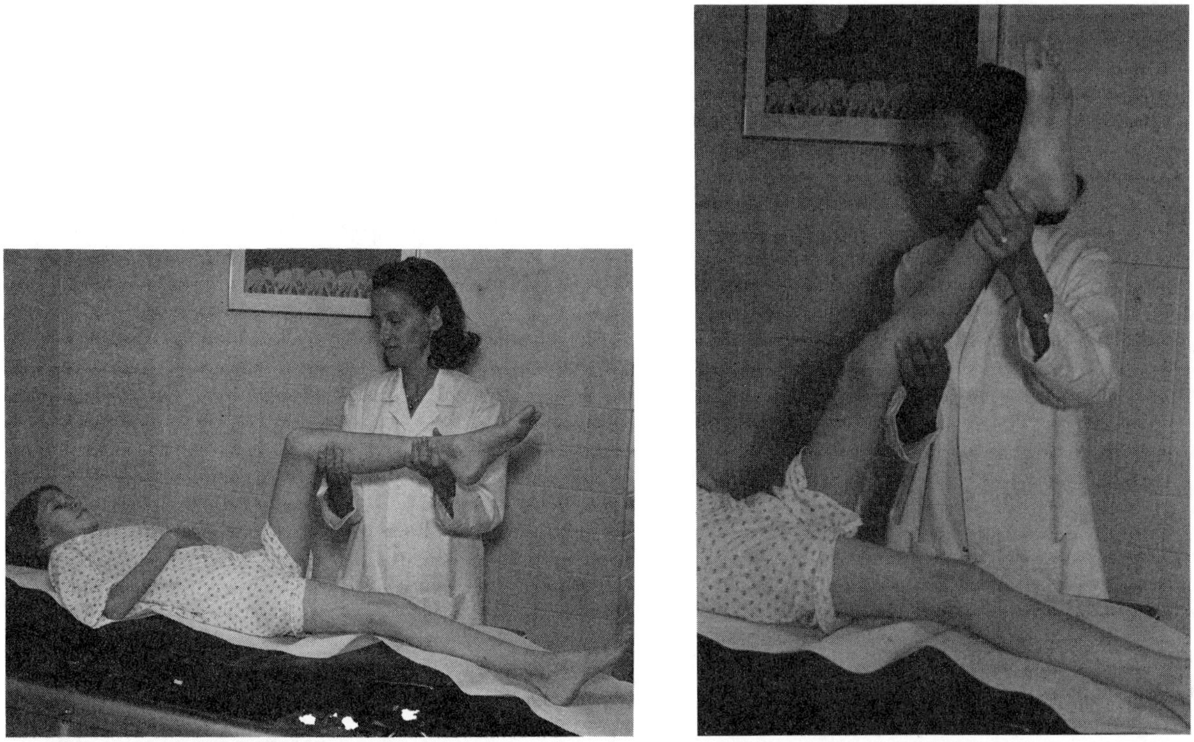

A

B

Fig. 7-59. A, Testing for Kernig sign. **B,** Pain or resistance on extension is abnormal.

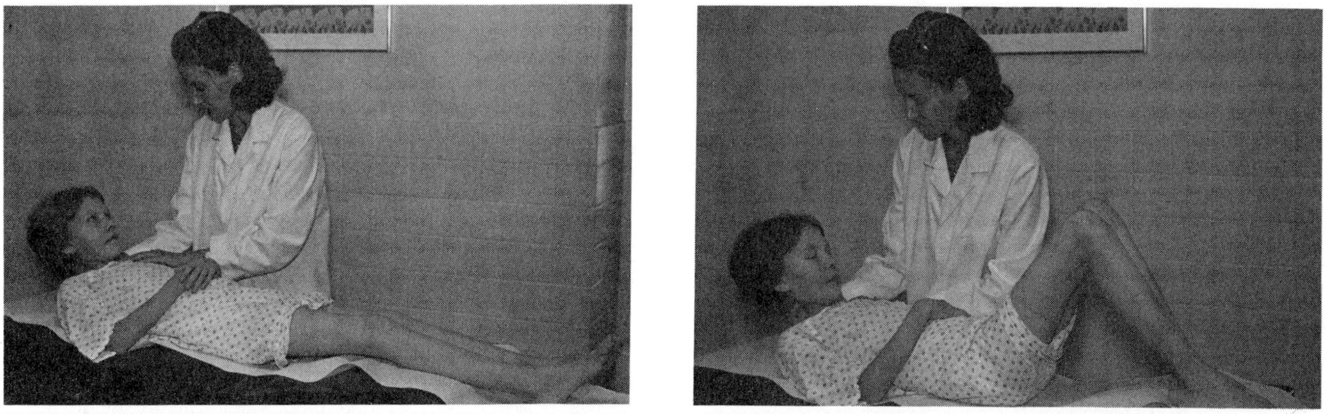

A

B

Fig. 7-60. A, Testing for Brudzinski sign. **B,** Pain or involuntary flexion of knees and hips is abnormal.

Cranial Nerves

The 12 cranial nerves arise directly from the brain and supply the structures of the head and neck. Parts of the tenth nerve, the vagus, branch off to supply structures of the trunk. Assessment of the cranial nerves is an important area of neurologic assessment (Table 7-18). With older children most of the tests can be presented as games and, because no traumatic equipment is used, may encourage trust and security at the beginning of the examination. However, much of the testing can be included when each "system" is examined, such as tongue movement and strength, gag reflex, swallowing, and position of the uvula during examination of the mouth.

"Soft" Signs

One of the difficulties in assessment of the nervous system is the clear-cut differentiation between normal and abnormal findings (sometimes referred to as "hard" signs). There is a gray area called "soft" signs, findings that are normal in a young child but that in the normal course of maturation disappear. They represent the persistence of a more primitive form of behavior or response and a failure to perform the age-specific activity. Although the list of soft signs is long and the controversy concerning their significance far from resolved, some of the classic signs are listed in Box 7-15.

Table 7-18 Assessment of cranial nerves

CRANIAL NERVE	DISTRIBUTION/FUNCTION	TEST
I—Olfactory (S)*	Olfactory mucosa of nasal cavity	With eyes closed, have child identify odors such as coffee, alcohol from a swab, or other smells; test each nostril separately
II—Optic (S)	Rods and cones of retina, optic nerve	Check for perception of light, visual acuity, peripheral vision, color vision, and normal optic disc
III—Oculomotor (M)*	Extraocular muscles (EOM) of eye: Superior rectus (SR)—Moves eyeball up and in Inferior rectus (IR)—Moves eyeball down and in Medial rectus (MR)—Moves eyeball nasally Inferior oblique (IO)—Moves eyeball up and out	Have child follow an object (toy) or light in the six cardinal positions of gaze (see Fig. 7-61)
	Pupil constriction and accommodation	Perform PERRLA
	Eyelid closing	Check for proper placement of lid
IV—Trochlear (M)	Superior oblique muscle (SO)—Moves eye down and out	Have child look down and in (Fig. 7-61)
V—Trigeminal (M, S)	Muscles of mastication	Have child bite down hard and open jaw; test symmetry and strength
	Sensory: face, scalp, nasal and buccal mucosa	With child's eyes closed, see if child can detect light touch in the mandibular and maxillary regions Test corneal and blink reflex by touching cornea lightly (approach from the side so that child does not blink before cornea is touched)
VI—Abducens (M)	Lateral rectus (LR) muscle—Moves eye temporally	Have child look toward temporal side (Fig. 7-61)
VII—Facial (M, S)	Muscles for facial expression	Have child smile, make funny face, or show teeth to see symmetry of expression
	Anterior two thirds of tongue (sensory)	Have child identify a sweet or salty solution; place each taste on anterior section and sides of protruding tongue; if child retracts tongue, solution will dissolve toward posterior part of tongue
	Nasal cavity and lacrimal gland, sublingual and submandibular salivary glands	Not tested
VIII—Auditory, acoustic, or vestibulocochlear (S)	Internal ear	Test hearing; note any loss of equilibrium or presence of vertigo

*S—sensory; M—motor.

Table 7-18 Assessment of cranial nerves—cont'd

CRANIAL NERVE	DISTRIBUTION/FUNCTION	TEST
IX—Glossopharyngeal (M, S)	Pharynx, tongue	Stimulate the posterior pharynx with a tongue blade; the child should gag
	Posterior one third of tongue (sensory)	Test sense of sour or bitter taste on posterior segment of tongue
X—Vagus (M, S)	Muscles of larynx, pharynx, some organs of gastrointestinal system, sensory fibers of root of tongue, heart, lung, and some organs of gastrointestinal system	Note hoarseness of the voice, gag reflex, and ability to swallow Check that uvula is in midline; when stimulated with a tongue blade, should deviate upward and to the stimulated side
XI—Accessory (M)	Sternocleidomastoid and trapezius muscles of shoulder	Have child shrug shoulders while applying mild pressure; with the hands placed on shoulders, have child turn head against opposing pressure on either side; note symmetry and strength
XII—Hypoglossal (M)	Muscles of tongue	Have child move tongue in all directions; have child protrude the tongue as far as possible; note any midline deviation Test strength by placing tongue blade on one side of tongue and having child move it away

Box 7-15 NEUROLOGIC "SOFT" SIGNS

Short attention span
Unusual body movements, such as mirroring
Poor coordination and sense of position
Excessive, sustained, and purposeless movement (hyperactivity)
Hypoactivity
Impulsiveness
Labile emotions
Distractibility
No established handedness
Language and articulation problems
Perceptual deficits (space, form, movement, time)
Problems with learning, especially reading, writing, and arithmetic

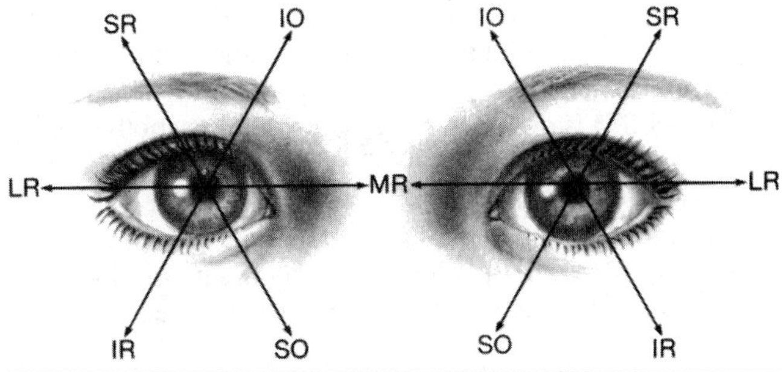

Fig. 7-61. Testing cardinal positions of gaze.

■ DEVELOPMENTAL ASSESSMENT

One of the most essential components of a complete health appraisal is assessment of developmental functioning. *Screening procedures* are designed to identify quickly and reliably those children whose developmental level is below normal for their age and who, therefore, require further investigation. They also provide a means of recording objective measurements of present developmental functioning for future reference. With the passage of P.L. 99-457, the Education of the Handicapped Act Amendments of 1986, much greater emphasis is placed on developmental assessment of children with disabilities, and nurses can play a vital role in providing this service. All of the procedures discussed in this section can be administered in a variety of settings—home, school, daycare center, hospital, practitioner's office, or clinic.

DENVER DEVELOPMENTAL SCREENING TEST

One of the most widely used screening tests for assessing a young child's development is the *Denver Developmental Screening Test* (DDST) (see Appendix B). It is composed of four major categories: personal-social, fine motor–adaptive, language, and gross motor and is applicable for children from birth through 6 years of age. The age divisions are monthly until 24 months and then every 6 months until 6 years of age. Up to 24 months of age, allowances are made for infants who were born prematurely by subtracting the number of weeks of missed gestation from their present age and testing them at the adjusted age. For example, a 16-week-old infant who was born 4 weeks early is tested at a 12-week adjusted age level.

The DDST and the revised DDST (DDST-R) have been subjected to several reliability and validity tests and have been found to yield normal, questionable, and abnormal results that correlate with psychometric tests, such as the Cattell Infant Intelligence Scale and the Revised Bayley Infant Scale. Weaknesses of the DDST include its lack of sensitivity in identifying children with speech and language delays (Borowitz and Glascoe, 1986) and identifying general delays in children of lower socioeconomic groups (Frankenburg, Dick, and Carland, 1975) and from different cultural backgrounds. For example, Southeast Asian children have demonstrated delays in the areas of personal-social development because of lack of familiarity with games such as pat-a-cake and in language because of differences in word usage, such as absence of plurals (Miller, Onotera, and Deinard, 1984). The more protective parental attitude of Southeast Asians toward the young child may also prevent early learning of self-help skills (Fung and Lau, 1985). Several of these variations were noted also in native African children (Olade, 1984). Such cultural differences must be considered when administering the test and scoring the results (Fig. 7-62).

The DDST* is designed for administration by both professionals and paraprofessionals and takes about 15 to 20 minutes to complete. The kits for testing include a red skein of wool, raisins, a small clear bottle with a 5/8-inch opening, a rattle with a narrow handle, eight 1-inch square blocks in red, blue, yellow, and green colors, a small bell, a tennis ball, and a pencil.

The major differences between the original DDST and the DDST-R are the arrangement of items on the form and the scoring. On the original form, items are scored as "P" for pass, "F" for fail, or "R" for refusal. On the DDST-R only the items passed are scored (Frankenburg and others, 1981).

Each item is designated by a bar that represents the ages at which 25%, 50%, 75%, and 90% of the tested population could perform the particular item. Scoring is based on the number of delays (Box 7-16).

Although it is not the purpose of this discussion to detail the instruction manual, there are some points concerning preparation, administration, and interpretation of the DDST (and the Denver II described on p. 291) that necessitate emphasis. Before beginning the screen, both the child and the parent need an explanation. For parents this means clarifying that the DDST is *not* an intelligence test but a method of helping the nurse observe what the child can do at a particular age. It is best to deemphasize the word *test* while emphasizing that the child is *not* expected to perform each item on the sheet.

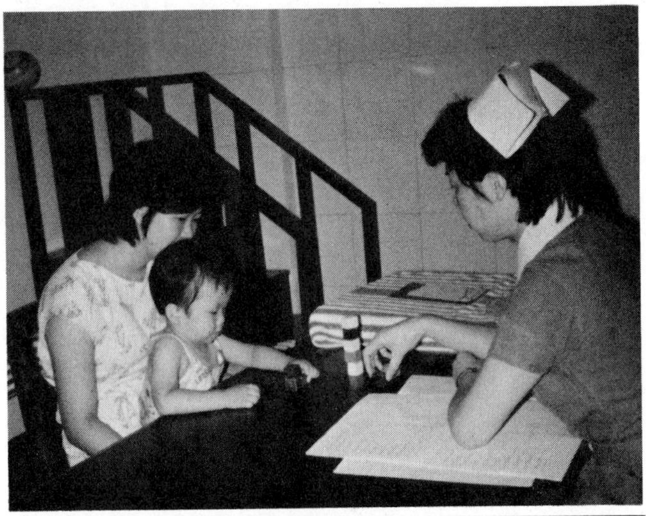

Fig. 7-62. When administering the DDST, the nurse must consider cultural variations that can erroneously label child delayed.

Box 7-16 SCORING OF THE DDST AND DDST-R

Scoring is based on the number of *delays,* defined as failure to perform an item that is passed by 90% of the children who are of the same age, or any item that falls completely to the left of the age line.

Abnormal score: Two or more sectors with two or more delays

or

One sector with two or more delays plus one or more sectors with one delay and, in that same sector, no passes through the age line

Questionable score: One sector with two or more delays

or

One or more sectors with one delay and in that same sector no passes through the age line

Untestable score: Number of refusals is large enough to cause the test result to be questionable or abnormal if they were scored as failures

Normal score: Any score that does not meet the above criteria

---

*Forms and instruction manual are available from Denver Developmental Materials, Inc., P.O. Box 6919, Denver, CO 80206-0919; (303) 355-4729.

NOTE: To ensure that the Denver Developmental Screening Test is administered and interpreted in the prescribed manner, it is recommended that those intending to administer the DDST first take the proficiency test, which can be obtained with the DDST forms and instructional manual.

The parent is told before the screening begins that the results of the child's performance will be explained after all the items have been concluded. It is the nurse's responsibility to properly inform parents of any testing or screening procedure before its administration so that they are fully aware of its purpose and intent.

The nurse can prepare toddlers and preschoolers for the procedure by presenting it as a game. Frequently the DDST is an excellent way to begin a health appraisal because it is nonthreatening, requires no painful or unfamiliar procedures, and capitalizes on the child's natural activity of play. Since children are easily distracted, it is best to perform each item quickly and to present only one toy from the kit at a time. After that toy's purpose is concluded, such as building a tower of blocks or identifying its color, the toy is replaced in the bag and another one is brought out for screening purposes. Other temporary factors that may interfere with the child's performance include fatigue, illness, fear, hospitalization, separation from the parent, or general unwillingness to perform activities asked of the child. In addition, undiagnosed mental retardation, hearing loss, vision loss, neurologic impairment, or a familial pattern of slow development greatly influences the child's performance.

Following completion of the DDST, the nurse asks the parent if the child's performance was typical of behavior at other times. If the parent replies affirmatively and the child's cooperation was satisfactory, the results are explained, emphasizing all successful items first, then those items failed but which the child was not expected to pass, and finally those items that were delays.

In explaining a normal score, the nurse focuses on how well the child performed and reinforces the parents' efforts in satisfactorily stimulating their child. In addition to assessing the child's present developmental level, the DDST can be used to guide parents toward those activities that are appropriate, although not necessarily expected, for the child's age.* Studies of parents' knowledge of developmental milestones indicate that parents have many misconceptions about normal development and either expect skills too early or fail to recognize delays (Shea and Fowler, 1983). By testing for items to the right of the age line (ones child is not expected to perform), children with advanced development, who may be gifted, can be identified (Fish and Burch, 1985).

In explaining delays, the parent's response is carefully noted, especially casual acceptance, such as "He'll catch up." Since all children with questionable or abnormal results should be rescreened before referral for diagnostic testing, some of the parents' more serious questions, such as "Does this mean my child is retarded?" can be deferred until the next screening session. The nurse must be aware of personal anxieties during these situations and refrain from giving glib reassurances, such as "I'm sure he will do better the next time." Rather, parents' questions are answered honestly yet with appropriate flexibility and concern by stating: "I need to observe your child again before I can give you any answers or even make assumptions concerning his developmental progress. I will rescreen him next week, and then possibly I will know more. What are your thoughts about how he performed the activities on the DDST?"

If the parents reply that the child's performance was not typical of usual behavior, it is best to defer any scoring or discussion of results with the parents, especially if the refusals yield a questionable or abnormal score. In this situation the DDST is rescheduled for a time when the child is more likely to cooperate.

DENVER II

The Denver II is a major revision and a restandardization of the DDST.† (See Appendix B.) It differs from the DDST in items included in the test, the test form, and the interpretation. The previous total of 105 items has been increased to 125, including an increase from 21 DDST to 39 Denver II language items. Previous items that were difficult to administer and/or interpret have been either modified or eliminated. Many items that were previously tested by parental report now require observation by the examiner.

Each item was evaluated to determine if significant differences exist on the basis of sex, ethnic group, maternal education, and place of residence. Items for which clinically significant differences exist were replaced, or if retained, are discussed in the Technical Manual. When evaluating children delayed on one of these items, the examiner can look up norms for the subpopulations to consider if the delay may be due to sociocultural or environmental differences.

The age scale of the Denver II is similar to the American Academy of Pediatrics' schedule for health supervision (see Box 7-1). The items on the test form are arranged in the same format as the DDST-R. The norms for the distribution bars were updated with the new standardization data but retain the 25th, 50th, 75th, and 90th percentile divisions. The test form contains a place to rate the child's behavioral characteristics (compliance, interest in surroundings, fearfulness, and attention span).

To determine relative areas of advancement and areas of delay, sufficient items should be administered to establish the basal and ceiling levels in each sector. By scoring appropriate items as "pass" or "fail" and relating such scores to the age of the child, each item can be interpreted as described in Box 7-17. To identify cautions, all items intersected by the age line are administered. To screen solely for developmental delays, only the items located totally to the *left* of the child's age line are administered. Scoring methods and criteria for referral are under investigation.

---

*Suggested Denver Developmental Activities are available from Denver Developmental Materials, Inc.

†The Denver II is available from Denver Developmental Materials, Inc. For those currently administering the DDST or DDST-R, using the Denver II requires only three new testing materials (doll, feeding bottle, and cup), the new manual, and new forms.

Box 7-17 INTERPRETATION OF DENVER II SCORES

Advanced—passed an item completely to the *right* of the age line (passed by less than 25% of children at an age older than the child)
OK—passed, failed, or refused an item intersected by the age line between the 25th and 75th percentile
Caution—failed or refused items intersected by the age line between the 75th and 90th percentile
Delay—failed an item completely to the *left* of the age line; refusals to the left of the age line may also be considered delays, since the reason for the refusal may be inability to perform the task

REVISED PRESCREENING DEVELOPMENTAL QUESTIONNAIRE

The Revised Prescreening Developmental Questionnaire (R-PDQ) is a revision of the original PDQ (Frankenburg, Fandal, and Thorton, 1987). Advantages of the R-PDQ include the addition and arrangement of items to be more age-appropriate, simplified parent scoring, and easier comparison with Denver Developmental Screening Test (DDST) norms for professionals. The R-PDQ is a parent-answered prescreen consisting of 105 questions from the DDST, although only a subset of questions are asked for each age-group. With less-educated parents, the form may need to be read to the caregiver.

Four different forms are available and are selected based on age: orange (0-9 months), purple (9-24 months), gold (2-4 years), and white (4-6 years) (see Appendix B). The caregiver answers the questions until (1) three "NOs" are circled (they do not have to be consecutive) or (2) all of the questions on both sides of the form have been answered. Scoring is based on the number of delays (Box 7-17). Children who have no delays are considered to be developing normally. If a child has one delay, the caregiver is provided with age-appropriate developmental activities* to pursue with the child and a rescreen with the R-PDQ is done 1 month later. If on rescreening, a child has one or more delays, the DDST or Denver II is administered as soon as possible. If a child has two or more delays on the first screening with the R-PDQ, the DDST or Denver II is administered as soon as possible. If a child receives other than normal DDST or Denver II results, a diagnostic evaluation is needed.

As of this writing, a new PDQ based on the Denver II items is being developed and should be available in the near future. In the meantime, the R-PDQ should be used (Frankenburg, 1990).

*Forms and complete instructions are available from Denver Developmental Materials, Inc., P.O. Box 6919, Denver, CO 80206-0919; (303) 355-4729.

DEVELOPMENTAL PROFILE

The Developmental Profile II is designed for use with children from birth through a functional age of 9½ years. With normal children it can be used appropriately from birth through 7 years. The following five scales are included: physical, self-help, social, academic, and communication. Administration time varies from 20 to 40 minutes depending on the child's age and the approach used, either interview, interview and direct testing, or self-interview. A detailed self-instructional manual is used for training (Alpern, Boll, and Shearer, 1985).*

McCARTHY SCALES OF CHILDREN'S ABILITIES

The McCarthy Scales of Children's Abilities (MSCA) is a developmental assessment tool for children 2½ to 8½ years old (McCarthy, 1972). It is based on six scales: verbal, perceptual-performance, quantitative, general cognition, memory, and motor. Administration time is from 45 minutes to 1 hour. Eighteen separate tests are administered to the child, and the scores from these tests contribute to one or more of the scores on the six scales. The final score correlates well with intelligence quotients from other accepted tests. It is a test that may be selected for follow-up when a child fails the DDST or is suspected of having retarded development (Hayes, 1981). A detailed self-instructional manual is used for training.†

WASHINGTON GUIDE TO PROMOTING DEVELOPMENT IN THE YOUNG CHILD

The Washington Guide to Promoting Development in the Young Child provides a framework for developmental assessment based on direct observation of a child's specific behaviors in eight categories: feeding, sleep, play, language, motor activities, discipline, toilet training, and dressing. In each category developmental accomplishments that would be expected for age-groups from birth to 5 years are grouped as "expected tasks" with an accompanying list of "suggested activities" for parental guidance. The Washington Guide differs from other developmental tools in that no score is obtained. It is used to observe the child on a systematic basis, to identify variations in development, and to provide suggestions regarding appropriate childrearing practices (Powell, 1981).

PRESCHOOL READINESS EXPERIMENTAL SCREENING SCALE

The Preschool Readiness Experimental Screening Scale (PRESS) is designed for screening 5-year-old children's readiness for school (Rogers and Rogers, 1972, 1975). It is a

*The Developmental Profile II Manual is available from Western Psychological Services, 12031 Wilshire Blvd., Los Angeles, CA 90025; (800) 222-2670 or (800) 423-7863 in California.

†The McCarthy Scales of Children's Abilities is available from Psychological Corporation, 555 Academic Ct., San Antonio, TX 78204-2498; (512) 299-1061 or (800) 228-0752.

simple test that can be integrated into the physical examination or administered separately. Five areas are assessed: knowledge of numbers, general knowledge, drawing coordination, and an overall assessment of performance and maturity. The scoring system rates children for school readiness as (1) high to above average, (2) average, (3) borderline, or (4) insufficient. The last score indicates a need for referral to a school psychologist or diagnostic center for further evaluation.

GOODENOUGH DRAW-A-PERSON TEST

A test that can be used to assess intellectual development is the Goodenough Draw-A-Person Test* (Goodenough, 1926; Harris, 1963). The child is given a pencil with an eraser and paper and simply asked to "draw a man or a person." No further directions are supplied regarding the drawing, other than that the child should draw the best picture of a person that he can. The child should be left alone and given as much time as needed to finish the picture.

The scoring is determined by giving 1 point for each item included in the drawing (Box 7-18). Each point is equal to 3 months. The number of points are converted to months and/or years and added to the base age of 3 years. The final score in months/years is approximately equal to the child's mental age. The child's intelligence quotient (IQ) can be found by the ratio of mental age to chronologic age multiplied by 100. For example, if a 5-year-old child scores 12 points on the test, he has a mental age of 6 years (3 years + [12 × 3 months] = 6 years) and an IQ of 120.

Although reports concerning the reliability of the Goodenough test vary, it is a valuable procedure for assessing intellectual development in children 3 to 10 years of age, particularly in screening for children with low scores who may require further measurement of mental functioning.

DEVELOPMENTAL SCREENING AND INTERPRETATION

Although screening tests are an effective method of applying the knowledge of children's expected rate of development to a large segment of the population, they are only as successful as the individual's expertise in administering them. Since many of the screening tests are devised to be used by paraprofessionals, there are inherent risks in screening if such individuals are not properly trained or supervised. For example, false-positives can label the child as developmentally delayed and cause problems that otherwise might not have existed. Nurses must ensure that screening tests are properly administered and the results correctly interpreted. The complexity of mental and physical health can never be measured by any one index. Evaluation of the child's total well-being is the result of evaluating data from a comprehensive history, physical examination, and developmental screening.

*The Goodenough Draw-A-Person Test is available from Psychological Corporation, 555 Academic Ct., San Antonio; TX 78204-2498, (512) 299-1061 or (800) 228-0752.

Box 7-18 METHOD OF SCORING GOODENOUGH DRAW-A-PERSON TEST*

1. Head present
2. Legs present
3. Arms present
4. Trunk present
5. Trunk longer than broad
6. Shoulder indicated
7. Both arms and legs attached to trunk
8. Legs and arms attached to trunk at proper level
9. Neck present
10. Outline of neck continuous with that of head or trunk or both
11. Eyes present
12. Nose present
13. Mouth present
14. Both nose and mouth in two dimensions; two lips shown
15. Nostrils indicated
16. Hair shown
17. Hair on more than circumference of head, nontransparent, better than scribble
18. Clothing present
19. Two articles of clothing, nontransparent
20. Entire clothing with sleeves and trousers shown, nontransparent
21. Four or more articles of clothing definitely indicated
22. Costume complete without incongruities
23. Fingers shown
24. Correct number of fingers
25. Fingers in two dimensions, length greater than breadth, angle subtended not greater than 180 degrees
26. Opposition of thumbs shown
27. Hands shown distinct from fingers and arms
28. Arm joints shown (elbow or shoulder or both)
29. Head in proportion
30. Arms in proportion
31. Legs in proportion
32. Feet in proportion
33. Arms and legs in two dimensions
34. Heel shown
35. Lines somewhat controlled
36. Lines well controlled
37. Head outline well controlled
38. Trunk outline well controlled
39. Outline of arms and legs well controlled
40. Outline of features well controlled
41. Ears present
42. Ears present in correct position
43. Eyebrows or lashes present
44. Pupil shown
45. Proportion of eyes correct
46. Glance directed to front in profile drawing
47. Both chin and forehead shown
48. Projection of shin shown
49. Profile with not more than one error
50. Correct profile

*In each item listed give the child 1 point. The number of points multiplied by 3 months plus 3 years equals the mental age.

KEY POINTS

- The most common approach to examining children follows a head-to-toe sequence.
- The four categories of assessment are inspection, palpation, percussion, and auscultation.
- Growth measurements during the physical examination focus on length, height, weight, skinfold thickness, and arm and head circumference. Assessment of growth is measured against standard growth charts to determine a child's status in comparison with other children of the same age.
- Measurements of temperature, pulse, respiration, and blood pressure constitute the physiologic approach to assessment.
- The general appearance of a child is a cumulative, subjective impression of physical appearance, state of nutrition, behavior, personality, interactions with parents and nurse, posture, development, and speech.
- Assessment of the skin, which primarily involves inspection and palpation, focuses on color, texture, temperature, moisture, and turgor. The nurse needs to be aware of both physiologic and ethnic factors that may affect these areas.
- In assessment of the lymph nodes, the nurse examines, by palpation, the part of the body in which the glands are located.
- The head is inspected for shape and symmetry.
- Assessment of the neck includes palpation of the trachea and thyroid gland.
- Examination of the eyes includes placement and alignment, inspection of external and internal structures, and vision testing.
- Ears are examined for placement and alignment, inspection of external and internal structures, and auditory testing.
- The lungs are examined by methods of inspection, palpation, percussion, and auscultation.
- Heart murmurs are classified as innocent, functional, and organic and should be evaluated for location, time, intensity, and loudness.
- Abdominal assessment follows an orderly sequence of inspection, auscultation, percussion, and palpation, since the latter may distort normal abdominal sounds.
- Examination of the genitalia may be anxiety-provoking in the child, and the nurse must avoid any transference of anxiety.
- Neurologic assessment addresses behavior, cognitive-perceptual development, motor functioning, sensory and cerebellar functioning, reflexes, cranial nerves, and soft signs.
- The Denver Developmental Screening Test, one of the most widely used assessment tools, is composed of four categories: personal-social, fine motor–adaptive, language, and gross motor.
- The Denver II, a major revision and a restandardization of the DDST, differs from the DDST in items included in the test, the test form, and the interpretation of scoring.

REFERENCES

Alpern, G., Boll, T., and Shearer, M.: Developmental Profile II Manual, Los Angeles, CA, 1985, Western Psychological Services.

American Academy of Pediatrics and American College of Obstetricians and Gynecologists: Guidelines for perinatal care, ed. 2, Elk Grove Village, IL, 1988, The Academy.

American Academy of Pediatrics, Committee on Early Childhood, Adoption, and Dependent Care: Health care of foster children, Pediatrics 79(4):644-646, 1987.

American Academy of Pediatrics, Committee on Practice and Ambulatory Medicine: Vision screening and eye examination in children, Pediatrics 77(6):918-919, 1986.

Arn, P., and others: Outcome of pectus excavatum in patients with Marfan syndrome and in the general population, J. Pediatr. 115(8):954-958, 1989.

Barber, N., and Kilmon, C.: Reactions to tympanic temperature measurement in an ambulatory setting, Pediatr. Nurs. 15(5):477-481, 1989.

Barrus, D.H.: A comparison of rectal and axillary temperatures by electronic thermometer measurement in preschool children, Pediatr. Nurs. 9(6):424-425, 1983.

Borowitz, K.C., and Glascoe, F.P.: Sensitivity of the Denver Developmental Screening Test in speech and language screening, Pediatrics 78(6):1075-1078, 1986.

Burke, S., Roberts, C., and Maloney, R.: Infant and child weights: reliability and validity of scales, Issues Compr. Pediatr. Nurs. 11(4):241-249, 1988.

Cavanaugh, R.M.: Pediatricians and the pneumatic otoscope: are we playing it by ear? Pediatrics 84(2):362-364, 1989.

Church, J.L., and Baer, K.J.: Examination of the adolescent: a practical guide, J. Pediatr. Health Care 1(2):65-72, 1987.

de Swiet, M., and others: Measurement of blood pressure in children, Br. Med. J. 299:107, 1989.

Dewey, K.G., and others: Infant growth and breastfeeding, Am. J. Clin. Nutr. 50:1116-1117, 1989.

Dressler, D.K., Smejkal, C., and Ruffolo, M.L.: A comparison of oral and rectal temperature measurement on patients receiving oxygen by mask, Nurs. Res. 32(6):373-375, 1983.

Eoff, M.J., and Joyce, B.: Temperature measurements in children, Am. J. Nurs. 81(5):1010-1011, 1981.

Erickson, R.: Oral temperature differences in relation to thermometer and technique, Nurs. Res. 29(3):157-164, 1980.

Fish, L.J., and Burch, K.J.: Identifying gifted preschoolers, Pediatr. Nurs. 11(2):125-127, 1985.

Frankenburg, W.K.: Personal communication, May 4, 1990.

Frankenburg, W.K., Dick, N.P., and Carland, J.: Development of preschool-aged children of different social and ethnic groups: implications for developmental screening, J. Pediatr. 87(1):125-232, 1975.

Frankenburg, W.K., Fandal, A., and Thornton, S.: Revision of Denver Prescreening Developmental Questionnaire, J. Pediatr. 110(4):653-657, 1987.

Frankenburg, W.K., and others: The newly abbreviated and revised Denver Developmental Screening Test, J. Pediatr. 99(6):995-999, 1981.

Frohlich, E., and others: Recommendations for human blood pressure determination by sphygmomanometers: report of a special task force appointed by the Steering Committee, American Health Association, Circulation 77:501A, 1988.

Fung, K., and Lau, S.: Denver Developmental Screening Test: cultural variables, J. Pediatr. 106(2):343, 1985.

Gemberling, C.: The adolescent gynecologic examination: an overview, J. Pediatr. Health Care 1(3):141-151, 1987.

Glasier, C., Mallory, G., and Steele, R.: Significance of opacification of the maxillary and ethmoid sinuses in infants, J. Pediatr. 114(1):45-50, 1989.

Goodenough, F.L.: Measurement of intelligence by drawings, New York, 1926, World Book Co.

Gray, D., Dixon, J., and Collin, J.: The closed eyes sign: an aid to diagnosing non-specific abdominal pain, Br. Med. J. 297:837, 1988.

Habicht, J., and others: Height and weight standards for preschool children: how relevant are ethnic differences in growth potential? Lancet 1(7858):611-615, 1974.

Haddock, R., Merrow, D., and Vincent, P.: Comparison of rectal and axillary temperatures, Neonatal Network 6(5):67-71, 1988.

Haddock, R., Vincent, P., and Merrow, D.: Axillary and rectal temperatures of full-term neonates: are they different? Neonatal Network 5(1):36-40, 1986.

Hancock, L.A.: FirstTemp, J. Pediatr. Health Care 1(3):163-164, 1987.

Harris, D.B.: Children's drawings as measures of intellectual maturity, San Diego, CA, 1983, Harcourt Brace Jovanovich, Inc.

Havener, W.H.: Synopsis of ophthalmology, ed. 6, St. Louis, 1984, Mosby–Year Book, Inc.

Hayes, J.S.: The McCarthy Scales of Children's Abilities: their usefulness in developmental assessment, Pediatr. Nurs. 7(4):35-37, 1981.

Heidenreich, T., and Giuffre, M.: Postoperative temperature measurement, Nurs. Res. 39(3):153-155, 1990.

Himes, J.H., and others: Parent-specific adjustments for evaluation of recumbent length and stature of children, Pediatrics 75(2):304-313, 1985.

Hoyt, C.S., Nickel, B.L., and Billson, F.A.: Ophthalmological examination of the infant: development aspects, Surv. Ophthalmol. 26(4):177-189, 1982.

Jaffe, B.F.: Pinna anomalies associated with congenital conductive hearing loss, Pediatrics 57(3):332-341, 1976.

Jellinek, M.S., and others: Pediatric symptom checklist: screening school-age children for psychosocial dysfunction, J. Pediatr. 112(2):201-209, 1988.

Jenista, J., and Chapman, D.: Medical problems of foreign-born adopted children, Am. J. Dis. Child. 141(3):20-33, 1987.

Jung, E., and others: Skinfold measurements in children: a comparison of Lange and McGaw calipers, Clin. Pediatr. 23(1):25-28, 1984.

Kovalesky, A: Nurses' guide to children's eyes, New York, 1985, Grune & Stratton, Inc.

Laestadius, N., Aase, J., and Smith, D.: Normal inner canthal and outer orbital dimensions, J. Pediatr. 74(3):465-468, 1969.

Looney, J.: Blood pressure by oscillometry, Med. Electronics, pp. 57-63, April 1978.

Lowry, P., and others: *Mycobacterium chelonae* causing otitis media in an ear-nose-and-throat practice, N. Engl. J. Med. 319:978-982, 1988.

Marks, A., and Fisher, M.: Health assessment and screening during adolescence, Pediatrics 80(1):135-158, 1987.

Martorell, R., Mendoza, F., and Castillo, R.: Genetic and environmental determinants of growth in Mexican-Americans, Pediatrics 84(5):864-871, 1989.

Martyn, K., and others: Comparison of axillary, rectal and skin-based temperature assessment in preschoolers, Nurse Pract. 13(4):31-36, 1988.

McCarthy, D.: Manual: McCarthy Scales of Children's Abilities, New York, 1972, The Psychological Corp.

Miller, V., Onotera, R., and Deinard, A.: Denver Developmental Screening Test: cultural variations in Southeast Asian children, J. Pediatr. 104(3):481-482, 1984.

Moore, W., and Roche, A.: Pediatric anthropometry, Columbus, OH, 1982, Ross Laboratories.

National Society to Prevent Blindness: Guide to testing distance visual acuity, Schaumburg, IL, 1988, The Society.

Neff, J., and others: Effect of respiratory rate, respiratory depth, and open versus closed mouth breathing on sublingual temperature, Res. Nurs. Health 12(3):195-202, 1989.

Neinstein, L., and others: Comfort of male adolescents during general and genital examination, J. Pediatr. 115(3):494-497, 1989.

Nelson, L.B., and others: Developmental aspects in the assessment of visual function in young children, Pediatrics 73(3):375-381, 1984.

Nichols, G.A., and others: Measuring oral and rectal temperatures of febrile children, Nurs. Res. 21(3):261-264, 1972.

Ogren, J.: The inaccuracy of axillary temperatures measured with an electronic thermometer, Am. J. Dis. Child. 144(1):109-111, 1990.

Olade, R.A.: Evaluation of the Denver Developmental Screening Test as applied to African children, Nurs. Res. 33(4):204-207, 1984.

O'Neill, T., and others: Diagnostic value of the apex beat, Lancet 1(8635):410-411, 1989.

Orlando, M., and Frank, T.: Audiometer and audioscope hearing screening compared with threshold test in young children, J. Pediatr. 110(2):261-263, 1987.

Park, J.K., and Guntheroth, W.G.: Accurate blood pressure measurement in children, Am. J. Noninvas. Cardiol. 3:297-309, 1989.

Park, M.: Pediatric cardiology for practitioners, ed. 2, St. Louis, 1988, Mosby–Year Book, Inc.

Park, M., and Menard, S.: Accuracy of blood pressure measurement by the Dinamap monitor in infants and children, Pediatrics 79(6):907-914, 1987.

Phillips, S., Bohannon, W., and Heald, F.: Teenagers' choices regarding the presence of family members during the examination of genitalia, J. Adolesc. Health Care 4(4):245-249, 1986.

Pickwell, S.: Primary health care of Indochinese refugee children, Pediatr. Nurs. 8(2):104, 1982.

Powell, M.L.: Assessment and management of developmental changes and problems in children, ed. 2, St. Louis, 1981, Mosby–Year Book, Inc.

Report of the Second Task Force on blood pressure control in children—1987, Pediatrics 79(1):1-25, 1987.

Rogers, W.B., and Rogers, R.A.: A new simplified Preschool Readiness Experimental Screening Scale (The PRESS): a preliminary report, Clin. Pediatr. 11:558-562, Oct. 1972.

Rogers, W.B., and Rogers, R.A.: A follow-up study of the preschool readiness experimental screening scale (The PRESS), Clin. Pediatr. 14:253-256, March 1975.

Ryan, A.: The accuracy of the Ross Laboratories Adipometer skinfold caliper, Clin. Pediatr. 24(3):174, 1985.

Sato-Viacrucis, K.: Personal communication, Jan. 8, 1986.

Schwartz, D., and Schwartz, R.: Validity of acoustic reflectometry in detecting middle ear effusion, Pediatrics 79(5):739-742, 1987.

Seymore, C., and others: Influence of position during examination, and sex of examiner on patient anxiety during pelvic examination, J. Pediatr. 108(2):312-317, 1986.

Shea, V., and Fowler, M.G.: Parental and pediatric trainee knowledge of development, Dev. Behav. Pediatr. 4(1):21-25, 1983.

Talbot, C.: The gynecologic examination of the pediatric patient, Pediatr. Ann. 15(7):501-508, 1986.

Terndrup, T., Allegra, J., and Kealy, J.: A comparison of oral, rectal, and tympanic membrane–derived temperature changes after ingestion of liquids and smoking, Am. J. Emerg. Med. 7(2):150-154, 1989.

Vessey, J., Braithwaite, K., and Wiedmann, M.: Teaching children about their internal bodies, Pediatr. Nurs. 16(1):29-33, 1990.

Watkins, S., Moore, T., and Phillips, J.: Clearing impacted ears, Am. J. Nurs. 84(9):1107, 1984.

Weir, M., and Weir, T.: Are 'hot' ears really hot? Am. J. Dis. Child. 143(7):763-764, 1989.

BIBLIOGRAPHY

Physical Assessment

Alexander, M.M., and Brown, M.S.: Physical examination. 12. Examining the chest and lungs, Nursing 75 5(1):44-48, 1975.

Alexander, M.M., and Brown, M.S.: Physical examination. 13. Examining the abdomen, Nursing 76 6(1):65-70, 1976.

Alexander, M.M., and Brown, M.S.: Physical examination. 14. Male genitalia, Nursing 76 6(2):39-43, 1976.

Alexander, M.M., and Brown, M.S.: Physical examination. 16. The musculoskeletal system, Nursing 76 6(4):51-56, 1976.

Alexander, M.M., and Brown, M.S.: Physical examination. 17. Performing the neurological examination, Nursing 76 6(6):38-43, 1976.

Alexander, M.M., and Brown, M.S.: Physical examination. 18. Neurological examination, Nursing 76 6(7):50-55, 1976.

Ashcroft, M.T., and Deshi, P.P.: Ethnic differences in growth potential of children of African, Indian, Chinese and European origin, Trans. R. Soc. Trop. Med. Hyg. 70:5-6, 1977.

Baker, N.C., and others: The effect of type of thermometer and length of time inserted on oral temperature measurements of afebrile subjects, Nurs. Res. 33(2):109-111, 1984.

Banco, L., Jayashekaramurthy, S., and Graffam, J.: The inability of a temperature-sensitive pacifier to identify fevers in ill infants, Am. J. Dis. Child. 142:171-172, 1988.

Barness, L.A.: Manual of pediatric physical diagnosis, ed. 5, St. Louis, 1980, Mosby–Year Book, Inc.

Bloch, B., and Hunter, M.L.: Teaching physiological assessment of black persons, Nurse Educ. 6:24-27, 1981.

Blondis, T.A., Snow, J.H., and Accardo, P.J.: Integration of soft signs in academically normal and academically at-risk children, Pediatrics 85:421-425, 1990.

Borders, C.F.: Strabismus/amblyopia: when to refer, Patient Care 18:21-52, 1984.

Bowers, A., and Thompson, J.: Clinical manual of health assessment, ed. 2, St. Louis, 1984, Mosby–Year Book, Inc.

Brown, M.S., and Alexander, M.M.: Physical examination. 15. Female genitalia, Nursing 76 6(3):39-41, 1976.

Brown, M.S., and Murphy, M.A.: Ambulatory pediatrics for nurses, ed. 2, New York, 1980, McGraw-Hill Book Co.

Browning, G., and Swan, I.: Sensitivity and specificity of Rinne tuning fork test, Br. Med. J. 297(6660):1381-1382, 1988.

Cibis, G., and Waeltermann, J.: Rapid strabismus screening for the pediatrician, Clin. Pediatr. 25(6):304-307, 1986.

Cross, A.W.: Health screening in schools, part I, J. Pediatr. 107(4):487-494, 1985a.

Cross, A.W.: Health screening in schools, part II, J. Pediatr. 107(5):653-661, 1985b.

Delancy, V.L., and North, C.: Skin assessment, Top. Clin. Nurs. 5(2):5-10, 1983.

DiChiara, E.: A sound method for testing children's hearing, Am. J. Nurs. 84(9):1104-1106, 1984.

Donham, J.: Rales and rhonchi: why do we use these terms? Focus Crit. Care 11(5):20-22, 1984.

Dunn, B.H.: Components of musculoskeletal examination, Orthop. Nurs. 1(6):33-36, 1982.

Egan, D., and Brown, R.: Vision testing of young children in the age range 18 months to 4-1/2 years, Child Care Health Dev. 10:381-390, 1984.

Forgacs, P.: The functional basis of pulmonary sounds, Chest 73(3):399-405, 1978.

Frary, T.: Pediatric examination pearls, J. Am. Acad. Physician Assist. 1(5):389-390, 1988.

Gammon, J.A.: Visual system screening in infants and young children, Pediatr. Rev. 4(3):71-73, 1982.

Gershel, J., and others: Accuracy of the Welch Allyn AudioScope and traditional hearing screening for children with known hearing loss, J. Pediatr. 106(1):15-20, 1985.

Greene, J.: Making adolescent space in a pediatric office, Pediatr. Nurs. 15(4):402-404, 1989.

Grimes, C.: Audiologic evaluation in infancy and childhood, Pediatr. Ann. 14(3):210, 1985.

Guo, S., Roche, A., and Houtkooper, L.: Fat-free mass in children and young adults predicted from bioelectric impedance and anthropometric variables, Am. J. Clin. Nutr. 50:435-443, 1989.

Guo, S., Roche, A., and Moore, W.: Reference data for head circumference and 1-month increments from 1 to 12 months of age, J. Pediatr. 113(3):490-494, 1988.

Hamill, B.: Comparing two methods of preschool and kindergarten hearing screening, J. Sch. Health 58(3):95-97, 1988.

Harris, J.A.: Pediatric abdominal assessment, Pediatr. Nurs. 12(5):355-362, 1986.

Hoekelmann, R.: An appraisal of the effectiveness of child health supervision, Curr. Opin. Pediatr. 1(1):146-155, 1989.

Johnson, A., Stayte, M., and Wortham, C.: Vision screening at 8 and 18 months, Br. Med. J. 299:545-549, 1989.

Johnson, J.L., and others: The school nurse's role in vision screening for the difficult-to-test student, J. Sch. Health 53(6):345-349, 1983.

Killam, P.: Orthopedic assessment of young children: developmental variations, Nurse Pract. 14(7):27-28, 1989.

Kirschen, D., Rosenbaum, A., and Ballard, E.: The dot visual acuity test—a new acuity test for children, J. Am. Optom. Assoc. 54(12):1055-1059, 1983.

Kresch, M.: Axillary temperature as a screening test for fever in children, J. Pediatr. 104(4):596-599, 1984.

Kronmiller, J.: Oral soft tissue abnormalities in children, Pediatr. Nurs. 13(3):161-165, 1987.

Lieber, M.T., and Taub, A.S.: Common foot deformities and what they mean for parents, MCN 13(1):47-50, 1988.

Linley, J.F.: Screening children for common orthopedic problems, Am. J. Nurs. 87(10):1312-1316, 1987.

Mancia, G., and others: Effects of blood pressure measurement by the doctor on patients' blood pressure and heart rate, Lancet 2(8352):695-698, 1983.

Marshall, W.A.: Geographical and ethnic variations in human growth, Br. Med. Bull. 37(3):273-279, 1981.

Mason, K.J.: Pediatric orthopaedics: developmental norms, Orthop. Nurs. 8(4):45-50, 1989.

McClellan, M.A.: The use of the physical examination to promote development of the preschooler, Child. Health Care 12(4):174-178, 1984.

Moss, J.R.: Helping young children cope with the physical examination, Pediatr. Nurs. 7(2):17-20, 1981.

Moss, J.R.: Predicting young children's cooperation with the physical examination, Pediatr. Nurs. 9(3):188-190, 1983.

O'Brien, E.: Clinical thermometry: in need of nursing research, J. Pediatr. Nurs. 3(3):207-208, 1988.

Olk, D.: Quieting the disruptive sibling, Contemp. Pediatr. 6(10):116, 1989.

Olness, K., and others: Height and weight status of Indochinese refugee children, Am. J. Dis. Child. 138:544-547, 1984.

Pulmonary terms and symbols: a report of the ACCP-ATS joint committee on pulmonary nomenclature, Chest 67(5):583-593, 1975.

Prior, J.A., Silberstein, J.S., and Stang, J.M.: Physical diagnosis: the history and examination of the patient, ed. 6, St. Louis, 1981, Mosby–Year Book, Inc.

Rieser, P.: Role of the school nurse in the assessment of linear growth, Community Nurs. Forum 4(1):1-12, 1987.
Roche, A., Guo, S., and Moore, W.: Weight and recumbent length from 1 to 12 mo of age: reference data for 1-mo increments, Am. J. Clin. Nutr. 49:599-607, 1989.
Roche, A., and others: Head circumference reference data: birth to 18 years, Pediatrics 79:(5):706-712, 1987.
Sanet, R., and Ellis, G.: What is the most effective vision screening tool to use with preschool-age children in early childhood programs? School Nurse 6:27-31, 1990.
Sato-Viacrucis, K.: The evolution of the Snellen E to the Blackbird, School Nurse, pp. 18-19, Spring 1985.
Schubiner, H.: Preventive health screening in adolescent patients, Prim. Care 16(1):211-230, 1989.
Seidel, H., and others: Mosby's guide to physical examination, St. Louis, 1987, Mosby–Year Book, Inc.
Shannon, D.A., and others: Hearing screening of high-risk newborns with brainstem auditory evoked potentials: a follow-up study, Pediatrics 73(1):22-26, 1984.
Shinozaki, T., Deane, R., and Perkins, F.: Infrared tympanic thermometer: evaluation of a new clinical thermometer, Crit. Care Med. 16(2):148, 1988.
Stata, K.: Improving hearing screening programs in the elementary school, School Nurse 4(3):16-19, 1988.
Sullivan, L.: How effective is preschool vision, hearing, and developmental screening? Pediatr. Nurs. 14(3):181-183, 1988.
Szydlo, V.: Approaching an adolescent about a pelvic exam, Am. J. Nurs. 88(11):1502-1506, 1988.
Tanner, J.M., and Davies, P.S.W.: Clinical longitudinal standards for height and height velocity for North American children, J. Pediatr. 107(3):317-329, 1985.
Thijs, C., and Leffers, P.: Sensitivity and specificity of Rinne tuning fork test, Br. Med. J. 298(6668):255, 1989.
Thomas, I., Gaitantzis, Y., and Frias, J.: Palpebral fissure length from 29 weeks gestation to 14 years, J. Pediatr. 111(2):267-268, 1987.
Thomson, L.R.: Understanding tympanometry, Pediatr. Nurs. 8(3):193-197, 1982.
Wagner, R.S.: Newer techniques in the evaluation of visual acuity in infants, J. Ophthalmic Nurs. Technol. 3(6):233-236, 1984.
Weststrate, J., and Deurenberg, P.: Body composition in children: proposal for a method for calculating body fat percentage from total body density of skinfold-thickness measurements, Am. J. Clin. Nutr. 50:1104-1115, 1989.
Wong, D.L.: The paper-doll technique, Pediatr. Nurs. 7(6):39-40, 1981.
Yoos, L.: A developmental approach to physical assessment, MCN 6(3):168-170, 1981.
Zerfas, A.: The insertion tape: a new circumference tape for use in nutritional assessment, Am. J. Clin. Nutr. 28:782-787, 1975.

Developmental Assessment

American Academy of Pediatrics, Committee on Children with Disabilities: Screening for developmental disabilities, Pediatrics 78(3):526-528, 1986.
Bradshaw, M.M.: Denver Developmental Screening Test. In Humenick, S.S., editor: Analysis of current assessment strategies in the health care of young children and childbearing families, Norwalk, CT, 1982, Appleton-Century-Crofts.
Burgess, D., and others: Parent report as a means of administering the Prescreening Developmental Questionnaire: an evaluation study, Dev. Behav. Pediatr. 5(4):195-200, 1984.
Casey, P., and others: Developmental intervention: a pediatric clinical review, Pediatr. Clin. North Am. 33(4):899-923, 1986.
Castiglia, P.T., and Petrini, M.A.: Selecting a developmental screening tool, Pediatr. Nurs. 11(1):8-17, 1985.
Dworkin, P.: British and American recommendations for developmental monitoring: the role of surveillance, Pediatrics 84(6):1000-1010, 1989.
Dworkin, P.: Developmental screening—expecting the impossible? Pediatrics 83(4):619-621, 1989.
Frankenburg, W.K., Chen, J., and Thornton, S.: Common pitfalls in the evaluation of developmental screening tests, J. Pediatr. 113(6):1110-1113, 1988.
Frankenburg, W.K., and Thornton, S.: A child development program for a busy office practice, Contemp. Pediatr. 6(2):90-106, 1989.
Koniak-Griffin, D.: Developmental assessment with the Denver Developmental Screening Test: an effective approach for clinical instruction and performance evaluation, J. Pediatr. Nurs. 2(2):102-110, 1987.
Meisels, S.J.: Uses and abuses of developmental screening and school readiness testing, Young Child. 42(2):4-9, 1987.
Meisels, S.J.: Can developmental screening tests identify children who are developmentally at risk? Pediatrics 83(4), 1989.
Sameroff, A.J.: Environmental context of child development, J. Pediatr. 109(1):192-200, 1986.
Schnelle, E.: Kindergarten neurodevelopmental screening: the school nurse's role, School Nurse 4(3):10-14, 1988.
Steele, S.M.: Assessing developmental delays in preschool children, J. Pediatr. Health Care 2(3):141-145, 1988.
Williams. P.: The Metro-Manila developmental screening test: a normative study, Nurs. Res. 33(4):208-212, 1984.

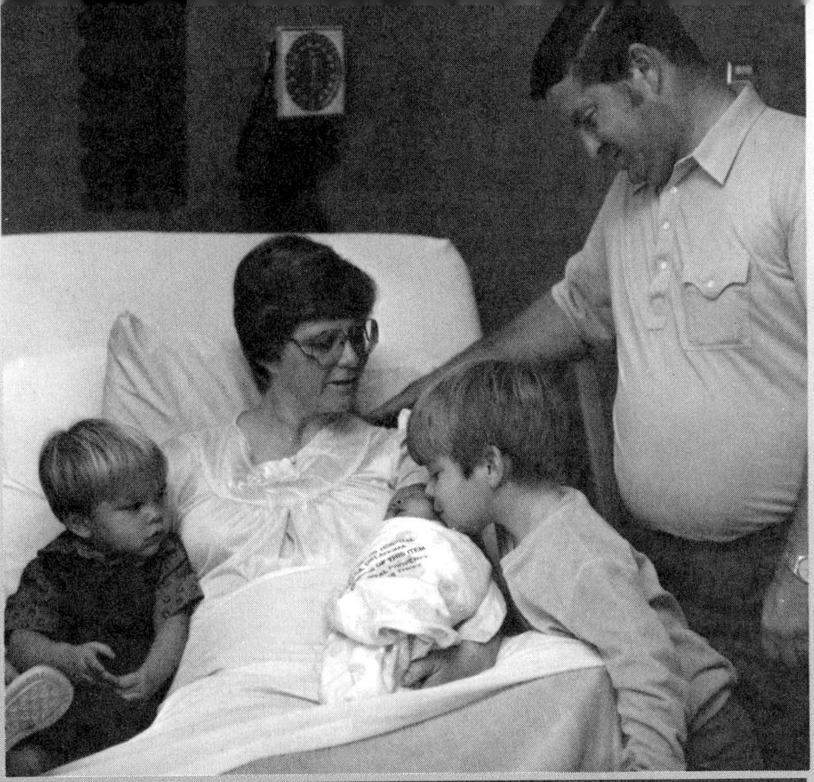

The Newborn

UNIT III

Probably no event is more dramatic or miraculous than the birth of a child. It is the culmination of a 9-month gestation period during which the fetus prepares for extrauterine existence and the parents prepare for the addition of a totally dependent member to their lives. At the time of delivery profound physiologic and psychologic reactions occur that further ready the child and parents for this experience.

In most instances the birth and the perinatal period are uneventful, and infants return home with their parents to begin developing as vital, healthy, and loved children. Chapter 8, *Health Promotion of the Newborn and Family,* is concerned with infants' normal adjustment to extrauterine life; their physiologic status at birth; and the nursing knowledge required to care for them at and immediately following delivery, to perform a newborn assessment, and to promote parent-infant attachment. Chapter 9, *Health Problems of the Newborn,* deals with problems related to physical status, environmental agents, birth injury, or metabolic errors that may occur in normal newborns at or during the perinatal period. The emphasis is on the nurse's recognition of, prevention of, and intervention for each of these problems.

Unfortunately not all neonates are born fully matured or perfectly developed. Chapter 10, *The High-Risk Newborn and Family,* focuses on identification and assessment of high-risk neonates, problems common to them because of their high-risk status, physiologic conditions requiring medical and nursing intervention, and supportive care of the child and family throughout this ordeal. Chapter 11, *Conditions Caused by Defects in Physical Development,* discusses the more common defects requiring immediate, temporary, or permanent intervention. Emphasis is on recognition of the abnormality, prevention of complications before and after correction, and emotional support of the family grieving over the loss of the anticipated perfect child.

CHAPTER 8

Health Promotion of the Newborn and Family

RELATED TOPICS

Aberrant sexual development, Ch. 11
Administration of medication, Ch. 27
Birth injuries, Ch. 9
Breast-feeding problems, Ch. 13
Cardiac development and function: embryologic development, Ch. 34
Changes in fluid volume related to growth, Ch. 28
Congenital heart disease, Ch. 34
Dermatologic problems in the newborn, Ch. 9
oride, Ch. 14
The high-risk newborn and family, Ch. 10
Motor vehicle injuries, Ch. 12
Multiple births, Ch. 3
Nutrition, Ch. 12
Physical examination, Ch. 7
Sibling rivalry, Ch. 14
The skin, Ch. 18

GLOSSARY

AGM Absorbent gelling material
attachment Emotional development from infant to parent
BNBAS Brazelton Neonatal Behavioral Assessment Scale
bonding Emotional development from parent to infant
circumcision Removal of the foreskin on the glans penis
engrossment Development of paternal attachment to infant
fontanels Spaces of unossified membranous tissue located on the cranium
multipara Woman who has had two or more pregnancies that resulted in viable fetuses
neonate Newborn infant
NPI Neonatal Perception Inventory
PMI Point of maximum intensity
primipara Woman who has had one pregnancy that resulted in one or more viable fetuses
sutures Bands of connective tissue between cranial bones
vertex Referring to the top of the head

Childbirth is an intense and exhausting physiologic and emotional experience for mothers and newborns (neonates). Even when this process progresses normally, neonates are required to withstand extreme changes as they leave a thermoconstant, aquatic, completely life-sustaining environment and enter a variable pressurized atmosphere that demands profound physiologic alteration for survival. The neonatal period, from birth to 27 days of life, presents the greatest risk to newborns. In the United States, for example, about three quarters of all deaths during the first year of life occur during these 4 weeks.

The nurse's role is one of supporting the family and infant through the birth process, preventing physiologic complications in the neonate's adjustment to extrauterine life, and promoting the attachment process between child and parents. Expert technologic and psychologic nursing care during the immediate postpartum period lays a strong foundation for healthy parent-child development.

ADJUSTMENT TO EXTRAUTERINE LIFE

The most profound physiologic change required of the newborn is transition from fetal or placental circulation to independent respiration. The loss of the placental connection means the loss of complete metabolic support, the most important and essential function being the supply of oxygen and the removal of carbon dioxide. The normal stresses of labor and delivery produce alterations of placental gas exchange patterns, acid-base balance in the blood, and cardiovascular activity in the neonate. Factors that interfere with this normal transition or increase fetal asphyxia (a condition of hypoxemia, hypercapnia, and acidosis) will affect the fetus's adjustment to extrauterine life.

IMMEDIATE ADJUSTMENTS

The newborn's adjustment to extrauterine life is a complex physiologic process. The first 24 hours are the most critical, since during this time respiratory distress and circulatory failure can occur rapidly and with little warning. There is a higher incidence of death during these initial 24 hours than during the entire succeeding perinatal period.

Respiratory System

The most critical and immediate physiologic change required of the newborn is the onset of breathing. The stimuli that help initiate the first respiration are primarily chemical and thermal. *Chemical* factors in the blood of low oxygen, high carbon dioxide, and low pH initiate impulses that excite the respiratory center in the medulla. The primary *thermal* stimulus is the sudden chilling of the infant who leaves a warm environment and enters a relatively cooler atmosphere. This abrupt change in temperature excites sensory impulses in the skin that are transmitted to the respiratory center.

The significance of *tactile* stimulation is questionable. Descent through the birth canal and normal handling during delivery, such as drying the skin, probably have some effect on initiation of respiration. Slapping the neonate's heel or buttocks has no beneficial effect; it can waste precious time in the event of respiratory difficulty and can cause additional damage if cerebral trauma has occurred.

The initial entry of air into the lungs is opposed by the surface tension of the fluid that filled the fetal lungs and alveoli. However, fetal lung fluid is removed by the pulmonary capillaries and lymphatic vessels. Some fluid is also removed during the normal forces of labor and delivery. As the chest emerges from the birth canal, fluid is squeezed from the lungs through the nose and mouth. Following complete emergence of the neonate's chest, a brisk recoil of the thorax occurs. Air enters the upper airway to replace the lost fluid. In cesarean birth the chest is not compressed, and the newborn may need additional respiratory support.

In the alveoli the surface tension of the fluid is reduced by *surfactant,* a substance produced by the alveolar epithelium that coats the alveolar surface. The effect of surfactant in facilitating breathing is discussed in relation to respiratory distress syndrome (see Chapter 10).

Circulatory System

Equally important as the initiation of respiration are the circulatory changes that allow blood to flow through the lungs. These changes occur more gradually and are the result of pressure changes in the lungs, heart, and major vessels. The transition from fetal circulation to postnatal circulation involves the functional closure of the fetal shunts: that is, the foramen ovale, the ductus arteriosus, and eventually the ductus venosus. (For a brief review of fetal circulation, see Chapter 34.)

Once the lungs are expanded, the inspired oxygen dilates the pulmonary vessels, which decreases pulmonary vascular resistance and consequently increases pulmonary blood flow. As the lungs receive blood, the pressure in the right atrium, right ventricle, and pulmonary arteries decreases. At the same time there is a progressive rise in systemic vascular resistance from the increased volume of blood through the placenta at cord clamping. This increases the pressure in the left side of the heart. Since blood flows from an area of high pressure to one of low pressure, the circulation of blood through the fetal shunts is reversed (see Fig. 34-2).

The most important factor controlling ductal closure is the increased oxygen concentration of the blood. Secondary factors are the fall in endogenous prostaglandins and acidosis. The foramen ovale closes functionally at or soon after birth from compression of the two portions of the atrial septum. The ductus arteriosus is closed functionally by the fourth day. Anatomic closure from deposition of fibrin and cell products takes considerably longer. Failure of the ducts to close results in various types of congenital heart defects (see Chapter 34).

Because of the reversible flow of blood through the ducts during the early neonatal period, functional murmurs are occasionally heard. In conditions such as crying or straining the increased pressure shunts unoxygenated blood from the right side of the heart across the ductal opening, causing transient cyanosis.

PHYSIOLOGIC STATUS OF OTHER SYSTEMS

The major life-dependent physiologic changes in the cardiovascular and respiratory systems of the newborn have already been discussed. However, all of the body systems undergo some change, and most systems are immature at birth. Each is observed closely for proper functioning and adjustment to extrauterine life.

Thermoregulation

Next to establishing respiration, heat regulation is most critical to the newborn's survival. Although the newborn's capacity for heat production is adequate, several factors predispose to excessive heat loss. First, the newborn's large surface area facilitates heat loss to the environment. The normal metabolic rate per unit weight of the newborn is about twice that of the adult, but the neonate's surface area per unit weight is about three times larger than that of the adult. Consequently, the infant produces only two thirds as much heat as an adult but loses twice as much heat per unit area. However, the large body surface is partially compensated by the newborn's usual position of flexion, which decreases the amount of surface area exposed to the environment.

The second factor that retards the conservation of body heat is the newborn's thin layer of subcutaneous fat. Since core body temperature is approximately 1° F higher than surface body temperature, this temperature gradient (difference) causes a heat transfer from a higher to lower temperature.

A third factor is the newborn's mechanism for producing heat. Unlike the adult, who can increase heat production through shivering, the chilled neonate cannot shiver but produces heat through nonshivering thermogenesis, which involves increased metabolism and oxygen consumption (see Thermoregulation, Chapter 10). The principal thermogenic sources are the heart, liver, and brain. However, there is an additional source unique to the newborn known as *brown adipose tissue* (BAT), or *brown fat.* Brown fat, which owes its name to its larger content of mitochondrial cytochromes, has a greater capacity for heat production through intensified metabolic activity than does ordinary adipose tissue. Heat generated in the brown fat is distributed to other parts of the body by the blood, which is warmed as it flows through the layers of this tissue. Superficial deposits of brown fat are located between the scapulae, around the neck, in the axillae, and behind the sternum. Deeper layers surround the kidneys, trachea, esophagus, some major arteries, and adrenals (Poissonnet, LaVelle, and Burdi, 1988). The location of the brown fat may explain why the nape of the neck often feels warmer than the rest of the infant's body.

Although concern is usually for newborns' ability to conserve heat, they also can have difficulty dissipating heat in an overheated environment. This increases the risk of hyperthermia.

Hemopoietic System

The blood volume of the newborn depends on the amount of placental transfer of blood. The blood volume of the full-term infant is about 80 to 85 ml/kg of body weight. Immediately after birth the total blood volume averages 300 ml, but, depending on how long the infant is attached to the placenta, as much as 100 ml can be added to the blood volume. The blood values for the newborn are listed in Appendix D.

Fluid and Electrolyte Balance

Changes occur in the total body water volume, extracellular fluid volume, and intracellular fluid volume during transition from fetal to postnatal life. Early in gestation the fetus is composed almost entirely of water and at term is 73% fluid, as compared to 58% in the adult. There is a higher level of extracellular fluid than intracellular fluid in the fetus, but this shifts progressively throughout postnatal life, probably because of the growth of cells at the expense of extracellular fluid. The infant has a proportionately higher ratio of extracellular fluid than the adult and consequently has a higher level of total body sodium and chloride and a lower level of potassium, magnesium, and phosphate (see Chapter 28).

A very important aspect of fluid balance is its relationship to other systems. Besides the rate of fluid exchange being seven times greater in the infant than in the adult, the infant's rate of metabolism is twice as great in relation to body weight. As a result, twice as much acid is formed, leading to more rapid development of acidosis. In addition, the immature kidneys cannot sufficiently concentrate urine to conserve body water. These three factors make the infant more prone to problems of dehydration, acidosis, and possible overhydration.

Gastrointestinal System

The ability of the newborn to digest, absorb, and metabolize foodstuff is adequate but limited in certain functions. Enzymes are available to catalyze proteins and simple carbohydrates (monosaccharides and disaccharides), but deficient production of pancreatic amylase impairs utilization of complex carbohydrates (polysaccharides). Deficiency of pancreatic lipase limits the absorption of fats, especially with ingestion of foods that have a high saturated fatty acid content, such as cow's milk.

The liver is the most immature of the gastrointestinal organs. The activity of the enzyme *glucuronyl transferase* is reduced, affecting the conjugation of bilirubin with glucuronic acid, which contributes to the physiologic jaundice of the newborn. The liver is also deficient in forming plasma proteins. The decreased plasma protein concentration probably plays a role in the edema usually seen at birth. Prothrombin and other coagulation factors are also low. The liver stores less glycogen at birth than later in life. Consequently the newborn is prone to hypoglycemia, which may be prevented by early and effective feeding, especially breast-feeding.

Some salivary glands are functioning at birth, but the majority do not begin to secrete saliva until about age 2 to 3 months, when drooling is common. The stomach capacity is limited to about 90 ml; thus the infant requires frequent small feedings. The colon also has a small volume for retention of contents, resulting in frequent bowel movements.

The infant's intestine is longer in relation to body size than that in the adult. Therefore there are a larger number of secretory glands and a larger surface area for absorption as compared to the adult's intestine. There are rapid peristaltic waves and simultaneous nonperistaltic waves along the entire esophagus. These waves, combined with an immature relaxed cardiac sphincter, make regurgitation a common occurrence.

Progressive changes in the stooling pattern indicate a properly functioning gastrointestinal tract. The infant's first stool is *meconium,* which is composed of amniotic fluid and its constituents, intestinal secretions, shed mucosal cells, and possibly blood (ingested maternal blood or minor bleeding of alimentary tract vessels). Passage of meconium should occur within the first 36 hours.

Usually by the third day after initiation of feedings, *transitional stools* appear. They are greenish brown to yellowish brown in color, thin, seeding, and less sticky than meconium, and may contain some milk curds. By the fourth day a typical *milk stool* is passed. In breast-fed infants the stools are yellow to golden in color and pasty in consistency. They have an odor similar to that of sour milk. In infants fed cow's milk formula, the stools are pale yellow to light brown, are firmer in consistency, and have a more offensive odor.

Breast-fed infants usually have more stools than do bottle-fed infants. The stool pattern can vary widely; six stools a day may be normal for one infant, whereas a stool every other day may be normal for another.

Renal System

All structural components are present in the renal system, but there is a functional deficiency in the kidney's ability to concentrate urine and to cope with conditions of fluid and electrolyte fluctuations, such as dehydration or a concentrated solute load.

Total volume of urine per 24 hours is about 200 to 300 ml by the end of the first week. However, the bladder involuntarily empties when stretched by a volume of 15 ml, resulting in as many as 20 voidings per day. The first voiding should occur within 24 hours. The urine is colorless and odorless and has a specific gravity of approximately 1.020.

Integumentary System

At birth all the structures within the skin are present, but many of the functions of the integument are immature. The two layers of the skin, the epidermis and dermis, are loosely bound to each other and are very thin. Slight friction across the epidermis, such as from rapid removal of adhesive tape, causes separation of these layers and blister formation. The transitional zone between the cornified and living layers of the epidermis is effective in preventing fluid from reaching the skin surface.

The *sebaceous glands* are very active late in fetal life and in early infancy because of high levels of maternal androgens. They are most densely located on the scalp, face, and genitalia and produce the greasy vernix caseosa that covers the infant at birth. Plugging of the sebaceous glands causes milia.

The *eccrine glands,* which produce sweat in response to heat or emotional stimuli, are functional at birth, and palmar sweating on crying reaches levels equivalent to those of anxious adults by 43 weeks of gestation. Observing palmar sweating is helpful in the assessment of pain (Harpin and Rutter, 1982). The eccrine glands produce sweat in response to higher temperatures than those required in adults, and the retention of sweat may result in miliaria.

The *apocrine glands* are another type of sweat gland that develop as an attachment to the hair follicle. They remain small and nonfunctional until puberty.

The growth phases of hair follicles usually occur simultaneously at birth. During the first few months the synchrony between hair loss and regrowth is disrupted, and there may be overgrowth of hair or temporary alopecia. Boys' hair grows faster than girls' hair, and in both sexes scalp hair growth is slower at the crown.

Because the amount of melanin is low at birth, newborns are lighter skinned than they will be as children. This also means that infants are more susceptible to the harmful effects of the sun.

Musculoskeletal System

At birth the skeletal system contains larger amounts of cartilage than ossified bone, although the process of ossification is fairly rapid during the first year. The nose, for example, is predominantly cartilage at birth and is frequently flattened by the force of delivery. The six skull bones are relatively soft and not yet joined. The sinuses are incompletely formed as well.

Unlike the skeletal system, the muscular system is almost completely formed at birth. Growth in the size of muscular tissue is caused by hypertrophy, rather than hyperplasia, of cells.

Defenses Against Infection

The infant is born with several defenses against infection. The first line of defense is the *skin* and *mucous membranes,* which protect the body from invading organisms. The second line of defense is the *cellular elements* of the immunologic system, which produces several types of cells capable of attacking a pathogen. The neutrophils and monocytes are phagocytes, cells that engulf, ingest, and destroy foreign agents. Eosinophils also probably have a phagocytic property, since in the presence of foreign protein they increase in number. The lymphocytes (T- and B-cells) are capable of being converted to other cell types, such as monocytes and antibodies. Although the phagocytic properties of the blood are present in the infant, the inflammatory response of the tissues to localize an infection is immature.

The third line of defense is the formation of specific *antibodies* to an antigen. This process requires exposure to various foreign agents for antibody production to occur. Infants are generally not capable of producing their own gamma globulins until the beginning of the second month of life, but they receive considerable passive immunity in the form of IgG from the maternal circulation and from human milk (see p. 333). They are protected against most major childhood diseases, including diphtheria, measles, poliomyelitis, infectious hepatitis, and rubella for about 3 months, provided the mother has developed antibodies to these illnesses.

Endocrine System

Ordinarily the endocrine system of the newborn is adequately developed, but its functions are immature. For example, the posterior lobe of the pituitary gland produces limited quantities of antidiuretic hormone (ADH), or vasopressin, which inhibits diuresis. This renders the newborn highly susceptible to dehydration.

The effect of maternal sex hormones is particularly evident in the newborn and it may cause a miniature puberty. The labia are hypertrophied, and the breasts may be engorged and secrete milk (witch's milk) during the first few days of life to as long as 2 months of age (Madlon-Kay, 1986). Female newborns may have pseudomenstruation (more often seen as a milky secretion than actual blood) from a sudden drop in progesterone and estrogen levels.

Neurologic System

At birth the nervous system is incompletely integrated but sufficiently developed to sustain extrauterine life. Most neurologic functions are primitive reflexes. The autonomic nervous system is crucial during transition because it stimulates initial respirations, helps maintain acid-base balance, and partially regulates temperature control.

Myelination of the nervous system follows the cephalocaudal-proximodistal laws of development and is closely related to the observed mastery of fine and gross motor skills. Myelin is necessary for rapid and efficient transmission of some, but not all, nerve impulses along the neural pathway. Tracts that develop myelin earliest are the sensory, cerebellar, and extrapyramidal. This accounts for acute senses of taste, smell, and hearing, as well as the perception of pain in the newborn. All cranial nerves are present and myelinated except the optic and olfactory nerves.

Sensory Functions

The newborn's sensory functions are remarkably well developed and have a significant effect on growth and development, including the attachment process. Unfortunately, minimal research has been done on evaluating the senses, mainly because of difficulty in accurate assessment.

Vision. At birth the eye is structurally incomplete. The fovea centralis is not yet completely differentiated from the macula. The ciliary muscles are also immature, limiting the ability of the eyes to accommodate and fixate on an object for any length of time. The pupils react to light, the blink reflex is responsive to a minimal stimulus, and the corneal reflex is activated by a light touch. Tear glands usually do not begin to function until the infant is 2 to 4 weeks of age.

The newborn has the ability to momentarily fixate on a bright or moving object that is within 20 cm (8 inches) and in the midline of the visual field. In fact the infant's ability to fixate on coordinated movement is greater during the first hour of life than during the succeeding several days. Visual acuity is reported to be between 20/100 and 20/400, depending on the vision measurement techniques (see Table 7-10).

The infant also demonstrates visual preferences: medium colors (yellow, green, pink) over dim or bright colors (red, orange, blue); black and white contrasting patterns, especially geometric shapes and checkerboards; large objects with medium complexity rather than small, complex objects; and reflecting objects over dull ones (Ludington-Hoe, 1983).

Hearing. Once the amniotic fluid has drained from the ears, the infant probably has auditory acuity similar to that of an adult. The newborn is able to detect a loud sound of about 90 decibels and reacts with a startle reflex. The newborn's response to sounds of low frequency and high frequency differs; the former, such as a heartbeat, metronome, or lullaby, tends to decrease an infant's motor activity and crying, whereas the latter elicits an alerting reaction.

There also seems to be an early sensitivity to the sound of human voices, although not to specific speech sounds. One study found that infants younger than 3 days of age can discriminate the mother's voice from that of other females (DeCasper and Fifer, 1980). As early as age 2 weeks the newborn may stop crying to listen to the sound of a voice. The cortical activity associated with hearing or with any other sense is still incomplete at this age because of the immature myelination of the various neural pathways beyond the midbrain. This lack of cortical integration is responsible for the infant's response to sound.

The internal and middle ear are larger at birth, but the external canal is small. The mastoid process and the bony part of the external canal have not yet developed. Consequently, the tympanic membrane and facial nerve are very close to the surface and can be easily damaged.

Smell. Research conducted on newborns' ability to smell demonstrates that they respond differently to various odors. Newborns react to strong odors such as alcohol or vinegar by turning their heads away. Breast-fed infants are able to smell breast milk and will cry for their mothers when the breasts are engorged and leaking. Infants are also able to differentiate the breast milk from their mother or from other females by the smell (Macfarlane, 1977). Such maternal odors are believed to influence the attachment process (Porter, Cernock, and Perry, 1983).

Taste. The newborn is able to distinguish between tastes, and various types of solutions elicit differing gustofacial reflexes. A tasteless solution elicits no facial expression, a sweet solution elicits an eager suck and a look of satisfaction, a sour solution causes the usual puckering of the lips, and a bitter liquid produces an angry, upset expression. For example, newborns prefer glucose and water to sterile water (Pete, 1989).

Touch. At birth the infant is able to perceive tactile sensation in any part of the body, although the face (especially the mouth), hands, and soles of the feet seem to be most sensitive. There is increasing documentation that touch and motion are essential to normal growth and development (Gunzenhauser, 1990). Gentle patting of the back or rubbing of the abdomen usually elicits a calming response from the infant. However, painful stimuli, such as a pinprick, will elicit an angry, upset response.

NEWBORN ASSESSMENT

The newborn requires thorough, skilled observation to ensure a satisfactory adjustment to extrauterine life. Assessment following delivery can be divided into three phases: (1) the initial assessment using the Apgar scoring system, (2) transitional assessment during the periods of reactivity, and (3) periodic assessment through systematic physical examination. Awareness of the expected normal findings during each assessment process helps the nurse recognize any deviation that may prevent the infant from progressing uneventfully through the early postnatal period.

INITIAL ASSESSMENT: APGAR SCORING

During the first seconds of the newborn's life, complex extensive physiologic changes occur. It is imperative that the nurse make astute observations during this time. One of the methods used to assess the newborn's immediate adjustment to extrauterine life is the Apgar scoring system, developed by Virginia Apgar in 1952. The score is based on observation of heart rate, respiratory effort, muscle tone, reflex irritability, and color (Table 8-1). Each item is given a score of 0, 1, or 2. Evaluations of all five categories are made 1 and 5 minutes after birth and are repeated until the infant's condition stabilizes. Total scores of 0 to 3 represent severe distress, scores of 4 to 6 signify moderate difficulty, and scores of 7 to 10 indicate absence of difficulty in adjusting to extrauterine life.

Low Apgar scores at 1 and 5 minutes are excellent indicators for determining newborns who require resuscitation. However, low scores at these times do not predict future neurologic outcome. The Apgar score is affected by the degree of prematurity, maternal sedation or analgesia, and neuromuscular disorders (American Academy of Pediatrics, Committee on Fetus and Newborn, 1986).

The *heart rate* is the most evaluative of the five items. For accuracy, the heart rate is counted for 1 minute and correlated with the infant's activity. The apical pulse is taken with a stethoscope, although palpation of the umbilical cord at its junction with the abdomen is reliable, and visible pulsations of the cord may be counted.

A heart rate less than 100 beats/minute indicates severe asphyxia and usually means that some form of resuscitation is necessary. Tachycardia, or heart rate greater than 160 beats/minute, indicates moderate, but recent, asphyxia and usually means that resuscitation is necessary.

Respiratory effort is evaluated as an index of adequate ventilation. This is assessed by listening to the lungs with a stethoscope and counting the respiratory rate for a full minute. If the respirations are slow, shallow, irregular, or gasping, they indicate respiratory distress.

Muscle tone refers to the degree of flexion and resistance offered when attempts are made to extend the newborn's extremities. The normal infant's position is one of flexion—the extremities are flexed and close to the body, and the fist is tightly clenched. Any attempt to alter this flexed position is met with resistance. At the other extreme, an asphyxiated infant is limp and offers no resistance to a change in position.

Reflex irritability is judged by the neonate's response to slapping the sole of the foot with the palm of the hand. The usual response from a healthy newborn is a loud, angry cry. A moderately depressed infant demonstrates annoyance by a facial grimace, but a severely depressed neonate has no behavioral response.

Color indicates central and peripheral tissue oxygenation. Few newborns are completely pink 1 minute after birth; most continue to have some blueness of the extremities, whereas the rest of the body is pink. Pallor and cyanosis all over the body indicate a severely asphyxiated neonate. In evaluating color, especially of dark-skinned newborns, it is important to inspect the color of the mucous membranes of mouth and conjunctiva as well as the color of the lips, palms of the hands, and soles of the feet.

TRANSITIONAL ASSESSMENT: PERIODS OF REACTIVITY

The newborn exhibits behavioral and physiologic characteristics that can at first appear to be signs of stress. However, during the initial 24 hours changes in heart rate, respiration, motor activity, color, mucus production, and bowel activity

Table 8-1 Infant evaluation at birth—Apgar scoring system

	0	1	2
Heart rate	Absent	Slow (less than 100 beats/minute)	Greater than 100 beats/minute
Respiratory effort	Absent	Slow or irregular	Good; crying lustily
Muscle tone	Limp	Some flexion of extremities	Active motion; well flexed
Reflex irritability	No response	Grimace	Cough or sneeze; vigorous cry
Color	Blue or pale	Body pink, extremities blue	Completely pink

occur in an orderly, predictable sequence, which is normal and indicates lack of stress. Distressed infants also progress through these stages but at a slower rate.

First Period

For 6 to 8 hours after birth the newborn is in the first period of reactivity. During the first 30 minutes the infant is very alert, cries vigorously, may suck a fist greedily, and appears very interested in the environment. At this time the neonate's eyes are usually open, suggesting that this is an excellent opportunity for mother, father, and child to see each other. Because the newborn has a vigorous suck reflex, this is an opportune time to begin breast-feeding. The newborn usually grasps the nipple quickly, satisfying both self and mother. This is particularly important for nurses to remember, since it is likely that after this initially highly active state the infant may be quite sleepy and uninterested in sucking. Physiologically the respiratory rate can be as high as 80 breaths/minute, rales may be heard, heart rate may reach 180 beats/minute, bowel sounds are active, mucus secretions are increased, and temperature may decrease slightly.

After this initial stage of alertness and activity the infant's responsiveness diminishes. Heart and respiratory rates decrease, temperature continues to fall, mucus production decreases, and urine or stool is usually not passed. The infant is in a state of sleep and relative calm. Any attempt at stimulation usually elicits a minimal response. This second stage of the first reactive period generally lasts 2 to 4 hours. Because of the decrease in body temperature, undressing or bathing the infant is avoided during this time.

Second Period

The second period of reactivity begins when the infant awakes from the deep sleep following the first period. The infant is again alert and responsive, heart and respiratory rates increase, the gag reflex is active, gastric and respiratory secretions are increased, and passage of meconium commonly occurs. This second period of reactivity lasts about 2 to 5 hours and provides another excellent opportunity for child and parents to interact. This period is usually over when the amount of respiratory mucus has decreased. Following this stage is a period of stabilization of physiologic systems and a vacillating pattern of sleep and activity.

After a discussion of the seemingly erratic patterns of behavior in the newborn, it is apparent that, in order to identify abnormalities or signs of distress in the respiratory, cardiovascular, or neurologic system, the nurse must thoroughly understand normal characteristics. Observation, not machinery, is the nurse's greatest tool for assessment, and the nursing goal is anticipation and prevention of neonatal stress. The timing of nursing care is based on observation of the neonate's physiologic status. For example, the infant should be dried immediately after delivery to minimize heat loss from evaporation; the initial bath should be postponed until after body temperature has stabilized; eye drops should be instilled after parents and child have established visual contact; and breast-feeding or bottle-feeding should be initiated during one of the two periods of reactivity.

PHYSICAL ASSESSMENT

An important aspect of the care of the newborn is a thorough physical assessment that includes estimation of gestational age and physical examination to identify normal characteristics and existing abnormalities. These initial and ongoing assessments are critical to establishing baseline data for planning, implementing, and evaluating care and should be one of the nurse's priorities in caring for the newborn. The discussion of physical examination focuses on normal findings, variations from the norm that require little or no intervention, and specific potential danger signs that require more careful observation. The reader is encouraged to review the material in Chapter 7 for further discussions of examination techniques. General guidelines for conducting a physical examination are presented in Box 8-1. See Table 8-3 for a summary of the physical examination of the newborn.

Assessment of Clinical Gestational Age

Assessment of gestational age is an important criterion because perinatal morbidity and mortality are related to gestational age and birth weight. One of the most frequently used methods of determining gestational age is based on physical and neurologic findings. Although several scales are in current use, the one commonly used is the Simplified Assessment of Gestational Age by Ballard, Novack, and Driver (1979) (Fig. 8-1, *A*). The scale is an abbreviated version of the assessment scale developed by Dubowitz, Dubowitz, and Goldberg (1970) and assesses six external physical and six neuromuscular signs. Each sign has a number score, and the cumulative score correlates with a maturity rating from 26 to 44 weeks (see Maturity rating box on scale). The maturity rating is accurate within ±2 weeks of the infant's true age and is valid, regardless of the infant's race (Stevens-Simon and others, 1989).

Assessments can be performed anytime from birth to 42 hours of age, but the greatest reliability is at 30 and 42

Box 8-1 GENERAL GUIDELINES TO PHYSICAL EXAMINATION OF THE NEWBORN

Provide a normothermic and nonstimulating examination area.
- Undress only body area examined to prevent heat loss.

Proceed in an orderly sequence (usually head to toe) with the following exceptions:
- Perform all procedures that require quiet first, such as auscultating the lungs, heart, and abdomen.
- Perform disturbing procedures, such as testing reflexes, last.
- Measure head, chest, and length at same time to compare results.

Proceed quickly to avoid stressing the infant.
- Check that equipment and supplies are working properly and are accessible.

Comfort the infant during and after the examination if upset.
- Talk softly.
- Hold infant's hands against chest.
- Swaddle and hold.
- Give pacifier or gloved finger to suck.

hours. By this time the infant has sufficiently stabilized and adjusted following birth, but changes resulting from rapid extrauterine maturation do not interfere with the findings. No matter what scale is used, the infant should be examined when alert and with strict adherence to the directions described by the original authors.

In order to facilitate the use of the assessment chart, the tests and relevant observations are further described in Table 8-2.

Weight related to gestational age. The weight of the infant at birth also correlates with the incidence of perinatal morbidity and mortality. Since many infants who weigh less than 2500 g (5½ pounds) are not premature by gestational age, there is often confusion between the preterm and the small-for-gestational-age infants; fetal growth, gestational age, and fetal maturity are closely related but are not synonymous. Maturity implies functional capacity—the degree to which the neonate's organ systems are able to adapt to the requirements of extrauterine life. Therefore gestational age is more closely related to fetal maturity than is birth weight. Some infants' heredity influences their size at birth. Oriental and black infants tend to be smaller than white newborns. Small parents have smaller infants and vice versa; therefore it is important to note the size of other family members as part of the assessment process.

Classification of infants at birth by both weight and gestational age provides a more satisfactory method for predicting mortality risks and providing guidelines for management of the neonate. The infant's birth weight, length, and head circumference are plotted on standardized graphs that identify normal values for gestational age (Fig. 8-1, *B*). The infant whose weight is appropriate for gestational age (between 10th and 90th percentile) can be presumed to have grown at a normal rate regardless of the time of birth—preterm, term, or postterm. The infant who is large for gestational age (above 90th percentile) can be presumed to have grown at an accelerated rate during fetal life; the small-for-gestational-age infant (below 10th percentile) can be assumed to have grown at a retarded rate during intrauterine life. Fig. 8-2 illustrates the disparity between birth weights of three preterm infants of the same gestational age; Fig. 8-3 shows associated risks of mortality.

General Measurements

There are several important measurements of the newborn that have significance when compared with each other as well as when recorded over time on a graph. For the full-term infant, average *head circumference* is between 33 and 35.5 cm (13 to 14 inches). Head circumference may be somewhat less immediately after birth because of the molding process that occurs during a normal vaginal delivery. Usually by the second or third day the normal size and contour of the skull have replaced the molded one.

Chest circumference is 30.5 to 33 cm (12 to 13 inches). Head circumference is usually about 2 to 3 cm (about 1 inch) greater than chest circumference. Because of the molding of the head during delivery, these measurements may initially appear equal. However, if the head is significantly smaller than the chest, microcephaly or premature closure of the sutures (craniostenosis) should be suspected. If the head is more than 4 cm (1¾ inches) larger than the chest in circumference and this relationship remains constant or increases over several days, then hydrocephalus must be considered. Other causes of increased head circumference are caput succedaneum, cephalhematoma, and subdural hematoma. Prematurity and malnutrition cause the head measurement to be significantly larger than the chest circumference, but this is because of

Table 8-2 Description of tests used in assessing gestational age

TEST	ASSESSMENT/DESCRIPTION
Posture	With the infant quiet and in a supine position, observe the degree of flexion in the arms and legs. Muscle tone and degree of flexion increase with maturity. Full flexion of the arms and legs = 4.
Square window	With the thumb supporting the back of the arm below the wrist, apply gentle pressure with index and third fingers on dorsum of hand without rotating the infant's wrist. Measure the angle between the base of the thumb and forearm. Full flexion (hand lies flat on ventral surface of forearm) = 4.
Arm recoil	With the infant supine, fully flex both forearms on upper arms, hold for 5 seconds; pull down on hands to fully extend and rapidly release arms. Observe the rapidity and intensity of recoil to a state of flexion. A brisk return to full flexion = 4.
Popliteal angle	With the infant supine and the pelvis flat on a firm surface, flex lower leg on thigh and then flex thigh on abdomen. While holding knee with thumb and index finger, extend lower leg with index finger of other hand. Measure the degree of the angle behind the knee (popliteal angle). An angle less than 90 degrees = 5.
Scarf sign	With the infant supine, support the head in the midline with one hand; use other hand to pull infant's arm across the shoulder so that infant's hand touches the shoulder. Determine location of elbow in relation to midline. Elbow does not reach midline = 4.
Heel to ear	With the infant supine and the pelvis flat on a firm surface, pull the foot as far as possible up toward the ear on the same side. Measure the distance of the foot from the ear and degree of knee flexion (same as popliteal angle). Knees flexed with a popliteal angle less than 10 degrees = 4.

ESTIMATION OF GESTATIONAL AGE BY MATURITY RATING

Symbols: X - 1st Exam O - 2nd Exam

NEUROMUSCULAR MATURITY

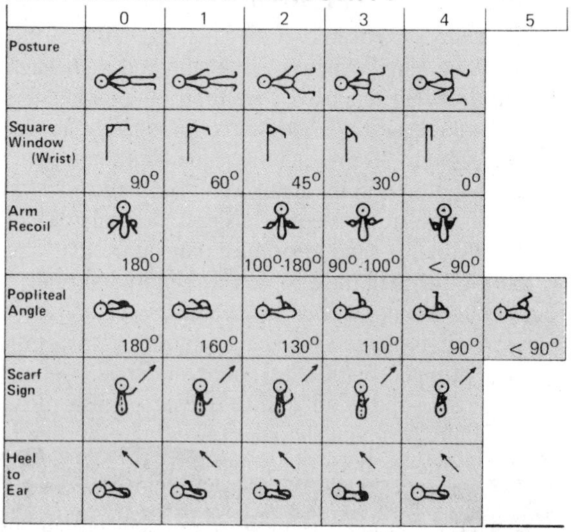

0 1 2 3 4 5
Posture
Square Window (Wrist)
90° 60° 45° 30° 0°
Arm Recoil
180° 100°-180° 90°-100° < 90°
Popliteal Angle
180° 160° 130° 110° 90° < 90°
Scarf Sign
Heel to Ear

A

Gestation by Dates ______________ wks

Birth Date __________ Hour __________ am pm

APGAR __________ 1 min __________ 5 min

PHYSICAL MATURITY

	0	1	2	3	4	5
SKIN	gelatinous red, trans-parent	smooth pink, visible veins	superficial peeling &/or rash, few veins	cracking pale area, rare veins	parchment, deep cracking, no vessels	leathery, cracked, wrinkled
LANUGO	none	abundant	thinning	bald areas	mostly bald	
PLANTAR CREASES	no crease	faint red marks	anterior transverse crease only	creases ant. 2/3	creases cover entire sole	
BREAST	barely percept.	flat areola, no bud	stippled areola, 1–2 mm bud	raised areola, 3–4 mm bud	full areola, 5–10 mm bud	
EAR	pinna flat, stays folded	sl. curved pinna, soft with slow recoil	well-curv. pinna, soft but ready recoil	formed & firm with instant recoil	thick cartilage, ear stiff	
GENITALS Male	scrotum empty, no rugae		testes descend-ing, few rugae	testes down, good rugae	testes pendulous, deep rugae	
GENITALS Female	prominent clitoris & labia minora		majora & minora equally prominent	majora large, minora small	clitoris & minora completely covered	

MATURITY RATING

Score	Wks
5	26
10	28
15	30
20	32
25	34
30	36
35	38
40	40
45	42
50	44

SCORING SECTION

	1st Exam=X	2nd Exam=O
Estimating Gest Age by Maturity Rating	______ Weeks	______ Weeks
Time of Exam	Date ______ Hour ______ am pm	Date ______ Hour ______ am pm
Age at Exam	______ Hours	______ Hours
Signature of Examiner	______ M.D.	______ M.D.

Fig. 8-1. A, Newborn maturity rating.

Courtesy Mead Johnson & Co., Evansville, IN. **A,** Scoring section modified from Ballard, J.L., and others: Pediatr. Res. 11:374, 1977. Figures modified from Sweet, A.Y.: Classification of the low-birth-weight infant. In Klaus, M.H., and Fanaroff, A.A.: Care of the high-risk infant, Philadelphia, 1977, W.B. Saunders Co.

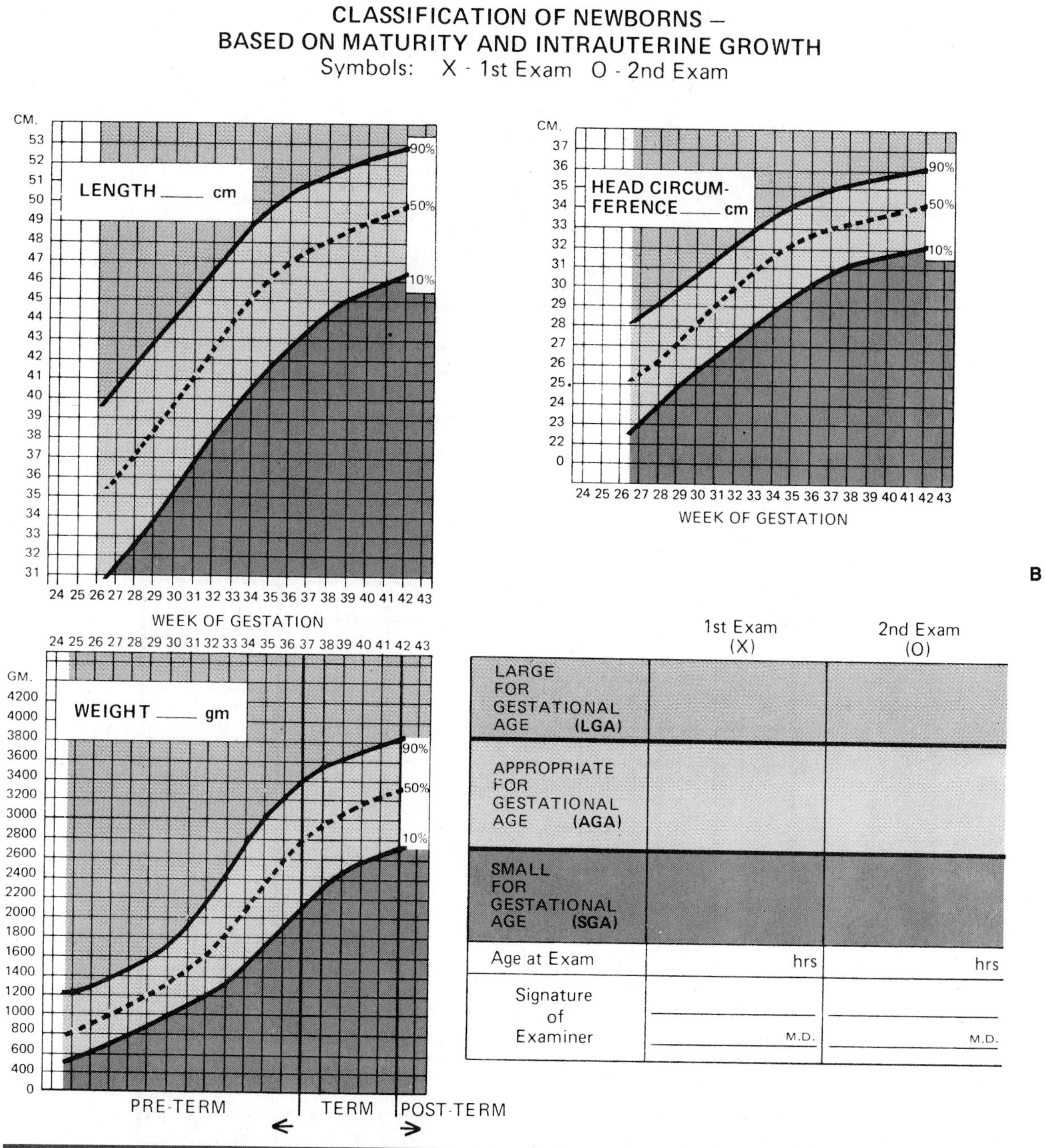

Fig. 8-1, cont'd. B, Newborn classification based on maturity and intrauterine growth.
B, Modified from Lubchenko, L.C., Hansman, C., and Boyd, E.: J. Pediatr. 37:403, 1966; Battagia, F.C., and Lubchenko, L.D.: J. Pediatr. 71:159, 1967.

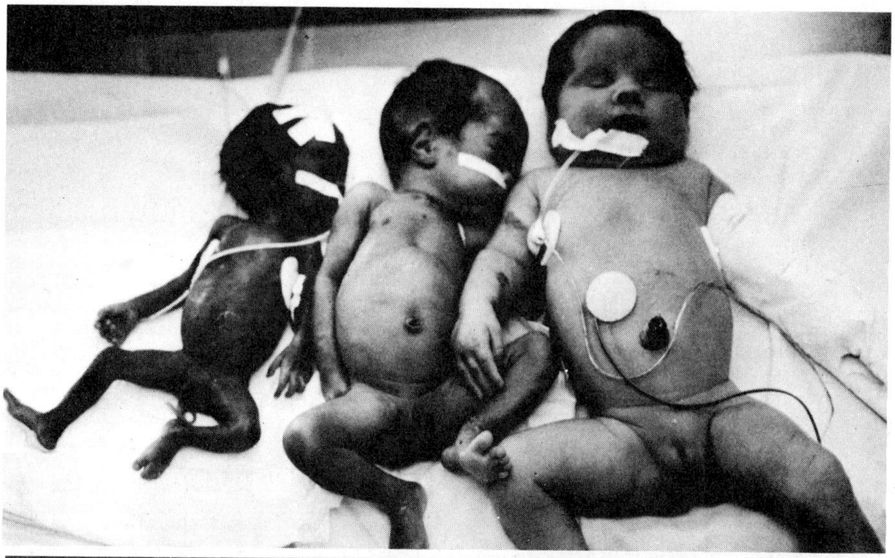

Fig. 8-2. Three babies, same gestational age, weight 600, 1400, and 2750 g, respectively, from left to right. They are plotted in Fig. 8-3 at points *A, B,* and *C.*

From Korones, S.B.: High-risk newborn infants: the basis for intensive nursing care, ed. 4, St. Louis, 1986, Mosby–Year Book, Inc., p. 118.

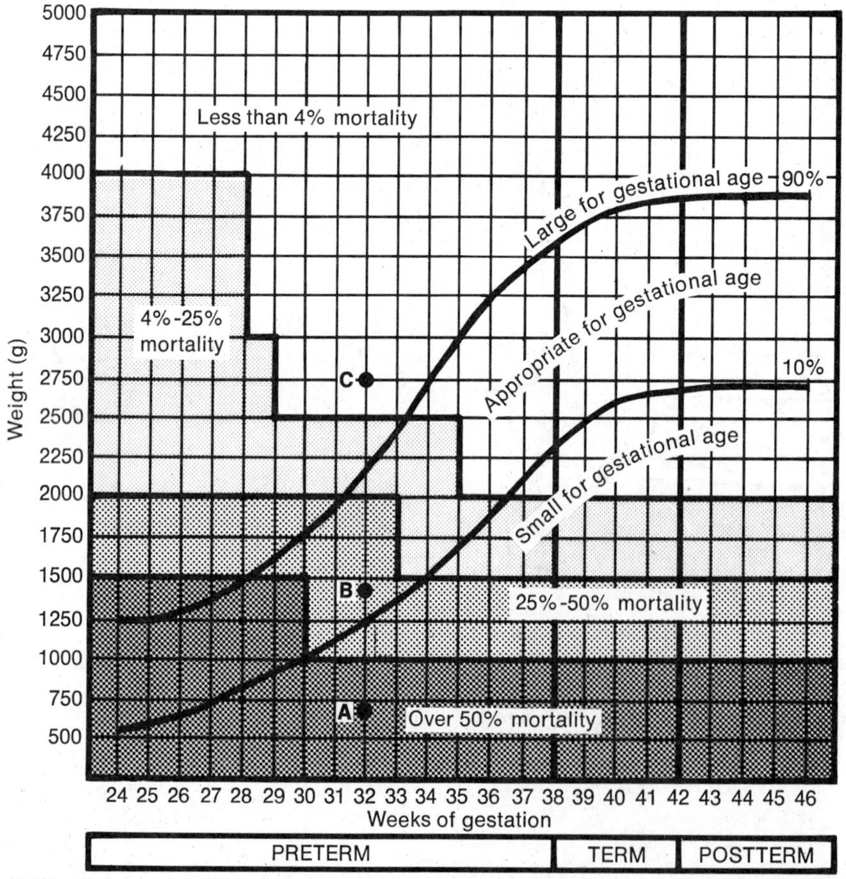

Fig. 8-3. Intrauterine growth status for gestational ages and according to appropriateness of growth.

Modified from Battaglia, F.C., and Lubchenco, L.C.: J. Pediatr. 71:159, 1967.

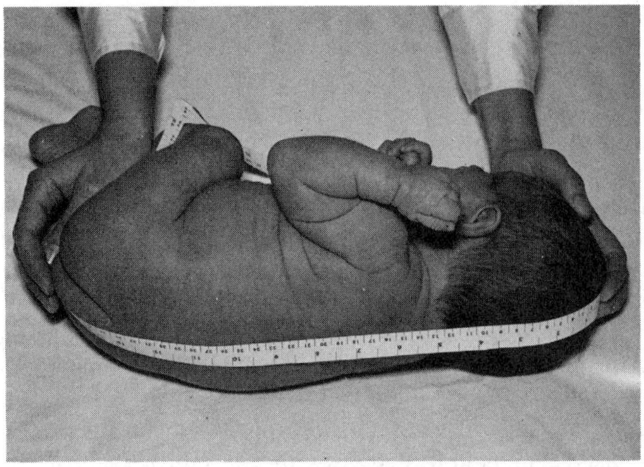

Fig. 8-4. Measurement of crown-to-rump length in newborn.

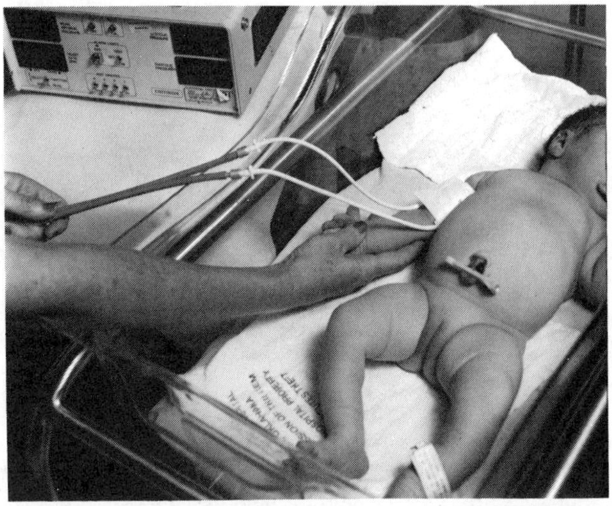

Fig. 8-5. Measurement of blood pressure using oscillometry.

decreased chest size, not increased head circumference.

Head circumference may also be compared with *crown-to-rump length,* or *sitting height* (Fig. 8-4). Crown-to-rump measurements are from 31 to 35 cm (12½ to 14 inches), approximately equal to head circumference. The relationship between the head and crown-to-rump measurements is more reliable than that between the head and chest.

Head-to-heel length is also measured. Because of the usual flexed position of the infant, the examiner must extend the leg completely when measuring total body length. The average length of the newborn is 48 to 53 cm (19 to 21 inches).

Body weight is taken soon after birth because weight loss occurs fairly rapidly. Normally the newborn loses about 10% of the birth weight by 3 to 4 days of age because of loss of excessive extracellular fluid and meconium, as well as limited food intake. The birth weight is regained by the tenth day of life. Most newborns weigh 2700 to 4000 g (6 to 9 pounds), the average weight being about 3400 g (7½ pounds). Accurate birth weights and lengths are important because they provide a baseline for assessment of risk status and future growth.

Another category of measurements is vital signs. *Axillary temperatures* are taken because insertion of a thermometer into the rectum can cause perforation of the mucosa (see Fig. 7-10, *B*). Core body temperature varies according to the periods of reactivity, but should be 36.5° to 37.6° C (97.7° to 99.7° F). Skin temperature is slightly lower than core body temperature. Therefore, axillary temperature may be less than rectal temperature, although the difference is small (as little as 0.2° F). There is no universal agreement on placement times for glass thermometers, although 3 to 5 minutes is probably adequate (Bliss-Holtz, 1989; Haddock, Vincent, and Merrow, 1986; Stephen and Sexton, 1987).

Pulse and *respirations* vary according to the periods of reactivity and to the infant's behaviors but are usually in the range of 120 to 140 beats/minute and 30 to 60 breaths/minute, respectively. Both are counted for a full 60 seconds to detect irregularities in rate, rhythm, and quality. Heart rate is taken apically with a stethoscope, although the brachial and femoral arteries are also palpated for equality of strength or fullness.

Measurement of blood pressure is recommended (American Academy of Pediatrics and American College of Obstetricians and Gynecologists, 1988); it provides useful baseline data and may indicate cardiac problems. Blood pressure is most easily and accurately assessed using oscillometry (Dinamap), although the device is less reliable when mean arterial pressure is below 40 mm Hg (Chia and others, 1990) (Fig. 8-5). The average oscillometric systolic/diastolic pressure is 65/41 at 1 to 3 days of age (Park and Menard, 1989). Comparisons should be made of the blood pressure in the upper and lower extremities.

✦ **NURSING ALERT** Systolic pressure in the calf that is 6 to 9 mm Hg less than systolic pressure in the upper arm is a sign of coarctation of the aorta and is reported for further evaluation (Park and Lee, 1989).

A suggested schedule for monitoring vital signs is upon admission to the nursery and at 4-hour intervals until the infant's condition is stable, and then once every 8 hours until discharge (American Academy of Pediatrics and American College of Obstetrics and Gynecologists, 1988). However, this schedule may vary according to institutional policy. Any change in the infant such as in color, muscle tone, or behavior necessitates more frequent monitoring.

General Appearance

Before each body system is assessed, it is important to describe the general posture and behavior of the newborn. The overall appearance yields valuable clues to the physical status of the infant.

Posture. In the full-term newborn the posture is one of flexion, a result of in utero position (Fig. 8-6). Most infants are born in a vertex (head first) presentation and keep the head flexed, with the chin resting on the upper chest. The

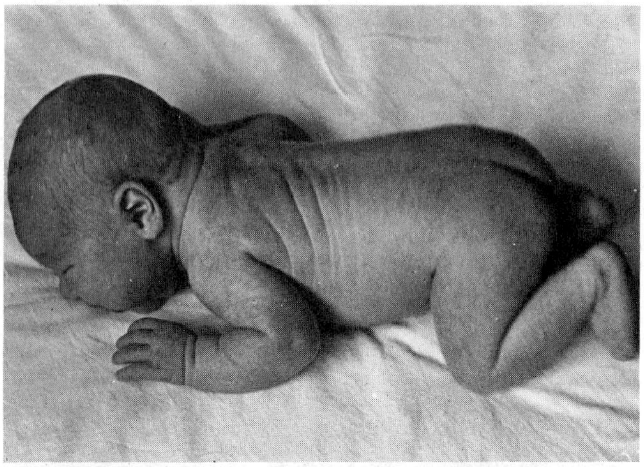

Fig. 8-6. Flexion position of neonate.

arms are flexed at the elbows and rest, folded, on the chest with hands clenched or fisted. The legs are flexed at the knees, the hips flexed with thighs resting on the abdomen, and the feet dorsiflexed against the anterior aspect of the legs. The vertebral column is also flexed.

Any deviation from this very characteristic fetal position must be recognized. For example, preterm as well as hypoxic infants do not assume an attitude of total flexion but rather one of limp extension. Nonvertex presentations also result in variations in posture. In breech presentations the posture will depend on the presenting part; for example, a frank breech presentation results in extended legs, abducted and fully rotated thighs, a flattened head on top, and a neck that appears elongated.

Behavior. The infant's behavior is carefully noted, especially the degree of alertness, drowsiness, and irritability, which are common signs of neurologic problems. Some questions to mentally ask when assessing behavior include:

- Is the infant awakened easily by a loud noise?
- Is the infant comforted by rocking, sucking, or cuddling?
- Do there seem to be periods of deep and light sleep?
- When awake, does the infant seem satisfied after a feeding?
- What stimuli elicit responses from the infant?
- When disturbed, how much does the infant protest?

Skin

The skin of the newborn is velvety smooth and puffy, especially about the eyes, the legs, the dorsal aspect of the hands and the feet, and the scrotum or labia.

At birth the skin is covered with a grayish white, cheeselike substance called *vernix caseosa,* a mixture of sebum and desquamating cells. If it is not removed during the bath, it will dry and disappear by about 24 to 48 hours. A fine, downy hair called *lanugo* is present on the skin, especially on the forehead, cheeks, shoulders, and back. *Milia,* distended sebaceous glands, appear as tiny white papules on the cheeks, chin, and nose. They usually disappear spontaneously in a few weeks. *Sudamina* or *miliaria* are distended sweat (eccrine) glands that cause minute vesicles on the skin surface, especially on the face.

Skin color depends on racial and familial background and varies greatly among newborns. In general, the white infant is usually pink to red; the black newborn may appear a pinkish or yellowish brown. Infants of Hispanic descent may have an olive tint or a slight yellow cast to the skin. Infants of Oriental descent may be a rosy or yellowish tan. The color of American Indian newborns depends upon the tribe and can vary from a light pink to a dark, reddish brown. By the second or third day the skin turns to its more natural tone and is drier and flakier.

General observations are made about the color of the skin in relation to activity, position, and temperature changes. In general the infant becomes redder when crying and may demonstrate transient periods of cyanosis. Decreased temperature increases the degree of cyanosis because of vasoconstriction. Several other color changes that may be noted on the skin are described in Table 8-3.

Head

General observation of the contour of the head is important, since molding occurs in almost all vaginal deliveries. In a vertex delivery the head is usually flattened at the forehead, with the apex rising and forming a point at the end of the parietal bones and the posterior skull or occiput dropping abruptly. The usual, more oval contour of the head is apparent by 1 to 2 days after birth. The change in shape occurs because the bones of the cranium are not fused, allowing for overlapping of the edges of these bones to accommodate to the size of the birth canal during delivery. Such molding does not occur in infants born by cesarean section.

Six bones—the frontal, occipital, two parietals, and two temporals—comprise the cranium. Between the junctions of these bones are bands of connective tissue called *sutures.* At the junction of the sutures are wider spaces of unossified membranous tissue called *fontanels.* The two most prominent fontanels are the *anterior fontanel,* formed by the junction of the sagittal, coronal, and frontal sutures, and the *posterior fontanel,* formed by the junction of the sagittal and lambdoidal sutures (Fig. 8-7, *A*).

Two other fontanels—the *sphenoidal* and *mastoid*—are normally present but are not usually palpable. An additional third fontanel located between the anterior and posterior fontanels along the sagittal suture is found in some normal neonates but is also found in some infants with Down syndrome. The presence of this sagittal or parietal fontanel is always recorded.

The skull is palpated for all patent sutures and fontanels, noting size, shape, molding, or abnormal closure. Sutures are felt as cracks between the skull bones; fontanels are felt as wider "soft spots" at the junction of sutures. These are

NURSING TIP: LOCATION OF SUTURES

The location of the suture is easily remembered because the coronal suture "crowns" the head and the sagittal suture "separates" the head.

Table 8-3 Summary of physical assessment of the newborn

ASSESSMENT	USUAL FINDINGS	COMMON VARIATIONS/MINOR ABNORMALITIES	POTENTIAL SIGNS OF DISTRESS/MAJOR ABNORMALITIES
General measurements	Head circumference 33-35 cm (13-14 inches) Chest circumference 30.5-33 cm (12-13 inches) Head circumference should be about 2-3 cm (1 inch) larger than chest circumference Crown-to-rump length 31-35 cm (12.5-14 inches) Crown-to-rump length approximately equal to head circumference Head-to-heel length 48-53 cm (19-21 inches) Birth weight 2700-4000 g (6-9 pounds)	Molding after birth may decrease head circumference Head and chest circumferences may be equal for first 1-2 days after birth Loss of 10% of birth weight in first week; regained in 10-14 days	Head circumference <10th or >90th percentile Birth weight <10th or >90th percentile
Vital signs			
Temperature	Axillary—36.5°-37° C (97.9°-98°F)	Crying may increase body temperature slightly Radiant warmer will increase axillary temperature	Hypothermia Hyperthermia
Heart rate	Apical—120-140 beats/minute	Crying will increase heart rate; sleep will decrease heart rate During first period of reactivity (6 to 8 hours), rate can reach 180 beats/minute	Bradycardia—Resting rate below 80-100 beats/minute Tachycardia—Rate above 160-180 beats/minute Irregular rhythm
Respirations	30-60 breaths/minute	Crying will increase respiratory rate; sleep will decrease respiratory rate During first period of reactivity (6 to 8 hours), rate can reach 80 breaths/minute	Tachypnea—Rate above 60 breaths/minute Apnea >15 seconds
Blood pressure	See inside front cover	Crying will increase blood pressure	Systolic pressure in calf 6-9 mm Hg less than in upper extremity
General appearance	*Posture*—Flexion of head and extremities, which rest on chest and abdomen	*Frank breech*—Extended legs, abducted and fully rotated thighs, flattened occiput, extended neck	Limp posture, extension of extremities
Skin	At birth, bright red, puffy, smooth Second to third day, pink, flaky, dry Vernix caseosa Lanugo Edema around eyes, face, legs, dorsa of hands, feet, and scrotum or labia Normal color changes: *Acrocyanosis*—Cyanosis of hands and feet *Cutis marmorata*—Transient mottling when infant is exposed to decreased temperature	Neonatal jaundice after first 24 hours Ecchymoses or petechiae caused by birth trauma *Milia*—Distended sebaceous glands that appear as tiny white papules on cheeks, chin, and nose *Miliaria* or *sudamina*—Distended sweat (eccrine) glands that appear as minute vesicles, especially on face *Erythema toxicum*—Pink papular rash with vesicles superimposed on thorax, back, buttocks, and abdomen; may appear in 24 to 48 hours and resolve after several days	Progressive jaundice, especially in first 24 hours Cracked or peeling skin Generalized cyanosis Pallor Grayness Plethora Hemorrhage, ecchymoses, or petechiae that persist *Sclerema*—Hard and stiff skin Poor skin turgor Rashes, pustules, or blisters *Café-au-lait spots*—Light brown spots *Nevus flammeus*—Port-wine stain

Continued.

Table 8-3 Summary of physical assessment of the newborn—cont'd

ASSESSMENT	USUAL FINDINGS	COMMON VARIATIONS/MINOR ABNORMALITIES	POTENTIAL SIGNS OF DISTRESS/MAJOR ABNORMALITIES
Skin—cont'd		*Harlequin color change*—Clearly outlined color change as infant lies on side; lower half of body becomes pink and upper half is pale *Mongolian spots*—Irregular areas of deep blue pigmentation, usually in the sacral and gluteal regions; seen predominantly in newborns of African, Asian, or Hispanic descent *Telangiectatic nevi ("stork bites")*—Flat, deep pink localized areas usually seen in back of neck	
Head	*Anterior fontanel*—Diamond-shaped, 2.5-4.0 cm (1-1.75 inches) (Fig. 1-2) *Posterior fontanel*—Triangular-shaped 0.5-1 cm (0.2-0.4 inch) Fontanels should be flat, soft, and firm Widest part of fontanel measured from bone to bone, not suture to suture	Molding following vaginal delivery Third sagittal (parietal) fontanel Bulging fontanel because of crying or coughing *Caput succedaneum*—Edema of soft scalp tissue *Cephalhematoma* (uncomplicated)—Hematoma between periosteum and skull bone	Fused sutures Bulging or depressed fontanels when quiet Widened sutures and fontanels *Craniotabes*—Snapping sensation along lambdoid suture that resembles indentation of Ping-Pong ball
Eyes	Lids usually edematous Eyes usually closed Color—Slate gray, dark blue, brown Absence of tears Presence of red reflex Corneal reflex in response to touch Pupillary reflex in response to light Blink reflex in response to light or touch Rudimentary fixation on objects and ability to follow to midline	Epicanthal folds in Oriental infants Searching nystagmus or strabismus *Subconjunctival (scleral) hemorrhages*—Ruptured capillaries, usually at limbus	Pink color of iris Purulent discharge Mongoloid slant in non-Orientals Hypertelorism (3 cm or greater) Hypotelorism Congenital cataracts Constricted or dilated fixed pupil Absence of red reflex Absence of pupillary or corneal reflex Inability to follow object or bright light to midline Blue sclera Yellow sclera
Ears	Position—Top of pinna on horizontal line with outer canthus of eye Startle reflex elicited by a loud, sudden noise Pinna flexible, cartilage present	Inability to visualize tympanic membrane because of filled aural canals Pinna flat against head Irregular shape or size Pits or skin tags	Low placement of ears Absence of startle reflex in response to loud noise Minor abnormalities may be signs of various syndromes
Nose	Nasal patency Nasal discharge—Thin white mucus Sneezing	Flattened and bruised	Nonpatent canals Thick, bloody nasal discharge Flaring of nares (alae nasi) Copious nasal secretions or stuffiness
Mouth and throat	Intact, high-arched palate Uvula in midline Frenulum of tongue Frenum of upper lip Sucking reflex—Strong and coordinated Rooting reflex Gag reflex Extrusion reflex Absent or minimal salivation Vigorous cry	Natal teeth (benign but may be associated with congenital defects) *Epstein pearls*—Small, white epithelial cysts along midline of hard palate	Cleft lip Cleft palate Large, protruding tongue or posterior displacement of tongue Profuse salivation or drooling *Candidiasis (thrush)*—White, adherent patches on tongue, palate, and buccal surfaces Inability to pass nasogastric tube Hoarse, high-pitched, weak, absent, or other abnormal cry

Table 8-3 Summary of physical assessment of the newborn—cont'd

ASSESSMENT	USUAL FINDINGS	COMMON VARIATIONS/MINOR ABNORMALITIES	POTENTIAL SIGNS OF DISTRESS/MAJOR ABNORMALITIES
Neck	Short, thick, usually surrounded by skin folds Tonic neck reflex Neck-righting reflex Otolith-righting reflex	*Torticollis* (wry neck)—Head held to one side with chin pointing to opposite side	Excessive skin folds Resistance to flexion Absence of tonic neck, neck-righting, or otolith-righting reflex Fractured clavicle
Chest	Anteroposterior and lateral diameters equal Slight sternal retractions evident during inspiration Xiphoid process evident Breast enlargement	Funnel chest (pectus excavatum) Pigeon chest (pectus carinatum) Supernumerary nipples Secretion of milky substance from breasts ("witch's milk")	Depressed sternum Marked retractions of chin, chest, and intercostal spaces during respiration Asymmetric chest expansion or overexpansion Redness and firmness around nipples Wide-spaced nipples
Lungs	Respirations chiefly abdominal Cough reflex absent at birth, present by 1-2 days Bilateral equal bronchial breath sounds	Rate and depth of respirations may be irregular, periodic breathing Crackles shortly after birth	Inspiratory stridor Expiratory grunt Retractions Persistent irregular breathing Periodic breathing with repeated apneic spells Deep sighing respirations Seesaw respirations Unequal breath sounds Persistent fine crackles Wheezing Diminished breath sounds Peristaltic sounds on one side, with diminished breath sounds on same side
Heart	Apex—Fourth to fifth intercostal space, lateral to left sternal border S_2 slightly sharper and higher in pitch than S_1	Sinus arrhythmia Transient cyanosis on crying or straining	Dextrocardia Displacement of apex Cardiomegaly Abdominal shunts Murmurs Thrills Persistent cyanosis
Abdomen	Cylindric in shape Liver—Palpable 2-3 cm below right costal margin Spleen—Tip palpable at end of first week of age Kidneys—Palpable 1-2 cm above umbilicus Umbilical cord—Bluish white at birth with two arteries and one vein Equal bilateral femoral pulses	Umbilical hernia *Diastasis recti*—Midline gap between recti muscles	Abdominal distention Localized bulging Distended veins Absent bowel sounds Enlarged liver and spleen Ascites Visible peristaltic waves Scaphoid or concave abdomen Green umbilical cord Presence of one artery in cord Urine or stool leaking from cord Palpable bladder distention following scanty voiding Absent femoral pulses
Female genitalia	Labia and clitoris usually edematous Urethral meatus behind clitoris Vernix caseosa between labia Urinates within 24 hours	Blood-tinged or mucoid discharge (pseudomenstruation) Hymenal tag	Enlarged clitoris with urethral meatus at tip Fused labia Absence of vaginal opening Fecal discharge from vaginal opening No urination within 24 hours Masses in labia

Continued.

Table 8-3 Summary of physical assessment of the newborn—cont'd

ASSESSMENT	USUAL FINDINGS	COMMON VARIATIONS/MINOR ABNORMALITIES	POTENTIAL SIGNS OF DISTRESS/MAJOR ABNORMALITIES
Male genitalia	Urethral opening at tip of glans penis Testes palpable in each scrotum Scrotum usually large, edematous, pendulous, and covered with rugae; usually deeply pigmented in dark-skinned ethnic groups Smegma Urinates within 24 hours	Urethral opening covered by prepuce Inability to retract foreskin Epithelial pearls Erection or priapism Testes palpable in inguinal canal Scrotum small	Hypospadias Epispadias Chordee Testes not palpable in scrotum or inguinal canal No urination within 24 hours Inguinal hernia Hypoplastic scrotum Hydrocele Masses in scrotum
Back and rectum	Spine intact, no openings, masses, or prominent curves Trunk incurvation reflex Anal reflex Patent anal opening Passage of meconium within 36 hours	Green liquid stools in infant under phototherapy	Anal fissures or fistulas Imperforate anus Absence of anal reflex No meconium within 36 hours Pilonidal cyst or sinus Tuft of hair along spine Spina bifida (any degree)
Extremities	Ten fingers and toes Full range of motion *Negative scarf sign*—Elbow does not reach midline Nail beds pink, with transient cyanosis immediately after birth Creases on anterior two thirds of sole Sole usually flat Symmetry of extremities Equal muscle tone bilaterally, especially resistance to opposing flexion Equal bilateral brachial pulses	Partial syndactyly between second and third toes Second toe overlapping into third toe Wide gap between hallux and second toe Deep crease on plantar surface of foot between first and second toes Asymmetric length of toes Dorsiflexion and shortness of hallux	*Polydactyly*—Extra digits *Syndactyly*—Fused or webbed digits *Phocomelia*—Hands or feet attached close to trunk *Hemimelia*—Absence of distal part of extremity Hyperflexibility of joints Persistent cyanosis of nail beds Yellowing of nail beds Sole covered with creases Simian crease Fractures Dislocated or subluxated hip Limitation in hip abduction Unequal gluteal or leg folds Unequal knee height (Allis or Galeazzi sign) Audible click on abduction (Ortolani sign) Asymmetry of extremities Unequal muscle tone or range of motion
Neuromuscular system	Extremities usually maintain some degree of flexion Extension of an extremity followed by previous position of flexion Head lag while sitting, but momentary ability to hold head erect Able to turn head from side to side when prone Able to hold head in horizontal line with back when held prone	Quivering or momentary tremors	*Hypotonia*—Floppy, poor head control, extremities limp *Hypertonia*—Jittery, arms and hands tightly flexed, legs stiffly extended, startles easily Asymmetric posturing (except tonic neck reflex) Opisthotonic posturing—Arched back Signs of paralysis Tremors, twitches, and myoclonic jerks Marked head lag in all positions

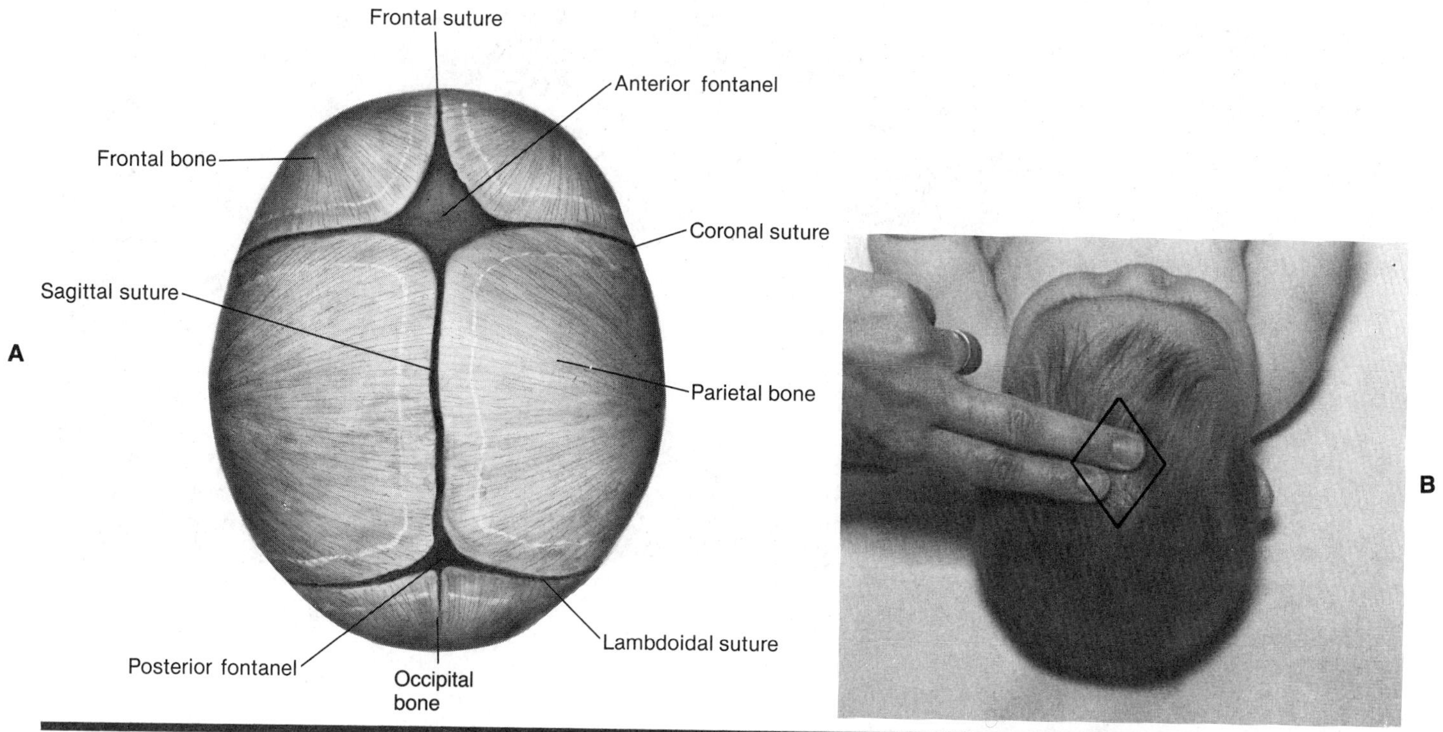

Fig. 8-7. A, Location of sutures and fontanels. **B,** Palpating anterior fontanel.

palpated by using the tip of the index finger and running it along the ends of the bones (Fig. 8-7, *B*).

The anterior fontanel is diamond shaped and measures 4 to 5 cm (about 2 inches) at its widest point (from bone to bone, rather than from suture to suture). The posterior fontanel is triangular shaped, measuring between 0.5 and 1 cm (less than ½ inch) at its widest part. It is easily located by following the sagittal suture toward the occiput.

The fontanels should feel flat, firm, and well demarcated against the bony edges of the skull. Frequently pulsations are visible at the anterior fontanel. Coughing, crying, or lying down may temporarily cause the fontanels to bulge and become more taut. However, a widened, tense, bulging fontanel is a sign of increased intracranial pressure. A markedly sunken, depressed fontanel indicates dehydration. Such findings are recorded and reported.

The skull is also palpated for any unusual masses or prominences, particularly those resulting from birth trauma, such as caput succedaneum or cephalhematoma (see Chapter 9). Because of the pliability of the skull, exerting pressure at the margin of the parietal and occipital bones along the lambdoid suture may produce a snapping sensation similar to the indentation of a Ping-Pong ball. This phenomenon, known as *physiologic craniotabes,* may be found normally, especially in newborns of breech birth, but also may indicate hydrocephalus or syphilis.

The degree of *head control* is assessed. Although *head lag* is normal in the newborn, the degree of ability to control the head in certain positions should be recognized. If the supine infant is pulled from the arms into a semi-Fowler position, head lag and hyperextension are noted (Fig. 8-8, *A*). However, as infants are brought forward into a sitting position, they attempt to control their heads in an upright position. As the head falls forward onto the chest, many infants attempt to right it into the erect position. If they are held in ventral suspension—that is, held prone above and parallel to the examining surface—the head is held in a straight line with the spinal column (Fig. 8-8, *B*). When lying on the abdomen, newborns have the ability to lift the head slightly, turning it from side to side. Marked head lag is seen in Down syndrome, hypoxic infants, and newborns with brain damage.

Eyes

Since newborns tend to keep their eyes tightly closed, it is best to begin the examination of the eyes by observing the lids for edema, which is normally present for the first 2 days after delivery. A *mongoloid slant,* the lateral upward slope of the eyes with an inner epicanthal fold, may indicate Down syndrome. The eyes are observed for symmetry and for hypertelorism. The distance between the inner canthi is usually not measured unless there is cause for further investigation.

Tears may be present at birth, but purulent discharge from the eyes shortly after birth is abnormal. It may signify *ophthalmia neonatorum* and should be reported.

In order to visualize the surface structures of the eye, the infant is held supine, and the head gently lowered. The eyes will usually open, similar to the mechanism of a doll's eyes. The sclera should be white and clear.

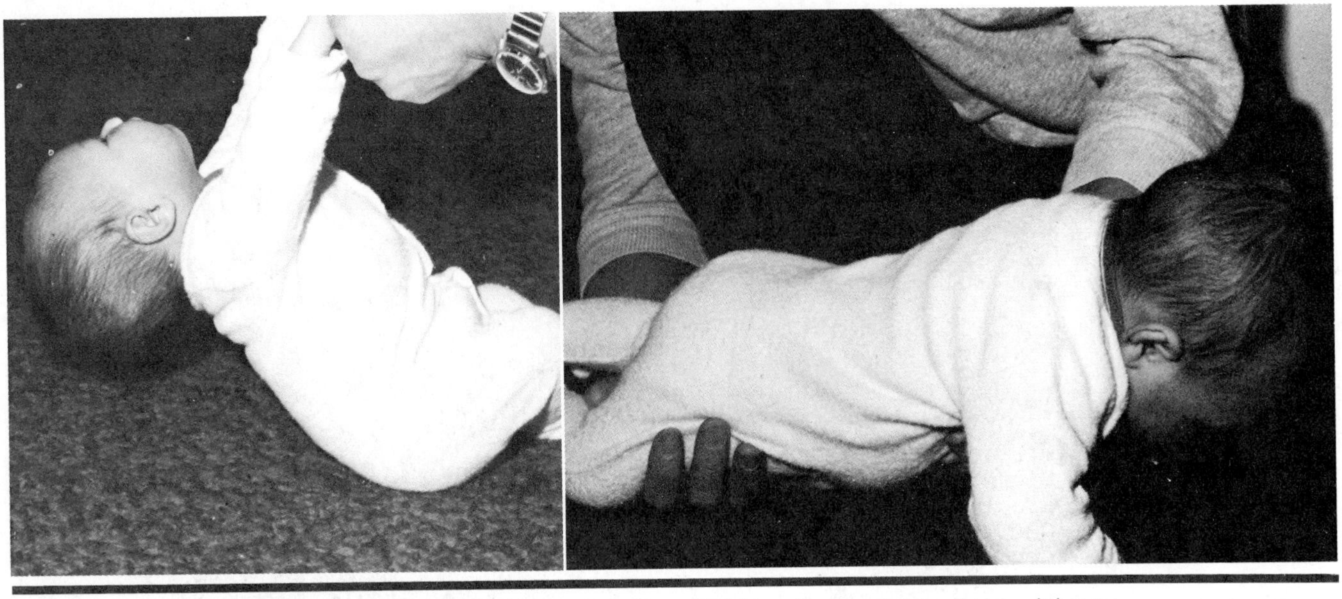

A

B

Fig. 8-8. Head control in infant. **A,** Inability to hold head erect when pulled to sitting position. **B,** Ability to hold head erect when placed in ventral suspension.

The cornea is examined for the presence of any opacities or haziness. The *corneal reflex* is present at birth but is generally not elicited unless brain or eye damage is suspected. The pupil usually responds to light by constricting. Absence of the *pupillary reflex,* particularly by 3 weeks of age, suggests blindness. A fixed, dilated, or constricted pupil may indicate anoxia or brain damage. A searching *nystagmus* is common after birth. *Strabismus* is a normal finding because of the lack of binocularity.

The color of the iris is noted. Most light-skinned newborns have slate gray or dark blue eyes, whereas dark-skinned infants have brown eyes. Absence of color is characteristic of albinism.

Although it is difficult to perform a complete funduscopic examination of the retina, a red reflex is easily elicited. Absence of the red reflex may indicate the presence of *retinal hemorrhages* or *congenital cataracts.*

Ears

The ears are examined for position, structure, and auditory function. The pinna is often flattened against the side of the head from pressure in utero. An otoscopic examination is ordinarily not performed because the canals are filled with vernix caseosa and amniotic fluid, making visualization of the drum difficult.

Auditory ability is assessed by making a sharp, loud noise close to the infant's head and noting the presence of the *startle reflex* (see Table 8-4) or twitching of the eyelids. In some nurseries hearing screening of newborns considered at risk for hearing loss may be performed (Box 8-2). Two tests currently used are the Crib-O-Gram and brainstem evoked auditory response (BEAR). The BEAR is more reliable (Cox, 1988). (See also Auditory Testing, Chapter 7.)

Box 8-2 INFANTS CONSIDERED AT RISK FOR HEARING LOSS

Family history of childhood hearing impairment
Congenital perinatal infection (e.g., cytomegalovirus, rubella, herpes, toxoplasmosis, syphilis)
Anatomic malformations involving the head or neck
Birth weight less than 1500 g
Hyperbilirubinemia at a level exceeding indications for exchange transfusion
Bacterial meningitis, especially that caused by *Haemophilus influenzae*
Severe asphyxia in the perinatal period
Ototoxic drugs

From American Academy of Pediatrics and American College of Obstetricians and Gynecologists: Guidelines for perinatal care, ed. 2, Elk Grove Village, IL, 1988, The Academy, p. 107.

✦ **NURSING ALERT** Absence of any behavioral response to a sudden noise may indicate congenital deafness and is always reported.

Nose

Patency of the nasal canals is assessed by holding the hand over the infant's mouth and one canal and noting the passage of air through the unobstructed opening. If nasal patency is questionable, it is reported because most newborns are obligatory nose breathers and are unable to breathe orally in response to nasal occlusion (Miller and others, 1985).

The nose is usually flattened after birth, and bruises are common, especially if forceps were used. Thin white mucus is very common in the newborn, but a thick, bloody nasal discharge without sneezing may suggest the snuffles of congenital syphilis. *Sneezing* is very common.

✦ **NURSING ALERT** Flaring of the nares is always noted because it is a serious sign of air hunger from respiratory distress.

Mouth and Throat

The mouth is inspected for its existing structures. The palate is normally high arched and somewhat narrow. The hard and soft palates are inspected for any clefts, which warrant further investigation. A common finding is *Epstein pearls*—small, white, epithelial cysts along both sides of the midline of the hard palate. They are insignificant and disappear in several weeks.

The *frenulum* of the upper lip is a band of thick, pink tissue that lies under the inner surface of the upper lip and extends to the maxillary alveolar ridge. It usually disappears as the maxilla grows. It is particularly evident when the infant yawns or smiles.

The *sucking reflex* is elicited by placing a nipple or tongue blade in the infant's mouth. The infant should exhibit a strong, vigorous suck. The *rooting reflex* is obtained by stroking the cheek and noting the infant's response of turning toward the stimulated side and sucking (Fig. 8-9). The *gag reflex* is elicited when using a tongue blade to visualize the oropharynx.

The *uvula* can be inspected while the infant is crying and the chin is depressed. However, it may be retracted upward and backward during crying. Tonsillar tissue is generally not seen in the newborn. Natal teeth (teeth present at birth as opposed to neonatal teeth—teeth that erupt during the first month of life) are seen infrequently and erupt chiefly at the position of the lower central incisors. They are reported because they are frequently found with developmental abnormalities and syndromes, including cleft lip and palate. Most natal teeth are loosely attached, but current thinking suggests preserving them until they exfoliate naturally (King and Lee, 1989; Leung, 1989).

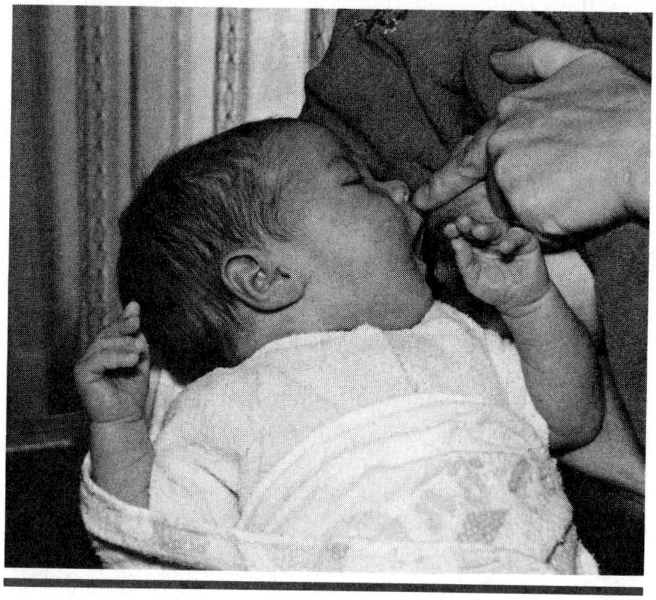

Fig. 8-9. Eliciting rooting reflex.

Neck

Since the newborn's neck is short and covered with folds of tissue, adequate assessment requires allowing the head to fall gently backward in hyperextension while the back is supported in a slightly raised position. The nurse observes for range of motion, shape, and any abnormal masses and palpates each clavicle for possible fractures.

Chest

The newborn's chest is almost circular because the anteroposterior and lateral diameters are equal. The ribs are very flexible, and slight intercostal retractions are normally seen on inspiration. The xiphoid process is commonly visible as a small protrusion at the end of the sternum. The sternum is generally raised and slightly curved.

The breasts are inspected for size, shape, and nipple formation, location, and number. Breast enlargement appears in many newborns of either sex by the second or third day and is caused by maternal hormones. Occasionally a milky substance sometimes called "witch's milk" is secreted by the infant's breasts. Infrequently, supernumerary nipples are present; if found, the kidneys should be evaluated because of the association of extra nipples with renal anomalies (Meggyessy and Méhes, 1987).

Lungs

The normal respirations of the newborn are irregular and abdominal, and the rate is between 30 and 60 breaths/minute. Periods of apnea lasting less than 15 seconds are considered normal. After the first forceful breaths required to initiate respiration, subsequent breaths should be easy and fairly regular in rhythm. Occasional irregularities occur in relation to crying, sleeping, and feeding.

Auscultation is best done when the infant is quiet. Bronchial breath sounds should be equal bilaterally. Any differences in auscultatory findings between symmetric sites is reported. *Crackles* soon after birth indicate areas of atelectasis, which represent the normal transition of the lungs to extrauterine life. However, persistence of crackles or presence of wheezing is also reported.

Heart

Heart rate is auscultated and may range from 100 to 180 beats/minute shortly after birth and, when the infant's condition has stabilized, from 120 to 140 beats/minute. The point of maximum intensity (PMI) may be palpated and is usually found in the fourth to fifth intercostal space, medial to the left midclavicular line. The PMI gives some indication of the location of the heart, which may be displaced in conditions such as diaphragmatic hernia or pneumothorax. If the heart is on the right side of the body, *dextrocardia* exists. This is reported, since the abdominal organs may also be reversed, with associated circulatory abnormalities.

Auscultation of the specific components of the heart sounds is difficult because of the rapid rate and effective transmission of respiratory sounds. However, the *first (S_1)* and *second (S_2) sounds* should be clear and well defined; the second sound is somewhat higher in pitch and sharper than the first. Murmurs are very frequently heard in the newborn, especially over the base of the heart or at the left sternal border in the third or fourth interspace. Ordinarily they are not associated with specific cardiac defects, since they more frequently represent the incomplete functional closure of fetal shunts. (Grading of heart murmurs is discussed in Chapter 7.) However, murmurs are always recorded and reported.

Abdomen

The normal contour of the abdomen is cylindric and usually prominent with visible veins. Bowel sounds are heard a few hours after birth. Visible peristaltic waves may be observed in thin newborns but should not be seen in well-nourished infants.

The umbilical cord is inspected to determine the presence of two arteries, which look like papular structures, and one vein, which has a larger lumen than the arteries and a thinner vessel wall. At birth the cord appears bluish white and moist. After clamping, it begins to dry and appears a dull, yellowish brown. It progressively shrivels in size and turns greenish black.

Palpation is done after inspection of the abdomen. The liver is normally palpable 3 cm (about 1 inch) below the right costal margin. The tip of the spleen can sometimes be felt, but a palpable spleen more than 1 cm below the left costal margin suggests enlargement and warrants further investigation.

Both kidneys should be palpated, although they are difficult to locate. Failure to palpate these organs is significant; generally it indicates that no abnormal masses are present in the area, but rarely it means that the kidneys are absent. Palpation is best done soon after delivery, when muscle tone is least. Supporting the infant in a semi-Fowler position with one hand and palpating the abdomen with the other hand usually causes the abdominal muscles to relax. Flexing the infant's knees toward the abdomen while the infant is supine will also increase relaxation. Both hands are used to locate the kidneys. As one hand palpates the abdominal area, the other hand provides countertraction by pushing upward from the posterior flank area. The lower half of the right kidney and the tip of the left kidney may be felt 1 to 2 cm (about ½ inch) above the umbilicus. The kidney is felt as an oval structure between the fingers of each hand.

The suprapubic area should also be palpated for evidence of a *distended bladder.* The neonate should void during the first 24 hours after birth. A distended bladder following a scanty voiding may indicate urethral obstruction.

During examination of the lower abdomen, it is particularly important to palpate for femoral pulses, which should be strong and bilaterally equal.

✦ **NURSING ALERT** Absence of the femoral pulses may indicate coarctation of the aorta, a congenital heart defect. Absent or weak femoral pulses are always reported for further evaluation.

Female Genitalia

Normally the labia minora and clitoris are edematous, especially following a breech delivery. However, the labia and clitoris must be carefully inspected to identify any evidence of ambiguous genitalia or other abnormalities. Normally in a female the urethral opening is located behind the clitoris. Any deviation from this may mistakenly suggest that the clitoris is a small penis, which can occur in conditions such as adrenal hyperplasia.

Virtually all female newborns have hymens, and this fact should be noted on the chart (Jenny, Kuhns, and Arakawa, 1987). A hymenal tag is occasionally visible from the posterior opening of the vagina. It is composed of tissue from the hymen and the labia minora. It usually disappears in several weeks. Generally the vaginal vault is not inspected. However, absence of the hymenal tag may indicate vaginal agenesis, and in this case further examination is warranted.

Vaginal discharge may be noted during the first week of life. This pseudomenstruation is a manifestation of the abrupt decrease of maternal hormones and usually disappears by 2 to 4 weeks. Fecal discharge from the vaginal opening indicates a rectovaginal fistula and is always reported. Vernix caseosa may be present in large amounts between the labia.

Male Genitalia

The penis is inspected for the urethral opening, which is located at the tip. However, the opening may be totally covered by the prepuce, or foreskin, which covers the glans penis. A tight prepuce is a very common finding in newborns and does not indicate phimosis. It should not be forcefully retracted. *Smegma,* a white cheesy substance, is commonly found around the glans penis, under the foreskin. An erection is not uncommon in the newborn. Small, white, firm lesions called *epithelial pearls* may be seen at the tip of the prepuce.

The scrotum may be large, edematous, and pendulous in the full-term neonate, especially in the infant born in breech position. It is more deeply pigmented in dark-skinned races. A noncommunicating *hydrocele* commonly occurs unilaterally and disappears within a few months. The scrotum should always be palpated for the presence of testes (see Chapter 7). In small newborns, particularly premature infants, the undescended testes may be palpable within the inguinal canal. Absence of the testes may also be a sign of ambiguous genitalia, especially when accompanied by a small scrotum and penis. *Inguinal hernias* may or may not be manifested immediately after birth. A hernia is more easily detected when the infant is crying. Palpable lymph nodes are most commonly found in the inguinal area (Bamji and others, 1986).

Back and Anus

The spine is inspected with the infant prone. The shape of the spine is gently rounded, with none of the characteristic S-shaped curves seen later in life. Any abnormal openings, masses, dimples, or soft areas are noted. A large, protruding sac anywhere along the spine, but most commonly in the sacral area, indicates some type of *spina bifida.* A small sinus, which may or may not be communicating with the spine, is a *pilonidal sinus.* It is frequently covered with a tuft of hair. Although it may have no pathologic significance, it may indicate the existence of spina bifida occulta or be a portal of entry into the spinal column. With the infant still prone, symmetry of the gluteal folds is carefully noted. Any evidence of asymmetry is reported, and tests for congenital hip dislocation are performed by trained (or skilled) examiners (see Chapter 11).

Passage of meconium during the first 24 to 48 hours of life indicates anal patency. If an imperforate anus is suspected and not readily visible, the little finger (gloved and lubricated) or a rubber catheter should be inserted into the anal opening. Rectal thermometers are not used because of the risk of mucosal perforation. In addition, the small diameter of the thermometer may pass through even a severely stenotic anus (El Haddad and Corkery, 1985).

With the infant still prone, the buttocks are gently separated to inspect the anal area for presence of *fissures,* or small cracks in the mucosa. Anal fissures are a common cause of constipation because the infant refuses to strain during defecation in order to avoid pain. Asymmetry of the mucosal folds around the sphincter also suggests fissures.

Extremities

The extremities are examined for symmetry, range of motion, and signs of malformation or trauma. The fingers and toes are counted, and supernumerary digits *(polydactyly)* or fusion of digits *(syndactyly)* is noted. A partial syndactyly between the second and third toes is a common variation seen in otherwise normal infants.

Range of motion of the extremities should be observed throughout the entire examination. *Hyperflexibility* of joints is characteristic of Down syndrome. Eliciting the *scarf sign* may be helpful in identifying abnormal flexion of joints (see Fig. 10-12).

The fingernails are examined; the nail beds should be pink, although slight blueness is evident in acrocyanosis. Persistent cyanosis of the nail beds indicates anoxia or vasoconstriction. Yellowing of the nail beds may indicate intrauterine distress, postmaturity, or hemolytic disease. Short or absent nails are seen in premature infants, whereas long nails, extending over the ends of the fingers, are characteristic of postmature newborns.

The palms of the hands should have the usual creases (see Fig. 7-13). A transverse palmar crease, called a *simian crease,* suggests Down syndrome. The full-term newborn usually has creases on the anterior two thirds of the sole of the foot. In postmature infants the sole is covered with deep creases, and in premature infants the creases are absent. The soles of the feet are flat with prominent fat pads. While examining the feet, the *grasp* and *Babinski reflexes* are elicited (Table 8-4 and Fig. 8-10). Any foot abnormalities are reported.

Table 8-4 Assessment of reflexes in the newborn

REFLEXES	EXPECTED BEHAVIORAL RESPONSES
▪ Localized	
Eyes	
Blinking or corneal reflex	Infant blinks at sudden appearance of a bright light or at approach of an object toward cornea; persists throughout life
Pupillary	Pupil constricts when a bright light shines toward it; persists throughout life
Doll's eye	As head is moved slowly to right or left, eyes lag behind and do not immediately adjust to new position of head; disappears as fixation develops; if persists, indicates neurologic damage
Nose	
Sneeze	Spontaneous response of nasal passages to irritation or obstruction; persists throughout life
Glabellar	Tapping briskly on glabella (bridge of nose) causes eyes to close tightly
Mouth and throat	
Sucking	Infant begins strong sucking movements of circumoral area in response to stimulation; persists throughout infancy, even without stimulation, such as during sleep
Gag	Stimulation of posterior pharynx by food, suction, or passage of a tube causes infant to gag; persists throughout life
Rooting	Touching or stroking the cheek along side of mouth causes infant to turn head toward that side and begin to suck; should disappear at about age 3-4 months, but may persist for up to 12 months (see Fig. 8-9)
Extrusion	When tongue is touched or depressed, infant responds by forcing it outward; disappears by age 4 months

Continued.

Table 8-4 Assessment of reflexes in the newborn—cont'd

REFLEXES	EXPECTED BEHAVIORAL RESPONSES
Mouth and throat—cont'd	
Yawn	Spontaneous response to decreased oxygen by increasing amount of inspired air; persists throughout life
Cough	Irritation of mucous membranes of larynx or tracheobronchial tree causes coughing; persists throughout life; usually present after first day of birth
Extremities	
Grasp	Touching palms of hands or soles of feet near base of digits causes flexion of hands and toes (see Fig. 8-10, *A*): palmar grasp lessens after age 3 months, to be replaced by voluntary movement; plantar grasp lessens by 8 months of age
Babinski	Stroking outer sole of foot upward from heel and across ball of foot causes toes to hyperextend and hallux to dorsiflex (see Fig. 8-10, *B*); disappears after age 1 year
Ankle clonus	Briskly dorsiflexing foot while supporting knee in partially flexed position results in one to two oscillating movements ("beats"); eventually no beats should be felt
▪ **Mass**	
Moro	Sudden jarring or change in equilibrium causes sudden extension and abduction of extremities and fanning of fingers, with index finger and thumb forming a C shape, followed by flexion and adduction of extremities; legs may weakly flex; infant may cry (Fig. 8-11); disappears after age 3-4 months, usually strongest during first 2 months
Startle	A sudden loud noise causes abduction of the arms with flexion of elbows; hands remain clenched; disappears by age 4 months
Perez	While infant is prone on a firm surface, thumb is pressed along spine from sacrum to neck; infant responds by crying, flexing extremities, and elevating pelvis and head; lordosis of the spine, as well as defecation and urination, may occur; disappears by age 4-6 months
Asymmetric tonic neck	When infant's head is quickly turned to one side, arm and leg extend on that side, and opposite arm and leg flex (Fig. 8-12); disappears by age 3-4 months, to be replaced by symmetric positioning of both sides of body
Trunk incurvation (Galant) reflex	Stroking infant's back alongside spine causes hips to move toward stimulated side; disappears by age 4 weeks
Dance or step	If infant is held so that sole of foot touches a hard surface, there is a reciprocal flexion and extension of the leg, stimulating walking (Fig. 8-13); disappears after age 3-4 weeks, to be replaced by deliberate movement
Crawl	When infant is placed on abdomen, he makes crawling movements with arms and legs; disappears at about age 6 weeks (Fig. 8-14)
Placing	When infant is held upright under arms and dorsal side of foot is briskly placed against hard object, such as table, leg lifts as if foot is stepping on table; age of disappearance varies

A

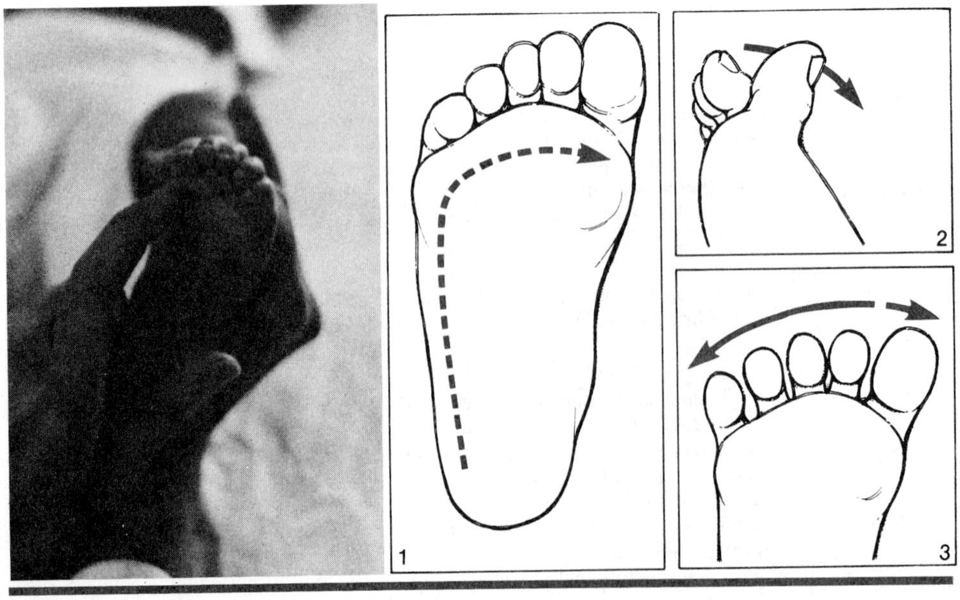

B

Fig. 8-10. A, Plantar or grasp reflex. **B,** Babinski reflex. *1,* Direction of stroke. *2,* Dorsiflexion of big toe. *3,* Fanning of toes.

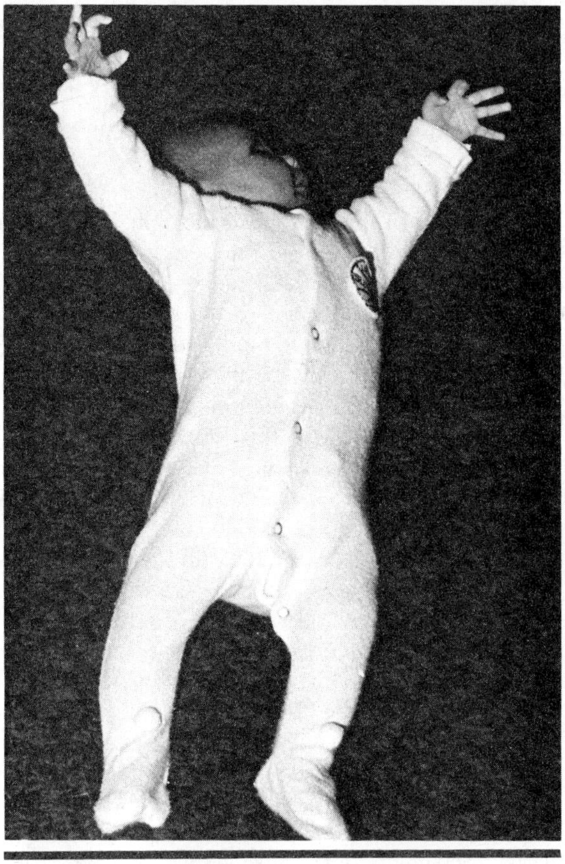

Fig. 8-11. Moro reflex.

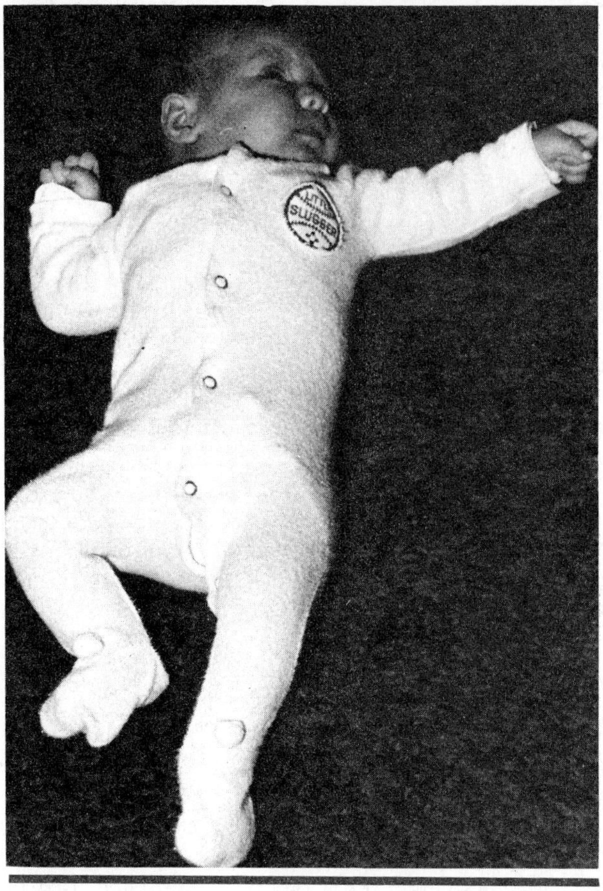

Fig. 8-12. Tonic neck reflex.

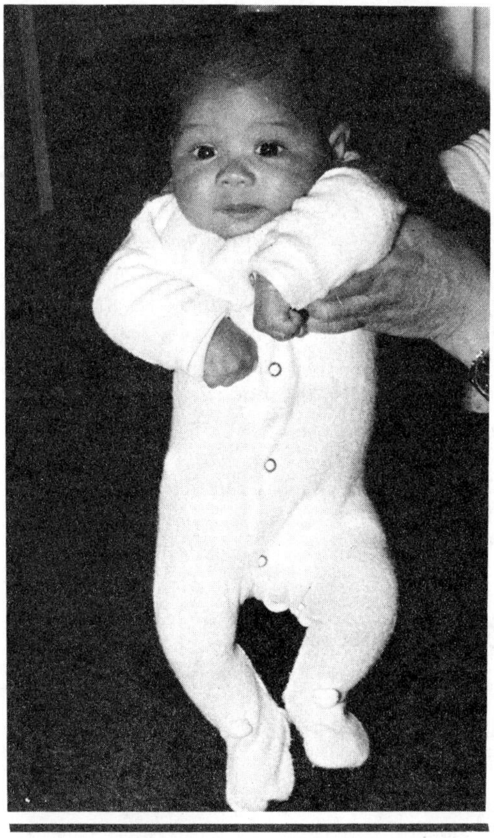

Fig. 8-13. Dance reflex.

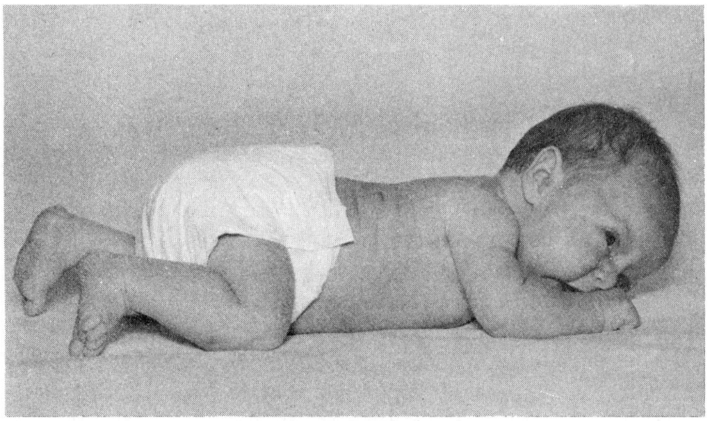

Fig. 8-14. Crawl reflex.

The extremities are inspected for evidence of fractures from birth trauma. The humerus and femur are most commonly involved. Limitation of movement, visible deformity, asymmetry of reflexes, and malposition of the site suggest a fracture.

Muscle tone is also assessed. By attempting to extend a flexed extremity, the nurse determines if tone is equal bilaterally. Extension of any extremity is usually met with resistance, and, when released, the extremity will return to its previous flexed position. *Hypotonia* suggests some degree of hypoxia, neurologic disorder, or Down syndrome. Asymmetric muscle tone may indicate a degree of paralysis from brain damage. Failure to move the lower limbs suggests a spinal cord lesion or injury. *Tremors, twitches,* and *myoclonic jerks* characterize neonatal seizures or may indicate neonatal narcotic withdrawal syndrome. Quivering or momentary tremors are usually normal (see Neonatal Seizures, Chapter 10).

NEUROLOGIC ASSESSMENT

Assessing neurologic status is a critical part of the physical examination of the newborn. Much of the neurologic testing takes place during evaluation of body systems, such as eliciting localized reflexes and observing posture, muscle tone, head control, and movement. However, several important mass (total body) reflexes also need to be elicited. They are usually left until the end of the examination because they may disturb the infant and interfere with auscultation. These reflexes, as well as several local reflexes, are described in Table 8-4. Deviations are indicated by absence, asymmetry, persistence, or weakness of a reflex.

BEHAVIORAL ASSESSMENT

Only about a decade ago, newborns were described as primitive beings who reacted to the environment through reflexes and had little ability to influence the environment around them. Now studies are increasingly demonstrating newborns' ability to react to various stimuli willfully and to greatly affect how others relate to them. The ability to respond to stimulation of all the senses and integrate them is collectively termed *behavior*. The Brazelton Neonatal Behavioral Assessment Scale is an instrument designed to objectively and systematically record behavior responses of newborns (see p. 340). The principal areas of behavior for newborns are sleep, wakefulness, and activity, such as crying.

Patterns of Sleep and Activity

Newborns begin life with a systematic schedule of sleep and activity that is initially evident during the periods of reactivity. For the first hour infants born of unmedicated mothers spend 60% of the time in the quiet alert state and only 10% of the time in the irritable crying state (Saigal and others, 1981). They are intensely alert, the eyes are wide open, and sucking behavior is vigorous. They then become quiet and relatively unresponsive to either internal or external stimuli and fall asleep for a few minutes to 2 to 4 hours. On awakening, they may be hyperresponsive to stimuli. For the next 2 to 3 days it is not unusual for infants to sleep almost constantly in order to recover from the exhausting birth process.

The infant's sleep comprises five distinct states,* which are summarized in Table 8-5. The cycle of these sleep states is highly variable and is based on the number of hours an infant sleeps per day, which may range anywhere from 10 to 23 hours (average of 16½ hours). About 50% of total sleep time is spent in irregular or rapid eye movement (REM) sleep. Sleep periods last 20 minutes to 6 hours with little day-night differentiation (Ferber, 1987).

States of sleep and periods of activity are highly influenced by environmental stimuli. As early as the immediate postbirth period, state is influenced by type of care. The sleep of infants in mothers' rooms is significantly more quiet, and they cry less than infants in the nursery (Keefe, 1987). It is especially important for parents to understand these states and the methods effective in altering them. An aware infant exhibits more motor activity before feeding than after. Feeding usually terminates the state of crying when hunger is the cause. Usually swaddling or wrapping an infant snugly in a blanket both promotes sleep and maintains body temperature. Some studies have focused on the effects of rocking on state. Intermittent, vertical rocking promotes more bright-alert behavior, whereas continuous, horizontal rocking induces more drowsy behavior (Byrne and Horowitz, 1981).

Cry

The newborn should begin extrauterine life with a strong, lusty cry. Variations in this initial cry can indicate abnormalities. A weak, groaning cry or grunt during expiration usually indicates severe respiratory disturbances. Absent, weak, or constant crying suggests brain damage. A high-pitched, shrill cry may be a sign of increased intracranial pressure.

The sounds produced by crying can be classified into two groups, those of discomfort and of comfort. Discomfort sounds consist initially of gasps and cries in which the consonant "H" is clearly distinguishable. Later the sounds of "W" and "L" are added. The almost universal "mama" sound is usually associated with much discomfort and is readily recognized by mothers.

The duration of crying is as highly variable in each infant as is the duration of sleep patterns. Some newborns may cry as little as 5 minutes or as much as 2 hours or more daily.

■ NURSING CARE OF THE NEWBORN AND FAMILY

The main nursing goal for newborns is provision of physical care, specifically the promotion and maintenance of ho-

**State* refers to an interaction between the infant and the environment in which the infant's behaviors form a continuum from arousal to consciousness (Keefe and others, 1989).

Table 8-5 States of sleep and activity

STATE/BEHAVIOR*	DURATION	IMPLICATIONS FOR PARENTING
Regular sleep		
Closed eyes Regular breathing No movement except for sudden bodily jerks	4-5 hours/day, 10-20 minutes/sleep cycle	External stimuli do not arouse infant Continue usual house noises Leave infant alone, if sudden loud noise awakens infant and child cries
Irregular sleep		
Closed eyes Irregular breathing Slight muscular twitching of body	12-15 hours/day, 20-45 minutes/sleep cycle	External stimuli that did not arouse infant during regular sleep may minimally arouse the child Periodic groaning or crying is usual; do not interpret as an indication of pain or discomfort
Drowsiness		
Eyes may be open Irregular breathing Active body movement	Variable	Most stimuli arouse infant Pick infant up during this time rather than leave in crib
Alert inactivity		
Responds to environment by active body movement and staring at close-range objects	2-3 hours/day	Satisfy infant's needs such as hunger Place infant in area of home where activity is continuous Place toys in crib or playpen Place objects within 17.5-20 cm (7-8 inches) of infant's view
Waking and crying		
May begin with whimpering and slight body movement Progresses to strong, angry crying, and uncoordinated thrashing of extremities	1-4 hours/day	Remove intense internal or external stimuli Stimuli that were effective during alert inactivity are usually ineffective Rock and swaddle to decrease crying

*Some classifications divide the fifth state into two states: alert with activity and crying.

meostasis or body equilibrium. For the family the principal objective is promotion of psychologic care—in particular, the promotion of parent-infant attachment and integration of the newborn into the family system.

PROVISION OF PHYSICAL CARE

Physical care for newborn includes: (1) maintenance of a patent airway, (2) maintenance of a stable body temperature, (3) protection from infection and injury, and (4) provision of optimum nutrition. The focus of care is in the nursery rather than the delivery room. Readers who are interested in a more detailed discussion of the immediate care of the neonate are referred to the many excellent maternity texts.

Maintain a Patent Airway

Establishing a patent airway is a primary objective in the delivery room and is the responsibility of the attending physicians and obstetric nurses. However, maintaining a patent airway continues to be a priority goal in the nursery with attention to proper positioning of the infant to facilitate drainage of secretions, especially after feeding (see Fig. 8-18). A bulb syringe is kept near the infant and is used if suctioning is required. Used bulb syringes should be replaced every 24 hours in the hospital and boiled for 10 minutes when used in the home to prevent bacterial contamination (Patel and others, 1988).*

NURSING ALERT To avoid aspiration of amniotic fluid or mucus, the pharynx is cleared first, then the nasal passages. The bulb is compressed *before* insertion to prevent forcing secretions into the bronchi.

If more forceful removal of secretions is required, mechanical suction is used. The use of the proper size catheter and correct suctioning technique is essential in order to prevent mucosal damage and edema. Gentle suctioning is necessary to prevent reflex bradycardia, laryngospasm, and cardiac arrhythmias from vagal stimulation. Suctioning is performed for 5 seconds to prevent depletion of the infant's oxygen supply.

In some nurseries the stomach is routinely lavaged to remove amniotic fluid that may cause abdominal distention and interfere with the establishment of respiration. Passing a catheter to the stomach also rules out esophageal atresia.

*Home care instructions for using a bulb syringe are available in Wong, D., and Whaley, L.: Clinical manual of pediatric nursing, ed. 3, St. Louis, 1990, Mosby–Year Book, Inc.

NURSING CARE PLAN
The Normal Newborn and Family

NURSING DIAGNOSIS: Ineffective airway clearance related to excess mucus, improper positioning

GOAL 1
Establish and maintain a patent airway

INTERVENTIONS
Suction mouth and nasopharynx with bulb syringe as needed
Lavage stomach of amniotic fluid and check for tracheoesophageal anomalies (not routinely done in all hospitals)
Position infant on side or abdomen with head slightly lower than chest (about 15 degrees) to facilitate drainage of secretions
Perform as few procedures as possible on infant during first hour and have oxygen ready for use if respiratory distress should develop
Take vital signs according to institutional policy and more frequently if necessary
Position infant on right side or abdomen after feeding to prevent aspiration
Keep diapers, clothing, and blankets loose enough to allow maximum lung (abdominal) expansion
Clean nares of any crusted secretions during bath or when necessary
Check for patent nares

EXPECTED OUTCOMES
Airway remains patent
Breathing is regular and unlabored
Respiratory rate is within normal limits (see inside front cover for normal limits)

NURSING DIAGNOSIS: Potential altered body temperature related to immature temperature control, change in environmental temperature

GOAL 1
Maintain stable body temperature

INTERVENTIONS
Wrap infant snugly in a warmed blanket
Place infant in a preheated environment (under radiant warmer or next to mother)
Place infant on a padded, covered surface
Take infant's temperature on arrival at nursery or mother's room; proceed according to hospital policy regarding method and frequency of monitoring
Maintain room temperature between 24° and 25.5° C (75° to 78° F) and humidity about 40% to 50%
Give initial bath according to hospital policy
  Prevent chilling of infant during daily bath
  Postpone bath if there is any question regarding stabilization of body temperature
Dress infant in a shirt and diaper and swaddle in a blanket or cover with blanket
Provide infant with a head covering if heat loss is a problem
Keep infant away from drafts, air conditioning vents, or fans
Place infant in a recessed cubicle with walls high enough to shield from cross ventilation
Warm all objects used to examine or cover infant, for example, place them under radiant warmer
Uncover only one area of body for examination or procedures
Postpone circumcision until after postnatal recovery period
Be alert to signs of hypothermia or hyperthermia

EXPECTED OUTCOME
Infant's temperature remains at optimum level (36.5° to 37.5° C [97.7° to 99.5° F])

NURSING DIAGNOSIS: Potential for infection related to deficient immunologic defenses, environmental factors

GOAL 1
Protect infant from infection

INTERVENTIONS
Wash hands before and after caring for each infant
Make certain appropriate eye prophylaxis has been carried out
Keep infant from potential sources of infection, e.g., persons with respiratory or skin infections, improperly prepared food sources, other unclean items
Clean vulva in posterior direction to prevent fecal contamination of vagina or urethra; stress this to parents
While cleaning penis, do not retract foreskin; gently wipe away smegma
Maintain asepsis during circumcision
*If infant has been circumcised, cover area with a petrolatum jelly gauze (if ordered)
Keep umbilical stump clean and dry
  Place diapers below umbilical stump
  Assess cord daily for odor, color, and drainage
Check eyes daily for evidence of inflammation or discharge
*Apply antibacterial agent or alcohol or both to cord as ordered

EXPECTED OUTCOMES
Infant exhibits no evidence of infection
Eyes remain clear with no evidence of irritation
Genital area is free of irritation
Cord appears dry, surrounding area free of infection

*Dependent nursing action.

NURSING DIAGNOSIS: Potential for trauma related to physical helplessness

GOAL 1

Ensure infant's identity

INTERVENTIONS

Make certain infant is properly identified
- Ensure that identification bracelet(s) properly and securely placed

Check often to ensure correct infant identity

EXPECTED OUTCOMES

Infant is identified
Identification bracelet remains in place

GOAL 2

Prevent physical injury

INTERVENTIONS

Never leave infant unsupervised on a raised surface without sides
Always close diaper pins and place them away from infant's body
Keep pointed or sharp objects out of infant's reach
Keep own fingernails short and trimmed; avoid jewelry that can scratch infant
Employ appropriate methods of handling and transporting infant

EXPECTED OUTCOME

Infant remains free of physical injury

GOAL 3

Prevent bleeding

INTERVENTIONS

*Administer vitamin K intramuscularly, using vastus lateralis muscle as site of injection
Check circumcision site; assess any oozing

EXPECTED OUTCOME

Infant exhibits no evidence of bleeding

NURSING DIAGNOSIS: Altered nutrition: less than body requirements (potential) related to immaturity, parental knowledge deficit

GOAL 1

Prepare for feeding

INTERVENTIONS

Determine parental feeding preference (breast or bottle)
Offer initial intake according to hospital policy, practitioner's protocol, and individual preference
Assess strength of suck and coordination with swallowing

EXPECTED OUTCOMES

Family determines feeding method
Infant demonstrates strong suck

GOAL 2

Provide optimum nutrition

INTERVENTIONS

Prepare for demand feeding of breast-fed infants; night feedings determined by condition and preferences of the mother
Offer bottle-fed infants 2 to 3 ounces of formula every 3 to 4 hours or on demand
Support and assist breast-feeding mothers during initial feedings
Avoid routine water or supplemental feedings for breast-feeding infants
Encourage father or other supportive person to remain with mother to help her and infant with positioning, relaxation, and reinforcement
Encourage father to participate in bottle-feeding
Place infant on right side after feeding to prevent regurgitation
Observe stool pattern

EXPECTED OUTCOMES

Infant retains feedings
Infant receives an adequate amount of nutrients (specify amount and frequency of feedings)
Infant loses less than 10% of birth weight

NURSING DIAGNOSIS: Altered family processes related to maturational crisis, birth of term infant, change in family unit

GOAL 1

Facilitate parent-infant attachment process

INTERVENTIONS

As soon after delivery as possible, encourage parents to see and hold infant; place newborn close to face of parents so that visual contact can be established
Ideally, perform eye care after initial meeting of infant and parents, within 1 hour after birth
Identify for parents specific behaviors manifested by infant, for example, alertness, ability to see, vigorous suck, rooting behavior, and attention to human voice
Discuss with parents their expectations of fantasy child vs real child, if indicated
Encourage parents to "talk out" their labor and delivery experience; identify any events that signify loss of control to either parent, especially mother
Identify behavioral steps in attachment process and evaluate those aspects that could be considered positive and those that may represent inadequate or delayed parenting
Encourage family to call for infant frequently if not rooming-in
Observe and assess the reciprocity of cues between infant and parent

*Dependent nursing action.

Continued.

NURSING CARE PLAN
The Normal Newborn and Family—cont'd

Assist parents in recognizing attention-nonattention cycles and in understanding their significance
Assess variables affecting development of attachment through observing infant and parent and interviewing each parent or other significant caregiver

EXPECTED OUTCOMES

Parents establish contact with infant immediately or soon after birth
Parents demonstrate attachment behaviors, such as touch, eye contact, naming and calling infant by name, talking to infant, participating in caregiving activities
Parents recognize attention-nonattention cycles

GOAL 2

Facilitate siblings' adjustment to newborn

INTERVENTIONS

Allow to visit and touch newborn when feasible
Explain physical differences in newborn, such as bald head, umbilical stump and clamp, circumcision
Explain to siblings realistic expectations regarding newborn abilities and needs
  Requires complete care
  Is not a playmate
Encourage siblings to participate in care at home
Encourage parents to spend individual time with other children at home

EXPECTED OUTCOME

Siblings express interest in newborn and realistic expectations for their age

GOAL 3

Prepare for discharge and home care

INTERVENTIONS

Instruct in newborn care
  Feeding (formula or breast)
  Bathing
  Umbilical and circumcision care
  Recognize states of activity for optimum interaction (see Table 8-5)
Encourage participation in parenting classes, if offered
Discuss importance and proper use of federally approved car restraints
  Refer to organizations that may rent car restraints
If parent-infant attachment is at risk, refer to appropriate agencies (social services, family and child services, at-risk programs)

EXPECTED OUTCOMES

Family demonstrates ability to provide care for infant
Family keeps appointments for follow-up care
Infant rides home in federally approved car restraint
Family members avail themselves of needed services

Vital signs are closely monitored, and any indication of respiratory distress is immediately reported.

Maintain Stable Body Temperature

Conserving the newborn's body heat is an essential nursing goal. Heat conservation requires an understanding of the causes of heat loss—evaporation, radiation, conduction, and convection. Nursing care is based on preventing heat loss through these mechanisms.

At birth a major cause of heat loss is *evaporation,* the loss of heat through moisture. The amniotic fluid that bathes the infant's skin favors evaporation, especially when combined with the cool atmosphere of the delivery room. Heat loss through evaporation is minimized by rapidly drying the skin and hair with a warmed towel and placing the infant in a heated environment.

Another source of heat loss is by way of *radiation,* the loss of heat to cooler solid objects in the environment that are not in direct contact with the infant. Loss of heat through radiation increases as these solid objects become colder and closer to the infant. The temperature of ambient or surrounding air in the Isolette or incubator essentially has no effect on loss of heat through radiation. This is a critical point to remember when attempting to maintain a constant temperature for the infant because, even though the temperature of the ambient air is optimum, the infant can be hypothermic.

An example of radiant heat loss is the placement of the incubator close to a cold window or air conditioning unit. The cold from either source will cool the walls of the incubator and subsequently the body of the neonate. To prevent this, the infant is placed as far away as possible from walls, windows, or ventilating units. If heat loss continues to be a problem, a radiant warmer may be placed over the infant or the infant and mother.

Heat loss can also occur through conduction and convection. *Conduction* involves loss of heat from the body from direct contact of skin with a cooler solid object; it is minimized by placing the infant on a padded, covered surface rather than directly on a hard table and by providing insulation through clothes and blankets. Placing the newborn very close to the mother, such as in her arms or on her abdomen immediately after delivery, is physically beneficial in terms of conserving heat, as well as fostering maternal attachment.

Convection is similar to conduction, except that heat

loss is aided by surrounding air currents. For example, placing the infant in the direct flow of air from a fan or air conditioner vent causes rapid heat loss through convection. Transporting the neonate in a crib with solid sides reduces airflow around the infant.

Protect from Infection and Injury

The most important practice for preventing cross-infection is through handwashing of all individuals involved in the infant's care. Although the use of cover gowns is a common nursing ritual, there is no evidence that cover gowns decrease infection (Rush and others, 1990). Several other procedures to prevent infection include eye care, bathing, and care of the circumcision or umbilical stump. Vitamin K is administered to protect against hemorrhage. In addition, several safety measures are practiced, particularly in terms of proper identification, and screening tests are used to detect genetic disorders such as phenylketonuria and hypothyroidism.

Identification. Proper identification of the newborn is the responsibility of the delivery room nurse. However, upon the infant's admission to the nursery, the nursery nurse *must* check that two identifying bands are securely fastened, usually on the wrist and ankle, and verify the information (name, sex, mother's admission number, date, and time of birth) against the birth records and the child's actual sex. When the infant is brought to the mother, she should also be asked to verify the information on the identification bands and the child's sex.

Eye care. Prophylactic eye treatment against *ophthalmia neonatorum,* infectious conjunctivitis of the newborn, includes the use of (1) silver nitrate (1%) solution, (2) erythromycin (0.5%) ophthalmic ointment or drops, or (3) tetracycline (1%) ophthalmic ointment or drops (preferably in single-dose ampules or tubes). The drug of choice has been either erythromycin or tetracycline because both were thought to afford protection against *Chlamydia trachomatis,* a major cause of ophthalmia neonatorum. Although silver nitrate is effective against gonococcal conjunctivitis, it is ineffective against *Chlamydia* and can cause a severe chemical conjunctivitis (American Academy of Pediatrics, Report of the Committee on Infectious Diseases, 1988). However, there is accumulating evidence that neither erythromycin nor tetracycline significantly reduces the incidence of chlamydial conjunctivitis. Effective prophylaxis may be better directed at treating maternal chlamydial infection (Hammerschlag and others, 1989; Recommendations and Reports, 1989).

Since studies on maternal attachment emphasize that in the first hour of life a newborn has a greater ability to focus on coordinated movement than at any other time during the next several days and since eye-to-eye contact is very important in the development of maternal-infant bonding, the routine administration of silver nitrate or antibiotics can be postponed up to 1 hour. However, there must be some kind of checklist to ensure that the drug is given within this time.

Bathing. The bath time can be an opportunity for the nurse to accomplish much more than general hygiene. It is an excellent time for observations of the infant's behavior, such as irritability, state of arousal, alertness, and muscular activity. Bathing is done after the vital signs have stabilized. There is no need to immediately wash a newborn, except to remove blood from the face and head. In addition, there may be some benefit to leaving the vernix on the skin. Proposed but unproven benefits include its insulating and lubricating properties. Cleansing only grossly soiled areas with soap and water rather than giving a daily bath does not increase infection rates in the hospital (Rush, 1986).

The bath time provides an opportunity for the nurse to involve the parents in the care of their child, to teach correct hygiene procedures, and to learn about their infant's individual characteristics (Fig. 8-15). The appropriate types of bathing supplies and the need for safety in terms of water temperature and supervision of the infant at all times during the bath are stressed. For example, if sponges are used, they need to dry thoroughly between each use (may require a clothes dryer) to prevent growth of organisms (Sheth and others, 1986).

Box 8-3 GUIDELINES FOR OPHTHALMIA NEONATORUM PROPHYLAXIS

1. Clean the eyelids with sterile cotton and sterile water if needed.
2. Separate lids and apply 2 drops or at least 1 to 2 cm (½ inch) of ointment in each conjunctival sac.
3. Massage lids to ensure spread of the medication.
4. Wipe excess medication from eye with sterile cotton 1 minute after application.
5. Do not rinse eyes with sterile normal saline.

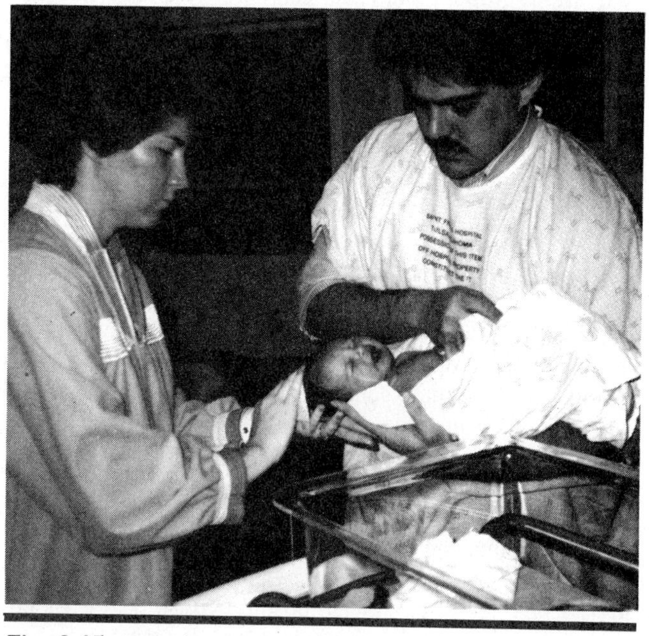

Fig. 8-15. Bath time is an excellent opportunity for parents to learn about their newborn.

Parents are encouraged to examine every finger and toe of their infant during bathing. Frequently normal variations such as Epstein pearls, mongolian spots, or "stork bites" cause parents much worry because they are unaware of the insignificance of such findings. Minor birth injuries may appear as major defects to them. Explaining how these occurred and when they will disappear reassures parents of their infant's normalcy. Common variations are discussed further in Chapter 9.

One of the most important considerations in skin cleansing is preservation of the skin's "acid mantle," which is formed from the uppermost horny layer of the epidermis, sweat, superficial fat, metabolic products, and external substances such as amniotic fluid, microorganisms, and cosmetics. The infant's skin surface has a pH of about 4.95 soon after birth, and the bacteriostatic effects of this pH are significant. Consequently, only plain warm water should be used for the bath. Alkaline soaps such as Ivory, oils, powder, and lotions are not used because they alter the acid mantle, thus providing a medium for bacterial growth. Talcum has the added risk of aspiration if it is applied too close to the infant's face (see Questions and Controversies, p. 623).

Cleansing proceeds in the cephalocaudal direction. A washcloth is used and turned so that a clean part touches the skin with each stroke. The eyes are carefully wiped from the inner to the outer aspect of the lid. The face is cleansed next. The nares are carefully inspected for any crusted secretions. The scalp is usually wiped, although it is sometimes necessary to shampoo the hair. Shampooing is best accomplished by positioning the infant's head over a small basin, lathering the scalp with a mild soap, and rinsing by pouring water from a small vessel over the head into the basin. The rest of the body should be covered during this procedure. The head is dried quickly in order to prevent heat loss from evaporation. The ears are cleaned with the twisted end of a washcloth.

The rest of the body is washed in a similar manner. Although the infant's skin requires little rubbing for adequate cleansing, certain areas (e.g., folds of neck, axillae, and creases at joints) need special attention. The area around the neck is especially prone to a rash from regurgitation of feeding and should be thoroughly washed and dried.

The genitalia of both sexes require careful cleansing. Cleansing of the vulva is done in a front-to-back direction. The bath is a perfect opportunity to stress this part of hygiene to the mother, for both the infant's and her protection against urinary tract infection.

Cleansing the male genitalia involves washing the penis and scrotum. Sometimes smegma needs to be removed by wiping around the glans. The foreskin is not retracted because it is normally tight in newborns. If the infant is not to be circumcised, the parents are taught how to cleanse under and around the foreskin by *retracting it gently only as far as it will go* and returning it to its normal position. Leaving the prepuce in a retracted position constricts the blood vessels supplying the glans penis, causing edema.

The buttocks and anal area are thoroughly cleansed of any fecal material. As with the rest of the body, the area is dried to prevent a warm, moist environment that fosters growth of bacteria.

Diapers are applied after the bath. They should fit snugly around the thighs and abdomen to prevent urine from leak-

QUESTIONS AND CONTROVERSIES

What are the advantages and disadvantages of disposable vs cloth diapers?

In the United States, the most commonly used diapers are disposable, home-laundered, or commercially laundered diapers. A number of factors—cost, convenience, skin care benefits, and environmental concerns—influence the relative merits of these three diaper types. Cost comparisons among cloth diapers and disposable diapers vary according to methods of comparison and sources of information (Lehrberger, 1989; Little, 1990). In general, home-laundered diapers are the least expensive when home labor cost is not included. Once home labor cost is included, the price difference between disposable diapers, diaper service reusable diapers, and home-laundered diapers is quite small. Disposable diapers are the most convenient, although a diaper service eliminates the need to shop for additional diapers.

Several studies provide considerable evidence that disposable diapers with absorbent gelling material (AGM) have benefits related to preserving healthy skin. In a comparison of infants wearing disposable diapers with AGM, conventional disposable diapers (no AGM), and home-laundered diapers, the AGM-diapered infants had the lowest degrees of diaper dermatitis (Campbell and others, 1987). Other studies that compared only AGM diapers with conventional disposable diapers also found significantly less diaper dermatitis in the AGM group (Campbell and others, 1988; Lane, Rehder, and Helm, 1990). Similar skin benefits with the use of AGM diapers have also been observed in infants with atopic dermatitis (Seymour and others, 1987).

The most controversial issue surrounding the discussion of disposable vs cloth diapers is their effect on the environment. Disposable diapers are discarded as solid waste in landfills, whereas waste from laundered diapers is disposed of as treated sewage. The main differences between solid waste and treated sewage are cost and possibly sanitation, with solid waste being more expensive. However, the manufacture and disposal of both kinds of diapers use energy resources and impact the environment differently, so that the issues are much more complex than simple comparisons make them appear. In addition, the infection transmission risks related to solid waste disposal are theoretic; to date, soiled diapers as solid waste have not caused a public health problem (Lehrberger, 1989; Little, 1990).* In the health care setting, cloth diapers might have unexpected disadvantages. Cloth diapers produce significantly more dust than disposable diapers—a factor that may be important to infants in closed environments, such as incubators (Hashimoto, 1987).

*A pamphlet for families is *Answers to Your Questions About the Environment,* available from The National Association of Pediatric Nurse Associates and Practitioners (NAPNAP), 1101 Kings Highway North, Suite 206, Cherry Hill, NJ 08034; (609) 667-1773; a similar pamphlet is available from Procter & Gamble, One Procter & Gamble Plaza, Cincinnati, OH 45202; (800) 543-0480 or (513) 983-1100.

ing. In males cloth diapers are folded with extra thickness in the front to provide greater absorbency. In females the placement of the extra fold depends on whether the infant is prone or supine. Diapers are fastened with the back side overlapping the front side to allow full flexion of the hips. The nurse should discuss the choice of cloth or disposable diapers with parents, stressing the advantages and disadvantages of the different types (see Questions and Controversies on opposite page).

Care of the umbilicus. Because the umbilical stump is an excellent medium for bacterial growth, various methods of cord care are practiced. None has proved to be superior, although one study found the topical application of triple dye (a solution of brilliant green, proflavine hemisulfate, and crystal violet) to be more effective than bacitracin ointment (Andrich and Golden, 1984). Also the use of povidone-iodine increases plasma iodide levels, which may suppress thyroid secretion (Newman, 1989; Ramsey and Svee, 1989). Regardless of the type of treatment, the diaper is placed below the cord to avoid irritation and wetness on the site.

Parents are instructed regarding stump deterioration and proper umbilical care. The stump deteriorates through the process of dry gangrene. Cord separation time is influenced by a number of factors, including type of cord care, type of delivery, and other perinatal events (Gladstone and others, 1988; Novack, Mueller, and Ochs, 1988; Oudesluys-Murphy and DeGroot, 1988):

- Average separation time of 14 days using triple dye daily during hospitalization; average time of 10 days using povidone-iodine applied daily until cord separation; average separation time of 7 days using only a dry gauze dressing
- Earlier separation in vaginal than in cesarean birth
- Delayed separation in infants with hyperbilirubinemia and septicemia

It takes a few more weeks for the cord base to heal completely following cord separation. During this time care consists of keeping the cord clean and dry and may include wiping the base with alcohol. Any signs of infection, such as presence of erythema and malodorous, purulent discharge, are reported.

Circumcision. Circumcision is the surgical removal of the foreskin on the glans penis. In the Jewish culture circumcision is performed during a highly significant ceremony called a *berith,* or *brit,* which takes place on the eighth day of life. A rabbi skilled in the procedure usually performs the circumcision. However, usually circumcision is routinely done in the hospital, although it is not a common practice in most countries. Despite the frequency of the procedure in the United States, there is much controversy regarding the benefits and risks (see Questions and Controversies at right).

In light of these arguments, parents must be allowed an *informed* consent regarding circumcision. Ideally prospective parents should have the opportunity to examine all the facts and to decide for themselves without unnecessary pressure from the educator or physician.

Circumcision is usually performed in the nursery. It

QUESTIONS AND CONTROVERSIES

What are the risks and benefits of neonatal circumcision?

Probably no routine surgical procedure has engendered more public and professional debate in the United States than neonatal circumcision. Since 1975 the American Academy of Pediatrics opposed routine neonatal circumcision on the grounds that there were no valid medical indications for the procedure and that a program of good personal hygiene offered all the advantages of circumcision without the attendant surgical risks. However, in 1989 the Academy reversed its position, stating that "newborn circumcision has potential medical benefits and advantages as well as disadvantages and risks." The statement does not recommend the procedure, but leaves the decision to the parents after they are "fully informed" of the risks and benefits (American Academy of Pediatrics, Task Force on Circumcision, 1989).

Arguments for circumcision include prevention of penile cancer, posthitis (inflammation of prepuce), and balanoposthitis (inflammation of glans and prepuce); decreased incidence of balanitis (inflammation of glans); and prevention of complications associated with later circumcision (Herzog and Alvarez, 1986; Kochen and McCurdy, 1980; Larsen and Williams, 1990). There is evidence that circumcision significantly decreases the incidence of urinary tract infection in infant males (Herzog, 1989; Wiswell and Geschke, 1989), as well as some sexually transmitted diseases later in life (Schoen, 1990). While these proposed medical benefits are widely publicized, not all authorities believe that they are completely substantiated (Lohr, 1989; Poland, 1990; Winberg and others, 1989). A nonmedical consideration is preservation of a male's body image that is consistent with his peers, since circumcision is such a common practice in the United States. For many parents the strongest motivating factor for deciding on circumcision for their newborn is the father's circumcision status (Brown and Brown, 1987).

Although neonatal circumcision is a relatively safe procedure when performed by skilled practitioners, it has its risks. Complications include hemorrhage, infection, dehiscence (separation of approximated skin edges), meatitis from loss of protective foreskin, adhesions, concealed penis, urethral fistula, and meatal stenosis. Most studies have used retrospective methods (chart reviews) to assess the incidence of postoperative complications, with one recent study reporting a rate of 0.19% (Wiswell and Geschke, 1989). However, the overall complication rate may be considerably higher. When data were collected prospectively (direct observation following the procedure), the overall rate was 7.7% (Infant circumcision, 1989). This difference in reported rates points out the need for more prospective studies, with emphasis on causes for various complications.

Another adverse effect of circumcision is the pain inflicted on the infant. Recent studies on the use of regional anesthesia document the distress exhibited in unanesthetized infants, such as increased heart rate, behavior changes, prolonged crying, increased cortisol levels, and decreased blood oxygenation (Dixon and others, 1984; Maxwell and others, 1987; Stang and others, 1988). In each of these studies the use of penile dorsal nerve block significantly reduced these signs of distress and produced no serious complications. Despite the favorable findings, the American Academy of Pediatrics did not endorse the use of a nerve block or any other type of anesthetic (American Academy of Pediatrics, Task Force on Circumcision, 1989). This is in contrast to their earlier statement on neonatal anesthesia, which recommends the use of anesthesia for newborns undergoing surgical procedures (American Academy of Pediatrics, 1987). Unfortunately, the use of nonpharmacologic pain reducers (pacifier, distraction) has not been found to be effective in reducing physiologic distress (Gunnar, Fisch, and Malone, 1984; Marchette, Main, and Redick, 1989).

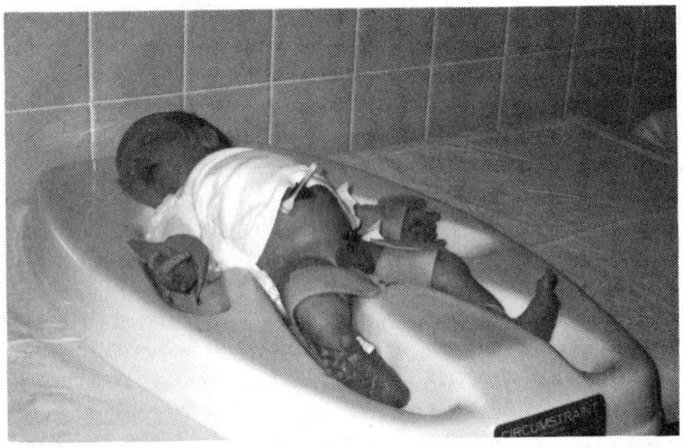

Fig. 8-16. Proper positioning of infant in circumstraint.

should not be performed immediately after delivery because of the neonate's unstabilized physiologic status and increased susceptibility to stress. Preoperative nursing care includes allowing the infant nothing by mouth before the procedure to prevent aspiration of vomitus (about 2 hours), checking for a signed consent form, and adequately restraining the infant, usually on a special board (Fig. 8-16). All the equipment used for the procedure, such as gloves, instruments, alcohol wipes, dressings, and draping towels, must be sterile.

The procedure involves freeing the foreskin from the glans penis by using a scalpel, Gomco clamp, or Hollister Plastibell. In the Gomco technique the foreskin is clamped and removed; the clamp crushes the nerve endings and blood vessels, promoting hemostasis. In the Plastibell procedure the foreskin is removed using a plastic ring and a string tied around the foreskin like a tourniquet. The excess foreskin is trimmed. In about 5 to 8 days the plastic ring separates and falls off.

As soon as the procedure is completed, the infant is released from the restraints and comforted. Since parents are often concerned about the infant's well-being during this time, they are informed of the infant's status. As soon as the infant is calmed and stabilized, he can be brought to the parents.

Care of the circumcision depends on the type of procedure. If a clamp was used, a petrolatum gauze dressing may be applied loosely to prevent adherence to the diaper. If the Plastibell was applied, no special dressing is required. Since the area is tender, the diaper is applied loosely to prevent friction against the penis; the first void is recorded (see Nursing Tip). Normally on the second day a yellowish-white exudate forms as part of the granulating process. This is not a sign of infection and should not be forcibly removed. As healing progresses, the exudate disappears. Parents are cautioned to report any evidence of bleeding or unusual swelling to the practitioner.

NURSING TIP: CHECKING FOR FIRST VOID AFTER CIRCUMCISION

To check for wetness in disposable diapers with absorbent gelling material, pinch crotch of diaper for "clumpy, doughy" feeling, since these diapers will feel dry despite voiding.

Vitamin K. Shortly after birth, vitamin K is administered intramuscularly to prevent hemorrhagic disease of the newborn (see Chapter 9). Normally, vitamin K is synthesized by the intestinal flora. However, since the infant's intestine is sterile at birth and since breast milk contains low levels of vitamin K, the supply is inadequate for at least the first 3 to 4 days. The major function of vitamin K is to catalyze the synthesis of prothrombin in the liver, which is needed for blood clotting and coagulation. The vastus lateralis muscle is the preferred injection site because of the absence of other well-developed muscle masses. Although injectable vitamin K is used in the United States, the oral form is as effective and less traumatic (Motohara and others, 1989; O'Connor and Addiego, 1986).

Screening for metabolic disease. A number of genetic metabolic disorders can be detected in the newborn period. There is no national policy in the United States; therefore the extent of neonatal screening is determined by state laws and voluntary guidelines. Most states require screening for phenylketonuria (PKU) and hypothyroidism (see Chapter 9). Other genetic diseases that may be tested for include galactosemia, maple syrup urine disease, homocystinuria, sickle cell anemia, and other hemoglobinopathies. The National Institutes of Health (1987) recommends the routine screening of all newborns for hemoglobinopathies to detect sickle cell anemia and initiate early treatment.

The nurse's responsibility is to educate parents regarding the importance of screening and to collect appropriate specimens at the recommended time. Follow-up of newborns discharged early or born at home is critical to prevent unidentified cases. (For information on several diseases that may be included in newborn screening, see American Academy of Pediatrics, Committee on Genetics, 1989).

Transportation after discharge. An important area of counseling is the safe transportation of the newborn home from the hospital. Ideally this counseling should occur *before* delivery to allow parents an opportunity to purchase a suitable infant care restraint. Hospitals and birthing centers should have policies regarding the safe discharge of a newborn in a car safety seat and provisions for parents to learn to use the device correctly (American Academy of Pediatrics, Committee on Accident and Poison Prevention, 1990.) Parents are more likely to use a restraint if the proper use of one is demonstrated and its necessity is stressed (Goodson, Buller, and Goodson, 1985). While federal safety standards do not specify the *minimum* weight of an infant and the appropriate type of restraint, newborns weighing 2 kg (4 pounds, 8 ounces) receive relatively good support in convertible seats with seat back to crotch strap height of 14 cm (5½ inches) or less. Rolled blankets and towels may be needed under the crotch to prevent slouching and can be placed along the sides to minimize lateral movement. Seats with shields (large padded surfaces in front of the child) and armrests (found on some other models) are unacceptable because of their proximity to the infant's face and neck (Bull and others, 1989). (For a discussion of appropriate car restraints for infants, see Chapter 14.)

Provide Optimum Nutrition

Selection of a feeding method is one of the major decisions faced by parents. In general there are three acceptable choices: human milk, commercially prepared cow's milk formula, and modified cow's milk. There are significant nutritional, economic, and psychologic advantages and differences among these methods (Box 8-4). Nurses need to be aware of the types of feeding to help parents choose the method that best meets their needs (see also Chapter 12).

Box 8-4 ADVANTAGES OF HUMAN MILK VS COW'S MILK

- Contains adequate (not excessive) protein; has greater quantities of certain amino acids, including cystine and taurine
- Contains more lactalbumin (produces easily digested curds) than casein (produces large, hard curds)
- Contains more lactose, which in the gut stimulates growth of microorganisms, which synthesize some B vitamins and produce organic acids that may retard growth of harmful bacteria
- Contains more monounsaturated fatty acids, which enhance absorption of fat and calcium
- Contains adequate (not excessive) minerals with exception of fluoride (low in both)
- Amounts of iron and zinc are low but more readily absorbed
- Contains less calcium and phosphorus but a more favorable ratio of the minerals, which prevents excessive calcium excretion
- Contains adequate amounts of vitamins A, B complex, and E; vitamin C content depends on maternal intake; vitamin D is low but more readily absorbed (vitamin C, D, and E are low in cow's milk, but K is higher)
- Contains growth modulators that modify growth or maturation
- Offers several immunologic benefits: contains various immunoglobulins (Ig), especially IgA; macrophages, granulocytes, T- and B-cell lymphocytes; and other factors that inhibit bacterial growth
- Has laxative effect
- Is economical, readily available, and sanitary
- Has psychologic benefits of close bond between infant and mother during feeding

Comparison of human milk and cow's milk. There are significant nutritional differences between human milk and whole cow's milk. Cow's milk contains much more available protein (3.5 g/dl) than human milk (0.7 g/dl), but more than the infant requires. The type of protein also differs. Human milk contains more whey proteins, especially lactalbumin, a more complete protein than casein protein. The higher percentage of casein in cow's milk results in formation of large, hard curds. Human milk is more easily digested because of the presence of soft, flocculent curds. Therefore, stomach emptying time is more rapid with human milk, necessitating more frequent feedings. Human milk also contains a higher amount of cystine, an amino acid essential during the first few weeks of life, because the enzyme cystathionase, which converts methionine to cystine, is very low in newborns. Taurine, a conditionally essential amino acid (necessary under certain conditions, such as fetal development and early infancy), is also present in larger amounts in human milk. Taurine is involved in fat metabolism, retinal development, and auditory maturation (Gaull, 1989; Tyson and others, 1989).

Cow's milk and human milk both provide 20 kcal/ounce, but human milk contains a higher amount of lactose, a disaccharide that is converted into the monosaccharides glucose and galactose. Galactose is essential for the formation of galactolipids, which are necessary for the growth of the central nervous system.

Although the amount of fat in both types of milk is similar, the type of fat differs. Human milk contains more monounsaturated fatty acids, especially linoleic acid, whereas cow's milk has more polysaturated fatty acids. Human milk has smaller fat globules than cow's milk, which enables the infant to absorb human milk fat more efficiently. In addition, the fat content of human milk varies during the feeding and with time of day. It is highest toward the end of feeding and at midday (Lawrence, 1989).

The mineral content of cow's milk is considerably greater than that of human milk, with the exception of iron and fluoride. Although the amount of iron is low in both types of milk, the iron in human milk is much better absorbed by the infant. Another difference is the amount of calcium and phosphorus, minerals especially needed by the rapidly growing infant. Cow's milk contains more of these minerals but a lower calcium/phosphorus ratio (1.5 to 1). Because of the infant's immature regulatory mechanisms, calcium is excreted, resulting in tetany. Human milk contains a smaller but more balanced proportion of these minerals and a higher calcium/phosphorus ratio (2 to 1), which are adequate to meet the infant's needs. Both types of milk contain adequate amounts of zinc, a mineral identified as essential to the human. However, the zinc in human milk is more readily absorbed. Both types of milk are low in fluoride and supplementation is recommended (see Fluoride, Chapter 14).

Both human and cow's milk provide adequate amounts of vitamins A and B complex. Vitamin C is low in cow's milk but higher in human milk, provided the mother's intake is adequate. Vitamin D is low in human milk but adequate, depending on the mother's intake and the infant's exposure to sunlight. Cow's milk and its preparations are usually fortified with vitamin D. Human milk contains only one quarter the amount of vitamin K as cow's milk, requiring supplementation at birth.

In addition to the nutritional differences between the two types of milk, other significant advantages to human milk exist. Recent evidence points to the presence of growth modulators, such as epidermal growth factor (EGF), that modify growth or differentiation. Although its role in human milk is still being defined, it appears that EGF stimulates DNA synthesis and intestinal tract maturation (Lawrence, 1989). Human milk also offers important immunologic advantages. It contains high levels of immunoglobulin A (IgA) and affords protection against several bacterial and viral diseases, especially those of the respiratory and gastrointestinal systems. IgA also probably protects against development of food allergies. In addition, human milk contains numerous other host defense factors, such as macrophages, granulocytes, and T- and B-lymphocytes (Hanson and others, 1985). Other physiologic benefits of human milk are its laxative effect and less irritation of the skin from stools. Nonphysiologic advantages are discussed under Breast-feeding.

Evaporated milk and commercially prepared formulas. The analysis of human and cow's milk shows that whole cow's milk is unsuitable for infant nutrition. It must be diluted to meet the lowered protein requirement, but, when dilute, it does not meet the caloric or fat requirement. Modified evaporated milk or commercially prepared formula is chosen as a substitute.

In the United States only a very small percentage of infants are fed evaporated milk formula. However, it has many advantages over whole milk. It is readily available in cans, needs no refrigeration if unopened, is less expensive than commercial formula, provides a softer, more digestible curd, and contains more lactalbumin and a higher calcium/phosphorus ratio. A common rule for preparing evaporated milk formula is diluting the 13-ounce can of milk with 17 ounces of water and adding 1 to 2 tablespoons of sugar or corn syrup.

Evaporated milk must not be confused with condensed milk, which is a form of evaporated milk with 45% more sugar. Because of its high carbohydrate concentration and disproportionately low fat and protein content, condensed milk is not used for infant feeding. Likewise, skim milk should not be used because it is deficient in caloric concentration, significantly increases the renal solute load and water demands, and deprives the body of essential fatty acids.

Commercially prepared formulas are milk-based formulas that have been modified to closely resemble human milk (Table 8-6). Although they are not an exact substitute, they do provide an optimum source of nutrition. The formu-

Table 8-6 Normal and special infant formulas

FORMULA (MANUFACTURER)	PROTEIN SOURCE	CARBOHYDRATE SOURCE	FAT SOURCE	INDICATIONS FOR USE	COMMENTS (NUTRITIONAL CONSIDERATIONS)
▪ Human and cow's milk formulas					
Human breast milk	Mature human milk; whey/casein ratio: 60:40	Lactose	Mature human milk	For all full-term infants except those with galactosemia; may be used with low-birth-weight infants	Recommended sole form of feeding for the first 5 to 6 months; nutritionally complete except for fluoride
Evaporated cow's milk formulas	Milk protein; whey/casein ratio: 18:82	Lactose, sucrose	Butterfat	For full-term infants with no special nutritional requirements; use of undiluted cow's milk after 6-12 months controversial	Supplement with iron and vitamin C; A and D if not fortified; fluoride if fluoridated water is not used for formula preparation
▪ Commercial infant formulas					
SMA (Wyeth)	Nonfat cow's milk, reduced mineral whey: whey/casein ratio: 60:40	Lactose	Oleo, coconut, oleic (safflower) and soy oils	For full-term and premature infants with no special nutritional requirements	Supplemented with iron, 12 mg/L

Modified from Kempe C., and others, editors: Current pediatric diagnosis and treatment, ed. 9, Copyright 1987 by Lange Medical Publications, Los Altos, CA. Modifications based on product information from Carnation 1988; Loma Linda 1988; Mead Johnson Nutritionals, 1988; Ross Laboratories, 1988; Wyeth Laboratories, 1989. For the most current information, consult product labels or package enclosures.

*MCT, medium chain triglycerides.

†L-Amino acids include L-cystine, L-tyrosine, and L-tryptophan, which are reduced in hydrolyzed, charcoal-treated casein.

‡Ross Laboratories and Mead Johnson manufacture several specialty formulas for metabolic disorders for infants.

Table 8-6 Normal and special infant formulas—cont'd

FORMULA (MANUFACTURER)	PROTEIN SOURCE	CARBOHYDRATE SOURCE	FAT SOURCE	INDICATIONS FOR USE	COMMENTS (NUTRITIONAL CONSIDERATIONS)
Enfamil (Mead Johnson)	Nonfat cow's milk, demineralized whey: whey/casein ratio: 60:40	Lactose	Soy, coconut oils	For full-term and premature infants with no special nutritional requirements	Available fortified with iron, 12 mg/L
Similac (Ross)	Nonfat cow's milk; whey/casein ratio: 18:82	Lactose	Soy and coconut oils, mono- and diglycerides	For full-term and premature infants with no special nutritional requirements	Available fortified with iron, 12 mg/L
Advance (Ross)	Nonfat cow's milk, soy protein isolate	Corn syrup	Corn and soy oils	For feeding of older infants	Lower-caloric content (16 cal/oz); fortified with iron, 12 mg/L
Good Start H.A. (Carnation)	Hydrolyzed whey	Lactose, maltodextrin	Palm, oleic, and coconut oils	For full-term infants	Manufacturer's claim regarding hypoallergenicity has been withdrawn
Good Nature (Carnation)	Nonfat cow's milk	Corn syrup solids	Palm, corn, and oleic oils	For feeding older infants	Contains more protein and calcium than "starter" formulas
Baby formula (Gerber)	Nonfat cow's milk; whey/casein ratio: 18:82	Lactose	Soy	For full-term and premature infants with no special nutritional requirements	Available fortified with iron, 11.5 mg/L
Similac Natural Care (Ross)	Nonfat cow's milk; whey protein concentrate	Hydrolyzed corn starch, lactose	MCT,* coconut, and soy oils	For low-birth-weight infants. Fed mixed with human milk or fed alternately with human milk. Improves vitamin/mineral content of human milk	Protein, 2.7 g/100 kcal. Osmolality, 24 cal/oz: 300 mOsm/kg water
Enfamil Human Milk Modifier (Mead Johnson)	Whey protein concentrate, casein	Corn syrup solids		For low-birth-weight infants; fed mixed with human milk; increases protein, calorie, calcium, phosphorus, and other nutrients	Used only as human milk fortifier, not as separate formula. One packet of powder supplies 3.5 kcal
▪ For milk protein–sensitive infants ("milk allergy"), lactose intolerance					
Prosobee (Mead Johnson)	Soy protein isolate	Corn syrup solids	Soy and coconut oils	With milk protein allergy, lactose intolerance, lactase deficiency, galactosemia	Hypoallergenic, zero band antigen; lactose and sucrose free
Isomil (Ross)	Soy protein isolate	Corn syrup, sucrose	Soy and coconut oils	With milk protein allergy, lactose intolerance, lactase deficiency, galactosemia	Lactose free
Isomil SF (Ross)	Soy protein isolate	Hydrolyzed corn starch	Soy and coconut oils	With milk protein allergy or sucrose intolerance	Sucrose and lactose free

Continued.

Table 8-6 Normal and special infant formulas—cont'd

FORMULA (MANUFACTURER)	PROTEIN SOURCE	CARBOHYDRATE SOURCE	FAT SOURCE	INDICATIONS FOR USE	COMMENTS (NUTRITIONAL CONSIDERATIONS)
▪ For milk protein–sensitive infants ("milk allergy"), lactose intolerance—cont'd					
Nursoy (Wyeth)	Soy protein isolate	Sucrose (liquid formula) Corn syrup solids (powdered formula)	Oleo, coconut, oleic, and soy oils	With milk protein allergy, lactose intolerance, lactase deficiency, galactosemia	Lactose free
Soyalac (Loma Linda)	Soybean solids	Sucrose, corn syrup	Soy oil	With milk protein allergy, lactose intolerance, lactase deficiency, galactosemia	Lactose free
I-Soyalac (Loma Linda)	Soy protein isolate	Sucrose tapioca dextrin	Soy oil	With milk protein allergy, lactose intolerance, lactase deficiency, galactosemia	Lactose and corn free
▪ For infants with malabsorption syndromes, milk allergy (hydrolysate formulas)					
RCF (Ross Carbohydrate Free) (Ross)	Soy protein isolate		Soy and coconut oils	With carbohydrate intolerance	Carbohydrate is added according to amount infant will tolerate
Portagen (Mead Johnson)	Sodium caseinate	Corn syrup solids, sucrose, lactose	MCT (coconut source) and corn oil	For impaired fat absorption secondary to pancreatic insufficiency, bile acid deficiency, intestinal resection, lymphatic anomalies	Nutritionally complete
Nutramigen (Mead Johnson)	Casein hydrolysate and L-amino acids†	Corn syrup solids, modified corn starch	Corn oil	For infants and children sensitive to food proteins; use in galactosemic patients	Nutritionally complete hypoallergenic formula; lactose and sucrose free
Pregestimil (Mead Johnson)	Casein hydrolysate and L-amino acids	Corn syrup solids, modified tapioca starch	Corn oil, MCT	Disaccharidase deficiencies, malabsorption syndromes, cystic fibrosis	Nutritionally complete, easily digestible protein, carbohydrate, and fat; lactose and sucrose free
Alimentum (Ross)	Casein hydrolysate and L-amino acids	Sucrose, modified tapioca starch	MCT, oleic and soy oils	For infants and children sensitive to food proteins or with cystic fibrosis	Nutritionally complete; hypoallergenic formula; lactose free
▪ Specialty formulas					
Lonalac (Mead Johnson)	Casein	Lactose	Coconut	For children with congestive cardiac failure, who require reduced sodium intake	For long-term management, additional sodium must be given; supplement with vitamins C and D and iron; Na = 1 mEq/L

*MCT, medium chain triglycerides.
†L-Amino acids include L-cystine, L-tyrosine, and L-tryptophan, which are reduced in hydrolyzed, charcoal-treated casein.
‡Ross Laboratories and Mead Johnson manufacture several specialty formulas for metabolic disorders for infants.

Table 8-6 Normal and special infant formulas—cont'd

FORMULA (MANUFACTURER)	PROTEIN SOURCE	CARBOHYDRATE SOURCE	FAT SOURCE	INDICATIONS FOR USE	COMMENTS (NUTRITIONAL CONSIDERATIONS)
▪ Specialty formulas—cont'd					
Similac PM 60/40 (Ross)	Whey protein concentrate, sodium caseinate (60:40 ratio)	Lactose	Coconut, corn oils	For newborns predisposed to hypocalcemia and infants with impaired renal, digestive, and cardiovascular functions	Low calcium, potassium, and phosphorus; relatively low solute load; Na = 7 mEq/L
▪ Diet modifiers					
Polycose (Ross)		Glucose polymers (corn syrup solids)		Used to increase calorie intake, as in failure-to-thrive infants	Carbohydrate only; a powdered or liquid calorie supplement; powder 23 kcal/tbsp
Moducal (Mead Johnson)		Hydrolyzed corn starch		Used to increase carbohydrate intake	Carbohydrate only. A powdered calorie supplement: 30 kcal/tbsp
Casec (Mead Johnson)	Calcium caseinate			Used to increase protein intake	Protein only; negligible fat and no carbohydrate
MCT Oil (Mead Johnson)			90% MCT (coconut source)	Supplement in fat malabsorption conditions	Fat only; 8.3 kcal/g; 115 kcal/tbsp
▪ For infants with phenylketonuria‡					
Lofenalac (Mead Johnson)	Casein hydrolysate, L-amino acids	Corn syrup solids, modified tapioca starch	Corn oil	For infants and children with phenylketonuria	111 mg phenylalanine per quart of formula (20 cal/qt); must be supplemented with other foods to provide minimal phenylalanine
Phenyl-free (Mead Johnson)	L-Amino acids	Sucrose, corn syrup solids, modified tapioca starch	Corn oil, coconut oil	For children over 1 year of age with phenylketonuria	Phenylalanine free; permits increased supplementation with normal foods
PKU 1 (Milupa)	L-Amino acids	Sucrose		For infants with phenylketonuria (available as PKU 2 for children over 1 year of age)	Phenylalanine- and fat-free; contains vitamins, minerals, and trace elements; must be supplemented with phenylalanine/protein, carbohydrate, and fat

las are available in three preparations: (1) a ready-to-use form in cans or bottles, (2) a concentrated liquid form that is diluted with an equal amount of water, and (3) a powdered form that must be prepared according to the manufacturer's directions. One consideration in the use of commercially prepared formulas is their cost. It is wise to advise parents to do comparison shopping, since one preparation can be considerably more expensive than another.

Breast-feeding. Human milk is the preferred form of nutrition for the infant. In the United States about 50% of newborns in hospitals are breast-fed, and about 20% are still breast-fed at 5 to 6 months (Ross Laboratories, 1989). The greatest incidence and duration of exclusive breast-feeding is among college-educated unemployed women at upper income levels (Ryan and others, 1990). The American Academy of Pediatrics (1982) and the National Association of Pediatric Nurse Associates and Practitioners (Fond and Wester, 1988) recommend breast-feeding for full-term infants.

Besides the physiologic qualities of human milk, the

most outstanding psychologic benefit of breast-feeding is the close maternal-child relationship. The infant is nestled very close to the mother's skin, can hear the rhythm of her heartbeat, feel the warmth of her body, and sense a peaceful security. The mother has a very close feeling of union with her child and feels a sense of accomplishment and satisfaction as the infant draws milk from her. Some mothers also experience a type of sensation similar to sexual excitement.

Breast-feeding is the most economical form of feeding, although it is not "free" milk because the lactating mother needs a high-protein, high-calorie diet. Breast milk is always available, ready to serve at room temperature, and free of contamination*; there is no need to sterilize bottles. Breast-feeding may also offer protection against obesity and atherosclerosis, although the evidence is inconclusive. Breast-fed infants, especially beyond 4 to 6 months of age, tend to grow at a satisfactory but slower rate than bottle-fed infants (Czajka-Narins and Jung, 1986; Ryan and Martinez, 1987).

Contraindications to breast-feeding include (American Academy of Pediatrics and American College of Obstetricians and Gynecologists 1988; Lawrence, 1989):

- Serious, debilitating maternal disease, such as heart disorder or advanced cancer
- Cytomegalovirus (CVM)—primary risk is to infants receiving CVM-infected donor milk, not to infected mother's infant
- Active tuberculosis
- Human-immunodeficiency virus (HIV)—if acceptable feeding substitutes exist
- Galactosemia in the infant

Mastitis is usually not a contraindication if the discomfort is tolerable. Rarely "breast milk jaundice" may require temporary cessation of breast-feeding (see Chapter 9).

The birth of twins need not create a breast-feeding problem. If both twins are full-term, they can begin feedings immediately after birth (Fig. 8-17).† Simultaneous feeding promotes the rapid production of milk needed for both infants and makes the milk that would normally be lost in the letdown reflex available to one of the twins. When only one infant is hungry, the mother should feed singly. She should also alternate breasts when feeding each infant and avoid favoring one breast for one infant. The sucking patterns of infants vary, and each infant needs the visual stimulation and exercise that alternating breasts provides.

Probably the greatest disadvantage of breast-feeding to many mothers is the perceived inconvenience of loss of freedom and independence. Being committed to feeding the infant every 2 to 3 hours can be overwhelming, especially to women with multiple responsibilities. Many women resume their careers shortly after their pregnancy and prefer to use bottle-feeding. However, breast-feeding and employment are possible, and suggestions for the mother are discussed in Chapter 12. Although breast-feeding is the preferred form of infant feeding, mothers' decisions regarding their preferences must be supported and respected.

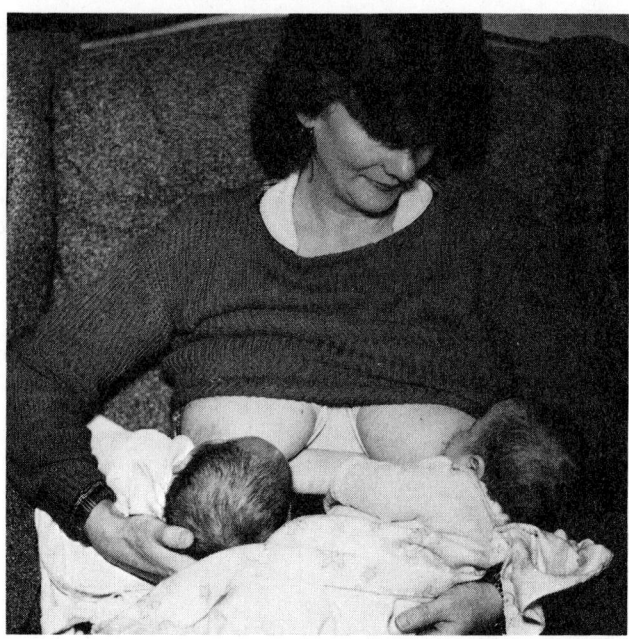

Fig. 8-17. Simultaneous breast-feeding of twins.

Successful breast-feeding probably depends more on the mother's desire to breast-feed, satisfaction with breast-feeding, and available support systems than on any other factors. Contrary to popular belief, breast-feeding is not instinctive. Mothers need support, encouragement, and assistance during their postpartum hospital stay to enhance their opportunities for success and satisfaction. Research increasingly supports the concept that the following hospital interventions promote breast-feeding (Bernard-Bonnin and others, 1989; Houston and Field, 1988; Reiff and Essock-Vitale, 1985):

- Increased information and support to mothers, especially phone follow-up
- Routines, such as frequent and early breast-feeding, especially during the first hour of life; immediate skin-to-skin contact, rooming-in, and careful control of drugs
- Direct modeling of the importance of breast-feeding by staff, such as implementing demand nursing with no formula supplementation and decreased emphasis on infant formula products

The influence of giving mothers complimentary formula samples as part of the "discharge pack" on duration of breast-feeding is controversial, although most studies demonstrate no significant negative effect (Feinstein and others, 1986; Ryan and others, 1990). Yet to be evaluated is the recent change in formula advertising. Traditionally in the United States formulas have not been advertised directly to the public, but this has changed, with some manufacturers

*NOTE: Human milk is not sterile; data suggest that healthy term infants can tolerate varying amounts of nonpathogenic and pathogenic organisms (Meier and Wilks, 1987).

†Excellent resources for breast-feeding twins are Sollid and others, 1989; Becker, 1986.

marketing infant formulas directly to families (Fleischman, 1990).

Dissatisfaction and the perception of "problems" with breast-feeding within the first 2 weeks have been identified as predictors of early weaning (Humenick and Van Steenkiste, 1983). Possibly if these mothers were identified early and received additional nursing support and encouragement, breast-feeding might be encouraged for extended periods. Certainly, nurses play a very significant role in the breast-feeding decision and must make themselves available to families for guidance and support. Several excellent books (Lawrence, 1989) and organizations* are available as resources for professionals and breast-feeding mothers (see also Lawrence, 1989, p. 598).

Bottle-feeding. With commercial formulas that closely approximate human milk and with greatly improved conditions of sanitation, bottle-feeding is an acceptable method of feeding. However, nurses should not assume that new parents automatically know how to bottle-feed their infant. These parents also need support and assistance in meeting their infant's needs.

Providing newborns with nutrition is only one aspect of the feeding. Holding them close to the body and rocking or cuddling them help to ensure the emotional component of feeding. Like breast-fed infants, bottle-fed infants need to be held on either side of the lap to expose them to different stimuli. The feeding should not be hurried. Even though they may suck vigorously for the first 5 minutes and seem to be satisfied, they are allowed to continue sucking. Infants need at least 2 hours of sucking a day. If there are six feedings per day, then about 20 minutes of sucking at each feeding provides for oral gratification.

After feedings infants are positioned on the right side to permit the feeding to flow toward the lower end of the stomach and to allow any swallowed air to rise above the fluid and through the esophagus (Fig. 8-18). This position prevents regurgitation and distention. To maintain the side-lying position, a pillow can be placed snugly behind the back.

Propping the bottle is discouraged for the following reasons:

1. It denies the infant the important component of close human contact
2. The infant may aspirate formula while sleeping
3. It may facilitate the development of middle ear infections. As the infant lies flat and sucks, milk that has pooled in the pharynx becomes a suitable medium for bacterial growth. Bacteria then enter the eustachian tube, which leads to the middle ear, causing acute otitis media
4. It encourages continuous pooling of formula in the mouth, which can lead to bottle caries when the teeth erupt (see Chapter 14).

Preparation of formula. The two traditional ways of preparing formula are the terminal heat method (all the utensils and formula are boiled together for 25 minutes) and the aseptic method (the equipment is boiled separately, after which the formula is poured into the bottles). Because of improved sanitary conditions in developed countries, neither of these methods is essential. The clean technique is satisfactory. Persons preparing the formula wash their hands well and then wash all the equipment used to prepare the formula, including the cans of formula or evaporated milk. The formula is prepared and bottled immediately before each feeding. Warming the formula is optional, although many parents prefer to warm it before feeding. Warming bottles in the microwave oven is not recommended because of the risk of burns from bottles exploding or the hot temperature of the fluid. Any milk remaining in the bottle after the feeding is discarded, since it is an excellent medium for bacterial growth. Opened cans of formula are covered and refrigerated until the next feeding.

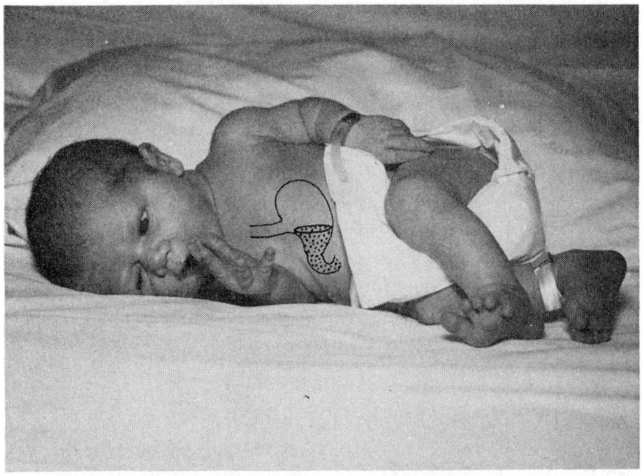

Fig. 8-18. Right-side-lying position after feeding.

Recent recommendations for labeling infant formulas require that the directions for preparation and use of the formula include pictures and symbols for nonreading individuals. In addition manufacturers are translating the directions into foreign languages, such as Spanish and Vietnamese, to prevent misunderstanding and errors in formula preparation. It is important to impress upon families that the proportions *must not be altered*—neither diluted to extend the amount of formula nor concentrated to provide more calories.

Feeding schedules. Ideally feeding schedules should be determined by the infant's hunger. Feeding infants when they signal readiness is called *demand feeding. Scheduled feedings* are arranged at predetermined intervals to meet family routines. Some hospitals routinely feed infants every 4 hours. Although this is satisfactory for bottle-fed infants, it hinders the breast-feeding process. Since breast-fed infants tend to be hungry every 2 to 3 hours, they should be fed on demand.

Supplemental feedings should *not* be offered to breast-fed infants in the nursery, because if the infants are satiated, they may not suck vigorously at the breast. Lactation depends on the breast being emptied at each feeding. If

*La Leche League International, Inc., P.O. Box 1209, Franklin Park, IL 60131-8209; (800) LA-LECHE. In Canada: 495 Main St., Winchester, Ontario, Canada KOC 2KO; (613) 774-2850.

milk is allowed to accumulate in the ducts, causing breast engorgement, ischemia results, suppressing the activity of the acini or milk-secreting cells. Consequently milk production is reduced. In addition, the process of sucking from a bottle is different from breast-nipple compression. The relatively inflexible rubber nipple prevents the tongue from its usual rhythmic action. Infants learn to put the tongue against the nipple holes to slow down the more rapid flow of fluid. When infants use these same tongue movements during breast-feeding, they may push the human nipple out of the mouth and may not grasp the areola properly (Lawrence, 1989).

Usually by 3 weeks of age, lactation is well established, and a feeding schedule has been formed. Bottle-fed infants retain about 2 to 3 ounces of formula at each feeding and are fed about six times a day. Breast-fed infants may feed as frequently as 10 to 12 times daily. Larger infants are able to retain increased amounts because of greater stomach capacity; as a result they generally sleep through the night sooner than smaller infants or breast-fed infants.

Feeding behavior. Five fairly distinct behavioral stages occur during successful feeding (O'Grady, 1971). Recognizing these steps can assist nurses in identifying potential feeding problems caused by improper feeding techniques. *Prefeeding behavior,* such as crying or fussing, demonstrates the infant's level of arousal and degree of hunger. *Approach behavior* is indicated by sucking movements or the rooting reflex. *Attachment behavior* includes those activities that occur from the time the infant receives the nipple until he grasps on and sucks. Attachment behavior is sometimes more pronounced during initial attempts at breast-feeding than bottle-feeding. *Consummatory behavior* consists of coordinated sucking and swallowing. Persistent gagging might indicate unsuccessful consummatory behavior. *Satiety behavior* is observed when infants let the mother know that they are satisfied. The most common expression of satiation is falling asleep.

PROMOTION OF PARENT-INFANT BONDING (ATTACHMENT)

The process of parenting is based on a mutual relationship between parent and infant. Much of past research on parent-child bonding has focused on the development of "mothering," or maternal attachment to the infant. Recently attention has focused on the infant's and father's role in this process. Although the words "bonding" and "attachment" are sometimes referred to as separate phenomena with *bonding* representing the development of emotional ties from parent to infant and *attachment* representing the emotional ties from infant to parent, in this discussion the words are used interchangeably to denote both processes.

As more is learned of the complexity of neonates and of their potential for influencing and shaping their environments, particularly their interaction with significant others, it is apparent that promoting positive parent-child relationships necessitates an understanding of factors involved in identifying behavioral steps in attachment, variables that enhance or hinder this process, and methods of teaching parents ways to develop a stronger relationship with their children, especially by recognizing potential problems.

Box 8-5 CLUSTERS OF NEONATAL BEHAVIORS IN BRAZELTON NEONATAL BEHAVIORAL ASSESSMENT SCALE

Habituation—ability to respond to and then inhibit responding to discrete stimulus (light, rattle, bell, pinprick) while asleep
Orientation—quality of alert states and ability to attend to visual and auditory stimuli while alert
Motor performance—quality of movement and tone
Range of state—measure of general arousal level or arousability of infant
Regulation of state—how infant responds when aroused
Autonomic stability—signs of stress (tremors, startles, skin color) related to homeostatic (self-regulating) adjustment of the nervous system
Reflexes—assessment of several neonatal reflexes

Infant Behavior

Nurses must appreciate the individuality and uniqueness of each infant. According to the individual temperament, the infant will change and shape the environment, which will undoubtedly influence future development. Obviously an infant who sleeps 20 hours a day will be exposed to fewer stimuli than one who sleeps 16 hours a day. In turn, each infant will likely effect a different response from parents. The infant who is quiet, undemanding, and passive may receive much less attention than the infant who is responsive, alert, and active. Such behavioral characteristics as irritability and consolability have been shown to influence the ease of transition to parenthood and the parent's perception of the infant (Roberts, 1983).

One method of systematically assessing the infant's behavior is the use of the *Brazelton Neonatal Behavioral Assessment Scale* (BNBAS) (Brazelton, 1984). The scale is designed to assess the infant's response to 28 items organized according to the clusters in Box 8-5.

Besides its use as an initial and ongoing tool to assess neurologic and behavioral responses, the scale can be used as an assessor of initial parent-child relationships, as a preventive instrument that identifies the caregiver as one who may benefit from a role model, and as a guide for parents to help them focus on their infant's individuality and to develop a deeper attachment to their child. Studies have demonstrated that by showing parents the unique characteristics of their infant, a more positive perception of the infant develops with increased interaction between infant and parent (Anderson, 1981; Beal, 1989; Liptak and others, 1983; Perry, 1983).

Nurses can intervene and positively influence the attachment of parent and child. The first step is recognizing individual differences and explaining to parents that such characteristics are normal. For example, most people believe that infants sleep throughout the day, except for feedings. For some newborns this may be true, but for many it is not.

Box 8-6 HOW TO MAKE THE INFANT'S WORLD MORE EXCITING*

Infant prefers animated and auditory objects.
Infant enjoys novelty, quickly tires of seeing same objects; mobile should be changed frequently.
Infant prefers to look at medium-intensity colors and contrasting colors, such as black and white.
Infant likes geometric shapes and checkerboards; prefers patterns over straight lines.
Contrasting lights and reflective surfaces such as mirrors are especially interesting.
But most of all, nothing is as fascinating as the human face and voice!

*Objects should be placed about 20 cm (8 inches) away from infant.

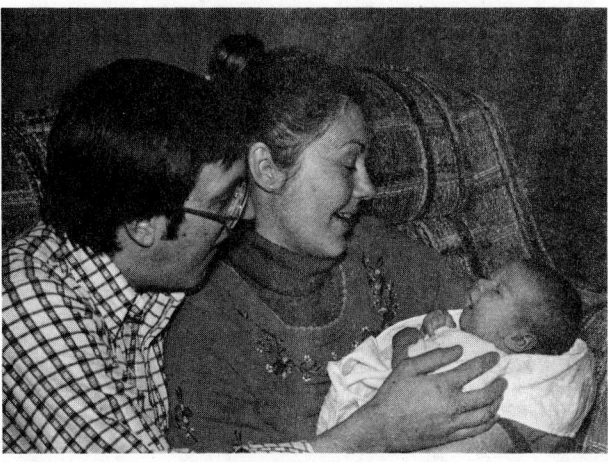

Fig. 8-19. En face position between parents and infant can be significant in attachment process.

Understanding that the infant's wakefulness is part of biologic rhythm and not a reflection of inadequate parenting can be crucial in promoting healthy parent-child relationships. Another aspect of helping parents concerns supplying guidelines on how to enhance the infant's development during awake periods. Placing the child in a crib to stare at the same mobile every day is not exciting, but carrying the infant into each room as one does daily chores can be fascinating. A few suggestions can make life more stimulating for the infant and gratifying for the parents (Box 8-6).

Maternal Attachment

During pregnancy, and often even before conception occurs, parents develop an image of the "ideal or fantasy infant." The unborn child has an imagined appearance, pattern of behavior, expected accomplishments, and predetermined effect on the life-style of the family. At birth the fantasy infant becomes the real infant. How closely the dream child resembles the real child influences the bonding process. Assessing such expectations during pregnancy and at the time of the infant's birth allows nurses to identify discrepancies in the parents' view of the fantasy vs real child syndrome.

The Neonatal Perception Inventory (NPI) (Broussard, 1979) is a screening tool that can be used to assess the mother's perception of her real infant as compared to her image of an "average" infant. It is hypothesized that for optimum mothering to occur the mother needs to see her infant as better than an "average" baby. Mothers who do not rate their infants as better than average may be at risk for developing parenting abilities that fail to meet the infant's needs. The NPI II (completed 4 weeks after delivery) was predictive of later childhood adjustment problems, whereas the NPI I (completed 1 to 2 days after infant's birth) was not (Broussard, 1976). In follow-up studies over a 19-year period, Broussard (1984) concluded that infants who were negatively perceived had the greatest risk for developing mental disorders.

The labor process also significantly affects the immediate attachment of mothers to their newborn children. Factors such as a long labor, feeling tired or "drugged" after delivery, and problems with breast-feeding can delay the development of initial positive feelings toward the newborn (Pascoe and French, 1989).

It is believed that there is a *maternal sensitive period* immediately and for a short time after birth when parents have a unique ability to attach to their infants (Klaus and Kennell, 1982). During the development of the attachment process, mothers demonstrated a predictable and orderly pattern of behavior. When they were presented with their nude infants, they began examining the infant with their fingertips, concentrating on touching the extremities. In about 4 to 8 minutes they proceeded to massage and encompass the trunk with their entire hands. They also found that the *en face* position, a position in which the mother's and the infant's eyes meet in visual contact in the same vertical plane, was significant in the formation of affectional ties (Fig. 8-19).

Similar patterns of touching have been observed by others (Rubin, 1963), which has led many clinicians to use assessment of touch as an indicator of maternal-infant attachment. However, other studies demonstrate different patterns for mothers, as well as the same pattern for nonmaternal persons, such as male and female nurses. Therefore, caution must be exercised in rigidly applying this parameter in assessing maternal attachment (Tulman, 1985; Templeton, Edgil, and Douglas, 1988).

Additional studies have attempted to substantiate the long-term benefits of providing parents with opportunities to optimally bond with their infant during the initial postpartum period. There is considerable controversy over the validity of the findings and concern with the emphasis on a "critical" period for bonding. These issues are reviewed in the Questions and Controversies on p. 342.

Another component of successful maternal attachment is the concept of *reciprocity* or reciprocal interaction. As the

QUESTIONS AND CONTROVERSIES

Does early and extended maternal-infant contact affect subsequent parenting and infant development?

Since Klaus and Kennell's initial research and postulation of a "maternal sensitive period," several investigators have sought to determine if early and extended maternal-infant contact has a significant influence on parenting and infant development. Among the more classic studies, researchers demonstrated that a total of 16 extra contact hours with their infant influenced mothers to be more reluctant to leave their infant with someone else, to show greater soothing behavior and fondling, and to engage in more eye-to-eye contact (Klaus and others, 1972; Kennell and others, 1974).

In a 2-year follow-up study the early contact group had better speech and communication patterns. In a 5-year follow-up, however, no differences were found between the groups in speech development, language comprehension, or intelligence. However, a correlation was noted in the early contact group between the mother's speech and communication patterns with the child at 2 years of age and the child's communication abilities at age 5 (Ringler and others, 1978).

There has been some evidence that increased parent-child contact at birth minimizes the risks of parenting disorders, such as abuse and neglect (O'Connor and others, 1980). However, not all studies support these findings, and when the influence of socioeconomic background variables is taken into consideration, they are more of a determinant of attachment than early and extended contact (Siegel and others, 1980). Another short-term benefit found by several investigators was prolonged breast-feeding (Goldberg, 1983; Taylor, Maloni, and Brown, 1986).

In light of these conflicting reports and the concerns regarding study design such as small sample sizes, lack of subject randomization, and different measures to assess attachment, some authorities claim that the emphasis on bonding has been unjustified and may lead to guilt and fear in those parents who did not receive early contact with their infant. There is also considerable concern over the literal interpretation of "sensitive" or "critical" to imply that without early contact optimum bonding cannot occur or, conversely, that early contact alone is sufficient to ensure competent parenting (Brown and Hellings, 1988; Lamb, 1989; Mitchell and Mills, 1983).

While the answer to whether early contact does affect parenting and child development is inconclusive, it is well known that Klaus and Kennell's work has had a major impact on the "humanization" of obstetric practices (Goldberg, 1983; McCall, 1982; Klaus and Kennell, 1983; Korsch, 1983). These alone have merit for creating a joyful and fulfilling experience for the family. Certainly it should be stressed to parents that while early bonding may be valuable, it does not represent an "all or none" phenomenon. Through the child's life there will be multiple opportunities for the development of parent-child attachment. Bonding is a complex process that develops gradually and is influenced by numerous factors, only one of which is the type of initial contact between the newborn and parent.

mother responds to the infant, the infant must respond to the mother by some signal such as sucking, cooing, eye contact, grasping, or molding (conforming to the other's body during close physical contact). Five steps are described in positive mother-infant reciprocity (Brazelton, 1974). The first step is *initiation,* in which interaction between infant and parent begins. Next is *orientation,* which establishes the partners' expectation of each other during the interaction. Following orientation is *acceleration* of the attention cycle to a peak of excitement. The infant reaches out and coos, both arms jerk forward, the head moves backward, the eyes dilate, and the face brightens. After a short time *deceleration* of the excitement and *turning away* occur, in which the infant's eyes shift away from the mother's and the child grasps his shirt. During this cycle of nonattention, repeated verbal or visual attempts to reinitiate the infant's attention are ineffective. This deceleration and turning away probably prevent the infant from being overwhelmed by excessive stimuli. In a good interaction both partners have synchronized their attention-nonattention cycles. Parents or other caregivers who do not allow the infant to turn away and who continually attempt to maintain visual contact encourage the infant to turn off the attention cycle and thus prolong the nonattention phase.

Although this description of reciprocal interacting behavior is usually observable in the infant by 2 to 3 weeks of age, nurses can use this information to teach parents how to interact with their infant. Recognizing the attention vs nonattention cycles and understanding that the latter is not a rejection of the parent helps parents develop competence in parenting.

Paternal Engrossment

Less attention and research have focused on father-infant bonding than on maternal bonding, although the important role fathers play in family development is being increasingly recognized. Like pregnant women, prospective fathers develop attachment behaviors to the fetus, such as talking to the unborn child, referring to the fetus by a nickname, and imagining caring for the newborn (Weaver and Cranley, 1983).

Fathers also show specific attachment behaviors to the newborn. This process of *paternal engrossment,* forming a sense of absorption, preoccupation, and interest in the infant, includes (1) visual awareness of the newborn, especially focusing on the beauty of the child, (2) tactile awareness, often expressed in a desire to hold the infant, (3) awareness of distinct characteristics with emphasis on those features of the infant that resemble the father, (4) perception of the infant as perfect, (5) development of a strong feeling of attraction to the child that leads to intense focusing of attention on the infant, (6) experiencing a feeling of extreme elation, and (7) feeling a sense of deep self-esteem and satisfaction. These responses are greatest during the early contacts with the infant and are intensified by the neonate's normal reflex activity, especially the grasp reflex and visual alertness (Greenberg and Morris, 1974). In addition to behavioral reactions, fathers also demonstrate physiologic responses such as increased heart rate and blood

THERAPEUTIC DIALOGUE

Encouraging Paternal Engrossment

The nurse brings the newborn to the parents shortly after birth and hands the infant to the father. The father carefully but somewhat unsteadily holds his son.

NURSE: Jonathan is so perfect and beautiful.

FATHER: Yes, but he is so small and fragile.

NURSE: He is small, but you think he is fragile?

FATHER: Yes. I never feel good around babies. They are cute and all, but I am always afraid I will drop them or hurt them.

NURSE: How do you think you could hurt them?

FATHER: I could squeeze them too hard or hurt that soft spot on the head.

NURSE: You are afraid of hurting them because you think they are fragile (nurse uses facilitative responding, p. 195).

FATHER: Yes, I already told my wife that she will have to do everything. She will be a good mother.

NURSE: Mrs. H., what do you think about all of this?

MOTHER: Well, I am a little afraid too but I would like to have some help with the baby. Do you think babies are so fragile?

NURSE: No. They look fragile because they are so small and, of course, they should be handled gently. But they don't break easily and they like firm hugging. Let's look at Jonathan's soft spot.

■ ■ ■

The nurse proceeds to show them the fontanels, explains their purpose, and has the parents feel the head. She explains that the skin over this area is not likely to tear or puncture. She demonstrates the grasp reflex and how the infant's grasp is strong enough for the nurse to pull him slightly forward. She encourages the parents, especially the father, to hold the infant in different positions.

■ ■ ■

FATHER: I never knew those things about the head. And I never knew you could pick up babies so many different ways. Jonathan seems to like being held against my shoulder. I guess that with practice this will feel more natural for me. He really is cute and he has strong hands. I bet he will be a good baseball player.

pressure during interactions with their newborns (Jones and Thomas, 1989).

The process of engrossment has significant implications for nurses. Initially it is imperative that nurses recognize the importance of early father-infant contact in releasing these behaviors. Fathers need to be encouraged to express their positive feelings, especially if such emotions are contrary to the cultural belief that fathers should remain stoic. If this is not clarified, fathers may feel confused and attempt to suppress the natural sensations of absorption, preoccupation, and interest in order to conform with societal expectations.

Mothers also need to be aware of the responses of the father toward the newborn, especially since one of the consequences of paternal preoccupation with the infant is less overt attention toward the mother. If both parents are able to share their feelings, each can appreciate the process of attachment toward their child and will avoid the unfortunate conflict of being insensitive and unaware of the other's needs. In addition, a father who is encouraged to form a relationship with his newborn is less likely to feel excluded and abandoned once the family returns home and the mother directs her attention toward caring for the infant.

Ideally the process of engrossment should be discussed with parents before the delivery, such as in prenatal classes, to reinforce the father's awareness of his natural feelings toward the expected child. Focusing on the future experience of seeing, touching, and holding one's newborn may also help expectant fathers become more comfortable in accepting their paternal feelings toward the unborn child. This in turn can assist them in being more supportive toward their wives, especially as the labor and delivery event draws near.

At the infant's birth the nurse can play a vital role in assisting the father to release or express engrossment by assessing the neonate in front of the couple; pointing out normal characteristics, especially the grasp reflex; encouraging identification through consistent referral to the child by name; encouraging the father to cuddle, hold, talk to, or feed the infant; and demonstrating whenever necessary the soothing powers of caressing, stroking, and rocking the child (Fig. 8-20) (see Therapeutic Dialogue). Fathers are encouraged to be with the mother during labor and delivery and to spend time alone with the mother and newborn after delivery. Whenever possible, the father should "room in" with the mother.

The nurse observes for the same indication of affectional ties from the father as those expected in the mother, such as visual contact in the en face position and embracing the infant close to the body. When present, such behaviors are reinforced. If such responses are not obvious, the nurse needs to assess the father's feelings regarding this birth, cultural beliefs that may prevent his emotional expression, and other factors in order to help him facilitate a positive attachment during this critical period. Literature can also be given to the parents to help them understand the process of attachment and its importance in parent-infant bonding.*

*A suggested book is Brazelton, T.B.: On becoming a family: the growth of attachment, New York, 1981, Dell Publishing Co., Inc.

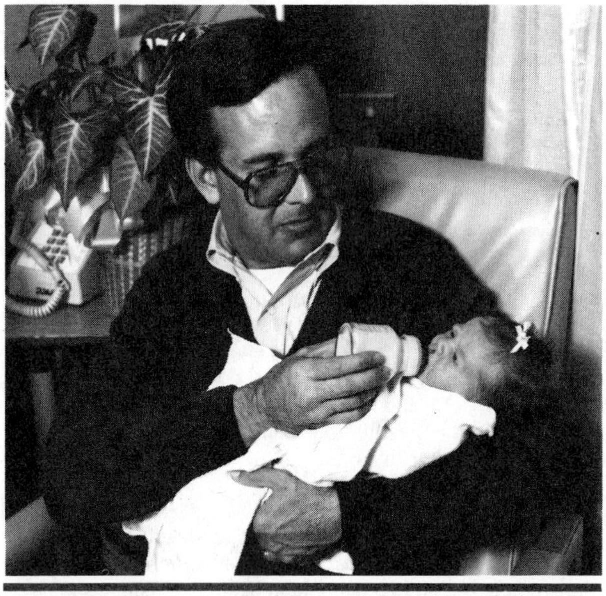

Fig. 8-20. A desire to hold the infant and participate in caregiving activities is an indication of paternal engrossment.

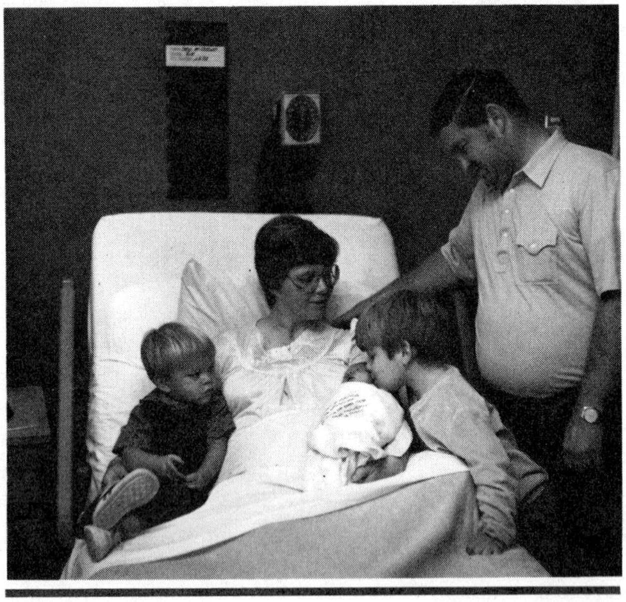

Fig. 8-21. Sibling visitation shortly after birth can be significant in the attachment process.

Siblings

Although the attachment process has been discussed almost exclusively in terms of the parents and infant, it is essential that nurses be aware of other family members, such as siblings and members of the extended family, who need preparation for the acceptance of this new child. Young children in particular need sensitive preparation for the birth to minimize sibling jealousy.

There is an increasing trend to allow siblings to visit the mother on the postpartum unit and to hold the newborn (Fig. 8-21). Research has demonstrated several benefits, such as more responsiveness of the visiting sibling to the mother and newborn (Schwab and others, 1983), less regressive behaviors after the birth (Kayiatos, Adams, and Gilman, 1984), and no adverse effects, such as increased bacterial infection of neonates (Solheim and Spellacy, 1988). In light of these findings, the American Academy of Pediatrics (1985) supports neonatal sibling visitation and has established guidelines for institutions.

Another trend has been siblings witnessing the birth. Unlike sibling visitation, the evidence supporting this practice is much more controversial and conflicting. Children exhibit different degrees of involvement in the birth process. Young children often fall asleep toward the end of delivery. Some reported benefits include children's increased knowledge of the birth process and less regressive behaviors following the birth (Daniels, 1983; Trause and Irvin, 1982). As research mounts, birthing centers that allow siblings at the birth are developing more definitive guidelines, such as age requirement of at least 4 to 5 years, the presence of a supportive person for the sibling only, and an adequate sequence of preparation in which parents explore all options for preparing their other children (Ballard and others, 1982; Daniels, 1983).

From preliminary observations during sibling visitation there is evidence that sibling attachment occurs and is not significantly affected by attendance at sibling preparation classes. The en face position is assumed much less often among the newborn and siblings than between mother and newborn, and, when this position is used, it is brief. Siblings focus more on the head or face than on touching or talking to the infant. The siblings' verbalizations are focused less on attracting the infant's attention and more on addressing the mother about the newborn (Marecki and others, 1985). Children who have established a prenatal relationship with the fetus have demonstrated more attachment behaviors, supporting the suggestion of encouraging prenatal acquaintance (Anderberg, 1988). Additional research is needed to establish theories on sibling bonding as have been constructed for parental bonding.

Multiple Births and Subsequent Children

Monotropy is a component of attachment that has special meaning for families with multiple births. Monotropy refers to the principle that a person can become optimally attached to only one individual at a time (Klaus and Kennell, 1982). If a parent can form only one attachment at a time, how then can all the siblings of a multiple birth receive optimum emotional care?

Minimal research is available on bonding and multiple births, and even less is known about paternal engrossment and sibling attachment. In regard to maternal-twin bonding, the conclusions of different authors vary. Some report that mothers bond equally to each twin at the time of birth, even if one twin is ill (Abbink, 1982). Others suggest that mothers of twins may take months or even years to form individual attachments to each child and even longer if the twins are identical. The mother's separation from a sick twin during the perinatal period can have devastating results, since attachment to the well child occurs quickly but may impede attachment to the other twin (Gromada, 1981).

Nurses can be instrumental in promoting bonding of multiple births. The most important principle is to assist the parents in recognizing the individuality of the children, especially in monozygotic (identical) twins. The BNBAS can be used to illustrate these differences and to stress effective strategies for dealing with multiple personalities at the same time. Other strategies for promoting individualism are discussed under Multiple Births in Chapter 3.

Another area of attachment that has received minimal attention is maternal bonding of multiparous mothers. Research suggests that there are several additional tasks to "taking on" a second child. These include (Walz, 1983):

- Promoting acceptance and approval of the first child for the second
- Grieving and resolving the loss of an exclusive dyadic relationship with the first child
- Planning and coordinating family life to include a second child
- Reformulating a relationship with the first child
- Identifying with the second child by comparing with the first child for physical and psychologic characteristics
- Assessing one's affective capabilities in providing sufficient emotional support and nurturance simultaneously to two children

Employed mothers who have a second child report fewer concerns regarding general aspects of separation from their child and the effect of separation on the child, but similar concerns regarding separation due to employment (Pitzer and Hock, 1989). It appears that while experience may decrease some concerns, it may not minimize other concerns.

Spacing of children appears to influence maternal stress following birth of a second child. Those mothers with children less than 2 years apart may experience the most stress, followed by mothers with children greater than 6 years apart. The least stress is likely to occur when children are spaced by 4 to 6 years (Lynch, 1982). Obviously multiparous mothers benefit from nursing support both in the hospital and at home. Unfortunately, they may be reluctant to admit concerns or problems because this is not a first-time experience. Providing sensitive care for their needs and fostering attachment behaviors, including in the siblings, is an essential component of nursing multiparous mothers.

Assessment of Attachment Behaviors

Unlike physical assessment of the neonate, which has concrete guidelines to follow, assessment of parent-child attachment requires much more skill in terms of observation and interviewing. The assessment process is even more challenging when one considers that postpartum hospital recovery is shorter and shorter. However, rooming-in of mother and infant and liberal visiting privileges for father, siblings, and grandparents facilitate recognition of behaviors that demonstrate positive or negative attachment.

What should the nurse observe when with the parents and the infant? Probably the most important activities to observe include feeding, bathing, and comforting. Guidelines for assessment of bonding behaviors are presented in Box 8-7.

Talking to the parents uncovers many variables that will affect the development of attachment and parenting (see also Chapter 16). What expectations do they have for this child? In other words, how similar are their predictions of the fantasy child and their realizations about the real child? They should be encouraged to talk about their relationship with their own parents. Mothering and fathering of a child probably depend more on the type of parenting that parents received as a child than on any other variable. Is this a planned birth, how do they see the addition of a dependent family member affecting their life-style, and what arrangements have they made in terms of such changes in life-style? What "support system" or significant others are available for assistance? What are their views regarding childrearing?

Assessing the family's bonding to the newborn is a complex process. The suggestions in Box 8-7 only serve as guidelines. Bonding behaviors vary greatly, and nurses must be cautious in judging the highly individual process. Certainly hospital routines and practitioners' interactions with the family should be sensitive to those strategies that enhance the bonding process.

Box 8-7 GUIDELINES FOR ASSESSING ATTACHMENT BEHAVIOR

When the infant is brought to the parents, do they reach out for the child and call the child by name?

Do the parents speak about the child in terms of identification—whom the infant looks like; what appears special about their child over other infants?

When parents are holding the infant, what kind of body contact is there—do parents feel at ease in changing the infant's position; are fingertips or whole hands used; are there parts of the body they avoid touching or parts of the body they investigate and scrutinize?

When the infant is awake, what kinds of stimulation do the parents provide—do they talk to the infant, to each other, or to no one; how do they look at the infant—direct visual contact, avoidance of eye contact, or looking at other people or objects?

How comfortable do the parents appear in terms of caring for the infant? Do they express any concern regarding their ability or disgust for certain activities, such as changing diapers?

What type of affection do they demonstrate to the newborn, such as smiling, stroking, kissing, or rocking?

If the infant is fussy, what kinds of comforting techniques do the parents use, such as rocking, swaddling, talking, or stroking?

DISCHARGE PLANNING AND CARE AT HOME

With increasingly shorter postpartum admissions and home delivery, discharge planning, referral, and home visiting are important components of comprehensive care. First-time, as well as "experienced," parents benefit from guidance and assistance with the infant's care, such as breast- or formula feeding, and with the family's integration of a new member, particularly sibling adjustment. To assess and meet these needs, discharge planning *must* begin immediately on admission to the hospital or birthing center. A nursing admission history assists in systematic collection of data to formulate nursing diagnoses and to plan care. This assessment continues throughout the admission and includes the family's support system. Nurses in the birthing, nursery, and postpartum units need to coordinate their assessments for the most effective interventions.

Ideally, the family should receive a home visit shortly after discharge. Some home care programs schedule three visits during the first 5 days if the mother is discharged the day of delivery and more frequently for families at risk, such as teenage parents. Other programs encourage telephone conversations. Common concerns or problems during this period are related to infant feeding, maternal fatigue and depression, bonding, neonatal jaundice, cord care, and excessive infant crying (Elmer and Maloni, 1988; Jansson, 1985).

Professional support for the new family should be continued from the hospital to the home through community services as needed. The concept of family-centered care is practiced when the family receives consistent comprehensive care, beginning with preventive prenatal care and continuing through child health maintenance.

KEY POINTS

- Transition from fetal or placental circulation to independent respiration is the most important physiologic change required of the newborn.
- Chemical and thermal factors help initiate the neonate's first respiration.
- Circulatory changes in the neonate result from shifts in pressure in the heart and major vessels and from functional closures of the fetal shunts.
- The newborn's large surface area, the thin layer of subcutaneous fat, and the newborn's unique mechanism for producing heat predispose the newborn to excessive heat loss.
- The infant's high rate of metabolism is closely correlated with the rate of fluid exchange, which is seven times greater in the infant than in the adult.
- The skin and mucous membranes, the reticuloendothelial system, and antibodies are the first, second, and third lines of defense against infection.
- Apgar scoring, the initial assessment of the newborn's heart rate, respiratory effort, muscle tone, reflex irritability, and color, is an excellent indicator of infants requiring resuscitation.
- Physical assessment of the newborn includes assessment of clinical gestational age, general measurements, general appearance, and head-to-toe assessment.
- Neurologic assessment focuses on localized reflexes and posture, muscle tone, head control, and movement and is best accomplished during the general physical examination.
- Behavioral assessment of newborns, with the Brazelton Neonatal Behavioral Assessment Scale, examines responses to seven categories: habituation, orientation, motor performance, range of state, regulation of state, autonomic regulation, and reflexes.
- Physical care for the newborn includes maintaining a patent airway, maintaining stable body temperature, protecting from infection and injury, and providing optimum nutrition.
- Although the attachment, or bonding, process primarily affects infants and parents, siblings also play an important role.

REFERENCES

Abbink, C.: Bonding as perceived by mothers of twins, Pediatr. Nurs. 8(6):411-413, 1982.

American Academy of Pediatrics: Neonatal anesthesia, Pediatrics 80(3):446, 1987.

American Academy of Pediatrics: Report of the Committee on Infectious Diseases, ed. 21, Elk Grove Village, IL, 1988, The Academy.

American Academy of Pediatrics and American College of Obstetricians and Gynecologists: Guidelines for perinatal care, ed. 2, Elk Grove Village, IL, 1988, The Academy.

American Academy of Pediatrics, Committee on Accident and Poison Prevention: Safe transportation of newborns discharged from the hospital, AAP News 6(7):12, 1990.

American Academy of Pediatrics, Committee on Fetus and Newborn: Postpartum (neonatal) sibling visitation, Pediatrics 76(4):650, 1985.

American Academy of Pediatrics, Committee on Fetus and Newborn: Use and abuse of the Apgar score, Pediatrics 78(6):1148-1149, 1986.

American Academy of Pediatrics, Committee on Genetics: Newborn screening fact sheets, Pediatrics 83(3):449-464, 1989.

American Academy of Pediatrics, Policy Statement Based on Task Force Report: The promotion of breast-feeding, Pediatrics 69(5):654-661, 1982.

American Academy of Pediatrics, Task Force on Circumcision: Report of the Task Force on Circumcision, Pediatrics 84(4):388-391, 1989.

Anderberg, G.J.: Initial acquaintance and attachment behavior of siblings with the newborn, JOGNN 17:49-54, 1988.

Anderson, C.J.: Enhancing reciprocity between mother and neonate, Nurs. Res. 30(2):89-93, 1981.

Anderson, S.: Siblings at birth: a survey and study, Birth Fam. J. 6:80-87, 1979.

Andrich, M.P., and Golden, S.M.: Umbilical cord care: a study of bacitracin ointment vs. triple dye, Clin. Pediatr. 23:342-344, 1984.

Ballard, J.L., Novak, K.K., and Driver, M.: A simplified score for assessment of fetal maturation of newly born infants, J. Pediatr. 95(5):769-774, 1979.

Ballard, R., and others: An alternative birth center in a hospital setting. In Klaus, M.H., and Kennell, J.H., editors: Maternal-infant bonding, ed. 2, St. Louis, 1982, Mosby–Year Book, Inc.

Bamji, M., and others: Palpable lymph nodes in healthy newborns and infants, Pediatrics 78(4):573-580, 1986.

Beal, J.: The effect on father-infant interaction of demonstrating the Neonatal Behavioral Assessment Scale, Birth 16(1):18-22, 1989.

Becker, P.: Counseling families with twins: birth to 3 years of age, Pediatr. Rev. 8(3):81-86, 1986.

Bernard-Bonnin, A., and others: Hospital practices and breastfeeding duration: a meta-analysis of controlled trials, Birth 16(2):64-66, 1989.

Bliss-Holtz, J.: Comparison of rectal, axillary, and inguinal temperatures in full-term newborn infants, Nurs. Res. 38(2):85-87, 1989.

Brazelton, T.B.: Mother-infant reciprocity. In Klaus, M., and others, editors: Maternal attachment and mothering disorders, New Brunswick, NJ, 1974, Johnson & Johnson Baby Products Co.

Brazelton, T.B.: Neonatal behavioral assessment scale, ed. 2, Philadelphia, 1984, J.B. Lippincott Co.

Broussard, E.R.: Neonatal prediction and outcome at 10/11 years, Child Psychiatry Hum. Dev. 7(2):85-93, 1976.

Broussard, E.R.: Assessment of the adaptive potential of the mother-infant system: the Neonatal Perception Inventories, Semin. Perinatol. 3(1):91-100, 1979.

Broussard, E.: The Pittsburgh first borns at age nineteen years. In Call, J., Galerson, E., and Tyson, R., editors: Frontiers of infant psychiatry, vol. 2, New York, 1984, Basic Books, Inc.

Brown, M.S., and Brown, C.A.: Circumcision decision: prominence and social concerns, Pediatrics 80(2):215-219, 1987.

Brown, M. and Hellings, P.: A case study of qualitative versus quantitative reviews: the maternal-infant bonding controversy, J. Pediatr. Nurs. 4(2):104-111, 1989.

Bull, M., and others: Special children, special car seats, Contemp. Pediatr. 6(11):122-136, 1989.

Byrne, J., and Horowitz, F.: Rocking as a soothing intervention: the influence of direction and type of movement, Infant Behav. Dev. 4:207-218, 1981.

Campbell, R.L., and others: Clinical studies with disposable diapers containing absorbent gelling materials: evaluation of effects on infant skin condition, J. Am. Acad. Dermatol. 17:978-987, 1987.

Campbell, R.L., and others: Effects of diaper types on diaper dermatitis associated with diarrhea and antibiotic use in children in day-care centers, Pediatr. Dermatol. 5(2):83-87, 1988.

Chia, F., and others: Reliability of the Dinamap noninvasive monitor in the measurement of blood pressure of ill Asian newborns, Clin. Pediatr. 29(5):262-267, 1990.

Cox, L.: Screening the high-risk newborn for hearing loss: the crib-o-gram v the auditory brainstem response, Inf. Young Child. 1(1):71-81, 1988.

Czajka-Narins, D., and Jung, E.: Physical growth of breastfed and formula fed infants from birth to age 2 years, Nutr. Res. 6:753-762, 1986.

Daniels, M.: The birth experience for the sibling: description and evaluation of a program, J. Nurs. Midwif. 28(5):15-22, 1983.

DeCasper, A.M., and Fifer, W.P.: Of human bonding: newborns prefer their mothers' voices, Science 208:1174-1176, June 1980.

Dixon, S., and others: Behavioral effects of circumcision with and without anesthesia, Dev. Behav. Pediatr. 5(5):246-250, 1984.

Dubowitz, L.M.S., Dubowitz, V., and Goldberg, C.: Clinical assessment of gestational age in the newborn infant, J. Pediatr. 77(1):1-10, 1970.

El Haddad, M., and Corkery, J.J.: The anus in the newborn, Pediatrics 76(6):927-928, 1985.

Elmer, E., and Maloni, J.A.: Parent support through telephone consultation, Matern. Child Nurs. J. 17(1):13-23, 1988.

Feinstein, J., and others: Factors related to early termination of breastfeeding in an urban population, Pediatrics 78(2):210-215, 1986.

Ferber, R.: Behavioral "insomnia" in the child, Psychiatr. Clin. North Am. 10(4):641-653, 1987.

Fleischman, D.: AAP raps Gerber for delivering formula samples, AAP News 6(5):1, 14, 1990.

Fond, K., and Wester, R.: NAPNAP policy statement on breastfeeding, J. Pediatr. Health Care 2(66):314, 1988.

Gaull, G.: Taurine in pediatric nutrition: review and update, Pediatrics 83(3):433-442, 1989.

Gladstone, I.M., and others: Randomized study of six umbilical cord care regimens, Clin. Pediatr 27(3):127-129, 1988.

Goldberg, S.: Parent-infant bonding: another look, Child Dev. 54:1355-1382, 1983.

Golub, H.L., and Corwin, M.J.: Infant cry: a clue to diagnosis, Pediatrics 69(2):197-201, 1982.

Goodson, J.G., Buller, C., and Goodson, W.H., III: Prenatal child safety education, Obstet. Gynecol. 65:312-315, 1985.

Greenberg, M., and Morris, N.: Engrossment: the newborn's impact upon the father, Am. J. Orthopsychiatry 44(4):520-531, 1974.

Gromada, K.: Maternal-infants attachment: the first step toward individualizing twins, MCN 6(2):129-134, 1981.

Gunnar, M.R., Fisch, R.O., and Malone, S.: The effects of pacifying stimulus on behavioral and adrenocortical responses to circumcision in the newborn, J. Am. Acad. Child Adolesc. Psychiatry 23(1):34-38, 1984.

Gunzenhauser, N., editor: Advances in touch: new implications in human development, Skillman, NJ, 1990, Johnson & Johnson Consumer Products, Inc.

Haddock, B., Vincent, P., and Merrow, D.: Axillary and rectal temperatures of full-term neonates: are the different? Neonatal Network 5(1):36-40, 1986.

Hammerschlag, M., and others: Efficacy of neonatal ocular prophylaxis for the prevention of chlamydial and gonococcal conjunctivitis, N. Engl. J. Med. 320(12):769-772, 1989.

Hanson, L.A., and others: Protective factors in milk and the development of the immune system, Pediatrics 75(suppl.):172-176, 1985.

Harpin, V.A., and Rutter, N.: Development of emotional sweating in the newborn infant, Arch. Dis. Child. 57:691-695, 1982.

Hashimoto, T.: A comparison of the amount of dust produced by disposable and cloth diapers in incubators, Pediatrician 14(suppl. 1):44-47, 1987.

Henningsson, A., and others: Bathing or washing babies after birth, Lancet 2:1401-1402, Dec. 1981.

Herzog, L.W.: Urinary tract infections and circumcision: a case-control study, Am. J. Dis. Child. 143(3):348-350, 1989.

Herzog, L.W., and Alvarez, S.R.: The frequency of foreskin problems in uncircumcised children, Am. J. Dis. Child. 140(3):254-256, 1986.

Houston, M., and Field, P.: Practices and policies in the initiation of breastfeeding, JOGNN 17(6):418-425, 1988.

Humenick, S.S., and Van Steenkiste, S.: Early indicators of breast-feeding progress, Issues Compr. Pediatr. Nurs. 6:205-215, 1983.

Infant circumcision: still debatable, Am. J. Nurs. 89(10):1268, 1989.

Jansson, P.: Early postpartum discharge, Am. J. Nurs. 85(5):547-550, 1985.

Jenny, C., Kuhns, M., and Arakawa, F.: Hymens in newborn female infants, Pediatrics 80:399-400, 1987.

Jones, L.C., and Thomas, S.A.: New fathers' blood pressure and heart rate: relationships to interaction with their newborn infants, Nurs. Res. 38(4):237-241, 1989.

Kayiatos, R., Adams, J., and Gilman, B.: The arrival of a rival: maternal perceptions of toddlers' regressive behaviors after the birth of a sibling, J. Nurs. Midwif. 29(3):205-213, 1984.

Keefe, M.: Comparison of neonatal nighttime sleep-wake patterns in nursery versus rooming-in environments, Nurs. Res. 36(3):140-144, 1987.

Keefe, M., and others: Development of a system for monitoring infant state behavior, Nurs. Res. 38(6):344-347, 1989.

Kennell, J.H., and others: Maternal behavior one year after early and extended post-partum contact, Dev. Med. Child Neurol. 16:172-179, April 1974.

King, N., and Lee, A.: Prematurely erupted teeth in newborn infants, J. Pediatr. 114(5):807-809, 1989.

Klaus, M.H., and Kennell, J.H., editors: Maternal-infant bonding, ed. 2, St. Louis, 1982, Mosby–Year Book, Inc.

Klaus, M., and Kennell, J.: Parent to infant bonding: setting the record straight, J. Pediatr. 102(4):575-576, 1983.

Klaus, M., and others: Maternal attachment—importance of the first postpartum days, N. Engl. J. Med. 286:460, 1972.

Kochen, M., and McCurdy, S.: Circumcision and the risk of cancer of the penis, Am. J. Dis. Child. 134(5):484-486, 1980.

Korsch, B.: More on parent-infant bonding, J. Pediatr. 102(2):249-250, 1983.

Lamb, M.E.: The bonding phenomenon: misinterpretations and their implications, J. Pediatr. 101(4):555-557, 1982.

Lane, A.T., Rehder, P.A., and Helm, K.: Evaluations of diapers containing absorbent gelling material with conventional disposable diapers in newborn infants, Am. J. Dis. Child. 144(3):315-318, 1990.

Larsen, G.L., and Williams, S.D.: Postneonatal circumcision: population profile, Pediatrics 85(5):808-811, 1990.

Lawrence, R.: Breast-feeding: a guide for the medical profession, ed. 3, St. Louis, 1989, Mosby–Year Book, Inc.

Lehrburger, C.: Diapers in the waste stream: a review of waste management and public policy issues, Philadelphia, 1989, National Association of Diaper Services.

Leung, A.: Incidence of natal and neonatal teeth, J. Pediatr. 115(6):1024, 1989.

Liptak, G.S., and others: Enhancing infant development and parent-practitioner interaction with the Brazelton Neonatal Assessment Scale, Pediatrics 72(1):71-78, 1983.

Little, A.D.: Disposable versus reusable diapers: health, environmental, and economic comparisons, Cincinnati, OH, 1990, Procter & Gamble Co.

Lohr, J.: The foreskin and urinary tract infections, J. Pediatr. 114(3):502-504, 1989.

Ludington-Hoe, S.M.: What can newborns really see? Am. J. Nurs. 83(9):1286-1289, 1983.

Lumley, J.: Preschool siblings at birth: short-term effects, Birth 10(1):11-16, 1983.

Lynch, A.: Maternal stress following the birth of a second child. In Klaus, M.H., and Robertson, M.O., editors: Birth, interaction and attachment, Skillman, NJ, 1982, Johnson & Johnson Baby Products Co.

Macfarlane, A.: The psychology of childbirth, Cambridge, MA, 1977, Harvard University Press.

Madlon-Kay, D.: "Witch's milk", Am. J. Dis. Child. 140(3):252-253, 1986.

Marchette, L., Main, R., and Redick, E.: Pain reduction during neonatal circumcision, Pediatr. Nurs. 15(2):207-210, 1989.

Marecki, M., and others: Early sibling attachment, JOGNN 14(5):418-423, 1985.

Maxwell, L.G., and others: Penile nerve block for newborn circumcision, Obstet. Gynecol. 70(3):415-419, 1987.

McCall, R.B.: A hard look at stimulating and predicting development: the cases of bonding and screening, Pediatr. Rev. 3(7):205-212, 1982.

Meggyessy, V., and Méhes, K.: Association of supernumerary nipples with renal anomalies, J. Pediatr. 3:412-413, 1987.

Meier, P., and Wilks, S.: The bacteria in expressed mothers' milk, MCN 12(6):420-423, 1987.

Miller, M.J., and others: Oral breathing in newborn infants, J. Pediatr. 107(3):465-469, 1985.

Miller, S.A., and Chopra, J.G.: Problems with human milk and infant formulas, Pediatrics 74(suppl.):639-647, 1984.

Mitchell, K., and Mills, N.M.: Is the sensitive period in parent-infant bonding overrated? Ped. Nurs. 9(2):91-94, 1983.

Motohara, K., and others: Relationship of milk intake and vitamin K supplementation to vitamin K status in newborns, Pediatrics 84(1):90-93, 1989.

National Institutes of Health Consensus Development Conference Statement: Newborn screening for sickle cell disease and other hemoglobinopathies, April 6-8, 1987.

Newman, N.M.: Use of povidone-iodine in umbilical cord care, Clin. Pediatr. 28:37, 1989.

Novack, A.H., Mueller, B., and Ochs, H.: Umbilical cord separation in the normal newborn, Am. J. Dis. Child. 142:220-223, Feb. 1988.

O'Conner, S., and others: Reduced incidence of parenting inadequacy following rooming-in, Pediatrics 66:176, 1980.

O'Connor, M., and Addiego, J.: Use of oral vitamin K to prevent hemorrhagic disease of the newborn infant, J. Pediatr., 1986.

O'Grady, R.: Feeding behavior in infants, Am. J. Nurs. 71(4):736-739, 1971.

Oudesluys-Murphy, A., and Degroot, C.: Perinatal factors and separation time of the umbilical cord, Am. J. Dis. Child. 142(12):1274-1275, 1988.

Paneth, N., and Fox, H.E.: The relationship of Apgar score to neurologic handicap: a survey of clinicians, Obstet. Gynecol. 61:547-550, 1983.

Park, M., and Lee, D.: Normative arm and calf blood pressure values in the newborn, Pediatrics 83(2):240-243, 1989.

Park, M., and Menard, S.: Normative oscillometric blood pressure values in the first 5 years in a office setting, Am. J. Dis. Child. 143(7):860-864, 1989.

Pascoe, J., and French, J.: Development of positive feelings in primiparous mothers toward their normal newborns, Clin. Pediatr. 28(10):452-456, 1989.

Patel, D., and others: Bacterial colonization of plastic bulb syringes, J. Pediatr. 112(3):466-468, 1988.

Perry, S.E.: Parents' perceptions of their newborn following structured interactions, Nurs. Res. 32(4):208-212, 1983.

Pete, J.: Newborn infants' preference for sterile water versus five-percent glucose and water, J. Pediatr. Nurs. 4(4):263-267, 1989.

Pitzer, M.S., and Hock, E.: Employed mothers' concerns about separation from the first- and second-born child, Res. Nurs. Health 12:123-128, 1989.

Poissonnet, C., LaVelle, M., and Burdi, A.: Growth and development of adipose tissue, J. Pediatr. 113(1):1-9, 1988.

Poland, R.: The question of routine neonatal circumcision, N. Engl. J. Med. 322(18):1312-1315, 1990.

Powell, M.: The Neonatal Behavioral Assessment Scale. In Powell, M.: Assessment and management of developmental changes and problems in children, ed. 2, St. Louis, 1981, Mosby–Year Book, Inc.

Ramsey, K.P., and Svee, R.L.: Povidone-iodine cord care, Pediatrics 82(6):951, 1988.

Recommendations and Reports: 1989 sexually transmitted diseases treatment guidelines, MMWR 38(S-8):25-28, 1989.

Reiff, M.I., and Essock-Vitale, S.M.: Hospital influences on early infant-feeding practices, Pediatrics 76(6):872-879, 1985.

Ringler, N., and others: The effects of extra postpartum contact and maternal speech patterns on children's IQs, speech, and language comprehension at five, Child Dev. 49:862-865, Sept. 1978.

Roberts, F.B.: Infant behavior and the transition to parenthood, Nurs. Res. 32(4):213-217, 1983.

Ross Laboratories Mothers' surveys: Recent trend in breast-feeding, Columbus, OH, 1989, Ross Laboratories.

Rubin, R.: Maternal touch, Nurs. Outlook 11:828-831, Nov. 1963.

Rush, J.: Does routine newborn bathing reduce *Staphylococcus aureus* colonization rates? A randomized controlled trial, Birth 13(3):176-180, 1986.

Rush, J., and others: A randomized controlled trial of a nursery ritual: wearing cover gowns to care for healthy newborns, Birth 17(1):25-30, 1990.

Ryan, A., and Martinez, G.: Physical growth of infants 7 to 13 months of age: results from a national survey, Am. J. Phys. Anthropol. 73:449-457, 1987.

Ryan. A., and others: Duration of breast-feeding patterns established in the hospital: influencing factors, Clin. Pediatr. 29(2):99-107, 1990.

Saigal, S., and others: Observations on the behavioral state of newborn infants during the first hour of life: a comparison of infants delivered by the Leboyer and conventional methods, Am. J. Obstet. Gynecol. 139:715-719, March 1981.

Schoen, E.: The status of circumcision of newborns, N. Engl. J. Med. 322(18):1308-1312, 1990.

Schwab, F., and others: Sibling visitation in neonatal intensive care unit, Pediatrics 71(4):835-838, 1983.

Seymour, J.L., and others: Clinical effects of diaper types on the skin of normal infants and infants with atopic dermatitis, J. Am. Acad. Dermatol. 17:988-997, 1987.

Sheth, K. and others: *Pseudomonas aeruginosa* otitis externa in an infant associated with a contaminated infant bath sponge, Pediatrics 77(6):920-921, 1986.

Siegel, E., and others: Hospital and home support during infancy: impact on maternal attachment, child abuse and neglect, and health care utilization, Pediatrics 66(2):183-190, 1980.

Solheim, K., and Spellacy, C.: Sibling visitation: effects on newborn infection rates, JOGNN 17:43-48, 1988.

Sollid, D., and others: Breast-feeding multiples, J. Perinat. Neonatal Nurs. 3(1):46-65, 1989.

Stang, H.J., and others: Local anesthesia for neonatal circumcision: effects on distress and cortisol response, JAMA 259(10):1507-1511, 1988.

Stephen, S., and Sexton, P.: Neonatal axillary temperatures: increases in readings over time, Neonatal Network 5(6):25-28, 1987.

Stevens-Simon, C., and others: Effects of race on the validity of clinical estimates of gestational age, J. Pediatr. 115(6):1000-1002, 1989.

Taylor, P., Maloni, J., and Brown, D.: Early suckling and prolonged breast-feeding, Am. J. Dis. Child. 140(2):151-154, 1986.

Templeton, J., Edgil, A., and Douglas, A.: Reva Rubin revisited, JOGNN 17(6):394-399, 1988.

Trause, M., and Irvin, N.: Care of the sibling. In Klaus, M.H., and Kennell, J.H., editors: Maternal-infant bonding, ed. 2, St. Louis, 1982, Mosby–Year Book, Inc.

Tulman, L.J.: Mothers' and unrelated persons' initial handling of newborn infants, Nurs. Res. 34(4):205-210, 1985.

Tyson, J., and others: Randomized trial of taurine supplementation for infants ≤ 1300-gram birth weight: effect on auditory brainstem-evoked responses, Pediatrics 83(3):406-415, 1989.

Walz, B.L.: Maternal tasks of taking on a second child in the postpartum period, Matern. Child Nurs. J. 12(3):185-216, 1983.

Weaver, R.H., and Cranley, M.S.: An exploration of paternal-fetal attachment behavior, Nurs. Res. 32(2):68-72, 1983.

Wilson, C.B., and others: When is umbilical cord separation delayed? J. Pediatr. 107(2):292-294, 1985.

Winberg, J., and others: The prepuce: a mistake of nature? Lancet 1(8638):598-599, 1989.

Wiswell, T.E., and Geschke, D.W.: Risks from circumcision during the first month of life compared with those for uncircumcised boys, Pediatrics 83(6):1011-1015, 1989.

BIBLIOGRAPHY

Physiologic Status of the Newborn/Assessment of the Neonate

Abrams L, and others: Effect of peripheral IV infusion on neonatal axillary temperature measurement, Pediatr. Nurs. 15(6):630-632, 1989.

Allen, M.C., and Capute, A.J.: Tone and reflex development before term, Pediatrics 85(suppl.):393-399, 1990.

Als, H.: Patterns of infant behavior: analogues of later organizational difficulties? In Duffy, F.H., and Geschwind, N., editors: Dyslexia, Boston, 1985, Little, Brown & Co., Inc.

Ashkenazi, S., and others: Size of liver edge in full-term, healthy infants, Am. J. Dis. Child. 138:377-378, 1984.

Baron, M., and Tafuro, P.: The extremes of age: the newborn and the elderly, Nurs. Clin. North Am. 20(1):181-190, 1985.

Becker, P.T., Lederman, R.P., and Lederman, E.: Neonatal measures of attention and early cognitive status, Res. Nurs. Health 12:381-388, 1989.

Catlin, E.A., and others: The Apgar score revisited: influence of gestational age, J. Pediatr. 109:865-868, 1986.

Coen, R.W., and others: A fast, efficient newborn exam, Patient Care 22(11):192-197, 200-204, 207, 1988.

Coen, R.W., and others: The detailed newborn examination, Patient Care 22(12):93-96, 99, 102, 1988.

Dodman, N.: Newborn temperature control, Neonatal Network 5(6):19-23, 1987.

Duffy, F.H., and others: Neural plasticity: a new frontier for infant development. In Fitzgerald, H.E., Lester, B.M., and Yogman, M.W., editors: Theory and research in behavioral pediatrics, vol. 2, New York, 1984, Plenum Press.

Fanaroff, A., and Martin, R., editors: Neonatal-perinatal medicine, ed 4, St. Louis, 1987, Mosby–Year Book, Inc.

Georgieff, M.K., and others: Mid-arm circumference/head circumference ratios for identification of symptomatic LGA, AGA, and SGA newborn infants, J. Pediatr. 109:316-321, 1986.

Haddock, B.J., Merrow, D.L., and Vincent, P.A.: Comparisons of axillary and rectal temperatures in the preterm infant, Neonatal Network 6(5):67-71, 1988.

Haith, M.M.: Sensory and perceptual processes in early infancy, J. Pediatr. 109(1):158-171, 1986.

Harpin, V.A., and Rutter, N.: Barrier properties of the newborn infant's skin. J. Pediatr. 102(3):419-425, 1983.

Hayes, J.S., Dreher, M.C., and Nugent, J.K.: Newborn outcomes with maternal marihuana use in Jamaican women, Pediatr. Nurs. 14(2):107-110, 1988.

Korones, S.B.: High-risk newborn infants: the basis for intensive nursing care, ed. 4, St. Louis, 1986, Mosby–Year Book, Inc.

Kunnel, M.T., and others: Comparisons of rectal, femoral, axillary, and skin-to-mattress temperatures in stable neonates, Nurs. Res. 37(3):162-164, 189, 1988.

Labson, L.H.: Newborn exam: evaluation in the nursery, Patient Care 17(10):95-98, 1983.

Lawhon, G.: Management of stress in premature infants. In Angelini, D.J., Whelan Knapp, C.W., and Gibes, R.M., editors: Perinatal/neonatal nursing: a clinical handbook, Boston, 1986, Blackwell Scientific Publications, Inc.

Lebenthal, E., Lee, P.C., and Heitlinger, L.A.: Impact of development of the gastrointestinal tract on infant feeding, J. Pediatr. 102(1):1-9, 1983.

Lebenthal, E., and Leung, Y.: The impact of development of the gut on infant nutrition, Pediatr. Ann. 16(3):211-222, 1987.

Linder, N., and others: Suckling stimulation test for neonatal tremor, Arch. Dis. Child. 64:44-52, 1989.

Lipsitt, L.P.: Learning in infancy: cognitive development in babies, J. Pediatr. 109(1):172-183, 1986.

Marchbanks, P.: Newborn assessment: physical examination. In Humenick, S.S., editor: Analysis of current assessment strategies in the health care of young children and childbearing families, Norwalk, CT, 1982, Appleton-Century-Crofts.

Medoff-Cooper, B., Weininger, S., and Zukowsky, K.: Neonatal sucking as a clinical assessment tool: preliminary findings, Nurs. Res. 38(3):162-165, 1989.

Moen, J.E., and others: Axillary versus rectal temperatures in preterm infants under radiant warmers, JOGNN, 16(5):348-352, 1987.

Parker, S., and others: Jitteriness in full-term neonates: prevalence and correlates, Pediatrics 85(1):17-23, 1990.

Ruchala, P.: The effect of wearing headcoverings on the axillary temperatures of infants, MCN 10(4):240, 1985.

Sasanow, S.R., Georgieff, M.K., and Pereira, G.R.: Mid-arm circumference and mid-arm/head circumference ratios: standard curves for anthropometric assessment of neonatal nutritional status, J. Pediatr. 109:311-315, 1986.

Scanlon, J.W., and others: A system of newborn physical examination, Baltimore, 1979, University Park Press.

Scharping, E.M.: Physiological measurements of the neonate, MCN 8(1):70-73, 1983.

Schiffman, R.F.: Temperature monitoring in the neonate: a comparison of axillary and rectal temperatures, Nurs. Res. 31(5):274-277, 1982.

Stevens, C.A., and others: Development of human palmar and digital flexion creases, J. Pediatr. 113:128-132, 1988.

Taylor, K.M.: The Apgar scoring system. In Humenick, S.S., editor: Analysis of current assessment strategies in the health care of young children and childbearing families, Norwalk, CT, 1982, Appleton-Century-Crofts.

Taylor, K.M.: Gestational age assessment. In Humenick, S.S., editor: Analysis of current assessment strategies in the health care of young children and childbearing families, Norwalk, CT, 1982, Appleton-Century-Crofts.

Wilson, C.B.: Immunologic basis for increased susceptibility of the neonate to infection, J. Pediatr. 108(1):1-12, 1986.

Nursing Care of the Neonate: General

Adam, H.M., Stern, E.K., and Stein, R.E.K.: Anticipatory guidance: a modest intervention in the nursery, Pediatrics 76(5):781-786, 1985.

American Academy of Pediatrics: Newborn screening for sickle cell disease and other hemoglobinopathies, Pediatrics 83(suppl.):entire issue, May 1989.

Caravella, S., Clark, D., and Dweck, H.: Health codes for newborn care, Pediatrics 80(1):1-5, 1987.

Greer, F.R., and others: Vitamin K_1 (phylloquinone) and Vitamin K_2 (menaquinone) status in newborns during the first week of life, Pediatrics 81(1):137-140, 1988.

Hammerschlag, M.R.: Chlamydial infections, J. Pediatr. 114(5):727-734, 1989.

Pang, S., and others: Worldwide experience in newborn screening for classical congenital adrenal hyperplasia due to 21-hydroxylase deficiency, Pediatrics 81(6):866-874, 1988.

Polichroniadis, M.: Parental understanding and attitudes towards neonatal biochemical screening, Midwives Chronicle Nurs. Notes 102(1213):42-43, 1989.

Wilkerson, N.N., and Barrows, T.L.: Synchronizing care with mother-baby rhythms, MCN 13(4):264-269, 1988.

Williams, J.K.: Screening for genetic disorders, J. Pediatr. Health Care 3(3):115-121, 1989.

Circumcision

Fergusson, D.M., Lawton, J.M., and Shannon, F.T.: Neonatal circumcision and penile problems: an 8-year longitudinal study, Pediatrics 81(4):537-541, 1988.

Harris, C.C.: Cultural values and the decision to circumcise, Image 18(3):98-104, 1986.

Kashani, I.A., and Faraday, R.: The risk of urinary tract infection in uncircumcised male infants, Int. Pediatr. 4(1):44-45, 1989.

Lindeke, L., Iverson, S., and Fisch, R.: Neonatal circumcision: a social and medical dilemma, Matern. Child Nurs. J. 12(1):31-37, 1986.

Wayland, J.R., and Higgins, P.G.: Newborn circumcision: father's involvement, Pediatr. Nurs. 9(1):41-42, 1983.

Williamson, P.S., and Evans, N.D.: Neonatal cortisol response to circumcision with anesthesia, Clin. Pediatr. 25(8):412-415, 1986.

Wirth, J.L.: Circumcision in Australia: an update, Aust. Paediatr. J. 22(3):225-226, 1986.

Wiswell, T.E., and others: Declining frequency of circumcision: implications for changes in the absolute incidence and male to female sex ratio of urinary tract infections in early infancy, Pediatrics 79(3):338-342, 1987.

Wiswell, T.E., and Roscelli, J.D.: Corroborative evidence for the decreased incidence of urinary tract infections in circumcised male infants, Pediatrics 78(1):96-99, 1986.

Wiswell, T.E., and others: Effect of circumcision status on periurethral bacterial flora during the first year of life, J. Pediatr. 113:442-446, 1988.

Nutrition

Beckholt, A.P.: Breast milk for infants who cannot breastfeed, JOGNN 19(3):216-222, 1990.

Benkov, K.J., and LeLeiko, N.S.: A rational approach to infant formulas, Pediatr. Ann. 16(3):225-230, 1987.

Boyes, S.M.: AIDS virus in breast milk: a new threat to neonates and donor breast milk banks, Neonatal Network 5(5):37-39, 1987.

Colebunders, R., and others: Breastfeeding and transmission of HIV, Lancet 2(8626/8627):1487, 1988.

Cunningham, A.S.: Breast-feeding and health, J. Pediatr. 110(4):658-659, 1987.

Evans, C.J., Lyons, N.B., and Killien, M.G.: The effect of infant formula samples on breastfeeding practice, JOGNN 15(5):401-405, 1986.

Frank, D.A., and others: Commercial discharge packs and breast-feeding counseling: effects on infant-feeding practices in a randomized trial, Pediatrics 80(6):845-854, 1987.

Gale, R., and others: Breast-feeding of term infants: three-hour vs. four-hour non-demand, Clin. Pediatr. 28(10):458-460, 1989.

Gray-Donald, K., and others: Effect of formula supplementation in the hospital on the duration of breast-feeding: a controlled clinical trial, Pediatrics 75(3):514-518, 1985.

Grossman, L.K., and others: The effect of postpartum lactation counseling on the duration of breast-feeding in low-income women, Am. J. Dis. Child. 144(4):471-474, 1990.

Grossman, L.K., and others: The infant feeding decision in low and upper income women, Clin. Pediatr. 29(1):30-37, 1990.

Hill, P.D.: Effects of education on breastfeeding success, Matern. Child Nurs. J. 16(2):145-156, 1987.

Howie, P.W., and others: Protective effect of breast feeding against infection, Br. Med. J. 300:11-16, 1990.

Hughes, R.B., and others: Outcome of teaching clean vs. terminal methods of formula preparation, Pediatr. Nurs. 13(4):275-276, 1987.

Kearney, M.H.: Identifying psychosocial obstacles to breastfeeding success, JOGNN 17(2):98-107, 1988.

Kerzner, B.: Breast-feeding: perspectives from 1988, Curr. Opin. Pediatr. 1:380-383, 1989.

Leventhal, J.M., and others: Does breast-feeding protect against infections in infants less than 3 months of age? Pediatrics 78(5):896-903, 1986.

Mathew, O.P., and Bhatia, J.: Sucking and breathing patterns during breast- and bottle-feeding in term neonates, Am. J. Dis. Child. 143:588-592, 1989.

McHarg, K.S.: Breastfeeding while employed, Res. Rev. 4(3):2, 1987.

Minchin, M.K.: Positioning for breastfeeding, Birth 16(2):67-73, 1989.

Moore, M.C.: Taurine supplementation: theoretical and practical considerations, Pediatr. Nurs. 14(6):489-491, 1988.

Nice, F.J.: Can a breast-feeding mother take medication without harming her infant? MCN 14:27-31, Jan./Feb. 1989.

Page-Goertz, S.: Discharge planning for the breastfeeding dyad, Pediatr. Nurs. 15(5):543-544, 1989.

Pipes, P.L.: Nutrition in infancy and childhood, ed. 4, St. Louis, 1989, Mosby–Year Book, Inc.

Report of the task force on the assessment of the scientific evidence relating to infant-feeding practices and infant health, Pediatrics 74(suppl.):579-762, 1984.

Rubin, D.H., and others: Relationship between infant feeding and infectious illness: a prospective study of infants during the first year of life, Pediatrics 85:464-471, 1990.

Ryan, A.S., and Martinez, G.A.: Breast-feeding and the working mother: a profile, Pediatrics 83(4):524-531, 1989.

Schlegel, A.M.: Observations on breast-feeding technique: facts and fallacies, MCN 8(3):204-208, 1983.

Shrago, L., and Bocar, D.: The infant's contribution to breastfeeding, JOGNN 19(3):209-215, 1990.

Task Force on Pediatric AIDS: Perinatal human immunodeficiency virus infection, Pediatrics 82(6):941-944, 1988.

Walker, M.: Commentary: another look at positioning for breastfeeding, Birth 16(2):74-80, 1989.

Winikoff, B., and others: Dynamics of infant feeding: mothers, professionals, and the institutional context in a large urban hospital, Pediatrics 77(3):357-365, 1986.

Wright, A.L., and others: Breast feeding and lower respiratory tract illness in the first year of life, Br. Med. J. 299:946-949, 1989.

Parent-Infant Bonding (Attachment)

Anderson, C.J.: Enhancing reciprocity between mother and neonate, Nurs. Res. 30(2):89-93, 1981.

Anderson, C.J.: Integration of the Brazelton Neonatal Behavioral Assessment Scale into routine neonatal nursing care, Issues Compr. Pediatr. Nurs. 9:341-351, 1986.

Avant, P.K.: A maternal attachment assessment strategy. In Humenick, S.S., editor: Analysis of current assessment strategies in the health care of young children and childbearing families, Norwalk, CT, 1982, Appleton-Century-Crofts.

Beal, J.A.: The Brazelton Neonatal Behavioral Assessment Scale: a tool to enhance parental attachment, J. Pediatr. Nurs. 1(3):170-177, 1986.

Berland, A.: Young fathers' support group, Pediatr. Nurs. 13(4):255-257, 1987.

Bristor, M.W., Helfer, R.E., and Coy, K.B.: Effects of perinatal coaching on mother-infant interaction, Am. J. Dis. Child. 138:254-257, 1984.

Buckner, E.B.: Use of Brazelton Neonatal Behavioral Assessment in planning care for parents and newborns, JOGNN 12:26-30, 1983.

Carter-Jessop, L.: Promoting maternal attachment through prenatal intervention, MCN 6(2):107-112, 1981.

Cronenwett, L.R., and Kunst-Wilson, W.: Stress, social support, and the transition to fatherhood, Nurs. Res. 30(4):196-201, 1981.

Cropley, C.: Assessment of mothering behaviors. In Johnson, S.H., editor: Nursing assessment and strategies for the family at risk, ed. 2, Philadelphia, 1986, J.B. Lippincott Co.

Davis, J.A.: Management of perinatal loss of a twin, Br. Med. J. 297(6663):1613, 1988.

Elsters, A.B., Lamb, M.E., and Kimmerly, N.: Perceptions of parenthood among adolescent fathers, Pediatrics 83(5):758-765, 1989.

Gaffney, K.F.: New directions in maternal attachment research, J. Pediatr. Health Care 2:181-188, 1988.

Gibes, R.M.: Clinical uses of the Brazelton Neonatal Behavioral Assessment Scale in nursing practice, Pediatr. Nurs. 7:23-26, May/June 1981.

Grace, J.T.: Does a mother's knowledge of fetal gender affect attachment? MCN 9:42-45, 1984.

Klaus, M.H., and Robertson, M.O., editors: Birth, interaction and attachment, Skillman, NJ, 1982, Johnson & Johnson Baby Products Co.

Murphy, C.M.: Assessment of fathering behaviors. In Johnson, S.H., editor: Nursing assessment and strategies for the family at risk, ed. 2, 1986, Philadelphia, J.B. Lippincott Co.

Novak, J., and Novak, R.: Facilitating fathering. In Craft, M., and Denehy, J.: Nursing interventions for infants and children, Philadelphia, 1990, W.B. Saunders Co.

Palkovitz, R.: Fathers' motives for birth attendance, Matern. Child Nurs. J. 16(2):123-129, 1987.

Palkovitz, R.: Sources of father-infant bonding beliefs: implications for childbirth educators, Matern. Child Nurs. J. 17(2):101-113, 1988.

Porter, L.S., and Sobong, L.C.: Differences in maternal perception of the newborn among adolescents, Pediatr. Nurs. 16(1):101-104, 1990.

Pressler, J.: Promoting attachment. In Craft, M., and Denehy, J.: Nursing interventions for infants and children, Philadelphia, 1990, W.B. Saunders Co.

Pridham, K.F.: The meaning for mothers of a new infant: relationship to maternal experience, Matern. Child Nurs. J. 16(2):103-122, 1987.

Pridham, K.F., and Chang, A.S.: What being the parent of a new baby is like: revision of an instrument, Res. Nurs. Health 12:323-329, 1989.

Ricks, S.S.: Father-infant interactions: a review of empirical research, Fam. Rel. 34(4):505-511, 1985.

Tomlinson, P.S.: Fathers' involvement with first-born infants: interpersonal and situational factors, Pediatr. Nurs. 13(2):101-105, 1987.

Tomlinson, P.S.: Verbal behavior associated with indicators of maternal attachment with the neonate, JOGNN 19(1):76-77, 1989.

Toney, L.: The effects of holding the newborn at delivery on paternal bonding, Nurs. Res. 32(1):16-19, 1983.

Walker, L.O.: Brazelton Neonatal Behavioral Assessment Scale. In Humenick, S.S., editor: Analysis of current assessment strategies in the health care of young children and childbearing families, Norwalk, CT, 1982, Appleton-Century-Crofts.

Walker, L.O.: Neonatal Perception Inventories. In Humenick, S.S., editor: Analysis of current assessment strategies in the health care of young children and childbearing families, Norwalk, CT, 1982, Appleton-Century-Crofts.

Weingarten, C.T.: Married mothers' perceptions of their premature or term infants and the quality of their relationships with their husbands, JOGNN 19(1):64-73, 1990.

Wieser, M.A., and Castiglia, P.T.: Assessing early father-infant attachment, MCN 9(2):104-106, 1984.

CHAPTER 9

Health Problems of the Newborn

RELATED TOPICS

Birth of a child with a physical defect, Ch. 11
The child with cognitive impairment, Ch. 24
Congenital adrenogenital hyperplasia, Ch. 38
Congenital defects caused by prenatal factors, Ch. 11
Diaper dermatitis, Ch. 13
Genetic counseling, Ch. 5
Health promotion of the newborn and family, Ch. 8
The high-risk newborn and family, Ch. 10
Impact of chronic illness or disability on the child and family, Ch. 22
Infants of diabetic mothers, Ch. 10

GLOSSARY

CH Congenital hypothyroidism
HDN Hemolytic disease of the newborn
hemolytic Related to destruction of red blood cells
heterozygous Having dissimilar genes at a given position (locus) on a pair of chromosomes
Hgb Hemoglobin
homozygous Having the same genes at a given position (locus) on a pair of chromosomes
hyperbilirubinemia Greater than normal amounts of bilirubin in the bloodstream
icterus Jaundice
IEM Inborn error(s) of metabolism
IRDS Idiopathic respiratory distress syndrome
jaundice Yellowish discoloration of skin, mucous membranes, and sclerae of the eyes
kernicterus (bilirubin encephalopathy) Toxic accumulation of bilirubin in central nervous system tissue
$NaHCO_3$ Sodium bicarbonate
PKU Phenylketonuria
RBC Red blood cell
Rh A blood factor contributing to blood incompatibility in the newborn infant
T_4 Thyroxine
TSH Thyroid-stimulating hormone

The newborn may experience a number of problems immediately or shortly after birth. Some, such as birth injuries, are caused by the forces of labor and delivery. Others, such as infections, are chiefly the result of environmental factors. Problems may also be related to the newborn's immature physiologic systems, particularly disorders related to jaundice. In addition, inborn errors of metabolism may be present at birth, and, if identified early, they can be successfully managed to prevent their deleterious effects.

Some conditions require no intervention other than careful assessment and continued observation to distinguish them from potential pathologic situations. Others require immediate identification and intervention to prevent future problems. The nurse's ability to recognize such conditions and institute appropriate care significantly affects newborns' immediate survival and later development.

BIRTH INJURIES

Birth injuries are injuries that occur during the birth process. The forces of labor and delivery may result in trauma, especially when the infant is large, the presentation is breech, forceful extraction is used, or inexperienced practitioners are in attendance. Birth trauma ranks ninth as a cause of neonatal mortality.

Many injuries are minor and resolve spontaneously in a few days; others, although minor, require some degree of intervention. Still others can be serious and even fatal. Part of the nurse's responsibility is identification of such injuries in order that appropriate intervention can be initiated as soon as possible. Birth injuries can be classified according to the type of body structure involved (Box 9-1).

SOFT TISSUE INJURY

Various types of soft tissue injury may be sustained during the birth process, primarily in the form of bruises and/or abrasions secondary to dystocia. Soft tissue injury usually occurs when there is some degree of disproportion between the presenting part and the maternal pelvis (cephalopelvic disproportion). Common types of soft tissue injury are listed in Box 9-2. These traumatic lesions generally fade spontaneously within a few days without treatment. However, petechiae that appear in areas other than the presenting part (during delivery) may be a manifestation of some underlying bleeding disorder and should be evaluated.

Nursing Considerations

Nursing care is primarily directed toward assessing the injury, maintaining asepsis of the area to prevent breakdown and infection, and providing an explanation and reassurance to the parents. Accurate descriptions of the injuries are recorded to facilitate subsequent comparative nursing evaluations (e.g., extent of petechiae).

Regardless of how benign the injury, parents are concerned and mourn the loss of the expected "perfect" infant. Explanations of the cause and treatment, if any, need to be thorough and repeated frequently. If the injury is disfiguring, such as extensive facial bruising, the parental feelings of revulsion should be respected. Nurses can demonstrate acceptance of the child through their example of sensitive, personal care of the infant. Even if the injuries are tempo-

Box 9-1 TYPES OF PHYSICAL INJURIES AT BIRTH

Soft Tissue Injury
Erythema
Abrasion
Petechiae
Ecchymoses
Subcutaneous fat necrosis
Subconjunctival (scleral) hemorrhage
Retinal hemorrhage
Hemorrhage into abdominal organ(s)

Head Injury
Skull molding
Caput succedaneum
Subgaleal hemorrhage
Cephalhematoma
Fracture (depressed or linear)
Intracranial hemorrhage
Subdural or epidural hematoma

Neurologic Injury
Facial paralysis
Brachial palsy (Erb-Duchenne paralysis, Klumpke palsy)
Phrenic nerve palsy (diaphragmatic paralysis)
Spinal cord injury

Box 9-2 COMMON TYPES OF SOFT TISSUE INJURY

Erythema and abrasions—usually the result of the application of forceps; discoloration is the same configuration as the instrument.
Petechiae—nonraised, pinpoint hemorrhages caused by a sudden increase and then release of pressure during passage through the birth canal; may be seen on the chest, face, and head.
Ecchymoses—small hemorrhagic areas (larger than petechiae) that may occur after traumatic, rapid (or "precipitate"), or breech delivery.
Subcutaneous fat necrosis—clearly outlined masses located in the subcutaneous tissues that are firm to the overlying skin but movable over the underlying tissue; most likely caused by traumatic manipulation during delivery.
Subconjunctival (scleral) hemorrhages—the result of rupture of capillaries in the sclera from pressure on the fetal head during delivery; most common location is the limbus of the iris.
Retinal hemorrhages—flame-shaped, irregular, or round areas of bleeding in the retina from excessive pressure on the fetal head during delivery; extensive areas may indicate subdural hematoma or brain trauma.

rary, the bonding process can be affected by the parents' initial feelings of shock, grief, and disappointment. Every effort should be made to facilitate bonding during the postpartum admission.

HEAD TRAUMA

Trauma to the head that occurs during the birth process is usually benign but occasionally results in more serious injury. The injuries that produce serious trauma, such as intraventricular hemorrhage and subdural hematoma, are discussed in relation to neurologic disorders in the newborn (see Chapter 10). Skull fractures are discussed in association with other fractures sustained during the birth process. The three most common types of extracranial hemorrhagic injury are caput succedaneum, subgaleal hemorrhage, and cephalhematoma.

Caput Succedaneum

The most commonly observed scalp lesion is caput succedaneum, a vaguely outlined area of edematous tissue situated over the portion of the scalp that presents in a vertex delivery (Fig. 9-1, *A*). The swelling consists of serum and/or blood, which accumulate in the tissues above the bone. Typically, the swelling extends beyond the bone margins and may be associated with overlying petechiae or ecchymosis. It is present at or shortly after birth. No specific treatment is needed, and the swelling subsides within a few days.

Subgaleal Hemorrhage

Subgaleal hemorrhage is bleeding into the subgaleal compartment (Fig. 9-1, *B*). The subgaleal compartment is a potential space that contains loosely arranged connective tissue; it is located beneath the galea aponeurosis, which is the tendinous sheath that connects the frontal and occipital muscles and forms the inner surface of the scalp. The injury occurs as a result of forces that compress and then drag the head through the pelvic outlet (Minarcik and Beachy, 1989). The bleeding extends beyond bone and can continue after birth, with potential for complications. Treatment is usually not needed, but it may be required for blood loss and shock. Resolution of the bleeding may cause hyperbilirubinemia.

Cephalhematoma

Infrequently a cephalhematoma is formed when blood vessels rupture during labor or delivery to produce bleeding into the area between the bone and its periosteum. The injury occurs most often with primiparous women, and it is often associated with forceps delivery. Unlike caput succedaneum, the boundaries of the cephalhematoma are sharply demarcated and do not extend beyond the limits of the bone (Fig. 9-1, *C*). The cephalhematoma may involve one or both parietal bones. Less commonly the occipital and rarely the frontal bones are affected. The swelling is usually minimal at birth and increases in size on the second or third day. Blood loss is not significant.

No treatment is indicated for uncomplicated cephalhematoma. Most lesions are absorbed within 2 weeks to 3 months. Lesions that result in severe blood loss to the area or that involve an underlying fracture require further evaluation. Hyperbilirubinemia may result during resolution of the hematoma. A local infection can develop and is suspected when a sudden increase in swelling occurs.

Nursing Considerations

Nursing care is directed toward assessment and observation of the common scalp injuries and vigilance in observing for possible associated complications such as infection, subdural hematoma, or intraventricular hemorrhage. Because these visible injuries resolve spontaneously, parents need reassurance of their usual benign nature (see also earlier discussion under Soft Tissue Injury).

FRACTURES

Fracture of the clavicle, or collarbone, is the most common birth injury. It is associated with difficult vertex or breech delivery of infants of above average weight. The fracture may be detected during delivery by an audible click or snap, although the newborn may be asymptomatic. The problem should be suspected in infants who demonstrate limited use of the affected arm, a malposition of the arm, asymmetric Moro reflex, or local swelling or tenderness, or who cry in pain when the arm is moved. Crepitus (the crackling sound produced by the rubbing together of fractured bone fragments) is often heard and/or felt on further examination, and radiographs usually reveal a complete fracture with overriding of the fragments.

Fractures of long bones, such as the femur or humerus, may be undetected because the epiphysis is mostly cartilage, which is usually not dense enough to show clearly on radiographs. Presence of fracture(s), especially in the absence of difficulty at birth, may be an indication to evaluate the infant for osteogenesis imperfecta (see Chapter 39).

Fractures of the neonatal skull are uncommon. The bones, which are less mineralized and more compressible, are separated by membranous seams that allow sufficient alteration in the head contour so that it can adjust to the birth canal during delivery. Skull fractures usually follow prolonged, difficult delivery or forceps extraction. Most fractures are linear, but some may be visible as depressed indentations resembling a Ping-Pong ball.

Nursing Considerations

Frequently, no intervention may be prescribed other than proper body alignment, careful dressing and undressing of the infant, and handling and carrying that support the affected bone. For example, when picking up the infant who has a fractured clavicle, it is important to support the upper and lower back rather than pull the infant up from under the arms. Occasionally, for immobilization and relief of pain, the arm on the side of the fractured clavicle is stabilized by pinning the sleeve to the shirt or by using a triangular sling or a figure-8 bandage.

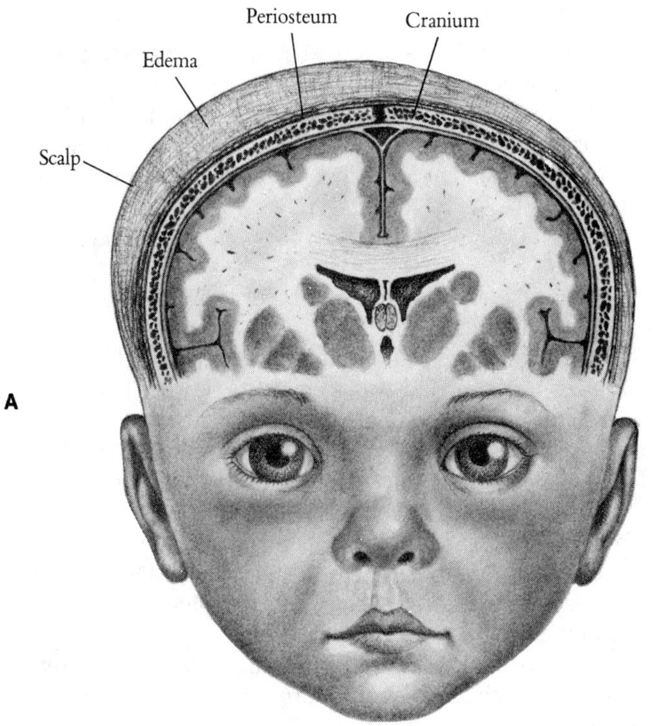

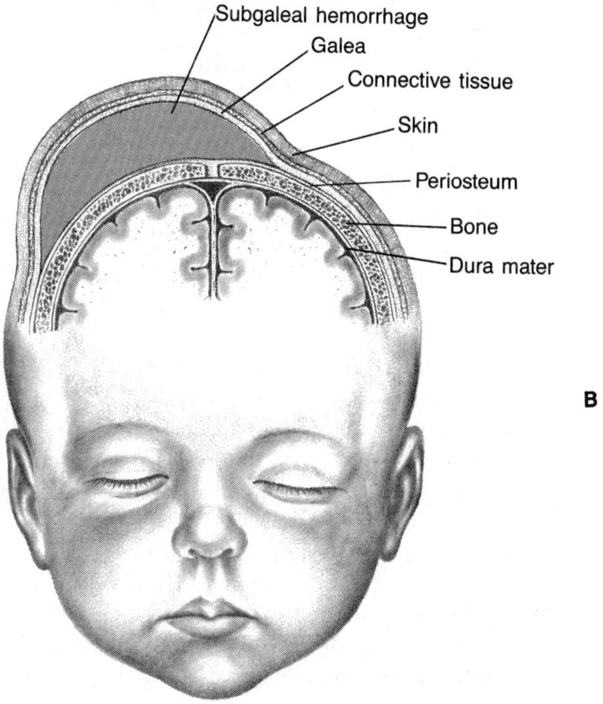

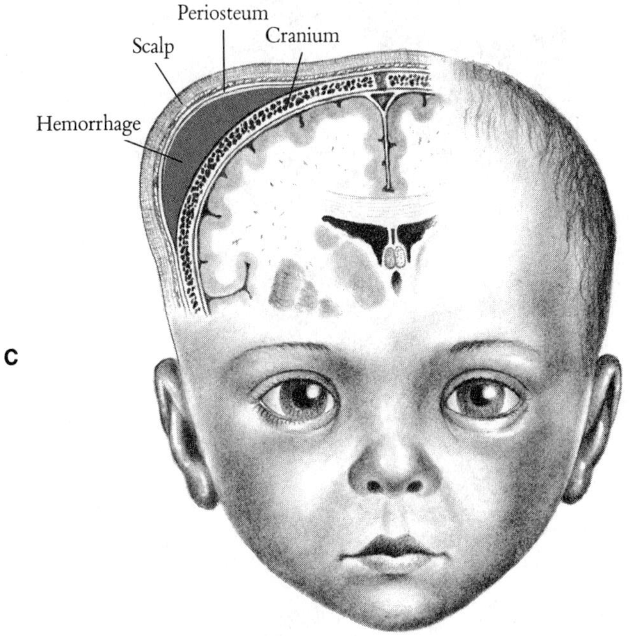

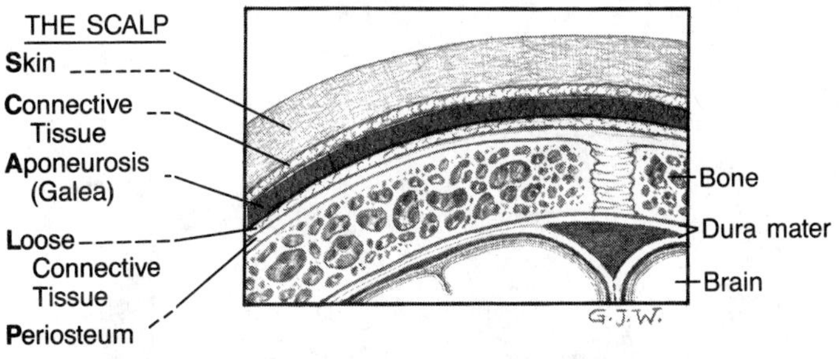

Fig. 9-1. A, Caput succedaneum. **B,** Subgaleal hemorrhage. **C,** Cephalhematoma.

A and **C** from Seidel, H.M., and others: Mosby's guide to physical examination, ed, 2, St. Louis, 1990, Mosby–Year Book, Inc.

✦ **NURSING ALERT** Examine more closely any infant who is reluctant to move an extremity. Fractures are often asymptomatic in the newborn; paralytic injuries are characterized by immobility of an extremity.

Skull fractures usually require no treatment, although a Ping-Pong fracture may be decompressed by nonsurgical methods. The infant is carefully observed for neurologic signs and evidence of cerebral complications. The parents of an infant with a fracture of any bone should be involved in caring for the infant during hospitalization as part of discharge planning for care at home. Family support is similar to that discussed on p. 353 for soft tissue injury.

PARALYSES

Pressure exerted on nerves during a difficult labor can cause injury and paralysis of muscles that the nerves supply. The most frequently observed nerve injuries are those involving the facial nerve and the brachial plexus.

Facial Paralysis

Pressure on the facial nerve during delivery may result in injury to cranial nerve VII. Clinical manifestations are primarily loss of movement on the affected side, such as inability to completely close the eye, drooping of the corner of the mouth, and absence of wrinkling of the forehead and nasolabial fold (Fig. 9-2). Paralysis is most noticeable when the infant cries. The mouth is drawn to the unaffected side, the wrinkles are deeper on the normal side, and the eye on the involved side remains open.

No medical intervention is necessary. The paralysis usually disappears spontaneously in a few days but may take up to 6 months.

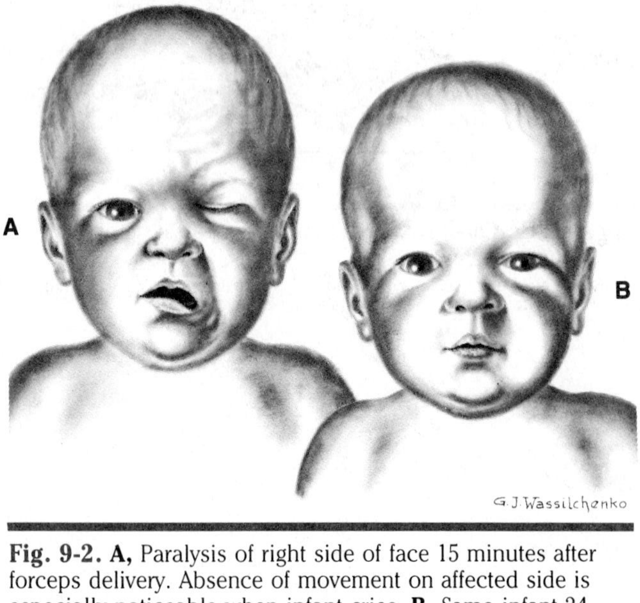

Fig. 9-2. A, Paralysis of right side of face 15 minutes after forceps delivery. Absence of movement on affected side is especially noticeable when infant cries. **B,** Same infant 24 hours later.

Brachial Palsy

Plexus injury results from forces that alter the normal position and relationship of the arm, shoulder, and neck. *Erb palsy* (Erb-Duchenne paralysis), caused by damage to the upper plexus, is usually a result of stretching or pulling away of the shoulder from the head. The less common lower plexus palsy, or *Klumpke palsy,* results from severe stretching of the upper extremity while the trunk is relatively less mobile.

The clinical manifestations of Erb palsy are related to the paralysis of the affected extremity and muscles. The arm hangs limp alongside the body and is internally rotated, and the wrist is pronated (Fig. 9-3). The muscles of the hand are paralyzed in lower plexus palsy with consequent wrist drop and relaxed fingers. In severe forms of brachial palsy, the entire arm is paralyzed and hangs limp and motionless at the side.

Treatment of an affected arm is aimed at preventing contractures of the paralyzed muscles and maintaining correct placement of the humeral head within the glenoid fossa of the scapula. Complete recovery from stretched nerves usually takes 3 to 6 months. Avulsion of the nerves may result in permanent damage, requiring surgical and orthopedic intervention.

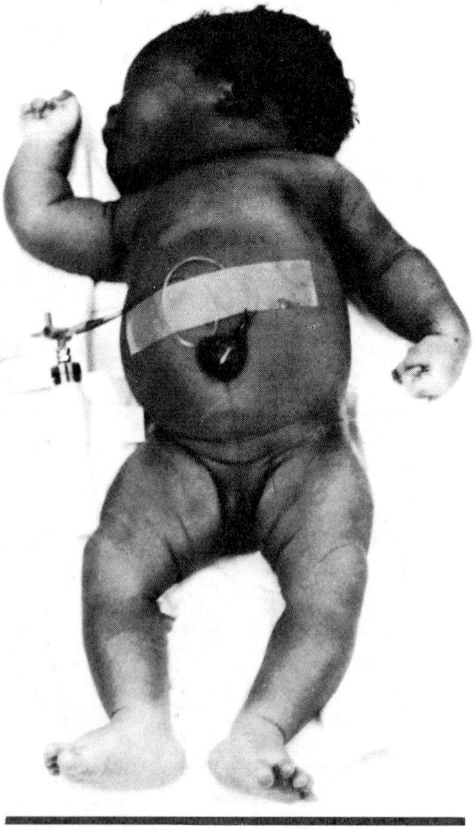

Fig. 9-3. Brachial plexus (Erb) palsy, left sided. Note extended, internally rotated arm and pronated wrist on affected side.

From Korones, S.B.: High-risk newborn infants: the basis for intensive nursing care, ed. 4, St. Louis, 1986, Mosby–Year Book, Inc.

Phrenic Nerve Paralysis

Phrenic nerve paralysis causes diaphragmatic paralysis as demonstrated on radiographic examination by a flattened appearing diaphragm on the affected side. The injury sometimes occurs in conjunction with brachial palsy. Respiratory distress is the most common and important sign of injury. Because injury to the phrenic nerve is usually unilateral, the lung on the affected side does not expand and respiratory efforts are ineffectual. To facilitate maximum expansion of the uninvolved lung, the infant is positioned on the affected side. Breathing is primarily thoracic, and cyanosis is a prominent sign. Pneumonia is a frequent complication.

Nursing Considerations

Nursing care of the infant with facial nerve paralysis involves aiding the infant in sucking and helping the mother with feeding techniques. Because part of the mouth cannot close tightly around the nipple, the use of a soft rubber nipple with a large hole is often helpful. Sometimes the infant needs to be gavage-fed to prevent aspiration. Breast-feeding is not contraindicated, but the mother will need additional assistance in helping the infant to grasp and compress the areolar area.

If the lid of the eye on the affected side does not close completely, artificial tears can be instilled daily to prevent drying of the conjunctiva, sclera, and cornea. The lid is often taped shut to prevent accidental injury. If eye care is needed at home, the parents are taught the procedure for administration of eye drops before the infant's discharge from the nursery (see Chapter 8).

Nursing care of the newborn with brachial palsy is concerned primarily with proper positioning of the affected arm. In upper arm paralysis the arm should be abducted 90 degrees with external rotation at the shoulder, 90-degree flexion at the elbow, full supination of the forearm, and slight extension of the wrist so that the palm of the hand is turned toward the face. The position may be maintained with intermittent splinting. The arm should also be put through complete passive range of motion exercises several times a day to maintain muscle tone and function. In dressing the infant, preference is given to the affected arm. Undressing begins with the unaffected arm, and redressing begins with the affected arm to prevent unnecessary manipulation and stress on the paralyzed muscles.

The infant with phrenic nerve paralysis requires the same nursing care as any infant with respiratory distress. As with other birth injuries, emotional needs of the family are similar to those discussed for soft tissue injury (see p. 353). Also, because of the extended length of recovery, follow-up is essential.

■ DERMATOLOGIC PROBLEMS IN THE NEWBORN

Numerous dermatologic problems may be encountered in the newborn period. Many are innocuous conditions that are of concern only to the parents; others require intervention to prevent complications. Some are discussed elsewhere as appropriate throughout the book; for example, skin manifestations and color changes in the newborn are discussed in Chapter 8. One of the most common observations in the newborn period is jaundice, which is discussed later in this chapter (see Problems Related to Physiologic Factors, p. 359).

ERYTHEMA TOXICUM NEONATORUM

Erythema toxicum neonatorum, also known as *flea bite dermatitis* or *newborn rash,* is a benign, self-limiting eruption that usually appears within the first 2 days of life. The lesions are firm, 1 to 3 mm, pale yellow or white papules or pustules on an erythematous base; they resemble flea bites. The rash appears most commonly on the face, proximal extremities, trunk, and buttocks, but it may be located anywhere on the body except the palms and soles. The rash is more obvious during crying episodes. There are no systemic manifestations, and successive crops of lesions heal without pigmentation. The rash usually lasts about 5 to 7 days.

The etiology is unknown. However, a smear of the pustule will show numerous eosinophils, which may be related to mechanical or thermal stimulation (Berg and Solomon, 1987). Although no treatment is necessary, parents are usually concerned about the rash and need to be reassured of its benign and transient nature.

CANDIDIASIS

Candida infections, also known as *moniliasis*, are not uncommon in the newborn. *Candida albicans*, the organism usually responsible, may cause disease in any organ system. It is a yeastlike fungus (producing yeast cells and spores) that can be acquired from a maternal vaginal infection during delivery, by person-to-person transmission (especially poor handwashing technique), or from contaminated hands, bottles, nipples, or other articles. Mucocutaneous, cutaneous, and disseminated candidiasis are all observed in this age-group. It is usually a benign disorder in the neonate, often confined to the oral and diaper regions.

Candidal Diaper Dermatitis

The warm, moist atmosphere created in the diaper area provides an optimum environment for candidal growth. The dermatitis appears in the perianal area, inguinal folds, and lower abdomen. The affected area is intensely erythematous with a sharply demarcated, scalloped edge, frequently with numerous satellite lesions that extend beyond the larger lesion (see Color Plate 15). The usual source of infection is through the gastrointestinal tract when organisms are swallowed from the birth canal during delivery. It may also appear 2 to 3 days after an oral infection.

Therapy consists of applications of an anticandidal ointment, such as nystatin, with each diaper change. Sometimes the infant also is given an oral antifungal preparation to eliminate any gastrointestinal source of infection (see following discussion).

Oral Candidiasis

Oral candidiasis (*thrush*) is characterized by white adherent patches on the tongue, palate, and inner aspects of the cheeks. It is often difficult to distinguish from coagulated milk (see Color Plate 13). The infant may refuse to suck because of pain in the mouth, but this is uncommon.

✦ **NURSING ALERT** Candidiasis can be distinguished from coagulated milk when attempts to remove the patches are unsuccessful, usually resulting in bleeding from the scraped surfaces.

The condition tends to be acute in the newborn, chronic in infants and young children, and to appear when the oral flora are altered as a result of antibiotic therapy. Although the disorder is usually self-limiting, spontaneous resolution may take as long as 2 months, during which time lesions may spread to the larynx, trachea, bronchi, and lungs and along the gastrointestinal tract. The disease is treated with good hygiene, application of a fungicide, and correction of any underlying disturbance. The source of infection, usually the mother, should be treated to prevent reinfection.

Topical application of 1 ml nystatin (Mycostatin) over the surfaces of the oral cavity four times a day or every 6 hours is usually sufficient to prevent spread of the disease or prolongation of its course. Another effective therapy is application of 1% aqueous gentian violet three times a day.

For candidiasis that is unresponsive to conventional treatment, several other drugs may be used, including amphotericin B (Fungizone), clotrimazole (Lotrimin), or miconazole (Monistat, Micatin). Various preparations may be given intravenously or applied topically. Clotrimazole or nystatin suppositories can also be inserted tightly into the tip of a split pacifier and given to the infant to suck. In older children the suppositories can be used as oral "lozenges" (Mansour and Gelfand, 1981).

Nursing Considerations

Nursing care is directed toward preventing spread of the infection and correct application of the prescribed topical medication. For candidiasis in the diaper area, the caregiver is taught to keep the diaper area as clean and dry as possible and to apply the medication to affected areas as prescribed. Good hygienic care is essential to prevent spread.

Oral nystatin is applied after feedings. The medication is distributed over the surface of the oral mucosa and tongue with an applicator, and the remainder of the dose is deposited in the mouth to be swallowed by the infant to treat any gastrointestinal lesions. Therapy is continued for about 1 week, even when lesions have disappeared within a few days.

When gentian violet is used, the solution is applied directly to the patches. The infant is not allowed to swallow any excess because the medication is irritating to trachea, larynx, and esophagus. After application of the solution, the infant is placed prone for a short time to allow secretions to flow from the mouth. Special care is taken when administering this preparation because gentian violet stains skin, clothing, bed linens, and other objects.

Other measures to control thrush, in addition to good hygienic care, include rinsing the infant's mouth with plain water after each feeding before applying the medication and boiling reusable nipples and bottles for at least 20 minutes after thorough washing (spores are heat-resistant). Pacifiers should be boiled for at least 20 minutes once daily, and the nipples of breast-feeding mothers should also be treated to prevent reinfection.

BULLOUS IMPETIGO

Bullous impetigo (impetigo neonatorum) is an infectious skin condition caused by various strains of group A beta-hemolytic streptococci or coagulase-positive *Staphylococcus aureus*. It is characterized by the eruption of bullous vesicular lesions on previously untraumatized skin. The lesions may appear on any body surface and sometimes become widespread, but the usual distribution involves the buttocks, perineum, trunk, and face. They vary in size from a few millimeters to several centimeters, contain turbid fluid, and are easily ruptured. The bullae rupture in 1 to 2 days, leaving a superficial red, moist, denuded area with very little crusting.

Warm saline compresses are applied to the lesions followed by gentle cleansing and application of a topical antibiotic several times a day. Systemic antibiotics and corticosteroids are sometimes administered to small infants and those with widespread lesions. Recovery is usually rapid and uneventful.

Nursing Considerations

Once the diagnosis is suspected, appropriate precautionary measures are instituted to prevent spread of the infection to other infants. Persons who have come in contact with the infant are investigated to determine a possible source of the infecting organism. Other infants in the nursery should be scrutinized for early detection of any evidence of infection. Parents and other visitors are instructed regarding precautions for prevention of infection.

The infant's arms may need to be restrained with elbow restraints or by pulling the undershirt sleeves over the hands and securing the openings with tape or by applying mittens. If restraints of any kind are used, the infant is allowed freedom of movement at supervised times. Rocking, cuddling, and holding during feeding are essential components of care.

"BIRTHMARKS"

Discolorations of the skin are common findings in the newborn infant. (See discussion on skin assessment of the newborn, Chapter 8.) Most, such as mongolian spots or telangiectatic nevi, involve no therapy other than reassurance to parents of the benign nature of these discolorations. Some can be a manifestation of a disease that suggests further examination of the child and other family members (e.g., the multiple flat, light brown *café au lait spots* that often characterize the autosomal-dominant hereditary disorder neurofibromatosis and are common findings in Albright syndrome).

Darker and/or more extensive lesions demand further scrutiny, and excision of the lesion is recommended when feasible or when excisional biopsy is performed. These lesions include the reddish-brown solitary nodule that appears on the face or upper arm and usually represents a spindle and epithelioid cell nevus (juvenile melanoma); a giant pigmented nevus (bathing trunk nevus); a dark brown to black irregular plaque that is at risk of transformation to malignant melanoma; and the dark brown or black macules that become more numerous with age (junctional or compound nevi).

Vascular birthmarks—orange or light red (salmon patch) or dark red or bluish-red (port wine stain) lesions—are permanent lesions that may become thicker and darker and grow proportionately larger with the child. Good results have been obtained with a series of laser treatments (Dicken, 1985). Lesions located in areas susceptible to trauma or injury and lesions on the face may be treated with laser therapy.

Strawberry hemangiomas, those red, rubbery nodules with a rough surface, may not be present at birth but may appear at 2 to 4 weeks of age. The parents can be reassured that the lesions (even very large ones) resolve spontaneously during childhood and usually require no treatment. If there is evidence of ulceration on the surface of the lesion (because of poor blood supply), the child should receive systemic antibiotics to prevent infection and subsequent scar formation.

Nursing Considerations

Although most birthmarks are benign, they can cause parents considerable anxiety if they are located on highly visible areas, such as the face. A complete explanation of the type of birthmark and treatment options is given, and parents may need advice regarding the use of cosmetic coverings (such as Covermark) at a later time when they feel that the child may be adversely affected by the defect.

■ PROBLEMS RELATED TO PHYSIOLOGIC FACTORS

Neonates are susceptible to a number of problems related to their immature physiologic status. Some can be attributed directly to mechanical injuries sustained during the birth process (intracranial hemorrhage [see Chapter 10], meconium aspiration [see Chapter 10]), some result from postdelivery disturbances (hypoglycemia and hypocalcemia), and others are pathologic variations of certain physiologic peculiarities in some newborn infants (blood incompatibilities). Three of these—hyperbilirubinemia, neonatal hypocalcemia, and neonatal hypoglycemia—are discussed here. Hyperglycemia related to maternal diabetes is discussed in Chapter 38.

HYPERBILIRUBINEMIA

The term *hyperbilirubinemia* refers to an excessive accumulation of bilirubin in the blood and is characterized by *jaundice,* or *icterus,* a yellowish discoloration of the skin and other organs. Hyperbilirubinemia is a common finding in the newborn and in most instances is relatively benign. However, it can also indicate a pathologic state. Following is a brief description of the classification of neonatal jaundice, pathophysiology of bilirubin production and excretion, complications of hyperbilirubinemia, and a discussion of several disorders that cause hyperbilirubinemia in the newborn.

Classification

Hyperbilirubinemia is classified according to the types of bilirubin responsible: *unconjugated* (indirect reacting) and *conjugated* (direct reacting). Special tests distinguish between the direct-reacting and indirect-reacting pigments. Hyperbilirubinemia that is characterized by elevation of unconjugated bilirubin is the type most commonly seen in newborns. Hyperbilirubinemia caused by increased levels of conjugated bilirubin (rare in newborns) implies a functioning liver but signifies serious hepatic problems, such as biliary atresia (see Chapter 11) or neonatal hepatitis. The following discussion of hyperbilirubinemia is limited to the unconjugated type.

Pathophysiology

Bilirubin is one of the breakdown products of hemoglobin (Hgb) that results from destruction of red blood cells (RBCs). Normal RBCs have a limited life span. At the end of their viability, they become fragile and the cell membranes rupture, releasing Hgb, which splits into two fractions, heme and globin. The globin (protein) portion is used by the body; the heme portion is converted to unconjugated bilirubin, an insoluble substance that is rapidly bound to serum albumin.

In the liver, bilirubin is detached from the plasma protein and, in the presence of the enzyme *glucuronyl transferase,* is conjugated with glucuronic acid to produce a highly soluble form, bilirubin glucuronide, which is then excreted into the bile. In the intestine, bacterial action reduces the conjugated bilirubin to urobilinogen and stercobilin, the pigment that gives stool its characteristic color. Most of the reduced bilirubin is excreted through the feces; a small amount is eliminated as urobilinogen in the urine (Fig. 9-4).

Normally the development and dissolution of jaundice follows a pattern. Levels peak at about 3 days after birth, decrease rapidly over the next 2 to 3 days, then gradually fall to normal levels. The normal newborn produces on an average twice as much bilirubin as does an adult because of higher concentrations of circulating erythrocytes and a shorter life span of RBCs (only 70 to 90 days, in contrast to 120 days in the older child and the adult). In addition, the ability of the liver to conjugate bilirubin is reduced because of limited glucuronyl transferase production.

Normally the body is able to maintain a balance between the destruction of RBCs and the use or excretion of by-products. However, when developmental limitations or a patho-

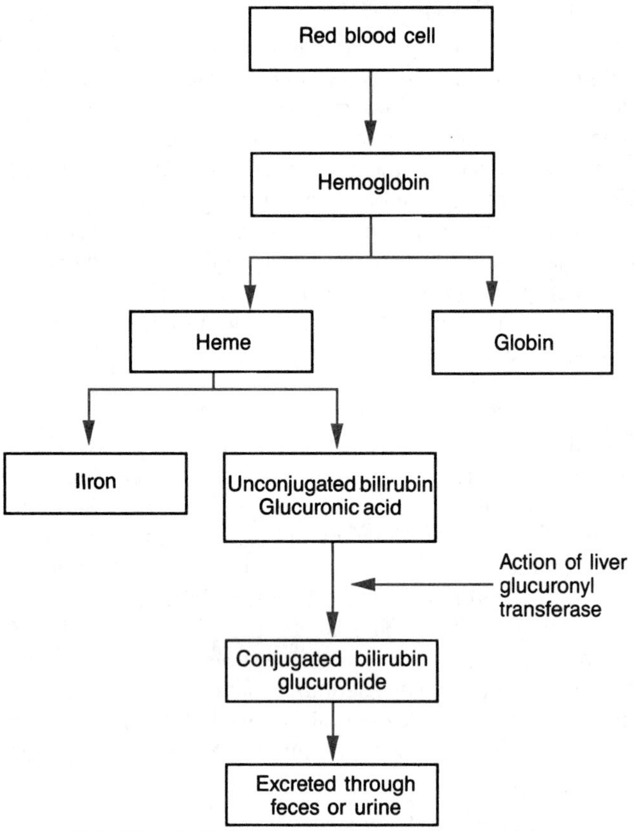

Fig. 9-4. Formation and excretion of bilirubin.

logic process interferes with this balance, bilirubin accumulates in the tissues to produce jaundice. Insoluble bilirubin appears as visible jaundice at serum concentrations greater than 5 mg/dl and is deposited in fatty subcutaneous tissue (Wilkerson, 1988).

In the newborn infant, hyperbilirubinemia may be the result of several factors (Box 9-3). Still other factors appear to influence the development of hyperbilirubinemia. Infants who pass their first meconium stool less than 12 hours after birth are less jaudiced than those who pass the first meconium stool more than 12 hours after delivery (Clarkson and others, 1984). Drugs may compete with bilirubin for binding to albumin, raising the levels of free bilirubin (Robertson, Fink, and Karp, 1988). Infants born at high altitudes demonstrate an increased bilirubin production accompanied by delayed bilirubin clearance in response to decreased oxygen availability (Leibson and others, 1989).

Complications. Unconjugated bilirubin is highly toxic to neurons; therefore an infant with severe jaundice is at risk of developing *bilirubin encephalopathy,* or *kernicterus,* severe brain damage resulting from the deposition of unconjugated bilirubin in brain cells. The damage occurs when the serum concentration reaches toxic levels, regardless of cause. A direct relationship exists between the total serum bilirubin concentration and the risk of kernicterus. In general, a serum bilirubin level of 20 mg/dl in full-term infants is considered the maximum level before the development of brain damage. Unconjugated bilirubin, bound to protein, is unable to cross the protective blood-brain barrier. When conditions lower the protein-binding capacity of plasma, free unconjugated bilirubin is available for cerebral entry.

Box 9-3 CAUSES OF HYPERBILIRUBINEMIA IN THE NEWBORN

Excess production of bilirubin (e.g., hemolytic disease, biochemical defects, bruises)
Disturbed capacity of the liver to secrete conjugated bilirubin (e.g., enzyme deficiency, bile duct obstruction)
Combined overproduction and undersecretion (e.g., sepsis)
Physiologic (developmental) factors (prematurity)
Association with breast-feeding or breast milk
Some disease states (e.g., hypothyroidism, galactosemia, infant of a diabetic mother)
Genetic predisposition to increased production (Native Americans, Asians, Eskimos)

Factors that enhance the development of kernicterus include metabolic acidosis, lowered albumin levels, free fatty acids, and drugs such as salicylates or sulfonamides that compete for attachment to the plasma protein. In addition, any condition that increases the metabolic demands for oxygen or glucose (such as fetal distress, hypoxia, hypothermia, or hypoglycemia) also increases the risk of brain damage despite lower serum levels of bilirubin.

The signs of kernicterus are those of central nervous system depression or excitation. Generally the clinical symptoms appear after the peak plasma bilirubin level has been established for several hours. Prodromal symptoms consist of decreased activity, lethargy, irritability, and a loss of interest in feeding. Within several hours these subtle findings are followed by rigid extension of all four extremities, opisthotonos, irritable cry, seizures, and gastric or pulmonary hemorrhage. Those who survive may eventually show evidence of neurologic damage, such as mental retardation, attention deficit disorder, delayed motor development or abnormal motor movement (especially ataxia or athetosis), behavior disorders, perceptual problems, or sensorineural hearing loss (Cashore and Stern, 1982).

Physiologic Jaundice

Physiologic or developmental jaundice *(icterus neonatorum)* results from the functional immaturity of the newborn liver combined with an increased bilirubin load from hemolysis of RBCs. It is not associated with any pathologic process, as is hemolytic disease of the newborn. Although almost all newborns experience elevated bilirubin levels, only about half demonstrate observable signs of jaundice.

The severity of physiologic jaundice differs markedly among different races. Infants of Oriental descent, including the American Indian and Eskimo, have mean bilirubin levels almost twice as high as those in whites. In addition, newborns from certain geographic locations, particularly areas around Greece, demonstrate an increased incidence of hyperbilirubinemia. Black infants have a lower incidence than white newborns. The reasons for these differences are unclear but may include environmental factors, such as maternal ingestion of certain ethnic foods, or a genetic predisposition for decelerated hepatic maturation (Gartner and Lee, 1987; Linn and others, 1985). A higher incidence of recurrence of hyperbilirubinemia has been observed in infants whose older siblings had hyperbilirubinemia at birth; this suggests the presence of genetic factors (Khoury, Calle, and Joesoef, 1988). The incidence is also associated with maternal diabetes mellitus, decreased gestational age, male sex, bruising, and induction of labor with oxytocin (Maisels and others, 1988).

Mechanisms involved in physiologic jaundice. Newborns have a rate of bilirubin production 2 to 2½ times that of adults and a relative deficiency of glucuronyl transferase. They also have a lower plasma-binding capacity for bilirubin because of reduced albumin concentrations as compared with older children. Normal changes in hepatic circulation following birth may contribute to reduced liver function. Circulatory function improves and enzyme activity increases rapidly after birth.

Normally conjugated bilirubin is reduced to urobilin by the intestinal flora and excreted in feces. However, the sterile newborn bowel is unable to convert bilirubin. Consequently, some unconjugated bilirubin is reabsorbed by the intestine and recirculated to the liver. Feeding (1) stimulates peristalsis and produces more rapid passage of meconium, thus diminishing the amount of reabsorption of unconjugated bilirubin, and (2) introduces bacteria to aid in reduction of bilirubin to urobilinogen. Colostrum, a natural cathartic, facilitates meconium evacuation.

Jaundice in Breast-Feeding Infants

Breast-feeding is associated with an increased incidence of jaundice. Two types have been identified: early-onset breast-feeding jaundice (or "jaundice associated with breast-feeding") and late-onset jaundice (or "breast-milk jaundice"). In late-onset jaundice, rising levels of bilirubin peak during the third week, then gradually diminish. Despite high levels of bilirubin that may persist for 3 to 12 weeks, these infants are well. The reason for the jaundice is unknown although it has been observed that infants with good functional nursing stimulate an earlier adequate supply of breast milk (Osborn, 1986). Early and frequent breast-feeding appears to reduce the likelihood of breast-feeding jaundice.

Breast-feeding–associated jaundice. Breast-feeding-associated jaundice (early-onset jaundice) begins at 2 to 4 days of age and occurs in approximately 10% to 25% of breast-fed newborns. The jaundice may be related to (1) decreased calorie and fluid intake by breast-fed infants before the milk supply is established, since fasting is associated with decreased hepatic clearance of bilirubin (Osborn, Reiff, and Bolus, 1984); or (2) abnormally large amounts of unsaturated fatty acids that inhibit conjugation through an ill-defined mechanism.

Breast milk jaundice. Breast milk jaundice (late-onset jaundice) begins at age 4 to 5 days and occurs in 2% to 3% of breast-fed infants (Maisels, 1985; Lascari, 1986). It may be caused by the presence of a factor in the breast milk (beta-glucuronidase) that breaks down bilirubin to a lipid-soluble form, which is reabsorbed in the gut. Less frequent stooling by breast-fed infants allows for extended time for reabsorption of bilirubin from stools.

Clinical Manifestations

Almost all newborns experience elevated bilirubin levels. However, about half demonstrate observable signs of jaundice—a yellowish discoloration observable principally in the sclera, nails, or skin. Jaundice caused by unconjugated bilirubin is bright yellow or orange; jaundice produced by conjugated bilirubin is a greenish, muddy yellow. As a rule, jaundice that appears within the first 24 hours is caused by hemolytic disease of the newborn, sepsis, or one of the maternally derived diseases, such as diabetes mellitus or infections. Jaundice that appears on the second or third day, peaks on the second to fourth days, and decreases between the fifth and seventh days is usually the result of physiologic jaundice. Jaundice appearing after the third day but within the first week suggests sepsis. The intensity of the jaundice is unrelated to the degree of hyperbilirubinemia. See Table 9-1 for a comparison of hemolytic and nonhemolytic jaundice.

Diagnostic Evaluation

The degree of jaundice is determined by serum bilirubin measurements. Normal values of unconjugated bilirubin are 0.2 to 1.4 mg/dl. In the newborn, levels must exceed 5 mg/dl before jaundice or icterus is observable. Hyperbilirubinemia is defined as a serum bilirubin value greater than 12.9 mg/dl in formula-fed infants and greater than 15 mg/dl in breast-fed infants (Frank, Turner, and Merenstein, 1989).

Noninvasive monitoring of bilirubin via cutaneous reflectance measurements (*transcutaneous bilirubinometry*) allows for repetitive estimations of bilirubin. These devices work well on dark- and light-skinned infants and correlate well with serum determinations of bilirubin level (Schumacher, Thornbery, and Gutcher, 1985; Smith and others, 1985).

Therapeutic Management

The aims of therapy for hyperbilirubinemia are to prevent kernicterus and, in any blood group incompatibility, to reverse the hemolytic process (see p. 366). The main forms of treatment involve phototherapy and pharmacologic management.

Phototherapy. Phototherapy consists of the application of fluorescent light on the infant's exposed skin. Light promotes excretion by photo-oxidation, or photoisomerization, a process that alters the structure of bilirubin to a soluble form for easier excretion. Sunlight also acts in the same way as fluorescent light.

Artificial light used for phototherapy includes any of the following: a single quartz halogen lamp or a bank of white daybright lights, special blue fluorescent light, or fluorescent green light (Frank, Turner, and Merenstein, 1989). Studies show varying results of comparisons of lights. Some findings are (1) no difference between effectiveness of blue and green lights (Vecchi and others, 1986), (2) green light

Table 9-1 Comparison of three types of unconjugated hyperbilirubinemia

	PHYSIOLOGIC JAUNDICE	BREAST-FEEDING–ASSOCIATED JAUNDICE	BREAST MILK JAUNDICE	HEMOLYTIC DISEASE
Cause	Immature hepatic function plus increased bilirubin load from red blood cell hemolysis	Poor milk intake related to fewer calories consumed by infant before mother's milk established	Possible factor in breast milk that breaks down bilirubin where it is reabsorbed from gut Less frequent stooling	Blood antigen incompatibility causes hemolysis of large numbers of erythrocytes Liver unable to conjugate and excrete excess bilirubin from hemolysis
Onset	After 24 hours (premature infants, before 48 hours)	2nd to 3rd day	4th to 5th day	During first 24 hours
Peak	72 hours	2nd to 3rd day	10 to 15 days	Variable
Duration	Decline 5th to 7th days		May remain jaundiced for weeks	
Therapy	Phototherapy Exposure to sunlight	Frequent breast-feeding Caloric supplements Phototherapy for bilirubin 18 to 20 mg/dl	Temporary discontinuation of breast-feeding for 48 hours	*Postnatal:* Exchange transfusion *Prenatal:* Transfusion (fetus) Prevent sensitization (Rh incompatibility) of Rh-negative mother with RhoGAM

appears to enhance the effectiveness of blue light (Hegyi and others, 1986), and (3) green light may be responsible for severe erythema and tanning (Tan, 1989). That phototherapy effectively reduces or prevents rising bilirubin levels is well documented; its long-term effects are unclear.

No universally accepted protocols exist for recommended uses of phototherapy. However, studies from the National Institute of Child Health and Human Development (NICHHD) demonstrated that phototherapy was most effective in the following situations (Brown and others, 1985):

1. Low-birth-weight infants (<2000 g) who received phototherapy at 24 ± 12 hours of life for 96 hours, regardless of bilirubin concentration
2. Infants of birth weight from 2000 to 2499 g who received phototherapy after serum bilirubin concentration had risen above 10 mg/dl and infants of birth weight >2500 g who received phototherapy after serum bilirubin concentration had risen above 13 mg/dl, provided there was no hemolytic disorder. (If hemolysis was present, phototherapy was not effective in controlling the hyperbilirubinemia.)

Black infants respond as well to phototherapy as white infants and phototherapy is most effective in the first 24 to 48 hours of its application. The effectiveness of phototherapy is determined by a decrease in bilirubin, usually to levels of 3 to 4 mg/dl after 8 to 12 hours of therapy. Concurrently, the infant's total physical status is assessed because the suppression of jaundice may mask signs of sepsis, hemolytic disease, or hepatitis.

A recent development and a promising alternative to traditional phototherapy is the *fiberoptic blanket*, which consists of a light-generating illuminator, a bundle of plastic fibers affixed to a panel that distributes the energy, and a soft, disposable, light-permeable cover to protect the infant. The blanket delivers therapeutic light consistently and continuously all around the infant and achieves the same photoisomerization as conventional phototherapy (Rose, 1990).

A trend in phototherapy is its use in the home to treat some types of neonatal hyperbilirubinemia. The controversy surrounding home phototherapy, especially its benefits and risks, is discussed in Questions and Controversies.

Pharmacologic management. Pharmacologic treatment of hyperbilirubinemia has focused mainly on the use of barbiturates, such as phenobarbital, which stimulate protein synthesis (increasing available albumin for binding with unconjugated bilirubin) and promote hepatic glucuronyl transferase synthesis (increasing conjugation of bilirubin and hepatic clearance of the pigment in bile). This therapy achieves best results in infants with hemolytic disease when it is given to the mother 1 to 2 weeks before delivery. However, its routine use in infants with hyperbilirubinemia does not achieve results rapidly enough to be effective.

Recommendations for prevention and management of jaundice in breast-fed infants (especially early-onset jaundice) include (Lascari, 1986):

1. Encourage frequent breast-feeding, preferably every 2 hours, and avoid supplementation.
2. Monitor rising bilirubin levels on an outpatient basis.
3. Temporarily discontinue breast-feeding for 48 hours and use formula when bilirubin levels reach 15 to 16 mg/dl.
4. Resume breast-feeding after a decrease in bilirubin level.

QUESTIONS AND CONTROVERSIES

What are the benefits and risks of home phototherapy?

Because jaundice is such a common occurrence among newborns, home phototherapy has been recommended as an alternative means of providing care. Studies of its benefits cite (1) cost savings from what otherwise would be prolonged hospitalizations and (2) prevention of parent-infant separation (Eggert and others, 1985; Slater and Brewer, 1984). Depending on the geographic location, savings are about 75% of the cost of hospitalization. Both studies demonstrated that the treatment was safe and effective.

However, home phototherapy is not universally endorsed. The American Academy of Pediatrics (1985) considers the available data on safety and efficacy inadequate. As guidelines for eligibility for home phototherapy, the Academy suggests considering as candidates only term infants who (1) are older than 48 hours; (2) are otherwise healthy as evidenced by the history, physical examination, and various blood and urine tests; and (3) have a serum bilirubin concentration greater than 14 mg/100 ml but less than 18 mg/100 ml with no elevation in conjugated bilirubin levels. In addition, the caretakers must be willing to assume the responsibilities and be capable of implementing the care. Risks, such as the possibility that a displaced eye patch may occlude the infant's airway, must be explained. Once serum bilirubin levels fall below 14 mg/100 ml, therapy should be discontinued with appropriate follow-up.

Nurses will obviously play an important role in establishing the risks and benefits of home phototherapy as they participate in the preparation, teaching, and supervision of these families.

Nursing Considerations

The primary nursing consideration is recognition of jaundice and helping to distinguish between a benign disorder and a life-threatening one.

Assessment

Part of the routine physical assessment includes observing for evidence of jaundice at regular intervals. Jaundice is most reliably assessed by observing the infant's skin color from head to toe and color of sclera and mucous membranes. When direct pressure is applied to the skin, especially over bony prominences such as the tip of the nose or the sternum, blanching occurs and the yellow coloration becomes more pronounced. For dark-skinned infants, the color of gums is the most reliable indicator. Also, bilirubin (especially at high levels) is not uniformly distributed in skin. Highest concentrations appear to be in the head areas (Rutledge and Ou, 1989).

NURSING ALERT Evidence of jaundice that appears before the infant is 24 hours of age is an indication for assessing bilirubin levels and prepare for implementing therapy.

The nurse observes the infant in natural daylight for a true assessment of color. When jaundice is observed, blood levels of bilirubin must be determined and monitored as necessary to establish the pattern of increase. Any neonate who becomes icteric during the first 24 hours of life and has rapidly rising bilirubin levels is referred to the physician for immediate evaluation.

The transcutaneous bilirubin meter is a useful screening device and is used to detect neonatal jaundice in full-term infants. However, phototherapy reduces the accuracy of the instrument; therefore its value is limited to the initial assessment in infants receiving phototherapy. Blood samples are also taken for measurement of bilirubin in the laboratory. When blood samples are taken for bilirubin measurement, the phototherapy unit should be turned off and the blood sample tube should be covered for transport to prevent a false reading from bilirubin destruction.

A careful history from the parents may reveal significant familial patterns of hyperbilirubinemia (older siblings of the infant). Other considerations in assessment include the ethnic origin of the family (e.g., higher incidence in Asian infants), type of delivery (e.g., induction of labor), and infant characteristics such as weight loss after birth, gestational age, sex, and presence of any bruising. The method of feeding and frequency of feeding are assessed. The blood types of both infant and mother are reviewed and any medications being given to the infant (e.g., cephalosporins) are noted.

Nursing Diagnoses

After the nursing assessment, a number of nursing diagnoses become evident. The most likely diagnoses are outlined and discussed in the Nursing Care Plan on p. 364. Others may be apparent in individual cases.

Planning

The broad objectives for management of hyperbilirubinemia are as follows:

1. Assist with measures to reduce serum bilirubin levels.
2. Prevent complications from therapy.
3. Support the family.

Implementation

Basic nursing care of the child with hyperbilirubinemia differs from that of any newborn infant only in management of specific therapy (see Nursing Care of the Newborn and Family, Chapter 8, and Nursing Care of High-Risk Newborns, Chapter 10).

Prevention of physiologic and breast-feeding jaundice may be possible with early introduction of feedings and frequent nursing. Every effort is made to provide an optimum thermal environment to reduce metabolic needs.

Phototherapy. The infant who receives phototherapy is placed nude under the light source and repositioned frequently to expose all body surface areas to the light. To be effective, light must come in contact with all the skin sur-

NURSING CARE PLAN
The Child with Hyperbilirubinemia

NURSING DIAGNOSIS: Potential for injury related to breakdown products of red blood cells in greater number than normal and immature blood-brain barrier

GOAL 1

Eliminate excess bilirubin

INTERVENTION

*Place infant under phototherapy lamp as prescribed

EXPECTED OUTCOME

Child is exposed to prescribed light source

GOAL 2

Protect infant during phototherapy

INTERVENTIONS

- Shield infant's eyes
  - Make certain that lids are closed before applying shield
  - Check eyes each shift for drainage or irritation
- Place infant nude under light; shield male genitalia (controversial)
- Change position frequently
- Monitor body temperature
  - Check axillary temperature with reading on servocontrolled unit
- Chart duration of therapy, type of lights, distance of lights to infant, use of open or closed bassinet, and shielding of infant's eyes
- Avoid the use of oily applications on the skin
- Ensure adequate fluid intake to prevent dehydration

EXPECTED OUTCOME

Infant displays no evidence of eye irritation, dehydration, elevated temperature

GOAL 3

Protect infant during and following exchange transfusion (if appropriate)

INTERVENTION

- Give infant nothing by mouth prior to procedure (usually for 3-4 hours)
- Check donor blood with physician for correct blood group and Rh type
- Assist physician during procedure; ensure asepsis
- Keep accurate records of amounts of blood infused and withdrawn
- Monitor vital signs, especially following infusion of calcium gluconate
- Maintain optimal body temperature of infant during procedure (blankets, radiant warmer)
- Observe for signs of exchange transfusion reactions
- Have resuscitative equipment (supplemental oxygen, airway, manual resuscitation bag, endotracheal tube, and laryngoscope) at bedside
- Apply sterile dressing to catheter site
- Check umbilical site for bleeding or infection
- Monitor vital signs following transfusion

EXPECTED OUTCOMES

- Infant exhibits no signs of adverse effects from transfusion
- Vital signs remain within normal limits (see inside front cover for normal variations)
- There is no evidence of infection or bleeding at infusion site

NURSING DIAGNOSIS: Altered family processes related to child with an adverse physiologic response

GOAL 1

Provide emotional support to family

INTERVENTIONS

- Discontinue phototherapy during family visiting; remove infant's eye shields
- Emphasize benign nature of physiologic jaundice
- Assure family that skin will regain normal pigmentation
- Advise breast-feeding mothers of possibility of prolonged jaundice

EXPECTED OUTCOME

Family demonstrates an understanding of the therapy and prognosis

GOAL 2

Prepare family for home phototherapy (if prescribed)

INTERVENTIONS

- Assess family's understanding of the disorder and the proposed therapy
- Instruct family regarding:
  - Placement and care of lamp unit
  - Proper eye care
    - Apply eye patches
    - Close lids before applying patches
    - Be certain patches fit snugly with no possibility of light leaks
    - Remove patches when light is discontinued—during feeding, while family is sleeping
  - Taking axillary temperature on infant
    - Every 15 minutes for initial hour
    - Every 4 hours thereafter while under lights
  - Proper positioning while under lamp
    - Rotate to expose all areas
    - Keep infant nude or dressed in mini-diaper according to unit policy
  - Providing increased fluid intake
  - Keeping a log of time spent under light, infant's color, feeding patterns, amount of feedings, diaper changes
  - Observing for signs of lethargy, change in sleeping pattern, any difficulty arousing infant, changes in stooling or voiding
  - Importance of bilirubin tests as prescribed
  - See Nursing Care Plan: The Low-Birth-Weight Infant, Chapter 10

EXPECTED OUTCOME

Family demonstrates the ability to provide home phototherapy for the infant (specify learning and methods of demonstration)

*Dependent nursing action.

QUESTIONS AND CONTROVERSIES

Should genitals be covered during phototherapy?

No consensus exists regarding protection of genitals. Some recommend covering the gonads with a shield, such as a bikini diaper fashioned from a face mask; others believe this precaution is unnecessary. Until a resolution to this controversy is achieved, the best approach is to follow individual institutional protocols. A small diaper may be needed if diarrhea is a problem. A light-permeable phototherapy diaper is currently under investigation (Millner, 1990).

face. Once phototherapy has been initiated, frequent (every 4 to 12 hours) serum bilirubin levels are necessary, since visual assessment of jaundice is no longer valid (Frank, Turner, and Merenstein, 1989).

Several precautions are instituted to protect the infant during phototherapy. The infant's eyes are shielded by an opaque mask to prevent exposure to the light (Fig. 9-5). The eye shield should be properly sized and correctly positioned to cover the eyes completely but prevent any occlusion of the nares. The infant's eyelids are closed before the mask is applied, since the corneas may become excoriated if they come in contact with the dressing. On each nursing shift the eyes are checked for evidence of discharge, excessive pressure on the lids, or corneal irritation. The eye patch is changed periodically, and the eyes are cleansed with sterile water. Eye shields are removed during feedings, and this opportunity is taken to provide visual and sensory stimulation.

✦ **NURSING ALERT** If the eye shield allows light to enter, the area of jaundice around the eyes will begin to disappear, indicating the need for better eye protection.

The phototherapy unit is often combined with a radiant heat warmer or servocontrolled incubator to provide an optimum thermal environment. The thermistor should be attached to the infant or covered with opaque tape so that it is not exposed to direct radiation. This may require changing the sensor from the abdomen to the back according to the infant's position. Placing the sensor on the infant's side reduces the need for frequent changes. Vital signs are taken at least every 4 hours to ensure that the infant's body temperature is normothermic. Sometimes it is necessary to regulate the temperature in the incubator to maintain proper body heat.

Infants who are in an open crib must have a protective Plexiglas shield between them and the fluorescent lights to minimize the amount of undesirable ultraviolet light reaching their skin and to protect them from accidental bulb breakage. Their temperature is closely monitored to prevent hyperthermia and, less often, hypothermia.

Accurate charting is another important nursing responsibility and includes (1) times that phototherapy is started and stopped, including intervals when no light was applied, (2) proper shielding of the eyes, (3) type of fluorescent lamp (by manufacturer), (4) number of lamps, (5) distance between surface of lamps and infant, (6) use of phototherapy in combination with an incubator or open bassinet, (7) photometer measurement of light intensity, and (8) occurrence of side effects.

Side effects of phototherapy. At present the long-term risks from phototherapy are not known. Although some minor side effects occur, there appears to be no increased mortality in infants treated with phototherapy (Lipsitz, Gartner, and Bryla, 1985). Minor side effects for which the nurse should be alert include loose, greenish stools; hyperthermia; increased metabolic rate; increased water loss (especially from increased bowel motility); electrolyte disturbances, such as hypocalcemia; and priapism. Although the effect of phototherapy on the eyes is uncertain, animal studies indicate that retinal degeneration may occur after several days of continuous exposure.

To prevent or minimize these effects, the temperature is closely monitored to detect early signs of hyperthermia and the skin is observed for evidence of dehydration and drying, which can lead to excoriation and breakdown. Oily lubricants or lotions are not used on the skin in order to prevent increased tanning, or a "frying" effect. Infants receiving phototherapy require 25% to 200% additional fluid volume to compensate for insensible and intestinal fluid loss (Adcock and Consolvo, 1989). There is some evidence that the use of a stockinette cap to cover the head prevents phototherapy-induced hypocalcemia in premature infants 37 gestational weeks or younger (Blake, 1983).

Another reaction to phototherapy is the *bronze-baby syndrome,* in which the serum, urine, and skin become blackish-brown in color several hours after the infant is placed under the light. This reaction is probably caused by retention of a bilirubin breakdown product of phototherapy (Frank, Turner, and Merenstein, 1989). This syndrome almost always occurs in infants who have elevated conjugated hyperbilirubinemia. The browning generally resolves following discontinuation of phototherapy.

Nurses caring for infants being treated with blue light may be subject to eye symptoms as evidenced by irritation, headaches, eye fatigue, distorted color vision, and difficulty adjusting to night vision. For nurses experiencing these symptoms protective goggles designed to filter light are available.*

Family support. Parents need constant reassurance concerning their infant's progress. All the procedures are explained to familiarize them with the benefits and risks.†

*Retina-Spec goggles—for information, contact Eye Communications, 870 S. Myrtle Ave., Monrovia, CA 91016; (800) 247-5731. In California, (800) 626-7694.

†A short description of "Jaundice in Newborns" is available from Wyeth Laboratories, P.O Box 8299, 145 King of Prussia, Radnor, PA 19087; (215) 383-0600.

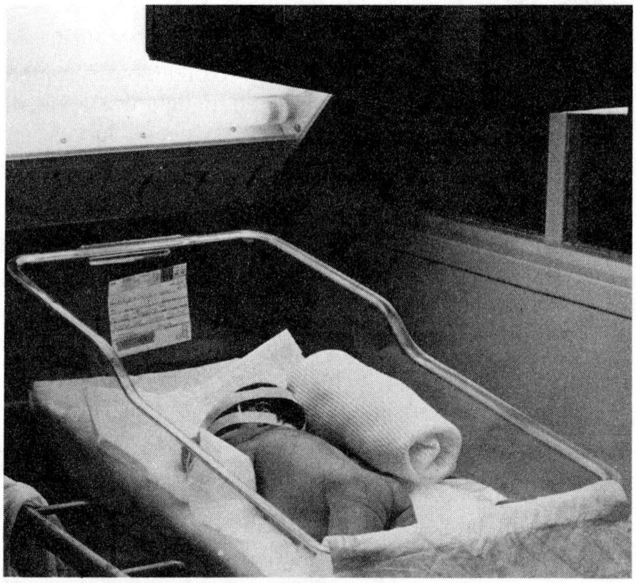

Fig. 9-5. Infant under phototherapy unit. Note that the eyes are shielded and the skin is exposed for maximum safety and therapeutic effect.

For example, they need to be reassured that the naked infant who is under the bilirubin light is warm and comfortable. Parents may be concerned about the blindfolds, since "blindness" is a frightening experience. Blindfolds are removed when the parents are visiting to facilitate the attachment process, and the parents can be reassured that the neonate is accustomed to darkness after months of intrauterine existence and benefits a great deal from auditory and tactile stimulation. If bronzing occurs, parents are informed that the discoloration disappears within 2 to 3 months.

One of the most important nursing interventions is recognition of breast-feeding jaundice. Lack of familiarity among health professionals has caused many newborns prolonged hospitalization, termination of breast-feeding, and unnecessary phototherapy. Supportive care of the new mother can encourage successful and frequent breast-feeding. Parents also need reassurance of the benign nature of the jaundice and encouragement to resume breast-feeding if temporary cessation is prescribed. Unfortunately, jaundice increases the risk of discontinuing breast-feeding and development of the vulnerable child syndrome, the belief of parents that their child has suffered a "close call" and is perceived as vulnerable to serious injury (Kemper, Forsyth, and McCarthy, 1989).

Discharge planning and home care. Discharge planning and home care depend on the type of jaundice and the treatment instituted. Most newborns are discharged after the bilirubin levels are near normal and no special care is needed. In jaundice associated with breast-feeding, follow-up blood studies are usually required to assess the progress of the jaundice. If temporary cessation of breast-feeding is prescribed, mothers should be taught to pump the breasts every 3 to 4 hours to maintain lactation; the expressed milk is frozen for use after breast-feeding is resumed. Most mothers resume breast-feeding if they are supported during this brief time. The infant should be fed formula with an orthodontic nipple, because this nipple requires the same sucking action as does breast-feeding. This prevents nipple confusion and difficulty in resuming breast-feeding (Gardner, O'Donnell, and Weismann, 1989).

If home phototherapy is instituted, the nurse is usually responsible for teaching family members and assessing their abilities to implement the treatment safely. General guidelines for home care preparation and education are discussed in Chapter 26. Written instructions and supervision of care, especially application of eye shields, are essential. The minor side effects of phototherapy are reviewed, and parents may need instruction in taking axillary temperatures,* and recording times and amounts of feedings and number of wet diapers and stools. Because of early discharge, adequate postpartal parent teaching is augmented by written instructions. These families require continued surveillance in the home, usually through referral to home care nursing agencies. Regardless of how benign the disorder or the therapy, these parents need support and understanding. Siblings also benefit from an explanation of the therapy to allay fears or misconceptions.

Evaluation

The effectiveness of nursing interventions is determined by continual reassessment and evaluation of care based on the following observational guidelines and expected outcomes:

1. Observe skin color; review bilirubinmometric and/or laboratory findings.
2. Observe for signs of neurologic impairment (see Box 10-1).
3. Check placement of eye shields; observe skin for signs of dehydration; take temperature.
4. Interview family members and observe parent-infant interactions.

Expected outcomes:
See Nursing Care Plan, p. 364.

HEMOLYTIC DISEASE OF THE NEWBORN

Hyperbilirubinemia in the first 24 hours of life is most often the result of hemolytic disease of the newborn (HDN) (*erythroblastosis fetalis*), an abnormally rapid rate of red cell destruction. Anemia caused by this destruction stimulates the production of red blood cells, which, in turn, provides increasing numbers of cells for hemolysis. Major causes of increased erythrocyte destruction are isoimmunization (primarily Rh) and ABO incompatibility.

Blood Incompatibility

The membranes of human blood cells contain a variety of antigens, also known as *agglutinogens*, which are substances capable of producing an immune response if recognized by the body as a foreign substance. It is the reciprocal

*Home care instructions for measuring temperature are available in Wong, D.L., and Whaley, L.F.: Clinical manual of pediatric nursing, ed. 3, 1990, Mosby–Year Book, Inc.

relationship between antigens on red blood cells and antibodies in the plasma that causes agglutination (clumping) to take place. In other words, antibodies in the plasma of one blood group (except the AB group, which contains no antibodies) will produce agglutination when mixed with antigens of a different blood group. In the ABO blood group system, the antibodies occur naturally. In the Rh system, the person must be exposed to the Rh antigen before significant antibody formation takes place to cause a sensitivity response.

Rh incompatibility (isoimmunization). The Rh blood group consists of several antigens, but for simplicity, only the terms *Rh-positive* (presence of antigen) and *Rh-negative* (absence of the antigen) are used in this discussion (see Autosomal Inheritance Patterns, Chapter 5). The presence or absence of the naturally occurring Rh factor determines the blood type. Ordinarily no problems are anticipated when the Rh blood types are the same in both mother and fetus or if the mother is Rh-positive and the infant Rh-negative. Difficulty may arise when the blood of the mother is Rh-negative and that of the infant is Rh-positive.

Although the maternal and fetal circulations are separate and distinct, sometimes fetal red blood cells (with antigens foreign to the mother) gain access to the maternal circulation through minute breaks in the placental vessels. The mother's natural defense mechanism responds to these alien cells by producing anti-Rh antibodies (isoimmunization).

Under normal circumstances, this process of isoimmunization has no effect on the fetus during the first pregnancy with an Rh-positive fetus because the initial sensitization to Rh antigens rarely occurs before the onset of labor. However, as larger amounts of fetal blood are transferred to the maternal circulation during placental separation, maternal antibody production is stimulated. During a subsequent pregnancy with an Rh-positive fetus, these previously formed maternal antibodies to Rh-positive blood cells enter the fetal circulation, where they attack and destroy fetal erythrocytes (Fig. 9-6). Because the disease begins in utero, the fetus attempts to compensate for the progressive hemolysis by accelerating the rate of erythropoiesis. As a result, immature red blood cells (erythroblasts) appear in the fetal circulation; hence the term *erythroblastosis fetalis.*

There is wide variability in the development of maternal sensitization to Rh-positive antigens. Sensitization may occur during the first pregnancy if the woman had previously received an Rh-positive blood transfusion. No sensitization may occur in situations in which a strong placental barrier prevents transfer of fetal blood into the maternal circulation. In about 10% to 15% of sensitized mothers there is no hemolytic reaction in the newborn.

In the most severe form of erythroblastosis fetalis, *hydrops fetalis,* the progressive hemolysis causes fetal hypoxia, cardiac failure, generalized edema (anasarca), and effusions in the pericardial, pleural, and peritoneal spaces. The fetus may be delivered stillborn or in severe respiratory distress.

ABO incompatibility. Hemolytic disease can also occur when the major blood group antigens of the fetus are different from those of the mother. The major blood groups are A, B, AB, and O. The incidence of these blood groups varies according to race and geographic location. In the North American white population, 46% have O blood group, 42% have A blood group, 9% have B blood group, and 3% have AB blood group.

The presence or absence of antibodies and antigens determines whether agglutination will occur (Table 9-2). Antibodies in the plasma of one blood group (except the AB group, which contains no antibodies) will produce an agglutination or clumping reaction when mixed with antigens of a different blood group. However, naturally occurring antibodies in the recipient's blood cause agglutination of the donor's red blood cells. The agglutinated donor cells become trapped in peripheral blood vessels where they hemo-

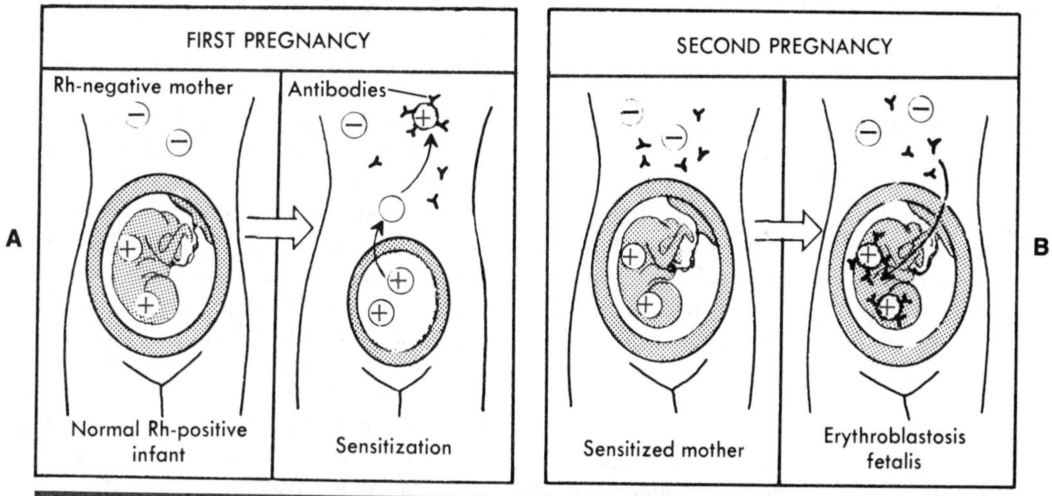

Fig. 9-6. Development of maternal sensitization to Rh antigens. **A,** Fetal Rh-positive erythrocytes enter maternal system. Maternal anti-Rh antibodies are formed. **B,** Anti-Rh antibodies cross placental barrier and attack fetal erythrocytes.

Table 9-2 ABO relationships of antigens/antibodies and donor-recipient compatibility

BLOOD GROUP (PHENOTYPE)	GENOTYPE	RED CELL ANTIGENS	PLASMA ANTIBODIES	RED CELL COMPATIBILITY: AS DONOR TO TYPE	RED CELL COMPATIBILITY: AS RECIPIENT FROM TYPE
A	AA,AO	A	B	AB,A	O,A
B	BB,BO	B	A	AB,B	O,B
AB	AB	A and B	None	AB	O,A,B,AB
O	OO	None	A and B	AB,A,B,O	O

Table 9-3 Potential maternal-fetal ABO incompatibilities

MATERNAL BLOOD GROUP	INCOMPATIBLE FETAL BLOOD GROUP
O	A or B
B	A or AB
A	B or AB

lyze, releasing large amounts of bilirubin into the circulation.

The most common blood group incompatibility in the neonate is between a mother with O blood group and an infant with A or B blood group (see Table 9-3 for possible ABO incompatibilities). Naturally occurring anti-A or anti-B antibodies already present in the maternal circulation cross the placenta and attack the fetal red blood cells, causing hemolysis. Usually the hemolytic reaction is less severe than in Rh incompatibility. Although the traditional thinking has been that the number of pregnancies is insignificant in the severity of ABO incompatibility, newer evidence suggests that the risk of hyperbilirubinemia is greater for subsequent offspring, especially if the first newborn had hyperbilirubinemia (Plotz, 1985).

Clinical Manifestations

Jaundice appears shortly after birth (during the first 24 hours) and serum levels of unconjugated bilirubin rise rapidly. Anemia results from the hemolysis of large numbers of erythrocytes and hyperbilirubinemia and jaundice from the liver's inability to conjugate and excrete the excess bilirubin. Most newborns with HDN are not jaundiced at birth. However, hepatosplenomegaly may be evident. If the infant is severely affected, signs of anemia (notably, marked pallor) and hypovolemic shock are apparent.

Diagnostic Evaluation

Maternal blood group and Rh typing is routine prenatally so that health professionals can be alert to the possibility of incompatibility at birth. The maternal blood group is compared with the infant's blood group and Rh type immediately after birth, and a direct Coombs test is performed on cord blood to rule out the possibility of the infant's developing HDN.

Antibody titer levels are measured periodically during pregnancy in Rh-negative mothers. Rising antibody titers (indirect Coombs test) indicate incompatibility. Diagnosis of Rh incompatibility before delivery is confirmed through amniocentesis and analysis of bilirubin levels in amniotic fluid. Increasing bilirubin levels represent progressive fetal hemolysis and may indicate the need for an intrauterine transfusion or immediate termination of the pregnancy. The disease can be confirmed postnatally by detecting antibodies attached to the circulating erythrocytes of affected infants (direct Coombs test).

Therapeutic Management

The primary aim of therapeutic management of isoimmunization is prevention. Postnatal therapy is usually exchange transfusion. Although phototherapy may control bilirubin levels in mild cases, the hemolytic disease can continue, causing severe anemia. Extracorporeal membrane oxygenation (see Chapter 10) has been successful in selected cases. Some investigators offer hope for pharmacologic management based on experiments with administration of metalloporphyrins, primarily tin-protoporphyrin, for ABO incompatibility (Delaney and others, 1988; Kappas and others, 1988). The drug decreases the conversion of heme to bilirubin by inhibiting the action of the enzyme heme oxygenase. Adverse reactions (acute photosensitivity) in some infants emphasize the need for more research before this option replaces phototherapy and exchange transfusion.

Prevention. The administration of Rh_o-immune globulin (RhoGAM*) to all unsensitized Rh-negative mothers after delivery or abortion of an Rh-positive infant or fetus prevents the development of maternal sensitization to the Rh factor. When RhoGAM is given to unsensitized mothers within 72 hours (but possibly as long as 3 to 4 weeks) after delivery or abortion, injected anti-Rh antibodies destroy the fetal erythrocytes that pass into the maternal circulation before these cells are able to exert an immunogenic effect. RhoGAM must be administered after the first delivery and repeated after subsequent ones. There is some evidence

*Ortho Diagnostic Systems, Inc., Raritan, NJ.

that prophylactic use of RhoGAM at 28 weeks of gestation further reduces the incidence of isoimmunization in those women sensitized during the first pregnancy (Bowman, 1985; Hammer, Bower, and Messina, 1984). RhoGAM is not effective against existing Rh-positive antibodies in the maternal circulation.

Exchange transfusion. Exchange transfusion, in which the infant's blood is removed in small amounts (usually 10 to 20 ml at a time) and replaced with compatible blood (such as Rh-negative blood), is a standard mode of therapy for treatment of severe hyperbilirubinemia and is the treatment of choice for hyperbilirubinemia caused by Rh incompatibility. Exchange transfusion removes the sensitized erythrocytes, lowers the serum bilirubin level to prevent kernicterus, corrects the anemia, and prevents cardiac failure.

The decision to perform an exchange transfusion must be individualized for each infant. General guidelines include: (1) an indirect serum bilirubin level of 20 mg/dl in full-term infants, (b) 15 mg/dl in high-risk infants weighing 1500 g, and (c) approximately 10 mg/dl for infants weighing 1000 g or less (Cashore and Stern, 1982). These guidelines may vary according to institutional practice and the newborn's gestational age and condition. Therapy may begin earlier when asphyxia, acidosis, hypothermia, hypoalbuminemia, sepsis, hemolysis, or hypoglycemia is present. An infant born with hydrops fetalis or signs of cardiac failure is a candidate for immediate exchange transfusion.

For exchange transfusion, fresh whole blood is typed and cross-matched to the mother's serum. The amount of donor blood used is usually double the blood volume of the infant, which is about 85 ml/kg body weight but is limited to no more than 500 ml. The two-volume exchange transfusion replaces approximately 85% of the neonate's blood.

Exchange transfusion is a sterile surgical procedure and requires 1 to 2 hours to complete. The umbilical cord is cut, and a catheter is inserted into the umbilical vein and threaded into the inferior vena cava. Depending on the infant's weight, 5 to 20 ml of blood is withdrawn within 15 to 20 seconds, and the same volume of donor blood is infused over 60 to 90 seconds.

Intrauterine transfusion. Infants of mothers already sensitized are sometimes treated by intrauterine transfusion, which consists of infusing blood into the peritoneal cavity or the umbilical vein of the fetus. The need for therapy is based on determinations of the optical density of amniotic fluid (via amniocentesis) as an index of the bilirubin concentration and degree of hemolysis. For a description of the procedure and the nursing care, the reader is referred to obstetric literature.

Nursing Considerations

The possibility of HDN can be anticipated from the prenatal and perinatal history. Prenatal evidence of incompatibility and the laboratory results of the Coombs test are cause for increased vigilance for early signs of jaundice in an infant. The cord is kept moist with a sterile saline-soaked dressing to preserve the umbilical vein for possible exchange transfusion. If an exchange transfusion is needed, the nurse prepares the infant and family and assists the practitioner with the procedure.

Exchange transfusions. In addition to assisting the practitioner during the initial stages of this procedure, the nurse keeps accurate records of blood volumes exchanged, including amounts of blood withdrawn and infused, time of each procedure, and cumulative record of the total volume exchanged. Vital signs that are monitored electronically are evaluated frequently and correlated with removal and infusion of blood. If signs of restlessness or cardiac arrhythmias occur, rate of infusion is slowed.

Throughout the procedure the infant requires attention to thermoregulation. The procedure is performed under a radiant warmer, and the blood is warmed before infusion. Hypothermia increases oxygen and glucose consumption, causing metabolic acidosis. Not only do these consequences hinder the infant's overall physical ability to withstand the long procedure, but they also inhibit the binding capacity of albumin and bilirubin and the hepatic enzymatic reactions, thus increasing the risk of kernicterus. Conversely, hyperthermia damages the donor erythrocytes, elevating the free potassium content and predisposing the infant to cardiac arrest.

After the procedure is completed, the nurse inspects the umbilical site for evidence of bleeding. Usually the catheter remains in place for use if needed for repeated exchanges. A sterile dressing is applied and checked periodically for evidence of bleeding or infection.

Exchange transfusion has many potential complications and a reported mortality of 0.5% to 3% (Keenan and others, 1985). Therefore conscientious care of the newborn is essential; this includes attention to asepsis to prevent infection and observation for signs of transfusion reactions (see Table 35-2). After the procedure is completed, the umbilical site is inspected for evidence of bleeding.

Unless kernicterus develops, most infants recover satisfactorily after HDN. If kernicterus has occurred, the family is apprised of the need for periodic assessments to detect sensorineural hearing loss, cerebral damage, or developmental lag in the child.

Family support. Parents frequently feel guilty because they think they have caused the blood incompatibility. Parents should never be made to feel responsible or negligent. They are encouraged to verbalize and express their thoughts. Actions that were taken to prevent any problems, such as frequent antepartum examinations and blood tests, should be referred to and praised.

HYPOGLYCEMIA

Hypoglycemia is said to be present when the infant's blood glucose concentration is significantly lower than that of the majority of infants of the same age and weight. In the full-term newborn, hypoglycemia is defined as plasma glucose concentrations of less than 35 mg/dl in the first 72 hours and 45 mg/dl thereafter; in low-birth-weight infants it is less than 25 mg/dl (Pildes and Lilien, 1983).

Pathophysiology

After birth the infant must supply nutrients to meet energy requirements for maintaining body temperature, respiration, muscular activity, and regulation of blood glucose, which is primarily derived from glycogen stores deposited in the liver, heart, and skeletal muscles during the last trimester of pregnancy. Under normal circumstances, the full-term infant usually has sufficient sources for the first 2 or 3 days. However, any condition that causes increased energy requirements can rapidly deplete these stores. The causes of hypoglycemia are categorized in Box 9-4.

Clinical Manifestations

The signs of hypoglycemia are usually vague and often indistinguishable from those observed in other conditions, such as hypocalcemia, septicemia, central nervous system disorders, or cardiorespiratory problems. Because the brain depends on glucose for energy, cerebral signs such as jitteriness, tremors, twitching, weak or high-pitched cry, lethargy, limpness, apathy, convulsions, and coma are prominent. Other clinical manifestations are cyanosis, apnea, rapid and irregular respirations, sweating, eye rolling, and refusal to feed. Frequently the symptoms are transient but recurrent.

BOX 9-4 CAUSES OF HYPOGLYCEMIA IN THE NEWBORN

Decreased substrate availability. Some infants exhibit hypoglycemia as a result of diminished glycogen and fat stores that are unable to provide sufficient energy to maintain glucose homeostasis until gluconeogenesis reaches adequate levels, e.g., preterm infants, infants with intrauterine growth retardation. Other infants are unable to use stored glycogen as a result of enzyme deficiencies, e.g., those with glycogen storage disease or other inborn errors of metabolism.

Endocrine disturbances. Hyperinsulinism is the most common endocrinologic disturbance resulting in hypoglycemia; it most commonly (15% to 75%) occurs in the infant of the diabetic mother. Other infants with hyperinsulinism include those with Beckwith-Wiedemann syndrome, erythroblastosis fetalis, islet cell dysplasia, those who have just had exchange transfusion, and those whose mothers have had tocolytic (labor-inhibiting) agents.

Increased use. Infants with normal energy stores at birth may be stressed by perinatal events such as asphyxia or hypothermia to the extent that available supplies are unable to meet the energy requirements of the neonate.

Miscellaneous and multiple mechanisms. Hypoglycemia caused by stimulation of glucose use by circulating endotoxins has been observed in infants with sepsis. Adrenal failure and hypoglycemia can occur as a result of adrenal hemorrhage in association with sepsis. Increased metabolism and a resultant need for increased caloric intake result from congestive heart failure secondary to congenital heart disease, which is compounded by feeding difficulties.

Diagnostic Evaluation

Diagnosis must be confirmed by direct analysis of blood glucose concentration. Two specimens of blood should be analyzed because of the many factors that can affect correct readings. Proper handling of the specimen is essential, since storage at room temperature increases glycolysis. Accurate readings can be facilitated by storing the blood sample in ice or removing the red blood cells by centrifugation.

Blood sugar level may also be determined with a drop of blood placed on a reagent strip such as Dextrostix or Chemstrip-BG, which may be read either manually or with a glucose reflectance meter. Although simple procedures, the tests are very sensitive and must be performed correctly to prevent false readings. For example, the blood must remain on the Dextrostix for exactly 1 minute and then be compared with the color chart. Inaccurate timing will produce varying stages of the reaction. Color changes that indicate a blood glucose level of less than 45 mg/dl should be confirmed by a laboratory analysis of whole blood. Because of poor correlations with capillary blood samples and high variability in values of blood glucose concentrations when reflectance meters are used, it has been recommended by researchers that this method should not be used in the high-risk infant (Lin and others, 1989). At least one other study found a reflectance meter (AccuChek II) to be accurate provided blood was collected and transferred to the strip using a capillary tube, and a tissue, not a cotton ball, was used to remove excess blood from the strip (Vitanza, Giacoia, and West, 1988).

Therapeutic Management

Intravenous infusion of glucose is the therapy for hypoglycemia. Infants who are at increased risk for developing hypoglycemia should have their blood glucose measured within 1 hour after birth. The procedure should be repeated every 1 to 2 hours for the first 6 to 8 hours, then every 4 to 6 hours for 2 days.

Oral glucose feedings are ineffective as a treatment for hypoglycemia, and in high concentrations can cause gastric irritation and osmotic diarrhea. Hypoglycemia can be prevented in most instances by the initiation of early feeding in normoglycemic newborns. Breast-fed infants should be put to breast as soon as possible after delivery. If feedings are poorly tolerated, intravenous glucose may be administered to these infants if they develop hypoglycemia. (See Infants of Diabetic Mothers, Chapter 10, for management of hypoglycemia related to hyperinsulinemia.)

Nursing Considerations

Much of the nursing responsibility for the hypoglycemic infant involves identification of the problem through careful observation of physical status. Another concern is to reduce environmental factors, such as cold stress and respiratory difficulty, that predispose the infant to the development of a decreased blood glucose level. Use of proper feeding techniques with the breast-fed or bottle-fed infant promotes adequate ingestion of nutrients, particularly carbohydrates.

Major nursing objectives also include preventing, anticipating, and recognizing potential dangers of concentrated dextrose infusion. Too-rapid infusion of the hypertonic solution can cause circulatory overload, hyperglycemia, and intracellular dehydration. Maintaining the ordered flow rate with an intravenous pump and checking and charting hourly intake decreases the chance of such hazards. If the intravenous transfusion has been temporarily discontinued, nurses should not try to "catch up" by increasing the rate to make up for the fluid lost during the interruption.

The infusion is administered through a large peripheral vein to increase hemodilution of the concentrated solution and to prevent irritation of the vessel walls. Extravasation of the fluid into the surrounding area can cause tissue sloughing. Termination of the glucose solution must be gradual to prevent hypoglycemia caused by hyperinsulinism.

Because hypoglycemia may be a symptom of some other underlying pathophysiologic process, parents are usually very concerned about their infant's progress, particularly since these infants do not feed well or behave responsively. Nurses need to be aware of parents' thoughts, to allow them to express their feelings, and to keep parents aware of the infant's progress.

HYPERGLYCEMIA

Hyperglycemia in the newborn is usually defined as a blood glucose concentration greater than 125 mg/dl in the term infant or greater than 150 mg/dl in the preterm infant. Affected infants are usually low-birth-weight infants who are unable to tolerate intravenous glucose infusions at the usual rate. The glucose intolerance is probably related to general immaturity of the usual regulatory mechanisms (DiGiacomo, Hagedorn, and Hay, 1989). Increased blood glucose levels may also occur in infants with sepsis or decreased insulin sensitivity (such as the infant with transient diabetes mellitus), infants receiving methylxanthines, and stressed infants (infants with respiratory distress syndrome, infants undergoing surgical procedures).

Hyperglycemia is usually asymptomatic but detected on routine screening. Most often, hyperglycemia is treated by reducing the infant's glucose intake. Insulin infusion is sometimes administered to very low-birth-weight infants who are unable to tolerate glucose solutions with concentrations greater than 5 g/dl. The additional insulin allows the infant to achieve adequate energy intake (Binder and others, 1989).

Nursing Considerations

Blood glucose is monitored frequently, especially in the infant receiving insulin. This requires numerous heel sticks, and sites should be rotated to minimize tissue damage (see Blood Specimens, Chapter 27). Urine output is carefully measured to detect any evidence of osmotic diuresis.

✦**NURSING ALERT** Any cerebral signs, such as jitteriness, twitching, seizure activity, or a diminished activity level, are indications for obtaining serum glucose and/or serum calcium levels immediately.

As in care of all infants, parents are given a careful explanation of the therapy and provided with frequent progress reports as well as support to reduce anxiety (see also Nursing Care of High-Risk Newborns, Chapter 10).

HYPOCALCEMIA

Hypocalcemia, like many conditions in the neonate, is difficult to differentiate from other disorders, and the etiology is ill defined. There are two times during the neonatal period when the incidence is highest. *Early-onset hypocalcemia,* which appears within the first 72 hours, is the more common form and typically affects the premature or small-for-date infant who has experienced perinatal hypoxia. Symptoms include jitteriness, apnea, cyanotic episodes, a high-pitched cry, and abdominal distention.

Late-onset hypocalcemia, which is not apparent until after the first 7 days of life, is commonly referred to as cow's milk–induced hypocalcemia or *neonatal tetany*. It is observed in well-nourished infants who are fed unmodified cow's milk. Cow's milk with a high phosphorus-to-calcium ratio depresses parathyroid activity, resulting in diminished serum calcium levels. The manifestations of neonatal tetany reflect neuromuscular irritation—twitching, tremors, and focal or generalized convulsive seizures that can be triggered by even minor stimuli and that vary in duration from a few seconds to 10 minutes. Neonatal tetany is rarely seen because of the prevalent use of commercial formula or human milk as the newborn's primary nutrition.

Diagnostic Evaluation

Diagnosis of hypocalcemia is confirmed with serum electrolyte determinations. Normal serum calcium values are between 8 and 10 mg/dl (4 to 5 mEq/L). Hypocalcemia is indicated at levels below 7 mg/dl or ionized calcium levels less than 3 to 3.5 mg/dl during the first 3 days of life.

Therapeutic Management

In most instances early-onset hypocalcemia is temporary and reverses itself in 1 to 3 days. Restoration of a normal calcium level is facilitated by early feedings, physiologic correction of the hypoparathyroidism, and sometimes administration of calcium supplements.

Treatment of hypocalcemia involves intravenous administration of 10% calcium gluconate. The drug is administered slowly for 2 to 3 minutes every 6 hours or continuously (Adcock and Consolvo, 1989) to prevent nausea, vomiting, bradycardia, and circulatory collapse. It is advisable to monitor the heart rate and blood pressure electronically. Care must be taken to ascertain that the needle is positioned within the vein because extravasation into surrounding tissue causes local necrosis, calcification, and sloughing. Intramuscular administration of calcium gluconate is contraindicated because it precipitates in the tissue, causing necrosis. If the infant can tolerate oral fluids, oral doses of calcium are given.

Nursing Considerations

Nursing care of the infant with hypocalcemia is directed toward identifying the cause of the manifestations observed and administration of calcium. The infant is monitored continuously during intravenous infusions. Calcium gluconate can cause tissue necrosis and scar formation; therefore it is recommended that the scalp veins be avoided. Calcium gluconate is also incompatible with a number of drugs, most notably sodium bicarbonate ($NaHCO_3$), which is often given for acidosis. To prevent tissue necrosis, the infusion site should be observed carefully and changed as needed. The needle is firmly secured to the skin by tape, and during removal gentle pressure is applied at the puncture site for at least 1 minute.

The nurse also observes for signs of acute hypercalcemia (nausea, vomiting, bradycardia). If such symptoms occur, the injection or infusion is discontinued and the practitioner is notified. Since convulsions are common, seizure precautions are instituted. Minor stimuli, such as picking the infant up for a feeding or a sudden jarring of the crib, can provoke tremors or seizures. During the acute phase, the environment around the infant is manipulated to allow for maximum rest and minimum activity.

The restlessness, irritability, and convulsive activity of the infant are of much concern to the parents. The nurse supports them during the hospitalization and emphasizes that the condition will subside rapidly with no subsequent ill effects. During the acute phase, parents are advised to disturb the infant as little as possible. However, as soon as the calcium level rises, they are encouraged to hold and feed the infant in order to reestablish parent-child attachment.

If the infant is discharged on formula feedings supplemented with calcium salts, the parents are taught the correct procedure for diluting the mineral in the formula and are advised to use only the prescribed formula.

HEMORRHAGIC DISEASE OF THE NEWBORN

Hemorrhagic disease of the newborn is a bleeding disorder that may appear within 1 to 5 days of life as a result of a deficiency of vitamin K. Newborn vitamin K stores are virtually absent, and there is a moderate deficiency of prothrombin activity, which decreases until approximately 72 hours after birth when it begins to increase. Consequently, vitamin K–dependent coagulation factors (II, VII, IX, X) are significantly reduced. In addition, the newborn's sterile intestinal tract is unable to synthesize the vitamin until feedings have begun. Breast-fed infants are particularly at risk because human milk is a poor source of vitamin K. Hemorrhagic manifestations rarely occur in infants fed fortified cow's milk formula from the first day of life because this formula is an adequate source of the vitamin.

Signs and symptoms of hemorrhagic disease typically appear 24 to 72 hours after birth and can include oozing from the umbilicus or circumcision site, bloody or black stools, hematuria, ecchymoses on skin and scalp, epistaxis, or bleeding from punctures. Diagnosis can be confirmed in the presence of prolonged prothrombin time (PT) and partial thromboplastin time (PTT) accompanied by normal platelet count and fibrinogen levels.

A late form (late-onset hemorrhagic disease) appears at about 4 to 7 weeks of age. This late-onset disease occurs in totally or predominantly breast-fed infants. It appears to be related to a factor in breast milk that inhibits vitamin K synthesis by the infant's bacterial flora. Manifestations of late-onset disease are evidence of intracranial hemorrhage, deep ecchymoses, bleeding from the gastrointestinal tract, and/or bleeding from mucous membranes, skin punctures, or surgical incisions.

Therapeutic Management

The goal of management is prevention of hemorrhagic disease of the newborn with prophylactic administration of vitamin K. In the United States, intramuscular administration of vitamin K (Aquamephyton, Mephyton) in a dose of 0.5 to 1 mg once during the first 24 hours of life is a standard practice. The use of prophylactic vitamin K is not routinely practiced in all countries.

In newborns with the disease, treatment is the same as the preventive measures, except that the vitamin may be given intravenously to prevent a hematoma at an intramuscular site. Bleeding usually ceases within 2 to 4 hours of vitamin K administration.

Some have reported success with daily oral administration of vitamin K to the infants (McNinch and others, 1985; Olson, 1987) or to the mothers during the last month of pregnancy (O'Connor and Addiego, 1986). To prevent late-onset disease it is recommended that mothers of breast-feeding infants receive oral vitamin K supplementation (von Kries and others, 1987). None of these is standard practice.

Nursing Considerations

Nursing care is primarily directed toward prevention and involves careful administration of the vitamin into the vastus lateralis muscle. In instances in which this procedure is not routinely carried out (e.g., home births or emergency deliveries), the nurse observes for signs of the disorder and notifies the practitioner for appropriate diagnosis and treatment.

Breast-feeding mothers are encouraged to increase their intake of foods containing vitamin K, primarily vegetables. The best sources are green vegetables, especially broccoli.

■ INBORN ERRORS OF METABOLISM

Inborn error(s) of metabolism (IEM) is a term applied to a large number of inherited diseases caused by the absence or deficiency of a substance essential to cellular metabolism, usually an enzyme, and most are characterized by abnormal protein, carbohydrate, or fat metabolism.

All biochemical processes are under genetic control, and each consists of a complex sequence of reactions. Fig. 9-7,

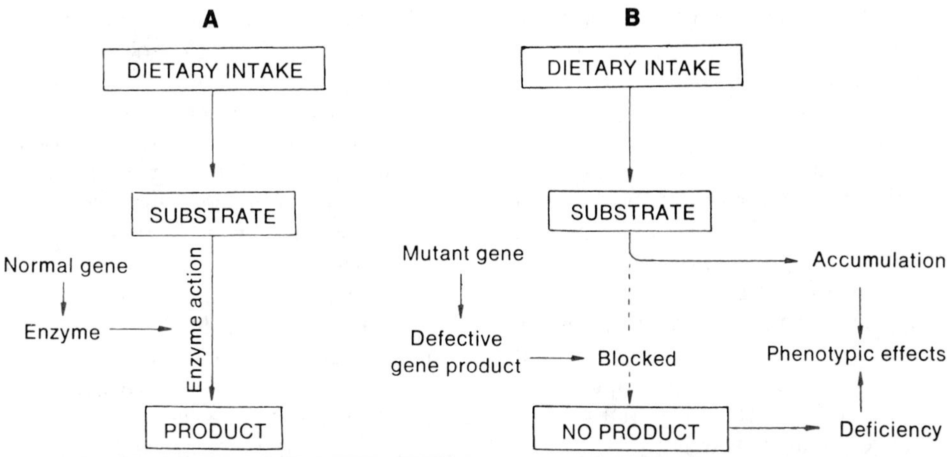

Fig. 9-7. Metabolic pathway. **A,** Normal metabolic pathway. **B,** Effect of defective gene action.

A, schematically represents a portion of a normal metabolic pathway. A substrate (the substance on which an enzyme acts) is converted to a product through the action of a specific enzyme. A metabolic pathway consists of many such reactions, or steps, each depending on the previous reaction and each catalyzed by a specific enzyme.

A specific gene is responsible for production of a specific enzyme in the metabolic pathway. Fig. 9-7, *B,* illustrates how a change in a gene that interferes with the synthesis of an essential enzyme interrupts this process. A block in the normal pathway can produce the following:

1. Accumulation of the substances preceding the block, such as galactose in galactosemia or phenylalanine in phenylketonuria
2. A deficiency in the product, such as thyroxine in familial hypothyroidism
3. An increase in the products of alternate metabolic pathways when these pathways are used, such as the production of phenylketones in phenylketonuria

These effects of defective gene action are observable in the individual as diseases.

The mode of inheritance in IEM is almost always autosomal recessive. This is best understood by considering the "double-dose effect" as it relates to the concept that one gene is responsible for one enzyme. If a specific gene controls the formation of an essential enzyme and each individual has two such genes (the normal homozygote), then the enzyme is produced in normal amounts. The heterozygote, having one gene with a normal effect, is still able to produce the enzyme in sufficient amounts to carry out the metabolic function under normal circumstances. Therefore the heterozygote does not exhibit symptoms of the disorder. However, the abnormal homozygote, who inherits a defective gene from both parents, has no functioning enzyme and thus is clinically affected.

Individually IEM are rare; collectively they account for a significant proportion of health problems in children. It is becoming possible to detect and screen for an increasing number of IEM—to detect the presence of the disease in the heterozygote, the newborn, and the fetus. In many IEM, early diagnosis and prompt treatment are essential to prevent a relentless course of physical and mental deterioration. Prenatal diagnosis provides for special care of the infant immediately after birth. Neonatal screening is useful in detecting some disorders after a few days of life, but it is less helpful in detecting symptoms early in the neonatal period.

Some nonspecific presenting manifestations—including lethargy, persistent vomiting, respiratory distress, hypothermia, coma, and seizures—are observed in a wide variety of both genetic and acquired disorders (Arn, Valle, and Brusilow, 1988; Burton, 1987). Time of onset may be important. Most IEM are symptom-free during the first 24 hours of life. Other manifestations that may indicate IEM include jaundice, hepatomegaly, coarse facial features, macroglossia, diarrhea, an abnormal odor, abnormal hair, dysmorphic features, and abnormal eye findings (e.g., cataracts, retinal changes) (Burton, 1987). A family history of neonatal deaths (within the same sibling group, in males, or among family members) alerts the observer to the possibility of a genetic disorder. Initial recognition of signs that might indicate an IEM is the responsibility of health professionals including nurses.

Although there are innumerable IEM only three are selected for discussion, because reasonable success has been achieved with treatment of these. Some IEM are also outlined in Table 5-4.

CONGENITAL HYPOTHYROIDISM

Congenital hypothyroidism (CH) (sometimes called by the undesirable term *cretinism*) is a deficiency of thyroid hormones believed to be present at birth. Results of screening tests in the United States indicate that CH occurs in one of every 4000 to 5000 births and females outnumber males 2 to 1 (Fanaroff and Martin, 1987). Infants with Down syndrome have a much higher rate of either permanent or transient forms of the disorder (Fort and others, 1984). Also, a higher incidence of other congenital abnormalities has been observed in infants with CH (New England Congenital Hypothyroidism Collaborative, 1988).

A number of etiologic factors are implicated in hypothyroidism and the condition may be permanent or transient. Permanent CH can result from defective thyroid gland development, an enzymatic defect in thyroxine synthesis, or (rarely) pituitary dysfunction. Transient hypothyroidism results from intrauterine transfer of goiter-inducing substances (such as the antithyroid drugs), which inhibit thyroid secretion. Although self-limiting, this type is potentially fatal because, once the maternal supply is terminated, the infant's thyroid is unable to produce its own hormones. In addition, regardless of etiology, a large goiter in a neonate may cause total obstruction of the airway.

Clinical Manifestations

The severity of the disorder depends on the amount of thyroid tissue present. Usually the newborn does not exhibit obvious signs of hypothyroidism, probably because of the exogenous source of prenatal thyroid hormone supplied by the maternal circulation. Clinical manifestations may be delayed in infants with a functional remnant of thyroid gland, infants with some types of familial hypothyroidism, and breast-fed infants, who may not display symptoms until weaned. Bone age is greatly retarded from birth. Reports of intellectual capacity are varied.

Classic features of untreated CH usually appear after about 6 weeks of life and include typical facial features (depressed nasal bridge, short forehead, puffy eyelids, and large tongue); thick, dry, mottled skin that feels cold to the touch; coarse, dry, lusterless hair; abdominal distention, umbilical hernia, hyporeflexia, bradycardia, hypothermia, hypotension with narrow pulse pressure, anemia, and widely patent cranial sutures. The infant displays difficulty feeding, decreased gastric motility, minimum crying, and excessive sleepiness. The most serious consequence is delayed development of the nervous system, which leads to severe mental retardation. The severity of the intellectual deficit is related to the degree of hypothyroidism and the duration of the condition before treatment. Other nervous system manifestations include slow, awkward movements and abnormal deep tendon reflexes (often referred to as "hung-up" because the relaxation phase after the contraction is slow).

Diagnostic Evaluation

Diagnosis is aimed at early identification of the disorder to prevent the serious effects on mental development resulting from delayed treatment. Neonatal screening consists of initial (T_4) measurement followed by measurement of thyroid-stimulating hormone (TSH) in specimens with low T_4 values (American Academy of Pediatrics and American Thyroid Association, 1987). Tests are routine and mandatory in most areas. Although a heel-stick blood sample for the spot test can be obtained at any time soon after birth, specimens are usually taken after 24 hours because the test is usually part of concurrent screen for other metabolic defects.

Screening results that show a low level of T_4 and a high level of TSH indicate CH and the need for further tests to determine the cause of the disease. Additional tests include serum measurement of thyroxine, triiodothyronine (T_3), protein-bound iodine (PBI), and thyrotropin-releasing factor to ascertain the amount of thyroid hormone secreted and the intactness of the homeostatic mechanisms. Tests of thyroid gland function (thyroid scan and uptake) usually involve oral administration of a radioactive isotope of iodine (^{131}I) and measurement of the iodine uptake by the thyroid, usually within 24 hours. In CH, protein-bound iodine, thyroxine, triiodothyronine, and free thyroxine levels are low and thyroid uptake of ^{131}I is decreased. Roentgenography is employed to assess bone age.

Therapeutic Management

Treatment involves thyroid hormone replacement therapy as soon as possible after diagnosis to abolish all signs of hypothyroidism and reestablish normal physical and mental development. The drug of choice is synthetic levothyroxine sodium (Synthroid or Levothroid). To prevent the risk of overdosage of thyroid hormones, thyroxine and triiodothyronine levels are measured regularly. Bone age surveys are also performed to ensure optimum growth. If adequate thyroid hormone replacement is begun shortly after birth, the chance for normal growth and intelligence appears to be excellent (Glorieux and others, 1985).

Nursing Considerations

The most important nursing objective is early identification of the disorder. Nurses caring for neonates must be certain that screening is performed, especially in infants who are discharged early or born at home. Although the screening test is very specific, some children may not be identified, and nurses in ambulatory settings for well-infant care need to be aware of the earliest signs of the disorder. Parental remarks about an unusually "quiet and good" baby together with any of the early physical manifestations should lead to a suspicion of hypothyroidism, requiring referral for specific tests. Unfortunately, many parents harbor guilt about their impressions of the infant before the diagnosis because the child's inactivity may not have alerted them to a problem, with the result that treatment is delayed.

Once the diagnosis is confirmed, parents need an explanation of the disorder and the necessity of lifelong treatment. The importance of compliance with the drug regimen must be stressed. Since the drug is tasteless, it can be crushed and added to formula, water, or food. If a dose is missed, twice the dose should be given the next day (Coody, 1984). Parents also need to be aware of signs indicating overdose, such as, rapid pulse, dyspnea, irritability, insomnia, fever, sweating, and weight loss. Signs of inadequate treatment are fatigue, sleepiness, decreased appetite, and constipation.

If the diagnosis was delayed past early infancy, the chance of permanent mental retardation is great. Parents need the same guidance in caring for their child as do others who have an offspring with cognitive impairment (see

Chapter 24). They need an opportunity to discuss their feelings regarding late recognition of the disorder. Although treatment will not reverse the intellectual deficit, it may prevent further damage. Genetic counseling is important, especially if the disorder is caused by an inborn error of thyroid hormone synthesis, which is autosomal recessive. (For a discussion of genetic counseling, see Chapter 5.)

PHENYLKETONURIA

Phenylketonuria (PKU) is a disease of protein metabolism, inherited as an autosomal-recessive trait, characterized by the inability to metabolize the essential amino acid phenylalanine. The disorder is detected in 1:10,000 to 15,000 live births and affects primarily white children, with the incidence highest in those living in the United States or Northern Europe. It is very rare in the African, Jewish, and Japanese populations.

In recent years it has become apparent that severe, classic PKU is at one end of a spectrum of conditions now known as *hyperphenylalaninemia.* Rarer forms, or *variants,* are the result of a deficiency of other enzymes, such as *dihydropteridine reductase* (DHPR) or *dihydrobiopterin synthetase* (DHBS) and are diagnosed and treated differently from classic PKU. The following discussion of PKU is limited to the severe, classic form.

Pathophysiology

The hepatic enzyme *phenylalanine hydroxylase,* which normally controls the conversion of phenylalanine to tyrosine, is absent in PKU. This results in the accumulation of phenylalanine in the bloodstream and urinary excretion of abnormal amounts of its metabolites, the phenyl acids (Fig. 9-8). One of these phenyl ketones, *phenylpyruvic acid,* gives urine the characteristic musty odor associated with this disease and is responsible for the term *phenylketonuria.*

Accumulation of phenylalanine and presumably the decreased levels of the neurotransmitters dopamine and tryptophan affect the normal development of the brain and central nervous system, resulting in defective myelinization, cystic degeneration of the gray and white matter, and disturbances in cortical lamination. Mental retardation occurs *before* the metabolites are detected in the urine and will progress if ingested phenylalanine levels are not lowered.

Amino acids produced by metabolism of phenylalanine are absent in PKU. One of these, tyrosine, is needed to form the pigment melanin and the hormones epinephrine and thyroxine. Decreased melanin production results in similar phenotypes of most children with phenylketonuria—blond hair, blue eyes, and fair skin that is particularly susceptible to eczema and other dermatologic problems. Children of genetically darker skin color may be red-haired or brunette.

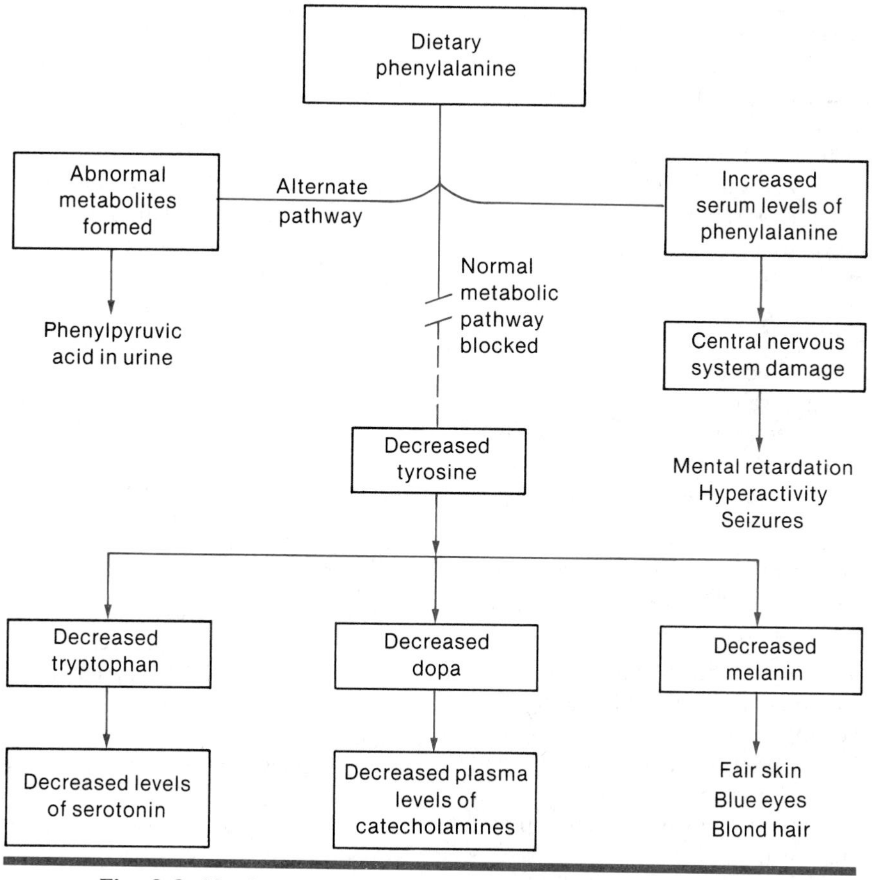

Fig. 9-8. Metabolic errors and consequences in phenylketonuria.

Clinical Manifestations

Clinical manifestations of PKU include failure to thrive, frequent vomiting, irritability, hyperactivity, and unpredictable, erratic behavior. Bizarre or schizoid behavior patterns are common in older children, such as fright reactions, screaming episodes, head banging, arm biting, disorientation, failure to respond to strong stimuli, and catatonia-like positions. Many of the severely retarded children have convulsions, and about 80% of untreated persons with PKU demonstrate abnormal electroencephalographs, regardless of whether overt seizures occur. Fortunately, this manifestation is rarely seen because of early detection and treatment.

Diagnostic Evaluation

The objective in diagnosing or treating the disorder is to prevent mental retardation. The most commonly used test for screening newborns is the *Guthrie blood test,* which is mandatory for all newborns in most states. If properly done, it detects serum phenylalanine levels greater than 4 mg/dl (normal value is 2 mg/dl). Only fresh heel blood, not cord blood, can be used for the test.

The screening test is most reliable if the blood sample is taken after the infant has ingested a source of protein. Because of early discharge, the American Academy of Pediatrics, Committee on Genetics (1982) recommends that the test be performed on all newborns before they leave the nursery, regardless of age, and that a repeat test be prepared by the third week of life on all infants in whom the initial specimen is taken within the first 24 hours of life. Because of the legal and ethical issues involved in taking blood samples before the disease can be detected, all institutions need to establish some mechanism for follow-up. Special consideration must be given to screening of infants born at home who have no hospital contact.

Because of the possibility of variant forms of hyperphenylalaninemia, a natural protein challenge test is recommended after about 3 months of dietary treatment to confirm the diagnosis of classic PKU.

Therapeutic Management

Treatment of PKU is dietary. Since the genetic enzyme is intracellular, systemic administration of phenylalanine hydroxylase is of no value. Phenylalanine cannot be eliminated because it is an essential amino acid in tissue growth. Therefore dietary management must do the following:

1. Meet the child's nutritional need for optimum growth.
2. Maintain phenylalanine levels within a safe range.

The diet is calculated to maintain serum phenylalanine levels between 2 and 8 mg/dl. Significant brain damage usually occurs when levels are greater than 10 to 15 mg/dl. At levels less than 2 mg/dl the body begins to catabolize its protein stores, resulting in growth retardation. The daily amounts are individualized for each child and require frequent changes based on appetite, growth and development, and blood phenylalanine levels.

Since all natural food proteins contain about 15% phenylalanine, specially prepared milk substitutes, such as Lofenalac,* or PKU-1,† are prescribed for the infant. These products are made from specially treated enzymatic casein hydrolysate, which provides only 0.4% phenylalanine (28.5 mg/8 ounces). They also contain minerals and vitamins to provide a balanced nutritional formula. Tyrosine deficiency and several other amino acids are supplied in the formula. Total or partial breast-feeding, because of the low phenylalanine content of breast milk, may be possible with close monitoring of phenylalanine levels (Lawrence, 1990).

Diet substitutes for older children, such as PKU 2,† and Phenyl-Free,* contain no phenylalanine and allow for greater exchanges with natural low-phenylalanine foods in the diet, leading to a more normal diet. These products are not recommended for children under 3 years of age (McCabe and others, 1987). Frequent monitoring of blood phenylalanine levels is necessary.

The low-phenylalanine diet is implemented as soon as possible after birth. It is not yet known how long the diet therapy must be continued. At present many centers discontinue the diet when the child is 6 to 8 years old. However, there is mounting evidence that increased phenylalanine levels beyond this age have neuropsychologic sequelae, such as lowered intelligence quotient, attentional and academic difficulties, especially in arithmetic, and visual-spatial problems (Brunner, Jordan, and Berry, 1983; Seashore and others, 1985). There is also the difficulty of compliance in resuming the diet, such as during pregnancy (Michals and others, 1985).

With improved dietary control of PKU, the increased life span of individuals with this disorder presents additional concerns. High phenylalanine blood levels in mothers with PKU affect the normal embryologic development of the fetus, leading to low birth weight, congenital malformations, microcephaly, and/or mental retardation in the infant. Since there is a strong correlation between maternal blood phenylalanine levels and improved fetal outcome, the low-phenylalanine diet should be resumed *prior to* pregnancy (Drogari and others, 1987; Rohr and others, 1987).

Nursing Considerations

The principal nursing consideration is teaching the family the dietary restrictions. The task of maintaining such a strict dietary regimen is very demanding. Foods with low phenylalanine levels, such as vegetables, fruits, juices, and some cereals, breads, and starches, must be measured to provide the prescribed amount of phenylalanine. Most high-protein foods, such as meat and dairy products, are either eliminated or restricted to small amounts. Also, the phenylalanine substitutes are quite expensive, adding financial burdens. Affected children are cautioned against the use of the artificial sweetener aspartame (NutraSweet) or consuming foods and beverages sweetened with this substance. Aspartame is converted to phenylalanine in the gut.

*Mead Johnson & Co., Evansville, IN.
†Milupa Corp., Darien, CT.

During infancy, maintaining the diet presents few problems. Solid foods, such as cereal, fruits, and vegetables, are introduced as usual to the infant. Difficulties arise as the child gets older. Decreased appetite and refusal to eat may reduce intake of the calculated phenylalanine requirement. The child's increasing independence may inhibit absolute control of what he or she eats. Either factor can result in decreased or increased phenylalanine levels. During the school years, peer pressure becomes a major force in deterring the child from eating the prescribed foods or abstaining from high-protein foods such as milkshakes or ice cream. Limitations of this diet are best illustrated by an example: a quarter-pound hamburger may be equal to a 2-day phenylalanine allowance for a school-age child. Illness and growth spurts will increase the body's need for this essential amino acid.

The assistance of a registered nutritionist is essential. Parents need a basic understanding of the disorder and practical suggestions regarding food selection and preparation.* Meal planning is based on an exchange list, and as soon as children are old enough, usually by early preschool, they should be involved in the daily calculation, menu planning, and formula preparation. Using a musical or voice-synthesizer calculator, cards, or colored beads can help children keep track of the daily allowance of phenylalanine foods (Messer, 1985).

Preparation of the formula can present some difficulties. It tends to be lumpy and has a distinctive odor and taste that has been described as similar to potato but more bitter. A blender or mixer dissolves the powder more easily, but this is inconvenient when traveling. Although the taste is virtually impossible to camouflage, adding orange Tang, fruit-flavored powdered punch, or strawberry or chocolate Quik helps vary the flavor somewhat without greatly altering the phenylalanine content. The chocolate-flavored formula can be heated and served as hot cocoa or frozen into popsicles.

Family support. In addition to the problems related to a child with a chronic disorder (see Chapter 22), the parents have the burden of knowing that they are carriers of the defect and must make serious decisions regarding future children. Prenatal testing is now available to detect the presence of the defective gene in heterozygotes. Genetic counseling is especially important for an affected child, who theoretically has a 50% chance of bearing an affected offspring (see Genetic Counseling, Chapter 5).

*A helpful resource is by Schuett, V., editor: Low-protein cookery for phenylketonuria, 1986, University of Wisconsin Press, 114 N. Murray St., Madison, WI 53715. For mothers who are breast-feeding, detailed information is presented by Ernest, A., and others: Guide to feeding the infant with PKU, Superintendent of Documents, U.S. Government Printing Office, Washington, DC 20402.

GALACTOSEMIA

Galactosemia is a rare autosomal-recessive disorder affecting approximately 1:50,000 births. It involves an inborn error of carbohydrate metabolism in which the hepatic enzyme *galactose-1-phosphate uridine transferase (UDP-galactose transferase)* is absent. The enzyme is one of three needed for the conversion of galactose to glucose (Fig. 9-9).

Clinical Manifestations

Infants with this disorder appear normal at birth. Within a few days after ingesting milk, as galactose accumulates in the blood, manifestations begin to appear. Affected infants appear jaundiced as a result of liver involvement, and they begin to vomit and lose weight. Hepatosplenomegaly and diarrhea may also occur. Cataracts are usually recognizable by 1 or 2 months of age, and cerebral damage is evidenced by drowsiness, lethargy, and hypotonia. Death during the first month of life is not uncommon in infants with untreated galactosemia.

Diagnostic Evaluation

Diagnosis is made on the basis of galactosuria, increased levels of galactose in the blood, or decreased levels of UDP-galactose transferase activity in erythrocytes. Newborn screening for this disease is required in many states. Heterozygotes can also be identified, since heterozygotic individuals have significantly lower levels of the essential enzyme. Although asymptomatic, such individuals have been noted to spontaneously dislike and therefore limit ingestion of galactose-containing foods.

Therapeutic Management

Treatment of galactosemia consists of eliminating all milk and lactose-containing foods, including breast milk. During

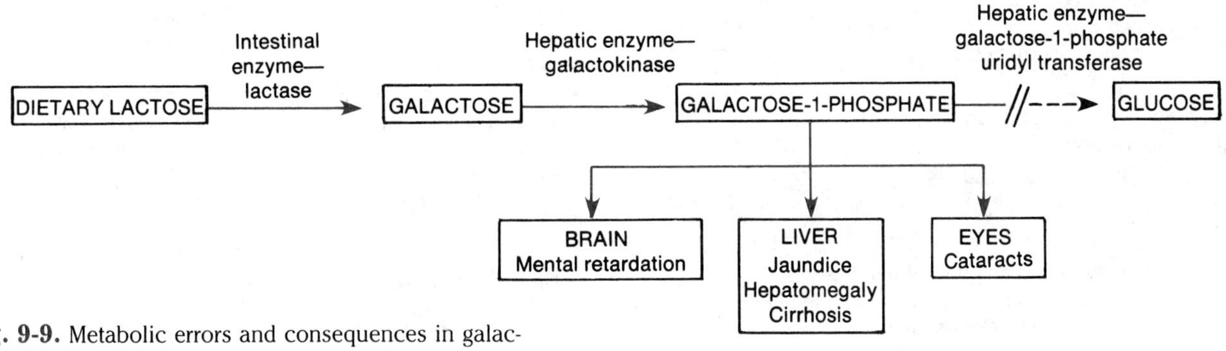

Fig. 9-9. Metabolic errors and consequences in galactosemia.

infancy, lactose-free formulas are used, with soy-protein formula being the feeding of choice (American Academy of Pediatrics, 1982).

Follow-up studies of children treated from birth or within the first month demonstrate that most of them have normal growth and intellectual functioning. However, they may have speech and language deficits (Waisbren and others, 1983), and some develop neurologic sequelae, such as mental retardation, tremors, and ataxia (Lo and others, 1984). Children treated later tend to have mental scores from normal to mildly retarded, but most have some degree of visual-perceptual handicap (Fishler and others, 1980).

Nursing Considerations

Nursing interventions are similar to those for PKU, except that dietary restrictions are easier to maintain because many more foods are allowed. However, reading food labels very carefully for the presence of any form of lactose, especially dairy products, is mandatory. Many drugs, such as penicillin, contain lactose as filler and must also be avoided. Unfortunately, lactose is an unlabeled ingredient in pharmaceuticals. Strict adherence to the diet is necessary for the first 7 to 8 years, followed by a modified regimen throughout life.

KEY POINTS

- Problems of the newborn may be attributed to birth injuries, infections, inborn errors of metabolism, and immature physiologic systems.
- The forces of labor and delivery may cause soft tissue injury, head trauma, fractures, and paralysis.
- The most common forms of paralysis in the newborn are facial nerve, brachial plexus, and phrenic nerve palsies.
- Common skin problems of the newborn include erythema toxicum, candidiasis, bullous impetigo, and discolorations of the skin.
- Because of immature physiologic status, infants may be predisposed to hyperbilirubinemia, neonatal hypocalcemia, and neonatal hypoglycemia.
- Hyperbilirubinemia is classified according to the two types of bilirubin: unconjugated and conjugated. In the newborn it may result from excess production of bilirubin, disturbed capacity of the liver to conjugate bilirubin, or bile duct obstruction resulting from biliary atresia.
- The primary treatment of unconjugated hyperbilirubinemia is phototherapy.
- Hemolytic disease of the newborn is characterized by abnormally rapid destruction of red blood cells as a result of blood incompatibility between mother and fetus.
- Categories of hypoglycemia are (1) decreased substrate availability, (2) endocrine disturbances, (3) increased utilization, and (4) other mechanisms.
- Hemorrhagic disease of the newborn is characterized by oozing from the umbilicus or circumcision site, bloody or black stools, hematuria, ecchymoses on skin and scalp, and epistaxis.
- The most significant inborn errors of metabolism are congenital hypothyroidism, phenylketonuria, and galactosemia.
- Thyroid replacement is required to treat congenital hypothyroidism.
- Dietary control is the treatment of choice for phenylketonuria and galactosemia.

REFERENCES

Adcock, E.W., and Consolvo, C.A.: Fluid and electrolyte management. In Merenstein, G.B., and Gardner, S.L.: Handbook of neonatal intensive care, ed. 2, St. Louis, 1989, Mosby–Year Book, Inc.

American Academy of Pediatrics and American Thyroid Association: Newborn screening for congenital hypothydroidism: recommended guidelines, Pediatrics 80:745-747, 1987.

American Academy of Pediatrics, Committee on Fetus and Newborn: Home phototherapy, Pediatrics 76:136, 1985.

American Academy of Pediatrics, Committee on Genetics: New issues in newborn screening for phenylketonuria and congenital hypothyroidism, Pediatrics 69(1):104-106, 1982.

Arn, P.H., Valle, D.L., and Brusilow, S.W.: Inborn errors of metabolism: not rare, not hopeless, Contemp. Pediatr. 5(12):47-63, 1988.

Berg, F.J., and Solomon, L.M.: Erythema neonatorum toxicum, Arch. Dis. Child. 62:327-328, 1987.

Binder, N.D., and others: Insulin infusion with parenteral nutrition in extremely low birth weight infants with hyperglycemia, J. Pediatr. 114:273-280, 1989.

Blake, S.J.: The bright side of phototherapy, MCN 8(1):23, 1983.

Bowman, I.M.: Controversies in Rh prophylaxis, Am. J. Obstet. Gynecol. 151:289-294, 1985.

Brown, A.K., and others: Efficacy of phototherapy in prevention and management of neonatal hyperbilirubinemia, Pediatrics 75(suppl.): 393-400, 1985.

Brunner, R.L., Jordan, M.K., and Berry, H.K.: Early-treated phenylketonuria: neuropsychologic consequences, J. Pediatr. 102(6):831-835, 1983.

Burton, B.K.: Inborn errors of metabolism: the clinical diagnosis in early infancy, Pediatrics 79:359-369, 1987.

Cashore, W.J., and Stern, L.: Neonatal hyperbilirubinemia, Pediatr. Clin. North Am. 29(5):1191-1203, 1982.

Clarkson, J.E., and others: Jaundice in full term healthy neonates—a population study, Aust. Paediatr. J. 20(11):303-308, 1984.

Coody, D.: Congenital hypothyroidism, Pediatr. Nurs. 10(5):342-345, 1984.

Delaney, J.K., and others: Photophysical properties of Sn-porphyrins: potential clinical implications, Pediatrics 81:498-504, 1988.

Dicken, C.H.: More on the treatment of port-wine stains with the argon laser, Mayo Clin. Proc. 60:115-117, 1985.

DiGiacomo, J.E., Hagedorn, M.I., and Hay, W.W., Jr.: Glucose homeostasis. In Merenstein, G.B., and Gardner, S.L.: Handbook of neonatal intensive care, ed. 2, St. Louis, 1989, Mosby–Year Book, Inc.

Drogari, E., and others: Timing of strict diet in relation to fetal damage in maternal phenylketonuria, Lancet 2:927-930, 1987.

Eggert, L., and others: Home phototherapy treatment of neonatal jaundice, Pediatrics 76:579-584, 1985.

Fanaroff, A.A., and Martin, R.J., editors: Neonatal-perinatal medicine: diseases of the fetus and infant, ed. 4, St. Louis, 1987, Mosby–Year Book, Inc.

Fishler, K., and others: Developmental aspects of galactosemia from infancy to childhood, Clin. Pediatr. 19:38-44, 1980.

Fort, P., and others: Abnormalities of thyroid function in infants with Down syndrome, J. Pediatr. 104(4):545-549, 1984.

Frank, C.G., Turner, B.S., and Merenstein, G.B.: Jaundice. In Merenstein, G.B., and Gardner, S.L.: Handbook of neonatal intensive care, ed. 2, St. Louis, 1989, Mosby–Year Book, Inc.

Gardner, S.L., O'Donnell, J.P., and Weismann, L.E.: Breastfeeding the sick neonate. In Merenstein, G.B., and Gardner, S.L.: Handbook of neonatal intensive care, ed. 2, St. Louis, 1989, Mosby–Year Book, Inc.

Gartner, L.M., and Lee, K.: Jaundice and liver disease. I. Unconjugated hyperbilirubinemia. In Fanaroff, A.A., and Martin, R.J., editors: Neonatal-perinatal medicine: diseases of the fetus and infant, ed. 4, St. Louis, 1987, Mosby–Year Book, Inc.

Glorieux, J., and others: Follow-up at ages 5 and 7 years on mental development in children with hypothyroidism detected by Quebec Screening Program, J. Pediatr. 107:913-919, 1985.

Hammer, R.M., Bower, E.J., and Messina, L.J.: The prenatal use of Rho (D) immune globulin, MCN 9:29-31, 1984.

Hegyi, T., and others: Transcutaneous bilirubinometry. III. Dermal bilirubin kinetics under green and blue light photography, Am. J. Dis. Child. 140:994-997, 1986.

Kappas, A., and others: Sn-protoporphyrin use in the management of hyperbilirubinemia in term newborns with direct Coombs-positive ABO incompatibility, Pediatrics 81:485-497, 1988.

Keenan, W.J., and others: Morbidity and mortality associated with exchange transfusion, Pediatrics 75(suppl.):417-421, 1985.

Kemper, K., Forsyth, B., and McCarthy, P.: Jaundice, terminating breastfeeding, and the vulnerable child, Pediatrics 84:773-778, 1989.

Khoury, M.J., Calle, E.E., and Joesoef, R.M.: Recurrence risk of neonatal hyperbilirubinemia in siblings, Am. J. Dis. Child. 142:1065-1069, 1988.

Lascari, A.D.: "Early" breast-feeding jaundice: clinical significance, J. Pediatr. 108(1):156-158, 1986.

Lawrence, R.A.: Breastfeeding: a guide for the medical profession, ed. 3, St. Louis, 1990, Mosby–Year Book, Inc.

Leibson, C., and others: Neonatal hyperbilirubinemia at high altitude, Am. J. Dis. Child. 143:983-987, 1989.

Lin, H.C., and others: Accuracy and reliability of glucose reflectance meters in the high-risk neonate, J. Pediatr. 116:998-1000, 1989.

Linn, S., and others: Epidemiology of neonatal hyperbilirubinemia, Pediatrics 75(4):770-774, 1985.

Lipsitz, P.J., Gartner, L.M., and Bryla, D.A.: Neonatal and infant mortality in relation to phototherapy, Pediatrics 75(suppl):422-426, 1985.

Lo, W., and others: Curious neurologic sequelae in galactosemia, Pediatrics 73(3):309-312, 1984.

Maisels, M.: Hyperbilirubinemia. In Nelson, N.M., editor: Current therapy in neonatal-perinatal medicine, St. Louis, 1985, Mosby–Year Book, Inc.

Maisels, M.J., and others: Jaundice in the healthy newborn infant: a new approach to an old problem, Pediatrics 81:505-511, 1988.

Mansour, A., and Gelfand, E.W.: A new approach to the use of antifungal agents in infants with persistent oral candidiasis, J. Pediatr. 98:161-162, Jan. 1981.

McCabe, E.R.B., and others: Evaluation of a phenylalanine-free product for treatment of phenylketonuria, Am. J. Dis. Child. 141:1327-1329, 1987.

McNinch, A.M., and others: Plasma concentrations after oral or intramuscular vitamin K1 in neonates, Arch. Dis. Child. 60:814-818, 1985.

Merenstein, G.B., and Gardner, S.L.: Handbook of neonatal intensive care, ed. 2, St. Louis, 1989, Mosby–Year Book, Inc.

Messer, S.S.: PKU: a mother's perspective, Pediatr. Nurs. 11:121-123, 1985.

Michals, K., and others: Return to diet therapy in patients with phenylketonuria, J. Pediatr. 106:933-936, 1985.

Millner, P.: Personal communication, 1990.

Minarcik, C.J., and Beachy, P.: Neurologic disorders. In Merenstein, G.B., and Gardner, S.L.: Handbook of neonatal intensive care, ed. 2, St. Louis, 1989, Mosby–Year Book, Inc.

New England Congenital Hypothyroidism Collaborative: Characteristics of infantile hypothyroidism discovered on neonatal screening, J. Pediatr. 104(4):539-544, 1984.

New England Congenital Hypothyroidism Collaborative: Neonatal hypothyroidism screening: status of patients at 6 years of age, J. Pediatr. 107(6):915-918, 1985.

New England Congenital Hypothyroidism Collaborative: Congenital concomitants of infantile hypothyroidism, J. Pediatr. 112:245-247, 1988.

O'Connor, M.E., and Addiego, J.E.: Use of oral vitamin K_1 to prevent hemorrhagic disease of the newborn infant, J. Pediatr. 108:616-619, 1986.

Olson, J.: Recommended dietary intakes (RDI) of vitamin K in humans, Am. J. Clin. Nutr. 45:687-690, 1987.

Osborn, L.M.: Management of neonatal jaundice. Nurse Pract. 11(4):41-52, 1986.

Osborn, L.M., Reiff, M.I., and Bolus, R.: Jaundice in the full-term neonate, Pediatrics 73(4):520-525, 1984.

Pildes, R.S., and Lilien, L.D.. Carbohydrate metabolism in the fetus and neonate. In Fanaroff, A., and Martin, R., editors: Behrman's neonatal-perinatal medicine, ed. 4, St. Louis, 1987, Mosby–Year Book, Inc.

Plotz, R.D.: Familial occurrence of hemolytic disease of the newborn due to AO blood group incompatibility, Hum. Pathol. 16:113-116, 1985.

Robertson, A., Fink, S., and Karp, W.: Effect of cephalosporins on bilirubin-albumin binding, J. Pediatr. 112:291-294, 1988.

Rohr, F.J., and others: New England maternal PKU project: prospective study of untreated and treated pregnancies and their outcomes, J. Pediatr. 110:391-398, 1987.

Rose, B.S.: Phototherapy: All wrapped up? Pediatr. Nurs. 16:57, 1990.

Rutledge, J.C., and Ou, C.: Bilirubin and the laboratory, Pediatr. Clin. North Am. 36:189-198, 1989.

Schumacher, R.E., Thornbery, J.M., and Gutcher, G.R.: Transcutaneous bilirubinometry: a comparison of old and new methods, Pediatrics 76(1):10-14, 1985.

Seashore, M.R., and others: Loss of intellectual function in children with phenylketonuria after relaxation of dietary phenylalanine restriction, Pediatrics 75(2):226-232, 1985.

Slater, L., and Brewer, M.: Home versus hospital phototherapy for term infants with hyperbilirubinemia: a comparative study, Pediatrics 73:515-519, 1984.

Smith, D., and others: Use of noninvasive tests to predict significant jaundice in full-term infants: preliminary studies, Pediatrics 75(2):278-280, 1985.

Tan, K.L.: Efficacy of fluorescent daylight, blue, and green lamps in the management of nonhemolytic hyperbilirubinemia, J. Pediatr. 114:132-137, 1989.

Vecchi, C., and others: Phototherapy for neonatal jaundice: clinical equivalence of fluorescent green and "special" blue lamps, J. Pediatr. 108(3):452-456, 1986.

Vitanza, A., Giacoia, G., and West, K.: Evaluation of a new glucose reflectance meter for use in the neonatal intensive care unit, J. Perinatol. 8(1):43-45, 1988.

von Kries, R., and others: Vitamin K_1 content of maternal milk: influence of the stage of lactation, lipid composition, and vitamin K_1 supplements, Pediatr. Res. 22:513-517, 1987.

Waisbren, S.E., and others: Speech and language deficits in early-treated children with galactosemia, J. Pediatr. 102(1):75-77, 1983.

Wilkerson, N.N.: A comprehensive look at hyperbilirubinemia, MCN 13:360-364, 1988.

BIBLIOGRAPHY

General

Fanaroff, A.A., and Martin, R.J., editors: Neonatal-perinatal medicine: diseases of the fetus and infant, ed. 4, St. Louis, 1987, Mosby–Year Book, Inc.

Korones, S.B.: High-risk newborn infants: the basis for intensive nursing care, ed. 4, St. Louis, 1986, Mosby–Year Book, Inc.

Birth Injuries

Cohen, A.W., and Otto, S.R.: Obstetric clavicular fractures: a three-year analysis, J. Reprod. Med. 25:119-122, Sept. 1980.

Feigin, F.D.: Postnatally acquired infections. In Fanaroff, A., and Martin, R., editors: Behrman's neonatal-perinatal medicine, ed. 4, St. Louis, 1987, Mosby–Year Book, Inc.

Greenwald, A.G., and others: Brachial plexus birth palsy: a ten year report on incidence and prognosis, J. Pediatr. Orthop. 4:689-692, 1984.

Ingardia, C.J., and Cetrulo, C.L.: Forceps—use and abuse, Clin. Perinatol. 8:63-66, Feb. 1981.

Jain, I.S., and others: Ocular hazards during birth, J. Pediatr. Ophthalmol. Strabismus 17:14-16, Jan./Feb. 1980.

Joseph, P.R., and Rosenfeld, W.: Clavicular fractures in neonates, Am. J. Dis. Child. 144:165-167, 1990.

Mangurten, H.H.: Birth injuries. In Fanaroff, A., and Martin, R., editors: Behrman's neonatal-perinatal medicine, ed. 4, St. Louis, 1987, Mosby–Year Book, Inc.

The first six hours of life: assessment of risk in the newborn—birth injuries, module 4, New York, 1982, March of Dimes–Birth Defects Foundation.

Dermatologic Problems

Abramovits, W.: Resistant oral candidiasis in an infant due to pacifier contamination, Clin. Pediatr. 20:393, June 1981.

Butler, K.M., and Baker, J.B.: Candida: an increasingly important pathogen in the nursery, Pediatr. Clin. North Am. 35:543-563, 1988.

Cohen, B.A.: Hemangiomas in infancy and childhood, Pediatr. Ann. 16:17-26, 1987.

Daftary, S.S., and others: Oral thrush in the new-born, Indian Pediatr. 17:287-288, March 1980.

Finn, M.C., Glowacki, J., and Mulliken, J.B.: Congenital vascular lesions: clinical application of a new classification, J. Pediatr. Surg. 18(6):894-900, 1983.

Larrow, L., and Noe, J.M: Port wine stain hemangiomas, Am. J. Nurs. 82:786-790, 1982.

Prendiville, J., and Esterly, N.B.: When congenital nevi signal underlying disease, Contemp. Pediatr. 4(3):24-52, 1987.

Tan, O.T., and Gilchrest, B.A.: Laser therapy for selected cutaneous vascular lesions in the pediatric population: a review, Pediatrics 82:652-661, 1988.

Hyperbilirubinemia

Adams, J.A., Hey, D.J., and Hall, R.T.: Incidence of hyperbilirubinemia in breast- vs. formula-fed infants, Clin. Pediatr. 24(2):69-73, 1985.

Bell, S.G.: Nonimmune hydrops fetalis, Neonatal Network 7(2):15-27, 1988.

Boyer, D.B., and Vidyasagar, D.: Serum indirect bilirubin levels and meconium passage in early fed normal newborns, Nurs. Res. 36:174-178, 1986.

Brucker, M.C., and MacMullen, N.J.: Neonatal jaundice in the home; assessment with a noninvasive device, JOGNN 16:355-358, 1987.

Costarino, A.T., and others: Bilirubin photoisomerization in premature neonates under low- and high-dose phototherapy, Pediatrics 75(3):519-522, 1985.

Costarino, A.T., Jr., and others: Effect of spectral distribution on isomerization of bilirubin in vivo, J. Pediatr. 107(1):125-128, 1985.

Curtis-Cohen, M., and others: Randomized trial of prophylactic phototherapy in the infant with very low birth weight, J. Pediatr. 107(1):121-124, 1985.

D'Epiro, P.: Neonatal jaundice: knowing when to treat, Patient Care 19(14):140-143, 1985.

deVries, L.S., Lary, L., and Dubowitz, L.M.S.: Relationship of serum bilirubin levels to ototoxicity and deafness in high-risk low-birth-weight infants, Pediatrics 76(3):351-354, 1985.

Dortch, E., and Spottiswoode, P.: New light on phototherapy: home use, Neonatal Network 4(4):30-34, 1986.

Dunn, P.A., and others: Care of the neonate with erythroblastosis fetalis, JOGNN 17:382-385, 1988.

Gannon, R.B., and Pickett, K.: Jaundice, Am. J. Nurs. 83(3):404-407, 1983.

Grossglauser, L.K.: Nonimmune hydrops fetalis: an overview, Neonatal Network 8(1):67-74, 1989.

Hartsell, M.B.: Home phototherapy, J. Pediatr. Nurs. 1:282-283, 1986.

Heiser, C.A.: Home phototherapy, Pediatr. Nurs. 13:425-427, 1987.

Hensleigh, P.A.: Preventing rhesus isoimmunization, Am. J. Obstet. Gynecol. 146:749-755, 1983.

Hill, A.S., Cochran, C.K., and Dickerson, C.: Nursing care of the infant with erythroblastosis fetalis, J. Pediatr. Nurs. 4:395-402, 1989.

Jaundiced babies bloom with home phototherapy, Am. J. Nurs. 84(7):871, 1984.

Kasprisin, D.O., and Kasprisin, C.A.: Introduction to transfusion therapy: a programmed text, New York, 1980, Medical Examination Publishing Co., Inc.

Kemper, K.J., Forsyth, B.W., and McCarthy, P.L.: Persistent perceptions of vulnerability following neonatal jaundice, Am. J. Dis. Child. 144:238-241, 1990.

Kivlahan, C., and James, E.J.P.: The natural history of neonatal jaundice, Pediatrics 74(3):364-370, 1984.

Levine, D.H., and Meyer, H.B.P.: Newborn screening for ABO hemolytic disease, Clin. Pediatr. 24:391-394, 1985.

Locklin, M.: Assessing jaundice in full-term newborns, Pediatr. Nurs. 13:15-19, 1987.

Maisels, M.J.: Jaundice in the newborn, Pediatr. Re. 3(10):305-320, 1982.

Maisels, M.J., and Gifford, K.: Normal serum bilirubin levels in the newborn and the effect of breast-feeding, Pediatrics 78:837-843, 1986.

Mauer, H.M., and others: Phototherapy for hyperbilirubinemia of hemolytic disease of the newborn, Pediatrics 75(suppl. 2):407-412, 1985.

Onishi, S., and others: Mechanism of development of bronze baby syndrome in neonates treated with phototherapy, Pediatrics 69(3):273-276, 1982.

Osborn, L.M., and others: Phototherapy in full-term infants with hemolytic disease secondary to ABO incompatibility, Pediatrics 74(3):371-374, 1984.

Page, S.: Rh hemolytic disease of the newborn, Neonatal Network 31(6):31-41, 1989.

Perry, L.E., Parer, J.T., and Inturrisi, M.: Intrauterine transfusion for severe isoimmunization, MCN 11:182-189, 1986.

Poland, R.L.: Breast milk jaundice, J. Pediatr. 99(1):86-87, 1981.

Rosenthal, P., Ramos, A., and Mungo, R.: Management of children with hyperbilirubinemia and green teeth, J. Pediatr. 108(1):103-105, 1986.

Shibley, B.: Now newborns can stay home for phototherapy, RN 5(2):69-71, 1988.

Slater, L., and Brewer, M.: Home versus hospital phototherapy for term infants with hyperbilirubinemia: a comparative study, Pediatrics 73(4):515-519, 1984.

Walther, F.J., Wu, P.Y.K., and Siassi, B.: Cardiac output changes in newborns with hyperbilirubinemia treated with phototherapy, Pediatrics 76(6):918-921, 1985.

Wilkerson, N.N.: Treating hyperbilirubinemia, MCN 14:32-36, 1989.

Wu, P.Y.K., and others: Metabolic aspects of phototherapy, Pediatrics 75(suppl. 2):427-433, 1985.

Metabolic Problems

Brown, D.R., Steranka, B.H., and Taylor, F.H.: Treatment of early-onset neonatal hypocalcemia, Am. J. Dis. Child. 135:24-28, Jan. 1981.

Carmen, S.: Neonatal hypoglycemia in response to maternal glucose infusion before delivery, JOGNN 15:319-323, 1986.

Lilien, L.D., and others: Treatment of neonatal hypoglycemia with minibolus and intravenous glucose infusions, J. Pediatr. 97(2):295-298, 1980.

McFadden, E.A., Zaloga, G.P., and Chernow, B.: Hypocalcemia: a medical emergency, Am. J. Nurs. 83:227-230, 1983.

Romagnoli, C., and others: Phototherapy-induced hypocalcemia, J. Pediatr. 94(5):815-816, 1979.

Salsbury, D.J., and Brown, D.R.: Effect of parenteral calcium treatment on blood pressure and heart rate in neonatal hypocalcemia, Pediatrics 69(5):605-609, 1982.

Schedewie, H.K., and others: Parathormone and perinatal calcium homeostasis, Pediatr. Res. 13:1-6, Jan. 1979.

Scott, S.M., and others: Effect of calcium therapy in the sick premature infant with early neonatal hypocalcemia, J. Pediatr. 104(5):747-751, 1984.

Sexson, W.R.: Incidence of neonatal hypoglycemia: a matter of definition, J. Pediatr. 105(1):149-150, 1984.

Shannon, L.F.: Insulin usage in the neonate, Neonatal Network 6(5):31-39, 1988.

Taur, K.M.: Physiologic mechanisms in childhood hypoglycemia, Pediatr. Nurs. 9(5):341-344, 1983.

Hemorrhagic Disease of the Newborn

Behrmann, B.A., and others: Resurgence of hemorrhagic disease of the newborn: a report of three cases, Can. Med. Assoc. J. 133(9):884-885, 1985.

Chaou, W., Chou, M., and Eitzman, D.V.: Intracranial hemorrhage and vitamin K deficiency in early infancy, J. Pediatr. 105(6):880-884, 1984.

Lane, P.A., and Hathaway, W.E.: Vitamin K in infancy, J. Pediatr. 106(3):351-359, 1985.

McNinch, A.W., and others: Hemorrhagic disease of the newborn returns, Lancet 1:1089-1090, 1983.

Motohara, K., and others: Severe vitamin K deficiency in breast-fed infants, J. Pediatr. 105(6):943-945, 1984.

Inborn Errors of Metabolism

American Academy of Pediatrics, Committee on Drugs: "Inactive" ingredients in pharmaceutical products, Pediatrics 76(4):635-643, 1985.

Applegarth, D.A., Dimmick, J.E., and Toone, J.R.: Laboratory detection of metabolic disease, Pediatr. Clin. North Am. 36:49-65, 1989.

Aronson, R, and others: Growth in children with congenital hypothyroidism detected by neonatal screening, J. Pediatr. 116:33-37, 1990.

Berger, L.R.: When should one discourage breast-feeding? Pediatrics 67:300-302, Feb. 1981.

Brown, A.L., and others: Racial differences in the incidence of congenital hypothyroidism, J. Pediatr. 9(6):934-936, 1981.

Brown, J.: The health hazard of unlabeled ingredients in pharmaceuticals, Pediatrics 73(3):402-404, 1984.

Burton, B.K.: Inborn errors of metabolism: the clinical diagnosis in early infancy, Pediatrics 79:359-369, 1987.

Coody, D.: Congenital hypothyroidism, Pediatr. Nurs. 10:342-345, 1984.

Fisher, D.A.: Effectiveness of newborn screening programs for congenital hypothyroidism: prevalence of missed cases, Pediatr. Clin. North Am. 34:881-898, 1987.

Kotzer, A.M., and McCabe, E.R.B.: Newborn screening for inherited metabolic disease: principles and practice, Neonatal Network 6(4):15-19, 1988.

LaFranchi, S.H., and others: Screening for congenital hypothyroidism with specimen collection at two time periods: results of the Northwest Regional Screening Program, Pediatrics 76(5):734-740, 1985.

Lechter, M.: "Hidden" lactose a source of GI distress, Patient Care 16(8):122, 1982.

New England Congenital Hypothyroidism Collaborative: Elementary school performance of children with congenital hypothroidism, J. Pediatr. 116:27-32, 1990.

Rovet, J.F.: Does breast-feeding protect the hypothyroid infant whose condition is diagnosed by newborn screening? Am. J. Dis. Child. 144:319-323, 1990.

Schmidt, K.: A primer to the inborn errors of metabolism for perinatal and neonatal nurses, J. Perinat. Neonatal Nurs. 2(4):60-71, 1989.

Smith, E.J.: Galactosemia: an inborn error of metabolism, Nurse Pract. 5:8-9, March/April 1980.

Phenylketonuria

American Academy of Pediatrics, Committee on Genetics: Maternal phenylketonuria, Pediatrics 76(2):313-314, 1985.

American Academy of Pediatrics, Committee on Nutrition: New developments in hyperphenylalaninemia, Pediatrics 65(4):844-846, 1980.

Barnico, L.M., and Cullinane, M.M.: Maternal phenylketonuria: an unexpected challenge, MCN 10:108-110, 1985.

Cederbaum, S.D., Koch, R., and Donnell, G.N.: Symposium on genetic engineering and phenylketonuria, Pediatrics 74(3):406-407, 1984.

Hayes, J.S., and others: Managing PKU: an update, MCN 12:119-123, 1987.

Holtzman, N.A.: Ethical issues in the prenatal diagnosis of phenylketonuria, Pediatrics 74(3):424-427, 1984.

Hurst, J.D., and Stullenbarger, B.: Implementation of a self-care approach in a pediatric interdisciplinary phenylketonuria (PKU) clinic, J. Pediatr. Nurs. 1:159-163, 1986.

Koch, R., and Friedman, E.G.: Accuracy of newborn screening programs for phenylketonuria, J. Pediatr. 98:267-269, Feb. 1981.

Levy, H.L., and Waisbren, S.E.: Effects of untreated maternal phenylketonuria and hyperphenylalaninemia, N. Engl. J. Med. 309:1269-1274, 1983.

Lott, J.W.: PKU: a nursing update, J. Pediatr. Nurs. 3:29-34, 1988.

Matalon, R.: Current status of biopterin screening, J. Pediatr. 104(4):579-581, 1984.

Meryash, D.L.: Prospective study of early neonatal screening for phenylketonuria, N. Engl. J. Med. 304:294-296, Jan. 1981.

Russell, F.F., Mills, B.C., and Zucconi, T.: Relationship of parental attitudes and knowledge to treatment adherence in children with PKU, Pediatr. Nurs. 14:514-516, 1988.

Sbravati, C., and Fischer, R.G.: What sugar substitutes are available and are there any differences between them? Pediatr. Nurs. 9(2):138, 1983.

Schor, D.P.: Phenylketonuria and temperament in middle childhood, Child. Health Care 14(3):163-167, 1986.

Steele, S.: Phenylketonuria: counseling and teaching functions of the nurse on an interdisciplinary team, Issues Compr. Pediatr. Nurs. 12:395-410, 1989.

Sturtevant, F.M.: Use of aspartame in pregnancy, Int. J. Fertil. 30(1):85-87, 1985.

Woo, S.L.C.: Prenatal diagnosis and carrier detection of classic phenylketonuria by gene analysis, Pediatrics 74(3):412-423, 1984.

CHAPTER 10

The High-Risk Newborn and Family

RELATED TOPICS

Administration of medications, Ch. 27
Assessment of clinical gestational age, Ch. 8
Birth of a child with a physical defect, Ch. 11
Birth injuries, Ch. 9
Bodily injury and pain, Ch. 26
Congenital defects caused by prenatal factors, Ch. 11
Diaphragmatic hernia, Ch. 11
Discharge planning and home care, Ch. 26
Esophageal atresia with tracheoesophageal fistula, Ch. 11
Fetal alcohol syndrome, Ch. 11
Gastroschisis, Ch. 11
Hiatal hernia, Ch. 11
Hyperbilirubinemia, Ch. 9
Hypocalcemia, Ch. 9
Hypoglycemia, Ch. 9
Infant mortality, Ch. 1
Malformations of the central nervous system, Ch. 11
Neonatal pain, Ch. 11
Newborn assessment, Ch. 8
Nursing care of the surgical neonate, Ch. 11
Omphalocele, Ch. 11
Pain assessment; pain management, Ch. 26
Promotion of parent-infant bonding (attachment), Ch. 8

GLOSSARY

AGA Appropriate for gestational age
AOP Apnea of prematurity
BPD Bronchopulmonary dysplasia
CNS Central nervous system
CPAP Continuous positive airway pressure
CPPB Continuous positive-pressure breathing
CPPV Continuous positive-pressure ventilation
ECG Electrocardiograph
ECMO Extracorporeal membrane oxygenation
ET Endotracheal
Fio_2 Fraction of inspired oxygen
HFJV High-frequency jet ventilation
HFO High-frequency oscillation
HFPPV High-frequency positive-pressure ventilation
HFV High-frequency ventilation
HgF Hemoglobin F
ICP Intracranial pressure
IDM Infant of diabetic mother
IMV Intermittent mandatory ventilation
IRDS Idiopathic respiratory distress syndrome
IUGR Intrauterine growth retardation
IVH Intraventricular hemorrhage
LBW Low birth weight; infant who weighs <2500 g
LGA Large for gestational age
NEC Necrotizing enterocolitis
NICU Neonatal intensive care unit
NNS Nonnutritive sucking
OFC Occipitofrontal circumference
$Paco_2$ Arterial carbon dioxide pressure
Pao_2 Arterial oxygen pressure (tension)
PDA Patent ductus arteriosus
PEEP Positive end-expiratory pressure
PFC Persistent fetal circulation
PIP Peak inspiratory pressure
PPHN Persistent pulmonary hypertension of the newborn
PVR Pulmonary vascular resistance
ROP Retinopathy of prematurity
Sao_2 Arterial oxygen saturation
SFD Small for dates
SGA Small for gestational age
VLBW Very low birth weight; infant who weighs <1500 g

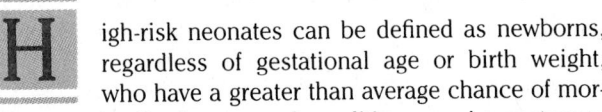

High-risk neonates can be defined as newborns, regardless of gestational age or birth weight, who have a greater than average chance of morbidity or mortality because of conditions or circumstances that are superimposed on the normal course of events associated with birth and the adjustment to extrauterine existence. This includes the periods in human growth and development from the time of viability until 28 days following birth and involves threats to life and health that occur during the prenatal, perinatal, and neonatal periods.

GENERAL MANAGEMENT OF HIGH-RISK NEWBORNS

In recent years there has been an increase in the survival rate of newborns that has coincided with the establishment of programs to improve the health of mothers and the timing of their pregnancies, and the introduction of important new techniques in neonatal care. The decreased neonatal mortality and the survival of low-birth-weight newborns has generated considerable debate and concern regarding the possibility of increased disability of survivors that might place additional demands on societal resources. Birth weight is the most important predictor of infant survival. Survival increases exponentially as birth weight increases to its optimum level (Hogue and others, 1989). When problems are anticipated, preparations can be made for intensive care during the periods of greatest threat; through this care the incidence of fetal and neonatal mortality can be significantly reduced.

IDENTIFICATION OF HIGH-RISK NEWBORNS

Nurses in a variety of settings play an important role in detection and intervention where high-risk factors are most likely to occur. Care begins in the preconception period when parents at risk for problems associated with procreation (usually genetic defects) are provided with information to make a judicious decision regarding childbearing. In the prenatal period the most important aspect in anticipating or averting problems is early and consistent prenatal care. Nurses in the community are in a position to detect families in need and to arrange opportunities for ongoing prenatal observation. During labor and delivery the obstetric nurse alert to signs of fetal distress and maternal conditions that contribute to neonatal morbidity can avert numerous problems. Assessment and prompt intervention in life-threatening emergencies often make the difference between a favorable outcome and a lifetime of disability. The nurse in the newborn nursery is familiar with the characteristics of neonates and recognizes the significance of serious deviations from expected observations. When the need for specialized care can be anticipated and planned for, the probability of successful outcome is increased.

Anticipation of Problems

Many of the factors that influence the outcome of these vulnerable periods occur simultaneously and in combination. For example, infants born prematurely often suffer from perinatal asphyxia, have cerebral hemorrhage during delivery, have associated congenital anomalies, and develop idiopathic respiratory distress syndrome. The list of factors associated with increased risk in the neonatal period con-

Box 10-1 HIGH-RISK SITUATIONS

Preconception

Hereditary diseases or abnormalities—inborn errors of metabolism, anomalies of heart and central nervous system, sickle cell anemia, and many others
Socioeconomic factors—poor nutrition and general health of mother; frequently teenage pregnancy
High altitude—associated with low-birth-weight infants
Parental age
Maternal—over 35 or under 16 years of age
Paternal—over 40 years of age
Maternal size—less than 5 feet; prepregnant weight greater than 20% over or under standards for height and weight
Grand multiparity—more than five, especially when the mother is over 35 years of age
History of obstetric complications—prolonged period of infertility, spontaneous abortion, placental accidents, previous larger-than-average or small-for-date newborns, eclampsia, isoimmunization, multiple pregnancies, previous birth of abnormal infant
Uterine abnormality—tumors (fibroid, myoma), developmental anomalies (uterus bicornis), incompetent cervix

Prenatal

Maternal disease—preeclampsia, hypertension, malignancy, heart disease, hemoglobinopathy, renal diseases, endocrine diseases (thyroid, diabetes)
Maternal infection—bacterial, viral, spirochetal, protozoal, chlamydia
Maternal disorders associated with pregnancy—preeclampsia, placental abnormalities, hyperemesis gravidarum
Socioeconomic problems—malnutrition, long-delayed or absent prenatal care
Maternal stress—physical, emotional
Maternal addiction—narcotics, barbiturates, amphetamines, hallucinogens, alcohol, cocaine, tobacco
Maternal medication—no drug is absolutely safe
Gases—maternal smoking, anesthesia
Multiple pregnancy—smaller fetal size and premature delivery
Isoimmunization—Rh or ABO blood incompatibility
Uterine accidents—abruptio placentae, placenta previa, ruptured uterus, trauma
Fetal size—larger or smaller than expected for age; over or under normal gestational age (preterm, postterm); cephalopelvic disproportion
Polyhydramnios or oligohydramnios—often associated with fetal anomalies
Diagnostic procedures—x-ray films or treatment, amniocentesis, chorionic villi sampling
Surgical procedures—incidental operation during course of pregnancy

Natal (Intrapartum)

Fever—may indicate maternal infection
Premature labor—preterm infant is at greater risk
Premature rupture of fetal membranes—associated with intrauterine infection and prolapse of umbilical cord
Fetal distress—tachycardia (fetal heart rate above 180 beats per minute), bradycardia (fetal heart rate below 120 beats per minute), irregular heart rate, meconium-stained amniotic fluid (in vertex presentation), abnormal deceleration curve (monitored), scalp vein pH 7.2 or less
Abnormalities of fetal position—transverse, breech, unengaged presenting part
Cesarean section—associated with higher neonatal morbidity; often performed because of adverse prenatal or natal conditions
Abnormal labor and/or delivery—precipitous, prolonged, breech, assisted (forceps), other complications
Uterine accidents—rupture, abruptio placentae
Cord accidents—knots, tight nuchal cord, prolapse, rupture
Maternal analgesia or anesthesia—may cause depression in fetus and newborn

Postnatal (Immediate)

Single umbilical artery—may be associated with fetal anomalies
Low Apgar score—especially 5-minute test
Abnormal placenta—massive infarction, evidence of separation, amnionitis, calcifications
Prematurity—newborn less able to withstand rigors of birth and transition
Multiple birth—newborn less able to withstand rigors of birth and transition
Disproportion between weight or length and gestation age—may indicate intrauterine growth retardation, intrauterine malnutrition, concomitant disorders (e.g., infant or diabetic mother)
Depression—may indicate central nervous system damage, hypoxia, maternal oversedation
Birth trauma—head injury, fractures, nerve damage
Presence of congenital anomalies—cleft palate, imperforate anus, choanal atresia, omphalocele, gastroschisis, diaphragmatic hernia, tracheoesophageal fistula, cardiovascular defect, etc.
Severe blood loss, sepsis, meconium aspiration—adversely influence adjustment

Neonatal (Warning Signs)

Abnormal respiration—may indicate congenital anomalies, lung syndromes, acidosis
Apneic episodes—may be caused by such factors as central nervous system disturbance, immaturity of regulatory mechanisms, congestion, sepsis, obstruction, drugs, cardiac anomalies, hypoglycemia, hypocalcemia, hypermagnesemia (maternal treatment for eclampsia or labor suppression)
Tremor and/or seizures—may indicate hypoglycemia, hypocalcemia, narcotic addiction, central nervous system hemorrhage or infection, postasphyxia
Limpness and/or lethargy—may be the result of sepsis, central nervous system damage, hypoxia, Down syndrome, hypothyroidism
Vomiting or difficulty in swallowing—central nervous system damage, immature reflexes, congenital defects, gastrointestinal infection
Abdominal distention—may indicate congenital anomalies, gastrointestinal infection
Failure to void or pass meconium in first 24 hours—associated with congenital anomalies
Pallow—may indicate anemia, hemorrhage, cold stress, or shock
Jaundice—especially serious when appears in first 24 hours
Petechiae—a sign of thrombocytopenia, infection
Thermal instability—iatrogenic factors, central nervous system damage, immaturity, environmental factors, sepsis
Failure to regain birth weight by 10 days of age—congenital anomalies, metabolic disorders, central nervous system damage, sepsis, feeding difficulties
Cyanosis—respiratory or cardiac disorders, apnea, hypoglycemia

tinues to grow as applied research in the fields of perinatology and neonatology adds new data. The major situations that contribute to perinatal morbidity, mortality in infancy, and possibly the future physical and intellectual qualities of the child, or that warn of impending difficulties are listed in Box 10-1.

Although not considered high-risk situations in the usual sense, difficulties in the ability of the mother to properly care for the child or disturbances in the mother-child relationship can have serious consequences—both immediate and long term—for the infant. These difficulties may be caused by neurologic, malignant, rheumatic, or other disorders that impair the mother's ability to physically care for her infant or by psychologic illness that interferes with her ability to provide proper care for the child. These situations are not discussed in depth here; however, nurses must be alert to indications of these special problems that may profoundly influence the well-being of the infant and place the infant at risk.

Classification of High-Risk Newborns

High-risk infants are most often classified according to size, gestational age, and predominant pathophysiologic problems. The more common problems related to physiologic status are closely associated with the state of maturity of the infant and usually involve chemical disturbances (e.g., hypoglycemia, hypocalcemia) and consequences of immature functioning organs and systems (e.g., hyperbilirubinemia, respiratory distress, hypothermia). Since high-risk factors are common to several specialty areas, particularly obstetrics, pediatrics, and neonatology, specific terminology is needed to describe the developmental status of the newborn (Box 10-2).

Formerly, weight at birth was considered to reflect a reasonably accurate estimation of gestational age. That is, if infants' birth weights exceeded 2500 g (5½ pounds), they were considered to be mature. However, accumulated data have shown that intrauterine growth rates are not the same for all infants and that other factors (e.g., heredity, placental insufficiency, and maternal disease) influence intrauterine growth and birth weight of the infant. From these data a more definitive and meaningful classification system that encompasses size, gestational age, and fetal outcome has been developed. It has also been determined that the lowest perinatal mortality is found in the full-term infant who weighs between 3000 and 4000 g (Fanaroff and Martin, 1987). (See Fig. 8-2 for size comparison of newborn infants.)

Many problems can be anticipated before delivery. Prenatal testing and labor monitoring have reduced the incidence of perinatal mortality, and specialized care of the distressed newborn is improving the survival rate. If the infant is likely to require special therapy at or soon after birth, plans can be made for the delivery to take place at or near a hospital that has the facilities to provide such care. In this way there is no delay in initiating needed care, and some of the hazards associated with transporting the sick newborn are averted.

Box 10-2 CLASSIFICATION OF HIGH-RISK INFANTS

Classification According to Size

Low-birth-weight (LBW) infant—an infant whose birth weight is less than 2500 g regardless of gestational age

Very-low-birth-weight (VLBW) infant—an infant whose weight is less than 1500 g

Moderately-low-birth-weight (MLBW)—an infant whose birth weight is 1501 to 2500 g

Appropriate-for-gestational-age (AGA) infant—an infant whose weight falls between the 10th and 90th percentiles on intrauterine growth curves

Small-for-date (SFD) or small-for-gestational-age (SGA) infant—an infant whose rate of intrauterine growth was slowed and whose birth weight falls below the 10th percentile on intrauterine growth curves

Intrauterine growth retardation (IUGR)—found in infants whose intrauterine growth is retarded (sometimes used as a more descriptive term for the SGA infant)

Large-for-gestational-age (LGA) infant—an infant whose birth weight falls above the 90th percentile on intrauterine growth curves

Classification According to Gestational Age

Premature (preterm) infant—an infant born before completion of 37 weeks of gestation, regardless of birth weight

Term infant—an infant born between the beginning of the 38 weeks and the completion of the 42 weeks of gestation, regardless of birth weight

Postmature (postterm) infant—an infant born after 42 weeks of gestational age, regardless of birth weight

Classification According to Mortality

Live birth—birth in which the neonate manifests any heartbeat, breathes, or displays voluntary movement, regardless of gestational age

Fetal death—death of the fetus after 20 weeks of gestation and before delivery, with absence of any signs of life after birth

Neonatal death—death that occurs in the first 27 days of life; early neonatal death occurs in the first week of life; late neonatal death occurs at 7 to 27 days

Perinatal mortality—describes the total number of fetal and early neonatal deaths per 1000 live births

Postnatal death—death that occurs at 28 days to 1 year

INTENSIVE CARE FACILITIES

Awareness of the unique characteristics of perinatal disorders has generated the provision of special care units in major medical facilities. Rapid advances in the understanding of the pathophysiology of the neonate and the increased capacity to apply this knowledge have emphasized the need for appropriate settings in which to care for the seriously ill infant. Advancements in electronics and biochemistry, new methods for monitoring cardiorespiratory function, microtechniques for biochemical determination from minute quantities of blood, noninvasive monitoring, and new methods for assisted ventilation and conservation of body heat have made it possible to effectively manage the newborn with serious illness.

Intensive care of the ill and immature newborn requires specialized knowledge and skill in a number of areas of expertise. Much of the equipment long used in the care of the critically ill adult is unsuited to the singular needs of the very small infant; therefore commonplace apparatus has been modified to meet these needs. Examples of modifications include respirators that deliver small volumes of oxygen in the proper concentration and pressure, infusion pumps that deliver very small amounts accurately, and crib units that provide a constant source of warmth and at the same time allow maximum access to the infant. Most important, intensive care has created a need for highly skilled personnel trained in the art of neonatal intensive care.

The diversity of special care needs requires that the unit be arranged for graduated care for the infant population. There should be adequate facilities and skilled personnel to provide one-to-one nursing care for each seriously ill infant, in addition to a means for graduation to one-to-three or one-to-four nursing care in a convalescent area where infants require less intensive care until they are ready to leave the unit.

Nurses in the neonatal intensive care unit (NICU) are highly trained in the management of a variety of sophisticated mechanical devices and educated in the art of recognizing subtle changes in infants' behavior, interpreting observations of others, and timing interventions appropriately. Proficiency is developed through daily observation and practice under the guidance of a skilled practitioner; in-service education is one of the prime objectives in the ongoing management of a successful NICU. The teaching activities of nurses in the NICU are extended to include not only new nurses but also residents, interns, and parents.

Organization of Services

The most efficient organization of services is a regionalized system consisting of facilities within a designated geographic area that provide three prescribed levels of care with special equipment, skilled personnel, and ancillary services concentrated in a centralized institution (Box 10-3).

Box 10-3 CHARACTERISTICS OF NEONATAL INTENSIVE CARE FACILITIES

Level I—a facility designed to provide management of normal maternal and newborn care but able to identify high-risk pregnancies and/or high-risk neonates early and implement emergency care in the event of complications. These are usually small community hospitals removed from urban areas but vital to health care in the area.

Level II—a facility that serves larger communities, usually is located in urban or suburban areas, and provides a full range of maternity and newborn care. It is equipped to manage the majority of maternal and neonatal complications, depending on the resources available.

Level III—a facility that offers the full range of maternal and newborn services of a level II facility. In addition, it has the capacity to provide care for the most complex neonatal complications. At least one full-time neonatologist is on the staff, as well as an impressive complement of pediatric subspecialists, including pediatric surgeons, geneticists, radiologists, anesthesiologists, and hospital epidemiologists who are at the disposal of the unit. All but some highly specialized types of cases are managed in a level III facility. Occasionally an infant requires specialized services not provided by all units, such as the infant with congenital heart disease or some other complex congenital anomaly.

Transporting High-Risk Newborns

When the infant at risk is identified or anticipated, arrangements are made for care in the intensive care facility. There is no question that the uterus is the ideal transport unit for the infant with anticipated difficulties; therefore whenever possible the mother is taken where special care is available for her delivery.

Many infants develop difficulties after a seemingly normal pregnancy and uncomplicated labor. Since it is impossible to predict when infants will require intensive care, a coordinated system is needed to ensure them an optimum opportunity for survival. Each hospital that delivers infants should be able to provide for appropriate stabilization and arrange for transport to a centralized facility. The infant must be warm, well oxygenated (including intubation if indicated), attached to a monitor, and when possible, receiving an intravenous infusion. It may be up to 4 hours before the infant is sufficiently stabilized for transfer. The infant is transported in a specially designed incubator unit containing a complete life-support system and other emergency equipment that can be carried by ambulance, van, or helicopter.

The transport team may consist of one or more of the highly trained persons from the NICU: a neonatologist (or a fellow in neonatology), a respiratory therapist, and one or more nurses. The professional assigned to accompany the infant must be constantly alert to every change in the infant's condition and be able to intervene appropriately. The neonate who must be moved from one place to another within the hospital (e.g., to surgery, from delivery room to nursery) is transported in an incubator or radiant warmer accompanied by necessary personnel and equipment.

NURSING CARE OF HIGH-RISK NEWBORNS

Nurses in an NICU are vital to the successful operation of the unit and the ultimate outcome of infant therapy. Neonatal intensive care nursing is a highly specialized area of knowledge and practice that requires lengthy supervised experience to reach a level of competence that permits independent nursing care. It involves an understanding of neonatal physiology and characteristics, a knowledge of the function and management of a number of mechanical devices and apparatus, the ability to recognize very subtle deviations from the expected, and the ability to implement a judicious course of action.

Nurses working in NICUs are subject to stresses not found in most nursing units. The critical nature of their patients' conditions generates a stressful atmosphere. The care demands constant observation and rapid evaluation and intervention. The infants are less responsive, physical eye contact is minimum or impossible, and even during the recovery phase infants remain less able to provide positive reinforcement because of their developmental level. Interaction with parents provides some positive feedback, but their own concerns and anxieties may impede such responses and more often place additional obligations on nurses (see p. 408). In addition, while the open environment (large expanses of glass and counters) enables maximum visibility of the infants, staff members are also exposed to constant observation.

Since the majority of infants who are admitted to intensive care facilities are born before the estimated date of delivery, the major discussion of problems related to the high-risk neonate will be directed toward the preterm infant. Low birth weight is generally accepted as the single largest factor contributing to infant mortality (see p. 413 for a description of the characteristics of preterm infants). The incidence of neonatal complications (e.g., hyperbilirubinemia and hyaline membrane disease) is highest in this group, and often other high-risk factors (e.g., severe congenital malformations) are found in association with prematurity. Nursing problems encountered in the intensive care nursery are discussed, followed by a consideration of common complications. Nursing care of high-risk infants with more serious disorders is examined in relation to specific high-risk conditions.

Assessment

At birth the newborn is given a rapid assessment to determine any apparent problems and identify those that demand immediate attention. This examination is primarily concerned with the evaluation of cardiopulmonary and neurologic functions. The assessment includes the assignment of an Apgar score (see Chapter 8) and an evaluation for pallor, cyanosis, prematurity, any obvious congenital anomalies, or evidence of disease. Delivery rooms are equipped with a special resuscitation area where infants with evidence of distress are resuscitated and evaluated before being transported to the NICU for therapy and more extensive assessment (see Assessment of Clinical Gestational Age, Chapter 8). During all activities a prime consideration is the conservation of body heat.

Maintaining detailed, ongoing records of all activities and observations is an important responsibility of nurses in the intensive care setting. Knowledge and operation of complex pieces of equipment and mechanical devices are inherent in the care of the ill neonate. However, sophisticated monitoring and life-support systems cannot replace the vigilance and constant scrutiny of the infants by experienced personnel.

Systematic Assessment

Subtle changes not apparent through the mechanical devices can be detected by alert nurses. Events, such as color changes, regurgitated formula, or misplaced eye pads, which will not register on a monitor until apnea develops, are quickly recognized and corrected by the nurse. Some of the crucial factors in observation of ill newborns cannot be detected by monitors, including feeding behaviors, tremulousness, abdominal distention and stool characteristics, behavior, skin manifestations, character and location of heart sounds, and respiratory data such as retractions, flaring nares, and grunting. These objective observations and the frequent observation by nurses that the infant looks "funny, strange, or different" cannot be measured by instruments (Maloni and others, 1986).

Primary nursing, in which nurses are responsible for the same infants each day, enables more accurate determination of day-to-day progress, as well as more continuity of care for parents. During the course of daily care the nurse makes frequent, systematic assessments of physical status, since vital signs of small infants change several times in the period of a very few hours. It has been said that the newborn undergoes as many changes in 4 to 6 hours as an adult does in 24 hours.

In the course of an assessment the nurse ascertains whether the life-support apparatus is functioning properly—that the respiratory equipment is at the correct pressure and volume setting and no leaks are apparent, that the monitors are set at the desired limits and tracings are within normal limits, and that the infusion pump is delivering the correct volume and type of fluid. The assessment of the infant should proceed in a systematic manner. Each nurse develops an approach that feels comfortable and follows the same pattern routinely. An observational assessment is usually performed hourly, or more frequently on very ill infants, and a synopsis is included in the charting. However, any assessment procedures that require that the infant be disturbed should be timed to allow for sufficient rest between assessments (Box 10-4).

The infant's position is changed every 1 to 2 hours, and any significant reaction to the changing process or to a specific position is noted. To conserve the infant's energy, the position changing and periodic treatments should be timed to coincide with an assessment. Much of the assessment can be accomplished without moving the child, but necessary handling is minimum and as atraumatic as possible.

Monitoring Physiologic Data

Most neonates under intensive observation are placed in a controlled thermal environment and monitored for heart rate, respiratory activity, and temperature. Routine monitoring of heart rate consists of a pulse rate indicator that signals each ventricular contraction by a flashing light and an electrocardiograph (ECG) tracing. The indicator is integrated with an alarm system so that when the heart rate falls below or rises above a preset rate, both audio and visual alarms alert the nurse. The limits for cardiac monitors are determined by the condition of the individual infant and the philosophy of the special care unit, but they are usually set to activate when below 100 beats per minute or above 180 beats per minute. Each alarm requires the nurse to observe, assess the situation, and make a decision regarding the infant's status.

Factors other than altered infant condition may trigger

Box 10-4 GUIDELINES FOR PHYSICAL ASSESSMENT

General Assessment

Weigh daily; or more often, if ordered.
Describe general body shape and size, presence and location of edema.
Describe any apparent deformities.

Respiratory Assessment

Describe shape of chest (barrel, concave), symmetry, presence of incisions, chest tubes, or other deviations, crepitus.
Describe use of accessory muscles: nasal flaring or substernal, intercostal, or subclavicular retractions.
Determine respiratory rate and regularity.
Describe breath sounds: stridor, crackles, wheezing, wet diminished sounds, areas of absence of sound, grunting, diminished air entry, equality of breath sounds.
Determine whether suctioning is needed.
Describe cry.
Describe ambient oxygen and method of delivery; if intubated, describe size of tube, type of ventilator, and settings.
Oxygen saturation by pulse oximetry.

Cardiovascular Assessment

Determine heart rate and rhythm.
Describe heart sounds, including any murmurs.
Determine the point of maximum intensity (PMI), the point where the heartbeat sounds loudest (a change in the point of maximum intensity may indicate a mediastinal shift).
Describe infant's color (may be of cardiac, respiratory, or hematopoietic origin): cyanosis, pallor, plethora, jaundice.
Assess color of nail beds, mucous membranes, lips.
Determine blood pressure (see Fig. 10-1). Indicate extremity used and cuff size (if Doppler used); use each extremity at least once.
Determine mean arterial pressure by indwelling arterial line.
Describe peripheral pulses, capillary filling, peripheral perfusion (mottling).
Describe monitors, their parameters, and whether alarms are in "on" position.

Gastrointestinal Assessment

Determine presence of abdominal distention: increase in circumference, shiny skin, evidence of abdominal wall erythema, visible peristalsis, visible loops of bowel, status of umbilicus.
Determine any signs of regurgitation, and time related to feeding; character and amount of residual if gavage fed; if nasogastric tube in place, describe type of suction, drainage (color, consistency, pH, guaiac).
Describe amount, color, consistency, and odor of any emesis.
Palpate liver margin.
Describe amount, color, and consistency of stools; check for occult blood and/or reducing substances if ordered or indicated by appearance of stool.
Describe bowel sounds: presence or absence.

Genitourinary Assessment

Describe any abnormalities of genitalia.
Describe amount (as determined by weight), color, pH, labstick findings, and specific gravity of urine (to screen for adequacy of hydration).
Check weight (the most accurate measure for assessment of hydration).

Neurologic-Musculoskeletal Assessment

Describe infant's movements: random, purposeful, jittery, twitching, spontaneous, elicited; level of activity with stimulation.
Describe infant's position or attitude: flexed, extended.
Describe reflexes observed: Moro, sucking, Babinski, and other expected reflexes.
Determine level of response, and consolability.
Determine changes in head circumference (if indicated); size and tension of fontanels, suture lines.
Determine pupillary responses.

Temperature

Determine skin and axillary temperature.
Determine relationship to environmental temperature.

Skin Assessment

Describe any discoloration, reddened area, or signs of irritation, especially where monitoring equipment, infusions, or other apparatus comes in contact with skin; also check and note any skin preparation used (e.g., povidone-iodine).
Determine texture and turgor of skin; dry, smooth, flaky, peeling, etc.
Describe any rash or skin lesion.
Determine whether intravenous infusion catheter or needle is in place and observe for signs of infiltration.
Describe parenteral infusion lines: location, type (arterial, venous, hyperalimentation, peripheral, and umbilical); type of infusion and relevant infusion; type of infusion pump and rate of flow; type of needle (butterfly, Quik-Cath); appearance of insertion site.

the alarm, for example, poor contact of electrodes with the skin, loose connections, poor placement, inadequate grounding, soiled electrodes, or movement. Cardiac monitors with the sensitivity set too high sometimes register more than one point of the QRS complex in the cardiac cycle, giving a falsely high pulse reading. Therefore it is essential to check the heartbeat and compare it with the monitor reading. Proper placement and maintenance of electrodes and their connections are nursing responsibilities. Adhesive electrodes are attached topically to the chest wall, usually one on each side, immediately below the clavicles at the midclavicular line with the electrode for the ground wire placed on the abdomen or leg (see Fig. 34-5).

Respiratory activity is also monitored, because the heart rate does not always drop with apnea, although bradycardia frequently follows an apneic spell. Apnea monitors consist of an impedance monitor that measures the electrical resistance across the chest as it changes with respiration. The alarm works in the same manner as the cardiac monitor. It is usually set at a 15- to 20-second delay for apnea. Apnea and cardiac monitors are often combined in the same monitoring equipment; electrode placement depends on the type of equipment used (see Apnea of Infancy, Chapter 13).

The placement of electrodes is a continual nursing problem because of the lack of flat areas on the neonate's chest and the limited space for alternating sites, the size of the electrodes, and irritation from the paste or tape. Electrodes for cardiac monitors can often be applied to the back or the

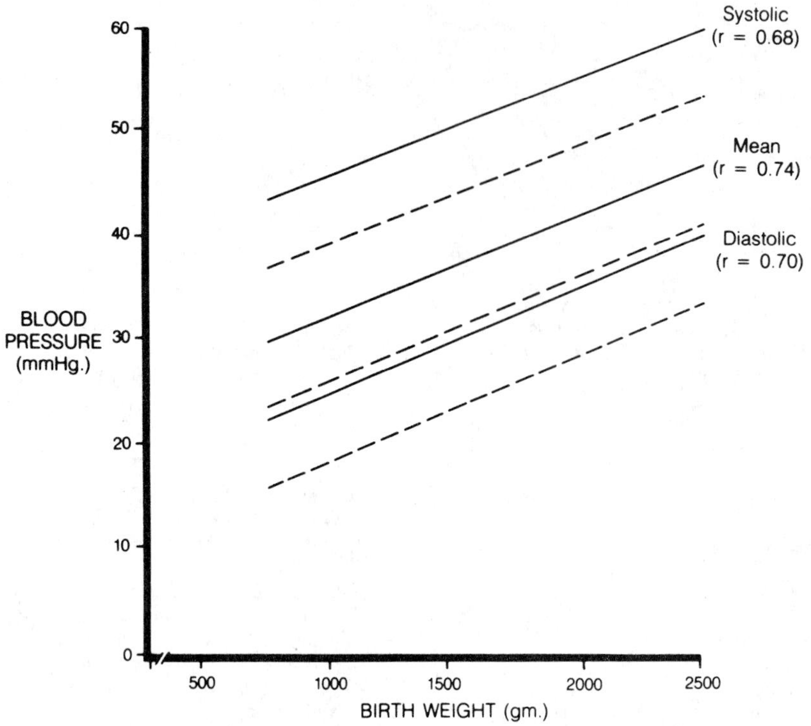

Fig. 10-1. Linear regression of systolic, mean, and diastolic blood pressure vs birth weights during the first 24 hours of life in 59 premature infants (n = 120). The dotted lines represent lowest systolic, diastolic, and mean pressures at 90% confidence level.
From Fanaroff, A.A., and Martin, R.J., editors: Neonatal-perinatal medicine, ed. 2, St. Louis, 1987, Mosby–Year Book, Inc., p. 128.

upper arms to provide relief for chest areas; nonadhesive limb electrodes eliminate possible skin irritation from tape. It is important to follow the manufacturer's directions for care and handling of electrodes to avoid malfunction or burns to sensitive skin.

Blood pressure is monitored routinely in the sick neonate by either internal or external means. Direct recording with arterial catheters is often employed but carries the risks inherent in any procedure in which a needle or other implement is introduced into a blood vessel. Oscillometry (Dinamap) or Doppler transcutaneous apparatus are simple, effective means for detecting hypotension (Fig. 10-1).

In the NICU, frequent laboratory examinations are an integral part of the ongoing assessment of infants' progress. Accurate intake and output records are kept on all infants. An accurate output can be obtained by collection of urine in a plastic urine collection bag (see Collection of Specimens, Chapter 27) or by weighing the diapers. Weighing the diapers is the simplest and least traumatic means of measuring urine output. The preweighed wet diaper is weighed on a gram scale, and the gram weight of the urine is converted directly to milliliters, for example, 25 g = 25 ml. Cotton balls inside the diaper next to the perineum absorb moisture that can be easily extracted with a syringe or weighed. Plastic collecting devices can be used when it is necessary to collect urine for laboratory examination. Specific gravity is often measured as a screening for renal function and adequacy of hydration. Since the volume normally voided is insufficient to float the standard urometer, a refractometer requiring only a single drop of urine is standard equipment in the NICU. A drop of urine can be easily aspirated from the wet diaper or cotton balls with a syringe.

Blood examinations are a necessary part of the ongoing assessment and monitoring of the sick neonate's progress. The tests performed most often are blood glucose, bilirubin, calcium, hematocrit, blood gases, and electrolytes. Samples may be obtained by taking blood from the heel, by venipuncture, or by an indwelling catheter in an umbilical vein, umbilical artery, or peripheral artery. The indwelling catheter is usually maintained at a slow drip with heparin infusion in order to prevent clotting of blood in the system. When the specimen is being collected, it is important to relate the type of test to the treatment the infant is receiving. For example, when an infant is receiving an intravenous infusion of glucose solution, collecting a sample of blood from the heel would provide a more accurate picture of the blood glucose level than would a sample from the intravenous catheter, and phototherapy must be discontinued when a blood sample is drawn for a bilirubin level test because the light will alter the bilirubin in the sample.

Capillary samples are usually collected from the heel after the foot has been warmed to approximately 45.5° C (110° F), which takes 5 to 10 minutes (see Blood Specimens, Chapter 27, for procedure). This is a stress-producing pro-

NURSING TIP: HEEL STICK

Wrapping the foot in a warm washcloth or disposable diaper is a simple way to create adequate vasodilation.

cedure, but research has indicated that nonnutritive sucking during the procedure produces a pacifying effect on the infant (Field and Goldson, 1984). When numerous samples must be drawn, it is important to keep a record of the amount of blood removed, since a tiny infant's blood supply can be seriously depleted over a period of time. Replacement should be considered at 10% total body water deficit.

Invasive and noninvasive methods are available for monitoring acid-base and oxygenation status. Arterial blood gas samples may be obtained from indwelling lines or from intermittent arterial punctures. Noninvasive techniques include transcutaneous monitors and pulse oximeters. Transcutaneous monitors provide continuous readings of oxygen (Pa_{O_2}) and carbon dioxide (Pa_{CO_2}) levels from sensors secured to the skin by electrodes. The device provides values from warmed skin that closely correlate with direct arterial oxygen and carbon dioxide values. Pulse oximeters provide continuous oxygen saturation (Sa_{O_2}) measurements from a sensor taped to an extremity (hand, foot, great toe). The nurse must note any changes in oxygenation associated with handling the infant and adjust care accordingly. Hourly readings are recorded with vital signs. Other monitoring devices may be employed in the care of the high-risk neonate, such as transcutaneous bilirubinometry.

Safety measures. The proliferation of equipment technology over the past few years has increased the dangers associated with its use, especially performance malfunction and electrical hazards. Malfunction includes such things as inaccurate monitor function, erratic delivery rates in infusion devices, and low or high suction in pumps. Electrical hazards are related to defective equipment, wiring, grounding, or improper use of equipment.

One of the most effective means for ensuring the safety of infant and staff is the nurse's knowledge, alertness, and common sense regarding the function of equipment. Electronic monitoring devices are checked to make certain that the alarms are not turned off, which negates their effectiveness. It is important to check equipment for all correct component parts, to remove from use and report equipment that is not performing according to specifications, and to obey the basic rules of electrical safety—handle equipment with care, be alert to signs of trouble, and follow electrical safety guidelines.

Parents need to be instructed regarding safety precautions and observations. They are usually uncomfortable around the equipment and atmosphere of an intensive care unit and therefore appreciate an explanation of the purposes and functions of the devices and pertinent safety aspects. Visiting siblings, especially toddlers, must be supervised closely to avoid their "playing" with the equipment and inadvertently causing harm to the neonate.

Nursing Diagnoses

Many nursing diagnoses may be evident after a careful assessment of the infant at risk. Some apply to all infants; others will vary according to the needs and characteristics of individual infants and their families. The nursing diagnoses that represent general guides for nursing intervention are found in the Nursing Care Plan on pp. 392–394. Since a number of health problems accompany infant immaturity, the nurse is also alert to the possibility of conditions and complications discussed later in this chapter and elsewhere in the book.

Planning

The nursing care plan for the high-risk infant depends to a large extent on the diagnosis of the health problem that places the infant at risk. However, the following are basic to the care of all high-risk infants:

1. Promote respiratory efforts.
2. Promote warmth.
3. Protect infant from infection.
4. Provide hydration and nutrition.
5. Conserve energy.
6. Prevent other complications—provide skin care, administer medications, relieve pain, and promote safety measures.
7. Provide developmental intervention.
8. Support family, promote parent-infant relationships, and prepare for home care.
9. Support family in the event of neonatal death.

Implementation

The naked infant is placed in the controlled microenvironment of an incubator. A Plexiglas top affords a clear view of the infant from all aspects. Easy access through portholes

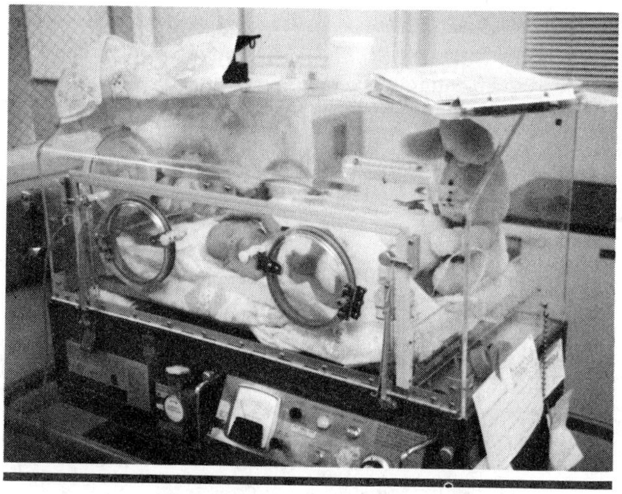

Fig. 10-2. Infant in incubator.

NURSING CARE PLAN
The Low-Birth-Weight Infant

NURSING DIAGNOSIS: Ineffective breathing pattern related to neuromuscular impairment (immature respiratory center), decreased energy, and fatigue

GOAL 1

Support respiratory efforts

INTERVENTIONS

Position for optimum air exchange
- Prone
- Neck roll when supine

Observe for deviations from desired functioning: recognize signs of distress
Suction as necessary to remove accumulated mucus from nasopharynx, trachea, and (where necessary) endotracheal tube
Carry out percussion, vibration, and postural drainage to loosen secretions in respiratory tree
Position prone or on side; turn head to side to prevent aspiration
Observe for signs of respiratory distress—nasal flaring, retractions, tachypnea
Maintain ambient oxygen at level to ensure satisfactory skin color with minimum respiratory effort and energy expenditure
Carry out regimen prescribed for supplemental oxygen therapy (maintain ambient oxygen concentration at minimum F_{IO_2} level to maintain good color and energy expenditure)
Apply and manage monitoring equipment correctly
Understand functioning of respiratory support apparatus
- Assisted ventilation apparatus
- Controlled ventilation apparatus
- Insufflation bags with masks and/or endotracheal adaptor
- Oxygen hoods
- Humidifier warmers

EXPECTED OUTCOMES

Breathing is regular and unlabored
Respiratory rate is within normal limits (specify)

NURSING DIAGNOSIS: Ineffective thermoregulation related to immature temperature control

GOAL 1

Provide neutral thermal environment

INTERVENTIONS

Place infant in humidified incubator, radiant warmer, or warmly clothed in open crib
Monitor temperature hourly in unstable infants (take skin and axillary temperature; check function of servocontrolled mechanism when used)
Check temperature of infant in relation to temperature of heating unit
Avoid situations that might predispose infant to chilling, such as exposure to cool air

EXPECTED OUTCOME

Infant's temperature remains within acceptable limits (specify)

NURSING DIAGNOSIS: Potential for infection related to deficient immunologic defenses

GOAL 1

Protect infant from infection

INTERVENTIONS

Carry out meticulous handwashing before handling infant
Ensure that all equipment in contact with infant is scrupulously clean or sterile
Prevent personnel with infections from coming into direct contact with infant
Isolate other infants who have infections according to agency policy
Instruct others in correct handwashing and other protective procedures
*Administer prophylactic antibiotics as ordered

EXPECTED OUTCOME

Infant exhibits no evidence of infection

NURSING DIAGNOSIS: Altered nutrition: less than body requirements (potential) related to inability to ingest nutrients because of weakness, helplessness

GOAL 1

Provide nutrition

INTERVENTIONS

*Maintain parenteral fluid or hyperalimentation therapy as ordered
Bottle-feed infant if strong sucking, swallowing, and gag reflexes are present (usually at gestational age of 33 to 35 weeks)
Follow unit protocol for advancing volume and concentration of formula
Gavage feed if infant tires easily or has weak sucking, gag, or swallowing reflexes
Assist mothers with breast-feeding if feasible and desirable
Follow unit protocols for advancing volume and concentration of formula

EXPECTED OUTCOMES

Infant receives an adequate amount of nutrients
Infant demonstrates a steady weight gain (approximately 20 to 30 g/day)

*Dependent or interdependent nursing actions.

NURSING DIAGNOSIS: Potential fluid volume deficit related to physiologic characteristics of preterm infant, helplessness

GOAL 1

Maintain hydration

INTERVENTIONS

Monitor therapies that increase insensible water loss, e.g., phototherapy, radiant warmers
Ensure adequate intake
Assess state of hydration, e.g., skin turgor, temperature, weight, mucous membranes, urine specific gravity
Regulate parenteral fluids
Avoid administering hypertonic fluids, e.g., undiluted medications
Monitor urine output and laboratory values for evidence of dehydration

EXPECTED OUTCOME

Infant exhibits no evidence of dehydration

NURSING DIAGNOSIS: Activity intolerance related to imbalance between oxygen supply and demand, physical weakness

GOAL 1

Conserve energy

INTERVENTIONS

Maintain neutral thermal environment
Concentrate activities to allow for longer periods of rest
Administer gavage feeding when infant tires easily
Ensure minimum handling of infant

EXPECTED OUTCOME

Infant rests 1 hour (uninterrupted) at regularly scheduled intervals (specify)

NURSING DIAGNOSIS: Potential impaired skin integrity related to immature skin structure, immobility

GOAL 1

Prevent skin breakdown

INTERVENTIONS

Cleanse skin with clear water or approved cleanser
Avoid use of alkaline-based or hexachlorophene cleansing products or lotions
Use only transpore tape to secure items to the skin
Apply protective preparation to skin on which tape or adhesive-backed items (e.g., electrodes) may be attached
Exert extreme care when performing activities involving skin, e.g., removing dressings, electrodes, tape
Place infant on water pillow or fleece
Turn at least every 2 hours

EXPECTED OUTCOME

Skin remains clean and intact with no evidence of irritation or injury

NURSING DIAGNOSIS: Altered growth and development related to preterm birth, unnatural environment, separation from parents

GOAL 1

Facilitate growth and development

INTERVENTIONS

Provide optimum nutrition
Provide developmental intervention as appropriate
Recognize signs of overstimulation (flaccidity, yawning, staring, eye floating, active averting, irritability, crying)
Promote parent-infant bonding

EXPECTED OUTCOMES

Infant exhibits a steady weight gain
Infant responds to appropriate stimuli

NURSING DIAGNOSIS: Altered family processes related to situational/maturational crisis, knowledge deficit (birth of a preterm and/or ill infant), interruption of bonding process

GOAL 1

Keep parents informed of infant's progress

INTERVENTIONS

Answer questions, encourage expression of concern regarding care and prognosis
Encourage mother and father to visit and/or call unit
Emphasize positive aspects of infant status
Be honest; respond to questions with correct answers

EXPECTED OUTCOME

Parents express feelings and concerns regarding the infant and his prognosis

GOAL 2

Facilitate parent-infant attachment process

INTERVENTIONS

Initiate parents' visit as soon as possible
Encourage parents to
- Visit infant frequently
- Touch, fondle, and caress infant

Continued.

NURSING CARE PLAN
The Low-Birth-Weight Infant—cont'd

- Become actively involved in infant's care
- Bring clothing to dress up infant as soon as condition permits

Reinforce parents' endeavors
Be alert to signs of tension in parents
Enable parents to spend time alone with infant
Help parents interpret infant responses; comment regarding any positive infant response
Help parents by demonstrating techniques and offer support

EXPECTED OUTCOMES

Parents visit infant soon after birth and at frequent intervals
Parents relate positively with infant
Parents provide care for the infant and demonstrate an attitude of comfort in relationships with the infant

GOAL 3

Facilitate sibling-infant attachment

INTERVENTIONS

Enable siblings to visit infant when feasible
Explain environment, events, and strange appearance of infant, e.g., why infant cannot come home, "special" bed
Provide photos of infant or other items if siblings unable to visit
Encourage siblings to make pictures, etc., for infant and place in incubator or bassinet

EXPECTED OUTCOMES

Siblings visit infant in nursery
Siblings exhibit an understanding of explanations (specify)
Siblings receive infant-related items (specify)

GOAL 4

Prepare for infant's discharge

INTERVENTIONS

Assess readiness of family (especially mother) to care for infant
Teach necessary techniques and observations
Arrange for public health referral if indicated
Reinforce follow-up care
Refer to appropriate agencies or services for needed assistance
Encourage and facilitate involvement with parent group
Teach family infant cardiopulmonary resuscitation technique and respond to choking incident
Refer to appropriate support group(s)

EXPECTED OUTCOMES

Family demonstrates the ability to provide care for the infant
Family members take advantage of available services
Family members keep appointments for follow-up care

NURSING DIAGNOSIS: Anticipatory grieving related to grave prognosis and/or death of infant

GOAL 1

Help parents understand reality of death

INTERVENTIONS

Provide family with the opportunity to hold their infant before death and, if possible, be present at the time of death
Arrange for or perform appropriate baptism rite for infant
Provide family with the opportunity to see, touch, hold, caress, examine, and talk to their infant privately after death
Allow family to bathe infant after death if they desire
Comply with family's wish regarding nurse's attendance
Keep baby's body available for a few hours to allow time for family who are hesitant an opportunity to see dead infant if they change their minds
Provide a photograph taken before and after infant's death to allow family to refer to at a later time to make infant seem more real

- Take photograph of infant being held or touched by an adult; avoid morgue-type photograph

Provide other tangible remembrances of child's death, e.g., name tags, armband, lock of hair (removed for intravenous insertion)
Encourage family to name the infant if they have failed to do so

EXPECTED OUTCOME

Family discuss the reality of the death and convey an attitude of acceptance

GOAL 2

Support family

INTERVENTIONS

Be available to family
Provide appropriate religious support, e.g., clergyman
Discuss the death with family
Talk with family openly and honestly about funeral arrangements

- Have information available regarding inexpensive services in the community
- Inform family of all options available

Provide opportunity for the family to call the unit if they have any questions
Contact family after the death to assess coping and status of grieving process
Refer family to appropriate support group(s)

EXPECTED OUTCOME

Family copes with infant's death appropriately

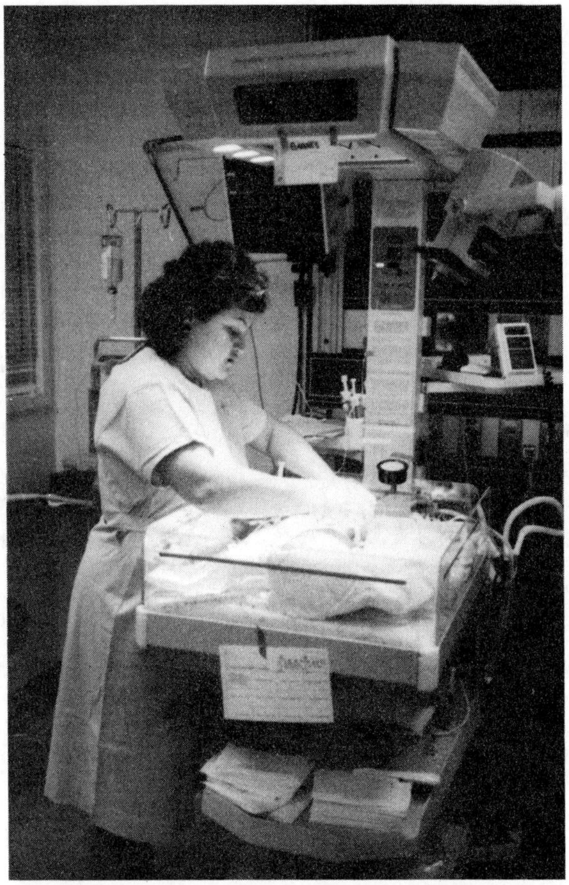

Fig. 10-3. Infant under overhead warming unit.

minimizes temperature and oxygen loss, and a large door provides a more extensive approach (Fig. 10-2). Maximum accessibility is provided by an open unit with an overhead radiant warming system. These units are employed for distressed infants who require a wide range of mechanical instrumentation, such as a ventilator, monitors, and intravenous infusions, and frequent manipulation, such as checking vital signs, suctioning, and chest percussion (Fig. 10-3).

Respiratory Support

The primary objective in the care of high-risk infants is to establish and maintain respiration. Many infants require supplemental oxygen and assisted ventilation. Infants with or without these supportive treatments are positioned to maximum airflow (see Idiopathic Respiratory Distress Syndrome, p. 417).

Thermoregulation

After the establishment of respiration, the most crucial need of the LBW infant is application of external warmth. Prevention of heat loss in the distressed infant is absolutely essential for survival, and maintaining a neutral thermal environment is a challenging aspect of neonatal intensive nursing care. Heat production is a complicated process that involves the cardiovascular, neurologic, and metabolic systems, and the immature neonate has all the problems related to heat production that are faced by the full-term infant (see Thermoregulation, Chapter 8). However, LBW infants are placed at further disadvantage by a number of additional problems. They have an even smaller muscle mass and deposits of brown fat for producing heat, lack insulating subcutaneous fat, and have poor reflex control of skin capillaries.

Pathophysiology. The immature neonate, unable to increase activity and lacking a shivering response, produces heat primarily through increased metabolic processes. Some heat continues to be generated by liver, heart, brain, and skeletal muscles, but the major source of increased production of heat during cold stress is *nonshivering thermogenesis.* Norepinephrine, secreted by the sympathetic nerve endings in response to chilling, stimulates fat metabolism in the richly vascularized brown adipose tissue to produce internal heat, which is then conducted through the blood to surface tissues. Significantly, an increase in metabolism requires an increase in oxygen consumption.

The consequences of cold stress that produce additional hazards to the neonate are hypoxia, metabolic acidosis, and hypoglycemia. Increased metabolism in response to chilling creates a compensatory increase in oxygen and calorie consumption. If available oxygen is not increased to accommodate this need, arterial oxygen tension is decreased. This is further complicated by a smaller lung volume in relation to metabolic rate that creates diminished oxygen in the blood and concurrent pulmonary disorders. A small advantage is gained by the persistence of fetal hemoglobin (HgF) because its increased capacity to carry oxygen allows the infant to exist for longer periods in conditions of lowered oxygen tension.

Norepinephrine, released in response to cold stress, causes pulmonary vasoconstriction, which further reduces the effectiveness of pulmonary ventilation. This decrease in oxygen diminishes the supply available for glucose metabolism. As a result, glucose is broken down by an alternate, hypoxic pathway (anaerobic glycolysis) that generates increased lactic acid formation. This, together with acid end products of brown fat metabolism, contributes to the acidotic state. Anaerobic metabolism dissipates glycogen at a greatly increased rate over aerobic metabolism, thus precipitating hypoglycemia. This condition is especially marked when glycogen stores are diminished at birth and when there is inadequate caloric intake after birth.

Maintaining thermoneutrality. To delay or prevent the effects of cold stress, newborns at risk are placed in a heated environment immediately following birth where they remain until they are able to maintain *thermal stability,* the capacity to balance heat production and conservation and heat dissipation. Since overheating produces an increase in oxygen and calorie consumption, the infant is also jeopardized in a hyperthermic environment. A *neutral thermal environment* is one that permits the infant to maintain a normal core temperature with minimum oxygen consumption and calorie expenditure. This means a deep body temperature that stays within a normal range of 36.5° to 37.5° C (97.7° to 99.5° F). A neutral thermal environment for newborns is 32.5° ± 1.4° C (90.5° ± 2.5° F) for larger infants and 35.4° ± 0.5° C (95.7° ± 1° F) for smaller infants (Merenstein, Gardner, and Blake, 1989).

The VLBW infant, with thin skin and almost no subcutaneous fat, can control body heat loss or gain only within a very limited range of environmental temperature. In these infants heat loss from radiation and evaporation is three to five times greater than in larger infants, and a decrease in body temperature is associated with an increase in mortality (Saur and Visser, 1984).

The three methods for maintaining a neutral thermal environment are by the use of a radiant warming panel, an incubator, and an open bassinet with cotton blankets. The dressed infant under blankets can maintain a temperature within a wider range of environmental temperatures; however, the close observations required by a high-risk infant are best accomplished if the infant remains unclothed. The incubator should always be prewarmed before placing an infant in it. The use of double-walled incubators significantly improves the infant's ability to maintain a desirable temperature and reduce energy expenditure related to heat regulation. The infant is clothed and warmly wrapped in blankets when removed from the warm environment of the incubator for feeding or cuddling. Inside or outside the incubator head coverings are effective in preventing heat loss (Fig. 10-4). A fabric-insulated bonnet is more effective than one fashioned from stockinette (Greer, 1988).

The most effective means for maintaining the desired range of temperature in the naked infant is by way of a manually adjusted or automatically controlled (servocontrolled) heat panel incubator. The latter mechanism, when set at the upper and lower limits of the desired circulating air temperature range, adjusts automatically in response to signals from a thermal sensor attached to the abdominal skin. If the infant's temperature drops, the warming device is triggered to increase heat output. The servocontrol is set to a desired skin temperature between 36° and 36.5° C (96.8° to 97.7° F) (Merenstein, Gardner, and Blake, 1989).

Disadvantages are always inherent in any mechanical device; therefore an important part of nursing assessment is to compare the infant's temperature with the temperature in the incubator. For example, if the infant's temperature fluctuates in response to sepsis or intracranial hemorrhage, the servocontrolled mechanism would respond by decreasing or increasing the ambient air temperature. Therefore a critical observation could be easily overlooked. A heat-sensing probe attached to the abdomen registers a falsely high temperature when the infant is in the prone position. Either the probe should be moved to the flank area of the back when the infant is placed in the prone position or the infant should remain on the back or side or in a partial side-lying position.

NURSING TIP: PREVENT HEAT LOSS

A cap can be fashioned from a piece of stockinette to help reduce heat loss from the head.

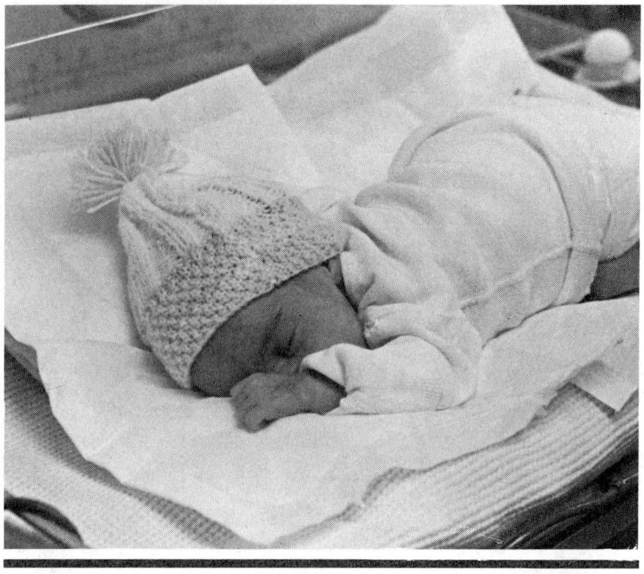

Fig. 10-4. Infant wearing cap knit by a loving mother. A satisfactory substitute can be fashioned from piece of stockinette.

NURSING ALERT Trends of increased or decreased ambient air temperature in response to fluctuations in the infant's body temperature should be assessed to rule out sepsis or other dysfunction.

Body temperature regulation can also be influenced by thermal sensors located in the trigeminal area of the face and on the forehead. When the infant's face is exposed to a cool environmental temperature, even though the body is adequately warmed, these temperature-stimulation zones respond as though the infant is cold stressed and may precipitate apnea. For this reason oxygen or any source of air, such as an oxygen mask or tube, should not blow directly on the infant's face. Oxygen concentrated around the head, such as that supplied to a hood, must be warmed.

The physical factors that effect temperature regulation operate to influence temperature regulation in incubators and radiant heat units. Loss of heat by convection is a constant problem in the open units, and the skin probe should be covered with a small foam or felt disk to avoid the effect of radiant heat acting directly on the sensor itself. Otherwise the heated sensor discontinues the heat source, and the infant remains cold.

First, the skin and then the axillary temperature provides the best indication of an infant's core temperature. Rectal temperature, in addition to the possibility of producing injury and vagal stimulation, is often misleading, since it reflects a drop in core temperature, a late response to cold stress. Heat production is activated by a lowered skin temperature; therefore core temperature drops only after body heat cannot be maintained by increased metabolic activity.

Nursing interventions to alleviate cold stress should be initiated with a drop in skin temperature (36.5° C) rather than when core temperature decreases.

Radiant heat loss is one of the greatest threats to temperature regulation in the incubator, since the temperature of circulating air within has no influence on heat loss to cooler surfaces without, such as windows, walls, or a lower nursery temperature. Lining the incubator (inside and outside) with aluminum foil may help prevent heat loss caused by radiation, but it must not extend so high that the view of the infant is obscured.

A high-humidity atmosphere contributes to body temperature maintenance by reducing *evaporative* heat loss. Humidity is provided in some incubators by air circulating over a heated water reservoir, which has the additional advantage of decreasing heat loss by convection as the air flows over the infant. Since stagnant, warm water provides an excellent breeding medium for microorganisms, the reservoir is emptied every 8 to 24 hours and replaced with sterile distilled water. The recommended humidity is 50% to 65%; higher humidity and a warmer environment are recommended for VLBW infants. Because of the ever-present danger of infection, most nurseries no longer use water in incubators. Heat and humidity are provided from an external source such as humidified oxygen or air.

Conductive heat loss can be reduced by warming all items that come in direct contact with the infant, such as scales, radiographic film, blankets, and the hands of caregivers. Warming the items before use can reduce this source of heat loss, for example, storing blankets in a warming unit ready for use, and placing a free-standing warming unit or a gooseneck lamp over a scale before weighing an infant. Some units place the infants on a water-heated pad in the crib to reduce heat loss (Topper and Stewart, 1984).

Two simple methods have been employed to reduce oxygen consumption, insensible water loss, and radiant heat demand, especially in VLBW infants under open radiant warmers. A heat shield of plastic wrap (such as Saran Wrap) stretched across the crib produces a microenvironment around the infant that reduces evaporative, convective, and radiant heat loss (Fig. 10-5). Use of a plastic heat shield, clothing, blankets, or incubating devices (e.g., bubble wrap) should NOT be used under radiant warmers, since these interfere with radiant heat delivery (Merenstein, Gardner, and Blake, 1989).

Protection from Infection

Protection from infection is an integral part of all newborn care, but preterm and sick neonates are particularly susceptible. The protective environment of a regularly cleaned and changed incubator provides effective isolation from airborne infective agents. However, thorough, meticulous, and frequent handwashing is the foundation of a preventive program. This includes *all* persons who come in contact with the infants and their equipment. After handling another infant or equipment, no one ever touches an infant without washing hands first.

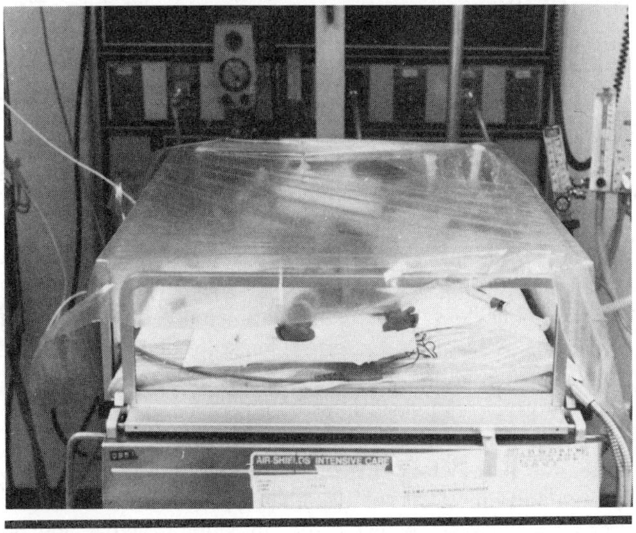

Fig. 10-5. Infant under plastic wrap, which produces a draft-free environment.

Personnel with communicable disorders are either barred from the unit until they are no longer infectious or are required to wear suitable shields (masks or gloves) to reduce the likelihood of contamination. In some areas annual influenza vaccination is recommended for NICU personnel. Most units have adopted universal precautions as a method of infection control (see Chapter 27).

Special clothing furnished by the institution is worn by everyone working in the unit. Fresh scrub dresses or suits are put on before entering the unit and are changed any time they become contaminated. When personnel leave the unit, the clothing is protected by a cover gown that is removed and discarded in the laundry hamper when reentering. Anyone entering the unit for a short time, whether or not they provide any care, must scrub thoroughly and either change to appropriate clothing or wear a cover gown. Parents are taught these precautionary measures and become willing and cooperative allies in protecting their infants from infection.

The use of gowns is not universal, however. As accumulated evidence indicates that special clothing and gowning are ineffective in preventing the spread of infection and are expensive, many institutions have abandoned the practice (Cloney and Donowitz, 1986).

The sources of infection rise in direct relationship to the number of persons and pieces of equipment coming in contact with the infants. All linen and equipment used in the care of infants is either sterile or scrupulously clean, and nondisposable items are cultured regularly for the presence of infectious organisms; protocol is established by each institution. Since organisms thrive best in water, plumbing and humidifying equipment are particularly hazardous. Disposable equipment used for water-related therapies, such as nebulizers and tubing, is changed regularly. For example, plastic tubes are discarded after 24 hours and water in humidifiers is changed every 8 hours or as recommended by the manufacturer.

Hydration

It is not uncommon for high-risk infants to receive supplemental parenteral fluids to supply additional calories, electrolytes, or water. Adequate hydration is particularly important in premature infants because extracellular water content is higher than that of a full-term infant (70% in full-term infants and up to 90% in preterm infants), and the capacity for osmotic diuresis is limited in premature infants' underdeveloped kidneys. Nephrogenesis is still taking place at a rapid rate during the later weeks of gestation, and early birth implies less than a full complement of functioning nephrons. As a result, preterm infants are highly vulnerable to water depletion, especially when there are increased losses through the gastrointestinal tract, lungs, and skin.

The preferred sites for intravenous (IV) infusions in neonates are peripheral veins on the dorsal surfaces of hands or feet and umbilical vessels; alternative but less frequently used sites are scalp veins and antecubital veins. Special precautions and frequent observations (at least once every hour) must accompany use of peripheral lines with hypertonic solutions (dextrose 10% to 12%) and hyperalimentation. The peripheral sites allow for maximum infant mobility except for the restrained IV site. If these sites are exhausted by long-term therapy, percutaneous central venous lines, Broviac catheters, or a venous cutdown (usually inserted in the saphenous or antecubital vein) may be employed. However, the increased use of small-gauge percutaneous catheters has reduced the need for the cutdown option (Cathas, 1986; Durand and others, 1986).

In most facilities NICU nurses insert percutaneous IV needles and catheters as well as maintain the infusions. IVs must always be delivered by continuous infusion pumps that deliver minute volumes at a preset flow rate. The needle is secured to the skin with transpore tape, with care taken not to cause undue pressure from the needle hub and tubing. Since very small infants are highly vulnerable to fluid shifts, the rates are very slow, carefully regulated, and checked hourly to prevent dehydration and detect inadvertent fluid overload that could cause congestive heart failure, pulmonary edema, or intraventricular hemorrhage.

Small, fragile peripheral blood vessels are subject to rupture and subsequent infiltration. This situation is compounded by the use of continuous infusion pumps that continue to infuse fluid into infiltrated tissues. Observations are especially important when using hypertonic solutions and IV drugs, which can cause severe tissue damage. Restraints are assessed frequently for tightness and to ascertain that they are accomplishing their purpose.

NURSING TIP: PERIPHERAL VENIPUNCTURE

A flashlight placed beneath the extremity helps illuminate tissues surrounding veins, thus outlining veins for better visualization.

✦ **NURSING ALERT** Nurses should be constantly alert for signs of infiltration (such as redness, edema, or color change of tissue; difficulty with the syringe or IV, and lack of blood return at site) and for signs of overhydration (see Chapter 28).

Infants who are tachypneic, receiving phototherapy, or under a radiant warmer have increased insensible water losses, which require appropriate fluid adjustments. Nurses must observe fluid status by daily (or more frequent) weights, accurate intake and output, specific gravity, dipstick measurements of urine, and evaluation of serum electrolyte levels.

A common problem observed in infants who have umbilical catheters in place is a reflex vasoconstriction of peripheral vessels, known as "cath toes," that can seriously impair circulation. The response is triggered by arterial vasospasm caused by the presence of the catheter, the infusion of fluids, or injection of medication. If the problem is not recognized promptly, the infant is in danger of losing the limb. The nurse must also observe for signs of thrombi in infants with arterial lines or in those receiving ampicillin.

✦ **NURSING ALERT** Circulatory effects are observed first in the toes but may extend to include the buttocks. The toes first flush, then turn a mulberry color, and, if the condition is not corrected, blanch. Warming the foot on the unaffected extremity causes a reflex vasodilation that relaxes the vessels in the affected extremity. If this treatment is ineffective, the catheter is removed to relieve the circulatory occlusion.

Nutrition

Optimum nutrition is critical in the management of LBW preterm infants, but there are difficulties in providing for their nutritional needs. The various mechanisms for ingestion and digestion of foods are not fully developed, and the younger the infant, the greater the problem. In addition, the nutritional requirements for this group of infants are not known with certainty. It is known that all preterm infants are at risk because of poor nutritional stores and several physical and developmental characteristics.

Physiologic characteristics. An infant's need for rapid growth and daily maintenance must be met in the presence of several anatomic and physiologic disabilities. Although some sucking and swallowing activities are demonstrated before birth and in premature infants, coordination of these mechanisms does not occur until approximately 32 to 34 weeks of gestation, and they are not fully developed until after birth. Initial sucking is not accompanied by swallowing, and esophageal contractions are uncoordinated. The gag reflex may not be developed until 36 weeks gestational age. Consequently infants are highly prone to aspiration and its attendant dangers. As infants mature, the suck-swallow pattern develops but is slow and ineffectual, and these reflexes may also become easily exhausted.

As with most full-term infants, preterm infants have poor

muscle tone in the area of the inferior esophageal (cardiac) sphincter. This causes milk in the stomach to be easily regurgitated into the esophagus, where it can trigger the chemoreceptors and cause apnea (vagal stimulation) and bradycardia, and increase the risk of aspiration. The stomach has a very limited capacity in preterm infants and is easily overdistended, further compromising respiration.

Physiologically preterm infants have approximately the same capacity to digest and absorb protein as full-term infants. However, carbohydrates and fats are less well tolerated. The secretion of lactase, a late-developing enzyme, is low in infants born before 34 weeks of gestation; therefore formulas containing lactose may not be well tolerated. Although amylase is deficient in preterm infants, an alternative enzyme (glucoamylase) is able to compensate in most neonates so that they are able to tolerate moderate amounts of starch (Lebenthal, 1982). Preterm infants are inefficient in digesting and absorbing lipids, especially the saturated triglycerides of cow's milk, because they have low levels of pancreatic lipase and low bile acid. Characteristics and problems related to immaturity are summarized in Table 10-1.

Nutritional needs. The demand for nutrients in LBW infants is much higher than that in larger infants, and individual infants vary in activity level, ease of achieving basal energy expenditure, thermoneutrality, physical condition, and efficacy of nutrient absorption. The American Academy of Pediatrics, Committee on Nutrition (1985) supports the caloric requirements of preterm infants shown in Table 10-2. Since most of the nutritional stores are accumulated in the final months of gestation, preterm infants are also hampered by low stores of calcium, iron, phosphorus, proteins, and vitamins A and C.

The amount and method of feeding are determined by the size and condition of the infant. Nutrition can be provided by either the parenteral or the enteral routes or by a combination of the two. Very small or ill infants are fed by the parenteral route until their condition is stabilized and their neurologic and physical state permits enteral feedings. Often enteral feedings must be supplemented by parenteral infusions to ensure an adequate intake of carbohydrates and water.

There is still some controversy regarding the type of enteral feeding that best meets the nutritional needs of LBW infants. The predominant view supports the use of milk from an infant's own mother or modified infant formulas. Commercial formulas have been designed specifically to meet the needs of small preterm infants (see Table 8-6) and provide for adequate growth and metabolic stability (studies reported by the American Academy of Pediatrics, Committee on Nutrition, 1985). Prepared formulas have the added advantage of allowing more concentrated feedings.

Table 10-1 Characteristics, problems, and management related to selected nutriments for the preterm infant

CHARACTERISTIC	PROBLEM	MANAGEMENT
Deficiency of proteolytic enzymes	Difficulty digesting casein protein	Feed whey-predominant formula or human milk
Low lactase activity	Poor digestion of lactose, providing substrate for bacterial growth in lower intestinal tract; distention from osmotic effect of lactose	Provide low lactose; feed glucose polymers
Pancreatic lipase; low bile salt levels	Unable to digest and absorb saturated triglycerides	Feed unsaturated medium-chain triglycerides, human milk; provide supplemental vitamin E
Poor sodium conservation	Hyponatremia	Feedings higher in sodium
Rapid bone growth and mineralization	Osteopenia; rickets	Feedings higher in calcium and phosphorus; supplemental vitamin D
Negative zinc balance	Skin lesions Related to poor fat absorption	Feed easily digested fats Feedings with zinc supplementation
Low iron	Anemia	Provide supplemental iron
Poor muscle tone of cardiac sphincter	Regurgitation: trigger chemoreceptors (apnea); vagal stimulation (bradycardia)	Semiupright position during feeding; feed small amounts Place prone, with head of bed elevated 30 to 45 degrees after feedings
Limited stomach capacity	Inadequate intake Distention	Small frequent feedings; continuous drip gavage feeding Nutrient supplementation
Noncoordination of suck/swallow/gag reflexes	Aspiration Inadequate intake	Alternative feeding methods Oral exercises
Muscle weakness	Exhaustion	Alternative feeding methods (such as bolus or continuous drip gavage)

Table 10-2 Estimated caloric requirement in typical, growing premature infants

CALORIC EXPENDITURE	Kcal/kg/d
Resting caloric expenditure	50
Intermittent activity	15
Occasional cold stress	10
Specific dynamic action	8
Fecal loss of calories	12
Growth allowance	25
TOTAL	120

Modified from Committee on Nutrition, American Academy of Pediatrics: Nutritional needs of low-birth-weight infants, Pediatrics 75:976-986, 1985.

Evidence indicates that milk produced by mothers whose infants are born before term contains higher concentrations of protein, sodium, and chloride (Gross and others, 1980; Anderson, Atkinson, and Bryan, 1981) and immunoglobulin A. Thus mothers appear to be the preferred source of milk for their preterm infants. The milk produced by mothers for their infants changes in content as the infants grow, so milk provided by mothers of older infants may not be appropriate for premature infants. Infants fed with their own mother's milk displayed a more rapid rate of growth in all parameters and a shorter length of time to regain birth weight (Gross, Oehler, and Eckerman, 1983). Human milk supplements are available for infants on breast milk who require additional calories and nutrients.

The antiinfectious attributes of human milk provide additional advantages for preterm infants. Secretory immunoglobulin A (IgA) concentration is higher in the milk from mothers of preterm infants than in the milk from mothers of full-term infants. Immunoglobulin A is important in the control of bacteria in the intestinal tract, where it inhibits adherence and proliferation of bacteria at epithelial surfaces (Gross and others, 1981). Finally, the psychologic advantages of using the milk from an infant's own mother cannot be overlooked.

Pooled human milk is less favored for preterm infants than it was previously. The composition of pooled milk does not meet all the nutritional requirements of preterm infants, resulting in a slower rate of growth than is achieved with the milk of the premature newborn's mother or commercial formula (Tyson and others, 1983). However, human milk protein supplements improve the growth of small premature infants fed human milk from banks (Rönnholm, Perheentupa, and Siimes, 1986). Also, breast milk contributed by donors is essentially raw milk and as such is a potential source of infection, especially for the transmission of cytomegalovirus and human immunodeficiency virus.

Although the timing of the first feeding has been a matter of controversy, most authorities now believe that early feeding, usually within 3 to 6 hours after birth, reduces the incidence of complicating factors such as hypoglycemia, dehydration, and the degree of hyperbilirubinemia. The feeding regimen employed varies from institution to institution. However, the initial enteral feeding is not attempted until infants have adapted to extrauterine existence as evidenced by temperature neutrality, normal breathing, and good color, tone, and cry.

Nipple feeding. Vigorous infants can be fed from a nipple with little difficulty, whereas weaker infants will require alternative methods. Sterile water may be offered first. The amount to be fed is determined largely by the infant's weight and is gradually and cautiously increased by increments of 1 to 2 ml per feeding each day, regulated by each infant's tolerance, until a satisfactory caloric intake is ensured. Sometimes supplementary calories are needed in the form of dietary additives, such as Lipomul-Oral* (which provides vegetable fat and carbohydrates), MCT oil† (which provides fat in the form of medium-chain triglycerides), Polycose, and human milk fortifier or formula with increased caloric density.

The rate of increase that is well tolerated varies from one infant to another, and determining this rate is often a nursing responsibility. Preterm infants require more time and patience to feed compared with full-term infants, and the oral-pharyngeal mechanism may be stressed by an attempt to feed too rapidly (Shaker, 1990). It is important not to tire the infants or overtax their capacity to retain the feedings. For example, infants with stomach capacities of 5 ml are unable to take enough formula to meet even the minimum daily requirements. When infants require more than 30 minutes to complete a feeding, the next one should be given by gavage. When infants are unable to tolerate bottle-feedings, intermittent feedings by gavage are instituted until they gain enough strength and coordination to use the nipple.

✦ **NURSING ALERT** Poor sucking in infants who have been feeding well may indicate serious illness and should be reported to the practitioner.

The nipple used should be relatively firm and stable. A high-flow pliable nipple, although it requires less energy to use, provides a flow rate too rapid for most preterm infants to manage without risk of aspiration. A firmer nipple facilitates a more "cupped" tongue configuration and allows for a more controlled, manageable flow rate. (Shaker, 1990).

The infant is positioned in the feeder's arms or placed semiupright in the lap (Fig. 10-6). The infant is held with the back curved slightly to simulate the position assumed naturally by most full-term newborns. Stroking the infant's lips, cheeks, and tongue before feeding helps promote oral sensitivity (Orr and Allen, 1986). Inward and upward support to the infant's cheeks and a slightly upward lift to the chin are provided by the fingers to assist nipple compression during feeding (Shaker, 1990).

Bottle-feedings are continued if infants are able to tolerate the feedings and take the required amount. The infant is best fed when fully alert. Drowsy infants feed more slowly, and liquid is more likely to fill the relaxed pharynx before

*The Upjohn Co., Kalamazoo, MI.
†Mead Johnson & Co., Evansville, IN.

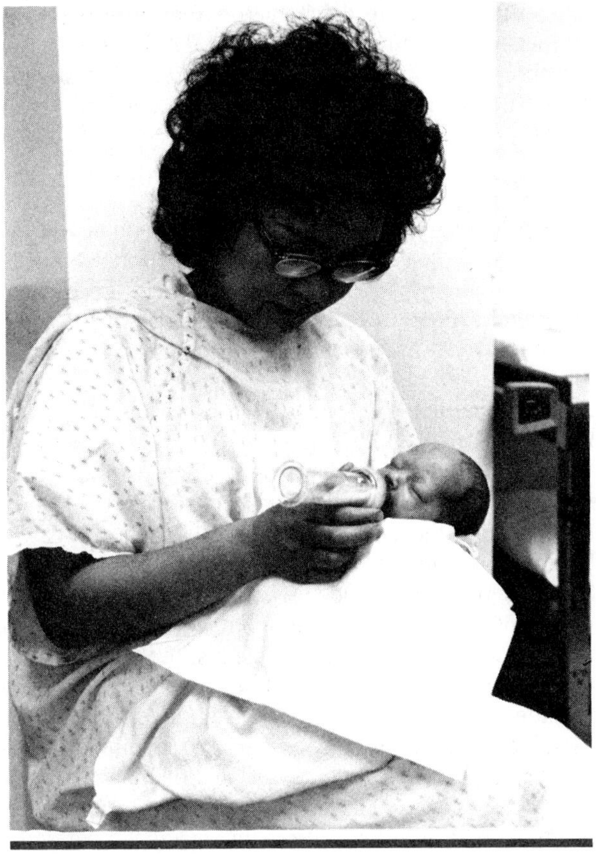

Fig. 10-6. Position for nipple-feeding premature infant.

the infant swallows, causing choking (Shaker, 1990). It is believed that many digestive powers require signal stimulation to respond. Some premature infants respond more slowly than full-term infants; therefore the feeding interval, as well as the amount of the feeding, is individualized. Some investigators have found that premature neonates fed on demand thrive better than those fed on a schedule and on the average can be discharged earlier (Collinge and others, 1982).

The complications of aspiration make it important that infants are not overfed. If infants take very little and appear to be tired, their feedings may have to be repeated in a short while and then at more frequent intervals. Preterm infants are often slow feeders and require periods of rest and frequent bubbling. To determine how well infants tolerate feedings, stomach contents may be aspirated before each feeding and the residual fluid recorded and replaced as part of the feeding.

✢ **NURSING ALERT** Residuals may indicate early necrotizing enterocolitis (NEC) and should be called to the attention of the practitioner.

Breast-feeding. Studies indicate that even small preterm infants are able to breast-feed if the infant has adequate sucking and swallowing reflexes and there are no other contraindications, such as facial defects, respiratory complications, or concurrent illness (Meier and Anderson, 1987; Meier and Pugh, 1985). Mothers who wish to breast-feed their preterm infants are encouraged to pump their breasts until their infants are sufficiently stable to tolerate breast-feeding. Premature infants are able to breast-feed when they (Gardner, O'Donnell, and Weisman, 1989):

- Experience wakeful periods and awaken prior to feedings
- Exhibit coordinated suck, swallow, and gag reflexes
- Have supplemental oxygen supplied by blow-by or nasal cannula
- Have adequate thermal support provided by swaddler, hat, or overhead radiant warmer

Time, patience, and dedication on the part of the mother and the nursing staff are needed to help infants with breast-feeding. The process is begun slowly—beginning with one feeding daily and gradually increasing the feedings as the infant tolerates them. Infants should not be placed on an empty breast to feed, since the infant will become exhausted, and nonnutritive sucking (NNS) does not stimulate milk production. The infant will become frustrated and refuse to feed without the reward of milk. Use of orthodontic nipples for bottle-feeding before the mother can effectively breast-feed provides the same sucking motion as used in breast-feeding. Supplementary bottle feeding is inefficient, since the baby expends energy and calories to feed twice. Feeding more often, supplementing by gavage feeding, or using a training nipple is more energy and calorically efficient (Gardner, O'Donnell, and Weisman, 1989).

Gavage feeding. Gavage feeding is one of the safest means of meeting the nutritional requirements of infants who are less than 32 weeks of gestation or infants who weigh less than 1650 g. These infants are usually too weak to suck effectively, are unable to coordinate swallowing, and lack a gag reflex. Gavage feedings may be provided by continuous drip regulated via infusion pump or by intermittent bolus feedings. For infants learning to nipple feed and who become excessively tired, are listless, or become cyanotic, intermittent gavage feeding is used as an energy-conserving technique.

A 15-inch (37.5 cm) size 5 or 8 French polyethylene feeding tube is used to instill the formula, and the usual methods for determining correct placement are employed (see Chapter 27 for technique). Although the more relaxed cardiac sphincter makes passage of the tube easier, there may be changes in heart rate and blood pressure in response to vagal stimulation. The procedure is best accomplished when an infant is in a prone or a right side-lying position with the head slightly elevated. It is preferable to insert the tube through the mouth rather than the nares. Nasal insertion obstructs nose breathing and may irritate the delicate nasal mucosa. Passage through the mouth also provides an opportunity to observe the sucking response. However, because of less stimulation of the gag reflex, nasal tube gavage may be used in certain situations, such as in older preterm infants who need supplementation after nipple feeding but who fight, gag, and vomit with oral tube management (Kaempf, Bonnabel, and Hay, 1989).

The stomach is aspirated, the contents measured, and the aspirant returned as part of the feeding. The amount of

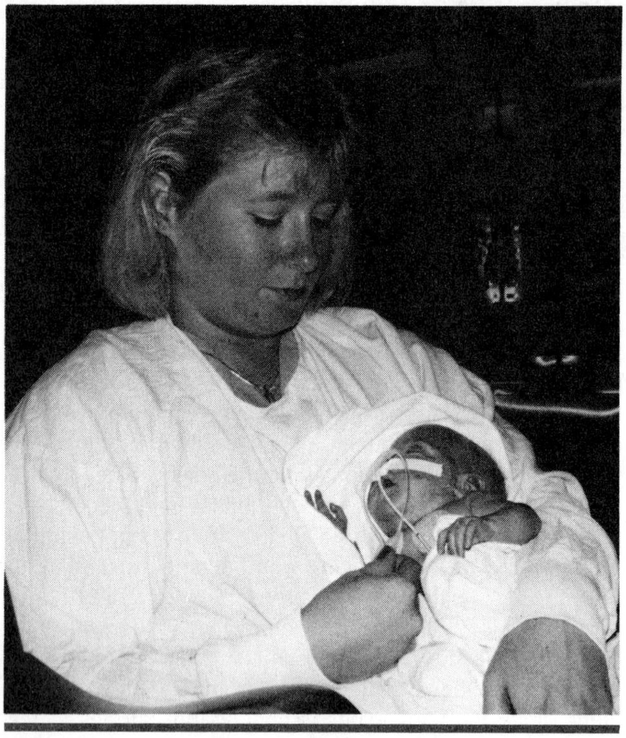

Fig. 10-7. Infant held during gavage feeding. Note oxygen source held in the vicinity of the face.

the aspirant depends on the length of time since the previous feeding or concurrent illness. Whether or not the amount of the aspirant is deducted from the total feeding varies among units. Some advocate deducting to avoid overdistending the stomach. For example, if a feeding is 25 ml and the aspirant is 5 ml, the aspirant is returned plus 20 ml of feeding for a total of 25 ml. In other units the amount is determined on an individual basis.

The formula is allowed to flow by gravity, and the length of time should approximate the time required for a nipple feeding. This procedure is not used as a timesaving method for the nurse. Complications of indwelling tubes include obstructed nares, mucous plugs, purulent rhinitis, epistaxis, and possible stomach perforation that sometimes occur with indwelling catheters.

The nurse needs to observe premature infants closely for behaviors that indicate readiness for bottle-feedings. These include: (1) a strong, vigorous suck; (2) coordination of sucking and swallowing; (3) a gag reflex; (4) sucking on the gavage tube, hands, or pacifier; and (5) rooting and wakefulness before and sleeping after feedings. When these behaviors are noted, infants can be challenged with nipple feedings introduced slowly.

The infant is held during feedings, even though the infant is unable to tolerate extended periods without oxygen (Fig. 10-7). Oxygen is supplied via either nasal cannula or through the oxygen source held in the vicinity of the nose. Also, NNS on a pacifier helps infants associate the sucking with the feeling of satiety. When compared with other LBW infants, those who are allowed NNS are ready for bottle-feeding earlier, require fewer tube feedings, demonstrate better weight gain, are discharged earlier, and have fewer complications (Bernbaum and others, 1983; Field and others, 1982). NNS also increases oxygenation during tube feeding (Bernbaum and others, 1983; Paludetto and others, 1984).

Feeding Resistance

Any feeding technique that bypasses the mouth precludes the opportunity for the affected child to "practice sucking and swallowing, or the opportunity to experience normal hunger and satiation cycles" (Orr and Allen, 1986). Infants may demonstrate aversion to oral feedings by such behaviors as averting the head to the presentation of the nipple, extruding the nipple by tongue thrust, gagging, or even vomiting (Geertsma and others, 1985).

Developmental delays have been noted in the areas of perceptual-motor performance as measured by standard tests, although the area of intellectual function measured within normal limits (O'Connor, Ralston, and Ament, 1988). Other observations include disinterest in or active resistance to oral play, diminished spontaneity and motivation, and shallow interpersonal relationships, probably related to the absence of some early incorporative patterns of normal oral experiences (Dowling, 1977). The longer the period of nonoral feeding, the more severe are the feeding problems, especially if this period occurs during the time when the infant progresses from reflexive to learned and voluntary feeding actions (Orr and Allen, 1986). Infancy is the period during which the mouth is the primary instrument for reception of stimulation and pleasure (see Oral Stage [Freud] Chapter 12).

Infants who are identified as at risk for feeding resistance should be provided with regular oral stimulation based on the child's developmental level. Those who exhibit feeding aversion should begin a stimulation program to overcome resistance and acquire the ability to take nourishment by the oral route. Since management requires long-term commitment, successful implementation of a plan for oral stimulation depends on maximum parental involvement and promotion of primary nursing (Orr and Allen, 1986). Key components and interventions are listed in Box 10-5.

Energy Conservation

One of the major goals of care for the high-risk infant is conservation of energy. Much of the care described in this section is directed toward this end, for example, disturbing the infant as little as possible, maintaining a neutral thermal environment, gavage feeding, easing respirations, and judicious application of stimulatory activities. When the infant is not required to expend energy to cope with efforts to breathe, eat, and alter body temperature, this energy can be used for growth and development. Diminishing environmental noise levels and shading the infant from bright lights also promote rest (See also Infant Stress, p. 404 and Developmental Intervention, p. 404).

The prone position is optimum for most preterm infants and results in improved oxygenation, better-tolerated feedings, and more organized sleep-rest patterns (Masterson,

Box 10-5 COMPONENTS OF A CARE PLAN TO OVERCOME FEEDING RESISTANCE

- Simulate normal feeding interactions.
  - Hold and cuddle infant in "en face" feeding position.
  - Engage in eye contact with infant.
  - Engage in verbal interaction with infant.
- Provide tactile stimulation.
  - Begin with torso and progress to head and neck.
  - Apply firm, consistent pressure.
  - Use palm or hand or textured object (e.g., wash cloth).
  - Gradually move toward mouth, cheeks, and lips.
  - Stroke oral area from cheeks to lips.
  - Pace according to child's tolerance.
- Overcome oral hypersensitivity (sensitivity to intraoral stimulation).
  - Provide oral stimulation as above.
  - When external oral stimulation is tolerated, attempt massage of gums and tongue (use finger or soft rubber item).
  - Massage gums from center and move toward molar region, and move gradually from anterior to posterior.
  - Withdraw stimulus and close child's mouth if child gags.
- Encourage oral exploration.
  - Assist child in mouthing hands, fingers, toes, or soft rubber toys.
  - Play oral games, e.g., blowing a kiss, kissing an object (toy animal).
- Provide oral feedings.
  - Introduce small volumes (even 3 to 5 ml) as early as possible.
  - Offer feedings consistently (water, formula).
  - Avoid force feeding.
- Provide feeding stimulation during tube feedings.
  - Hold child in feeding position.
  - Provide oral stimulation during bolus feedings.
  - Give oral feedings before tube feedings.
  - Give bolus feedings in response to hunger when possible rather than on predetermined schedule.
- Provide nonnutritive sucking to encourage use of oral musculature.

Data from Orr, M.J., and Allen, S.S.: Optimal oral experiences for infants on long-term total parenteral nutrition, Nutr. Clin. Pract. 9:288-295, 1986.

QUESTIONS AND CONTROVERSIES

Should procedures be "clustered" to allow sufficient time for rest between disturbances, or should procedures be scattered to reduce the time spent at each disturbance?

The environment of the NICU has been shown to be highly disturbing and stress producing to infants. In an effort to reduce the number of times an infant is disturbed, nurses have been performing a number of procedures (clustering) at one time. A number of authorities are advocating lengthy periods of rest without disturbance for these infants (Brazelton, 1986). Alterations in the infant's daily routine are made to accommodate a more flexible or structured schedule—whichever is better for the individual infant (Shields and Tenorio, 1988).

Researchers have found that many routine nursing procedures, especially tracheal suctioning, are highly stressful to vulnerable infants. Norris, Campbell, and Brenkert (1982) demonstrated that infants with respiratory distress syndrome reacted to nursing procedures with decreased $tcPo_2$ measurements, and the longer the disturbance the sharper was the decrease and the longer the recovery time. Perlman and Volpe (1983) also noted a marked increase in blood pressure following suctioning, which places vulnerable infants at risk for intraventricular hemorrhage.

NURSING TIP: TAPE REMOVAL

Adhesive tape is best removed by applying a water-soaked cotton ball to the tape, then lifting the tape *carefully* while applying pressure on the skin directly beneath the tape.

Zucker, and Schulze, 1987; Orenstein and Whitington, 1983). Infants exhibit less physical activity and energy expenditure when they are placed in the prone position (Fox and Molesky, 1990; Masterson, Zucker, and Schulze, 1987). Others appear to prefer a side-lying posture. Supine positioning for preterm infants is not desirable because they appear to lose their sense of equilibrium when supine and use up vital energy in attempts to recover balance by postural changes (Cole and Frappier, 1985).

Skin Care

The skin of premature infants is characteristically immature relative to that of full-term infants. Because of the increased sensitivity and fragility of premature skin, it is recommended that no alkaline-based soap or detergent be used that might destroy the "acid mantle" of the skin. The skin is cleansed with plain, clear water or mild, nonalkaline cleanser only two to three times per week. Any topical preparation (including creams, lotions, or medicated ointments) should be carefully assessed for possible toxic effects before application. The increased permeability of the skin facilitates absorption of ingredients. Hexachlorophene has been discontinued as a cleansing agent because of its proven toxic effect. Other germicides (e.g., alcohol or povidone-iodine) are used with caution, and the skin is rinsed after their use (Kuller, Lund, and Tobin, 1983). These substances may cause severe irritation and chemical burns in VLBW infants.

The skin is easily excoriated and denuded; therefore care must be taken to avoid damage to the delicate structure. The total thickness of the skin is less than that of full-term infants and has fewer elastic fibers, and there is less cohesion between the thinner skin layers. Adhesives used after heel sticks or to secure monitoring equipment or intravenous infusions may excoriate the skin or adhere to the skin surface so well that the skin can be separated from understructures and pulled away with the tape. Paper tape is contraindicated, since it adheres tightly, does not stretch, and is difficult to remove after application. Transpore tape is a safer tape to apply directly to the skin of small infants. It is best to use as little tape as possible. Applying a coating of a protective substance (such as the pectin-based barrier Hollihesive) between the skin and adhesive objects is effective in preventing excoriation (Lund and others, 1986). When correctly applied, polyurethane elastic film has been used with success in many units to protect the skin and reduce water loss (Knauth and others, 1989; Kuller, Lund, and Tobin, 1983). The film serves as a protective layer on which adhesive can be attached and serves as a protective layer over abrasions and excoriations.

Eucerin cream creates a satisfactory moisture barrier and is frequently used under tape and applied to denuded areas. Many NICUs now use limb bands rather than adhesive-backed electrodes for attaching monitor equipment. These consist of wires encased in plastic tubing with saline or other electrolyte solution used to activate the connection. This eliminates the need for adhesives. When dressings or adhesive tape is removed from the extremities of very small and immature infants, it is unsafe to use scissors because it is easy to snip off tiny extremities or nick loosely attached skin. Solvents used to remove tape tend to dry and burn the delicate skin.

The area of skin care in LBW infants has not been investigated extensively. Therefore, the foregoing discussion reflects only some of the efforts to prevent skin trauma, and no definitive management practice can be wholeheartedly endorsed at this time. Hopefully, research in this important area will be forthcoming.

During skin assessment of preterm infants, nurses are also alert to the subtle signs that indicate zinc deficiency, a common problem in these infants. Breakdown usually occurs in the areas around the mouth, buttocks, fingers, and toes. In VLBW infants it may also occur in the creases of the neck, wrists, ankles, and around wounds. Zinc deficiency is most likely to appear in infants with sepsis, those experiencing nasogastric losses, or those who had surgery. Any suspicious lesions are reported to the physician so that zinc supplements can be prescribed.

Administration of Medications

Administration of therapeutic agents, such as drugs, ointments, intravenous infusions, and oxygen, requires judicious handling and meticulous attention to details. The computation, preparation, and administration of drugs in minute amounts often requires collaboration between nurses to reduce the chance of error. In addition, the immaturity of an infant's detoxification mechanisms and inability to demonstrate symptoms of toxicity (e.g., signs of auditory nerve involvement from ototoxic drugs such as gentamycin) complicate drug therapy and require that nurses be particularly alert for signs of adverse reaction. (See Administration of Medications, Chapter 27.)

Recently warnings have been issued regarding the hazards of administering bacteriostatic and hyperosmolar solutions to infants. Benzyl alcohol, a common preservative in bacteriostatic water and saline, has been shown to be toxic to newborns and should not be used to flush intravenous catheters or to dilute or reconstitute medications. It is recommended that medications with preservatives be avoided whenever possible (American Academy of Pediatrics Committee on Fetus and Newborn, 1983; Food and Drug Administration, 1982). Nurses must read labels carefully to detect the presence of preservatives in any medication to be administered to an infant.

Hyperosmolar solutions present a potential danger to preterm infants. Hyperosmolar solutions given orally to infants can produce clinical, physiologic, and morphologic alterations, the most serious of which is necrotizing enterocolitis (Atakent and others, 1984). Medications (oral or parenteral) should be sufficiently diluted to prevent complications related to hyperosmolality.

Infant Stress

Preterm infants are subject to stress just as other human beings are, but are biologically deficient in their capacity to cope with or adapt to environmental stresses. It is known that stress affects hypothalmus function, causing adverse effects on growth, heat production, and neurologic mechanisms (Gunderson and Kenner, 1987). Interventions designed to reduce stress in premature infants produced improvement in sleeping behavior and growth (see Developmental Intervention, which follows). Nurses can have a profound influence in creating an environment by modifying behaviors and environmental factors that produce infant stress in the NICU, for example, gentle handling, correct positioning, and reduction of noxious stimuli. Alert observation to evidence of stress and providing appropriate intervention help to reduce disorganized behavior.

Developmental Intervention

Recently attention has been focused on the effects of early intervention, or its lack, on both normal and preterm infants. Findings indicate that infants are able to respond to a greater variety of stimuli than was previously thought. Numerous studies have been based on the assumption that premature infants receive inadequate stimulation. Others have observed that the atmosphere and activities of the NICU are overstimulating. More current studies suggest that infants are not necessarily understimulated but instead are subjected to *inappropriate* stimulation (Barnard and Bee, 1983; VandenBerg, 1985).

The present approach to developmental intervention is one of tailoring the interaction to the developmental level and tolerance of each infant. The standard for assessing the premature infant's behavior is the Assessment of Preterm Infants' Behavior (APIB), which tests the current status and organization of the infant's subsystems of functioning and their interplay (Als and others, 1982).

Three stages of developmental organization have been identified for preterm infants (Box 10-6). During the early stages of development, stimulation produces uncoordinated, random activity, such as jerky limb extension, hyperflexion, and irregular vital signs. At this stage infants need to have minimum environmental stimulation. They are han-

Box 10-6 STAGES OF ORGANIZATION IN PREMATURE INFANTS

1. **Physiologic organization** (infants less than 33 weeks of gestation)—primary need is for stabilization and integration of autonomic functions, such as respiration, heart rate, and temperature.
2. **Coming out** (between 34 and 36 weeks of gestation)—development of motor systems; infants are able to respond to visual and auditory stimuli if interaction begins when they are in an alert state.
3. **Reciprocity** (36 to 40 weeks of gestation and beyond)—emergence of defined states of consciousness, such as sleeping, waking, crying, and alertness; infants can benefit from individualized stimulation programs.

Modified from Gorski, P.A., Davison, M.F., and Brazelton, T.B.: Stages of behavioral organization in the high-risk neonate: theoretical and clinical considerations, Semin. Perinatol. 3:61-72, 1979.

dled with slow, controlled movements (some infants are unstable if moved abruptly), and their random movements are controlled with limbs held close to their bodies during turning or other position changes. This containment prevents or diminishes motor disorganization and reduces stress (VandenBerg, 1985). Additional containment measures include support with blanket rolls, if medically feasible. A nest constructed by placing blanket rolls underneath the bed sheet helps infants in maintaining an attitude of flexion when prone or side-lying (Cole and Frappier, 1985). This is believed to approximate the normal intrauterine position in which preterm infants would lie at this stage of gestation. A flexed position facilitates hand-to-mouth behaviors, stimulates visual activity, facilitates symmetric posture, enhances comfort, and decreases stress (Pelletier and Palmieri, 1985).

Although it must be individually adjusted, skin contact has been demonstrated to improve the clinical course and behavior of LBW infants (Field, Scafidi, and Schanberg, 1987). Short periods of gentle massage, based on behavioral clues from the infant and proceeding in a cephalocaudal direction, have exhibited positive physiologic responses (White-Traut and Goldman, 1988). Regular passive skin-to-skin contact (kangaroo care) between parents and LBW infants helps alleviate stress. The parent wears a loose-fitting, open-front top that provides a modified marsupial-like pocket carrier for the infant. The undressed (except for diaper) infant is placed in a vertical position on the parent's bare chest, which permits direct eye-to-eye contact, skin-to-skin sensations, and close proximity (Affonso, Wahlberg, and Persson, 1989).

When infants have reached sufficient developmental organization and stability, interventions are designed and implemented to support their growing abilities (Box 10-7). Nurses become adept at learning to read infants' behavioral clues and supplying appropriate intervention. Behavioral clues include both approach and avoidance behaviors (Cole, 1985). Approach behaviors that should be supported

Box 10-7 BEHAVIORAL MANIFESTATIONS OF DEVELOPMENTAL ORGANIZATION

Motor Stability Behaviors

Smooth, well-modulated posture and well-modulated tone
Synchronous smooth movements with efficient motoric strategies:
- Hand clasping
- Foot clasping
- Finger folding
- Hand-to-mouth maneuvers
- Grasping
- Suck searching and sucking
- Handholding
- Tucking

State Stability and Attention Regulation Behaviors

Clear, robust sleep states
Rhythmic, robust crying
Good self-quieting or consolability
Robust, focused, shiny-eyed alertness with intent or animated facial expressions, including:
- Frowning
- Cheek softening
- Mouth pursing to "ooh" face
- Cooing
- Attentional smiling

Data from Lawhon, G.: Management of stress in premature infants. In Angelini, D.J., Whelan Knapp, C.W., and Gives, K.M., editors: Perinatal/neonatal nursing: a clinical handbook, Boston, 1986, Blackwell Scientific Publications, Inc.

and enhanced are positive movements, such as tongue extension, handclasp, hand-to-mouth movements, sucking, looking, and cooing.

NURSING ALERT See Box 10-8 for avoidance behaviors that signal the infant's need for "time-out."

Any intervention program for premature or convalescing infants must be individualized. When infants are recovering and are free of support systems, medically stable, and on room air or smaller amounts of oxygen, they are assessed to document their behavioral styles. An effective program may be designed to provide limited sensory stimulation involving one or two senses or multisensory experiences that include tactile, visual, auditory, vestibular, olfactory, and gustatory stimuli. The objective of any intervention program is to avoid stressing infants—overstimulation is as detrimental as understimulation.

When the condition of an infant is sufficiently advanced to begin developmental intervention, some activities are individualized according to each infant's cues, temperament, state, behavioral organization, and particular needs. Intervention periods are short, for example, 1 to 2 minutes of visual stimulation, 2 to 3 minutes of voices, and 5 minutes of quiet music. One type of intervention at a time is applied to document the infant's tolerance and response (Box 10-9). However, the types and duration of any stimuli should be adjusted based on individual infant cues. When intervention is implemented, the parents should be involved as early as

Box 10-8 BEHAVIORAL MANIFESTATIONS OF STRESS IN THE PRETERM INFANT

Autonomic and Visceral Signs
Seizures
Respiratory pauses, tachypnea
Color change to mottled, webbed, cyanotic, gray, flushed
Gagging, gasping
Spitting up
Hiccoughing
Straining; producing a bowel movement
Tremors and startling; twitching
Coughing
Sneezing
Yawning
Sighing

Motor Signs
Flaccidity ("tuning out") of trunk, extremities, face (gape face)
Hypertonicity
- Hyperextensions:
  - Legs (sitting on air, leg bracing)
  - Arms (airplaning, salutes)
  - Trunk (arching, opisthotonos)
  - Finger splaying
  - Facial grimacing
  - Tongue extensions
  - Protective maneuvers (e.g., hand on face, high guard arm position, fisting)
- Hyperflexion of trunk and extremities (fetal tuck)

Frantic, diffuse activity

State-Related Signs
Diffuse sleep or awake states
- Accompanied by whimpering sounds, facial twitches, and discharge smiling
- Eye floating
- Strained fussing or crying
- Staring
- Active averting
- Panicked or worried alertness
- Glassy-eyed or strained alertness
- Rapid-state oscillation
- Irritability and diffuse arousal
- Crying

Box 10-9 GUIDELINES FOR DEVELOPMENTAL INTERVENTION

General Guidelines
Individualize interventions for each infant.
Offer only during periods of alertness.
Limit to one or two types of stimulus per session.
Provide intervention for short periods.
Space periods according to infant's tolerance.
Titrate interventions according to infant's cues.
Terminate stimulation if infant displays evidence of overstimulation*:
- Color changes—mottled, gray, flushed
- Gagging, gasping, spitting up
- Straining as if or actually producing a bowel movement
- Yawning, sighing
- Flaccidity—truncal, extremity, facial
- Hyperextensions—leg, arm, trunk, finger
- Facial grimacing, tongue extension
- Hyperflexion—trunk, extremity
- Frantic, diffuse activity

Visual
Place and magazine photographs (black-and-white schematic faces) in visual range (19 to 22 cm) in "en face" position.
Cover mattress with black-and-white patterned material for length of intervention (may be too stimulating for some infants).
Provide black-and-white mobiles with varied hanging shapes.
Initiate eye-to-eye contact; repeat as tolerated.
Alternate holding black-and-white pattern still and moving it across the infant's visual field.

Tactile
Press skin appropriately.
Stroke skin slowly and gently in head-to-toe direction; begin with trunk and move to more sensitive areas such as face.
Provide alternate textures, e.g., sheep-skin, satin, velvet.
Provide boundaries, foot bracing, blankets.

Auditory
Play tape of parents' voices.
Play classical music recording or music box (jazz or rock is less effective).
Speak with a variety of voice inflections; alternate adult and baby talk.
Call infant by name at each interaction.

Vestibular
Place on water bed with oscillations and waves per minute determined on an individual basis; alternate oscillation with rest periods (may not be acceptable intervention in some units).
Rock in chair.
Place in sling (hammock) and rock.
Provide passive range-of-motion exercises to knee and hip joints.
Close infant's fist around cloth toy.
Lift head to upright position, tip to right and then to left, stopping at midline.
Slowly change position during handling.

Olfactory
Pass open breast milk or formula container under nose.
Pass various sweet smelling items under nose, e.g., cherry syrup, cinnamon, nutmeg, strawberry extract.

Gustatory
Place infant's hand or a pacifier in mouth when sucking movements are observed or during gavage feeding.
Place 2 drops of milk in infant's mouth with each tube feeding.

Modified from Chaze, B.A., and Ludington Hoe, S.M.: Sensory stimulation in the NICU, Am. J. Nurs. 84:68-71, 1984.
*Als, H.: Toward a synactive theory of development: promise for the assessment and support of infant and individuality, Infant Mental Health J 3:229-243, 1982.

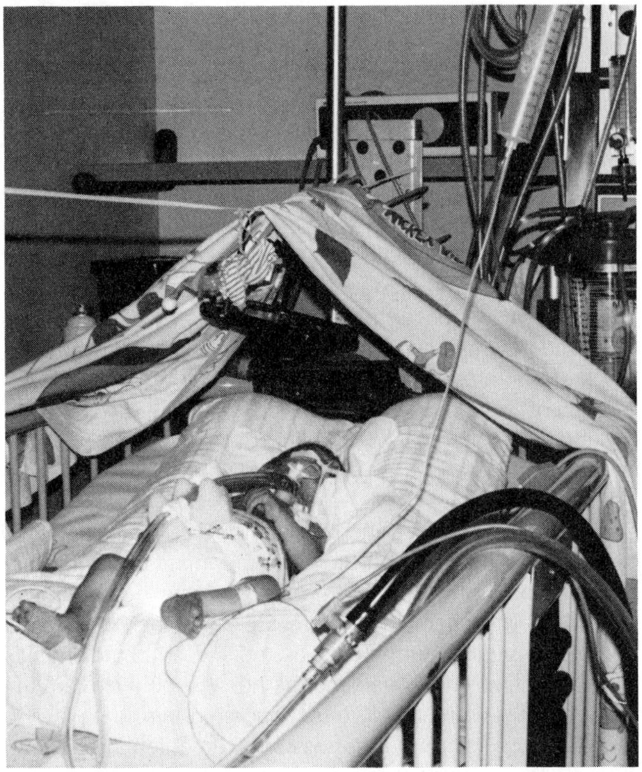

Fig. 10-8. Infant shaded from overhead lights.

possible. Appropriate interventions may have the additional benefit of enhancing early parent-infant relationships that contribute to growth and development at later stages of infancy (Field, Scafidi, and Schanberg, 1987).

NICU environment. A hazard to infants that has been of concern to nurses and others who work in the intensive care units is the noise level that results from monitoring equipment, alarms, and general unit activity. Although a relationship of noise levels and deafness in surviving infants has not been proved and risk criteria have not been established, personnel are cautioned to reduce noise-generating activities such as closing doors (including incubator portholes), listening to loud radios or talking loudly, and handling equipment (e.g., trash containers). Noise levels have been correlated with the incidence of intracranial hemorrhage, especially in the VLBW infant, as determined by auditory brainstem potentials (Marshall and others, 1980).

Twenty-four-hour surveillance of sick infants implies maximum visibility. However, many units have instigated a program to help establish a night-day sleep pattern by either darkening the room, if the infants' condition allows it, covering cribs with blankets, or placing eye patches over the infants' eyes at night. Others believe that rest for these infants is so vital to their growth that they are provided with total rest for 1 of every 3 hours. The light should be diminished, cribs or incubators are covered with blankets, and the infants are not disturbed for handling of any kind during this rest period (Brazelton, 1984) (Fig. 10-8). Experiments have indicated that infants in a "night and day" nursery, in which the nursery was darkened (except for low-intensity light) and noise significantly reduced or eliminated, spent more time sleeping, less time feeding, and gained more weight than similar infants in a nursery lighted 24 hours per day (Mann and others, 1986).

Family Involvement

Often professional health workers are so absorbed in the lifesaving physical aspects of care that the emotional needs of infants and their families are ignored. The significance of early parent-child interaction and infant stimulation has been documented by reliable research, and nurses, aware of these infant and family needs, must incorporate activities that facilitate family interaction into the nursing care plan.

The birth of a preterm infant is an unexpected and stressful event for which families are emotionally unprepared. They find themselves simultaneously coping with their own needs, the needs of their infant, and the needs of their families (especially when there are other children). To compound the situation, the precarious nature of their infant's condition engenders an atmosphere of apprehension and uncertainty. They are faced with multiple crises and overwhelming feelings of responsibility, expense, and frustration.

All parents have some anxieties about the outcome of a pregnancy, but following a premature birth the concern is heightened about both the viability and the intactness of their infant. Mothers see their infant only briefly before the newborn is removed to the intensive care unit or even to another hospital, leaving them with just the recollection of the infant's very small size and unusual appearance. They usually feel alone or lost in the maternity ward, belonging neither with mothers who have lost their infants nor with those who delivered healthy, full-term infants. The staff and physicians are often guarded in discussing the infant's condition; mothers are continually expecting to hear that their infant has died, and they are sensitive to the anxieties of other mothers and staff members. Leaving their infant and going home empty-handed only serves to compound their feelings of disappointment, failure, and deprivation.

When an infant is to be transported from the hospital, the parents need a description of the facility where the infant is going. They need to know the location, reputation, and nature of the facility and the care that the infant is expected to receive. The name of the infant's physician and the telephone number of the nursery should be given to them, and unfamiliar terms explained to them, such as *neonatologist, ventilator, infusion,* and *incubator.* Explanations are made simple, and parents are given the opportunity to ask questions. If booklets are available that describe the facility, they are given to the family.

Perhaps most important of all, the parents, especially the mother, should have some contact with the infant before the transport. To be able to see, touch, and (if possible) hold their infant facilitates the attachment process. Often a photograph, or even a videotape, of their infant can serve as a bond until the parents are able to travel to the regional facility. When possible, it is often advisable to transfer the mother to the same institution as her infant.

Parents need to be informed of their infant's progress

Box 10-10 TASKS OF PARENTS OF A HIGH-RISK INFANT

Work through the crisis events surrounding labor and delivery.
Acknowledge that the infant's life is endangered and that the infant might die, and begin the grief process.
Confront and recognize feelings of inadequacy and guilt in not delivering a healthy child.
Adapt to the neonatal intensive care environment.
Resume parental relationships with infant and initiate the caregiving role, *or*
Adapt to the loss in the event of neonatal death.

Modified from Siegel, R., Gardner, S.L., and Merenstein, G.B.: In Merenstein, G.B., and Gardner, S.L.: Handbook of neonatal intensive care, ed. 2, St. Louis, 1989, Mosby–Year Book, Inc.

and reassured that the infant is receiving proper care. They need to understand the smallest aspects of the infant's condition and treatment. Parents need a realistic assessment of the situation that is honest and direct. Using nonmedical terminology, moving at a pace that is comfortable for parents to assimilate the information, and avoiding lengthy technical explanations facilitate communication with family members (Siegel, Gardner, and Merenstein, 1989). Tasks that must be accomplished by parents during their infant's care are presented in Box 10-10.

Facilitating Parent-Infant Relationships

Because of their physiologic instability, infants are separated from their mothers immediately and surrounded by a complex, impenetrable barrier of glass windows, mechanical equipment, and special caregivers. There is increasing evidence to indicate that the emotional separation that accompanies the physical separation of mothers and infants interferes with the normal maternal-infant attachment process discussed in Chapter 8. Maternal attachment is a cumulative process that begins before conception, is strengthened by significant events during pregnancy, and matures through maternal-infant contact during the neonatal period.

When an infant is sick, the necessary physical separation appears to be accompanied by an emotional estrangement on the part of parents that may seriously damage the capacity for parenting their infant. This detachment is further hampered by the tenuous nature of the infant's condition. When survival is in doubt, parents may be reluctant to establish a relationship with their infant. They prepare themselves for the death of the infant while continuing to hope for recovery. This anticipatory grief (Chapter 23) and hesitancy to embark on a relationship are evidenced by behaviors such as delay in giving the infant a name, reluctance in visiting the nursery, or when they do visit, focusing on equipment and treatments rather than on their infant, and hesitancy to touch or handle the infant when they are provided with the opportunity.

Comprehensive management of high-risk newborns includes encouraging and facilitating parental involvement rather than isolating parents from their infant and associated care. This is particularly important in relation to mothers; and to reduce the effects of physical separation, mothers are united with their newborn at the earliest opportunity. Preparing the parents to see their infant for the first time is a nursing responsibility.

Before the first visit the parents should be prepared for their infant's appearance, the equipment that is attached to the child, and some indication of the general atmosphere of the unit. The initial encounter with the intensive care unit is a stressful experience, and the frightening array of people, equipment, and activity is likely to be overwhelming. A book of photographs or pamphlets describing the NICU environment (infants in incubators or under radiant warmers, monitors, mechanical ventilators, and intravenous equipment) provides a useful and nonthreatening introduction to the NICU.

Parents should be encouraged to visit their infant as soon as possible. Even if they saw the infant at the time of transport or shortly after birth, the infant may have changed considerably, especially if there are a number of medical and equipment requirements associated with the infant's hospitalization. At the bedside the nurse should explain the function of each piece of equipment and the role it plays in facilitating recovery. When possible, some items related to therapy can be removed; for example, phototherapy can be temporarily discontinued and eye patches removed to permit eye-to-eye contact.

Parents appreciate the support of a nurse during the initial visit with their infant, but they may also appreciate some time alone with the infant for a short while. It is important during the early visits to emphasize positive aspects of their infant's behavior and development so that parents can focus on their infant as an individual rather than on the equipment that surrounds the child. For example, the nurse may describe the infant's spontaneous behaviors during care, such as grasp, swallowing, and movement, or make comments about the infant's biologic functions. Most institutions have open visiting policies so that parents and siblings may visit their infant as often as they wish.

Parents vary greatly in the degree to which they are able to interact with their infant. Some may wish to touch or hold their infant during the first visit, whereas others may not feel comfortable enough even to enter the nursery. These reactions depend on a variety of prenatal and postnatal factors, such as the parity of the mother and her preparation before birth; the size, condition, and physical appearance of the infant; and the type of treatment the infant is receiving. It is essential to recognize that the individualized pacing and quality of the interactions are more important than early onset of these interactions. Parents may not be receptive to early and extended infant contact, since they need time to adjust to the impact of an infant with birth problems and must be helped to grieve before acceptance of their infant can take place.

The parents' inability to focus on their infant is a clue for the nurse to assist the parents in expressing feelings of guilt, anxiety, helplessness, inadequacy, anger, and ambivalence. Nurses can help parents deal with these distressing

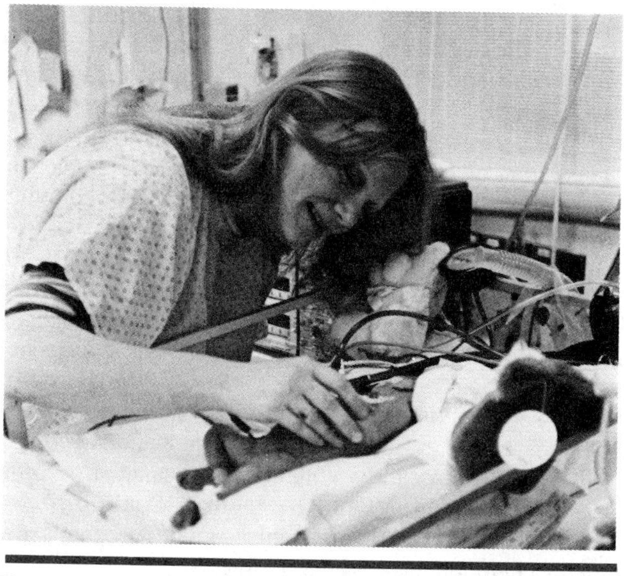

Fig. 10-9. Encouraging interaction of mother and her premature infant in intensive care unit facilities mother-infant attachment process.

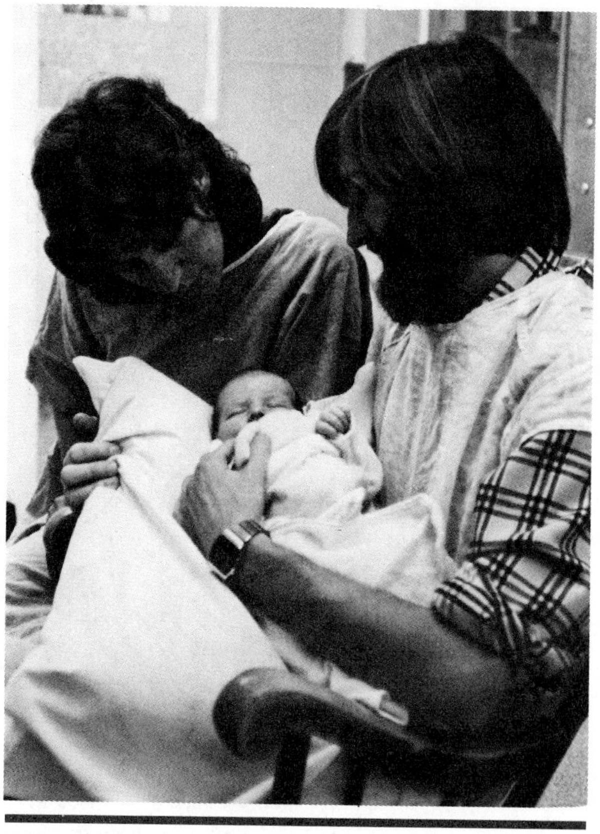

Fig. 10-10. Mother and father visit their newborn infant.

feelings and recognize that they are normal responses shared by other parents. It is important to point out and reinforce the positive aspects of parents' behavior and interactions with their infant.

Most parents feel shaky and insecure about initiating interaction with their infant. Nurses can sense parents' level of readiness and offer encouragement in these initial efforts. Parents of premature infants follow the same acquaintance process as do parents of term infants. They may quickly proceed through the process or may require several days or even weeks to complete the process. Parents begin by touching their infant's extremities with their fingertips and poking the infant tenderly, then proceed to caresses and fondling (Fig. 10-9). Touching is the first act of communication between parents and their child. Parents need to be prepared for their infant's exaggerated and generalized startle responses to a touch so that they will not interpret these as negative reactions to their overtures. It may be necessary to limit tactile stimuli when the infant is critically ill and labile, but the nurse can offer other options—speaking softly or sitting at the bedside.

Eventually parents begin to endow their infant with an identity—a part of the family. When an infant no longer appears as a foreign object and begins to take on aspects of family members, such as the father's chin or the sister's nose, nurses can facilitate this incorporation. Parents are encouraged to bring in clothes and toys for their infant (based on developmental level), and the nurse can help parents set goals for themselves and for the infant. Feeding schedules are discussed, and parents are encouraged to visit at times when they can become involved in the care of their infant (Fig. 10-10).

Throughout the parental-infant acquaintance process, the nurse listens carefully to what the parents say in order to assess their concerns and their progress toward incorporating their infant into their lives. The manner in which parents refer to their infant and the questions they ask reveal their worries and feelings and can serve as valuable clues to future relationships with the infant. The alert nurse is attuned to these subtle indications of parents' needs that provide guidelines for nursing intervention. Often all that parents need is reassurance that the behaviors about which they are concerned are normal reactions and will disappear as the infant matures (e.g., an exaggerated Moro reflex or inability to coordinate swallowing) and that they will have the support of the nurse during caregiving activities.

Parents need guidance in their relationships with their infant and assistance in their efforts to meet their infant's physical and developmental needs. The nursing staff must help parents understand that their preterm infant offers few behavioral rewards and show them how to accept small rewards from their infant. The infant's reactions and behaviors are explained to parents, who take their infant's jerky, rejective behavior personally. They need reassurance that these behaviors are not a reflection on their parenting skills. Parents are taught to recognize their infant's cues regarding stimulation, handling, and other interaction, especially aversive behaviors that indicate a need for rest. Nurses need to include parents in planning their infant's care and sensory stimulation materials, such as a music box or recording.

Above all, nurses must encourage and reinforce parents during their caregiving activities and interactions with their infant in order to promote healthy parent-child relationships. The importance of facilitating the parental-infant at-

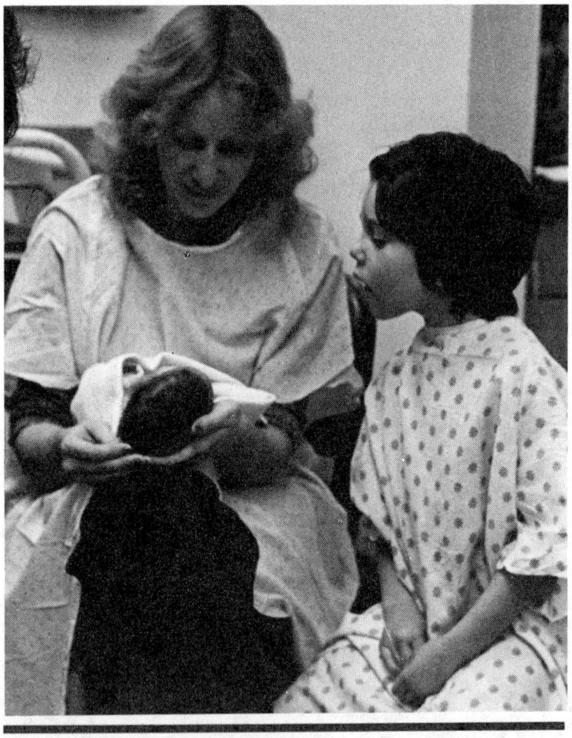

Fig. 10-11. Big sister gets acquainted with the new baby.

tachment process cannot be overemphasized, since studies indicate that lack of early attachment in premature infants may contribute to problems such as child abuse later on.

Siblings. In the past concerns about sibling visitation in the NICU focused on fear of infection and disruption of nursing routines. These fears have not been substantiated (Kowba and Schwirian, 1985; Scrimshaw and March, 1984), and sibling visits are now part of the normal operation of most NICUs (Fig. 10-11).

Birth of a preterm infant is a difficult time for siblings, who rely on the support of understanding parents. When the happy anticipation is changed to sadness, worry, and altered routines, siblings are bewildered and deprived of their parents' attention. They know something is wrong, but they have only a dim understanding of what it is. Concern about negative effects of seeing the ill newborn on visiting siblings has not been confirmed. Children have not hesitated to approach or touch the infant, and children less than 5 years of age have been less reluctant than older children (Schwab and others, 1983); in addition, there have been no measurable differences between previsit and postvisit behaviors (Trause and others, 1981).

Potential benefits of sibling visits must be weighed against exposure of the child to the environment of the NICU. Children must be prepared for the unfamiliar NICU atmosphere, but contact with the infant appears to have a positive effect on siblings by helping them to deal with the reality rather than the bizarre fantasies that are characteristic of young children. It also helps to bond the family as a unit.

Support groups. Parents need to feel that they are not alone. Parent support groups have been of immeasurable value to families of infants in the NICU. Some groups consist of parents who have infants in the hospital who share the same anxieties and concerns. Other groups include parents who have had infants in the NICU and who have dealt with the crisis effectively. The groups are usually under the leadership of a staff person and involve physicians, nurses, and social workers, but it is the parents who can offer other parents something that no one else can provide.

A relatively new national organization evolved from a local parent's group. **Parent Care, Inc.*** provides information, referrals, and support to parents and professionals concerned with the care of high-risk infants. It also publishes a national newsletter and a resource directory that provide information on items useful to parents, such as "preemie" clothing, and hosts local and national conferences. Information can be obtained by contacting or forming a local group. The **Family Resource Coalition†** is a North American network of family support programs designed to help families of preterm infants.

Discharge Planning and Home Care

Parents become very apprehensive and excited as time for discharge approaches. They have many concerns and insecurities regarding the care of their infant. They fear the child may still be in danger, that they will be unable to recognize signs of distress or illness in their infant, and that the infant may not yet be ready for discharge. Nurses need to begin early to assist parents in acquiring or increasing their skills in the care of their infant. Appropriate instruction must be provided and sufficient time allowed for the family to assimilate the information and learn the continuing special care requirements. Where rooming-in or other live-in arrangements are available, parents can stay for a few days and assume the care of their infant under the supervision and support of the nursery staff.

There should be appropriate medical and nursing follow-up and referrals to services that can benefit the family, including developmental follow-up. Public health agencies provide nursing supervision, counseling, and referral for nursing visits. Organized support groups are part of many communities, including those discussed previously and those designed for parents of infants who require special care because of specific defects or disabilities, and those for parents of multiple births (see Chapter 3). Some manufacturers provide for the special needs of such infants. For example, premature size disposable diapers are available from the manufacturers of Pampers.‡

Car seat safety is an essential aspect of discharge planning, and infants less than 37 weeks of gestation should have a period of observation in an appropriate car seat to monitor for possible apnea, bradycardia, and decreased Sa_{O_2}. Several models can be adapted for small infants with the placement of blanket rolls on each side of the infant to support the head and trunk. For adequate support without slumping, the seat-back-to-crotch strap distance must be 14

*1010 South Union Street, Alexandria, VA 22314; (703) 836-4678.
†230 N. Michigan Ave., Suite 1625, Chicago, IL 60601.
‡Procter & Gamble; phone toll free: (800) 543-4932; in Ohio: (800)582-2623.

cm or less (Bull and Stroup, 1985). Other researchers have found that "premature infants, both with and without apnea, are at risk for significant hypoxia while placed in a recommended car seat" (Willett and others, 1986, 1989). LBW infants are best transported lying prone in infant-only child safety seats with harness designed to fit small bodies (Richards, 1989) or well supported in a car bed restraint (Mini Swinger*) (Bull, Weber, and Stroup, 1988). The American Academy of Pediatrics (1990) has published guidelines for the safe transportation of premature infants. (See Chapter 12 for a discussion of infant car restraints.)

Knowing that members of the staff (especially the primary nurse) are available for telephone or personal contact when the parents take the infant home provides a measure of security to anxious parents. Most NICU facilities maintain a policy of open communication between staff and parents both during the infant's hospitalization and following discharge. It is the responsibility of the NICU staff to make certain that parents are prepared to care for their infant—emotionally and physically.

Vulnerable child. The term *vulnerable child syndrome* is applied to physically healthy children who are perceived by their parents to be at high risk for medical or developmental problems (Culley, Perrin, and Chaberski, 1989). The syndrome has been observed in parents of children who have had an earlier illness or injury from which they had not been expected to recover. The family continues to perceive the child as fragile, vulnerable, "different," and having needs that warrant special status in the family, which adversely affects the child's and family's behavior. The parents may lack confidence in their parenting ability persisting beyond the illness. The parents may also become overly indulgent and have difficulty setting limits, resulting in interference with normal development. Consequently the child becomes dependent, demanding, and out of control (Bernbaum and Hoffman-Williamson, 1986). Overprotection and frequent visits to the health care provider are characteristic.

Problems that may arise in the high-risk newborn include overfeeding, underfeeding, and difficulty separating the child from the parent. To help parents deal with the stress of home care for the infant, nurses can help families to discuss their fears and anxieties, which are exaggerated in parents of preterm infants, and encourage the family to create a normal routine in caring for the infant. Parents need to learn the normal developmental delays expected of premature infants and the importance of setting disciplinary limits and schedules. Continued explanations and clarification of the infant's true health status and ongoing support of the parents' efforts are important aspects of follow-up care.

Developmental Outcome

Some physiologic systems in preterm infants mature earlier than they would have if the infant had remained within the uterus; for example, the function of some enzyme and immunologic systems and organs, such as the kidneys and gastrointestinal system efficiency; others slow down, such as growth in height and weight; still others keep pace with the development of fetuses still in utero, for example, reflex behaviors.

Box 10-11 FACTORS THAT AFFECT GROWTH AND DEVELOPMENT OF PRETERM INFANTS

Past history
Gestational age at birth
Head circumference, weight, and length at birth
Length of growth delay
Days necessary to regain birth weight
Measurements at term date
Head circumference, weight, length at discharge from hospital
Medical diagnosis, its severity, treatment, and response
Length of hospitalization

Longitudinal studies of infants born prematurely indicate that there are differences in many aspects of development that may be a consequence of the immaturity at birth and related perinatal problems. Preterm infants remain in a lower percentile range for height, weight, and head circumference, although they follow the same general growth pattern as infants born at term (Ross, Lipper, and Auld, 1985; Westwood and others, 1983). There is a rapid increase in growth during the first 6 months, and growth remains somewhat accelerated until the normal growth curve is reached by age 2 to 3 years. See Box 10-11 for factors that affect growth and development of preterm infants.

Neurologic impairment (such as intraventricular hemorrhage) and serious sequelae correlate with the size and gestational age of infants at birth and with the severity of neonatal complications (Hack and others, 1984). The greater the degree of immaturity, the greater the degree of disability. A greater incidence of cerebral palsy, attention deficit disorder, visual-motor deficits, and altered intellectual functioning is observed in preterm than in full-term infants. However, behavioral development can be enhanced when families are provided with support and infants are referred to appropriate services for neurologic and developmental interventions (Slater and others, 1988). Parental interest and involvement are very important variables in developmental progress of infants.

All infants at risk seem to benefit from special care, since undesirable sequelae appear to be decreased in infants who receive intensive medical and nursing care as opposed to those whose care is delayed or less than intensive. Although the risk of perinatal complications is highest in VLBW infants and the mortality is higher, a positive outcome is believed to be possible even for these survivors of extremely low birth weight (Bennett, Robinson, and Sells, 1983).

A concern of personnel in NICUs is the incidence of sensory impairment in surviving premature infants. Retinopathy of prematurity, a dreaded complication of oxygen therapy, is discussed on p. 433. More difficult to anticipate and de-

*Distributed by Shinn and Associates, 2853 W. Jolly, Okemos, MI 48864; (517) 332-0211.

tect is a hearing deficit. Because LBW infants show significant visual-motor deficits compared with full-term infants at a later time, many NICUs routinely screen infants for hearing acuity. The brainstem-evoked auditory response (BEAR), one method of screening, monitors stimulus-related changes in the electrical activity of the auditory pathway by way of noninvasive electrodes applied to the scalp. Follow-up testing is a vital part of ongoing care.

Neonatal Loss

The precarious nature of many high-risk infants makes death a very real and ever-present possibility. Although infant mortality has been reduced sharply with improved technology, the mortality rate is still greatest in the neonatal period of life. Nurses in the NICU are the persons who must prepare the parents for an inevitable death and facilitate a family's grieving process after an expected or an unexpected death.

The loss of an infant has special meaning for the grieving parents. It represents a loss of a part of themselves (especially for mothers), a loss of the potential for immortality that offspring represent, and the loss of the dream child that has been fantasized throughout the pregnancy. There is a sense of emptiness and failure. In addition, when an infant has lived for such a short time, there are few, if any, pleasant memories to serve as a basis for identification and idealization that are part of the resolution of a loss.

To help the parents understand that the death is a reality, it is important that the parents are encouraged to hold their infant before death and if possible be present at the time of death so that their infant can die in their arms if they choose. Many who deny the need to hold the infant later regret the decision (Null, 1989). Parents should be provided with an opportunity to see, touch, hold, caress, examine, and talk to their infant privately after death and to bathe their infant if they desire as a final act of caring. If parents are hesitant about seeing their dead infant, it is advisable to keep the body in the unit for a few hours, since many parents change their minds after the initial shock of the death.

Parents may need to see and hold the infant more than once: the first time to say "hello" and the last time to say "goodbye." If parents wish to see the infant after the body has been taken to the morgue, the infant should be retrieved, wrapped in a blanket, and taken to the mother's room or other private place. The nurse should stay with the parents and provide them an opportunity for private time alone with their dead infant.

Some units have implemented a hospice approach for families with infants for whom the decision has been made not to prolong life and who are receiving only palliative care. A special "family" room is set aside that contains all supportive equipment needed for the care of the infant and also provides a homelike atmosphere for the family (Landon-Malone, Kirkpatrick, and Stull, 1987). All hospice services are available to the family, and the infant remains under the care and supervision of a primary nurse on the NICU staff. (See Chapter 23 for further discussion of hospice care.)

A photograph of the infant taken before or after death is highly desirable. The parents may not wish to see the photograph at the time of death, but the chance to refer to it later will help make their infant seem more real, which is a part of the normal grief process. A photograph of their infant being held by the hand or touched by an adult offers a more positive image than a morgue type of photograph. Other tangible remembrances of the child can be provided, such as name tags, armbands, and locks of hair shaved for intravenous insertion or other procedures. If the parents have not done so, they should be encouraged to name their infant.

At least one nurse who is familiar to the family should be present during the discussion about a dead or dying infant. The nurse should talk with parents openly and honestly about funeral arrangements, since few of them have had experience with this aspect of death. Many funeral homes now offer inexpensive arrangements for these special cases. Someone from the NICU should take the responsibility for acquiring this type of information. Families need to be informed of options available, but it is preferable to encourage a funeral because the ritual provides an opportunity for parents to feel the support of friends and relatives. A clergyman of the appropriate faith may be notified if the parents wish.

Before the parents leave the hospital, they are given the telephone number of the unit (if they do not have it) and invited to call any time they have any further questions. Many intensive care units make it a point to contact the parents following a neonatal death to assess the parents' coping mechanisms, evaluate the grieving process, and provide support as needed. Several organizations are available to offer support and understanding to families who have lost a newborn, including **Compassionate Friends,*** **S.H.A.R.E. (Source of Help in Airing & Resolving Experiences),†** and **A.M.E.N.D. (Aiding Mothers & Fathers Experiencing Neo-Natal Death).‡** (See also Chapter 23 for further discussion of the family and the grief process.)

Baptism. Since many Christian parents wish to have their child baptized if death is anticipated or a decided possibility, this becomes a nursing responsibility. Whenever possible, it is most desirable that a representative of the parents' faith—that is, a Roman Catholic priest or a Protestant minister—perform such a ritual. When death is imminent, a nurse or a physician can perform the baptism by simply pouring water on the infant's forehead (a medicine dropper is a convenient means) while repeating the words, "I baptize you in the name of the Father and of the Son and of the Holy Spirit." This includes a birth of any gestational age, particularly when the parents are of the Roman Catholic faith.

*P.O. Box 3696, Oak Brook, IL 60522-3696; (312) 323-5010; in Canada, 685 William Ave., Winnipeg, Canada, R3E 022.

†St. John's Hospital, 800 Carpenter, Springfield, IL 62769; (217) 544-6464, Ext. 5275.

‡Contact Maureen Connelly, 4324 Berrywick Terrace, St. Louis, MO 63128; (314) 487-7582.

When the faith of the parents is uncertain, a conditional baptism can be carried out by saying, "If you are capable of receiving baptism, I baptize you in the name of the Father and of the Son and of the Holy Spirit." The fact of the baptism is recorded in the infant's chart and a notice placed on the crib or incubator. Parents are informed at the first opportunity.

Evaluation

The effectiveness of nursing interventions is determined by continual reassessment and evaluation of care based on the following observational guidelines and expected outcomes:

1. Take vital signs and perform respiratory assessments at time intervals based on infant's condition and needs; observe infant's respiratory efforts and response to therapy; check functioning of equipment; review laboratory test results.
2. Measure abdominal skin and axillary temperatures at specified intervals.
3. Observe infant's behavior and appearance for evidence of sepsis.
4. Assess for hydration; assess and measure fluid intake; observe infant during feeding, measure amount of formula or parenteral intake; weigh daily.
5. Observe infant's behavior for evidence of fatigue.
6. Observe infant for evidence of complications (follow assessment guide in Box 10-4); observe infant's reaction to medical therapies.
7. Observe infant's response to developmental intervention.
8. Observe parental interaction with the infant; interview family regarding their feelings, concerns, and readiness for home care.
9. Interview family and observe their behaviors during and after the death of their infant.

Expected outcomes:
See Nursing Care Plan, pp. 392-394.

HIGH-RISK CONDITIONS RELATED TO DYSMATURITY

In any newborn, various disease states and congenital abnormalities are associated with increased risk in the neonatal period and may or may not be related to the state of maturity. This segment of the chapter is devoted to a description of the dysmature states, prematurity and postmaturity. Although prematurity is encountered more frequently and is a greater threat to life, postmaturity is not without problems.

PRETERM INFANTS

Prematurity accounts for the largest number of admissions to an NICU. Not only does the immaturity of these infants place them at risk for neonatal complications (e.g., hyperbilirubinemia and idiopathic respiratory distress syndrome, which is highest in the preterm infant), but also other high-risk factors (e.g., congenital abnormalities in association with prematurity).

Etiology

Most of the aspects concerning high-risk neonates listed in Box 10-1 are related to the incidence of prematurity; however, the actual cause of prematurity is not known in most instances. The incidence of prematurity is lowest in the middle to high socioeconomic classes, in which pregnant women are generally in good health, are well nourished, and receive prompt and comprehensive prenatal care; the incidence is highest in the low socioeconomic class, in which a combination of deleterious circumstances is present. Other factors, such as multiple pregnancies, preeclampsia, and placental accidents that interrupt the normal course of gestation prior to completion of fetal development, are responsible for a large number of premature births.

The outlook for premature infants is largely, but not entirely, related to the state of physiologic and anatomic immaturity of the various organs and systems at the time of birth. Infants at term have advanced to a state of maturity sufficient to allow a successful transition to the extrauterine environment. Infants born prematurely must make the same adjustments but with functional immaturity proportional to the stage of development reached at the time of birth. The degree to which infants are prepared for extrauterine life can be predicted to some extent by weight and estimated gestational age (see Assessment of Clinical Gestational Age, Chapter 8). An understanding of prenatal development provides some concept of the status of the systems at various stages of development that must cope with functional changes that occur with birth.

Characteristics

Preterm infants have a number of characteristics that are distinctive at various stages of development. Identification of these characteristics provides valuable clues to the gestational age and hence to the physiologic capabilities of infants. The general, outward physical appearance changes as the fetus progresses to maturity. Characteristics of skin, general attitude (or posture) when supine, appearance of hair, and amount of subcutaneous fat provide cues to a newborn's physical development. Observation of spontaneous, active movements and response to stimulation and passive movement contributes to the assessment of neurologic status. The appraisal is made as soon as possible after admission to the nursery, since much of the observation and management of infants depends on this information.

On inspection premature infants are very small and appear scrawny because they lack or have only minimum subcutaneous fat deposits, with a proportionately large head in relation to the body, which reflects the cephalocaudal direction of growth. Of all the body measurements, the head is reduced least, and sucking pads in the cheeks are strikingly prominent. The skin is bright pink, smooth, and shiny (may be edematous), with small blood vessels clearly visible underneath the thin, transparent epidermis. The fine lanugo hair is abundant over the body but is sparse, fine, and fuzzy on the head. The ear cartilage is soft and pliable, and the soles and palms have minimum creases, resulting

CLINICAL EVALUATION

PRETERM | **TERM**

The preterm infant lies in a "relaxed attitude," limbs more extended; his body size is small, and his head may appear somewhat larger in proportion to the body size. The term infant has more subcutaneous fat tissue and rests in a more flexed attitude.

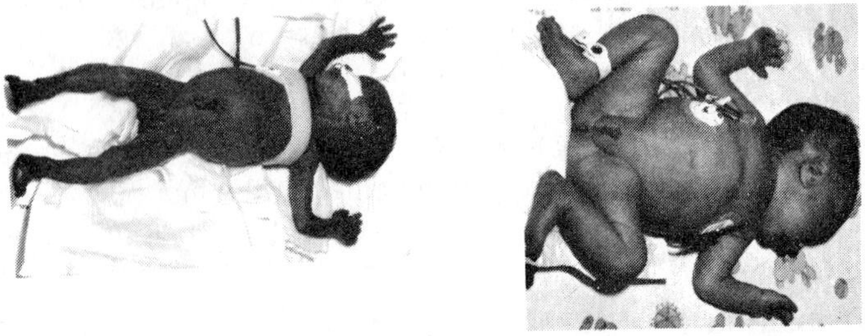

The preterm infant's ear cartilages are poorly developed, and the ear may fold easily; the hair is fine and feathery, and lanugo may cover the back and face. The mature infant's ear cartilages are well formed, and the hair is more likely to form firm separate strands.

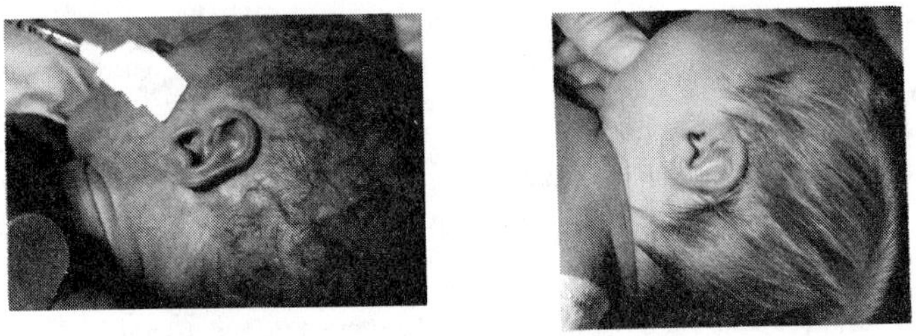

The sole of the foot of the preterm infant appears more turgid and may have only fine wrinkles. The mature infant's sole (foot) is well and deeply creased.

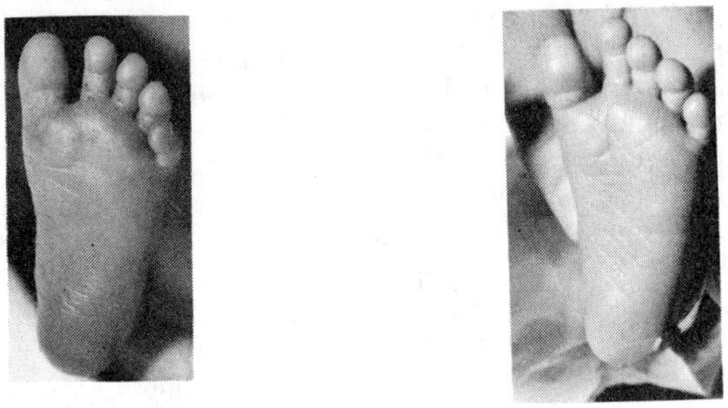

The preterm female infant's clitoris is prominent, and labia majora are poorly developed and gaping. The mature female infant's labia majora are fully developed, and the clitoris is not as prominent.

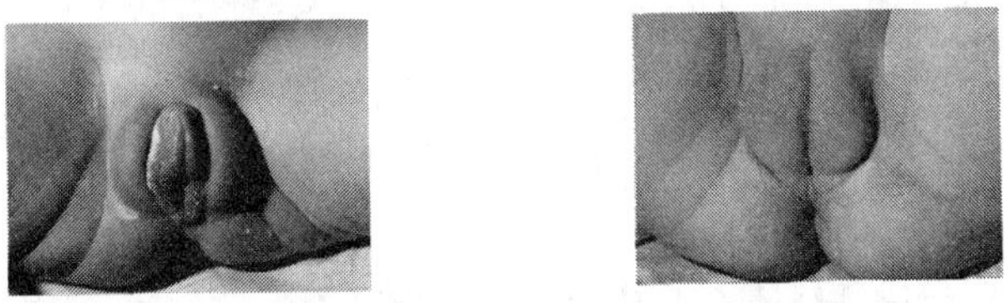

The preterm male infant's scrotum is undeveloped and not pendulous; minimal rugae are present, and the testes may be in the inguinal canals or in the abdominal cavity. The term male infant's scrotum is well developed, pendulous, and rugated, and the testes are well down in the scrotal sac.

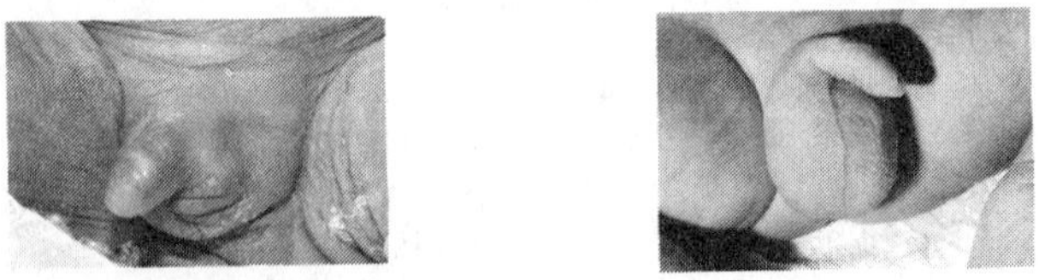

Scarf sign—The preterm infant's elbow may be easily brought across the chest with little or no resistance. The mature infant's elbow may be brought to the midline of the chest, resisting attempts to bring the elbow past the midline.

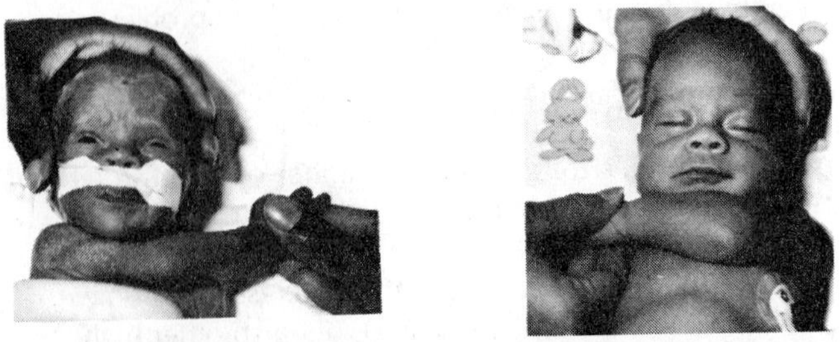

Fig. 10-12. Clinical and neurologic examinations comparing preterm and full-term infants.
Data from Pierog, S.H., and Ferrara, A.: Medical care of the sick newborn, ed. 2, St. Louis, 1976, Mosby-Year Book, Inc.

NEUROLOGIC EVALUATION

PRETERM **TERM**

Grasp reflex—The preterm infant's grasp is weak; the term infant's grasp is strong, allowing the infant to be lifted up from the mattress.

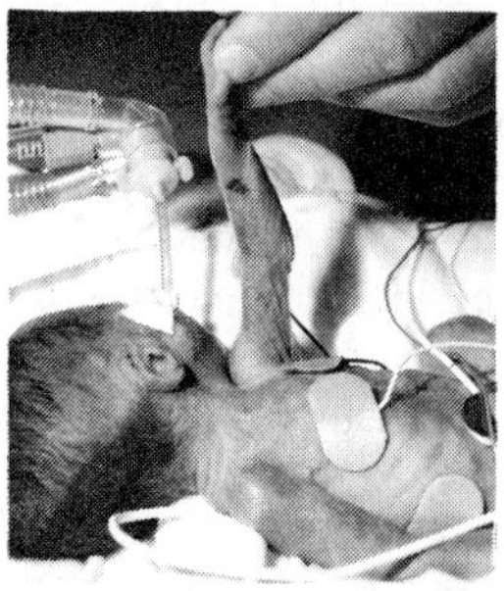

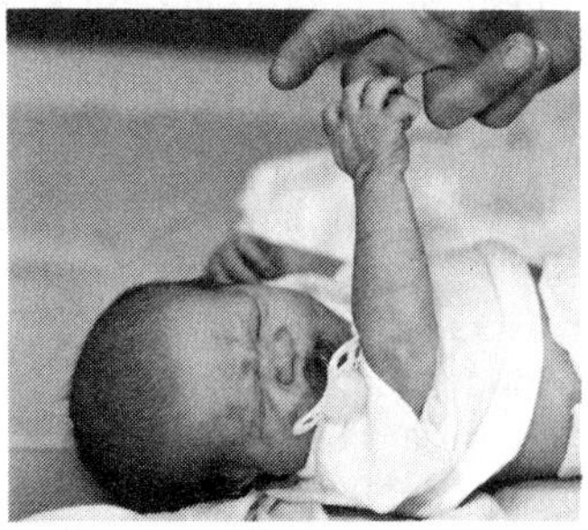

Heel-to-ear maneuver—The preterm infant's heel is easily brought to the ear, meeting with no resistance. This maneuver is not possible in the term infant, since there is considerable resistance at the knee.

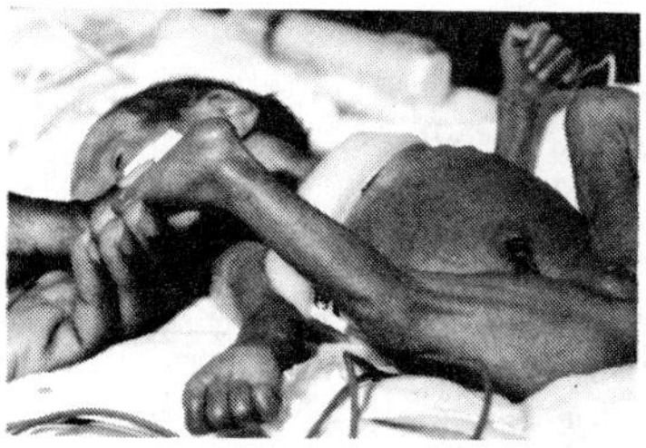

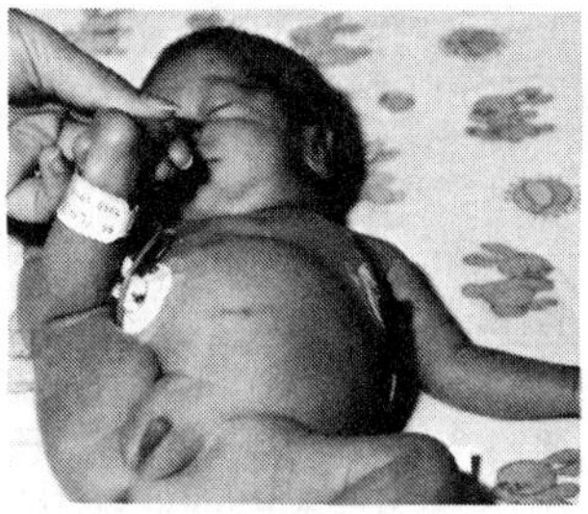

Fig. 10-12, cont'd. For legend see opposite page.

in a smooth appearance. The bones of the skull and the ribs feel soft, and the prominent eyes may be closed. Male infants have few scrotal rugae, and the testes are undescended; the labia and clitoris are prominent in females. (See Fig. 10-12 for a comparison of the features of normal and premature infants.)

In contrast to full-term infants' overall attitude of flexion and continuous activity, premature infants are inactive and torpid. The extremities maintain an attitude of extension and remain in any position in which they are placed. Reflex activity is only partially developed—sucking is absent, weak, or ineffectual; swallowing, gag, and cough reflexes are weak; and other neurologic signs are absent or diminished. Physiologically immature, preterm infants are unable to maintain body temperature, have limited ability to excrete solutes in the urine, and have increased susceptibility to infection. A pliable thorax along with immature lung tissue and regulatory center lead to periodic breathing, hypoventilation, and frequent periods of apnea. They are more susceptible to biochemical alterations such as hyperbilirubinemia and hypoglycemia (see Chapter 9), and they have a higher extracellular water content that renders them more vulnerable to fluid and electrolyte derangements. Premature infants will exchange fully half their extracellular fluid volume every 24 hours as compared with one seventh in adults.

The soft cranium is subject to characteristic nonintentional deformation, or "preemie head," caused by positioning from one side to the other on a mattress. The head looks disproportionately longer from front to back, is flattened on both sides, and lacks the usual convexity seen at the temporal and parietal areas (Budreau, 1987). This positional molding is frequently a concern to parents and may influence the parents' perception of the infant's attractiveness and their responsiveness to the infant. Positioning the infant on a waterbed mattress can reduce or minimize cranial molding.

Therapeutic Management

When preterm infants are anticipated, the intensive care nursery is alerted and a pediatrician, ideally a neonatologist, is present for their delivery. Infants who do not require resuscitation are transferred immediately to the NICU in a heated incubator where they are weighed, and intravenous lines, oxygen therapy, and other therapeutic interventions are initiated as determined by the needs of the infants. Resuscitation is conducted in the delivery area until infants can be safely transported to the NICU. Ongoing care is described elsewhere in the chapter and is not repeated in this section.

Nursing Considerations

The nursing care, like the therapeutic management, is individualized for each infant. See appropriate discussions under Nursing Care of High-Risk Infants for details of care.

POSTMATURE INFANTS

Infants born of a gestation that extends beyond 42 weeks as calculated from the mother's last menstrual period are considered to be postmature or postterm, regardless of birth weight. This constitutes approximately 12% of all births. The cause of delayed birth is unknown. Some infants are appropriate for gestational age, but many show the characteristics of progressive placental dysfunction. Others—often called postmature infants—display the characteristics of infants who are 1 to 3 weeks of age, such as absence of lanugo, little if any vernix caseosa, abundant scalp hair, long fingernails, and whiter skin than term newborns. Frequently the skin is cracked, parchmentlike, and desquamating. A common finding in postmature infants is a wasted physical appearance that reflects intrauterine deprivation. Depletion of subcutaneous fat gives them a thin, long appearance. The little vernix caseosa that remains in the skin folds is usually stained a deep yellow or green.

There is a significant increase in fetal and neonatal mortality in postterm infants compared with those born at term. They are especially prone to intrauterine hypoxia associated with the decreasing efficiency of the placenta and to the meconium aspiration syndrome. The greatest risk occurs during the stresses of labor and delivery, particularly in infants of *primigravidas,* women delivering their first child. Cesarean section or induction of labor is usually recommended when infants are significantly overdue.

HIGH RISK RELATED TO DISTURBED RESPIRATORY FUNCTION

The lungs are critical to the early adaptation to extrauterine life and must be prepared to assume independent respiration as soon as the placental blood supply is interrupted. To support respiration, it is essential that sufficient prenatal maturation takes place in order to ensure adequate surface area, blood supply, and metabolic capability to maintain ventilation and tissue oxygenation. Deficiencies relative to this vital function can seriously impair respiratory efforts, and most of the neonates who require neonatal intensive care have respiratory problems.

APNEA OF PREMATURITY

Apnea of prematurity (AOP), or recurrent idiopathic AOP, is a common phenomenon in the preterm infant. Rarely observed in full-term infants, the prevalence of apneic spells increases the younger the gestational age. Approximately one third of infants less than 32 weeks of gestation and almost all apparently healthy infants less than 30 weeks of gestation have apneic spells. Characteristically, premature infants are periodic breathers; they have periods of rapid respiration separated by periods of very slow breathing and often short periods during which there are no visible or audible respirations. Apnea is primarily an extension of this periodic breathing and can be defined as a lapse of spontaneous breathing for 20 or more seconds, which may or may not be followed by bradycardia and color change. Apnea of prematurity should not be confused with apnea of infancy (see Chapter 13).

Box 10-12 POSSIBLE CAUSES OF NEONATAL APNEA

- Airway obstruction with mucus or poor position
- Anemia
- Dehydration
- Cooling
- Overheating
- Hypercapnia
- Hypocapnia
- Hypoglycemia
- Hypocalcemia
- Sepsis, meningitis
- Seizures
- Increased vagal tone (frequently observed in infants with very full stomachs after eating)
- Prolonged periodic breathing
- Central nervous system depression from pharmacologic agents
- Intracranial hemorrhage
- Heart failure
- Depression following maternal obstetric sedation
- Respiratory-distressed infants who are tiring

Pathophysiology

Although the cause of AOP is unknown, it probably reflects the immature and poorly refined neurologic and chemical respiratory control mechanisms. These infants are not as responsive to oxygen and carbon dioxide, and their neurons have fewer dendritic associations than those of the more mature infant. The respiratory reflexes of these infants are significantly more immature, which may be a contributing factor in the etiology (Gerhardt and Bancalari, 1984). In addition, apnea is characteristically observed during periods of rapid eye movement in sleep.

Clinical Manifestations

A number of factors that appear to promote the incidence of apnea in preterm neonates can be treated. Apnea can be anticipated in infants with any of a variety of circumstances (Box 10-12); conversely, one of these disorders may be suspected in infants with persistent apneic spells. Although apnea is an expected event in preterm neonates, it should not be designated as such until all other causes are ruled out. The observation of apnea is cause to screen for any of the causes listed in Box 10-12.

Therapeutic Management

It has been found that oral administration of theophylline is often effective in reducing the frequency of primary apnea-bradycardia spells in newborns. Theophylline and caffeine act as central nervous system (CNS) stimulants to breathing. Neonates who receive these drugs have serum theophylline levels measured regularly and must be closely observed for symptoms of toxicity. Serum theophylline is determined by the size and response of the infant and is maintained within a therapeutic range, which varies among NICUs.*

✦ **NURSING ALERT** Signs of theophylline toxicity are tachycardia (rate greater than 180 to 190 beats per minute) and (later) vomiting.

Nursing Considerations

Management of periodic apnea consists of monitoring respiration and heart rate routinely in all small preterm infants and prevention of conditions that might precipitate it. Mechanical apnea monitors provide a means to alert the staff to cessation of respiration according to a preset delay time, usually 15 to 20 seconds. Effective monitoring devices do not make alert nursing observation unnecessary. Any mechanical device is subject to malfunction. Without close observation, even of monitored infants, many unidentified episodes of prolonged apnea and severe bradycardia occur (Southall and others, 1983). Nursing observation combined with monitoring is the most effective means of identifying neonatal apnea (Muttitt and others, 1988).

✦ **NURSING ALERT** When the alarm sounds, infants are first assessed for color and for presence of respiration. If they display the usual color and respirations, the nurse should investigate possible causes of a false alarm, such as faulty lead placement, detached or disconnected leads, improper alarm setting, or mechanical failure.

If it is begun early, gentle tactile stimulation, such as rubbing the back or chest gently or turning the infant over, will stop most apneic spells. If stimulation fails to reinstitute respiration, the nose and oropharynx are suctioned, and if breathing does not begin, the chin is raised gently and sufficient pressure is applied with mask and bag to lift the rib cage. The infant is never shaken. After breathing is restored, the infant is assessed for possible precipitating factors, such as temperature, humidity, distention (if not observed earlier), and ambient oxygen content of the incubator. It is important for nurses to document episodes of apnea. A careful record is maintained of the number of apneic spells, the appearance of the infant during and after attacks, and whether the infant self-stimulates or if exogenous stimulation is needed to restore breathing. Persistent and repeated periods of apnea are treated by mechanical ventilation with the respirator set at low pressure and rate.

Various methods devised to provide an intermittent stimulus for breathing, such as oscillating water beds, have achieved variable success. A water bed providing continuous, gentle, irregular, head-to-foot oscillations by way of a small, inflatable bladder connected to an electronic oscillator supplies very subtle vestibular-proprioceptive stimulation for breathing. Although in one study LBW infants on water beds were found to sleep more, to be less restless during sleep, and to display fewer jittery or unsmooth movements, the incidence of apnea was not affected (Korner, Ruppel, and Rho, 1982). VLBW infants were more distressed on water beds than were larger LBW infants.

*Therapeutic ranges for theophylline have been described as 6 to 12 μg/ml, 7 to 14 μg/ml, and 8 to 11 μg/ml in NICUs polled.

IDIOPATHIC RESPIRATORY DISTRESS SYNDROME

Respiratory distress is a name applied to respiratory dysfunction in neonates and is primarily a disease related to developmental delay in lung maturation. The terms *respiratory distress syndrome* (RDS), *idiopathic respiratory distress syndrome* (IRDS), and *hyaline membrane disease* (HMD) are most often applied to the severe lung disorder that is not only responsible for more infant deaths than any other disease but also carries the highest risk in terms of long-term respiratory and neurologic complications (see Chapter 32 for a discussion of adult RDS). It is seen almost exclusively in preterm infants. The disorder is rare in infants of narcotic-addicted mothers or infants who have been subjected to intrauterine stress (e.g., maternal preeclampsia or hypertension). *Pneumonia* in the neonatal period is respiratory distress caused by pathogenic organisms and may occur alone or as a complication of IRDS.

Pathophysiology

Preterm infants are born before the lungs are fully prepared to serve as efficient organs for gas exchange. This appears to be a critical factor in the development of RDS. Although the precise cause is still undetermined, several features in the development of the disorder are established, and there are a number of interdependent relationships that complicate the situation.

Before birth there is evidence of fetal respiratory activity. The lungs make feeble respiratory movements, and fluid is excreted through the alveoli. Since the final unfolding of the alveolar septa, which increases the surface area of the lungs, takes place during the last trimester of pregnancy, premature infants are born with numerous underdeveloped and many uninflatable alveoli. There is limited pulmonary blood flow, resulting from the collapsed state of the fetal lungs and from poor vascular development in general and an immature capillary network in particular. Because of the increased pulmonary vascular resistance, the major portion of fetal blood is shunted from the lungs by way of the ductus arteriosus and foramen ovale (see Cardiac Development and Function, Chapter 34).

At the time of birth, infants must initiate breathing and then keep the previously fluid-filled lungs inflated with air. At the same time the pulmonary capillary blood flow must be increased approximately tenfold to provide for adequate lung perfusion and to alter the intracardiac pressure that closes the fetal cardiac structures. Most full-term infants successfully accomplish these adjustments; preterm infants with respiratory distress are unable to do so. Although numerous factors are involved, most authorities believe that the central factor responsible for this adaptation is normal development of the surfactant system.

Surfactant is a surface-active phospholipid secreted by the alveolar epithelium. Acting much like a detergent, this substance reduces surface tension of fluids that line the alveoli and respiratory passages, resulting in uniform expansion and maintenance of lung expansion at low intraalveolar pressure. Immature development of these functions produces consequences that seriously compromise respiratory efficiency. Deficient surfactant production causes unequal inflation of alveoli on inspiration and collapse of alveoli on end expiration. Without surfactant, infants are unable to keep their lungs inflated and therefore exert a great deal of effort to reexpand the alveoli with each breath. It has been estimated that each breath requires as much negative pressure (60 to 75 cm H_2O) as the initial lung expansion at birth. As a result, infants use more oxygen to expend this energy than they take in, which rapidly leads to exhaustion. With increasing exhaustion they are able to open fewer and fewer alveoli. This inability to maintain lung expansion produces widespread atelectasis.

In the absence of alveolar stability (normal functional residual capacity) and with progressive atelectasis, the pulmonary vascular resistance (PVR) increases, whereas with normal lung expansion it would decrease. Consequently there is hypoperfusion to the lung tissue with a decrease in effective pulmonary blood flow. The increase in PVR causes partial reversion to the fetal circulation with a right-to-left shunting of blood through the persisting fetal communications—the ductus arteriosus and foramen ovale.

Inadequate pulmonary perfusion and ventilation produce hypoxemia and hypercapnia. Pulmonary arterioles, with their thick muscular layer, are markedly reactive to diminished oxygen concentration. Thus a decrease in oxygen tension causes vasospasm in the pulmonary arterioles that is further enhanced by a decrease in blood pH. This vasoconstriction contributes to a marked increase in PVR. In normal ventilation with increased oxygen concentration, the ductus arteriosus constricts and the pulmonary vessels dilate to decrease PVR (Fig. 10-13).

Prolonged hypoxemia activates anaerobic glycolysis, which produces increased amounts of lactic acid. An increase in lactic acid causes metabolic acidosis; inability of the atelectatic lungs to blow off excess carbon dioxide produces respiratory acidosis. Lowered pH causes further vasoconstriction. With deficient pulmonary circulation and alveolar perfusion, the Pa_{O_2} continues to fall, the pH falls, and materials needed for surfactant production are not circulated to the alveoli.

Pulmonary edema observed in the early stages of IRDS also contributes to impaired gas exchange. Factors believed to facilitate this fluid accumulation in the lungs include renal immaturity or insufficiency resulting from hypoxemia, high fluid intake and patent ductus arteriosus, left ventricular dysfunction associated with papillary muscle necrosis, low serum protein concentration and low colloid osmotic pressure, increased alveolar surface tension that enhances the shift of interstitial fluid to alveolar spaces, oxygen toxicity, and high plasma vasopressin (summarized by Yeh and others, 1982).

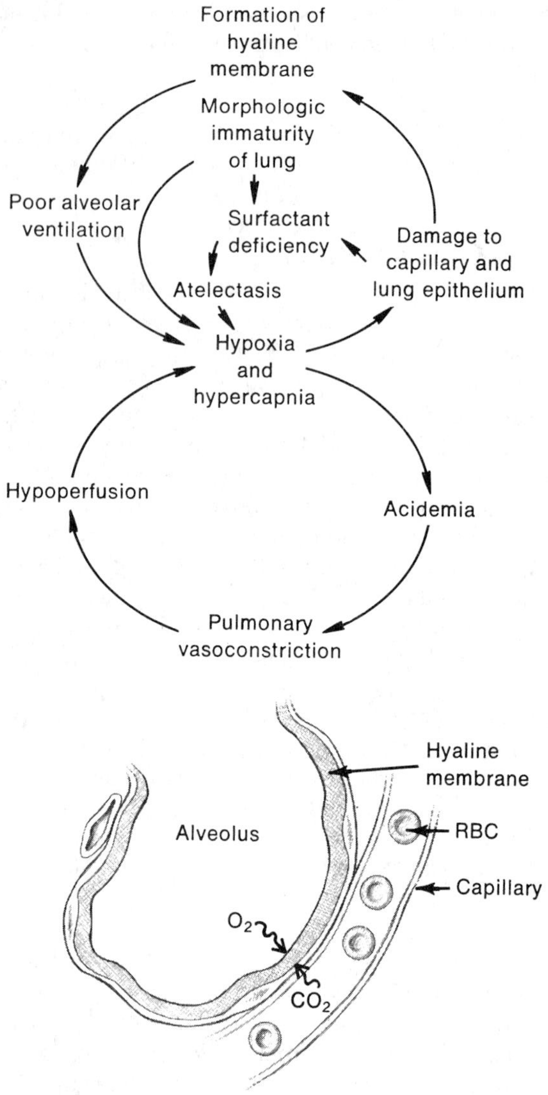

Fig. 10-13. Interdependent relationship of factors involved in pathology of idiopathic respiratory distress syndrome.
From Pierog, S.H., and Ferrara, A.: Medical care of the sick newborn, ed. 2, St. Louis, 1976, Mosby–Year Book, Inc.

Deficiencies in other systems contribute to respiratory distress. For example, a high threshold of the respiratory center to afferent stimuli and weak gag and cough reflexes reflect the immaturity of the nervous system. In addition, the persistence of fetal hemoglobin, so beneficial in prenatal existence, may place the infant at a disadvantage during respiratory distress. Although the binding power of fetal hemoglobin for oxygen is much greater than in adult hemoglobin, this increased affinity also causes less oxygen to be released to the tissues at normal oxygen tension. In the newborn the arterial oxygen concentration must fall to a lower level for bound oxygen to be released from fetal hemoglobin.

A hyaline membrane is formed as hypoxemia and the in-

Table 10-3 Major factors in respiratory distress

CAUSE	EFFECT
Increased surface tension of alveoli (surfactant deficiency)	Alveolar collapse; atelectasis; increased difficulty of breathing
Impaired gas exchange	Hypoxemia and hypercapnia with respiratory acidosis
Increased pulmonary vascular resistance	Hypoperfusion of pulmonary circulation
Hypoperfusion (with hypoxemia)	Tissue hypoxia and metabolic acidosis
Increased transudation of fluid into lungs	Hyaline membrane formation; impaired gas exchange

creased pulmonary vascular pressure cause transudation of fluid into the alveoli. Necrotic cells from damaged alveoli plus the fibrin in the transudate form a membranous layer that lines the alveoli and inhibits gas exchange. Presence of the membrane contributes to respiratory difficulties by greatly diminishing lung distensibility, or *compliance,* the elastic quality of lung tissue that permits expansion in response to a given amount of applied pressure during inspiration. Affected lungs are stiffer and require far more pressure than do normal lungs to achieve an equal amount of expansion. The major factors that produce respiratory distress in immature infants are summarized in Table 10-3.

IRDS is a self-limiting disease, and following a period of deterioration (approximately 48 hours) and in the absence of complications, affected infants begin to improve by 72 hours. Often heralded by the onset of diuresis, this improvement has been attributed primarily to increased production and greater availability of surface-active material.

Clinical Manifestations

Infants with IRDS can develop respiratory insufficiency either acutely or over a period of hours. Usually the observable signs produced by the pulmonary changes begin to appear in infants who apparently achieve normal breathing and color soon after birth. In 30 minutes to 2 hours breathing gradually becomes more rapid (greater than 60 breaths per minute). Infants may display retractions—suprasternal or substernal; supracostal, subcostal, or intercostal—which result from a compliant chest wall. Weak chest wall muscles and the highly cartilaginous nature of the rib structure produce an abnormally elastic rib cage. Thus considerable negative pressure is wasted as the infant attempts to produce higher intrathoracic pressure changes. During this early period the infant's color remains satisfactory and auscultation reveals good air entry. Some of the criteria for evaluating respiratory distress in infants are illustrated in Fig. 10-14.

Within a few hours, respiratory distress becomes more obvious. The respiratory rate continues to increase (to 80 to 120 breaths per minute), and breathing becomes more labored. It is significant to note that infants will increase the *rate* rather than the *depth* of respiration when in distress. Substernal retractions become more pronounced as the diaphragm works hard in an attempt to fill collapsed air sacs. Fine inspiratory rales can be heard over both lungs, and there is an audible expiratory grunt. This grunt, a useful mechanism observed in the earlier stages of IRDS, serves to increase end-expiratory pressure in the lungs, thus maintaining alveolar expansion and allowing gas exchange for an additional brief period. Flaring of the nares is also a sign that accompanies tachypnea, grunting, and retractions in respiratory distress. Central cyanosis (a bluish discoloration of oral mucous membranes and generalized body cyanosis) is a late and serious sign of respiratory distress. Initially cyanosis may be abolished by supplemental oxygen.

At this point the respiratory distress may gradually decrease over 12 to 24 hours with eventual recovery, or it may increase in severity. In distressed infants cyanosis becomes more marked despite increases in ambient oxygen concentration. Often there is pallor caused by peripheral vasoconstriction, but it is frequently masked by cyanosis. The infants become flaccid and unresponsive and begin to display frequent apneic episodes. Chest auscultation reveals diminished breath sounds. The chances of recovery without assisted ventilation are then very small. Severe IRDS is often associated with a shocklike state, as manifested by diminished cardiac inflow and low arterial blood pressure.

Infants with IRDS who survive the first 96 hours have a reasonable chance of recovery. Complications of IRDS include those described as complications of oxygen therapy (see Chapter 31), patent ductus arteriosus and congestive heart failure, persistent pulmonary hypertension, intraventricular hemorrhage, bronchopulmonary hyperplasia, retinopathy of prematurity, necrotizing enterocolitis, and neurologic sequelae.

Diagnostic Evaluation

Laboratory data are nonspecific, and abnormalities observed are identical to those observed in numerous biochemical abnormalities of the newborn, that is, the findings of hypoxemia, hypercapnia, and acidosis. To determine complicating factors, specific tests are carried out, such as blood, urine, and spinal fluid cultures (to rule out sepsis), blood glucose (to test for hypoglycemia), serum calcium (to test for hypocalcemia), blood gas measurements for serum pH (to test for acidosis), and Pa_{O_2} (to test for hypoxia). Other special examinations may be employed to diagnose or rule out complications.

Radiographic findings characteristic of IRDS include (1) a diffuse granular pattern over both lung fields closely resembling ground glass that represents alveolar atelectasis, and (2) dark streaks, or bronchograms, within the ground glass areas that represent dilated air-filled bronchioles (Fig. 10-15). It is important to distinguish between IRDS and pneumonia in infants with respiratory distress.

Prenatal diagnosis. Fetal lung maturity depends on

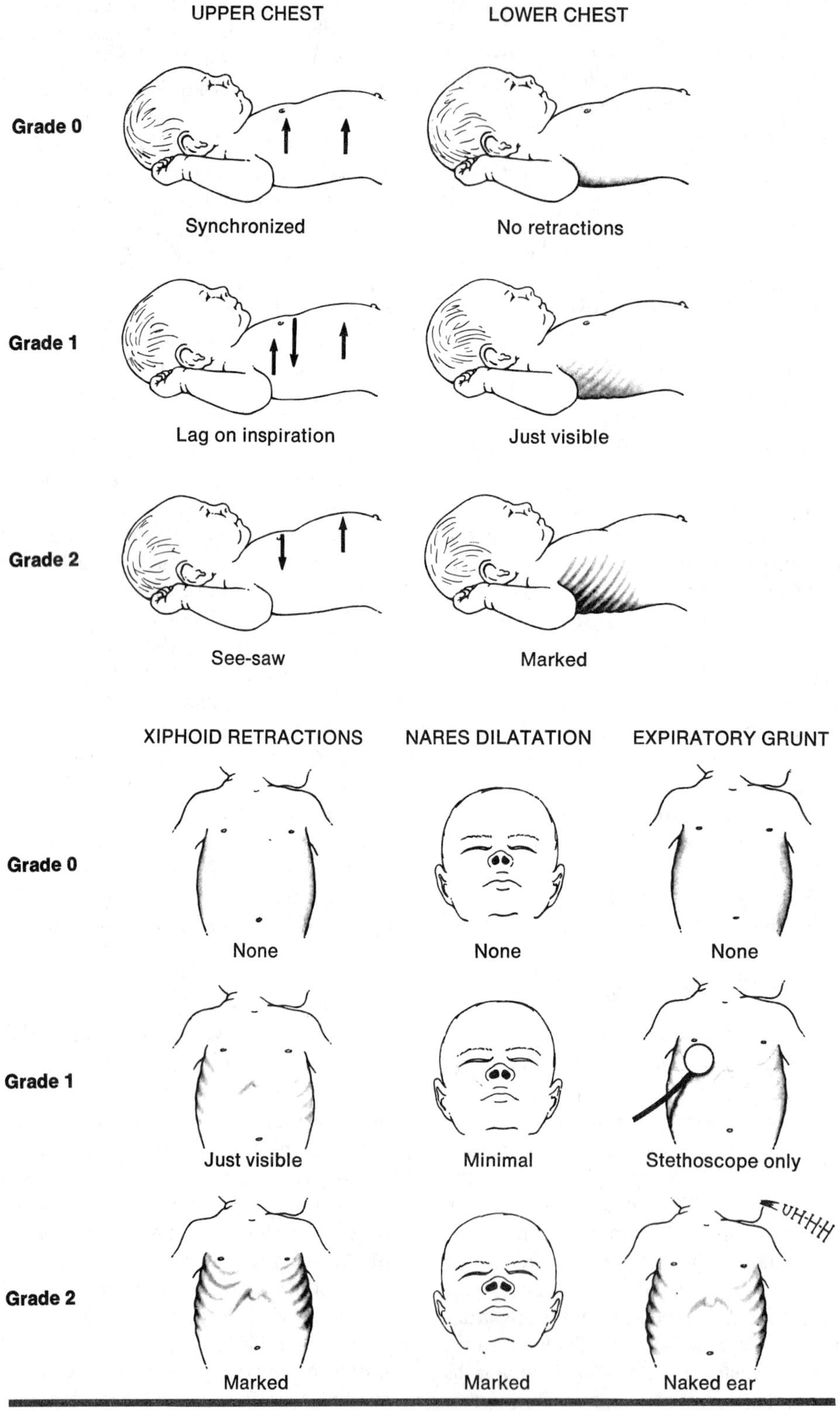

Fig. 10-14. Criteria for evaluating respiratory distress.

Adapted from Silvermann, W.A., and Anderson, D.H.: Pediatrics 17:1, 1956. Copyright American Academy of Pediatrics, 1956.

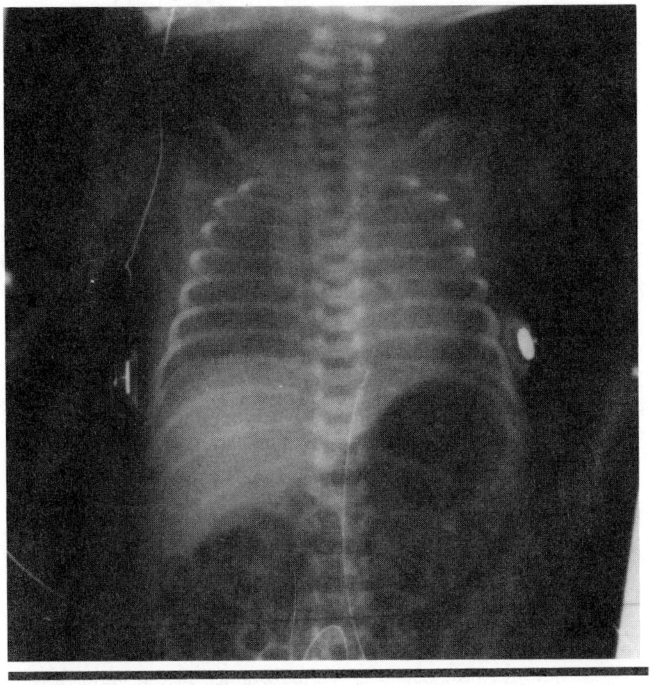

Fig. 10-15. Reticulogranular infiltrate and air bronchogram in hyaline membrane disease. Note air in stomach.

gestational age, except in some specific instances that may not be known until the time of labor or delivery. Functional maturity of the fetal lung can be determined by using surfactant phospholipids in amniotic fluid as indicators of maturity. The most commonly tested is the lecithin/sphingomyelin (L/S) ratio, which measures the relationship between these two lipids during gestation. Phospholipids are synthesized by fetal alveolar cells, and the concentrations in amniotic fluid change during gestation. Initially there is more sphingomyelin, but at about 32 to 33 weeks the concentrations become equal, and then sphingomyelin diminishes and lecithin increases significantly until the fetus has developed sufficient surface-active material to maintain alveolar stability at about 35 weeks.

Other key surfactant compounds (also phospholipids) that are needed to stabilize surfactant are phosphatidylinositol (PI) and phosphatidylglycerol (PG). Without these compounds lecithin is not functional as a surfactant. Concentrations of PI parallel those of lecithin, peaking at 35 weeks and gradually decreasing. At 36 weeks PG appears in amniotic fluid and increases until term. By measuring these phospholipids—L/S ratio, PI, and PG—the maturity of the lungs can be estimated with a high degree of accuracy. Abnormal pregnancies may be associated with acceleration (before 33 weeks) or delay (later than 37 weeks) in fetal lung maturation.

Other, but less frequently employed, methods have been devised to provide rapid, inexpensive, and accurate measures of lung maturity. These include the "shake" or "bubble" test, in which stable foam or bubbles form when amniotic fluid is shaken in the presence of ethanol, and the tap tests, in which abundant bubbles appear in a test tube of amniotic fluid with 6N hydrochloric acid and diethyl ether (Socol, Sing, and Depp, 1984).

Therapeutic Management

The treatment of IRDS is largely supportive and includes all the general measures required for any premature infant, as well as those instituted to correct imbalances. The supportive measures that are most crucial to a favorable outcome are (1) maintain a neutral thermal environment to conserve utilization of oxygen, (2) provide additional fraction of inspired oxygen (Fio_2) content by increasing ambient oxygen concentration or by assisted ventilation, (3) prevent hypotension and hypovolemia, (4) correct respiratory acidosis by assisted ventilatory support, and (5) correct metabolic acidosis by intravenous administration of sodium bicarbonate, which also dilates pulmonary vessels and reduces the constriction response. Nipple and gavage feedings are contraindicated in any situation that creates a marked increase in respiratory rate because of the greater hazards of aspiration. Nutrition is provided by parenteral therapy during the acute stage of the disease.

Oxygen therapy. The goals of oxygen therapy are to provide adequate oxygen to the tissues, prevent lactic acid accumulation resulting from hypoxia, and at the same time avoid the toxic effects of oxygen. Numerous methods have been devised to improve oxygenation (Table 10-4). All require that the gas be warmed and humidified before entering the respiratory tract. If the infant does not require mechanical ventilation, oxygen can be supplied to a plastic hood placed over the infant's head to supply variable concentrations of humidified oxygen (see Oxygen Therapy, Chapter 31). If oxygen saturation of the blood cannot be maintained at a satisfactory level and the carbon dioxide level ($Paco_2$) rises, infants will require ventilatory assistance.

Continuous positive airway pressure (CPAP) or *continuous positive pressure breathing* (CPPB), the application of 3 to 10 cm of water (positive) pressure to the airway, uses the infant's spontaneous respiration to improve oxygenation by helping prevent alveolar collapse and increasing diffusion time. If oxygenation is not improved, or if infants require assisted ventilation to decrease $Paco_2$ levels, *intermittent mandatory ventilation* (IMV) or *continuous positive pressure ventilation (CPPV)* is used with *positive end-expiratory pressure (PEEP)*. This allows infants to breathe at their own rate but provides positive pressure at regular preset intervals and end-expiratory pressure to prevent alveolar collapse and overcome tube resistance.

If the Pao_2 cannot be maintained or the $Paco_2$ level rises, infants may require one of three high-frequency ventilation (HFV) modalities. HFV delivers gas at very rapid rates to provide adequate minute volumes using lower proximal airway pressures by way of *high-frequency positive-pressure ventilation* (HFPPV), *high-frequency oscillation* (HFO), or *high-frequency jet ventilation* (HFJV). HFV is recommended for intractable respiratory failure, especially for infants with pulmonary air leaks. It is primarily a short-term therapy (Kercsmar and others, 1988), and it is believed to reduce

Table 10-4 Common methods for assisted and controlled ventilation in respiratory distress syndrome

METHOD	DESCRIPTION	HOW PROVIDED
Common methods		
Continuous positive airway pressure (CPAP) or continuous distending pressure (CDP)	Provides constant distending pressure to airway in spontaneously breathing infant	Nasal prongs Nasopharyngeal tubes Endotracheal tube
Positive end-expiratory pressure (PEEP)	Provides increased end-expiratory pressure that prevents alveolar collapse during controlled ventilation	Endotracheal intubation
Continuous positive-pressure ventilation (CPPV)	Maintains continuous positive pressure to airways in infant attached to ventilator	Endotracheal intubation and either volume- or pressure-controlled ventilators
Intermittent mandatory ventilation (IMV)	Allows infant to breathe spontaneously at own rate but provides mechanical cycled respirations and pressure at regular preset intervals	Endotracheal intubation and ventilator
Alternative methods		
High-frequency ventilation (HFV):		
High-frequency positive-pressure ventilation (HFPPV)	Low-compliant circuit provides high gas flow through the circuit: operates at rates between 60 and 150 breaths/minute	Conventional infant ventilators: endotracheal tube
High-frequency oscillation (HFO)	Application of high-frequency, low-volume, sine-wave flow oscillations to the airway at rates between 480 to 1200 breaths/minute	Variable-speed piston pump (or loudspeaker, fluidic oscillator); endotracheal tube
High-frequency jet ventilation (HFJV)	Uses a separate, parallel, low-compliant circuit and injector port to deliver small pulses or jets of fresh gas deep into airway at rates between 250 and 900 breaths/minute	May be used alone or with low-rate IMV with endotracheal tube

Table 10-5 Medications used in the treatment of respiratory distress syndrome

MEDICATION	PURPOSE	COMMENTS
Antibiotics	Treat pneumonia and/or septicemia Pneumonia prophylaxis	Observe for adverse response Check serum blood levels for selected medications
Aminoglycosides	Therapy for sepsis	Nephrotoxic; observe urine output and electrolytes Ototoxic; test for possible hearing impairment Check serum drug levels
Pancuronium	Muscle paralysis to prevent additive pressures generated when infant is breathing spontaneously during mechanical ventilation, to prevent air leaks, to provide better oxygenation and ventilation	Close observation of infant for muscle involvement and need for repeat dose Causes relaxed arterioles and pooling of blood Ventilator alarms in "on" position in case of accidental disconnection; infant unable to make any respiratory effort Eyes taped closed; eye drops to prevent corneal irritation
Furosemide	Facilitates renal excretion of fluid; reduces pulmonary edema Especially valuable when spontaneous diuresis does not occur	Observe for onset of diuresis Requires observation and fluid regulation to prevent dehydration Assess electrolyte status; K^+ replacement may be necessary Long-term use may result in calculi and hydronephrosis
Vitamin E	Decreases oxygen-derived free radical production Given prophylactically to infants on oxygen therapy to prevent or reduce the severity of retinopathy of prematurity, intraventricular hemorrhage, and bronchopulmonary dysplasia	Oxygen-free radicals believed to cause oxidative damage to tissues Use of drug is experimental

the incidence of barotrauma, which frequently complicates oxygen therapy (Boros and others, 1985; Carlo and others, 1984; Pokora and others, 1983). However, there is an increased incidence of necrotizing tracheitis reported with HFJV (Boros and others, 1986; Wiswell and others, 1988).

Complications of oxygen therapy. Although lifesaving, oxygen therapy is not without hazards. Positive pressure introduced by mechanical apparatus has caused an increased incidence of air leaks that produce complications, such as *pneumothorax* and *pneumomediastinum* (see discussion on p. 425). Other complications directly related to oxygen therapy include *retinopathy of prematurity* (p. 433), *bronchopulmonary dysplasia* (p. 425), and various problems associated with intubation, such as nasal, tracheal, or pharyngeal perforation, stenosis, inflammation, palatal grooves, subglottic stenosis, tube obstruction, and infection.

Medical therapies. In addition to the establishment of one or more intravenous lines to maintain hydration and nutrition, infants with respiratory distress syndrome receive a variety of medications. Those that are usually administered are outlined in Table 10-5.

A relatively recent addition to the medical therapies for IRDS is the administration of artificial surfactant or surfactant obtained from exogenous sources, such as human amniotic fluid following cesarean section, human pulmonary lavage, or animal lungs. The surfactant is given prophylactically at birth or on diagnosis of IRDS at 16 to 24 hours of age. Treatment prevents atelectasis and contributes to fluid clearance from alveoli, thereby increasing compliance and decreasing the work of breathing. In addition, the patent alveoli decrease pulmonary vascular resistance and increase blood flow to improve gas exchange. A single dose lasts approximately 72 hours. A dramatic improvement may take place with a single dose, but most infants require multiple doses (Kendig and others, 1988). Treated infants exhibit fewer respiratory complications (Collaborative European Multicenter Study Group, 1988; Lang and others, 1990).

Prevention. Since IRDS is a maturational disorder primarily related to the production of pulmonary surfactant, one approach to prevention is through stimulation of surfactant production. Some experiments with administration of corticosteroids to mothers from 24 hours to 7 days before delivery have demonstrated a significant reduction in the incidence of IRDS in their infants when compared with controls (Collaborative Group on Antenatal Steroid Therapy, 1981). No beneficial effects have been found in prevention of IRDS by administration of corticosteroids to infants after birth.

The most successful approach to prevention of IRDS is prevention of premature delivery, especially in elective early delivery and cesarean section. Improved methods for assessing the maturity of the fetal lung by amniocentesis, although not a routine procedure, allow a reasonable prediction of adequate surfactant formation (see Diagnostic Evaluation). Since estimation of a date of delivery can be miscalculated by as much as 1 month, these tests are particularly valuable when scheduling elective cesarean section. An aggressive approach using tocolysis (ritadine administration) to delay delivery and maternal administration of corticosteroids to induce surfactant production appears to reduce the incidence of IRDS in preterm infants (Kwong and Egan, 1986; Papageorgiou and others, 1989).

Nursing Considerations

Care of infants with IRDS involves all the observations and interventions described for high-risk infants. In addition, the nurse is concerned with the complex problems related to respiratory therapy and the constant threat of hypoxemia and acidosis that complicates the care of patients in respiratory difficulty.

The respiratory therapist, an important member of the neonatal intensive care team, is responsible for the maintenance of respiratory equipment. Although it is the responsibility of the respiratory therapist to regulate the apparatus, nurses should understand the equipment and be able to recognize when it is not functioning correctly. The most essential nursing function is to observe and assess the infant's response to therapy. Since oxygen concentration and ventilation parameters are prescribed according to the infant's blood gas measurements and transcutaneous oxygen ($TcPo_2$) and pulse oximeter readings and because an infant's status can change rapidly, continuous monitoring and close observation are mandatory.

Changes in oxygen concentration are based on these observations. The amount of oxygen administered, expressed as the fraction of inspired air (Fio_2), is determined on an individual basis according to pulse oximeter and/or direct or indirect measurement of arterial oxygen concentration. Capillary samples, collected from the heel (see Chapter 27 for the procedure), are useful for pH and $Paco_2$ determinations but *not* for oxygenation status. Continuous transcutaneous or pulse oximetry readings are recorded at least hourly. Blood sampling is necessary 15 to 30 minutes after ventilator changes for the acutely ill infant and every 2 to 4 hours for sick infants (Parry and Gunnell, 1989).

Thick, tenacious mucus may form in the respiratory tract as a result of the infant's pulmonary condition. Pulmonary debris interferes with gas flow and predisposes the infant to obstruction of the passages, including the endotracheal (ET) tube. Suctioning should be performed as often as necessary (every 15 minutes, every 1 to 2 hours, or once daily) based on individual infant assessment, which includes auscultation of the chest, evidence of decreased oxygenation, excess moisture in the ET tube, or increased infant irritability. Instillation of 0.25 to 0.5 ml of sterile normal saline in the ET tube before insertion of the suction catheter aids in loosening mucus and removing secretions.

✦ **NURSING ALERT** Suctioning is not an innocuous procedure (may cause bronchospasm, bradycardia due to vagal nerve stimulation, hypoxia, and increased intracranial pressure [ICP], predisposing to intraventricular hemorrhage) and should *never* be carried out on a routine basis (Hagedorn, Gardner, and Abman, 1989). Improper suctioning technique can also cause infection, airway damage, or even pneumothoraces.

When suctioning nasopharyngeal passages, the trachea, or ET tube, the catheter should be inserted gently but quickly, and then intermittent suction applied as the catheter is withdrawn. It is imperative that the time the airway is obstructed by the catheter be limited to no more than 5 seconds because continuous suction removes air from the lungs along with the mucus. The object of suctioning an artificial airway is to maintain patency of that airway, not the bronchi. Suction applied beyond the ET tube can cause traumatic lesions of the trachea. The Fio_2 should be increased by 10% before suctioning to compensate for a decrease in (Fio_2) during the procedure (see Chapter 31).

✦ **NURSING ALERT** The oxygenation monitor or pulse oximeter is observed before, during, and after the suctioning to provide an ongoing assessment of oxygenation status and to prevent hypoxemia.

Research indicates that suctioning to a point where the catheter meets resistance and is then withdrawn causes trauma to the tracheobronchial wall. A suction catheter premeasured to a point that extends 0.5 cm beyond the end of the ET tube and inserted to a matching mark on the ET tube provides effective removal of secretions without damage to tracheobronchial mucosa (Brodsky, Reidy, and Stanievich, 1987; Kleiber, Krutzfield, and Rose, 1988).

Removal of secretions can be further facilitated by positioning and application of percussion and vibration to the thoracic wall. The technique and positioning for postural drainage, percussion, and vibration are outlined in Chapter 31. However, the Trendelenburg position should not be used with these infants, since it can contribute to increased intracranial pressure. The principles are the same, but the cupped hand is much too large to be used on very small infants. Commercial devices are available for this purpose. Vibration is difficult to accomplish on infants whose respiratory rate is 60 to 80 breaths per minute. Commercial vibrators are also available that are safe in an O_2 environment (modified battery-operated devices, such as an electric toothbrush, pose shock hazards).

Percussion and vibration are performed as needed with rotation of segments of the lungs that are percussed. Preterm infants are unable to tolerate a full regimen each time. In those with a respiratory rate over 60 breaths per minute the procedures interfere with the expiratory phase, causing air trapping, hypoxemia, or hypercarbia. The length of time allotted to any given segment is also subject to the individual infant's tolerance and the degree of lobar involvement, which is best determined through radiologic evaluation.

The most advantageous positions for facilitating an infant's open airway are on the side with the head supported in alignment by a small folded towel or, when on the back, positioned to keep the neck slightly extended. With the head in the "sniffing" position, the trachea is opened at its maximum; hyperextension reduces the tracheal diameter in neonates. The supported side-lying position can also be used effectively (Bozynski and others, 1988).

Inspection of the skin is part of routine infant assessment. Position changes and use of water pillows or fleece are helpful in guarding against skin breakdown.

Mouth care is especially important when infants are receiving nothing by mouth, and the problem is often aggravated by the drying effect of oxygen therapy. Drying and cracking can be prevented by good oral hygiene using saline swabs. Irritation to the nares or mouth that occurs from appliances used to administer oxygen may be reduced by the use of a water-soluble ointment.*

MECONIUM ASPIRATION SYNDROME

Meconium aspiration is a serious condition that accounts for a substantial number of neonatal fatalities. It occurs when fetuses have been subjected to fetal asphyxia or other intrauterine stress that causes increasing peristalsis, relaxing of the anal sphincter, and passage of meconium into the amniotic fluid. The majority of meconium aspiration takes place with the first breath. However, a severely compromised fetus may aspirate in utero. At delivery of the chest and initiation of the first breath, infants inhale fluid and meconium in the nasoorophargynx.

Pathophysiology

Meconium-stained amniotic fluid is graded in severity from 1+ to 4+. Meconium that discolors the amniotic fluid to a "tea" color is 1+. The grade and the property to produce disease increase in direct relationship to the particulate matter in the fluid. Fresh meconium is very sticky and tenacious and, when inhaled, adheres to airways and alveoli, producing uneven obstruction and inhibiting normal airflow to and from gas-exchanging surfaces. This uneven ventilation, perfusion, and decreased lung compliance result in respiratory distress.

Affected infants increase respiratory efforts in order to create greater negative intrathoracic pressures and improve gas flow into the lungs. Hyperinflation plus hypoxemia and acidemia cause increased pulmonary vascular resistance. Right-to-left shunting (intrapulmonary, atrial, or ductus arteriosus) often follows. Air trapping associated with meconium obstructions of multiple airways causes overdistention of portions of the lungs and contributes to air leaks, which are common.

Clinical Manifestations

Infants who have been stressed for some time are stained from passage of green meconium stools (those with more recent meconium passage are not stained), tachypneic, hypoxic, and depressed at birth. They develop expiratory grunting and retractions similar to those experienced by infants with IRDS. Infants usually hyperventilate early in the course of the disease; later hypoventilation is noted. Cardiovascular hypoxemia, acidemia, hyperinflation, and pulmonary cardiovascular involvement contribute to cyanosis. The infants are often stressed, hypothermic, hypoglycemic, and hypocalcemic. Severe meconium aspiration progresses to respiratory failure.

---

*For Nursing Care Plan: The Infant with Respiratory Distress Syndrome, see Wong, D.L., and Whaley, L.F.: Clinical manual of pediatric nursing, St. Louis, 1990, Mosby–Year Book, Inc.

Diagnostic Evaluation

At birth, meconium can often be visualized in the respiratory passages and vocal cords. Chest radiographs show uneven distribution of patchy infiltrates, air trapping, and hyperexpansion.

Therapeutic Management

Prevention of meconium aspiration includes vigorous suctioning of the hypopharynx before delivery of the shoulders. Suctioning the trachea is controversial, although a frequently employed modality. Resuscitation is initiated and maintained until the infant is breathing spontaneously and has good color.

Infants with respiratory distress are admitted to the NICU. Management of chemical pneumonitis consists of ventilatory support, intravenous fluids, and chest percussion and postural drainage. Since these infants are prone to develop persistent pulmonary hypertension, they are maintained somewhat hyperoxic as a precautionary measure and may be candidates for extracorporeal membrane oxygneation therapy (see Persistent Pulmonary Hypertension of the Newborn, p. 432). Complications are managed symptomatically or as described under the specific disorder.

Nursing Considerations

Nursing considerations are the same as for any neonates. See nursing care in oxygen therapy, persistent pulmonary hypertension, and other complications.

EXTRANEOUS AIR SYNDROMES (AIR LEAKS)

Extraneous air syndromes, extraalveolar air accumulation, and *air leaks* are names applied to various clinically recognized disorders produced as a result of alveolar rupture and subsequent escape of air to tissues in which air is not normally present (Korones, 1986). Extraneous air collection (1) may occur spontaneously in normal neonates, (2) can result from congenital renal/pulmonary malformations, and (3) often complicates underlying respiratory disease and its therapy.

Following alveolar rupture, air often vents directly into the pleural space to create *pneumothorax*. It may vent into the perivascular interstitium, the *perivascular emphysema* space, where it can dissect along the perivascular sheaths to eventually enter the mediastinum and cause *pneumomediastinum*. More extensive leaks involve the pericardium, manifested as *pneumopericardium*, or emphysema in the cervical, subcutaneous, or retroperitoneal soft tissues.

Clinical Manifestations

Spontaneous pneumothorax usually occurs during the first few breaths after birth, primarily in term or postterm infants, and is evident by the gradual onset of symptoms of respiratory distress after arrival in the nursery. Positive pressure resuscitation and mechanical respiratory support have created an increase in the incidence of ruptured alveoli. It can be suspected on the basis of respiratory manifestations and a shift in location of maximum intensity of heart sounds and absent or diminished breath sounds (although breath sounds may not be altered because of the small diameter of the chest and auscultation of referred breath sounds). These may proceed to the more severe signs. Pneumothorax, predominantly tension pneumothorax, during ventilatory assistance is common.There may also be chest asymmetry, altered cardiac sounds (diminished, shifted, or muffled), palpable liver and spleen, and subcutaneous emphysema.

✦ **NURSING ALERT** Early manifestations of pneumothorax include tachypnea, restlessness and irritability, lethargy, grunting, flaring nares, and retractions. Pneumothorax during ventilatory assistance is evident from abrupt and profound duskiness or cyanosis, significant declines in heart rate, arterial blood pressure, and pulse pressure, and poor peripheral perfusion.

Therapeutic Management

Diagnosis is confirmed by transillumination of the chest with a fiberoptic probe and/or radiographic examination. Treatment is urgent. Evacuation of trapped air is accomplished by chest tube insertion into the pleural space through a small chest incision that is then attached to continuous suction via water-seal drainage. Needle aspiration serves as an emergency measure until chest tubes can be inserted. Pneumomediastinum seldom requires treatment, but pneumopericardium is managed by needle aspiration or tube drainage.

Nursing Considerations

The most important nursing function is close vigilance for the possibility of air leak in susceptible infants, which is most effective for early detection. Nurses maintain a high level of suspicion in (1) infants with IRDS with or without positive pressure ventilation, (2) infants with meconium-stained amniotic fluid, (3) infants with radiographic evidence of interstitial or lobar emphysema, (4) infants who required resuscitation at birth, or (4) infants receiving CPAP or positive-pressure ventilation. For infants at risk, needle aspiration equipment (30 ml syringe, three-way stopcock, and 19- to 25-gauge butterfly needles) should be at the bedside for emergency use.

The general nursing care of the infant with an exogenous air syndrome is the same as that for all high-risk neonates. Respiratory management is similar to that for infants with IRDS. Frequent assessment of breath sounds, monitoring efficacy of gas exchange, and regulating oxygen therapy according to the needs of the infants are vital nursing functions. Care of chest tubes is an additional responsibility and is not significantly different from care in older children and adults.

BRONCHOPULMONARY DYSPLASIA

Bronchopulmonary dysplasia (BPD), also known as *chronic* or *respirator lung disease,* is a pathologic process that may develop in the lungs of infants, primarily VLBW infants, with lung disorders (e.g., IRDS, meconium aspiration, and persistent pulmonary hypertension). BPD is an iatrogenic disease caused by therapies used to treat lung disease: exposure to high oxygen concentrations, use of positive-pressure ventilation (CPAP or PEEP), endotracheal intubation; prolonged use of these therapies; fluid overload; and patent ductus arteriosus (PDA). The reported incidence of the disorder in survivors of IRDS is between 20% and 30% (Koops, Abman, and Accurso, 1984), and the incidence of infants surviving with milder forms of chronic lung disease is much higher (Bancalari and Gerhardt, 1986). The infants who survive are at risk for frequent hospitalization because of their borderline respiratory reserve, hyperactive airway, and increased susceptibility to respiratory infection.

Pathophysiology

The pulmonary changes are characterized by interstitial edema and epithelial swelling followed by thickening and fibrotic proliferation of the alveolar walls and squamous metaplasia of the bronchiolar epithelium. Areas of atelectasis and cystlike foci of hyperaeration are visible on radiographs between 10 and 20 days of life and persist for weeks; however, some infants may not demonstrate cystic foci. In addition, the ciliary activity is paralyzed by high oxygen concentrations that interfere with the ability to clear the lung of mucus, thus aggravating airway obstruction and atelectasis.

As survival of immature preterm infants (less than 28 weeks of gestation) increases, the occurrence of BPD also increases. Despite the fact that management of O_2 therapy, barotrauma, fluids, and PDA has improved, BPD is still on the rise in VLBW and early-gestational-age infants (Hagedorn, Gardner, and Abman, 1989).

The marked similarity between BPD and the *Wilson-Mikity syndrome,* in which the lungs of premature infants exhibit alveolar thickening and cystlike patterns of hyperventilation, has led some investigators to theorize that the two disorders may be part of a continuous spectrum of the same lung disease. Other diseases associated with similar radiographic findings include congenital heart disease, viral pneumonia caused by cytomegalovirus, and pulmonary interstitial emphysema. There are no specific clinical signs or laboratory alterations that confirm a diagnosis, which is made on the basis of radiographic findings.

Therapeutic Management

The first approach to management is prevention of the disorder in susceptible infants. To reduce the risk of barotrauma when mechanical ventilation is being used, the lowest peak inspiratory pressure (PIP) necessary to obtain adequate ventilation is maintained and the lowest level of inspired oxygen is used to maintain adequate oxygenation. Fluid administration is carefully controlled and restricted. Drug or surgical intervention is indicated when there is a PDA.

There is no specific treatment for BPD except to maintain adequate arterial blood gases with the administration of oxygen and avoid progression of the disease. Some have reported improvement in infants administered dexamethasone (Gladstone, Ehrenkranz, and Jacobs, 1989; Harkavy and others, 1989), although the infants exhibited significant delay in weight gain. Weaning infants from the ventilator is difficult and must be accomplished gradually. These infants do not tolerate excessive or even normal amounts of fluid well and have a tendency to accumulate interstitial fluid in the lungs, which aggravates the condition.

Oral diuretics are used to control interstitial fluid. Bronchodilators may be effective and promote improvement in infants with chronic lung disease. Theophylline improves lung compliance and reduces expiratory resistance in BPD ventilated infants.

Growth and development are delayed in some infants with BPD, related in part to the difficulties in providing adequate nutrition and in part to the lack of normal sensory stimulation due to prolonged hositalization. Children with BPD have metabolic needs far greater than those of the average child (Kurzner and others, 1988). This can create a problem for the caregiver who must meet the goals of adequate nutrition while avoiding overhydration, especially if the child is ill, eats poorly, or has cardiopulmonary instability (Goldson, 1990). The infant may be further compromised by gastroesophageal reflux, a frequent complication in premature infants (see Chapter 33).

Prognosis. Reports vary regarding the mortality rate for this disorder. The hospital stay is frequently long because of the infant's need for supplemental oxygen, although home oxygen therapy provides selected infants the opportunity for discharge. However, a significant proportion of deaths occur after discharge from the hospital. Use of nasal cannulas provides an acceptable way to administer oxygen for the dependent infant to promote development of motor and social skills (Hagedorn, Gardner, and Abman, 1989). A large percentage of survivors have significant disabilities, such as cerebral palsy, mental retardation, deafness, and blindness, which is consistent with the VLBW infant population and probably unrelated to the BPD.

Nursing Considerations

Infants with BPD expend considerable energy in their efforts to breathe; therefore it is important that they receive plenty of opportunities for rest and additional calories. Growth records provide clues to the need for change in their diets, and some infants require nutritional supplements. Since they tire easily and large quantities of formula might compromise respiration, small frequent feedings are better tolerated.

NURSING ALERT Observe children for signs of respiratory distress.

Adequate hydration is extremely important because greater amounts of fluid are lost through respiration, and secretions must be thinned sufficiently to facilitate removal by coughing and suctioning. However, since BPD increases lung permeability, some infants are subject to pulmonary edema and require fluid restriction.

NURSING ALERT Nurses must be alert to signs of both overhydration and underhydration, such as weight changes, skin turgor, output measurements, urine specific gravity, and signs of edema.

Parents are extremely anxious regarding the prognosis when their infant has BPD. In addition, the lengthy hospitalization interferes with parent-child relationships and deprives the infant of parental stimulation. The nurses should encourage the parents to visit the infant and become involved in the routine care. The parents need to be informed regarding medical care, equipment, and procedures related to their infant and taught procedures, such as suctioning and chest physiotherapy.

Home care. Since the availability of home cardiac/apnea monitors and home oxygen therapy has increased, many of these infants can be discharged when they are gaining weight, oxygen need is low (less than 1 L/min) and they pass "room air challenge" (i.e., are able to keep O_2 saturation greater than 85% for 20 to 30 minutes in room air). Home care is desirable to promote parent-infant bonding, minimize health care costs, and prevent nosocomial infections. Preparation for home care requires education and considerable reassurance (see Chapter 26). Management of home monitoring equipment and home oxygen therapy is stress-provoking, but most families become comfortable with the machinery while their infant is still in the hospital. Families must be reminded about their infant's increased risk of infection and cautioned regarding contact with persons who have respiratory infections. Because of their minimum respiratory reserve, these infants can be threatened by even a minor illness.

Because of the high mortality rate in the first year, parents are taught cardiopulmonary resuscitation* and how to manage any other emergency that might be anticipated for their infant. Helping families cope with their anxieties and reassuring them of their ability to manage the care of their infant are important nursing functions. Parents need follow-up in the home and the comfort of knowing that help is only a telephone call away.

HIGH RISK RELATED TO INFECTIOUS PROCESSES

Newborns are highly susceptible to infection. Their immature immune systems and their inability to localize infection render them especially vulnerable to infectious organisms. Prevention of infection in neonates, particularly in infants who are already compromised by physiologic or structural disorders, is a primary nursing function. The nurse must be aware of potential sources of transmission and recognize those infants who are at risk.

*Home care instructions are available in Wong, D.L, and Whaley, L.F.: Clinical manual of pediatric nursing, ed. 3, St. Louis, 1990, Mosby–Year Book, Inc.

SEPSIS

Sepsis, or *septicemia*, refers to a generalized bacterial infection in the bloodstream. Neonates are highly susceptible to infection as a result of diminished nonspecific (inflammatory) and specific (humoral) immunity, such as impaired phagocytosis, delayed chemotactic response, minimum or absent IgA and IgM, and decreased complement levels. Because of the infant's poor response to pathogenic agents, there is usually no local inflammatory reaction at the portal of entry to signal an infection and the resulting symptoms tend to be vague and nonspecific. Consequently diagnosis and treatment may be delayed.

Although the mortality from sepsis has diminished, the incidence of septicemia has not diminished. Nursery epidemics are not infrequent, and the high-risk infant has a four times greater chance of developing septicemia than does the normal neonate. The frequency of infection is almost twice as great in male infants as in females and carries a higher mortality for males as well. Other factors increasing the risk of infection are prematurity, bottle-feeding, and use of steroids for treating lung disease. Bottle-feeding can introduce pathogens from environmental contamination of formula or equipment. However, with a proper surveillance program and good technique in handling and preparing formula this is usually not a major problem.

Breast-feeding has a protective benefit against infection. Colostrum contains agglutinins that are effective against gram-negative bacteria. Human milk contains large quantities of IgA and iron-binding protein that exert a bacteriostatic effect on *Escherichia coli.* Human milk also contains macrophages and lymphocytes that promote a local inflammatory reaction.

Pathophysiology

The premature withdrawal of the placental barrier leaves infants vulnerable to most common viral, bacterial, fungal, and parasitic infections. Normally, immune substances, primarily immunoglobulin G (IgG), are acquired from the maternal system and stored in fetal tissues during the final weeks of gestation to provide newborns with passive immunity to a variety of infectious agents. Early birth interrupts this transplacental transmission; thus preterm infants have a low level of circulating IgG; the concentrations of immune substances directly relate to the length of gestation. Immunoglobulin A (IgA), which plays a role in defense against viral infections, and immunoglobulin M (IgM), with properties that are most efficient in dealing with gram-negative organisms, are not transferred to fetuses, leaving infants highly vulnerable to invasion by these organisms.

Defense mechanisms of neonates are further hampered by a low level of complement, diminished opsonic ability, monocyte dysfunction, and reduced number and inefficient functioning of circulating leukocytes. Furthermore, these leukocytes, with diminished motility and phagocytic capacity, are unable to concentrate their limited numbers selectively at the site of infection. In addition, a hypofunctioning adrenal gland contributes only a meager antiinflammatory response. Consequently these deficiencies permit rapid invasion, spread, and multiplication of organisms.

Sources of Infection

Sepsis in the neonatal period can be acquired prenatally across the placenta from the maternal bloodstream or during labor from ingestion or aspiration of infected amniotic fluid. Prolonged rupture of the membranes always presents a risk of this type from maternal-fetal transfer of pathogenic organisms. In utero transplacental transfer of organisms can occur, such as cytomegalovirus, *Toxoplasma,* and *Treponema pallidum* (syphilis), which cross the placental barrier during the latter half of pregnancy.

Early sepsis (less than 3 days) is acquired at birth; infection can occur from direct contact with organisms from the maternal gastrointestinal and genitourinary tracts. The most common infecting organisms are *Streptococcus agalactiae* and *Escherichia coli,* which may be present in the vagina from fecal contamination. *E. coli* accounts for about two thirds of all cases of sepsis caused by gram-negative organisms. Proper hygiene of the perineum is one method of preventing this mode of transmission. Other pathogens that are harbored in the vagina and that may infect the infant include gonococci, *Candida albicans,* herpes simplex virus (type II), *Listeria* organisms, chlamydia, and β-hemolytic streptococci.

Late sepsis (1 to 3 weeks following birth) is primarily nosocomial, and the offending organisms are usually the staphylococci, *Klebsiella,* enterococci, and sometimes *Pseudomonas.* The infant is at risk for self-infection because of the proximity of the umbilical wound to the perineum. Bacterial invasion can also occur through sites other than the umbilical stump, such as the skin; mucous membranes of the eye, nose, pharynx, and ear; and internal systems such as the respiratory, nervous, urinary, and gastrointestinal systems.

Postnatal infection is acquired by cross-contamination from other infants, personnel, or objects in the environment. Bacteria that are frequently called "water bugs" (because they are able to grow in water) are found in water supplies, humidifying apparatus, sink drains, suction machines, most respiratory equipment, and indwelling venous and arterial catheters used for infusions, blood sampling, and monitoring vital signs. Neonatal sepsis is most common in the infant at risk, particularly the preterm infant or the infant born following a difficult or traumatic labor and delivery, who is least capable of resisting such bacterial invasion. Frequently these organisms are transmitted by the personnel from person to person or object to person by poor handwashing and inadequate housecleaning.

Clinical Manifestations

A few neonatal infections (e.g., pyoderma, conjunctivitis, omphalitis, and mastitis) are easily recognized. However, systemic infections are characterized by subtle, vague, nonspecific, and almost imperceptible physical signs. Often the only complaint concerning an infant's progress is "failure to do well," not looking "right," or nonspecific respiratory distress. Rarely is there any indication of a local inflammatory response, which would suggest the portal of entry into the bloodstream. The presence of some bacteria is indicated by a specific characteristic, for example, *Pseudomonas* organisms, which produce necrotic purplish skin lesions, or group B β-hemolytic streptococci, which usually result in severe respiratory distress, periods of apnea, and a chest radiograph identical to IRDS.

All body systems tend to show some indication of sepsis, although often there is little correlation between the manifestations and the etiologic factors involved. For example, convulsions may not represent CNS infection, and fever, a universal feature of infection in older children, may be absent in neonates. It is usually nursing observation of subtle changes in the appearance and behavior of infants that leads to the detection of infection. The nonspecific, early signs are hypothermia and changes in color, tone, activity, and feeding resulting in unabsorbed formula with abdominal distention, jaundice, lethargy, and apnea. Significantly, similar signs may be manifestations of a number of clinical conditions unrelated to sepsis, such as hypoglycemia, hypocalcemia, heroin withdrawal, or CNS disorders. Since meningitis is a frequent sequela of sepsis, signs of increased intracranial pressure (ICP) may also be evident. Clinical signs that may indicate possible neonatal sepsis are listed in Box 10-13.

Diagnostic Evaluation

Because sepsis is so easily confused with other neonatal disorders, the definitive diagnosis is established by laboratory and radiographic examination. Isolation of the specific organism is always attempted through cultures of blood, urine, and cerebrospinal fluid. Direct (conjugated) hyperbilirubinemia often occurs in infants with sepsis, particularly sepsis of gram-negative origin. Blood studies may show signs of anemia, leukocytosis, or leukopenia. Leukopenia is usually an ominous sign because of its frequent association with high mortality.

Therapeutic Management

Early recognition and diagnosis with institution of vigorous therapeutic measures are essential to increase the infant's chance for survival and reduce the likelihood of permanent neurologic damage. Often diagnosis of sepsis is based on suspicion, and antibiotic therapy is initiated before laboratory results are available for confirmation and identification of the exact organism. Treatment consists of circulatory support, respiratory support, aggressive administration of antibiotics, and immunotherapy.

Supportive therapy usually involves administration of oxygen if respiratory distress or cyanosis is evident, careful regulation of fluids and correction of electrolyte or acid-base imbalance, and temporary discontinuation of oral feedings. Blood transfusions may be needed to correct anemia and shock, and electronic monitoring of vital signs and regulation of the thermal environment are mandatory.

Antibiotic therapy is continued for 7 to 10 days if cultures are positive, discontinued in 3 days if cultures are negative, and most often administered via intravenous infusion. Transfusions with fresh, irradiated granulocytes or polymorphonuclear leukocytes obtained from adult donors by con-

Box 10-13 MANIFESTATIONS OBSERVED IN NEONATAL SEPSIS

General Signs
Infant generally "not doing well"
Poor temperature control—hypothermia, hyperthermia (rare)

Circulatory System
Pallor, cyanosis, or mottling
Cold, clammy skin
Hypotension
Edema
Abnormal heartbeat—bradycardia, tachycardia, arrhythmia

Respiratory System
Irregular respirations, apnea, or tachypnea
Cyanosis
Grunting
Dyspnea
Retractions

Central Nervous System
Diminished activity—lethargy, hyporeflexia, coma
Increased activity—irritability, tremors, seizures
Full fontanel
Increased or decreased tone
Abnormal eye movements

Gastrointestinal System
Poor feeding
Vomiting, increased stomach residual after feeding
Diarrhea or decreased stool
Abdominal distention
Hepatomegaly

Hematopoietic System
Jaundice
Pallor
Purpura, petechiae, ecchymosis
Splenomegaly
Bleeding

tinuous-flow centrifugation leukapheresis have been introduced as therapy for bacterial sepsis. The results have proved to be highly effective in lowering mortality from this disease. Intravenous gammaglobulin has also proved effective as a prophylactic measure against nosocomial infections (Chirico and others, 1987; Clapp and others, 1989).

Prognosis is variable. Before the discovery of antibiotics the mortality from bacterial sepsis was 95% to 100%, but early recognition, antibiotics, and supportive therapy have reduced mortality to less than 50% (Bruhn and Jones, 1985). However, mental retardation can occur with late diagnosis of meningitis or inadequate length of treatment.

Nursing Considerations

Nursing care of the infant with sepsis involves observation and assessment as outlined for any high-risk infant. Recognition of the existing problem is of paramount importance; it is usually the nurse who observes and assesses infants and who identifies that "something is wrong" with them. Awareness of the potential modes of infection transmission also helps the nurse identify those at risk for developing sepsis. Much of the care of infants with sepsis involves the medical treatment of the illness. Knowledge of the side effects of the specific antibiotic and proper regulation and administration of the drug are vital. Because the volume of fluid required to administer antibiotics via Soluset would seriously compromise a small infant, antibiotics are usually administered via a heparin lock system or special injection cap near the infusion site. The medication is administered slowly by mechanical pump.

Prolonged antibiotic therapy poses additional hazards for affected infants. Oral antibiotics destroy intestinal flora responsible for synthesis of vitamin K, which can reduce blood coagulability. In addition, they predispose the infants to growth of resistant organisms and superinfection from fungal or mycotic agents, such as *Candida albicans.* Nurses must be alert for evidence of such complications.

A number of specimens may be needed to help identify the cause and source of the infection. For obtaining spinal fluid for examination, the time-honored positioning in the side-lying, flexed posture has been recently challenged (Gleason and others, 1983). The investigators found that although Po_2 decreased and heart rate increased with infants in any of three positions (lateral recumbent with full flexion, lateral recumbent with partial neck extension, and sitting with head support and spine flexion), the Pco_2 increased only in the fully flexed position. It is recommended that the fully flexed position be avoided and that the side-lying position (modified with neck extension) or the sitting position be used for obtaining spinal fluid specimens. Continual cardiorespiratory and pulse oximetry monitoring provides an ongoing assessment of the infant's condition during the procedure.

Part of the total care of infants with sepsis is to decrease any additional physiologic or environmental stress. This includes providing an optimum thermoregulated environment and anticipating potential problems, such as dehydration or hypoxia. Precautions are implemented to prevent spread of infection to other newborns, but to be effective, activities must be carried out by all caregivers. Proper handwashing, use of disposable equipment (e.g., linens, catheters, feeding utensils, and intravenous equipment), disposing of excretions (e.g., vomitus and stool), and adequate housekeeping of the environment and equipment are essential. Since nurses are the most consistent caregivers involved with sick infants, it is usually their responsibility to oversee that all phases of isolation are maintained by everyone.

Another aspect of caring for infants with sepsis involves observation for signs of complications including meningitis and shock, a severe complication caused by the release of toxins into the bloodstream.

NURSING ALERT Observe for signs of complications such as meningitis (full or bulging anterior fontanel or presence of seizure behavior) or shock (rapid, irregular respirations and pulse). Blood pressure usually falls when an infant is in septic shock, and therefore this measurement should be a part of the monitoring of all infants' routine vital signs.

Other complications of sepsis include pyarthrosis (which may affect any joint but most commonly localizes in the hip) and osteomyelitis. Local inflammation of the involved area is again uncommon, so identification is difficult. Limited movement of the affected joint and/or extremity may be one of the few indications of infection.

NECROTIZING ENTEROCOLITIS

Necrotizing enterocolitis (NEC) is an acute inflammatory disease of the bowel with increased incidence in preterm and other high-risk infants, but it is most common in those who weigh less than 2000 g. Three factors appear to play an important role in its development: intestinal ischemia, colonization by pathogenic bacteria, and excess substrate (formula feeding) in the intestinal lumen.

Pathophysiology

The precise cause of the disorder is still uncertain, although it appears to occur in infants whose gastrointestinal tract has suffered vascular compromise. Intestinal ischemia in fetuses is most commonly a consequence of decreased cardiac output as a result of asphyxia. In newborns enteric vascular ischemia is an effect of an earlier oxygen depletion in the brain and heart that triggered the "diving reflex." To meet the oxygen needs of these vital organs, blood is shunted away from the organs that are better able to withstand prolonged anoxia, such as the intestines. As a result of this circulatory shunting, there is convulsive vasoconstriction of the mesenteric vessels with a severe reduction of blood supply to the intestines.

The damage to mucosal cells lining the bowel wall is great—diminished blood supply to these cells causes their death in large numbers, they stop secreting protective, lubricating mucus, and the thin, unprotected bowel wall is attacked by proteolytic enzymes. Thus the bowel wall continues to swell and break down. In addition, it is unable to synthesize protective immunoglobulin M (IgM), and the mucosa is permeable to macromolecules, such as exotoxins, which further hampers intestinal defenses. Gas-forming bacteria invade the damaged areas to produce *pneumatosis intestinales,* the presence of air in the submucosal or subserosal surfaces of the bowel.

A consistent relationship has been observed between the development of NEC and enteric feeding of hypertonic substances, for example, formula and hyperosmolar medications. It is unclear whether this connection is the result of the formula imposing a stress on an ischemic bowel, serving as a substrate for bacterial growth, or both.

Clinical Manifestations

The prominent clinical signs of NEC are a distended (often shining) abdomen, gastric retention, and blood in the stools or gastric contents. Nonspecific signs include lethargy, poor feeding, hypotension, apnea, vomiting (often bile-stained), decreased urine output, and unstable temperature. The onset is usually between 4 and 10 days, but signs may be evident as early as 4 hours and as late as 30 days. NEC in full-term infants almost always occurs in the first 10 days when the gut is least mature; late-onset NEC is confined primarily to preterm infants (Wilson and others, 1982).

Diagnostic Evaluation

Radiographic studies show a sausage-shaped dilation of the intestine that progresses to marked distention and the characteristic pneumatosis intestinales—"soapsuds" or bubbly appearance of thickened bowel wall and ultralumina. There may be air in the portal circulation or free air observed in the abdomen, indicating perforation. Laboratory findings may include anemia, leukopenia, leukocytosis, and electrolyte imbalance. In severe cases coagulopathy and/or thrombocytopenia may be evident. Organisms are often cultured from blood, although bacteremia or septicemia may not be prominent early in the course of the disease. Breath hydrogen measurements are suggested as an aid to diagnosis of NEC and have proved to be 99% effective in detecting absence of the disease, thereby preventing prolonged withholding of feedings from these infants (Cheu, Brown, and Rowe, 1989).

Therapeutic Management

Treatment of NEC begins with prevention. Oral feedings are withheld for at least 24 to 48 hours from infants who are believed to have suffered birth asphyxia and as long as deemed necessary from VLBW infants. Breast milk is the preferred enteral nutrient because it confers some passive immunity (IgA), macrophages, and lysozymes.

Treatment of confirmed NEC consists of discontinuation of all oral feedings, institution of abdominal decompression via nasogastric suction, administration of intravenous antibiotics, and correction of extravascular volume depletion, electrolyte abnormalities, acid-base imbalances, and hypoxia. Replacing oral feedings with parenteral fluids decreases the need for oxygen and circulation to the bowel.

Prognosis. With early recognition and treatment, medical management is increasingly successful. If there is progressive deterioration under medical management or evidence of perforation, surgical resection and anastomosis are carried out. Extensive involvement may necessitate establishment of an ileostomy, jejunostomy, or colostomy. Sequelae in surviving infants include short-gut syndrome (see Chapter 33), colonic stricture with obstruction, fat malabsorption, and failure to thrive secondary to intestinal dysfunction.

Nursing Considerations

Nursing responsibilities begin with early recognition. Because the signs are similar to those observed in many other disorders of the newborn, nurses must constantly be aware of the possibility of this disease.

✢ **NURSING ALERT** Observe for indications of early development of NEC by checking the abdomen frequently for distention (palpating and measuring abdominal girth, measuring residual gastric contents before feedings, and listening for presence of bowel sounds), serial hematocrit measurements, and performing all routine assessments for high-risk neonates.

When the disease is suspected, the nurse assists with diagnostic procedures and implements the therapeutic regimen. Vital signs, including blood pressure, are monitored for changes that might indicate impending sepsis or cardiovascular shock, and measures are instituted to prevent transmission to other infants. It is especially important to avoid rectal temperatures because of the increased danger of perforation. To avoid pressure on the distended abdomen and to facilitate continuous observation, infants are frequently left undiapered and positioned supine or on the side.

Conscientious attention to nutritional and hydration needs is essential, and antibiotics are administered as prescribed. The time at which oral feedings are reinstituted varies considerably but is usually at least 7 to 10 days following diagnosis and treatment. Sterile water or electrolyte solution may be given initially and followed by dilute human milk (if available) or elemental predigested formula. The concentration is gradually increased as tolerated until the infant is again taking full-strength feedings.

Since NEC is an infectious disease, one of the most important nursing functions is control of infection. Strict handwashing is the primary barrier to spread, and confirmed cases are isolated with the use of cohort nursing, the same nurses caring for the infected infants. No one with symptoms of a gastrointestinal disorder should care for these or any other infants.

The infant who requires surgery requires the same careful attention and observation as any infant with abdominal surgery, including ostomy care. This disorder is one of the most frequent reasons for performing ileostomies on newborns. Throughout the medical and surgical management of infants with NEC, the nurse is continually alert to signs of complications, such as sepsis, disseminated intravascular coagulation, hypoglycemia, and other metabolic derangements.

■ HIGH RISK RELATED TO CARDIOVASCULAR COMPLICATIONS

LBW infants and those who are otherwise physically compromised are subject to complications in all major systems. This segment is not concerned with congenital cardiac anomalies or the complications that result from these lesions (see Chapter 34). The disorders described here are observed in the neonatal period, usually as complications of pulmonary dysfunction and respiratory therapy.

PERSISTENT PATENT DUCTUS ARTERIOSUS

A common complication of severe respiratory disease in preterm infants is persistent patent ductus arteriosus (PDA). It occurs in the majority of preterm infants under 1200 g, and the incidence diminishes in direct relationship to increasing birth weight. During fetal life the ductus remains patent through the vasodilatory action of prostaglandins within its tissues. Postnatally the increase in oxygen tension has a constricting effect on the ductus, but it may reopen in these small infants in response to the lowered oxygen tension associated with respiratory impairment. It is still unknown whether PDA is a contributing factor in the development of respiratory distress or whether respiratory distress contributes to the development of PDA.

Clinical Manifestations

Signs of PDA may appear within the first week of life. Early signs of PDA are increased $Paco_2$, decreased Pao_2, increased Fio_2, and recurrent apnea. Other signs include bounding peripheral pulses, wide pulse pressure with decreased diastolic blood pressure, pericardial hyperactivity, cardiomegaly, and a systolic or continuous murmur. If the PDA is wide open, a murmur may not be heard. Spontaneous closure usually takes place (usually within 12 weeks), but in infants with severe lung involvement the left-to-right shunting of blood leads to life-threatening pulmonary insufficiency. Confirmation of the diagnosis may be determined by echocardiography.

Therapeutic Management

Therapy consists of careful fluid regulation, respiratory support, and administration of indomethacin, a prostaglandin synthetase inhibitor that has been successful in constricting the ductus in critically ill, preterm infants. However, the drug has been found to inhibit platelet function, and its use has been questioned, especially in the presence of intraventricular hemorrhage. If a ductus reopens following cessation of therapy, reinstitution of the medication may produce a favorable response. Other therapies may be given before indomethacin is tried. These might include furosemide to prevent fluid overload and promote diuresis, Since indomethacin competes with albumin for binding sites, its use is controversial in infants with hyperbilirubinemia or compromised renal function. Digoxin is given to promote cardiac function. Surgical ligation may be necessary if medical therapy is unsuccessful after 48 hours.

Nursing Considerations

Nursing observations are important in the recognition and management of PDA. Assisting in early detection, assessing cardiovascular status carefully, and monitoring for complications following implementation of therapy are nursing responsibilities. The focus of activities related to therapy includes collection of specimens for laboratory examination, continued assessment of renal function (adequate urine output, any abnormal laboratory findings), and observation for any bleeding tendencies (hematest-positive stools or gastric aspirate, oozing from heel sticks or venipuncture sites, and laboratory evidence of clotting abnormalities) (Cohen, 1983).

Other nursing observations and management are the

same as for the high-risk infant and the infant with PDA (see Chapter 34).

PERSISTENT PULMONARY HYPERTENSION OF THE NEWBORN

Persistent pulmonary hypertension of the newborn (PPHN), or *persistent pulmonary hypertension* (PPH), formerly known as *persistent fetal circulation* (PFC), is a condition in which affected infants display severe pulmonary hypertension, with pulmonary artery pressure levels equal to or greater than systemic pressure, and large right-to-left shunts through both the foramen ovale and the ductus arteriosus. Since full development of pulmonary arterial musculature occurs late in gestation, PPHN is primarily a condition of full-term or postterm infants, many of whom were products of complicated pregnancies or deliveries. The condition is often associated with massive aspiration (especially meconium aspiration), cold stress, and/or respiratory distress (e.g., IRDS or pneumonia) and is believed to be precipitated by perinatal factors, such as perinatal asphyxia, that cause or contribute to vasospasm.

PPHN can be either primary or secondary: primary PPHN occurs when the pulmonary vascular system fails to open with the initial respiration at birth; secondary PPHN results from stress that increases pulmonary vascular resistance and causes a return to fetal cardiopulmonary circulation. PPHN is most frequently observed in infants at 35 to 44 weeks of gestation who have a history of perinatal asphyxia, polycythemia, acidosis, or sepsis and respiratory distress within the first 24 hours. The infants become hypoxic when agitated and display marked cyanosis, tachypnea with grunting and retractions, and decreased peripheral perfusion. A loud pulmonary component of the second heart sound and sometimes a systolic ejection murmur are present. Mild cases may display only minimum tachypnea and cyanosis during stressful episodes, such as crying or feeding.

Diagnosis is established from clinical signs and diagnostic tests including chest radiography, electrocardiography, echocardiography, and sometimes cardiac catheterization.

Therapeutic Management

Treatment includes careful fluid regulation and evaluation of intravascular fluid volume. Supplemental oxygen is administered to reduce hypoxia and decrease pulmonary vasoconstriction. Assisted ventilation may be needed if hypoxia is not corrected by noninvasive methods, often by airway hyperventilation, and is accompanied by paralysis with pancuronium to minimize opposition to the respirator (Fox and Duara, 1983). Vasopressors are frequently prescribed to decrease PVR thereby decreasing right-to-left shunting and increasing cardiac output.

Another approach to management of infants with pulmonary complications is the use of *extracorporeal membrane oxygenation* (ECMO) with a modified heart-lung machine. Blood is shunted from the right atrium to a servoregulated roller pump, pumped through a membrane lung and a small heat exchanger, and returned to the systemic circulation via the aorta. The ECMO provides oxygen to the circulation and allows the lungs to rest (Bartlett and others, 1985). The goal of ECMO is to "buy time" for the severely injured lung to heal while diminishing its exposure to oxygen and barotrauma (Fig. 10-16). However, recent reports of serious complications render its use less attractive.

Nursing Considerations

The nursing care is the same as for infants with respiratory difficulties and infants supported by mechanical respirators. Because handling for any reason causes a decrease in arterial oxygen concentration, the stresses imposed by routine care must be weighed against the risk of iatrogenic hypoxia. It is important to decrease noxious stimuli that cause crying and struggling and to employ nursing interventions, such as giving pacifiers, that keep nonsedated infants calm. Continuous monitoring of central venous pressure, vital signs, blood pressure, and $tcPo_2$, and pulse oximetry monitoring of oxygenation decrease the need for physical manipulation and disturbance. Infants are assessed for pulmonary vascular response, for example, increased Pao_2 and signs of systemic hypotension, gastrointestinal bleeding, or pulmonary hemorrhage.

ANEMIA

Preterm infants tend to develop anemia that is more severe and appears earlier than in more mature infants. It may be the result of hemorrhage during the course of labor and delivery (into brain, liver, spleen, or kidneys), blood disorders (hemolytic disease, thrombocytopenia), conditions that produce swelling or distention of abdominal organs, or iatrogenic from blood withdrawn in the NICU for laboratory tests. Physiologic characteristics of prematurity tend to contribute to development of anemia, that is, a drop in the production of fetal hemoglobin and shortened survival time of the red blood cells. This lag in hematopoiesis during continued growth results in physiologic anemia, probably as a consequence of diminished erythropoietin values (Stockman and others, 1984).

Fortunately, even VLBW infants are able to accommodate the gastrointestinal absorption of iron required for their high needs. Iron is supplied in iron-fortified formulas or iron supplements as both a preventive and therapeutic measure. Transfusions with packed red blood cells are often required for severe anemia, usually for replacement of blood loss resulting from iatrogenic measures. At 4 to 12 weeks of age a "physiologic anemia" reaches a peak, at which time infants sometimes display signs that suggest true anemia.

Nursing Considerations

One of the most common causes of anemia in preterm infants is blood loss associated with frequent sampling for blood gas and metabolic analyses. Therefore an important nursing responsibility is careful monitoring and recording of all blood drawn for tests. It is surprising how easily and rapidly the small total blood volume of premature infants is depleted by repeated withdrawals. Replacement is generally considered at 10% total blood volume deficit.

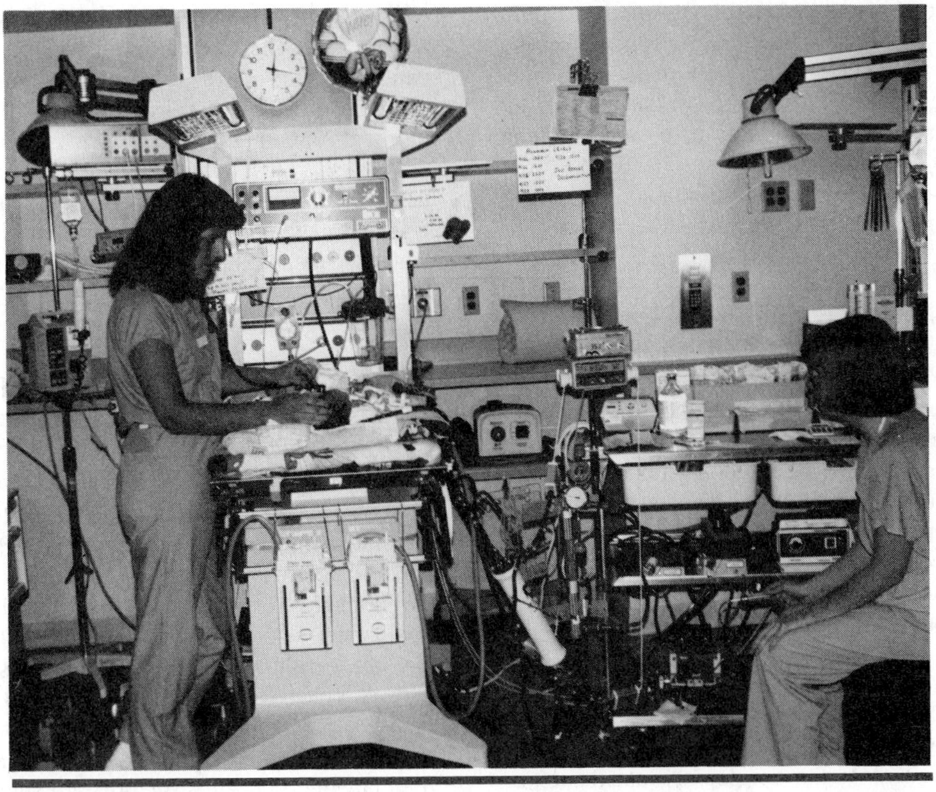

Fig. 10-16. Infant on extracorporeal membrane oxygenation. Two nurses are needed: one to monitor the infant and the other to monitor functioning of equipment.

Observation for signs of anemia is a vital nursing function. The traditional signs of anemia in the child are often observed in the preterm infant: feeding difficulties, dyspnea, tachycardia, tachypnea, diminished activity, and pallor. However, some infants may not display all of these signs. Poor weight gain may be an indication of a lowered hemoglobin level. Nursing precautions and observations during blood transfusion for the preterm infant are similar to those for any child.

POLYCYTHEMIA/HYPERVISCOSITY SYNDROME

The current definition of polycythemia is a venous hematocrit of 65% or more. Above a hematocrit of 65%, blood flow becomes increasingly sluggish and hyperviscous, resulting in hypoperfusion of organs. Polycythemia results from in utero twin-to-twin transfusion and maternal-fetal transfusion, prolonged emptying of placental blood to the infant at birth, or increased red blood cell production after birth. Among infants with polycythemia a high incidence of cardiopulmonary distress symptoms (persistent fetal circulation, cyanosis, and apnea), seizures, hyperbilirubinemia, and gastrointestinal abnormalities exists. However, there is confusion regarding which infants will display neonatal symptoms, which infants will have persistent neurologic and developmental abnormalities, and whether treatment affects the clinical course.

Therapy is equally controversial. However, appropriate therapy for correcting metabolic disturbances (e.g., hypoxia, hypoglycemia, and hyperbilirubinemia) is implemented, and lowering blood viscosity by partial plasma exchange transfusion may be considered in symptomatic cases.

Nursing considerations

Nursing care involves watching for signs of polycythemia (e.g., plethora, peripheral cyanosis, respiratory distress, lethargy, jitteriness or seizure activity, hypoglycemia, hyperbilirubinemia) and assisting with diagnostic tests and therapeutic procedures. Care of the infant with hyperbilirubinemia is discussed in Chapter 9.

RETINOPATHY OF PREMATURITY

Although often discussed in relation to respiratory dysfunction, *retinopathy of prematurity* (ROP) is a disorder involving blood vessels. ROP is a term used to describe all phases of retinal changes in the eye observed in preterm infants. The older term, *retrolental fibroplasia* (RLF), describes the cicatricial changes that characterize the later stages in the most severely affected infants. ROP is primarily, but not exclusively, a disease of premature infants. The incidence of the disease correlates with the degree of the infant's maturity—the younger the gestational age, the greater the likelihood of the development of ROP.

Numerous factors have been implicated in the cause of ROP in addition to immaturity, including hyperoxemia and hypoxemia, hypercarbia and hypocarbia, patent ductus arteriosus, prostaglandin synthetase inhibitors, apnea, intraventricular hemorrhage, infection, vitamin E deficiency, lactic acidosis, maternal diabetes, prenatal complications, and genetic factors. Previously considered to be an iatrogenic disease related to hyperoxia, ROP is now believed to be a complex disease of prematurity with multiple causes and therefore difficult to prevent and manage.

Pathophysiology

The disorder is characterized by severe vascular constriction in the immature retinal vasculature followed by hypoxia in those areas. This appears to stimulate vascular proliferation of retinal capillaries into the hypoxic areas where veins become numerous and dilate. As new vessels proliferate toward the lens, the aqueous humor and then the vitreous humor become turbid. The retina becomes edematous, and hemorrhages separate the retina from its attachment. Advanced scarring occurs from the retina to the lens, destroying the normal architecture of the eye. This extensive retinal detachment and scarring result in irreversible blindness.

Diagnostic Evaluation

A system of classification has been established to describe the location and extent of the developing vasculature involved. Normal vascular growth proceeds in an orderly fashion from the disc toward the *ora serrata,* the irregular anterior margin of the retina. The four stages of ROP are outlined in Box 10-14.

Therapeutic Management

Although judicious use and careful monitoring of supplemental oxygen have reduced the incidence of ROP, the disease has not been eradicated. Prophylactic administration of vitamin E has been used in some units but is still considered to be an experimental drug by the American Academy of Pediatrics Committee on Fetus and Newborn (1985); its use is not without complications.

Although prevention is the primary goal of therapeutic management, treatment of retinal pathology is directed toward arresting the proliferation process. Cryotherapy is the best treatment when performed by a pediatric ophthalmologist.

Box 10-14 FOUR STAGES OF RETINOPATHY OF PREMATURITY

1. A demarcation line (separates the avascular retina anteriorly from the vascularized retina posteriorly)
2. A ridge (formed from the demarcation line with the height and width, occupies volume, and extends beyond the plane of the retina)
3. A ridge with extraretinal fibrovascular proliferation
4. Retinal detachment

From An international classification of retinopathy of prematurity, Pediatrics 74:127-133, 1984.

Nursing Considerations

Adherence to the principles of oxygen administration and careful monitoring of oxygenation status are the first lines of defense against development of ROP (Hagedorn, Gardner, and Abman, 1989). Constant assessment and vigilance are necessary just as for any high-risk neonate. When the infant suffers partial or complete visual impairment, the parents will need a considerable amount of support and assistance in meeting the special developmental needs of the infant (see Chapter 25).

HIGH RISK RELATED TO NEUROLOGIC DISTURBANCE

Neurologic complications are observed with increased frequency in preterm infants and in infants born following a difficult labor and delivery. A disproportionately high incidence of perinatal encephalopathy, or cerebral palsy, and psychomotor retardation is found in the high-risk infant population, especially VLBW infants. Preterm infants are also more vulnerable to cerebral insults, such as hypoxia and chemical alterations. In addition, fragility and increased permeability of capillaries and prolonged prothrombin time predispose the brain of the preterm infant to trauma when delicate structures are subjected to increased pressure, such as the forces of labor, high mechanical ventilatory pressures, and seizure activity. All of these factors contribute to intracranial insults, including traumatic bleeding in the newborn, which consists of four major types: intraventricular, subdural, primary subarachnoid, and intracerebellar.

PERINATAL HYPOXIC-ISCHEMIC BRAIN INJURY

Hypoxic-ischemic brain injury is the most common cause of neurologic impairment of a nonprogressive type observed in infants and children. The brain damage usually results from intrauterine asphyxia, either before or during delivery, but it can happen postnatally as well. Ischemia and hypoxemia occur together, although one or the other predominates. The major causes of serious hypoxemia are listed in Box 10-15.

Newborns are particularly vulnerable to ischemic injury caused by decreased cerebral blood flow following asphyxia. Most infants who have suffered intrauterine oxygen deprivation have low Apgar scores; thus postnatal hypoxia is superimposed on an already existing problem.

Clinical Manifestations

The neurologic signs that indicate encephalopathy appear within the first hours after the hypoxic episode with manifestations of bilateral cerebral dysfunction. The infant is stuporous or comatose. Seizures begin after 6 to 12 hours in about 50% of the infants, and they become more frequent and severe by 12 to 24 hours. Between 24 and 72 hours there may be deterioration in the level of consciousness, and after 72 hours persistent stupor, abnormal tone (usually

Box 10-15 PRIMARY CAUSES OF PERINATAL HYPOXEMIA AND CEREBRAL ISCHEMIA

Perinatal Hypoxemia
1. Intrauterine asphyxia with respiratory failure at the time of birth
2. Postnatal respiratory insufficiency secondary to severe IRDS or recurrent apnea
3. Severe cyanotic heart defects (right-to-left shunts) or persistent pulmonary hypertension

Primary Cerebral Ischemia
1. Intrauterine asphyxia with cardiac insufficiency
2. Postnatal cardiac insufficiency secondary to severe congenital heart disease or recurrent apnea
3. Postnatal cardiovascular collapse secondary to sepsis

Data from Hill, A., and Volpe, J.J.: Seizures, hypoxic-ischemic brain injury, and intraventricular hemorrhage in the newborn, Ann. Neurol. 10:109-121, 1981.

hypotonia), and disturbances of sucking and swallowing are evident. Muscular weakness of the hips and shoulders is observed in full-term infants, and lower limb weakness occurs in premature infants. Apneic episodes are seen in approximately 50% of the affected infants.

Improvement in the neurologic deficiencies is highly variable and difficult to predict, although infants who demonstrate the most rapid initial improvement appear to have the best prognosis. Myocardial failure and acute tubular necrosis are frequent complications. The major long-term sequelae of hypoxic-ischemic injury are mental retardation, seizures, and cerebral palsy.

Therapeutic Management

Treatment involves vigorous supportive care to provide adequate ventilation to prevent aggravating the existing hypoxia and measures to maintain cerebral perfusion and prevent cerebral edema. Seizures are managed as described in the discussion on p. 436. Prevention is the most important therapy, however, and every effort should be made to recognize high-risk pregnancies, monitor the fetuses, and initiate appropriate therapy early.

Nursing Considerations

Nursing care is primarily the same as for any high-risk infant: careful assessment and observation for signs that might indicate cerebral hypoxia or ischemia, monitoring of ventilatory and intravenous therapy, observation and management of seizures, and general supportive care to infants and parents, including guidelines for management in the event of cognitive impairment (see Chapter 24). These infants are usually on intravenous alimentation.

PERIVENTRICULAR-INTRAVENTRICULAR HEMORRHAGE

Periventricular-intraventricular hemorrhage (PVH/IVH) is known by a variety of terms according to the locus of bleeding: *periventricular hemorrhage* (PVH), *intraventricular hemorrhage* (IVH), *germinal matrix hemorrhage–intraventricular hemorrhage* (GMH/IVH), and *subependymal-intraventricular hemorrhage* (SE/IVH). Most authorities use the term IVH to describe this disorder, which is responsible for a significant percentage of seriously ill infants and neonatal mortality. IVH is extremely common in preterm infants, especially VLBW infants less than 32 weeks of gestation and less than 1500 g (Minarcik and Beachy, 1989).

Pathophysiology

During the early months of prenatal development there is an extensive but fragile vascular network in the region of the ventricles that receives a disproportionately large amount of cerebral blood flow. Toward term, more blood is directed to the germinal matrix located in the periventricular region near the caudate nuclei of the cerebrum. Therefore premature infants are subject to rupture in this heavily vascularized region, especially during an event that is likely to increase cerebral blood flow, such as hypoxic episodes and the associated increased venous pressure. In PVH the bleeding originates in these capillaries. The blood may rupture through the ependymal lining of the ventricles and fill all or part of the ventricular system. Under pressure the ventricular system can dilate and cause acute hydrocephalus. Eventually obliterative arachnoiditis may develop and obstruct the flow of cerebrospinal fluid. In severe cases the hemorrhage extends into the cerebral parenchyma.

Several clinical features are associated with IVH, such as birth asphyxia, early gestational age, low birth weight, respiratory distress, metabolic derangements, and hypertension.

Clinical Manifestations

An increase in intracranial pressure (ICP) from hemorrhage is manifested by a sudden deterioration in condition—apnea, bradycardia, cyanosis, hypotonia, drop in hematocrit, full anterior fontanel, increased occipitofrontal circumference (OFC), separated sutures, and neurologic signs, such as twitching, stupor, apnea, and convulsions. Consumption of clotting factors during PVH may contribute to further bleeding and ventricular hemorrhage. Survivors of IVH may develop hydrocephalus, a variety of motor deficits, and mental retardation.

Diagnostic Evaluation

When intracranial hemorrhage is suspected, studies of intracranial stuctures are performed by ultrasonography, computed tomography (CT), or magnetic resonance imaging (MRI). A classification based on the extent of germinal matrix hemorrhage is listed in Box 10-16.

Therapeutic Management

Treatment of IVH is confined to supportive care, including ventilatory support, maintenance of oxygenation, regulation of fluid and acid-base balance, suppression of seizures, and any attendant complications. Although a number of therapies have been proposed, including spinal and ventricular taps, diuretics, indomethacin, phenobarbital, vitamin E, and steroids, none has received wide medical acceptance. Mus-

Box 10-16 CLASSIFICATION OF BRAIN HEMORRHAGE

0—no bleeding
1—germinal matrix only
2—germinal matrix with blood in the ventricles
3—germinal matrix with blood in the ventricles and ventricular dilatation
4—intraventricular and parenchymal bleeding (other than germinal matrix)

cle paralysis has been used to prevent intracranial hypertension precipitated by suctioning (Fanconi and Duc, 1987). The prognosis of infants suffering from IVH is based on the grade of injury; however, long-term outcome is unpredictable.

Nursing Considerations

In addition to the routine observations and management, nursing care is directed toward prevention of increased cerebral blood pressure. It has been observed that some nursing procedures increase ICP. For example, there is a marked increase in blood pressure during suctioning (Perlman and Volpe, 1983), and head positioning produces measurable changes in ICP. It has been found that ICP is highest when infants are in the dependent position and decreases when the head is elevated 30 degrees (Emery and Peabody, 1983). However, this finding is not universally supported.

Cerebral pressure is lower when infants are in a midline position as opposed to a right side-lying position. When the head is turned to the right without body alignment, the resulting venous congestion creates hydrostatic pressure fluctuations that increase ICP (Goldberg and others, 1983). Infants encumbered with tubes and monitoring equipment are more difficult to turn while maintaining head-body alignment.

Other interventions that may reduce the risk of increased ICP include avoiding interventions that cause crying (such as painful procedures). Crying can impede venous return, increase cerebral blood volume, and compromise cerebral oxygenation in LBW infants. These consequences must be considered when nursing care includes activities that precipitate crying. Care includes evaluating manipulations and handling, and administering analgesics to reduce discomfort. "Each intervention should be preceded by the questions, 'How stressful will this be for the infant?' and 'Is it necessary?' " (Kling, 1989).

INTRACRANIAL HEMORRHAGE

Intracranial hemorrhage (ICH) in neonates, although manifested in the same ways as those described in older children, occurs with different frequencies and different degrees of severity.

Subdural Hematomas

Subdural hematomas, life-threatening collections of blood in the subdural space, are most often produced by the stretching and tearing of the large veins in the *tentorium cerebelli,* the dural membrane that separates the cerebrum from the cerebellum. With improved obstetric care these have become relatively uncommon; however, they are especially serious because of the inaccessibility of the hematoma to aspiration by subdural tap. Less frequently, hemorrhage occurs when veins in the subdural space over the surface of the brain are torn (see also Head Injury, Chapter 37).

Subarachnoid Hemorrhage

Subarachnoid hemorrhage, the most common type of intracranial hemorrhage, occurs in term infants as a result of trauma and in preterm infants as a result of hypoxia. Small hemorrhages are the most common. Bleeding is of venous origin, and underlying contusion may also occur.

Intracerebellar Hemorrhage

Intracerebellar hemorrhage is a common finding on postmortem examination of the premature infant and can be a primary hemorrhage in the cerebellum associated with skull compression during abrupt, precipitous delivery, or it may occur secondary to extravasation of blood into the cerebellum from a ventricular hemorrhage. In the full-term infant the bleeding may follow a difficult delivery.

Nursing Considerations

Nursing care is the same as care of the infant with periventricular-intraventricular hemorrhage or with perinatal hypoxic-ischemic brain injury.

NEONATAL SEIZURES

Seizures in the neonatal period are usually the clinical manifestation of a serious underlying disease. Although not life threatening as an isolated entity, seizures constitute a medical emergency because they signal a disease process that may produce irreversible brain damage. Consequently it is imperative to recognize a seizure and its significance so that the cause as well as the seizure, can be treated (Box 10-17).

Pathophysiology

The features of neonatal seizures are different from those observed in the older infant or child. For example, the well-organized, generalized tonic-clonic seizures seen in older children are rare in infants, especially preterm infants. The newborn brain, with its immature anatomic and physiologic status and less cortical organization and myelination, is insufficient to allow ready development and maintenance of a generalized seizure. The advanced degree of development of limbic structures with connections to the diencephalon and brainstem probably accounts for the higher frequency of seizure manifestations that originate in these structures, such as oral movements, oculomotor deviations, and apnea.

Box 10-17 CAUSES OF NEONATAL SEIZURES

Metabolic
Hypoglycemia; hyperglycemia
Hypocalcemia
Hypomagnesemia
Pyridoxine deficiency
Aminoacidurias (e.g., phenylketonuria, maple syrup urine disease)

Toxic and Electrolyte
Hypernatremia
Hyponatremia
Narcotic withdrawal
Uremia
Bilirubin encephalopathy (kernicterus)

Prenatal Infections
Toxoplasmosis
Syphilis
Cytomegalic inclusion disease
Herpes simplex
Hepatitis

Postnatal Infections
Bacterial meningitis
Viral meningoencephalitis
Sepsis
Brain abscess

Trauma at Birth
Hypoxic encephalopathy
Intracranial hemorrhage
Subarachnoid, epidural hemorrhage
Intraventricular hemorrhage of prematurity

Malformations
Central nervous system agenesis
Hydroencephalopathy
Parencephalopathy
Tuberous sclerosis

Miscellaneous
Degenerative disease
Benign familial neonatal seizures

Table 10-6 Classification of neonatal seizures

TYPE	CHARACTERISTICS
Clonic	Rhythmic jerking movements About 1 to 3 per second May migrate randomly from one part of the body to another Simultaneous involvement of separate areas Movements may start at different times and at different rates
Tonic	Extensions of all four limbs (similar to decerebrate rigidity) Upper limbs are maintained in a stiffly flexed position (resembles decorticate rigidity) Appear more frequently in preterm infants Commonly associated with IVH
Myoclonic	Single or multiple flexion jerks of limbs Often indicate a metabolic etiology
Subtle	May develop in either full-term or preterm infants Often overlooked by inexperienced observer Signs: Clonic horizontal eye deviation Repetitive blinking or fluttering of the eyelids, staring Twitching Drooling, sucking, or other oral-buccal-lingual movements Arm movements resemble rowing or swimming Leg movements described as pedaling or bicycling Apnea (common) Signs may appear alone or in combination

Clinical Manifestations

Seizures in newborns may be subtle and barely discernible or grossly apparent. Since most neonatal seizures are subcortical, they do not have the etiologic and prognostic significance of seizures in children. The type of seizure is seldom important, since one may produce any of a variety of manifestations. Neonatal seizures can be divided into four major types. In order of frequency, these classifications are outlined in Table 10-6 and consist of clonic, tonic, myoclonic, and subtle seizures (Volpe, 1989). Clonic, multifocal clonic, and migratory clonic seizures are more common in term infants.

Jitteriness or tremulousness in the newborn is a repetitive shaking of an extremity or extremities that may be observed with crying, may occur with changes in sleeping state, or may be elicited with stimulation. Jitteriness is relatively common in newborns, affecting 44% of healthy full-term newborns in one study (Parker and others, 1990), and in a mild degree may be considered normal during the first 4 days of life. Jitteriness can be distinguished from seizures by several characteristics: jitteriness is not accompanied by ocular movement as are seizures; the dominant movement in jitteriness is tremor, whereas seizure movement is clonic jerking that cannot be stopped by flexion of the affected limb; and jitteriness is highly sensitive to stimulation, whereas seizures are not. If jittery movements persist beyond the fourth day, if the movements are persistent and prolonged after a stimulus, or if they are easily elicited with minimum stimulus, further evaluation is indicated.

A *tremor* is defined as repetitive movements of both hands (with or without movement of legs or jaws) at a frequency of 2 to 5 per second and lasting more than 10 minutes (Linder and others, 1989). It is common in newborn infants and has a variety of causes, including neurologic damage, hypoglycemia, and hypocalcemia. In most instances tremors are of no pathologic significance.

Diagnostic Evaluation

Early evaluation and diagnosis of seizures is urgent. In addition to a careful physical examination, the pregnancy and family histories are investigated for familial and prenatal causes. Blood is drawn for glucose and electrolyte examination, and cerebrospinal fluid is obtained for examination for gross blood, cell count, protein, glucose, and culture. Electroencephalography may help identify subtle seizures but is less helpful in establishing a diagnosis. Other diagnostic procedures, such as computed tomography and echoencephalography, may be indicated.

Therapeutic Management

Treatment is directed toward prevention of cerebral damage and involves correction of metabolic derangements, respiratory and cardiovascular support, and suppression of the seizure activity. The underlying cause is treated, for example, glucose infusion for hypoglycemia, calcium for hypocalcemia, and antibiotics for infection. If needed, respiratory support is provided for hypoxia, and anticonvulsants may be administered, especially when the other measures fail to control the seizures. Phenobarbital is the drug of choice given orally or intravenously and is used if seizures are severe and persistent. Other drugs that may be employed are phenytoin (Dilantin), paraldehyde, and diazepam (Valium).

Nursing Considerations

The major nursing responsibilities in the care of infants with seizures are to recognize when the infant is having a seizure so that therapy can be instituted, to carry out the therapeutic regimen, and to observe the response to the therapy and any further evidence of seizures or other symptomatology (see Nursing Tip). Assessment and other aspects of care are the same as for all high-risk infants. Parents need to be informed of their infant's status, and the nurse should reinforce and clarify the explanations of the practitioner. The infant's behaviors need to be interpreted for the parents, and the infant's responses to the treatment must be anticipated and their significance explained. Parents are encouraged to visit their infant and perform the parenting activities consistent with the plan of care. Seizures are a frightening phenomenon and generate a great deal of anxiety and fear, which is easily compounded by the justifiable concern of the staff. Providing support and guidance is an important nursing function.

NURSING TIP: DIFFERENTIATE TREMORS FROM SEIZURES

A simple test to rule out pathology in neonatal tremors is to stimulate sucking in the infant. The test consists of placing a pacifier or the examiner's gloved finger in the mouth of the infant, who is lying supine with both hands free. The test is considered to be a tremor if the activity stops instantly with sucking and returns after the finger or pacifier is removed (Linder and others, 1989).

HIGH RISK RELATED TO MATERNAL CONDITIONS

Conditions in the maternal system can have a significant effect on the fetus that extends into the postnatal period. A number of these conditions that are congenital malformations and disorders and can cause permanent disability are discussed in Chapter 11. Maternal diabetes and drug addiction are presented in the following section.

A number of maternal infections are detrimental to both the mother and the fetus. Some produce permanent physical or mental defects; others cause illness in the newborn period. It is important to be aware of a possible infection in the mother in order to be alert for evidence of the illness in the newborn, and to be aware of signs in the newborn that indicate intrauterine exposure to a maternal infection. (For further discussion see Chapter 11.)

INFANTS OF DIABETIC MOTHERS

Before insulin therapy, few diabetic women were able to conceive; for those who did, the mortality rate for both mother and infant was high. As a result of effective control of maternal diabetes and an increased understanding of fetal disorders, the morbidity and mortality of infants of diabetic mothers (IDMs) have been significantly reduced.

The severity of the maternal diabetes affects infant survival. Severity of maternal diabetes is determined by the duration of the disease before pregnancy, the age of onset, the extent of vascular complications, and abnormalities of the current pregnancy, such as pyelonephritis, diabetic ketoacidosis, pregnancy-induced hypertension, and noncompliance. The single most important factor influencing fetal well-being is the euglycemic status of the mother. It has been found that reasonable metabolic control started before conception and continued during the first weeks of pregnancy can prevent malformations in IDMs (Fuhrmann and others, 1983).

Effects of Diabetes on the Fetus

Hypoglycemia, defined as a blood sugar level below 35 mg/dl in the first 72 hours, 45 mg/dl thereafter for full-term newborns, and below 25 mg/dl for premature LBW infants, appears a short time after birth and is associated with increased insulin activity in the blood. It has been demonstrated that IDMs have hypertrophy and hyperplasia of the pancreatic islet cells and that they are actually in a state of hyperinsulinism.

It is generally agreed that during fetal life high maternal blood sugar levels provide a continual stimulus to the fetal islet cells for insulin production. This sustained state of hyperglycemia promotes fetal insulin secretion that ultimately leads to excessive growth and deposition of fat, which probably accounts for the infants who are large for gestational age (LGA). When the glucose supply is removed abruptly at the time of birth, the continued production of insulin soon depletes the blood of circulating glucose, creating a state of hyperinsulinism and hypoglycemia within ½ to 4 hours, especially in infants of mothers with class C diabetes or beyond. Precipitous drops in blood glucose levels can cause serious neurologic damage or death.

Tests of fetal well-being are performed routinely on the expectant mother with diabetes during pregnancy. Ultrasonography is performed at 18 to 20 weeks to determine fetal size and to rule out the presence of fetal anomalies. It may be repeated periodically during the course of fetal development. Urinary estriol, protein, and creatinine are measured weekly after 30 weeks of gestation, and nonstress or oxytocin challenge tests for assessment of fetal and placental function are performed after 33 weeks. Before delivery, fetal lung maturation tests via amniocentesis are carried out, including lecithin/sphingomyelin ratio, phosphatidylglycerol, and disaturated phosphatidylcholine measurements.

Some mothers are hospitalized at 36 to 37 weeks of gestation for management. Insulin and dietary alterations are made in accordance with blood glucose determinations. Techniques such as closed- or open-loop continuous insulin infusion devices may be employed to maintain a satisfactory blood glucose concentration.

Clinical Manifestations

Infants of well-controlled diabetic mothers are essentially no different from other infants, but infants of poorly controlled diabetic mothers have a characteristic appearance. They are usually macrosomic for their gestational age, very plump and full-faced, liberally coated with vernix caseosa, and plethoric. The placenta and umbilical cord are also larger than average. However, infants of mothers with advanced diabetes may be small for gestational age (SGA) or appropriate for gestational age (AGA) because of the maternal vascular involvement. There is an increase in congenital anomalies in this group in addition to a high susceptibility to hypoglycemia, hypocalcemia, hyperbilirubinemia, and IRDS. Abnormalities in these infants are the result of exposure to elevated glucose and ketone levels, placental insufficiency, and prematurity. Although they are large, these infants are often prematurely born in an elective early delivery or because of complications.

Therapeutic Management

The most effective management appears to be careful observation of all IDMs, often in the special care nursery. The infants are examined for the presence of any anomalies or birth injuries, and blood studies for initial determinations of glucose, calcium, hematocrit, and bilirubin are obtained on a regular basis.

Since the hypertrophied pancreas is so sensitive to blood glucose concentrations, the administration of oral glucose may trigger a massive insulin release resulting in rebound hypoglycemia. Therefore feedings of breast milk or formula are begun within the first hour after birth. Some practitioners prefer early feedings of nonglucose carbohydrates, such as invert sugar or galactose, because they are less insulinogenic. Approximately half of these infants do very well and adjust without complications. Critically ill infants require IV infusions. Oral and intravenous intake may be titrated to maintain adequate blood sugar levels. Frequent blood glucose determinations are needed for the first 2 days of life to assess the degree of hypoglycemia present at any given time. Testing blood taken from the heel with reagent strips is a simple and effective screening evaluation that can then be confirmed by laboratory examinations several times a day.

Nursing Considerations

Because some IDMs are born prematurely, they are subject to the problems discussed in relation to the preterm infant. In addition to the routine care of the newborn, the infants require observation for signs of complications.

✦ **NURSING ALERT** Nurses caring for IDMs are alert to signs of hypoglycemia (Chapter 9), hyperbilirubinemia (Chapter 9), polycythemia (p. 433), and IRDS (p. 417).

NARCOTIC-ADDICTED INFANTS

Narcotics, which have a low molecular weight, readily cross the placental membrane and enter the fetal system. When the mother is a habitual user of narcotics, especially heroin or methadone, the unborn child also becomes passively addicted to the drug, which places such infants at risk during the early neonatal period.

Clinical Manifestations

Most passively addicted infants of drug-dependent mothers appear normal at birth but begin to exhibit signs of drug withdrawal within 12 to 24 hours if the mother has been taking heroin by itself. If mothers have been taking methadone, the signs appear somewhat later, anywhere from 1 or 2 days to 2 to 3 weeks or more after birth. The manifestations become most pronounced between 48 and 72 hours of age and may last anywhere from 6 days to 8 weeks, depending on the severity of the withdrawal (Box 10-18).

The clinical manifestations of withdrawal in neonates, which are predominantly those of autonomic nervous system hyperirritability, may persist for 3 or 4 months. The most common acute signs are tremors, restlessness, hyperactive reflexes, increased muscle tone, sneezing, tachypnea, and a high-pitched, shrill cry. Although these infants suck avidly on fists and display an exaggerated rooting reflex, they are poor feeders with uncoordinated and ineffectual sucking and swallowing reflexes. Regurgitation and

Box 10-18 SIGNS OF NARCOTIC WITHDRAWAL IN THE NEONATE

Irritability	Tachypnea (>60/min)
Tremors	Excoriations (knees, face)
Shrill cry	Frequent sneezing
Hypertonicity of muscles	Frequent yawning
Frantic sucking of hands	Vomiting
Poor feeding	Temperature instability
Hyperactivity	Diarrhea
Little sleeping	Convulsions
Sweating	

vomiting after feedings are common, and diarrhea is a later manifestation.

An unusual observation in a large percentage of these infants is generalized sweating, the incidence of which is unusual in newborn infants. It is significant that although passively addicted infants have some tachypnea, cyanosis, and/or apnea, they rarely develop respiratory distress syndrome. Apparently, heroin or stress factors in the intrauterine environment cause accelerated lung maturation even with a high incidence of prematurity.

Not all infants of heroin-addicted mothers will show signs of withdrawal. Because of irregular and varying degrees of drug use, quality of drug, and mixed drug usage by the mother, some infants display mild or variable manifestations. Most manifestations are the vague, nonspecific signs characteristic of all infants in general; therefore it is important to differentiate between drug withdrawal and other disorders before specific therapy is instituted. Often other states (e.g., hypocalcemia, hypoglycemia, or sepsis) coexist with the drug withdrawal.

Infants who do not display the signs of fetal alcohol syndrome but are born to mothers who are also heavy alcohol drinkers have significantly more tremors, hypertonia, restlessness, excessive mouthing movements, crying, and inconsolability than infants of addicted mothers who do not drink (Coles and others, 1984). An added concern regarding narcotic users is that many of the mothers often use other drugs, such as tranquilizers, sedatives, narcotics, amphetamines, phencyclidine (PCP), and other psychotropic agents.

Therapeutic Management

The treatment of the passively addicted infant initially consists of modulating the environment to decrease external stimuli. Drug therapies include parenteral and/or oral administration of phenobarbital, chlorpromazine, diazepam, or paregoric.

Nursing Considerations

When possible, the nursery personnel are alerted to the likelihood of drug-addicted infants. If the mother has had good prenatal care, the practitioner is aware of the problem and therapy has been instituted before delivery. However, a number of mothers deliver their infants without the benefit of adequate care, and the addiction is unknown to health care personnel at the time of delivery. The degree of narcosis or withdrawal is closely related to the amount of drug the mother has habitually taken, the length of time she has been taking the drug, and the drug level of the mother at the time of delivery. The most severe symptoms are observed in the infants of mothers who have taken large amounts of drugs over a long period. In addition, the nearer to the time of delivery that the mother takes the drug, the longer it takes for the child to develop withdrawal and the more severe are the manifestations. The infant may not exhibit withdrawal symptoms until 7 to 10 days after delivery.

Once the presence of withdrawal is identified in an infant, nursing care is directed toward reducing the stimuli (such as dimmed lights and decreased noise levels) that might trigger hyperactivity and irritability, providing adequate nutrition and hydration, and promoting maternal-infant relationships. Irritable and hyperactive infants have been found to respond to comforting, movement, and close contact. Wrapping infants snugly, as well as rocking, and holding them tightly, limits their ability to self-stimulate. Infants who were placed on water beds showed fewer withdrawal symptoms, were released from the hospital sooner, and gained weight more rapidly and earlier when compared with a control group sleeping in conventional bassinets (Oro and Dixon, 1988). Arranging nursing activities to reduce the amount of disturbance helps to decrease exogenous stimulation.

Loose stools and poor intake and regurgitation following feeding predispose the infants to malnutrition, dehydration, and electrolyte imbalance. Frequent weighing, careful monitoring of intake and output, and supplemental parenteral fluids may be necessary. In addition, the infants burn up energy with continual activity and increase oxygen consumption at the cellular level. It takes considerable time and patience to ensure that they receive a sufficient caloric and fluid intake.

Hyperactive infants must be protected from skin abrasions on the knees, toes, and cheeks that are caused by rubbing on bed linens when lying on their abdomens. Monitoring and recording the activity level and its relationship to other activities, such as feeding and preventing complications, are important nursing functions.

A valuable aid to anticipating problems in newborns is recognizing drug addiction in the mothers. Unless the mothers are enrolled in a methadone rehabilitation program, they seldom risk calling attention to their habit by seeking prenatal care. Consequently infants and mothers are exposed to the additional hazards of obstetric and medical complications. Moreover, the nature of heroin addiction makes the user susceptible to disorders such as infection (hepatitis, acquired immune deficiency syndrome [AIDS]), foreign body reaction, and the hazards of inadequate nutrition and premature birth. Methadone treatment does not prevent withdrawal reaction in neonates, but the clinical course may be modified. Also, the intensive psychologic support of mothers is a factor in the treatment and reduction of perinatal mortality. Experience has indicated that mothers are usually anxious and depressed, lack confidence, have poor self-images, and have difficulty with interpersonal relationships. They may have a psychologic need for the pregnancy and an infant.

Initial symptoms or recurrence of withdrawal symptoms may develop after discharge from the hospital; therefore it is important to establish rapport and maintain contact with the family so that they will return for treatment if this occurs. The demands on the caregiver of the narcotic-addicted infant are enormous and nonrewarding in terms of positive feedback. The infants are difficult to comfort and cry for long periods, which can be especially trying for the caregiver following the infant's discharge from the hospital. Long-term follow-up to evaluate the status of the infant and the family is very important. Sudden infant death syndrome (SIDS) and AIDS are observed more frequently in infants born to users of methadone and heroin (Oleske and others, 1983).

There are many problems in relation to the disposition of infants of drug-dependent mothers. Those who advocate separation of mothers and children argue that the mothers are not capable of assuming responsibility for their infant's care, that child care is frustrating to them, and that their existence is too disorganized and chaotic. Others encourage the maternal-infant bond and recommend a protected environment such as a therapeutic community, a halfway house, or continuous, ongoing, supportive services in the home after discharge. Each situation requires careful evaluation and the cooperative efforts of a variety of health professionals, whether the choice is foster home placement or supportive follow-up care of mothers who keep their infants.

COCAINE EXPOSURE

Cocaine, the number one illicit drug used in the United States, has multiple modes of use. However, use of the relatively inexpensive and easily administered "crack" form is increasing alarmingly, especially among women (Hadeed and Siegel, 1989). Because crack vaporizes at relatively low temperatures, it is smoked and absorbed in large quantities through the pulmonary vasculature. The drug readily crosses the placenta, placing the fetus at risk.

Cocaine is a CNS stimulant and peripheral sympathomimetic, and the effects on the fetus are secondary to maternal effects—increased blood pressure, decreased uterine blood flow, and increased vascular resistance. Consequently the fetus suffers decreased blood pressure and hypoxia. The difficulties encountered by cocaine-exposed infants are compounded when the mother is taking the drug in conjunction with other illicit drugs. Also, prenatal exposure to cocaine has been implicated as a risk for SIDS in infancy (Bauchner and others, 1988).

Clinical Manifestations

Infants born to cocaine users have decreased birth weight, length, and occipitofrontal circumference. Teratogenic effects, possible genitourinary malformations, are less clear and still debated. The infants are jittery, cranky, feed poorly, and often remain intolerant to cuddling and inattentive to cooing and other comforting behaviors. Scores on the Brazelton Neonatal Assessment Scale have shown infants to be low in responding appropriately to arousal, auditory, and visual stimuli (Lewis, Bennett, and Schmeder, 1989).

Therapeutic Management

Treatment of these infants is similar to that for narcotic-addicted infants—sedation and reduction of external stimuli.

Nursing Considerations

Nursing care of cocaine-exposed infants is the same as that for narcotic-addicted infants. Since they have increased flexor tone, these infants respond to swaddling in a semi-flexed position (Schneider, Griffith, and Chasnoff, 1989). Effects of the drug from breast milk (Chasnoff, Lewis, and Squires, 1987) and topical cocaine applications to nipples (Chaney, Franke, and Wadlington, 1988) have been reported; therefore mothers should be cautioned regarding this hazard to their infants.

INFANTS OF MOTHERS WHO SMOKE

Cigarette smoking during pregnancy is clearly associated with significant birth weight deficits up to 440 g in full-term newborns and there is a definite dose-response relationship between the number of cigarettes smoked by the mother and these deficits (Haddow and others, 1987). This dose-related response also affects the Apgar scores—the number of infants with low Apgar scores (whose mothers smoked three packs per day) is nearly four times that of infants whose mothers smoked none or only one pack per day (Garn and others, 1981). Also, reviews of large studies indicate that 21% to 39% of the incidence of low birth weight is attributable to maternal cigarette smoking (Department of Health and Human Services [DHHS], 1983).

The rate of preterm births is increased in mothers who smoke, but the infants are smaller at *all* stages of gestation. They show fetal growth retardation in length, weight, and chest and head circumference, and these deficits are not related to maternal appetite or weight gain (DHHS, 1983). Concentrations of two pharmacologically active substances found in tobacco, nicotine and cotinine, have been found to be higher in newborns of mothers who smoke than in their mothers. In addition, these substances secreted in breast milk have a half-life of 70 to 80 minutes (Luck and others, 1982). It has also been shown that cigarette smoking has detrimental effects beyond the neonatal period with deficits in growth, intellectual and emotional development, and behavior (DHHS, 1983; Naeye and Peters, 1984). (See also Passive Smoking, Chapter 32.)

The overwhelming evidence of the detrimental effects of maternal cigarette smoking on newborns has led some investigators to suggest the diagnostic term *fetal tobacco syndrome* for infants who fit the key features listed in Box 10-19. The purpose of this suggestion is to focus attention on

Box 10-19 KEY FEATURES OF "FETAL TOBACCO SYNDROME"

1. The mother smoked five or more cigarettes a day throughout pregnancy.
2. The mother had no evidence of hypertension during pregnancy, specifically: (a) no preeclampsia, and (b) documentation of normal blood pressure at least once after the first trimester.
3. The newborn has symmetric growth retardation at term (up to or greater than 37 weeks), defined as: (a) a birth weight less than 2500 g, and (b) a ponderal index ([weight in g]/[length in m^3]) greater than 2.32.
4. There is no other obvious cause of intrauterine growth retardation (e.g., congenital infection or anomaly).

Modified from Nieburg, P., and others: The fetal tobacco syndrome (commentary), JAMA 253:2998-2999, 1985.

this important health problem that is directly related to maternal behavior.

Nursing Considerations

Nurses are prime candidates for disseminating information to expectant mothers about the risks related to smoking. Mothers who stop or substantially reduce smoking during pregnancy improve the quality of life for their unborn infants. In one study, infants of expectant mothers who were given information, support, encouragement, practical guidance, and behavior modification during pregnancy delivered infants with significantly higher birth weights than controls (Sexton and Hebel, 1984). If mothers continue to smoke while breast-feeding, they should be told to do so *immediately after* breast-feeding to reduce the amount of nicotine and cotinine in the breast milk (Luck and others, 1982).

KEY POINTS

- High-risk neonates may be defined as newborns, regardless of gestational age or birth weight, who have a greater than average chance of morbidity or mortality because of conditions or circumstances superimposed on the normal course of events associated with birth and adjustment to extrauterine existence.
- Identification of high-risk newborns may occur during any one of the following stages: preconceptual, prenatal, natal, or postnatal.
- High-risk infants may be classified according to size, gestational age, and mortality.
- Newborn intensive care units are categorized according to the population served and degree of treatment.
- General management of the newborn entails immediate care; protection from infection; monitoring physiologic data, including heart rate, respiratory activity, temperature, and blood pressure; laboratory data; and systematic assessment of the high-risk infant.
- Assessment of the newborn includes a general assessment, respiratory assessment, cardiovascular assessment, gastrointestinal assessment, genitourinary assessment, neurologic-musculoskeletal assessment, skin assessment, and temperature.
- Because their metabolic processes are immature, high-risk newborns are placed in a heated environment to help control thermoneutrality.
- Because of the immature, fragile skin of premature infants, the nurse should use caution when applying topical preparations and when removing bandages or dressings.
- Meeting the high-risk infant's nutritional needs requires specific knowledge of physiologic characteristics, the infant's particular needs, and methods of feeding.
- Delayed development in high-risk neonates is a concern; developmental interventions are individualized to ameliorate the effects.
- Parental involvement in the care of high-risk infants is important, and nurses should help to facilitate parent-infant relationships by guiding them to support groups and home health teaching.
- Prematurity accounts for the largest number of admissions to an NICU.
- Several severe respiratory conditions place the infant at high risk: apnea of prematurity, IRDS, meconium aspiration syndrome, extraneous air syndromes, and BPD. Therapeutic management of IRDS includes oxygen therapy and assisted ventilation.
- Newborns are highly susceptible to infection, particularly sepsis.
- Cardiovascular complications in the high-risk infant may include persistent patent ductus arteriosus, persistent pulmonary hypertension, anemia, and polycythemia/hyperviscosity syndrome.
- Neurologic disturbances in the high-risk newborn may include perinatal hypoxic-ischemic brain injury, periventricular-intraventricular hemorrhage, intracranial hemorrhage, and neonatal seizures.
- Maternal conditions that pose a threat to the newborn include diabetes, drug addiction, and smoking.

REFERENCES

Affonso, D.D., Wahlberg, V., and Persson, B.: Exploration of mothers' reactions to the kangaroo method of prematurity care, Neonatal Network 7:43-51, 1989.

Als, H., and others: Toward a research instrument for the assessment of preterm infants' behavior. In Fitzgerald, H., Lester, B.M., and Yogman, M.W., editors: Theory and research in behavioral pediatrics, vol. I, New York, 1982, Plenum Publishing Corp.

American Academy of Pediatrics: Safe transportation of premature infants, AAP News 6(7):11, 1990.

American Academy of Pediatrics, Committee on Fetus and Newborn, Committee on Drugs: Benzyl alcohol: toxic agent in neonatal units, Pediatrics 72:356-358, 1983.

American Academy of Pediatrics, Committee on Fetus and Newborn: Vitamin E and the prevention of retinopathy of prematurity, Pediatrics 76:315-316, 1985.

American Academy of Pediatrics, Committee on Nutrition: Nutritional needs of low-birth-weight infants, Pediatrics 75:976-986, 1985.

Anderson, G.H., Atkinson, S.A., and Bryan, M.H.: Energy and macronutrient content of human milk during early lactation from mothers giving birth prematurely and at term, Am. J. Clin. Nutr. 34:258-265, 1981.

Atakent, Y., and others: The adverse effects of high oral osmolal mixtures in neonates, Clin. Pediatr. 23:487-490, Sept. 1984.

Bancalari, E., and Gerhardt, T.: Bronchopulmonary dysplasia, Pediatr. Clin. North Am. 33:1-23, 1986.

Barnard, K.E., and Bee, H.L.: The impact of temporally patterned stimulation on the development of preterm infants, Child Dev. 54:1156-1167, 1983.

Bartlett, R.H., and others: Extracorporeal circulation in neonatal respiratory failure: a prospective randomized study, Pediatrics 76:479-487, 1985.

Bauchner, H., and others: Risk of sudden infant death syndrome among infants with in utero exposure to cocaine, J. Pediatr. 113:831-835, 1988.

Baumgart, S.: Reduction of oxygen consumption, insensible water loss, and radiant heat demand with use of a plastic blanket for low-birth-weight infants under radiant warmers, Pediatrics 74:1022-1028, 1984.

Bennett, F.C., Robinson, N.M., and Sells, C.J.: Growth and development of infants weighing less than 800 grams at birth, Pediatrics 71:319-323, 1983.

Bernbaum, J., and Hoffman-Wiliamson, M.: Following the NICU graduate, Contemp. Pediatr. 3:22-37, 1986.

Bernbaum, J.C., and others: Nonnutritive sucking during gavage feeding enhances growth and maturation in premature infants, Pediatrics 71:41-45, 1983.

Boros, S.J., and others: Neonatal high-frequency jet ventilation: four years' experience, Pediatrics 75:657-663, 1985.

Boros, S.J., and others: Necrotizing tracheobronchitis: a complication of high-frequency ventilation, J. Pediatr. 109:95-100, 1986.

Bozynski, M.E.A., and others: Lateral positioning of the stable ventilated very-low-birth-weight infant, Am. J. Dis. Child. 142:200-202, 1988.

Brazelton, T.B.: Personal communication, 1984.

Brodsky, L., Reidy, M. and Stanievich, J.F.: The effects of suctioning techniques on the distal tracheal mucosa in intubated low birth weight infants, Int. J. Pediatr. Otorhinolaryngol. 14:1-14, 1987.

Bruhn, F.W., and Jones, B.: Infection in the neonate. In Merenstein, G.B., and Gardner, S.L.: Handbook of neonatal intensive care, St. Louis, 1985, Mosby–Year Book, Inc.

Budreau, G.K.: Postnatal cranial modeling and infant attractiveness: implications for nursing, Neonatal Network 5(5):13-19, 1987.

Bull, M.J., and Stroup, K.B.: Premature infants in car seats, Pediatrics 75:336-339, 1985.

Bull, M.J., Weber, K., and Stroup, K.B.: Automotive restraint systems for premature infants, J. Pediatr. 112:385-388, 1988.

Carlo, W.A., and others: Decrease in airway pressure during high-frequency jet ventilation in infants with respiratory distress syndrome, J. Pediatr. 104:101-105 1984.

Cathas, M.K.: Percutaneous central venous catheters, JOGNN 15:324-332, 1986.

Chaney, N.E., Franke, J., and Wadlington, W.B.: Cocaine convulsions in a breast-feeding baby, J. Pediatr. 112:134-135, 1988.

Chasnoff, I.J., Lewis, D.E., and Squires, L.: Cocaine intoxication in a breast-fed infant, Pediatrics 80:836-838, 1987.

Cheu, H.W., Brown, D.R., and Rowe, M.I.: Breath hydrogen excretion as a screening test for the early diagnosis of necrotizing entercolitis, Am. J. Dis. Child. 143:156-159, 1989.

Chirico, G., and others: Intravenous gammaglobulin therapy for prophylaxis of infection in high-risk neonates, J. Pediatr. 110:437-442, 1987.

Clapp, D.W., and others: Use of intravenously administered immune globlulin to prevent nosocomial sepsis in low birth weight infants: report of a pilot study, J. Pediatr. 115:973-978, 1989.

Cloney, D.L., and Donowitz, L.G.: Overgrown use for infection control in nurseries and neonatal intensive care units, Am. J. Dis. Child. 140:680-683, 1986.

Cohen, M.A.: The use of prostaglandins and prostaglandin inhibitors in critically ill neonates, MCN 8:194-199, 1983.

Cole, J.G.: Infant stimulation reexamined: an environmental- and behavioral-based approach, Neonatal Network 3(5):24-31, 1985.

Cole, J.G., and Frappier, P.A.: Infant stimulation reassessed: a new approach to providing care for the preterm infant, JOGNN 14:471-477, 1985.

Coles, C.D., and others: Neonatal ethanol withdrawal: characteristics in critically normal nondysmorphic neonates, J. Pediatr. 105:445-451, 1984.

Collaborative European Multicenter Study Group: Surfactant replacement therapy for severe neonatal respiratory distress syndrome: an international clinical trial, Pediatrics 82:683-691, 1988.

Collaborative Group on Antenatal Steroid Therapy: Effect of antenatal dexamethasone administration on the prevention of respiratory distress syndrome, Am. J. Obstet. Gynecol. 141:276, 1981.

Collinge, J.M., and others: Demand vs. scheduled feedings for premature infants, JOGNN 11:362-367, 1982.

Culley, B.S., Perrin, E.C., and Chaberski, M.J.: Parental perceptions of vulnerability of formerly premature infants, J. Pediatr. Health Care 3:237-245, 1989.

Department of Health and Human Services: The health consequences of smoking for women: a report of the surgeon general, Washington, DC, 1983, publication 410-889/1284.

Dowling, S.: Seven infants with esophageal atresia, Psychoanal. Study Child 32:215-256, 1977.

Durand, M., and others: Prospective evaluation of percutaneous central venous Silastic catheters in newborn infants with birth weights of 510 to 3,920 grams, Pediatrics 78:245-250, 1986.

Emery, J.R., and Peabody, J.L.: Head position affects intracranial pressure in newborn infants, J. Pediatr. 103:950-953, 1983.

Fanconi, S., and Duc, G.: Intratracheal suctioning in sick preterm infants: prevention of intracranial hypertension and cerebral hypoperfusion by muscle paralysis, Pediatrics 79:538-543, 1987.

Field, T., and Goldson, E.: Pacifying effects of nonnutritive sucking on term and preterm neonates during heelstick procedures, Pediatrics 74:1012-1015, 1984.

Field, T., and others: Nonnutritive sucking during tube feedings: effects on preterm neonates in an intensive care unit, Pediatrics 70:381-384, 1982.

Field, T., Scafidi, F., and Schanberg, S.: Massage of preterm newborns to improve growth and development, Pediatr. Nurs. 13:385-387, 1987.

Field, T., and others: Tactile/kinesthetic stimulation effects on preterm neonates, Pediatrics. 77:654-658, 1986.

Food and Drug Administration: Benzyl alcohol may be toxic to newborns, FDA Drug Bull. 12:10-11, 1982.

Fox, M.D., and Molesky, M.G.: The effects of prone and supine positioning on arterial oxygen pressure, Neonatal Network 8:25-29, 1990.

Fox, W.W., and Duara, S.: Persistent pulmonary hypertension in the neonate: diagnosis and management, J. Pediatr. 103:505-514, 1983.

Fuhrmann, K., and others: Prevention of congenital malformations in infants of insulin-dependent diabetic mothers, Diabetes Care 6:219-223, 1983.

Gardner, S.L., O'Donnell, J.P., and Weisman, L.E.: Breastfeeding the sick neonate. In Merenstein, G.B., and Gardner, S.L.: Handbook of neonatal intensive care, ed. 2, St. Louis, 1989, Mosby–Year Book, Inc.

Garn, S.M., and others: Effect of maternal cigarette smoking on Apgar scores, Am. J. Dis. Child. 135:503-506, 1981.

Geertsma, M.A., and others: Feeding resistance after parenteral hyperalimentation, Am. J. Dis. Child. 139:255-256, 1985.

Gerhardt, T., and Bancalari, E.: Apnea of prematurity. II. Respiratory reflexes, Pediatrics 74:63-64, 1984.

Gladstone, I.M., Ehrenkranz, R.A., and Jacobs, H.C.: Pulmonary function tests and fluid balance in neonates with chronic lung disease during dexamethasone treatment, Pediatrics 84:1072-1076, 1989.

Gleason, C.A., and others: Optimal position for a spinal tap in preterm infants, Pediatrics 71:31-35, 1983.

Goldberg, R.N., and others: The effect of head position on intracranial pressure in the neonate, Crit. Care Med. 11:428-430, 1983.

Goldson, E.: Bronchopulmonary dysplasia, Pediatr. Ann. 19:13-18, 1990.

Greer, P.S.: Head coverings for newborns under radiant warmers, JOGNN 17(4):265-271, 1988.

Gross, S.J., Oehler, J.M., and Eckerman, C.O.: Head growth and developmental outcome in very low-birth-weight infants, Pediatrics 71:70-75, 1983.

Gross, S.J., and others: Nutritional composition of milk produced by mothers delivering preterm, J. Pediatr. 96:641-644, 1980.

Gross, S.J., and others: Elevated IgA concentration in milk produced by mothers delivered of preterm infants, J. Pediatr. 99:389-393, 1981.

Gunderson, L.P., and Kenner, C.: Neonatal stress: physiologic adaptation and nursing implications, Neonatal Network 6(1):37-42, 1987.

Hack, M., and others: Catch-up growth in very-low-birth-weight infants, Am. J. Dis. Child. 138:370-375, 1984.

Haddow, J.E., and others: Cigarette consumption and serum cotinine in relation to birthweight, Br. J. Obstet. Gynecol. 94:678-681, 1987.

Hadeed, A.J., and Siegel, S.R.: Maternal cocaine use during pregnancy: effect on the newborn infant, Pediatrics 84:205-210, 1989.

Hagedorn, M.I., Gardner, S.L., and Abman, S.H.: Respiratory diseases. In Merenstein, G.B., and Gardner, S.L.: Handbook of neonatal intensive care, ed. 2, St. Louis, 1989, Mosby–Year Book, Inc.

Harkavy, K.L., and others: Dexamethasone therapy for chronic lung disease in ventilator- and oxygen-dependent infants: a controlled trial, J. Pediatr. 115:979-983, 1989.

Hogue, C.J.R., and others: Overview of the National Infant Mortality Surveillance (NIMS) Project, MMWR 38(No. SS-3):1-46, 1989.

Kaempf, J.W., Bonnabel, C., and Hay, W.W., Jr.: Neonatal nutrition. In Merenstein, G.B., and Gardner, S.L.: Handbook of neonatal intensive care, ed. 2, St. Louis, 1989, Mosby–Year Book, Inc.

Kendig, J.W., and others: Surfactant replacement therapy at birth: final analysis of a clinical trial and comparisons with similar trials, Pediatrics 82:756-762, 1988.

Kercsmar, C.M., and others: Bronchoscopic findings in infants treated with high-frequency jet ventilation versus conventional ventilation, Pediatrics 82:884-887, 1988.

Kleiber, C., Krutzfield, N., and Rose, E.F.: Acute histologic changes in the tracheobronchial tree associated with different suction catheter insertion techniques, Heart Lung 17(1):10-14, 1988.

Kling, P.: Nursing interventions to decrease the risk of periventricular-intraventricular hemorrhage, JOGNN 18:457-464, 1989.

Knauth, A., and others: Semipermeable polyurethane membrane as an artificial skin for the premature neonate, Pediatrics 83:945-950, 1989.

Koops, B., Abman, S., and Accurso, F.: Outpatient management and followup of BPD, Clin. Perinatol. 11:101-122, 1984.

Korner, A.F., Ruppel, E.M., and Rho, J.M.: Effects of water beds on the sleep and motility of theophylline-treated preterm infants, Pediatrics 70:864-869, 1982.

Korones, S.B.: High-risk newborn infants: the basis for intensive nursing care, ed. 4, St. Louis, 1986, Mosby–Year Book, Inc.

Kowba, M.D., and Schwirian, P.M.: Direct sibling contact and bacterial colonization in newborns, JOGNN 14:412-417, 1985.

Kuller, J.M., Lund, C., and Tobin, C.: Improved skin care for premature infants, MCN 8:200-203, 1983.

Kurzner, S.I., and others: Growth failure in infants with bronchopulmonary dysplasia: nutrition and elevated resting metabolic expenditure, Pediatrics 81:379-384, 1988.

Kwong, M.S., and Egan, E.A.: Reduced incidence of hyaline membrane disease in extremely premature infants following delay of delivery in mother with preterm labor: use of ritodrine and betamethasone, Pediatrics 78:767-774, 1986.

Landon-Malone, K.A., Kirkpatrick, J.M, and Stull, S.P.: Incorporating hospice care in a community hospital NICU, Neonatal Network 6(1):13-19, 1987.

Lang, M.J., and others: A controlled trial of human surfactant replacement therapy for severe respiratory distress syndrome in very low birth weight infants, J. Pediatr. 116:295-300, 1990.

Lebenthal, E.: Physiologic considerations in the feeding of the premature and compromised infant, Child Care Newsletter 1(3):5-8, 1982.

Lewis, K.D., Bennett, B., and Schmeder, N.H.: The care of infants menaced by cocaine abuse, MCN 14:324-329, 1989.

Linder, N., and others: Suckling stimulation test for neonatal tremor, Arch. Dis. Child. 64:44-46, 1989.

Luck, W., and others: Nicotine and cotinine—two pharmacologically active substances as parameters for the strain on fetuses and babies of mothers who smoke, J. Perinat. Med. 10:107-108, 1982.

Lund, C., and others: Evaluation of a pectin-based barrier under tape to protect neonatal skin, JOGNN 15:39-43, 1986.

Maloni, J.A., and others: Validation of infant behavior identified by neonatal nurses, Nurs. Res. 35:133-138, 1986.

Mann, N.P., and others: Effect of night and day on prematures in the nursery, Br. J. Med. 293:1265-1267, 1986.

Marshall, R.E., and others: Auditory function in newborn intensive care unit patients revealed by auditory brain-stem potentials, J. Pediatr. 96:731-735, 1980.

Masterson, J., Zucker, C., and Schulze, K.: Prone and supine positioning effects on energy expenditure and behavior of low birth weight neonates, Pediatrics 80:689-692, 1987.

Meier, P., and Anderson, G.C.: Responses of small preterm infants to bottle- and breast-feeding, MCN 12:97-105, 1987.

Meier, P., and Pugh, E.J.: Breast-feeding behavior of small preterm infants, MCN 10:396-401, 1985.

Merenstein, G.B., Gardner, S.L., and Blake, W.W.: Heat balance. In Merenstein, G.B., and Gardner, S.L.: Handbook of neonatal intensive care, ed. 2, St. Louis, 1989, Mosby–Year Book, Inc.

Minarcik, C.J., Jr., and Beachy, P.: Neurologic disorders. In Merenstein, G.B., and Gardner, S.L.: Handbook of neonatal intensive care, ed. 2, St. Louis, 1989, Mosby–Year Book, Inc.

Muttitt, S.C., and others: Neonatal apnea: diagnosis by nurse versus computer, Pediatrics 82:713-720, 1988.

Naeye, R.L., and Peters, E.C.: Mental development of children whose mothers smoked during pregnancy, Obstet. Gynecol. 64:60-107, 1984.

Null, S.: Nursing care to ease parents' grief, MCN 14:84-89, 1989.

O'Connor, M.J., Ralston, C.W., and Ament, ME.: Intellectual and perceptual-motor performance of children receiving prolonged home total parenteral nutrition, Pediatrics 81:231-236, 1988.

Oleske, J., and others: Immune deficiency syndrome in children, JAMA 249:2345-2347, 1983.

Oro, A.S., and Dixon, S.D.: Waterbed care of narcotic-exposed neonates, Am. J. Dis. Child. 12:186-188, 1988.

Orr, M.J., and Allen, S.S.: Optimal oral experiences for infants on long-term total parenteral nutrition, Nutr. Clin. Pract., 9:288-295, 1986.

Paludetto, R., and others: Transcutaneous oxygen tension during non-nutritive sucking in preterm infants, Pediatrics 74:539-542, 1984.

Papageorgiou, A.N., and others: Reduction of mortality, morbidity, and respiratory distress syndrome in infants weighing less than 1,000 grams by treatment with betamethasone and ritodrine, Pediatrics 83:493-497, 1989.

Parker, S., and others: Jitteriness in full-term neonates: prevalence and correlates, Pediatrics 85:17-23, 1990.

Parry, W.H, and Gunnell, O.R.: Acid-base homeostasis and oxygenation. In Merenstein G.B., and Gardner, S.L.: Handbook of neonatal intensive care, St. Louis, 1989, Mosby–Year Book, Inc.

Pelletier, J.M., and Palmeri, A.: Infants at risk. In Clark, P.N., and Allen, A.S., editors: Occupational therapy for children, St. Louis, 1985, Mosby–Year Book, Inc.

Perlman, J.M., and Volpe, J.J.: Suctioning in the preterm infant: effects on cerebral blood flow velocity, intracranial pressure, and arterial blood pressure, Pediatrics 72:329-334, 1983.

Pokora, T., and others: Neonatal high-frequency jet ventilation, Pediatrics 72:27-32, 1983.

Rönnholm, K.A., Perheentupa, J., and Siimes, M.A.: Supplementation with human milk protein improves growth of small premature infants fed human milk, Pediatrics 77:649-655, 1986.

Richards, D.D: The challenge of transporting children with special needs, American Academy of Pediatrics, Safe Ride News, pp. 1-4, Spring, 1989.

Ross, G., Lipper, E.G., and Auld, P.A.M.: Physical growth and developmental outcome in very low birth weight premature infants at 3 years of age, J. Pediatr. 107:284-286, 1985.

Sauer, P.J.J., and Visser, H.K.A.: The neutral temperature of very low-birth-weight infants, Pediatrics 74:288-289, 1984.

Schneider, J.W., Griffith, D.R., and Chasnoff, I.J.: Infants exposed to cocaine in utero: implications for developmental assessment and intervention, Inf. Young Child. 2(1):25-36, 1989.

Schwab, F., and others: Sibling visiting in a neonatal intensive care unit, Pediatrics 71:835-838, 1983.

Scrimshaw, S.C.M., and March, D.M.: I had a baby sister but she only lasted one day, JAMA 251:732-733, 1984.

Sexton, M., and Hebel, J.R.: A clinical trial of change in maternal smoking and its effect on birth weight, JAMA 251:911-915, 1984.

Shaker, C.S.: Nipple feeding premature infants: a different perspective, Neonatal Network 8(5):9-17, 1990.

Shields, P.I., and Tenorio, K.E.: Cluster care nursing: Maricela's story (case study), Pediatr. Nurs. 14:125-127, 1988.

Siegel, R., Gardner, S.L., and Merenstein, G.B.: Families in crisis: theoretical and practical considerations. In Merenstein, G.B., and Gardner, S.L.: Handbook of neonatal intensive care, ed. 2, St. Louis, 1989, Mosby–Year Book, Inc.

Slater, M.A., and others: Neurodevelopment of monitored versus nonmonitored very low birth weight infants: the importance of family influences, J. Dev. Behav. Pediatr. 8(5):278-285, 1988.

Socol, M.L., Sing, E., and Depp, O.R.: The tap test: a rapid indicator of fetal pulmonary maturity, Am. J. Obstet. Gynecol. 148:445-450, 1984.

Southall, D.P., and others: Undetected episodes of prolonged apnea and severe bradycardia in preterm infants, Pediatrics 72:541-551, 1983.

Stockman and others: Anemia of prematurity: determinants of the erythropoietin response, J. Pediatr. 105:786-795, 1984.

Topper, W.H., and Stewart, T.P.: Thermal support for the very-low-birth-weight infant: role of supplemental conductive heat, J. Pediatr. 105:810-814, 1984.

Trause, M.A., and others: Separation for childbirth: the effect on the sibling, Child Psychiatry Hum. Dev. 12:95-104, 1983.

Tyson, J.E., and others: Growth, metabolic response, and development in very-low-birth-weight infants fed banked human milk or enriched formula. I. Neonatal findings, J. Pediatr. 103:95-104, 1983.

VandenBerg, K.A.: Revising the traditional model: an individualized approach to developmental interventions in the intensive care nursery, Neonatal Network 3(5):32-38, 1985.

Volpe, J.J.: Neonatal seizures: current concepts and revised classification, Pediatrics 84:422-428, 1989.

Westwood, M., and others: Growth and development of full-term nonasphyxiated small-for-gestational-age newborns: follow-up through adolescence, Pediatrics 71:376-382, 1983.

White-Traut, R.C., and Goldman, M.B.C.: Premature infant massage: is it safe? Pediatr. Nurs. 14:285-289, 1988.

Willett, L.D., and others: Risk of hypoventilation in premature infants in car seats, J. Pediatr. 109:245-248, 1986.

Willett, L.D., and others: Ventilatory changes in convalescent infants positioned in car seats, J. Pediatr. 115:451-455, 1989.

Wilson, R., and others: Age onset of necrotizing enterocolitis: an epidemiologic analysis, Pediatr. Res. 12:82-84, 1982.

Wiswell, T.E., and others: Tracheal and bronchial injury in high-frequency oscillatory ventilation and high-frequency flow interruption compared with conventional positive pressure ventilation, J. Pediatr. 112:249-253, 1988.

Yeh, T.F., and others: Furosemide prevents the renal side effects of indomethacin therapy in premature infants with patent ductus arteriosus, J. Pediatr. 101:433-437, 1982.

BIBLIOGRAPHY

General

Bernbaum, J., and D'Agostino, J.: The NICU graduate: managing the major complications, Contemp. Pediatr. 3(8):69-82, 1986.

Bethea, S.W.: Primary nursing in the infant special care unit, JOGNN 14:202-208, 1985.

Brooke, O.G., and others: Effects on birth weight of smoking, alcohol, caffeine, socioeconomic factors, and psychosocial stress, Br. Med. J. 298:795-801, 1989.

Burch, S.M., and Chadwick, J.V.: Use of a retroset in the delivery of intravenous medications in the neonate, Neonatal Network 6(2):51-54, 1987.

Chathas, M.K.: Percutaneous central venous catheters in neonates, JOGNN 15:324-332, 1986.

Cole, C.H.: Prevention of prematurity: can we do it in America, Pediatrics 76:310-312, 1985.

Costarino, A., and Baumgart, S.: Modern fluid and electrolyte management of the critically ill premature infant, Pediatr. Clin. North Am. 33:153-176, 1986.

Cunningham, N., and Hutchinson, S.: Neonatal nurses and issues in research ethics, Neonatal Network 8(5):29-48, 1990.

Duara, S., and others: Neonatal screening with auditory brainstem responses: results of follow-up audiometry and risk factor evaluation, J. Pediatr. 108:276-281, 1986.

Elhassani, S.B.: Preventing neonatal exposure to toxins, Contemp. Pediatr. 6(4):60, 65-70, 79-82, 1989.

Fanaroff, A., and Martin, R.J.: Behrman's neonatal-perinatal medicine, ed. 4, St. Louis, 1987, Mosby–Year Book, Inc.

Fay, M.J.: The positive effects of positioning, Neonatal. Network 6(5):23-28, 1988.

Fonner, C.J., Rushton, C.H., and Fletcher, A.B.: Preparation for neonatal emergencies: a neonatal emergency medication sheet, Pediatr. Nurs. 15:527-530, 1989.

Glass, S.M., and Giacoia, G.P.: Intravenous drug therapy in premature infants: practical aspects, JOGNN 16(5):310-315, 1987.

Grassi, L.C.: Life, money, quality: the impact of regionalization on perinatal/neonatal intensive care, Neonatal Network 6(4):53-58, 1988.

Hargrove, C.: Administration of IV medications in the NICU: the development of a procedure, Neonatal Network 6(2):41-49, 1987.

Harpin, V.A., and Rutter, N.: Barrier properties of the newborn infant's skin, J. Pediatr. 102:419-425, 1983.

Hazinski, M.F.: New guidelines for pediatric and neonatal cardiopulmonary resuscitation and advanced life support. III. Neonatal advanced life support, Pediatr. Nurs. 13:57-60, 1987.

Hyde, B.B., and McCown, D.E.: Classical conditioning in neonatal intensive care nurseries, Pediatr. Nurs. 12:11-14, 1986.

Ifft, D.L., and others: Reliability of head circumference measurements for preterm infants, Neonatal Network 8(3):41-45, 1989.

Jhaveri, M.K., and Kumar, S.P.: Passage of the first stool in very low birth weight infants, Pediatrics 79:1005-1007, 1987.

Kelting, S., and Johnson, C.: Erythropoiesis and neonatal blood transfusion, MCN 12:172-177, 1987.

Kitchen, W.H., and others: Health and hospital readmissions of very-low-birth-weight and normal-birth-weight children, Am. J. Dis. Child. 144:213-218, 1990.

LaRossa, M.M., and Brown, J.V.: Foster grandmothers in the premature nursery, Am. J. Nurs. 82:1834-1835, 1982.

Lynch, T.M.: Invasive and noninvasive pressure monitoring in neonates, J. Perinat. Neonatal Nurs. 1(1):58-71, 1987.

Marshall, R.E.: Neonatal pain associated with caregiving procedures, Pediatr. Clin. North Am. 36:885-903, 1989.

Mattson, D., and O'Connor, M.: Transilluminator assistance in neonatal venipuncture, Neonatal Network 5(1):42-45, 1986.

Merenstein, G.B., and Gardner, S.L.: Handbook of neonatal intensive care, ed. 2, St. Louis, 1989, Mosby–Year Book, Inc.

Mitchell, S.H., and Najak, Z.D.: Low-birthweight infants and rehospitalization: what's the incidence? Neonatal Network 8(3):27-30, 1989.

Mulligan, K.S., and Webb, L.Z.: Developing an evacuation procedure for a nursery complex, Neonatal Network 6(6):47-52, 1988.

Nelson, D., and Heitman, R.: Factors influencing weight change in preterm infants, Pediatr. Nurs. 12:425-428, 1986.

Oehler, J.M., Peter, M.A., and Seyler, S.: Support groups: are they really helpful in dealing with NICU stress? Neonatal Network 8(2):21-25, 1989.

Pinelli, J., and Ferguson, M.K.: Transporting high-risk newborns: the importance of communication, Neonatal Network 3(6):23-26, 1985.

Sammons, W.A.H., and Lewis, J.M.: Premature babies: a different beginning, St. Louis, 1985, Mosby–Year Book, Inc.

Thigpen, J.L.: Neonatal mortality: early prediction using a neonatal status score, Neonatal Network 6(6):33-39, 1988.

Tobin, C.R.: The Teflon intravenous catheter: incidence of phlebitis and duration of catheter life in the neonatal patient, JOGNN 17(1):35-42, 1988.

Tribotti, S.: Admission to the neonatal intensive care unit: reducing the risks, Neonatal Network 8(4):17-22, 1990.

Troiano, N.H.: Applying principles to practice in maternal-fetal transport, J. Perinat. Neonatal Nurs. 2(3):20-30, 1989.

Urtis, J.M., Clayton, D., and Jay, S.S.: Infant morbidity: a measurement of severity and occurrence of illness in preterm and term infants, J. Pediatr. Nurs. 3:110-117, 1988.

Webb, A.A.: Methods of intravenous therapy in preterm infants, Issues Compr. Pediatr. Nurs. 10:215-221, 1987.

Wen, S.W., and others: Smoking, maternal age, fetal growth, and gestational age at delivery, Am. J. Obstet. Gynecol. 162:5-58, 1990.

Wise, B.V., and Lawrence-Nolan, L.: A risk of blood transfusions for premature infants, MCN 15:86-89, 1990.

General Nursing Care

Bellig, L.L., and Tomasulo-Roborecky, F.: The expanded neonatal nursing role and the high-risk family, Neonatal Network 2:20-24, 1983.

Blackburn, S.: The neonatal ICU: a high-risk environment, Am. J. Nurs. 82:1708-1712, 1982.

Budreau, G., and Kleiber, C.: Nursing management of the infant with an intraoral appliance, JOGNN 16(1):23-29, 1987.

Carey, B.E.: Major complications of central lines in neonates, Neonatal Network 7(6):17-28, 1989.

Chaze, B.A., and Ludington-Hoe, S.M.: Sensory stimulation in the ICU, Am. J. Nurs. 84:68-71, 1984.

DesRosier, M.B.: Taking a baby, Am. J. Nurs. 88:67, 1988.

Donowitz, L.G.: Failure of the overgrown to prevent nosocomial infection in a pediatric intensive care unit, Pediatrics 77:35-38, 1986.

Donowitz, L.G.: Handwashing technique in a pediatric intensive care unit, Am. J. Dis. Child. 141:683-685, 1987.

Experience and reason—briefly recorded: urine output measurements in premature infants, Pediatrics 83:116-118, 1989.

Gordin, P.C.: Assessing and managing agitation in a critically ill infant, MCN 15:26-32, 1990.

Harper, R.G., Little, G.A., and Sia, C.G.: The scope of nursing practice in level III neonatal intensive care units, Pediatrics 70:875-878, 1982.

Hermansen, M.C., and Buches, M.: Urine output determination from superabsorbent and regular diapers under radiant heat, Pediatrics 81:428-431, 1988.

Jacobson, G., and others: Handwashing: ring-wearing and number of microorganisms, Nurs. Res. 34:186-188, 1985.

Kennedy, J.: Evacuation of a neonatal unit, Can. Nurse 79:26-29, 1983.

Kunnl, M.T., and others: Comparisons of rectal, femoral, axillary, and skin-to-mattress temperatures in stable neonates, Nurs. Res. 37:162-164, 1988.

Norris, S., Campbell, L.A., and Brenkert, S.: Nursing procedures and alterations in transcutaneous oxygen tension in premature infants, Nurs. Res. 31:330-336, 1982.

Reams, P.K., and Deane, D.M.: Bagged versus diaper urine specimens and laboratory values, Neonatal Network 6(6):17-20, 1988.

Reedy, N.J., and others: Maternal fetal transport: a nurse team, JOGNN 13:91-100, 1984.

Thompson, C.E.: Going the distance as a neonatal nurse, Neonatal Network 7(3):11, 1988.

Updyke, C., and others: Positional support for premature infants, J. Occup. Ther. 40:712-715, 1986.

Thermoregulation

Haddock, B.J., Merrow, D.L., and Vincent, P.A.: Comparisons of axillary and rectal temperatures in the preterm infant, Neonatal Network 6(5):67-71, 1988.

Kaplan, M., and Eidelman, A.I.: Improved prognosis in severely hypothermic newborn infants treated by rapid rewarming, J. Pediatr. 105:468-469, 1984.

Malin, S.W., and Baumgart, S.: Optimal thermal management for low birth weight infants nursed under high-powered radiant warmers, Pediatrics 79:47-54, 1987.

Marks, K.H., Nardis, E.E., and Momin, M.N.: Energy metabolism and substrate utilization in low birth weight neonates under radiant warmers, Pediatrics 78:465-472, 1986.

Marks, K.H., and others: Thermal head wrap for infants, J. Pediatr. 107:956-959, 1985.

Mayfield, S.R., and others: Temperature measurement in term and preterm neonates, J. Pediatr. 104:271-275, 1984.

Moen, J.E., and others: Axillary versus rectal temperatures in preterm infants under radiant warmers, JOGNN 16(5):348-352, 1987.

Ruchala, P.: The effect of wearing headcoverings on the axillary temperatures of infants, MCN 10:240, 1985.

Schiffman, R.F.: Temperature monitoring in the neonate: a comparison of axillary and rectal temperatures, Nurs. Res. 31:274-278, 1982.

Vaughlans, B.: Early maternal-infant contact and neonatal thermoregulation, Neonatal Network 8(5):19-21, 1990.

Feeding and Nutrition

Boggs, K.R., and Rau, P.K.: Breastfeeding the premature infant, Am. J. Nurs. 83:1437-1439, 1983.

Churella, H.R., Bachhuber, W.L., and MacLean, W.C.: Survey: methods of feeding low-birth-weight infants, Pediatrics 76:243-249, 1985.

Costarino, A., and Baumgart, S.: Modern fluid and electrolyte management of the critically ill premature infant, Pediatr. Clin. North Am. 33:153-178, 1986.

Feher, S.D.K., and others: Increasing breast milk production for premature infants with a relaxation/imagery audiotape, Pediatrics 83:57-60, 1989.

Forte, A., Mayberry, L.J., and Ferketich, S.: Breast milk collection and storage practices among mothers of hospitalized neonates, J. Perinatol. 7(1):35-39, 1987.

Gavage tube insertion in the premature infant, MCN 12:24-27, 1987.

Gill, N.E., and others: Effect of nonnutritive sucking on behavioral state in preterm infants before feeding, Nurs. Res. 37(5):347-350, 1988.

Hopkinson, J.M., Schanler, R.J., and Garza, C.: Milk production by mothers of premature infants, Pediatrics 81:815-820, 1988.

Jain, L., and others: Energetics and mechanics of nutritive sucking in the preterm and term neonate, J. Pediatr. 111:894-898, 1987.

Lebenthal, E., Lee, P.C., and Heitlinger, L.A.: Impact of development of the gastrointestinal tract on infant feeding, J. Pediatr. 102:1-9, 1983.

Lebenthal, E., and Leung, Y.K.: Feeding the premature and compromised infant: gastrointestinal considerations, Pediatr. Clin. North Am. 35:215-238, 1988.

Lefrak-Okikawa, L.: Nutritional management of the very low birth weight infant, J. Perinat. Neonatal Nurs. 2(1):66-77, 1988.

McCoy, R., and others: Nursing management of breast feeding for preterm infants, J. Perinat. Neonatal Nurs. 2(1):42-55, 1988.

Measel, C.P.: A practical popular pacifier, Pediatr. Nurs. 8(3):199-200, 1982.

Meier, P.: Bottle- and breast-feeding: effects on transcutaneous oxygen pressure temperature in preterm infants, Nurs. Res. 37:36-41, 1988.

Meier, P., and Pugh, E.J.: Breast-feeding behavior of small preterm infants, MCN 10:396-401, 1985.

Meier, P., and Wilks, S.: The bacteria in expressed mothers' milk, MCN 12:420-423, 1987.

Moore, A.C.: Total parenteral nutrition for infants, Neonatal Network 6(2):33-40, 1987.

Moran, J.R., and others: Epidermal growth factor in human milk: daily production and diurnal variation during early lactation in mothers delivering at term and at premature gestation, J. Pediatr. 103:402-405, 1983.

Pereira, G.R., and Barbosa, M.M.: Controversies in neonatal nutrition, Pediatr. Clin. North Am. 33:65-89, 1986.

Pete, J.M.: Newborn infants' preference for sterile water versus five-percent glucose and water, J. Pediatr. Nurs. 4:263-267, 1989.

Tietjen, S.D.: Starting an infant's IV, Am. J. Nurs. 90(5):44-47, 1990.

Weaver, K.A., and Anderson, G.C.: Relationship between integrated sucking pressures and first bottle-feeding scores in premature infants, JOGNN 17(2):113-120, 1988.

Wilks, S., and Meier, P.: Helping mothers express milk suitable for preterm and high-risk infant feeding, MCN 13:121-123, 1988.

Wink, D.M.: Better breast milk for preemies? Am. J. Nurs. 89:48-50, 1989.

Developmental Outcome

Aylward, G.P.: Environmental influences on the developmental outcome of children at risk, Inf. Young Child. 2:1-9, 1990.

Bauchner, H., Brown, E., and Peskin, J.: Premature graduates of the newborn intensive care unit: a guide to follow-up, Pediatr. Clin. North Am. 35:1207-1226, 1988.

Knutson, M.G., Biro, P.J., and Padgett, D.: Tracking infants at risk: Washington State's high priority infant tracking system, J. Pediatr. Health Care 1:180-189, 1987.

Krywanio, M.L., and Jones, L.C.: Developing an early intervention program for infants at risk, J. Pediatr. Nurs. 3:375-382, 1988.

Lawhon, G., and Melzar, A.: Developmental care of the very low birth weight infant, J. Perinat. Neonatal Nurs. 2(1):56-65, 1988.

Rice, B.R., and Feeg, V.D.: First-year developmental outcomes for multiple-risk premature infants, Pediatr. Nurs. 11(1):30-35, 1985.

Saigal, S., and others: Intellectual and functional status at school entry of children who weighed 1000 grams or less at birth: a regional perspective of births in the 1980s, J. Pediatr. 116:409-416, 1990.

Schraeder, B.D., Rappaport, J., and Courtwright, L.: Preschool development of very low birthweight infants, J. Nurs. Sch. 9(4):174-178, 1987.

Termini, L., and others: Reasons for acute care visits and rehospitalization in very low-birthweight infants, Neonatal Network 8(5):23-26, 1990.

Villar, J., and others: Heterogeneous growth and mental development of intrauterine growth-retarded infants during the first 3 years of life, Pediatrics 74:783-791, 1984.

Developmental Intervention

Anderson, G.C.: Skin to skin: kangaroo care in Western Europe, Am. J. Nurs. 89:662-666, 1989.

Anderson, G.C., Marks, E.A., and Wahlberg, V.: Kangaroo care for premature infants, Am. J. Nurs. 86:807-809, 1986.

Barb, S.A., and Lemons, P.K.: The premature infant: toward improving neurodevelopmental outcome, Neonatal Network 7(6):7-15, 1989.

Brinker, R.P., and others: Identifying infants from the inner city for early intervention, Inf. Young Child. 2(1):49-58, 1989.

Eyler, F.D., and others: Effects of developmental intervention on heart rate and transcutaneous oxygen levels in low-birthweight infants, Neonatal Network 8(3):17-23, 1989.

Field, T.M., and others: Tactile/kinesthetic stimulation effects on preterm neonates, Pediatrics 77:654-658, 1986.

Harrison, L.L.: Teaching stimulation strategies to parents of infants at high risk, MCN 14:125, 1989.

Heriza, C.B., and Sweeney, J.K.: Effects of NICU intervention on preterm infants. 1. Implications for neonatal practice, Inf. Young Child. 2(3):31-47, 1990.

Heriza, C.B., and Sweeney, J.K.: Effects of NICU intervention on preterm infants. 2. Implications for movement research, Inf. Young Child. 2(4):29-41, 1990.

Horn, M.H.: Alerting an infant in brightly lit room, Crit. Care Nurse 6:84, 1986.

Lawhon, G.: Management of stress in premature infants. In Angelini, D.J., Whelan-Knapp, C.M., and Gibes, R.M.: Perinatal neonatal nursing: a clinical handbook, Boston, 1986, Blackwell Scientific Publications, Inc.

Lawhon, G., and Melzar, A.: Developmental care of the very low birth weight infant, J. Perinat. Neonatal Nurs. 2(1):56-65, 1988.

Long, T., Katz, K., and Pokorni, J.: Developmental intervention with the chronically ill infant, Inf. Young Child. 1(4):78-88, 1989.

Lott, J.W.: Developmental care of the preterm infant, Neonatal Network 7(4):21-28, 1989.

Nelson, D.B., and Clements, C.: Preterm infant stimulation: the analysis of a concept, J. Pediatr. Health Care 2:79-88, 1988.

Nelson, D., Heitman, R., and Jennings, C.: Effects of tactile stimulation on premature infant weight gain, JOGNN 15(3):262-267, 1986.

Resnick, M.B., and others: Developmental intervention for low birth weight infants: improved early developmental outcome, Pediatrics 80:68-74, 1987.

Robinson, J., and others: Eyelid opening in preterm neonates, Arch. Dis. Child. 64:943-948, 1989.

Rushton, C.H.: Promoting normal growth and development in the hospital environment, Neonatal Network 4(6):21-30, 1986.

Thoman, E.B., and Graham, S.E.: Self-regulation of stimulation by premature infants, Pediatrics 78:855-860, 1986.

Thomas, K.A.: How the NICU environment sounds to a preterm infant, MCN 14:249-251, 1989.

Weibley, T.T.: Inside the incubator, MCN 14:96-100, 1989.

Whitelaw, A.: Kangaroo baby care: just a nice experience or an important advance for preterm infants (commentary)? Pediatrics 85:604-605, 1990.

Whitelaw, G., and others: Skin-to-skin contact helps mothers bond with low birth weight babies, Arch. Dis. Child. 63:1377-1381, 1988.

White-Traut, R.C., and Nelson, M.N.: Maternally administered tactile, auditory, visual, and vestibular stimulation: relationship to later interactions between mothers and premature infants, Res. Nurs. Health 11:31-39, 1988.

White-Traut, R.C., and Pate, C.M.H.: Modulating infant state in premature infants, J. Pediatr. Nurs. 2:96-101, 1987.

White-Traut, R.C., and Tubeszewski, K.A.: Multimodal stimulation of the premature infant, J. Pediatr. Nurs. 1:90-95, 1986.

Family Support

Able-Boone, H., Dokecki, P.R., and Smith, M.S.: Parent and health care provider communication and decision making in the intensive care nursery, Child. Health Care 18:133-141, 1989.

Affleck, G., and others: Effects of formal support on mothers' adaptation to the hospital-to-home transition of high-risk infants: the benefits and costs of helping, Child Dev. 60:488-501, 1989.

Anderberg, G.J.: Initial acquaintance and attachment behavior of siblings with the newborn, JOGNN 17(1):49-54, 1988.

Arenson, J.: Discharge teaching in the NICU: the changing needs of NICU graduates and their families, Neonatal Network 6(4):29, 47-51, 1988.

Barrera, M.E., Rosenbaum, P.L., and Cunningham, C.E.: Early home interventions with low-birth-weight infants and their parents, Child Dev. 57:20-23, 1986.

Blackburn, S., and Lowen, L.: Grandparents in NICUs, MCN 11:190-192, 1986.

Blackburn, S., and Lowen, L.: Impact of an infant's premature birth on the grandparents and parents, JOGNN 15:173-178, 1986.

Blank, D.M.: Relating mothers' anxiety and perception to infant satiety, anxiety, and feeding behavior, Nurs. Res. 35(6):347-351, 1986.

Brooten, D., and others: Anxiety, depression, and hostility in mothers of preterm infants, Nurs. Res. 37(4):213-216, 1988.

Bull, M.J., Weber, K., and Stroup, K.B.: Automotive restraint systems for premature infants, J. Pediatr. 112:385-388, 1988.

Bull, M.J., and others: Establishing special needs car seat loan program, Pediatrics 85:540-547, 1990.

Butts, P.A., and others: Concerns of parents of low birthweight infants following hospital discharge: a report of parent-initiated telephone calls, Neonatal Network 7(2):37-42, 1988.

Cagan, J.: Weaning parents from intensive care unit care, MCN 13:275-277, 1988.

Campbell, L.A.: The very low birth weight infant: sensory experience and development, Top. Clin. Nurs. 6(4):19-33, 1985.

Censullo, M.: Home care of the high-risk newborn, JOGNN 15:146-153, 1986.

Consolvo, C.A.: Relieving parental anxiety in the care-by-parent unit, JOGNN 5:154-159, 1986.

Consolvo, C.A.: Siblings in the NICU, Neonatal Network 5(5):7-12, 1987.

Edwards, K.A., and Allen, M.E.: Nursing management of the human response to the premature birth experience, Neonatal Network 6(5):82-86, 1988.

Edwards, L.D., and Saunders, R.B.: Symbolic interactionism: a framework for the care of parents of preterm infants, J. Pediatr. Nurs. 5:123-128, 1990.

Eiker, S.: Dealing with long-term problems: a parent's perspective, Neonatal Network 5(2):45-49, 1986.

Fajardo, B.: Brief intervention with parents in the special care nursery, Neonatal Network 6(6):23-30, 1988.

Fleischman, A.R.: The immediate impact of the birth of a low birth weight infant on the family, National Center for Clinical Infant Programs 6(4):1-19, 1986.

Gennaro, S.: Maternal anxiety, problem-solving ability, and adaptation to the premature infant, Pediatr. Nurs. 11:343-348, 1985.

Gennaro, S.: Anxiety and problem-solving ability in mothers of premature infants, JOGNN 15:160-164, 1986.

Gottwald, S.R., and Thurman, S.K.: Parent-infant interaction in neonatal intensive care units: implications for research and service delivery, Inf. Young Child. 2(3):1-9, 1990.

Harrison, L.L., and Twardosz, S.: Teaching mothers about their preterm infants, JOGNN 15:165-172, 1986.

Hayward, E.A., Janes-Kelly, S., and Sikora, M.: Rooming-in: a preventative health care measure in the neonatal intensive care unit, Neonatal Network 7(3):29-34, 1988.

Huckabay, L.M.D.: The effect of bonding behavior of giving a mother her premature baby's picture, Nurs. Pract. 1:115-119, 1987.

Jacknik, M., Gumerman, S., and Parker, C.: Evaluating public health nursing follow-up of the high-risk infant, MCN 8:251-256, 1983.

Jenkins, R.L., and Tock, M.K.S.: Helping parents bond to their premature infant, MCN 11:32-34, 1986.

Johnson, S.H.: The premature infant. In Johnson, S.H., editor: Nursing assessment and strategies for the family at risk, ed. 2, Philadelphia, 1986, J.B. Lippincott Co.

Kavanaugh, K.: Infants weighing less than 500 grams at birth: providing parental support, J. Perinat. Neonatal Nurs. 2(2):58-66, 1988.

Kelting, S.: Supporting parents in the NICU, Neonatal Network 4(6):14-18, 1986.

Kowba, M.D., and Schwirian, P.M.: Direct sibling contact and bacterial colonization in newborns, JOGNN 14:412-417, 1985.

Levy-Shiff, R., Sharir, H., and Mogilner, M.B.: Mother- and father-preterm infant relationships in the hospital preterm nursery, Child Dev. 60:93-102, 1989.

Magyary, D.: Early social interactions: preterm infant-parent dyads, Issues Compr. Pediatr. Nurs. 7:233-254, 1984.

McBurney, B.H.: The role of the community hospital nurse in supporting parents of transported infants, Neonatal Network 6(4):60-64, 1988.

McCain, G.C.: Family functionng 2 to 4 years after preterm birth, J. Pediatr. Nurs. 5:97-104, 1990.

Montgomery, L.A.V.: An anticipatory support program for high-risk parents: follow-up results, Neonatal Network 8(3):31-33, 1989.

Montgomery, L.A.V., and Williams-Judge, S.: An anticipatory support program for high-risk parents, Neonatal Network 8(3):31-33, 1989.

Murphy, K.M.: Interactional styles of parents following the birth of a high-risk infant, J. Pediatr. Nurs. 5:33-41, 1990.

Mussell, G., and others: Use of live video transmission in the NICU, Neonatal Network 8(4):37, 1990.

Oehler, J.M.: The very low-birthweight infant as an early social partner: exploring maternal reactions, expectations, and attitudes, Neonatal Network 9(2):79, 1990.

Raff, B.S.: The use of homemaker—home health aides' perinatal care of high-risk infants, JOGNN 15:142-145, 1986.

Rivers, A., Caron, B., and Heck, M.: Experience of families with very low birthweight children with neurologic sequelae, Clin. Pediatr. 26:223-230, 1987.

Salitros, P.H.: Transitional infant care: a bridge to home for high-risk infants, Neonatal Network 4(4):35-41, 1986.

Satariano, H.J., Briggs, N.J., and O'Neal, C.: Discharges from neonatal intensive care: how satisfied are parents? Pediatr. Nurs. 13:352-353, 1987.

Sherwen, L.N.: The nursing role in helping the high-risk mother in crisis master maternal tasks, J. Perinatol. 6:75-78, 1986.

Sims-Jones, N.: Back to the theories: another way to view mothers of prematures, MCN 11:394-397, 1986.

Smith, S.M.: Primary nursing in the NICU: a parent's perspective, Neonatal Network 5(4):25-27, 1987.

Solheim, K., and Spellacy, C.: Sibling visitation: effects on newborn infection rates, JOGNN 17(1):43-48, 1988.

Steele, K.H.: Caring for parents of critically ill neonates during hospitalization: strategies for health care professionals, MCN 16(1):13-27, 1987.

Troy, P., and others: Sibling visiting in the NICU, Am. J. Nurs. 88:68-70, 1988.

Turley, M.A.: A meta-analysis of informing mothers concerning the sensory and perceptual capabilities of their infants: the effects on maternal-infant interaction, MCN 14(3):183-198, 1985.

Whetsell, M.V., and Larrabee, M.J.: Using guilt constructively in the NICU to affirm parental coping, Neonatal Network 7(4):21-27, 1988.

Yoos, L.: Applying research in practice: parenting the premature infant, Appl. Nurs. Res. 2(1):30-34, 1989.

Neonatal Loss

Amadeo, D.M.: A time for tears, Am. J. Nurs. 967-969, 1988.

Baird, S.F.: Helping the family through a crisis, Nursing '87 17(6):66-67, 1987.

Beckey, R.D., and others: Development of a perinatal grief checklist, JOGNN 14:194-199, 1985.

Bright, P.D.: Adolescent pregnancy and loss, Matern. Child. Nurs. J. 16(1):1-12, 1987.

Brown, S.E.,: A case study in death with dignity, Neonatal Network 5(2):51-53, 1986.

Bryan, E.M.: When a twin dies, Nurs. Times 80(10):24-26, 1984.

Butler, N.C.: The NICU culture versus the hospice culture: can they mix? Neonatal Network 5(2):35-42, 1986.

Eich, W.F.: When is emergency baptism appropriate? Am. J. Nurs. 87:1680-1681, 1987.

Evans, M.L., and Englebardt, S.P.: Evaluation of a multidisciplinary perinatal bereavement program, Neonatal Network 8(4):31-35, 1990.

Furrh, C.B., and Copley, R.: What you can offer when a newborn infant dies? Nursing '89 19(9):52-54, 1989.

Gardner, S.L., and Merenstein, G.B.: Helping families deal with perinatal loss, Neonatal Network 5(2):17-22, 1986.

Gardner, S.L., and Merenstein, G.B.: Perinatal grief and loss: an overview, Neonatal Network 5(2):7-15, 1986.

Glassman-Feibusch, B.: Extremely uncaring (letters to the editor), MCN 8:442, 1983.

Harden, M.: God bless the child and the keepers, Am. J. Nurs. 88:654-655, 1988.

Ilse, S., and Furrh, C.B.: Development of a comprehensive follow-up care plan after perinatal and neonatal loss, J. Perinat. Neonatal Nurs. 2(2):23-33, 1988.

Johannsen, L.: As birth and death coincide, MCN 14:89-92, 1989.

Jost, K.E., and Haase, J.E.: At the time of death: help for the child's parents, Child. Health Care 18:146-152, 1989.

Klingbeil, C.G.: Extended nursing care after a perinatal loss: theoretical implications, Neonatal Network 5(3):21-28, 1986.

Krone, C., and Harris, C.C.: The importance of infant gender and family resemblance with parents' perinatal bereavement process: establishing personhood, J. Perinat. Neonatal Nurs. 2(2):1-11, 1988.

Maguire, D.P., and Skoolicas, S.J.: Developing a bereavement follow-up program, J. Perinat. Neonatal Nurs. 2(2):67-77, 1988.

Malcolm, N., and Wooten, B.: It's hard to say goodbye, Can. Nurse 83(4):26-28, 1987.

Mina, C.: A program for helping grieving parents, MCN 10:118-121, 1985.

Novak, S.: In moments of crisis, MCN 13:349-351, 1988.

Shwartz, D.: When the baby doesn't come home, Child. Today 13:21-24, 1984.

Swanson-Kauffman, K.: There should have been two: nursing care of parents experiencing the perinatal death of a twin, J. Perinat. Neonatal Nurs. 2(2):78-86, 1988.

Szgalsky, J.B.: Perinatal death, the family, and the role of the health professional, Neonatal Network 8(2):15-19, 1989.

Thomas, N., and Cordell, A.: The dying infant: aiding parents in the detachment process, Pediatr. Nurs. 9:355-357, 1983.

Trouy, M.B., and Ward-Larson, C.: Sibling grief, Neonatal Network 5(4):35-40, 1987.

VanPutte, A.W.: Perinatal bereavement crisis: coping with negative outcomes from prenatal diagnosis, J. Perinat. Neonatal Nurs. 2(2):12-22, 1988.

Walker, L.J., and McDonough-Tuccillo, C.A.: Family support following infant death, Neonatal Network 2:41-43, 1983.

Wilson, A.L., and others: Parental responses to perinatal death: mother-father differences, Am. J. Dis. Child. 139:1235-1241, 1985.

Windau, V., and Dewitt, P.J.: Emergency baptism by nurses in an NICU: answering a spiritual need, Neonatal Network 7(1):57-62, 1988.

Work, R.B.: When we cannot cure, care (letters to the editor), MCN 8:111-112, 1983.

Idiopathic Respiratory Distress Syndrome

Avery, M.E.: The argument for prenatal administration of dexamethasone to prevent respiratory distress syndrome, J. Pediatr. 104:240, 1984.

Bancalari, E.: Transcutaneous oxygen monitoring: a new wave in newborn care, Comtemp. Pediatr. 4(1):107-110, 1987.

Birdsall, C.: How do you measure transcutaneous oxygen? Am. J. Nurs. 87(10):1273, 1987.

Boynton, B.R., and others: Combined high-frequency oscillatory ventilation and intermittent mandatory ventilation in critically ill neonates, J. Pediatr. 105:297-300, 1984.

Bucher, H., and others: Hyperoxemia in newborn infants: detection by pulse oximetry, Pediatrics 84:226-230, 1989.

Carter, J.M., and others: High-frequency oscillatory ventilation and extracorporeal membrane oxygenation for the treatment of acute neonatal respiratory failure, Pediatrics 85:159-164, 1989.

Cheng, M., and Williams, P.D.: Oxygenation during chest physiotherapy of very-low-birth-weight infants: relations among fraction of inspired oxygen levels, number of hand ventilations, and transcutaneous oxygen pressure, J. Pediatr. Nurs. 4(6):411-418, 1989.

Clancy, G.T.: Blood gas monitoring and management of neonates with respiratory distress, J. Perinat. Neonatal Nurs. 1(1):72-83, 1987.

Doyle, L.W., and others: Effects of antenatal steroid therapy on mortality and morbidity in very low birth weight infants, J. Pediatr. 108:287-292, 1986.

Erenberg, A., and Nowak, A.J.: Palatal groove formation in neonates with orotracheal tubes, Am. J. Dis. Child. 134:974, 1984.

Few, B.J.: Neonatal update: surfactant replacement therapy, MCN 12:129, 1987.

Few, B.J.: Corticosteroids and repiratory distress syndrome, MCN 13:17, 1988.

Garland, J.S., and others: Increased risk of gastrointestinal perforations in neonates mechanically ventilated with either face mask or nasal prongs, Pediatrics 76:406-410, 1985.

Gitlin, J.D., and others: Randomized controlled trial of exogenous surfactant for the treatment of hyaline membrane disease, Pediatrics 79:31-37, 1987.

Gruden, M.: High-frequency ventilation: an overview, Crit. Care Nurs. 5:36-40, 1985.

Gunderson, L.P., and Kenner, C.: Transcutaneous oxygen monitoring: description and clinical application, Neonatal Network 6(6):7-14, 1988.

Harbold, L.A.: A protocol for neonatal use of pulse oximetry, Neonatal Network 8(1):41-42, 56-57, 1989.

Hartsell, M.: Noninvasive oxygen monitoring, J. Pediatr. Nurs. 87(1):54-64, 1987.

Hay, W.W., Brockway, J.M., and Eyzaguirre, M.: Neonatal pulse oximetry: accuracy and reliability, Pediatrics 83:717-722, 1989.

Henderson, C.: Overwhelmed by infant resuscitation? Remember your "ABCDEs," Neonatal Network 7(3):35-39, 1988.

Inwood, S., Finley, G.A., and Fitzhardinge, P.M.: High-frequency oscillation: a new mode of ventilation for the neonate, Neonatal Network 4(5):53-58, 1986.

Ioli, J.G., and Richardson, M.J.: Giving surfactant to premature infants, Am. J. Nurs. 90:59-60, 1990.

Jennis, M.S., and Peabody, J.L.: Pulse oximetry: an alternative method for the assessment of oxygenation in newborn infants, Pediatrics 79:524-528, 1987.

Kaplow, R., and Fromme, L.R.: Nursing care plan for the patient receiving high-frequency jet ventilation, Crit. Care Nurs. 5:25-27, 1985.

Karp, T.B., and others: High frequency jet ventilation: a neonatal nursing perspective, Neonatal Network. 4(5):42-50, 1986.

Kling, P.: Respiratory distress syndrome in the tiny baby, Neonatal Network 4(5):7-13, 1986.

Lapido, M.: Respiratory distress syndrome, Neonatal Network 8(3):9-14, 1989.

Loper, D.L.: Surfactant replacement therapy, Neonatal Network 4(5):14-17, 1986.

McMillan, D.D., and others: Benefits of orotracheal and nasotracheal intubation in neonates requiring ventilatory assistance, Pediatrics 77:39-44, 1986.

Neumann, M.: Surfactant administration: an ethical dilemma, JOGNN 17(2):80-82, 1988.

Oellrich, R.G.: Pneumothorax, chest tubes, and the neonate, MCN 10:29-35, 1985.

Polak, M.J., Donnelly, W.H., and Bucciarelli, R.L.: Comparison of airway pathologic lesions after high-frequency jet or conventional ventilation, Am. J. Dis. Child. 143:228-232, 1989.

Richardson, C.: Hyaline membrane disease: future treatment modalities, J. Perinat. Neonatal Nurs. 2(1):78-88, 1988.

Riedel, K.: Pulse oximetry: a new technology to assess patient oxygen needs in the neonatal intensive care unit, J. Perinat. Neonatal Nurs. 1(1):49-57, 1987.

Runkle, B., and Bancalari, E.: Acute cardiopulmonary effects of pancuronium bromide in mechanically ventilated newborn infants, J. Pediatr. 104:614-617, 1984.

Walsh, C.M., and others: Controlled supplemental oxygenation during tracheobronchial hygiene, Nurs. Res. 36:211-215, 1987.

Respiratory Conditions

American Academy of Pediatrics, Committee on Fetus and Newborn: Recommendations on extracorporeal membrane oxygenation, Pediatrics 85:618-619, 1990.

Cunningham, A.S., and others: Tracheal suction and meconium: a proposed standard of care, J. Pediatr. 115:153-154, 1990.

Gregory, S.E.B.: Air leak syndromes, Neonatal Network 5(4):40-46, 1987.

Kleiber, C., and Hummel, P.A.: Factors related to spontaneous endotracheal extubation in the neonate, Pediatr. Nurs. 15:347-351, 1989.

Marecki, M.A.: *Chlamydia trachomatis:* a developing perinatal problem, J. Perinat. Neonatal Nurs. 1(4):1-11, 1988.

Martin, R.J., Miller, M.J., and Carlo, W.A.: Pathogenesis of apnea in preterm infants, J. Pediatr. 109:733-741, 1986.

Murphy, J.D., Vawter, G.F., and Reid, L.M.: Pulmonary vascular disease in fetal meconium aspiration, J. Pediatr. 104:785-789, 1984.

Perehudoff, B.: Newborn resuscitation in the delivery room, J. Perinat. Neonatal Nurs. 3(2):81-90, 1989.

Swaminathan, S., and others: Long-term pulmonary sequelae of meconium aspiration syndrome, J. Pediatr. 114:356-361, 1989.

Turnage, C.S.: Meconium aspiration syndrome, J. Perinat. Neonatal Nurs. 3(2):69-80, 1989.

Wood, A.F.: Sequelae of perinatal analysis, Neonatal Network 5(5):21-23, 1987.

Bronchopulmonary Dysplasia

Abman, S.H., Accurso, F.J., and Koops, B.L.: Experience with home oxygen in the management of infants with bronchopulmonary dysplasia, Clin. Pediatr. 23:471-474, 1984.

Adams, D.: Kasey's story, Neonatal Network 7(3):19-23, 1988.

Avery, G.B., and others: Controlled trial of dexamethasone in respirator-dependent infants with bronchopulmonary dysplasia, Pediatrics 75:106-107, 1985.

Boyzynski, M.E.A.: Comprehensive management of the infant with bronchopulmonary dysplasia: a growing challenge, Inf. Young Child. 2(1):14-24, 1989.

Frank, M.: Theophylline: a closer look, Neonatal Network 6(2):7-13, 1987.

Hagedorn, M.I., and Gardner, S.L.: Physiologic sequelae of prematurity: the nurse practitioner's role. 1. Respiratory issues, J. Pediatr. Health Care 3:288-297, 1989.

Harvey, C., and others: Training parents for home care of babies who have bronchopulmonary dysplasia: the role of the parenting specialist, Zero to Three, pp. 19-22, 1988.

Jackson, D.F.: Nursing care plan: home management of children with BPD, Pediatr. Nurs. 12:342-348, 1986.

Loisel, D.B., Smith, M.M., and MacDonald, M.G.: Plasma theophylline levels as related to toxicity in infants with severe chronic lung disease, Neonatal Network 6(2):15-19, 1987.

McElheny, J.E.: Parental adaptation to a child with bronchopulmonary dysplasia, J. Pediatr. Nurs. 4:346-352, 1989.

Paulson, P.R.: Nursing considerations for discharging children home on low-flow oxygen, Issues Compr. Pediatr. Nurs. 10:109-214, 1987.

Perry, M.A., and Hayes, N.M.: Bronchopulmonary dysplasia: discharge planning and complex home care, Neonatal Network 7(3):13-17, 1988.

Pridham, K.F., and others: Parental issues in feeding young children with bronchopulmonary dysplasia, J. Pediatr. Nurs. 4:177-185, 1989.

Steele, N.F., and Harrison, B.: Technology-assisted children: assessing discharge preparation, J. Pediatr. Nurs. 1:150-158, 1986.

Young, L.Y., Creighton, D.E., and Sauve, R.S.: The needs of families of infants discharged home with continuous oxygen therapy, JOGNN 17(3):187-193, 1988.

Sepsis

Amspacher, K.A.: Necrotizing enterocolitis: the never-ending challenge, J. Perinat. Neonatal Nurs. 3(2):58-68, 1989.

Becker, L., and Lagomarsino, W.: Isolation guidelines for perinatal patients: creating a new protocol, MCN 12:400-404, 1987.

Cerase, P.A.: Neonatal sepsis, J. Perinat. Neonatal Nurs. 3(2):48-57, 1989.

Cohen, S.P.: Bacterial sepsis in the very low birth weight infant, J. Perinat. Neonatal Nurs. 1(4):66-77, 1988.

Cushing, A.H.: Omphalitis: still potential for disaster, Contemp. Pediatr. 4(5):61-73, 1987.

Gaffney, S.E, and Salinger, L.: Group B streptococcus: the pregnant woman and her neonate, JOGNN 16(2):91-96, 1987.

Gordin, P.C.: Candida infection in the very low birth weight infant, J. Perinat. Neonatal Nurs. 1(4):47-55, 1988.

Henneberry, C.: Candida sepsis in the very low birthweight infant, Neonatal Network 5(6):39-45, 1987.

Larson, E.: Rituals in infection control: what works in the newborn nursery? JOGNN 16(6):411-416, 1987.

Larson, E.: Trends in neonatal infections, JOGNN 16(6):404-409, 1987.

Poulsen, N.: Candidiasis in the premature infant, Neonatal Network 8(4):9-14, 1990.

Stegagno, M., and others: Immunologic follow-up of infants treated with granulocyte transfusion for neonatal sepsis, Pediatrics 76:508-511, 1985.

Walsh, M., and Kliegman, R.M.: Necrotizing enterocolitis: treatment based on staging criteria, Pediatr. Clin. North Am. 33:179-201, 1986.

Whiteman, L., Wuethrick, M., and Egan, E.: Infants who survive necrotizing enterocolitis, Matern. Child. Nurs. J. 14(3):123-134, 1985.

Cardiovascular Conditions

Dallman, P.R.: Erythropoietin and the anemia of prematurity, J. Pediatr. 105:756-757, 1984.

Dooley, K.J.: Management of the premature infant with a patent ductus arteriosus, Pediatr. Clin. North Am. 31:1159-1174, 1984.

Dudell, G.G., and Gersony, W.M.: Patent ductus arteriosus in neonates with severe respiratory disease, J. Pediatr. 104:915-919, 1984.

Fuller, R.: Cardiac function and the neonatal EKG. I. Introduction to neonatal EKGs, Neonatal Network 7(4):47-51, 1989.

Fuller, R.: Cardiac function and the neonatal EKG. II. Bradycardia, Neonatal Network 7(6):61-63, 1989.

Fuller, R.: Cardiac function and the neonatal EKG. III. Tachycardia, Neonatal Network 7(6):65-67, 1989.

Fuller, R.: Cardiac function and the neonatal EKG. IV. Chamber enlargement and axis determination, Neonatal Network 8(1):77-81, 1989.

Gerraughty, A.B., and Younie, L.J.: The artificial lung for gravely ill newborns, Am. J. Nurs. 87:655-658, 1987.

Goble, M.M., and Rocchini, A.P.: Neonatal hypertension: why it happens, what to do about it, Contemp. Pediatr. 7(2):89-100, 104-108, 113-118, 1990.

Hageman, J., Adams, A., and Gardner, T.: Persistent pulmonary hypertension of the newborn, Am. J. Dis. Child. 138:627-695, 1984.

Henry, G.W.: Noninvasive assessment of PPHN, Clin. Perinatol. 2:627-639, 1984.

Krueger, E., and others: Prevention of symptomatic patent ductus arteriosus with a single dose of indomethacin, J. Pediatr. 111:749-754, 1987.

Lawson, M.: Persistent pulmonary hypertension of the newborn: current trends in classification and diagnosis, Neonatal Network 6(1):27-35, 1987.

Nugent, J.: Extracorporeal membrane oxygenation in the neonate, Neonatal Network 4(50):27-38, 1986.

Sell, E., and others: Persistent fetal circulation—neurodevelopment outcome, Am. J. Dis. Child. 139:25-28, 1985.

Southwell, S.: Update on the treatment of persistent pulmonary hypertension of the newborn, Neonatal Network 4(50):19-25, 1986.

Stockman, J.A.: Anemia of prematurity, Pediatr. Clin. North Am. 33:111-128, 1986.

Retinopathy of Prematurity

Bancalari, E., and others: Influence of transcutaneous oxygen monitoring on the incidence of retinopathy of prematurity, Pediatrics 79:663-669, 1987.

Brown, D.R., and others: Retinopathy of prematurity, Am. J. Dis. Child. 141:154-160, 1987.
Few, B.J.: Pharmacologic use of vitamin E, MCN 13:283, 1988.
Gardner, S.L., and Hagedorn, M.I.: Physiologic sequelae of prematurity: the nurse practitioner's role. II. Retinopathy of prematurity, J. Pediatr. Health Care 4:72-76, 1990.
George, D.S., and others: The latest on retinopathy of prematurity, MCN 13:254-258, 1988.
An international classification of retinopathy of prematurity. II. The classification of retinal detachment, Pediatrics 82:37-43, 1988.
Long, C.A.: Cryotherapy: a new treatment for retinopathy of prematurity, Pediatr. Nurs. 15:269-272, 1989.
Lucey, J.F., and Dangman, B.: A reexamination of the role of oxygen in retrolental fibroplasia, Pediatrics 73:82-96, 1984.
Multicenter trial of cryotherapy for retinopathy of prematurity: preliminary results, Pediatrics 81:697-706, 1988.
Noerr, B.: Vitamin E (alpha-tocopherol), Neonatal Network 9(2):85-87, 1990.
Purohit, D.M., and others: Risk factors for retrolental fibroplasia: experience with 3,025 premature infants, Pediatrics 76:339-344, 1985.
Shapiro, C.: Retrolental fibroplasia: what we know and what we don't know, Neonatal Network 4(6):33-44, 1986.

Neurologic Disturbances

Allan, W.C., and Volpe, J.J.: Periventricular-intraventricular hemorrhage, Pediatr. Clin. North Am. 33:47-63, 1986.
Brann, A.W.: Hypoxic ischemic encephalopathy (asphyxia), Pediatr. Clin. North Am. 33:451-464, 1986.
Calciolari, G., Perlman, J.M., and Volpe, J.J.: Seizures in the neonatal intensive care unit of the 1980s, Clin. Pediatr. 27:119-123, 1988.
Cunningham, M.: Intraventricular hemorrhage in the premature, Dimens. Crit. Care Nurs. 6:20-27, 1987.
Gilman, J.T., and others: Rapid sequential phenobarbital treatment of neonatal seizures, Pediatrics 83:674-678, 1989.
Guzzetta, F., and others: Periventricular intraparenchymal echodensities in the premature newborn: critical determinant of neurologic outcome, Pediatrics 78:995-1006, 1986.
Kuban, K., and Teele, R.L.: Rationale for grading intracranial hemorrhage in premature infants, Pediatrics 74:358-363, 1984.
MacDonald, N.P.: Motor development in premature infants with intracranial hemorrhage, Pediatr. Nurs. 12:263-267, 1986.
Painter, M.J., Bergman, I., and Crumrine, P.: Neonatal seizures, Pediatr. Clin. North Am. 33:91-109, 1986.
Scher, M.S., and Painter, M.J.: Controversies concerning neonatal seizures, Pediatr. Clin. North Am. 36:281-310, 1989.
Torrence, C.: Neonatal seizures. I. A developmental and clinical understanding, Neonatal Network 4(8)9-15, 1985.

Conditions Related to Maternal Conditions

Alexander, L.L.: The pregnant smoker: nursing implications, JOGNN 16(3):167-173, 1987.
Berk, M.A., and others: Macrosomia in infants of insulin-dependent diabetic mothers, Pediatrics 83:1029-1034, 1989.
Berman, S.M., Hogue, C.J.R., and Marks, J.S.: Maternal cigarette smoking: effect on infant birth weight (letter), JAMA 253:911-915, 1984.
Calciolari, G., Perlman, J.M., and Volpe, J.J.: Seizures in the neonatal intensive care unit of the 1980s: types, etiologies, timing, Clin. Pediatr. 27:119-123, 1988.
Chavez, G.F., Mulinare, J., and Cordero, J.F.: Maternal cocaine use during early pregnancy as a risk factor for congenital urogenital anomalies, JAMA 262:796-798, 1989.
Committee on Drugs: Neonatal drug withdrawal, Pediatrics 102:895-902, 1983.
Flandermeyer, A.A.: A comparison of the effects of heroin and cocaine abuse upon the neonate, Neonatal Network 6(3):42-47, 1987.
Fulroth, R., Phillips, B., and Durand, D.J.: Perinatal outcome of infants exposed to cocaine and/or heroin in utero, Am. J. Dis. Child. 143:905-910, 1989.
Hayes, J.S., Dreher, M.C., and Nugent, J.K.: Newborn outcomes with maternal marihuana use in Jamaican women, Pediatr. Nurs. 14:107-110, 1988.
Kennard, M.J.: Cocaine use during pregnancy: fetal and neonatal effects, J. Perinat. Neonatal Nurs. 3(4):53-63, 1990.
Merker, L., Higgins, P., and Kinnard, E.: Assessing narcotic addiction in neonates, Pediatr. Nurs. 11:177-181, 1985.
Mulinare, J., and Carders, J.F.: Maternal cocaine use during early pregnancy as a risk factor for congenital urogenital anomalies, JAMA 262:795-798, 1989.
Perlman, R.H.: The infant of the diabetic mother: pathophysiology and management, Primary Care 10:751-760, 1983.
Rhodes, A.M.: Maternal liability for fetal injury? MCN 15:41, 1990.
Smith, J.E., and Deitch, K.V.: Cocaine: a maternal, fetal, and neonatal risk, J. Pediatr. Health Care 1:120-124, 1987.
Torrance, C.R., and Horns, K.M.: Appraisal and caregiving for the drug-addicted infant, Neonatal Network 8(3):49-59, 1989.
Verklan, M.T.: Safe in the womb? Drug and chemical effects on the fetus and neonate, Neonatal Network 8(10):59-65, 1989.
White, E.E.: Developmental abnormalities in the chemically dependent newborn, Home Healthc. Nurs. 5(4):26-31, 1987.

CHAPTER 11

Conditions Caused by Defects in Physical Development

RELATED TOPICS

Autosomal inheritance patterns, Ch. 5
Birth injuries, Ch. 9
"Birthmarks," Ch. 9
Bodily injury and pain, Ch. 26
Cerebral palsy, Ch. 40
Gastric feeding techniques, Ch. 27
Health promotion of the newborn and family, Ch. 8
The high-risk newborn and family, Ch. 10
Hypertrophic pyloric stenosis, Ch. 33
Multifactorial disorders, Ch. 5
Newborn assessment, Ch. 8
Osteogenesis imperfecta, Ch. 39
Preparation for procedures: surgical procedures, Ch. 27
Promotion of parent-infant bonding (attachment), Ch. 8

GLOSSARY

ACM Arnold-Chiari malformation
AFP Alpha fetoprotein
agenesis Absence of a body part caused by lack of primordial tissue
anomaly Marked deviation from the normal; anything structurally unusual, irregular, or contrary to a general rule
aplasia Absence of a body part caused by failure of the normal primordia to develop
association A nonrandom occurrence of multiple malformations for which no specific or common etiology has been identified

atrophy Decreased development of a mass of tissue or an organ as a result of a decrease in cell size or number
CDH Congenital dislocated hip
CHD Congenital hip dysplasia
CIC Clean intermittent catheterization
CL Cleft lip
CLP Cleft lip and palate
CL(P), CL/P Cleft lip with or without cleft palate
CNS Central nervous system
congenital Present at birth
CP Cleft palate
CSF Cerebrospinal fluid
CT Computed tomography
deformity Abnormal form, shape, or position of a part caused by mechanical forces
differentiation Process whereby embryonic cells acquire individual characteristics and function
dysplasia Abnormal organization of cells into tissue(s) and its morphologic result(s)
EA Esophageal atresia
ET Endotracheal
FAS Fetal alcohol syndrome
GI Gastrointestinal
GU Genitourinary
hyperplasia, hypoplasia Overdevelopment or underdevelopment of an organ or tissue that results from an increase or decrease in the number of cells
hypertrophy Increase in the size of organs, tissues, or cells
ICP Intracranial pressure
malformation Morphogenic defect of an organ, part of an organ, or larger region of the body resulting from an intrinsically abnormal developmental process
MRI Magnetic resonance imaging
MZ Monozygotic
NG Nasogastric
nociception Perception by nerve endings of traumatic or painful stimuli
NTD Neural tube defect
OFC Occipital frontal circumference
pathogenesis Mechanisms leading to an abnormal structure, form, or function
SB Spina bifida
syndrome A recognized pattern of malformations with a single, specific etiology
TEF Tracheoesophageal fistula
teratogen A substance, agent, or process that interferes with normal prenatal development, producing one or more developmental abnormalities in the fetus
TEV Talipes equinovarus
TORCH Toxoplasmosis, other, rubella, cytomegalovirus, herpes
VP ventriculoperitoneal

Congenital malformations constitute a large percentage of the health problems of infants and children, and although many severe disorders of childhood can be either prevented or effectively treated, very little progress has been achieved in prevention of congenital defects. Birth defects are listed as the underlying cause of death in 20.5% of reported infant deaths, making birth defects the leading cause of infant mortality (Centers for Disease Control, 1989). It is calculated that approximately one third of hospitalized children suffer from a congenital abnormality or its sequelae.

DEFECTS IN PHYSICAL DEVELOPMENT

Congenital malformations may be caused by genetic or environmental factors, and not all congenital defects are considered to be malformations—for example, inborn errors of metabolism and mental retardation. However, this chapter is primarily concerned with structural abnormalities, most of which are apparent at birth, and with the impact on the family of the birth of a child with a physical defect. The genetic basis of physical defects is discussed in Chapter 5, and specific disorders are presented as appropriate throughout the book.

The period from conception to birth is a mysterious and little known phase of the life cycle. It is the period when the fewest outside demands are placed on the organism, but at the same time it is fraught with dangers that may have lifelong consequences. Recognition of the importance of this period of rapid growth and change has focused interest on fetal development, the relationship between prenatal events and infant health, and the factors that influence the well-being of the individual during this and subsequent stages of life.

PRENATAL DEVELOPMENT

When they begin their existence, human beings bear no resemblance to the complex organisms into which they will develop. In fact, during the very early stages they are indistinguishable from any other animal species. The early zygote contains no structures that remotely correspond to any of the organs and tissues that will make up the fully developed individual. Development consists of two distinct but interrelated processes: growth and differentiation.

Fetal Growth

Growth results when cells divide and synthesize new proteins and is reflected in increased size and weight. It is accomplished by two mechanisms: (1) *hyperplasia* and (2) *hypertrophy.* Hyperplasia is the predominant form of growth during the embryonic period; although the rate decreases during later stages of gestation, cell division continues in variable degrees throughout childhood. Hypertrophy is more prominent during later periods of growth.

Each organ and tissue has a typical growth pattern, and all organs progress from a stage characterized by increase in cell number to one of growth by increase in cell size. Any interference with this pattern of growth results in a reduction in the size and weight of that organ. However, the consequences of the inhibiting factor depend on whether the insult is inflicted during a period of hyperplasia or a period of hypertrophy. Interruption of growth during cell enlargement is usually only temporary and can be overcome with proper intervention. Interference with growth during a period of cell proliferation is likely to cause irreversible growth retardation of that organ with permanent deficit in overall cell numbers.

Differentiation

Differentiation is the process by which early cells are systematically modified and specialized to form all the tissues that are necessary to ensure an organized, coordinated individual. Each step in this process depends on successful completion of a previous step. Anything that interferes with one of these steps, such as a mutant gene or environmental agent, will cause an arrest in the development of that particular tissue or organ. Divergence from the normal course of development will result in maldevelopment of a part or, if it occurs at an early age, a sequence of distortions causing more severe or multiple malformations.

There appears to be a relationship between the incidence of one congenital anomaly and the presence of additional anomalies in an affected child. For example, there is a striking association between malformed ears and kidney abnormalities that reflects a common developmental stage. The knowledge of the stage of development for a variety of organs and systems provides a valuable clue for the examiner. When one defect is observed, closer scrutiny may reveal defects in another organ or system related to the same stage of development.

Organogenesis

Extremely rapid development and change take place during the first 8 to 12 weeks of fetal life, and the beginnings of all major organ systems are formed. The embryo begins to acquire the specific functions needed to integrate these organs and organ systems into an organized, coordinated whole. It is also the period during which the organism is most vulnerable to structural disturbance from environmental hazards.

Sensitive Periods in Prenatal Development

Every organ, system, and body part goes through a period during which it experiences the most rapid cell division and differentiation. During this time the organism displays a marked susceptibility to injurious influences. These specific stages of crucial developmental advancement are termed *sensitive,* or *critical periods,* and the major impact of environmental factors on development always coincides with these periods.

The sensitive periods for all organs or parts do not occur simultaneously. A part that is susceptible to adverse influences at one particular time may be resistant to the same influences at other periods of development. At the same time, another part may be highly sensitive at that moment. Susceptibility to environmental influences decreases as organ formation advances—the younger the organism and the fewer the number of cells, the greater the extent of involvement when an adverse influence is applied.

During the period of intensive differentiation most teratogenic agents are highly effective and may produce a variety of deformities. The type of defect that is produced depends on which organ is most susceptible at the time of application. The susceptibility of most tissues to teratogenic influences decreases rapidly in the later periods of development, which are characterized by growth and elaboration of established organs. However, some tissues, particularly the central nervous system, are sensitive to varying degrees throughout fetal life and even beyond. Fig. 11-1 illustrates the approximate times of critical differentiation for some of the major organs and systems.

The origin or method by which prenatal growth processes are disturbed to produce a structural or functional defect is termed teratogenesis (from the Greek *teratos,* monster, and *genesis,* production). An agent capable of producing such an effect is a *teratogen.* (See Congenital Defects Caused by Prenatal Factors, p. 519.)

BIRTH OF A CHILD WITH A PHYSICAL DEFECT

Parents are the most significant influence in the life of the child, and the initial parent-infant attachment is the relationship on which future interactions are based. The birth of any child is considered by some to constitute a crisis situation, but when the newborn suffers from a physical or mental defect, the parents' need for understanding and supportive care from health professionals is magnified. The manner in which nurses and other health personnel work with the parents immediately after the birth profoundly influences the situation for all persons concerned.

Parental Responses

Part of the preparation for childbirth involves fantasies and images of the expected infant. Normally, every parent wishes for a perfect child, but at the same time the parents fear that the infant will be abnormal. This fear is often expressed by the expectant parents when they state that their concern is not whether the child is a girl or a boy, just that the infant is healthy. One of the first things the mother wishes confirmed at the time of birth is: "Is my baby all right?" In many instances there is some discrepancy between the parents' idealized child and the infant the mother delivers, as, for example, the birth of a boy when they had hoped for a girl. Resolution of this discrepancy is a developmental task of parenthood and is essential to the estab-

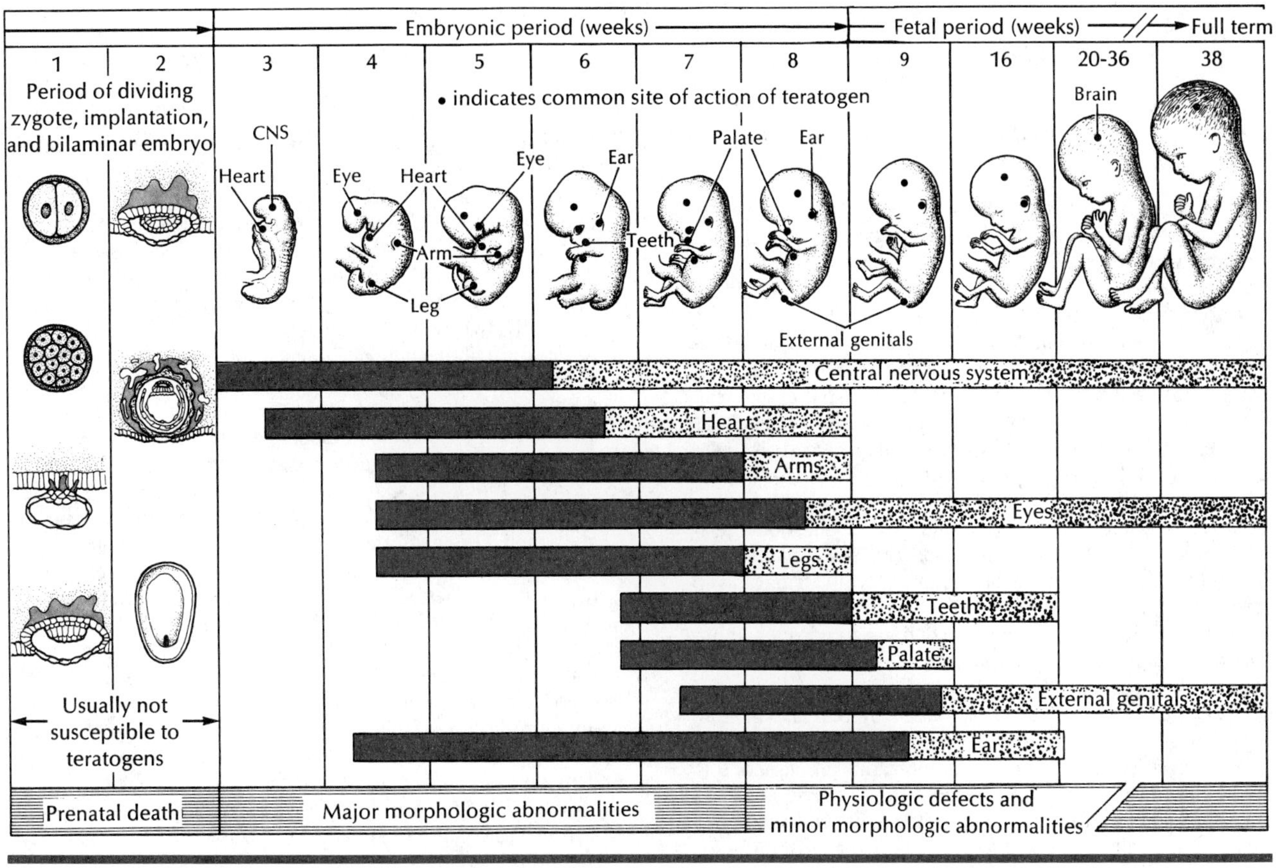

Fig. 11-1. Sensitive, or critical, periods in human development. Solid red line denotes highly sensitive periods; stippled color indicates stages when embryo is less sensitive to teratogens.

From Moore, K.L.: The developing human: clinically oriented embryology, ed. 4, Philadelphia, 1988, W.B. Saunders Co.

lishment of a healthy parent-child relationship. If this discrepancy is too great, as with the birth of an infant with a gross defect, or when the wishes of the parents are unrealistic, the resulting emotional stress may be overwhelming.

The more severe the defect, the greater the impact of the experience, especially for the mother. The birth of a child with a physical defect abruptly ends the psychologic attachment the mother has formed during pregnancy with the idealized child. She and the father must now deal with loss of the anticipated healthy child while they face meeting the demands of the abnormal child for care and affection. The birth of an infant with a defect evokes the same psychologic reaction as the death of a child. The need for the parents to grieve for the loss of the expected child while adapting to the care of the child with a disability places overwhelming demands on them at a time when their own psychologic and physiologic resources have been depleted by the birth experience (Solnit and Stark, 1963). The impact of this new and unexpected burden inhibits the accomplishment of the grief work that normally follows a loss.

The grief reaction experienced by parents at the birth of a child with a physical disability is the same as the response that follows the loss of any valued or significant object. The parents experience shock, frustration, and anger at what has happened to them, and they ask themselves, "Why? Why me?" Parents may feel shame and embarrassment, often with feelings of personal failure and guilt. Frequently the mother believes that she might have caused harm to the unborn child, and she may associate the condition with wrongdoing or evil thoughts, especially if the pregnancy was unwanted initially. She may believe the defect to be the result of passive or active attempts to terminate the pregnancy, such as deliberate attempts to induce abortion or failure to obtain prenatal care or comply with the practitioner's instructions.

There is a phase of overwhelming *shock,* accompanied by weeping and feelings of helplessness. To deal with stress and anxiety, parents use defense mechanisms that have provided protection in the past. A very common response is *disbelief* and *denial,* which may be short-lived or may last for many months. They do not appear to "hear" what is told to them about their child, and they behave as though nothing is wrong with the child. However, denial during the shock phase of the grief process can serve as a constructive means for parents to deal with the sudden and profound impact of the initial stress until they are better able to cope with the situation.

When parents are unable to face the reality of the infant's condition, they may *withdraw* from the situation either physically or emotionally. They frequently become incapac-

QUESTIONS AND CONTROVERSIES

Are there times or circumstances under which certain infants should be denied medical care?

One of the most painful dilemmas faced by families and health professionals is the decision regarding the care of children with severe defects, including decisions for life or death. In most cases there is no problem; infants are treated and deformities corrected as early as possible. The ethical, moral, and legal dilemmas are encountered when decisions must be made for children with lethal or borderline prognoses. Most parents and professionals resist keeping children alive who have universally fatal disorders, such as anencephaly or trisomy 13. The usual management is sedation and skilled nursing and parental care. No heroic measures are attempted. With infants who are borderline—that is, those for whom the quality of life may be questionable—the problem becomes more complex. These are infants with conditions such as severe prematurity, brain damage, and severe spina bifida.

As knowledge and technology continue to advance, more and more high-risk and borderline children are surviving neonatal hazards, but the incidence of severe developmental defects and chronic sequelae also increases (Britton, Fitzhardinge, and Ashby, 1981). The prevailing philosophy is to treat these children. However, the reasons are varied: it is morally right; to treat is best because the outcome is uncertain; it is hospital or nursery policy; it is a way to learn about treatment; to allow a child to die sets a poor example for staff; and it avoids legal entanglements.

Most of the reasons have little to do with the interests of the child (Duff, 1981). The wisdom of these rescue efforts is being questioned. Do the benefits of treatment outweigh the burdens of treatment to the infant? Will treatment achieve for that child a state of functioning that is satisfactory to the infant who has never experienced the advantages and disadvantages of a normal world (Penticuff, 1988)? Is existence, or life, an end in itself regardless of the quality of that life?

Likewise, the question has arisen regarding who has the right to deny treatment for severely afflicted children. All too often health professionals, oriented toward aggressive treatment and saving lives, impose their values on families who are aware of the long-term implications but who are made to feel guilty if they resist therapeutic efforts on the child's behalf. Many times salvaging the lethally impaired or marginally viable child places such an emotional and financial burden on the family that both the child and the family suffer.

The Committee on Bioethics of the American Academy of Pediatrics (1983) has stated that "while the needs and interests of parents, as well as the larger society, are proper concerns . . . (the) primary moral and legal obligation is to the child-patient. Withholding or withdrawing life-sustaining treatment is justified only if such a course serves the interests of the patient." The Academy (1984) has provided some principles on which care and treatment of disabled infants can be based. Both the Academy and the President's Commission for the Study of Ethical Problems in Medicine and Biomedical and Behavioral Research (1983) recommend establishment of infant bioethics committees to aid parents and treating physicians in making ethical decisions.

Ideally decisions regarding care of a child who is severely disabled should be shared by both family and health professionals. Parents need to know the long-term personal and social implications of the decision, and, even when greatly stressed, the parents are capable of sharing these difficult decisions (Benfield, Lieb, and Vollman, 1978). Parents are expressing concern regarding their perceptions that prolonged care imposes undue stress and suffering on the infant (Harrison, 1986). Families of neonates for whom life support was withdrawn expressed no guilt about their decision on follow-up; nor did they suffer prolonged or pathologic grieving (Walwork and Ellison, 1985). Whether this can be applied to denying treatment is questionable.

When families are forced into a position of helplessness and professionals are unable to assume the responsibility, the ultimate decision is turned over to a committee or to the courts. It is becoming increasingly important for families of children who are severely disabled to "have a major voice in deciding what constitutes practical, sensible help and minimal tyranny" (Duff, 1981). However, some parents accept decision making by others and sometimes openly welcome the relinquishment of responsibility (Pinch and Spielman, 1989).

The controversy will not be resolved to the satisfaction of all, and each situation must be determined by the principal persons involved. Unfortunately, the person central to the issues (the child) is unable to have a voice in the matter. Whether later repercussions, such as lawsuits related to right to a life of questionable quality, become a reality, is only hinted at presently. The debate will undoubtedly continue for some time. However, "physicians, parents, hospital bioethical review committees, and society as a whole must deal realistically, and compassionately, with the complex issues at hand to provide the proper treatment for affected infants (Strain, 1983)."

itated and unable to function in their usual manner. They may avoid interpersonal contacts. Unable to face relatives and friends for fear of the reactions they may encounter, parents choose the protection of isolation. They feel as though they are alone in a world all their own. Avoidance behaviors on the part of others, including health workers, contribute to this withdrawal and compound the feelings of loneliness that are so common in parents of an abnormal infant.

Parents often extend this avoidance behavior to include the infant. They seem to be unable to face the infant, and visiting patterns become sporadic or nonexistent. Sometimes it takes time for the parents to master their own feelings before they are able to deal constructively with the situation. A more subtle form of isolation is seen in parents who are very objective in their behavior toward the infant and the defect. They are intellectually concerned with the infant's medical care but display no emotional involvement. Their attention is focused on the abnormality, not on the infant.

Parental reactions may be quite varied, including guilt, anger, anxiety, and sadness, which often extend for years and which depend to a large extent on the type and severity of the defect. A gross, visible anomaly, especially one involving the face, usually elicits a more intense emotional response than one that is less apparent, such as a heart defect. The extent of the impairment cannot be used as a criterion to determine the degree of parental depressive reactions. Because of their limited contact with congenital defects, parents' perception of the abnormality and its implications may be distorted, and much depends on previous feelings they may have experienced with a similar abnormality. Therefore their reactions may seem out of proportion to the actual extent and severity of the impairment as viewed by health professionals.

Nursing Considerations

The attitudes and behaviors of nurses and other health personnel at the birth of a child with a defect significantly influence the effect that the situation has on the parents. During this time parents are particularly sensitive and responsive to the behaviors of those with whom they are in contact. Therefore the reactions of health professionals toward the infant and the parents provide cues to the parents that can affect their feelings toward the infant and themselves. Parents are the persons who exert the greatest influence on the growth and development of the child, and the initial relationship with the child significantly affects the subsequent course of interaction.

Initial contact. The first indication that all is not well often occurs at the time of delivery. The atmosphere of happy anticipation suddenly changes to one laden with anxiety. Even when the mother is unable to see the infant, she may sense with terrifying awareness the heightened and prolonged tension in the room, which conveys to her that something is seriously wrong. Personnel, unprepared for this disturbing experience, find it difficult to cope with their own feelings and react with frustration and resentment toward a situation that they are powerless to change. As a result they may forget about or retreat from the parents, who at this moment are suffering the most.

Most physicians believe that it is their responsibility to inform the parents of a congenital anomaly. At the time of delivery, unless a pediatrician is in attendance, there is a delay while the physician is involved with the mother's care. During this period the mother, unable to see her child and feeling the tense atmosphere, will believe either that the child is normal but that others do not share her enthusiasm or that the child has a defect that is so terrible that the professional people in the room are unable to talk about it. A nurse, the person who is most likely to be free to support the mother and who is familiar with most common congenital anomalies, can make truthful statements about the defect.

The manner in which nurses present the infant to the parents may well set the tone for the early parent-child relationship. It is probably best to explain briefly, in simple language, the nature of the defect and to reinforce and help clarify information given by the practitioner before the infant is shown to them. At this time they are more apt to "hear" what is said. Parents attach a great deal of meaning to the behavior of others during this critical period and will watch the facial expressions of others closely for signs of revulsion or rejection. Presenting the infant as something precious, although incomplete, and emphasizing the well-formed aspects of the infant's body provide some reassurance to parents in this crisis period.

It is important to allow time and opportunity for the parents to express their initial response to the situation. Many issues may surface, such as the importance placed on this particular infant or the cultural significance of one sex over the other. They need to be encouraged to ask questions and to receive honest, straightforward answers without undue optimism or pessimism.

Family support. Parents must be allowed ample time to grieve for the loss of the expected child before they are able to form an emotional attachment to the child they have. However, as long as the disabled child remains a living reminder of their loss, parents may never be able to totally resolve their grief. It is a nursing responsibility to help parents with their grief work and to facilitate the formation of a satisfactory adjustment to the child with a defect. They need help to see their infant as a *person,* support in coping with their situation, and guidance in physical care of the child.

Nurses who understand the grief response will be prepared to support the parents through this necessary process. This is particularly important with the birth of a child with a defect, because the parents cannot begin to invest any feeling for the child until they are able to talk about and work through their feelings of disappointment, resentment, guilt, and helplessness. Parents need to talk, and the supportive nurse is one who creates and maintains an atmosphere that encourages expression of feelings. Open expression is difficult for many people, and the parent(s) may hesitate to display intense feelings. Containing those feelings expends considerable energy that would be better used later on to develop a relationship with the infant. Nurses, therefore, need to listen closely for cues that indicate areas of discomfort or readiness to talk.

Parents may not be ready to talk about their feelings during the first few days following the birth. Their dream has vanished, and when others avoid them it is often interpreted as another abandonment. Staying near and available tells them that they are not alone and that someone cares about them and their feelings. What is said to them is also important. Cliches such as "You will be able to have more children" or "It could be a lot worse" are not a comfort to the parents. Such behavior implies that this infant is not important, and this behavior may lose the parents' trust (Paparella, 1982).

Initiating a discussion about matters that were of concern to others in a similar situation may help the parents to know that their feelings are natural. Parents need to be allowed silence and solitude if this is their wish. The parents are likely to be angry and will often direct this anger at anyone at hand—physicians, nurses, friends, and families who have normal children. Serving as a nonjudgmental target for their frustrations helps parents to relieve some of their distress. Nurses must be prepared to accept any or all of the parental reactions and defenses—anger, hostility, rejection, dependency—without anger and without withdrawing from the situation. If nurses make themselves available to the parents for support, they can often find nonthreatening ways to help, comfort, and support. Most important, nurses need to promote communication and understanding within the family and help strengthen family interpersonal relationships. Family disintegration is a sequela that is all too common to the birth of a child with a physical disability.

Care of the infant. Many parents are very uneasy about handling their infant and require support and encouragement in their caregiving tasks. A longer period of dependency is needed by these parents to regroup their resources for coping. Although they should not feel forced to care for the infant until they are ready for the responsibility, they can be given opportunities to assume care of the infant as soon as possible to help them deal with the reality of the infant's condition. Parents' responses are highly individual and must be evaluated on this premise. However, all parents need sympathetic, patient, and understanding help to gain feelings of adequacy in the care of their child and to facilitate development of a positive relationship with the infant later on. As anxiety and the intensity of emotional responses abate, parents begin to feel more comfortable with the infant and more confident in their ability to provide needed care.

Supplying information. Parents need to have accurate, up-to-date information given to them early and in language they can understand. Since they do not hear all that is said the first time it is told to them, they want careful explanations about the child's defect, the treatments outlined, and what will be expected of them. Parents often misinterpret information and therefore require repeated explanations. Often the nurse's responsibility is to explain, interpret, and clarify information that has been given by the physician and to answer questions. Following basic concepts of interviewing, the nurse determines what the parents know and proceeds from that point. One cannot assume that the parents' failure to ask questions means they understand. Most parents have little or no knowledge of basic anatomy or physiology; therefore, pictures and other visual aids can be used effectively to explain both normal and deviant structures.

Teaching the parents to provide the special care that is frequently required for an infant with a physical defect is an important nursing responsibility. Special feeding, holding, and positioning techniques need to be explained and demonstrated. Anticipatory guidance regarding problems that are peculiar to each abnormality reduces apprehension and stimulates the parents to institute preventive measures and to make alert observations.

Numerous agencies and organizations offer services to families of children with congenital defects. Some provide services for a variety of defects; others are devoted to specific disorders. They help families with ongoing problems and with anticipating problems they will encounter in raising a child with a defect, including financial burdens. Many have local support groups. All have unique and specialized services designed to help support the family and aid parents in their problem solving. Among those that include most types of defects and diseases are the **National Easter Seal Society for Crippled Children and Adults,*** the **March of Dimes–Birth Defects Foundation,†** and the **Association of Birth Defects in Children,‡** most of which have branches in all major cities and communities. The state **Program for Children with Special Health Needs** (formerly Crippled Children's Services) is also a prime source of assistance. (See Nursing Care Plan: The Child with a Chronic Illness or Disability, Chapter 22).

NURSING CARE OF THE SURGICAL NEONATE§

Advances in early detection of defects (including prenatal diagnosis), surgical techniques, and anesthesia have made it possible for correction or amelioration of many physical defects in the newborn period. Approximately 2% to 3% of newborn infants have anomalies that require surgery during the neonatal period (Rosenbaum, 1986), often as emergencies. Fortunately most are correctable with a high degree of success, even those that are dramatic in their presentation.

Preoperative Care

Most of the problems encountered with the infant undergoing surgery have been discussed in relation to the high-risk infant (e.g., airway maintenance, cardiovascular support, thermoregulation, fluid and electrolyte balance, and nutritional needs). Electronic monitoring of cardiovascular and respiratory status is implemented and maintained, as well as regular comprehensive assessments (see Systematic Assessment, Chapter 10). Monitoring and assessments are continued in the postoperative period in addition to problems related to specific surgery. Some congenital defects are often associated with other anomalies; therefore assessment should include careful observation for evidence of these.

Fluid and electrolyte disturbances are corrected and the infant is stabilized before surgery. Prophylactic antibiotic administration may begin before surgery, and the infant is observed for any evidence of infection. In addition to routine care, special attention is directed to specific defects, such as abdominal decompression, management of open lesions, and specific measurements (e.g., abdominal girth, head dimensions). (See also discussion of specific defects.)

---

*2023 West Ogden Ave., Chicago, IL 60612; (312) 243-8400.

†1275 Mamaroneck Ave., White Plains, NY 10605; (914) 428-7100.

‡3526 Emerywood Lane, Orlando, FL 32812; (305) 859-2821.

§The information in this section was derived almost exclusively from Rushton, C.H.: The surgical neonate: principles of nursing management, Pediatr. Nurs. 14:141-151, 1988.

Postoperative Care

Surgery imposes significant stresses on the neonate, especially the preterm or ill infant. The assessment and observations remain much the same as for preoperative care, with the additional problems related to surgery, such as anesthesia and pain. It is essential to maintain physiologic stability to avoid undesirable consequences (Rushton, 1988). Because the neonate is subject to many adverse effects of stress in all physiologic parameters, continual vigilance is mandatory.

Many of the physiologic problems to which the neonate is vulnerable have been discussed in relation to assessment and nursing care of the normal newborn (Chapter 8) and the high-risk infant (Chapter 10). Optimum ventilation, thermoregulation, fluid regulation, and immaturity are primary concerns. Some of the possible reactions, their probable cause, and the nursing responsibilities are outlined in Table 11-1.

Because of the respiratory characteristics of newborns some compromising responses may be anticipated. The newborn's poor chest wall stability, smaller and more reactive airways, fewer and smaller alveoli, and poorly developed accessory muscles contribute to respiratory dysfunction. Compression by intrapleural fluid, air, or blood or a distended abdomen can further compromise pulmonary efforts. Respiratory distress is a common problem in preterm infants. Most postoperative neonates require mechanical ventilation, which may be further influenced by the type, duration, and urgency of the surgery. Neonates are highly subject to acidosis and hypoxia and require continuous monitoring of oxygen. (See also Idiopathic Respiratory Distress Syndrome, Chapter 10.)

Table 11-1 Possible effects of surgery on selected systems

PHYSIOLOGIC RESPONSE	NURSING RESPONSIBILITIES
▪ Cardiovascular system	
Hypotension related to: Large doses of anesthesia Vasodilation (narcotics) Myocardial depression (anesthetic agents) Impaired venous return Hypertension related to: Hypervolemia, pain, hypercarbia Increased ICP, vasoconstrictor drugs Tachycardia related to: Compensation for hypovolemia Pain Certain drugs Bradycardia related to: Hypoxemia (most commonly) Vagal stimulation Increased ICP (certain drugs) Vasoconstriction related to: Hypothermia	Observe for signs of low cardiac output: tachycardia, poor perfusion (slow capillary filling), weak peripheral pulse, decreased intensity of heart sounds, decreased urinary specific gravity Observe for signs of congestive heart failure: tachycardia, increased peripheral vasoconstriction (skin changes), pulmonary venous engorgement (respiratory distress) Monitor laboratory data Administer blood products, vasoactive drugs, cardiotonics as prescribed Monitor and maintain fluid balance, including blood loss Provide ventilatory support as needed
▪ Respiratory system	
Increased respiratory rate related to physiologic characteristics Airway obstruction related to: Bronchospasm Laryngeal edema Mucus plugs Compressed lung tissue related to: Air, fluid, or blood in pleural cavities Anatomic defects of diaphragm Intrinsic pulmonary lesions Ventilation/perfusion imbalance related to: Atelectasis Inadequate respiratory effort Pulmonary edema Pneumothorax Hypoventilation related to: Termination of anesthesia Administration of narcotics, hypocarbia, cold stress, lack of the surgical stimulus	Observe respiratory rate, symmetry; breath sounds (pitch, intensity, quality, duration, location), color, use of accessory muscles, signs of airway obstruction (decreased breath sounds, decreased Po_2, respiratory distress, improper head alignment), signs of respiratory distress (marked retractions, nasal flaring, grunting, tachypnea, cyanosis), signs of impaired diaphragmatic movement (distended abdomen, constrictive dressings) Monitor oxygenation/ventilation, laboratory data Administer oxygen in amount and manner prescribed Position for optimum ventilation Alleviate any impediment to diaphragm exursion

Data from Rushton, C.H.: The surgical neonate: principles of nursing management, Pediatr. Nurs. 14:141-151, 1988.

Continued.

Table 11-1 Possible effects of surgery on selected systems—cont'd

PHYSIOLOGIC RESPONSE	NURSING RESPONSIBILITIES
▪ Immune system	
Subject to infection related to: Inability to generate rapid and effective immune defenses Effects of anesthesia and surgery may mask assessment data	Observe for evidence of sepsis (bradycardia, temperature instability, poor feeding, change in activity level, irregular respiration or apnea), GI disturbances, evidence of abnormal clotting (bleeding from punctures, surgical sites) Monitor for signs of pulmonary or cardiovascular compromise Monitor fluid administration to maintain vascular volume Administer antibiotics as ordered
▪ Endocrine system	
Hypoglycemia related to: Surgical stress Rapid depletion of glycogen stores Decreased gluconeogenesis with stress Hypothermia Hypocalcemia related to: Immaturity Stress Decreased parathyroid hormone secretion Hypomagnesemia related to: Hypocalcemia	Observe for apnea, tachypnea, lethargy, pallor, tremors or seizures Monitor serum glucose levels (Dextrosticks/chemstrips); verify abnormal values Administer supplemental glucose as described Maintain neutral thermal environment Monitor serum calcium levels Observe for lethargy, vital sign instability, apnea, irritability, jitteriness, seizures Administer supplemental calcium if prescribed Observe for neuromuscular excitability (tetany, seizures) Monitor serum magnesium levels in infants with above signs
▪ Hepatic system	
Jaundice related to: Immature enzyme systems Edema related to: Diminished oncotic pressure Inability to maintain albumin levels	Observe for evidence of jaundice, edema Monitor serum albumin levels Meticulous skin care Albumin supplementation if prescribed
▪ Renal system	
Inability to concentrate urine and excrete waste related to: Immature renal function	Observe for amount and characteristics of urinary output Monitor renal function, drug levels, intravascular volume
▪ Gastrointestinal system	
Abdominal distention related to: Hypoactive bowel Obstruction Hypoactivity related to: Bowel surgery Peritonitis Perforation Hyperactivity related to: Obstruction Feeding modification related to: GI surgery (see specific GI surgeries)	Observe for skin color and integrity (erythema of abdominal wall, prominent veins), abdominal distention, (e.g., serial abdominal girth measurements) Palpate abdomen for tenderness Percuss abdomen for organomegaly, evidence of masses Monitor bowel sounds (hyperactivity or hypoactivity) Observe frequency, volume, and characteristics of vomiting and vomitus; frequency, volume, and characteristics of stools Delay enteral feedings if prescribed Monitor parenteral feedings and fluid therapy Provide alternative enteral feedings as prescribed (gavage, gastrostomy) Begin and monitor oral feedings as prescribed Provide ostomy care if indicated
▪ Neurologic system	
Hypothermia related to: Immaturity of thermoregulation Seizures related to: Hypoxemia Hypoglycemia Hypocalcemia Unresponsiveness Stress related to: Surgical procedure Pain (see discussion on p. 462)	See Thermoregulation below. Monitor blood calcium, glucose Observe for any seizure activity, unresponsiveness, evidence of pain (see Box 11-1), signs of hypoglycemia or hypocalcemia (see above) Administer sedatives, analgesics, anticonvulsives, glucose, calcium as prescribed

Table 11-1 Possible effects of surgery on selected systems—cont'd

PHYSIOLOGIC RESPONSE	NURSING RESPONSIBILITIES
▪ Hemopoietic system	
Anemia related to: Blood loss Hyperviscosity related to: Polycythemia Decreased RBC deformability Plasma protein abnormalities Polycythemia related to: Chronic hypoxia Coagulation defects related to: Inherited coagulation defects Physiologic coagulation factor defects Transitory coagulation disturbances Platelet abnormalities	Monitor any blood loss Monitor laboratory data Administer blood and/or blood products as ordered Observe for complications related to hemopoietic dysfunction and blood administration
▪ Fluid and electrolyte disturbances	
Abnormal fluid losses related to: Blood loss Fluid shifts, e.g., losses to interstitial tissues (third space) Transudated fluid GI, renal, wounds, drains Membrane injury from sepsis or injury Insensible losses from open wounds, exposed viscera	Observe for evidence of dehydration (see Chapter 28) Monitor laboratory data Monitor blood pressure, central venous pressure Weigh daily or as ordered Measure vital signs Monitor fluid and electrolyte administration Administer albumin, electrolytes
▪ Acid-base balance	
Acid-base disturbance related to: Cold stress Respiratory embarrassment GI disturbances Infectious processes Surgery Immature buffering mechanisms Acidosis related to: Ventilatory insufficiency (respiratory acidosis) Ischemic tissue damage Cold stress	Monitor acid-base status Monitor respirations (see above) Administer bicarbonate or other buffer as prescribed Maintain neutral thermal environment (see Thermoregulation below)
▪ Thermoregulation	
Hypothermia related to: Unstable regulatory mechanisms Heat loss from large surface area, open wounds, defects Depletion of glycogen stores and metabolism of brown fat See Thermoregulation, Chapter 10	Monitor environmental and infant's skin temperatures Maintain optimum thermal environment Observe for evidence of hypothermia: peripheral vasoconstriction, apnea, cyanosis, decreased body temperature, respiratory distress, tachycardia Minimize heat loss Conserve heat and provide external warmth as needed, including coverings for head and extremities Warm any blood and irrigating solutions Observe for any seizure

Cardiovascular support is of particular importance because the immature sympathetic innervation of the myocardium makes the neonate particularly sensitive to vagal stimulation induced by many postoperative procedures, such as nasogastric (NG) tubes, endotracheal (ET) tubes, and suctioning (Rushton, 1988). The infant may be given atropine preoperatively to block these responses. Any evidence of early compensation for diminished cardiac output is noted and interventions are implemented before decompensation occurs.

Careful management of fluid and electrolyte status is vital to surgical care. The natural tendency for rapid fluid shifts related to characteristics of the neonate (see Chapter 28) may be aggravated by stress and any abnormal losses associated with some surgical procedures. (See also Hydration, Chapter 10).

The reader should refer to Chapter 10, The High-Risk Newborn and Family, for more information on managing the ill and/or low-birth-weight infant and for preoperative and postoperative care of neonates with specific defects.

NEONATAL PAIN

It has long been believed that the nerve pathways of newborn infants are not sufficiently myelinated to transmit painful stimuli, that the infant does not possess sufficiently integrated cortical function to interpret or recall pain experiences, and that the risk of anesthesia is too great to justify any possible benefit of pain relief (Anand and Hickey, 1987; Shapiro, 1989). Consequently, invasive procedures (including some types of surgery) were performed on infants without anesthesia. This traditional view has been refuted by a number of research studies, which indicate that infants, both preterm and full term, perceive and react to pain in much the same manner as children and adults. Evidence indicates that pain pathways, cortical and subcortical centers needed for pain perception, and neurochemical systems associated with pain transmission and modulation are intact and functional in the neonate. Slower conduction speed is offset by shorter interneuron distances traveled by the impulse (Anand and Hickey, 1987).

Pain perception has both physiologic and psychologic components, and it is accepted that newborns recognize and respond to painful stimuli. However, because pain is a sensation with strong emotional associations, it is difficult to differentiate between pain perception and nociceptive activity in neonates. Consequently, the term *nociception* (the perception by nerves of injurious influences or painful stimuli) is frequently used to discuss pain in the neonate.

Physiologic responses to painful stimuli have been well documented by numerous studies. The summary of these observations indicate that painful stimuli cause a global stress response in infants undergoing surgery with minimal or no analgesia. This response is evidenced by cardiorespiratory changes (marked increases in heart rate and blood pressure, and decreased $tcPo_2$), palmar sweating, and hormonal and metabolic changes (release of catecholamines, growth hormone, glucagon, cortisol, other corticosteroids, and aldosterone). Breakdown of carbohydrate and fat stores leads to severe and prolonged hyperglycemia and increases in plasma lactate, pyruvate, ketone bodies, and some fatty acids. Increased protein breakdown has been measured by changes in plasma amino acids and elevated nitrogen excretion (these and other observations are summarized by Anand and Hickey, 1987).

The stress response to surgery was found to be shorter in duration than that observed in adults but was three to five times greater, perhaps as a result of lack of deep anesthesia (Anand, 1986). It was also observed that the response was decreased by appropriate anesthesia, indicating that the nociceptive stimuli of surgery were responsible for the stress response (Anand and Aynsley-Green, 1988; Anand, Sippell, and Aynsley-Green, 1987). Various reports and assumptions regarding memory of pain in the neonate have not been substantiated.

It has also been found that neonates release endorphins in response to stress and that the supply may become depleted (Hindmarsh, Sankaran, and Watson, 1984). It is now recommended that infants receive appropriate analgesia or anesthesia for potentially painful procedures. Relatively safe local or systemic pharmacologic agents are available to permit anesthesia or analgesia to neonates and are indicated for those undergoing surgical procedures (American Academy of Pediatrics, Committee on Fetus and Newborns, 1987).

Other effects of pain may include increased wakefulness and irritability, as well as alterations in feeding, vomiting, loss of appetite, and loss of interest in or energy for sucking. Interruptions in sleep-wake patterns, behavioral states, and parent-infant interactions also occur and may interfere with recovery from surgery (Shapiro, 1989).

Pain Assessment

Assessment of pain in the preverbal child is difficult, especially in the neonate, because evaluative tools and verbal responses do not apply. Evaluation must be based on physiologic changes and behavioral observations. Several studies have been devoted to assessing infant's responses to nociception (Brown, 1987; Dale, 1989; Franck, 1986; Johnston and Strada, 1986). Although behaviors including vocalizations, facial expressions, body movements, and general state are common to all infants, they vary with different situations. Crying associated with pain is more intense and sustained. Facial expression is the most consistent characteristic, and most infants respond with increased body movements. However, the infant may be experiencing pain even when lying quietly with eyes closed (Shapiro, 1989). Nursing assessment for evidence of pain is indicated any time the infant suffers tissue damage. Observable manifestations identified as indicators of acute pain in neonates are listed in Box 11-1.

Pain Management

Nonpharmacologic measures used to alleviate pain are discussed extensively in Chapter 26. Those employed to reduce discomfort in the neonatal intensive care unit (NICU) include repositioning, swaddling, containment, cuddling, rocking, music, reducing environmental stimulation, tactile comfort measures, and nonnutritive sucking (D'Apolito, 1984; Field and Goldson, 1984; Franck, 1987; Shapiro, 1989).

Morphine is the most widely used narcotic analgesic for pharmacologic management of neonatal pain, with fentanyl as an effective alternative (Maguire and Maloney, 1988). Fentanyl is also used as an anesthetic during surgery, especially in the preterm, low-birth-weight infant (Anand, Sippell, and Aynsley-Green, 1987; Collins and others, 1985). (See Pain Management, Chapter 26, for more information on pharmacologic management of pain in the infant.)

Family Support

Parents are universally concerned that their infants are suffering pain during procedures. Nurses need to address

Box 11-1 MANIFESTATIONS OF ACUTE PAIN IN THE NEONATE

Physiologic Responses
- Vital signs: observe for variations
  - Increased heart rate
  - Increased blood pressure
  - Rapid, shallow respirations
- Oxygenation
  - Decreased $tcPo_2$
  - Decreased Sao_2
- Skin: observe color and character
  - Pallor or flushing
  - Diaphoresis
  - Palmar sweating
- Other observations
  - Increased muscle tone
  - Dilated pupils
  - Laboratory evidence of metabolic or endocrine changes
    - Hyperglycemia
    - Lowered pH
    - Elevated corticosteroids

Behavioral Responses
- Vocalizations: observe quality, timing, and duration
  - Crying
  - Whimpering
  - Groaning
- Facial expression: observe characteristics, timing, orientation of eyes and mouth (see Fig. 26-3)
  - Grimaces
  - Brow furrowed
  - Chin quivering
  - Eyes tightly closed
  - Mouth open and squarish
- Body movements and posture: observe type, quality, and amount of movement or lack of movement; relationship to other factors
  - Limb withdrawal
  - Thrashing
  - Rigidity
  - Flaccidity
  - Fist clenching
- Changes in state: observe sleep, appetite, activity level
  - Changes in sleep/wake cycles
  - Changes in feeding behavior
  - Changes in activity level
  - Fussiness, irritability
  - Listlessness

these concerns and encourage the parents to speak with the professionals involved. Parents have the right to withhold consent for invasive procedures and are entitled to honest answers from those responsible for the infant's care. When permissible, they can also help provide comfort measures for the infant. It is important that parents are aware that nurses are sensitive to the infant's pain and are reassured that the infant will not suffer unduly (Butler, 1988; Shapiro, 1989).

MALFORMATIONS OF THE CENTRAL NERVOUS SYSTEM

Defects of the central nervous system (CNS) are usually the result of embryologic developmental failures. Some can be attributed to genetic factors; others may be a result of postnatal infections. However, in most cases the etiology is obscure. The defects discussed in this section are abnormalities of neural tube closure and hydrocephalus, which is characterized by an increase of free fluid in the cranial cavity.

DEFECTS OF NEURAL TUBE CLOSURE

Abnormalities that are derived from the embryonic neural tube (neural tube defects [NTDs]) constitute the largest group of congenital anomalies that is consistent with multifactorial inheritance. Normally the spinal cord and cauda equina are encased in a protective sheath of bone and meninges (Fig. 11-2, *A*). Failure of neural tube closure produces defects of varying degrees. They may involve the entire length of the neural tube or may be restricted to a small area. Terms applied to these abnormalities are listed in Box 11-2.

Etiology

Two of the defects, anencephaly and spina bifida (SB), occur in association with one another more often than would be expected by chance, suggesting a common origin. The CNS defects may alternate in siblings, which also tends to support the theory of a common origin. In a family who has had a child with either anencephaly or SB, the possibility of having a subsequent child with either anomaly is higher than in the general population—approximately 4% to 8% (McKusick, 1988). Environmental influences that have been implicated, based on animal experiments or observed in human beings, include radiation, maternal hyperthermia, gestational diabetes mellitus, vitamin A deficiency or excess, valproic acid deficiency, and folic acid deficiency (Swaiman, 1989). Recent evidence supports the hypothesis that NTDs may be caused by the interaction of a genetic predisposition with an essential nutrient deficiency (folic acid), and that multivitamins containing folic acid taken during the first 6 weeks of pregnancy will prevent (by more than 50%) their occurrence (Milunsky and others, 1989).

The following discussion of NTDs is limited to the two most common types—SB occulta and myelomeningocele, an abnormality that causes significant childhood disability—and anencephaly because of current ethical issues.

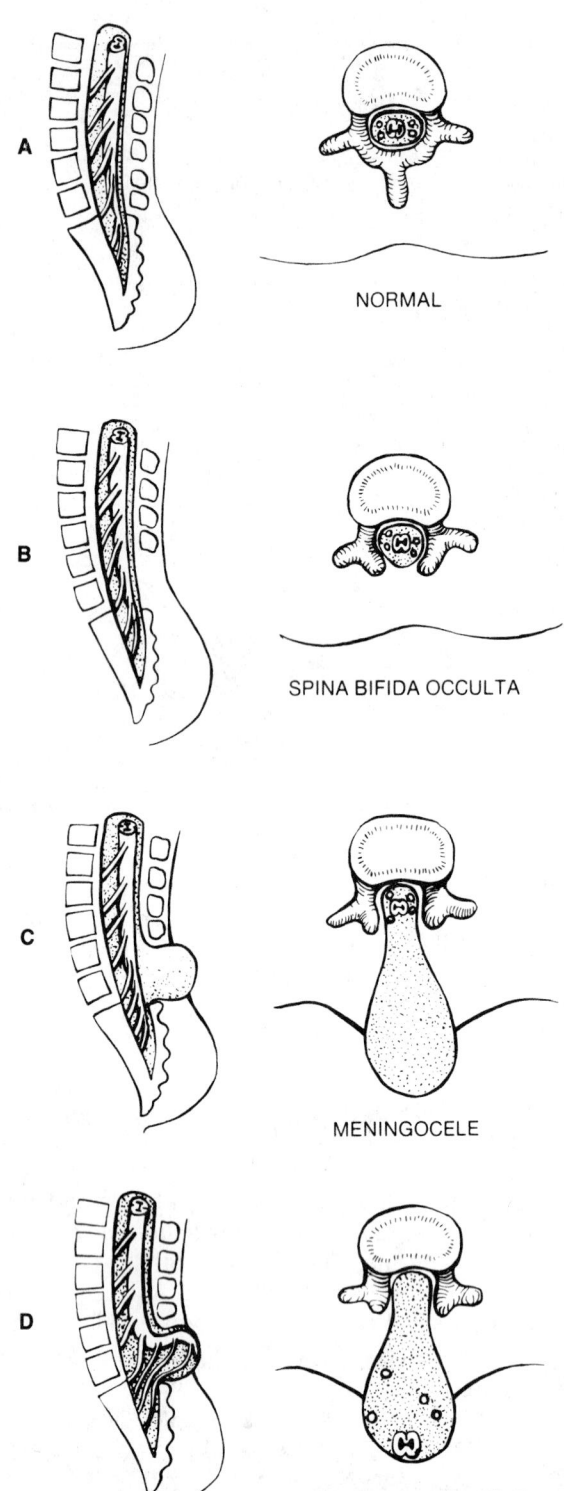

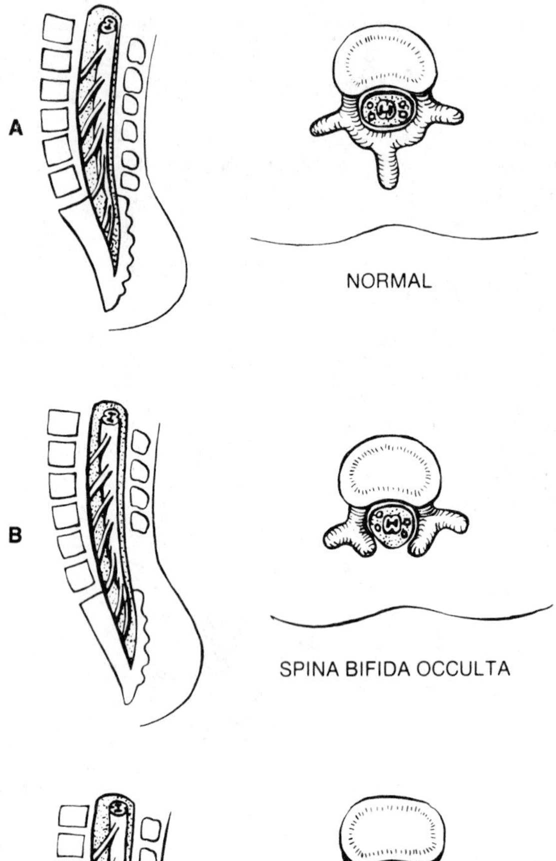

Fig. 11-2. Midline defects of osseous spine with varying degrees of neural herniations. **A,** Normal. **B,** Spina bifida occulta. **C,** Meningocele. **D,** Myelomeningocele.

Box 11-2 ABNORMALITIES OF NEURAL TUBE CLOSURE

Myelodysplasia—all-inclusive term that refers to defective development of any part of the spinal cord; usually used to describe abnormalities without gross superficial defects

Rachischisis—fissure in the spinal column that leaves the meninges and spinal cord exposed

Spinal dysrhaphia—defect in closure of the vertebral column with varying degrees of tissue protrusion through the bony cleft

Spina bifida—synonymous with spinal dysraphia

Spina bifida occulta—fusion failure of posterior vertebral arches without accompanying herniation of spinal cord or meninges; usually not visible externally (Fig. 11-2, *B*)

Spina bifida cystica—defect in closure with external saccular protrusion through the bony spine with varying degrees of nerve involvement

Meningocele—form of spina bifida; consists of a saclike cyst of meninges filled with spinal fluid (Fig. 11-2, *C*)

Myelomeningocele (meningomyelocele)—hernial protrusion of a saclike cyst containing meninges, spinal fluid, and a portion of the spinal cord with its nerves (Fig. 11-2, *D*)

Encephalocele—herniation of brain and meninges through a defect in the skull producing a fluid-filled sac in the occipital region

Anencephaly—absent brain; this anomaly consists of only an exposed vascular mass with no bony covering; incompatible with life

SPINA BIFIDA OCCULTA

Noncystic SB is failure of the spinous processes to join posteriorly in the lumbosacral area (L5 and S1). Routine radiographic examinations indicate that the disorder is quite common, but it may not be apparent unless there are associated cutaneous manifestations or neuromuscular disturbances. The incidence is estimated to occur in up to 25% of younger children, in whom there is eventual fusion of the vertebral arches, and in approximately 5% to 10% of the population (Scarff and Fronczak, 1981).

Superficial indications include a skin depression or dimple (which may also mark the outlet of a dermal sinus tract that extends to the subarachnoid space), port-wine angiomatous nevi, dark tufts of hair, or soft, subcutaneous lipomas. These signs may be absent, appear singly, or be present in combination.

Neuromuscular disturbances are not uncommon in children with SB occulta and usually consist of progressive disturbance of gait with foot weakness and/or bowel and bladder sphincter disturbances. The usual cause is abnormal adhesion, or *tethering*, to a bony or fixed structure, resulting in traction on the spinal cord and cauda equina. (See Fig. 4-8 for spinal cord development and Fig. 40-7 for areas innervated by specific spinal nerves.) Manifestations may not be evident during periods of slow growth but tend to arise during periods of rapid growth, especially during the adolescent growth spurt at the end of the first decade and beginning of the second decade of life (Anderson, 1989).

Plain radiography is employed to disclose the precise bony defect in the symptomatic lesion and to establish the diagnosis in the suspected, nonsymptomatic occult variety. Magnetic resonance imaging (MRI) is the most sensitive tool for evaluating NTDs. Computed tomography (CT) scan, ultrasound, and myelography are also used to differentiate between SB occulta and other spinal disorders.

MYELOMENINGOCELE (MENINGOMYELOCELE)

The cystic defect myelomeningocele affects about 1 of every 1000 live births (Khoury, Erickson, and James, 1982), but the incidence may be as high as 4.2 per 1000 live births in some parts of the world (Owens and others, 1981). It is detected at birth, accounts for 90% of spinal cord lesions, and may be located at any point along the spinal column. Usually the sac is encased in a fine membrane that is prone to tears through which cerebrospinal fluid leaks. In other instances the sac may be covered by dura, meninges, or skin, in which instances there is rapid and spontaneous epithelialization.

Since the lumbar segment is the last portion of the neural tube to close, the largest number of myelomeningoceles is found in the lumbar or lumbosacral area (Fig. 11-3). The location and magnitude of the defect determine the nature and extent of neurologic impairment. When the defect is located below the second lumbar vertebra, the nerves of the cauda equina are involved, giving rise to symptoms such as flaccid, areflexic partial paralysis of the lower extremities and varying degrees of sensory deficit.

The anomaly most frequently associated with myelomeningocele is hydrocephalus; and 90% to 95% of children with SB have hydrocephalus (Anderson, 1989). In myelomeningocele obstruction to CSF is caused by downward displacement of the brainstem and cerebellum through the foramen magnum secondary to a defect known as the *Arnold-Chiari malformation (ACM),* usually type 2. In most cases hydrocephalus is apparent at birth; in other children it appears shortly thereafter (see p. 471 for manifestations and discussion of hydrocephalus).

Pathophysiology

The pathophysiology of SB is best understood when related to the normal formative stages of the nervous system. At approximately 20 days of gestation a decided depression, the neural groove, appears in the dorsal ectoderm of the embryo. During the fourth week of gestation the groove deepens rapidly, and its elevated margins develop laterally and then fuse dorsally to form the neural tube. Neural tube formation begins in the cervical region near the center of the embryo and advances in both directions—caudally and cephalically—until by the end of the fourth week of gestation the ends of the neural tube, the anterior and posterior neuropores, are closed.

The primary defect in neural tube malformations is believed by most authorities to be a failure of neural tube closure. However, there is evidence to indicate that the defects are a result of splitting of the already closed neural tube as a result of an abnormal increase in cerebrospinal fluid pressure during the first trimester.

Clinical Manifestations

The manifestations of SB vary widely according to the degree of the spinal defect. The defect is readily apparent on inspection. The degree of neurologic dysfunction is directly related to the anatomic level of the defect and thus the nerves involved. Sensory disturbances usually parallel motor dysfunction. The upper level of sensory and motor impairment can be determined by observation of the infant's response to a pinprick over the legs and trunk. The infant will respond to the sensory stimulus with limb movement, arousal, and crying. When withdrawal activity is used to determine the lowest level of spinal cord function, the response to pinprick should begin above the lesion.

Defective nerve supply to the bladder affects both sphincter and detrusor tone, which often causes constant dribbling of urine or produces overflow incontinence in childhood. However, some infants void in a stream. Frequently there is poor anal sphincter tone and poor anal skin reflex, which result in lack of bowel control and sometimes

A

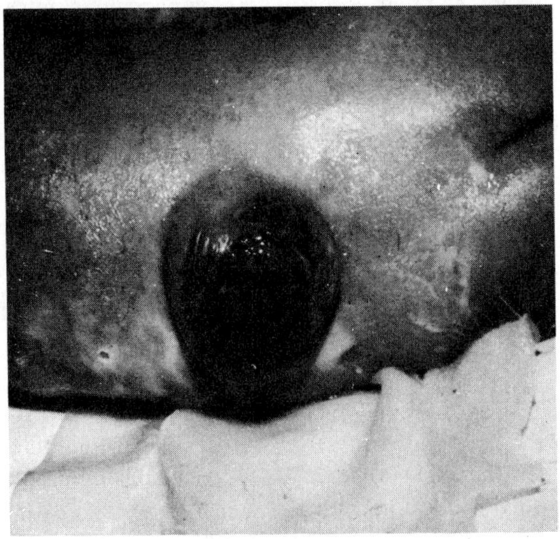

B

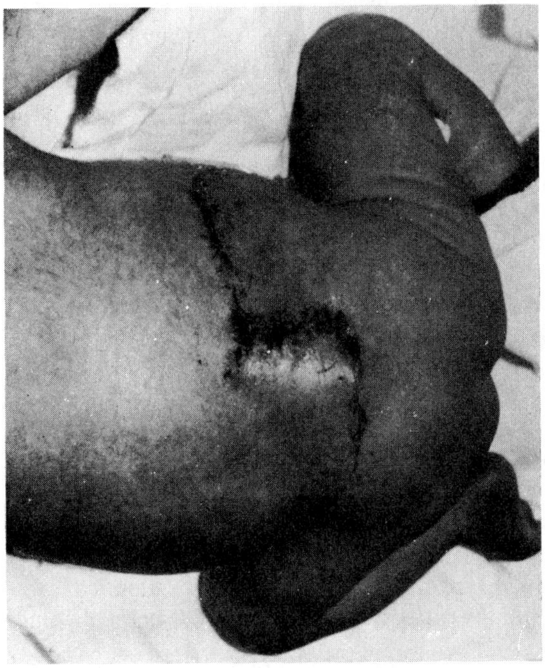

Fig. 11-3. A, Meningomyelocele before surgery. (An antibacterial dressing was used.) **B,** Repair of same patient.

Courtesy M.C. Gleason, M.D., San Diego, CA. From Ingalls, A.J., and Salerno, M.C.: Maternal and child health nursing, ed. 6, St. Louis, 1987, Mosby–Year Book, Inc.

rectal prolapse. If the defect is located below the third sacral vertebra, there is no motor impairment but there may be saddle anesthesia with bladder and anal sphincter paralysis.

Sometimes the denervation to the muscles of the lower extremities will produce joint deformities in utero. These are primarily flexion or extension contractures, talipes valgus or varus contractures, kyphosis, lumbosacral scoliosis, and hip dislocations. The extent and severity of these associated deformities again depend on the degree of nerve involvement. Most flexion deformities result from the pull of stronger, fully innervated muscles acting without the counterpull of their nonfunctioning paralyzed antagonists.

Diagnostic Evaluation

The diagnosis is made on the basis of clinical manifestations and examination of the meningeal sac. If the mass can be transilluminated (i.e., becomes translucent when a light is held behind it), the defect is probably a meningocele. In these cases neurologic function is rarely disturbed even though the nerve roots are somewhat displaced. If the mass does not transilluminate, it is more likely a myelomeningocele. Other diagnostic measures used to evaluate the brain and spinal cord include MRI, ultrasound, CT, and myelography.

Laboratory examinations are used primarily to determine causative organisms in the major complications of myelomeningocele—meningitis and urinary tract infections. Children with urinary tract incontinence require urinalysis, culture, blood urea nitrogen (BUN) evaluation, and creatinine clearance evaluation.

Prenatal detection. It is possible to determine the presence of some major open NTDs prenatally. Ultrasonic scanning of the uterus and elevated concentrations of alpha-fetoprotein (AFP), a fetal-specific gamma-1 globulin, in amniotic fluid may indicate the presence of anencephaly or myelomeningocele. The optimum time for performing these diagnostic tests is between 16 and 18 weeks of gestation (American Academy of Pediatrics, Committee on Genetics, 1987), before AFP concentrations normally diminish and in sufficient time to permit a therapeutic abortion. It is recommended that such diagnostic procedures be considered for all mothers who have borne an affected child, and testing is offered to all pregnant women. Only 5% are detected in this manner; 95% of affected children are born to parents anticipating a normal child (Myers, 1984).

Therapeutic Management

Management of the child who has a myelomeningocele requires a multidisciplinary approach involving the specialties of neurology, neurosurgery, pediatrics, urology, orthopedics, rehabilitation, and physical therapy, as well as intensive nursing care in a variety of specialty areas. The collaborative efforts of these specialists are focused on (1) the myelomeningocele and the problems associated with the defect—hydrocephalus, paralysis, orthopedic deformities, genitourinary abnormalities; (2) possible acquired problems that may or may not be associated, such as meningitis, hypoxia, and hemorrhage; and (3) other abnormalities, such as cardiac or gastrointestinal malformations.

Infancy. Initial care involves prevention of infection, neurologic assessment, including observation for associated anomalies, and dealing with the impact of the anomaly on the parents. Although meningoceles are repaired early, especially if there is danger of rupture of the sac, the philosophy regarding skin closure of myelomeningocele varies radically. Most authorities believe that early closure, within the first 24 to 48 hours, offers the most favorable outcome, especially in regard to morbidity and mortality from serious infection. Proponents argue that early closure, preferably in the first 12 to 18 hours, not only prevents local infection and trauma to the exposed tissues but also avoids stretching of other nerve roots, which may occur as the meningeal sac expands during the first 24 hours after birth, thus preventing further motor impairment (Reigel, 1982).

There are those who recommend that surgical repair is best delayed for further assessment of neurologic function, intellectual potential, and extent of complications (Charney and others, 1985). They believe that, in addition to increased ability of the infant to tolerate the surgical procedure, delay allows for better epithelialization of the sac (thus reducing the risk of infection) and permits easier mobilization of skin for closure. Delay is also thought to be beneficial by some because early closure contributes to the development of hydrocephalus by reducing the absorptive surface provided by the meningocele (Linder and others, 1984). It is also argued that delay frees the family from immediate decision making and allows time to hear all the facts and weigh the consequences of decisions.

A variety of plastic surgical procedures are employed for skin closure without disturbing the neural elements or removing any portion of the sac. The objective is satisfactory skin coverage of the lesion and meticulous closure. Wide excision of the large membranous covering may damage functioning neural tissue. Where the skin over the defect is intact, as often occurs with meningocele, surgical intervention may be performed to prevent tethering of the spinal cord.

Associated problems are assessed and managed by appropriate surgical and supportive measures. Shunt procedures provide relief from imminent or progressive hydrocephalus (see p. 471). Meningitis, urinary tract infection, and pneumonia are treated with vigorous antibiotic therapy and supportive measures.

Outcome. The early prognosis for the child with myelomeningocele depends on the neurologic deficit present at birth, including motor ability and bladder innervation and the presence of associated cerebral anomalies. Early surgical repair of the spinal defect, antibiotic therapy to reduce the incidence of total meningitis and ventriculitis, and correction of hydrocephalus have significantly increased the survival rate.

There are those who question whether operative procedures should be considered for children with overwhelming neurologic deficit or whether the disorder should be allowed to assume its natural course. Considerable research is directed toward selection of infants for surgical repair and infants for supportive care only (Gross and others, 1983; Lorber and Salfield, 1981). There are supporters and critics of this philosophy (Letters to the editors, 1984). Criteria for selection or nonselection are based on the prognosis for quality of life. Such controversies present serious ethical problems (see Questions and Controversies, p. 456).

Improved surgical techniques do not alter the major physical disability and deformity or chronic urinary tract and pulmonary infections that affect the quality of life for these children. Superimposed on these physical problems are the effects that the disorder has on family life and finances and on school and hospital services.

Orthopedic considerations. According to most orthopedists, musculoskeletal problems that will affect later locomotion should be evaluated early, and treatment, where indicated, should be instituted without delay. In collaboration with appropriate members of the team, the child is evaluated in regard to the true level of neurologic functioning, and corrective measures are carried out in coordination with the activities of the neurosurgeon. Casting, bracing, traction, and surgical techniques for correction of hip, knee, and foot deformities are employed when they may aid later ambulation. The minimum degree of future disability can usually be ascertained, although the maximum degree of disability is impossible to predict.

Great diversity is observed in patterns of musculoskeletal involvement. The hip flexors and adductors are innervated by L1 to L3, whereas extensors and abductors are innervated by L5 to S1. Consequently there is often an imbalance in muscle pull around a joint. Children with lesions at L2 or above have some hip flexion and are usually confined to a wheelchair for mobility. Children with lesions at L2 to L5 have strong hip flexors and are candidates for crutches and braces, although the majority use a wheelchair most of the time. At levels L3 and L4 there is usually an imbalance between sensory and motor nerve involvement, and hip dislocation is often a problem. Children with sacral lesions are able to walk, but some require ankle bracing.

A variety of devices are available to provide mobility to children with spinal cord lesions, including lightweight braces, special "walking" devices, and custom-built wheelchairs (see also Chapter 39). Corrective procedures, when indicated, are best initiated at an early age so that the child will not lag significantly behind age-mates in developmental progress. Where there is little hope for lower extremity functioning, surgery is seldom recommended.

Management of genitourinary function. Myelomeningocele is one of the most common causes of neuropathic (or neurogenic) bladder impairment in childhood, and the prognosis for children who survive the early hazards of meningitis and hydrocephalus ultimately depends on the severity of their renal disease. Not only does renal failure pose a threat to life, but the lack of bladder control is important to the development of self-image and the social acceptability of the child. Ongoing assessment and monitoring of urologic status are lifelong problems in management of the myelodysplastic child with or without surgical repair of the spinal defect. Since the majority of these children suffer from incontinence and are subject to recurrent or persistent pyuria, prevention and treatment of renal complications are a constant goal.

Innervation of the lower urinary tract musculature is complex and controlled by several areas in the nervous system. Neurologic impairment can cause these various components to fail to act in unison, resulting in impaired urinary storage, altered bladder tone (increased or decreased), and inadequate or increased resistance of the bladder neck and urethra. In children with myelomeningocele decreased bladder tone produces the *flaccid* bladder with incomplete emptying. Increased tone causes a *spastic* bladder in which there are uninhibited bladder contractions. When coordination is faulty, high intravesical pressure may be created, predisposing the bladder to vesicoureteral reflux and incomplete emptying. The residual urine predisposes to infection, and the vesicoureteral reflux can lead to hydronephrosis. This combination can cause progressive renal damage and eventual renal failure.

Urination is also influenced by physical maturation. In the normal infant urination is a simple cord reflex with automatic emptying at a specific bladder volume. The bladder increases in size and capacity with growth, and the child develops voluntary control of muscles related to urination. The child with bladder neuropathy has little or no sensation of bladder fullness, poor bladder capacity, no awareness of urine passing through the urethra, and no ability to stop urinary flow (Lozes, 1988).

Treatment of renal problems includes regular urologic care with periodic imaging studies of the kidneys and bladder with prompt and vigorous treatment of infections. Regular emptying of the bladder is established, usually by clean intermittent catheterization (CIC). Catheterization can be performed easily by parents, even in neonates, and self-catheterization can be taught successfully to children as young as 4 to 6 years of age. It is particularly valuable when urinary retention, overflow incontinence, and reflux are problems (Shoenberg and Meador, 1982). Although many children achieve dryness for 2 hours or more with CIC, the technique is not successful for others.

Medications are often used to improve bladder storage and continence. The most commonly prescribed are oxybutynin chloride (Ditropan) and propantheline bromide (Pro-Banthine), which increase bladder capacity and lower intravesicular pressure. At times alpha-adrenergic drugs, such as ephedrine, are used to increase urethral resistance to achieve continence.

When continence cannot be attained by CIC and medication, surgical intervention may be necessary. Surgical procedures include implantation of an artifical urinary sphincter, bladder augmentation, creating a continent ileal reservoir (Kropp procedure), or creating a urinary diversion, such as ureteroileostomy, ureterostomy, or cystostomy.

Bowel control. Some degree of fecal continence can usually be achieved in most children with myelomeningocele with diet modification, regular toilet habits, and prevention of constipation and impaction. It is frequently a lengthy process. Medications to increase stool firmness and decrease peristalsis often help when used in conjunction with other methods.

Prevention. Numerous observers have noted that there appears to be a relationship between vitamin deficiency (especially vitamins C, A, and folic acid) and the incidence of NTDs. This provides additional evidence to support a balanced diet in women who anticipate becoming pregnant. It has also been suggested that infants with NTD suffer less trauma to nerve roots if they are delivered by cesarean section. However, data are incomplete in both observations.

Nursing Considerations

Care of the infant or child with myelomeningocele requires both immediate and long-term nursing and medical supervision. Long-term management involves an interdisciplinary team effort to help the child and family with the multitude of problems associated with this disability. The following discussion is limited to care of the infant. Some of the problems related to bowel, bladder, and lower extremity impairment are discussed in Chapter 40.

Assessment

At the time of delivery an examination is performed to assess the intactness of the membranous cyst. During transport to the nursery every effort is made to prevent trauma to this protective covering. In addition to the routine assessment of the newborn (see Chapter 8) the infant is assessed for level of neurologic involvement. Movement of extremities or skin response, especially an anal reflex, that might provide clues to the degree of motor or sensory impairment is noted. It is important to observe the infant's behavior in conjunction with the stimulus, since limb movements can be induced in response to spinal cord reflex activity that has no connection with the higher centers. The head circumference is measured daily (see Chapter 7), and the fontanels are examined for signs of tension or bulging.

Nursing Diagnoses

Following the nursing assessment a number of nursing diagnoses become evident. The most likely diagnoses are outlined and discussed in the Nursing Care Plan on p. 469. Others may be apparent in individual cases.

Planning

The goals of nursing care for the infant with myelomeningocele are as follows:

1. Prevent damage to the myelomeningocele sac.
2. Prevent complications.
3. Support and educate family.

Implementation

The basic needs of the infant with a myelomeningocele are essentially the same as for any newborn infant (see Chapter 8). Special needs related to the defect and potential complications are discussed in the following section. As the child matures, the problems increase and involve all aspects of daily living; therefore care is directly related to the child's habilitation at each stage of development.

Care of myelomeningocele sac. The infant is usually placed in an incubator or warmer so that temperature can be maintained without clothing or covers that might irritate the delicate lesion. When an overhead warmer is used, the dressings over the defect require more frequent moistening because of the dehydrating effect of the dry heat.

Before surgical closure the myelomeningocele is prevented from drying by the application of a sterile, moist, nonadherent dressing over the defect. The moistening solution is usually sterile normal saline, although soaks with antibacterial drugs such as silver nitrate or bacitracin are also advocated. Dressings are changed frequently (every 2 to 4 hours), and the sac is closely inspected for leaks, abrasions, irritation, or any signs of infection. It must be carefully cleansed if it becomes soiled or contaminated. Most sacs rupture during delivery or transport, and any opening in the sac greatly increases the risk of infection to the CNS.

NURSING ALERT The nurse should be alert to early signs of infection, such as elevated temperature (axillary), irritability, lethargy, and nuchal rigidity, and to signs of increased intracranial pressure (ICP), which might indicate developing hydrocephalus.

Since the exposed meningeal sac constitutes a sizable area, the potential for accelerated fluid and heat loss is a nursing concern. Therefore special efforts are extended to prevent hypothermia and to compensate for fluid loss with additional intake if needed.

Special measures to toughen the skin or membrane may be indicated, but care must be taken to prevent a dressing from adhering to and damaging the sac. Prolonged use of ointments or moist dressings is usually contraindicated to avoid maceration and breakdown of the tissues. A large doughnut-shaped piece of foam rubber or other spongy material can be fashioned to provide a protective shield for the sac. The edges should be left sufficiently wide to allow for adequate anchoring with strips of bandage or tape. A sterile drape, gauze, or other protective cover can form a roof over the opening but should not come in contact with the sac.

Positioning. One of the most difficult, important, and challenging aspects in the early care of the infant with myelomeningocele is positioning. Before surgery the infant is kept in the prone position to minimize tension on the sac and the risk of trauma. The prone position allows for optimum positioning of the legs, especially in cases of associated hip dysplasia. Ideally, the infant is placed in a low Trendelenburg position to reduce spinal fluid pressure in the sac, with the hips only slightly flexed to reduce tension on the defect. The legs are maintained in abduction with a pad between the knees to counteract hip subluxation, and a small roll is placed under the ankles to maintain a neutral foot position. A variety of aids, including diaper rolls, pads,

NURSING CARE PLAN
The Infant with Myelomeningocele

NURSING DIAGNOSIS: Potential for infection related to presence of infective organisms, nonepithelialized meningeal sac, paralysis

GOAL 1
Prevent infection

INTERVENTIONS
Position infant to prevent contamination from urine and stool
Cleanse myelomeningocele carefully with sterile saline
*Apply sterile dressings, moisten with sterile solution as ordered (saline, silver nitrate, antibiotic)
*Administer antibiotics as prescribed
Administer similar care to operative site postoperatively

EXPECTED OUTCOME
Meningeal sac remains clean, intact, and exhibits no evidence of infection

GOAL 2
Prevent urinary tract infection

INTERVENTIONS
Avoid urethral contamination with stool
Carry out meticulous perineal hygiene
*Administer antibiotics as prescribed
*Administer urinary tract antiseptics if prescribed
Ensure adequate fluid intake

EXPECTED OUTCOME
Infant exhibits no evidence of urinary tract infection

NURSING DIAGNOSIS: Potential for trauma related to delicate spinal lesion

GOAL 1
Prevent local trauma

INTERVENTIONS
Handle infant carefully
Place infant in prone position or side-lying position, if permitted
Apply protective devices (around sac) if appropriate
Modify routine nursing activities, e.g., feeding, making bed, comforting activities

EXPECTED OUTCOME
Meningeal sac remains intact

NURSING DIAGNOSIS: Potential impaired skin integrity related to paralysis, continual dribbling of urine and feces

GOAL 1
Prevent skin irritation

INTERVENTIONS
Change diapers as soon as soiled, if diapered
Keep perianal area clean and dry

EXPECTED OUTCOME
Perianal area remains clean and dry with no evidence of irritation

NURSING DIAGNOSIS: Potential for trauma related to impaired cerebrospinal fluid circulation

GOAL 1
Prevent increased intracranial pressure

INTERVENTIONS
Measure occipitofrontal circumference daily
Observe for signs of increased intracranial pressure (see Chapter 37)

EXPECTED OUTCOME
Evidence of increased intracranial pressure is detected early and appropriate interventions implemented†

NURSING DIAGNOSIS: Potential for injury related to neuromuscular impairment

GOAL 1
Prevent or minimize hip and lower extremity deformity

INTERVENTIONS
Carry out passive range of motion exercises; do not push past point of resistance
Carry out muscle stretching when indicated
Maintain hips in slight to moderate abduction to prevent dislocation and feet in neutral position

EXPECTED OUTCOMES
Lower extremities maintain flexibility
Maintain hips and lower extremities in correct articulation and alignment

See also:
- Nursing Care Plan: The Child with a Chronic Illness or Disability, Chapter 22
- Nursing Care Plan: The Child in the Hospital, Chapter 26
- Nursing Care Plan: The Family of the Ill or Hospitalized Child, Chapter 26

*Dependent nursing action.
†Nursing outcome.

small sandbags, or specially designed frames and appliances, can be used to maintain the desired position.

The prone position affects other aspects of the infant's care. For example, in this position the infant is more difficult to keep clean, pressure areas are a constant threat, and feeding becomes a problem. The infant's head is turned to one side for feeding. Fortunately, most defects are repaired early, and the infant can be held for feeding as soon as the surgical site is sufficiently healed to permit handling. Physical therapy consultation may be sought for difficult positioning problems.

General care. Diapering the infant is contraindicated until the defect has been repaired and healing is well advanced or epithelialization has taken place. The padding beneath the diaper area is changed as needed to keep the skin dry and free of irritation. When urinary retention is detected (the bladder is still an abdominal organ in early infancy), CIC* is employed. Since the bowel sphincter is frequently affected, there is continual passage of stool, often misinterpreted as diarrhea, which is a constant irritant to the skin and a source of infection to the spinal lesion. This provides another rationale for closure before the infant's first feeding while the meconium is still free of organisms. A protective drape is applied to minimize stool contamination of the lesion.

Areas of sensory and motor impairment are subject to skin breakdown and therefore require meticulous care. Placing the infant on a soft foam or fleece pad reduces pressure on the knees and ankles. Periodic cleansing, application of lotion, and gentle massage aid circulation. Changing linen is best accomplished by two persons—one changes the linen while the other holds the infant, ensuring that the spine is maintained in good alignment without tension in the area of the defect.

Gentle range of motion exercises are sometimes carried out to prevent contractures, and stretching of contractures is performed when indicated. However, these exercises may be restricted to the foot, ankle, and knee joint. Where the hip joints are unstable, stretching against tight hip flexors or adductor muscles, which act much like bowstrings, may aggravate a tendency toward subluxation. A physical therapy consultation is usually obtained.

Since infants with unrepaired myelomeningocele are unable to be held in the arms and cuddled as unaffected infants are, their need for tactile stimulation is met by fondling, stroking, and other comfort measures. To facilitate handling and reduce parental anxiety, the infant reclines on a pillow placed in the parent's lap. Bright mobiles or other objects can be placed within the infant's view, and other stimulating activities usually provided for infants are appropriate. All infants respond to pleasant sounds (see Developmental Intervention, Chapter 10).

Postoperative care. Postoperative care of the infant with myelomeningocele involves the same basic care as that of any postsurgical infant—monitoring vital signs, monitoring intake and output, nourishment, and observation for signs of infection. Wound management is carried out according to the directions of the surgeon, and general care is continued as preoperatively.

The prone position is maintained after operative closure, although many neurosurgeons allow a side-lying or partial side-lying position unless it aggravates a coexisting hip dysplasia or permits undesirable hip flexion. This offers an opportunity for position changes, which reduces the risk of pressure sores and facilitates feeding. If permitted by the physician, the infant can be held upright against the body, with care taken to avoid pressure on the operative site.

The nurse is in a position to aid the physician in determining the extent of neuromuscular involvement. Movement of the extremities or skin response, especially an anal reflex, that might provide cues to the degree of motor or sensory status is noted. The head circumference is measured daily (see Chapter 7), and the fontanels are examined for signs of tension or bulging. The nurse is also alert to early signs of infection, such as elevated temperature (axillary), irritability, lethargy, and nuchal rigidity, and to signs of increased ICP. The infant is also assessed and catheterized for urine retention. Although it may not have been a problem preoperatively, swelling around the operative site may cause transient urine retention, which resolves in 1 to 2 days.

Family support and home care. As soon as the parents are able to cope with the infant's condition, they are encouraged to become involved in care. They need to learn how to continue at home the care that has been initiated in the hospital—positioning, feeding, skin care, and range of motion exercises when appropriate. Parents are taught clean catheterization technique when prescribed. The family needs to know the signs of complications and how to reach assistance when needed. In cases in which the defect has not been repaired, they are taught to care for the lesion.

As the child grows and develops, it is important that the parents encourage and stimulate the infant to accomplish age-appropriate developmental tasks within the limits imposed by the disabilities. Upper limb movement can be stimulated early by placing the infant on the floor in a prone position with toys within reach. Activities that encourage body consciousness, such as rolling over and pulling to a sitting position, should be encouraged at the appropriate times. Creeping and crawling, even in a limited way, help the child to explore the environment. The parents may need help to modify appliances and activities normally expected of a growing child. For example, the paraplegic infant should be encouraged to use arms and shoulders as much as possible. When sitting in an infant seat, stroller, high chair, or feeding table, the infant's hips can be supported, a footrest provided, and hard-soled shoes worn to maintain the feet in correct alignment and to protect the insensitive feet from trauma. A standing table is helpful for a variety of activities, and it is best for the child to begin supported weight bearing and standing as close as possible to the time expected for normal children.

It is important for the family to understand the nature of

---

*For home care instructions see Wong, D.L., and Whaley, L.F.: Clinical manual of pediatric nursing, ed. 3, St. Louis, 1990, Mosby–Year Book, Inc.

sensory deficit in a child with a spinal defect. The child will be insensitive to pressure or other sources of tissue injury. Therefore the family must be alert to hot or cold items that could cause thermal injury to tissues and to inspect the skin regularly for signs of pressure, especially over bony prominences. Because of sensory impairment, the child is unaware of bladder discomfort; therefore signs of urinary tract infections may be easily overlooked. Urinary tract infection is often considered when the child becomes ill.

Prognosis. The long-range planning with and support of the parents and child begin in the hospital and extend throughout childhood and even beyond. Long-term care of these children is of uncertain length. Nurses assume an important role as a central member of the health team. As a coordinator the nurse reviews information with the family, takes responsibility for family teaching, and acts as a liaison between inpatient and outpatient services. The child will need numerous hospitalizations over the years, and each one will be a source of stress to which the younger child is especially vulnerable.

Habilitation involves solving not only problems of self-help and locomotion but also the most distressing problem of incontinence, which threatens the child's social acceptability. Assistance with preparing the child and the school regarding the special needs of children with disabilities helps provide a better initial adjustment to broader social experiences. It would be difficult to enumerate all that the condition entails in terms of suffering, frustration, family stress, and economic burden. Numerous organizations and agencies are able to offer assistance and support to children and families. The **Spina Bifida Association of America*** is organized to provide services and support for families of children with spinal lesions. Special reading materials are also available from other sources.† Organizations whose services extend to all children with physical disabilities are listed in Appendix E.

The multiple aspects of care of the child with a disability are discussed in Chapter 22 and need not be elaborated on here; nor are complex problems associated with partial or complete lower extremity paralysis dealt with here. These are discussed in Chapter 40 and include bowel and bladder control, orthopedic appliances, and the observation and management of complications, especially urinary tract infections and pressure necrosis.

Evaluation

The effectiveness of nursing interventions is determined by continual reassessment and evaluation of care based on the following observational guidelines and expected outcomes:

1. Inspect the spinal lesion, take appropriate measurements (weight, vital signs, head circumference), observe the child's general health status, and check completed care against the preoperative checklist.
2. Take vital signs, inspect the operative site (or preoperative lesion), inspect skin (especially dependent areas), measure head circumference, and assess range of motion of lower extremities.
3. Observe parent-infant interactions, behavior of family members, and interview family members regarding their feelings and concerns.

Expected outcomes:
See Nursing Care Plan, p. 469.

ANENCEPHALY

Anencephaly, the most serious NTD, is a congenital malformation in which both cerebral hemispheres are absent. The condition is incompatible with life, and most affected infants are stillborn. For those who survive, no specific treatment is available. The infants have intact brainstems and are able to maintain vital functions (such as temperature regulation and cardiac and respiratory function) for a few hours to several days but eventually die of respiratory failure (Erlen and Holzman, 1988).

Traditionally these infants have been provided comfort measures, but with no effort at resuscitation. Directives to withdraw all support (e.g., feeding) were met with universal resistance by nursery personnel, whose primary function is nurturance. Recently the practice of allowing these infants to die peacefully has been questioned as the need for organ donors continues to expand (see Questions and Controversies, p. 472).

HYDROCEPHALUS

Hydrocephalus is a condition caused by an imbalance in the production and absorption of cerebrospinal fluid (CSF) in the ventricular system. When production is greater than absorption, CSF accumulates within the ventricular system, usually under increased pressure, producing passive dilation of the ventricles. The disorder occurs in association with a number of anomalies.

Pathophysiology

To appreciate the condition, an understanding of the dynamics of CSF and the relationship between the various structures that make up the ventricular and subarachnoid spaces is necessary (Fig. 11-4). The primary site of CSF formation is believed to be the choroid plexuses of the lateral ventricles, although CSF is also believed to be produced by the brain parenchyma.

Ventricular circulation. The fluid flows from the lateral ventricles through the *foramen of Monro* to the third ventricle, where it combines with fluid secreted into the third ventricle. From there it flows through the *aqueduct of Sylvius* into the fourth ventricle, where more fluid is formed; it then leaves the fourth ventricle by way of the lateral *foramen of Luschka* and the midline *foramen of Magendie* into the *cisterna magna*. From there it flows to the cerebral and cerebellar subarachnoid spaces where it is absorbed by some mechanism that is not entirely clear. A large portion is absorbed through the arachnoid villi, but the sinuses,

*1700 Rockville Pike, Suite 540, Rockville, MD 20852; (800) 621-5141. (Also provides general information and referrals.) In Maryland, (301) 770-7222.
†Recommended: *Spina Bifida,* available from Medic Publishing Co., P.O. Box 89, Redmond, WA 98073-0089; (206) 881-2883.

QUESTIONS AND CONTROVERSIES

Should infants with anencephaly be kept alive for use as organ donors?

With advances in surgical technology and development of immunosuppressive agents, major organ transplantation has become an acceptable alternative treatment for a number of otherwise healthy children with developmental defects and a variety of end-stage disease processes. It is anticipated that continued improvement in survival will create a concomitant increase in a demand for donor organs. This anticipated shortage has prompted the proposal that anencephalic infants be considered as a viable source of organ donors (Harrison, 1986). In the United States approximately 1800 infants with anencephaly are born each year; aside from the neurologic malformation, their organs are presumed suitable for transplantation (Fletcher, Robertson, and Harrison, 1986); and of the 25% to 45% of these infants born live, 95% die within 1 week (Baird and Sadovinick, 1984).

This suggestion raises several issues. The uniform Determination of Death Act defines death as (1) the irreversible cessation of circulatory and respiratory function or (2) the irreversible cessation of all functions of the entire brain, including the brainstem. The Uniform Anatomical Gift Act states that anatomic gifts can be made only after the donor has been declared dead. In their definition of death the President's Commission for the Study of Ethical Problems in Medicine and Biomedical and Behavioral Research (1981) did not take into consideration prognostic uncertainty. Since higher centers are absent, these infants can be defined as "brain absent," but they are not dead in a legal sense. Brainstem activity serves as the source of integration of vital physiologic processes, thereby producing the appearance of being alive.

Proxy consent for organ donation can be obtained after a patient is dead. In the case of infants and children this right has been relegated to the parents. Using anencephalic infants amounts to removing the organs from an individual who is legally still alive. The question is: Do the parents have the right to sacrifice the life of the infant for the benefit of another? Utilitarians argue that anencephalic infants are oblivious to what life they have and that early termination would do them no conceivable harm. Also, because of their limited life expectancy, significant others would have little opportunity to "bond" with these infants, and earlier death would shorten their grieving process.

Also at stake is the highly valued idea of respect for persons and individual rights to self-determination, regardless of level of competence, mental capacity, or life expectancy. Some classify these infants as "nonpersons" who lack the ability to experience a "personal" life. Others insist that they are "persons" and, as such, deserve to be treated with respect. This right may at times conflict with the principle of beneficence. That is, should individual rights of a dying, brain-absent infant take precedence over the well-being of an infant or child for whom organ transplantation may be lifesaving? Christian and Judaic ethics stand firmly against taking a human life no matter how great the benefit to others. From a moral standpoint what is accomplished would be good; the means of accomplishment would not.

Data from Arras and Shinnar, 1988; Baird and Sadovinick, 1984; Botkin, 1988; Fletcher, Robertson, and Harrison, 1986; Harrison, 1986; Landwirth, 1988; Shewmon and others, 1989.

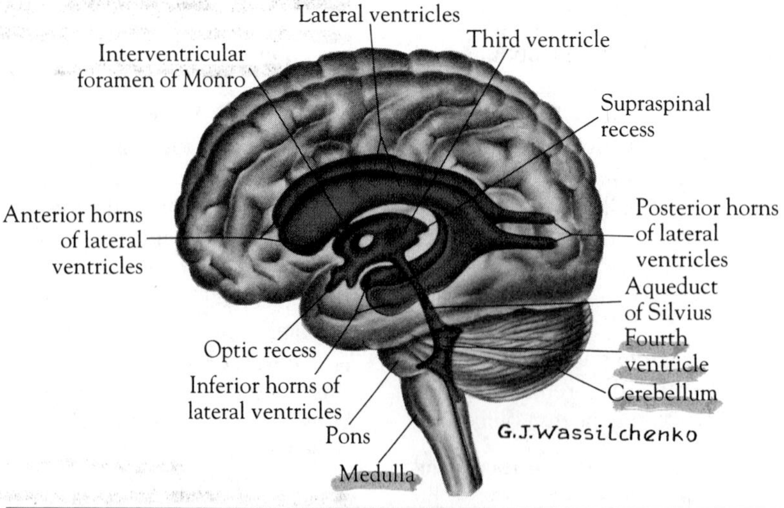

Fig. 11-4. Cerebral ventricular system.

From Thompson, J., and others: Mosby's manual of clinical nursing, ed. 2, St. Louis, 1989, Mosby–Year Book, Inc.

veins, brain substance, and dura also participate in absorption.

Mechanisms of fluid imbalance. The causes of hydrocephalus are varied, but the result is either (1) impaired absorption of CSF fluid within the subarachnoid space *(communicating hydrocephalus)* or (2) obstruction to the flow of CSF through the ventricular system *(noncommunicating hydrocephalus)*. Rarely, a tumor of the choroid plexus causes increased CSF secretion. Any imbalance of secretion and absorption causes an increased accumulation of CSF in the ventricles, which become dilated and compress the brain substance against the surrounding rigid bony cranium. When this occurs before fusion of the cranial sutures, it produces enlargement of the skull as well as dilation of the ventricles.

Most cases of noncommunicating hydrocephalus are a result of developmental malformations. Although the defect usually is apparent in early infancy, it may become evident at any time from the prenatal period to late childhood or early adulthood. Other causes include neoplasms, infections, and trauma. An obstruction to the normal flow can occur at any point in the CSF pathway to produce increased pressure and dilation of the pathways proximal to the site of obstruction. Table 11-2 describes the most frequent sites of obstruction and the consequences.

Developmental defects—for example, Arnold-Chiari mal-

Table 11-2 Sites and types of hydrocephalus

SITE AND TYPE	CAUSES AND COMMENTS
▪ Noncommunicating hydrocephalus	
Site: Agueduct of Sylvius	Accounts for 20% of hydrocephalus
Type: Stenosis or atresia	Congenital (X-linked recessive in small number) Insidious onset of symptoms from birth to adulthood
Gliosis	Postinflammatory, usually secondary to perinatal infection or hemorrhage Prenatal maternal infection (toxoplasmosis)
Obstructive	Tumors of third ventricle or midbrain Ependymitis from maternal toxoplasmosis Congenital aneurysm of vein of Galen
Site: Fourth ventricle and foramen magnum	Accounts for 50% of all hydrocephalus
Type: Chiari malformations	Accounts for 40% of fourth ventricle obstructions
Type 1	A neural tube defect with herniation of medulla through foramen magnum; may be asymptomatic; similar to type 2, but more mild
Type 2 (Arnold-Chiari malformation)	A more severe defect; downward displacement of brainstem, fourth ventricle, and lower parts of cerebellum through foramen magnum with fixed attachment of spinal cord at site of a myelomeningocele
Type 3	High cervical or occipitocervical myelomeningocele with cervical herniation through body defect
Absence or occlusion of ventricles	Congenital (Dandy-Walker syndrome) caused by obstruction of foramina of Luschka and Magendie Tumors of posterior fossa (e.g., medulloblastoma) cause pressure on surrounding tissues to produce obstruction Less often: subdural hematoma, bacterial or granulomatous meningitis
▪ Communicating hydrocephalus	
Site: Arachnoid villi and cisterna magna	Obstruction by thick arachnoid membrane or meninges
Type: Meningitis	Bacterial or granulomatous Acute phase: clumping of purulent fluid in drainage channels Chronic phase: organization of blood and exudate that results in fibrosis of subarachnoid spaces
Prenatal maternal infections	Toxoplasmosis, cytomegalic inclusion disease, mumps
Meningeal malignancy	Secondary to leukemia or lymphoma
Arachnoid cyst	Located in basal cistern or (uncommon) over cerebral cortex
Tuberculosis, fungal, or parasitic infection	More common in children age 2 to 10 years

formations (ACMs) (see discussion below), aqueduct stenosis, aqueduct gliosis, and atresia of the foramina of Lushcka and Magendie (Dandy-Walker syndrome)—account for most cases of hydrocephalus from birth to 2 years of age. Hydrocephalus is so often associated with myelomeningocele that all such infants should be observed for its development. In the remainder of cases there is a history of intrauterine infection, perinatal hemorrhage (anoxic or traumatic), and neonatal meningoencephalitis (bacterial or viral). In older children hydrocephalus is most often the result of intracranial masses (vascular anomalies, cysts, tumors), preexisting developmental defects, intracranial infections, or hemorrhage.

Arnold-Chiari malformations. ACM is a brain defect involving posterior fossa contents; the major types are described in Table 11-2. The type II malformation, seen almost exclusively with myelomeningocele, is characterized by caudal displacement of a small cerebellum, medulla, pons, and fourth ventricle into the cervical spinal canal through an enlarged foramen magnum. The resulting obstruction of CSF flow causes the hydrocephalus.

Clinical Manifestations

The two factors that influence the clinical picture in hydrocephalus are the acuity of onset and the presence of preexisting structural lesions. In infancy before closure of the cranial sutures, head enlargement is the predominant sign, whereas in older infants and children the lesions responsible for hydrocephalus produce other neurologic signs through pressure on adjacent structures before causing CSF.

Infancy. In infants the head grows at an abnormal rate, although the first signs may be bulging fontanels without head enlargement (Fig. 11-5). The anterior fontanel is tense, often bulging, and nonpulsatile. Scalp veins are dilated and markedly so when the infant cries. With the increase in intracranial volume the bones of the skull become thin and the sutures become palpably separated to produce the "cracked-pot" sound (Macewen sign) on percussion of the skull. There may be frontal enlargement or "bossing" with depressed eyes and a "setting-sun" sign, in which the sclera is visible above the iris because of pressure on a thinned orbital roof or the third ventricle on the tectum of the mesencephalon. Pupils are sluggish with unequal response to light.

The infant is irritable and lethargic and may display changes in level of consciousness, opisthotonos (often extreme), and lower extremity spasticity. The infant will cry when picked up or rocked and quiet when allowed to lie still. Early infantile reflex acts may persist, and normally expected responses fail to appear, indicating failure in the development of normal cortical inhibition.

Infants with ACM may exhibit behaviors that reflect cranial nerve dysfunction as a result of brainstem compression, including swallowing difficulties, stridor, apnea, aspiration, respiratory difficulties, and arm weakness. There may be absent or diminished gag reflex (Anderson, 1989).

If hydrocephalus is allowed to progress, development of lower brainstem functions is disrupted, as manifested by difficulty in sucking and feeding and a shrill, brief, high-pitched cry. Eventually the skull becomes enormous and the cortex is destroyed. If the hydrocephalus is rapidly progressive, the infant may display emesis, somnolence, seizures, and cardiopulmonary embarrassment. Severely affected infants usually do not survive the neonatal period.

Childhood. The signs and symptoms in early to late childhood are caused by increased ICP, and specific manifestations are related to the focal lesion. Most commonly resulting from posterior fossa neoplasms and aqueduct stenosis, the clinical manifestations are primarily those associated with space-occupying lesions, that is, headache on

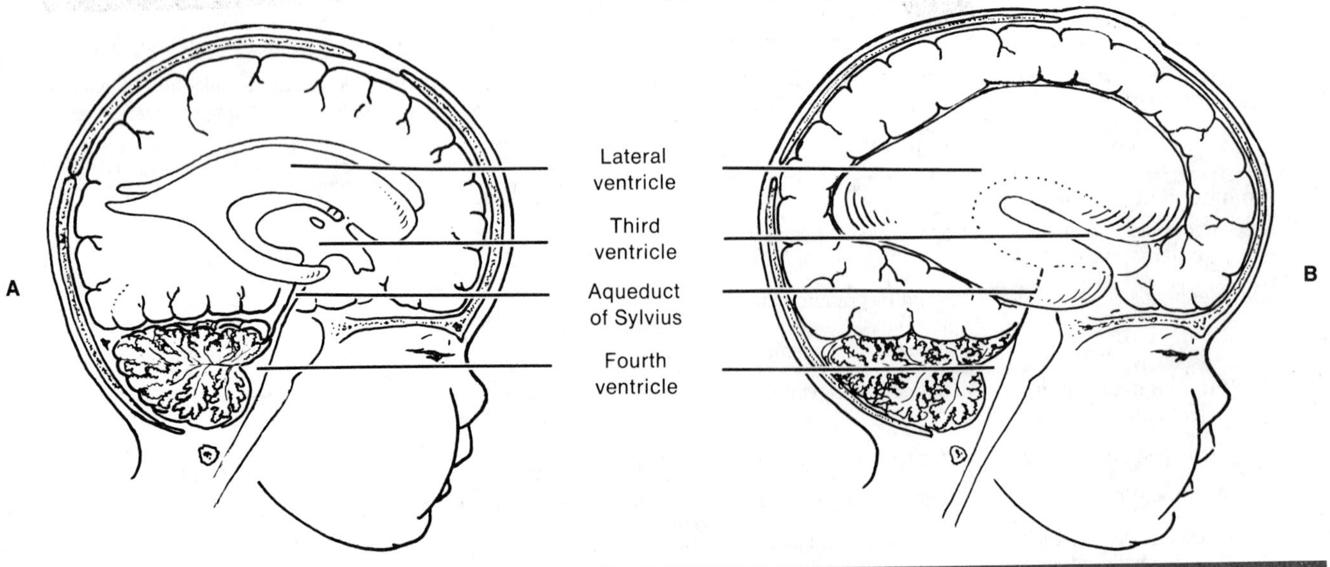

Fig. 11-5. Hydrocephalus: a block in flow of cerebrospinal fluid. **A,** Patent cerebrospinal fluid circulation. **B,** Enlarged lateral and third ventricles caused by obstruction of circulation—stenosis of aqueduct of Sylvius.

awakening with improvement following emesis or upright posture, papilledema, strabismus, and extrapyramidal tract signs such as ataxia (see Chapter 37). As with infants, the child will be irritable, lethargic, apathetic, confused, and often incoherent. In one of the congenital defects with later onset, the Dandy-Walker syndrome, characteristic manifestations are bulging occiput, nystagmus, ataxia, and cranial nerve palsies.

Manifestations of ACM in children over 3 years of age are related to spinal cord dysfunction rather than brainstem compression as observed in infants. Commonly seen are scoliosis proximal to the level of the myelomeningocele (usually associated with ACM) and development of upper extremity spasticity, which may progress to weakness and atrophy. Cranial nerve deficits are rare (Anderson, 1989).

Diagnostic Evaluation

In infancy the diagnosis of hydrocephalus is based on head circumference that crosses one or more grid lines on the measurement chart within a period of 2 to 4 weeks and on associated neurologic signs that are present and progressive. However, other diagnostic studies are needed to localize the site of CSF obstruction. Routine daily head circumference measurements are carried out in infants with myelomeningocele and intracranial infections. In evaluation of a premature infant, specially adapted head circumference charts are consulted to distinguish abnormal head growth from rapid head growth that takes place normally.

The primary diagnostic tools for detecting hydrocephalus are CT and MRI (Fig. 11-6). Sedation is required, since the child must remain absolutely still for an accurate picture. Diagnostic evaluation of children who have symptoms of hydrocephalus after infancy is similar to that employed in those with a suspected intracranial tumor. In the neonate echoencephalography is useful in comparing the ratio of lateral ventricle to cortex. Sometimes isotope ventriculograms are used to assess the flow and patency of existing shunts and check the size of the ventricles.

Problems in differential diagnosis are related to the child whose head circumference is greater than the 97th percentile but whose head growth parallels the normal growth curve. It is sometimes valuable to measure parental occipitofrontal circumference (OFC) to detect a possible normal familial characteristic (benign familial megalencephaly). (See Table 37-4 for diagnostic tests for neurologic evaluation.)

Therapeutic Management

The treatment of hydrocephalus is directed toward (1) relief of the hydrocephalus, (2) treatment of complications, and (3) management of problems related to the effect of the disorder on psychomotor development. The treatment is, with few exceptions, surgical.

Medical therapy has been largely disappointing. Many newborn infants with progressive cranial enlargement secondary to intracranial hemorrhage demonstrate spontaneous stabilization and resolution. Serial lumbar punctures and medications have been used with varying success. The administration of acetazolamide and isosorbide or furosemide has proved beneficial in decreasing the production of CSF in selected cases of slowly progressive disease. The medication reduces the ICP until spontaneous arrest of hydrocephalus takes place (Shinnar and others, 1985) or as a temporizing measure when surgery is contraindicated.

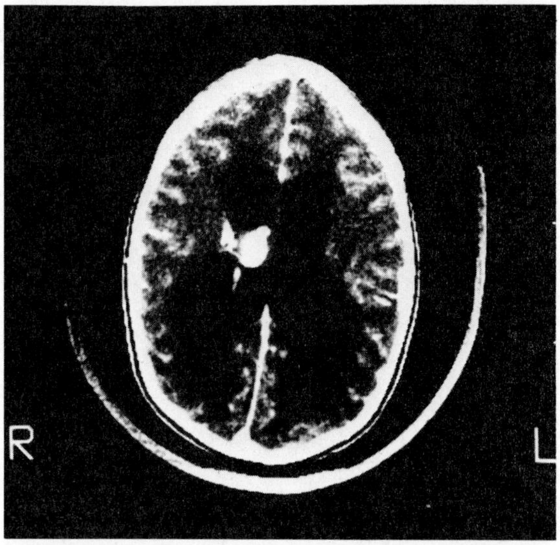

Fig. 11-6. CT scan reveals enlarged ventricles of child with hydrocephalus.

Surgical treatment. Improved techniques have established surgical treatment as the therapy of choice in almost all cases of hydrocephalus. This is accomplished by direct removal of an obstruction, for example, resection of a neoplasm, cyst, or hematoma or, in rare instances of fluid overproduction, by choroid plexus extirpation (plexectomy or electric coagulation). However, most children require a shunt procedure that provides primary drainage of the CSF from the ventricles to an extracranial compartment, usually the peritoneum. See Handbook of Therapeutic Interventions

Most shunt systems consist of a ventricular catheter, a flush pump, a unidirectional flow valve, and a distal catheter. All are radiopaque for easy visualization after placement, and all are tested for accuracy before insertion. A reservoir is frequently added to allow direct access to the ventricular system for administration of medications and removal of fluid. In all models the valves are designed to open at a predetermined intraventricular pressure and close when the pressure falls below that level, thus preventing backflow of secretions. High-pressure valves are used to prevent complications from rapid decompression of the ventricles. Medium-pressure valves are used in most children, especially those with long-standing hydrocephalus. Low-pressure valves are used in small infants.

The preferred procedure is the ventriculoperitoneal (VP) shunt, especially in neonates and young infants (Fig. 11-7). There is greater allowance for excess tubing, which minimizes the number of revisions needed as the child grows. Since it requires repeated lengthening, the ventriculoatrial (VA) shunt (ventricle to right atrium) is reserved for older children who have attained most of their somatic growth and children with abdominal pathology. The VA shunt is

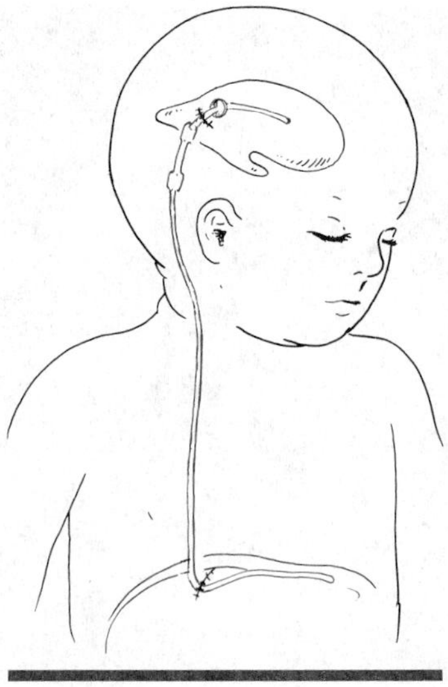

Fig. 11-7. Ventriculoperitoneal shunt. Catheter is threaded beneath the skin.

contraindicated in children with cardiopulmonary disease or elevated CSF protein.

A ventricular bypass into intracranial channels may be used in older children with noncommunicating hydrocephalus caused by aqueduct stenosis or posterior fossa masses (e.g., medulloblastoma). Technical difficulties preclude its use in infants, since these spaces are poorly developed in the infant. Ventriculopleural shunts are sometimes used in children over 5 years of age. Other sites that are used occasionally for shunting include the facial vein and the subgaleal or subarachnoid spaces.

The initial shunt is placed when indicated based on individual assessment. There is wide variation in the time of revisions. In most instances revisions are performed when physical signs indicate shunt malfunction. Sometimes revisions are planned for specific times during development. In all mechanisms the initial success rate is relatively high; however, shunts are associated with complications that interfere with continued shunt function or that threaten the life of the child.

Complications. The major complications of VP shunts are infection and malfunction. All shunts are subject to mechanical difficulties, such as kinking, plugging, or separation and migration of tubing. Malfunction is most often caused by mechanical obstruction either within the ventricles from particulate matter (tissue or exudate) or at the distal end from thrombosis or displacement as a result of growth. The child with a shunt obstruction often presents as an emergency with clinical manifestations of increased ICP, frequently accompanied by worsening neurologic status.

The most serious complication, shunt infection, can occur at any time, but the period of greatest risk is 1 to 2 months following placement. The infection is generally the result of intercurrent infections at the time of shunt placement. Infections include septicemia, bacterial endocarditis, wound infection, shunt nephritis, meningitis, and ventriculitis. Meningitis and ventriculitis are of greatest concern, since any complicating CNS infection is a significant predictor of intellectual outcome. Infection is treated with massive doses of antibiotics administered by the intravenous route. A persistent infection requires removal of the shunt until the infection is controlled. External ventricular drainage (EVD) is used until CSF is sterile.

A serious shunt-related complication is subdural hematoma caused by too rapid reduction of ICP and size. This usually can be averted by careful assessment of ICP prior to insertion of the shunt and use of correct valvular pressure. Other complications that may occur include peritonitis, abdominal abscesses, perforation of abdominal organs by catheter or trochar (at time of insertion), fistulas, hernias, and ileus.

Prognosis. The prognosis of children with treated hydrocephalus depends largely on the rate at which hydrocephalus develops, the duration of raised ICP, the frequency of complications, and the cause of the hydrocephalus. For example, malignant tumors may have a high mortality regardless of other complicating factors.

Untreated, hydrocephalus has a 50% to 60% mortality rate caused by the disorder or intercurrent illnesses. In the survivors there is a high incidence of subnormal intellectual capacity, and a large majority have major physical and/or disabling neurologic handicaps such as ataxia, spastic diplegia, poor fine motor coordination, and perceptual deficits. Spontaneous arrest occurs occasionally in approximately 40% of those with near-normal intelligence.

Surgically treated hydrocephalus with continued neurosurgical and medical management has a survival rate of about 80%, with the highest incidence of mortality occurring within the first year of treatment. Of the surviving children approximately one third are both intellectually and neurologically normal and one half have neurologic disabilities. However, the intelligence is in the lower ranges of normal, with deficits more pronounced in nonverbal intellectual skills. These children are also at greater risk for developing an emotional problem, such as anxiety neurosis or antisocial-conduct disorder (Noetzel, 1986).

Hydrocephalus complicating a meningomyelocele carries a less favorable prognosis. In some children irreversible damage may have been produced by the hydrocephalus or from the original infection; in addition, there are sometimes coincidental cerebral defects. Generally, noninfective hydrocephalus appears to carry the best prognosis.

Nursing Considerations

Care of the child with hydrocephalus involves both preoperative and postoperative management. It is also important to carefully assess the child with myelomeningocele (p. 465) for signs of increasing ICP, since hydrocephalus is commonly associated with that anomaly.

Assessment

Preoperatively the infant with diagnosed or suspected hydrocephalus is observed carefully for signs of increasing

ICP. In infants the head is measured daily at the point of largest measurement—the OFC (see Chapter 7 for technique). To avoid the likelihood of wide discrepancies, the point at which the measurements are taken is indicated on the head with a marking pen. Fontanels and suture lines are gently palpated for size, signs of bulging, tenseness, and separation. An infant with hydrocephalus and normal ICP will display bulging under certain circumstances such as straining or crying; therefore such accompanying behavior should be noted. Irritability, lethargy, or seizure activity, as well as altered vital signs and feeding behavior, may indicate advancing pathology.

In older children, who are usually admitted to the hospital for elective or emergency shunt revision, the most valuable indicator of increasing ICP is an alteration in the child's level of consciousness and the way in which the child interacts with the environment. Changes are identified by observation and by comparing present behavior with customary behavior, sleep patterns, developmental capabilities, and habits obtained through a detailed history and a baseline assessment. This baseline information serves as a guide for postoperative assessment and evaluation of shunt function.

Nursing Diagnoses

Following the nursing assessment a number of nursing diagnoses become evident. The most likely diagnoses are outlined and discussed in the Nursing Care Plan on p. 478. Others may be apparent in individual cases.

Planning

The goals of nursing care of the child with hydrocephalus include:

1. Prevent complications of hydrocephalus and/or corrective surgery.
2. Provide education and emotional support to the family.

Implementation

General nursing care of the infant with hydrocephalus may present special problems. Maintaining adequate nutrition often requires flexible feeding schedules to accommodate diagnostic procedures, since feeding before or after handling can precipitate an episode of vomiting. Small feedings at more frequent intervals are often better tolerated than larger ones spaced farther apart. These infants are often difficult to feed and require extra time and innovation.

The nurse is responsible for preparation of the child for diagnostic tests such as tomography and for assisting the physician with procedures such as a ventricular tap, which is often performed to relieve excessive pressure during the preoperative period, and CSF examination. (See Chapter 27 for preparing children for procedures.) If surgery is anticipated, intravenous infusions should not be placed in a scalp vein.

Fortunately, almost all children with hydrocephalus are recognized, and treatment is begun early. For those children with significant head enlargement care must be exercised to see that the head is well supported when the infant is fed or moved to prevent extra strain on the infant's neck, and measures must be taken to prevent development of pressure areas. Not infrequently infants with irreversible brain damage or with severe developmental defects such as hydroencephaly, in which both cerebral hemispheres fail to develop and are replaced with a membranous sac filled with CSF, are placed in long-term institutions specially designed for care of these infants.

Postoperative care. In addition to routine postoperative care and observation, the infant or child is positioned carefully on the unoperated side to prevent pressure on the shunt valve and pressure areas. The child is kept flat to help avert complications resulting from too rapid reduction of intracranial fluid. When the ventricular size is reduced too rapidly, the cerebral cortex may pull away from the dura and tear the small interlacing veins, producing a subdural hematoma. This is not a problem in children with elective shunt revision, since their intraventricular size and pressure have been normal. The surgeon indicates the position to be maintained and the extent of activity allowed. If there is increased ICP, the surgeon will prescribe the head of the bed to be elevated and/or allow the child to sit up to enhance gravity flow through the shunt. Sedation is avoided because the level of consciousness is an important observation (see Chapter 26 for pain management).

Observation for signs of increased ICP, which indicate obstruction of the shunt, is continued. Neurologic assessment includes pupil dilation (pressure causes compression or stretching of the oculomotor nerve, producing dilation on the same side as the pressure) and blood pressure (hypoxia to the brainstem causes variability in these vital signs). Sometimes the valve can be tested for patency and flushed to maintain patency by pumping several times to relieve the pressure. This is done by compressing the reservoir or antechamber of the valve mechanism, thus forcing a bolus of fluid from the reservoir into the distal catheter. Fluid that moves out of the chamber indicates a patent peritoneal catheter; ready refilling of the chamber with CSF is evidence of a patent ventricular catheter. The procedure is repeated when indicated or routinely as ordered. If these measures are unsuccessful, the shunt may require replacement.

Intake and output are carefully monitored. Children are often placed on fluid restriction with nothing by mouth (NPO) for 24 to 48 hours. The intravenous infusion is closely monitored to prevent fluid overload. Routine feeding is resumed after the prescribed NPO period, but the presence of bowel sounds is determined before feeding children with VP shunts.

Since infection is the greatest hazard of the postoperative period, nurses are continually on the alert for the usual manifestations of CSF infection, which may include elevated vital signs, poor feeding, vomiting, decreased responsiveness, and seizure activity. There may be signs of local

NURSING CARE PLAN
The Infant with Hydrocephalus

NURSING DIAGNOSIS: Potential for injury related to increased intracranial pressure

GOAL 1

Prevent increased intracranial pressure

INTERVENTIONS

Carry out postoperative care of shunt as prescribed
Position to facilitate drainage of cerebrospinal fluid
Observe for early signs of increasing ICP:
- Irritability
- Lethargy
- Infant:
  - Cries when picked up or handled; quiets when lies still
  - Increased OFC measurement
  - Separated sutures
  - Change in level of consciousness
- Child:
  - Headache (especially in morning)
  - Apathy
  - Confusion

EXPECTED OUTCOME

Child exhibits no evidence of increased intracranial pressure

NURSING DIAGNOSIS: Potential for infection related to presence of mechanical drainage system

GOAL 1

Prevent infection

INTERVENTIONS

Provide wound care as prescribed

EXPECTED OUTCOME

Child exhibits no evidence of infection (fever, lethargy, heat, redness, swelling at site)

NURSING DIAGNOSIS: Altered family processes related to a child with a chronic defect

GOAL 1

Support family

INTERVENTIONS AND EXPECTED OUTCOMES

See Nursing Care Plan: The Family of the Ill or Hospitalized child, Chapter 26

See also:
Nursing Care Plan: The Low-Birth-Weight Infant, Chapter 10
Nursing Care Plan: The Child with a Chronic Illness or Disability, Chapter 22

inflammation at the operative sites and along the shunt tract. Antibiotics are administered by the intravenous route as ordered, and the nurse may also need to assist the physician with intraventricular instillation. The incision site is inspected for leakage, and any suspected drainage is tested for glucose, an indication of CSF.

Meticulous skin care is continued postoperatively, with extra care taken to prevent tissue damage from pressure. A sheepskin pad underneath the child and a doughnut for the head help prevent pressure on prominent areas. Skin is inspected regularly for any signs of pressure, irritation, or infection.

Family support. Specific needs and concerns of parents during periods of hospitalization are related to the reason for the child's hospitalization (shunt revision, infection, diagnosis) and the diagnostic and/or surgical procedures to which the child must be subjected. Often parents have very little understanding of anatomy; therefore they need further exploration and reinforcement of information that was given to them by the physician and neurosurgeon, as well as information about what they can expect. They are especially frightened of any procedure that involves the brain, and the fear of retardation or brain damage is very real and pervasive. Nurses can do much to allay their anxiety with explanations of the rationale underlying the various nursing and medical activities such as positioning or testing and by simply being available and willing to listen to their concerns.

To prepare for the child's discharge and home care, the parents are instructed on how to recognize signs that indicate shunt malfunction or infection and how to pump the shunt, if necessary. Active children may have accidents, such as a fall, that can damage the shunt, and the tubing may pull out of the distal insertion site or become disconnected during normal growth.

The management of hydrocephalus in a child is a demanding task for both family and health professionals, and helping a family cope with the child is an important nursing responsibility. It is important to emphasize that hydrocephalus is a lifelong problem and that the child will require evaluation on a regular basis. The overall aim is to establish realistic goals and an appropriate educational program that will assist the child in achieving the optimum potential. Families can be referred to community agencies for support and guidance. The **National Hydrocephalus Foundation**

(NHF)* provides information on the condition for families and assists interested groups in establishing local organizations. Helpful booklets are available from this and other sources.

Anticipatory guidance will prepare parents for possible problems and help them to avoid being overprotective of the child. There need be few restrictions placed on the child's activities (mainly contact sports), and the child should be encouraged to live as would any other of the same age and abilities. Parents need support and encouragement in coping with the child and problems the child may encounter in relationships with peers and others. Reactions of other children when the child has a noticeably enlarged head or requires shaving at times of revision are stress situations for both child and parents (see Chapter 22 for problems and coping with the child with a disability).

Evaluation

The effectiveness of nursing interventions is determined by continual reassessment and evaluation of care based on the following observational guidelines and expected outcomes:

1. Measure OFC, take vital signs, observe incision site and skin over pressure points, and observe behavior.
2. Interview and observe family members.

Expected outcomes:
See Nursing Care Plan, p. 478.

CRANIAL DEFORMITIES

In the normal newborn the cranial sutures are separated by membranous seams several millimeters wide. For the first few hours to 1 to 2 days after birth, the cranial bones are highly mobile, which allows the cranial bones to mold and slide over one another, adjusting the circumference of the head to accommodate to the changing shape and character of the birth canal. The principal sutures in the infant's skull are the sagittal, coronal, and lambdoidal sutures, and the major soft areas at the juncture of these sutures are the anterior and posterior fontanels (see Fig. 8-7).

Following birth, growth of the skull bones occurs in a direction *perpendicular* to the line of the suture, and normal closure occurs in a regular and predictable order. Although there are wide variations in the age at which closure takes place in individual children, solid union of all sutures is not completed until very late childhood. Normally sutures and fontanels are ossified by the following ages:

8 weeks—posterior fontanel closed
6 months—fibrous union of suture lines and interlocking of serrated edges
18 months—anterior fontanel closed
12 years—sutures unable to be separated by ICP

*Route One, River Road, Box 210 A, Joliet, IL 60436; (815) 467-6548.

Closure of a suture before the expected time inhibits the perpendicular growth. Since normal increase in brain volume requires expansion, the skull is forced to grow in a direction *parallel* to the fused suture. This alteration in skull growth always produces a distortion of the head shape when the underlying brain growth is normal. The small head with closed and normal shape is the result of deficient brain growth; the suture closure is secondary to this brain growth failure. Failure of brain growth is not secondary to suture closure.

Various types of cranial deformities are encountered in early infancy. These include the enlarged head with frontal protrusion, or bossing, characteristic of hydrocephalus, the parietal bossing that is seen in chronic subdural hematoma, the small head, and a variety of skull deformities (Fig. 11-8). Some occur during prenatal development; in others, head circumference is usually within normal limits at birth and the deviation from normal development becomes apparent with advancing age.

MICROCEPHALY

Primary microcephaly reflects a small brain and may be caused by an autosomal-recessive disorder, a chromosomal abnormality, or application of a toxic stimulus during the period of induction and major cell migration in prenatal development. These stimuli may be irradiation (especially between 4 and 20 weeks of gestation), maternal infection (notably toxoplasmosis, rubella, or cytomegalovirus), or chemical agents. *Secondary microcephaly* can result from a variety of insults that occur during the third trimester of pregnancy, the perinatal period, or early infancy. Infection, trauma, metabolic disorders, and anoxia are all capable of causing decreased brain growth and early closure of cranial sutures.

In both types the neurologic manifestations range from decerebration, complete unresponsiveness, and/or autistic behavior to mild motor impairment, educable mental retardation, and/or mild hyperkinesis. There appears to be a decided relationship between microcephaly and mental retardation of varying degrees.

Nursing Considerations

There is no treatment. Nursing care is directed toward helping parents adjust to rearing a child with cognitive impairment (see Chapter 24).

CRANIOSYNOSTOSIS (CRANIOSTENOSIS)

In craniosynostosis, contrasted with microcephaly, suture closure is the primary defect and is not the result of impaired brain growth. As a consequence, brain growth continues, and the clinical picture depends on which sutures close, the duration of the closure process, and the success or failure of the other sutures to compensate by expansion. Usually the skull growth is inhibited in a direction at right angles to the closed sutures (see Fig. 11-8).

The most common form is premature closure of the sag-

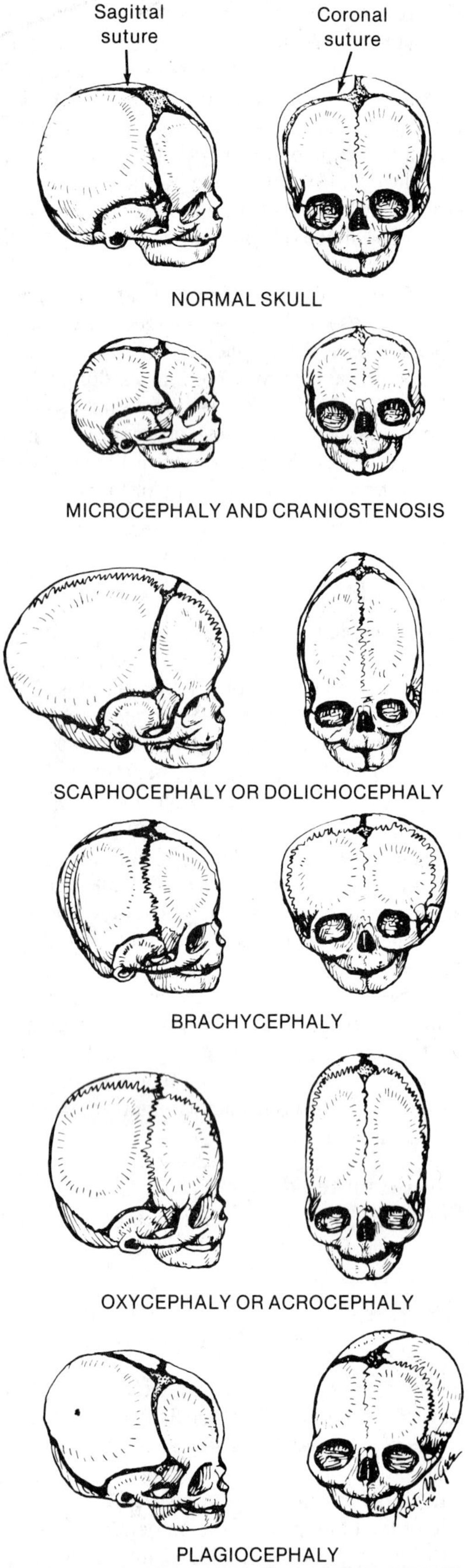

Fig. 11-8. Craniostenosis. Abnormal head configuration resulting from premature closing of cranial sutures.

ittal suture with resulting elongation of the skull in the anteroposterior direction. (A similar head shape is seen as a result of postnatal position maintenance in some premature infants.) Craniosynostosis causes some increase in ICP, which may or may not cause mental retardation but can result in progressive papilledema, optic atrophy, and eventual blindness.

Therapeutic Management

Treatment, if any, involves surgical excision of long bars of bone along or parallel to the fused suture. Various surgical procedures are employed in an effort to release the fused suture and direct growth. Lining the bony margins of the suture with silicone to delay closure is infrequently used. Surgery is performed to achieve the best possible cosmetic effect and, in severe cases, to relieve cerebral pressure symptoms and complications. The advised timing of suture release is before 6 months of age for best cosmetic results.

Nursing Considerations

Nursing care is primarily observation for signs of hemorrhage or infection. Following cranial surgery pressure bandages are applied and carefully maintained to reduce swelling. Providing emotional support to families is an important nursing function.

CRANIOFACIAL ABNORMALITIES

Craniofacial abnormalities are those deformities involving the skull and facial bones. They have a low incidence rate in the population, but their effects can be psychologically devastating to affected children and their families. Deformities caused by abnormal growth of cranial bone(s) are listed in Box 11-3.

The disorders are compatible with life; therefore unless they are corrected or modified, affected children go through their growing period under the burden of a grotesque, freaklike appearance often so severe that parents keep their chil-

Box 11-3 CRANIAL ABNORMALITIES CAUSED BY ABNORMAL BONE GROWTH

Hypertelorism—wide spacing between the eyes
Crouzon disease—craniofacial dysostosis (abnormal ossification of fetal cartilages) with shallow orbits and underdevelopment of the middle third of the face
Apert syndrome—craniostenosis resulting in a pointed head; may be extracranial abnormalities, such as syndactyly (webbing) of fingers and toes and cardiac defects
Treacher Collins syndrome—asymmetric facial deformity including absent cheekbones, underslung jaw, and small chin; there is also antimongoloid slant of the eyes and other minor defects
Pierre Robin syndrome—displacement of the chin as a result of micrognathia (mandibular hypoplasia) or retrognathia (normal-sized mandible positioned posteriorly); there is also glossoptosis with obstruction of the airway, and a cleft palate may be present

dren away from school, playmates, and sometimes even siblings (Koop, 1981).

Therapeutic Management

Surgical correction of defects involves peeling the patient's face away from the skull and remolding the understructures. Parts can be brought together, the skull reshaped, and pieces removed. The procedures are performed at various ages, depending on the anomaly, in centers specializing in this pediatric problem. The timing of surgery is determined on an individual basis to ensure normal growth and before school entry. Depending on the abnormality, other surgeries are performed, such as mandibular and digit correction. Following surgery, continued growth conforming to the inborn abnormality is unlikely.

Nursing Considerations

Nursing efforts are directed toward preparation for surgery (there may be several surgical procedures over a period of time), postoperative care similar to care of any child with cranial surgery, and support of the child and family. There is frequently adjustment to the unfamiliar body image, which may be as traumatic as the previous deformity. A helmet is worn to protect the operative site and bone grafts for varying lengths of time, from 6 months to 2 years. Follow-up care is very important.

PLAGIOCEPHALY

Plagiocephaly is a rhomboid-shaped deformity that occurs in at least 1 of 300 live births and is rarely caused by brain malformation or unilateral suture stenosis (Clarren, 1981). The rapidly growing infant head is easily molded by continued pressure against a surface, such as the uterine wall or a mattress. As a result the skull is progressively flattened. There is usually a history of the infant lying on the flattened aspect of the head with limited head movement when lying down.

Therapeutic Management

Surgical correction of cosmetically disfiguring plagiocephaly is performed according to the nature and extent of the deformity. A recent innovation involves application of a helmet constructed of polypropylene shaped normally but large enough to fit the largest diameter of the head. Treatment is begun at 4 to 10 months of age, and the helmet is worn until the head conforms to the shape of the helmet.

Nursing Considerations

An important nursing function is helping to identify children with significant deformity and referring them for evaluation. Nursing care of the surgical patient is the same as that for other children with similar surgery. Care of the child with helmet therapy involves teaching parents the importance of making certain that the child wears the device as prescribed. Mild unpleasant scalp odors that develop are controlled by daily washing of both scalp and helmet (Clarren, 1981).

■ SKELETAL DEFECTS

The types and variations of deformity in developmental skeletal defects are numerous and display an equally diverse spectrum of physical disability. Some skeletal deformities constitute one or more of the manifestations associated with a syndrome, for example, the short extremities of the various forms of dwarfism, the long, thin extremities and sternal deformities of arachnodactyly (Marfan syndrome), and somatic defects in chromosomal aberrations. Many are isolated defects with hereditary (clawhand, polydactyly), environmental (thalidomide phocomelia or amelia), or multifactorial (congenital hip dysplasia) etiology. This discussion is limited to those defects in development that are most common, that are amenable to therapy, and that involve nurses to a considerable extent. Less common defects and disorders are listed in Table 11-3.

CONGENITAL HIP DYSPLASIA

The broad term *congenital hip dysplasia* describes imperfect development of the hip that can affect the femoral head, the acetabulum, or both. More commonly known as congenital hip dislocation (CHD) or congenital dislocated hip (CDH), the disorder is apparent at birth and displays various degrees of deformity. The condition is reversible with early treatment but can rapidly progress to dislocation as the child begins to walk. The cause of hip dysplasia is unknown, but it is one of the most common congenital defects, with an incidence of about 1:500 to 1:1000 births.

The disorder occurs more frequently in females than in males (7:1) and occurs 25 to 30 times more often in first-degree relatives than in the general population. The concordance in monozygotic twins is 40% but only 3% in dizygotic twins, which suggests that genetic factors play a role in the etiology. One fourth of cases involve both hips, and when only one hip is involved, the left hip is affected three times more often than the right. CDH is frequently associated with other conditions, such as SB.

Pathophysiology

Intrauterine, racial, and cultural factors are associated with congenital hip disorders. There appears to be a striking relationship between the development of dislocation and methods of handling infants. Among the cultures with the highest incidence of dislocation (Navajo Indians and Canadian Eskimos), newly born infants are tightly wrapped in blankets or other swaddling material or are strapped to cradle boards. In cultures where mothers carry infants on their backs or hips in the widely abducted straddle position, such as in the Far East and Africa, the disorder is virtually unknown.

Prenatal factors that are considered to influence development of hip abnormalities are maternal hormone secretion and mechanical factors of intrauterine posture. Toward the end of pregnancy there is increased maternal pelvic laxity mediated by maternal hormone secretion (principally estrogen), which affects the fetal joints as well. All joints are more lax in the newborn period, and the greater incidence

Table 11-3 Congenital defects involving the skeleton

DISORDER	DESCRIPTION AND ANATOMIC VARIATION	THERAPY
Achondroplasia	Inherited (autosomal dominant) Defect in ossification at the epiphyseal plate, resulting in very short limbs, large head, and lordosis	None
Osteogenesis imperfecta	Inherited (autosomal dominant, autosomal recessive) Characterized by brittle, fragile, and easily fractured bones Intrauterine fractures may produce congenital deformities	Reduction of fractures Careful handling of extremities
Pes planus (flatfoot)	Normal finding in infancy May be result of muscular weakness in older child	Rarely indicated Wedge on inner side of heel and sole for persistent or severe cases
Pes valgus	Eversion of entire foot but sole rests on ground	Exercises
Pes varus	Inversion of entire foot but sole rests on ground	Exercises
Metatarsus valgus	Eversion of forefoot while heel remains straight Also called toeing out or duck walk	Passive exercises
Talipes deformities	See Box 11-5	
Supernumerary digits (polydactyly)	Excessive number of fingers, toes, or both; usually inherited (autosomal dominant)	No treatment, or amputation of extra digits to improve function or for cosmetic reasons
Genu varum (bowleg)	May be congenital, result of rickets, or caused by osteochondrosis of proximal tibial epiphysis	Corrective splinting Osteotomy in severe or neglected cases
Genu recurvatum (back knee)	Congenital, result of prenatal developmental defect or abnormal intrauterine position Developmental, result of postnatal trauma or infection	Repeated corrective casting Exercises
Klippel-Feil syndrome	Absence of one or more cervical vertebrae and two or more fused together Neck short and limited in motion Sometimes kyphosis and scoliosis	Rarely indicated Scapula brought down and fixed if marked deformity or loss of function Bracing of spinal deformities
Arachnodactyly (Marfan syndrome)	Inherited (autosomal dominant) Abnormal length of fingers, toes, and extremities; hypermobility of joints; defects of spine and chest (pigeon breast); other associated abnormalities	Supportive measures
Congenital spine deformities	Kyphosis, scoliosis, lordosis, or a combination of these	Prevention of progression of defect with growth Casting and/or bracing Operative stabilization of affected vertebrae
Arthrogryposis multiplex congenita	Incomplete fibrous ankylosis of many or all joints (except spine and jaw) associated with hypoplasia of attached muscles Contracture deformities—some extension, others flexion	Bracing, splinting, correcting surgery, and rehabilitation efforts

of hip dislocation in females may be explained by their greater reactivity to the maternal hormones.

Reliable evidence indicates an association between a higher incidence of congenital hip deformities with breech presentations and cesarean section (often necessitated by abnormal intrauterine position). The position of the legs in frank breech position—that is, with the hips acutely flexed and knees extended—is an important factor in the etiology of hip dislocation. The larger number of firstborn children may be related to this factor, since the breech position in first deliveries is nearly always a frank breech. Other prenatal factors that contribute to hip dysplasia include twinning and large infant size.

Three degrees of CDH are illustrated in Fig. 11-9 and outlined in Box 11-4. Also, mounting evidence lends support to the suggestion that there are two types of CDH: the common type due to laxity of the supporting capsule and another type as a result of an abnormality of the acetabulum. The excessive laxity of the joint may prevent detection in early infancy. The femoral head remains in contact with the acetabulum until additional stress (such as standing) moves it away (Bialik and others, 1986).

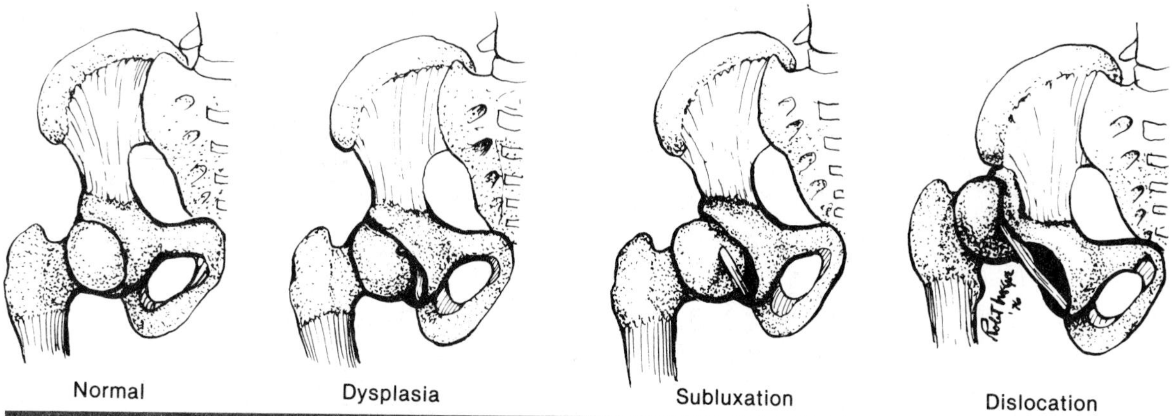

Fig. 11-9. Configuration and relationship of structures in congenital hip deformities.

Box 11-4 DEGREES OF CONGENITAL HIP DYSPLASIA

Acetabular dysplasia (or preluxation)—the mildest form, in which there is neither subluxation nor dislocation. The dysplasia reflects an apparent delay in acetabular development evidenced by osseous hypoplasia of the acetabular roof, which is oblique and shallow, although the cartilaginous roof is comparatively intact. The femoral head remains in the acetabulum.

Subluxation—accounts for the largest percentage of congenital hip dysplasias. Subluxation implies incomplete dislocation or dislocatable hip and is sometimes regarded as an intermediate state in the development from primary dysplasia to complete dislocation. The femoral head remains in contact with the acetabulum, but a stretched capsule and ligamentum teres cause the head of the femur to be partially displaced. Pressure on the cartilaginous roof inhibits ossification and produces a flattening of the socket.

Dislocation—the femoral head loses contact with the acetabulum and is displaced posteriorly and superiorly over the fibrocartilaginous rim. The ligamentum teres is elongated and taut.

Clinical Manifestations

The diagnosis of CDH should be made in the newborn period if possible, since treatment initiated before 2 months of age achieves the highest rate of success. In the newborn period dysplasia usually appears as hip joint laxity rather than as outright dislocation. Subluxation and the tendency to dislocate can be demonstrated by the Ortolani or Barlow tests. With the infant relaxed in the supine position and the legs facing the examiner, the hips are flexed at right angles and the knees are flexed. The examiner places the middle finger of each hand over the greater trochanter and the thumbs on the inner side of the thigh at a point opposite the lesser trochanter. The knees are carried to midabduction, and each hip joint in turn is submitted first to forward pressure exerted behind the trochanter and second to backward pressure exerted from the thumbs in front as the opposite joint is held steady. If the femoral head can be felt to slip forward into the acetabulum on pressure from behind, it has been dislocated *(Ortolani test)* (Fig. 11-10, *D*). Sometimes an audible click can be heard on exit or entry of the femur out of or into the acetabulum. If, on pressure from the front, the femoral head is felt to slip out over the posterior lip of the acetabulum and immediately slips back in place when pressure is released, the hip is said to be dislocatable or "unstable" *(Barlow test)*.

The Ortolani and Barlow tests are most reliable from birth to 2 months of age and must be performed by experienced operators to prevent fracture or other damage to the hip. For example, when these tests are performed too vigorously in the first 2 days of life, when the hip subluxates freely, persistent dislocation may occur (Cheetham and others, 1983). Adduction contractures develop at about 6 to 10 weeks, and the Ortolani sign disappears. After this time the most sensitive test is limited abduction (Fig. 11-10, *B*). Other signs are shortening of the limb on the affected side *(Galleazzi sign, Allis sign)* (Fig. 11-10, *C*), asymmetric thigh and gluteal folds (Fig. 11-10, *A*), and broadening of the perineum (in bilateral dislocation). Weight bearing may precipitate a transition from subluxation to dislocation in unrecognized cases. Often the disorder is not apparent at birth.

In the older infant and child the affected leg will be shorter than the other with telescoping or piston mobility, that is, the head of the femur can be felt to move up and down in the buttock when the extended thigh is pushed first toward the child's head and then pulled distally. Instability of the hip on weight bearing delays walking and produces a characteristic limp. When the child stands first on one foot and then on the other (holding onto a chair, rail, or someone's hands), bearing weight on the affected hip, the pelvis tilts downward on the normal side instead of upward as it would with normal stability *(Trendelenburg sign)* (Fig. 11-10, *E*). In both unilateral and bilateral dislocations the greater trochanter is prominent and appears above a line from the anterosuperior iliac spine to the tuberosity of the ischium. The child with bilateral dislocations has marked lordosis and a peculiar waddling gait.

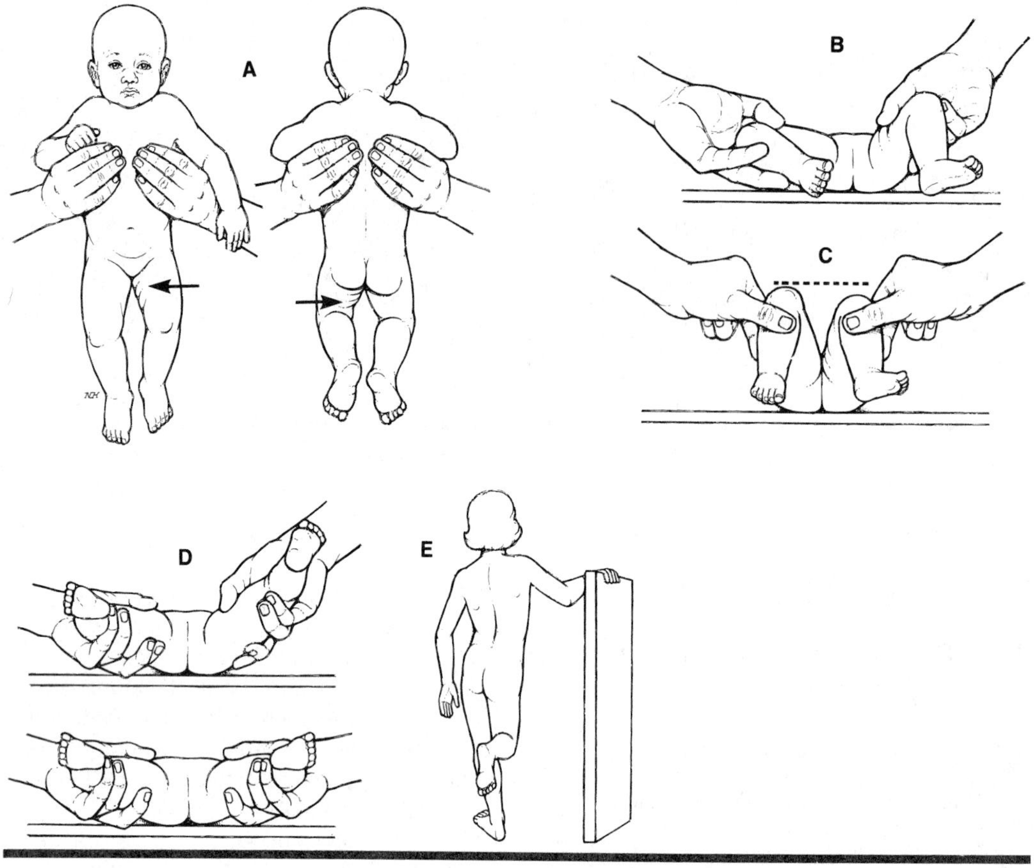

Fig. 11-10. Signs of congenital dislocation of the hip. **A,** Asymmetry of gluteal and thigh folds. **B,** Limited hip abduction, as seen in flexion. **C,** Apparent shortening of the femur, as indicated by the level of the knees in flexion. **D,** Ortolani click (if infant is under 4 weeks of age). **E,** Positive Trendelenburg sign or gait (if child is weight bearing).

Diagnostic Evaluation

The primary diagnostic tools in the newborn period are the assessment techniques just described. Although the disorder is usually identified in early infancy, there is also a category that cannot be detected at birth. Therefore ruling out CDH at birth does not provide security, and examination of the hip is carried out at each well-child visit in the event that a late-onset dislocation becomes evident. In older infants and children radiographic examination is useful in confirming the diagnosis. An upward slope in the roof of the acetabulum (the acetabular angle) greater than 40 degrees with upward and outward displacement of the femoral head is a frequent finding in older children. Radiographic examination in early infancy is not reliable, because ossification of the femoral head does not normally take place until the third to sixth month of life. However, the cartilaginous head can be visualized directly with real-time high-resolution ultrasonography.

Therapeutic Management

Treatment is begun as soon as the condition is recognized, since early intervention is more favorable to the restoration of normal bony architecture and function. The longer treatment is delayed, the more severe the deformity, the more difficult the treatment, and the less favorable the prognosis. The treatment varies with the age of the child and the extent of the dysplasia.

Newborn to six months. The hip joint is maintained by dynamic splinting in a safe position with the proximal femur centered in the acetabulum in an attitude of flexion. A variety of abduction devices are available for maintaining the femur in the acetabulum. Of these the Pavlik harness is the most widely used device, and with time, motion, and gravity the hip works into a more abducted, reduced position (Fig. 11-11). The harness is worn continuously until the hip is clinically and radiographically stable, usually about 3 to 6 months. It is highly effective when the device is well constructed, follow-up care is adequate, and the parents follow instructions in its use.

When adduction contracture is present, other devices (such as skin traction) are employed to slowly and gently stretch the hip to full abduction, after which wide abduction is maintained until stability is attained. When there is difficulty in maintaining stable reduction, a hip spica cast is applied and changed periodically to accommodate the child's growth. After 3 to 6 months, sufficient stability is acquired

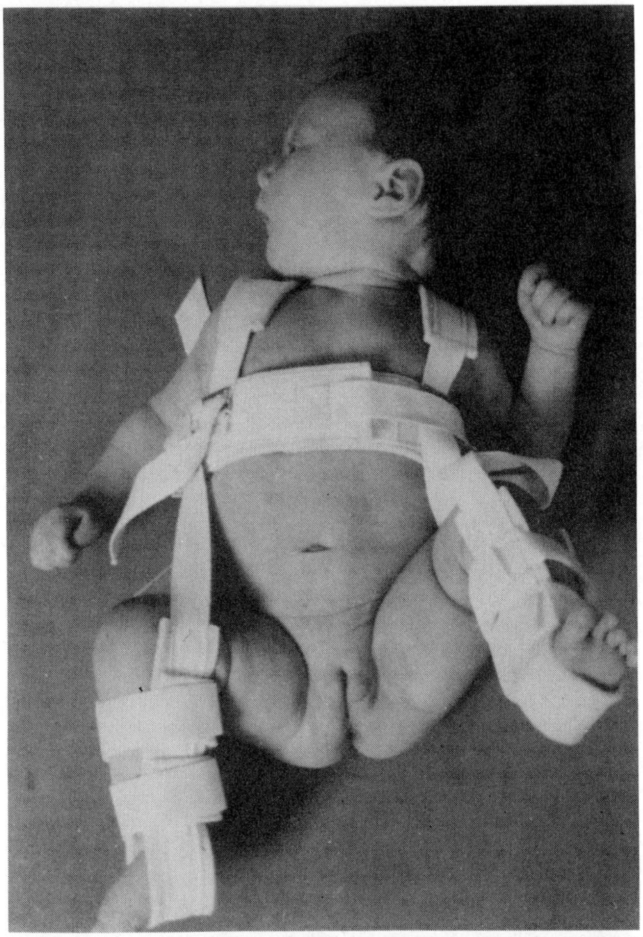

Fig. 11-11. Child in Pavlik harness.

to allow transfer to a removable protective abduction brace. The duration of treatment depends on development of the acetabulum but is usually accomplished within the first year.

Six to eighteen months. In this age-group the dislocation is not recognized until the child begins to stand and walk, when attendant shortening of the limb and contractures of hip adductor and flexor muscles become apparent. Gradual reduction by traction is followed by plaster cast immobilization, which is maintained until radiographic examination confirms a stable joint. Often soft tissue may obstruct and complicate reduction and subsequent joint development. In this case open reduction is performed to remove the obstruction, followed by postoperative spica cast immobilization and, later, replacement with an abduction splint.

Older child. Correction of the hip deformity in the older child is inherently more difficult than in the preceding age-groups because secondary adaptive changes and other etiologic factors (such as juvenile rheumatoid arthritis or nonambulatory cerebral palsy) complicate the condition. Operative reduction, which may involve preoperative traction, tenotomy of contracted muscles, and any one of several innominate osteotomy procedures designed to construct an acetabular roof, is usually required. After cast removal and before weight bearing is permitted, range of motion exercises help restore movement. Next, rehabilitative measures are instituted. Successful reduction and reconstruction become increasingly difficult after the age of 4 years and are usually impossible or inadvisable after age 6 because of severe shortening and contracture of muscles and deformity of the femoral and acetabular structures.

Nursing Considerations

Nurses are in a unique position to detect CDH in the newborn. During the infant assessment process and routine nurturing activities the hips and extremities are inspected for any deviations from normal. Usually only nurses specially trained in the technique are permitted to perform Ortolani and Barlow tests, but any nurse can be alert to other signs of CDH. These observations are reported to the attending practitioner, and the ambulatory child who displays a limp or an unusual gait should be referred for evaluation. This may indicate an orthopedic or neurologic problem. Nonambulatory children with cerebral palsy should also be assessed for evidence of dislocation.

✦ **NURSING ALERT** Observations during routine care, such as diapering, provide an excellent opportunity to observe the infant for limited movement and a wide perineum, which is an indication to assess for leg shortening, gluteal folds, and limited abduction.

Care of the child in a reduction device. The major nursing problems in the care of an infant or child in a cast or other device are related to maintenance of the device and adapting nurturing activities to meet the needs of the infant or child. Generally treatment and follow-up care of these children are carried out in a clinic, physician's office, or outpatient unit. Hospitalization may be necessary for cast application or brace fitting but seldom exceeds 24 to 48 hours. Longer hospitalization is required for open reduction or if the child is hospitalized for a concurrent illness.

Family support and home care. The primary nursing goal is teaching parents to apply and maintain the reduction device. The Pavlik harness allows for easy handling of the infant and usually produces less apprehension in the parent than heavy braces and casts. It is important that parents understand the correct use of the appliance, which may or may not allow for its removal during bathing. When the infant has a harness that is not removed, a sponge bath is recommended and the skin beneath the harness is assessed daily for irritation. Powders and lotions are not used because they tend to cake or "ball" underneath straps or clothing.

The parents are permitted to pad shoulder straps at pressure points if desired, but unbuckling or removal is determined individually based on the family's level of understanding and the degree of deformity in the hip. In general, parents are not encouraged to adjust the harness without supervision. The child should be examined by the practitioner before any adjustment is attempted to make certain the hips are in correct placement before the harness is resecured.

Casts and braces offer more challenging nursing problems, since they cannot be removed for routine care, although sometimes the physician allows a brace to be removed for bathing. Care of an infant or small child with a cast requires nursing innovation to reduce irritation and to maintain cleanliness of both the child and the cast, particularly in the diaper area. Cast care and observation are discussed in Chapter 39 and therefore are not elaborated on here. However, inasmuch as CDH is almost the exclusive reason for application of casts in early infancy, some of the problems specific to that age-group are mentioned.

Parents are taught the proper care of the cast (or brace) and are helped to devise means for maintaining cleanliness. A disposable diaper (newborn size) is tucked beneath the entire perineal opening of the cast. A larger (toddler size) diaper can be applied and fastened over the small diaper and cast (Holland, 1983).

For tightly fitting casts transparent sheeting can be cut into strips as for petalling (see Chapter 39) and one edge applied to the cast edge and the other directly to the perineum; this forms a continuous waterproof bridge between the perineum and the cast to prevent leakage. An additional advantage to the use of this dressing material is that it keeps both the skin and the cast dry while allowing for observation of the skin beneath the dressing.

Older infants and small children may stuff bits of food, small toys, or other items under the cast; parents should be alerted to this possibility so that suitable preventive measures can be instigated.

Feeding the infant in a hip spica cast or brace offers problems of positioning. Very young infants can be fed in the supine position with the head elevated, and, with the infant's hips and legs supported on a pillow at the side, the parent can cuddle the infant during feeding. A somewhat similar position can be used for breast-feeding, that is, with the infant supported on pillows or held in a "football" hold facing the mother with the legs behind her. An alternate position is to hold the infant upright on the mother's lap with the legs of the infant astride the mother's leg.

Infants who are able to sit up can be fed in a feeding table or modified high chair. Parents may be able to fashion a tilt board with padded seat or an adjustable chair. The table or chair provides an excellent place for the child to play in an upright position. The child's car seat is also a vital consideration. Modifications can be made on several standard, government-approved car seats (Shesser, 1985), and instructions can be obtained for modification of one model, which has been tested (Feller and others, 1986).* A specially designed car restraint for a young child in a spica cast is shown in Fig. 11-12.

It is important for nurses, parents, and other caregivers to understand that these children need to be involved in all the activities of any child in the same age-group. Toys are chosen that can be used in a prone position on the floor or in the seats devised for feeding and other activities. Confinement in a cast or appliance should not exclude children from family (or unit) activities. They can be held astride a lap for comfort and transported to areas of activity. The child may be allowed to walk in a cast or brace. An adapted wheelchair, stroller, or scooter can offer mobility to the older infant or child. (See Chapter 39 for further discussion of care of a child in a spica cast. Also, inexpensive booklets can be obtained from several sources.† See Nursing Care Plan: The Child with Congenital Hip Dysplasia [Congenital Dislocated Hip] and Home Care Instructions: Caring for the Child in a Cast.‡)

*Automobile Safety for Children Program, James Whitcomb Riley Hospital for Children, Indiana School of Medicine, 702 Barnhill Drive, P-121, Indianapolis, IN 46223; (317) 274-2977; Indiana, 1-800-KID-N-CAR.

†Recommended: *Spina Bifida,* available from Medic Publishing Co., P.O. Box 89, Redmond, WA 98073-0089; (206) 881-2883.

‡In Wong, D.L., and Whaley, L.F.: Clinical manual of pediatric nursing, ed. 3, St. Louis, 1990, Mosby–Year Book, Inc.

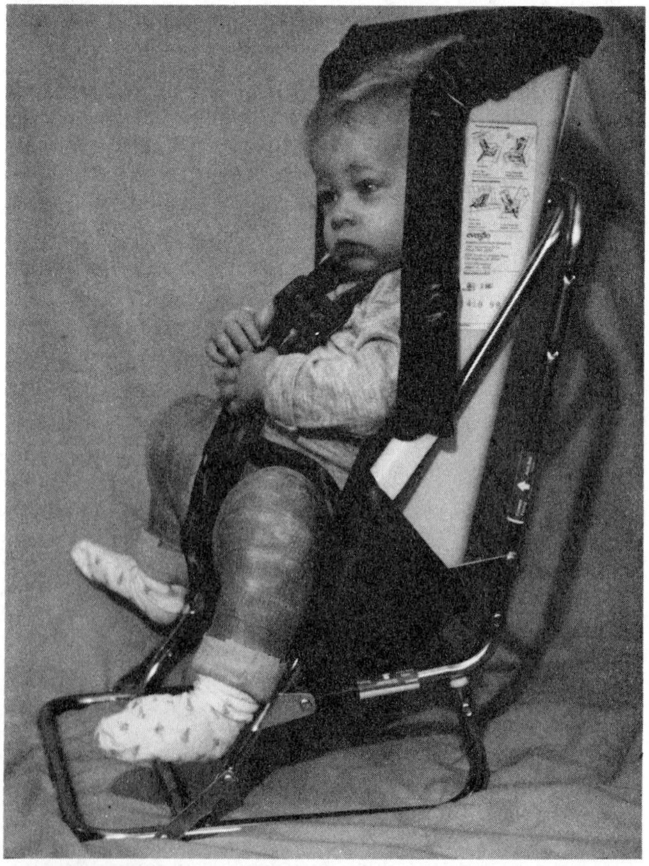

Fig. 11-12. Child in specially designed car restraint (Spelcast).

NURSING TIP: REDUCING WETNESS

For heavy wetters or for night use, a sanitary napkin can be placed inside the small diaper for added absorbency. Both diapers are changed at each wetting. Another alternative is the newer diapers with absorbent gel material that holds moisture.

Box 11-5 VARIATIONS IN ANKLE AND FOOT DEFORMITIES

Talipes varus—an inversion or a bending inward
Talipes valgus—an eversion or bending outward
Talipes equinus—plantar flexion in which the toes are lower than the heel
Talipes calcaneus—dorsiflexion, in which the toes are higher than the heel

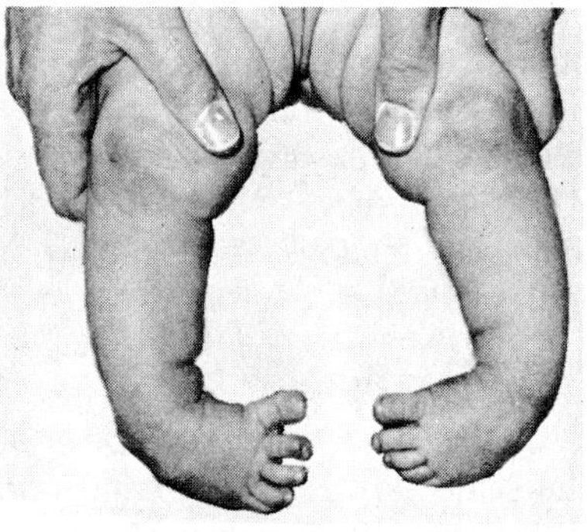

Fig. 11-13. Bilateral congenital talipes equinovarus (congenital clubfoot) in 2-month-old infant.
From Brashear, H.R., Jr., and Raney, R.B.: Handbook of orthopaedic surgery, ed. 10, St. Louis, 1986, Mosby–Year Book, Inc.

CONGENITAL CLUBFOOT

Clubfoot is a general term used to describe a common deformity in which the foot is twisted out of its normal shape or position. Any foot deformity involving the ankle is called *talipes,* derived from *talus,* meaning ankle, and *pes,* meaning foot. Deformities of the foot and ankle are conveniently described according to the position of the ankle and foot. The more common talipes deformities are listed in Box 11-5.

Most clubfeet are a combination of these positions, and the most frequently occurring type of clubfoot (approximately 95%) is the composite deformity *talipes equinovarus (TEV),* in which the foot is pointed downward and inward in varying degrees of severity (Fig. 11-13). Unilateral clubfoot is somewhat more common than bilateral clubfoot and may occur as an isolated defect or in association with other disorders or syndromes such as chromosomal aberrations, arthrogryposis (a generalized immobility of the joints), or SB.

The frequency of clubfoot in the general population is 1:700 to 1:1000 live births, with boys affected twice as often as girls. There is a 35% concordance in monozygotic twins as opposed to a 3% concordance in dizygotic twins, which indicates a hereditary component.

Pathophysiology

The precise cause of clubfoot is unknown. Some authorities attribute the defect to abnormal positioning and restricted movement in utero, although the evidence is not conclusive. Other experts implicate arrested or anomalous embryonic development, since the foot normally goes through flexion and eversion during early development and gradually assumes a normal attitude by the seventh month. Arrested development during this early stage tends to result in a rigid deformity, whereas mechanical pressures from intrauterine position are more likely to be operating in the more flexible deformities. Embryologists are divided in acceptance of the embryonic arrest theory.

Diagnostic Evaluation

The deformity is readily apparent and easily detected at birth. However, it must be differentiated from some positional deformities that can be passively corrected or overcorrected. The true clubfoot is fixed, whereas paralytic changes in the lower extremities of children with neuromuscular involvement often produce equinovarus deformity.

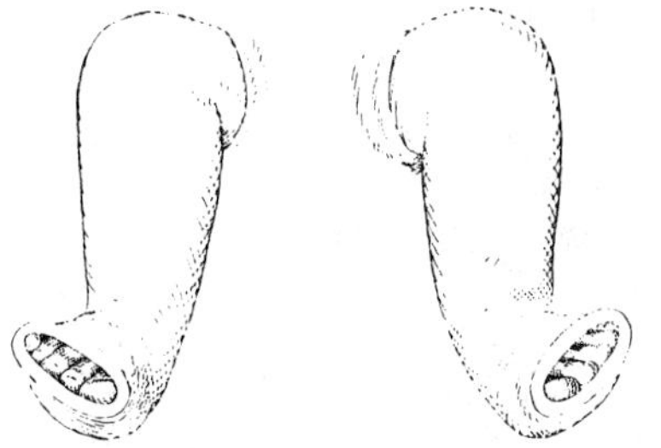

Fig. 11-14. Feet casted for correction of bilateral congenital talipes equinovarus.
From Brashear, H.R., Jr., and Raney, R.B.: Handbook of orthopaedic surgery, ed. 10, St. Louis, 1986, Mosby–Year Book, Inc.

Therapeutic Management

The rapid growth during infancy is a potent remodeling force. When treatment is indicated, this rapid growth will improve the result, facilitate the quality of correction, and decrease the time required for treatment (Bunch, 1979). Treatment is begun as soon as the deformity is recognized and involves three stages: (1) correction of the deformity, (2) maintenance of the correction until normal muscle balance is regained, and (3) follow-up observation to avert possible recurrence of the deformity. Some feet respond to treatment readily, some respond only to prolonged, vigorous, and sustained efforts, and the improvement in others remains disappointing even with maximum effort on the part of all concerned.

Correction of TEV is most reliably accomplished by manipulation and the application of a series of casts begun immediately or shortly after birth and continued until marked overcorrection is reached (Fig. 11-14). Successive casts allow for gradual stretching of tight structures on the medial side and gradual contraction of lax structures on the lateral side of the foot. Manipulation and casting are repeated frequently (every few days for 1 to 2 weeks, then at 1- to 2-

week intervals) in order to accommodate the rapid growth of early infancy. Because of strong, thickened ligaments, cartilaginous anlages of the bone may become distorted. If manipulation is ineffective, surgical correction is performed to correct bony deformity, release tight ligaments, or lengthen or transplant tendons. The extremity or extremities are casted until the desired result is achieved.

Nursing Considerations

Nursing care of the child with nonsurgical correction of clubfoot is the same as it is for any child who has a cast (see Chapter 39). The child will spend a considerable time in a corrective device; therefore, nursing care plans include both long-term and short-term goals. Conscientious observation of skin and circulation is particularly important in young infants because of their normally rapid growth rate. Since treatment and follow-up care are handled in the orthopedist's office, clinic, or outpatient department, parent education and support are important in nursing care of these children.

Parents need to understand the overall treatment program, the importance of regular cast changes, and the role they play in the long-term effectiveness of the therapy. Reinforcing and clarifying the orthopedist's explanations and instructions, teaching parents about care of the cast or appliance, including vigilant observation for potential problems, and encouraging parents to facilitate normal development within the limitations imposed by the deformity or therapy are all part of nursing responsibilities. A helpful and inexpensive booklet is available to help families understand the disorder.* (See Nursing Care Plan: The Child with Congenital Clubfoot.†)

METATARSUS ADDUCTUS (VARUS)

Metatarsus adductus, or metatarsus varus, is probably the most common congenital foot deformity. In most instances it is the result of abnormal intrauterine positioning and is usually detected at birth. The deformity is characterized by medial adduction of the toes and forefoot, frequently associated with inversion, and convexity of the lateral border of the foot. Unlike TEV, with which it is often confused, the angulation occurs at the tarsometatarsal joint while the heel and ankle remain in a neutral position. This deformity often causes a pigeon-toed gait in the child.

Management depends on the rigidity of the deformity. Correction can usually be accomplished by gentle manipulation and passive stretching of the foot, which the parent is taught to perform. Repeated and consistent stretching is continued for the first 6 weeks, after which the treatment is based on the flexibility of the foot. Those feet that do not respond to the manipulation require orthopedic intervention. If the child is able to actively overcorrect the deformity voluntarily on stimulation, continued stretching is generally sufficient. If the foot cannot be actively or passively overcorrected, the feet are stretched and manipulated and held with casts.

Nursing Considerations

The nursing role primarily involves identifying the defect, so that early therapy and instruction of the parents can be instigated. The nurse teaches the parents how to hold the heel firmly and to stretch only the forefoot; otherwise, undue force on the heel may produce a valgus deformity. If casting is needed, the nurse instructs the parents in cast care and observation (see Chapter 39).

SKELETAL LIMB DEFICIENCY

Congenital limb deficiencies, or reduction malformations, are manifest by a variety of degree of loss of functional capacity. They are characterized by underdevelopment of skeletal elements of the extremities. The range of malformation can extend from minor defects of the digits to serious abnormalities such as *amelia,* absence of an entire extremity, or *meromelia,* partial absence of an extremity, which includes *phocomelia* (seal limbs), an intercalary deficiency of long bones with relatively good development of hands and feet attached at or near the shoulder or the hips.

In rare instances prenatal destruction of limbs has been reported, but most reduction deformities are primary defects of development (agenesis, aplasia). Therefore, congenital amputations, in the literal sense, are not amputations, since nonexistent limbs cannot be amputated.

Pathophysiology

Limb deficiencies can be attributed to both heredity and environment. The upper limb appears first as a limb bud in the fourth week of gestation, and its entire skeleton can be recognized in its early stages by the fifth week of gestation. During the sixth week of gestation cartilage forms the structural model of the bones, and ossification from humerus to phalanges begins between the sixth and seventh weeks of gestation. The development of the upper limbs precedes that of the lower limbs slightly, and the cartilaginous structure appears in a proximodistal sequence. By 8 weeks of gestation the digits are well formed and their number determined; by 12 weeks of gestation primary centers of ossification can be detected in nearly all bones of the extremities.

Malformations can originate at any stage of limb development. Formation of limbs may be suppressed at the time of limb bud formation, or there may be interference in later stages of differentiation and growth. Heredity appears to play a prominent role, and prenatal environmental insults have been implicated in a number of cases. The well-publicized thalidomide tragedy is a dramatic illustration of the effects of environmental interference with limb development. Children damaged by maternal ingestion of the drug displayed a variety of serious limb anomalies that demonstrated a clear relationship between the time of exposure and the presence and type of limb deformity.

**Club Foot,* available from Medic Publishing Co., P.O. Box 89, Redmond, WA 98073-0089; (206) 881-2883.

†In Wong, D.L., and Whaley, L.F.: Clinical manual of pediatric nursing, ed. 3, St. Louis, 1990, Mosby–Year Book, Inc.

Therapeutic Management

It is generally agreed that children with congenital limb deficiencies should be fitted with prosthetic devices whenever possible and that such a functional replacement should be applied at the earliest possible stage of development in an attempt to match the motor readiness of the infant. This favors natural progression of prosthetic use. For example, an infant with an upper extremity deficiency is fitted with a simple passive device, such as a mitten prosthesis, between 3 and 6 months of age when limb exploration is active, sitting is beginning with the extremities needed for support, and bilateral hand activities are to be encouraged. Lower limb prostheses are applied when the infant is ready to pull to a standing position. In preparation for prosthetic devices surgical modification is often necessary to ensure the most favorable use of the device, since severe deformity can interfere with its effective use. Phocomelic digits are preserved for controlling switches of externally powered appliances in upper extremities. Digits (in both upper and lower extremities) provide the child with surfaces for tactile exploration and stimulation. Prostheses are replaced to accommodate growth and increasing capabilities of the child.

Nursing Considerations

Prosthetic application training and habilitation are most successfully carried out in a center that specializes in meeting the special needs of these children, especially very young children and those with multiple amputations. It involves a team of health professionals and the parents, who must encourage the child in making age-commensurate adjustments to the environment. Although these children need assistance, excessive overprotection may produce overdependency with later maladjustment to school and other situations.

■ DISORDERS OF THE GASTROINTESTINAL TRACT*

Congenital defects of the gastrointestinal (GI) tract can involve any portion from the mouth to the anus. Most are apparent at birth or shortly after and are anomalies in which normal growth ceased at a crucial stage of embryonic development, leaving the structure in an embryonic form or only partially completed. The result may be atresia, malposition, nonclosure, or any number of variations.

Atresia is absence or closure of a normal body orifice. Closure at any point along the length of the GI tract creates an obstruction to the normal progress of nutrients and secretions. Most common anomalies are atresias of the esophagus, intestine, and anus, requiring surgical intervention.

Other defects of development include *annular pancreas,* in which the head of the pancreas surrounds and constricts the second segment of duodenum, and *malrotation of the colon,* in which associated structures remain in abnormal positions. For example, the cecum remains in the upper right quadrant and the posterior fixation of the mesentery is inadequate and allows twisting of the small intestine, or *volvulus,* to create an obstruction.

Obstruction can also be caused by *peritoneal bands* or *folds* that cross the duodenum as they attach the abnormally placed cecum to the right peritoneum. Thus the duodenum is partially obstructed by the external pressure of the bands. In *meconium ileus* the intestine becomes obstructed by thick, inspissated, impacted meconium—the earliest manifestation of cystic fibrosis. *Congenital megacolon (Hirschsprung disease)* is caused by the absence or deficiency of innervation to the musculature of the rectum and distal colon, which inhibits propulsive peristalsis and creates a functional obstruction.

The diagnosis and management of most intestinal atresias and obstructions are similar to the diagnosis and management of intestinal obstruction from other factors, most of which are discussed in Chapter 33. The congenital defects considered in this chapter include abnormalities of the lip and palate, esophagus, anus, and biliary tree. Biliary atresia is also considered here because the liver is part of the digestive system, although the condition does not interfere with the passage of food. Some malformations of the gastrointestinal tract are considered here, since they are identified at birth and are cause for considerable parental concern.

CLEFT LIP AND/OR PALATE

Clefts of the lip and palate are facial malformations that are common to all human populations and constitute a severe handicap to the affected individual. The defects are classified into two major groups. The first includes those clefts that involve the lip and anterior maxilla regardless of whether the defect involves the remaining portions of the hard and soft palate (sometimes called harelip). The second group consists of those clefts that involve only the hard and soft palate. Although there are differences in the severity and extent of deformities within each category, the terms and the abbreviations associated with these groups are defined in Box 11-6. The term *complete cleft* indicates the maximum degree of clefting.

Etiology

Many factors appear to be involved in the etiology of CL/P, and evidence indicates that CL(P), is developmentally and

Box 11-6 CLEFT LIP AND/OR PALATE

CL—clefts that involve the lip
CLP—clefts that involve the lip and palate
CL(P)—clefts that involve the lip with or without cleft palate
CP—clefts that involve the hard and soft palate only
CL/P—all types of clefts that involve the lip and/or palate

*Cindy Hylton Rushton, R.N.C, M.S.N., assisted in the revision of this section.

genetically different from CP. Defective development of the embryonic *primary* palate may result in clefts of the lip and anterior maxilla; clefts of the hard and soft palate are caused by defective development of the embryonic *secondary* palate and often appear in persons with CL. There are no less than 50 recognized syndromes that include CL(P) as a feature: some are caused by mutant genes, others result from chromosomal abnormalities, and teratogens have been implicated in a very small number.

The great majority of cases appear to be consistent with the concept of multifactorial inheritance as evidenced by an increased incidence in relatives and a higher concordance in monozygotic (MZ) than in dizygotic twins. However, there is apparently no relationship between the incidence of CL(P) and the incidence of CP among relatives; that is, relatives of persons with CP have an increased incidence of CP but not CL(P) and vice versa. A low concordance rate in MZ twins with CP suggests that the environmental influence in development of CP is stronger than in CL(P) (Nora and Fraser, 1989).

Isolated CP is rarer than CL(P) and affects more females than males. The incidence of some form of clefting is 1:700 births (American Cleft Palate Education Foundation, 1985) and shows a wide variation among races. The defect appears more often in certain tribes of American Indians and Orientals than in whites and less frequently in American blacks. There is less racial difference in the specific defects. More males than females have CL(P), particularly the more severe defects, but CP occurs more often in females. CLP is the most common of the facial malformations (40%) (March of Dimes–Birth Defects Foundation, undated).

Pathophysiology

Development of the primary and secondary palates takes place at different times and involves different developmental processes. Cleft lip with or without cleft palate results from failure of the maxillary processes to fuse with the nasal elevations on the frontal prominence, which normally occurs during the sixth week of gestation (Fig. 11-15, *A*). Merging of the upper lip at the midline is completed between the seventh and eighth weeks of gestation. There is evidence, however, that in some cases separation may be the result of rupture subsequent to fusion.

Fusion of the secondary palate (hard and soft palate) takes place later in development, between the seventh and twelfth weeks of gestation (Fig. 11-15, *B* to *D*). At the time the primary palate is completed, the two lateral palatine processes are situated in a vertical position at the side of the tongue. In the process of migrating to a horizontal position they are, for a short time, separated by the tongue. With development of the neck and jaws, the tongue moves downward, allowing the palatine processes to fuse with each other and with the primary palate to form the roof of the mouth. If there is delay in this movement or if the tongue fails to descend soon enough, the remainder of development proceeds but the palate never fuses.

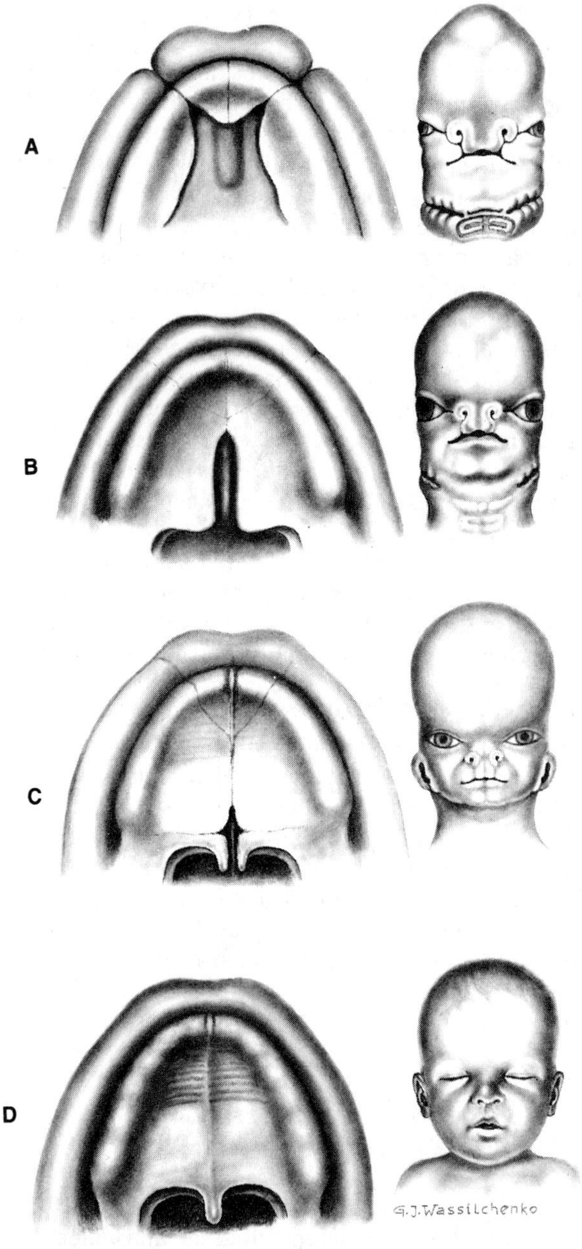

Fig. 11-15. Stages in palatine development.

Diagnostic Evaluation

A cleft that involves the lip with or without CP is readily apparent at birth and is one of the defects that elicit the most severe emotional reactions in parents. Incomplete fusion of the primary palate produces a variation in the degree of malformation (Fig. 11-16). Clefts of the lip may be unilateral or bilateral and may range from a notch in the vermilion border of the lip to complete separation extending to the floor of the nose. Where the cleft is unilateral, about two thirds is on the left side, and an associated CP is found more often with bilateral than with unilateral CL. Varying degrees of nasal distortion usually accompany CL, and the defect frequently involves supernumerary, deformed, or absent teeth.

Clefts of the palate may occur as an isolated defect or in association with CL. Less obvious than CL, the defect may not be detected without a thorough assessment of the mouth. The deformity can be identified by placing the examiner's fingers directly on the palate. Without a proper evaluation, the defect may not be detected until the infant has difficulty with initial feedings. As with CL, the degree of deformity varies and may involve only the uvula or may extend through both the soft and hard palates to the incisive foramen. The isolated CP occurs in the midline, but, when associated with CL, the defect may involve the midline of the soft palate and extend into the hard palate on the side of the lip cleft or on both sides in bilateral clefts. Clefts of the hard palate form a continuous opening between the mouth and the nasal cavity. This creates special feeding problems. The infant is unable to develop suction because of the defect and has difficulty in swallowing. The open pathway must be closed in order to provide sufficient pressure for the swallowing sequence.

Therapeutic Management

Treatment of the child with CLP involves the cooperative efforts of a number of specialists—pediatrician, nurses, plastic surgeon, orthodontist, prosthodontist, otolaryngologist, speech therapist, and sometimes a psychiatrist. Treatment continues over a long time, but even after completion of a program of health care the child will probably retain defects of speech, facial appearance, or other problems related to the cleft. Management is directed toward closure of the cleft(s), prevention of complications, habilitation, and facilitation of normal growth and development of the child.

Surgical correction: cleft lip. Closure of the lip defect precedes that of the palate, although the optimum times for surgery are still being debated. Those who favor immediate repair of the lip argue that it makes the infant more acceptable to the parents before discharge from the hospital, thereby improving establishment of satisfactory parent-child relationships. Others prefer to wait until the infant shows a steady weight gain and a satisfactory hemoglobin level. They believe that the delay allows for more symmetric development of facial structures, offers time to detect any associated serious anomalies unrecognized at birth, and reduces parental disappointment with surgical repair. That is, parents ordinarily adjust to the defect during this time and more fully appreciate the cosmetic effects of the surgical correction. Technical repair of the CL/P can be accomplished quite successfully at any age.

The method of repair of the CL involves one of several staggered suture lines to minimize notching of the lip from retraction of scar tissue. Surgeons use any of a variety of devices to protect the suture line from undue tension, such as tape or a Logan bow (Fig. 11-17). Regardless of the method used, generally measures are instituted to reduce crying and the arms are restrained at the elbows to prevent the infant's hands from rubbing the incision.

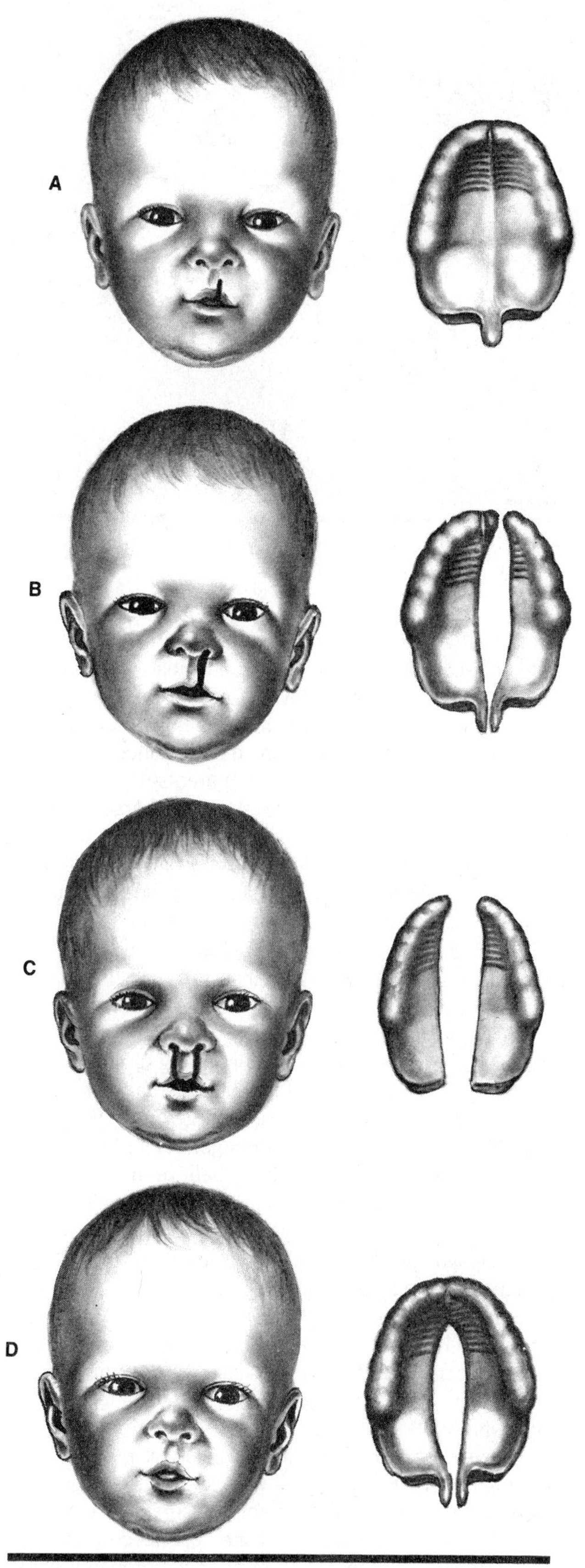

Fig. 11-16. Variations in clefts of lip and palate at birth. **A,** Notch in vermilion border. **B,** Unilateral cleft lip and palate. **C,** Bilateral cleft lip and cleft palate. **D,** Cleft palate.

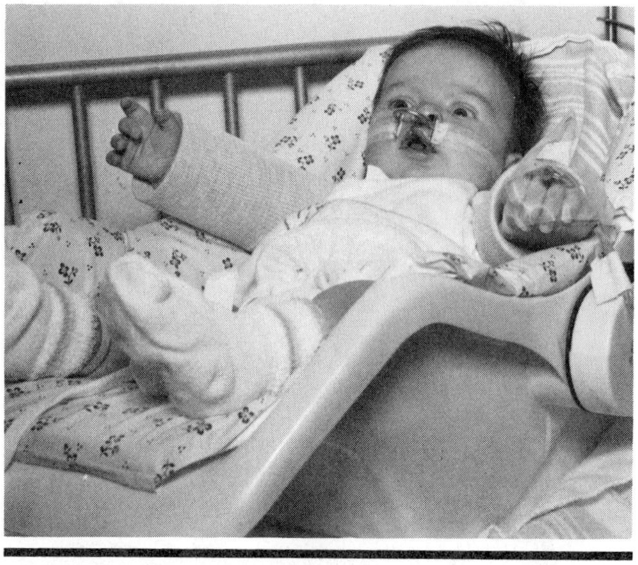

Fig. 11-17. Infant with Logan bow in place to prevent tension on suture line. Note elbow restraints.

Improved surgical techniques have minimized deformity related to scar retraction, but good cosmetic results are difficult to obtain in defects that are more severe initially. In the absence of infection or trauma, healing takes place with little scar formation; however, in some instances the results are less than satisfactory from the parents' (and, later, the child's) viewpoint. Undesirable physical characteristics of the older child are residual nasal deformity, mildly protruding lower lip, and a somewhat flattened lower third of the upper lip usually with an abnormally shaped red lip margin. Not infrequently, revisions may be required at a later age.

Surgical correction: cleft palate. CP repair is generally postponed until a later age than repair of the CL in order to take advantage of palatal changes that occur with normal growth. Since clefts vary considerably in size, shape, and degree of deformity, the timing of repair is individualized but is usually performed sometime between the ages of 6 months and 5 years. Most surgeons prefer to close the cleft between 1 and 2 years of age, before the child develops faulty speech habits. Others believe that best results are obtained when surgery is delayed until 4 years of age. If surgery is delayed beyond 3 years of age, a special denture plate helps occlude the cleft to assist in development of normal speech patterns. In addition, it is inadvisable to remove the tonsils because they trap air and thus allow for better speech.

Long-term problems. The team concept in the delivery of health care is exemplified in the habilitation of the child with CL/P. Treatment of individual patients is integrated by a group of specialists who meet periodically to examine the child and consult with each other and with the parents. Even with good anatomic closure, the majority of children with CL/P have some degree of speech impairment that requires speech therapy. The physical problems are the result of inefficient functioning of the muscles of the soft palate and nasopharynx, improper tooth alignment, and varying degrees of hearing loss.

Improper drainage of the middle ear, as a result of inefficient function of the eustachian tube, causes increased pressure in the middle ear and contributes to recurrent otitis media with scarring of the tympanic membrane. This scarring plus the additional accumulation of fluid under pressure hampers the movement of the eardrum and the small bone of the middle ear, which leads to hearing impairment in a large proportion of children with palatal clefts. The problem may be easily overlooked in the infant and young child, thereby contributing to permanent impairment. Upper respiratory tract infections require immediate and meticulous attention, and pressure-equalizing drainage tubes may be inserted to facilitate drainage in chronic serous otitis media.

Extensive orthodontics and prosthodontics are usually needed to correct problems of malposition of teeth and maxillary arches. Changes take place in the structures of the teeth next to the cleft. There may be extra teeth present, or the teeth may be malformed or malpositioned, which can interfere with feeding. In addition a significant number of these children have an inadequate nasal airway that forces them to breathe through their mouths, which also contributes to oral deformity. Children with clefts of both lip and palate require four stages of orthodontic therapy. The first stage (birth to 18 months) is concerned with aligning the maxillary segments into a near-normal relationship. This is frequently done before lip closure in severely expanded segments to facilitate a primary lip closure.

The second stage (2 to 5 years) consists of repositioning maxillary segments and/or correcting a dental crossbite (a condition in which the upper teeth close inside the lower teeth) in an attempt to allow the primary teeth to develop in a normal relationship. Third stage therapy (10 to 11 years) takes place during the mixed dentition stage and involves correction of faulty occlusion. In the fourth stage (12 to 18 years) treatment of the permanent teeth is accomplished in much the same manner as for any teenage child except for alignment and spacing in the cleft area.

Often temporary or permanent dental prostheses are necessary to replace missing teeth; these assist in chewing and produce a more pleasing cosmetic effect. Special dental plates, or obturators, are sometimes used to mechanically close clefts in the palate to facilitate feeding and speech until permanent closure is attempted. However, any appliance must be checked periodically to ensure a proper fit and to see that it is performing its intended function.

The major potential handicap for a child with a CP is defective speech. This can occur as a result of any or all of the previously discussed complications: insufficient palate function, faulty dentition, and hearing loss. A cleft palate interferes with speech sounds in the mouth that are normally made through interaction of the throat and palatine muscles. Improper tooth alignment can pose a mechanical hazard to development of clear speech, and hearing loss from middle ear infection is an additional impediment because of difficulty in interpreting sounds. With isolated CL no speech problem should be anticipated. However, children without mouth defects develop undesirable speech habits, and children with CL may develop speech problems unrelated to the defect. The child with a CP usually requires the services of a competent speech therapist.

Some of the more difficult long-term problems are related to social adjustment of the child. The better the physical habilitation, the better the chance for emotional and social adjustment, although the presence of the defect and the degree of residual disability are not directly related to a satisfactory adjustment. Physical defects are always a threat to the self-image, and abnormal speech quality is an impediment to social expression.

Nursing Considerations

The management of the child with CL/P offers some special challenges to both nurses and families in relation to modification of feeding techniques and long-term management. Otherwise, unless there are associated complicating anomalies, other aspects of nursing care of these children offer no significant differences from that of any newborn.

Assessment

Since the lip defect is readily visible at birth, assessment consists of describing the location and extent of the defect, and the palatine cleft is estimated by visualization during crying. CP without CL is detected by palpating the palate with the finger during the newborn assessment.

The emotional impact of the birth of a child with a cosmetic as well as a functional disability is especially traumatic to the family. Consequently, the nursing assessment is also concerned with the emotional reaction of the family to the child and the defect.

Nursing Diagnoses

Following the nursing assessment a number of nursing diagnoses become evident. The most likely diagnoses are outlined and discussed in the Nursing Care Plan on pp. 494-495. Others may be apparent in individual cases.

Planning

The goals of care for the infant with CL/P include preoperative care, short-term postoperative care, and long-term management. The major goals of care include:

Preoperative care:
1. Help families cope with the impact of a child with a defect.
2. Implement and carry out a feeding method.
3. Prepare infant for surgery.

Postoperative care:
1. Prevent injury to operative site.
2. Provide nutrition.
3. Prevent complications.
4. Support family.

Implementation

The immediate nursing problems in the care of an infant with CL/P deformities are related to feeding the infant and dealing with the severe parental reaction to the defect. Facial deformities are particularly disturbing to parents. A CL is the most disfiguring of the visible defects and generates strong negative responses in both nurses and parents. It is especially important for nurses to emphasize the positive aspects of the infant's physical appearance and to express optimism regarding surgical correction. The manner of the nurse in handling the infant should convey to the parents that the infant is indeed a precious human being (see also Birth of a Child with a Physical Defect, p. 454)

Feeding. Feeding the infant offers a special challenge to nurses, and the process is often time consuming and laborious. Clefts of lip or palate reduce the infant's ability to suck, which interferes with compression of the areola or nipple and usually renders both breast-feeding and bottle-feeding difficult. Liquid taken into the mouth has a tendency to escape via the cleft through the nose. Feeding is usually best accomplished with the infant's head in an upright position, either held in the nurse's hand or cradled in the arm. The type of feeding equipment and rate of feeding must be individualized for each infant.

Normal nipples are often unsuitable for these infants, who are unable to generate the suction required; therefore special nipples or other feeding devices are needed. A variety of special "cleft palate" nipples and nurser units have been devised and used with some success. Many satisfactory brands are readily available; most are relatively inexpensive. Some allow formula to be deposited directly into the pharynx in much the same manner as with a bulb syringe. In others the nipple is equipped with a flange to partially cover the palatal cleft. The sides of a regular plastic bottle can be compressed to facilitate flow, allowing the feeder to control the flow of formula. It also reduces the amount of negative pressure exerted by the infant, which frequently increases the amount of ingested air.

Success has also been achieved by the modification of a standard nipple or a red "preemie" nipple. A single small slit or a crosscut is made in the end of the nipple with a sharp surgical blade or a pair of scissors with sharp, thin blades. This allows the infant to express the formula readily. The size of the slit is adjusted to the needs of the infant. If the formula dribbles from the sides of the nipple or the nostrils during the feeding, the slit is too long; if it takes longer than 30 minutes to feed, the slit is too short.

Using these various types of nipples for feeding also has the advantage of helping to meet the infant's sucking needs and, when placed in the normal sucking position (not through the cleft), encouraging use of the sucking muscles. Muscle development is especially important for later development of speech. The nipple should be positioned in such a way that the end is situated well back in the infant's mouth and can be compressed by the infant's tongue and existing palate. If a single-slit nipple is used, the slit should be placed vertically so that the infant will be able to produce and stop a flow of milk by alternately opening and closing the opening. No matter which type of nipple is used, gentle, steady pressure on the base of the bottle reduces the chance of choking or coughing, and the person feeding should resist the temptation to remove the nipple

NURSING CARE PLAN
The Infant with Cleft Lip and/or Palate Repair

Preoperative care (cleft lip)

NURSING DIAGNOSIS: Altered nutrition: less than body requirements related to difficulty eating

GOAL 1
Provide adequate nutritional intake

INTERVENTIONS
Administer diet appropriate for age (specify)
Modify feeding techniques to adjust to defect
  Hold child in upright (sitting) position
  Use special feeding appliances
  Bubble frequently
Assist mother with breast-feeding if this is mother's preference

EXPECTED OUTCOMES
Infant consumes an adequate amount of nutrients (specify amount)
Infant exhibits appropriate weight gain

NURSING DIAGNOSIS: Potential altered parenting related to infant with a highly visible physical defect

GOAL 1
Facilitate family's acceptance of infant

INTERVENTIONS
Allow expression of feelings
Convey attitude of acceptance of infant and family
Indicate by behavior that child is a valuable human being
Describe results of surgical correction of defect
  Use photographs of satisfactory results
Arrange meeting with other parents who have experienced a similar situation and coped successfully

EXPECTED OUTCOMES
Family discusses feelings and concerns regarding the child's defect, its repair, and future prospects
Family exhibits an attitude of acceptance of infant

See also Nursing Care Plan: The Child Undergoing Surgery, Preoperative Care, Chapter 27

Postoperative care (cleft lip)

NURSING DIAGNOSIS: Potential for trauma related to surgical procedure, immature reasoning

GOAL 1
Prevent trauma to suture line

INTERVENTIONS
Position on back or side
Maintain lip protective device
Use nontraumatic feeding techniques
Restrain arms to prevent access to operative site
  Use jacket restraints on older infant
Avoid placing objects in the mouth following cleft palate repair (suction catheter, tongue depressor, straw, pacifier, small spoon)
Prevent vigorous and sustained crying
Cleanse suture line gently after feeding and as necessary in manner ordered by surgeon
Teach cleansing and restraining procedures, especially when infant will be discharged before suture removal

EXPECTED OUTCOME
Operative site remains undamaged

GOAL 2
Prevent aspiration of secretions

INTERVENTIONS
Position to allow for mucus drainage (partial side-lying position, semi-Fowler position)

EXPECTED OUTCOME
Child manages secretions without aspiration

NURSING DIAGNOSIS: Altered nutrition: less than body requirements related to physical defect, surgical procedure

GOAL 1
Provide adequate nutritional intake

INTERVENTIONS
Administer diet appropriate for age
Involve family in determining best feeding methods
Modify feeding techniques to adjust to defect
  Feed in sitting position
  Use special appliances
  Encourage frequent bubbling
  Assist with breast-feeding if method of choice
Teach feeding and suctioning techniques to family
Monitor IV fluids (if prescribed)

EXPECTED OUTCOMES
Infant consumes an adequate amount of nutrients (specify amounts)
Family demonstrates ability to carry out postoperative care

NURSING CARE PLAN
The Infant with Cleft Lip and/or Palate Repair—cont'd

NURSING DIAGNOSIS: Pain related to surgical procedure

GOAL 1

Relieve discomfort

INTERVENTIONS:

*Administer analgesics and/or sedatives as ordered
See Nursing Care Plan: The Child in Pain, Chapter 26

EXPECTED OUTCOME

Infant appears comfortable and rests quietly

NURSING DIAGNOSIS: Sensory-perceptual alterations (gustatory, tactile) related to feeding methods (some types), arm restraints

GOAL 1

Provide comfort measures

INTERVENTIONS

Remove restraints periodically while supervised
Provide cuddling and tactile stimulation
Involve parents in infant's care
Apply developmental interventions appropriate for infant's level and tolerance (see Chapter 10)

EXPECTED OUTCOME

Child rests quietly, is not irritable, and responds appropriately

NURSING DIAGNOSIS: Altered family processes related to child with a physical defect

GOAL 1

Support family

INTERVENTIONS AND EXPECTED OUTCOMES

See Nursing Care Plan: The Family of the Ill or Hospitalized Child, Chapter 26
Refer family to appropriate agencies and support groups

See also Nursing Care Plan: The Child with a Chronic Illness or Disability, Chapter 22

*Dependent nursing action.

frequently because of the noise the infant makes or for fear that the infant will choke.

Feedings that extend beyond 20 to 30 minutes can deplete the infant's energy (Curtin, 1990). When the infant has trouble with nipple feeding, either a rubber-tipped medicine dropper, Asepto syringe, or Breck feeder often provides an efficient, safe feeding device. The rubber extension or thin nipple should be sufficiently long to extend well back into the mouth to reduce the likelihood of regurgitation through the nose. The formula is deposited on the back of the tongue and the flow controlled by bulb compression that is adjusted to the infant's capacity to handle it. Gavage feedings may be needed occasionally to supplement oral feedings.

✦ **NURSING ALERT** The nurse should be alert for evidence of nutritional deprivation (e.g., weight loss, signs of hunger before expected feeding times, wasted appearance). These infants should be referred to a dietitian for formula calorie adjustment or supplementation.

Success has been reported with the use of a custom-made plastic palate constructed of rapid setting acrylic from a mold of the infant's mouth. With the device the infant is able to feed more normally. The device prevents food from being expelled from the nasal cavity and has an added advantage of allowing for more normal "speech" sounds, which is reassuring to the parents (Learning to close the cleft, 1982). However, the device is quite expensive and must be replaced as the infant grows.

Because of their difficulty generating suction and occluding the oral cavity, these infants have a tendency to swallow more air than infants with normal oral cavities. Consequently, the infant must be fed slowly and bubbled more frequently and may require more frequent feedings.

With some infants, spoon feeding of formula works best. The parents should begin to feed the infant as soon as possible, preferably after the initial nursery feeding. In this way they are able to help determine the method best suited to them and the infant and to become adept in the technique before the infant is discharged from the hospital. Contrary to previous thought, the infant can be successfully breastfed. The nipple is positioned and stabilized well back in the oral cavity so that tongue action facilitates milk expression. However, the suction required to stimulate milk may be absent initially; therefore a breast pump may be useful before nursing to stimulate the let-down reflex (Curtin, 1990)

Preoperative care. In preparation for surgical repair, the parents are frequently instructed to accustom the infant to some of the needs of the early postoperative period, particularly if surgery is delayed several months. Since it is mandatory for the infant to avoid prone positioning postoperatively, it is helpful to accustom the infant to lie on the back or side to reduce the irritability and resistance associated with any change in routine. It is also helpful to place the infant or child in arm restraints periodically before admission and, after admission, to feed the infant in the manner to be used postoperatively. No special formula is required, and the infant is usually allowed to eat up to about 6 hours preoperatively. Preoperative preparation, including medication, is determined by the surgeon and anesthesiologist.

Postoperative care: cleft lip. The major efforts in the postoperative period are directed toward protecting the operative site. Before the infant leaves the operating room, the lip protective device (if used) or the butterfly closure is taped securely to the cheeks to relax the operative site and prevent tension on the suture line caused by crying or other facial movement. Arm restraints are applied to prevent the infant from rubbing or otherwise disturbing the suture line and are ready at the bedside for immediate application on arrival at the unit. It is advisable to pin the cuff of the restraints to the infant's clothing or bed to prevent rubbing the face with the upper arms.

An older infant who is able to roll over will require a jacket restraint in addition to arm restraints, to prevent rolling on the abdomen and rubbing the face on the sheet. It is important to remove the restraints periodically to allow for exercising the arms, to provide relief from restrictions, and to observe the skin for signs of irritation. It is advisable to release the restraints one at a time, especially in a very vigorous, active infant or child. Removing restraints also offers an opportunity for cuddling and body contact. Sitting the child in an infant seat provides a change of position and a different perspective of the environment. Adequate analgesia is recommended to relieve postoperative pain; sedation is sometimes needed for a very restless, anxious infant.

Feeding is essentially the same as before surgery. It is safe to offer clear liquids when the infant has fully recovered from the anesthesia, and formula feeding is usually resumed when tolerated. The surgeon will specify any preferences or restrictions in feeding method. The mouth should be rinsed with water before and after each feeding.

The suture site is carefully cleansed of formula or serosanguineous drainage as needed with a gauze- or cotton-tipped swab dipped in saline or other solution, depending on the preference of the surgeon. Medicated ointments, such as bacitracin, may be prescribed for application to the suture line after cleansing. Meticulous care of the suture line is a nursing responsibility, since inflammation or sloughing will interfere with optimum healing and the ultimate cosmetic effect of the surgical repair. The area is carefully inspected at each feeding. A broad spectrum antibiotic may be prescribed for several days postoperatively.

Gentle aspiration of mouth and nasopharynx secretions is necessary to prevent aspiration and minimize the chances of respiratory complications. A side-lying or partial side-lying position is helpful for the infant in the immediate postoperative period and for one who has difficulty in handling secretions. As with any infant, the child with cleft lip repair is placed on the right side after feedings to reduce the chance of aspirating regurgitated formula.

Preparation for discharge and home care. Parents are encouraged to participate in the care of the infant as soon as feasible following surgery. They can resume the preoperative feeding method with the infant in a sitting position. The infant should be fed slowly and carefully and bubbled at frequent intervals. Parents are taught to follow each feeding with water (in the same manner as the feeding) and to cleanse the suture line to free any crusts that might form. This promotes healing and helps prevent undue scarring. If the surgeon approves, ointment (such as A and D Ointment) or mineral oil may be applied to keep the area lubricated.

Parents are cautioned to continue with elbow restraints until the suture line is well healed. The infant should not be allowed to cry, if possible, to prevent undue stress on the suture line. Cuddling, holding, and other comfort measures usually are effective, in addition to the time spent during feedings.

Postoperative care: cleft palate. The child with a CP repair is allowed to lie on the abdomen, especially immediately postoperatively. The child with a CP repair may be fed with a wide-bowl spoon (such as a soup spoon) or from the side of the spoon, with the nurse or parent taking care not to insert the spoon into the mouth where it might damage the suture line. Fluids are best taken from a cup.

✦ **NURSING ALERT** The nurse should avoid the use of suction or other objects in the mouth, such as a tongue depressor when the suture lines are being checked or straws when the child is given liquids. Forks are contraindicated, and thermometers are not placed in the mouth.

Sometimes the child will have difficulty breathing following surgery, since it is often necessary to alter an established pattern of breathing and adjust to breathing through the nose. This is frustrating but seldom requires more than positioning and support. Sometimes the infant or child is placed in a mist tent for a short period after surgery. Some surgeons place a single suture at the end of the tongue to facilitate extending the tongue if the airway should become obstructed. It is usually removed after the first 24 hours.

The elbows are restrained to keep the hands away from the mouth, and the parents are instructed to maintain this precaution at home until the palate is healed, usually in 4 to 6 weeks. They should be instructed to remove the restraints (usually one at a time) at frequent intervals to allow the child to exercise the arms. As with the infant with a CL, the child should be kept from crying, if possible, by giving attention and affection and providing diversional activities.

The child is usually discharged on a soft diet, which parents are instructed to continue until the surgeon directs them otherwise. They should be cautioned against allowing the child to eat hard items such as toast, hard cookies, and potato chips, which could damage the newly repaired palate. The nurse might suggest that the parents not offer the child any food harder than mashed potatoes.

Long-term parental guidance. The problems of parents and the child with a CP extend beyond the initial adjustment to the defect, acceptance of the child, and surgical correction of the defect. These families need support and encouragement by health professionals and guidance in activities that facilitate the most normal outcome for the child. With the combined efforts of family and the health team, the majority of these children achieve a satisfactory habilitation. Parents need to understand the function of therapy and the purpose of any appliance. They are taught proper care and placement of any device, and establishing good mouth care and proper brushing habits is especially important for these children.

Because of the increased risk of middle ear infection, the ears are examined regularly and hearing tests are scheduled early and repeated periodically throughout childhood. It is particularly important to emphasize the need for an ear examination when the child has a cold in the nose, throat, or chest. When treatment can be implemented early, the chances are greater that permanent changes in the ear can be avoided. Parents can be alert to signs of any hearing impairment in the child in order to obtain needed help and prevent progression of any deficit (see Chapter 25).

The parents are also provided with guidance in helping the child to develop normal speech. They should encourage the child's early attempts to make sounds. Some parents erroneously believe that the child may form poor speech habits if he tries to speak before the palate is repaired. However, attempting to delay speech further hampers its development. Activities that encourage the child to use the natural inclination to imitate sounds, including his own, are valuable aids; these include singing, repeating rhymes, and speaking games such as "pat-a-cake." The child with a CP is able to produce many sounds clearly, and parents should try to understand what the child is saying without correcting the speech during these early attempts. As with any toddler who is learning to use speech communication, "baby talk" is discouraged. Parents can use simple speech with short two- to three-word sentences. Parents should also understand that normal children at this age often leave out final sounds of words and should not attribute this characteristic to the defect.

Following surgery parents can assist palatal function by stimulating the child to use simple words that require coordination of the speech apparatus, encouraging chewing and frequent swallowing to exercise throat and palatine muscles, and engaging in blowing games to help close off the posterior palate. The speech therapist evaluates the individual needs of the child and directs the parents in specific activities to facilitate speech development. The more the child is encouraged to use speech, the sooner he will gain self-confidence and assurance in social situations. Some children may require additional surgery to correct defective speech that cannot be managed with speech therapy alone.

Throughout the child's habilitation the ultimate goal should be the development of a healthy personality and self-esteem. Several agencies provide services and information for children with CL/P and their families. These include the **American Cleft Palate Association** and **The Cleft Palate Foundation,*** the **March of Dimes–Birth Defects Foundation,†** and state **Program for Children with Special Health Needs** (formerly Crippled Children's Services).

Evaluation

The effectiveness of nursing interventions is determined by continual reassessment and evaluation of care based on the following observational guidelines and expected outcomes:

Preoperative care:

1. Observe and interview family members relative to their understandings, feelings, and concerns regarding the defect and anticipated surgery and their interactions with the infant.
2. Observe infant during feeding.
3. Check preoperative checklist.

Postoperative care:

4. Inspect operative site, including the protective tape or device.
5. Observe infant during feeding; measure intake and output; weigh infant daily.
6. Observe operative site for evidence of infection, bleeding, sloughing, or irritation.
7. Observe and interview family regarding their understandings and concerns about the infant, including long-term needs.

Expected outcomes:

See Nursing Care Plan, pp. 494-495.

ESOPHAGEAL ATRESIA WITH TRACHEOESOPHAGEAL FISTULA

Congenital esophageal atresia (EA) and tracheoesophageal fistula (TEF) are rare malformations that represent a failure of the esophagus to develop as a continuous passage and of the trachea and esophagus to separate into distinct structures. These defects may occur as separate entities or in combination, and without early diagnosis and treatment they are rapidly fatal.

The incidence of EA and TEF is not known. Various authorities have estimated the incidence to be from 1:800 to 1:5000 live births. There appear to be no sex differences, but the birth weight of most affected infants is significantly lower than average and there is an unusually high percentage of prematurity. A history of maternal polyhydramnios is common, and approximately half the infants with esophageal defects have associated anomalies, especially congenital heart disease, anorectal malformations, and genitourinary (GU) anomalies. The possibility of VATER association of congenital defects (vertebral defects, imperforate anus, and EA with TEF) should be considered in infants

---

*1218 Grandview Ave., Pittsburgh, PA 15211; (800) 24-CLEFT or (412) 481-1376.

†1275 Mamaroneck Ave., White Plains, NY 10605; (914) 428-7100. In Canada: **Canadian Cleft Lip and Palate Family Association,** 170 Elizabeth St., Toronto, Ontario, Canada M5G1E8; **AboutFace,** 123 Edward Street, Suite 1405, Toronto, Ontario, Canada M5G 1E2; (416) 593-1488.

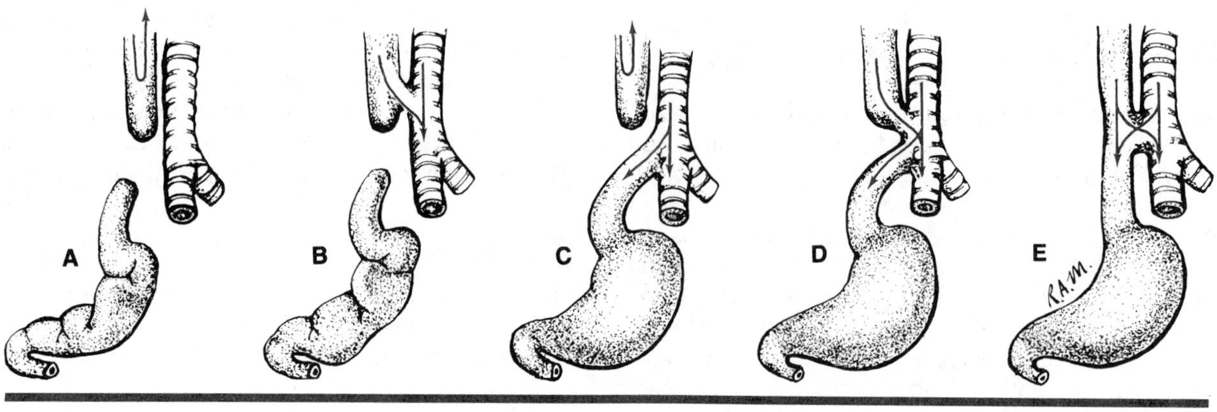

Fig. 11-18. Five most common types of esophageal atresia and tracheoesophageal fistula.

with EA and TEF. There is little evidence to implicate heredity as a factor.

Pathophysiology

The esophagus develops from the first segment of the embryonic gut. During the fourth and fifth weeks of gestation, this foregut normally lengthens and separates longitudinally and each longitudinal portion fuses to form two parallel channels (the esophagus and the trachea) that are joined only at the larynx. Anomalies involving the trachea and esophagus are caused by defective separation, incomplete fusion of the tracheal folds following this separation, or altered cellular growth during the process. The resulting esophageal defect may consist merely of two blind pouches, one at the pharyngeal end and one at the gastric end. More often one portion ends in a blind pouch and the other is connected to the trachea by way of a fistula.

The most commonly encountered form of EA and TEF (80% to 95% of cases) is one in which the proximal esophageal segment terminates in a blind pouch and the distal segment is connected to the trachea or primary bronchus by a short fistula at or near the bifurcation (Fig. 11-18, *C*). The second most common type or "pure" EA (5% to 8%) consists of a blind pouch at each end, widely separated and with no communication to the trachea (Fig. 11-18, *A*). Less frequently an otherwise normal trachea and esophagus are connected by a fistula (Fig. 11-18, *E*). Extremely rare anomalies involve a fistula from the trachea to the upper esophageal segment (Fig. 11-18, *B*) or to both the upper and lower segments (Fig. 11-19, *D*).

Clinical Manifestations

The presence of EA is suspected in an infant with excessive salivation and in a newborn with drooling that is frequently accompanied by choking, coughing, and sneezing. If fed, the infant swallows normally but suddenly coughs and struggles, and the fluid returns through the nose and mouth. The infant becomes cyanotic and may stop breathing as the overflow of fluid from the blind pouch is aspirated into the trachea or bronchus. The cyanosis is the result of laryngospasm, the protective mechanism that operates to prevent aspiration into the trachea, and, over time, respiratory distress develops.

In the infant with EA with a distal TEF (type C) the stomach becomes distended with air, and thoracic and abdominal compression (especially during crying) cause the gastric contents to be regurgitated through the fistula into the trachea, producing a chemical pneumonitis. When the upper segment of the esophagus opens directly into the trachea (types B and D), the infant is in danger of aspirating any swallowed material. Cyanosis or choking during feeding may be the only symptom of type E fistula.

Diagnostic Evaluation

To establish a diagnosis of EA, a catheter is gently passed into the esophagus. It will meet with resistance if the lumen is blocked but will pass unobstructed if the lumen is patent. A moderately stiff catheter is used to avoid coiling in the esophageal pouch. Aspiration of stomach contents or auscultation over the stomach as air is introduced through the catheter confirms a patent esophagus. Gastric lavage immediately after delivery, although not a universal practice, offers earlier diagnosis of EA.

Although the diagnosis is established on the basis of clinical signs and symptoms, the exact type of anomaly is determined by radiographic studies. A radiopaque catheter is inserted into the hypopharynx and advanced until it encounters an obstruction. Chest films are taken to ascertain whether the tube reaches the stomach and whether it appears to pass through the normal or abnormal channels. Films that show air in the stomach indicate a connection between the trachea and the distal esophagus in types C and D. No gas is observed in the bowel in types A and B. Occasionally fistulas are not patent, which makes their presence more difficult to diagnose. A careful esophagraphic or bronchoscopic examination may be performed to visualize the fistula.

The presence of polyhydramnios prenatally is a clue to the possibility of EA in the unborn infant, especially if the defect is type A or C. Amniotic fluid, normally swallowed by the fetus, is unable to reach the GI tract.

Therapeutic Management

The treatment of EA and TEF includes prevention of pneumonia, supportive therapy, and surgical repair of the anomaly. Since type C is the most common, the discussion is directed primarily toward that anomaly.

When EA with a TEF is suspected, the infant is immediately deprived of oral intake, intravenous fluids are begun, and the infant is positioned to facilitate drainage of secretions and decrease the likelihood of aspiration. For example, the head is elevated in type C anomaly. Accumulated secretions are suctioned frequently from the mouth and pharynx. A catheter is placed into the upper esophageal pouch and attached to continuous suction, and the infant's head is kept in an upright position so that fluid collected in the pouch is easily removed and to prevent aspiration of gastric contents. A gastrostomy is usually performed to decompress the stomach and prevent further aspiration of gastric contents by way of the fistula. Since aspiration pneumonia is almost inevitable and appears early, broad-spectrum antibiotic therapy is instituted.

Surgical correction. Most malformations can be corrected surgically in one operation or staged with two or more procedures. The success depends on early diagnosis before complicating factors (pneumonia, dehydration, and inanition) have progressed to an irreversible stage, skilled nursing care, and the technical skill and judgment of the surgeon. With measures instituted to prevent aspiration pneumonia and to ensure adequate hydration and nutrition, surgery can be postponed to allow for more effective treatment of pneumonia so that the infant can better withstand the complex surgery. The delay also offers an opportunity for further evaluation and assessment to rule out any associated anomalies, optimize respiratory support, and treat problems associated with prematurity.

The surgery consists of a thoracotomy with division and ligation of the TEF and an end-to-end anastomosis of the esophagus. A chest tube is inserted to drain chest fluid. For infants who are premature, have multiple anomalies, or are in very poor condition, a staged operation is preferred that involves palliative measures, including gastrostomy, ligation of the TEF, and provision of constant drainage of the esophageal pouch.

There are rare instances in which a primary anastomosis cannot be accomplished because of insufficient length of the two segments of esophagus. In these cases an esophageal replacement procedure using bowel or gastric tube esophagostomy may be necessary to bridge the missing esophageal segment. When the stomach is used, a tube is fashioned from the greater curvature of the stomach, tunneled into the chest, and anastomosed to the esophagus. Alternatively a segment of either the right or the transverse colon is dissected and transplanted, along with its undisturbed blood and nerve supply, through a surgical opening in the diaphragm and ligated to the esophageal pouches, maintaining the proximodistal orientation. At this time the gastrostomy and esophagostomy are closed. In both types of repair, peristalsis is largely ineffective and food is conducted to the stomach by gravity.

Esophageal replacement is usually deferred until the child is 18 to 24 months old. In the meantime the fistula is closed and the child fed directly by gastrostomy, and the upper esophageal segment is drained by means of a cervical esophagostomy.

Prognosis. In all surgical procedures involving the esophagus there may be problems with stricture caused by scar tissue contraction that require evaluation by barium x-ray studies, esophagoscopy, and mechanical dilation. Many surgeons routinely perform dilation at regularly scheduled intervals for some time after surgery. The procedure may need to be repeated several times during growth. Strictures that do not respond to dilation require surgical intervention.

Nursing Considerations

Anomalies associated with the trachea and esophagus are relatively rare but, when present, constitute a serious threat to the infant and require immediate nursing intervention.

Assessment

Nursing responsibility for detection of this serious malformation begins *immediately* after birth. The defect is suspected in any infant who has an excessive amount of mucus or difficulty with secretions and unexplained episodes of cyanosis. Ideally the condition is diagnosed before the initial feeding, but often it is not. Poor handling of mucus is characteristic of other problems, for example, the infant with CNS damage and the preterm infant with weak or absent cough and swallowing reflexes. This is often a cause of confusion, especially with the premature infant who may also have a TEF. Cyanosis is usually the result of laryngospasm caused by overflow of saliva into the larynx from the proximal esophageal pouch, and it normally clears after removal of the secretions from the oropharynx by suctioning. Any suspicion of a TEF fistula or EA is reported to the practitioner immediately.

Nursing Diagnoses

Following the nursing assessment a number of nursing diagnoses become evident. The most likely diagnoses are outlined and discussed in the Nursing Care Plan on p. 500. Others may be apparent in individual cases.

Planning

The broad objectives for management of an infant with EA and TEF are as follows:

1. Prevent respiratory distress.
2. Provide nutrition.
3. Prevent complications.
4. Support the infant and family.

Implementation

The infant is placed in an incubator or under a radiant warmer, and humidified oxygen is administered to help re-

NURSING CARE PLAN
The Child with Esophageal Atresia and Tracheoesophageal Fistula

NURSING DIAGNOSIS: Ineffective airway clearance related to abnormal opening between esophagus and trachea or obstruction to swallowing secretions

GOAL 1
Maintain patent airway and prevent aspiration

INTERVENTIONS

Remove accumulated secretions from oropharynx
Position for patent airway, lung expansion, and prevention of aspiration of saliva or stomach contents (depends on type of defect)
  Supine with head elevated on an inclined plane (at least 30 degrees)
Administer nothing by mouth

EXPECTED OUTCOMES

Airway remains patent
Infant does not aspirate secretions
Respiration remains within normal limits (see inside front cover)

NURSING DIAGNOSIS: Impaired swallowing related to mechanical obstruction

GOAL 1
Provide nutrition

INTERVENTIONS

Administer gastrostomy feedings when tolerated
Progress to oral feedings as prescribed according to child's condition
Provide for nonnutritive sucking

EXPECTED OUTCOME

Child receives sufficient nourishment and exhibits a satisfactory weight gain

GOAL 2
Teach child to take oral feedings (following late repair)

INTERVENTIONS

Introduce foods one at a time
Provide foods with various textures and flavors
Teach child to chew foods well
Begin with slightly liquid feedings and progress to more solid food
Cut food in small noncylindric pieces
Avoid foods such as whole hot dogs or large pieces of meat
See Box 10-5 for interventions related to the infant who resists oral feedings

EXPECTED OUTCOME

The child takes an adequate amount of nourishment and displays no evidence of malnourishment

*Dependent nursing action.

NURSING DIAGNOSIS: Potential for injury related to surgical procedure

GOAL 1
Prevent trauma to surgical site

INTERVENTIONS

Suction only with catheter premeasured to a distance that does not reach to surgical site

EXPECTED OUTCOME

Child does not exhibit evidence of injury to surgical site

NURSING DIAGNOSIS: Anxiety related to inability to swallow, discomfort from surgery

GOAL 1
Provide comfort and security

INTERVENTIONS

Provide tactile stimulation
Position comfortably postoperatively
Avoid restraints where possible
Administer mouth care
Offer pacifier frequently
*Administer analgesics as prescribed (see Nursing Care Plan: The Child in Pain, Chapter 26)

EXPECTED OUTCOMES

Child rests calmly, is alert when awake, and engages in nonnutritive sucking
Mouth remains clean and moist

NURSING DIAGNOSIS: Altered family processes related to the child with a physical defect

GOAL 1
Educate parents for home care

INTERVENTIONS

Teach family skills and observations needed for home care
  Positioning
  Signs of respiratory distress
  Signs of contracture—refusal to eat, dysphagia, increased coughing
  Assist in acquiring needed equipment and services
  Care of gastrostomy and esophagostomy when infant has staged surgery, including techniques such as suctioning, care of operative site and/or ostomies, dressing changes, and so on

EXPECTED OUTCOME

Family demonstrates the ability to provide care to the infant, an understanding of signs of complications, and appropriate actions

See also:
Nursing Care Plan: The Family of the Ill or Hospitalized Child, Chapter 26
Nursing Care Plan: The Low-Birth-Weight Infant, Chapter 10

lieve respiratory distress. Although intubation may be necessary if the infant is in severe respiratory distress, positive pressure is contraindicated because it may add to air pressure in the stomach and compound the distress.

Preoperative care. The mouth and nasopharynx are carefully suctioned, and the infant is placed in an optimum position to facilitate drainage. Depending on the type of malformation, the infant should be positioned to facilitate drainage and avoid aspiration. The most desirable position for a newborn who is suspected of having the typical EA with TEF (e.g., type C) is supine with the head elevated on an inclined plane of at least 30 degrees. This positioning serves to minimize the reflux of gastric secretions up the distal esophagus into the trachea and bronchi, especially when intraabdominal pressure is elevated during episodes of crying. Head-down positioning would be indicated for type A or B anomaly.

It is imperative that any secretions that can be a source of aspiration be removed at once. Until surgery the blind pouch is kept empty by intermittent or continuous suction through an indwelling nasal or oral catheter that extends to the end of the pouch. The catheter has a tendency to become clogged with mucus; therefore it must be irrigated frequently with normal saline and replaced daily or as needed. Initially the gastrostomy tube is inserted and left open so that any air that enters the stomach through the fistula can escape, thus minimizing the danger of gastric contents being regurgitated into the trachea. The tube empties by gravity drainage. Gastrostomy buttons are frequently inserted after the gastrostomy is well established. (See Chapter 27 for management of gastrostomy feeding.)

Feedings through the gastrostomy tube and irrigations with fluid are contraindicated before surgery unless a TEF is not present. Nursing interventions include frequent respiratory assessment, optimum thermoregulation, fluid management, and nutritional support.

Often the infant must be transferred to a hospital with specialized care units. Care is exercised to maintain the desired position and continue suctioning during transport. Specially designed units are equipped for transporting infants to critical care facilities. During transport the infant is accompanied by a physician, nurse, or a physician/nurse team. Parents are advised of the infant's condition and provided with necessary support and information.

Postoperative care. Postoperative care for these infants is essentially the same as for any high-risk newborn. The infant is returned to the warm, high-humidity atmosphere of the incubator, the chest tube is attached to suction, nutrition is supplied by hyperalimentation, and the gastrostomy tube is returned to gravity drainage until the infant can tolerate feedings, usually on the second or third postoperative day. Drainage from the gastrostomy is inspected and measured, since saliva in the collection container is evidence of a patent esophagus.

The gastrostomy tube is elevated and secured at a point above the level of the stomach. This allows gastric secretions to pass to the duodenum, while swallowed air can escape through the open tube. If tolerated, gastrostomy feedings may be initiated and continued until the esophagus anastomosis is healed, on about the tenth to fourteenth day. Before oral feedings are initiated and the chest tube removed, a barium swallow is performed to verify the integrity of the esophageal anastomosis.

The initial attempt at oral feeding must be carefully observed to make certain that the infant is able to swallow without choking. Oral feedings are begun with glucose water followed by frequent, small feedings of formula. Until the infant is able to take a sufficient amount by mouth, oral intake may need to be supplemented by bolus or continuous drip gastrostomy feedings. Ordinarily the infant is not discharged until oral fluids are taken well. The gastrostomy tube may be removed before discharge or maintained for supplemental feedings at home. However, the infant who has undergone palliative surgery will be discharged with the gastrostomy tube in place.

Special problems. Upper respiratory complications are a threat to life in both the preoperative and the postoperative periods. In addition to pneumonia, there is a constant danger of respiratory embarrassment resulting from atelectasis, pneumothorax, and laryngeal edema. Tracheal suctioning should only be done using a premeasured catheter to avoid injury to the suture line. Any persistent respiratory difficulty after removal of secretions is reported to the surgeon immediately. The infant is monitored for anastomotic leaks as evidenced by saliva or purulent chest tube drainage, increased white blood count, and temperature instability.

In the infant awaiting esophageal replacement surgery, the catheter is removed and the upper esophageal segment is drained by means of an artificial opening in the neck (cervical esophagostomy), which allows escape of the swallowed saliva. This is a source of annoyance, since the skin may become irritated by moisture from the continual discharge of saliva. Frequent removal of drainage and application of a thin layer of protective ointment are usually sufficient treatment. The enterostomal therapist may provide helpful guidance in the event of skin breakdown.

For the infant who requires esophageal replacement, nonnutritive sucking is provided by a pacifier. Sometimes small amounts of water are given orally under the guidance of an occupational or speech therapist. In this case the water drains from the esophagostomy but allows the infant to develop mature sucking patterns.

The child who has corrective surgery delayed until 18 to 24 months of age may have a different problem. Children who must remain NPO for an extended period have not been able to go through the processes of eating in the normal manner. They frequently have difficulty with this new task and may become extremely resistant to learning it (Dixon, 1987). They require patient, firm guidance in learning the techniques of taking food into the mouth and swallowing after repair (see Feeding Resistance, Chapter 10). A referral to an occupational or speech therapist may be necessary.

Family support, discharge planning, and home care. Preparing parents for discharge of their infant involves teaching the techniques that will be continued in home care, such as careful suctioning, gastrostomy feeding, and skin care. The parents are taught child or infant behaviors that might be expected after corrective surgery, such as those that indicate that the child needs to be suctioned, signs of respiratory difficulty, and signs that indicate constriction of the esophagus (poor feeding, dysphagia, drooling, or regurgitating small amounts).

Parents are reminded that it is particularly important to guard against the child swallowing foreign objects. They are instructed to cut solid food into small pieces, teach the child to chew thoroughly, and avoid foods such as whole hot dogs or large pieces of meat that may become lodged in the esophagus. With a child in any of the stages of locomotion, this is no simple problem.

Most infants will have some tracheomalasia; therefore parents should be reassured that their infant's "barky" cough is normal and will gradually diminish as the infant grows and trachea becomes stronger. Since over one half of the infants with EA/TEF will develop gastroesophageal reflux, precautions should be initiated (see Gastroesophageal Reflux, Chapter 33). Parents will also need help in acquiring needed equipment, such as a suction machine, and special services.

Evaluation

The effectiveness of nursing interventions is determined by continual reassessment and evaluation of care based on the following observational guidelines and expected outcomes:

1. Observe infant's respiratory behavior.
2. Weigh daily; observe infant's eating behavior.
3. Inspect surgical site; observe infant's behavior; take vital signs.
4. Observe and interview family members.

Expected outcomes:
See Nursing Care Plan, p. 500.

ANORECTAL MALFORMATIONS

Malformations in the anorectal region of the GI tract are manifested in several variations, often termed *imperforate anus.* They are among the more common congenital malformations caused by abnormal development (approximately 1:5000) (Fig. 11-19). A large number of infants with anorectal defects will have another serious associated congenital anomaly, the most common of which are those involving the GU tract, heart, and esophagus.

Clinically anorectal malformations are classified on the basis of sex and the relationship of the rectum to the pub-

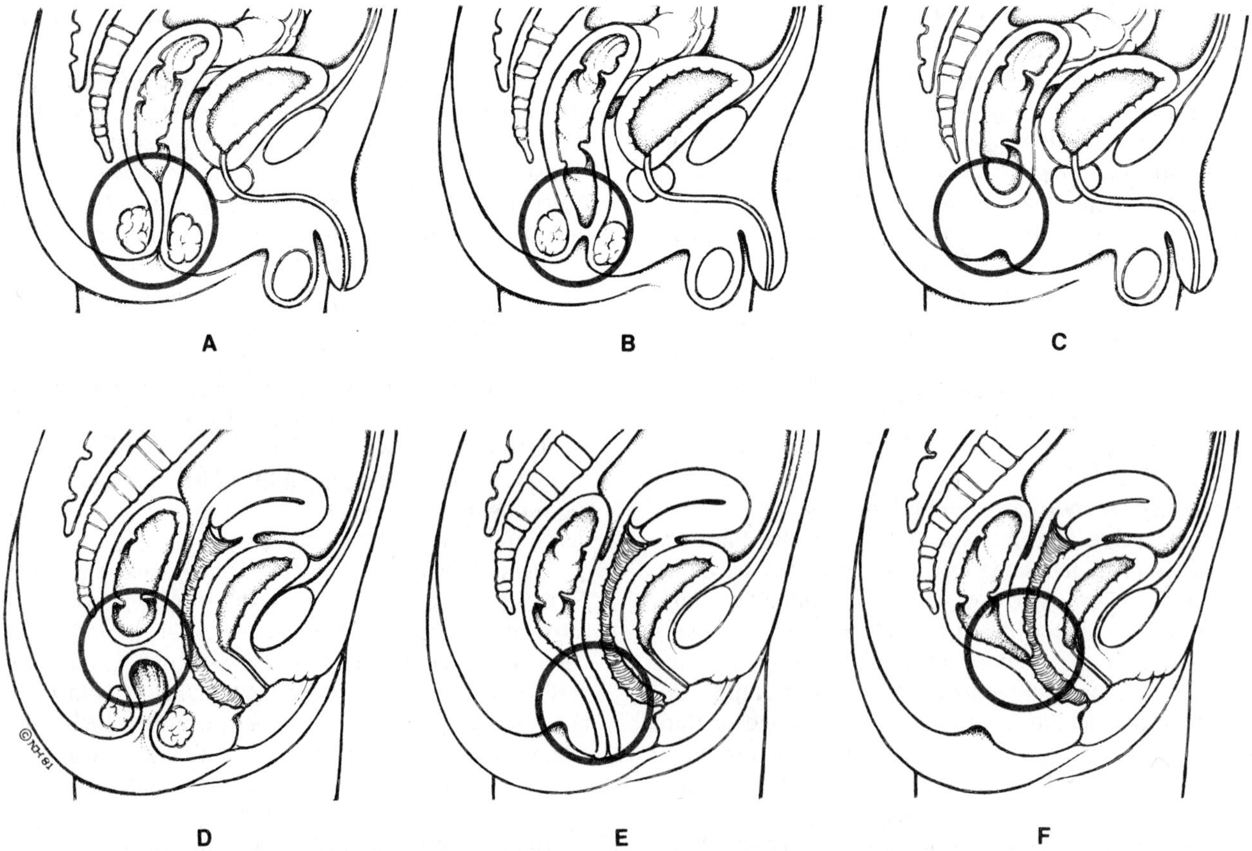

Fig. 11-19. Anorectal stenosis and imperforate anus. **A,** Congenital and stenosis. **B,** Anal membrane atresia. **C,** Anal agenesis. **D,** Rectal atresia. **E,** Rectoperoneal fistula. **F,** Rectovaginal fistula.

Box 11-7 CLASSIFICATION OF ANORECTAL MALFORMATIONS

Low anomalies—rectum has descended normally through the puborectalis muscle, the internal and external sphincters are present and well developed with normal function, and there is no connection to the genitourinary tract. These may be anal stenosis with or without an obstructive membrane (see Fig. 11-19, *A* or *B*), frequently with an external fistula to the perineum or vestibule through which meconium is passed.

Intermediate anomalies—rectum is at or below the level of the puborectalis muscle, the anal dimple and external sphincter are positioned normally, but the anal opening is located anteriorly in the perineum. There may be a persistent connection to the genitourinary tract.

High anomalies—rectum ends above the puborectalis muscle. There is absence of internal and external sphincters, and the puborectalis muscle is relatively ineffectual. These anomalies occur almost exclusively in males, where there is usually a rectourethral fistula; a rectovaginal communication is found in females (see Fig. 11-19, *F*). Wide variations are found in high anomalies; these are often associated with maldevelopment of the sacrum, which interferes with innervation to anal and urethral musculature.

orectalis muscle (Box 11-7). A distinction between these categories is important for planning therapy and determining a prognosis (Seashore, 1986).

Pathophysiology

About the seventh week of gestation the future rectum and anus develop from an expanded portion of the caudal hindgut, the *cloaca,* which is subsequently divided by downward growth of a urorectal septum into a urogenital sinus and a rectum. At about the same time the lower urogenital portion has acquired an external opening, whereas the rectum is separated from the exterior by the *anal membrane.* This membrane breaks down by the beginning of the eighth week of gestation to form a continuous patent communication between the outside and the remainder of the gut. Most anorectal malformations result from abnormal partitioning of the cloaca by the urorectal septum.

Diagnostic Evaluation

Checking for patency of the anus and rectum is a routine part of the newborn assessment and includes observation or inquiries regarding the passage of meconium. Inspection of the perineal area reveals absence of an anal opening or the thin, translucent membrane of anal membrane atresia. The appearance of the perineum alone does not accurately predict the level of the lesion. However, complete absence of anal features, a flat perineum, and absence of external sphincter contraction when stimulated generally indicate an intermediate or high lesion. TEF is a common finding in association with anorectal malformations and should be considered in the assessment when an anorectal anomaly is noted.

Digital and endoscopic examination identify constriction or the blind pouch of rectal atresia. Stenosis may not become apparent until 1 year of age or older when the child has a history of difficult defecation, abdominal distention, and ribbonlike stools. Fistulas may not be apparent at birth, but as peristalsis gradually forces the meconium through the fistula, they can be identified by careful examination. A rectourinary fistula is suspected on the basis of meconium in the urine and confirmed by radiographs of contrast media injected through a tiny catheter into the fistula.

Definitive diagnosis of the extent and location of the high lesion is made by radiographic examination. Abdominal ultrasound or tomography may be performed to verify the infant's anatomy. Renal ultrasound and voiding cystourethrography are recommended for the infant with a high lesion to identify or rule out the possibility of associated anomalies of the urinary tract. Further examination is also indicated if there is evidence of urinary tract infection or other symptoms. In addition, cardiac evaluation and skeletal films may be done to rule out other anomalies.

Therapeutic Management

Successful treatment for anal stenosis is generally accomplished by manual dilations. The procedure, begun by the physician, is repeated on a regular basis by the nurses in the hospital and continued at home by the parents, after they are carefully instructed in the technique. An imperforate anal membrane is excised and followed by daily anal dilations.

Reconstruction of an anus in the proper position is the goal of surgical treatment of intermediate anorectal malformations. The most important consideration in the probable success of reconstruction is the level at which the rectum terminates, especially in its relationship to the puborectalis sling of the levator ani muscle. Where the bowel has come through this structure, surgical correction often can be accomplished in the neonatal period by way of an abdominal-perineal pull-through procedure and/or anoplasty.

Infants with high anomalies require a divided sigmoid colostomy in the newborn period. This allows time for the infant to gain weight, for a more leisurely evaluation of the anomaly, and for protection of the GU tract from fecal contamination if a fistula is present. Antibiotics are usually administered prophylactically. Final correction of higher defects is usually postponed for a year. The most common procedure is the posterior sagittal anorectoplasty. When children, after a pull-through procedure, fail to achieve bowel control at a reasonable age, a permanent colostomy may be necessary.

Nursing Considerations

The first nursing responsibility is identification of undetected anorectal malformations. A poorly developed anal dimple, a rounded perineum, or vertebral abnormality suggests a high lesion. A newborn who does not pass a stool within 24 hours of birth requires further assessment, and meconium that appears at an inappropriate orifice is reported. Preoperative care includes diagnostic evaluation, gastrointestinal decompression, and intravenous fluids.

Postoperative nursing care ordinarily presents few problems and is primarily directed toward healing of the anoplasty without infection or other complications. Where the infant has undergone a pull-through procedure with anoplasty, special nursing care involves maintaining the anal area as clean as possible with scrupulous perineal care. Initially there may be continuous passage of stool. There may or may not be a temporary dressing and drain, but when the infant is passing stool, dressings are of little value. The preferred placement is a side-lying prone position with the hips elevated or a supine position with the legs suspended at a 90-degree angle to the trunk to prevent pressure on perineal sutures. Frequent perineal cleansing in a tub and measures to reduce friction on skin are initiated. If skin irritation becomes problematic, an enterostomal therapist should be consulted.

The infant is given regular infant formula as soon as peristalsis returns. In the meantime there may be a nasogastric tube for abdominal decompression and intravenous feedings. Care of the infant with a colostomy involves frequent dressing changes, meticulous skin care, and correct application of a collection device.

Nursing care of children with permanent colostomies is the same as for any child with a colostomy (see Chapter 27).

Family support, discharge planning, and home care. Long-term follow-up is essential for children with high lesions. Following a definitive pull-through procedure, toilet training is delayed. Complete continence is seldom achieved at the usual ages of 3 to 4 years. Bowel habit training, diet modification, and administration of stool softeners help children slowly improve bowel management, but optimum results may not be achieved until later childhood or adolescence. Support and reassurance during the slow progression to normal function are essential, and any type of coercive toilet training is discouraged. Approximately 80% will ultimately achieve normal or at least socially acceptable continence (Seashore, 1986).

Parents are instructed in perineal and wound care or care of the colostomy. Anal dilations may be necessary for some infants. Parents are advised to observe stooling patterns and signs of anal stricture or complications. Information on dietary modifications and/or administration of medications is included in counseling. For infants with high lesions, plans for corrective surgery should be discussed.

BILIARY ATRESIA

Biliary atresia is the obstruction or absence of a portion of the bile ducts. Blockage may be either *intrahepatic,* the absence of bile ducts within the liver, or *extrahepatic,* in which there is absence or obstruction of the main bile passages outside the liver. Numerous variations are encountered, but the most common abnormality is complete atresia of the extrahepatic structures. The cause is unknown. It is generally considered to be a developmental anomaly, but recent evidence implicates a viral infection before or shortly after birth (Glaser, Balistreri, and Morecki, 1984). The predictable course of the disease terminates in irreversible obliteration of the extrahepatic bile ducts.

Clinical Manifestations

Jaundice is usually the earliest evidence of biliary atresia and is the most striking feature of the disorder. It is first observed in the sclera. It may be present at birth but is not usually apparent until the child is 2 to 3 weeks of age. The urine becomes dark and stains the diaper, and the stools are lighter than expected. Hepatomegaly and abdominal distention are common, and splenomegaly occurs later. Poor fat metabolism results in poor weight gain and general failure to thrive. As the disease progresses, the child becomes irritable and difficult to comfort.

Diagnostic Evaluation

No single test or combination of tests is diagnostic. The disease is suspected on the basis of clinical signs, including a steady increase in *conjugated* hyperbilirubinemia. Percutaneous or open surgical liver biopsy with cholangiogram is performed to identify the presence or absence of intrahepatic bile ducts. Presence of intrahepatic bile ducts indicates that the atresia is of extrahepatic origin and amenable to surgical exploration. Hepatobiliary scans and a complete workup for other causes of neonatal jaundice may be undertaken.

Therapeutic Management

The major hope in care of these children is that the condition will benefit from surgery. Surgical reconstruction is possible in about 10% of cases of extrahepatic atresia when the lesion is either a distal atresia with patent proximal hepatic duct or a cystic dilation of ducts adjacent to the hilum of the liver. Surgery is most successful when performed early; therefore diagnosis is urgent.

In the more common atresias there are no patent extrahepatic ducts. In these cases a hepatic portoenterostomy (Kasai procedure) is employed, in which a substitute duct is formed from a segment of jejunum if there are any hepatic duct remnants. The procedure provides effective palliation for some patients; for others complications of progressive liver disease occur despite initially satisfactory bile secretion (Lally and others, 1989).

Liver transplantation has become a more encouraging alternative for children with uncorrectable atresia. The 1-year survival rate has improved from 25% to 75% with the use of the newer immunosuppressive agent, cyclosporine, and low doses of steroids (Iwatsuki and Starzl, 1986). Pettitt, Zitelli, and Rowe (1984) report an 84% survival rate. The recent success with partial liver transplants and those from living donors offers an encouraging alternative to scarce cadaver donors. As a result, liver transplant is rapidly becoming the surgical treatment of choice, although the Kasai procedure is often performed in these children to provide relief and prevent nutritional deficiencies while they are awaiting a donor liver.

Medical management is primarily supportive. It is the method of choice for intrahepatic atresia and supplemental to surgical therapy in extrahepatic atresia. Medical management consists of a high-calorie formula containing fats that can be digested without bile (Pregestimil, Portagen) and water-miscible vitamins. The bile acid–binding drug cholestyramine is sometimes useful to prevent reabsorption of bile from the intestines. However, it is not effective where bile is not excreted into the intestines. Phenobarbital helps reduce irritability and enhances bile flow. A low-salt diet and diuretics may reduce ascites formation.

Nursing Considerations

Nursing care of the infant with biliary atresia is primarily supportive. Initially the infant is not uncomfortable and requires care suited to any infant of the same age. Cool or tepid soaks sometimes help ease the intense itching that accompanies jaundice. Rubbing or massaging the skin promotes vasodilation, which aggravates the itching. As the disease progresses, the accumulation of toxic products causes the child to become irritable, restless, and difficult to comfort. Efforts are extended to allow as much sleep and rest as possible. The child is cared for on awakening and given sedatives and comforting measures as tolerated.

During the diagnostic phase of the illness the nurse assists with tests and procedures as ordered. The child who has undergone exploratory or corrective surgery is given the same care as any infant following abdominal surgery. Infants with the Kasai operation require care of the double stoma and collection, measurement, and replacement of bile via the stomal openings. A modified Kasai procedure eliminates the external stoma and obviates the need for refeeding bile. Parental teaching includes this practice, administration of medications, and observation for signs of cholangitis.

The child who is selected for transplantation is transferred to an institution where the procedure is to be performed. It is an anxious period, as well as one of hope. Families need a great deal of support. The **Children's Liver Foundation, Inc.*** provides educational materials, programs, and support systems for parents of children with liver disease. Other agencies that provide services for children with congenital disabilities are listed in Appendix E.

HERNIAS

A hernia is a protrusion of a portion of an organ or organs through an abnormal opening. The danger from herniation arises when the organ protruding through the opening is constricted to the extent that circulation is impaired or when the protruding organs encroach on and impair the function of other structures. The herniations of concern here are those that protrude through the diaphragm, the abdominal wall, or the inguinal canal. Because they involve the GU tract, inguinal and femoral hernias are discussed in the next section.

*76 South Orange Ave., Suite 202, South Orange, NJ 07079; (201) 761-1111.

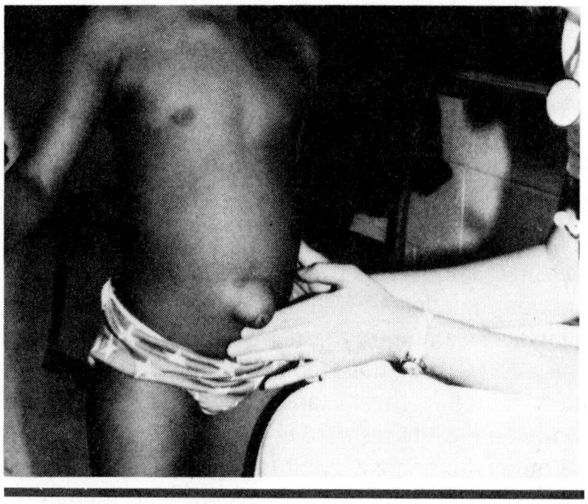

Fig. 11-20. Child with an umbilical hernia.

UMBILICAL HERNIA

Ordinarily the umbilical ring, through which the umbilical blood vessels provide essential elements to the developing fetus, undergoes spontaneous, gradual closure after birth. Incomplete closure of this fascial ring results in the protrusion of portions of omentum and intestine through the opening. The size of the defect varies from less than 1 cm (½ inch) to 4 or 5 cm (about 2 inches) (Fig. 11-20). The hernias are seen as soft swellings or protrusions covered by skin that are readily reducible with the finger, and small defects usually close spontaneously by 3 to 4 years of age. However, very large hernias often persist. Those that have not disappeared by school age require surgical closure. Strangulation or incarceration of herniated bowel is rare but requires immediate surgical intervention.

Nursing Considerations

Because the sight of an umbilical hernia is very disconcerting to parents, they need reassurance regarding the innocuous nature of the defect. Taping or strapping appears to be of no value in expediting closure and may even retard it. The application can also cause troublesome skin irritation; when done improperly, it may cause strangulation.

DIAPHRAGMATIC HERNIA

In congenital diaphragmatic hernia the abdominal contents herniate through the diaphragm into the pleural cavity, seriously compromising respiration. The defect is associated with an exceptionally high mortality and constitutes a surgical emergency in the immediate newborn period.

Pathophysiology

The herniation represents failure of the pleuroperitoneal canal to close completely during embryonic development, which allows various degrees of protrusion of abdominal viscera through the defect into the thoracic cavity. It is not unusual to find most of the abdominal organs (stomach, small intestine, spleen, left lobe of liver, left kidney, and all but the descending colon) in the thorax. The more severe defects occur with herniation through the foramen of Bochdalek; less severe are herniations through the foramen of Morgagni.

Respiration is compromised by hypoplasia and compression of the lung, including airways and blood vessels, on the affected side. Ineffective motion of the leaf of the diaphragm on the affected side interferes with the normal diaphragmatic breathing of the neonate. Respiration is further compromised when the stomach and intestine (generally found within the chest) rapidly become distended with swallowed air as the result of crying. Negative thoracic pressure from crying tends to pull the intestines into the chest and further distends those already there. This increased volume in the chest cavity displaces the mediastinum to the unaffected side to produce a partial collapse of the opposite lung.

Clinical Manifestations

Severe respiratory distress, including dyspnea and cyanosis, is often present at birth, but signs may appear at any time in the neonatal period or even later. There is a 50% to 70% mortality when the signs of the defect are evident at delivery and a 40% mortality when the defect is identified within 24 hours; mortality approaches 0% when signs appear after 24 hours (Ramenofsky, 1986). In addition to dyspnea the infant may display vomiting, signs of severe colicky pain, discomfort after feeding, and constipation. The chest is barrel shaped and the abdomen markedly scaphoid (sunken). Less frequently the defect (usually a Morgagni type) is asymptomatic and is discovered by radiographic examination.

Diagnostic Evaluation

The diagnosis is usually established by radiographic examination, which shows fluid- and air-filled loops of intestine in the affected side of the chest (80% are present on the left side). The mediastinum is shifted to the unaffected side, causing a similar shift in the point of maximum intensity on auscultation. Auscultation also reveals absence of breath sounds on the affected side of the thorax, and bowel sounds may be present. Blood gas and pH determinations are made to assess the status of oxygenation and acidosis.

Therapeutic Management

The affected infant requires immediate respiratory support, which includes positioning with the head and thorax higher than the abdomen and feet to facilitate downward displacement of abdominal organs, nasogastric suction for decompression of the stomach, and conscientious efforts to prevent the infant from crying. Oxygen is provided, but positive-pressure ventilation, if needed, is administered cautiously by endotracheal tube to prevent pneumothorax, a constant danger because of the uneven distribution of intrapulmonary pressures in the hypoplastic, atelectatic, and compressed lung tissue. Low ventilatory pressure with rapid ventilatory rate is preferred; positive end-expiratory pressure is contraindicated (Ramenofsky, 1986).

Intravenous fluids are begun by way of an umbilical artery catheter, metabolic and respiratory acidosis is corrected, and antibiotics are usually administered prophylactically. Traditional management has been early surgical repair of the defect; however, increased survival rates have been reported with surgery delayed following a period of preoperative stabilization (Cartlidge, Mann, and Kapilar, 1986; Sakai and others, 1987). If the infant is to be transported to a special facility, stabilization and transport are accomplished as quickly as possible.

Postoperative management involves continuation of ventilatory therapy, acid-base stabilization, and attention to pulmonary arterial pressure and mediastinal positioning. Right-to-left shunting frequently occurs in these infants through the foramen ovale, through the ductus arteriosus, or within the lung, and all are associated with development of pulmonary hypertension. These complications are managed symptomatically.

Following surgery for severe defects there is usually a period of relative pulmonary stability that lasts up to 18 hours. After this "honeymoon" period the infant often develops progressive pulmonary insufficiency secondary to persistent pulmonary hypertension. The deterioration is the result of several factors, one of which is overexpansion of the normal lungs into the empty space on the affected side created by the undeveloped lung. This causes a shift in the mediastinum, which is mobile in the neonate. Additional factors include circulatory problems secondary to a mediastinal shift and pulmonary infection. Extracorporeal membrane oxygenation (ECMO) is a rescue technique for infants who are unresponsive to conventional medical therapy (see Chapter 10).

Nursing Considerations

Preoperative nursing care is primarily supportive. Upright positioning is maintained, and measures are implemented to decrease crying, such as performing distressing procedures at one time. Oxygen therapy, abdominal decompression, and intravenous fluids are maintained, and the infant is prepared for surgery.

Postoperative care includes the routine observations discussed in the care of the high-risk infant. The infant should be positioned on the affected side to take advantage of gravity, which facilitates expansion of the unaffected lung and reduces the likelihood of overexpansion into the unaffected side. Close observation to detect signs of respiratory embarrassment or fluid and electrolyte imbalances is crucial. The infant is closely monitored for signs of mediastinal shift, pulmonary hypertension, and infection.

Because of the serious nature of the condition and urgency of treatment, the parents are in great need of support and guidance. Because the condition is one of high risk, the interventions outlined for the high-risk infant are appropriate here.

HIATAL HERNIA

Congenital herniations through the normal esophageal hiatus in the newborn are usually of the sliding type. Because the muscular ring of the hiatus is not snug, it permits the cardiac end of the stomach to slide above the diaphragm and back into the abdomen. This produces the symptoms seen with associated incompetent or relaxed cardiac sphincter *(chalasia),* that is, reflux of gastric contents into the esophagus with subsequent regurgitation.

Therapeutic management is directed toward treatment of the esophageal reflux. When conservative management, such as upright posture and feeding modification, is disappointing, the defect is repaired surgically. Nursing considerations are the same as for gastroesophageal reflux (Chapter 33).

ABDOMINAL WALL DEFECTS

Omphalocele and gastroschisis, the most common abdominal wall defects, have been considered for some time to be embryologically distinct disorders. The distinction at birth has been that an omphalocele is a covered defect of the umbilical ring with a sac into which intraabdominal contents may herniate. Gastroschisis is a defect in the anterior abdominal wall, uncovered, and with a normally inserted umbilical cord. This distinction is being questioned (Glick and others, 1985). Because the controversy is unresolved, the two disorders are considered separately in this discussion.

Omphalocele

Omphalocele is a serious congenital malformation in which a variable amount of the abdominal contents protrudes into the base of the umbilical cord. As the embryonic midgut grows and elongates, it projects from the abdomen, which is too small to contain it, into the umbilical cord. This migration takes place from the sixth to the tenth week of fetal life. Normally the intestines return rapidly into the abdomen by the eleventh week of gestation; failure to return produces an omphalocele.

In contrast to an umbilical hernia, the omphalocele is covered only by a translucent sac of amnion to which the umbilical cord inserts. The sac may contain only a small loop of bowel or most of the bowel and other abdominal viscera. If the sac ruptures, the abdominal contents eviscerate through the opening in the abdominal wall. The abdomen is smaller than usual, making replacement of the bowel more difficult. Omphalocele may be associated with other anomalies, such as trisomies 13 and 18, cardiac defects, TEF, imperforate anus, and GU anomalies.

Since the advent of prenatal ultrasonography, an increasing number of these defects are detected before birth. This has created a debate regarding the optimum mode of delivery—vaginal vs surgical. At present the majority favor surgical delivery, especially when the defect is a large one (Pomerance, 1986).

The omphalocele is covered immediately with moist gauze and kept moist until the infant is taken to the operating room. The moist dressing is covered with plastic wrap to avoid loss of heat and moisture. Small lesions are repaired as soon as possible to prevent infection or tissue damage. Larger lesions may require gradual reduction by way of plastic material sewn to the margins of the defect and pulled together at the top to form a chimney, with steady pressure applied to the protruding mass over a course of days to gradually enlarge the intraabdominal space to accommodate the intestinal contents.

Rarely, nonoperative treatment, consisting of repeated application of a cicatrizing or toughening solution to the sac, is used with excessively large omphaloceles; surgical repair is postponed for 6 to 12 months. Management of ruptured omphalocele is similar to that for gastroschisis. Complications include infection, rupture, and intestinal obstruction.

Gastroschisis

Gastroschisis is herniation through a defect of the abdominal wall that permits extrusion of abdominal contents without involving the umbilical cord. The defect is usually located to the right of the intact umbilicus and is not encased in a protective sac. Herniation through the defect can take place prenatally or perinatally. If the evisceration is of long standing, the abdominal cavity will be small and the protruding bowel thickened as a result of poor blood return and irritation from amniotic fluid. The bowel is almost normal and the abdominal cavity adequate in eviscerations that take place just before birth. Major anomalies outside the GI tract are uncommon in children with gastroschisis.

Therapy is directed toward prevention of infection, nutrition, and surgical closure of the defect. A primary closure is preferred but is not always possible. When the abdomen is too small to accommodate the extruded contents, a Silastic pouch is placed over the herniated viscera to contain the bowel and to aid in reduction until surgical closure is attempted (Fig. 11-21). When the bowel has returned to the abdominal cavity with the aid of gravity, the opening is sur-

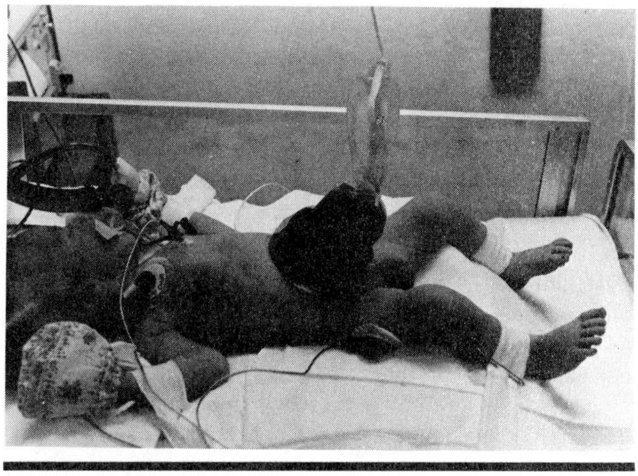

Fig. 11-21. Gastroschisis enclosed in a Silastic pouch.

gically closed. The return may take a few hours to a few days, depending on the size of the abdominal cavity relative to the amount of viscera.

Some of the problems that may be encountered postsurgically when the abdomen is unable to accommodate the viscera are respiratory embarrassment caused by the increased pressure on the diaphragm, decreased venous return to the heart because of pressure on the vena cava, and possible bowel necrosis from excessive crowding and prolonged ileus. If the infant develops respiratory distress, the sutures may need to be released and the pouch replaced until adequate respiratory function can be reinstated.

Nursing Considerations

Nursing care is the same as for any high-risk infant. Infection is a constant threat before surgery, and careful positioning and handling are needed to prevent rupture of the intact omphalocele sac or disturbance of the Silastic bag used for gradual reduction. Viscera should be protected with saline-soaked sponges and Kling dressings wrapped around the defect. Heat and fluid losses from the exposed viscera are major concerns in the preoperative period; therefore thermoregulation is critical, and fluid resuscitation may be massive to compensate for losses. The gastrointestinal tract is decompressed via nasogastric tube before surgery to aid in reduction. Postsurgical care includes particular attention to observation for signs of complications and assessment to detect indications that the replaced bowel is functioning. Nutritional support may be necessary when ileus persists. It may require several weeks for normal function to return.

Family support, discharge planning, and home care. Educational needs of the family depend on the presence of associated anomalies, particularly in the infant with omphalocele. Some infants may require special feeding regimens. If necessary, parents should be aware of possible wound complications, feeding intolerance, or bowel obstruction.

■ DEFECTS OF THE GENITOURINARY TRACT*

External defects of the genitourinary (GU) tract are usually obvious at birth. Several, such as hypospadias, epispadias, and undescended testes (cryptorchidism), do not necessitate immediate repair but may require one or more staged repairs during early childhood. Others, such as exstrophy of the bladder, require initial intervention at birth with repeated medical and surgical treatment for several years. The anatomic location of these defects frequently causes more psychologic concern to children and parents than does the actual condition or treatment. Hernias are common in young children and are usually repaired as soon as diagnosis is established.

*Cindy Hylton Rushton, R.N.C, M.S.N., assisted in the revision of this section.

PSYCHOLOGIC PROBLEMS RELATED TO GENITAL SURGERY

It has long been observed that hospitalization and separation can have a traumatic effect on children. Also, the location and site of the defect and the need for repeated surgery cause some children more emotional concern than does the actual defect. Observations have also shown that the timing of medical and surgical procedures has wide-ranging effects on later adult behavior. Surgery involving sexual organs can be particularly disruptive to children, especially preschoolers fearing punishment, retaliation, body mutilation, or castration. More emotional disturbances have been noted in children who had GU surgery than in those who had ear, nose, or throat surgery (Blotcky and Grossman, 1978), and profound problems with concepts of body image and sexuality have developed.

There are four areas that appear to influence the reaction of children to genital surgery (Manley, 1982): (1) separation anxiety, (2) the hospital experience, (3) the anxiety of the parents, and (4) body image and castration anxiety. The problem of separation anxiety has been diminished through short-term hospitalization, ambulatory surgery, and unrestricted visiting by parents. The same practices have also reduced the effects of the hospital experience (see Chapter 26). It is the presence of the attachment object(s) that is most important for reducing anxiety. Children are less distressed in a strange environment when a familiar person is present to provide a secure base for their adaptive responses. The child is particularly vulnerable at approximately 15 to 22 months of age, when separation is incomplete and the child requires frequent reunion with a parent.

The body image of a child is largely derived as a result of feedback from the primary caregivers, and parental anxiety regarding an acceptable physical appearance and adequate future sexual competency is readily communicated to the affected child. Therefore children with birth defects are at risk for developing a distorted body image that reflects the caregivers' subtly communicated evaluation of their bodies (Schultz, Klykylo, and Wacksman, 1983). The trend toward early repair of visible genital defects is based in large part on these psychologic variables. The earlier a repair can be achieved, the more likely the development of a normal body image. Also, the earlier the repair, the shorter the time that the parents must look at the defect and risk transferring their anxiety and concern to the child.

During the years from 3 to 6, the phallico-oedipal period, children show a strong interest and concern about the genital area, sex differences, and genital normality or its lack. This is especially true if there is an older male sibling or playmate with whom to make comparisons. It is also a time when children are frightened of what they perceive to be threats to their body, especially the sex organs. They also view any untoward happening as a punishment for real or imagined wrongdoing or unacceptable sexual feelings, such as masturbation, sex play, or erotic feelings. Surgical repair is recommended before the development of these fears and anxieties. Postoperative withdrawal and aggressive behavior have been observed in 2- to 6-year-old boys who had hypospadias repair (Lepore and Kesler, 1979).

PHIMOSIS

Phimosis is a narrowing or stenosis of the preputial opening of the foreskin that prevents retraction of the foreskin over the glans penis. It is a normal finding in infants and very young boys and usually disappears as the child grows and the distal prepuce dilates. Occasionally the narrowing obstructs the flow of urine, resulting in a dribbling stream or even ballooning of the foreskin with accumulated urine during voiding.

Inflammation or infection of the phimotic foreskin occurs occasionally and is managed as any other inflammation or infection. Severe phimosis is treated surgically by circumcision.

Nursing Considerations

Proper hygiene of the phimotic foreskin in infants and young boys consists of external cleansing during routine bathing. The foreskin should not be forcibly retracted, because it may create scarring, which can prevent future retraction. Furthermore, retraction of the tight foreskin can result in paraphimosis, a condition in which the retracted foreskin cannot be replaced in its normal position over the glans. This causes edema and venous congestion created by constriction by the tight band of foreskin—a urologic emergency that requires immediate evaluation.

INGUINAL HERNIA

Inguinal hernias account for approximately 80% of all hernias and are the most common surgical procedures performed in infancy (with the possible exception of circumcision). Inguinal hernias occur more frequently in boys (90%) than in girls; femoral hernias occur more often in females but are uncommon in children.

Pathophysiology

Inguinal hernia is derived from persistence of all or part of the processus vaginalis, the tube of peritoneum that precedes the testicle through the inguinal canal into the scrotum during the eighth month of gestation. Following descent of the testicle, the proximal portion of the processus vaginalis normally atrophies and closes, whereas the distal portion forms the tunica vaginalis, which envelops the testicle in the scrotum. When the upper portion fails to atrophy, the abdominal fluid or an abdominal structure can be forced into it, creating a palpable bulge or mass. The persistent sac may end at any point along the inguinal canal; it may stop at the inguinal ring or extend all the way into the scrotum (Fig. 11-22). The hernial sac is present at birth but does not usually become apparent until the infant is able to

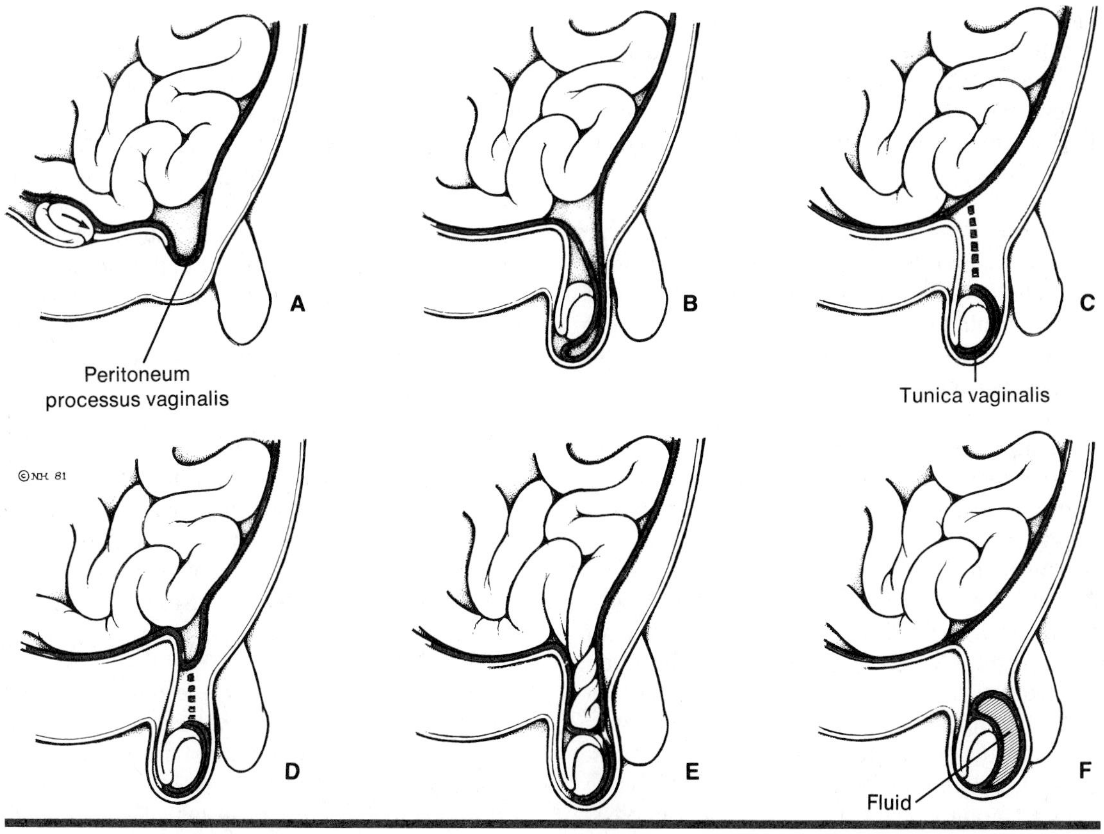

Fig. 11-22. Development of inguinal hernias. **A** and **B,** Prenatal migration of processus vaginalis. **C,** Normal. **D,** Partially obliterated processus vaginalis. **E,** Hernia. **F,** Hydrocele.

build up sufficient intraabdominal pressure to open the sac, usually at 2 to 3 months of age. Since the inguinal canal is short, hernias occur relatively early.

Clinical Manifestations

This very common defect is asymptomatic unless the abdominal contents are forced into the patent sac. Most often it appears as a painless inguinal swelling that varies in size. It disappears during periods of rest or is reducible by gentle compression; it appears when the infant cries or strains or when the older child strains, coughs, or stands for a long period. The defect can be palpated as a thickening of the cord in the groin, and the "silk glove" sign can be elicited by rubbing together the sides of the empty hernial sac.

Sometimes the herniated loop of intestine becomes partially obstructed, producing variable symptoms that may include fretfulness and irritability, tenderness, anorexia, abdominal distention, and difficulty in defecating. Occasionally the loop of bowel becomes incarcerated (irreducible), with symptoms of complete intestinal obstruction that, left untreated, will progress to strangulation and gangrene. Incarceration occurs more often in infants under 10 months of age and is more common in girls.

Therapeutic Management

The treatment for hernias is prompt, elective surgical repair in healthy infants and children as soon as the defect is diagnosed. Since there is a significant incidence of bilateral involvement, many physicians advocate exploration of both sides. This practice of exploration remains controversial, however. It is preferable to attempt reduction of a recently incarcerated hernia in order that surgery can be delayed to allow the injured tissues to recover somewhat, but irreducible or strangulated hernias are treated as emergencies.

Nursing Considerations

Both infants and children tolerate surgery very well. There is usually no restriction placed on their activities, and it is not uncommon for the child to be discharged from the hospital on the day of surgery. Every attempt is made to keep the wound clean and reasonably dry. With infants and small children who are not yet toilet trained, the wound is left without a dressing. Changing diapers as soon as they become damp helps reduce the chance of irritation or infection of the incision, or the child may be left undiapered. It is unnecessary to apply a urine-collecting device.

Parents are instructed to give the child sponge baths instead of tub baths for 2 to 5 days and to change diapers more frequently than usual during the day and once or twice during the night. There are no restrictions placed on the infant's or toddler's activity, but older children are cautioned against lifting, pushing, wrestling and fighting, bicycle riding, and athletics for about 3 weeks (Gans and Austin, 1986). School children are permitted to attend classes as soon as they are comfortable but are excused from physical education activities for the same length of time as specified for restricting physical activity.

If surgery is postponed because of acute illness, failure to thrive, exposure to communicable disease, or a temporary family psychologic problem, the parents need to be taught the signs of incarcerated hernia, simple measures to reduce it (a warm bath, avoidance of upright positioning, and comfort measures to reduce crying), and where to call for assistance if relief is not obtained in a reasonably short time.

FEMORAL HERNIA

Femoral hernias are rare in children. When they occur, there is a higher incidence in girls than in boys. The disorder is suspected from a swelling in the groin area associated with severe pain. Treatment and management are the same as for inguinal hernia. Strangulation is a frequent complication.

HYDROCELE

Hydrocele is the presence of fluid in the persistent processus vaginalis and is the result of the same developmental process as inguinal hernia (Fig. 11-22, *F*). When the upper segment of the processus vaginalis has been obliterated but the tunica vaginalis still contains peritoneal fluid, this is called a *noncommunicating hydrocele.* This type of hydrocele is common in newborns and often subsides spontaneously as fluid is gradually absorbed.

A *communicating hydrocele* is one in which the processus vaginalis remains open and into which peritoneal fluid may be forced by intraabdominal pressure and gravity. The length of the hydrocele depends on the length of the processus vaginalis and may extend into the tunica vaginalis within the scrotum. The hydrocele is asymptomatic except for a palpable bulge in the inguinal or scrotal areas. Unlike a hernia, the hydrocele may not be reducible and may not be produced by a sudden increase in intraabdominal pressure (such as straining). The scrotum appears to be larger after an active day and smaller in the morning. Since a communicating hydrocele represents a patent processus vaginalis, it can predispose to herniation; therefore, surgical repair is indicated if spontaneous resolution does not take place by 1 year of age.

Nursing Considerations

The nursing care of the infant with a hydrocele is essentially the same as that for inguinal hernia. Parents are advised that there is often temporary swelling and discoloration of the scrotum that resolves spontaneously.

CRYPTORCHIDISM (CRYPTORCHISM)

Cryptorchidism is failure of one or both testes to descend normally through the inguinal canal into the scrotum. Absence of testes within the scrotum can be the result of (1) *undescended (cryptorchid)* testes, (2) *retractile* testes, or (3) *anorchia* (absence of testes). Undescended testes can be categorized further according to location (Box 11-8). The incidence of cryptorchidism is 3% to 4% of full-term infants and falls to approximately 1% at age 1 year. The rate does

Box 11-8 CLASSIFICATION OF CRYPTORCHID TESTES

Abdominal—located proximal to the internal inguinal ring
Canalicular—located between the internal and external inguinal rings
Ectopic—located outside the normal pathways of descent between the abdominal cavity and the scrotum

not change in the years that follow (reported in Saggese and others, 1989).

Pathophysiology

Normally the testes descend from the abdomen, where they develop, into the scrotum during the seventh to ninth month of gestation. The progress is aided by the gubernaculum, a mass of tissue containing smooth muscle that is attached to the lower pole of the testes. The process is poorly understood, and the role of hormones in facilitating and/or initiating the descent is also unclear. The testes descend to the scrotum behind the processus vaginalis, a peritoneal outpocketing that retains a communication with the peritoneal cavity and projects down through various muscle and fascial planes before the testes enter the inguinal canal (see Fig. 11-22, *A* to *D*).

Normally the upper part of the processus vaginalis atrophies and closes, and the lower part is pinched off to form the tunica vaginalis of the testes. Cryptorchidism occurs when one or both testes fail to descend through the inguinal canal. The descent can be arrested at any point along its normal path. Congenital inguinal hernias frequently accompany the defect. *Ectopic testis* is a testis that has progressed normally through the inguinal canal but, after passing through the external inguinal ring, has become lodged in superficial tissue of the abdominal wall, upper thigh, or perineum. The role of androgens in promoting testicular descent remains uncertain and controversial (Koyle, Rajfer, and Ehrlich, 1988).

Retractile testes are normally descended testes that are pulled back into the inguinal canal as a result of a hyperactive cremasteric reflex. The cremasteric reflex is very active after 6 months of age and peaks by 4 to 5 years. This reflex (the drawing up of the scrotum and testicle when the skin over the front and inside of the thigh is stimulated) is particularly sensitive to touch and cold.

Clinical Manifestations

Undescended testes are rarely a cause of discomfort. The entire scrotum, or one side of it, appears smaller than normal and incompletely developed, an observation made by concerned parents who often bring the child for medical evaluation.

Diagnostic Evaluation

It is important to differentiate the true undescended testis from the more common retractile testis. Retractile testes can be "milked" or pushed back into the scrotum, but truly undescended ones cannot. For examination the cremasteric reflex can be obviated by placing the child in a squatting position or by applying firm finger pressure on the external ring before palpating the abdomen or genitalia (see Fig. 7-48).

NURSING TIP: TESTICULAR EXAMINATION

An undescended testis is usually smaller and softer than its descended mate.
A well-developed rugous scrotum usually indicates normal testicular descent (may be confused by presence of a hydrocele or inguinal hernia).
A retractile testis is usually bilateral (the cremasteric reflex is equally brisk on both sides).
A testicle can usually be distinguished from a lymph node by its elastic nature. A testicle is mobile and can be massaged down into the scrotum, although it will spring back into the canal.
Application of soap, cornstarch, or talcum powder to the tip of the examiner's fingers facilitates massaging the inguinal canal.

Undescended testes may be felt along the inguinal canal, but those in the abdominal cavity usually cannot. Ultrasonography, tomography, and laparoscopy are sometimes employed to verify cryptorchidism in children undergoing orchiopexy. See Nursing Tip for suggestions to employ in diagnostic examination.

There have been recent reports of undescended testes in children who had been found to have normally descended testes (acquired undescended testis) (Schiffer and others, 1987). Although acquired undescended testes are relatively uncommon, evaluation of the testes should continue to be a part of the routine physical assessment.

Therapeutic Management

A retractile testis that can be manipulated into the scrotum will eventually assume a satisfactory scrotal position without medical or surgical intervention. The diagnosis is not made at a single examination, and parents are asked if they have observed the testes in the scrotum at some time. If so, the anomaly probably represents the retractile variety and the parents can be reassured. By 1 year of age the cryptorchid testes will descend spontaneously in approximately 75% of cases in both term and preterm infants (Penny, 1986). In contrast true undescended testes rarely descend spontaneously after 1 year of age.

Some authorities favor a trial of human chorionic gonadotropin (HCG) therapy in older children. This requires a series of injections over a few weeks. Recent studies that excluded retractile testes report a success rate of less than 30% with HCG therapy (Rajfer and others, 1986). If the testes do not descend spontaneously, orchiopexy is performed before the child's second birthday, preferably between 1 and 2 years of age. Surgical repair is done to (1) prevent damage to the undescended testicle by exposure to the higher degree of body heat in the undescended location, (2) decrease the incidence of tumor formation, which is higher in undescended testicles, (3) avoid trauma and torsion, (4) close the processus vaginalis, and (5) prevent the cosmetic and psychologic handicap of an empty scrotum. Because of increased propensity toward neoplastic changes (even after orchiopexy), cryptorchid testes are better observed in the scrotal position.

The timing of the surgery is important, as it is in any genital surgery. The repair is not attempted in the first year unless there is an accompanying hernia. Fewer psychologic effects and a higher rate of fertility may be achieved when repair takes place at an early age. Having both testes in the scrotum by school age prevents psychologic problems related to body image and peer group embarrassment, since the empty scrotum is smaller in size and altered in shape.

In the routine procedure for undescended testes, the testes are brought down into the scrotum and secured in that position without tension or torsion. A simple orchiopexy for a palpable testis can usually be performed in an outpatient surgical unit without the need for overnight hospitalization. Intraabdominal testes require considerable surgical skill because of technical problems resulting from variations in the length of the spermatic cord, and overnight hospitalization may be necessary.

In most cases the family can be reassured of normal function in adulthood; however, untreated children are at high risk for developing testicular cancer eventually.

Nursing Considerations

The postoperative nursing care is directed toward prevention of infection and instructing parents in home care of the child. Infection is prevented by carefully cleansing the operative site of stool and urine. Observation of the wound for complications and activity restrictions are discussed. Parents are concerned about the future fertility of the child. Therefore the prognosis for fertility is determined, and the family is counseled regarding this eventuality and the optimum time for discussing the probabilities with the child—ideally as a part of sex education.

HYPOSPADIAS

Hypospadias refers to a condition in which the urethral opening is located below the glans penis or anywhere along the ventral surface of the penile shaft (Fig. 11-23). In very mild cases the meatus is just below the tip of the penis. In the most severe malformations the meatus is located on the perineum between the halves of the scrotum. Chordee, or ventral curvature of the penis, results from the replacement of normal skin with a fibrous band of tissue and usually accompanies more severe forms of hypospadias. In addition, the foreskin is usually absent ventrally and, when combined with chordee, gives the organ a hooded and crooked appearance (Fig. 11-24). In severe cases the altered appearance may leave the sex in doubt at birth, since the perineal position of the meatus may be mistaken for a female urethra. Since undescended testes may also be present, the small penis may appear to be an enlarged clitoris. In any case of ambiguous genitalia, further study, such as chromosomal analysis, is essential.

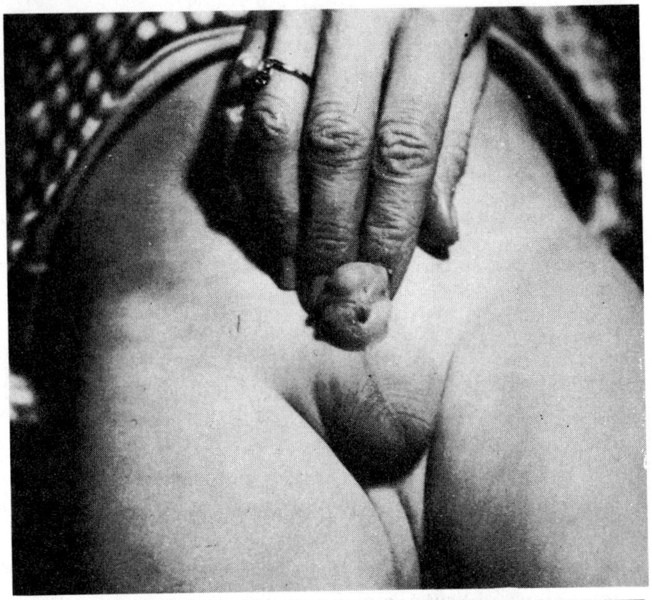

Fig. 11-23. Hypospadias.
Courtesy M.C. Gleason, M.D., San Diego, CA. From Ingalls, A.J., and Salerno, M.C.: Maternal and child health nursing, ed. 6, St. Louis, 1987, Mosby–Year Book, Inc.

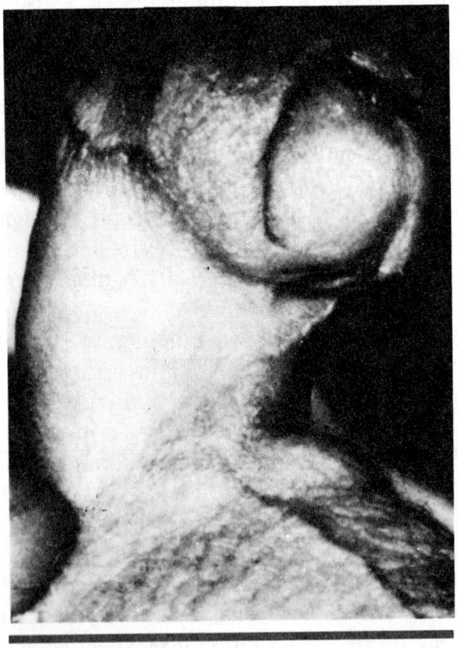

Fig. 11-24. Hypospadias with significant chordee.
From Shirkey, H.C.: Pediatric therapy, ed. 6, St. Louis, 1980, Mosby–Year Book, Inc.

Surgical Correction

The principal objectives in surgical correction are (1) to enable the child to void in the standing position by voluntarily directing the stream in the usual manner, (2) to improve the physical appearance of the genitalia for psychologic reasons, and (3) to produce a sexually adequate organ. The procedure involves releasing the chordee (when present), extending the length of the urethra, and constructing a new meatal opening. Since the prepuce is valuable skin for the reconstructive surgery, circumcision should not be done on these infants.

A mild defect without chordee is usually corrected for psychologic and cosmetic reasons. When the meatus is located on the glans penis, no intervention may be required except if chordee is present or there is upward deflection of the urinary stream. In most instances the surgical repair can be accomplished with one-stage procedures, even as outpatient surgery. When hypospadias is more severe, repair often requires more than one surgical procedure to progressively extend the length of the urethra.

The preferred time for surgical repair is 6 to 18 months, before the child has developed body image and castration anxiety. Occasionally a short course of testosterone is administered preoperatively to achieve additional penile size to facilitate the surgery. Microscopic optical magnification and delicate instruments are used during surgery. Sometimes repairs for more severe cases of hypospadias may result in fistulas and strictures, necessitating additional surgical intervention.

Nursing Considerations

Preparation of parents and child for the type of procedure to be done and the expected cosmetic result helps avert later problems. Frequently parents are informed of what is to be surgically corrected but are not advised of what to expect as a reasonable consequence. As a result they are greatly disappointed to see a physically imperfect penis. If children are old enough to understand what is occurring, they are also prepared for the operation and the expected outcome.

Hypospadias repair may require some type of urinary diversion to promote optimum healing and to maintain the position and patency of the newly formed urethra. Following repair of more severe hypospadias the child is often placed under a bed cradle and immobilized with arm and leg restraints. Restraints can be removed periodically when the child is awake and under supervision, and appropriate diversional activities provided. Sedation may be required for the excessively irritable or restless child, and pain may be controlled with analgesics. Parental rooming-in is recommended to reduce the child's anxiety.

Parents are taught to care for the indwelling catheter or stent and irrigation technique if indicated. They need to know how to empty the urine bag and how to avoid kinking, twisting, or blockage of the catheter or stent. Often the child is discharged with a catheter or stent dripping directly into the diaper. In older children a urine collection device can be used. Parents are taught how to tape the drainage bag to the leg to allow the child to be mobile and to *never* clamp off a catheter. An extra bag is sent home with the family in case of tears or leakage. The family is advised to encourage the child to increase fluid intake. Twice-daily bathing is recommended, as is loose clothing. Straddle toys, sandboxes, swimming, and rough activities are avoided until allowed by the surgeon.

EPISPADIAS

Epispadias is a rare defect in which the meatal opening is located on the dorsal surface of the penis. As in hypospadias, the defect can occur in differing degrees of severity. The treatment is surgical and usually includes penile and urethral lengthening plus bladder neck reconstruction for continence when necessary. The nursing considerations are similar to those discussed for hypospadias.

EXSTROPHY OF BLADDER

Exstrophy of the bladder is an obvious and serious congenital defect that occurs three times more frequently in males than in females (Fig. 11-25). There is no familial tendency, but it rarely occurs in siblings. There are varying degrees of the defect.

Pathophysiology

Exstrophy results from failure of the abdominal wall and underlying structures, including the ventral wall of the bladder, to fuse in utero. As a result the lower urinary tract is exposed and the everted bladder appears bright red through the abdominal opening. This is accompanied by a constant seepage of urine from the exposed ureteral orifices, making the area malodorous and susceptible to infection. The constant accumulation of urine on the surrounding skin pro-

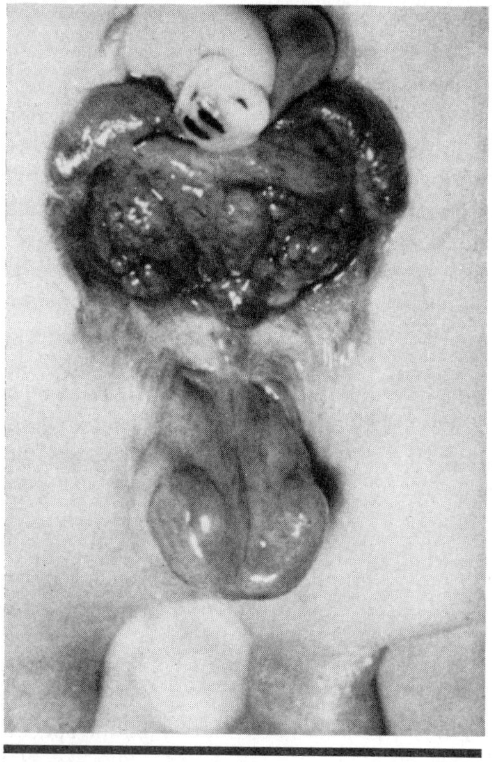

Fig. 11-25. Exstrophy of bladder.
Courtesy E.S. Tank, M.D., Division of Urology, University of Oregon Health Sciences Center, Portland, OR.

duces tissue ulceration and further infection. Progressive renal damage from infection and obstruction may terminate in renal failure if left untreated.

In males the defect is almost always associated with epispadias and may include other problems, such as undescended testes, a short penis, or inguinal hernia. The sexual handicap in males may be severe because the penis protrudes inadequately. In females the genitalia may be affected, with a cleft or bifid clitoris, completely separated labia, and absent vagina. In either sex, separation of the pubic bones causes difficulty in walking, such as a waddling gait.

Therapeutic Management

The objectives of treatment include (1) preservation of renal function, (2) attainment of urinary control, (3) adequate reconstructive repair for psychologic benefit, and (4) improvement of sexual function, particularly in males. Closure of the bladder is ideally accomplished within the first 48 hours of life when the circulating maternal hormones allow the pelvis to be approximated anteriorly without the need for iliac osteotomies. To promote optimum healing, the infant is usually maintained in traction or elastic external compression for a few weeks until adequate union of the separated pubis takes place.

Final repair is completed before school age. Essentially all patients with exstrophy have vesicoureteral reflux that requires antireflux surgery, usually accompanied by bladder neck reconstruction in an attempt to produce urinary continence. These initial procedures are ordinarily performed at 2½ to 3 years of age, and penile lengthening, release of dorsal chordee, and urethral construction with advancement of the urinary meatus at about 4 to 6 years of age.

In females the urethroplasty and other reconstruction are performed at the same time as the antiincontinence procedure, but vaginoplasty is delayed until puberty. Both boys and girls in whom surgery is delayed may require a temporary urinary diversion procedure. Those with complications or continued problems with continence are candidates for an artificial genitourinary sphincter or antirefluxing intestinal diversion, such as ureteral sigmoid implant, bilateral ureterostomy, or ileal conduit.

Nursing Considerations

Physical care of the unrepaired defect includes meticulous hygiene of the bladder area to prevent infection and excoriation of the surrounding tissue. A sterile nonadherent dressing is placed over the exposed bladder area to prevent infection and to keep the diaper from adhering to the mucosa. An ointment may be prescribed for the surrounding skin to protect it from the constantly draining urine. If external compression is used, the skin is inspected periodically for evidence of pressure necrosis.

Other aspects of preoperative care are similar to those for any major abdominal surgery. Since a routine urinalysis is part of most admission procedures, a urine specimen can be obtained by allowing urine to drip into a container by holding the child prone over a basin or by aspirating some urine directly from the bladder area into a medicine dropper or syringe. If a sterile specimen is needed for evaluation of existing infection, the former procedure is preferable, but a sterile container must be used. A mechanical and/or bowel preparation may be required.

Postoperative nursing care following bladder neck reconstruction and antireflux surgery (ureteral reimplantation) includes routine wound care and careful monitoring of urine output from the bladder and/or ureteral drainage tubes. Care following a penile lengthening, chordee release, and urethral reconstruction is similar to care following hypospadias repair.

In addition to routine postsurgical care, nursing following a continent diversion includes wound care, observation of nasogastric suction (surgery requires bowel resection), and measurement and observation of urinary output. In most cases a continent urinary diversion can be created. Regular emptying of the urinary reservoir by clean intermittent catheterization is needed but preferable to permanent urinary conduits, which require a drainage appliance. Therefore permanent urinary conduits are rarely performed.

Family support and prognosis. One of the most devastating aspects of exstrophy of the bladder is its gross appearance. Although the actual physical care is not difficult, it is not easy for parents to assume responsibility for what to them seems an enormous task because of the emotional impact of the defect.

Parents and child should be instructed regarding a realistic outcome of surgery, since unrealistic expectations of the cosmetic and functional result may leave them very disappointed and discouraged. When possible, continuous care by one nurse helps the family adjust to all aspects of recovery. As difficult as it was for parents to adjust to the defect at the time of the child's birth, it may be equally disturbing for them to accept the fact that surgical closure does not ensure normal urination and that urinary diversion may be necessary.

The prospect of a permanent urinary diversion procedure provokes powerful emotional responses. Parents often worry about the child's sexual adjustment, even though they may not voice such thoughts. Part of the nursing admission history is directed toward evaluating the parents' and child's expectation of the surgical repair, knowledge of the possibility of eventual urinary diversion, and feelings concerning this permanent change in body function.

It is not unusual for parents to be ambivalent in their feelings toward surgical creation of a urinary diversion, especially if they have become accustomed to the general care, which for infants differs little from diapering an unaffected child. In such situations it is good to discuss the long-range advantages of a permanent urinary diversion in contrast to the ever-present danger of infection and kidney damage and the constant inconvenience of seeping urine. A well-fitting ileostomy bag allows the child almost unrestricted freedom in activities enjoyed by other children and results in no major alteration in toileting, except emptying the bag at periodic intervals. This is extremely important to older children and adolescents, who want to be accepted as one of the group and deplore any stigma of being different.

When the infant is discharged with an unrepaired defect, ordinarily diapers are placed over the defect in the usual manner. Diapers are changed frequently to prevent infection, ulceration, and odor and after a bowel movement to prevent contamination of the exposed area. General infant care remains unchanged except for sponge baths rather than immersion in water. A public health referral is an important component of discharge planning, and ideally home visits should begin immediately after the infant's release from the hospital.

Even with improved reconstructive surgery for these patients, substantial psychologic support and guidance are needed to help them adjust to their fears of inadequate penile size, ugliness of genitalia, potential inability to procreate, and rejection by peers, especially the opposite sex. Ongoing discussion groups for parents and children are particularly useful in promoting resolution of these fears and allowing for optimum psychologic adjustment, particularly during adolescence.

OBSTRUCTIVE UROPATHY

Structural or functional abnormalities of the urinary system that obstruct the normal flow of urine can produce renal disorders. When there is interference with urine flow, the collecting system above the obstruction causes *hydronephrosis* (the collection of urine in the renal pelvis to the point of cyst formation from the distention) with eventual pressure destruction to renal parenchyma, although the dilating ureters form a reservoir that reduces the effect on the kidneys for a long time.

Obstruction may be congenital or acquired, unilateral or bilateral, complete or incomplete, and the manifestations acute or chronic. The obstruction can occur at any level of the upper or lower urinary tract (Fig. 11-26). Partial obstruction may not be symptomatic unless there is a water or solute diuresis. Boys are affected more commonly than girls, and malformations should be suspected when patients have some other congenital defects (e.g., prune belly syndrome, chromosome anomalies, hypospadias, anorectal malformations, and aural defects).

Pathophysiology

The pathologic changes depend on the location and nature of the defect, the site of obstruction, the duration of the obstruction, and complications such as infection or urinary calculi. With hydronephrosis, glomerular filtration ceases when intrapelvic pressure equals the filtration pressure in glomerular capillaries. However, a pressure gradient usually is established because of some flow beyond the obstruction as a result of periodic relaxation of ureteral wall musculature. There is also an exchange of solutes and water between the pooled urine in the renal pelvis and fluid in the adjoining tissues and fluid compartments (such as interstitial fluid in the pelvic wall and inner kidney medulla), resulting from an intrarenal vascular adjustment caused by a corresponding increase in peritubular capillary pressure.

Damage to distal nephrons in chronic uropathy alters the

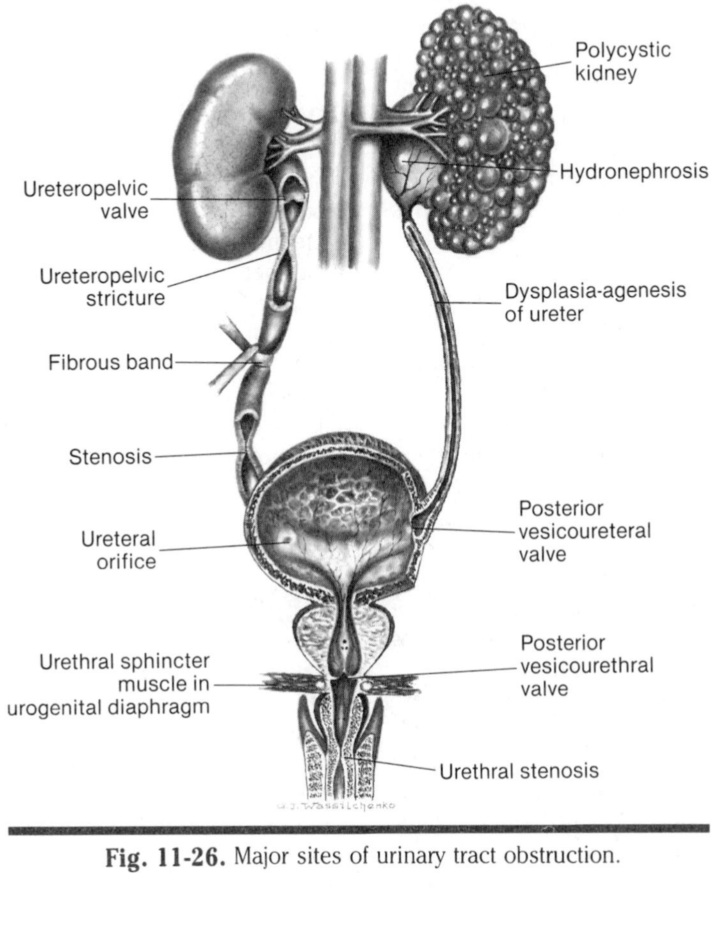

Fig. 11-26. Major sites of urinary tract obstruction.

ability to concentrate urine, contributing to increased urine flow and metabolic acidosis occurring from decreased excretion of acid secondary to impaired ability of the distal nephron to secrete hydrogen ions. Partial obstruction results in progressive loss of renal function as a result of irreversible damage to the nephrons. Pooled urine serves as a medium for bacterial growth; therefore, urinary tract infections further increase the extent of renal damage.

Clinical Manifestations

The clinical manifestations depend on whether the obstruction is acute or chronic, partial or complete, and the extent of complications (e.g., infection). There may be pain or strangury (slow and painful urination, drop by drop) and hematuria (if caused by calculi). The type and location of pain are related to the area of obstruction (e.g., abdominal, flank, suprapubic, or radiating to the testicle or inguinal region).

Chronic obstruction may cause polyuria and polydipsia as a result of inability to concentrate urine, anemia caused by renal damage that impairs the secretion of erythropoietin, failure to thrive, unexplained febrile episodes caused by urinary infection, frequent voiding, weak or forceful urinary stream, and daytime and nocturnal enuresis. A full bladder and/or enlarged kidney may be evident on examination of the abdomen (Kaplan, 1983).

Diagnostic Evaluation

Laboratory examination reveals findings of acute or chronic renal failure. A voiding cystoureterogram may demonstrate the presence of posterior ureteral valves or vesicoureteral reflux, and ultrasonography may help identify and localize the site of obstruction. Prenatal diagnosis and postnatal screening for urinary tract abnormalities by ultrasonography is advocated by some authorities (Elder and Duckett, 1988; Helin and Persson, 1986; Steinhart and others, 1988) and is being used with increasing frequency. Early identification of affected infants permits early management of abnormalities that otherwise may not be recognized until later in life after irreversible renal damage.

Therapeutic Management

Early diagnosis and surgical correction or bypass procedures, such as ileal conduit or cutaneous ureterostomy, that divert the flow of urine are essential in order to prevent progressive renal damage. Often a percutaneous nephrostomy tube or tubes are inserted through the skin and underlying tissues into the renal pelvis to relieve intrarenal pressure until an alternative diversion is established. Medical complications of acute or chronic renal failure and/or infection are managed as described for those disorders.

Prognosis. The prognosis depends on the type of obstruction, the degree of irreversible renal damage, presence of renal dysplasia, the age at which the diagnosis was established, and the severity of complications. Despite the improvements in corrective surgery, some patients develop renal failure, which may evolve over a highly variable period of time that can extend into adulthood. Renal failure can result from hypoplasia-dysplasia, pyelonephritic scarring, and other proposed mechanisms that cause progressive nephron loss (Warshaw, Hymes, and Woodard, 1982). Careful follow-up of children should extend throughout childhood and adolescence, especially when any degree of renal insufficiency is present.

Nursing Considerations

Nursing goals in urinary tract obstruction include helping to identify cases, assisting with diagnostic procedures, and caring for children with complications (described elsewhere). Preparing parents and children for procedures is a major nursing responsibility, especially preparation for urinary diversion procedures (see Preparation for Procedures, Chapter 27).

Parents and children need emotional support and counseling during the lengthy management of these disorders. Parents are the primary target during infancy and very early childhood when most reparative surgery is performed. They will need assistance in managing the apparatus that accompanies many temporary and permanent repair procedures. Many children are discharged with ureteral drainage systems in place that must be protected from damage, and the danger of infection is a constant concern. Parents are taught to care for the equipment and recognize the signs of possible obstruction or infection within the system (see Discharge Planning and Home Care, Chapter 26).

Children with external diversional systems will need psychologic support and guidance, especially as they reach adolescence and body image concerns assume more prominence. Those with progressive renal deterioration may face the prospect of dialysis and/or transplantation and the emotional aspects that accompany these procedures.

ABERRANT SEXUAL DEVELOPMENT

The birth of a child with ambiguous genitalia is a situation that constitutes a crisis quite different from that of many other congenital anomalies. Uncertain sex is a potential lifetime social tragedy for the child and family. Furthermore, the electrolyte disturbances that accompany conditions in which sex is doubtful can be life threatening. Thus the problem of appropriate sex must be solved quickly and accurately and requires no less speed and skill than life-threatening anomalies such as tracheoesophageal fistula. There are studies that can be carried out during the first few days of life that help guide those involved in making a correct gender choice. Even a brief delay in gender assignment can generate rumors that can be a source of distress to a child and family for years.

Etiology

Genetic sex is determined at the time of conception and depends on whether the ovum is fertilized by a sperm bearing an X chromosome or one bearing a Y chromosome. The phenotypic evidence of sex depends on whether subsequent processes proceed normally: differentiation of primitive gonads, differentiation and development of internal duct systems, and differentiation and development of external genitalia. The normal order of events can be altered by abnormalities of the chromosomal complement, defects of embryogenesis, or biochemical (hormonal) abnormalities. Disturbances in any of these processes will lead to abnormal sexual development evidenced by the presence of ambiguous genitalia at birth.

Normal sexual development. For the first 6 weeks of life the developing embryo is morphologically neutral, neither male nor female. The primitive, bipotential (able to form either a testicle or an ovary) gonad consists of an outer layer, the cortex, and an inner medulla. Differentiation into testes and ovary takes place during the seventh and eighth weeks of gestation. At this time, in the male the medullary portion develops and the cortical zone regresses; in the female the cortex is preserved while the medulla regresses. Active factors from the male testes cause the müllerian duct system to regress. Without these factors the primitive gonad has an inherent tendency to feminize. The embryonic ovary develops in the absence of male hormone stimulation.

The final stage of sexual development is differentiation of the external genitalia, which in the early embryo consists of a urogenital sinus, two lateral labioscrotal swellings, and an anteriorly situated genital tubercle. Depending on the presence or absence of male hormones, the genital tubercle differentiates into a penis or a clitoris. In response to testicular androgens, the labiosacral folds fuse to form a scrotum and ventral skin of the penis; the urethral folds form the perineal and penile urethra. Without the influence of masculinizing secretions, the urethral folds do not fuse and instead become the labia minora, the labiosacral folds remain unfused to separate into the labia majora, and the urogenital sinus differentiates into a lower vagina and the vaginal and urethral openings (Fig. 11-27).

Abnormal sexual development. Disturbances in the

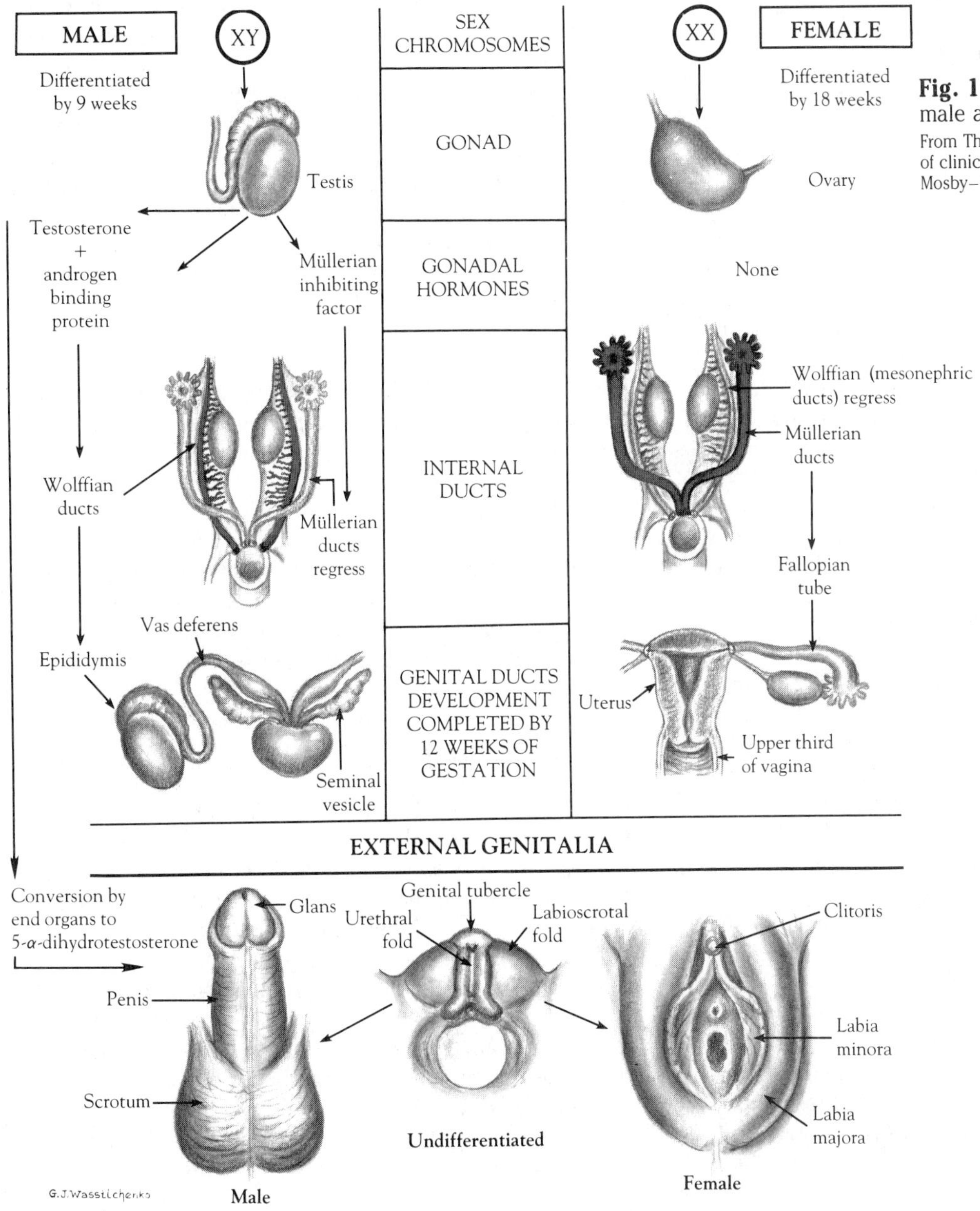

Fig. 11-27. Sex differentiation in male and female.

From Thompson, J. and others: Mosby's manual of clinical nursing, ed. 2, St. Louis, 1989, Mosby–Year Book, Inc.

Box 11-9 MECHANISMS AND SITES OF DEFECTIVE SEXUAL DEVELOPMENT

Abnormal sex determination—chromosomal abnormalities result in disturbance of sexual development (see Chapter 5).

Abnormal differentiation of gonads—when induction of the bipotential gonad fails, sex differentiation proceeds in the direction of the female phenotype, regardless of genetic sex.

Abnormal differentiation of ductal systems—biologic inactivity of androgenic male organizer substances or insensitivity of ductal tissue to its action results in a persistent female duct system, which leads to the presence of a uterus and uterine tubes.

Abnormal secretion of or tissue insensitivity to testicular androgen—complete failure of male hormone secretion produces female external genitalia in a genetic male. Partial or incomplete failure results in incomplete masculinization with ambiguity of external genitalia. The genetic female fetus exposed to large amounts of androgenic hormone may exhibit varying degrees of masculinization of the external genitalia (congenital adrenal hyperplasia).

normal order of events in sex determination will produce abnormal sexual development with the presence of ambiguous or inappropriate external genitalia at birth. Ambiguous genitalia can be variable and may often closely conform to one sex or the other. In some forms the external sexual structures represent those of a perfectly normal male or female, whereas the genetic sex is the direct opposite. A situation in which the phenotypic sex differs from the chromosomal sex is often termed *intersex.*

A failure or abnormality in any of the four steps of sexual development can lead to abnormal development in subsequent stages. The mechanisms and sites of defective development are summarized in Box 11-9.

Types of Abnormalities

Some disorders with abnormal sexual development are not characterized by ambiguous genitalia in the newborn period. For example, the most common sex chromosomal disorders do not become apparent until later childhood, adolescence, or even young adulthood when the individual seeks medical attention because of problems of delayed development or infertility. The four conditions producing ambiguous genitalia in the newborn that require prompt and accurate evaluation are the masculinized female (female pseudohermaphrodite), the incompletely masculinized male (male pseudohermaphrodite), the true hermaphrodite, and mixed gonadal dysgenesis.

Ambiguous genitalia in the newborn is most often the result of virilization in the female by adrenal androgens after the time of early gonadal differentiation. The most common type, congenital adrenal hyperplasia (CAH), is an inherited deficiency of adrenal corticoid hormones (see also Chapter 38). The resulting decrease in cortisol stimulates pituitary secretion of corticotropin (ACTH), which causes the adrenal cortex to increase production of adrenal hormones, including the androgens. Since the adrenal gland differentiates later than the gonadal duct systems but before differentiation of the external genitalia, the masculinization of the external genitalia is the predominant feature. Internal female anatomy is normal. CAH is the only intersex problem that is life-threatening and should be considered in any situation where sex is doubtful.

External genitalia in the incompletely masculinized male may be incompletely male, ambiguous, or completely female. The complex nature of virilization offers numerous opportunities for disturbance in the process. Defects may be the result of deficient production of fetal androgen, deficiency in any of the enzymes needed for testosterone biosynthesis, or unresponsiveness or subresponsiveness of genital structures to testosterone. True hermaphrodites are rare and may be either genetic males or females with *both* ovarian and testicular tissues, with an ovary on one side and a testis on the other, or a combination of ovotestis. The external genitalia may be male, usually cryptorchid, or normal female, but in the majority of cases are ambiguous.

Mixed gonadal dysgenesis is the second most common disorder, in which affected infants are sex chromosomal mosaics (see Maldistribution of Chromosomes, Chapter 5). Genitalia vary greatly, but in those who appear predominantly female, the dysplastic testis may cause masculinization at puberty. External appearance of genitalia is described in Table 11-4.

Diagnostic Evaluation

Diagnostic tools and their significant findings that help determine sex and assist in making a gender assignment are outlined in Box 11-10.

Therapeutic Management

The assignment of a gender sex to the infant whose sex is doubtful constitutes a social emergency. The long-term implications are such that a hasty decision based on appearance alone may be disastrous, and the optimum sex of rearing may not be the same as the genetic or gonadal sex. The infant's anatomy rather than genetic sex is the primary criterion on which the choice of gender should be based. An incomplete female is better able to adjust than is an inadequate male. A functional vagina can be constructed surgically, and with appropriate administration of hormones the anatomically incomplete female can lead a relatively normal life, but it is as yet impossible to construct a satisfactory penis from an inadequate phallus for an equally satisfactory adjustment of the incomplete male.

In most instances of ambiguous genitalia it is recommended that the infant be reared as a female. Genetic males with a phallus of adequate size that will respond to testosterone at the time of puberty can be considered for male rearing. Adequate studies should be carried out early to assist in gender selection, even though they may delay final sex assignment for several days or even weeks. Supportive measures, such as appropriate surgical reconstruction techniques, that provide normal-appearing external

Table 11-4 Ambiguous genitalia

NORMAL FINDINGS	AMBIGUOUS FINDINGS
Male	
Penile shaft protrudes from perineum and hangs freely	Small penis (less than 2 to 3 cm [0.8 to 1.2 inches] in newborn) may be enlarged clitoris
Urethral meatus centered at tip of glans penis	Urethral meatus anywhere along dorsal or ventral surface of penis, especially on perineum
Two scrotal sacs hang freely, covered with loose, wrinkled skin	Small scrotum with smooth, tight skin and any degree of separation in midline may be enlarged labia
Palpable testes in each scrotum	Absent testes may be undescended; if combined with small scrotum, may be evidence of enlarged labia
Female	
Small clitoris at anterior end of labia	Enlarged clitoris that protrudes from labia may be small penis
Urethral meatus located between clitoris and vagina	Urethral meatus located in clitoris may suggest small penis
Labia minora prominent in newborn but atrophied and almost absent in prepubertal female; completely separated from clitoris to posterior vault of vagina; on palpation, no masses in labia	Prominent labia, partially or completely fused with palpable masses on each side, may be small scrotum with testes

Box 11-10 ASSESSMENT TO DETERMINE A GENDER ASSIGNMENT

History—previous abortions (may help identify chromosomal aberrations); ingestion of steroids; relatives with ambiguous genitalia or who died in the first weeks of life
Physical examination—presence of palpable gonads strongly suggests a male genotype
Chromosomal analysis—detects chromosomal abnormalities and precise genetic sex; results are available in 2 to 3 days
Endoscopy, ultrasonography, and radiographic contrast studies—reveal presence, absence, or nature of internal genital structures
Biochemical tests—include 17-ketosteroids, 17-hydroxycorticoids, and urinary pregnanediol; urinary steroid excretion patterns help detect several of the adrenal cortical syndromes
Laparotomy or gonad biopsy—in some instances is the only way to arrive at a definitive diagnosis

structures are carried out. Removal of inappropriate internal structures and dysgenic gonads is recommended.

Nursing Considerations

Families need a great deal of support and encouragement from nurses and other members of the health team to cope with this emotionally charged situation. Parents are confused, anxious, and overwhelmed by feelings of guilt and shame. They may pressure for immediate sex assignment because they are concerned about the child and the child's future, and because they must face questioning relatives and friends. The best approach is honesty. The disorder should be treated as any other disorder, and no attempt should be made to camouflage the problem. The sequence of embryologic events leading to the defect can be explained using correct terminology to describe sexual deviations. An understanding of the anomaly assists parents in explaining the defect to others, just as with any other physical defect. It requires sympathy and understanding to deal with parental anxiety during this trying period and to guide them throughout the long-term management (see also Chapter 22).

CONGENITAL DEFECTS CAUSED BY PRENATAL FACTORS

Before birth the maternal host determines the well-being of the fetus by the manner in which she protects, favors, or deprives it. An unfavorable maternally imposed environment may produce effects on the fetus that are of a transient nature with few, if any, deleterious consequences or effects serious enough to cause long-range health problems in the infant or child. Several syndromes involving a variety of malformations have been attributed to an adverse prenatal environment.

As a result of data gathered from retrospective studies and animal experiments, a few basic principles have emerged that present some insight into the probability of children being affected by specific teratogens (Box 11-11).

DEFECTS CAUSED BY INFECTIOUS AGENTS

The range of pathologic conditions produced by infectious agents is large, and the difference between the maternal and fetal effects caused by any one agent is also great. Some maternal infections, especially during early gestation, can result in fetal loss or malformations because the ability of the fetus to handle infectious organisms is limited and the fetal immunologic system is unable to prevent the dissemination of infectious organisms to the various tissues.

Not all prenatal infections produce teratogenic effects. Further, the clinical picture of disorders caused by transplacental transfer of infectious agents is not always well-defined. One group of microbial agents can cause remarkably similar manifestations, and it is not uncommon to test for all when a prenatal infection is suspected. This is the so-called TORCH complex, an acronym outlined in Box 11-12.

To determine the causative agent in a symptomatic infant, tests are performed to rule out each of these infections. The "O" category may involve testing for several viral infections (e.g., hepatitis, varicella zoster, measles, mumps) and listeriosis. Sometimes "S" is added (TORCHS) to include congenital syphilis. Bacterial infections are not included in the TORCH workup, because they are usually identified by clinical manifestations and readily available laboratory tests. Gonococcal conjunctivitis (ophthalmia neonatorum) and chlamydial conjunctivitis have been eliminated or significantly reduced by prophylactic measures at birth (see Chapter 8). AIDS, a growing prenatal and postnatal concern, is discussed in Chapter 35. The major maternal infections, their possible teratogenic effects, and specific nursing considerations are outlined in Table 11-5.

Box 11-11 PRINCIPLES OF TERATOLOGY

The susceptibility of the organism to teratogenic factors is determined by the stage of development.

The effect of a teratogen depends on genetic predisposition.

There are indications that a teratogenic agent accentuates the incidence of those defects that occur sporadically, implying underlying genetic instabilities.

A single teratogen may produce a variety of anomalies. For example, it has been established that rubella infection of the mother can produce a variety of defects, including cataracts, deafness, heart anomalies, and mental retardation.

A variety of teratogenic agents may produce similar anomalies; for example, viruses, chemicals, and radiation can all produce a mental deficit.

Teratogenic anomalies may be indistinguishable from hereditary malformations (phenocopies), for example, inherited deafness and deafness caused by maternal rubella.

Many teratogenic agents have little or no adverse effect on the maternal system and may even be beneficial to the mother. For example, the drug thalidomide, an effective hypnotic drug, nontoxic to the mother, is severely teratogenic to the fetus.

Nursing Considerations

One of the major goals in care of infants suspected of having an infectious disease is identification of the causative

Box 11-12 TORCHS COMPLEX

T Toxoplasmosis
O Other (e.g., hepatitis)
R Rubella
C Cytomegalovirus infection
H Herpes simplex
S Syphilis

Table 11-5 Infections acquired from mother before, during, or after birth

FETAL OR NEWBORN EFFECT	COMMENTS AND NURSING CONSIDERATIONS*
▪ Acquired immune deficiency syndrome (AIDS) (human i nmunodeficiency virus [HIV])	
No significant difference between infected and uninfected infants at birth in some instances Embryopathy reported by some observers Depressed nasal bridge Mild upward or downward obliquity of eyes Long palpebral fissures with blue sclerae Patulous lips Ocular hypertelorism Prominent upper vermilion border	Transmitted transplacentally; during delivery; in breast milk No treatment currently available other than supportive care IV gamma globulin when diagnosed Average age of onset of clinical signs is 4 to 6 months; mean age of diagnosis is 12 months
▪ Chickenpox (varicella-zoster virus)	
First trimester exposure—congenital varicella syndrome: limb dysplasia, microcephaly, cortical atrophy, chorioretinitis, cataracts, cutaneous scars, other anomalies, auditory nerve palsy, mental retardation	Transmitted: first trimester (fetal varicella syndrome); intrapartum (infection) Treatment: exposed infants—varicella-zoster immune globulin (VZIG) to infants born to mothers with onset of disease within 5 days before or 2 days after delivery (7 days before and 7 days after in United Kingdom) Isolation precautions 21 days after birth (if hospitalized)
▪ Chlamydia infection *(Chlamydia trachomatis)*	
Conjunctivitis, pneumonia	Transmitted: last trimester or intrapartum Apply prophylactic medication to eyes at time of birth Treatment: antibiotics
▪ Coxsackie virus (group B)	
Poor feeding, vomiting, diarrhea, fever; cardiac enlargement, arrhythmias, congestive heart failure; lethargy, seizures, meningeal involvement	Transmitted: first trimester or late in pregnancy

*Isolation precautions depend on institutional policy (see Chapter 26).

Table 11-5 Infections acquired from mother before, during, or after birth—cont'd

FETAL OR NEWBORN EFFECT	COMMENTS AND NURSING CONSIDERATIONS*
▪ Cytomegalic inclusion disease—CID (cytomegalovirus [CMV])	
Microcephaly, cerebral calcifications, chorioretinitis Jaundice, hepatosplenomegaly Petechial or purpuric rash Neurologic sequelae: seizure disorders, sensorimotor deafness, mental retardation	Transmitted: throughout pregnancy Affected individuals excrete virus Virus detected in urine by electron microscopy Avoid kissing affected child Pregnant women should avoid close contact with known cases Treatment: antimetabolites, antiviral agent
▪ Erythema infectiosum (parvovirus B19)	
Fetal hydrops and death from anemia and heart failure, early exposure Anemia from later exposure No teratogenic effects established Ordinarily, low risk of ill effect to fetus	Transmitted: transplacentally First-trimester infection most serious effects Pregnant health care workers should not care for patients who might be highly contagious (e.g., aplastic crisis) Routine exclusion of pregnant women from workplace where disease is occurring not recommended
▪ Gonococcal disease *(Neisseria gonorrhoeae)*	
Ophthalmitis Neonatal gonococcal arthritis, septicemia, meningitis	Transmitted: last trimester or intrapartum Apply prophylactic medication to eyes at time of birth Obtain smears for culture Treatment: penicillin
▪ Hepatitis B (virus)	
May be asymptomatic Acute hepatitis, changes in liver function	Transmitted: transplacentally, contaminated maternal secretions during delivery Treatment: hepatitis B immune globulin to all infants of HBsAG-positive mothers
▪ Herpes, neonatal (herpes simplex virus)	
Cutaneous lesions: vesicles at 6 to 10 days of age; may be no lesions Disseminated disease resembles sepsis Visceral involvement: granulomas Early nonspecific signs: fever, lethargy, poor feeding, irritability, vomiting May include hyperbilirubinemia, seizures, flaccid or spastic paralysis, apneic episodes, respiratory distress, lethargy, or coma	History of genital infection in mother/partner in 50% of cases Transmitted: intrapartum either ascending and/or direct contact, especially primary infection Cesarean section sometimes a preventive measure for mothers with active lesions Vaginal delivery of infants of mothers with recurrent infection thought to be at lower risk Suggest infants room-in with mother in private room
▪ Listeriosis *(Listeria)*	
Acquired in late pregnancy: stillborn or acutely ill: may die within an hour after birth Late onset: septicemia; meningitis	Transmitted: transplacentally or by aspiration of secretions at birth Segregate infants until cultures are negative
▪ Lyme disease *(Borrelia burgdorferi)*	
Stillbirth Congenital defects reported: congenital heart disease, syndactyly, cortical blindness Prematurity Rash	Transmitted: transplacentally Immediate treatment of affected pregnant women with appropriate antibiotic Advise pregnant women to avoid tick exposure in endemic areas
▪ Rubella, congenital (rubella virus)	
Eye defects: cataracts (unilateral or bilateral), microphthalmia, retinitis, glaucoma CNS signs: microcephaly, seizures, severe mental retardation Congenital heart defects: patent ductus arteriosus Auditory: high incidence of delayed hearing loss Intrauterine growth retardation Hyperbilirubinemia, spinal fluid abnormalities, thrombocytopenia, hepatomegaly	Transmitted: first trimester; early second trimester Pregnant women should avoid contact with all affected persons, including infants with rubella syndrome Emphasize vaccination of all unimmunized prepubertal children, susceptible adolescents, and adult females of childbearing age Caution women against pregnancy for at least 3 months after vaccination

Continued.

Table 11-5 Infections acquired from mother before, during, or after birth—cont'd

FETAL OR NEWBORN EFFECT	COMMENTS AND NURSING CONSIDERATIONS*
▪ Syphilis, congenital *(Treponema pallidum)*	
Copper-colored maculopapular cutaneous lesions (after 7th day), mucous membrane patches, hair loss, nail exfoliation, sniffles (syphilitic rhinitis), profound anemia, poor feeding, pseudoparalysis of one or more limbs, dysmorphic teeth (older child)	Transmitted: transplacentally, usually after 18th week of pregnancy Most severe form of syphilis Strict isolation of infant Treatment: penicillin
▪ Toxoplasmosis *(Toxoplasma gondii)*	
Hydrocephaly, cerebral calcifications, chorioretinitis (classic triad) Microcephaly, seizures, mental retardation, deafness Encephalitis, myocarditis, hepatosplenomegaly, anemia, jaundice, diarrhea, vomiting, purpura	Transmitted: throughout pregnancy Predominant host for organism is cats May be transmitted through cat feces, poorly cooked or raw infected meat Caution pregnant women to avoid contact with cat feces, e.g., emptying cat litter boxes Treatment: sulfonamides, pyrimethamine

organism. Until the diagnosis is established, appropriate precautions are implemented according to institutional policy. In suspected cytomegalovirus and rubella infections, pregnant personnel are cautioned to avoid contact with the infant. Herpes simplex is easily transmitted from one infant to another; therefore risk of cross-contamination is reduced or eliminated by wearing gloves and gowns for patient contact. Masks may be required for personnel when caring for infants with an infection such as congenital rubella. The hospital infection control department provides guidelines for the type and duration of precautions. Careful handwashing is always an important nursing intervention in reducing spread of any infection.

Special feeding techniques may need to be implemented for infants with feeding difficulties, and infants subject to seizures are protected from adverse environmental stimuli. Specimens need to be obtained for laboratory examinations, and the infant and parents need to be prepared for diagnostic procedures. When possible, long-term disabilities are prevented by early evaluation and implementation of therapy. The family is taught any special handling techniques needed for the care of their infant and signs of complications or possible sequelae. If sequelae are inevitable, the family will need assistance in determining how they can best cope with the problems, such as assistance with home care, referral to appropriate agencies, or placement in an institution for care.

The major goal of nursing care is prevention of these disorders with provision of adequate prenatal care for the expectant mother and precautions regarding exposure to teratogenic infections (Fig. 11-28).

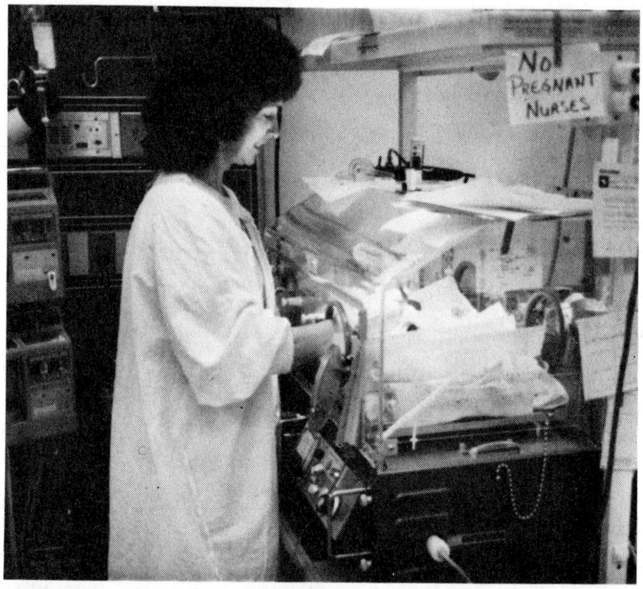

Fig. 11-28. Hospital personnel practice preventive measures when caring for affected infants.

DEFECTS CAUSED BY CHEMICAL AGENTS

In the wake of the thalidomide tragedy of the early 1960s, in which hundreds of malformed children were born, chemical agents have been implicated in a number of congenital defects. The relationship of the fetal and maternal circulations allows for the interchange of chemical substances across the placental membrane. The limited metabolic capabilities of the fetal liver and its immature enzyme and transport systems render the unborn child ill equipped for maintaining homeostasis when chemical disturbances are imposed by the mother. This includes both substances produced by the mother in response to a disease state (such as diabetes) and exogenous substances ingested or inhaled by the mother.

The teratogenic effect of drugs is not believed to have an effect on developing tissue until day 15 of gestation, when tissue differentiation begins to take place. Before that time drugs usually have little effect on the embryo, because drugs are not believed to have a significant affinity for undifferentiated tissue. Also, until implantation takes place, at approximately 7 days after conception, the embryo is not exposed to maternal blood that contains the drug. However some drugs may affect the uterine lining, making it unsuitable for implantation. Drugs administered between days 15 and 90 may produce an effect if the tissue for which it has an affinity is in the process of differentiation at that time. After 90 days, when differentiation is complete, most fetal tissues are believed to be relatively resistant to teratogenic effects of drugs (Luery, 1985). However, the impact on ongoing neurologic development is not known.

Nursing Considerations

It has been estimated that women take an average of four or five drugs—either prescription or over-the-counter preparations—during their pregnancy. In addition, hormones, frequently administered as drugs, are often classified as such. Consequently expectant mothers are cautioned against ingesting any medication without first consulting their practitioners. To help ensure that fewer women will inadvertently take some chemical that might be harmful to the fetus, labels on medications are now required to include information regarding the possible teratogenic effects of the drug. Excessive use of some very commonplace drugs, such as alcohol (see below), valproic acid (Jager-Roman and others, 1986), and isotretinoin (Accutane) (Lammer and others, 1985) have been shown to produce some characteristic malformations in the fetus.

Nurses should be aware of the **Association for Birth Defect Children,*** which offers help and information to families with children with defects caused by maternal exposure to drugs, chemicals, radiation, and other environmental agents.

FETAL ALCOHOL SYNDROME

The term *fetal alcohol syndrome (FAS)* is now widely used to describe infants with characteristic facial and associated features attributed to excessive ingestion of alcohol by the mother during pregnancy. It is now known that alcohol (ethanol and ethyl alcohol) definitely interferes with normal pregnancy, that the effects on the fetus are permanent, and that even moderate use of alcohol during pregnancy may impair the mother-child bonding process. Observers have concluded that there is no safe level of alcohol consumption in pregnancy (Davis, Partridge, and Storrs, 1982) and that women who plan to become pregnant should stop consuming alcohol at least 3 months before they plan to become pregnant.

It is unclear to what extent the defects of FAS are related to the amount of alcohol consumed. It is not the degree of alcoholism in the mother that is related to the presence of abnormalities in the fetus; rather, it is the amount consumed in excess of the liver's ability to detoxify that places the fetus at risk. The liver's capacity to detoxify is limited and inflexible—when the liver receives more alcohol than it is able to handle, the excess is continually recirculated until the organ is able to reduce it to carbon dioxide and water. This circulating alcohol has a special affinity for brain tissue. Other factors that contribute to the teratogenic effects include toxic acetyl aldehyde (a degradation byproduct of ethanol) and other substances that may be added to the alcohol. The poor nutritional state of the alcoholic mother further compromises the fetus.

The effects on the fetal brain are reflected in the central nervous system manifestations of fetal alcohol syndrome. The major features of FAS are outlined in Box 11-13. Mental retardation, hearing disorders, and a variety of defects in craniofacial development are prominent features (Fig. 11-29). Affected infants display the physical features of the syndrome and the characteristic behaviors beginning in the first 24 hours of life (Lemons, 1983). These include difficulty in establishing respirations, irritability, lethargy, seizure activity, tremulousness, opisthotonos, poor suck reflex, and abdominal distention. Affected infants frequently develop metabolic problems.

The initial difficulties in the newborn period are managed by preventing stimulation that might precipitate seizures, sedation and/or anticonvulsant therapy, and general supportive measures. The defects and their effects are irreversible, so the major emphasis must be aimed at prevention.

Nursing Considerations

The nursing care of affected infants involves the same assessment and observations that are employed for any high-

Box 11-13 MAJOR FEATURES OF FETAL ALCOHOL SYNDROME

Facial Features
Short palpebral fissures
Hypoplastic philtrum (vertical ridge in upper lip)
Thinned upper lip
Short, upturned nose
Hypoplastic maxilla
Micrognathia or prognathia in adolescence
Retrognathia in infancy

Neurologic
Mental retardation
Motor retardation
Microcephaly
Poor coordination
Hypotonia
Hearing disorders

Behavior
Irritability (infancy)
Hyperactivity (child)

Growth
Prenatal growth retardation
Persistent postnatal growth lag

*3526 Emerywood Lane, Orlando, FL 32812; (305) 859-2821.

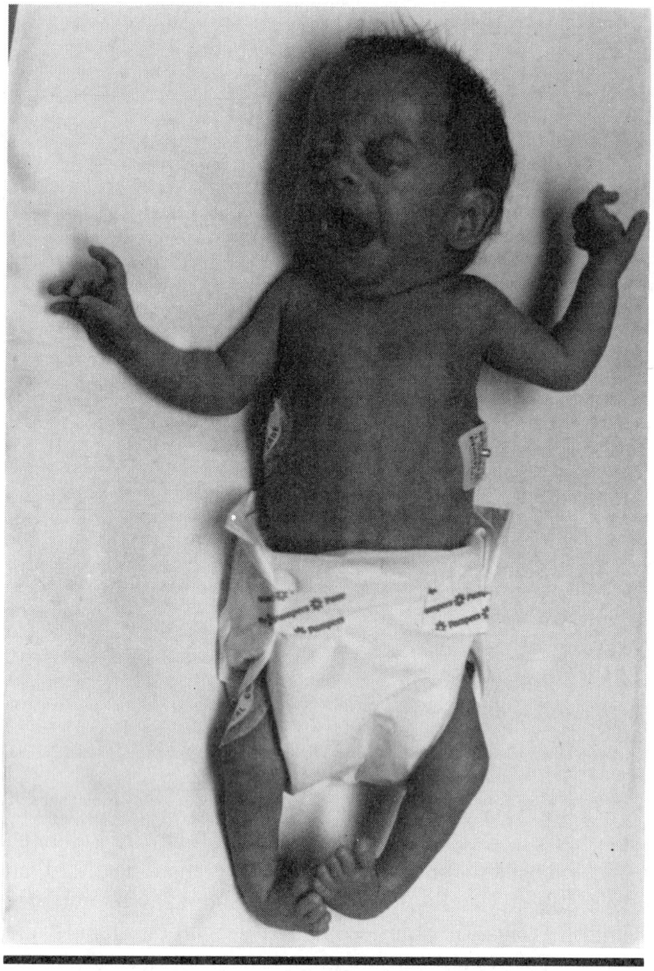

Fig. 11-29. Infant with fetal alcohol syndrome.

risk infant (see Chapter 10). Poor feeding is characteristic of infants with FAS and can be a significant problem throughout infancy. Special emphasis should be placed on monitoring weight gain, analyzing feeding behaviors, and devising strategies to promote nutritional intake.

Identifying and treating the alcoholic mother provide a greater challenge. As with all pregnant women, the pregnant alcoholic mother is urged to obtain prenatal care and to abstain from consuming alcohol. In general, light to moderate drinking throughout pregnancy does not appear to have any markedly adverse effects on the offspring. However, the dangers of heavy drinking are known, and women with histories of excessive alcohol ingestion should be counseled regarding the risks to the fetus. A change in drinking habits even as late as the third trimester (when brain growth in the fetus is greatest) is associated with improved fetal outcome, although adverse effects have been reported with alcohol exposure during the first 2 months of pregnancy (Day and others, 1989).

RADIATION

Ionizing radiation in large doses has been shown to be both mutagenic and teratogenic in humans. Pelvic irradiation of pregnant women—from natural background radiation that is present everywhere in varying degrees, from occupational exposure, or from diagnostic or therapeutic procedures—is believed to be hazardous to the embryo, although the extent of teratogenicity and the exact dosage required to induce somatic change are still under consideration. Radiation may damage the conceptus at any time during its prenatal existence, and it is known that rapidly dividing and differentiating cells, such as those of the embryo, have increased radiosensitivity. As with other teratogens, the type of effect produced is closely correlated with the stage of development at which the radiation exposure occurs.

Although data are incomplete, there are indications that a larger number of chromosome abnormalities occur in children born to parents who have been exposed to increased preconception radiation. This finding is consistent with the observation that chromosome abnormalities are highest in infants of older mothers, and there is an increased frequency of chromosomally abnormal fetuses born to parents with occupational exposure to radiation. To help prevent the possibility of radiation damage, it is advisable (1) to avoid unnecessary radiation exposure, such as elective radiographs, in women of childbearing age except during the 2 weeks immediately following menstruation, (2) to ask if pregnancy is a possibility, and (3) to advise both men and women who have lower abdominal or pelvic radiographs to avoid conception for several months (Cohen, 1984). Also, the harmful effects of maternal radioactive iodine (RAI) therapy on the fetal thyroid gland have led to the conclusion that termination of pregnancies that occur during RAI therapy should be considered.

NUTRITION

The human conceptus has no store of nutrients to sustain vital functions during the prenatal period; therefore it must rely on the mother as its single source of nutrition. A number of related factors, acting alone or in combination, influence fetal access to nutrients. These include reduction of maternal intake of specific nutrients and the general nutritional state of the mother. The chronically malnourished mother has few nutritional reserves available for fetal use, and the accumulated effects of lifetime nutritional deficiency may produce physiologic and anatomic structural defects that impair the mother's ability to support pregnancy and contribute to difficulties during labor. The teenage mother who has special nutritional requirements for meeting her own growth needs may compete with the fetus for available nutrients. Diet fads, such as the Zen macrobiotic diet and some of the new restrictive diets, seriously compromise the health of both the mother and the fetus (see Chapter 13).

Current information indicates that the restriction of calories and protein during prenatal development profoundly affects the size, viability, postnatal growth, and behavior of children. The timing and duration of nutritional deprivation appear to be crucial. Of greatest concern are the consequences of dietary restriction at the time the brain is undergoing the most rapid growth and development. Insufficient nutrients to the fetus during the time of rapid brain cell division result in permanent deficiency in brain cell numbers. The long-term consequences of nutritional deficiency may be manifest as cognitive, behavioral, and language retardation. There is a highly complicated relationship between maternal intake, postnatal environmental conditions, and the intellectual functions of offspring that is worthy of further exploration.

OTHER FACTORS

The intrauterine environment minimizes the possibility of trauma to the fetus; however, during the later months of gestation, maintaining an attitude of complete flexion in the cramped quarters of the uterus predisposes the fetus to a number of deformities, for example, metatarsus varus, torticollis, and CDH.

Defects sometimes occur as a result of amniotic bands or adhesions between the amnion and the fetus. Bands of amniotic tissue can constrict the blood supply to fetal limbs, inhibiting the growth of distal segments and altering their configuration. A decrease in the production of amniotic fluid may create deformities of varying degrees as a result of the restriction of intrauterine space, for example, malformations of the jaw and ribs, asymmetry of the head, and compression marks on the body.

There is increasing evidence to indicate that fetuses may be adversely affected by the high temperatures to which they are subjected when expectant mothers indulge in the environment of a hot tub or sauna. With the increasing popularity of these innovations, nurses should advise pregnant women to seek the advice of their practitioners before extensive use of such items. Trauma, diagnostic and therapeutic procedures, and living at a very high altitude may also cause adverse effects in the fetus.

KEY POINTS

- Approximately one third of hospitalized children suffer from a congenital abnormality or its sequelae.
- Prenatal development consists of growth by hyperplasia and hypertrophy, differentiation into specialized cells, and organogenesis.
- Typical reactions of parents to an infant with a physical defect include grief over "loss" of a perfect child, shock, and withdrawal.
- The nurse's primary roles in care of an infant with a physical defect are caregiver, provider of family support, and supplier of information.
- Surgery initiates a number of physiologic responses, including cardiovascular, respiratory, endocrine, renal, gastrointestinal, immune, neurologic, and fluid and electrolyte.
- Nurses must be sensitive to pain in the neonate, be alert for signs of pain, and intervene appropriately.
- One of the largest groups of congenital anomalies includes those associated with the embryonic neural tube, the most common of which are spina bifida occulta and myelomeningocele.
- Care of the infant and child with myelomeningocele requires both immediate and long-term professional supervision. Associated problems include infection, neurologic damage, impaired renal function, and musculoskeletal impairment.
- Therapeutic management of hydrocephalus focuses on relief of intracranial pressure, treatment of complications, and management of problems related to the effect of the disorder on psychomotor development.
- Three degrees of congenital hip dysplasia are acetabular dysplasia, subluxation, and dislocation.
- Treatment of congenital hip dysplasia involves maintaining the head of the femur correctly positioned in the acetabulum by means of an external mechanical device, usually the Pavlik harness.
- Treatment of clubfoot involves manual overcorrection of the deformity, maintenance of the correction until normal muscle balance is gained, and follow-up observation to detect possible recurrence of the deformity.
- Cleft lip deformities are repaired at the earliest opportunity; cleft palate repair is usually delayed to take advantage of growth changes.
- Management of cleft lip and/or palate involves a multidisciplinary approach to care involving professionals from surgery, medicine, nursing, dentistry, and speech therapy.
- Tracheoesophageal fistula consists of an abnormal connection between the esophagus and the trachea, placing the untreated infant at risk for life-threatening aspiration.
- Anorectal defects are often associated with other congenital anomalies, such as those involving the gastrointestinal tract and heart.
- Defects involving herniation through the abdominal wall range from a simple umbilical hernia to complex gastroschisis.
- Genitourinary tract defects are repaired as early as possible to restore normal function and prevent psychologic problems in childhood.
- Obstructive uropathy can result in significant renal damage unless it is recognized and managed early.
- Ambiguous genitalia constitute a social emergency; therefore an appropriate gender should be established as early as possible.
- Prenatal development can be modified by a variety of environmental factors, including chemicals, infectious agents, radiation, mechanical factors, nutrition, temperature, and maternal health.

REFERENCES

American Academy of Pediatrics, Committee on Bioethics: Treatment of critically ill newborns, Pediatrics 72:565-566, 1983.

American Academy of Pediatrics, Committee on Genetics: α-Fetoprotein screening, Pediatrics 80:444-445, 1987.

American Academy of Pediatrics, Infant Bioethics Task Force and Consultants: Guidelines for infant bioethics committees, Pediatrics 74:306-310, 1984.

American Cleft Palate Education Foundation: Information about cleft lip and palate, Pittsburgh, 1985, Cleft Palate Foundation.

Anand, K.J.: Hormonal and metabolic functions of neonates and infants undergoing surgery, Curr. Opin. Cardiol. 1:681-689, 1986.

Anand, K.J., and Aynsley-Green, A.: Measuring the severity of surgical stress in newborn infants, J. Pediatr. Surg. 23:297-305, 1988.

Anand, K.J., and Hickey, P.: Pain and its effects in the human neonate and fetus, N. Engl. J. Med. 317:1321-1329, 1987.

Anand, K.J., Sippell, W.G., and Aynsley-Green, A.: Randomized trial of fentanyl anaesthesia in preterm babies undergoing surgery: effects on the stress response, Lancet 31:243-247, 1987.

Anderson, S.M.: Secondary neurologic disability in myelomeningocele, Inf. Young Child. 1(4):9-21, 1989.

Arras, J.D., and Shinnar, S.: Anencephalic newborns as organ donors: a critique, JAMA 259:2284-2285, 1988.

Baird, P.A., and Sadovinick, A.D.: Survival in infants with anencephaly, Clin. Pediatr. 23:268-271, 1984.

Benfield, D.G., Lieb, S.A., and Vollman, J.H.: Grief responses of parents to neonatal death and parent participation in deciding care, Pediatrics 62:171, 1978.

Bialik, V., and others: Clinical assessment of hip instability in the newborn by an orthopedic surgeon and a pediatrician, J. Pediatr. Orthop. 6:703-706, 1986.

Blotcky, M.J., and Grossman, I.: Psychological implications of childhood genitourinary surgery, J. Am. Acad. Child Psychiatry 17:488-492, 1978.

Botkin, J.R.: Anencephalic infants as organ donors, Pediatrics 82:250-256, 1988.

Britton, S.B., Fitzhardinge, P.M., and Ashby, S.: Is intensive care justified for infants weighing less than 801 gm at birth? J. Pediatr. 99:937-943, 1981.

Brown, L.: Physiologic responses to cutaneous pain in neonates, Neonatal Network 6(3):18-22, 1987.

Bunch, W.H.: Common deformities of the lower limb, Pediatr. Nurs. 5(4):18-22, 1979.

Butler, N.C.: How to raise professional awareness of the need for adequate pain relief for infants, Birth 15(1):38-41, 1988.

Cartlidge, P.H., Mann, N.P., and Kapilar, L.: Preoperative stabilization in congenital diaphragmatic hernia, Arch. Dis. Child. 61:1226-1228, 1986.

Centers for Disease Control: Contribution of birth defects to infant mortality—United States, 1986, MMWP 38:633-635, 1989.

Charney, E.B., and others: Management of the newborn with myelomeningocele: time for a decision-making process, Pediatrics 75:58-64, 1985.

Cheetham, C.H., and others: Congenital dislocation of the hip (letter), Br. Med. J. 286:277, 1983.

Clarren, S.K.: Plagiocephaly and torticollis: etiology, natural history, and helmet treatment, J. Pediatr. 98:92-95, 1981.

Cohen, F.L.: Clinical genetics in nursing practice, Philadelphia, 1984, J.B. Lippincott Co.

Collins, C., and others: Fentanyl pharmacokinetics and hemodynamic effects in preterm infants during ligation of patent ductus arteriosus, Anesth. Analg. 64:1078-1080, 1985.

Curtin, G.: The infant with cleft lip or palate: more than a surgical problem, J. Perinat. Neonatal Nurs. 3(3):80-89, 1990.

Dale, J.C.: A multidimensional study of infants' behaviors associated with assumed painful stimuli: phase II, J. Pediatr. Health Care 3(1):34-38, 1989.

D'Apolito, K.: The neonate's response to pain, MCN 9:256-257, 1984.

Davis, P.J.M., Partridge, J.W., and Storrs, C.N.: Alcohol consumption in pregnancy: how much is safe? Arch. Dis. Child. 57:940-943, 1982.

Day, N.L., and others: Prenatal exposure to alcohol: effect on infant growth and morphologic characteristics, Pediatrics 84:536-541, 1989.

Dixon, A.G.: Jeff's story: a unique approach to the care of an infant with esophageal atresia and a cervical esophagostomy, Neonatal Network 4(6):7-12, 1986.

Duff, R.S.: Counseling families and deciding care of severely defective children: a way of coping with "medical Vietman," Pediatrics 67:315-320, 1981.

Elder, J.S, and Duckett, J.W.: Management of the fetus and neonate with hydronephrosis detected by prenatal ultrasonography, Pediatr. Ann. 17:19-28, 1988.

Erlen, J.A., and Holzman, I.R.: Anencephalic infants: should they be organ donors? Pediatr. Nurs. 14:6-64, 1988.

Feller, N., and others: A multidisciplinary approach to developing safe transportation for children with special needs, Orthop. Nurs. 5(5):25-27, 1986.

Field, T., and Goldson, E.: Pacifying effects of nonnutritive sucking on term and preterm neonates during heelstick procedures, Pediatrics 74:1012-1015, 1984.

Fletcher, J.C., Robertson, J.A., and Harrison, M.R.: Primates and anencephalics as sources for pediatric organ transplant: medical, legal, and ethical issues, Fetal Ther. 1:150-164, 1986.

Franck, L.S.: A new method to quantitatively describe pain behavior in infants, Nurs. Res. 35:28-31, 1986.

Franck, L.S.: A national survey of the assessment and treatment of pain and agitation in the neonatal intensive care unit, JOGNN 16(6):387-393, 1987.

Gans, S.L., and Austin, E.: Hernias and hydroceles. In Gennis, S.S., and Kagan, B.M.: Current pediatric therapy 12, Philadelphia, 1986, W.B. Saunders Co.

Glaser, J.H., Balistreri, W.F., and Morecki, R.: Role of reovirus type 3 in persistent infantile cholestasis, J. Pediatr. 105:912-915, 1984.

Glick, P.L., and others: The missing link in the pathogenesis of gastroschisis, J. Pediatr. Surg. 20:406-409, 1985.

Gross, R.H., and others: Early management and decision making for the treatment of myelomeningocele, Pediatrics 72:450-458, 1983.

Harrison, M.R.: Organ procurement for children: the anencephalic as donor, Lancet 2:1383-1385, 1986.

Helin, I., and Persson, P.: Prenatal diagnosis of urinary tract abnormalities by ultrasound, Pediatrics 78:879-883, 1986.

Hindmarsh, K.W., Sankaran, K., and Watson, V.G.: Plasma beta-endorphin concentrations in neonates associated with acute stress, Dev. Pharmacol. Ther. 7:198-204, 1984.

Holland, S.H.: Up-to-date home care of a baby in a hip spica cast, Pediatr. Nurs. 9(2):114-115, 1983.

Iwatsuki, S., and Starzl, T.E.: Disorders of the biliary tree. In Gellis, S.S., and Kagan, B.M.: Current pediatric therapy 12, Philadelphia, 1986, W.B. Saunders Co.

Jager-Roman, E, and others: Fetal growth, major malformations, and minor anomalies in infants born to women receiving valproic acid, J. Pediatr. 108:997-1004, 1986.

Johnston, C.C., and Strada, M.E.: Acute pain response in infants: a multidimensional description, Pain 24:373-382, 1986.

Kaplan, M.R. Hematuria in childhood, Pediatr. Rev. 5:99-105, 1983.

Khoury, M.J., Erickson, J.D., and James, L.M.: Etiologic heterogeneity of neural tube defects: clues from epidemiology, Am. J. Epidemiol. 115:538-548, 1982.

Koop, C.E.: The most important advances of the last 10 years, Pediatr. Consult. 12(1):1-6, 1981.

Koyle, M.A., Rajfer, J., and Ehrlich, R.M.: The undescended testis, Pediatr. Ann. 17:39-46, 1988.

Lally, K.P., and others: Preoperative factors affecting the outcome following repair of biliary atresia, Pediatrics 83:723-726, 1989.

Lammer, E.J., and others: Retinoic acid embryopathy, N. Engl. J. Med. 313:837-841, 1985.

Landwirth, J.: Should anencephalic infants be used as organ donors? Pediatics 82:257-259, 1988.

Learning to close the cleft, Time Magazine, April 12, 1982.

Lemons, P.K.M.: The sequelae to addiction, Crit. Care Update 10(6):7-10, 1983.

Lepore, A.G., and Kesler, R.W.: Behavior of children undergoing hypospadias repair, J. Urol. 122:68-72, 1979.
Letters to the editors: Care of the child with myelomeningocele, Pediatrics 74:162-167, 1984.
Linder, M., and others: Effects of meningomyelocele closure on the intracranial pulse pressure, Child's Brain 11:176-182, 1984.
Lorber, J., and Salfield, S.A.: Results of selective treatment of spina bifida cystica, Arch. Dis. Child. 56:822-830, 1981.
Lozes, M.H.: Bladder and bowel management for children with myelomeningocele, Inf. Young Child. 1(1):52-62, 1988.
Luery, N.M.: Drugs in pregnancy, Am. Druggist 192:102-104, 1985.
Maguire, D.P, and Maloney, P.: A comparison of fentanyl and morphine use in neonates, Neonatal Network 7(1):27-32, 1988.
Manley, C.B.: Elective genital surgery at one year of age: psychological and surgical considerations, Surg. Clin. North Am. 62(6):941-953, 1982.
March of Dimes–Birth Defects Foundation: Public health information sheet: cleft lip and palate, White Plains, NY, undated material, March of Dimes–Birth Defects Foundation.
McKusick, V.A.: Mendelian inheritance in man, ed. 8, Baltimore, 1988, Williams & Wilkins.
Milunsky, A., and others: Multivitamin/folic acid supplementation in early pregnancy reduces the prevalence of neural tube defects, JAMA 262:284-287, 1989.
Myers, G.J.: Myelomeningocele: the medical aspects, Pediatr. Clin. North Am. 31:165-175, 1984.
Noetzel, M.J.: Hydrocephalus. In Gellis, S.S., and Kagan, B.M.: Current pediatric therapy 12, Philadelphia, 1986, W.B. Saunders Co.
Nora, J.J., and Fraser, F.C.: Medical genetics: principles and practice, ed. 3, Philadelphia, 1989, Lea & Febiger.
Owens, J.R., and others: 19-year incidence of neural tube defects in area under constant surveillance, Lancet, pp. 1032-1035, Nov. 7, 1981.
Paparella, B.H.: Caring for the severely handicapped newborn, Nursing '82 12(12):61-64, 1982.
Penny, R.: Undescended testes. In Gellis, S.S., and Kagan, B.M.: Current pediatric therapy 12, Philadelphia, 1986, W.B. Saunders Co.
Penticuff, J.H.: Neonatal intensive care: parental prerogatives, J. Perinat. Neonatal Nurs. 1(3):77-86, 1988.
Pettitt, B.J., Zitelli, B.J., and Rowe, M.I.: Patients with biliary atresia coming to liver transplantation, J. Pediatr. Surg. 19:779-785, 1984.
Pinch, W.J., and Spielman, M.L.: Parental voices in the sea of neonatal ethical dilemmas, Issues Compr. Pediatr. Nurs. 12:423-435, 1989.
Pomerance, J.J.: Disorders of the umbilicus. In Gellis, S.S., and Kagan, B.M.: Current pediatric therapy 12, Philadelphia, 1986, W.B. Saunders Co.
President's Commission for the Study of Ethical Problems in Medicine and Biomedical and Behavioral Research: Defining death, Washington, DC, 1981, U.S. Government Printing Office.
President's Commission for the Study of Ethical Problems in Medicine and Biomedical and Behavior Research: Deciding to forego life-sustaining treatment, Bethesda, MD, 1983, U.S. Government Printing Office.
Rajfer, J., and others: Hormonal therapy for cryptorchidism: a randomized, double-blind study comparing human chorionic gonadotropin and gonadotropin-releasing hormone, N. Engl. J. Med. 314:466-470, 1986.
Ramenofsky, M.L.: Congenital diaphragmatic hernia. In Gellis, S.S., and Kagan, B.M.: Current pediatric therapy 12, Philadelphia, 1986, W.B. Saunders Co.
Reigel, D.H.: Spina bifida. In McLauren, R.L.: Pediatric psychology, New York, 1982, Grune & Stratton, Inc.
Rosenbaum, K.: Genetics and dysmorphology. In Welch, K., and others, editors: Pediatric surgery, ed. 4, St. Louis, 1986, Mosby–Year Book, Inc.
Rushton, C.H.: The surgical neonate: principles of nursing management, Pediatr. Nurs. 14:141-151, 1988.
Saggese, G., and others: Hormonal therapy for cryptorchidism with a combination of human chorionic gonadotropin and follicle-stimulating hormone, Am. J. Dis. Child. 143:980-982, 1989.
Sakai, H., and others: Effect of surgical repair on respiratory mechanics in congenital diaphragmatic hernia, J. Pediatr. 111:432-438, 1987.
Scarff, T.B., and Fronczak, S.: Myelomeningocele: a review and update, Rehab. Lit. 42(5-6):143-146, 192, 1981.
Schiffer, K.A., and others: Acquired undescended testes, Am. J. Dis. Child. 141:106-107, 1987.
Schultz, J.R., Klykylo, W.M., and Wacksman, J.: Timing of elective hypospadias repair in children, Pediatrics 71:342-351, 1983.
Seashore, J.H.: Disorders of the anus and rectum. In Gellis, S.S., and Kagan, B.M.: Current pediatric therapy 12, Philadelphia, 1986, W.B. Saunders Co.
Shapiro, C.: Pain in the neonate: assessment and intervention, Neonatal Network 8(1):7-21, 1989.
Shesser, L.K.: Car seat modification for children under treatment for congenital dislocated hip, Orthop. Nurs. 4(6):11-13, 1985.
Shewmon, D.A., and others: The use of anencephalic infants as organ sources, JAMA 261:1773-1781, 1989.
Shinnar, S., and others: Management of hydrocephalus in infancy: use of acetazolamide and furosemide to avoid cerebrospinal fluid shunts, J. Pediatr. 107:31-37, 1985.
Shoenberg, W.H., and Meador, M.: Analysis of 48 children with myelodysplasia, J. Urol. 127:749-750, 1982.
Solnit, A., and Stark, M.: Mourning and the birth of a defective child, Psychoanal. Study Child. 16:523-537, 1963.
Steinhart, J.M., and others: Ultrasound screening of healthy infants for urinary tract abnormalities, Pediatrics 82:609-614, 1988.
Strain, J.E.: The decision to forgo life-sustaining treatment for seriously ill newborns, Pediatrics 72:572-573, 1983.
Swaiman, K.F.: Pediatric neurology, St. Louis, 1989, Mosby–Year Book, Inc.
Walwork, E., and Ellison, P.H.: Follow-up of families of neonates in whom life support was withdrawn, Clin. Pediatr. 24:14-20, 1985.
Warshaw, B.L., Hymes, L.C., and Woodard, J.R.: Long-term outcome of patients with obstructive uropathy, Pediatr. Clin. North Am. 29:815-826, 1982.

BIBLIOGRAPHY

The Child with a Physical Defect

Brenner, V.M.: Unilateral pulmonary hypoplasia/agenesis in the neonate: a case report, Neonatal Network 6(3):49-57, 1987.
Bucciarelli, R.L., and Eitzman, D.V.: Baby Doe: where we stand now, Contemp. Pediatr. 5(1):116-128, 1988.
Bull, M.J., and others: Special children, special car seats, Contemp. Pediatr. 6(1):122-134, 1989.
Friedman, J.M.: A practical approach to dysmorphology, Pediatr. Ann. 19:95-101, 1990.
Heller, A., and others: Birth defects and psychosocial adjustment, Am. J. Dis. Child. 139:257-263, 1985.
Jackson, P.L.: When the baby isn't "perfect," Am. J. Nurs. 85:396-399, 1985.
Jones, K.L.: Smith's recognizable patterns of human malformation, ed. 4, Philadelphia, 1988, W.B. Saunders Co.
Kilgo, J.L., Richard, N., and Noonan, M.J.: Teaming for the future: integrating transition planning with early intervention services for young children with special needs and their families, Inf. Young Child. 2(2):37-48, 1989.
Lemons, P.M.: Beyond the birth of a defective child, Neonatal Network 5(3):13-20, 1986.
Lynch, M.E.: Congenital defects: parental issues and nursing supports, J. Perinat. Neonatal Nurs. 2(4):53-59, 1989.
Mitchell, C., and Rutherford, P.A.: The fragile survivor, Am. J. Nurs. 87:603-606, 1987.
Porter, F.L.: Pain in the newborn, Clin. Perinatol. 16:549-564, 1989.

Ramp, J.B., and others: Conjoined twins: a multidisciplinary approach, Neonatal Network 8(1):29-39, 1989.

Romney, M.C.: Congenital defects: implications on family development and parenting, Issues Compr. Pediatr. Nurs. 7:1-15, 1984.

Shaw, N.: Common surgical problems in the newborn, J. Perinat. Neonatal Nurs. 3:50-65, 1990.

Wasserman, G.A., and others: Contributors to attachment in normal and physically handicapped infants, J. Am. Acad. Child Adolesc. Psychiatry 26(1):9-15, 1987.

Williams, J.K.: Evaluating the dysmorphic child, Pediatr. Nurs. 9(4):241-248, 1983.

Winter, R.M.: A combinational method for grouping cases with multiple malformations, J. Med. Genet. 25:118-122, 1988.

Ethical Issues

Archer-Duste, H.: Clinical ethics: a mandate for nursing, J. Perinat. Neonatal Nurs. 1(3):49-56, 1988.

Ashwal, S., and Schneider, S.: Brain death in the newborn, Pediatrics 84:429-437, 1989.

Aumann, G.M.E.: New changes, new choices: problems with perinatal technology, J. Perinat. Neonatal Nurs. 1(3):1-9, 1988.

Bailey, C.F.: Withholding or withdrawing treatment on handicapped newborns, Pediatr. Nurs. 12:413-416, 1986.

Bator, A.: Subjectively speaking . . . , Am. J. Nurs. 84:883, 1984.

Bowden, V.R.: Selective nontreatment of handicapped newborns: how do we decide? Child. Health Care 17:12-17, 1988.

Cerase, P.A.: Ethical dilemmas in resuscitation of the very-low-birth-weight infant, J. Perinat. Neonatal Nurs. 1(3):69-76, 1988.

Chitwood, L.: A lesson in living, Nursing '84 14(1):55-56, 1984.

Coulter, D.L.: Neurologic uncertainty in newborn intensive care, N. Engl. J. Med. 316:840-844, 1987.

Cushing, M.: Do not feed . . . , Am. J. Nurs. 83:602-604, 1983.

Cushing, M.: The implications of withdrawing nutritional devices, Am. J. Nurs. 84:191-192, 1984.

Davidhizar, R.M., and Monhaut, N.: Giving bad news by phone, Nursing '85 15(4):58-59, 1985.

Davis, A.J.: A newborn's right to life vs. death, Am. J. Nurs. 81:1035, 1981.

Drane, J.F.: The defective child: ethical guidelines for painful dilemmas, JOGNN 13:42-48, 1984.

Elsea, S.B.: Ethics in maternal-child nursing, MCN 10:303-308, 1985.

Fost, N.: Ethical issues in pediatrics, Curr. Opin. Pediatr. 1:176-178, 1989.

Fotion, N.C.: Ethics and the afflicted child, Crit. Care Q. 8(12):75-83, 1985.

Fries, E.S.: The ethical issues of transplanting organs from anencephalic newborns, MCN 14:412-414, 1989.

Fromer, M.J.: Solving ethical dilemmas in nursing practice. In Chinn, P.L., editor: Ethical issues in nursing, Rockville, MD, 1986, Aspen Systems Corp.

Fry, S.T.: Ethical issues in organs retrieved from anencephalic infants, Issues. Compr. Pediatr. Nurs. 12:437-445, 1990

Gates, E.: Obstetrical decision making in the delivery of the extremely premature infant, Neonatal Network 5(1):7-14, 1986.

Hall, L.F., and Stoops, P.M.: Acquainting a new mother with her less-than-perfect baby, MCN 9:136, 1984.

Hazinski, M.: Organ donation and the new "required request" law, Pediatr. Nurs. 13:370-371, 1987.

Homer, M.B.: Selective treatment, Am. J. Nurs. 84:309-312, 1984.

Joint Policy Statement: Principles of treatment of disabled infants, Pediatrics 73:559-560, 1984.

Kraft, L.A., and Wilson, C.J.: Dilemmas in the care of impaired infants: effects on nursing and health care, Neonatal Network 6(5):73-81, 1988.

Kraybill, E.N.: Parental autonomy in situations of moral ambiguity, J. Pediatr. 113:327, 1988.

Lantos, J.D.: The Hastings Center project on imperiled newborns: Supreme Court, jury, or Greek chorus? (commentary), Pediatrics 83:615-616, 1989.

Lantos, J.D.: Survival after cardiopulmonary resuscitation in babies of very low birth weight. Is CPR futile therapy? N. Engl. J. Med. 318:91-95, 1988.

Leikin, S.: A proposal concerning decisions to forgo life-sustaining treatment for young people, J. Pediatr. 115:17-22, 1989.

Marchwinski, S.: The dilemma of moral and ethical decision making in the intensive care nursery, Neonatal Network 6(5):17-20, 1988.

McClowry, S.G.: Research and treatment: ethical distinctions related to the care of children, J. Pediatr. Nurs. 2:23-29, 1987.

Minogue, J.P., and Reedy, N.J.: Companioning parents in perinatal decision making, J. Perinat. Neonatal Nurs. 1(3):25-35, 1988.

Murphy, M.A.: What price success: can we afford "saved" babies? J. Pediatr. Health Care 3(6):285-286, 1989.

Nelson, R.M.: Decisions concerning the care of very low birthweight infants, Neonatal Network 5(1):16-21, 1986.

Novak, J.: An ethical decision-making model for the neonatal intensive care unit, J. Perinat. Neonatal Nurs. 1(3):57-67, 1988.

Olson, V.T., and Hooke, M.M.: The complexities of do not resuscitate orders, MCN 13:157-162, 1988.

Rothenberg, L.S.: To feed or not to feed: that is the question and the ethical dilemma, J. Pediatr. Nurs. 1:226-229, 1986.

Rushton, C.H.: Ethical decision-making in critical care. 2. Strategies for nurse preparation, Pediatr. Nurs. 14:497-499, 1988.

Saga, M.J.: Dilemmas in practice, Am. J. Nurs. 88:29-30, 1988.

Sandelowski, M.: The politics of patienthood, MCN 11:235-238, 1986.

Short-DeGraff, M.A., and Healey, S.M.: Postpartum depression related to care for the child with special needs, Inf. Young Child. 2(2):24-36, 1989.

Smith, J.B.: Ethical issues raised by new treatment options, MCN 14:183-187, 1989.

Symposium: Would you let this infant die? Am. J. Dis. Child. 7(3):71-72, 77-78, 83, 86, 88, 1990.

Thompson, J.E., and Thompson, H.O.: Living with ethical decisions with which you disagree, MCN 13:245-250, 1988.

Verzemnieks, I.L., and Nash, D.: Ethical issues related to pediatric care, Nurs. Clin. North Am. 19:319-328, 1984.

Walters, J.W.: Approaches to ethical decision making in the neonatal intensive care unit, Am. J. Dis. Child. 142:825-830, 1988.

Watchko, J.F.: Decision making on critically ill infants by parents, Am. J. Dis. Child. 137:795-798, 1983.

West, M.: The mother, the developmentally disabled child and the nurse, Top. Clin. Nurs. 6(3):19-29, 1984.

Winslow, G.R.: Anencephalic infants as organ sources: should the law be changed? J. Pediatr. 115:824-832, 1989.

Youngner, S.J.: Do-not-resuscitate orders: no longer a secret, but still a problem, Hastings Center Report 17(1):24-33, 1987.

Surgery and Pain

American Academy of Pediatrics: Committee on Fetus and Newborn, Committee on Drugs, Section on Anethesiology, and Section on Surgery: Neonatal anesthesia, Pediatrics 80:446, 1987.

Anand, K.J.S., and Aynsley-Green, A.: Measuring the severity of surgical stress in newborn infants, J. Pediatr. Surg. 23(4):297-305, 1988.

Anand, K.J.S., and Carr, D.B.: The neuroanatomy, neurophysiology, and neurochemistry of pain, stress and analgesia in newborns and children, Pediatr. Clin. North Am. 36:795-821, 1989.

Beaver, P.K.: Premature infants' response to touch and pain: can nurses make a difference? Neonatal Network 6(3):13-17, 1987.

Butler, N.B.: The ethical issues involved in the practice of surgery on unanesthetized infants, AORN J. 46(6):1136-1144, 1987.

Butler, N.B.: How to raise professional awareness of the need for adequate pain relief for infants, Birth 15(1):38-41, 1988.

Butler, N.B.: More on neonatal pain, Perinatal Press 11(2):19-20, 1988.

Dale, J.C.: A multidisciplinary study of infants' behaviors associated with assumed painful stimuli: phase I, Pediatr. Nurs. 12:27-31, 1986.

Field, T., and Goldson, E.: Effects of nonnutritive sucking on neonates during heelstick procedures, Pediatrics 74:1012-1015, 1984.

Fitzgerald, M., Millard, C., and MacIntosh, N.: Hyperalgesia in premature infants, Lancet 6(8580):292, 1988.

Franck, L.S.: Pain in the nonverbal patient: advocating for the critically ill neonate, Pediatr. Nurs. 15:65, 1989.

Grunau, R.V., and Craig, K.D.: Pain expression in neonates: facial action and cry, Pain 28:395-410, 1987.

Jones, M.A.: Identifying signs that nurses interpret as indicating pain in newborns, Pediatr. Nurs. 15:76, 1989.

Lawson, J.R.: Standards of practice and the pain of premature infants, Zero to Three 9:1-5, 1988.

Marshall, R.E.: Neonatal pain associated with caregiving procedures, Pediatr. Clin. North Am. 36:885-903, 1989.

Paxton, J.M.: Transport of the surgical neonate, J. Perinat. Neonatal Nurs. 3(3):43-49, 1990.

Pigeon, H.M., and others: How neonatal nurses report infants' pain, Am. J. Nurs. 89:1529-1530, 1989.

Porter, F.L.: Pain in the newborn, Clin. Perinatol. 16(2):549-564, 1989.

Powers, L., and others: Pediatric surgery, In Merenstein, G.B., and Gardner, S.L.: Handbook of neonatal intensive care, ed. 2, St. Louis, 1989, Mosby–Year Book, Inc.

Roberts, P.: A cry for research: pain in the neonate, Can. Nurse 84(6):17-19, 1988.

Schechter, N.L.: The undertreatment of pain in children: an overview, Pediatr. Clin. North Am. 36:781-794, 1989.

Shaw, N.: Common surgical problems in the newborn, J. Perinat. Neonatal Nurs. 3(3):50-65, 1990.

Shearer, M.H.: Surgery on the paralyzed, unanesthetized newborn, Birth 13(2):79, 1986.

Wise, B.V., and Lawrence-Nolan, L.: A risk of blood transfusions for premature infants, MCN 15:86-89, 1990.

Yaster, M.: Analgesia and anesthesia in neonates, J. Pediatr. 111:394-396, 1987.

Neurologic Defects

Arsenault, L.: Delayed onset symptomatic hydrocephalus related to aqueductal stenosis, J. Neurosurg. Nurs. 15(5):291-297, 1983.

Bernardo, M.L.: Craniosynostosis: the child's care from detection through correction, MCN 4:234-237, 1979.Brown, J.P., and Reichenbach, M.A.: Screening children with myelodysplasia for readiness to learn self-catheterization, Rehab. Nurs. 14:334-337, 1989.

Burton, B.K.: Maternal serum α-fetoprotein screening, Pediatr. Ann. 18:687-697, 1989.

Charney, E.B.: Parental attitudes toward management of newborns with myelomeningocele, Dev. Med. Child. Neurol. 32:14-19, 1990.

Charney, E.B., and others: Management of Chiari II complications in infants with myelomeningocele, J. Pediatr. 111:364-371, 1987.

Clark, L.W.: The importance of touch with an anencephalic baby, MCN 7:336-337, 1982.

Cohen, F.L.: Neural tube defects: epidemiology, detection, and prevention, JOGNN 16(2):105-115, 1987.

Gardner, K.L.: Etiology of open neural tube defects, Genet. Pract. 5(2):1-2, 1988.

Graham, J.M.: Craniostenosis: a new approach to management, Pediatr. Ann. 10:258-264, 1981.

Graham, J.M., deSaxe, M., and Smith, D.W.: Sagittal craniostenosis: fetal head constraint as one possible cause, J. Pediatr. 95:747-750, 1979.

Grant, L.: Hydrocephalus: an overview and update, J. Neurosurg. Nurs. 16(6):313-318, 1984.

Guertin, S.R.: Cerebrospinal fluid shunts, evaluation, complications, and crisis management, Pediatr. Clin. North Am. 34:203-217, 1987.

Hanus, S.H., Bernstein, N.R., and Kapp, K.A.: Immigrants into society: children with craniofacial anomalies, Clin. Pediatr. 20(1):37-41, 1981.

Humphrey, P.A., Britt, P.H., and Peters, C.R.: Craniofacial malformations, Am. J. Nurs. 79:1230-1234, 1979.

Jackson, P.L.: Peritoneal shunting for hydrocephalus, Crit. Care Update 10(4):33-39, 1983.

Jeffries, J.S., Killam, P.E., and Varni, J.W.: Behavioral management of fecal incontinence in a child with myelomeningocele, Pediatr. Nurs. 8:267-270, 1982.

Joseph, D.B., and others: Clean, intermittent catheterization of infants with neurogenic bladder, Pediatrics 84:78-82, 1989.

Killam, P.E., and others: Behavioral pediatric weight rehabilitation for children with myelomeningocele, MCN 8:280-286, 1983.

Macbriar, B.R.: Self-concept of preadolescent and adolescent children with a meningomyelocele, Issues Compr. Pediatr. Nurs. 6:1-11, 1983.

Macedo, A., and Posel, L.F.: Nursing the family after the birth of a child with spina bifida, Issues Compr. Pediatr. Nurs. 10:55-65, 1987.

Myhre, C.M., Richards, T., and Johnson, J.: Maternal serum α-fetoprotein screening: an assessment of fetal well-being, J. Perinat. Neonatal Nurs. 2(4):13-20, 1989.

Noetzel, M.J.: Neural tube defects and other congenital and genetic disorders, Curr. Opin. Pediatr. 1:308-314, 1989.

Odio, C., McCracken, G.H., and Nelson, J.D.: CSF shunt infections in pediatrics, Am. J. Dis. Child. 138:1103-1108, 1984.

Pinyerd, B.J.: Siblings of children with myelomeningocele: examining their perceptions, MCN 12(1):61-70, 1983.

Richardson, K., and others: Biofeedback therapy for managing bowel incontinence caused by meningomyelocele, MCN 10:388-392, 1985.

Scheinblum, D.T., and Hammond, M.: The treatment of children with shunt infections: extraventricular drainage system care, Pediatr. Nurs. 16:139-143, 1990.

Shesser, L.K.: Car seat modification for children under treatment for congenital dislocated hips, Orthop. Nurs. 4(6):11-13, 1985.

Shesser, L.K., and Kling, T.F.: Practical considerations in caring for a child in a hip spica cast: an evaluation using parental input, Orthop. Nurs. 5(3):11-15, 1986.

Steele, S.: Young children with meningomyelocele, with special reference to handling, positioning, and child-adult play interactions, Issues Compr. Pediatr. Nurs. 11:213-225, 1988.

Tilem, D., and Greenberg, C.S.: Nursing care of the child with a ventriculostomy, J. Pediatr. Nurs. 3:188-193, 1988.

Van Cleve, L.: Parental coping in response to their child's spina bifida, J. Pediatr. Nurs. 4:172-176, 1989.

Skeletal Defects

Aiello, D.H.: Congenital dysplasia of the hip, diagnosis, treatment, nursing care, AORN J. 49:1566-1606, 1989.

Bull, M.J., and others: Special children, special car seats, Contemp. Pediatr. 6(1):122-134, 1989.

Coleman, S.S.: When a child is born with hip problems, Patient Care 17(14):68-98, 1983.

Feller, N., and others: A multidisciplinary approach to developing safe transportation for children with special needs, Orthop. Nurs. 5(5):25-27, 1986.

Garbarino, J.: Maltreatment of young children with disabilities, Inf. Young Child. 2(2):49-57, 1989.

Hall, J.G.: When a child is born with congenital anomalies, Contemp. Pediatr. 5(8):78-87, 1988.

Hirsch, P.J., and others: Treatment of hip dysplasia in the first nine months, Orthop. Clin. North Am. 13(3):605-618, 1982.

Lieber, M.T., and Taub, A.S.: Common foot deformities and what they mean for parents, MCN 13:47-50, 1988.

Linley, J.F.: Screening children for common orthopaedic problems, Am. J. Nurs. 87:1312-1316, 1987.

Mulley, D.A.: Harnessing babies' dysplastic hips, Am. J. Nurs. 84:1006-1008, 1984.

Short-DeGraff, M.A., and Healey, S.M.: Postpartum depression related to care for the child with special needs, Inf. Young Child. 2(2):24-36, 1989.

Staheli, L.T.: Management of congenital hip dysplasia, Pediatr. Ann. 18:24-32, 1989.

Stout, J.D., Bull, M.J., and Stroup, K.B.: Safe transportation for infants and preschoolers with special needs, Inf. Young Child. 2(2):67-73, 1989.

Swagman, A.: Caring for limb-deficient children and their families, MCN 11:46-52, 1986.

Swanson, A.B.: Congenital limb deformities: classification and treatment, Clin. Symp. 33(3):3-32, 1981.

Thurman, S.K., Cornwell, J.R., and Korteland, C.: The liaison infant family team (LIFT) project: an example of case study evaluation, Inf. Young Child. 2(2):74-82, 1989.

Trott, A.W.: Children's foot problems, Orthop. Clin. North Am. 13:641-655, 1982.

Wenger, D.R., and Leach, J.: Foot deformities in infants and children, Pediatr. Clin. North Am. 33:1411-1427, 1986.

Gastrointestinal Defects

Balluff, M.A.: Nutritional needs of an infant or child with a cleft lip or palate, Ear Nose Throat J. 65:44-49, 1986.

Barss, V.A., Benacerraf, B.R., and Frigoletto, F.D.: Antenatal sonographic diagnosis of fetal gastrointestinal malformations, Pediatrics 76:445-450, 1985.

Burgess, D.B., Martin, H.P., and Lilly, J.R.: The developmental status of children undergoing the Kasai procedure for biliary atresia, Pediatrics 70:624-629, 1982.

Colburn, N., and Cherry, R.S.: Community-based team approach to the management of children with cleft palate, Child. Health Care 13:122-128, 1985.

Curtin, G.: The infant with cleft lip or palate: more than a surgical problem, J. Perinat. Neonatal Nurs. 3(3):80-89, 1990.

Dixon, A.G.: Jeff's story: a unique approach to the care of an infant with esophageal atresia and cervical esophagostomy, Neonatal Network 4(6):7-12, 1986.

Erikson, I., and Mitchell, C.: Which child gets the transplant? Am. J. Nurs. 88:287-288, 1988.

Fentner, S.: Abdominal wall defects: omphalocele and gastroschisis, Neonatal Network 6(3):29-41, 1987.

Fria, T.J., and others: Conductive hearing loss in infants and young children with cleft palate, J. Pediatr. 111:84-88, 1987.

Geggel, R.L., and others: Congenital diaphragmatic hernia: arterial structural changes and persistent pulmonary hypertension after surgical repair, J. Pediatr. 107:457-464, 1985.

Habal, M.B.: The team approach: comprehensive care of patients born with cleft lips and/or cleft palate, Basics 24:4-7, 1986.

Hall, D.E., Roberts, K.B., and Charney, E.: Umbilical hernia: what happens after age 5 years? J. Pediatr. 99:415-417, 1981.

Hazle, N.: An infant who survived gastroschisis, MCN 6:35-40, 1981.

Heller, A., Tidmarsh, W., and Pless, I.B.: The psychosocial functioning of young adults born with cleft lip or palate, Clin. Pediatr. 20:459-465, 1981.

Huth, M.M., and O'Brien, M.E.: The gastrostomy feeding button, Pediatr. Nurs. 13:241-245, 1987.

Karrer, F.M., and Lilly, J.R.: Corticosteroid therapy in biliary atresia, J. Pediatr. Surg. 20:693-695, 1985.

Kobayashi, A., Itabashi, F., and Ohbe, Y.: Long-term prognosis in biliary atresia after hepatic portoenterostomy: analysis of 35 patients who survived beyond 5 years of age, J. Pediatr. 105:243-246, 1984.

Konigs, K.: Application of an ostomy pouch to a preterm infant, Neonatal Network 5(5):49-51, 1987.

Lilly, J.R.: Biliary atresia and liver transplantation: the National Institutes of Health point of view, Pediatrics 74:159-160, 1984.

Lilly, J.R., and Karrer, F.M.: Contemporary surgery of biliary atresia, Pediatr. Clin. North Am. 32:1233-1246, 1985.

Loukimo, I., and Lindahl, H.: Esophageal atresia: primary results of 500 consecutively treated patients, J. Pediatr. Surg. 18:217-229, 1983.

Lynch, M.E.: Congenital defects: parental issues and nursing supports, J. Perinatal Neonatal Nurs. 2(4):53-59, 1989.

Malatack, J.J., and others: The who, when, and how of liver transplants, Contemp. Pediatr. 5(2):152-160, 1988.

McNichol, J.: When eating doesn't come naturally, MCN 14:23-26, 1989.

Moynihan, P., and Gerraughty, A.: Diaphragmatic hernia: low stress = higher survival, Am. J. Nurs. 85:662-665, 1985.

Oellrich, R.G., and Cusumano, M.M.: Biliary atresia, Neonatal Network 5(5):25-32, 1987.

Paradis, K.J.G., Freese, D.K., and Sharp, H.L.: A pediatric perspective on liver transplantation, Pediatr. Clin. North Am. 35:409-433, 1988.

Pashayan, H.M., and McNab, M.: Simplified method of feeding infants born with cleft palate with or without cleft lip, Am. J. Dis. Child. 133:145-147, 1979.

Pate, C.M.H.: Care of the family following the birth of a child with a cleft lip and/or palate, Neonatal Network 5(6):30-37, 1987.

Scheurerle, J., and others: A survey of nursing care for parents and infants with cleft lip and palate, Cleft Palate J. 21:110-114, 1984.

Short, B.L., Miller, M.K., and Anderson, K.D.: Extracorporeal membrane oxygenation in the management of respiratory failure in the newborn, Clin. Perinatol. 14:737-747, 1987.

Smith-Blair, N., and Stephenson, C.: Gastroschisis: a nursing perspective, Focus Crit. Care 13(2):9-19, 1986.

Styer, G.W., and Freeh, K.: Feeding infants with cleft lip and/or palate, JOGNN 10:329-331, 1981.

Theorell, C.J.: Congenital diaphragmatic hernia: a physiologic approach to management, J. Perinat. Neonatal Nurs. 3(3):66-79, 1990.

Torfs, C., Curry, C., and Roeper, P.: Gastroschisis, J. Pediatr. 116:1-6, 1990.

Williams, L.: Care of the pediatric liver transplant patient in the ICU, Crit. Care Q. 8(1):13-25, 1985.

Williams, R.: Congenital diaphragmatic hernia: a review, Heart Lung 11:532-538, 1982.

Zissermann, L.: Feeding problems: weaning an infant from a transpyloric tube, Pediatr. Nurs. 12:33-37, 1986.

Zitelli, B.J., and others: Evaluation of the pediatric patient for liver transplantation, Pediatrics 78:559-565, 1986.

Genitourinary Defects

American Academy of Pediatrics: Summary of annual meeting of the section on pediatric urology, Pediatrics 83:591-596, 1989.

Belman, A.B.: Acquired undescended (ascended) testis: effects of human chorionic gonadotropin, J. Urol. 140:1189-1190, 1988.

Bernhardt, J.: Percutaneous nephrostomy tubes in the neonate with obstructive uropathy, Neonatal Network 4:51-53, 1986.

Cassani, V.: Tracheoesophageal anomalies, Neonatal Network 3(2):20-29, 1983.

Castiglia, P.T.: Ambiguous genitalia, J. Pediatr. Health Care 3(6):319-321, 1989.

deVries, P., and Pena, A.: Posterior sagittal anoplasty, J. Pediatr. Surg. 17:638, 1982.

DiGrande, A.: The child born with ambiguous genitalia: family assessment and nursing intervention, Issues Compr. Pediatr. Nurs. 7:307-318, 1984.

Donahoe, P.K.: The diagnosis and treatment of infants with intersex abnormalities, Pediatr. Clin. North Am. 34:1333-1348, 1987.

Huddleston, K., and others: MIC or foley: comparing gastrostomy tubes, MCN 14:20-22, 1989.

Hulbert, W.C., and Duckett, J.W.: Current views on posterior urethral valves, Pediatr. Ann. 17:31-36, 1988.

Jeffs, R.D.: Exstrophy, epispadias, and cloacal and urogenital sinus abnormalities, Pediatr. Clin. North Am. 34:1233-1257, 1987.

Kaplan, B.S., and others: Polycystic kidney diseases in childhood, J. Pediatr. 115:867-880, 1989.

Khoury, A.E., and Churchill, B.M.: The artificial urinary sphincter, Pediatr. Clin. North Am. 34:1175-1185, 1987.
Levitt, S.B., and Reda, E.F.: Hypospadias, Pediatr. Ann. 17:48-57, 1988.
Loper, D.L.: Gastrointestinal development: embryology, congenital anomalies and impact on feedings, Neonatal Network 2(1):27-36, 1983.
Marshall, D.G.: Femoral hernias in children, J. Pediatr. Surg. 18:160-162, 1983.
Mazur, T.: Ambiguous genitalia: detection and counseling, Pediatr. Nurs. 9:417-422, 1983.
Mitchell, M.E., and Rink, R.C.: Pediatric urinary diversion and undiversion, Pediatr. Clin. North Am. 34:1319-1332, 1987.
Pagon, R.A.: Diagnostic approach to the newborn with ambiguous genitalia, Pediatr. Clin. North Am. 34:1019-1031, 1987.
Pappis, C.H., and others: Unsuspected urological abnormalities in cryptorchid boys, Pediatr. Radiol. 18:51-53, 1988.
Peevy, K.J., Speed, F.A., and Hoff, C.J.: Epidemiology of inguinal hernia in preterm neonates, Pediatrics 77:246-247, 1986.
Reinburg, Y.U., and Gonzalez, Y.: Upper urinary tract obstruction in children: current controversies in diagnosis, Pediatr. Clin. North Am. 34:1291-1304, 1987.
Rezvani, I.: Cryptorchidism: a pediatrician's view, Pediatr. Clin. North Am. 34:735-746, 1987.
Saenger, P.: Abnormal sex differentiation, J. Pediatr. 104:1-17, 1984.
Sheldon, C.A., and Duckett, J.W.: Hypospadias, Pediatr. Clin. North Am. 34:1259-1272, 1987.
Stevens, M.S., and Reinitz, M.: Nursing a child through exstrophic bladder reconstruction surgery, MCN 5:265-270, 1980.
Welsh, S. and Gatch, G.C.: Imperforate anus: diagnosis and surgical treatment, AORN J. 42:692-698, 1985.

Prenatal Influences: General

Bank, K.M., and others: Reproductive hazards in the work place, Fam. Community Health 6(1):44-56, 1983.
Benirschke, K., and others: Developmental terms—some proposals: first report of an international working group, Am. J. Med. Genet. 3:297-302, 1979.
Brent, R.L.: The effects of embryonic and fetal exposure to x-ray, microwave and ultrasound, Clin. Obstet. Gynecol. 26:484-510, 1983.
Brent, R.L.: The effects of ionizing radiation, microwaves, and ultrasound on the developing embryo: clinical interpretations and applications of the data, Curr. Probl. Pediatr. 14(9):1-87, 1984.
Jacobson, H.N.: Advances in knowledge of fetal and maternal nutrition, Food Nutr. News 58:22-24, 1986.
Jankowski, C.B.: Radiation and pregnancy: putting the risks in proportion, Am. J. Nurs. 86:260-265, 1986.
Kalter, H., and Warkany, J.: Congenital malformations: etiologic factors and their role in prevention, part I, N. Engl. J. Med. 308:424-431, 1983.
Kalter, H., and Warkany, J.: Congenital malformations, part II, N. Engl. J. Med. 308:491-497, 1983.
Miao, C.Y., Zuberbuhler, J.S., and Zuberbuhler, J.R.: Prevalence of congenital anomalies at high altitude, J. Am. Coll. Cardiol., 12:224-228, 1988.
Rhodes, A.M.: Legal alternatives for fetal injury, MCN 15:111, 1990.
Rivera, J., and Villar, J.: Nutritional supplementation during two consecutive pregnancies and the interim lactation period: effect on birth weight, Pediatrics 81:51-57, 1988.
Shepard, T.H.: Counseling pregnant women exposed to potentially harmful agents during pregnancy, Clin. Obstet. Gynecol. 26:478-483, 1983.
Warkany, J.: Teratogen update: hyperthermia, Teratology 33:365-369, 1986.
Yip, R.: Altitude and birth weight, J. Pediatr. 111:869-876, 1987.

Prenatal Influences: Infectious Agents

Adler, S.P., and others: Cytomegalovirus infections in neonates due to blood transfusions, Pediatr. Infect. Dis. 2:114-118, 1983.
Alford, C.A., Pass, R.F., and Stagno, S.: Chronic congenital infections: common environmental causes for severe and subtle birth defects, Birth Defects 19(5):187-192, 1983.
Alkalay, A.L., Pomerance, J.J., and Rimoin, D.L.: Fetal varicella syndrome, J. Pediatr. 111:320-323, 1987.
Alpert, G., and Plotkin, S.A.: A practical guide to the diagnosis of congenital infections in the newborn infant, Pediatr. Clin. North Am. 33:465-479, 1986.
American Academy of Pediatrics Committee on Infectious Diseases: Parvovirus B19, erythema infectiosum (fifth disease and pregnancy), Pediatrics 85:131-133, 1990.
Beasley, R.P., and others: Prevention of perinatally transmitted hepatitis B virus infections with hepatitis B immune globulin and hepatitis B vaccine, Lancet 2:1099-1102, 1983.
Brady, M.: Preventing the perinatal spread of hepatitis B, J. Pediatr. Health Care 3(1):49-51, 1989.
Bromberg, M.H., and Hsia, L.S.Y.: Rubella in the perinatal period, J. Perinat. Neonatal Nurs. 1(4):24-32, 1988.
Brown, Z.A., and others: Effects on infants of a first episode of genital herpes during pregnancy, N. Engl. J. Med. 317:1246-1251, 1987.
Butt, W., and others: Intracranial lesions of congenital cytomegalovirus infection detected by ultrasound scanning, Pediatrics 73:611-614, 1984.
Centers for Disease Control: Congenital syphilis—New York City, 1986-1988, MMWR 38:825-829, 1989.
Centers for Disease Control: Prevention of perinatal transmission of hepatitis B virus: prenatal screening of all pregnant women for hepatitis b surface antigen, MMWR 37:341-346, 1988.
Centers for Disease Control: Rubella and congenital rubella syndrome—United States, 1985-1988, MMWR 38:173-182, 1989.
Centers for Disease Control: Rubella vaccination during pregnancy, MMWR 38:289-293, 1989.
Committee on Infectious Diseases: Report of the Committee on Infectious Diseases, Elk Grove Village, IL, 1988, American Academy of Pediatrics.
Conboy, T.J., and others: Early clinical manifestations and intellectual outcome in children with symptomatic congenital cytomegalovirus infection, J. Pediatr. 111:343-348, 1987.
Delaplane, D., and others: Fatal hepatitis B in early infancy: the importance of identifying HBsAg-positive pregnant women and providing immunoprophylaxis to their newborns, Pediatrics 72:176-180, 1983.
DeVore, N.E., Jackson, V.M., and Piening, S.L.: TORCH infections, Am. J. Nurs. 83:1660-1665, 1983.
Dworsky, M.E., and others: Cytomegalovirus infection of breast milk and transmission in infancy, Pediatrics 72:295-299, 1983.
Dworsky, M.E., and others: Occupational risk for primary cytomegalovirus infection among pediatric health-care workers, N. Engl. J. Med. 309:950, 1983.
Faix, R.G.: Survival of cytomegalovirus on environmental surfaces, J. Pediatr. 106:649-652, 1985.
Frinkel, J.K.: Toxoplasmosis, Pediatr. Clin. North Am. 32:917-932, 1985.
Gauntt, C.J., and others: Coxsackievirus Group B antibodies in the ventricular fluid of infants with severe anatomic defects in the central nervous system, Pediatrics 76:64-68, 1985.
Griffin, M.P., and others: Cytomegalovirus infection in a neonatal intensive care unit, Am. J. Dis. Child. 142:1188-1193, 1988.
Hinman, A.R.: Prevention of congenital rubella infection: symposium summary, Pediatrics 75:1162-1165, 1985.
Hutto, C., and others: Intrauterine herpes simplex virus infections, J. Pediatr. 110:97-101, 1987.
Kaplan, K.M., and others: A profile of mothers giving birth to infants with congenital rubella syndrome, Am. J. Dis. Child. 1144:118-123, 1990.
Klein, M.E.: Hepatitis B virus: perinatal management, J. Perinat. Neonatal Nurs. 1(4):12-23, 1988.
Koskiniemi, M., Lappalainen, M., and Hedman, K.: Toxoplasmosis needs evaluation, Am. J. Dis. Child. 143:724-728, 1989.
Kumar, M.L., and others: Congenital and postnatally acquired cytomegalovirus infections: long term follow-up, J. Pediatr. 104:674-679, 1984.

Kumar, M.L., and others: Postnatally acquired cytomegalovirus infection in infants of CMV-excreting mothers, J. Pediatr. 104:669-679, 1984.

Leland, D., and others: The use of TORCH titers, Pediatrics 72:41-43, 1983.

Lin, H., and others: Transplacental leakage of HBeAg-positive maternal blood as the most likely route in causing intrauterine infection with hepatitis B virus, J. Pediatr. 111:877-881, 1987.

MacDonald, A.B., and others: Stillbirth following maternal Lyme disease, NY State J. Med. 87:615-616, 1987.

Mascola, L., and others: Congenital syphilis, JAMA 252:1719-1722, 1984.

Miller, E., and others: Outcome in newborn babies given anti-varicella-zoster immunoglobulin after perinatal maternal infection with varicella-zoster virus, Lancet 2:371-373, 1989.

Nankervis, G.A., and others: A prospective study of maternal cytomegalovirus infection and its effect on the fetus, Am. J. Obstet. Gynecol. 149:435-440, 1984.

Paryani, S.G., and Arvin, A.M.: Intrauterine infection with varicella-zoster virus after maternal varicella, N. Engl. J. Med. 314:1542-1546, 1986.

Paryani, S.G., and others: Sequelae of acquired cytomegalovirus infection in premature and sick term infants, J. Pediatr. 107:451-456, 1985.

Pass, R.F., and others: Young children as a probable source of maternal and congenital cytomegalovirus infection, N. Engl. J. Med. 316:1366-1370, 1987.

Prober, C.G., and others: Low risk of herpes simplex virus infections in neonates exposed to the virus at the time of vaginal delivery to mothers with recurrent genital herpes simplex virus infections, N. Engl. J. Med. 316:240-244, 1987.

Ritter, S.E., and Vermund, S.H.: Congenital toxoplasmosis, JOGNN 14:435-439, 1985.

Rubella vaccination during pregnancy: United States, 1971-1988, MMWR 38:2889, 1989.

Samson, L.F.: Perinatal viral infections and neonates, J. Perinat. Neonatal Nurs. 1(4):56-65, 1988.

Schalm, S.W., and others: Prevention of hepatitis B infection in newborns through mass screening and delayed vaccination of all infants of mothers with hepatitis B surface antigen, Pediatrics 83:1041-1047, 1989.

Sever, J.L., and others: Toxoplasmosis: maternal and pediatric findings in 23,000 pregnancies, Pediatrics 82:181-192, 1988.

Tedberg, A.J., and others: Clinical manifestations of epidemic neonatal listeriosis, Pediatr. Infect. Dis. J. 6:817-820, 1987.

Withers, J., and Bradshaw, E.: Preventing neonatal hepatitis-B infection, MCN 11:270-272, 1986.

Prenatal Influences: AIDS

American Academy of Pediatrics, Task Force on Pediatric AIDS: Perinatal human immunodeficiency virus infection, Pediatrics 82:941-944, 1988.

Boland, M.G., and Klug, R.M.: AIDS: the implications for home care, Am. J. Nurs. 86:404-411, 1986.

Boyes, S.M.: AIDS virus in breast milk: a new threat to neonates and donor breast milk banks, Neonatal Network 5(5):37-39, 1987.

Edmondson, K.S.: Acquired immune deficiency syndrome in the neonate, Neonatal Network 6(4):7-12, 1988.

Grippi, C., Ward, L., and Roncoli, M.: The case of baby Alice: AIDS/ARC in infancy, Neonatal Network 6(5):9-15, 1988.

Iazzeti, L.: Nursing management of the pediatric AIDS patient, Issues Compr. Pediatr. Nurs. 9:119-129, 1986.

Inglis, A.D., and Lozano, M.: AIDS and the neonatal ICU, Neonatal Network 5(3):39-43, 1986.

Iosub, S., and others: More on human immunodeficiency virus embryopathy, Pediatrics 80:512-516, 1987.

Ippolito, C., and Gibes, R.M.: AIDS and the newborn, J. Perinat. Neonatal Nurs. 1(4):78-86, 1988.

Johnson, J.P., and others: Natural history and serologic diagnosis of infants born to human immunodeficiency virus—infected women, Am. J. Dis. Child. 143:1147-1153, 1989.

Kennedy, K.I., Fortney, J.A., and Sokal, D.C.: Breastfeeding and HIV, Lancet 1:333, 1989.

Marion, R.W., and others: Fetal AIDS syndrome score, Am. J. Dis. Child. 141:429-431, 1987.

Nicholas, S.W., and others: Human immunodeficiency virus infection in childhood, adolescence, and pregnancy: a status report and national research agenda, Pediatrics 83:293-308, 1989.

Qazi, Q.H., and others: Lack of evidence for craniofacial dysmorphism in perinatal human immunodeficiency virus infection, J. Pediatr. 12:7-11, 1988.

Scott, G.B., and others: Survival in children with perinatally acquired human immunodeficiency virus type 1 infection, N. Engl. J. Med. 321:1791-1796, 1989.

Stear, L.A., and Elinger, S.S.: Understanding acquired immunodeficiency syndrome: implications for pregnancy, J. Perinat. Neonatal Nurs. 1(4):33-46, 1988.

Wiley, K., and Grohar, J.: Human immunodeficiency virus and precautions for obstetric, gynecologic, and neonatal nurses, JOGNN 17:165-168, 1988.

Prenatal Influences: Chemical Agents

Barbour, B.G.: Is fetal alcohol syndrome completely irreversible? MCN 14:44-46, 1989.

Chavez, G.F., Mulinare, J., and Cordero, J.F.: Maternal cocaine use during early pregnancy as a risk factor for congenital urogenital anomalies, JAMA 262:795-798, 1989.

Church, M.W., and Gerkin, K.P.: Hearing disorders in children with fetal alcohol syndrome: findings from case reports, Pediatrics 82:147-154, 1988.

Coles, C.D., and others: Persistence over the first month of neurobehavioral differences in infants exposed to alcohol prenatally, Behav. Dev. 10:23-37, 1987.

Council on Scientific Affairs: Fetal effects of maternal alcohol use, JAMA 249:2517, 1983.

Eliason, M.J., and Williams, J.K.: Fetal alcohol syndrome and the neonate, J. Perinat. Neonatal Nurs. 3(4):64-72, 1990.

Ernhart, C.B., and others: Alcohol teratogenicity in the human: a detailed assessment of specificity, critical period, and threshold, Am. J. Obstet. Gynecol. 156:33-39, 1987.

Graham, J.M., and others: Independent dysmorphology evaluations at birth and 4 years of age for children exposed to varying amounts of alcohol in utero, Pediatrics 81:772-778, 1988.

Hanold, K.C.: Teratogenic potential of valproic acid, JOGNN 15:111-116, 1986.

Kuller, J.M.: Effects on the fetus and newborn of medications commonly used during pregnancy, J. Perinat. Neonatal Nurs. 3(4):73-87, 1990.

Luke, B.: Megavitamins and pregnancy: a dangerous combination, MCN 10:18-23, 1985.

Michaelis, J., and others: Prospective study of suspected associations between certain drugs administered during early pregnancy and congenital malformations, Teratology 27:57, 1983.

Miller, P.K.: Vitamin A during pregnancy, Teratology 35:269-274, 1987.

Mills, J., and Graubard, B.I.: Is moderate drinking during pregnancy associated with an increased risk for malformations? Pediatrics 80:309-314, 1987.

Mills, J., and others: Maternal alcohol consumption and birth weight: how much drinking during pregnancy is safe? JAMA 252:1875-1879, 1984.

Pregnancy categories for prescription drugs, FDA Drug Bull. 12(3):24, 1982.

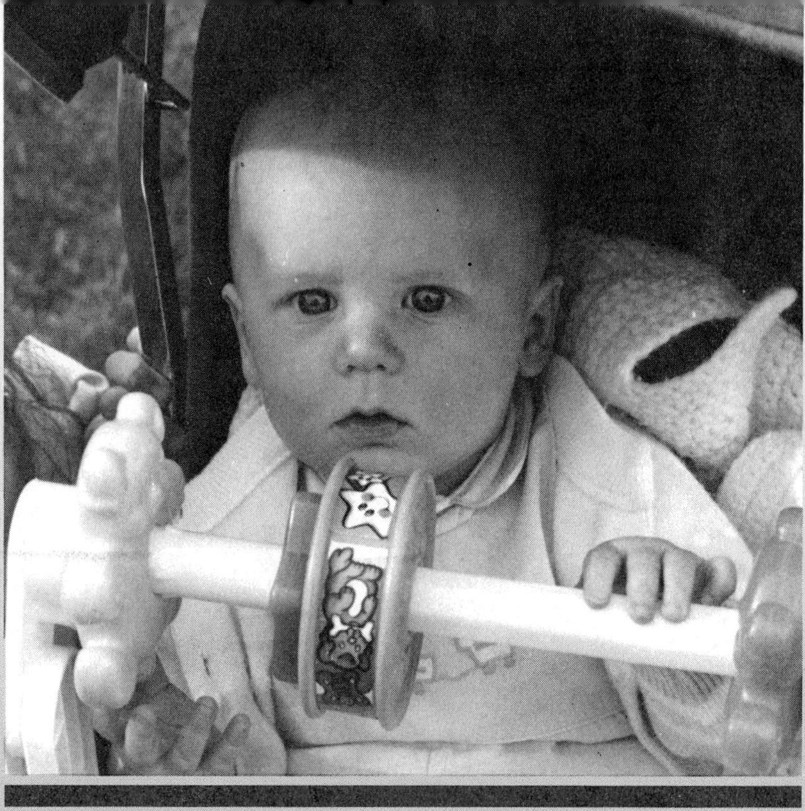

Infancy

UNIT IV

The first 12 months of childhood is the period of most rapid gain in physical size and most dramatic achievement of developmental milestones in an individual's entire life. It is marked by an orderly progression of physical, intellectual, and social maturation. It is also a highly vulnerable period for both positive and negative influences governing optimum growth and development.

Chapter 12, *Health Promotion of the Infant and Family,* investigates the infant's biologic, psychosocial, cognitive, and social development. It is concerned with fostering optimum health through anticipatory guidance regarding nutrition, prevention of disease and injury, and promotion of parent-child attachment. Chapter 13, *Health Problems During Infancy,* deals with health problems that commonly occur during the first year, usually as a result of environmental rather than pathologic processes, and that therefore can be prevented. It is also concerned with conditions of unknown cause, such as sudden infant death syndrome, which has profound emotional consequences on the developing family.

CHAPTER 12

Health Promotion of the Infant and Family

RELATED TOPICS

Animal bites, Ch. 18
Dental health, Ch. 14
Growth and development of children, Ch. 4
Ingestion of injurious agents, Ch. 16
Injuries—the leading killer, Ch. 1
Injury prevention, Ch. 14
Intramuscular administration of medication, Ch. 27
Preschool or daycare experience, Ch. 15
Provision of optimum nutrition, Ch. 8
Promotion of parent-infant bonding (attachment), Ch. 8
Separation anxiety, Ch. 26
Sunburn, Ch. 18

GLOSSARY

ACIP Advisory Committee on Immunization Practices
acquired immunity Immunity from exposure to the invading agent, either bacteria, virus, or toxin
active immunity Immune bodies are actively formed against specific antigens, either *naturally* by having had the disease clinically or subclinically or *artificially* by introducing the antigen (vaccine) into the individual
adjuvant Substance added to the vaccine to keep the antigen at the injection site and to enhance the antigenic process
antibody A protein, found mostly in serum, that is formed in response to exposure to a specific antigen
antigen A variety of foreign substances, including bacteria, viruses, toxins, and foreign proteins, that stimulate the formation of antibodies
antitoxin Antibody formed in response to a toxin (antigen)
attenuate Reduce the virulence (infectiousness) of a pathogenic microorganism by such measures as treating it with heat or chemicals or cultivating it on a certain medium
deciduous (primary) teeth Initial teeth that are eventually shed
DT Diphtheria, tetanus (full dose)
DTP Diphtheria, tetanus, pertussis
Hib *Haemophilus influenzae* type b
HIV Human immunodeficiency virus
Ig Immunoglobulin
immunity An inherited or acquired state in which an individual is resistant to the occurrence or the effects of a specific disease, particularly an infectious agent
IPV Inactivated polio virus
ITQ Infant Temperament Questionnaire
MMR Measles, mumps, rubella
narcissism Self-love; concerned only with self
natural immunity Innate immunity or resistance to infection or toxicity
NCVIA National Childhood Vaccine Injury Act
object permanence Realization that objects exist outside of visual field
OPV Oral polio virus
passive immunity Temporary immunity by transfusing plasma proteins either *artificially* from another human or an animal that has been actively immunized against an antigen or *naturally* from the mother to the fetus via the placenta
physiologic anemia Depression of hemopoietic system from high level of fetal hemoglobin
PRP-D Diphtheria toxoid conjugate
PRP-HbOC Diphtheria CRM_{197} protein conjugate
PRP-OMP Meningococcal protein conjugate
schema Pattern of action and/or thought
sensorimotor cognition Learning primarily through senses and movement
solitary play Play that is centered on own activities
stereopsis Depth perception
Td Tetanus, diphtheria (reduced dose)
TIG Tetanus immune globulin
toxin A poisonous substance, usually produced by the invading microorganism
toxoid A toxin that has been treated to destroy its toxic properties but retain its antigenic quality
vaccine Collectively, a term to denote any type of active immunization agent, such as toxoids or attenuated live viruses; specifically, a suspension of disease-causing bacteria or viruses that acts like an antigen, stimulates antibody production, and produces active acquired immunity
weaning Process of relinquishing bottle-feeding or breast-feeding

The miracle of birth is surpassed only by the wonder of growth and development unfolding over the succeeding months and years. The biologic growth and developmental maturation of the infant are a study of perfection in nature. The nurse's understanding of these processes is essential to the optimum care of the child and family. To present relevant data for appreciation of growth and development, it is necessary to systematize and categorize the facts into various levels of maturation and age-groups. However, we must always bear in mind that no child will be represented in any one table or chart, because each child is as much an individual as the number of variables that influence his or her existence.

PROMOTING OPTIMUM GROWTH AND DEVELOPMENT

General concepts of growth and development, such as stages and patterns of development and individual differences, are discussed extensively in Chapter 4. This chapter is primarily concerned with biologic, psychosocial, cognitive, body image, and social development of the child from 1 to 12 months of age. It also includes a discussion of common parental concerns that are typical of the developmental characteristics of this age-group.

BIOLOGIC DEVELOPMENT

At no other time in life are physical changes and developmental achievements so dramatic as during infancy. All major body systems undergo progressive maturation, and there is concurrent development of skills that increasingly allows infants to respond to and cope with the environment. Acquisition of these fine and gross motor skills occurs in an orderly sequence, following usual cephalocaudal-proximodistal laws.

Proportional Changes

During the first year growth is very rapid, especially during the initial 6 months. Infants gain 680 g (1½ pounds) per month until age 6 months, when the birth weight has at least doubled. An average weight for a 6-month-old child is 7.26 kg (16 pounds). Weight gain decreases by half that amount during the second 6 months. By 1 year of age the infant's birth weight has tripled, with an average weight of 9.75 kg (21½ pounds).

Height increases by 2.5 cm (1 inch) per month during the first 6 months, and by half that amount monthly during the second 6 months. Average height is 65 cm (25½ inches) at 6 months and 74 cm (29 inches) at 12 months. By 1 year the birth length has increased by almost 50%. The increase in length occurs mainly in the trunk, rather than in the legs, and contributes to the characteristic physique of the older infant (see Fig. 12-9, *A*).

Head growth is also rapid. During the first 6 months head circumference increases approximately 1.5 cm (½ inch) per month, but decreases to only 0.5 cm (¼ inch) per month during the second 6 months. The average size is 43 cm (17 inches) at 6 months and 46 cm (18 inches) at 12 months. By 1 year head size has increased by almost 33%. Closure of the cranial sutures occurs, with the posterior fontanel fusing by 6 to 8 weeks of age and the anterior fontanel closing by 12 to 18 months of age, with the average age at 14 months (Duc and Largo, 1986).

Expanding head size reflects the growth and differentiation of the nervous system. By the end of the first year the brain has increased in weight about two and one half times. The maturation of the brain is exhibited in the dramatic developmental achievements of infancy (see Table 12-3). The primitive reflexes (see Table 8-4) are replaced by voluntary, purposeful movement, and new reflexes that influence motor development appear (Box 12-1).

The chest assumes a more adult contour, with the lateral diameter becoming larger than the anteroposterior diameter. The chest circumference approximately equals head circumference by the end of the first year. The heart grows less rapidly than does the rest of the body. Its weight is usually doubled by 1 year of age, in comparison with body weight, which triples during the same period. The size of the heart is still large in relation to the chest cavity; its width is about 55% of the width of the chest.

Sensory Changes

During infancy visual acuity gradually improves, and binocular fixation is established. The major developmental characteristics of vision during infancy are listed in Box 12-2.

Binocularity, or the fixation of two ocular images into one cerebral picture (fusion), begins to develop by 6 weeks of age and should be well established by age 4 months. Lack of binocular vision results in strabismus and must be detected early to prevent permanent blindness.

Depth perception (stereopsis) begins to develop by age 7 to 9 months but may exist earlier as an innate safety mechanism. Studies have demonstrated that even 2- to 3-month-old infants distinguish depth. At about 7 months the parachute reflex appears, which may be a protective response during a fall (Fig. 12-1 and Box 12-1).

Infants also have a *visual preference* for looking at the human face, which also has a developmental sequence. For example, at age 6 weeks they show more interest in a picture of a face with eyes than without. By 10 weeks of age a picture with both eyes and eyebrows elicits more response, and by 20 weeks of age the mouth is also necessary. By age

Box 12-1 NEUROLOGIC REFLEXES THAT APPEAR DURING INFANCY

Reflex	Expected Behavioral Response	Age of Appearance (Months)
Labyrinth-righting	Infant in prone or supine position is able to raise head	2, strongest at 10
Neck-righting	While infant is supine, head is turned to one side; shoulder, trunk, and finally pelvis will turn toward that side	3, until 24-36
Body-righting	A modification of the neck-righting reflex in which turning hips and shoulders to one side causes all other body parts to follow	6, until 24-36
Otolith-righting	When body of an erect infant is tilted, head is returned to upright, erect position	7-12, persists indefinitely
Landau	When infant is suspended in a horizontal prone position, the head is raised, legs and spine are extended	6-8, until 12-24
Parachute	When infant is suspended in a horizontal prone position and suddenly thrust downward, hands and fingers extend forward as if to protect against falling (see Fig. 12-1)	7-9, persists indefinitely

Box 12-2 MAJOR DEVELOPMENTAL CHARACTERISTICS OF VISION

Age (Weeks)	Development
Birth	Visual acuity 20/100-20/400* Pupillary and corneal (blink) reflexes present Able to fixate on moving object in range of 45 degrees when held 20-25 cm (8-10 inches) away Cannot integrate head and eye movements well (doll's eye reflex—eyes lag behind if head is rotated to one side)
4	Can follow in range of 90 degrees Can watch parent intently as he or she speaks to infant Tear glands begin to function Visual acuity is hyperoptic because of less spheric eyeball than in adult
6-12	Has peripheral vision to 180 degrees Binocular vision begins at age 6 weeks, is well established by age 4 months Convergence on near objects begins by age 6 weeks, is well developed by age 3 months Doll's eye reflex disappears
12-20	Recognizes feeding bottle Able to fixate on a 1.25 cm (½ inch) block Looks at hand while sitting or lying on back Looks at mirror image Able to accommodate to near objects
20-28	Adjusts posture to see an object Able to rescue a dropped toy Develops color preference for yellow and red Able to discriminate between simple geometric forms Prefers more complex visual stimuli Develops hand-eye coordination Pats image of self in mirror
28-44	Can fixate on very small objects Depth perception begins to develop Lack of binocular vision indicates strabismus
44-52	Visual acuity, 20/40-20/60 Visual loss may develop if strabismus is present Can follow rapidly moving objects

*Measurement of visual acuity differs according to testing procedures (see also Table 7-10).

6 months infants respond to facial expressions and can distinguish between familiar and strange faces. This is about the same time as stranger anxiety is manifested (see p. 549).

With progressive myelination of the auditory pathway, the specific responses of locating sound replace the generalized response of the neonate (Fig. 12-2). The major developmental characteristics of hearing are listed in Box 12-3. (For a further discussion of hearing and the senses of smell, taste, and touch, see Chapter 8.)

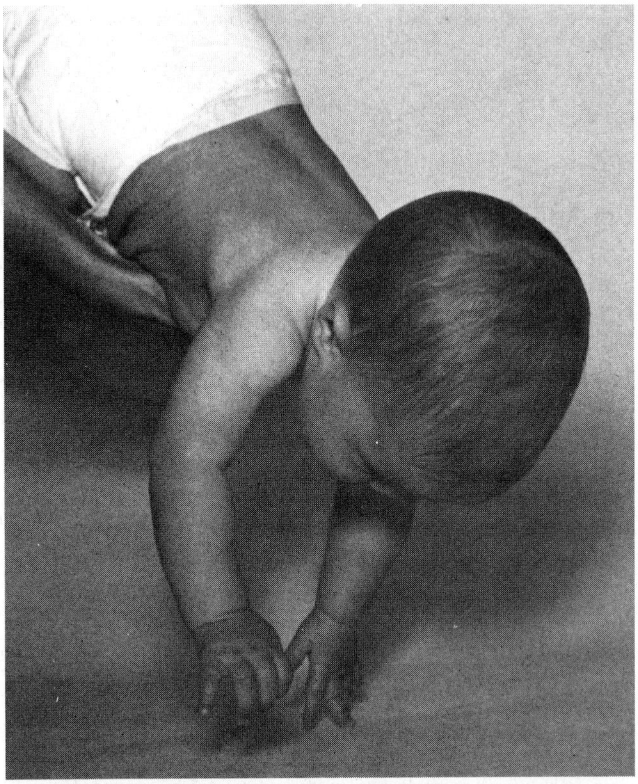

Fig. 12-1. Parachute reflex.

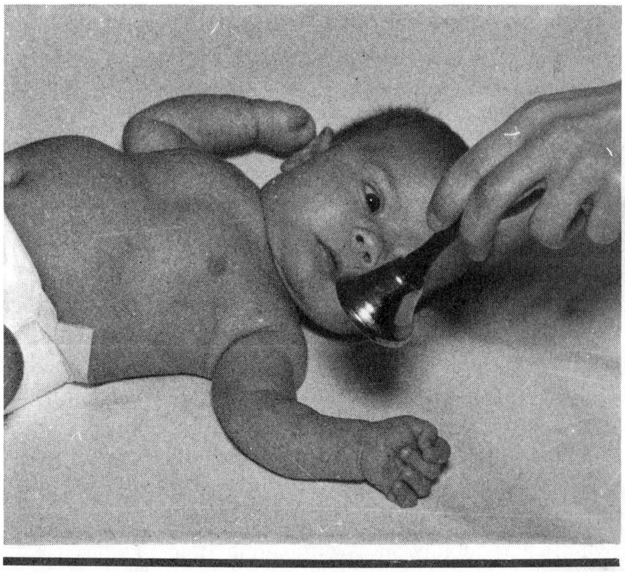

Fig. 12-2. Three-month-old infant locates sound by turning head to side and looking in direction of the sound.

Maturation of Systems

Other organ systems also change and grow during infancy. The respiratory rate slows somewhat (see inside front cover) and is relatively stable. Respiratory movements continue to be abdominal. Several factors predispose the infant to more severe and acute respiratory problems. The close proximity of the trachea to the bronchi and its branching structures rapidly transmits an infectious agent from one anatomic location to another. The short, straight eustachian

Box 12-3 MAJOR DEVELOPMENTAL CHARACTERISTICS OF HEARING

Age (Weeks)	Development
Birth	Responds to loud noise by startle reflex Responds to sound of human voice more readily than to any other sound Low-pitched sounds, such as lullaby, metronome, or heartbeat, have quieting effect
8-12	Turns head to side when sound is made at level of ear
12-16	Locates sound by turning head to side and looking in same direction (Fig. 12-2)
16-24	Can localize sounds made below ear, which is followed by localization of sound made above ear; will turn head to the side and then look up or down Begins to imitate sounds
24-32	Locates sounds by turning head in a curving arc Responds to own name
32-40	Localizes sounds by turning head diagonally and directly toward sound
40-52	Knows several words and their meaning, such as "no," and names of members of the family Learns to control and adjust own response to sound, such as listening for the sound to occur again

tube closely communicates with the ear, allowing infection to ascend from the pharynx to the middle ear. In addition, the immunologic ability of the mucosal lining provides less protection against infection in infancy than during later childhood.

Although the lumen of the trachea and bronchi enlarges during infancy, it remains small in comparison with the total size of the lung, maintaining low resistance to the volume of air inspired. The ability of the entire respiratory tract to produce mucus is diminished, decreasing the humidification of the large volume of inspired air. In addition, the volume of dead space, that amount of air needed to fill the respiratory passages with each breath, is large, requiring the infant to breath about twice as fast as the adult to provide the body with the needed amount of oxygen.

The heart rate slows (see inside front cover), and the rhythm is frequently sinus arrhythmia (rate increases with inspiration and decreases with expiration). Blood pressure also changes during infancy (see inside front cover). Systolic pressure rises during the first 2 months as a result of the increasing ability of the left ventricle to pump blood into the systemic circulation. Diastolic pressure decreases during the first 3 months, then gradually rises to values close to those at birth. Fluctuations in blood pressure occur during varying states of activity and emotion.

Significant hemopoietic changes occur during the first year (see Appendix D). Fetal hemoglobin is present for the first 5 months, with adult hemoglobin forming at about 13 weeks of age. Maternal iron stores are present for the first 5 to 6 months in full-term newborns and then gradually diminish, which partially accounts for lowered hemoglobin levels toward the end of the first 6 months.

Physiologic anemia is seen at 2 to 3 months of age because of the decreasing number of red blood cells. This phenomenon is thought to be caused by the depression of the hemopoietic system because of the high level of fetal hemoglobin, which suppresses the production of erythropoietin, a hormone released by the kidney. The occurrence of physiologic anemia is not affected by an adequate supply of iron. However, when erythropoiesis is stimulated, iron supplies are then necessary for formation of hemoglobin.

The digestive processes are immature at birth. Saliva is secreted in small amounts, but the majority of the digestive processes do not begin functioning until age 3 months, when drooling is common because of the poorly coordinated swallowing reflex. The enzyme *ptyalin* (also called amylase) is present in small amounts but usually has little effect on the foodstuff because of the small amount of time the food stays in the mouth. Gastric digestion in the stomach consists primarily of the action of hydrochloric acid and rennin, an enzyme that acts specifically on the casein in milk to cause the formation of curds, coagulated semisolid particles of milk. The curds cause the milk to be retained in the stomach long enough for digestion to occur. The amount of rennin decreases throughout life. This enzyme functions best in a moderately acidic medium; the child's stomach has less acidity than the adult's, which enhances the action of rennin.

Digestion also takes place in the duodenum, where pancreatic enzymes and bile begin to break down protein and fat. Secretion of the pancreatic enzyme *amylase,* which is needed for digestion of complex carbohydrates, is deficient until about the fourth to sixth month of life. *Lipase* is also limited, and infants do not achieve adult levels of fat absorption until 4 to 5 months of age. *Trypsin* is secreted in sufficient quantities to catabolize protein into polypeptides and some amino acids.

The immaturity of the digestive processes is evident in the appearance of stools. During infancy solid foods, such as peas, carrots, corn, and raisins, are passed incompletely broken down in the feces. An excess quantity of fiber easily disposes the child to loose, bulky stools.

During infancy the stomach enlarges to accommodate a greater volume of food. By the end of the first year the infant is able to tolerate three meals a day and an evening bottle and may have one or two bowel movements daily. However, with any type of gastric irritation the infant is vulnerable to diarrhea, vomiting, and dehydration (see Chapters 28 and 29).

The liver is the most immature of all the gastrointestinal organs throughout infancy. The ability to conjugate bilirubin and to secrete bile is achieved after the first couple of weeks of life. However, the capacities for gluconeogenesis, formation of plasma protein and ketones, storage of vitamins, and deaminization of amino acids remain relatively immature for the first year of life.

Maturation of suckling, sucking, and swallowing reflexes

parallels the changes in the gastrointestinal tract and prepares the infant for the introduction of solid foods. *Suckling,* which is first seen at birth, denotes extension and a pulling-in pattern of tongue movements as in licking. During breastfeeding the lips gently clamp the areola in place as the mandible and tongue thrust forward to grasp the nipple and areola. The sucking fat pads in the cheeks fill the mouth and help maintain negative pressure. The tongue then moves rhythmically forward to the gums and lips and back toward the hard palate, compressing the areola between itself and the palate to "milk" the collecting ductules. As milk flows from the nipple, it stimulates the swallowing reflex and is ejected into the esophagus.

In bottle-feeding the *sucking* action is different. Consequently breast-fed infants may become confused if given a bottle. The relatively inflexible rubber nipple may prevent the tongue from moving rhythmically forward and backward. In addition, the flow of milk may be too rapid, causing choking. Infants learn to control the stream of milk by pushing the tongue against the rubber nipple holes. When given the breast again, they may use the same action and push the human nipple out of the mouth (Lawrence, 1989).

Swallowing (deglutition) is the ability to collect the food (bolus) and propel it into the esophagus. Mature sucking and swallowing are acquired with development of the orofacial muscles. During the *infantile (visceral) swallow reflex* (Fig. 12-3, *A*) food lies in a shallow groove on the dorsum of the tongue. As the tongue is pressed upward toward the palate, the milk flows by gravity down the sloping tongue to the pharynx. The milk also flows along the sides of the mouth in lateral furrows between the tongue and cheek pads. As the bolus moves downward, the posterior wall of the pharynx comes forward to displace the soft palate. The larynx is then elevated, and the epiglottis diverts the flow to either side of the pharynx so that the food passes around, but not over, the larynx and into the laryngopharynx. The bolus is then propelled by pharyngeal peristaltic movement into the esophagus (Pipes, 1989).

As the infant grows, the tongue becomes smaller in proportion to the oral cavity and attains greater motility. Consequently the *mature (somatic) swallow reflex* (Fig. 12-3, *B*) is significantly different. The tongue remains behind the central incisors, and the mandible no longer thrusts forward. The dorsum of the tongue is less concave and remains higher and parallel, not inclined, against the palate, and the lateral furrows are absent because of tooth eruption. Tongue pressure and movement against the hard palate pushes the bolus back into the pharynx, where the food is passed over the epiglottis to enter the laryngopharynx and esophagus. The development of mature sucking is thought to develop after the first 6 months.

Infants also exhibit a special reflex called the *Santmyer swallow.* When a puff of air is directed at the face, the infant has a reflex swallow (Orenstein and others, 1988).

The immunologic system undergoes numerous changes during the first year. The newborn receives significant amounts of maternal immunoglobulin (Ig) G, which confers immunity for about 3 months against antigens to which the mother was exposed. During this time the infant begins to synthesize IgG, and about 40% of adult levels are reached by 1 year of age. Significant amounts of IgM are produced at birth, and adult levels are reached by 9 months of age. The production of IgA, IgD, and IgE is much more gradual, and maximum levels are not attained until early childhood.

During infancy the ability of the skin to contract and shiver in response to cold increases. The peripheral capillaries respond to change in ambient temperature to regulate heat loss. In response to cold, the capillaries constrict, conserving core body temperature and decreasing potential evaporative heat loss from the skin surface. In response to heat the capillaries dilate, decreasing internal body temperature through evaporation, conduction, and convection. Shivering causes the muscles and muscle fibers to contract, generating metabolic heat, which is distributed throughout the body. Accumulation of adipose tissue during the first 6 months serves to insulate the body against heat loss.

The shift in the total body fluid at birth—from a higher level of intracellular fluid to extracellular fluid—continues during the first year, resulting in about 35% extracellular fluid and 40% intracellular fluid, or a total body fluid of 75%. The proportionally higher ratio of extracellular fluid, which is composed of blood plasma, interstitial fluid, and lymph, predisposes the infant to a more rapid loss of total body fluid and consequently dehydration.

The immaturity of the renal structures also predisposes the infant to dehydration. Complete maturity of the kidney occurs during the latter half of the second year, when the cuboidal epithelium of the glomeruli becomes flattened.

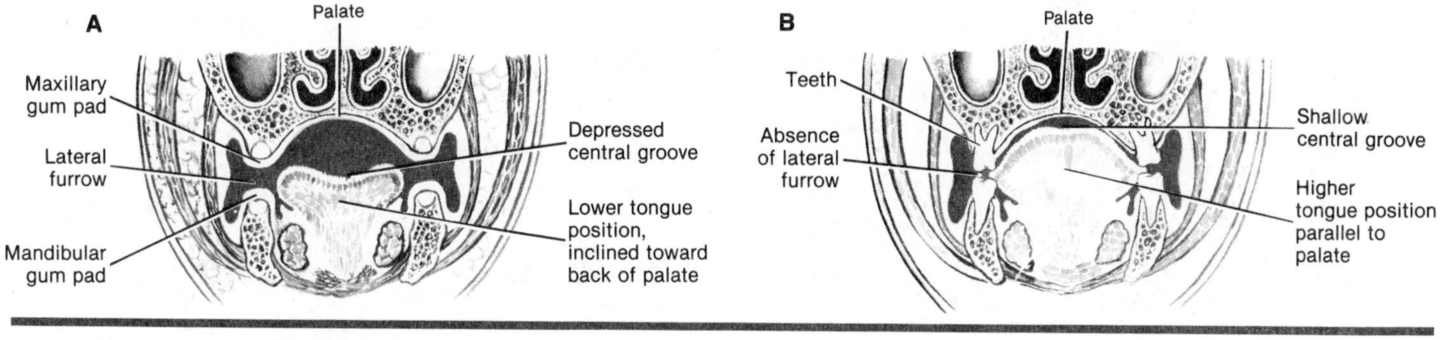

Fig. 12-3. Comparison of, **A,** infantile (visceral) swallow reflex and, **B,** mature (somatic) swallow reflex.

Before this time the filtration capacity of the glomeruli is reduced.

The endocrine system is adequately developed at birth, but its functions are immature. The interrelatedness of all the endocrine organs has a major effect on the function of any one gland. The lack of homeostatic control because of various functional deficiencies renders the infant especially vulnerable to imbalances in fluid and electrolytes, glucose concentration, and amino acid metabolism.

For example, corticotropin (ACTH) is produced in limited quantities during infancy. ACTH acts on the adrenal cortices to produce their hormones, particularly the glucocorticoids and aldosterone. Because the feedback mechanism between ACTH and the adrenal cortex is immature during infancy, there is much less tolerance for stressful conditions, which affect fluid and electrolytes and the metabolism of fats, proteins, and carbohydrates. In addition, although the islets of Langerhans produce insulin and glucagon during fetal life and early infancy, blood sugar levels tend to remain labile, particularly under conditions of stress.

Fine Motor Development

Fine motor behavior includes the use of the hands and fingers in the prehension (grasp) of an object. Grasping occurs during the first 2 to 3 months as a reflex and gradually becomes voluntary. At 1 month the hands are predominantly closed, and by 3 months they are mostly open. By this time the infant demonstrates a desire to grasp an object, but "grasps" more with the eyes than with the hands. By 4 months the child regards a small pellet and the hands and looks from the object to the hands and back again. Hand regard is common at this age because of the limitation of symmetric positioning, which prevents the infant from exploring the periphery. Hand regard occurs in children who are blind, because it is a developmental process that occurs without visual stimulation. The fingering usually includes pulling at blankets and clothes and sucking on the fists or fingers.

By 5 months the infant is able to voluntarily grasp an object, but prehension is two-handed. The palmar grasp begins with grasping the object in the ulnar side of the palm (toward the fourth and fifth fingers) for the first 6 months. From 6 to 8 months, grasping occurs on the radial side (second and third fingers) and the base of the thumb. From 8 to 10 months the index, fourth, and fifth fingers form a crude pincer grasp with the lower part of the thumb (Fig. 12-4). By 12 months the index finger and thumb are used in apposition for a neat pincer grasp (Fig. 12-5).

By 6 months infants have increased manipulative skill. They hold the bottle, grasp their feet and pull them to the mouth, feed themselves a cracker. They enjoy tearing and crumbling paper and explore it thoroughly in the mouth. If given two objects, they will hold one and drop the other. By 7 months they transfer objects from one hand to the other (see Fig. 12-8, *E*) and use one hand for grasping. They enjoy banging objects and explore movable parts of a toy.

By 10 months pincer grasp is established, and infants are able to pick up a raisin and other finger foods. They can deliberately let go of an object and will offer it to someone, but true casting, deliberate throwing of objects, one after the other, is not evident until 12 to 15 months of age. By 11 months they put objects into a container and like to remove them. By 1 year of age infants try to build a tower of two blocks, but fail. Deliberately releasing an object has advanced; they now release a cube into a cup following a demonstration.

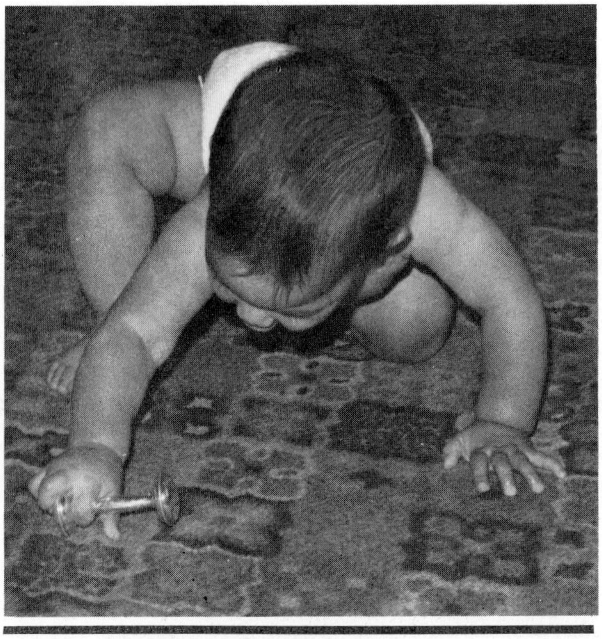

Fig. 12-4. Crude pincer grasp.

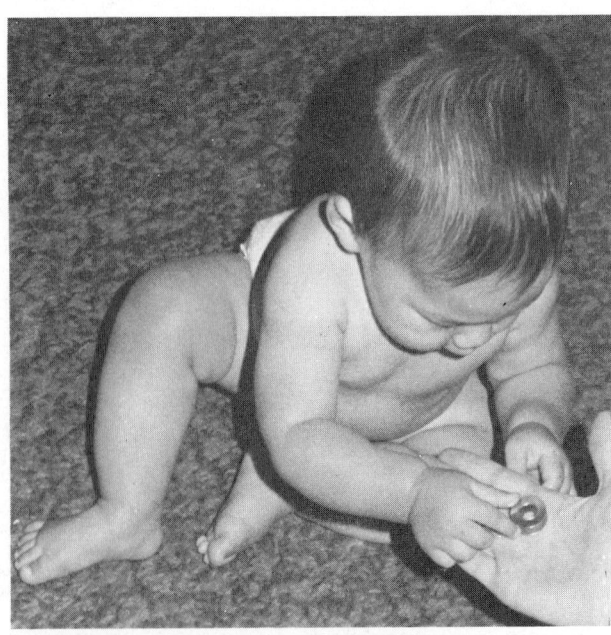

Fig. 12-5. Neat pincer grasp.

Gross Motor Development

Gross motor behavior includes developmental maturation in posture, head balance, sitting, creeping, standing, and walking. The full-term neonate is born with some ability to hold the head erect and reflexly assumes the postural tonic neck position when supine. Several of the primitive reflexes have significance in terms of development of later gross motor skills. The *righting reflexes* elicit certain postural responses, particularly of flexion or extension. They are responsible for certain motor activities, such as rolling over, assuming the crawl position, and maintaining normal head-trunk-limb alignment during all activities. The neck-righting reflex, which turns the body to the same side as the head, enables the child to roll over from supine to prone. Other reflexes, such as the otolith-righting and labyrinth-righting reflexes, enable the infant to raise the head (see Box 12-1).

The asymmetric tonic neck reflex, which persists from birth to 3 months, prevents the infant from rolling over. The symmetric tonic neck reflex, which is evoked by flexing or extending the neck, helps the infant to assume the crawl position. When the head and neck are extended, the extensor tone of the upper extremities and the flexor tone of the lower extremities increase. The child extends the arms and bends the knees. Because of the strong flexor tone of the lower extremities, the infant may initially crawl backward before forward. This reflex disappears when neurologic maturity allows actual crawling to occur because independent limb movement is required.

Head control. The full-term newborn can momentarily hold the head in midline and parallel when the body is suspended ventrally and can lift and turn the head from side to side when prone. However, marked head lag is evident when the infant is pulled from a lying to a sitting position. By 3 months the infant can hold the head well beyond the plane of the body and by 4 months can lift the head and front portion of the chest about 90 degrees above the table, bearing weight on the forearms. Only slight head lag is evident when the infant is pulled from a lying to a sitting position. By 6 months the infant can raise the chest and upper part of the abdomen off the table, maintaining weight on the hands. By 7 months the child can bear weight on one hand while exploring with the other. Figs. 12-6 and 12-7 illustrate development of head control.

✦ **NURSING ALERT** Any child who displays head lag at 6 months of age should have a developmental/neurologic evaluation.

Rolling over. The newborn may accidentally roll over because of the rounded back. The neck-righting reflex enables the infant to roll from back to side at 4 months. The ability to willfully turn from the abdomen to the back occurs at 5 months, and from the back to the abdomen at 6 months. It is noteworthy that the parachute reflex, which elicits a protective response to falling, appears at 7 months.

Sitting. The ability to sit follows progressive head control and straightening of the back, as shown in Fig. 12-8. Although there is marked head lag in the sitting position at birth, the neck, shoulder, and arm muscles contract, enabling infants to raise the head when pulled halfway to a sitting position. They will make attempts to lift the chin and right the head while sitting. At 3 months head lag is slight; at 4 months it is absent; by 6 months they lift the head when about to be pulled into a sitting position. By the next month they spontaneously raise the head in an attempt to sit up by themselves.

For the first couple of months the back is uniformly rounded. As the spinal column straightens, infants are able to be propped in a sitting position. By 7 months they can sit alone, leaning forward on the hands for support. By 8 months they can sit well unsupported and begin to explore their surroundings in this position rather than in a lying position. By 10 months they can maneuver from a prone to a sitting position.

Locomotion. If young infants are placed in a standing position, the body is usually limp at the hips and knees. By 6 to 7 months they are able to bear all their weight. By 9 months they stand holding onto furniture and can pull

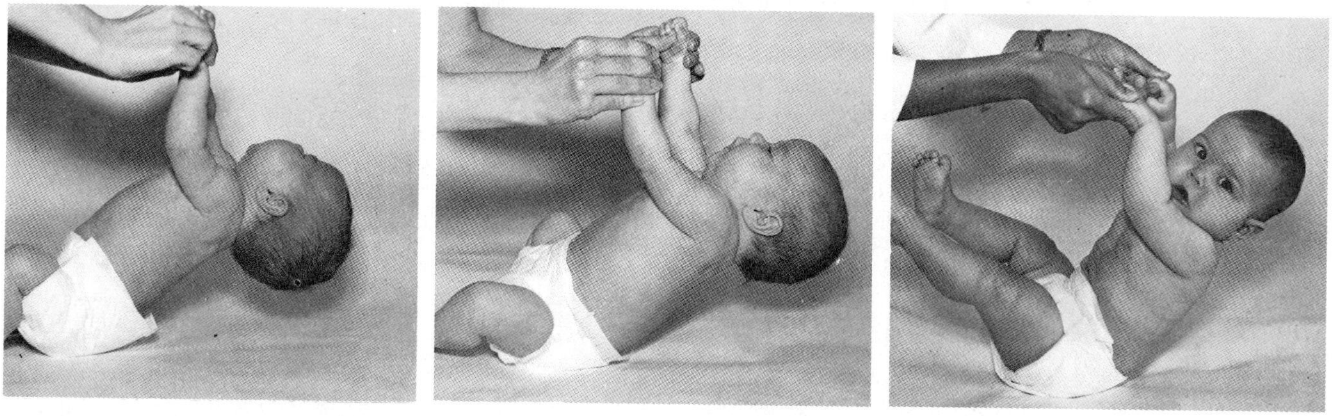

A B C

Fig. 12-6. Head control while pulled to sitting position. **A,** Complete head lag at 1 month. **B,** Partial head lag at 2 months. **C,** Almost no head lag at 4 months.

A

B

C

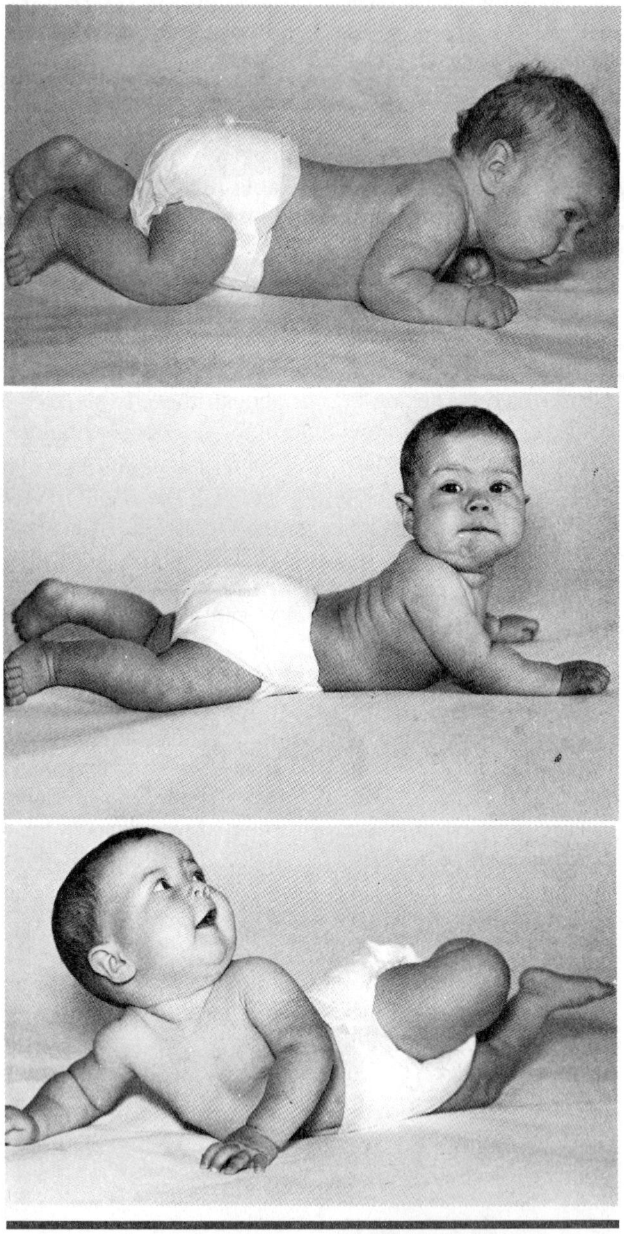

Fig. 12-7. Head control while prone. **A,** Momentarily lifts head at 1 month. **B,** Lifts head and chest 90 degrees and bears weight on forearms at 4 months. **C,** Lifts head, chest, and upper abdomen and can bear weight on hands at 6 months. Note how this position facilitates turning from abdomen to back.

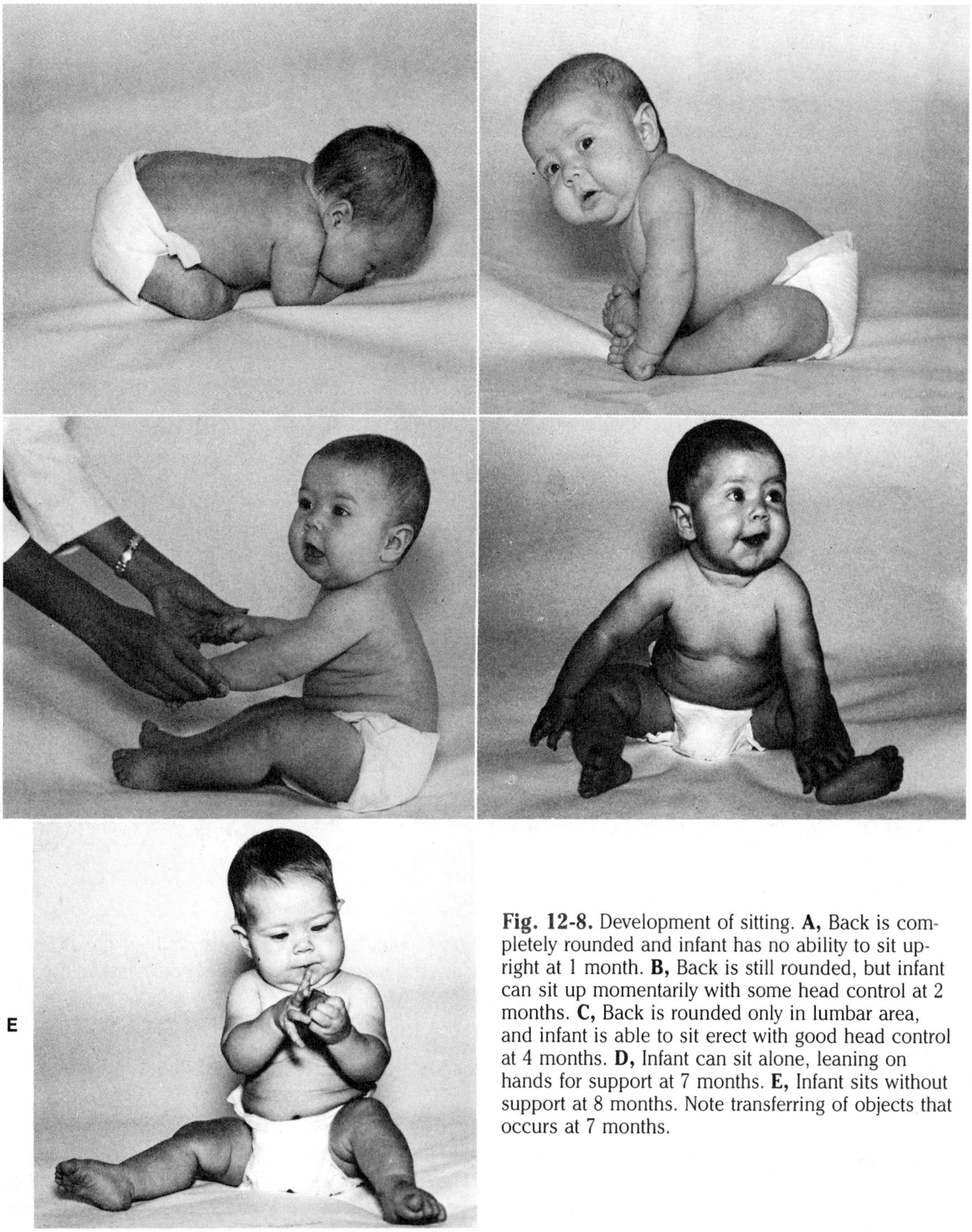

Fig. 12-8. Development of sitting. **A,** Back is completely rounded and infant has no ability to sit upright at 1 month. **B,** Back is still rounded, but infant can sit up momentarily with some head control at 2 months. **C,** Back is rounded only in lumbar area, and infant is able to sit erect with good head control at 4 months. **D,** Infant can sit alone, leaning on hands for support at 7 months. **E,** Infant sits without support at 8 months. Note transferring of objects that occurs at 7 months.

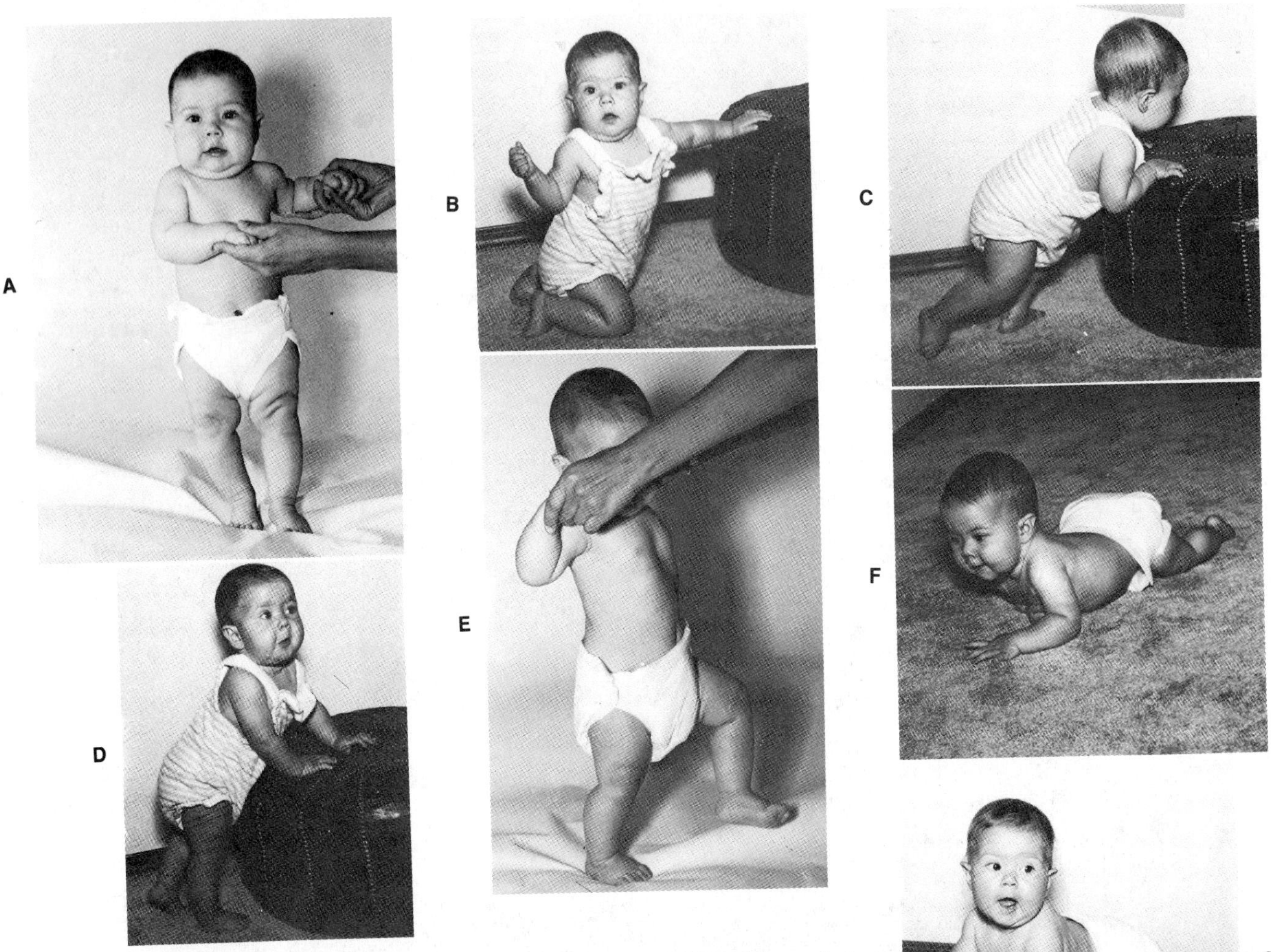

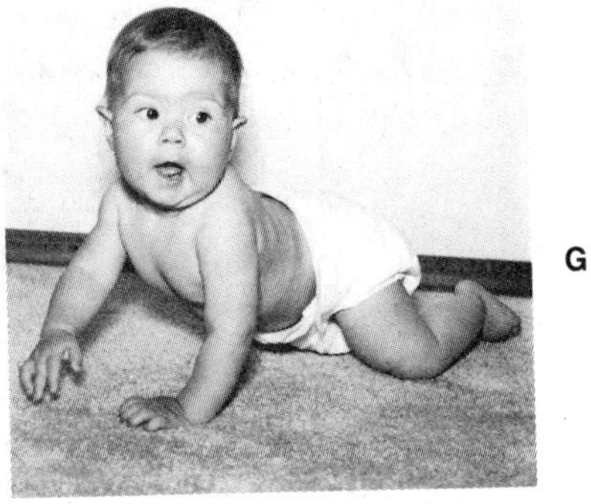

Fig. 12-9. Development of locomotion. **A,** Infant bears full weight on feet by 7 months. **B,** Infant can maneuver from sitting to kneeling position. **C,** Infant can pull self to standing position. **D,** Infant can stand holding onto furniture at 9 months. **E,** While standing, infant takes deliberate step at 10 months. **F,** Infant crawls with abdomen on floor and pulls self forward with hands at 10 months. **G,** Infant creeps on hands and knees at 11 months.

themselves to the standing position but are unable to maneuver back down, except by falling. At 10 months they can step with one foot and crawl well. At 11 months they can creep and cruise or walk while holding onto furniture or with both hands held. By 52 weeks walking with one hand held is achieved. Fig. 12-9 illustrates development of locomotion.

PSYCHOSOCIAL DEVELOPMENT

Infants are born with the basic abilities needed for extrauterine survival, such as respiration, thermoregulation, and digestion. However, they cannot survive without a caregiver to provide for their essential needs, such as food, warmth, and security. In addition to their basic needs, which must be supplied for them, infants have certain tasks that they must achieve for themselves during the first year of life. How their needs are met by others greatly determines to what degree they accomplish their tasks. The stages of development have been studied and described by several noted psychoanalysts, including Erikson and Freud.

Developing a Sense of Trust (Erikson)

Erikson's phase I (birth to 1 year) is concerned with *acquiring a sense of trust* while overcoming a sense of *mistrust.* The trust acquired in infancy is foundational for all the succeeding phases. It allows the infant a feeling of physical comfort and security, which assists him in experiencing unfamiliar, unknown situations with a minimum of fear. The crucial element for the achievement of this task is the *quality* of the parent (caregiver)–child relationship. The provision of food, warmth, and shelter is alone inadequate for the development of a strong ego. The infant and parent must jointly learn to satisfactorily meet their needs in order for mutual regulation of frustration to occur. When this synchrony fails to develop, mistrust is the eventual outcome.

The acquisition of trust involves the libidinal or psychologic energy of the erotic centers of the body, namely the mouth. Erikson has described particular stages in the oral phase. The first social modality is primarily *oral.* During the first 3 to 4 months food intake is the most important social activity in which the infant engages. The id processes are most evident; the newborn can tolerate little frustration or delay of gratification. Primary *narcissism* is at its height. However, as bodily processes such as vision, motor movements, and vocalization are more cortically controlled, the id processes, which operate on the *pleasure principle,* become a component of the ego structure, which operates on the *reality principle.* The infant gradually learns to accept delayed gratification and alternative methods of eliciting a positive response from the environment.

Either extreme in terms of "delayed gratification" leads to mistrust. If caregivers always meet children's needs before they signal readiness, infants will never learn to test their ability to control the environment. If the delay is prolonged, infants will experience constant frustration and eventually mistrust others in their efforts to satisfy them.

The next social modality involves an incorporative mode of reaching out to others through *grasping.* Initially grasping is reflexive, but it has a powerful social meaning to the parents. The reciprocal response of the infant's grasping is the parents' holding on and touching.

Tactile stimulation is significant in the total process of acquiring trust. During the newborn period the parent's exploration of the infant's body is considered an important aspect of bonding. Continued physical contact becomes an important (if not crucial) determinant of attachment of the caregivers. Rejection of physical contact by *attachment figures,* not mere acquaintances or strangers, eventually leads to anger and conflict in the child (Biggar, 1984). Therefore the degree of parenting skill, the quantity of food, or the length of sucking does not determine the quality of the experience; rather, it is the total nature of the interpersonal relationship, including the component of touch, that regulates the infant's formulation of trust.

During the second incorporative stage, the more active and aggressive modality of *biting* occurs. Infants learn that they can hold on to what is their own and can more fully control the environment. During this stage they are confronted with one of their first conflicts of breast-feeding as they quickly learn that biting causes withdrawal of the nipple and anxiety in the mother. Yet biting also brings internal relief from teething discomfort and a sense of power or control. The successful resolution of this conflict strengthens the mother-child relationship at a time when the infant is recognizing her as the most significant person in his or her life.

At about the same time (6 months of age), stranger anxiety is evident. Infants have formed strong attachments to the most significant people in their world, the parents. Separation can be devastating and, if prolonged, can affect future personality development. Although unpleasant for parent and child to experience, demonstration of stranger anxiety is an important component of parent-infant attachment.

Oral Stage (Freud)

Freud's oral stage during infancy involves id gratification through oral satisfaction. Before the teeth erupt, usually during the first 6 months of life, the infant is in the *oral-passive,* or *oral-dependent, stage.* Pleasure is derived through sucking, eating, and rooting. During and after teething the infant is in the *oral-aggressive stage* and can bite as well as suck for gratification.

The erogenous zones are the mouth and lips; any object that comes in contact with this zone is potentially pleasurable. The "mouthing activity" of the infant is very evident during the first year, when everything is explored by sucking or biting. The sucking needs of infants vary, just as the "oral needs" of adults differ. Some infants are satisfied by the amount of sucking supplied through feeding, whereas others require additional opportunities for sucking pleasure, such as the use of a pacifier or thumb.

COGNITIVE DEVELOPMENT

Intellectual development is concurrent with biologic, motor, language, and personal-social achievements, many of which must occur before learning can take place. For example, visual ability must be sufficient for the infant to see objects clearly before associations about the object can be made. Learning occurs when behavior changes as a result of experience or growth. As motor function progresses, learning occurs through the infant's more active participation in the environment. The theory most frequently quoted to explain cognition, or the ability to know, is that of Piaget.

Sensorimotor Phase (Piaget)

The period of birth to 24 months is termed the sensorimotor phase and is composed of six stages; however, inasmuch as this discussion is concerned with ages birth to 12 months, only the first four stages are discussed (Table 12-1; see Table 14-1 for the stages from 13 to 24 months).

During the sensorimotor phase infants progress from reflex behaviors to simple repetitive acts to imitative activity. Three crucial events take place during this phase. First, infants learn to separate themselves from other objects in the environment. They realize that others besides themselves control the environment and that certain readjustments must take place for mutual satisfaction to occur. This coincides with Erikson's concept of the formation of trust and mutual regulation of frustration. Piaget also believes in a "conflict" during each phase. The goal during one phase is to establish a balance between the desire to function at a higher level while recognizing the limitations created by the environment. He believes that achieving a near equilibrium in a constantly changing environment is the goal of biologic, affective (emotional), and mental functions.

The second major accomplishment is achieving the concept of *permanency,* or the realization that objects that leave the visual field still exist.

Table 12-1 Sensorimotor phase during infancy*

STAGE	AGE (MONTHS)	COGNITIVE DEVELOPMENT	BEHAVIOR
I. Use of reflexes	Birth-1	Repetitious use of reflexes establishes a pattern of experiences Totally autistic (self-centered) being	Mostly reflexive (sucking, swallowing, rooting, grasping, crying) Little or no tolerance for frustration or delayed gratification
II. Primary circular reactions	1-4	Use of reflexes is gradually replaced by voluntary activity Recognition of causality occurs when repetition of events causes one stimulus to produce a consistent response Beginning notion of temporal space or time occurs as infant realizes the progression of an orderly sequence of events Beginning separation of self from others Learns from type of interaction between object or individual rather than from object itself Engages in an activity for the pleasure of the activity more than for its result	Recognizes familiar faces and objects (for example, bottle) Shows anticipation before feeding Awareness of strange surroundings indicates memory Discovers parts of own body—plays with hands, fingers, feet Becomes bored when left alone Shows no stranger anxiety unless caregiver's skill differs from usual routine
III. Secondary circular reactions	4-8	Intentional activity replaces repetitious activity that did not produce a desired result Beginning of object permanency when object is beyond perceptual range Progressive idea of time, awareness of before and after in a sequence of events Able to imitate selective activity from several events Further separation of self from environment Idea of quality and quantity Beginning recognition of symbols as type of communication	Secures objects by pulling on a string Searches for objects that have fallen Shows stranger anxiety Able to tolerate some frustration and delayed gratification Imitates sounds and simple gestures Great interest in mirror image (see Fig. 12-11) Beginning independence in self-feeding Shows displeasure if activity is inhibited Language development, attracts attention by methods other than crying Realizes that parents are present even if not in visual field
IV. Coordination of secondary schemas and their application to new situations	9-12	Concept of object permanence advances, beginning of intellectual reasoning Associates symbols with events, but classification is based on own experience Distinguishes objects from the related activity and perceives them as objects Distinguishes end products from their means, attempts to remove barriers to achieve the end	Actively searches for a hidden object (Fig. 12-10) Comprehends meanings of words and simple commands Knows that gestures (bye-bye, kiss) have certain meanings Is able to put objects in a container Works to get toy that is out of reach Ventures away from mother to explore surroundings

*For phases during toddlerhood see Table 14-1.

The last major intellectual achievement of this period is the ability to use *symbols* or "mental representation." The use of symbols allows the infant to think of an object or situation without actually experiencing it. The recognition of symbols is the beginning of understanding of time and space.

Use of reflexes. The first stage, from birth to 1 month, is identified by the infant's use of reflexes. At birth the infant's individuality and temperament are expressed through the physiologic reflexes of sucking, rooting, grasping, and crying. The repetitious nature of the reflexes is the beginning of associations between an act and a sequential response. When infants cry because they are hungry, a nipple is put in the mouth, and they suck, feel satisfaction, and sleep. They are assimilating this experience while perceiving auditory, tactile, and visual cues. This experience of perceiving certain patterns, or "ordering," is foundational for the subsequent stages.

Primary circular reactions. This stage marks the beginning of the replacement of reflexive behavior with voluntary acts. During the period from 1 to 4 months, activities such as sucking or grasping become deliberate acts that elicit certain responses. The beginning of accommodation is evident. Infants incorporate and adapt their reactions to the environment and recognize the stimulus that produced a response. Previously they would cry until the nipple was brought to the mouth. Now they associate the nipple with the sound of the parent's voice. They accommodate this new piece of information and adapt by ceasing to cry when they hear the voice, before receiving the nipple. A realization of causality and a recognition of an orderly sequence of events is taking place. The environment is taken in with all the senses and with whatever motor ability is present.

Secondary circular reactions. The secondary circular reaction stage is a continuation of primary circular reactions and lasts until 8 months of age. In this stage the primary circular reactions are repeated and prolonged for the response that results. Grasping and holding now become shaking, banging, and pulling. Shaking is performed to hear a noise, not solely for the pleasure of shaking. Quality and quantity of an act become evident. "More" or "less" shaking produces different responses. Causality, time, deliberate intention, and separateness from the environment begin to develop.

Three new processes of human behavior—imitation, play, and affect—occur. *Imitation* requires the differentiation of selected acts from several events. By the second half of the first year infants can imitate sounds and simple gestures. *Play* becomes evident as they take pleasure in performing an act after they have mastered it. Much of infants' waking hours are absorbed in sensorimotor play. *Affect* (outward manifestation of emotion and feeling) is seen as infants begin to develop a sense of permanency. During the first 6 months infants believe that an object exists only for as long as they can visually perceive it. In other words, out of sight—out of mind. When the object continues to be present or remembered even though it is beyond the range of perception, affect to external objects is evident. Object permanence is a critical component of parent-child attachment and is seen in the development of stranger anxiety at 6 to 8 months of age (p. 549).

Coordination of secondary schemas and their application to new situations. During the fourth sensorimotor stage, infants use previous behavioral achievements primarily as the foundation for adding new intellectual skills to their expanding repertoire. This stage is largely transitional. Increasing motor skills allow for greater exploration of the environment. They begin to discover that hiding an object does not mean that it is gone but that removing an obstacle will reveal the object. This marks the beginning of intellectual reasoning. Furthermore, they can experience an event by *observing* it, and they begin to associate symbols with events, such as "bye-bye" with "Daddy goes to work," but the classification is purely their own. Unlike the second stage, where infants learned from the type of interaction between objects or individuals, in this stage they learn from the object itself. Intentionality is further developed in that now they will actively attempt to remove a barrier to the desired (or undesired) action (Fig. 12-10). If something is in their way, they will attempt to climb over it or push it away. Previously an obstacle would cause them to give up any further attempt to achieve the desired goal.

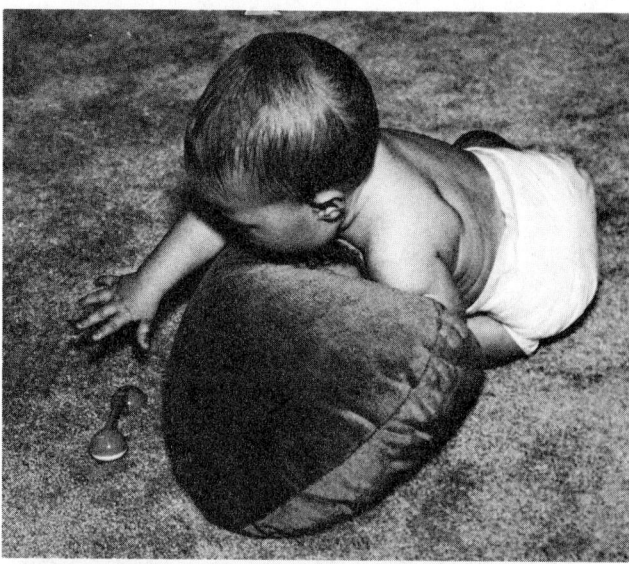

Fig. 12-10. Nine-month-old infant actively searches for object hidden behind pillow.

DEVELOPMENT OF BODY IMAGE

The development of body image parallels sensorimotor development. Infants' kinesthetic and tactile experiences are the first perceptions of their body, and the mouth is the principal area of pleasurable sensations. Other parts of the body are primarily objects of pleasure—the hands and fingers to suck and the feet to play with. As physical needs are met, they feel comfort and satisfaction with their body. Messages conveyed by the caregivers reinforce these feelings. For example, when infants smile, they receive emotional satisfaction from others who smile back.

Achieving the concept of object permanence is basic to the development of self-image. By the end of the first year infants recognize that they are distinct from their parents. At the same time there is increasing interest in their image, especially in the mirror (Fig. 12-11). As motor skills develop, they learn that parts of the body are useful; for example, the hands bring objects to the mouth, and the legs help them move to different locations. All of these achievements transmit messages to them.

DEVELOPMENT OF SEXUALITY

A sexual identity begins at birth, when the child is named and significant others, especially the parents, act certain ways toward the infant because of the respective gender. Touch is crucial to infant development and plays a primary role in sexual development. Infants have a great oral sensitivity, manifest through sucking and mouthing. They enjoy skin-to-skin contact and explore their own body for pleasure. Infants are capable of genital self-stimulation to orgasm; erections in male infants are common. Parents' re-

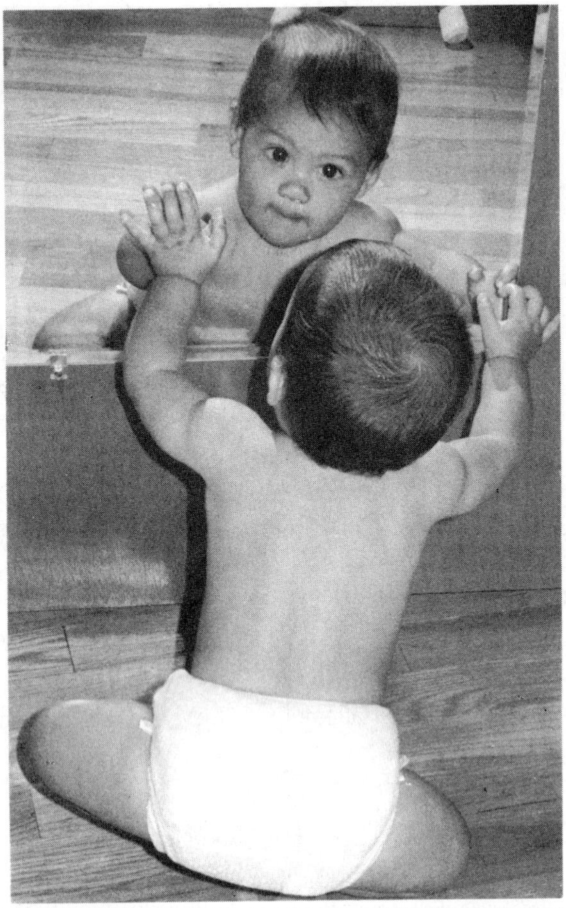

Fig. 12-11. Eight-month-old infant enjoying her image in mirror.

sponses to these early manifestations of sexuality influence children's evolving attitude; therefore, a healthy, accepting response by parents is important.

SOCIAL DEVELOPMENT

Infants' social development is initially influenced by their reflexive behavior, such as the grasp, and eventually depends primarily on the interaction between them and the principal caregivers. Attachment to the parent is increasingly evident during the second half of the first year. In addition, tremendous strides are made in communication and personal-social behavior. Play is a major socializing agent and provides stimulation needed to learn from and interact with the environment.

Attachment

The importance of human physical contact cannot be overemphasized. Parenting is not an instinctual ability but a learned acquired process. The attachment of parent and child, which probably begins before birth and assumes even more importance at birth (see Chapter 8), continues during the first year. In the following discussion of attachment, the word "mother" is used in the broad context of the consistent caregiver with whom the child relates more than anyone else. However, in society's changing social climate and sex role stereotypes, this may very well be the father. Studies on father-child attachment demonstrate that similar stages occur as with mother attachment (Lincoln, 1984).

During infancy attachment progresses with the child assuming an increasingly significant role. Two components of cognitive development are required for attachment: (1) the ability to discriminate the mother from other individuals and (2) the achievement of object permanence. Both of these processes prepare the infant for an equally important aspect of attachment—separation from the parent. Separation-individuation should occur as a harmonious, parallel process with emotional attachment (Sherwen, 1983).

During the formation of attachment to the parent the infant progresses through four distinct but overlapping stages. For the first few weeks infants respond indiscriminately to anyone. Beginning at about 8 to 12 weeks of age, they cry, smile, and vocalize more to the mother than to anyone else but continue to respond to others, whether familiar or not. At age 6 months or so infants show a distinct preference for the mother. They follow her more, cry when she leaves, enjoy playing with her more, and feel most secure in her arms. About 1 month after showing attachment to the mother, many infants begin attaching to other members of the family, most often the father.

Infants acquire other developmental behaviors that influence the attachment process. These include (1) differential crying, smiling, and vocalization (more to mother than to anyone else), (2) visual-motor orientation (looking more at mother even if she is not close), (3) crying when mother leaves the room, (4) approach through locomotion (crawling, creeping, or walking), (5) clinging (especially in presence of a stranger), and (6) exploring away from mother while using her as a secure base.

Effects of prolonged separation. Attachment is considered so critical to optimum child development that many researchers have documented the effects of prolonged and early separation on infants in the absence of quality mother substitutes. Some of the most famous research on emotional deprivation has been done by John Bowlby, John Robertson, and René Spitz. Bowlby (1969) studied the effects of the infant's separation from the mother and noted severe mental and physical retardation, particularly if emotional deprivation occurred during the first 3 years of life. He observed that the progressive retardation could be arrested or reversed if no further emotional deprivation occurred after the first 2 years but that prolonged severe deprivation beginning early in the first year and lasting for 3 years led to severe permanent effects. Among these were the inability to form trusting, intimate interpersonal relationships, language impairment, and deficiency in abstract thinking. Robertson (1953) and Bowlby (1969) found typical behavioral reactions of infants who were hospitalized and separated from their mothers (see Separation Anxiety, Chapter 26).

Spitz (1945) studied the effects of emotional deprivation of children raised in foundling homes or institutions. The infants were cared for by one nurse who had responsibility for eight children. Although the caregiver might be a loving, motherly person, she lacked the time necessary to devote individual attention and stimulation to each child. As a result the children were retarded in physical growth, were more susceptible to disease, and demonstrated decreasing developmental quotients over a 2-year period. Spitz found that children who were given one-to-one attention by a mother substitute developed normally.

Although these studies represent extreme examples of young children reared in environments essentially devoid of quality mothering, rather than temporary separation, such as daycare, the question remains regarding the long-term effects of separation and other stresses on children. The present findings and conclusions are controversial but are focusing more on the *resiliency* of children to adapt than on the inevitable negative consequences (see Questions and Controversies). Based on such findings nurses need to assess each family with the understanding that stress is not necessarily harmful and that even under adverse conditions children can adapt. Individual risk factors that influence a child's coping ability are evaluated, and tools such as the Infant Temperament Questionnaire (see p. 552) are used to assess "goodness of fit." When parental separation occurs, every effort is made to help the family provide suitable mothering substitutes for the child. The child's plasticity and resiliency to cope are stressed to the family to minimize their feelings of responsibility and guilt (Nelms, 1985).

QUESTIONS AND CONTROVERSIES

How detrimental and permanent are stressful events, such as maternal deprivation, during infancy?

Much of the present research on the effects of stress during childhood demonstrates that children have an incredible ability to adapt despite adversity. Thomas and Chess (1984) revealed a very high rate of recovery in children with adjustment problems and found that parent separation, divorce, or death was not predictive of early adult status. Extensive reviews of research regarding the effects of stress on children, such as maternal deprivation, hospitalization, birth of a sibling, and parental death, confirmed similar findings (Rutter, 1981). Such studies have identified risk factors that increase children's vulnerability to stress, such as "difficult" temperament, lack of "fit" between child and parent, age (especially between 6 months and 5 years), male gender, genetics, below-average intelligence, multiple and continuing stresses such as frequent hospital admissions or foster care placements and homes marked by discord or divorce, and lack of social supports.

However, the basic conclusion is that stress alone does not dictate inevitable negative consequences. Rather, emphasis must be placed on individual differences in vulnerability to deprivation and stress. Significant separation or lack of attachment to the mother figure must be viewed in light of other substitutes in the child's life, such as fathers, siblings, relatives, neighbors, and teachers, who also can significantly influence development (Garmezy and Rutter, 1983).

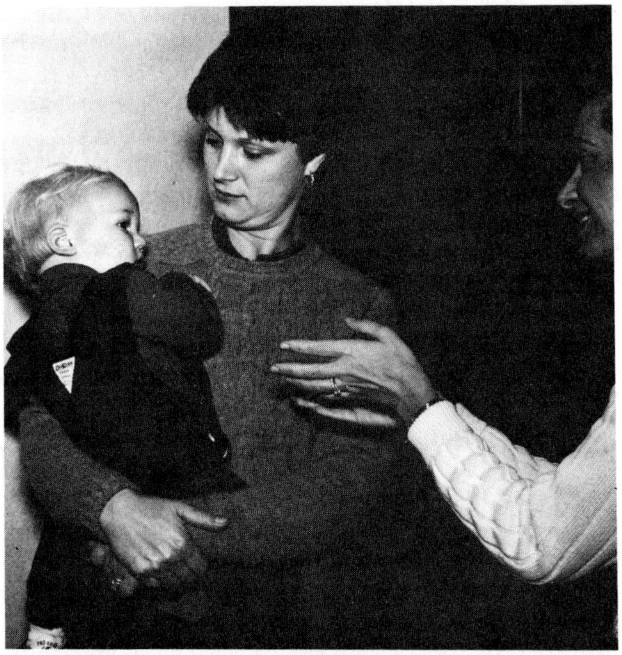

Fig. 12-12. Stranger fear behaviors include clinging to the parent and turning away from a stranger.

Separation anxiety. Between 4 and 8 months the infant progresses through the first stage and separation-individuation and begins to have some awareness of self and mother as separate individuals. At the same time object permanence is developing, and the infant is aware that the parent can be absent. Consequently, separation anxiety develops and is manifest through a predictable sequence of behaviors.

During the early second half of the first year infants protest when placed in their crib, and a short time later object when the mother leaves the room. Subsequently infants may not notice the mother's absence if they are absorbed in an activity. However, when they realize her absence, they protest. From this point onward they become very alert to her activities and whereabouts. By 11 to 12 months they are able to anticipate her imminent departure by watching her behaviors and begin to protest *before* she leaves. At this point many parents learn to postpone alerting the child to their departure until just before leaving (Bowlby, 1969).

Stranger fear. As infants demonstrate attachment to one person, they correspondingly exhibit less friendliness to others. Between ages 6 and 8 months fear of strangers and stranger anxiety become prominent and are related to infants' ability to discriminate between familiar and nonfamiliar people. Such behaviors as clinging to the parent, crying, and turning away from the stranger are common (Fig. 12-12). Suggestions for coping with stranger fear and separation anxiety are discussed on p. 558.

Language Development

The infant's first means of verbal communication is crying. Crying as a biologic sign conveys a message of urgency and signals displeasure, such as hunger. However, crying is also a social event that affects the development of the parent-infant relationship, either by its absence, which usually has a positive effect on parents, or its presence, which may evoke a negative response or persuade parents to minister to the child's physical or emotional needs.

In the first few weeks of life crying has a reflexive quality and is mostly related to physiologic needs. Infants cry for a period of 1 to 1½ hours a day up to 3 weeks of age, then build up to 2, and even 4, hours by 6 weeks. Crying tends to decrease by 12 weeks. It is thought that the increase in crying for no apparent reason during the first few months may be related to the discharge of energy and the maturational changes in the central nervous system. During the end of the first year infants cry for attention, from fear, especially stranger fear, and from frustration, usually in response to their developing but inadequate motor skills (Brazelton, 1987; Lester, 1985).

Many parents state that they can distinguish between different types of cry and from these messages are able to interpret the infant's needs. However, crying can be a source of acute distress for parents, especially the unconsolable crying of colic (see Chapter 13). Parents benefit from an explanation of the variability of crying among infants and assurance that periods of "unexplained fussiness" are normal. Some parents may need guidance in consoling techniques, such as holding, swaddling, massaging, caressing, rocking, walking, or stimulating sucking.

Vocalizations heard during crying eventually become syllables and then words, for example, the "mama" heard during vigorous crying. Infants vocalize as early as 5 to 6 weeks by making small throaty sounds. By 2 months they make single vowel sounds, such as *ah, eh,* and *uh.* By 3 to 4 months the consonants *n, k, g, p,* and *b* are added and infants coo, gurgle, and laugh aloud. By 8 months they add the consonants *t, d,* and *w* and combine syllables, such as "dada," but do not ascribe meaning to the word until 11 to 12 months. They make sounds, such as coughing or snorting, to attract attention. By 9 to 10 months they can comprehend the meaning of the word "no," obey simple commands, and respond to their name. By 1 year they can say two to three words with meaning.

During the acquisition of new language skills it is not unlikely for the child to temporarily give up other recently learned sounds or words. This is often distressing for parents after waiting in anticipation for the words "dada" or "mama." However, these sounds are frequently abandoned for other vocalizations and may not be repeated for several weeks. It is reassuring for parents to know that the child will again say these words, probably with meaning.

Personal-Social Behavior

Personal-social behavior includes the child's personal responses to the environment. It is the area most influenced by external stimuli but, as in the other fields of behavior, follows certain developmental laws. Personal-social behavior implies communication with one's self and with others. It is foundational for the successful mastery of skills such as feeding, control of bodily functions, independence, and cooperativeness in play.

Infants have the ability to shape their environment and to elicit certain responses. Newborns show visual preference for the human face and, as early as 1 week of age, begin to watch the parent intently as he or she speaks to them. As they regard the parent's face, activity diminishes, their head bobs up and down, and their mouth moves almost as if trying to say something.

By 6 to 8 weeks a social smile in response to pleasurable stimuli is present. This has a profound effect on family members and is a tremendous stimulus for evoking continued responses from others. By 3 months infants show considerable interest in the environment: excitement when a toy is presented, refusal to be left alone, recognition of parent, and demonstration of pleasure by squealing. By 4 months they laugh aloud and enjoy strange, novel stimuli.

By 6 months infants are very personable. They play games such as peekaboo when their head is hidden in a towel, they signal their desire to be picked up by extending their arms, and they show displeasure when a toy is removed or their face is washed. There is increasing demonstration of their ability to control the environment. The acquisition of fine and gross motor skills allows much more independence in movement.

By the second half of the first year infants understand simple discipline, such as the meaning of the word "no" or a scolding remark. They comprehend different facial expressions and are sensitive to emotional changes in others. Imitation is developing during this time. By 7 months they imitate actions and noises, by 8 months sounds, and by 10 months games such as pat-a-cake and peekaboo.

From 11 months onward they are increasingly independent. They are learning to feed themselves, using fingers, spoon, and cup (with much spilling), and can help with dressing by putting the foot out for a shoe or pushing the arm through the sleeve. They not only comprehend the meaning of "no," but shake their head to signal understanding. They can follow simple directions and will gladly perform for others to attract and prolong attention.

Play

Play during infancy represents the various social modalities observed during cognitive development. Infants' activity is primarily narcissistic, revolving around their own body. As discussed under development of body image, parts of the body are primarily play and pleasure objects.

During the first year play becomes more sophisticated and interdependent. From birth to 3 months infants' responses to the environment are global and largely undifferentiated. Play is dependent; pleasure is demonstrated by a quieting attitude (1 month), later by a smile (2 months), and then by a squeal (3 months). From 3 to 6 months infants show more discriminate interest in stimuli and begin to play alone with a rattle or soft stuffed toy or to play with someone else. There is much more interaction during play. By 4 months of age they laugh aloud, show preference for certain toys, and become excited when food or a favorite object is brought to them. They recognize an image in a mirror, smile at it, and vocalize to it.

By 6 months to 1 year play involves sensorimotor skills.

Actual games are played, such as peekaboo, pat-a-cake, verbal repetition, and imitation of simple gestures in response to demonstration. Play is much more selective, not only in terms of specific toys but also in terms of "playmates." Although play is solitary or one-sided, infants choose with whom they will interact. At 6 to 8 months they usually refuse to play with strangers. Parents are definite favorites, and infants know how to attract their attention. At 6 months they extend the arms to be picked up, at 7 months cough to make their presence known, at 10 months pull the parent's clothing, and at 12 months call them by name. This represents a tremendous advance from the newborn who signaled biologic needs by crying to express displeasure.

Stimulation is as important for psychosocial growth as food is for physical growth. Knowledge of developmental milestones allows nurses to guide parents regarding proper play for infants. It is not sufficient to place a mobile over a crib and toys in a playpen for a child's optimum social, emotional, and intellectual development. Play must provide interpersonal contact as well as recreational and educational stimulation. Infants need to be *played with,* not merely *allowed to play.* Although the type of play infants engage in is called *solitary,* this is only a figurative, not literal, term to denote one-sided play. The kind of toys given to the child is much less important than the quality of personal interaction that occurs.

Table 12-2 lists play activities that are appropriate for the developmental level of the infant in view of motor, language, and personal-social achievements. Although the activities are grouped according to the major mode of stimulation provided, there is overlap in many instances. In addition, play activities suggested for one age-group may be appropriate for older infants but inappropriate for younger infants.

TEMPERAMENT

The infant's temperament or behavioral style influences the kind of interaction that occurs between the child and parents, and other family members (see general discussion of

Table 12-2 Play during infancy

AGE (MONTHS)	VISUAL STIMULATION	AUDITORY STIMULATION	TACTILE STIMULATION	KINETIC STIMULATION
Suggested activities				
Birth-1	Look at infant within close range Hang bright, shiny object within 20-25 cm (8-10 inches) of infant's face and in midline	Talk to infant, sing in soft voice Play music box, radio, television Have ticking clock or metronome nearby	Hold, caress, cuddle Keep infant warm May like to be swaddled	Rock infant, place in cradle Use carriage for walks
2-3	Provide bright objects Make room bright with pictures or mirrors on walls Take infant to various rooms while doing chores Place infant in infant seat for vertical view of environment	Talk to infant Include in family gatherings Expose to various environmental noises other than those of home Use rattles, wind chimes	Caress infant while bathing, at diaper change Comb hair with a soft brush	Use cradle gym or swing Take in car for rides Exercise body by moving extremities in swimming motion
4-6	Place infant in front of mirror Place in front of television with family Give brightly colored toys to hold (small enough to grasp)	Talk to infant, repeat sounds infant makes Laugh when infant laughs Call infant by name Crinkle different papers by infant's ear Place rattle or bell in hand, show how to shake them	Give infant soft squeeze toys of various textures Allow to splash in bath Place nude on soft furry rug and move extremities	Use swing or stroller Bounce infant in lap while holding in standing position Help infant roll over Support infant in sitting position, let lean forward to balance self Put infant in an open box and tilt gently
Suggested toys				
Birth-6	Nursery mobiles Unbreakable mirrors See-through crib bumpers Contrasting-colored sheets Tracking tube* Visual panels*	Music boxes Musical mobiles Crib dangle bells Small-handled clear rattle Spin-a-round*	Stuffed animals Soft clothes Soft or furry quilt Soft mobiles	Rocking crib/cradle Weighted or suction toy

*These toys are from a specially designed series called Child Development Toys produced as part of the Johnson & Johnson Baby Products Child Development Program. They are available for purchase; information can be obtained by calling (800) 678-2686.

Continued.

Table 12-2 Play during infancy—cont'd

AGE (MONTHS)	VISUAL STIMULATION	AUDITORY STIMULATION	TACTILE STIMULATION	KINETIC STIMULATION
▪ Suggested activities				
6-9	Give infant large toys with bright colors, movable parts, and noisemakers Place unbreakable mirror where infant can see self Play peekaboo, especially hiding face in a towel Make funny faces to encourage imitation Give paper to tear, crumble Give ball of yarn or string to pull apart	Call infant by name Repeat simple words such as "dada," "mama," "bye-bye" Speak clearly Name parts of body, people, and foods Tell infant what you are doing Use word "no" only when necessary Give simple commands Show infant how to clap hands, bang a drum	Let infant play with various textures of fabric Have bowl with foods of different size and textures to feel Let infant "catch" running water Encourage "swimming" in large bathtub or shallow pool Give wad of sticky tape to manipulate	Place infant on floor to crawl, roll over, sit Hold upright to bear weight and bounce Pick up—say "up" Put down—say "down" Place toys out of reach; encourage infant to get them Play pat-a-cake
9-12	Show infant large pictures in books Take infant to places where there are animals, many people, different objects (shopping center) Play ball by rolling it to child, demonstrate "throwing" it back Demonstrate building a two-block tower	Read infant simple nursery rhymes Point to body parts and name each one Imitate sounds of animals	Give infant finger foods of different textures Let infant mess and squash food Let infant feel cold (ice cube) or warm objects, say what temperature each is Let infant feel a breeze (fan blowing)	Give large push-pull toys to encourage walking Place furniture in a circle to encourage cruising Encourage "rough-house" play Turn infant in different positions
▪ Suggested toys				
6-12	Various colored blocks Nested boxes or cups Books with rhymes and bright pictures Strings of big beads and snap beads Simple take-apart toys Large ball Cup and spoon Fitting forms* Large puzzles Jack-in-the box	Rattles of different sizes, shapes, tones, and bright colors Squeaky animals and dolls Records with light, rhythmic music Balls in a bowl*	Soft, different-textured animals and dolls Sponge toys, floating toys Squeeze toys Teething toys Books with textures/objects, such as fur and zipper	Activity box for crib Push-pull toys Swing

Temperament in Chapter 4 and Questions and Controversies). In assessing a child's temperament, it is the parents' perception of the child and the degree of *fit* between their expectations and the child's actual temperament that are important. The more dissonance or lack of harmoney between the child's temperament and the parent's ability to accept and deal with the behavior, the more risk for subsequent parent-child conflicts.

The Infant Temperament Questionnaire (ITQ) (Carey and McDevitt, 1978) can be used as a screening tool with parents. The questionnaire focuses on nine temperament variables, but the questions relate specifically to activities such as sleep, feeding, play, diapering, and dressing. The scores from the ITQ help identify the child's temperamental style. Use of the ITQ is well accepted by parents and should be accompanied by an adequate explanation of the results (Little, 1983, 1985). In discussing the results it is best to avoid terms such as "difficult" and describe the child in terms of characteristics, such as intense or irregular.

With knowledge of the infant's temperament, nurses are better able to (1) provide parents with background information that will help them see their child in a better perspective, (2) offer a more organized picture of their child's behavior and possibly reveal distortions in their perceptions of the behavior, and (3) guide parents regarding appropriate childrearing techniques (Blosser, 1979; Carey, 1981; Chess and Thomas, 1985).

Childrearing Practices Related to Temperament

Most parents realize that their infant is born with unique characteristics, and few parents of difficult infants need to

QUESTIONS AND CONTROVERSIES

What effect does infant temperament have on parenting?

Although the importance of temperament is generally acknowledged, its influence on parenting is less clear, and studies often report conflicting findings. However, there is evidence that infant temperament does affect parenting, at least in terms of parents' perception of their parenting role.

An "easy" child is apt to make parents feel more thankful and content in their parenting role, whereas a less soothable, more fussy infant may cause parents to be depressed and anxious (Ventura, 1982). Infants who are less predictable in their behavior, such as sleeping, feeding, and general satisfaction, cause parents to feel less competent and to experience less ease in transition to parenthood (Roberts, 1983). Mothers have been noted to react less and be less responsive to infants who demonstrate "difficult" behavior (Campbell, 1979). Mothers, especially of first-born children, report having major concerns regarding the behavior of "difficult" infants and of having to make large family adjustments because of their infants (Kronstadt and others, 1979).

Infants with "difficult" temperament also tend to have more colic, injuries, and night waking (Carey, 1972, 1974). These children sleep about 2 hours less a night and 1 hour less during the day than the "easy" child (Weissbluth, 1981). Exactly what effect these variables have on parenting is unclear. There is evidence that having a "difficult" child mobilizes parents to provide a more responsive home environment (Houdlin, 1987). One study found that, among the various temperament types, the "difficult" group had higher intelligence quotients if the family was of higher socioeconomic status. It might be that, in order to deal with the child's negative behaviors, the parents pay greater attention to the child, which eventually forms more rapid development (Maziade and others, 1987). Such findings emphasize the tremendous challenge, as well as the opportunity, that exists in rearing these children.

be told of the challenge of caring for them. However, very few parents are aware of the significance of the temperamental characteristics and of constructive approaches to dealing with them. The following are examples of interventions that promote more positive parenting of infants with different temperament styles.*

"Difficult" children may respond better to scheduled feedings and structured caregiving routines than demand feedings and frequent changes in daily routines. These children sleep less and may need more structured approaches to bedtime to prevent bedtime problems. "Highly distractible children" may require additional soothing measures such as swinging, rocking, or being carried in a pack that the parent wears across the chest or back. Children with "high activity" levels require vigilant watching, and parents need to take extra precautions in safeguarding the home. These children benefit from increased opportunities for gross motor activity to constructively channel their energy.

The child who is "slow to warm up" may demonstrate more stranger fear than other children and may require more gradual and frequent preparation for new situations, such as substitute child care. Even the "easy child" can present problems in that the parents may need reminders to feed the child who sleeps for prolonged intervals and rarely signals needs by crying. They may have to "retrain" the child because of the ease of developing troublesome habits, such as keeping the child up late or allowing frequent television watching.

Appropriate counseling based on awareness of the child's temperament can greatly enhance the quality of interaction between parents and infant. Even just letting parents know that "difficult" traits are innate can greatly relieve feelings of guilt and incompetence.

SUMMARY OF GROWTH AND DEVELOPMENT DURING INFANCY

Knowledge of the developmental sequence allows the nurse to assess normal growth and minor or abnormal deviations, helps parents gain realistic expectations of their child's ability, and provides guidelines for suitable play and stimulation. Several studies document that parents lack knowledge of child growth and development, are apt to set inappropriate behavioral expectations for their children, and desire information about developmental landmarks (Kliman and Vukelich, 1985; Shea and Fowler, 1983). Emphasizing the child's *developmental age* rather than chronologic age strengthens the parent-child relationship by fostering trust and lessening frustration. Therefore, the importance of a thorough understanding and appreciation of the growth and development of children cannot be overemphasized.

Because of the complexity of the developmental process during the first 12 months, Table 12-3 is presented to help organize and clarify the data already discussed. Although all milestones are important, some represent essential integrative aspects of development that lay the foundation for the achievement of more advanced skills. These essential milestones are designated by a square (■) in the chart. The table represents the *average* monthly age at which various skills are attained. It must be remembered that, although the sequence is the same, the rate will vary among children.

COPING WITH CONCERNS RELATED TO NORMAL GROWTH AND DEVELOPMENT

New parents, and some who are experienced, have many concerns about childrearing during the first year. Fears, day-care, discipline, thumb or pacifier sucking, and teething are just a sampling of topics that parents have questions about. Nurses must be aware of these concerns and provide answers that give guidance and help decrease anxiety.

---

*Recommended references for parents are Turecki, S., and Tonner, L.: The difficult child, Toronto, 1985, Bantam Books; and Chess, S., and Thomas, A.: Know your child: an authoritative guide for today's parents, New York, 1987, Basic Books, Inc.

Table 12-3 Growth and development during infancy

AGE (MONTHS)	PHYSICAL	GROSS MOTOR	FINE MOTOR
1	Weight gain of 150 to 210 g (5 to 7 ounces) weekly for first 6 months Height gain of 2.5 cm (1 inch) monthly for first 6 months Head circumference increases by 1.5 cm (½ inch) monthly for first 6 months Primitive reflexes present and strong Doll's eye reflex and dance reflex fading Obligatory nose breather (most infants)	■ Assumes flexed position with pelvis high, but knees not under abdomen when prone (at birth, knees flexed under abdomen) ■ Can turn head from side to side when prone, lifts head momentarily from bed (see Fig. 12-7, *A*) Has marked head lag, especially when pulled from lying to sitting position (see Fig. 12-6, *A*) Holds head momentarily parallel and in midline when suspended in prone position Assumes asymmetric tonic neck reflex position when supine Makes crawling movements when prone When held in standing position, body limp at knees and hips In sitting position back is uniformly rounded, absence of head control (see Fig. 12-8, *A*)	Hands predominantly closed Grasp reflex strong Hand clenches on contact with rattle
2	Posterior fontanel closed Crawling reflex disappears	■ Assumes less flexed position when prone—hips flat, legs extended, arms flexed, head to side Less head lag when pulled to sitting position (see Fig 12-6, *B*) Can maintain head in same plane as rest of body when held prone and parallel to floor When prone, can lift head almost 45 degrees off table When held in sitting position, holds head up but head bobs forward (see Fig. 12-8, *B*) Assumes asymmetric tonic neck reflex position intermittently	Hands frequently open Grasp reflex fading
3	Primitive reflexes fading	Able to hold head more erect when sitting, but still bobs forward Has only slight head lag when pulled to sitting Assumes symmetric body position Able to raise head and shoulders from prone position to a 45- to 90-degree angle from table; bears weight on forearms When held in standing position, able to bear slight fraction of weight on legs Regards own hand	■ Actively holds rattle but will not reach for it Grasp reflex absent Hands kept loosely open Clutches own hand, pulls at blankets and clothes
4	■ Moro, tonic neck, rooting, and Perez reflexes have disappeared Drooling begins	■ Has almost no head lag when pulled to sitting position (see Fig. 12-6, *C*) ■ Balances head well in sitting position (see Fig. 12-8, *C*) Back is less rounded, curved only in lumbar area Able to sit erect if propped up Able to raise head and chest off couch to angle of 90 degrees (see Fig. 12-7, *B*) Assumes predominant symmetric position Rolls from back to side	■ Inspects and plays with hands, pulls clothing or blanket over face in play Tries to reach objects with hand but overshoots Grasps object with both hands Plays with rattle placed in hand, shakes it, but cannot pick it up if dropped Can carry objects to mouth

Milestones that represent essential integrative aspects of development that lay the foundation for the achievement of more advanced skills are indicated by a square.

SENSORY	VOCALIZATION	SOCIALIZATION/COGNITION
Visual acuity approaches 20/100* ■ Able to fixate on moving object in range of 45 degrees when held at a distance of 20-25 cm (8-10 inches) Follows light to midline Quiets when hears a voice	Cries to express displeasure Makes small throaty sounds Makes comfort sounds during feeding	Is in sensorimotor phase—stage I, use of reflexes (birth–1 month) and stage II, primary circular reactions (1–4 months) Watches parent's face intently as she or he talks to infant
Binocular fixation and convergence to near objects beginning When supine, follows dangling toy from side to point beyond midline Visually searches to locate sounds Turns head to side when sound is made at level of ear	■ Vocalizes, distinct from crying Crying becomes differentiated Coos Vocalizes to familiar voice	■ Demonstrates social smile in response to various stimuli
■ Follows object to periphery (180 degrees) ■ Locates sound by turning head to side and looking in same direction (see Fig. 12-2) Begins to have ability to coordinate stimuli from various sense organs	■ Squeals aloud to show pleasure Coos, babbles, chuckles Vocalizes when smiling "Talks" a great deal when spoken to Cries less during periods of wakefulness	Displays considerable interest in surroundings Ceases crying when parent enters room Can recognize familiar faces and objects, such as feeding bottle Shows awareness of strange situations
Able to accommodate to near objects Binocular vision well established Can focus on a 1.25 cm (½-inch) block Beginning eye-hand coordination	Makes consonant sounds *n*, *k*, *g*, *p*, *b* Laughs aloud Vocalization changes according to mood	Is in stage III, secondary circular reactions Demands attention by fussing: becomes bored if left alone Enjoys social interaction with people Anticipates feeding when sees bottle Shows excitement with whole body, squeals, breathes heavily Shows interest in strange stimuli Begins to show memory

*Degree of visual acuity varies according to vision measurement procedures (see Table 7-10).

Continued.

Table 12-3 Growth and development during infancy—cont'd

AGE (MONTHS)	PHYSICAL	GROSS MOTOR	FINE MOTOR
5	Growth rate may begin to decline Beginning signs of tooth eruption	Has no head lag when pulled to sitting position When sitting, able to hold head erect and steady Able to sit for longer periods when back is well supported Back is straight When prone, assumes symmetric positioning with arms extended Can turn over from abdomen to back When supine, puts feet to mouth	■ Able to grasp objects voluntarily Uses palmar grasp, bidextrous approach Plays with toes Takes objects directly to mouth Holds one cube while regarding a second
6	Birth weight doubled Weight gain of 90 to 150 g (3 to 5 ounces) weekly for next 6 months Height gain of 1.25 cm (½ inch) monthly for next 6 months Teething may begin with eruption of two lower central incisors ■ Chewing and biting occur Landau reflex appears—when infant is suspended in a horizontal prone position, the head is raised, legs and spine are extended	When prone, can lift chest and upper abdomen off table, bearing weight on hands (see Fig. 12-7, *C*) When about to be pulled to a sitting position, lifts head Sits in high chair with back straight Rolls from back to abdomen When held in standing position, bears almost all of weight Hand regard is absent	Resecures a dropped object Drops one cube when another is given Grasps and manipulates small objects Holds bottle Grasps feet and pulls to mouth
7	Eruption of upper central incisors	■ When supine, spontaneously lifts head off table ■ Sits, leaning forward on both hands (see Fig. 12-8, *D*) When prone, bears weight on one hand Sits erect momentarily Bears full weight on feet (see Fig. 12-9, *A*) When held in standing position, bounces actively	■ Transfers objects from one hand to the other (Fig. 12-8, *E*) Has unidextrous approach and grasp Holds two cubes more than momentarily Bangs cube on table Rakes at a small object
8	Begins to show regular patterns in bladder and bowel elimination Parachute reflex appears (see Fig. 12-1); when infant is suspended in a horizontal prone position and suddenly thrust downward, hands and fingers extend forward as if to protect self from falling	■ Sits steadily unsupported (see Fig. 12-8, *E*) Readily bears weight on legs when supported, may stand holding on Adjusts posture to reach an object	Has beginning pincer grasp using the index, fourth, and fifth fingers against the lower part of the thumb Releases objects at will Rings bell purposely Retains two cubes while regarding the third cube Secures an object by pulling on a string Reaches persistently for toys out of reach
9	Eruption of upper lateral incisor may begin	Crawls, may progress backward at first Sits steadily on floor for prolonged time (10 minutes) Recovers balance when leans forward but cannot do so when leaning sideways Pulls self to standing position and stands holding onto furniture (Fig. 12-9, *B-D*)	■ Uses thumb and index finger in crude pincer grasp (see Fig. 12-4) Preference for use of dominant hand now evident Grasps third cube Compares two cubes by bringing them together

SENSORY	VOCALIZATION	SOCIALIZATION/COGNITION
Visually pursues a dropped object Able to sustain visual inspection of an object Can localize sounds made below the ear	■ Squeals Has vowel-like cooing sounds interspersed with consonantal sounds (for example, ah-goo)	Smiles at mirror image Pats bottle with both hands More enthusiastically playful, but may have rapid mood swings Able to discriminate strangers from family Vocalizes displeasure when object taken away Discovers part of body
Visual acuity 20/60 to 20/40 Adjusts posture to see an object Prefers more complex visual stimuli Can localize sounds made above the ear Will turn head to the side, then look up or down	■ Begins to imitate sounds ■ Babbling resembles one-syllable utterances such as *ma, mu, da, di, hi* Vocalizes to toys, mirror image Laughs aloud Takes pleasure in hearing own sounds (self-reinforcement)	Recognizes parents; begins to fear strangers Holds arms out to be picked up Has definite likes and dislikes Begins to imitate (coughs, protrudes tongue) Excites on hearing footsteps Laughs when head is hidden in a towel Has frequent mood swings—from crying to laughing with little or no provocation Briefly searches for a dropped object (object permanence beginning)
■ Can fixate on very small objects Responds to own name Localizes sound by turning head in a curving arch Has beginning awareness of depth and space Has taste preferences	■ Produces vowel sounds and chained syllables—*baba, dada, kaka* Vocalizes four distinct vowel sounds "Talks" when others are talking	■ Is increasingly fearful of strangers, shows signs of fretfulness when parent disappears Imitates simple acts and noises Tries to attract attention by coughing or snorting Plays peekaboo Demonstrates dislike of food by keeping lips closed Exhibits oral aggressiveness in biting and mouthing Demonstrates expectation in response to repetition of stimuli ■ Looks briefly for toy that disappears
	Makes consonant sounds *t, d,* and *w* Listens selectively to familiar words Utterances signal emphasis and emotion Combines syllables, such as dada, but does not ascribe meaning to them	Has increasing anxiety over loss of parent, particularly mother, and fear of strangers Responds to word "no" Dislikes dressing, diaper change
Localizes sounds by turning head diagonally and directly toward sound Depth perception is increasing	Responds to simple verbal commands Comprehends "no-no"	Is in stage IV, coordination of secondary schemata Parent (mother) is increasingly important for own sake Shows increasing interest in pleasing parent Begins to show fears of going to bed and being left alone Puts arms in front of face to avoid having it washed ■ Searches for an object if sees it hidden

Continued.

Table 12-3 Growth and development during infancy—cont'd

AGE (MONTHS)	PHYSICAL	GROSS MOTOR	FINE MOTOR
10	Labyrinth-righting reflex is strongest—when infant is in prone or supine position, is able to raise head	Crawls by pulling self forward with hands (see Fig. 12-9, *F*) Can change from prone to sitting position Pulls self to sitting position Stands while holding onto furniture, sits by falling down Recovers balance easily while sitting While standing, lifts one foot to take a step (Fig. 12-9, *E*)	Crude release of an object is beginning Grasps bell by handle
11	Eruption of lower lateral incisors may begin	■ Creeps with abdomen off floor (Fig. 12-9, *G*) When sitting, pivots to reach toward back to pick up an object Cruises or walks holding onto furniture or with both hands held	Can hold crayon to make a mark on paper Explores objects more thoroughly (for example, clapper inside bell) Drops object deliberately for it to be picked up Puts one object after another into a container (sequential play) Able to manipulate an object to remove it from tight-fitting enclosure
12	Birth weight tripled Birth length increased by 50% Head and chest circumference equal (head circumference 46.5 cm [18½ inches]) Has total of six to eight deciduous teeth Anterior fontanel almost closed Landau reflex fading Babinski reflex disappears Lumbar curve develops, lordosis evident during walking	Walks with one hand held Cruises well May attempt to stand alone momentarily Can sit down from standing position without help	Has neat pincer grasp (Fig. 12-5) Releases cube in cup Attempts to build two-block tower but fails Tries to insert a pellet into a narrow-neck bottle but fails Can turn pages in a book, many at a time

Separation and Stranger Fear

During infancy a number of fears can appear. However, the fear that causes parents most concern is fear related to strangers and separation. Although erroneously interpreted by some as a sign of undesirable, antisocial behavior, stranger fear and separation anxiety are important components of a strong, healthy parent-child attachment. However, this period can present difficulties for parent and child. Parents may be more confined to the home because baby-sitters are violently protested by the infant. To accustom the infant to new people, parents are encouraged to have close friends or relatives visit often. This provides for other persons with whom the child is comfortable and who can give parents time for themselves.

Infants also need opportunities to safely experience strangers. Usually toward the end of the first year infants begin to venture away from the parent and demonstrate curiosity about strangers. If allowed to explore at their own rate, many infants will eventually "warm up." If parents hold the child away from their face, the infant can observe while maintaining close physical contact.

A number of factors influence the child's intensity of fear of strangers (Vasta, 1982):

SENSORY	VOCALIZATION	SOCIALIZATION/COGNITION
	■ Says "dada," "mama" with meaning Comprehends "bye-bye" May say one word (for example, "hi," "bye," "what," "no")	Inhibits behavior to verbal command of "no-no" or own name Imitates facial expressions, waves bye-bye Extends toy to another person but will not release it Repeats actions that attract attention and are laughed at Pulls clothes of another to attract attention Plays interactive games such as pat-a-cake Reacts to adult anger, cries when scolded Demonstrates independence in dressing, feeding, locomotive skills, and testing of parents Looks at and follows pictures in a book Looks around a corner or under a pillow for an object
	Imitates definite speech sounds Uses jargon	Experiences joy and satisfaction when a task is mastered Reacts to restrictions with frustration Rolls ball to another on request Anticipates body gestures when a familiar nursery rhyme or story is being told (for example, holds toes and feet in response to "This little piggy went to market") Plays game up-down, "so-big," or peekaboo by covering face
Discriminates simple geometric forms (for example, circle) Amblyopia may develop with lack of binocularity Can follow rapidly moving object Controls and adjusts response to sound; listens for sound to recur	■ Says two or more words besides dada, mama Comprehends meaning of several words (comprehension always precedes verbalization) Recognizes objects by name Imitates animal sounds Understands simple verbal commands (for example, "Give it to me," "Show me your eyes")	Shows emotions such as jealousy, affection (may give hug or kiss on request), anger, fear Enjoys familiar surroundings and explores away from parent Is fearful in strange situation, clings to parent May develop habit of "security blanket" or favorite toy Has unceasing determination to practice locomotor skills ■ Searches for an object even if has not seen it hidden, but searches only where object was last seen

- Sex, age, and size of the stranger—female, younger age, and smaller size (including kneeling or sitting rather than standing) being less stressful
- Approach—loud, sudden, intrusive approach causing more distress
- Child's proximity to parent—closer to parent (on parent's lap rather than in infant seat) being less stressful

Consequently, the best approach for the stranger (who may be the nurse) is to talk softly, meet the child at eye level (to appear smaller), maintain a safe distance from the infant, and avoid sudden, intrusive gestures, such as holding the arms out and smiling broadly.

Parents also may wonder whether they should encourage the child's clinging, dependent behavior, especially if there is pressure from others who view this as "spoiling" (see discussion below). Parents need to be reassured that such behavior is healthy, desirable, and necessary for the child's optimum emotional development. If parents can reassure the infant of their presence, the infant will learn to realize that they are still there even if not physically present. Talking to infants when leaving the room, allowing them to hear one's voice on the telephone, and using transitional objects, such as a favorite blanket or toy, reassures them of the parent's continued presence.

This is a no less trying but necessary time for infants, because parents cannot always be with the child. An excellent example of necessary separation is bedtime. Fear of going to bed or being left alone in the dark commonly occurs during the second half of the first year. Fear at bedtime is only one of the many bedtime problems that can occur in young children, and is discussed in Chapter 15.

Spoiled Child Syndrome

A common concern of parents is that too much attention can "spoil" a child. Many of the recommendations for promoting attachment, such as attending to the infant's needs to establish trust, accepting fear of strangers and separation from parent, and holding and rocking the crying child, are described by parents as methods of spoiling (Wilson, Witzke, and Volin, 1981). However, research on parents' response to crying during early infancy does not support the contention that "picking up a crying baby" leads to spoiling. Ainsworth (1982) found that the amount an infant cried during the first 3 months had no correlation with the frequency of crying during the rest of the first year. However, the degree of maternal responsiveness to crying did. Parents who were less responsive, such as not picking up the infant immediately on crying, had infants who cried *more* than those of parents who responded promptly to crying. Parents of colicky infants less than 3 months old who responded to the crying with increased attention successfully decreased the overall crying time (Taubman, 1984).

If "too much attention" does not cause spoiling in early infancy, parents need to understand what "spoiling" really is and how it differs from normal behavior that may mimic aspects of spoiling. The *spoiled child syndrome* has been defined as "excessive self-centered and immature behavior, resulting from the failure of parents to enforce consistent, age-appropriate limits" (McIntosh, 1989). Spoiled children demand to have their own way, are inconsiderate of others, and have intrusive, obstructive, and manipulative behavior. Indulging children combined with clear expectations and limits does not cause spoiling. But indulgence with failure to provide guidelines for acceptable behavior can result in a "spoiled brat" (McIntosh, 1989).

Several age-related normal behaviors and child characteristics can be mistaken for evidence of spoiling, such as:

- Crying during early infancy that may or may not be associated with colic
- Toddler behaviors such as negativism, persistent exploration, and temper tantrums
- Children with difficult temperaments or attention deficits
- Children experiencing extreme stress from marital discord, abuse, substance abuse, or mental illness in a parent

With anticipatory guidance regarding expected but challenging behaviors and situations that may produce extreme stress in children, parents should feel comfortable in loving their infant without fear of spoiling. However, as the infant gets older, parents need assistance in providing limits that prevent normal, disruptive behaviors, such as temper tantrums, from becoming problems.

Limit-Setting and Discipline

As infants' motor skills advance and mobility increases, parents are faced with the need to set safe limits (see discussion of nurse's role in injury prevention on p. 585). Although there are numerous disciplinary techniques, some are more appropriate for this age than others. Parents can begin discipline using a negative voice and stern eye-to-eye contact. When more definitive measures must be used, one of the most effective approaches is time-out. The basic principles are the same as those discussed in Chapter 14, except that the place for time-out needs to be commensurate with the child's abilities. For example, the playpen is better for most infants than a chair. Although parents may be concerned with instituting discipline during infancy, it is important to stress that the earlier effective disciplinary methods are employed, the easier it is to continue these approaches.

Alternate Child Care Arrangements

For many parents, especially working mothers, the need for locating safe and competent child care facilities for the infant is an increasingly difficult problem—one that is compounded by the number of women with children working outside the home. Over the past 25 years there has been a marked shift in child care arrangements, with fewer children cared for at home and more children cared for in group centers or other settings.

Types of child care. The basic types of care are in-home care, either in the parent's or caregiver's home (family daycare), and center-based care, usually in a daycare center. In-home care may consist of a full-time baby-sitter who lives in the home, a full-time baby-sitter who comes to the home, cooperative arrangements such as exchange baby-sitting, and family daycare. A licensed family daycare home typically provides care and protection for up to five children for part of a 24-hour day and does not include informal arrangements such as exchange baby-sitting or caregivers in the child's own home. The five children include the family daycare parents' own children younger than 5 years of age living in the home. Unfortunately, many family daycare homes operate without a license and may care for large numbers of infants without adequate staff and facilities.

Center-based care usually refers to a licensed daycare facility that provides care for six or more children, for 6 or more hours in a 24-hour day. Work-based group care is another option that is becoming increasingly popular as employers recognize the benefit of quality and convenient child care to their employees.

Nurses have an important role in providing guidance to parents in selecting suitable, well-qualified facilities or individuals to care for their child. The decision to leave an infant in another's care often engenders doubt and guilt in the parent. Therefore any assistance is often appreciated.*

Guidelines for selecting daycare facilities are discussed

*A recommended resource is *Finding the Best Care for Your Infant and Toddler* from National Center for Clinical Infant Programs, 2000 14th St., North, Arlington, VA 22201; (703) 528-4300.

in Chapter 15. Issues of particular concern with infant care are staff-child ratio, nurturing qualities of the caregivers, consistency of staff, and safety and cleanliness of the facility. The same conscientious attention should be applied to locating competent baby-sitters. References from other employers are essential, and there is no substitute for observing the interaction between the individual and the child. Although very young infants need little if any preparation for the introduction of a new caregiver, older infants may benefit from a gradual placement to reduce stranger fear. At all times the parent should have the right to visit the child, and regular conferences should be established to review the child's progress. The American Academy of Pediatrics, Committee on Early Childhood, Adoption, and Dependent Care (1984) also recommends that health professionals expand their role to include establishing a system for exchanging information about the child with the daycare provider as well as with the parent.

Thumb-Sucking and Use of Pacifier

Sucking is the infant's chief pleasure, and it may not be satisfied by breast- or bottle-feeding. It is such a strong need that infants who are deprived of sucking, such as those with a cleft lip repair, will suck on their tongue. Some newborns are born with sucking pads on their fingers from in utero sucking activity. Several benefits of nonnutritive sucking have been documented, such as increased weight gain in premature infants and decreased crying (Anderson, 1986).

Problems arise when parents are concerned about sucking of fingers, thumb, or pacifier and attempt to restrain this natural tendency. Before giving advice, nurses should investigate the parents' feelings and base guidance on this information (see Therapeutic Dialogue).

During infancy and early childhood there is no need to restrain sucking of fingers or pacifier. Malocclusion may occur if thumb-sucking persists past 4 years of age or when the permanent teeth erupt. There is probably less dental displacement with the use of pacifier than with the use of a hard, rigid finger. Pacifiers may be relinquished earlier than thumbs because they are less readily available. The effect of continual use of a pacifier on early speech and language development is unknown, but it is possible that the pacifier may decrease the child's desire to imitate sounds and affect intelligibility. Parents need to be alerted that continual dependency on a pacifier may influence speech development (Merrifield and Ryberg, 1985). If the child uses a pacifier, safety considerations in purchasing one must be stressed (see p. 578).

To decrease dependence on nonnutritive sucking, sucking pleasure can be increased by prolonging feeding time. A small-holed, firm nipple causes stronger sucking and slower feeding. Also, the parent's excessive use of the pacifier to calm the child should be explored. It is not unusual for parents to place a pacifier in the infant's mouth as soon as crying begins, thus reinforcing a pattern of distress-relief.

Thumb-sucking reaches its peak at ages 18 to 20 months and is most prevalent when the child is hungry or tired. Persistent thumb-sucking in a listless, apathetic child always warrants investigation. It may be a sign of an emotional problem between parent and child or of boredom, isolation, and lack of stimulation.

Treatment for continued sucking of fingers or pacifier in an older child is controversial. Some of the available methods include the use of a bitter substance on the finger (Friman, Barone, and Christopherson, 1986); contracting with the child—using a formal agreement with rewards for meeting a mutually agreed on goal (Cipes, Miraglia, and Gaulin-Kremer, 1986); and paradoxical therapy—reframing the sit-

THERAPEUTIC DIALOGUE

Thumb-Sucking

During a well-child visit the nurse observes that the mother persistently takes the thumb out of her 10-month-old daughter's mouth.

NURSE: I can see that Annie likes to suck her thumb.

MOTHER: Too much. I am always trying to discourage her from this habit.

NURSE: You have concerns about her thumb-sucking?

MOTHER: Of course. Her teeth are coming in so nice and straight, and I don't want the thumb to make them crooked.

NURSE: Tell me about the thumb making the teeth crooked.

MOTHER: My mother feels that it does. My brother sucked his thumb until he was 2 years old, and as a teenager he needed braces. Now, I never sucked my thumb, and my teeth are straight.

NURSE: I understand how your mother could make that connection. Do you think that teeth can become crooked for other reasons?

MOTHER: I guess so. Why?

NURSE: I asked because your mother is partially right. Thumb-sucking after age 4 can cause dental problems, but teeth can need braces for many other reasons. Babies enjoy sucking. Sometimes, making an issue of the sucking can cause it to last longer. Sucking on a thumb or pacifier is very common in young children, especially in infants. It satisfies their need to suck and helps them to comfort themselves. Let's talk about thumb-sucking at your next visit.

MOTHER: OK. I appreciate our talking about this because my taking the thumb out of her mouth doesn't stop the habit. She often gets angry and cries, and I feel upset. For now, I'll just let her suck her thumb.

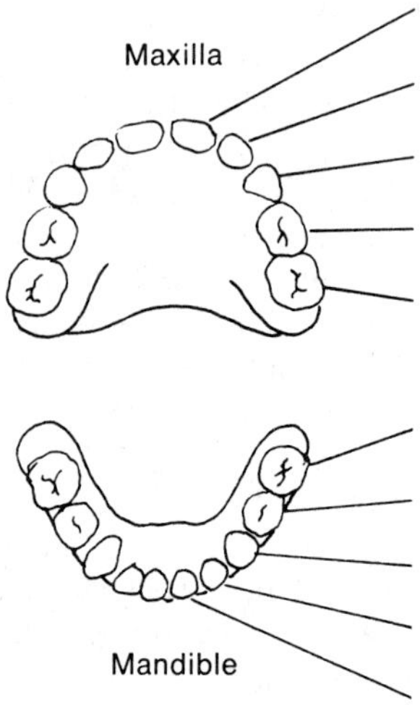

	Average age of eruption (mo)	Average age of shedding (yr)
Maxilla	9.6	7.5
	12.4	8
	18.3	11.5
	15.7	10.5
	26.2	10.5
Mandible	26.0	11
	15.1	10
	18.2	9.5
	11.5	7
	7.8	6

Fig. 12-13. Sequence of eruption and shedding of primary teeth.

uation so that the child finds it unsatisfactory (MacKenzie, 1987).

Teething

One of the more difficult periods in the infant's (and parents') life is the eruption of the deciduous (primary) teeth, often referred to as teething. The age of tooth eruption shows considerable variation among children, but the order of their appearance is fairly regular and predictable (Fig. 12-13). The first primary teeth to erupt are the lower central incisors, which appear at approximately 6 to 8 months of age. These are followed closely by the upper central incisors. A quick guide to assessment of deciduous teeth during the first 2 years is: *age of the child in months* − 6 = *number of teeth.*

The exact mechanisms responsible for the eruption of teeth are not fully understood. The growth of the root, dentin, and pulp of the tooth, the pressure exerted against the periodontal tissue, and hormonal control of pituitary growth hormone and thyroid hormone are some of the theories under investigation.

Teething is a physiologic process, and as the crown of the tooth breaks through the periodontal membrane, some discomfort may be experienced. Some children show minimum evidence of teething, such as drooling, increased finger-sucking, or biting on hard objects. Others are very irritable, have difficulty sleeping, and refuse to eat. Generally signs of illness such as fever, vomiting, or diarrhea are not symptoms of teething but of illness. Continued irritability may be a clue to disturbances other than teething and warrants further investigation.

Since teething pain is a result of inflammation, cold is soothing. Giving the child a cold metal spoon, a frozen teething ring, or an ice cube wrapped in a washcloth helps relieve the inflammation. Several nonprescription topical anesthetic ointments are available, such as Baby Ora-Jel. The active ingredient in most of them is benzocaine. If these are used, parents are advised to apply them correctly.

In the event of persistent irritability that affects sleeping and feeding, systemic analgesics, such as acetaminophen, can be given judiciously. Parents should know that this is a temporary measure. The use of teething powders or procedures such as cutting or rubbing the gums with aspirin are discouraged, because ingestion of the powder, infection or irritation of the tissue, or aspiration of the aspirin can occur.

Infant Shoes

Many parents are unaware of the type of shoes that are appropriate for the older infant and buy expensive infant shoes because of misleading advertising claims. Inflexible shoes that have hard soles can be detrimental by delaying walking, aggravating intoeing and outtoeing, and impeding the development of supportive foot muscles. Therefore counseling parents regarding footwear should begin when infants are 6 months old, well before they are walking (Glendon, 1987).

It is helpful to begin by explaining to parents that changes in the feet occur during infancy and early childhood as locomotion and weight bearing progress. At birth the feet are flat because the arches are protected by fat pads on the soles of the feet. As the bones in the arches develop, the pads disappear and the feet begin to assume a mature shape. A normal arch is determined by proper alignment of all the bones and development of the surrounding musculature, not by the height of the arch.

When children begin walking, the main reason for shoes is *protection.* To provide protection, the shoe should retain its fit, be made of durable material with a smooth interior and few construction seams to irritate the skin, and be soft and flexible, especially in the toe area. A high-top shoe is not necessary for support but may be helpful in keeping the foot in the shoe.

A good shoe conforms to the anatomic shape of the foot, with a rounded toe and sufficient toe room. During weight bearing there should be at least the space of half the width of the thumbnail, or 1.25 cm (½ inch), between the end of the longest toe and the shoe. Roomy and square-toed socks allow for proper growth and alignment. Inexpensive but well-constructed sneakers or soft-leather moccasin-type shoes are suggested as adequate footgear for walking infants.

Even if the shoes are fitted properly, frequent changes are needed to accommodate the infant's rapidly growing feet. Shoe size changes at approximately 3-month intervals between 12 to 36 months; during this time the child's foot should be measured every 3 months (Chong, 1987). Curled toes when shoes are removed and redness and irritation of the skin on the bottom of the toes indicate the need for a larger size.

PROMOTING OPTIMUM HEALTH DURING INFANCY

The infant's first year is a time of monumental change and achievement, and the rapidity of the changes can easily overwhelm parents. Each month and phase of development have implications for care of the child. Health promotion during this time involves nutritional guidance, appropriate sleep and activity, proper dental care, prevention of disease through immunization, and provision of a safe environment.

NUTRITION

Ideally, discussion of optimum nutrition should begin prenatally with the decision to breast- or bottle-feed the infant. The choice for either is highly individual and is discussed in Chapter 8. This section is primarily concerned with infant nutrition during the next 12 months, when growth needs and developmental milestones ready the child for introduction of solid foods. Frequently the nurse is asked when to begin feeding solid foods, how to introduce new foods, and what foods are best. A thorough understanding of each of these areas is needed to answer these questions so that the nutritional needs of infants are met.

Infant Feeding

Much controversy has existed regarding infant feeding and the need for solid foods. Before 1920 solid foods were seldom offered until 1 year of age. After that time there was a trend to add solid foods at increasingly earlier ages. However, clinical studies have not offered substantial proof of superior nutritional states over breast milk, commercially prepared formula, or modified cow's milk when solids are fed to infants younger than 4 months of age. In addition, introducing foods too early may have adverse effects, such as allergies.

The first 6 months. Human milk is the most desirable complete diet for the infant for the first 6 months. The normal infant receiving breast milk from a well-nourished mother needs no specific vitamin and mineral supplements, with the exceptions of fluoride in a dose of 0.25 mg daily (regardless of the fluoride content of the local water supply) and iron by 6 months of age (when fetal iron stores are depleted). Supplements of 400 IU of vitamin D daily may be indicated if the mother's vitamin D intake is inadequate; some authorities also suggest supplements if the infant does not benefit from adequate ultraviolet light because of dark skin color or little exposure to light (American Academy of Pediatrics, Committee on Nutrition, 1980). However, current concern is focused on too much sun exposure, and some studies provide evidence that vitamin D supplementation may not be necessary (Greer and Marshall, 1989). Even in hot climates, additional fluids are not needed (Brown and others, 1986).

Employed mothers can continue breast-feeding with guidance and encouragement. Most mothers find that a program of breast-pumping when away from home and bottle-feeding of breast milk, with or without supplemental formula feedings, is successful. Milk can be expressed by hand or pump and safely refrigerated for up to 24 hours. After that time freezing is suggested (Lawrence, 1989). However, in addition to efficient breast-pumping, these mothers also cite the need for child care by a trusted agency or individual and support and assistance from significant others (MacLaughlin and Strelnick, 1984; Reifsnider and Myers, 1985). Like all breast-feeding mothers, these women must have proper nutrition and rest for lactation. With a schedule of work and child care, careful planning is required to successfully manage the demands of both responsibilities.*

An acceptable alternative to breast-feeding is commercial iron-fortified formula (American Academy of Pediatrics, Committee on Nutrition, 1989b). Like human milk, it supplies all the nutrients needed by the infant for the first 6 months. The only supplementation required is 0.25 mg of fluoride if the local water supply is not fluoridated or if the infant is given ready-to-feed formula, which eliminates the use of fluoridated tap water.

If evaporated milk formula is given, supplemental iron, vitamin C, and fluoride (depending on local water supply) are required. Commercially prepared vitamin/iron preparations with or without fluoride are available to meet the specific needs of the infant. The nurse needs to assess the type of formula given and the fluoride content of local water before advising the parent. Unmodified cow's milk, low-fat milk, or imitation milks are not acceptable as a major source of nutrition for infants (American Academy of Pediatrics, Committee on Nutrition, 1983, 1984).

The amount of formula per feeding and the number of feedings per day vary among infants, but general guidelines are given in Table 12-4. Usually infants on demand feeding

*A recommended resource for working mothers is Eiger, M., and Olds, S.: The complete book of breastfeeding, New York, 1987, Workman Publishing.

Table 12-4 Volume of formula per feeding and number of feedings per day*

AGE IN MONTHS (MIDPOINT)	FORMULA CONSUMED PER FEEDING (ml)†	(oz)	FEEDINGS PER DAY
1	94.6	3.2	6.6
2	124.2	4.2	6.4
3	162.7	5.5	5.4
4	162.7	5.5	5.5
5	162.7	5.5	4.8
6	177.4	6.0	4.7
7	171.5	5.8	4.4
8	180.4	6.1	4.5
9	168.6	5.7	4.0
10	183.4	6.2	4.0
11	201.1	6.8	4.0
12	174.5	5.9	3.9

From Ross Laboratories, 1989.
*Infants fed human milk or a combination of cow's milk, human milk, and formula excluded.
†1 fluid ounce = 29.573 ml.

determine their own feeding schedule, but some infants, especially those with "easy" temperaments, may need a more planned schedule based on average feeding patterns to ensure sufficient nutrients.

The addition of solid foods before 4 to 6 months of age is not recommended. Solid foods during the early months are not yet compatible with the ability of the gastrointestinal tract and nutritional needs of the infant. For example, feeding solids exposes infants to food antigens that may produce food protein allergy.

Developmentally, infants are not ready for solid food. The extrusion (protrusion) reflex is strong and often pushes food out of the mouth. Infants instinctively suck when given food. Because of their limited motor abilities, infants are unable to deliberately push food away or avoid feeding. Therefore, early introduction of solids is a type of forced feeding.

The second 6 months. During the second half of the first year human milk or formula continues to be the primary source of nutrition. If breast-feeding is discontinued, commercial iron-fortified formula should be substituted. The American Academy of Pediatrics, Committee on Nutrition (1986) suggests that whole cow's milk can be given if the infant is consuming one third of the calories as supplemental foods consisting of a balanced mixture of cereal, vegetables, fruits, and other foods to ensure adequate sources of iron and vitamin C. However, this recommendation is not universally accepted. A large proportion of infants who receive a diet of solid food and cow's milk do not consume adequate amounts of iron and some vitamins, but excessive amounts of sodium, potassium, chloride, and protein (Anderson and others, 1989; Montalto, Benson, and Martinez, 1985). Consequently, many authorities suggest the use of iron-fortified formula (Tunnessen and Oski, 1987; Ziegler and others, 1990).

Formulas specially marked for older children (Advance by Ross Laboratories and Good Nature by Carnation Nutritional Products) offer no advantages for infants and provide excessive protein; Good Nature provides less than the recommended amounts of calories from fat (American Academy of Pediatrics, Committee on Nutrition, 1989a; Foman, Sanders, and Ziegler, 1990).

The major change in feeding habits is the addition of solid foods to the infant's diet. Physiologically and developmentally the infant 4 to 6 months of age is in a transition period. By this time the gastrointestinal tract has matured sufficiently to handle more complex nutrients and is less sensitive to potentially allergenic foods. Tooth eruption is beginning and facilitates biting and chewing. The extrusion reflex has disappeared, and swallowing is more coordinated to allow the infant to easily accept solids. Head control is well developed, permitting infants to sit with support and purposely turn the head away to communicate disinterest in food. Voluntary grasping and improved eye-hand coordination gradually allow infants to pick up finger foods and feed themselves. Their increasing sense of independence is evident in their desire to hold the bottle and try to "help" during feeding. The major developmental milestones associated with feeding are listed in Box 12-4.

Box 12-4 DEVELOPMENTAL MILESTONES ASSOCIATED WITH FEEDING

Age (Months)	Behavior
Birth	Sucking, rooting, and swallowing reflexes Feels hunger and indicates desire for food by crying; expresses satiety by falling asleep Extrusion reflex is strong
3-4	Extrusion reflex is fading Beginning eye-hand coordination
4-5	Can approximate lips to the rim of a cup
5-6	Can use fingers to feed self a cracker
6-7	Chews and bites May hold own bottle, but may not drink from it (prefers for it to be held)
7-9	Refuses food by keeping lips closed; has preferences Holds a spoon and plays with it during feeding May drink from a straw Drinks from a cup with assistance
9-12	Picks up small morsels of food (finger foods) and feeds self Holds own bottle and drinks from it Drinks from a cup but spills some of the contents Uses a spoon with much spilling

Selection of Foods

The choice of foods to introduce first is variable but should meet the reasons for feeding solids, such as supplying nutrients not found in formula or breast milk. Cereal is generally introduced first because of its high iron content (7 mg/3 tablespoons of prepared dry cereal). Commercially prepared ready-to-serve dry cereals include rice, barley, oatmeal, and high-protein cereals, but rice is usually suggested as an initial food because of its easy digestibility and low allergenic potential. Cereals such as Cream of Farina are not used because infant commercial cereals are a better source of iron. Some of the commercial baby cereals are combined with fruit. There is little nutritional benefit from these preparations, and they are more expensive. Inasmuch as all new foods should be added one at a time, mothers should avoid cereal combinations when beginning a new grain.

Cereal is mixed with formula until whole milk is given. If the infant is breast-fed, the cereal is mixed with expressed breast milk or water rather than with cow's milk because the child may be sensitive to cow's milk. If fruit juices have been started, they can be mixed with the dry cereal. The vitamin C content of the juice enhances the absorption of iron in the cereal.

The addition of other foods is arbitrary. A common sequence is strained fruits followed by vegetables and finally meats. At 6 months foods such as a cracker, heel of french bread, or zwieback can be offered as a type of finger and teething food. By 8 to 9 months junior foods and nutritious finger foods such as a firmly cooked vegetable, raw pieces of fruit, or cheese can be given. By 1 year well-cooked table foods are served. General guidelines for feeding and introducing solid foods to infants are listed in Parent Guidelines: Introducing Solid Foods to Infants and Parent Guidelines: Feeding During the First Year.

Food Preparation

Commercially prepared baby foods are the most commonly used types of food served to infants in the United States. They are convenient and contain no added salt or sugar, but are relatively expensive. An alternative is preparing baby foods at home, which is a simple and inexpensive process.

PARENT GUIDELINES
Introducing Solid Foods to Infants

Introduce solids when infant is hungry.
Begin spoon feeding by pushing food to back of tongue because of infant's natural tendency to thrust tongue forward.
Use a small spoon with straight handle; begin with 1 or 2 teaspoons of food; gradually increase to a couple of tablespoons per feeding.
Introduce one food at a time, usually at intervals of 4 to 7 days to allow for identification of food allergies.
As the amount of solid food increases, decrease the quantity of milk to prevent overfeeding.
Do not introduce foods by mixing them with formula in the bottle.

PARENT GUIDELINES
Feeding During the First Year

Birth to 6 months

Breast-feeding
Most desirable complete diet for first half of year.*
Requires supplements of fluoride (0.25 mg), regardless of the fluoride content of the local water supply, and iron by 6 months of age.
Requires supplements of vitamin D (400 units) if mother's diet is inadequate

Formula
Iron-fortified commercial formula is a complete food for the first half of the year.*
Requires fluoride supplements (0.25 mg) when the concentration of fluoride in the drinking water is below 0.3 parts per million (ppm).
Evaporated milk formula requires supplements of vitamin C, iron, and fluoride (in accordance with the fluoride content of the local water supply).

6 to 12 months

Solid foods
May begin to add solids by 5 to 6 months of age.
First foods are strained, pureed, or finely mashed.
Finger foods such as teething crackers, raw fruit, or vegetables can be introduced by 6 to 7 months.
Chopped table food or commercially prepared junior foods can be started by 9 to 12 months.
With the exception of cereal, the order of introducing foods is variable; a recommended sequence is weekly introduction of other foods, beginning with fruit, then vegetables, and then meat.
As the quantity of solids increases, the amount of formula should be limited to approximately 900 ml (30 oz) daily.

METHOD OF INTRODUCTION:

Introduce solids when infant is hungry.
Begin spoon feeding by pushing food to back of tongue because of infant's natural tendency to thrust tongue forward.
Use small spoon with straight handle; begin with 1 or 2 teaspoons of food; gradually increase to 2 to 3 tablespoons per feeding.
Introduce one food at a time, usually at intervals of 4 to 7 days; identify food allergies.
As the amount of solid food increases, decrease the quantity of milk to prevent overfeeding.
Never introduce foods by mixing them with the formula in the bottle.

Cereal
Introduce commercially prepared iron-fortified infant cereals and administer daily until 18 months.
Rice cereal is usually introduced first because of its low allergenic potential.
Can discontinue supplemental iron once cereal is given.

Fruits and vegetables
Applesauce, bananas, and pears are usually well tolerated.
Avoid fruits and vegetables marketed in cans that are not specifically designed for infants because of variable and sometimes high lead content and addition of salt, sugar, and/or preservatives.
Offer fruit juice only from a cup, not a bottle, to reduce the development of "nursing caries."

Meat, fish, and poultry
Avoid fatty meats.
Prepare by baking, broiling, steaming, or poaching.
Include organ meats such as liver, which has a high iron, vitamin A, and vitamin B complex content.
If soup is given, be sure all ingredients are familiar to child's diet.
Avoid commercial meat/vegetable combinations because protein is low.

Eggs and cheese
Serve egg yolk hard boiled and mashed, soft cooked, or poached.
Introduce egg white in small quantities (1 tsp) toward end of first year to detect an allergy.
Use cheese as a substitute for meat and as finger food.

*Breast-feeding or commercial formula feeding for up to 12 months of age is recommended. After 1 year whole cow's milk can be given.

Fruits and vegetables can be steamed in a small amount of water and pureed in a blender or food processor. Many of them can be mashed fine with a fork, such as ripe banana. Fruits such as apples or pears require little or no water in the cooking process. Vegetables such as carrots, potatoes, or string beans require additional water in the cooking and blending process.

No water used in cooking should be discarded, because the water-soluble vitamins will be lost. Vitamin C is naturally destroyed by heat; therefore cooked fruits or vegetables do not supply this essential nutrient. Orange juice should not be warmed for this reason. Vitamin C is also destroyed by oxidation and alkaline solutions. Containers used for juice should always be light resistant, kept covered, and refrigerated to prevent oxidative loss.

Meats can easily be prepared by steaming, boiling, baking, or poaching but not by frying. Meat should be lean, because the infant's ability to handle saturated fats is limited. Meat can be pureed in a blender with liquid, such as leftover vegetable broth or meat broth. Baby food grinders are also available that finely grind small portions of cooked table food. Inasmuch as the food is ground dry, some type of liquid or other pureed ingredient, such as mashed potatoes, squash, carrots, or other vegetable to which the infant has already been introduced, must be added. When chewing is fairly well established, table food can be chopped finely and placed on the high-chair tray for the child to pick up and eat.

Generally any foods served in the home can be given to an infant. However, because the precise relationship between salt intake and high blood pressure has not been established and the safety of "extremes" in children's diets is unknown, it is recommended that salt or sugar be used in moderation in preparing food (American Academy of Pediatrics, 1983b). If sweetening is needed, refined sugar can be used, but honey and corn syrup are avoided because of the risk of infant botulism (Wilkinson and Clore, 1988). Preferably, foods prepared for the infant should be fresh or frozen, because canned foods other than those prepared for infants may have excessive sodium or sugar or be a source of lead from the container.

Food Storage

Storage of commercial baby food requires a few simple rules. Unopened jars can remain on the shelf indefinitely. Opened jars are refrigerated and can be used for a couple of days. If the infant does not finish a jar of food at one time, a portion of the food is removed from the jar using a clean spoon. If this is not done, bacteria are introduced, and the salivary enzymes on the feeding spoon begin to digest unused portions of the food. The dried baby foods (manufactured by Heinz) are prepared in individual portions, thus eliminating storage problems and waste of unused food.

For convenience home-prepared baby foods can be made in advance and frozen in small jars or in special plastic bags that are sealed by heat and can be reheated by placing them in boiling water. If microwave heating is used, the food is mixed thoroughly and checked to ensure a safe temperature before feeding. The temperature of the container may not indicate the heat intensity of the food (see also p. 584). Individual portions of food can be frozen in ice cube trays, transferred to a large container, and individually defrosted as needed. With reasonable care in the preparation and storing of foods there is little need to worry about bacterial contamination.

Method of Introduction

When the spoon is first introduced, infants often push it away and appear dissatisfied. Some patience and skill are required to overcome this initial response. A small-bowled, straight, long-handled spoon, similar to a demitasse spoon, allows a small portion of food to be placed toward the back of the tongue. If food is placed on the front of the tongue and pushed out, it is simply scooped up and refed. As infants become accustomed to the spoon, they will more eagerly accept the food and eventually open the mouth in anticipation (or keep it closed in dislike). Since the first introduction of food is a new experience, spoon feeding should be attempted after ingestion of some breast milk or formula to associate this activity with a pleasurable and satisfying experience. Trying to introduce a food *after* the entire milk feeding is usually useless because the infant is satiated and has no inclination to try something new.

After several spoon feedings, food can be introduced at the beginning of a meal. It is best to introduce many foods during the first year when the infant is more likely to eat them because of a hearty appetite resulting from a rapid growth rate. During the toddler years eating becomes less of an adventure, and strong food preferences become evident.

One food item is introduced at intervals of 4 to 7 days to allow for identification of food allergies. New foods are fed in small amounts, from 1 teaspoon to a few tablespoons. As the amount of solid food increases, the quantity of milk is decreased to less than 1 L daily to prevent overfeeding.

Because feeding is a learning process as well as a means of nutrition, new foods are given alone to allow the child to learn new tastes and textures. Sometimes it is necessary to camouflage a new food by mixing it with another favorite food to encourage the child to try it, although this should not become a routine. Food should not be mixed in the bottle and fed through a nipple with a large hole. This deprives the child of the pleasure of learning new tastes and developing a discriminating palate. It can also cause problems with poor chewing of food later in life because this experience is lacking. Guidelines for the introduction of new foods are given in the Parent Guidelines on p. 565.

Introducing solid foods can be an exciting time for parent and child. Most infants are good eaters and enjoy eating from a spoon and later feeding themselves. However, the transition from "parent doing it" to "baby doing it" can be a trying experience, particularly for those who value a clean house or who view cleaning up the mess as a waste of time. The infant's first, second, and often twentieth try at self-feeding or cup feeding is a sloppy experience. Finger foods such as soft fruits or vegetables are just as good playthings as food; they can be squeezed, smeared, squashed, and thoroughly painted on oneself, others, and the surrounding environment. However, all of this is part of learning, and mastery follows many accidents.

If parents find this experience distressing, a few suggestions may prove helpful. The feeding area should have a floor that can be easily wiped and is relatively far from walls, upholstered furniture, or drapes. A hand-held portable vacuum is helpful in cleaning up crumbs. Messes are confined to one area if the child is seated in a high chair rather than allowed to crawl or walk around while drinking or eating. Infants should be expected to get themselves covered with food; therefore a large bib (plastic can be wiped easily but needs to be removed after feeding) should be used, and washable clothes that are easily removed. High chairs can be thoroughly cleaned in a shower. Outdoor dining provides an excellent opportunity for practicing with a cup, spoon, or fingers because accidents are simple to hose or sweep away. Children cannot be pressured into eating neatly or developing table manners before manipulative skill is acquired.

If older infants suddenly refuse to eat, the feeding process should be investigated. It is not unusual for an 11-month-old infant to become stubborn, push the spoon away, and refuse to open the mouth. He or she may not be content with having a spoon to play with while someone else does the feeding. Helping parents understand the child's growing need for independence may prevent many temper tantrums and power struggles later on.

Weaning

Weaning, the process of giving up one method of feeding for another, usually refers to relinquishing the breast or bottle for a cup. In Western societies this is generally regarded as a major task for infants and is frequently seen as a potentially traumatic experience. It is psychologically significant because the infant is required to give up a major source of oral pleasure and gratification.

There is no one time for weaning that is best for every child, but generally most infants show signs of readiness during the second half of the first year. They have learned that good things come from a spoon. Their increasing desire for freedom of movement may lessen their desire to be held close for feedings. They are acquiring more control over their actions and can easily manipulate a cup to their lips (even if it is held upside down!). Imitation becomes a powerful motivator by age 8 or 9 months, and they enjoy using a cup or glass like others do.

Weaning should be gradual by replacing one bottle- or breast-feeding at a time. The last feeding to be discontinued is usually the nighttime feeding. It is advisable to never begin allowing a child to take a bottle of milk to bed, because this is a major cause of dental caries in deciduous teeth. If breast-feeding must be terminated before 5 or 6 months of age, weaning should be to a bottle to provide for the infant's continued sucking needs. If discontinued later, weaning can be directly to a cup.

SLEEP AND ACTIVITY

Sleep patterns vary among infants, and active infants typically sleep less than placid children. Generally by 3 to 4 months of age most infants have developed a nocturnal pattern of sleep lasting from 9 to 11 hours. The total daily sleep is about 15 hours. The number of naps per day varies, but by the end of a year infants may take one or two naps. Breast-fed infants usually sleep for less prolonged periods, with more frequent waking, especially during the night, than do bottle-fed infants. Because of the trend toward breast-feeding, sleep norms such as those described above, which were based primarily on bottle-fed infants, may no longer be relevant (Butte, Smith, and Garza, 1990; Elias and others, 1986).

Most infants are naturally active and need no encouragement to be mobile. However, problems can arise when devices such as playpens, strollers, commercial swings, and walkers are used excessively. These restrict movement and prevent infants from exploring and developing gross motor skills. Contrary to popular belief, walkers do not enhance coordination and have inherent hazards, especially the possibility of falls (Stoffman and others, 1984).

Formal infant exercise programs do not provide any long-term benefit to normal infants, and the possibility for damage to the infant's skeletal system exists. For these reasons, such programs are not recommended (American Academy of Pediatrics, Committee on Sports Medicine, 1988).

Sleep Disturbances

Concerns regarding sleep are common during infancy. Sometimes they are as basic as parents' questioning if the infant needs additional sleep. In this case it is best to investigate the reason for their concern, stressing the individual needs of each child. Infants who are active during wakeful periods and who are growing normally are sleeping a sufficient amount of time.

However, there are a number of more serious concerns that require intervention. Sleep disturbances caused by organic dysfunction are rare with the exception of colic, which is discussed in Chapter 13. The more common sleep disturbances are a learned pattern or developmental characteristic of some infants (Table 12-5). Although many families may report sleep problems that are typical of these patterns, interventions are offered *only* when the pattern is disruptive to the family. For example, co-sleeping or the "family bed," in which parents allow the children to sleep with them, is a relatively common and accepted practice, especially among black, Hispanic, and Asian families, such as the Japanese (Schachter and others, 1989; Lozoff, Wolf, and Davis, 1984). Other groups that are adopting co-sleeping include (1) single parents, whose need for company may encourage this practice; (2) working parents, who desire the closeness at night that was lost during the day, and (3) parents who have had an issue about sleep or separation in their own past (Brazelton, 1990).

However, when a sleeping problem is presented, a careful assessment is essential (see Box 6-15). Charting sleep

Table 12-5 Selected sleep disturbances during infancy and early childhood

DISORDER/DESCRIPTION	MANAGEMENT
▪ Nighttime feeding*	
Child has a prolonged need for middle-of-night bottle- or breast-feeding Child goes to sleep at the breast or with a bottle Awakenings are frequent (may be hourly) Child returns to sleep after feeding; other comfort measures (e.g., rocking or holding) are usually ineffective	Increase daytime feeding intervals to 4 hours or more (may need to be done gradually) Offer last feeding as late as possible at night; may need to gradually reduce amount of formula or length of breast-feeding Offer no bottles in bed Put to bed *awake* When child is crying, check at progressively longer intervals each night; reassure child but do not hold, rock, take to parent's bed, or give bottle or pacifier
▪ Developmental night crying	
Child aged 6-12 months with undisturbed nighttime sleep now awakes abruptly; may be accompanied by nightmares	Reassure parents that this is temporary phase Enter room immediately to check on child but keep reassurances *brief* Avoid feeding, rocking, taking to parent's bed, or any other routine that may initiate trained night crying
▪ Trained night crying* (inappropriate sleep associations)	
Child typically falls asleep in place other than own bed, e.g., rocking chair or parent's bed, and is brought to own bed while asleep; upon awakening, cries until usual routine is instituted, e.g., rocking	Put child in own bed when *awake* If possible, arrange separate sleeping area from other family members When child is crying, check at progressively longer intervals each night; reassure child but do not resume usual routine
▪ Refusal to go to sleep*	
Child resists bedtime and comes out of room repeatedly Nighttime sleep may be continuous, but frequent awakenings and refusal to return to sleep may occur and become a problem if parent allows child to deviate from usual sleep pattern	Evaluate if hour of sleep is too early (child may resist sleep if not tired) Assist parents in establishing consistent before-bedtime routine and enforcing consistent limits regarding child's bedtime behavior If child persists in leaving bedroom, close door for progressively longer periods Use reward system with child to provide motivation
▪ Nighttime fears	
Child resists going to bed or wakes during the night because of fears Child seeks parent's physical presence and with parent nearby, falls asleep easily, unless fear is overwhelming	Evaluate if hour of sleep is too early (child may fantasize when nothing to do but think in dark room) Calmly reassure the frightened child; keeping a nightlight on may be helpful Use reward system with child to provide motivation to deal with fears Avoid patterns that can lead to additional problems, e.g., sleeping with child or taking child to parent's room If child's fear is overwhelming, consider desensitization, e.g., progressively spending longer periods of time alone; consult professional help for protracted fears Distinguish between nightmares and sleep terrors (confused partial arousals) (see Table 15-3)

Modified from Ferber R: Behavioral "insomnia" in the child, Psychiatr Clin North Am 10(4):641-653, 1987.
*Guidelines for parents in dealing with these sleep problems are in Wong, D.L., and Whaley, L.F.: Clinical manual of pediatric nursing, ed. 3, St. Louis, 1990, Mosby–Year Book, Inc.

habits both before and after interventions is also an important strategy.* Questions regarding the frequency and duration of waking, the usual bedtime routine, the number of nighttime feedings, the perceived problem (e.g., how much disruption the behavior generates), and the attempted interventions are important in planning effective approaches designed for the specific sleep problem. A common suggestion given for any type of sleep problem—"let the child cry until falling asleep"—is very difficult to implement and inappropriate for certain conditions. Once the parents relent and console the child, they have only reinforced the crying. An equally effective but more practical approach for trained night crying is to let the child cry for progressively longer times between *brief* parental interventions that consist only of reassurance, not rocking, holding, or using the bottle or pacifier. For example, the parents may check on the child every 5 minutes during the first night and progressively extend this interval by 5 minutes on successive nights (Ferber, 1985).

*A 2-week sleep record for families is available in Wong, D., and Whaley, L.: Clinical manual of pediatric nursing, ed. 3, St. Louis, 1990, Mosby–Year Book, Inc.

The best way to prevent sleep problems is to encourage parents to establish bedtime rituals that do not foster problematic patterns. One of the most constructive is placing infants *awake* in their own crib. When infants are accustomed to falling asleep somewhere else, such as their parent's arms, and then being transferred to their crib, they awaken in unfamiliar surroundings and are unable to fall asleep until the routine is repeated. Also, the bed should be used for sleeping only—not as a playpen. It is advisable not to hang playthings over or on the bed; in this way the child associates the bed with sleep—not with activity. Although these interventions described above and in Table 12-5 are usually successful, it is much easier to prevent the problem with appropriate counseling during the early months of the infant's life.*

DENTAL HEALTH†

Good dental hygiene begins as soon as the primary teeth erupt. The teeth and gums are initially cleaned by wiping them with a damp cloth; toothbrushing is too harsh for the tender gingiva. The infant can be stabilized by cradling with one arm and using the free hand to cleanse the teeth. Oral hygiene can be made pleasant by singing or talking to the infant. There are no clear guidelines as to when toothbrushing should begin. However, it is generally recommended that, as more teeth erupt and the infant adjusts to the routine of cleaning, a small, soft-bristled toothbrush can be used. Water is preferred to paste, since infants are unable to effectively expectorate.

Fluoride, an essential mineral for building caries-resistant teeth, is needed during infancy when unerupted teeth are developing. Fluoride supplements are prescribed as appropriate for:

- All infants 2 weeks of age or older who live in areas with suboptimum levels of fluoride in the local water supply.
- Exclusively breast-fed infants, regardless of the fluoride content of the local water supply.
- Infants who consume relatively little fluoridated tap water, such as those receiving ready-to-serve formula.

Dietary considerations are also important because habits begun during infancy tend to continue into later years. Foods with concentrated sugar are used sparingly (if at all) in the infant's diet. The practice of coating pacifiers with honey or using commercially available hard-candy pacifiers is discouraged. Besides being cariogenic, honey also may cause infant botulism, and parts of the candy pacifier can be aspirated (Ramsey, Goldbach, and Stephenson, 1989). Parents need to be counseled regarding the detrimental effects of frequent and prolonged bottle- or breast-feeding during sleep, when the sweet milk or other fluid, such as juice, bathes the teeth, producing *nursing caries.* (See also Chapter 14 for a more extensive discussion of dental care, including nursing caries.)

*An excellent resource for parents is Ferber, R.: Solve your child's sleep problems, New York, 1985, Simon & Schuster.

†Caryn Stoermer Hess, R.N., M.S., assisted in the revision of this section.

IMMUNIZATIONS

One of the most dramatic advances in pediatrics has been the decline of infectious diseases over the past 50 years because of the widespread use of immunization for preventable diseases. Although many of the presently available immunizations can be given to individuals of any age, the recommended primary schedule begins during infancy and, with the exception of boosters, is completed during early childhood. Therefore the discussion of childhood immunizations for diphtheria, tetanus, pertussis (DTP); polio; measles, mumps, rubella (MMR); and *Haemophilus influenzae* type b (Hib) is included under health promotion during the first year. Selected vaccines that are generally reserved for children considered at high risk for the disease are discussed on p. 570 and as appropriate throughout the text.

Current Status of Immunizations

The routine use of immunizations has dramatically altered the morbidity and mortality from once common and feared childhood diseases. Unfortunately, with success have come both complacency and unwarranted fears. For example, in some urban areas up to 50% of children under 2 years of age are underimmunized—a factor that contributed to measles epidemics in 1989 and promoted current recommendations for a second dose of measles vaccine during childhood (see p. 573) (Measles, 1989).

Unfounded fears regarding side effects of vaccines, especially DTP, have also had an impact on immunization rates and vaccine production. Concerns about DTP vaccine causing sudden infant death syndrome (SIDS) and pertussis vaccine resulting in permanent neurologic damage are unsubstantiated (Cherry, 1990; Griffin and others, 1990; Hoffman and others, 1987). However, public awareness of initial reports caused many families to bring lawsuits against vaccine producers, causing a drastic increase in vaccine costs and at one time prompting some manufacturers to stop vaccine production. In response to the concerns of manufacturers, practitioners, and parents of vaccine-injured children, the National Childhood Vaccine Injury Act (NCVIA) of 1986 and the Vaccine Compensation Amendments of 1987 were passed. Basically these laws are designed to provide fair compensation for children who are inadvertently injured and provide greater protection from liability for vaccine manufacturers and providers. The NCVIA is concerned with DTP, MMR, and oral and inactivated polio vaccines (IPVs). Practitioners are required to fully inform families of the risks and benefits of the vaccines and to record certain information (see p. 578) and report selected postvaccine events such as anaphylaxis, encephalopathy, or paralytic poliomyelitis (Clayton and Hickson, 1990; National Childhood Vaccine Injury Act, 1988).

Several advances in the area of vaccines have been significant, especially the introduction of Hib vaccines (see discussion on p. 573 and Appendix G) and the varicella (chickenpox) vaccine. At this writing the varicella vaccine is under investigation for use in immunization of high-risk children, such as those who are immunosuppressed, and in healthy children. Findings demonstrate that the vaccine is effective, is well tolerated, and produces few reactions and that viral spread to siblings is mild and infrequent (Tsolia and others, 1990). Promising results have been obtained in a combination vaccine of varicella and MMR (Englund and others, 1989). An improved pertussis vaccine is being tested that appears to be effective with fewer side effects (Morgan and others, 1990). Enhanced potency IPVs are available that may one day replace or be used with oral poliovirus (OPV) (Modlin and others, 1990).

Health professionals need to be aware of the importance of education in addressing parents' concerns and dispelling unfounded fears. Since nurses frequently administer vaccines during health supervision visits, they may have the responsibility for adequately informing parents of the nature, prevalence, and risks of the disease; the type of immunization product to be used; expected benefits; the risk of side effects; and the need for accurate immunization records. Referring to immunizations as "baby shots" and limiting the discussion to a vague statement about their benefit are unacceptable.

Materials designed for patient education should be available to the family; information sheets should include a section that the parents sign in order to confirm their understanding of the benefits and risks of the vaccine. In essence, the sheet is a signed informed consent that the vaccine can be given.

Schedule for Immunizations

Two organizations—the Advisory Committee on Immunization Practices (ACIP) of the U.S. Public Health Service and the Committee on Infectious Diseases of the American Academy of Pediatrics (AAP)—govern the recommendations for immunization policies and procedures. Because ACIP is concerned primarily with national health issues and the Committee on Infectious Diseases formulates its recommendations for infants and children who receive regular health care, there are occasionally different perspectives in each group's recommendations. The policies of each committee are recommendations, not rules, and they change as a result of advances in the field of immunology. Nurses need to realize the purpose of each organization, to view immunization practices in light of the needs of an individual child as well as a community, and to keep informed of the latest advances and changes in policy.

The recommended age for beginning primary immunizations of infants is 2 months (Table 12-6). Children born prematurely should receive the full dose of each vaccine at the appropriate chronologic age. If the infant is hospitalized, OPV is initiated after discharge to prevent transmission of OPV in the nursery. Recommended schedules for children not immunized during infancy are included in Table 12-7. Tables 12-8 and 12-9 describe immunization schedules for Canadian children. Children who began primary immunization at the recommended age but who fail to receive all the

Table 12-6 Recommended schedule for active immunization of normal infants and children (United States)*

RECOMMENDED AGE	IMMUNIZATION(S)†	COMMENTS
2 months	DTP, OPV	Can be initiated as early as age 2 weeks in areas of high endemicity or during epidemics
4 months	DTP, OPV	2-month interval desired for OPV to avoid interference from previous dose
6 months	DTP	A third dose of OPV is not indicated in the U.S. but is desirable in geographic areas where polio is endemic
15 months	Measles, mumps, rubella (MMR)	MMR preferred to individual vaccines; tuberculin testing may be done at the same visit
	Hib	Any of the Hib conjugate vaccines may be used
18 months	DTP,‡§ OPV‖	See footnotes
4-6 years	DTP,¶ OPV	At or before school entry
11-12 years	MMR	Second dose of measles on entrance to middle or junior high school
14-16 years	Td	Repeat every 10 years throughout life

Modified from American Academy of Pediatrics: Report of the Committee on Infectious Diseases, ed. 21, Elk Grove Village, IL, 1988, The Academy.

*For all products used, consult manufacturer's package insert for instructions for storage, handling, dosage, and administration. Biologics prepared by different manufacturers may vary, and package inserts of the same manufacturer may change from time to time. Therefore, the practitioner should be aware of the contents of the current package insert.

†DTP, diphtheria and tetanus toxoids with pertussis vaccine; OPV, oral poliovirus vaccine containing attenuated poliovirus types 1, 2, and 3; MMR, live measles, mumps, and rubella viruses in a combined vaccine; Hib, *Haemophilus influenzae* type b conjugate vaccines (PRP-D, HbOC, or PRP-OMP); Td, adult tetanus toxoid (full dose) and diphtheria toxoid (reduced dose) for adult use. DTP, Td, and Hib vaccines are given intramuscularly; MMR vaccine is given subcutaneously.

‡Should be given 6 to 12 months after the third dose.

§May be given simultaneously with MMR and Hib at age 15 months.

‖May be given simultaneously with MMR and Hib at 15 months of age or at any time between 12 and 24 months of age.

¶Up to the seventh birthday.

Author's note: Updates based on following references: (1) American Academy of Pediatrics, Committee on Infectious Diseases: *Haemophilus influenzae* type b vaccines: immunization of children at 15 months of age, Pediatrics 86(5):794-796, 1990; and (2) American Academy of Pediatrics, Committee on Infectious Diseases: Measles: reassessment of the current immunization policy, Pediatrics 84(6):1110-1113, 1989. **Prior to publication, additional recommendations for Hib vaccines were made; these are discussed in Appendix G.**

Several exceptions to the schedules on pp. 570-572 exist (i.e., in high-risk areas or during outbreaks of a disease) and changes in recommendations occur frequently. Nurses must update their information to keep abreast of specific circumstances warranting exceptions to these guidelines and new vaccine recommendations.

Table 12-7 Recommended immunization schedules for children not immunized in first year of life (United States)

RECOMMENDED TIME	IMMUNIZATION(S)	COMMENTS
Less than 7 years old		
First visit	DTP, OPV, MMR	MMR if child ≥15 months old; tuberculin testing may be done at same visit
Interval after first visit: 1 month	Hib	For children aged 18-60 months; can be given concurrently with DTP (at separate sites) and other vaccines*
2 months	DTP, OPV	
4 months	DTP	A third dose of OPV is not indicated in the United States, but is desirable in geographic areas where polio is endemic
10-16 months	DTP, OPV	OPV is not given if third dose was given earlier
4-6 years (at or before school entry)	DTP, OPV	DTP is not necessary if the fourth dose was given after the fourth birthday; OPV is not necessary if recommended OPV dose at 10-16 months following first visit was given after the fourth birthday
10 years later	Td	Repeat every 10 years throughout life
Entrance to middle or junior high school	MMR	
7 years old and older		
First visit	Td, OPV, MMR	
Interval after first visit: 2 months	Td, OPV	
8-14 months	Td, OPV	
10 years later	Td	Repeat every 10 years throughout life
Entrance to middle or junior high school	MMR	

Modified from American Academy of Pediatrics: Report of the Committee on Infectious Diseases, ed. 21, 1988, Elk Grove Village, IL, The Academy.
*The initial three doses of DTP can be given at 1- to 2-month intervals: so, for the child in whom immunization is initiated at age 24 months or older, one visit could be eliminated by giving DTP, OPV, and MMR at the first visit; DTP and Hib at the second visit (1 month later); and DTP and OPV at the third visit (2 months after the first visit). Subsequent DTP and OPV 10 to 16 months after the first visit is still indicated. Hib, MMR, DTP, and OPV can be given simultaneously at separate sites if return of vaccine recipient for future immunizations is doubtful. See author's note, Table 12-6.

Table 12-8 Routine immunization schedule for infants and children (Canada)

AGE	IMMUNIZATION AGAINST			
2 months	Diphtheria	Pertussis	Tetanus	Poliomyelitis
4 months	Diphtheria	Pertussis	Tetanus	Poliomyelitis
6 months	Diphtheria	Pertussis	Tetanus	Poliomyelitis[1]
12 months	Measles	Mumps	Rubella[2]	
18 months	Diphtheria	Pertussis	Tetanus	Poliomyelitis
	Haemophilus influenzae			
4-6 years	Diphtheria	Pertussis	Tetanus	Poliomyelitis
14-16 years	Diphtheria[4]		Tetanus[4]	Poliomyelitis[1]

From National Advisory Committee on Immunization: Canadian immunization guide, ed. 3, Canada, 1989, Authority of the Minister of National Health and Welfare, Health Protection Branch, Laboratory Centre for Disease Control.

Notes:

1. This dose may be omitted if live (oral) polio vaccine is being used exclusively.
2. Rubella vaccine is also indicated for all girls and women of childbearing age who lack proof of immunity. At all medical visits, the opportunity should be taken to check whether girls and women need rubella vaccine.
3. A single dose of *Haemophilus influenzae* b (Hib) conjugate vaccine should be administered to all children ages 18 to 24 months. Children ages 25 to 60 months should also be considered for vaccination, particularly those in daycare centers and at increased risk of invasive Hib disease. Conjugate vaccine should be given at the first visit for children over 18 months of age who are unlikely to return for further immunization. Conjugate vaccine and diphtheria pertussis tetanus (DPT) vaccines may be given simultaneously at different sites.
4. Diphtheria and tetanus toxoid (Td), a combined adsorbed "adult type" preparation for use in persons 7 years of age or more, contains less diphtheria toxoid than preparations given to younger children and is less likely to cause reactions in older persons.

Table 12-9 Routine immunization schedules for children not immunized in early infancy (Canada)

TIMING	IMMUNIZATION AGAINST			
▪ For children 1 through 6 years of age				
First visit[3,5]	Diphtheria	Pertussis	Tetanus	Poliomyelitis
Interval after 1st visit				
1 month	Measles	Mumps	Rubella[2]	
2 months	Diphtheria	Pertussis	Tetanus	Poliomyelitis
4 months	Diphtheria	Pertussis	Tetanus	Poliomyelitis[1]
16 months	Diphtheria	Pertussis	Tetanus	Poliomyelitis
Preschool[6]	Diphtheria	Pertussis	Tetanus	Poliomyelitis
See Note 3	Haemophilus influenzae b			
At age 14-16 years	Diphtheria[4]	Tetanus[4]	Poliomyelitis[1]	
▪ For children 7 years of age and over				
First visit[5]	Diphtheria[4]		Tetanus[4]	Poliomyelitis
Interval after 1st visit				
1 month	Measles	Mumps	Rubella[2]	
2 months	Diphtheria		Tetanus	Poliomyelitis
14 months	Diphtheria		Tetanus	Poliomyelitis
10 years	Diphtheria		Tetanus	Poliomyelitis[1]

From National Advisory Committee on Immunization: Canadian immunization guide, ed. 3, Canada, 1989, Authority of the Minister of National Health and Welfare, Health Protection Branch, Laboratory Centre for Disease Control.

Notes:

1-4. See Table 12-8.

5. Measles, mumps, and rubella vaccines may also be given at the first visit if it is considered likely that a child will not return for further immunization.

6. If the last dose of the primary series for diphtheria, pertussis, tetanus, and poliomyelitis is given after the 4th birthday, this dose may be omitted.

doses do not have to begin the series again, but receive only the missed doses. In situations when there is doubt that the child will return for immunization according to the optimum schedule, DTP, OPV, MMR, and Hib vaccine can be administered simultaneously. DTP, MMR, and Hib vaccine are given in separate syringes in different injection sites (American Academy of Pediatrics, Report of the Committee on Infectious Diseases, 1988).

Recommendations for Routine Immunizations

Several vaccines are administered to all children in the United States according to the schedules listed in Tables 12-6 and 12-7. The following is a brief description of the immunizations.

Diphtheria. Diphtheria vaccine is commonly administered (1) in combination with tetanus and pertussis vaccines (DTP) for children younger than 7 years of age, (2) in a combined vaccine with tetanus (DT) for children younger than 7 years of age who have some contraindication for receiving pertussis vaccine, (3) in smaller doses (15% to 20% of that in DTP or DT) with tetanus vaccine (Td) for use in children age 7 years and older, or (4) as a single antigen when combined antigen preparations are not indicated. Although the diphtheria vaccine does not produce absolute immunity, when given according to the recommended schedule, protective antitoxin persists for 10 years or more.

Tetanus. Three forms of tetanus vaccine—tetanus toxoid, tetanus immune globulin (TIG) (human), and tetanus antitoxin (usually horse serum)—are available. Tetanus toxoid is used for routine primary immunization, usually in one of the combinations listed above, and provides protective antitoxin levels for 10 years or more.

For wound management, passive immunity is available with TIG or animal-source antitoxin. However, because the risk of severe reaction, such as anaphylactic shock or serum sickness, is always greater to the foreign substances of animal serum, the choice is TIG. In persons with a history of two previous doses of tetanus toxoid, a booster dose of the toxoid can be given. When tetanus toxoid and TIG are given concurrently, separate syringes and different sites are used. Table 12-10 presents a summary of the recommended procedure for tetanus prophylaxis in wound management.

Pertussis. Pertussis is recommended for all children 6 weeks through 6 years of age (up to the seventh birthday) who have no neurologic contraindications to its use. It is not given to children 7 years or older because the risk of receiving the vaccine increases as the incidence, severity, and fatality of the disease decrease.

Polio. The trivalent oral form of poliovirus (OPV) (developed by Sabin) is recommended for all children younger than 18 years of age who have no specific contraindications to its use, regardless of the number of administrations of inactivated poliovirus vaccine (IPV) (developed by Salk) they have received. OPV is used in the United States because the live virus can be shed to contacts, who become immunized through this exposure. However, OPV has caused vaccine-associated paralysis in both recipients and contacts. Because of the greater risk of vaccine-associated paralysis in children with immunodeficiency diseases, IPV is the vaccine of choice for these children and any close contacts be-

Table 12-10 Guide to tetanus prophylaxis in wound management

HISTORY OF TETANUS IMMUNIZATION (DOSES)	CLEAN, MINOR WOUNDS*		ALL OTHER WOUNDS†	
	Td	TIG	Td	TIG
Uncertain or less than 3	Yes	No	Yes	Yes
3 or more‡	No§	No	No‖	No

*Td = adult-type tetanus and diptheria toxoids. If the patient is younger than 7 years, DT or DTP is given (see text). TIG = tetanus immune globulin.
† Including but not limited to wounds contaminated with dirt, feces, soil, saliva, etc; puncture wounds, avulsions; and wounds resulting from missiles, crushing, burns, and frostbite.
‡If only three doses of fluid toxoid have been received, a fourth dose of toxoid, preferably an absorbed toxoid, should be given.
§Yes, if more than 10 years since last dose.
‖Yes, if more than 5 years since last dose.

cause it has no reported history of causing vaccine-associated paralysis. However, IPV has the disadvantage of being given by subcutaneous injection.

Measles. Because of the presence of maternal antibodies, measles (rubeola) virus vaccine should be delayed until 15 months of age for infants who live in communities where the disease is not prevalent. However, during the course of measles outbreaks, the vaccine can be given any time after 6 months of age, followed by a second inoculation after age 15 months.

Recent outbreaks of measles among unvaccinated preschool-age children and among vaccinated school-age children and college students have prompted new recommendations regarding measles immunization. The American Academy of Pediatrics, Committee on Infectious Diseases (1989) recommends a second dose of MMR at entrance to middle school or junior high school (approximately age 11 to 12 years). ACIP, however, recommends that the second dose be given when children enter kindergarten or first grade (at 4 to 6 years) (Measles Prevention, 1989a). Revaccination should include all individuals born after January 1, 1957, who have not received two doses of measles vaccine after 12 months of age. Individuals born before this date are thought to be immune because of exposure to natural measles virus. However, evidence suggests that a significant number of these individuals may be susceptible to measles (Braunstein, Thomas, and Ito, 1990).

Mumps. Mumps virus vaccine is recommended for children over 12 months of age and is typically given at 15 months in combination with measles and rubella. It should not be administered to infants younger than 12 months because persisting maternal antibodies can interfere with the immune response.

Because of recent outbreaks of the disease, especially in children 10 to 19 years, mumps immunization is recommended for all individuals born after 1957 who may be susceptible to mumps, that is, those who have no history of having had the disease or vaccine or when there is no laboratory evidence of immunity (Recommendations, 1989b).

Rubella. Rubella is a relatively mild infection in children, but in a pregnant woman it presents serious risks to the developing fetus. Therefore the aim of rubella immunization is actually protection of the unborn child rather than the recipient of the immunization.

Rubella immunization is recommended for all children at 12 months of age or older. If administered in a combined form with measles vaccine, it should be given to children at about 15 months of age. Increased emphasis should also be placed on vaccinating all unimmunized prepubertal children and susceptible adolescents and adult women in the childbearing age-group.

Because the live attenuated virus may cross the placenta and present a risk to the developing fetus, rubella vaccine is not given to any pregnant woman or to any woman who may become pregnant in the 3 months following the immunization. Although the precaution of maintaining adequate contraception for this 3-month period following the vaccination is standard practice, current evidence from women who received the vaccine while pregnant and delivered unaffected offspring indicates that the risk to the fetus is negligible (Rubella, 1989). In addition, there is no reported danger of administering rubella vaccine to a child if the mother is pregnant.

***Haemophilus influenzae* type b.** As of this writing, four vaccines have been developed for *Haemophilus influenzae* type b (Hib) infection. The first vaccine, Hib capsular polysaccharide (PRP), was licensed in 1985 and recommended for children 2 years of age. The vaccine was unsatisfactory because it did not protect children at greatest risk—those under 2 years. The immunogenicity of the vaccine was improved by coupling it to a protein. These new conjugate vaccines are able to induce immunity in infants as young as 2 to 3 months of age (Eskola, 1990). Three Hib conjugate vaccines are currently available:

- Diphtheria toxoid conjugate (PRP-D) (ProHIBit)
- Diphtheria CRM_{197} protein conjugate (PRP-HbOC) (HibTITER)
- Meningococcal protein conjugate (PRP-OMP) (PedvaxHIB)

Both the American Academy of Pediatrics, Committee on Infectious Diseases (1990) and the ACIP recommend any of the three conjugate vaccines at 15 months of age (Recommendations, 1990). As of this writing both groups are considering lowering the recommended age, since the vaccine is effective in younger infants (see Appendix G).

Table 12-11 Recommendations for selected nonmandated vaccines

IMMUNIZATION	DESCRIPTION	ADMINISTRATION/PRECAUTIONS
Influenza virus vaccine	Affords protection against strains of influenza Recommended for children 6 months and older with chronic disorders of cardiovascular or pulmonary systems, including asthma, whose severity warranted regular medical care or hospitalization during preceding year; other eligible children include those with diabetes mellitus, renal dysfunction, anemia, immunosuppression, human immunodeficiency virus (HIV) infection, or those on long-term aspirin therapy (because of risk of developing Reye syndrome after influenza infection)	Administered in fall, preferably November; repeated yearly Intramuscular injection; 2 doses of split vaccine at least 4 weeks apart for children 12 years or younger; 1 dose of split or whole vaccine for children over 12 years Contraindicated in persons with anaphylactic hypersensitivity to eggs May be given simultaneously with other childhood immunizations but at separate site
Pneumococcal polysaccharide vaccine (Pneumovax; Pnu-Imune)	Affords protection against 23 types of *Streptococcus pneumoniae* Recommended for children 2 years and older with sickle cell disease, functional or anatomic asplenia, nephrotic syndrome, human immunodeficiency virus (HIV) infection, and Hodgkin disease before beginning cytoreduction therapy	Subcutaneous or intramuscular injection Revaccination is not recommended Should be deferred during pregnancy
Meningococcal polysaccharide vaccine (Menomune)	Affords protection against *Neisseria meningitidis*, serogroups A, C, Y, and W-135 Recommended for children 2 years and older with terminal complement deficiencies and anatomic or functional asplenia	Subcutaneous injection Duration of protection unknown Safety during pregnancy not established
Hepatitis B vaccine (Recombivax HB; Engerix-B)	Affords protection against hepatitis B virus (HBV) Recommended for several high-risk groups, especially adults at risk for infection from contaminated blood products; among children, infants born to mothers who are hepatitis B surface antigen (HBsAg)–positive	Infants: combined hepatitis B immune globulin (HBIG) and HB vaccine; intramuscular injections at separate sites Administered within 12 hours of birth, with second and third doses given 1 and 6 months after the initial dose

References
American Academy of Pediatrics: Report of the Committee on Infectious Diseases, ed. 21, Elk Grove Village, IL, 1988, The Academy.
Recommendation of the Immunization Practices Advisory Committee (ACIP): Prevention and control of influenza. 1. Vaccines, MMWR 38(17):297-309, 1989.
Recommendation of the Immunization Practices Advisory Committee (ACIP): Protection against viral hepatitis, MMWR 39(RR-2):1-26, 1990.

Recommendations for Selected Immunizations

Several additional vaccines are recommended for children at high risk for particular diseases. Most of these children have chronic disorders or impaired immune systems that make them more susceptible to certain infections than the general population. Selected immunizations are presented in Table 12-11. Others, such as the rabies vaccine, are discussed elsewhere in this text.

Reactions

Vaccines for routine immunizations are among the safest and most reliable drugs available. However, minor side effects do occur following many of the immunizations, and rarely a serious reaction may result from the vaccine (Table 12-12).

With inactivated antigens, such as DTP, side effects are most likely to occur within a few hours or days of administration and are usually limited to local tenderness, erythema, and swelling at the injection site; low-grade fever; and behavioral changes (drowsiness, fretfulness, eating less, prolonged or unusual cry) (Long and others, 1990). Local reactions tend to be less severe when the deltoid site is used rather than the vastus lateralis and when a needle of sufficient length to deposit the vaccine in the muscle is used (see Nursing Tips, p. 577). Rarely more severe reactions may occur, especially with pertussis (see Table 12-10). Reactions to DTP tend to be more severe if they occurred with a previous immunization.

Hib vaccine is one of the safest vaccines available but may be associated with low-grade fever and mild local reactions at the site of subcutaneous injection, which resolve rapidly. Fever (temperature more than 38.5° C) may rarely occur (American Academy of Pediatrics, Committee on Infectious Diseases, 1985).

Unlike the inactivated antigens, live attenuated virus vaccines such as measles, mumps, rubella, and oral poliovirus multiply for days or weeks, and unfavorable reactions and "vaccine-associated" disorders can occur for a period of 30 to 60 days. However, they are usually mild, although reac-

Table 12-12 Possible side effects of recommended childhood immunizations and nursing responsibilities*

IMMUNIZATION	REACTION	NURSING RESPONSIBILITIES
Diphtheria	Fever usually within 24-48 hours Soreness, redness, and swelling at injection site Behavioral changes: drowsiness, fretfulness, anorexia, prolonged or unusual crying	Nursing responsibilities for DTP apply to immunizations for diphtheria, tetanus, and pertussis Instructions for DTP: advise parents of possible side effects Recommend prophylactic use of acetaminophen at time of DTP immunization and every 4-6 hours for a total of 3 doses Advise parents to notify practitioner *immediately* of any unusual side effects, such as those listed under pertussis in Table 12-13 Before administering next dose of DTP, inquire about reactions, especially those listed under pertussis in Table 12-13
Tetanus	Same as for diphtheria but may include urticaria and malaise All may have delayed onset and last several days Lump at injection site may last for weeks, even months, but gradually disappears	
Pertussis	Same as for tetanus but may include loss of consciousness, convulsions, persistent inconsolable crying episodes, generalized or focal neurologic signs, fever (temperature at or above 40.5° C [10.5° F]), systemic allergic reaction	
Poliovirus (OPV)	Essentially no immediate side effects Vaccine-associated paralysis rarely occurs within 2 months of immunization (estimated risk 1:7.8 million doses); more likely to occur in close contact than in OPV recipient	Assess presence of family members at risk from trivalent OPV because of immune deficiency states
Measles	Anorexia, malaise, rash, and fever may occur 7 to 10 days after immunization Rarely (estimated risk 1:1 million doses) encephalitis may occur	Advise parents of more common side effects and use of antipyretics for fever If a persistent fever with other obvious signs of illness occurs, have them notify physician immediately
Mumps	Essentially no side effects other than a brief, mild fever	See general comment to parents*
Rubella	Fever, lymphadenopathy, or mild rash that lasts 1 or 2 days within a few days after immunization Arthralgia, arthritis, or paresthesia of the hands and fingers may occur about 2 weeks after vaccination and is more common in older children and adults	Advise parents of side effects, especially of time delay before joint swelling and pain; assure them that these symptoms will disappear May recommend use of mild analgesics for pain
Haemophilus influenzae type b	Low-grade fever Mild local reactions at injection site Rarely fever above 40° C (105° F)	Advise parents of possible mild side effects

*General comment to parents regarding each immunization: the benefit of being protected by the immunization is believed to greatly outweigh the risk from the disease.

tions to rubella tend to be more troublesome in older children and adults.

Contraindications

Nurses need to be aware of the reasons for withholding immunizations—both for the child's safety in terms of avoiding reactions and for the child's maximum benefit from receiving the vaccine. Unfounded fears and lack of knowledge regarding contraindications can needlessly prevent a child from having protection from life-threatening diseases. The contraindications to the usual childhood vaccines are presented in Table 12-13. A general discussion of specific concerns follows.

The general contraindication for all immunizations is a severe febrile illness. This precaution is to avoid adding the risk of adverse side effects from the vaccine on an already ill child or mistakenly identifying a symptom of the disease as having been caused by the vaccine. The presence of minor illnesses such as the common cold is *not* a contraindication. Live virus vaccines are generally not administered to anyone with an altered immune system, because multiplication of the virus may be enhanced, causing a severe vaccine-induced illness. In addition, household contacts of such children should not receive OPV because the virus multiplies in the gastrointestinal tract and excreted virus in the stool can be communicated to the immunosuppressed child. Exceptions are made when the risks of contracting the disease outweigh the risks of the immunization, as in children with HIV who should receive MMR, but not OPV.

Another contraindication to live virus vaccines is the presence of recently acquired passive immunity through blood transfusions, immunoglobulin, or maternal antibodies. Administration of such vaccines should be postponed until 3 months after passive immunization with immuno-

Table 12-13 Contraindications to routine immunizations

CONTRAINDICATIONS (EXCEPTIONS)	RATIONALE	NURSING CONSIDERATIONS
Diphtheria, tetanus, pertussis (DTP)		
Febrile illness (Minor, nonfebrile illness is not a contraindication)	Signs and symptoms associated with the illness may be erroneously attributed to the vaccine	Explain reason for postponement to family and reschedule immunization at earliest return visit
Immediate, severe, anaphylactic reaction to previous administration of one of these vaccines	Hypersensitivity to some component in the vaccine may result in a severe reaction during reimmunization	Take a careful history of reactions to previous vaccines or a component in the vaccine, e.g., the preservative thimerosal
Pertussis		
Neurologic disorder, e.g., infantile spasms, uncontrolled epilepsy, or progressive encephalopathy, characterized by progressive developmental delay or changing neurologic findings	Danger of serious reaction to pertusis vaccination is possibly increased if any of these conditions are present when receiving the vaccine and may result in confusion about causation of neurologic findings	Take a detailed neurologic history including past convulsions, fainting spells, tremors, and specific reactions to DTP; report any such findings to practitioner before administering the vaccine
Personal (not family) history of convulsions Have or suspected of having neurologic conditions, e.g., tuberous sclerosis, certain inherited metabolic or degenerative diseases, that predispose to seizures or neurologic deterioration Any of the following reactions *after* receiving pertussis vaccine: Encephalopathy within 7 days A convulsion, with or without fever, occurring within 3 days Persistent, inconsolable screaming or crying for 3 or more hours or an unusual high-pitched cry within 48 hours Collapse or shocklike state within 48 hours Temperature of 40.5° C (104.9° F) or greater, unexplained by another cause, within 48 hours An immediate severe or anaphylactic reaction to vaccine (extremely rare)		
Measles, mumps, and rubella (MMR); oral poliovirus (OPV)		
Febrile illness (Minor, nonfebrile or febrile illness is not a contraindication)	Signs and symptoms associated with the illness may be erroneously attributed to the vaccine	Explain reason for postponement to family and reschedule immunization at earliest return visit
Anaphylactic egg hypersensitivity (Milder forms of allergy to egg or chicken feathers are not a contraindication)	Severe egg hypersensitivity may result in systemic anaphylactic reactions in allergic person receiving measles and mumps vaccine containing trace amounts of egg antigens	Take a careful history of allergic reactions to egg Report positive findings to practitioner before administering vaccine
Anaphylactic reaction to neomycin (Minor, delayed reaction of an erythematous pruritic papule after MMR inoculation is not a contraindication to a second dose)	Severe neomycin sensitivity can result in systemic anaphylactic reactions in allergic person receiving MMR vaccines containing trace amounts of neomycin	Take a careful history of allergic reactions to neomycin Report positive findings to practitioner before administering vaccine
Pregnancy Live oral poliovirus vaccine may be given if substantial risk of exposure is present (inactivated poliovirus [IPV] is preferred if immunization can be completed before anticipated exposure)	Theoretic risk to fetus	Take careful history of all women of childbearing age for possibility of pregnancy or conception within next 3 months

From American Academy of Pediatrics: Report of the Committee on Infectious Diseases, ed. 21, Elk Grove Village, IL, 1988, The Committee. For more detailed information consult the Report, the vaccine manufacturers' package insert, and the child's health care practitioner.

Table 12-13 Contraindications to routine immunizations—cont'd

CONTRAINDICATIONS (EXCEPTIONS)	RATIONALE	NURSING CONSIDERATIONS
Congenital disorders of immune function Immunosuppressive therapy (except investigational varicella vaccine); may immunize 3 months after immunosuppressive therapy is discontinued	Depressed immune functions prevent antibody-response to vaccines: fatal vaccine-associated infections can occur	Emphasize to family need to avoid child's exposure to these viral infections Stress importance of regular immunoglobulin therapy to provide passive protection in selected children
Children on steroid therapy are evaluated for the risk of live virus vaccines (IPV may be given)	Duration and dosage of steroids affect immune system differently	Advise family that household contacts should not receive oral poliovirus vaccine because the virus can be transmitted to the immunocompromised child
Children with symptomatic or asymptomatic human immunodeficiency virus (HIV) infection should receive all routine vaccines except oral poliovirus vaccine (IPV can be given)	Reports of severity of actual infection are thought to outweigh potential risks from vaccines	Advise family that household contacts should not receive oral poliovirus vaccine because the virus can be transmitted to the immunocompromised child

globulin. At times the vaccine and immunoglobulin are given simultaneously because of imminent exposure to disease. Vaccination should be repeated in 3 months, unless there is serologic evidence of antibody production (Recommendations, 1989a).

Pregnancy is a contraindication to mumps, measles, and rubella vaccines, although the risk of fetal damage is primarily theoretic. As a precaution these vaccines should not be given to women who are likely to become pregnant within 3 months after vaccination. Oral poliovirus is also withheld unless there is risk of exposure during an outbreak of polio.

A final contraindication is a known allergic response to a previously administered vaccine or a substance in the vaccine (see DTP in Table 12-13). Measles, mumps, and rubella virus vaccines contain minute amounts of neomycin, and measles and mumps vaccines, which are grown on chick embryo tissue cultures, may contain substances allergenic to egg-sensitive individuals. However, only a history of anaphylactoid reaction to neomycin or to egg is considered a contraindication to their use. To identify the rare child who may not be able to receive the vaccines, a careful allergy history is taken (see Box 6-13). If the child has a history of anaphylaxis, it is reported to the physician before administering the vaccine. Although rare, severe reactions to measles vaccine have occurred in children with egg allergy, and as a precaution such children should be skin tested for sensitivity and, if they react positively, be given incremental doses of vaccine (American Academy of Pediatrics, Report of the Committee, 1988).

Administration/Precautions

The principal precautions in administering immunizations include proper storage of the vaccine to protect its potency and institution of recommended procedures for injection. The nurse must be familiar with the manufacturer's directions for storage and reconstitution of the vaccine. For example, if the vaccine is to be refrigerated, it should be stored on a center shelf, not on the door where frequent temperature increases from opening the refrigerator can alter the vaccine's potency. For protection against light the vial can be wrapped in aluminum foil. Periodic checks are established to ensure that no vaccine is used after its expiration date.

The DTP vaccines contain the adjuvant alum to retain the antigen at the depot site and prolong the stimulatory effect. Because subcutaneous or intracutaneous injection of the adjuvant can cause local irritation, inflammation, or abscess formation, attention to excellent intramuscular injection technique must be used (see Nursing Tips). The total series requires a number of injections, and every attempt is made to rotate the sites and administer the injections as

NURSING TIPS: DTP INJECTION

To minimize local reactions from DTP vaccines:

- Select a needle of adequate length (1 inch in infants) to deposit the antigen deep in the muscle mass (Hick and others, 1989)
- Inject into the vastus lateralis or ventrogluteal muscle; the deltoid may be used in children 18 months or older (Ipp and others, 1989)
- Use an air bubble to clear the needle after injecting the vaccine (theoretically beneficial but unproven)

Note: Changing the needle on the syringe after drawing up the vaccine and before injecting it has not been shown to be effective (Salomon and others, 1987).

painlessly as possible (see discussion on intramuscular injections in Chapter 27). When two or more injections are given at separate sites, the order of injections is arbitrary. Some practitioners suggest injecting the less painful one first (MMR or Hib vaccine), then DTP, whereas others advocate injecting at two sites simultaneously (requires two operators). Research is needed to determine which sequence is least painful. Since allergic reactions can occur after injection of vaccines, appropriate precautions are taken (see Nursing Alert under Chemotherapy, Chapter 36).

Another important nursing responsibility is accurate documentation. Each child should have an immunization record for parents to keep, especially for families who move frequently. The NCVIA requires that the following information be documented on the medical record: day, month, and year of administration; manufacturer and lot number of vaccine; and the name, address, and title of the person administering the vaccine (National Childhood Vaccine Injury Act, 1988). Additional data to record are the site and route of administration and evidence that the parent or legal guardian gave informed consent before the immunization was administered.

INJURY PREVENTION

Injuries are a major cause of death during infancy, especially for children 6 to 12 months old. Constant vigilance, awareness, and supervision are essential as the child gains increased locomotor and manipulative skills that are coupled with an insatiable curiosity about the environment. Injuries can be grouped into the following categories: aspiration of foreign objects, suffocation, motor vehicle injuries, falls, poisoning, burns, and bodily damage. Table 12-14 lists the major developmental achievements of each period during infancy and the appropriate injury prevention plan.

Aspiration of Foreign Objects

Asphyxiation by foreign material in the respiratory tract, combined with mechanical suffocation, is the leading cause of fatal injury in children younger than 1 year of age. The size, shape, and consistency of foods or objects are important determinants of fatal obstruction. For example, small objects (less than 3.2 cm, or 1¼ inches) are more likely to completely obstruct the airway. A spheric or cylindric object plugs the airway more completely than any other shaped object. Pliable objects are less likely to be expelled than rigid ones. Unfortunately, common household items can be deadly to infants.

Nonfood items cause the majority of deaths in young children. Balloons, whether partially inflated, uninflated, or popped, cause more deaths in children than any other kind of small object and should be kept from infants and young children. Even the practice of inflating latex gloves to amuse children in health settings may pose a danger (Slasor, 1989). Another hazard is plastic lining from diapers; the accessibility of the plastic diaper lining is especially dangerous to young children.

As soon as infants can place objects in the mouth, they are vulnerable to aspiration of small objects, such as those left within reach or removable parts of objects that may on initial inspection appear safe. Rattles, for example, have small beads in them to produce noise. A broken or cracked rattle can be dangerous because the beads can easily be swallowed while the infant has the toy in the mouth. Stuffed animals are another potentially dangerous toy if any of the parts, such as the eyes or nose, are removable buttons or plastic pieces.

All toys must be carefully inspected for potential danger. An active infant can grab a low-hanging mobile and quickly chew off a small piece. As soon as the infant crawls or plays on the floor, the floor must be kept free of any small articles that can be picked up and swallowed, such as coins.

When infant clothes are purchased, the type of closure used should be considered. A front button can easily be pulled off and swallowed. Safety pins for diapers should be kept closed and away from the dressing table. Even though a young infant may not search for them, practicing this good habit from the beginning prevents future injuries.

Food items are the second most common cause of aspiration, and the most frequent offenders are hot dogs, candy, nuts, and grapes (Harris and others, 1984). When new foods are given to the child, nuts, hard candies, or fruits with pits or seeds should be avoided. When traveling, especially in airplanes, or entertaining, snack foods such as peanuts and popcorn should be kept away from young children. If given to young children, hot dogs must be cut into small, irregular pieces rather than served whole or sliced into sections, because their size (diameter), round shape, and consistency allow for complete occlusion of the airway.

Pacifiers can also be dangerous because the entire object may be aspirated if it is small or the nipple and shield may become detached from the handle and become lodged in the pharynx. Improvised pacifiers, such as those commonly made in hospitals from a padded nipple, also present dangers. The nipple may separate from the plastic collar and be aspirated (Millunchick and McArtor, 1986). In addition, candy pacifiers pose dangers because the candy portion can dislodge from the circular base and be aspirated (Ramsey, Goldbach, and Stephenson, 1989). To be safe, pacifiers should be of sturdy construction, have a shield or flange with at least two ventilation holes and be large enough to prevent entry into the mouth, and preferably have a handle that can be grasped.

Another commonly aspirated substance is baby powder, which is usually a mixture of talc (hydrous magnesium silicate) and other silicates. Although the use of talc has been discouraged, it is a common baby care product and can cause severe and often fatal aspiration pneumonia. One of the factors involved in talc aspiration is the similar appearance of baby powder containers and nursing bottles. Talc containers often become favorite playthings and are placed in the mouth (Mofenson and others, 1981). Improper use of powder by sprinkling it directly on the skin creates a cloud of talc dust that is easily inhaled. Parents are advised of the danger of baby powder and discouraged from using it. If

Table 12-14 Injury prevention during infancy

▪ Age: Birth–4 months

Major developmental accomplishments

Involuntary reflexes, such as the crawling reflex, may propel infant forward
May roll over
Increasing eye-hand coordination and voluntary grasp reflex

Injury prevention

Aspiration
Not as great a danger to this age-group, but should begin practicing safeguarding early (see under 4-7 Months)
Know emergency procedures for choking*
Never shake baby powder directly on infant; place powder in hand and then on infant's skin; store container closed and out of infant's reach
Hold infant for feeding; do not prop bottle

Suffocation
Keep all plastic bags stored out of infant's reach; discard large plastic garment bags after tying knots
Do not cover mattress with plastic; no pillows or loose blankets
Make sure crib design follows federal regulations (distance between crib slats no more than 2⅜ inches) and mattress fits snugly†
Position crib away from other furniture
Avoid sleeping in bed with infant
Use pacifier with safe design; do not use stuffed bottle nipple for pacifier
Do not tie pacifier on a string around infant's neck
Remove bibs at bedtime
Drowning—never leave infant alone in bath
Keep playpen sides up

Motor vehicles
Transport infant in federally approved rearward-facing car seat*
Do not place infant on the seat or in one's lap
Do not place a child in a carriage or stroller behind a parked car

Falls
Always raise crib rails
Never leave infant on a raised, unguarded surface
When in doubt where to place child, use the floor
Restrain child in the infant seat, and never leave child unattended while the seat is resting on a raised surface
Use high chair when child is old enough to sit well
Hold rail when carrying infant downstairs

Poisoning
Not as great a danger to this age-group, but should begin practicing safeguards early (see under 4-7 Months)

Burns
Have fire extinguisher in home
Install smoke detectors in home on each floor near bedrooms
Avoid or use caution when warming formula in microwave oven; always check temperature of liquid before feeding
Always check bath water; adjust hot-water heater temperature to 49° C (120° F)
Do not pour or drink hot liquids when infant is close by, such as sitting on lap
Do not smoke near infant
Do not leave infant in the sun for more than a few minutes; keep exposed areas covered, e.g., wide-brim hat
Use flame-retardant sleepwear and wash according to label directions
Use cool mist vaporizers
Do not keep child in parked car (risk of overheating)
Check surface heat of car restraint before placing child in seat

Bodily damage
Avoid sharp, jagged-edged objects
Keep diaper pins closed and away from infant
Protect infant from young children and animals, especially dogs

▪ Age: 4-7 months

Major developmental accomplishments

Rolls over
Sits alone momentarily
May stand while holding onto support
Grasps and manipulates small objects
Resecures a dropped object
Has well-developed eye-hand coordination
Can focus on and locate very small objects
Mouthing very prominent

*Home care instructions for care of the choking infant and for use of child safety seats are available in Wong, D. and Whaley, L.: Clinical manual of pediatric nursing, ed. 3, St. Louis, 1990, Mosby–Year Book, Inc.
†Information is available from U.S. Consumer Product Safety Commission; (800) 638-CPSC.

Continued.

Table 12-14 Injury prevention during infancy—cont'd

▪ Age: 4-7 months—cont'd

Injury prevention

Aspiration
Keep buttons, beads, and other small objects out of infant's reach, including sibling's small toys
Use pacifier with safe design; do not use candy pacifier
Keep floor and carpet free of any small objects
Do not feed infant hard candy, nuts, food with pits or seeds, whole or circular pieces of hot dogs or grapes, or other large pieces of food
Do not feed infant while child is lying down
Inspect toys for removable parts
Avoid balloons as playthings
Keep baby powder, if used, out of reach

Suffocation
May begin to teach swimming as part of water safety
Do not tie toys across crib or playpen

Motor vehicles
(See under Birth–4 Months)

Falls
Use lap/crotch belt to restrain in a high chair
Keep crib rails raised to full height
Remove bumper pads when child can stand in crib

Poisoning
Make sure that paint for furniture or toys does not contain lead
Place toxic substances on a high shelf and/or in locked cabinet
Hang plants or place on high surface rather than on floor
Avoid storing large quantities of cleaning fluids, paints, pesticides, and other toxic substances
Discard used containers of poisonous substances
Do not store toxic substances in food containers
Discard used button-sized batteries; store new batteries in safe area
Know telephone number of local poison control center (usually listed in front of telephone directory)
Keep syrup of ipecac in home; use only if advised

Burns
Always check bath water; adjust hot-water heater temperature to 49° C (120° F) or lower
Keep faucets out of reach
Cover tub spout or run cold water after using hot water
Place hot objects (cigarettes, candles, incense) on high surface; do not drink hot liquids or smoke near infant
Limit exposure to sun; apply sunscreen

Bodily damage
Give toys that are smooth and rounded, preferably made of wood or plastic
Avoid long, pointed objects as toys
Keep sharp objects out of infant's reach

▪ Age: 8-12 months

Major developmental accomplishments

Crawls
Stands, holding onto furniture
Stands alone
Cruises around furniture
Walks
Climbs
Pulls on objects
Throws objects
Able to pick up small objects
Explores by putting objects in mouth
Dislikes being restrained
Explores away from parent
Increasing understanding of simple commands and phrases
Helpless in water

Injury prevention

Aspiration
(See under 4-7 Months)

Suffocation
Keep doors of ovens, dishwashers, refrigerators, and front-loading clothes washers and dryers closed at all times
If storing an unused appliance, such as a refrigerator, remove the door
Fence swimming pools
Always supervise when near any source of water, such as cleaning buckets, drainage areas, toilets
Eliminate unnecessary pools of water
Keep bathroom doors closed

Motor vehicles
Transport infant over 17 to 20 lbs in federally approved forward-facing car seat
Do not allow to crawl behind a parked car
If infant plays in a yard, have the yard fenced or use a playpen

Burns
Place guards in front or around any heating appliance, fireplace, or furnace
Keep electrical wires hidden or out of reach
Place plastic guards over electrical outlets; place furniture in front of outlets
Keep hanging tablecloths out of reach
Do not allow infant to play with electrical appliance, cigarette lighter
Apply a sunscreen when infant is exposed to sunlight

Bodily damage
Do not allow infant to use a fork for self-feeding
Use plastic cups or dishes
Check safety of toys and toy box
Protect from young children and animals, especially dogs

Table 12-14 Injury prevention during infancy—cont'd

Age: 8-12 months—cont'd
Injury prevention—cont'd
Falls Place gates at top and bottom of stairs if child has access to either end Dress in safe shoes and clothing (soles that do not "catch" on floor, tied shoelaces, pant legs that do not hang on floor) Keep large toys and bumper pads out of crib or playpen (child can use these as "stairs" to climb out) Avoid using walkers, especially near stairs
Poisoning Administer medications as a drug, not as a candy Do not administer medications unless so prescribed by a physician Replace medications and poisons immediately after use Replace child-protector cap properly Have syrup of ipecac in home; use only if advised

they prefer to use a powder, a cornstarch preparation can be substituted (see Questions and Controversies, p. 623). Whenever a powder is used, it is placed in the hand and then applied to the skin, never shaken directly from the container to the skin. The container is kept closed and immediately stored in a safe place, especially away from curious toddlers who often imitate caregiving activities and may accidentally shake it on the infant.

Suffocation

Mechanical suffocation is another important cause of death by asphyxiation and includes asphyxiation by covering the mouth and nose, by pressure on the throat and chest, and by exclusion of air, such as by refrigerator entrapment.

An infant who is placed in a bed under blankets and sheets that are tucked in can be caught under them and be unable to wriggle free. Baby pillows filled with plastic foam beads that make them resemble small bean bags are dangerous; very young infants are suffocated when the pillow contours to the face and blocks the airway (Rollins, 1990). There are potential dangers in adults sleeping with a small infant because of the possibility of their rolling over and smothering the child. Even though this possibility is slight, the consequent parental guilt accompanying the death can be devastating.

Another cause of suffocation is plastic bags. Large plastic bags used over garments are very lightweight and can easily and quickly be wrapped around the head of an active infant or pressed against his face. Pillows and mattresses should not be covered with plastic for this reason. Older infants may play with a plastic bag and accidentally pull it over their heads. Because plastic is nonporous, suffocation takes place in a matter of minutes.

Anything tied around the infant's neck can potentially cause strangulation. Bibs should be removed at bedtime, and objects such as pacifiers should never be hung on a string around the infant's neck. This is a common practice in some cultures that can be remedied by attaching a short string tied to a pacifier and pinning the string on the child's shirt.

Toys that have strings attached, such as a telephone, or toys that are tied to cribs or playpens can be hazards because the string can become wrapped around the child's neck or the child can become entrapped in the toy. As a precaution, all cords should be less than 30 cm (12 inches) long. Crib toys should be hung high enough that the infant cannot become entangled in them or should no longer be used once the child is able to reach them.

Restraining straps, if applied too loosely or left unfastened, can be a hazard. For example, a child may slide off a high chair beneath the tray and become strangled on the loose strap. All straps should be fastened securely.

Infant strangulation may occur if the infant's head becomes caught between the crib slats and mattress or objects close to the crib. Suffocation deaths are not confined to cribs; ill-fitting mattresses in adult or youth beds, bunk beds, and waterbeds have also been reported. According to federal regulation the distance between crib slats should not be more than 2⅜ inches (about 6 cm), roughly the width of three adult fingers. Mattresses and bumper pads should fit snugly against the slats. A general rule is that if two adult fingers can be placed between the mattress and crib or bed side, the mattress is too small. A temporary solution is to place large, rolled towels in the space to create a snug fit. Ideally, information regarding correct crib design should be given prenatally before parents have purchased or borrowed a crib.*

The crib design should have no protrusions; children

*The booklet *It Hurts When They Cry* gives basic information on hazards, safety features, and proper use of nursery furniture and equipment. It is available at no charge from U.S. Consumer Product Safety Commission, Publication Request, Washington, DC 20207; additional free information is available by calling the Danny Foundation at (800) 83-DANNY.

have died when clothing caught on raised corner posts as the child climbed out of the crib.

Mesh-sided playpens and cribs can result in death if the sides are left in the lowered position. Infants have suffocated when they fell off the edge of the mattress and the head or chest was compressed between the floorboard and mesh side. Parents should be advised of this danger and encouraged to *always* keep the sides locked securely in the up position whenever the child is in the playpen or crib.

The crib should be positioned away from large furniture, because children who crawl out of the crib may become caught between the two objects. Cribs should also be located away from windows, where drape cords can become wrapped around the infant's neck.

Motor Vehicle Injuries

Automobile injuries are the leading cause of accidental death in children older than 1 year of age. However, a significant number of infants are injured or die from improper restraint within the vehicle. All infants must be secured in a federally approved restraint rather than held or placed on the seat of the car.

Infant restraints are either designed as an infant-only model (Fig. 12-14, *A*) or as a convertible infant-toddler model (Fig. 12-14, *B*). Either restraint is a semi-reclined seat that faces the *rear* of the car. In this position the most dangerous forces in a crash are absorbed by the infant's back. The restraint is anchored to the vehicle with the car seat belt and has a harness system for restraining the infant. Some harness systems require a clip to keep the shoulder straps correctly positioned (see inset, Fig. 12-14, *A*).

Generally the middle of the back seat is considered the safest area of the car. However, with an infant restraint it is preferable to position the child in the front seat, where the driver can observe the infant without having to turn around, provided the front seat can be locked in position.

For restraints to be effective they must be used properly. Dressing the infant in an outfit with sleeves and legs allows the harness to securely hold the child in the seat. A small blanket or towel rolled tightly can be placed on either side of the head to minimize movement and keep the infant's hips against the back of the seat. Padding between the infant's legs and crotch is added to prevent slouching. Thick soft padding should not be placed under the infant or behind the back because, during an impact, the padding will compress, leaving the harness straps loose. Although many infant restraints can be recliners, they should only be used in the car in the position specified by the manufacturer. (For further discussion of restraints see Chapter 14.)

Falls

Falls are most common after 4 months of age when the infant has learned to roll over, but they can occur at any age. Newborns are normally active, assume a flexed position, and have crawling and Moro reflexes that can propel them forward. The best advice is never to place a child unattended on a raised surface that has no type of guardrails. When in doubt, the safest place is the floor. Even though young infants cannot climb over a partially raised crib rail, it is best to form a habit of raising the side rail all the way, because someday that infant will be able to climb out. Crib sides should have a latching device that cannot be easily released. Ideally cribs should be placed on carpeted, not hard, floors.

Another danger area for falling is a changing table, which is usually high and narrow. Although these tables have a restraining belt, children are never left unattended, even when restrained. The best way to avoid having to leave is to arrange the area with all necessary articles within easy reach so the child is always in full sight of the caregiver. It only takes a fraction of a second for an infant to fall off. During the latter half of the first year, infants usually resist dressing and diapering and may be difficult to manage. If there is danger that the child is strong enough to resist restraining, the infant should be changed on the floor.

Infant seats, high chairs, walkers, and swings present additional opportunities for falls. If the infant seat is placed on a table, the child should never be left unrestrained or unat-

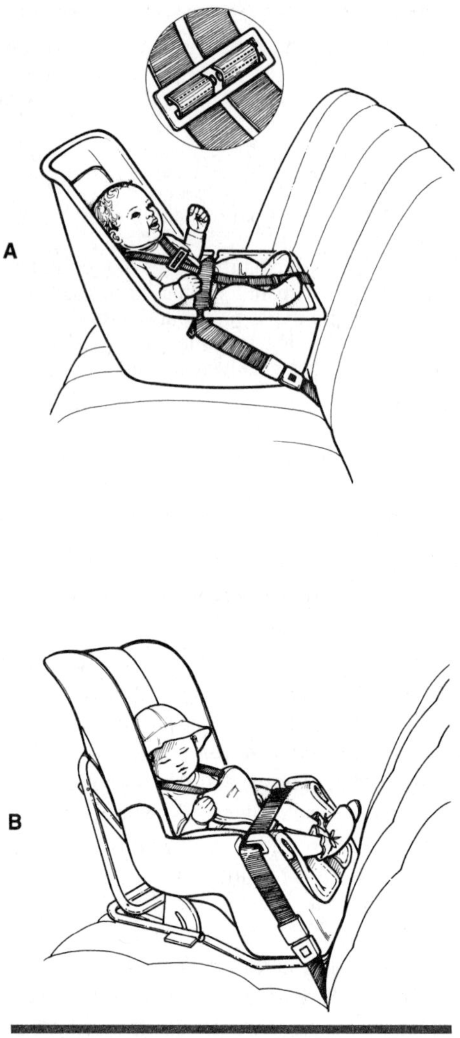

Fig. 12-14. Infant car safety seats. **A,** Rear-facing infant-only safety seat. *Inset:* Harness retainer (clip). **B,** Convertible seat in rear-facing position for use with infants.

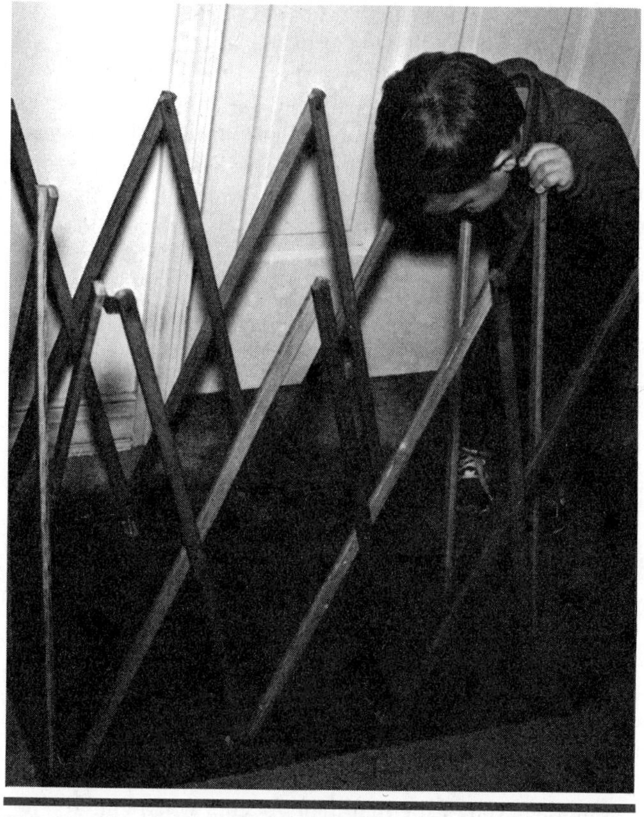

Fig. 12-15. Freestanding enclosures can cause head entrapment, but when secured to the floor they provide a protective barrier from heaters such as this floor furnace.

tended. The same rule is essential for other baby equipment, particularly when the child has learned to crawl and to stand up. Small infants can slip through a high chair if a protective harness is not used. High chairs are designed for older infants who can sit well and who are tall enough to have the tray at the level of their chest or abdomen. Walkers are responsible for a number of different types of injuries that occur because the walker tipped over or fell down stairs (Rieder, Schwartz, and Newman, 1986). Parents need to be warned of these dangers and encouraged to keep a constant vigil on their child's activities; the use of walkers should be discouraged.

Once infants are mobile, they should not be allowed to crawl unsupervised on any raised surface, near stairs, or near any water reservoir. Gates should be used at the *bottom* and *top* of stairs, because both present dangers to the crawling and climbing infant. However, certain types of gates can present hazards. Freestanding enclosures constructed of criss-crossed wood slats that expand and contract can trap the head or neck when children attempt to climb over them (Fig. 12-15). If these types of gates are used, they must be securely fastened to prevent mobility of the slats.

Sometimes even when the environment is made safe infants may literally trip over their own feet. Slippery socks; hard, slick soles on shoes or rubber soles that can catch, especially on a carpet; and long pants or pajama bottoms can easily upset a child's balance. Such dangers need to be pointed out to parents, especially when infants are taking their first steps.

Poisoning

Poisoning is one of the major causes of death in children younger than 5 years of age. The highest incidence occurs in those in the 2-year-old group, with the second highest incidence in 1-year-old children. Infants who do not crawl are relatively free from danger of poisonous agents by virtue of immobility. However, once locomotion begins, danger from poisoning is present almost everywhere. There are more than 500 toxic substances in the average home, and about 34% of all poisonings occur in the kitchen.

The major reason for ingestion of poisons is improper storage. To protect the infant, toxic agents should not be placed on a low shelf, table, or floor. Drugs that are kept in a purse pose additional dangers; if the purse is given to infants to play with, they may open it and ingest the drug. Another unrecognized hazard is during diaper changes when infants are near many toxic substances such as ointments, creams, oils, and talc. Parents may even hand the infant a potentially poisonous object to quiet him or her. Such dangers need to be stressed to parents and toys kept at diapering areas to minimize risks.

Poisoning is almost always the result of inadequate supervision, but it may not represent neglect. Children are very fast, and it takes only seconds to eat a bar of soap or a handful of cleanser or detergent. Although infants usually do not possess the manipulative skill to open closed jars, they are amazingly persistent and inventive. For example, an ant trap placed in an out-of-the-way corner is easy for a crawling infant to find.

Plants are another source of poisoning for infants. Plants are frequently placed on the floor, and the leaves or flowers are attractive and easy to pull off. More than 700 species of plants are known to have caused illness or death.

Another danger is ingestion of button-sized batteries that are used in devices such as hearing aids, calculators, watches, and cameras. Because they are bright and shiny, they are attractive to children. However, they can cause severe morbidity, even death, if lodged in the esophagus. The strong alkali in a battery can leak and cause a severe caustic burn. As a precaution small batteries must be safely stored and discarded when young children cannot easily retrieve them.

Not all poisonings result from ingestion—inhalation is another possible route, such as inhaling chlorine vapors from household cleaning or pool supplies (Wood and others, 1987). Recent concern has addressed passive cocaine toxicity in young children exposed to freebase cocaine ("crack") smoking by adults (Bateman and Heagarty, 1989). Children should be protected from environments where these toxins exist (for a discussion of passive cigarette smoking, see Chapter 32).

The only sure way to prevent poisoning is to remove toxic agents, which means placing them high out of the infant's reach. However, because crawling infants soon become climbing toddlers, it is best to keep all toxic agents, especially drugs, in a locked cabinet. Special plastic hooks can be attached to the inside of cabinet doors to keep them securely closed (see Fig. 12-16). Firm thumb pressure is required to unlatch the hook, and small children are usually unable to manipulate them. Locks are best, but for cleaning agents frequently used, such as under a kitchen sink, hooks are a practical alternative.

With several hundred toxic substances in each house, locking up all potentially toxic substances could present a problem; however, careful planning can help. A large surplus of cleaning agents, furniture polishes, laundry additives, paints, insecticides, and solvents should be avoided. Used poison containers should be promptly discarded and not used to store another poison without adequately marking the package. Any potentially hazardous substance should not be stored in any type of food container. A popular container used to store toxic liquids is a soda bottle. A child who is unaware of the dangerous contents is a vulnerable victim for poisoning. Parents should know the location of local poison control centers and call them in the event of a suspected poisoning. Emergency measures for poisoning are discussed in Chapter 16.

Burns

Burns such as scalding from water that is too hot, excessive sunburn, and burns from house fires, electrical wires, sockets, and heating elements such as radiators, registers, and floor furnaces cause a significant number of deaths and many more injuries in infants. The infant's skin is particularly sensitive to irritation, and the mechanisms for temperature perception are not completely developed. As a general precaution all homes should have smoke alarms installed near the bedroom areas.

Scald burns from hot tap water can be prevented by lowering the hot water heater to a safe temperature of 49° C (120° F). In addition, the bathwater should be checked before the infant is immersed. If formula or food is warmed in a microwave oven, it must be checked before feeding because the container may remain cool while the contents are hot (Smelt and Cawdry, 1989). Another danger is explosion of the bottle from the buildup of steam. Because of these dangers, microwaving infant formula or food should be avoided or done with heat convection. The handles of cooking utensils should be turned toward the back of the stove. When the infant is underfoot, pouring hot liquids and cooking with hot oil are avoided. Hanging tablecloths are also placed out of the infant's reach.

Sunburn can be a source of a first- or second-degree burn. Exposure to direct sunlight should be avoided. When infants are in the sun, the body, especially the face and head, should be covered. Sunscreen can be used on older infants (see Sunburn, Chapter 18). Although black-skinned infants burn less readily, their thin skin can become sunburned and needs protection.

Electrical outlets should be covered with protective plastic caps that prevent the child from sucking on the outlet or putting objects such as hairpins into it (see Fig. 12-16). Live wires are placed out of reach so that curious infants cannot chew on them and break the rubber coating (Fig. 12-16). Infants should not be allowed to play near television sets, stereo units, or other appliances, whether these units are on or off; infants cannot determine when the appliance is safe.

Any heat-producing element should have a guard placed in front of it. Fireplaces should be well screened because they are very appealing and within easy access. Small portable heaters should be placed on a high surface. Floor furnaces should have barrier gates to prevent children from crawling or walking over them (see Fig. 12-15). Burning cigarettes, candles, and incense are kept out of reach, and infants should not be held by a smoking adult, because falling ashes are a hazard, especially to the eyes. Heated-mist vaporizers are a source of burns and should not be used. If humidity is needed, only cool-mist vaporizers are safe.

By law all infant sleepwear must be flame retardant. Unfortunately this does not apply to all infant clothing. Flame-retardant fabric must never be viewed as the ultimate protection against burns. Repeated washing reduces the flame-retardant properties, and the use of soap or bleach destroys the protection. Inasmuch as detergent should be used for washing flame-retardant clothing, infants who are sensitive to such wash agents are unprotected when their clothing is washed even with a mild soap. If sleepwear is home sewn, parents are advised to look for specially treated flame-retardant fabric.

Another type of thermal injury occurs when children are exposed to excessive heat during confinement in poorly ventilated cars. The practice of leaving the windows open a couple of inches is not protective. The nurse should caution parents never to leave children in parked cars, especially when the automobile is in direct sunlight.

Children can also be burned by overheated metal hardware and vinyl seats in cars parked in the sun. As a precaution the surface heat of car restraints should be determined before placing children in them. Covering the restraints and hardware (such as metal latches on seat belts) may be necessary to prevent skin burns. An additional safeguard is buying a light-colored restraint, which absorbs less heat.

Drowning

Drowning in this age-group can occur in only inches of water. Consequently, infants should never be left unsupervised in a bathtub, hot tub, or near a source of water such as a swimming pool, lake, toilet, or bucket. Organized swimming instruction is not recommended for children under 3 years of age (American Academy of Pediatrics, 1987). Infants and toddlers are at increased risk of infection and convulsions from swallowing large amounts of water. Even if young children are taught to swim, no infant can be expected to learn the elements of water safety or to react appropriately in an emergency. Therefore all young children need to be considered at risk when near water.

Bodily Damage

Injuries can occur in numerous ways. Sharp, jagged-edged objects can cause wounds in the skin. Long, pointed articles, such as the common toothpick or fork, can be poked into the eye or ear, causing serious damage (Budnick, 1984). Such articles should be safely stored away from the infant's reach; forks are best avoided for self-feeding until the child has mastered the spoon, usually by age 18 months.

In addition to hazards such as aspiration from toys, small articles can be placed in the ear or nose, and excessive noise from toys can result in sensorineural hearing loss. Although toys with the highest noise levels are model airplanes, air guns, toy cap guns, and firecrackers, even common squeaking toys used by young children may be harmful if placed close to the ear (Axelsson and Jerson, 1985).

Even clothes and hair can present dangers to infants who cannot call attention to the problem. For example, constriction injuries can occur from excessively tight bands on socks, as well as fibers of hair or thread wrapping tightly around appendages, usually toes or fingers (Barton and others, 1988; Rosen, 1983).

Another frequently unrecognized danger to infants is animal attacks. Helpless infants, as newcomers to the home, can provoke jealousy in animals, especially dogs and cats. However, unprovoked attacks by ferrets and roosters have also been reported (Paisley and Lauer, 1988; Pinckney and Kennedy, 1982; Prieser and Lavell, 1987). Parents must be constantly vigilant to protect the child from household pets and farm animals (see Animal Bites, Chapter 18).

Nurse's Role in Injury Prevention

When the potential environmental dangers to which infants are vulnerable are considered, the task of preventing these injuries only begins to be appreciated. Nurses must be aware of the possible causes of injury in each age-group in order for *anticipatory* preventive teaching to occur. For example, the guidelines for injury prevention during infancy presented in Table 12-10 should be discussed *before* the child reaches the susceptible age-group. Preventive teaching ideally occurs during pregnancy. Inasmuch as two thirds of all injuries to children occur in the home, the importance of safety cannot be overemphasized. Parent Guidelines summarizes a home safety checklist that can be presented to parents to increase their awareness of danger areas in the home and assist them in implementing safety devices and practices *before* their absence can inflict injury on infants. In addition, displays such as a safety demonstration board (Fig. 12-16) can be helpful in familiarizing parents with inexpensive, commercial devices that can be used in the home to prevent injuries.

PARENT GUIDELINES
Child Safety Home Checklist

Safety: fire, electrical, burns

- ☐ Guards in front of or around any heating appliance, fireplace, or furnace (including floor furnace)*
- ☐ Electrical wires hidden or out of reach*
- ☐ No frayed or broken wires
- ☐ No overloaded sockets
- ☐ Plastic guards or caps over electrical outlets, furniture in front of outlets*
- ☐ Hanging tablecloths out of reach and away from open fires*
- ☐ Smoke detectors tested and operating properly
- ☐ Kitchen matches stored out of child's reach*
- ☐ Large, deep ashtrays throughout house (if used)
- ☐ Small stoves, heaters, and other hot objects (cigarettes, candles, coffee pots, slow cookers) placed where they cannot be tipped over or reached by children
- ☐ Hot water heater set 49° C (120° F) or lower
- ☐ Pot handles turned toward back of stove
- ☐ No loose clothing worn near stove
- ☐ No cooking or eating hot foods or liquids with child standing nearby or sitting in lap
- ☐ All small appliances, such as iron, turned off, disconnected, and placed out of reach when not in use
- ☐ Cool, not hot, mist vaporizer used
- ☐ Fire extinguisher available on each floor and checked periodically
- ☐ Electrical fuse box and gas outlet accessible
- ☐ Family escape plan in case of a fire and practiced periodically; fire escape ladder available on upper level floors
- ☐ Telephone number of fire or rescue squad and address of home with nearest cross street posted near phone

Safety: poisoning

- ☐ Toxic substances, including batteries, placed on a high shelf and preferably in locked cabinet
- ☐ Toxic plants hung or placed on high surface rather than on floor*
- ☐ Excess quantities of cleaning fluid, paints, pesticides, drugs, and other toxic substances not stored in home
- ☐ Used containers of poisonous substances discarded where child cannot obtain access
- ☐ Telephone number of local poison control center and address of home with nearest cross street posted near phone
- ☐ Syrup of ipecac in home containing 2 doses per child
- ☐ Medicines clearly labeled in childproof containers and stored out of reach
- ☐ Household cleaners, disinfectants, and insecticides kept in their original containers, separate from food and out of reach
- ☐ Smoking in areas away from children

Safety: falls

- ☐ Nonskid mats, abrasive strips, or texture surfaces in tubs and showers
- ☐ Exits, halls, and passageways in rooms kept clear of toys, furniture, boxes, or other items that could be obstructive
- ☐ Stairs and halls well lighted, with switches at both top and bottom
- ☐ Sturdy handrails for all steps and stairways
- ☐ Nothing stored on stairways
- ☐ Treads, risers, and carpeting in good repair
- ☐ Glass doors and walls marked with decals

PARENT GUIDELINES
Child Safety Home Checklist—cont'd

- [ ] Safety glass used in doors, windows, and walls
- [ ] Gates on top and bottom of staircases and elevated areas, such as porch, fire escape*
- [ ] Guardrails on upstairs windows with locks that limit height of window opening and access to areas such as fire escape*
- [ ] Crib side rails raised to full height; mattress lowered as child grows*
- [ ] Restraints used in high chairs, walkers, or other baby furniture; walkers not used near stairs*
- [ ] Scatter rugs secured in place or used with nonskid backing
- [ ] Walks, patios, and driveways in good repair

Safety: suffocation and aspiration

- [ ] Small objects stored out of reach*
- [ ] Toys inspected for small removable parts or long strings*
- [ ] Hanging crib toys and mobiles placed out of child's reach*
- [ ] Plastic bags stored away from young child's reach, large plastic garment bags discarded after tying in knots*
- [ ] Mattress or pillow not covered with plastic or in manner accessible to child*
- [ ] Crib design according to federal regulations with snug-fitting mattress*†
- [ ] Crib positioned away from other furniture or windows*
- [ ] Portable playpen gates up at all times while in use*
- [ ] Accordion-style gates not used*
- [ ] Bathroom doors kept closed and toilet seats down*
- [ ] Faucets turned off firmly*
- [ ] Pool fenced with locked gate
- [ ] Proper safety equipment at poolside
- [ ] Electric garage door openers stored safely and adjusted to raise when door strikes object
- [ ] Doors of ovens, trunks, dishwashers, refrigerators, and front-loading clothes washers and dryers closed at all times*
- [ ] Unused appliance, such as a refrigerator, securely closed with lock or doors removed*
- [ ] Food served in small noncylindric pieces to young children*
- [ ] Toy chests without lids or with lids that securely lock in open position*
- [ ] Pails, buckets, and wading pools kept empty when not in use*
- [ ] Clothesline above head level
- [ ] At least one member of household trained in basic life support (CPR), including first aid for choking‡

Safety: bodily injury

- [ ] Knives, power tools, and unloaded firearms stored safely or placed in locked cabinet
- [ ] Garden tools returned to storage racks after use
- [ ] Pets properly restrained and immunized for rabies
- [ ] Swings, slides, and other outdoor play equipment kept in safe condition
- [ ] Yard clear of broken glass, nail-studded boards, and other litter
- [ ] Cement birdbaths placed where young child cannot tip them over*
- [ ] Telephone number of ambulance or rescue squad and address of home with nearest cross street posted near phone

*Safety measures are specific for homes with young children. All safety measures should be implemented in homes where children reside and visit frequently, such as those of grandparents or baby-sitters.
†Federal regulations available from U.S. Consumer Product Safety Commission; (800) 638-CPSC.
‡Home care instructions for infant cardiopulmonary resuscitation and infant/child choking are available in Wong, D.L., and Whaley, L.F.: Clinical manual of pediatric nursing, ed 3, St. Louis, 1990, Mosby–Year Book, Inc.

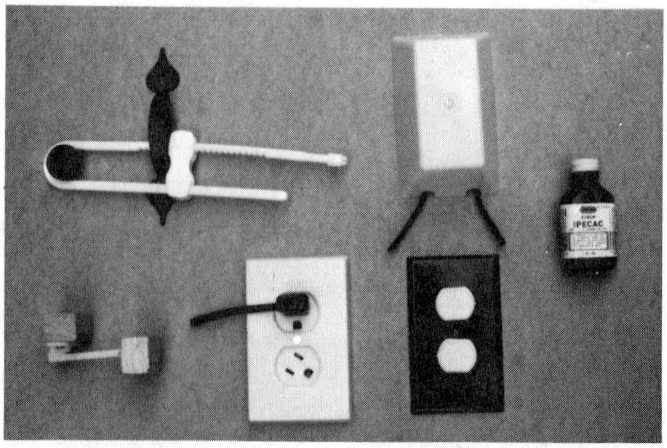

Fig. 12-16. Safety demonstration board *(clockwise from lower left):* cabinet latch, shock guard for electrical outlet, syrup of ipecac, and two types of outlet covers (white cover is passive device that automatically covers outlet when plug is removed).

Injury prevention requires *protection* of the child and *education* of the parents or caregiver. Nurses in ambulatory care settings, health maintenance centers, or visiting nurse agencies are in a most favorable position for injury education. This does not exclude nurses in inpatient facilities, who could use visiting times as an excellent opportunity for discussing this topic.

One approach to teaching injury prevention is to relate why children in various age-groups are prone to specific types of injuries. Stressing prevention is just as important as emphasizing the *why* of the injury. However, injury prevention must also be practical. Asking parents for their ideas leads to realistic suggestions that can be followed. For instance, bathroom cleaning agents, cosmetics, and personal care items can be placed on a top shelf in the linen closet, and towels or sheets can be stored on the lower shelves and floor.

If an injury has occurred, the nurse should not be too quick to admonish the parent. Injuries do not always indicate neglect. It is a difficult task to watch children carefully without overprotecting or unnecessarily confining them. Small falls help children learn the dangers of heights. Touching a hot object once can emphasize to the child the pain of a burn. Allowing children to explore while maintaining *consistent, age-appropriate limits* is sound advice.

Parents need to remember that infants and young children cannot anticipate danger or understand when it is or is not present. A dead electrical wire may present no actual harm, but, if the child is allowed to play with it, a poor behavior is enforced and will be practiced when the child encounters a live wire. Although it is always wise to explain why something is dangerous, it must be remembered that small children need to be physically removed from the situation.

It is not easy to teach safety, supervise closely, and refrain from saying "no" a hundred times a day. Parents become acutely aware of this dilemma as soon as the infant learns to crawl. Preventing injuries to children is usually the first reason for limit-setting and discipline, but limits are also set to prevent damage to valuable household objects. When small children are in the home, dangerous objects must be removed or guarded and valuable articles placed out of reach.

When children are taught the meaning of "no," they should also be taught what "yes" means. Children should be praised for playing with suitable toys, their efforts at behaving or listening should be reinforced, and recreational toys that are innovative and creative should be provided for them. Infants love to tear paper and avidly pursue books, magazines, or newspapers left on the floor. Instead of always scolding them for destroying a valued book, old, discarded reading material can be kept available for them to play with. If they enjoy pots and pans, a cabinet can be arranged with safe utensils for them to explore.

One additional factor must be stressed concerning injury prevention and education. Children are imitators; they copy what they see and hear. *Practicing safety teaches safety,* which applies to parents and their children and to nurses and their clients. Saying one thing but doing another confuses children and can lead to difficulties as the child grows older.

ANTICIPATORY GUIDANCE—CARE OF FAMILIES

Childrearing is no easy task; it presents challenges to new parents as well as to "seasoned" parents. With society's changing roles and mores, combined with a highly mobile population, there is little stability for traditional role models and time-honored methods of raising children. As a result, parents look more to professionals for guidance. Nurses are in an advantageous position to render assistance and suggestions. Every phase of a child's life has its particular traumas—toilet training for toddlers, unexplained fears for preschoolers, or identity crises for adolescents. For parents of an infant some challenges center around dependency, discipline, increased mobility, and safety. Major areas for parental guidance during the first year are listed in Box 12-5.

At birth the major task for parents and infant is attachment. Nursing interventions to promote parent attachment to the infant are discussed in Chapter 8. In addition, during

Box 12-5 GUIDANCE DURING INFANT'S FIRST YEAR

First 6 Months

Understand each parent's adjustment to newborn, especially mother's postpartal emotional needs.
Teach care of infant and assist parents to understand his or her individual needs and temperament and that the infant expresses wants through crying.
Reassure that infant cannot be spoiled by too much attention during the first 4 to 6 months.
Encourage parents to establish a schedule that meets needs of child and themselves.
Help parents understand infant's need for stimulation in environment.
Support parents' pleasure in seeing child's growing friendliness and social response, especially smiling.
Plan anticipatory guidance for safety.
Stress need for artificial immunization.
Prepare for introduction of solid foods.

Second 6 Months

Prepare parents for child's "stranger anxiety."
Encourage parents to allow child to cling to mother or father and avoid long separation from either.
Guide parents concerning discipline because of infant's increasing mobility.
Encourage use of negative voice and eye contact rather than physical punishment as a means of discipline; if unsuccessful, use one slap on the hand.
Encourage showing most attention when infant is behaving well, rather than when crying.
Teach accident prevention because of child's advancing motor skills and curiosity.
Encourage parents to leave child with suitable mother substitute to allow some free time.
Discuss readiness for weaning.
Explore parents' feelings regarding infant's sleep patterns.

the first 6 months there are several important areas of teaching. Parents may not realize the infant's need for stimulation or be aware of how to provide it, and suggestions for suitable toys may be needed (see Table 12-2). During the early months the infant's social responses, such as smiling, grasping, and vocalizing, should be supported. It is most important that during these first few months parent and child develop reciprocal relationships and meet each other's needs.

During the second 6 months the child's increasing stranger anxiety and increasing independence through locomotion present major challenges. Preparing parents for the child's fear of strangers and encouraging them to allow the clinging dependent behavior helps minimize potential conflicts. Stressing that such behavior indicates a strong parental attachment focuses on the *positive* aspects of stranger anxiety. Encouraging parents to find a suitable baby-sitter, particularly someone who can visit often, allows them freedom and enjoyment together without feelings of guilt. This is important not only for the child, who learns how to adjust to a crisis, but also for the parents, who need to spend time alone with each other to communicate, to love, and to enjoy one another's company. Time for one another can easily be lost in the responsibilities of raising a family.

As the infant achieves greater skill in all areas of development, safety becomes a major problem. Helping parents *anticipate* potential dangers in the home decreases the possibility of injuries occurring. Limit-setting is part of teaching safety, and establishing certain "rules" early helps children learn what is acceptable behavior. Neither a laissez-faire nor a dictator approach to discipline is advisable. A commonsense approach that incorporates understanding, firmness, and consistency by both parents usually yields the best results.

KEY POINTS

- Biologic development of the child encompasses proportional changes; sensory changes, including binocularity, depth perception, and visual preference; maturation of biologic systems; fine motor development; and gross motor development.
- Erikson's theory of psychosocial development (birth to 1 year) is concerned with acquiring a sense of trust while overcoming a sense of mistrust.
- Freud's oral stage during infancy involves gratification of the id through oral satisfaction.
- Piaget's theory of cognitive development, as it applies to the infant, focuses on the sensorimotor phase, which includes the use of reflexes, primary circular reactions, secondary circular reactions, and coordination of secondary schemata and their application to new situations.
- Development of body image begins in infancy; by 1 year of age infants recognize that they are distinct from their parents.
- Social development of the infant is guided by attachment, language development, personal-social behavior, and participation in play.
- Temperament influences the kind of interaction that occurs between the child and parents and siblings.
- Parents are faced with many concerns, including infant fears, daycare, limit-setting and discipline, thumbsucking and pacifier use, teething, and choice of infant shoes.
- Breast milk or formula is the most desirable food for the infant during the first 6 months, followed by gradual introduction of solid food during the second 6 months.
- Infants may be prone to sleep disturbances, and the nurse should instruct the parents, after careful assessment, in strategies to deal with the specific problem.
- Fluoride supplements, dietary intake, and cleaning the teeth promote good dental hygiene.
- Recommended routine immunizations include those for diphtheria, tetanus, pertussis, polio, measles, mumps, rubella, and *Haemophilus influenzae* type b.
- Recommended immunizations for selected groups of children are influenza virus, pneumococcal polysaccharide, and hepatitis B vaccines.
- Because injuries are a major cause of death during infancy, parents should be alerted to aspiration of foreign objects, suffocation, falls, poisoning, burns, motor vehicle injuries, and bodily damage, and preventive actions needed to be taken to make the environment safe for infants.

REFERENCES

Ainsworth, M.: Early caregiving and later patterns of attachment. In Klaus, M., and Robertson, M., editors: Birth, interaction, and attachment, Skillman, N.J., 1982, Johnson & Johnson Baby Products Co.

American Academy of Pediatrics: Report of the Committee on Infectious Diseases, ed. 21, Elk Grove Village, IL, 1988, The Academy.

American Academy of Pediatrics, Committee of Accident and Poison Prevention: Injury control for children and youth, Elk Grove Village, IL, 1987, The Academy.

American Academy of Pediatrics, Committee on Early Childhood, Adoption, and Dependent Care: The pediatrician's role in promoting the health of a patient in day care, Pediatrics 74(1):157-158, 1984.

American Academy of Pediatrics, Committee on Infectious Diseases: *Haemophilus* type b polysaccharide vaccine, Pediatrics 76(2):322-323, 1985.

American Academy of Pediatrics, Committee on Infectious Diseases: Measles: reassessment of the current immunization policy, Pediatrics 84(6):1110-1113, 1989.

American Academy of Pediatrics, Committee on Infectious Diseases: *Haemophilus influenzae* type b conjugate vaccines: immunization of children at 15 months of age, Pediatrics 86(5):794-796, 1990.

American Academy of Pediatrics, Committee on Nutrition: Vitamin and mineral supplement needs in normal children in the United States, Pediatrics 66(6):1015-1020, 1980.

American Academy of Pediatrics, Committee on Nutrition: Toward a prudent diet for children, Pediatrics 71(1):78-80, 1983.

American Academy of Pediatrics, Committee on Nutrition: Imitation and substitute milks, Pediatrics 73(6):876, 1984.

American Academy of Pediatrics, Committee on Nutrition: Prudent lifestyle for children: dietary fat and cholesterol, Pediatrics 78(3):521-525, 1986.

American Academy of Pediatrics, Committee on Nutrition: Follow-up or weaning formulas, Pediatrics 83(6):1067, 1989a.

American Academy of Pediatrics, Committee on Nutrition: Iron-fortified infant formulas, Pediatrics 84(6):1114-1115, 1989b.

American Academy of Pediatrics, Committee on Sports Medicine: Infant exercise programs, Pediatrics 82(5):800, 1988.

Anderson, G.: Pacifiers: the positive side, MCN 11(2):122-124, 1986.

Anderson, K., and others: Water-soluble vitamin intakes of infants consuming mixed diets, J. Am. Diet. Assoc. 89(5):688-689, 1989.

Axelsson, A., and Jerson, T.: Noisy toys: a possible source of sensorineural hearing loss, Pediatrics 76(4):574-578, 1985.

Barton, D., and others: Hair-thread tourniquet syndrome, Pediatrics 82(6):925-928, 1988.

Bateman, D., and Heagarty, M: Passive freebase cocaine ("crack") inhalation by infants and toddlers, Am. J. Dis. Child. 143(1):25-27, 1989.

Biggar, M.: Maternal aversion to mother-infant contact. In Brown, C., editor: The many facets of touch, 1984, Skillman, N.J., Johnson & Johnson Baby Products Co.

Blosser, C.: Avoiding potential behavior problems in children, Pediatr. Nurs. 5(3):11-15, 1979.

Bowlby, J.: Attachment and loss, vol. 1, New York, 1969, Basic Books, Inc.

Braunstein, H., Thomas, S., and Ito, R.: Immunity to measles in a large population of varying age, Am. J. Dis. Child. 144(3):296-298, 1990.

Brazelton, T.: Parent-infant cosleeping revisited, Ab Initio 2(1):1-7, 1990.

Brazelton, T.: What every baby knows, Menlo Park, CA, 1987, Addison-Wesley Publishing Co., Inc.

Brown, K., and others: Milk consumption and hydration status of exclusively breast-fed infants in a warm climate, J. Pediatr. 108:677-680, 1986.

Budnick, L.D.: Toothpick-related injuries in the United States, 1979 through 1982, JAMA 252(6):796-797, 1984.

Butte, N., Smith, E., and Garza, C.: Energy utilization of breast-fed and formula-fed infants, Am. J. Clin. Nutr. 51:350-358, 1990.

Campbell, S.B.G.: Mother-infant interaction as a function of maternal ratings of temperament, Child Psychiatry Hum. Dev. 10(2):67-76, 1979.

Carey, W.B.: Clinical applications of infant temperament measurements, J. Pediatr. 81(4):823-828, 1972.

Carey, W.B.: Night waking and temperament in infancy, J. Pediatr. 84(5):756-758, 1974.

Carey, W.B.: Intervention strategies using temperament data. In Brown, C.C., editor: Infants at risk: assessment and intervention, Skillman, N.J., 1981, Johnson & Johnson Baby Products Co.

Carey, W.B., and McDevitt, S.C.: Revision of the infant temperament questionnaire, Pediatrics 61(5):735-739, 1978.

Cherry, J.: Pertussis vaccine encephalopathy: it is time to recognize it as the myth that it is, JAMA 263(12):1679-1680, 1990.

Chess, S., and Thomas, A.: Temperamental differences: a critical concept in child health care, Pediatr. Nurs. 11(3):167-171, 1985.

Chong, A.: Selecting shoes for children, Baby Talk 52(3):40-42, 1987.

Cipes, M., Miraglia, M., and Gaulin-Kremer, E.: Monitoring and reinforcement to eliminate thumbsucking, J. Pediatr. Nurs. 1(5):361, 1986.

Clayton, E., and Hickson, G.: Compensation under the national childhood vaccine injury act, J. Pediatr. 116:508-513, 1990.

Duc, G., and Largo, R.: Anterior fontanel: size and closure in term and preterm infants, Pediatrics 78(5):904-908, 1986.

Elias, M., and others: Sleep/wake patterns of breast-fed infants in the first 2 years of life, Pediatrics 77(3):322-329, 1986.

Englund, J., and others: Placebo-controlled trial of varicella vaccine given with or after measles-mumps-rebella vaccine, J. Pediatr. 114:37-44, 1989.

Eskola, J.: Recent advances in the development and use of childhood vaccines, Curr. Opin. Pediatr. 2(1):73-80, 1990.

Ferber, R.: Solve your child's sleep problems, New York, 1985, Simon & Schuster.

Fomon, S., Sanders, K., and Ziegler, E.: Formulas for older infants, J. Pediatr. 116(5):690-696, 1990.

Friman, P., Barone, V., and Christophersen, E.: Aversive taste treatment of finger and thumb sucking, Pediatrics 78(1):174-176, 1986.

Fulginiti, V.A.: Patient education for immunizations, Pediatrics 74(suppl. 5):961-963, 1984.

Garmezy, N., and Rutter, M., editors: Stress, coping, and development in children, New York, 1983, McGraw-Hill Book Co.

Glendon, M.: If the shoe fits . . . wear it, Pediatr. Nurs. 13(4):230-271, 1987.

Greer, F., and Marshall, S.: Bone mineral content, serum vitamin D metabolite concentrations, and ultraviolet B light exposure in infants fed human milk with and without vitamin D2 supplements, J. Pediatr. 114(2):203-212, 1989.

Griffin, M., and others: Risk of seizures and encephalopathy after immunization with the diphtheria-tetanus-pertussis vaccine, JAMA 263(12):1641-1645, 1990.

Harris, C.S., and others: Childhood asphyxiation by food, JAMA 251:2231-2235, 1984.

Hick, J., and others: Optimum needle length for diphtheria-tetanus-pertussis inoculation of infants, Pediatrics 84(1):136-137, 1989.

Hoffman, H., and others: Diphtheria-tetanus-pertussis immunization and sudden infant death: results of the national institute of child health and human development cooperative epidemiological study of sudden infant death syndrome risk factors, Pediatrics 79(4):598-611, 1987.

Houldin, A.: Infant temperament and the quality of the childrearing environment, Matern. Child Nurs. J. 16(2):131-143, 1987.

Ipp, M., and others: Adverse reactions to diphtheria, tetanus, pertussis-polio vaccination at 18 months of age: effect of injection site and needle length, Pediatrics 83(5):679-682, 1989.

Kliman, D.S., and Vukelich, C.: Mothers and fathers: expectations for infants, Fam. Rel. 34:305-313, 1985.

Kronstadt, D., and others: Infant behavior and maternal adaptations in the first six months of life, Am. J. Orthopsychiatry 49(3):454-464, 1979.

Lawrence, R.A.: Breast-feeding, ed. 3, St. Louis, 1989, Mosby–Year Book, Inc.

Lester, B.M.: There's more to crying than meets the ear. In Lester, B.M., and Boukydis, C.F., editors: Infant crying, New York, 1985, Plenum Publishing Corp.

Lincoln, L.M.: Fathering and the separation-individuation process, Matern. Child Nurs. J. 13(2):103-111, 1984.

Little, D.L.: Parent acceptance of routine use of the Carey and McDevitt Infant Temperament Questionnaire, Pediatrics 71:104-106, 1983.

Little, D.L.: Written explanation of temperament scores, Pediatrics 75(2):275-277, 1985.

Long, S.S., and others: Longitudinal study of adverse reactions following diphtheria-tetanus-pertussis vaccine in infancy, Pediatrics 85(3):294-302, 1990.

Lozoff, B., Wolf, A.W., and Davis, N.S.: Cosleeping in urban families with young children in the United States, Pediatrics 74(2):171-182, 1984.

MacKenzie, E.: Thumb-sucking debate, Pediatrics 79(3):485-486, 1987.

MacLaughlin, S., and Strelnick, E.G.: Breast-feeding and working outside the home, Issues Compr. Pediatr. Nurs. 7(1):67-81, 1984.

Maziade, M., and others: Temperament and intellectual development: a longitudinal study from infancy to four years, Am. J. Psychiatry 144(2):144-150, 1987.

McIntosh, B.: Spoiled child syndrome, Pediatrics 83(1):108-114, 1989.

Measles prevention: recommendations of the immunization practices advisory committee (ACIP), MMWR 38(S-9):1-17, 1989a.

Measles—United States, first 26 weeks, 1989, MWWR 38(50):863-872, 1989b.

Merrifield, E.B., and Ryberg, J.W.: What parents should know about pacifiers, Child. Nurs. 3(4):1-3, 1985.

Millunchick, E., and McArtor, R.: Fatal aspiration of a makeshift pacifier, Pediatrics 77(3):369-370, 1986.

Modlin, J., and others: The humoral immune response to type 1 oral poliovirus vaccine in children previously immunized with enhanced potency inactivated poliovirus vaccine or live oral poliovirus vaccine, Am. J. Dis. Child. 144(4):480-484, 1990.

Mofenson, H.C., and others: Baby powder—a hazard! Pediatrics 68(2):265-266, 1981.

Montalto, M.B., Benson, J.D., and Martinez, G.A.: Nutrient intakes of formula-fed infants and infants fed cow's milk, Pediatrics 75(2):343-351, 1985.

Morgan, C., and others: Comparison of acellular and whole-cell pertussis-component DTP vaccines, Am. J. Dis. Child. 144:41-45, 1990.

National Childhood Vaccine Injury Act: requirements for permanent vaccination records and for reporting of selected events after vaccination, MMWR 37(13):197-200, 1988.

Nelms, B.C.: Attachment versus spoiling, Pediatr. Nurs. 9(1):49-51, 1983.

Nelms, B.C.: Stress during childhood: long-lasting effects? Pediatr. Nurs. 11(2):95-98, 1985.

Orenstein, S., and others: The Santmyer swallow: a new and useful infant reflex, Lancet 1(8581):345-346, 1988.

Paisley, J., and Lauer, B.: Severe facial injuries to infants due to unprovoked attacks by pet ferrets, JAMA 259:2005-2006, 1988.

Pinckney, L.E., and Kennedy, L.A.: Traumatic deaths from dog attacks in the United States, Pediatrics 69(2):193-196, 1982.

Pipes, P.L.: Nutrition in infancy and childhood, ed. 4, St. Louis, 1989, Mosby–Year Book, Inc.

Preiser, G., and Lavell, T.: Rooster attacks on children, Pediatrics 79(3):426-427, 1987.

Ramsey, K., Goldbach, R., and Stephenson, S.: Near fatal aspiration of a candy pacifier, Pediatrics 84(1):126-127, 1989.

Recommendations of the Immunization Practices Advisory Committee (ACIP): general recommendations on immunization, MMWR 38(13):205-227, 1989a.

Recommendations of the Immunization Practices Advisory Committee (ACIP): mumps prevention, MMWR 38(22):388-400, 1989b.

Recommendations of the Immunization Practices Advisory Committee (ACIP): supplementary statement: change in administration schedule for *Haemophilus* b conjugate vaccines, MMWR 39(14):232-233, 1990.

Reifsnider, E., and Myers, S.T.: Employed mothers can breast-feed, too! MCN 10:256-259, 1985.

Rieder, M., Schwartz, C., and Newman, J.: Patterns of walker use and walker injury, Pediatrics 78(3):488-493, 1986.

Roberts, F.B.: Infant behavior and the transition to parenthood, Nurs. Res. 32(4):213-217, 1983.

Robertson, J.: Some responses of young children to the loss of maternal care, Nurs. Times 49:382-386, 1953.

Rollins, J.: Recall of baby pillows likely, Pediatr. Nurs. 16(3):282, 1990.

Rosen, R.: Stocking constriction injuries, J. Pediatr. 103(6):937, 1983.

Rubella vaccination during pregnancy—United States, 1971-1988, MMWR 38(17):289-293, 1989.

Rutter, M.: Stress, coping and development: some issues and some questions, J. Child Psychol. Psychiatry 22(4):323-356, 1981.

Salomon, M., and others: Evaluation of the two-needle strategy for reducing reactions to DPT vaccination, Am. J. Dis. Child. 141(7):796-798, 1987.

Schachter, F., and others: Cosleeping and sleep problems in Hispanic-American urban young children, Pediatrics 84(3):522-530, 1989.

Shea, V., and Fowler, M.G.: Parental and pediatric trainee knowledge of development, Dev. Behav. Pediatr. 4(1):21-25, 1983.

Sherwen, L.N.: Separation: the forgotten phenomenon of child development, Top. Clin. Nurs. 5(1):1-11, 1983.

Slasor, R.: Word of caution, Point of View 26(1):23, 1989.

Smelt, G., and Cawdry, H.: Burns from fluid heated in a microwave oven, Br. Med. J. 298:1452, 1989.

Spitz, R.A.: Hospitalism: an inquiry into the genesis of psychiatric conditioning in early childhood. In Fenechel, D., and others, editors: Psychoanalytic studies of the child, vol. 1, New York, 1945, International University Press.

Stoffman, J.M., and others: Injuries to children from vehicles with wheels: baby walkers . . . , Can. Med. Assoc. J. 131:573-575, 1984.

Taubman, B.: Clinical trial of the treatment of colic by modification of parent-infant interaction, Pediatrics 74:998-1003, 1984.

Thomas, A., and Chess, S.: Genesis and evolution of behavioral disorders: from infancy to early adult life, Am. J. Psychiatry 141(1):1-9, 1984.

Tsolia, M., and others: Live attenuated varicella vaccine: evidence that the virus is attenuated and the importance of skin lesions in transmission of varicella-zoster virus, J. Pediatr. 116:184-189, 1990.

Tunnessen, W., and Oski, F.: Consequences of starting whole cow milk at 6 months of age, part 1, J. Pediatr. 111(6):813-816, 1987.

Vasta, R., editor: Strategies and techniques of child study, New York, 1982, Academic Press, Inc.

Ventura, J.N.: Parent coping behaviors, parent functioning, and infant temperament characteristics, Nurs. Res. 31(5):269-273, 1982.

Wagner, T.J., and Hindi-Alexander, M.: Hazards of baby powder? Pediatr. Nurs. 10(2):124-125, 1984.

Weissbluth, M.: Sleep duration and infant temperament, J. Pediatr. 99(5):817-819, 1981.

Wilkinson, W., and Clore, E.: Infant botulism: a dilemma for nursing, J. Pediatr. Nurs. 3(3):164-168, 1988.

Wilson, A.L., Witzke, D.B., and Volin, A.: What it means to "spoil" a baby: parents' perception, Clin. Pediatr. 20(12):798-802, 1981.

Wood, B., and others: Chlorine inhalation toxicity from vapors generated by swimming pool chlorinator tablets, Pediatrics 79(3):427-430, 1987.

Ziegler, E., and others: Cow milk feeding in infancy: further observations on blood loss from the gastrointestinal tract, J. Pediatr. 116(1):11-18, 1990.

BIBLIOGRAPHY

Growth and Development

Baumann, S.: Physical aspects of the self: a review of some aspects of body image development in childhood, Psychiatr. Clin. North Am. 4(3):455-470, 1981.

Belfer, M., and Lukens, P.: Body image: impacts and distortions. In Levine, M., and others, editors: Developmental-behavioral pediatrics, Philadelphia, 1983, W.B. Saunders Co.

Erikson, E.: Childhood and society, ed. 2, New York, 1963, W.W. Norton & Co., Inc.

Knobloch, H., and Pasamanick, B.: Gesell and Amatruda's developmental diagnosis, New York, 1974, Harper & Row, Publishers, Inc.

Lombardino, L., and others: Evaluating communicative behaviors in infancy, J. Pediatr. Health Care 1(5):240-246, 1987.

Lowrey, G.H.: Growth and development of children, ed. 8, St. Louis, 1986, Mosby–Year Book, Inc.

Maier, H.: Three theories of child development, ed. 3, New York, 1988, Harper & Row, Publishers, Inc.

Marino, B.: Assessments of infant play: applications to research and practice, Issues Compr. Pediatr. Nurs. 11(4):227-240, 1988.

Papalia, D., and Olds, S.: A child's world, infancy through adolescence, ed. 4, New York, 1987, McGraw-Hill Book Co.

Piaget, J.: The construction of reality in the child, New York, 1975, Ballantine Books, Inc.

Seligman, S.: Emotional and social development in infancy and early childhood, Early Child. Update 5(4):1-2, 1989.

Whitehouse, H.: How infants achieve self-organization and self-confidence: implications for health care professionals and parents, part 1, Matern. Child Nurs. Curr. 34(5):17-22, 1987.

Whitehouse, H.: How infants achieve self-organization and self-confidence: implications for health care professionals and parents, part 2, Matern. Child Nurs. Curr. 35(1):1-6, 1988.
Zigler, E., and Lang, M.E.: The emergence of "superbaby": a good thing? Pediatr. Nurs. 11(5):337-342, 1985.

Attachment/Temperament

Als, H.: Assessing infant individuality. In Brown, C.C., editor: Infants at risk, Skillman, N.J., 1981, Johnson & Johnson Baby Products Co.
Barret, R., and Robinson, B.: Adolescent fathers: often forgotten parents, Pediatr. Nurs. 12(4):273-277, 1986.
Belsky, J., and Rovine, M.: Nonmaternal care in the first year of life and the security of infant-parent attachment, Child Dev. 59:157-167, 1988.
Blank, D.M.: Development of the infant tenderness scale, Nurs. Res. 34(4):211-216, 1985.
Brewer, J.M.H.: The revised infant temperament scale. In Humenick, S.S., editor: Analysis of current assessment strategies in the health care of young children and childbearing families, Norwalk, CT, 1982, Appleton-Century-Crofts.
Carey, W.B.: Measuring infant temperament, J. Pediatr. 96(3):423-425, 1980.
Carey, W.B., and McDevitt, S.C.: Stability and change in individual temperament diagnoses from infancy to early childhood, Am. Acad. Child Psychiatry 17:331-337, Spring 1978.
Chamberlin, R.: Behavioral problems and their prevention, Pediatr. Rev. 2(1):13-18, 1980.
Harris, C.H.: Assessment of children's behavior. In Johnson, S.M., editor: Nursing assessment and strategies for the family at risk, New York, 1986, J.B. Lippincott Co.
Harris, E., Weston, D., and Lieberman, A.: Quality of mother-infant attachment and pediatric health care use, Pediatrics 84(2):248-254, 1989.
Klaus, M., and Kennell, J.: Parent-infant bonding, ed. 2, St. Louis, 1982, Mosby–Year Book, Inc.
Koniak-Griffin, D., and Ludington-Hoe, S.: Developmental and temperament outcomes of sensory stimulation in healthy infants, Nurs. Res. 37(2):70-76, 1988.
Koniak-Griffin, D., and Rummell, M.: Temperament in infancy: stability, change, and correlates, Matern. Child Nurs. J. 17(1):25-40, 1988.
Lamb, J.: The rapproachement subphase of the separation-individuation process, Matern. Child Nurs. J. 15(3):129-138, 1986.
Skerrett, K., Hardin, S.B., and Puskar, K.R.: Infant anxiety, Matern. Child Nurs. J. 12(1):51-59, 1983.
Thomas, A., and Chess, S.: Temperament and development, New York, 1977, Brunner/Mazel, Inc.
Wasserman, R., and others: Infant temperament and school age behavior: 6-year longitudinal study in the pediatric practice, Pediatrics 85(5):801-807, 1990.
Zahr, L.: Lebanese mother and infant temperaments as determinants of mother-infant interaction, J. Pediatr. Nurs. 2(6):418-427, 1987.

Concerns Related to Growth and Development

For bibliography on daycare, see Chapter 15.
Castiglia, P.: Thumb sucking, J. Pediatr. Health Care 2(6):322-323, 1988.
Clutter, L.: Helping parents prepare for travel and vacations with children, Pediatr. Nurs. 14(3):211-215, 1988.
Friman, P.: Thumb-sucking in childhood, Feelings Med. Signif. 29(3):11-14, 1987.
McDonald, R.E., and Avery, D.R.: Dentistry for the child and adolescent, ed. 4, St. Louis, 1987, Mosby–Year Book, Inc.

Nutrition

American Academy of Pediatrics, Committee on Nutrition: Pediatric nutrition handbook, ed. 2, Elk Grove Village, IL, 1985, The Academy.
Barness, L.A.: Infant feeding: formula, solids, Pediatr. Clin. North Am. 32(2):355-362, 1985.
Beaton, G.H.: Nutritional needs during the first year of life: some concepts and perspectives, Pediatr. Clin. North Am. 32(2):275-288, 1985.
Bishop, W.S.: Weaning the breast-fed toddler or preschooler, Pediatr. Nurs. 11(3):211-214, 1985.
Blank, D.: Relating mothers' anxiety and perception to infant satiety, anxiety, and feeding behavior, Nurs. Res. 35(6):347-351, 1986.
Current issues in feeding the normal infant, Pediatrics 75(suppl. 1):135-181, 1985.
Dusdieker, L.B., and others: Effect of supplemental fluids on human milk production, J. Pediatr. 106(2):207-211, 1985.
Filer, L., editor: Assessment of bone mineralization in infants, J. Pediatr. 113(suppl. 1, pt. 2), 1988.
Fomon, S.: Bioavailability of supplemental iron in commercially prepared dry infant cereals, J. Pediatr. 110(4):660-661, 1987.
Hillman, L., and others: Vitamin D metabolism, mineral homeostasis, and bone mineralization in term infants fed human milk, cow milk-based formula, or soy-based formula, J. Pediatr. 112(5):864-874, 1988.
Katcher, A.L., and Lanese, M.G.: Breast-feeding by employed mothers: a reasonable accommodation in the work place, Pediatrics 75(4):644-647, 1985.
Martinez, G.A., and Ryan, A.S.: Nutrient intake in the United States during the first 12 months of life, J. Am. Diet. Assoc. 85(7):826-830, 1985.
Martinez, G.A., Ryan, A.S., and Malec, D.J.: Nutrient intakes of American infants and children fed cow's milk or infant formula, Am. J. Dis. Child. 139:1010-1018, 1985.
Nelson, S., and others: Lack of adverse reactions to iron-fortified formula, Pediatrics 81(3):360-364, 1988.
Nemethy, M., and Clore, E.: Microwave heating of infant formula and breast milk, J. Pediatr. Health Care 4(3):131-135, 1990.
Picciano, F.: Nutrient needs of infants, Nutr. Today 22(1):8-13, 1987.
Rogers, C., Morris, S., and Taper, L.: Weaning from the breast: influences on maternal decisions, Pediatr. Nurs. 13(5):341-345, 1987.
Ross, L.: Weaning practices, J. Nurse Midwife 26(1):9-14, 1981.
Ryan, A., Martinez, G., and Krieger, F.: Feeding low-fat milk during infancy, Am. J. Phys. Anthropol. 73:539-548, 1987.
Satter, E.: Developmental guidelines for feeding infants and young children, Food Nutr. News 56(4):21-26, 1984.
Schmitt, B.D.: When weaning is delayed, Contemp. Pediatr. 7(6):67-68, 1990.
Stuff, J., and Nichols, B.: Nutrient intake and growth performance of older infants fed human milk, J. Pediatr. 115(6):959-968, 1989.
Tsang, R., and Nichols, B., editors: Nutrition during infancy, St. Louis, 1988, Mosby–Year Book, Inc.
Tseng, E., Potter, S., and Picciano, M.: Dietary protein source and plasma lipid profiles of infants, Pediatrics 85(4):548-552, 1990.
Turick-Gibson, T.: Infant botulism, Pediatr. Nurs. 14(4):280-283, 1988.
Williams, K., and Morse, J.: Weaning patterns of first-time mothers, MCN 14(3):188-192, 1989.

Sleep and Activity

Adams, L., and Rickert, V.: Reducing bedtime tantrums: comparison between positive routines and graduated extinction, Pediatrics 84(5):756-761, 1989.
Edgil, A.E., Wood, K.R., and Smith, D.P.: Sleep problems of older infants and preschool children, Pediatr. Nurs. 11(2):87-89, 1985.
Ferber, R.: Assessment procedures for diagnosis of sleep disorders in children. In Noshpitz, J., editor: Sleep disorders for the clinician, London, 1987, Butterworths.
Ferber, R.: Behavioral insomnia in the child, Psychiatr. Clin. North Am. 10(4):641-653, 1987.
Ferber, R.: Sleep disorders in children, Pediatr. Consultant 7(2):1-12, 1988.

Ferber, R.: Sleeplessness, night awakening, and night crying in the infant and toddler, Pediatr. Rev. 9(3):1-14, 1987.

Guilleminault, C., editor: Sleep and its disorders in children, New York, 1987, Raven Press.

Keener, M. and others: Infant temperament, sleep organization, and nighttime parental interventions, Pediatrics 81(6):762-771, 1988.

Lozoff, B., Wolf, A.W., and Davis, N.S.: Sleep problems seen in pediatric practice, Pediatrics 75(3):477-483, 1985.

Osterholm, P., Lindeke, L.L., and Amidon, D.: Sleep disturbance in infants aged 6 to 12 months, Pediatr. Nurs. 9(4):269-271, 1983.

Rickert, V., and Johnson, C.: Reducing nocturnal awakening and crying episodes in infants and young children: a comparison between scheduled awakenings and systematic ignoring, Pediatrics 81(2):203-212, 1988.

Schmitt, B.: The prevention of sleep problems and colic, Pediatr. Clin. North Am. 33(4):763-774, 1986.

Schmitt, B.: When your child refuses to go to bed, Contemp. Pediatr. 6(7):70-71, 1989.

Weissbluth, M., Davis, A.T., and Poncher, J.: Night waking in 4- to 8-month-old infants, J. Pediatr. 104(3):477-480, 1984.

Dental Health

For bibliography, see Chapter 14.

Immunizations

Ada, G.: The immunological principles of vaccination, Lancet 335(8687):523-526, 1990.

Baraff, L., and others: Infants and children with convulsions and hypotonic-hyporesponsive episodes following diphtheria-tetanus-pertussis immunization: follow-up evaluation, Pediatrics 81(6):789-794, 1988.

Bellanti, J.A., editor: Pediatrics vaccination: update 1990, Pediatr. Clin. North Am. 37(3):513-784, 1990.

Berkowitz, C., and others: Persistence of antibody and booster responses to reimmunization with *Haemophilus influenzae* type b polysaccharide and polysaccharide diphtheria toxoid conjugate vaccines in children initially immunized at 15 to 24 months of age, Pediatrics 85(3):288-293, 1990.

Bernbaum, J., and others: Half-dose immunization for diphtheria, tetanus, pertussis: response of preterm infants, Pediatrics 83(4):471-476, 1989.

Blennow, M., and Granstrom, M.: Adverse reactions and serologic response to a booster dose of acellular pertussis vaccine in children immunized with acellular or whole-cell vaccine as infants, Pediatrics 84(1):62-67, 1989.

Brunell, P., and others: Combined vaccine against measles, mumps, rubella, and varicella, Pediatrics 81(6):779-784, 1988.

Campion, J., and Casto, D.: *Haemophilus influenzae* type b–conjugate vaccine, J. Pediatr. Health Care 2(4):215-218, 1988.

Current status of *Haemophilus influenzae* type b vaccines, Pediatrics 85(suppl. 4, pt. 2):631-704, 1990.

Daum, R., and others: Decline in serum antibody to the capsule of *Haemophilus influenzae* type b in the immediate postimmunization period, J. Pediatr. 114(5):742-747, 1989.

Engel, N.: The National Vaccine Injury Compensation Program, MCN 15:109, 1990.

Griffin, M., and others: Risk of seizures and encephalopathy after immunization with the diphtheria-tetanus-pertussis vaccine, JAMA 263(12):1641-1645, 1990.

Grimes, D., and Woolbert, L.: Measles outbreaks: who are at risk and why, J. Pediatr. Health Care 3(4):187-193, 1989.

Gross, T., Milstein, J., and Kuritsky, J.: Bulging fontanelle after immunization with diphtheria-tetanus-pertussis vaccine and diphtheria-tetanus vaccine, J. Pediatr. 114(3):423-425, 1989.

Hayden, G., and others: Progress in worldwide control and elimination of disease through immunization, J. Pediatr. 114(4):520-527, 1989.

Hinman, A., and others: Live or inactivated poliomyelitis vaccine: an analysis of benefits and risks, Am. J. Public Health 78(3):291-295, 1988.

Hutchins, S., and others: Measles outbreak among unvaccinated preschool-aged children: opportunities missed by health care providers to administer measles vaccine, Pediatrics 83(3):369-374, 1989.

Johnson, C., and others: Humoral immunity and clinical reinfections following varicella vaccine in healthy children, Pediatrics 84(3):418-421, 1989.

Johnson, C., and others: Live attenuated varicella vaccine in healthy 12- to 24-month-old children, Pediatrics 81(4):512-518, 1988.

Katz, S.: Poliovirus vaccine policy, Am. J. Dis. Child. 143(9):1007-1009, 1989.

Kemp, A., Van Asperen, P., and Mukhi, A.: Measles immunization in children with clinical reactions to egg protein, Am. J. Dis. Child. 144(1):33-35, 1990.

Klein, N., Morgan, K., and Wansbrough-Jones, M.: Parents' beliefs about vaccination: The continuing propagation of false contraindications, Br. Med. J. 298:1687, 1989.

Krantz, I., and others: Immunogenicity and safety of a pertussis vaccine composed of pertussis toxin inactivated by hydrogen peroxide, in 18- and 23-month-old children, J. Pediatr. 116(4):539-543, 1990.

Krasinski, K., and Borkowsky, W.: Measles and measles immunity in children infected with human immunodeficiency virus, JAMA 261(17):2512-2516, 1989.

Lavi, S., and others: Administration of measles, mumps, and rubella virus vaccine (live) to egg-allergic children, JAMA 263(2):269-271, 1990.

Lepow, M.: Recent advances in *Haemophilus influenzae* b and pertussis immunization, Curr. Opin. Pediatr. 1(1):74-78, 1989.

Livengood, J., and others: Family history of convulsions and use of pertussis vaccine, J. Pediatr. 115:527-531, 1989.

Madore, D., and others: Safety and immunologic response to *Haemophilus influenzae* type b oligosaccharide-CRM conjugate vaccine in 1- to 6-month-old infants, Pediatrics 85(3):331-337, 1990.

Marcuse, E.: Why wait for DTP-E-IPV? Am. J. Dis. Child. 143(9):1006-1007, 1989.

Markowitz, L., and others: Patterns of transmission in measles outbreaks in the United States, 1985-1986, N. Engl. J. Med. 320(2):75-81, 1989.

Marshall, G., and Barbour, S.: Meaningful immunization for the immune-deficient child, Contemp. Pediatr. 6(9):109-124, 1989.

Moxon, E.R.: The scope of immunisation, Lancet 335(8687):448-451, 1990.

Nelson, W., and Granoff, D.: Protective efficacy of *Haemophilus influenzae* type b polysaccharide-diphtheria toxoid-conjugate vaccine, Am. J. Dis. Child. 144:292-295, 1990.

Recommendations of the Immunization Practices Advisory Committee: Pneumococcal polysaccharide vaccine, MMWR 38(5):64-76, 1989.

Recommendations of the Immunization Practices Advisory Committee (ACIP): Protection against viral hepatitis, MMWR 39(S-2):1-26, 1990.

Recommendations of the Immunization Practices Advisory Committee (ACIP): Prevention and control of influenza. 1. Vaccines, MMWR 38(17):297-309, 1989.

Rubella and congenital rubella syndrome—United States, 1985-1988, MMWR 38(11):173-182, 1989.

Salerno, C., and Jackson, M.: What does the National Childhood Vaccine Injury Act require of nurses? Am. J. Nurs. 88(7):1019-1020, 1988.

Salk, D.: Polio immunization policy in the United States: a new challenge for a new generation, Am. J. Public Health 78(3):296-300, 1988.

Starr, S.: Status of varicella vaccine for healthy children, Pediatrics 84(6):1097-1099, 1989.

Stiehm, E.R.: Skin testing prior to measles vaccination for egg-sensitive patients, Am. J. Dis. Child. 144(1):32, 1990.

Injury Prevention

Bass, J.L., and others: Educating parents about injury prevention, Pediatr. Clin. North Am. 32(1):233-243, 1985.

Bausell, R.B.: A national survey assessing pediatric preventive behaviors, Pediatr. Nurs. 11:438-442, 1985.

Bee, D., and others: Delayed death from ingestion of a toothpick, N. Engl. J. Med. 320(10):673, 1989.

Berger, L.R., and others: Promoting the use of car safety devices for infants: an intensive health education approach, Pediatrics 74(1):16-19, 1984.

Berger, L.R., and Kalishman, S.: Floor furnance burns to children, Pediatrics 71(1):97-99, 1983.

Cotton, W.H., and Davidson, P.J.: Aspiration of baby powder, N. Engl. J. Med. 313:1662, 1985.

Dershewitz, R.A., and Christophersen, E.R.: Childhood household safety, Am. J. Dis. Child. 138:85-88, 1984.

DeSwarte, J.: Nursing's responsibility in promoting the use of car safety seats for children, Home Health Care 2(1):23-25, 1984.

Gallagher, S.S., Hunter, P., and Guyer, B.: A home injury prevention program for children, Pediatr. Clin. North Am. 32(1):95-112, 1985.

Greensher, J., and Mofenson, H.C.: Injuries at play, Pediatr. Clin. North Am. 32(1):127-139, 1985.

Johnson, G.: Aspiration of makeshift pacifier, Pediatrics 79(1):170, 1987.

Katcher, M., Landry, G., and Shapiro, M.: Liquid-crystal thermometer use in pediatric office counseling about tap water burn prevention, Pediatrics 83(5):766-771, 1989.

Lipe, H.P.: Prevention of nervous system trauma from travel in motor vehicles, J. Neurosurg. Nurs. 17(2):77-82, 1985.

Miller, R.E., and others: Pediatric counseling and subsequent use of smoke detectors, Am. J. Public Health 72:392-393, 1982.

Moss, J., and Tobin, S.: The relationship of parental perceptions and experiences to car seat use in rural children, J. Pediatr. Nurs. 3(2):103-109, 1988.

Nachem, B., and Bass, R.A.: Children still aren't being buckled up, MCN 9(5):320-323, 1984.

Nyman, G.: Infant temperament, childhood accidents, and hospitalization, Clin. Pediatr. 26(8):398-404, 1987.

Puczynski, M., Rademaker, D., and Gatson, R.L.: Burn injury related to the improper use of a microwave oven, Pediatrics 72:714-715, 1983.

Rivera, F., Kamitsuka, M., and Quan, L.: Injuries to children younger than 1 year of age, Pediatrics 81(1):93-97, 1988.

Rumack, B.H.: Diapers and poisons, JAMA 248:2164, 1982.

Temple, D.M., and McNeese, M.C.: Hazards of battery ingestion, Pediatrics 71(1):100-103, 1983.

Tron, V.A., Baldwin, V.J., and Pirie, G.E.: Hot tub drownings, Pediatrics 74(4):789-790, 1985.

Wagner, T.J., and Hindi-Alexander, M.: Hazards of baby powder? Pediatr. Nurs. 10(2):124-125, 1984.

Yanofsky, N.N., and Morain, W.D.: Upper extremity burns from woodstoves, Pediatrics 73(5):722-726, 1984.

CHAPTER 13

Health Problems During Infancy

RELATED TOPICS

Anaphylaxis, Ch. 29
Apnea of prematurity, Ch. 10
Bronchial asthma, Ch. 32
Candidiasis, Ch. 9
Cardiopulmonary resuscitation, Ch. 31
The child with cognitive impairment, Ch. 24
Disorders affecting the skin, Ch. 18
Feeding resistance, Ch. 10
Gastroesophageal reflux, Ch. 33
Impact of chronic illness or disability on the child and family, Ch. 22
Impact of life-threatening illness on the child and family, Ch. 23
Nutritional assessment, Ch. 6
Obesity, Ch. 21

GLOSSARY

AD Atopic dermatitis
AGM Absorbent-gelling material
allergens or **allergic antigens** Usually proteins that are capable of inducing IgE antibody formation ("sensitization") when ingested, injected, or inhaled
ALTE Apparent life-threatening event
AOI Apnea of infancy
apnea (pathologic) Respiratory pause of more than 20 seconds or shorter pause associated with cyanosis, marked pallor, hypotonia, or bradycardia
atopy Allergy with tendency to be inherited
CPR Cardiopulmonary resuscitation
deficiency Inadequate intake of a nutrient that causes adverse clinical effects
fat-soluble vitamins Refer to A, D, E, and K
food allergy or **hypersensitivity** Refers to adverse reactions involving immunologic mechanisms, usually IgE
food intolerance Refers to adverse reactions involving known or unknown nonimmunologic mechanisms
food sensitivity Refers to any type of adverse reaction to food or food additives
FTT Failure to thrive
hypervitaminosis Excessive intake of a vitamin that causes adverse clinical effects
IgE Immunoglobulin E
kwashiorkor Protein deficiency with low or adequate energy sources
macrominerals Minerals whose daily requirement are greater than 100 mg
marasmus State of semistarvation from inadequate protein and energy
microminerals (trace elements) Minerals whose daily requirements are less than 100 mg
NCAFS Nursing Child Assessment Feeding Scale
NFTT Nonorganic failure to thrive
OFTT Organic failure to thrive
PEM Protein-energy malnutrition
RDA Recommended dietary allowance

sensitization Initial exposure of an individual to allergen, resulting in an immune response; subsequent exposure induces a much stronger response
SIDS Sudden infant death syndrome
U.S. RDA United States Recommended Daily Allowance
vegan General term referring to individuals who exclude all animal products from the diet
vegetarian General term referring to individuals who exclude meat from the diet but may include dairy and poultry products and fish
water-soluble vitamins Refer to B complex and C

The infant's immature physiologic system predisposes to several potential health problems during the first year. This chapter deals primarily with health problems that are influenced by environmental factors affecting the physical or psychologic development of the child. Some of the problems, such as nutritional disturbances, have special implications for nurses because they are preventable. Others, such as sudden infant death syndrome (SIDS), are uncontrollable and unpredictable, but the intervention needed after the death of the child is crucial for the reintegration of the family. Although several of the topics discussed here can occur in age-groups other than infancy, the greatest significance of these disorders is evident during the early months and years of life. Prompt awareness and identification of health problems hopefully will avert complications in later life. Prevention, whenever possible, rather than treatment should be every health professional's goal in the care of children.

NUTRITIONAL DISTURBANCES

Malnutrition is a general term that refers to poor or inadequate nutrition. Although it is generally thought of in terms of undernutrition, it also includes overnutrition, which may be manifested as obesity or hypervitaminosis. Inadequate nutrition is most commonly seen as iron deficiency anemia (see Chapter 35), vitamin deficiencies, or failure to thrive. The most severe states of malnutrition, involving protein and energy deficiencies, are kwashiorkor and marasmus. Each of these is related to a wide variety of factors—economic, social, and cultural. While poverty is the economic precursor of malnutrition, it is usually when certain cultural and social factors coincide with poverty that malnutrition becomes a threat. Culture influences food selection and may limit certain nutritious foods because of preference, not availability. Social factors include a detached parenting style, often seen in nonorganic failure to thrive, and an inability of the family to independently take advantage of food assistance programs (Karp, Scholl, and Greene, 1985).

Since all of these nutritional disturbances are amenable to some degree of alteration through intervention, the nutritional disturbances to be discussed could potentially be eliminated. However, adequate food supplies alone are not the answer, especially when sociocultural factors that affect food consumption are considered. Therefore nutritional counseling becomes a complex process that must take into account all the variables affecting the physical and psychologic makeup of the family.

VITAMIN DISTURBANCES

Vitamins are an essential food element and function in small quantities by regulating specific metabolic activity, usually by acting as *coenzymes*. When vitamin coenzymes enter the body, they are combined with a protein *apoenzyme* that has been synthesized within the cell to form a *holoenzyme*. The quantity of apoenzymes any cell can produce limits the body's ability to make use of excessive vitamins (Jarvis, 1984). A deficiency of the vitamin directly affects the metabolic activity it regulates. However, regular ingestion of excessive amounts of vitamins may produce a toxic effect.

True vitamin disturbances are rare in the United States, but subclinical deficiencies are commonly seen, especially in lower socioeconomic groups where proper dietary intake may be unbalanced. In a study of children ages 7 to 18 years, approximately a third of the children and two thirds of adolescent girls consumed less than the recommended amount of vitamin B_6 (Study of calcium intake, 1984). Vitamin D–deficient rickets, once rarely seen because of vitamin D–fortified milk, has increased. Populations at risk include (1) children born of mothers who are vitamin D deficient, (2) individuals who are exposed to minimal sunlight because of distinctive clothing, housing in areas of high pollution, or dark skin pigmentation, (3) adherence to vegetarian diets that are low in sources of vitamin D, and (4) use of milk products, such as yogurt or raw cow's milk, that are not supplemented with vitamin D as the primary source of milk (Saal, Ratzan, and Carey, 1985). Children may also be at risk secondary to disorders or their treatment. For example, vitamin deficiencies of the fat-soluble vitamins A and D may occur in malabsorptive disorders. Children on high doses of salicylates, such as for rheumatoid arthritis, may have impaired vitamin C storage (Olness, 1985).

Of equal, if not greater concern, is the overuse of vitamins. An excessive dose of a vitamin is generally defined as 10 or more times the recommended dietary allowance (RDA), although the fat-soluble vitamins, especially A and D, tend to cause toxic reactions at lower doses (Council on Scientific Affairs, 1987). With the addition of vitamins to commercially prepared foods, the potential for hypervitaminosis has increased, especially when combined with the injudicious use of vitamin supplements. Hypervitaminosis of

A and D presents the greatest problems, because these fat-soluble vitamins are stored in the body. Vitamin D is the most likely of all vitamins to cause toxic reactions in relatively small overdoses. However, there appears to be variance in the tolerance to different vitamin intakes. For example, two children ingesting excessive amounts of vitamin A may not both demonstrate clinical features of intoxication (Carpenter and others, 1987).

It is now well documented that the water-soluble vitamins, primarily niacin, B_6, and C, can also cause toxicity by

Table 13-1 Vitamins and their nutritional significance

PHYSIOLOGIC FUNCTIONS/SOURCES	RESULTS OF DEFICIENCY OR EXCESS	NURSING CONSIDERATIONS
▪ Vitamin A (retinol)*		
Functions	***Deficiency***	
Necessary component in formation of pigment rhodopsin (visual purple) Formation and maintenance of epithelial tissue Normal bone growth and tooth development Needed for growth and spermatogenesis Involved in thyroxine formation	Night blindness Keratinization (hardening and scaling) of epithelium Xerophthalmia (hardening and scaling of cornea and conjunctiva) Phrynoderma (toad skin) Drying of respiratory, gastrointestinal, and genitourinary tracts Defective tooth enamel Retarded growth Impaired bone formation Decreased thyroxine formation	Encourage foods rich in vitamin A, such as whole cow's milk As milk consumption decreases, encourage foods rich in vitamin A
Sources	***Excess***	
Natural form—liver, kidney, fish oils, milk and nonskimmed milk products, egg yolk Provitamin A (carotene)—carrots, sweet potatoes, squash, apricots, spinach, collards, broccoli, cabbage, artichokes	Early signs—irritability, anorexia, pruritus, fissures at corners of nose and lips Later signs—hepatomegaly, jaundice, retarded growth, poor weight gain, thickening of the cortex of long bones with pain and fragility, hard tender lumps in extremities and occiput of the skull May cause birth defects from excessive maternal intake	Emphasize correct use of vitamin supplements and potential hazards of excess Investigate child's dietary habits to calculate approximate intake; if excessive, remove supplemental source (e.g., daily feeding of liver)
	NOTE: Overdose only results from ingestion of large quantities of the vitamin, not the provitamin; large amounts of carotene (carotenemia) cause yellow or orange discoloration of the skin (not the sclera, urine, or feces as in jaundice), but none of the above symptoms	Advise parents of the benign nature of carotenemia; treatment is avoidance of excess pigmented fruits or vegetables, especially carrots; skin color returns to normal in 2 to 6 weeks
▪ Vitamin B_1 (thiamin)†		
Functions	***Deficiency***	*Vitamin B complex*
Coenzyme (with phosphorus) in carbohydrate metabolism Needed for healthy nervous system	Gastrointestinal—anorexia, constipation, indigestion Neurologic—apathy, fatigue, emotional instability, polyneuritis, tenderness of calf muscles, partial anesthesia, muscle weakness, paresthesia, hyperesthesia, decreased or absent tendon reflexes, convulsions, and coma (in infants) Cardiovascular—palpitations, cardiac failure, peripheral vasodilation, edema	Encourage foods rich in B vitamins Stress proper cooking and storage techniques to preserve potency, such as minimum cooking of vegetables in small amount of liquid; storage of milk in opaque container Advise against fad diets that severely restrict groups of food, such as vegetarianism (vegans or macrobiotics) Explore need for vitamin supplements when dieting or when using goat milk exclusively for infant feeding (deficient in folic acid) or when the breast-feeding mother is a strict vegetarian (vitamin B_{12}) Emphasize correct use of vitamin supplements and potential hazards of excesses
Sources	***Excess***	
Pork, beef, liver, legumes, nuts, whole or enriched grains and cereals, green vegetables, fruits, milk, brown rice	Headache Irritability Insomnia Rapid pulse Weakness	

*Fat soluble.
†Water soluble.

Table 13-1 Vitamins and their nutritional significance—cont'd

PHYSIOLOGIC FUNCTIONS/SOURCES	RESULTS OF DEFICIENCY OR EXCESS	NURSING CONSIDERATIONS
▪ Vitamin B_2 (riboflavin)†		
Functions Coenzyme (with phosphorus) in carbohydrate, protein, and fat metabolism Maintains healthy skin especially around mouth, nose, and eye ***Sources*** Milk and its products, eggs, organ meat (liver, kidney, and heart), enriched cereals, some green leafy vegetables,‡ legumes	***Deficiency*** **Ariboflavinosis** Lips—cheilosis (fissures at corners of lips), perlèche (inflammation at corners of lips) Tongue—glossitis Nose—irritation and cracks at nasal angle Eyes—burning, itching, tearing, photophobia, corneal vascularization, cataracts Skin—seborrheic dermatitis, delayed wound healing and tissue repair ***Excess*** Paresthesia, pruritus	Same as vitamin B complex
▪ Niacin (nicotinic acid, nicotinamide)†		
Functions Coenzyme (with riboflavin) in protein and fat metabolism Needed for healthy nervous system, skin, and normal digestion May lower cholesterol ***Sources*** Meat, poultry, fish, peanuts, beans, peas, whole or enriched grains except corn and rice Milk and its products are sources of tryptophan (60 mg of tryptophan = 1 mg of niacin)	***Deficiency*** **Pellagra** Oral—stomatitis, glossitis Cutaneous—scaly dermatitis on exposed areas Gastrointestinal—anorexia, weight loss, diarrhea, fatigue Neurologic—apathy, anxiety, confusion, depression, dementia Death ***Excess*** Release of vasodilator, histamine (flushing, decreased blood pressure, increased cerebral blood flow; aggravates asthma) Dermatologic problems (pruritus, rash, hyperkeratosis, acanthosis nigricans) Increased gastric acidity (aggravates peptic ulcer disease) Hepatotoxicity Increased serum uric acid levels Elevated plasma glucose levels Certain cardiac arrhythmias	Same as vitamin B complex If used as hypolipidemic agent, stress safe dosage to prevent child's accidental ingestion
▪ Vitamin B_6 (pyridoxine)†		
Functions Coenzyme in protein and fat metabolism Needed for formation of antibodies, hemoglobin Needed for utilization of copper and iron Aids in conversion of tryptophan to niacin ***Sources*** Meats, especially liver and kidney, cereal grains (wheat and corn), yeast, soybeans, peanuts, tuna, chicken, salmon	***Deficiency*** Scaly dermatitis, weight loss, anemia, retarded growth, irritability, convulsions, peripheral neuritis ***Excess*** Peripheral nervous system toxicity (unsteady gait, numb feet and hands, clumsiness of hands, sometimes perioral numbness) May cause peptic ulcer disease or seizures	Same as vitamin B complex Stress proper cooking and storing techniques to preserve potency Cook food covered in small amount of water Do not soak food in water Store in light-resistant container

*Fat soluble.
†Water soluble.
‡Green leafy vegetables include spinach, broccoli, kale, turnip greens, mustard greens, collards, dandelion greens, and beet greens.

Continued.

Table 13-1 Vitamins and their nutritional significance—cont'd

PHYSIOLOGIC FUNCTIONS/SOURCES	RESULTS OF DEFICIENCY OR EXCESS	NURSING CONSIDERATIONS
▪ Folic acid (folacin; reduced form is called folinic acid or citrovorum factor)†		
Functions Coenzyme for single-carbon transfer (purines, thymine, hemoglobin) Necessary for formation of red blood cells ***Sources*** Green leafy vegetables, cabbage, asparagus, liver, kidney, nuts, eggs, whole grain cereals, legumes, bananas	***Deficiency*** Macrocytic anemia, bone marrow depression, glossitis, intestinal malabsorption ***Excess*** Rare because megadoses not available over the counter May cause insomnia and irritability	Same as vitamin B complex Stress proper cooking and storing techniques to preserve potency Cook food covered in small amount of water Do not soak food in water Store in light-resistant container
▪ Vitamin B_{12} (cobalamin)†		
Functions Coenzyme in protein synthesis; indirect effect on formation of red blood cells (particularly on formation of nucleic acids and folic acid metabolism) Needed for normal functioning of nervous tissue ***Sources*** Meat, liver, kidney, fish, shellfish, poultry, milk, eggs, cheese, nutritional yeast, sea vegetables	***Deficiency*** **Pernicious anemia** (one form of deficiency from absence of intrinsic factor in gastric secretions) General signs of severe anemia Lemon yellow tinge to skin Spinal cord degeneration ***Excess*** Excess is rare	Same as vitamin B complex
▪ Biotin		
Functions Coenzyme in carbohydrate, protein, and fat metabolism Interrelated with functions of other B vitamins ***Sources*** Liver, kidney, egg yolk, tomatoes, legumes, nuts	***Deficiency*** Deficiency is uncommon because synthesized by bacterial flora ***Excess*** Unknown	Same as vitamin B complex
▪ Pantothenic acid†		
Functions Coenzyme in carbohydrate, protein, and fat metabolism Synthesis of amino acids, fatty acids, and steroids ***Sources*** Liver, kidney, heart, salmon, eggs, vegetables, legumes, whole grains	***Deficiency*** Deficiency is uncommon because of its multiple food sources and synthesis by bacterial flora ***Excess*** Minimum toxicity (occasional diarrhea and water retention)	Same as vitamin B complex

*Fat soluble.
†Water soluble.

Table 13-1 Vitamins and their nutritional significance—cont'd

PHYSIOLOGIC FUNCTIONS/SOURCES	RESULTS OF DEFICIENCY OR EXCESS	NURSING CONSIDERATIONS
▪ Vitamin C (ascorbic acid)†		
Functions Essential for collagen formation Increases absorption of iron for hemoglobin formation Enhances conversion of folic to folinic acid Affects cholesterol synthesis and conversion of proline to hydroxyproline Probably a coenzyme in metabolism of tyrosine and phenylalanine May play role in hydroxylation of adrenal steroids May have stimulating effect on phagocytic activity of leukocytes and formation of antibodies Antioxidant agent (spares other vitamins from oxidation) ***Sources*** Citrus fruits, strawberries, tomatoes, potatoes, melon, cabbage, broccoli, cauliflower, spinach, papaya, mango	***Deficiency*** **Scurvy** Skin—dry, rough, petechiae, perifollicular hyperkeratotic papules (raised areas around hair follicles) Musculoskeletal—bleeding muscles and joints, pseudoparalysis from pain, swelling of joints, costochondral beading (scorbutic rosary) Gums—spongy, friable, swollen, bleed easily, bluish red or black color, teeth loosen and fall out General disposition—irritable, anorexic, apprehensive, in pain, refuses to move, assumes semi-froglike position when supine (scorbutic pose) Signs of anemia Decreased wound healing Increased susceptibility to infection ***Excess*** Diarrhea Increased excretion of uric acid and acidification of urine (may cause urate precipitation and formation of oxalate stones) Hemolysis Impaired leukocytosis activity Damage to beta cells of pancreas and decreased insulin production Reproductive failure "Rebound scurvy" from withdrawal of large amounts	Encourage foods rich in vitamin C Investigate infant's diet for sources of vitamin, especially when cow's milk is principal source of nutrition Stress proper cooking and storing techniques to preserve potency Wash vegetables quickly; do not soak in water Cook vegetables in covered pot with minimum water and for short time; avoid copper or cast iron cookware Do not add baking soda to cooking water Use fresh fruits and vegetables as soon as possible; store in refrigerator Store juice in airtight opaque container Wrap cut fruit or eat soon after exposing to air In caring for child with scurvy: Position for comfort and rest Handle very gently and minimally Administer analgesics as needed Prevent infection Provide good oral care Provide soft, bland diet Emphasize rapid recovery when vitamin is replaced Emphasize correct use of vitamin supplement and potential hazards of excess Identify groups at risk for vitamin C supplements: those with thalassemia; those on anticoagulant or aminoglycoside antibiotic therapy
▪ Vitamin D_2 (ergocalciferol) and D_3 (cholecalciferol)*		
Functions Absorption of calcium and phosphorus and decreased renal excretion of phosphorus ***Sources*** Direct sunlight Cod liver oil, herring, mackerel, salmon, tuna, sardines Enriched food sources—milk, milk products, too much cereals, margarine, breads, many breakfast drinks	***Deficiency*** **Rickets** Head—craniotabes (softening of cranial bones, prominence of frontal bones), deformed shape (skull flat and depressed toward middle), delayed closure of fontanels Chest—rachitic rosary (enlargement of costochondral junction of ribs), Harrison groove (horizontal depression in lower portion of rib cage), pigeon chest (sharp protrusion of sternum) Spine—kyphosis, scoliosis, lordosis Abdomen—potbelly, constipation	Encourage foods rich in vitamin D, especially fortified cow's milk In breast-fed infants encourage use of vitamin D supplements if maternal diet inadequate or infant exposed to minimal sunlight In caring for child with rickets: Maintain good body alignment Reposition frequently to prevent decubiti and respiratory infection Handle very gently and minimally

*Fat soluble.
†Water soluble.

Continued.

Table 13-1 Vitamins and their nutritional significance—cont'd

PHYSIOLOGIC FUNCTIONS/SOURCES	RESULTS OF DEFICIENCY OR EXCESS	NURSING CONSIDERATIONS
	Extremities—bowing of arms and legs, knock-knee, saber shins, instability of hip joints, pelvic deformity, enlargement of epiphysis at ends of long bones Teeth—delayed calcification, especially of permanent teeth Rachitic tetany—seizures	Prevent infection Institute seizure precautions Have 10% calcium gluconate available in case of tetany Observe for possibility of overdose from supplements If prescribed, supervise proper use of orthopedic splints or braces
	Excess Acute—vomiting, dehydration, fever, abdominal cramps, bone pain, convulsions, and coma Chronic—lassitude, mental slowness, anorexia, failure to thrive, thirst, urinary urgency, polyuria, vomiting, diarrhea, abdominal cramps, bone pain, pathologic fractures Calcification of soft tissue—kidneys, lungs, adrenal glands, vessels (hypertension), heart, gastric lining, tympanic membrane (deafness) Osteoporosis of long bones Elevated serum levels of calcium and phosphorus	Same as vitamin A; may include low-calcium diet during initial therapy
▪ Vitamin E (tocopherol)*		
Functions Production of red blood cells and protection from hemolysis Muscle and liver integrity Coenzyme factor in tissue respiration Minimizes oxidation of polyunsaturated fatty acids and vitamins A and C in intestinal tract and tissues	***Deficiency*** Hemolytic anemia from hemolysis caused by shortened life of red blood cells, especially in premature infants, and focal necrosis of tissues Causes infertility in rats, but not in humans (does *not* increase human male virility or potency)	Initiate early feeding in premature infants; may need supplementation (some evidence that vitamin E may prevent severe intracranial hemorrhage in high-risk neonates)
Sources Vegetable oils, wheat germ oil, milk, egg yolk, muscle meats, fish, whole grains, nuts, legumes, spinach, broccoli	***Excess*** Little is known: less toxic than other fat-soluble vitamins but excess of water-soluble preparations has been fatal in premature infants	
▪ Vitamin K*		
Functions Catalyst for production of prothrombin and blood-clotting factors II, VII, IX, and X by the liver ***Sources*** Pork, liver, green leafy vegetables (spinach, kale, cabbage), tomatoes, egg yolk, cheese	***Deficiency*** Hemorrhage ***Excess*** Hyperbilirubinemia in infants Hemolytic anemia in individuals who are deficient in glucose-6-phosphate dehydrogenase	Administer prophylactically to newborns Other indications include intestinal disease, lack of bile, prolonged antibiotic therapy; may be used in management of blood-clotting time when anticoagulants such as warfarin (Coumadin), and dicumarol (bishydroxycoumarin), which are vitamin K antagonists, are used

*Fat soluble.

the following mechanisms (Alhadeff, Gualtieri, and Lipton, 1984):

1. May have direct toxic effects, especially niacin and B_6
2. May lead to dependency states with development of deficiency symptoms when the vitamin is abruptly discontinued, such as ascorbic acid
3. May mask signs of a disease, such as vitamin C and interference with Clinitest results (common test used to detect glucose or acetone in urine) in diabetes
4. May interact with drugs or other vitamins, such as folic acid's effect on reducing serum phenytoin levels
5. May be combined with high doses of fat-soluble vitamins, such as high-dose multisupplement preparation

Deficiencies and excesses of vitamins A, B complex, C, D, E, and K are summarized in Table 13-1. General nursing considerations are discussed on p. 606, and specific interventions are presented in Table 13-1.

MINERAL DISTURBANCES

A number of minerals are essential nutrients. The *macrominerals* refer to those with daily requirements greater than 100 mg and include calcium, phosphorus, magnesium, sodium, potassium, chloride, and sulfur. *Microminerals* or *trace elements* have daily requirements less than 100 mg and include several essential minerals and those whose exact role in nutrition is still unclear. The greatest concern with minerals is deficiency, especially iron deficiency anemia (see Chapter 35). However, other minerals that may be inadequate in children's diets, even with supplementation, include calcium, phosphorus, magnesium, and zinc (Moss and others, 1989). Low levels of zinc can cause nutritional failure to thrive (Walravens, Hambidge, and Koepfer, 1989).

The regulation of mineral balance in the body is a complex process. Dietary extremes of mineral intake can cause a number of mineral-mineral interactions that could result in unexpected deficiencies or excesses. For example, excessive amounts of one mineral, such as zinc, can result in a deficiency of another mineral, such as copper, even if sufficient amounts of copper are ingested. This is thought to be the result of competition in the process of absorption because of (1) displacement of one mineral by another on the molecule necessary for their uptake from the lumen in the intestinal cell or (2) competition for pathways through the intestinal wall or into the bloodstream. Therefore megadose therapy with one mineral may not cause toxicity from an excess but rather from a deficiency in a competing mineral.

Deficiencies can also occur when various substances in the diet interact with minerals. For example, iron, zinc, and calcium can form insoluble complexes with phytates and/or oxalates (substances found in plant proteins), which affect the bioavailability of the specific mineral. An example of a food interaction is the poor absorbability of calcium from spinach (Heaney, Weaver, and Recker, 1988). Food interactions of this type are particularly significant in vegetarian diets because high-fiber foods are rich in phytates (Brune, Rossander, and Hallberg, 1989).

Deficiencies and excesses of the essential macro- and microminerals are summarized in Table 13-2. General nurs-

Table 13-2 Minerals and their nutritional significance

PHYSIOLOGIC FUNCTIONS/SOURCES	RESULTS OF DEFICIENCY OR EXCESS	NURSING CONSIDERATIONS
▪ Calcium*		
Functions	***Deficiency***	
Bone and tooth development and maintenance (in combination with phosphorus) Muscle contractions, especially the heart Blood clotting Absorption of vitamin B_{12} Enzyme activation Nerve conduction Integrity of intracellular cement substances and various membranes	**Rickets** Tetany Impaired growth, especially of bones and teeth	Encourage foods rich in calcium, especially dairy products Caution that oxalates in leafy vegetables (spinach), oxalates in chocolates, and a high phosphorus intake (especially from carbonated beverages) can decrease calcium absorption Discourage use of whole cow's milk in newborns because the phosphorus-to-calcium ratio favors excretion of calcium Advise against fad diets, especially those that restrict dairy products
Sources	***Excess***	
Dairy products, egg yolk, sardines, canned salmon with bones, dark-green leafy vegetables (except spinach), soybeans, dried beans, and peas	Drowsiness, extreme lethargy Impaired absorption of other minerals (iron, zinc, manganese) Calcium deposits in tissues (renal failure)	Emphasize correct use of calcium supplement, especially the possible interaction between megadoses of calcium and resulting deficiency states of other minerals
▪ Chloride*		
Functions	***Deficiency***	
Acid-base and fluid balance Enzyme activation in saliva Component of hydrochloric acid in stomach	Acid-base disturbances (hypochloremic alkalosis, dehydration); occurs mostly in combination with sodium loss	Deficiency and excess are unusual; most diets supply adequate chloride (usually in combination with sodium) Disease states such as excessive vomiting can necessitate chloride replacement
Sources	***Excess***	
Salt, meat, eggs, dairy products, many prepared and preserved foods	Acid-base disturbance	

*Macrominerals—required intake >100 mg/day.

Continued.

Table 13-2 Minerals and their nutritional significance—cont'd

PHYSIOLOGIC FUNCTIONS/SOURCES	RESULTS OF DEFICIENCY OR EXCESS	NURSING CONSIDERATIONS
▪ Chromium†		
Functions	***Deficiency***	
Involved in glucose metabolism and energy production	Possible abnormal glucose metabolism	No specific recommendations are needed
Sources	***Excess***	
Meat, cheese, whole grain breads and cereals, legumes, peanuts, brewer's yeast, vegetable oils	Unknown	
▪ Copper†		
Functions	***Deficiency***	
Production of hemoglobin Essential component of several enzyme systems	Anemia, leukopenia, neutropenia	Deficiency from inadequate food sources is less likely than from excess intake of other minerals, especially zinc and possibly iron; therefore emphasize the correct use of any vitamin supplement
Sources	***Excess***	
Organ meats, oysters, nuts, seeds, legumes, corn oil margarine	Severe vomiting and diarrhea Hemolytic anemia	Caution against cooking acid foods in unlined copper pots, which can lead to chronic and toxic accumulation of copper
▪ Fluorine†		
Functions	***Deficiency***	
Formation of caries-resistant teeth Strong bone development	Increased susceptibility to tooth decay	In areas with optimally fluoridated water, encourage sufficient intake to supply recommended amount of fluoride (see Chapter 14) In areas of unfluoridated water or when ready-to-use formula, bottled water, or breast milk is used, stress the importance of fluoride supplements
Sources		
Fluoridated water and foods or beverages prepared with fluoridated water; fish, tea, commercially prepared chicken for infants		
	Excess	
	Fluorosis (mottling and/or pitting of enamel) Severe bone deformities	In areas with excess fluoride in the water consider the use of bottled water in drinking and possibly cooking to reduce the fluoride intake to safe levels Fluorine has the narrowest range of safe and adequate intake; therefore, stress the importance of storing supplements in a safe area
▪ Iodine†		
Functions	***Deficiency***	
Production of thyroid hormone Normal reproduction	**Goiter** (enlarged thyroid from decreased thyroxine formation)	Encourage use of iodized salt for individuals living far from the sea
Sources	***Excess***	
Seafood, kelp, iodized salt, sea salt, enriched bread, milk (from dairy processing)	Unknown from food sources; may occur from ingestion of iodine preparations, such as saturated solutions of potassium iodide (SSKI)	If iodine preparations are in the home, stress the importance of safe storage

*Macrominerals—required intake >100 mg/day.
†Microminerals or trace elements—required intake <100 mg/day.

Table 13-2 Minerals and their nutritional significance—cont'd

PHYSIOLOGIC FUNCTIONS/SOURCES	RESULTS OF DEFICIENCY OR EXCESS	NURSING CONSIDERATIONS
▪ **Iron†**		
Functions	***Deficiency***	
Formation of hemoglobin and myoglobin Essential part of several enzymes and proteins	**Anemia** (see Chapter 35)	Encourage foods rich in iron Discourage excessive milk consumption, especially more than 1 liter per day (milk is a very poor source of iron) If iron supplements are prescribed, teach parents factors that affect absorption (see box below)

FACTORS THAT AFFECT IRON ABSORPTION

Increase	*Decrease*
Acidity (low pH)—administer iron between meals (gastric hydrochloric acid)	Alkalinity (high pH)—avoid any antacid preparation
Ascorbic acid (vitamin C)—administer iron with juice, fruit, or multivitamin preparation	Phosphates—milk is unfavorable vehicle for iron administration
Vitamin A	Phytates—found in cereals
Calcium	Oxalates—found in many fruits and vegetables (plums, currants, green beans, spinach, sweet potatoes, tomatoes)
Tissue need	Tannins—found in tea, coffee
Meat, fish, poultry	Tissue saturation
Cooking in cast iron pots	Malabsorptive disorders
	Disturbances that cause diarrhea or steatorrhea
	Infection

PHYSIOLOGIC FUNCTIONS/SOURCES	RESULTS OF DEFICIENCY OR EXCESS	NURSING CONSIDERATIONS
Sources	***Excess***	
Liver, especially pork, followed by calf, beef, and chicken; kidney, red meat, poultry, shellfish, whole grains, iron-enriched infant formula and cereal, enriched cereals and bread, legumes, nuts, seeds, green leafy vegetables (except spinach), dried fruits, potatoes, molasses	Hemosiderosis (excess iron storage in various tissues of the body, especially the spleen, liver, lymph glands, heart, and pancreas) Hemochromatosis (excess iron storage with cellular damage)	Stress the importance of storing iron supplements in a safe area
▪ **Magnesium***		
Functions	***Deficiency***	
Bone and tooth formation Production of proteins Nerve conduction to muscles Activation of enzymes needed for carbohydrate and protein metabolism	Tremors, spasm Irregular heartbeat Muscular weakness Lower extremity cramps Convulsions, delirium	Deficiency and excess are unusual, except in disease states such as prolonged vomiting or diarrhea or kidney dysfunction, where replacement may be needed
Sources	***Excess***	
Whole grains, nuts, soybeans, meat, green leafy vegetables (uncooked), tea, cocoa, raisins	Nervous system disturbances due to imbalance in calcium-to-magnesium ratio	

*Macrominerals—required intake >100 mg/day.
†Microminerals or trace elements—required intake <100 mg/day.

Continued.

Table 13-2 Minerals and their nutritional significance—cont'd

PHYSIOLOGIC FUNCTIONS/SOURCES	RESULTS OF DEFICIENCY OR EXCESS	NURSING CONSIDERATIONS
■ Manganese†		
Functions Activation of enzymes involved in reproduction, growth, and fat metabolism Normal bone structure Nervous system functioning ***Sources*** Nuts, whole grains, legumes, green vegetables, fruit	***Deficiency*** Unknown ***Excess*** Unknown	No specific recommendations are needed
■ Molybdenum†		
Functions Essential component of several oxidative enzymes ***Sources*** Legumes, whole grains, organ meats, some dark green vegetables	***Deficiency*** Very rare; diagnosed in patients on complete total parenteral alimentation ***Excess*** Produces secondary copper deficiency (growth failure, anemia, and disturbed bone development)	No specific recommendations are needed
■ Phosphorus*		
Functions Bone and tooth development (in combination with calcium) Involved in numerous chemical reactions, including protein, carbohydrate, and fat metabolism Acid-base balance ***Sources*** Dairy products, eggs, meat, poultry, legumes, carbonated beverages	***Deficiency*** Weakness, anorexia, malaise, bone pain ***Excess*** Produces secondary calcium deficiency from disturbed calcium-to-phosphorus ratio	Dietary deficiency is uncommon, although prolonged use of antacids can produce deficiency, in which case supplementation is recommended To preserve calcium-to-phosphorus ratio in newborns, discourage use of whole cow's milk
■ Potassium*		
Functions Acid-base and fluid balance (major extracellular fluid areas) Nerve conduction Muscular contraction, especially the heart Release of energy ***Sources*** Bananas, citrus fruit, dried fruits, meat, fish, bran, legumes, peanut butter, potatoes, coffee, tea, cocoa	***Deficiency*** Cardiac arrhythmias Muscular weakness Lethargy Kidney and respiratory failure Heart failure ***Excess*** Cardiac arrhythmias Respiratory failure Mental confusion Numbness of extremities	Dietary deficiency and excess are unlikely, although disease states such as prolonged nausea and vomiting, or the use of diuretics can result in hypokalemia; in such instances, encourage replacement with supplements of rich food sources, such as bananas

*Macrominerals—required intake >100 mg/day.
†Microminerals or trace elements—required intake <100 mg/day.

Table 13-2 Minerals and their nutritional significance—cont'd

PHYSIOLOGIC FUNCTIONS/SOURCES	RESULTS OF DEFICIENCY OR EXCESS	NURSING CONSIDERATIONS
▪ Selenium†		
Functions Antioxidant, especially protective of vitamin E Protects against toxicity of heavy metals Associated with fat metabolism ***Sources*** Seafood, organ meats, egg yolk, whole grain, chicken, meat, tomatoes, cabbage, garlic, mushrooms, milk	***Deficiency*** Keshan disease—cardiomyopathy in children (found in China) ***Excess*** Eye, nose, and throat irritation Increased dental caries Liver and kidney degeneration	Deficiency and excess are uncommon in North America, although selenium deficiency can occur in patients on prolonged total parenteral alimentation; in these instances supplementation is required
▪ Sodium*		
Functions Acid-base and fluid balance (major extracellular fluid cation) Cell permeability; absorption of glucose Muscle contraction ***Sources*** Table salt, seafood, meat, poultry, numerous prepared foods	***Deficiency*** Dehydration Hypotension Convulsions Muscle cramps ***Excess*** Edema Hypertension Intracranial hemorrhage	Deficiency intake is very rare, although losses secondary to nausea, vomiting, excessive sweating, and use of diuretics can occur and require replacement Encourage parents to limit excessive use of salt in preparing foods and commercial foods with high sodium content, such as smoked meats
▪ Sulfur*		
Functions Essential component of cell protein, especially of hair and skin Enzyme activation Associated with energy metabolism Detoxification of certain chemical reactions ***Sources*** Dairy products, eggs, meat, fish, nuts, legumes	***Deficiency*** Unknown ***Excess*** Unknown	No specific recommendations are needed
▪ Zinc†		
Functions Component of about 100 enzymes Synthesis of nucleic acids and protein in immune system and coagulation Release of vitamin A from liver Improved wound healing with vitamin C ***Sources*** Seafood (especially oysters), meat, poultry, eggs, wheat, legumes	***Deficiency*** Loss of appetite Diminished taste sensation Delayed healing Skin lesions—erythematous, crusted lesions around body orifices Alopecia Diarrhea Growth failure Retarded sexual maturity	Encourage food sources rich in zinc, especially protein Caution that fiber, phytates, oxalates, tannins (in tea or coffee), iron, and calcium adversely affect zinc absorption Recognize groups at risk for zinc deficiency, such as vegetarians and Mexican-Americans, whose diets may have restricted or low meat content and high fiber, phytate content; and patients with malabsorption syndromes
	Excess Vomiting and diarrhea Malaise, dizziness Anemia, gastric bleeding Impaired absorption of calcium and copper	Emphasize correct use of zinc supplements and the possible interaction with other minerals

*Macrominerals—required intake >100 mg/day.
†Microminerals or trace elements—required intake <100 mg/day.

ing considerations are discussed below (at right), and specific interventions are presented in the table.

VEGETARIAN DIETS

The importance of vegetarian diets and their relationship to potential nutritional deficiencies in children cannot be overemphasized. The stricter the vegetarian diet, the more difficult it becomes to ensure adequate nutrition for infants and children. The major types of vegetarianism are described in Box 13-1.

Many individuals who are concerned about healthful diets subscribe to vegetarian diets that are not typified by the above categories. Therefore during nutritional assessment it is necessary to clearly list exactly what the diet includes and excludes.

The lacto-ovovegetarian diet is associated with the least deficiencies, although protein intake needs to be monitored. The lactovegetarian diet may be low in protein, as well as iron. The major deficiencies in the stricter vegetarian diets are inadequate protein for growth, inadequate calories for energy and growth, poor digestibility of many of the natural, unprocessed foods, especially for infants, and deficiencies of vitamin B_{12}, niacin, thiamine, riboflavin, vitamin D, iron, calcium, and zinc. In the United States vegetarian diets are common among members of Black Muslim or Seventh Day Adventist faiths.

Because vegetarian diets eliminate the major sources of complete proteins (those proteins with all the essential amino acids in amounts needed to support physiologic functions), protein deficiency can occur. Fortunately, this problem is easily remedied by selecting foods with complementary amino acids and consuming them at the same meal (Box 13-2).

Achieving a nutritionally adequate vegetarian diet is not difficult, but it requires careful planning and knowledge of nutrient sources. For children, the lacto-ovovegetarian diet is nutritionally adequate; however, the vegan diet requires supplementation with vitamins D and B_{12}, particularly for children ages 2 to 12 years. Infants on a vegan diet should be breast-fed for the first 6 months and preferably for 1 year, fed solid foods after about 4 months, and receive iron-fortified cereal for at least 18 months. The use of vitamin C juices with foods high in iron will further improve iron absorption. If cow's or human milk is not given, fortified soy milk is recommended (Fanelli and Kuczmarski, 1983). Other approaches toward increasing vitamin D and calcium intake in the diet that may be accepted by the macrobiotic teachers are inclusion of fatty fish (herring, salmon, sardines, trout, tuna) and less fiber, since high fiber intake limits mineral absorption by decreasing intestinal transit time and binding calcium, iron, and other minerals (Dagnelie and others, 1990).

When solid foods are introduced, the safety and digestibility of the selections must be considered. Raw fruits with seeds, vegetables, and nuts are hazardous for young children because of the danger of aspiration. Beans, grain cereals, and vegetables should be served well cooked and mashed during infancy. A variety of foods should be introduced during the early years to ensure a more well-balanced intake.

Box 13-1 TYPES OF VEGETARIAN DIETS

Lacto-ovovegetarians exclude meat from their diet but eat milk and eggs and sometimes fish.
Lactovegetarians exclude meat and eggs but drink milk.
Pure vegetarians (vegans) eliminate any food of animal origin, including milk and eggs.
Macrobiotics are even more restrictive than pure vegetarians in that cereals, especially brown or polished rice, are the mainstay of the diet.

Box 13-2 FOOD COMBINATIONS FOR COMPLEMENTARY AMINO ACIDS

Grains (cereal, rice, pasta) and **legumes** (beans, peas, lentils, peanuts)
Grains and **milk products** (milk, cheese, yogurt)
Seeds (sesame, sunflower) and **legumes**

NURSING CONSIDERATIONS

Identification of nutrient imbalance is the initial nursing goal and requires assessment, based on a dietary history and physical examination, for signs of deficiency or excess (see Chapter 6). Once assessment data are collected, they should be evaluated against standard intakes to identify areas of concern. The most widely used standard is the Recommended Dietary Allowances (RDA), developed by the National Academy of Sciences, Food and Nutrition Board. The RDA are not average requirements but recommendations intended to meet the physiologic needs of almost every healthy person. To meet the needs of those with the highest requirements, the RDA will exceed most people's requirements. Therefore children consuming less than the RDA are not necessarily consuming an inadequate diet but are more likely at risk for deficiency than those who are consuming nutrients in amounts equal to the RDA.

The RDA are used primarily by professionals involved in nutrition. To provide consumers with reliable information about the nutrient content of the foods they purchase, the U.S. Recommended Daily Allowances (U.S. RDA) were developed and provide information about nutrition on package labels. Eight nutrients must be listed—protein, vitamin A, vitamin C, thiamin, riboflavin, niacin, calcium, and iron, as well as caloric density. Listing of other minerals and vitamins is optional unless they are added to a food. Since the U.S. RDA are based on the RDA, they also include a margin of safety and are generally higher than the needs of most people.

Several organizations have published dietary advice for the public; most well-known are the Dietary Guidelines for Americans, which encourage eating a variety of foods, maintaining ideal body weight, consuming adequate starch and fiber, and limiting intake of fat, cholesterol, sugar, salt, and alcohol (U.S. Department of Agriculture, 1985). The American Academy of Pediatrics, Committee on Nutrition (1986) advises following these guidelines for children, especially eating a varied diet and maintaining ideal body weight. However, they caution that limiting fat should be done in moderation, with fat providing 30% to 40% of calories.

Since one of the best assurances of nutritional adequacy is eating a variety of foods, families need guidelines for selecting foods that provide essential nutrients without exceeding energy requirements. Commonly eaten foods are often grouped together on the basis of similarity and composition and nutritional value. One classification is the basic four food groups: fruits/vegetables, bread/cereal, milk/cheese, and meat/poultry/fish/beans. Several other classification systems exist; for example, a fifth group of fats/sweets/alcohol is often added to the basic four groups, as well as a sixth group of combination foods (soup/stew/pizza/casseroles). Counseling families about nutritionally adequate diets should emphasize the importance of selecting foods from each food group (see Table 4-5) and an explanation of the U.S. RDA on food labels.

Unfortunately there are no restrictions on the availability of toxic doses of vitamins or minerals. With the unsubstantiated claims for megadose therapy in curing ailments from the common cold to cancer, many individuals consume large amounts of nutrients. Nurses need to inform families of the potential dangers from excess vitamins or minerals. The idea that "more is better" is incorrect and is probably best dispelled by a simple explanation of the body's inability to use more than the needed requirement.

PROTEIN AND ENERGY MALNUTRITION

Hunger is one of the world's gravest and most prevalent health problems. In the Third World, where 75% of children live, more than half of the children are short and underweight for their age. An even more serious consequence is the infant mortality rate, which may be 10 times higher than that in the United States (Guthrie, 1988). Children often suffer from the most extreme forms of protein-energy malnutrition (PEM)—marasmus and kwashiorkor.

In the United States milder forms of PEM are seen, although the classic cases of marasmus and kwashiorkor also occur. Unlike developing countries where the main reason for PEM is inadequate food, in the United States PEM occurs despite ample dietary supplies (see Failure to Thrive, p. 616).

Kwashiorkor

Kwashiorkor is a deficiency of protein with low or an adequate supply of calories. The word comes from the Ghan language and means "the sickness the older child gets when the next baby is born." It is an appropriate name because the syndrome develops in the first child, usually between 1 and 4 years of age, when weaned from the breast once the second child is born. The first child is fed a diet consisting mainly of starch grains or tubers. Such a diet provides adequate calories in the form of carbohydrates but an inadequate amount of high-quality proteins.

Pathophysiology and clinical manifestations. The pathophysiology of kwashiorkor results from protein deficiency, both in quantity and quality (Rossouw, 1989). Since protein is essential for tissue growth and cell repair, all body systems are affected, but rapidly growing cells, such as those of the epithelium and mucosa, are most severely damaged. The skin is scaly and dry and has areas of depigmentation. Several dermatoses may be evident, partly resulting from the vitamin deficiencies. Permanent blindness results from the severe lack of vitamin A. Immunity is severely affected and is of considerable importance in the development of infections.

Mineral deficiencies are common, especially iron, calcium, and zinc. Acute zinc deficiency is a common complication of severe PEM and results in skin rashes, loss of hair, impaired immune response and susceptibility to infections, digestive problems, night blindness, changes in affective behavior, defective wound healing, and impaired growth. Its depressant effect on appetite further limits food intake (Solomons, 1982).

With kwashiorkor the hair is thin, dry, coarse, and dull. Depigmentation is common, and patchy alopecia may occur. There is loss of weight in conjunction with edema (ascites) from the hypoalbuminemia. The edema often masks the severe muscular atrophy, making the children appear less debilitated than they actually are (Fig. 13-1). Total body water increases, but total body potassium decreases with

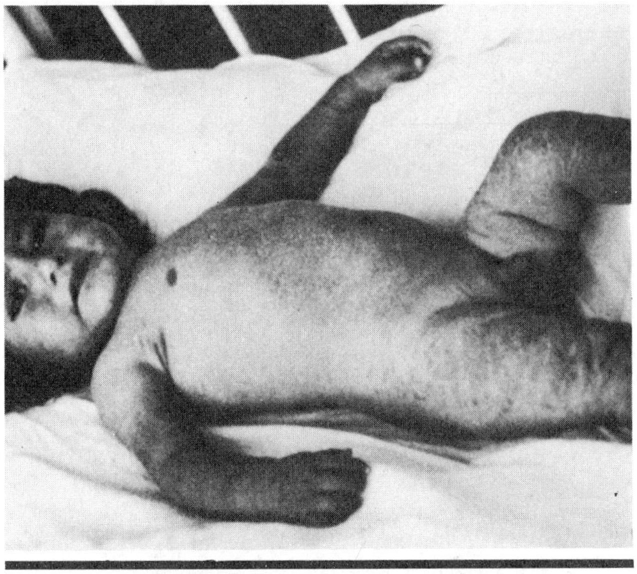

Fig. 13-1. Child with kwashiorkor. Note the edema, which masks muscle wasting.

From Guthrie, H.A.: Introductory nutrition, ed. 6, St. Louis, 1986, Mosby–Year Book, Inc. Courtesy Dr. John Beard, Pennsylvania State University.

retention of sodium, causing signs of hypokalemia and hypernatremia.

Diarrhea frequently occurs from a lowered resistance to infection and further complicates the electrolyte imbalance. Gastrointestinal disturbances occur, such as fatty infiltration of the liver and atrophy of the acini cells of the pancreas. Behavioral changes are evident as the child grows progressively more irritable, lethargic, withdrawn, and apathetic. Fatal deterioration may be caused by diarrhea and infection or as the result of circulatory failure.

Marasmus

Marasmus is the result of general malnutrition of both calories and protein. It is a common occurrence in underdeveloped countries during times of drought, such as Ethiopia. Because children are fed last in these cultures, there is seldom enough food remaining for the younger ones.

Marasmus is usually a syndrome of physical and emotional deprivation and is not confined to geographic areas where food supplies are inadequate. It may be seen in failure-to-thrive children, where the cause is not solely nutritional but primarily emotional.

Pathophysiology and clinical manifestations. Marasmus is characterized by gradual wasting and atrophy of body tissues, especially subcutaneous fat (Fig. 13-2). Children with the condition appear to be very old; their skin is flabby and wrinkled, unlike children with kwashiorkor, who appear more rounded from the edema. Fat metabolism is less impaired than in kwashiorkor, so that vitamin A deficiency is usually minimal or absent.

In general, the clinical manifestations of marasmus are similar to those seen in kwashiorkor with the following exceptions: no edema from hypoalbuminemia or sodium retention, which contributes to a severely emaciated appearance; no dermatoses caused by vitamin deficiencies; little or no depigmentation of hair or skin; more normal fat metabolism and lipid absorption; and smaller head size and slower recovery following treatment.

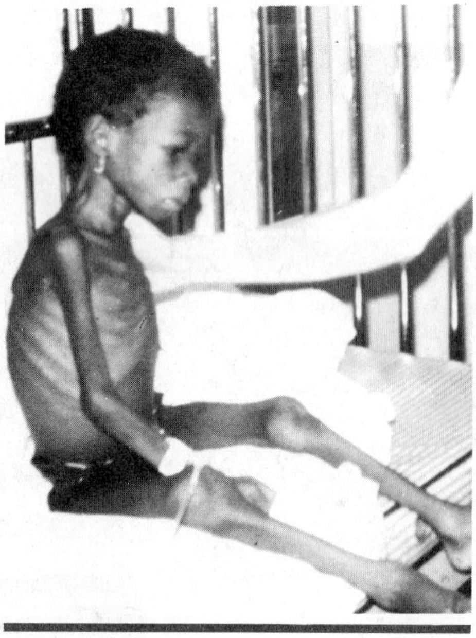

Fig. 13-2. Child with marasmus.
From Dodge, P.R., Prensky, A.L., and Feigin, R.D.: Nutrition and the developing nervous system, St. Louis, 1975, Mosby–Year Book, Inc. Courtesy Donald Anderson, M.D., Travis Air Force Base, CA.

As in kwashiorkor, body metabolism is minimal, and maintaining body temperature is complicated by lack of subcutaneous fat. The child is fretful, apathetic, withdrawn, and so lethargic that prostration frequently occurs. Intercurrent infection with debilitating diseases such as tuberculosis, parasitosis, and dysentery is common. Severe, chronic malnutrition in infancy results in decreased brain growth and has implications for the child's future mental capacity.

Therapeutic Management

Treatment of kwashiorkor and marasmus includes providing a diet high in quality proteins and/or carbohydrates as well as vitamins and minerals. Electrolyte imbalance requires immediate attention, and parenteral fluid replacement may be necessary initially to correct the dehydration and restore renal function. Occasionally oral fluids are not tolerated, necessitating the use of hyperalimentation. Coexisting problems such as infection, diarrhea, parasitic infestation, and anemia necessitate prompt attention for optimum recovery.

A recent recommendation is the addition of psychosocial stimulation to the treatment of severely malnourished children. A long-term structured play program involving parents has been shown to result in marked developmental improvements. However, these children continued to be behind in nutritional status and locomotor development (Grantham-McGregor, Schofield, and Harris, 1983).

Nursing Considerations

Provision of essential physiologic needs such as rest, individually tailored activity, and protection from infection is paramount. Since children are usually weak and withdrawn, they depend on others to feed them. Hygiene may be distressing because of the poor integrity of the skin, and decubiti are a constant threat. Appropriate developmental stimulation should also be provided.

A larger problem is prevention of these conditions through education concerning the importance of high-quality proteins and adequate carbohydrates. Since children with marasmus may suffer from emotional starvation as well, care should be consistent with care of the failure-to-thrive child (p. 616).

OBESITY

Obesity is a complex condition that may or may not be related to the chronic ingestion of more calories than are needed to supply the body's energy requirement. Genetic factors play a significant role, since there is a strong correlation of obesity among biologic family members that is not evident among parents and adopted children (Stunkard and others, 1986, 1990).

Firm evidence links obesity in adolescence to obesity in

adulthood (see Obesity, Chapter 21); the evidence for obesity in infancy remaining a risk factor for adult obesity is controversial. Although recent studies have examined the role of infant feeding methods and subsequent overweight, these results are also conflicting. One study found that infants who were breast-fed beyond 6 months of age had slower growth rates than bottle-fed infants during the second half of the first year (Dewey and others, 1989). However, another study found that infants described as vigorous feeders who were breast-fed and had delayed introduction of solid foods were heavier at 6 years of age (Agras and others, 1990). A factor that may influence the effect of breast-feeding on infant weight gain is the mother's attitude—mothers who breast-feed tend to prefer leaner infants than mothers who bottle-feed (Kramer and others, 1983).

Despite the conflicting data on exactly what causes infant obesity, all authorities agree that *prevention* holds greater promise than treatment. Besides the physiologic component of increased numbers of fat cells, there are also the psychologic disadvantages of firmly entrenched food habits and dependency on food. Consequently, evaluation of overnutrition *early* in life is essential, with attention to those factors that may prevent obesity.

Nursing Considerations

The principal nursing goal is prevention of obesity. If infants are overweight for their height, the goal is to slow weight gain, not cause weight loss. During infancy the development of obesity is influenced by parental practices. Therefore intervention involves helping the parent establish appropriate feeding habits for the infant or change inappropriate ones. This involves much more than dietary counseling. Psychologic factors play an important role, particularly the philosophy that a fat baby is a healthy baby, or, more subconsciously, that a fat "healthy" baby is a sign of good mothering (Sherman and Alexander, 1990). Such beliefs are difficult to dispel, and counseling may need to include other family members, such as grandmothers, who can greatly influence the mother's practices (Dietz, 1989).

Although the exact role breast-feeding has on the development of subsequent obesity is unclear, its protective effect may be related to self-regulation of intake. With bottle-feeding, parents may encourage the infant to finish all of the formula, establishing a habit of eating beyond the initial feeling of satiety. During nutritional counseling the nurse should discuss with parents appropriate feeding habits, such as allowing the child to regulate the need for formula and solid food. With proper education parents can come to understand that a "good eater" is not a big eater but one who eats moderately without necessarily "cleaning the plate."

The addition of solid foods is another important aspect of nutritional counseling. When solid foods are added, the quantity of milk should be decreased to less than 1 liter to maintain the proper caloric balance. If the infant seems unsatisfied with fewer bottle feedings and refuses water, the milk or formula can be diluted to yield fewer calories per ounce. Other alternatives are substituting water for a bottle

Table 13-3 Nutritive values of milk (per 8 oz)

	WHOLE MILK	NONFAT OR SKIM MILK	LOW-FAT OR PARTIALLY SKIM MILK
Calories	150	86	121
Protein (g)	8	8	8
Fat (g)	8	0.5	5
Percent milk fat	3.25 (min.)	0.5 (max.)	2 (avg.)
Carbohydrates (g)	11	12	12
Calcium (mg)	291	302	297
Iron (mg)	0.12	0.10	0.12
Vitamin A (IU)	307	500	500
Thiamine (mg)	0.09	0.09	0.10
Riboflavin (mg)	0.4	0.3	0.4
Niacin (mg)	0.2	0.2	0.2
Vitamin C (mg)	2	2	2

Data from Newer knowledge of milk and other fluid dairy products, Rosemont, IL, 1979, National Dairy Council.

of formula or using a smaller-hole nipple to prolong sucking with less intake. A commercial formula, Advance, is also available and provides 20% fewer calories than regular formula or whole cow's milk. Substituting skim or low-fat milk for whole milk or formula is unacceptable. Although they contain a significant reduction in calories, they are not nutritionally sound for infants. Their low fat content deprives the infant of essential fatty acids, significantly increased amounts of solids and electrolytes elevate the renal solute load and water demands, and their vitamin A content is reduced. A comparison of whole, nonfat (skimmed), and low-fat (partially skimmed) milk is presented in Table 13-3.

The selection of solid foods should also be considered. Approximately 20% of commercial baby foods contain less than 50 kcal/100 g, whereas another 20% contain more than 100 kcal/100 g. Choosing low-calorie foods can significantly lower the daily calorie intake without actually decreasing the total quantity of food. Food charts can be used to familiarize parents with the calorie content of foods, as well as encouraging reading of food labels. Sweet foods are kept to a minimum. This includes not adding additional sugar to the formula or cereal and avoiding finger foods such as cookies. Other foods rich in calories that are restricted in serving size rather than eliminated include butter, cream, ice cream, pudding, and chocolate.

Parents are also encouraged to interpret the infant's signals of discomfort and intervene in ways other than through feeding. Crying, fussiness, or sucking does not necessarily indicate hunger. Rocking, stroking, holding, and offering a pacifier may be more appropriate than automatically responding with food (Wishon and Kinnick, 1986).

Since activity is also an important factor in maintaining appropriate weight, parents are encouraged to promote exercise in their child. Although infants are naturally active, placing them in confined areas, such as cribs or playpens, and in front of televisions establishes poor habits. There is a direct relationship between time spent viewing television and the tendency toward obesity (Dietz and Gortmaker, 1985).

FOOD SENSITIVITY

Food sensitivity is a general term that includes any type of adverse reaction to food or food additives. Food sensitivities can be divided into two broad categories (Anderson, 1986):

Food allergy or **hypersensitivity,** which refers to those reactions involving immunologic mechanisms, usually immunoglobulin E (IgE); the reactions may be immediate or delayed and mild or severe, such as an anaphylactic reaction

Food intolerance, which refers to those reactions involving known or unknown nonimmunologic mechanisms; lactose intolerance is an example of a reaction that looks like allergy but is due to deficiency of the enzyme lactase

However, this classification is not universally accepted; therefore, the terms *food sensitivity, hypersensitivity, allergy,* and *intolerance* are often used interchangeably.

Food allergy is caused by exposure to *allergens,* also called *allergic antigens,* usually proteins (but not the smaller amino acids) that are capable of inducing IgE antibody formation ("sensitization") when ingested. Sensitization refers to the initial exposure of an individual to an allergen, resulting in an immune response; subsequent exposure induces a much stronger response that is clinically apparent. Consequently, food hypersensitivity typically occurs after the food has been ingested one or more times. In infants an allergic response can occur with the first ingestion because of transplacental sensitization in utero or because of sensitization to the substance passed through breast milk (Wilson, Self, and Hamburger, 1990). Allergens can also produce an allergic response when inhaled or injected, but these routes rarely apply to food allergens (see also discussion of asthma in Chapter 32). The most common food allergens are eggs, cow's milk, peanuts, soy, wheat, corn, and fish (Box 13-3) (Zeiger and others, 1986).

Food allergies can occur at any time, but are common during infancy because the immature intestinal tract is more permeable to proteins than the mature intestinal tract, thus increasing the likelihood of an immune response. Allergies in general demonstrate a genetic component: children who have one parent with allergy have a 50% to 58% risk of developing allergy; children who have both parents with allergy have up to a 100% risk of developing allergy (cited in Zeiger and others, 1986). Allergy with a hereditary tendency is referred to as *atopy.* Some infants with atopy can be identified at birth from elevated levels of IgE in cord blood.

Although the reason is unknown, many children "outgrow" their food allergies. Children who are allergic to more than one food may develop tolerance to each food at different times. The most common allergens, such as soy, are outgrown less readily than other food allergens. Because of the tendency to lose the hypersensitivity, allergic foods should be reintroduced into the diet after a period of abstinence (usually a year or more) to evaluate if the food can be safely added to the diet (Sampson and Scanlon, 1989).

There is evidence that food allergies can be prevented. The protective role of exclusive breast-feeding and avoidance of hyperallergenic foods is controversial, but most authorities recommend the guidelines in Box 13-4 for infants with a family history of atopy.

Box 13-3 HYPERALLERGENIC FOODS/SOURCES

Milk*: Ice cream, butter, margarine (if it contains dairy products), yogurt, cheese, pudding, baked goods, wieners, bologna, canned creamed soups, instant breakfast drinks, powdered milk drinks, milk chocolate
Eggs*: Mayonnaise, creamy salad dressing, baked goods, egg noodles, some cake icing, meringue, custard, pancakes, French toast, root beer
Wheat*: Almost all baked goods, wieners, bologna, pressed or chopped cold cuts, gravy, pasta, some canned soups
Legumes: Peanuts,* peanut butter or oil, beans, peas, lentils
Nuts*: Some chocolates, candy, baked goods, cherry soda (may be flavored with a nut extract), walnut oil
Fish or shellfish*: Cod liver oil, pizza with anchovies, Caesar salad dressing, any food fried in same oil as fish
Soy*: Soy sauce, teriyaki or worcestershire sauce, tofu, baked goods using soy flour or oil, soy nuts, soy infant formulas or milk, soybean paste, tuna packed in vegetable oil, many margarines
Chocolate: Cola beverages, cocoa, chocolate-flavored drinks
Buckwheat: Some cereals, pancakes
Pork, chicken: Bacon, wieners, sausage, pork fat, chicken broth
Strawberries, melon, pineapple: Gelatin, syrups
Corn: Popcorn, cereal, muffins, cornstarch, corn meal, corn bread, corn tortilla
Citrus fruits: Orange, lemon, lime, grapefruit; any of these in drinks, gelatin, juice, or medicines
Tomatoes: Juice, some vegetable soups, spaghetti, pizza sauce, and catsup
Spices: Chili, pepper, vinegar, cinnamon

*Most common allergens.

Cow's Milk Allergy

Cow's milk allergy is a multifaceted disorder representing adverse systemic and local gastrointestinal reactions to cow's milk protein. The hypersensitivity may be manifest through a variety of signs and symptoms (Box 13-5) that may appear within 45 minutes of milk ingestion or after a period of several days (Hill and others, 1986, 1989). The diagnosis is initially made from the history, although the practitioner needs a high index of suspicion, since the timing and diversity of clinical manifestations vary greatly. For example, cow's milk allergy may be manifest as colic (see discussion on p. 614) or sleeplessness in an otherwise healthy infant (Kahn and others, 1989).

Box 13-4 GUIDELINES FOR PREVENTING ATOPY IN CHILDREN

Identify Children at Risk
Family history of allergy
Increased IgE in cord blood and postnatal serum

Prenatal Precautions (Last Trimester)
Avoid any known food allergens
Avoid milk and other dairy products, peanuts, and eggs
Minimize ingestion of other hyperallergenic foods (see Box 13-3)

Postnatal Precautions
Breast milk or casein/whey hydrolysate formula (e.g. Nutramigen, Pregestimil, Alimentum) exclusively for at least 6 months
No solid food for 6 months
No cow's milk or soy formula for 12 months
No egg, fish, corn, citrus, peanuts, nuts, or chocolate for 12 months
One new food added at 5-day intervals to identify possible reaction

Environmental Control
Limited exposure to dust, molds, animals, and cigarette smoke

Data from Johnstone, D.: Strategy for intervention of food allergy in infants, Int. Pediatr. 4(4):319-325, 1989; and Zeiger R., and others: Effectiveness of dietary manipulation in the prevention of food allergy in infants, Part 2, J. Allergy Clin. Immunol. 78(1, pt. 2):224-238, 1986.

Box 13-5 CLINICAL MANIFESTATIONS OF COW'S MILK SENSITIVITY

Gastrointestinal
*Diarrhea
*Vomiting
*Colic
*Abdominal pain
Hematochezia (bloody stools)
Malabsorption
Enteropathy
Constipation
Anorexia
Colitis

Respiratory
*Rhinitis
*Bronchitis
*Asthma
*Sneezing
*Coughing
*Chronic nasal discharge
Recurrent croup
Serous otitis media

Dermatologic
*Eczema
Urticaria
Hives

Central Nervous and Behavioral
*Excessive crying
Excessive night waking; sleeplessness
Excessive sweating
Headache
Hyperirritability
Hyperactivity
Lethargy

Vascular
Facial pallor
Infraorbital edema (swelling under eyes)

Constitutional
Failure to thrive
Retarded growth
Malnutrition

*Most common.

Diagnostic evaluation. A number of diagnostic tests may be performed, including stool analysis for blood (both frank and occult bleeding can occur from the colitis), serum IgE levels, skin-prick testing, and radioallergosorbent test (RAST) (measures IgE antibodies to specific allergens in serum by radioimmunoassay). Both skin testing and RAST help identify the offending food, but the results are not always conclusive.

The most definitive diagnostic strategy is elimination of milk, followed by challenge testing after improvement of symptoms. Challenge testing involves reintroducing small quantities of milk in the diet to detect resurgence of symptoms; at times challenge testing involves the use of a placebo so that the parent is unaware of or "blind" to the timing of allergen ingestion.

✦ **NURSING ALERT** Careful observation of the child is required during a challenge test because of the possibility of anaphylactic reaction.

Therapeutic management. Treatment of cow's milk allergy is elimination of all dairy products. For infants fed cow's milk formula, this primarily involves changing the formula to a casein or whey hydrolysate milk formula, in which the protein has been broken down (or "predigested") into its amino acids through enzymatic hydrolysis. Soy-based formula is not recommended, because as many as 20% of these infants are also allergic to soy (American Academy of Pediatrics, 1989). Goat's milk is not an acceptable substitute, since it cross-reacts with cow's milk protein and is deficient in folic acid. Infants who are breast-fed but have symptoms of cow's milk hypersensitivity are treated by eliminating all dairy products from the lactating mother's diet. These women need vitamin D and calcium supplementation to prevent deficiency. Infants are maintained on the dairy-free diet for 1 or 2 years, at which time very small quantities of milk are reintroduced.

Nursing considerations. The principal nursing objectives are identification of potential milk allergy and appropriate counseling of parents regarding substitute formulas. The protein hydrolysate formulas are less palatable than milk-based formulas. Consequently, reluctance to accept the new formula may be a problem. This can be overcome by introducing the formula gradually over a few days using 1 ounce of new formula to 7 ounces of old formula, then 2 to 6 ounces, 3 to 4, and as needed. Parents also need to be reassured that the infant will receive complete nutrition from the new formula and will suffer no ill effects from the absence of cow's milk.

Once solid foods are started, parents need guidance in avoiding all associated milk products (see Box 13-3). This requires carefully reading all food labels to avoid potential addition of milk products to the prepared food.

Lactose Intolerance

Lactose intolerance refers to at least two different entities that involve a deficiency of the enzyme lactase, which is needed for the digestion of lactose. *Congenital lactose intolerance* appears soon after birth when the diet contains

Box 13-6 GUIDELINES FOR REDUCING OR ELIMINATING SYMPTOMS OF LACTOSE INTOLERANCE

Limit milk consumption to one glass at a time.
Drink milk with other foods rather than alone.
Eat hard cheese, cottage cheese, or yogurt instead of milk (frozen yogurt may be less well tolerated than certain brands of fresh yogurt).
Use enzyme tablets (LactAid, Lactrase) to predigest the lactose in milk or supplement the body's own lactase (add tablets to milk or sprinkle on dairy products such as ice cream).
Eat small amounts of dairy foods daily to help colonic bacteria adapt to ingested lactose.

From Savaiano, D., and Kotz, C.: Recent advances in the management of lactose intolerance, Contemp. Nutr. 13(9,10):4, 1988.

lactose from milk. *Late-onset lactose intolerance* is similar to the congenital type but manifests later in life. Ethnic groups with a high incidence of lactose intolerance include Orientals, southern Europeans, Arabs, Jews, and blacks. The principal manifestations include diarrhea, abdominal pain, distension, and flatus shortly after ingesting milk products.

In older children, lactose intolerance may be diagnosed on the basis of the history and improvement following a lactose-free diet. In infants the hydrogen-breath test is frequently used. Undigested carbohydrate, such as lactose, in the colon causes gas production by bacteria. Breath samples are analyzed for the amount of hydrogen.

Treatment of lactose intolerance is elimination of many dairy products. In infants soy-based formula can be substituted for cow's milk formula or human milk. Some children are able to tolerate small amounts of lactose (see guidelines in Box 13-6). Since dairy products are a major source of calcium and vitamin D, supplementation of these nutrients is needed to prevent deficiency.

Nursing considerations. Nursing care is similar to the interventions discussed for cow's milk allergy: explaining the dietary restrictions to the family; identifying alternate sources of calcium, such as yogurt and green leafy vegetables, and the need for supplementation; and discussing sources of lactose, especially hidden sources, such as its use as a bulk agent in certain medications. Parents are advised to check with the pharmacist regarding this possibility when obtaining medication.

FEEDING DIFFICULTIES

A number of feeding difficulties can occur during the infant's first year. Minor breast-feeding problems are common and often cause mothers considerable concern and discomfort. Some, such as spitting up, require little more than parental reassurance. Others, such as colic, can tremendously disrupt a family, although the problem resolves spontaneously. Still other disorders, such as rumination, can be fatal, even though there is no organic cause. (See also Feeding Resistance, Chapter 10.)

BREAST-FEEDING PROBLEMS

Many mothers have concerns regarding breast-feeding, and with earlier discharge from postpartum units, common problems, such as engorgement and painful nipples, may occur after the mother is at home. New mothers are often concerned about their milk supply, and excessive anxiety can affect successful lactation. There is increasing evidence that some exclusively breast-fed infants gain weight more slowly than bottle-fed infants, especially after the first 4 to 6 months, but that their growth is adequate (Dewey and others, 1989). However, failure to thrive from insufficient milk supply has been documented in breast-feeding infants (Lawrence, 1989). Observation of growth during the first year is essential, and evidence of delayed growth may necessitate intervention to increase the frequency and amount of breast-feeding and/or the use of supplementation.

NURSING ALERT Provide anticipatory guidance to lactating mothers regarding "growth" or "appetite" spurts that occur at:
3 weeks, 6 weeks, and 3 months.
Encourage more frequent feedings to increase milk production rather than use of supplemental formula or solid foods (Neifert and Seacat, 1986).

The more common breast-feeding problems and their interventions are summarized in Table 13-4. Most of them are easily remedied, provided the mother receives the attention needed to identify the concern. Assessment includes a detailed history of the complaint, examination of the breasts, and observation of breast-feeding (Box 13-7).

Many breast-feeding problems respond rapidly to simple interventions, such as correcting the infant's feeding position. However, the mother needs continual reassurance of success and support that allow her the needed rest and re-

Box 13-7 GUIDELINES FOR OBSERVING THE BREAST-FEEDING COUPLE

Position of mother, her body language, and tension
Position of infant: child's ventral (front) surface should be next to mother's ventral surface with the face directly in front of the breast; the infant cannot swallow if the head has to turn to the breast
Position of mother's hand on breast: using two fingers to compress areola and support breast facilitates infant's ability to grasp areola properly
Position of infant's lips on areola: lips should gently clamp the *entire* areola; lower lip should not be folded in so infant sucks lip
Use of alternate breasts and feeding time on each breast
Technique to break suction: should release suction using fingers between areola and lips; should not pull infant from the breast

Table 13-4 Common breast-feeding problems

PROBLEM	COMMENTS/INTERVENTIONS
Engorgement	Best intervention is prevention with frequent nursing on both breasts for complete emptying of ducts If engorgement occurs, infant is unable to properly grasp the distended areola Interventions: Express manually small amount of milk; electric pump may be beneficial for some Use warm compresses or a warm shower; for severely engorged breasts, cold compresses may be helpful to reduce vascularity Compress areola with fingers to facilitate infant's grasp Use well-fitting nursing brassiere and wear 24 hours a day For excessive discomfort, take aspirin or acetaminophen 30 minutes before feeding
Painful nipples	Most common causes are poor feeding technique, improper care of breasts, excessive moisture from milk leaking If left untreated, discomfort may cause mother to terminate breast-feeding Interventions for care of breasts: Avoid soaps, oils, or self-prescribed treatments Apply small amount of breast milk to areola after feeding and let dry Air nipples as much as possible; use heat (60-watt bulb placed 18 inches away or hair dryer on low setting) Change breastpads frequently Interventions related to feeding: Start the let-down reflex before putting infant to breast Begin nursing with less affected breast, then nurse on affected side Position infant properly at breast; check that entire areola is grasped Change infant's position; use football hold For excessive discomfort, take analgesics 30 minutes before feeding; apply ice to nipples
Let-down reflex	Let-down (ejection) reflex is essential to delivery of milk from alveoli and smaller milk ducts into larger lactiferous ducts and sinuses Controlled primarily by release of prolactin and oxytocin Pain, stress, and anxiety can interfere with reflex Interventions: Provide quiet, relaxing atmosphere for nursing; for example, soothing music, privacy, pillows for positioning, decreased distractions Stroke the breast gently Apply warmth to the breast May need to use oxytocin nasal spray to induce a reflex
Inadequate milk supply	Production of milk depends on supply and demand Rarely is related to organic causes, such as decreased glandular tissue Interventions: Reassure mother that her milk supply is probably adequate and depends on frequent nursing Encourage more frequent nursing (at least six times daily at both breasts) Encourage adequate rest, nutrition, and fluids (increased fluids, however, have not been shown to increase milk production) Avoid use of supplemental formula feedings before breast-feeding is well established to prevent nipple confusion Monitor the infant's growth; in some cases formula supplementation may be indicated; an alternative to bottle-feeding is the use of a supplemental feeding device consisting of a plastic bag or syringe for formula and a thin feeding tube that is placed next to the mother's nipple during nursing

laxation to nurse her infant. Referral to supportive agencies, such as local groups of **La Leche League,*** or a lactation specialist, may be beneficial.

REGURGITATION AND "SPITTING UP"

The return of small amounts of food after a feeding is a common occurrence during infancy. It should not be confused with actual vomiting, which can be associated with a number of disturbances that may be insignificant or serious. It is usually benign, although persistent regurgitation necessitates medical evaluation to rule out gastroesophageal reflux. For clarification the following terms are defined:

Regurgitation—return of undigested food from the stomach, usually accompanied by burping
Spitting up—dribbling of unswallowed formula from the infant's mouth immediately after a feeding

The insignificance of regurgitation or spitting up should be explained to parents, especially to those who are unduly concerned about it. It can be reduced by some simple mea-

*For information call (800) LA-LECHE.

NURSING TIP: BURPING THE INFANT

To check if an infant has burped, place one hand on the infant's abdomen and the other hand on the back and gently jiggle the child. If a splashing sound is not heard, the infant has burped (Temple and Farley, 1983).

sures, such as frequent burping during and after feeding (see Nursing Tip), minimum handling at feeding and after, and positioning the child on the right side with the head slightly elevated after feeding. The inconvenience of spitting up can be managed with the use of absorbent bibs on the infant and protective cloths on the parent.

Sometimes frequent dribbling of formula causes excoriation of the corners of the mouth, chin, and neck. Keeping the area dry promotes healing but can be difficult to maintain. Helpful suggestions include applying a thin film of petrolatum or A and D ointment to the affected areas after cleansing and using absorbent nonplastic-lined terry-cloth bibs, which are changed frequently.

PAROXYSMAL ABDOMINAL PAIN (COLIC)

Colic is generally described as paroxysmal abdominal pain or cramping that is manifested by loud crying and drawing the legs up to the abdomen. Other definitions include variables such as duration of cry greater than 3 hours a day and parental dissatisfaction with the child's behavior. It is more common in young infants under the age of 3 months than in older infants, and infants with "difficult" temperaments are more likely to be colicky (Barr and others, 1989). Despite the obvious behavioral indications of pain, the child tolerates the formula well, gains weight, and thrives.

Many theories have been investigated as potential causative factors but currently no one theory is supported universally. In fact, much controversy exists over the etiology of the condition, and some authorities question if colic merely represents a maturational stage (see Questions and Controversies).

While colic is considered a minor ailment, the presence of a colicky, crying, irritable infant can have an intense emotional impact on parent-child attachment and family relationships. Parents, especially mothers, often relate histories of a daily routine that is laden with feelings of frustration, anger, despair, and helplessness. A vicious cycle ensues in which the parent's own anxiety may be transferred to the infant, further increasing the tension, irritability, and crying.

Therapeutic Management

Management of colic should begin with an investigation of diagnosable causes, such as cow's milk allergy. If a sensitivity to cow's milk is strongly suspected, a trial substitution of another formula, such as a casein hydrolysate (Nutramigen), is warranted. Soy formulas are avoided because of the possibility of sensitivity to soy protein as well. When no specific inciting agent can be found, the supportive measures discussed under Nursing Considerations are employed.

The use of drugs, including sedatives, antispasmodics, antihistamines, and antiflatulents, is sometimes recommended. The most commonly used sedatives are phenobarbitol and hydroxyzine hydrochloride (Atarax). The antispasmodic dicyclomine hydrochloride (Bentyl) is not recommended for infants under 6 months of age because of rare instances of death (Pinyerd and Zipf, 1989).

Nursing Considerations

The initial step in managing colic is to take a thorough, detailed history of the usual daily events. Areas that should be

QUESTIONS AND CONTROVERSIES

What are the causes of colic?

Among the theories that have been investigated as potential causes are too rapid feeding, overeating, swallowing excessive air, improper feeding technique (especially in positioning and burping), and emotional stress or tension between parent and child. While all of these may occur, there is no evidence that one factor is consistently present. Recent research indicates that colic may be a sign of cow's milk allergy or intolerance and that eliminating cow's milk products from the infant's diet and the diet of lactating mothers can reduce the symptoms (Forsyth, 1989; Lothe and Lindberg, 1989; Moore, Robb, and Davidson, 1988). Parental smoking has also been associated with colic and it is hypothesized that gastrointestinal contractions are triggered by olfactory or gustatory stimulation through a vagal reflex mechanism (Said, Patois, and Lellouch, 1984).

Some investigators discount the biologic causes of colic and attribute the problem to parents' ineffective responses to the infant's crying or too little carrying of the infant (Hunziker and Barr, 1986; Taubman, 1984, 1988). It is of interest that the incidence of colic differs markedly among social classes—with more parents from a higher socioeconomic status reporting colic. A possible explanation may be greater acceptance of an infant's crying behavior among lower social groups (Hide and Guyer, 1982). Increase in crying over the first several weeks is normal and is thought to represent maturation of the nervous system. It may be that some parents are particularly sensitive to crying, particularly if it occurs in infants who also demonstrate difficult temperament.

A biologic theory and the interaction theory present two opposing viewpoints, yet each theory has substantial research to support its tenets. To explain this dichotomy, Geertsma and Hyams (1989) propose that colic has multiple causes and that the intensity of cry may be significant in distinguishing between them (previous studies have only considered duration of cry). They found that infants who passed more flatus cried more intensely and inconsolably than infants with less flatus, who cried less intensely and responded to comforting measures. They suggest that the "high-intensity group" may have pain due to organic causes, such as milk sensitivity, and the "lower-intensity group" may have no organic cause but require greater soothing measures than noncolic infants.

stressed include (1) diet of the breast-feeding mother, (2) time of day when attacks occur, (3) relationship of the attacks to feeding time, (4) presence of specific family members during attacks and habits, such as smoking, (5) activity of the mother or usual caregiver before, during, and after the crying, (6) characteristics of the cry (duration, intensity), and (7) measures used to relieve the crying and their effectiveness. Of special emphasis is a careful assessment of the feeding process via *demonstration* by the parent.

If milk sensitivity is suspected, breast-feeding mothers should follow a milk-free diet (see Box 13-3) for a minimum of 5 days in an attempt to reduce symptoms in the infant. Mothers need to be cautioned that some nondairy creamers may contain calcium caseinate, a cow's milk protein. If this approach is helpful, lactating mothers may need calcium supplements to meet the body's requirement. Bottle-fed infants may improve with the same dietary modifications as for the child with cow's milk allergy (see p. 611).

More often than not, no change is required in feeding practices. When no cause can be identified, it is preferable to determine the time of the onset of crying and attempt to manipulate the circumstances associated with it. For example, some infants have episodes of colic around the family's dinner time, when all household members are home and the mother is preoccupied with cooking. The overstimulating, more tense atmosphere may upset the infant. Encouraging someone else to prepare dinner or the mother to prepare dinner earlier in the day and feed the infant in a more quiet area of the house may help reverse the environmental conditions that may have provoked the attack of colic. Other approaches for relieving colic are listed in Parent Guidelines. Parents are encouraged to try as many of them as possible because not all are effective for every infant.*

*A booklet that may be helpful is *Coping with Infant Colic: A Guide for Parents,* available from Ross Laboratories, Columbus, OH.

One of the most important areas of nursing concern is the support of parents during the colic period. It should be stressed that despite the crying and obvious pain, the infant is doing well. Colic disappears spontaneously, usually by 3 months of age, although guarantees should never be given

PARENT GUIDELINES
Relieving Colic

Place infant prone over a covered hot-water bottle, heated towel, or covered heating pad.
Massage abdomen.
Respond immediately to the crying.
Change the infant's position frequently; walk with child's face down with body across the parent's arm and hand under the abdomen applying gentle pressure (Fig. 13-3).
Use a front carrier for transporting the infant; carry infant more frequently.
Swaddle tightly with a soft, stretchy blanket.
Place in a wind-up swing.
Take for car rides or outside for a change in environment.
Use a commercial device in the crib that simulates the vibration and sound of a car ride or plays soothing "noise" or in utero sounds.
Provide smaller, frequent feedings; burp during and after feedings using the shoulder position, and place in an upright seat after feedings.
Introduce a pacifier for added sucking.
In breast-fed infants, have mother avoid all milk products for a trial period.
If household members smoke, avoid smoking near infant; preferably confine smoking activity to outside of home.
If nothing reduces the crying, place infant in crib and allow to cry; periodically hold and comfort child and put down again.

THERAPEUTIC DIALOGUE
Colic

During a routine clinical visit, the nurse is taking a history from the parents of a 2-month-old male infant. While both parents look tired, they have mentioned no concerns until the nurse inquires about the infant's habits.

NURSE: Tell me about the baby's daily habits, such as his routine for feeding, sleeping, awake time, and crying.
MOTHER: He eats about every 4 hours and usually falls asleep after each meal except at dinner. Then he decides it is time to cry and cry and cry.
NURSE: He cries a lot at this time of the day?
FATHER: That's an understatement. Quite frankly, we are at the point where we don't know what to do. Some friends have told us this is colic and not to worry, but just try to live with a screaming baby!
NURSE: It sounds like it has been a difficult time.
MOTHER: Yes. My husband says he hates to come home after work, and yet I cannot wait for him to walk in the door to take the baby for a little while. Is this colic, or are we doing something wrong?
NURSE: From what you have told me about the baby's vigorous eating and good weight gain, I think it is colic. Tell me about your thoughts regarding doing something wrong.
FATHER: This is our first child, and we know we have a lot to learn. But when nothing you do comforts your child, you cannot help feeling inadequate as a parent.
NURSE: Your feelings are so understandable and typical of parents with a colicky infant. Let's talk more about what you have tried and some things that may help you survive this temporary misery.
MOTHER: Just hearing you say that the colic is temporary and other parents feel the way we do is helpful.

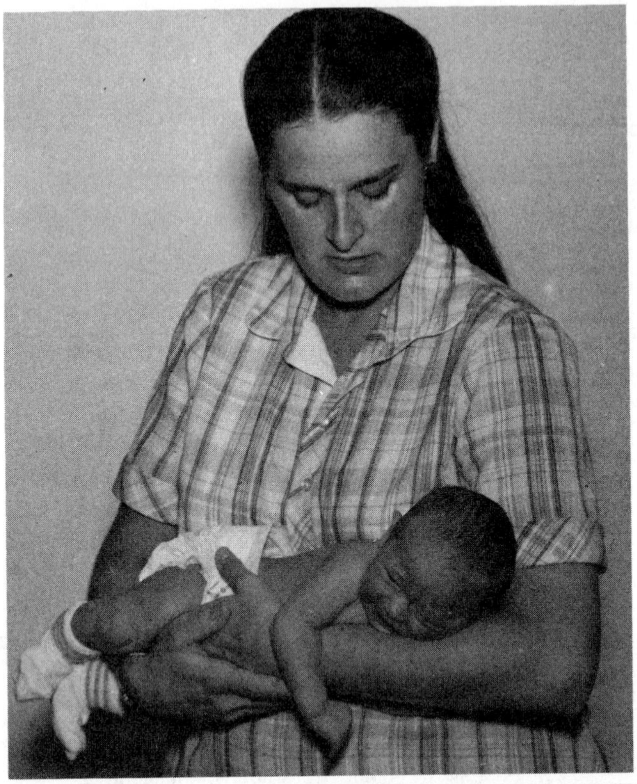

Fig. 13-3. The "colic carry" may be comforting to an infant with colic.

because it may continue for much longer. The parent, especially the mother, should be encouraged to leave the house and arrange for some free time. Most important, it should be emphasized that colic does not indicate poor or inadequate parenting. Parents' negative feelings toward the infant and insecurities regarding their parenting abilities are normal. Parents are encouraged to talk about such feelings, since active listening may do more to relieve the colic syndrome than offering stereotyped advice, remedies, and glib statements such as, "Don't worry about it; your child will eventually outgrow the colicky spells." (See Therapeutic Dialogue, p. 615.)

RUMINATION

Rumination is the active, voluntary return of swallowed food into the mouth. The food is then rechewed, partially or completely reswallowed, or expelled. Technically, this is not a feeding problem since infant ruminators usually have hearty appetites. However, in some instances rumination may lead to progressive malnutrition and even death, since considerable food and fluid loss can occur.

Rumination differs from regurgitation, which is involuntary. The ruminating infant makes purposeful movements of the mouth, tongue, and stomach in an attempt to force food back into the oropharynx. On successful regurgitation the infant is obviously satisfied with the activity.

Organic causes for rumination are rarely found, although the possibility of gastroesophageal reflux should be investigated in the differential diagnosis. It may also be seen in profoundly retarded children. However it is most often considered a result of a disturbed parent-child relationship. The factors culminating in the disorder may be similar to those described in nonorganic failure to thrive. Some authorities believe rumination is a conditioned behavioral response to an increased need for self-stimulation or parental attention (Linscheid, 1985).

Treatment typically involves psychotherapy to improve parenting ability or behavior modification techniques to modify eating patterns. Behavioral approaches vary, but may include increased attention, such as holding before, during, and after meals, or the use of time-out (Whitehead and others, 1985).

Nursing Considerations

The primary objective is to terminate the ruminating behavior and restore normal feeding patterns. This is accomplished through a structured feeding plan. Generally the same guidelines apply to feeding the ruminating child as apply to feeding the failure-to-thrive child (see p. 621). In addition, emphasis should be placed on the following areas:

1. Have the same person feed the child as often as possible. This is even more critical than in failure to thrive.
2. Continue *positive* attention immediately after the feeding, since ruminating infants often vomit after a feeding once they are left unattended.
3. Introduce new foods, with emphasis on texture, consistency, and flavor. These children are often "picky eaters," and new foods introduced too quickly can increase rumination.
4. If acceptance of solids is a problem, give the child a small quantity of milk (or juice), immediately followed by 1 teaspoon of solid food. Begin with pureed food and, once accepted, advance to junior and adult foods. Gradually give fewer sips of milk and more spoonfuls of food until a regular diet for the child's age is achieved.

These children may require prolonged inpatient intervention to reduce their rumination. Positive stimulation programs must accompany the feeding plan, since loneliness has been known to trigger ruminating episodes (Fleisher, 1979). Parents need to be included in learning how to feed the child, and follow-up after discharge is essential to prevent a recurrence of the behavior.

FAILURE TO THRIVE

The term *failure to thrive (FTT)* refers to a state of inadequate growth from inability to obtain and/or use calories required for growth. It is a symptom, not a disease, but regardless of the etiology, all children have malnutrition (see discussion of PEM, p. 607). Failure to thrive has no universal definition, although one of the more common parameters is a weight and sometimes height that fall below the 5th percentile for the child's age. Some authorities use the 3rd percentile as a criterion, but the widely used National Center for Health Statistics growth charts include only the 5th, not the 3rd, percentile in their measurements. Growth measurements alone are not used to diagnose children with FTT. Rather, the finding of a persistent deviation from an established growth curve is cause for concern.

Three general categories of failure to thrive have been defined:

Organic failure to thrive (OFTT), which is the result of a physical cause, such as congenital heart defects, neurologic lesions, microcephaly, chronic urinary tract infection, gastroesophageal reflux, renal insufficiency, malabsorption syndrome, endocrine dysfunction, or cystic fibrosis. This category accounts for less than half of all FTT.

Nonorganic failure to thrive (NFTT), which has a definable cause that is unrelated to disease. NFTT is most often the result of psychosocial factors, such as inadequate nutritional information by the parent; deficiency in maternal care or a disturbance in maternal-child attachment; or a disturbance in the child's ability to separate from the parent, leading to food refusal to maintain attention (Chatoor and others, 1985). NFTT has been described under a variety of less acceptable names, including maternal deprivation, environmental deprivation, and deprivation dwarfism.

Idiopathic failure to thrive, which is unexplained by the usual organic and environmental etiologies but may also be classified as NFTT. Both categories of NFTT account for the majority of cases of FTT.

Traditionally the category of NFTT has implied a disturbance in the parent-child interaction. However, this is not always the case. Many other factors can lead to inadequate feeding of the infant (Box 13-8). In these instances parent education and provision of necessary supports (financial or psychosocial) are successful in correcting the reason for the malnutrition. Dealing with families in which a child has NFTT because of a parent-child disturbance is much more difficult and is the focus of the nursing care discussion on p. 618.

Box 13-8 SELECTED CAUSES OF NFTT USUALLY UNRELATED TO DISTURBED PARENT-CHILD INTERACTIONS

Poverty—lack of funds to buy sufficient food; may dilute formula to extend available supply

Health beliefs—use of fad diets; excessive concern with preventing conditions such as obesity, hypercholesterolemia, or nursing caries

Inadequate nutritional knowledge—cultural confusion of newly arrived immigrants who are unaware of appropriate food selections in American markets; parents with cognitive impairment

Family stress—overwhelming involvement with another chronically ill child; lack of energy to deal with feeding problems in addition to other needs of child with OFTT; any number of other stresses (financial, marital, excessive parenting and employment responsibilities, depression, chemical abuse, acute grief)

Feeding resistance—result of nonoral nutritional therapy early in life (see Feeding Resistance, Chapter 10)

Insufficient breast milk—result of a number of different causes (fatigue, illness, poor release of milk, insufficient glandular tissue, lack of confidence)

References: Callaran and Hiner, 1987; Frank and Zeisel, 1988; Lansky and others, 1982; Lawrence, 1989; Lifshitz and Moses, 1989; McJunkin, Bithoney, and McCormick, 1987; Pugliese and others, 1987.

Diagnostic Evaluation

Diagnosis is initially made on anthropomorphic findings documenting growth retardation. If FTT is recent, the weight, but not the height, is below accepted standards (usually the 5th percentile); if FTT is long-standing, both weight and height are depressed, indicating chronic malnutrition (Frank and Zeisel, 1988).

Additional diagnostic procedures include a dietary history; a complete history and physical examination for signs of serious chronic illness or other conditions known to cause growth retardation, such as lead poisoning (Bithoney, 1986); developmental assessment; and a family assessment. Other tests are selected only as indicated to rule out organic problems. Unfortunately, many of these children undergo exhausting, traumatic, and expensive diagnostic procedures that are unnecessary. To prevent the overuse of diagnostic procedures, NFTT should be considered *early* in the differential diagnosis.

Therapeutic Management

Regardless of the cause of FTT, the treatment is directed at reversing the malnutrition. The goal is to provide sufficient calories to support "catch-up" growth—a rate of growth greater than the expected rate for age. Depending on the severity of the malnutrition, the approaches used for PEM may be instituted (see p. 608). Any coexisting medical problems, such as lead poisoning, are treated.

In cases of NFTT due to a disturbed parent-child relationship, a multidisciplinary team of physician, nurse, dietitian, child-life specialist, and social worker or mental health professional is needed to deal with the multiple psychologic problems. Efforts are made to relieve any additional stresses on the family, such as referrals to welfare agencies or supplemental food programs (Women, Infants, and Children [WIC]).

Prognosis

The prognosis for NFTT is related to the cause. If the parents have simply been ignorant of the infant's needs, teaching may remedy the child's limited caloric intake and permanently reverse the growth failure. However, when the family dysfunction is extensive, the prognosis is uncertain. Factors related to poor prognosis are severe feeding resistance, lack of awareness in and cooperation from the parent(s), low family income, low maternal educational level, and early age of onset of NFTT (Ayoub and Milner, 1985; Drotar and Sturm, 1988). Many of these children are below normal in intellectual development, have poorer language development and less well-developed reading skills, attain lower social maturity, and have a higher incidence of behavioral disturbances (Oates, Peacock, and Forrest, 1985). Such findings indicate that a long-term plan is needed for the optimum development of these children.

Nursing Considerations

Caring for the child with NFTT presents many nursing challenges, both when treatment takes place in the hospital or home. Providing a positive feeding environment, teaching the parent successful feeding strategies, and supporting the child and family are essential components of care.

Assessment

Nurses play a critical role in the diagnosis of NFTT through their assessment of the child, parents, and family interaction. Knowledge of the characteristics of children with NFTT and their families is essential in helping identify these children and hastening the confirmation of a correct diagnosis (Box 13-9). Accurate assessment of initial weight and height and daily weight is mandatory, as well as recording of all food intake. The feeding behavior of the child is documented, as well as the parent-child interaction during feeding, other caregiving activities, and play.

An excellent feeding observation instrument is the Nursing Child Assessment Feeding Scale (NCAFS), which is designed to assess the feeding interaction of infants up to 12 months of age (Barnard and others, 1989).* (See also Nutritional Assessment, Chapter 6.) The approximate developmental age should be assessed on admission by administering an appropriate developmental test. Only after objective measurements are available is a plan of care for stimulation outlined.

The nursing admission history and ongoing assessment should also focus on the following characteristics that have been identified in many of these children and their parents.

The child. Besides the obvious signs of malnutrition and delayed development, children with NFTT may interact differently from children with OFTT (Box 13-9). They display intense interest in inanimate objects, such as a toy, but much less interest in social interactions. They are vigilant of people at a distance but become increasingly distressed as they come closer. They dislike being touched or held and avoid face-to-face contact. However, when held, they protest briefly on being put down and are apathetic when left alone.

Frequently there is a history of difficult feeding, vomiting, sleep disturbance, and excessive irritability. Difficulties in infant feeding may include poor appetite, poor suck, crying during feedings, vomiting, hoarding food in the mouth, ruminating after feeding, refusal to switch from liquids to solids, and aversion behavior such as turning from food or spitting food. Ultimately these habit patterns become attention-seeking mechanisms to prolong the attention received at mealtime. In addition, chronic reduction in calories can lead to appetite depression, which compounds the problem.

An outstanding feature of children with NFTT is their irregularity (low rhythmicity) in activities of daily living. Some of these children typify the "difficult" temperament pattern. However, another type is the passive, sleepy, lethargic infants who do not wake up for feedings. Parents who have been advised of "demand feeding schedules" may be unsure of whether to wake the child or let the child sleep. Because of their inexperience and lack of guidance, parents may develop a pattern of infrequent feeding that is inadequate to meet the infant's nutritional needs. Such a pattern is particularly detrimental with the breast-feeding infant, in whom frequent nursing is essential to an adequate milk supply.

It cannot be assumed that such characteristics in a child result in NFTT. Rather, there is probably a complex set of variables that are significant. One may be the degree of *fit* between the child's temperament and that of the parents. Since the personalities of infants can have definite effects on the parent-child attachment process, identifying such situations of disharmony may be one approach toward prevention and anticipatory guidance.

The parents. Some parents are at increased risk for attachment problems because of (1) isolation and social crisis, (2) inadequate support systems, and (3) poor parenting as a child. Other factors that should be considered are lack of education; physical and mental health problems, such as retardation, depression, or drug dependence; immaturity, especially in adolescent parents; and lack of commitment to parenting, such as giving higher priority to career goals.

Frequently these parents and their families are under stress and in multiple chronic emotional, social, and financial crises. Of particular significance is the prevalence of marital discord, including frequent arguments, separations, and reconciliations (Altemeier and others, 1985).

Many of these parents display negative maladaptive feelings toward the infant (Box 13-10). Inadequate feeding and caregiving may be part of an abuse cycle. Ambivalence toward pregnancy can be an early clue when combined with other characteristics of high-risk parents. Being alert to such clues may avert a potential NFTT situation by identifying these parents prenatally and planning interventions aimed at increasing satisfying parenting skills.

*Training is required to use the NCAFS, and information on the training program is available from Georgina Sumner, Director, NCAST, WJ-10, University of Washington, Seattle, WA 98195; (206) 543-8526.

Box 13-9 CLINICAL MANIFESTATIONS OF NONORGANIC FAILURE TO THRIVE

- Growth failure—below 5th percentile in weight only or weight and height
- Developmental retardation—social, motor, adaptive, language
- Apathy
- Poor hygiene
- Withdrawn behavior
- Feeding or eating disorders, such as vomiting, anorexia, pica, rumination
- No fear of strangers (at age when stranger anxiety is normal)
- Avoidance of eye-to-eye contact
- Wide-eyed gaze and continual scan of the environment ("radar gaze")
- Stiff and unyielding or flaccid and unresponsive
- Minimum smiling

Box 13-10 PARENTAL MALADAPTIVE BEHAVIORS TOWARD INFANT

Persistent ambivalence or negative feelings about the fetus and the pregnancy during the prenatal period
Makes no plans for obtaining basic infant supplies
Appears indifferent to infant at time of delivery; may appear sad or angry; is expressionless
Makes no effort to establish eye-to-eye contact with infant
Handles infant only when necessary
Does not talk to infant
Makes few or no spontaneous movements with infant
Asks few questions about care
Sees infant as ugly, fat, or unattractive
Displays disgust with infant's drooling and sucking sounds; is revolted by infant's body fluids
Annoyed with diaper changing
Perceives infant's odor as revolting
Holds infant with little support to head and body
Holds infant away from body during feeding or props bottle for feeding; seldom cuddles infant
Does not coo or talk to infant
Refers to infant in an impersonal manner
Develops inappropriate responses to infant's needs, such as leaving infant in one place for long periods, leaving child alone in room, overfeeding or underfeeding, overstimulating or understimulating infant, forcing or refusing eye contact, bouncing or tickling infant when child is fatigued
Cannot discriminate between infant's signals for hunger, comfort, rest, body contact
Is convinced the infant has a defect or disease even when reassured to the contrary
Makes negative statements regarding parenting role
Believes the infant is judging him/her and efforts as an adult
Believes the infant does not love him/her
Develops paradoxical attitudes and behaviors toward the infant

Nursing Diagnoses

A number of nursing diagnoses are prominent in the nursing care of the child with NFTT. The most common nursing diagnoses are outlined in the Nursing Care Plan on p. 620. If an organic cause is found, additional nursing diagnoses may be related to care specific for that disorder, such as heart disease.

Planning

Planning needs to begin as soon as possible on admission. The priority nursing goal is providing the infant with sufficient nutrients for growth. More specific nursing care depends on the identified cause of FTT. If an organic etiology is confirmed, care is related primarily to management of the disorder. If the problem is one of inadequate knowledge regarding child feeding, parental education is required. When serious psychosocial factors are involved, hospitalization is needed and additional interventions are required to meet the needs of both the child and family. The following are goals for the hospitalized child with NFTT:

1. Structure a feeding environment that encourages the child to consume adequate calories; provide age-appropriate foods.
2. Provide appropriate developmental stimulation for the child.
3. Teach parents feeding techniques and other caregiving activities, such as suitable play, that are successful in the hospital.
4. Provide a nurturing environment for the parent; make appropriate referrals for supportive services.

Implementation

Since part of the difficulty between parent and child is dissatisfaction and frustration, the child should have a consistent primary nurse for all three shifts (Fig. 13-4). Only the same nurse caring for the child over a period of time can learn to perceive the child's cues and reverse the cycle of dissatisfaction, especially in the area of feeding. Since these children are not ill with any physical disorder but debilitated from general malnutrition, they should be placed in a room with noninfectious children of a similar age.

Since many of these children are responding to stimuli that have led to the negative feeding patterns, the first goal is to structure the feeding environment to encourage eating. Initially staff members may need to feed these children to assess thoroughly the difficulties encountered during the feeding process and to devise strategies that eliminate or minimize such problems. General guidelines for the feeding process are outlined in Box 13-11.

Foods appropriate to the child's age are selected. To increase caloric intake, supplements, such as Polycose or powdered milk, can be added to foods, and powdered commercial formula can be prepared to yield 24 cal/oz, rather than 20 cal/oz. Often, these children have been exclusively bottle-fed and refuse all solids. In these situations, introduction of solids begins with pureed foods, then junior foods, finger foods, and finally regular table food.

Besides attending to the physical needs of the child, the nurse must plan care for appropriate developmental stimulation. The word "appropriate" is emphasized because it refers to the child's developmental, not chronologic, age. Once an approximate developmental age is established, a planned program of play is instituted. Ideally a child life specialist should be involved to implement and supervise the stimulation program. Every effort is made to teach the parent how to play and interact with the child.

Nursing care of these children involves a "systems" approach. In other words, for the entire family to become healthy, each member must be helped to change. To nurture the child back to physical, developmental, and emotional health during hospitalization while neglecting the emotional needs of the parents does not solve the problem. Therefore, nursing care must also be directed to the parents and siblings. Other significant persons, who can be helped to be more emotionally, physically, and financially supportive to the family unit, can become the emotional reservoir needed by parents to nurture their child. Some hospitals have special programs, such as volunteer foster grandparents. They spend scheduled, consistent periods of time with the infant as a kind of surrogate parent. Mental health services, such as individual or group therapy, may also be beneficial.

NURSING CARE PLAN
The Child with Nonorganic Failure to Thrive

NURSING DIAGNOSIS: Altered nutrition: less than body requirements related to deprivation of necessities, emotional deprivation

GOAL 1

Make feeding a priority goal

INTERVENTIONS

Provide unlimited feedings of a regular diet for the age of the child (preferably foods to which the child is accustomed)
Avoid interruption of feedings with other activities, such as laboratory examinations or radiography
Keep accurate record of intake to ensure ingestion of calculated daily calories
Weigh daily and record to ascertain weight gain

EXPECTED OUTCOME

Child gains 1 to 2 ounces per day (minimum)

GOAL 2

Introduce a positive feeding environment

INTERVENTIONS

Assign one nurse for feeding
Maintain calm, even temperament; be persistent
Provide a quiet, unstimulating environment
Hold young child for feeding
Maintain eye-to-eye contact with child
Talk to child by giving appropriate directions and praise for eating
Follow the child's rhythm of feeding
Establish a structural routine and follow it consistently

EXPECTED OUTCOME

Infant responds positively to feeding practices (specify)

NURSING DIAGNOSIS: Altered growth and development related to socially restricted environment (infant deprivation), physical neglect

GOAL 1

Provide a nurturing environment for the hospitalized child

INTERVENTIONS

Apply primary care concepts to ensure continuity of care with a minimum number of caregivers
Provide gentle, confident, and loving handling
Perform physical care with as much holding, rocking, and cuddling as the child will respond to
Encourage eye-to-eye contact
Employ consistent schedule in meeting child's needs for food, hygiene, care, and rest
Assign a foster grandparent or child life specialist to child
Provide sensory stimulation and play appropriate to the child's developmental level

EXPECTED OUTCOME

Child displays a positive response to interventions (e.g., social smile)

NURSING DIAGNOSIS: Altered parenting related to (specify, e.g., knowledge deficit, poverty)

GOAL 1

Reduce parental anxiety and provide education

INTERVENTIONS

Welcome parents and encourage, but do not pressure, them to become involved in the child's care
Teach parents about the child's physical care, developmental skills, and emotional needs through example, not lecture
Afford parents the opportunity to discuss their lives and feelings toward the child
Supply emotional nurturance without encouraging dependency
Promote parents' self-esteem and confidence by praising their achievements with the child
Prepare parents for adjustments with anticipatory guidance

EXPECTED OUTCOME

Parents demonstrate the ability to provide appropriate care to the child

GOAL 2

Prepare for discharge

INTERVENTIONS

Assess home environment and relationships
Continue interventions begun in the hospital
Establish a consistent contact system through public health nurse
Establish an infant stimulation program
Provide for stress-relieving services to the family
Refer to appropriate agencies for assistance with financial, social, mental health, or other family needs

EXPECTED OUTCOMES

Child exhibits continued weight gain appropriate for age
Family follows through on programs and activities

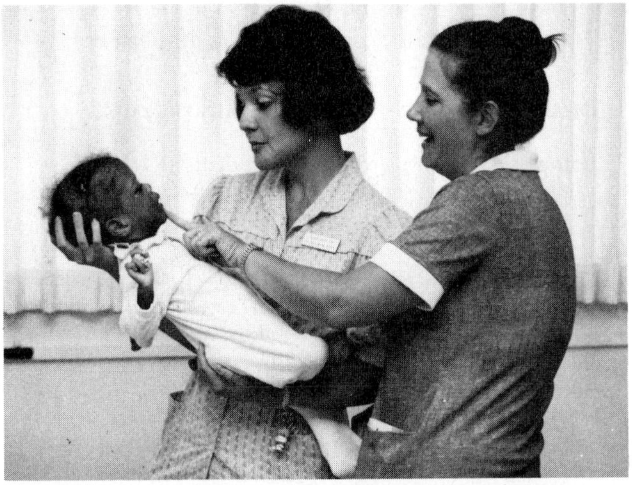

Fig. 13-4. A consistent core of nurses is important in developing trust with infants with nonorganic failure to thrive.

Box 13-11 GUIDELINES FOR FEEDING CHILDREN WITH NONORGANIC FAILURE TO THRIVE

Provide a quiet, unstimulating atmosphere. A number of these children are very distractible, and their attention is diverted with minimal stimuli. Older children do well at a feeding table; younger children should always be held. A single adult in the feeding situation is recommended.

Maintain a calm, even temperament throughout the meal. Negative outbursts may be commonplace in this child's habit formation. Limits on eating behavior definitely need to be provided, but they should be stated in a firm, calm tone. If the nurse is hurried or anxious, the feeding process will not be optimized.

Talk to the child by giving directions about eating. "Take a bite, Lisa" is appropriate and directive. The more distractible the child, the more directive the nurse should be to refocus attention on feeding. Positive comments about feeding are actively given.

Follow the child's rhythm of feeding. The child will set a rhythm when the previous conditions are met.

Develop a structured routine. NFTT children are in particular need of routine feeding patterns. Disruption in their other activities of daily living has great impact on feeding responses, so these should be structured also. The same nurse should feed the child in the same way and place as often as possible. The length of the feeding should also be established (usually 30 minutes).

Be persistent. This is perhaps one of the most important guidelines. Parents often give up when the child begins negative feeding behavior. Calm perseverance through 10 to 15 minutes of food refusal will eventually diminish negative behavior. Although forced feeding is avoided, "strictly encouraged" feeding is essential.

Maintain a face-to-face posture with the child when possible. Encourage eye contact and remain with the child throughout the meal.

Care of the parents is aimed at helping them increase their feelings of self-esteem through positive, successful parenting skills. Initially this necessitates providing an environment in which they feel welcomed and accepted. Because these parents are often distrustful of authority figures, it may take some time before they develop any trust toward the nurse. One approach is to empathize with the parent about the difficulties of childrearing. For example, the nurse may state that many parents find adjusting to parenthood a trying time or that the demands of caring for an infant can become overwhelming.

Once the parents feel comfortable enough to visit with their infant, teaching infant care techniques is begun through *example* and *demonstration,* not by lecturing. As the nurse perceives the infant's cues, these are emphasized to the parents. For example, during a feeding the nurse might comment that the infant is still hungry because the child sucks vigorously and looks at the nurse. When the infant is satisfied, the nurse points out that the infant is signaling this by releasing the strong suck, closing the eyes, and breathing deeply and more slowly. By example, the child is gently placed in the crib for a nap.

At the same time the parents are offered an opportunity to care for the infant without making demands on them. For example, the nurse suggests that at the next feeding one of the parents offer the child the bottle. Whenever the parents participate, they are praised for their efforts and encouraged to continue caring for the child.

Before discharge, plans are made to continue these interventions at home. A public health referral is made, and if a foster grandparent was included, this person should also visit the family. Social agencies that can provide financial or housing assistance to lessen the stress of everyday life are also contacted.

Evaluation

The effectiveness of nursing interventions is determined by continual reassessment and evaluation of care based on the following observational guidelines and expected outcomes:

1. Record weight and calorie intake daily; document child's reaction to feeding environment; review notes to see if changes were made as necessary to improve eating and if consistent group of nurses fed child.
2. Perform periodic developmental screening tests.
3. Document parents' relationship with staff or other supportive individuals. Note length of time parents visit with these people, appointments kept with referral services, and any requests for help.
4. Keep a record of all teaching and compare taught skills with parent's actual skills.

Expected outcomes:
See Nursing Care Plan, p. 620.

SKIN DISORDERS

A number of skin problems manifest themselves during infancy. The most common is diaper dermatitis; others that occur during infancy are seborrheic dermatitis and atopic dermatitis. While these conditions can be benign, they are often of considerable concern to parents. The nurse is in an advantageous position to counsel parents regarding care of these common skin problems.

DIAPER DERMATITIS

Dermatitis in the diaper area is encountered frequently by nurses in all pediatric settings. Approximately 50% of young children demonstrate some degree of diaper dermatitis, and about 5% have severe rash (intense erythema, scaling, papules, and ulcerations). The peak age for diaper dermatitis is 9 to 12 months and may be associated with decreased frequency of diaper changes and modifications in diet, such as change from breast milk to formula and introduction of solids. The incidence is generally reported as greater in bottle-fed than in breast-fed infants (Jordan and others, 1986), although other studies report no difference (Austin and others, 1988; Lane, Rehder, and Helm, 1990).

Pathophysiology and Clinical Manifestations

Diaper dermatitis is caused by prolonged and repetitive contact with an irritant, principally urine, feces, soaps, detergents, ointments, and friction. Although the obvious irritant in the majority of incidences is urine and feces, the specific components that contribute to irritation include a combination of factors (Fig. 13-5).

Prolonged contact of the skin with diaper wetness affects several skin properties. It produces higher friction, greater abrasion damage, increased transepidermal permeability, and increased microbial counts (Zimmerer, Lawson, and Calvert, 1986). Therefore healthy skin becomes less resistant to potential irritants.

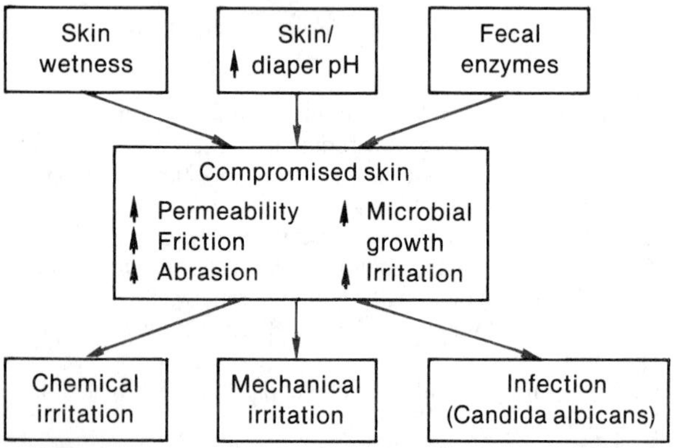

Fig. 13-5. Principal factors involved in development of diaper dermatitis.

Modified from a model developed by L. Benjamin, R.W. Berg, W.E. Jordan, A.M. Marrer, and R.E. Zimmerer. Reproduced with permission of the Procter & Gamble Co.

Table 13-5 Skin eruptions in the diaper area

AREA INVOLVED	USUAL DIAGNOSIS/CAUSE
Convex surfaces involved; folds spared	Contact dermatitis Allergic or irritant dermatitis/ chemical irritants (urine, feces, detergents, soaps)
Folds involved, sharply demarcated	Intertrigo/heat, moisture, and sweat retention Seborrheic dermatitis/inborn trait
Folds involved with satellite lesions	Seborrheic dermatitis with secondary candidiasis/ inborn trait plus *Candida albicans* infection
Perianal	Chemical and mechanical irritation/chemical irritants (fecal enzymes)
Perianal with satellite lesions	Primary candidiasis/*C. albicans* infection
Band of erythema at diaper margins	"Tide mark" dermatitis/plastic or rubber border on diaper and sweat retention
Small, sterile vesicopustules	Miliaria "Heat rash," "prickly heat"/hot, humid climate in diaper area
Vesicles or bullae	Bullous impetigo/usually *Staphylococcus aureus* or combined with streptococcus Herpes (less common)/herpes simplex

Modified from Jacobs, A.H.: Eruptions in the diaper area, Pediatr. Clin. North Am. 25(2):209-224, 1978.

While ammonia has long been thought to cause diaper rash because of the association between the strong odor on diapers and dermatitis, ammonia alone is not sufficient. The important function of urine is related to an increase in pH from the breakdown of urea in the presence of fecal urease. The increased pH promotes the activity of fecal enzymes, principally proteases and lipases, which act as irritants. Fecal enzymes also increase the permeability of skin to bile salts, another potential irritant in feces. The decreased incidence of diaper dermatitis in breast-fed infants is felt to be related to this interaction between pH and fecal enzymes, since feces from breast-fed infants have lower fecal enzyme activity and lower pH (Berg, Buckingham, and Steward, 1986; Buckingham and Berg, 1986).

The eruption of diaper dermatitis can be manifested primarily on convex surfaces or in the folds, and the lesions can represent a variety of types and configurations (Table 13-5). Eruptions involving the skin in most intimate contact with the diaper (e.g., the convex surfaces of buttocks, inner thighs, mons pubis, and scrotum) but sparing the folds are likely to be caused by chemical irritants, especially from urine and feces (see Color Plate 14). Other causes are detergents or soaps from inadequately rinsed cloth diapers or the fragrance added to some diapers or disposable wipes.

Perianal involvement is usually the result of chemical irritation from feces, especially diarrheal stools. *Candida albicans* infection produces perianal inflammation with satellite lesions (see Color Plate 15). Whether *C. albicans* initiates or aggravates diaper dermatitis is not known. Risk factors for development of *Candida* infection are an altered immune status and antibiotic therapy (Honig and others, 1988).

Therapeutic Management

Treatment is primarily related to the measures discussed under Nursing Considerations. For stubborn inflammations that do not respond to these interventions, topical glucocorticoid preparations are sometimes required. If steroids are prescribed, their use is generally limited to low-potency preparations such as 1% hydrocortisone cream. Potent fluorinated steroids are avoided because of the potential side effects of striae, epidermal atrophy, suppression of the pituitary-adrenal axis, cessation of longitudinal growth, and frank Cushing syndrome from chronic use. The common use of triamcinolone-containing preparations combined with antiyeast and antibacterial agents such as Mycolog is not recommended, because all of the ingredients may not be needed and certain agents can cause a contact dermatitis (Liptak, 1987).

Candida infections are treated with nystatin ointment. Where *Candida* is the causative agent, oral administration of a fungicide is advised because the gastrointestinal tract is usually the source of infection (see Candidiasis, Chapter 9).

Nursing Considerations

Nursing interventions are aimed at altering the three factors considered to produce dermatitis—wetness, pH, and fecal irritants. The most significant factor amenable to intervention is the moist environment created in the diaper area. Changing the diaper as soon as it becomes wet eliminates a large part of the problem, and removing the diaper entirely for extended periods to expose the area to light and air facilitates drying and healing. Occlusive diaper coverings, such as plastic pants, prevent evaporation and should not be used except for brief social occasions. During the nighttime the diaper should be changed at least once, such as before the parents retire. Double diapering (the use of two cotton or disposable diapers *without* the plastic lining) or the use of disposable diapers with absorbent gelling material (AGM) increases absorbency, and diapers with AGM draw wetness away from the skin.

After soiling, the perineal area should be cleansed, preferably with plain water and, if needed, a mild soap. Wiping with a wet cloth is usually sufficient to remove urine. However, after stooling, the area, especially the skin folds, needs to be thoroughly cleansed, rinsed, and dried. In some instances, especially with diarrheal stools and irritated skin, a sponge bath may be given. Exposing the skin to warm, dry air for a few minutes before applying the diaper is helpful (see Nursing Tip). Parents are advised that the use of disposable wet "wipes" can aggravate the dermatitis because the child may be sensitive to one or more agents in the product.

Occasionally applying an occlusive ointment, such as zinc oxide or petrolatum, to noninflamed skin can prevent the development of diaper dermatitis, provided good hygiene is also practiced. During cleansing, the ointment is removed and then reapplied. Zinc oxide is most easily removed with mineral oil. These ointments are not usually applied to inflamed areas, because they tend to contribute to sweat retention. The use of talcum powder is of questionable benefit and poses the hazard of accidental aspiration (see Questions and Controversies). Despite the known risks of talc, it is a common baby care product. The majority of

NURSING TIP: DRYING THE SKIN

After towel drying the skin, use a hair dryer set on the cool or low setting for a few minutes to thoroughly dry the diaper area.

QUESTIONS AND CONTROVERSIES

What are the benefits and risks of talc vs cornstarch?

Talc and cornstarch are common ingredients in baby powders, and the majority of parents routinely use such products to keep the diapered area dry, to make the baby smell nice, and to prevent or treat diaper rash (Hayden and Sproul, 1984). However there is considerable concern with the safety of using talc and cornstarch and controversy regarding their benefits.

Talc is a soft, flexible, crystalline magnesium-silicate that is chemically related to several asbestos group minerals (Lockey and Parry, 1984). Mined talc is seldom pure and may contain several other mineral fibers, including asbestos. Epidemiologic studies have clearly linked lung cancer and other pleural disorders to asbestos exposure, including the amount found in talc. There is also evidence that talc may be linked to ovarian cancer (Cramer and others, 1982). However, the greatest risk among young children is aspiration pneumonia from accidental inhalation (see Aspiration of Foreign Objects, Chapter 12).

Cornstarch is an absorbable starch. Unlike talc, it is not associated with pulmonary complications. However, traditionally it has been assumed that cornstarch promotes the growth of *Candida albicans.* A study comparing cornstarch and talc found that neither product supports growth of the fungi under conditions normally found in the diaper area (Leyden, 1984).

The benefits of both products are related to their ability to absorb moisture and reduce friction. Cornstarch is somewhat more effective in reducing friction and tends to cake less than talc when the skin is wet (Leyden, 1984). Based on these properties and its safety in terms of inhalation injury, cornstarch is the preferred product if the parents choose to apply a powder.

parents are likely to receive a free sample of the product in the nursery and to continue using that brand (Hayden and Sproul, 1984). While no known research exists to substantiate whether the practice of free talc samples influences the incidence of inhalation injury, nurses have a responsibility to inform parents of the risks and to instruct them in the correct application and safe storage of powders (see Aspiration of Foreign Objects, Chapter 12).

The selection and care of diapers are very important aspects in preventing inflammation or further irritation. There is also evidence that the type of diaper can influence the development of dermatitis (see Questions and Controversies, p. 330).* If diapers are laundered at home, they should be soaked in a quaternary ammonium compound (such as Diaparene) or dilute hypochlorite (bleach), washed in hot water with a simple laundry soap (such as Ivory), and run through the rinse cycle twice.

SEBORRHEIC DERMATITIS

Seborrheic dermatitis is a chronic, recurrent, inflammatory reaction of the skin that occurs most commonly on the scalp (cradle cap), but may involve the eyelids (blepharitis), external ear canal (otitis externa), nasolabial folds, and inguinal region. The cause is unknown, although it is more common in early infancy when sebum production is increased. The lesions are characteristically thick, adherent, yellowish, scaly, oily patches that may or may not be mildly pruritic. If pruritus is present, the infant may be irritable. Unlike atopic dermatitis, seborrheic dermatitis is not associated with a positive family history for allergy and is very common in infants shortly after birth and after puberty. Diagnosis is made primarily by the appearance and location of the crusts or scales.

Nursing Considerations

Cradle cap may be prevented with adequate scalp hygiene. Not infrequently parents omit shampooing the infant's hair from fear of damaging the "soft spots" or fontanels. The nurse should discuss how to shampoo the infant's hair and emphasize that the fontanel is like skin anywhere else on the body—it does not puncture or tear with mild pressure.

When seborrheic lesions are present, the treatment is mainly directed at removing the crusts. Parents are taught the appropriate procedure to clean the scalp, which may necessitate a demonstration. Shampooing should be done daily with a mild soap or commercial baby shampoo; medicated shampoos are not needed. The shampoo is applied to the scalp and allowed to remain on until the crusts are softened, and then the scalp is thoroughly rinsed (Morelli and Weston, 1987). Using a fine-tooth comb or a soft facial brush after shampooing helps remove the loosened crusts from the strands of hair.

*A pamphlet, *Diaper Rash*, which describes the development of diaper rash related to kinds of diapers, is available from the American Academy of Pediatrics, 141 Northwest Point Blvd., P.O. Box 927, Elk Grove Village, IL 60007; (800) 433-9016.

ATOPIC DERMATITIS (ECZEMA)

Eczema or eczematous inflammation of the skin refers to a descriptive category of dermatologic diseases and not to a specific etiology. Atopic dermatitis (AD) is a type of pruritic eczema that usually begins during infancy and is associated with allergy with a hereditary tendency (atopy). AD presents in three forms based on the age of the child and the distribution of lesions:

1. **Infantile (infantile eczema)**—usually begins between 2 and 6 months of age and generally undergoes spontaneous remission by 3 years of age.
2. **Childhood**—may follow the infantile form; it occurs at 2 to 3 years of age, and 90% of the children will manifest the disease by the age 5 years.
3. **Preadolescent and adolescent**—begins at about 12 years of age and may continue into the early adult years or indefinitely.

Because the disease occurs predominantly in infancy, this discussion is restricted to the infantile form of atopic dermatitis.

The diagnosis of AD is based on a combination of history and morphologic findings (Box 13-12). The victims of the disease have a lower threshold for cutaneous itching, and many authorities believe the dermatologic manifestations appear subsequent to scratching of the intense pruritus. For example, infants will rub their faces against bed linen, and crawling (a form of scratching) results in irritation of knees and elbows. Lesions will disappear if the scratching is stopped.

The majority of children with infantile AD have a family history of atopy (eczema, asthma, or allergic rhinitis), which strongly supports a genetic predisposition. The cause is unknown but appears to be related to abnormal function of the skin, including alterations in sweating, peripheral vascular function, and heat tolerance. The disease is better in humid climates and worse in fall and winter, when homes are heated and environmental humidity is lower. The disorder can be controlled but not cured.

Therapeutic Management

The major goals of management are to (1) relieve pruritus, (2) hydrate the skin, (3) reduce inflammation, and (4) prevent or control secondary infection. Most of the general measures for managing AD serve to reduce pruritus as well as other aspects of the disease. General management includes avoiding exposure to skin irritants, avoiding overheating, improving skin hydration, and administration of medications such as antihistamines, topical steroids, and (sometimes) mild sedatives as indicated. There is some evidence that increased doses of vitamin C reduce the severity of AD (Kline as cited by Krowchuk and others, 1990).

Differing philosophies regarding cleansing and hydrating the skin of the child with AD generally embrace two methods—the wet and the dry methods. In the dry method baths are infrequent, and skin is cleansed with a nonlipid, hydrophilic agent such as Cetaphil. The wet method consists of frequent baths (up to 4 times per day) followed immediately by the application of a lubricant (while the skin is still

Box 13-12 CLINICAL MANIFESTATIONS OF ATOPIC DERMATITIS

Distribution of Lesions

Infantile form—generalized, especially cheeks, scalp, trunk, and extensor surfaces of extremities (see Color Plate 11)
Childhood form—flexural areas (antecubital and popliteal fossae, neck), wrists, ankles, and feet
Preadolescent and adolescent form—face, sides of neck, hands, feet, face, and antecubital and popliteal fossae (to a lesser extent)

Appearance of Lesions

Infantile form
- Erythema
- Vesicles
- Papules
- Weeping
- Oozing
- Crusting
- Scaling
- Often symmetric

Childhood form
- Symmetric involvement
- Clusters of small erythematous or flesh-colored papules or minimally scaling patches
- Dry and may be hyperpigmented
- Lichenification (thickened skin with accentuation of creases)
- Keratosis pilaris (follicular hyperkeratosis) common

Adolescent/adult form
- Same as childhood manifestations
- Dry, thick lesions (lichenified plaques) common
- Confluent papules

Other Manifestations

Intense itching
Unaffected skin dry and rough
Black children likely to exhibit more papular and/or follicular lesions than white children
May exhibit one or more of the following:
- Lymphadenopathy, especially near affected sites
- Increased palmar creases (many cases)
- Atopic pleats (extra line or groove of lower eyelid)
- Prone to cold hands
- Pityriasis alba (small, poorly defined areas of hypopigmentation)
- Facial pallor (especially around nose, mouth, and ears)
- Bluish discoloration beneath eyes ("allergic shiners")
- Increased susceptibility to unusual cutaneous infections (especially viral)

damp) to trap moisture in the skin. No soap or a very mild, nonperfumed soap (such as Dove, Lowila, or Neutrogena) is used. Some advocate oil or oilated oatmeal baths with light drying so that a protective, oily film remains on the skin. Showers are avoided because of their drying effect.

Enhancing skin hydration can be accomplished by application of preparations that occlude the skin to prevent evaporation and retain moisture in the upper skin layers and/or by replacement of natural moisturizing substances in the skin. A variety of emollients containing petrolatum or lanolin have occlusive properties and are prescribed according to the degree of occlusion desired. For the majority of patients lotions applied twice or three times daily maintain satisfactory hydration. The frequency may be increased if greater hydration is required. Creams or ointments provide more occlusion, and those that contain urea or lactic acid improve the binding of water in the skin as well as prevent evaporation of moisture.

Sometimes colloid baths, such as the addition of 2 cups of cornstarch to a tub of warm water, provide temporary relief of itching and may help the child sleep if given before bedtime. Cool wet compresses are soothing to the skin and provide antiseptic protection.

Moderate or severe pruritus is usually relieved by administration of oral antihistamine drugs (hydroxyzine [Atarax] or diphenhydramine [Benadryl]), and the amount is tailored to the individual child. Since pruritus increases at night, a mild sedative may be needed.

Occasional flare-ups require the use of topical steroids to diminish inflammation. Low-, moderate-, or high-potency topical corticosteroids are prescribed, depending on the degree of involvement, the area of the body to be treated, the age of the child, and the type of vehicle to be used (e.g., cream, lotion, ointment). Secondary infection is managed with appropriate antibiotic therapy.

There is much controversy regarding prevention of atopic dermatitis by limiting the exposure of high-risk infants to allergens both prenatally and postnatally. Although conclusive evidence for preventive strategies is lacking, the guidelines in Box 13-4 may be recommended.

Nursing Considerations

Long-term treatment of AD is usually established on an outpatient basis. As a result, the major burden of responsibility and physical care rests on the parents in the home. A vicious cycle of exacerbations–scratching–infection–irritability–frustration is the usual course unless the initial phase can be altered.

Assessment

Assessment of the child with AD includes a family history for evidence of atopy, a history of previous involvement, and any environmental or dietary factors associated with the present and previous exacerbations. The skin lesions are examined for type, distribution, and evidence of secondary infection. The parents are interviewed regarding the child's behavior, especially in relation to the child's scratching, irritability, and sleeping patterns. The interview should also include exploration of the family's feelings and methods of coping with the situation.

Nursing Diagnoses

A number of nursing diagnoses may be identified for the child with AD. The most common nursing diagnoses are outlined in the Nursing Care Plan on p. 626. Others will be apparent in individual cases.

NURSING CARE PLAN
The Child with Atopic Dermatitis (Infantile Eczema)

NURSING DIAGNOSIS: Impaired skin integrity related to eczematous lesions

GOAL 1

Relieve itching

INTERVENTIONS

Eliminate any woolen or rough garment or furry stuffed toys; nylon garments promote sweating
Launder all clothes or bedsheets in mild detergent and rinse very well
Provide colloid bath (e.g., cornstarch in warm water) for temporary relief at bedtime
Apply cool compresses if needed
*Administer oral antihistamines, if prescribed
*Administer mild sedative, if prescribed

EXPECTED OUTCOME

Child does not scratch and rests or plays quietly

GOAL 2

Promote healing

INTERVENTIONS

*Carry out prescribed therapeutic regimen
- Dry method:
  - Bathe infrequently
  - Cleanse skin with nonlipid, hydrophilic agent (e.g., Cetaphil)
- Wet method:
  - Bathe frequently, up to 4 times per day
  - Follow immediately with application of lubricant
  - Use no soap or very mild soap (e.g., Neutrogena, Lowila, Dove)
  - Provide oil or oilated oatmeal baths, if prescribed
  - Avoid showers
  - *Apply hydrating preparations as prescribed

*Provide hypoallergenic diet as prescribed

EXPECTED OUTCOME

Child appears comfortable and rests and plays quietly

GOAL 3

Provide hygienic care without aggravating lesions

INTERVENTIONS

Administer good personal hygiene—cleansing method as prescribed; no bubble bath, bath oil, perfume, or powder
Dress in loose-fitting, one-piece, long-sleeve and long-pants outfit (if appropriate for weather conditions)

EXPECTED OUTCOME

Child is clean, well groomed, and exhibits no evidence of irritation

GOAL 4

Prevent or minimize scratching

INTERVENTIONS

Keep fingernails and toenails short and clean
Wrap hands in soft cotton gloves or stockings; pin to shirt cuff
Avoid overheating, high humidity, and perspiration
Use elbow restraints when absolutely necessary, but allow supervised periods of unrestricted movement

EXPECTED OUTCOME

Affected areas remain free of irritation or infection

GOAL 5

Promote rest

INTERVENTIONS

Plan meals, baths, medications, and treatments around nap or bedtime
Make child as comfortable as possible before sleep to enhance restfulness (for example, give sedation and then bathe before bedtime)

EXPECTED OUTCOME

Child receives an adequate amount of rest for age

NURSING DIAGNOSIS: Altered family processes related to child's discomfort and lengthy therapy

GOAL 1

Prepare family for home care

INTERVENTIONS

Encourage play activities that are suitable to skin condition and child's developmental age
Demonstrate proper procedure for dilution of soaks and applying wet dressings
Suggest applying dressings at quiet times when child is well rested and has received medication for itching

EXPECTED OUTCOME

Family demonstrates correct performance of procedures (specify procedures)

GOAL 2

Assist parents in avoiding causative allergens

INTERVENTIONS

Avoid any furry, hairy stuffed toys or dolls
- Avoid play materials that contain allergens (e.g., wheat-based paste or finger paint)
- Provide kinesthetic, moving toys, large toys, which require less fine motor skills if hands are covered, and quiet musical or visual toys

Stress reason for hypoallergenic diet or removal of inhalants, especially that positive results are not immediate
Give written list of foods restricted as well as those allowed
Assess home environment *before* suggesting ways to eliminate inhalants
Make public health referral for long-term home care follow-up

EXPECTED OUTCOME

Family eliminates irritating substances from diet and environment of child

*Dependent nursing action.

Planning

The objectives for nursing care of the child with AD are similar to those for medical management as follows:

1. Relieve pruritus.
2. Improve skin hydration.
3. Prevent secondary infection.
4. Support child and family.

Implementation

The child with AD presents a nursing challenge. Controlling the intense pruritus is imperative if the disorder is to be successfully managed, since scratching leads to the formation of new lesions and may cause secondary infection. In addition to the medical regimen, other measures can be taken to prevent or minimize the scratching. Fingernails and toenails are cut short, kept clean, and filed frequently to prevent sharp edges. Gloves or cotton stockings may have to be placed over the hands and pinned to shirtsleeves. To prevent any contact with the skin, elbow restraints are sometimes necessary. One-piece outfits with long sleeves and long pants also decrease direct contact with the skin. Whether gloves or elbow restraints are used, the child needs time to be free from such restrictions. An excellent time to remove any protective devices is during the bath or after receiving sedative or antipruritic medication.

NURSING ALERT Do not remove elbow restraints during sleep because of the likelihood that the child will scratch while asleep.

Conditions that increase itching are eliminated when possible. Woolen clothes or blankets, rough fabrics, and furry stuffed animals are removed. Since heat and humidity cause perspiration, which intensifies the itching, proper dress for climatic conditions is essential. Pruritus is often precipitated by exposure to the irritant effects of certain components of common products such as soaps, detergents, fabric softeners, perfumes, and powders. Most children experience less itching when soft cotton fabrics are worn next to the skin. During cold months, synthetic fabrics (not wool) should be used for overcoats, hats, gloves, and snowsuits.

Clothes and sheets are laundered in a mild detergent and rinsed thoroughly in clear water (without fabric softeners and antistatic chemicals). Putting the clothes through a second complete wash cycle without using detergent minimizes the amount of residue remaining in the fabric.

Preventing infection is usually secondary to preventing scratching. Personal hygiene is accomplished as described previously. Baths are given as prescribed, the water kept tepid, and soaps (except as indicated) and bubble baths are avoided, as well as the use of oils and powders. Skinfolds and diaper areas need frequent cleansing with plain water. A room humidifier or vaporizer may benefit children with extremely dry skin. The lesions are examined for signs of infection, usually the presence of honey-colored crusts with surrounding erythema. Any signs of infection are reported to the practitioner.

NURSING ALERT If the child is being treated with frequent baths for hydration, it is imperative that the emollient preparation be applied immediately following bathing (while the skin is still slightly moist) to prevent drying.

Soaks and compresses are applied and medications for pruritus or infection are administered as directed. The family is given *explicit written* instructions on the preparation and use of soaks, special baths, and topical medications, including the order of application if more than one is prescribed. Directions are worded in language the family understands. For example, if a solution is to be diluted in the ratio of 1 to 20 parts of water, it is preferable to express the ratio concretely, such as 1 cup of solution mixed with 20 cups of water. It is important to emphasize that one thick application of a topical medication is *not* equivalent to several thin applications, and that excessive use of an agent, particularly steroids, can be hazardous. If children have difficulty remaining still for a 10- or 15-minute soak, bath, or dressing application, these can be carried out at naptime or when the child is engrossed in television or a story.

Since adequate rest is also important for these children, who are usually fretful and irritable, planning meals, baths, medications, and treatments during awake periods is paramount. Sleepy, tired children are normally cranky, and such behavior only intensifies the urge to scratch. During periods of irritability, these children tend to be anorectic, which is worsened by restriction of their usual foods.

Diet modification is another source of frustration to parents. When a hypoallergenic diet is prescribed, parents need help in understanding the reason for the diet and guidelines for avoiding hyperallergenic foods (see Box 13-4).

Since hypoallergenic diets take time before visible effects are apparent, parents need reassurance that results may not be seen immediately. If airborne allergens also worsen the eczema, the family is counseled regarding measures to "allergy proof" the home (see Bronchial Asthma, Chapter 32).

Family support. Parents can be assured that the lesions will not produce scarring (unless secondarily infected) and that the disease is not contagious. However, the child will be subject to repeated exacerbations and remissions. Spontaneous and permanent remission takes place at approximately 2 to 3 years of age in most children with the infantile disorder.

Perhaps it is because the physical problems seem insurmountable during periods of acute exacerbation that the emotional stress becomes so intense for the family members. They need time to discuss negative feelings and to be reassured that these feelings are expected, normal, acceptable, and healthy, provided there is an emotional outlet to dissipate the invested energy. During acute phases, relieving as much anxiety as possible in both parents and child has a beneficial emotional and physical effect, since stress tends to aggravate the severity of the condition.

Evaluation

The effectiveness of nursing interventions is determined by continual reassessment and evaluation of care based on the following observational guidelines and expected outcomes:

1. Observe the child's behavior, clothing, and activities.
2. Examine the skin surface for evidence of dryness.
3. Examine skin lesions for evidence of secondary infection.
4. Interview the family and encourage dialogue regarding the child and aspects of care.

Expected outcomes:
See Nursing Care Plan, p. 626.

DISORDERS OF UNKNOWN ETIOLOGY

A number of disorders may occur during early childhood in which the etiology is unknown or speculative. However, two of the disorders, sudden infant death syndrome and autism, occur almost exclusively during infancy and generate tremendous stress for the family. In one, the family must cope with the loss of an infant; in the other, the family must deal with the stresses of caring for a severely disturbed child. Competent and sensitive nursing care can relieve some of the emotional burden.

SUDDEN INFANT DEATH SYNDROME

Sudden infant death syndrome (SIDS), also known by outdated terms such as cot or crib death, is defined as "the sudden death of an infant under 1 year of age that remains unexplained after a complete postmortem examination, including an investigation of the death scene and a review of the case history" (cited by Zylke, 1989). It is the leading cause of death in children between the ages of 1 month and 1 year and claims the lives of 7000 infants annually. Table 13-6 summarizes the major epidemiologic characteristics of SIDS.

Table 13-6 Epidemiology of SIDS

FACTORS	OCCURRENCE
Incidence	2:1000 live births
Peak age	2 to 4 months; 90% occur by 6 months
Sex	Higher percentage of males affected
Time of death	During sleep
Time of year	Increased incidence in winter; peak in January
Racial	Greater incidence in Native Americans and blacks, followed by whites; lower in Chinese
Socioeconomic	Increased occurrence in lower socioeconomic class
Birth	Higher incidence in: Premature infants, especially infants of low birth weight Multiple births* Neonates with low Apgar scores Infants with central nervous system disturbances and respiratory disorders such as bronchopulmonary dysplasia Increasing birth order (subsequent siblings as opposed to firstborn child)
Feeding habits	Not significant; breast-feeding does not prevent SIDS
Siblings	May have greater incidence
Maternal	Younger age Cigarette smoking Drug addiction (opioids and possibly cocaine)

*Although a rare event, simultaneous death of twins from SIDS can occur (Smialek, 1986).

Etiology

Numerous theories have been proposed regarding the etiology of SIDS; however, the cause is unknown. The most compelling hypothesis is that SIDS is related to a brainstem abnormality in the neurologic regulation of cardiorespiratory control. Abnormalities include prolonged sleep apnea, increased frequency of brief inspiratory pauses, excessive periodic breathing, and impaired arousal responsiveness to increased carbon dioxide or decreased oxygen. A prominent aspect of the respiratory control hypothesis was the apnea hypothesis, which proposed that SIDS victims experienced periods of prolonged apnea during sleep and eventually died during one of these episodes because of a failure in the autonomic regulation of breathing (Hunt and Brouillette, 1987). However, apnea of infancy is not the cause of SIDS. The vast majority of infants with apnea do not die, and only a minority of SIDS victims have documented apparent life-threatening events (ALTE) (see Apnea of Infancy, p. 630). A theory that has been disproved associates SIDS with diphtheria, tetanus, and pertussis vaccines (Hoffman and others, 1987).

Although the etiology is unknown, autopsies reveal consistent pathologic findings, such as pulmonary edema and intrathoracic hemorrhages, that confirm the diagnosis of SIDS. Consequently, all infants with suspected SIDS death should be autopsied, and these findings shared with the parents as soon as possible after the death.

Children at Risk for SIDS

Certain groups of children are at increased risk for SIDS. These groups include (National Institutes, 1987):

1. Infants with one or more severe ALTEs requiring cardiopulmonary resuscitation (CPR) or vigorous stimulation
2. Preterm infants who continue to have pathologic apnea at the time of hospital discharge
3. Siblings of two or more SIDS victims
4. Infants with certain types of diseases or conditions, such as central hypoventilation

Home monitoring and/or the use of respiratory stimulant drugs is recommended for these groups of children. No diagnostic tests exist to predict which infants, including those in the above groups, will survive or die, and home monitoring is no guarantee of survival (Bentele and Albani, 1988; Ward and others, 1986). At the present time, strategies to prevent SIDS are best directed at decreasing known risk factors, such as mothers seeking adequate prenatal care and avoiding cigarette smoking and drug abuse both before and after the child's birth.

Whether subsequent siblings of the SIDS infant are at increased risk for SIDS is unclear. Some studies report a fivefold greater risk (Guntheroth, Lohmann, and Spiers, 1990), whereas others report that the risk in the SIDS family is virtually the same as that in families of like size and maternal age (Peterson, Sabotta, and Daling, 1986). Even if the increased risk is correct, families have a 99% chance that their subsequent child will *not* die of SIDS. Home monitoring is not recommended for this group of children (National Institutes, 1987).

Nursing Considerations

Loss of a child from SIDS presents several crises with which the parents must cope. In addition to grief and mourning for the death of their child, the parents must face a tragedy that was extremely sudden, unexpected, and unexplained. The psychologic intervention for the family must deal with these additional variables. This discussion focuses primarily on the objectives of care for families experiencing SIDS, rather than on the process of grief and mourning, which is explored in Chapter 23.

One approach toward delineating the nursing care plan for these families is to base it on the usual sequence of events that occurs after the infant is found. This approach encompasses the different areas in which nurses may be involved with the family.

Finding the infant. Usually it is the mother who finds the child dead in the crib. Typically the child is in a disheveled bed, with blankets over the head, and huddled into a corner. Frothy, blood-tinged fluid fills the mouth and nostrils, and the infant may be lying face down in the secretions, suggesting that he or she bled to death. The diaper is wet and full of stool, which is consistent with a cataclysmic type of death. The hands may be clutching the sheets, as if the child were in distress before death. The initial appearance of the child combined with the shock of such an unexpected event adds to the horror that the parents must face.

Frequently the mother is alone and must deal with her initial shock, panic, grief, questions of the other siblings, and the decision of where to find help. The first persons to arrive may be the police and ambulance attendants. Hopefully they will handle the situation by asking few questions, giving *no* indication of wrongdoing, abuse, or neglect, making sensitive judgments concerning the resuscitation efforts for the child, and comforting the members of the family as much as possible. These individuals should be properly informed about SIDS in order to recognize its characteristic signs and tell parents that their child probably died from a disease called sudden infant death syndrome, which cannot be predicted or prevented. A compassionate, sensitive approach to the family during the very first few minutes can help spare them some of the overwhelming guilt and anguish that frequently follow this type of death.

Arriving at the emergency room. The first contact that nurses typically have with these families is in the emergency room, when the infant is seen by a physician in order to be pronounced dead. Usually there is no attempt at resuscitation. During the time in the emergency room several aspects warrant special consideration. Parents are asked only factual questions, such as when they found the infant, how he or she looked, and who they called for help. Any remarks that may suggest responsibility, such as why didn't they go in earlier, didn't they hear the infant cry out, was the head buried in a blanket, or were the other siblings jealous of this child, are avoided.

The events that took place when help arrived are discussed. If resuscitation was attempted, the infant may have fractured ribs, internal bleeding, and traumatic bruising, which can simulate physical abuse. Also if statements were made that were misguided, such as, "This looks like suffocation," they can be corrected before parents harbor them in their minds as indications of their guilt. The discussion of an autopsy should be presented at this time, emphasizing that a diagnosis cannot be confirmed until the postmortem examination is completed. Instructions about the autopsy and funeral arrangements may need to be repeated or put in writing. If the mother was breast-feeding, she needs information about abrupt discontinuation of lactation (Lawrence, 1989).

Another very important aspect of compassionate care toward these parents is allowing them to say good-bye to their child. Before they go into the examining room, any blood or emesis is removed from the child, the body is covered partially with a sheet or blanket, and the room is put in order, especially if instruments and equipment were used. These are the parents' last moments with their child, and they should be as quiet, meaningful, peaceful, and undisturbed as possible. The child's belongings are packaged for the parents to take home if they wish. Because the parents leave the hospital without their infant, it is helpful to accompany them to the car or arrange for someone else to take them home (Woolsey, 1988).

Returning home. When the parents return home, they should be visited by a competent, qualified professional as soon after the death as possible. A referral should also be made to the local **SIDS Foundation.** Printed material that contains excellent information about SIDS (available from the national* or local organizations*) should be provided.

During the initial home visit one of the nursing objectives is to assess what the parents have been told, what they think happened, and how they have explained this to the other siblings. If parents have been told about SIDS, they may answer the questions factually and seem to understand and accept the diagnosis. Although this might be so, it is unusual for parents not to have second thoughts, doubts, and feelings of guilt. Pursuing the factual answer by asking

---

***National Sudden Infant Death Syndrome Foundation,** 10500 Little Patuxent Parkway, Suite 420, Columbia, MD 21044, (800) 221-5105; **Sudden Infant Death Syndrome Clearinghouse,** 8201 Greensboro Drive, Suite 600, McLean, VA 22102, (703) 821-8955; **American Sudden Infant Death Syndrome Institute,** 275 Carpenter Dr., Suite 100, Atlanta, GA 30328, (800) 232-SIDS (in Georgia, [800] 847-SIDS).

about feelings or emotions may uncover repressed thoughts that, when once said aloud, can be dealt with.

The nurse cannot deal with all the issues related to the child's death in one visit. During the initial visit the nurse may be doing most of the talking, as the parents are helped to gain an understanding of the disease. If the visit is made within a day or two of the death, the parents are in the impact phase of crisis, in which their thinking abilities are disorganized and distracted. It is difficult for them to deal with the crisis in concrete terms, especially in exploring problem-solving approaches. During the turmoil phase, which is usually the first week following the death, there is more structured thinking, although it is global rather than specific.

During the second visit the goal is to help the parents bring their feelings out into the open. This may require "precipitating" emotions by asking about crying and feeling sad, angry, or guilty. It is an attempt to provoke a display of emotions, not just an admission of a feeling. During this session the parents are helped to explore their usual coping mechanisms and, if these are ineffectual, to investigate new approaches. It may be a time when parents are making rash decisions such as moving away to avoid questions or deciding never to have another child. This is not the time to decide these issues rationally and logically but rather to acknowledge that they are unable to deal with them.

Because questions like these do arise and must be answered eventually, the number of visits and plan for intervention must be flexible. For example, the needs of the siblings must be considered. Although they may initially appear accepting of the explanation and well-adjusted, subsequent problems are common and may include (1) changes in the parent-child interaction, such as increased anger toward the parent or increased discipline problems; (2) altered sleep patterns, including resistance to going to bed and bedtime fears; and (3) changes in social patterns, from withdrawn to aggressive behavior (Mandell, McAnulty, and Carlson, 1983). Children need an opportunity to talk about their perception of the death. With young children, the use of stories about death, drawing, or play is recommended (see Chapter 6 for communication techniques). Even if they express no concerns, their safety and the inability to have predicted, prevented, or caused the death *must* be emphasized. Parents should be aware that sibling grief often lasts as long as adult grief—typically longer than a year (Burns, House, and Ankenbauer, 1986).

One of the important decisions for many parents is the question of a subsequent pregnancy and their concern regarding recurrent SIDS. The optimum timing for a subsequent pregnancy is not known, and many families have a strong desire to rebuild the family, often within the first year (Swoiskin-Schwartz, Deatrick, and Hanson, 1988). If another pregnancy occurs before both parents are ready, they may be forced to deal with an additional crisis before resolution of the first. One of the dangers of having another child soon after the other's death is that this infant may become a "replacement" child. Even when parents are well prepared for the birth of a subsequent child, they may have difficulty conceiving, have doubts about the child's well-being, be overprotective and view the child as more vulnerable, especially near the age of the other infant's death, and need support that these responses are normal. Nurses can help families assess their readiness for another child and support them in their decision.

APNEA OF INFANCY

Apnea, the cessation of respirations, can be of three types (Brazy, Kinney, and Oakes, 1987):

- **Central**—absence of airflow and respiratory effort
- **Obstructive**—absence of airflow but presence of respiratory effort
- **Mixed**—absence of airflow and respiratory effort (central apnea), followed by resumption of respiratory effort without airflow (obstructive apnea)

Short periods of central apnea (≤15 seconds) can be normal at any age.

Pathologic apnea is a respiratory pause that is prolonged (≥20 seconds) or associated with cyanosis, marked pallor or hypotonia, or bradycardia. Apnea of infancy (AOI) generally refers to pathologic apnea in infants greater than 37 weeks of gestation (see also discussion of apnea of prematurity in Chapter 10). The clinical presentation of AOI is an apparent life-threatening event (ALTE) (previously referred to by the inaccurate and misleading expression, near-miss SIDS) (Box 13-13). AOI can be a symptom of many disorders, including sepsis, seizures, upper airway abnormalities, gastroesophageal reflux, hypoglycemia or other metabolic problems, and impaired regulation of breathing during sleep or feeding. In rare instances, the ALTE may be the result of intentional poisoning by a caregiver (Hickson and others, 1989). However, in about half the cases no cause is identified. Infants with a history of ALTE are at increased risk for SIDS, but these children constitute less than 7% of all SIDS victims (National Institute, 1987).

Diagnostic Evaluation

Diagnostic procedures generally include a number of tests (blood chemistry, chest radiograph, electrocardiography,

Box 13-13 DEFINITION OF AN APPARENT LIFE-THREATENING EVENT

Frightening to the observer, who fears child died or would have died without vigorous intervention

Some combination of:

- *Apnea*—usually central but occasionally obstructive
- *Color change*—cyanosis or pallor, but sometimes plethora
- *Marked change in muscle tone*—usually extreme limpness
- *Choking or gagging*

Data from National Institutes of Health Consensus Development Conference on Infantile Apnea and Home Monitoring, Sept. 29 to Oct. 1, 1986, Pediatrics 79(2):292-299, 1987.

and electroencephalography) to rule out specific, sometimes treatable causes, such as seizures. The most widely used test, however, is continuous recording of cardiorespiratory patterns (cardiopneumogram or pneumocardiogram). Four channel pneumocardiograms are commonly used; the four monitor channels are heart rate, respirations (chest impedance), nasal air flow, and oxygen saturation. A more sophisticated test, polysomnography ("sleep test"), also records brain waves, eye and body movements, esophageal manometry, and end-tidal carbon dioxide measurements. However, none of these tests can predict risk. Some children with normal results may still have subsequent apneic episodes.

Therapeutic Management

Treatment usually involves continuous home monitoring of cardiorespiratory rhythms and/or the use of methylxanthines (respiratory stimulant drugs, such as theophylline or caffeine). Theophylline is more widely used because it is available in oral form and blood levels are easily obtained. However, side effects are greater with theophylline than with caffeine. Therapeutic levels of theophylline are typically 6 to 10 μg/ml, and of caffeine 10 to 20 μg/ml (Davis and Sweeney, 1989). The criteria for discontinuing the monitoring is based on the infant's clinical condition. A general guideline for discontinuation is when infants with ALTE have gone 2 or 3 months without significant numbers of alarms or apneic episodes that did not require intervention. A normal pneumogram is not required (National Institutes, 1987). Some practitioners use event recorders (apnea monitors with internal memories that record cardiorespiratory events associated with alarms) to evaluate whether alarms are real or false (Weese-Mayer and others, 1989).

Nursing Considerations

The diagnosis of AOI engenders great anxiety and concern in parents, and the institution of home monitoring presents additional physical and emotional burdens. If monitoring is required, the nurse can be a major source of support to the family in terms of education about the equipment, observation of the infant's status, and immediate intervention during apneic episodes, including cardiorespiratory resuscitation (CPR). To help the family cope with the numerous procedures they must learn, adequate preparation before discharge and written instructions are essential.*

Before the actual teaching begins, parents need an opportunity to discuss their feelings about the diagnosis, especially if another child has died from SIDS. Excessive fears and concerns, especially since monitoring offers no guarantees of survival, can block their readiness to learn (Duncan and Webb, 1983).

Box 13-14 GUIDELINES FOR USING APNEA MONITORS

- Use the monitor despite its shortcomings, such as false alarms.
- Do not adjust the monitor to eliminate false alarms. Adjustments could compromise the monitor's effectiveness.
- Place monitor on firm surface away from crib and drapes; plug directly into wall socket with three-pronged outlet.
- Do not sleep in the same bed as a monitored infant. Moving the infant monitor could cause malfunctions.
- Keep pets and children away from the monitor and infant.
- Keep the monitor away from possible electrical interferences such as appliances (e.g., electric blankets, televisions, air conditioners, remote telephones).
- Check the monitor several times a day to be sure the alarm is working and that it can be heard from room to room. Be sure caregiver can reach the monitor quickly (in less than 10 seconds).
- Periodically check the monitor's breath detection indicator and battery or charger connections.
- Be aware that strong signals from nearby radio and television stations, airports, ham radios, or police stations could interfere with the monitor. Check for interference if the monitor is to be operated in these areas.
- Read the monitor's user manual carefully; report problems promptly.
- Inform local utility and rescue squads of home monitoring.
- Keep emergency numbers near all phones in home.
- Practice safety precautions:
  - Remove leads when infant is not attached to monitor.
  - Unplug power cord from electrical outlet when cord is not plugged into monitor.
  - Use safety covers on electrical outlets to discourage children from inserting objects into a socket.

Data primarily from FDA safety alert: important tips for apnea monitor users, Department of Health and Human Services, Rockville, MD, 1990.

Several types of home monitors are available, and most hospitals select the model that the infant will use at home. Nurses, especially those involved in the care at home, must become familiar with the equipment, including its advantages and disadvantages. Safety is a major concern, since monitors can cause electrical burns and electrocution (see guidelines in Box 13-14).

Caregivers need detailed information regarding proper attachment of the electrodes to the infant's chest with impedance monitors that detect chest movement. The electrodes are placed in the midaxillary line, at a space 1 or 2 fingerbreadths below the nipple (Fig. 13-6). Adhesive electrodes are attached directly to the skin. For home use, electrodes attached to a belt that is placed around the child's trunk are preferred. The belt is positioned so that the electrodes contact the skin in the same area as shown in Fig. 13-6.

Monitors are effective only if they are used. They do not prevent death but alert the caregiver to the ALTE in time to intervene. The need to use the monitor and to respond appropriately to alarms must be stressed. Noncompliance can result in the infant's death (Meny, Blackman, and Fleischmann, 1988).

*Home care instructions for apnea monitoring and CPR are available in Wong, D.L., and Whaley, L.F.: Clinical manual of pediatric nursing, ed. 3, St. Louis, 1990, Mosby–Year Book, Inc. Educational materials may also be obtained from the National Sudden Infant Death Syndrome Foundation, the American Sudden Infant Death Syndrome Institute (see p. 629), and the Homegoing Education and Literature Program (Helping Hand Program), Children's Hospital, 700 Children's Dr., Columbus, OH 43205, (614) 461-2361.

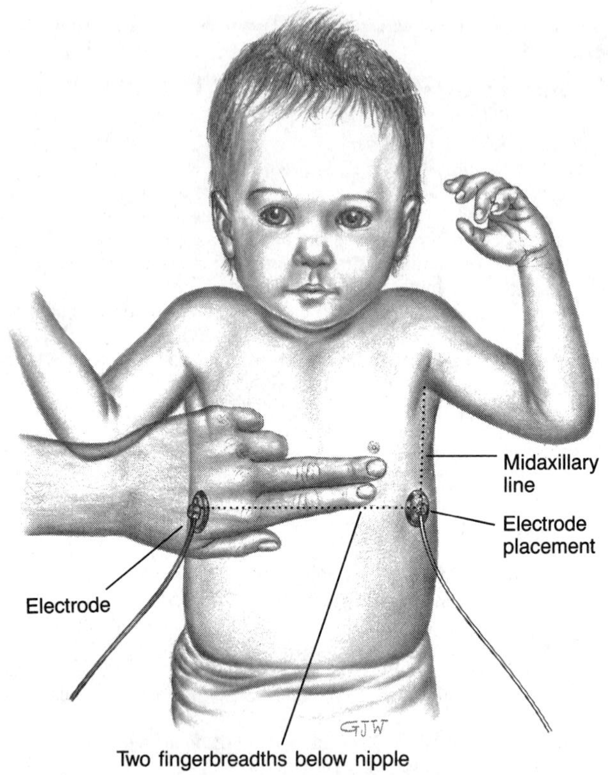

Fig. 13-6. Electrode placement for apnea monitoring. In small infants one fingerbreadth may be used.

✦ **NURSING ALERT** If the infant is apneic, never vigorously shake the child. Gently stimulate the trunk by patting or rubbing. If there is no response, turn the infant over and flick the feet. If there is still no response, begin CPR.

Family support. Although AOI is not a chronic illness, many of the stresses observed during the monitoring period are characteristic of those families with chronically ill children. Parents report increased stress, anxiety, and fatigue, especially mothers who typically have to respond 24 hours a day and feel responsible for the infant's survival (DiMaggio and Sheetz, 1983). However, serious health hazards in mothers appear infrequent, especially when support is available (McElroy, Steinschneider, and Weinstein, 1986). Stress is not limited to those families with a child on a monitor; families with a child who is not being monitored but who is receiving drug treatment also exhibit high anxiety levels (Sweeney, 1988).

Siblings are affected, and behavioral problems, regression, or anxiety are not uncommon. Apnea and/or the monitoring can be detrimental to the affected child, who may be characterized as "spoiled" and have developmental delays, decreased attention span, or hyperactivity (Wasserman, 1984; Deykin and others, 1984). However, these negative effects may be temporary (Kahn and others, 1989). To deal with these potential effects, nurses need to use the same interventions as those discussed for children with chronic illness (see Chapter 22) and be aware of the need for referral when difficulties are suspected.

To lessen the continuous responsibility of monitoring, other family members such as grandparents should be taught how to manipulate the equipment, read and interpret the signals, and administer CPR. They are encouraged to stay with the infant for regular periods to allow parents respite. Support groups of other families who have successfully completed monitoring can also be of benefit. Since babysitters are difficult to locate, nurses can help provide parents with qualified sitters; support group members or nursing students may be potential sources of qualified caregivers (Nuttall, 1988).

INFANTILE AUTISM

Autism is a complex developmental disorder accompanied by severe and usually permanent intellectual and behavioral deficits. It occurs in 1:2500 children, is about four times more common in males than in females, although females are more severely affected, and is not related to socioeconomic level, race, or religion (Ritvo and others, 1989).

Etiology

The etiology of autism is an unsolved and controversial question. However, considerable evidence supports a biologic cause. Individuals with autism may have abnormal electroencephalograms, seizures, delayed development of hand dominance, persistence of primitive reflexes, metabolic abnormalities (elevated blood serotonin), and cerebellar vermal hypoplasia (part of the brain involved in regulating motion and some aspects of memory) (Courchesne and others, 1988; Volkmar and Cohen, 1988).

There is also strong evidence for a genetic basis. Twin studies demonstrate a very high concordance (96%) for monozygotic (identical) twins and a 24% concordance for dizygotic (nonidentical) twins. These concordances are consistent with an autosomal recessive pattern of inheritance (Ritvo and others, 1985a, 1985b). In addition, between 5% and 16% of males with autism are positive for the fragile X chromosome (Chudley and Hagerman, 1987).

Clinical Manifestations/Diagnostic Evaluation

Children with autism demonstrate several peculiar and bizarre characteristics, primarily in social interactions, communication, and behavior. Diagnosis is based on the criteria from the Diagnostic and Statistical Manual of Mental Disorders (Box 13-15). Since the clinical manifestations typically seen in children with autism are described in Box 13-15, they are not repeated here. The majority of children with autism are mentally retarded, with scores typically in the moderate to severe range. More females than males tend to have very low intelligence scores. Despite relatively severe mental retardation, some children with autism excel in particular areas, such as art, music, memory, mathematic calculation, or perceptual skills, such as puzzle building. Instances of exceptional ability despite a low overall mental capacity are know as the *savant syndrome.* However, even those children with exceptional abilities are rarely able to productively use their talents, because of their other severe deficits.

Prognosis

Autism is a severe disabling condition. Only about 1% to 2% of the autistic population ultimately achieve independence, with the majority requiring lifelong supervision. Aggravation of psychiatric symptoms occurs in about half the children during adolescence, with girls having a tendency for continued deterioration. Prognosis is most favorable for children with communicative speech development by age 6 years and an intelligence quotient above 50 at the time of diagnosis (Gillberg and Steffenburg, 1987).

Nursing Considerations

Therapeutic intervention for children with autism is a specialized area, involving professionals with advanced preparation in care of these children. While various therapeutic approaches have been used, behavior modification, which demands a highly structured and intensive educational treatment program, is considered the most effective treatment modality. In general, the objective is to increase social interaction, teach verbal communication and educational skills, and decrease unacceptable behavior by positive reinforcement. In severely self-abusive cases, aversive treatment, including the use of electric shock, has been used; however, aversive approaches have generated many controversial arguments from the standpoint of human rights and

Box 13-15 DIAGNOSTIC CRITERIA FOR AUTISTIC DISORDER

At least eight of the following sixteen items are present, these to include at least two items from A, one from B, and one from C.

A. Qualitative impairment in reciprocal social interaction as manifested by the following:
   (1) Marked lack of awareness of the existence or feelings of others (e.g., treats a person as if he or she were a piece of furniture; does not notice another person's distress; apparently has no concept of the need of others for privacy)
   (2) No or abnormal seeking of comfort at times of distress (e.g., does not come for comfort even when ill, hurt, or tired; seeks comfort in a stereotyped way, e.g., says "cheese, cheese, cheese" whenever hurt)
   (3) No or impaired imitation (e.g., does not wave bye-bye; does not copy mother's domestic activities; mechanical imitation of others' actions out of context)
   (4) No or abnormal social play (e.g., does not actively participate in simple games; prefers solitary play activities; involves other children in play only as "mechanical aids")
   (5) Gross impairment in ability to make peer friendships (e.g., no interest in making peer friendships; despite interest in making friends, demonstrates lack of understanding of conventions of social interaction, for example, reads phone book to uninterested peer)

B. Qualitative impairment in verbal and nonverbal communication, and in imaginative activity, as manifested by the following:
   (1) No mode of communication, such as communicative babbling, facial expression, gesture, mime, or spoken language
   (2) Markedly abnormal nonverbal communication, as in the use of eye-to-eye gaze, facial expression, body posture, or gestures to initiate or modulate social interaction (e.g., does not anticipate being held, stiffens when held, does not look at the person or smile when making a social approach, does not greet parents or visitors, has a fixed stare in social situations)
   (3) Absence of imaginative activity, such as playacting of adult roles, fantasy characters, or animals; lack of interest in stories about imaginary events
   (4) Marked abnormalities in the production of speech, including volume, pitch, stress, rate, rhythm, and intonation (e.g., monotonous tone, questionlike melody, or high pitch)
   (5) Marked abnormalities in the form or content of speech, including stereotyped and repetitive use of speech (e.g., immediate echolalia or mechanical repetition of television commercial); use of "you" when "I" is meant (e.g., using "You want cookie?" to mean "I want a cookie"); idiosyncratic use of words or phrases (e.g., "Go on green riding" to mean "I want to go on the swing"); or frequent irrelevant remarks (e.g., starts talking about train schedules during a conversation about sports)
   (6) Marked impairment in the ability to initiate or sustain a conversation with others, despite adequate speech (e.g., indulging in lengthy monologues on one subject regardless of interjections from others)

C. Markedly restricted repertoire of activities and interests, as manifested by the following:
   (1) Stereotyped body movements (e.g., hand-flicking or -twisting, spinning, head-banging, complex whole-body movements)
   (2) Persistent preoccupation with parts of objects (e.g., sniffing or smelling objects, repetitive feeling of texture of materials, spinning wheels of toy cars) or attachment to unusual objects (e.g., insists on carrying around a piece of string)
   (3) Marked distress over changes in trivial aspects of environment (e.g., when a vase is moved from usual position)
   (4) Unreasonable insistence on following routines in precise detail (e.g., insisting that exactly the same route always be followed when shopping)
   (5) Markedly restricted range of interests and a preoccupation with one narrow interest (e.g., interested only in lining up objects, in amassing facts about meteorology, or in pretending to be a fantasy character)

D. Onset during infancy or childhood (after 36 months of age).

Note: Consider a criterion to be met *only* if the behavior is abnormal for the person's developmental level. The examples within parentheses are arranged so that those first mentioned are more likely to apply to younger or more handicapped, and the later ones, to older or less handicapped, persons with this disorder.

Slightly modified from Diagnostic and statistical manual of mental disorders, ed. 3, revised (DSM-III-R), Washington, DC, 1987, American Psychiatric Association.

the value of potential treatment goals. Although the prognosis for most children with autism is poor, early diagnosis of the child's problem and early educational treatment positively influence the child's future development.

Autism, like so many other chronic conditions, involves the entire family and often becomes "a family disease." Unfortunately, the psychogenetic theory, popular in the 1960s especially among psychoanalysts, had portrayed the parents as the detached, refrigerator-type individuals. Although the psychogenetic theory is unsupported by current findings, the theory has caused many public misconceptions about these families and greatly intensified many parents' guilt (Seifert, 1990). Nurses can help alleviate the guilt and shame often associated with this disorder by stressing what is known from a biologic standpoint, as well as how little is known about the cause of autism. Careful questioning of the parents about the infant's very early behavior usually yields evidence of autistic tendencies before any significant parental or environmental factors could have negatively influenced the child.

Parents need expert counseling early in the course of the disorder and should be referred to the **Autism Society of American (ASA).*** ASA is the most efficient clearinghouse for information about education, treatment programs and techniques, and facilities such as camps and group homes. There is also a siblings group called SHARE (Siblings Helping Persons with Autism Through Resources and Energy).

When these children are hospitalized, they usually present many management problems. Decreasing stimulation by using a private or semiprivate room, avoiding extraneous auditory and visual distraction, and encouraging parents to bring in possessions the child is attached to may lessen the disruptiveness of hospitalization. Since physical contact frequently upsets these children, minimum holding may be necessary to prevent temper tantrums.

Care must be taken when performing procedures on, administering medicine to, or feeding these children, since they are either fussy eaters who may willfully starve themselves or gag to prevent eating, or they are indiscriminate hoarders, swallowing any available edible or inedible items, such as a thermometer. Their disturbing sleep patterns may also pose problems in a hospital setting. A thorough assessment of the child's usual routine and activities can help maintain an environment that is more manageable and conducive to physical recovery.

A key principle in working with these children is establishing trust. They need to be introduced slowly to new situations, with visits with caregivers kept short whenever possible. Because these children have difficulty organizing their behavior and redirecting their energy, they need to be told directly what to do. Communication should be brief and concrete, such as, "sit on bed" (Zoltak, 1986).

As much as possible, the family is encouraged to care for the child in the home. With the help of family support programs in many states, families are often able to provide the home care and assist with the educational services the child needs. As the child approaches adulthood, the family may require assistance in locating a long-term placement facility for the affected adult (see also Chapter 24).

*8601 Georgia Ave., Suite 503, Silver Springs, MD 20910; (301) 565-0433. Another helpful book is *An Introduction to Your Child Who Has Autism,* available from the Medic Publishing Co., P.O. Box 89, Redmond, WA 98073-0089; (206) 881-2883.

KEY POINTS

- Common nutritional disturbances of infancy include vitamin and mineral disturbances, some types of vegetarian diets, protein and calorie malnutrition, obesity, and food intolerance.
- Malnutrition refers to poor or inadequate nutrition and may result from undernutrition or overnutrition. Common manifestations of undernutrition in the infant include iron deficiency anemia, vitamin deficiencies, and failure to thrive. Manifestations of overnutrition are hypervitaminosis and obesity.
- Mineral disturbances may be caused by mineral-mineral interactions and mineral-diet interactions.
- Vegetarians may be classified into four groups: lacto-ovovegetarians, lactovegetarians, pure vegetarians, and zen macrobiotics.
- Protein and energy malnutrition may occur as a complication of underlying disease, or as a result of fad diets, lack of parental education about infant nutrition, inappropriate management of food allergy, and incorrect preparation of formula.
- Calorie consumption, method of feeding, birth weight, sex, age at introduction of solid foods, and activity level all play a part in infant obesity.
- Food intolerance encompasses food allergies and food sensitivities, the most serious of which are cow's milk allergy and lactose intolerance.
- Common feeding difficulties in the infant include breast-feeding problems, regurgitation and "spitting up," and paroxysmal abdominal pain (colic). Less frequent but serious feeding problems include rumination and failure to thrive.
- Treatment of colic may involve change in feeding practices, correction of stressful environment, and support of parent.
- Failure to thrive may be classified as organic, resulting from some physical cause, and nonorganic, resulting from psychosocial factors involving the child and caregiver (e.g., maternal deprivation), environmental causes (e.g., inadequate parental knowledge of child feeding), or unexplained causes.
- Common skin disorders of infancy are diaper dermatitis, seborrheic dermatitis, and atopic dermatitis.
- Sudden infant death syndrome is the leading cause of death in children between the ages of 1 month and 1 year.
- The primary nursing responsibility in care associated with SIDS and other conditions of unknown etiology is emotional support of the family.
- Children with apnea of infancy receive home monitoring to alert the family to an apparent life-threatening event.

■ Autism is a severely disabling condition characterized by deficits in social interaction, communication, and behavior.

REFERENCES

Agras, W., and others: Influence of early feeding style on adiposity at 6 years of age, J. Pediatr. 116(5):805-809, 1990.

Alhadeff, L., Gualtieri, T., and Lipton, M.: Toxic effects of water-soluble vitamins, Nutr. Rev. 42(2):33-40, 1984.

Altemeier, W.A. III, and others: Prospective study of antecedents for nonorganic failure to thrive, J. Pediatr. 106(3):360-365, 1985.

American Academy of Pediatrics, Committee on Nutrition: Prudent life-style for children: dietary fat and cholesterol, Pediatrics 78(3):521-525, 1986.

American Academy of Pediatrics, Committee on Nutrition: Hypoallergenic infant formulas, Pediatrics 83(6):1068-1069, 1989.

Anderson, J.: The establishment of common language concerning adverse reactions to foods and food additives, J. Allergy Clin. Immunol. 78(1, pt. 2):140-144, 1986.

Austin, A., and others: A survey of factors associated with diaper dermatitis in thirty-six pediatric practices, J. Pediatr. Health Care 2(6):295-299, 1988.

Ayoub, C., and Milner, J.: Failure to thrive: parental indicators, types, and outcomes, Child Abuse Neglect 9:491-499, 1985.

Barnard, K., and others: Measurement and meaning of parent-child interaction. In Morrison, F., Lord, C., and Keating, D., editors: Applied developmental psychology, vol. 3, New York, 1989, Academic Press, Inc.

Barr, R., and others: Feeding and temperament as determinants of early infant crying/fussing behavior, Pediatrics 84(3):514-521, 1989.

Bentele, K., and Albani, M.: Are there tests predictive of prolonged apnoea and SIDS? A review of epidemiological and functional studies, Acta. Paediatr. Scand. 342(suppl):1-21, 1988.

Berg, R.W., Buckingham, K.W., and Steward, R.L.: Etiologic factors in diaper dermatitis: the role of urine, Pediatr. Dermatol. 3(2):102-106, 1986.

Bithoney, W.: Elevated lead levels in children with nonorganic failure to thrive, Pediatrics 78(5):891-895, 1986.

Brazy, J., Kinney, H., and Oakes, W.: Central nervous system structural lesions causing apnea at birth, J. Pediatr. 3(2):163-175, 1987.

Brune, M., Rossander, L., and Halberg, L.: Iron absorption: no intestinal adaptation to a high-phytate diet, Am. J. Clin. Nutr. 49:542-545, 1989.

Buckingham, K.W., and Berg, R.W.: Etiologic factors in diaper dermatitis: the role of feces, Pediatr. Dermatol. 3(2):107-112, 1986.

Burns, E., House, J., and Ankenbauer, M.: Sibling grief in reaction to sudden infant death syndrome, Pediatrics 78(3):485-487, 1986.

Callaran, D., and Hiner, L.: Vulnerable sibling: hyponatremia from caries prevention, Pediatrics 79(4):637-639, 1987.

Carpenter, T., and others: Severe hypervitaminosis A in siblings: evidence of variable tolerance to retinol intake, J. Pediatr. 111(4):507-512, 1987.

Chatoor, I., and others: A developmental classification of feeding disorders associated with failure to thrive: diagnosis and treatment, In Drotar, D., editor: New directions in failure to thrive, New York, 1985, Plenum Press.

Chudley, A., and Hagerman, R.: Fragile X syndrome, J. Pediatr. 110(6):821-831, 1987.

Council on Scientific Affairs: Vitamin preparations as dietary supplements and as therapeutic agents, JAMA 257(14):1929-1936, 1987.

Courchesne, E., and others: Hypoplasia of cerebellar vermal lobules VI and VII in autism, N. Engl. J. Med. 318(21):1349-1354, 1988.

Cramer, D.W., and others: Ovarian cancer and talc, Cancer 50:372-376, 1982.

Dagnelie, P., and others: High prevalence of rickets in infants on macrobiotic diets, Am. J. Clin. Nutr. 51:202-208, 1990.

Davis, N., and Sweeney, L.: Infantile apnea monitoring and SIDS, J. Pediatr. Health Care 3(2):67-75, 1989.

Dewey, K., and others: Infant growth and breast feeding, Am. J. Clin. Nutr. 50:1116-1118, 1989.

Deykin, E., and others: Apnea of infancy and subsequent neurologic, cognitive, and behavioral status, Pediatrics 73(5):638-645, 1984.

Dietz, W.H., Jr.: The overweight child: psychosocial effects and treatment, Feelings Med. Signif. 31(1):1-4, 1989.

Dietz, W.H., Jr., and Gortmaker, S.L.: Do we fatten our children at the television set? Obesity and television viewing in children and adolescents, Pediatrics 75(5):807-812, 1985.

DiMaggio, G.T., and Sheetz, A.H.: The concerns of mothers caring for an infant on an apnea monitor, MCN 8(4):294-297, 1983.

Drotar, D., and Sturm, L.: Prediction of intellectual development in young children with early histories of nonorganic failure-to-thrive, J. Pediatr. Psychol. 13(2):281-296, 1988.

Duncan, J.A., and Webb, L.Z.: Teaching families home apnea monitoring, Pediatr. Nurs. 9(3):171-175, 1983.

Fanelli, M.T., and Kuczmarski, R.J.: Food selection for vegetarians, Diet. Curr. 10(1):1-6, 1983.

Fleisher, D.R.: Infant rumination syndrome, Am. J. Dis. Child. 133:266-269, March 1979.

Forsyth, B.: Colic and the effect of changing formulas: a double-blind, multiple-crossover study, J. Pediatr. 115(4):521-526, 1989.

Frank, D., and Zeisel, S.: Failure to thrive, Pediatr. Clin. North Am. 35(6):1187-1206, 1988.

Geertsma, M., and Hyams, J.: Colic—a pain syndrome of infancy? Pediatr. Clin. North Am. 36(4):905-919, 1989.

Gillberg, C., and Steffenburg, G.: Outcome and prognostic factors in infantile autism and similar conditions: a population-based study of 46 cases followed through puberty, J. Autism Dev. Disord. 17:273-287, 1987.

Grantham-McGregor, S., Schofield, W., and Harris, L.: Effect of psychosocial stimulation on mental development of severely malnourished children: an interim report, Pediatrics 72(2):239-243, 1983.

Guntheroth, W., Lohmann, R., and Spiers, P.: Risk of sudden infant death syndrome in subsequent siblings, J. Pediatr. 116(4):520-524, 1990.

Guthrie, G.: Six to eighteen—the perilous months, Nutr. Today 23(3):4-11, 1988.

Hayden, G.F., and Sproul, G.T.: Baby powder use in infant skin care: parental knowledge and determinants of powder usage, Clin. Pediatr. 23:163-165, 1984.

Heaney, R., Weaver, C., and Recker, R.: Calcium absorbability from spinach, Am. J. Clin. Nutr. 47:707-709, 1988.

Hickson, G., and others: Parental administration of chemical agents: a cause of apparent life-threatening events, Pediatrics 83(5):772-776, 1989.

Hide, D.W., and Guyer, B.M.: Prevalence of infant colic, Arch. Dis. Child. 57:559-560, 1982.

Hill, D., and others: Manifestations of milk allergy in infancy: clinical and immunologic findings, J. Pediatr. 109(2):270-276, 1986.

Hill, D., and others: Recovery from milk allergy in early childhood: antibody studies, J. Pediatr. 114(5):761-766, 1989.

Hoffman, H., and others: Diphtheria-tetanus-pertussis immunization and sudden infant death: results of the National Institute of Child Health and Human Development Cooperative Epidemiological Study of sudden infant death syndrome risk factors, Pediatrics 79(4):598-611, 1987.

Honig, P., and others: Amoxicillin and diaper dermatitis, J. Am. Acad. Dermatol. 19:275-279, 1988.

Hunt, C., and Brouillette, R.: Sudden infant death syndrome: 1987 perspective, J. Pediatr. 110(5):669-678, 1987.

Hunziker, U., and Barr, R.: Increased carrying reduces infant crying: a randomized controlled trial, Pediatrics 77(5):641-648, 1986.

Jarvis, W.T.: Vitamin use and abuse, Contemp. Nutr. 9(10):1-2, 1984.

Johnstone, D.: Strategy for intervention of food allergy in infants, Int. Pediatr. 4(4):319-325, 1989.

Jordan, W.E., and others: Diaper dermatitis: frequency and severity among a general infant population, Pediatr. Dermatol. 3(3):198-207, 1986.

Kahn, A., and others: Long-term development of children monitored as infants for an apparent life-threatening event during sleep: a 10-year follow-up study, Pediatrics 83(5):668-673, 1989.

Kahn, A., and others: Milk intolerance in children with persistent sleeplessness: a prospective double-blind crossover evaluation, Pediatrics 84(4):595-603, 1989.

Karp, R.J., Scholl, T.O., and Greene, G.W.: Precursors of malnutrition in children, Public Health Curr. 25(3):11-14, 1985.

Kramer, M., and others: Maternal psychological determinants of infant obesity: development and testing of two new instruments, J. Chron. Dis. 36(4):329-335, 1983.

Krowchuk, D., and others: Pediatric dermatology update, Pediatrics 86(1):126-127, 1990.

Lane, A., Rehder, P., and Helm, K.: Evaluations of diapers containing absorbent gelling material with conventional disposable diapers in newborn infants, Am. J. Dis. Child. 144(3):315-318, 1990.

Lansky, S., and others: Failure to thrive during infancy in siblings of pediatric cancer patients, Am. J. Pediatr. Hematol. Oncol. 4(4):361-366, 1982.

Lawrence, R.A.: Breastfeeding: a guide for the medical profession, ed. 3, St. Louis, 1989, Mosby–Year Book, Inc.

Leyden, J.J.: Cornstarch, Candida albicans, and diaper rash, Pediatr. Dermatol. 1(4):322-325, 1984.

Lifshitz, F., and Moses, N.: A complication of dietary treatment of hypercholesterolemia, Am. J. Dis. Child. 143:537-542, 1989.

Linscheid, T.R.: Feeding disorders during infancy and early childhood, Feelings Med. Signif. 27(3):11-14, 1985.

Liptak, G.: Diaper dermatitis. In Hoekelman, R.A., and others, editors: Primary pediatric care, St. Louis, 1987, Mosby–Year Book, Inc.

Lockey, J.E., and Parry, W.T.: Health implications of naturally occurring mineral fibers, Fam. Community Health 7(3):1-7, 1984.

Lothe, L., and Lindberg, T.: Cow's milk whey protein elicits symptoms of infantile colic in colicky formula-fed infants: a double-blind crossover study, Pediatrics 83(2):262-266, 1989.

Mandell, F., McAnulty, E.H., and Carlson, A.: Unexpected death of an infant sibling, Pediatrics 72(5):652-657, 1983.

McElroy, E., Steinschneider, A., and Weinstein, S.: Emotional and health impact of home monitoring on mothers: a controlled prospective study, Pediatrics 78(5):780-786, 1986.

McJunkin, J., Bithoney, W., and McCormick, M.: Errors in formula concentration in an outpatient population, J. Pediatr. 111(6, pt. 1):848-850, 1987.

Meny, R., Blackmon, L., and Fleischmann, D.: Sudden infant death and home monitors, Am. J. Dis. Child. 142:1037-1040, 1988.

Moore, D., Robb, T., and Davidson, G.: Breath hydrogen response to milk containing lactose in colicky and noncolicky infants, J. Pediatr. 113(6):979-984, 1988.

Morelli, J., and Weston, W.: Soaps and shampoos in pediatric practice, Pediatrics 80(5):634-637, 1987.

Moss, A., and others: Use of vitamin and mineral supplements in the United States: current users, types of products, and nutrients. Advance data from vital and health statistics, No. 174, Hyattsville, MD: National Center for Health Statistics, 1989.

National Institutes of Health Consensus Development Conference on Infantile Apnea and Home Monitoring, Sept. 29 to Oct. 1, 1986, Pediatrics 79(2):292-299, 1987.

Neifert, M., and Seacat, J.: Medical management of successful breastfeeding, Pediatr. Clin. North Am. 33(4):743-762, 1986.

Nuttall, P.: Maternal responses to home apnea monitoring of infants, Nurs. Res. 37(6):354-357, 1988.

Oates, R.K., Peacock, A., and Forrest, D.: Long-term effects of nonorganic failure to thrive, Pediatrics 75(1):36-40, 1985.

Olness, K.N.: Nutritional consequences of drugs used in pediatrics, Clin. Pediatr. 24(8):417-420, 1985.

Peterson, D., Sabotta, E., and Daling, J.: Infant mortality among subsequent siblings of infants who died of sudden infant death syndrome, J. Pediatr. 108(6):911-914, 1986.

Pinyerd, B., and Zipf, W.: Colic: idiopathic, excessive, infant crying, J. Pediatr. Nurs. 4(3):147-161, 1989.

Pugliese, M., and others: Parental health beliefs as a cause of nonorganic failure to thrive, Pediatrics 80(2):175-182, 1987.

Ritvo, E., and others: Concordance for the syndrome of autism in 40 pairs of afflicted twins, Am. J. Psychiatry 142(1):74-77, 1985a.

Ritvo, E., and others: Evidence for autosomal recessive inheritance in 46 families with multiple incidences of autism, Am. J. Psychiatry 142(2):187-192, 1985b.

Ritvo, E., and others: The UCLA–University of Utah epidemiologic survey of autism: prevalence, Am. J. Psychiatry 146(2):194-199, 1989.

Rossouw, J.: Kwashiorkor in North America, Am. J. Clin. Nutr. 49:588-592, 1989.

Saal, H.M., Ratzan, S.K., and Carey, D.E.: Yogurt: contributory factor in development of nutritional rickets, Clin. Pediatr. 24:452-454, 1985.

Said, G., Patois, E., and Lellouch, J.: Infantile colic and parental smoking, Br. Med. J. 289(6446):660, 1984.

Sampson, H., and Scanlon, S.: Natural history of food hypersensitivity in children with atopic dermatitis, J. Pediatr. 115(1):23-27, 1989.

Seifert, C.: Case studies in autism: a young child and two adolescents, Lanham, MD, 1990, University Press of America, Inc.

Sherman, J., and Alexander, M.: Obesity in children: a research update, J. Pediatr. Nurs. 5(3):161-167, 1990.

Smialek, J.: Simultaneous sudden infant death syndrome in twins, Pediatrics 77(6):816-821, 1986.

Solomons, N.W.: Mineral interactions in the diet, Contemp. Nutr. 7(7):1-2, 1982.

A study of the calcium intake of children and teenagers, Minneapolis, MN, 1984, General Mills, Inc.

Stunkard, A., and others: An adoption study of human obesity, N. Engl. J. Med. 314(4):193-198, 1986.

Stunkard, A., and others: The body-mass index of twins who have been reared apart, N. Engl. J. Med. 322(21):1483-1487, 1990.

Sweeney, L.: Impact on families caring for an infant with apnea, Compr. Pediatr. Nurs. 11:1-15, 1988.

Swoiskin-Schwartz, S., Deatrick, J., and Hanson, D.: Parents' views about having a child after a SIDS death, J. Pediatr. Nurs. 3(1):24-28, 1988.

Taubman, B.: Clinical trial of the treatment of colic by modification of parent-infant interaction, Pediatrics 74(6):998-1003, 1984.

Taubman, B.: Parental counseling compared with elimination of cow's milk or soy milk protein for the treatment of infant colic syndrome: a randomized trial, Pediatrics 81(6):756-761, 1988.

Temple, W.J., and Farley, D.H.: The succussion splash as an infant "burp" sign, N. Engl. J. Med. 308(26):1604, 1983.

U.S. Department of Agriculture, U.S. Department of Health and Human Services: Nutrition and your health: dietary guidelines for Americans, Home and Garden Bulletin No. 232, ed. 2, U.S. Government Printing Office, 1985.

Volkmar, F., and Cohen, D.: Neurobiologic aspects of autism, N. Engl. J. Med. 318(21):1390-1392, 1988.

Walravens, P., Hambidge, M., and Koepfer, D.: Zinc supplementation in infants with a nutritional pattern of failure to thrive: a double-blind, controlled study, Pediatrics 83(4):532-538, 1989.

Ward, S., and others: Sudden infant death syndrome in infants evaluated by apnea programs in California, Pediatrics 77(4):451-458, 1986.

Wasserman, A.L.: A prospective study of the impact of home monitoring on the family, Pediatrics 74(3):323-329, 1984.

Weese-Mayer, D., and others: Assessing validity of infant monitor alarms with event recording, J. Pediatr. 115(5, pt. 1):702-708, 1989.

Whitehead, W.E., and others: Rumination syndrome in children treated by increased holding, J. Pediatr. Gastroenterol. Nutr. 4:550-556, 1985.
Wilson, N., Self, T., and Hamburger, R.: Severe cow's milk–induced colitis in an exclusively breast-fed neonate, Clin. Pediatr. 29(2):77-80, 1990.
Wishon, P.M., and Kinnick, V.G.: Helping infants overcome the problem of obesity, MCN 11(2):118-121, 1986.
Woolsey, S.: Support after sudden infant death, Am. J. Nurs. 88(10):1347-1348, 1988.
Zeiger, R., and others: Effectiveness of dietary manipulation in the prevention of food alergy in infants, J. Allergy Clin. Immunol. 78(1, pt. 2):224-238, 1986.
Zimmerer, R.E., Lawson, K.D., and Calvert, C.J.: The effects of wearing diapers on skin, Pediatr. Derm. 3(2):95-101, 1986.
Zoltak, B.: Autism: recognition and management, Pediatr. Nurs. 12(2):90-94, 1986.
Zylke, J.: Sudden infant death syndrome: resurgent research offers hope, JAMA 262(12):1565-1566, 1989.

BIBLIOGRAPHY

Vitamin and Mineral Disturbances

American Academy of Pediatrics, Committee on Nutrition: Vitamin and mineral supplement needs in normal children in the United States, Pediatrics 66(6):1015-1020, 1980.
Chesney, R.: Requirements and upper limits of vitamin D intake in the term neonate, infant, and older child, J. Pediatr. 116(2):159-165, 1990.
Crombie, I., and others: Effect of vitamin and mineral supplementation on verbal and non-verbal reasoning of schoolchildren, Lancet 355:744-7447, 1990.
Dixon, A.: Think zinc, Neonatal Network 5(4):29-33, 1987.
Dwyer, J.: Promoting good nutrition for today and the year 2000, Pediatr. Clin. North Am. 33(4):799-822, 1986.
Erdman, J.: Nutrient interactions involving vitamins and minerals, Contemp. Nutr. 13(2):1-2, 1988.
Few, B.: Pharmacologic use of vitamin E, MCN 13(4):283, 1988.
Fish, W., and others: Effect of intramuscular vitamin E on mortality and intracranial hemorrhage in neonates of 1000 grams or less, Pediatrics 85(4):578-584, 1990.
Gibson, R.S.: Dietary intakes of trace elements in infants during their first year, Food Nutr. News 57(10):1-6, 1985.
Golden, N.H.N.: Trace elements in human nutrition, Human Nutr. Clin. Nutr. 36C:185-202, 1982.
Goldstein, M.: Potential problems with the widespread use of niacin, Am. J. Med. 85:881, 1988.
Hathcock, J.N., and others: Evaluation of vitamin A toxicity, Am. J. Clin. Nutr. 52:183-202, 1990.
Heaney, R., and Weaver, C.: Oxalate: effect on calcium absorbability, Am. J. Clin. Nutr. 50:830-832, 1989.
Holland, P., and others: Prenatal deficiency of phosphate, phosphate supplementation, and rickets in very-low-birthweight infants, Lancet 335:697-701, 1990.
Hurrell, R., and others: Iron absorption in humans as influenced by bovine milk proteins, Am. J. Clin. Nutr. 49(3):546-662, 1989.
Mahaffey, K., Gartside, P., and Glueck, C.: Blood lead levels and dietary calcium intake in 1- to 11-year-old children: the second National Health and Nutrition Examination Survey, 1976-1980, Pediatrics 78(2):257-262, 1986.
Mahoney, C.P., and others: Chronic vitamin A intoxication in infants fed chicken liver, Pediatrics 65(5):893-896, 1980.
Mertz, W.: The significance of trace elements for health, Nutr. Today 18(5):26-31, 1983.
Mertz, W.: The essential elements: nutritional aspects, Nutr. Today 19(1):22-30, 1984.
Murphy, S.P., Subar, A.F., and Block, G.: Vitamin E intakes and sources in the United States, Am. J. Clin. Nutr. 52:361-367, 1990.
Nestle, M.: Promoting health and preventing disease: National Nutrition Objectives for 1990 and 2000, Nutr. Today 23(3):26-30, 1988.
Patel, P., and others: Intoxication from vitamin A in an asthmatic child, Can. Med. Assoc. J. 139:755-756, 1988.
Pennington, J.: The Food and Drug Administration and the dietary guidelines, Fam. Community Health 12(1):1-13, 1989.
Poland, R.: Vitamin E for prevention of perinatal intracranial hemorrhage, Pediatrics 85(5):865-867, 1990.
Prestridge, L., and Shulman, R.: Vitamin excesses and deficiencies, Curr. Opin. Pediatr. 1:397-402, 1989.
Sauberlich, H.: Vitamins—how much is for keeps? Nutr. Today 22(1):20-28, 1987.
Shapiro, A., and others: Vitamin K deficiency in the newborn infant: prevalence and perinatal risk factors, J. Pediatr. 109(4):675-680, 1986.
Sorenson, A.W., and Butrum, R.R.: Zinc and copper in infant diets, J. Am. Diet. Assoc. 83(3):291-297, 1983.
Specker, B., and Tsang, R.: Cyclical serum 25-hydroxyvitamin D concentrations paralleling sunshine exposure in exclusively breast-fed infants, J. Pediatr. 110(5):744-747, 1987.
Specker, B., and others: Increased urinary methylmalonic acid excretion in breast-fed infants of vegetarian mothers and identification of an acceptable dietary source of vitamin B-12, Am. J. Clin. Nutr. 47:89-92, 1988.
Thomas, K.: Folic acid deficiency related to the use of goat milk for infant feeding, Issues Compr. Pediatr. Nurs. 4:37-43, 1980.
Vrchota, K., Oberg, C., and Harris, K.: Beriberi in a Southeast Asian adolescent, Am. J. Dis. Child. 143(3):270-272, 1989.
Williams, S.R.: Nutrition and diet therapy, ed. 6, St. Louis, 1989, Mosby–Year Book, Inc.
Wyatt, D., Noetzel, M., and Hillman, R.: Infantile beriberi presenting as subacute necrotizing encephalomyelopathy, J. Pediatr. 110(6):888-892, 1987.

Vegetarian Diets

Dietz, W.H., and Dwyer, J.T.: Nutritional implications of vegetarianism for children. In Suskind, R.M., editor: Textbook of pediatric nutrition, New York, 1981, Raven Press.
Hanning, R.M., and Zlotkin, S.H.: Unconventional eating practices and their health implications, Pediatr. Clin. North Am. 32(2):429-445, 1985.
Johnston, P.K.: Getting enough to grow on, Am. J. Nurs. 84(3):336-339, 1984.
O'Connell, J., and others: Growth of vegetarian children: the farm study, Pediatrics 84(3):475-481, 1989.
Rudy, C.A.: Vegetarian diets for children, Pediatr. Nurs. 10(5):329-333, 1984.
Rudy, C.A.: Teaching families about the well-balanced vegetarian diet, Child. Nurse 3(5):1-3, 1985.
Trahms, C.: Vegetarian diets for children. In Pipes, P.: Nutrition in infancy and childhood, ed. 4, St. Louis, 1989, Mosby–Year Book, Inc.

Protein and Energy Malnutrition

Benjamin, D.: Laboratory tests and nutritional assessment: protein-energy status, Pediatr. Clin. North Am. 36(1):139-161, 1989.
Cameron, N., and others: Timing and magnitude of adolescent growth in height and weight in Cape coloured children after kwashiorkor, J. Pediatr. 109(3):548-555, 1986.
Graham, G., Lembcke, J., and Morales, E.: Quality-protein maize as the sole source of dietary protein and fat for rapidly growing young children, Pediatrics 85(1):85-91, 1990.
Grantham-McGregor, S., Schofield, W., and Powell, C.: Development of severely malnourished children who received psychosocial stimulation: six-year follow-up, Pediatrics 79(2):247-254, 1987.
Keusch, G.T., and others: Impairment of hemolytic complement activation by both classical and alternative pathways in serum from patients with kwashiorkor, J. Pediatr. 105(3):434-436, 1984.
Kulkarni, M., and others: Age-independent anthropometric criteria in

the assessment of PEM, Am. J. Dis. Child. 142(12):1268-1270, 1988.
McFarlane-Ferreira, Y., and LeLeiko, N.: Altered nutritional states: the effects of primary malnutrition, Curr. Opin. Pediatr 1:394-396, 1989.
Viteri, F.E.: Primary protein-energy malnutrition: clinical, biochemical, and metabolic changes. In Suskind, R.M., editor: Textbook of pediatric nutrition, New York, 1981, Raven Press.

Obesity

Agras, W., and others: Does a vigorous feeding style influence early development of adiposity? J. Pediatr. 110(5):799-804, 1987.
Bouchard, C., and others: The response to long-term overfeeding in identical twins, N. Engl. J. Med. 322(21):1477-1482, 1990.
Castiglia, P.: Obesity in infants and toddlers, J. Pediatr. Health Care 1(4):218-220, 1987.
Dietz, W.H., Jr.: Childhood obesity: susceptibility, cause, and management, J. Pediatr. 103(5):676-686, 1983.
Dietz, W.H., Jr.: Prevention of childhood obesity, Pediatr. Clin. North Am. 33(4):823-833, 1986.
Epstein, L.H., Wing, R.R., and Valoski, A.: Childhood obesity, Pediatr. Clin. North Am. 32(2):363-379, 1985.
Griffiths, M., and others: Metabolic rate and physical development in children at risk of obesity, Lancet 336(8707):76-78, 1990.
Kaplan, K., and Wadden, T.: Childhood obesity and self-esteem, J. Pediatr. 109(2):367-370, 1986.
Korsch, B.: Childhood obesity, J. Pediatr. 109(2):299-300, 1986.
Kramer, M.S.: Breast-feeding, solid foods and subsequent obesity, J. Pediatr. 98:883-887, June 1981.
Morgan, J.: Prevention of childhood obesity, Issues Compr. Pediatr. Nurs. 9(1):33-38, 1986.
Mossberg, H.: 40-year follow-up of overweight children, Lancet 2(8661):491-493, 1989.
Newmann, C.: Obesity in childhood. In Levine, M.D., and others, editors: Developmental-behavioral pediatrics, Philadelphia, 1983, W.B. Saunders Co.
Satter, E.: The feeding relationship, J. Am. Diet. Assoc. 86(3):352-356, 1986.
Woolston, J.: Obesity in infancy and early childhood, J. Am. Acad. Child Adolesc. Psychiatry 26:123-126, 1987.

Food Sensitivity

American Academy of Pediatrics, Committee on Nutrition: Soy-protein formulas: recommendations for use in infant feeding, Pediatrics 72(3):359-363, 1983.
Anderson, J.A.: Food allergy and food intolerance, Contemp. Nutr. 9(9):1-2, 1984.
Berezin, S.: Gastrointestinal milk intolerance of infancy, Am. J. Dis. Child. 143(3):361-362, 1989.
Bierman, C.W., and Furukawa, C.T.: Food allergy, Pediatr. Rev. 3(7):213-220, 1982.
Biller, J., and others: Efficacy of lactase-treated milk for lactose-intolerant pediatric patients, J. Pediatr. 111(1):91-94, 1987.
Bock, S.A.: Food sensitivity, a critical review and practical approach, Am. J. Dis. Child. 134:973-982, Oct. 1980.
Bock, S.A.: Prospective appraisal of complaints of adverse reactions to foods in children during the first 3 years of life, Pediatrics 79(5):683-688, 1987.
Brill, B.: Oral rehydration, food allergy, and specialized nutrition, Curr. Opin. Pediatr. 1:384-393, 1989.
Institute of Food Technologists' Expert Panel on Food Safety and Nutrition: Food allergies and other food sensitivities, Contemp. Nutr. 10(11):1-2, 1985.
Kahn, A., and others: Insomnia and cow's milk allergy in infants, Pediatrics 76(6):880-884, 1985.
Lee, B., Geha, R., and Leung, D.: IgE response and its regulation in allergic disease, Pediatr. Clin. North Am. 35(5):953-967, 1988.
Proujansky, R., Winter, H., and Walker, A.: Gastrointestinal syndromes associated with food sensitivity, Adv. Pediatr. 35:219-238, 1988.
Savaiano, D., and Kotz, C.: Recent advances in the management of lactose intolerance, Contemp. Nutr. 13(9,10):1-4, 1988.
Stern, M., and Walker, W.A.: Food allergy and intolerance, Pediatr. Clin. N. Am. 32(2):471-492, 1985.
White, J.E., and Owsley, V.B.: Helping families cope with milk, wheat, and soy allergies, MCN 8:423-428, 1983.
Wytock, D., and DiPalma, J.: All yogurts are not created equal, Am. J. Clin. Nutr. 47(3):454, 1988.
Yunginger, J.: Allergens: recent advances, Pediatr. Clin. North Am. 35(5):981-993, 1988.

Feeding Difficulties: General

Edgehouse, L., and Radzyminski, G.: A device for supplementing breast-feeding, MCN 15(1):34-35, 1990.
Finney, J.: Preventing common feeding problems in infants and young children, Pediatr. Clin. North Am. 33(4):775-788, 1986.
Frappier, P., Marino, B., and Shishmanian, E.: Nursing assessment of infant feeding problems, J. Pediatr. Nurs. 2(1):37-44, 1987.
Hill, P., and Humenick, S.: Insufficient milk supply, Image 21(3):145-148, 1989.
Humphrey, N.M.: Minor breast-feeding problems, Child. Nurse 3(7):1-4, 1985.
Lierman, C., and others: Multidisciplinary treatment of feeding disorders in the home, Pediatr. Nurs. 13(4):266-270, 1987.
Loughlin, H.H., and others: Early termination of breast-feeding: identifying those at risk, Pediatrics 75(3):508-513, 1985.
Neifert, M.R., Seacat, J.M., and Jobe, W.E.: Lactation failure due to insufficient glandular development of the breast, Pediatrics 76(5):823-828, 1985.
Pittard, W.: Practical advice for the nursing mother, Pediatr. Basics, 43:10-15, 1986.
Satter, E.: Childhood feeding problems, Feelings Med. Signif. 32(2):5-10, 1990.
Walker, M.: Functional assessment of infant breast-feeding patterns, Birth 16(3):140-147, 1989.
Walker, M., and Driscoll, J.: Sore nipples: the new mother's nemesis, MCN 14:260-265, 1989.

Failure to Thrive

Ayoub, C., Pfeifer, D., and Leichtman, L.: Treatment of infants with nonorganic failure to thrive, Child Abuse Neglect 3:937-941, 1979.
Bithoney, W.G., and Newberger, E.H.: Child and family attributes of failure-to-thrive, Dev. Behav. Pediatr. 8(1):32-36, 1987.
Bithoney, W., and Rathbun, J.: Failure to thrive. In Levine, M.D., and others, editors: Developmental-behavioral pediatrics, Philadelphia, 1983, W.B. Saunders Co.
Blank, D.: Relating mothers' anxiety and perception to infant satiety, anxiety, and feeding behavior, Nurs. Res. 35(6):347-351, 1986.
Casey, P.H., Bradley, R., and Wortham, B.: Social and nonsocial home environments of infants with nonorganic failure to thrive, Pediatrics 73(3):348-353, 1984.
Castiglia, P.: Failure to thrive, J. Pediatr. Health Care 2(1):50-57, 1988.
Endert, C., and Wooldridge, N.: Nonorganic failure to thrive, Diet. Curr. 14(1):1-6, 1987.
Handen, B., Mandell, F., and Russo, D.: Feeding induction in children who refuse to eat, Am. J. Dis. Child. 140(1):52-54, 1986.
Harrison, L.: The failure-to-thrive child. In Johnson, S., editor: Nursing assessment and strategies for the family at risk, ed. 2, Philadelphia, 1986, J.B. Lippincott Co.
Hilton, A.: Approaches for feeding the young child with anorexia, J. Pediatr. Nurs. 2(1):45-49, 1987.
Klein, M.: The home health nurse clinician's role in the prevention of nonorganic failure to thrive, J. Pediatr. Nurs. 5(2):129-135, 1990.
Showers, J., and others: Nonorganic failure to thrive: identification and intervention, J. Pediatr. Nurs. 1(4):240-246, 1986.

Singer, L.: Long-term hospitalization of failure-to-thrive infants: developmental outcome at three years, Child Abuse Negl. 10:479-486, 1986.

Singer, L.: Long-term hospitalization of nonorganic failure-to-thrive infants: patient characteristics and hospital course, J. Dev. Behav. Pediatr. 8(1):25-31, 1987.

Steele, S.: Nonorganic failure to thrive: a pediatric social illness, Issues Compr. Pediatr. Nurs. 9(1):47-58, 1986.

Stickler, G.B.: 'Failure to thrive' or failure to define, Pediatrics 74(4):559, 1984.

Wilcox, W., Neiburg, P., and Miller, D.: Failure to thrive: a continuing problem of definition, Clin. Pediatr. 28(9):391-394, 1989.

Yoos, L.: Taking another look at failure to thrive, MCN 9(1):32-36, 1984.

Colic

Barr, R.: Infantile colic and lactose intolerance (letter to the editor), J. Pediatr. 115(3):501-502, 1989.

Carey, W.B.: "Colic" or excessive crying in young infants. In Levine, M.D., and others, editors: Developmental-behavioral pediatrics, Philadelphia, 1983, W.B. Saunders Co.

Carey, W.B.: Colic: exasperating but fascinating and gratifying, Pediatrics 84(3):568-569, 1989.

Gillies, C.: Infant colic: is there anything new? J. Pediatr. Health Care 1(6):305-312, 1987.

Hartsell, M.: New product to quiet baby's crying spells, J. Pediatr. Nurs. 2(6):438-439, 1987.

Hartsell, M.: Sleeptight infant soother and colic, J. Pediatr. Nurs. 15(1):59-60, 1990.

Hyams, J., and others: Colonic hydrogen production in infants with colic, J. Pediatr. 115(4):592-594, 1989.

Loadman, W., and others: Reducing the symptoms of infant colic by introduction of a vibration/sound-based intervention, Pediatr. Res. 21:182A, 1987.

Romanko, M.V., and Brost, B.A.: Swaddling: an effective invention for pacifying infants, Pediatr. Nurs. 8:259-261, 1982.

Sampson, H.: Infantile colic and food allergy: fact or fiction? J. Pediatr. 115(4):583-584, 1989.

Schmitt, B.: The prevention of sleep problems and colic, Pediatr. Clin. North Am. 33(4):763-774, 1986.

Schmitt, B.: When your baby has colic, Contemp. Pediatr. 7(2):85-86, 1990.

Spencer, J., and others: White noise and sleep induction, Arch. Dis. Child. 65(1):135-137, 1990.

Skin Disorders

Antherton, D.: Controversies in therapeutics: role of diet in treating atopic eczema: elimination diets can be beneficial, Br. Med. J. 297(6661):1458-1460, 1988.

Berg, R.: Etiology and pathophysiology of diaper dermatitis, Adv. Dermatol. 3:75-98, 1988.

Broadbent, J., and Sampson, H.: Food hypersensitivity and atopic dermatitis, Pediatr. Clin. North Am. 35(5):1115-1130, 1988.

Buckley, R.H., and Mathews, K.P.: Common 'allergic' skin diseases, JAMA 248(2):2611-2622, 1982.

Burks, A., and others: Atopic dermatitis: clinical relevance of food hypersensitivity reactions, J. Pediatr. 113(3):447-451, 1988.

Campbell, R., and others: Effects of diaper types on diaper dermatitis associated with diarrhea and antibiotic use in children in day-care centers, Pediatr. Dermatol. 5(2):83-87, 1988.

Chandra, R., Puri, S., and Hamed, A.: Influence of maternal diet during lactation and use of formula feeds on development of atopic eczema in high risk infants, Br. Med. J. 299:228-230, 1989.

David, T.J., and Longson, M.: Eczema and herpes simplex infection, Arch. Dis. Child. 60:338-343, 1985.

Gonzalez, J., and Hogg, R.J.: Metabolic alkalosis secondary to baking soda treatment of a diaper rash, Pediatrics 67(6):820-822, 1981.

Hide, D., and Guyer, B.: Clinical manifestations of allergy related to breast- and cow's milk-feeding, Pediatrics 76(6):973-975, 1985.

Hurwitz, S.: Eczematous eruptions in childhood, Pediatr. Rev. 3(1):23-30, 1981.

Kramer, M.: Does breast-feeding help protect against atopic disease? Biology, methodology, and a golden jubilee of controversy, J. Pediatr. 112(2):181-190, 1988.

Krusinski, P., and Flowers, F.: Handbook of pediatric dermatology, St. Louis, 1990, Mosby–Year Book, Inc.

Leung, D., and Kamada, M.: Developments in allergy, Curr. Opin. Pediatr. 1(1):27-34, 1989.

Lucas, A., and others: Early diet of preterm infants and development of allergic or atopic disease: randomised prospective study, Br. Med. J. 300:837-840, 1990.

Munz, D., Powell, K.R., and Pai, C.H.: Treatment of candidal diaper dermatitis: a double-blind placebo-controlled comparison of topical nystatin with topical plus oral nystatin, J. Pediatr. 101(6):1022-1025, 1982.

Nicol, N.: Atopic dermatitis: the (wet) wrap-up, Am. J. Nurs. 87(12):1560-1563, 1987.

Rasmussen, J.E.: Diseases of the scalp, Pediatr. Rev. 7(4):109-116, 1985.

Sampson, H.A., and Jolie, P.L.: Increased plasma histamine concentrations after food challenges in children with atopic dermatitis, N. Engl. J. Med. 311(6):372-376, 1984.

Apnea of Infancy

Andrews, M., and others: Home apnea: monitoring in the Intermountain West, J. Pediatr. Health Care 1(5):255-260, 1987.

Bairam, A., and others: Theophylline versus caffeine: comparative effects in treatment of idiopathic apnea in the preterm infant, J. Pediatr. 110(4):636-639, 1987.

Graber, H.P., and Balas-Stevens, S.: A discharge tool for teaching parents to monitor infant apnea at home, MCN 9(3):178, 1984.

Hartsell, M.: Selecting home monitors, J. Pediatr. Nurs. 1(1):54-57, 1986.

Hunt, C.E., and others: Home pneumograms in normal infants, J. Pediatr. 106(4):551-555, 1985.

Katcher, M., Shapiro, M., and Guist, C.: Severe injury and death associated with home infant cardiorespiratory monitors, Pediatrics 78(5):775-779, 1986.

Kelly, D., and others: Apnea and periodic breathing in normal infants, Pediatr. Pulmonol. 1:215-219, 1985.

Muttitt, S., and others: Neonatal apnea: diagnosis by nurse versus computer, Pediatrics 82(5):713-720, 1988.

Norris-Berkemeyer, S., and Hutchins, K.: Home apnea monitoring, Pediatr. Nurs. 12(4):259-262, 1986.

Orlowski, J.: Cerebrospinal fluid endorphins and the infant apnea syndrome, Pediatrics 78(2):233-237, 1986.

Orr, W.C., and others: Effect of sleep state and position on the incidence of obstructive and central apnea in infants, Pediatrics 75(5):832-835, 1985.

Rodriguez, A., Warburton, D., and Keens, T.: Elevated catecholamine levels and abnormal hypoxic arousal in apnea of infancy, Pediatrics 79(2):269-274, 1987.

Saylor, C., and others: Anxiety in mothers of infants on apnea monitors, Child. Health Care 18(2):117, 1989.

Spitzer, A., and Fox, W.: Infant apnea, Pediatr. Clin. North Am. 33(3):561-581, 1986.

Toubas, P., and others: Effects of maternal smoking and caffeine habits on infantile apnea: a retrospective study, Pediatrics 78(1):159-163, 1986.

Webb, L.Z., and Duncan, J.A.: Selecting the right home apnea monitor, Pediatr. Nurs. 9(3):179-182, 1983.

Sudden Infant Death Syndrome

Balarajan, R., Raleigh, V., and Botting, B.: Sudden infant death syndrome and postneonatal mortality in immigrants in England and Wales, Br. Med. J. 298(6675):716-720, 1989.

Bass, M., Kravath, R., and Glass, L.: Death-scene investigation in sudden infant death, N. Engl. J. Med. 35(6):100-105, 1986.

Bauchner, H., and others: Risk of sudden infant death syndrome among infants with in utero exposure to cocaine, J. Pediatr. 113(5):831-834, 1988.

Bergman, A.: Twenty-fifth anniversary of the National Sudden Infant Death Syndrome Foundation, Pediatrics 82(2):272-274, 1988.

Black, L., and others: Effects of birth weight and ethnicity on incidence of sudden infant death syndrome, J. Pediatr. 108(2):209-214, 1986.

Buck, G.: When the bough breaks: fresh clues to the cause of crib death, Sciences 28(4):32-37, 1988.

Chan, M.: Sudden infant death syndrome and families at risk, Pediatr. Nurs. 13(3):166-168, 1987.

de Jonge, G., and others: Cot death and prone sleeping position in the Netherlands, Br. Med. J. 298(6675):722, 1989.

Dunne, K., and Matthews, T.: Near-miss sudden infant death syndrome: clinical findings and management, Pediatrics 79(6):889-893, 1987.

Einspieler, C., and others: The predictive value of behavioural risk factors for sudden infant death, Early Human Dev. 18:101-109, 1988.

Farrar, H., and Kearns, G.: Cocaine: clinical pharmacology and toxicology, J. Pediatr. 115(5, Part 1):665-675, 1989.

Gilbert, R., and others: Signs of illness preceding sudden unexpected death in infants, Br. Med. J. 300(6734):1237-1239, 1990.

Gino, C.: SIDS research that causes pain, Am. J. Nurs. 88(10):1353-1354, 1988.

Giulian, G., Gilbert, E., and Moss, R.: Fetal hemoglobin levels in sudden infant death syndrome, N. Engl. J. Med. 316:1122-1126, 1987.

Grether, J., and Schulman, J.: Sudden infant death syndrome and birth weight, J. Pediatr. 114(4, pt. 1):561-567, 1989.

Grether, J., Schulman, J., and Croen, L.: Sudden infant death syndrome among Asians in California, J. Pediatr. 116(4):525-528, 1990.

Guilleminault, C., and others: Five cases of near-miss sudden infant death syndrome and development of obstructive sleep apnea syndrome, Pediatrics 73(1):71-78, 1984.

Guilleminault, C., and others: Near-miss sudden infant death syndrome in eight infants with sleep apnea-related cardiac arrhythmias, Pediatrics 76(2):236-242, 1985.

Haglund, B., and Cnattingius, S.: Cigarette smoking as a risk factor for sudden infant death syndrome: a population-based study, Am. J. Public Health 80:29-32, 1990.

Jezierski, M.: Infant death: guidelines for support of parents in the emergency department, J. Emerg. Nurs. 15(6):475-476, 1989.

Kahn, A., and others: Sudden infant death syndrome in a twin: a comparison of sibling histories, Pediatrics 78(1):146-150, 1986.

Kahn, A., and others: Polysomnographic studies of infants who subsequently died of sudden infant death syndrome, Pediatrics 82(5):721-727, 1988.

Kaplan, D.W., Bauman, A.E., and Krous, H.F.: Epidemiology of sudden infant death syndrome in American Indians, Pediatrics 74(6):1041-1046, 1984.

Kelly, D., and others: Pneumograms in infants who subsequently died of sudden infant death syndrome, J. Pediatr. 109(2):249-254, 1986.

Krongrad, E., and O'Neill, L.: Near miss sudden infant death syndrome episodes? A clinical and electrocardiographic correlation, Pediatrics 77(6):811-815, 1986.

Lee, N., and others: Sudden infant death syndrome in Hong Kong: confirmation of low incidence, Br. Med. J. 298(6675):721, 1989.

Lewis, N., McBride, J., and Brooks, J.: Ventilatory chemosensitivity in parents of infants with sudden infant death syndrome, J. Pediatr. 113(2):307-311, 1988.

Milner, A., and Ruggins, N.: Sudden infant death syndrome: recent focus on the respiratory system, Br. Med. J. 198(6675):689-690, 1989.

Nelson, E., Taylor, B., and Weatherall, I.: Sleeping position and infant bedding may predispose to hyperthermia and the sudden infant death syndrome, Lancet 1(8631):199-204, 1989.

Nikolaisen, S.M.: The impact of sudden infant death on the family: nursing intervention, Top. Clin. Nurs. 3(3):45-53, 1981.

Nikolaisen, S.M., and Williams, R.A.: Parent's view of support following the loss of their infant to sudden infant death syndrome, West. J. Nurs. Res. 2(3):593-601, 1980.

Oren, J., Kelly, D., and Shannon, D.: Familial occurrence of sudden infant death syndrome and apnea of infancy, Pediatrics 80(3):355-358, 1987.

Price, M., and others: Maternal perceptions of sudden infant death syndrome, Child. Health Care 14(1):22-31, 1985.

Rehm, R.S.: Teaching cardiopulmonary resuscitation to parents, MCN 8(6):411-414, 1983.

Southall, D.: Role of apnea in the sudden infant death syndrome: a personal view, Pediatrics 80(1):73-84, 1988.

Southall, D., and others: Cardiorespiratory function in 16 full-term infants with sudden infant death syndrome, Pediatrics 78(5):787-796, 1986.

Sudden infant death syndrome as a cause of premature mortality—United States, 1984-1985, MMWR 37(42):644-645, 1988.

Swoiskin, S.: Sudden infant death: nursing care for the survivors, J. Pediatr. Nurs. 1(1):33-39, 1986.

Vigevano, F., Capua, M., and Bernardina, B.: Startle disease: an avoidable cause of sudden infant death, Lancet 1(8631):216, 1989.

Ward, S., and others: Predicting SIDS: evaluation of apnea programs, Pediatrics 77:451-455, 1986.

Williams, R.A., and Nikolaisen, S.M.: Sudden infant death syndrome: parents' perceptions and responses to the loss of their infant, Res. Nurs. Health 5:55-61, 1982.

Infantile Autism

Campbell, M., and others: Naltrexone in autistic children: an acute open dose range tolerance trial, J. Am. Acad. Child Adolesc. Psychiatry 28:200-206, 1989.

Christian, W.P.: Childhood autism. In Levine, M., and others, editors: Developmental-behavioral pediatrics, Philadelphia, 1983, W.B. Saunders Co.

Cruz, V.K., Andron, L., and Sammons, C.: Cookie monster is autistic . . . help younger children with developmentally disabled siblings cope, Child. Today 13(2):18-20, 1984.

Dudziak, D.: Parenting the autistic child, J. Psychosoc. Nurs. Ment. Health Services 20(1):11-16, 1982.

Gualtieri, C.: Fenfluramine and autism: careful reappraisal is in order, J. Pediatr. 108(3):417-419, 1986.

Ho, H.H., and others: Blood serotonin concentrations and fenfluramine therapy in autistic children, J. Pediatr. 108(3):465-469, 1986.

Killion, S., and McCarthy, S., Hospitalization of the autistic child. I. Assessment. II. Autistic children, intervention, MCN 5(6):412-423, 1980.

Lewis, M.: Gifted or dysfunctional: the child savant, Pediatr. Ann. 14(10):733-742, 1985.

Omity, E.: Neurophysiology of infantile autism, J. Am. Acad. Child Psychiatry 24:251-262, 1985.

Ritvo, E., and others: Fenfluramine therapy for autism: promise and precaution, Psychol. Bull. 22(1):133-140, 1986.

Seifert, C.: Holistic interpretation of autism: a theoretical framework, Lanham MD, 1990, University Press of America, Inc.

Seifert, C.: Theories of autism, Lanham MD, 1990, University Press of America, Inc.

Stone, W.L., and others: Play and imitation skills in the diagnosis of autism in young children, Pediatrics 86(2):267-272, 1990.

Treffert, D.: An unlikely virtuoso: Leslie Lemke and the story of savant syndrome, Sciences 29(1):28-35, 1988.

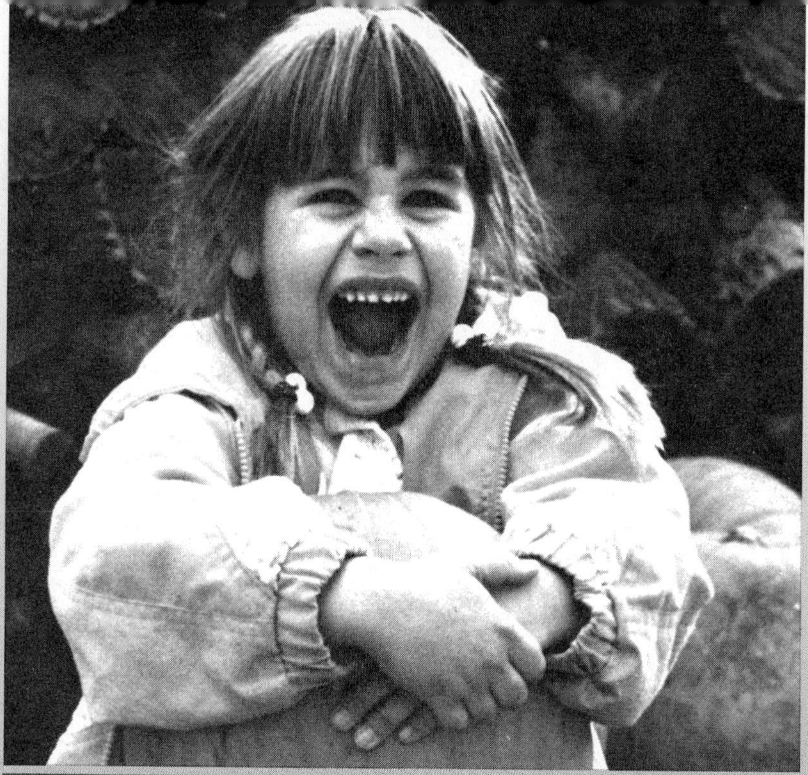

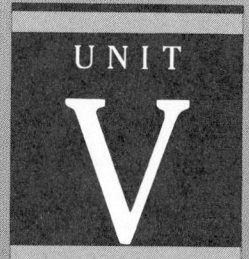

Early Childhood

UNIT

V

Early childhood comprises the period of toddlerhood and the preschool years. It is primarily a time of physical development and refinement, attainment of social skills, and achievement of independent behavior. Dramatic changes occur in the child as he leaves the dependent world of infancy and readies himself for the self-sufficient life of a school-age child. Chapters 14 and 15, *Health Promotion of the Toddler and Family* and *Health Promotion of the Preschooler and Family,* are concerned with the biologic growth and psychologic development of the toddler and preschooler. However, the family is the focus of nursing care to provide for the child an environment that fosters mental and physical health. Emphasis is placed on promoting optimum development during each phase of early childhood, especially through anticipatory guidance regarding nutrition, achievement of self-care activities, prevention of injury, and specific parental concerns.

Chapter 16, *Health Problems of Early Childhood,* deals with health problems that commonly occur during early childhood. Although many of the disorders typical of this period are caused by infectious processes, most of the child's care is implemented in the home, necessitating nursing guidance rather than direct intervention. The other conditions discussed are environmental and social factors to which toddlers and preschoolers are especially vulner able or by which they are greatly influenced. In the discussion of each of these health problems, emphasis is placed on prevention, recognition, and nursing interventions that return the child to an optimum physical and mental status following recovery.

CHAPTER 14

Health Promotion of the Toddler and Family

RELATED TOPICS

Animal bites, Ch. 18
Attachment, Ch. 12
Dental disorders, Ch. 18
Enuresis, Ch. 18
Family influences on child health promotion, Ch. 3
Fears, Ch. 15
Growth and development of children, Ch. 4
Ingestion of injurious agents, Ch. 16
Injuries—the leading killer, Ch. 1
Injury prevention: infant, Ch. 12; preschooler, 15
Sleep disturbances, Ch. 12
Social, cultural, and religious influences on child health promotion, Ch. 2
Spiritual development, Ch. 15
Stress in childhood, Ch. 4

GLOSSARY

AGM Absorbent gelling material
animism Ascribing lifelike qualities to inanimate objects
caries Decayed areas on teeth
centration Tendency to focus on one aspect of object or event rather than all aspects
egocentrism Inability to take another's viewpoint
global organization of thought Changing any part of whole changes the whole
irreversibility Unable to undo mentally an action that is initiated physically
negativism Persistent negative response to requests
operations Ability to cognitively manipulate objects
parallel play Playing alongside but not with other children
physiologic anorexia Decreased appetite resulting from decreased nutritional need
plaque Soft bacterial deposits that form on the teeth

preoperational thought Phase of cognition before ability to use operations
regression Retreat from present pattern of functioning to past levels of behavior
temper tantrums Sudden, explosive outbursts of anger
toddler Child ages 12 to 36 months
transductive reasoning Reasoning from the particular to the particular

The *terrible twos* has often been used to describe the toddler years, a period from 12 to 36 months of age. It is a time of intense exploration of the environment as children attempt to find out how things work, what the word *no* means, and how to control others with temper tantrums, negativism, and obstinacy. The phrase "they get into everything" actually underestimates toddlers' voracity for adventure, but the very adventure of getting into things is the means of acquisition of learning and knowledge.

Although this can be a difficult time for parents and child as each learns to know the other better, it is also an extremely important period for developmental achievement and intellectual growth. Successful mastery of the tasks of this age requires a strong foundation of trust during infancy and frequently necessitates guidance from others when parent and toddler face the struggles of toilet training, limit-setting and discipline, and sibling rivalry. Nurses who understand the dynamics of growth and development of the toddler can help families deal effectively with the developmental needs of this age.

PROMOTING OPTIMUM GROWTH AND DEVELOPMENT

General concepts of growth and development, such as stages and patterns of development and individual differences, have been extensively discussed in Chapter 4. This chapter is primarily concerned with biologic, psychosocial, cognitive, and social development of toddlers. It also includes a discussion of common parental concerns typical of the developmental characteristics of this age-group.

BIOLOGIC DEVELOPMENT

Biologic development and maturation of body systems is less dramatic during early childhood than in infancy. However, maturation of body systems continues, and many organs achieve mature functioning. The acquisition of fine and gross motor skills is dramatic and allows toddlers to master a wide variety of activities.

Proportional Changes

Growth slows considerably during toddlerhood. The average weight gain is 1.8 to 2.7 kg (4 to 6 pounds) per year. The average weight at 2 years is 12 kg (27 pounds). The birth weight is quadrupled by 2½ years of age. The rate of increase in height also slows. The usual increment is an addition of 7.5 cm (3 inches) per year and occurs mainly in elongation of the legs rather than the trunk. The average height of a 2-year-old is 86.6 cm (34 inches). In general, adult height is about twice the child's height at 2 years of age. Accurate measurement of height and weight during the toddler years should reveal a steady growth curve that is *steplike* in nature rather than linear (straight), which is characteristic of the growth spurts during the early childhood years.

The rate of increase in head circumference slows somewhat by the end of infancy, and head circumference is usually equal to chest circumference by 1 to 2 years of age. The usual total increase in head circumference during the second year is 2.5 cm (1 inch). Then the rate of increase slows until at age 5 years the increase is less than 1.25 cm (½ inch) per year. The anterior fontanel closes between 12 and 18 months of age.

Chest circumference continues to increase in size and exceeds head circumference during the toddler years. Its shape also changes as the transverse or lateral diameter exceeds the anteroposterior diameter. After the second year the chest circumference exceeds the abdominal measurement, which, in addition to the growth of the lower extremities, gives the child a taller, leaner appearance. However, the toddler retains a squat, "pot-bellied" appearance because of the less well developed abdominal musculature and short legs (Fig. 14-1). The legs retain a slightly bowed or curved appearance during the second year from the weight of the relatively large trunk.

Sensory Changes

Visual acuity of 20/20 is achieved during the toddler years, although 20/40 is considered acceptable. Full binocular vision is well developed by 12 months of age, and any evidence of persistent strabismus should receive professional attention as early as possible to prevent amblyopia. Depth perception continues to develop but, because of the child's lack of motor coordination, falls from heights remain a persistent danger.

The senses of hearing, smell, taste, and touch become increasingly well developed, coordinated with each other, and associated with other experiences. All of the senses are used to explore the environment. Toddlers will visually inspect an object by turning it over; they may taste it, smell it, and touch it several times before they are satisfied with

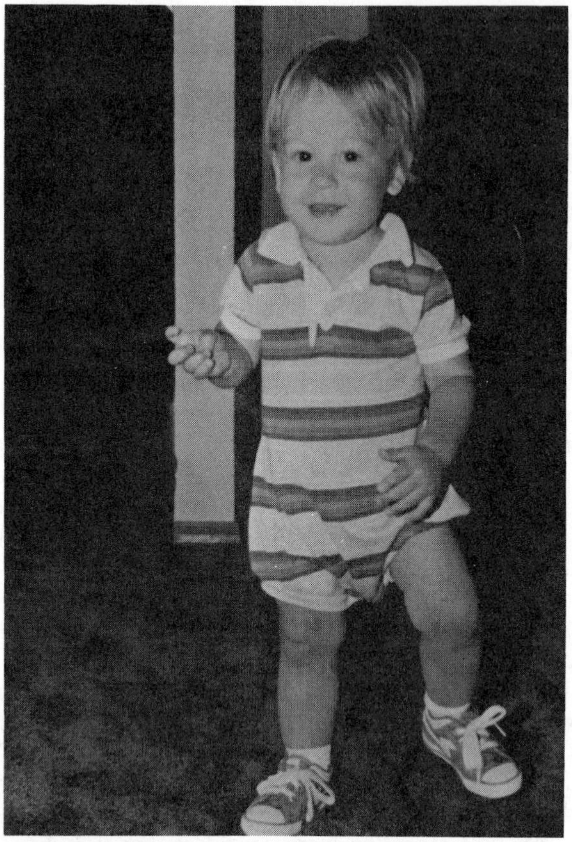

Fig. 14-1. Typical toddling gait.

their investigation. They will shake it to see if it makes noise and vigorously test its durability.

Another example of the integrated function of the senses is the toddler's development of specific taste preferences. The child is much less likely than infants to try a new food because of its appearance or smell, not only its taste. Nonsensory associations with objects also take on significance. For example, if parents refuse a particular food because of their dislike, they will transfer this negative connotation to the child before the child has had an opportunity to taste it. Awareness of these factors is important in several areas of childrearing, such as feeding, teaching socially acceptable habits, and reinforcing appropriate behavioral responses to various situations.

Touch continues to be important to the toddler. Descending development of the spinal tract is evidenced by increased sensation in the lower extremities, such as tickling the feet. Pleasant tactile sensations soothe and comfort the toddler, especially in times of stress or fatigue.

Maturation of Systems

Most of the physiologic systems are relatively mature by the end of toddlerhood. By the end of the first year all the brain cells are present but continue to increase in size. Myelination of the spinal cord is almost complete by 2 years of age, which parallels the completion of most of the gross motor skills associated with locomotion. Brain growth is 75% completed by the end of 2 years.

Development of various areas of the brain seems to correspond with the progressive intellectual capacity of the child. Various areas of the cerebral cortex undergo specific changes as developmental progress occurs, such as Broca area for speech and cortical areas for control of the legs, hands, feet, and sphincters. Because this neuromotor organization is so inclusive, complex, and intricate, the child is limited in the ability to attend to any one aspect of behavior for more than a few minutes.

Between 2 and 3 years of age coordination and consolidation of these voluntary functions allow the toddler to listen better, look longer, and have an extended span of attention. Although postural control is increasingly developed as myelination of the spinal cord advances, the immaturity of this control, combined with the child's limited experiences and the lack of visual perception, makes simple acts such as seating oneself in a chair or climbing down stairs difficult tasks.

Volume of the respiratory tract and growth of associated structures continue to increase during early childhood, lessening some of the factors that predisposed the child to frequent and serious infections during infancy. However, the internal structures of the ear and throat continue to be short and straight, and the lymphoid tissue of the tonsils and adenoids continues to be large. As a result, otitis media, tonsillitis, and upper respiratory tract infections are common. The respiratory and heart rates slow, and the blood pressure increases (see inside front cover). Respirations continue to be abdominal.

The digestive processes are fairly complete by the beginning of toddlerhood. The acidity of the gastric contents continues to increase and has a protective function, since it is capable of destroying many types of bacteria. Stomach capacity increases to allow for the usual schedule of three meals a day.

One of the more prominent changes of the gastrointestinal system is the voluntary control of elimination. With complete myelination of the spinal cord, control of anal and urethral sphincters is gradually achieved. Urination and defecation are controlled by a visceral reflex. For example, as urine accumulates in the bladder, the proprioceptors within the muscle tissues are activated by the stretching of the walls. Impulses are sent by the visceral afferent fibers to the spinal cord and then to the autonomic nervous system, which in turn causes the smooth muscle of the bladder wall to contract and expel the urine. The physiologic ability to control the sphincters probably occurs somewhere between ages 18 and 24 months. Bladder capacity also increases considerably. By 14 to 18 months of age the child is able to retain urine for up to 2 hours or longer.

The skin functionally matures during early childhood. The epidermis and dermis are more tightly bound together, increasing their resistance to infection and irritation and creating a more effective barrier against fluid loss. Production of sebum is minimum, which contributes to the development of dry skin. The eccrine glands are functional during early childhood and react to changes in temperature, but they produce very minimal amounts of sweat. Hair grows thicker and coarser and usually darkens and loses some curliness. Fine hair is evident on the lower arms and legs. Production of adipose tissue declines as hyperplasia of muscle cells increases. With the concurrent growth of the lower extremities, the child assumes more adultlike proportions.

Under conditions of moderate variation in temperature, the toddler rarely has the difficulties of the young infant in maintaining body temperature. The capillaries are able to conserve core body temperature by constricting in response to cold and dilating in response to heat. Shivering is much more effective as a source of thermogenesis. Shivering is an involuntary act that results in rhythmic muscle contraction, which increases cellular metabolism, producing heat. The child also learns mechanisms to control body temperature—by putting on clothing when cold or removing it when warm.

The defense mechanisms of the tissues and blood, particularly phagocytosis, are much more efficient in the toddler than in the infant. The production of antibodies is well established. Immunoglobulin G (IgG), which neutralizes microbial toxins, reaches adult levels by the end of the second year of life. Passive immunity from maternal transfer during fetal life disappears by the beginning of toddlerhood. Immunoglobulin M (IgM), which responds to artificial immunizing techniques and combats serious infection, attains adult levels during late infancy. Immunoglobulins A, D, and E increase gradually, not reaching eventual adult levels until later childhood. Many young children demonstrate a sudden increase in colds and minor infections when entering nursery school because of the exposure to new antigens.

Gross and Fine Motor Development

The major gross motor skill during the toddler years is the development of location. By 15 months toddlers walk alone; by age 18 months they try to run but fall easily; and by 2 years they walk well and run fairly well, using a wide stance for extra balance. Between 2 and 3 years of age, refinement of the upright, biped position is evident in improved coordination and equilibrium. By 2 years toddlers can walk up and down stairs, and by age 2½ years they jump, using both feet, stand on one foot for a second or two, and manage a few steps on tiptoe. By the end of the second year they stand on one foot, walk on tiptoe, and climb stairs with alternate footing.

Fine motor development is demonstrated in increasingly skillful manual dexterity. Once the pincer grasp is achieved, usually at 9 to 10 months of age, toddlers combine this skill with other developing sensory and cognitive abilities. For example, by age 12 months they are able to grasp a very small object but are unable to release it at will. At 15 months they can drop a pellet into a narrow-necked bottle. Casting, or voluntarily throwing objects, and retrieving them become almost obsessive activities around 15 months of age. By 18 months they can throw a ball overhand without losing their balance.

Visual perception of geometric shapes is also evident at this time. At age 12 months children selectively look at a round hole in a special form board but are unable to insert a round object. By age 15 months they promptly place the round object in the hole, even if the board is revised or turned upside down. Spatial relations also are evident in their ability to build a tower with blocks; by age 18 months, a tower of three to four blocks; by age 24 months, a tower of six to seven blocks; and by age 30 months, a tower of eight blocks or more.

Fine motor skill and visual ability are demonstrated in toddlers' progressive adeptness in manipulating a pencil or crayon. By age 15 months they will scribble spontaneously and by 24 months of age will imitate a circular stroke and a vertical line. By the end of the toddler period copying a circle and imitating a cross are possible.

Mastery of gross and fine motor skills is evident in all phases of the child's activity, such as play, dressing, language comprehension, response to discipline, social interaction, and proneness to injuries. Activities occur less in isolation and more in conjunction with other physical and mental abilities to produce a purposeful result. For example, the toddler walks to reach a new location, releases a toy to pick it up or to choose a new one, and scribbles to look at the image produced. The possibilities of the exploration, investigation, and manipulation mastery of the environment—and its hazards—are endless.

PSYCHOSOCIAL DEVELOPMENT

Toddlers are faced with the mastery of several important tasks. If the need for basic trust has been satisfied, they are ready to give up dependence for control, independence, and autonomy. Some of the specific tasks to be dealt with include the following:

- Differentiation of self from others, particularly the mother
- Toleration of separation from parent
- Ability to withstand delayed gratification
- Control over bodily functions
- Acquisition of socially acceptable behavior
- Verbal means of communication
- Ability to interact with others in a less egocentric manner

Mastery of these goals is only begun during late infancy and the toddler years, and such tasks as developing interpersonal relationships with others may not be completed until adolescence. However, crucial foundations for successful completion of such developmental tasks are laid during these early formative years.

Developing a Sense of Autonomy (Erikson)

According to Erikson, the developmental task of toddlerhood is acquiring a sense of *autonomy* while overcoming a sense of *doubt* and *shame.* As infants gain trust in the predictability and reliability of their parents, environment, and interaction with others, they begin to discover that their behavior is their own and that it has a predictable, reliable effect on others. However, although they realize their will and control over others, they are confronted with the conflict of exerting autonomy and relinquishing the much enjoyed dependence on others. Exerting their will has definite negative consequences, whereas retaining dependent, submissive behavior is generally rewarded with affection and approval. However, continued dependency creates a sense of doubt regarding their potential capacity to control their actions. This doubt is compounded by a sense of shame for feeling this urge to revolt against others' will and a fear that they will exceed their own capacity for manipulating the environment. The latter fear is a basis for instituting limit-setting and consistent discipline at this age. Without appropriate limits on what is acceptable vs nonacceptable behavior, children have no guidelines for establishing the end points of their ability to control.

Just as the infant has the social modalities of grasping and biting, the toddler has the newly gained modality of holding on and letting go. To hold on and let go is evident with the use of the hands, mouth, eyes, and eventually, the sphincters, when toilet training is begun. These social modalities are expressed constantly in the child's play activities, such as casting or throwing objects away, taking objects out of boxes, drawers, or cabinets, holding on tighter when someone says, "No, don't touch," and spitting out food as taste preferences become very strong.

Several characteristics, especially negativism and ritualism, are typical of toddlers in their quest for autonomy. As toddlers attempt to express their will, they often act contrary to everything around them. The words "no" or "me do" can be the sole vocabulary. Emotions become very strongly expressed, usually in rapid mood swings. One minute toddlers can be engrossed in an activity, and the next minute they might be violently angry because they were unable to manipulate a toy or open a door. If scolded for doing something wrong, they can have a temper tantrum and almost instantaneously pull at the parent's legs to be picked up and comforted. Often these swift changes are difficult for parents to understand and cope with. Many parents find the negativism exasperating and, instead of dealing constructively with it, give into it, which further threatens children in their search for learning acceptable methods of interacting with others (see p. 660).

In contrast to negativism, which frequently disrupts the environment, ritualism becomes the needed buffer to maintain sameness and reliability. Toddlers can venture out with security when they know that there still exist familiar people, places, and routines. One can easily understand why change, such as hospitalization, represents such a threat to these children. Without the comfortable rituals, there is little opportunity to exert autonomy. Consequently dependency and regression occur (see p. 661).

Erikson focuses on the development of the *ego* during this phase of psychosocial development. There is a struggle as the child deals with the impulses of the id and attempts to tolerate frustration and learns socially acceptable ways of interacting with the environment. The ego, which may be thought of as reason or common sense, is evident as the child is able to tolerate delayed gratification. It operates on the *reality principle,* whereas the id operates on the *pleasure principle.*

There is also a rudimentary beginning of the *superego,* or conscience, which is the incorporation of the morals of society and the process of acculturation. With the development of the ego children further differentiate themselves from others and expand their sense of trust within themselves. But as they begin to develop awareness of their own will and capacity to achieve, they also become aware of their ability to fail. This ever-present awareness of potential failure creates fear of doubt and shame. Successful mastery of the task of autonomy necessitates opportunities for self-mastery while withstanding the frustration of necessary limit-setting and delayed gratification. Opportunities for self-mastery are present in appropriate play activities, toilet training, the crisis of sibling rivalry, and successful interactions with significant others.

Anal Stage (Freud)

Freud's anal stage roughly corresponds with Erikson's stage of autonomy, or the period from 18 months to 3 years of age. Within this psychosexual framework the anal zone becomes the center of the child's physical, emotional, and psychologic efforts. Pleasure comes from moving the bowels, but the child is also met with the conflict of gaining physical satisfaction from involuntary evacuation vs gaining emotional reinforcement by holding on and letting go at the parent's will. The process of toilet training is regarded as the resolution of this conflict.

COGNITIVE DEVELOPMENT

By the beginning of the second year it is quite clear that the toddler "thinks" and "reasons" things out. There is deliberate trial-and-error experimentation to produce certain results. The mental abstracts of time, space, and causality begin to have meaning, but the child's conception of each is different from that of the adult's. The main cognitive achievement of early childhood is the acquisition of language, which represents mental symbolism.

Sensorimotor and Preconceptual Phase (Piaget)

The period of 12 to 24 months of age is a continuation of the final two stages of the sensorimotor phase (Table 14-1). During this time the cognitive processes develop rapidly and at times seem similar to mature thinking. However, reasoning skills are still quite primitive and need to be understood to effectively deal with the typical behaviors of this age child.

Tertiary circular reactions. In the fifth stage (from 13 to 18 months), the child uses active experimentation to achieve previously unattainable goals. Newly acquired physical skills are increasingly important for the function they serve rather than for the acts themselves. The child incorporates the old learning of secondary circular reactions and applies the combined knowledge to new situations, with emphasis on the results of the experimentation. In this way there is the beginning of rational judgment and intellectual reasoning. During this stage there is further differentiation of oneself from objects. This is evident in the child's increasing ability to venture away from the parent and to tolerate longer periods of separation.

Awareness of a causal relationship between two events is apparent. After flipping a light switch, toddlers are aware that a reciprocal response occurs. However, they are not

Table 14-1 Sensorimotor and preconceptual phases during toddlerhood*

STAGE	AGE	COGNITIVE DEVELOPMENT	BEHAVIOR
Sensorimotor			
V. Tertiary circular reactions	13-18 months	Active experimentation to achieve previously unattainable goals Increased concept of object permanence Differentiation of oneself from objects Early traces of memory Beginning awareness of spatial, causal, and temporal relationships Able to enter into an action at any point without reproducing the entire sequence	Insatiable curiosity about the environment Uses all sensory cures for exploration Ventures away from parent for longer periods Uses physical skills to achieve a particular goal Can find hidden objects, but only in first location Able to insert a round object into a hole Fits smaller objects into each other (nesting) Gestures "up" and "down" Puts objects into a container and takes them out Realizes that "out of sight" is not out of reach; opens doors and drawers to find objects Gains comfort from parent's voice even if the parent is not visually present
VI. Invention of new means through mental combinations	19-24 months	Awareness of object permanence regardless of the number of invisible displacements Can infer a cause while only experiencing the effect Imitation is increasingly symbolic Beginning sense of time in terms of anticipation, memory, and ability to wait Egocentricism in thought and behavior Global organization of thought	Searches for an object through several hiding places Will infer a cause by associating two or more experiences (such as candy missing, sister smiling) Imitates words and sounds of animals Imitates adult behavior (domestic mimicry) Follows directions and understands requests Uses words "up," "down," "come," and "go" with meaning Has some sense of time; waits in response to "just a minute"; may use word "now" May sit and wait for meals at the table for short period of time Refers to self by name Engages in parallel play; demonstrates awareness of ownership Very concerned with ritualistic, routinized schedule
Preconceptual	2-4 years†	Increased use of language as mental symbolization Egocentricism still present in thought, play, and behavior Increased sense of time, space, causality Global organization of thought Transductive reasoning Concept of animism Unable to conceptualize two aspects of one object Magical thinking	Uses two- to three-word phrases Increased vocabulary Refers to self by pronoun Possessive of own toys, uses word "mine" Begins to use past tense of verbs Uses phrases "going to," "in a minute," "today," "all done" Uses many future-oriented words, such as "tomorrow," "next day," "afternoon," but poor conception of passage of time Follows directions using prepositions—up, behind, under, in back of, and so on Transfers knowledge of one object to same object in another location (e.g., electrical outlet) Very traditional and ritualistic, small change in routine represents a drastic change in entire schedule Reasoning of causal relationships is directly by proximity of two or more events

*For the previous four stages during early infancy see Table 12-1.
†Cognitive development and behavior apply primarily to ages 24 to 36 months.

able to transfer that knowledge to new situations. Therefore every time they see what appears to be a light switch, they must reinvestigate its function. Such behavior demonstrates the beginning of categorizing data into distinct classes, subclasses, and so on. There are innumerable examples of this type of behavior as toddlers continuously explore the same object each time it appears in a new place. A classic example is their curiosity about electrical outlets. Even if they receive a shock from one of them, they will adamantly poke, taste, and inspect every other outlet. This inability to transfer information leaves toddlers particularly vulnerable to accidents. However, traces of memory are evident because they will usually avoid the outlet where the shock occurred.

Since classification of objects is still rudimentary, the appearance of an object denotes its function. For example, if the child's toys are stored in a paper bag or large container, that toy receptacle is no different than the garbage pail or laundry basket. If allowed to turn over the toy receptacle, the child will just as quickly do the same to other similar objects because, in the child's mind, there is no difference. Expecting toddlers to judge which receptacles are permissible to explore and which are not is inappropriate for this age-group. Instead, the forbidden object, such as the garbage pail, should be placed out of reach.

The discovery of objects as objects leads to the awareness of their spatial relationships. Children are able to recognize different shapes and their relationship to each other. For example, they can fit slightly smaller boxes into each other (nesting) and can place a round object into a hole, even if the board is turned around, upside down, or reversed. However, not until 2 years of age can they do the same thing with a square. Children are also aware of space and the relationship of their body to dimensions such as height. They will stretch, stand on a low stair or stool, and pull a string to reach an object.

Object permanence has also advanced. Although they still cannot find an object that has been invisibly displaced or moved from under one pillow to another pillow without their seeing the change, toddlers are increasingly aware of the existence of objects behind closed doors, in drawers, and under tables. Parents are usually acutely aware of this developmental achievement because they find high places and locked cabinets the only areas inaccessible to toddlers. Parents also experience toddlers' protest behaviors when the parents leave, since toddlers are aware that their parents are absent when they cannot see them.

Invention of new means through mental combinations. During ages 19 to 24 months the child is in the final sensorimotor stage. This stage completes the more primitive, autistic thought processes of infancy and prepares the way for more complex mental operations during the phase of preoperational thought. One of the most dramatic achievements of this stage is in the area of object permanence. Children will now actively search for an object in several potential hiding places. In addition, they can infer a cause when only experiencing the effect. They can infer that an object was hidden in any number of places even if they only saw the original hiding place.

Imitation displays deeper meaning and understanding. Earlier, imitation was very concrete and action oriented. For example, "bye-bye" was a behavioral response more than a conceptual gesture of departure. Now it has a broader meaning, such as Daddy is going to work, it is time for a walk, or something is no longer present. There is greater symbolization to imitation.

One type of symbolic imitation is *domestic mimicry,* the imitation of household activity. Toddlers are acutely aware of others' actions and attempt to copy them in gestures and in words. They can imitate the parents' performance of a household task both physically and verbally. Parents often remark how accurately they see themselves in their child when the child engages in domestic mimicry. Such activity is part of the child's learning sex-role behavior.

The conception of time is still embryonic, but children have some sense of timing in terms of anticipation, memory, and the limited ability to wait. They may listen to the command, "Just a minute," and behave appropriately. However, their sense of timing is exaggerated—1 minute can last an hour. Toddlers' limited attention spans also indicate their sense of immediacy and concern for the present.

Egocentrism, or the inability to envision situations from perspectives other than one's own, is evident in all aspects of toddlers' behavior. They see, experience, and live every event in reference to themselves. For example, if a person is positioned between the toddler and another child, the toddler, who is facing the person, will explain that both children can see the middle person's face. The young child is unable to realize that the other person views the middle person from a different perspective, the back. A common example of egocentric behavior is the toddler who takes a toy away from another child. The child is concerned only with playing with the toy and is unable to conceptualize that taking the toy away will make the other child unhappy.

Preconceptual phase. At approximately 2 years of age the child enters the preconceptual phase of cognitive development, which lasts until about 4 years. The preconceptual phase is a subdivision of the *preoperational phase,* which spans ages 2 to 7 years. The preconceptual phase is primarily one of transition, which bridges the purely self-satisfying behavior of infancy and the rudimentary socialized behavior of latency. The principal characteristics of this stage are egocentric use of language and dependence on perception in problem solving (Thomas, 1985).

During 2 to 4 years children learn a variety of words and there is an increasing use of language. In fact, toddlers talk a lot. Speech is primarily of two types—egocentric or socialized. *Egocentric speech* consists of repeating words and sounds for the pleasure of hearing oneself and is not intended to communicate. This *collective monologue* reflects the child's lingering self-centeredness.

Socialized speech is for communication; however, it is still egocentric in that children communicate about themselves to others. Before age 3 most speech is directed at self-fulfillment or self-reference, such as, "Want drink," or "I do," and is directed mostly to adults. Since children think that everyone else's world is the same as theirs, they expect others to understand their verbal messages even when limited information is conveyed.

Preoperational thinking implies that children cannot think in terms of "operations"—the ability to manipulate objects in relation to each other in a logical fashion. Rather, toddlers think primarily based on their perception of an event. Problem solving is based on what they see or hear directly rather than on what they recall about objects and events. Critical to this type of thought is the concept of *centration*—the tendency to focus on one aspect rather than consider all the possible alternatives. Another aspect of their thinking relates to reasoning. Toddlers' reasoning is neither deductive, from the general to the specific, nor inductive, from the specific to the general, but *transductive,* from the particular to the particular. For example, if they did not like one food on the table, they may not like any other food. This prelogic is often very difficult to understand and confusing for parents, who will respond to the previous example by stating, "What does this food have to do with that food?" As far as toddlers are concerned, the decision is logical because it is based on their frame of reference. No amount of "reasoning" will reverse this logic.

Typical of toddlers' thinking is *global organization* of thought processes, or the idea that changing any part of the whole changes the entire whole. Behaviorally this is repeatedly demonstrated in the toddler's ritualistic and rigidly traditional world. Everything must remain the same for the entire event to remain constant. Changing the smallest detail disrupts the entire experience. For example, moving the crib a few inches upsets the entire room. Substituting a new dish for the usual one spoils the entire meal. Rescheduling one part of the day's activity ruins the whole day. Such preoccupation with sameness is usually not evident in every phase of the child's life. It may center around a "security blanket" or a favorite teddy bear, but the ritualism represents a secure and reassuring foundation. When one realizes the importance of tradition and routine, the great disruption that illness and hospitalization represent to toddlers can be appreciated.

Another peculiarity of preconceptual thought is the concept of *animism,* in which children attribute lifelike qualities to inanimate objects. For example, after falling down the stairs, the child blames the stairs for causing the accident and will frequently "scold" the stairs. Cause and effect is more related to proximity of events than to anything else. In some instances this is a correct assumption, such as flicking the light switch turns the lamp on. But in other circumstances two simultaneous events do not cause each other, such as turning the light off at bedtime and the parent leaving the room. Fears of darkness are not unlikely when, in the child's mind, darkness is the "cause" of separation. Being aware of this type of causal thinking is especially important when young children are subjected to painful or frightening procedures. For example, when lights are turned off in a radiology room, the x-ray machine is turned on. The sudden darkness and loud noise can be frightening even though no pain is inflicted. Explaining the procedures by turning the machine and lights on with people present will help the child disassociate the two events of darkness and loud noise.

Another significant cognitive characteristic is *irreversibility*—children are unable to undo or reverse mentally the actions they initiate physically. Therefore when told to stop doing something, they are unable to conceive of the opposite behavior. Consequently, directions should be phrased *positively* in terms of what is expected, such as "Put the toy down," rather than "Don't throw the toy."

Within the second year the child increasingly uses language symbolically and is concerned with the "why" and "how" of things. For example, a pencil is "something to write with" and food is "something to eat." However, such mental symbolization is closely associated with prelogical reasoning. For instance, a needle is "something that hurts." Such painful experiences take on new significance, since memory is associated with the specific event and fears are likely to develop, such as resistance to people who wear white uniforms or rooms that look like the practitioner's office. Sometimes the child's ability to recall events is underestimated, and little thought is given to the preparation for visits to a hospital or other health facility, resulting in fears that can last a lifetime. Because of the vulnerability of these early years, it is essential to prepare children for new experiences, whether it is a new baby-sitter or a visit to the dentist.

MORAL DEVELOPMENT

Moral development is usually viewed as one aspect of socialization, as children learn to conform to the expectations of their culture. Several theorists incorporate moral development into their theoretical frameworks, and most view its progress as paralleling that of cognitive development. One of the more prominent theories is that of Lawrence Kohlberg.

Preconventional or Premoral Level (Kohlberg)

Toddlers' development of moral judgment is at the most basic level. There is little, if any, concern for why something is wrong. Young children behave because of the freedom or restriction that is placed on actions. In the *punishment and obedience orientation* whether an action is good or bad depends on whether it results in reward or punishment. If children are punished for it, the action is bad. If they are not punished, the action is good, regardless of the meaning of the act. For example, if parents allow hitting, the child will perceive that hitting is good because it is not associated with punishment (Thomas, 1985).

The type of discipline also affects children's moral development. When parents use power to control behavior, such as physical punishment or withholding privileges, children receive a negative view of morals, especially toward authority figures, such as law enforcement agencies. When parents withdraw love or attention, children behave primarily because of guilt, rather than from an internalization of morals. However, when parents give explanations for the misbehavior and try to help children change through positive approaches, such as consequences or rewards, children feel less hostility and are more likely to base their actions on an analysis of why an act may be wrong (Schuster and Ashburn, 1986). Of course, the effect of discipline is not limited to the toddler years, and the sole use of explanation is inappropriate. However, parents usually establish discipline techniques at this time, and the use of constructive approaches should begin early (see p. 658).

SPIRITUAL DEVELOPMENT

Because of their immature cognitive processes, toddlers have only a vague idea of God and religious teachings. However, routines, such as saying prayers before meals or at bedtime, can be very important and comforting. Toward the end of toddlerhood, when children are in preoperational thought, there is some advancement of their understanding of God. Religious teachings may influence their behavior, such as reward or fear of punishment (heaven or hell) and moral development (see also discussion in Chapter 15.)

DEVELOPMENT OF BODY IMAGE

As in infancy, the development of body image closely parallels cognitive development. With increasing motor ability toddlers recognize the usefulness of body parts and gradually learn their respective names.

Once they begin preoperational thought, toddlers can use symbols to represent objects, but their thinking may lead to inaccuracies. For example, if someone who is pregnant is called "fat," they will describe all "fat" ladies as having babies. There is a beginning recognition of words used to describe physical appearance, such as "pretty," "handsome," or "big boy." Such expressions eventually influence how children view their own bodies, and such labeling (negative or positive) becomes part of their body image.

Although there has been little research done on body image development in young children, it is evident that body integrity is poorly understood and that intrusive experiences are threatening. For example, during a physical assessment toddlers forcefully resist procedures such as examining the ear or mouth and taking a rectal temperature. Toddlers also have unclear body boundaries and may associate nonviable parts, such as feces, with essential body parts. This can be seen in the toddler who is upset by flushing the toilet and watching the stool disappear (Griffiths, 1983).

DEVELOPMENT OF SEXUALITY

Just as toddlers explore their environment, they also explore their bodies and find that touching certain body parts is pleasurable. Genital fondling (masturbation) can occur and involves manual stimulation, as well as posturing movements (especially in young girls) such as tightening of the thighs or mechanical pressure applied to the pubic or suprapubic area (Fleisher and Morrison, 1990). Other demonstrations of sensual activities include rocking, swinging, and hugging people and toys. Parental reactions to toddlers' sexual behavior will influence the children's own attitudes and should be accepting rather than critical.

Children in this age-group are learning vocabulary associated with anatomy, elimination, and reproduction. Certain associations between words and functions become significant and can influence future sexual attitudes. For example, if parents refer to the genitals as dirty, especially in the context of elimination, this association between "genitals" and "dirty" may be transferred to sexual functions by the child.

Sex-role differences become obvious to children and are evident in much of their imitative play. Early attitudes are formed about affectional behaviors between adults from observing parental and other adult sexual/sensual activities. (See also Sex Education, Chapter 15.)

Nurses can assist parents in fostering a positive body image in their child by encouraging them to avoid negative labels, such as "skinny arms" or "chubby legs"—self-perceptions that can last a lifetime. Body parts, especially those related to elimination and reproduction, should be called by their correct names. Respect for the body should be practiced.

SOCIAL DEVELOPMENT

Toddlers are very social beings. As they begin to develop a sense of separateness, they are increasingly able to explore away from the parent, although anxiety related to imposed separations and strangers is at a peak. Major advances occur in language ability and personal-social behavior, although social skills, such as waiting a turn or manners, are extremely rudimentary. Play continues to be a major socializing agent and provides toddlers with invaluable opportunities to learn about the environment.

Individuation-Separation

A major task of the toddler period is differentiation of self from significant others, usually the mother. The differentiation process consists of two phases: *separation*, the children's emergence from a symbiotic fusion with the mother, and *individuation,* those achievements that mark children's assumption of their own individual characteristics in the environment (Mahler, Pine, and Bergman, 1975). Although the process begins during the latter half of infancy, the major achievements occur during the toddler years.

Toddlers have an increased understanding and awareness of object permanence and some ability to withstand delayed gratification and tolerate moderate frustration. They begin to lose some of the previous resistance to separation, yet appear to become even more concerned about the parent's whereabouts. They have learned from experience that parents exist when physically absent. Repetition of events such as going to bed without the parents but waking to find them again reinforces the reliability of such brief separations. Consequently toddlers are able to venture away from their parents for brief periods because of the security of knowing that the parent will be there when they return. Verbal and visual reassurance from the parent gradually replaces some of the previous need to be physically close for comfort.

Toddlers also show less fear of strangers, but only when their parents are present. When left alone with a stranger, they are very fearful; acutely anxious; manifest depressive behavior, such as crying and withdrawal; and may become restless, hyperactive, or passive, reverting to regressive behaviors. Such reactions may be evident when a child is left with a baby-sitter or during the initial days of nursery school or daycare.

These behaviors are not pathologic or harmful if parents realize how desperately their children need them. In fact, indiscriminate friendliness toward strangers and lack of anxiety during separation from parents is reason for concern. Sensitive, perceptive parents will be aware of the child's need for increased love, affection, and attention when they are together. An attitude such as "They will get used to the baby-sitter" will not help young children positively tolerate separation.

Parents often need help in realizing the necessity of preparing children for an inevitable separation. Particularly with the firstborn, parents tend to overprotect children, shield them from any anxiety-producing experience, and insulate them from less than immediate gratification. Although this is not necessarily harmful, especially if opportunities for independence are allowed later, it does not prepare children for unexpected events. A typical example is the birth of a sibling. The child is faced with the crisis of sibling rivalry as well as separation from the parent. No wonder the child will not welcome the infant—the intruder caused mother to leave! Allowing children to experience brief periods of separation early during infancy prepares them for such experiences later. Indeed, they may still manifest the typical behaviors of protest, but they will also have learned that mother or father always returns. Therefore it is easy to appreciate the tremendous loss that the death of a parent represents for young children; unlike their other experiences with separation, this time the parent will not return. (For a discussion of the controversy regarding long-term consequences of separation, see Questions and Controversies, p. 549.)

Transitional objects, such as a favorite blanket or toy, provide security for young children, especially when they are separated from parents, dealing with a new stress, or just fatigued (Fig. 14-2). Security objects often become so important to toddlers that they refuse to have them taken away. Such behavior is normal; there is no need to discourage this tendency. During separations, such as daycare, hospitalization, or even overnight with a relative, transitional objects should be provided to minimize any feelings of fear or loneliness.

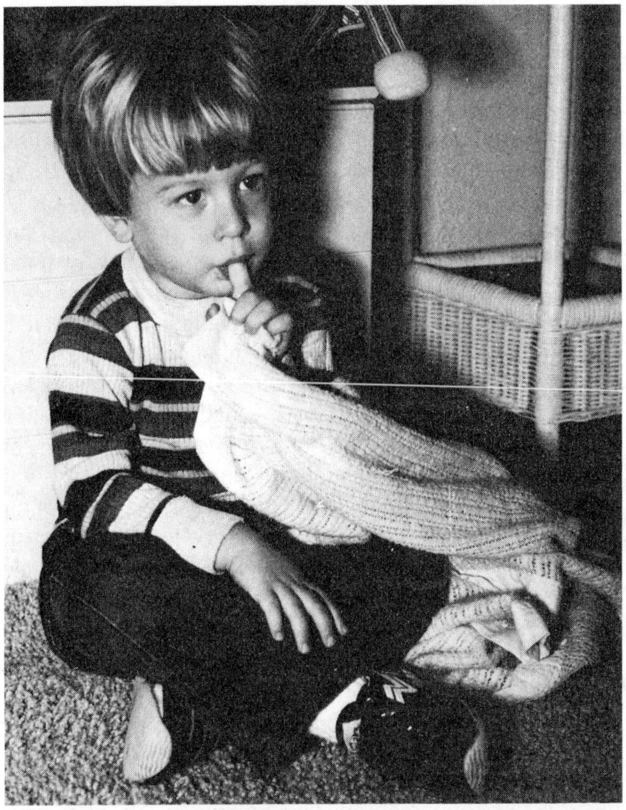

Fig. 14-2. Transitional objects, such as a warm and fuzzy blanket and a finger, are sources of security to toddlers.

Learning to tolerate and master brief periods of separation is an important developmental task of children in this age-group. In addition, it is a necessary component of parenting, since brief periods of separation from their children allow parents to recoup their energy and patience and to minimize directing their irritations and frustrations at the children.

Language Development

The most striking characteristic of language development during early childhood is the increasing level of comprehension. Although the number of words acquired—from about 4 at 1 year of age to approximately 300 at age 2 years—is notable, the ability to comprehend and understand speech is much greater than the number of words the child can say. This is particularly evident in bilingual families where the vocabulary may be delayed, but comprehension in either language is appropriate.

At age 1 year the child uses one-word sentences or holophrases. The word "up" can mean "pick me up" or "look up there." For the child the one word conveys the meaning of a sentence, but to others it may mean many things or nothing. During this age about 25% of the vocalizations are intelligible. By the age of 2 years the child uses multiword sentences by stringing together two or three words, such as the phrases, "mama go bye-bye" or "all gone," and approximately 65% of the speech is understandable.

Personal-Social Behavior

One of the most dramatic aspects of development in the toddler is personal-social interaction. Parents frequently wonder why their manageable, docile, lovable infant has turned into a determined, strong-willed, volatile-tempered little tyrant. In addition the tyrant of the terrible twos can swiftly and unpredictably revert back to the adorable infant. All of this is part of "growing up" and is evident in such areas as dressing, feeding, playing, and establishing self-control.

Toddlers are developing skills of independence, which are evident in all areas of behavior. By 15 months children feed themselves, drink well from a cup, and manage a spoon, with considerable spilling. By 18 months they use a spoon well and may be using a fork. Between ages 2 and 3 years they eat with the family and like to help with chores such as setting the table or removing dishes from the dishwasher, but lack table manners and may find it difficult to sit through the family's entire meal.

In dressing, toddlers also demonstrate strides in independence. The 15-month-old child helps by putting the arm or foot out for dressing and pulls shoes and socks off. The 18-month-old child removes gloves, helps with pullover shirts, and may be able to unzip. By age 2 years the toddler removes most articles of clothing and puts on socks, shoes, and pants without regard for right or left and back or front. Help is still needed to fasten clothes.

Table 14-2 Play during toddlerhood

PHYSICAL DEVELOPMENT	SOCIAL DEVELOPMENT	MENTAL DEVELOPMENT AND CREATIVITY
▪ Suggested activities		
Provide space in which to encourage physical activity Provide sandbox, swing, and other scaled-down playground equipment	Provide replicas of adult tools and equipment for imitative play Permit child to "help" with adult tasks Encourage imitative play Provide toys and activities that allow for expression of feelings Allow child to play with some actual items used in the adult world; for example, let child help wash dishes or play with pots and pans and other utensils (check for safety)	Provide for water play Encourage building, drawing, and coloring Provide various textures in objects for play Provide large boxes and other safe containers for imaginative play Read stories appropriate to age Monitor television viewing
▪ Suggested toys		
Push-pull toys Rocking horse, stick horse Balls Blocks (unpainted) Pounding board Low gym and slide Pail and shovel Containers Play dough	Music and a record player or tape recorder Purse Housekeeping toys (broom, dishes) Toy telephone Dishes, stove, table and chairs Mirror	Wooden puzzles Cloth picture books Paper, finger paint, thick crayons Blocks Large beads to string Wooden shoe for lacing Appropriate TV programs

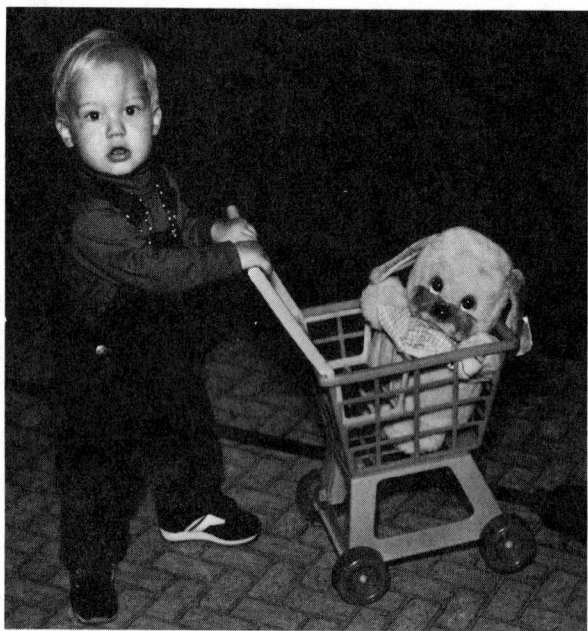

Fig. 14-3. Imitative play is common during toddler years.

Play

Play magnifies toddlers' physical and psychosocial development. Interaction with people becomes increasingly important. The solitary play of infancy progresses to *parallel* play. The toddler plays alongside, not with, other children. Although sensorimotor play is still prominent, there is much less emphasis on the exclusive use of one sensory modality. The toddler inspects the toy, talks to the toy, tests its strength and durability, and invents several uses for it.

Play assumes many forms and serves several functions (Table 14-2). Imitation is one of the most distinguishing characteristics of play and enriches children's opportunity to engage in fantasy. With less emphasis on sex-stereotyped toys, play objects such as dolls, carriages, dollhouses, dishes, cooking utensils, child-sized furniture, trucks, and dress-up clothes are suitable for both sexes (Fig. 14-3).

Increased locomotive skills make push-pull toys, stick horses, straddle trucks or cycles, a small, low gym and slide, varied size-balls, and rocking horses appropriate for the energetic toddler. Finger paints, thick crayons, chalk, blackboard, paper, and puzzles with large simple pieces use the child's developing fine motor skills. Interlocking blocks in varied sizes (but large enough to avoid aspiration) and shapes provide hours of fun and, during later years, are useful objects for creative and imaginative play.

Talking is a form of play for the toddler, who enjoys musical toys such as play record players, "talking" dolls and animals, and play telephones. Appropriate children's television programs are excellent for children in this age-group, who learn to associate words with visual images. Toddlers also enjoy "reading" stories from a picture book and imitating the sounds of animals.

Tactile play is also important for the exploring toddler. Water toys, a sandbox with pail and shovel, finger paints, soap bubbles, and clay provide excellent opportunities for free creative and manipulative recreation. Parents sometimes forget the fascination of feeling slippery cream, catching airy bubbles, squeezing and reshaping clay, or smearing paints. These types of unstructured activities are as important as educational play to allow children freedom of expression.

Selection of appropriate toys must involve safety factors, especially in relation to size and sturdiness. The oral activity of toddlers makes them at risk for aspirating small objects. Parents need to be especially vigilant of toys played with in other children's homes or those of older siblings. Toys are a potential source of serious bodily damage to toddlers, who may have the physical strength to manipulate them but not the knowledge to appreciate their danger (see Parent Guidelines: Toy Safety, Chapter 4).

TEMPERAMENT

Temperamental characteristics of children during infancy tend to predominate during toddlerhood. Most difficult infants remain difficult during early childhood, but the easy infants also become less easy (Carey and McDevitt, 1978). In addition, mothers are more likely to rate children as difficult at 1 to 3 years than earlier (McDevitt and Carey, 1981). It is not surprising for parents to see toddlers as more challenging, especially considering the typical negativistic traits of this age-group. Parents of easy infants may be particularly distressed by the behavior change, whereas parents of difficult children may be more prepared, because of a previously troublesome year, or be overwhelmed by the additional behaviors. The use of the Toddler Temperament Scale can assist in identifying temperamental characteristics that benefit from individualized approaches to childrearing (Fullard, McDevitt, and Carey, 1984). For practitioners in a busy setting, asking parents about their impression of the child's temperament yields reliable data that can help professionals gain a greater understanding of the parent-child interactional process (Houldin, Fullard, and Heverly, 1989).

While temper tantrums are common in toddlers, certain temperament characteristics make some children more prone to such outbursts. Active, intensely responding children are apt to have yelling, screaming, and flinging behavior during tantrums. Parents benefit from forewarning of extreme outbursts and the knowledge that the intensely negative behavior is not abnormal and is tempered by the child's intensely happy moods (Zuckerman and Frank, 1983).

Discipline is also influenced by temperament. Easy children generally respond well to mild forms of discipline, including a stern voice and sustained eye contact. However, difficult children often need more structured types of discipline such as time-out or rewards, and the effectiveness of one approach may be short-lived. Efforts at preventing misbehavior are especially important with children who have persistent natures (see Parent Guidelines, p. 658). Without "friendly warnings" such children often have difficulty terminating an activity. These children may be punished for behavior that is merely typical of their temperament, and if allowed to continue, the pattern can develop into a behavior problem (Chess and Thomas, 1985). Slow-to-warm-up children may also present challenges, especially when combined with toddlers' usual fear of strangers. These children require gradual introduction to new situations, such as daycare and babysitters. (See also Temperament, Chapter 4.)

SUMMARY OF GROWTH AND DEVELOPMENT DURING TODDLERHOOD

Developmental achievements during the toddler years occur in physical, gross and fine motor, language, and social areas. The key developmental ages are 18 and 24 months, although the chronologic ages of 15 and 30 months are also significant. Fifteen months of age is a particularly integrative period of developmental achievement, since it represents the completion or fruition of many skills that were unperfected at 1 year of age. Table 14-3 presents a summary of the major features of growth and development for the age-groups of 15, 18, 24, and 30 months.

COPING WITH CONCERNS RELATED TO NORMAL GROWTH AND DEVELOPMENT

The toddler years can be one of the most trying and confusing periods for parents. Behaviorally the toddler can be described as untiringly energetic, insatiably inquisitive, annoyingly negative, and obstinately ritualistic. Understanding these behaviors helps parents realize their necessity and allows them to effectively deal with the developmental tasks of children in this age-group.

Toilet Training

One of the major tasks of toddlerhood is toilet training. Voluntary control of the anal and urethral sphincters is achieved sometime after the child is walking, probably between ages 18 and 24 months. However, complex psychophysiologic factors are required for readiness. The child must be able to recognize the urge to let go and hold on and be able to communicate this sensation to the parent. In addition, there is probably some necessary motivation in the desire to please the parent by holding on, rather than pleasing oneself by letting go.

Usually physiologic and psychologic readiness is not complete until ages 18 to 24 months. By this time the child has mastered the majority of essential gross motor skills, can communicate intelligibly, is less in conflict with self-assertion and negativism, and is aware of the ability to control the body and please the parent. One of the most important responsibilities of nurses is to help parents identify the readiness signs in their child (Box 14-1).*

A number of techniques can be helpful when initiating training. One is the selection of a potty-chair and/or use of the toilet. A free-standing potty-chair allows children a feeling of security (Fig. 14-4). Planting the feet firmly on the floor also facilitates defecation (Stadler, 1989). Another option is a portable seat attached to the regular toilet, which may ease the transition from potty-chair to regular toilet. Placing a small bench under the feet helps to stabilize the

---

*A helpful brochure is *Toilet Training: A Parent's Guide,* available from the American Academy of Pediatrics, 141 Northwest Point Blvd., P.O. Box 927, Elk Grove Village, IL 60009-0927; (800) 433-9016.

Table 14-3 Growth and development during toddler years

AGE (MONTHS)	PHYSICAL	GROSS MOTOR	FINE MOTOR
15	Steady growth in height and weight Head circumference 48 cm (19 inches) Weight 11 kg (24 pounds) Height 78.7 cm (31 inches)	Walks without help (usually since age 13 months) Creeps up stairs Kneels without support Cannot walk around corners or stop suddenly without losing balance Assumes standing position without support Cannot throw ball without falling	Constantly casting objects to floor Builds tower of two cubes Holds two cubes in one hand Releases a pellet into a narrow-necked bottle Scribbles spontaneously Uses cup well but rotates spoon
18	Physiologic anorexia from decreased growth needs Anterior fontanel closed Physiologically able to control sphincters	Runs clumsily, falls often Walks up stairs with one hand held Pulls and pushes toys Jumps in place with both feet Seats self on chair Throws ball overhand without falling	Builds tower of three to four cubes Release, prehension, and reach well developed Turns pages in a book two or three at a time In drawing, makes stroke imitatively Manages spoon without rotation
24	Head circumference 49 to 50 cm (19.5 to 20 inches) Chest circumference exceeds head circumference Lateral diameter of chest exceeds anteroposterior diameter Usual weight gain of 1.8 to 2.7 kg (4 to 6 pounds) Usual gain in height of 10 to 12.5 cm (4 to 5 inches) Adult height approximately double height at 2 years of age May have achieved readiness for beginning daytime control of bowel and bladder Primary dentition of 16 teeth	Goes up and down stairs alone with two feet on each step Runs fairly well, with wide stance Picks up object without falling Kicks ball forward without overbalancing	Builds tower of six to seven cubes Aligns two or more cubes like a train Turns pages of book one at a time In drawing, imitates vertical and circular strokes Turns doorknob, unscrews lid
30	Birth weight quadrupled Primary dentition (20 teeth) completed May have daytime bowel and bladder control	Jumps with both feet Jumps from chair or step Stands on one foot momentarily Takes a few steps on tiptoe	Builds tower of eight cubes Adds chimney to train of cubes Good hand-finger coordination; holds crayon with fingers rather than fist Moves fingers independently In drawing, imitates vertical and horizontal strokes, makes two or more strokes for cross

child's position. It is probably best to keep the potty in the bathroom and to let the child observe the excreta being flushed down the toilet to associate these activities with usual practices. If a potty-seat is not available, having the child sit *facing* the toilet tank provides added support (Fig. 14-5). Practice sessions should be limited to 5 or 10 minutes, a parent should stay with the child, and sanitary habits should be employed after every session. Children should be praised for cooperative behavior and/or successful evacuation. Dressing children in easily removed clothing, using training pants, "pull-on" diapers, or panties, and encouraging imitation by watching others are other helpful suggestions. Forcing children to sit on the potty for long periods, spanking them for having accidents, and other methods of negative control are avoided.

Parents need to be very clear in the instructions given to

SENSORY	VOCALIZATION	SOCIALIZATION
Able to identify geometric forms; places round object into appropriate hole Binocular vision well developed Displays an intense and prolonged interest in pictures	Uses expressive jargon Says four to six words, including names "Asks" for objects by pointing Understands simple commands May use head-shaking gesture to denote "no" Uses "no" even while agreeing to the request	Tolerates some separation from parent Less likely to fear strangers Beginning to imitate parents, such as cleaning house (sweeping, dusting), folding clothes, mowing lawn Feeds self using cup with little spilling May discard bottle Manages spoon but rotates it near mouth Kisses and hugs parents, may kiss pictures in a book Expressive of emotions, has temper tantrums
	Says 10 or more words Points to a common object, such as shoe or ball, and to two or three body parts	Great imitator ("domestic mimicry") Manages spoon well Takes off gloves, socks, and shoes and unzips Temper tantrums may be more evident Beginning awareness of ownership ("my toy") May develop dependency on transitional objects, such as "security blanket"
Accommodation well developed In geometric discrimination, able to insert square block into oblong space	Has vocabulary of approximately 300 words Uses two- to three-word phrases Uses pronouns I, me, you Understands directional commands Gives first name; refers to self by name Verbalizes need for toileting, food, or drink Talks incessantly	Stage of parallel play Has sustained attention span Temper tantrums decreasing Pulls people to show them something Increased independence from mother Dresses self in simple clothing
	Gives first and last name Refers to self by appropriate pronoun Uses plurals Names one color	Separates more easily from mother In play, helps put things away, can carry breakable objects, pushes with good steering Begins to notice sex differences; knows own sex May attend to toilet needs without help except for wiping

toddlers to encourage elimination. For example, one mother used the phrase "Put pee in potty," when the child sat on the toilet. Several hours later, the child brought the potty to the mother with plastic letters of "P" in it. Also, it may be helpful to stress to children that when they feel the urge to eliminate, they have the time to get to the toilet and then urinate or defecate. The entire process of elimination is new to toddlers, and relationships between body functions and habits that adults take for granted may not be clear to children. (See also Fears, Chapter 15.)

Bowel training is usually accomplished before bladder training because of its greater regularity and predictability. There is a stronger sensation for defecation than urination, and the sensation of defecation can be brought to the child's attention. In fact, nighttime bladder training may not be completed until 4 or 5 years of age, and even later train-

Box 14-1 GUIDELINES FOR ASSESSING TOILET TRAINING READINESS

Physical Readiness
Voluntary control of anal and urethral sphincters, usually by 18 to 24 months
Ability to stay dry for 2 hours; decreased number of wet diapers; waking dry from nap
Regular bowel movements
Gross motor skills of sitting, walking, and squatting
Fine motor skills to remove clothing

Mental Readiness
Recognizes urge to defecate or urinate
Verbal or nonverbal communicative skills to indicate when wet or has urge to defecate or urinate
Cognitive skills to imitate appropriate behavior and follow directions

Psychologic Readiness
Expresses willingness to please parent
Able to sit on toilet for 5 to 10 minutes without fussing or getting off
Curiosity about adults' or older sibling's toilet habits
Impatience with soiled or wet diapers; desire to be changed immediately

Parental Readiness
Recognizes child's level of readiness
Willing to invest the time required for toilet training
Absence of family stress or change, such as a divorce, moving, new sibling, or imminent vacation

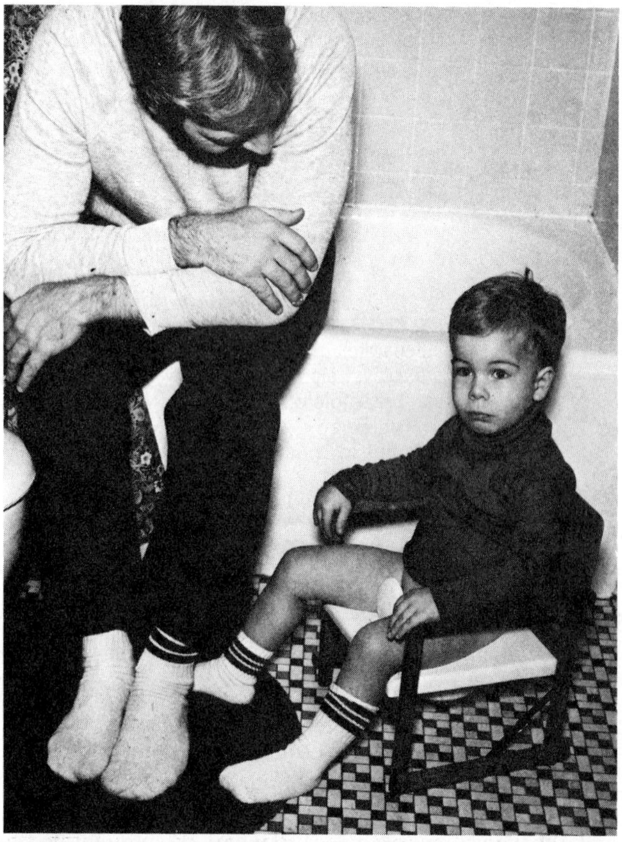

Fig. 14-4. Toddler on free-standing potty-chair, while father stays with child.

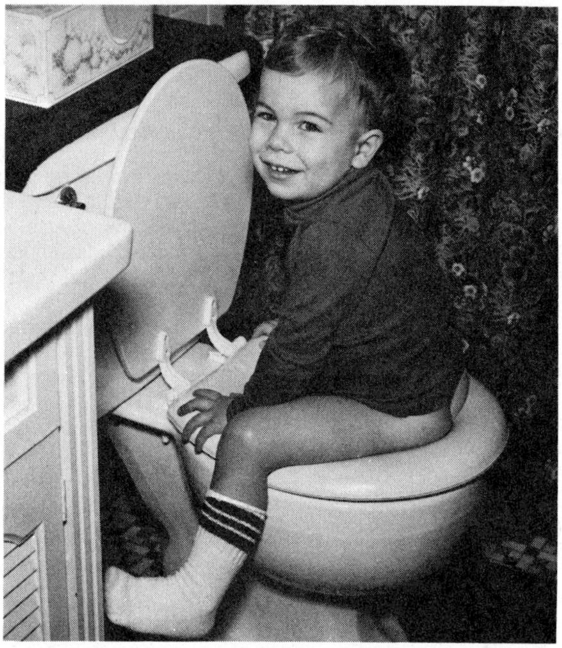

Fig. 14-5. Sitting in reverse fashion on regular toilet provides additional security to young child.

ing is normal (Fergusson and others, 1986). Limiting fluid intake before the children's hour of sleep and waking them once around midnight may help decrease the incidence of bed-wetting but do not teach voluntary control. Boys may begin toilet training in the stand-up position or by sitting on a potty-chair or toilet. Imitating father during the preschool years is a powerful motivating force.

Daytime accidents are also common, particularly during periods of intense activity. Young children become so engrossed in play activity that if they are not reminded they will wait until it is too late to reach the bathroom. The following example illustrates appropriate intervention:

> Three-year-old Susan had been toilet trained during the day for the last 4 months. Occasional accidents had decreased to almost zero. Now that the weather was warmer, her mother had been allowing her to play outside for a few hours each afternoon, but she noticed that Susan's pants were wet each time. She did not scold Susan for the accidents but reminded herself to bring the child into the house every hour and to show her how to open the door and call for her mother. She also brought the potty-chair downstairs where Susan could reach it quickly. After the first day of the hourly reminders, Susan called her mother and came in on her own. She still needed to be reminded at least once during the afternoon, but the accidents were few. (For other suggestions regarding toilet training, refer to Chapter 24.)

Sibling Rivalry

Sibling rivalry refers to the natural jealousy and resentment of children to a new child in the family. The arrival of a new infant represents a crisis for even the best prepared toddlers. Toddlers do not hate or resent the infant but despise the changes that this additional sibling produces, especially the separation from mother during the birth. The parents now share their love and attention with someone else, the usual routine is disrupted, and toddlers may lose their crib and/or room—all at a time when they thought they were in control of their world. It is not so difficult to understand the child's unwelcomed feelings toward this intruder when one considers the kinds of ambivalent feelings that surround the experience of parenting. Parents will ventilate feelings of jealousy concerning loss of independence and freedom. The difference between both types of jealousy is that the adult can rationalize and understand the change, but toddlers cannot.

Sibling rivalry tends to be most pronounced in the first-born, who experiences "dethronement," loss of sole parental attention. It also seems to be most difficult for children under 2 years old, particularly in terms of mother-child interaction (Feiring, Lewis, and Jaskir, 1983). Three- and 4-year-old children are more secure within themselves and have other interpersonal attachments besides their mother. They have achieved a greater degree of independence in dressing, feeding, toileting, and playing; therefore they are less dependent on the parent for physical comfort and psychologic fulfillment. Five-year-olds may again have difficulty in accepting a new sibling because they are adjusting to the separation from home imposed by entering school.

Preparation of children for the birth of a sibling is quite individual, but age dictates some important considerations. Time for toddlers is a vague concept. Tomorrow could be yesterday or next week, and a month from now could be never. Preparing children too soon for the birth may lessen their interest by the time the event occurs. A good time to start talking about the new baby is when toddlers become aware of the pregnancy and the changes taking place in the home in anticipation of the new member.

Older children need to be prepared earlier because frequently they are aware of the expected sibling from overhearing adults' conversation. Jealousy can develop from feeling left out, and, since fantasy dictates reality, fear of the unknown can lead to fear of abandonment, separation anxiety, and insecurity.

Children can benefit from "siblings'" classes that may be part of prenatal sessions. They learn about the characteristics of infants and are taught simple tasks of caring for the new baby (Honig, 1986; MacLaughlin and Johnston, 1984; Spadt, Martin, and Thomas, 1990). Books can help children prepare for birth and cope with sibling rivalry (Gates, 1979; Grossman, 1982; Honig, 1986).*

Toddlers need to have a realistic idea of what the newborn will be like. Telling them that a new playmate will come home soon sets up unrealistic expectations. Rather, parents should stress the activities that will take place when the baby arrives home, such as diapering, bottle- or breast-feeding, bathing, and dressing. At the same time parents should emphasize which routines will stay the same, such as reading stories or going to the park. If toddlers have had no contact with an infant, it is a good idea to introduce

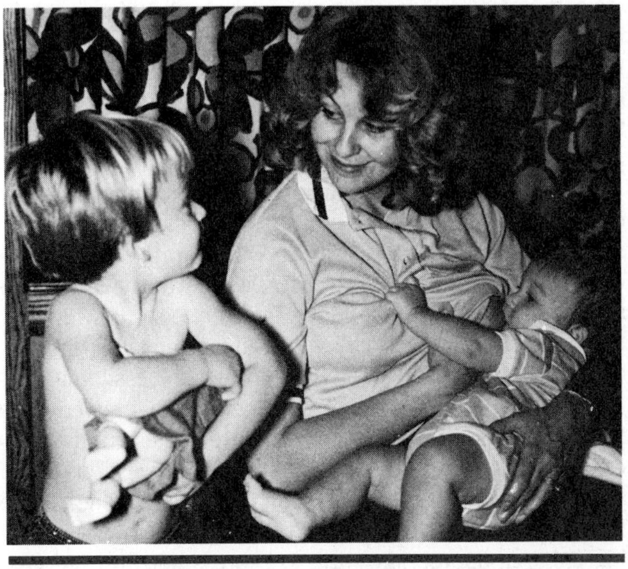

Fig. 14-6. Toddlers enjoy participating in caregiving activities for new sibling, such as this toddler who is "breast-feeding" his doll.

them to one, if feasible. Providing a doll on which toddlers can imitate parental behaviors is another excellent strategy. They can tend to the doll's needs (diapering, feeding) at the same time the parent is performing similar activities for the infant (Fig. 14-6).

Since a new sibling in the home is stressful, any additional stresses for the toddler are avoided or minimized. For example, moving the toddler to a regular bed or to a different room should be done well in advance of the infant's arrival.

When the new baby arrives, toddlers keenly feel the changed focus of attention. Visitors may initiate problems when they inadvertently shower the infant with attention and presents while neglecting the older child. Parents can minimize this by alerting visitors to the toddler's needs, having small presents on hand for the toddler, and including the child in the visit as much as possible.

How children exhibit jealousy is complex. Some will overtly hit the infant, push the child off mother's lap, or pull the bottle or breast from the infant's mouth. More often the expressions of hostility and resentment are much more subtle and covert. Toddlers may verbally express a wish that the infant "go back inside mommy," or they will revert to more infantile forms of behavior, such as demanding a bottle, soiling their diaper, clinging for attention, using baby talk, or aggressively acting out toward others. The latter is particularly common in preschoolers who may seem accepting of the new sibling at home but behave poorly in nursery school. This is a form of displacement that says, "I can't let my parents know how I feel, so I will tell you." Encouraging parents to explore how their older child is acting with other caregivers is an important aspect of intervention.

Regardless of how well adjusted and accepting toddlers or preschoolers appear, infants must be protected by supervising the interaction between siblings. Other safety considerations are "baby proofing" the house and instructing children regarding the dangers of small, sharp, or pointed ob-

*Another excellent book is Rogers, F.: The new baby, New York, 1985, G.P. Putnam's Sons.

jects to infants. Side rails on cribs should be kept fully raised and the mattress lowered to discourage toddlers from picking up the infant. Infant seats or bassinets should be placed on the floor so that young children cannot pull them off a raised surface "to see the baby" (MacLaughlin and Johnston, 1984).

The first few weeks at home with a newborn and toddler can be challenging for parents. Assuring them that this period will pass, that the toddler will learn to accept the changes in life-style, and that the newborn will sleep through the night is part of the intervention. Allowing parents to talk about their feelings of ambivalence and frustration and suggesting ways of dealing with the sibling jealousy help all members of the family with this experience. Indeed, sibling rivalry is so common regardless of the children's ages that it is a part of family life. Suggestions, such as spending time with each child, letting children settle their arguments, and accepting angry feelings while teaching children appropriate ways to express hostility, are general guidelines for dealing with the eventual conflicts between brothers and sisters.

Limit-Setting and Discipline

In its broadest sense, *discipline* means to teach or refers to a set of rules governing conduct and may be used interchangeably with *limit-setting.* However, these terms can also refer to different concepts: *limit-setting* referring to establishing the rules or guidelines for behavior and *discipline* being the action taken to enforce the rules following noncompliance. Generally, the clearer the limits are set and consistently enforced, the less need there is for discipline.

Therefore the initial nursing goal is to help parents establish realistic and concrete "rules." Limit-setting and discipline are positive, necessary components of childrearing and serve several useful functions as they help children:

- Test their limits of control.
- Achieve in areas appropriate for mastery at their level.
- Channel undesirable feelings into constructive activity.
- Protect themselves from danger.
- Learn socially acceptable behavior.

Children want and need limits. Unrestricted freedom is a tremendous threat to their security and safety. Through testing the limits imposed on them, children learn the extent to which they can manipulate their environment, as well as gain reassurance from knowing that others will be there to protect them from potential harm.

Minimizing misbehavior. The best approach toward discipline is to structure interactions with children so that unacceptable behavior is prevented or minimized. While many parents devise strategies that are most effective for their child, general guidelines include those listed in Parent Guidelines.

PARENT GUIDELINES
Minimizing Misbehavior

Praise children for desirable behavior with attention and verbal approval.

Structure the environment to prevent unnecessary difficulties; for example, place fragile objects in inaccessible area.

Set clear and reasonable rules; expect the same behavior regardless of the circumstances, and if exceptions are made, clarify that the change is for one time only.

Teach desirable behavior through own example, such as using a quiet, calm voice rather than screaming.

Review expected behavior before special or unusual events, such as visiting a relative or dinner in a restaurant.

Phrase requests for appropriate behavior positively, such as "Put the book down," rather than "Don't touch the book."

Call attention to unacceptable behavior as soon as it begins; use distraction to change the behavior or offer alternatives to annoying actions, such as a quiet toy for one that is excessively noisy.

Give advance notice or "friendly reminders," such as "When the TV program is over, it is time for dinner" or "I'll give you to the count of three and then we have to go."

Be attentive to situations that increase the likelihood of misbehaving, such as overexcitement or fatigue, or decreased personal tolerance to minor infractions.

Offer sympathetic explanations for not granting a request, such as "I am sorry I can't read you a story now, but I have to finish dinner. Then we can spend time together."

Keep any promises made to children.

Avoid outright conflicts; temper discussions with statements such as "Let's talk about it and see what we can decide together" or "I have to think about it first."

General guidelines for implementing discipline. Regardless of the type of discipline used, certain principles are essential in ensuring the efficacy of the approach (Box 14-2). Many strategies, such as behavior modification, can only be implemented effectively when principles of consistency and timing are followed. A pattern of intermittent or occasional enforcement of limits actually prolongs the undesired behavior because toddlers learn that if they are persistent, the behavior is permitted eventually. Delaying punishment weakens its intent, and practices such as telling the child, "Wait until your father comes home," are not only ineffectual, but also convey negative connotations about the other parent.

Types of discipline. To deal with misbehavior, parents need to implement appropriate disciplinary action. Numerous approaches are available, and some have definite advantages over others. The following discussion presents the more common strategies.

Corporal punishment. Corporal punishment most often takes the form of spanking. Based on the principles of aversive therapy, inflicting pain through spanking causes a dramatic short-term decrease in the behavior. However, there are some serious flaws in this approach: (1) it teaches children that violence is acceptable; (2) many times the spanking is the result of parental rage and may physically harm

Box 14-2 GENERAL GUIDELINES FOR IMPLEMENTING DISCIPLINE

Consistency—implement disciplinary action exactly as agreed on and for each infraction.
Timing—initiate discipline as soon as the child misbehaves; if delays are necessary, such as to avoid embarrassment, verbally disapprove of the behavior and state that disciplinary action will be implemented.
Commitment—follow through with the details of the discipline, such as timing of minutes; avoid distractions that may interfere with the plan, such as telephone calls.
Unity—make certain that all caregivers agree on the plan and are familiar with the details to prevent confusion and alliances between child and one parent.
Flexibility—choose disciplinary strategies that are appropriate to the child's age, temperament, and the severity of the misbehavior.
Planning—plan discipline strategies in advance and prepare child if feasible, for example, explaining the use of time-out; for unexpected misbehavior, try to discipline when you are calm.
Behavior-orientation—always disapprove of the behavior, not the child, with such statements as "That was a wrong thing to do. I am unhappy when I see behavior like that."
Privacy—administer discipline in private, especially with older children who may feel ashamed in front of others.
Termination—once the discipline is administered, consider the child as having a "clean slate" and avoid bringing up the incident or lecturing.

the child; and (3) children become "accustomed" to spanking, requiring more severe corporal punishment each time. Consequently parents may use paddles, whips, or other objects, or they may eliminate a spanking because of their unwillingness to "hit the child harder," a practice that may prolong the behavior.

Reasoning and scolding. Reasoning involves explaining why an act is wrong and is usually appropriate for older children, especially when moral issues are involved. However, young children cannot be expected to "see the other side" because of their egocentricity. Sometimes children use the "reasoning" as a way of gaining attention. For example, they may misbehave in order for the parents to give them a lengthy explanation of the wrongdoing because negative attention is better than none. When children use this technique, parents may have to end the explanation with a statement of, "This is the rule, and this is how I expect you to behave. I won't explain it any further."

Unfortunately, reasoning is frequently combined with scolding, which sometimes takes the form of shame or criticism. For example, the parent may state, "You are a bad boy for hitting your brother." Unfortunately, children take such remarks seriously and personally, believing that *they* are bad. It is important to focus only on the misbehavior, not on the child. Use of "I" messages rather than "you" messages expresses personal feelings without accusation or ridicule. For example, an "I" message attacks the behavior—"I am upset when Johnny is punched. I don't like to see him hurt"—not the child.

Reward. Reward is based on behavior modification theory—if an act is consistently rewarded, the desired behavior will be strengthened. Using rewards is a positive approach; by encouraging children to behave in specified ways, the tendency to misbehave is lessened. With young children using paper stars is a very effective method. For older children the "token system" is appropriate, especially if a certain number yields a special reward, such as a trip to the movies or a new book. In planning a reward system, the expected behaviors must be clearly explained to the child and the rewards must be reinforcing. A chart should be used to record the stars or tokens, and every earned reward should be promptly given. Verbal approval should always accompany extrinsic rewards. (A more formal reward system involving a contract, which is appropriate for older children, is discussed in Chapter 27 under Compliance).

Ignoring or extinction. Ignoring also uses behavior modification theory—if an act is consistently ignored, the unreinforced behavior will eventually be extinguished. Although this approach sounds very simple, it is often difficult to implement consistently. Parents frequently "give in" and resort to previous patterns of discipline. Consequently the behavior is actually reinforced because the child learns that persistence gains parental approval.

For this approach to be effective, health professionals must devote a fair amount of time toward (1) explaining the approach in detail, (2) recording behavior before the extinction process is instituted to see if a problem exists and to compare results after ignoring is begun, (3) making certain that the parent's attention is the reinforcer, and (4) warning parents of a phenomenon called "response burst," which refers to an *increase* in the child's behavior soon after the process is initiated because the child is "testing" the parents to see if they are serious about the plan.

Time-out. Time-out is actually a refinement of the common practice of "sending the child to his or her room." It is also based on the premise of removing the reinforcer, that is, the satisfaction or attention the child is receiving from the activity. When placed in an unstimulating and isolated place, children become bored and consequently agree to behave in order to reenter the family group. Time-out avoids many of the problems of other disciplinary approaches because no physical punishment is involved, no reasoning or scolding is given, and the parent is usually not present for all of the time-out, facilitating his or her ability to consistently apply the punishment. It also offers both the child and the parent a "cooling off" time. To be effective, time-out must be planned in advance (see Parent Guidelines, p. 660).

Consequences. The strategy of consequences involves allowing children to experience the results of their misbehavior and includes three types:

Natural—those that occur without any intervention, such as being late and missing dinner
Logical—those that are directly related to the rule, such as not being allowed to play with another toy until the used ones are put away
Unrelated—those that are imposed deliberately, such as no playing until homework is completed

PARENT GUIDELINES
Using Time-Out

Select an area for time-out that is safe, convenient, and unstimulating, but where the parent can monitor the child, such as the bathroom, hallway, or laundry room.
Determine what behaviors warrant a time-out.
Make sure children understand the "rules" and how they are expected to behave.
Explain to children the process of time-out:
- When they misbehave, they will be given *one* warning.
- If they do not obey, they will be sent to the place designated for time-out.
- They are to sit there for a specified period of time.
- If they cry, refuse, or display any disruptive behavior, the time-out period will begin *after* they quiet down.
- When they are quiet for the duration of the time, they can then leave the room.

A rule for the length of time-out is *1 minute per year of age;* use a kitchen timer with an audible bell to record the time rather than a watch.
Implement time-out in a public place by selecting a suitable area or explain to children that time-out will be spent immediately upon returning home and mark their hand with a felt-tip pen as a reminder.

Natural or logical consequences are preferred but are effective only when they are meaningful to children. For example, the natural consequence of living in a messy room may do little to encourage cleaning up, but no friends over until the room is neat can be very motivating! The use of withdrawing privileges is often a form of unrelated consequences. After the child experiences the consequence, the parent should refrain from any comment, because the usual tendency is for the child to try to place blame for imposing the rule.

Temper Tantrums

Toddlers may assert their independence by violently objecting to attempts at restricting their behavior. They may lie down on the floor, kick their feet, and scream at the top of their lungs. Head-banging, head-rolling, and breath-holding are other behaviors some children use. While these mannerisms are very disturbing to observe, they usually do not become behavior problems (Abe, Oda, and Amatomi, 1984). Breath-holding and fainting from lack of oxygen cause no physical harm because the accumulation of carbon dioxide stimulates the respiratory control center to initiate breathing. However, head-banging results in self-inflicted injury, and the child requires protection, such as holding or being placed in a protected environment.

The best approach toward extinguishing attention-seeking behavior is to ignore it (no verbal or eye contact with the child), provided the behavior is not inflicting injury. The parent should remain close by and after the tantrum has subsided offer a toy or a favorite activity to substitute for the ungranted request and to reward the posttantrum behavior. When tantrums occur because the child refuses to comply, the parent can ignore it for a few minutes but may have to physically carry the child if the request must be met, such as getting in the car or going to bed (Schmitt, 1989).

Box 14-3 GUIDELINES FOR IDENTIFYING CHILDREN WITH PROBLEM TANTRUMS

Parents express concern; feel angry, sad, and helpless; and/or report nothing positive about the child.
Child is younger than 1 year or older than 4 years.
Tantrums occur regularly in school.
Tantrums are associated with aggressive, violent behavior.
There is a history of other concerns, such as sleep disorders, food refusal, or extreme diffficulty with separation.
Child displays unusual flirtatiousness or extreme modesty (suggests possible sexual abuse).

Modified from Needlman, R., Howard, B., and Zuckerman, B.: Temper tantrums: when to worry, Contemp. Pediatr. 6(8):12-14, 1989.

When tantrums do occur, it is important for the parent to intervene *immediately* to prevent the buildup of angry feelings and being unable to calmly ignore the behavior. Frequently temper tantrums can be avoided by using the approaches on p. 658; time-out is an effective discipline approach for dealing with the unacceptable behavior (see Parent Guidelines).*

Temper tantrums are common during the toddler years and essentially represent normal developmental behaviors. However, temper tantrums can be signs of serious problems. Nurses should be alert to situations that require further evaluation (Box 14-3).

Negativism

One of the more difficult aspects of rearing toddlers is related to their persistent negative "no" response to every request. The negativism is not an expression of being fresh or disrespectful, but a necessary assertion of self-control. One method of dealing with the negativism is by reducing the opportunities for a "no" answer. Asking the child, "Do you want to go to sleep now?" is almost certain to be met with an emphatic "no." A more appropriate approach is to tell the child that it is time to go to sleep and proceed accordingly.

In their attempt to exert control, children like to make choices. When confronted with appropriate choices, such as, "You can have a peanut butter and jelly sandwich or chicken noodle soup for lunch," they are more likely to choose one than automatically say no. However, if their response is negative, parents should make the choice for the child. Many of the suggestions for preventing misbehavior in Parent Guidelines, p. 658, also help minimize negativism.

*A helpful brochure is *Temper Tantrums: A Normal Part of Growing Up,* available from American Academy of Pediatrics, 141 Northwest Point Blvd., P.O. Box 927, Elk Grove Village, IL 60009-0927; (800) 433-9016.

Coping with Stress

Adults rarely think of young children as being exposed to stress or suffering its consequences. However the normal demands of growing up coupled with the usual pressures most families experience mean that few, if any, young children are reared stress free. Minimum amounts of stress are beneficial during the early years to help children develop effective coping skills. However, excessive stress is destructive, and young children are especially vulnerable because of their limited capacity to cope.

To help parents deal with stress in their children's life, they must be aware of signs of stress (see Box 4-7) and be helped to identify the source. The normal stresses during toddlerhood are listed in Box 14-4. In addition, any number of other stresses may be imposed on children, such as alternate caregiving arrangements, birth of a sibling, marital discord, relocation, or illness. Watching children at play can identify stressors. For example, one child was seen pounding on a doll, yelling "Go away! Go away!" The parent was quick to observe that the child's recent irritability was probably caused by the stress of a new sibling.

The best approach to dealing with stress is prevention—monitoring the amount of stress in children's lives so that levels exceeding their coping ability do not occur. In many instances this is as simple as increasing the child's rest periods to allow for quiet recovery time. Often it involves adequately preparing the child for change, such as daycare or a new sibling. It also requires helping the child cope with stress. Play is an excellent vehicle for venting anger or frustration, and toys such as drums, play nails and hammer, clay, and playdough provide alternative methods of dissipating anxiety. They also begin to teach socially acceptable ways of dealing with such feelings. Another approach is the use of relaxation and imagery. Even young children can learn to "let their bodies go limp like a rag doll" or "imagine floating on a cloud."

Box 14-4 SOURCES OF STRESS IN TODDLERS

Negativism—does not like to take orders; may be downright contrary
Rigidity—wants own way; is upset when rituals are disrupted; dislikes interference
Lack of sociability—engages in solitary or parallel play but is generally disinterested in socializing
Self-centeredness—believes the world revolves around her or him; does not want to share; may dawdle
Separation anxiety—fears strangers; is shy
Stranger anxiety—fears strangers; is shy
Toilet training—especially if begun before the child is ready
Bedtime—dislikes being ordered to bed; may fear bed-wetting or separation from parents; may have terrifying dreams
Tantrums—may revert to temper tantrums or destructive behavior; may hit or bite
Security object—may have a security object that, if lost or misplaced, leads to great emotional upset
Overdoing—may become overstimulated or overtired
Fears—in particular, may include animals or anything that makes a loud noise
Medical facilities—visits to health practitioners may prove extremely stressful

Modified from Kuczen, B.: Childhood stress: don't let your child be a victim, New York, 1982, Delacorte Press, p. 15.

Regression. Regression is a retreat from a present pattern of functioning to past levels of behavior. It usually occurs in instances of stress, when one attempts to cope by reverting to patterns of behavior that were successful in earlier stages of development. Regression is common in toddlers because almost any additional stress lessens their ability to master present developmental tasks. At first such regression appears acceptable and comfortable for children, but on closer inspection it becomes evident that the loss of newly acquired achievements is frightening and threatening, since children are aware of their total helplessness in the recent past. Parents, too, become concerned about regressive behavior and frequently in their efforts to deal with it force the child to cope with an additional source of stress—the pressure to live up to expected standards.

When regression does occur, the best approach is to ignore it, while praising existing patterns of appropriate behavior. The child is saying, "I can't cope with this present stress and accomplish this new skill as well, but I will eventually if given patience and understanding." For this reason it is not advisable to introduce new areas of learning when an additional crisis is present or expected, such as beginning toilet training shortly before a sibling is born or during a brief period of hospitalization.

Fears. Fears are very common during this age and include fear of annihilation, going to sleep, animals, and engines, especially the vacuum cleaner, with the greatest fear continuing to be fear of strangers and separation from parents or other usual caregivers. Because fear of strangers and separation begins in infancy, it is discussed in Chapter 12. The other fears often escalate in the preschool period and consequently are discussed in Chapter 15.

PROMOTING OPTIMUM HEALTH DURING TODDLERHOOD

Physical and psychosocial changes in toddlers affect several areas of health maintenance and promotion, namely, nutrition, sleep and activity, dental health, and injury prevention. Nursing intervention, especially anticipatory guidance, can positively affect the optimum development of the child and family during this exciting, but often troublesome, period of childhood.

NUTRITION

During the period from 12 to 18 months of age the growth rate slows, resulting in a slight adjustment from a previous caloric requirement of 108 kcal/kg (50 kcal/pound) of body weight during early infancy to 102 kcal/kg (46 kcal/pound) during the next 2 years. Protein requirements also decrease slightly from 2.2 to 1.5 g/kg for infants to 1.2 g/kg for toddlers but are still higher than at succeeding ages to meet the demands of muscle tissue growth (Food and Nutrition Board, 1989). Fluid needs drop from an infant requirement of approximately 140 ml/kg to a toddler requirement of 115 ml/kg. The reduced fluid requirement represents a decrease in the total body water and an increase in fluid within the cells (intracellular fluid).

The requirements for most vitamins and minerals increase slightly during toddlerhood. The need for minerals such as iron, calcium, and phosphorus may be difficult to meet considering the characteristic food habits of children in this age-group. Milk intake, the chief source of calcium and phosphorus, should average 2 to 3 cups a day. More than a quart of milk consumption daily considerably limits the intake of solid foods, resulting in deficient dietary iron, as well other nutrients.

At approximately 18 months of age most toddlers manifest this decreased nutritional need in a phenomenon known as *physiologic anorexia.* They become picky, fussy eaters with strong taste preferences. They may eat voraciously one day and almost nothing the next. They are increasingly aware of the nonnutritive function of food: the pleasure of eating, the social aspect of mealtime, and the control of refusing food. They are influenced by factors other than taste when choosing food. If a family member refuses to eat something, children are likely to imitate that response. If the plate is overfilled, they are likely to push it away, overwhelmed by its size. If food does not appear or smell appetizing, they will probably not agree to try it. Conversely, if food is served attractively and referred to in appealing ways, such as calling an apple slice an "apple cookie" or half a hard-boiled egg a "canoe," children will often try new foods. In essence, mealtime is more closely associated with psychologic components that nutritional ones, and nutritional counseling must address the characteris tics of this age-group.

Nutritional Counseling

Eating habits established in the first 2 or 3 years of life tend to have lasting effects on subsequent years. If food is used as a regard or sign of approval, a child may overeat for nonnutritive reasons. If food is forced and mealtime is consistently unpleasant, the usual pleasure associated with eating may not develop. Mealtimes should be enjoyable rather than times for discipline or family arguments. The social aspect of mealtime may be distracting for young children; therefore an earlier feeding hour may be appropriate. Young children are unable to sit through a long meal and become fidgety and disruptive. This is particularly common when children are brought to the table just after active play. Calling them in from play 15 minutes before mealtime allows them ample opportunity to get ready for eating while settling down their active minds and bodies.

For some young children, sitting at the table may be more disruptive than functional. Frequent nutritious snacks can replace a meal. "Grazing"—nibbling and snacking—is a good way to ensure proper nutrition, provided appropriate foods are offered.

The method of serving food also takes on more importance during this period. Toddlers need to feel control and achievement in their abilities. Giving them large, adult-size portions contributes to their feeling overwhelmed. In general, what is eaten is much more significant than how much is consumed. Small amounts of meat and vegetables supply greater food value than a large consumption of bread or potato. Serving sizes need to be appropriate for age (see Nursing Tips). It is often a good idea to offer less than toddlers may eat and let the child ask for more. Young children tend to like less spicy, bland foods, although this is a culturally determined preference. Substitutions should be provided for foods that they do not enjoy, but this practice should be used sparingly to avoid catering to all toddlers' eating requests.

NURSING TIPS: SERVING SIZE FOR YOUNG CHILDREN

A general guide to the serving size of food is 1 tablespoon of solid food per year of age or one fourth to one third of the adult portion size.
Use the tablespoon guide for easily measured food such as vegetables or rice.
Use the fraction guide for bread or milk.

The ritualism of this age also dictates certain principles in feeding practices. Toddlers like the same dish, cup, or spoon every time they eat. They may reject a favorite food simply because it is served in a different utensil. If one food touches another they often refuse to eat it. Mixed foods, such as stews or casseroles, are also rarely favorites. Since toddlers are unpredictable in their table manners, it is best to use plastic dishes and cups, both for economic and for safety reasons. For some children a regular mealtime schedule also contributes to their desire and need for predictability and ritualism.

Appetite and food preferences are sporadic during these years. A child may enjoy one food for 3 days in a row and then suddenly refuse to eat it again for days. Such food fads or "jags" do not ensure a well-balanced diet, but attempts to alter them are met with bitter resentment and unwavering obstinacy. It is preferable to accept such extremes and offer other foods in small portions. Generally, the child will choose another "favorite food" that may compensate for the nutritional inadequacy. Introducing at least three items from the basic four food groups at each meal helps develop a variety of taste preferences and well-balanced habits. When offering snacks, several small pieces of food (carrot sticks, cheese blocks, raisins, crackers, sliced cold meat, apple slices) can be placed in an ice cube tray for a pick-and-choose menu. A sample menu for toddlers is given in Box 14-5.

Developmentally, most children by 12 months of age are eating the same food prepared for the rest of the family. Some may have mastered using a cup with occasional spilling, although most cannot adeptly use a spoon until 18 months of age or later (Table 14-4) and generally prefer using their fingers (Fig. 14-7). Some children find weaning

Box 14-5 SAMPLE MENUS FOR TODDLERS BASED ON BASIC FOOD GROUPS*

Breakfast	⅓ cup dry, unsweetened cereal 4 oz lowfat milk ½ cup orange juice
Snack	½-1 whole banana
Lunch	1 tbsp peanut butter 1 slice whole wheat bread ½ apple 4-6 oz lowfat milk
Snack	1 graham cracker 4-6 oz lowfat milk
Dinner	1 chicken leg ¼ cup rice 2 tbsp green beans 4-6 oz lowfat milk

DAILY TOTAL:

Milk:	24 ounces
Meat:	2 ounces
Fruits/veg:	4 servings (½ piece or ¼ cup is a serving)
Breads/cereal:	4 servings (½ slice or ¼ cup is a serving)

Prepared by Cecilia L. Davis, R.D., L.D.,
*Fats and simple carbohydrates should be served sparingly to meet caloric needs. Serving sizes are minimums for nutritional adequacy. Many children eat more.

Table 14-4 Developmental milestones associated with feeding

AGE (MONTHS)	DEVELOPMENT
12-18	Drools less Drinks well from a household cup but may drop it when finished Holds cup with both hands Begins to use a spoon but turns it before reaching mouth
24	Can use a straw Chews food with mouth closed and shifts food in mouth Distinguishes between finger and spoon foods Holds small glass in one hand; replaces glass without dropping Uses spoon correctly but with some spilling
36	Spills small amount from spoon Begins to use fork; holds it in fist Uses adult pattern of chewing, which involves rotary action of jaw

easy and voluntarily relinquish the bottle by the first birthday. Others are unable to sacrifice that pleasure and require a bottle at nighttime or occasionally during the day. Allowing children to give up the bottle when they are ready is preferable to forcing the issue.

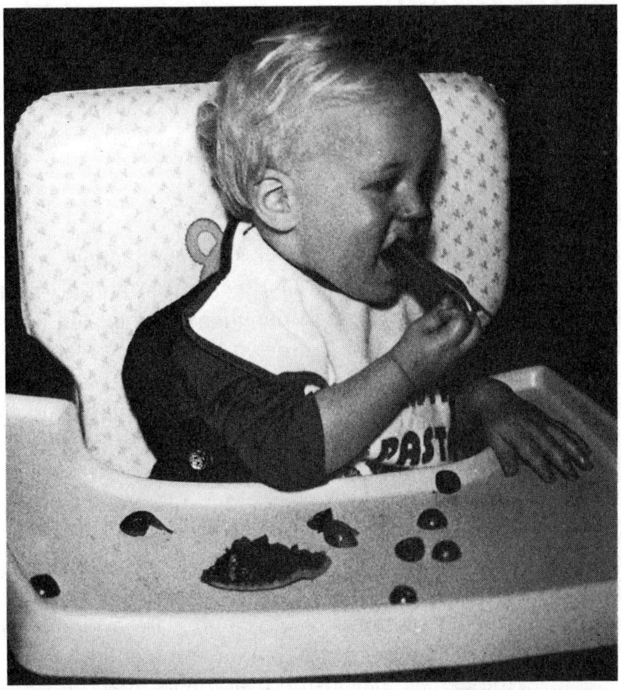

Fig. 14-7. Toddlers enjoy "finger feeding."

Some toddlers reject all solid food in preference for the bottle, a practice that can be discouraged by gradually diluting the milk with water to make it less satisfying and introducing foods at times when the child is most likely to be hungry, such as on awakening. Occasionally it may be necessary to withhold bottle-feedings, as well as other in-between-meal foods and fluids other than water, until the child is hungry enough to eat solid foods. Forcing the child to eat solid foods usually results in conflicts and does little to establish healthy eating habits.

SLEEP AND ACTIVITY

Total sleep decreases only slightly during the second year and averages about 12 to 13 hours. Most children take one nap a day, and by the end of the second or third year many relinquish this habit. The activity level is high, and there is rarely a problem with too little physical exercise, provided inappropriate restrictions are not instituted. With increasing numbers of young children cared for outside the home, attention to the kinds of activity provided is important. For example, children with high activity levels may benefit from an environment in which outdoor play is encouraged.

Sleep problems, especially going to bed and falling asleep, are common and are probably related to fears of separation. Bedtime rituals (same hour of sleep, snack, quiet activity) are helpful, and transitional objects, such as a favorite stuffed animal or blanket, can ease the insecurity at bedtime. For problems that persist, the interventions outlined in Table 12-5 should be employed.

DENTAL HEALTH*

The importance of oral hygiene in preserving the teeth and maintaining healthy gums cannot be overemphasized or begun too early. Nurses are in an optimum position to promote dental hygiene in their care of both well children and ill children during hospitalization.

Regular Dental Examinations

Ideally the child should see a dentist (or pedodontist, a pediatric dentist) soon after the first teeth erupt and no later than by 2½ years when primary dentition is completed. During these visits the dentist can begin to develop a relationship with the child, assess oral health, teach parents correct methods of dental hygiene, and provide nutritional counseling, especially in relation to preventing nursing bottle caries.

Initial visits to the dentist should be nontraumatizing. Since toddlers react negatively to new and potentially frightening experiences, the initial visit can center around meeting the dentist, seeing the equipment, and sitting in the chair. Statements such as "It won't hurt," are avoided because they suggest possible discomfort. If the child is uncooperative, the dentist may just look at the teeth and reserve a more thorough examination for another visit. Modeling can also be effective—the child can observe procedures performed on the parent or a cooperative sibling. This type of conditioning is very important in preparing the child for future experiences.†

Removal of Plaque

The objective of oral hygiene is removal of *plaque,* soft bacterial deposits that adhere to the teeth and cause dental caries (decay) and periodontal (gum) disease. The most effective methods for plaque removal are brushing and flossing. Several brushing techniques exist, although there is no universal agreement regarding the best method. One that is suitable for cleaning the primary teeth is the *scrub* method. The tips of the bristles are placed firmly at a 45-degree angle against the teeth and gums and moved back and forth in a vibratory motion. The ends of the bristles should be wiggling but not moving forcefully back and forth, which can damage the gums and enamel. All the surfaces of the teeth are cleaned in this manner except the lingual (inner or tongue side) surfaces of the anterior teeth. To clean these surfaces, the toothbrush is placed vertical to the teeth and moved up and down. Only a few teeth are brushed at one time, using six to eight strokes for each section. A systematic approach is used so that all surfaces are thoroughly cleaned.

For young children the most effective cleaning is done by parents. Several positions can be used that facilitate access to the mouth and help stabilize the head for comfort:

- Stand with child's back toward adult. (When done in front of a bathroom mirror, both child and adult can see what is being done in the mirror.)
- Sit on a couch or bed with child's head resting in adult's lap.
- Sit on the floor or a stool with child's head resting between adult's thighs (Fig. 14-8).

With all positions, use one hand to cup the chin and one to brush the teeth. Brushing the child's teeth from behind is easier because it is similar to brushing one's own teeth. For easier access to back teeth, the mouth is held partially open; fully opening the mouth causes the masseter muscle to contract, narrowing the space near the back molars (see Nursing Tips).

For effective cleaning, a small toothbrush with soft, rounded, multitufted nylon bristles that are short and uniform in length is recommended. Nylon bristles dry more rapidly after use and retain their shape better than natural bristles. Toothbrushes are replaced as soon as the bristles are frayed or bent. With young children, brushing may be more easily accomplished using only water, since many children dislike the foam from toothpaste and the foam interferes with visibilty. There is also the danger of swallowing fluoridated toothpaste (see following discussion under Fluoride). When using toothpaste, children should select the flavor they like to encourage the brushing habit.

After the teeth have been cleaned, flossing with dental floss is done to remove plaque and debris from between the teeth and below the gum margin where brushing is ineffective. Even if the teeth are widely spaced, flossing is necessary to remove debris below the gum line to prevent *gingivitis,* inflammation of the gums. Since young children do not have the dexterity to manipulate the floss, parents are taught the procedure. A length of dental floss about 45 cm (18 inches) long can either be tied in a circle or wrapped around the fingers. The circle method may be easier for children to learn. Floss holders are also available and offer the advantage of only one hand being needed for flossing, freeing the other hand to stabilize the child's head (McDonald and Avery, 1987).

With about 2.25 cm (1 inch) of floss held tautly against the thumbs, the floss is gently inserted between two teeth, wrapped around the base of the tooth in a C shape, and directed *below* the gingival margin to remove plaque. The floss is then moved toward the occlusal (biting) surface of the tooth to remove plaque between the teeth as well. This sweeping motion is repeated a few times on every tooth surface, using a clean segment of floss.

NURSING TIPS: ENCOURAGING YOUNG CHILDREN'S COOPERATION DURING TOOTHBRUSHING

To encourage children to open their mouth, ask them to "tweet like a bird" to brush the front teeth and to "roar like a lion" to brush the back teeth.

Sing, tell stories, or talk to children during teeth cleaning to prevent boredom.

*Caryn Stoermer Hess, R.N., M.S., assisted in the revision of this section.

†A book to help prepare the child is *When Your Child Goes to the Dentist,* by Fred Rogers, Family Communications, 4802 Fifth Avenue, Pittsburgh, PA 15213; (412) 687-2990.

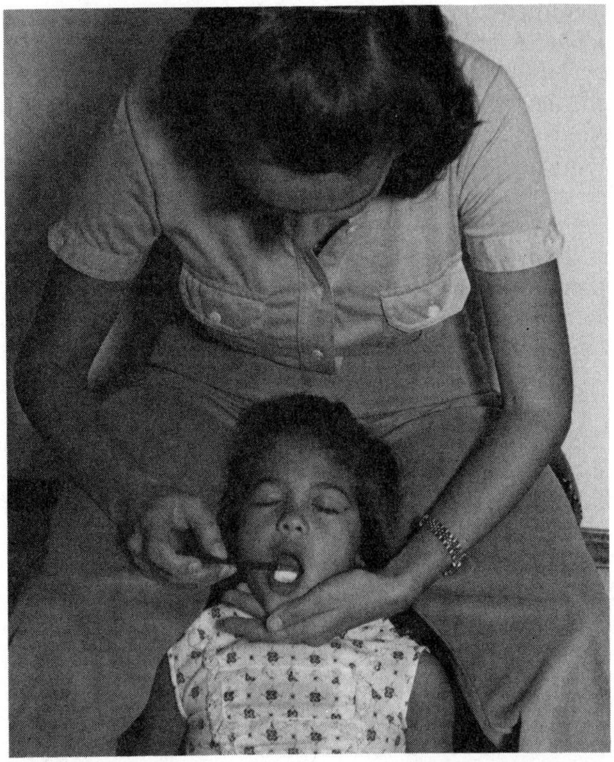

Fig. 14-8. Position that facilitates parent's brushing of child's teeth.

A disclosing agent is helpful in identifying those areas of the teeth where plaque accumulates. It also helps motivate children to clean their teeth, because plaque is difficult to see. After cleaning, the mouth is inspected to ensure that all traces of plaque have been removed. Where plaque remains, the teeth are rebrushed until the red color is gone.

Although it is generally recognized that thorough plaque removal once a day is sufficient, cleaning the teeth more frequently increases the probability of effective cleaning (McDonald and Avery, 1987). Ideally the teeth should be cleaned after each meal and especially before bedtime, and the child given nothing to eat or drink after the night brushing except water. At those times when brushing is impractical, the "swish-and-swallow" method of cleaning the mouth is taught: with a mouthful of water the child rinses the mouth and swallows, repeating the procedure three or four times. When children want to begin brushing their own teeth, they are encouraged to do so before or after brushing by an adult. Supervision is needed, but children can begin to start taking some responsibility for their dental habits.

Fluoride

Numerous studies have documented the effectiveness of fluoride in reducing the incidence of tooth decay. Children who drink water containing 1 part per million (ppm) fluoride when their teeth are forming may have a 50% to 65% decrease in caries (Crall, 1986). When adequate amounts of fluoride are ingested before eruption of the teeth and to a lesser extent after tooth eruption, the enamel is more resistant to caries. Fluoride replaces the hydroxyl ion in the calcium hydroxyapatite molecule to form calcium fluorapatite, which alters the crystal of the tooth, making it more resistant to acid solubility. The changes in crystalline structure also affect the anatomy of the tooth—the cusps are shorter and the crevices smaller—thus facilitating plaque removal.

Despite the proven benefits of fluoride, only about half of the population in the United States have naturally or artificially fluoridated water. The National 1990 Objectives for Fluoridation and Dental Health proposed that at least 95% of the population would receive fluoridated water. Unfortunately, this objective has not been met (Progress, 1989). Numerous controversies exist regarding the proposed dangers of mass fluoridation, and antifluoridationists have been successful in preventing communities from instituting this public health benefit (see Questions and Controversies).

In communities where the water supply is not fluoridated, oral fluoride supplements are recommended (Table 14-5). Nurses have a responsibility to ensure an optimal fluoride regimen for children and to counsel families regarding correct use of supplements (Box 14-6). One advantage

QUESTIONS AND CONTROVERSIES

Is mass fluoridation harmful?

Among the arguments against mass fluoridation the following have generated the most public concern: increased incidence of cancer, Down syndrome, and allergies among those living in fluoridated areas (Margolis and Cohen, 1985). However, none of these claims has been substantiated. Researchers have found that the rate of cancer is no greater in fluoridated areas than in comparable locations without fluoridation (Hoover, McKay, and Fraumeni, 1976). The same conclusion was reached regarding Down syndrome (Needleman, Pueeschel, and Rothman, 1974). The American Academy of Allergy's statement (1971) on allergy and fluoride concludes that there is no evidence to support this association.

The one well-known effect of excessive fluoride ingestion is *fluorosis,* which can cause staining (chalky white to yellow or brown) of the teeth and in more severe forms, loss and decreased resistance of the enamel to decay. Very mild fluorosis is not a public health hazard, nor a major cosmetic concern for affected children. Moderate and severe fluorosis is directly related to the fluoride dosage and occurs predominantly in areas with high levels of natural fluoridation, not in areas of artificial fluoridation where optimum fluoride levels are provided. Ingesting excessive fluoride after age 5 or 6 years does not result in fluorosis because of complete calcification of the permanent teeth, except for the third-year molars. As with any drug, acute toxicity can occur from ingestion of large quantities of the mineral. A lethal dose for children is estimated to be 32 to 64 mg/kg (Heifetz and Horowitz, 1986). However, this is not a contraindication to its use. The same precautions must be practiced as with any drug—store out of reach of children and avoid large supplies of the drug in the home (Hess and others, 1984).

Table 14-5 Supplemental fluoride dosage schedule (mg/day*)

	CONCENTRATION OF FLUORIDE IN DRINKING WATER (PPM)		
AGE	<0.3	0.3-0.7	>0.7
2 weeks-2 years	0.25	0	0
2-3 years	0.50	0.25	0
3-16 years	1.00	0.50	0

From American Academy of Pediatrics, Committee on Nutrition: Fluoride supplementation, Pediatrics 77(5):758-761, 1986.
*2.2 mg sodium fluoride contains 1 mg fluoride.

Box 14-6 GUIDELINES FOR AN OPTIMUM FLUORIDE REGIMEN

Base recommendations on the fluoride content of the drinking water, including bottled or well water, with the exception of amounts for breast-feeding infants, who should receive fluoride supplements regardless of fluoride content of the water supply.

If the water is fluoridated, encourage consumption of tap water either through supplemental feedings to infants or through preparation of frozen-concentrated juice, powdered drinks, soup, gelatin, or other foods made with fluoridated water.

If impractical and the child ordinarily drinks little tap water, consider a fluoride supplement.

In areas with excessive fluoride levels, suggest the use of bottled unfluoridated water.

Encourage parents to supervise the young child's toothbrushing, to use a pea-sized amount of fluoridated toothpaste or to substitute a nonfluoridated brand, and to teach children not to eat toothpaste.

If the water is unfluoridated, instruct in proper administration of supplements:
- Place drops directly on the tongue to allow it to mix with saliva and come in contact with the teeth.
- Encourage older children to chew the tablet and swish it in the mouth for 30 seconds before swallowing.
- Give nothing to eat or drink afterward for 30 minutes.
- Administer supplements on an empty stomach without calcium-rich products, such as milk.

Recommend the daily use of a fluoridated mouthrinse in children 6 years and older and instruct in proper technique:
- Use only the recommended amount.
- Expectorate after a timed 1-minute rinse.
- Avoid food or fluid for 30 minutes afterward.

Advise parents to store fluoridated dentifrice, mouthrinse, and supplements in a safe place away from small children and to keep no more than a 4-month supply of supplements in the home.

Encourage compliance by administering the supplement at same time each day and posting reminders, such as fluoride sticker on bathroom mirror.

Modified from Hess, C., and others: Fluoride: too much or too little, Pediatr. Nurs. 10(6):397-403, 1984.

of supplements is that the child receives a known quantity of fluoride daily. This is in contrast to fluoridated water, where the supply depends on the amount of water consumed and where parents need to be encouraged to use water to prepare drinks and foods. A major disadvantage of supplementation is compliance and cost. The supplements are considerably more expensive than community fluoridation, and adhering to a daily administration schedule for 16 years is difficult for many families.

Another consideration is the type of toothpaste. A fluoride dentifrice reduces caries even further when the water supply is fluoridated, because it imparts a topical benefit to the teeth. However, a concern with fluoride toothpaste is excess ingestion by young children and the possibility of *fluorosis,* a condition characterized by an increase in the degree and extent of the enamel's porosity. As a safeguard, the child's use of toothpaste should be supervised to prevent swallowing of excessive amounts. Fluoride rinses, which also offer topical benefits, are not recommended for children under 6 years of age because of their likelihood of swallowing the liquid (American Dental Association, 1984).

Low-Cariogenic Diet

Diet is critical to developing good teeth because the carious process depends primarily on fermentable sugars, especially sucrose. Refined table sugar is not the only concentrated sweet food that is cariogenic. Natural foods, including honey, molasses, corn syrup, and dried fruits such as raisins, are highly cariogenic. Complex carbohydrates, such as breads, potato, and pasta, also contribute to caries because they lower the plaque pH (see Dental Disorders, Chapter 18).

Ideally such foods should be eliminated. However, since this is impractical, some suggestions can be helpful. The first is that *the frequency with which sugar is consumed is more important than the total amount eaten.* Therefore when sweets are eaten, they are less damaging if consumed immediately after a meal rather than as a snack between meals. When sweets are served as the dessert, the teeth can be cleaned afterward, decreasing the amount of time the sugar is in the mouth.

The form of sugar is also important. The more cariogenic foods are those that are sticky or hard, since they remain in the mouth longer. Consequently sucking on lollipops is more cariogenic than eating a chocolate bar.

These suggestions can help parents plan "treats" in a way that is less damaging to the teeth. In addition, parents should be aware of foods that are good snacks without contributing to tooth decay (Table 14-6). Substitutes for cariogenic sweets can also include sugarless gum and candy. Sugarless gum chewed after eating may actually protect against cavities by stimulating saliva that neutralizes acid (Jensen and Wefel, 1989). The artificial sweeteners saccharin and aspartame are noncariogenic; sorbitol has low cariogenic potential (Institute of Food Technologists, 1987). Likewise, parents should know about hidden sources of sugar, such as numerous prescription and nonprescription drugs, and many popular cereals, including the "all-natural" variety (Table 14-7). Reading food labels is essential in eliminating sources of sucrose.

A special form of tooth decay in children between 18 months and 3 years of age is *nursing caries* (also called *nursing bottle caries* or *bottle-mouth caries*), which occurs

Table 14-6 Low-cariogenic snack foods

BASIC FOOD GROUP	GOOD SNACKS EATEN ALONE	SNACKS BETTER SERVED WITH MEALS
Bread and cereal	Popcorn and other seeds	Bread and cereals, pasta, crackers, potato products, pretzels, all sweet baked goods
Fruit and vegetable	All raw, fresh, frozen, or waterpack fruits or vegetables or their juices prepared without addition of sugars*	All items prepared or used with the addition of sugars,* dried fruits such as raisins, catsup, gelatin
Meat	Meat of all kinds, including luncheon meats, leftovers, and smoked meat; nuts of all kinds; peanut butter*; bean dips*	Meats prepared with sugars,* candy-coated nuts
Dairy	Milk—whole, low-fat, skim, or buttermilk; all cheeses, especially cheddar; plain yogurt; dips and spreads*; flavored drinks*; hard-boiled eggs	Chocolate milk, malts, shakes, cocoa, ice cream, ice milk, sherbet, other dairy desserts, flavored yogurt

Modified from Madsen, K.O.: Advances in dietary counseling for the prevention of dental caries. In Wei, S.H.: National symposium on dental nutrition, Iowa City, 1978, University of Iowa.

*Check labels for added sugars. Look for (cane, maple, brown) sugar (sucrose), molasses, invert sugar, honey, dextrose (glucose), (modified) corn (sugar, syrup, sweetener, solids), lactose, levulose (fructose), and carob.

Table 14-7 Sucrose content of selected cereals

CEREAL (1-OUNCE SERVING)	SUCROSE (GRAMS/1-OUNCE SERVING)
Shredded Wheat	0
Cheerios	1
Cornflakes	2
Total	3
Rice Krispies	3
Quaker 100% Natural Cereal	6
Raisin Bran (Post)	9
Raisin Bran (Kellogg)	12
Honey Nut Cheerios	10
Frosted Flakes	11
Frosted Rice	11
Froot Loops	13
Apple Jacks	14
Honey Smacks	15

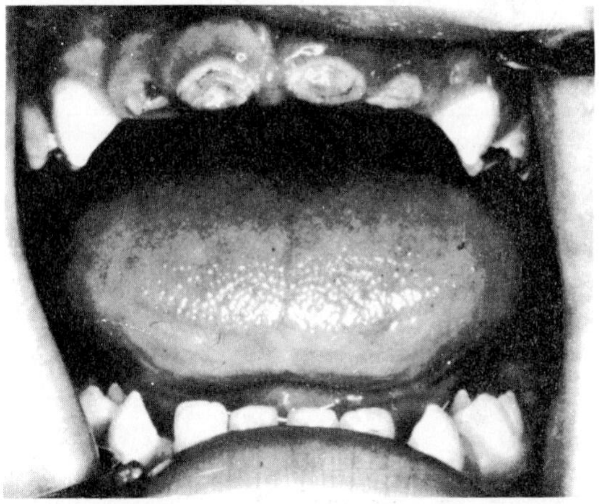

Fig. 14-9. Nursing caries. Note the extensive carious involvement of maxillary primary incisors.

From McDonald R., and Avery D.: Dentistry for the child and adolescent, ed. 5, St. Louis, 1987, Mosby–Year Book, Inc.

when the child is routinely given a bottle of milk or juice at nap or bedtime, or uses the bottle as a pacifier while awake. Frequent nocturnal breast-feeding for prolonged periods also leads to extensive destruction of the teeth (Ripa, 1988). The practice of coating pacifiers in honey can also contribute to caries and may be a potential source of botulism poisoning. Other factors that may contribute to nursing caries include sleep difficulties, a strong-tempered child, single parenting, and less fluoride supplementation or professional counseling (Marino and others, 1989). As the sweet liquid pools in the mouth, the teeth are bathed for several hours in this cariogenic environment. The maxillary (upper) incisors and molars are affected most, since the mandibular (lower) incisors are thought to be protected by the lower lip, tongue, and saliva (Fig. 14-9). Severely decayed teeth may require the application of stainless steel bands to preserve the spacing until the permanent teeth erupt.

Prevention involves eliminating the bedtime bottle completely, feeding the last bottle before bedtime, substituting a bottle of water for milk or juice, not using the bottle as a pacifier, and never coating pacifiers in sweet substances. Juice in bottles, especially commercially available ready-to-use bottles, is discouraged, since the beverage is especially damaging because the sugar is more readily converted to acid. Juice should always be offered in a cup in order to avoid prolonging the bottle-feeding habit.

Nurses are in an excellent position to counsel parents regarding this habit, especially if it occurs during a hospitalization. Although the child may need the comfort of the bottle at this stressful time, parents can be shown photographs depicting the typical tooth destruction and given literature about the condition.* Over an extended hospital stay children can be gradually weaned from the bedtime bottle or given a bottle of water. Health professionals should never contribute to the habit by propping bottles for convenience during feedings.

INJURY PREVENTION

Injuries cause more deaths in children 1 to 4 years of age than in any other childhood period except adolescence. In addition, the injury death rate has remained relatively unchanged during the past decade, whereas the corresponding rates from all other causes of death combined have declined significantly. Injury's prominence as the leading cause of death among toddlers and preschoolers underscores the need to emphasize safety awareness among parents. Child protection and parent education are key determinants in injury prevention.

A major factor in the critical increase of injuries during early childhood is the unrestricted freedom achieved through locomotion combined with an unawareness of danger within the environment. Specific categories of injuries and appropriate prevention are best understood by associating them with the major developmental achievements of young children (Table 14-8). The discussions of injuries in Chapters 1 and 12 are also relevant to safety concerns at this age.

*Sources of information about nursing bottle caries and other aspects of child dental health include **National Institute of Dental Research,** Westwood Building, 5333 Westbard Ave., Bethesda, MD 20816, (301) 496-2883; **American Society of Dentistry for Children,** 211 E. Chicago Ave., Suite 1036, Chicago, IL 60611, (312) 337-2169; **American Dental Association,** 211 E. Chicago Ave., Chicago, IL 60611, (312) 440-2593; and **Canadian Dental Association,** 1815 Alta Vista Dr., Ottawa, Ontario K1G 3Y6, (613) 523-1770. Guidelines for children's dental care are available in Wong, D., and Whaley, L.: Clinical manual of pediatric nursing, ed. 3, St. Louis, 1990, Mosby–Year Book, Inc.

Table 14-8 Injury prevention during early childhood

DEVELOPMENTAL ABILITIES RELATED TO RISK OF INJURY	INJURY PREVENTION
Walks, runs, and climbs Able to open doors and gates Can ride tricycle Can throw ball and other objects	**Motor vehicles** Use federally approved car restraint; if restraint is not available, use lap belt Supervise child while playing outside Do not allow child to play on curb or behind a parked car Do not permit child to play in pile of leaves, snow, or large cardboard container in trafficked area Supervise tricycle riding Lock fences and doors if not directly supervising children Teach child to obey pedestrian safety rules Obey traffic regulations; cross only at crosswalks and only when the traffic signal indicates it is safe to cross Stand back a step from the curb until it's time to cross Look left, right, and left again and check for turning cars before crossing the street Use sidewalks; when there is no sidewalk, walk on the left, facing the traffic Wear light colors at night, and attach fluorescent material to clothing
Able to explore if left unsupervised Has great curiosity Helpless in water; unaware of its danger; depth of water has no significance	**Drowning** Supervise closely when near any source of water Keep bathroom doors closed Have fence around swimming pool and lock gate Teach swimming and water safety
Able to reach heights by climbing, stretching, and standing on toes Pulls objects Explores any holes or opening Can open drawers and closets Unaware of potential sources of heat or fire Plays with mechanical objects	**Burns** Turn pot handles toward back of stove Place electric appliances, such as coffee maker and popcorn machine, toward back of counter Place guardrails in front of radiators, fireplaces, or other heating elements Store matches and cigarette lighters in locked or inaccessible area; discard carefully Place burning candles, incense, hot foods, and cigarettes out of reach Do not let tablecloth hang within child's reach Do not let electric cord from iron or other appliance hang within child's reach Cover electrical outlets with protective plastic caps Keep electrical wires hidden or out of reach Do not allow child to play with electrical appliance, wires, or lighters Stress danger of open flames; teach what "hot" means Always check bathwater temperature; adjust hot-water heater temperature to 120° F or lower; do not allow children to play with faucets Apply a sunscreen when child is exposed to sunlight

Table 14-8 Injury prevention during early childhood—cont'd

DEVELOPMENTAL ABILITIES RELATED TO RISK OF INJURY	INJURY PREVENTION
Explores by putting objects in mouth Can open drawers, closets, and most containers Climbs Cannot read labels Does not know safe dose or amount	**Poisoning** Place all potentially toxic agents out of reach or in a locked cabinet Caution against eating nonedible items, such as plants Replace medications and poisons immediately; replace child-protector caps properly Administer medications as a drug, not as a candy Do not store large surplus of toxic agents Promptly discard empty poison containers; never reuse to store a food item or other poison Teach child not to play in trash containers Never remove labels from containers of toxic substances Have syrup of ipecac in home; use only if advised Know number and location of nearest poison control center (usually listed in front of telephone directory)
Able to open doors and some windows Goes up and down stairs Depth perception unrefined	**Falls** Keep screen in window, nail securely, and use guardrail Place gates at top and bottom of stairs Keep doors locked or use child-proof doorknob covers at entry to stairs, high porch, or other elevated area Remove unsecured or scatter rugs Apply nonskid decals in bathtub or shower Keep crib rails fully raised and mattress at lowest level Place carpeting under crib and in bathroom Keep large toys and bumper pads out of crib or playpen (child can use these as "stairs" to climb out), then move to youth bed when child is able to crawl out of crib Avoid using walkers, especially near stairs Dress in safe clothing (soles that do not "catch" on floor, tied shoelaces, pant legs that do not hang on floor) Keep child restrained in vehicles; never leave unattended in shopping cart Supervise at playgrounds; select play areas with soft ground cover and safe equipment (see Box 14-7)
Puts things in mouth May swallow hard or nonedible pieces of food	**Choking and suffocation** Avoid large, round chunks of meat, such as whole hot dogs (slice lengthwise into short pieces) Avoid fruit with pits, fish with bones, dried beans, hard candy, chewing gum, nuts, popcorn, grapes Choose large sturdy toys without sharp edges or small removable parts Discard old refrigerators, ovens, and so on If storing an old appliance, remove the doors Keep automatic garage door transmitter in inaccessible place Select safe toy boxes or chests without heavy, hinged lids
Still clumsy in many skills Easily distracted from tasks Unaware of potential danger from strangers or other people	**Bodily damage** Avoid giving sharp or pointed objects—such as knives, scissors, or toothpicks—especially when walking or running Do not allow lollipops or similar objects in mouth when walking or running Teach safety precautions, for example, to carry knife or scissors with pointed end away from face Store all dangerous tools, garden equipment, and firearms in locked cabinet Be alert to danger of supervised animals and household pets Use safety glass and decals on large glassed areas, such as sliding glass doors Teach name, address, and phone number and to ask for help from appropriate people (cashier, security guard, policeman) if lost: have identification on child (shown in clothes, inside shoe) Teach stranger safety: Avoid personalized clothing in public places Never go with a stranger Tell parents if anyone makes child feel uncomfortable in any way Always listen to child's concerns regarding others' behavior Teach child to say "no" when confronted with uncomfortable situations

Motor Vehicle Injuries

Motor vehicle injuries cause more accidental deaths in all pediatric age-groups after age 1 year than any other type of injury or disease and are responsible for almost one half of all accidental deaths among children ages 1 to 4 years. Many of the deaths are caused by injuries within the car when restraints have not been used or have been used improperly. Approved restraints properly installed and applied can reduce fatalities by 71% and injuries by 61% (Kahane, 1986).

Nurses have a responsibility for educating parents regarding the importance of car restraints and their proper use. Three basic types of federally approved restraints are available: (1) infant-only device, (2) convertible models for both infants and toddlers, and (3) boosters. Several other types of restraints are available for children with special needs (see Chapter 22 and Fig. 11-12). The infant-type restraints are discussed in Chapter 12; the convertible restraints and boosters are included here.

The convertible restraint is suitable for infants in the rearward-facing position and for toddlers in the forward-facing position (Fig. 14-10). The transition point for switching to the forward-facing position is defined by the manufacturer, but is generally at a body weight of 7.7 to 9 kg (17 to 20 pounds). Authorities suggest using the upper weight limit. The restraint consists of a molded hard plastic or metal frame with energy-absorbing padding and a special harness system designed to hold the child firmly in the seat and distribute the forces to body areas that can withstand the impact.

Convertible restraints use different types of harness systems:

- **Five-point harness,** consisting of a strap over each shoulder, one on each side of the pelvis, and one between the legs; all five come together at a common buckle
- **Padded shield,** consisting of shoulder straps attached to a shield that is held in place by a crotch strap
- **T-shield,** consisting of retracting shoulder straps attached to a flat chest shield with a rigid stalk that attaches to a restraint between the legs (Fig. 14-10)

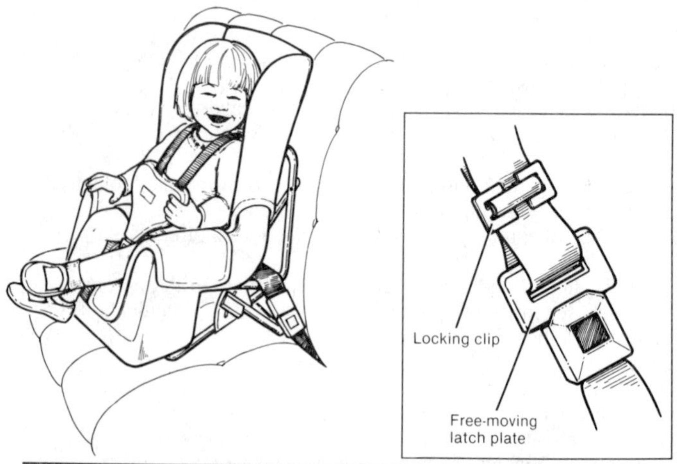

Fig. 14-10. Convertible seat in forward-facing position for older infants and children. *Inset:* Use of locking clip.

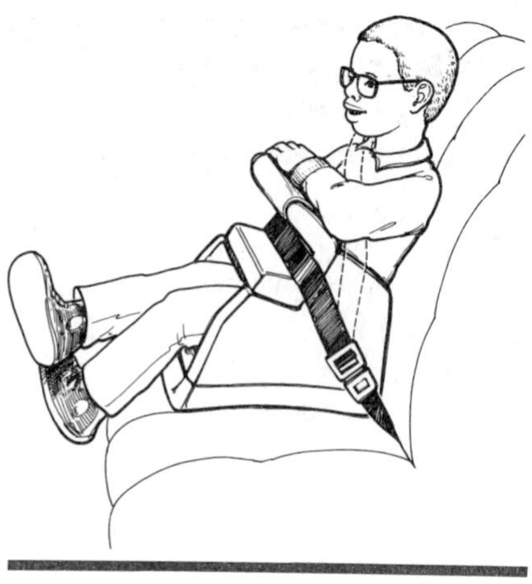

Fig. 14-11. Automobile booster seat. Dashed lines indicate placement of shoulder strap (away from neck or face) for models that can accommodate both lap and shoulder belts.

Boosters are not restraint systems like the convertible devices, because they depend on the vehicle belts to hold the child and booster in place. Boosters are of two types:

- **Low-shield model** that primarily uses a lap belt (Fig. 14-11)
- **Belt-positioning model** that uses the lap/shoulder belt

Some older model restraints require the use of a top anchor (tether) strap to prevent the child from pitching forward in a crash. If the tether strap is not used, up to 90% of the restraint's protection is lost. Instructions for proper installation of the tether strap and permanent bracket are included with the car restraint. Cars with free-sliding latchplates on the lap/shoulder belt require the use of a metal locking clip to keep the belt in a tight-holding position. The locking clip is threaded onto the belt above the latchplate (see inset, Fig. 14-10). If parents have newer cars with automatic lap/shoulder belts, they need to have additional lap belts installed to properly secure the restraint.

Children should use car restraints until they have outgrown them. The "rule of fours" serves as a guide: if the child either weighs about 40 pounds (18 kg) or is 40 inches (100 cm) tall, then the restraint can be replaced by a regular car restraint system. Children who outgrow the convertible restraint may still be able to ride safely in a booster seat until the midpoint of the head is higher than the vehicle seat back. If a car safety seat is not available, the lap belt provides more protection than no restraint (except for infants, where there is no safe alternative to approved restraint devices). A shoulder belt is used *only* if it does not cross the child's neck or face. The safest area of the car for children is the middle of the back seat.

When purchasing a restraint, parents should consider cost and convenience. The convertible-type seats are more expensive initially but cost less than two separate systems. Convenience is a major factor because a cumbersome restraint may be used less and improperly. Before buying a restraint, it is best to try out different models. For example, some types are too large for subcompact cars. Asking neighbors about the advantages and disadvantages of their restraints is helpful. Some service clubs and hospitals have loan programs for restraints. Information about approved models and other aspects of car restraints is available from several organizations and sources.*

For any restraint to be effective it must be used consistently and properly. Reasons for decreased compliance during the toddler years include removal of straps by the child, inability to attach straps over heavy winter clothing, and child's crying, fussing, and boredom (Arneson and others, 1985). Examples of misuse include misrouting of the vehicle seat belt through the restraint, failing to use the vehicle seat belt to secure the restraint, failing to use a tether strap, failing to use the restraint's harness system, and incorrectly positioning the child, especially facing infants forward instead of rearward (Bull, Stroup, and Gerhart, 1988). To address these issues, nurses must stress correct use of car restraints and rules that ensure compliance (see Parent Guidelines). Children riding in car safety seats are generally much better behaved than children left unrestrained, which can be a major benefit to parents and should be emphasized as an additional advantage of restraints (Christophersen, 1977).

Injuries may also occur during sudden stops when objects are left unrestrained. On sudden impact a loose ball becomes a projectile missile. Therefore, all items should be secured or stored in the trunk.

Children over 3 years of age are often involved in pedestrian traffic injuries, with the majority occurring between noon and 6 PM (Guyer, Talbot, and Pless, 1985). Because of their gross motor skills of walking, running, and climbing and their fine motor skills of opening doors and fence gates, they are able to leave most restricted areas when unsupervised. Unaware of danger and unable to approximate the speed of a car, they are hit by moving vehicles. Running after a ball, playing in a pile of leaves or snow or inside a cardboard box, riding a tricycle, and playing behind a parked car or near the curb are common activities that may result in a vehicular tragedy. A precaution when children are playing in driveways is to attach to the tricycle a pole with a bright flag that is high enough to be visible through an automobile's back window.

Preventing vehicular injuries involves protecting and educating children about the danger from moving or parked vehicles. Although preschool children are too young to be trusted to always obey, emphasis on looking for moving vehicles before crossing the street, recognizing the color of traffic lights for stop and go, and following traffic officers' signals emphasizes a good habit. Most important, what is preached must be practiced. Children learn through imitation, and consistency reinforces learning.

*****American Academy of Pediatrics**, 141 Northwest Point Blvd., P.O. Box 927, Elk Grove, IL 60007, (800) 433-9016; and local division of traffic safety or **Department of Transportation, National Highway Traffic Safety Administration**, (800) 424-9393. Guidelines for car seat safety are available in Wong, D., and Whaley, L.: Clinical manual of pediatric nursing, ed. 3, St. Louis, 1990, Mosby–Year Book, Inc.

PARENT GUIDELINES
Using Car Safety Seats

Read the manufacturer's directions and follow them exactly.

Anchor the safety seat securely to the car's seat and apply harness snugly to child.

Do not start the car until *everyone* is properly restrained.

Always use the restraint, even for short trips.

If the child begins to climb out or undo the harness, firmly say, "No." It may be necessary to stop the car to reinforce the expected behavior. The use of rewards, such as stars or stickers, for cooperative behavior is very effective.

Encourage the child to help attach buckles, straps, and shields.

Decrease boredom on long trips. Keep special toys in the car for quiet play; talk to the child; point out objects and teach the child about them. Stop periodically. If the child wishes to sleep, make sure child stays in the restraint.

Insist that others who transport children also follow these safety rules.

Drowning

Drowning, not including drowning from water transportation, ranks second among boys and third among girls ages 1 to 4 years as a cause of accidental death. With well-developed skills of locomotion, toddlers are able to reach potentially dangerous areas, such as bathtubs, swimming pools, hot tubs, and lakes. Even unlikely sources of water, such as toilets and buckets, are dangerous. As inquisitive toddlers lean over the rim of the receptacle, their high center of gravity and poor coordination make it difficult for them to extricate themselves (Jumbelic and Chambliss, 1990). Their intense drive for exploration and investigation, combined with an unawareness of the danger of water and their helplessness in water, makes drowning always a viable threat. It is also one category of injuries that results in death within minutes, diminishing the chance for rescue and survival. Supervising children when near any source of water is essential; teaching swimming and water safety can be helpful but cannot be regarded as sufficient protection.

Burns

Burns rank second to motor vehicle injuries among girls and third among boys in this age-group as a cause of accidental death. A major contributing factor to the sex difference is that girls tend to play indoors and imitate sex-related functions, such as cooking at the stove. Their ability to climb, stretch, and reach objects above their head makes any hot surface a potential source of danger. Scalds from pulling pots on top of themselves are a major source of burns. As a precaution, pot handles should be turned toward the back of the stove. Ideally the knobs for controlling the range burners should be out of reach, not on the front panel where nimble fingers can turn them on and accidentally touch the hot burner. Oven doors should be closed whenever the oven is turned on or when it is cooling. The outside of doors of automatic self-cleaning ovens may become hot and, if touched, could cause a burn. Other sources of heat, such as radiators, fireplaces, accessible furnaces, kerosene heaters, or wood-burning stoves, should have guards placed in front of them. The tops of some of these heaters are designed to become hot enough to boil water to provide humidity. They are hazardous if touched or if the pan of water is spilled (Rissmiller, 1983). Portable electric heaters must be placed in a high area, well out of reach of climbing young children.

Hot objects such as candles, incense, cigarettes, pots of tea or coffee, or irons must be placed away from children. The flame of a candle and the smoke of a cigarette invite investigation. Ashtrays with a center well are preferred to prevent the cigarette from falling off the rim, and adults should try not to smoke, cook, or drink hot liquids when children are physically close. If tablecloths are used, the edges should be placed out of reach to prevent injuries from both burns and falling objects.

Flame burns represent one of the most fatal types of burns and commonly occur when children play with matches and accidentally set themselves (and the home) on fire (Fig. 14-12). All matches must be stored safely away from children, and parents need to teach children the dangers of playing with matches. In addition, all homes should have smoke detectors installed to alert the occupants to fire and a safety plan for immediate escape.

Electrical burns also represent an immediate danger to children. With preschoolers' ability to manipulate small, thin objects, they are able to insert hairpins or other conductive articles into electrical sockets. Young toddlers may explore outlets and wires by mouthing them. Since water is an excellent conductor, the chance for a severe circumoral electrical burn is great. An unusual electrical burn occurred when a toddler placed a small battery in a wet diaper (Mecrow, 1988). Electrical outlets should have protective guards plugged into them when not in use or be made inaccessible by placing furniture in front of them when feasible. Children should not be allowed to play with electrical cords, appliances, or batteries, which should be kept out of reach as much as possible.

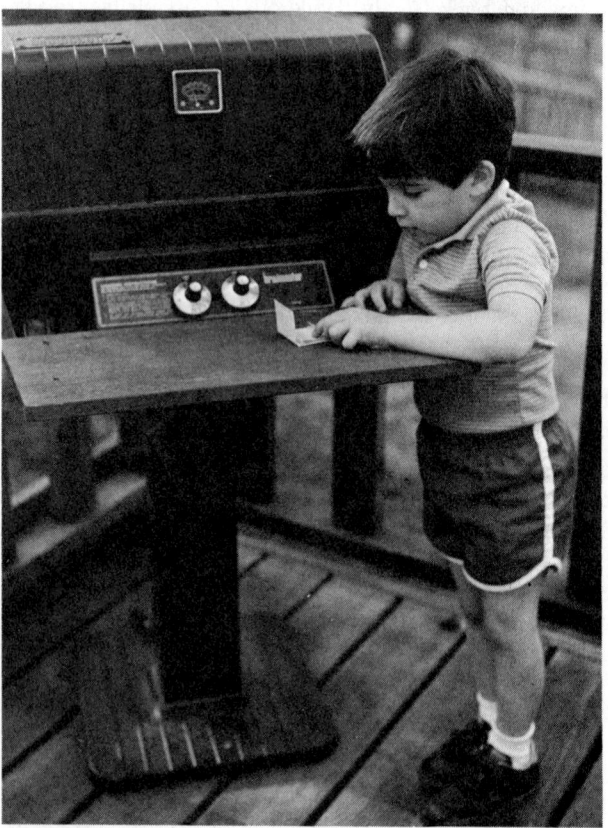

Fig. 14-12. Matches are potentially deadly hazard for young children.

An example of an appliance that interests children and can present a hazard is an electric popcorn popper. Children can become so excited by the popping that they may inadvertently pull the electric cord and popper off the table, resulting in a burn from contact with the hot oil, corn, or appliance.

Scald burns are the most common type of thermal injury in children. Among young children a significant type of scalding burn is caused by high-temperature tap water, which children come in contact with either as a result of turning on the hot-water faucet, falling into a bathtub of hot water, or deliberate abuse. Besides the obvious prevention of always supervising youngsters when they are near tap water and checking bathwater temperatures, a recommended passive prevention is to limit household water temperatures to less than 49° C (120° F). At this temperature it takes 10 minutes for exposure to the water to cause a full-thickness burn. Conversely, water temperatures of 54° C (130° F), the usual setting of most water heaters, expose household members to the risk of full-thickness burns within 30 seconds. Nurses can help prevent such burns by advising parents of this common household danger and recommending that they readjust the water heater to a safe temperature. A meat or candy thermometer is a convenient way to measure water temperature. An easy-to-read hot-water gauge that changes color to show water temperatures between 120° and 150° is available. To measure bath water, special "Frog Prince" or "Bath Bear" thermometers that change color to show "hot," "cool," or "OK" water temperature are convenient for home use.*

Poisoning

Ingestion of toxic agents is extremely common during early childhood. The highest incidence occurs in children in the 2-year-old group. Although in many instances poisoning does not result in mortality, it may cause significant morbidity, such as esophageal stricture from lye ingestion. Although mouthing activity decreases after 1 year of age, exploring objects by tasting them is part of children's curious investigation. Young children's taste is not refined and discriminating. Children under 6 years of age are more likely to eat "disgusting" substances (Rozin and others, 1985). While young children may be able to identify some items as poisonous, they do not understand the toxic effects of ingesting excessive amounts of a familiar drug, such as vitamins.

*Clinitemp, Inc., PO Box 681130, Indianapolis, IN 46268; (317) 872-4155.

In addition, the apparent safety of such drugs is reinforced by their daily administration (Osborne and Garrettson, 1985). Almost every nonfood substance is potentially harmful, including many house plants, and by 2 years of age toddlers are able to climb most heights, open most drawers or closets, and unscrew most lids. By trial and error younger children also manage to undo tops of bottles, plastic containers, aerosol cans, and jars.

However, they are most likely to ingest substances that are on their level, such as plants, cleaning agents stored under sinks, rat poison, or diaper pail deodorants. Child-guard tops are required on some substances, such as prescription drugs, but many young children have outwitted such "safe" caps. In addition, pharmacists often transfer drugs to regular containers for the elderly, who may have difficulty with child-guard closures. Newer forms of drugs, such as transdermal patches (Corneli and others, 1989; Reed and Hamburg, 1986) and cough-suppressant lozenges, have created additional dangers, since they are not packaged with safety caps, and in the case of lozenges look like candy.

Many potentially toxic substances are not protected with safety caps and must be stored properly. Even common household items, such as mouthwash that contains ethanol (alcohol), can be toxic to young children (Weller-Fahy, Berger, and Troutman, 1980).

The major reason for poisoning is improper storage. The guidelines suggested in Chapter 12 are applicable to children in this age-group as well. However, unlike the infant who was confined to certain heights and unable to unlatch inventive locks, young children manage to find access to many high-level, tight-security places (Fig. 14-13). For this age-group only a locked cabinet is safe.

Parents should have two doses of ipecac syrup for each child in the home, know its proper use and administration, and have the phone number and location of the nearest poison control center. Emergency and preventive measures for accidental poisoning are discussed in Chapter 16.

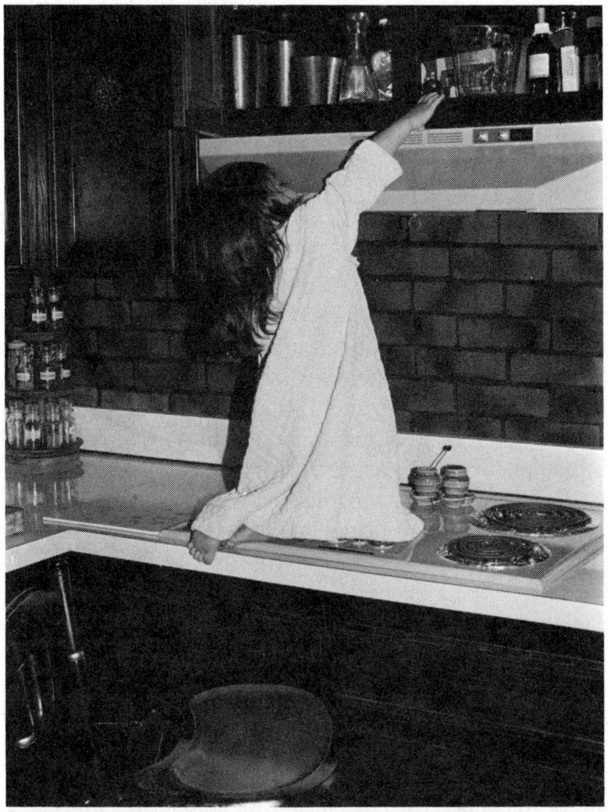

Fig. 14-13. No unlocked cabinet can be considered safe with young children. This 3-year-old child used her high chair to climb on to the counter to open high storage area. Note additional danger of stepping on stove, where accidental burns can occur.

Falls

During this age playground injuries become common, and many of the injuries are related to playground equipment and occur at home or at daycare (Playground, 1988). Children need to be taught safety at play areas, such as no horseplay on high slides or jungle gyms, *sitting* on swings, and staying away from moving swings. Other guidelines for playground safety are listed in Box 14-7.

Box 14-7 PLAYGROUND SAFETY

Be certain there are no sharp edges, corners, or projections.
Make sure that concrete footings are not exposed.
Examine area for a safe resilient surface under the equipment, such as sand to reduce the impact from a fall.
Be certain that the scale of the equipment matches the child's size.
There should be no holes where fingers, arms and legs, and necks could get caught.
The incline of a slide should not exceed 30 degrees.
"S" hooks on swings must be closed.
Check for litter, broken glass, exposed wires, or electrical outlets.

From American Association for Leisure and Recreation, National Survey of Elementary School Playground Equipment.

The climbing and running activity of the typical toddler is complicated by total neglect for and lack of appreciation of danger combined with immature coordination and a high center of gravity. Falling from stairs is a major cause of injury, with more children in this age-group sustaining head injury than older children (Joffe and Ludwig, 1988). Gates must be placed at both ends of stairs. Accessible windows that are left open during warm weather must be screened or guarded with a rail. Falling from open windows is a major cause of accidental death in urban lower socioeconomic groups. Doors leading to stairwells or porches must be locked, since preschool children can easily open them. A convenient type of lock is a sliding bar or hook that can be attached to the door and frame at a level higher than the child can reach, provided that inventive youngsters do not pull a chair over to unlatch the hook or bar.

Another source of falls is from cribs and vehicles. In addition to crib rails being fully raised, the mattress should be kept at the lowest position, and toys or bumper pads that may be used as steps to climb out should be removed. Ideally the floor should be carpeted. Once children reach a height of 89 cm (35 inches), they should sleep in a bed rather than a crib. If a bunk bed is selected, parents should be aware of possible dangers: falls and head entrapment between the mattress and guardrail or between the supporting mattress slats. Children who sleep on the top bunk should be 6 years or older (Concerns, 1987).

To prevent falls from vehicles, children must always be properly restrained. They should never ride in the open back of a truck; the danger of falls can be compounded by another vehicle striking the child. Another hazard is grocery shopping carts. Children left unattended can easily fall out.

Clothing can also increase the chance of falling. Slippery shoes or socks, rubber-soled shoes that "catch" on the floor and rug, and loose or cuffed pants can easily make a child fall. Simple safety measures, such as checking clothing and shoes, keeping shoelaces tied with double knots, or using Velcro closures, can prevent such needless injuries.

Aspiration and Suffocation

Usually by 1 year of age children chew well, but they may have difficulty with large pieces of food such as meat or whole hot dogs and with hard foods such as nuts or dried beans. Young children cannot discard pits from fruit or bones from fish like older children. It takes practice to learn how to chew gum without swallowing it. Therefore the same precautions as discussed for infants regarding food selection must be implemented (see Chapter 12).

Play objects for toddlers must still be chosen with an awareness of the danger of small parts. Large, sturdy toys without sharp edges or removable parts are safest. Coins, paper clips, pull-tabs on cans, thumbtacks, nails, screws, jewelry (especially pierced earrings), and all types of pins are common household objects that can cause significant harm if swallowed or aspirated. Because of the danger of aspiration, parents should be taught emergency procedures for choking (see Fig. 31-23).

Another cause of death by traumatic asphyxiation is from electrically operated garage doors (Satran, 1981). Young children playing in the garage may become trapped under the door. Although the automatic doors should reverse when striking an object, they may not do so when hitting a flexible object or one that is very close to the ground. Precautions include placing controls where they are inaccessible to children, such as high on a wall and in a locked car, and instructing children that the transmitter is not a toy. Periodically the door should be checked to be certain it returns when striking an object.

Suffocation is less frequent from causes seen during infancy but is an ever-present threat from old refrigerators, ovens, and other large appliances. Toddlers can climb inside these appliances and if they close the door behind them will be trapped inside. Discarding old appliances and removing all doors during storage prevent such tragic injuries.

Bodily Damage

Toddlers are still clumsy in many of their skills and can seriously harm themselves when walking while holding a sharp or pointed object or having food or objects such as spoons in their mouths. Preventing such occurrences is the best approach with toddlers. With preschoolers teaching safety is most important. The child should be taught that when walking with a pointed object such as a knife or scissors, the pointed end is held away from the face. Dangerous garden or workshop equipment and all firearms should be stored in a locked cabinet. Power lawn mowers are especially dangerous, and young children should not be allowed in an area where a mower is being used; nor should they be taken for a ride on a mower or allowed to operate the device (American Academy of Pediatrics, Committee on Accident and Poison Prevention, 1990). Safety education should include respect for firearms and their proper and appropriate use including nonpowder guns, such as air guns and rifles, that cause serious penetrating injuries (American Academy of Pediatrics, Committee on Accident and Poison Prevention, 1987). In addition, the child should be warned of and protected against potential danger from animals (see Bodily Damage, Chapter 12, and Animal Bites, Chapter 18).

Toys can be a source of danger, and safety must be a prime consideration when selecting toys (see Parent Guidelines: Toy Safety, Chapter 4). Most toys have age ranges written on them to designate their safety, but this must be tempered with knowledge of the specific child's readiness.

Household safety should be practiced and includes the usual precautions recommended for any age-group (see Parent Guidelines: Child Safety Home Checklist, Chapter 12). An additional safeguard for young children is the use of safety glass in doors and windows and the application of decals on glassed areas to lessen the likelihood of running through glass.

ANTICIPATORY GUIDANCE—CARE OF FAMILIES

Understanding toddlers is fundamental to successful childrearing, regardless of the approach used. Nurses, particularly those in ambulatory or child health centers, are in a most favorable position to assist parents in meeting the tasks and needs of children in this age-group. It seems to be an almost universal phenomenon that prevention yields better results than treatment. Anticipatory guidance in each of the areas presented in Box 14-8 is paramount if one wishes to prevent future problems. Advice is sometimes not the sole answer. Actual assistance, such as being available for home visiting or telephone consulting, should be part of the nurse's flexible repertoire of interventions. Whether parents are experiencing the rearing dilemmas of a first or a subsequent child, they benefit from sharing their feelings, frustrations, and satisfactions. They need adult companionship, freedom from childrearing responsibilities, and periodic separations from their children. Sometimes they lose perspective of the needs of each other in the marital relationship and fail to communicate effectively. Part of a nurse's responsibility is to provide opportunities for ventilation of parents' feelings and guidance in areas such as marital needs, career fulfillment, and peer companionship.

Box 14-8 GUIDANCE DURING TODDLER YEARS

Age 12 to 18 Months

Prepare parents for expected behavioral changes of toddler, especially negativism and ritualism.
Assess present feeding habits and encourage gradual weaning from bottle and increased intake of solid foods.
Stress expected feeding changes of physiologic anorexia, presence of food fads and strong taste preferences, need for scheduled routine at mealtimes, inability to sit through an entire meal, and lack of table manners.
Assess sleep patterns at night, particularly habit of a bedtime bottle, which is a major cause of dental caries, and procrastination behaviors that delay hour of sleep.
Prepare parents for potential dangers of the home, particularly motor vehicle, poisoning, and falling injuries; give appropriate suggestions for safeproofing the home.
Discuss need for firm but gentle discipline and ways in which to deal with negativism and temper tantrums: stress positive benefits of appropriate discipline.
Emphasize importance for both child and parents of brief, periodic separations.
Discuss new toys that use developing gross and fine motor, language, cognitive, and social skills.
Emphasize need for dental supervision, types of basic dental hygiene at home, and food habits that predispose to caries: stress importance of supplemental fluoride.

Age 18 to 24 Months

Stress importance of peer companionship in play.
Explore need for preparation for additional sibling; stress importance of preparing child for new experiences.
Discuss present discipline methods, their effectiveness, and parents' feelings about child's negativism; stress that negativism is important aspect of developing self-assertion and independence and is not a sign of spoiling.
Discuss signs of readiness for toilet training; emphasize importance of waiting for physical and psychologic readiness.
Discuss development of fears, such as darkness or loud noises, and of habits, such as security blanket or thumbsucking; stress normalcy of these transient behaviors.
Prepare parents for signs of regression in time of stress.
Assess child's ability to separate easily from parents for brief periods of separation under familiar circumstances.
Allow parents opportunity to express their feelings of weariness, frustration, and exasperation; be aware that it is often difficult to love toddlers at times when they are not asleep!
Point out some of the expected changes of the next year, such as longer attention span, somewhat less negativism, and increased concern for pleasing others.

Age 24 to 36 Months

Discuss importance of imitation and domestic mimicry and need to include child in activities.
Discuss approaches toward toilet training, particularly realistic expectations and attitude toward accidents.
Stress uniqueness of toddlers' thought processes, especially through their use of language, poor understanding of time, causal relationships in terms of proximity of events, and inability to see events from another's perspective.
Stress that discipline still must be quite structured and concrete and that relying solely on verbal reasoning and explanation leads to injuries, confusion, and misunderstanding.
Discuss investigation of nursery school or daycare center toward completion of second year.

KEY POINTS

- The toddler stage, extending from 12 months to 36 months, is a period of intense exploration of the environment.
- Biologic development during the toddler years is characterized by the acquisition of fine and gross motor skills that allow children to master a wide variety of activities.
- Although most of the physiologic systems are mature by the end of toddlerhood, development of certain areas of the brain is still occurring, allowing for greater intellectual capacity.
- Locomotion is the major gross motor skill acquired during toddlerhood, followed by increased eye-hand coordination.
- Specific tasks in the psychosocial development of a toddler include differentiating self from others, tolerating separation from parent, coping with delayed gratification, controlling bodily functions, acquiring socially acceptable behavior, verbally communicating, and interacting with others in a less egocentric manner.
- According to Erikson, the major developmental task of toddlerhood is acquiring a sense of autonomy while overcoming a sense of doubt and shame.
- Language is the major cognitive achievement in toddlerhood.
- In Piaget's sensorimotor and preconceptual phases of development, the toddler experiments by incorporating the old learning of secondary circular reactions with new skills and applies this knowledge to new situations. There is the beginning of rational judgment, an understanding of causal relationships, and discovery of objects as objects.
- Preconceptual thought is characterized by global organization of thought processes, animism, and irreversibility.
- Discipline, or a punishment-obedience orientation, aids in children's moral development.
- Development of body image occurs with increasing motor ability, at which point toddlers recognize the importance and capacity of body parts.
- The two phases of differentiation of self from significant others are separation and individuation.
- The most striking characteristic of language development during early childhood is the increasing level of comprehension.

- Parental concerns during the toddler years include toilet training, coping with sibling rivalry, limit-setting and discipline, dealing with temper tantrums and negativism, and coping with stress.
- Effective discipline techniques for toddlers include reward, ignoring or extinction, and time-out.
- Nutrition is important at this stage because eating habits established in toddlerhood tend to have lasting effects in subsequent years.
- Regular dental examinations, fluoride supplementation, removal of plaque, and provision of a low-cariogenic diet promote optimum dental health.
- Because of increased locomotion, toddlers are at high risk for sustaining injuries. Fatal injuries are primarily the result of motor vehicle accidents, drownings, and burns.

REFERENCES

Abe, K., Oda, N., and Amatomi, M.: Natural history and predictive significance of head-banging, head-rolling, and breath-holding spells, Dev. Med. Child Neurol. 26 (5):644-648, 1984.

American Academy of Allergy: A statement of the question of allergy to fluoride as used in the fluoridation of community water supplies, J. Allergy 45:347-348, 1971.

American Academy of Pediatrics, Committee on Accident and Poison Prevention: Injuries related to "toy" firearms, Pediatrics 79(3):473-474, 1987.

American Academy of Pediatrics, Committee on Accident and Poison Prevention: Ride-on mower injuries in children, Pediatrics 86(1):141-143, 1990.

American Dental Association, Council on Dental Therapeutics: Accepted dental therapeutics, ed. 40, Chicago, 1984, American Dental Association.

Arneson, S., and others: Factors affecting parental use of child automobile safety restraints, J. Assoc. Care Child. Health 13(4):181-186, 1985.

Bull, M.J., Stroup, K.B., and Gerhart, S.: Misuse of car safety seats, Pediatrics 81(1):98-101, 1988.

Carey, W.B., and McDevitt, S.: Stability and change in individual temperament diagnoses from infancy to early childhood, Am. Acad. Child Psychiatry 17(2):331-337, 1978.

Chess, S., and Thomas, A.: Temperamental differences: a critical concept in child health care, Pediatr. Nurs. 11(3):167-171, 1985.

Christophersen, E.R.: Children's behavior during automobile rides: do car seats make a difference? Pediatrics 60(1):69-74, 1977.

Concerns about the safety of bunk beds, Pediatr. Alert, Nov. 19, 1987.

Corneli, H., and others: Toddler eats clonidine patch and nearly quits smoking for life (letter), JAMA 261:42, 1989.

Crall, J.J.: Promotion of oral health and prevention of common pediatric dental problems, Pediatr. Clin. North Am. 33(4):887-899, 1986.

Feldman, K.W., and others: Tap water scald burns in children, Pediatrics 62(1):1-7, 1978.

Fergusson, D.M., Horwood, L.J., and Shannon, F.T.: Factors related to the age of attainment of nocturnal bladder control: an 8-year longitudinal study, Pediatrics 78(5):884-890, 1986.

Fleisher, D.R., and Morrison, A.: Masturbation mimicking abdominal pain or seizures in young girls, J. Pediatr. 116:810-814, 1990.

Food and Nutrition Board, National Research Council: Recommended Dietary Allowances, ed. 10, Washington, DC, 1989, National Academy Press.

Fullard, W., McDevitt, S., and Carey, W.: Assessing temperament in one- to three-year-old children, J. Pediatr. Psychol. 9:205-217, 1984.

Gates, S.: Children's literature: it can help children cope with sibling rivalry, MCN 5(5):351-352, 1979.

Griffiths, S.S.: The role of the pediatric nurse clinician in promoting the development of body image in children. In Beal, J.A., editor: Issues and advanced practice in pediatric nursing, Reston, VA, 1983, Reston Publishing Co., Inc.

Grossman, C.S.: Using children's books to foster acceptance of a new sibling into a one-child family, Clin. Pediatr. 21(8):502, 1982.

Guyer, B., Talbot, A.M., and Pless, I.B.: Pedestrian injuries to children and youth, Pediatr. Clin. North Am. 32(1):163-174, 1985.

Heifetz, S., and Horowitz, H.: Amounts of fluoride in self-administered dental products: safety considerations for children, Pediatrics 77(6): 876-882, 1986.

Hess, C.S., and others: Fluoride: too much or too little, Pediatr. Nurs. 10(6):397-403, 1984.

Honig, J.C.: Preparing preschool-aged children to be siblings, MCN 11(1):37-43, 1986.

Hoover, N., McKay, F., and Fraumeni, J.: Fluoridated drinking water and the occurrence of cancer, J. Natl. Cancer Inst. 57(4):757-768, 1976.

Houldin, A., Fullard, W., and Heverly, M.A.: Toddler temperament and quality of child-rearing environment, Pediatr. Nurs. 15(5):491-496, 544, 1989.

The Institute of Food Technologists' Expert Panel on Food Safety and Nutrition: Sweeteners: nutritive and non-nutritive, Contemp. Nutr. 12(9):1-4, 1987.

Jensen, M.E., and Wefel, J.S.: Human plaque pH responses to meals and the effects of chewing gum, Br. Dent. J. 167:204-208, 1989.

Joffe, M., and Ludwig, S.: Stairway injuries in children, Pediatrics 82(3, part 2):457-461, 1988.

Jumbelic, M.I., and Chambliss, M.: Accidental toddler drowning in 5-gallon buckets, JAMA 263:1952-1953, 1990.

Kahane, C.J.: An evaluation of child passenger safety: the effectiveness and benefits of safety seats, U.S. Department of Transportation, No. DOT HS 806 890, Washington, DC, National Highway Traffic Safety Administration, Feb. 1986.

MacLaughlin, S.M., and Johnston, K.B.: The preparation of young children for the birth of a sibling, J. Nurs.-Midwif. 29(6):371-376, 1984.

Mahler, M.S., Pine, F., and Bergman, A.: The psychological birth of the human infant: symbiosis and individuation, New York, 1975, Basic Books.

Margolis, F.J., and Cohen, S.N.: Successful and unsuccessful experiences in combating the antifluoridationists, Pediatrics 76(1):113-118, 1985.

Marino, R.V., and others: Nursing bottle caries: characteristics of children at risk, Clin. Pediatr. 28(3):129-131, 1989.

McDevitt, S., and Carey, W.: Stability of ratings vs. perceptions of temperament from early infancy to 1-3 years, Am. J. Orthopsychiatry 51(2):342-345, 1981.

McDonald, R., and Avery, D.: Dentistry for the child and adolescent, ed. 5, 1987, Mosby–Year Book, Inc.

Mecrow, I.K.: Burn to toddler's penis from an electrochemical battery, Br. Med. J. 297(6659):1315, 1988.

Needleman, H., Pueschel, S., and Rothman, K.: Fluoridation and occurrence of Down's syndrome, N. Engl. J. Med. 291:821-823, 1974.

Needlman, R., Howard, B., and Zuckerman, B.: Temper tantrums: when to worry, Contemp. Pediatr. 6(8):12-34, 1989.

Osborne, S., and Garrettson, L.: Perception of toxicity and dose by 3- and 4-year-old children, Am. J. Dis. Child. 139(8):790-792, 1985.

Playground-related injuries in preschool-aged children—United States, 1983-1987, MMWR 37(41):629, 1988.

Progress toward achieving the National 1990 Objectives for Fluoridation and Dental Health, Clin. Pediatr. 28(11):543-544, 1989.

Reed, M., and Hamburg, E.: Person-to-person transfer of transdermal drug-delivery systems: a case report (letter), N. Engl. J. Med 314:1120-1121, 1986.
Ripa, L.W.: Nursing caries: a comprehensive review, Pediatr. Dent. 10(4):268-282, 1988.
Rissmiller, R.: Kerosene heaters—a new burn threat to children, Clin. Pediatr. 22(3):203, 1983.
Rozin, P., and others: Children's concept of food; the development of contamination sensitivity to disgusting substances, Dev. Psychol. 21(6):1075-1079, 1985.
Satran, L.: Fatalities caused by electrically operated garage doors, Pediatrics 68(3):422-423, 1981.
Schmitt, B.D.: Parents' guide to behavior problems: how to deal with temper tantrums, Contemp. Pediatr. 6(8):39-40, 1989.
Schuster, C.S., and Ashburn, S.S.: The process of human development: a holistic approach, ed. 2, Boston, 1986, Little, Brown & Co, Inc.
Spadt, S.K., Martin, K.R., and Thomas, A.M.: Experiential classes for siblings-to-be, MCN 15:184-186, 1990.
Stadtler, A.C.: Preventing encopresis, Pediatr. Nurs. 15(3):282-284, 1989.
Thomas, R.M.: Comparing theories of child development, ed. 2, Belmont, CA, 1985, Wadsworth Publishing Co.
Weller-Fahy, E., Berger, L., and Troutman, W.: Mouthwash: a source of acute ethanol intoxication, Pediatrics 66(2):302-304, 1980.
Zuckerman, B.S., and Frank, D.A.: Infancy. In Levine, M.D., and others, editors: Developmental-behavioral pediatrics, Philadelphia, 1983, W.B. Saunders Co.

BIBLIOGRAPHY

For additional citations relevant to toddlerhood, refer to Chapter 12.

Growth and Development

Ames, L.B., and Ilg, F.L.: Your two-year-old: terrible or tender, New York, 1979, Delacorte Press.
Howard, B.T.: Growing together: the toddler years need not be turbulent, Contemp. Pediatr. 7(6):21-40, 1990.
Lamb, J.M.: The rapprochement subphase of the separation-individuation process, Matern. Child Nurs. J. 15(3):129-138, 1986.
Larzelere, R.E., Martin, J.A., and Amberson, T.G.: The toddler behavior checklist: a parent-completed assessment of social-emotional characteristics of young preschoolers, Fam. Rel. 38:418-425, 1989.
Lee, J., and Fowler, M.D.: Merely child's play? Developmental work and playthings, J. Pediatr. Nurs. 1(4):260-270, 1986.
Lincoln, L.M.: Fathering and the separation-individuation process, Matern. Child Nurs. J. 13(2):103-111, 1984.
Oberklaid, F., and others: Assessment of temperament in the toddler age group, Pediatrics 85(4):559-566, 1990.
Pontious, S.L.: Practical Piaget: helping children understand, Am. J. Nurs. 82(1):114-117, 1982.
Selekman, J.: The development of body image in the child: a learned response, Top. Clin. Nurs. 5(1):12-21, 1983.
Shelly, J.A., and others: The spiritual needs of children, Downers Grove, IL, 1982, Inter-Varsity Press.

Toilet Training

The age of mastery: a multi-disciplinary roundtable discusion on toilet training and enuresis, New York, Kimberly-Clark Corp., April 14, 1989.
Berk, L., and Friman, P.: Epidemiologic aspects of toilet training, Clin. Pediatr. 29(5):278-282, 1990.
Euler, M.M., and McClellan, M.A.: Toilet training: ready or not? Pediatr. Nurs. 7(1):15-20, 1981.
Euler-Horner, M.M.: The challenge of toilet training—bowel management for the child with psychogenic encopresis or neurogenic deficit, Pediatr. Basics 32:4-10, 1982.

Sibling Rivalry

Castiglia, P.T.: Sibling rivalry, J. Pediatr. Health Care 3(1):52-54, 1989.
Dunn, J., Kendrick, C., and MacNamee, R.: The reaction of first-born children to the birth of a sibling: mothers' reports, J. Child Psychol. Psychiatry 22(1):1-18, 1981.
Merrill, J.: Announcing the newcomer, Baby Talk 52(3):16-20, 1987.
Schmitt, B.D.: Sibling rivalry toward a new baby, Contemp. Pediatr. 7(3):111-112, 1990.
Wilford, B., and Andrews, C.: Sibling preparation classes for preschool children, Matern. Child Nurs. J. 15(3):171-185, 1986.

Limit-Setting and Discipline/Temper Tantrums

American Academy of Pediatrics, Committee on Psychosocial Aspects of Child and Family Health: The pediatrician's role in discipline, Pediatrics 72(3):373-374, 1983.
Campbell, S.B., and others: A multidimensional assessment of parent-identified behavior problem toddlers, J. Abnorm. Child Psychol. 10(4):569-592, 1982.
Castiglia, P.T.: Temper tantrums, J. Pediatr. Health Care 2(5):267-268, 1988.
Christophersen, E.R.: Incorporating behavioral pediatrics into primary care, Pediatr. Clin. North Am. 29(2):261-296, 1982.
Christophersen, E.R.: Anticipatory guidance on discipline, Pediatr. Clin. North Am. 33(4):789-798, 1986.
Farber, J.M.: Mild 'punishment' works, Pediatrics 68(2):298, 1981.
Gonzalez-Mena, J.: A positive approach to discipline, Twins 1(5):44-45, 1985.
Hirsch, D.L.O., and Russo, D.C.: Behavior management. In Levine, M.D., and others, editors: Developmental-behavioral pediatrics, Philadelphia, 1983, W.B. Saunders Co.
Kvols-Riedler, K., and Kvols-Riedler, B.: Redirecting children's misbehavior, Pediatrics: Nursing Update 1(3), Princeton, NJ, 1985, Continuing Professional Education Center.
Schmitt, B.D.: The stubborn toddler who just says "No," Contemp. Pediatr. 7(4):71-72, 1990.

Stress

Busen, N.H.: Societal values: a cause of stress in children, J. Pediatr. Health Care 2(6):300-306, 1988.
Garmezy, N., and Rutter, M., editors: Stress, coping, and development in children, New York, 1983, McGraw-Hill, Inc.
Grey, M., and Hayman, L.L.: Assessing stress in children: research and clinical implications, J. Pediatr. Nurs. 2(5):316-327, 1987.
Kuczen, B.: Childhood stress: don't let your child be a victim, New York, 1982, Delacorte Press.
Lamontagne, L.L., Mason, K.R., and Hepworth, J.T.: Effects of relaxation on anxiety in children: implications for coping with stress, Nurs. Res. 34:289-292, 1985.
Medeiros, D.C., Porter, B.J., and Welch, I.O.: Children under stress, Englewood Cliffs, NJ, 1983, Spectrum Books.
Saunders, A., and Remsberg, B.: The stress-proof child: a loving parent's guide, New York, 1984, Holt, Rinehart & Winston, Inc.
Scandrett, S., and Uecker, S.: Relaxation training. In Bulechek, G.M., and McCloskey, J.C., editor: Nursing interventions: treatment for nursing diagnoses, Philadelphia, 1985, W.B. Saunders Co.

Nutrition

American Academy of Pediatrics, Committee on Nutrition: Pediatric nutrition handbook, ed. 2, Elk Grove Village, IL, 1985, The Academy.
Brock, D.T.: Decreasing toddlers' sodium intake, Pediatr. Nurs. 11(1):47-50, 1985.
La Leche League: Toddler grazing, Baby Talk, pp. 20-45, May 1989.
Lucas, B.: Nutrition in childhood. In Krause, M.V., and Mahan, L.K.: Food, nutrition, and diet therapy, ed. 7, Philadelphia, 1984, W.B. Saunders Co.

Pipes, P.: Nutrition in infancy and childhood, ed. 4, St. Louis, 1989, Mosby–Year Book, Inc.

Rosenthal, S.R., and Padron, C.Z.: Nutrition assessment of the young child (two through six years). In Simko, M.D., Cowell, C., and Hreha, M.S.: Practical nutrition: a quick reference for the health care practitioner, Rockville, MD, 1989, Aspen Publishers, Inc.

Satter, E.: Developmental guidelines for feeding infants and young children, Food Nutr. News 56(4):21-26, 1984.

Satter, E.: Child of mine: feeding with love and good sense, Palo Alto, CA, 1986, Bull Publishing Co.

Satter, E.: How to get your kid to eat . . . but not too much, Palo Alto, CA, 1987, Bull Publishing Co.

Schmitt, B.D.: When your toddler or preschooler won't eat, Contemp. Pediatr. 6(9):127-128, 1989.

Wurtman, J.J.: What do children eat? Eating styles of the preschool, elementary school, and adolescent child. In Suskind, R.M., editor: Textbook of pediatric nutrition, New York, 1981, Raven Press.

Dental Health

Alvarez, J.O., and Navia, J.M.: Nutritional status, tooth eruption, and dental caries: a review, Am. J. Clin. Nutr. 49:417-426, 1989.

American Academy of Pediatrics, Committee on Nutrition: Fluoride supplementation, Pediatrics 77(5):758-761, 1986.

Bullen, C., and others: Improving children's oral hygiene through parental involvement, J. Dent. Child. 55(2):125-128, 1988.

Committee on Research, The American Academy of Periodontology: Gum disease affects most young people in varying degrees, Point of View 26(2):10, 1989.

Council on Dental Therapeutics: Guidelines for the acceptance of fluoride-containing dentifrices, J. Am. Dent. Assoc. 110:545-547, 1985.

Feigal, R.J.: Common oral diseases of children, Pediatr. Ann. 14(2):133-138, 1985.

Goepferd, S.J.: Infant oral health: a protocol, J. Dent. Child. 53(4):261-266, 1986.

Goepferd, S.J.: Infant oral health: a rationale, J. Dent. Child. 53(4):257-260, 1986.

Goepferd, S.J.: An infant oral health program: the first 18 months, Pediatr. Dent. 9(1):8-12, 1987.

Grytten, J., and others: Longitudinal study of dental health behaviors and other caries predictors in early childhood, Community Dent. Oral Epidemiol. 16(6):356-359, 1988.

Guide to dental health, J. Am. Dent. Assoc. 112:20-30, 1986.

Herrmann, H.J., and Roberts, M.W.: Preventive dental care: the role of the pediatrician, Pediatrics 80(1):107-110, 1987.

Hess, C., and others: Fluoride and caries prevention, Child. Nurse 4(2):1-4, 1986.

Hess, C., and others: Preventing tooth decay in children, Baby Talk 52(3):30-31, 1987.

Hitchens-Serota, J.A.: Assessing parents' knowledge of pediatric dental disease, Pediatr. Nurs. 12(6):435-438, 1986.

Kronmiller, J.E., and Nirschl, R.F.: Preventive dentistry for children, Pediatr. Nurs. 11:446-449, 1985.

Kuster, C.G.: The modern pediatric dental office experience, Pediatr. Ann. 14(2):148-158, 1985.

McDermott, R., and McCormack, K.: Nursing caries syndrome: implications for children's health care professionals, Child. Health Care 15(1):49-54, 1986.

National Center for Health Statistics: Use of dental services and dental health: United States, 1986, Vital and Health Statistics, Series 10, No. 165. DHHS Pub. No. (PHS) 88-1593. Public Health Service, Washington, DC, 1988, U.S. Government Printing Office.

Nirschl, R.F., and Kronmiller, J.E.: Evaluating oral health needs in preschool children, Clin. Pediatr. 25(7):358-362, 1986.

Sheridan, P.G.: NIDR—40 years of research advances in dental health, Public Health Rep. 103(5):493-499, 1988.

Speedie, G.: Nursology of mouth care: preventing, comforting and seeking activities related to mouth care, J. Adv. Nurs. 8(1):33-40, 1983.

Injury Prevention

Agran, P., Winn, D., and Dunkle, D.: Injuries among 4- to 9-year-old restrained motor vehicle occupants by seat location and crash impact site, Am. J. Dis. Child. 143:1317-1321, 1989.

American Academy of Pediatrics, Committee on Accident and Poison Prevention: Automatic passenger protection systems, Pediatrics 74(1):146-147, 1984.

Arneson, S.W., and Triplett, J.L.: Riding with Bucklebear: an automobile safety program for preschoolers, J. Pediatr. Nurs. 5(2):115-122, 1990.

Becker, P.G., and Turow, J.: Earring aspiration and other jewelry hazards, Pediatrics 78(3):494-496, 1986.

Bodiwala, G.G., Thomas, P.D., and Otubushin, A.: Protective effect of rear-seat restraints during car collisions, Lancet 1(8634):369-371, 1989.

Bull, M.J., and others: Establishing special needs car seat loan program, Pediatrics 85(4):540-547, 1990.

Fuchs, S., and others: Cervical spine fractures sustained by young children in forward-facing car seats, Pediatrics 84(2):348-354, 1989.

Gunnip, A., and others: Car seats: helping parents do it right! J. Pediatr. Health Care 1:190-195, 1987.

Halpern, J.S.: How safe are child safety seats? J. Emerg. Nurs. 16(3, pt. 1):151-155, 1990.

Kidwell-Udin, P., Jacobson, D., and Jensen, R.: It's never too soon to teach car safety, MCN 12(5):344-345, 1987.

Killam, P., and Smith, K.: Getting kids into car seats, MCN 13(2):124-126, 1988.

Okstein, C.J., Odal, M., and Kelly, R.W.: Odontoid fracture in a child occupying a child restraint seat, Pediatrics 82(1):117-121, 1988.

Paulson, J.A.: Seat restraint contamination and cleaning, Pediatrics 78(1):113-114, 1986.

Ros, S.P.: Lawn mower injuries in children, Int. Pediatr. 4:59-60, 1989.

Tay, J.S., and Garland, J.S.: Serious head injuries from lawn darts, Pediatrics 79(2);261-263, 1987.

Tong, T.: Falls from pickup trucks during childhood, Am. J. Dis. Child. 143:997-998, 1989.

Tron, V.A., Baldwin, V.J., and Pirie, G.E.: Hot tub drownings, Pediatrics 75:789-790, 1985.

Wilson, M.: Injury prevention: protecting the under-6 set, Contemp. Pediatr. 5(5):19-34, 1988.

CHAPTER 15

Health Promotion of the Preschooler and Family

RELATED TOPICS*

Alternate child care arrangements, Ch. 12
Communication impairment, Ch. 25
Drawing, p. 197
Goodenough Draw-a-Person Test, Ch. 7
Limit-setting and discipline, Ch. 14
School phobia, Ch. 18
Sibling rivalry, Ch. 14
Television, Ch. 4
Working mothers, Ch. 3

GLOSSARY*

associative play Group play of similar or identical activities but without rigid rules

magical thinking Belief that thoughts are powerful and cause events

preschooler Child ages 3 to 5 years

The preschool years, a period from 3 to 5 years of age, comprise the end of early childhood. This is an age of discovery, inventiveness, curiosity, and developing sociocultural patterns of behavior. In some ways it is a time of ease and comfort for parents, particularly when many of the childrearing tasks, such as toileting, independence, and self-care have been mastered.

The years from birth until the child enters school are considered the most critical period for emotional and psychologic development. It is also the time of greatest parental influence on the formation of the child. Once children enter school, their environment widens beyond the home. School becomes a major contributing factor, and peers, teachers, and other authority figures, as well as selected "idols" from the mass media, greatly influence their thinking and behavior. Helping families realize and understand the pliability and malleability of young children as early as possible is an important nursing responsibility.

*See also Related Topics and Glossary in Chapter 14.

PROMOTING OPTIMUM GROWTH AND DEVELOPMENT

The combined biologic, psychosocial, cognitive, spiritual, and social achievements of children in this age-group prepare preschoolers for their most significant change in lifestyle—entrance into school. Their control of bodily systems, experience of brief and prolonged periods of separation, ability to interact cooperatively with other children and adults, use of language for mental symbolization, and increased attention span and memory ready them for the next major period—the school years. Successful achievement of previous levels of growth and development is essential for preschoolers to refine many of the tasks that were mastered during the toddler years.

BIOLOGIC DEVELOPMENT

The rate of physical growth slows and stabilizes during the preschool years. Average weight gain remains about 2.3 kg (5 pounds) per year. The average weight at 3 years is 14.6 kg (32 pounds), at 4 years 16.7 kg (36.75 pounds), and at 5 years 18.7 kg (41.25 pounds).

Growth in height also remains steady at a yearly increase of 6.75 to 7.5 cm (2.5 to 3 inches) and generally occurs in elongation of the legs rather than of the trunk. The average height at 3 years is 95 cm (37.25 inches), at 4 years 103 cm (40.5 inches), and at 5 years 110 cm (43.25 inches).

Physical proportions no longer resemble those of the squat, potbellied toddler. The preschooler is slender but sturdy, graceful, agile, and posturally erect. There is little difference in physical characteristics according to sex, except as dictated by such factors as dress and hairstyle.

Most bodily systems are mature and stable and can adjust to moderate stress and change. Motor development consists for the most part of increases in strength and refinement of previously learned skills, such as walking, running, and jumping. However, muscle development and bone growth are still far from mature. Excessive activity and overexertion can injure delicate tissues. Properly fitted shoes, good posture, appropriate exercise, and adequate rest are essential for optimum development of the musculoskeletal system.

Gross and Fine Motor Behavior

Walking, running, climbing, and jumping are well-established by 36 months. Refinement in eye-hand and muscle coordination is evident in several areas. At age 3 the preschooler rides a tricycle, walks on tiptoe, balances on one foot for a few seconds, and broad jumps. By age 4 the child skips and hops proficiently on one foot (Fig. 15-1) and catches a ball reliably. By age 5, the child skips on alternate feet, jumps rope, and begins to skate and swim.

Drawing. Drawing shows several advancements in perception of shape and development of fine muscle coordination. The 3-year-old child copies a circle and imitates a cross and vertical and horizontal lines. The writing instrument is held with the fingers rather than in the fist. The child scribbles or scrawls but names what has been drawn. The 3-year-old is not able to draw a complete stick figure but draws a round circle, later adds facial features, and by age 5 or 6 can draw several parts (head, arms, legs, body, and facial features). Between 4 and 5 years the child can trace a cross and copy a square. The triangle and diamond are usually the last geometric figures to be mastered, sometime between 5 and 6 years.

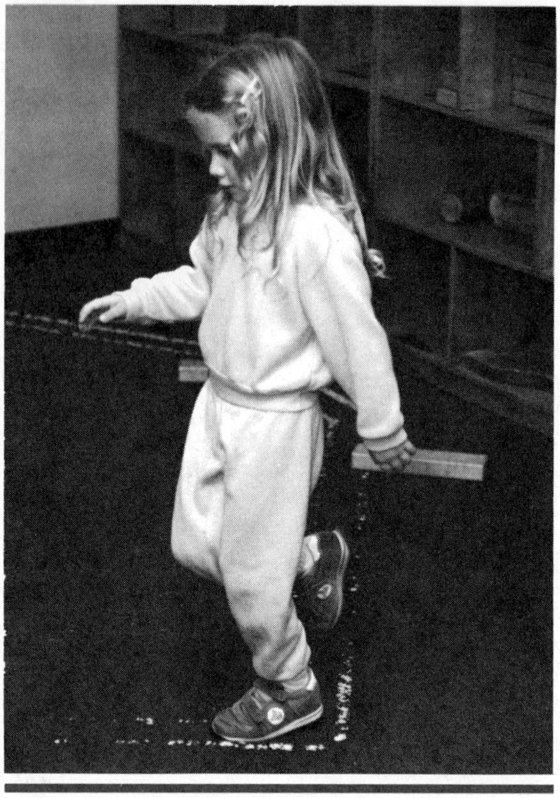

Fig. 15-1. A 4-year-old child has sufficient balance to walk or hop on one foot.

Children's drawings have been studied extensively. As children progress from scribbling to picture making, they advance through four distinguishable stages (Kellogg, 1969). In the *placement stage* 15-month-old children place their very earliest spontaneous scribblings on the paper in a specific placement pattern, such as in the center, all over, across the lower half, or across the page in a diagonal direction (Fig. 15-2). Approximately 17 different placement patterns appear by age 2 years and once developed are never lost.

By 3 years of age, children are in the *shape stage.* They draw single-line outline forms, such as rectangles, circles, ovals, crosses, and other odd shapes. As soon as they draw diagrams, they almost immediately progress to the *design stage,* in which simple forms are drawn together to make structured designs. When two diagrams are united, the resulting design is called a *combine.* Three or more united diagrams produce an *aggregate.* Between the ages of 4 and 5 most children enter the *pictorial stage,* in which their designs are recognizable as familiar objects. Early pictorial

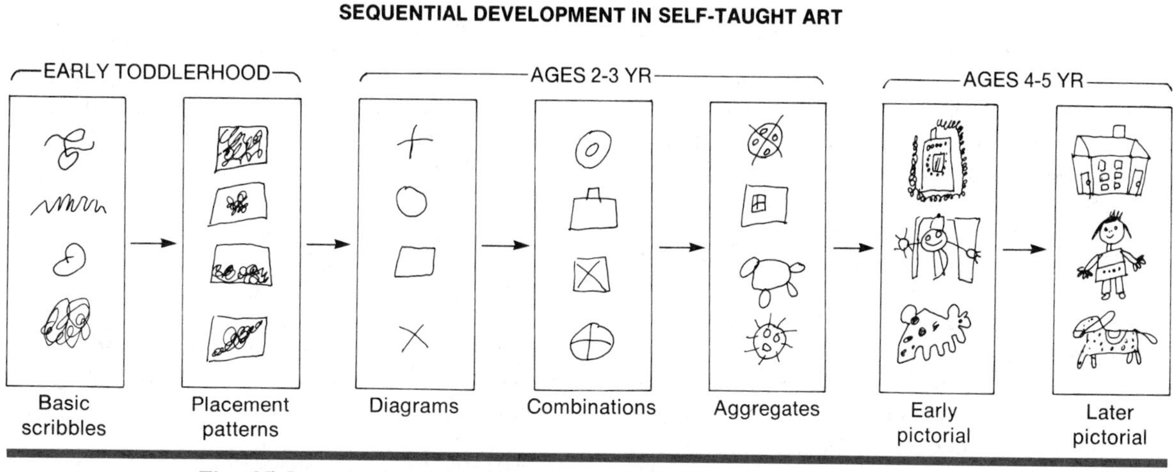

Fig. 15-2. Sequential development in self-taught art.
From Kellogg, R.: Understanding children's art. In Readings in Psychology Today, Del Mar, CA, 1969, Communications/Research/Machines/Inc.

drawings are suggestive of such things as human figures, houses, animals, and trees. Later pictorial drawings are more clearly defined and recognizable; they are not representations of the actual object but esthetically satisfying structures that *resemble* familiar objects. For example, the initial human figure drawing is a circle with arms attached to the head. It is more an aggregate drawing than any attempt to copy a human figure. Drawings of animals follow the human figure drawing but are only a slight modification, such as attaching ears to the top of the head.

Children's drawings before age 6 are strikingly similar universally, suggesting that some inherent neurologic mechanisms influence the type of self-taught art forms. After age 6 environmental influence, particularly from parents and teachers, shapes much of what children draw. Kellogg suggests that uninhibited scribbling and drawing are necessary for children to learn to read, and that children who have been free to experiment and produce abstract forms have developed the mental set required for learning symbolic language. Scribbling and drawing also help develop the fine muscle skills and eye-hand coordination eventually required for making precise letters and numbers.

Drawing is also a tool used for assessing intelligence, personality development, and psychosocial adjustment. The precise value of using drawing to measure such concepts is still an inexact science. However, children do reveal thoughts about themselves in their drawings, especially school-age children. It is generally not necessary to have in-depth knowledge of children's drawings to make assumptions about their significance. Being receptive to all the clues, both verbal and nonverbal, is essential to understand how and what children are communicating to others.

PSYCHOSOCIAL DEVELOPMENT

By the time children reach 3 years of age their gross and fine motor abilities are sufficiently developed to enable them to pursue almost limitless activities. If they have been allowed to express their independence and negativism constructively, they are ready to direct their energy toward new learning. They learn how to interact and relate to other children and adults; they learn appropriate sex-role functions and socially acceptable behavior; they learn right and wrong and the types of reward or punishment associated with each. However, learning does not necessarily imply success. Without guidance and reinforcement, children can learn unacceptable behavior and instead of feeling accomplishment will feel inadequacy, guilt, and inferiority.

Developing a Sense of Initiative (Erikson)

If preschoolers have mastered the tasks of the toddler period, they are ready to face the developmental endeavors of this stage. Erikson maintains that the chief psychosocial task of the preschool period is acquiring a sense of initiative. Children are in a stage of energetic learning. They play, work, and live to the fullest and feel a real sense of accomplishment and satisfaction in their activities. Conflict arises when children overstep the limits of their ability and inquiry and experience a sense of *guilt* for not having behaved or acted appropriately. Feelings of guilt, anxiety, and fear may also result from thoughts that differ from expected behavior.

A particularly stressful thought is wishing one's parent dead. As a sense of rivalry or competition develops between the same-sex child and parent, the child may think of ways to get rid of the interfering parent. In most situations this contest is resolved when the child strongly identifies with the same-sex parent and peers during the school years. However, if that same-sex parent dies before the identification process is completed, the preschooler can be overwhelmed with feelings of guilt for having wished and therefore causing (he thinks) the death. Clarifying for children that wishes cannot and do not make events occur is essential in helping them overcome their guilt and anxiety.

Development of the *superego,* or *conscience,* starts toward the end of the toddler years and is a major task for preschoolers. Learning right from wrong and good from bad is the beginning of morality. Children in this age-group are generally unable to understand the reasons why something is acceptable or unacceptable. They are aware of appropriate behavior primarily through punishment or reward and rely almost completely on parental principles for developing their own moral judgment. However, verbal enforcement of limits is much more effective. For example, in order to prevent injuries, parents need to supervise toddlers, keep them fenced in, and tell them not to run into the street. The preschooler is much more aware of danger and can be relied on to listen and obey in most instances. If allowed to disagree and question, they will develop socially acceptable behavior and independence in thought and action.

Developing a conscience implies learning the *sociocultural mores* of the family's heritage. Depending on the type of attitudes conveyed, children will learn not only appropriate behaviors but also tolerant, biased, or prejudiced values concerning their ethnic, religious, and social background and those of other groups. Much of this influence may remain dormant until they associate with children or adults of a different heritage. Then, depending on the particular group, they may be accepted or ostracized for their attitudes.

Oedipal Stage (Freud)

As soon as children comprehend their separateness as persons, they begin to realize that there are categories of objects, such as things, people, males, females, children, and adults. One of the principal goals in further differentiation of oneself from others is learning sex differences and sexually appropriate behavior.

Freud has long recognized this task by describing the period as the *oedipal,* or *phallic* stage. Conflict arises when the male child realizes that his father is much stronger and more powerful than he. Subconsciously he wishes that his father were dead. Concurrently he has noticed physical sexual differences, in specific that boys have a penis but that girls do not. In his mind he surmises that girls have lost their penis for some wrongdoing. His guilt regarding his feelings toward his father makes him fear the same punishment of mutilation, resulting in the *castration complex.*

Girls have similar wishes to marry their father and kill their mother, a phenomenon sometimes called the *Electra complex.* However, females do not fear castration because they have no penis to be removed; rather they experience *penis envy* (desire to have a penis). Freud has developed the female role in the phallic stage less fully than the male's role.

The resolution of the Oedipus or Electra complex is identification with the same-sex parent. *Sex typing,* or the process by which an individual develops the behavior, personality, attitudes, and beliefs that are appropriate for his or her culture and sex, occurs through several mechanisms during this period. Probably the most powerful are childrearing practices and imitation. The ways in which parents dress, hold, cuddle, caress, discipline, and talk to their child all express some aspect of sexually oriented behavior. Studies increasingly demonstrate that gender identification is not solely biologic or genetic but primarily a result of complex postnatal psychologic factors and that most children are aware of their sex and the expected set of related behaviors by 1½ to 2½ years of age. Although toddlers might be aware of their particular sex, they do not possess the language and cognitive skills to investigate sexual identity as fully as preschoolers.

COGNITIVE DEVELOPMENT

One of the tasks related to the preschool period is readiness for school and scholastic learning. Many of the thought processes of this period are crucial for achieving such readiness, and it is intentional that the child begins school when 5 to 6 years old rather than at an earlier age.

Preoperational Phase (Piaget)

Piaget's cognitive theory actually does not include a period specifically for children 3 to 5 years old. The preoperational phase comprises the age span from 2 to 7 years and is divided into two stages, the *preconceptual phase,* ages 2 to 4, and the phase of *intuitive thought,* ages 4 to 7.

One of the main transitions during these two phases is the shift from totally egocentric thought to social awareness and the ability to consider other viewpoints. This transition is very closely associated with the development of the superego. Children are able to think and verbalize their mental processes without having to act out their thinking. However, they can only think of one idea at a time, a concept known as *centration.* They are unable to think of all parts in terms of the whole. Outside influences or perceptions direct their understanding of a visual concept.

The concept of *conservation,* or the idea that a mass can be changed in size, shape, volume, or length without losing or adding to the original mass, is not understood by prelogical children (below age 7 years). Preschoolers judge what they see by the immediate perceptual clues given them. For example, if two lines of equal length are presented in such a way that one appears longer than the other, children will state that one line is longer, even if they measure both lines with a ruler or yardstick and find that each has the same length. Children therefore judge experiences by outside appearances and results, not by intrinsic, logical indicators.

Understanding this prelogical thinking in young children can help nurses interact with them in an effective manner. One example of how the manipulation of matter according to the child's understanding can facilitate the performance of an activity concerns the administration of drugs. If the child is to receive 5 ml of liquid medication, it is advisable to give it in a small medicine cup rather than a large cup, since the child will imagine that the large vessel contains more liquid. Being unable to perceive the two dimensions of height and width simultaneously, the child will choose one dimension and measure the amount according to that standard. If the child refuses the medicine in the small cup, he or she may accept it once it is poured into a large cup because the liquid will appear less in a tall, wide container.

There are many everyday examples of how the young child's inability to understand conservation of matter influences his behavior. Probably one of the most common situations involves eating and the amount of food placed on a dish. If the same amount of food is placed on a small and a large plate, the child may state that the large plate contains more food and may feel overwhelmed by the apparently large quantity. Parents are usually "taught" this by their children and "learn" ways to use this thinking to encourage compliance. Meat that is cut thin and flat appears to be larger in quantity than the same amount of meat that is cut thick, and the child will generally consume more of the thicker portion. The opposite also has its advantages. Giving a child a large, flat cookie may be more satisfying than a small, thick one.

Children develop logical thought processes and understanding of conservation of numbers, substance, and length during the school-age years (see Chapter 17). It is no accident that learning subjects such as mathematics or science is begun at age 6 and later. Although some younger children might comprehend the meaning, reversibility, and symbolization of numbers, most do not until age 6 or 7.

Language continues to develop during the preschool period. Speech remains primarily a vehicle of egocentric communication. Preschoolers assume that everyone thinks as they do and that a brief explanation of their thinking makes them understood by others. Because of this self-referenced, egocentric verbal communication, it is frequently necessary to explore and understand young children's thinking through other, nonverbal approaches. For children in this age-group, the most enlightening and effective method is *play*. Play becomes the child's work of understanding, adjusting to, and working out life's experiences. Because of children's rich imagination and unlimited ability to invent and imitate, all kinds of play hold therapeutic and communicative value. At this age children's egocentricity dominates their interactions. Expressions about others, such as a doll, puppet, truck, and dog, are actually descriptions of themselves. To know what children are really thinking demands skill, time, and patience of those willing to learn to look beyond the words and into the hearts and minds of children.

Preschoolers afford adults, particularly parents, teachers, and nurses, the richest opportunity for comprehending the uniqueness, innocence, and genuineness of children. Children's conversation with their toys can tell more in a few minutes than many long hours of conversation between two adults, which is illustrated in the following example:

> Five-year-old Ann is playing mommy and has her family of dolls nearby. She is "talking" on her telephone, exclaiming to her doll children, "Be quiet! Can't you see that I am busy? This is an important business call. Go away and play somewhere else." She hangs up the phone and becomes the little girl at whom she had just yelled. She pretends she is crying and says, "I always do bad things. I wish Mommy wouldn't yell at me all the time."
>
> Ann's mother has overheard this play conversation and is acutely aware of the similarity between the play session and real-life experiences in the home. She had never before realized how the child must have felt when she was preoccupied with other business. She had always been irritated by her daughter's inconsiderateness. As she analyzed the example more closely, she realized that this was happening a few times a day and that, with her working part-time, she never really gave the child her undivided attention. She planned to set aside 1 hour every morning before leaving for work to play or read to Ann and to confine her business telephone calls to the evening when Ann's father was home.

This mother was perceptive to clues regarding the child's feelings. However, not all parents are as aware and frequently negate what they hear, believing it to be unimportant or irrelevant. To understand children is to listen to their spoken and nonspoken language. Communicating messages to them may also necessitate using their methods, such as play, imitation, and role-playing. Unlike toddlers who respond less favorably to anticipatory explanation or preparation for a potentially frightening experience, preschoolers have the ability to comprehend simple explanations, can enjoy preparation such as seeing or playing with equipment, and can relate how they feel and think by using puppets or dolls.

Preschoolers increasingly use language without comprehending the meaning of words, particularly concepts such as time. Time is best explained in relation to an event, such as "Your mother will visit you after you finish your lunch." Avoiding terms such as *yesterday, tomorrow, next week,* and *Tuesday* to express when an event is expected to occur and associating time with usual expected daily occurrences help children learn about temporal relationships and increase their trust in others' predictions. Children are usually not able to tell time on a clock until 7 or 8 years of age.

Age is another concept that is judged by one set of criteria, such as size or physical appearance. A 5-year-old child's question, "Was the baby just born?" illustrates that the small 10-month-old infant could be a newborn to the preschooler. Children gradually develop the ability to judge age based on multiple factors other than size when they are approximately 8 years old.

Preschoolers' thinking is often described as *magical*. Because of their egocentrism and transductive reasoning (association of one event with a simultaneous event), they believe that thoughts are all-powerful. Such thinking places them in the vulnerable position of feeling guilty and responsible for bad thoughts, which may coincide with the occurrence of a wished event. A typical example is wishing a new sibling dead. If that sibling does die, young children think their wish caused the death. Their inability to logically reason the cause and effect of illness or an accident makes it especially difficult for them to understand such events.

Preschoolers believe in the power of words and accept their meaning literally. A significant example of this type of thinking is calling children "bad" because they did something wrong. In their minds telling children that they are bad means that they are bad. For this reason it is better to relate such words to the act by saying, for example, "That was a bad thing to do."

MORAL DEVELOPMENT

Moral development continues to advance and is influenced by the cognitive processes typical of the preschool years. Although many theorists incorporate moral development within their theoretic framework, one of the more prominent theorists whose work deals primarily with moral development is Lawrence Kohlberg.

Preconventional or Premoral Level (Kohlberg)

Moral issues are based on preschoolers' egocentric, limited, and cognitively biased considerations. Three-year-old children continue to behave according to the punishment-obedience orientation typical of toddlers. From approximately 4 to 7 years of age children are in the stage of *naive instrumental orientation,* in which actions are directed toward satisfying their needs and less frequently the needs of others. There is a very concrete sense of justice. Reciprocity or fairness involves the philosophy of "You scratch my back and I'll scratch yours," with no thought of loyalty or gratitude (Thomas, 1985).

SPIRITUAL DEVELOPMENT

Children's knowledge of faith and religion is learned from significant others in their environment, usually from the parents and their religious practices. However, young children's understanding of spirituality is influenced by their cognitive level. Preschoolers have a concrete conception of a God with physical characteristics who is often like an imaginary friend. They understand simple Bible stories and memorize short prayers, but their understanding of the meaning of these rituals is limited. They benefit from concrete representations of religious practices, such as picture Bible books, and small statues, such as those of the Nativity scene (Shelley and others, 1982).

Development of the conscience is strongly linked to spiritual development. At this age children are learning right from wrong and behave correctly to avoid punishment. Wrongdoing provokes feelings of guilt, and preschoolers often misinterpret illness as a punishment for real or imagined transgressions. It is important that children view God as one who bestows unconditional love, rather than as a judge of good or bad behavior. Praying to God and observing religious traditions, for example, prayers before meals or bedtime, can help children through stressful periods, such as hospitalization.

DEVELOPMENT OF BODY IMAGE

The preschool years play a significant role in the development of body image. With increasing comprehension of language, preschoolers recognize that individuals have undesirable and desirable appearances. They recognize differences in skin color and racial identity and are vulnerable to learning prejudices and biases. They are aware of the meaning of words, such as *pretty* or *ugly,* and reflect the opinions of others regarding their own appearance. By 5 years of age children compare their size to their peers' and can become conscious of being large or short, especially if others refer to them as "so big" or "so little" for their age.

Despite the advances in body image development, preschoolers have poorly defined body boundaries and little knowledge of their internal anatomy. Intrusive experiences are frightening, especially those that disrupt the integrity of the skin, such as injections and surgery. There is a fear that if the skin is "broken" all their blood and "insides" can leak out. Therefore, bandages are critical to "keeping everything from coming out."

DEVELOPMENT OF SEXUALITY

Sexual development during these years is a very important phase to a person's overall sexual identity and beliefs. Preschoolers are forming strong attachments to the opposite sex parent while identifying with the same sex parent.

Sexual identity is developing beyond gender recognition, and modesty may become a concern, as well as fears of mutilation. There is sex-role imitation, and "dressing up" like Mommy or Daddy is an important activity. Attitudes and responses of others to role-playing can condition the child to views of self or others. For example, comments such as "Boys shouldn't play with dolls" can influence a boy's self-concept of masculinity. This may be a time when children begin forming ideal images of how they would want to look as adults (Selekman, 1983).

Sexual exploration may be more pronounced now than ever before, particularly in terms of exploring and manipulating the genitals. Questions about sexual reproduction may come to the forefront in the preschooler's search for understanding (see Sex Education, p. 692).

SOCIAL DEVELOPMENT

Dramatic advancements in social development occur during the preschool period. The individuation-separation process is complete. Language allows for greater communication of needs and feelings, and personal-social skills are improving to the point of almost complete independence.

Individuation-Separation

Preschoolers have relinquished much of the anxiety with strangers and the fear of separation of earlier years. They relate to unfamiliar people easily and tolerate brief separations from parents with little or no protest. However, they still need parental security, reassurance, guidance, and approval, especially when entering nursery school or elementary school. Prolonged separation, such as that imposed by illness and hospitalization, is difficult, but preschoolers respond very well to anticipatory preparation and concrete explanation. They can cope with changes in daily routine much better than toddlers; however, they may develop more imaginary fears. They gain security and comfort from familiar objects, such as toys, dolls, or photographs of family members. They are able to work through many of their unresolved fears, fantasies, and anxieties through play, especially if guided with appropriate play objects, for example, dolls or puppets, that represent family members, medical and nursing staff, and other children.

Language

Language during the preschool years is quite sophisticated and complex. It also becomes a major mode of communication and social interaction. Vocabulary increases dramatically, from 300 words at age 2 to over 2100 words at the end of 5 years. Sentence structure, grammatical usage, and intelligibility also advance to a more adult level (Lowrey, 1986).

Children between the ages of 3 and 4 form sentences of about three to four words and include only the most essential words to convey a meaning. Such speech is often termed *telegraphic* for its brevity in length. Three-year-old children ask many questions and use plurals, correct pronouns, and the past tense of verbs. They name familiar objects, such as animals, parts of the body, relatives, and friends. They can give and follow simple commands. They talk incessantly, regardless of whether anyone is listening or answering them. They enjoy musical or talking toys or dolls and imitate new words proficiently.

From ages 4 to 5 preschoolers use longer sentences of four to five words and use more words to convey a message, such as prepositions, adjectives, and a variety of verbs. They follow simple directional commands, such as "Put the ball on the chair," but can carry out only one request at a time. They answer questions, such as "What do you do when you are hungry?" by describing the appropriate action. The pattern of asking questions is at its peak, and children usually repeat the question until they receive an answer.

By the end of age 5 children use all parts of speech correctly, except for deviations from the rule. They can define simple words by describing their use, shape, or general category of classification, not only by stating their outward appearance. For example, they define a ball as "round, something you bounce, or a toy," rather than by its color. They can give some opposites, such as "If Mommy is a woman, Daddy is a man." By the time they are 6 years old, they can describe an object according to its composition, such as "A spoon is made of metal."

Personal-Social Behavior

The pervasive ritualism and negativism of toddlerhood gradually diminish during the preschool years. Although self-assertion is still a major theme, preschoolers demonstrate their sense of autonomy differently. They are able to verbalize their request for independence and perform independently because of their much refined physical and cognitive development. They fully care for themselves by 4 or 5 years of age, needing little if any assistance with dressing, eating, or toileting (Fig. 15-3). They can also be trusted to obey warnings of danger, although 3- or 4-year-old children may exceed their boundaries at times.

They are also much more sociable and willing to please. They have internalized many of the standards and values of the family, and their conscience dictates many of their actions. By the end of early childhood they begin to question parental values and compare them to those of their peer group and other authority figures; as a result, they may be less willing to abide by the family's code of conduct. Preschoolers become increasingly aware of their position and role within the family. Although this is a more secure age for experiencing the addition of another sibling, relinquishing the position of first or youngest is still difficult and requires appropriate preparation (see Sibling Rivalry, Chapter 14).

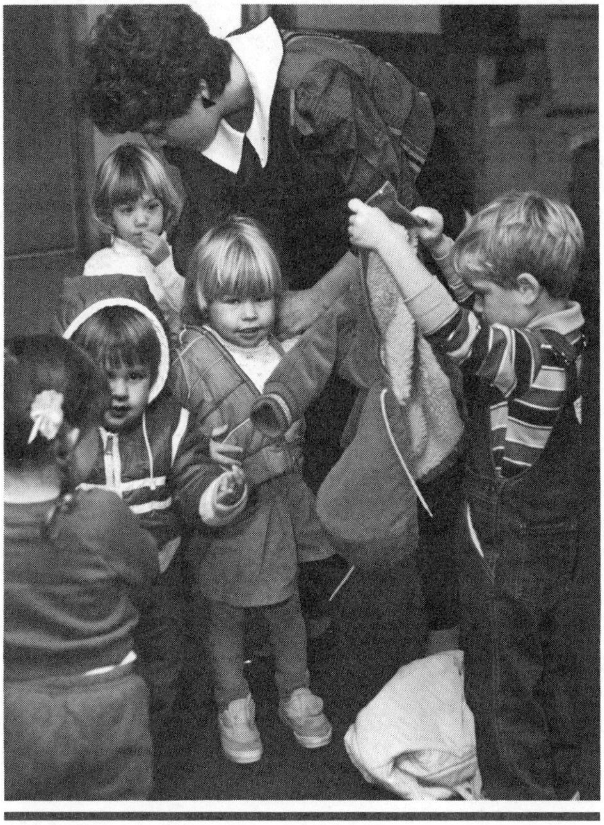

Fig. 15-3. Most preschoolers are able to dress themselves, needing help only for more difficult items of clothing.

Play

Various types of play are typical of this period, but preschoolers especially enjoy both parallel and associative play—group play in similar or identical activities but without rigid organization or rules. Play should provide for physical, social, and mental development (Table 15-1).

Play activities for physical growth and refinement of motor skills include jumping, running, and climbing. Tricycles, trucks, wagons, gym and sports equipment, sandboxes, wading pools, and winter sleds can help develop muscles and coordination. Activities such as swimming, ice skating, and skiing teach safety as well as muscle development and coordination.

Manipulative, constructive, creative, and educational toys provide for quiet activities, fine motor development, and self-expression. Easy construction sets, large blocks of various sizes and shapes, a counting frame, alphabet or number flash cards, paints, crayons, simple carpentry tools, musical toys, illustrated books, simple sewing or handicraft sets, large puzzles, and clay are suitable toys. Electronic games and educational computer programs are especially valuable in helping children learn basic skills, such as letters and simple words. Although their attention span is still short, preschoolers are beginning to enjoy crafts, especially

Table 15-1 Play during preschool years

PHYSICAL DEVELOPMENT	SOCIAL DEVELOPMENT	MENTAL DEVELOPMENT AND CREATIVITY
▪ Suggested activities		
Provide space for the child to run, jump, and climb	Encourage interaction with neighborhood children	Encourage creative efforts with raw materials
Teach child to swim	Intervene when children become destructive	Read stories
Teach simple sports and activities	Enroll child in nursery school	Monitor television viewing
		Attend theater and other cultural events appropriate to child's age
		Take short excursions to park, seashore, museums
▪ Suggested toys		
Seesaw	Sailboat	Books
Medium-height slide	Cash register, toy typewriter	Jigsaw puzzles
Adjustable swing	Child-size playhouse	Musical toys (xylophone, toy piano, drum, horns)
Vehicles to ride	Dolls, stuffed toys	Picture games
Tricycle	Dishes, table	Blunt scissors, paper, paste
Wading pool	Ironing board and iron	Newsprint, crayons, poster paint, large brushes, easel, finger paint
Wheelbarrow	Trucks, cars, trains, airplanes	Musical and rhythmic toys
Sled	Play clothes for dress-up	Flannel board and pieces of felt in colors and shapes
Wagon	Doll carriage, bed, high chair	Pregummed geometric shapes (colored)
Roller skates, speed-graded to skill	Doctor and nurse kits	Records, tapes
	Nails, hammer, saw	Blackboard and chalk (colored and white)
	Grooming aids, makeup or shaving kits	Wooden and plastic construction sets
		Magnifying glass, magnet

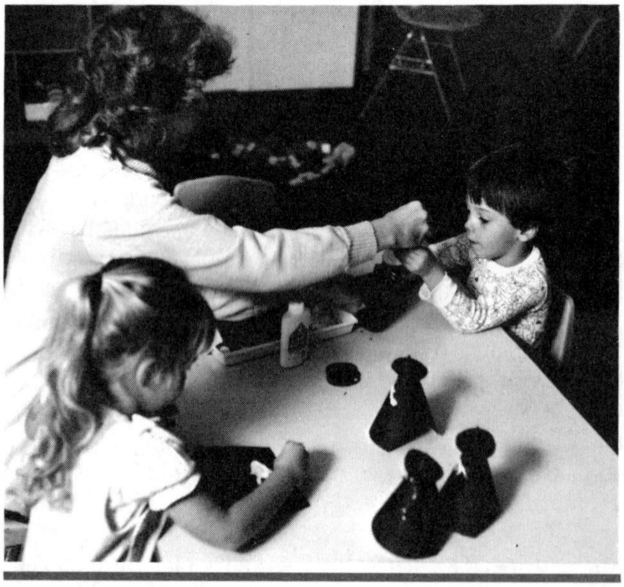

Fig. 15-4. Preschoolers are beginning to enjoy creative activities and appreciate the attention and assistance of adults.

with the guidance and assistance of adults (Fig. 15-4). A helpful rule in planning creative activities is one simple project per year of age. For example, 3-year-old children usually have the patience to decorate three eggs, but become bored and restless with more.

Probably the most characteristic and pervasive preschooler activity is *imitative, imaginative,* and *dramatic play.* Dress-up clothes, dolls, housekeeping toys, dollhouses, play-store toys, telephones, farm animals and equipment, village sets, trains, trucks, cars, planes, hand puppets, and doctor and nurse kits provide hours of self-expression. Probably at no other time is the reproduction of the behavior of significant adults so faithful and absorbing as in 4- and 5-year-old children. Toward the end of the preschool period, children are less satisfied with make-believe or pretend objects and enjoy actually doing the activity, such as cooking and carpentry.

Television and video also have their places in children's play, although each should only be one part of children's total repertoire of social and recreational activities. Parents are encouraged to supervise selection of programs, preview programs for appropriateness, and schedule hours for television viewing. Children enjoy and learn from educational children's programs, which are purposely shown before dinner or after meals to provide a quiet activity. Television can become an interactive activity when parents view programs with children and discuss program content (see Television, Chapter 4).

Imaginary playmates. Play is so much a part of the young child's life that reality and fantasy become blurred. The make-believe is reality during play and only becomes fantasy when the toys are put away or the dress-up clothes are removed. It is no wonder that imaginary playmates are so much a part of this age period. The appearance of imaginary companions usually occurs between the ages of 2½ and 3 years, and for the most part such playmates are relinquished when the child enters school. There seems to be a relationship between the level of intelligence and the presence of the imaginary companion. The more intelligent children tend to have the most vivid and complex pretend playmates (Fish and Burch, 1985).

Imaginary companions serve many purposes—they become friends in times of loneliness, they accomplish what the child is still attempting, and they experience what the child wants to forget or remember. It is not unusual for the "friend" to have a myriad of vices and to be blamed for wrongdoing. Sometimes the child hopes to escape punishment by saying, "My friend George broke the glass." At other times the preschooler may fantasize that the "companion" misbehaved, and the child plays the role of parent. This becomes a way of assuming control and authority in a safe situation.

Parents often worry about their child having imaginary playmates, not realizing how normal and useful they are. They need to be reassured that children's fantasy is a sign of health that helps them differentiate between make-believe and reality. Parents can acknowledge the presence of imaginary companions by calling them by name and even agreeing to simple requests such as setting an extra place at the table, but they should not allow the child to use the playmate to avoid punishment or responsibility. For example, if the child blames the companion for upsetting the room, the parents need to state clearly that the child is the only person they see and therefore the child is responsible for cleaning up.

TEMPERAMENT

Temperament influences children's social development and interactions. In Chapters 4, 12, and 14 the importance of temperament during early childhood has been discussed. Since temperamental characteristics tend to remain stable, the same considerations in terms of childrearing apply during the preschool years. One major concern in this age-group is the effect of temperament on adjustment in group situations, especially school, and the long-term consequences of temperamental characteristics. In particular the degree of adaptability to new situations, intensity of response, distractibility, amount of persistence, mood, and activity level may influence a child's chances for success in school (Schor, 1985). There is some evidence that preschoolers born at very low weights are more likely to have temperamental characteristics related to behavior problems and learning skills (Schraeder, Heverly, and Rappaport, 1990). Consequently, parents can benefit from suggestions that can promote preschoolers' adjustment. For example, children who are slow to warm up need gradual introduction to new situations and may benefit from the parent's presence until they have settled in. Children with high activity levels tend to adjust better to environments that allow freedom of movement, rather than a structured or regimented classroom. The more awareness parents have of their children's unique behaviors, the better able they are to inform teachers or other caregivers of the children's needs and successful approaches to handling the youngsters. The Behavioral Style Questionnaire can be used to identify temperamental characteristics in children who are in the age range of 3 to 7 years (McDevitt and Carey, 1978).

SUMMARY OF GROWTH AND DEVELOPMENT DURING THE PRESCHOOL YEARS

By the age of 3 the child has made tremendous strides from the dependency and callowness of infancy and the negativism and clumsiness of toddlerhood. The preschooler has excellent gross and fine motor control. He is a very social and domesticated being and cares for himself almost completely. Language use is a vehicle of communication, learning, and self-expression. These and other major developmental achievements for children 3, 4, and 5 years old are summarized in Table 15-2.

COPING WITH CONCERNS RELATED TO NORMAL GROWTH AND DEVELOPMENT

In many respects the preschool years present few childrearing problems. However, there are special situations during this period that require parental guidance. They include preschool or daycare experience, sex education, speech problems, and stress. In addition, parents may need counseling regarding children who exhibit signs of giftedness or aggressive behavior. The issue of divorce, which has a significant impact on preschoolers, is discussed in Chapter 3.

Preschool or Daycare Experience

During the preschool years many children attend some type of early childhood program, usually nursery school or a daycare center. Group care has become commonplace with the large number of mothers presently employed outside the home (see Alternate Child Care Arrangements, Chapter 12). The effects of early education and stimulation on children have increasingly gained recognition and importance, although recent concern has focused on programs that stress formal academics (Howes, 1989) (for a discussion of the effects of daycare on young children, see Working Mothers, Chapter 3). Since social development widens to include age-mates and other significant adults, preschool provides an excellent vehicle for expanding children's experiences with others.

In nursery school or daycare centers children are exposed to opportunities for learning group cooperation, adjusting to various sociocultural differences, and coping with frustration, dissatisfaction, and anger. If activities are tailored to provide mastery and achievement, children increasingly feel success, self-confidence, and personal competence. Whether or not structured learning is imposed is less important than the social climate, type of guidance, and attitude toward the children that is fostered by the teacher or leader. With a teacher who is aware of preschoolers' developmental abilities and needs, the children will learn from any activity that is provided. Most nursery schools incorpo-

Table 15-2 Growth and development during preschool years

AGE (YEARS)	PHYSICAL	GROSS MOTOR	FINE MOTOR	LANGUAGE
3	Usual weight gain of 1.8 to 2.7 kg (4 to 6 pounds) Usual gain in height of 7.5 cm (3 inches) May have achieved night-time control of bowel and bladder	Rides tricycle Jumps off bottom step Stands on one foot for a few seconds Goes up stairs using alternate feet, may still come down using both feet on the step Broad jumps May try to dance, but balance may not be adequate	Builds tower of nine or ten cubes Builds bridge with three cubes Adeptly places small pellets in narrow-necked bottle In drawing, copies a circle, imitates a cross, names what he has drawn, cannot draw stickman but may make circle with facial features	Has vocabulary of about 900 words Uses primarily "telegraphic" speech Uses complete sentences of three to four words Talks incessantly, regardless of whether anyone is paying attention Repeats sentence of six syllables Constantly asks questions
4	Pulse and respiration decrease slightly Growth rate is similar to that of previous year Length at birth is doubled Maximum potential for development of amblyopia	Skips and hops on one foot Catches ball reliably Throws ball overhand Walks down stairs using alternate footing	Imitates a gate with cubes Uses scissors successfully to cut out picture following outline Can lace shoes, but may not be able to tie bow In drawing, copies a square, traces a cross and diamond, adds three parts to stick figure	Has vocabulary of 1500 words or more Uses sentences of four to five words Questioning is at peak Tell exaggerated stories Knows simple songs May be mildly profane if associates with older children Obeys four prepositional phrases, such as "under," "on top of," "beside," "in back of," or "in front of" Names one or more colors Comprehends analogies, such as, "If ice is cold, fire is ______" Repeats four digits Uses words liberally but frequently does not comprehend meaning
5	Pulse and respiration decrease slightly Eruption of permanent dentition may begin, especially if deciduous tooth eruption was early (before age 6 months) First permanent teeth to erupt are four molars, which come in behind the last temporary teeth (often mistaken for temporary molars)	Skips and hops on alternate feet Throws and catches ball well Jumps rope Skates with good balance Walks backward with heel to toe Jumps from height of 12 inches, lands on toes Balances on alternate feet with eyes closed	Ties shoelaces Uses scissors, simple tools, or pencil very well In drawing, copies a diamond and triangle; adds seven to nine parts to stickman; prints a few letters, numbers, or words, such as first name	Has vocabulary of about 2100 words Uses sentences of six to eight words, with all parts of speech Names coins (nickel, dime, and so on) Names four or more colors Describes drawing or pictures with much comment and enumeration Asks meaning of words Asks inquisitive questions

SOCIALIZATION	COGNITION	FAMILY RELATIONSHIPS
Dresses self almost completely if helped with back buttons and told which shoe is right or left Buttons and unbuttons accessible buttons Pulls on shoes Has increased attention span Feeds self completely Pours from a bottle or pitcher Can prepare simple meals, such as cold cereal and milk Can help to set table, dry dishes without breaking any Likes to "help" entertain by passing around food May have fears, especially of dark and going to bed Knows own sex and appropriate sex of others Play is parallel and associative Begins to learn simple games and meaning of rules, but follows them according to self-interpretation Speaks to doll, animal, truck, and so on Begins to work out social interaction through play Able to share toys, although expresses idea of "mine" frequently	Is in preconceptual phase Is egocentric in thought and behavior Has beginning understanding of time; uses many time-oriented expressions, talks about past and future as much as about present, pretends to tell time Has improved concept of space as demonstrated in understanding of prepositions and ability to follow directional command Has beginning ability to view concepts from another perspective	Attempts to please parents and conform to their expectations Is less jealous of younger sibling; may be opportune time for birth of additional sibling Is aware of family relationships and sex role functions Boys tend to identify more with father or other male figure Has increased ability to separate easily and comfortably from parents for short periods
Very independent Tends to be selfish and impatient Aggressive physically as well as verbally Takes pride in accomplishments Has mood swings Boasts and tattles Shows off dramatically, enjoys entertaining others Tells family tales to others with no restraint Still has many fears Play is associative Imaginary playmates are common Uses dramatic, imaginative, and imitative devices Works through unresolved conflicts, such as jealousy toward sibling, anger toward parent, or unconquered fear in himself Sexual exploration and curiosity demonstrated through play, such as being "doctor" or "nurse"	Is in phase of intuitive thought Causality is still related to proximity of events Understands time better, especially in terms of sequence of daily events Is unable to conserve matter Judges everything according to one dimension, such as height, width, or first Immediate perceptual clues dominate judgment Can choose longer of two lines or heavier of two objects Is beginning to develop less egocentrism and more social awareness May count correctly but has poor mathematic concept of numbers Still believes that thoughts cause events Obeys because parents have set limits, not because of understanding of reason behind right or wrong	Rebels if parents expect too much, such as perfect table manners Takes aggression and frustration out on parents or siblings Do's and don'ts become important May have rivalry with older or younger siblings, may resent older's privileges and younger's invasion of privacy and possessions May run away from home Identifies strongly with parent of opposite sex Is able to run simple errands outside the home
Is less rebellious and quarrelsome than at age 4 years Is more settled and eager to get down to business Is not as open and accessible in thoughts and behavior as in earlier years Is independent but trustworthy, not foolhardy, more responsible Has fewer fears, relies on outer authority to control the world Is eager to do things right and to please; tries to "live by the rules"	Begins to question what parents think by comparing them to age-mates and other adults May notice prejudice and bias in outside world Is more able to view other's perspective, but tolerates differences rather than understands them Tends to be matter-of-fact about differences in others May begin to show understanding of conservation of numbers through counting objects regardless of arrangement	Gets along well with parents Does not try to run away from home May seek out parent more often than at age 4 years for reassurance and security, especially when entering school Is upset not to find parent, for example, when arriving home from school Tolerates siblings, but finds 3-year-old children a special nuisance Begins to question parents' thinking and principles Strongly identifies with parent of same sex, especially boys with their fathers

Continued.

Table 15-2 Growth and development during preschool years—cont'd

AGE (YEARS)	PHYSICAL	GROSS MOTOR	FINE MOTOR	LANGUAGE
5—cont'd	Handedness is established (about 90% are right-handed)			Can repeat sentence of ten syllables or more Knows names of days of week, months, and other time-associated words Defines words using action as well as description Knows composition of articles, such as, "A shoe is made of ________" Can follow three demands in succession

rate a similar daily schedule of quiet play, active outdoor activity, group activities such as games and projects, creative or free play, and snack and rest periods.

Nursery school is particularly beneficial for children who lack a peer-group experience, such as an only child, and for children from culturally deprived homes. Nursery school provides extensive stimulation for language, physical, and social development. It also is an excellent preparation for entrance into elementary school. For a child from a poor home, elementary school can be so overwhelming that all learning is impeded by the sensory overload. Regular school places many more demands on children for prolonged attention, self-disciplined behavior, and demonstrated progress in performance and achievement than the less-structured atmosphere of preschool. Nursery school and kindergarten are a transitional preparation for the demands of academic learning in later years.

Guiding parents in selecting a preschool program. A major nursing responsibility is guiding parents in locating suitable facilities with a well-qualified staff. State licensing agencies can help parents identify daycare centers that accept children of specific age-groups and are conveniently located to home and work. Their records are available to the public and provide reports from the health, safety, and fire departments, periodic evaluations from the licensing agency, complaints filed against the center, and qualifications of the center's employees. State-licensed programs are supposed to abide by established standards, which represent the *minimum* requirements and safeguards. However, enforcement of the standards is sometimes inadequate. Early childhood programs may also belong to a voluntary accreditation system, the National Academy of Early Childhood Programs, which serves as a model for *optimum* care.* References from other parents are also helpful, provided they have investigated the center carefully and have remained involved with the agency's activities.

Other areas for parents to evaluate are the center's daily program, teacher qualifications, student-to-staff ratio, discipline policy, environmental safety precautions, provision of meals, sanitary conditions, adequate indoor/outdoor space per child, and fee schedule. Although fees vary considerably, it should be kept in mind that a program that charges a minimum fee may also be providing minimum services. In terms of an overall evaluation there is *no substitute for a personal observation of the facility.* Parents should arrange to meet the director and some of the employees, especially those who would be caring for the child. Checklists are helpful to systematically evaluate the center and make comparisons with other facilities (Green, 1986; Wong, 1986).

*Information about the accreditation criteria and procedures of the National Academy of Early Childhood Programs is available from the **National Association for the Education of Young Children**, 1834 Connecticut Avenue, N.W., Washington, DC 20009; (800) 424-2460; (202) 232-8777. These criteria are excellent guidelines for evaluating nursery or daycare centers.

SOCIALIZATION	COGNITION	FAMILY RELATIONSHIPS
Acts "manly" or "womanly" Has fairly consistent and polished manners Cares for self totally, occasionally needing supervision in dress or hygiene May complain over minor injuries but tries to be brave for major pain Play is associative Likes rules and tries to follow them but may cheat to avoid losing Begins to notice group conformity and sense of belonging Is very industrious, tries to accomplish a goal, and feels pride and satisfaction, as well as unhappiness and discontent May demand to watch television more now that understands programs better Is not ready for concentrated close work or small print because of slight farsightedness and still unrefined eye-hand coordination Imitative play mimics the portrayed adult like a mirror image Wants to use real objects during play, such as actual ingredients to make cookies rather than sand or mud	Uses time-oriented words with increased understanding Is very curious about factual information regarding the world	Enjoys doing activities, such as sports, cooking, shopping, and so on, with parent of same sex

Several resources are also available to familiarize parents with characteristics of quality child care (see Suggested Readings, p. 703, and Hobbie, 1989).

One of the areas that is increasingly important in selecting child care centers is the agency's health practices. Substantial evidence shows that children, especially those under 3 years, in daycare centers have more illnesses, especially diarrhea, hepatitis A, meningitis, otitis media, respiratory tract infections, and cytomegalovirus, than children not in daycare centers (Haskins and Kotch, 1986; Wald and others, 1988). The strongest predictor of risk of illness is the number of children in the room (Bell and others, 1989).

Another concern is the frequency of injuries in daycare centers and daycare homes. One report of daycare homes found a high rate of safety hazards (Wasserman and others, 1989), and other reports indicate that injuries, especially falls on playgrounds, occur frequently in daycare centers (Lee and Bass, 1990; Sacks and others, 1989). What is less clear is whether these risks are greater than those in the child's own home; preliminary data suggest that the risk is not greater (Rivara and others, 1989).

Nurses play an important role in infection control and injury prevention. Not only can they advise parents regarding the evaluation of a center's sanitary and safety practices, but they can also take an active part in educating staff and children (Gillis and others, 1989). Measures to minimize infection transmission include handwashing of children and employees (Fig. 15-5); changing diapers as soon as they are soiled; properly disposing of diapers, preferably placing them in a plastic bag and discarding them in a closed container stored away from children; thoroughly cleaning the diaper-changing surface and accessory items that may become contaminated during a diaper change; never using di-

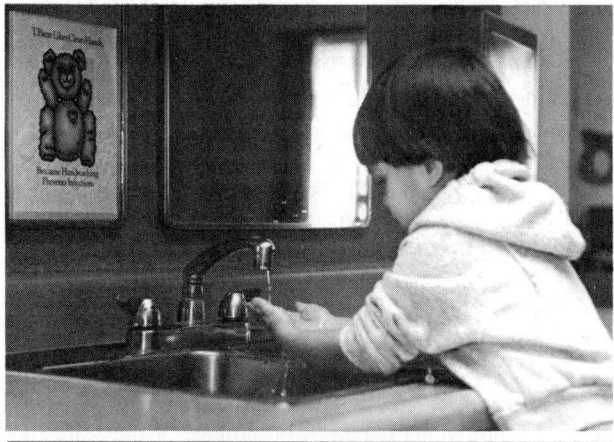

Fig. 15-5. Thorough handwashing is the single most effective method of preventing infection. Note the poster on the mirror; the T. Bear symbol is part of the national infection control campaign sponsored by U.S. Department of Health and Human Services.

aper-changing areas for food preparation; not permitting staff who care for children to prepare food; excluding children who are ill from school or caring for them in a separate area; and limiting the number of children in one room. In many areas special centers provide daycare for children while they are ill (Smith, Shillam, and Zimmerman, 1989). Injury prevention strategies are presented in Table 14-8 and Parent Guidelines: Child Safety Home Checklist, Chapter 12.

Preparing the child. Children need preparation for the preschool experience, whether it is a formal nursery school, organized daycare center, or family daycare home. The following suggestions are also appropriate for children entering kindergarten. For young children these programs represent a change from their usual home environment and prolonged separation from parents. Even if children have been cared for by a baby-sitter, preschool or daycare differs because the individualized attention is not as intense or sustained.

The nurse helps the parents assess the children's readiness in terms of age, physical ability, and social development. For example, a group experience may be difficult for young children with short attention spans. These children may require a different type of preschool experience that provides for more individualized attention.

Before children begin the school experience, the parents should present the idea as exciting and pleasurable. Talking to them about activities such as painting, building with blocks, or enjoying swings and other outdoor equipment allows the children to fantasize about the forthcoming event in a positive manner. When the day arrives to begin school, the parents should behave confidently. Such behavior requires the parents to have resolved their own feelings regarding the nursery or daycare experience.

Parents should introduce their child to the teacher and the school. In some instances it is helpful to remain for at least some part of the first day until the child is comfortable and at ease. If parents do stay, they should be available to the child but inconspicuous. Frequently a full-day routine is too overwhelming for a child and needs to be shortened to a morning or afternoon session. This is particularly important to remember for children beginning in a daycare center. Another action that can facilitate children's adjustment is providing the school with detailed information about the home environment, such as familiar routines, favorite activities, food preferences, names of siblings or pets, and personal habits. Such information helps the child feel familiar in the strange surroundings. When schools automatically request this information, the parent has a valuable clue to evaluating the quality of the program, since it represents the staff's awareness of each child's needs. Transitional objects, such as a favorite toy or blanket, may also help the child bridge the gap from home to school.

The nurse should also encourage parents to discuss their feelings regarding the child's separation from home, particularly guilt about leaving the child in someone else's care when the parent returns to work. Practical ways of alleviating anxiety and improving the quality of time spent with the child include planning a household schedule that divides major chores into smaller ones, combining household duties with a childcare activity, such as cleaning the bathroom while the child is bathing, and providing time for relaxation and activity with the child.

Sex Education

Preschoolers have absorbed a tremendous amount of information and experienced many things during their short lifetimes. Although their thinking may not be adultlike, they search constantly for explanations and reasons that are logical and reasonable to them. The word *why* seems to supplant the word *no,* which was common in toddlerhood. One of their major developmental achievements has been severing the psychologic "placenta" from their mother as they discover their sense of self apart from others. It is only natural that as they learn about "me," they will also want to know such things as "why me," and "how me." Questions such as "Where do babies come from?" are sexual in content but informational in intent. Such inquiries are as casual as "Why is the sky blue?" "What makes it rain?" or "Who is that?" It is the *way* in which questions about procreation are answered that conditions even the youngest children to separate these questions from others about their world. If these questions are answered honestly and as matter-of-factly as any other inquiry, children will continue to search for answers. If they are answered with a "tall tale" or an anxious "You are too young to know about that," children will learn to keep such questions to themselves. Unfortunately as they harbor these silent mysteries, they are formulating their own theories to explain birth. Since magical thinking need not be based on logic or fact, any fantastic, often terrifying explanation can substitute for truth.

Regardless of whether children are given sex education, they will engage in games of sexual curiosity and exploration. By 3 years of age children are aware of the anatomic differences between the sexes and are very concerned with how the other sex "works." This is not really "sexual" curiosity, because many children are still unaware of the reproductive function of the genitals. Their curiosity concerns the eliminative function of the anatomy. Boys watch girls urinate because they wonder how they can without a penis. Since they cannot see anything but a stream coming out, they want to observe further for where it comes out. "Doctor play" is often a game invented for just such investigation. Girls are no less curious about boys' anatomy. It is intriguing to have a closer inspection of this "thing" that girls do not have.

Even if children's curiosity is satisfied about the eliminative differences, once they are told about the "special place where babies come out," they are more mystified and determined to find that opening. Unfortunately investigation often yields even fewer answers and may result in anxiety and shame if they are caught and scolded for their behavior. When considering the facts of reproduction and viewing them in terms of the young child's thinking processes, it becomes clear how absurd and incredible the "facts of life" really are. Think about the "special place where the baby grows," "the seed or egg that grows when the father's seed or sperm meets it," and "the special opening" that is so small it cannot be found but through which a fairly large person emerges. And most fantastic of all is how the father's sperm meets the mother's egg! Surely this is more preposterous than any fairy tale about witches, princesses, or monsters!

As children absorb these facts, no matter how expertly they are explained, they will form their own theories. Since the only framework they have for "special place," "growing," "seed or egg," and "opening" is eating and eliminating, they fit all the new information into this understandable explanation. Children need the correct information repeated several times as they attempt to assimilate it as logical and reasonable.

Parents' role in sex education. Preschoolers do not have the benefit of potential sex education in school or from their peer group as older children do. They rely on parental information or misinformation in their search for "how me" (how they came to be). Although sexual mores have seen a kind of liberation movement in the past several decades, parents still may feel uncomfortable when faced with their child's probing questions. Usually overanxious parents' close communication by reacting in one of two ways: either by giving no answers or by giving too much information. Should parents err in the direction of too much information, children will simply become bored or end the conversation with an irrelevant question. Parents worry a great deal about whether they can "harm" their children with "too much" information or tell their children things that they will not understand. Generally, knowledge is not harmful. In fact, the experts advise parents to tell their children a bit more than they think their children can understand (Gordon and Snyder, 1989). It does not matter if children do not understand everything parents say. What matters is that parents are approachable people.

Two rules govern answering questions about sex or other sensitive issues, such as death, divorce, or adoption. The first is to *find out what children know and think.* By investigating the theories they have conjured in their minds as a reasonable explanation, parents can not only give correct information but also help children understand why their explanation is inaccurate. For example, before children ever ask about where babies come from, they usually have imagined that the mother "ate" something that made the baby grow in her stomach. Therefore the baby will come out like a bowel movement. When parents give the appropriate information, they can also correct this "eating-elimination" theory. The following example illustrates how uncorrected misconceptions can lead to unexpected problems:

> Five-year-old John knew his mother was to have a baby soon. He saw how large her abdomen was becoming and, when he asked why, was told that the baby was growing inside mother's stomach. At about the same time, John began eating excessively and became extremely constipated. He would violently object to any measures directed at relieving the constipation and if he evacuated, he would become very upset. During a visit to a nurse friend's home, his mother related these events. The nurse asked about John's understanding of the baby's conception and birth. Mother offered the same limited explanation that she had given her son. The nurse pointed out that based on the information that the "baby grows in the stomach," John probably thought he did understand. According to his logic, he was having a baby by eating a lot and did not want it to come out in the only way he knew body products to exit. Mother saw the logic behind this theory and agreed to explore it with John.
>
> John related almost precisely the story as predicted by the nurse. If his mother could have a baby, so could he by eating so much that his belly would enlarge. As he saw himself grow bigger, he was sure that he was pregnant, and he greatly feared that the baby would come out "prematurely" (as he had overheard) if he had a bowel movement. When the nurse explained the correct facts, John was relieved, although somewhat disappointed to learn of his inability to bear children. He asked about the father's role and was given the appropriate explanation. He wondered about "Daddy entering Mommy in a special place and giving her a sperm that made the egg grow," and stated, "I guess for now I won't make any babies. Can I go out and play?" The overeating and constipation resolved without any further intervention.

Another reason for ascertaining what the child thinks and knows before offering any information is that the "unasked for" answer may be given. For example, 4-year-old Sally asked her father, "Where did I come from?" Both parents quickly took this inquiry as a clue for offering sex education. After the explanation, the child exclaimed, "I don't want to know about all that! All I know is Mary came from New York and I want to know where I was born."

The second rule for giving information is *honesty.* It is true that much of the correct information will be forgotten or misunderstood by the preschooler, but what is more important is that the correct information be restated over time until the child absorbs and comprehends the facts. Even though the correct anatomic words may be hard to pronounce and even more difficult to remember, they become foundational content for explaining other concepts later on. They also reinforce the fact that procreation is not associated with ingestion or elimination but that it occurs in a place that is near but not the same as where the child urinates or defecates. Parental honesty also shows children that parents will be truthful in other phases of inquiry and learning. This approach avoids the establishment of a "double standard," whereby parents can tell "little white lies" but children must always be straightforward.

Honesty does not imply imparting to children every fact of life or allowing excessive permissiveness in sexual curiosity. When children ask one question, they are looking for one answer, not the entire procreation cycle. When they are ready, they will ask about the other "unfinished" parts of the story. Sooner or later they will wonder how the "sperm meets the egg" and "how the baby gets out," but it is best to wait until they ask.

When children do not ask questions, parents should take advantage of natural opportunities to discuss reproduction, such as talking about someone who is pregnant or discussing a television program or movie about biologic aspects. Many excellent books on sex education are available for preschool children at public libraries, and the **Sex Information and Education Council of the United States (SIECUS)*** and local chapters of **Planned Parenthood Federation of America†** have bibliographies of suggested reading material. Parents should read any book *before* giving it or reading it to the child.

The question usually arises as to how much sexual curiosity should be satisfied. Developmentally, children progress through different stages of sexual exploration. The infant who finds the genitals is exploring another pleasurable part of the body. The 3-year-old brother who peeks into the bathroom to watch his sister urinate is not perverted but is finding out how she urinates without a penis. Five-year-old children engaged in doctor play are not promiscuous but are trying to find concrete evidence to support explanations about birth. Regardless of how normal these activities are, many parents are bewildered by them and do not know what to say or do when confronted with such behavior.

One positive approach is to neither condone nor condemn the sexual curiosity but to answer questions the child may have and then encourage the child to engage in some other activity. In this way children can be helped to understand that there are ways that their sexual curiosity can be satisfied other than through playing investigative games. This in no way condemns the activity but stresses alternative methods to seek solutions and answers. Allowing children unrestricted permissiveness only intensifies their anxiety and concern, since exploring and searching usually yield little evidence to satisfy their sexual curiosity.

Occasionally parents are faced with special dilemmas, for example, when children ask to see "how Mommy and Daddy do it" or accidentally witness sexual intercourse. When such events occur, parents must remember that sex education is much more than textbook facts. It is part of a greater concept called *sexuality*. Two people unite intimately because of the special relationship they have together. Intercourse is not a physical act apart from feeling or emotion but a private act that two people share in caring and pleasure. Such an explanation does not deny children's right to be curious, nor does it deny them the request because their wish is bad or dangerous. On the contrary, it teaches appropriate social behavior and in particular stresses the meaningful, intimate relationship between man and woman. When children witness sexual acts, parents should use the opportunity immediately to communicate that sex is healthy and natural. However, to prevent subsequent interruptions, children are cautioned to always knock first, or, if they are too young to understand or comply, a lock on the door is appropriate (Goldsmith, 1986).

Masturbation. Parents' attitudes toward masturbation closely parallel their view toward sex education for their children. Much of what has been discussed under sexual curiosity applies to masturbation as well. Masturbation, or self-stimulation of the genitals, occurs at any age for a variety of reasons and, if not excessive, is normal and healthy. Masturbation may be considered excessive when it interferes with children's regular activities or causes soreness, pain, or sufficient tissue damage to create a potential for infections. For preschoolers masturbation is a part of sexual curiosity and exploration.

Many individuals have certain beliefs about masturbation. Traditionally people have believed it to be sinful and harmful to health. A common myth was that masturbation led to insanity, probably from the observation that mentally ill people masturbate excessively. However, this behavior is a symptom—not a cause—of mental illness. Some people with strong religious beliefs think that masturbation distracts people from the true ideal of sexuality: primarily procreation within a marital relationship. Others who think of themselves as neutral regard masturbation as a subject that requires further study, but they do not encourage it as something positive or healthy. Finally, those who take a liberal view hold that it is not only harmless but positively good, healthy, and at times necessary. They believe that it helps young people grow up sexually in a natural way.

If parents are concerned with masturbation by their children, it is essential for nurses to assess which belief the parents hold as doctrine for acceptable moral conduct. Individuals who view any form of masturbation as negative and unacceptable will need more help in understanding it as a natural, healthy expression of sexual development. In all cases it is advisable to investigate the circumstances associated with so-called masturbation, because all genital stimulation is not masturbation for sexual stimulation but may be an expression of anxiety, boredom, or unresolved conflicts. For example, a boy who repeatedly touches his penis all day is not masturbating for pleasure but may be reassuring himself that it is intact. This may be an expression of castration anxiety and should be investigated further. Children who openly and publicly masturbate are inviting a reaction, such as discipline, punishment, or criticism. They may be overwhelmed by their sexual feelings and asking others to help them channel their emotions into more constructive outlets. As part of teaching their children socially acceptable behavior, parents should emphasize that masturbation, like other forms of sex play, is a private act.

Gifted Children

The importance of the identification of gifted children and their needs is increasingly being recognized. Although the definition of *gifted* varies, the most widely used criterion is superior intelligence—usually defined as an intelligence quotient (IQ) of 130 or above, although this depends on the test. A broader view considers specific academic aptitude, creative or productive thinking, leadership ability, visual and performing arts, and psychomotor ability either singly or in combination as signs of giftedness (Goldsmith and Feldman, 1985; Landesman, 1985). Most children are identified as gifted when they enter school and receive IQ tests; no valid tests exist for predicting giftedness in infancy (Shapiro and others, 1989). However, not all gifted children are identified, and the tragic loss of the opportunity to develop their potential may result. Consequently, nurses who are aware of the behavioral and developmental characteristics

*130 W. 42nd St., Suite 2500, New York, NY 10036; (212) 819-9770.

†National office: 810 Seventh Avenue, New York, NY 10019; (212) 541-7800; (800) 829-7732.

Box 15-1 CHARACTERISTICS OF GIFTED CHILDREN

Birth weight and head circumference above 50th percentile
Early developmental milestones, especially walking
Early development of language and complex usage of speech
Temperamental characteristics of persistence, intensity, extreme self-confidence, sensitivity, and responsiveness to stimulation
Constant questioning and curiosity
Rich fantasy, such as imaginary playmates
Highly developed sense of humor
Strong interest in special areas, such as music, science, or mechanical skills

Modified from Fish, L., and Burch, K.: Identifying gifted preschoolers, Pediatr. Nurs. 1(2):125-127, 1985; Goldsmith, L.T., and Feldman, D.H.: Identifying gifted children: the state of the art, Pediatr. Ann 14(10):709-716, 1985.

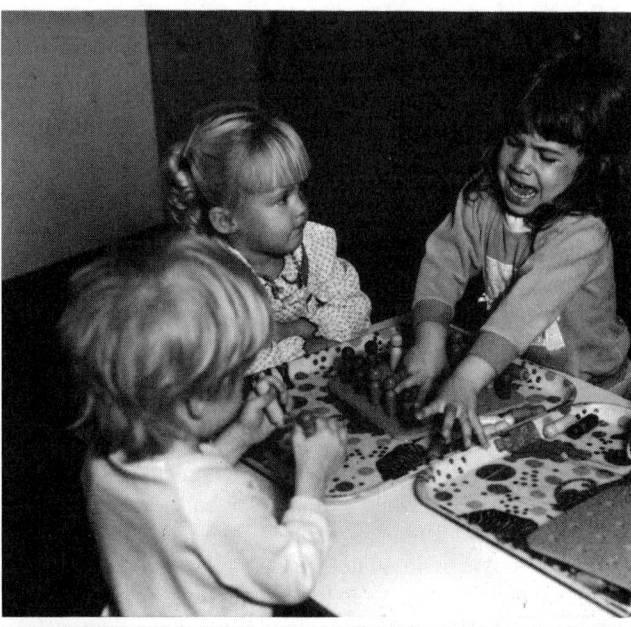

Fig. 15-6. Preschoolers generally direct their aggression toward peers, especially when their desires are frustrated.

of giftedness can assess children's mental and physical capabilities and assist in early identification (Box 15-1).

Gifted children can present unique challenges to parents. They often demand increased stimulation as infants and continue to seek a great deal of attention from their parents. Their high energy level and persistence can lead to discipline problems similar to those seen in children with difficult temperaments. Parents may be intimidated by having a child smarter than themselves and be hesitant to set limits. However, gifted children are children first and have the same needs for love, security, and consistent controls as other youngsters. Sometimes children's above-average skills in one area cause adults to exaggerate their abilities in all areas and thus expect excessively mature behavior. Parents may mislabel slower achievement in a particular skill as lack of trying, when it really represents children's natural progression of abilities (McGuffog, 1985). These children also benefit from academic settings that provide enrichment and accelerated learning commensurate with their capabilties (Robinson, 1985). Consequently, early identification of giftedness and appropriate parental guidance can be critical to the optimum development of giftedness and the children's emotional adjustment. A number of organizations provide information, testing, and other services to families with gifted children and to professionals.

Aggression

Aggression refers to behavior that attempts to hurt a person or destroy property. It differs from anger, which is a temporary emotional state, but anger may be expressed through aggression. Aggression is influenced by a complex set of biologic, sociocultural, and familial variables. There is evidence that gender differences exist and that males are more aggressive than females (Maccoby and Jacklin, 1980). Preschool children are most often aggressive to peers (Fig. 15-6). Other factors that tend to increase aggressive behavior are frustration, modeling, and reinforcement.

Frustration, or the continual thwarting of self-satisfaction by parental disapproval, humiliation, punishment, and insults, can lead children to act out their frustration on others as a means of release. Especially if they fear their parents, these children will displace their anger on others, particularly peers and other authority figures. This type of aggression frequently applies to the "well-behaved child" at home who is a discipline problem at school or a "bully" among playmates.

Modeling, or imitating behavior of significant others, is a powerful influencing force in preschoolers. Children who see their parents fighting, both physically or verbally, are observing behavior that they come to know as acceptable. Another aspect of modeling is establishing a double standard for acceptable conduct. For example, in some families aggression is synonymous with masculinity, and boys are encouraged to defend themselves. Although defending one's rights is to be encouraged for both sexes, at times the principle of "toughness" or "standing up for yourself" is not tempered with judgment, fairness, or equality but becomes an excuse for ruling and dominating others. Such permissive aggression can be extremely anxiety producing for children because it makes them feel out of control, even though they outwardly may appear to be the "boss" or "bully."

Another significant source for modeling is television. Numerous studies have found a positive correlation between viewing violent programs and immediate aggression (Singer, 1985). These findings received widespread attention when the National Institute of Mental Health concluded that violence on television does lead to aggression by children who watch the programs (Pearl, 1982). Consequently, parents need encouragement to supervise programming, especially for those children with aggressive tendencies (see discussion under Television, Chapter 4).

Reinforcement can also shape aggressive behavior and is closely associated with modeling "masculine" behavior. Sometimes the reward for aggressive behavior is negative, such as punishment or disapproval, but is reinforcing because it represents attention. For example, children who are ignored by their parents until they hit a sibling learn that such acts are forceful attention mechanisms. In addition, parents who permit aggressive behavior by not interfering communicate silent, implicit approval of such acts.

One of the tasks of preschoolers is learning socially acceptable behavior and the ability to control and redirect aggression toward the appropriate source. Parents can help children by modeling appropriate behavior and encouraging children to express themselves verbally. For example, rather than condoning hitting another child for taking a toy, parents can suggest that the child state how he or she feels, such as "I am angry when you take my ball. Give it back."

Children should not be made to feel guilty or ashamed for being angry or frustrated. When they recognize these feelings, they are better able to channel them into constructive, not destructive, outlets. One of the earliest demonstrations of aggression is temper tantrums. If parents handle them constructively by not attending to or reinforcing them and by helping children find control through appropriate play situations, young children will learn to acknowledge such feelings and express them in alternative ways, such as pounding on clay or hitting a punching bag. When children are out of control, they may need to be physically restrained or removed from the scene to prevent them from hurting themselves or others (Barlow, 1989).

Sometimes the type of discipline used to extinguish other forms of unacceptable behavior actually promotes aggressive behavior. For example, if the child is spanked for the act, aggression is used to "teach" a lesson against aggression! Parental permissiveness and lack of discipline may also foster aggressiveness (Shonkoff, 1983). The combined use of time-out and reinforcement for solitary play is an effective intervention for aggression. In addition, minimizing anger and frustration can lead to fewer opportunities for acting out behavior (see Parent Guidelines: Minimizing Misbehavior, Chapter 14).

When extreme behaviors, such as aggression, are present in children, parents are often concerned about the need for professional help. Generally, the difference between "normal" and "problematic" behavior is not the actual behavior, but the *quantity* (number of occurrences), *severity* (interfering with social or cognitive functioning), *distribution* (different manifestations), and *duration* (at least 4 weeks) of the activity. In addition, any *sudden change* in behavior should be taken seriously (Phillips, Sarles, and Friedman, 1980). When aggressive tendencies are evaluated, these factors are assessed to distinguish between behaviors typically seen at various ages and those that may represent an underlying problem.

Speech Problems

The most critical period for speech development occurs between 2 and 4 years of age. During this period children are using their rapidly growing vocabulary to interact with the environment. However, the rate of vocabulary acquisition does not parallel the advancing mental ability or the degree of comprehension. This failure to master sensorimotor integrations results in stuttering or stammering as children try to say the word they are already thinking about. This hesitancy or nonfluency in speech pattern is a *normal* characteristic of language development. However, when parents or other significant caregivers place undue emphasis or stress on this pattern, a real speech problem can occur. Children who are pressured into producing sounds ahead of schedule may cope by reverting to baby speech or stuttering.

The best therapy for speech problems is prevention and early detection. One of the most essential factors involves anticipatory preparation of parents for the expected hesitation in speech during the preschool period and discussion of developmental achievements characteristic of children in each age-group. Each of these is discussed in Chapter 25 and should be included in the health promotion of preschoolers.

Coping with Stress

Although the preschool years generally are less troublesome than toddlerhood for parents, this period of life presents children with many unique stresses. Many are innate and stem from their unique understanding of the world, such as fears. Others are imposed, such as beginning school. Although minimum amounts of stress are beneficial during the early years to help children develop effective coping skills, excessive stress is harmful, and young children are especially vulnerable because of their limited capacity to cope.

To help parents deal with stress in their child's life, they must be aware of signs of stress (see Box 4-7) and be helped to identify the source (Box 15-2). In addition, any number of other stresses may be present, such as the birth of a sibling, marital discord, relocation, or illness. The best approach to dealing with stress is prevention—monitoring the amount of stress in children's lives so that levels exceeding their coping ability do not occur. In many instances structuring children's schedules to allow rest and preparing them for change, such as entering school, are sufficient measures. Because stress is such a constant aspect of daily living, the preschool years are not too young to help children learn to cope with stress. They can learn the meaning of the word *stress* and recognize physical signs of stress reaction, such as rapid pulse, pounding heart, or fatigue. Teaching children relaxation and imagery is very effective. Young children can learn to "let their bodies go limp like a rag doll" or "imagine flying like bird." Parents can use stories to help children imagine pleasurable events. As language skills improve, preschoolers should be encouraged to talk about their feelings and to explore other ways of expressing emotions. Play is an excellent vehicle for venting anger or frustration, and toys such as drums, clay, and punching bags provide alternative methods of dissipating anxiety. Toys also begin to teach socially acceptable ways of dealing with such feelings.

Box 15-2 SOURCES OF STRESS IN PRESCHOOLERS

Three-Year-Old

Infantile behavior—reverts to babyish ways; can't completely let go of babyhood
Stubbornness—although the child is developing an interest in social relationships and a concept of "we," the child may lapse into uncooperative behvior
Possessiveness—guards belongings and may be bossy about them
Jealousy—particularly when it comes to parents' love
Separation anxiety
Stranger anxiety
Confusion—can't always discriminate between fantasy and reality
White lies—may result from wishful thinking, fantasy, and desire to please or impress
Imaginary playmate—often blamed in the white lies
Fears—may be precipitated by imagination; may also fear dogs or other animals
Speech—may stutter or stumble over words
Activity level—seems to be in perpetual motion; may exhaust himself or herself
Eating—may forget to eat or lose interest in food
Nap or bedtime—may fear bad dreams, the dark, or missing out on some fun while asleep
Destructiveness—may enjoy wrecking or destroying
Questions—continually asks "why," and is upset if trusted adults do not respond or do not know the answer

Four-Year-Old

Insecurity—may develop nervous habits such as nail biting, facial tic, thumb-sucking, genital manipulation, eye-blinking, or nose-picking; may insist on bringing a familiar item from house to preschool
Exaggerations—may attempt to boost self-image with boasts
Companionship—enjoys interacting with friends, although there may be many quarrels
Silliness—tends to engage in rambunctious, silly play; likes words and is fascinated by rhyming syllables or foul language; is disciplined for lack of control
Property rights—protects belongings; may become bossy
Sex—interested in the human body; may engage in exhibitionism
Activity level—enjoys running, jumping, and slamming doors; may be punished for disruptive behavior
Fears—picks up fears from adults; may fear dark room, snakes and lizards, or anything perceived as "creepy"
Attention—likes to talk and is frustrated if ignored or put off; whines to get own way

Five-Year-Old

Approval—parents' love and acceptance are vital; seeks praise
School—may have difficulty adjusting to kindergarten
Separation anxiety—particularly fears loss of mother
Infantile behavior—may occasionally lapse into babyish behavior as a result of realizing that babyhood is ended
Worrying—may develop irrational fears, take information out of context, or fret over a misinterpreted, overheard conversation
Masturbation—is concerned about being "bad"
Belongings—protects possessions
Showing off—performs in order to gain praise
Procrastination—may dillydally now and then
Name calling—insults others to boost self-image, but is upset when she or he is the victim of mockery

From Kuczen, B.: Childhood stress: don't let your child be a victim, New York, 1982, Delacorte Press, pp. 15-17.

Fears

The greatest number and variety of real and imagined fears are present during the preschool years and include fear of the dark, being left alone (especially at bedtime), animals (particularly large dogs and snakes), ghosts, sexual matters (castration), and objects or persons associated with pain. The exact cause of children's fears is unknown. Freudians believe that the upsurge of fears during the preschool years results from the anxiety of being injured and mutilated (castration complex). Piaget views fears as a product of the type of thinking of children in this age-group. Preschoolers are caught between the egocentric thinking of infants, which protects them from imagined fears, and the more logical thought processes of school-age children, which help explain and dispel potential fears. Children in the preconceptual stage still engage in egocentric thought but are now able to imagine an event without actually experiencing it. For example, seeing someone hurt is sufficient for realizing what the hurt must be like and for consequently fearing that hurt. In medical practice this is frequently observed. When watching another child getting an injection, the preschooler may become very upset, almost as if he or she received the injection. The concept of animism (ascribing lifelike qualities to inanimate objects) explains why children fear objects. For example, one child refused to move his bowels after watching a television commercial in which the toilet bowl was portrayed as turning into a monster, with the seat cover making a chomping movement. The child was afraid the toilet "would get him" if he sat on it (Pilapil, 1990).

A fear that is peculiar to this age is fear of annihilation. Because of poorly defined body boundaries and improved cognitive abilities, toddlers develop concerns related to loss of body parts, such as feces being flushed away or bath water going down the drain. Although they are now aware that objects can disappear, preschool children cannot understand concepts of size, for example, that they cannot disappear down the drain because they are too large.

Preschoolers are also likely to develop parent-induced fears—fears that stem from imitating their parents. When parents demonstrate their fears, the concerns are communicated to the children. Such fears tend to be long-lasting and difficult to dispel (Wolman, 1978).

The best way to help children overcome their fears is by actively involving them in finding practical methods to deal with experiences that frighten them. This may be as simple as keeping a dim night-light on in the bedroom to assure the child that no monsters lurk in the dark or letting the child bathe a doll or play with toys in a tub of water and then opening the drain with the toys still in the tub to demonstrate that large objects cannot go down the drain. In this way the experience that created the fear in the child can be reconstructed without involving the child directly as the victim. The child is allowed alternative methods to feel in control and powerful while overcoming fear.

Exposing children to the feared object in a safe situation provides a type of conditioning or desensitization. For instance, children who are afraid of dogs should never be forced to approach or touch one, but they may be gradually introduced to the experience by watching other children play with the animal. This type of modeling, demonstrating fearlessness in others, can be very effective if children are allowed to progress at their own rate.

Sometimes fears do not subside with simple measures or developmental maturation. When children experience severe fears that disrupt family life, professional help is required. Successful training programs may include (1) muscle relaxation, (2) imagining a pleasant scene, and (3) reciting brave statements. Rewards or "tokens" may be given for "bravery" and not being afraid (Graziano and Mooney, 1980). Such interventions can be applied in clinical settings to reduce fears (e.g., of being alone or of painful procedures).

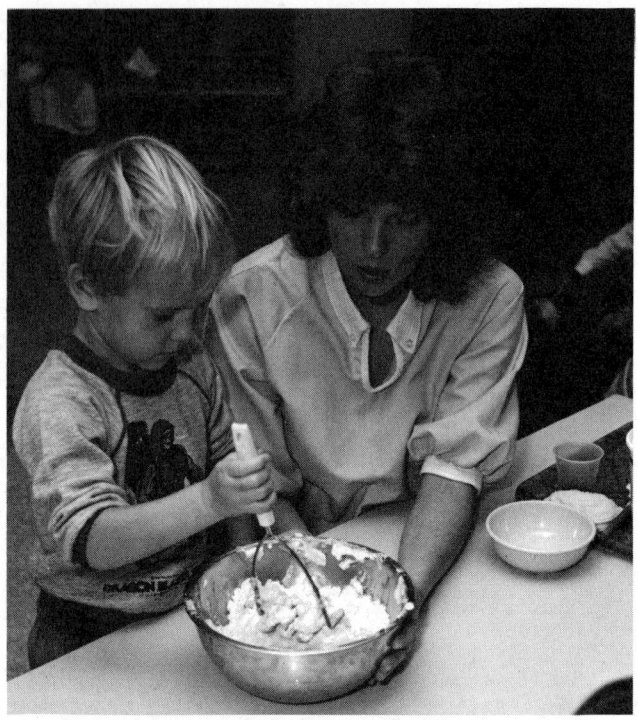

Fig. 15-7. Preschool children enjoy helping adults and are more likely to try new foods if they can assist in the preparation.

PROMOTING OPTIMUM HEALTH DURING THE PRESCHOOL YEARS

Health promotion mainly involves guidance regarding nutrition, sleep, dental health, and injury prevention. A brief discussion of each subject is presented to emphasize the particular needs or differences of preschoolers vs toddlers. (For a more comprehensive understanding the reader is urged to also review the material presented in Chapter 14 under Promoting Optimum Health During Toddlerhood.)

NUTRITION

Nutritional requirements for preschoolers are fairly similar to those for toddlers. The requirement for calories per unit of body weight continues to decrease slightly to 90 kcal/kg for an average daily intake of 1800 calories. Fluid requirements may also decrease slightly to about 100 ml/kg daily but depend on activity level, climatic conditions, and state of health. Protein requirements are 1.2 g/kg for an average daily consumption of 24 g (Food and Nutrition Board, 1989).

Some preschoolers still have food habits that are typical of toddlers, such as food fads and strong taste preferences. When children reach 4 years of age, they seem to enter another period of finicky eating, which is generally characteristic of the more rebellious and rowdy behavior of children in this age-group. By age 5 years children are more agreeable to trying new foods, especially if encouraged by an adult who allows the child to help with food preparation or experiments with a new taste or different dish (Fig. 15-7).

Box 15-3 SAMPLE MENUS FOR PRESCHOOLERS BASED ON BASIC FOOD GROUPS*

Breakfast	½-1 cup dry, unsweetened cereal 4-6 oz lowfat milk ½ cup orange juice
Lunch	1 tbsp peanut butter 1-2 slices whole wheat bread 1 apple 6-8 oz lowfat milk
Snack	8 oz carton fruited yogurt 1 graham cracker
Dinner	1 broiled chicken leg ½ cup rice 2 tbsp-½ cup green beans 6-8 oz lowfat milk
Snack	1 banana
DAILY TOTAL:	
Milk:	24 ounces or equivalent
Meat:	2-3 ounces
Fruits/veg:	4 servings (1 piece or ½ cup is a serving)
Breads/cereal:	4 servings (½ slice or ¼ cup is a serving)

Prepared by Cecilia L. Davis, R.D., L.D.

*Fats and simple carbohydrates should be served sparingly to meet caloric needs. Serving sizes are minimums for nutritional adequacy. Many children eat more.

Mealtimes can become battlegrounds if parents expect impeccable table manners. Usually the 5-year-old child is ready for the "social" side of eating, but the 3- or 4-year-old child still has difficulty sitting quietly through a long family meal.

Parents sometimes worry about the quantity of food preschoolers consume. In general, the quality is much more important than the quantity, a fact that should be stressed during nutritional counseling. Young children often consume more food than parents realize. One approach toward lessening this parental concern is advising parents to keep a weekly record of everything the child eats. In particular, the need for measuring the amount of food, such as setting aside ½ cup of vegetables and serving the child from this premeasured amount, is stressed to provide a more accurate estimate of food intake at each meal. Usually by the end of the week, when they look at the food chart, parents are amazed at how much the child has consumed, even though at each meal the amount seemed minimal. In general, preschoolers consume only slightly more than toddlers, or about half of an adult's portion. Sample menus for preschoolers are given in Box 15-3.

SLEEP AND ACTIVITY

Sleep patterns vary widely, but the average preschooler sleeps about 12 hours a night and infrequently takes daytime naps. Children with reported sleep problems sleep less than those without sleeping difficulties (Edgil, Wood, and Smith, 1985). Activity levels continue to be high, although quiet activities, such as television, are increasingly appealing and can become an unhealthy substitute for active play.

Table 15-3 Comparison of nightmares vs sleep terrors

NIGHTMARES	SLEEP TERRORS
▪ Description	
A scary dream; takes place within REM sleep and is followed by full waking	A partial arousal from very deep (stage IV, non-REM) nondreaming sleep
▪ Time of distress	
After the dream is over and child wakes and cries or calls; not during the nightmare itself	During the terror itself, as child screams and thrashes; afterward is calm
▪ Time of occurrence	
In the second half of the night, when dreams are most intense	Usually 1 to 4 hours after falling asleep, when nondreaming sleep is deepest
▪ Child's behavior	
Crying in younger children, fright in all; these persist even though the child is awake	Initially the child may sit up, thrash, or run in a bizarre manner, with eyes bulging, heart racing, and profuse sweating; may cry, scream, talk, or moan; there is apparent fright, anger, and/or obvious confusion, which *disappears* when child is fully awake
▪ Responsiveness to others	
Child is aware of and reassured by other's presence	Child is not very aware of another's presence, is not comforted, and may push person away and scream and thrash more if held or restrained
▪ Return to sleep	
May be considerably delayed because of persistent fear	Usually rapid; often difficult to keep child awake
▪ Description of dream	
Yes (if old enough)	No memory of a dream or of yelling or thrashing
▪ Interventions	
Accept dream as real fear Sit with child; offer comfort, assurance, and sense of protection May lie down with child or take to own bed *only* if child is not calmed by other measures and understands this is special occasion Consider professional counseling for recurrent nightmares unresponsive to above approaches	Observe child for a few minutes, *without interfering,* until child becomes calm or wakes fully Intervene only if necessary to protect child from injury Guide child back to bed if needed Stress to parents that sleep terrors are a normal, common phenomenon in preschoolers that requires relatively no intervention

Modified from Ferber, R.: Solve your child's sleep problems, New York, 1985, Simon & Schuster, Inc.

Preschoolers' increased gross motor abilities and coordination provide them the opportunity to engage in many sports, if only at a novice level. Whether young children should begin formalized training in an activity at this early age is controversial. The consensus is to expose children to a wide variety of physical activities rather than concentrate on one area. However, children's interest in specific events should be respected, since early training can be advantageous.

Sleep Disturbances

The preschool years are a prime time for sleep disturbances. Young children sometimes have trouble going to sleep, especially after so much activity and stimulation during the day. Others may develop bedtime fears, wake during the night, or have nightmares or sleep terrors. Still others may prolong the inevitable through elaborate rituals.

Recommendations for sleep disturbance are offered only *after* a thorough assessment of the problem has been completed (see Box 6-15). Interventions can differ greatly; for example, nightmares and sleep terrors require very different approaches (Table 15-3). For children who delay going to bed, a recommended approach involves counseling parents about the importance of a consistent bedtime ritual and emphasizing the normalcy of this type of behavior in young children. Attention-seeking behavior is ignored, and the child is not taken into the parents' bed or allowed to stay up past a reasonable hour. Other measures that may be helpful include keeping a light on in the room, providing transitional objects, such as a favorite toy, or leaving a drink of water by the bed.

Helping children slow down before bedtime also contributes to less resistance to going to bed. One approach is to establish limited rituals that signal readiness for bed, such as a bath or story. Parents can reinforce the pattern by stating, "After this story it is bedtime," and consistently carrying through the routine. If extra stimulation such as having visitors arrive at bedtime is disruptive to children's routine, it is advisable to settle children in bed beforehand.

DENTAL HEALTH

By the beginning of the preschool period, the eruption of the deciduous (primary) teeth is complete. Dental care is essential to preserve these temporary teeth and to teach good dental habits (see Chapter 14). Although preschoolers' fine motor control is improved, they still require assistance and supervision with brushing, and flossing should be done by parents. Professional care and prophylaxis, especially fluoride supplements, should be continued. If children are cared for away from home, parents are encouraged to monitor the dental care provided by others, including the diet, to keep cariogenic foods to a minimum.

Trauma to teeth during this period is not uncommon, and appropriate care of an evulsed tooth is important (see Chapter 18). Even though the evulsed tooth is not permanent, preservation of the space is necessary for proper eruption of the secondary teeth and prevention of abnormal tongue habits (Greene, Louie, and Wycoff, 1990).

INJURY PREVENTION

Because of improved gross and fine motor skills, coordination, and balance, preschoolers are less prone to falls than toddlers. They tend to be less reckless, listen more to parental rules, and are aware of potential danger, such as hot objects, sharp instruments, and dangerous heights. Putting objects in the mouth as part of exploration has all but ceased, although poisoning is still a danger. Pedestrian motor vehicle injuries increase from activities such as playing in the street, riding tricycles, running after balls, or forgetting safety regulations when crossing streets. In general, the guidelines suggested for injury prevention in Table 14-8 apply to children in this age-group as well.

Box 15-4 GUIDANCE DURING PRESCHOOL YEARS

Age 3 Years

- Prepare parents for child's increasing interest in widening relationships.
- Encourage enrollment in nursery school.
- Emphasize importance of setting limits.
- Prepare parents to expect exaggerated tension-reduction behaviors, such as need for "security blanket."
- Encourage parents to offer the child choices when the child vacillates.
- Expect marked changes at 3½ years when the child becomes less coordinated (motor and emotional), becomes insecure, exhibits emotional extremes, and develops behaviors such as stuttering.
- Prepare parents to expect extra demands on their attention as a reflection of the child's emotional insecurity and fear of loss of love.
- Warn parents that the equilibrium of the 3-year-old will change to the aggressive out-of-bounds behavior of the 4-year-old.
- Anticipate a more stable appetite with more expansive food selection.
- Stress need for protection and education of child to prevent injury (see Injury Prevention, Chapter 14)

Age 4 Years

- Prepare for more aggressive behavior, including motor activity and shocking language.
- Expect resistance to parental authority.
- Explore parental feelings regarding child's behavior.
- Suggest some kind of respite for primary caregivers, such as placing the child in nursing school for part of the day.
- Prepare for increasing sexual curiosity.
- Emphasize importance of realistic limit setting on behavior and appropriate discipline techniques.
- Prepare parents for the highly imaginary 4-year-old who indulges in "tall tales" (to be differentiated from lies) and for the child's acquisition of imaginary playmates.
- Suggest swimming lessons if not begun earlier.
- Expect nightmares or an increase in them and suggest they make sure child is fully awakened from a frightening dream.
- Provide reassurance that a period of calm begins at 5 years of age.

Age 5 Years

- Expect a tranquil period at 5 years.
- Prepare child for entrance into school environment.
- Make sure immunizations are up to date before entering school.

However, emphasis is now on *education* for safety and potential hazards, in addition to appropriate protection. Because preschoolers are great imitators, it is essential that parents set a good example by "practicing what they preach." Children are quick to observe discrepancies in what they are told to do. Establishing habits at this time, such as wearing bicycle helmets with the first bicycle, can create long-term safety behaviors.

ANTICIPATORY GUIDANCE—CARE OF FAMILIES

The preschool years present fewer childrearing difficulties than earlier years, and this stage of development is facilitated by appropriate anticipatory guidance in the areas already discussed (Box 15-4). There is also a shift in childrearing practices from one mainly of protection to one primarily of education, especially in terms of injury prevention.

During this period an emotional transition between parent and child occurs. Although children are still attached to their parents and accept all their values and beliefs, they are nearing the period of life when they will question previous teachings and prefer the companionship of peers. Entry into school marks a separation for parents, as well as for children. Parents need help in adjusting to this change, particularly if the mother has focused her daily activity on home responsibilities. As preschoolers begin nursery or elementary school, mothers may need to seek activities beyond the family, such as community involvement or pursuing a career. In this way all family members are adjusting to change, which is part of the process of growing and developing.

KEY POINTS

- The preschool years comprise the period from 3 to 5 years of age, a time that is considered critical for emotional and psychologic development.
- Biologic development in the preschool period is characterized by mature body systems and refinement in gross and fine motor behavior, as evidenced by participation in activities such as running, riding a tricycle, and drawing.
- According to Erikson, acquiring a sense of initiative is the chief psychosocial task of the preschooler. Development of the superego occurs during this period, and conscience begins to emerge.
- In Freudian theory, preschoolers are in the oedipal stage. Resolution of this stage occurs when children strongly identify with their parent of the same sex.
- According to Piaget, the preschool age is characterized by intuitive or prelogical thinking and a move toward logical thought processes through advanced, complex learning, language, and understanding of causality.
- The seeds of moral development are planted during the preschool period. According to Kohlberg, children are in the stage of naive instrumental orientation, in which they are concerned with satisfying their own needs and, less frequently, the needs of others.
- Social development booms in this period with individuation-separation, more sophisticated language, greater independence, and more complex, imaginative forms of play.
- Four areas of special concern to parents during the preschool period are preschool or daycare experience, sex education, speech problems, and stress.
- In selecting a daycare facility parents should inquire about daily programs, teacher qualifications, accreditation, student-to-staff ratio, discipline policies, meals, fees, and health practices.
- Two rules that govern answering questions about sex and other sensitive issues are to find out what the child thinks and to be honest.
- Preschool aggression may result from frustration, modeling behavior, and reinforcement.
- Fears constitute a great part of the preschool period; objects, potential annihilation, and parent-induced fears are common sources.
- Health promotion continues to be directed toward proper nutrition, adequate sleep, proper dental care, and injury prevention.

REFERENCES

Bell, D.M., and others: Illness associated with child day care: a study of incidence and cost, Am. J. Public Health 79(4):479-484, 1989.

Edgil, A., Wood, K., and Smith, D.: Sleep problems of older infants and preschool children, Pediatr. Nurs. 11(2):87-89, 1985.

Fish, L., and Burch, K.: Identifying gifted preschoolers, Pediatr. Nurs. 1(2):125-127, 1985.

Food and Nutrition Board, National Research Council: Recommended Dietary Allowances, ed. 10, Washington, DC, 1989, National Academy Press.

Gilliss, C.L., and others: A health-education program for day-care centers, MCN 14:266-268, 1989.

Goldsmith, L.T., and Feldman, D.H.: Identifying gifted children: the state of the art, Pediatr. Ann. 14(10):709-716, 1985.

Goldsmith, S.: Human sexuality: the family source book, St. Louis, 1986, Mosby–Year Book, Inc.

Gordon, S., and Snyder, C.W.: Better sexual health, Boston, 1989, Allyn & Bacon, Inc.

Graziano, A.M., and Mooney, K.C.: Family self-control instruction for children's nighttime fear reduction, J. Consult. Clin. Psychol. 48(2):206-213, 1980.

Green, M.: Helping parents make the right child-care choice, Contemp. Pediatr. 3(6):40-49, 1986.

Greene, J.C., Louie, R., and Wycoff, S.J.: Preventive dentistry. II. Periodontal diseases, malocclusion, trauma, and oral cancer, JAMA 263(3):421-425, 1990.

Haskins, R., and Kotch, J.: Day care and illness: evidence, cost, and public policy, Pediatrics 77(6, Pt. 2):951-982, 1986.

Hobbie, C.: Choosing quality child care programs, J. Pediatr. Health Care 3(5):270-271, 1989.

Howes, C.: Pressuring children to learn versus developmentally appropriate education, J. Pediatr. Health Care 3(4):181-186, 1989.

Kellogg, R.: Understanding children's art. In Readings in Psychology Today, Del Mar, CA, 1969, Communications/Research/Machines/Inc.
Landesman, S.: Defining giftedness, Pediatr. Ann. 14(10):698-706, 1985.
Lee, E.J., and Bass, C.: Survey of accidents in a university day-care center, J. Pediatr. Health Care 4:18-23, 1990.
Lowrey, G.: Growth and development of children, ed. 8, St. Louis, 1986, Mosby–Year Book, Inc.
Maccoby, E.E., and Jacklin, C.N.: Sex differences in aggression: a rejoinder and reprise, Child Dev. 51:964-980, 1980.
McDevitt, S., and Carey, W.: The measurement of temperament in 3-7 year old children, J. Child Psychol. Psychiatry 19:245-253, 1978.
McGuffog, C.: Problems of gifted children, Pediatr. Ann. 14(10):719-726, 1985.
Pearl, D., editor: Television and behavior: ten years of scientific progress and implications for the eighties, U.S. Department of Health and Human Services, No. ADH82-1195, 1982.
Phillips, S., Sarles, R., and Friedman, S.: Consultation and referral: when, why, and how, Pediatr. Ann. 9(7):36-45, 1980.
Pilapil, V.: A horrifying television commercial that led to constipation, Pediatrics 85(4):592-593, 1990.
Rivara, F.P., and others: Risk of injury to children less than 5 years of age in day care versus home care settings, Pediatrics 84(6):1011-1016, 1989.
Robinson, N.M.: Educational options for gifted children, Pediatr. Ann. 14(10):745-756, 1985.
Sacks, J.J., and others: The epidemiology of injuries in Atlanta day-care centers, JAMA 266(12):1641-1645, 1989.
Schor, D.P.: Temperament and the initial school experience, Child. Health Care 13(3):129-134, 1985.
Schraeder, B.D., Heverly, M.A., and Rappaport, J.: Temperament, behavior problems, and learning skills in very low birth weight preschoolers, Res. Nurs. Health 13:27-34, 1990.
Selekman, J.: The development of body image in the child: a learned response, Top. Clin. Nurs. 5(1):12-21, 1983.
Shapiro, B.K., and others: Giftedness: can it be predicted in infancy? Clin. Pediatr. 28(5):205-209, 1989.
Shelly, J., and others: The spiritual needs of children, Downer's Grove, IL, 1982, Inter-Varsity Press.
Shonkoff, J.P.: Preschool. In Levine, M.D., and others, editors: Developmental-behavioral pediatrics, Philadelphia, 1983, W.B. Saunders Co.
Singer, D.G.: Does violent television produce aggressive children? Pediatr. Ann. 14(12):804-810, 1985.
Smith, K.D., Shillam, P.J., and Zimmerman, F.A.: Standards and criteria: group child care for sick children, Pediatr. Nurs. 15(6):600-602, 1989.
Thomas, R.M.: Comparing theories of child development, ed. 2, Belmont, CA, 1985, Wadsworth Publishing Co.
Wald, E.R., and others: Frequency and severity of infections in day care, J. Pediatr. 112(4):540-546, 1988.
Wasserman, R.C., and others: Injury hazards in home day care, J. Pediatr. 114(1, P. 1):591-593, 1989.
Wolman, B.B.: Children's fears, New York, 1978, Grossett & Dunlap.
Wong, D.: Guiding parents in selecting day-care centers, Pediatr. Nurs. 12(3):181-187, 1986.

BIBLIOGRAPHY

References specific to preschoolers are included here; additional references can be found in Chapters 12 and 14.

Growth and Development

Ames, L.B., and Ilg, F.I.: Your three-year-old: friend or enemy, New York, 1980, Delacorte Press.
Ames, L.B., and Ilg, F.I.: Your four-year-old: wild and wonderful, New York, 1981, Delacorte Press.
Ames, L.B., and Ilg, F.I.: Your five-year-old: sunny and serene, New York, 1981, Delacorte Press.
Betz, C.: Faith development in children, Pediatr. Nurs. 7(2):22-25, 1981.
Food and Nutrition Board, National Academy of Sciences, National Research Council, Washington, DC, 1989.
Garbarino, J., and others: What children can tell us, San Francisco, 1989, Jossey-Bass, Inc., Publishers.
Gelman, R., and Baillargem, R.: A review of Piagetian concepts. In Flavell, J., and Markham, E., editors: Handbook of child psychology, vol. 3, New York, 1984, John Wiley & Sons, Inc.
Kay, P.: The imaginary companion: review of the literature, Matern. Child Nurs. J. 9:8-11, 1980.
Larson, C.P., Pless, B., and Miettinen, O.: Preschool behavior disorders: their prevalence in relation to determinants, J. Pediatr. 113:278-285, 1988.
Lowrey, G.: Growth and development of children, ed. 8, St. Louis, 1986, Mosby–Year Book, Inc.
Mitchell, S.: Imaginary companions: friend or foe? Pediatr. Nurs. 6(6):29-30, 1980.
Schickendanz, J., and Schickendanz, D.: Toward understanding children, Boston, 1983, Little, Brown & Co., Inc.
Schraeder, B.D., and Tobey, G.Y.: Preschool temperament of very-low-birth-weight infants, J. Pediatr. Nurs. 4(2):119-126, 1989.
Thomas, A., and Chess, S.: Genesis and evolution of behavioral disorders from infancy to early adult life, Am. J. Psychiatry 141:1-9, 1984.

Preschool or Daycare Experience

American Academy of Pediatrics, Committee on Early Childhood, Adoption, and Dependent Care: The pediatrician's role in promoting the health of a patient in day care, Pediatrics 74(1):157-158, 1984.
American Academy of Pediatrics, Committee on Psychosocial Aspects of Child and Family Health: The mother working outside the home, Pediatrics 73(6):874-875, 1984.
Anderson, L.J., and others: Day-care center attendance and hospitalization for lower respiratory tract illness, Pediatrics 82(3):300-308, 1988.
Bartlett, A.V., Reeves, R.R., and Pickering, L.K.: Rotavirus in infant-toddler day care centers: epidemiology relevant to disease control strategies, J. Pediatr. 113:435-441, 1988.
Birchfield, M.: Illnesses and children in a preschool center, Matern. Child Nurs. J. 15(3):187-197, 1986.
Bonner, A., and Dale, R.: *Giardia lamblia* day care diarrhea, Am. J. Nurs. 86:818-820, 1986.
Child Welfare League of America, Standards for Day Care Service, New York, 1984, The League.
Crowley, A.A.: The child care dilemma: expanding nurse practitioner involvement, J. Pediatr. Health Care 2(3):128-134, 1988.
Dashefsky, B., Wald, E., and Li, K.: Management of contacts of children in day care with invasive *Haemophilus influenzae* type b disease, Pediatrics 78(5):939-940, 1986.
Fleming, D.W., and others: Childhood upper respiratory tract infections: to what degree is incidence affected by day-care attendance? Pediatrics 79(1):55-60, 1987.
Kopac, C.A., and Price, D.: Bringing together the young and old with intergenerational day care, Pediatr. Nurs. 13(4):227-229, 1987.
Makintubee, S., Istre, G.R., and Ward, J.I.: Transmission of invasive *Haemophilus influenzae* type b disease in day care settings, J. Pediatr. 111:180-186, 1987.
Marks, M.I., and Dorchester, W.L.: Secondary rates of *Haemophilus influenzae* type b disease among day care contacts, J. Pediatr. 111(2):305-306, 1987.
Novak, J., and Pecoraro, N.: Policy and position statement: child care, J. Pediatr. Health Care 3(3):158-159, 1989.
Passarelli, C.: Marketing the PNP to day-care centers, Pediatr. Nurs. 13(1):11-14, 1987.

Rapp, G.S., and Lloyd, S.A.: The role of "home as haven" ideology in child care use, Fam. Relations 38:426-430, 1989.

Roberts, M.C., and Broadbent, M.H.: Increasing preschoolers' use of car safety devices: an effective program for day care staff, Child. Health Care 18(3):157-162, 1989.

Schmelzer, M., Reeves, S.R., and Zahner, S.J.: Health services in day-care centers: a public health nursing design, Public Health Nurs. 3(2):120-125, 1986.

Smith, D.: Myths about day care: fact or fantasy? Pediatr. Nurs. 10(4):278-280, 1984.

Smith, D.: Common diseases children contract in day care: patterns and prevention, Pediatr. Nurs. 12(3):175-179, 1986.

Sterne, G.G.: Day care for sick children, Pediatrics 79(3):445-446, 1987.

Summers, K.: Establishment of a hospital based children's sick room, Pediatr. Nurs. 14(1):38-39, 1988.

Wilson, D., and Bess, C.: Establishing a community-based sick child center, Pediatr. Nurs. 12(6):439-441, 1986.

Zigler, E., and Hall, N.W.: Day care and its effect on children: an overview for pediatric health professionals, J. Dev. Behav. Pediatr. 9:38-46, 1988.

Sex Education

Aquilino, M.L., and Ely, J.: Parents and the sexuality of preschool children, Pediatr. Nurs. 11(1):41-46, 1985.

Bullough, V., and Bullough, B.: PNPs, patients, parents, and sexuality, Pediatr. Nurs. 8(3):177-182, 1982.

Calderone, M.S.: Sexual health and the child, Compr. Ther. 6(12):3-7, 1980.

Calderone, M.S.: Adolescent sexuality: elements and genesis, Pediatrics (suppl.) 76(4):699-703, 1985.

Castiglia, P.T.: Masturbation, J. Pediatr. Health Care 2(2):111-112, 1988.

Children's books on sex and siblings, Am. J. Nurs. 79(11):1968, 1979.

Gallo, A.: Early childhood masturbation, Pediatr. Nurs. 5(5):47-49, 1979.

Goldsmith, S.: Human sexuality: the family source book, St. Louis, 1986, Mosby–Year Book, Inc.

Greydanus, D.E., and Geller, B.: Masturbation, N.Y. State J. Med. 80(12):1892-1896, 1980.

Malinowski, J.S.: Answering a child's questions about sex and a new baby, Am. J. Nurs. 79(11):1965-1968, 1979.

Masters, W.H., Johnson, V.E., and Kolodny, R.C.: Human sexuality, ed. 3, Glenview, Ill., 1988, Scott, Foresman & Co.

Aggression

Bloomfield, I.: Psychological aspects of violence and aggression, Int. J. Soc. Psychiatry 26(3):218-221, 1980.

Hayes, S.C., Rincover, A., and Volosin, D.: Variables influencing the acquisition and maintenance of aggressive behavior: modeling versus sensory reinforcement, J. Abnorm. Psychol. 89(2):254-262, 1980.

Jacklin, C.N., and Maccoby, E.E.: Issues of gender differentiation. In Levine, M.D., and others, editors: Developmental-behavioral pediatrics, Philadelphia, 1983, W.B. Saunders Co.

Fears

Derevensky, J.L.: Children's fears: a developmental comparison of normal and exceptional children, J. Genet. Psychol. 135:11-21, 1979.

DuPont, R.L.: Phobias in children, J. Pediatr. 102(6):999-1002, 1983.

Graziano, A.M., Degiovanni, I.S., and Garcia, K.A.: Behavioral treatment of children's fears: a review, Psychol. Bull. 86(4):804-830, 1979.

Miller, S.R.: Children's fears: a review of the literature with implications for nursing research and practice, Nurs. Res. 28(4):217-223, 1979.

Sleep Disturbances

Beltramini, A., and Hertzig, M.: Sleep and bedtime behavior in preschool-aged children, Pediatrics 71(2):153-158, 1983.

Crawford, W., Bennet, R., and Hewitt, K.: Sleep problems in pre-school children, Health Visit 62(3):79-81, 1989.

DiMario, F., and Emery, E.S., III: The natural history of night terrors, Clin. Pediatr. 26(10):505-511, 1987.

Edgil, A., and others: Sleep problems of older infants and preschool children, Pediatr. Nurs. 11(2):87-89, 1985.

Gates, D., and Morwessel, N.: Night terrors: strategies for family coping, J. Pediatr. Nurs. 4(1):48-53, 1989.

McMenamy, C., and Katz, R.C.: Brief parent-assisted treatment for children's nighttime fears, J. Dev. Behav. Pediatr. 10(3):145-148, 1989.

Pagel, J.: Nightmares, Am. Fam. Physician 39(3):145-148, 1989.

Rieger, I.: Sleep disorders in children, Aust. Fam. Physician 18(6):699, 701, 1989.

SUGGESTED READINGS FOR PARENTS ON DAYCARE

Child sexual abuse prevention: tips to parents, U.S. DHHS, National Center on Child Abuse and Neglect, 1984. (Includes an excellent section on choosing a child care center; copies are free from NCCAN Clearinghouse, P.O. Box 1182, Washington, DC 20013.)

Clark-Stewart, A.: Daycare, Cambridge, MA, 1982, Harvard University Press.

Coleman, M., and Priner, P.: What about day care? Columbia, MO, 1980, Missouri Cooperative Extension Service, University of Missouri–Lincoln University. (Single copies are $1.00 and may be ordered from Cooperative Extension Service, 1408 I. 70 Drive, S.W., Columbia, MO 65203.)

Endsley, R.G., and Bradbard, M.: Quality day care: a handbook of choices for parents and caregivers, Englewood Cliffs, NJ, 1981, Prentice-Hall, Inc.

How to choose a good early childhood program, Washington, DC, 1984, National Association for the Education of Young Children. (Single copies are free with a self-addressed, stamped, business-size envelope from NAEYC, 1834 Connecticut Avenue, N.W., Washington, DC 20009; [800] 424- 2460; [202] 232-8777.)

Mitchell, G.: The day care book, Briarcliff Manor, NY, 1979, Stein Day Publishers, Scarborough House.

Plain talk about when your child starts school, Rockville, MD, 1980, National Institute of Mental Health, US DHHS Pub. No. (ADM)80-1021.

Rogers, F.: Going to day care, New York, 1985, G.P. Putnam's Sons. (Recommended for preparing young children for daycare.)

Rogers, F: When your child goes to school, Pittsburgh, Family Communications, Inc.

Scarr, S.: Mother care/other care, New York, 1984, Basic Books, Inc., Publishers.

Seigel-Gorelick, B: The working parent's guide to child care, Boston, 1983, Little, Brown & Co., Inc.

Tips on selecting the "right" day care facility, Elk Grove Village, IL, 1985, American Academy of Pediatrics. (Single copies are $.50 and may be ordered from the Academy, 141 Northwest Point Blvd., Elk Grove Village, IL 60007; [800] 433-9016; [708] 228-5005.)

CHAPTER 16

Health Problems of Early Childhood

RELATED TOPICS

GLOSSARY

airborne Dissemination of microbial aerosols, usually into the respiratory tract; may be droplets or dust

BAL British anti-Lewisite (dimercaptopropanol, dimercaprol)

$CaNa_2EDTA$ Calcium disodium edetate

carrier Person or animal that harbors an infectious agent without apparent clinical disease and serves as a potential source of infection

catarrhal Refers to inflamed mucosa with free discharge

chelation Use of a chemical compound to firmly bind a metal

child maltreatment Broad term that includes intentional physical abuse or neglect, emotional abuse or neglect, or sexual abuse of children, usually by an adult

child molester Older person whose conscious sexual desires or responses are directed toward developmentally immature children or adolescents who do not fully comprehend sexual actions and are unable to give informed consent

child pornography Arranging and photographing in any media sexual acts that involve children, alone or with adults or animals, regardless of consent by legal guardians; also may denote distribution of such material

child prostitution Involving children in sex acts for profit and usually with changing partners

CNS Central nervous system

communicable disease Illness caused by a specific infectious agent or its toxic products through a direct or indirect mode of transmission of that agent from a reservoir

contact Person or animal that has been in association with an infected person, animal, or contaminated environment that might transfer the infective agent

control measures Methods used to prevent spread of an organism

CPS Child Protective Services

direct transmission Direct and immediate transfer of infectious agents either by direct contact (touching, biting, kissing, or sexual intercourse) or by droplet spread usually limited to a distance of about 1 meter or less (sneezing, coughing, spitting, singing, or talking)
EI Erythema infectiosum
emetic Drug that induces vomiting
emotional abuse Deliberate attempt to destroy or significantly impair a child's physical and/or psychologic development
emotional neglect Failure to meet a child's needs for affection, attention, and emotional nurturance
enanthema Eruption on mucous surface
endemic Disease occurring regularly within a geographic location
EP Erythrocyte protoporphyrin
epidemic Disease affecting more than the expected number of persons in a community
exanthema Eruptive rash, fever
exhibitionism Indecent exposure, usually exposure of genitals by an adult male to children or female adults
HGS Herpetic gingivostomatitis
host Living person or animal that provides subsistence or lodging for an infectious agent under natural conditions
HPV Human parvovirus
HSV Herpes simplex virus
incest Any physical sexual activity between family members; blood relationship is not required (can include stepparents, nonrelated siblings); does not include sexual relations between legally sanctioned partners, such as spouses
incubation period Time between infection or exposure to disease and appearance of initial symptoms
indirect transmission Contact with contaminated objects or other infected source
infectious agent Organism capable of producing infection or infectious disease
isolation Separation of infected persons from noninfected persons for the period of communicability under conditions that prevent transmission of the etiologic agent
mode of transmission Mechanism by which an infectious agent is transported from reservoir to susceptible human host
molestation Vague term that includes "indecent liberties" (e.g., touching, fondling, kissing, self-pleasuring, oral-genital contact)
MSP Munchausen syndrome by proxy
NAC *N*-Acetylcysteine
pandemic Disease affecting large portions of the world population
PCC Poison Control Center
pedophilia Literally means "love of child"; does not denote type of sexual activity but the preference of an adult for prepubertal children as a means of achieving sexual excitement
period of communicability Time or times during which an infectious agent may be transferred directly or indirectly from an infected person to another person
physical abuse Deliberate infliction of physical injury
physical neglect Omission of a direct act or behavior with resulting detrimental effects on a child's physical and/or psychologic development
plumbism Chronic lead poisoning
prodromal period Interval between early manifestations of disease and overt clinical syndrome
quarantine Restriction of activities of persons who have been exposed to a communicable disease until the incubation period has expired
reservoir Environment in which an infectious agent lives and multiplies and on which it depends for survival
salicylism Chronic salicylate poisoning
sexual abuse Contacts or interactions between a child and an adult when the child is being used for sexual stimulation of that adult or another person
source of infection Person, object, or substance from which an infectious agent passes immediately to the host
vector Arthropods or other invertebrates that transmit infection by inoculation or deposition of infectious agents on skin, food, or other objects
vehicle Anything serving as an intermediate means by which an infectious agent is transported from reservoir to host, usually objects (fomites), water, soil, food, or biologic products such as plasma
VZIG Varicella zoster immune globulin

This chapter is concerned with health problems that occur most frequently during the early childhood years, such as poisoning and child abuse, and with disease or illness that requires intervention, such as communicable disease. The influence of growth and development on each health problem is of special concern, since the etiology or the treatment may be directly affected by the child's age. Knowledge of the pathologic, psychologic, developmental, and familial variables of the health problem is necessary to plan and provide optimum care that is individualized to meet each child's particular needs.

INFECTIOUS DISORDERS

Young children are especially susceptible to infectious disease, and a number of disorders occur predominantly during these early years. At this age children's resistance to infectious agents may still be low, but their exposure to such agents is beginning to increase as a result of social involvement outside the home. These disorders include typical childhood communicable diseases, conjunctivitis, stomatitis, and intestinal parasitic diseases. Other common infectious diseases, such as otitis media, are discussed in those chapters devoted to specific biologic system disorders.

COMMUNICABLE DISEASES

The incidence of common childhood communicable diseases has declined greatly since the advent of immunizations. Serious complications resulting from such infections have been further reduced through the use of antibiotics and antitoxins. However, infectious diseases do occur, and nurses must be familiar with the infectious agent in order to recognize the disease and institute appropriate preventive and nursing interventions. To facilitate understanding of communicable diseases, several terms are defined in the Glossary at the beginning of this chapter.

Nursing Considerations

The more common communicable diseases of childhood, their therapeutic management, and specific nursing care are described in Table 16-1. The following is a general dis-

Table 16-1 Communicable diseases of childhood

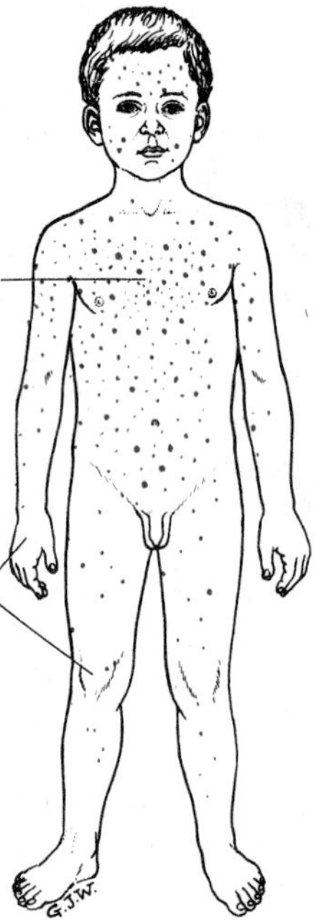

Fig. 16-1. Chickenpox (varicella). (See also Color Plate 1.)

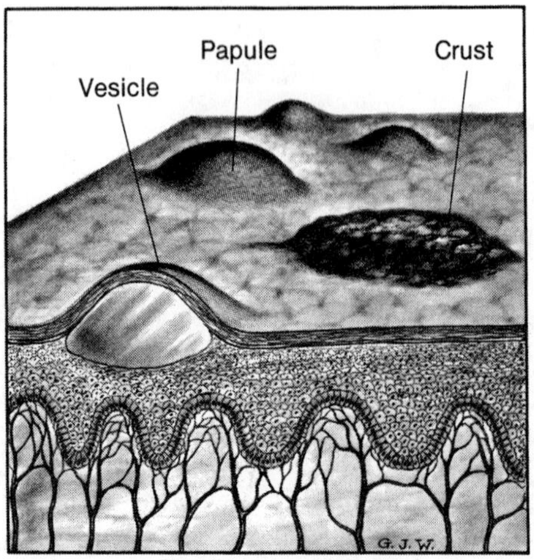

Simultaneous stages of lesions in chickenpox

DISEASE

CHICKENPOX (varicella) (Fig. 16-1)
Agent: varicella zoster
Source: primary secretions of respiratory tract of infected persons; to a lesser degree skin lesions (scabs not infectious)
Transmission: direct contact, droplet spread, and contaminated objects
Incubation period: 2 to 3 weeks, usually 13 to 17 days
Period of communicability: probably 1 day before eruption of lesions (prodromal period) to 6 days after first crop of vesicles when crusts have formed

DIPHTHERIA
Agent: *Corynebacterium diphtheriae*
Source: discharges from mucous membranes of nose and nasopharynx, skin, and other lesions of infected person
Transmission: direct contact with infected person, a carrier, or contaminated articles
Incubation period: usually 2 to 5 days, possibly longer
Period of communicability: variable; until virulent bacilli are no longer present (identified by three negative cultures); usually 2 weeks but as long as 4 weeks

cussion of nursing considerations for communicable diseases. The reader is also referred to Chapter 18 for a discussion of nursing care for dermatologic conditions.

Assessment

Identification of the infectious agent is of primary importance in order to prevent exposure to susceptible individuals. Nurses in ambulatory care settings, such as emergency rooms, health maintenance centers, nursery or regular schools, and physicians' offices, are often the first persons to see signs of a communicable disease, such as a rash or sore throat. The nurse must operate under a high index of suspicion for common childhood diseases in order to identify potentially infectious cases and to recognize diseases that require medical intervention. An example is the com-

Text continued on p. 715.

Table 16-1 Communicable diseases of childhood—cont'd

CLINICAL MANIFESTATIONS	THERAPEUTIC MANAGEMENT/COMPLICATIONS	NURSING CONSIDERATIONS
Prodromal stage: slight fever, malaise, and anorexia for first 24 hours; rash highly pruritic; begins as macule, rapidly progresses to papule and then vesicle (surrounded by erythematous base, becomes umbilicated and cloudy, breaks easily and forms crusts); all three stages (papule, vesicle, crust) present in varying degrees at one time **Distribution:** centripetal, spreading to face and proximal extremities but sparse on distal limbs **Constitutional signs and symptoms:** elevated temperature from lymphadenopathy, irritability from pruritus	**Specific:** usually none; antiviral agent (acyclovir) for infected high-risk children; varicella-zoster immune globulin (VZIG) after exposure in high-risk children **Supportive:** diphenhydramine hydrochloride or antihistamines to relieve itching; skin care to prevent secondary bacterial infection **Complications:** Secondary bacterial infections (abscesses, cellulitis, pneumonia, sepsis) Encephalitis Varicella pneumonia Hemorrhagic varicella (tiny hemorrhages in the vesicles and numerous petechiae in the skin) Chronic or transient thrombocytopenia	Maintain *strict* isolation in hospital Isolate child in home until vesicles have dried (usually 1 week after onset of disease) and isolate high-risk children from infected children Administer skin care: give bath and change clothes and linens daily; administer topical application of calamine lotion; keep child's fingernails short and clean; apply mittens if child scratches Lessen pruritus; keep child occupied Remove loose crusts that rub and irritate skin Teach child to apply pressure to pruritic area rather than scratch it If older child, reason with child regarding danger of scar formation from scratching Avoid use of aspirin; use of acetaminophen controversial
Vary according to anatomic location of pseudomembrane **Nasal:** resembles common cold, serosanguineous mucopurulent nasal discharge without constitutional symptoms; may be frank epistaxis **Tonsillar/pharyngeal:** malaise; anorexia; sore throat; low-grade fever; pulse increased above expected for temperature within 24 hours; smooth, adherent, white or gray membrane; lymphadenitis possibly pronounced (bull's neck); in severe cases, toxemia, septic shock, and death within 6 to 10 days **Laryngeal:** fever, hoarseness, cough, with or without previous signs listed; potential airway obstruction, apprehensive, dyspneic retractions, cyanosis	Antitoxin (usually intravenously); preceded by skin or conjunctival test to rule out sensitivity to horse serum Antibiotics (penicillin or erythromycin) Complete bed rest (prevention of myocarditis) Tracheostomy for airway obstruction Treatment of infected contacts and carriers **Complications:** Myocarditis (second week) Neuritis: abnormal condition characterized by inflammation of a nerve. (neuralgia, hyperesthesia, anesthesia, paralysis, MD, & defective reflexes.	Maintain *strict* isolation in hospital Participate in sensitivity testing; have epinephrine available Administer antibiotics; observe for signs of sensitivity to penicillin Administer *complete* care to maintain bed rest Use suctioning as needed Regulate humidity for optimum liquefaction of secretions Observe respirations for signs of obstruction

Prodrome: an early sign of a developing condition or disease.

The earliest phase of a developing condition or disease.

Continued.

Table 16-1 Communicable diseases of childhood—cont'd

DISEASE

ERYTHEMA INFECTIOSUM (fifth disease)
Agent: human parvovirus B19 (HPV)
Source: infected persons
Transmission: unknown; possibly respiratory secretions and blood
Incubation period: 4 to 14 days, maybe as long as 20 days
Period of communicability: uncertain but before onset of symptoms in most children; also for about 1 week after onset of symptoms in children with aplastic crisis

EXANTHEMA SUBITUM (roseola)
Agent: human herpes virus type 6
Source: unknown
Transmission: unknown (virtually limited to children between 6 months and 2 years of age)
Incubation period: unknown
Period of communicability: unknown

MEASLES (rubeola) (Fig. 16-2)
Agent: virus
Source: respiratory tract secretions, blood, and urine of infected person
Transmission: usually by direct contact with droplets of infected person
Incubation period: 10 to 20 days
Period of communicability: from 4 days before to 5 days after rash appears but mainly during prodromal (catarrhal) stage

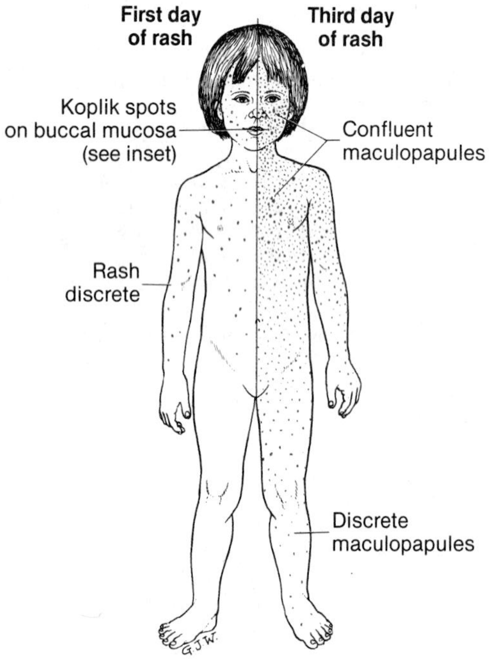

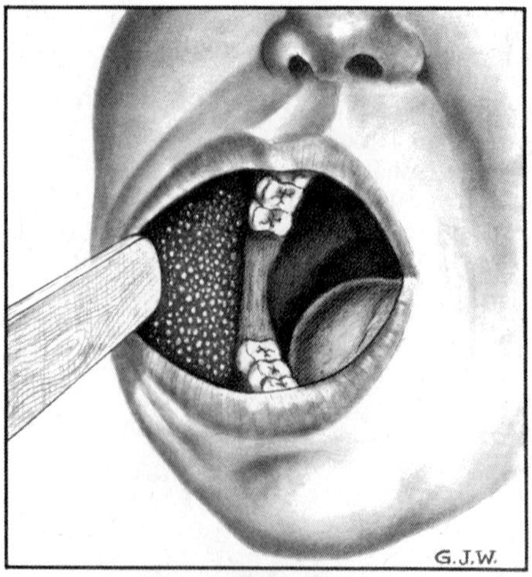

Fig. 16-2. Measles (rubeola). (See also Color Plate 2.)

CLINICAL MANIFESTATIONS	THERAPEUTIC MANAGEMENT/COMPLICATIONS	NURSING CONSIDERATIONS
Rash appears in three stages: *I*—erythema on face, chiefly on cheeks, "slapped face" appearance; disappears by 1 to 4 days (see Color Plate 4) *II*—about 1 day after rash appears on face, maculopapular red spots appear, symmetrically distributed on upper and lower extremities; rash progresses from proximal to distal surfaces and may last a week or more *III*—rash subsides but reappears if skin is irritated or traumatized (sun, heat, cold, friction) In children with aplastic crisis rash is usually absent and prodromal illness includes fever, myalgia, lethargy, nausea, vomiting, and abdominal pain	None necessary **Complications:** Self-limited arthritis and arthralgia May result in fetal death if mother infected during pregnancy but no evidence of congenital anomalies Aplastic crisis in children with hemolytic disease or immune deficiency	Reassure parents regarding benign nature of condition in affected child; isolation of child not necessary Place hospitalized child (immunosuppressed or with aplastic crises) suspected of HPV infection on respiratory and contact isolation Pregnant women: need not be excluded from workplace where HPV infection; should not care for patients with aplastic crises; explain low risk of fetal death to those in contact with affected children
Persistent high fever for 3 to 4 days in child who appears well Precipitous drop in fever to normal with appearance of rash **Rash:** discrete rose-pink macules or maculopapules appearing first on trunk, then spreading to neck, face, and extremities; nonpruritic, fades on pressure, lasts 1 to 2 days (see Color Plate 5) **Associated signs and symptoms:** cervical/postauricular lymphadenopathy, injected pharynx, cough, coryza	Nonspecific Antipyretics to control fever Anticonvulsives for child with history of febrile seizures **Complications:** Febrile seizures	Teach parents measures for lowering temperature (antipyretic drugs) If child is prone to seizures, discuss appropriate precautions Reassure parents regarding benign nature of illness
Prodromal (catarrhal) stage: fever and malaise, followed in 24 hours by coryza, cough, conjunctivitis, Koplik spots (small, irregular red spots with a minute, bluish white center first seen on the buccal mucosa opposite the molars 2 days before rash); symptoms gradually increase in severity until second day after rash appears, when they begin to subside **Rash:** appears 3 to 4 days after onset of prodromal stage, begins as erythematous maculopapular eruption on face and gradually spreads downward; more severe in earlier sites (appears confluent) and less intense in later sites (appears discrete); after 3 to 4 days assumes brownish appearance, and fine desquamation occurs over areas of extensive involvement **Constitutional signs and symptoms:** anorexia, malaise, generalized lymphadenopathy	Vitamin A supplementation **Supportive:** bed rest during febrile period; antipyretics Antibiotics to prevent secondary bacterial infection in high-risk children **Complications:** Otitis media Pneumonia Bronchiolitis Obstructive laryngitis and laryngotracheitis Encephalitis	Isolation until fifth day of rash; if hospitalized, institute respiratory precautions Maintain bed rest during prodromal stage; provide quiet activity **Fever:** instruct parents to administer antipyretics; avoid chilling; if child is prone to seizures, institute appropriate precautions (fever spikes to 40° C [104° F] between fourth and fifth days) **Eye care:** dim lights if photophobia present; clean eyelids with warm saline solution to remove secretions or crusts; keep child from rubbing eyes; examine cornea for signs of ulceration **Coryza/cough:** use cool mist vaporizer; protect skin around nares with layer of petrolatum; encourage fluids and soft bland foods **Skin care:** keep skin clean; use tepid baths as necessary

coryza = runny nose (rhinitis).

Continued.

Table 16-1 Communicable diseases of childhood—cont'd

DISEASE

MUMPS
Agent: paramyxovirus
Source: saliva of infected persons
Transmission: direct contact with or droplet spread from an infected person
Incubation period: 14 to 21 days
Period of communicability: most communicable immediately before and after swelling begins

PERTUSSIS (whooping cough)
Agent: *Bordetella pertussis*
Source: discharge from respiratory tract of infected persons
Transmission: direct contact or droplet spread from infected person; indirect contact with freshly contaminated articles
Incubation period: 5 to 21 days, usually 10
Period of communicability: greatest during catarrhal stage before onset of paroxysms and may extend to fourth week after onset of paroxysms

paroxysm: episodic increase in symptoms. A convulsion, fit, seizure or spasm.

POLIOMYELITIS
Agent: enteroviruses, three types; type 1—most frequent cause of paralysis, both epidemic and endemic, type 2—least frequently associated with paralysis, type 3—second most frequently associated with paralysis
Source: feces and oropharyngeal secretions of infected persons, especially young children
Transmission: direct contact with persons with apparent or inapparent active infection; spread is via fecal-oral and pharyngeal-oropharyngeal routes
Incubation period: usually 7 to 14 days, with range of 5 to 35 days
Period of communicability: not exactly known; virus is present in throat and feces shortly after infection and persists for about 1 week in throat and 4 to 6 weeks in feces

CLINICAL MANIFESTATIONS	THERAPEUTIC MANAGEMENT/COMPLICATIONS	NURSING CONSIDERATIONS
Prodromal stage: fever, headache, malaise, and anorexia for 24 hours, followed by "earache" that is aggravated by chewing **Parotitis:** by third day, parotid gland(s) (either unilateral or bilateral) enlarges and reaches maximum size in 1 to 3 days; accompanied by pain and tenderness **Other manifestations:** submaxillary and sublingual infection, orchitis, and meningoencephalitis	**Symptomatic and supportive:** analgesics for pain and antipyretics for fever Intravenous fluid may be necessary for child who refuses to drink or vomits because of meningoencephalitis **Complications:** Sensorineural deafness Postinfectious encephalitis Myocarditis Arthritis Hepatitis Epididymo-orchitis Sterility (extremely rare in adult males)	Isolation during period of communicability; institute respiratory precautions during hospitalization Maintain bed rest during prodromal phase until swelling subsides Give analgesics for pain; if child is unwilling to chew medication, use elixir form Encourage fluids and soft, bland foods; avoid foods requiring chewing Apply hot or cold compresses to neck, whichever is more comforting To relieve orchitis, provide warmth and local support with tight-fitting underpants (stretch bathing suit works well)
Catarrhal stage: begins with symptoms of upper respiratory infection, such as coryza, sneezing, lacrimation, cough, and low-grade fever; symptoms continue for 1 to 2 weeks, when dry, hacking cough becomes more severe **Paroxysmal stage:** cough most often occurs at night and consists of short, rapid coughs followed by sudden inspiration associated with a high-pitched crowing sound or "whoop"; during paroxysms cheeks become flushed or cyanotic, eyes bulge, and tongue protrudes; paroxysm may continue until thick mucous plug is dislodged; vomiting frequently follows attack; stage generally lasts 4 to 6 weeks, followed by convalescent stage	Antimicrobial therapy (e.g., erythromycin) Administration of pertussis-immune globulin **Supportive treatment:** hospitalization required for infants, children who are dehydrated, or those who have complications Bed rest Increased oxygen intake and humidity Adequate fluids Intubation possibly necessary **Complications:** Pneumonia (usual cause of death) Atelectasis Otitis media Convulsions Hemorrhage (subarachnoid, subconjunctival, epistaxis) Weight loss and dehydration Hernia Prolapsed rectum	Isolation during catarrhal stage; if hospitalized, institute respiratory precautions Maintain bed rest as long as fever present Keep child occupied during day (interest in play associated with fewer paroxysms) Reassure parents during frightening episodes of whooping cough Provide restful environment and reduce factors that promote paroxysms (dust, smoke, sudden change in temperature, chilling, activity, excitement); keep room well ventilated Encourage fluids; offer small amount of fluids frequently; refeed child after vomiting Provide high humidity (humidifier or tent); suction gently but often to prevent choking on secretions Observe for signs of airway obstruction (increased restlessness, apprehension, retractions, cyanosis) Involve public health nurse if child cared for at home
May be manifest in three different forms: **Abortive or inapparent**—fever, uneasiness, sore throat, headache, anorexia, vomiting, abdominal pain; lasts a few hours to a few days **Nonparalytic**—same manifestations as abortive but more severe, with pain and stiffness in neck, back, and legs **Paralytic**—initial course similar to nonparalytic type, followed by recovery and then signs of central nervous system paralysis	No specific treatment, including antimicrobials or gamma globulin Complete bed rest during acute phase Assisted respiratory ventilation in case of respiratory paralysis Physical therapy for muscles following acute stage **Complications:** Permanent paralysis Respiratory arrest Hypertension Kidney stones from demineralization of bone during prolonged immobility	Maintain complete bed rest Administer mild sedatives as necessary to relieve anxiety and promote rest Participate in physiotherapy procedures (use of moist hot packs and range of motion exercises) Position child to maintain body alignment and prevent contractures or decubiti; use footboard Encourage child to move; administer analgesics for maximum comfort during physical activity Observe for respiratory paralysis (difficulty in talking, ineffective cough, inability to hold breath, shallow and rapid respirations); report such signs and symptoms to practitioner; have tracheostomy tray at bedside

Continued.

Table 16-1 Communicable diseases of childhood—cont'd

DISEASE

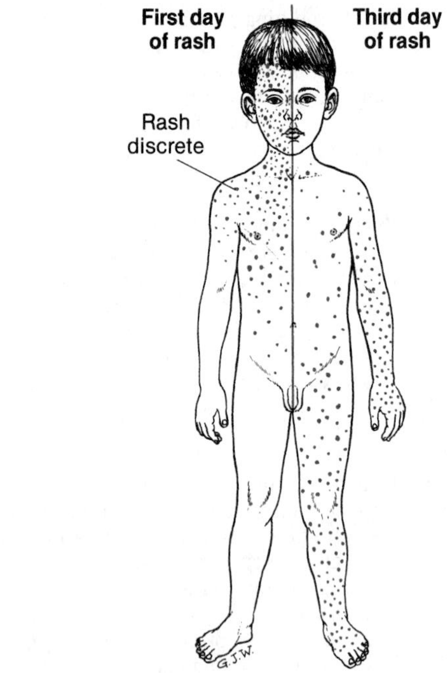

Fig. 16-3. Rubella (German measles). (See also Color Plate 3.)

RUBELLA (German measles) (Fig. 16-3)
Agent: rubella virus
Source: primarily nasopharyngeal secretions of person with apparent or inapparent infection; virus also present in blood, stool, and urine
Transmission: direct contact and spread via infected person; indirectly via articles freshly contaminated with nasopharyngeal secretions, feces, or urine
Incubation period: 14 to 21 days
Period of communicability: 7 days before to about 5 days after appearance of rash

SCARLET FEVER (Fig. 16-4)
Agent: group A β-hemolytic streptococci
Source: usually from nasopharyngeal secretions of infected persons and carriers
Transmission: direct contact with infected person or droplet spread; indirectly by contact with contaminated articles, ingestion of contaminated milk or other food
Incubation period: 2 to 4 days, with range of 1 to 7 days
Period of communicability: during incubation period and clinical illness approximately 10 days; during first 2 weeks of carrier phase, although may persist for months

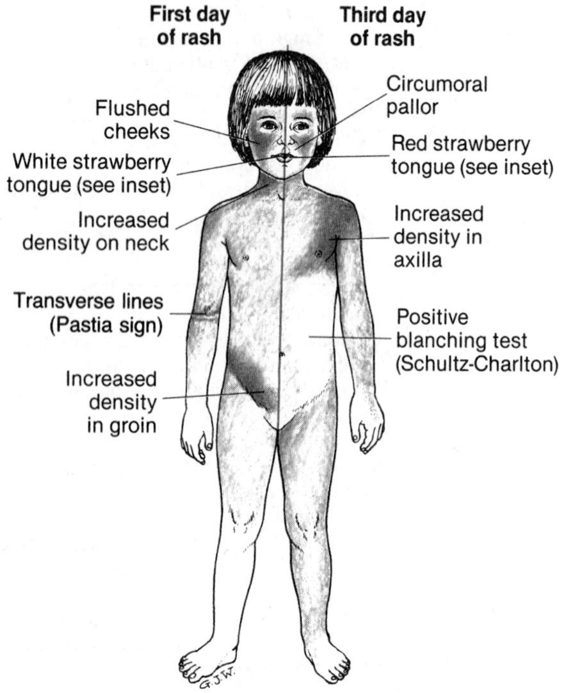

Fig. 16-4. Scarlet fever.

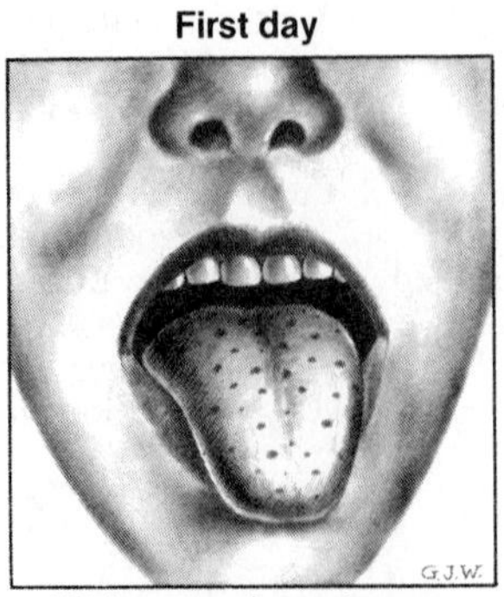

White strawberry tongue

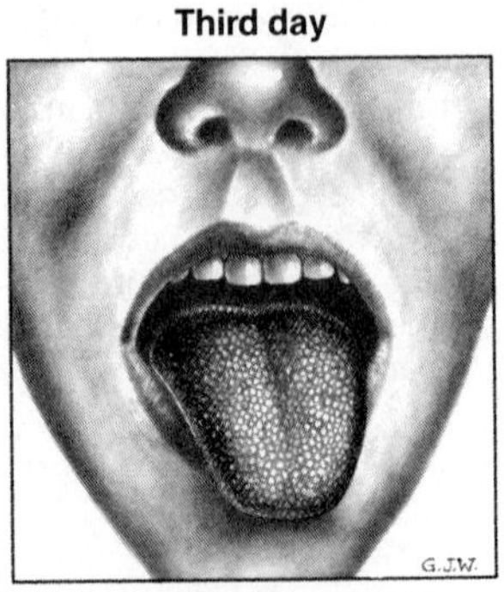

Red strawberry tongue

CLINICAL MANIFESTATIONS	THERAPEUTIC MANAGEMENT/COMPLICATIONS	NURSING CONSIDERATIONS
Prodromal stage: absent in children, present in adults and adolescents; consists of low-grade fever, headache, malaise, anorexia, mild conjunctivitis, coryza, sore throat, cough, and lymphadenopathy; lasts for 1 to 5 days, subsides 1 day after appearance of rash **Rash:** first appears on face and rapidly spreads downward to neck, arms, trunk, and legs; by end of first day body is covered with a discrete, pinkish red maculopapular exanthema; disappears in same order as it began and is usually gone by third day **Constitutional signs and symptoms:** occasionally low-grade fever, headache, malaise, and lymphadenopathy	No treatment necessary other than antipyretics for low-grade fever and analgesics for discomfort **Complications:** Rare (arthritis, encephalitis, or purpura); most benign of all childhood communicable diseases; greatest danger is teratogenic effect on fetus	Reassure parents of benign nature of illness in affected child Employ comfort measures as necessary Isolate child from pregnant women
Prodromal stage: abrupt high fever, pulse increased out of proportion to fever, vomiting, headache, chills, malaise, abdominal pain **Enanthema:** tonsils enlarged, edematous, reddened, and covered with patches of exudate; in severe cases appearance resembles membrane seen in diphtheria; pharynx is edematous and beefy red; during first 1 to 2 days tongue is coated and papillae become red and swollen (white strawberry tongue); by the fourth or fifth day white coat sloughs off, leaving prominent papillae (red strawberry tongue); palate is covered with erythematous punctate lesions **Exanthema:** rash appears within 12 hours after prodromal signs; red pinhead-sized punctate lesions rapidly become generalized but are absent on the face, which becomes flushed with striking circumoral pallor; rash is more intense in folds of joints; by end of first week desquamation begins (fine, sandpaper-like on torso; sheetlike sloughing on palms and soles), which may be complete by 3 weeks or longer	Treatment of choice is a full course of penicillin (or erythromycin in penicillin-sensitive children); fever should subside 24 hours after beginning therapy Antibiotic therapy for newly diagnosed carriers (nose or throat cultures positive for streptococci) **Supportive measures:** bed rest during febrile phase, analgesics for sore throat **Complications:** Otitis media Peritonsillar abscess Sinusitis Glomerulonephritis Carditis, polyarthritis (uncommon)	Institute respiratory precautions until 24 hours after initiation of treatment Ensure compliance with oral antibiotic therapy (intramuscular benzathine penicillin G [Bicillin] may be given if parents' reliability in giving oral drugs is questionable) Maintain bed rest during febrile phase; provide quiet activity during convalescent period Relieve discomfort of sore throat with analgesics, gargles, lozenges, antiseptic throat sprays (Chloraseptic), and inhalation of cool mist Encourage fluids during febrile phase; avoid irritating liquids (citrus juices) or rough foods; when child is able to eat, begin with soft diet Advise parents to consult practitioner if fever persists after beginning therapy Discuss procedures for preventing spread of infection

NURSING CARE PLAN
The Child with a Communicable Disease

NURSING DIAGNOSIS: Potential for infection related to susceptible host and infectious agents

GOAL 1
Prevent disease

INTERVENTIONS
Operate under a high index of suspicion for children who are susceptible to infectious diseases
Identify high-risk children to whom communicable disease may be fatal; in case of an outbreak, advise parents to confine child to the home
Participate in public education regarding prophylactic immunizations, method of spread of communicable diseases, proper preparation and handling of food and water supplies, and control of animal vectors in regard to reservoirs of disease (not a factor in childhood communicable disease but in other infectious illness such as malaria)
Participate in immunization programs or screening programs to identify streptococcal infections

EXPECTED OUTCOME
Susceptible children do not contract the disease

GOAL 2
Prevent spread of disease

INTERVENTIONS
Institute appropriate infection control practices (see Chapter 27)
Make referral to public health nurse when necessary to ensure appropriate procedures in the home
Work with families to ensure compliance with therapeutic regimens
Identify close contacts who may require prophylactic treatment (specific immune globulin or antibiotics)
Report disease to local health department

EXPECTED OUTCOME
Infection remains confined to original source

GOAL 3
Prevent complications

INTERVENTIONS
Ensure compliance with therapeutic regimen (bed rest, antibiotics, adequate hydration)
Institute seizure precautions if febrile convulsions are a possibility
Monitor temperature; unexpected elevations may signal an infection
Attend to good body hygiene
Ensure adequate hydration with small, frequent sips of water or favorite drinks and soft, bland foods (gelatin, pudding, ice cream, soups); feed again after vomiting; observe for signs of dehydration

EXPECTED OUTCOME
Child exhibits no evidence of complications such as infection or dehydration

NURSING DIAGNOSIS: Potential impaired skin integrity related to child's propensity to scratch

GOAL 1
Prevent scratching

INTERVENTIONS
Keep nails short and clean
Apply mittens or elbow restraints
Dress in lightweight, loose, and nonirritating clothing
Cover affected areas (long sleeves, pants, one-piece outfit)
Bathe in cool water with no soap or apply cool compresses
Apply soothing lotions (sparingly on open lesions)
Avoid exposure to heat or sun

EXPECTED OUTCOME
Skin remains intact

NURSING DIAGNOSIS: Pain related to skin lesions, malaise

GOAL 1
Relieve discomfort

INTERVENTIONS
Keep mucous membranes moist with use of cool-mist vaporizer, gargles, and lozenges
Apply petrolatum to chapped lips or nares
Cleanse eyes with physiologic saline solution
Keep skin clean (change bedclothes and linens at least daily)
Administer oral hygiene
Assess need for pain medication (Chapter 26)
Employ nonpharmacologic pain reduction techniques
*Administer analgesics, antipyretics, and antipruritics as needed

EXPECTED OUTCOMES
Skin and mucous membranes are clean and free of irritants
Child exhibits minimal evidence of discomfort (specify)

NURSING DIAGNOSIS: Impaired social interaction related to isolation from peers

GOAL 1
Prepare child for restriction of activities

*Dependent nursing action.

NURSING CARE PLAN
The Child with a Communicable Disease—cont'd

INTERVENTIONS

Explain reason for confinement and use of any special precautions
Allow child to play with gloves, mask, and gown (if used)

EXPECTED OUTCOME

Child demonstrates understanding of restrictions

GOAL 2

Promote social interaction

INTERVENTIONS

Always introduce self to child; allow to see face before donning protective clothing, if required
Provide diversionary activity
Encourage parents to remain with child during hospitalization
Encourage contact with friends via telephone (in hospital can use intercom between room and nurse's station)
Prepare child's peers for altered physical appearance, such as with chickenpox

EXPECTED OUTCOME

Child engages in suitable activities and interactions
Peers accept child

NURSING DIAGNOSIS: Altered family processes related to child with an acute illness

GOAL 1

Provide emotional support

INTERVENTIONS

Reinforce family's effort to carry out plan of care
Provide assistance when necessary, such as visiting nurse to help with home care
Keep family aware of child's progress
Stress rapidity of recovery in most cases

EXPECTED OUTCOMES

Family continues to comply with expectations

mon complaint of sore throat. Although most often a symptom of a minor viral infection, it can signal diphtheria or a streptococcal infection, such as scarlet fever. Each of these bacterial conditions requires appropriate medical treatment to prevent serious sequelae.

Assessment of the following is helpful in identifying potentially communicable diseases: (1) recent exposure to a known case, (2) prodromal symptoms or evidence of constitutional symptoms, such as a fever or rash (see Table 16-1), (3) immunization history, and (4) history of having the disease. Since immunizations are available for several of the diseases and usually an attack confers lifelong immunity, the possibility of many infectious agents can be eliminated based on these two criteria.

The nurse should also be familiar with tests commonly used to confirm or rule out the diagnosis of infectious diseases. The hemagglutination inhibition test is used to detect rubella antibodies; a high antibody titer indicates immunity. Specific tests for scarlet fever include a throat culture and the anti–streptolysin O, which detects rising antibody titer to streptolysin O. A test for diagnosing diphtheria is the Schick test, which detects a reaction to inoculation with diphtheria toxin. Knowledge of test results allows for appropriate decision making regarding the need for treatment or isolation. For example, rubella is a benign childhood disease that requires no special intervention. Ordinarily the recommendation is to confine the child to the home for about 7 days after the appearance of the rash. However, if the mother is in the first trimester of pregnancy, immediate steps need to be taken to isolate the child from the mother if her antibody titer is low. In addition, any pregnant visitors should avoid close contact with the child.

Nursing Diagnoses

A number of nursing diagnoses are prominent in the nursing care of the child with a communicable disease; others are specific to individual cases. The most common nursing diagnoses are presented in the Nursing Care Plan (opposite page and above).

Planning

The principal nursing goals in addition to identification of the communicable disease (see Assessment) are as follows:

1. Prevent spread of infection to others.
2. Prevent complications.
3. Provide comfort measures.
4. Support the child and family.

Implementation

Many of the diseases require only supportive measures until the illness runs its course. Children are usually cared for at home until the disease is no longer communicable and until they feel well enough to resume normal activity.

Prevent spread. Prevention consists of two components: prevention of the disease and control of its spread to others. Primary prevention rests almost exclusively on immunization. (The nurse's role in immunization of children is discussed in Chapter 12.)

Control measures to prevent spread of the disease include appropriate techniques to reduce risk of cross-transmission of infectious organisms between patients and to protect health care workers from organisms harbored by patients. If the child is hospitalized, the facility's policies for isolation precautions are instituted (see Infection Control, Chapter 27). The most important procedure to stress is handwashing. Persons directly caring for the child or handling contaminated articles must wash their hands before beginning care of another patient. The child is instructed to practice good handwashing technique after toileting and before eating. For those diseases spread by droplets, the nurse instructs the family in measures aimed at reducing airborne transmission. The child who is old enough should use a tissue to cover the face during coughing or sneezing; otherwise the parent should cover the child's mouth with a tissue and then discard the tissue. The usual hygiene measures of not sharing eating and drinking utensils should be stressed to the family.

✚ **NURSING ALERT** If a child is admitted to the hospital with an undiagnosed exanthema, strict isolation is instituted until a diagnosis is confirmed. Childhood communicable diseases requiring strict isolation are diphtheria and chickenpox.

Prevent complications. While most youngsters recover without any difficulty, certain groups of children are at risk for serious, even fatal, complications from communicable diseases, especially the viral diseases of chickenpox and erythema infectiosum (EI). Children with an immunodeficiency—those receiving steroid or other immunosuppressive therapy, those with a generalized malignancy such as leukemia or lymphoma, or those with an immunologic disorder—are at risk for viremia from replication of the virus in the blood. Children with hemolytic disease, such as sickle cell disease, are at risk for aplastic anemia from EI. The human parvovirus (HPV) infects and lyses red blood cell precursors, thus interrupting the production of red blood cells. Therefore, in patients who need increased red blood cell production to maintain normal cell volumes, the virus may precipitate a severe aplastic crisis (Gowda and others, 1987). Because of dependence on a high rate of red blood cell production and an immature immune system, the fetus is also vulnerable to severe anemia as a result of HPV infection in the mother.

High-risk children who have signs of these communicable diseases are referred to the practitioner immediately. School nurses who are aware of such susceptible children are responsible for warning the parents about recent outbreaks of these communicable diseases in order to prevent the children's exposure to known cases. In most instances high-risk children are kept out of school until the outbreak is over.

Prevention of complications from diseases such as diphtheria and scarlet fever necessitates parental compliance with antibiotic therapy. Oral preparations are usually prescribed to prevent the trauma of an injection. With oral preparations the need to complete the entire course of therapy is stressed (see Compliance, Chapter 27). Varicella-zoster immune globulin (VZIG) may be given to high-risk children after exposure to chickenpox to prevent the development of varicella. The antiviral agents acyclovir and vidarabine may also be used to treat varicella infections in children with immunodeficiency. Both of these drugs have been shown to decrease the rate and severity of complications from varicella-zoster infections (Balfour and Englund, 1989). Antiviral treatment of chickenpox in healthy children has also been effective in decreasing the number of lesions and promoting faster healing (Balfour and others, 1990). Recent evidence suggests that vitamin A supplementation reduces both morbidity and mortality in measles and that all children with severe measles should be given vitamin A supplements (Hussey and Klein, 1990).

Provide comfort. Many of the communicable diseases cause skin manifestations that are bothersome to the child. The chief discomfort from most of the rashes is itching, and measures such as cool baths (usually without soap) and lotions, such as calamine, are helpful.

✚ **NURSING ALERT** When lotions with active ingredients such as diphenhydramine in Caladryl are used, they are applied sparingly, especially over open lesions where excessive absorption can lead to drug toxicity, and in children simultaneously receiving oral diphenhydramine (Schunk and Svendsen, 1988; Tomlinson, Helfaer, and Weiderman, 1987).

To avoid overheating, which increases itching, children should wear lightweight, loose, nonirritating clothing and keep out of the sun. If the child persists in scratching, the nails are kept short and smooth; mittens and clothes with long sleeves or legs may be needed. For severe itching, antipruritic medication, such as diphenhydramine (Benadryl) or hydroxyzine (Atarax), may be required, especially when the child desires to sleep.

An elevated temperature is common, and both antipyretic medicine (acetaminophen) and environmental manipulation are implemented (see Controlling Elevated Temperatures, Chapter 27). The antipyretic is effective in lowering the fever, but evidence suggests that in chickenpox the medication does not significantly reduce the symptoms of itching, anorexia, abdominal pain, fussiness, or vomiting and that it may delay scabbing of the lesions (Doran and others, 1989).

A sore throat, another frequent symptom, is managed with lozenges, saline rinses (if the child is old enough to cooperate), and analgesics. Since most children are anorectic during an illness, bland foods and increased liquids are usually preferred. During the early stages of the disease children voluntarily curtail their activity, and while bed rest is beneficial, it should not be imposed unless specifically indicated (e.g., in pertussis). During periods of irritability, quiet activity (e.g., reading, music, television, puzzles, coloring) helps distract children from the discomfort.

Support the child and family. Most communicable diseases are benign, but they produce considerable concern and anxiety for some parents. Often the occurrence of a disease such as chickenpox is the first time the child is acutely uncomfortable. Parents need assistance to cope effectively with manifestations of the illness, such as intense itching. Sometimes a visiting nurse may be beneficial to help the family develop a plan of care and encourage compliance with any treatments.

The family and child need reassurance that recovery from the disease is generally rapid. However, visible signs of the dermatosis may be present for some time after the child is well enough to resume usual activities. When the disease involves noticeable signs, such as the crusts of chickenpox, the child benefits from preparation before returning to school. For example, the parent can discuss the child's physical appearance with the teacher and/or school nurse and request that they explain the child's condition to classmates.

Evaluation

The effectiveness of nursing interventions is determined by continual reassessment and evaluation of care based on the following observational guidelines and expected outcomes:

1. Observe or inquire about family members' use of control measures; observe for signs of disease in household contacts.
2. Monitor vital signs, especially temperature; inquire about the identification of high-risk contacts and appropriate isolation of the contact; observe or inquire about compliance with antibiotic therapy.
3. Inquire about effectiveness of comfort measures.
4. Interview family and child regarding their feelings and concerns, especially when child returns to school.

Expected outcomes:
See Nursing Care Plan, pp. 714-715.

CONJUNCTIVITIS

Acute conjunctivitis, inflammation of the conjunctiva, is a common condition in children. It occurs from a variety of causes that are typically age related. In newborns conjunctivitis can occur from infection during birth, most often from *Chlamydia trachomatis* (inclusion conjunctivitis). In infants recurrent conjunctivitis may be a sign of nasolacrimal duct obstruction. In children the usual causes are viral, bacterial, allergic, or related to a foreign body. Bacterial infection accounts for most instances of acute conjunctivitis in children. Diagnosis is made primarily from the clinical manifestations (Box 16-1), although cultures of purulent drainage may be needed to identify the specific infecting agent.

Therapeutic Management

Treatment of conjunctivitis depends on the cause. Viral conjunctivitis and bacterial conjunctivitis are self-limited. However, because bacterial conjunctivitis is highly contagious, it is usually treated with topical antibacterial agents such as polymyxin and bacitracin (Polysporin), which shorten the duration of clinical disease and enhance eradication of the organism (Gigliotti and others, 1984). Drops may be used during the day and an ointment at bedtime because the ointment preparation remains in the eye longer. Ointments are usually not used in the daytime because they blur vision. Corticosteroids are avoided because they reduce ocular resistance to bacteria. Supportive treatment includes removal of the accumulated secretions. (Prevention of neonatal conjunctivitis, or ophthalmia neonatorum, is discussed in Chapter 8.)

Box 16-1 CLINICAL MANIFESTATIONS OF CONJUNCTIVITIS

Bacterial Conjunctivitis ("Pink Eye")
Purulent drainage
Crusting of eyelids, especially on awakening
Inflamed conjunctiva
Swollen lids
Usually both eyes infected

Viral Conjunctivitis
General
Usually occurs with upper respiratory infection
Serous (watery) drainage
Inflamed conjunctiva
Swollen lids

Hemorrhagic
Caused by specific virus, enterovirus 70
Severe inflammation
Subconjunctival hemorrhage
Photophobia

Allergic Conjunctivitis
Itching
Watery to viscous stringy discharge
Inflamed conjunctiva
Swollen lids

Conjunctivitis Caused by Foreign Body
Tearing
Pain
Inflamed conjunctiva
Usually only one eye affected

Nursing Considerations

Nursing goals include keeping the eye clean and properly administering ophthalmic medication. Accumulated secretions are always removed by wiping from the inner canthus downward and outward, away from the opposite eye. Warm, moist compresses, such as a clean washcloth wrung out with hot tap water, are helpful in removing the crusts. Compresses are *not* kept on the eye because an occlusive covering promotes bacterial growth. Medication is instilled immediately after the eyes have been cleaned and according to correct procedure (see Chapter 27).

Prevention of infection in other family members is an important consideration with bacterial conjunctivitis. The child's washcloth and towel are kept separate from those used by others. Tissues used to clean the eye are disposed of properly. The child should not rub the eyes and is instructed in correct handwashing technique.

STOMATITIS

Stomatitis refers to inflammation of the oral mucosa, which may include the buccal (cheek) and labial (lip) mucosa, tongue, gingiva, palate, and floor of the mouth. It may be due to local or systemic factors. In healthy children aphthous stomatitis and herpetic stomatitis are typically seen. Children with immunosuppression and those receiving chemotherapy or head and neck radiotherapy are at high risk for developing mucosal ulceration and herpetic stomatitis (see Management of Problems Related to Irradiation and Drug Toxicity: Mucosal Ulceration, Chapter 36).

Aphthous Stomatitis

Aphthous stomatitis (aphthous ulcer, canker sore) is a benign but painful condition whose cause is unknown. Its onset is usually associated with mild traumatic injury (biting the cheek, hitting the mucosa with a toothbrush, or a mouth appliance rubbing on the mucosa), allergy, and emotional stress. In some children aphthous stomatitis, fever, and pharyngitis occur periodically (usually at 4- to 6-week intervals), although the children grow normally and exhibit no long-term sequelae (Marshall and others, 1987). The lesions are painful, small, whitish ulcerations surrounded by a red border. They are distinguished from other types of stomatitis by healthy adjacent tissues, absence of vesicles, and no systemic illness. The ulcers persist for 4 to 12 days and heal uneventfully.

Herpetic Gingivostomatitis

Herpetic gingivostomatitis (HGS) is caused by the herpes simplex virus (HSV), most often type 1, and may occur as a primary infection or recur in a less severe form known as recurrent herpes labialis (commonly called "cold sores" or "fever blisters"). The primary infection usually begins with a fever; the pharynx becomes edematous and erythematous; and vesicles erupt on the mucosa, causing severe pain (see Color Plate 20). Cervical lymphadenitis often occurs, and the breath has a distinctly foul odor. The disease can last 5 to 14 days with varying degrees of severity.

In the recurrent form the vesicles appear on the lips usually singly or in groups. The precipitating factors for the cold sores include emotional stress, trauma (often related to dental procedures), or exposure to excessive sunlight.

Therapeutic Management

Treatment for both types of stomatitis is aimed at relief of symptoms, primarily pain. Acetaminophen is usually sufficient for mild cases, but with more severe HGS, stronger analgesics such as codeine may be needed. Topical anesthetics are helpful and include over-the-counter preparations, such as Orabase, Anbesol, and Kanka, or prescription formulas, such as viscous xylocaine. A mixture of equal parts of diphenhydramine (Benadryl) elixir and Kaopectate provides mild analgesia, antiinflammatory properties, and a protective coating for the lesions.

Specific treatment for children with severe cases of HGS is the use of acyclovir (Zovirax). Application of tetracycline directly to the lesions can prevent secondary bacterial infection in HGS and may reduce the pain and shorten the course of aphthous stomatitis. The tetracycline tablets are opened, and the powder is applied to the lesions with a cotton-tipped applicator. There is little or no risk of staining of the teeth from the topical use of tetracycline (McDonald and Avery, 1987).

Nursing Considerations

The chief nursing goals for children with stomatitis are relief of pain and prevention of spread of the herpes virus. Analgesics and topical anesthetics are used as needed to provide relief, especially before meals to encourage food and fluid intake. Drinking bland fluids through a straw is helpful in avoiding the painful lesions. Mouth care is encouraged; the use of a very soft bristle toothbrush or disposable foam-tipped toothbrush provides gentle cleaning near ulcerated areas.

Careful handwashing is essential when caring for children with HGS. Since the infection is autoinoculable, children should keep their fingers out of the mouth; contaminated hands also can infect other body parts. Very young children may need elbow restraints to ensure compliance. All articles placed in the mouth are cleaned thoroughly. Newborns and individuals with immunosuppression should not be exposed to infected children.

✦ **NURSING ALERT** When examining herpetic lesions, wear gloves. The virus easily enters breaks in the skin and can cause herpetic whitlow of the fingers.

Because herpes infection is often associated with sexual transmission, the nurse should explain to parents and older children that HGS is usually caused by type 1 HSV, the type not associated with sexual activity (Feldman and Aretakis, 1986).

■ INTESTINAL PARASITIC DISEASES

Intestinal parasitic diseases, including helminths (worms) and protozoa, constitute the most frequent infections in the world, and although many are concentrated in the tropical regions, others are not. A number of these infections are encountered with relative frequency in the United States and are of importance in children in the pediatric age-groups. Young children are especially at risk because of typical hand-mouth activity and uncontrolled fecal habits.

Intestinal parasitic infections in humans are caused by various infecting organisms. This discussion is limited to the two most common parasitic infections among children in the United States—giardiasis and pinworms. Table 16-2 describes the outstanding features of other helminths that belong to the family of nematodes. Most nematodes, with the exception of threadworm and *Toxocara*, are effectively treated with mebendazole, pyrantel pamoate, or piperazine citrate (Table 16-3).

GENERAL NURSING CONSIDERATIONS

Nursing responsibilities related to intestinal parasitic infections involve assisting with identification of the parasite, treatment of the infection, and prevention of initial infection

Table 16-2 Common intestinal parasites

LIFE CYCLE, PATHOGENESIS, TRANSMISSION	CLINICAL MANIFESTATIONS	COMMENTS
▪ **Ascariasis—*Ascaris lumbricoides* (common roundworm)**		
Adult lays eggs in small intestine; eggs deposited in stool; incubation in soil 2-3 weeks; swallowed eggs hatch in small intestine, larvae penetrate intestinal villi, enter portal vein to liver, proceed to lungs, rupture capillaries into respiratory system, ascend to upper passages to be swallowed, proceed to small intestine, and mature into adult worms (total time 2-3 months) Transferred to mouth by way of contaminated food, fingers, toys, etc.	Light infections: asymptomatic Heavy infections: anorexia, irritability, nervousness, enlarged abdomen, weight loss, fever, intestinal colic Severe infections: intestinal obstruction, appendicitis, perforation of intestine with peritonitis, obstructive jaundice, lung involvement—pneumonitis	Largest of the intestinal helminths Affects principally young children 1-4 years of age Prevalent in warm climates
▪ **Hookworm disease—*Necator americanus***		
Worms live in small intestine and feed on villi; process of attachment produces bleeding; ova deposited in bowel, expelled in feces; hatch in damp, shaded soil; larvae attach to skin, penetrate and enter bloodstream, migrate to lungs, exit into alveoli, migrate to upper passages to be swallowed; develop in upper intestine Transmitted by discharging eggs on the soil and in turn pick up infection from direct skin contact with contaminated soil	Light infections in well-nourished individuals; no problems Heavier infections: mild to severe anemia, malnutrition May be itching and burning ("ground itch") followed by erythema and a papular eruption in areas to which organism migrates	Wearing shoes is recommended, although children playing in contaminated soil expose many skin surfaces
▪ **Strongyloidiasis—*Strongyloides stercoralis* (threadworm)**		
Life cycle similar to that of hookworm, except that worm is not attached to intestinal mucosa and feeding larvae (not eggs) may be deposited in soil; also sometimes penetrate colonic mucosa and enter systemic circulation, migrate to respiratory structures, and are subsequently swallowed Transmission is same as for hookworm except autoinfection common	Light infection: asymptomatic Heavy infection: respiratory signs and symptoms; abdominal pain, distention; nausea and vomiting; diarrhea—large, pale stools, often with mucus Threat to life in children with weakened immunologic defenses	Older children and adults affected more often than young children Severe infections may lead to severe nutritional deficiency
▪ **Visceral larva migrans—*Toxocara canis* (dogs)** **Intestinal toxocariasis—*Toxocara cati* (cats)**		
In natural host (dog or cat), larvae migrate to liver and lungs and reach maturity in intestines; when ingested by immature host (human), larvae migrate aimlessly to become encapsulated in muscles and organs such as liver, lungs, kidney, eye, and brain; most serious are those in eye and central nervous system Transmitted by direct contamination of hands from contact with dog, cat, or objects or ingestion of soil	Depends on reactivity of infected individual May be asymptomatic except for eosinophilia Specific diagnosis difficult	Dogs and cats should be kept away from areas where children play; sandboxes especially important transmission areas Periodic deworming of diagnosed dogs and cats Control of dog population Continued education and laws to prevent indiscriminate canine defecation
▪ **Trichuriasis—*Trichuris trichiura* (whipworm)**		
Adult worms live in the cecum; in heavy infections, also in the colon and rectum; passed in feces, slow development in soil (3-4 weeks); eggs swallowed, larvae hatch in small intestine, penetrate villi and mature; return to lumen and migrate to cecum Transmitted from contaminated soil, vegetables, toys, and other objects	Light infections: asymptomatic Heavy infections; abdominal pain and distention; diarrhea	Most frequent in warm, moist climates Occurs most often in undernourished children living in unsanitary conditions

Table 16-3 Drugs used to treat intestinal parasitic infections

DRUG/PEDIATRIC DOSAGE	SIDE EFFECTS	COMMENTS
Furazolidone (Furoxone) 1.25 mg/kg q.i.d. × 10 days (maximum 100 mg q.i.d.)	Nausea Vomiting Headache Hemolysis possible in glucose-6-phosphate dehydrogenase (G-6-PD) deficiency	Drug of choice for giardiasis if cost is not a factor Contraindicated during pregnancy
Mebendazole (Vermox) 100 mg b.i.d. × 3 days 100 mg × 1 dose (repeat in 2 weeks for pinworm)	Occasional, transient abdominal pain Diarrhea in massive infection with expulsion of worms	Drug of choice of hookworm, roundworm, pinworm, and whipworm Tablets may be chewed, crushed, or mixed with food Not recommended during pregnancy Recommended for children over 2 years
Metronidazole (Flagyl) 15 mg/kg/day (maximum 750 mg) t.i.d. × 10 days	Nausea Diarrhea Vomiting Metallic taste Abdominal cramps Headache	May be ineffective in children receiving phenobarbital Not recommended during pregnancy
Piperazine citrate (Antepar) 75 mg/kg/day (maximum 3.5 g) × 2 days (repeat in 2 weeks for pinworm)	Nausea Vomiting Diarrhea Abdominal cramping Urticaria	Side effects are rare with recommended dose May exacerbate seizures in children with seizure disorders
Pyrantel pamoate (Antiminth) 11 mg/kg × 1 dose (maximum 1 g) (repeat in 2 weeks for pinworm)	Nausea Vomiting Diarrhea Abdominal cramps Tenesmus	Side effects are rare with recommended dose Little published data on safety in pregnant women and children under 2 years of age Protect drug from light
Pyrvinium pamoate (Povan) 5 mg/kg × 1 dose (maximum 350 mg) (repeat in 2 weeks for pinworm)	Nausea Vomiting Diarrhea Abdominal cramping	Alternative drug for pinworms Warn parents that drug stains stool and vomitus bright red, as well as clothing or skin if in contact with drug Swallow tablets whole to avoid staining teeth
Quinacrine (Atabrine) 6 mg/kg/day (maximum 300 mg) t.i.d. × 7 days	Nausea Vomiting Temporary discoloration of skin, sclera, and urine	Highest frequency of side effects Take with meals to decrease gastric upset Advise parents of benign discoloration which may take 3 months to fade Crush tablets and mix with strong flavoring (e.g., jam) to disguise bitter taste
Thiabendazole (Mintezol) 25 mg/kg b.i.d. (maximum 3 g/day) × 2 days	Drowsiness Dizziness Giddiness Headache Impaired alertness and coordination	Treatment for severe cases of *Toxocara;* also used for threadworm Use with caution in patients with renal or hepatic dysfunction Warm parents of drowsiness and dizziness in child Administer after meals

or reinfection. Identification of the organism is accomplished by laboratory examination of substances containing the worm, its larvae, or embryonated ova. Most are identified by examining feces smears from the stools of persons suspected of harboring the parasite. Stool specimens should be large enough to obtain an ample sampling, not merely a fecal fragment. Specimens are easily obtained from diapers, although the stool should not be contaminated with urine. (For toilet-trained children, see Nursing Tip.) Fresh specimens are best for revealing parasites or larvae; therefore collected specimens should be taken directly to the laboratory for examination. If this is not feasible, the specimen is placed in a container with a preservative. Parents need clear instructions on obtaining an adequate sam-

NURSING TIP: STOOL SPECIMEN

To obtain a stool specimen for identification of ova and parasites, place plastic wrap over the toilet bowl to collect the stool. Use a tongue depressor or disposable spoon or knife to collect the stool and place the specimen in a covered disposable cup or plastic bag.

ple and the number of samples required (see Collection of Specimens, Chapter 27).

In most parasitic infections, examination of other family members, especially children, may be carried out to identify those who are similarly affected. Nurses frequently assume the responsibility for directing and instructing the families in the collection and disposition of specimens. The treatment regimen may need further explanation and reinforcement, particularly when it involves other household members and care of clothing and bed linen. When other members are treated, the family needs to understand the nature of transmission and that in some cases the medication must be repeated in 2 weeks to 1 month to kill organisms hatched since initial treatment.

The nurse's most important function in relation to these parasites is preventive education of children and families regarding good hygiene and health habits. Careful handwashing before eating or handling food and after using the toilet is the most important precautionary method. Other preventive practices are listed in the Parent Guidelines on p. 722.

GIARDIASIS

Giardiasis is caused by the protozoan, *Giardia lamblia* (also called *G. intestinalis, G. duodenalis,* and *Lamblia intestinalis*). It is the most common intestinal parasitic pathogen in the United States, and its prevalence among children in daycare centers has been reported to be as high as 47% (Steketee and others, 1989). Risk factors for children attending daycare centers include longer duration of total attendance, increased weekly attendance, low family income, and large family size (four or more members) (Novotny and others, 1990). Breast milk plays a protective role in infants exposed to these organisms (Pickering and Engelkirk, 1988).

Life Cycle, Pathogenesis, and Transmission

Infection begins with ingestion of the cysts, the nonmotile stage of the protozoa. The stomach acid activates the cysts, which then pass into the duodenum. Following completion of excystation, trophozoites (parasites in their active feeding stage) emerge and colonize the distal duodenum and proximal jejunum. As the cycle continues, cysts are passed in feces; they are not infective initially but must complete a process of maturation requiring hours to days. Cysts can survive in the environment for months (Craft, 1985). The mechanism of pathogenesis is not known.

Chief modes of transmission are person-to-person; water, especially mountain lakes, streams, and pools frequented by diapered infants; food; and animals, possibly puppies. In children, person-to-person transmission is the most likely cause.

Clinical Manifestations

Although individuals infected with giardiasis may be asymptomatic, young children, especially infants, usually manifest symptoms such as diarrhea, vomiting, anorexia, and failure to thrive. Children over 5 years of age most often complain of abdominal cramps with intermittent loose stools and constipation. The stools may be malodorous, watery, pale, and greasy. Most infections resolve spontaneously in 4 to 6 weeks, except in rare instances in which the infection becomes chronic and may last for months or years. The chronic form is usually associated with intermittent loose, foul-smelling stools with or without abdominal bloating, flatulence, sulfur-tasting belches, epigastric pain, vomiting, headache, and weight loss.

Diagnostic Evaluation

Unlike most other intestinal parasites, *G. lamblia* is not easily diagnosed from stool specimens. Since *Giardia* organisms are excreted in a highly variable pattern, six or more stool specimens collected over several weeks may be necessary to identify the trophozoites or cysts.

Since the organism lives in the upper intestine, aspiration or biopsy of the duodenum or upper jejunum may be performed. The string test may be used to aspirate duodenal fluid directly. A nylon string is attached to a gelatin capsule, which is swallowed; several hours later the string is withdrawn and the contents are examined microscopically for trophozoites (Pickering and Engelkirk, 1988). Other tests that may be used to detect *Giardia* antigen in the stool are counterimmunoelectrophoresis (CIE) and enzyme-linked immunosorbent assay (ELISA).

Therapeutic Management

Three drugs are available for treatment of giardiasis (see Table 16-3). The drug of choice is quinacrine, based on economics (it is less than one-tenth the cost of furazolidone) and inadequate knowledge of the long-term safety of metronidazole. Unfortunately, quinacrine has the highest frequency of side effects, especially nausea and vomiting; causes temporary yellow staining of the skin, sclera, and urine; and has a very bitter taste (Turner, 1985).

Nursing Considerations

The most important nursing consideration is prevention of giardiasis, especially among children attending daycare centers and the staff. Attention to meticulous sanitary practices, especially during diaper changes, is essential (see Parent Guidelines on p. 722 and Fig. 16-5). Nurses can play an important role in educating daycare staff regarding appropriate sanitation.

Once children are infected, compliance with the treatment is essential and the interventions suggested in Table

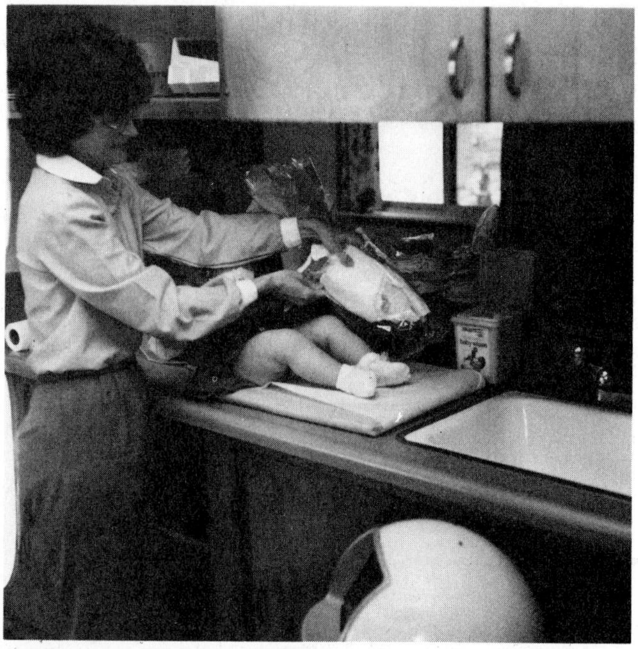

Fig. 16-5. Prevention of giardiasis, especially in daycare centers, requires sanitary practices during diaper changes such as wrapping diapers in plastic bags and discarding in a covered receptacle.

PARENT GUIDELINES
Preventing Intestinal Parasitic Disease

Always wash hands and fingernails with soap and water before eating and handling food and after toileting.
Avoid placing fingers in mouth and biting nails.
Discourage children from scratching bare anal area.
Change diapers as soon as soiled and dispose of in plastic bags in closed receptable out of children's reach.
Disinfect toilet seats and diaper changing areas; use dilute household bleach (1:10 solution) or Lysol and wipe clean with paper towels.
Drink water that is specially treated, especially if camping.
Wash all raw fruits and vegetables or food that has fallen on the floor.
Avoid growing foods in soil fertilized with human excreta.
Teach children to defecate only in a toilet, not on the ground.
Keep dogs and cats away from playgrounds or sandboxes.
Avoid swimming in pools frequented by diapered children.
Wear shoes outside.

16-3 for the administration of quinacrine are given to parents. If other household members are infected, the nurse should inquire about any pregnant members, since treatment for giardiasis is contraindicated during pregnancy.

ENTEROBIASIS (PINWORMS)

Enterobiasis, or pinworms, caused by the nematode *Enterobius vermicularis,* is reported to be the most common helminthic infection in the United States. It is universally present in temperate climatic zones, and may infect 32% of all U.S. children at any one time (Cheng, 1986). However, some evidence suggests that the incidence is declining (Vermund and MacLeod, 1988). Crowded conditions, such as in classrooms and daycare centers, favor transmission.

Life Cycle, Pathogenesis, and Transmission

Infection begins when the eggs are ingested or inhaled. The eggs hatch in the upper intestine, mature in 2 to 4 weeks, and migrate to the cecal area. The females then mate, migrate out the anus, and lay up to 17,000 eggs (Cheng, 1986). The movement of the worms on skin and mucous membrane surfaces causes intense itching, and since the surface of the eggs is durable and adhesive, they easily adhere to almost any surface. As the child scratches, eggs are deposited on the hands and under the fingernails. The typical hand-to-mouth activity of youngsters makes them especially prone to continual reinfection. Pinworm eggs also persist in the environment for up to a week or longer, contaminating anything they contact, such as toilet seats, doorknobs, bed linen, underwear, and food. Since they float in the air, they are also easily inhaled.

Clinical Manifestations

The principal symptom of pinworms is intense perianal itching. However, in young children who have difficulty verbalizing this discomfort, general irritability, restlessness, poor sleep, bed-wetting, distractibility, and short attention span should arouse suspicion that the disorder is present. In females the worms may migrate to the vagina and urethra to cause infection.

Diagnostic Evaluation

The most common test for diagnosing pinworms is the tape test (see Nursing Considerations). The worms may also be identified by using a flashlight to inspect the anal area while the child sleeps. It is best not to place underpants on the child to avoid disturbing the child as much as possible. If worms are found, this can be very upsetting to parents, a fact that should be considered before recommending this procedure.

Therapeutic Management

Four drugs are available for treatment of pinworms (see Table 16-3). The drug of choice is mebendazole, which is safe, effective, convenient, and has few side effects. However, it is not recommended for children under 2 years of age or for pregnant women. Since pinworms are easily transmitted, all household members are treated. Any of the drugs is repeated in 2 weeks to prevent reinfection.

Nursing Considerations

Nursing care is directed at identifying the parasite, eradicating the organism, and preventing reinfection. Parents need clear, detailed instructions for the tape test. A loop of transparent (not "frosted") tape, sticky side out, is placed around the end of a tongue depressor, which is then firmly pressed against the child's perianal area. A convenient commercially prepared tape is also available for this purpose. Pinworm specimens are collected in the morning as soon as the child awakens and *before* the child has a bowel movement or bathes. The procedure may need to be repeated more than once before eggs are collected. Parents are instructed to place the tongue blade in a glass jar or loosely in a plastic bag so that it can be brought in for microscopic examination. For specimens collected in the hospital, practitioner's office, or clinic, the tape is placed smoothly on a glass slide, sticky side down, for examination.

Compliance with the drug regimen is usually excellent because the duration of treatment is typically only one dose. However, the family is reminded of the need to take a second dose in 2 weeks. Posting a reminder on the refrigerator door or bathroom mirror is helpful.

To prevent reinfection, certain cleaning practices, such as washing all clothes and bed linen in hot water and vacuuming the house, may be recommended. However, there is little documentation of their effectiveness, since pinworms survive on so many surfaces. Helpful suggestions include handwashing after toileting and before eating, disposing of diapers in a closed receptacle as soon as they are soiled, and keeping the child's fingernails short to minimize the chance of ova collecting under the nails, dressing children in one-piece sleeping outfits, and daily showering rather than tub bathing.

INGESTION OF INJURIOUS AGENTS

Since the passage of the Poison Prevention Packaging Act of 1970, which provides that certain potentially hazardous drugs and household products be sold in child-resistant containers, the incidence of poisonings in children has decreased dramatically. However, despite these advances, poisoning remains a significant health concern, with most cases occurring in children under 4 years of age (Unintentional poisoning, 1989). Children are poisoned by a variety of substances (Box 16-2), although not all common household items are toxic (Box 16-3; see also Box 16-6). Knowledge of nontoxic substances prevents unnecessary crises in the family and overtreatment. More than 90% of poisonings occur in the home (Litovitz, Schmitz, and Holm, 1989), although a significant number take place elsewhere, especially in a grandparent's or friend's home (Polakoff and others, 1984).

The developmental characteristics of young children predispose them to poisoning by ingestion. Infants and toddlers explore their environment through oral experimentation. Since the sense of taste is less discriminatory at this age, many unpalatable substances are ingested. In addition, toddlers and preschoolers are developing autonomy and initiative, which increase their curiosity and exploration. Imitation is also a powerful motivator, especially when combined with lack of awareness of danger.

This section is primarily concerned with the immediate emergency treatment of ingestion of injurious agents and the specific management of plant, corrosive, hydrocarbon, acetaminophen, salicylate, iron, and lead poisoning. Appropriate suggestions for prevention are discussed briefly on p. 726 and in Chapter 14 under Poisoning.

Box 16-2 MOST FREQUENTLY REPORTED POISONING IN CHILDREN LESS THAN 6 YEARS OF AGE

Nonpharmaceuticals	Total Number*
Cosmetics/personal care products (perfume, cologne, aftershave)†	92,560
Cleaning products (hypochlorite ["household"] bleach)	87,393
Plants (pothos, devil's ivy)	79,350
Hydrocarbons (gasoline)	26,317
Insecticides, pesticides, rodenticides	31,542
Arts, crafts, and office supplies	19,163
Chemicals (alkali)	16,215
Alcohols (isopropanol ["rubbing"] alcohol)	15,463
Pharmaceuticals	
Analgesics (pediatric acetaminophen)	77,241
Cough and cold preparations	58,899
Topicals (diaper care products)	40,069
Vitamins (pediatric multiple vitamins with iron, no fluoride)	30,326
Antimicrobials (antibiotics)	28,058
Gastrointestinal preparations (antacids)	22,426

Data from Litovitz, T., Schmitz, B., and Holm, K.: 1988 annual report of the American Association of Poison Control Centers National Data Collection System, Am. J. Emerg. Med. 7(5):495-545, 1989.
*In 1 year; represents categories with more than 15,000 ingestions reported.
†Most common substances in each category are in parentheses. Substances ingested are not necessarily most toxic but often represent ready availability.

Box 16-3 COMMON NONTOXIC INGESTIONS

Antacids	Makeup (some types)
Antibiotics	Pencil lead
Ballpoint pen inks	Petroleum jelly
Calamine lotion	Play-Doh and modeling clay
Candles	Sachets (essential oils, powders)
Chalk	Shampoos
Crayons	Suntan products
Deodorants	Thermometer mercury (ingested only)
Fabric softeners	Toothpaste (without fluoride)
Glues and pastes	Vitamins without iron
Hair products	Zinc oxide
Hand lotions and creams	
Lubricants	

From Barkin, R., and Rosen, P.: Emergency pediatrics, ed. 3, St. Louis, 1990, Mosby–Year Book, Inc.

PRINCIPLES OF EMERGENCY TREATMENT

A poisoning may or may not require emergency intervention, but in every instance medical evaluation is necessary to initate appropriate action. Parents are advised to call the Poison Control Center (PCC) *before* initiating any intervention, since instructions on labels of many household products are not correct treatment measures. The local PCC telephone number (usually listed in the front of the telephone directory*) should be posted near each phone in the house.

Based on the initial telephone assessment, the PCC counsels the parents to begin treatment at home and/or to bring the child to an emergency facility. When a call is taken, the caller's name and telephone number is recorded to reestablish contact if the connection is interrupted. Since most poisonings are managed outside health care facilities, usually at the patient's home, expert advice is essential in minimizing adverse effects. When the exact quantity or type of ingested toxin is not known, admission to a hospital for laboratory evaluation and surveillance for signs of poisonings (Table 16-4) is critical during the postingestion period.

General guidelines for emergency home treatment of poisoning are listed on p. 725. Selected interventions, especially those that require professional intervention, are discussed next.

*Also available by calling (800) 555-1212 for any state in the United States.

Table 16-4 Common signs of poisoning

GENERAL SIGNS	SPECIFIC SIGNS
Gastrointestinal system Abdominal pain Vomiting Diarrhea Anorexia **Respiratory/circulatory system** Depressed respirations Labored respirations Unexplained cyanosis Signs of shock: increased, weak pulse; decreased blood pressure; increased, shallow respiration; pallor; cool, clammy skin **Central nervous system** Convulsions Overstimulation Sudden loss of consciousness Dizziness Stupor, lethargy Coma	**Corrosives** Severe burning pain in mouth, throat, stomach White, swollen mucous membranes; edema of lips, tongue, pharynx (respiratory obstruction) Violent vomiting, hemoptysis Drooling and inability to clear secretions Signs of shock Anxiety and agitation **Hydrocarbons** Gagging, choking, coughing Nausea Vomiting Alterations in sensorium, e.g., lethargy Weakness Respiratory symptoms of pulmonary involvement Tachypnea Cyanosis Retractions Grunting **Salicylates** Nausea Disorientation Vomiting Dehydration Diaphoresis Hyperpnea Hyperpyrexia Oliguria Tinnitus Coma Convulsions

Assessment

The first and most important principle in dealing with a poisoning is to treat the child first, not the poison. This necessitates an immediate concern for life support; vital signs are taken and respiratory and/or circulatory support instituted as needed. The victim's condition is routinely reevaluated. The increased recovery rate from acute poisonings is largely attributable to vigorous use of supportive measures after symptoms appear. Since shock is a complication of several types of household poisons, particularly corrosives, measures to reduce the effects of shock, such as elevation of legs and head to the level of the heart to promote venous drainage and provision of warmth and rest, are important. Maintenance of respiratory function may require mouth-to-mouth resuscitation or insertion of an airway and/or mechanical ventilation.

The emergency room nurse's responsibility is to be prepared for immediate intervention with any of the necessary equipment. Since time and speed are critical factors in recovery from serious poisonings, anticipation of potential problems and complications may mean the difference between life and death.

Gastric Decontamination

In general, the immediate treatment is to remove the ingested poison by inducing vomiting. The preferred method for use at home is to administer ipecac syrup, an emetic that exerts its action by direct stimulation of the vomiting center and through an irritant effect on the gastric mucosa.

✦ **NURSING ALERT** The use of an emetic is generally contraindicated in conditions that increase the risk of aspiration and when emesis of the poison, such as a corrosive, redamages the mucosa of the esophagus and pharynx.

Proper administration of ipecac is essential (see Emergency Treatment). Ipecac is available in 1-ounce (30 ml) vials. However, the label information does not include directions for a second dose if the child fails to vomit after the first dose. Therefore parents need clear instructions for proper use and dose. As a precaution, parents are advised to have full doses of ipecac for *each child* in the home, to carry the emetic when traveling, and to be certain that other caregivers (baby-sitters or relatives) have the emetic available. Because children share activities, it is not uncommon for more than one child to ingest the toxic substance. In an emergency ipecac can be obtained from an all-night pharmacy, convenience store, emergency squad, or emergency department. It is inexpensive and has a shelf life of 16 years (Boehnert and others, 1985). Neither milk, fluid volume, food, nor activity level alter ipecac's effectiveness (Grbcich and others, 1987a, 1987b; Rodgers and Matyunas, 1986). Therefore the common suggestions of forcing fluids and encouraging movement are unnecessary. Despite the fact that ipecac is highly effective, its use as a home emetic is a

QUESTIONS AND CONTROVERSIES

Should ipecac be available by prescription only, and should activated charcoal be used in the home?

Ipecac is considered the emetic of choice for removal of toxic substances from the stomach. However, concern exists over its ready availability, specifically its abuse by individuals with anorexia nervosa and bulimia and by parents who intentionally poison their children with ipecac (Munchausen syndrome by proxy) (Friedman, 1984; McClung and others, 1988; Sutphen and Saulsbury, 1988). In some countries other than the United States, ipecac is available only with a prescription. This practice, however, severely limits its timely use during home management of poisonings.

Prompt administration of ipecac (within 30 minutes) results in significantly less absorption of the poison than delayed administration of ipecac (about 80 minutes) (Amitai and others, 1987b). When ipecac is administered in the home, many children avoid a visit to an emergency department. It has been estimated that 100,000 unnecessary emergency department visits can be avoided using ipecac in the home. As one author states, "Anorexia nervosa, bulimia, and Munchausen syndrome by proxy are complex psychologic problems that will not be solved by restricting the sale of ipecac syrup" (Litovitz, 1988). Unfortunately, surveys of households with children reveal that ipecac is not widely available. Some experts suggest that not only should ipecac remain a nonprescription drug, but that practitioners should regularly dispense it while providing pediatric care to increase its availability in the home (Malloy and Rhoads, 1988).

Some professionals question the effectiveness of ipecac in preventing absorption of ingested toxins. Some believe that activated charcoal is significantly more effective for many more poisons than can be removed by ipecac-induced vomiting (Vale, Meredith, and Proudfoot, 1986). For example, one study showed that using activated charcoal alone resulted in lower plasma levels of the poison than using ipecac before arrival at the emergency room followed by activated charcoal in the emergency room (Albertson and others, 1989).

Some also suggest that activated charcoal should be replaced as the home remedy. Activated charcoal is safe and highly effective in preventing absorption of many poisons. However, the many arguments against its home use include (1) availability—not a stock item in all stores; (2) dosage—must be based on kilograms of body weight, which is more difficult for parents; (3) compliance—children often refuse to drink the black liquid; and (4) interference with an emetic—if used with ipecac, activated charcoal must be given after the emetic, and parents may not remember the correct sequence (Dockstader, Lawrence, and Bresnick, 1986; Greensher and others, 1987). In addition, commercial preparations of activated charcoal are not without risks. Premixed suspensions of activated charcoal and 70% sorbitol (used to improve its palatability and to act as a cathartic) have caused severe dehydration in young infants (Farley, 1986; McCord and Okun, 1987).

EMERGENCY TREATMENT
Poisoning

1. Assess the victim:
   a. Take vital signs; reevaluate routinely.
   b. Initiate cardiorespiratory support if needed.
   c. Treat other symptoms, such as seizures.
2. Terminate exposure:
   a. Empty mouth of pills, plant parts, or other material.
   b. Flush eyes continuously for 15 to 20 minutes.
   c. Flush skin and wash with soap and a soft cloth; remove contaminated clothes, especially if a pesticide, acid, alkali, or hydrocarbon is involved.
   d. Bring victim of an inhalation poisoning into fresh air.
   e. Give water to dilute ingested poison.
3. Identify the poison:
   a. Question the victim and witnesses.
   b. Save all evidence of poison (empty bottle, opened container, vomitus, urine).
   c. Be alert to signs and symptoms of potential poisoning in absence of other evidence (see Table 16-4).
   d. Call Poison Control Center or other competent emergency facility for immediate advice regarding treatment.
4. Remove poison and prevent absorption:
   a. Induce vomiting; administer ipecac if ordered:
      —6 to 12 months: 10 ml; do not repeat.
      —1 to 12 years: 15 ml; repeat dosage *once* if vomiting has not occurred within 20 minutes.
      —Over 12 years: 30 ml; repeat dosage *once* if vomiting has not occurred within 20 minutes.
      —Give 10 to 20 ml/kg of clear fluids after ipecac.
   b. Do not induce vomiting if:
      —Victim is comatose, in severe shock, or convulsing or has lost the gag reflex.
      —Poison is a low-viscosity hydrocarbon (unless it contains a more toxic substance, e.g., pesticide or heavy metal) or a strong acid or alkali.
   c. Place child in side-lying, sitting, or kneeling position with head below chest to prevent aspiration.
   d. Administer activated charcoal (usual dose 1 g/kg) 30 to 60 minutes *after* vomiting from ipecac, if ordered.

source of dispute (see Questions and Controversies).

If the child is admitted to an emergency facility, gastric lavage may also be done to empty the stomach of the toxic agent. Lavage is indicated for young infants in whom ipecac is contraindicated; if the patient is comatose or convulsing or requires a protected airway; or if the ingested poison is rapidly absorbed (strychnine or cyanide). The use of lavage in petroleum distillate poisoning remains controversial because of the danger of aspiration. When lavage is performed, the largest-diameter tube that can be inserted is used to facilitate passage of gastric contents.

Another method of decontaminating the stomach is the use of activated charcoal, an odorless, tasteless, fine black powder that adsorbs many compounds, creating a stable complex. It is used within 1 hour of the poisoning but *after* giving an emetic, to avoid the charcoal also adsorbing the emetic and preventing its pharmacologic effect. It is mixed with water or saline cathartic to form a slurry. Slurries are

NURSING TIP: ACTIVATED CHARCOAL

To increase the child's acceptance of activated charcoal, mix it with flavoring or a sweetener and serve through a straw and in an opaque glass with a cover, such as a disposable coffee cup and lid or an ordinary cup covered with aluminum foil or placed inside a small paper bag.

neither gritty nor distasteful but resemble black mud. (To increase their acceptability, see Nursing Tip.) Sorbitol, an artificial sweetener, is added to many commercial preparations (SuperChar, Actidose) as a flavoring and a cathartic. However, concentrated amounts of sorbitol have been known to cause severe dehydration in infants (see Questions and Controversies). Cathartics, such as sodium or magnesium, may be administered to stimulate evacuation of the bowel, thus decreasing systemic absorption of the poison and aiding in removal of the charcoal. However, the use of cathartics is controversial.

Activated charcoal is also used in multiple doses to reduce systemic absorption of many toxic agents, even overdoses of intravenous drugs. The presence of activated charcoal in the gut is thought to create "gastrointestinal dialysis." The gut mucosa assumes the properties of a dialysis membrane, permitting drugs to diffuse from the vascular space into the gut lumen, where they can be bound by activated charcoal and excreted in the stool (Mofenson and others, 1985).

In a minority of poisonings specific antidotes are available to counteract the poison. They are highly effective and should be available in all emergency facilities. The supply of antidotes should be checked routinely and replaced as used or according to expiration dates. Among the more commonly employed antidotes are *N*-acetylcysteine for acetaminophen poisoning, oxygen for carbon monoxide inhalation, naloxone for opioid overdose, Digibind for digoxin toxicity, and antivenin for certain poisonous bites.

Family Support

A poisoning is more than a physical emergency for the child. It usually represents an emotional crisis for the parents, particularly in terms of guilt, self-reproach, and insecurity in the parenting role. The emergency room is no place to admonish the family for negligence, lack of appropriate supervision, or failure to safe-proof the home. Rather it is a time to calm and support the child and parents, while unaccusingly exploring the circumstances of the injury. If the nurse prematurely attempts to discuss ways of preventing such an incident from recurring, the parents' anxiety will block out any suggestions or offered guidance. Therefore it is preferable for the nurse to delay the discussion until the child's condition is stabilized or, if the child is discharged immediately after emergency treatment, to make a public health referral.

Box 16-4 QUESTIONNAIRE FOR POISON PREVENTION

1. Where do I store cleaning products, medicines, laundry aids, and garden supplies?
2. What do I keep under the sink in the kitchen and bathroom?
3. Do I have any medicines (e.g., pain relievers, tranquilizers, birth control pills, antacids) in my purse?
4. Are all the medicines and household products clearly labeled and in their original container?
5. Do I refer to medicine as candy to encourage my child to take it?
6. Are any medications left on the table or kitchen counter for handy use?
7. Do I keep drugs prescribed for previous illnesses?
8. Is my child out of sight when I take medicine?
9. When using any medicine or household product, do I keep my eye on it at all times, put it away immediately after use, or put it down where my child cannot get it?
10. Are any of my garden plants or houseplants poisonous?
11. Do all cabinets that store toxic products have a lock on them?
12. What is stored in the garage or basement?
13. Are paints, gasoline, solvents, insecticides, poisons, and fertilizers either on a high shelf or locked in a cabinet?
14. Do I teach my child never to touch any nonfood item without asking me first?

NURSING TIP: PREVENTING POISONING

Encourage parents to bend down to the child's eye level and survey the home environment for potential hazards. Have the parents try to open cabinets and reach shelves to access poisons.

Prevention of Recurrence

The ultimate objective is to prevent poisonings from occurring or recurring. One effective counseling method is first to discuss the difficulties of constantly watching and safeguarding young children. In this way the monumental task of raising children is shared as a common problem, with injury prevention as one part of the parental role, not as the central issue. This approach also incorporates other contributory causes for the incident, such as inadequate support systems, marital discord, discipline techniques (especially use of physical punishment), and maternal distress (Bithoney and others, 1985). A visit to the home, especially after a repeat poisoning situation, is recommended as part of the follow-up care to assess hazards, including family factors, and to evaluate appropriate safe-proofing measures. One method of identifying risk areas is to ask specific questions or to have the parent complete a questionnaire designed to isolate factors that predispose children to poisoning. (See Nursing Tip.)

Box 16-4 is a sample questionnaire of items that may de-

Box 16-5 TEACHING STRATEGY FOR PARENT EDUCATION AND PREPARATION FOR ACCIDENTAL POISONING

Question	Intervention
If you suspected that your child had ingested (eaten) a poison, what would you do first?	If answer is correct, ask for more specifics, such as telephone number of local poison control center If answer does not include knowledge of local poison control center, supply information Stress necessity of not wasting time and of saving all evidence of poisoning
Do you have ipecac syrup in your home?	If answer is yes, ask for specific directions concerning its dosage and readministration If answer is no, supply correct information
Should you always make the child vomit?	If answer is no, ask for specific poisons that are treated differently, such as turpentine and drain cleaner If answer is yes, supply correct information Emphasize that instructions on container of household products are minimum and sometimes inaccurate emergency treatment; medical advice should *always* be sought before relying on that information alone
If you suspected that your child had taken a poison, but there were no signs of illness and the child denied doing so, what would you do?	Emphasize need to always seek medical advice rather than waiting for signs or believing the child

termine what environmental manipulation is needed to "poison-proof" homes. A teaching plan designed to assess parents' preparedness in case of an accidental poisoning and to supply appropriate strategy and instruction where necessary is presented in Box 16-5. Such tools enable nurses to counsel families systematically and efficiently in the area of injury prevention.

Passive measures (those that do not require active participation) have been the most successful in preventing poisoning and include child-resistant closures and a limited number of tablets in one container, such as bottles of baby aspirin. Other preventive methods include the use of warning labels, such as Mr. Yuk or a skull and crossbones, to alert children to potential dangers. However, the effectiveness of such labels is questionable. One study found that children actually preferred to touch labeled containers after undergoing education incorporating Mr. Yuk stickers (Vernberg, Culver-Dickinson, and Spyker, 1984). If labeling is used, it must be combined with parental counseling and emphasis on proper storage of poisonous agents. Poison warning stickers with information about the local PCC should be placed by each telephone in the house. Other important information to include by the telephone is the home address with the nearest cross street in case an ambulance is needed. In an emergency family members may not remember the house address, and baby-sitters may not be aware of the information.

Even in the busiest health care facilities, poison prevention can be effective. Reminding parents of the telephone number of the local PCC, encouraging them to have ipecac in the home for emergency use, and counseling them on correct use of the emetic can increase their readiness in the event of a poisoning (Woolf and others, 1987). (See Nursing Care Plan: The Child with Poisoning.*)

PLANT POISONING

Plant parts are one of the most common foreign substances ingested by children. Fortunately, most of these children are not seriously affected and do not require hospitalization. However, some are severely, even fatally, poisoned. Given the abundance of plants both in and outside the home, it is essential that parents be advised of this danger. Some of the more common poisonous plants as well as nontoxic varieties that can be safely grown are listed in Box 16-6. Preventive measures include (1) placing houseplants out of young children's reach, such as on high shelves or in hanging baskets; (2) teaching children *never* to eat anything without parental permission; and (3) avoiding making teas or homemade medicines from plants. Treatment is usually symptomatic and supportive. If the plant ingested cannot be identified, careful observation without aggressive intervention is recommended (McGuigan, 1984).

CORROSIVE POISONING

Corrosive or caustic substances include strong acids or alkalis that cause chemical burns of mucosal surfaces (see Table 16-4 for signs of poisoning). Numerous household products are corrosive, including drain, toilet, or oven cleaners; electric dishwasher detergents; some detergents or cleansers; mildew remover; batteries; Clinitest tablets; and denture cleaners. Household bleach, the most frequent corrosive material ingested, is considered an irritant because it does not cause mucosal ulceration. Disk batteries can cause severe esophageal perforations if the strong alkaline liquid in the battery leaks following ingestion. Liquid products cause more damage than granular substances because they are swallowed more easily and can damage the mucosa as far down as the duodenum, whereas granular material adheres to the oral mucosa and causes burns limited to the oropharyngeal area. Alkaline products have a neutral taste and may be swallowed in greater quantity than acids. The very unpleasant taste of acids frequently causes

*In Wong, D.L., and Whaley, L.F.: Clinical manual of pediatric nursing, ed. 3, St. Louis, 1990, Mosby–Year Book, Inc.

Box 16-6 POISONOUS AND NONPOISONOUS PLANTS

Poisonous Plants	Toxic Parts	Nonpoisonous Plants
Apple	Leaves, seeds	African violet
Apricot	Leaves, stem, seed pits	Aluminum plant
Azalea	Foliage and flowers	Asparagus fern
Buttercup	All parts	Begonia
Cherry (wild or cultivated)	Twigs, seeds, foliage	Boston fern
Chrysanthemum	All parts	Christmas cactus
Daffodil	Bulbs	Coleus
Dumb cane, dieffenbachia	All parts	Gardenia
Elephant ear	All parts	Grape ivy
English ivy	All parts	Jade plant
Foxglove	Leaves, seeds, flowers	Piggyback begonia
Holly	Berries	Piggyback plant
Honeysuckle	All parts	Poinsettia†
Hyacinth	Bulbs	Prayer plant
Ivy	Leaves	Rubber tree
Mistletoe*	Berries, leaves	Snake plant
Oak tree	Acorn, foliage	Spider plant
Philodendron	All parts	Swedish ivy
Plum	Pit	Wax plant
Poison ivy, poison oak	Leaves, fruit, stems, smoke from burning plants	Weeping fig
Pothos	All parts	Zebra plant
Rhubarb	Leaves	
Tulip	Bulbs	
Water hemlock	All parts	
Wisteria	Seeds, pods	
Yew	All parts	

*Eating one or two berries or leaves is probably nontoxic (Hall, Spoerke, and Rumack, 1986).
†Mildly toxic if ingested in massive quantities.

early gagging and choking. Chemical epiglottitis from acid contacting the mucosa can occur and cause airway occlusion from the resulting edema (Friedman, 1989).

Vomiting is contraindicated in the treatment of corrosives, since emesis can cause repeated damage to the mucosal wall. Emergency care is aimed at preventing further damage by diluting the corrosive agent with water, if it does not induce vomiting. Milk is not recommended by some authorities because it coats the mucous membranes and may obscure the surface for evaluation of burns. Neutralization with vinegar or lemon juice is contraindicated because the neutralizing reaction may produce heat, thus causing a thermal burn in addition to the chemical burn. Other aspects of care include providing a patent airway if necessary, administering analgesics for pain, and giving the child either nothing by mouth or only a liquid diet if tolerated. Long-term care may involve repeated dilatation or surgery to correct an esophageal stricture. A potential sequela is the development in adulthood of squamous cell carcinoma at the site of the stenosis. These children need to be instructed as young adults to seek medical advice immediately if dysphagia develops.

HYDROCARBON POISONING

Hydrocarbons refer to organic compounds that contain carbon and hydrogen; many, but not all, hydrocarbons are distillates of petroleum. Hydrocarbons of concern if ingested include gasoline, kerosene, lamp oil, mineral seal oil (a product found in furniture polish), lighter fluid, turpentine, many paint thinners and removers, and certain furniture polishes and cleaning agents—all products that may be found in the home and garage. Because they are frequently stored incorrectly in unmarked containers and may have a pleasant aroma, they are often ingested by young children (Klein and Simon, 1986).

The immediate danger from most hydrocarbons is aspiration, since even small amounts aspirated into the lungs can cause severe, sometimes fatal, chemical pneumonitis (see Table 16-4 for signs of poisoning). However, adverse systemic effects from gastrointestinal absorption are usually mild. High-viscosity (thick) hydrocarbons, such as Vaseline, vegetable oil, or mineral oil, are nontoxic and may have a laxative effect if large amounts are ingested. Distillates that have high volatility (evaporate quickly), low viscosity, and low surface tension, such as gasoline, kerosene, lighter fluid, mineral seal oil, or turpentine, cause the most severe pneumonitis because they tend to spread easily over a large surface area.

The initial management of the child with hydrocarbon poisoning includes stabilization of vital signs, administration of oxygen as needed, and decontamination of the child by removing clothing and washing skin that has come in contact with the poison. Treatment of the ingestion is controversial. Gastric emptying is generally not attempted because of the risk of further aspiration of the hydrocarbon. However, gastric emptying using lavage may be indicated for severe gastrointestinal symptoms or when hydrocarbons contain other toxic chemicals, such as camphor (causes central nervous system [CNS] excitement or depression); halogenated hydrocarbons (produce hepatitis, nephritis, diarrhea, and CNS excitement or depression); aromatics (result in aplastic anemia, dysrhythmias, and CNS and respiratory depression); heavy metals (result in gastrointestinal bleeding, renal failure, and neurologic sequelae); and pesticides (cause cholinergic signs and symptoms). These toxic additives may be collectively referred to as CHAMP (Barkin and Rosen, 1990).

ACETAMINOPHEN POISONING

Acetaminophen is increasingly used as a mild analgesic/antipyretic drug, especially as a substitute for aspirin, and is the most common source of drug poisoning among children. It is available in many palatable forms that are well accepted by youngsters and in many drug dosages that are easily misused by parents (causing both underdosing and overdosing) (Gribetz and Cronley, 1987).

Acetaminophen poisoning occurs primarily from acute overdose. A toxic dose is 150 mg/kg of body weight, but in children that dose may not produce severe toxicity (Barkin and Rosen, 1990). Toxicity from chronic therapeutic use is rare but has been reported in children. Ingestion of approximately 150 mg/kg/day, or about double the recommended maximum therapeutic dose (90 mg/kg/day) of acetaminophen, for several days results in toxicity (Henretig and others, 1989).

Pathophysiology and Clinical Manifestations

Acute overdose of acetaminophen results in hepatic damage. The damage is not from the drug itself but from one of its metabolites, which in large quantities is toxic to the liver cells. Normally the liver produces the substance glutathione, which combines with the metabolite to negate its toxic effect; the detoxified combination is excreted through the kidneys. However, large doses of acetaminophen exceed the liver's supply of glutathione, allowing the metabolite to cause hepatic necrosis. Signs and symptoms occur in four stages if the poisoning is untreated (Box 16-7).

Diagnostic Evaluation

Because of the initially mild symptoms, diagnosis is confirmed by serum acetaminophen levels drawn at least 4 hours after ingestion; toxic levels are 150 μg/ml at 4 hours and 37.5 μg/ml at 12 hours (Barkin and Rosen, 1990). Liver and kidney function tests are performed to assess the pathologic effect of toxicity on these two organs.

Therapeutic Management

Initial management depends on the amount presumed ingested and the serum acetaminophen level. Emesis or lavage may be indicated, with or without the subsequent use of activated charcoal. A definitive treatment for acetaminophen toxicity is the use of the antidote *N*-acetylcysteine (NAC) (concentrated form of Mucomyst). NAC functions as a glutathionine substitute and binds with the metabolite so that the liver is protected. It may be given orally (mixed with cola or fruit juice) every 4 hours for a total of 18 doses. Because of its offensive odor (similar to rotten eggs), the nasogastric route may be used. When activated charcoal is administered, the charcoal is removed by lavage before administering the antidote either orally or nasogastrically. NAC may also be given intravenously over 20 hours. Available data indicate that the oral administration of the antidote is as effective as the intravenous regimen and that oral NAC may be superior when treatment is delayed (Smilkstein and others, 1988).

Box 16-7 STAGES OF CLINICAL MANIFESTATIONS IN ACETAMINOPHEN POISONING

1. **Initial period** (2 to 4 hours after ingestion)
   Nausea
   Vomiting
   Sweating
   Pallor
2. **Latent period** (24 to 36 hours)
   Patient improves
3. **Hepatic involvement** (may last up to 7 days)
   Pain in right upper quadrant
   Jaundice
   Confusion
   Stupor
   Coagulation abnormalities
4. **Recovery**
   Patients who do not die in hepatic stage gradually recover

Nursing Considerations

Nursing goals are essentially the same as those discussed for salicylate poisoning (see p. 730). If oral NAC is ordered, acceptance by the child is a nursing challenge. With continued resistance, passing a nasogastric tube may be less stressful to the child than trying to administer the oral preparation.

As with any poisoning, the primary goal is prevention. With the present emphasis on acetaminophen as a "safe" substitute for aspirin, it is important to stress that in excess this drug, as with any other, is capable of toxic and lethal side effects.

SALICYLATE POISONING

Aspirin (acetylsalicylic acid), the most common salicylate, can cause both acute and chronic poisoning in children. In recent years the incidence of acute salicylate poisoning has declined, primarily because of child-resistant closures, limited quantity of the drug per container, and the association of Reye syndrome with aspirin ingestion (Arrowsmith and others, 1987).

Chronic poisoning (salicylism) occurs from administration of multiple doses of the drug in dosages that are excessive but below acute toxic levels. The most frequent causes for misuse of aspirin are parents' misunderstanding of health professional's instructions, incorrect dosage information from health professionals, use of aspirin without medical supervision, and use of several aspirin-containing products simultaneously (McGuigan, 1983).

Another source of acute salicylate intoxication is methyl salicylate, which is commercially available in oil of wintergreen, a flavoring agent. One teaspoon of oil of wintergreen, which is about one "swallow," contains the equivalent of 5 g of salicylate or 21.7 adult aspirin tablets–an amount that can be fatal to a child (Howrie, Moriarty, and Breit, 1985). Toxicity occurs more rapidly because of increased absorption.

Salicylate toxicity is dose related. Acute ingestions of less than 150 mg/kg are mildly toxic; ingestion of 150 to 300 mg/kg constitutes moderate toxicity. Severe toxicity results when 300 to 500 mg/kg or more is ingested (Temple, 1981). Chronic ingestions of more than 100 mg/kg/day for 2 days or more may produce toxicity (the usual therapeutic dose of aspirin is 65 mg/kg/day) (McGuigan, 1983).

Pathophysiology and Clinical Manifestations

Toxic amounts of salicylates directly affect the respiratory system. Hyperventilation, the most obvious clinical manifestation of salicylate overdose, causes loss of carbon dioxide and respiratory alkalosis. Signs of respiratory alkalosis include confusion, loss of consciousness, and, if not treated, coma and death from respiratory failure. Salicylates also increase metabolism, resulting in greater oxygen consumption, carbon dioxide production, and heat production, which is manifest as hyperpyrexia. Metabolic acidosis occurs from the accumulation of ketones and other organic acids and results in symptoms of anorexia, vomiting, and diaphoresis.

In a chronic overdose, salicylates can cause bleeding tendencies because aspirin inhibits platelet aggregation and prothrombin production. The other symptoms of chronic poisoning are similar to acute overdose but are more subtle during onset, tend to be more severe, especially dehydration, coma, and/or seizures (Gaudreault, Temple, and Lovejoy, 1982), and may be confused with the illness being treated. Therefore chronic poisoning can be a more serious intoxication than with acute ingestions.

Diagnostic Evaluation

Aspirin exerts its peak effect in 2 to 4 hours, and its effects may last for as long as 18 hours. There is usually a delay of up to 6 hours before evidence of toxicity is noted. This delay represents a serious diagnostic problem, because by the time symptoms are evident, pathophysiologic disturbances are fairly advanced. Since the manifestation of symptoms is delayed, laboratory tests to determine serum salicylate levels are essential. These levels are compared to a special chart (nomogram) that determines the degree of toxicity from the time of ingestion.

Therapeutic Management

Treatment depends on the amount of the drug ingested. Salicylate ingestions of less than 300 mg/kg can be managed at home by inducing vomiting if treatment is not delayed. When a substantial amount of time passes between ingestion and initiation of treatment, the child should be brought to a health care facility.

Severe intoxications are managed in a health care facility. The immediate treatment is removal of the drug from the stomach either by forced emesis or gastric lavage, followed by the administration of activated charcoal and a cathartic. Further therapy depends on serum salicylate levels and clinical manifestations. The acid-base disturbances are treated with appropriate electrolyte transfusions. Intravenous administration of sodium bicarbonate facilitates salicylate excretion. Calories and fluids are supplied to meet the increased metabolic rate. The hyperpyrexia is controlled with cool sponges and hypothermia blankets to reduce the possibility of convulsions. Vitamin K may be administered to decrease bleeding tendencies. In extreme cases of salicylate poisoning, external removal of the drug may be attempted through peritoneal dialysis or hemodialysis, but such intervention is usually reserved for life-threatening intoxication.

Nursing Considerations

The major nursing objectives are removal of the poison, observation of latent effects from the overdose, assistance with any medical treatments of the complications, prevention of recurrence of the poisoning, and emotional support of the child and parents. Relevant interventions are discussed under Principles of Emergency Treatment and in Box 16-5.

Prevention of acute ingestion involves the same precautions as recommended for any toxic substance. However, many parents are unaware of the danger of methyl salicylate, especially since oil of wintergreen is sold as a food additive and may not be perceived as potentially toxic. Therefore public education is essential to prevent this uncommon but life-threatening poisoning.

Of special concern is prevention of chronic salicylate poisoning. Parents need education regarding the current recommendation of avoiding aspirin use in children. When purchasing nonprescription remedies, such as cold preparations, parents must check labels for the addition of aspirin to the product.

HEAVY METAL POISONING

Heavy metal poisoning can occur from the ingestion of a variety of substances, the most common being lead. Other sources that are important in terms of children are iron (see following section) and mercury. Mercury, a rare form of heavy metal poisoning, has occurred in children from a variety of sources, such as broken thermometers or thermostats, broken fluorescent lights, and use of interior latex house paint (Mack, 1989; Mercury exposure, 1990). Elemental mercury (also called metallic mercury or quicksilver) is nontoxic if ingested. However, mercury is volatile at room temperature and enters the bloodstream after it is inhaled, causing toxicity (tremors, memory loss, insomnia, gingivitis, diarrhea, anorexia, weight loss). The classic form of mercury poisoning is called *acrodynia* (or "painful extremities"). To prevent inhalation, spilled mercury must be cleaned up quickly, using disposable towels and rubber gloves and washing the hands well after removing the spill.

Heavy metals have an affinity for certain essential tissue chemicals, which must remain free for adequate cell functioning. When metals are bound to these substances, cellular enzyme systems are inactivated. Consequently the pathologic effects and treatment are similar to those for lead poisoning. Differences involve the body systems affected and the choice of chelating agent.

IRON POISONING

The most frequent source of iron poisoning in young children is pediatric formulations of multiple vitamins with iron. Factors thought to be responsible for the frequency of these iron ingestions include widespread availability, large number of tablets prescribed and packaged, failure of parents to recognize the potential lethality of iron, and failure of safety closures (Banner and Tong, 1986). The similarity between enteric-coated iron tablets and candy-coated choc-

Box 16-8 STAGES OF CLINICAL MANIFESTATIONS IN IRON POISONING

1. **Initial period** (½ to 6 hours after ingestion)
   Vomiting
   Hematemesis
   Diarrhea
   Hematochezia (bloody stools)
   Gastric pain
2. **Latency** (2 to 12 hours)
   Patient improves
3. **Systemic toxicity** (4 to 24 hours)
   Metabolic acidosis
   Fever
   Hyperglycemia
   Bleeding
   Shock
   Death (may occur)
4. **Hepatic injury** (48 to 96 hours)
   Seizures
   Coma
5. **Late sequelae**
   Rarely pyloric stenosis develops at 2 to 5 weeks

olate, such as M&Ms, contributes to their attractiveness to children.

The toxic dose of an iron ingestion is based on the amount of elemental iron in various salts (sulfate, gluconate, fumarate), which ranges from 20% to 33%. Ingestions of 60 mg/kg are considered dangerous (Barkin and Rosen, 1990).

Iron is toxic to several body systems, and intoxication produces five distinct stages of clinical manifestations (Box 16-8).

Diagnostic Evaluation

Diagnosis is based on the calculation of ingested elemental iron and the child's clinical status, especially presence of spontaneous vomiting, diarrhea, and epigastric pain. Specific tests include serum iron, total iron-binding capacity (TIBC), blood glucose, and abdominal radiographs for presence of iron masses. A serum concentration of greater than 500 μg/dl strongly supports the need for aggressive therapy.

Therapeutic Management

Initial management consists of forced emesis or lavage; the administration of sodium bicarbonate via lavage is controversial. For severe intoxication, chelation therapy with deferoxamine is instituted. In rare instances surgical removal of large amounts of iron tablets may be warranted. Supportive care includes preventing shock and maintaining adequate renal function by correcting plasma and volume deficiencies, since blood and fluid losses in the gastrointestinal tract caused by mucosal injury from the corrosive effects of iron can rapidly progress to life-threatening hypovolemia.

Nursing Considerations

Nursing interventions are similar to those for any drug ingestion (see Salicylate Poisoning), with the main emphasis on supportive care during the critical stages of the intoxication and family counseling to prevent recurrence.

For children receiving chelation therapy, careful observation of vital signs is essential. In children with symptoms of iron poisoning, deferoxamine often causes the urine to turn an orange or red color (Klein-Schwartz and others, 1990). Parents should be alerted to this possibility to avoid needless worry.

✦ **NURSING ALERT** If intravenous deferoxamine is given too rapidly, hypotension, facial flushing, rash, urticaria, tachycardia, and shock may occur. Stop the infusion, maintain the intravenous line with normal saline, and notify the practitioner immediately.

LEAD POISONING (PLUMBISM)

Lead poisoning is a prevalent and significant pediatric problem. Although symptomatic lead poisoning with its associated life-threatening encephalopathy is rarely seen today, many asymptomatic young children have lead levels sufficiently elevated to cause irreversible neurologic and intellectual damage. The prevalence of lead poisoning among children in the United States depends on the criteria used to define abnormal blood lead levels. At blood lead levels considered a health hazard (>15 μg/dl), but below the current abnormal level of >25 μg/dl, between 3 and 4 million children may be affected. An additional 400,000 fetuses may be exposed to excessive maternal blood lead levels (Agency for Toxic Substances, 1988). Although the greatest risk is to poor children under 6 years of age living in urban areas, lead poisoning affects children of all social strata. For example, children of wealthier families living in old homes in restored urban areas are at risk (Needleman, 1988).

Factors Related to Lead Ingestion

Several factors influence the ingestion of lead-containing substances, and successful long-term cure and prevention of lead poisoning involves change in all the variables.

Environmental characteristics. The most important contributing factor is the availability of lead in the environment. Lead enters the system either by ingestion or inhalation. The six major environmental sources of lead are paint, gasoline, stationary sources (e.g., lead smelters), dust and soil, food, and water (Box 16-9) (Agency for Toxic Substances, 1988). Lead-based paint from old housing remains the most frequent high-dose source of lead. A lead paint chip about the size of a nickel can contain 50,000 μg of lead; the safe upper limit of daily lead ingestion for children is 5 μg/kg. Almost all cases of symptomatic lead poisoning result from the ingestion of lead paint chips (American Academy of Pediatrics, Committee on Environmental Hazards and Committee on Accident and Poison Prevention, 1987). The deleading process (sanding, scraping, and burning of painted surfaces) also contributes significant amounts of ingested and inhaled lead to inhabitants (Amitai and others, 1987a; Rey-Alvarez and Menke-Hargrave, 1987).

Not until the late 1970s did the U.S. Consumer Product

Box 16-9 POTENTIAL SOURCES OF LEAD

Common Sources
Interior and exterior lead-based paint
Dust (household)
Interior and exterior paint removal (deleading)
Soil contaminated by automobile exhaust
Industrial sources (lead smelters)
Food
Air
Drinking water

Uncommon Sources
Metallic objects (shot from shotgun shells, fishing weights)
Lead-glazed ceramics
Old toys, furniture (cribs), and utensils
Storage battery casings (especially if burned)
Gasoline sniffing
Exposed lead solder in food cans
Imported canned foods and toys
Folk medicines (e.g., azarcon, Greta, Paylooah)*
Imported cosmetics
Leaded glass artwork
Antique pewter cookware or containers
Farm or maritime equipment (painted with lead-based paint)
Colored newsprint or food wrappers
Bonemeal- and dolomite-based calcium supplements

Modified from American Academy of Pediatrics, Committee on Environmental Hazards and Committee on Accident and Poison Prevention: Statement on childhood lead poisoning, Pediatrics 79(3):457-465, 1987.
*Fine powders fed to young children as a cure for fever or rash.

Safety Commission finally ban the addition of lead to paints for residential use. Consequently, substantial amounts of lead remain on the painted interior and exterior surfaces of older homes. Although the child's home environment is usually the source of lead, other buildings, such as nursery or daycare centers, can contribute to lead exposure.

Another significant source of lead in the child's environment is dust and soil that become contaminated by automobile exhaust, deteriorated lead paint, and emission from lead smelters. Food in lead-soldered cans and drinking water supplied in lead pipes or in plumbing with lead-soldered joints can also contribute to ingested sources of the heavy metal.

Characteristics of the child. Developmentally young children are at risk for lead poisoning because of their high level of oral activity. Particularly during late infancy and toddlerhood, children explore their environment by putting objects in their mouth. This normal hand-to-mouth activity contributes to the amount of lead they ingest in dust and dirt. Because of their size, young children inhale air that is closer to the ground, which is more heavily contaminated with lead. In addition, the child who ingests lead often practices *pica,* the habitual, purposeful, and compulsive ingestion of nonfood substances (Laraque and others, 1990).

In addition, three to five times more lead is absorbed in children than in adults. Absorption is also enhanced by dietary deficiencies of iron, calcium, and zinc. The greatest risk appears to be from iron deficiency, even in the absence of anemia (Clark, Royal, and Seeler, 1988).

Lead poisoning is not confined to the young child who ingests the substance. It can also occur in older children who habitually sniff leaded gasoline. The nurse must be aware of children experimenting with drugs or other psychotropic substances and the possibility of gasoline sniffing, which is especially prevalent among American Indian children on reservations (Coulehan and others, 1983).

Parental characteristics. Parent-child interaction has been reported as a significant variable in the ingestion of high levels of lead. Children with symptomatic lead poisoning generally receive less adequate child care than children without plumbism, including poor hygienic practices, insufficient feeding to promote adequate nutrition, infrequent use of medical facilities, and insufficient rest. Parents use few resources to stimulate the child, tend to be less affectionate, and have an immature attitude toward maintaining discipline. These findings are *not* related to differences in income, educational level, age of parents, or number of household occupants—factors usually thought to be associated with lead poisoning (Hunt, Hepner, and Seaton, 1982). The correlation between parental behavior and lead levels is significant after children are 6 months of age, when their mobility and oral activity make lead accessible (Dietrich and others, 1985). Characteristics related to inadequate parenting have not been found to be significant in low-level lead exposure (Bellinger and others, 1986).

Mothers also play a role in exposing their fetuses to lead. Infants who had umbilical cord lead levels of 10 to 25 μg/dl (levels below the current acceptable criteria of less than 25 μg/dl) scored lower on developmental tests than infants with lead levels below 10 μg/dl (Bellinger and others, 1987). The detrimental neurologic effects of prenatal lead exposure appear to be greatest for males and infants from very poor families (Dietrich and others, 1987).

Pathophysiology and Clinical Manifestations

Normally, ingested lead is very slowly excreted via the kidneys, alimentary tract, and, to a small extent, sweat. Retained lead is stored chiefly in the bone, where it is inert. However, with chronic ingestion the rate of absorption exceeds the rate of excretion, and excess lead is deposited in the tissues and circulatory system, with about 90% attached to the erythrocytes. Even when the chronic ingestion stops, it takes the body twice as long to excrete the stored lead as it did to accumulate it. As a result, several body systems continue to be affected after the environmental removal of the poison (Fig. 16-6).

Hematologic system. Lead is extremely toxic to the biosynthesis of heme, preventing the formation of hemoglobin and causing its precursors, especially erythrocyte protoporphyrin (EP), coproporphyrin, and delta-aminolevulinic acid (ALA), to increase in the body. EP is elevated in the blood when the blood-lead concentration is only minimally increased (5 to 10 μg/dl) and is a sensitive, but not specific, indicator of abnormal lead levels. The latter two intermediary metabolites are found in the urine in excessive amounts when the blood-lead concentration reaches 80 μg/dl of whole blood. Reduction of the heme molecule in the red

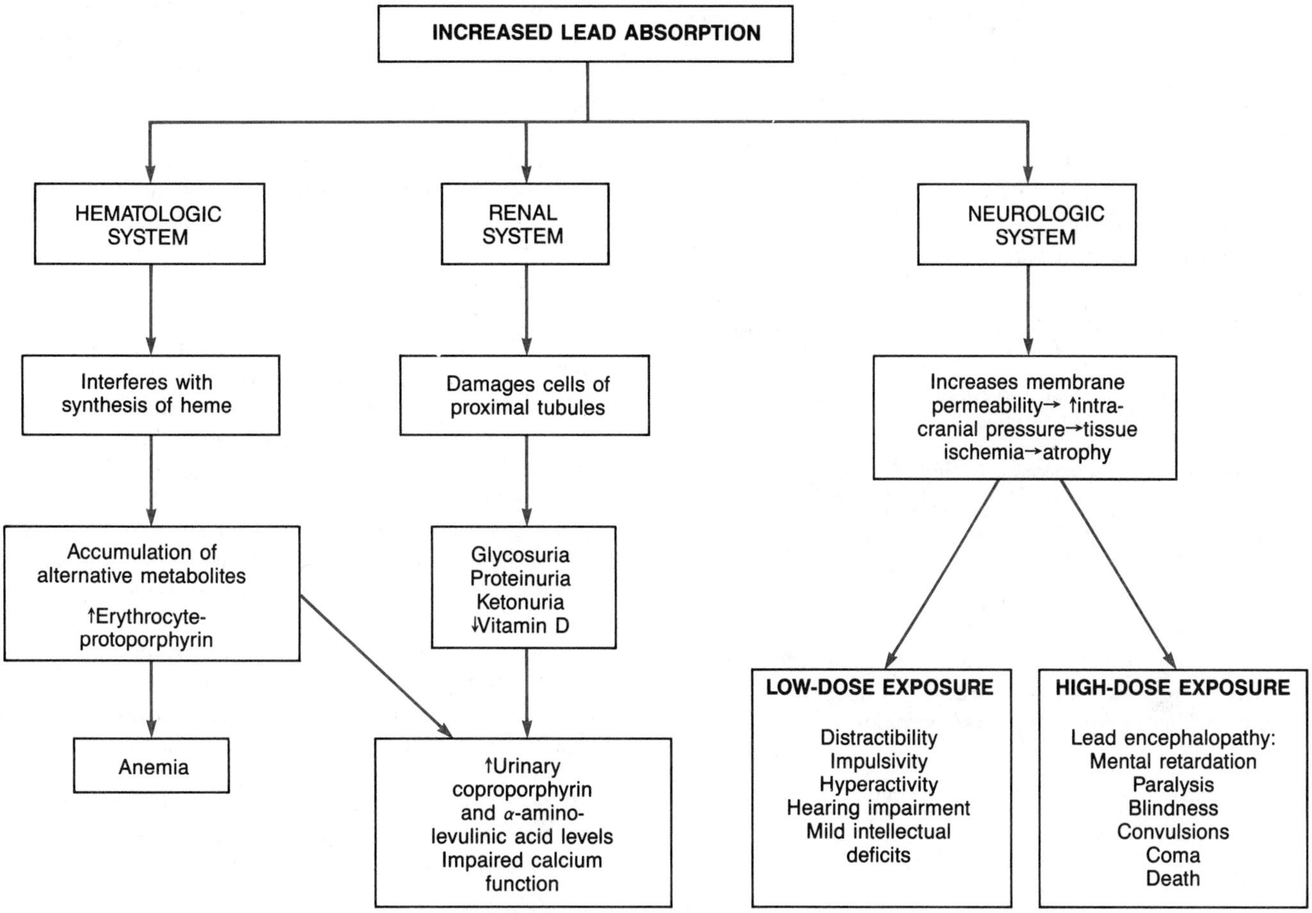

Fig. 16-6. Main effects of lead on body systems.

blood cell results in anemia, one of the initial signs of the disease.

Renal system. Lead damages the cells of the proximal tubules, resulting in abnormal excretion of glucose, protein, amino acids, and phosphate and interference with the synthesis of vitamin D. With adequate treatment, kidney damage is usually reversible. Severe irreversible lead nephropathy is probably limited to protracted childhood plumbism.

Central nervous system. The most serious and irreversible side effects of lead intoxication are on the nervous system. Initially, membrane permeability increases, with a shift of fluid into the interstitial spaces of the brain. As a result, increased intracranial pressure causes cortical atrophy and *lead encephalopathy*—convulsions, mental retardation, paralysis, blindness, and ultimately coma and death. Lead encephalopathy is almost always associated with a blood-lead concentration greater than 100 μg/dl.

However, before lead encephalopathy occurs, low-dose exposure to lead causes neurologic and intellectual deficits. Hyperactivity, aggression, impulsiveness, decreased interest in play, lethargy, irritability, hearing impairment, learning difficulties, short attention span, and distractibility are common signs of asymptomatic poisoning. Studies demonstrate that as prenatal and postnatal lead levels increase, the child's intelligence quotient decreases (Bellinger and others, 1987; Faust and Brown, 1987). Such manifestations of behavioral disturbance are important clues to the identification of children with early poisoning.

Prominent clinical signs of gasoline sniffing are mainly those of central nervous system toxicity: irritability, tremor, hallucinations, confusion, lack of impulse control, depression, delirium, chorea, ataxia, and sleep disturbances.

Other manifestations. Other vague symptoms of plumbism are acute crampy abdominal pain, vomiting, constipation, anorexia, headache, and fever. Some evidence suggests that in young children lead affects growth, especially infants with elevated prenatal and postnatal blood lead levels (Schwartz, Angle, and Pitcher, 1986; Shukla and others, 1989). However, other researchers have found no effect on stature in young adults who had both low and high levels of lead exposure during childhood (Sachs and Moel, 1989).

Diagnostic Evaluation

Several tests are available to detect the presence of toxic amounts of lead in the body. The most frequently used procedures for routine screening are the blood-lead concentration and the erythrocyte protoporphyrin (EP) level. Blood lead levels reflect absorption from exposure to lead, while EP determinations measure the adverse metabolic effect of

Box 16-10 GUIDELINES FOR LEAD SCREENING

All preschool children, or children at risk for lead poisoning, ages 9 months to 6 years who:
—Live in or frequently visit old, dilapidated housing
—Associate with individuals who have known lead toxicity
—Live near lead-smelting plants
—Have household members involved in lead-related occupation or hobby (e.g., stained glass work)
Children of any age living in older housing under renovation
Initial screen with EP test at 9 to 15 months of age at time of hematocrit test
Additional screens as indicated at 18 months of age and at frequent intervals (3 to 6 months)

Modified from American Academy of Pediatrics, Committee on Environmental Hazards and Committee on Accident and Poison Prevention: Statement on childhood lead poisoning, Pediatrics 79(3):457-465, 1987.

Table 16-5 Erythrocyte protoporphyrin (EP) by extraction: risk classification of asymptomatic children for priority medical evaluation

BLOOD LEAD (μg/dl)	EP (μg/dl) <35	35-109	110-249	>250
Not done	I	*	*	*
<24	I	Ia	Ia	EPP+
25-49	Ib	II	III	III
50-69	†	III	III	IV
>70	†	†	IV	IV

From Centers for Disease Control: Preventing lead poisoning in young children, DHHS Pub. No. 99-2230, Washington, DC, 1985, U.S. Government Printing Office.
EPP+, Erythropoietic protoporphyria. Iron deficiency may cause elevated EP levels up to 300 μg/dl, but this is rare.
*Blood lead test needed to estimate risk.
†In practice, this combination of results is not generally observed; if it is observed, immediately retest with venous blood.
NOTE: Diagnostic evaluation is more urgent than the classification indicates for:
1. Children with any symptoms compatible with lead toxicity
2. Children under 36 months of age
3. Children whose blood lead and EP levels place them in the upper part of a particular class
4. Children whose siblings are in a higher class

These guidelines refer to the interpretation of screening results, but the final diagnosis and disposition rest on a more complete medical and laboratory examination of the child.
AUTHOR'S NOTE: EP can also be measured by hematofluorometer methods, which result in values different from those above using extraction.

lead on heme synthesis. Toxic blood lead levels are 25 μg/dl when accompanied by an EP level of 35 μg/dl or more (American Academy of Pediatrics, 1987). However, with increasing evidence that blood lead levels less than 25 μg/dl cause irreversible neurologic damage, acceptable limits may be defined by a lower blood lead content in the future. Guidelines for screening young children for abnormal lead levels are listed in Box 16-10.

Based on the results on the blood lead and EP screening tests (Table 16-5), the Centers for Disease Control (1985) has established a classification that suggests the relative risk and the priority for medical evaluation and environmental intervention. The classification for medical evaluation is defined as follows:

Class IV: Urgent risk of lead toxicity; need for medical evaluation within 24 hours and not later than 48 hours
Class III: High risk; **Class II:** Moderate risk — Need for diagnostic tests but child not in immediate danger
Class I: Low risk; no need for diagnostic tests

Class I is subdivided into two additional categories. Class Ia includes children with iron deficiency, and these children should have further testing of their iron status. Class Ib includes children with transient, stable, declining, or increasing blood lead levels. These children should be carefully followed.

Screening tests are not diagnostic tests. The diagnosis is based on findings from a complete history and physical examination. Additional findings include radiographic evidence of "lead lines" in long bones or lead deposits in the abdomen, increased levels of urinary coproporphyrin and delta-aminolevulinic acid (ALA), and evidence of anemia (not a specific finding). A calcium disodium edetate ($CaNa_2EDTA$) mobilization (or provocative) test may also be performed to assess the amount of lead that can be "mobilized" or removed by chelation therapy. After an intramuscular injection of calcium disodium, urine is collected for a specified period and urine lead levels are measured.

Therapeutic Management

The most important aspect of treatment is removing the source of lead. In addition, medical conditions such as iron deficiency are corrected. More definitive therapy, using chelating agents that remove the lead by combining it with another substance, is determined by the risk category (Box 16-11).

$CaNa_2EDTA$ is the chelating agent of choice. It forms a fairly stable, highly soluble compound and increases the urinary excretion of lead by 20 to 50 times. It may be used alone or in combination with the chelating drug dimercaptopropanol (dimercaprol), also called BAL (British anti-Lewisite). Lead excreted in urine is initially mobilized from bone; changes in lead levels in other organs vary. One of the dangers during the initial rapid loss of lead (including the $CaNa_2EDTA$ mobilization test) is the redistribution of lead, which may cause a temporary increase in brain lead levels. In symptomatic children, lead encephalopathy can worsen and potentially be fatal (Chisolm, 1987). Because BAL is more effective than $CaNa_2EDTA$ in removing lead from the brain, it is administered as the initial dose of chelation therapy in children with blood lead levels greater than 70 μg/dl (Piomelli and others, 1984).

D-Penicillamine (Cuprimine, Depen) is the only commercially available oral chelating drug, although others are under investigation. It enhances urinary excretion of lead, but less effectively than $CaNa_2EDTA$. It is sometimes used on an outpatient basis, but patients must be carefully monitored for side effects and reactions (transient decrease in white

Box 16-11 CLASSIFICATION OF RISK AND SUGGESTED MEDICAL TREATMENT FOR LEAD POISONING

Urgent risk—children with confirmed lead poisoning require inpatient chelation therapy
High risk—children whose repeat screening tests fall in class II and III but who also have positive confirmatory diagnostic tests and positive calcium disodium edetate mobilization test may receive inpatient or outpatient chelation therapy
Moderate risk—children whose repeat screening tests fall in class II but who have negative diagnostic tests do not require chelation therapy but removal of lead sources and careful follow-up
Low risk—children in class I require only periodic rescreening until they are 6 years old

Modified from Centers for Disease Control: Preventing lead poisoning in young children, DHHS Pub. No. 99-2230, Washington, DC, 1985. U.S. Government Printing Office.

blood cells and platelets, rash, enuresis, abdominal pain) (Shannon, Graef, and Lovejoy, 1988).

NURSING ALERT D-Penicillamine is not given to anyone with a history of penicillin allergy.

The exact protocol for chelation therapy differs according to practitioner preference, but it generally includes a schedule of $CaNa_2EDTA$ and BAL six times a day for 5 days. If encephalopathy is present, fluid volume is restricted to prevent additional cerebral edema and the drugs are administered intramuscularly. Children without encephalopathy can receive $CaNa_2EDTA$ intravenously.

Symptomatic treatment largely involves controlling seizures, which are often severe and protracted, since the anoxia that accompanies the convulsions compounds the brain damage from lead. Hepatic and renal function is carefully monitored; nephrotoxicity is a side effect of plumbism and $CaNa_2EDTA$. Daily serum electrolyte levels should be taken. Cleansing enemas are ordered for episodes of acute lead ingestion or when lead is visible on radiologic examination in the gastrointestinal tract. Every effort is made to prevent infection and maintain adequate hydration. If iron deficiency anemia coexists with plumbism, it is treated after chelation therapy because iron increases the toxicity of BAL.

Prognosis

Although most of the pathophysiologic effects of lead are reversible, the most serious consequences of both high and low lead exposure are the permanent effects on the central nervous system. In children with lead encephalopathy, brain damage results in mental retardation, behavior changes, possible paralysis, and seizures. However, low-dose exposure may also cause permanent neurologic deficits. Young children with low blood lead levels (average 43 µg/dl), when tested as young adults, had more academic problems (reading disabilities, school failures), poor coordination (hand-eye movements, finger tapping), and a higher incidence of minor delinquency than children with lower blood lead levels (Needleman and others, 1990).

Nursing Considerations

The primary nursing goal in lead poisoning is to prevent the child's further exposure to lead. For children with low-level exposure, this often requires identifying the sources of lead in the environment. Careful history taking is one of the most useful and valuable tools and should concentrate on the areas listed in Box 16-12.

When old, dilapidated housing is the major source of lead in the environment, the family needs instruction regarding correct deleading procedures. As much of the flaking pain as possible is scraped or sanded from the walls, ceilings, and floors. However, when these procedures are employed, children and pregnant women must not remain in the home, day or night, until the process is completed. Following deleading, the house must be thoroughly cleaned using wet mopping before the inhabitants return. Household members employed in occupations such as lead-smelting work should shower and change into clean clothing before leaving work. Members of cultures using folk remedies that contain lead must be advised of the danger and encouraged to avoid such practices.

In addition, the children must be supervised and guided toward activity other than pica. Helping parents learn methods of stimulating their children, locating preschool or day-care centers, or helping parents organize a play group are methods of improving parenting and consequently lessening those factors that contribute to plumbism. If nutritional deficiencies coexist, parents need guidance in planning meals that provide sufficient minerals or instruction regarding administration of supplements, such as iron. Consistent mealtimes should be planned with instructions that the child eat only at these times to reduce the practice of pica. As in any situational crisis, parents need support and understanding if their child is treated for plumbism. Many of the families at highest risk for lead poisoning have the few-

Box 16-12 GUIDELINES FOR ASSESSING POTENTIAL FOR LEAD POISONING

Sources of lead in the child's environment, especially old dilapidated housing and other frequented sites, such as day-care center, relatives' homes, or play areas near heavily trafficked areas; living near lead smelter
Occupation of household members and hobbies that may include the use of lead
Folk remedies or art supplies that may contain lead
History of pica and hand-mouth habits, such as sucking thumb or fingers, mouthing objects, and biting nails
Change in behavior or behavioral problems, such as hyperactivity, aggression, and excessive irritability
Developmental delay
Other risk factors, such as crowded urban living conditions, poverty, and inadequate maternal care
Eating habits that may cause nutritional deficiencies (iron, calcium, zinc)

est resources to comply with measures, such as relocation or deleading the home. Appropriate referrals are essential in locating assistance for parents.

For children who must undergo chelation therapy, the nurse must attempt to reduce the pain from multiple intramuscular injections if the intravenous route cannot be used. Children need to be prepared for the injections and allowed to express their pain and anger. Needle play and aggressive play, such as pounding or throwing bean bags, provides an excellent outlet for frustrations. Children also deserve an explanation of the need for treatment; the nurse should emphasize that it is not a punishment for eating lead or paint. All the injections should be administered when children are in an area other than their rooms to maintain a "safe" environment.

Chelating agents are administered deeply into a large muscle mass. To lessen the pain from $CaNa_2EDTA$, the local anesthetic procaine is injected with the drug. Rotation of sites is essential to prevent the formation of painful areas of fibrotic tissue. Since $CaNa_2EDTA$ and lead are toxic to the kidneys, records are kept of intake and output and the results of urinalysis are assessed to monitor renal functioning. Because of the risk of seizures, appropriate precautions are instituted at the bedside of children with high blood lead levels.

✚ **NURSING ALERT** $CaNa_2EDTA$ is never given in the absence of an adequate urine output. Children receiving the drug intramuscularly must be able to maintain adequate oral intake of fluids.

Health professionals have an even broader responsibility in terms of educating the public regarding the signs and symptoms of the disease, especially in children with lead levels that are clinically borderline. The most frequent behavior deviations of negativism, distractibility, and hyperactivity may be mistakenly diagnosed as other problems, with labels such as learning disorder, delinquency, or behavior problem, when in reality the child is suffering from the physical effects of a toxic substance. If such children were detected earlier, the chance for optimum development would probably be greater. However, until lead poisoning is attacked as a social problem as well as a physical problem, its high incidence and irreversible sequelae may not be significantly altered. (See Nursing Care Plan: The Child with Lead Poisoning.*)

■ CHILD MALTREATMENT

Child maltreatment is a broad term that includes intentional physical abuse or neglect, emotional abuse or neglect, or sexual abuse of children, usually by adults. It is one of the most significant social problems affecting children. Although statistics only partially reflect the true incidence of child maltreatment, it is estimated that more than 2 million children are reported yearly to child protective services in the United States (Highlights, 1989).

Although the following discussion is concerned with abuse against children, parent-child abuse may be only one type of violence in the family. Violence between parents also often occurs; the abusing parent may also be the abused spouse (McKibben, DeVos, and Newberger, 1989). Family violence also increases the risk of physical and sexual abuse in youngsters who leave the home to avoid maltreatment. Ironically, these "runaways" often encounter continued abuse "on the streets" as they try to survive. Runaways comprise about 95% of missing children; the remaining children are those abducted by noncustodial parents, relatives, or strangers (American Academy of Pediatrics, Committee on Early Childhood, Adoption, and Dependent Care, 1986).

CHILD NEGLECT

Child neglect involves more children than any other form of maltreatment—55% of maltreated children are reported for neglect (not including emotional abuse), and 46% of all maltreatment-related fatalities are associated with deprivation of necessities (Highlights, 1989). Neglect is generally considered an omission, rather than a commission, of a direct act or behavior that has a detrimental effect on the child's physical and psychologic development. It can be defined as the failure of a parent or other person legally responsible for the child's welfare to provide for the child's basic needs and an adequate level of care (Council on Scientific Affairs, 1985).

Unlike the study of physical abuse, relatively little research has been done on the etiology of neglect, although it appears that many risk factors identified with physical abuse apply to neglect as well (see discussion on p. 738). For example, neglectful parents often demonstrate a lack of knowledge of parenting skills. They may be unaware that an infant needs to be fed every 3 to 4 hours, be unable to cook a meal, or not know what constitutes a nutritious meal. The most serious lack of knowledge is failure to recognize emotional nurturing as an essential need of children. The reader is also encouraged to review the discussion on failure to thrive in Chapter 13, which may result from physical or emotional neglect.

Types of Neglect

Neglect takes many forms and can be classified broadly as physical or emotional maltreatment. *Physical neglect* involves the deprivation of necessities, such as food, clothing, shelter, supervision, medical care, and education. *Emotional neglect* generally refers to the failure to meet the child's needs for affection, attention, and emotional nurturance. It may also include lack of intervention for or fostering maladaptive behavior, such as delinquency or substance abuse. Overprotection may also be included, since it deprives children of the opportunity to develop to their maximum potential (Snyder, Hampton, and Newberger, 1983). *Emotional abuse* is an even more difficult aspect of

*In Wong, D.L., and Whaley, L.F.: Clinical manual of pediatric nursing, ed. 3, St. Louis, 1990, Mosby–Year Book, Inc.

Box 16-13 CLINICAL MANIFESTATIONS OF POTENTIAL CHILD MALTREATMENT

Physical Neglect

Suggestive physical findings

Failure to thrive
Signs of malnutrition, such as thin extremities, abdominal distention, lack of subcutaneous fat
Poor personal hygiene, especially of teeth
Unclean and/or inappropriate dress
Evidence of poor health care, such as nonimmunized status, untreated infections, frequent colds
Frequent injuries from lack of supervision

Suggestive behaviors

Dull and inactive; excessively passive or sleepy
Self-stimulatory behaviors, such as finger sucking or rocking
Begging or stealing food, Absenteeism from school, Drug or alcohol addiction, Vandalism or shoplifting — in older child

Emotional Abuse and Neglect

Suggestive physical findings

Failure to thrive
Feeding disorders, such as rumination
Enuresis
Sleep disorders

Suggestive behaviors

Self-stimulatory behaviors, such as biting, rocking, sucking
During infancy, lack of social smile and stranger anxiety
Withdrawal
Unusual fearfulness
Antisocial behavior, such as destructiveness, stealing, cruelty
Extremes of behavior, such as overcompliant and passive or aggressive and demanding
Lags in emotional and intellectual development, especially language
Suicide attempts

Physical Abuse

Suggestive physical findings

Bruises and welts
- On face, lips, mouth, back, buttocks, thighs, or areas of torso
- Regular patterns descriptive of object used, such as belt buckle, hand, wire hanger, chain, wooden spoon, squeeze or pinch marks
- May be present in various stages of healing

Burns
- On soles of feet, palms of hands, back, or buttocks
- Patterns descriptive of object used, such as round cigar or cigarette burns, "glovelike" sharply demarcated areas from immersion in scalding water, rope burns on wrists or ankles from being bound, burns in the shape of an iron, radiator, or electric stove burner
- Absence of "splash" marks and presence of symmetric burns

Fractures and dislocations
- Skull, nose, or facial structures
- Injury may denote type of abuse, such as spiral fracture or dislocation from twisting of an extremity or whiplash from shaking the child
- Multiple new or old fractures in various stages of healing

Lacerations and abrasions
- On backs of arms, legs, torso, face, or external genitalia
- Unusual symptoms, such as abdominal swelling, pain, and vomiting from punching
- Descriptive marks such as from human bites or pulling the hair out

Chemical
- Unexplained repeated poisoning, especially drug overdose
- Unexplained sudden illness, such as hypoglycemia from insulin administration

Suggestive behaviors

Wary of physical contact with adults
Apparent fear of parents or going home
Lying very still while surveying environment
Inappropriate reaction to injury, such as failure to cry from pain
Lack of reaction to frightening events
Apprehensive when hearing other children cry
Indiscriminate friendliness and displays of affection
Superficial relationships
Acting-out behavior, such as aggression, to seek attention
Withdrawal behavior

Sexual Abuse

Suggestive physical findings

Bruises, bleeding, lacerations or irritation of external genitalia, anus, mouth, or throat
Torn, stained, or bloody underclothing
Pain on urination or pain, swelling, and itching of genital area
Penile discharge
Sexually transmitted disease, nonspecific vaginitis, or venereal warts
Difficulty in walking or sitting
Unusual odor in the genital area
Recurrent urinary tract infections
Pregnancy in young adolescent

Suggestive behaviors

Sudden emergence of sexually related problems, including excessive or public masturbation, age-inappropriate sexual play, promiscuity, or overtly seductive behavior
Withdrawn, excessive daydreaming
Preoccupied with fantasies, especially in play
Poor relationships with peers
Sudden changes, such as anxiety, loss or gain of weight, clinging behavior
In incestuous relationships, excessive anger at mother for not protecting daughter
Regressive behavior, such as bed-wetting or thumb-sucking
Sudden onset of phobias or fears, particularly fears of the dark, men, strangers, or particular settings or situations (e.g., undue fear of leaving the house or staying at the daycare center or the baby-sitter's house)
Running away from home
Substance abuse, particularly of alcohol or mood-elevating drugs
Profound and rapid personality changes, especially extreme depression, hostility, and aggression (often accompanied by social withdrawal)
Rapidly declining school performance
Suicidal attempts or ideation

maltreatment to define but refers to an adult's concerted attack on a child's development of self and social competence; it is a pattern of psychically destructive behavior. Emotional abuse may take the following forms: rejecting, isolating, terrorizing, ignoring, and corrupting the child (Garbarino, Guttmann, and Seeley, 1986).

Identification of Neglect

Neglect from deprivation of necessities is easier to identify than emotional neglect or abuse, because physical signs of neglect are usually evident (Box 16-13). While emotional maltreatment may be readily suspected, it is very difficult to substantiate. Physical signs are often nonspecific, and nurses must rely on suggestive behaviors, which range from depression to acting-out behavior, to help identify a possible abuse situation. Unfortunately, none of these behaviors is diagnostic of neglect, and caution is necessary to avoid false accusations. Although primary caregivers are generally responsible for instances of emotional maltreatment, this is not always the case. School teachers also can inflict emotional abuse on students. Indications of teacher abuse in children include excessive worry about school performance; expressed fear of the teacher; negative perception of self and of school; excessive crying, nightmares, headaches, and stomachaches; and decreased attendance (Krugman and Krugman, 1984).

Nursing Considerations

Nursing goals are similar to those discussed under physical abuse, with identification and prevention as priorities (see p. 741). Often neglect is caused by ignorance, and early education of caregivers regarding children's basic physical and emotional needs can avert serious problems. Parents must also be aware that emotional abuse can occur outside the home, such as in substitute care facilities or school. Any persistent change in children's behavior is a clue to unsatisfactory situations and must be taken seriously. Nurses can be alert to such problems by routinely incorporating questions about children's activities into their assessment and by investigating, either directly or through referral, any suspicious complaints.

PHYSICAL ABUSE

Physical abuse has received more attention than any other type of child maltreatment and is reported in about 22% of all maltreatment cases. In one report physical injury accounted for 62% of all fatalities from child maltreatment (Highlights, 1988).

As pervasive as the problem is, not one definition of child abuse is universally accepted. Kempe and others (1962) coined the term *battered child syndrome* (BCS) to refer to "a clinical condition in young children who have received serious physical abuse, generally from a parent or foster parent." However, this definition restricts abuse to the most severe forms and is less appropriate than broader definitions that include the spectrum of abuse, such as "the nonaccidental injury of a child ranging from minor bruises and lacerations to severe neurologic trauma and death" (Council on Scientific Affairs, 1985). In addition to this definition, each state in the United States defines abuse according to its individual reporting laws.

Factors Predisposing to Physical Abuse

The exact cause of child abuse is not known, but three major criteria—parental characteristics, characteristics of the child, and environmental characteristics—seem to predispose children to physical injury by their parents or other caregivers. Despite numerous research studies that have attempted to isolate specific attributes of the parent, child, or environment that cause abuse, no single etiologic factor is responsible for abuse. Rather, an *interaction* between several variables appears to create a high-risk situation for maltreatment to occur; the greater number of variables, the greater the risk. Different variables may be responsible for certain types of maltreatment. For example, poverty may be more strongly associated with neglect, whereas parental characteristics may be more strongly related to physical abuse. One combination of risk factors predisposing to physical abuse is poor nurturing during the parent's own childhood, negative feelings toward the pregnancy, and birth of a temperamentally difficult child who is developmentally delayed and/or in poor physical health (Sherrod and others, 1985).

In the following discussion nurses must be careful to avoid stereotyping parents and children in an attempt to predict or diagnose abuse (Krowchuk, 1989). No test has sufficient sensitivity to predict abuse without falsely accusing many individuals (false positives) and missing some abusers (false negatives) (Kotelchuck, 1982).

Parental characteristics. Extensive research has focused on parental characteristics that distinguish abusive parents from nonabusive parents. Unfortunately, the findings from most of these studies provide conflicting evidence. For example, it is commonly believed that abusive parents were abused as children. However, few studies support this relationship (Widom, 1989). While physical punishment tends to occur often in abusive parents' childhood, most of the parents were not physically abused as children. However, abusive parents who report that they were severely punished as children are much more likely to injure their own children (Kotelchuck, 1982). If the abuse was not overt physical violence, abusive parents typically recall their punishment as unfair and severe and characterize their relationship with their parents as negative. Abusive parents tend to have difficulty controlling aggressive impulses, and the free expression of violence is one of the most consistent qualities of these families (Altemeier and others, 1982).

Another finding is that abusive families are often more socially isolated and have fewer supportive relationships than nonabusive parents. With little or no available support system and the presence of concurrent stresses imposed by the child or environment, these parents are extremely vulnerable to additional crises of any nature. They literally strike out at the child as a method of releasing their increasing frustration and anxiety. Some studies suggest that the level of social support is an important factor in identifying potential abusers, and that enhancement of the person's support system may be a prevention or intervention strategy for abuse (Turner and Avison, 1985).

Another characteristic of some abusing parents is inadequate knowledge of normal developmental expectations. Thus they expect their children to nurture and parent them, in the same way their parents demanded similar behavior. This concept of *role reversal,* or the parent acting as the child and expecting the child to become the parent, is an important reason why some children escape abuse, whereas others become the victims.

Other factors identified in abusing parents include low self-esteem, less adequate maternal functioning, untruthfulness, poor rapport in the interviewing situation, and negative attitude toward pregnancy.

Characteristics of the child. The child also *unintentionally* contributes to the abusing situation. In families of two or more children, only one child is usually the victim of abuse. This child's temperament, position in the family, additional physical needs if ill or cognitively impaired, activity level, or degree of sensitivity to parental needs all contribute to the potential for physical abuse. For example, the firstborn may not be abused if he or she fits into the "easy-child pattern" and demands little other than routine feeding and diapering. During the early years, the docile child may learn how to meet the parent's needs by being quiet, playing alone, showing the parent affection, and acting as grown up and self-sufficient as possible. However, this situation is never safe for the child. Any added stress, such as illness, pregnancy, birth of a sibling, or financial need, can upset this precarious balance between the parent and child.

Not infrequently the abused child is illegitimate, unwanted, brain damaged (especially in situations where the parents cannot accept the retardation), hyperactive, physically disabled, or from a broken home. Sometimes children are abused because they remind the parent of someone the parent dislikes, such as a younger brother or sister who received all the attention from their own parents. Premature infants may be at risk for maltreatment because of the failure of parent-child bonding during early infancy. Often a difficult pregnancy, labor, or delivery is a predisposing factor in abuse, especially when the infant is born prematurely or with congenital anomalies.

Although one child is usually the victim in an abusing family, removing that child from the home often places the other siblings at risk for abuse. Child maltreatment usually is not confined to one child because of a disturbed parent-child relationship but is a result of a family in distress (Jean-Gilles and Crittenden, 1990). Therefore, no child is safe if left in the abusing environment unless the parents can be helped to learn new parenting skills and to meet their needs and release their frustration through alternatives other than attacking their children.

Environmental characteristics. The environment is an integral part of the potential abusing situation. Typically the environment is one of chronic stress, including problems of divorce, extramarital relations, financial deficit, unemployment, poor housing, alcoholism, and drug addiction.

The social milieu of the abusive family is one devoid of adequate support systems. The environment becomes a trap from which there is no emotional exit except to direct the anger and frustration toward a helpless victim, the child.

Although most reporting of abuse has been from lower socioeconomic populations, child abuse is not a problem of any one societal group. It spans all educational, social, and economic levels. Certainly stresses imposed by poverty predispose lower socioeconomic families to abusive situations, and abuse in these groups is more apt to be reported. However, concealed crises can also be present in upper-class families. For example, a wealthy family experiencing major life changes, such as rehousing, the birth of an additional child, or marital discord, may have sufficient environmental stressors imposed on them to produce a potentially abusing situation. Wealthy families may be so overinvolved with commitments outside the home that abuse may be inflicted by substitute caregivers. Nurses need to be aware of such factors in order to identify the hidden sources of child abuse and neglect.

Identification of Physical Abuse

One of the most critical responsibilities of health professionals is identifying abusive situations as early as possible. The characteristics just discussed can serve as a framework to assess the vulnerability of families to abuse but never to predict actual abuse. Rather, a thorough physical examination and a careful, detailed history are the diagnostic tools to identify abuse. Nurses have a very special role as members of a multidisciplinary team. The nurse may be the first person to see the child and parent and may be the consistent caregiver if the child is hospitalized.

Evidence of maltreatment. Recognition of abuse or neglect necessitates a familiarity with both physical and behavioral signs suggestive of maltreatment (see Box 16-13). No one indicator is exclusively diagnostic of maltreatment; a pattern or combination of indicators should arouse suspicion and further investigation. In addition, signs of possible abuse must be coupled with an understanding of cultural practices and medical disorders that may resemble abuse and tragically result in a false accusation (see Questions and Controversies). Not all forms of physical abuse demonstrate obvious signs. Violent shaking of children can cause fatal intracranial trauma without signs of external head injury (Alexander and others, 1990).

Munchausen syndrome by proxy. One of the more unusual and perplexing types of abuse is the Munchausen syndrome by proxy (MSP), which refers to illness that one person fabricates or induces in another person. In children, it is usually the mother who fabricates signs and symptoms of illness in her child, the proxy, to gain attention from the medical staff. Rarely the father may be the perpetrator (Makar and Squier, 1990). MSP can take many forms, such as adding maternal blood to the child's urine to simulate hematuria (Salmon and others, 1988), presenting a fictitious medical history (Guandolo, 1985), chronic poisoning of the child (Sutphen and Saulsbury, 1988), or suffocating the child to cause apnea and seizures (Makar and Squier, 1990). Another form of MSP is alleging that the child has been sexually abused by someone else to gain recognition as the child's protector (Rand, 1989).

Such cases are often very difficult to confirm and require a high index of suspicion to protect the children (Box 16-14). Nurses play an important role in monitoring the parent's activities to identify instances of causing the children's symptoms. Some report using a hidden video camera to

QUESTIONS AND CONTROVERSIES

How serious is the problem of "mistaken" diagnosis of child abuse?

Although most concern among health professionals is to detect child abuse early and to protect the child from further abuse, one must also recognize the possibility of a mistaken diagnosis of child maltreatment. Incidence data indicate that approximately 60% of the 2.2 million reports in 1987 were unsubstantiated for child abuse and neglect by child protective services (Highlights, 1989). Although some degree of overreporting is to be expected because the law requires the reporting of suspected maltreatment, the present level of overreporting is considered unreasonably high. Some of the increase is most likely due to the practice of "defensive" medicine—health professionals are legally required to report suspected maltreatment, but there is no penalty for reporting unsubstantiated cases. Therefore playing it "safe" is preferable to failing to report and facing criminal prosecution. Another negative effect of the overreporting is that the protective child services are so overburdened with minor cases that children in real danger of serious maltreatment may be poorly investigated (Besharov, 1985).

There are numerous reports of mistaken diagnosis in the literature. Some of them involve lack of understanding of cultural traditions, such as the Oriental practices of coin rubbing and cupping, which produce welts or bruises (Asnes and Wisotsky, 1981; Saulsbury and Hayden, 1985), or the use of heat (moxibustion), which causes circular burns (Feldman, 1984). Several diseases may be erroneously attributed to abuse, such as hemophilia, meningitis, sudden infant death syndrome, osteogenesis imperfecta, and erythema multiforme (Adler and Kane-Nussen, 1983; Kirschner and Stein, 1985). Unintentional injuries may also be wrongly diagnosed as abuse, such as burns from metal buckles on car seats (Schmitt, Gray, and Britton, 1978), lacerations from seat belts (Baker, 1986), or retinal hemorrhage after cardiopulmonary resuscitation (Goetting and Sowa, 1990). Normal variants, such as mongolian spots and congenital anomalies of genitalia, can be mistaken for abuse (Adams and Horton, 1989; Koblenzer, 1989). Such wrongful accusations can cause families tremendous grief, including removal of the child from the home.* Mistaken diagnoses of child abuse can be minimized by being knowledgeable of situations mimicking abuse, by performing a careful history and physical examination, and by giving parents every opportunity to present their account of the situation (Wong, 1987). Parents should be involved in every phase of the investigative process, including the initial proceedings of suspected child abuse and neglect (SCAN) teams at hospitals (Reid, 1985).

*An organization of victims wrongfully accused of abuse is the **National Association of State VOCAL (Victims of Child Abuse Laws) Organizations,** 1030 G. St., Sacramento, CA 95814; (916) 863-7470

document the parent's behavior (Epstein and others, 1987). Consequences for children with MSP can be serious. They often undergo needless and painful medical procedures and treatments. The parent's actions may induce a serious illness in children, one that may even be fatal. Children may develop chronic invalidism, accepting the illness story and believing themselves to be ill. Finally, they may develop MSP as an adult (Meadow, 1989). Even when some of these children are removed from the home, they continue to suffer severe psychologic trauma. Other siblings remaining in the home may become substitute victims (McGuire and Feldman, 1989).

Box 16-14 WARNING SIGNS OF MUNCHAUSEN SYNDROME BY PROXY

- Unexplained, prolonged, recurrent, or extremely rare illness
- Discrepancies between clinical findings and history
- Illness unresponsive to treatment
- Signs and symptoms occur only in parent's presence
- Parent knowledgeable about illness, procedures, and treatments
- Parent very interested in interacting with medical staff
- Parent very attentive toward child (refuses to leave hospital)
- Family members with similar symptoms

Box 16-15 WARNING SIGNS OF PHYSICAL ABUSE

- Physical evidence of abuse and/or neglect, including previous injuries
- Conflicting stories about the "accident" or injury from the parents or others
- Cause of injury blamed on sibling or other party
- An injury inconsistent with the history, such as a concussion and broken arm from falling off a bed
- History inconsistent with child's developmental level; such as a 6-month-old turning on the hot water
- A complaint other than the one associated with signs of abuse; for example, a chief complaint of a cold when there is evidence of first- and second-degree burns
- Inappropriate parental concern for the degree of the injury, such as an exaggerated or absent emotional response
- Refusal of the parents to sign for additional tests or agree to necessary treatment
- Excessive delay in seeking treatment
- Absence of the parents for questioning
- Inappropriate response of child, such as little or no response to pain, fear of being touched, excessive or lack of separation anxiety, indiscriminate friendliness to strangers
- Previous reports of abuse in the family
- Repeated visits to emergency facilities with injuries

History pertaining to the incident. Besides observable evidence of physical abuse, the type of history revealed by the parents or other caregiver, such as the baby-sitter or mother's boyfriend, is a significant diagnostic factor. Those areas of the history that should arouse suspicion of abuse are summarized in Box 16-15.

NURSING ALERT Incompatibility between the history and the injury is probably the most important criterion on which to base the decision to report suspected abuse (Krugman, 1989a, 1989b).

An important point to remember when taking a history is that maltreated children rarely betray their parents by confessing to the abuse they received. If questioned, they will repeat the same story as the parents and try to defend their parents' actions. If the interviewer directly accuses the parents of abuse, the child may accept responsibility for the act in an attempt to vindicate the parents from the accusation. Whether children respond in this way out of fear is uncertain. However, children do fear losing whatever security and love they have. Between abusive acts children may receive some measure of attention and love from the parents. If they betray the parents, they may lose this and be uncertain or fearful of the consequences, such as foster care. Preserving the present situation may be less frightening than the unknown future.

Parental behaviors. Certain behavioral responses of the parents to their child and to the interviewer may alert the nurse to the possibility of maltreatment. Some parents have difficulty in showing concern toward their child. They are unable to comfort the youngster and give no indication of realizing how the child may feel, physically or emotionally. Instead they are critical of and angry with the child for being injured. They maintain that the child was responsible for the injury. If asked any question regarding their responsibility of protecting or supervising the child, they become hostile and aggressive. They act as if the child's injury is an assault on them. Their entire perception of the incident is in terms of how it affects them, not the child, which indicates their preoccupation with their own needs and their inability to give any support to others.

In cases of family violence where the wife is also abused, the battered wife may appear to be more concerned about her mate's needs in order to keep him happy and may be less focused on the child. The couple even may appear to be very loving. In these instances the abused child may also appear to be very attached to the mother to protect the mother from being battered when she returns home. In these situations, inquiries should be made regarding spouse abuse as well as child abuse.

In contrast to parents who seem overtly aloof, many abusive parents also show great concern for their children. Some may be overprotective and excessively concerned in relationship to the severity of the injury. It is often difficult to determine if parents have abused their child by watching how they interact with the child in front of others. Therefore, while certain behavioral characteristics of parents may arouse suspicion, their attitude toward the child is not diagnostic of abuse.

Child behaviors. Abused children's response to their parents or the injury may also support the suspicion of abuse. Although no one pattern is typical, extremes of behavior may be observed. Children may be very unresponsive to the parent or excessively clinging and intolerant of separation. There may be overattachment to the abusing parent, possibly in the hope of preventing any upset that may precipitate anger and another attack. During care of the injury, children may be passive and accepting of the discomfort or uncooperative and fearful of any physical contact. Some children shy away from strangers as if frightened, whereas others are unusually affectionate and outgoing.

Nursing Considerations

Nursing care involves several important areas, ideally beginning with prevention of abuse and, following an abusive act, the identification and protection of the child from further abuse.

Prevention. Prevention of child maltreatment has been an extremely difficult goal. Programs aimed at identifying potential abusers and instituting supportive intervention before the occurrence of a physically abusive act have met with variable success. However, nurses have played an important role in such programs. For example, prenatal and infancy home visiting by nurses to primiparas who were either teenagers, unmarried, or of low socioeconomic status resulted in significantly fewer reports of child abuse during the first 2 years of life (Olds and others, 1986; Olds and Kitzman, 1990). The nurses provided information on normal child growth and development and routine health care needs, served as informal support persons, and referred families to appropriate services when a need for assistance was identified.

Such programs provide models that can be used to reduce factors known to increase the risk of abuse. However, nurses in a variety of settings can implement similar activities. Nurses in prenatal clinics can prepare expectant families for the adjustment to parenthood and can be alert to signs that may indicate a parent in need of help (Box 16-16). Nursery and postpartum nurses can foster the attachment process by encouraging parents to hold and look at their infant and observing the interactions (Box 16-17). In neonatal intensive care units nurses can minimize the effects of separation by encouraging parents to visit and help

Box 16-16 OBSERVATIONS OF PARENTS-TO-BE DURING PRENATAL CARE

1. Are the parents overconcerned with the baby's sex?
2. Are the parents overconcerned with the baby's performance? Do they worry that the infant will not meet the standard?
3. Is there an attempt to deny that there is a pregnancy (mother not willing to gain weight, no plans whatsoever, refusal to talk about the situation)?
4. Is this child going to be one child too many? Could he or she be the "last straw"?
5. Is there great depression over this pregnancy?
6. Is the mother alone and frightened, especially by the physical changes caused by the pregnancy? Do careful explanations fail to dissipate these fears?
7. Is support lacking from husband and/or family?
8. Where are the parents living? Do they have a listed telephone number? Are their relatives and friends nearby?
9. Did the mother and/or father formerly want an abortion but not go through with it or wait until it was too late?
10. Have the parents considered relinquishment of their child? Why did they change their minds?

Modified from Kempe, C.N.: Approaches to preventing child abuse, Am. J. Dis. Child. 130:941-947, Sept. 1976. Copyright 1976, American Medical Association.

Box 16-17 OBSERVATIONS TO BE MADE AT POSTPARTUM AND PEDIATRIC CHECKUPS

1. Do the parents have fun with the baby?
2. Do the parents establish eye contact (direct en face position) with the baby?
3. How do the parents talk to the baby? Is everything they express a demand?
4. Are most of their verbalizations about the child negative?
5. Do they remain disappointed over the child's sex?
6. What is the child's name? Where did the name come from? When was the child named?
7. Are the parents' expectations for the child's development far beyond the child's capabilities?
8. Are the parents very bothered by the baby's crying? How do they feel about the crying?
9. Do the parents see the baby as too demanding during feedings? Are they repulsed by the messiness? Do they ignore the baby's demands to be fed?
10. What are the parents' reactions to the task of changing diapers?
11. When the baby cries, are the parents able to comfort him or her?
12. What are other family members' reactions to the baby?
13. What types of support is the mother receiving?
14. Are there sibling rivalry problems?
15. Is the husband jealous of the baby's drain on the mother's time and affection?
16. When the parents bring the child to the practitioner's office, do they get involved and take control over the baby's needs and what's going to happen (during the examination and while in the waiting room), or do they relinquish control to the physician or nurse (e.g., undressing, holding, or allowing the child to express fears)?
17. Can attention be focused on the child in the parents' presence? Can the parents see something positive for them in that?
18. Do the parents make nonexistent complaints about the baby? Do they call with strange stories that the child has, for example, stopped breathing, turned color, or is doing something "on purpose" to aggravate the parent?
19. Do the parents make emergency calls for very small things, not major things?

Modified from Kempe, C.N.: Approaches to preventing child abuse, Am. J. Dis. Child. 130:941-947, Sept. 1976. Copyright 1976, American Medical Association.

them become comfortable in the child's care. Those in ambulatory settings can teach parents appropriate methods of bathing, feeding, toileting, disciplining, and preventing injuries, while stressing children's normal needs and developmental characteristics. Nurses must be sensitive to the parents' needs for attention, reassurance, and reinforcement. Nurses need to know what community services are available, including self-help groups, and make timely referrals.

Identification and protection from further abuse. Initially, identification of instances of suspected abuse or neglect is essential. The nurse may come in contact with abused children in an emergency room, practitioner's office, or school. Signs that indicate possible abuse (see Box 16-13) must be recognized.

✦ **NURSING ALERT** The priority is to remove the child from the abusive situation to prevent further injury.

All states and provinces in North America have laws for mandatory reporting of child maltreatment. Suspected child abuse is reported to the local authorities.* Referrals usually come to the Bureau of Child Welfare and are assigned to a caseworker in an agency such as the Child Protective Services (CPS). Once a referral has been made, a caseworker is assigned to investigate the report. Based on the findings, the child may be left in the home or temporarily removed.

A court proceeding may be necessary before the child can be placed outside the home or when parental rights may be terminated. When the courts are involved, they usually require firsthand testimony by the referring parties. This may mean that nurses in the school, hospital, or public health agency are subpoenaed or that their records are introduced as evidence. In either situation nurses have a great responsibility in reporting facts, not hearsay or subjective opinion, to present evidence of abuse or to vindicate individuals wrongfully accused of abuse. (See Questions and Controversies, p. 740.)

Accurate nurses' notes are critical in any suspected abuse situation. A suggested outline for recording pertinent assessment data is presented in Box 16-18. In addition, color photographs (preferably, instant developing type) should be taken; color of bruises can be important in evaluating time of injury (Table 16-6). Behaviors are described, not interpreted, and are recorded daily to establish a progress record. Conversations between the nurse, child,

*Telephone numbers are usually listed under "Child abuse" in the business white pages of the local directory, or call the emergency child abuse hotline: (800) 422-4453 ([800] 4-A-CHILD).

Box 16-18 GUIDELINES FOR ASSESSMENT DATA IN SUSPECTED ABUSE

History of Injury
1. Date, time, and place of occurrence
2. Sequence of events with recorded times
3. Presence of witnesses
4. Time lapse between injury's occurrence and initiation of treatment
5. Interview with child when appropriate, including verbal quotations and information from drawing or other play activities
6. Interview with parent, witnesses, or other significant persons, including verbal quotations
7. Description of parent-child interactions (verbal interactions, eye contact, touching, parental concern)

Physical Examination
1. Location, size, shape, and color of bruises; approximate location, size, and shape on drawing of body outline
2. Distinguishing characteristics, such as a bruise in the shape of a hand; round burn (possibly caused by cigarette)
3. Symmetry or asymmetry of injury; presence of other injuries
4. Degree of pain; any bone tenderness
5. Evidence of past injuries; general state of health and hygiene
6. Developmental level of child; perform screening test (see Developmental Assessment, Chapter 7)

Table 16-6 Stages of healing noted in bruises

COLOR	AGE OF BRUISE
Red to red-blue	Less than 24 hours
Purple to dark blue	1 to 4 days
Green to yellow-green	5 to 7 days
Yellow to brown	7 to 10 days
Disappearance	1 to 3 weeks

and parent are recorded in quotation form as much as possible. The nurse must bear in mind that the record of the hospital admission or home visit may be the most supporting evidence available. Nurses must be willing to take an active, responsible part in reporting and testifying to child abuse. Part of the long-term plan is help for parents, but the priority must be protection of the child.

Care of child. Frequently children suspected of abuse are hospitalized for medical management of their injuries. Most abuse cases are managed by a multidisciplinary team, including at least a physician, nurse, and social worker. These children's needs are the same as those of any hospitalized child but are multiplied by their situation. Even though they tend to adjust easily to their new environment and make friends quickly, they need a consistent caregiver. At times the child's indiscriminate affection for any adult seems to diminish the necessity of consistency. However, such behavior is a learned response from previous relationships with others. Children want to love and attach themselves to one special person, but their efforts to do so with their parents often were met with frustration and physical punishment or neglect. Therefore they are no longer inclined to assume the same risk, unless the effort comes from the other person.

The nurse has the obligation of demonstrating acceptance and affection for these children, while not expecting the same in return, until they begin to trust that the nurse will not turn against them for not meeting the nurse's needs. This can be made very difficult by the children's behavior, such as clinging for attention.

The nurse is placed in the position of showing the child acceptance while attempting to modify the negative behavior. Using anger or any aggressive act is avoided. Instead, the nurse plans a program of attention based on play, group interaction with other children, and quiet time with the child. Behavior modification is employed to foster positive behavior and may include praise or tokens for rewards. Through such modeling, alternate ways of interacting and disciplining their child can be demonstrated to parents.

Hospitalization is often extended as eventual placement is arranged. Frequently this is longer than necessary for recovery from the injury or neglect. These children must be guided toward physical and mental wellness during this period. They are treated as children with the usual physical needs, developmental tasks, and play interests—not as dramatic victims of abuse. The nurse is their advocate in this goal. Others who want to question them without justified reason are intercepted by the nurse.

The nurse also encourages the children to continue their relationships with the parents. The nurse does not become a substitute parent to the exclusion of the children's natural parents. Such an intent only intensifies the parents' feelings of inadequacy, worthlessness, and isolation. It in no way helps them understand their child or promotes their trust in health professionals. The goal of the consistent nurse-child relationship is to provide a role model for the parents. The nurse helps them to relate positively and constructively to their child and to foster a therapeutic environment during the child's reprieve from the abusing situation.

Discharge planning should begin as soon as the legal disposition for placement has been decided, which may be temporary foster home placement, return to the parents, or permanent termination of parental rights. The latter is the most drastic resolution, but it is necessary in situations of repeated abuse. Whenever children are remanded to a foster home or juvenile institution, they must be allowed the opportunity to express their feelings. No matter how severe the abuse, they usually mourn the loss of their parents. They need help to understand why they must not return home and that this new home is in no way a punishment. Whenever possible, foster parents should be encouraged to visit, and the nurse should take an active role in helping these parents understand the child. It is unfortunate that some abused children live in torment as they are sent from one foster home to another, sometimes enduring worse circumstances than existed in their original home. Only through constant evaluation of the placement residence and the child's adjustment to a new environment can the vicious cycle of abuse, abandonment, and neglect be stopped.

Care of family. One of the most difficult, yet essential, components of success with abusing parents is the quality of the therapeutic relationship. It must be one of genuine concern and treatment, not one of accusation and punishment. Nurses must examine their personal feelings toward these parents, particularly when sexual abuse is present. Some see the act of abuse as disgusting and totally without justification, whereas others can identify with it, at least in the sense of realizing the exasperation and frustration occasionally felt toward their own children. In some way, such as group discussion, nurses must come to an understanding of their feelings to be effective with abusing parents. For example, viewing the parent as the patient and the child as the victim of abuse places the emphasis on "treatment" rather than "punishment." Unless the nurse's attitude is positive, abusing parents will not be motivated to change, since they will not be working with a trusting person who demonstrates the behavior being asked of them.

These parents cannot be fooled. Their survival as a child depended on their perception of other people's needs, and they are very skillful at saying what is expected of them while not making any attempts to change. This may be why self-help groups such as **Parents Anonymous*** (a group for parents who have abused or fear that they may abuse their child, but only in terms of physical abuse, not sexual abuse) are so successful. The members cannot be deluded

*7120 Franklin Ave., Los Angeles, CA 90046; (800) 421-0353.

because they know the "game" so well. Such groups also are very accepting and nonjudgmental because everyone has been in the same position. Group peer pressure and commitment are important motivating factors that keep parents from reverting to previous behaviors. The group also provides a release mechanism; when parents are angry, they can call a fellow member and vent their feelings over the phone rather than on the child.

Since some parents may have unrealistic expectations of children's capabilities, the nurse also fosters knowledge and understanding of normal growth and development. The nurse demonstrates how to handle children, how to teach them at their age level, and what realistically to expect from them. Since these parents are often very sensitive to criticism or domination and may already possess a low self-esteem, teaching is implemented through demonstration and example rather than through lecturing. Any competent parenting abilities they demonstrate are praised in an attempt to promote their sense of parental adequacy. Abusing parents desperately need "mothering" to be able to mother or father their own children. The nurse attends to their needs for security, trust, and release from responsibility. Home visits may be planned at times when the children are at school, with a friend, or asleep to allow maximum attention to the parent.

SEXUAL ABUSE

Sexual abuse is one of the most devastating types of child maltreatment, and current estimates indicate that it has increased tremendously during the past decade. This is not only because of growing public awareness. It is also associated with the (1) expansion of definitions to include extrafamilial abuse, (2) increase in the numbers of programs to treat sexual abusers and victims, and (3) shifts in state and local policy emphasis on reporting and investigating sexual maltreatment. The number of reported occurrences was approximately 16% of all child maltreatment cases in 1987 (Highlights, 1989). This is probably a small percentage of the actual incidence, since many instances are never reported because the victim, female or male, is afraid, feels guilty or ashamed, thinks he or she will not be believed, or fears the loss of love from someone, such as a parent. Sexual abuse may include physical abuse, both as part of sexual arousal for the abuser and to force compliance from the child (Hobbs and Wynne, 1990).

As with all forms of child maltreatment, no universal definition for sexual abuse exists. The Child Abuse and Prevention Act (Public Law 100-294) defines sexual abuse as "the use, persuasion, or coercion of any child to engage in sexually explicit conduct (or any simulation of such conduct) for producing any visual depiction of such conduct, or rape, molestation, prostitution, or incest with children."

To be considered child abuse, these acts have to be committed by a person responsible for the child's care, such as a parent or baby-sitter. If a stranger commits the act, it is considered sexual assault and is handled solely by the police and criminal courts (National Center on Child Abuse and Neglect, 1989).

Sexual abuse includes several types of sexual maltreatment, including incest, molestation, exhibitionism, child pornography, child prostitution, and pedophilia. The Glossary at the beginning of this chapter defines these terms (see also *child molester*) (Kempe and Kempe, 1984; Fuller, 1989). Definitions of rape are presented in Chapter 20.

Characteristics of Abusers and Victims

Much less is known about the characteristics of sexual abusers and their victims than in any other type of child maltreatment. However, some significant differences exist depending on whether the abuse occurs outside or within the family context.

Extrafamilial sexual abuse. In the majority of incidences of extrafamilial sexual abuse the offender is known to the victims or their families and is often a friend, neighbor, or someone in a position of authority. In a significant number of situations the sexual abuse has taken place repeatedly over weeks or months. Families are often ambivalent about reporting abuse to avoid disgrace, or they may not believe the victim. Offenders come from all levels of society and may even be prominent persons in the community.

Exhibitionists are usually younger men from late adolescents through their 20s and 30s. Unlike the stereotype of "dirty old men," their numbers decline after age 40. They usually have normal intelligence with a good work history, and may appear socially intact. They are often described as shy and immature but may be married and have children. They prefer younger girls as victims because of their more frightened response. Exhibitionism rarely includes sex acts or violence, but the potential does exist (Kempe and Kempe, 1984).

Pedophiliacs, often called "child molesters," may force a child to engage in different sex acts. Other pedophiliacs, however, may love the child without physical contact. The principal characteristic of these individuals is that they prefer children to adults as sex objects. The sexual activity tends to be a fairly immature form of sexual gratification (undressing and looking at the child, touching, kissing, fondling, perhaps masturbation) and reveals a desire to dominate the sexual activity. Pedophiliacs may be men or women, and their preference may be the same- or the opposite-sex child. Most prefer children in certain age-groups. Pedophilia is a way of life; most pedophiliacs see no harm in what they are doing, since they believe they have a genuine love of children. They may be in careers that cater to children, such as coaching or teaching, and may be known and respected by the community. They tend to frequent child-oriented places, such as skating rinks, video arcades, or amusement parks. They are very sensitive to identifying youngsters in need of love and attention, such as those from unhappy homes, runaways, and missing children. The sexual activity may begin after a rather lengthy relationship with the offender that has engendered the child's trust. Children are pressured to participate in sexual activity and to keep it a secret by many of the same ploys used by most offenders (see Box 16-19).

Pornography and prostitution may involve strangers as

well as the children's own parents. These offenders have no typical characteristics, although the abused children tend to be runaways—young adolescents who engage in these activities to provide money for food, shelter, drugs, and alcohol.

Intrafamilial sexual abuse. About three fourths of all reported instances of incest occurs between father or stepfather and daughter. Mother-son, mother-daughter, and sibling incest account for most of the remaining cases. Sexual play or experimentation is common among young siblings and usually stops as the children become older. In most instances sibling abuse has less disturbing emotional consequences for the victims than other types of incestuous relationships, but this is not always so, especially when the victim is forced to submit. However, these cases are less likely to come to the attention of authorities.

Incestuous relationships between father and daughter are generally prolonged, and the victims are usually reluctant to report the situation because of fear of retaliation and fear that they will not be believed. Typically, incestuous relationships begin later than other forms of child abuse; in general, the average age of the sexual abuse victim is 9 years (Highlights, 1988). The eldest daughter is usually abused, but in her absence another sister is substituted. Sexual abuse by relatives, especially those with a strong emotional bond to the victim, is the most devastating to the child (Feinauer, 1989).

Sexual abuse is not limited to girls. Boys are also victims of both intrafamilial and extrafamilial abuse. Incidence rates are at best inaccurate and range from conservative estimates of 5 to 6:1000 to liberal estimates of 1:6 (Krugman, 1989b; Zaphiris, 1986). Males are much less likely to report abuse, and available research indicates that they suffer greater emotional harm from incestuous relationships, especially between mother-son, than female victims. The reason for the greater emotional damage is not known but may be related to the lack of opportunity for identification with the father. Boys are more likely than girls to be subjected to anal penetration and oral-genital contact, to have subtle physical findings, and to be abused by a father, stepfather, or mother's boyfriend (Spencer and Dunklee, 1986).

Initiation and Perpetuation of Sexual Abuse

The cycle of sexual abuse often starts innocently, unless it involves an isolated attack, such as rape. Often offenders spend time with the victims to gain their trust before initiating any sexual contact. Most victims are then pressured into being an accessory to the sexual activity through various means. The methods of pressure are such that the child may be totally unaware that sexual activity is part of the offer (Box 16-19).

Children may reveal the fear that their parents would not believe them, especially if the offender is a trusted member of the family. Some fear they will be blamed for the situation. Many young children with limited vocabulary have difficulty describing the activity when they do have the courage or opportunity to complain. Consequently the abuse is perpetuated over a prolonged period.

Seductiveness by the child does not initiate incest. Most young females experiment in seduction, especially during the preschool years, but the father's response normally differentiates this playfulness from overt sexual invitation. Although the reasons for incest are complicated and can occur in various family types, it does not occur in healthy families (Kempe and Kempe, 1984). Most incestuous relationships are directly tied to sexual maladjustment and estrangement between husband and wife. Most begin following the cessation of sexual relationships with the usual partner. Most fathers experience little guilt, and many wives at some level are aware of the incestuous affair. The wife may react by tolerating the situation or may resort to use of denial; some remain unaware of the activity (Hogan and Juhasz, 1984). Consequently the home offers little protection to young victims, since abusers have easy access to their victims and the children feel they cannot reveal their secret to other family members.

Box 16-19 METHODS USED TO PRESSURE CHILDREN INTO SEXUAL ACTIVITY

The child is offered material goods, such as special favors or privileges.
The adult misrepresents moral standards by telling the child that it is "okay to do." Children grow up believing that if an adult tells them to do something, they should do it.
Isolated and emotionally and socially impoverished children are enticed by adults who meet their needs for warmth and human contact.
The successful sex offender pressures the victim into secrecy regarding the activity by describing it as a "secret between us" that other people may take away if they find out.
The offender also plays on the child's fears, including fear of punishment by the offender, fear of repercussions if the child tells, and fear of abandonment or rejection by the family.

Identification of Sexual Abuse

Unlike physical abuse or neglect, sexual abuse may occur with few if any obvious physical indications of the activity. Also, many individuals are hesitant to believe children and unwilling to report incidents. Even health professionals are sometimes at fault when they perform cursory physical examinations of the genitalia and ignore behavior or verbal comments that suggest abuse. When sexual abuse is suspected, other children in the family should also be checked, since multiple victims may be involved.

Unfortunately, no typical profile of the victim exists, and one must have a high index of suspicion to identify these children. Physical signs vary and may include any of those listed in Box 16-13 for sexual abuse (see Questions and Controversies, p. 746).

The victim may exhibit various behavioral manifestations. Unfortunately, none of these behaviors is diagnostic of sexual abuse (Legrand, Wakefield, and Underwager, 1989). When abused children exhibit these behaviors, the signs may be incorrectly attributed to the normal stresses of childhood, especially in older school-age children or ado-

QUESTIONS AND CONTROVERSIES

How valid are the findings from the genital examination in diagnosing sexual abuse in children?

Unlike physical abuse, in which signs of maltreatment are often apparent, little or no evidence of sexual activity may be found in sexual abuse. To help substantiate accusations of molestation, several investigators have attempted to define characteristics of genitalia in males and females that are "diagnostic" of sexual abuse. Of the many findings that have been reported as conclusive or "highly suspect," the following are often considered the most significant: vaginal opening greater than 4 mm (Cantwell, 1983; White, Ingram, and Lyna, 1989), hymenal tears and synechiae (tissue bands) inside the vagina (Emans and others, 1987), reflex anal dilatation (Hobbs and Wynne, 1989), and condylomata acuminata (anogenital or venereal warts) (Hanson and others, 1989).

However, most subjects in these studies were children suspected of sexual abuse; without a control group of nonabused children, it is impossible to be certain that the same findings are not present in all children. Even the few studies with control groups found the same genital signs in the nonabused children, although not as often. Surprisingly, little is known about the normal range of genital characteristics in children. What is known casts serious doubt on the diagnostic validity of any of the "highly suspect" signs. McCann and others (1990a) conducted studies on prepubertal children who had been carefully screened to rule out sexual abuse. They found that the size of the vaginal opening varied greatly; an opening greater than 4 mm was not unusual. The size was influenced by the examination position, amount of traction applied to the labia, degree of relaxation during the examination, and the child's age. In examining the anal and vaginal areas, the researchers found that any findings often associated with sexual abuse, including reflex anal dilatation (opening of the anal sphincters during knee-chest position), hymenal tears, and vaginal synechiae, also were not unusual in nonabused children (McCann and others, 1989, 1990b). Another study investigated the likelihood of condylomata acuminata occurring in children who were not sexually abused; only 11% of the children (none under 3 years of age) with the warts were judged to be victims of molestation (Cohen, as cited by Krowchuk and others, 1990).

In light of these findings, proof of sexual abuse does not rest on the physical examination. The only definitive physical evidence of sexual assault is presence of sperm (Aiken, 1990). In reviewing cases of sexual abuse with successful conviction of the perpetrator, experts contend that the most important evidence is the quality of the history (including the medical record) and the ability of children to tell their story (De Jong and Rose, 1989).

lescents. Even those signs considered most predictive of sexual abuse, such as sexually inappropriate behavior for age, enactment of adult sexual activity, and intense focus on sexual activity (e.g., masturbation), do not always indicate that sexual abuse has occurred. Conversely, abused children may not demonstrate more knowledge of sexual activity than nonabused children. However, one difference in the abused children's explanation of sexual activity may be unusual affective responses. For example, abused children may relate stories that include fear of going to sleep or of being with a parent (Gordon, Schroeder, and Abrams, 1990).

The disclosure of the secret comes about in a variety of ways—the act is observed by others, resulting in a direct confrontation; the child tells someone, such as a parent of a friend; visible clues of the relationship are observed, such as an accumulation of coins, gifts, or candy; or more obvious clues are seen, such as a child coming home disheveled or becoming pregnant; and physical or behavioral signs and symptoms are observed. Children usually describe the experience in terms of whether it was unpleasant or hurt or was pleasurable (usually a response to hand-genital contact); some indicate no reaction. Young children often feel no guilt or shame because the act is pleasurable and they are unaware of its inappropriateness.

Response of families. Families respond to sexual abuse with a variety of emotional reactions that may be as intense and disruptive as they are for the victim, regardless of the type of abuse. The immediate reactions range from not believing the child to being very supportive (De Jong, 1988). A common reaction is denial of the child's accusation. The parents may be surprisingly unable to provide adequate emotional support to the child at this time, even when their attitude toward the child has been supportive in the past.

Parents and other family members may display the same type of emotional responses as the victim, such as inability to eat or sleep and somatic complaints of headache or backache. In the acute emotional phase, parents have a need to blame someone. The three common targets are the offender, the child, and themselves. The parents typically express anger at the child for "stupid" behavior and may even restrict the child's privileges as punishment. When the victim is a female, the parents may question her sexual provocation of the event. Self-blaming parents assume full responsibility, believing that they have been inadequate parents or should not have allowed the child to go out. When a baby-sitter or trusted relative is involved in the assault and the child's complaint has not been believed until obvious evidence is presented, the parents are often devastated by guilt.

Nursing Considerations

Nursing care of sexually abused children involves the same objectives as those discussed for physically maltreated victims: prevention, identification, and protection from further abuse. Many of the interventions are identical, such as reporting the abuse and caring for the child in the hospital if admission is required, and are discussed on p. 742. Because evidence of sexual maltreatment may be less obvious than in other types of abuse, nurses must have a high index of suspicion and be aware of clues to sexual abuse (see Box 16-13). When the child has sustained physical harm, the care is consistent with that provided a rape victim, with the same considerations for the child's preparation and psychologic needs during the examination (see Rape, Chapter 20).

Prevention. One aspect of sexual abuse that is receiving increasing attention is prevention. Most of the prevention programs are directed at teaching children to recognize situations that increase the risk of sexual abuse and to respond in ways that reduce the risk. Currently there is much controversy regarding the effectiveness of these programs. The main issue is whether young children should be expected to participate in their own protection. Some experts suggest that in the struggle between sexual offender and potential child victim, most factors favor the adult, who has superior knowledge, strength, and skill to overcome most children's efforts at self-protection (Conte, Wolf, and Smith, 1989). At least one review of child sexual abuse prevention programs have found them to be largely ineffective in teaching young children about sexual abuse or its prevention (Gilbert and others, 1989). Such research clearly indicates that sexual abuse prevention is more than teaching children to say "no" or to recognize their right not to be touched in "private places." It is equally important to teach children safety in terms of potential risk situations. Several suggestions for parents regarding protecting and educating children against possible molestation are presented in the Parent Guidelines.

The nurse is frequently in a position to discuss this topic with parents as part of health maintenance and to provide guidelines. Books are available for parents that describe sexual abuse and its prevention.* Helpful games such as "What if the baby-sitter wants to wrestle and hug but tells you to keep it a secret?" can be used to explore dangerous situations in advance and help children learn the importance of saying "No." They need reassurance that no matter what the other person says or does, the parents want to know and will not punish them. Even if children do participate in the activity before telling the parents, they must be reassured that it was not their fault.

In addition, parents need to be made aware that "nice" people, including friends and relatives, can be offenders; parents should carefully observe how others act toward the child. A sudden change in the child's behavior and a response such as "I don't like uncle anymore" are clues to investigate the relationship. In the event of any doubt, further solitary encounters with this person and the child should be prevented. It is sometimes to the child's great misfortune that parents do not take certain comments seriously, such as "He hugs me too tight" or "I don't want to go with him." Casual parental statements such as "He just loves you" or "You do whatever adults tell you to do" can place children in jeopardy. Health professionals can alert parents to such dangers and guide them toward an appreciation of the

PARENT GUIDELINES
Preventing or Dealing with Sexual Abuse

Sexual assault of children occurs more frequently than most of us realize. It may be preventable if children have good preparation. *To provide protection and preparation,* as parents we can:

- Pay careful attention to who is around our children. (Unwanted touch *may* come from someone we like and trust.)
- Back up a child's right to say "No."
- Encourage communication by taking seriously what our children *say.*
- Take a second look at signals of potential danger.
- Refuse to leave our children in the company of those we do not trust.
- Include information about sexual assault when teaching about safety.
- Provide specific definitions and examples of sexual assault.
- Remind children that even "nice" people sometimes do mean things.
- Urge children to tell us about *anybody* who causes them to be uncomfortable.
- Prepare children to deal with bribes and threats, as well as possible physical force.
- Eliminate secrets between us and our children.
- Teach children how to say "No," ask for help, and control who touches them and how.
- Model self-protective and limit-setting behavior for our children.

Should it ever become necessary *to help a child recover from a sexual assault,* as parents we can:

- Listen carefully and understand how children tell us.
- Support the child for telling by praise, belief, sympathy, and lack of blame.
- Know local resources, and choose help carefully.
- Provide opportunities to talk about the assault.
- Provide opportunities for the entire family to go through a recovery process.

Sexual assault affects all of us, whether or not our own children are assaulted. *To help deal with this social problem,* all of us can:

- Provide sympathetic care and support to those who have been victimized.
- Recognize that offenders do not change without intervention.
- Organize neighborhood programs to support each other's efforts to protect children.
- Encourage schools to provide information about sexual assault as a problem of health and safety.
- Organize community groups to support educational, treatment, and law enforcement programs.

From Adams, C., and Fay, J.: No more secrets: protecting your child from sexual assault, San Luis Obispo, CA, 1981, Impact Publishers, Inc.

*Additional sources of information are the **National Committee for Prevention of Child Abuse,** Publishing Department, 332 S. Michigan Ave., Suite 950, Chicago, IL 60604-4357, (312) 663-3520; **Clearinghouse on Child Abuse and Neglect,** P.O. Box 1182, Washington, DC 20013, (703) 821-2086; **C. Henry Kempe National Center for the Prevention and Treatment of Child Abuse and Neglect,** 1205 Oneida St., Denver, CO 80220, (303) 321-3963; **American Association for Protecting Children, American Humane Association,** 63 Inverness Dr. E., Englewood, CO 80112, (800) 227-5242 (outside Colorado) or (303) 792-9900; and **National Resource Center on Child Sexual Abuse,** 11141 Georgia Ave., Wheaton, MD 20902, (800) 543-7006.

problem, providing concrete guidelines for child education and protection.

Care of child. The type of care needed by the child depends on the circumstances of the sexual abuse. It varies from reassurance and support when the act involves exhibitionism to long-term counseling in incestuous situations. When children report potentially sexually abusive experiences, their reports need to be taken seriously, but also cautiously to avoid alarming the child or falsely accusing a person. Children's reports may vary from contradictory stories to unwavering versions of the experience. While their stories may sound contradictory, this may reflect the child's experiences in several instances of abuse. Also, children who repeatedly tell identical facts may have been prompted to do so (Kempe and Kempe, 1984). Increasing evidence suggests that the types of interrogation children are exposed to following reports of sexual abuse shape their thinking. In addition, a parent may persuade a child to believe that abuse occurred for a particular purpose, such as gaining custody in a divorce dispute (Yates and Musty, 1988). Consequently, children may falsely accuse individuals of abuse, not because the children are lying but because they are affirming what the interviewer or parent wants to hear. Through the use of leading questions, closed questions (those requiring yes or no answers), intimidation, prodding, and selective reinforcement for certain answers, children begin to tell stories that never occurred. Eventually they may come to experience the tale as reality (Wakefield and Underwager, 1989).

When questioning children who may be victims of abuse, nurses must be very skillful interviewers to avoid biasing the interaction. Courts may allow a hearsay declaration (an out-of-court statement) to be used as legal evidence. Medical records should include verbatim statements made by the child and interviewer that reflect appropriate nonleading questions and statements (Myers, 1986). Nurses should clarify their role in the child abuse investigation process. Some experts suggest that health professionals limit the interview to the child's physical and mental health concerns and leave the topics of the family's social, legal, or other problems to the police or CPS personnel (Koop, 1988).

In preparation for an interview, every effort is made to make the child feel comfortable with appropriate introductions and to avoid duplicating the behaviors typically used by offenders, such as touching the child without permission. The interview is conducted in a quiet and private location, preferably a neutral place, such as a school playroom or office, and not where the abuse occurred. Neutral questions are asked first, such as the child's reaction to the hospital (if appropriate). Then the incident is discussed in general terms. The interview should include such nonleading questions as "Do you know why you were brought to the hospital?" "Do you know what will happen here?" or "How do you feel about being here?" Later the question "Can you tell me what happened?" and other questions may then elicit an account of the incident. Sometimes the parents are able to help the child to describe the incident, and questions can then be directed to the circumstances of the assault. Questions should progress chronologically and proceed from the nonsexual to the more sexual content. If the child shows evidence of becoming too upset, the focus is redirected toward more neutral and less emotionally charged areas.

Children are given the opportunity to ask questions, but if they are reticent, they are never pressured into talking. Young children in particular lack the verbal skills to describe body parts adequately. These children may benefit from play situations that provide opportunities for disclosure, such as drawing, using puppets or anatomically correct dolls, and doll houses.

Considerable controversy exists regarding the use of children's drawings and anatomically correct dolls as *diagnostic* tests for sexual abuse. Two studies that investigated the type of human figure drawings made by allegedly sexually abused and by nonsexually abused children found that those in the abuse group included more details about genitalia than the other group (Hibbard and Hartman, 1990; Hibbard, Roghmann, and Hoekelman, 1987). In these studies it is not known if the interview process with the sexual abuse group influenced the subsequent drawings. Also, in one of these studies the difference between the groups was not statistically significant. The authors caution that the presence of genitalia on a human figure drawing does not prove sexual abuse; the children's description and explanation of the drawing are more relevant than its content. Genitalia on drawings may raise suspicion of abuse but are not diagnostic. The use of drawings as an assessment technique is not supported by scientific research (Conoley and Kramer, 1989; Wakefield and Underwager, 1988).

The controversy regarding the validity of anatomically correct dolls is of even more concern, because some professionals are using the dolls as diagnostic tools in the investigation of suspected sexual abuse. Research on the dolls' diagnostic value has yielded conflicting results. One study that examined the behavioral responses of abused and nonabused children found no difference between the groups playing with the dolls. The finding that the interviewer could easily influence the children to demonstrate sexual acts with the dolls was a special concern (McIver, Wakefield, and Underwager, 1989). Other researchers who observed only the behavior of nonabused children with the dolls have reported that many of these children's activities were similar to those described by professionals who use the dolls in sexual abuse investigations (Gabriel, 1985). Other studies, however, have shown that the frequency of sexual behavior with the dolls differs among sexually abused and nonsexually abused children. In one study significantly more children who had been sexually abused demonstrated sexual behavior in their play (Jampole and Weber, 1987). While it appears that the use of anatomically correct dolls is not diagnostic of sexual abuse, some professionals believe that the dolls help children communicate what happened and are a useful method of opening up communication, especially with young children (Leventhal and others, 1989). Others maintain that there is no way to

NURSING CARE PLAN
The Child Who Is Maltreated

NURSING DIAGNOSIS: Potential for trauma related to characteristics of child, caregiver(s), environment

GOAL 1
Protect from further abuse

INTERVENTIONS
Implement measures to prevent abuse
- Report suspicions to appropriate authorities
- Assist in removing child from unsafe environment and establishing in a safe environment
- Establish protective measures for the hospitalized child as indicated

Keep factual, objective records of
- Child's physical condition
- Child's behavioral response to parents, others, and environment
- Interviews with family members

EXPECTED OUTCOME
Suspected child abuse victim is removed from abusive environment

GOAL 2
Prevent recurrence

INTERVENTIONS
Collaborate efforts of multidisciplinary team to continually evaluate progress of child in foster home or in return to own family
Be alert for signs of continued abuse or neglect
Help parents identify those circumstances that precipitate an abusive act and alternative ways to deal with the release of anger other than attacking child
Refer for alternative placement when indicated

EXPECTED OUTCOME
Child is free of injury or neglect

NURSING DIAGNOSIS: Fear/anxiety related to negative interpersonal interaction, repeated maltreatment, powerlessness

GOAL 1
Relieve or reduce anxiety and stress

INTERVENTIONS
Provide consistent caregiver and therapeutic environment during hospitalization
Demonstrate acceptance of child while not expecting same in return
Show attention while not reinforcing inappropriate behavior
Plan appropriate activities for attention with nurse, other adults, and other children; use play to work through relationships
Avoid displacing anger on child, such as shouting or yelling, as method of dealing with own frustration toward child's negative behavior
Praise child's abilities in order to promote self-esteem
Treat child as one who has a specific physical problem for hospitalization, not as "abused" victim
Avoid asking too many questions
Use play, especially family or doll house activity, to investigate type of relationships perceived by child
Provide one consistent person to whom child relates regarding events of abuse

EXPECTED OUTCOMES
Child exhibits minimal or no evidence of distress
Child engages in positive relationships with caregivers

NURSING DIAGNOSIS: Altered parenting related to child, caregiver, or situational characteristics that precipitate abusive behavior

GOAL 1
Prevent abuse

INTERVENTIONS
Identify families at risk for potential abuse
Promote parental attachment to child
Emphasize child-rearing practices, especially effective methods of discipline
Increase parents' feeling of adequacy and self-esteem
Encourage support systems that lessen stress and total responsibility of child care on one or both parents
Teach children to recognize situations that place them at risk for sexual abuse and teach assertive responses

EXPECTED OUTCOME
Families exhibit evidence of positive interaction with children

GOAL 2
Support parents

INTERVENTIONS
Provide "mothering" by directing attention to parent, taking over child care responsibilities until parent feels ready to participate, and focusing on parent's needs
Refer parents to special support groups and/or counseling
Help identify a support group for parents, such as extended family or nearby neighbors; help these significant others understand their important role in also preventing further abuse

EXPECTED OUTCOMES
Parents demonstrate appropriate parenting activities
Parents seek group and individual support

Continued.

NURSING CARE PLAN
The Child Who Is Maltreated—cont'd

GOAL 3

Educate parents regarding normal child growth and development

INTERVENTIONS

Teach realistic expectations of child's behavior and capabilities

Emphasize alternate methods of discipline, such as reward and verbal disapproval

Suggest methods of handling developmental problems or goals, such as toddler negativism, toilet training, and independence

Teach through demonstration and role modeling, rather than lecture; avoid authoritarian approach

EXPECTED OUTCOME

Parents demonstrate an understanding of normal expectations for their child

GOAL 4

Reduce environmental crises

INTERVENTIONS

Refer to social agencies that can provide assistance in areas such as financial support, adequate housing, and employment

EXPECTED OUTCOME

Parents receive assistance with problems

use the dolls to obtain reliable evidence about past events (Wakefield and Underwager, 1988).

In interviewing the child, every effort is made to coordinate the number of interviewers and to assign a primary professional to work with the child. Videotaping or audiotaping is ideal for limiting the number of traumatic events. If nurses are not the primary professional, they can serve as the child's advocate to prevent excessive questioning and embarrassment by others.

Care of family. Care of the family also depends on the circumstances of the sexual abuse. With a nonparent offender the family may be more able to support the child than if incest was involved. Family members are encouraged to express their feelings of anger, guilt, shame, and/or embarrassment, but are also cautioned to avoid displacing such feelings on the child. For example, it is easy for parents to admonish the child with statements, such as "We told you never to go with strangers," that make the child feel responsible.

Family members are advised to encourage the child to resume normal activities and to observe the child for signs of distress (see Posttraumatic Stress Disorder, Chapter 18). Children express their feelings primarily through behavior. Parents should be alert for changes in behavior that indicate distress resulting from the incident, such as remaining in the house, refusing to go to school, changes in sleeping patterns, and frequency of dreams and nightmares. Children are encouraged to talk about these feelings and nightmares, since the more they can talk about the experience, the more they will be able to gain control over it.

In incestuous relationships the goal is to protect the child. The preferred approach is to remove the offender, not the child, from the home. However, this is not always possible, especially when the offender refuses to admit responsibility or the other parent, usually the mother, sides with the offender, usually the father, and prefers that the child leave the home. If the child is placed in a foster home, the same interventions are appropriate as those discussed under physical abuse (see p. 738). However, the child may feel even more responsible for the family breakup than in other situations of maltreatment because of the intimate part the child played in the abuse.

Numerous treatment programs exist for sex offenders, but currently no one approach has proved successful. Research indicates that a combination of individual and group therapy for at least 2 years is needed for treatment of incest; even less is known about treatment of other types of perpetrators. Groups such as **Parents United International, Inc.,*** have been successful in helping sexually abused families, and nurses can be instrumental in making referrals to local chapters. The primary goal of Parents United is to break the cycle of child sexual abuse. Parents United helps the following groups: child victims, siblings, AMACs (adults molested as children), offenders (men and women), and nonoffending parents. All groups are led by professionally trained therapists. A condition of membership is that the person must be receiving one-on-one therapy.

There is no way to predict which families will be successfully rehabilitated. With father-daughter incest, however, the best results occur when the father accepts full responsibility for the act, the mother acknowledges her role in failing to protect the child, and the child is able to understand and forgive the parents and develop a positive self-image despite the traumatic experience (Kempe and Kempe, 1984).

*P.O. Box 952, San Jose, CA 95108-0952; (408) 453-7616.

KEY POINTS

- Common disorders during early childhood include communicable diseases, intestinal parasitic infections, conjunctivitis, and stomatitis.
- Nursing goals in the treatment of a communicable disease are identification, provision of comfort, prevention of spread to others, and prevention of complications.
- Intestinal parasitic diseases constitute the most common infections in the world; giardiasis and enterobiasis are the most widespread parasitic infections among children in the United States.
- Although the incidence of poisoning has decreased in the last 20 years as a result of more stringent packaging regulations, childhood poisoning remains a serious health concern.
- The major principles of emergency treatment for poisoning are assessment, supportive measures, gastric decontamination, family support, and prevention of recurrence.
- Ipecac is an effective and safe emetic for home use in poisonings but is contraindicated in situations that increase the risk of aspiration and that involve ingestion of corrosives, wherein vomiting redamages the mucosa.
- Three simple measures that can reduce the severity of a poisoning are knowing the telephone number of the Poison Control Center, having ipecac in the home (two doses per child), and administering it correctly.
- Acetaminophen poisoning is the most common drug poisoning among children and occurs primarily from acute overdose.
- Potential sources of heavy metal poisoning in children are lead, iron, and mercury.
- The most important factor contributing to lead poisoning is its availability in the child's environment. Lead-based paint is the most toxic source of lead.
- Child maltreatment may take the form of physical abuse or neglect, emotional abuse or neglect, and sexual abuse.
- Parental, child, and environmental characteristics are criteria that singly or together predispose children to physical abuse.
- Identification of physical abuse entails securing evidence of maltreatment, taking a history pertaining to the incident, and assessing parental and child behaviors.
- Sexual abuse has soared in the last decade; common forms are incest, molestation, rape, exhibitionism, child pornography, child prostitution, and pedophilia.

REFERENCES

Adams, J., and Horton, M.: Is it sexual abuse? Confusion caused by a congenital anomaly of the genitalia, Clin. Pediatr. 28(3):146-148, 1989.

Adler, R., and Kane-Nussen, B.: Erythema multiforme: confusion with child battering syndrome, Pediatrics 72(5):718-720, 1983.

Agency for Toxic Substances and Disease Registry: The nature and extent of lead poisoning in children in the United States: a report to Congress, Atlanta, July 1988, U.S. Department of Health and Human Services, Public Health Service.

Aiken, M.M.: Documenting sexual abuse in prepubertal girls, MCN 15:176-177, 1990.

Albertson, T., and others: Superiority of activated charcoal alone compared with ipecac and activated charcoal in the treatment of acute toxic ingestions, Ann. Emerg. Med. 18:56-59, 1989.

Alexander, R., and others: Incidence of impact trauma with cranial injuries ascribed to shaking, Am. J. Dis. Child. 144:724-726, 1990.

Altemeier, W.A., III, and others: Antecedents of child abuse, J. Pediatr. 100(5):823-829, 1982.

American Academy of Pediatrics, Committee on Early Childhood, Adoption, and Dependent Care: Missing children, Pediatrics 78(2):370-372, 1986.

American Academy of Pediatrics, Committee on Environmental Hazards and Committee on Accident and Poison Prevention: Statement on childhood lead poisoning, Pediatrics 79(3):457-465, 1987.

Amitai, Y., and others: Hazards of "deleading" homes of children with lead poisoning, Am. J. Dis. Child. 141(7):758-760, 1987a.

Amitai, Y., and others: Ipecac-induced emesis and reduction of plasma concentrations of drugs following accidental overdose in children, Pediatrics 80(3):364-367, 1987b.

Arrowsmith, J., and others: National patterns of aspirin use and Reye syndrome reporting, United States, 1980 to 1985, Pediatrics 79(6):858-863, 1987.

Asnes, R.S., and Wisotsky, D.H.: Cupping lesions simulating child abuse, J. Pediatr. 99:267-268, 1981.

Baker, R.B.: Seat belt injury masquerading as sexual abuse, Pediatrics 77(3):435, 1986.

Balfour, H., and Englund, J.: Antiviral drugs in pediatrics, Am. J. Dis. Child. 143:1307-1316, 1989.

Balfour, H.H., and others: Acyclovir treatment of varicella in otherwise healthy children, J. Pediatr. 116(4):633-639, 1990.

Banner, W., Jr., and Tong, T.G.: Iron poisoning, Pediatr. Clin. North Am. 33(2):393-409, 1986.

Barkin, R.M., and Rosen, P., editors: Emergency pediatrics, ed. 3, St. Louis, 1990, Mosby–Year Book, Inc.

Bellinger, D., and others: Correlates of low-level lead exposure in urban children at 2 years of age, Pediatrics 77(6):826-833, 1986.

Bellinger, D., and others: Longitudinal analysis of prenatal and postnatal lead exposure and early cognitive development, N. Engl. J. Med. 316(17):1037-1043, 1987.

Besharov, D.J.: "Doing something" about child abuse: the need to narrow the grounds for state intervention, Harvard J. Law Public Policy 8(3):539-589, 1985.

Bithoney, W.G., and others: Childhood ingestions as symptoms of family distress, Am. J. Dis. Child. 139(3):456-459, 1985.

Boehnert, M.T., and others: Advances in clinical toxicology, Pediatr. Clin. North Am. 32(1):193-211, 1985.

Cantwell, H.B.: Vaginal inspection as it relates to child sexual abuse in girls under thirteen, Child Abuse Negl. 7:171-176, 1983.

Centers for Disease Control: Preventing lead poisoning in young children, DHHS Pub. No. 99-2230, Washington, DC, 1985, U.S. Government Printing Office.

Cheng, T.C.: General parasitology, Orlando, FL, 1986, Academic Press, College Division.

Chisolm, J.J.: Mobilization of lead by calcium disodium edetate: a reappraisal, Am. J. Dis. Child. 141(12):1254-1256, 1987.

Clark, M., Royal, J., and Seeler, R.: Interaction of iron deficiency and lead and the hematologic findings in children with severe lead poisoning, Pediatrics 81(2):247-254, 1988.

Conoley, J.C., and Kramer, J.J., editors: Tenth mental measurements yearbook, Lincoln, NB, 1989, University of Nebraska Press.

Conte, J., Wolf, S., and Smith, T.: What sexual offenders tell us about prevention strategies, Child Abuse Negl. 13:293-301, 1989.

Coulehan, J.L., and others: Gasoline sniffing and lead toxicity in Navajo adolescents, Pediatrics 71(1):113-117, 1983.

Council on Scientific Affairs: AMA diagnostic and treatment guidelines concerning child abuse and neglect, JAMA 254(6):796-800, 1985.

Craft, J.C.: Giardiasis in childhood. In Nelson, J.D., and McCracken, G.H., editors: Clinical reviews in pediatric infectious disease, St. Louis, 1985, Mosby–Year Book, Inc.

De Jong, A.: Maternal responses to the sexual abuse of their children, Pediatrics 81(1):14-21, 1988.

De Jong, A., and Rose, M.: Frequency and significance of physical evidence in legally proven cases of child sexual abuse, Pediatrics 84(6):1022-1026, 1989.

Dietrich, K.N., and others: Contribution of social and developmental factors to lead exposure during the first year of life, Pediatrics 75(6):1114-1119, 1985.

Dietrich, K.N., and others: Low-level fetal lead exposure effect on neurobehavioral development in early infancy, Pediatrics 80(5):721-730, 1987.

Dockstader, L., Lawrence, R., and Bresnick, H.: Home administration of activated charcoal: feasibility and acceptance, Vet. Hum. Toxicol. 28(5):471, 1986.

Doran, T., and others: Acetaminophen: more harm than good for chickenpox? J. Pediatr. 114(6):1045-1048, 1989.

Emans, S., and others: Genital findings in sexually abused symptomatic and asymptomatic girls, Pediatrics 79(5):778-785, 1987.

Epstein, M., and others: Munchausen syndrome by proxy: considerations in diagnosis and confirmation by video surveillance, Pediatrics 80(2):220-224, 1987.

Farley, T.: Severe hypernatremic dehydration after use of an activated charcoal-sorbitol suspension, J. Pediatr. 109(4):719-722, 1986.

Faust, D., and Brown, J.: Moderately elevated blood lead levels: effects on neuropsychologic functioning in children, Pediatrics 80(5):623-629, 1987.

Feinauer, L.L.: Comparison of long-term effects of child abuse by type of abuse and by relationship of the offender to the victim, Am. J. Fam. Ther. 17:48-56, 1989.

Feldman, A., and Aretakis, D.: Herpetic gingivostomatitis in children, Pediatr. Nurs. 12(2):111-113, 1986.

Feldman, K.W.: Pseudoabusive burns in Asian refugees, Am. J. Dis. Child. 138(8):768-769, 1984.

Friedman, E.J.: Death from ipecac intoxication in a patient with anorexia nervosa, Am. J. Psychiatry 141:702-703, 1984.

Friedman, E.M.: Caustic ingestions and foreign bodies in the aerodigestive tract of children, Pediatr. Clin. North Am. 36(6):1403-1410, 1989.

Fuller, A.K.: Child molestation and pedophilia, JAMA 261(4):602-606, 1989.

Gabriel, R.: Anatomically correct dolls in the diagnosis of sexual abuse of children, J. Melanie Klein Soc. 3:40-51, 1985.

Garbarino, J., Guttmann, E., and Seeley, J.: The psychologically battered child, San Francisco, 1986, Jossey-Bass, Inc., Publishers.

Gaudreault, P., Temple, A.R., and Lovejoy, F.H.: The relative severity of acute versus chronic salicylate poisoning in children: a clinical comparison, Pediatrics 70(4):566-569, 1982.

Gigliotti, F., and others: Efficacy of topical antibiotic therapy in acute conjunctivitis in children, J. Pediatr. 104(4):623-626, 1984.

Gilbert, N., and others: Protecting young children from sexual abuse: does preschool training work? Lexington, MA, 1989, Lexington Books.

Goetting, M.G., and Sowa, B.: Retinal hemorrhage after cardiopulmonary resuscitation in children: an etiologic reevaluation, Pediatrics 85(4):585-588, 1990.

Gordon, B., Schroeder, C., and Abrams, M.: Children's knowledge of sexuality: a comparison of sexually abused and nonabused children, Am. J. Orthopsychiatry 60(2):250-257, 1990.

Gowda, N., and others: Human parvovirus infection in patients with sickle cell disease with and without hypoplastic crisis, J. Pediatr. 110(1):81-84, 1987.

Grbcich, P., and others: Effect of fluid volume on ipecac-induced emesis, J. Pediatr. 110(6):970-972, 1987a.

Grbcich, P., and others: Effect of milk on ipecac-induced emesis, J. Pediatr. 110(6):973-975, 1987b.

Greensher, J., and others: Ascendency of the black bottle (activated charcoal), Pediatrics 80(6):949-950, 1987.

Gribetz, B., and Cronley, S.: Underdosing of acetaminophen by parents, Pediatrics 80(5):630-633, 1987.

Guandolo, V.L.: Munchausen syndrome by proxy: an outpatient challenge, Pediatrics 75(3):526-530, 1985.

Hall, A., Spoerke, D., and Rumack, B.: Assessing mistletoe toxicity, Ann. Emerg. Med. 15(11):1320-1323, 1986.

Hanson, R., and others: Anogenital warts in childhood, Child Abuse Negl. 13:225-233, 1989.

Henretig, F., and others: Repeated acetaminophen overdosing causing hepatotoxicity in children, Clin. Pediatr. 28(11):525-528, 1989.

Hibbard, R., and Hartman, G.: Genitalia in human figure drawings: childrearing practices and child sexual abuse, J. Pediatr. 116(5):822-828, 1990.

Hibbard, R., Roghmann, K., and Hoekelman, R.: Genitalia in children's drawings: an association with sexual abuse, Pediatrics 79(1):129-136, 1987.

Highlights of official child neglect and abuse reporting 1986, Denver, 1988, The American Humane Association.

Highlights of official aggregate child neglect and abuse reporting 1987, Denver, 1989, The American Humane Association.

Hobbs, C., and Wynne, J.: Sexual abuse of English boys and girls: the importance of anal examination, Child Abuse Negl. 13:195-210, 1989.

Hobbs, C., and Wynne, J.: The sexually abused battered child, Arch. Dis. Child. 65(4):423-427, 1990.

Hogan, N.S., and Juhasz, A.M.: The detection of incest, Home Healthcare Nurse 2(4):20-26, 1984.

Howrie, D.L., Moriarty, R., and Breit, R.: Candy flavoring as a source of salicylate poisoning, Pediatrics 75(5):869-871, 1985.

Hunt, T.J., Hepner, R., and Seaton, K.W.: Childhood lead poisoning and inadequate child care, Am. J. Dis. Child. 136:538-542, 1982.

Hussey, G., and Klein, M.: A randomized, controlled trial of vitamin A in children with severe measles, N. Engl. J. Med. 323(3):160-164, 1990.

Jampole, L., and Weber, M.: An assessment of the behavior of sexually abused and non-sexually abused children with anatomically correct dolls, Child Abuse Negl. 11:187-192, 1987.

Jean-Gilles, M., and Crittenden, P.: Maltreating families: a look at siblings, Fam. Relations 39(3):232-329, 1990.

Kempe, C.H., and others: The battered child syndrome, JAMA 181:17-24, 1962.

Kempe, R.S., and Kempe, C.H.: The common secret: sexual abuse of children and adolescents, New York, 1984, W.H. Freeman and Co., Publishers.

Kirschner, R.H., and Stein, R.J.: The mistaken diagnosis of child abuse: a form of medical abuse? Am. J. Dis. Child. 139:873-875, 1985.

Klein, B.L., and Simon, J.E.: Hydrocarbon poisonings, Pediatr. Clin. North Am. 33(2):411-419, 1986.

Klein-Schwartz, W., and others: Assessment of management guidelines: acute iron ingestion, Clin. Pediatr. 29(6):316-321, 1990.

Koblenzer, P.J.: Dermatologic conditions misdiagnosed as evidence of child abuse (letter), JAMA 261(24):3547-3548, 1989.

Koop, C.E.: The surgeon general's letter on child sexual abuse, Rockville, MD, 1988, U.S. Dept. of Health and Human Services, Public Health Service, Health Resources and Services Administration, Bureau of Maternal and Child Health and Resources Development, Office of Maternal and Child Health.

Kotelchuck, M.: Child abuse and neglect: prediction and misclassification. In Starr, R.H., editor: Child abuse prediction policy implications, Cambridge, MA, 1982, Ballinger Publishing Co.

Krowchuk, D., and others: Pediatric dermatology update, Pediatrics 86(1):128, 1990.

Krowchuk, H.: Child abuser stereotypes: consensus among clinicians, Appl. Nurs. Res. 2(1):35-39, 1989.

Krugman, R.: Advances and retreats in the protection of children, N. Engl. J. Med. 320(8):531-532, 1989a.

Krugman, R.: New light on a dark area: an update on child abuse and neglect, Curr. Opin. Pediatr. 1(1):168-171, 1989b.

Krugman, R.D., and Krugman, M.K.: Emotional abuse in the classroom, Am. J. Dis. Child. 138(3):284-286, 1984.

Laraque, D., and others: Blood lead, calcium status, and behavior in preschool children, Am. J. Dis. Child. 144(2):186-189, 1990.

Legrand, R., Wakefield, H, and Underwager, R.: Alleged behavioral indicators of sexual abuse, Issues Child Abuse Accus. 1(2):1-5, 1989.

Leventhal, J., and others: Anatomically correct dolls used in interviews of young children suspected of having been sexually abused, Pediatrics 84(5):900-906, 1989.

Litovitz, T.: In defense of retaining ipecac syrup as an over-the-counter drug, Pediatrics 82(3):514-515, 1988.

Litovitz, T., Schmitz, B., and Holm, K.: 1988 annual report of the American Association of Poison Control Centers National Data Collection System, Am. J. Emerg. Med. 7(5):495-545, 1989.

Mack, R.: Mercury—a true healer, a wicked murderer, Contemp. Pediatr. 6(8):139-148, 1989.

Makar, A.F., and Squier, P.J.: Munchausen syndrome by proxy: father as a perpetrator, Pediatrics 85(3):370-373, 1990.

Malloy, M., and Rhoads, G.: Syrup of ipecac: the case for distribution from physicians' offices, Am. J. Dis. Child. 142(6):640-642, 1988.

Marshall, G., and others: Syndrome of periodic fever, pharyngitis, and aphthous stomatitis, J. Pediatr. 110(1):43-46, 1987.

McCann, J., and others: Perianal findings in prepubertal children selected for nonabuse: a descriptive study, Child Abuse Negl. 13:179-193, 1989.

McCann, J., and others: Comparison of genital examination techniques in prepubertal girls, Pediatrics 85(2):182-187, 1990a.

McCann, J., and others: Genital findings in prepubertal girls selected for nonabuse: a descriptive study, Pediatrics 86(3):428-439, 1990b.

McClung, H.J., and others: Intentional ipecac poisoning in children, Am. J. Dis. Child. 142(6):637-639, 1988.

McCord, M., and Okun, A.: Toxicity of sorbitol-charcoal suspension, J. Pediatr. 111(2):307-308, 1987.

McDonald, R.E., and Avery, D.R.: Dentistry for the child and adolescent, ed. 5, St. Louis, 1987, Mosby–Year Book, Inc.

McGuigan, M.A.: Chronic salicylate poisoning: when therapy turns into intoxication, Pediatr. Consult. 2(3):1-8, 1983.

McGuigan, M.A.: Treatment of poisoning, Clin. Symp. 36(5):1-32, 1984.

McGuire, T., and Feldman, K.: Psychologic morbidity of children subjected to Munchausen syndrome by proxy, Pediatrics 83(2):289-292, 1989.

McIver, W., Wakefield, H., and Underwager, R.: Behavior of abused and non-abused children in interviews with anatomically correct dolls, Issues Child Abuse Accus. 1(1):39-48, 1989.

McKibben, L., DeVos, E., and Newberger, E.: Victimization of mothers of abused children: a controlled study, Pediatrics 84(3):531-535, 1989.

Meadow, R.: Munchausen syndrome by proxy, Br. Med. J. 299:248-250, 1989.

Mercury exposure from interior latex paint—Michigan, MMWR 39(8):125, 1990.

Mofenson, H., and others: Gastrointestinal dialysis with activated charcoal and cathartic in the treatment of adolescent ingestions, Clin. Pediatr. 24:678-684, 1985.

Myers, J.: Role of physician in preserving verbal evidence of child abuse, J. Pediatr. 109(3):409-411, 1986.

National Center on Child Abuse and Neglect: Child abuse and neglect: a shared community concern, Washington, DC, 1989, DHHS Pub. No. (OHDS) 89-30531.

Needleman, H.L.: Why we should worry about lead poisoning, Contemp. Pediatr. 5(3):34-55, 1988.

Needleman, H., and others: The long-term effects of exposure to low doses of lead in childhood, N. Engl. J. Med. 322(2):83-88, 1990.

Novotny, T., and others: Prevalence of *Giardia lamblia* and risk factors for infection among children attending day-care facilities in Denver, Public Health Rep. 105(1):72-75, 1990.

Olds, D., and Kitzman, H.: Can home visitation improve the health of women and children at environmental risk? Pediatrics 86(1):108-116, 1990.

Olds, D.L., and others: Preventing child abuse and neglect: a randomized trial of nurse home visitation, Pediatrics 78(1):65-78, 1986.

Pickering, L., and Engelkirk, P.: *Giardia lamblia,* Pediatr. Clin. North Am. 35(3):565-577, 1988.

Piomelli, S., and others: Management of childhood lead poisoning, J. Pediatr. 105(4):523-532, 1984.

Polakoff, J., and others: The environment away from home as a source of potential poisoning, Am. J. Dis. Child. 138:1014-1017, 1984.

Rand, D.C.: Munchausen syndrome by proxy as a possible factor when abuse is falsely alleged, Issues Child Abuse Accus. 1(4):32-34, 1989.

Reid, D.: Pitfalls in determining child abuse, Lancet 1(8441):1316-1317, 1985.

Rey-Alvarez, S., and Menke-Hargrave, T.: Deleading dilemma: pitfall in the management of childhood lead poisoning, Pediatrics 79(2):214-217, 1987.

Rodgers, G.C., Jr., and Matyunas, N.J.: Gastrointestinal decontamination for acute poisoning, Pediatr. Clin. North Am. 33(2):261-285, 1986.

Sachs, H., and Moel, D.: Height and weight following lead poisoning in childhood, Am. J. Dis. Child. 143(7):820-822, 1989.

Salmon, R., and others: Factitious hematuria with underlying renal abnormalities, Pediatrics 82(3):377-379, 1988.

Saulsbury, F.T., and Hayden, G.F.: Skin conditions simulating child abuse, Pediatr. Emerg. Care 1(3):147-150, 1985.

Schmitt, B., Gray, J., and Britton, H.: Car seat burns in infants: avoiding confusion with inflicted burns, Pediatrics 62(4):607-609, 1978.

Schunk, J., and Svendsen, D.: Diphenhydramine toxicity from combined oral and topical use, Am. J. Dis. Child. 142(10):1020-1021, 1988.

Schwartz, J., Angle, C., and Pitcher, H.: Relationship between childhood blood lead levels and stature, Pediatrics 77(3):281-288, 1986.

Shannon, M., Graef, J., and Lovejoy, F.: Efficacy and toxicity of D-penicillamine in low-level lead poisoning, J. Pediatr. 112(5):799-804, 1988.

Sherrod, K.B., and others: Toward a semispecific, multidimensional, threshold model of maltreatment. In Drotar, D., editor: New directions in failure to thrive: implications for research and practice, New York, 1985, Plenum Press.

Shukla, R., and others: Fetal and infant lead exposure: effects on growth in stature, Pediatrics 84(4):604-612, 1989.

Smilkstein, M., and others: Efficacy of oral *N*-acetylcysteine in the treatment of acetaminophen overdose, N. Engl. J. Med. 319(24):1557-1562, 1988.

Snyder, J.C., Hampton, R., and Newberger, E.H.: Family dysfunction: violence, neglect, and sexual misuse. In Levine, M.D., and others, editors: Developmental-behavioral pediatrics, Philadelphia, 1983, W.B. Saunders Co.

Spencer, M.J., and Dunklee, P.: Sexual abuse of boys, Pediatrics 78(1):133-138, 1986.

Steketee, R.W., and others: Recurrent outbreaks of giardiasis in a child day care center, Wisconsin, Am. J. Public Health 79(4):485-490, 1989.

Sutphen, J.L., and Saulsbury S.T.: Intentional ipecac poisoning: Munchausen syndrome by proxy, Pediatrics 82(3, pt. 2):453-456, 1988.

Temple, A.R.: Acute and chronic effect of aspirin toxicity and their treatment, Arch. Intern. Med. 141:364-369, 1981.

Tomlinson, G., Helfaer, M., and Wiedermann, B.: Diphenhydramine toxicity mimicking varicella encephalitis, Pediatr. Infect. Dis. J. 6(2):220-221, 1987.

Turner, J.A.: Giardiasis and infections with *Dientamoeba fragilis,* Pediatr. Clin. North Am. 32(4):865-880, 1985.
Turner, R.J., and Avison, W.R.: Assessing risk factors for problem parenting: the significance of social support, J. Marriage Fam. 47(4):881-892, 1985.
Unintentional poisoning mortality—United States, 1980-1986, MMWR 38(10):153-157, 1989.
Vale, J., Meredith, T., and Proudfoot, A.: Syrup of ipecacuanha: is it really useful? Br. Med. J. 293(6558):1321-1322, 1986.
Vermund, S., and MacLeod, S.: Is pinworm a vanishing infection? Am. J. Dis. Child. 142:566, 1988.
Vernberg, K., Culver-Dickinson, P., and Spyker, D.A.: The deterrent effect of poison-warning stickers, Am. J. Dis. Child. 138:1018-1020, 1984.
Wakefield, H., and Underwager, R.: Interrogation of children, Issues Child Abuse Accus. 1(1):14-28, 1989.
White, S.T., Ingram, D.L., and Lyna, P.R.: Vaginal introital diameter in the evaluation of sexual abuse, Child Abuse Negl. 13:217-224, 1989.
Widom, C.S.: Does violence beget violence: a critical examination of the literature, Psychol. Bull. 106(1):3-28, 1989.
Wong, D.L.: False allegations of child abuse: the other side of the tragedy, Pediatr. Nurs. 13(5):329-333, 1987.
Woolf, A., and others: Prevention of childhood poisoning: efficacy of an educational program carried out in an emergency clinic, Pediatrics 80(3):359-363, 1987.
Yates, A., and Musty, T.: Preschool children's erroneous allegations of sexual molestation, Am. J. Psychiatry 145:989-992, 1988.
Zaphiris, A.G.: The sexually abused boy, Prev. Sex. Abuse 1(1):1-4, 1986.

BIBLIOGRAPHY

Communicable Diseases

Alkalay, A., Pomerance, J., and Rimoin, D.: Fetal varicella syndrome, J. Pediatr. 111(3):320-323, 1987.
American Academy of Pediatrics: Report of the Committee on Infectious Diseases, ed. 21, Elk Grove Village, IL, 1988, The Academy.
American Academy of Pediatrics, Committee on Infectious Diseases: Parvovirus, erythema infectiosum, and pregnancy, Pediatrics 85(1):131-133, 1990.
Asano, Y., and others: Human herpesvirus type 6 infection (exanthem subitum) without fever, J. Pediatr. 115(2):264-268, 1989.
Baba, K., and others: Increased incidence of herpes zoster in normal children infected with varicella zoster virus during infancy: community-based follow-up study, J. Pediatr. 108(3):372-377, 1986.
Bell, L.M., and others: Human parvovirus B19 infection among hospital staff members after contact with infected patients, N. Engl. J. Med. 321(8):485-491, 1989.
Chiriboga-Klein, S., and others: Growth in congenital rubella syndrome and correlation with clinical manifestations, J. Pediatr. 115(2):251-255, 1989.
English, P.C.: Diphtheria and theories of infectious disease: centennial appreciation of the critical role of diphtheria in the history of medicine, Pediatrics 76(1):1-9, 1985.
Fitzgerald, M.G., Pullen, G.R., and Hosking, C.S.: Low affinity antibody to rubella antigen in patients after rubella infection in utero, Pediatrics 81(6):812-814, 1988.
Fleming, J.W.: How to differentiate dermatologic conditions—often confusing and difficult—in infants and school-age children, MCN 6(5):346-354, 1981.
Jones, S., and Jenista, J.: Fifth disease: role for nurses in pediatric practice, Pediatr. Nurs. 16(2):148-150, 1990.
Josephson, A., and Gombert, M.: Airborne transmission of nosocomial varicella from localized zoster, J. Infect. Dis. 158(1):238-241, 1988.
Koch, W., and others: Manifestations and treatment of human parvovirus B19 infection in immunocompromised patients, J. Pediatr. 116(3):355-359, 1990.
Krugman, S., and others: Infectious diseases of children, ed. 8, St. Louis, 1985, Mosby–Year Book, Inc.
Labson, L.H.: Doctor, I can't stand this itching! Patient Care 18(17):89-121, 1984.
Rasmussen, J.E.: Recent advances in pediatric dermatology, Curr. Opin. Pediatr. 1(1):57-60, 1989.
Relief for that persistent itch, Patient Care 18(17):185, 1984.
Report of the Task Force on Pertussis and Pertussis Immunization—1988, Pediatrics 81(6, pt. 2), 1988.
Risks Associated with human parvovirus B19 infection, MMWR 38(6):18-20, 1989.
Suga, S., and others: Human herpesvirus-6 infection (exanthem subitum) without rash, Pediatrics 83(6):1003-1006, 1989.
Ware, R.: Human parvovirus infection, J. Pediatr. 114(3):343-348, 1989.
Ware, R., and others: Chronic immune-mediated thrombocytopenia after varicella infection, J. Pediatr. 112(5):742-744, 1988.
Williams, H., and Douglass, C.: Nursing implications for post-polio sequelae, Orthop. Nurs. 5(6):18-21, 1986.

Intestinal Parasitic Diseases

Birkhead, G., and Vogt, R.: Epidemiologic surveillance for endemic *Giardia lamblia* infection in Vermont, Am. J. Epidemiol. 129(4):762-768, 1989.
Borgatti, R.: When protozoa invade the GI tract, Patient Care 17(14):226-253, 1983.
Carroll, M.J.: Routine procedures for examination of stool and blood for parasites, Pediatr. Clin. North Am. 32(4):1041-1046, 1985.
Common-source outbreak of giardiasis—New Mexico, MMWR 38(23):405-407, 1989.
Getting rid of pinworms, roundworms, scabies mites, or lice, Patient Care 18(17):189-190, 1984.
Greensmith, C., and others: Giardiasis associated with the use of a water slide, Pediatr. Infect. Dis. J. 7:91-94, 1988.
Harter, L., and others: Giardiasis in an infant and toddler swim class, Am. J. Pub. Health 74(2):155-156, 1984.
Henley, M., and Sears, J.R.: Pinworms: a persistent pediatric problem, MCN 10(6):111-113, 1985.
Hood, C.: *Enterobius vermicularis,* Practitioner 233(1466):503, 1989.
Hotez, P.: Hookworm disease in children, Pediatr. Infect. Dis. J. 8(8):516-520, 1989.
Jones, J.E.: Pinworms, Am. Fam. Physician 38(3):159-164, 1988.
Katzman, E.M.: What's the most common helminth infection in the U.S.? MCN 14(3):193-195, 1989.
Markell, E.K.: Intestinal nematode infections, Pediatr. Clin. North Am. 32(4):971-986, 1985.
McIntyre, P., and others: Chemotherapy in giardiasis: clinical responses and in vitro drug sensitivity of human isolates in axenic culture, J. Pediatr. 108(6):1005-1010, 1986.
Rauch, A., and others: Longitudinal study of *Giardia lamblia* infection in a day care center population, Pediatr. Infect. Dis. J. 9(3):186-189, 1990.
Sears, J.R.: To prevent reinfestation (letters to the editor), MCN 10(6):377, 1985.
Seidel, J.S.: Treatment of parasitic infections, Pediatr. Clin. North Am. 32(4):1077-1095, 1985.
Sokol, R., Lichtenstein, P., and Farrell, M.: Quinacrine hydrochloride–induced yellow discoloration of the skin in children, Pediatrics 69(2):232-233, 1982.
Stehr-Green, J., and others: Intestinal parasites in pet store puppies in Atlanta, Public Health Briefs 77(3):345-346, 1987.
Unger, B., and others: Enzyme-linked immunosorbent assay for the detection of *Giardia lamblia* in fecal specimens, J. Infect. Dis. 149(1):90-97, 1984.
Vinayak, V.K., and others: Detection of *Giardia lamblia* antigen in the feces by counterimmunoelectrophoresis, Ped. Infect. Dis. 4(4):383-386, 1985.

Conjunctivitis/Stomatitis

Bodor, F.F., and others: Bacterial etiology of conjunctivitis–otitis media syndrome, Pediatrics 76(1):26-28, 1985.

Corey, L.: First-episode, recurrent, and asymptomatic herpes simplex infections, J. Am. Acad. Dermatol. 18(1, pt. 2):169-172, 1988.

Friedlaender, M.H., Okumoto, M., and Kelley, J.: Diagnosis of allergic conjunctivitis, Arch. Ophthalmol. 102:1198-1199, 1984.

Hammerschlag, M.: Conjunctivitis in infancy and childhood, Pediatr. Rev. 5(9):285-290, 1984.

Howes, D.S.: The red eye, Emerg. Med. Clin. North Am. 6(1):43-56, 1988.

Kovalesky, A.: Nurse's guide to children's eyes, Orlando, FL, 1985, Grune & Stratton, Inc.

Lewis, L., Glauser, T., and Joffie, M.: Gonococcal conjunctivitis in prepubertal children, Am. J. Dis. Child. 144(5):546-548, 1990.

Nirschi, R., and Kronmiller, J.: Evaluating oral health needs in preschool children, Clin. Pediatr. 25(7):358-362, 1986.

Reed, D.B.: Viral and bacterial conjunctivitis: prevention of disastrous results, Postgrad. Med. 86(4):103-114, 1989.

Scully, C., and Porter, S.: Recurrent aphthous stomatitis: current concepts of etiology, pathogenesis and management, J. Oral Pathol. Med. 18(1):21-27, 1989.

Sheahan, S.L., and Seabolt, J.P.: *Chlamydia trachomatis* infections: a health problem of infants, J. Pediatr. Health Care 3(3):144-149, 1989.

Stanker, P., and others: Protocol—conjunctivitis, School Nurse 5(2):34-36, 1989.

Ingestion of Injurious Agents

Edgerton, P.H.: Symptoms of digitalis-like toxicity in a family after accidental ingestion of lily of the valley plant, J. Emerg. Nurs. 15(3):220-223, 1989.

Edmonson, M.B.: Caustic alkali ingestions by farm children, Pediatrics 79(3):413-416, 1987.

Edwards, I.R.: Labelling toxic plants, N.Z. Med. J. 103(891):275, 1990.

Edwards, N.: Local toxicity from a poinsettia plant: a case report, J. Pediatr. 102(3):404-405, 1983.

Einhorn, A., and others: Serious respiratory consequences of detergent ingestions in children, Pediatrics 84(3):472-474, 1989.

Keim, K.A.: Preventing and treating plant poisonings in young children, MCN 8(4):287-289, 1983.

Kunkel, D.B.: Plant poisoning in children, Pediatr. Ann. 16(11):927-932, 1987.

Kurt, T.L.: The (internal) dangers of acrylic fingernails, JAMA 263(16):2181, 1990.

Moulin, D., and others: Upper airway lesions in children after accidental ingestion of caustic substances, J. Pediatr. 106(3):408-410, 1985.

Peterson, R., and Peterson, L.: Cleansing the blood: hemodialysis, peritoneal dialysis, exchange transfusion, charcoal hemoperfusion, forced diuresis, Pediatr. Clin. North Am. 33(3):675-689, 1986.

Rothstein, F.C.: Caustic injuries to the esophagus in children, Pediatr. Clin. North Am. 33(3):665-674, 1986.

Rumack, B.H.: Acetaminophen overdose in children and adolescents, Pediatr. Clin. North Am. 33(3):691-701, 1986.

Shannon, M., Amitai, Y., and Lovejoy, F.: Multiple dose activated charcoal for theophylline poisoning in young infants, Pediatrics 80(3):368-370, 1987.

Steel, P., and Spyker, D.A.: Poisonings, Pediatr. Clin. North Am. 32(1):77-86, 1985.

Vertrees, J., McWilliams, B., and Kelly, H.: Repeated oral administration of activated charcoal for treating aspirin overdose in young children, Pediatrics 85(4):594-598, 1990.

Walton, W.W.: An evaluation of the poison prevention packaging act, Pediatrics 69(3):363-370, 1982.

Wong, D.: Dispelling some myths about ipecac, Am. J. Nurs. 88(7):952, 1988.

Wood, B., Colombo, J., and Benson, B.: Chlorine inhalation toxicity from vapors generated by swimming pool chlorinator tablets, Pediatrics 79(3):427-430, 1987.

Zwiener, R.J., and Ginsburg, C.M.: Organophosphate and carbamate poisoning in infants and children, Pediatrics 81(1):121-126, 1988.

Heavy Metal Poisoning

Bellinger, D.C., and Needleman, H.L.: Lead and the relationship between maternal and child intelligence, J. Pediatr. 102(4):523-527, 1983.

Berger, O., Gregg, D., and Succop, P.: Using unstimulated urinary lead excretion to assess the need for chelation in the treatment of lead poisoning, J. Pediatr. 116(1):46-51, 1990.

Brown, M., Bellinger, D., and Matthews, J.: In utero lead exposure, MCN 15(2):94-96, 1990.

Centers for Disease Control: Folk remedy-associated lead poisoning in Hmong children—Minnesota, MMWR 32(42):555-556, 1983a.

Centers for Disease Control: Lead poisoning from Mexican folk remedies—California, MMWR 32(42):554-555, 1983b.

Centers for Disease Control: Preventing lead poisoning in young children, Atlanta, 1985.

Colliver, J.A., Kolm, P., and Verhulst, S.J.: Dentine lead and IQ: interpretation of results of residuals analysis, J. Pediatr. 102(4):573-574, 1983.

Elemental mercury poisoning in a household—Ohio, 1989, MMWR 39(25):424-425, 1990.

Graziano, J., Lolacono, N., and Meyer, P.: Dose-response study of oral 2,3-demercaptosuccinic acid in children with elevated blood lead concentrations, J. Pediatr. 113(4):751-757, 1988.

Hudson, P., and others: Elemental mercury exposure among children of thermometer plant workers, Pediatrics 79(6):935-938, 1987.

Klein-Schwartz, W., and others: Assessment of management guidelines: acute iron ingestion, Clin. Pediatr. 29(6):316-321, 1990.

Landrigan, P., and Graef, J.: Pediatric lead poisoning in 1987: the silent epidemic continues, Pediatrics 79(4):582-583, 1987.

Lead poisoning following ingestion of homemade beverage stored in a ceramic jug—New York, MMWR 38(21):379-380, 1989.

Lee, J.S.: Cadmium, mercury, and lead—the heavy metal gang, Fam. Community Health 7(3):8-14, 1984.

Markowitz, M.E., and Rosen, J.F.: Assessment of lead stores in children: validation of an 8-hour $CaNa_2EDTA$ provocative test, J. Pediatr. 104(3):337-341, 1984.

Markowitz, M., Rosen, J., and Bijur, P.: Effects of iron deficiency on lead excretion in children with moderate lead intoxication, J. Pediatr. 116(3):360-364, 1990.

Miller, S.J.: Nursing care of the lead-burdened child: a problem oriented approach, Pediatr. Nurs. 7(5):47-52, 1981.

Miller, S.: Lead in calcium supplements (response to letter), JAMA 257:1810, 1987.

Moutinho, M., and others: Acute mercury vapor poisoning, Am. J. Dis. Child. 135(1):42-44, 1981.

Occupational and environmental lead poisoning associated with battery repair shops—Jamaica, MMWR 38(27):474-481, 1989.

Rudner, N.: Children with elevated lead levels, J. Pediatr. Health Care 2(1):46-49, 1988.

Sayre, J.W.: Deleading houses: dangers in the dust, Am. J. Dis. Child. 141(7):727-728, 1987.

Shannon, M., and Graef, J.: Lead intoxication from lead-contaminated water used to reconstitute infant formula, Clin. Pediatr. 28(8):380-382, 1989.

Tunnessen, W., McMahon, K., and Baser, M.: Acrodynia: exposure to mercury from fluorescent light bulbs, Pediatrics 79(5):786-789, 1987.

Child Maltreatment

Alexander, P.C.: A systems theory conceptualization of incest, Fam. Proc. 24:79-88, 1985.

Alexander, R., Surrell, J., and Cohle, S.: Microwave oven burns to children: an unusual manifestation of child abuse, Pediatrics 79(2):255-260, 1987.

Alexander, R., and others: Serial abuse in children who are shaken, Am. J. Dis. Child. 144(1):58-60, 1990.

American Academy of Pediatrics, Committee on Adolescence: Role of the pediatrician in management of sexually transmitted diseases in children and adolescents, Pediatrics 79(3):454-456, 1987.

American Academy of Pediatrics, Committee on Bioethics: Religious exemptions from child abuse statutes, Pediatrics 81(1):169-171, 1988.

American Academy of Pediatrics, Committee on Early Childhood, Adoption, and Dependent Care: Oral and dental aspects of child abuse and neglect, Pediatrics 78(3):537-539, 1986.

American Academy of Pediatrics, Committee on Hospital Care: Medical necessity for the hospitalization of the abused and neglected child, Pediatrics 79(2):300, 1987.

American Academy of Pediatrics, Task Force on Child Abuse and Neglect: Public disclosure of private information about victims of abuse, Pediatrics 82(3):387, 1988.

Baum, E., and others: Child sexual abuse, criminal justice, and the pediatrician, Pediatrics 79(3):437-439, 1987.

Berkner, P., Kastner, T., and Skolnick, L.: Chronic ipecac poisoning in infancy: a case report, Pediatrics 82(3):384-385, 1988.

Boyd, A.: Condylomata acuminata in the pediatric population, Am. J. Dis. Child. 144(7):817-824, 1990.

Browne, E., Davies, C., and Wiley, C.: Early prediction and prevention of child abuse, Br. Med. J. 298(6683):1326-1327, 1989.

Burgess, A., Hartman, C., and Kelley, S.: Assessing child abuse: the triads checklist, J. Psychosoc. Nurs. 28(4):6-14, 1990.

Cantwell, H.B.: Update on vaginal inspection as it relates to child sexual abuse in girls under thirteen, Child Abuse Negl. 2:545-546, 1987.

Chan, J., and Leff, P.: Play and the abused child: implications for acute pediatric care, Child. Health Care 16(3):169-176, 1988.

Claytor, R., Barth, K., and Shubin, C.: Evaluating child sexual abuse: observations regarding ano-genital injury, Clin. Pediatr. 28(9):419-422, 1989.

Cohle, S., and others: Fatal pepper aspiration, Am. J. Dis. Child. 142(6):633-636, 1988.

Coleman, L.: Learning from the McMartin hoax, Issues Child Abuse Accus. 1(2):68-71, 1989.

Coleman, L.: Medical examination for sexual abuse: have we been misled? Issues Child Abuse Accus. 1(3):1-9, 1989.

Crittenden, P., and Morrison, A.: An early parental indicator of potential maltreatment, Pediatr. Nurs. 14(5):415-417, 1988.

Davis, A., and Emans, J.: Human papilloma virus infection in the pediatric and adolescent patient, J. Pediatr. 115(1):1-9, 1989.

de Young, M.: Issues in determining the veracity of sexual abuse allegations, Child. Health Care 17(1):50-57, 1988.

Dubowitz, H.: Prevention of child maltreatment: what is known, Pediatrics 83(4):570-577, 1989.

Ellerstein, N.S., editor: Child abuse and neglect: a medical reference, New York, 1981, John Wiley & Sons, Inc.

Elvik, S.L.: From disclosure to court: the facets of sexual abuse, J. Pediatr. Health Care 1:136-140, 1987.

English, P.C.: Pediatrics and the unwanted child in history: foundling homes, disease, and the origins of foster care in New York City, 1860 to 1920, Pediatrics 73(5):699-711, 1984.

Enos, W., Conrath, T., and Byer, J.: Forensic evaluation of the sexually abused child, Pediatrics 78(3):385-398, 1986.

Faller, K.C.: Characteristics of a clinical sample of sexually abused children: how boy and girl victims differ, Child Abuse Negl. 13:281-291, 1989.

Finkel, M.A.: Anogenital trauma in sexually abused children, Pediatrics 84(2):317-322, 1989.

Flaherty, E., and Weiss, H.: Medical evaluation of abused and neglected children, Am. J. Dis. Child. 144(3):330-334, 1990.

Fontana, V.J., and Robison, E.: Observing child abuse, J. Pediatr. 105(4):655-660, 1984.

Friedman, S.R.: What is child sexual abuse? J. Clin. Psychol. 46(3):372-375, 1990.

Fulginiti, V., and Krugman, R.: Cleveland, England: child abuse in the public eye, Am. J. Dis. Child. 143(6):651-652, 1989.

Fuster, C., and Neinstein, L.: Vaginal *Chlamydia trachomatis* prevalence in sexually abused prepubertal girls, Pediatrics 79(2):235-238, 1987.

Gage, R.B.: Consequences of children's exposure to spouse abuse, Pediatr. Nurs. 16(3):258-260, 1990.

Gale, J., and others: Sexual abuse in young children: its clinical presentation and characteristic patterns, Child Abuse Negl. 12:163, 1988.

George, J., and Quattrone, M.: Reporting child abuse: duties and dangers, J. Emerg. Nurs. 14(1):34-35, 1988.

Gill, F.T.: Caring for abused children in the emergency department, Holistic Nurs. Pract. 4(1):37-43, 1989.

Goff, C., and others: Vaginal opening measurement in prepubertal girls, Am. J. Dis. Child. 143:1366-1368, 1989.

Greenfield, M.: Disclosing incest: the relationships that make it possible, Psychosoc. Nurs. 28(7):20-23, 1990.

Griest, K., and Zumwalt, R.: Child abuse by drowning, Pediatrics 83(1):41-46, 1989.

Gutman, L.T.: Sexual abuse and human papillomavirus infection, J. Pediatr. 116(3):495-496, 1990.

Hanigan, W., Peterson, R., and Njus, G.: Tin ear syndrome: rotational acceleration in pediatric head injuries, Pediatrics 80(5):618-622, 1987.

Heger, A., and Emans, S.: Introital diameter as the criterion for sexual abuse, Pediatrics 85(2):222-223, 1990.

Herman-Giddens, M., and Berson, N.: Harmful genital care practices in children: a type of child abuse, JAMA 261(4):577-579, 1989.

Hickson, G., and others: Parental administration of chemical agents: a cause of apparent life-threatening events, Pediatrics 83(5):772-776, 1989.

Jenny, C., Sutherland, S., and Sandahl, B.: Developmental approach to preventing the sexual abuse of children, Pediatrics 78(6):1034-1038, 1986.

Johnson, C., Kaufman, K., and Callendar, C.: The hand as a target organ in child abuse, Clin. Pediatr. 29(2):66-72, 1990.

Kanter, R.K.: Retinal hemorrhage after cardiopulmonary resuscitation or child abuse, J. Pediatr. 108(3):430-432, 1986.

Kauffman, C.K., Neill, M.K., and Thomas, J.N.: The abusive parent. In Johnson, S.J., editor: Nursing assessment and strategies for the family at risk, ed. 2, Philadelphia, 1986, J.B. Lippincott Co.

Keefe, M.R.: Intervening with families of infants and child abuse, Springhouse, PA, 1987, Springhouse Corp.

Kelley, S.J.: Drawings: critical communications for sexually abused children, Pediatr. Nurs. 11(6):421-426, 1985.

Kelley, S.J.: Parental stress response to sexual abuse and ritualistic abuse of children in day-care centers, Nurs. Res. 39(1):25-29, 1990.

Kempe, C.H., and Helfer, R.E., editors: The battered child, ed. 3, Chicago, 1982, University of Chicago Press.

Kharasch, S., Vinci, R., and Reece, R.: Esophagitis, epiglottitis and cocaine alkaloid ("crack"): "accidental" poisoning or child abuse? Pediatrics 86(1):117-119, 1990.

Kiefer, L.: Defense considerations in the child as witness in allegations of sexual abuse. II. The child witness: legal competency, Issues Child Abuse Accus. 1(2):48-57, 1989.

Kleinman, P., and others: Radiologic contributions to the investigation and prosecution of cases of fatal infant abuse, N. Engl. J. Med. 320(8):507-511, 1989.

Klevan, J., and De Jong, A.: Urinary tract symptoms and urinary tract infection following sexual abuse, Am. J. Dis. Child. 144:242-244, 1990.

Krivacska, J.J.: Primary prevention of child sexual abuse: alternative, non-child directed approaches, Issues Child Abuse Accus. 1(4):1-9, 1989.

Landwirth, J.: Children as witnesses in child sexual abuse trials, Pediatrics 80(4):585-589, 1987.

Leahey, M., and Wright, L.: Families and psychosocial problems, Springhouse, PA, 1987, Springhouse Corp.

Leventhal, J.M.: Have there been changes in the epidemiology of sexual abuse of children during the 20th century? Pediatrics 82(5):766-773, 1988.

Leventhal, J., Berg, A., and Egerter, S.: Is intrauterine growth retardation a risk factor for child abuse? Pediatrics 79(4):515-519, 1987.

Lewin, L.: Establishing a therapeutic relationship with an abused child, Pediatr. Nurs. 16(3):263-264, 1990.

Malatack, J.J., and others: Munchausen syndrome by proxy: a new complication of central venous catheterization, Pediatrics 75(3):523-525, 1985.

Margolin, L., and Craft, J.: Child sexual abuse by caretakers, Fam. Relations 38:450-455, 1989.

Marshall, W., Puls, T., and Davidson, C.: New child abuse spectrum in an era of increased awareness, Am. J. Dis. Child. 142(6):664-667, 1988.

Martinez, J., and others: High prevalence of genital tract papillomavirus infection in female adolescents, Pediatrics 82(4):604-608, 1988.

McCauley, J., Gorman, R., and Guzinski, G.: Toluidine blue in the detection of perineal lacerations in pediatric and adolescent sexual abuse victims, Pediatrics 78(6):1039-1043, 1986.

Meadow, R.: ABC of child abuse: epidemiology, Br. Med. J. 298(6675):727-730, 1989.

Meadow, R.: Poisoning, Br. Med. J. 298(6685):1445-1446, 1989.

Miller, E.L.: Interviewing the sexually abused child, MCN 10:103-105, 1985.

Mittleman, R., Mittleman, H., and Wetli, C.: What child abuse really looks like, Am. J. Nurs. 87(9):1185-1188, 1987.

Muchlinski, E., Boonstra, C., and Johnson, J.: Planning and implementing a pediatric sexual assault evidentiary examination program, J. Emerg. Nurs. 15(3):249-255, 1989.

Muram, D.: Child sexual abuse—genital tract findings in prepubertal girls. I. The unaided medical examination, Am. J. Obstet. Gynecol. 160(2):328-333, 1989.

Muram, D., and Elias, S.: Child sexual abuse—genital tract findings in prepubertal girls. II. Comparison of colposcopic and unaided examinations, Am. J. Obstet. Gynecol. 160(2):333-335, 1989.

Newbern, V.B.: Sexual victimization of child and adolescent patients, Image 21(1):10-13, 1989.

Orenstein, D., and Wasserman, A.: Munchausen syndrome by proxy simulating cystic fibrosis, Pediatrics 78(4):621-624, 1986.

Osborn, M., and Bryan, S.: Patient care guidelines: evidentiary examination in sexual assault, J. Emerg. Nurs. 15(3):284-290, 1989.

Paradise, J.E.: Predictive accuracy and the diagnosis of sexual abuse: a big issue about a little tissue, Child Abuse Negl. 13:169-176, 1989.

Paradise, J., Rostain, A., and Nathanson, M.: Substantiation of sexual abuse charges when parents dispute custody or visitation, Pediatrics 81(6):835-839, 1988.

Post, C.A.: Play therapy with an abused child: a case study, Child Adolesc. Psychiatr. Ment. Health Nurs. 3(1):34-36, 1990.

Rand, D.C.: Munchausen syndrome by proxy: integration of classic and contemporary types, Issues Child Abuse Accus. 2(2):83-89, 1990.

Reece, R.M., and Grodin, M.A.: Recognition of nonaccidental injury, Pediatr. Clin. North Am. 32(1):41-60, 1985.

Reinhart, M.A.: Child abuse: cocaine absorption by rectal administration, Clin. Pediatr. 29(6):357, 1990.

Rew, L., and Sapp, A.: A family- and community-based health-promotion group for sexually abused children, Fam. Community Health 11(4):41-51, 1989.

Riggs, S., Alario, A., and McHorney, C.: Health risk behaviors and attempted suicide in adolescents who report prior maltreatment, J. Pediatr. 116(5):815-821, 1990.

Rosenthal, P.A., and Doherty, M.B.: Serious sibling abuse by preschool children, J. Am. Acad. Child Psychiatry 23(2):186-190, 1984.

Runyan, D.K., and Gould, C.L.: Foster care for child maltreatment. I. Impact on delinquent behavior, Pediatrics 75(3):562-568, 1985.

Runyan, D.K., and Gould, C.L.: Foster care for child maltreatment. II. Impact on school performance, Pediatrics 76(5):841-847, 1985.

Runyan, D., and others: Impact of legal intervention of sexually abused children, J. Pediatr. 113(4):647-653, 1988.

Saucier, B.L.: The effects of play therapy on developmental achievement levels of abused children, Pediatr. Nurs. 15(1):27-30, 1989.

Saulsbury, F., Chobanian, M., and Wilson, W.: Child abuse: parenteral hydrocarbon administration, Pediatrics 73(5):719-722, 1984.

Scherb, B.J.: Standardized care plans: suspected abuse and neglect of children, J. Emerg. Nurs. 14(1):44-47, 1988.

Schwab, N.C.: Child abuse and neglect: legal and clinical implications for school nursing practice, School Nurse 5(4):17-28, 1989.

Senner, A., and Ott, M.: Munchausen syndrome by proxy, Issues Compr. Pediatr. Nurs. 12(5):345-357, 1989.

Sink, F.: Child sexual abuse: comprehensive assessment in the pediatric health care setting, Child. Health Care 15(2):108-113, 1986.

Skuse, D.H.: Emotional abuse and neglect, Br. Med. J. 298:1692-1694, 1989.

Soditus, C., and Mock, D.: Interrupting the cycle of child abuse, MCN 13(3):196-199, 1988.

Stahler, G., DuCette, J., and Povich, E.: Using mediation to prevent child maltreatment: an exploratory study, Fam. Relations 39(3):317-322, 1990.

Starr, R.H., Jr., editor: Child abuse prediction: policy implications, Cambridge, MA, 1982, Ballinger Publishing Co.

Subramanian, K.: Reducing child abuse through respite center intervention, Child Welfare 64(5):501-509, 1985.

Switzer, J.V.: Reporting child abuse, Am. J. Nurs. 86(6):663-664, 1986.

Underwager, R., and Wakefield, H.: The real world of child interrogations, Springfield, IL, 1990, Charles C Thomas, Publisher.

Velasquez, J., Christensen, M.L., and Schommer, B.L.: Intensive services help prevent child abuse, MCN 9(2):113-117, 1984.

Wakefield, H., and Underwager, R.: Accusations of child sexual abuse, Springfield, IL, 1988, Charles C Thomas, Publisher.

Wakefield, H., and Underwager, R.: Manipulating the child sexual abuse system, Issues Child Abuse Accus. 1(2):58-67, 1989.

Weber, S.: Munchausen syndrome by proxy, J. Pediatr. Nurs. 2(1):50-54, 1987.

Welldon, E.V.: Women who sexually abuse children, Br. Med. J. 300:1527-1528, 1990.

West, R., Davies, A., and Fenton, T.: Accidental vulval injuries in childhood, Br. Med. J. 298:1002-1003, 1989.

Wheeler, D., and Hobbs, C.: Mistakes in diagnosing non-accidental injury: 10 years' experience, Br. Med. J. 296(6631):1233-1236, 1988.

White, S., and others: Interviewing young sexual abuse victims with anatomically correct dolls, Child Abuse Negl. 10:519-529, 1986.

Wild, N.J.: Prevalence of child sex rings, Pediatrics 83(4):553-558, 1989.

Yates, A., and Terr, L.: Anatomically correct dolls: should they be used as the basis for expert testimony? J. Am. Acad. Child Adolesc. Psychiatry 27(3):387-388, 1988.

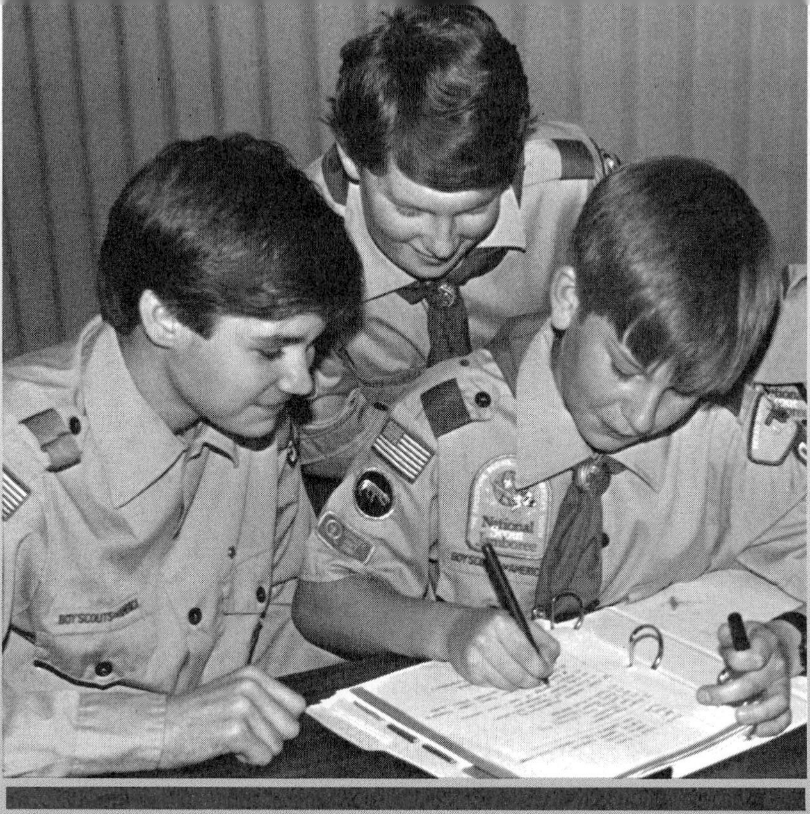

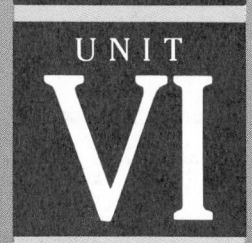

Middle Childhood

UNIT VI

Children in the middle childhood years enjoy a relatively stable period of slow but steady growth and maturation with few physical or emotional stresses. It is a comfortable period of adjustment with a developmental pace sufficiently slow to meet the physical and psychologic demands placed on them. It becomes a period of broadening horizons as children encounter a wider sphere of influence—school, peers, and multiple opportunities for social interaction. During this period children learn the fundamental skills of their culture and develop inner resources for coping with larger social units. The emphasis during this period is on competence in physical and mental tasks and on equally important changes in social relationships.

Chapter 17, *Health Promotion of the School-Age Child and Family,* provides a brief overview of the developmental changes that take place in middle childhood, including a lengthy summary of the major characteristics of each age within the period of middle childhood. Chapter 18, *Health Problems of Middle Childhood,* outlines the more common health problems encountered during these years. Few major illnesses are associated with middle childhood, although children during this time are still subject to many of the problems that characterize the earlier childhood years, such as injuries, and, with wider social relationships, communicable diseases that continue to be prevalent.

CHAPTER 17

Health Promotion of the School-Age Child and Family

RELATED TOPICS

Discipline: Shaping behavior, Ch. 3
Growth and development of children, Ch. 4
Guidelines for assessing sleep problems in children, p. 206
Health problems of middle childhood, Ch. 18
Injuries—the leading killer, Ch. 1
Physical and developmental assessment of the child, Ch. 7
Psychosocial history, Ch. 6
Injuries and health problems related to sports participation, Ch. 39

GLOSSARY

ATV All-terrain vehicle

concrete operations More logical thought about real objects and experiences

conservation Recognition that properties of an object or substance do not change when its appearance is altered in some superficial way

egocentric The tendency to view the world from one's own perspective

operation An action performed on an object or set of objects; mental operations act on thought

preoperation Thinking on a symbolic level; unable to use cognitive operations

prepubescence The state of being prepubertal; the years preceding puberty (lasting approximately 2 years) in which preliminary physical changes (accelerated growth, appearance of secondary sex characteristics) leading to sexual maturity take place

REM Rapid eye movement

The segment of the life span that extends from age 6 to approximately age 12 has been endowed with a variety of labels, each of which describes an important characteristic of the period. The middle years are most often referred to as *school-age* or the *school years.* This period begins with entrance into the wider sphere of influence represented by the school environment, which has a significant impact on development and relationships. The term *gang age* describes children's affiliation with age-mates and with learning the culture of childhood. Within peer groups children establish the first close relationships outside the family group.

From a psychoanalytic point of view this is the period of *latency,* which has been considered to be a time of sexual tranquility between the oedipal phase of early childhood and the eroticism of adolescence. It is during this time that children experience the intimacy of relationships with same-sex peers following the indifference of earlier years and preceding the heterosexual fascination that accompanies the changes of puberty. However, the concept of sexual latency is now being questioned in the light of early sexual exploration and the exploitation of sex in the media.

PROMOTING OPTIMUM GROWTH AND DEVELOPMENT

Physiologically the middle years begin with shedding the first deciduous tooth and end at puberty with the acquisition of final permanent teeth (with the exception of the wisdom teeth). During the preceding 5 to 6 years, children have progressed from helpless infants to sturdy, complicated individuals with the capacity to communicate, conceptualize in a limited way, and become involved in complex social and motor behavior. Physical growth has been equally rapid. In contrast, the period of middle childhood, between the rapid growth of early childhood and the turmoil of the prepubescent growth spurt, is a time of gradual growth and development, with steadier and more even progress in both its physical and emotional aspects.

Children's physical health is generally good, and it is a comfortable period of physical adjustment. Physiologic processes in general have developed to the point that they can be maintained at stable levels under ordinary conditions or can be readily adjusted to meet changing needs and stresses. Under normal circumstances these children are usually well able to meet the physical and psychologic demands that are placed on them.

There is a special quality about the middle childhood years. This is the period of childhood the adult remembers with fond recollection. School-age children like this age period, and it is the one to which preschoolers eagerly look forward and for which adolescents yearn. In the Western world school-age children have considerable freedom and few responsibilities.

With a firm foundation of trust, autonomy, and initiative, school-age children are ready and eager for the wider world of learning and competition associated with developing a sense of industry and the successful acquisition of earlier, simpler skills. These skills are accompanied by the mild but persistent expectations of the society in which the children live, which serve as guidelines for behavior. Children who succeed in achieving the tasks of early childhood are able to move into middle childhood with the skills of locomotion, language, and control of body functions. They move from the egocentricity of early childhood to the subperiod of cognitive domain described as *concrete operations* and are now ready to undertake the tasks associated with the school experience. These tasks are characterized by three outward thrusts: the interpersonal push from home and family into the peer group, the physical thrust into the world of active games and work that requires neuromuscular skills, and the mental thrust into the world of mature concepts, logic, symbolism, and communication.

Until recently middle childhood generated the least interest and preoccupation among psychologists and others concerned with the effects of childhood experiences on later adjustments. However, it has been found that this period makes an important contribution to children's learning the fundamental skills of their culture and developing competence and self-esteem. It is a time of intellectual growth, investment in work, and the first real commitment to a social unit outside of and larger than the family.

BIOLOGIC DEVELOPMENT

During middle childhood, growth in height and weight assumes a slower but steady pace as compared with the earlier years and the years immediately ahead. Between ages 6 and 12, children will grow an average of 5 cm (2 inches) per year to gain 30 to 60 cm (1 to 2 feet) in height and will almost double in weight, increasing 2 to 3 kg (4½ to 6½ pounds) per year. The average 6-year-old child is about 116 cm (45 inches) tall and weighs about 21 kg (46 pounds); the average 12-year-old child stands about 150 cm (59 inches) tall and weighs approximately 40 kg (88 pounds). During this age period girls and boys differ very little in size, although boys tend to be slightly taller and somewhat heavier than girls. Toward the end of the school-age years both boys and girls begin to increase in size, although most girls begin to surpass boys in both height and weight, to the acute discomfort of both.

Proportional Changes

School-age children are more graceful than they were as preschoolers, and they are steadier on their feet. Their body proportions take on a slimmer look with longer legs, varying body proportion, and a lower center of gravity. Posture improves over that of the preschool period to facilitate locomotion and efficiency in using the arms and trunk. These proportions make climbing, bicycle riding, and other activities much easier. Fat gradually diminishes, and its distribution patterns change, contributing to the thinner appearance of children during the middle years.

Accompanying the skeletal lengthening and fat diminution is an increase in the percentage of body weight repre-

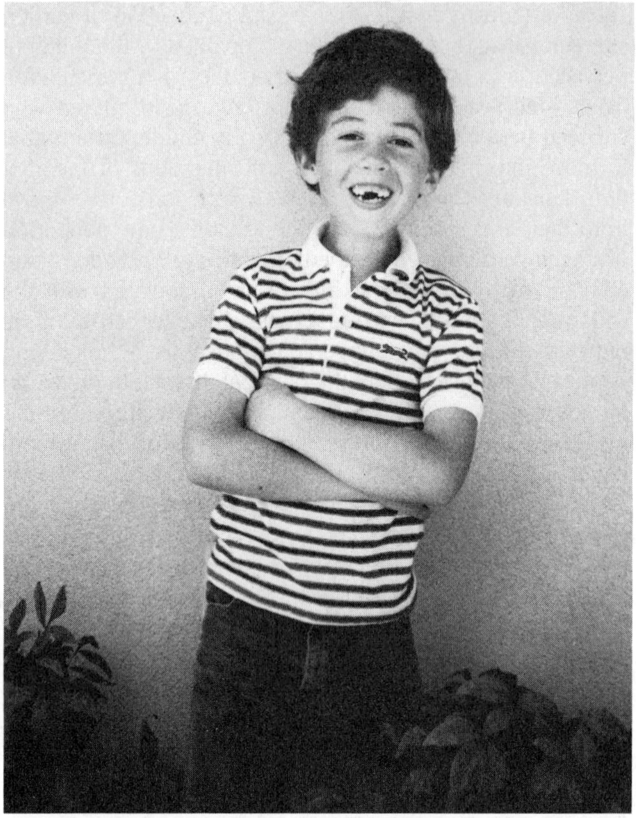

Fig. 17-1. Middle childhood is the stage of development when deciduous teeth are shed.

sented by muscle tissue. By the end of this age period both boys and girls will double their strength and physical capabilities, and their steady and relatively consistent acquisition of refined coordination will increase their poise and skill. However, this increased strength can be misleading. Although strength increases, muscles are still functionally immature when compared with those of the adolescent and are more readily damaged by muscular injury caused by overuse.

The most pronounced changes and those that seem best to indicate increasing maturity in children are a decrease in head circumference in relation to standing height, a decrease in waist circumference in relation to height, and an increase in leg length related to height. These observations often provide a clue to a child's degree of maturity that has proved useful in predicting readiness for meeting the demands of school. There appears to be a correlation between physical indications of maturity and success in school.

Certain physiologic and anatomic characteristics are typical of children in the years of middle childhood. Facial proportions change as the face grows faster in relation to the remainder of the cranium. The skull and brain grow very slowly during this period and increase little in size thereafter. Since all of the primary (deciduous) teeth are lost during this age span, middle childhood is sometimes known as the *age of the loose tooth* (Fig. 17-1) and the early years of middle childhood as the *ugly duckling stage,* when the new secondary (permanent) teeth appear to be much too large for the smaller face.

Maturation of Systems

Maturity of the gastrointestinal system is reflected in fewer stomach upsets, better maintenance of blood sugar levels, and an increased stomach capacity, which permits retention of food for longer periods. The school-age child does not need to be fed as carefully, as promptly, or as frequently as before. Caloric needs in relation to stomach size are less than they were in the preschool years and less than they will be during the coming adolescent growth spurt.

Physical maturation is evidenced in other body tissues and organs. Bladder capacity, although differing widely among individual children, is generally greater in girls than in boys. There are individual variations in frequency of urination and differences in one child according to circumstances such as temperature, humidity, time of day, amount of fluids ingested, and emotional state.

The heart grows more slowly during the middle years and is smaller in relation to the rest of the body than at any other period of life. Consequently, many believe that strongly competitive sports with prolonged, intense physical exertion may be damaging to school-age children. The heart and respiratory rates steadily decrease, and the blood pressure increases during ages 6 to 12 (see inside front cover).

Bones continue to ossify throughout childhood, but, since mineralization is not completed until maturity, children's bones resist pressure and muscle pull less than mature bones. Consequently care must be taken to prevent alterations in bone structure, and children should be provided with well-fitted shoes, chairs, and desks that allow correct sitting posture with the feet able to reach the floor and the hips able to fit well back in the seat. Children should have ample opportunity to move around and should observe appropriate caution in carrying heavy loads. For example, they should shift books and/or tote bags from one arm to the other. Back packs distribute weight more evenly.

Wider differences between children are observed at the end of middle childhood than at the beginning—and the differences are sometimes striking. These differences become increasingly apparent and, if extreme or unique, may create emotional problems unless the associated characteristics of height and weight relationships, rapid or slow growth, and other important features of development are recognized and explained to the children and their families. In addition, physical maturity is not necessarily correlated with emotional and social maturity. Seven-year-old children who look like 10-year-old children will think and act like 7-year-old children. To expect behavior appropriate for 10-year-old children from them is unrealistic and can be detrimental to their development of competence and self-esteem. Conversely, to treat 10-year-old children as though they were 7 years old is an equal disservice to them.

Prepubescence

Toward the end of middle childhood the discrepancies in growth and maturation between boys and girls become more apparent. On the average there is a difference of approximately 2 years between girls and boys in the age at which observable signs of pubescence appear. Preadolescence is, for some, a period of rapid growth, especially for girls; for others, mostly boys, it is generally a period of continued steady growth in height and weight. On the whole it is a healthy period of childhood—the period between childhood diseases and the diseases of adulthood.

There is no universal age at which children assume the characteristics of preadolescence. The first physiologic signs begin to appear at about 9 years (particularly in girls) and are usually clearly evident in 11- to 12-year-old children. Although preadolescent children do not want to be different, at this age the variability in physical growth and physiologic changes between children of the same sex, between the two sexes, and even within each individual child is often striking. This variability, especially in relation to the onset of secondary sex characteristics, is of utmost concern to the preadolescent. Either early or late appearance of these characteristics is a source of embarrassment and uneasiness to both sexes.

Preadolescence is a time when there is considerable overlapping of developmental characteristics with elements of both middle childhood and early adolescence. However, there are sufficient unique characteristics to set this period apart as an age category, even with the wide range of variability in ages 11 and 12 (or even 9 to 13) in some children. Generally the earliest age at which puberty begins is 10 years in girls and 12 years in boys, although there has been an increase in the number of girls reaching puberty at age 9. The average age of puberty in girls is 12, and in boys it is 14. Boys experience little sexual maturation during preadolescence.

PSYCHOSOCIAL DEVELOPMENT

There is no concept more difficult to assess or more elusive than that of the personality or the "self." Most persons draw inferences regarding children's personalities from observation of their behaviors. These behaviors are based on many different innate and acquired characteristics, the way in which these characteristics are organized, and the manner in which each characteristic modifies or alters the other to contribute to the unique quality of each child. Personality is reflected in the way in which children react to themselves and others, the way in which others react to them, and the way in which they adjust to their environment. Evolution of the personality involves a number of different types of development—physical, intellectual, social, and emotional—all of which are profoundly influenced by the environment in which children grow and develop.

Latency (Freud)

Middle childhood is the period in psychosexual development that Freud has described as the *latency period.* He maintains that this time of life involves consolidation and elaboration of previously acquired traits and skills with the assumption that no new significant conflicts or impulses will arise. Growth and development patterns follow the lines established in earlier stages. The primary personality development is the development of the superego. It is a time of preparation for the important and dramatic psychosexual changes that take place during the genital stage of adolescence.

Developing a Sense of Industry (Erikson)

Successful mastery of Erikson's first three stages of psychosocial development is probably the most important accomplishment in terms of development of a healthy personality (Erikson, 1963). With a foundation of trust, autonomy, and initiative, children are fairly certain to progress through subsequent stages with relative ease. Successful completion of these stages implies confidence in an environment of loving relationships within a stable family unit that has prepared the child to engage in experiences and relationships beyond these intimate groups. It has been suggested that the individual's fundamental attitude toward work is established during middle childhood. It is during this time that children receive the systematic instruction prescribed by their individual cultures and develop the skills needed to become useful, contributing members of their social communities.

A sense of industry, for which a more descriptive term is the *stage of accomplishment,* is achieved somewhere between age 6 and adolescence. The goal of this stage of development is to achieve a sense of personal and interpersonal competence by the acquisition of technologic and social skills. School-age children are eager to build skills and participate in meaningful and socially useful work. Interests expand in the middle years, and, with a growing sense of independence, children want to engage in tasks that can be carried through to completion (Fig. 17-2). Failure to develop a sense of accomplishment results in a sense of *inferiority.*

There are many attributes of industry that contribute to the child's sense of competence and mastery. Intrinsic motivation is associated with increased competence in mastering new skills and assuming new responsibilities. Children gain a great deal of satisfaction from independent behavior in exploring and manipulating their environment and from interaction with peers. Extrinsic sources of reinforcement in the form of grades, material rewards, additional privileges, and recognition provide encouragement and stimulation. Often the acquisition of skills is a means for achieving success in special activities such as athletics or social organizations such as scouting. Peer approval is a strong motivating power.

The danger inherent in this period of personality development is the imposition of situations that might result in a sense of inadequacy or inferiority. This may happen if the previous stages have not been successfully achieved or if a child is incapable of or unprepared for assuming the responsibilities associated with developing a sense of accomplishment. Feelings of inferiority or lack of worth can be derived from children themselves or from the social environment. Children with physical or mental limitations are at a disadvantage for acquisition of certain skills, and, when the reward structure is based on evidence of mastery, children

A 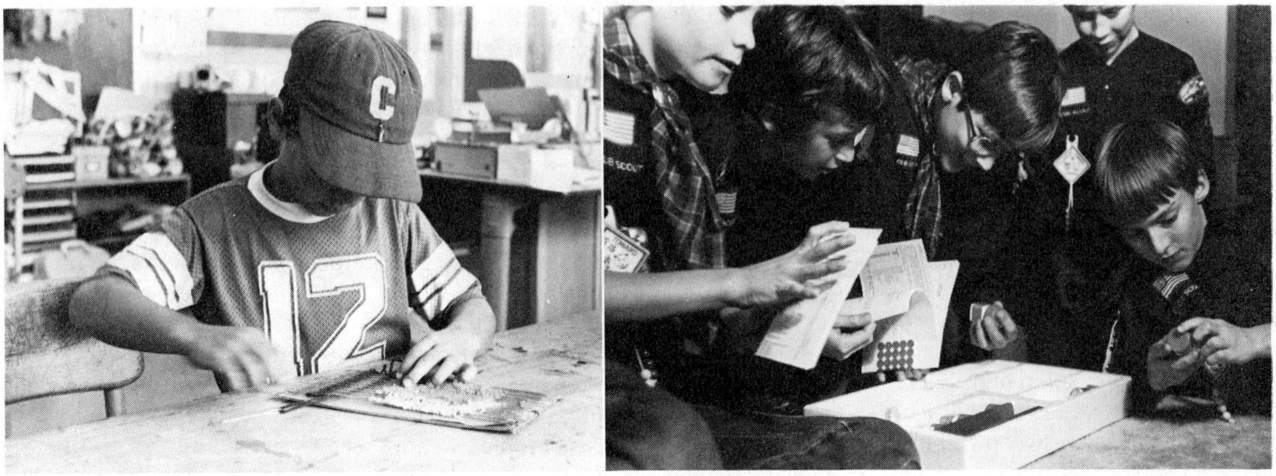 B

Fig. 17-2. School-age children are motivated to complete tasks. **A,** Working alone. **B,** Working with others.

who are incapable of developing these skills are bound to feel inadequate and inferior.

Even children without chronic disabilities represent such a wide range of individual differences in capabilities and preferences that they will experience feelings of inadequacy in some areas. No child is able to do well in everything, and children must learn that they will not be able to master each skill that they attempt. All children, even children who in most instances have positive attitudes toward work and their own capabilities, will feel some degree of inferiority in regard to a specific skill that they cannot master.

To some extent, success or aptitude in one area may compensate for failure or ineptitude in another. However, the differences in reinforcement provided for success in various areas have a very significant effect on feelings of adequacy. For example, in the United States reading proficiency is more highly rewarded than mechanical aptitude such as tinkering with broken automobile engines. A higher social value is placed on success in team sports than on success in operating a ham radio. However, compensating for the inability to excel in more socially valued skills through mastery of other less valued skills is difficult for the child. Also, as a corollary to this, the social environment places a negative value on any kind of failure, and this serves to further stimulate feelings of inferiority in the less capable child. Repeated failures often generate such strong feelings in the child that eventually he is reluctant to attempt any new task that may bring failure or is fearful that he will not be able to perform as well as his peers. Thus intrinsic motivation toward engaging in a task for the pleasure of the challenge conflicts with the external forces that cause feelings of doubt and inferiority. Consequently, the child may no longer try.

Much depends on the child's concept of success or failure. Children who aspire for more than they are capable of will usually experience failure. In contrast, children who set their aspirations lower than their level of achievement are more likely to experience success. Most accomplishments during the school years are very public. Success or failure in school is known to family, teachers, peers, and others. In the social environment of school and sometimes at home, feelings of inferiority may be produced through comparison with others, suggesting that the child is not as good as some peer, sibling, or another subcultural group. This inadequacy becomes a source of embarrassment. The child may even be shamed for the failure. These earlier conflicts of doubt and guilt are very closely associated with feelings of inferiority.

A sense of accomplishment also involves the ability to cooperate and to compete with others—to cope more effectively with people. Middle childhood is the time when children learn the value of doing things alongside and with others and the benefits derived from division of labor in the accomplishment of goals. Children need and want real achievement. When they have access to tasks that need to be done, that they are able to do well despite individual differences in their innate capacities and emotional development, and that they are suitably rewarded for, children will be able to achieve a sense of industry and accomplishment that prepares them for establishing a stable identity later in life.

TEMPERAMENT

The enduring reactivity patterns or temperamental traits identified in infancy continue to be important in middle childhood as determinants of some aspects of behavior. Analyzing behavioral patterns observed in past situations can provide clues to the way that a child may react to new situations, although long-range projections are not always successful. Through interaction with environment, experiences, motives, and abilities, many children change. Major temperamental characteristics persist into adolescence in many children; in others they do not.

Parents and teachers are persons who are in the best position to assess a child's behavioral style and try to make their demands and expectations consonant with the individual child's temperamental characteristics. With easy children this rarely poses a problem. They adapt readily to almost any childrearing program and new situation. School entry or other experiences are usually smooth and accomplished with minimum stress. Difficulties arise with difficult, slow-to-warm-up children and children who are easily distracted.

Slow-to-warm-up children who usually exhibit discomfort when introduced to new situations need time to become accustomed to a new environment, authority figures, and expectations. These children may respond with tears, somatic complaints, or other maneuvers to avoid the event. They should be encouraged to try new experiences but also should be allowed to adapt to their surroundings at their own speed. Pressure to move quickly into new situations only strengthens the tendency to withdraw. Even afterschool activities can be cause for reaction, but attending with a friend or contracting for permission to withdraw after a trial of a specified number of times may provide them with sufficient incentive to try.

Difficult or easily distracted children may benefit from "practice" sessions in which they are prepared for the event by role-playing, visiting the site, stories, or other methods of getting them acquainted with what to expect. Children who are very persistent need to know when they are expected to stop what they are doing so that the signal to stop will not come as a surprise, thus triggering a reaction. Children with difficult temperaments need to be handled with exceptional patience, firmness, and understanding so they can learn appropriate behavior in their interactions with others. It is important for teachers to be matched to the temperament of children whenever possible to ensure a "good fit." Although teachers should be sensitive and understanding of children with all temperaments, there are some who are better able to cope with difficult children.

COGNITIVE DEVELOPMENT

Somewhere around the beginning of the school years, children begin to acquire the ability to relate a series of events and actions to mental representations that can be expressed both verbally and symbolically. This is the stage in development that Piaget describes as *concrete operations,* wherein children are able to use their thought processes to experience events and actions. Since the word "operation" implies an action that is performed on an object or set of objects, a mental operation is an alteration or transformation that is carried out in thought rather than in action. Toddlers or preschool children can perform acts that involve ordering, such as correctly arranging a graduated set of circles from largest to smallest on a stick, or they can find their way to a friend's house, but they are unable to verbalize the action or actions involved in the process. School-age children are able to articulate the process and can perform the action mentally without the need to carry out the behaviors.

Developing Concrete Operations (Piaget)

As children move from the preschool years into the world of wider relationships, their conceptual abilities become increasingly more flexible. During the *concrete-operational* period children rapidly acquire cognitive operations and apply these new skills when thinking about objects, situations, and events. Their rigid, egocentric outlook is replaced by thought processes that allow them to see things from the point of view of another. They become aware of a variety of perspectives and become more sensitive to the fact that others do not always perceive events exactly as they do. They are able to delay an action until they have evaluated alternative responses to situations, and their steady reduction in egocentricity helps form the basis for logical thought and the development and maturation of morality.

The concrete-operational stage takes place between the years 7 and 11. During this stage children develop an understanding and use for relationships between things and ideas. They progress from making judgments based on what they see (perceptual) to making judgments based on what they reason (conceptual). They are increasingly able to master symbols and to use their memory store of past experiences in evaluating and interpreting the present. They gain insight into the basic components of concrete operational thought: conservation, classification, and combinational skills.

Conservation. One of the major cognitive tasks of school-age children is learning that physical matter does not appear and disappear by magic. They learn that certain properties of the environment are not changed simply by altering their disposition in space. They are able to resist perceptual cues that suggest such alterations in the physical state of an object.

Conservation of liquid, mass, number, length, area, and volume can be demonstrated by the use of commonplace items (Fig. 17-3). To explain the observations that the mass has been unaltered, the child may use one of the three concepts outlined in Box 17-1.

When children are able to use the concepts of identity, reversibility, and reciprocity, they can conserve along any physical dimension. They perceive the concept of volume in relation to container size and shape, recognize that size is not necessarily related to weight or volume, and are able to manipulate or "see" in a concrete manner. They recognize that logical operations move in two directions (such as addition and subtraction or multiplication and division) and that certain properties are invariant (e.g., 7 remains 7 whether it is represented by 3 + 4, 2 + 5, or seven buttons, seven stars, or seven boys).

Children learn that a given number of objects such as pennies will remain the same no matter how far apart they are spaced. When younger school-age children are presented with two rows of pennies, they will declare that a row of six pennies closely aligned is not equivalent to a row of six pennies spaced apart (conservation of length). As they advance in development, they see that the numbers remain the same no matter how they are related to one another in space.

There appears to be a developmental sequence in children's capacity to conserve matter. Children usually grasp conservation of numbers (ages 5 to 6) before conservation of substance. Conservation of liquids, mass, and length

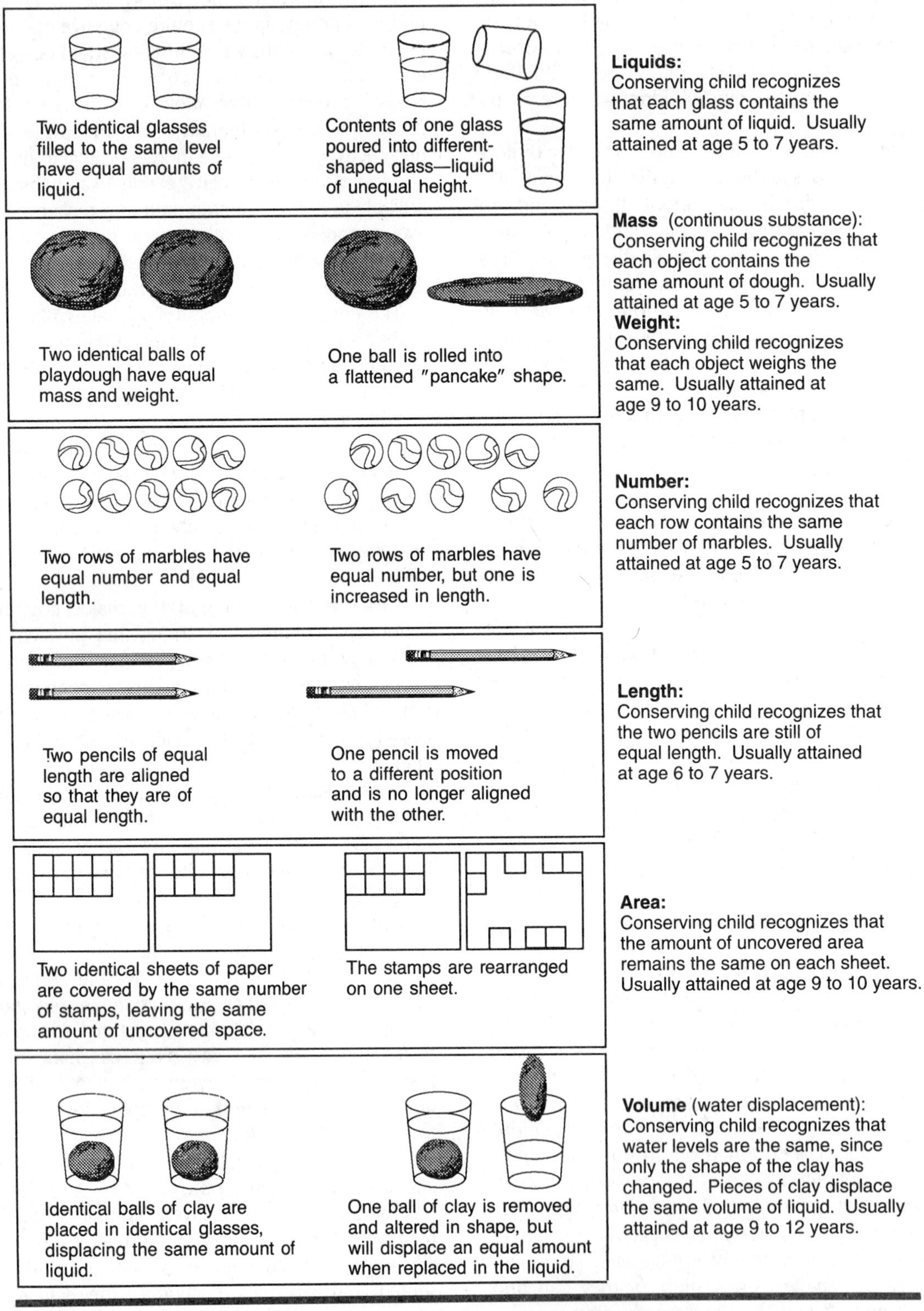
Two identical glasses filled to the same level have equal amounts of liquid.
Contents of one glass poured into different-shaped glass—liquid of unequal height.
Liquids:
Conserving child recognizes that each glass contains the same amount of liquid. Usually attained at age 5 to 7 years.
Two identical balls of playdough have equal mass and weight.
One ball is rolled into a flattened "pancake" shape.
Mass (continuous substance):
Conserving child recognizes that each object contains the same amount of dough. Usually attained at age 5 to 7 years.
Weight:
Conserving child recognizes that each object weighs the same. Usually attained at age 9 to 10 years.
Two rows of marbles have equal number and equal length.
Two rows of marbles have equal number, but one is increased in length.
Number:
Conserving child recognizes that each row contains the same number of marbles. Usually attained at age 5 to 7 years.
Two pencils of equal length are aligned so that they are of equal length.
One pencil is moved to a different position and is no longer aligned with the other.
Length:
Conserving child recognizes that the two pencils are still of equal length. Usually attained at age 6 to 7 years.
Two identical sheets of paper are covered by the same number of stamps, leaving the same amount of uncovered space.
The stamps are rearranged on one sheet.
Area:
Conserving child recognizes that the amount of uncovered area remains the same on each sheet. Usually attained at age 9 to 10 years.
Identical balls of clay are placed in identical glasses, displacing the same amount of liquid.
One ball of clay is removed and altered in shape, but will displace an equal amount when replaced in the liquid.
Volume (water displacement):
Conserving child recognizes that water levels are the same, since only the shape of the clay has changed. Pieces of clay displace the same volume of liquid. Usually attained at age 9 to 12 years.

Fig. 17-3. Common methods for testing the child's ability to conserve.

usually is accomplished at about ages 6 to 7, weight sometime later (ages 9 to 10), and volume displacement last (ages 9 to 12).

Reversibility is used by children in selecting a course of action, thus providing greater control over themselves and their environment. They have the ability to think through an action sequence, anticipate the consequences, and, if needed, return to the beginning and rethink the action in a different direction. They no longer need to experience an action before they can anticipate the results. Reversibility

Box 17-1 CONCEPTS USED TO EXPLAIN CONSERVATION

Identity—since nothing has been added and nothing has been taken away, the pancake is still the same clay with nothing changed but the shape.
Reversibility—the clay can be reshaped into its original form, that of a ball.
Reciprocity—although the pancake appears larger in circumference, the ball is much thicker. In this instance the child demonstrates the ability to deal with two dimensions at the same time and comprehend that a change in one dimension compensates for a change in another.

allows mental action to replace physical action and provides the children with the ability to disassemble and reassemble certain kinds of things in their thoughts.

Classification. Classification skills involve the ability to group objects according to the attributes that they share in common. School-age children now have the ability to place things in a sensible and logical order, to group and sort, and, in doing so, to hold a concept in their minds while they make decisions based on that concept. It is characteristic of middle childhood that children derive a great deal of enjoyment from classifying and ordering their environment. They become occupied with numerous and varied collections of objects, such as wrappers, stamps, shells, dolls, cars, stones, and anything that is classifiable (Fig. 17-4). They even begin to order friends and relationships (e.g., first best friend, second best friend).

As children mature, they progress from collecting simply for the sake of collecting and become more selective and discriminating. Their classification systems become more complex and are based on abstract ideas rather than on perception and experience. Much of the pleasure of collections is the appraising, ordering, and reordering of the parts.

School children are able to *serialize,* that is, to arrange objects according to some ordinal scale or quantified dimension such as size, weight, or color. They develop the ability to understand relational terms and concepts, such as bigger and smaller; darker and paler; heavier and lighter; to the right of and to the left of; first, last, and intermediate (e.g., fourth, second); and more than and less than. They can see family relationships in terms of reciprocal roles; for example, in order to be a brother, one must have a sibling. It is common for a preschool child to refer to the adult female in a family as "your mother" even when discussing the relationship with the woman's husband.

Combinational skills. It is during the school-age years that children develop the ability to manipulate numbers and to learn the skills of addition, subtraction, multiplication, and division. They learn to apply the basic operations to any object or quantity. They learn the alphabet and the ever-widening world of symbols called words that can be arranged in terms of structure and their relationship to the alphabet. They learn to tell time, to see the relationship

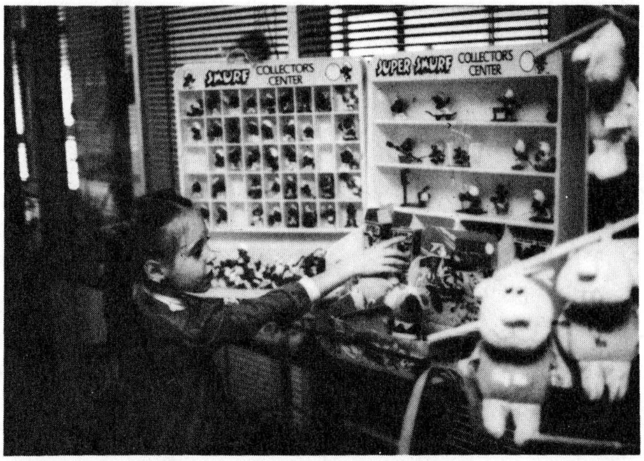

Fig. 17-4. School-age children are often avid collectors.

of events in time (history) and places in space (geography), and to combine time and space relationships (geology and astronomy).

School-age children are able to entertain a hypothesis through use of conceptual principles and perceived events and to evaluate evidence that might support or disprove a hypothesis. These capabilities allow them to expand beyond the limits of their own experience and to consider events that happened before, will happen in the future, and are hypothesized to be happening in the present.

The most significant skill, the ability to read, is acquired during the school years and becomes the most valuable tool for independent inquiry. Children's capacity for exploration, imagination, and expansion of knowledge is enhanced with the ability to read as they progress from the repetition and confusion of early efforts to increasing facility and comprehension.

It is through no accident that the schools are prepared to meet the essentials of children's intellectual capabilities at the time that their cognitive processes are ready to assume appropriate intellectual achievements. The increase in capacity for logical thinking during this stage of concrete operations is based on the sensorimotor schemes of infancy and the representational abilities of preschool children. Children are now able to move into the formal operations that characterize the period of adolescence.

MORAL DEVELOPMENT (KOHLBERG)

As children move from egocentrism to more logical patterns of thought, they also move through stages in the development of conscience and moral standards. The beginning of this development is evident during the preschool years when children, to some extent, adopt and internalize the moral values of their parents and their standards for evaluating the behavior of themselves and others. Adopting parental standards makes children feel similar to the parents, thereby strengthening their identification.

Growth in moral thought and judgment progresses between ages 6 and 12. Young children do not believe that standards of behavior come from within themselves but that rules are established and set down by others. At first rules are perceived as definite, covering limited situations, and requiring no reason or explanation. Children learn the standards for acceptable behavior, act according to these standards, and feel guilty when they violate the standards. Although children 6 or 7 years old know the rules and what they are supposed to do, they do not understand the reasons behind them. Young children usually judge an act by its consequences. Rewards and punishment guide their judgment; a "bad act" is one that breaks a rule or does harm. When a child and an adult conflict in judging an act, the adult is right. Children may believe that what other people tell them to do is right and that what they think themselves is wrong. Consequently children 6 or 7 years old are more likely to interpret accidents and misfortunes as punishment for misdeeds.

Older school-age children are able to judge an act by the intentions that prompted it rather than just by the consequences. Rules and judgments become less absolute and authoritarian and begin to be founded more on the needs and desires of others. Rules of conduct are more readily considered in terms of mutual agreement and based on cooperation and respect for others. For older children a rule violation is apt to be viewed in relation to the total context in which it appears; reactions are influenced by the situation, as well as by the morality of the rule itself. However, it is not until adolescence or beyond that children are able to view morality on an abstract basis with sound reasoning and principled thinking. Whereas a younger child can judge an act only according to whether it is right or wrong, older children will take into account a different point of view to make a judgment. They are able to understand and accept the concept of doing as they would have others do to them.

SPIRITUAL DEVELOPMENT

Children at this age think in very concrete terms but are avid learners and have a great desire to learn about their God. They picture God as human and tend to describe him in terms of character traits such as loving and helping. He is a very important person in the lives of many children. They are fascinated by heaven and hell and, with a developing conscience and concern about rules, they fear going to hell for misbehavior. School-age children want and expect to be punished for misbehavior but, if given the option, tend to choose a punishment that "fits the crime." Often they view illness or injury as a punishment for a real or imagined misdeed. The beliefs and ideals of family and religious personages are more influential than their peers in matters of faith.

School-age children begin to learn the difference between the natural and the supernatural but have difficulty understanding symbols. Consequently, religious concepts must be presented to them in concrete terms. They try to relate phenomena in the world in a logical, systematic manner, which is at once both satisfying and occasionally disheartening. Religion affords a means whereby children can relate themselves to their deity in a direct and personal way.

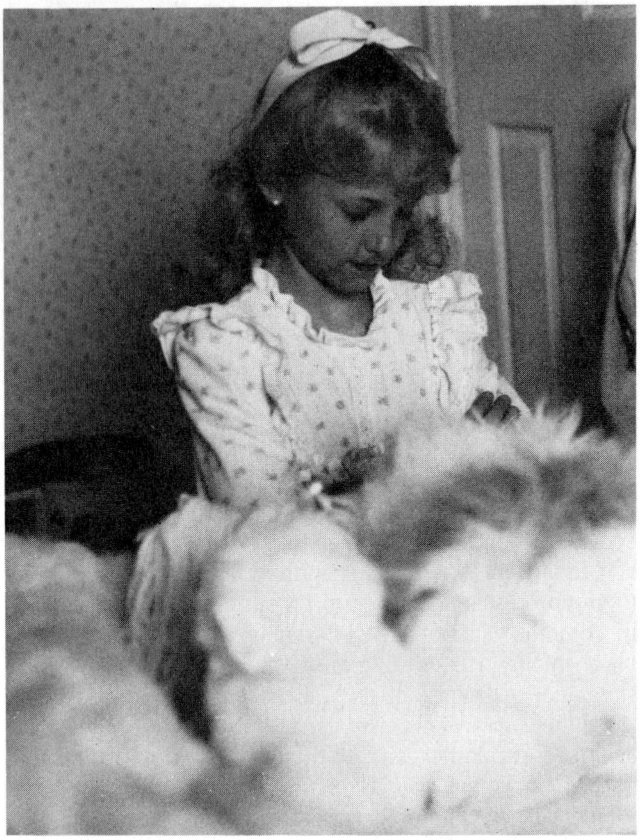

Fig. 17-5. Children are comforted by prayer or other religious rituals.

Children are comforted by prayer or other religious rituals and, if this is a part of their daily lives, these activities can help them cope with threatening situations (Fig. 17-5). Their petitions to their God in prayers tend to be for very tangible rewards and, although younger children expect their prayers to be answered, as they get older they begin to recognize that this does not always occur and become less concerned when prayers are not answered. They are able to discuss their feelings about their faith and how it relates to their lives.

LANGUAGE DEVELOPMENT

Children enter middle childhood with remarkably efficient language skills, but they will achieve many important linguistic accomplishments during the school-age years. During the elementary school years they learn to correct previous syntactic errors and begin to use more complex grammatical forms, such as correct past tenses for irregular verbs, correct plurals for irregular nouns, and correct use of personal pronouns.

Word usage, as well as the ability to find and retrieve words quickly when called upon to produce what they know in a relatively short period of time, grows considerably during the school years. Children learn to apply the minimum distance principle—the rule that the subject of a verb in an active sentence is the noun or pronoun that immediately precedes it. For example, a 6-year-old child will understand the sentence "Ask Mary her last name" but until age 9 or 10 years will be confused by the sentence "Ask Mary what to bring to the party."

Narrative skills improve markedly. School-age children are increasingly able to provide directives that others can correctly interpret without visual data, for example, explaining directions over the telephone. By age 10 to 12 years the child should be able to use factitive words (such as know, think, and believe) and complex pronouns and conjunctions, and be able to form grammatically correct sentences. School-age children gradually become more proficient at making inferences about meanings and learn the subtle exceptions to grammatical rules, which make them less likely to engage in literal interpretation of messages.

They rapidly develop *metalinguistic awareness*—an ability to think about language and to comment on its properties. This enables them to appreciate jokes, riddles, and puns because of their play on words, sounds, or double meanings. They are beginning to understand metaphors and proverbial meaning to figurative statements such as, "A stitch in time saves nine." The acquisition of cognitive skills enables them to think about the quality of their own and others' speech and to evaluate and clarify messages.

SOCIAL DEVELOPMENT

Children at the beginning of the middle childhood years normally enter a period of less intense emotions, secure in their dependency on their parents and family and with self-confidence tempered by a more realistic perspective. Their energies are now available to explore the environment beyond the family, to gradually increase the scope of interpersonal interactions, and to invest their curiosity in a greater understanding of the world.

Identification with peers appears to be a strong influence in children's gaining independence from parents. The aid and support of the group provide children with enough security to risk the moderate parental rejection brought about by each small victory in their development of independence.

Questions of masculinity and femininity take on importance as sex-role learning assumes more prominence. Boys associate with boys, and girls with girls, each pursuing their own interests, with communication between the sexes confined to that which is necessary. Much of the child's concept of the appropriate sex role is acquired through relationships with peers. During the early school years there is little difference relative to sex in the play experiences of children. Games and many other activities are shared by both girls and boys. However, in the later school years the differences become marked. Boys and girls grow more intolerant of each other, especially on the surface.

Social Relationships and Cooperation

Daily relationships with age-mates provide the most important social interactions in the life of school-age children. For the first time children are able to join in group activities with unrestrained enthusiasm and steady participation, when formerly interactions had been limited to short periods under considerable adult supervision. With increased skills and wider opportunities, children are able to become involved with one or several peer groups in which they can gain status as respected members.

There are valuable lessons to be learned from daily interaction with age-mates. First, children learn to appreciate the numerous and varied points of view that are represented in the peer group. As they play together, children discover that there are numerous occupations for fathers and mothers, perhaps more than one version of the same song, different rules for the same game, and different customs for celebrating the same holiday. As children interact with peers who see the world in ways that are somewhat different from the way they see it, they become aware of the limits of their own point of view. Because age-mates are peers and are not forced to accept one another's ideas as they are expected to accept those of adults, other children have a significant influence on decreasing the egocentric outlook of the individual child. Consequently, they learn to argue, persuade, bargain, cooperate, and compromise in order to maintain friendships.

Second, children become increasingly sensitive to the social norms and pressures of the peer group. The peer group establishes standards for acceptance and rejection, and children may be willing to modify their behavior in order to be accepted by the group. They are judged by the physical impression they convey, the skills they can perform, and other abilities they can demonstrate. This need for peer approval becomes a powerful influence toward conformity. The child learns to dress, talk, and otherwise behave in a manner acceptable to the group. A variety of roles, such as class joker or class hero, may be assumed by the individual child in order to gain approval from the group. However, no child will be able to adapt perfectly to all the requirements made by the peer group. If some children find that the discrepancies between the values of the peer group and the values of their families are too great, they may be forced to relinquish the pleasure of interaction with the group in order to abide by the regulations established in the home. Thus, to diminish conflict within the family, some children may be forced into a position outside the peer group.

Third, the interaction among peers leads to the formation of intimate friendships between same-sex peers (Fig. 17-6). School age is the time when children have "best friends" with whom they share secrets, private jokes, and adventures and come to one another's aid in times of trouble. In the course of these friendships children also fight, threaten, break up, and reunite. These dyadic relationships, in which children experience love and closeness for a peer, seem to be important as a foundation for heterosexual relationships in adulthood. The conflicts encountered in the relationship are usually resolved in terms that the children are able to control. Since neither child has authority over the other, as in an adult-child relationship, the children must work through their differences within the framework of their commitment to each other. Friendships between children of different races are common during early childhood but tend to decline in preadolescence (Sandler, 1989).

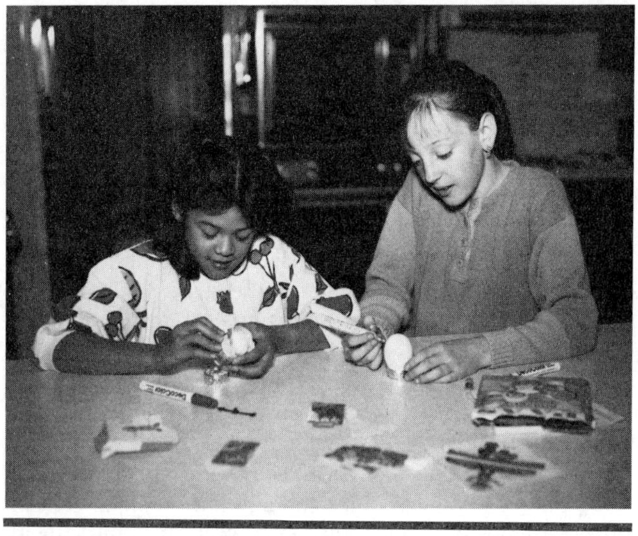

Fig. 17-6. School-age children enjoy engaging in activities with a "best friend."

Peer groups. One of the outstanding characteristics of middle childhood is the formation of formalized groups. Initially children in the early middle years merely hang around the periphery of the formalized group watching, learning, practicing various skills, and participating in group activities whenever the members of the gang allow them to do so. In a year or two, as they advance in age, children eventually take their places as full-fledged participating members. The process is facilitated if they have a buddy.

One of the prominent features of middle childhood groups is the code of rigid rules imposed on the members. There is an exclusiveness in the selection of persons who have the privilege of joining. They often adopt a "uniform" and special words that signify membership in the group. Acceptance in the group is often determined on a pass-fail basis that is based on social or behavioral criteria. Conformity is the core of the group structure. There are often secret codes, shared interests, and special modes of dress, and each child must abide by a standard of behavior established by the group. Understanding of and conformity to the rules provide children with feelings of security and relieve them of the responsibility of making decisions.

Membership in the group provides children with a comfortable place in society. Many of the values of the group, such as physical strength, daring, ingenuity, and comradeship, have not been stressed in the family, but these, too, are worthy values and contribute to an individual child's total personality. By merging their identities with that of their peers, children are able to move from the family group to an outside group as a step toward seeking further independence. They substitute conformity to a peer-group pattern for conformity to a family pattern while they are still too shaky and insecure to function independently.

During the early school years gangs are rather small, loosely organized groups with changing membership and little formal structure and without the more prolonged cohesiveness characteristic of gangs in later school years. They do not demonstrate the elements of give-and-take, cooperation, and order that are seen in groups of older children. As a rule girls' groups are less formalized than boys' groups, and although there may be a mixture of both sexes in the earlier school years, the groups of later school years are composed predominantly of children of the same sex. Common interests are a frequent basis around which a group is structured.

Children's strong desire not to be different creates problems for those who are, for various reasons, unable to meet the accepted standards of the peer group. Children with disabilities or those who are in some way so deprived that they are unable to compete have a difficult time. Self-consciousness results when children are unable to dress as other children dress, do not have spending money like other children, or appear different from other children, such as the child who has numerous freckles, red hair, or such minor physical defects as strabismus. Any of these differences will set a child apart from the group and often make the child a target for the criticism and ridicule of the peer group.

Although peer group identification and association are essential to a child's emergence into the world, there can be dangers inherent in strong peer-group attachment. Peer pressures may force children into taking risks, even against their better judgment. Minor infractions and immoralities, such as stealing apples from the neighbor's tree, smoking, or sexual exposure, are disturbing to adults but seem to be a normal part of gang activity. However, acts of violence or destruction and foolhardy risks to safety are sometimes the outgrowth of overzealous group cohesiveness.

Relationships with Families

Although the peer group is highly influential and necessary to normal child development, parents are still the primary influence in shaping children's personalities, setting standards for behavior, and establishing value systems. It is the family values that usually predominate when parental and peer value systems come into conflict. Although children may appear to reject parental values while testing the new values of the peer group, ultimately they will retain and incorporate into their own value systems the parental values they have found to be of worth. Peer associations seem to remain within the social class system, and not infrequently there may be discriminate membership on the basis of ethnic or racial origin.

As children move into the wider world of peer-group relationships, parents are faced with the task of relinquishing their hold. They may find it difficult to face the rejection that is demonstrated as their children stand solidly with the peer group. During this time children will want to spend more time in the company of their peers and may seem eager to leave the house; they will often prefer activities of the group to family activities. This can be very disturbing to parents. During this time parents can best serve the interests of their children through tolerant understanding and support even when there may be intolerance and criticism of the parents and their ways when those ways deviate from that of the group. In the child's eyes the parents no longer assume the stature they previously enjoyed. Children discover that parents can be wrong, and they begin to question the knowledge and authority of the parents who previously were considered to be all-knowing and all-powerful.

Although increased independence is the goal of middle childhood, children are not yet prepared to reject parental control. Children need and want restrictions placed on their behavior; they are not yet prepared to cope with all the problems of their expanding environment. They feel more secure knowing that there is an authority greater than themselves to implement such controls and restrictions. Children may complain loudly about the restrictions and try their best to break down parental barriers, but they are uneasy if they can succeed in doing so. Children feel secure with reasonable, consistent controls. They respect the adults on whom they can rely to prevent them from acting on each and every urge. Children sense in this behavior an expression of love and concern for their welfare.

Children also need their parents as adults, not as pals. Sometimes parents, hurt at their children's rejection, attempt to maintain their love and gratitude by assuming the role of "pals." Children need the stable, secure strength provided by mature adults to whom they can turn during troubled relationships with peers or stressful changes in their world. During a disruption in their lives, such as times of failure, periods of illness, or a move that separates them from the security of friends, children need the firm, secure anchor of parental interest and concern. With a secure base in a loving family, children are able to develop confidence in themselves and gain the maturity needed to break loose from the group and stand independently.

Research by Vandell, Minnett, and Santrock (1987) indicates that children's relationships with siblings change during the middle years. With age, siblings become more equal in power and status. Whereas in earlier years older siblings were influential in the younger siblings' learning, the previous instruction/help relationship becomes one of companionship. Positive emotional tone increases, but sibling conflict increases as the siblings get older. The researchers believe that middle childhood is a period of transition for sibling relationships, a juncture between the open bickering of early childhood and the supportive relationship observed in adult siblings.

DEVELOPMENT OF SELF-CONCEPT

Closely associated with developing a sense of industry is developing a concept of one's value and worth. With the emphasis on skill building and broadened social relationships, children are continually occupied in the process of self-evaluation. Children's self-concepts are composed of their own critical self-assessment plus what they interpret as the opinions of family members and outside social contacts—the mental picture they have of themselves, including their bodies. Although each child is different and unique, some aspects of the self-concept are common to others.

Body Image

Body image is the thoughts children entertain about their bodies. School-age children are quite knowledgeable about the human body, and social development during this period focuses to a large extent on the body and its capabilities. School-age children are able to draw a recognizable human figure, although individually their portrayal of body parts may vary considerably. They are acutely aware of bodies—their own, those of their peers, and those of adults. It is important that children know body functions and that adults correct misinformation children may have about the body (e.g., what is fat).

Social development during the school years, with emphasis on peer relationships, prescribes that children conform to group norms. They evaluate themselves to determine how their physical appearance, body configuration, and coordination compare to those of their peers. The head is the most noticeable and, to them, important part of the body. They also model themselves after their parents and compare themselves to favored peers and images observed in the media.

It is not unusual for children in middle childhood to be curious about their own bodies and the bodies of other children. They often experiment, and it is a common occurrence for two or more children to unclothe (to varying degrees) and play "doctor." Such experimentations and explorations allow children to pursue an investigation of similarities and differences as one means of acquiring norms. Fortunately, such self-investigations are not observed by others, but if children are surprised in the act, the best approach is to provide reassurance that the behavior is normal, thus relieving any anguish or guilt they may feel. It is only when these activities are carried to the extreme or when parents overreact to them that they become clinical problems (Levine, 1983).

Children are acutely aware of physical disabilities in others, and it is not unusual for them to believe that their own bodies are not all right, are not the right size or the right shape, or that they are in some way defective. They respond to such concerns in a variety of ways. For example, they will conceal perceived shortcomings of body or performance, such as the obese child who refrains from going swimming, the child who conveniently forgets a gym suit, the child who conceals an imagined defect, or the child with enuresis who declines invitations to slumber parties. Children seldom express these concerns to families. However, they need to be reassured about both the uniqueness and the sameness of their bodies while respecting their privacy and allowing them appropriate protective strategies. Children who are different become acutely aware of the differences and may find themselves excluded from the group. When children are teased or criticized about being different, the effect will be lasting. They remember the teasing well into adulthood.

Self-Esteem

Self-esteem is children's picture of their individual worth and consists of both positive and negative qualities. Children actively strive to achieve internalized goals or levels of attainment. At the same time they continually receive feedback on the quality of their performance from those whom they consider to be authorities. By the time they reach school age, children have already received messages regarding the extent to which they are able to accomplish tasks that have been delegated to them. For example, one child may have been given prestigious responsibilities at home or at school or received special commendation for an achievement. On the other hand, another child may have been sent to a special class for slow learners or may have been the last person chosen when children choose up sides for a game. These and other signs serve as clues to social evaluation that children then incorporate as part of their self-evaluation.

Children approach the process of self-evaluation from a framework of either self-confidence or self-doubt. Children who during the preschool years have mastered the maturational crises of autonomy and initiative are able to face the world with feelings of pride rather than shame. At first children's self-concepts are formed exclusively from what they perceive to be their parents' evaluation of them. During middle childhood the opinions of peers and teachers further complicate the process. Criticisms and peer approval are sources of data for evaluation. Parents and other adults are no longer the only persons who respond to their skills, talents, and abilities. Peers also identify skills and capabilities, and each child soon begins to internalize these outside opinions. If children regard themselves as worthwhile or satisfactory persons, they are considered to have high self-esteem, self-confidence, or a positive self-concept. If they view themselves as worthless, they are said to have poor or low self-esteem.

Pets have also been observed to influence a child's self-esteem. Pets can be important in making a child feel loved, accepted, and secure (Davis, 1985). However, it has been found that children who "bond" with a pet before the age of 6 years or after the age of 10 years scored higher on tests of self-concept than children who acquire animals in middle childhood (Poresky and others, 1988).

The difficulty that children encounter in the attempt to assess their own abilities is their inclination to rely on their own expectations or on the expectations expressed by others regarding their performance. They depend almost entirely on external evidence of worth, such as school grades, teachers' comments, and parental and peer approval. Children do not yet have the capacity to develop their own, independent criteria by which they can evaluate their own accomplishments, and it is especially difficult for them to assess their achievement in abstract skills.

Nothing succeeds like success. The significant adults in children's lives can often manage, unseen, to manipulate the their environment so that they meet with success. Each small success increases a child's self-image a little. The more positive children feel about themselves, the more confident they feel in trying again for success. All children profit from feelings that they are in some way special to significant adults. A positive self-image makes them feel likable, worthwhile, and persons with a valuable contribution to make in their world. Such feelings lead to self-respect, self-confidence, and a general feeling of happiness. Parents can assist their school-age children in developing self-esteem by helping to increase their self-confidence, by being honest, providing opportunities for creativity, helping them succeed in activities, and providing positive reinforcement. Nurses can enhance self-esteem by fostering supportive relationships between children and members of their families and by emphasizing children's strengths and positive aspects of their behavior (Winkelstein, 1989).

DEVELOPMENT OF SEXUALITY

Evidence indicates that many children experience some form of sex play during or before preadolescence as a response to normal curiosity, not as a result of love or sexual urge. Children are experimentalists by nature, and this play is incidental and transitory. Any adverse emotional consequences or guilt feelings depend on how the behavior is managed by the parents, if it is discovered, or whether children view their actions as wrong in the eyes of significant persons, particularly the parents.

Much of children's attitude toward sex that is acquired indirectly at a very early age affects the way in which they respond to sexual information presented at a later time. Many parents discourage sex exploration either through subtle substitution of activities that divert their children's attention from the genitalia or by expressions of anger or disgust at their behavior. These tactics clearly communicate to children that they should not engage in such activities nor ask questions about sex or their genitals, which limits the children's sources of information.

In addition, parents seldom teach young children the correct terminology for sexual organs or sexual feeling; therefore, the only vocabulary available to them is the one that identifies sexual organs with excretory functions. Thus these parental attitudes influence the children's perception of the cleanliness of their genitalia. If they learn that excretory organs and functions are dirty, they may associate the "dirtiness" with the reproductive organs and functions. If children learn the correct terminology for the organs and their functions, this association should be reduced or eliminated.

Sex Education

Because parents often either repress or avoid their children's sexual curiosity, the sexual information that they receive in childhood is acquired almost entirely from their peers. When peers are the primary source of sexual information, it is transmitted and exchanged in secret, clandestine conversation and contains a large amount of misinformation. The context in which these communications take place creates anxiety in children and barriers to trust; therefore, they continue to keep sexuality a secret. These reactions inhibit spontaneous expressions or questioning of the parents.

The subject of where sex education should be taught and by whom arouses a good deal of controversy. Many individuals and groups are unconditionally opposed to the inclusion of sex education in the schools. Others believe that sex information should not be taught separately from other information but should be presented as naturally as information about other body functions and natural phenomena such as the solar system, the changing seasons, and the migratory habits of birds. Children's questions about sex should be answered to the same extent as their questions about any other topic—honestly and at their level of understanding. During the preschool years children will be satisfied with simple answers, but as they gain more knowledge and understanding of the world, their curiosity about everything will be deeper. When sex is treated as though it is a normal part of growth and development and questions are answered matter-of-factly, parental responses are less apt to contain overtones of guilt and anxiety that in turn produce anxiety in children.

Middle childhood appears to be an ideal time for formal sex education, and many authorities believe that the topic is best presented from a life-span approach. Initial curiosity about differences in body structure between boys and girls and between children and adults occurs in the preschool years, and the next stage, adolescence, arouses both anxiety and excitement about sexual encounters. Information about sexual maturation and the process of reproduction presented during middle childhood helps to minimize a child's uncertainty, embarrassment, and feelings of isolation that often accompany the events of puberty.

Although sex education programs are not universally a part of the elementary school curriculum, some progressive educators have successfully incorporated sex education into a number of school programs. Because of the natural social orientation of this period of development, structured group learning situations can be successfully used for discussion of sexuality. Children are more comfortable if boys and girls are segregated for discussions, but each needs information about both sexes.

An approach that has been advanced suggests that sexuality can best be presented in the context of its central role as a biologic mechanism for the survival of the culture. Children can learn that sexual maturation and reproduction are each individual's contribution to the natural order of things. This approach provides a natural entry into discussion of sexuality as a basis for family units, marriage, and attitudes toward children, as well as into a presentation of the biologic facts of sexuality. More difficult, but equally important, is for children to view sexual intimacy as a close, personal relationship and a means of conveying love, as well as a means for assuring the survival of the species.

Preadolescents need more precise information. They are interested in concrete information, such as "What if I start my period in the middle of class?" or "How can I keep people from telling I have an erection?" It is important to tell them what they want to know and what they can expect to happen as they become mature sexually.

Nurse's Role in Sex Education

No matter where nurses practice, they can provide information on human sexuality to both parents and children. Nurses can help parents by first becoming knowledgeable about human sexuality themselves, including the common myths and misconceptions associated with sex and the reproductive process. They need to know their own attitudes and feelings toward sexuality and to feel comfortable with these feelings.

During encounters with parents, nurses can be open and available for questions and discussion. They can set an example by the language they use in discussing body parts and their function and by the way in which they deal with problems that have emotional overtones, such as exploratory sex play and masturbation. Parents need to be helped to understand normal behaviors and to view sexual curiosity in their children as a part of the developmental process. Assessing the parents' level of knowledge and understanding of sexuality provides cues to their need for supplemental information that will better prepare them for the increasingly complex explanations that will be needed as their children grow older.

Sometimes short classes or group discussions for parents are helpful for discussing disturbing behaviors and anticipating the questions and forthcoming learning needs of the children. When possible, it is wise to include both parents. Sex education in the home should be assumed by both parents so that the children will not acquire a distorted view of either the male or the female role that may alter relationships with the opposite sex in later life. Most important, nurses should take an active role in encouraging, developing, and providing sex education to children at all levels as an integral part of their learning.

PLAY

As children enter the school years, their play takes on new dimensions that reflect a new stage of development. Not only does play involve increased physical skill, intellectual ability, and fantasy, but, as they form groups and cliques, children begin to evolve a sense of team or club. To belong to a group is of vital importance. Each individual child must abide by the rules of the group, which may be extremely rigid, and energy is devoted to team success as well as personal success.

Rules and Rituals

The need for conformity in middle childhood is strongly manifested in the activities and games so important in the life of school-age children. Up to this point they have either played games they have invented themselves or have played in the company of a friend or an adult when rules more or less evolved with the game. Now they begin to see the need for rules, and the games they play have fixed and unvarying rules that may be bizarre and extraordinarily rigid (especially those made up by the group). But part of the enjoyment of the game is to know the rules, since knowing means belonging. Once the rules are established and agreed on, the demand for conformity is vigorous (Fig. 17-7).

Conformity and ritual permeate the play of school-age children. Not only do they dominate in games, but they are also evident in much of the children's behavior and language. Childhood is full of chants and taunts such as, "Eeny, meeny, miney, mo," "Johnny's mad and I'm glad," "Last one is a rotten egg," and "Step on a crack, break your mother's back." Children derive a great deal of pleasure from such sayings that have been handed down with few

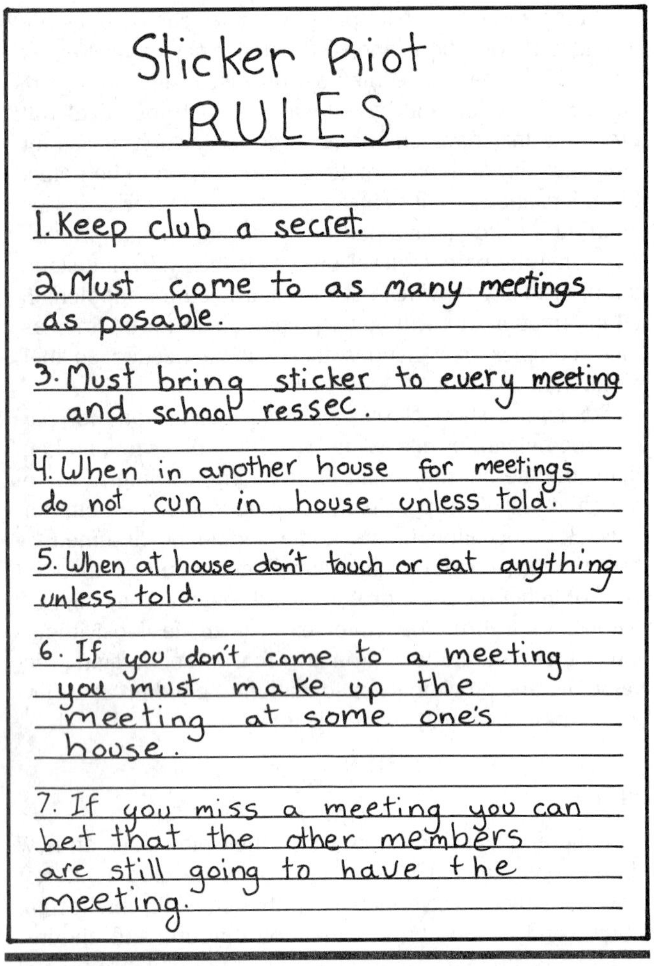
Sticker Riot
RULES

1. Keep club a secret.
2. Must come to as many meetings as posable.
3. Must bring sticker to every meeting and school ressec.
4. When in another house for meetings do not run in house unless told.
5. When at house don't touch or eat anything unless told.
6. If you don't come to a meeting you must make up the meeting at some one's house.
7. If you miss a meeting you can bet that the other members are still going to have the meeting.

Fig. 17-7. A list of club rules compiled by a group of 9-year-old children.

changes through generation after generation of children. Sometimes these sayings are elaborated on with particular variations to meet the special attributes of a particular group. The undeviating ritual frequently is invested with some magical quality that serves to give the children involved a sense of power over the unconquerable world about them.

Team play. A more complex form of group play that evolves from group games is the team game and those sports that form part of the life of the early school years. The rules of such games may even require the presence of a referee, umpire, or person of authority in order that they can be followed more accurately. Team membership has three significant characteristics that promote child development during the middle years (Newman and Newman, 1984).

First, children learn to subordinate personal goals to group goals. Team membership means that each child is accountable to the other team members and carries with it the responsibility that each member's acts may affect the success or failure of the entire group. Each member's behavior is open to public evaluation, and children risk ostracism or ridicule if they contribute to a team loss. Team accomplishments reflect on all the players. Although individual skills are recognized, team successes and failures are shared by all members—the best and the poorest alike. In this way children learn the concept of interdependence, that all players must rely on one another. Unfortunately instead of the better members helping the weaker members to improve, all too often the poorer members are scorned and scapegoated, especially when the team loses.

Second, children learn about division of labor as an effective strategy for the attainment of a goal. They learn that each position on a team has a specific function and that the team has a greater chance of winning if each person performs a specific function instead of the work of all the other members. Once children learn this concept in team play, they can transfer the knowledge to other aspects of life. Once they learn that certain goals are best accomplished by dividing tasks among several individuals, they begin to see a relationship to principles of organization in other social structures. A corollary to this is the concept that some children are best equipped to perform one part of the task, whereas other children are best suited to another aspect of the task.

Third, team play helps children to learn about the nature of competition and the importance of winning—an attribute highly valued in the United States. In all team play there is a winning and losing side. Since losing is often interpreted as failure, children will go to great lengths to avoid the public embarrassment and personal shame that accompany failure. The more a child identifies with the team and values membership in the group, the more distasteful losing becomes. Fear of losing and the failure it implies are strong incentives for group commitment. The importance of winning is not universally valued however. Some cultures and subcultures place emphasis on the game and consideration for one's companions rather than on the outcome.

Team play can also contribute to children's social, intellectual, and skill growth. Children will work hard to develop the skills needed to become members of a team, to improve their contribution to the group effort, and to anticipate the consequences of their behavior for the group. Team play helps stimulate cognitive growth, as children are called on to learn many complex rules, make judgments about those rules, plan strategies, and assess the strengths and weaknesses of members of their own team and the opposing team (Fig. 17-8).

Quiet Games and Activities

Although the play of school-age children is highly active, they also enjoy many quiet and solitary activities (Fig. 17-9). The middle childhood years are the time for collections, which constitute another ritual. Young school-age children's collections are an odd assortment of unrelated objects in messy, disorganized piles. Collections of later years are more orderly and selective, and they are organized neatly in scrapbooks, on shelves, or in boxes.

School-age children become fascinated with increasingly complex board or card games, such as Monopoly and rummy, that they can play with a best friend or a group. As in all games, their adherence to rules is fanatic. There is

Fig. 17-8. Activities engaged in by school-age children, such as Little League baseball, vary according to the child's interest and opportunity.

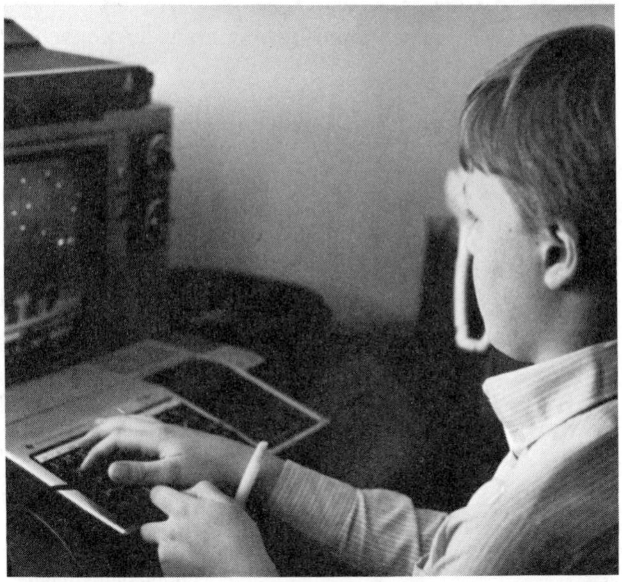

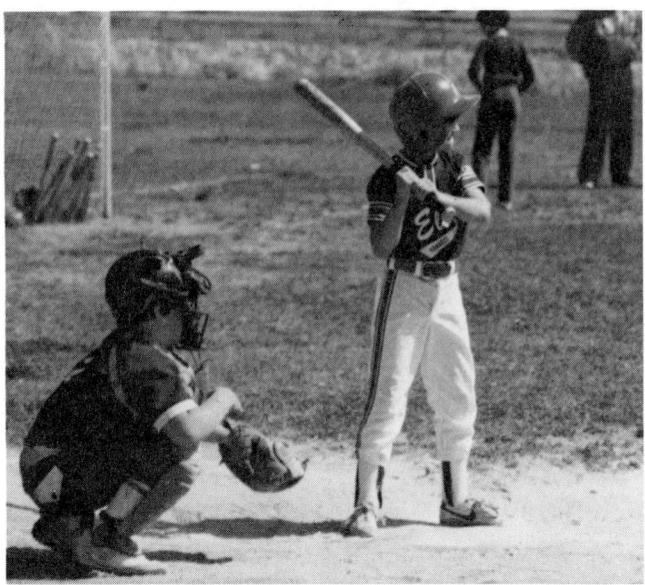

Fig. 17-9. A home computer provides educational and recreational activity.

usually much discussion and argument, but the disagreement is easily resolved through reading the appropriate rule of the game.

The newly acquired skill of reading becomes increasingly satisfying as school-age children begin to expand their knowledge of the world through books. School-age children never tire of stories and, just like preschool children, they love to have stories read aloud. Sewing, cooking, carpentry, gardening, and creative endeavors such as painting are other activities children enjoy. Many of these creative skills, as well as athletic skills such as swimming, riding, hiking, dancing, and skating, that are acquired and delighted in during childhood continue to be enjoyed into adolescence and adulthood.

Hero worship is another characteristic of children and adolescents. The object of the adoration can be any of a variety of persons, such as a friend, relative, teacher, or national sports or entertainment figure (Fig. 17-10). The difficulty arises when the idol provides an inappropriate role model.

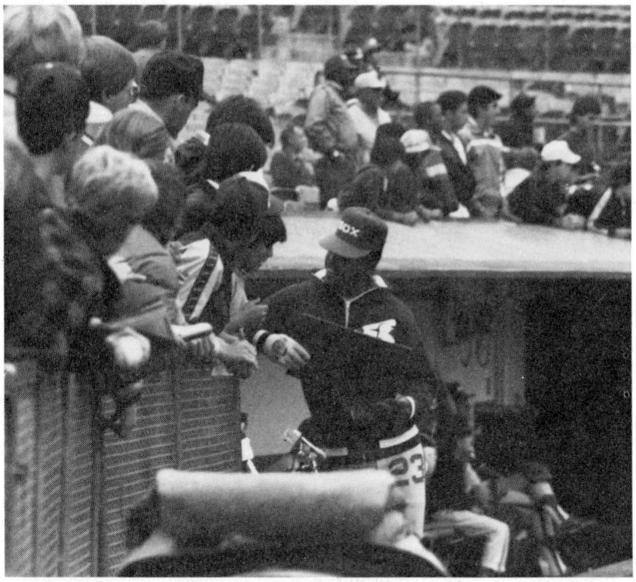

Fig. 17-10. Hero worship is a characteristic of middle childhood.

Ego Mastery

Play also affords children the means to acquire representational mastery over themselves, their environment, and other persons. Through play children can feel as big, as powerful, and as skillful as their imaginations will allow, and they can attain vicarious mastery and power over whomever and whatever they choose. They need to feel in control in their play. School children still need the opportunity to use large muscles in exuberant outdoor play and the freedom to exert their newfound autonomy and initiative. They need space in which to exercise large muscles and to work off tensions, frustrations, and hostility. Physical skills practiced and mastered in play help them develop a feeling of personal competence, which contributes to a sense of accomplishment and helps provide a place of status in the peer group.

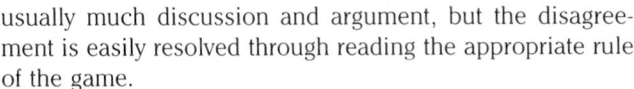

SUMMARY OF GROWTH AND DEVELOPMENT IN MIDDLE CHILDHOOD

The preceding stages of child development increasingly demonstrate individuality in the patterns of development. As children grow and mature, these differences become more pronounced. Although the rate generally slows, devel-

Table 17-1 Growth and development during school-age years

AGE (YEARS)	PHYSICAL AND MOTOR	COGNITION	ADAPTIVE	SOCIALIZATION
6	Height and weight gain slower; 5 cm (2 inches) and 2.3 kg (5 pounds) Central mandibular incisors erupt Gradual increase in dexterity Active age; constant activity Often returns to finger feeding More aware of hand as a tool Likes to draw, print, and color	Attends first grade Counts 13 pennies Knows whether it is morning or afternoon Defines common objects such as fork and chair in terms of their use Obeys triple commands in succession Shows personal right hand and left ear Says which is pretty and which is ugly of a series of drawings of faces Describes the objects in a picture rather than simply enumerating them Reads from memory; enjoys oral spelling game Is in period of more tension, but is intellectually more stimulating	At table, uses knife to spread butter or jam on bread At play, cuts, folds, pastes paper toys, sews crudely if needle is threaded Cannot tie knot Enjoys making simple figures in clay Takes bath without supervision; performs bedtime activities alone Likes table games, checkers, simple card games Is more independent, probably influence of school Has own way of doing things Tries out own abilities	Can share and cooperate better Has great need for children of own age Often engages in rough play Is often jealous of younger brother or sister Does what child sees adults doing Often has temper tantrums Is a boaster Will cheat to win Has difficulty owning up to misdeeds Sometimes steals money or attractive items Giggles a lot Has increased socialization, such as tattling
7	Continues to grow 5 cm (2 inches) and 2.5 kg (5.5 pounds) a year Maxillary central incisors and lateral mandibular incisors erupt Gross motor actions are cautious but not fearful More cautious in approaches to new performances Repeats performances to master them Posture more tense and unstable; maintains one position longer	Attends second grade Notices that certain parts are missing from pictures Can copy a diamond Repeats three numbers backward Reads ordinary clock or watch correctly to nearest quarter hour; uses clock for practical purposes More mechanical in reading; often does not stop at the end of a sentence, skips words such as it, the, he, and so on	Uses table knife for cutting meat; may need help with tough or difficult pieces Brushes and combs hair acceptably without help or "going over"	Is becoming a real member of the family group Likes to help and have a choice Is less resistant and stubborn Spends a lot of time alone; does not require a lot of companionship Stealing may still be a problem Boys take part in group play with boys; girls prefer playing with girls
8-9	Continues to grow at 5 cm (2 inches) and 3 kg (6.6 pounds) a year Movement fluid; often graceful and poised Always on the go; jumps, chases, skips Increased smoothness and speed in the motor control Dresses self completely Eyes and hands are well coordinated	Attends third and fourth grades Gives similarities and differences between two things from memory Counts backward from 20 to 1 Repeats days of the week and months in order; knows the date Describes common objects in detail, not merely their use Makes change out of a quarter Reads classic books but also enjoys comics	Makes use of common tools such as hammer, saw, or screwdriver Uses household and sewing utensils Helps with routine household tasks such as dusting, sweeping Assumes responsibility for share of household chores Looks after all of own needs at table Buys useful articles; exercises some choice in making purchases Goes about home and community freely, alone or with friends	Easy to get along with at home; better behaved Likes the reward system Dramatizes Is more sociable Is better behaved Is interested in boy-girl relationships but will not admit it Likes to compete and play games More critical of self

Table 17-1 Growth and development during school-age years—cont'd

AGE (YEARS)	PHYSICAL AND MOTOR	COGNITION	ADAPTIVE	SOCIALIZATION
		Is more aware of time; can be relied on to get to school on time Is afraid of failing a grade; ashamed of bad grades	Runs useful errands Likes pictorial magazines Likes school; wants to answer all the questions Great reader; may plan to wake up early just to read Enjoys school Likely to overdo; hard to quiet down after recess	
10-12	Slow growth in height and rapid weight gain (6.25 cm [2.5 inches] and 4.5 kg [10 pounds]), may become obese in this period Posture is more similar to an adult's; will overcome lordosis Pubescent changes may begin to appear, especially in females Body lines soften and round out in females Rest of teeth (except wisdom teeth) will erupt and tend toward full development	Attends fifth to seventh grades Writes occasional short letters to friends or relatives on own initiative Uses telephone for practical purposes Responds to magazines, TV, or other advertising by mailing coupons Reads for practical information or own enjoyment stories or library books of adventure or romance, or animal stories	Does occasional or brief work on own initiative around home and neighborhood Is sometimes left alone at home or at work for short period Is successful in looking after own needs or those of other children left in own care Makes useful articles or does easy repair work Cooks or sews in small way Raises pets Writes brief stories Produces simple paintings or drawings Washes and dries own hair Is responsible for a thorough job of cleaning hair, but may need reminding to do so	Likes family; family really has meaning Likes mother and wants to please her in many ways Demonstrates affection Likes dad too; he is adored and idolized Respects parents Loves friends; talks about them constantly Chooses friends more selectively Loves conversation Has beginning interest in opposite sex Is more diplomatic

opment continues to be uneven, with periods of acceleration in some areas followed by a leveling-off period. At the same time, other areas progress normally. In addition, each child has a unique developmental pattern; therefore, any attempt to describe the typical child of any age-group can only represent an average and should not be considered as absolute criteria for any given child (Table 17-1).

COPING WITH CONCERNS RELATED TO NORMAL GROWTH AND DEVELOPMENT

Middle childhood is not a period of latent development. It is a period of searching, goal-directed exploration, and increasingly complex decision making. It is a time of preparation, trying new experiences, testing abilities, and refining performance. When difficult problems arise, most school-age children have developed sufficient coping skills to be ready to confront them and to persevere until they are solved.

SCHOOL EXPERIENCE

The school serves as the agent for transmitting the values of the society to each succeeding generation of children and as the setting for much of their relationship with peers. As a socializing agent second only to the family, the school exerts a profound influence on the social development of children. Until school entrance at approximately 5 or 6 years, the primary sphere of influence over children is the family, in which their major interactions are with parents and siblings. Neighborhood children, daycare, and nursery school provide broader relationships, but parents serve as the only continuous adult contact for most children—those with whom they are most intimately involved and who set the pattern of their daily lives. School entrance marks a sharp change in the children's experiences. Their world at once becomes more complex, requiring adjustments to a new set of relationships and expectations.

School entrance constitutes a sharp break in the structure of a child's world. For some children it is their first experience in conforming to a group pattern imposed by an adult who is not a parent and who has responsibility for too

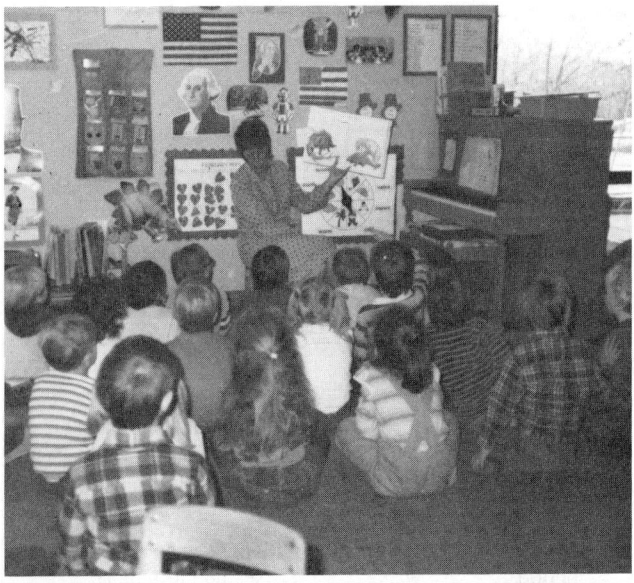

Fig. 17-11. School represents an important change in a child's life, and teachers exert a significant influence on the child.

many children to be constantly aware of each child as an individual (Fig. 17-11). Children want to go to school and usually adapt to the new condition with little difficulty. Successful adjustment is directly related to the child's physical and emotional maturity and the parent's readiness to accept the separation associated with school entrance. Cooperation among parents and support for the child are successful ways of coping with school entry stress (Elizur, 1986). Unfortunately some parents express their unconscious attempts to delay their child's maturity by clinging behavior, particularly with their youngest child.

Anticipatory Socialization

By the time they enter school, the majority of children have a fairly realistic concept of what school involves. They receive information regarding the role of pupil from parents, playmates, and the communication media. In addition, most children have had some experience with daycare, nursery school, and kindergarten.

Children's attitudes toward school and the extent of their adjustment are strongly influenced by the attitudes of their parents. Middle-class children have fewer adjustments to make and less to learn about expected behavior, since the school tends to reflect dominant middle-class customs and values. Parents who view school as a place that they have helped to create and support and that is directed toward the same objectives for socialization as their own usually prepare their children with useful anticipatory socialization and furnish them with confidence to meet the challenge. Parents who view the school as an agency of an alien culture and one that they have little, if any, power to affect may unknowingly teach their children to be fearful of school, even though they agree with its purposes and objectives.

Anticipatory socialization is also provided by television, the power of which cannot be overestimated in the acquisition of information and attitudes. Whether programming has socialization as the primary objective (such as the children's program, "Sesame Street") or general entertainment (including commercials), most observers believe that television viewing increases a child's vocabulary, extends the child's horizons, and helps pave the way for the school experience. This is particularly true among children in poorer families.

Although most children have had some experience with schooling before they enter first grade, the extent to which early childhood education prepares children for primary school varies. Some preschool programs merely provide custodial care; others emphasize emotional, social, and intellectual development as well. The type of early childhood programming that stresses a cognitive over a social emphasis appears to be more effective in facilitating later academic performance, particularly in children from low-income families.

Role of the Teacher

To facilitate transition from home to school, educators select teachers with personality characteristics that allow them to deal with potential problems of young children. Because they react to the teacher on the basis of past experience, children respond best to teachers with attributes that they would desire in a warm, loving parent. As a parent surrogate, the teacher in the early grades performs many of the activities formerly assumed by the parents (usually the mother), such as recognizing the children's personal needs (such as a need to go to the bathroom or for help with clothing) and helping to develop their social behavior (such as manners).

Teachers, like parents, are concerned about the psychologic and emotional welfare of children. Although the functions of teachers and parents differ, both place constraints on behavior, and both are in a position to enforce standards of conduct. However, the teacher's primary responsibility is stimulating and guiding children's intellectual development, as opposed to providing for their physical welfare beyond the school setting.

Teachers share the parental influence in shaping a child's attitudes and values. They serve as models with whom children can identify and whom they try to emulate. Teacher approval is sought; teacher disapproval is avoided. The teacher is a very significant person in the life of a child during the early school years, and hero worship of a teacher may extend into late childhood and preadolescence. It is not uncommon for the first or second grader to be heartbroken and tearful at leaving a familiar teacher at the end of the school term or to be upset when faced with a substitute teacher for even a short period.

Children's interest in school and learning and much of their social interaction and self-concept are related to interactions with the teacher. The differential systems of reward and punishment administered by the teachers affect the emotional adjustment and self-concept of children, as well as how they respond to school in general. The interaction between the teacher and individual pupils affects the pupil's acceptance by other children, which in turn affects the child's self-concept. Behaviors praised by the teacher usually acquire a positive value, whereas those viewed negatively by the teacher are similarly devalued by the children. In this way the teacher exerts considerable influence in a number of areas, such as attitudes toward minority groups, the disabled, or less favorably endowed children. Teacher approval of and self-acceptance in children are very closely related.

The teacher sets the emotional tone of the classroom. Those who are able to establish a positive social climate are usually concerned about the mental health and social dynamics of the children. Feeling a responsibility for personality development in their pupils, they are alert and sensitive to a child's anxieties, peer-group relationships, self-concepts, and general attitudes toward school. Learner-centered behaviors, such as supportive statements that reassure or commend children, accepting and clarifying statements that help them refine ideas and feelings to provide a sense of being understood, and constructive assistance that aids them with their own problem solving, all contribute to the expansion and development of a positive self-concept.

Role of the Parents

Parents share responsibility with the schools for helping children achieve their maximum potential. There are numerous ways in which parents can supplement the school program. Some general and specific guidelines for parents are outlined in Parent Guidelines.

LIMIT-SETTING AND DISCIPLINE

Numerous factors influence the amount and manner of discipline and limit-setting imposed on school-age children: the psychosocial maturity of the parents, childhood childrearing experiences of the parents, temperament of the children, context of the children's misconduct, and response of the children to rewards and punishments. The purpose of discipline is (1) to help the child interrupt or inhibit a forbidden action, (2) to point out a more acceptable form of behavior so that the child knows what is right in a future situation, (3) to provide some reason, understandable to the child, that explains why one action is inappropriate and another action is more desirable, and (4) to stimulate the child's ability to empathize with the victim of a misdeed (Newman and Newman, 1984).

As children are increasingly able to see a situation from the point of view of another, they are able to understand the effects of their reactions on others and themselves. Disciplinary techniques should help children control their own behavior. Reasoning is an effective technique for this age-group. With advancing cognitive skills they are able to benefit from more complex types of disciplinary strategies. For example, withholding privileges, requiring recompense, imposing penalties, and contracting can be used with great success. Problem solving is the best approach to limit-setting, and children themselves can be included in the process of determining appropriate disciplinary measures.

PARENT GUIDELINES
Helping Children in School

General guidelines

Be supportive—through companionship share ideas and thoughts.
Be positive—every child should experience some success each day.
Share an interest in reading—use the library, discuss books they are reading.
Support and encourage activity rather than passivity.
Encourage originality—help children make their own projects from discarded articles or other available materials.
Foster the development of hobbies and collections.
Encourage children to wonder and reflect during free time.
Encourage family experiences and trips to places of interest.
Encourage questions—help children discover sources for information or places in which to explore and investigate.
Stimulate creative thinking and problem solving—help children try out new solutions to problems without fear of making mistakes.
Use rewards rather than punishment.

Specific guidelines

Meet the teacher at the beginning of school and plan to visit the school to see what is taught and expected.
Send the child to school every day—teachers are concerned when parents make other plans for their children; it conveys the impression that school is unimportant.
Demonstrate an interest in what the child is learning.
Demonstrate an interest in content and growth more than in grades.
Set goals that the child can achieve.
Take advantage of situations that support and reinforce school learning.
Share information with teachers that will help them understand the child better.
Communicate with the teacher if there appears to be a problem—avoid waiting for a scheduled conference.
Provide a quiet, well-lighted area for study that is safe from interruption; do not allow television, radio.
Enforce regular study time—some children can do their work at a single session; others do best in 20- to 30-minute sessions with breaks between study times.
Support the child in home study; offer guidance for finding answers but do not give the answers; before providing explanations, determine what the child understands about the problem, read the material aloud, and discuss it briefly with the child.
Teach the child to break large tasks (such as a report) into smaller manageable tasks spread over the allotted time rather than attempt the entire project the night before it is to be completed.

Dishonest Behavior

During middle childhood it is not uncommon for children to engage in what is considered to be antisocial behavior. Lying, stealing, and cheating may become manifest in previously well-behaved children. It is especially disturbing to parents who may have difficulty coping with this behavior.

Lying. Preschool children often have difficulty distinguishing between fact and fantasy. They do not as yet have the cognitive capacity to deliberately mislead. Sometimes they misperceive or fail to remember an event. By the time they reach school age they still tell stories but can distinguish between what is real and what is make-believe. If not, they need to be taught to distinguish between fantasy and reality. Often children will exaggerate a story or situation as a means to impress their family or friends.

Young children will lie to escape punishment or get out of some difficulty, even when the evidence of their misbehavior is before their eyes. Lying is more common in families in which punishment is severe. Also, the honesty and veracity modeled by the parents is repeated in the children. If parents lie, the children will emulate their behavior. Older children may lie in order to meet expectations set by others to which they have been unable to measure up. They may lie because of a low self-esteem, as a means for getting ahead or acquiring something with little effort, or for a variety of other reasons. However, most children are very concerned with the wrongfulness of lying and cheating—especially in their friends. They are quick to tell on others when they detect them in the act of cheating.

Parents need to be reassured that all children lie sometimes and that they often have difficulty separating fantasy from reality. Parents should be helped to understand the importance of their own behavior as role models and being truthful in their relationships with children. The issue can be discussed with the children directly to impress upon them how much of their own security and respect is lost when they are not believed (Schowalter, 1983).

Cheating. Cheating is most common in young children, ages 5 to 6. They find it difficult to lose at a game or contest and cheat in order to win. They have not yet acquired the full realization of the wrongfulness of this behavior and do it almost automatically. It usually disappears as they mature. However, when children observe parental behaviors, such as boasting about cheating on income taxes or some transaction, they assume this to be appropriate behavior. Parents need to be aware of the types of behaviors they model for their children. When they set examples of honesty, children are more likely to conform to these standards.

Stealing. Like other ethically related behavior, stealing is not an unexpected event in the younger child. Between 5 and 8 years, children's sense of property rights is limited, and they tend to take something simply because they are attracted to it, or they take money for what it will buy. They are equally likely to give away something valuable that belongs to them. When young children are caught and punished, they are penitent—"didn't mean to," and promise "never to do it again," but it is quite likely that they will repeat the performance the following day. Often they not only steal, but will lie about it as well or attempt to justify the act with excuses. It is seldom helpful to trap children into admission by asking directly if they did the offensive thing. Children do not take on such responsibility until nearer the end of middle childhood.

There are several reasons why children steal: lack of a sense of property rights, trying to acquire the means with which to bribe favors from other children, a strong desire to own the coveted item, or as a means for revenge in order to "get back at someone" (usually a parent) for what they consider to be unfair treatment. Older children may steal to supplement an inadequate income from other sources. Sometimes stealing is an indication that something is seriously wrong or lacking in the child's life. For example, a child may steal to make up for love or another satisfaction that he feels is lacking.

In the lower socioeconomic levels where living arrangements are crowded and children have little privacy and much of the family property is communal, children may fail to develop a sense of property rights. Also, sometimes parents unintentionally confuse children with seemingly conflicting values. In the attempt to teach unselfishness, they may force children to share belongings with others, with the result that the children fail to develop a true sense of property rights.

If children are told not to take money from their mother's purse or their father's pocket, but observe the parents doing the same thing, they receive conflicting messages. Parents may go through a child's pockets or other private areas at night and even discard, without explanation, items of which they do not approve. Children should have some place that is private to them alone and is respected by other family members. If children's personal rights are respected, they are more likely to respect the rights of others.

It is difficult for many parents to cope with stealing in their children. However, in most situations it is best not to attempt to find a hidden or deep meaning to the stealing. An admonition, together with an appropriate and reasonable punishment, such as having the older child pay back the money or return the stolen items, will take care of the majority of cases. Most children can be taught to respect the property rights of others with little difficulty, despite the temptations and opportunities presented to them. Some children simply need more time to learn the importance of the culture's rules regarding private property.

COPING WITH STRESS

Children of today are under a tremendous amount of stress, and they are pressured from a variety of directions. It is impossible to describe all the stressors to which children are subjected. Some are discussed elsewhere in this book under specific types of stresses, especially those in which nurses assume a major role, such as hospitalization, illness, abuse, crippling injuries, and death or the threat of death.

In the normal course of growing up, children are pressured by their peers to identify with their friends; to eat, dress, and look like their friends; to talk about the same things that their friends talk about; to engage in the same activities as their friends and yet to compete with them. They are pressured by parents to excel in school, in athletics, or other activities and socially at ever younger ages. Children in middle-class America today face more stresses in their effort to live up to greater expectations than have children in previous generations. They are overprogrammed with activities such as ballet lessons, music lessons, athletics, and other activities until the cumulative effect is overwhelming.

Although children receive better treatment than in earlier times when beatings and child labor were commonplace, their physical and emotional well-being is threatened by different stresses. Children are stressed by conflict within the home and are in constant anxiety regarding the separation that these disruptions can engender. The divorce rate, and the number of single-parent families, is higher than ever before, resulting in altered relationships and increasing responsibilities. The stress of the arms race and the impact of the nuclear threat on children is beginning to be investigated; even very young children know about the threat and fear a nuclear disaster (Beardslee and Mack, 1982).

The school environment is often a stressful experience for some children and a threat to their self-image. A report by Krugman and Krugman (1984) describes a number of children who were emotionally abused by an elementary school teacher whose behavior included harassment, labeling ("stupid"), screaming at the children until they cried, inappropriate threats to obtain class control, unrealistic academic goals, fear-inducing techniques, and physical punishments. The students displayed behaviors noticeably different from previous school years, symptoms of stress, expressions of excessive worry about school, change from positive to negative self-perception, and verbalizations of fear of physical harm from the teacher. Although parents and nurses should be cautious in attempts to interpret such behaviors (they are in many ways similar to school phobia; see Chapter 18), a high degree of suspicion might be justified if the symptoms are not explained by other factors or represent a marked change from previous patterns.

Children are also being encouraged to feel, think, and behave at a level of maturity far beyond what could reasonably be expected of persons their age (Elkind, 1981). They are expected to take on many adult-type responsibilities, to make decisions they are not really able to make, and to achieve more. They have little time for being *children*. Children need time for the spontaneous activities of childhood.

The sources of such problems can be categorized as (1) inner feelings, such as being angry, embarrassed, feeling jealous, or being unable to fall asleep; (2) the behavior of others, such as fights with friends, being teased, being ignored, not being listened to, parents traveling or fighting, teachers getting angry; and (3) objective situations, such as school, moving, hospitalization, auditions, sports, being left alone (Saunders and Remsberg, 1984). The responses are those observed in any stress situation: doing nothing, acting impulsively without thought, or problem solving. Potentiated sources of stress are listed in Box 17-2.

Many variables contribute to children's ability to cope with stress. Masten and others (1988) found that children ages 8 to 13 with low IQ, low socioeconomic status, and poor family relationships displayed disruptive behavior in school when faced with a stressful life event (e.g., parental separation or a death in the family). Under similar circumstances, more advantaged children did not exhibit such behavior, although they were less interested in school than nonstressed peers. Boys appeared to be more susceptible than girls. It was speculated that boys experienced less social support at school than did girls.

✦NURSING ALERT The nurse who observes the following signs of stress in a child should explore the situation further:

- Stomach pains or headache
- Sleep problems
- Bed-wetting
- Changes in eating habits
- Aggressive or stubborn behavior
- Reluctance to participate

To help children cope with the stresses in their lives, the parent, teacher, or health worker must be able to recognize signs that indicate a child is undergoing stress (see Box 4-7) and identify the source promptly. Children need to be taught how to recognize signs of stress in themselves, such as a pounding heart, rapid breathing, or butterflies in the stomach. Once they are able to recognize that they are stressed, they can employ techniques for managing their stress. Probably the most useful technique is to help them plan a means for dealing with any stress through problem solving (Kuczen, 1982).

First, they need to learn relaxation techniques such as deep-breathing exercises, progressive relaxation of muscle groups, and positive imagery (see Box 26-6). Encouraging them to "blow off steam" through physical activity reduces tension and anxiety. Second, they must identify the problem. Those involving situations or actions of others are relatively simple to identify. Feelings within themselves are sometimes more difficult. Third, alternative actions must be explored. Children should list all possibilities, including those that they know will not work. Fourth, they need to examine what might happen as a consequence of each alternative they have listed. By this time they are relaxed and ready for the final step, to select what they perceive to be the best option. It is sometimes helpful to have children model their behavior after someone they know who has successfully coped with a similar problem. When children are assisted with the process a few times, they are able to apply problem solving automatically.

Fears

School-age children are afraid of a number of things. They are less fearful of body safety than they were as preschoolers, although they still fear being hurt, poisoned, kidnapped, or having to undergo surgery. There is also a lessening of the fear of noises, darkness, storms, and dogs. Most of the new fears that trouble school-age children are related to school and family—for example, fear of failing, of teachers, and bullies. There are some differences between the sexes in fears. Girls are proportionately more fearful than boys of bugs, snakes, cemeteries, tornadoes and strong winds, strangers, getting lost, war, and something bad happening to their parents (Moracco and Camilleri, 1983).

Box 17-2 POTENTIAL SOURCES OF STRESS IN MIDDLE CHILDHOOD

Sources of Stress for the Six-Year-Old:

Expectations—parents, teachers, and other adults begin to demand more
School—first grade introduces the child to the more formal, academic setting; it may be the child's first experience away from home all day
Activity level—may find it difficult to sit still for long periods of time; may have frequent accidents, such as spilling milk
Competition—the child wants to be "first" or best
Shyness—may initially be shy in a new situation, but usually recovers quickly
Aggression—may become hostile or aggressive; temper tantrums peak
Sensitivity—begins to read body language or facial expressions and becomes upset when disapproval is sensed
Teasing—engages in teasing, but becomes upset when on the receiving end
Decisions—has difficulty coping with increasing independence
Jealousy—sibling rivalry is common
Fears—usually center around newly found independence and might include fear of getting lost or fear of making an embarrassing social blunder

Sources of Stress for the Seven-Year-Old:

Moodiness—is often moody, unhappy, or pensive
Approval—continues to need praise and approval from peer group and parents
Modesty—demands privacy when in the bathroom or dressing
Organization—is comfortable with rules, regulations, routines, and order; becomes upset when they are disrupted
Interruptions—hates to be disturbed when intensely involved in an activity
Idols—has a desire to be more like an admired idol
Friendship—becomes more selective about playmates

Sources of Stress for the Eight-Year-Old:

Self-criticism—is very critical of personal ability and performance
Parental authority—is beginning to resent parenteral authority
Loneliness—likes frequent interaction with friends; may hate to miss school
Praise—continues to seek approval but can identify when praise is not genuine
Independence—may begin to stay alone for brief periods of time while parents run errands, with resulting feelings of uneasiness

Sources of Stress for the Nine-Year-Old:

Rebelliousness—occasionally tests independence by rebelling
Opposite sex—engages in sex-segregated play; expresses an aversion to the opposite sex
Fair play—has a keen sense of what is fair and is vehement in demanding personal rights when a situation is perceived as unfair
Interruptions—continues to dislike interruptions but will usually resume an activity after an interruption
Propriety—has a sense of propriety and will often be upset if siblings or parents offend the child's notion of decorum or dignity

Sources of Stress for the Ten- to Twelve-Year-Olds:

Sexual maturation—girls, in particular, may become self-conscious regarding obvious signs of development
Social issues—a new level of awareness can generate concern regarding pressing societal problems
Size—both boys and girls may be upset by the fact that the girls are taller; the extremely small or extremely large child may be concerned about his or her size
Shyness—if the child already has a problem in this area, it is likely to become more pronounced at this stage
Opposite sex—may become interested, yet shy, around members of the opposite sex
Confusion—too much freedom can cause the child to flounder
Health—it is not uncommon for a child to become a hypochondriac during this period of development
Money—child is anxious to earn and handle money, but often uses poor judgment
Competition—continues to be highly competitive and looks to peer group for prestige
Burnout—child may become vigorously involved in so many activities that he or she finally becomes exhausted
Self-concept—may engage in teasing, scapegoating, or vicious attacks to temporarily boost his or her self-image; guilt often ensues; may be self-conscious about attempting a new skill
Parents—often becomes highly critical or intolerant of parents
Idols—continues hero worshipping
Fair play—continues to have a highly developed sense of fair play
Drugs and sex—may be tempted to experiment with drugs or sex because everyone is doing it
Peer pressure—becomes a powerful motivating force
Self-criticism—child may be highly critical of personal performance

From Kuczen, B.: Childhood stress: don't let your child be a victim, New York, 1982, Delacorte Press.

Parents and other persons involved with children should discuss children's fears with them individually or through group activities. Their viewpoints must be respected, and their need to communicate their concerns recognized. Sometimes children of this age are often inclined to hide their fears to avoid being ridiculed or labeled "a baby" or "chicken." Hiding fears does not end them; therefore children who are afraid to communicate them may develop displaced fears, or phobias. Children need to know that their concerns are listened to and understood. Parents who convey this to their children without becoming overprotective will help them feel less lonely and, therefore, less frightened.

Latchkey Children

The term *latchkey children* is used to describe children who are left to care for themselves or whose care arrangements are so loose that they are ineffective (Long and Long, 1982) (Fig. 17-12). The increasing numbers of single-parent families and working mothers, together with the lack of available child care, has created a stress-provoking situation for as many as 10 million school-age children in the United States (McClellan, 1984).

Inadequate adult supervision after school leaves children at greater risk for injury and delinquent behavior. Latchkey children feel more lonely, isolated, and fearful than children who have someone to care for them—fully one fourth

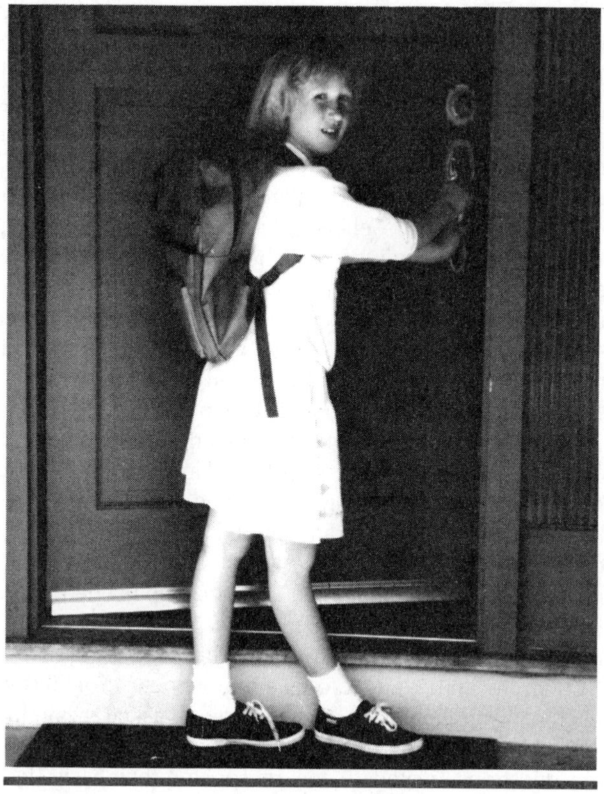

Fig. 17-12. A child unlocks the door to let herself into her home after school.

of children interviewed in one study lived in constant fear, some to the point of absolute terror (Long and Long, 1982). To cope with their fears and anxieties while alone, these children devised several strategies—hiding (in a bathroom, closet, shower, or under a bed), playing the television at loud volume as a distraction to drown out noises and indicate that someone was at home, and using pets as a comfort.

Many communities and persons concerned about their welfare are trying to help children and their parents deal with this potentially serious problem. School-age care programs have been implemented by some communities and employers. Some guidelines appropriate for presentation to parents and/or children to help alleviate their stress and increase the children's safety are listed in Box 17-3. Other types of programs include those designed to teach self-help skills to children and those that provide telephone check-in and reassurance programs for children. One such program involves soliciting the assistance of volunteer "grandmas" (Ehrman, 1986), a hotline program that links latchkey children to reassuring older persons.

Nurses should be aware of services in their communities designed to meet the needs of latchkey children and include this information in anticipatory guidance of school-age children and their families. It is vital that children have adequate supervision and companionship. Services for latchkey children should be part of every pediatric nurse's resources so they can provide parents with information on

Box 17-3 GUIDELINES FOR LATCHKEY CHILDREN

Safety

Teach the child not to display keys and to always lock doors.
Tell the child not to enter the house after school if the door is ajar, a window is open, or anything appears unusual.
Walk through the after-school routine with the child.
Consult with public safety officials about burglar-proofing and fireproofing the home.
Teach the child first-aid procedures.
Teach safety rules to the child who is expected to cook (microwave ovens are safest).
Emphasize fire safety rules and conduct practice fire drills.
Teach and reinforce traffic and bicycle safety.
Teach the child weather-related safety (e.g., stay inside but do not take a bath during an electrical storm, go to and stay in a storm cellar during a tornado warning).
Teach and reinforce water safety practices (e.g., do not go swimming alone, caution about safe bathing methods and keeping the toilet lid down when infants or toddlers are in their care).
Keep firearms securely locked away and teach the child that they are for adult use only.
Teach the child not to open the door to anyone.

Telephone Use

Be certain that the child knows home telephone number, address, and the parents' names.
Teach the child to tell callers that the parents are "busy"; do not tell a caller that parents are not at home.
Teach the child not to tell casual callers the home address. Tell the caller that the parent is not able to come to the phone right now and to call back later.
Keep a list of emergency numbers by the telephone. Make certain the child knows how to report emergencies.
Have a list of telephone numbers of friends or neighbors who will be at home and available for help with emergencies.
Ask public safety officials to offer classes about when and how to call them.
If a "telephone hotline" for latchkey children exists, teach the child how to use it.

After-School Activities

Arrange for the child to spend some afternoons with friends.
Provide structured activities for the child.
Have the child attend a public library–sponsored activity rather than watch television at home.
Discuss with the child things to do after school.
Emphasize the positive aspects of independence and resourcefulness but do not demand too much from the child.
Help the child feel successful in self-care.
Counsel parents to consider the potential problems of an older child assuming care of younger ones before the child is developmentally ready.

Loneliness

Help the child talk about experiences and feelings about being alone after school.
Consider a pet to help comfort and provide company for the child.
Be punctual in arriving home. A child's anxiety level accelerates when parents are not home when expected.
Call the child if there is to be a delay in arriving home.
Leave a tape-recorded message for the child to play on arrival home from school.
Form a group of parents with flex-time so that their children can be cared for by one of the group after school.

Modified from McClellan, M.A.: On their own: latchkey children, Pediatr. Nurs. 10:198-202, 1983.

programs available in the community, other possible care arrangements, and call-in services.

PROMOTING OPTIMUM HEALTH DURING THE SCHOOL YEARS

Health supervision of children, begun in early childhood, is continued in middle childhood; it includes the periodic ongoing health assessment and guidance advised for children 6 to 12 years of age. Since regular health checkups and prophylactic measures such as immunizations are a routine function of health supervision, this need not be reiterated. The frequency of checkups is usually reduced to yearly assessment of growth progress and screening for vision, hearing, posture, and general health status.

When children enter school, they leave the relatively protected environment of home and neighborhood and experience interpersonal contacts with a larger number of children. Although the incidence of childhood disease has declined significantly in recent times, some diseases are not as yet controlled. Many childhood illnesses can be prevented by careful health supervision. For example, most of the communicable diseases, formerly a cause of high morbidity in school children, can be prevented by immunization (see Chapter 12). The body's natural defenses against illness should be supported through careful attention to diet, rest, exercise, and protection from extreme mental and physical stress.

It is not uncommon for school-age children to complain of assorted physical symptoms that are particularly apparent at age 9 and during preadolescence. The more common somatic complaints are headaches, dizziness, or sudden, unexpected pains in various part of the body, most often localized in the head or stomach but occasionally in the leg. Sometimes the discomfort can be directly related to an unpleasant situation at school or a distasteful task at home, but often the desire for play overpowers the demands of the symptoms. In the preadolescent period children may suffer periods of extreme fatigue when they are so "out of sorts" that they hate everything and everybody. At this time they may benefit from a day home from school in which to rest and recoup their resources. When school officials are aware of this need, they are ready to cooperate and allow absence when it is desirable. Children of this age do not like to miss school and usually will not take undue advantage of the situation.

HEALTH BEHAVIORS

Children should begin to learn good health practices at an early age and be able to actively and responsibly participate in their health care. It is during the early years that lifelong habits and beliefs are established. With increased cognitive skills children are capable of making decisions about what health behaviors they will pursue and selecting from alternatives. By the end of middle childhood, children should be able to assume personal responsibility for self-care in the areas of hygiene, nutrition, exercise and recreation, sleep, and safety. Competence involves the ability to make decisions based on evaluation of internal strengths and weaknesses and external environmental influences. Children need education, involvement, and reinforcement from caregivers and health professionals who support and encourage positive health behaviors (Koster, 1983).

Studies on causal beliefs of children about illness and wellness have determined that they rank self-controlled or self-initiated actions (such as eating and exercise) ahead of uncontrollable elements (such as germs and bad weather) as causes of illness. Older but not younger school-age children are able to understand health and illness as reciprocal aspects of the wellness concept (Green and Bird, 1986).

Health education is a primary element in comprehensive health care, and programs should be designed to promote desired health behavior through guided learning and modeling. An optimum program should help children learn about their bodies and how their behavior affects their health and recognize that adaptation may be needed to protect health (Lasky, Gulbrandsen, and Scoblic, 1981). The program should emphasize health rather than illness.

Children can be taught to take a more active role in relationships with health care providers. If asked what they would like to ask the practitioner, most children have specific questions related to the reason for their visit (Igoe, 1989). At least one program has been successful in teaching assertive and participatory behavior. The behaviors encouraged in the children were (1) asking questions, (2) telling about themselves, (3) listening and learning about new ways to take care of themselves, (4) helping decide what to do, and (5) doing those things that promote health (Igoe, 1988). (See also Health Education, p. 792.)

NUTRITION

Although calorie needs are diminished in relation to body size during middle childhood, resources are being laid down for the increased growth needs of the adolescent period. It is important to impress on children and their parents the value of a diet balanced to promote growth (see Box 17-5). When children enter school, they develop an eating style that is increasingly independent of parental influence and scrutiny. Parents do not know what their children eat when they are away from home. A parent may pack a lunch to be eaten at school but be unaware of how much is eaten, traded, sold, or thrown away.

Mealtime continues to be a central issue in many families. Although it should be a pleasant part of a child's day, parents' concern and emphasis on manners often make it a battleground. Likes and dislikes established at an early age continue in middle childhood, although the propensity for single food preferences begins to end and children acquire a taste for an increasing variety of foods. Since children usually eat as the family does, the quality of their diet depends to a large extent on their family's pattern of eating. Other interests and participation in outside activities often compete with mealtime.

Outside Influences

Influenced by the mass media and the temptation of an immense variety of "junk food," it is all too easy for children to fill up on empty calories—foods that do not promote growth, such as sugars, starches, and excess fats. They have more freedom to move without parental supervision and often have small amounts of money to spend on candy, soft drinks, and other easily accessible treats. Midafternoon snacks are common, and it is wise to encourage fruit, nuts, and other wholesome finger foods to meet this need. Nutrition is a joint responsibility of both the child and the family.

The popularity of fast-food restaurants has aroused the interest of nutritionists and other health professionals concerned with children's nutrition. The restaurants are fast, relatively inexpensive, and appealing to children, and their convenience is attractive to busy parents as an alternative to eating at home. Because the nutritional content of fast-foods is usually unknown, it is difficult for nutrition-conscious parents to help children select appropriate items from the available menu. Nurses can support consumer groups and parents in advocating more of these restaurants to offer items higher in nutritional value (such as skimmed milk, broiled meats, and fresh fruits and vegetables) and listing ingredients on the menu as required for packaged foods. A recent report by the Massachusetts Medical Society Committee on Nutrition (1989) offers consumer guidelines for fast-foods. See also Table 21-2.

The threat of childhood obesity is an increasingly prevalent health problem in school-age children today in the United States. The easy availability of high-calorie foods, combined with the tendency toward more sedentary activities such as watching television and the trend away from walking or cycling and toward transportation by automobile and bus have reduced caloric expenditure. The problem of childhood obesity is discussed further in Chapter 21. Given the threat of obesity and a diet-conscious society, however, many school-age children attempt to diet either in an effort to prevent obesity or to lose weight because of imagined overweight or to conform to peer behaviors and pressures. Children need to be educated about food selection and the importance of body-building nutrients as opposed to empty caloric intake.

School Programs

Working parents who assume their children to be sufficiently mature frequently leave the responsibility of meal preparation to them. Although most older school-age children are capable of preparing simple fare, all too often breakfast and/or lunch may be inadequate, makeshift, or nonexistent. In recognition of this problem, the federal government has established the National School Lunch Program (NSLP) and the School Breakfast Program (SBP) in many areas. These meals must meet specified nutritional requirements and furnish one third of the daily recommended dietary allowance for children in the United States. Most schools subscribe to the programs, and, although it is difficult to measure directly, it is believed that these school feeding programs positively influence the behavior and learning capacity of children. Improvement in comprehensive tests of basic skills was documented in a study by Meyers and others (1989). However, children who purchase school lunches often select only the items they want, or, if they must take all the items in the lunch, no one insists that they eat them.

Nutrition education. Nutrition education can and should be integrated throughout a child's school years as part of classroom learning. In school the basic food groups, serving sizes, and the elements of a wholesome diet can be taught, as well as how food products are grown, processed, and prepared. School projects often include growing vegetables in the classroom or at home, and science projects in the more advanced grades might include some simple animal experiments. Some learning activities appropriate to school-age children are outlined in Box 17-4. The school nurse can take an active role in nutrition education by working with teachers to plan and implement units of nutrition instruction and with parents and children to give nutritional guidance (Box 17-5).

SLEEP AND REST

The amount of sleep and rest required during middle childhood is a highly individual matter. There is no specific amount needed by a child at any given age. The amount depends rather on the child's age, activity level, and other factors such as health status. The growth rate has slowed; therefore, less energy is expended in growth than was expended during the preceding periods and than will be required during the adolescent growth spurt.

During the school years children usually do not require a nap, but they spend 8 to 9.5 hours in bed and sleep approximately 95% of that time (Coble and others, 1987). Fewer bedtime problems are observed with advancing years, but occasional difficulties are still associated with the necessary bedtime ritual. Usually there is little problem for children 6 and 7 years old, and the task of going to bed can be facilitated by encouraging quiet activity before bedtime, such as coloring and reading. For many children bedtime is improved considerably by allowing them a small radio to which they can listen for a specified time.

Although most children in middle childhood must frequently be reminded to go to bed, 8- to 9-year-old children and 11-year-old children are particularly resistant. Often children are unaware that they are tired; if they are allowed to remain up later than usual, they are fatigued the following day. Sometimes bedtime resistance can be resolved by allowing a later bedtime in deference to their advancing age. However, it should be made clear that this privilege depends on compliance—going to bed without stalling and without complaints. A firm approach to bedtime is usually the most successful. Parents can help children by giving them a little advance warning, but the children should realize that when the final bedtime is announced, the parents really mean it. Twelve-year-old children usually offer no difficulty in relation to bedtime. Some even retire early in or-

Box 17-4 ACTIVITIES FOR NUTRITION TEACHING OF SCHOOL-AGE CHILDREN

Have children collect pictures of snack foods from magazines and categorize as good, sometimes good, or not good (can be made into a poster for display).
Collect articles about nutrition issues related to health and disease prevention.
Conduct nutrition discussions helping children brainstorm and express what they know about topics such as:
- Vitamins
- Sugar
- Cholesterol
- Proteins
- Exercise
- Basic food groups
- Minerals
- Fiber
- Sodium
- Fast foods
- Reading labels

Ask each child to keep a record of foods eaten for a 24-hour period; then have the children discuss the records either in pairs or small groups.
Ask each child to keep an exercise diary to become aware of how active or inactive they are.
Bring and/or have the children bring labels from grocery items and discuss the contents of the product, including the ingredients and percentages of each in the product.
Take a walk or field trip to a local produce market (or department of supermarket). Ask the manager to show children how to select fresh, ripe items and introduce them to new or less popular fruits and vegetables with which they may be unfamiliar.
Show films or film strips available through state and local health departments.
Arrange for someone to speak on a selected topic related to nutrition. This may be someone from a local hospital, college, health department, or a parent.
Help the children assemble recipes for health snacks and prepare a booklet to be presented to parents, teachers, or others.
Bring, or have the children bring, items with which to assemble a chef's salad, a healthy drink, or other nutritious item.
Teach awareness of media messages by having children:
- Note television commercial advertisements.
- Bring pictures from magazines.
- Discuss the ways in which the advertisers entice viewers or readers to buy the product.

Have the children devise a commercial for a healthy snack or meal, using the tactics they observed and discussed.

Compiled from Loschiavo, J.P.: Modifying the eating behavior of young children, School Nurse 3(6):30-35, 1987.

Box 17-5 SAMPLE MENUS FOR A SCHOOL-AGE CHILD*

Breakfast	2 4-inch waffles 2 tbsp. syrup ½ cup orange juice
Lunch	1 cheeseburger 1 medium soft drink
Snack	1 cup frozen yogurt *or* 1 cup cereal with lowfat milk
Dinner	1 cup spaghetti with tomato sauce 1 piece garlic bread Green salad with romaine lettuce and dressing 1 banana 1 cup lowfat milk
Snack	2 cups plain popcorn
Daily total:	
Milk:	24 ounces
Meat:	4 ounces
Fruits/vegetables:	4 servings (1 piece or ½ cup is a serving)
Breads/cereal:	4 servings (1 slice or ½ cup cooked is a serving)

Prepared by Cecilia L. Davis, R.D., L.D.
*Fats and simple carbohydrates should be served sparingly to meet caloric needs. Serving sizes are minimum for nutritional adequacy. Many children eat more.

der to enjoy slow preparations for bed, to read, or to listen to their radio or tape recorder.

Sleep Disorders

During middle childhood there is a marked reduction in the need for sleep initiation and maintenance. The child is in control of sleep associations, and the major causes of sleep disturbances of younger children are not present. Nighttime sleep is usually continuous, and the child has developed a repertoire of tactics (such as reading or playing quietly without involving the parents) to deal with occasional difficulties in falling asleep. If a child's sleep problem concerns the family, a thorough assessment is needed to plan appropriate interventions (see Box 6-15).

Bedtime resistance. The cause of bedtime resistance is not always clear. For some children it is related to normal fears of their age, such as fear of the dark, strange noises, intruders, or other imagined phenomena. Children who are subject to frightening dreams are hesitant to retire, and their sleep is more apt to be disturbed following emotional stimulation before bedtime. Sometimes children are loath to give up some exciting or interesting activity in which they are involved, or they are reluctant to leave the protective social circle of the family. Another factor associated with time for retirement is related to status. For example, older children are given the privilege of a later bedtime than younger children. Promotion to a later bedtime is highly prestigious, and age-mates compare their bedtimes. This may explain why parental decisions are often hotly contested by children who believe that playmates enjoy a more privileged position in this area. In some situations going to bed is used as a method of control. When going to bed early is imposed as a punishment or staying up a little longer is a reward, children may view bedtime as punitive or status-degrading.

Some children resort to multiple "curtain calls," such as wanting a drink of water, one more story, needing to go to the bathroom, or wanting to watch television. Often children persist in coming out of their rooms repeatedly after being put back to bed. Some voice fears, such as someone outside their window. The parents may have difficulty determining whether or not the fear is legitimate or the behavior a bid for attention. Consistent reassurance and limit-setting usually resolve the problem. Children feel tense and insecure when limits are applied inconsistently, such as granting permission one night and punishing the next for the same behavior (Ferber, 1987).

Sleepwalking. The night terrors of preschool children are replaced by sleepwalking (somnambulism) and sleeptalking. Like night terrors, sleepwalking is associated with transition from stage 4 to stage 1 of non-REM sleep and occurs approximately 90 to 120 minutes following the onset of sleep. The phenomenon is more common in boys than in girls, and there is evidence to indicate that there may be a hereditary basis to its occurrence (Abe and others, 1984; Guilleminault, 1987).

The episodes are characterized by a lack of responsiveness to the environment, automatic actions, and retrograde amnesia of variable severity (Guilleminault, 1987). The episodes begin when the child sits up abruptly and walks. During sleepwalking, movements are clumsy and repetitive; finger and hand movements are often observed. Most commonly children move about restlessly, then lie down and return to sleep. However, they may get out of bed and engage in nonpurposeful walking. They rarely perform purposeful acts during sleepwalking. Any attempts to communicate with a child elicit only mumbled and slurred responses. Sleeptalking, like sleepwalking, is not purposeful, and speech is usually incomprehensible and monosyllabic (Anders and Keener, 1983)

The best approach is to leave sleepwalking children alone unless they are in danger or may endanger others. However, clumsiness and stereotyped movements can make sleepwalking very dangerous. If the environment is not safe, a child can get hurt. Usually children complete their mission and return quietly to bed. If they must be wakened, it is best to call them by name slowly and softly, orient them to where they are, explain that they were walking in their sleep, and assure them that it will not happen when they are more relaxed. Preventive measures include avoiding overfatigue, getting adequate rest, employing relaxation techniques, and relieving any stress the children may be experiencing.

Approximately 15% of children between ages 5 and 12 walk at least once (Anders and Keener, 1983). The problem is usually self-limiting and requires no treatment. Children who sleepwalk persistently must be protected from harm during their wandering, and some troublesome cases may require low-dose sedation, such as diazepam before retiring. Persistent sleepwalking occurs in only a small percentage of children, some of which may benefit from hypnosis and psychotherapy.

Nightmares. Nightmares are a part of the normal developmental process, although they are less common in children ages 6 to 12 than the bad dreams of younger children. However, nightmares at this more tranquil age may indicate a specific underlying conflict that strongly influences the child's behavior and thought (Terr, 1987). Children have numerous worries, and nightmares are not an unusual accompaniment to daytime worries. Resolving worries will frequently reduce nightmares.

A traumatic event will often produce posttraumatic nightmares, which are anxiety-provoking and literal in their depiction of the trauma. As time goes on, the dreams of affected children may consist of "modified repetitions"; that is, they may add more current material to the recurrent dreams (e.g., involving others who were not a part of the traumatic event). Some even believe these dreams are predictive. Current external stresses, movies, or stories may also precipitate a nightmare by reactivating old traumas (Terr, 1987). For a comparison of nightmares and night terrors see Table 15-3.

PHYSICAL ACTIVITY

Exercise is essential for developmental progress in a number of areas, including muscle development and tone, refinement of balance and coordination, gaining strength and endurance, and stimulating body functions and metabolic processes. Throughout middle childhood children's increasing capabilities and adaptability permit greater speed and effort in motor activities, and larger, stronger muscles with greater efficiency and skill permit longer and increasingly strenuous play without exhaustion. During this period children acquire the necessary coordination, timing, and concentration that are required to participate in adult-type activities, even though they may lack the strength, stamina, and control of the adolescent and adult. Consequently, a larger amount of physical activity is expected and encouraged during the school years.

Children should be afforded opportunities of various kinds that provide satisfying experiences to meet individual likes and dislikes. Children need ample space in which to run, jump, skip, and climb and safe facilities and equipment to use both inside and outside. Appropriate activities that promote coordination and development during the school-age years include running, skipping rope, swimming, roller skating, ice skating, and bicycle riding. Positive reinforcement achieved by experiencing increasingly smooth, rhythmic, and efficient use of the body conditions the child toward regular physical activity. However, it must be kept in mind that although school-age children are large and appear to be strong, they may not be prepared yet for strenuous competitive athletics.

Most children need little encouragement to engage in

physical activity. They have so much energy that they seldom know when to stop. However, children with disabilities or those who hesitate to become involved in active play, such as obese children, require special assessment and help in determining activities that will appeal to them, that are compatible with their limitations, and that at the same time meet their developmental needs. Also, parents need to limit television viewing to encourage outside activities.

Physical Fitness

In the past, physical fitness has been considered to be the physical prowess needed to engage in competitive sports. Today the term is applied to optimal functioning of all physical systems of the body and includes five components: muscle strength, endurance, flexibility, body composition, and cardiorespiratory endurance (American Academy of Pediatrics, Committee on Sports Medicine and Committee on School Health, 1987). Enhanced cardiorespiratory endurance can be achieved by engaging in aerobic activities that maintain the heart rate at 75% of maximum for 20 to 25 minutes and performed three times a week. Suitable activities include swimming, running, bicycling, field hockey, aerobic dancing, and fast walking.

Concern has been generated by the diminishing level of physical fitness in school-age children and the decrease in funding for school physical education programs. In addition, the perception that aerobic activities are not pleasurable and the increasing attraction of television as a spare time activity are believed to contribute to the lack of motivation in children to a lifelong habit of maintaining physical fitness. Nurses can support efforts to include physical fitness as an integral part of school programs and encourage children in finding and engaging in activities they find both pleasurable and beneficial. Nurses should help the children develop an enjoyment of activities that have the potential to contribute to lifelong fitness.

Sports. A great deal of controversy has surrounded the trend toward earlier participation in competitive athletics and determining the amount and type of competitive sports that are appropriate for children in the elementary grades. The current view is that virtually every child is suited for some type of sport, and authorities do not discourage participation if children are matched to the type of sport appropriate to their abilities and to their physical and emotional constitution. School-age children enjoy competition and, when those involved with children in this age-group understand each child's physical limitations and teach them the proper techniques and safety to avoid injury to developing bones and muscles, a safe and appropriate sport can be found for even the most unskilled and nonaggressive child.

During middle childhood girls have the same basic structure as boys and thus have a similar response to systematic exercise training. At puberty, when boys become larger and have more muscle mass, it is usually recommended that girls compete only against other girls. Before puberty there is no essential difference in strength and size between girls and boys, making these precautions unnecessary (Shaffer, 1980).

Enjoyment of sports and fitness in childhood can be encouraged by well-organized extracurricular sports programs based in the community or school (Box 17-6). The American Academy of Pediatrics, Committee on Sports Medicine and Committee on School Health (1989) recommends that preadolescent years is a time to teach fundamental motor skills, develop fitness in a practical, safe, and gradual manner, and promote desired attitudes and values. Activities should include both practice sessions and unstructured play; the actual game or event should be managed in a manner that stresses mastery of the sport and enhancing self-image rather than winning or pleasing others. All children should have an opportunity to participate; and special ceremonies should recognize all participants rather than individuals.

Box 17-6 GOALS OF ORGANIZED ATHLETICS FOR PREADOLESCENT CHILDREN

Organized extracurricular athletic programs for preadolescent children should focus on assisting children to develop:

- Enjoyment of sports and fitness that will be sustained through adulthood
- Physical fitness
- Basic motor skills
- A positive self-image
- A balanced perspective on sports in relation to the child's school and community life
- A commitment to the values of teamwork, fair play, and sportsmanship

Modified from American Academy of Pediatrics, Committee on Sports Medicine and Committee on School Health: Organized athletics for preadolescent children, Pediatrics 84:583-584, 1989.

Box 17-7 SAFEGUARDS FOR ATHLETIC PROGRAMS

Every athletic program should require the following:

- Participation physical examinations at least every 2 years
- Warm-up procedures
- The availability of a medically trained person who is competent in recognizing significant injuries during practices and games of contact sports
- The establishment of policies for first aid, referral of injured participants, treatment, rehabilitation, and certification for return to participation
- Suitable and well-maintained sports facilities
- Appropriate protective equipment
- Strict enforcement of rules concerning safety
- A formal surveillance method to ensure that goals are met

Modified from American Academy of Pediatrics, Committee on Sports Medicine and Committee on School Health: Organized athletics for preadolescent children, Pediatrics 84:583-584, 1989.

In addition to ensuring the interest, suitability, and safety (Box 17-7) of the sport, parents must make certain that coaches (if involved in the sport) are skillful in managing children and do not engage in abusive types of behavior. Coaches, parents, and others involved in children's sports play critical roles in shaping children's self-esteem (American Academy of Pediatrics, Committee on Sports Medicine and Committee on School Health, 1989). Any sport for children should emphasize the pleasure of the activity, which more often involves individual rather than team sports. It is wise to expose children to a variety of individual sports. The overall emphasis of both team and individual sports should be on playing and learning. Parents who pressure their children to perform beyond their capabilities run the risk of the child being injured, developing a distaste for the activity, and developing a lowered self-image (American Academy of Pediatrics, Committee on School Health, 1983).

The same principles described in the preceding paragraphs apply to children with chronic illnesses such as diabetes, epilepsy, asthma, or allergies if the disorder is mild and can be controlled with medication. Children with mental retardation need not be excluded from sports competition if they are matched evenly against other children of equal abilities and provided with skilled supervision and coaching. Sometimes the activities need to be modified to accommodate the limitations of these children.

Acquisition of Skills

School-age children also demonstrate increasing capacity in fine muscle facility and complex artistic skills. Handedness is well established by the beginning of the school years, and the child makes great strides in writing and drawing during this age period. It is a period of energetic and vibrant creative productivity. With the tools of language and reading, children can create poems, stories, and plays. With more advanced fine motor skills, they are able to master an unlimited variety of handicrafts, such as ceramics, needlework, wood carving, and beadwork. They avidly pursue these skills in solitude, with a friend, or in programs offered through organizations such as boys' or girls' clubs, scouting, or the YWCA and YMCA, which use crafts as a means to occupy, entertain, and educate children.

Music is a favorite form of expression in middle childhood (Fig. 17-13). School-age children are stimulated and invigorated by music. They can sing in harmony, play instruments in orchestras and bands, and otherwise manage music at a more complex level. They can compose original songs, learn lyrics almost effortlessly, and turn any empty moment into an occasion for singing, to which any family, bus driver, or group leader can attest.

School-age children are capable of assuming responsibility for their own needs, although their distaste for soap and water and "dress" clothes is legendary. School-age children can and want to assume their share of household tasks, which usually are related to the male and female roles that have been defined by their culture, and many assume responsibility for tasks outside the home, such as babysitting, yard tending, or paper routes (Fig. 17-14).

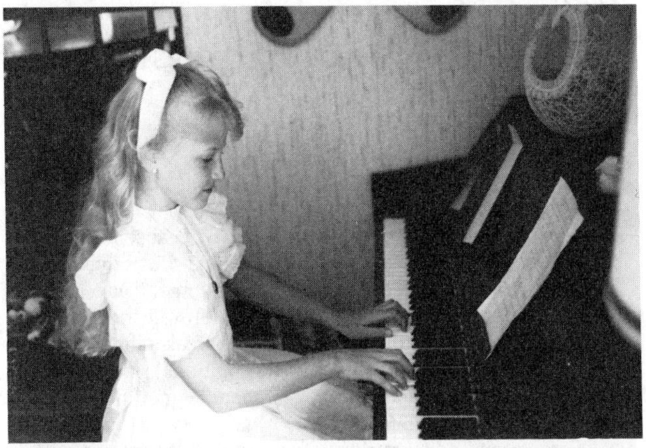

Fig. 17-13. Music is a favorite form of expression for school-age children.

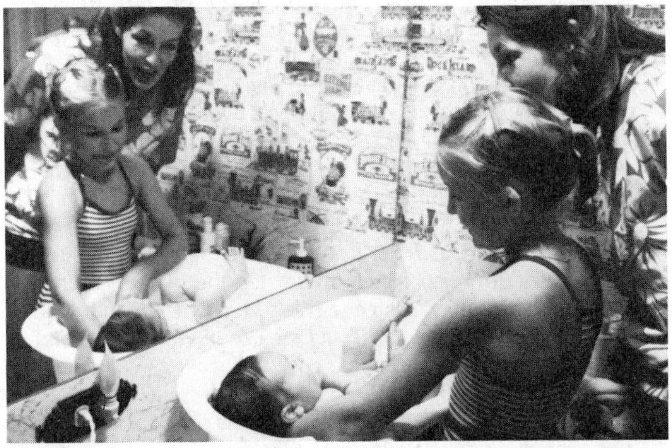

Fig. 17-14. Children can assume responsibility for a variety of household tasks.

Television

For some time child development specialists and parents have been concerned about the effect that television has on child development and behavior. There is no doubt that children learn from television, but the values and attitudes are not always realistically displayed and often conflict with those they have been taught. School-age children are better able to distinguish fantasy from reality, and some have had sufficient life experience to be able to view much of television fare with skepticism. However, television rarely depicts the reality of day-to-day situations that confront children. For example, the concept of work is distorted. Children on television do not perform household tasks; frequently there is no evidence of work in the television family. (See Chapter 4 for a discussion of children and television.)

QUESTIONS AND CONTROVERSIES

Is playing video games bad for school-age children?

Video games have been criticized and supported in relation to their effect on children and adolescents. They have been reputed to keep children from school and to cause tension, sleeplessness, and violence. Others support the activity as a means for improving eye-hand coordination and as a substitute for the inactivity of passive television viewing. Other benefits include development of inductive reasoning (drawing generalizations from specific observations), improving spatial perception, and learning to handle multiple variables that interact simultaneously.

Parents and educators have expressed concern regarding the effects of video games on children and complain that games are addictive, distract students from homework, reduce involvement in sports, provide less opportunity to develop social skills, and promote criminal activity (Soper and Miller, 1983). There has been no confirmation of these suggested effects. At least one observer finds that relatively few children are led to deviant behavior by playing video games, even in arcades (Ellis, 1984). Other researchers found support, on a short-term basis, for the notion that playing video games affects children's aggression fantasies (Graybill and others, 1985). Although there are some compulsive aspects in the play, no identifiable problems were correlated with the amount of time spent playing (Egli and Meyers, 1984).

At least one researcher suggests that the ability to suspend reality in video games dissipates the dilemmas and conflicts of everyday existence (Klein, 1984). There is interest among educators concerning the use of video games as a means of improving reading speed, as well as skimming and scanning skills, but the habitual use of short, incomplete sentences without punctuation does not provide positive writing models (Radencich, 1984).

In some instances children play video games in arcades for much the same reason that they watch television: escape, a sense of personal involvement in the action, and a source of (or substitute for) companionship (Selnow, 1984).

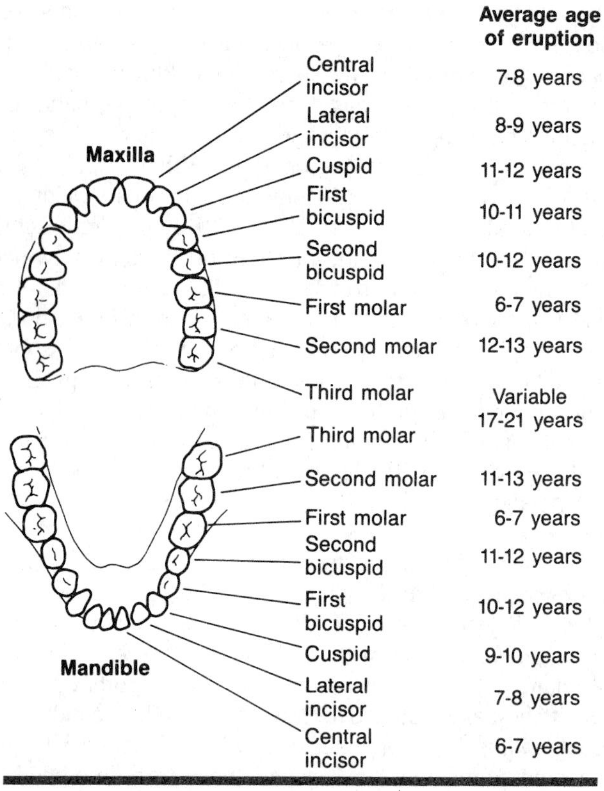

Fig. 17-15. Sequence of eruption of secondary teeth.
Data from McDonald, R.E., and Avery, D.R.: Dentistry for the child and adolescent, ed. 5, St. Louis, 1987, Mosby–Year Book, Inc.

DENTAL HEALTH

The first permanent (secondary) teeth erupt at about 6 years of age. Before their appearance they have been developing in the jaw beneath the deciduous (primary) teeth. Meanwhile, the roots of the latter are gradually being absorbed, so that at the time a deciduous tooth is shed, only the crown remains. At 6 years of age all the primary teeth are present, and those of the secondary dentition are relatively well formed. At this time eruption of the permanent teeth begins, usually starting with the 6-year molar, which erupts posterior to the deciduous molars. The others appear in approximately the same order as eruption of the primary teeth and follow shedding of the deciduous teeth (Fig. 17-15).

The pattern of shedding primary teeth and the eruption of secondary teeth are subject to wide variation among children. To allow the larger permanent teeth to occupy the limited space left by shed primary teeth, a series of complicated changes must take place in the jaws. It is at this time that many of the difficulties created by crowding of teeth become apparent. With the appearance of the second permanent (12-year) molars, most of the permanent teeth are present. The third permanent molars, or wisdom teeth, may erupt from 18 to 25 years of age or later. Permanent dentition, as in other aspects of development, is somewhat more advanced in girls than it is in boys.

Since it is during the school-age years that the permanent teeth erupt, good dental hygiene and regular attention to dental caries are a vital part of health supervision during this period. Children of this age tend to become lax and allow oral hygiene to taper off unless carefully supervised. Children are assuming more responsibility for their own care but are not sufficiently motivated by improved appearance and odor as they will be during adolescence.

Correct brushing and flossing techniques should be taught or reinforced, and the role that fermentable carbohydrates play in production of dental caries should be emphasized. It is also important to be alert to possible malocclusion problems that may result from irregular eruption of permanent teeth and that may impair function.

Comprehensive dental supervision is as essential as regular medical supervision and should be an integral part of the overall health maintenance program. Regular dental prophylaxis (teeth cleaning) by a dentist or dental hygienist is an important aspect of dental care. Fluoride application should be continued to decrease the susceptibility of the tooth enamel to acid breakdown. (See Chapter 14 for a discussion of fluoride and other aspects of dental care.)

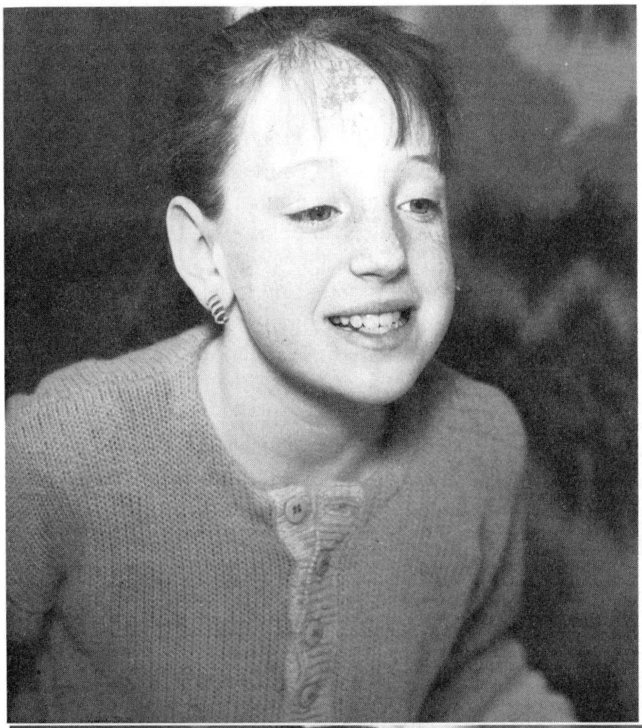

A

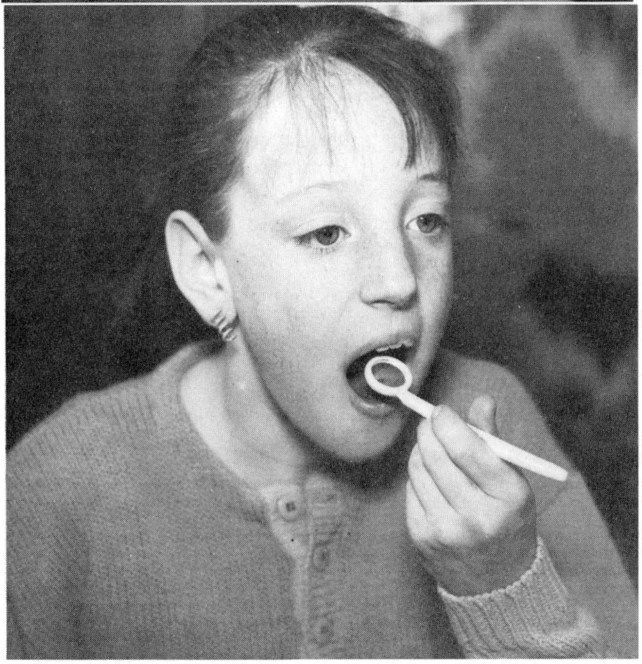

B

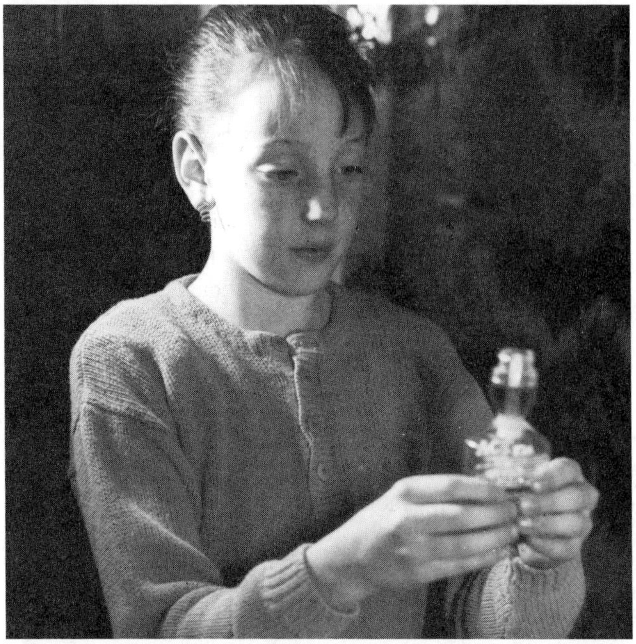

C

Fig. 17-16. Dental care. **A,** Inspection after using a disclosing tablet. **B,** Continued inspection. **C,** Using fluoride rinse.

Brushing

One of the most effective means of preventing dental caries is a regimen of proper oral hygiene tailored to the individual child by the dentist. Children should be taught to carry out their own dental care under the supervision and guidance of parents. Parents should learn proper brushing technique along with their children and should supervise their children's efforts until the children can assume full responsibility for their own care.

Most practitioners believe that the majority of children do not possess the fine motor skills needed to brush their teeth properly until they are able to write in script—at approximately 7 years (Boraz, 1981). Ideally, teeth should be brushed after meals, after snacks, and at bedtime. (See Tables 14-6 and 14-7 for sucrose content of snack foods and cereals.) The bedtime brushing is especially important because there is more time for interaction between oral bacteria and unremoved substrate on the tooth substance. Children who brush their teeth frequently and become accustomed to the feel of a clean mouth at an early age usually maintain the habit throughout life.

The thoroughness of plaque removal (cleaning) can be checked using a plaque-disclosing agent that stains any remaining plaque red. The child should inspect the teeth closely with the aid of a mirror and under adequate light. The teeth are again cleansed with a fluoridated dentifrice to remove the remaining plaque and provide further protection. This procedure may be carried out regularly or occasionally, according to instructions from the child's dentist. Toothpastes recommended by the American Dental Association Council on Dental Therapeutics carry a seal of approval, easily identified on the package. They have been submitted to exhaustive testing and demonstrate the ability to reduce the incidence of dental caries when used correctly (Council on Dental Therapeutics, 1985).

For school-age children with mixed and permanent dentition the best toothbrush is one of soft nylon bristles with an overall length of about 21 cm (6 inches). The design of the brush is of little importance; it is usually left to a child's preference. Numerous methods of brushing the teeth have been described and recommended for children, but there is no conclusive evidence that one method is superior over another. The thoroughness of the cleaning is more important than the specific technique used (Fig. 17-16). The dentist will assess all factors, such as manipulative skills and special needs of a child, and suggest the most appropriate brushing technique and regimen. Brushing is followed by flossing. Flossing is done by the parents until children acquire the manual dexterity needed. Most children are not able to floss properly until about 8 or 9 years of age.

SCHOOL HEALTH

Child health maintenance is ultimately the responsibility of parents; however, public schools and health departments in the United States have contributed to the improvement of child health by providing a healthful school environment, health services, and health education functions that emphasize sound health practices. Most of these constitute major components of community health services and involve large amounts of public funds and large numbers of health professionals, including nurses, on either a full-time or part-time basis. School health programs contribute to the goals of the community toward education and the development of children.

A safe and healthful school environment is the first essential element of any school health program. Conditions within the school setting should make a positive contribution to the physical, mental, and social development of the children. See Boxes 17-8 and 17-9 for factors that contribute to healthful school living and the characteristics of an ongoing school health program of health maintenance through assessment, screening, and referral activities.

Health Education

Health education of school children is primarily directed toward providing knowledge of health and influencing habits, attitudes, and conduct in relation to health and accident prevention. The Committee on School Health of the American Academy of Pediatrics believes that community health programs can be instrumental in changing poor health practices and makes the recommendations outlined in Box 17-10 (American Academy of Pediatrics, Committee on School Health, 1985).

A viable health education program is based on sound health concepts but should be adjusted to meet specific local needs, objectives, and legal requirements. Parents must understand and approve the health education curriculum so that its teaching will be reinforced at home. A comprehensive approach to health education is more successful in developing positive health practices than one in which the subjects are taught in isolation. The American Academy of Pediatrics, Committee on School Health (1985) recommends integration of health subjects appropriate to the age and maturity of children at each level. There are some top-

Box 17-8 FACTORS THAT CONTRIBUTE TO HEALTHFUL SCHOOL LIVING

A clean, safe, and wholesome school and classroom environment that provides suitable lighting, seating, heating, ventilation, furniture, equipment, and a safe play area
A health program that is concerned about the physical and mental health of children, teachers, and other staff members involved in the school operation
A schedule of activities that is suited to the capabilities and maturational level of each child
A regular physical education program
A planned food service program that provides both meal services and an example of good nutrition practices

Box 17-9 CONTENT OF SCHOOL HEALTH SERVICES

Health appraisal—screening tests (vision, hearing), measurements (height, weight), and medical, dental, and psychologic examinations
Emergency care and safety—emergency treatment (first aid), notification of parents, and transportation of the ill or injured child to home or hospital
Communicable disease control—detection and exclusion of affected children and policies for readmission and attendance at school (immunizations required in most states before school entry)
Counseling and guidance—health guidance, referral, and follow-up for parents and children with special health needs
Adjustment to individual student needs

Box 17-10 RECOMMENDATIONS FOR SCHOOL HEALTH PROGRAMS

Health education is a subject that should be taught as part of basic education and deserves the same priority in the curriculum as traditional subjects.
Planned integrated programs of comprehensive health education should be a requirement for students from kindergarten through grade 12 and should be taught by specially qualified teachers or those certified to teach health education.
Health education should include the active participation of students for the most effective learning of sound health concepts.
Financial support for health education programs must be ensured. Proper funding is critical to the development of effective programs, and the agencies responsible must be convinced to continue or increase funding.
Comprehensive health education programs should be directed by qualified health educators who function in consultation and cooperation with school personnel and administrators.
The programs should be monitored by a well-organized school health committee composed of representative parents, students, pediatricians, and health agencies (e.g., public health nurses) in the community.
Health education should be a part of every elementary school and secondary school teachers' training program.
School districts, other public agencies, the medical community, and private agencies should intensify their health education program for adults as part of a coordinated community health education effort, and pediatricians should make health education a regular component of the child health supervision and routine illness visits.
Research studies to evaluate the impact of such programs on students must be carried out at local and national levels.

From American Academy of Pediatrics, Committee on School Health: Health education and schools, Pediatrics 75:1160-1165, 1985.

ics that may be associated with differing social and cultural attitudes and should be presented accurately but with sensitivity to those attitudes.

School Nursing Services

School nurses assume a major role in the school health program. Working in collaboration with others in the school and community, their service consists of three interrelated aspects of child health care: health supervision, health counseling, and health education. These functions are not necessarily limited to the confines of the school environment but also extend into the community in which the students live. As a health practitioner the school nurse is in a position to promote and evaluate health services throughout the community as they affect children and to collaborate with agencies in planning for health and safety.

Traditionally school nurses have been viewed from a limited perspective that placed them in the role of disease detector, applier of Band-Aids, and official caregiver in cases of illness and injury. Although these are still important functions and their importance should not be minimized, this traditional role has acquired much broader dimensions. School nurses are being prepared to provide primary health care on a broader scale that includes assessment of physical, psychomedical, psychoeducational, behavioral, and learning disorder problems and to provide comprehensive well-child care. The school nurse practitioner is also concerned with development, implementation, and evaluation of health care plans and programs.

Some school districts have hired paraprofessionals (health aides, licensed vocational nurses) to meet the needs of students and staff. These paraprofessionals are trained to assist a professional and are not equipped to "recognize, assess, manage, or make appropriate referrals for the myriad health problems now being handled in schools" (American Academy of Pediatrics, Committee on School Health, 1987). The competence of the paraprofessional must be determined and documented by the health practitioner, and the paraprofessional must be provided with regular supervision, preferably direct supervision, by a licensed professional school nurse.

Since the passage of Public Laws 94-142 and 99-457, which require the integration of children with chronic illness or disability into the regular classrooms, school nurses are responsible for the medical and nursing needs of these children in the school setting. School nurses assess and monitor all health problems that come into the school and compile a health care list of all such problems and their associated therapies. Nurses usually call the parent of the child and arrange for a visit to the home, made by either themselves or a public health nurse, where they gather information and determine if a nursing care plan is needed at the school. They collaborate with the family, including their suggestions in the care plan. The plan is discussed with the child's teachers and any needed education provided. School nurses are the only ones in the school system qualified to deal with medical problems.

Sometimes all that is required is an assessment and making the teacher aware that the child has a health problem. In other cases more complex teaching is needed, such as how to observe for certain signs (e.g., insulin reaction), techniques that must be learned (e.g., tracheostomy suctioning, gastrostomy or nasogastric tube feedings), and management of emergencies (care of a child during a seizure). School nurses instruct teachers in the necessary procedures and review their performance approximately every 4 weeks. Most teachers are required to demonstrate competence in cardiopulmonary resuscitation.

Children who must take medications at school need written authorization from the child's attending physician and/or written permission from the parents allowing the nurse to administer or supervise the administration of the medication. The medication must be brought to the school in a container appropriately labeled by the pharmacist or physician (American Academy of Pediatrics, Committee on School Health, 1984). Medications are kept locked up in the nurse's office; the child is not allowed to carry them at school. This may vary in some school districts or situations involving children who usually have the responsibility for taking their own medications. The children are allowed to do so provided the physician and a parent provide the required authorization. Guidelines for administration of medications in schools can also be obtained from the **National Association of School Nurses, Inc.***

The preparation, qualifications, and utilization of school nurses and school nurse practitioners vary throughout the United States. Some communities consider the school nurse an essential member of the school organization with a full-time school commitment; in other communities school health practice is merely a part of the total community health program assumed by the health department. The relative merits of the two types of services are a matter of controversy. It has been shown that screening programs and physical examinations by a competent nurse practitioner maximize the identification and resolution of health problems (DeAngelis and others, 1983; Oda and others, 1985).

INJURY PREVENTION

Because school-age children have developed more refined muscular coordination and control and can apply their cognitive capacities to a more judicious course of action, the incidence of unintentional injury is diminished in children in this age-group when compared with the incidence in early childhood. School-age children have a wider environment and more environments in which they need protection, they acquire skills and interest that expose them to new perils, they have less supervision, they take more responsibility, and begin to participate in the adult world.

As previously described, the type of injuries most prevalent in children in any age-group largely reflects the child's developmental stage. Table 17-2 outlines some of the developmental characteristics and accomplishments of middle childhood that predispose such children to physical injury and guidelines for injury prevention.

*Lamplighter Lane, P.O. Box 1300, Scarborough, ME 04074; (207) 883-2117.

Table 17-2 Injury prevention during school-age years

DEVELOPMENTAL ABILITIES RELATED TO RISK OF INJURY	INJURY PREVENTION
Is increasingly involved in activities away from home Is excited by speed and motion Is easily distracted by environment Can be reasoned with	**Motor vehicles** Educate child regarding proper use of seat belts while a passenger in a vehicle Maintain discipline while a passenger in a vehicle, for example, keep arms inside, do not lean against doors or interfere with driver Emphasize safe pedestrian behavior Insist on wearing safety apparel (e.g., helmet) where applicable, such as riding motorcycle, moped
Is apt to overdo May work hard to perfect a skill Has cautious, but not fearful, gross motor actions Likes swimming	**Drowning** Teach child to swim Teach basic rules of water safety Select safe and supervised places to swim Check sufficient water depth for diving Swim with a companion Use an approved flotation device in water or boat
Has increasing independence Is adventuresome Enjoys trying new things	**Burns** Instruct child in behavior in the areas involving contact with potential burn hazards (e.g., gasoline, matches, bonfires or barbecues, lighter fluid, firecrackers, cigarette lighters, cooking utensils, chemistry sets); avoid climbing or flying kites around high-tension wires Instruct child in proper behavior in the event of fire (e.g., fire drills at home, school, and so on) (see Chapter 29) Teach child safe cooking (use low heat, avoid any frying, be careful of steam burns especially from microwaving)
Adheres to group rules May be easily influenced by peers Strong allegiance to friends	**Poisoning** Educate child regarding hazards of taking nonprescription drugs and chemicals, including aspirin and alcohol Teach child to say "no" if offered illegal or dangerous drugs or alcohol Keep potentially dangerous products in properly labeled receptacles—preferably out of reach
Has increased physical skills Needs strenuous physical activity Is interested in acquiring new skills and perfecting attained skills Is daring and adventurous, especially with peers Frequently plays in hazardous places Confidence often exceeds physical capacity Desires group loyalty and has strong need for friends' approval Attempts hazardous feats Accompanies friends to potentially hazardous facilities Delights in physical activity Is likely to overdo Growth in height exceeds muscular growth and coordination	**Bodily damage** Help provide facilities for supervised activities Encourage playing in safe places Keep firearms safely locked up except during adult supervision Teach proper care of, use of, and respect for devices with potential danger (power tools, firecrackers, and so on) Stress eye protection when using potentially hazardous objects or devices or when engaged in potentially hazardous sports Teach safety regarding use of corrective devices (glasses); if child wears contact lenses, monitor duration of wear to prevent corneal damage Stress careful selection and maintenance of sports and recreation equipment Emphasize proper conditioning, safe practices, and use of safety equipment for sports or recreational activities Caution against engaging in hazardous sports, such as those involving trampolines Use safety glass and decals on large glassed areas, such as sliding glass doors Teach name, address, and phone number and to ask for help from appropriate people (cashier, security guard, policeman) if lost; have identification on child (sewn in clothes, inside shoe) Teach stranger safety: Avoid personalized clothing in public places Never go with a stranger Tell parents if anyone makes child feel uncomfortable in any way Always listen to child's concerns regarding others' behavior Teach child to say "no" when confronted with uncomfortable situations

The incidence of injury during middle childhood is significantly higher in school-age boys than in school-age girls, and their death rate is twice that of girls (see Chapter 1). Most injuries occur in or near the home or school. The prevalence of injury depends on the dangers present in the environment, protection offered by adults, and the behavior patterns of the children. Also school-age children, although conscious of rules and frequently imposing them in relationships with peers, tend to challenge established rules. It is often difficult to maintain a balance between the level of supervision and restriction needed by children and the children's need for freedom and independence.

The incidence of transportation-related injuries in school-age children is higher than that of younger children, and the incidence of non–motor vehicle–involved bicycle injury is higher than that of teenagers and preschool children. The incidence of injuries from burns and poisonings is lowest in school-age children. However, physically active school-age children are highly susceptible to cuts and abrasions, and the incidence of childhood fractures, strains, and sprains is impressive.

Risk-Taking Behavior

Achieving social acceptance is a primary objective for school-age children, and they will often attempt dangerous acts (sometimes extreme behaviors) to prove themselves worthy of acceptance and improve their status in the peer group (Levine, 1983). Peer pressure is a normal part of psychologic development, but at the same time it is a major contributor to risk-taking behaviors. In one study approximately 50% of peer challenges encouraged problem behavior that placed children at risk for injury or hazardous habits (Lewis and Lewis, 1984). School-age children are in the process of moving from preoperational to concrete operational thinking and are only beginning to understand causal relationships. Therefore they may attempt certain activities without planning or evaluating the consequences.

Risk takers often are persons with inadequate self-regulatory behavior. They are "impulsive rather than constrained, uninhibited rather than shy: they flout rules from an early age, and they covet adoration from their peers" (Lipsitt, 1988). These children need to learn the motivation or the incentives for such behavior and to visualize the consequences if the risk-taking behavior ends in a tragic outcome. More deaths occur in young children from injuries due to poor behavior control than from all diseases combined (Lipsitt, 1987) (see Questions and Controversies).

Motor Vehicle Injury

As in all other age-groups, the most common cause of severe accidental injury and death in school-age children is motor vehicle accidents—either as pedestrian or passenger. Pedestrian fatalities are two and a half times more frequent than occupant deaths in school-age children, and the peak incidence is in the 5- to 9-year-old age-group (Rivara and Barber, 1985). Half occur at night. Most of the injuries are caused by children who misinterpret traffic signs or disobey common traffic safety regulations, cross the street

QUESTIONS AND CONTROVERSIES

Are some children "injury-prone" or at increased risk of injury?

There is some controversy regarding whether or not there is an entity that has been labeled the "accident-prone (injury-prone) child." Some investigators have found child characteristics to be important in recurrent injuries (Bijur, Stewart-Brown, and Butler, 1986; Gallagher and others, 1984; Sims, 1985). The temperament of some children seems to render them at increased risk for injury. This includes children who are stubborn, easily frustrated, overreactive, restless, careless, overly aggressive, or lacking in self-control. In situations of stress some children become increasingly impulsive and disorganized to the point that they are unable to recognize or heed danger signals. The resentful, hostile child and the immature or mentally subnormal child who attempts to compete with others beyond his capacity in a hazardous environment represent other types of children who have many injuries. Some children are less able than others to negotiate their environment safely, and this disability is due, in part, to aspects of their own behavior (Bijur and others, 1988).

Other investigators question previous findings and attribute the concept of "accident-proneness" to a misinterpretation of statistical data (Langley, 1982; Sass and Crook, 1981). Injuries appear to be more common in boys, frequently related to sports, and in some age-groups; for example the peak rate of injuries occurs in junior high school boys (Boyce and Soboewski, 1989; Feldman and others, 1983; Sheps and Evans, 1987). There is also evidence to indicate family influences. A small number of families accounted for a disproportionately large number of injuries, and members of the families tended to have similar rates of injury (Schor, 1987). Family stressors are often related to childhood injuries. Supervision of children suffers, and individual members are less cautious when families are stressed. Also, a negative attitude toward health care providers by mothers has been a factor in childhood injury (Horwitz and others, 1988).

Left-handed children are twice as likely as right-handed children to have an injury requiring medical attention, which may reflect the fact that they must live in an environment designed for right-handed persons (Coren, 1989). As a result, left-handed children must either use the nondominant hand or adopt body postures and manipulation patterns that are at variance with the design and implementation of structures.

It is not established to what extent repeated injuries may be self-motivated. Certainly with the overreactive and impulsive child whose characteristics are those of a child with an attention deficit disorder, as well as with the immature child, this is doubtful. It has also been shown that children undergoing stressful changes in their lives are more susceptible to accidents. There is concern regarding some accidental injuries in school children, such as poisoning, that are considered to be nonaccidental unless specifically reported otherwise. The "accident" may be a manifestation of a significant mental health problem. It has also been found that the number of injuries before 5 years of age were the best predictors of injuries reported between 5 and 10 years of age (Bijur, Golding, and Haslum, 1988).

against a red light, cross in other than designated crosswalks, dart into the street, and walk in the same direction as the traffic. Teaching and modeling correct pedestrian behavior can reduce the incidence of these injuries.

Use of restraint systems, door-lock mechanisms, and appropriate passenger seating and behavior are simple but effective measures for eliminating noncrash injuries and reducing the severity of crash injuries. The importance of emphasizing the correct use of seat restraints cannot be overemphasized. Children in this age-group do not usually require special car seats, and, despite evidence that safety belt use saves life and injury, estimates of seat belt use in children ages 5 to 13 are still discouragingly low: 15% in 1984 and 39% in 1988 (Agran, Winn, and Dunkle, 1989).

Injuries to children ages 5 to 9 years restrained in adult-type seat belts are related to anatomic differences between adults and children. Although booster seats are available for these children, low usage has been reported (Agran, Winn, and Dunkle, 1989). Children's sitting height is less than the adult, and the center of gravity is located above the level of the lap belt. Consequently, the greater proportion of body mass above the belt may cause more forward motion and jackknifing over the belt, increasing the risk of head injury from impact with interior vehicle parts. Lap/shoulder belts may lie over the face and neck of a small-sized child. The child's smaller and less developed iliac crests are not suited to serve as an anchor for belts designed to restrain adults, and their intraabdominal organs are less protected by the bony pelvis (reported by Agran, Winn, and Dunkle, 1989). The natural behavior of children (such as readjusting the seating position, moving about, and otherwise altering the fit of the restraint) influences the effectiveness of the restraint.

Studies support the effectiveness of education in increasing compliance with seat belt use (Roberts and Fanurik, 1986; Roberts and Turner, 1986). Parents should make certain that the restraints are fitted to their children and fastened correctly. To reduce risk of sliding beneath the standard seat belt during a collision, children should sit up straight and well back in the seat, and the seat should be moved forward until the feet fit firmly against the toe board. Children should be cautioned against assuming alternate seating positions, such as tailor fashion, while riding in the car. (See Chapter 14 for a comprehensive discussion of safety restraints.) See Questions and Controversies.

All-terrain vehicles. All-terrain vehicles (ATVs), designed for off-road use by children and adolescents, are increasingly popular with children under 16 years of age but are responsible for a significant number of childhood injuries. The two- and four-wheeled motorized vehicles are unlicensed and require no advanced training (three-wheeled ATVs are no longer being sold). They all have a short wheelbase and low profile, which makes them relatively unstable and unable to be seen easily. The vehicles can also achieve substantial speed. Most injuries occur when the driver loses control of the vehicle, is thrown from the vehicle, or collides with fixed objects or other vehicles (Rivara, 1982; American Academy of Pediatrics, Committee on Accident and Poison Prevention, 1987a). Immature judgment and/or motor skills are the most common factors contributing to injury (Dolan, Knapp, and Andres, 1989).

The Committee views ATVs as a major hazard to the health of children, opposes their use by children, and states that "the safe use of these vehicles requires skill, judgment, and experience." However, for parents who allow their use, the Committee provides safety guidelines (Box 17-11).

QUESTIONS AND CONTROVERSIES

Should seat belts be mandatory in school buses?

Although it is established that seat belts reduce motor vehicle injuries, most school buses are not equipped with seat restraints. Advocates argue that seat belts in buses would serve two purposes: (1) reduce the risk of injury, and (2) serve to teach and reinforce the importance of seat belt use while riding in any motor vehicle (Spital, Spital, and Spital, 1986). Seat belts specifically designed for school buses can also keep children from being ejected from their seats and colliding with hard interior surfaces (Widome, 1988)

It is argued that school bus interiors, contrasted with passenger cars, have no dashboards, knobs, or other projections into which a child can collide and that most are equipped with energy-absorbing high-backed seats. Also, unlike automobile collisions, school buses have more weight and length to help absorb impact. Some argue that belted children may be at greater risk of injury than passengers thrown against the energy-absorbing seat backs. An investigation by the National Transportation Safety Board (1987) revealed that fatalities and serious injuries were largely attributable to the occupants' seating position being in direct line with the crash forces and, therefore, unlikely to be mitigated by the presence of a lap belt. However, the board had stated several times that seat belts would reduce the severity of injuries (Spital, Spital, and Spital, 1986).

All the arguments for seat belt use that are advocated for automobile passengers can be applied to school buses. However, it can be pointed out that the number of injuries from school bus collisions is almost negligible when compared to automobile collision injuries.

Bicycle Injury

The majority of school-age children have bicycles, and their penchant for riding them increases the risk of injury on streets and byways. Bicycle injuries account for approximately 574,000 emergency room visits annually (Bicycle-related injuries, 1987), and the bicycle leads the Consumer Product Safety Commission's list of causes of product-related injuries. Most childhood bicycle injuries (approximately 480,000 per year) occur in children ages 5 to 14 (Hancock, 1987). Deaths are usually caused by head injuries and almost always are the result of bicycle/motor vehicle collision (Friede and others, 1985).

Most bicycle injuries do not involve collision with an automobile. They occur when the rider loses control as a re-

Box 17-11 GUIDELINES FOR SAFE USE OF ALL-TERRAIN VEHICLES

Vehicles should be sturdy and stable; quality construction is essential.
Riders should receive instruction from a mature, experienced cyclist.
Riding should be supervised and allowed only after the rider has demonstrated competence in handling the machine on familiar terrain (preferably require licensing).
Riders should wear approved helmets and protective clothing (e.g., trousers, boots, gloves).
Riders should avoid public roadways.
Riding should be restricted to familiar terrain.
Nighttime riding should not be allowed.
Vehicle should not carry more than one person.

Based on and modified from Committee on Accident and Poison Prevention of the American Academy of Pediatrics, Pediatrics 79:306-307, 1987.

sult of riding too fast, performing stunts, or encountering hazards in the road (Karp, 1987). One study found that collisions between motor vehicles and bicycles occurred during afternoon rush hour (4 PM to 6 PM) and all bicycle injuries, whether or not a car was involved, occurred between 4 PM and 8 PM (Selbst, Alexander, and Ruddy, 1987). Many injuries are related to violations of traffic laws by the bicyclist, including wrong-way riding (facing traffic), failure to yield right-of-way, and turning violations (Paulson, 1983). Some are caused by "dashing out" type behavior (Pless and Stulginskas, 1982). Others have been related to road conditions described as hazardous—bumps, potholes, and gravel (Selbst, Alexander, and Ruddy, 1987).

In addition to major injuries, cuts and bruises from falls and collisions account for a large number of injuries. Other injuries include trauma to internal organs from bicycle handlebars (Sparnon and Ford, 1986). These injuries initially seem to be trivial, but injured children develop serious symptoms (e.g., pain, vomiting, or collapse) hours later. Hematuria has also been reported as a result of improperly fitted bicycle seats (Nichols, 1984).

Many of the difficulties of school-age children can be attributed to their developmentally related limited range of vision and their inability to process perceptions of road situations sufficiently well and quickly enough to ride safely in traffic. Other important factors are lack of instruction in use of the equipment, lack of safety equipment, and riders who are unfamiliar with the bicycle, for example, having ridden for less than a month.

To prevent bicycle injuries, both parents and children should learn and periodically review bicycle safety. Children need bicycles that are suited to their size and age—they should be able to stand with the balls of both feet on the ground when seated on the bicycle, be able to place both feet flat on the ground when straddling the center bar, and be able to grasp the brake lever comfortably and easily enough to apply sufficient pressure to brake the bicycle (American Academy of Pediatrics, Committee on Accident and Poison Prevention, 1978). Parents should be discouraged from buying their child a bicycle that the child can "grow into." Children should be able to demonstrate to parents a basic competence in handling themselves on the bicycle before they are allowed to use it without supervision (Betz, 1983).

Since head injury is the major cause of bicycle-related fatalities (Weiss and Duncan, 1986), probably the single most important aspect of bicycle safety is to encourage the rider to wear a protective helmet (Fig. 17-17). Hard-shelled helmets lined with expanded polystyrene (Styrofoam) provide the best head protection (Weiss, 1986). The helmet should be one that can be adjusted to the individual child's head, fits securely, and does not limit the child's vision or hearing. A brightly colored helmet improves visibility. The helmet should carry the seal indicating it has passed the safety standards of the American National Standards Institute. Since children's head sizes have nearly reached adult size before their full skeletal height is reached, a helmet purchased at age 7 or 8 may be worn through adolescence with a few alterations in the fitting pads (Weiss, 1987).

In a study of serious head injuries in bicycle riders only 4% wore helmets (Thompson, Rivara, and Thompson, 1989). Although most young riders acknowledge that wearing a helmet is important for safety, reasons for not wearing them include because they forgot, because their friends do

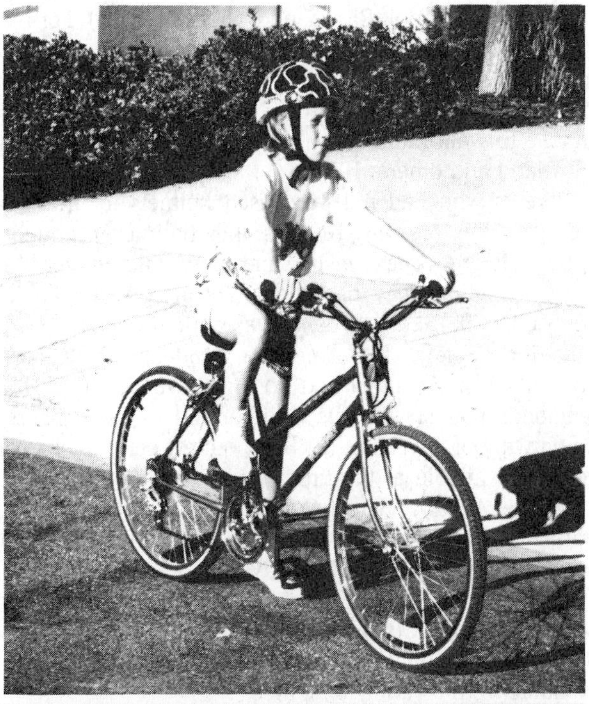

Fig. 17-17. The right-size bike is important; the child should be able to sit on the bike and place the balls of both feet on the ground. The foot should comfortably reach and manipulate the pedal in the down position. Wearing a protective helmet is mandatory.

Box 17-12 GUIDELINES FOR BICYCLE SAFETY

Ride bicycles with traffic and away from parked cars.
Ride single file.
Walk bicycles through busy intersections only at crosswalks.
Give hand signals well in advance of turning or stopping.
Keep as close to the curb as practical.
Watch for drain grates, potholes, soft shoulders, and loose dirt or gravel.
Keep both hands on handlebars, except with signaling.
Never ride double on a bicycle.
Do not carry packages that interfere with vision or control; do not drag objects behind bike.
Watch for and yield to pedestrians.
Watch for cars backing up or pulling out of driveways; be especially careful at intersections.
Look left, right, then left before turning into traffic or roadway.
Never hitch a ride on a truck or other vehicle.
Learn rules of the road and respect for traffic officers.
Obey all local ordinances.
Wear well-fitted helmet.
Wear shoes while riding.
Wear light colors at night and attach fluorescent material to clothing and bicycle.
Be certain the bicycle is the correct size for rider.
Equip bicycle with proper lights and reflectors.
Have the bicycle inspected to ensure good mechanical condition.

not wear them, and because they find the helmets uncomfortable (DiGuiseppi, Rivara, and Koepsell, 1990). For many it is primarily one of personal appearance. Taunts of schoolmates are powerful deterrents, and some children who are not allowed to ride a bicycle without a helmet choose to walk rather than incur the ridicule of age-mates (Howland and others, 1989).

Parents who had not purchased helmets for their children gave the following reasons: they had never thought of it, helmets are too expensive, and their children would not wear helmets if they had them (DiGuiseppi, Rivara, and Koepsell, 1990). Parents as well as children need to be educated on safety. The American Academy of Pediatrics, Committee on Accident and Poison Prevention (1990) recommends that (1) parents be informed of the dangers of riding without a helmet, (2) retail outlets carry inexpensive helmets available at the time of bicycle purchase, (3) the Consumer Product Safety Commission develop mandatory standards for helmets, (4) parents and community-based programs promote bicycle safety and helmet use, and (5) the media depict helmet use in all programs and promotional materials. Guidelines for bicycle safety are listed in Box 17-12. Informational pamphlets on bicycle safety are available from a variety of sources.*

*_The Bike Book_, published by the National Safety Council, 444 N. Michigan Ave., Chicago, IL 60611; _Bicycling Is Great Fun for Wise Bicycle Drivers_, AAA, Traffic Safety Dept., 8111 Gatehouse Road, Falls Church, VA 22047; handouts are available from the American Academy of Pediatrics, Publications Department, P.O. Box 927, Elk Grove Village, IL 60009-0927.

Other Vehicles

Serious injuries are also associated with other moving conveyances, including injuries on skateboards, roller skates, skis, and other sports equipment (see also Chapter 39).

Skateboards. After a short period of decline, skateboards are again assuming popularity, with an accompanying resurgence of related injuries. Although severe injuries are uncommon and moderate injuries are reported frequently, the severity of injuries increased with the decreasing age of the children (Retsky, Jaffe, and Christoffel, 1987). School-age children often use their skateboards on streets and highways, increasing the likelihood of high-speed collisions with objects or vehicles. The American Academy of Pediatrics, Committee on Accident and Poison Prevention (1989) has published recommendations for skateboard use (Box 17-13). Bicycle helmets may provide adequate protection, but a special skateboard helmet has been designed and is available.*

Roller skates. Like skateboard injuries, roller skate injuries involve predominantly the upper extremities (especially the wrist and forearm) as children attempt to break the fall with outstretched arms (see Fig. 39-8). Safety measures that decrease the likelihood of injury include protective headgear, instruction in correct technique, learning in an uncongested area on level, familiar terrain, and learning to fall properly. The skill level of the child should be carefully evaluated before the child is allowed to use these conveyances. Younger children sustain injuries more frequently than older children. Some authorities believe that children should not be encouraged to engage in these activities (roller skating) until their bone strength and skills are sufficiently mature to decrease the risk of fracture—in most cases this occurs between 9 and 10 years of age (Inkelis and others, 1988).

Ride-on mowers. Twenty-five percent of the 19,100 ride-on mower injuries and 30% of the deaths reported by the Consumer Product Safety Commission (Smith, 1988) were children. The children were either run over or backed over by another driver or fell either from the mower on

*Pro-Tec, Inc., Kent, WA.

Box 17-13 RECOMMENDATIONS FOR SKATEBOARD USE

Children younger than 5 years of age should not use skateboards. They are not developmentally prepared to protect themselves from injury.
Children who ride skateboards should wear helmets and protective padding to prevent injury.
Skateboards should never be ridden near traffic. Their use should be prohibited on streets and highways. Activities that bring skateboards together (e.g., "catching a ride") are especially dangerous.
Some types of use, such as riding homemade ramps on hard surfaces, may be particularly hazardous.

Modified from American Academy of Pediatrics, Committee on Accident and Poison Prevention: Pediatrics 83:1070-1071, 1989.

which they were riding or from a trailer being pulled by a mower. Fourteen percent of the injuries were sustained by children between the ages of 5 and 16 who were operating the mower. Similar injuries and problems can be attributed to snowmobiles.

Injuries at School

The risk of injury at school is relatively low, despite the amount of time children spend in that environment. The injuries occur in the gyms, shops, laboratories, and on the playing fields. Most injuries occur on the way to and from school. Many are related to sports activities (see Chapter 39). Persons concerned for child safety should be alert to hazards in the school environment and should become involved in efforts to make the environment safe from every aspect—physical facilities, equipment, training practices, and supervision (see also Physical Fitness, p. 788).

Farm Injuries

Recently, attention has been focused on injuries related to farm animals, equipment, and structures (Cogbill, Busch, and Stiers, 1985; Rivara, 1985). Agriculture is reported as the second most dangerous occupation in the United States (underground mining is first) (National Safety Council, 1983), and school-age children are involved in most of the farm activities and play in the farm environment. Many, including children of migrant workers, constitute a significant proportion of agricultural workers. Most injuries take place during the summer when children are home from school and in the autumn when farming activity is brisk (Swanson and others, 1987). Health facilities are also more scattered and less accessible for emergency treatment than they are in urban areas.

Health workers need to be aware of the problems and to emphasize to the farm family the hazards related to their environment and ways to prevent injuries, especially when children are present. Rural schools should provide safety awareness for children regarding machinery operating, safety procedures, and injury prevention (Salmi and others, 1989; Swanson and others, 1987). Nurses in rural areas can be advocates for farm safety programs and revision of the current farm safety legislation.

Other Injuries

Falls are still a source of injury but less so than in preschool children and toddlers. Injuries at public playgrounds, amusement parks (especially water slides), around the home (power tools, ladders, fireworks), and at school are ongoing concerns of parents and health care providers. Sharp missiles (including toothpicks) must be handled with care to prevent puncture wounds.

Injuries to eyes are a constant threat to school-age children involved in rough play (see Prevention, Chapter 25). The normally shallow bony orbit of children in this age-group makes them particularly vulnerable to eye trauma, especially during contact sports or activities.

Injuries have been reported for a variety of toys (slingshots, water balloons, lawn darts, chemistry sets, sleds) and household equipment (mowers, lawn trimmers). Gunshot wounds, previously a major problem in older children, has become a significant problem during the past few years, particularly in the inner city (Ordog and others, 1988). In a survey of 50 families it was found that 38% kept at least one gun at home, more than half of these kept a gun loaded at all times, and 10% kept it loaded, unlocked, and within a child's reach (Patterson and Smith, 1987). Also, the so-called "toy" firearms (air guns and air rifles) cause frequent firearm injuries to children, many less than 12 years of age (American Academy of Pediatrics, Committee on Accident and Poison Prevention, 1987b; Christoffel, Tanz, and Sagerman, 1984).

Nurse's Role in Injury Prevention

Nurses are primary advocates for preventive care and guidance. Safety education can be incorporated in all aspects of nursing care, and anticipatory guidance for both parents and school-age children is part of nursing interventions. The most effective means of prevention is education of the child and family regarding the hazards of risk-taking behavior and improper use of equipment. No piece of equipment is safe unless a child is physically and mentally equipped to use it. A careful history and a knowledge of normal growth and development serve as guidelines for both planned and impromptu consultation.

It is especially important for nurses to be conscientious regarding preventive teaching and guidance. Parents are often unaware of hazards to their children at various ages, especially those related to normal developmental progress. Primary physicians vary considerably in the efforts they expend in educating parents regarding preventive care. In one study related to automobile safety, it was found that only 29% of physicians always or usually ask if child restraints are used (Faber, Hoppe, and Diehl, 1985).

A major function of school nurses is preventive education and safety. They should be alert to hazards in the school and instrumental in evaluating safety risks and implementing safety programs. Preventive education for children, parents, and school personnel is an ongoing part of the school nurse's responsibility. Characteristics of the school-age child and preventive measures are listed in Table 17-2.

ANTICIPATORY GUIDANCE—CARE OF FAMILIES

The parents of the school-age child find themselves in the position of sharing their child's time and interests with the increasingly important peer group. As a child feels the need to fit into a peer group and gain a sense of industry through individual and cooperative production and performance, he moves away from the close, familiar relationships of the family group. It is through these early peer relationships that children begin to prepare for moving from narrow, sheltered family relationships to a broader world of relationships and increased independence. Parents must learn to provide support as unobtrusively as possible without feeling rejected, hurt, or angry. The nurse can help parents of the school-age child by providing anticipatory guidance and reassurance throughout this period of child development and maturation (Box 17-14).

Box 17-14 GUIDANCE DURING MIDDLE CHILDHOOD

Age 6 Years
Expect strong food preferences and frequent refusals of specific food items.
Expect increasingly ravenous appetite.
Prepare parents for emotionality as child experiences erratic mood changes.
Anticipate increase in susceptibility to illness and more sickness than at previous ages.
Teach injury prevention and safety, especially bicycle safety.
Respect the child's need for privacy; provide a room of his own if possible.
Prepare for increasing interests outside the home.
Encourage interaction with peers.

Age 7 to 10 Years
Expect improvement in health with fewer illnesses; however, allergies may increase or become apparent.
Prepare for increase in minor injuries.
Emphasize caution in selection and maintenance of sports equipment and reemphasize teaching safety.
Expect increased involvement with peers and interest in activities outside the home.
Encourage independence but maintain limit-setting and discipline.
Expect more demands upon mother at 8 years.
Expect increasing admiration for father at 10 years; encourage father-child activities.
Prepare for prepubescent changes in girls.

Age 11 to 12 Years
Prepare child for body changes of pubescence.
Expect a growth spurt in girls.
Make certain the child's sex education is adequate with accurate information.
Expect energetic but stormy behavior at 11 to become more even-tempered at 12.
Encourage child's desire to "grow up" but allow regressive behavior when needed.
Expect an increase in masturbation.
Child may need increased amount of rest.
Educate child regarding experimentation with potentially harmful activities.

Health Guidance
Provide for regular health and dental care.
Teach and model sound health practices—including diet, rest, activity.
Encourage children to engage in appropriate physical activities.
Provide a safe physical and emotional environment.
Teach and model safety practices.

KEY POINTS

- Middle childhood, ages 6 to 12 years, is a period when the school environment exercises a profound influence on development and relationships. It is an important period when children venture outside the family group, learn about their culture, and develop feelings of competence and self-esteem.
- Skeletal lengthening, higher ratio of muscle mass to fat, and maturation of the gastrointestinal system are major components in biologic development during middle childhood.
- Developing a sense of industry, or accomplishment, is a major task during the middle years (Erikson).
- Freud described middle childhood as a latency period, a period of consolidation and elaboration of previously acquired traits and skills and development of the superego.
- Piaget's theory of concrete operations refers to the school-age period, when children are able to use their thought processes to experience events and actions and make judgments based on what they reason.
- Through identity, reversibility, and reciprocity, children master the cognitive task of conservation.
- Moral development progresses with the move to more logical thought, although much is still attributed to parental influence and standards.
- Spiritual development entails a curiosity about deities, a knowledge of the difference between the natural and supernatural, and reliance on prayers or other religious rituals.
- Entertaining different points of view, becoming sensitive to social norms of peers, and forming peer friendships are the most important features of social development in the middle years.
- Children develop a self-concept from their own self-assessment and feedback from others.
- Because of advanced intellectual activity, middle childhood may be the ideal time for formal sex education.
- Play takes the form of rules and ritual, team activity, quiet games and activities, and ego mastery.
- Providing optimum nutrition may be hampered by availability of junk foods and coordinating meal schedules with working parents.
- Typical parental concerns during middle childhood include dishonest behavior, lying, cheating, stealing, and school-related stress.
- The school years are an ideal time for children to begin to take responsibility for their own health.
- School health programs commonly offer health appraisal, emergency care and safety, communicable disease control, counseling and guidance, adjustment to individual student needs, and health education.
- The major sources of accidental injury during middle childhood involve a variety of conveyances including motor vehicles, bicycles, skateboards, and roller skates.

REFERENCES

Abe, K., and others: Sleepwalking and recurrent sleeptalking in children of childhood sleepwalkers, Am. J. Psychiatry 141:800-801, 1984.

Agran, P., Winn, D., and Dunkle, D.: Injuries among 4- to 9-year-old restrained motor vehicle occupants by seat location and crash impact site, Am. J. Dis. Child. 143:1317-1321, 1989.

American Academy of Pediatrics: Child safety suggestions: choosing the right size bicycle for your child, 1978, Evanston, IL.

American Academy of Pediatrics, Committee on Accident and Poison Prevention: All-terrain vehicles: two-, three-, and four-wheeled unlicensed motorized vehicles, Pediatrics 79:306-308, 1987a.

American Academy of Pediatrics, Committee on Accident and Poison Prevention: Injuries related to "toy" firearms, Pediatrics 79:473-474, 1987b.

American Academy of Pediatrics, Committee on Accident and Poison Prevention: Skateboard injuries, Pediatrics 83:1070-1071, 1989.

American Academy of Pediatrics, Committee on Accident and Poison Prevention: Bicycle helmets, Pediatrics 85:229-230, 1990.

American Academy of Pediatrics, Committee on School Health: Sports medicine: health care for young athletes, Evanston, IL, 1983, American Academy of Pediatrics.

American Academy of Pediatrics, Committee on School Health: Administration of medication in school, Pediatrics 74:433, 1984.

American Academy of Pediatrics, Committee on School Health: Health education and schools, Pediatrics 75:1160-1161, 1985.

American Academy of Pediatrics, Committee on Sports Medicine and Committee on School Health: Physical fitness and the schools, Pediatrics 80:449-450, 1987.

American Academy of Pediatrics, Committee on School Health: Qualifications and utilization of nursing personnel delivering health services in schools, Pediatrics 79:647-648, 1987.

American Academy of Pediatrics, Committee on Sports Medicine and Committee on School Health: Organized athletics for preadolescent children, Pediatrics 84:583-584, 1989.

Anders, T.F., and Keener, M.A.: Sleep-wake state development and disorders of sleep in infants, children, and adolescents. In Levine, M.D., and others: Developmental-behavioral pediatrics, Philadelphia, 1983, W.B. Saunders Co.

Beardslee, W., and Mack, J.: The impact of nuclear developments on children and adolescents. In Task Force Report No. 20, Washington, DC, 1982, American Psychological Association.

Betz, C.L.: Bicycle safety: opportunities for family education, Pediatr. Nurs. 9:109-111, 1983.

Bicycle-related injuries: data from the National Electronic Injury Surveillance System, MMWR 36:269-271, 1987.

Bijur, P.E., Golding, J., and Haslum, M.: Persistence of injury: can injuries of preschool children predict injuries of school-aged children? Pediatrics 82:707-712, 1988.

Bijur, P.E., Stewart-Brown, S., and Butler, N.: Child behavior and accidental injury in 11,966 preschool children, Am. J. Dis. Child. 140:487-492, 1986.

Bijur, P.E., and others: Behavioral predictors of injury in school-age children, Am. J. Dis. Child. 142:1307-1312, 1988.

Boraz, R.A.: Preventive dentistry for the pediatric patient, Issues Compr. Pediatr. Nurs. 5:89-97, 1981.

Boyce, W.T., and Sobolewski, S.: Recurrent injuries in school children, Am. J. Dis. Child. 143:338-342, 1989.

Christoffel, K.K., Tanz, R., and Sagerman, S.: Childhood injuries caused by nonpowder firearms, Am. J. Dis. Child. 138:557-561, 1984.

Coble, P.A., and others: EEG sleep of healthy children 6 to 12 years of age. In Guilleminault, C. editor: Sleep and its disorders in children, New York, 1987, Raven Press.

Cogbill, T.H., Busch, H.M., and Stiers, G.R.: Farm accidents in children, Pediatrics 76:562-566, 1985.

Council on Dental Therapeutics: Guidelines for the acceptance of fluoride-containing dentifrices, J. Am. Dent. Assoc. 110:545-547, 1985.

Davis, J.H.: Children and pets: a therapeutic connection, Pediatr. Nurs. 11:377-379, 1985.

DeAngelis, C., and others: Comparative values of school physical examinations and mass screening tests, J. Pediatr. 102:477-481, 1983.

DiGuiseppi, C.G., Rivara, F.P., and Koepsell, T.D.: Attitudes toward bicycle helmet ownership and use by school-age children, Am. J. Dis. Child. 144:83-86, 1990.

Dolan, M.A., Knapp, J.F., and Andres, J.: Three-wheel and four-wheel all-terrain vehicle injuries in children, Pediatrics 84:694-698, 1989.

Egli, E.A., and Meyers, L.S.: Bull. Psychonomic Soc. 22:309-312, 1984.

Ehrman, D.: Hotline provides latchkey children phone link to retirees, Child. Teens Today 7(4):5, 1986.

Elizur, J.: The stress of school entry: parent coping behaviors and children's adjustment to school, J. Child Psychol. Psychiatry 27:625-638, 1986.

Elkind, D.: The hurried child, growing up too fast too soon, Menlo Park, CA, 1981, Addison-Wesley Publishing Co., Inc.

Ellis, D.: Video arcades, youth, and trouble, Youth Soc. 16(1):47-65, 1984.

Erikson, E.H.: Childhood and society, ed. 2, New York, 1963, W.W. Norton & Co., Inc.

Faber, M.M., Hoppe, S.K., and Diehl, A.K.: Physician knowledge and clinical behavior regarding automobile safety for children, Pediatrics 75:248-253, 1985.

Feldman, W., and others: Prospective study of school injuries: incidence, types, related factors and initial management, Can. Med. Assoc. J. 129:1279-1283, 1983.

Ferber, R.: The sleepless child. In Guilleminault, C., editor: Sleep and its disorders in children, New York, 1987, Raven Press.

Friede, A.M., and others: The epidemiology of injuries to bicycle riders, Pediatr. Clin. North Am. 32:141-151, 1985.

Gallagher, S.S., and others: The incidence of injuries among 87,000 Massachusetts children and adolescents: results of the 1980-81 Statewide Childhood Injury Prevention Program Surveillance System, Am. J. Public Health 74:1340-1347, 1984.

Graybill, D., and others: Effects of playing violent versus nonviolent video games on the aggressive ideation of aggressive and nonaggressive children, Child Study J. 15:199-205, 1985.

Green, K.E., and Bird, J.E.: The structure of children's beliefs about health and illness, J. School Health 56:325-328, 1986.

Guilleminault, C.: Disorders of arousal in children: somnambulism and night terrors. In Guilleminault, C., editor: Sleep and its disorders in children, New York, 1987, Raven Press.

Hancock, L.A.: Safe biking—a bike helmet, J. Pediatr. Health Care 1:334-335, 1987.

Horwitz, S.M., and others: Determinants of pediatric injuries, Am. J. Dis. Child. 142:605-611, 1988.

Howland, J., and others: Barriers to bicycle helmet use among children, Am. J. Dis. Child. 143:741-744, 1989.

Igoe, J.B.: Healthy long-term attitudes on personal health can be developed in school-age children, Pediatrician 15:127-136, 1988.

Igoe, J.B.: HealthPACT helps youngsters to be more active in their health care, Child Behav. Dev. Lett. 5(4):1-2, 1989.

Inkelis, D.H., and others: Roller skating injuries in children, Pediatr. Emerg. Care 4:127-132, 1988.

Karp, S.: A 10-point program for bicycle safety, Contemp. Pediatr. 4(6):16-27, 1987.

Klein, M.H.: The bite of Pac-Man, J. Psychohistory 11:395-401, 1984.

Koster, M.K.: Self-care: health behavior for the school-age child, Top. Clin. Nurs. 5(1):29-40, 1983.

Krugman, R.D., and Krugman, M.K.: Emotional abuse in the classroom, Am. J. Dis. Child. 138:284-286, 1984.

Kuczen, B: Childhood stress, New York, 1982, Delacorte Press.

Langley, J.: The "accident prone" child: the perpetration of a myth, Aust. Paediatr. J. 16:243-246, 1982.

Lasky, P.A., Gulbrandsen, M., and Scoblic, M.: Health education translated into health behavior, Issues Compr. Pediatr. Nurs. 5:167-175, 1981.

Levine, M.D.: Middle childhood. In Levine, M.D., and others: Developmental-behavioral pediatrics, Philadelphia, 1983, W.B. Saunders Co.

Lewis, C.E., and Lewis, M.A.: Peer pressure and risk-taking behaviors in children, Am. J. Publ. Health 74:580-584, 1984.

Lipsitt, L.P.: Risk-taking: more a threat to development then most of us realize (editorial), Child Behav. Dev. Lett. 3(9):8, 1987.
Lipsitt, L.P.: On teaching skills to risk takers (editorial), Child Behav. Dev. Lett. 5(5):8, 1988.
Long, T.J., and Long, L.: Latchkey children: the child's view of self care, U.S. Educational Resources Information Center, ERIC Document ED 214 666, 1982.
Massachusetts Medical Society Committee on Nutrition: Fast-food fare: consumer guidelines, N. Engl. J. Med. 321:752-756, 1989.
Masten, A.S., and others: Many variables determine the effects of stress, J. Child Psychol. Psychiatry 29:745-762, 1988.
McClellan, M.A.: On their own: latchkey children, Pediatr. Nurs. 10:198-202, 1984.
Meyers, A.F., and others: School breakfast program and school performance, Am. J. Dis. Child. 143:1234-1239, 1989.
Moracco, J.C., and Camilleri, J.: A study of fears in elementary school children, Elementary School Guid. Counsel. 18:82-87, 1983.
National Safety Council: Accident facts, Chicago, 1983, National Safety Council.
National Transportation Safety Board: Crashworthiness of large post-standard school buses, Washington, DC, 1987, National Transportation Safety Board.
Newman, B.M., and Newman, P.R.: Development through life: a psychosocial approach, ed. 3, Homewood, IL, 1984, Dorsey Press.
Nichols, T.W., Jr.: Bicycle-seat hematuria (letter), N. Engl. J. Med. 311:1128, 1984.
Oda, D.S., and others: Nurse practitioners and primary care in schools, MCN 10:127-131, 1985.
Ordog, G.J., and others: Gunshot wounds in children under 10 years of age, Am. J. Dis. Child. 142:618-622, 1988.
Patterson, P.J., and Smith, L.R.: Firearms in the home and child safety, Am. J. Dis. Child. 141:221-223, 1987.
Paulson, J.A.: Accidental injuries. In Behrman, R.E., and Vaughan, V.C. III: Textbook of pediatrics, ed. 12, Philadelphia, 1983, W.B. Saunders Co.
Pless, I.B., and Stulginskas, J.: Accidents and violence as a cause of morbidity and mortality in childhood, Adv. Pediatr. 29:471-495, 1982.
Poresky, R.H., and others: Pets influence self-concept, J. Psychol. 122:463-469, 1988.
Radencich, M.C.: From Dick and Jane to Tron? Reading World 24(2):1-3, 1984.
Retsky, J., Jaffe, D., and Christoffel, K.K.: Child injuries due to skateboards: recurrence in the 1980s (abstract), Clin. Res. 35:915A, 1987.
Rivara, F.P.: Minibikes: a case study in underregulation. In Bergman, A.B., editor: Preventing childhood injuries, Report of the 12th Ross roundtable on critical approaches to common pediatric problems, Columbus, OH, 1982, Ross Laboratories.
Rivara, F.P.: Fatal and nonfatal farm injuries to children and adolescents in the United States, Pediatrics 76:567-573, 1985.
Rivara, F.P., and Barber, M.: Demographic analysis of childhood pedestrian injuries, Pediatrics 76:375-381, 1985.
Roberts, M., and Fanurik, D.: Rewarding elementary school children for their use of safety belts, Health Psychol. 5:185-196, 1986.
Roberts, M., and Turner, D.: Rewarding parents for their children's use of safety seats, J. Pediatr. Psychol. 11:25-36, 1986.
Salmi, L.R., and others: Fatal farm injuries among young children, Pediatrics 83:267-271, 1989.
Sandler, A.: Social development in middle childhood, Pediatr. Ann. 18:380-387, 1989.
Sass, R., and Crook, G.: Accident proneness: science or non-science? Int. J. Health Serv. 11:175-190, 1981.
Saunders, A., and Remsberg, B.: The stress-proof child, New York, 1984, Holt, Rinehart, & Winston.
Schor, E.L.: Unintentional injuries: patterns within families, Am. J. Dis. Child. 141:1280-1284, 1987.
Schowalter, J.E.: Common topics of parental concern: developmental considerations, Columbus, OH, 1983, Ross Laboratories.
Selbst, S.M., Alexander, D., and Ruddy, R.: Bicycle-related injuries, Am. J. Dis. Child. 141:140-144, 1987.
Selnow, G.W.: Playing videogames: the electronic friend, J. Communication 34:148-156, 1984.
Shaffer, T.E.: The young athlete: new guidelines in sports medicine, Pediatr. Consult. 1(5):1-12, 1980.
Sheps, S.B., and Evans, G.D.: Epidemiology of school injuries: a two-year experience in a municipal health department, Pediatrics 79:69-75, 1987.
Sims, A.C.P.: Head injury, neurosis and accident proneness, Adv. Psychosom. Med. 13:49-70, 1985.
Smith, E.V.: Hazard analysis of ride-on mowers, Consumer Product Safety Commission, May 1988.
Soper, W.B., and Miller, M.J.: Junk-time junkies: an emerging addiction among students, School Counselor 31:40-43, 1983.
Sparnon, A.L., and Ford, W.D.A.: Handlebar injuries in children, J. Pediatr. Surg. 21:118-119, 1986.
Spital, M., Spital, A., and Spital, R.: The compelling case for seat belts on school buses, Pediatrics 78:928-932, 1986.
Swanson, J.A., and others: Accidental farm injuries in children, Am. J. Dis. Child. 141:1276-1279, 1987.
Terr, L.C.: Nightmares in children. In Guilleminault, C., editor: Sleep and its disorders in children, New York, 1987, Raven Press.
Thompson, R.S., Rivara, F.P., and Thompson, D.C.: A case-control study of the effectiveness of bicycle safety helmets, N. Engl. J. Med. 320:1361-1367, 1989.
Vandell, D., Minnett, A., and Santrock, J.: Sibling relationships change during middle childhood, J. Appl. Dev. Psychol. 8:247-257, 1987.
Weiss, B.D.: Bicycle helmet use by children, Pediatrics 77:677-679, 1986.
Weiss, B.D.: Bicycle helmets, N.Y. State J. Med. 87:319-320, 1987.
Weiss, B.D., and Duncan, B.: Bicycle helmet use by children, Am. J. Public Health 76:1022-1023, 1986.
Widome, M.D.: School bus seat belts? (letter), Pediatrics 82:134-135, 1988.
Winkelstein, M.L.: Fostering positive self-concept in the school-age child, Pediatr. Nurs. 15:229-233, 1989.

BIBLIOGRAPHY

General

Adger, H., and DeAngelis, C.: Sexuality education: our schools can do better, Contemp. Pediatr. 6(10)56-67, 1989.
Betz, C.L.: Faith development in children, Pediatr. Nurs. 7(2):22-25, 1981.
Cameron, C.L., Juszczak, L., and Wallace, N.: Using creative arts to help children cope with altered body image, Child. Health Care 12:108-112, 1984.
Chess, S., and Thomas, A.: Temperamental differences: a critical concept in child health care, Pediatr. Nurs. 11:167-171, 1985.
Dworkin, P.H.: Behavior during middle childhood: developmental themes and clinical issues, Pediatr. Ann. 18:347-355, 1989.
Feldman, H.: The development of thinking skills in school-age children, Pediatr. Ann. 18:356-362, 1989.
Ferber, R.: Sleep schedule-dependent causes of insomnia and sleepiness in middle childhood and adolescence, Pediatrician 17:13-20, 1990.
Flavell, J.H.: Cognitive development, ed. 2, Englewood Cliffs, NJ, 1985, Prentice-Hall, Inc.
Goldsmith, H.H., and Gottesman, I.I.: Origins of variation in behavioral style: a longitudinal study of temperament in young twins, Child Dev. 2:91-99, 1981.
Guilleminault, C., editor: Sleep and its disorders in children, New York, 1987, Raven Press.
Hartley, R.: Imagine you're clever, J. Child Psychol. Psychiatry 27:383-398, 1986.

Hegvik, R.L., McDevitt, S.C., and Carey, W.B.: The middle childhood temperament questionnaire, Dev. Behav. Pediatr. 3(6):197-200, 1982.
Humphreys, A.P., and Smith, P.K.: Rough and tumble, friendship, and dominance in school children: evidence for continuity and change with age, Child Dev. 58:201-212, 1987.
Kaluger, G., and Kaluger, M.F.: Human development: the span of life, ed. 3, St. Louis, 1984, Mosby–Year Book, Inc.
Landman, G.B.: Language development from six to twelve, Pediatr. Ann. 18:373-379, 1989.
Maccoby, E.E.: Social development: psychological growth and the parent-child relationship, New York, 1980, Harcourt Brace Jovanovich, Inc.
Mahowald, M.W., and Rosen, G.M.: Parasomnias in children, Pediatrician 17:21-31, 1990.
Marsman, J.C., and Herold, E.S.: Attitudes toward sex education and values in sex education, Fam. Relations 35:357-369, 1986.
Mason, K.J.: Pediatric orthopaedics: developmental norms, Orthop. Nurs. 8(4):45-50, 1989.
McCown, D.E.: Moral development in children, Pediatr. Nurs. 10:42-44, 1984.
Rauckhorst, L.M., and Aroian, J.F.: Camp nursing: a way to season your summer? J. Pediatr. Nurs. 2:167-173, 1987.
Reasoner, R.W.: Enhancement of self-esteem in children and adolescents, Fam. Community Health 6(2):51-64, 1983.
Schor, D.P.: Temperament and the initial school experience, Child Health Care 13:129-134, 1985.
Selekman, J.: The development of body image in the child: a learned response, Top. Clin. Nurs. 5(1):12-21, 1983.
Shaffer, D.R.: Developmental psychology: theory, research, and applications, Monterey, CA, 1985, Brooks/Cole Publishing Co.
Shelly, J.A.: The spiritual needs of children, Downers Grove, IL, 1982, InterVarsity Press.
Sherwin, L.N.: Separation: the forgotten phenomenon of child development, Top. Clin. Nurs. 5(1):1-11, 1983.
Stanwyck, D.J: Self-esteem through the life span, Fam. Community Health 6(2):11-28, 1983.
Stone, L.J., and Church, J.: Childhood and adolescence, ed. 5, New York, 1983, Random House, Inc.
Weir, R., Rideout, E., and Crook, J.: Pediatric use of emergency departments, J. Pediatr. Nurs. 3:204-210, 1989.
Zaichkowsky, L.D., Zaichkowsky, L.B., and Martinek, T.J.: Growth and development: the child and physical activity, St. Louis, 1980, Mosby–Year Book, Inc.

Stress and Coping

Allen, M.T.: An overview of the type A behavior pattern in children and adolescents, Pediatr. Nurs. 9:407-412, 1983.
Coolsen, P., Seligson, M., and Garbarino, J.: When school's out and nobody's home, Chicago, 1985, National Committee for Prevention of Child Abuse.
DuPont, R.L.: Phobias in children, Pediatrics 102:999-1002, 1983.
Garmezy, N.: Stressors of childhood. In Garmezy, N., and Rutter, M.: Stress, coping, and development in children, New York, 1983, McGraw-Hill, Inc.
Guerney, L., and Moore, L.: Phone Friend: a prevention-oriented service for latchkey children, Child. Today 12(6):5-10, 1983.
LaMontagne, L.L.: Three coping strategies used by school-age children, Pediatr. Nurs. 10:25-28, 1984.
Lewis, C.E., Siegel, J.M., and Lewis, M.A.: Feeling bad: exploring sources of stress among pre-adolescent children, Am. J. Public Health 74:117-122, 1984.
McClellan, M.A.: On their own: latchkey children, Pediatr. Nurs. 10:198-202, 1984.
Minde, K.K.: Effect of social change on the behavior of school-age children, Pediatrician 15:170-175, 1988.
Nelms, B.C.: Corporal punishment in the schools: sanctioned abuse? (editorial), J. Pediatr. Health Care 3:219-220, 1988.
Nelms, B.C.: Children feel the pressure too (editorial), J. Pediatr. Health Care 3:229, 1989.
Nowicki, S., and Oxenford, C.: The relation of hostile nonverbal communication styles to popularity in preadolescent children, J. Genet. Psychol. 150:39-44, 1989.
Rodman, H., Pratto, D.J., and Nelson, R.S.: Child care arrangements and children's functioning: a comparison of self-care and adult-care children, Dev. Psychol. 212:413-418, 1985.
Rowland, B.H., Robinson, B.E., and Coleman, M.: A survey of parents' perceptions regarding latchkey children, Pediatr. Nurs. 12:278-283, 1986.
Valenti, S.M.: Stressors at school age, Fam. Community Health 2(4):15-29, 1980.
Williams, R.L., and Fosarelli, P.D.: Telephone call-in services for children in self-care, Am. J. Dis. Child. 141:965-968, 1987.

Health Promotion

Altman, D.G., and Revenson, T.A.: Children's understanding of health and illness concepts: a preventive health perspective, J. Primary Prevent. 6(1):53-67, 1985.
American Academy of Pediatrics, Committee on School Health: School health: a guide for health professionals, Elk Grove Village, IL, 1987, American Academy of Pediatrics.
Andersen, A.R., and Clore, E.R.: Asbestos in schools: reducing pediatric risk factors, Pediatr. Nurs. 12:296-321, 1986.
Bailey-Britton, A.M.: The relationship between health and academic performance in school-age children, Issues Compr. Pediatr. Nurs. 10:273-289, 1987.
Baldwin, J., and Davis, L.L.: Assessing parents as health educators, Pediatr. Nurs. 15:453-462, 1989.
Bausell, R.B.: A national survey assessing pediatric preventive behaviors, Pediatr. Nurs. 11:438-444, 1985.
Belkengren, R.B., and Sapala, S.: Physical fitness from infancy through adolescence, Pediatr. Nurs. 8:A-I, 1982.
Bruhn, J.G., and Nader, P.R.: The school as a setting for health education, health promotion, and health care, Fam. Community Health 4(1):57-69, 1982.
Courtnage, L.: The use of prescribed medication in the schools: a status report on the state policies and guidelines, J. School Health 52:543-548, 1982.
Cross, A.W.: Health screening in schools, part I, J. Pediatr. 107:487-494, 1985.
Cross, A.W.: Health screening in schools, part II, J. Pediatr. 107:653-661, 1985.
Czupryna, L.: Primary prevention in a camp setting, MCN 9:197-199, 1984.
Dailey, C.P.: Teaching parents and children preventive health behaviors, Fam. Community Health 7(1):34-43, 1985.
DeAngelis, C.: Health care for the elementary school age child. In Green, M., and Haggerty, R.J.: Ambulatory pediatrics, Philadelphia, 1984, W.B. Saunders Co.
Denehy, J.: What do school-age children know about their bodies? Pediatr. Nurs. 290-292, 1984.
Eiden, H., Thomas, M., and Fosarelli, P.: A teaching tool for children in self-care, J. Pediatr. Health Care 1:292-297, 1987.
Gulbrandsen, M., Lasky, P.A., and Scoblic, M.: Translating health knowledge into health behavior, Issues Compr. Pediatr. Nurs. 5:177-184, 1981.
Hester, N.D.: Health concerns of school-age children, Issues Compr. Pediatr. Nurs. 10:251-262, 1987.
Hull, H.F., and others: Risk factors for measles vaccine failure among immunized students, Pediatrics 76:518-523, 1985.
Hussey, C.G., and Hirsh, A.M.: Health education for children, Top. Clin. Nurs. 5(1):22-28, 1983.

Igoe, J.B.: Children as future health consumers: teaching them to take a more active role, School Nurse Network 1:1-9, 1986.
Kaufman, D.H.: An interview guide for helping children make health-care decisions, Pediatr. Nurs. 11:365-367, 1985.
Kornguth, M.L.: School illnesses: who's absent and why? Pediatr. Nurs. 16:95-99, 1990.
Korsch, B.: What do patients and parents want to know? What do they need to know? Pediatrics 74:917, 1984.
Lasky, P.A., and Eichelberger, K.M.: Health-related views and self-care behaviors of young children, Fam. Rel. 34:13-18, 1985.
Lewis, C.E., and Lewis, M.A.: Determinants of children's health-related beliefs and behaviors, Fam. Community Health 4(4):85-97, 1982.
Lindsey, C.N., and others: Children on medication: a guide for teachers, Rehabil. Lit. 41(5-6):124-126, 1980.
Meeker, R., and others: A comprehensive school health initiative, Image 18:86-91, 1986.
Mickalide, A.D.: Children's understanding of health and illness: implications for health promotion, Health Values 3:5-21, 1986.
Moore, J.B.: Determining the relationship of autonomy to self-care agency of locus of control in school-age children, Matern. Child Nurs. J. 16(1):47-60, 1987.
Morris, N.M.: Pediatric health promotion through risk reduction, Fam. Community Health 3(1):63-76, 1980.
Murray, R., and Zentner, J.: Nursing assessment and health promotion through the life span, ed. 2, Englewood Cliffs, NJ, 1980, Prentice-Hall, Inc.
O'Brien, R.W., Bush, P.J., and Parcel, G.S.: Stability in a measure of children's health locus of control, J. School Health 59(4):161-164, 1989.
Oda, D.: A viewpoint on school nursing, Am. J. Nurs. 81:1677-1678, 1981.
Oda, D.S., and others: Nurse practitioners and primary care in schools, MCN 10:127-131, 1985.
Otto, J.: Be prepared for camp nursing, Am. J. Nurs. 80:906-907, 1980.
Perrin, E.C., and Perrin, J.M.: Clinician's assessments of children's understanding of illness, Am. J. Dis. Child. 13:874-878, 1983.
Robinson, T.: School nurse practitioners on the job, Am. J. Nurs. 81:1674-1676, 1981.
Rose, D.A., Chen, S.C., and Souter, C.M.: Development of an in-service education program by school nurses, J. Community Health Nurs. 4(3):171-178, 1987.
Seybold, S.A., and Klisch, M.L.: Preparing grade school faculty to teach family life education, MCN 7:50-54, 1982.
Smith, N.J.: Sports participation: current developmental considerations in childhood and adolescence, Columbus, OH, 1985, Ross Laboratories.
Switzer, K.H., and Kelly, J.T.: The nurse: a member of the school team, MCN 6:289-293, 1981.
Vessey, J.A., Braithwaite, K.B., and Wiedmann, M.: Teaching children about their internal bodies, Pediatr. Nurs. 16:29-33, 1990.
Wold, S.J.: School nursing: a framework for practice, St. Louis, 1981, Mosby–Year Book, Inc.
Wood, S.P.: School-aged children's perceptions of the causes of illness, Pediatr. Nurs. 9:101-104, 1983.

Nutrition

Lowenberg, M.E.: The development of food patterns in young children. In Pipes, P.L.: Nutrition in infancy and childhood, ed. 3, St. Louis, 1985, Mosby–Year Book, Inc.
Pipes, P.L.: Nutrition in infancy and childhood, ed. 4, St. Louis, 1989, Mosby–Year Book, Inc.
Williams, S.R.: Nutrition and diet therapy, ed. 5, St. Louis, 1985, Mosby–Year Book, Inc.
Wurthman, J.J.: What do children eat? Eating styles of the preschool, elementary school, and adolescent child. In Suskind, R.M., editor: Textbook of pediatric nutrition, New York, 1981, Raven Press.

Injury Prevention

Agran, P.A., and Dunkle, D.E.: Motor vehicle occupant injuries to children in crash and noncrash events, Pediatrics 70:993-996, 1982.
American Academy of Pediatrics, Committee on Accident and Poison Prevention: Child safety suggestions: safe bicycling, Evanston, IL, 1978, American Academy of Pediatrics.
American Academy of Pediatrics, Committee on Accident and Poison Prevention: Automatic passenger protection systems, Pediatrics 74:146-147, 1984.
American Academy of Pediatrics, Committee on Research, and Committee on Accident and Poison Prevention: Reducing the toll of injuries in childhood requires support for a focused research effort, Pediatrics 72:736-737, 1983.
Arenson, S., and others: Factors affecting parental use of child automobile safety restraints, Child. Health Care 13(4):181-186, 1985.
Berger, L.R., Kaishman, S., and Rivara, F.P.: Injuries from fireworks, Pediatrics 75:877-882, 1985.
Bergman, A.B.: Use of education in preventing injuries, Pediatr. Clin. North Am. 29:331-338, 1982.
Christoffel, K.K.: Child passenger safety, Am. J. Dis. Child. 143:1271-1272, 1989.
Greensher, J.: How anticipatory guidance can improve control of childhood "accidents," Pediatr. Consult. 3(2):1-5, 1984.
Greensher, J., and Mofenson, H.C.: Injuries at play, Pediatr. Clin. North Am. 32:127-139, 1985.
Guyer, B., Talbot, A.M., and Pless, I.B.: Pedestrian injuries to children and youth, Pediatr. Clin. North Am. 32:163-174, 1985.
Holland, S.H.: Car safety for school children and adolescents, Child. Nurse 4(4):1-4, 1986.
Kellermann, A.L., and Realy, D.T.: Protection or peril? An analysis of firearm-related deaths in the home, N. Engl. J. Med. 314:1557-1560, 1986.
Lee, E.J.: Accident reports: survey of high school injuries, Pediatr. Nurs. 13:151-154, 1987.
Lyons, J.F., and Hester, N.O.: Research-generated nursing diagnoses for healthy school-age children, Issues Compr. Pediatr. Nurs. 10:149-150, 1987.
Micik, S., and Miclette, M.: Injury prevention in the community: a systems approach, Pediatr. Clin. North Am. 32:251-265, 1985.
Pless, I., and Arsenault, A.: The role of health education in the prevention of injuries to children, J. Soc. Issues 43:87-103, 1987.
Pless, I.B., Verreault, R., and Tenina, S.: A case-control study of pedestrian and bicyclist injuries in childhood, Am. J. Public Health 79:995-998, 1989.
Ridenour, M.V.: Elementary school playgrounds: safe play areas or inherent dangers, Percept. Mot. Skills 64:447-451, 1987.
Righi, F.C., and Krozy, R.E.: The child in the car: what every nurse should know about safety, Am. J. Nurs. 83:1421-1424, 1983.
Rivara, F.P.: Fatal and nonfatal farm injuries to children and adolescents in the United States, Pediatrics 76:567-573, 1985.
Rivara, F.P., and others: Attitudes and practices toward children as pedestrians, Pediatrics 84:1017-1021, 1989.
Scheidt, P.C.: Behavioral research toward prevention of childhood injury, Am. J. Dis. Child. 142:612-617, 1988.
Schetky, D.H.: Children and handguns—a public health concern, Am. J. Dis. Child 139:229-231, 1985.
Sheps, S.B., and Evans, G.D.: Epidemiology of school injuries: a 2-year experience in a municipal health department, Pediatrics 79:69-75, 1987.
Tay, J.S., and Garland, J.S.: Serious head injuries from lawn darts, Pediatrics 79:261-263, 1987.
Westman, J.A., and Morrow, G.: Moped injuries in children, Pediatrics 74:820-822, 1984.
Wilson, M.H.: Preventing injury in the "middle years," Contemp. Pediatr. 6(6):20-54, 1989.
Wintemute, G.J., and others: When children shoot children: eighty-eight unintended deaths in California, JAMA 257:3107-3109, 1987.
Zuckerman, B.S., and Duby, J.C.: Developmental approach to injury prevention, Pediatr. Clin. North Am. 32:17-29, 1985.

CHAPTER 18

Health Problems of Middle Childhood

RELATED TOPICS

GLOSSARY

AD-HD Attention deficit–hyperactivity disorder
ecchymoses (bruises) Localized red or purple, discolorations caused by extravasation of blood into dermis and subcutaneous tissues
ECM Erythema chronicum migrans
erythema A reddened area caused by increased amounts of oxygenated blood in the dermal vasculature
NF1 Neurofibromatosis, type 1
PABA *p*-Aminobenzoic acid
petechiae Pinpoint tiny and sharply circumscribed spots in the superficial layers of the epidermis
primary lesions Skin changes produced by some causative factor
PTSD Posttraumatic stress disorder
RAP Recurrent abdominal pain
secondary lesions Skin changes that result from alteration in primary lesions
SJS Stevens-Johnson syndrome
SPF Sun protective factor
TS Tourette syndrome
UVA Ultraviolet A
UVB Ultraviolet B

As a group school-age children are fairly healthy when compared with children in infancy and early childhood, and ages 9 to 12 are usually the healthiest years. As would be expected, respiratory illnesses (the leading cause of morbidity) and gastrointestinal upsets are most common. A factor contributing to this overall health state is the quantity of lymphoid tissue, at its height during this stage, which helps to fight infection and ward off disease. An eleven-year-old child has almost twice the amount of a young adult.

Most children in this age-group have either contracted the communicable diseases of childhood or been immunized against them. Their excellent appetites, adequate rest, and sufficient physical exercise further contribute to their general good health. The common health problems of school-age children are not illnesses of serious import as individual entities and all are amenable to therapy. Conditions that are not uncommon in middle childhood are dental problems and emotional or behavior disorders. Allergic manifestations, especially asthma, may reach a peak during the middle childhood years, and a variety of other serious disorders make a significant contribution to childhood morbidity. These will be considered as appropriate in relation to ill children.

■ DISORDERS AFFECTING THE SKIN

Skin disorders are common at all ages; therefore many that are usually limited to a specific age-group are discussed in relation to children in that age category, for example, birthmarks in the newborn, diaper rash and eczema in infancy, and acne during adolescence. Chemical dermatitis caused by poisons is included in the discussion of poisoning in Chapter 16.

THE SKIN

The skin and its component and associated structures constitute the integumentary system. The largest organ in the body, the skin is a thin structure (only about 1 mm thick at birth, increasing to approximately twice that thickness at maturity) that serves primarily as an insulator, not as an organ of exchange.

Anatomically and physiologically the skin differs markedly in various areas of the body, and each variation is adapted to meet special stresses. Regions such as the soles of the feet, the eyelids, and the back vary in skin thickness and looseness and in the kinds and quantities of appendages they contain, such as sweat glands and hair follicles. These variations are the basis for the localization of many disorders to specific areas and for the distribution of certain eruptions in characteristic patterns.

Purposes of the Skin

This functionally simple but morphologically complex structure serves several physical functions essential to life.

Protection. The skin serves as a protection against trauma, including mechanical, thermal, chemical, and radiant. The intact tough outer layer is a mechanical barrier. Organisms and chemicals penetrate it with difficulty, and it is further protected by the oily and slightly acid secretions of its sebaceous glands, which limit the growth of bacteria.

Impermeability. Very few substances are able to penetrate the skin with ease. It seals the body from the environment. The outer side of the upper layer, with its low water content, is in equilibrium with the viable cells underneath. It protects against loss of essential body constituents to the environment. The effectiveness of this impermeable membrane is demonstrated by the profuse fluid loss that follows damage to the epidermis by superficial burns, injury, poison ivy, or other agents. Loss of water and some electrolytes takes place only through pores in this effective barrier.

Heat regulation. The skin also adjusts heat loss to heat production to maintain the thermal balance of the body. This is accomplished primarily through functioning of cutaneous blood vessels and sweat glands. The vascular supply to the skin, much more extensive than needed for tissue nourishment, is regulated by way of central and local neural and hormonal processes.

Sensation. As a sensory organ, perceptions (touch,

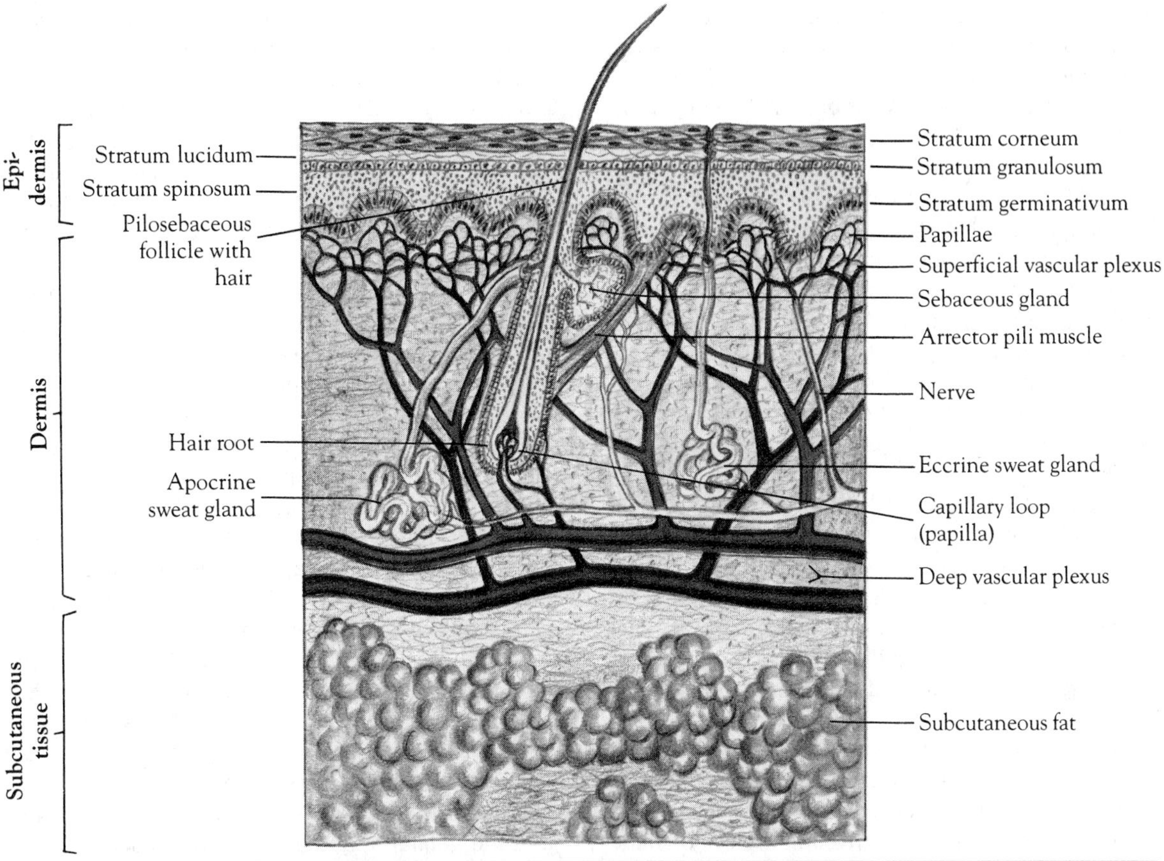

Fig. 18-1. Cross-section of normal skin.
From Thompson, J.M., and others: Mosby's manual of clinical nursing, ed. 2, St. Louis, 1989, Mosby–Year Book, Inc., p. 544.

pain, heat, and cold) are registered through the nerves that permeate the skin. To some extent, skin is also an organ of expression that betrays strong feelings: blushing (shame or embarrassment), redness (anger), blanching (fear), and sweating (anxiety).

Skin Structure

The skin consists of three layers: the epidermis, the corium or dermis, and an inner layer composed of fatty tissue of varying thickness that separates the skin from the subcutaneous tissues. The activity of the skin is controlled by the autonomic nervous system and the endocrine glands (Fig. 18-1).

The efficiency with which the skin layers prevent evaporative loss of water (independent of sweat) increases with development. A transitional zone between the epidermal layers allows more of the larger fluid content (70%) of the lower layers to enter the outer, drier layers (15% water), where it is lost in greater or lesser amounts, depending on environmental temperature and humidity. In the young child the transitional zone is less effective than that in an older child or adult. The fluid loss is most marked in the prematurely born infant.

Epidermis. The epidermis, the outermost portion of relatively uniform thickness, consists of five layers, the lowest of which is composed of specialized cells called basal cells that are continually replacing the cell population. As they multiply, the older cells are displaced outwardly by the constant stream of new cells. The older cells progressively flatten and alter until they form dead, scalelike, or horny flakes with no cellular details and composed of *keratin.* These flakes are constantly sloughed off the surface of the body. This continual epidermal renewal is nourished by fluid from blood vessels in the dermis. The intact epidermis provides a relatively impenetrable barrier to the loss of body contents and the entrance of environmental hazards.

Elaborating this outer layer are specialized cellular invaginations of epidermal origin, the glandular appendages and hair follicles. Although they are situated mainly in the dermis, these structures are lined with epithelial cells and are derived from the epithelial skin layer. This has significance when a large area of epidermis is damaged. It is from the cells lining these structures that new epithelium is derived.

Diseases of the skin focus sharply on the epidermis, which is the site of many distinctive patterns, ranging from the vesiculation of contact dermatitis to common superficial tumors. Clearly visible, these morphologic changes produce the varied patterns on which a dermatologic diagnosis is made.

Dermis. The dermis, or *corium,* constitutes the bulk of the skin. It is a firm, fibrous, and elastic connective tissue network containing an elaborate system of blood vessels, lymphatics, and nerves and varies throughout the body from 1 to 4 mm in thickness. In addition, it is invaded by the epidermal downgrowth of hair follicles and glands. Functionally the corium has a major protective role for these varied essential components of the skin.

More hidden than the epidermis, changes in the corium are more difficult to interpret on inspection. Biopsy and histologic studies are more often needed to confirm a diagnosis based on manifestations in the corium. Since it is composed predominantly of connective tissue, the dermis frequently permits an awareness and observation of many diffuse systemic disorders of connective tissue—the "collagen" diseases.

Subcutaneous tissue. A thick layer of subcutaneous tissue lies beneath the dermis and is composed of a looser type of connective tissue that varies greatly in extent in various parts of the body. In addition to larger blood vessels, lymph channels, and nerve trunks, the subcutaneous tissue serves as a depot for the storage of fat that acts as a cushion, insulates the body against cold, and largely determines its contours.

Hair. The various skin appendages develop at different times and at different rates. An extensive growth of fine body hair, lanugo, begins to appear at the end of the second intrauterine month, reaches its maximum development between the seventh and eighth months of fetal life, and begins to decrease before birth. It continues to regress steadily during early infancy and is replaced by a less extensive distribution of hair. Hair follicles are fully developed at birth, but the amount and texture of scalp hair vary between individual infants. The scalp hair is lost during the first few months after birth, then is slowly replaced by permanent hair, which gradually thickens and often darkens as the child grows.

At puberty the secretion of androgenic hormones stimulates an increase in the thickening and darkening of scalp hair, the growth of hair in the axilla and pubic regions of both sexes, and the growth of facial hair in boys. Late in adolescence some boys acquire additional amounts and distribution of body hair, such as on the chest.

Sebaceous glands. The sebaceous glands form in connection with hair follicles. Their function is to produce a fatty secretion called sebum that helps keep the skin supple by decreasing water loss. The sebaceous activity is maintained at a relatively constant rate by the secretion of androgens; an increase in androgens causes an increase in sebum production. Sebaceous glands have a regional distribution and are most abundant on the scalp, the face, and the genitals; are less numerous on the trunk; are sparse on the extremities; and do not appear on the palms and soles.

Sebaceous glands begin to form during the fifth month of fetal life and are very active during the month before birth, when they produce the protective vernix caseosa observed on newborn infants. The sebaceous activity slowly subsides after birth and continues to decrease throughout infancy. In the newborn period and early infancy sebaceous secretion may cause minor problems such as "cradle cap" in some infants. The secretion remains low during early childhood, which contributes to dryness and susceptibility to chapping, especially during the winter months. Sebaceous secretion gradually rises in childhood to increase markedly at puberty, where it remains constant and contributes greatly to the disturbing skin problems of adolescence.

Sweat glands. The sweat glands, both eccrine and apocrine, are present at birth. They appear between the fifth and seventh months of fetal life, but their activity is scant. The eccrine sweat glands function primarily as part of the body heat–regulating mechanism and to some extent in maintaining electrolyte balance. At birth the density of the eccrine glands is greater than at any other time of life (because of the smaller skin surface area) because no new glands are formed after birth. The sweat glands are equivalent in size, structural maturity, and position within the dermis in the full-term newborn and the adult (Shalita, 1981). They function at birth but produce more sweat as childhood advances, to reach full potential at puberty. There are individual differences in the amount of sweat produced, and there are no sex differences until after puberty, when males sweat more than females. Numerous factors influence the amount and chemical content of the sweat, for example, emotions and some disease states such as congestive heart failure in infancy and cystic fibrosis.

Apocrine sweat glands, located primarily in the axilla and the genital and anal areas, are inactive throughout infancy and childhood and mature during puberty. When the secretions from these glands are acted upon by bacteria, they cause the unpleasant odor associated with sweating.

Skin of younger children. The major skin layers arise from different embryologic origins. Early in the embryonic period, a single layer of epithelium forms from the ectoderm, while simultaneously the corium develops from the mesenchyme. In the infant and small child the epidermis is still loosely bound to the corium. This poor adherence causes the layers to separate readily during an inflammatory process to form blisters. This is especially true in preterm infants, who have an even greater propensity to blister formation and separation during careless handling (such as removal of adhesive tape). The skin is thinner than in older children, and the cells of all strata are more compressed.

Several characteristics influence skin responses in infants and young children. Their skin is far more susceptible to superficial bacterial infection. They are more likely to have associated systemic symptoms with some infections and are more apt to react to a primary irritant than to a sensitizing allergen. Infants and young children are more frequently affected by chronic atopic dermatitis (eczema). The infant's skin is much more prone to develop a toxic erythema as a result of skin eruptions or drug reactions and is subject to maceration, infection, and the sweat retention associated with diaper rash.

SKIN LESIONS

Lesions of the skin can be a result of a wide variety of specific etiologic factors. In general, skin lesions originate from

(1) contact with injurious agents such as infectious organisms, toxic chemicals, and physical trauma, (2) hereditary factors, (3) some external factor that produces a reaction in the skin (for example, allergens), or (4) or a systemic disease of which the lesions are a cutaneous manifestation (e.g., measles, lupus erythematosus, nutritional deficiency diseases). Such responses are highly individual. An agent that may be harmless to one individual may be damaging to another, and a single agent may produce various types of responses in different individuals.

Among other factors involved in the etiology of skin manifestations is the age of the child. For example, infants are subject to "birthmark" malformations and atopic dermatitis that appears early in life, the school-age child is susceptible to ringworm of the scalp, and acne is a characteristic skin disorder of puberty. Contact dermatitis, such as poison ivy, is seen only where the noxious agent is a feature of the area. Similarly, reactions to insect bites are associated with life cycle and seasonal activities. Although less common in children, tension and anxiety may produce, modify, or prolong many skin conditions.

Pathophysiology of Dermatitis

Over half of dermatologic problems are various forms of dermatitis. This implies a sequence of inflammatory changes in the skin that are grossly and microscopically similar but diverse in course and causation. Acute responses produce intercellular and intracellular edema, the formation of intradermal vesicles, and an initial minimum infiltration of inflammatory cells into the epidermis. In the dermis there is edema, vascular dilation, and early perivascular cellular infiltration. The location and manner of these reactions produce the lesions characteristic of each disorder. The changes are reversible, and the skin ordinarily recovers without blemish and completely intact unless complicating factors such as ulceration from the primary irritant, scratching, and infection are introduced or underlying vascular disease develops. In chronic conditions permanent effects are seen that vary according to the disorder, the general condition of the affected individual, and available therapy.

Subjective symptoms. Many cutaneous lesions are associated with local symptoms, the most common being itching, which varies in kind and intensity. Pain or tenderness often accompanies some skin lesions, and other sensations may be described as burning, prickling, stinging, or crawling. Alterations in local feeling or sensation include anesthesia (absence of sensation), hyperesthesia (excessive sensitivity), and hypesthesia or hypoesthesia (diminished or lessening of sensation). These symptoms may remain localized or may migrate, may be constant or intermittent, and may be aggravated by a specific activity or circumstance, such as exposure to sunlight.

Clinical Manifestations

One of the advantages of skin disorders is that often the diagnosis is readily established by a thorough health history. A simple, careful inspection can determine the distribution, size, and arrangement of lesion components and the morphology of individual lesions. In addition, intrinsic causes must be distinguished from extrinsic causes. Extrinsic causes usually result from physical, chemical, or allergic irritants or from an infectious agent such as bacteria, fungi, viruses, or animal parasites. Skin manifestations can be produced by such intrinsic causes as a specific infection, drug sensitization, or other allergic phenomena.

Lesion. According to the nature of the pathologic process, lesions assume more or less distinct characteristics. They are usually the result of disturbance of function, inflammation, or growth. Although the names that have been applied to these lesions are of little value in themselves, they are important for descriptive purposes in the processes of record keeping and communication. To examine the various aspects of the lesion, the inspection must take place under natural or adequate artificial light. A low-powered magnifying lens serves as a useful adjunct and, in diseases with abnormalities of pigmentation or those associated with fluorescence, a Wood light may be useful.

Skin lesions are classified as:

Primary lesions—skin changes produced by some causative factor (Fig. 18-2)

Secondary lesions—changes that result from alteration in the primary lesions, such as those caused by rubbing, scratching, medication, or involution and healing (Fig. 18-3)

Distribution pattern. How lesions are distributed over the body is a useful aid in diagnosis. Local processes are distinguished from generalized ones. Many lesions are primarily associated with specific areas, such as extensor areas in atopic dermatitis or uncovered areas that allow exposure to sun or noxious agents such as poison ivy; others are related to location of specific cutaneous appendages, such as the unique sebaceous gland distribution of acne.

Configuration and arrangement. The size, shape, and arrangement of a lesion or groups of lesions assist in diagnosis. *Discrete* (individually distinct) lesions are distinguished from *clustered* (appear close together), *diffuse* (scattered), or *confluent* (running together) configurations. Grouped or clustered lesions are characteristic in herpes eruptions; *annular* (ringed) or *arciform* lesions are typical of ringworm and diseases resulting from vascular reactions, such as urticaria or drug reaction; linear arrangements usually represent an exogenous influence that has either caused the process or contributed to its spread, such as scratching.

Diagnostic Evaluation

It is important to determine whether the child has had an allergic condition such as asthma or hay fever or has had previous skin disease. Eczema, often associated with allergies, frequently begins in infancy. It should be determined when the lesion or symptom first became apparent, as well as whether it is related to ingestion of a food or other substance, including any medication the child might be taking. It may be related to some activity, such as contact with plants, insects, or chemicals.

When it is suspected that a skin problem might be related to a systemic disease, such as one of the collagen diseases or immune deficiency disease, studies to rule out

PRIMARY SKIN LESIONS

Flat circumscribed area of color change (red, brown, purple, white, tan); less than 1 cm in diameter; nonpalpable
Example: Freckle, nevus, measles, flat mole

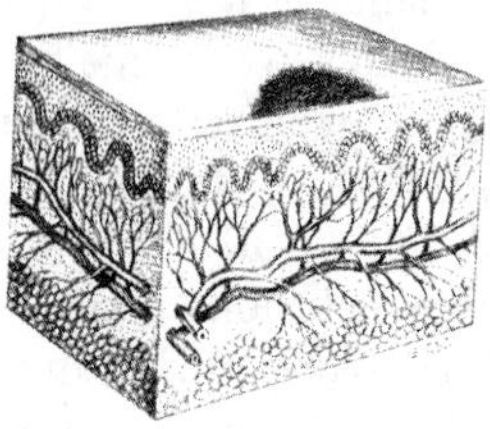

Macule

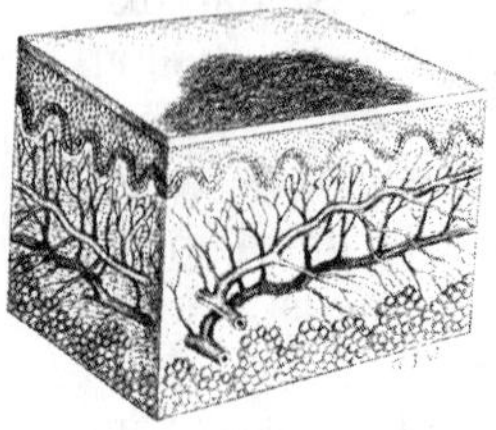

Patch

Flat, circumscribed, irregularly shaped, discoloration; nonpalpable; greater than 1 cm in diameter
Example: Mongolian spot, vitiligo, port-wine stain

Small, circumscribed, firm, elevated, discoloration (red, pink, tan, brown, bluish); less than 1 cm in diameter; the more superficial it is, the more distinct are the borders
Example: Wart, ringworm, milia, pigmented nevi

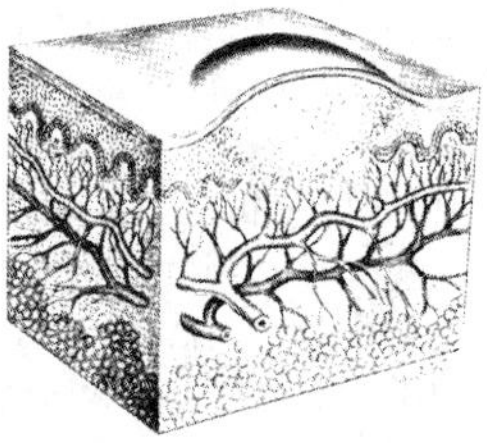

Papule

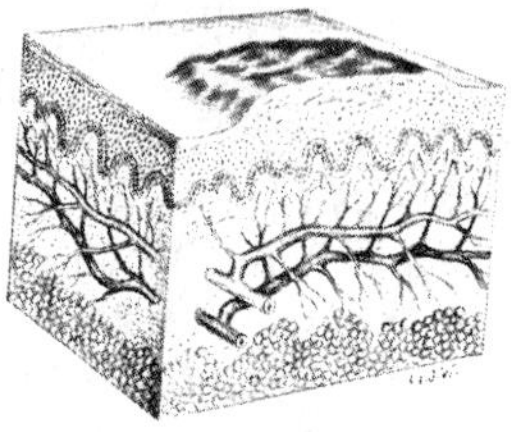

Plaque

Flattened, raised, firm, surface area relatively large in relation to height; greater than 1 cm in diameter
Example: Psoriasis

Solid, circumscribed, firm elevation; round or ellipsoid; located deep in dermis or subcutaneous tissue
Example: Dermatofibroma, dermoid cyst, lipoma

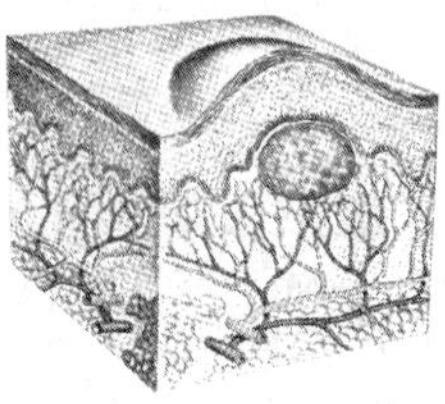

Nodule

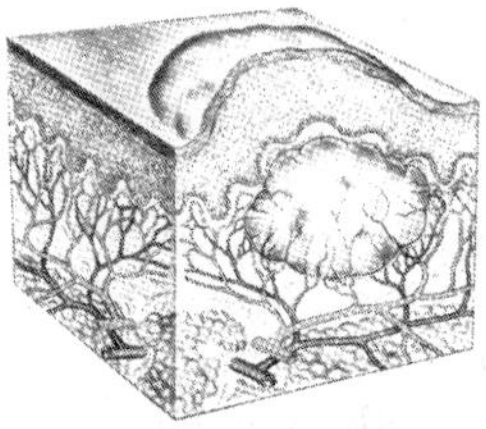

Tumor

Elevated, solid; may or may not be clearly demarcated; greater than 1 cm in diameter; and deeper than nodule
Example: Cavernous hemangioma, neoplasm

Elevated, circumscribed, palpable, encapsulated semisolid or fluid-filled mass in dermis or subcutaneous tissue
Example: Epidermoid cyst, sebaceous cyst

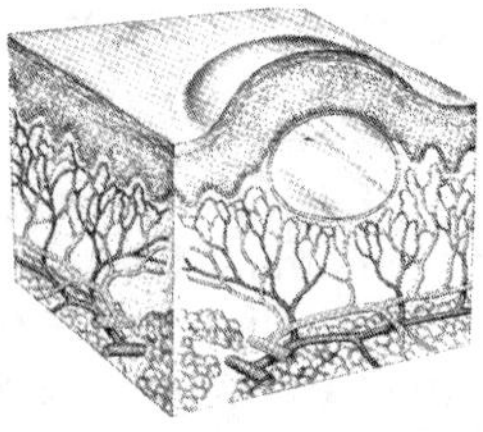

Cyst

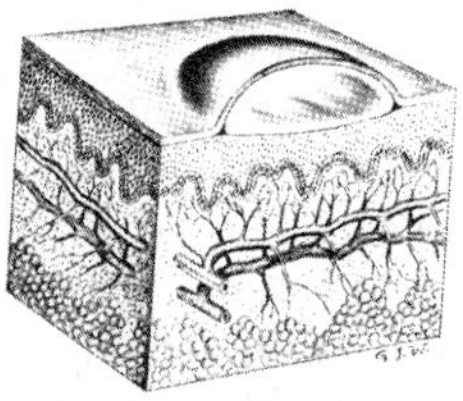

Vesicle

Small (less than 1 cm in diameter), superficial circumscribed elevation; contains serous or blood-tinged fluid
Example: Chicken pox, herpes, poison ivy

Vesicle filled with pus; may or may not be caused by infection
Example: Acne, impetigo, folliculitis

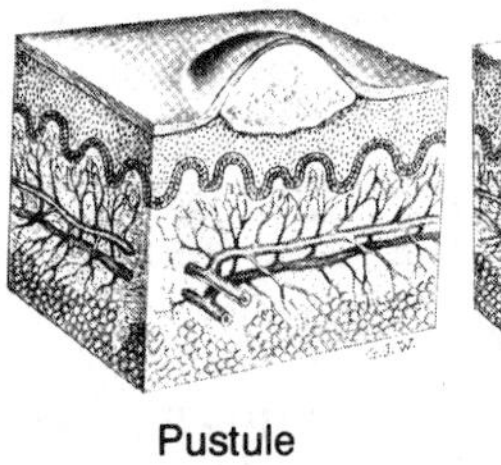

Pustule

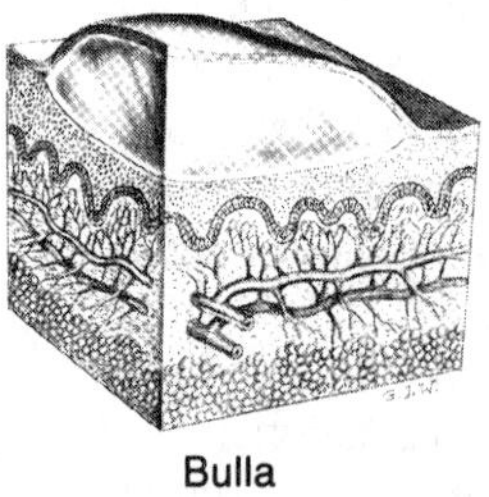

Bulla

Fluid-filled vesicle greater than 1 cm in diameter; a large vesicle; bleb; blister
Example: Second-degreee burn, bullous impetigo

Elevated, round or flat topped, irregularly shaped; transient, changing; variable diameter; pale pink in color
Example: Insect bites, urticaria

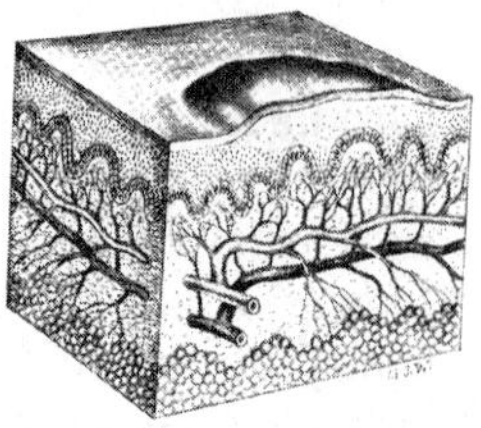

Wheal

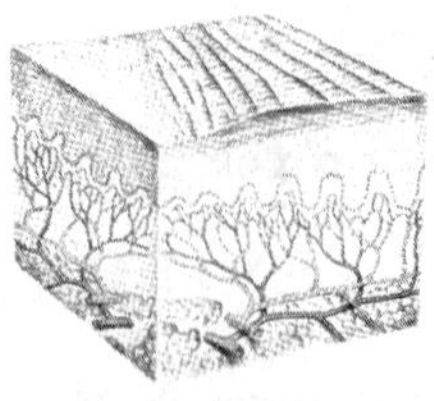

Lichenification

Loss of superficial epidermis, linear or punctate
Example: Scratch, abrasion

Fig. 18-2. Primary skin lesions.

SECONDARY SKIN LESIONS

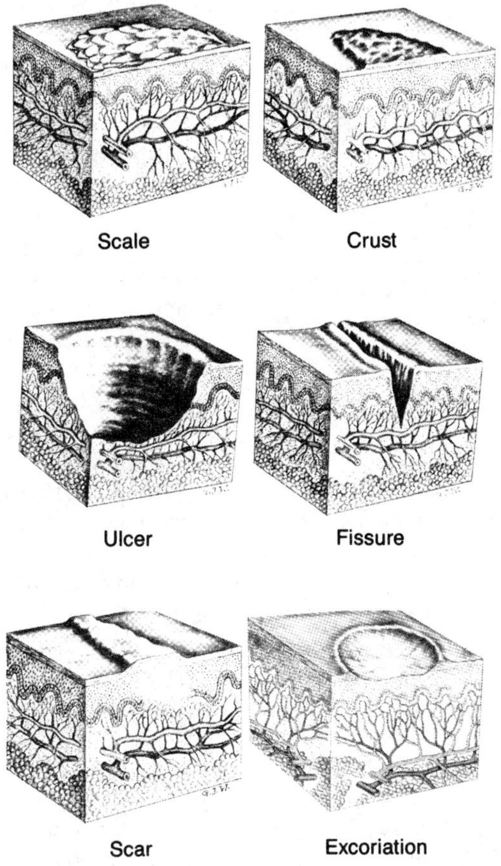

Scale: Mound of flaky, dead, cornified tissue shed from the skin; irregular shape; variable thickness and diameter; dry or oily; silver, white, or tan color
Example: Psoriasis, ringworm

Crust: Dried masses of serum, pus, dead skin, and debris that can be found surmounting any lesion; slightly elevated; brown, black, tan, or straw-colored
Example: Impetigo, scab, eczema

Ulcer: Irregularly shaped, concave, excavation with loss of epidermis and dermis; variable size; exudative; red or reddish blue
Example: Decubiti

Fissure: Deep linear split through epidermis into dermis; small; deep; red
Example: Chapping, tinea pedis

Scar: Permanent thick to thin fibrous tissue that replaces damaged corium by production and deposition of collagen; irregular shape; red, pink, or white; atrophic or hypertrophic
Example: Vaccination, healed wound, abrasion, laceration

Excoriation: Rough, thickened, and hardened epidermis with accentuated skin markings
Example: Result of chronic dermatitis, such as eczema

Fig. 18-3. Secondary skin lesions.

these possibilities are carried out. Diagnostic modalities include microscopic examination, cultures, skin biopsy, cytodiagnosis, patch testing, and examination under Wood light. Allergic skin testing and various other laboratory tests (blood count, sedimentation rate) are employed when indicated.

Therapeutic Management

The human body tends to heal; therefore treatment is directed toward eliminating or ameliorating influences that interfere with normal healing processes. Some disorders may demand aggressive therapy, but by and large the major aim of any treatment is to prevent further damage, eliminate the cause, prevent complications, and provide relief from discomfort while tissues undergo healing. Factors that contribute to the dermatitis and prolong the course of the disease must be eliminated when possible. The most common offenders in pediatrics are environmental factors (such as soaps, bubble baths, shampoos, rough or tight clothing, blankets, and toys) and the natural elements (such as dirt, sand, heat, cold, moisture, and wind). Dermatitis can also be aggravated by home remedies and medications.

Dressings are frequently applied to skin lesions and are universally used for wound management. Dressings serve several useful functions. They are used to (1) protect the wound from infection, (2) protect the wound from trauma, (3) provide compression in the event of anticipated bleeding or swelling, (4) apply medication, (5) absorb drainage, and/or (6) debride necrotic tissue (Sieggreen, 1987).

Most skin disorders will respond to topical therapy, that is, application of an active ingredient directly to the affected areas. This is applied by way of a pharmacologically inert vehicle that contributes to the therapy with physical properties that protect, soothe, or cleanse. However, there are oc-

Box 18-1 CHARACTERISTICS OF TOPICAL MEDICATIONS

The active ingredient of choice must be safe and suited to the specific disorder.
The proper vehicle must be used to apply the active ingredient to the area. It must reach and maintain sufficient contact with the affected area; it must be nonirritating to affected and healthy skin.
The cosmetic effect of the preparation should not be more unsightly than the lesion.
The cost must be maintained within the means of the family.
Instructions for use of the preparation must be clear.

casions when therapeutic agents are systemically administered. Since the type of medication and the active ingredient vary with the preference of individual practitioners, in the discussions of the various types of skin disorders only a representative example of some of the preferred therapeutic regimens is included.

Topical applications. A variety of topical agents are available for treatment of dermatologic problems. Characteristics of a topical agent are listed in Box 18-1. In addition, several basic concepts are kept in mind. Overtreatment should be avoided. For example, when the dermatitis is acute, the applications should be mild and bland to avoid further irritation. Broken or inflamed skin, especially in children, is more absorbent than intact skin, and chemicals that are nonirritating to intact skin may be quite irritating to inflamed skin. The dermatitic skin is also more likely to develop allergic contact-type sensitization to substances applied as medication or base. Infants and small children are particularly sensitive to topical antihistamines and the "caine" type of anesthetics, both of which are potent allergic sensitizers. Phenol, often incorporated into medications as an antipruritic, is avoided with children.

Topical applications may be applied to treat the disorder, reduce the itching associated with many diseases, decrease external stimuli, or apply external heat or cold. The emollient action of soaks, baths, and lotions provides a soothing film over the skin surface that reduces external stimuli. Application of heat tends to aggravate most conditions, and its use is usually reserved for reducing specific inflammatory processes, such as folliculitis and cellulitis. Ordinarily applications offer greatest relief when they are lukewarm, tepid, or cool.

The most frequent means for topical treatment of skin disorders are wet dressings, soaks, lotions and shake solutions, baths, creams and ointments, sprays and aerosols, pastes, powders, occlusive dressings, soaps and shampoos, other topical treatments, and topical glucocorticoid therapy.

Topical corticosteroid therapy. The glucocorticoids are the therapeutic agents used most widely for skin disorders. Their local antiinflammatory effects are merely palliative so that the medication must be applied until the disease state undergoes a remission or the causative agent is eliminated. Corticosteroids are applied directly to the affected area, and, because they are essentially nonsensitizing and have only minor side effects, they can be applied over prolonged periods with continuing effectiveness. As with the use of any steroids, in large amounts they may mask signs of infection, and there may be exacerbation of symptoms following termination of the drug.

Hydrocortisone preparations are available in sprays, lotions, creams, ointment, gels, suspension, and powders. Many can be purchased without a prescription. Families should be cautioned that the medication cannot be used for all skin disorders. The concentrations available without prescription are not adequate for some stubborn conditions (e.g., psoriasis) and may cause worsening of inflammation caused by fungus or bacteria. It has also been found that users apply too much topical hydrocortisone; therefore they should be counseled that it is both effective and economical to apply only a thin film and massage it into the skin.

Other topical therapies. Other topical treatments include chemical cautery (especially useful for warts), cryosurgery, electrodesiccation (chiefly used for warts, granulomas, and nevi), ultraviolet therapy (primarily used in psoriasis and acne), laser therapy, and special acne therapies such as dermabrasion and acne "surgery."

Systemic therapy. Therapeutic agents are often used as an adjunct to topical therapy in dermatologic disorders, and those most frequently used therapeutically are the corticosteroids and the antibiotics. The corticosteroid hormones with their capacity to inhibit inflammatory and allergic reactions are valuable in the treatment of severe skin disorders. Dosage is carefully adjusted and gradually tapered to the minimum that is effective and tolerated. In infants and children, dosage is larger than is usually calculated from body-weight ratios. Protracted use may temporarily suppress growth, however.

Antibiotics, which interfere with the growth of microorganisms, are used in severe or widespread skin infections. The danger inherent in the use of antibiotics is their tendency to produce a hypersensitivity in the patient; therefore they are used with caution. Antifungal agents are the only means for treating systemic fungal infections.

Nursing Considerations

Skin disorders present nurses with some of their most challenging problems. In children the identification of skin disorders requires a familiarity with various types of lesions in order to accurately describe them and to advise parents regarding medical consultation. Removal of foreign objects (such as small splinters), mild sunburn, and scratches pose no problem, but lesions, lacerations, and bites need careful evaluation and referral.

Assessment

To assist in establishing a diagnosis, it is important for nurses to accurately describe any deviation in the character of the skin, using both inspection and palpation. The color, shape, and distribution of the lesions are noted, including absence of pigment (vitiligo). The individual lesions are described according to the accepted terminology and may involve more than one type, such as a maculopapular rash.

To confirm or amplify the findings made by inspection, the skin is gently palpated to detect characteristics such as temperature, moisture, texture, elasticity, and the presence of edema. It should be indicated whether the findings are restricted to the area of the lesion(s) or are generalized.

The child's subjective symptoms provide additional information. Older children are able to describe the condition as painful, itching, tingling, or in other descriptive terms. However, much can be determined by observation of the younger child's behavior and the parents' account of these reactions. Does the child scratch? Is the child restless or irritable? Does the child favor or avoid using a part? A careful history may provide clues. Has the child had access to chemicals? Has the child been in the woods or around a woodpile? Has the child eaten a new food? Is the child taking medication? Has the child any known allergy? Do any playmates have a similar lesion? A doubtful diagnosis is frequently confirmed on the basis of history.

Nursing Diagnosis

Nursing diagnoses are determined following an assessment of the child and the skin lesions. The major diagnoses identified for the child with a skin disorder are outlined in the Nursing Care Plan on pp. 814-815.

Planning

The goals of care for the child with a skin condition are:

1. Prevent secondary damage to the lesions(s).
2. Relieve discomfort.
3. Educate and support the child and family.

Implementation

Therapeutic programs are usually designed to provide general measures such as rest, protection, and relief of discomfort and specific treatments such as a definitive medication or physical technique. Since only a few skin diseases are contagious, it is usually not necessary to isolate the affected child unless there is a danger of acquiring a secondary infection, for example, the child who is receiving large doses of corticosteroids or other immunosuppressant drugs or the child with an immunologic deficiency disorder. If the skin manifestation is caused by a viral exanthem, such as measles or chicken pox, the child should be prevented from exposing other susceptible children.

Autoinoculation is a constant hazard in some disorders such as impetigo or (to a lesser extent) warts. Measures are implemented to lessen the itching sensation and reduce scratching. Such methods, along with general cleanliness and hygiene, also serve to reduce the likelihood of secondary infection of a primary lesion.

NURSING TIP: DRYING SKIN SURFACES

A hair dryer, on the cool or low setting, is an excellent means for drying skin areas prone to collect moisture, such as the neck (under the chin), axilla, groin, and between the buttocks.

Relief of symptoms. Most of the therapeutic regimens are directed toward relief of pruritus, the most common subjective complaint. Itching is believed to result from stimulation of C fibers at the dermoepidermal junction. These fibers are similar to but distinct from pain fibers. Substances released within the skin, histamine and endopeptidases, also elicit itching, although their release triggers are unknown (Barnett, 1987).

Cooling the affected area and increasing the skin pH make conditions for enzymatic action less favorable (Madden, 1986). Such measures include cool baths or compresses to reduce external stimuli to the area and alkaline applications, such as baking soda baths, to increase skin pH. Maintenance of cleanliness and good aeration improve comfort. Clothing and bed linen should be soft and lightweight to decrease the irritation from friction and stimulation.

During any type of treatment, both affected and unaffected skin is protected from damage and secondary infection. Preventing scratching is of primary importance. The cooperation of older children can be obtained, although they may need reminding to stop scratching or rubbing, but in smaller and uncooperative children, the use of techniques and devices such as mittens, restraints (especially during sleep), or special coverings is required. Keeping fingernails short, well-trimmed, and clean helps reduce the chance of secondary infection.

Antipruritic medications may be prescribed for severe itching, especially if it disturbs the child's rest. Pain and discomfort are usually managed with nonpharmacologic measures and mild analgesia; severe pain may require more potent medication (see Pain Management, Chapter 26).

Topical therapy. Therapy usually involves some type of topical treatment, and the mode of application depends on the nature and location of the lesion being treated. For example, soothing lotions, creams, and intermittent wet dressings or soaks help cool and dry; ointments, lotions, and creams soften and lubricate dry, scaling areas. Nurses and parents are responsible for the application of topical therapeutic agents and the administration of systemic medications. Therefore an understanding of the various methods of application, the type and consistency of the preparation, and their purposes and uses is needed for effective application.

NURSING CARE PLAN
The Child with a Skin Disorder

NURSING DIAGNOSIS: Impaired skin integrity related to environmental agents, somatic factors, immunologic deficit

GOAL 1
Promote healing

INTERVENTIONS

Carry out therapeutic regimens as prescribed or support and assist parents in carrying out treatment plan
*Administer topical treatments and applications
*Administer systemic medications, if ordered
Prevent secondary infection and autoinoculation
Encourage rest
Reduce external stimuli that aggravate condition
Encourage well-balanced diet
Administer skin care and general hygiene measures

EXPECTED OUTCOME

Affected area exhibits signs of healing

NURSING DIAGNOSIS: Potential impaired skin integrity related to mechanical trauma, body secretions, increased susceptibility to infection

GOAL 1
Maintain skin integrity

INTERVENTIONS

Keep skin clean and dry; cleanse skin at least once daily
Inspect total skin area frequently for evidence of irritation or breakdown
Protect skinfolds and surfaces that rub together
Keep clothing and linen clean and dry
Apply protective lotion to areas where excoriation is most likely (e.g., anal and perineal areas, knees, elbows, ankles, and chin)
Carry out good perineal care under urine collection device, when applicable
Keep suture line dry, especially in areas subject to moisture (e.g., mouth, perineum)

EXPECTED OUTCOME

Skin remains clean, dry, and free of irritation

GOAL 2
Prevent secondary infection

INTERVENTIONS

Maintain careful handwashing before handling affected child
Wear surgical gloves when handling or dressing affected parts if indicated by nature of lesion
Teach child and family hygienic care and medical asepsis
Devise methods to prevent secondary infection of lesion in small or uncooperative children
- Keep nails short and clean
- Apply mittens or elbow restraints
- Dress in one-piece outfit with long sleeves and legs

EXPECTED OUTCOME

Skin lesions remain confined to primary sites

GOAL 3
Protect healthy skin surface

INTERVENTIONS

Teach and impress on child importance of keeping hands away from lesion(s)
Help child determine ways of preventing autoinoculation
Devise means for keeping small or uncooperative children from spreading infection to other areas
Protect healthy skin from maceration by keeping it dry

EXPECTED OUTCOME

Healthy skin remains clean and intact

NURSING DIAGNOSIS: Potential for infection related to presence of infective organisms

GOAL 1
Prevent spread of infection to self and others

INTERVENTIONS

Implement universal precautions (see Chapter 27)
Isolate affected child from susceptible individuals if indicated
Maintain careful handwashing after caring for child
Avoid unnecessary close contact with affected child during infective stage of disease
Use correct technique for disposal of dressings, solutions, and other fomites in contact with lesion(s)
Teach and reinforce positive habits of hygienic care

EXPECTED OUTCOMES

Infection remains confined to primary site
Child and family comply with preventive measures

NURSING DIAGNOSIS: Potential impaired skin integrity related to allergenic factors

GOAL 1
Prevent occurrence and/or recurrence

*Dependent nursing action.

NURSING CARE PLAN
The Child with a Skin Disorder—cont'd

INTERVENTIONS

Avoid or reduce contact with agents or circumstances known to precipitate skin reaction
Teach child to recognize agents or circumstances that produce reaction

EXPECTED OUTCOME

Child avoids precipitating agents

NURSING DIAGNOSIS: Pain related to skin lesions, pruritus

GOAL 1

Relieve discomfort

INTERVENTIONS

Avoid or reduce external stimuli that aggravate discomfort, such as clothing and bed linen
Implement other appropriate nonpharmacologic pain reduction techniques (see Chapter 26)
*Apply soothing treatments and topical applications as ordered
*Administer medications to relieve discomfort and/or restlessness and irritability
See Nursing Care Plan: The Child in Pain, Chapter 26

EXPECTED OUTCOME

Child remains calm and exhibits no evidence of discomfort

NURSING DIAGNOSIS: Body image disturbance related to perception of appearance

GOAL 1

Promote a positive self-image

INTERVENTIONS

Encourage child to express feelings about personal appearance and perceived reactions of others

EXPECTED OUTCOME

Child verbalizes feelings and concerns

GOAL 2

Provide tactile contact

INTERVENTIONS

Hold child
Remember that there is no substitute for the stimulation and comfort of human contact
Touch and caress unaffected area

EXPECTED OUTCOMES

Child exhibits signs of comfort
Child responds positively to tactile stimulation

GOAL 3

Support child

INTERVENTIONS

Teach self-care where appropriate
Involve child in planning treatment schedules
Support and encourage child in efforts to deal with multiple problems that may be associated with disorder, including discomfort, rejection, discouragement, and feelings of self-revulsion
Encourage child to maintain usual activities

EXPECTED OUTCOMES

Child collaborates in determining means for improving appearance
Child maintains customary activities and relationships

NURSING DIAGNOSIS: Altered family processes related to having a child with a severe skin condition (e.g., eczema, psoriasis, ichthyosis)

GOAL 1

Support family

INTERVENTIONS

Teach family skills needed to carry out therapeutic program
Inform family of expected and unexpected results of therapy and a course of action to follow
Help devise special techniques to carry out therapy
Be aware of overprotectiveness and restrictiveness, which can stifle child's emotional growth
Allow and encourage family members, particularly the one who cares for the child most of the time, to express negative feelings, such as anger, frustration, and perhaps guilt
Stress that negative feelings are normal, acceptable, and expected but that they must have an outlet in order for family members to remain healthy
Encourage family in efforts to carry out plan of care
Provide assistance when appropriate
Refer to agencies and services that assist with social, financial, and medical problems

EXPECTED OUTCOME

Family demonstrates necessary skills (specify)

*Dependent nursing action.

NURSING TIP: APPLYING LOTION

Children love to be "painted." Therefore lotion applications can be fun when an ordinary paintbrush is used.

NURSING TIP: TOPICAL APPLICATIONS

Apply topical applications systematically with the contour of the body surface (not simply up and down).

It is especially important to wash the hands before and after application of topical therapies. The skin is assessed before the treatment or application of medication and reassessed after the treatment is completed. Any observed changes are noted and described. Nursing responsibilities related to specific disorders are discussed in relation to those disorders.

Wet compresses. Wet compresses or dressings are probably the mildest form of topical therapy. They cool the skin by evaporation, relieve itching and inflammation, and cleanse the area by loosening and removing crusts and debris. Any of a variety of ingredients, such as the time-honored Burow solution (available without a prescription), can be applied on Kerlix gauze, plain gauze, or (preferably) soft cotton cloths such as freshly laundered handkerchiefs or strips from diaper, sheeting, or pillowcase material.

Dressings immersed in the desired solution are wrung out slightly and applied to the affected area wet but not dripping. They are applied flat and smooth and in such a way that motion is not totally restricted—fingers are wrapped separately, and arms and legs are wrapped so that elbows and knees can bend. Dressings are kept in place by Kerlix or other cotton wrap, tubular stockinette, mittens, and socks (two pair—one to hold the dressings in place, the other to take up movement) but are left uncovered. When evaporation begins to dry them, the dressings are removed, rewet in the solution, and reapplied to the area using aseptic technique. The solution is not poured or syringed directly over the dressings. As fluid evaporates, the solution becomes increasingly concentrated and thus stronger, which may be damaging to sensitive lesions.

Water is the most important ingredient in wet dressings, and evaporation is primarily responsible for the symptomatic relief experienced by the patient. The most common solutions used for wet dressings are aluminum acetate (Burow solution) and normal saline, which are applied to cleanse and disinfect open, oozing, crusting, and/or secondarily infected lesions. Sometimes fresh warm or tepid tap water is used alone or in conjunction with topical steroids.

Fresh solution at room temperature is applied at 2-, 3-, or 4-hour intervals and is allowed to remain on the lesion from 30 minutes to 1½ hours. Wet dressings are seldom continued after about 48 hours. The child must be guarded against chilling during treatment, and no more than 20% of the body should be covered at one time to avoid the risk of hypothermia. After treatment the skin is dried thoroughly by patting with a towel. Application of lotion or other medication may be ordered at this time.

Moist dressings. Dry dressings are commonly used only on wounds that produce considerable exudate. Dry dressings adhere to the wound surface, damaging newly forming tissue. Skin lesions heal in a moist environment. The dressing is squeezed or wrung to remove excess moisture before application and changed before it dries to ensure continuous moisture. The dressings may be gauze or cotton saturated with the desired solution. Transparent dressings also function as moist dressings. The adhesive sticks to intact epithelium but not to new epithelium. Because they are transparent, they allow for wound assessment and require fewer changes than traditional moist dressings.

Occlusive dressings. Used primarily in association with topical steroids, occlusive dressings are usually restricted to treatment of chronic dermatoses. A thin application of ointment or cream is covered with a thin, transparent, pliable plastic film anchored with adhesive. Occlusive dressings promote moisture retention, nonevaporation of the vehicle, and maceration of the epidermis, all of which increase the penetration of medications. Although of value in certain situations, the dangers are bacterial and candidal infections, sweat retention, and increased likelihood of side effects from the medication used. The treatment consists of an 8- to 10-hour period, usually overnight, and covers no greater than 10% of the body.

Small children may need some type of restraint, depending on the location of the dressing. Often clothing can be worn that covers the area; for example, leg dressings are covered with pants legs. If the child attempts to remove or disturb the dressings, elbow restraints may be needed. Diversional activities are always a useful nursing tool.

Soaks. When young children are uncooperative in the use of wet dressings, soaks are often employed for removal of crusts and for their mild astringent action, using the same solution employed for wet compresses. Gaining young children's cooperation for hand or foot soaks is difficult unless the procedure is made attractive to them through play (see Nursing Tips: Water Play Activities). The

NURSING TIPS: WATER PLAY ACTIVITIES

Older infants and toddlers delight in playing with brightly colored objects or poker chips scattered over the bottom of the receptacle, and preschoolers can be challenged to hold a floating item beneath the water's surface. These activities require supervision; infants and small children will often place items in their mouths, and children can easily lose control with water play.

Washing dishes, cars, dolls, or doll clothes will occupy many children for quite some time.

older child is able to cooperate but may need something to do during the procedure such as listening to music, a story, or watching television.

NURSING TIP: SOAKING AN EXTREMITY

Soaking a single extremity (a foot or a hand) can be easily accomplished by placing the solution and the extremity in a plastic sealable bag. The closure is then zipped snugly around the limb. This method for soaking fingers or toes can be highly entertaining to young children (Perelson and Seyler, 1985).

Baths. Baths are especially useful in the treatment of widespread dermatitis by evenly distributing the soothing antipruritic and antiinflammatory effects of the solution, usually oatmeal or mineral oil preparations. The solution is added to a tub of lukewarm water. The temperature of the bath is tepid, and the duration of treatment is usually 15 to 30 minutes. Therapeutic baths are always more interesting when the child is accompanied by toy boats or other items for water play.

Topical applications. Various applications are applied to skin lesions to ease discomfort, prevent further injury, and facilitate healing. The most frequently used applications are described in Table 18-1.

Table 18-1 Topical preparations

DESCRIPTION	CHARACTERISTICS	APPLICATION	COMMENTS
Lotions Powder suspended in solution	Liquid evaporates, cools the skin Provides a coating of soothing, lubricating, protective, drying powder	Apply evenly over skin with hands or gauze "Paint" on with brush or cotton ball	Not applied to oozing surfaces Ordinarily not washed off between applications Removed by soaking with solution used for soaks or dressings
Creams and gels Thick liquid or soft solid	Contain oil with a high melting point (cream) Tend to disappear when rubbed into skin	Place a teaspoonful in palm of hand and rub briskly between hands until thin and smooth Apply to skin area	Less occlusive than other preparations Esthetically more pleasing Nongreasy, easily applied Readily removed with soap and water
Ointment Oil is main constituent: animal (lanolin), petrolatum, vegetable oil	Those with high water content disappear on application Water-repellent ointments retain heat for increased absorption of medication Can cause maceration when used with occlusive dressings Absorbent ointments contain no water but absorb water	Not applied to hairy, intertriginous, or macerated areas	Greasy sensation Difficult to remove with water (except those with high water content) Absorbent ointments are more lubricating than water-in-oil
Pastes Powders mixed with ointment base	Medications incorporated into pastes are released more slowly than from creams and ointments More porous and less occlusive than ointments	Apply with a tongue depressor and "butter" on	More difficult to apply Must be removed with mineral oil
Powders Chemically inert	Soothing Absorb moisture Reduce friction Chiefly prophylactic Applied to intertriginous areas	Apply in fine film to prevent caking and lumping when wet Sprinkle powder in palm, then apply to skin	Use is controversial in pediatrics Exert care to prevent inhalation by child
Sprays and aerosols Active agents suspended in alcohol-base spray	Alternative method of delivering a solution to skin	Shake container thoroughly before application Shield child's face from spray to avoid inhalation	Useful when direct application is difficult or uncomfortable for the child Uncomfortable for patient
Soaps and shampoos Bacterial agents	Effective in eliminating common pathogens and parasites	Bathe or shampoo as usual	Useful adjunctive treatment Those containing hexachlorophene used with caution
Sunscreen agents (see p. 834)			

Discharge planning and family support. Childhood dermatologic conditions always involve the family. Since few situations require hospitalization and children who are hospitalized will complete a therapy program at home, the family must carry out the treatment plan; therefore their cooperation is essential. Child and parents are more apt to be motivated if they are told why something is being done in a certain way. Success of treatment depends on the correct interpretation of instructions, and it is often the nurse's responsibility to teach the parent how to carry out the instructions and offer encouragement, support, and assistance with problem solving.

Regimens that are simple to accomplish in the hospital or office situation may be frustrating and baffling at home. The family often needs assistance in adapting equipment available in the home to the therapy, for example, dressings from clean scraps and rags and the use of utensils for soaks. One of the most difficult areas to deal with is the child's irritability and tendency to disturb dressings and scratch or pick at lesions. Nurses can help parents devise protective restraining devices and distracting activities for the child. Treatments at home, in the clinic, or in the clinician's office that are scheduled and arranged to accommodate the child's schooling, as well as the parents' activities, are more apt to be carried out.

It is important that parents and child be given as much explanation as possible about both the expected and the unexpected results of treatment, including any ill effects that might occur. Although a treatment plan is chosen for its probability of being beneficial without doing harm, using medications that contain the fewest and safest ingredients, persons with skin disorders are highly susceptible to irritation. They are directed to discontinue treatment and report any unexpected reactions to the appropriate person(s). Skin changes bother people so that they often try anything, including home remedies and patent medicines. The use of patent medicines is discouraged unless this has first been discussed with the practitioner and has received approval.

Since the skin is the most visible portion of the body, defects in its surface that alter its appearance are sometimes an additional source of distress to the affected child and the family. Unsightly lesions or medicinal preparations applied to the skin are often sources of revulsion and rejection by others. Other children will make derogatory comments and may even reject the affected child. Parents of other children may fear that their children will "catch" the disorder. Occasionally the affected child's own family will reduce their interaction with him, especially close physical contact, or otherwise demonstrate a distaste for the condition that the child may interpret as rejection. This is seldom a difficulty with dermatitis of short duration, but chronic conditions can create problems in development of a positive self-concept.

Evaluation

The effectiveness of nursing interventions is determined by continual reassessment and evaluation of care based on the following observational guidelines and expected outcomes:

1. Observe if reasonable care is used in performing nursing activities, monitor lesions, and observe child's reactions to therapies.
2. Use assessment techniques to recognize relief of discomfort as described in Chapter 26.
3. Reassess skin lesions; observe and interview child and family regarding compliance with therapy.

Expected outcomes:
See Nursing Care Plan, pp. 814-815.

WOUNDS

Wounds are produced in a variety of ways, and the manner and extent of the injury determines the manner of healing and the form of management. In general, wounds are classified as *open* if the skin has been divided or disrupted and *closed* if the skin surface remains intact (Box 18-2). Wounds can also be superficial, involving only the epidermis, or deep, involving the dermis, subcutanous tissue, and even deeper structures.

Epidermal Injuries

Abrasions are the most common epidermal wounds of childhood, usually in the form of a skinned knee or elbow. In most injuries the margins of the abraded area are superficial, involving only the outer layers of epidermis, although the central portion may extend into the dermis. Initially the defect is filled by a blood clot and necrotic debris, which subsequently dehydrate to form a scab. Epithelial tissue is composed of *labile* cells, which are constantly destroyed and replaced throughout life. Injury to these tissues is accomplished by *regeneration,* that is, rapid replacement by similar cells.

The epithelial wound heals by migration and proliferation of epithelial cells from the wound margin and from cells surviving in transected skin appendages. This response begins within 24 to 48 hours after the wound is incurred. Cell migration ceases when migrating cells make

Box 18-2 TYPES OF WOUNDS

Closed Wounds
Blister—raised circumscribed area of epidermis containing serum
Contusion—injury to subcutaneous tissues without disrupting the skin
Sprain—disruption in continuity of a ligament
Fracture—discontinuity of bone tissue

Open Wounds
Abrasion—removal of the superficial layers of skin by rubbing or scraping
Evulsion—forcible pulling out or extraction of tissue
Laceration—torn or jagged wound; accidental cut wound
Incision—a division of the skin made with a sharp object; cut
Penetrating wound—disruption of the skin surface that extends into underlying tissue or into a body cavity
Puncture—a wound with relatively small opening compared to the depth

contact with epithelial cells migrating from all other sites. Fixed basal cells adjacent to the wound edge and in skin appendages begin to divide rapidly to replace the migrated cells. As resurfacing is accomplished, the migrated cells begin to divide and thicken the new epithelial layer. When coverage of the wound surface is completed, the scab sloughs off, and keratinization begins.

To prevent possible tattooing, an abrasion from which the dirt cannot be removed will require abrading under topical anesthesia, and those covering a very large area (over 15% of the body) will need medical attention.

Injury to Deeper Tissues

Tissues composed of *permanent* cells, such as muscle and nerve cells, are unable to regenerate. Therefore these tissues *repair* themselves by substituting fibrous connective tissue for the injured tissue. This fibrous tissue, or scar, serves as a patch to preserve or restore the continuity of the tissue. Wounds involving permanent cells include surgical incisions, lacerations, ulcers, evulsions, and full-thickness burns. Injured cells of glandular organs and bones, composed of *stable* cells, multiply less vigorously and heal more slowly (see Bone Healing and Remodeling, Chapter 39).

Process of wound healing. The nonspecific repair mechanism of wound healing with scar formation involves the processes of *inflammation, fibroplasia, contraction,* and *scar maturation.* Table 18-2 sums up the healing process.

Inflammation. The initial response at the site of injury is inflammation, a vascular and cellular response, which prepares the tissues for subsequent repair process. There is a transient constriction of transected blood vessels, lasting 5 to 10 minutes, followed by active vasodilation of all local small vessels and increased blood flow to the area. This is accompanied by increased permeability of small venules, allowing plasma to leak into surrounding tissues (edema). A blood clot is formed along wound edges, forming a framework for future growth of capillaries and epithelial cells.

At the same time vessel walls become lined with leukocytes, which pass through the walls and concentrate at the injured site, where they ingest bacteria and debris (phagocytosis). Fibroblasts attracted to the area from blood vessels deposit fibrin throughout the clot. Adjacent capillaries begin to form buds that stretch across the supporting fibrin threads, and epithelial cells secrete a fibrolytic enzyme that allows their advancement across the wound. This initial phase of wound healing takes place during the first 3 to 5 days following injury.

Fibroplasia. Fibroplasia (*granulation* or *proliferation*), the second phase of healing, lasts from 5 days to 4 weeks. Fibroblasts, immature connective tissue cells, migrate to the healing site and begin to secrete collagen into the meshwork spaces. Granulation tissue is highly vascular, reddish-colored connective tissue that organizes and restructures, forming thicker, stronger fibers arranged in orderly layers. A thin layer of epithelial tissue is regenerated over the surface of the wound, and leukocytes gradually disappear from the area.

Contraction and maturation. During the third and fourth phases of wound healing *(differentiation, maturation)* collagen continues to be deposited and organized into layers, compressing the new blood vessels and gradually ceasing blood flow across the wound. Fibroblasts disappear as the wound becomes stronger. Fibroblast movement causes contraction of the healing area, helping to bring wound edges closer together. A mature scar is then formed. The maturation process may continue for years, and the extent to which the scar remodels and matures varies among individuals.

Table 18-2 Summary of wound healing process

PHASE	ACTIVITY	COMMENTS
1. Inflammation (3 to 5 days)	Clot formation as meshwork for capillary growth Inflammation with phagocytosis; wound debris removed Epithelial cell migration	Wound weakest during this phase
2. Fibroplasia (5 days to 4 weeks)	Granulation tissue formed Migration of fibroblasts Secretion of collagen Abundant capillary buds	Wound fragile Granulation tissue bleeds profusely if disturbed
3. Scar contracture (1 to 6 weeks)	Continued deposition of collagen Further organization and remodeling Blood vessels compressed Healing area contracts Blood flow across wound gradually ceases	Appears as broad, pinkish, raised scar Heavy use of any affected muscles is discouraged
4. Scar maturation (several months)	Formation of mature scar Shrinkage of wound Contracture deformity can occur if wound is near a joint	Scar is acellular and avascular tissue Pale in color Does not tan when exposed to sunlight Will not sweat or produce hair May cause itching

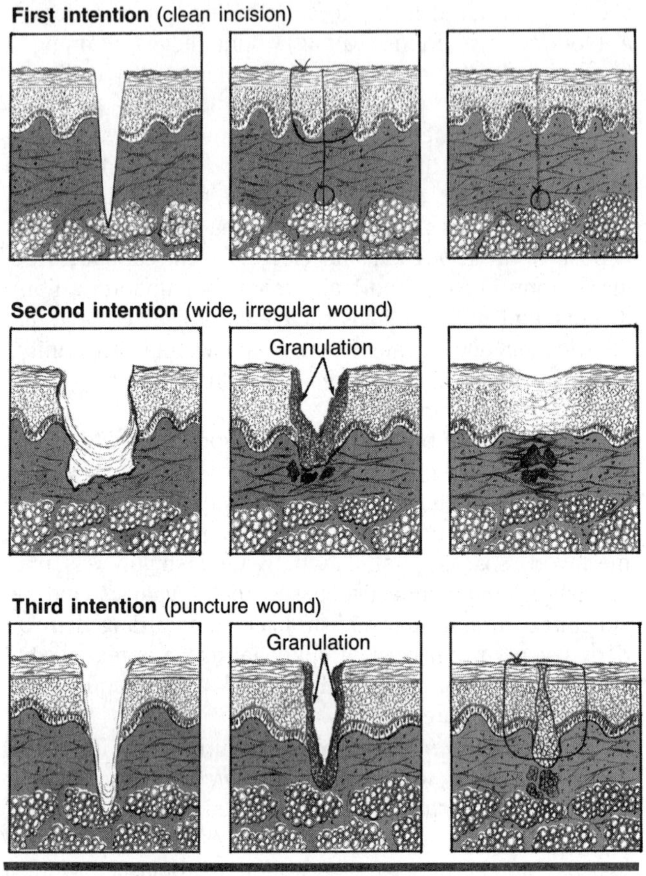

Fig. 18-4. Types of wound healing.

Types of wound healing. Repair healing takes place in one of three ways: by *primary, secondary,* or *tertiary intention* (Fig. 18-4). Primary intention healing takes place when all layers of the wound (skin, subcutaneous tissue, and muscle) margins are neatly approximated, as in a surgical incision. Unless infection interferes or the wound edges separate, these wounds heal with a minimum of scarring.

Repair by secondary intention takes place in wounds that occur from ulceration and lacerations in which the edges cannot be approximated, such as an evulsion or a third-degree burn. The inflammatory reaction may be greater, and the chance of infection increased. Often debris, cells, and exudate must be cleaned away (debrided) before healing can take place. Healing takes place from the edges inward and from the bottom of the wound upward until the defect is filled. More granulation tissue and a larger scar are formed than in healing by primary intention.

Repair by tertiary intention takes place when suturing is delayed after injury or the wound later breaks down and is sutured or resutured when granulation is present. More granulation tissue is formed than in healing by primary intention, and there is greater chance of microorganisms invading the wound. Frequently suturing a contaminated wound is deliberately delayed to afford better removal of infection before closing. Wounds healed by tertiary intention result in a larger and deeper scar than in primary intention.

Children heal aggressively with abundant scar tissue, especially during growth spurts. The highly elastic quality of children's skin pulls on wounds, which defend against the pull by aggressive scarring. Consequently, the child's skin heals with more scar tissue than the less elastic skin of the adult (Jobe, 1990).

Factors That Influence Healing

Numerous factors can influence the rate and efficiency of wound healing. In general, wounds in children heal more rapidly than those in older persons because of their increased metabolism and good circulation. Factors that delay wound healing are outlined in Table 18-3. Some research has indicated that a topical application of epidermal growth factor (EGF) significantly accelerated the rate of wound healing (Brown and others, 1989).

Nursing Considerations

Cuts, scratches, scrapes, and abrasions are all part of growing up. No child escapes them. Small injuries to the skin are managed by the parents at home with only a few simple guidelines from the nurse. Cuts on the face, a gaping cut

Table 18-3 Factors influencing wound healing

FACTOR	EFFECT ON HEALING
Nutritional deficiencies	
Vitamin C	Inhibits formation of collagen fibers and capillary development
Protein	Reduces supply of amino acids for tissue repair
Zinc	Impairs epithelialization
Impaired circulation	Reduces supply of nutrients to wound area Inhibits inflammatory response and removal of debris from wound area
Corticosteroids	Impair phagocytosis Inhibit fibroblast proliferation Depress formation of granulation tissue Inhibits wound contraction
Foreign bodies	Inhibit wound closure Increase inflammatory response
Infection	Increases inflammatory response Increases tissue destruction
Mechanical friction	Damages or destroys granulation tissue
Fluid accumulation	Accumulation in area inhibits tissues from approximating
Radiation	Inhibits fibroblastic activity and capillary formation May cause tissue necrosis
Diseases	
Diabetes mellitus	Inhibits collagen synthesis Impairs circulation and capillary growth Hyperglycemia impairs phagocytosis
Anemia	Reduces oxygen supply to tissues

longer than 1/4 inch, or one that bleeds persistently should be evaluated for possible suturing. Those covering a very large area (over 15% of the body) will need medical attention. There is also a high risk of contamination from wounds sustained in a bicycle injury. Since abrasions are often painful, analgesics such as acetaminophen are advised.

Parents are instructed to wash their hands, then wash the wound vigorously but gently with soap and water for at least 5 minutes, and rinse the wound well. If possible, the wound is left exposed to air, since wounds heal faster without a dressing. However, if the area is one that will probably get dirty, it can be covered with a Band-Aid sterile dressing. Ointments, sprays, alcohol, or antiseptic preparations are not needed; some sting and can damage normal tissue.

Abrasions are cleaned in the same manner as wounds, except that any foreign matter must be removed with clean tweezers, and loose skin cut off with sterile scissors. Small abrasions are left exposed; larger ones are covered with Telfa or other nonstick dressing that is changed in 12 hours, and the wound left uncovered after 24 hours. Bruises are managed with ice applications for 20 to 30 minutes.

Lacerations present a special challenge to nurses. The injured child and family are usually very distressed by the bleeding, variable degrees of shock, and the guilt that usually accompany the injury. Because scalp lacerations bleed so profusely, they are especially frightening. The initial nursing intervention is to apply pressure to the area and attempt to calm the child before undertaking further examination. Unless there is bleeding from a severed artery, the wound can be cleansed with a forced jet of sterile tepid water or saline (via syringe) and examined for extent, depth, and presence of foreign material such as dirt, glass, or fabric fragments. The location of the wound also dictates assessment. For example, wounds over bony areas may contain bone chips, and clear fluid seeping from severe head wounds may indicate cerebrospinal fluid. (See also Trauma Management, Chapter 39, and Head Injury, Chapter 37.) A pressure dressing is applied for transfer to medical care; the child in a medical facility is prepared for suturing.

Hydrogen peroxide and povidone-iodine are contraindicated for cleaning fresh open wounds. Hydrogen peroxide can cause formation of subcutaneous gas when applied under pressure (Schneider and Hebert, 1987). Both solutions can be toxic to freshly injured tissues (Oberg and Lindsey, 1987). For many children the use of topical anesthesia for repair of lacerations has reduced the discomfort and anxiety generated by injected anesthesia (Bonadio and Wagner, 1988). The topical solution of tetracaine, epinephrine, and cocaine (TAC) is most often mentioned. However, the safety of this topical anesthetic appears to be site- and dose-related and has not been established for very young children. Therefore it is to be used on nonmucosal surfaces and in minimal doses and used cautiously (if at all) in infants. Sutured lacerations are managed the same as surgical incisions. (See Chapter 26 for nonpharmacologic and pharmacologic pain management.)

Puncture wounds that do not require a tetanus booster (see Chapter 39) are soaked in warm water and soap for 15 minutes. Causing the wound to rebleed may be helpful. A Band-Aid can be applied if desired. The wound is carefully observed for signs of infection from dirt and bacteria that might be trapped beneath the wound surface. Puncture wounds of the head, chest, or abdomen or those that could still contain a portion of the puncturing object must be evaluated.

Parents are cautioned against opening blood blisters and against kissing the wound "to make it better." The wound can easily become contaminated from germs in the human mouth. Also, scabs would be allowed to slough off without assistance; picking or early removal may cause scarring. Parents are advised to seek medical help if there is evidence of infection.

Surgical incisions. Care of a surgical incision is directed toward maintaining the integrity of the site, promoting the healing process, and preventing complications. The current postsurgery management is to remove the original dressing 24 to 48 hours after surgery so the incision can be exposed to air. Nurses, or parents if they desire, cleanse the skin and apply the dressing while the child is in the hospital, and parents continue the procedure at home.

Parents are instructed to wash their hands thoroughly with soap and water and clean under their fingernails. They then remove the dressing and wash the wound gently with mild soap and water. If the dressing adheres to the stitches, they can wet it with lukewarm water until it can be removed without difficulty. Because a washcloth might catch on stitches, the parents are advised to use their hands for washing the wound. The wound is then rinsed with clear, lukewarm water and dried with a clean, soft towel. A dry sterile dressing or adhesive bandage is applied, or the wound is left uncovered, according to specific instructions. The child is usually allowed to shower after 48 hours but is advised not to bathe.

Open wounds. Open wounds, such as denuded areas, excoriations, pressure ulcers, or evulsed wounds are managed by application of moist dressings or synthetic plastic-film dressings. Because dehydration damages tissues in the wound bed, the injured tissues are not allowed to dry completely. Crusts impede epithelial migration and thus delay healing. (See Burns, Chapter 29.)

A number of therapies have been advocated for treatment of pressure necrosis, depending on the stage of sore development and the philosophy of the therapist or institution protocol. For management of this important problem, the reader is directed to the extensive literature available on the topic.

FOREIGN BODIES

Small wooden splinters can be removed by parents with a needle and tweezers that have been sterilized with alcohol or a flame. The area around the sliver is washed with soap and water before attempting the removal. The sliver is exposed with the needle and then grasped firmly by the tweezers and pulled in the same direction in which it entered. Some foreign bodies should have medical evaluation; these include a fishhook, a deeply imbedded object such as a needle in a foot or near a joint, glass splinters, or other difficult-to-see objects. A small hand vacuum cleaner is effective in removing loose items such as glass splinters, gravel, dirt, or leaves from the surface of the skin before they become imbedded. This is especially valuable for trauma victims.

Cactus Spines

Small cactus prickles or spines are often troublesome to remove, and attempts are distressing to the child and family. Large spines or clumps can be removed with tweezers. To remove very fine spines, a number of options are available. In a study using a variety of methods on animal models, Martinez and others (1987) found that the most effective method involved an application of a thin layer of water-soluble household glue covered with a single layer of gauze. The application was allowed to dry, then removed. Other methods reported as highly successful include the following:

- Apply hair removal wax, let dry, and remove (Hennes, 1988). Takes less time to dry than glue.
- Place cellophane tape, sticky side down, over the spines and lift off (Cooper, 1988).

Table 18-4 Bacterial infections

DISORDER/ ORGANISM	MANIFESTATIONS	MANAGEMENT	COMMENTS
Impetigo contagiosa (Fig. 18-5; see also Color Plate 17)—*Staphylococcus, Streptococcus*	Begins as a reddish macule Becomes vesicular Ruptures easily, leaving superficial, moist erosion Tends to spread peripherally in sharply marginated irregular outlines Exudate dries to form heavy, honey-colored crusts Pruritus common Systemic effects: minimal or asymptomatic See Chapter 9 for bullous impetigo	Careful removal of undermined skin, crusts, and debris by softening with 1:20 Burow solution compresses Topical application of bactericidal ointment Systemic administration of oral or parenteral antibiotics (penicillin) in severe or extensive lesions	Tends to heal without scarring unless secondary infection Autoinoculable and contagious Very common in toddler, preschooler
Pyoderma—*Staphylococcus, Streptococcus*	Deeper extension of infection into dermis Tissue reaction more severe Systemic effects: fever, lymphangitis	Soap and water cleansing Wet compresses Bathing with antibacterial soap as prescribed	Autoinoculable and contagious May heal with or without scarring
Folliculitis (pimple), furuncle (boil), carbuncle (multiple boils)—*Staphylococcus aureus*	Folliculitis: infection of hair follicle Furuncle: larger lesion with more redness and swelling at a single follicle Carbuncle: more extensive lesion with widespread inflammation and "pointing" at several follicular orifices Systemic effects: malaise, if severe	Skin cleanliness Local warm moist compresses Topical application of antibiotic agents Systemic antibiotics in severe cases Incision and drainage of severe lesions, followed by wound irrigations with antibiotics or suitable drain implantation	Autoinoculable and contagious Furuncle and carbuncle tend to heal with scar formation A lesion should *never* be squeezed
Cellulitis—*Streptotoccus, Staphylococcus, Haemophilus influenzae*	Inflammation of skin and subcutaneous tissues with intense redness, swelling, and firm infiltration Lymphangitis "streaking" frequently seen Involvement of regional lymph nodes common May progress to abscess formation Systemic effects: fever, malaise	Oral or parenteral antibiotics Rest and immobilization of both affected area and child Hot moist compresses to area	Hospitalization may be necessary for child with systemic symptoms Otitis media may be associated with facial cellulitis
Staphylococcal scalded skin syndrome—*Staphylococcus aureus*	Macular erythema with "sandpaper" texture of involved skin Epidermis becomes wrinkled (in 2 days or less) and large bullae appear	Systemic administration of antibiotics Gentle cleansing with saline, Burow solution, or 0.25% silver nitrate compresses	Infant subject to fluid loss, impaired body temperature regulation, and secondary infection, such as pneumonia, cellulitis, and septicemia Heals without scarring

- Drop wax from a lighted candle over the affected area (from a sufficient height to avoid burning the skin), then cool by immersing in cold water and lift off.
- Apply facial beauty mask gel (Gelbard, 1984; Putnam and Lawton, 1985).

INFECTIONS OF THE SKIN

Dermatologic infections and other disorders of the skin constitute a significant portion of children's visits to offices and clinics. The social nature of school children and their proximity to other children render them highly susceptible to communicable diseases, including those caused by parasites. Most are troublesome ailments and are the source of considerable physical and emotional discomfort. For most of the disorders the diagnosis and treatment are relatively simple; for others the management is more complex and puzzling.

BACTERIAL INFECTIONS

Normally the skin harbors a variety of bacterial flora, including the major pathogenic varieties of staphylococci and streptococci. The degree of their pathogenicity depends on the specific organism's invasiveness and toxigenicity, the integrity of the skin, the barrier of the host, and the immune and cellular defenses of the host. Children with immune deficiency states are highly susceptible to bacterial invasion. This includes infants, children with congenital immune deficiency disorders, children in a debilitated condition, those on immunosuppressive therapy, and those with a generalized malignancy such as leukemia or lymphoma.

Because of the characteristic "walling-off" process of the inflammatory reaction (abscess formation), staphylococci are more difficult to treat, and the local infected area is associated with an increase in numbers of bacteria all over the skin surface that serve as a source of continuing infection. Staphylococcal infections occur most often in children in the younger age-groups, and the incidence decreases with advancing age. All of these factors emphasize the importance of careful handwashing and cleanliness when caring for infected children and their lesions to prevent spread of the infection and as an essential prophylactic measure when caring for infants and small children. Common bacterial skin disorders are outlined in Table 18-4.

Nursing Considerations

The major nursing functions related to bacterial skin infections are to prevent the spread of infection and to prevent complications. Handwashing is mandatory before and after contact with an affected child. Handwashing is also emphasized to both the child and the family, and the child should be provided with towels separate from other family members. Impetigo contagiosa is easily spread by self-inoculation; therefore the child must be cautioned against touching the involved area. This is difficult to accomplish. Distraction or reminders are useful but are not helpful when the child is alone, such as bedtime.

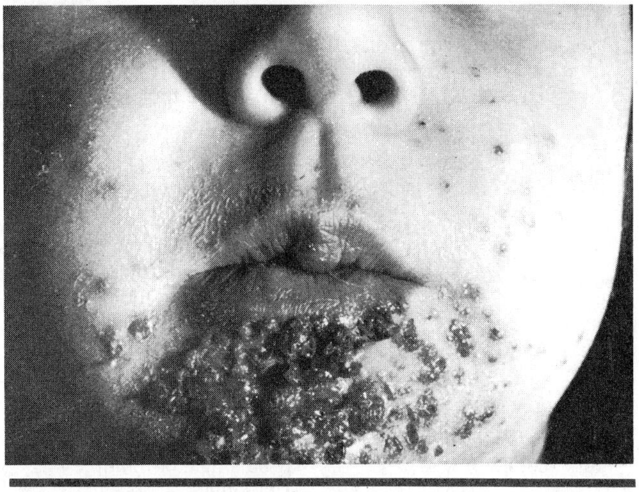

Fig. 18-5. Impetigo contagiosa. (See also Color Plate 17.)
From Stewart, W.D., Dantos, J.L., and Maddin, S.: Dermatology: diagnosis and treatment of cutaneous disorders, ed. 4, St. Louis, 1978, Mosby–Year Book, Inc.

Children and parents are often tempted to squeeze follicular lesions. They must be warned that squeezing will not hasten the resolution of the infection and that there is a risk of making the lesion worse or spreading the infection. No attempt should be made to puncture the surface of the pustule with a needle or sharp instrument. A child with a sty may waken with the eyelids of the affected eye sealed shut with exudate. The child or the parents are instructed to gently wipe the lid with clear warm water and a clean washcloth until the exudate has been removed.

The child with limited cellulitis of an extremity is usually managed at home on oral antibiotics and warm compresses. The parents are taught the procedures and instructed in administration of the medication. Children with more extensive cellulitis, especially around a joint with lymphadenitis or on the face, are usually admitted to the hospital for parenteral antibiotics. Nurses are responsible for administering the medication, applying compresses, and maintaining the intravenous infusion.

VIRAL INFECTIONS

Viruses are intracellular parasites that produce their effect by using the intracellular substances of the host cells. Composed of only a DNA or RNA core enclosed in an antigenic protein shell, viruses are unable to provide for their own metabolic needs or to reproduce themselves. After a virus penetrates a cell of the host organism, it sheds the outer shell and disappears within the cell, where the nucleic acid core stimulates the host cell to form more virus material from its intracellular substance. In a viral infection the epidermal cells react with inflammation and vesiculation (as in herpes simplex) or by proliferating to form growths (warts).

Most of the communicable diseases of childhood are associated with rashes, and each rash is characteristic. The type of lesion and the configuration of the viral exanthems of rubeola, rubella, scarlet fever, and chickenpox are described in Table 16-1. Other common viral disorders of the skin are outlined in Table 18-5.

Table 18-5 Viral infections

DISEASE	MANIFESTATIONS	MANAGEMENT	COMMENTS
Verruca (warts)	Small, benign tumors Usually well-circumscribed, gray or brown, elevated firm papules with a roughened, finely papillomatous texture Occur anywhere but usually appear on exposed areas such as fingers, hands, face, and soles May be single or multiple Asymptomatic	Not uniformly successful Local destructive therapy, individualized according to location, type, and number—surgical removal, electrocautery, curettage, cryotherapy (liquid nitrogen), caustic solutions (lactic acid and salicylic acid in flexible collodion, retinoic acid, salicylic acid plasters), x-ray treatment Hypnotherapy may be effective	Common in children Tend to disappear spontaneously Course unpredictable Most destructive techniques tend to leave scars Autoinoculable Repeated irritation will cause to enlarge
Variants: Verruca vulgaris (common wart)	A skin-colored to brown, rough-surfaced epithelial growth May be single or multiple Asymptomatic Most frequent sites are dorsal and palmar surfaces of hands, fingers, and around nails		
Verruca plana juvenilis (juvenile wart)	Flat, skin-colored to brown, slightly raised, smooth lesion Asymptomatic Lesions multiple Commonly located on face and dorsum of hands		
Verruca plantaris (plantar wart)	Located on plantar surface of feet and, because of pressure, are practically flat; may be surrounded by a collar of hyperkeratosis	Apply caustic solution to wart, wear foam insole with hole cut to relieve pressure on wart; soak 20 min after 2-3 days. Repeat until wart comes out	Destructive techniques tend to leave scars, which may cause problems with walking
Human papillomavirus	See Chapter 20		
Herpes simplex virus Type 1 (cold sore, fever blister) Type II (genital)	Grouped, burning, and itching vesicles on inflammatory base, usually on or near mucocutaneous junctions (lips, nose, genitals, buttocks) Vesicles dry, forming a crust, followed by exfoliation and spontaneous healing in 8-10 days May be accompanied by regional lymphadenopathy	Avoidance of secondary infection Burow solution compresses during weeping stages Topical therapy has proved to have effect on recurrences Oral antiviral (Acyclovir) for initial infection or to reduce severity in recurrence	Heal without scarring unless secondary infection Aggravated by corticosteroids Positive psychologic effect from treatment May be fatal in children with depressed immunity
Varicella zoster virus (herpes zoster; shingles)	Caused by same virus that causes varicella (chickenpox) Virus has affinity for posterior root ganglia, posterior horn of spinal cord, and skin; crops of vesicles usually confined to dermatome following along course of affected nerve Usually preceded by neuralgic pain, hyperesthesias, or itching May be accompanied by constitutional symptoms	Symptomatic Analgesics for pain Mild sedation sometimes helpful Local moist compresses Drying lotions may be helpful Ophthalmic variety: systemic corticotropin (ACTH) and/or corticosteroids Acyclovir	Pain in children usually minimal Postherpetic pain does not occur in children Chickenpox may follow exposure; isolate affected child from other children in a hospital or school May occur in children with depressed immunity; can be fatal
Molluscum contagiosum Cause: pox virus	Flesh-colored papules with a central caseous plug (umbilicated) Usually asymptomatic	Cases in well children resolve spontaneously in about 18 months Treatment reserved for troublesome cases Curettage or cryotherapy	Common in school-age children Spread by skin-to-skin contact, including autoinoculation and fomite-to-skin contact

DERMATOPHYTOSES (FUNGAL INFECTIONS)

The dermatophytoses (ringworm) are infections caused by a group of closely related filamentous fungi that invade primarily the stratum corneum, hair, and nails. These are superficial infections that live on, not in, the skin. They are confined to the dead keratin layers but are unable to survive in the deeper layers. Since the keratin is being desquamated constantly, the fungus must multiply at a rate that equals the rate of keratin production to maintain itself; otherwise the infection would be shed with the discarded skin cells. Common dermatophytoses are outlined in Table 18-6.

Table 18-6 Dermatophytoses (ringworm)

DISEASE/ ORGANISM	MANIFESTATIONS	MANAGEMENT	COMMENTS
Tinea capitis—*Trichophyton tonsurans, Microsporum audouini, M. canis* (see Fig. 18-6, *A*, and Color Plate 7)	Lesions in scalp but may extend to hairline or neck Characteristic configuration of scaly, circumscribed patches and/or patchy, scaling areas of alopecia Generally asymptomatic, but severe, deep inflammatory reaction may occur that manifests as boggy, encrusted lesions (kerions) Pruritic Microscopic examination of scales is diagnostic	Oral griseofulvin Oral ketoconazole for difficult cases Selenium sulfide shampoos Topical antifungal agents, e.g., clotrimazole, haloprogin, miconazole	Person-to-person transmission Animal-to-person transmission Rarely, permanent loss of hair *M. audouini* transmitted from one human being to another directly or from personal items; *M. canis* usually contracted from household pets, esp. cats Atopic individuals more susceptible
Tinea corporis—*Trichophyton rubrum, T. mentagrophytes, Microsporum canis, Epidermophyton* (see Fig. 18-6, *B*, and Color Plate 8)	Generally round or oval, erythematous scaling patch that spreads peripherally and clears centrally; may involve nails (tinea unguium) Diagnosis: direct microscopic examination of scales Usually unilateral	Oral griseofulvin Local application of antifungal preparation such as tolnaftate, haloprogin, miconazole, clotrimazole; apply 1 inch beyond periphery of lesion; continual application 1 to 2 weeks after no sign of lesion	Usually of animal origin from infected pets Majority of infections in children caused by *M. canis* and *M. audouini*
Tinea cruris ("jock itch")—*Epidermophyton floccosum, T. rubrum, T. mentagrophytes*	Skin response similar to tinea corporis Localized to medial proximal aspect of thigh and crural fold; may involve scrotum in males Pruritic Diagnosis: same as for tinea corporis	Local application of tolnaftate liquid Wet compresses or sitz baths may be soothing	Rare in preadolescent children Health education regarding personal hygiene
Tinea pedis ("athlete's foot")—*T. rubrum, T. interdigitale, E. floccosum*	On intertriginous areas between toes or on plantar surface of feet Lesions vary: Maceration and fissuring between toes Patches with pinhead-sized vesicles on plantar surface Pruritic Diagnosis: direct microscopic examination of scrapings	Oral griseofulvin Local applications of tolnaftate liquid and antifungal powder containing tolnaftate Acute infections: compresses or soaks followed by application of glucocorticoid cream Elimination of conditions of heat and perspiration by clean, light socks and well-ventilated shoes; avoidance of occlusive shoes	Most frequent in adolescents and adults; rare in children, but are an increase with wearing of plastic shoes Transmission to other individuals rare despite general opinion to contrary Ointments not successful
Candidiasis (moniliasis)—*Candida albicans*	Grows in chronically moist areas Inflamed areas with white exudate, peeling, and easy bleeding Pruritic Diagnosis: characteristic appearance	Amphotericin B or nystatin ointment to affected areas	Common form of diaper dermatitis (see Color Plate 15) Oral form common in infants (see Chapter 9 and Color Plate 13)

A

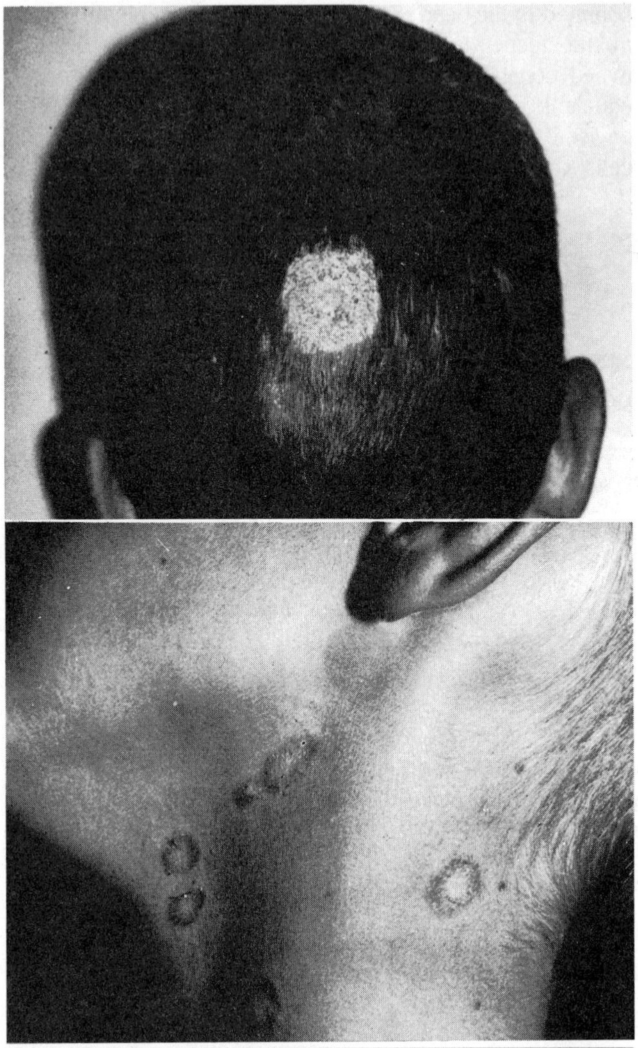

B

Fig. 18-6. A, Tinea capitis. **B,** Tinea corporis. Both infections caused by *Microsporum canis,* the "kitten" or "puppy" fungus. (See also Color Plates 7 and 8.)

From Stewart, W.D., Danto, J.L., and Maddin, S.: Dermatology: diagnosis and treatment of cutaneous disorders, ed. 4., St. Louis, 1978, Mosby–Year Book, Inc.

Three principal types of fungi are responsible for dermatophyte infections: *Trichophyton, Microsporum,* and *Epidermophyton.* They are designated by the Latin word *tinea,* with further designation related to the area of the body where they are found, for example, tinea capitis (ringworm of the scalp) (Fig. 18-6, *A*). Dermatophyte infections are most often transmitted from one person to another or from infected animals to humans. Atopic individuals are more susceptible to dermatophyte infections. Fungi exert their effect by means of an enzyme that digests and hydrolyzes the keratin of hair, nails, and the stratum corneum. Dissolved hair breaks off to produce the bald spots characteristic of tinea capitis. In the annular lesions the fungi are found principally in the edge of the inflamed border as they move outward from the inflammation. Diagnosis is made from microscopic examination of scrapings taken from the advancing periphery of the lesion, which almost always produces scale.

Nursing Considerations

When teaching families regarding the care of children with ringworm, it is important to emphasize good health and hygiene. Because of the infectious nature of the disease, several basic hygienic measures are particularly pertinent. Affected children are not to exchange with other children any grooming items, headgear, scarves, or other articles of apparel that have been in proximity to the infected area. Affected children are provided with their own towel and directed to wear a protective cap at night to avoid transmitting the fungus to bedding, especially if they sleep with another person. Since the infection can be acquired by animal-to-human transmission, all household pets should be examined for the presence of the disorder. Other sources of infection are seats with headrests, such as theater seats or seats in public transportation.

Treatment with the drug griseofulvin frequently lasts for weeks or months, and, because subjective symptoms subside, children or parent may be tempted to decrease or discontinue the drug. The nurse should impress on members of the family the importance of maintaining the prescribed dosage schedule. They are also instructed regarding the possibility of side effects from the drug such as headache, gastrointestinal upset, fatigue, insomnia, and photosensitivity. For children who take the drug over many months, periodic testing is required to monitor leukopenia and assess liver and renal function.

SCABIES

Scabies is an endemic infestation caused by the scabies mite, *Sarcoptes scabiei,* which becomes pandemic at 30-year cyclic intervals, with each incidence lasting approximately 15 years. The current pandemic is nearing completion. Lesions are created as the impregnated female scabies mite burrows into the stratum corneum of the epidermis (never into living tissue) where she deposits her eggs and fecal material. These burrows form minute, linear, grayish-brown threadlike lesions that are often difficult to see.

Clinical Manifestations

The reaction causes intense pruritus that leads to punctate discrete excoriations secondary to the itching. Maculopapular lesions are characteristically distributed in intertriginous areas: interdigital surfaces (see Color Plate 10), axillary-cubital area, popliteal folds, and inguinal region. However, there is large variability in type of lesions. Infants often develop an eczematous eruption; therefore the observer must look for discrete papules, burrows, or vesicles. A mite is identified as a black dot at the end of a burrow. In children over 2 years of age the largest percentage of eruptions are found in the hands and wrists and, in children less than 2 years, on feet and ankles. Children with Down syndrome do not complain of itching, and therefore they can get a severe infestation before it is recognized.

The inflammatory response and itching occur after the host becomes sensitized to the mite, approximately 30 to 60 days following initial contact. (In persons previously sensitized to the mite the inflammatory response occurs within

48 hours after exposure.) After this time, anywhere the mite has traveled will begin to itch and develop the characteristic eruption. Consequently mites will not necessarily be located at all sites of eruption. Also, a person needs prolonged contact with the mite to become infested. Since it takes about 45 minutes for the mite to burrow under the skin, transient body contact is less likely to cause transfer of the mite.

Therapeutic Management

The diagnosis is made by microscopic identification from scrapings of the burrow. Treatment is application of 1% lindane (gamma benzene hexachloride—Kwell, Scabene) in a vanishing cream base. A recent study found 5% permethrin cream to be more effective and less toxic than the Kwell (Schultz and others, 1990). Permethrin (Nix), a standard therapy for pediculosis, is not approved for use for scabies; however, a newer permethrin product (Elimite) is approved for children over age 2 months. A widely used but less effective alternative is crotamiton (Eurax). Because of the length of time between infestation and physical symptoms (30 to 60 days), all persons who were in close contact with the affected child will need treatment. This may include persons such as boyfriends or girlfriends, baby-sitters, and grandparents, as well as immediate family members. The objective is to treat as thoroughly as possible the first time.

Nursing Considerations

Nurses instructing families in use of the scabicide should emphasize the importance of following the directions accurately. Lindane lotion is applied to cool, dry skin—not following a hot bath. It is applied over the entire cutaneous surface from the neck down and left on for the recommended time, usually 4 hours for infants and 6 hours for older children and adults. Since it is a superficial skin disorder, penetration need not be promoted. One liberal application is sufficient. The physician usually prescribes enough medication for the entire family, allowing 2 ounces for adults and 1 ounce for each child.

Crotamiton is usually applied at bedtime for 2 consecutive days. However, to take advantage of its antipruritic properties, some advocate its application for at least five consecutive 24-hour periods (Stein, 1987).

Touching and holding the affected child should be minimized until treatment is completed, and hands should be washed carefully after contact is made. Nurses in hospitals are to wear gloves when caring for an affected child. Following treatment, freshly laundered bed linen and underclothing are used, and previously worn clothing is washed in very hot water and ironed. Families need to know that, although the mite will be killed, the rash and the itch will not be eliminated until the stratum corneum is replaced, which takes approximately 2 to 3 weeks. Soothing ointments or lotions can be used for pruritus.

PEDICULOSIS CAPITIS

Pediculosis capitis (head lice, or "cooties") is an infestation of the scalp by *Pediculus humanus capitis*, a very common parasite, especially in school-age children. These lice infestations are not a major health threat, but they are highly communicable and create embarrassment and a panic reaction in the family and community. They can also cause a child to be ridiculed by other children.

The louse is a blood-sucking organism that requires approximately five meals a day. The adult louse lives only about 48 hours when away from a human host, and the life span of the average female is only 1 month. The female lays her eggs at night at the junction of a hair shaft and close to the skin because the eggs need a warm environment.

Nurses or parents should carefully inspect the head of a child who scratches the head more than usual for bite marks, redness, and nits. The hair is systematically spread with two flat-sided sticks or tongue depressors, and the scalp observed for any movement that indicates a louse. Lice are visible to the naked eye. The nits, or eggs, hatch in approximately 7 to 10 days; therefore the egg is about 4 mm, or ¼ inch, from the scalp at the time of hatching and appears as a tiny whitish oval speck adhering to the hair shaft. The adherent nature of the nits distinguish them from dandruff, which falls off readily. Empty nit cases, indicating hatched lice, are translucent rather than white and are usually located more than ¼ inch from the scalp.

Clinical Manifestations

Itching, caused by the crawling insect and insect saliva on the skin, is usually the only symptom. The most common sites of involvement are the occipital area, behind the ears, at the nape of the neck, and (occasionally) the eyebrows and eyelashes. Diagnosis is made by observation of the white eggs (nits) firmly attached to the base of the hair shafts. Because of their brief life span and mobility, adult lice are more difficult to locate. Nits must be differentiated from dandruff, lint, hair spray, and other items of similar size and shape. On inspection nits are attached to the hair shaft. Scratch marks and/or inflammatory papules caused by secondary infection may also be found on the scalp in the vulnerable areas (see Color Plate 12).

Therapeutic Management

A number of pediculocides are available that are highly effective. Lindane shampoo (1%) (Kwell, Scabene) is applied as prescribed and repeated in 7 to 10 days to kill the hatching nymphs. However, lindane is not effective against nits and, if not used properly, is potentially toxic, especially in infants. Permethrin (1%) creme rinse kills both lice and nits after one application. Both lindane and permethrin must be obtained by prescription. Pyrethrin preparations (RID, A-200 Pyrinate, R & C Shampoo, Pronto, and Triple X) can be obtained without a prescription and appear to be as effective as lindane.

A commercial preparation of 0.5% malathion lotion (Ovide Lotion) is again available for treatment of pediculosis. Malathion was shown to be superior to other preparations because of its effectiveness and low toxicity, but it was removed from the market because it was commercially unprofitable. Also available is a creme rinse containing a chemical that loosens the natural adhesive bonding of nits to hair shafts. It is designed to ease removal of nits with a metal comb that accompanies the product. However, to be effective, any treatment should be accompanied by an educational and reinfestation-prevention program.

Nursing Considerations

Management of pediculosis infection consists of a three-step process: (1) application of pediculocidal product, (2) manual removal of nit cases, (3) and preparation of the environment (Clore, 1989).

Application. It is important to apply the pediculocide according to the directions described on the label of the pediculocide. The treatment should not be administered after a warm bath or shower because vasodilation from the heat increases skin absorption of chemicals. For the same reason, use of a hair dryer is avoided.

Parents are advised to read the directions several times in a quiet room before beginning treatment (McLaury, 1983). The child should be made as comfortable as possible during the application process because the pediculocide must remain on the scalp and hair for several minutes. The child is placed face up with the head extended over a sink, basin, or wash tray. To prevent the drug from getting onto other body parts, a plastic drape is placed over the child and secured around the neck, and the child is instructed to close the eyes tightly during application. The child can be provided with a towel or washcloth with which to cover the eyes. If eye irritation occurs, the eyes must be flushed well with tepid water. Because most of the application times are 10 minutes, some diversional activity should be provided for the child.

Nit removal. Instructions on the labels indicate that dead lice and remaining nits are removed with an extra fine–tooth comb while the hair is still damp. Most preparations include a comb to dislodge the firmly adhered nits. If the comb is ineffective in removing the nit cases, they must be removed with tweezers or between the fingernails. All detectable nits and nit cases are removed because it is almost impossible to distinguish viable from nonviable nits with the naked eye. It is unsafe to assume that nit cases farther than ¼ inch from the scalp are incapable of hatching (Clore, 1989). The child is examined daily for evidence of newly laid nits for at least 2 weeks following treatment.

Environmental management. Live lice will survive for up to 48 hours away from the host but nits are shed into the environment and capable of hatching in 7 to 10 days. Therefore measures must be taken to prevent further infestation (see Parent Guidelines). Spraying with insecticide is not recommended because of the danger to children and animals (Editorial comment, 1984). Families should also be advised that the pediculocide is relatively costly, especially when several members of the household require treatment.

Prevention. The increasing incidence of pediculosis in school children has become a serious concern for school nurses, parents, and community health agencies. School nurses are constantly on the coordinate school-community prevention control programs for pediculosis. The **National Pediculosis Association*** has been organized by a group of parents frustrated by repeated infestations of their children. They have developed an approach to the problem to encourage vigorous effort on the part of parents and the community to reduce the epidemics in children. Some of their suggestions include encouraging parents to notify others if a child becomes infected and preventing children from reentering school until they are completely free of nits.

Psychologic aspects. There are several things that nurses should be aware of in order to successfully manage or to assist parents in coping with the problem. It should be emphasized that *anyone* can get pediculosis. It has no respect for age, socioeconomic level, or cleanliness. The louse does not jump or fly, but it can be transmitted from one person to another on personal items. Therefore children are cautioned against sharing combs, hats, caps, scarves, coats, and other items used on or near the hair. Children who share lockers are more likely to contract an infestation, and slumber parties and contact sports place

NURSING TIP: SHAMPOO

Playing "beauty parlor" during the shampoo is a useful strategy. The child lies supine, with the head over a sink or basin, and covers the eyes with a dry towel or washcloth. This prevents medication, which can cause chemical conjunctivitis, from splashing into the eyes.

NURSING TIP: NIT REMOVAL

A dilute rinse (equal parts vinegar and water) may help loosen the nits for easier removal. Soak hair in vinegar solution, and then wrap in a towel for 15 minutes. Rinse thoroughly (Reeves, 1987).

PARENT GUIDELINES
Preventing the Spread and Recurrence of Pediculosis

Machine wash all washable clothing, towels, and bed linens in hot water and dry in a hot dryer for at least 20 minutes. Dry-clean nonwashable items.
Thoroughly vacuum carpets, car seats, pillows, stuffed animals, rugs, mattresses, and upholstered furniture.
Seal nonwashable items in plastic bags for 14 days if parents are unable to afford dry cleaning and do not have a vacuum cleaner.
Soak combs, brushes, and hair accessories in lice-killing products for 1 hour or in boiling water for 10 minutes.

From Clore, E.R.: Dispelling the common myths about pediculosis, J. Pediatr. Health Care 3:28-33, 1989.

*P.O. Box 149, Newton, MA 02161; (617) 449-6487.

children at risk. Lice are not carried or transmitted by household pets.

The psychologic effects of lice infestations can be highly stressful to children. They are influenced by the reactions of others, including their parents, and may be made to feel ashamed or guilty. Parents are strongly cautioned against cutting a child's hair or, worse, shaving a child's head. Lice infest short hair as readily as long hair, and these actions only compound the child's distress and serve as a continual reminder to peers, who are always ready to taunt another with something out of the ordinary (McLaury, 1983). See Nursing Care Plan: The Child with Pediculosis Capitis.*

■ SYSTEMIC DISORDERS RELATED TO SKIN LESIONS

Numerous disorders have skin manifestations as part of the clinical picture of the disease. Many of these have been discussed in relation to communicable diseases (Chapter 16) and others as appropriate throughout the book. With the exception of fungal infections, the following are primarily systemic disorders associated with contact with animals or insects.

SYSTEMIC MYCOTIC (FUNGAL) INFECTIONS

Mycotic (systemic or deep fungal) infections have the capacity to invade the viscera as well as the skin. The best known of these are primarily lung diseases, which are usually acquired by inhalation. They produce a variable spectrum of disease, and some are quite common in certain geographic areas. They are not transmitted from person to person but appear to reside in the soil, from which their spores are airborne. The cutaneous lesions are granulomatous and appear as ulcers, plaques, nodules, fungating masses, and abscesses. The course of deep fungal diseases is chronic, with slow progression that favors sensitization (Table 18-7).

RICKETTSIAL INFECTIONS

Rickettsiae are intracellular parasites, similar in size to bacteria, that inhabit the alimentary tract of a wide range of natural hosts. With the exception of Q fever, mammals become infected only through the bites of infected insects (lice and fleas) or arachnids (ticks and mites), which serve as both infectors and reservoirs. Rickettsial diseases are more common in temperate and tropical climates and in areas where humans live in association with arthropods. Infection in humans is incidental (except epidemic typhus) and not necessary for the survival of the rickettsial species. However, once the organism invades a human, it causes a disease that varies in intensity from a benign self-limiting illness to a fulminating and frequently fatal one. Some rickettsial infections are outlined in Table 18-8.

*In Wong, D.L., and Whaley, L.F.: Clinical manual of pediatric nursing, ed. 3, St. Louis, 1990, Mosby–Year Book, Inc.

LYME DISEASE

Lyme disease, relatively recently recognized and the most common tick-borne disorder in the United States, is believed to affect 1500 to 3000 people annually (Hurwitz, 1988). Although the disease is being reported with increasing frequency, the exact incidence is unknown.

Etiology and Pathophysiology

Lyme disease is caused by the spirochete, *Borrelia burgdorferi,* which enters the skin and bloodstream through the saliva and feces of ticks. The most commonly known vectors of the disease are the deer tick *Ixodes dammini* in the Midwest and Northeast and *Ixodes pacificus* in the Pacific Northwest regions of the United States. The ticks are very small, 2 to 4 mm in length, making detection difficult. The preferred hosts of *I. dammini* are white-tailed deer and white-footed mice. Any wild or domestic animal can act as intermediary host, and birds are frequent carriers (Eichenfield, 1986).

Clinical Manifestations

The disease may present in any of three stages, which may be distinct or isolated, overlapping, or absent. Exacerbations and remission are common.

Stage 1 consists of the tick bite at the time of inoculation, followed in 3 to 32 days by the development of erythema chronicum migrans (ECM) at the site of the bite. The lesion begins as a small erythematous papule that enlarges radially over a period of days to weeks, resulting in a large circumferential ring with a raised, edematous doughnutlike border. The thigh, groin, and axilla are common sites. The lesion is described as "burning," feels warm to the touch, and occasionally is pruritic.

Many patients develop multiple, smaller secondary annular lesions without the indurated center. They may occur anywhere, except the palms and soles, and in untreated patients they disappear in 3 to 4 weeks. Constitutional symptoms, including headache, malaise, fatigue, anorexia, stiff neck, generalized lymphadenopathy, splenomegaly, conjunctivitis, sore throat, abdominal pain, and cough, are often observed.

Stage 2, the most serious stage of the disease, is characterized by systemic involvement of neurologic, cardiac, and musculoskeletal systems that appears 2 to 11 weeks after the cutaneous phase is completed. Headache is the most frequent symptom, but in early stages it is not associated with neurologic abnormalities. Later neurologic features include meningoencephalitis, cranial nerve palsies, and peripheral radiculoneuritis.

Cardiac complications, which may appear in a smaller number of persons 4 to 5 weeks after ECM, are commonly atrioventricular conduction abnormalities and may result in severe heart block. Patients may be asymptomatic but can develop syncope, palpitations, dyspnea, chest pain, and severe bradycardia.

Stage 3 begins 4 to 6 weeks following the rash, but it may develop months or years later. Musculoskeletal pains that involve the tendons, bursae, muscles, and synovia can

Table 18-7 Systemic mycoses

DISORDER/ORGANISM	SKIN MANIFESTATIONS	SYSTEMIC MANIFESTATIONS	MANAGEMENT	COMMENTS
North American blastomycosis—*Blastomyces dermatitidis*	Chronic granulomatous lesions and microabscesses in any part of body Initial lesion is a papule; undergoes ulceration and peripheral spread	Pulmonary symptoms such as cough, chest pain, weakness, and weight loss May have skeletal involvement, with bone destruction and formation of cutaneous abscesses	Intravenous administration of amphotericin B	Usual portal of entry is lungs Source of infection unknown Noninfectious Pulmonary infections may be mild and self-limiting and require no treatment Progressive disease, often fatal
Cryptococcosis—*Cryptococcus neoformans (Torula histolytica)*	Usually on face; acneiform, firm, nodular, painless eruption	Central nervous system (CNS) manifestations; headache, dizziness, stiff neck, and signs of increased intracranial pressure Low-grade fever, mild cough, lung infiltration	Intravenous amphotericin B; may be administered intrathecally for CNS involvement 5-Fluorocytosine for meningitis Excision and drainage of local lesions	Acquired by inhalation of dust, but may enter through skin Prognosis serious Noninfectious Increased incidence in persons receiving corticosteroids with lymphoreticular malignancies, or type II diabetes
Histoplasmosis—*Histoplasma capsulatum*	Not distinctive or uniform, but most appear as punched-out or granulomatous ulcers	General systemic symptoms may include pallor, diarrhea, vomiting, irregular spiking temperature, hepatosplenomegaly, and pulmonary symptoms Any tissue of body may be involved with related symptoms	Intravenous amphotericin B for severe cases Oral ketoconazole	Organism cultured from soil, especially where contaminated with fowl droppings Fungus enters through mouth and respiratory tract Endemic in Mississippi and Ohio River valleys Disseminated diseases most common in infants and children
Coccidioidomycosis (valley fever)—*Coccidioides immitis*	Erythema nodosum Erythema multiforme Erythematous maculopapular rash	Primary lung disease, usually asymptomatic May be sign of acute febrile illness Disseminated disease is very serious	Intravenous amphotericin B Intravenous miconazole (synthetic imidazole) Intravenous miconazole plus oral ketoconazole for CNS involvement Surgical resection of persistent pulmonary cavities	Inhalation of aerospores from soil Endemic in southwestern United States Usually resolves spontaneously Increased incidence in dark-skinned races (Filipino, black, Mexican, Asian)

begin at the same time as the cutaneous ECM, but the pauciarticular arthritis usually does not develop until later. Arthritis is the presenting symptom in 50% of cases (Culp and others, 1987). In children the arthritis is characterized by intermittently painful swollen joints (primarily the knees), with spontaneous remissions and exacerbations. Recurrences do not always involve the same joint.

Diagnostic Evaluation

The diagnosis is based primarily on history, observation of the lesion, and development of subsequent manifestations. Many persons do not remember a tick bite or the rash. Laboratory diagnosis is usually established in later stages through serologic testing, either by indirect immunofluorescence (IFA) or enzyme-linked immunosorbent assays

Table 18-8 Eruptions caused by rickettsiae

DISORDER/ORGANISM/HOST	MANIFESTATIONS	MANAGEMENT	COMMENTS
Rocky Mountain spotted fever—*R. rickettsii* Arthropod: tick Transmission: tick Mammal source: wild rodents; dogs	Gradual onset: fever, malaise, anorexia, myalgia Abrupt onset: rapid temperature elevation, chills, vomiting, myalgia, severe headache Maculopapular or petechial rash primarily on extremities (ankles and wrists) but may spread to other areas, characteristically on palms and soles	Control: protection from tick bite by proper wearing apparel, tick repellent Tetracycline or chloramphenicol Vigorous supportive therapy	Usually self-limited in children Onset in children may resemble any infectious disease Severe disease rare in children Children and dogs should be inspected regularly if they play in wooded areas See Table 18-11 for management of ticks
Epidemic typhus—*R. prowazekii* Arthropod: body louse Transmission: infected feces into broken skin Mammal source: humans	Abrupt onset of chills, fever, diffuse myalgia, headache, malaise Maculopapular rash becomes petechial 4 to 7 days later, spreading from trunk outward	Control: immediate destruction of vectors Tetracycline or chloramphenicol	Patient should be isolated until deloused See discussion on p. 827 for management of pediculosis Excreta from infected lice also in dust—disinfect patient's clothing, bedding, and possessions with DDT and wash in hot water
Endemic typhus—*R. typhi* Arthropod: rat fleas, or lice Transmission: flea bite; inhaling or ingesting flea excreta Mammal source: rats	Headache, arthralgia, backache followed by fever; may last 9-14 days Maculopapular rash after 1-8 days of fever begins in trunk and spreads to periphery; rarely involves face, palms, soles	Control; eliminate rat reservoir, insect vectors, or both Supportive treatment: Tetracycline or chloramphicol	Fairly common in United States Shorter duration than epidemic typhus A mild, seldom fatal illness Difficult to distinguish from epidemic typhus
Rickettsialpox—*R. akari* Arthropod: mouse mite Transmission: mite Mammal source: house mouse	Maculopapular rash following primary lesion and eschar at site of bite, fever, chills, headache	Control: eradication of rodent reservoir and mite vector Tetracycline or chloramphenicol Supportive treatment	Self-limited nonfatal disease Endemic in New York City Found in many cities in United States

(ELISA) (Eichenfield, 1986). A new specific laboratory technique, polymerase chain reaction (PCR), has been developed, enabling identification of spirochetes with a high degree of accuracy (Rosa and Schwan, 1989).

Therapeutic Management

Symptomatic relief is attained with aspirin or prednisone. Children over 9 years of age are treated with tetracycline, and children under 9 years are given penicillin for 10 to 20 days (American Academy of Pediatrics, Committee on Infectious Diseases, 1988). The treatment is effective in preventing second-stage manifestations in most cases.

Neurologic manifestations are managed with intravenous penicillin. Cardiac problems are treated the same as neurologic symptoms, with the addition of acetylsalicylic acid (aspirin) and daily prednisone. A temporary pacemaker may be needed for heart block. Lyme arthritis is managed with symptomatic use of aspirin or other nonsteroidal anti-inflammatory drugs and penicillin. Most children with Lyme disease recover in a reasonable period (Hurwitz, 1988).

Nursing Considerations

The major thrust of nursing care, especially in endemic areas, is prevention. Prevention of the disorder involves educating the parents to protect their children from exposure to the ticks with simple measures (see p. 842). In endemic areas tick habitats can include yards and parks as well as wooded areas. Many ticks have been found in lawns (Falco and Fish, 1988).

Parents or other caregivers should examine their children carefully for ticks if they have been in areas where ticks are likely to be found and remove them promptly (see Table 18-11). Parents should also be alert for signs of the skin lesion, especially if their children are known to have been exposed to the tick vector.

Some recommend the use of insect repellents such as DEET (*N,N,*-diethyl-*m*-toluamide) or permethrin (Permanone Tick Repellent) as a clothing spray to protect against insects. Parents should be advised to use them judiciously. DEET is absorbed through the skin; therefore repeated, heavy applications may cause toxicity in infants and children.

Information about Lyme disease, especially Lyme disease during pregnancy, can be obtained from the **National Lyme Borreliosis Foundation.*** Information is also available from the Lyme disease hotline.†

CAT SCRATCH DISEASE

Cat scratch disease (CSD) is a subacute regional adenitis that follows the scratch or bite of an animal, especially a cat (99% of cases) and is caused by a pleomorphic gram-negative bacillus. The disease is usually a benign, self-limiting illness that resolves spontaneously in about 2 to 4 months.

The usual manifestations are a painless, nonpruritic erythematous papule at the site of inoculation, followed by regional lymphadenitis. The disease may persist for several months before gradual resolution. In some children the adenitis progresses to suppuration, and a few children may be very ill with various symptoms, including a prolonged high temperature. The diagnosis is made on the basis of three of the following: (1) cat contact (usually a kitten), (2) lymphadenopathy, (3) an inoculation site, and (4) a positive CSD skin test (Carithers, 1985). Some children have been reported to develop granulomatous hepatitis secondary to CSD.

The treatment is primarily supportive. Antibiotics do not appear to shorten the duration or prevent progression to suppuration, although some have reported improvement with administration of trimethoprim-sulfamethoxazole (Collip, 1989; Flessner, 1989). Activity is limited to prevent trauma to the large lymph nodes, and bed rest is indicated for children who have fevers. Analgesics may be needed for discomfort and fever. Most children can continue normal activities during the course of the disease. The animals are not ill during the time they transmit the disease, and most authorities do not recommend disposal of a cherished pet.

■ SKIN DISORDERS RELATED TO CHEMICAL OR PHYSICAL CONTACTS

Children come in contact with an endless variety of substances and objects in day-to-day activities, including sunshine. Some children are troubled very little by these encounters; others are sensitive to many commonplace substances. The following discussion is restricted to the more frequently observed dermatides or reactions.

CONTACT DERMATITIS

Contact dermatitis is an inflammatory reaction of the skin to chemical substances, natural or synthetic, that evoke a hypersensitivity response or to those agents that cause direct irritation. The initial reaction occurs in an exposed region, most commonly the face and neck, backs of the hands, forearms, male genitalia, and lower legs. There is characteristically a sharp delineation between inflamed and normal skin early in the reaction that ranges from a faint, transient erythema to massive bullae on an erythematous swollen base. Itching is a constant symptom.

The cause may be a *primary irritant* or a *sensitizing agent*. A primary irritant is one that irritates any skin. A sensitizing agent produces an irritation on those who have met the irritant or something chemically related to it, have undergone an immunologic change, and have become sensitized. Prior exposure is not a necessarily factor in the reaction. A sensitizer irritates in relatively low concentrations only persons who are allergic to it.

The clinical course is relatively short (1 to 4 weeks) if the causative agent is eliminated, and whether or not there are complications from secondary invasion or reactions to topical therapy depends on the severity of the original reaction.

Sensitizing reactions are acquired by repeated or prolonged exposure, and the sensitizing capacity of different substances varies widely. Strong sensitizers require only one or two exposures and occur in a higher percentage of individuals; weak sensitizers require numerous exposures, and a smaller percentage of those exposed will be sensitized. The length of time from exposure to development of sensitivity varies considerably and may be as short as a week or much longer. Sometimes with repeated exposure and reactions the skin loses its capacity to return to normal, or secondary factors become predominant to produce a chronic inflammatory process.

The major goal in treatment is to prevent further exposure of the skin to the offending substance. Providing there is no further irritation, the normal recuperative powers of the skin will produce satisfactory results without treatment. The most frequent offenders are plant and animal irritants, the prototype of which is poison ivy (see next page).

The most common contact dermatitis in infants occurs on the convex surfaces of the diaper area as a result of chemical irritation from ammonia, putrefactive enzymes acting on urinary amino acids, or, less often, laundry products (see Diaper Dermatitis, Chapter 13). Other agents that frequently produce dermatologic responses from contact are animal irritants such as wool, feathers, and furs; vegetable irritants such as oleoresins, oils, and turpentine; and chemicals of all kinds, including synthetic fabrics (e.g., shoe components), dyes, metals, cosmetics, perfumes, and soaps (including bubble baths). The list is endless.

Several cosmetic products advertised as safe for children may be responsible for skin irritation in children. These include a cream hair relaxer marketed especially for children that contains lye and must be used with extreme care. Because children's hair is more resistant to artificial curling or straightening, pediatric preparations contain chemicals as strong as or stronger than those intended for use on adults.

Nursing Considerations

Nurses frequently detect evidence of contact dermatitis during routine physical assessments. Skin manifestations in

*Box 462, Tolland, CN 06084; (203) 871-2900 or (203) 872-6346.
†(914) 285-LYME.

specific areas suggest limited contact, such as around the eyes (mascara), areas of the body covered by clothing but not protected by undergarments (wool), or areas of the body not covered by clothing (ultraviolet injury). Generalized involvement is more likely to be bubble bath or soap. Often nurses are able to elicit the offending agent and counsel families regarding management. If the lesions persist, are extensive, or show evidence of infection, medical evaluation is indicated.

POISON IVY, OAK, AND SUMAC

Contact with the dry or succulent portions of any of three poisonous plants produces localized, streaked or spotty, oozing, and painful impetiginous lesions. Poison ivy grows almost everywhere east of the Rockies, poison oak is mainly found west of the Rockies, and poison sumac is usually restricted to swamp areas of the Southeast. Only Nevada, Hawaii, and Alaska (and regions above 4000 feet) appear to be free of the plants (Fig. 18-7).

The offending substance in these plants is an oil, urushiol, that is extremely potent. Sensitivity to urushiol is not inborn but is developed after one or two exposures and may change over a lifetime. Repeated exposures appear to lower the reaction; exposure after long periods away from it may elicit a heightened response. Some highly sensitive persons may suddenly become resistant and vice versa. All parts of the plants contain urushiol; thus dried leaves and stems contain the irritant. Even smoke from burning brush piles can produce a reaction. There is widespread contact with the skin from the smoke of burning plants, and lung reactions from smoke inhalation can be life-threatening.

Animals do not seem to be affected by the oil; dogs or other animals who have run or played in the plants may carry the sap on their fur, and animals who eat the plants can transfer the oil in saliva. Shoes, tools, and toys can transfer the oil. Golf balls that have been in the rough are sources of contact.

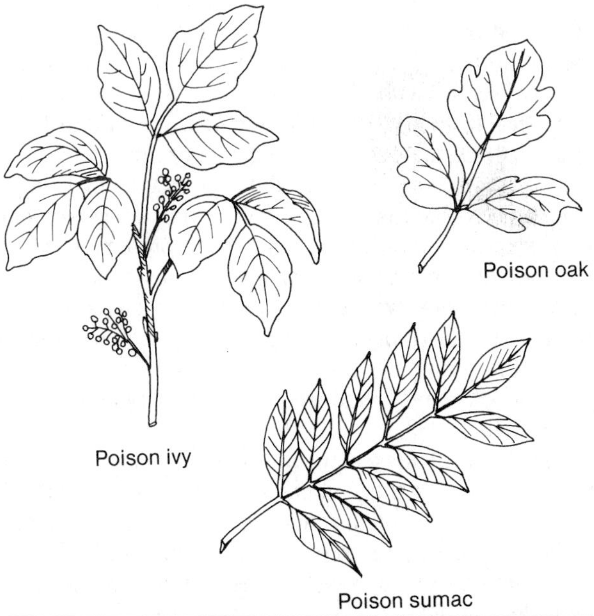

Fig. 18-7. Poison ivy, poison oak, and poison sumac.

Clinical Manifestations

The substance begins to take effect as soon as it touches the skin. It penetrates through the epidermis and bonds with the dermal layer, where it initiates an immune response. The full-blown reaction is evident after about 2 days with redness, swelling, and itching at the site of contact. Several days later, streaked or spotty blisters oozing serum from damaged cells produce the characteristic impetiginous lesions (see Color Plate 9). The lesions dry and heal spontaneously, and itching stops by 10 to 14 days.

Therapeutic Management

Treatment of the lesions include calamine lotion, soothing Burow solution compresses, and/or Aveeno baths to relieve discomfort. Topical corticosteroid gel is very effective for prevention or relief of inflammation, especially when applied before formation of blisters. Oral corticosteroids may be needed for several reactions, and a sedative such as diphenhydramine (Benadryl) may be ordered.

Nursing Considerations

When it is known that the child has made contact with the plant, the area is immediately flushed (within 15 minutes) with *cold* running water to neutralize the urushiol not yet bonded to the skin. If there is a stream nearby, an effective method is to have the child enter the water (clothes and all) and allow the water to rinse the oil from both skin and clothing. Soap is contraindicated because it removes protective skin oils and dilutes the urushiol, allowing it to spread, and hard scrubbing irritates the skin. All clothing that has come in contact with the plant is removed with care and thoroughly laundered in hot water and detergent. Every effort should be made to prevent the child from scratching the lesions. Although the lesions do not spread by contact with the blister serum or from scratching, the lesions can become secondarily infected.

Prevention. Prevention is best accomplished by avoidance of contact and removal of the plant from the environment when feasible. All children, especially those known to be sensitive, should be taught to recognize the plant. Information regarding means for destroying plants can be obtained from the U.S. Departments of Agriculture or Forestry.

SUNBURN

Sunburn is a very common skin injury caused by overexposure to ultraviolet light waves—either sunlight or artificial light in the ultraviolet range. The sun emits a continuous spectrum of visible and nonvisible light rays that range in length from very short to very long. The shorter, higher-frequency waves are more damaging than longer wavelengths, but much of the light is filtered out as it travels through the atmosphere. Of the light that does filter through, ultraviolet

A (UVA) waves are the longest and cause only minimum burning but play a significant role in photosensitive and photoallergic reactions. They are also responsible for premature aging of the skin and potentiate the effects of UVB. Ultraviolet B (UVB) waves are shorter and responsible for tanning, burning, and most of the harmful effects attributed to sunlight, especially skin cancer.

Numerous factors influence the amount of UVB exposure. Radiation is strongest at midday (10 AM to 3 PM), when the distance from the sun to a given spot on the earth is shortest. Solar intensity also varies with seasons, time zones, and altitude. Exposure is greater at higher altitudes and less when the sky is hazy (although its effect is easily underestimated). Window glass effectively screens out UVB but not UVA. Fresh snow and water reflect ultraviolet rays, especially when the sun is directly overhead; some are reflected by sand.

Some persons are more susceptible to sunburn than others. Protection from effects of the sun is provided by the fibrous keratin of the outer epidermis and the pigment melanin, produced by the melanocytes of the innermost, or basal, layer of the epidermis. Areas of the body with thick keratin layers (palms and soles) offer the greatest protection. The protective pigment layer decreases the intensity of all ultraviolet light by physically blocking and scattering the radiation. Ultraviolet rays stimulate the melanocytes to produce more melanin, turning the skin darker. After several days of exposure, the dark melanin is able to absorb most of the incoming ultraviolet radiation before the rays can cause further damage.

Persons with light skin and eyes produce melanin slowly and are more prone to burn, while very dark-skinned people are able to tolerate more rays without damage. A high altitude increases the risk of burning, sun becomes stronger near the equator, and sunlight is reflected from the surfaces of sand, snow, and water. Sunlight penetrates the atmosphere even on hazy days.

Other factors can play a role in sensitivity to ultraviolet rays. People with certain diseases (e.g., porphyria, lupus erythematosus) are more sensitive to the sun's rays. Some substances increase the skin's sensitivity, for example, numerous medications (e.g., barbiturates, oral contraceptives, sulfonamides, anticonvulsants), topical products (e.g., antiseptic soap, after-shave lotions, colognes), and certain foods containing photosensitizing chemicals (e.g., carrots, parsley, limes).

The ultraviolet rays penetrate the skin surface, where they precipitate a chemical change in the cell molecules, producing toxic by-products that irritate surrounding tissues. The result is redness, tissue swelling, increased capillary permeability, and the tenderness characteristic of superficial (first-degree) burns and the coagulation, necrosis, and blistering of partial thickness (second-degree) burns (see Burns, Chapter 29). Sunburned skin is exquisitely sensitive, and severe sunburn may be accompanied by nausea, chills, fever, abdominal cramping, and headache. Dehydration may occur.

Excessive or long-term exposure to the sun causes permanent damage to the skin. Ninety percent of skin cancers occur in areas that are exposed to sunlight, and rates of skin cancers are higher in parts of the world where sunlight is more intense. Studies have also shown that childhood is a crucial time for sun exposure. Children who immigrate to sunny climates after 10 years of age develop cancer at lower rates than native-born children. In general, children receive three times as much sun exposure as adults, and teenagers are a high-risk group, with their emphasis on the desirability of a tan skin (Hurwitz, 1989).

Nursing Considerations

Treatment involves stopping the burning process, decreasing the inflammatory response, and rehydrating the skin. Local application of cool tap water soaks or immersion in a tepid water bath for 20 minutes or until the skin is cool limits tissue destruction and relieves the discomfort. After the cool applications, a bland oil-in-water moisturizing lotion can be applied, but petrolatum-based products that trap radiant heat in the tissues are avoided (Anders and Leach, 1983). Acetaminophen is recommended for relief of discomfort. Partial thickness burns are treated the same as those from any heat source.

Prevention. Protection from sunburn is the major goal of management, and the harmful effects of the sun on the delicate skin of infants and children are receiving increased attention. Protection can be achieved by physical means, that is, protective clothing and a hat, or by chemical means. Two types of products are available for sun protection: topical sunscreens, which partially absorb ultraviolet light, and sun blockers, which block out ultraviolet rays by reflecting sunlight. The most frequently recommended sun blockers are zinc oxide and titanium dioxide ointments.

Some chemicals have the capacity to absorb certain wavelengths of light and thus provide protection to the cutaneous surface when applied to the skin. Sunscreens are products containing a sun protective factor (SPF) based on evaluation of effectiveness against ultraviolet rays. The SPF is indicated by number, such as 15, which indicates that, if a person normally burns in 10 minutes without a sunscreen, use of sunscreen with SPF 15 will allow them to remain in the sun for 15 times 10 or 150 minutes (2½ hours) before acquiring the same degree of erythema or burn.

There is disagreement regarding the frequency of application. One opinion is that reapplication of sunscreen does not extend the period of protection; the protection will remain the same no matter how many times it is reapplied (Nicol, 1989). However, the predominant view is that sunscreen should be applied 15 to 20 minutes before exposure (so that the protective chemicals can penetrate the upper skin layers) and reapplied frequently and liberally (Coody, 1987; Hurwitz, 1989).

Most chemical sunscreens are available with SPF ranging from 2 to over 30; the higher the number, the greater the protection. The American Academy of Pediatrics recommends waterproof sunscreens with a minimum SPF of 15. The maximum SPF approved by the Federal Drug Administration (FDA) is 15.

The most effective sunscreens are those containing *p*-aminobenzoic acid (PABA) and PABA-esters, effective

NURSING TIP: AVOIDING HARMFUL SUN EXPOSURE

Observe the length of one's shadow to assess the time when the sun's rays are most damaging. Seek protection from the sun when the shadow is shorter than one's height (Holloway, 1990).

against UVB. PABA is more effective, penetrates the outer layer of skin, and may accumulate with repeated use, thus providing protection even when the child is swimming or sweating. PABA may stain clothing; PABA-esters are less likely to stain clothing but are less effective than PABA. However, PABA can cause an allergenic response in sensitive persons, manifest as redness and itching 24 hours after application. Benzophenones also offer protection against UVA but are less effective than the PABA preparations and wash off easily. For best results, the sunscreen should be effective against both UVA and UVB.

The range of sunscreens available offer the consumer access to a type and combination to meet any need. Preparations made specifically for children are marketed especially for infants and children (Nicol, 1989). Sunscreens are applied evenly to all exposed areas, with special attention to skin folds and areas that might become exposed as clothing shifts. Parents are directed to read labels of sunscreen products carefully for the SPF and follow the manufacturer's directions for application.

It is wise to avoid direct sun exposure when solar radiation is assumed to be of maximum intensity. The strongest radiation occurs when the sun is at its highest (directly overhead). Earlier or later in the day with the sun at a 45-degree angle, the earth's atmosphere provides protection equivalent to a SPF of 2.4 (Holloway, 1990).

Persons who care for or work with children, such as teachers, daycare workers, coaches, youth group leaders, and relatives, should be made aware of sun safety for children. An excellent pamphlet, *For Every Child Under the Sun: A Guide to Sensible Sun Protection,* provides helpful information and is endorsed by the American Academy of Pediatrics. It is available from the **Skin Cancer Foundation.*** Sun damage is cumulative. Although most long-term effects (cancer, wrinkling) are not evident until adulthood, skin care must begin in childhood. Application of a sunscreen product is recommended for children after 6 months of age; infants less than 6 months of age should be kept out of the sun. It should be the goal of every nurse to teach skin care as a basic practice that becomes a routine part of a child's life, much the same as tooth care (see Parent Guidelines).

PARENT GUIDELINES
Sun Exposure

Remember that tanning indicates sun injury and risks of skin cancer begin in childhood.
Keep infants and children out of the sun as much as possible.
- Use carriage with hood when taking infants outdoors.
- Use canopy on stroller for older infants.

Schedule child's activities to avoid sun exposure between 10 AM and 3 PM whenever possible.
Take increased precautions when living or vacationing in the mountains or the tropics.
Protect child when outdoors with clothing (sun hat, long-sleeved shirt, long pants).
Apply sunscreen with SPF of at least 15.
Apply sunscreen to exposed areas:
- Before every exposure
- On cloudy as well as sunny days
- Even when child plays in shade; sun reflects from sand, snow, cement, and water

Reapply liberally every 2 to 3 hours and whenever child goes in the water or sweats heavily.
Check with child's practitioner regarding any medications the child is taking and observe for any evidence of side effects (rash, redness, swelling).
Examine skin regularly for signs of any change in pigmented nevi (rapid growth, crusting, ulceration, bleeding, change in pigmentation, development of inflamed satellite lesions, loss of normal skin lines) or subjective symptoms (tenderness, pain, itching).
Prohibit child from using sun lamps or tanning parlors.
Set a good example by following the above guidelines.

Modified from For every child under the sun, The Skin Cancer Foundation, 245 Fifth Ave., Suite 2402, New York, NY 10016.

COLD INJURY

Cold injuries are most commonly seen in very cold regions. The nature of the heat-regulating mechanisms of the body are such that the inner portion of the body, or core, produces heat and the periphery, or outer area, conserves or dissipates the heat. When the body attempts to conserve heat, the outer tissues are subjected to low temperatures, and local trauma may result.

Chilblain, redness and swelling of the skin, occurs when extremities, usually the hands, are exposed intermittently to temperatures 30° to 60° F. The response may vary but is characterized by intense vasodilation that increases the temperature of involved tissues above unaffected tissue and produces edematous, reddish-blue patches that itch and burn. As warming takes place, the sensations become more intense but ordinarily subside in a few days.

Frostbite is the term used to describe tissue damage caused when excessive heat loss to local tissues allows ice crystals to form in tissues. The mechanisms of slow or rapid freezing differ. Slow freezing causes ice crystals to form in the extracellular fluid, leading to increased osmolality and movement of water from the cells. This causes cellular dehydration and destruction. Rapid freezing produces both extracellular and intracellular freezing and immediate cellular destruction. Rapid freezing takes place at high altitudes or with high conductivity from cold water immersion.

*P.O. Box 561, New York, NY 10156; (212) 725-5176.

When frozen tissues thaw, the tissue damage is like that from a high-temperature burn—red blood cell aggregation, stasis, venous thrombosis, tissue edema and ischemic damage, increased tissue pressure, and death and necrosis of surrounding tissues.The frostbitten part appears white or blanched, feels solid, and is without sensation.

Rapid rewarming is associated with less tissue necrosis than slow thawing. It restores blood flow and shortens the period of cellular damage. Rewarming produces a flush (sometimes deep purple) and a return of sensation, which is extremely painful. Large blisters may appear 24 to 48 hours after rewarming and begin to reabsorb within 5 to 10 days, followed by formation of a hard black eschar. Superficial injury often heals without incident.

Therapeutic Management

Rewarming is accomplished by immersing the part in well-agitated water at 100° to 108° F, and discomfort is managed with analgesics and sedatives. Care of blistered skin is similar to that described for burns. It is seldom possible to estimate the extent of tissue loss until new skin layers are revealed after the eschar layer separates; therefore amputation of extremities is usually delayed for 60 to 90 days unless there is evidence of gangrene.

Nursing Considerations

The frostbite victim should be transferred to the nearest emergency treatment center; the injured parts should be protected from trauma. The injured areas are handled gently, and the patient is prevented from ambulating on injured feet. Rubbing injured tissues is contraindicated and can cause damage by rupture of crystallized cells. After rewarming, a loose dressing is applied. Dry heat is not applied. (See Burns, Chapter 29, and Pain Management, Chapter 26).

HYPOTHERMIA

Hypothermia is defined as the cooling of the body's core temperature (rectal or esophageal) to injurious levels, usually identified as below 35° C (95° F). Hypothermia occurs in environmental settings when heat production by exercise and metabolism is less than heat lost by convection, conduction, or radiation. There is a 6% drop in blood flow for each 1° C decrease in core temperature (Coln and Emmrich, 1989). Very young children with a large surface area relative to body mass, and thin persons are at the greatest risk for hypothermia.

The body in positive heat balance attempts to conserve heat by alternate vasoconstriction and vasodilation in extremities. Threat of prolonged or severe cold exposure causes the body to conserve core temperature at the expense of the extremities by shunting warm blood to the core after passing through the muscles of the extremities. Shivering contributes to warming by raising the metabolic rate to increase the heat of blood before it returns to the core (Coln and Emmrich, 1989). Clinical manifestations related to degree of hypothermia are outlined in Table 18-9.

Therapeutic Management

Rewarming is the major objective of therapy. For mild hypothermia (30° to 35° C) only external application of heat lamps or immersion in water (38° to 42° C) is necessary to restore core temperature with little risk of complications. Lower temperatures require core rewarming by any of several modalities—warm humidified oxygen, intravenous fluids, rectal lavage, peritoneal lavage (dialysis) with warm fluids, hemodialysis, application of external warmth to core circulation areas (groin, axilla, posterior neck region), and/or extracorporeal blood rewarming.

Supportive therapy includes maintenance of ventilation, cardiac monitoring, monitoring renal function, and correct-

Table 18-9 Physical effects of hypothermia

TEMPERATURE	CHARACTERISTICS
35° C (95° F)	Increased respiratory rate, decreased intestinal motility; vigorous shivering; may be conscious and alert; task performance often impaired
32° C (90° F)	May continue uncontrollable shivering or may begin to show muscular rigidity; decreased respiratory rate; atrial fibrillation; may still be conscious but sensorium changes evident; impaired cognition, reasoning, and speech; loss of manual skills and dexterity; brief vasodilation that causes flushes and warm sensation and possible confusion
30° C (86° F)	Decreased cerebral blood flow; may show increased blood pressure (may be difficult to obtain), tachycardia, and tachypnea; may have supraventricular arrhythmia, PCVs, and T-wave inversion; usually conscious, but a loss of consciousness is preceded by irritability
27° C (80° F)	Bradycardia and slowed respiratory rate; metabolic rate decreased by 50%; decreased oxygen uptake, CO_2 production; ventricular fibrillation; rigid extremities
25° C (77° F)	Hypotension; glomerular filtration and blood flow to kidneys reduced by 30%
20° C (68° F)	Unconscious; nonfunctioning reflexes; unresponsive pupils; respirations barely detectable or undetectable; extremities and trunk cold to touch; abnormal ECG; pulse may decrease to 4 per minute, progressing to cardiac standstill; flat EEG; dead appearance
18° C (65° F)	Injury to peripheral tissue

ing fluid and acid-base imbalances. Prognosis is directly correlated with the degree of hypothermia, method of rewarming, and presence of underlying medical conditions.

Nursing Considerations

Nursing care consists of monitoring vital functions and assisting with therapies. Obtaining a history from family or other observers, including outside environmental temperature, length of exposure to elements, location of exposure site (e.g., outside or inside a vehicle or structure), and any care that may have been given, is essential (McGuire, 1987). If trauma is associated with the hypothermia, the mechanism and circumstances of injury are ascertained.

Prevention. Anticipation of cold conditions and knowledge of cold survival techniques are the basis of prevention. Children living in cold climates should have adequate protection when outdoors. Multiple layers of warm clothing are more effective than a single heavy layer for reducing the rate of heat loss, although they do not prevent it. Families living in cold climates should take precautions against unexpected prolonged exposure to cold, for example, store extra blankets, food rations, and other equipment in their vehicles in the event of an unexpected mechanical breakdown.

Loss of central core temperature can be reduced by 50% when an individual assumes the fetal position. A person suspected of hypothermia should be moved to a sheltered area, and wet clothing removed and replaced with dry, warm garments. Warm, high-calorie liquids are important if the person is conscious.

SKIN DISORDERS RELATED TO DRUG SENSITIVITY

Adverse reactions to drugs are seen more often in the skin than in any other organ, although any organ of the body can be affected. The reaction may be a result of toxicity related to drug concentration, individual intolerance to the average dosage of the drug, or an allergic or idiosyncratic response. The manifestations may be associated with side effects or secondary effects of a drug, either of which are unrelated to its primary pharmacologic actions.

DRUG REACTIONS

Although any drug is capable of producing almost any form of reaction in the susceptible individual, some have a tendency to produce a particular reaction consistently, and some are more likely than others to produce an untoward effect. Many are allergenic responses following a prior administration of the drug, even a topical application. Other factors influence a drug response in a particular individual. For example, drug eruptions occur with less frequency in children than in adults, the incidence increases with the number of drugs being given, climate may be a factor when light sensitivity produces a response on sun-exposed surfaces, and it is well known that genetic factors affect the way in which some individuals are able to metabolize specific drugs.

Manifestations of drug reactions may be delayed or immediate. Seven days are usually required for a child to develop sensitivity to a drug that has never been administered previously. With prior sensitivity the manifestations appear almost immediately. Rashes are the most common manifestation of adverse drug reactions in children—exanthematous, urticarial, or eczematoid. However, individual drug reactions may vary from a single lesion to extensive, generalized epidermal necrosis. Cutaneous manifestations can resemble almost any skin disease and can be seen in almost any degree of severity. With few exceptions, the distribution of a drug eruption is widespread, since it results from a circulating agent, appears as an inflammatory response with itching, is sudden in onset, and may be associated with constitutional symptoms such as fever, malaise, gastrointestinal upsets, anemia, or liver and kidney damage.

Drug reactions are also related to the amount of drug administered and the route of administration. For example, larger amounts precipitate a more severe response than a small amount, and drugs taken orally are less sensitizing than those administered intravenously. Another common response is a fixed eruption, that is, a recurrent eruption at the same site with each readministration of the drug. The lesion, a purplish-red round or oval plaque with a sharp border seen most frequently on the extremities, disappears slowly, and the pigmentation deepens with each episode.

In most cases treatment for simple cutaneous reactions consists of discontinuation of the drug. Sometimes a decision is made to continue the drug (such as an antibiotic in an infant or small child) until the cause of the rash is clearly indicated. In urticarial-type eruptions antihistamines may be ordered, and for widespread and severe lesions corticosteroids are beneficial. Severe anaphylactic reactions are a medical emergency (see Anaphylaxis, Chapter 29).

Nursing Considerations

The most effective means of management is prevention. Parents always remember a severe response. A careful history will elicit evidence of a previous drug reaction. The history should include the name of the drug, nature of the reaction, drug dose, and how soon after administration the reaction occurred (see Box 6-13).

Nurses who suspect that a rash is caused by a medication should withhold any further dose and report the eruption to the practitioner. The most frequent offenders in drug reactions are penicillin and sulfonamides, and nurses must be alert to this possibility. However, even commonplace drugs, including aspirin, barbiturates, chemical agents in a number of foods, flavoring agents, and preservatives, are capable of producing an undesired response. Persons who have severe reactions are reminded to obtain and wear an identification bracelet or chain in case of emergency or inadvertent administration of the offending drug.

ERYTHEMA MULTIFORME

Erythema multiforme is an acute, cutaneous disorder most often resulting from infections (usually viruses) or drug reactions. The characteristic lesion consists of an urticarial plaque with a dusky or vesicular center, which appears primarily on the palms, soles, and extensor surfaces.

Treatment involves discontinuing the drug, applying wet compresses for erosive lesions, and administering analgesics for discomfort. Antihistamines may be prescribed for pruritus.

ERYTHEMA MULTIFORME EXUDATIVUM (STEVENS-JOHNSON SYNDROME)

Erythema multiforme exudativum (Stevens-Johnson syndrome) (SJS) is the severe form of erythema multiforme and is characterized by lesions of the skin and mucous membranes, fever, and multiple systemic symptoms. The disease is presumed to be primarily a hypersensitivity reaction to certain drugs, although the reaction may follow an upper respiratory tract infection. The disorder is relatively rare, occurs at any age, and is more common in males than in females.

The syndrome usually begins with flulike symptoms—malaise, sore throat, fever, and severe headache. Balanitis, conjunctivitis, or stomatitis appears next, followed in a few days by an erythematous papular rash. The lesions can involve any cutaneous surface, including the palms and soles, but usually spare the scalp. They can be scattered or confluent. The initial lesions enlarge by peripheral expansion with a vesicular center that often becomes bullous. Mucous membrane ulceration often becomes severe enough to interfere with eating, and many patients have pulmonary involvement.

Mild disease requires only symptomatic treatment. However, severe disease requires hospitalization with protective isolation. Fluid and nutritional requirements are high, and most patients respond well to viscous lidocaine and a liquid diet. Intravenous feedings may be needed for extensive oral involvement. Meticulous mouth care is important, and skin care frequently requires management in a burn unit (see Stomatitis, Chapter 16). Daily ophthalmologic examination is advised. Dry eyes are a problem as well as risk of chronic mild symblepharon (adhesion of lids to the eyeball). Antibiotics are administered to patients with positive cultures, but the use of corticosteroids is controversial, and its efficacy unproven.

The mortality is estimated to be from 10% to 15% during the acute phase, especially in patients with pulmonary involvement. The disease is self-limiting, and the skin lesions gradually disappear without scarring in 2 to 3 weeks but may recur on reexposure to an offending drug. Since these patients are usually managed in a burn unit, the nursing care is the same as for a burned child. The family needs emotional support to cope with the life-threatening nature of the disease.

TOXIC EPIDERMAL NECROLYSIS

Toxic epidermal necrolysis (Lyell disease) (TEN) is a drug-induced injury to the skin characterized by a generalized erythematous rash that rapidly evolves into bullae and peeling. It appears to be a hypersensitivity reaction with precipitating factors similar to those responsible for erythema multiforme. The more common offending drugs are phenobarbital, phenytoin, allopurinol, sulfonamides, and penicillin. The clinical appearance is the same as that seen in the more common (in children) staphylococcal scalded skin syndrome (SSSS).

The disease begins with a prodromal period of fever and malaise and a generalized erythematous rash that rapidly evolves into bullae and extensive epidermal peeling. Oral lesions are similar to those observed in SJS. Treatment consists of withdrawal of the offending drug, fluid and electrolyte replacement, and skin management as for severe burns. The disease can be protracted, and mortality rate can range from 25% to 50%. It is essential that families of children receiving anticonvulsants or sulfonamides be informed of the significance of a rash and the importance of reporting it to their health professional promptly.

MISCELLANEOUS SKIN PROBLEMS

A number of skin lesions are caused by extrinsic or intrinsic factors. Some of these are listed in Table 18-10. Others are discussed briefly in the following discussion and elsewhere in the book as appropriate.

CONGENITAL SKIN DISORDERS

There are a number of congenital skin disorders, usually inherited as autosomal dominant traits. Psoriasis in children less than 16 years of age is uncommon (Table 18-10), and photosensitivity eruptions associated with other inherited diseases appear early in childhood. Ichthyoses are a heterogeneous group of disorders characterized by scaling that create a challenging problem in treatment. Because of wide variability, these disorders are not discussed in detail.

NEUROFIBROMATOSIS-1

Neurofibromatosis-1 (NF1), or von Recklinghausen disease, is a relatively common genetic disorder with an autosomal dominant inheritance pattern. It occurs in 1:3000 persons and has one of the highest mutation rates known (Cohen, 1984). The manifestations are highly variable and appear to result from some defect that alters peripheral nerve differentiation and growth.

There is marked clinical variability in manifestations which first appear as small, discrete, flat, pigmented skin lesions with smooth edges (café-au-lait spots, pigmented nevi; see Color Plate 16) and/or axillary or inguinal freckling that develops in early infancy or childhood. Slow-growing cutaneous and subcutaneous neurofibromas that grow along the course of a peripheral nerve may appear in later childhood or adolescence and increase in number with age. Lisch nodules, dome-shaped clear–to–yellow or brown elevations on the iris surface, develop prior to pu-

Table 18-10 Miscellaneous skin disorders

DISEASE/CAUSATIVE AGENT	LOCAL MANIFESTATIONS	MANAGEMENT	COMMENTS
Urticaria—usually allergic response to drugs or infection	Development of wheals Vary in size and configuration and tend to appear quickly, spread irregularly, and fade within a few hours May be constant or intermittent, sparse or profuse, small or large, discrete or confluent May be acute, chronic, or recurrent in acute attacks	Local soothing and antipruritic applications Antihistamines Epinephrine or ephedrine Cortisone or corticotropin (ACTH) in severe cases Severe upper respiratory involvement may require tracheostomy	Known etiology agents should be avoided May be accompanied by malaise, fever, lymphadenopathy Severe cases may involve mucous membranes, internal organs, and joints Obstruction to air passages constitutes medical emergency (see Chapter 31)
Intertrigo—mechanical trauma and aggravating factors of excessive heat, moisture, and sweat retention	Red, inflamed, moist, partially denuded, marginated areas, the shape of which is determined by location Appears where opposing skin surfaces rub together, such as intergluteal folds, groin, neck, and axilla Hyperhydrosis and obesity are often factors	Affected areas kept clean and dry Skin folds kept separated with a generous supply of nonmedicated powder Area exposed to air and light Remove excess clothing	A form of diaper irritation Prevent recurrence by keeping susceptible areas clean and dry Frequently associated with overheating from too much clothing
Psoriasis—unknown; hereditary predisposition; may be triggered by stress	Round, thick, dry, reddish patches covered with coarse, silvery scales over trunk and extremities; first lesions commonly appear in scalp; facial lesions more common in children than adults Affected cells proliferate at a much more rapid rate than normal cells	Exposure to sunlight, ultraviolet light Topical corticosteroids Tar derivates Trihydroxyanthracine Keratolytic agents (salicylic acid) Psoralin—ultraviolet A (PUVA)* Emollients may provide relief	Uncommon in children under age 6 years Persons are otherwise healthy individuals Coal tar and psoralin act synergistically with ultraviolet light Keratolytic agents enhance absorption of corticosteroids Humidifiers may help in winter
Alopecia			
Alopecia areata	Sudden onset of asymptomatic, noninflammatory, round, bald patches in hairy parts of body	Psychologic support Inducement of allergic contact dermatitis to stimulate growth of hair Minoxidil (peripheral vasodilator)	Family history in 10%-26% of cases Some concern regarding drug therapy safety Refer to support groups†
Traumatic alopecia	Traction alopecia around scalp margins from tight hair styles (e.g., braids, pony tails, corn rows)	Counseling regarding hair styling, use of hair cosmetics, hot combs, rollers	More prevalent in black children and adolescents Prolonged traction can produce fibrosis of hair root and permanent loss
Trichotillomania	Compulsive hair pulling	Determine and treat cause	Chronic hair pulling may require psychologic therapy
Tinea capitis	See Table 18-6	See Table 18-6	See Table 18-6
Numerous other causes			

*Still considered investigational.
†**National Alopecia Areata Foundation,** P.O. Box 5027, Mill Valley, CA 94941.

berty in most affected individuals. Elephantiasis (thickening and enfolding of the skin) occurs in some individuals.

Other characteristics may include developmental delay or retardation, seizures, scoliosis or kyphosis, short stature, macrocephaly, speech defects, learning disabilities, or a variety of congenital malformations. The severity varies considerably and can vary within the same family. One family may have only café-au-lait spots or axillary freckling, whereas another has more severe manifestations.

The diagnosis is established by physical findings based on National Institutes of Health (NIH) Consensus Conference guidelines (Box 18-3). In doubtful cases nodule biopsy may be performed. A family history is elicited to determine if the specific case is inherited or if it represents a new mutation. Risk for transmitting the disorder to offspring is 50%. Therapy is limited to excision of tumors, which produce pain or impair function, and symptomatic management of other manifestations.

Box 18-3 CRITERIA FOR DIAGNOSIS OF NF1

An individual with two or more of the following clinical signs meets the criteria for NF1:

Six or more café-au-lait spots larger than 5 mm in diameter in prepubertal children and larger than 15 mm in postpubertal individual

Two or more neurofibromas of any type or one plexiform neurofibroma

Freckling in the axillary or inguinal region

Optic glioma

Two or more Lisch nodules

A distinctive osseous lesion, e.g., sphenoid dysplasia or thinning of long bone cortex with or without pseudoarthrosis

A first-degree relative with NF1 according to the criteria listed above

Nursing Considerations

Nursing care is primarily recognition of signs that indicate a possibility of the disease, referral for diagnosis, and family counseling and support. It is important that a diagnosis be made, even when the only manifestations are a few café-au-lait spots. The family will need to know the genetic implications and be alert for signs that indicate the child is developing any of the more serious characteristics at a later time. Cancer occurs to excess in patients with the disorder, although the rates vary widely. Other members of the family should be assessed for possible evidence of the disorder.

Families can be referred to the **National Neurofibromatosis Foundation, Inc.,*** an organization with the purpose of increasing public awareness of NF1 to provide help and support to families affected by the disorder and stimulating research. Professionals involved with persons with the disease can get recent information and technical help in treatment, lists of meetings, and funding sources from a new computerized telecommunications network, NFORMATION.† Also a helpful and inexpensive booklet is available to help families understand the disease.‡

BITES AND STINGS

Children come in contact with a variety of other animal and insect species. Usually the contact is of no consequence, but children might be injured by the encounter and receive a physical injury (such as an animal bite or insect sting). Because they spend considerable time outdoors and in fields and vacant lots, children often come in contact with insects. Consequently children are frequently the victims of insects that puncture the skin for the purpose of sucking blood, injecting venom, or laying their eggs. In the process of these activities, substances foreign to the victim may create an allergic sensitivity in that individual to produce pruritus, urticaria, or systemic reactions of greater or lesser degree, depending on the child's sensitivity.

Ordinarily insect bites are of little significance and cause only minor inconvenience. However, they can attain importance if:

- They cause symptoms that interfere with the child's normal activities, such as the effects of a spider bite.
- They signify the presence of a contagious skin disease, such as scabies.
- The parasite is able to transmit other diseases, for example, ticks that transmit Rocky Mountain spotted fever.
- The venom causes a response that can be life-threatening, such as bee stings.

INSECT STINGS AND BITES

Children come in contact with a variety of insects during their play. Some of the stinging or biting insects (such as mosquitoes, fleas, and gnats) are found almost everywhere; others seem to be more common to specific areas. For example, honeybees are more prevalent in suburbs and rural areas. Hornets, wasps, and yellow jackets are more often found in the cities. Being scavengers, they often feed on garbage. The fire ant is located predominantly in the Southeast. Insect bites are high-morbidity but, fortunately, low-mortality disorders.

The more common classes of insects, their method of producing a reaction, and the management are outlined in Table 18-11. Some proteins in insect venom are species specific, others are common to a number of species; therefore crossover reactivity is common. The usual local response to a sting is sharp pain, a local wheal (less than 2 inches in diameter), and erythema accompanied by intense itching at the site, lasting less than 24 hours. The reaction is produced by enzymes, cytotoxic proteins, and vasoactive compounds, primarily histamine and kinins (Schuberth, 1989).

Systemic reactions can occur and, although a rare occurrence, in some instances can be life-threatening. Non-life-threatening systemic reactions begin several minutes to several hours after the sting and consist of simple urticaria, erythema, pruritus, and angioedema. Serious, life-threatening reactions usually begin within 5 to 10 minutes after the sting and can include airway obstruction secondary to laryngeal edema, bronchospasm, hypotension, and cardiovascular collapse (Schuberth, 1989).

To prevent contact with stinging and biting insects, children are taught behaviors that reduce the likelihood of injury. In addition, topical insect repellents are generally believed to provide safe and effective protection for several hours. The best all-purpose repellents contain the active ingredient diethyltoluamide (DEET), which has proved to be effective for a variety of insects, including mosquitoes, chiggers, ticks, fleas, and biting flies. Protection can last from 1 to several hours, but the effectiveness is affected by the concentration of active ingredients and the product must be reapplied after sweating, swimming, wiping, or exposure to

*141 Fifth Avenue, Suite 7-S, New York, NY 10010; (800) 323-7938, (212) 460-8980.

†**Neurofibromatosis Institute, Inc.,** 715 Bison Dr., Houston, TX 77079.

‡Recommended: *Neurofibromatosis,* available from Medic Publishing Co., P.O. Box 89, Redmond, WA 98073-0089, (206) 881-2883.

Table 18-11 Skin lesions caused by insect bites and stings

MECHANISM/CHARACTERISTICS	MANIFESTATIONS	MANAGEMENT
▪ Insect bites—flies, gnats, mosquitoes, fleas		
Mechanism: Foreign protein in insects' saliva introduced when skin penetrated for a bloodsucking meal Distribution: Almost everywhere—fleas, mosquitoes, ants Suburbs and rural areas—bees Urban areas—hornets, wasps, yellow jackets	Hypersensitivity reaction Papular urticaria Firm papules; may be capped by vesicules or excoriated Little or no reaction in nonsensitized person	Treatment: Antipruritic agents and baths Antihistamines Prevention of secondary infection Prevention: Avoid contact Remove focus, such as treating furniture, mattresses, carpets, and pets, where insects may live Apply insect repellent when exposure is anticipated
▪ Chiggers—harvest mite		
Mechanism: Creeps into skin pores and hair follicles to feed Manifestations: Erythematous papules Intense itching	Same as insect bites May require systemic steroids for extensive bites	Favor warm areas of body, especially intertriginous areas and areas covered with clothing Avoid contact, especially in areas of tall grass and underbrush Apply insect repellent when exposure is anticipated
▪ Hymenoptera stings—bees, wasps, hornets, yellow jackets, fire ants		
Mechanism: Injection of venom through stinging apparatus Venom contains histamine, allergenic proteins, and often a spreading factor, hyaluronidase Severe reactions caused by hypersensitivity and/or multiple stings Hypersensitive children should wear identifying tag to indicate allergy and therapy needed; family should keep emergency medication and be taught its administration	Local reaction: small red area, wheal, itching, and heat Systemic reactions: may be mild to severe, including generalized edema, pain, nausea and vomiting, confusion, respiratory embarrassment, and shock	Treatment: Carefully scrape off stinger if present Cleanse with soap and water Apply cool compresses or ice packs Apply common household product, e.g., lemon juice, paste made with aspirin, baking soda, or Adolph's Meat Tenderizer Elevate involved extremity Antihistamines Severe reactions: administer epinephrine, corticosteroids; treat for shock Prevention: Child taught to wear shoes, to avoid wearing bright clothing and flowery prints, shiny jewelry, or perfumed grooming products that might attract the insect (cologne, scented hair spray) and to avoid places where the insect may be contacted
▪ Black widow spider		
Mechanism: Venom injected through a clawlike appendage; has neurotoxic action Characteristics: Spider is recognized by red or orange hourglass-shaped marking on underside Avoids light and bites in self-defense	Mild sting at time of bite Area becomes swollen, painful, and erythematous Dizziness, weakness, and abdominal pain May produce delirium, paralysis, convulsions, and (if large amount of venom absorbed) death	Treatment: Cleanse wound with antiseptic Apply ice packs Muscle relaxant, such as calcium gluconate Analgesics and/or sedatives Hydrocortisone or diazepam IV Prevention: Teach children to avoid places that harbor the spider, e.g., woodpiles
▪ Brown recluse spider		
Mechanisms: Venom injected via fangs Venom contains powerful necrotoxin Characteristics: Spider is fawn to dark brown and recognized by fiddle-shaped mark on head Shy; bites only when annoyed or surprised Prefers dark areas where seldom disturbed	Mild sting at time of bite Transient erythema followed by bleb or blister; mild to severe pain in 2-8 hours; purple, star-shaped area in 3-4 days; necrotic ulceration in 7-14 days Systemic reactions may include fever, malaise, restlessness, nausea and vomiting, and joint pain Generalized petechial eruption Wounds heal with scar formation	Treatment: Local application of cool compresses Antibiotics Corticosteroids Relief of pain Wound may require skin graft Some advocate early excision of necrotic area and surrounding tissue Prevention: Teach children to avoid possible nesting sites

Continued.

Table 18-11 Skin lesions caused by insect bites and stings—cont'd

MECHANISM/CHARACTERISTICS	MANIFESTATIONS	MANAGEMENT
▪ Scorpions		
Mechanism: Sting by means of a hooked caudal stinger that discharges venom Venom of more venomous species contains hemolysins, endotheliolysins, and neurotoxins Characteristics: Usual habitat is southwestern United States	Intense local pain, erythema, numbness, burning, restlessness, vomiting Ascending motor paralysis with convulsions, weakness, rapid pulse, excessive salivation, thirst, dysuria, pulmonary edema, coma, and death Some species produce only local tissue reaction with swelling at puncture site (distinctive) Symptoms subside in a few hours Deaths occur among children under 4 years of age, usually in first 24 hours	Treatment: Delay absorption of venom by application of tourniquets for 10-15 minutes Administer of antivenin Surveillance in PICU Prevention: Teach children to avoid possible nesting sites
▪ Ticks		
Mechanism: In process of sucking blood, head and mouth parts are buried in skin Characteristics: Feed on blood of mammals Significant in humans because of pathologic organism carried May be vectors of various infectious diseases, such as Rocky Mountain spotted fever, Q fever, tularemia, relapsing fever, Lyme disease, tick paralysis Must attach and feed 1-2 hours to transmit disease Usual habitat is very wooded area	Tick usually attached to skin, head embedded Produce firm, discrete, intensely pruritic nodules at site of attachment May cause urticaria or persistent localized edema	Treatment: Grasp tick with fingers protected by gloves or tissues as close as possible to point of attachment Pull straight up with steady, even pressure Remove any remaining part (e.g., head) with sterile needle Cleanse wounds with soap and disinfectant If bare hands touch tick during removal, wash hands thoroughly with soap and water Prevention: Teach children to avoid areas where prevalent Inspect skin (especially scalp) after being in wooded areas

rain. Since some adverse effects have been reported in young children and because long-term effects of diethyltoluamide are unknown, caution is advised against excessive application or prolonged use, especially those of high concentration (Fischer and Parks, 1986).

Most bites are managed by simple symptomatic measures such as cool compresses, calamine lotion, and prevention of secondary infection. The emergency treatment or specific suggestions for some of their bites or stings are discussed briefly. Often treatment consists of applications of a substance that relieves the swelling and discomfort and can be made from common household products.

Hymenoptera Stings

When an insect stings, its stinger often remains imbedded in the skin. Since bees have barbed stingers that penetrate the skin, any pressure on the venom sac at the tip of the barb pushes more venom into the skin. The best approach is to flick the stinger off with the fingernail or knife blade—never squeeze the area. Another method is to cover the area with transparent tape and then peel the tape off. The stinger should come off with the tape (Gorrell, 1985).

Children are taught to avoid contact with bees and to recognize the insect (e.g., it is not part of the flower). For those who have become sensitized to hymenoptera bites and demonstrate a severe life-threatening systemic response, intramuscular administration of epinephrine provides immediate relief and must be available for emergency use. For hypersensitive children a kit must be available that contains epinephrine, a hypodermic syringe, and perhaps ephedrine and an antihistamine preparation (a tourniquet is included in the kit, but its use is not recommended). Hypersensitive children should wear a Medic Alert bracelet, and the families are reminded to check the expiration date on the kit and replace an outdated one. Families should determine if a school nurse is available at the school; if not, someone at the school should be designated to inject the epinephrine in case of an emergency.

Some authorities recommend that children with a history of generalized reactivity to an insect sting undertake a program of skin testing and desensitization to prevent serious or fatal reactions. Others believe that the risk of systemic reactions is so low that it does not justify subjecting these children to a protracted and expensive treatment regimen.

Arachnid Bites

Most arachnids in the United States, including tarantulas, are relatively harmless. All spiders produce venom that is injected via fangs. Some are able to pierce skin; in others the venom is insufficiently toxic. There is a local tissue reaction that is relieved by cool compresses or the methods described for hymenoptera stings.

Only scorpions and two spiders—the brown recluse and black widow—inject venom deadly enough to require immediate attention. Children bitten by any of these arachnids must receive medical attention as soon as possible.

Ticks

Ticks are troublesome creatures because they become partially imbedded in the skin as they feed. Numerous methods have been suggested for their removal, but the only really effective method is to grasp the tick with curved forceps as close as possible to the point of attachment and pull straight up with a steady, even pressure (Needham, 1985). If a portion of the body (e.g., the head) remains, it can be removed with a sterile needle in the same manner as a sliver. The bite is cleansed with soap and a disinfectant after removal. If the hands have touched the tick, they are washed thoroughly with soap and water.

To avoid ticks, children should wear long pants tucked into the socks and a long-sleeved shirt when walking in infested areas, especially in the spring and summer. Whenever possible, children should avoid grass and shrubbery where ticks may be lurking. Ticks can also be picked up by dogs and other household pets. Parents are advised to check their children carefully for the organisms when their children have been in areas where they might be acquired. Light clothing makes ticks more visible.

ANIMAL BITES

Animal bites are common injuries and include both wild and domestic animals. Over 2 to 3.5 million persons are bitten by animals each year (March, 1982), and young adults are the most frequent victims (Chun, Berkelhamer, and Herold, 1982). Younger children are more defenseless and more vulnerable. Wild animal bites are discussed in relation to rabies, and the local wounds are treated the same as domestic animals, such as dogs, cats, hamsters, and mice; therefore this discussion is directed primarily toward dog bites.

Over half the victims of dog bites are less than 4 years of age, and boys are bitten more frequently than girls. Contrary to accepted belief, stray dogs are seldom involved in the attacks; most of the dogs are owned by the family of the victim or a neighbor (Elliot and others, 1985). Most dog attacks occur in or adjacent to the owners' yards, and the attack is usually preceded by verbal or physical contact with the animal (Wright, 1985). The problem is unlikely to diminish as the animal population is increasing rapidly, and a there is a growing trend to acquire large, aggressive guard dogs (Baker, 1989). For example, the proportion of deaths resulting from attacks by pit bull dogs increased from 20% to 62% in the last 10 years (Sacks, Sattin, and Bonzo, 1989).

About 90% of animal bites are caused by dogs and less than 10% by cats (Esposito and Adam, 1989). However, cat scratches are extremely common (see Cat Scratch Disease, p. 832). Most dog or cat injuries are to the upper extremities. Small children are more likely to receive bites or scratches to the head, face, and neck because of their tendency to put their heads near the animal's head and flail their arms rather than protecting their heads.

Deaths from dog bite–related injuries in the United States over the past 10 years have been predominantly in the pediatric age-group (Sacks, Sattin, and Bonzo, 1989). Of reported cases 70% were in children less than 10 years of age and, where the breed of dog was known, pit bulls were implicated almost three times as often as German shepherds, previously reported as the most dangerous breed. Also, pit bull attacks were almost twice as likely to be caused by strays.

Animal bites are potentially serious because of the likelihood of significant infection—5% of dog bites and 20% to 50% of cat bites (Baker, 1989). Injuries vary in intensity from small puncture wounds to complete evulsion of tissue that can be associated with significant crush injury. Dog bites generally present as lacerations or evulsions; cats exert less biting force, but their sharp teeth penetrate more deeply inoculating organisms deep into tissues.

The location of a bite influences the incidence of infection. Injuries to the arm and hand tend to become infected more often than those on legs, scalp, and face. Redness, swelling, and tenderness develop around the site of injury, often accompanied by purulent or serosanguineous drainage. It may be difficult to assess hand infection, since most lymphatic drainage is contained in the dorsal subcutaneous space, and swelling occurs in this area when the injury may be elsewhere (Baker, 1989).

Therapeutic Management

General wound care consists of rinsing the wound with copious amounts of saline or Ringer's lactate delivered under pressure via a large syringe and washing the surrounding skin with mild soap. A clean pressure dressing is applied, and the extremity is elevated if the wound is bleeding. Medical evaluation is advised because there is danger of tetanus and rabies, although dogs in most urban areas are required to be immunized against rabies. Bites from wild animals, such as squirrels, bats, and raccoons, are potentially dangerous (see Rabies, Chapter 37).

Prophylactic antibiotics are indicated for puncture wounds and wounds in areas that may prove to be cosmetically or functionally impaired if infected. Extensive lacerations are debrided and loosely sutured to allow for drainage in the event of infection. Primary closure of jagged irregular wounds with associated crush injury and devitalized tissue is contraindicated, except for facial wounds because of cosmetic reasons (Avery and First, 1989). Tetanus toxoid is administered according to standard guidelines (see Chapter 12), and rabies protocol followed. Injuries to poorly vascularized areas such as the hands are more likely to become infected than those in more vascularized areas such as the face; puncture wounds are more apt to become infected than lacerations.

Nursing Considerations

The most important aspect related to animal bites is prevention. It is important that children understand animal behavior and develop an honest respect for all animals. It is vital that they learn how to treat animals and how to react to them. Suggestions about what families can do and tell children about animals is outlined in Parent Guidelines. Meeting a strange dog can be both frightening and a danger to a child (Fig. 18-8). The child should remain calm and follow the suggestions outlined.

Parents who are contemplating a pet, especially a dog, for themselves or their children should receive some advice about the dog that is least likely to be a danger to their children. The level of sociability with children is the key to a selection, and dogs range from dangerous, bad, and unsuitable to tolerant of children to exceptionally good with children—some under certain conditions. For example, dogs that are too clumsy, impetuous, or vigorous are not suitable for small children, and some dogs must be raised with the children. Small dogs are usually recommended for children, but if a large dog is desired, a Labrador retriever is a good choice (Lauer, White, and Lauer, 1982). A categorization of dogs related to their potential interaction with chil-

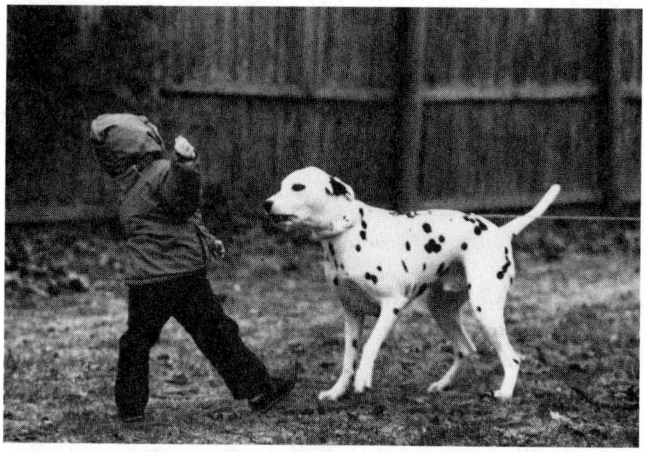

Fig. 18-8. Children need to be taught how to behave around both strange and familiar dogs.

PARENT GUIDELINES
Animal Safety

Avoid all strange animals, especially wild, sick, or injured ones. The same techniques employed in teaching children not to talk to strangers should be used to teach them not to approach strange animals.

Notify the Health Department or police of any wild, sick, or injured animals.

Never permit a child to break up an animal fight, even when his own pet is involved. Use a rake, broom, or garden hose to separate the animals.

Become aware, and make children aware, of the danger of mistreating or teasing pets. Pets are not toys, but living creatures who will bite if mauled, annoyed, or frightened.

Alert your child to dangerous and nervous animals in your neighborhood and do not permit him to enter yards or houses that harbor them.

Do not allow a child to disturb an animal that is eating or sleeping. Set a good example by your own behavior.

Do not let your pet come into indiscriminate contact with other animals.

Avoid the indiscriminate contact between your pet and human beings.

Do **not** purchase or obtain pets for your children until such time as they demonstrate their maturity and ability to handle and care for the pets. This ability is rare in a child under 4 years of age and unusual in a child under 6. Factors to be considered at any age are the maturity and disposition of the child and the animal. Some people never develop this maturity.

From Mofenson, H.C., Greensher, J., and Teitelbaum, H.: How to avoid animal bites, Med. Times 100:92, 1972.

Stress to children the importance of avoiding routes, when riding bicycles of tricycles, where dogs are known to chase vehicles.

Teach children that each animal has the right to a free existence and freedom from man-inflicted pain. Set a good example by your own behavior.

Under your supervision or that of some other adult, have children make friends with pets, in the immediate neighborhood, with which the children will be in contact.

Never hold your face close to an animal.

Do not permit a child or young person to lead a large dog.

Never tease, pull the tail, or take away food, bone, or toy with which an animal is playing.

Do not run, ride a bicycle, or skate in front of a dog. It will startle the dog.

Do not touch a dog while the dog is asleep or unaware of your presence. Always speak to any dog that has not seen you approach so that the dog becomes aware of your presence and will not be startled.

Avoid all unnecessary contact with wild animals—now an important spreader of rabies.

Do not overexcite an animal, even in play.

Do not keep animals confined with short ropes or chains. This may make them aggressive and vicious, especially when teased.

Have children avoid dogs raised in a home without children. Such animals may resent children.

Do not allow an inexperienced child or adult to feed a dog. Such persons may pull back when the animal moves to take the food, frightening the animal. This practice is dangerous.

dren can be found in the publication *The Right Dog for You.**

SNAKEBITES

Most snakes in the United States are harmless, and few poisonous snakebites are reported each year. Of the estimated 8000 bites from poisonous snakes, fewer than 20 are fatal (Avery and First, 1989), or 0.25%. Asian and African snakes are far more dangerous than those in the United States and Europe. The major species in the United States are the *Crotilidae* (pit vipers), which include the rattlesnakes, copperheads, and cottonmouths, and the *Elapidae,* which include coral snakes and cobras. Almost all bites are attributed to the *Crotilidae.*

The manifestations and morbidity are highly variable and depend on the species and size of the snake, the amount of venom injected, the time of year, the age and size of the child, and the location of the bite. Also, injection of venom is not an invariable consequence of a bite; 20% to 25% of all bites by poisonous snakes are not associated with injection of venom (Ginsburg and Gädeke, 1989).

The initial action after snakebite is to move the victim away from the area, to attempt to calm the child, and to place the child at rest. A loose tourniquet applied proximal to the bite delays the flow of lymph, which can carry the venom to the systemic circulation. It should not be tight enough to occlude circulation; a pulse distal to the bite should be palpable. Any constricting items of clothing or jewelry should be removed from the affected limb, a splint applied to immobilize the limb, and the victim transported to the nearest medical facility. Ice or cold is not applied because it may increase ischemia.

If the child has been bitten by a large snake, if less than 30 minutes (some authorities say 5 minutes) have elapsed since the child was bitten, and if medical help is more than 30 minutes away, incision and suction may be beneficial, although there is controversy regarding its efficacy. Two small parallel incisions (¼ inch long by ⅛ inch deep) are made along the fang marks, and suction is applied by a suction device from a snakebite kit or an empty syringe. Mouth suction is discouraged because of danger of infection from organisms in the mouth. If possible, the dead snake should be transported with the patient for identification.

HUMAN BITES

Children often acquire lacerations from the teeth of other humans in rough play, during fights, or as victims of child abuse. Many preschool children bite others out of frustration or anger. Most childhood bites by humans are superficial and rarely become infected when the child receives early treatment (Baker and Moore, 1987; Esposito and Adams, 1989). Because human dental plaque and gingiva harbor pathogenic bacteria, all human bites should receive attention. Also delayed treatment increases the risk of infection.

If the laceration is less than ¼ inch in length, the wound can be treated at home. The wound is washed vigorously with soap and water, and a pressure dressing applied to stop bleeding. Ice applications minimize discomfort and swelling. Increased pain or redness at the wound site is an indication that the child should receive medical attention for antibiotic therapy. Tetanus toxoid is needed if more than 5 years has elapsed since the last immunization. Wounds greater than ¼ inch should receive medical attention.

*Tortora, D.F.: The right dog for you, New York, 1980, Simon & Schuster.

DENTAL DISORDERS

Since all of the permanent teeth (except the wisdom teeth) erupt during middle childhood, dental health is of particular importance. Ideally children should receive regular preventive dental care and supervision in daily hygienic care from the time the teeth begin to erupt (see Chapters 14 and 17). The importance of dental care is undisputed; however, limited or inadequate dental care results in the most prevalent of all childhood health problems, chiefly dental caries, malocclusion, periodontal disease, and trauma. Although these conditions are not considered illnesses, they have harmful long-range effects on children's health.

DENTAL CARIES

Dental caries is one of the most common chronic diseases that affect individuals at all ages. Although 100% preventable, dental caries is the principal oral problem in children and adolescents. Although the overall incidence of dental caries in children has decreased since the introduction of fluoridation, it is still an important health problem. Reducing the incidence and consequences of the disorder is of primary importance in childhood because dental caries, if untreated, results in total destruction of involved teeth. The ages of greatest vulnerability are 4 to 8 years for the primary dentition and 12 to 18 years for the secondary or permanent dentition (see Figs. 12-13 and 17-15 for sequence of tooth eruption).

Pathophysiology

Dental caries is a multifactorial disease. The incidence of lesions and the likelihood of progressive invasion vary considerably and depend on a number of factors being present in the right combination: (1) the host, (2) microorganisms, (3) substrate, and (4) time.

Host. The prevalence of caries is directly related to the tooth size and morphology and to the consistency, composition, and amount of saliva. Improperly developed, crowded, or deeply fissured teeth increase the incidence of caries. The areas most subject to attack by bacteria are (in order of difficulty of complete cleansing) grooves and fissures, interdermal areas, gum margins, and other smooth surfaces. Newly erupted teeth that have not yet acquired sufficient surface minerals are more susceptible to decay than those that have been erupted for 2 or more years. Undoubtedly hereditary factors influence resistance and susceptibility, since similar patterns and anatomic characteristics are seen in successive generations. Salivary flow can mechanically clean away bacteria and food debris. It also contains buffering systems, lysozymes, peroxidases, and immunoglobulins that influence the development of caries.

Microorganisms. Three types of microflora that produce different effects contribute to the formation of dental caries. Acidogenic bacteria act on fermentable carbohydrates in dental plaque to produce organic acids that decalcify hard surface tooth enamel. With the inner organic matrix exposed, proteolytic organisms and acids digest and destroy the inner tooth structure. These destructive organisms are harbored and protected in a gelatinous plaque formed on the tooth surface by still another group of bacteria that are thought to play no primary role in production of decay.

Substrates. Caries formation is strongly influenced by the two concurrent processes that continually operate on enamel surfaces—acid production and acid neutralization by saliva. The material on which the acid-forming bacteria act consists essentially of carbohydrates. Among the fermentable carbohydrates, sucrose has been consistently implicated as the most cariogenic. Sucrose-containing substances, especially in tenacious forms that cling (such as chewy candy) or that promote prolonged contact with the teeth (such as chewing gum, hard candy, and lollipops), when ingested between meals, contribute markedly to the development of dental caries. Saliva and other foods that are ingested at mealtime tend to help neutralize much of the acid formed from sucrose.

Time and other factors. Bacterial enzymes act on salivary glycoproteins to produce a tenacious protein matrix on the tooth surface. This substance, along with the microorganisms, forms *dental plaque*. If plaque removal is inadequate or nonexistent for a significant length of time (a few days), the plaque is metabolized by the bacteria to form acid, which initiates the demineralization of enamel (Rule, 1982).

Other factors that contribute to caries formation are heredity, the amount of fluoride in drinking water, lack of or ineffectual oral hygiene, and the child's general state of health. Hereditary factors appear to influence both resistance and susceptibility to dental caries. For example, structural defects, such as deep fissures on occlusive surfaces, predispose to decay, and persons in whom acid formation exceeds neutralization are more prone to caries. The effectiveness of the buffering action of saliva is highly variable among individuals.

Fluoride incorporated into the crystallites of the surface enamel increases the resistance to acid dissolution. Poor oral hygiene that permits the accumulation of food debris on tooth surfaces provides for proliferation of acid-forming bacteria that thrive in this environment. Removal of food particles and bacteria-laden plaque inhibits destructive acid formation.

The susceptibility to dental decay may be influenced by the general health of the child. Children who suffer from chronic debilitating disease show increased caries activity, as do children with systemic conditions that alter the quality and quantity of saliva produced.

Diagnostic Evaluation

Because the permanent teeth erupt during middle childhood, children are more susceptible to development of dental caries during this time than at any other age. Caries penetrate the vulnerable teeth rapidly at this age, as opposed to the slower, intermittent activity characteristic at later ages.

Caries on visible surfaces are easily detected by oral inspection. Large, extensive caries are apparent even to the untrained eye, but small, beginning lesions are best identified by trained professionals. Caries between the teeth may not be located without x-ray examination.

Therapeutic Management

Well-informed health care professionals can provide dental information and make periodic dental assessments. However, dentists are best prepared to provide both of these services and are the only ones qualified to treat most dental problems. Prophylaxis is the major thrust of dental therapy, including hygiene and fluoride treatment (see Chapter 14). Plasticized sealant, applied to deep fissures and grooves of healthy teeth, is effective in blocking cavity formation. Ismail (1989) reported 46% fewer cavities in sealed teeth than in unsealed teeth 4 years after application.

Treatment of dental caries involves removal of all carious portions of teeth as soon as detected, preparation of a retentive cavity, and replacement of the lost portion of the tooth with a material that is durable in the mouth environment. This restoration of involved teeth not only prevents progression of established caries but also reduces the number of bacteria in the oral cavity to decrease the danger to uninvolved teeth.

Nursing Considerations

Oral inspection is an integral part of the nursing assessment of the child in any setting. If there is any evidence of dental caries or other unhealthy state, the child is referred for dental services. The family may have a family dentist or a pedodontist who can provide needed care. An alarming number of children do not receive regular dental supervision, and a significant number reach adulthood without having been examined or treated by a dentist. Nurses can be active members of preventive educational programs and serve as counselors to families regarding the importance of regular dental care, oral hygiene, and dietary management.

Nurses can encourage good oral hygiene by teaching correct tooth cleaning to both children and their parents. The random brushing allowed during the early childhood years should be replaced by more careful and methodic cleansing techniques. Children are taught to brush the teeth according to the method recommended by their dentist and the proper use of dental floss (see Chapter 14). The importance of regular administration of fluoride is emphasized (see Chapter 14). This includes the knowledge of the fluoride content of the drinking water, including bottled water if this is the family practice. School-age children can usually manage the chewable tablets, which have both a topical and a systemic effect. It is often difficult for parents to give medications on a daily basis over a period of years; therefore the children are taught to assume responsibility for taking fluoride as part of their daily dental hygiene.

Restriction of cariogenic foods is also important in the preventive management of dental caries, but this should be viewed as an activity in which all family members are involved and not simply a directive for the child to obey. It should not be communicated in such a way that the child interprets the withholding of sweets as a punishment.

Concern has been generated about the sugar content of children's pharmaceutical products, especially since children with chronic conditions, such as seizure disorders, asthma, and recurrent urinary tract or ear infections, must take medications over a period of years. Evidence indicates a significant association between intake of sucrose-based medications and an increased incidence of dental caries (Shaw and Glenwright, 1989). Children with chronic illness who regularly take medications containing sugar are cautioned to brush their teeth after taking the medication just as they would after eating any carbohydrate substance. Also, children taking tricyclic antidepressants are more prone to develop dental caries.

Sometimes the greatest task for nurses is not teaching dental care but counseling children and families to be motivated to develop sound dental hygiene and nutritional practices. School nurses have an excellent opportunity to engage in detection of dental needs, educating children in dental hygiene and preventing dental problems, making referrals, and motivating children to comply with prophylaxis and treatment.

Children should be prepared for dental services in such a way that visits to the dentist are a positive experience. Keeping appointments and following through on recommended treatments and practices are habits that extend beyond childhood.

PERIODONTAL DISEASE

Periodontal disease, inflammatory and degenerative conditions involving the gums and tissues supporting the teeth, often begins in childhood and accounts for a significant amount of tooth loss in adulthood. The more common periodontal problems are *gingivitis* (simple inflammation of the gums) and *periodontitis* (inflammation of the gums and loss of connective tissue and bone in the supporting structures of the teeth). An uncommon condition is *acute necrotizing ulcerative gingivitis* ("trench mouth").

The most prevalent periodontal disease, gingivitis, is a reversible inflammatory disease that begins very early in many children and is most often associated with the buildup of plaque on the teeth. Changes take place in the plaque bacteria, in both type and number of organisms, causing them to release a variety of destructive exotoxins, enzymes, and other noxious agents. They act to produce an inflammatory reaction in the gingival tissues, causing the gums to become red, edematous, tender, and subject to bleeding at the slightest irritation.

Management is directed toward prevention by conscientious brushing and flossing and by depriving the bacteria of the substrates required to produce the disease. The implementation and maintenance of preventive dental practice, including use of fluoride, plus good dental hygiene are effective in preventing both caries and periodontal disease.

Nursing Considerations

Nursing care of the child with periodontal disease is primarily supportive and preventive; it includes education regarding dental hygiene and regular inspection of the gingival tissues for signs of early inflammation. The child should be directed to see the dentist at any signs of inflammation or irritation.

Nurses caring for teenagers should observe for evidence of chewing tobacco use. The easily detectable clinical lesions appear as tooth erosion, periodontal destruction, and red or white mucosal alterations. The primary site of lesions is the anterior mandibular mucobuccal fold region.

MALOCCLUSION

When teeth of the upper and lower dental arches approximate in the proper relationships, the physiologic function of mastication is more effective, and the cosmetic effect is more pleasing. Teeth that are uneven, crowded, or overlapping or that otherwise interfere with their ability to meet their opponents in the opposite jaw in the appropriate relationships may be predisposed to dental disease (Fig. 18-9). More than half of children 12 to 17 years of age suffer from malocclusions that could be corrected (Guide to Dental Health, 1985).

The most common cause of malocclusion is hereditary

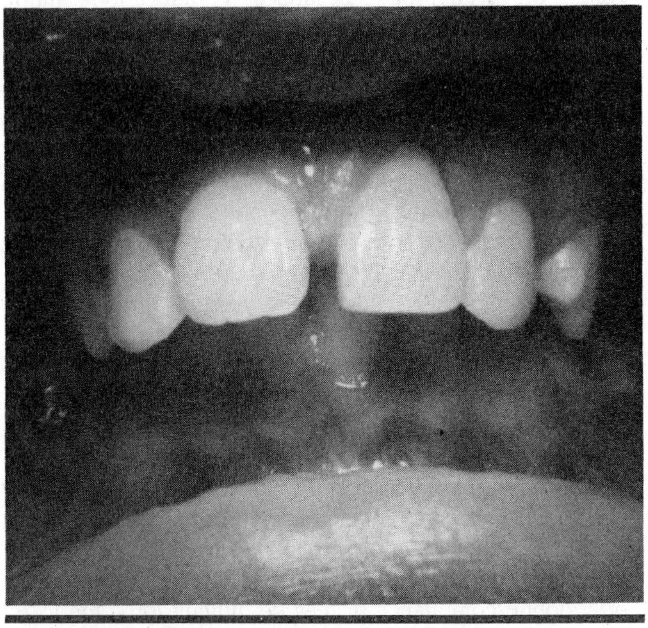

Fig. 18-9. Malocclusion in a school-age child.

factors, but abnormal growth and habits such as thumb-sucking and tongue thrusting also contribute to the disordered alignment and occlusion of the teeth. The important aspects in treatment of malocclusion are elimination of habits that aggravate the deformity and corrective therapy at the optimum time. Orthodontic treatment is usually most successful when it is started in the later school-age years or the early adolescent years, after the last primary teeth have been shed and before growth ceases. However, the trend is toward early correction to prevent problems if the irregularity interferes with normal function and speech; therefore referral should be made as soon as malocclusion is evident. For example, removal of extra teeth, impacted teeth, or prosthetic replacement of missing teeth can prevent problems from developing.

Nursing Considerations

The nurse who detects evidence of malocclusion in a child is obligated to recommend that the teeth be examined by a dentist for possible orthodontia. With the trend toward earlier correction, the sooner the child is evaluated, the better will be the chance for receiving needed treatment. Dealing with habits that predispose to malocclusion, such as thumb- or finger-sucking, is more difficult to manage.

Although orofacial appearance is a subjective phenomenon, there may be a risk of adverse effect on a child's self-esteem and body image. Poorly aligned teeth can be a source of psychologic as well as physical stress to affected children. Many children with malocclusion suffer from teasing from peers or siblings if the irregularities are severe enough. However, it is usually the parents who initiate an orthodontic examination.

After fixed appliances, or braces, have been applied, the child is advised that there will be some discomfort for a few days. During the orthodontic treatments, which average 18 to 30 months, proper oral hygiene is vital. Although the bands or brackets protect the teeth they cover, plaque can collect on the unprotected surfaces or under loose-fitting bands. The teeth are to be brushed with a fluoride toothpaste after every meal and snack and at bedtime, using the method recommended by the dentist. Some orthodontists recommend using an oral irrigating device to remove food from between the teeth and around the braces. However, the device does not remove plaque and is not a substitute for thorough brushing. The orthodontist cautions the child about foods that should not be eaten. Some can damage the braces; others may be difficult to remove from the teeth during cleaning. Forbidden items include chewing gum, ice, nuts, toffee, hard candy, corn-on-the-cob, uncut apples, hard taco shells, nachos, and popcorn.

Occasionally tooth movement or poking at braces with a pencil or other object may cause an arch wire to break or protrude. If this happens the child is instructed to cover the broken portion with a special wax provided by the dentist and schedule an appointment as soon as possible. Regular visits are usually scheduled every 3 to 6 weeks.

Sometimes children need considerable reinforcement for orthodontic compliance. It may be difficult for some to relate the present barriers of discomfort, inconvenience, and embarrassment with the future reinforcers of improved appearance and dental health. Teenagers with a heightened awareness of body image and physical attractiveness are especially at risk for noncompliance (see Chapter 26 for a discussion of noncompliance).

Box 18-4 PERIODS FOR INCREASED FREQUENCY OF DENTAL TRAUMA

Preschool (1 to 3 years)—injury usually secondary to falls or child abuse
School age (7 to 10 years)—injury more often following bicycle and playground accidents
Adolescence (16 to 18 years)—injury generally sustained secondary to fights, athletic injury, and automobile accidents

Data from Berkowitz, R., Ludwig, S., and Johnson, R.: Dental trauma in children and adolescents, J. Pediatr. 19:166-171, 1980.

TRAUMA

Injury to the teeth is not an uncommon occurrence in childhood (Box 18-4). This includes fractures of varying degrees of severity, chipping, dislocation, or evulsion. All tooth injuries require prompt treatment by a competent dentist in order to prevent permanent displacement or loss. Delayed examination and diagnosis of tooth damage all too frequently result in infection or pulp involvement that can be avoided by early attention. Also, because it can affect the remaining teeth, loss of a permanent tooth requires professional attention to maintain normal alignment and position of teeth.

Boys experience injury to permanent teeth much more frequently than girls, although this observation is not supported in all studies. Trauma usually involves the maxillary incisors, and children with protruding teeth, craniofacial abnormalities, or neuromuscular disorders are more likely to sustain dental injuries. A tooth that is avulsed (evulsed, exarticulated, or "knocked out") can be reimplanted and retained permanently if replaced without delay (Krasner, 1990).

Nursing Considerations: Tooth Evulsion

A permanent tooth that is avulsed should be replanted by the child, parent, or nurse and stabilized as soon as possible so that the blood supply to the tooth can be reestablished and the tooth kept alive. If the tooth is replaced within 30 minutes, there is a 70% chance that it will become reattached and roots will not resorb or the crown exfoliate. Evulsed primary teeth are usually not reimplanted.

Before reimplantation it is important to carefully rinse a dirty tooth in milk, saline solution, or under running water to avoid disturbing the adhering periodontal membrane, which is essential to the success of the reimplantation. The tooth is held by the crown, not the root, while rinsing, with the drain plugged. The tooth is then fit back into its socket the best way possible, even if it means placing it backward or at an angle (Kochman, 1989). If the tooth is reimplanted almost immediately, excessive pressure is not needed; however, it becomes extremely difficult after clot formation (in approximately 10 minutes). The tooth is held in place by the child during transportation to a dentist. Care is taken to avoid sudden stops or turns that might cause the child to swallow or aspirate the loose tooth.

If the child or parents are reluctant to reimplant the tooth, the next best alternative is to place the tooth in cold milk, contact lens solution, or saline for transport to the dentist. Cold milk has precisely the osmolality to maintain fluid balance within the tissues surrounding the tooth. Tap water is not recommended (Kochman, 1989). The third alternative for transport is to place the tooth under the child's tongue, or under the parent's tongue if the child is too young or too anxious. After implantation the tooth will usually become firmly attached, although endodontic therapy is often required. If reimplantation is not permanent, the tooth may be retained anywhere from 6 months to 12 years and serves to facilitate normal development and occlusion, since loss of teeth during the period of permanent tooth eruption may adversely affect such development.

As with all mouth trauma, an evulsed tooth causes a large amount of bleeding, which is most distressing to the child. Bleeding is frightening to children and their families; therefore the nurse or anyone who is faced with dental trauma should be prepared to cope with the emotionality that accompanies a tooth evulsion. Using a calm approach and providing gentle reassurance to the child requires only a moment and goes a long way toward reducing anxiety.

EMERGENCY TREATMENT
Evulsed Tooth

Recover tooth.
Hold tooth by crown; avoid touching root area.
If tooth is dirty, rinse it gently under running water or saline; be sure to insert stopper in sink or basin (to avoid tooth loss).
Insert tooth into socket.
Have child maintain tooth in place.
Transport child to dentist immediately.
Avoid sudden stops or sharp turns to prevent dislodging tooth.

If reluctant to reimplant tooth:

Place evulsed tooth in suitable medium for transport:
a. Cold milk
b. Saliva—under the child's or parent's tongue
If child is holding tooth in the mouth, avoid sudden stops to prevent swallowing tooth.
DON'T FORGET TO TAKE TOOTH

DISORDERS OF CONTINENCE

Disorders involving elimination and continence are common in childhood, especially diarrhea; constipation is observed less frequently (see also Chapter 33). More troublesome problems of elimination are enuresis and encopresis.

ENURESIS

Enuresis (bed-wetting) is a common and troublesome disorder that is difficult to define because of the variable ages at which children achieve bladder control. Bladder control depends on a number of factors, including the individual child's developmental tempo, the manner in which training is carried out, the personality makeup of the child, and the emotional climate of the home environment. In a broad sense enuresis can be defined as repeated involuntary urination (usually nocturnal) in children who are beyond the age when voluntary bladder control should normally have been acquired. Some authorities place 4 years as an arbitrary age by which diurnal and nocturnal bladder control is normally accomplished, although 5 years of age is probably more accurate.

Enuresis can also be defined as *primary,* bed-wetting in children who have never been dry for extended periods, or *secondary,* the onset of wetting after a continuous dry period of more than 1 year (American Psychiatric Association, 1987). The incidence is approximately 5% to 17% in otherwise normal children between 3 and 15 years of age.

No clear-cut etiology for enuresis as a distinct entity has been determined. A high frequency of bed-wetting has been observed in parents, siblings, and other near relatives of symptomatic children, and these observations are supported by a high concordance rate in enuretic monozygotic twins. Family studies indicate that the closer the relationship, the higher the incidence of enuresis (Friman, 1986). Approximately 75% of all children with functional enuresis have a first-degree relative who has, or has had, the disorder (American Psychiatric Association, 1987). It appears that these persons have difficulty in inhibiting the mechanisms that regulate the emptying of the bladder.

Enuresis is more common in boys than in girls, but the reason for this higher frequency is not altogether clear. Other factors that have been observed include a higher frequency in children in the lower socioeconomic groups and a higher frequency in black children than in white children. An increased prevalence has also been observed among late-maturing adolescents, both male and female, than early or midmaturers, and the children describe themselves as tense, having difficulty sleeping, and having bad dreams. Children ages 6 through 11 have temperaments described as high strung and lost their temper easily (Levine, 1983). Enuretic children are more likely to be afraid of the dark.

Pathophysiology

Enuresis is primarily a problem of delayed or incomplete neuromuscular maturation of the bladder and as such is benign and self-limiting. There are children who exhibit temporary regressive behavior after the birth of a sibling or who have occasional "accidents" when they become involved in play to such an extent that they are unaware of a full bladder, become excited, or "forget" to empty the bladder. In other children enuresis may be caused by problems associated with toilet training that are related to the age at which training is begun, the emotional atmosphere that surrounds the training situation, or an excessive amount of emotional dependence on the mother. In some children enuresis is one behavioral manifestation of a personality disorder. However, behavioral problems associated with enuresis are probably a result rather than a cause of the enuresis.

A significant number of nocturnal enuretic episodes are related to deep sleep. These children seem to sleep more soundly than others and to waken from either external or internal stimuli. Many of these children demonstrate increased frequency and magnitude of spontaneous bladder contractions during the non-rapid-eye-movement (N-REM) stage of sleep preceding bed-wetting. Bed-wetting appears to occur as the child moves from the deeper stages of non-REM sleep into the REM stage.

Enuresis has a strong familial tendency and seems to be associated with a developmental delay that causes such intense urgency that the child is unable to inhibit bladder contraction after the bladder is distended beyond a certain volume. Such children acquire bladder control with difficulty and, even after control, are more prone to enuresis when subjected to stress than are other children. In addition, most of these children have a borderline functional bladder capacity. The small bladder is unable to hold a full night's urine excretion.

Clinical Manifestations

The predominant symptom is urgency that is immediate and accompanied by acute discomfort, restlessness, and sometimes urinary frequency. Nocturnal enuresis is most common and is occasionally accompanied by diurnal wetting; diurnal bed-wetting without nocturnal bed-wetting is unusual. In most affected children nocturnal bed-wetting is a primary maturational problem and usually ceases between ages 6 and 8, although it may continue into adolescence.

Diagnostic Evaluation

Organic causes that may be related to enuresis should be ruled out before psychogenic factors are considered. These include structural disorders of the urinary tract, urinary tract infection, major neurologic deficits, nocturnal epilepsy, disorders such as diabetes mellitus and diabetes insipidus that increase the normal output of urine, and disorders such as chronic renal failure or sickle cell disease that impair the concentrating ability of the kidneys. In other cases the enuresis is influenced by emotional factors, although it is doubtful that they are etiologic factors.

In older children routine examinations are carried out to rule out infection, and bladder capacity is determined by having the children hold off voiding until they feel urgency, at which time they void into a measured container. A bladder volume of 300 to 350 ml is sufficient to hold a night's urine.

Therapeutic Management

Enuresis not resulting from organic causes can be approached in several ways. No method is so successful as to achieve universal endorsement; however, some have proved helpful in keeping the child dry during the night. Frequently more than one technique is employed.

Bladder retention training. Most children with enuresis have smaller functional bladder capacities. Bladder training is aimed at stretching the bladder to accommodate increasingly larger volumes of urine. After forcing fluids the child is instructed to postpone voiding as long as can be tolerated before emptying the bladder. The heightened threshold for retention allows the child to remain dry throughout the night.

Motivational therapy. Motivational therapy involves a series of counseling interviews designed to encourage the child to assume responsibility for the disorder and the necessary learning. Approaches include reassurance, guilt removal, and emotional support by the family and health personnel. The emphasis is on promoting the development of positive parent-child relationship and reinforcement for progress, ranging from works of praise to material rewards. Punishment for bed-wetting is discouraged.

This responsibility-reinforcement therapy emphasizes "sensation awareness" of bladder fullness and positive reinforcement for progressive steps toward the ultimate goal of being dry. Such response shaping requires considerable input by a supportive family and health professionals (Rushton, 1989).

Behavior modification (conditioning) therapy. A number of electrical devices are available that are based on the conditioned reflex response. These consist of a wire pad attached to a bell or buzzer that wakens the child as soon as the first drops of urine create a closed circuit. The child is thus conditioned to waken at the initiation of micturition or to the stimulus of the bell or buzzer. Most have reported a substantial success rate with the device. There appear to be no undesirable emotional effects, although this is debatable.

There are disadvantages to the use of electrical devices. A practical problem is the disturbance it may create when other children sleep in the same room or in the same bed. The child may be too sleepy or forget to reset the alarm following its activation to render it effective for the remainder of the night. There may be a risk of ulceration and scarring caused by slow electrolysis of tissue cells when the child does not hear the alarm or turns the alarm off without waking while the current continues to flow or when the batteries have run down to a feeble point where the alarm is insufficiently loud.

Drug therapy. A number of pharmacologic agents can be used in the treatment of enuresis, either alone or in combination with other techniques. The selection depends on the interpretation of the cause. The drug used most frequently is the tricyclic antidepressant drug imipramine (Tofranil), which exerts an anticholinergic action on the bladder to inhibit urination. The dosage and time of administration are individualized, and the drug is given in amounts sufficient to lighten sleep but not to cause wakefulness. The suggested length of treatment is 6 to 8 weeks, followed by gradual withdrawal over 4 weeks. Since this drug is dangerous in overdosage, parents must be cautioned about judicious use and keeping supplies of the drug far from the reach of younger siblings.

Anticholinergic drugs, especially oxybutynin, reduce uninhibited bladder contractions and may be helpful for children with daytime urinary frequency. Some success has also been achieved with desmopressin (DDAVP) nasal spray, an analog of vasopressin, which reduces nighttime urine output to a volume less than functional bladder capacity.

Miscellaneous therapies. Restricting or eliminating fluids after the evening meal is aimed at decreasing the output of urine during the night. This method has proved to be of questionable value.

Having the child void before retiring and then wakened and taken to the bathroom has met with limited success. Favorable responses are probably a result of the focused concern by both parents and child and of the positive behavioral reinforcement it provides. For this to be effective, the parent should be sure that the child is fully awake when the bladder is emptied.

Other therapies include psychotherapy, hypnotherapy, and diet therapy. These therapies have been used in special cases and with varying success.

Nursing Considerations

No matter which of the various techniques are used, the nurse can help both children and parents to understand the problem of enuresis, the treatment plan, and the probable difficulties they may encounter in the process. Essential to the success of any method is the supportive management of parents and their children. Both need encouragement and patience. The problem is discussed with the parents, and, since any treatment involves and requires the child's active participation, children are included as well. The most important predictor for the outcome of treatment is family difficulties. Family disturbances influence the initial arrest of the enuresis, the relapse rate, and the long-term success rate (Dische and others, 1983).

Many parents believe that enuresis is caused by an emotional disturbance and fear that they have somehow produced the situation by imprudent childrearing practices. They need reassurance that the bed-wetting is not a manifestation of emotional disturbance nor does it represent willful misbehavior. They should be informed about the nature of enuresis and cautioned against scolding, shaming, threatening, and punishing a child, which are useless and harmful.

Communication with children is directed toward eliminating the emotional impact of the problem by relieving them of feelings of shame, guilt, and the burden of parental disapproval and toward building up their self-confidence and motivating them toward independent control. More important, the nurse can provide consistent support and encouragement to help sustain them through the inconsistent and unpredictable treatment process. Children need to believe that they are helping themselves and to sustain feelings of confidence and hope. Children who have mastered bed-wetting demonstrate an improvement in self-concept (Moffatt, Kato, and Pless, 1987.)

ENCOPRESIS

Encopresis is repeated voluntary or involuntary passage of feces of normal or near-normal consistency into places not appropriate for that purpose in the individual's own sociocultural setting (American Psychiatric Association, 1987). The disorder is less common than enuresis, but the two may coexist. It may not be an isolated symptom, but clustered with other somatic symptoms—social withdrawal, antisocial-aggressive behaviors, affective-dependent behaviors, and somatic manifestations. Although many children demonstrate significant behavior problems, most children with encopresis do not (Friman, 1988).

A child who has never achieved fecal incontinence by 4 years of age is said to have primary, or continuous, encopresis. This type is more frequently observed as a result of neglect, lax training methods, mental subnormalities, and familial causes. Secondary, or discontinuous, encopresis is fecal incontinence occurring in a child over 4 years of age preceded by at least 1 year of fecal continence (American Psychiatric Association, 1987). The disorder is more common in males than in females.

Because chronic soiling is now considered to be physiologic as well as behavioral, the term *idiopathic fecal incontinence (IFI)* has been suggested as a more descriptive term and should be used except when psychiatric dysfunction contributes to the soiling (Stroh, Stern, and McCarthy, 1989).

Etiology

One of the most common causes of encopresis is constipation, which may be precipitated by environmental change, such as birth of a new sibling, moving to a new house, changing schools, or even having to use new or unfamiliar toilet facilities (Johns, 1985). Voluntary retention usually follows a painful incident with voluntary suppression of defecation (e.g., a child with anal fissures). Involuntary retention may be produced by emotional problems caused by the encopresis that sets up a fear-pain cycle and results in a learned process of abnormal defecation patterns. Psychogenic encopresis, in which the soiling is caused by the emotional problems, is often related to a disturbed mother-child relationship.

Normally children and adolescents have one or two soft-formed stools per day. Children with soiling problems tend to form large-bore stools, which are painful to excrete. Therefore they tend to avoid defecation and withhold stooling. Stool held in the rectum and sigmoid colon loses water, progressively hardens, causing successively more painful bowel movements. Thus a pain-retention-pain cycle is established. Many children have diarrhea or loose leakage in their clothing and pass small amounts of hard stool, suggesting leakage around an impaction (Rappaport and Levine, 1986; Stroh, Stern, and McCarthy, 1989).

During school years children may experience exacerbations at the transition to school. Some of the reasons for developing retentive tendencies at this time are fear of using school bathrooms, a busy schedule, and the interruption of an established time schedule for bowel evacuation. Children at any age may react to stress with bowel dysfunction.

Clinical Manifestations

The manifestation of simple constipation is painful expulsion of hard, pelletlike stools. Voluntary retention is usually temporary, and there is a history of a painful precipitating episode and blood-streaked stools. Involuntary retention is associated with a history of abdominal pain, distention, moodiness, poor appetite, and accumulation of stools with periodic passage of voluminous stools. Children display a characteristic posturing during suppression of colonic signals to defecate—stiffening, standing in a corner with straight legs and a bright-red face, "doing a little dance," "crawling," or hiding behind furniture or a tree when playing outdoors (Rappaport and Levine, 1986; Younger and Hughes, 1983). They typically hide soiled underwear. It is not unusual for soiling to take place after bathing because of reflex stimulation.

School performance and attendance are affected as the child's offensive odor becomes a target for scorn and derision from classmates. The child is not well liked by peers because of it and may be severely rejected by the parents as a result of the symptom. The rejection by peers and parents causes further withdrawal and other behavioral manifestations.

Therapeutic Management

Treatment is directed toward the cause of the soiling. Diet, lubricants, and a toilet ritual that encourages the child to establish normal defecation are used (Younger and Hughes, 1983). Fecal impaction is relieved by catharsis, suppositories, and/or mineral oil. Customary dosages are usually insufficient. Dietary changes may be helpful, such as elimination of milk and dairy products and increased amounts of high-fiber foods, such as fruits, vegetables, and cereals, as well as increased fluids. Behavior therapy may be indicated to eliminate any fear that has developed as a result of painful defecation. Frequently psychotherapeutic intervention with the child and the family becomes necessary.

Nursing Considerations

The prevailing attitude of nurses toward the family of a child with encopresis is one of no-fault, thus relieving the guilt of both parents and child. A thorough history of the soiling is essential—when soiling began, how often it occurs, under what circumstances, and if the child uses the toilet successfully at all (Stroh, Stern, and McCarthy, 1989). Since parents and child are reluctant to volunteer information, direct questioning about the soiling is more successful. Following a history a complete physical assessment is performed.

Education regarding the physiology of normal defecation, toilet training as a developmental process, and the treatment outlined for the particular family is prerequisite to a successful outcome. Parents are relieved to know that other parents share this problem and are surprised to know that functional changes that take place as the condition develops make control of seepage impossible. Many parents complain that their children soil because they are do not take time from play for a bowel movement. Actually the child may be unaware of a prior sensation and unable to control the urge once it begins. They may be so accustomed to bowel accidents that they are unable to smell or feel it and even deny soiling when it occurs (Stroh, Stern, and McCarthy, 1989).

The regimen prescribed for stimulating elimination is outlined and explained to parents. Sitting the child on the toilet at routine intervals is not recommended because it may intensify parent-child conflict and result in a power play. Enemas may be needed for impactions, but long-term use prevents the child from assuming responsibility for defecation (Johns, 1985). Initially lubricants are given liberally, but stimulant cathartics often cause abdominal cramps that can be a frightening experience for a child.

Family counseling is directed toward reassurance that most problems resolve successfully, although the child may have relapses during periods of stress, such as vacation or illness. If encopresis persists beyond occasional relapses, the condition will need to be reevaluated. Behavior modification techniques are explained, and the family is assisted with a plan suited to their particular situation.

BEHAVIORAL DISORDERS IN SCHOOL-AGE CHILDREN

A number of classification systems have been employed to outline the various problems of middle childhood that interfere with development, learning, and social relationships. Although there is no universal categorization, most authorities seem to broadly classify behavioral disorders in some manner that identifies mental subnormality, learning disabilities, neuroses, psychoses, and antisocial behavior. Many disorders have a major organic or developmental component, whereas others are seen almost exclusively in children of school age. Still others are primarily problems of adolescence, and many extend throughout the course of childhood. Very often a change in behavior is one of the manifestations of an organic disease; at other times emotional problems produce somatic symptoms of greater or lesser seriousness.

The variety and extent of emotional and behavioral disorders of childhood are much too numerous to be considered here; some are discussed elsewhere (for example, mental retardation in Chapter 24 and sensory impairment in Chapter 25).

ATTENTION DEFICIT–HYPERACTIVITY DISORDER

Attention deficit–hyperactivity disorder (AD-HD) is the latest term applied to various behavior problems that in some way impair the child's capacity to profit from new experiences. The syndrome of manifestations affects a significant number of children and is 10 times more frequent in boys than in girls. The difficulties are most often school related, behavioral or academic, and difficulties with social relationships in general are often manifested by aggressive behavior and mood lability that interferes with peer relationships and makes disciplining difficult.

Considerable confusion and disagreement exist regarding AD-HD, previously known as attention deficit disorder (ADD) with or without hyperactivity, hyperactivity, minimal brain damage (MBD), and hyperkinesis. Not all children display hyperactivity. In addition there are individuals who evidenced AD-HD at an earlier age but who no longer demonstrate the hyperactivity. Many of the children have specific learning disabilities.

Early identification of affected children is needed, since the characteristics of the disorder significantly interfere with the normal course of emotional and psychologic development. In an attempt to cope with attention deficit, many of these children develop maladaptive behavior patterns that are a deterrent to psychosocial adjustment. Their behavior evokes negative responses from others, and repeated exposure to negative feedback adversely affects the child's self-concept.

The term *specific learning disabilities* refers to the behavioral outcomes of impaired functioning in central processing such as dyslexia, dysphasia, and inability to calculate or draw. It is primarily an educational concern and mentioned briefly at the conclusion of this segment.

Etiology

The etiology of AD-HD is uncertain, obscure, and often speculative. As the definition implies, it may be related to virtually any illness or trauma affecting the brain that occurs at any stage of development—before, during, or after birth. Multiple causes, including psychosocial factors, are probably involved.

Behavioral and learning disorders have been noted in children with some of the sex chromosomal abnormalities. For example, in girls with Turner syndrome there is a high incidence of impaired spatial abilities and right-left directional sense, and a large number of boys with Klinefelter syndrome have learning, behavioral, or peer problems. A sex-linked factor may be operating because the hyperkinetic syndrome is much more common in boys than in girls.

A popular theory is the concept of a developmental lag. Distractibility, short attention span, and impulsiveness are all normal characteristics of children at a much younger developmental level. Since the symptoms tend to diminish with age, it is postulated that this may have an anatomic basis, that is, a maturational lag in myelination of the prefrontal cortex that takes place through adolescence. In addition, hyperactivity may be merely a normal variant of innate temperament in some children who represent the extreme end of the normal distribution curve for activity.

Support for a biochemical etiology is suggested by the way in which a majority of hyperactive children respond to central nervous system stimulant drugs. In these hyperactive children there appears to be an absence or insufficiency of norepinephrine, a neurotransmitter that normally appears in high concentrations in areas of the brain that have much to do with activity level, mood, and awareness. Another theory suggests some alteration in the reticular activating system of the midbrain, a key area for controlling consciousness and attention, that interferes with its function of filtering out extraneous stimuli. Consequently these children are unable to focus on one stimulus but are compelled to respond to every stimulus in the environment. Central nervous system stimulants that increase the level of norepinephrine and/or activate the reticular activating system cause a reduction in the undesired behavior. The fact that these children show few, if any, symptoms in a stress situation (such as the clinician's or principal's office) provides additional support to this hypothesis, because stress increases the level of norepinephrine.

Interest in diet as a factor in hyperactivity continues to generate controversies. There are those who believe that the observed behavioral patterns are related to an innate sensitivity to certain food items and/or food additives. Although this theory does not have wholehearted support, some children do show improvement when certain foods are eliminated from their diet, particularly those containing salicylates and those with specific additives such as artificial coloring, sweetening, and preservatives.

Clinical Manifestations

The behaviors exhibited by the child with AD-HD are not unusual aspects of child behavior. The difference lies in the quality of motor activity and developmentally inappropriate inattention, impulsivity, and hyperactivity the child displays. The manifestations may be numerous or few, mild or severe, and will vary with the developmental level of the child. Any given child will not have every manifestation that is characteristic of a syndrome, and the degree of severity is highly variable. Mild manifestations of the symptoms may not be apparent in a good educational and family environment, whereas severe symptomatology will be recognizable even in the most healthy and accommodating environment. Every dysfunctional child is, in some respects, different from all other children with AD-HD.

Most behavioral manifestations are apparent at an early age, but the learning disabilities may not become evident until the child enters school. The symptoms are more prominent before age 10, after which they become more subtle, tending to diminish with advancing age. The disorder is unpredictable; it may remit spontaneously at any age, and the number of years a child will require treatment is unknown. Although it appears that most characteristics of AD-HD do not extend into adolescence, increasing evidence indicates that hyperactive children do not necessarily outgrow their symptoms (Brown, 1986). Concomitant emotional difficulties are frequent, and there are indications of continued difficulties in school, difficulties with peers and authority figures, and continued aggressive behavior.

Children who are unable to function normally in their home and school environment will meet with constant failure and rejection and will react with hostility or other inappropriate behaviors. Their frequent recognition that they are "bad" or not "right inside" will produce a negative self-concept and reactive hostility.

The basic characteristics outlined in Box 18-5 reflect disturbances in central processing. These criteria are the basis for establishing a diagnosis of AD-HD. Research has found that children with AD-HD exhibit attention, behavioral, and cognitive impairments, whereas children with AD-HD with-

Box 18-5 DIAGNOSTIC CRITERIA FOR ATTENTION DEFICIT–HYPERACTIVITY DISORDER

Note: Consider a criterion met only if the behavior is considerably more frequent than that of most people of the same mental age.

A. A disturbance of a least 6 months during which at least eight of the following are present:
  (1) Often fidgets with hands or feet or squirms in seat (in adolescents, may be limited to subjective feelings of restlessness)
  (2) Has difficulty remaining seated when required to do so
  (3) Is easily distracted by extraneous stimuli
  (4) Has difficulty awaiting turn in games or group situations
  (5) Often blurts out answers to questions before they have been completed
  (6) Has difficulty following through on instructions from others (not due to oppositional behavior or failure of comprehension), e.g., fails to finish chores
  (7) Has difficulty sustaining attention in tasks or play activities
  (8) Often shifts from one uncompleted activity to another
  (9) Has difficulty playing quietly
  (10) Often talks excessively
  (11) Often interrupts or intrudes on others, e.g., butts into other children's games
  (12) Often does not seem to listen to what is being said to him or her
  (13) Often loses things necessary for tasks or activities at school or at home (e.g., toys, pencils, books, assignments)
  (14) Often engages in physically dangerous activities without considering possible consequences (not for the purpose of thrill-seeking), e.g., runs into street without looking

  Note: The above items are listed in descending order of discriminating power based on data from a national field trial of the DSM-III-R criteria for Disruptive Behavior Disorders.

B. Onset before the age of seven

C. Does not meet the criteria for a Pervasive Developmental Disorder

Criteria for Severity of Attention Deficit–Hyperactivity Disorder:

Mild: Few, if any symptoms in excess of those required to make the diagnosis and only minimal or no impairment in school and social functioning

Moderate: Symptoms or functional impairment intermediate between "mild" and "severe"

Severe: Many symptoms in excess of those required to make the diagnosis and significant and pervasive impairment in functioning at home and school and with peers

From Diagnostic and statistical manual of mental disorders, ed. 3—revised (DSM-III-R), Washington, DC, 1987, American Psychiatric Association.

out hyperactivity show deficits in an attention/cognitive dimension (Berry, Shaywitz, and Shaywitz, 1985). Management problems and antisocial behavior are associated with hyperactivity; increased impulsivity is not associated with attention deficits in the absence of hyperactivity.

The same researchers found that there are sex differences in children with AD-HD. Disruptive, uncontrolled behaviors are more frequent among boys; girls with AD-HD without hyperactivity display poor self-esteem and are significantly older than boys with the same type of AD-HD. Girls with AD-HD with or without hyperactivity are more likely to suffer peer rejection than boys. Girls may not be diagnosed as readily as boys, and cognitive deficits play a more prominent role with girls; behavioral disturbances increase the likelihood of identification for boys.

Diagnostic Evaluation

Neurologic and psychologic examinations are useful in detecting specific defects, and observations made in a familiar environment may help confirm suspicions. However, it is the history that ultimately determines the diagnosis. The child seldom displays symptoms in the practitioner's office and acts reasonably normal in a one-to-one relationship.

A history, both medical and developmental, and description of the child's behavior should be obtained from as many observers of the child as possible, especially parents and teachers, as well as the observations of the health professionals involved. It should include descriptions of the child's behavior in home and school situations. In obtaining descriptive material, the interviewer must question the observers carefully because some persons, especially parents, may be so concerned with gross behaviors that they overlook less distressing but equally important symptoms. For example, parents may report a "colicky" infant, a child who began to run as soon as he walked, a toddler who is compelled to touch everything in sight, and a child who resists sleep until exhausted. A history of delayed or atypical language development is associated with specific learning disabilities. A pregnancy and birth history may provide clues to a situation that might have produced an episode of hypoxia.

A physical examination, including a detailed neurologic evaluation, will help rule out any severe neurologic disorders. Psychologic testing, especially projective tests, is valuable in determining visual-perceptual difficulties, problems with spatial organization, and other phenomena that suggest cortical or diencephalic involvement, and it helps to identify the child's intelligence and achievement levels. Psychiatric and other disorders are ruled out, including lead poisoning, petit mal seizures, partial hearing loss, psychosis, and witnessing sexual activity (common in children in lower socioeconomic groups).

Therapeutic Management

Management of the child with AD-HD usually involves a multiple approach that includes family education and counseling, medication, proper classroom placement, environmental manipulation, and sometimes psychotherapy for the child.

Behavioral therapy and psychotherapy. Behavioral therapy is often successful for the child whose behavior, mood, and reality-perception disturbances are not severe. This consists of a relatively controlled environment in conjunction with behavior modification techniques, family counseling, and/or psychotherapy (see Nursing Considerations). Diet modification has proved to be effective for some children but is not a standard therapeutic modality.

Pharmacologic therapy. Many drugs have been advocated for management of the symptoms of AD-HD. The most frequently prescribed medications are the sympathomimetic amines methylphenidate or dextroamphetamine (Dexedrine). They produce strong effects on central nervous system dopamine and norepinephrine. Methylphenidate is preferred because of its less marked effect on prolactin and growth hormone. The child is begun on a small dose that is gradually increased until the desired response is achieved. Less often prescribed are magnesium pemoline (Cylert) and the tricyclic antidepressants. Pemoline is a mild central nervous system stimulant with a slower onset, and its effect appears less marked. Tricyclic antidepressants, principally imipramine (Tofranil) and desipramine (Norpramin), have proved to be effective in some children, but cardiac side effects must be monitored.

Nursing Considerations

Nurses, especially school nurses, are active participants in all aspects of management of the child with AD-HD. Nurses in the community setting work with families in the home on a long-term basis to help plan and implement therapeutic regimens and to evaluate the effectiveness of therapy. They are in the best position to coordinate services and serve as liaison between other health and education professionals directly involved in a child's therapy program. School nurses have an understanding of the child's special needs and work with teachers. The nurse in any setting (community, school, hospital, practitioner's office) can provide support and guidance to children and families during the difficult tasks associated with growing up with a disabling condition.

The management of the child with AD-HD begins with an explanation to the parents and the child about the diagnosis, including the nature of the problem and the practitioner's concept of the underlying central nervous system basis for the disorder. Most parents are confused and feel some measure of guilt. To some it is confirmation of the fear that the child may be "crazy" or has some irreversible, serious disease; to others it is a relief. They need the opportunity to vent their feelings and suspicions. A common complaint of parents is that health professionals have not listened to what they have to say about their child.

The parents need information about the prognosis and an understanding of the treatment plan. The greater their understanding of the disorder and its effects, the more likely they will be to carry out the recommended program of therapy. It is important that they understand that the therapy is not necessarily a panacea and that it will extend over a long period. This has particular significance for changes they need to make in environmental management. Reading material to help the child and family can be obtained from a variety of sources.

Medication. Parents are reminded that some medications (pemoline) require 2 to 3 weeks to achieve an effect. Others are begun at low dosage and increased until the desired effect is attained. When evaluating the child's response to the medication, it is helpful to obtain reports from the teacher as well as from the parents, since the parents may see the child when the effects of the drug are wearing off. Observing the child's behavior through visits to home and school is useful for assessing attention span, interactional patterns with others at school, and behaviors with academic tasks. The nurse can consult with the teacher about the child's behavior in general. This information provides data needed to regulate dosage based on recorded, systematic observations of the child's behaviors in at least two settings.

Parents need to be informed of the possible side effects of the medication—anorexia, blurred vision, and sleeplessness—which usually disappear after several weeks. A common complaint is that the child becomes quiet and very sensitive, crying at the slightest provocation. Sleeplessness is reduced by administering the medication early in the day. It has also been found that the absorption of methylphenidate is accelerated when administered with meals and impeded when given before meals (Chan and others, 1983). Another troublesome side effect is depressed growth, probably caused by interference with the release of growth hormone; therefore the physician may sometimes discontinue the drug on weekends or on vacations to allow for some catch-up growth, although some believe there is no theoretic or practical advantage to the practice (Brown, 1986).

Children on tricyclic antidepressants display a dramatic increase in the incidence of dental caries (Slome, 1984). The marked anticholinergic action of the drugs increases saliva viscosity and produces a dry mouth. Emphasis on rigorous dental hygiene, conscientious home fluoride treatment, regular visits to the dentist, limited intake of refined carbohydrates, and artificial saliva is an important nursing function. The child should be kept well hydrated.

Parents may express concern that the child may become addicted to antidepressant drugs. There is always the possibility of abuse, including suicide attempts; however, usually the child is no longer interested in the drug once the need is past—particularly since the effect of the drug in these children is opposite that produced in normal individuals. However, parents are cautioned to keep the drugs safely stored away from children who may inadvertently ingest them.

In those children in whom a salicylate-free diet relieves the disordered behavior, which is caused by an allergic reaction to food additives, the parents may need help with the child's diet; for example, it is the nurse's responsibility to find out what the child *can eat* and help the parents find sources for the proper foods, especially if the child is on a special metabolic diet.

Environmental manipulation. The child's environment is simplified by decreasing external stimuli, reducing alternatives, encouraging desired patterns of behavior, and sometimes diet control. The parents may need assistance to determine firm but reasonable limits and support in their efforts to provide a stable and predictable environment with regular routines of sleeping, eating, working, and playing. The child needs an environment in which distractions are reduced to a minimum and that is relatively free of external stimuli. In addition, the more the environment is controlled, the less medication is required.

Appropriate classroom placement. Special training activities in the schools are designed to offer a direct attack on such areas of deficit as visual perception, auditory perception, and other areas involving integration and coordination. These may be accomplished in self-contained classes with a limit of six to eight children, special resource rooms with equipment and teaching teams, mobile consultants who move from room to room to provide assistance to teachers and children, and special first-grade programs in which high-risk children receive special attention to prevent or reduce the need for services as they progress. The purpose of programs for children with special learning disabilities is to assist them toward more successful achievement, personal adjustment, and eventual retention in the regular classroom. However, because a true perceptual problem exists, improvement is noted by an increased attention span, allowing the child to focus on one stimulus while blocking out others; refinement of fine motor control; and advancement in other areas of disability.

Psychiatric, psychologic, and social therapies. On the whole, psychotherapy is relatively unsuccessful in the treatment of the basic characteristics of AD-HD. However, psychotherapy is sometimes useful in children who have experienced negative experiences to the extent that their self-image is threatened. Often children with this disorder describe themselves as stupid or "mentally retarded." They are different from the other children, and they know it. Although they have strengths, they seldom have an opportunity to demonstrate them. Consequently they develop coping mechanisms to deal with their negative self-image. They are restless and disruptive, resort to clowning, and develop somatic symptoms. They may become apathetic, resort to daydreaming, appear "not to care," or display perfectionistic perseverance in the attempt to do well. Shy children may withdraw. The child with behavior problems is the one who will get help earlier than the quiet child. Therefore the quiet child may not receive help until the problem is well advanced, which is a disadvantage because remediation takes longer when it is begun with older children. Both child and family may need help during certain periods of stress.

SPECIFIC LEARNING DISABILITY

Learning-disabled children are those who exhibit a disorder in one or more of the basic psychologic processes involved in understanding or in using spoken or written language. The disability may be manifested in disorders of listening, thinking, talking, reading, writing, spelling, or calculating. They include conditions that have been referred to as perceptual disabilities and developmental aphasia. They do not include learning problems, which result primarily from visual, hearing, or motor disabilities, mental retardation, emotional disturbances, or environmental disadvantage.

QUESTIONS AND CONTROVERSIES

Should school children be placed on medication to improve classroom behavior?

The controversy surrounding the use of methylphenidate (Ritalin) for hyperactivity and inattentiveness has gained considerable attention among lay persons (including educators) and health professionals. Parents and other lay persons hear about therapies and their effectiveness from lay magazines, newpapers, or on television news or talk show discussions (Silver, 1986) and begin to pressure practitioners to prescribe the medication in the hope that the child's disruptive behavior can be modified.

Drug therapy has been shown to improve attentiveness of many children diagnosed as having AD-HD. Many clinicians imply that the educational problems of these children are caused by their attention deficit and that medication is effective in 70% to 80% of affected children (Shaywitz and Shaywitz, 1984). Teacher ratings report that 90% of medicated students evinced 50% improvement initially and 76% continued to exhibit improvement (Safer and Krager, 1989). These observations have prompted harassed teachers to press for controlling the behavior of these children with medication. Parents feel pressured by school authorities to place their children on medication (Steinberg, 1988). Researchers in one study found that 6% of students in one elementary school were receiving medication for hyperactivity or inattentiveness, many of whom were described as learning impaired, not hyperactive (Safer and Krager, 1988). However, the drug has been found to be ineffective in improving classroom behavior and performance in 20% to 30% of children with AD-HD. Also, researchers have questioned the reliability of casually recruited raters such as parents and classroom teachers (McBride, 1988).

Children do not become addicted to the medications or exhibit withdrawal symptoms when the drugs are discontinued nor do they require increasing doses with age (Castiglia, 1990). The drugs serve as replacement rather than additive therapy with children with AD-DH (Baren, 1989). However, health practitioners are often hesitant to recommend medication for behavior problems. Serious side effects have been reported from the use of stimulants: growth retardation and precipitation of Tourette syndrome (Shaywitz and Shaywitz, 1984). The Committee on Children with Disabilities and the Committee on Drugs of the American Academy of Pediatrics (1987) state that "medication for children with attention deficit disorder should never be used as an isolated treatment" and should be used only when it is "clearly indicated for a child with an attention problem that significantly affects school performance or that is associated with significant behavior disorder."

Malpractice suits have been filed against physicians for failing to make a diagnosis early enough so that the drug can be prescribed; other physicians have been sued because the drug produced psychotic episodes in children (Cowart, 1988).

These learning disabilities occur frequently in children diagnosed with AD-HD with or without hyperactivity. *Learning disability* is an educational term, and schools, recognizing this disability, provide services for affected children.

The types of disabilities include *dyslexia* (difficulty with reading), *dysgraphia* (difficulty with writing), *dyscalculia* (difficulty with calculation), right-left confusion, and short attention span. Most affected children are hypoactive, and their needs are frequently overlooked or their behavior is mistaken for retardation. Special education classes offer help and encouragement for these children and their parents, and early recognition facilitates the process of gaining the special assistance needed to function in the school situation. The **Association for Children and Adults with Learning Disabilities*** provides information and support to families with a child with a learning disability.

TIC DISORDERS

A tic is an involuntary, recurrent, random, rapid, highly stereotyped movement or vocalization, occurring in 10% to 35% of all children (Table 18-12). Tics can be simple or complex and involve motor movements, eye movements, or vocalizations (Box 18-6). Tics decrease during concentration, are markedly diminished during sleep, and become more exaggerated when the affected children are under stress or excitement. Obsessive-compulsive behaviors, in the form of ritualistic activities, also may be present and can occur in individuals free of tics. No major psychologic components are evident (Golden, 1987). A number of medications can precipitate tics.

Almost all mild *transient tic disorders* of childhood are self-limited and disappear within a few months, usually less than a year. The most common tics involve the eyes, head, and face and treatment does not affect recovery. Tic disorders can begin at any time during childhood. Boys are affected at least three times as often as girls and, in over 50% of cases, tics are observed in other family members (Avery and First, 1989).

Tic disorders that persist beyond 1 year are considered to be chronic and consist of one form of either motor or vocal manifestations but not both (Erenberg, 1988). The most severe of the chronic tics is Gilles de la Tourette's syndrome. Diagnosis of a tic disorder is based on clinical observations.

Most tic disorders resolve by late childhood or adolescence without treatment and cause no physical harm to the child. Therapeutic management consists primarily of support to the child and family, reassurance about prognosis, and education regarding expectations (of the child) for control. Although the child is able to suppress the manifestations to some degree, persistent pressure for control constitutes an additional stress to an affected child. Haloperidol or pimozide may provide relief of symptoms of chronic tics, and genetic counseling is also advised for families of children with chronic tics.

*4156 Library Road, Pittsburgh, PA 15234; (412) 341-1515. Also recommended: *Learning Disability*, available from Medic Publishing Co., P.O. Box 89, Redmond, WA 98073-0089; (206) 881-2883.

Table 18-12 Spectrum of tic disorders

	MILD	⟷	CHRONIC
Duration	Acute	Subacute	Chronic
Motor tics	Simple	Complex	Obscene gestures
	Few		Multiple
Vocal tics	None	Noises	Coprolalia
Suppressible	Yes		No

Box 18-6 TYPES OF TICS

Simple motor—eye blinking, grimacing, neck jerking, shoulder jerking
Complex motor—jumping, squatting, stamping the foot, thrusting out an arm, hitting or biting self, ritualistic movements (smelling an object, touching own or another's body, obsessive or compulsive patterns of behavior), grooming behaviors
Simple vocal—throat clearing, sniffing, grunting, coughing, snorting, lip noises
Complex vocal—echolalia (repeating last-heard sound, word, or phrase of another), palilalia (repeating own sounds or words), coprolalia (use of socially unacceptable words, often obscene), shouting words out of context

TOURETTE SYNDROME

Tourette disorder (Gilles de la Tourette's syndrome; TS) is the most complex and severe of the tic disorders. It begins between ages 2 and 16, persists throughout life, and is characterized by rapidly repetitive multiple motor and vocal movements. The etiology is uncertain, although most theories implicate abnormalities of various neurotransmitters. Support for a genetic origin, based on family studies, suggests that the disorder is inherited as a autosomal-dominant, sex-influenced trait (Pauls and Leckman, 1986).

The manifestations of TS wax and wane in intensity and exhibit a continuing pattern of change in which old tics disappear and new tics develop (Box 18-7). The onset is usually mild, and the initial tic of brief duration. The minor tics then come and go, becoming more intense and lasting longer (Erenberg, 1988). Some tics may be severe from the onset, often with no symptom-free periods. Diagnosis is based on clinical observations, especially if other family members are affected. The tics do not lead to physical deterioration or affect the child's life expectancy.

Therapeutic Management

Treatment of TS is primarily symptomatic and consists of child and family education and support. Children with more severe tics sometimes obtain symptomatic relief from medications. Haloperidol, a dopamine-blocking agent, is the most widely prescribed drug. Pimozide and fluphenazine, with similar action to haloperidol, or clonidine, an alpha-2-adrenergic drug, may also be prescribed. Genetic counseling is advised.

Box 18-7 DIAGNOSTIC CRITERIA FOR TOURETTE DISORDER

A. Both multiple motor and one or more vocal tics have been present at some time during the illness, although not necessarily concurrently.
B. The tics occur many times a day (usually in bouts), nearly every day or intermittently throughout a period of more than 1 year.
C. The anatomic location, number, frequency, complexity, and severity of the tics change over time.
D. Onset is before age 21.
E. Occurrence does not occur exclusively during Psychoactive Substance Intoxication or known central nervous system disease, such as Huntington's chorea and postviral encephalitis.

From Diagnostic and statistical manual of mental disorders, ed. 3—revised (DSM-III-R), Washington, DC, 1987, American Psychiatric Association.

Nursing Considerations

Nurses are important in the management of TS. Education of children, families, teachers, and others involved in children's everyday life is a major aspect of therapy. Punishment for the behaviors is inappropriate, since they are involuntary. Affected children are often quick to anger, have a low frustration tolerance, and may engage in temper tantrums. These children need to be guided toward acceptable substitute behaviors in order to develop normally, socially and emotionally (Comings and Comings, 1985). For example, suggest a child retire to a quiet area to gain control of emotions or provide a pillow, stuffed toy, or punching bag on which to vent feelings.

Influential persons in the children's lives must help foster feelings of self-esteem. Children with TS demonstrate a constant, ongoing battle over the control of their impulses, which becomes more difficult with controlling behaviors of parents. Children with TS are more likely to be well-adjusted if they perceive parental relationships as positive (Edell and Motta, 1989). A child's self-concept can be damaged if parents react to the disability with guilt or anger, which they usually manifest as hostility.

Nurses may assist families engaged in long-term monitoring of symptoms, which includes establishing the waxing and waning and whether or not they interfere with development and adaptation in an important way, requiring more intense therapy. Families of children on medication need to be alert to possible side effects, including lethargy, personality change, increased appetite and overweight, depression, Parkinsonian symptoms (tremor, muscle rigidity, shuffling gait, hypokinesia, and difficulty chewing, swallowing, and speaking), and anticholinergic symptoms (confusion, excitement, dilated pupils, blurred vision, dry mouth, and dysphagia).

The family may benefit from referral to health agencies such as the local health departments, social services, and parent groups. The **Tourette Syndrome Association*** is active in research and education and provides services to affected children and their families.

■ EMOTIONAL DISORDERS OF CHILDHOOD

Some disorders affecting children produce distress to both children and their families. No organic basis can be detected in most situations. Some are amenable to interventions by health professionals.

POSTTRAUMATIC STRESS DISORDER

It is now believed that children do not outgrow the fear that follows a traumatic shock (Terr, 1989). Seemingly all right following a traumatic event, children tend to relive or visualize these experiences for years and retain some fear specific to the event. They continue to function in school as always but have a feeling of foreboding regarding the future. It is important for children to talk about their experience and fears and to be reassured regarding the randomness of an event such as a playground shooting, rape, attack, or natural disaster (e.g., hurricane, earthquake).

Posttraumatic stress disorder (PTSD) is frequently observed following an overwhelming stimulus, for example, a sibling dying while in the child's care. The way in which children react depends on what resources the individual child brings to the situation— coping strategies used, defense mechanisms summoned, and the child's social environment. PTSD has also been observed in physically abused children (McCormack, Burgess, and Hartman, 1989). Each individual reacts differently. Although most children rapidly adapt, studies indicate that children do not outgrow the trauma but that they can be helped to overcome their sense of hopelessness (Terr, 1989).

The response to the event, invariant and uniform in all persons, takes place in a sequence of three stages. The initial response to the stressor is intense arousal, which usually lasts for a few minutes to 1 or 2 hours, depending on the stressor and the individual. The stress hormones are at the maximum as the individual prepares for "fight" or "flight." A prolonged arousal phase may indicate psychosis.

The second phase, which lasts approximately 2 weeks, is one in which defense mechanisms are mobilized. It is a period of quiescence in which the event appears to have produced no impression. The victims feel numb, and stress hormone secretion is absent. The reaction is outside their awareness, not well controlled, and involves some type of behavioral pattern. Defense mechanisms are less adaptive to specific situations and may not be what the situation demands. Denial that anything is wrong is a frequently observed defense mechanism.

The third phase is one of coping, which normally extends over 2 to 3 months. It is one of consciously directed

*42-40 Bell Blvd., Bayside, NY 11361; (718) 224-2999.

inquiry. The victims want to know what happened and appear to be getting worse, when actually they are getting better. Numerous psychologic symptoms may be apparent, such as depression, repetitive phenomenon, phobic symptoms, anxiety symptoms, and conversion reactions. Children frequently display repetitive actions. They play out the situation over and over again in an attempt to come to terms with their fear. Flashbacks are common. This phase can be self-perpetuating, and a prolonged reaction can develop into an obsession with the traumatic event. Some traumatic effects remain indefinitely (Terr, 1989). Researchers have also found that children with PTSD have impaired startle inhibition, indicating long-lasting alteration in the brainstem circuits that help startle modulation (Ornitz and Pynoos, 1989).

Nursing Considerations

Children need to deal with any traumatic event; much depends on the intensity of the event and their reaction to it. Their reactions depend heavily on their social environment and the way in which their caretaking adults react to the event. Children usually react in much the same manner as their caregivers (contagious pathology); therefore it is important to be aware of these reactions also. In the second, or defense, phase of the PTSD the appropriateness of the defense mechanism must be assessed, and children must be assisted in application of their defense. If children do not engage in some catharsis or if their defense phase is prolonged, they may need referral for special psychologic help.

Coping is a learned response, and children in the third phase can be helped to use their coping strategies to deal with their fear. Children usually are willing to accept reasoning. Those who are assisted in their catharsis and allowed expression will survive without serious lasting effects. They should be encouraged to play out the stress and/or discuss their feelings about the event. If they are unable to do this, they may become obsessed with the traumatic event and need professional help. Conversion reactions are common obsessive behaviors in children.

Children need professional help if any of the phases of PTSD are prolonged. Boys tend to be more apt to have a prolonged defense phase than girls. Occasionally the event will be unrecognized, and the affected child will engage in what is considered to be unusual behavior. In the case of any sudden change in behavior, the child needs to be assessed for a traumatic event—"Did something happen?" When the change in behavior is determined to be a traumatic event, treatment can be implemented.

SCHOOL PHOBIA

School phobia is a term used to describe children, other than beginning students, who resist going to school because of dread of the school situation, concerns with leaving home, or both. As a rule children below the age of 13 who fear school tend to be separation-anxious—children who are afraid of leaving the people they love. For these children the term "school refuser" is rapidly replacing "school phobia," which is more accurate after the age of 13 years. By this time children have worked through immature separation fears (Last and others, 1987).

Anxiety that frequently verges on panic is a constant manifestation, and children can develop symptoms as a protective mechanism to keep them from facing the situation that distresses them. Physical symptoms are prominent and may affect any part of the body—anorexia, nausea, vomiting, diarrhea, dizziness, headache, leg pains, or abdominal pains, to name a few. They may even develop a low-grade fever. A striking feature of school phobia is the prompt subsiding of symptoms when it is evident that the child can remain at home. Another significant observation is absence of symptoms on weekends and holidays, unless they are related to other places such as Sunday school or parties. Occasional mild reluctance is not uncommon among school children, but if the fear continues for longer than a few days, it must be considered a serious problem—a warning of an important personality problem.

Unlike most other behavior problems of children, school phobia is more common in girls than in boys, there is no relationship to socioeconomic status, ethnic origin, or other subcultural affiliation, and no particular age predominates. The onset is usually sudden and precipitated by a school-related incident. A poor attendance record for trivial reasons can be elicited by a careful history.

Etiology

School phobia can be caused by a number of factors. Sometimes the complaints can be related to a transient, specific cause such as fear of a mismatched or overcritical teacher, fear of failing an examination or giving an oral recitation for a painfully shy child, or discrimination based on race, dress, or physical defect. Sometimes it may be related to a school bully or threatening gang. An insecure home situation in which the child fears that he may be deserted by a parent while he is gone may be the basis of anxiety, especially if the parent has previously threatened to leave for some reason.

A frequent source of fear is separation anxiety based on a strong dependent relationship between the mother and child in which the child is reluctant to leave the mother and she is equally reluctant (even though this may be unconscious) to have him leave her. The intense need for closeness between mother and child is normal in infancy, but the persistence of this type of relationship into childhood is totally inappropriate. Characteristically these children are not afraid to go to school, but rather they are afraid to leave home. They fear something dreadful might happen while they are separated from their families. No event is required to trigger the associated behaviors. However, symptoms may be precipitated by a situation that intensifies the mutual dependency between the mother and the child, such as illness, arrival of a new baby, move to a strange neighborhood or a new school, or parental discord.

In some instances children have an unrealistic, exaggerated view of their abilities and achievements. When they feel threatened by incidents that challenge their estimate of themselves, such as a minor episode that leads to embarrassment, return to school after an absence, transfer to another class, or even imagined social or academic failure, they become anxious and withdraw, frequently seeking proximity to the mother. Sometimes the step-up in expectations at school or change of important personnel at school (e.g., teacher or principal) is a contributing factor. Occasionally the child may be suffering from an undiagnosed learning disability.

Therapeutic Management

The treatment for school phobia depends on the cause. The children really *want* to go to school but just cannot force themselves to do so; they are not delinquent children. They are anxious, tense, and distressed because they are unable to muster enough courage to attend school. If the cause of the problem is an examination, relationships with a bully, or a mismatch between teacher and child, it can be dealt with accordingly. When the child is helped to understand and cope with the fear, the symptoms usually disappear. In severe cases when returning to school is unsuccessful, professional psychiatric consultation is usually desirable to help identify possible distorted family relationships or a personality disturbance in the child and to help both child and family understand the sources of the problem.

Nursing Considerations

The primary goal for the child with school phobia is to *return the child to school.* The longer the child is permitted to stay out of school, the more difficult it is to reenter. Well-meaning parents or others who permit the child to stay away from school and support any efforts with written excuses only confirm the child's feelings of worthlessness and inability to cope. Parents must be convinced gently but firmly that *immediate* return is essential and that they, the parents, are the ones who must insist upon the child's return for it to be effective.

Some modifications in school attendance might be necessary for the child with severe symptoms. The child who is unable to return to regular classes may be allowed to go to school on a part-time basis, spending the time in the counselor's office or nurse's office and getting homework from the teacher after class. It may be necessary to transport the child to and from school or even have a parent attend class with the child. However, this practice is not allowed to continue for an unlimited time, and the time limit should be agreed on beforehand. The essential factor is that the child must return to school right away, maintain the pattern of going, and remain there even while a solution is being worked out. The school nurse can provide both teacher and parents with support in carrying out this plan.

Prevention. Prevention of school phobia as well as other dependency problems can be developed by the encouragement of independence at appropriate times during infancy and early childhood. For example, by 6 months of age children are left with a baby-sitter during a parents' night out. Two-year-olds can be left home (while awake) with a sitter. By 3 years of age children should experience being left somewhere other than their home (e.g., grandparents' home). As soon as they are able, they are allowed to feed, dress, and wash themselves. By 3 to 4 years of age children can be allowed to play in the yard by themselves, and later they should be allowed to play in the neighborhood by themselves.

Certain clues indicate that a child may be subject to first-time fear; thus children can be helped to adjust to it. Extra preparation may be needed for children who are very fearful, have trouble adjusting to new situations, or are very clinging (Last and others, 1987). Many individuals continue to manifest some form of fear throughout their school careers. When the problem is identified early and effectively treated and negative emotions surrounding school minimized, a child is less likely to carry residual fears throughout life.

For most first-time school fears, as for any new and potentially frightening experience, simple reassurances and a little advance preparation are all that is needed. Direct contact with the school and teachers is an excellent means of allaying anticipatory anxiety. Parents can take children to visit the school about a month before school starts, introduce them to the teacher, and let them experience the classroom firsthand.

Bedtime, when the family is usually relaxed, is an excellent time to help children resolve first-day day jitters. Bedtime stories and books suited to the occasion are available from bookstores and libraries. Another option is a tape entitled "I Can Take Care of Myself,"* one of a series designed to help children cope with a variety of common fears (dark, nightmares, baby-sitters, doctors, dentists, monsters).

Parents who suspect that their child may be especially frightened may want to accompany the child to school and wait outside the classroom the first day. A gradual breakaway over succeeding days should relieve their child's and their own anxiety. If the distress extends beyond 2 weeks, professional help may be needed (Last and others, 1987).

RECURRENT ABDOMINAL PAIN

Recurrent abdominal pain (RAP) is one of the somatic complaints of childhood that is almost always attributed to a psychogenic etiology, although it can be a symptom of either psychosomatic or organic disease. RAP is traditionally defined as three or more separate episodes of abdominal pain during a 3-month period. Similar to the "spastic" or "irritable colon syndrome" of adulthood, the disorder affects 10% to 20% of school-age children at some time in their childhood. It is rarely seen in children less than 5 years of age; its peak incidence is in children ages 10 to 12 years. Girls are affected slightly more often than boys (Coleman and Levine, 1986).

Etiology and Pathophysiology

Only a minority of youngsters with RAP have an organic basis for their pain, which includes inflammatory bowel dis-

**Happy Heart Tapes* by J. Thomas can be obtained from the Center for Attitude Modification, P.O Box 2886, Del Mar, CA 92014; (619) 453-7310.

ease, peptic ulcer disease, lactose intolerance, pelvic inflammatory disease, urinary bladder infection, and pancreatitis. Psychiatric disorders such as depression and school avoidance account for a small number of these cases. In 90% to 95% no organic cause can be found (Farrell, 1984; Poole, 1984). The bulk of children with RAP suffer from functional abdominal pain, which is ill-defined and often misinterpreted to mean fictitious or imagined pain (Olson, 1987).

The most plausible etiologic theories describe functional abdominal pain as dyskinesia (Davidson, 1986) or dysmotility (Coleman and Levine, 1986) and as multifactorial (Levine and Rappaport, 1984). Normally intestinal contents arrive at the distal portion of the intestine with a relatively high fluid content where fluid is extracted to a greater degree in the distal colon and rectum. In dysmotility (dyskinesia) the normally relaxed distal intestine fails to relax, preventing the flow of its contents toward the rectum. The resulting excessive distention in the proximal bowel and spasms of the distal intestinal musculature produce the dysmotility. Pressure on nerve endings causes pain.

The basis for a multifactorial etiology describes both causative and predisposing factors: (1) somatic predisposition, dysfunction, or disorder; (2) life-style and habit, including routines, diet, and life tempo; (3) temperament and learned response patterns, such as the child's behavior style, personality, and learned coping skills; and (4) milieu and critical events, that is, the child's intimate surroundings (familial, social, and cultural norms) and unexpected sources of stress or gratification (Coleman and Levine, 1986).

Children at risk for RAP tend to be high achievers who have great personal goals or whose parents have unusually high expectations. They are described as more mature and sensitive than others or as worriers. At risk are children who are overly concerned about what others think about them but have difficulty meeting the expectations of parents, teachers, and others. They are uncomfortable with expressions of anger or argument, especially in those persons who are significant in their lives. School attendance is adversely affected, and these children generally exhibit poor learning performance. It is not uncommon for symptoms to be aggravated during school days.

Clinical Manifestations

Children with RAP have real pain that the child usually locates in the periumbilical and/or epigastric area. However, on palpation the pain is more likely to be experienced in the epigastric area or in the lower right or left quadrant and is accompanied by vague tenderness without muscle guarding. Other symptoms that may accompany the abdominal pain are headache, flushing, pallor, dizziness, and fatigue. Nausea, vomiting, and diarrhea are sometimes part of the syndrome. The symptoms reflect the heightened intensity of response to stimulation of the autonomic bowel sites. The loose stools are the result of the exaggerated propulsive motility, and the pain is caused by the sharply increased mechanical tension in the gut.

Diagnostic Evaluation

Diagnosis consists of a complete family history and the child's health history, physical examination, and laboratory tests. The family history may provide evidence of a hereditary disorder or mimicry of adult symptoms. The child is evaluated for evidence of an organic basis for symptoms such as pain that radiates to the back, pain that awakens the child from sleep, recurrent fever, and weight loss. The pain is assessed for location, quality, frequency, duration, any associated symptoms, alleviating factors, and exacerbating factors (Olson, 1987).

Therapeutic Management

Treatment is difficult. Hospitalization may be necessary, and the child frequently shows improvement in the hospital environment. Initial efforts are directed toward ruling out organic causes of the pain, relieving discomfort, and attempting to determine the situations that precipitate attacks.

Most authorities recommend a high-fiber diet (including fiber-containing cookies), psyllium bulk agents, and lubricants such as mineral oil to help colonic emptying. If these are not effective, they are discontinued. Bowel training to establish regular bowel habits is encouraged. When simple measures are ineffective, an antispasmodic drug such as propantheline bromide may be prescribed to relieve the muscle spasm.

Nursing Considerations

The nurse can be instrumental in assessment and management of recurrent abdominal pain in children. Many of the techniques used in a routine assessment can elicit information that might help identify those factors that contribute to the child's symptomatology. The child's social and psychologic adjustment should be evaluated, and details of the pain should be obtained directly from the child when possible.

Questions that provide clues to parent-child relationships and how the family deals with angry feelings provide useful information for diagnosis and management. Relationships with peers, school problems, and other concerns of the child need to be explored, and any evidence of depression should be noted. It is also significant that psychogenic somatic symptoms generally do not awaken the child from sleep.

Once the diagnosis has been established, the parents and the child need an explanation of the pain, which can be compared to a skeletal muscle cramp or "charley horse" for easier comprehension. Reassurance that the symptoms are not unique to their child and that the pain can be expected to subside is helpful in relieving parental fears and anxieties.

High-fiber diet is discussed with the child and family (see Chapter 33), and bowel training is emphasized. The child is encouraged to establish a pattern of sitting on the toilet for 10 to 15 minutes immediately after breakfast to take advantage of the increased colonic activity following meals. If necessary, stimulatory suppositories can be used to induce early morning defecation.

When parents are reassured that there is no organic

cause of the pain, they will need some guidance regarding what they can do during a pain episode. All too often they feel helpless and anxious, which tends to compound the child's distress. The simple expedient of putting the child at rest by having him or her lie down in a peaceful, quiet environment and providing comfort will often relieve the symptoms in a short time. A heating pad may also help ease the discomfort. (See also Nonpharmacologic Pain Management, Chapter 26). If pain is not relieved by these simple measures, the parents are taught how to administer antispasmodics. For example, if pain is precipitated by meals, having the child take the medication 20 to 30 minutes before mealtime may prevent an episode.

The most valuable assistance that the nurse can provide is support and reassurance to the family. One of the most difficult aspects of therapy is helping parents and child understand the cause of the pain. When open communication is established and families are able to see a relationship between stress-provoking situations and the child's symptoms, the chance for remedial action is enhanced. Follow-up care and continued support are essential because the symptoms tend to remit and exacerbate; therefore the availability of a supportive health professional can be a source of comfort to the child and family.

CONVERSION REACTION

Conversion reaction, also known as hysteria, hysterical conversion reaction, conversion symptoms, and childhood hysteria, is a psychophysiologic disorder with a sudden onset that can usually be traced to a precipitating environmental event. The manifestations involve primarily the voluntary musculature and special senses and include abdominal pain, fainting, pseudoseizures, paralysis, headaches, and visual field restriction. Once considered rare in childhood, the diagnosis occurs more frequently than has generally been acknowledged. In childhood the disorder is observed with equal frequency in both sexes, but girls outnumber boys during adolescence. The most commonly observed symptom is seizure activity, which can be differentiated from symptoms of neurogenic origin by formal tests, the most useful of which is the finding of a normal electroencephalogram.

It has been observed that nearly all children with conversion reaction have experienced a major family crisis before the onset of symptoms. Particularly traumatic is an unresolved grief reaction in the child, such as loss of a parent or other significant person through death, divorce, or moving (Maloney, 1980). It is not uncommon for the child to exhibit symptoms of the lost person. The families of children with conversion reaction characteristically display problems in communication, and depression or hypochondriasis in a parent is a common finding.

Educating the child and family regarding the cause underlying emotional stresses or feelings and alternative approaches to coping with stress may alleviate the child's symptoms, although families are not always receptive to the intervention. If deep personality problems are evident, psychiatric consultation is usually indicated. Nursing care is similar to that for the child with recurrent abdominal pain.

CHILDHOOD DEPRESSION

Depression in childhood is often difficult to detect because children may be unable to express their feelings and tend to act out their problems and concerns. Authorities agree that childhood depression exists but they do not agree whether or not it is the same as adult depression. The characteristics of depression are largely determined by parallel developments in symbolism, language, and cognitive development (Aylward, 1985). Younger children demonstrate a more cause-and-effect relationship between the stressors and the depressive manifestations, which are primarily the biologic deprivation syndromes. As children develop, the relationships between stressful events and depression are less clear. Their reactions are less physiologic and more cognitively complex, and the observed behaviors tend to be age specific (Herzog and Rathburn, 1982). Depressed children exhibit a distinctive style of thinking characterized by low self-esteem, hopelessness, and a tendency to explain negative events in terms of personal shortcomings (McCauley and others, 1988).

Some states of depression are of a temporary nature, for example, acute depression precipitated by a traumatic event. This might include a period of hospitalization, loss of a parent through death or separation, or loss of a significant relationship with something (a pet), someone (a friend or family member), or a place (move from a familiar home, neighborhood, or city). The easily identified manifestations include a sad, downcast face, tearfulness, irritability, and withdrawal from previously enjoyed activities and relationships. The child tends to spend more time in solitary activities, especially television viewing, and schoolwork is impaired. Some children become more dependent and clinging; others become more aggressive and disruptive. Sleeplessness and/or loss of appetite are not common reactions. Responses are not sustained and can be modified with social and family support.

More serious and less common are depressive responses to more chronic stress and loss; these are frequently observed in children with chronic illness or disability. There is no apparent precipitating event, but there is often a history of frequent disruptions in important relationships. Commonly there is also a history of depressive illness in one or both parents during the child's lifetime. The manifestations are similar to responses to acute reactions. Some of the primary and associated symptoms that are observed in depressed children and the DSM-III criteria currently used for establishing a diagnosis of major depression are outlined in Box 18-8. There are a number of similarities among major depressive disorders in childhood and several other psychologic disorders.

Therapeutic Management

Depressed children are managed by a health team especially prepared in the care of children with mental disor-

Box 18-8 PRIMARY AND ASSOCIATED SYMPTOMS OF DEPRESSION IN CHILDREN

Primary Symptoms
Depressed affect (dysphoric mood)
Anhedonia (loss of pleasure)
Self-deprecatory ideation
Tearfulness
Low sense of self-worth/self-esteem
Social withdrawal
Impairment of schoolwork
Psychomotor retardation
Difficulty with biologic functions (sleeping, eating)
Morbid ideation/suicide attempts

Associated Symptoms
Irritability
Moodiness
Social interactive difficulties
Pathologic guilt
Fatigue
Somatic complaints
Anxiety, decreased concentration
Obsessive rumination and thoughts
Attention deficit
Feelings of helplessness/hopelessness
Enuresis/encopresis
Aggressive and explosive behaviors

From Aylward, G.P.: Understanding and treatment of childhood depression, J. Pediatr. 107:1-9, 1985; as modified from Diagnostic and statistical manual of mental disorders, ed. 3 (DSM-III), Washington, DC, 1980, American Psychiatric Association.

ders. Treatment of depression should be undertaken in the least constrictive environment, usually outpatient management. Suicidal children are admitted to the hospital for protection if the family is unable to provide constant monitoring. For children with associated disruptive behavior, such as fighting with peers or family, hospitalization may be advised. Most therapeutic regimens focus on pharmacotherapy with tricyclic antidepressants as the most commonly prescribed medication. Others are monoamine oxidase inhibitors and lithium (Weller and Weller, 1989).

Nursing Considerations

The management of childhood depression is usually psychotherapeutic and highly individualized. Nurses should be aware that depression is a problem that can easily be overlooked in the school-age child and one that can interrupt normal growth and development. Recognizing depression and making appropriate referrals is an important nursing function. Identification of the depressed child requires a careful history (health, growth and development, social, and family health), interviews with the child, and observations by the nurse, parents, and teachers. If the child is placed on antidepressants, the child and family need to be instructed to monitor the child for side effects of the specific drug prescribed. See Chapter 21 for a more definitive discussion of depression and suicide.

CHILDHOOD SCHIZOPHRENIA

There is considerable disagreement regarding the cause of schizophrenia, whether the onset is in adulthood or childhood. Some authorities favor a biochemical basis, whereas others support the theory of a complex combination of psychosocial and environmental stresses. Support for an interpersonal theory of schizophrenia comes from a number of sources. The major theories point to disturbed family or parent-child relationships as an etiologic basis. There is evidence to indicate that genetic factors contribute significantly to its development. The likelihood of children born to a schizophrenic parent developing the disorder is 15 times greater than that for children in the general population—even when they are separated from the parent at an early age. There is also a high concordance rate (40% to 60%) in monozygotic (identical) twins. Of children genetically predisposed to schizophrenia, those with poor family relationships are the most likely to develop full-blown symptoms of the disease (Berman, 1987).

The symptomatology among children shows wide variation according to each affected child's developmental level, the age of onset, the nature of early childhood experiences, and the type of defense mechanisms used. However, the basic core disturbance is a lack of contact with reality and the subsequent development of a world of the child's own. Unlike the abrupt onset of the adult disorder, childhood schizophrenia is characterized by a gradual onset of neurotic symptoms followed by any of more than 100 different abnormal manifestations, including those in Box 18-9.

Nursing Considerations

Nursing care is directed toward identifying children and referral for specialized care. Consistent application of a therapeutic plan is mandatory for a successful program of care, and nurses with special skills work with these children on a long-term basis. Since it is a specialized area of nursing

Box 18-9 SOME CHARACTERISTICS OF CHILDHOOD SCHIZOPHRENIA

Bizarre behavioral patterns and stereotyped movements such as robotlike walking, whirling, or graceful gyrations
Periods of hypoactivity alternating with periods of hyperactivity
Inappropriate affect that ranges from flatness to explosiveness
Common occurrences of temper tantrums
Language disturbances such as speaking in fragmented sentences, parrotlike repetition of words, development of a private language, and altered tone of voice; some schizophrenic children are mute or will only utter a single word on rare occasions
Distorted time orientation with a blending of past, present, and future
Distorted sense of and use of their bodies
Apparent denial of the human quality in people, such as attempting to use a person as a step stool to reach an object
Conveying a nonhuman identity by action, sounds, or posture, such as barking or calling self a vacuum cleaner
Frequent occurrences of compulsive behavior and phobias

practice, the reader is directed to seek further information from textbooks on child psychiatry.

KEY POINTS

- Middle childhood is a relatively healthy period and most problems encountered are not considered serious.
- The skin serves several important functions: protection, prevention of loss of body fluids, heat regulation, and sensation.
- It is important for nurses to be able to describe skin lesions accurately.
- The stages of wound healing consist of inflammation, fibroplasia, scar contraction, and scar maturation.
- Wound healing occurs by primary, secondary, or tertiary intention.
- Bacterial, viral, and fungal infections are common in childhood.
- Prevention of infection or reinfection is the primary goal in management of pediculosis.
- Contact dermatitis may involve a reaction to a primary irritant or sensitization.
- Teaching prevention of thermal injury, especially sunburn, is an important nursing function.
- Adverse reactions to drugs occur more often in the skin than in any other organ.
- Dental care continues to be important; most frequent problems that arise are dental caries and malocclusion.
- The behavioral disorders of childhood are primarily attention deficit–hyperactivity disorder and tic disorders.
- Some of the major emotional disorders involving school-age children include school phobia, recurrent abdominal pain, conversion reaction, depression, and schizophrenia.

REFERENCES

American Academy of Pediatrics, Committee on Children with Disabilities and Committee on Drugs: Medication for children with an attention deficit disorder, Pediatrics 80:758-760, 1987.

American Academy of Pediatrics, Committee on Infectious Diseases: Report of the Committee on Infectious Disease, ed. 21, Elk Grove, IL, 1988, American Academy of Pediatrics.

American Psychiatric Association: Diagnostic and statistical manual of mental disorders, ed. 3 (DSM-III-R), Washington, DC, 1987, American Psychiatric Association.

Anders, J.E., and Leach, E.E.: Sun versus skin, Am. J. Nurs. 83:1015-1020,1983.

Avery, M.E., and First, L.R., editors: Pediatric medicine, Baltimore, 1989, Williams & Wilkins.

Aylward, G.P.: Understanding and treatment of childhood depression, J. Pediatr. 107:1-9, 1985.

Baker, M.D.: Bites and scratches: when pets fight back, Contemp. Pediatr. 6(6):76-84, 1989.

Baker, M.D., and Moore, S.E.: Human bites in children, Am. J. Dis. Child. 141:1285-1290, 1987.

Baren, M: The case for Ritalin: a fresh look at the controversy, Contemp. Pediatr. 6(1):16-28, 1989.

Barnett, N.K.: Pruritus. In Hoekelman, R.A., editor-in-chief: Primary pediatric care, St. Louis, 1987, Mosby–Year Book, Inc.

Berman, B.: Children at high risk for schizophrenia: parent and offspring perceptions of family relationships, J. Abnorm. Psychol. 96:364-366, 1987.

Berry, C.A., Shaywitz, S.E., and Shaywitz, B.A.: Girls with attention deficit disorder: a silent minority? A report on behavioral and cognitive characteristics, Pediatrics 76:801-809, 1985.

Bonadio, W.A., and Wagner, V.: Efficacy of TAC anesthetic for repair of pediatric lacerations, Am. J. Dis. Child. 142:203-205, 1988.

Brown, G.L.: Attention deficit disorder. In Gellis, S.S., and Kagan, B.M.: Current pediatric therapy 12, Philadelphia, 1986, W.B. Saunders Co.

Brown, G., and others: Enhancement of wound healing by topical treatment with epidermal growth factor, N. Engl. J. Med. 321:76-79, 1989.

Carithers, H.A.: Cat-scratch disease—an overview based on a study of 1,200 patients, Am. J. Dis. Child. 139:1124-1133, 1985.

Castiglia, P.T.: Hyperactivity, J. Pediatr. Health Care 4:42-45, 1990.

Chan, Y-P.M., and others: Methylphenidate hydrochloride given with or before breakfast. II. Effects on plasma concentration of methylphenidate and ritalinic acid, Pediatrics 72:56-59, 1983.

Chun, Y-T., Berkelhamer, J.E., and Herold, T.E.: Dog bites in children less than 4 years old, Pediatrics 69:119-120, 1982.

Clore, E.R.: Dispelling the common myths about pediculosis, J. Pediatr. Health Care 3:28-33, 1989.

Cohen, F.L.: Clinical genetics in nursing practice, Philadelphia, 1984, J.B. Lippincott Co.

Coleman, W.L., and Levine, M.D.: Recurrent abdominal pain: the cost of the aches and the aches of the cost, Pediatr. Rev. 8:143-151, 1986.

Collipp, P.J.: Cat-scratch disease therapy (letter), Am. J. Dis. Child. 143:1261, 1989.

Coln, D., and Emmrich, P.: Hypothermia and frostbite. In Eichenwald, H.F., and Ströder, J., editors: Current therapy in pediatrics—2, Toronto, 1989, B.C. Decker, Inc.

Comings, D.E., and Comings, B.G.: Tourette syndrome: clinical and psychological aspects of 250 cases, Am. J. Genet. 37:435-450, 1985.

Coody, D.: There is no such thing as a good tan, J. Pediatr. Health Care 1:125-132, 1987.

Cooper, L.I.: Removing cactus spines (letter), Am. J. Dis. Child. 142:1140, 1988.

Cowart, V.S.: The Ritalin controversy: what's made this drug's opponents hyperactive? JAMA 259:2521-2523, 1988.

Culp, R.W., and others: On the arthritis of Lyme disease, J. Bone Joint Surg. 69A:96-99, 1987.

Davidson, M.: Recurrent abdominal pain: look to dyskinesia as the culprit, Contemp. Pediatr. 3(12):16-42, 1986.

Dische, S., and others: Childhood nocturnal enuresis: factors associated with outcome of treatment with an enuresis alarm, Dev. Med. Child Neurol. 25:67-80, 1983.

Edell, B.H., and Motta, R.W.: The emotional adjustment of children with Tourette's syndrome, J. Psychol. 123:51-57, 1989.

Editorial comment: Pediatr. Alert 9:22, 1984.

Eichenfield, A.H.: Diagnosis and management of Lyme disease, Pediatr. Ann. 15:583-594, 1986.

Elliot, D.L., and others: Pet-associated illness, N. Engl. J. Med. 313:985-987, 1985.

Erenberg, G.: Identification and management of patients with tics/Tourette syndrome, Feelings 30:21-24, 1988.

Esposito, A.L., and Adams, D.: Infection of skin and subcutaneous tissue. In Eichenwald, H.F., and Ströder, J., editors: Current therapy in pediatrics–2, Toronto, 1989, B.C. Decker, Inc.

Falco, R.C., and Fish, D.: Prevalence of Ixodes dammini near the homes of Lyme disease patients in Westchester County, NY, Am. J. Epidemiol. 127:826-830, 1988.

Falco, R.C., and Fish, D.: Lyme disease ticks on well-kept lawns, Am. J. Epidemiol. 127:826-830, 1988.

Farrell, M.K.: Abdominal pain, Pediatrics 74(suppl.):955-957, 1984.

Fischer, R.G., and Parks, B.R.: Using insect repellents effectively, Pediatr. Nurs. 12:212, 1986.

Flessner, M.F.: A tough diagnosis in a neutropenic patient: it's cat-scratch disease, JAMA 261:991, 1989.

Friman, P.C.: A preventive context for enuresis, Pediatr. Clin. North Am. 33:871-886, 1986.

Friman, P.C., and others: Do encopretic children have clinically significant behavior problems? Pediatrics 82:407-409, 1988.

Gelbard, M.K.: Removal of small cactus spines from the skin, JAMA 252:3368, 1984.

Ginsburg, C.M. and Gädeke, R.: Snakebites. In Eichenwald, H.F., and Ströder, J., editors: Current therapy in pediatrics–2, Toronto, 1989, B.C. Decker, Inc.

Golden, G.S.: Movement disorders: sorting the benign from the serious, Contemp. Pediatr. 4(5):77-92, 1987.

Gorrell, R.: Practical pointers, Consultant 25:154, 1985.

Guide to dental health, J. Am. Dent. Assoc. (suppl.) pp. 37-46, 1985.

Hennes, H.: Removal of cactus spines from the skin, Am. J. Dis. Child. 142:587, 1988.

Herzog, G.B., and Rathburn, J.M.: Childhood depression, Am. J. Dis. Child. 136:115-119, 1982.

Holloway, L.: Shadow method for sun protection (letter), Lancet 335:484, 1990.

Huessy, H.R.: Adolescents and Ritalin, Pediatrics 75:614, 1985.

Hurwitz, S.: That summer rash could be Lyme disease, Contemp. Pediatr. 5(6):74-82, 1988.

Hurwitz, S.: There's no such thing as "a good tan," Contemp. Pediatr. 5(5):55-66, 1989.

Ismail, A.I., and others: Effect of sealants to children's teeth, J. Publ. Health Dent. 49:206-211, 1989.

Jobe, R.: Personal communication, 1990.

Johns, C.: Encopresis, Am. J. Nurs. 85:153-156, 1985.

Kochman, Doron: What to do about facial trauma, Contemp. Pediatr. 6(7):72-83, 1989.

Krasner, P.R.: The treatment of avulsed teeth, J. Pediatr. Health Care 4:86-90, 1990.

Last, C.G., and others: Separation anxiety and school phobia: a comparison using DSM-III criteria, Am. J. Psychiatry 144:653-657, 1987.

Lauer, E.A., White, W.C., and Lauer, B.A.: Dog bites—a neglected problem in accident prevention, Am. J. Dis. Child. 136:202-204, 1982.

Levine, M.D.: Disordered processes of elimination. In Levine, M.D., and others: Developmental-behavioral pediatrics, Philadelphia, 1983, W.B. Saunders Co.

Levine, M.D., and Rappaport, L.A.: Recurrent abdominal pain in school children: the loneliness of the long-distance physician, Pediatr. Clin. North Am. 31:969-991, 1984.

Madden, E.J.A: Itch, J. Pain Sympt. Manag. 1(2):97-99, 1986.

Maloney, M.J.: Diagnosing hysterical conversion reactions in children, J. Pediatr. 97:1016-1020, 1980.

March, S.M.: Infections due to dog and cat bites, Pediatr. Infect. Dis. 1:351-355, 1982.

Martinez, T.T., and others: Removal of cactus spines from the skin, Am. J. Dis. Child. 141:1291-1292, 1987.

McBride, M.C.: An individual double-blind crossover trial for assessing methylphenidate response in children with attention deficit disorder, J. Pediatr. 113:137-145, 1988.

McCauley, E., and others: Cognitive attributes of depression in children and adolescents, J. Consult. Clin. Psychol. 56:903-908, 1988.

McCormack, A., Burgess, A.W., and Hartman, C.: Familial abuse and post-traumatic stress disorder, J. Traumatic Stress 1:231-242, 1989.

McGuire, M.A.: Think hypothermia, Point of View 24(3):12-14, 1987.

McLaury, P.: Head lice—pediatric social disease, Am. J. Nurs. 83:1300-1303, 1983.

Moffatt, M.E.K., Kato, C., and Pless, I.B.: Improvements in self-concept after treatment of nocturnal enuresis: randomized controlled trial, J. Pediatr. 110:647-652, 1987.

National Institutes of Health: Neurofibromatosis: National Institutes of Health consensus Developmental Conference Statement, Bethesda, MD, 1987, National Institutes of Health, p. 6.

Needham, G.R.: Evaluation of five popular methods for tick removal, Pediatrics 75:997-1002, 1985.

Nicol, N.H.: What's new with sunscreens? choices—choices—choices, Pediatr. Nurs. 15:417-418, 1989.

Oberg, M., and Lindsey, D.: Do not put hydrogen peroxide or povidone iodine into wounds! Am. J. Dis. Child. 141:27-28, 1987.

Olson, A.: Recurrent abdominal pain: an approach to diagnosis and management, Pediatr. Ann. 16:834-842, 1987.

Ornitz, E.M., and Pynoos, R.S.: Startle modulation in children with post-traumatic stress disorder, Am. J. Psychiatry 146:866-869, 1989.

Pauls, D.L., and Leckman, J.F.: The inheritance of Gilles de la Tourette's syndrome and associated behaviors: evidence for autosomal dominant transmission, N. Engl. J. Med. 315:993-997, 1986.

Perelson, A.M., and Seyler, M.F.: First aid: soaking an injured finger or toe, Emerg. Med. 16:158, 1985.

Poole, S.R.: Recurrent abdominal pain in childhood and adolescence, Am. Fam. Physician 30:131-137, 1984.

Putnam, M.H., and Lawton, M.B.: Resourceful women unmask cactus spines, JAMA 253:2830, 1985.

Rappaport, L.A., and Levin, M.D.: The prevention of constipation and encopresis: a developmental model and approach, Pediatr. Clin. North Am. 33:859-869, 1986.

Reeves, J.R.: Head lice and scabies in children, Pediatr. Infect. Dis. 6:598-602, 1987.

Rosa, P.A., and Schwan, T.G.: A specific and sensitive assay for the Lyme disease spirochete *Borrelia burgdorferi* using the polymerase chain reaction, J. Infect. Dis. 160:1018-1029, 1989.

Rule, J.T.D: Recognition of dental caries, Pediatr. Clin. North Am. 29:439-456, 1982.

Rushton, H.G.: Nocturnal enuresis: epidemiology, evaluation, and currently available treatment options, J. Pediatr. 114(suppl.):691-696, 1989.

Sacks, J.J., Sattin, R.W., and Bonzo, S.E.: Dog bite–related fatalities from 1979 through 1988, JAMA 262:1489-1492, 1989.

Safer, D.J., and Krager, J.M.: A survey of medication treatment for hyperactive/inattentive students, JAMA 260:2256-2258, 1988.

Schneider, D, and Hebert, L.: Subcutaneous gas from hydrogen peroxide administration under pressure, Am. J. Dis. Child. 141:10-11, 1987.

Schuberth, K.C.: How dangerous are insect stings? Contemp. Pediatr. 6(5):69-88, 1989.

Schultz, M.W., and others: Comparative study of 5% permethrin cream and 1% lindane lotion for the treatment of scabies, Arch. Dermatol. 126:167-170

Shalita, A.R.: Principles of infant skin care, Skillman, NJ, 1981, Johnson & Johnson Baby Products Co.

Shaw, L., and Glenwright, H.D.: The role of medications in dental caries formation: need for sugar-free medications for children, Pediatrician 16:153-155, 1989.

Shaywitz, S.E., and Shaywitz, B.A.: Neurochemical correlates of attention deficit disorder, Pediatr. Clin. North Am. 31:387-397, 1984.

Sieggreen, M.Y.: Healing of physical wounds, Nurs. Clin. North Am. 22:439-447, 1987.

Silver, L.B.: Controversial approaches to treating learning disabilities and attention deficit disorder, Am. J. Dis. Child. 140:1045-1052, 1986.

Slome, B.: Rampant caries: a side effect of tricyclic antidepressant therapy, Genet. Dent. 32:494-496, 1984.

Stein, D.H.: Problems with ectoparasites. I. Scabies, Child Care Newsletter 6(1):1-2, 1987.

Steinberg, A.: Do drugs substitute for discipline? AIM Report 17(24), 1988.

Stroh, S.E., Stern, H.P., and McCarthy, S.G.: Fecal incontinence in children: a clinical update, MCN 14:252-254, 1989.

Taplin, D., and others: Malathion for treatment of Pediculus humanus capitis infestation, JAMA 247:3103-3105, 1982.

Terr, L.: Traumatic events in childhood have lasting effects, AAP News 5(5):1, 1989.

Weller, E.B., and Weller, R.A.: Pediatric management of depression, Pediatr. Ann. 18:104-113, 1989.

Wright, J.C.: Severe attacks by dogs: characteristics of the dogs, the victims, and the attack settings, Public Health Rep. 100:55-61, 1985.

Younger, J.B., and Hughes, L.S.: No-fault management of encopresis, Pediatr. Nurs. 9:185-187, 1983.

BIBLIOGRAPHY

Skin Disorders: General

A check list of summer safety tips, Contemp. Pediatr. 5(6):68-73, 1988.

Cerrato, P.L.: What diet does for wound healing, RN 51(6):73-75, 1988.

Chauvin, V.G.: Common skin rashes in children and adolescents, School Nurse 5(1):23-38, 1989.

Cohen, B.A.: Common dermatoses of childhood, Am. Fam. Physician 32(4):186-203, 1985.

Engebo, D.A.: Safe and effective use of tetracaine, adrenaline, and cocaine (TAC) solution anesthetic for anesthetizing of lacerations, J. Emerg. Nurs. 16:100-101, 1990.

Gelfant, B.B.: Healing skin wounds, Point of View 23(3):6-8, 1986.

Heimbach, D.M., and others: Suiting the dressing to the wound, Patient Care 21(11):164-166, 1987.

Lester, R.S.: Topical formulary for the pediatrician, Pediatr. Clin. North Am. 30:749-765, 1983.

McBurney, E.I.: Diagnostic dermatologic methods, Pediatr. Clin. North Am. 30:419-434, 1983.

Neuberger, G.B.: Wound care, Nursing '88 17(2):34-37, 1987.

Obringer, A.C., Meadows, A.T., and Zackai, E.H.: The diagnosis of neurofibromatosis-1 in the child under the age of 6 years, Am. J. Dis. Child. 143:717-721, 1989.

Parker, F: The skin and the elements: sun, plants, and stinging and biting organisms, Emerg. Care Q. 4(3):21-31, 1988.

Sieggreen, M.Y.: Healing of physical wounds, Nurs. Clin. North Am. 22:439-447. 1987.

Weston, J.A., Hawkins, K., and Weston, W.L.: Foot dermatitis in children, Pediatrics 72:824-827, 1983.

Infections

Blackman, J.A., and others: Management of young children with recurrent herpes simplex skin lesions in special education programs, Pediatr. Infect. Dis. 4:221-224, 1985.

Brady, M.: Common viral skin problems of childhood: warts and molluscum, J. Pediatr. Health Care 2:208-210, 1988.

Caputo, R.V.: Fungal infections in children, Dermatol. Clin. North Am. 4:137-150, 1986.

Carter, S.: Etiology and treatment of facial cellulitis in pediatric patients, Pediatr. Infect. Dis. 2:222, 1983.

Coskey, R.J., and Coskey, L.A.: Diagnosis and treatment of impetigo, J. Am. Acad. Dermatol. 17:62-63, 1987.

Frieden, I.J.: Diagnosis and management of tinea capitis, Pediatr. Ann. 16:39-48, 1987.

Gellis, S.E.: Warts and molluscum contagiosum in children, Pediatr. Ann. 16:69-76, 1987.

Goldberg, G.N.: An individualized approach to wart therapy, Contemp. Pediatr. 3(11):123-133, 1986.

Guess, H.A., and others: Epidemiology of herpes zoster in children and adolescents: a population-based study, Pediatrics 76:512-517, 1985.

Krugman, S., and others: Infectious diseases of children, ed. 8, St. Louis, 1985, Mosby–Year Book, Inc.

Notarangelo, P.R., and Dixon, D.M.: Opportunistic systemic mycoses and the critical care patient, Crit. Care Update 10:7-11, 1983.

Putnam, C.D., and Reynolds, M.S.: Mupriocin: a new topical therapy for impetigo, J. Pediatr. Health Care 3:224-227, 1989.

Rees, P.L., and Dixon, D.M.: Opportunistic mycoses, Am. J. Nurs. 81:1160-1165, 1981.

Stein, D.H.: Superficial fungal infections, Pediatr. Clin. North Am. 30:545-561, 1983.

Scabies and Pediculosis

Bowerman, J.G., and others: Comparative study of permethrin 1% creme rinse and lindane shampoo for the treatment of head lice, Pediatr. Infect. Dis. J. 6:252-255, 1987.

Brimhall, C.L., and Esterly, N.B.: Uninvited guests: skin infestations of childhood, Contemp. Pediatr. 7(1):18-57, 1990.

Clore, E.R.: Lice: ancient pest with new resistance, Pediatr. Nurs. 9:347-350, 1983.

Kuffel, J.: Treating a child with head lice, RN 50(9):32, 1987.

Lane, A.T.: Scabies and head lice, Pediatr. Ann. 16:51-54, 1987.

Malathion for head lice, Med. Lett. Drugs Ther. 31:110-111, 1989.

Mocsny, N.: What's wrong with this patient? RN 52(5):61-63, 1989.

Park, B.R., and Smith, D.: Treatment of head lice and scabies in children, Pediatr. Nurs. 15:522-524, 1989.

Sanford-Driscoll, M.: Pharmacotherapy of head lice in children: an update, J. Pediatr. Health Care 1:284-287, 1987.

Systemic Disorders

Elliot, D.L., and others: Pet-associated illness, N. Engl. J. Med. 313:985-995, 1985.

Ginsburg, C.M.: Cat-scratch adenitis, Pediatr. Infect. Dis. 3(5):437-438, 1984.

Hahn, D.B., and others: Lyme disease: an increasing health risk for school-age children, J. School Health 57:221-223, 1987.

Lee, B.C.: Be ready for Lyme disease in your own backyard, RN 52(4):26-29, 1989.

Maran, J.N., and Crispell, K.A.: Lyme disease: an elusive diagnosis, J. Pediatr. Health Care 3:60-66, 1989.

Margileth, A.M.: Cat-scratch disease update, Am. J. Dis. Child. 138:711-713, 1984.

Thompson, S.: Summertime and ticks, Am. J. Nurs. 83:768-769, 1983.

Wear, D.J., and others: Cat scratch disease: a bacterial infection, Science 221:1403-1408, 1983.

Woodward, W.E.: What clinicians should know about Rocky Mountain spotted fever, Drug Ther. 12:106-114, 1982.

Chemical and Physical Injuries

Beyea, S.C.: What people expect you to know about poison ivy, RN 52(8):23-25, 1989.

Brown, F.E., and others: Frostbite: long term effects on bone growth, Pediatrics 71:955-959, 1983.

Hurwitz, S., Rhodes, A., and Wiley, H.: For every child under the sun: a guide to sensible sun protection, New York, 1986, The Skin Cancer Foundation.

LaVoy, K.: Dealing with hypothermia and frostbite, RN 48(1):53-56, 1985.

Leach, J.: How to recognize photosensitivity disorders, Contemp. Pediatr. 6(6):56-74, 1989.

Lewis, R.M., and Fischer, R.G.: Sunscreen agents, Pediatr. Nurs. 13:200, 1987.

Moss, J.R.: Playing it safe in the sun, Child. Nurse 4(3):1-3, 1986.

Ramsay, C.A.: Photosensitivity in children, Pediatr. Clin. North Am. 30:687-699, 1983.

Robinson, L.A.: Sun exposure and sun protection, Pediatr. Nurs. 8:272-273, 1982.

Robinson, M., and Seward, P.H.: Environmental hypothermia in children, Pediatr. Emerg. Care 2:254, 1986.
Weinstock, M.A., and others: Nonfamilial cutaneous melanoma incidence in women associated with sun exposure before 20 years of age, Pediatrics 84:199-204, 1989.
Wingate, E.: A nursing perspective on frostbite, Crit. Care Update 10:8-15, 1983.

Miscellaneous Skin Disorders

Datloff, J., and Esterly, N.B.: A system for sorting out pediatric alopecia, Contemp. Pediatr. 3(10):53-72, 1986.
Dunn, M.L., Cockerline, E.B., and Rice, M.R.: Treatment options for psoriasis, Am. J. Nurs. 88:1082-1087, 1988.
Eldridge, R., and others: Neurofibromatosis type 1 (Recklinghausen's disease), Am. J. Dis. Child. 143:833-837, 1989.
Pau, A.K., and others: Drug allergy documentation by physicians, nurses, and medical students, Am. J. Hosp. Pharm. 46:558-560, 1989.
Prendiville, J.S., and others: Management of Stevens-Johnson syndrome and toxic epidermal necrolysis in children, J. Pediatr. 115:881-887, 1989.
Rasmussen, J.E.: Psoriasis in childhood, Dermatol Clin. North Am. 4:99-106, 1986.
Riccardi, V.M.: The multiple forms of neurofibromatosis, Pediatr. Rev. 3:293-298, 1982.
Stephenson, C.: Diagnosing and dealing with neurofibromatosis in children, MCN 7:387-390, 1982.
Stroud, J.D.: Hair loss in children, Pediatr. Clin. North Am. 30:641-657, 1983.
Taylor, J.A., and others: Toxic epidermal necrolysis, Clin. Pediatr. 28:404-407, 1989.
Tunnessen, W.W.: What's new in pediatric dermatology? In Oski, F.A., and Stockman, J.A., III: The yearbook of pediatrics, St. Louis, 1985, Mosby–Year Book, Inc.
Twarog, F.J.: Urticaria in childhood: pathogenesis and management, Pediatr. Clin. North Am. 30:887-897, 1983.

Bites and Stings

Adamski, D.B: Assessment and treatment of allergic response to stinging insects, J. Emerg. Nurs. 16:77-80, 1990.
Amitai Y., and others: Scorpion sting in children, Clin. Pediatr. 24:136-140, 1985.
Cardoni, A.A.: Meat tenderizer and bee stings (letter), Pediatrics 74:447, 1984.
Eitzen, E.M., and Seward, P.L.N.: Arthropod envenomations in children, Pediatr. Emerg. Care 4:266-270, 1988.
Ginsburg, C.M.: Fire ant envenomation in children, Pediatrics 73:689-692, 1984.
Graft, D.F., and Schuberth, K.C.: Hymenoptera allergy in children, Pediatr. Clin. North Am. 30:873-886, 1983.
Graft, D.F., and others: A prospective study of the natural history of large local reactions after hymenoptera stings in children, J. Pediatr. 104:664-668, 1984.
Hainer, B.L.: Cat scratch disease, J. Fam. Pract. 25:497-503, 1987.
Honig, P.J.: Bites and parasites, Pediatr. Clin. North Am. 30:563-581, 1983.
Jaffe, A.C.: Animal bites, Pediatr. Clin. North Am. 30:405-413, 1983.
King, R.C., and Giles, J.: Dealing with insect bites, RN 47(5):53-55, 1984.
Rich, J.: Snakebite, Nursing '87 17(6):33, 1987.
Schuberth, K.C., and others: An epidemiologic study of insect allergy in children. I. Characteristics of the disease, J. Pediatr. 100:546-551, 1982.

Dental Problems

Babington, M.A., and Spadaro, D.C.: Cariogenic medications, Pediatr. Nurs. 8:165-171, 1982.
Crall, J.J.: Promotion of oral health and prevention of common pediatric dental problems, Pediatr. Clin. North Am. 33:887-898, 1986.
Featherstone, J.D.B.: The mechanism of dental decay, Nutr. Today 22(3):10-16, 1987.
Feldman, A.L., and Aretakis, D.A.: Herpetic gingivostomatitis in children, Pediatr. Nurs. 12:111-113, 1986.
Herrmann, H.J. and Roberts, M.W.: Preventive dental care: the role of the pediatrician, Pediatrics 80:107-110, 1987.
Hess, C.S., and others: Fluoride: too much or too little? Pediatr. Nurs. 10:397-403, 1984.
Kronmiller, J.E.: Oral soft tissue abnormalities in children, Pediatr. Nurs. 13:161-165, 1987.
Jenkins, N.: Diet and dental caries, Food Nutr. News 56:29-32, 1984.
Josell, S.D., and Abrams, R.G.: Traumatic injuries to the dentition and its supporting structures, Pediatr. Clin. North Am. 29:717-711, 1982.
Kilmon, C., and Helpin, M.L.: Recognizing dental malocclusion in children, Pediatr. Nurs. 9:204-208, 1983.
Kronmiller, K.E., and Nirschl, R.F.: Preventive dentistry for children, Pediatr. Nurs. 11:446-449, 1985.
McDonald, R.E., and Avery, D.R.: Dentistry for the child and adolescent, ed. 8, St. Louis, 1988, Mosby–Year Book, Inc.
McGuire, S.: Fluoride content of bottled water, N. Engl. J. Med. 321:836-837, 1989.
Mertz-Fairhurst, E.J.: Current status of sealant retention and caries prevention, J. Dent. Educ. 48(suppl. 2):80-85, 1984.
Robertson, J.S., and Maddux, J.E.: Compliance in pediatric orthodontic treatment: current research and issues, Child. Health Care 15:40-48, 1986.
Starr, R.M., and Gravitz, R.F.: Pit and fissure sealants in the prevention of tooth decay, Pediatr. Nurs. 11:289-291, 1985.
Weinstein, L.B., Abrams, R.A., and Ayers, C.S.: Increasing awareness of sugar ingestion among children, Pediatr. Nurs. 14:277-279, 1988.

Elimination Disorders

Ack, M., Norman, M.E., and Schmitt, B.D. (in discussion): Enuresis: the role of alarms and drugs, Patient Care 19:75-90, 1985.
Castiglia, P.T.: Encopresis, J. Pediatr. Health Care 1:335-337, 1987.
Castiglia, P.T.: Nocturnal enuresis, J. Pediatr. Health Care 1:280-282, 1987.
Crowley, A.A.: A comprehensive strategy for managing encopresis, MCN 9:395-400, 1984.
Friman, P.C., and Warzak, W.J.: Nocturnal enuresis: a prevalent, persistent, yet curable parasomnia, Pediatrician 17:38-45, 1990.
Gibson, L.Y.: Bedwetting: a family's recurrent nightmare, MCN 14:270-272, 1989.
Johns, C.: Encopresis, Am. J. Nurs. 85:153-156, 1985.
Levine, M.D.: Encopresis: its potentiation, evaluation, and alleviation, Pediatr. Clin. North Am. 29:315-330, 1982.
Novello, A.C., and Novello, J.R.: Enuresis, Pediatr. Clin. North Am. 34:719-733, 1987.
O'Regan, S., and others: Constipation: a commonly unrecognized cause of enuresis, Am. J. Dis. Child. 140:260-261, 1986.
Rushton, H.: Nocturnal enuresis: epidemiology, evaluation, and current available treatment options, J. Pediatr. 114:691-696, 1989.
Schmitt, B.D.: Encopresis, Primary Care 11:497-511, 1984.
Schmitt, B.D.: Nocturnal enuresis, Primary Care 11:485-495, 1984.
Shapiro, S.R.: Enuresis: treatment and overtreatment, Pediatr. Nurs. 11(3):203-207, 1985.
Stadtler, A.C.: Preventing encopresis, Pediatr. Nurs. 15:282-284, 1989.
Younger, J.B., and Huges, L.S.: No-fault management of encopresis, Pediatr. Nurs. 9:185-187, 1983.

Attention Deficit–Hyperactivity Disorder

Anderson, V., and Oberklaid, F.: Developmental dysfunction: learning disabilities and attention deficits in children and adolescents, Curr. Opinion Pediatr. 1:156-161, 1989.

Brown, R.T., and Wynne, M.E.: Sustained attention in boys with attention deficit disorder and the effect of methylphenidate, Pediatr. Nurs. 10:35-39, 1984.

Dulcan, M.K.: Attention deficit disorder: evaluation and treatment, Pediatr. Ann. 14:383-398, 1985.

Eichlseder, W.: Ten years of experience with 1,000 hyperactive children in a private practice, Pediatrics 76:176-184, 1985.

Golden, G.S.: A hard look at fad therapies for developmental disorders, Contemp. Pediatr. 4(10):47-60, 1987.

Howell, D.C., Huessy, H.R., and Hassuk, B.: Fifteen-year follow-up of a behavioral history of attention deficit disorder, Pediatrics 76:185-190, 1985.

Kelly, P.C., and others: Self-esteem in children medically managed for attention deficit disorder, Pediatrics 83:211-217, 1989.

Levine, M.D., and Melmed, R.D.: The unhappy wanderers: children with attention deficits, Pediatr. Clin. North Am. 29:105-120, 1982.

Niebuhr, V.N., and Smith, K.E.: Simple tests to assess behavior problems, Contemp. Pediatr. 7(1):117-138, 1990.

Safer, D.J., and Krager, J.M.: Trends in medication treatment of hyperactive school children, Clin. Pediatr. 22:500-503, 1983.

Schultz, F.R., and others: Methylphenidate treatment of hyperactive children: effects of the hypothalamic-pituitary-somatomedin axis, Pediatrics 70:987-992, 1982.

Varley, C.K.: A clinical nurse specialist's role in the comprehensive management of attention deficit disorder, Child. Health Care 13:139-142, 1985.

Behavior Disorders

Adkins, A.S.: Helping your patient cope with Tourette syndrome, Pediatr. Nurs. 15:135-137, 1989.

Barabas, G.: Tourette's syndrome: an overview, Pediatr. Ann. 17:391-393, 1988.

Bassett, L.B., Gudas, L.J., and McAnulty, E.H.: The learning-disabled child: recognition, evaluation, and management, Pediatr. Nurs. 8:325-329, 1982.

Cowell, J.M.: Dilemmas in assessing the health status of children with learning disabilities, J. Pediatr. Health Care 4:24-31, 1990.

Epstein, M., and Cullinan, D.: Depression in children, J. School Health 56:10-12, 1986.

Erenberg, G., Cruse, R.P., and Rothner, A.D.: The natural history of Tourette syndrome: a follow-up study, Ann. Neurol. 22:383-385, 1987.

Feagans, L.: A current view of learning disabilities, J. Pediatr. 102:487-494, 1983.

Finn, P.A.: Self-destructive behavior in school-age children: a hidden problem? Pediatr Nurs. 12:198-199, 1986.

Gilligan, J.: Understanding learning disabilities, School Nurse 3(4):22-25, 1987.

Golden, G.S.: Movement disorders in children: Tourette syndrome, Dev. Behav. Pediatr. 3:209-212, 1982.

Kenealy, P.: Children's strategies for coping with depression, Behav. Ther. 27:27-34, 1989.

Parker, K.: Helping school-age children cope with Tourette syndrome, J. School Health 74(1):30-32, 1985.

Roddy, S.M.: Bad habit, simple tic, or Tourette syndrome? Contemp. Pediatr. 6(11):22-36, 1989.

Shaywitz, S.E., Grossman, H.J., and Shaywitz, B.A., editors: Symposium on learning disorders, Pediatr. Clin. North Am. 31:1, 1984.

Shaywitz, S.E., and others: Current status of the neuromaturational examination as an index of learning disability, J. Pediatr. 104:819-823, 1984.

Stefl, M.E.: Mental health needs associated with Tourette syndrome, Am. J. Public Health 74:1310-1313, 1984.

White, J.E.: Special nursing needs of hospitalized children with learning disabilities, MCN 8:209-212, 1983.

Emotional Disorders

Brady, M.A., and others: Childhood depression: development of a screening tool, Pediatr. Nurs. 10:222-227, 1984.

Bumbalo, J.A., and Siemon, M.K.: Nursing assessment and diagnosis: mental health problems of children, Top. Clin. Nurs. 5(1):41-54, 1983.

Child, A.A., Murphy, C.M., and Rhyne, M.C.: Depression in children: reasons and risks, Pediatr. Nurs. 6(4):9-13, 1980.

Dolgan, J.I.: Depression in children, Pediatr. Ann. 19:45-50, 1990.

Extended sleep (hypersomnia) in young depressed patients, Am. J. Psychiatry 142:905-910, 1985.

Fond, K., and Brosnan, J.: School phobia: the school anxiety syndrome, Pediatr. Nurs. 6(5):9-13, 1980.

Gartner, J.C.: Recurrent abdominal pain—who needs a workup? Contemp. Pediatr. 6(9):62-82, 1989.

Gaylord, N., and Carson, S.: Assessing recurrent abdominal pain in children, Nurs. Pract. 8:9-22, 1983.

Herman, S.P., and Schowalter, J.E.: Depression, suicide, and the young child, Emerg. Med. 13(16):61-68, 1981.

Korup, U.L.: Parent and teacher perception of depression in children, J. School Health 55:367, 1985.

Maisami, M., and Freeman, J.M.: Conversion reactions in children as body language: a combined child psychiatry/neurology team approach to the management of functional neurologic disorders in children, Pediatrics 80:46-52, 1987.

McConville, B.J.: The causes and treatment of depression in young children, J. Child. Contemp. Soc. 15(6):61-68, 1982.

McGrath, P.J., and Feldman, W.: Clinical approach to recurrent abdominal pain in children, J. Dev. Behav. Pediatr. 7:56-60, 1986.

Mitchell, J., Varley, C., and McCauley, E.: Depression in children and adolescents, Child. Health Care 16:290-293, 1988.

Nelms, B.C.: Assessing childhood depression: do parents and children agree? Pediatr Nurs. 12:23-26, 1986.

Nelms, B.C., and Brady, M.A.: Assessment and intervention: the depressed school-age child, Pediatr. Nurs. 6(4):15-19, 1980.

Page-Goertz, S.: Recurrent abdominal pain in children, Issues Compr. Pediatr. Nurs. 11:179-191, 1988.

Pineiro-Carrero, V.M., and others: Abnormal gastroduodenal motility in children and adolescents with recurrent functional abdominal pain, J. Pediatr. 113:820-825, 1988.

Porter, E.: The school nurse's role in school phobia, School Nurse 3(4):8-11, 1987.

Promoting emotional health—role of the nurse practitioner, J. Pediatr. Health Care 2:1-2, 1988.

Rhyne, M.C., and others: Children at risk for depression, Am. J. Nurs. 12:1379-1382, 1986.

Rutter, M.: Prevention of children's psychosocial disorders: myth and substance, Pediatrics 70:883-894, 1982.

Ryan, N.M.: Recurrent abdominal pain among school-age children, MCN 11:102-106, 1986.

Schmitt, B.D.: School refusal, Pediatr. Rev. 8:99-101, 1986.

Simmons, J.E.: When to refer to a child psychiatrist, Contemp. Pediatr. 4(2):77-94, 1987.

Sledden, E.A., Maddux, J.E., and Katnick, R.J.: Psychological assessment and consultation in pediatric neurology, Child. Health Care 16:43-50, 1987.

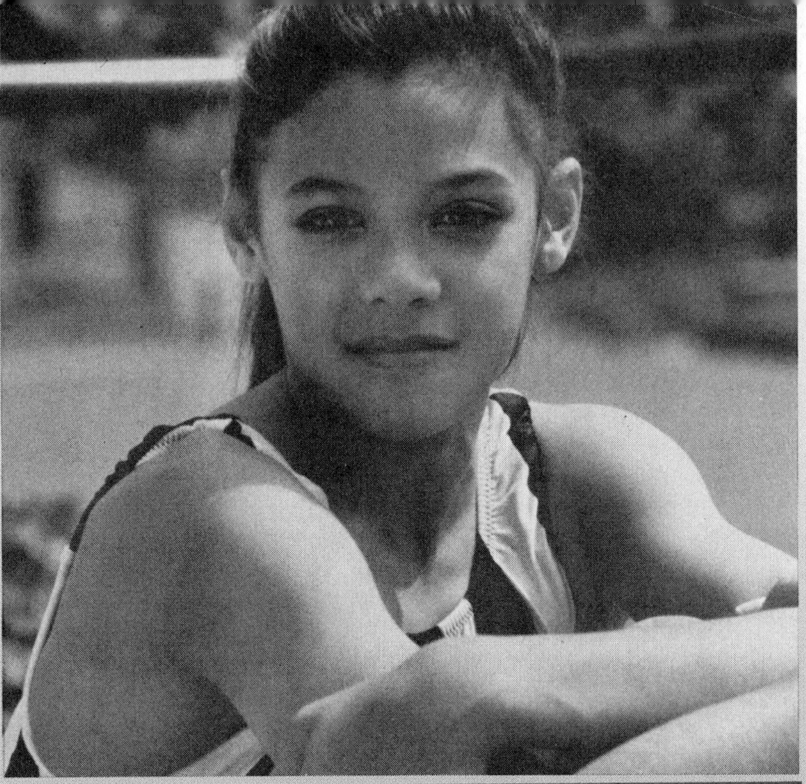

Adolescence

UNIT VII

Adolescence is a period of transition that is based on childhood experiences and accomplishments and ultimately aspires to mature, independent, and responsible functioning. This transition is a biologic, emotional, and social process, a preparatory period requiring the accomplishment of defined developmental tasks in order to attain satisfactory adjustment to adulthood. The early years of adolescence are concerned with individuation from previous dependency roles and a gradual movement toward peer-group identity. The focus of an adolescent's world is the peer group—the persons the adolescent knows who are going through the same transition and who understand the adolescent's problems and frustrations. Later years of adolescence are centered around acquiring a personal identity, completing the separation process from family, and career-directed activity.

The physiologic changes that take place during puberty have both psychologic and social significance for adolescent boys and girls, and the rate and degree of equanimity with which adolescents grow and mature varies widely among individuals. Although it is a relatively healthy period of life, most of the health and emotional problems of teenagers are directly related to the biologic alterations and the emotional responses associated with this tumultuous period of life.

Chapter 19, *Health Promotion of the Adolescent and Family,* provides an overview of the transitional adolescent period during which young people must adjust to rapid body changes, establish a personal identity, gain emotional and (for some) economic freedom from their parents, and evolve a set of values uniquely their own. Chapters 20 and 21 are concerned with some of the health problems associated with adolescence as a result of either the changes related to biologic maturation or the psychologic adjustments imposed by these changes and societal expectations of society. Chapter 20, *Physical Health Problems of Adolescence,* is devoted primarily to physical problems of this age-group, including problems related to sexuality; Chapter 21, *Behavioral Health Problems of Adolescence,* focuses on health problems that are related to the multiple changes of adolescence and that impose a serious threat to health and well-being.

CHAPTER 19

Health Promotion of the Adolescent and Family

RELATED TOPICS

Adolescent pregnancy, Ch. 20

Alterations in growth and maturation, Ch. 20

Growth and development of children, Ch. 4

Health problems of the female reproductive system, Ch. 20

Health problems of the male reproductive system, Ch. 20

Injuries and health problems related to sports participation, Ch. 39

Injury prevention, Ch. 17

Precocious puberty, Ch. 38

Sexually transmitted diseases, Ch. 20

GLOSSARY

adolescence Psychologic, social, and maturational process initiated by pubertal changes

adrenarche Pubertal changes caused by increased secretion of androgenic hormones or their precursors.

ATV All-terrain vehicle

heterosexual Sexual preference for persons of the opposite sex

homosexual Sexual attraction to persons of the same sex

identity The condition of being a specific person

menarche Establishment of menstrual function.

MVA Motor vehicle accident

primary sex characteristics External and internal reproductive organs

puberty Achievement of sexual maturity

SBC School-based clinic

secondary sex characteristics Physical features that distinguish the sexes but play no direct part in reproduction

thelarche Beginning of breast development in the female

Adolescence begins at puberty, and accompanying the pubertal changes there are corresponding changes in the personality. There is considerable variation in the time of the onset of puberty and in the manner in which different individuals cope with the multiple developmental events associated with pubertal changes. Adolescence is a period of transition and a time of physical, social, and emotional maturing as the girl prepares for womanhood and the boy readies for manhood. During this period of development the individual makes the most significant progress in learning to live effectively in society.

PROMOTING OPTIMUM GROWTH AND DEVELOPMENT

The precise boundaries of adolescence are difficult to define, but this period is customarily viewed as beginning with the gradual appearance of secondary sex characteristics at about 11 or 12 years of age and ending with cessation of somatic growth at 18 to 20 years. However, there are such wide individual and cultural variations that, more than in any other age category, no sharp age delineation can be made. Adolescence tends to begin and end earlier in girls than in boys.

There are several terms that are commonly used in reference to this particular stage of growth and development. *Puberty* primarily refers to the maturational, hormonal, and growth process that occurs when the reproductive organs begin to function and the secondary sex characteristics develop. This process is sometimes further delineated as *pubescence,* the period of about 2 years immediately before puberty characterized by the prepubertal growth spurts, when the child is developing preliminary physical changes that herald sexual maturity; *puberty,* the point at which sexual maturity is achieved, marked by the first menstrual flow in girls and by less obvious indications in boys; and *postpubescence,* a 1- to 2-year period following puberty during which skeletal growth is completed and reproductive functions become fairly well established. Puberty ends with the ability to reproduce, which in girls is soon after the onset of menstruation with the establishment of regular ovulation and in boys is soon after the first nocturnal emission when spermatogenesis is established. *Adolescence,* less firmly fixed, literally means "to grow into maturity" and is generally regarded as the psychologic, social, and maturational process initiated by pubertal changes. The term *teenage years* is used synonymously with *adolescence* to describe the years between ages 13 and 19.

Although the changes that take place during adolescence are primarily those affecting the body and personality, children in this period are highly influenced by the culture in which they grow and develop. In some of the more primitive societies the transition to adulthood is recognized soon after or simultaneously with puberty. The event is solemnized by some type of ritual, ceremony, or other "rite of passage." From that point on, the young people assume the privileges, responsibilities, and status accorded adults in the society. Decisions regarding the future are made when they are young, and the psychologic turmoil is relatively brief. The youngsters know from early childhood what is expected; prepared for their roles in adult activities, they slip easily into the new position accepted by parents, society, and themselves.

In more complex societies this transition is less clearly delineated, and society is equally vague about attainment of adult status. School years are legally over at 16 to 18 years but may continue to age 25 or beyond for many young people. Adolescents are legally permitted to drive at as young an age as 14 in some states and at a later age in others, but adult insurance premiums are not granted until age 25. In many states adolescents are not allowed to gamble or purchase liquor until age 21. Many activities in which young people are allowed to participate are considered to be those of adults, such as wars, voting, marriage, and childbearing, while at the same time they are considered youngsters in relation to social status and control of resources in the adult community. This ambiguity of society and parents contributes to adolescents' own confusion and uncertainty about themselves.

In addition to this prolonged period of cultural maturation, adolescents' ultimate goals and adult roles are less defined and clear-cut in advanced societies than they are in primitive societies. In advanced cultures there are choices to be made regarding occupation, marriage, and even social and religious values. Although adolescents want to achieve adult status and privileges, they are faced with so many possibilities and choices that they are often reluctant to assume the associated responsibilities. They are eager to grow up yet fearful of the implications. It is no wonder that adolescence is a time of confusion and turmoil.

BIOLOGIC DEVELOPMENT

The physical changes of puberty are primarily the result of hormonal activity influenced by the central nervous system, although all aspects of physiologic functioning are mutually interacting. Growth and change are more dramatically and visibly demonstrated at this time than at any other period in life. The very obvious physical changes are noted in increased physical growth and the appearance and development of secondary sex characteristics; less obvious are physiologic alterations and neurogonadal maturity accompanied by the ability to procreate. Physical distinction between the sexes is determined on the basis of differential characteristics: *primary sex characteristics* are the external and internal organs that carry on the reproductive functions; *secondary sex characteristics* are the characteristics that distinguish the sexes from each other but play no direct part in reproduction. Because most of the physical changes that take place during adolescence are directly related to the hormonal changes of that period, a discussion of these

Jeanette M. Broering, R.N., M.S., C.P.N.P., assisted in the revision of this chapter.

changes is presented first, followed by a consideration of general growth trends and development of secondary sex characteristics.

Hormonal Changes of Puberty

It is generally accepted that the events of puberty are caused by hormonal influences and are controlled by the anterior pituitary gland (adenohypophysis) in response to a stimulus from the hypothalamus. Probably in some way related to brain maturation, hypothalamic stimulation causes the anterior pituitary to release gonadotropins that in turn stimulate the gonads. Stimulation to the gonads results in fulfillment of a dual function: (1) production and release of gametes—production of sperm in the male and maturation and release of ova in the female—and (2) secretion of sex-appropriate hormones—estrogen and progesterone from the female ovaries and testosterone from the male testes.

The dynamics of the reproductive hormone system include both neural and endocrine functions involving principally the hypothalamus, the adenohypophysis, and the gonads. The chain of reactions that causes ripening of the ovum in the female and production of sperm in the male begins in the region of the hypothalamus. Neurosecretory hormones, the *gonadotropin-releasing factors (GnRF)*, synthesized and discharged by the hypothalamus, are carried via the hypophyseal portal vessels to the adenohypophysis, where they trigger the release of the gonadotropins *follicle-stimulating hormone (FSH)* and *luteinizing hormone (LH)*, also known in the male as *interstitial cell–stimulating hormone (ICSH)*. Increasing levels of these gonadotropic hormones in the blood stimulate the appropriate responses in the gonads.

Inhibition, or *negative feedback*, in the reproductive endocrine system refers to diminished gonadotropin secretion as a result of increasing serum levels of sex hormones. When sex hormone levels increase, GnRF secretion is diminished; when sex hormone levels decrease, the hypothalamus is stimulated to release GnRF, again initiating the sequence that produces the appropriate gonadal responses (Fig. 19-1).

Initiation of puberty. The precise mechanism that institutes the changes at puberty is not completely understood. Evidence suggests that bone age is the somatic marker that best correlates with readiness to initiate puberty (Kaplan, 1982). Although the pituitary and gonads are capable of mature function and can respond to stimuli at any age, the hypothalamic-pituitary-gonadal system is maintained in a dormant state throughout prepubescent childhood by some central nervous system inhibitory factor in the region of the hypothalamus. It is believed that the receptor sites in the hypothalamus are so highly sensitive that the most minute quantities of circulating sex hormones are sufficient to inhibit the secretion of GnRF during childhood. The hypothalamus loses this negative sensitivity at puberty and allows the hypothalamic-pituitary-gonadal mechanism to attain full secretory function. As puberty progresses, a powerful amplification process causes the pituitary and gonads to become increasingly sensitive to positive stimulation.

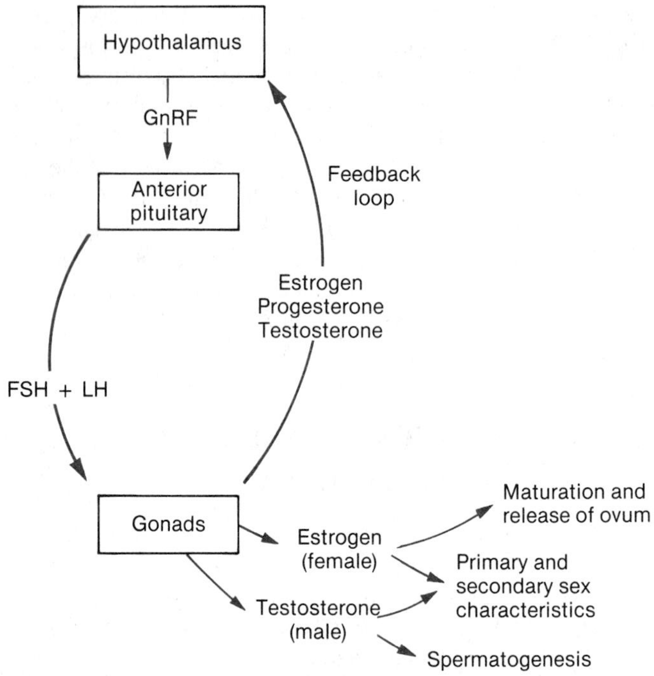

Fig. 19-1. Hormonal interaction between hypothalamus, pituitary, and gonads.

Sex hormones. Sex hormones are secreted by the ovaries, testes, and adrenal glands; they are produced in varying amounts in both sexes throughout life. The adrenal cortex is responsible for the small amounts secreted during the prepubescent years, but the sex hormone production that accompanies maturation of the gonads is responsible for the variety of biologic changes observed during pubescence and puberty. (See Table 38-1 for the major somatic effects produced by the sex hormones.)

Estrogen, the feminizing hormone, is found in low quantities during childhood and is secreted in slowly increasing amounts until about age 11. In males this gradual increase continues through maturation. In females the onset of estrogen production in the ovaries causes a pronounced estrogen increase that continues to rise until about 3 years after the onset of menstruation, at which time it reaches a maximum level that is then maintained throughout the reproductive life of the female.

Androgens, the masculinizing hormones, are also secreted in small and gradually increasing amounts until approximately ages 7 to 9, when there is a rapid increase in output in both sexes, especially boys, until about age 15. These hormones appear to be responsible for most of the rapid growth changes of early adolescence. With onset of testicular function, the level of androgens (principally testosterone) in males increases over that in females and continues to increase until a maximum is attained at maturity.

Pubertal Growth Spurt

A constant phenomenon associated with sexual maturation is a dramatic increase in growth. The relatively uniform physical growth of childhood shifts to markedly diverse

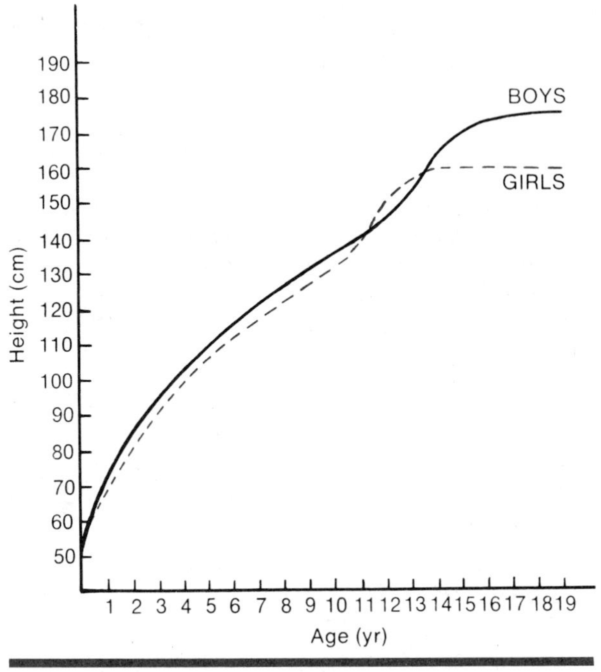

Fig. 19-2. Linear growth throughout childhood.
From Tanner, J.M., Whitehouse, R.H., and Takaishi, M.: Arch. Dis. Child. 41:454-471, 1966.

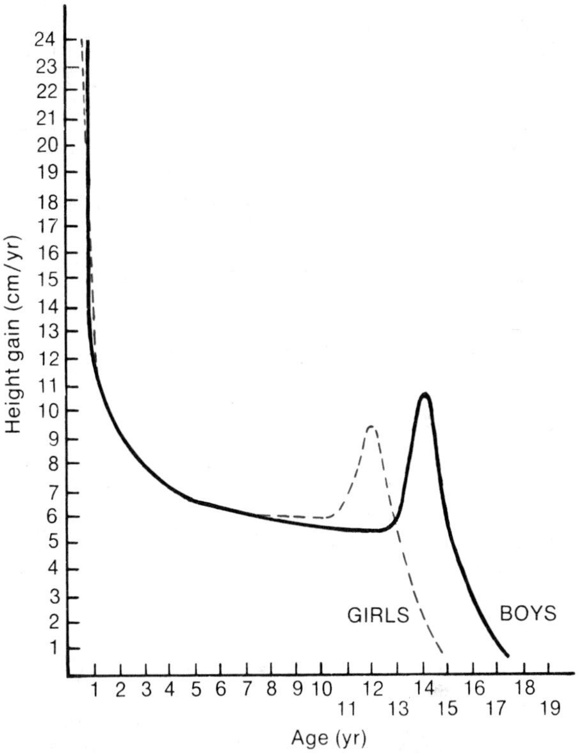

Fig. 19-3. Linear growth in centimeters per year.
From Tanner, J.M., Whitehouse, R.H., and Takaishi, M.: Arch. Dis. Child. 41:454-471, 1966.

rates of growth in adolescence. The final 20% to 25% of linear growth is achieved during puberty, and most (but not all) of this growth occurs during a 24- to 36-month period—the adolescent *growth spurt* (Fig. 19-2 and Fig. 19-3). This accelerated growth occurs in all children but, as in other areas of development, is highly variable in age of onset, duration, and extent. Visible signs of puberty are the development of secondary sex characteristics.

Puberty in girls can begin any time between 8 and 14 years of age and, once initiated, usually is completed within 3 years. The average girl, in whom the growth spurt is slower and less extensive than in boys, will gain 5 to 20 cm (2 to 8 inches) in height and 7 to 25 kg (15 to 55 pounds) in weight. Menarche, the onset of menstruation, occurs about 2½ years after the onset of puberty. At this time girls will have achieved 90% to 95% of adult height. Growth in height ceases in girls at 16 or 17 years of age (Fig. 19-4).

On the average, puberty begins about 1½ to 2 years later in boys—between 9½ and 16 years of age. During this period the average boy will gain 10 to 30 cm (4 to 12 inches) in height and 7 to 30 kg (15 to 65 pounds) in weight. In boys growth in height commonly ceases at 18 or 20 years of age. The major developmental changes of puberty are the growth and maturation of the gonads and the appearance of secondary sex characteristics (Fig. 19-5).

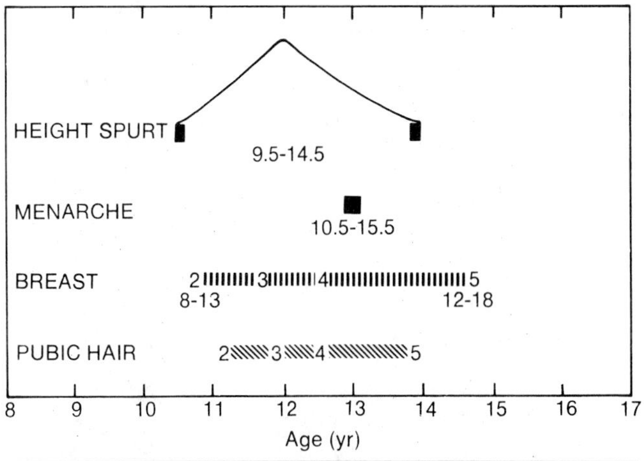

Fig. 19-4. Approximate timing of developmental changes in girls. Number indicates stages of development. Range of ages during which some of the changes occur is indicated by inclusive numbers below them. See Figs. 19-6 and 19-7 for explanation.
From Marshall, W.A., and Tanner, J.M.: Arch. Dis. Child. 44:291, 1969.

Sexual Maturation

The visual evidence of sexual maturation is achieved in orderly sequence, and the state of maturity can be estimated on the basis of the appearance of these external manifestations. The age at which the changes are observed and the time required to progress from one stage to another may vary considerably among individual children.

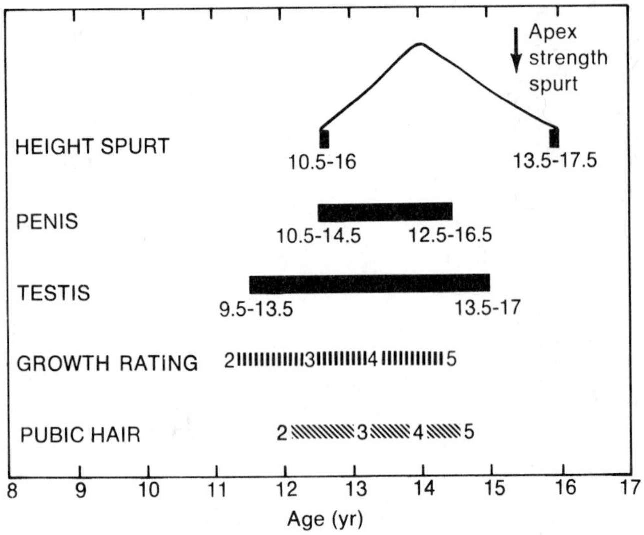

Fig. 19-5. Approximate timing of developmental changes in boys. Numbers indicate stages of development. Range of ages during which some of the changes occur is indicated by inclusive numbers below them. See Fig. 19-8 for explanation.
From Marshall, W.A., and Tanner, J.M.: Arch. Dis. Child. 45:13, 1970.

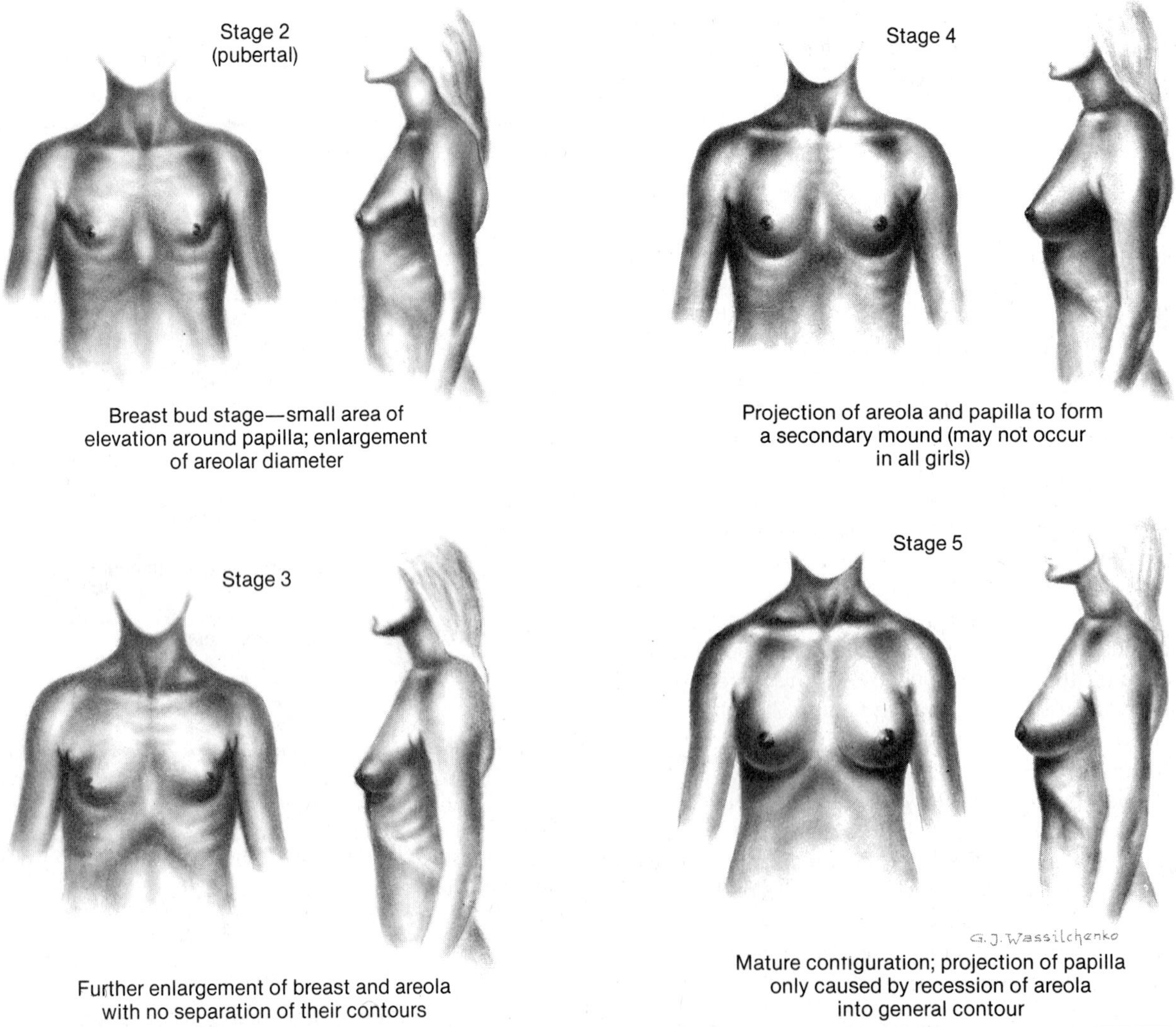
Stage 2
(pubertal)
Breast bud stage—small area of elevation around papilla; enlargement of areolar diameter
Stage 4
Projection of areola and papilla to form a secondary mound (may not occur in all girls)
Stage 3
Further enlargement of breast and areola with no separation of their contours
Stage 5
G. J. Wassilchenko
Mature configuration; projection of papilla only caused by recession of areola into general contour

Fig. 19-6. Development of the breast in girls—average age span, 11 to 13 years. Stage 1 (prepubertal—elevation of papilla only) is not shown.
Modified from Marshall, W.A., and Tanner, J.M.: Arch. Dis. Child. 44:291, 1969; and Daniel, W.A., and Paulshock, B.Z.: Patient Care, pp. 122-124, May 13, 1979.

Sexual maturation in girls. In most girls the initial indication of puberty is a broadening of the pelvic girdle. A benign physiologic leukorrhea occurs as the vaginal and uterine tissues begin to mature and expand. However, the most dramatic evidence of pubertal development is the appearance of breast buds, an event known as *thelarche* (Fig. 19-6). This is followed in approximately 2 to 6 months by growth of pubic hair on the mons pubis, known as *adrenarche* (Fig. 19-7).

The initial appearance of menstruation, or *menarche*, occurs about 2 years after the appearance of the first pubescent changes, approximately 1 year after attainment of peak height velocity and 6 months after attainment of peak weight velocity. Menarche has been related to a critical gain in body fat content, although this is controversial (Garn, LaVelle, and Pilkington, 1983) (see Chapter 39). The normal age range of menarche is usually considered to be 10 to 15 years, with the average age being 12½ years for North American girls. During the establishment of the ovarian cycle, the menstrual periods are usually scanty and irregular and may not be accompanied by ovulation. Ovulation usually occurs 12 to 24 months after menarche.

Sexual maturation in boys. Early pubertal changes in boys begin with testicular enlargement and growth of internal structures but minimum enlargement of the penis (phallus). The scrotal skin becomes wrinkled and red, penile and testicular enlargement continues, spermatogenesis begins, and pubic hair growth starts (Fig. 19-8). As puberty advances, there is an increase in length and width of the penis, scrotal skin becomes darkly pigmented, and the characteristic male hair distribution pattern is evident. As serum testosterone levels rise over a 12-month period, the peak height and weight velocities are attained concurrently during late adolescence.

For boys there is no sudden physical change to indicate puberty such as the menarche in girls. The overt signal in boys is the beginning of nocturnal emissions of seminal fluid, which occur spontaneously during sleep at periodic intervals. Unlike cyclic germ cell production in the female, spermatogenesis is a continuous process that is usually well established by 17 years of age. As with girls, mature germ cells may not be produced for several months. The average age range at which boys attain puberty is 12½ to 16½ years, with a mean of 14 years.

Changes in Body Systems

Concurrent with pubertal changes, other organ systems are altered through the influence of hormone secretion and growth. Almost every system is affected, some strikingly so, and the changes differ between boys and girls.

Skeletal growth. Skeletal growth differences between boys and girls are primarily reflected in limb length and are apparently a function of hormonal effects at puberty. The earlier cessation of growth in girls is caused by epiphyseal unity under the potent effect of estrogen secretion, and the hormonal effect on female bone growth is much stronger than the similar effect of testosterone in males. In boys the prolonged growth period before puberty and the less rapid

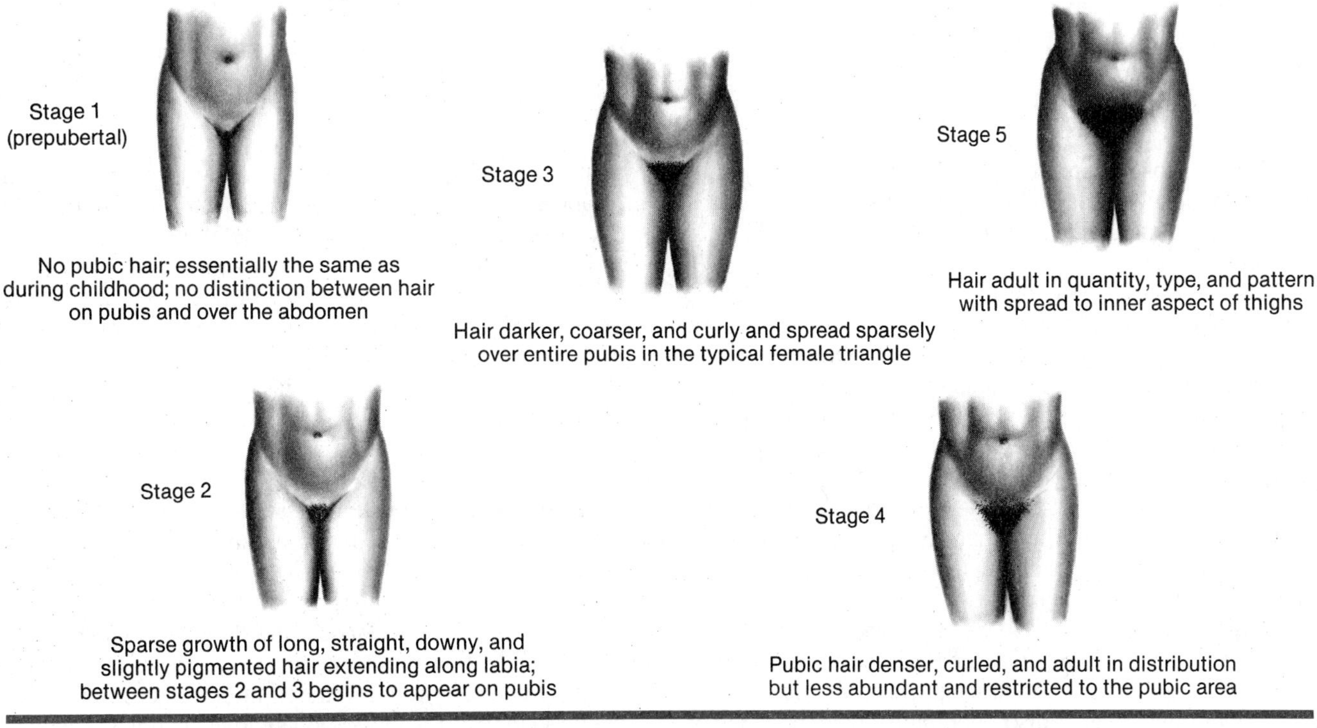
Stage 1
(prepubertal)
No pubic hair; essentially the same as during childhood; no distinction between hair on pubis and over the abdomen
Stage 3
Hair darker, coarser, and curly and spread sparsely over entire pubis in the typical female triangle
Stage 5
Hair adult in quantity, type, and pattern with spread to inner aspect of thighs
Stage 2
Sparse growth of long, straight, downy, and slightly pigmented hair extending along labia; between stages 2 and 3 begins to appear on pubis
Stage 4
Pubic hair denser, curled, and adult in distribution but less abundant and restricted to the pubic area

Fig. 19-7. Growth in pubic hair in girls—average age span for stages 2 through 5, 11 to 14 years.

Modified from Marshall, W.A., and Tanner, J.M.: Arch. Dis. Child. 44:291, 1969; and Daniel, W.A., and Paulshock, B.Z.: Patient Care, pp. 122-124, May 13, 1979.

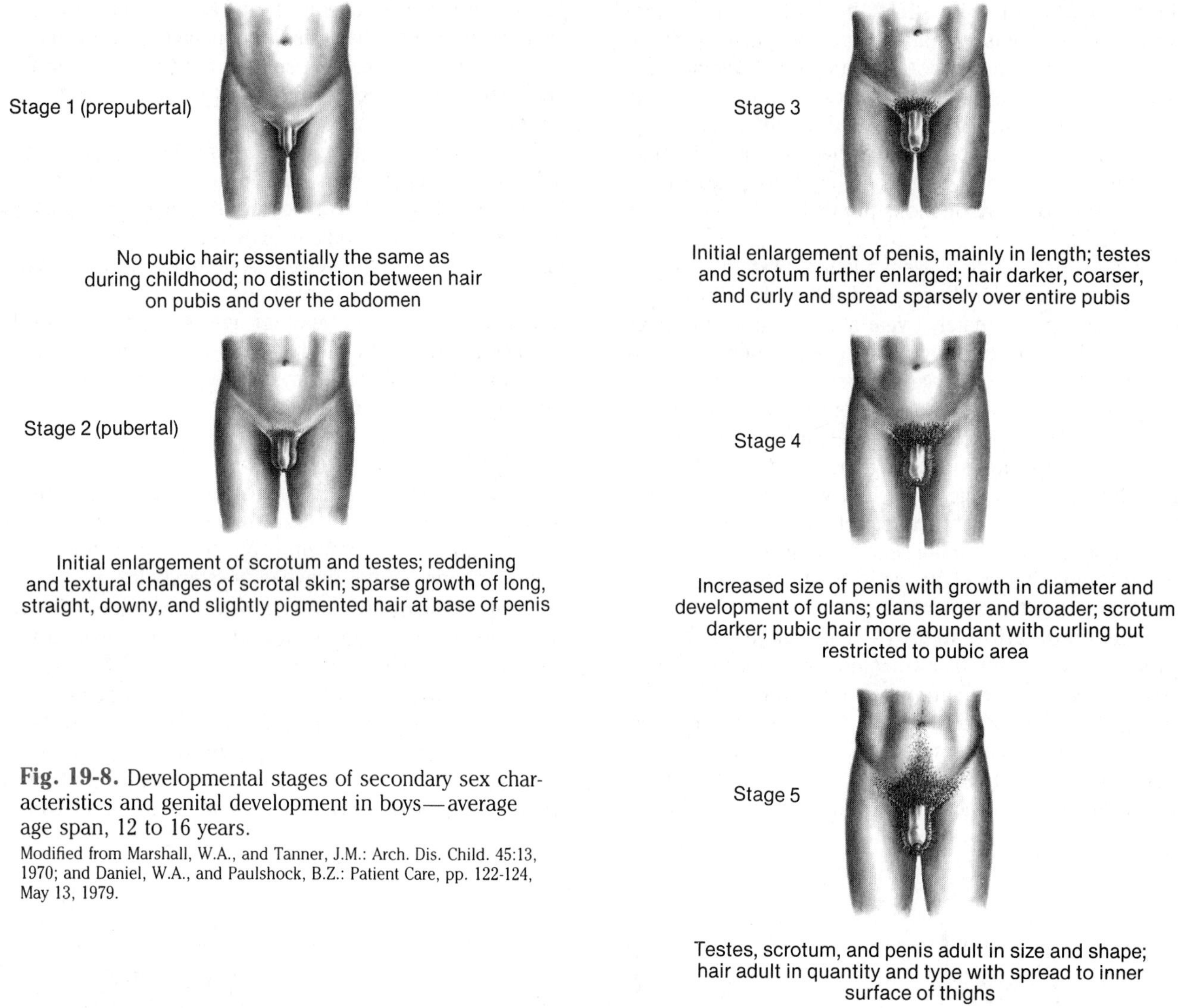
Stage 1 (prepubertal)
No pubic hair; essentially the same as during childhood; no distinction between hair on pubis and over the abdomen
Stage 2 (pubertal)
Initial enlargement of scrotum and testes; reddening and textural changes of scrotal skin; sparse growth of long, straight, downy, and slightly pigmented hair at base of penis
Stage 3
Initial enlargement of penis, mainly in length; testes and scrotum further enlarged; hair darker, coarser, and curly and spread sparsely over entire pubis
Stage 4
Increased size of penis with growth in diameter and development of glans; glans larger and broader; scrotum darker; pubic hair more abundant with curling but restricted to pubic area
Stage 5
Testes, scrotum, and penis adult in size and shape; hair adult in quantity and type with spread to inner surface of thighs

Fig. 19-8. Developmental stages of secondary sex characteristics and genital development in boys—average age span, 12 to 16 years.
Modified from Marshall, W.A., and Tanner, J.M.: Arch. Dis. Child. 45:13, 1970; and Daniel, W.A., and Paulshock, B.Z.: Patient Care, pp. 122-124, May 13, 1979.

epiphyseal closure are reflected in their greater overall height and longer arms and legs. Other skeletal differences are increased shoulder width in boys and broader hip development in girls.

This increase in size develops in a characteristic sequence of changes. Growth in length of extremities and the neck precedes growth in other areas, and since these parts are the first to reach adult length, the hands and feet appear larger than normal during adolescence. Increases in hip and chest breadth take place in a few months, followed several months later by an increase in shoulder width. These changes are followed by an increase in length of the trunk and depth of the chest. This sequence of changes is responsible for the characteristic long-legged, gawky appearance of the early adolescent child.

Head. Although the brain has achieved the major portion of its growth before adolescence, proportional changes in the skull occur as the face lengthens concurrently with other body alterations. A disproportion is noted in the facial features as the forehead becomes higher and wider, and the nose appears large as it lengthens before puberty. Later the mouth and lips become fuller, and, last, the jaw reaches adult size and configuration. The baby face of childhood disappears, and the large head, characteristic of childhood, becomes smaller in relation to the total body size.

Hypertrophy of the laryngeal mucosa and enlargement of the larynx and vocal cords occur in both boys and girls to produce voice changes. Girls' voices become slightly deeper and considerably fuller, but the effect in boys is striking. The "change of voice" in adolescent boys is one of the most noticeable traits of puberty, causing the voice to shift uncontrollably from deep to high tones in the middle of a sentence.

Body mass. Growth of lean body mass, principally muscle, tends to occur during adolescence after the bone growth spurt and is both quantitatively and qualitatively greater in males than in females at comparable stages of pubertal development. Muscle development, under the influence of androgenic hormones, increases steadily. Muscles become very well developed in boys, but in girls muscle mass increase is proportionate to general tissue growth.

Nonlean mass, primarily fat, also increases but follows a less orderly pattern of growth. There may be a transient increase in subcutaneous fat just before the skeletal growth spurt, especially noted in boys, followed 1 to 2 years later by a modest to marked decrease, again more noticeable in boys. Variable amounts of fat are then deposited to fill out and contour the mature physique in patterns characteristic of the adult of the appropriate sex. In both sexes, fat on the trunk increases at a fairly steady rate, but under the influence of ovarian hormones, the overall fatty tissue deposition in girls is more pronounced. Adipose tissue is distributed over the entire body, particularly in the regions over the thighs, hips, and buttocks and around the breast tissue, altering the angular childhood figure to the smoother, rounded body contours of the mature female.

Skin changes. Hormonal influences in puberty cause acceleration in growth and maturation of the skin and its structural appendages. Secretion of estrogen causes the skin of the female to develop a soft, smooth, but thicker texture with increased vascularity; androgenic hormones produce increased thickness and some darkening of the skin. *Sebaceous* glands are extremely active at this time, especially on genitals and in "flush areas" of the body (face, neck, shoulders, and upper back and chest). This increased activity and the structural nature of the glands are important in the pathogenesis of a common problem of puberty, acne (see Chapter 20).

Eccrine sweat glands, present almost everywhere on the human skin, become fully functional during puberty. Under sympathetic control these glands produce sweat over the entire body where evaporation helps eliminate body heat. The eccrine glands respond to emotional, as well as thermal, stimulation. Heavy sweating appears to be more pronounced in boys than in girls. The palms and soles ordinarily produce sweat on emotional stimulation but may cause sweating with more intense thermal heating. This also applies to the forehead and axillae.

Apocrine sweat glands, larger than eccrine glands and nonfunctional in childhood, reach secretory capacity during puberty. Unlike the eccrine glands, the apocrine glands are limited in distribution and grow in conjunction with hair follicles in the axillae, around the areola of the breast, around the umbilicus, on the external auditory canal, and in the genital and anal regions. Apocrine glands release a thick secretion as a result of emotional stimulation that, when acted on by surface bacteria, becomes highly odoriferous. The pH of the axillae, acidic during childhood, shows a progressive rise to a distinctly alkaline level during adolescence when the apocrine glands begin to function.

Body hair assumes characteristic distribution patterns and texture changes during puberty. Some are common to both boys and girls; others appear to be related entirely to male androgen secretion. Estrogens seem to produce no consistent effect. Under the influence of gonadal and adrenal androgens, hair coarsens, darkens, and lengthens at sites related to secondary sex characteristics. Pubic and axillary hair appears in both sexes, although pubic hair is more extensive in males than in females. Beard and mustache hair normally depends on testicular androgens but can be increased in hirsute women. Body hair that usually appears on the chest, upward along the linea alba, and sometimes on other areas (such as the back and shoulders) appears in males and is androgen dependent. Extremity hair appears in varying amounts in both males and females but is also more prolific in the male. There is a strong genetic influence on the degree of extremity hirsutism in both sexes.

Cardiopulmonary system. The size and strength of the heart, blood volume, and systolic blood pressure increase, whereas the pulse rate and basal heat production decrease (see inside front cover). Consistent with the general developmental timetable, these changes appear earlier in girls, who establish a slightly higher pulse rate and a slightly lower systolic blood pressure than boys. Blood volume, which has increased steadily during childhood, reaches a higher value in boys than in girls, a fact that may be related to the increased muscle mass in pubertal boys. Adult values are reached for all formed elements of the blood, but hematocrit levels are higher in boys, platelet count and sedimentation rate are increased in girls, and white blood cell numbers are decreased in both boys and girls.

Respiratory rate, decreasing steadily throughout childhood, reaches the adult rate in adolescence. However, respiratory volume, vital capacity, and other physiologic properties related to respiratory function are increased, and to a far greater extent in males than in females. The differences between the sexes are a result of the greater lung growth associated with the increased shoulder and chest size in boys.

Other changes. Other changes relative to the attainment of mature physiologic capacity are evident in body fluid volume and composition and in basal metabolic rate; declining throughout life, they reach adult levels during the adolescent years. The slightly higher metabolic rate in boys is thought to be a function of androgenic hormones.

Through progressive maturation of the body as it reaches adult size, the adolescent develops the ability to respond to physical stresses and strains equal to or in excess of adult competence. During this period physiologic responses to exercise change drastically: performance improves, especially in boys, and the body is able to make the physiologic adjustments needed for normal function after exercise is completed. These capabilities are a result of the increased size and strength of muscles and the increased level of cardiac, respiratory, and metabolic functioning. Adolescents enjoy physical activity, and there appears to be a positive relationship between regular exercise and physical conditioning activities and improved general health, endurance, and appearance.

PSYCHOSOCIAL DEVELOPMENT

Adolescence is a time when young people are learning how to use their developing mental capacities. Their ability to reason, to assess and evaluate, and to use divergent thinking to come up with new ideas increases during this period of life. The adolescent begins to think beyond the present and into the future. However, these capacities and the ability to make good judgments are still limited by inexperience and as yet insufficient knowledge from which to gain an adequate perspective for problem solving.

Whereas the changes that take place during the middle childhood years are relatively gradual and regular, during early adolescence the alterations occur quickly. Adolescents experience rapid body changes, a shift from the homogeneous uniformity of grade school to the heterogeneous world of classmates, teachers, and courses in high schools, and expanding relationships and expectations for behavior. These fast-paced changes undoubtedly are responsible for much of the inner turmoil that finds external expression in the adolescent.

Developing a Sense of Identity (Erikson)

The traditional psychosocial theory identifies the developmental crisis of adolescence as establishing a sense of identity (Erikson, 1963). Throughout childhood, individuals go through the process of identification as they concentrate on various parts of the body at specific times. During infancy children identify themselves as separate from the mother, during early childhood they establish a gender role identification with the appropriate sex parent, and in later childhood they establish who they are in relation to others. In adolescence they come to see themselves as distinct individuals, somehow unique and separate from every other individual.

The early period of adolescence with its rapid physical growth and maturational changes causes youngsters to experience new and unfamiliar feelings and a heightened sensitivity to peer approval. During this time adolescents are faced with the crisis of *group identity* vs alienation. In the period that follows, the individual hopes to attain autonomy from the family and develop a sense of *personal identity* as opposed to role diffusion. A sense of group identity appears to be essential as a prelude to a sense of personal identity. Young adolescents must resolve questions concerning relationships with a peer group before they are able to resolve questions about who they are in relation to family and society.

Group identity. During the early stage of adolescence the pressure to belong to a group is intensified (Fig. 19-9). For teenagers it is essential to find a group to which they feel that they can belong and that provides them with status. Belonging to a crowd helps adolescents to define the differences between themselves and their parents. They dress as the group dresses and wear makeup and hairstyles according to group criteria—all of which are different from those of the parental generation. Language, music, and dancing reflect a culture that belongs exclusively to the adolescent. When adults begin to emulate these fashions and interests, the style changes immediately. Evidence of adolescent conformity to the peer group and nonconformity to the adult group provides teenagers with a frame of reference in which they can display their own self-assertion while they reject their identity with their parents' generation.

The peer group offers an identity to the young adolescent in terms of acceptance and of the roles it defines. Within the group the young person can try out and experiment with a variety of roles while surrounded by the security and warmth of those who face the same problems, feel the

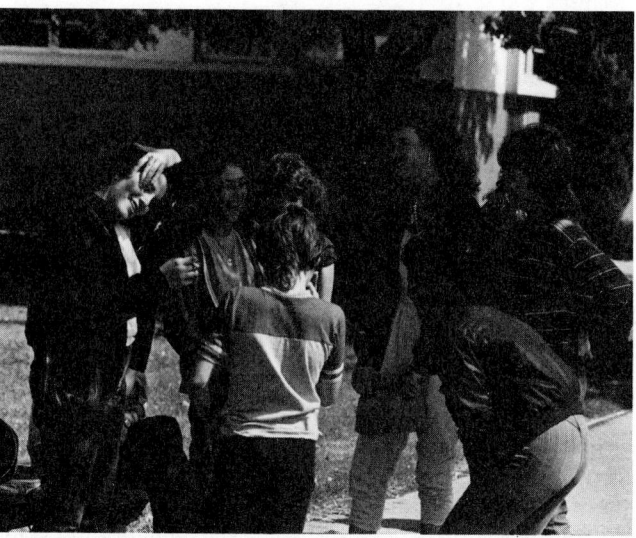

Fig. 19-9. The peer group is a major influence in adolescent development.

same way, behave the same way, and wear the same symbols of belonging. There is comfort in standing together against those who do not understand—to giggle, shout, and act silly in the company of those with whom they share an emotional attachment. To be different is to be unaccepted and alienated from the group.

Individual identity. The quest for personal identity is part of the ongoing identification process. As youngsters establish an identity within a group, they are also attempting to incorporate multiple body changes into a concept of the self. Body awareness is part of self-awareness, and for some time the adolescent will engage in assimilating the self represented by this physical dimension. In this search for identity, adolescents take into consideration the relationships that have developed between themselves and others in the past, as well as the directions they hope to be able to take in the future.

Significant others hold certain expectations for the behavior of the adolescent. Often these expectations or demands are persistent enough to induce certain decisions that might be made differently or not at all if the individual could be solely responsible for identity formation. It is all too easy to slip into the roles that are expected by these external influences without incorporating personal goals or questioning these decisions in relation to the developing personality. Thus the individual becomes what parents or others wish the individual to be based on these premature decisions. In addition, a young person might form a negative identity when society or the culture provides a self-image that is contrary to the values of the community. Labels such as "juvenile delinquent," "hood," or "failure" are applied to certain adolescents who then accept and live up to these labels with behaviors that validate and strengthen them.

The process of evolving a personal identity is time-consuming and fraught with periods of confusion, depression, and discouragement. To determine an identity and a place in the world is a critical and perilous feature of adolescence. However, as the pieces gradually shift and settle into place, a positive identity will eventually emerge from the confusion. *Role diffusion* results when the individual is unable to formulate a satisfactory identity from the multiplicity of aspirations, roles, and identifications.

Sex-role identity. Adolescence is the time for consolidation of a sex-role identity. In the preschool and early school years children learn to apply an appropriate gender label to themselves, acquire information about sex-associated expectations, and develop a sex-role preference. The establishment of close relationships with same-sex peers, which begins in later childhood, is intensified during early adolescence. Through these relationships children learn about the possibility of intimacy between equals and are exposed to peer standards for appropriate sex-role behavior. In early adolescence the peer group begins to communicate some expectations regarding sexual relationships, and as development progresses, adolescents encounter expectations for mature sex-role behavior from both peers and adults. Expectations such as these vary from culture to culture, among geographic areas, and among socioeconomic groups.

Adolescents are urged to make a career choice, and the decision about an occupation has important implications for their sex-role identity. Although most occupations or careers are now viewed as appropriate for either sex, some members of society still categorize jobs according to how they relate to sex-role expression. If the choice is considered "sex appropriate," the work environment will support the sex-role identity. To enter a career that is not generally selected by one's own sex may lead to constant tension as a result of challenges directed toward the individual's competence and sex-role identity. The trend toward equalizing career opportunities and minimizing the sex-role connotations of many occupations ideally will eliminate much of this source of antagonism.

Genital Stage (Freud)

The genital period, the longest and last of Freud's psychosexual stages, begins with puberty and extends to old age. It is the stage in which the individual arrives at full sexual potency. Throughout adolescence and young adulthood the libido is invested in activities that prepare the individual to satisfy the mature sex instinct through procreation. The activities are primarily those of forming friendships, preparing for a career, courting, and marriage.

Unlike the phallic stage of early childhood when sexuality is primitive and mainly self-centered, sexuality in the genital stage is primarily heterosexual. Sexual interests increase markedly in vigor and intensity and are focused on members of the opposite sex. New problems arise as adolescents find social disapproval and prohibitions of their own consciences conflicting with intense sexual desires.

COGNITIVE DEVELOPMENT

In the final stage of cognitive development the child is no longer limited to the concrete or the observable. Like the preceding stages the advanced stage of cognitive development determines what young people learn when they interact with other people and how they will behave toward others.

Developing Formal Operations (Piaget)

Progression in the realm of cognitive thinking culminates with the capacity for abstract thinking. This stage, the period of *formal operations,* is Piaget's fourth and last stage and is attained at different ages, depending on the individual child's motivation, practice, opportunities, and cultural differences.

Young people can begin thinking about the world in new ways. Living in the nonpresent as well as the present, they are no longer restricted to the real and actual, which was typical of the period of concrete thought—they are also concerned with the possible. They now think beyond the present. At this time their thoughts can be influenced by more logical principles than by their own perceptions and experiences. They become capable of scientific reasoning and formal logic. Without having to center attention on the immediate situation, they can imagine the possible—a sequence of events that might occur, such as college and occupational possibilities, how things might change in the future, such as relationships with parents, and the consequences of their actions, such as dropping out of school.

They are capable of mentally manipulating more than two categories of variables at the same time. For example, they can consider the relationship between speed, distance, and time in planning a trip. They can detect logical consistency or inconsistency in a set of statements and evaluate a system or set of values in a more analytic manner. For instance, they question the parent who insists on honesty in the youngster but at the same time cheats on an income tax report or expense account.

Young people can consider their own thinking, as well as the thinking of others. They wonder what opinion others have of them, and they are increasingly able to imagine the thoughts of others. With this capacity comes the ability to differentiate between others' thoughts and their own and to interpret the thoughts of others more accurately. Thus they see themselves and the world in more relativistic ways. As they come to know that other cultures and communities have different norms and standards from their own, it becomes easier to accept members of these other cultures, and the decision to behave in their own culture in an accepted manner becomes a more conscious commitment to that culture.

Idealism

With the capacity for abstract thinking and the use of deductive reasoning, young people are concerned about gaining a clear understanding of life and its purpose. They often become disillusioned with the world they see and search for an ideal and decent world to which their ideal and decent selves can respond. This part of the self is hidden from view and may not be revealed to any but the closest friends. Adolescents are continually discarding old illusions and constructing new ones to take their place. Consequently, they may embrace idealistic movements and causes. Many turn to religion—their own or a new one—as a source of comfort and reassurance.

Most adolescents accept society as it exists and attempt to adjust as best they can to things as they are. Some devote themselves to a life of pleasure and seek to extend this existence as long as they possibly can. Others, convinced that injustice and repression have reached an intolerable point, become revolutionaries or radical reformers in an attempt to create a better place in which to live.

As a whole, adolescents are able to maintain the conviction that virtue and decency are possible, and they are seldom totally disillusioned. They are able to discern in others the idealism that they feel. They are prone to setbacks with feelings of helplessness and depression, and few are able to carry their idealism beyond adolescence in careers and organizational activities. They have established a personal value system that reaches within themselves and is externally imposed on them by parents or adult authority figures. By late adolescence most have come to terms with things as they are. They have evaluated their capabilities in relation to their ambitions and economic realities and have either entered the work force or the armed forces or embarked on the pursuit of an educational goal.

Moral Development

As children move through the stages of cognition and logical thought, they also progress through sequential stages of moral development. As with other developmental processes, moral development approaches or achieves adult levels during adolescence.

Conventional and postconventional level (Kohlberg). Kohlberg's theory of development of moral judgment and thought (1975) proposes that, at the conventional level, which includes youngsters of preadolescence and adolescence ages 10 to 16, the major concern is to act or behave in such a way that will gain or maintain the approval of others. There is obedience of rules and respect for authority.

The shift from conventional to postconventional morality that takes place during late adolescence is characterized by serious questioning of existing moral values and their relevance to society and the individual. Adolescents can easily take the role of another. They understand duty and obligation based on reciprocal rights of others, as well as the concept of justice that is founded on making amends for misdeeds and repairing or replacing what has been spoiled by wrongdoing. However, they seriously question established moral codes, often as a result of observing that adults verbally ascribe to a code but do not adhere to it. Their advanced cognitive development makes adolescents more aware of moral questions and values and closely parallels the general process of identity formation. Coincident with these advancements are rapidly changing social demands that require continual reappraisal of these values and beliefs. They are aware of the contradictions in the existing social and value structures in which they participate.

Adolescent boys and girls must make choices. They are changing, as is their social world. They find that there are many ways to live their lives, their behavioral domain is expanded, and they encounter situations that they have never before faced that require decisions about actions to be taken and decisions based on moral evaluation and judgment. Whereas younger children merely accept the decisions or point of view of adults, adolescents must substitute their own set of morals and values in order to gain autonomy from adults. When old principles are challenged but new and independent values have not yet emerged to take their place, young people search for a moral code that preserves their personal integrity and guides their behavior, especially in the face of strong pressure to violate the old values. Their decisions involving moral dilemmas must be based on an internalized set of principles that provides them with the resources to evaluate the demands of the situation and to plan a course of action consistent with their ideals.

New perspectives (Gilligan). Kohlberg's approach to conceptualizing moral development is being reexamined. Concerns have been raised about differences in the way males and females make moral decisions. Using Kohlberg's framework, Gilligan introduced a feminine perspective on emergence of moral development. He observed that females rarely progressed any further than midway in their capacity for moral decision making, whereas males were more likely to advance to the highest level of postconventional reasoning. Traditional moral decision making relies exclusively on principles of justice, preserving rights, and obeying rules. This process fosters making abstract independent moral decisions regardless of the outcome or impact on others who may be affected by the ruling or decision.

Gilligan's assumption states that, although females are no less capable of high-level moral decision making, they approach ethical situations from a different perspective. Females appear to carry on an internal dialogue between the two moral voices of justice on one hand and caring and connectedness on the other. Therefore moral decisions are made with consideration of the responsibility to maintain interpersonal connectedness and uphold the community moral standard (Gilligan, 1982; Muuss, 1988). Development of a holistic theory of moral reasoning has relevance for nursing so that both constructs of caring and justice become valued and translated into nursing practice (Nokes, 1989).

Spiritual Development

As youngsters move toward independence from parents and other authorities, some begin to question the values and ideals of their families. Others cling to these values as a stable element in their lives as they struggle with the conflicts of this turbulent period. Adolescents need to work out these conflicts for themselves, but they also need support from authority figures and peers for their resolution. Often the peer group is more influential than parents, although values acquired during the formative years are usually maintained.

Adolescents are capable of understanding abstract concepts and interpreting analogies and symbols. They are able to empathize, philosophize, and think logically. Most are searching for ideals and speculate about illogical statements and conflicting ideologies. Their tendency toward introspection and emotional intensity at this age often makes it difficult for others to know what they are thinking. They tend to keep their thoughts private, fearing that no one will understand these feelings that they perceive to be unique and special. Young people may reject the formal worship service but engage in individual worship in the privacy of their rooms. It is not uncommon for them to reveal deep spiritual concerns and then become silly and deny these feelings (Shelly, 1982). They need support and encouragement in their struggle for understanding and the freedom to question without censure.

Youth today appear to be placing more emphasis on personal than on institutionalized religion (Dickinson, 1982). This is consistent with the greater stress young people place on personal values, relationships, and moral standards and their lessening reliance on traditional social beliefs and institutions. Evangelistic types of worship are increasingly attractive to younger persons. Many adolescents are attracted to the new religious sects (e.g., the so-called Jesus Movement, Hare Krishna, and Children of God) (Galanter, 1980). These affiliations may be a response to disillusionment with conventional religious structures, an anchor following a period of rootlessness and identity confusion, or a source of satisfying values in a chaotic society. For some, joining a particular movement represents a fad with the adventure of confounding conventional parents (Conger and Peterson, 1984).

SOCIAL DEVELOPMENT

To achieve full maturity, adolescents must free themselves from family domination and define an identity independent of parental authority. However, this process is fraught with ambivalence on the part of both teenagers and their parents. Adolescents want to grow up and be free of parental restraints, yet they are fearful as they try to comprehend the responsibilities that are linked with independence. A predominant theme of discussions with teenagers involves the escape from parental dominance. However, this is usually an attempt to conceal the feelings of dependence and anxiety that are generated by the preparation for leaving the sanctuary of the family—the final separation-individuation process of childhood.

Part of this emancipation process involves developing social relationships outside the family that help teenagers identify their role in society. Increasing absence from home through frequent contacts with peers is essential to this socialization process. Adolescence is a time of intense sociability and often a time of equally intense loneliness. Acceptance by peers, a few close friends, and the secure love of a supportive family are requisites for the interpersonal maturation process.

Relationships with Parents

During adolescence the parent-child relationship changes from one of protection-dependency to one of mutual affection and equality. The process of achieving independence often involves turmoil and ambiguity as both parent and adolescent learn to play new roles and work toward this end, while at the same time resolving the often painful series of rifts essential to establishing the ultimate relationships.

Most of the behavior observed in adolescents is related to the external restrictions and checks that are placed on this spontaneous maturation process. On one hand, adolescents are accepted as maturing preadults. They are allowed privileges formerly denied, and they are provided with increasing responsibilities. On the other hand, because of their unpredictability and insecurity in evaluating situations and making sound judgments, they must conform to regulations and restrictions set by adults. This state of affairs is particularly exemplified by the struggle between parents and adolescents concerning the hour of curfew.

During adolescence the behavior observed in the toddler is relived as the individual again seeks autonomy. If what occurred during the toddler period is known, it is possible to make some predictions regarding the probable behavior of the adolescent (Blos, 1979). The teenager's earliest attempts to achieve emancipation from parental controls are manifested in a period of rejection of the parents. Adolescents are critical, argumentative, and generally remote with both parents. They are frequently absent from home and family activities and spend an increasing amount of time with the peer group. They are less close and confiding in relationships with parents. This rejection is not consistent, however, and varies with mood changes. At times young teenagers feel highly competent and demand their "rights"; at other times, after being hurt in battles with the world, they may accept parental guidance and security.

As teenagers assert their rights for grown-up privileges, they frequently create tensions within the home. They resist parental control, and conflicts can arise from almost any situation or any subject. Some of the favorite topics of dispute include use of the telephone, manners, dress, chores and duties, homework, disrespectful behavior, friendships, dating, money, automobiles, and time schedules. Present in these areas of conflict are the overriding argument that "Everyone else has one" or is allowed the desired item or privilege and the ever-present assertion that "You don't understand me" and "You always treat me like a baby." Spoken or unspoken, parents' reactions consist of "Is this all the thanks I get for what I have done, or am doing, for you?"

With advancing adolescence, teenagers become more competent, and with this competence comes a need for more autonomy. However, although they are psychologically better prepared for independence, they are often thwarted in their efforts by lack of money or by other parental barriers. Much conflict arises from the teenager's outside activities and the elements of privacy and trust. Too many parents believe that they must know all of their adolescent's activities and feelings; they may go through the teenager's belongings in an attempt to find out what the youngster is doing. To gain the respect and trust of their adolescents, parents must respect their privacy and show an honest and sincere interest in what they believe and feel. Teenagers need not only guidance and support from their parents but also enough leeway to establish their own individuality.

Sometimes teenagers prove to be a source of pleasure and fulfillment beyond the parents' expectations. The adolescent may be one who is of a particularly happy disposition or one whose talents and abilities in areas such as music, art, scholastic achievement, or athletics provide the parents with pleasure and gratification. Most parental disappointments in adolescent children are related to the parents' own expectations for success or failure.

The recent trends in society in terms of equality and relaxation of previous moral standards have made the adjustments of teenagers and parents increasingly difficult. The so-called generation gap is widening in relation to a number of attitudes, values, and beliefs. Parents can no longer find guidance from their own experiences in understanding the needs of today's teenager. Consequently, in their frustration, bewilderment, and disappointment, they are forced to undertake a painful reevaluation of a number of their previously held attitudes and beliefs.

Peer Relationships and Influence

Although parents remain the primary influence in the lives of adolescents, most adolescents find that peers assume a more significant role at this time than they did during childhood. The peer group serves as a strong support to teenagers, individually and collectively providing them with a sense of belonging and a feeling of strength and power. It forms that transitional world between dependence and autonomy. As adolescents spend increasing amounts of time among their peers and have less contact with their parents, the peer group becomes an important socializing agent. It acts as a support for conformity and for questioning and challenging adult values and societal institutions; the peer group is a new frame of reference from which to reject the old.

Peer group. Adolescents have always been social, gregarious, and group oriented. Although there are a few who remain outside, either from preference or rejection, the majority seek the safety, companionship, and reciprocal reinforcement of a group. The peer group has an intense influence on adolescents' self-evaluation and behavior. In order to gain acceptance by a group, younger teenagers tend to conform completely in such things as modes of dress, hairstyle, taste in music, and vocabulary, often at the expense of individuality and self-assertion. The teenagers' entire being is measured by the reactions of their peers. Since most teenagers are still insecure and lacking in confidence, they are unable to tolerate differences between themselves and their peers; therefore conformity is the rule within primary friendship groups. To belong is of utmost importance; thus adolescents behave in a way that will ensure their establishment in a group. Adolescents are highly susceptible to social approval, acceptance, and demands. To be ignored or criticized by peers creates feelings of inferiority, inadequacy, and incompetence.

Except in a few small, homogeneous high schools, teenagers distribute themselves into a relatively predictable social hierarchy. The largest social division is the *set.* Both boys and girls can be members of a set, but for some occasions and activities they separate into like-sex crowds. The adolescents know to which set they and others belong, although in large schools they may not all know each other. Thus the circle of acquaintances is broadened, and within their set adolescents develop the adult social skill of exchanging breezy, pert greetings with people they know only slightly.

Based on common tastes, interests, and background, smaller, distinct, and rather exclusive crowds or cliques of selected close friends who are emotionally attached to each other exist within the set. Although cliques may become formalized, most remain informal and small. Each clique has an identifying feature that proclaims its difference from others and its solidarity within itself in much the same way the adolescent generation as a whole sets itself apart from the adult generation. Although the criteria for membership may not be publicly voiced, the groups tend to include or exclude persons according to consistent standards.

Cliques are usually made up of one sex, and girls tend to be more cliquish than boys and to have a greater need for close friendships. Groups congregate at lunch, at a favorite hangout (such as a shopping mall), or in the intimacy of someone's bedroom to talk about things that are of utmost concern to teenage girls, such as clothes, makeup, and, especially, boys. Boys' groups tend to revolve around sports, hobby activities, and rough games, although they, too, gossip and discuss the opposite sex. Within the intimacy of the group adolescents gain support in learning about themselves, consideration for the feelings of others, and increased ego development and self-reliance.

The school is psychologically important to adolescents as a focus of social life, a setting in which to define and elaborate relationships with peers. In addition, most teenagers have a selected gathering place or hangout to which they can go alone or preferably with others of the same sex for the purpose of mingling with a group of persons from the opposite sex without the formalities or financial obligations of a date.

Best friends. Personal friendships of the one-to-one variety usually develop between like-sex adolescents. This relationship is closer and more stable than it is in middle childhood, and it is important in the quest for identity. A best friend is the best audience on whom to try out possible roles and identities that the adolescent wants to test. Best friends may try a role together, each providing support for the other. Each cares about what the other thinks and feels. Since a sense of intimacy grows within a permanent relationship, the stability of this like-sex friendship is an important link in the progress toward an intimate heterosexual relationship in young adulthood.

Heterosexual Relationships

During adolescence, relationships with members of the opposite sex take on new importance. The increased interest in heterosexual relationships is a natural outgrowth of the physical maturation of the reproductive organs that is taking place at this time. The interaction between body development and cultural expectations helps adolescents incorporate ideas about mature sexuality. As they begin to assimilate and integrate the changes of puberty, adolescents turn with increasing frequency toward the opposite sex, not motivated by a need to find a permanent partner but rather as a means to enhance their own sex-role identity. Early dating is usually closely related to peer-group membership and social status and, like other phases of development, follows a predictable, sequential pattern. However, the time and rapidity of progress are influenced by many cultural factors, such as the philosophy of the community, traditions, parents' wishes, and the teenagers themselves.

Typically, 12-year-old children still maintain same-sex friendships, although there are increasing opportunities for mixed-group activities. Although there seems to be a trend toward earlier dating, on the *average*, dating activities begin in the seventh and eighth grades and are usually "crowd" dates at organized school functions. For example, a group of girls just happen to be around a certain group of boys at most activities. There is seldom pairing off within the group, although a few boys and girls may see each other on a paired-off basis. By the ninth grade, crowd dates are still popular, but now there is more pairing off of couples. In the tenth grade paired crowd dates, in which some boys and girls come as couples and join the crowd consisting of several couples and perhaps a few unattached friends, are the rule (Kaluger and Kaluger, 1988).

Double-dating follows group dating and is the more common practice in the eleventh grade; both double-dating and single-pair dating are common by the twelfth grade. Most adolescents are dating to some degree by the time they leave high school. The group dating patterns provide a means whereby the potential stress and anxiety associated with heterosexual relationships are buffered by the peer group. When the focus is on group activities rather than on dyadic contacts, heterosexual friendships are less threatening.

The type and degree of seriousness of heterosexual relationships vary. The initial stage is usually noncommittal, extremely mobile, and seldom characterized by any deep romantic attachments. Crushes, those strong feelings of attachment to an important or well-liked adult in the youngster's life who embodies the qualities considered most valuable by the adolescent, are common in early adolescence; they constitute one of the earliest "love" attachments. During early midadolescence, as their sexual capacity is evolving, young boys frequently feel the need to test out the power of their sexuality by numerous exploits and conquests. It may be a response to inner sexual pressures or a need to conform to group expectations. With advancing adolescence and more firm sexual identities, steady dating and boy-girl love relationships with deeper commitment become more numerous among teenage youngsters.

Steady dating is evidence of adolescent insecurity and uncertainty—an escape from loneliness and being left out—and provides a sense of belonging (Fig. 19-10). The relationship continues until misunderstanding or boredom ends the association, and the process is often repeated with another partner. During this time the relationship between love and sexuality is brought into focus. Boys and girls in the middle teens find it hard to believe that sex can exist without love; therefore each boy-girl attachment is viewed as real love. Parental attempts to break up these early heterosexual relationships may only cause the youngsters to prolong the attachments as a further expression of defiance. Hasty marriages based on such rebellion are therefore usually doomed to failure.

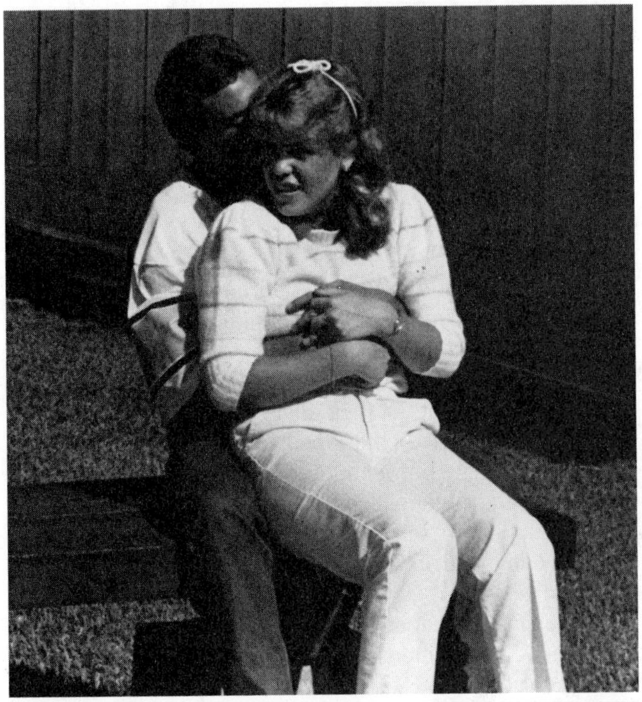

Fig. 19-10. Heterosexual relationships are an important part of adolescence.

DEVELOPMENT OF SELF-CONCEPT

Development of a personal identity is the major psychosocial task of adolescence (see p. 878) and is necessary to the process of final separation from parents. The self-concept becomes more differentiated as adolescents evolve a more complex picture of themselves, one that takes situational factors into account. The self-concept becomes more individuated, more distinct from the concepts of others. Whereas younger children describe themselves in terms of similarities with peers, as adolescence advances, youngsters describe themselves more in terms of their special characteristics. They begin to view themselves from a more abstract perspective and less from a physical and concrete aspect. Self-reflection is evident. Teenagers are acutely aware of their appearance as they begin to acquire an image of themselves as adults, but they see discrepancies between their ideal and actual skills and abilities.

Every aspect of adolescence influences the self-concept. Relationships with family and peers are profound influences. Family support is found to have a significant influence on the self-concept in both girls and boys (Hoelter and Harper, 1987), and there is a strong relationship between teenagers' self-concept and the feedback they receive from others (Street, 1988). It has also been found that sexually active girls reported lower self-esteem than their sexually inexperienced peers. This difference was not observed in boys (Orr and others, 1989).

Body Image Development

Physical growth and maturation during adolescence occur so rapidly that young people have difficulty adjusting to the changes, which creates feelings of confusion about their bodies. They have lost the security of a familiar body and feel a strangeness about their altered bodies. Consequently, they may try either to hide them or to advertise them, or they may alternate between the two extremes.

Strange and unfamiliar feelings press on them as inner urges announce a sexual awakening. These feelings must also be integrated into the self-image. Sexuality is not the same for boys as it is for girls, and it has different psychic overtones that influence behavior and adaptation. Although it appears that the intensity of the sexual drive is different in adolescent boys and girls, this has not been conclusively demonstrated. Current findings indicate that the difference may be related to the biologic nature of the sex drive and the hormonal influence of androgens in males (Udry and others, 1985).

Adolescents are continually comparing themselves with their peers and making judgments of their own normality based on these observations. Pubertal children feel most comfortable when they are just like their friends and agemates. Perceived defects or deviations from the group average are threatening to their idealized image. Any blemish is likely to be magnified out of proportion, and any delay of the visible evidence of maturity is cause for worry. Unfortunately, this is also the time when the hormonal effect of the sebaceous glands produces acne that creates problems for many youngsters. To the adolescent, even the most insignificant pimple may be viewed as a colossal disfigurement; every blemish is a major catastrophe. The advent of chronic disease or a permanent physical disability has very special significance during adolescence and creates additional stresses for both the affected youngster and health workers.

It has been determined that the body image established during adolescence is the one that individuals retain throughout life. Much of adolescents' search for identity takes place before a mirror as they try to read from the reflected features just who they are and what they look like to other people. Adolescents practice facial expressions and postures, try out hair arrangements, worry about a pimple, and in other ways attempt to assess the best means to achieve a maximum effect—to reveal the "true self."

Although many of the changes of puberty have features common to both girls and boys, the implications and responses are different in the two sexes, and many of these adjustments are influenced by the values and prohibitions of the culture. Often the body changes per se may be less significant than the meaning and importance that these changes have for adolescents and other persons in their lives.

Boys' responses to puberty. The early adolescent increases in height and muscle mass are welcomed by the adolescent boy, whose timing of pubertal events can be significantly slower, by 1 to 2 years, when compared with the same-age female peers. Although his more mature physique brings highly valued increase in strength and greater athletic skills, this rapid growth is uneven, and therefore he has some trouble adjusting. When bones grow faster than muscles, muscles are taut and respond with quick, jerky movements; when muscles grow faster than bones, they become somewhat loose and sluggish. For a time he is awkward and uncoordinated. Often his size outstrips his strength, and he tires more easily. Fatigue, lack of coordination, and appearing "funny" and "out of shape" are sources of embarrassment, self-consciousness, and feelings of inadequacy. He has difficulty accepting his new body image at first, and accusations of clumsiness, laziness, or stupidity do little to strengthen his self-concept during a time that offers such strong challenges to his self-esteem.

The development of secondary sex characteristics, especially the growth of facial and body hair, has psychologic and social meaning to the adolescent boy. This, more than any other secondary characteristic, is associated with the masculine sex role, and the ritual act of shaving at the slightest evidence of growth is a means for the young boy to validate his identification with this role (Fig. 19-11). Shaving also provides a legitimate excuse to gaze at and admire the broadening shoulders and altered features of his changing body image. Unfortunately with many adolescent boys the appearance of acne and an awkward appearance when assuming adult poses often interfere with the pleasure of this experience. See Development of Sexuality, p. 885.

Girls' responses to puberty. As girls begin to experience pubertal changes, they also become body conscious. Since the onset of puberty in girls is almost 2 years in advance of that in boys, their initial reaction to increased

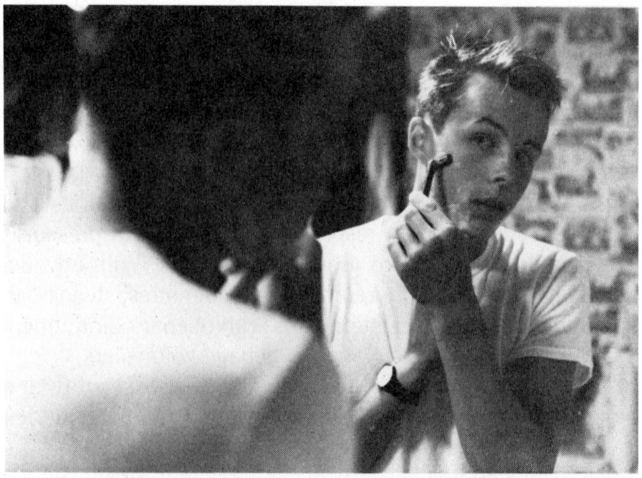

Fig. 19-11. The act of shaving offers the adolescent male the opportunity to study his changing appearance.

height may be embarrassment as they find themselves towering above their male classmates. They worry about becoming too tall. Adolescent girls often slouch or adopt a hunched posture in an attempt to minimize this increased height, especially early-maturing girls who are normally of above-average height. The increase in weight and the normal plumping of features with fat deposition are predominant concerns of pubescent girls. They often perceive these changes as evidence of a tendency toward obesity, and many attempt to avoid such alterations by strict and faddish dieting. This ill-timed strategy can deprive their bodies of essential nutrients during a period of rapid body development.

The young girl is interested in her changing form and feminine curves. The average girl looks on her budding breasts with pleasure as a sign of approaching maturity and evidence of her femininity. She observes and may even measure the growth of her developing breasts and continually compares her own progress with that of her friends and classmates. She begins to wear a brassiere. Some girls are sensitive about their breast development and attempt to hide it, whereas others are delighted with their new figures and wear tight sweaters and clothes that accentuate their curves.

Development of some of the secondary sex characteristics may be less pleasing to girls than it is to boys, particularly the growth of body hair. A culture in which smooth-skinned females are preferred makes it necessary for the girl to shave her underarms and legs regularly to meet the standards for feminine appearance. Although this practice is another indication of maturity, it does not have the same sex-role significance as face shaving does for the adolescent boy. The girl becomes increasingly conscious of the feminine ideal, and in an effort to approach this standard, she experiments with a variety of cosmetics and hairstyles. Alone and together, she and her friends spend endless hours before the mirror posing, applying cosmetics, and combing their hair. This practice provides the same narcissistic outlet for the girl that is available to the boy through shaving.

The advent of menstruation, that exclusive feature of female puberty, provides the greatest impetus toward full realization and acceptance of female sexuality. Menstruation is positive evidence of womanhood and the potential for pregnancy and childbearing. Most girls are adequately prepared for the event and take this new function in stride, looking forward to menstruation, feeling satisfaction at its onset, and seeing it as the symbol of their passage from childhood to womanhood. Others find it distressing, frightening, and difficult to accept. In some it reawakens old fears of body injury and castration. Still others accept it matter-of-factly. Because of its sudden onset, the first menstruation can be a traumatic experience for the girl who has not been taught what to expect. As a rule, if the young girl has established a positive gender role during childhood, the transition to womanhood, with all its ramifications, is accepted as the normal phenomenon that it is.

A difficulty faced by the pubescent girl is related to the discrepancy in the onset of puberty in girls and in boys. She is often placed in the position where she must explain or hide the fact of her own body changes from her male peers. The dissemination of information to boys about these changes lags significantly behind; therefore the girl finds it difficult to accept the changes she is experiencing while attempting to hide or mask them from the boys whose attention and approval she is seeking.

DEVELOPMENT OF SEXUALITY

Among the many developmental events that characterize puberty, none is more dramatic or more challenging to youngsters' emerging sense of identity than changes associated with sexual development. All the physical changes described at the beginning of the chapter require physical adjustments and lead to a changed self-image.

The tension between sexuality as pleasure and sexuality for reproduction is universal. Traditionally societies have attempted to control premarital sexual activity in order to protect fertility and its associated preservation of economic welfare and continuation of a viable work force (Brooks-Gunn and Furstenberg, 1989). The onset of masturbatory activity occurs during puberty. Although both genders engage in this behavior, it is more commonly reported by males. Masturbation provides an opportunity for sexual self-exploration prior to development of regular social-sexual interaction with another individual. Participation in this behavior is greatly influenced by learned cultural attitudes, religion, and sex-role expectations; therefore variable rates of this behavior have been observed (Gagnon, 1977).

Current enlightenment accepts that to engage in the practice from time to time is normal and temporarily helps provide the young man with important information about how his body works and how adult physical sexuality and reproduction are accomplished. He learns that organ responses to sexual excitement can be initiated at will and that orgasmic climax with a predictable release of tension, or repeatedly deferred at will, contributes to a developing sense of mastery over sexual impulses and new sexual capacities. Without guilt and worry, the adolescent boy can incorporate this aspect of his masculinity into a more positive self-concept.

Males

Self-perceived sex drive in males reaches a peak during adolescence and tends to be genitally oriented. The frequency of erections is increased in response to a variety of stimuli, as is the frequency of sexual outlet through masturbation or intercourse.

Primary sex characteristics of genital growth, the appearance in size and shape of the penis and testes, can be an area of great concern for adolescent males. Although the ability for penile erection is present at birth, during puberty the maturation of male genital function allows the male to produce seminal emission through the process of ejaculation. This may occur spontaneously as a "nocturnal emission" or "wet dream." However, the majority of males experience first ejaculation through masturbation (Katchadorian, 1980).

Adolescent boys are generally not well prepared for the maturation of the reproductive organs (Gaddis and Brooks-Gunn, 1985). Spontaneous ejaculations are frequently puzzling, troublesome, and embarrassing events. Unless he has been prepared in advance for this eventuality, the boy often finds it difficult to seek an explanation from his parents; therefore he turns to friends or reading material to gain information or he may puzzle about the meaning in his own mind.

Females

Unlike the adolescent boy, strong sexual feelings in the adolescent girl are not usually centered in the genital region but are more generalized and ill defined. Her reproductive apparatus, less obvious than that of the boy, contributes in only a vague way to sexual awareness. The girl in early adolescence may experience pleasant sensations and even tingling in the genital area, but these feelings are diffuse and difficult to separate from other body sensations. In the adolescent girl the urge for self-stimulation is not as strong as it is in the male.

Although many girls handle the genitalia for the pleasant sensation that is evoked, not all carry the activity to a climax. Sexual feelings are centered less on the genitalia and erotic gratification with release of tension than on the manipulation of a pleasant state with romantic feelings about love. However, with the more open, liberal views regarding female sexual responses, it is being revealed that much of the nature of the adolescent girl's sexual arousal may have more of a cultural than a biologic basis.

Heterosexual Relationships

Authorities disagree regarding the value of early opposite sex relationships in the development of a sexual identity. Some believe that longer like-sex relationships are necessary to fully develop the characteristics of the individual's own sex, whereas others believe that dating provides adolescents with experience in human relationships, promotes social skills, and enhances their ability to choose a mate wisely. Having a variety of dating partners and experiences undoubtedly promotes a wiser mate selection and favors earlier and longer dating practices; however, early dating can involve an adolescent pair in a close sexual relationship before they are ready for intimacy. The sense of intimacy, the developmental crisis of early adulthood, must be built on a firm sense of identity, which early adolescents lack.

Heterosexual codes among teenage youngsters have undergone a notable change in recent years. The extent to which adolescents engage in intimate sexual relationships is not known precisely. Studies indicate that casual sexual relationships are generally not acceptable. Some degree of permanent commitment is needed before sexual intimacy is considered appropriate. Many adolescents have indulged in petting, including transient, exploratory homosexual petting, and petting is generally more acceptable than intercourse as a form of sexual expression.

QUESTIONS AND CONTROVERSIES

Do the various media adversely affect adolescent sexuality?

Considerable concern has been expressed regarding the effect of the various media on sexuality in teenagers. It has been said that television (TV) and other media have become the leading source of sex education in the United States today (Sprafkin and Silverman, 1981). As a source of information, television ranks close behind peers (Thornburg, 1981). TV offers teenagers an opportunity to glimpse the secretive world of adult sex before they can learn from firsthand experience. It teaches them about gender roles and patterns of courtship and sexual gratification that they might be unable to observe anywhere else (Gagnon and Simon, 1987; Silverman-Watkins, 1983).

Some family shows have handled the issue of teenage sexual activity responsibility and have depicted married couples acting affectionately toward one another (Strasburger, 1989). Specific topics (such as AIDS) may also be more intensively discussed on TV than elsewhere (Harris and others, 1988). However, studies have found a relationship between TV viewing and sexual activity among teenagers; soap operas have received the most criticism. The main message they convey is that adults do not use contraception nor plan for sex. To be "swept away" is the natural way to have sex (Wattleton, 1987), which is consistent with the views and explanations for nonuse of contraception by adolescents (Harris and others, 1986).

R-rated movies, whether viewed in theaters or at home on videocassettes, are providing messages about sexuality. When compared with TV, the frequency of sex acts or reference in movies is seven times higher, and, not uncommonly, the depiction of sexual acts is much more explicit (Strasburger, 1989). Although observers have found that pregnant teens had spent more time watching TV than nonpregnant teens, both soap operas and the prime-time series they watched had fewer sexual references than did the movies they viewed (Soderman, 1988).

Sexually explicit lyrics are heard on records and tapes, although these are subject to variable interpretation. Certainly, today's song lyrics are considered to be the most sexually graphic ever written (Fedler, Hall, and Tanzi, 1982). However, some studies indicate that teenagers' knowledge and comprehension of lyrics is age dependent and limited (Faelten, 1988).

Of greater concern is the impact of music television (MTV). Teenagers watch MTV programming frequently (Sun and Lull, 1986), and it seems to appeal to teenagers who are ordinarily light viewers of regular TV (Strasburger, 1989). Performance videos display gyrating and posturing, but concept music (strongly male oriented) tells stories that depict sex and violence combined with sexual imagery (Sherman and Dominick, 1986). In addition, rock stars serve as role models for impressionable children and young adolescents (Strasburger, 1989).

Much of advertising includes tantalizing provocative innuendos. "Sex sells" is the watchword of advertising, and sexy ads are used to sell every type of product—except birth control. Also, beer and wine commercials tend to exploit female sexuality. Combining sexual enticement and alcohol is especially unfortunate in view of the health risks that teenagers face from both.

Kissing and petting are the traditional first steps in the sequence of heterosexual activity for most adolescents (Grant and Demetriou, 1988). A greater proportion of adolescents are sexually experienced with each successive year of adolescence. A recent report indicates that 17% of boys and 5% of girls had had intercourse by 15 years of age; 48% of boys and 27% of girls had done so by their seventeenth birthday, and 83% of boys and 74% of girls by 20 years of age (Hayes, 1987).

In general, males experience sexual relationships with a number of females, whereas most females restrict their experiences to steady boyfriends, most often their future mates. For girls such intimacy is closely allied to an affectionate commitment. The overall major sexual codes in adolescence appear to be (1) petting with affection, in which the couple stops short of full sexual intercourse; (2) permissiveness with affection, which permits coitus in a stable relationship, usually between a steady-dating pair of older adolescents; and (3) the double standard of male sexual behavior, in which the majority of boys feel justified in engaging in coitus with other girls to demonstrate and enhance their virility while expecting abstinence from the girl to whom they are romantically committed.

Adolescents engage in sexual relationships to experience pleasurable sensations, to satisfy sexual drives, to satisfy curiosity, to achieve conquests, to express some degree of affection, or to conform. Often the urge to belong and gain reassurance and the wish to really belong to someone provoke a series of increasingly intimate physical contacts with a favored boyfriend or girlfriend, with each contact being more sexually provocative than the last. Eventually sexual intercourse can become established as a behavior pattern and a method for ensuring social participation or even as an end in itself.

Society places the responsibility on the girl for inhibiting the boy's sexual advances; therefore if she concedes through a need to conform or for acceptance, she is faced with fears of disease, pregnancy, and being labeled "fast" or "bad." Often the experience can be psychologically harmful, especially when it produces a conflict of values, resulting in feelings of guilt and worthlessness. The increasing incidence of sexual activity among teenagers has important implications for health professionals because of the associated health-related problems.

The current trend toward greater permissiveness regarding adolescent sexual behavior will undoubtedly have an effect on the adolescent developmental experience. It is likely that young people will be accorded progressively more decision-making authority concerning control over their bodies. These alterations in the attitudes and value systems toward sex will have important implications for health professionals. It has been predicted that attitudes toward sex will shift from a moral context to a predominantly health context within a few years.

Homosexuality in Adolescents

The development of homosexuality during childhood or adolescence has been greatly ignored, thought to be either a transient experience on the way to becoming a heterosexual adult or a pathologic event (Bidwell, 1988). The pediatric community has recognized the special needs of these adolescents in order to foster a healthy transition during this period (American Academy of Pediatrics, 1983).

To fully understand the unique needs of gay and lesbian youth, it is essential to understand the components of human sexuality. Four dimensions of childhood sexual learning and identity have been described (see Development of Sexuality, Chapter 4). Biosexual identity is established at birth, and gender identity, the internal awareness of being either male or female, occurs during toddler and preschool years. Sex-role identity usually refers to how the person appears as either feminine or masculine. Sexual orientation, the feelings of attraction to another relative to love (Woods, 1987), is established during late childhood through adulthood and occurs along a continuum from exclusively heterosexual to exclusively homosexual. Several theories have been advanced in an attempt to understand the origins of sexual orientation involving genetic, hormonal, psychologic, or sociologic factors (Savin-Williams, 1988).

In addition to all the normal tasks of adolescence, gay males and females have their own unique issues of identity formation. This process has been called "coming out" and does not refer to any particular event or time, but rather to a series of events that lead adolescents to establish an integrated sense of who they are.

The identity process involves four steps (Troiden, 1988). Initially the preadolescent or adolescent becomes sensitized to feeling different in relation to stereotyped gender activities (e.g., all boys play sports and girls are always feminine) from their same-sex peers. Second, by middle to late adolescence the young person begins to feel that he or she probably is homosexual. This occurs at about age 17 in males and age 18 in females (Troiden, 1988). For some this recognition occurs in young adulthood as they reflect on their childhood feelings. This is a period of identity confusion, which can result in feelings of isolation and depression. Gay males and lesbian females may choose to respond to these feelings through a variety of coping strategies such as denial, avoidance, repair by seeking a cure, or redefinition (e.g., "this is only a phase" or "only with this specific person" or "only when I'm drunk do I feel this way").

Identity assumption is the third stage, in which youths begin to acknowledge their homosexual identity and begin to experiment with their sexuality and to socialize within the homosexual subculture. This usually occurs during the early to mid twenties. The last stage is commitment, during which individuals acknowledge to themselves and to the external community that they are homosexual.

Adolescence is a crucial time when teenagers may begin to question their sexual orientation. Nurses need to recognize the potential for same-gender attraction and to be sensitive to the fact that not all youths will be involved in heterosexual relationships. Nurses need to evaluate their own attitudes and beliefs about homosexuality to determine their own comfort level in providing health care to gay or lesbian youths.

Obtaining a health history demands special attention.

Because nurses may not be aware of sexual preference before an interview, questions regarding sex should be phrased in a nonjudgmental fashion to allow either response. Frequently youths may have feelings about the same sex but may not feel comfortable in disclosing or discussing these feelings. However, health professionals who are open and nonjudgmental about sexual orientation may offer the adolescents their initial opportunity to talk about this sensitive topic.

Gay and lesbian youths need a variety of special services. Because of long-standing biases against homosexuality in society, there may not be social support or positive adult role models for these youths. Family members may have concerns about the young person being homosexual but are unable to discuss it or may be supportive of the homosexuality but reject the youngster.

Frequently youths disclose their feelings about being gay to a health professional. Those who question their sexual identity should not be reassured that these feelings are only a passing phase. Instead, referral to an agency sensitive to the counseling and support services necessary is essential for gay adolescents and their families. In addition to their special needs, gay and lesbian youths need the same health education and health care services that all teenagers need, including sex education, information on sexually transmitted disease, and AIDS prevention. Health professionals who care for gay and lesbian youths are encouraged to obtain additional education regarding health care for these youths (Bidwell, 1988; Sanford, 1989).

EMOTIONALITY

The pubertal changes in physical appearance are accompanied by alterations in emotional control and response. The stability of the prepubescent period is replaced by the turmoil precipitated by the physical and psychologic changes that teenagers experience. They are deluged with new sensations and feelings they cannot understand. The behavior of adolescents is bewildering to others and often to the adolescents themselves. They are frequently labeled as unstable, inconsistent, and unpredictable. The behaviors they exhibit have even been described as pseudopathologic or as representing a normal psychosis. It is true that many of the transient symptoms that are relatively common in adolescence resemble pathologic syndromes in the adult, such as mood swings, depression, periodic regression to childhood, and mild antisocial behavior.

Most feelings in early adolescence seem to originate from within the individual rather than from the environment. Adolescents characteristically exhibit alternating and recurrent episodes of disturbed behavior with periods of relative tranquility. There is an increase in moods and sentiments. They vacillate between emotional ups and downs and between considerable maturity and childlike behavior. One minute they are exuberant and enthusiastic; the next minute they are depressed and withdrawn. Unpredictable but essentially normal outbursts of primitive behavior appear as the teenager loses control over instinctual drives.

Little things can cause an emotional upheaval and, depending on the teenager's interpretation, can mean a great deal. As the tension is relieved, emotion is brought under control, and the individual retreats in order to work over what has happened, to attempt to master anger, and in the overall process to grow in the ability to control emotions and gain from the new experience. These emotional outbursts and ensuing periods of calm may last only a few minutes or hours or may extend over a period of weeks. Adolescents are given to extensive daydreaming that may be so intense that they do not hear another person speaking to them. On the other hand, they may become hostile or ready to fight, complain, or resist everything.

The cyclic pattern that has been apparent throughout childhood continues in adolescence. The outgoing, balanced child is replaced by the withdrawn, pensive, and moody early adolescent child who is often unhappy and humorless. Adolescents again shift to a more vigorous, expansive state during the middle teens. They are less apt to have their feelings hurt and are less inclined to cry at the least provocation as was evident earlier. Teenagers again retreat into a phase of withdrawal, moodiness, and introspection. They often feel excessively tired. For many it is a troubled time. Teenagers are better able to control their emotions in later adolescence. They can approach problems more calmly and rationally, and, although they are still subject to periods of depression, their feelings are less vulnerable, and they are beginning to demonstrate the more mature emotions of later adolescence.

In later adolescence sources of emotion are more apt to come from the external environment than from within. Anger is the most disruptive emotion, often a consequence of interruption or restriction of activities. However, whereas early adolescents react immediately and emotionally, older adolescents can control their emotions until they can be expressed in a socially acceptable time and place. They are still subject to heightened emotion, and, when it is expressed, their behavior reflects feelings of insecurity, tension, and indecision.

INTERESTS AND ACTIVITIES

During early adolescence the interests and activities of girls and boys are in sharp contrast. Boys spend a great deal of time in active outdoor sports or "just going out with the guys." They enjoy hobbies and clubs, television takes up a good part of their time, and school-related activities are increasingly important (Fig. 19-12). Girls and mixed-sex activities occupy the interest and concern of boys, but they do not become prominent concerns until their development more nearly approaches that of the more rapidly maturing girls. As their bodies gain strength and size, "making the team" is a major concern for many youths, and a boy may spend an excessive amount of time in attempting to perfect athletic skills. The essential bicycle of middle childhood is replaced by the automobile, the symbol of status to the adolescent (Fig. 19-13). If a car cannot be acquired, a motorcycle or motor bike is preferable to walking, riding the bus,

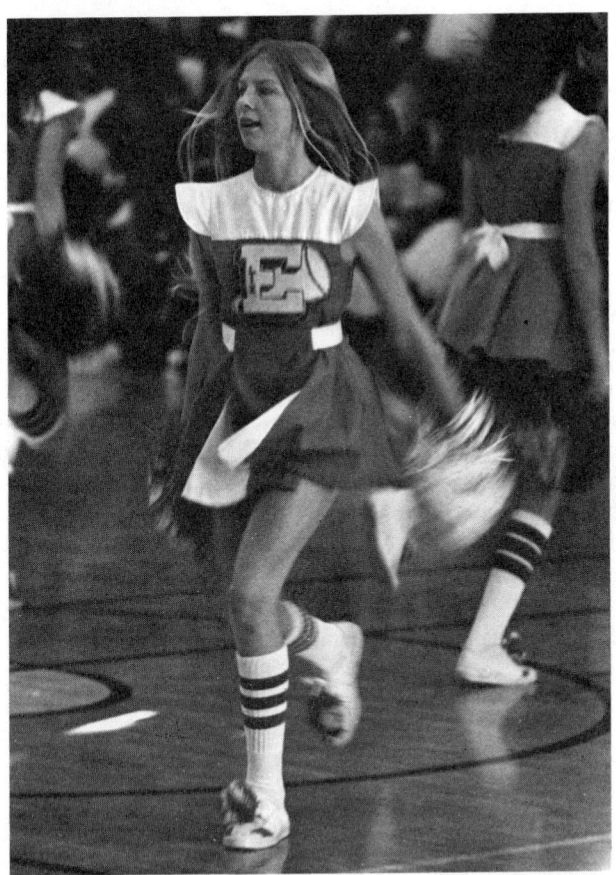

Fig. 19-12. School-related activities occupy an important role in early adolescence.

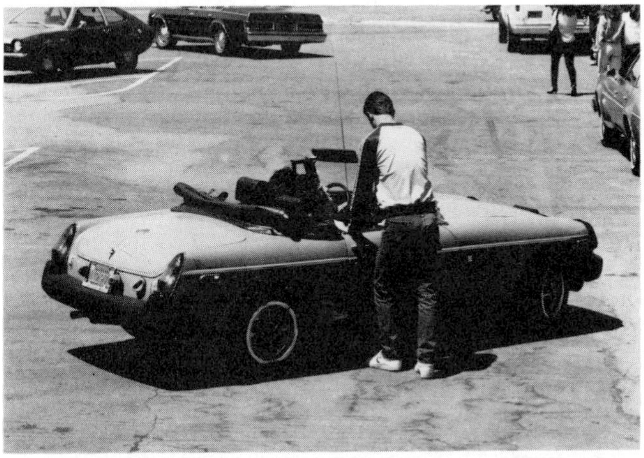

Fig. 19-13. The automobile becomes an important status symbol of adolescence.

or the humiliation of being chauffeured by a parent or sibling. Most boys avidly seek part-time employment, many because of economic necessity.

Although girls' leisure interests involve many outdoor activities, a greater interest in parties and social activities is evident. They are interested in hobbies, self-improvement

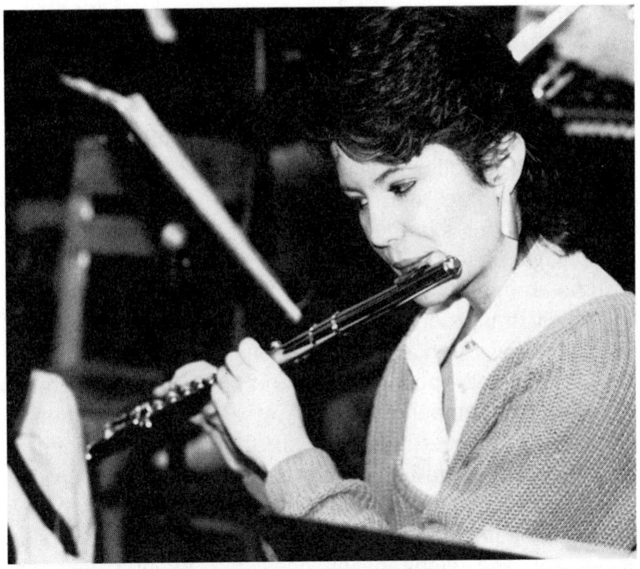

Fig. 19-14. Developing skills and abilities is a prime interest of the young adolescent.

(Fig. 19-14), and volunteer activities, and many seek part-time jobs out of economic need or in order to purchase more clothes and other teenage "necessities." A large number of girls, and some boys, assume the responsibility for the care of small children as baby-sitters, a common means of earning money during adolescence. However, teenage baby-sitters need some basic guidelines.*

Teenagers are avid conversationalists and spend much of their time in the company of other girls, talking, listening to records, and experimenting with makeup, hairstyles, and clothes. They enjoy shopping for clothes, but there is seldom agreement between mother and daughter regarding types and styles of clothing. Many of their thoughts and feelings are confessed in a diary. Daydreaming is a prominent characteristic of the adolescent.

Members of both sexes enjoy movies, rock concerts, dancing, and other communal activities and entertainment. Girls seem to prefer sentimental, romantic films when they are available, whereas boys would rather see sports, mystery, or action films. X-rated movies are crowded with adolescents. With the availability of a variety of videocassette films, adolescents are congregating in small groups to watch films on home videocassette recorders. However, there is little research on the types of videocassette films teenagers watch. Teenage girls and boys begin to appreciate and enjoy the theater and to share in the experience of audience reaction to the performance. They increasingly progress toward enjoyment of more adult activities and interests, and their developing social competence makes them more willing to accompany adults on occasion to share in the fun and activity.

Reading is still a favorite occupation of teenagers and

*A suggested resource is *Guide for the First-Time Baby-Sitter,* available from Johnson & Johnson, Grandview Rd., Skillman, NJ 08558.

may serve to satisfy some of their needs for vicarious experiences. Reading is more purposeful at this stage than at earlier ages, and most adolescents prefer to read magazines rather than books. Boys read magazines of a scientific or technical nature, and girls prefer women's magazines. The avid interest in collections that was so prominent in middle childhood declines during adolescence to be replaced by individual hobbies in the areas of the arts and sciences.

Teenagers have an affinity for stereo tape players, which assume an important role in their lives, and they are avidly addicted to transistor radios, which accompany many of their other activities, such as studying, walking, or working. Much of their money is spent on tapes and compact discs, which are collected in much the same way as books are. Often a favorite recording is regarded with the feeling accorded a well-loved book and is played over and over again.

When not engaged in other activities, they are probably participating in "rap sessions" or in endless telephone conversations. The telephone provides that essential link between peers when they are physically removed from one another. It is a way to fulfill the need for flight from parents to peers without leaving the home. The conversations may consist of gossip, plans, experiences, or an account of the activities of the day. The topics vary greatly, but the amount of time so engaged is often measured in hours. For boy-girl conversations, the telephone provides a means for closeness without fear of complications that physical proximity may engender.

Teenage interests and activities are subject to rapid change. Each succeeding generation of teenagers has its own peculiar characteristics evidenced by their behavior, vocabulary, dress, and other external manifestations that reflect and establish a clear line of separateness, although superficial, between the peer and the adult cultures. The rapidity with which these external trappings change is often astonishing.

The adolescent age-group is a major force in the economic marketplace. Today's adolescents have more money to spend than any previous generation of teenagers, and the advent of television and movies for some ethnic groups has made adolescents a much more visible and identifiable group. Symbols of their identity are brought to their attention through the media by advertisers of cosmetics, radios, tapes, and fad clothing. Members of this easily impressionable group are readily persuaded to part with money in their ever-present quest for acceptance and popularity, even though based on superficial values.

SUMMARY OF GROWTH AND DEVELOPMENT

Growth and development during adolescence is both physically and psychologically rapid and dramatic. At the end of this turbulent period young people are able to verbalize conceptually, establish independence, become comfortable with their bodies, build new and meaningful relationships, seek economic and social stability, and develop a workable value system.

The characteristics described throughout the chapter are summarized as *early adolescence,* during which youngsters cast off childhood, emerge as adolescents, and find a new self; *middle (or mid) adolescence,* when teenagers belong to an adolescent subculture and begin to find a place in the large community; and *late adolescence,* when they crystallize an identity and emerge as adults. These periods represent an *average* pattern and may not necessarily apply to any single individual (Table 19-1).

COPING WITH CONCERNS RELATED TO NORMAL GROWTH AND DEVELOPMENT

The stresses encountered during adolescence are continual and affect almost every aspect of a youngster's daily life. Normal body changes in relation to attainment of sexual maturity and the process of adjustment to an altered body image are prime sources of stress and anxiety. Early-maturing females and late-maturing children are especially sensitive to the stresses of being different from their peers. Many feel intense anxiety over their sense of self and identity. The major areas of stress during adolescence are listed in Box 19-1. See Peterson and Spiga (1982) for a review of adolescence and stress.

Coping with Stress

A common stress of adolescence is the "cultural shock" of the high school milieu. The youngster moves from the familiar and relatively narrow sphere of relationships with neighborhood children and homogeneous subgroups to a wider representation of peers. The peer group now represents geographic, cultural, and socioeconomic groups different from those with which the youngster is familiar. The teenager is confronted with behaviors of other adolescents that are entirely unanticipated.

The structure of social relationships is different. Whereas school-age relationships are determined mainly by who lives nearby, in the high school setting the groups are often determined by ethnic background, intelligence, or social status. The members of these groups organize themselves into clubs or exclusive groups that emphasize likenesses and exclude those who do not meet the criteria for inclusion. Thus young people who have felt accepted in groups in the past are now faced with the impact of social prejudice and the shock of *exclusion* (Elkind, 1984).

Box 19-1 AREAS OF STRESS IN ADOLESCENCE

Body image
Sexuality conflicts
Scholastic pressures
Competitive pressures
Relationships with parents
Relationships with siblings
Relationships with peers
Finances
Decisions about present and future roles
Career planning
Ideologic conflicts

Table 19-1 Growth and development during adolescence

DIMENSION	EARLY ADOLESCENCE (11-14 YEARS)	MIDDLE ADOLESCENCE (14-17 YEARS)	LATE ADOLESCENCE (17-20 YEARS)
Growth	Rapidly accelerating growth Reaches peak velocity Secondary sex characteristics appear	Growth decelerating Stature reaches 95% of adult height Secondary sex characteristics well advanced	Physically mature Structure and reproductive growth almost complete
Cognition	Limited ability for abstract thinking Explores newfound ability for abstract thought Clumsy groping for new values and energies Comparison of "normality" with peers of same sex	Developing capacity for abstract thinking Enjoys intellectual powers, often in idealistic, altruistic terms Concern with philosophic, political, and social problems	Established abstract thought Can perceive and act on long-range options Able to view problems comprehensively Intellectual and functional identity established
Identity	Preoccupied with rapid body changes Trying out of various roles Measurement of attractiveness by acceptance or rejection of peers Conformity to group norms	Reestablishes body image as growth decelerates Very self-centered; increased narcissism Tendency toward inner experience and self-discovery Has a rich fantasy life Idealistic Able to perceive future implications of current behavior and decisions; variable application	Body image and gender role definition nearly secured Irreversible sexual identity Phase of consolidation of identity Stability of self-esteem Comfortable with physical growth Social roles defined and articulated
Relationships with parents	Defining independence-dependence boundaries Strong desire to remain dependent on parents while trying to detach No major conflicts over parental control	Major conflicts over independence and control Low point in parent-child relationship Greatest push for emancipation; disengagement Final and irreversible emotional detachment from parents; mourning	Emotional and physical separation from parents completed Independence from family and less conflict Emancipation nearly secured Extension of independence without conflict
Relationships with peers	Seeks peer affiliations to counter instability generated by rapid change Upsurge of close idealized friendships with members of the same sex Struggle for mastery takes place within peer group	Strong need for identity to affirm self-image Behavioral standards set by peer group Acceptance by peers extremely important—fear of rejection Exploration of ability to attract the opposite sex	Recedes in importance in favor of individual friendship Testing of male-female relationships against possibility of permanent alliance Relationships characterized by giving and sharing
Sexuality	Self-exploration and evaluation Limited dating Limited intimacy	Multiple plural relationships Decisive turn toward heterosexuality (if is homosexual, knows by this time) Exploration of "sex appeal" Feeling of "being in love" Tentative establishment of relationships	Forms stable relationships and attachment to another Growing capacity for mutuality and reciprocity Preeminence of individual as dating partner Intimacy involves commitment rather than exploration and romanticism
Emotionality	Most ambivalence Wide mood swings Intense daydreaming Anger outwardly expressed with moodiness, temper outbursts, and verbal insults and name-calling	Tendency toward inner experiences; more introspective Tendency to withdraw when upset or feelings are hurt Vacillation of emotions in time and range Feelings of inadequacy common; difficulty in asking for help	More constancy of emotion Anger more apt to be concealed

Unlike the socialization of school-age children that consists of cooperative activities centered on a common goal, the new relationships and social interactions of teenagers are based on mutual trust and loyalty. Inexperienced youth now encounter complex and multilayered relationships. When they find their loyalty used and exploited, they experience another form of shock, *betrayal*. Youngsters also discover that the objects of their idealization, that is, persons whom they admire or on whom they develop "crushes," are merely human, which produces another type of shock, *disillusionment* (Elkind, 1984).

According to research there are negative consequences for adolescents who must cope with several transitions at once (Simmons and others, 1987). Transitions include beginning puberty, starting to date, and enrolling in a new school (high school). Other major transitions, such as moving to a new neighborhood or a divorce in the family, can produce an additive effect. Cumulative stresses affect both males and females, as exhibited by declines in grade point average and an increase in extracurricular involvement.

The adolescent is faced with pressures from peers to conform, which often involve flaunting adult authority and even serious health risks. Health risks include pressures for sexual experimentation and use of hard drugs, alcohol, and cigarettes, as well as potentially dangerous physical activities (see Chapter 21 and Injury Prevention, p. 899). The likelihood of rape is greatest at this time (for further information, see Sexual Abuse, Chapter 16, and Rape, Chapter 20).

Fears

Teenagers are not afraid of darkness, loud noises, bogeymen, or separation, but they are fearful that they may not be able to live up to what they believe to be their roles and responsibilities as adults. The intense adolescent sexual urge generates fear and anxieties about the size and appearance of primary and secondary sexual characteristics and the ability to perform. Many adolescents fear relationships with persons of the opposite sex. Youngsters who are shy and afraid to relate to persons of the opposite sex may develop a hatred to compensate for the craving they are unable to satisfy. Some fear losing self-control.

Many young people are worried about homosexuality. Most teenagers go through a brief phase, usually during early adolescence, when they are attracted to members of the same sex. Sexual experimentation commonly occurs between same-sex individuals or groups and is a temporary defense against the fears associated with full heterosexual relationships. For most youngsters the phase passes with only the temporary concerns regarding the possible implications.

Teenagers are fearful regarding their ability to assume the responsibilities expected of an adult. They worry that they will be unable to make a living or to cope with the independence that adulthood implies. All teenagers live with the fear of nuclear war and the possible end of existence as they know it. Boys especially are worried about having to serve in the armed forces.

Limit-Setting and Discipline

Adolescence is probably the most difficult period of development for both the child and the parents. Parents are confused about how much freedom to allow their teenager, and the youngster is torn between the desire for independence and the security of dependence. Conflicts between parents and teenagers are not unexpected (see Relationships with Parents, p. 881). Teenagers need firm but reasonable limitations to protect them from behaviors that place them in jeopardy.

With their capacity for abstract thought and reasoning, teenagers are able to understand limits imposed by parents. They often rebel against restrictions but feel more secure with the protection they afford, especially when a parental mandate provides a face-saving means for avoiding a situation they do not feel competent to manage. It is much easier for an adolescent to place the onus on parents rather than on themselves when they decline to engage in an activity with peers in which they may feel insecure or fearful.

Teenagers need firm limits in areas such as curfews, minimum activities on school nights, and chaperoned activities. Privileges should balance limitations, and teenagers should be allowed increasing privileges as they demonstrate mature behavior worthy of more freedom. Discipline, as always, must be fair and suitable to the offense. Unusually harsh limitations only serve to stimulate rebellion. Many of the strategies employed earlier are appropriate for this age-group, such as withholding privileges, contracting, and negotiating. Also, it is vitally important that a youngster not be chastised in the presence of peers.

PROMOTING OPTIMUM HEALTH DURING ADOLESCENCE

Adolescents are, on the whole, healthy individuals. The disease level is low during this age period, but there is heightened concern about the body. Most of the health problems and the more common illnesses are in some way related to the physical changes of puberty. The disorders associated with adolescent development are discussed in Chapter 20; health promotion in persons in this age-group is primarily one of health teaching and guidance.

Adolescents as a group are eager to learn about themselves, and nurses who are truly interested in them, who respect them as persons, and who are willing to listen to them will be able to gain their confidence and trust. It is important to establish rapport with the adolescent, at the first interview if possible. Overidentification is avoided. Relating naturally and honestly, acting neither as a young person nor as a parent, is the best approach. Nurses should be prepared to talk to parents following the time spent with the youngster, and the young person should be invited to stay during the discussion.

During this period of gaining independence from families and the strong peer-group influences, teenagers are vulnerable to practices that may be hazardous to their health and well-being. They need someone to whom they can turn for guidance, with whom they can test out ideas, and with whom they feel free to express their fears and feelings. Nurses as health professionals and respected adults have the opportunity to provide adolescents with factual information about what is taking place in their bodies and to clarify misconceptions about menstruation, nocturnal emissions, pregnancy, and other physical changes of puberty.

Both individual and group conferences with teenagers provide excellent opportunities to discuss actual or potential health problems such as pregnancy, sexually transmitted disease, and the hazards of smoking and experimenting with drugs, including alcohol. Adolescents are frequently confused about the information they receive from parents, friends, and written material to which they have access. Very often teenagers feel more comfortable in a group situation. With peer support they are better able to explore ideas that they may not be able to express individually. Individual counseling provides adolescents with a knowledgeable adult in whom they can confide without the threat of an intimate relationship.

Adolescents are able to assume the major responsibility for their own health, including maintaining health practices (e.g., toothbrushing, caring for appliances), taking prescribed medications, keeping appointments, and performing procedures when necessary. Laws and practices regarding medical care of adolescents without consent of their parents vary (see Informed Consent, Chapter 27). This is especially relevant in relation to the youngster seeking guidance regarding possible sexually transmitted diseases, contraception, and pregnancy (see Chapter 20).

SCHOOL-BASED CLINICS

School-based clinics (SBCs) were originally designed in an attempt to reduce the adolescent pregnancy rate and related health problems. They have expanded to meet a variety of health needs and concerns of adolescents and are gaining rapid acceptance throughout the nation. SBCs differ from traditional school health services in that they function as integral parts of the mainstream health system (Keenan, 1986). As part of established health-care institutions (e.g., health department, hospital, medical schools, or other organizations) responsible for their operations, SBCs offer more comprehensive care than is available through school health services and have access to a wider range of services.

Many children live in households in which families, under heavy social and economic stresses, have less time to supervise health care. Since children usually receive health care at the initiative and discretion of parents, these circumstances hamper regular access to care (Black, 1989). Because of the location of SBCs, they are able to reach most adolescents regularly. Teenagers spend more time at school than anywhere else; they need not be transferred elsewhere to get care, and time from class for the teenager and from work for a parent are minimized.

A clinical nurse specialist plays a prominent role in SBCs and serves as manager, coordinator, and liaison between the clinic and the parent institution. Referrals to the clinic come from a variety of sources—school personnel (counselors, teachers, school nurses), peer referrals, and self-referrals. Often appointments are managed through school personnel. SBCs are filling a need, especially for a medically disadvantaged youth.

NUTRITION

The rapid and extensive development in height, weight, muscle mass, and sexual maturity of adolescence is accompanied by new and greater nutritional requirements. Since nutritional needs are closely related to the increase in body mass, the peak requirements occur in the year of maximum growth, during which time the body mass almost doubles. This period occurs between the tenth and twelfth years in girls and about 2 years later in boys. The calorie and protein requirements during this year are high, and as a result of this anabolic need, the adolescent is highly sensitive to caloric restrictions. Adolescents want food, their appetites soar, and their capacity to consume food is often awe inspiring, as any parent of a teenage boy can attest. A fast-growing boy may never get enough. His stomach may be too small to accommodate the amount of food he requires to meet his growth needs unless he eats at very frequent intervals. Failure to consume an adequate diet at this time can potentially retard growth and delay sexual maturation.

Not only do teenagers eat at every pause in the day's activities, but they enjoy food and the pleasures related to its consumption. Food is part of the attraction of the "hangouts" and gathering places that teenagers frequent. For example, the corner deli or fast-food diner provides such favored items as hamburgers, ice cream, soft drinks, and the company of equally hungry peers. Large bags of assorted snacks are an essential part of beach gatherings, rock concerts, and other outdoor get-togethers.

The nutritional needs of adolescents are difficult to determine because of the meager nutritional information on members of this age-group. Defining dietary requirements is further complicated by the influence of emotional and other stress factors that affect nutrient utilization and the psychologic factors that influence adolescent eating habits. In addition, the diverse variations in growth rates during adolescence and the equally wide range in ages at which these changes take place complicate any attempt to set minimum dietary standards for this age-group. Consequently, the recommended dietary allowances for teenagers include a safety factor that attempts to allow for these differences under average circumstances. Energy needs are highly variable; nutrition should be adjusted to meet increased energy requirements during physical activity. Inactive teenagers are subject to obesity even though their energy intake is below the recommended level, whereas extremely active youngsters will require more than the recommended amounts. Therefore food required for energy must be balanced with energy expenditure.

Protein intake remains a constant need throughout childhood and adolescence to meet continual growth needs. There is usually sufficient intake well above the recommended dietary allowance, except in those young people who limit their food intake because of economic problems or in an attempt to lose weight. When the supply is limited, dietary protein will be used to meet energy requirements at the expense of new tissue synthesis. Consequently a reduction in the growth rate can occur despite what appears to be an adequate protein intake.

Minerals that are most likely to be deficient in the adolescent diet are calcium, iron, and zinc. There is a substantial increase in the need for these minerals during the period of rapid growth—calcium for skeletal growth, iron for expansion of muscle mass and blood volume, and zinc for the generation of both skeletal and muscle tissue (Marino and King, 1980). Calcium retention varies considerably with the growth rate of the adolescent. On the average, boys accumulate a greater amount during peak periods of growth than girls, and fast-growing youngsters retain more than slow-growing youngsters. Increased amounts of milk are usually required to supplement an average diet to ensure an adequate calcium intake during this time. Evidence indicates that boys are more likely than girls to eat foods that meet calcium requirements (Marino and King, 1980).

Iron is essential for meeting the needs of the increased muscle and soft tissue growth and the rapid growth demands of an expanding red cell mass. Although this expansion occurs more quickly in adolescent boys, adolescent girls have an additional iron loss from menstruation. Consequently, the need is probably equivalent in both sexes. An inadequate iron intake is reflected in the high incidence of anemia in the adolescent population at all socioeconomic levels. Few adolescents consume sufficient amounts of iron and therefore should be advised to include good sources of iron in their diet, such as red meats, dried beans, green vegetables, iron-fortified cereals, and snacks that include peanuts, raisins, and other dried fruits. It has also been determined that ascorbic acid improves the absorption of iron from nonheme iron sources. Zinc is now recognized as essential for growth and sexual maturation of the adolescent. American adolescents tend to consume less than the recommended intake of this mineral. Sources rich in zinc include animal products such as meat, seafood, eggs, and milk.

Eating Habits and Behaviors

Eating and behavior toward food are primarily family-centered during early and middle childhood, and food habits are largely related to cultural and individual family preferences and patterns. With adolescence and the move toward independence, family influences on the child change. Teenagers' interests, attitudes, and routines are altered as an increasing number of meals are eaten away from home. These changes are largely a result of the high value that teenagers place on peer acceptability and sociability; therefore their eating habits are easily influenced by their associates. In addition, family criticism about food habits tends to have a negative effect on a wise selection of an adequate diet.

Omitting breakfast or eating a breakfast that is nutritionally poor in quality is frequently a problem. Often adolescent youngsters are sleepy in the morning, hate to get up, and delay getting up as long as possible; consequently, they have no time to eat. Many do not like breakfast food items. Other reasons for skipping breakfast are that they are not hungry, there is no one with whom to eat, or no breakfast is prepared for them. The youngster who dislikes traditional breakfast fare may react favorably to a peanut butter sandwich or a hamburger, both of which are nutritionally good and often more acceptable to the teenager. The goal of an adequate, good-tasting breakfast requires that someone prepare it and that the youngster arrange the time to eat it.

Pressure for time and their commitments to activities adversely affect the teenager's eating habits. Snacks, usually selected on the basis of accessibility rather than nutritional merit, become more and more a part of the habitual eating pattern during adolescence. Adolescents characteristically reject or only infrequently eat a sufficient amount of fresh fruits and vegetables, especially those that are rich in ascorbic acid. Fast-food items, to which they are especially attracted, contain few fruits and vegetables, thus contributing to a low dietary intake of vitamins C and A, and folic acid. Fast foods are also high in energy, fat, and sodium but low in fiber, all of which have been implicated in the etiology of degenerative diseases in later life (Marino and King, 1980). Milk is usually passed over in favor of soft drinks, the appropriate social drink of the peer culture.

Overeating or undereating during adolescence presents special problems. As they experience the normal increase in weight and fat deposition of the growth spurt, teenage girls often resort to dieting. The desire for the admired slim figure and a fear of becoming "fat" prompt teenage girls to embark on nutritionally inadequate reducing regimens that sap their energy and deprive their growing bodies of essential nutrients. They resort to diets on their own or with peers in an effort to conform. Many adopt the current fad diets and are victims of food misinformation. Vegetarian diets are becoming increasingly popular among teenagers and are a source of concern; unless they are carefully planned to provide sufficient dairy products and eggs, optimum growth and development may be compromised. Boys are less inclined to undereat. They are more concerned about gaining in size and strength. However, they tend to eat foods high in calories but low in other essential nutrients.

Iron deficiency anemia is relatively common in undernourished teenage girls, and the severe form of malnutrition, anorexia nervosa, occurs most frequently during adolescence when the girl becomes obsessed with self-denial of eating pleasures. Obesity from either overeating or underactivity is another form of inadequate nutrition that occurs often in adolescence.

Nursing Considerations

Nothing can *make* adolescents eat wisely. Since their food habits reflect many influences and conditions, these must be considered when planning nutritional education and guidance. Food habits begun in early childhood are difficult to break. In some families, failure to develop the habits of eating nutritious foods and a habitual lack of variety in a family's diet contribute to a lack of adequate nutrition. The quality of a diet is related to the number of different food items eaten in a day, and consistently skipped meals are associated with a poor diet.

When helping teenagers select a nutritious diet, the nurse should begin with their present diet and actively involve them in the process. It is important to remember that there are many ways to achieve an adequate diet, and that no pattern should be prejudged as inadequate until it is determined that it is indeed deficient in essential nutrients (see Box 19-2 for a sample menu). Adolescents do not re-

Box 19-2 SAMPLE MENUS FOR THE ADOLESCENT (13-19 YEARS)*

Breakfast	2 4-inch waffles ¼ cup syrup ¼ cup orange juice 1 cup lowfat milk
Lunch	1 "quarter pounder" hamburger with cheese 1 small order french fries 1 medium soft drink
Snack	1 cup frozen yogurt with fruit and nut topping *or* 1 peanut butter sandwich 1 cup lowfat milk
Dinner	1½ cups lasagna 1-2 pieces garlic bread Green salad with romaine lettuce and dressing 1 apple Iced tea
Snack:	3-4 cookies 1 cup lowfat milk
DAILY TOTAL:	
Milk:	32 ounces or equivalent
Meat:	4 ounces
Fruits/vegs:	4 servings (1 piece or ½ cup is a serving)
Breads/cereal:	4 servings (1 slice or ½ cup cooked is a serving)

Prepared by Cecilia L. Davis, R.D., L.D.
*Fats and simple carbohydrates should be served sparingly to meet caloric needs. Serving sizes are minimums for nutritional adequacy. Many children eat more.

spond well to judgmental attitudes. It is not unusual to discover that their diet patterns, although unusual by adult standards, are actually satisfactory. Teenagers dislike being talked down to or preached at, but they do respond when their independence is respected and they are given the opportunity to make their own decisions regarding food choices.

In general, adolescents are body conscious and concerned about their appearance. When diet is associated with clear skin, firm flesh, and glossy hair, the teenager is more likely to be receptive to nutritional education. However, helping young persons arrive at a decision for change is more difficult than providing information. They respond best when the counselor provides straightforward information, talks with them and not at them, and listens to what they have to say. Listening objectively to their ideas, clarifying misconceptions without ridicule, and involving them in diet planning are necessary if essential knowledge is to be translated into action. It is best to begin at the nutritional level where the individual is. A current food fad may be a good point from which to build a nutritious diet, taking into consideration other factors (cultural, social, economic) without prohibitions or declaring any food to be "bad."

As snacks become more a part of adolescents' eating patterns, it is important that they contribute something other than calories to their diet. Although "empty calorie" snacks are not a desirable substitute for nutritious foods, because adolescents' energy requirements are so high, they are able to consume some of these foods without compromising their nutrition, provided that high-quality foods are eaten the rest of the day. More often than not, what adolescents eat is determined by what is available. When made readily accessible, items such as fruits, vegetables, and dairy products are excellent and nutritious snack foods. A refrigerator shelf stocked by parents with good-tasting snack items especially for their youngsters can contribute significantly to improving adolescents' diets and giving them a feeling that they are important and worthwhile persons. Similarly, schools might provide nutritious snack foods in cafeterias and on-campus vending machines to encourage the purchase of these items by the teenage population.

It is often necessary to work with parents to help them understand the dietary needs and eating behaviors of their teenagers. Many are conscious of their responsibility for the nutrition of their children, whereas others are indifferent. Family influence on adolescents is likely to change as the teenagers move toward independence and the peer group exerts a greater influence. Poorer food practices appear to result when status, sociability, independence, and enjoyment are predominant influences. Diets tend to be better when adolescents consider health to be an important factor. Good family relationships, emotional stability, and adjustment to reality are also characteristics associated with better food habits.

SLEEP AND REST

Teenagers vary in their need for sleep and rest. Rapid physical growth, the tendency toward overexertion, and the overall increased activity of this age contribute to fatigue in adolescents. Their propensity for staying up late makes it very difficult for them to get out of bed in the mornings, and they sleep late at every opportunity. Adequate sleep and rest at this time are important to a total health regimen.

EXERCISE AND ACTIVITY

Adolescents probably spend more time and energy practicing and participating in sports activities than members of any other age-group. The practice of sports and games contributes significantly to growth and development, the educational process, and better health. It provides exercise for growing muscles, interactions with peers, and a socially acceptable means to enjoy stimulation and conflict. In addition, competitive activities help the teenager in the process of self-appraisal, development of self-respect, and concern for others (Fig. 19-15). Sports for young people are discussed further in relation to sports injuries (see Chapter 39).

Dancing has always occupied a central place in the customs of many cultures. There is delight in physical movement and a feeling of relief that comes from release of tension in activity. Dancing can also serve as a means of

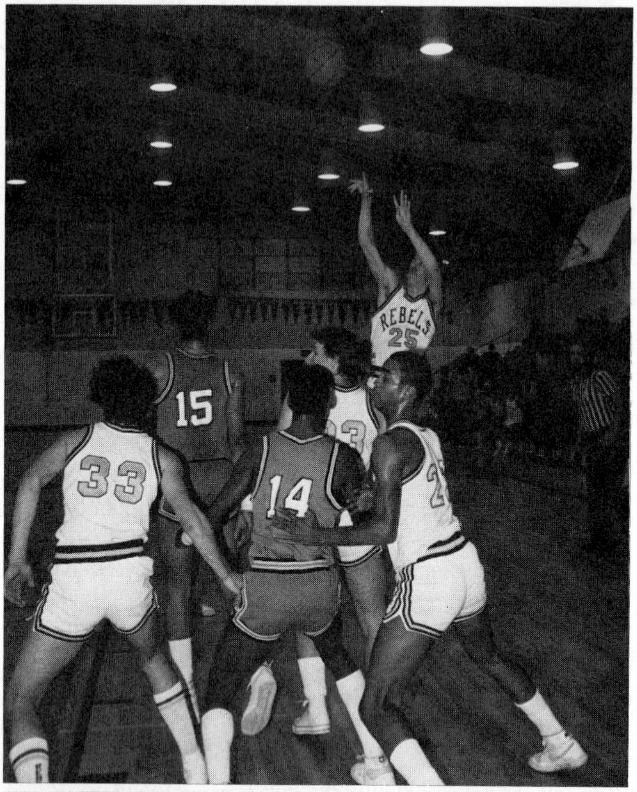

Fig. 19-15. Most adolescents aspire to become a member of a school athletic team.

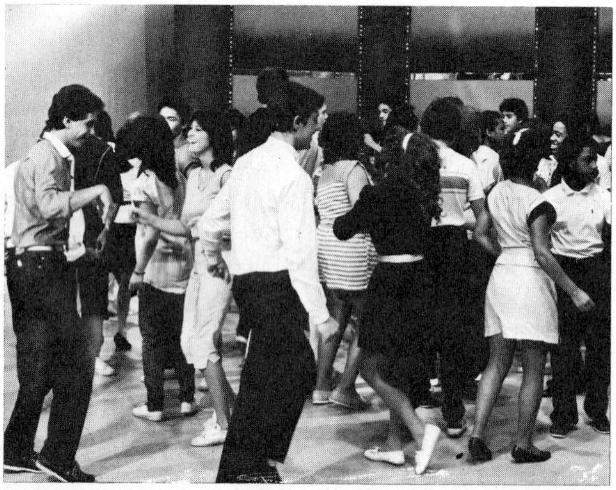

Fig. 19-16. Adolescents enjoy the activity and social aspects of dancing.

expressing specific sexual and aggressive urges in symbolic form and action. Many of the popular dances have decided sexual overtones and erotic movements. At the same time, the structure of the dance is such that dancers seldom touch one another. In this way the urges can be expressed without the danger of close physical contact (Fig. 19-16).

DENTAL HEALTH

Dental health should not be neglected during adolescence, although the rate of caries formation is not as great as it was in childhood. Early adolescence is usually the time when corrective orthodontic appliances are worn, and these are frequently a source of embarrassment and concern to the youngster. Reassurance regarding the temporary nature of the annoyance and anticipation of an improved appearance help to make the inconvenience tolerable. It is also important to reinforce the orthodontist's directions regarding use and care of the appliances and to emphasize careful attention to toothbrushing during this time.

PERSONAL CARE

The body-conscious teenager is highly receptive to discussion and counseling about personal care and hygiene. Body changes associated with puberty bring with them special needs for cleanliness. The hyperactive sebaceous glands and newly functioning apocrine glands make the daily bath imperative, and underarm deodorants assume an important place in personal care. The adolescent will find that hair requires more frequent shampooing, and girls will have questions about hair removal, use of cosmetics, and menstrual hygiene. Many group discussions center around the virtues of particular products or methods. Adolescents are continually bombarded with messages from the media regarding the best means to enhance their popularity and appeal to the opposite sex. Nurses are in a position to help them evaluate the relative merits of commercial products.

Vision

Regular vision testing is a vital part of health care and supervision during adolescence. At this time the incidence of visual refractive difficulties reaches a peak that is not exceeded until the fifth decade of life. Adolescents may not have poorer vision than children or adults, but the increased demands of schoolwork make good vision important for academic success. Consequently, teenagers are more likely to be referred for visual evaluation. The need for corrective lenses can create psychologic problems for teenagers if they believe that glasses spoil their appearance or do not fit their body image. For those who are able to tolerate and afford them, contact lenses are a happy solution. For some the impact of a visual defect, no matter how slight, may prove to be a great personal concern.

Hearing

There has been considerable concern regarding current teenage practices causing possible damage to the hearing of youngsters. Cochlear damage from relatively continuous exposure to the loud sound levels of rock music, especially from stereos and radios, has been documented. The popularity of portable FM radios and stereo cassette players with lightweight earphones, which enable the listener to adjust the volume, are of particular concern to health care professionals. When these units are used for extended periods, the potential for permanent hearing loss is undisputed. Appealing to individual youngsters for more judicious use is of doubtful benefit, although they should be informed of the risk. Efforts directed toward legislating legal limits to the noise exposure that can be achieved through the sets and widespread education may be possible solutions. (See Chapter 25 for a discussion of noise-related hearing loss.)

Posture

The process of normal development during adolescence does little to promote good posture in the teenage girl or boy. The rapid skeletal growth that is usually associated with a significant lag in muscular growth leads to weakness, easy fatigability, and awkwardness. These characteristics predispose youngsters to slumping and make them less inclined to stand or sit erectly. A relative reduction in physical activity, which often accompanies rapid skeletal growth, aggravates the situation, especially in teenage girls. The adolescent who is routinely engaged in vigorous physical activity appears to have fewer problems with posture.

Many adolescents, especially those early-maturing few who gain additional height in advance of their peers, feel conspicuous and attempt to disguise their height by adopting a slouching posture. Early pubescent breast development may cause shy girls to hunch forward and drop their heads. This is usually a transient phase that disappears as they develop confidence and maturity. Most of these postural problems resolve as the adolescent matures.

A few preexisting musculoskeletal problems, such as lateral spine deviation, or scoliosis, are likely to become exaggerated during the growth spurt and require treatment. However, most postural problems do not require special attention and treatment, and poor posture is not a source of pain. Actually the teenager's posture is primarily of concern to the parents, who continually admonish the youngster to "sit up" or "stand up straight." The teenager, unaware of any postural defect, fails to see or understand the problem. Consequently, parental nagging only creates additional hostility and resistance on the part of the adolescent.

The best approach to counseling teenagers about posture is to show, not tell, them and to serve as a proper model. Good posture can be demonstrated best when the adolescent stands before a full-length mirror. Postural defects and desired alterations can be pointed out in full view of both the young person and the nurse. A sunken chest, winged scapulas, a swayback, protuberant abdomen, and drooping head and shoulders are clearly visible, and the nurse can demonstrate the simple corrections that can transform the youngster into a more attractive and ultimately healthier person. Adolescents will need reassurance that the fatigue they feel when attempting to maintain correct posture is a transient effect caused by weak muscles, especially those of the back, and that they will soon acquire the strength and endurance to maintain the desired posture. If they concentrate on assuming correct positioning several times each day, with regular practice it will eventually become a permanent aspect of their person.

Serious postural defects detected in the process of a physical assessment will require early medical intervention. Scoliosis is usually intensified during adolescence. Nurses can refer the youngster to the appropriate source, such as the family physician, pediatrician, or health clinic, for evaluation and implementation of corrective therapy. Nurses are important sources of support and reassurance to the teenager and the parents throughout lengthy bracing, casting, and exercise programs.

Ear Piercing

The popular trend of ear piercing may sometimes create a health problem for the uninformed teenager. It is a nursing responsibility to caution girls or boys against the practice of having their ears pierced by friends, mothers, or themselves. Although in most cases there are few if any serious side effects, there is always a danger of such complications as infection, cyst or keloid formation, bleeding, dermatitis, or metal allergy. Therefore the procedure should be performed by a physician or qualified nurse using proper sterile technique. This is especially important if the youngster has a history of diabetes, allergies, or skin disorders. Teenagers are prone to the development of keloids, particularly if there is a history of keloid formation.

Suntanning

The continuous quest for an attractive appearance leads many teenagers to excessive sunbathing and artificial means for acquiring a tan. Emphasis on "tan is beautiful" has gained wide acceptance because it is associated with appearing healthy, attractive, and leading a leisurely lifestyle. However, the practice is not without risk. The incidence of skin cancer has increased greatly and at an alarming rate, mostly the result of excessive sun exposure. Long-term effects include premature aging of the skin and phototoxic reactions in susceptible individuals.

The increasing popularity of artificial suntanning has prompted concern on the part of health professionals regarding the use of sun lamps and suntanning machines. In addition to commercial tanning salons, tanning bulbs can be purchased through local department stores, making these devices easily and readily available. Although these devices are required to carry a warning from the Food and Drug Administration regarding their danger, nurses need to educate adolescents about the hazards of exposure to ultraviolet light. There is no such thing as a "good tan." Emphasis on premature aging, which threatens the body image, may have more immediate impact on the teenager than will a discussion of future development of cancer. Education on the use of sunscreens, including hypoallergenic products, with a sun protective factor (SPF) of at least 15 is important health teaching. Those who insist on using suntanning equipment should be warned that goggles must be worn in tanning booths to prevent serious corneal burning. See Sunburn, Chapter 18, for a discussion of sun exposure and protection.

Slow Maturation

Both early- and late-maturing children feel out of place among their classmates, but the slow-maturing children appear to suffer the most pronounced inner turmoil and may be hesitant to voice their concerns. The rate of maturation is important during the school years, but at puberty it assumes gigantic proportions to these children and often to their parents. Late-maturing youngsters are painfully aware of their shortcomings and find themselves being left out of private discussions about body changes experienced by the group; some are ostracized, and some, especially boys, are objects of scorn and ridicule. They feel cheated and may well believe that they are doomed to a permanent position outside the group. Such fears and failures only serve to accentuate the normal doubts and concerns about the self that are part of this critical age period.

The girl feels out of place among her companions whose hips and bosoms are developing, feels cheated because she has not yet menstruated, and feels that she is not a part of the giggling and boy talk of her friends. The boy feels weak and small compared with his muscular companions with whom he can no longer compete, and his high voice sounds childish compared with the deep tones around him. Slow-maturing youngsters need support and reassurance that they are not abnormal and need only to be patient until the time comes when they, too, will develop the characteristics for which they yearn. Early-maturing boys are less at a disadvantage than early-maturing girls or late-maturing boys. Late-maturing boys usually suffer most. The child with endocrine or genetic disorders that interfere with the maturation process needs special help, which is discussed in Chapter 20.

SEX EDUCATION AND GUIDANCE

Contemporary adolescents are constantly exposed to sexual symbolism and erotic stimulation from the mass media. At the same time, the development of primary and secondary sex characteristics and the increased sensitivity of the genitalia generate thoughts and fantasies about heterosexual relationships. In addition, the culture expects that adolescents will date, flirt, and experience sexual or romantic feelings. As a result, teenagers are often confused and ambivalent about sexuality and heterosexual relationships.

Although many adolescents have received sex education from parents and school throughout childhood, they are not always adequately prepared for the impact of puberty. A large portion of their knowledge is acquired from peers, television, movies, and magazines. Consequently, much of the sex information they accumulate is incomplete, inaccurate, riddled with cultural and moral issues, and usually not very helpful. Adolescents need to know the emotional aspects of their sexuality, as well as the need to take responsibility for their sexual behavior.

The questions of who is responsible for teaching and how the teaching can be best accomplished must be considered. Responsibility for sex education is and has been assumed by parents, schools, churches, community agencies such as **Planned Parenthood Federation of America, Inc.,*** and health professionals. Among this last group, nurses should—and many do—take an active role in talking to young people about their sexuality. To be able to discuss the topic with teenagers adequately, nurses must have not only an understanding of the physiologic aspects of sexuality and a knowledge of cultural and societal values but also an awareness of their own attitudes, feelings, and biases about sexuality. One cannot give information without simultaneously conveying attitudes. These attitudes in turn influence the behavior of young people.

Sex education should incorporate three steps: (1) an understanding of the facts and consequences of sex, (2) establishing values for behavior and relationships, and (3) learning to be aware of one's emotions. This implies that there are important questions that adolescents must consider and that "ignoring any of the three components can result in serious difficulties. Inattention to the facts makes one vulnerable to the serious consequences of pregnancy or a sexually transmitted disease. Ignoring values can lead to guilt and low self-esteem. Ignoring feelings can leave one deeply scarred by hurt, anger, and fear." (Voss, 1988).

The most comprehensive approach to sex education is offered by the **Sex Information and Education Council of the United States (SIECUS),*** an interdisciplinary organization founded to establish sexuality as a health entity and to dignify it by openness of approach, study, and scientific research. SIECUS maintains that every sex education program should present the topic from six aspects: biologic, social, health, personal adjustments and attitudes, interpersonal associations, and the establishment of values.

Whether nurses counsel young people on an individual basis, in mixed groups, or in groups segregated by sex makes little difference. Some nurses and teenagers are uneasy in mixed groups for discussions of sexuality, and no hard-and-fast rule prevails. Ideally boys and girls should be able to discuss sex objectively with one another and in groups, but this is not always possible. The difference in the rate of maturation between boys and girls and between different members of the same sex often makes it desirable to discuss certain aspects of sexuality in segregated groups. Sometimes individuals or small groups will deliberately seek the opportunity to talk over some subjects in the security of unmixed company. As a general rule, the need for separate discussion groups diminishes as young people progress toward maturity.

Sex education should consist of instructions concerning normal body function and associated feelings and emotions. Information should be presented in a straightforward manner using correct terminology. When discussing sex and sexual activities, nurses should use simple but correct language—not street language, highly scientific terminology, or evasive jargon. For example, the term *sexual intercourse* is usually understood by teenagers, whereas few are familiar with the terms *coitus* or *copulation;* the term *sexual relationships* is too vague, and the four-letter street terms

*Education Department, 810 Seventh Ave., New York, NY 10019; (212) 541-7800 or (800) 829-7732.

*130 W. 42nd St., Suite 2500, New York, NY 10036; (212) 819-9770.

are inappropriate. Once the meaning of biologic terms such as *uterus, testicles,* and *vagina* is understood, teenagers prefer to use them in their discussions.

Both boys and girls need to know more about what is going on in their bodies than they are able to see. Although most girls are adequately prepared for menstruation, they do not always understand its relationship to the total process of reproduction. Many are under the erroneous impression that the "safe" time for sexual intercourse is midway between menstrual periods. Whether they are sexually active or not, adolescents should receive accurate information about pregnancy, including when and how it occurs and ways by which it can be avoided. They need to know about sexually transmitted diseases, the manner in which they are transmitted, symptoms, and how to get treatment if anyone becomes infected.

Teenagers as a whole are limited in their knowledge and understanding of the sexuality of the opposite sex. Unless they are taught differently, each assumes that members of the other sex feel as they do. When girls understand the directness of the drive for sexual release that is experienced by young boys, they are better able to conduct themselves appropriately. This same knowledge will help boys to understand that girls do not feel the same urges as they do. Both need to recognize that they have a responsibility for their own behavior.

It is also important for teenagers to know that the thoughts and fantasies that may be disturbing to them are a normal part of the developmental process and should not be a source of guilt feelings. Adolescents, girls in particular, will want answers to questions such as, "What is it like?" "Does it hurt?" "What happens when . . .?" and "Is it all right if you . . .?" Boys are often concerned about the fallacy that there is a relationship between penis size and sexual function. They need reassurance that masturbation is a normal and common practice, that pornography is not harmful (Gordon and Snyder, 1989), that some degree of homosexuality is not unusual in early adolescence, and that oral-genital relations are normal substitutes for intercourse in certain situations.

Young people are at the stage of life when the sexual aspects of interpersonal relationships become particularly important. Societal expectations push them toward dating, and their own inner sex drive urges them toward exploration. Teenagers' curiosity and desire for information extend beyond the need for anatomic and physiologic knowledge. They need to know more than the mechanics of conception, gestation, and birth. They need to know about the sexuality of the opposite sex and to be helped to view the nature of sex as a powerful life force—a force to be used as an intense, vital human experience that is earned by maturity—not as a childhood game at which to play.

An excellent resource for sex education is *Sex Education for Adolescents. A Bibliography of Low-Cost Materials* available from the Committee on Adolescence of the American Academy of Pediatrics.*

*141 Northwest Point Blvd, P.O. Box 927, Elk Grove Village, IL; (413) 532-3374.

INJURY PREVENTION

Physical injuries are the greatest single cause of death in the adolescent age-group and claim more lives than all other causes combined. The most vulnerable ages are the years 15 to 24, when accidental injuries account for 61% of deaths in boys and 39% of deaths in girls. The tragedy of this is that the figures remain fairly constant from year to year, and almost all fatal injuries are preventable. (See Chapter 1 for statistics.)

As in all age-groups, injury is closely related to the developmental characteristics associated with normal growth and maturation. During adolescence, peak physical, sensory, and psychomotor function gives teenagers a feeling of strength and confidence that they have never experienced before, and the physiologic changes of puberty give impetus to many basic instinctual forces. One manifestation of this is an increase in energy that simply must be discharged through action, often at the expense of logical thinking and other control mechanisms. Because of this need for action, adolescents are prone to act impulsively. Their propensity for risk-taking behavior plus a feeling of indestructibility makes adolescents especially prone to injury (Fig. 19-17).

The care and management of specific types of injuries are discussed where appropriate throughout the book and are not considered here. These include head injuries, spinal cord injuries, burns, near-drowning, and fractures.

Bicycle Injuries

Bicycle use is common in early adolescence. Nine out of 10 adolescents report riding a bicycle and 92% report never wearing a helmet; 72% report never using a light at night (Vance and others, 1989). The overwhelming majority of deaths from bicycle injuries involve teenagers, and many youths are intoxicated at the time of the injury. For a more

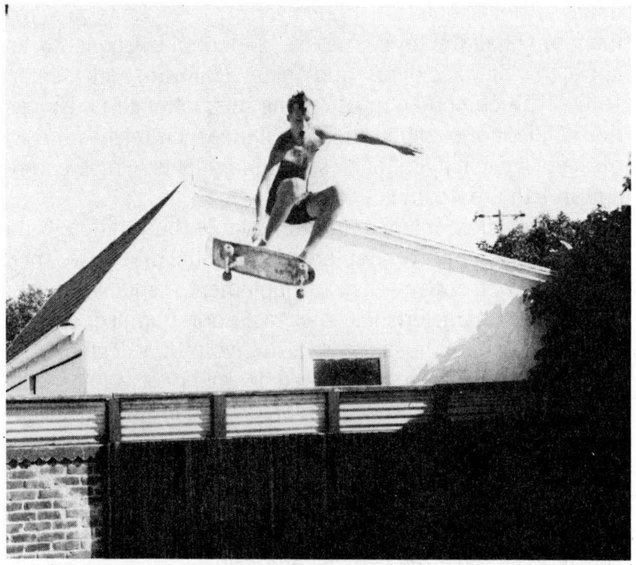

Fig. 19-17. Teenager riding a skateboard from the roof of a neighbor's house into a backyard swimming pool.

extensive discussion of bicycle injuries and bicycle safety, see Chapter 17.

Motor Vehicle–Related Injuries

Teenage drivers contribute substantially to vehicular fatalities, both their own and those of others. Almost half the fatalities in the 16- to 19-year-olds are related to motor vehicles (Rivara, 1988). The adolescent's newly acquired ability to drive and the normal developmental need for independence and freedom make the automobile an attractive if not necessary part of adolescent life. A significant number of fatal teenage injuries involve vehicles that were being driven too fast for the existing conditions. Almost all are related to the actions of the driver and are disproportionately high among young drivers—often caused by ignorance of or disregard for sound and defensive driving principles. Most fatal injuries involving adolescent drivers occur because of improper driving or poor judgment on the part of the driver. These young people, delighted with the freedom that a driver's license affords them, are less concerned about the new responsibilities associated with this freedom. They have yet to learn behavioral patterns that are gained with experience and maturity.

Teenagers have a natural proclivity for experimentation with new behaviors. Unfortunately, they exhibit poor judgment in weighing the expected gain or utility against the possible harm when engaging in a risky behavior. Developmentally their behavior appears very self-centered; their concern is only for themselves. They act irresponsibly and have difficulty understanding how their behavior might cause injury to other persons.

Characteristics of motor vehicle accidents (MVAs) among adolescents have been identified. More than half of MVAs among adolescents occur at night between the hours of 8 PM and 4 AM (Vance and others, 1989). Males are twice as likely to be involved in a serious MVA at night as females. Adolescents are poor users of seat belts and use them only half the time. The use of alcohol is frequently associated with accidents and injury (Runyan and Gerken, 1989). The combination of driving inexperience and ingestion of alcohol or other illicit substances diminishes the adolescent's capacity to make sound judgments, which can result in lethal outcomes.

Motor vehicle injuries are preventable, but, although the implications for prevention are obvious, the preventive measures are not always easy to implement, especially when behavioral characteristics such as poor impulse control, recklessness, and hostility are also involved. A degree of social experimentation is involved in much of adolescents' behavior. Young men feel pressured to be brave and exhibit a "macho" image, which often involves disregarding speed limits and other safety laws, as well as intentional failure to use passenger restraints (Brown, Sanders, and Schonberg, 1986). Young drivers are also encouraged by peers to speed, overcrowd the vehicle, and drink.

The role that nurses can play in prevention of motor vehicle injuries is to become active proponents of driver education and safety programs in the school and community that emphasize the use of good driving habits and judgment. They can encourage teenagers to obtain such instruction and encourage parents to determine the quality of this instruction and to take measures to improve the quality if it is found lacking.

Nonautomotive Vehicle Injuries

The increasing use of other motorized vehicles, such as all-terrain vehicles (ATVs), mopeds, and snowmobiles, has caused an increase in injuries related to these vehicles, especially among youngsters below the legal age for driving automobiles. The mean age of children sustaining moped injuries is 12.8 years (Westman and Morrow, 1984). The injuries are more serious than bicycle injuries, although mopeds are often considered to be deluxe bicycles rather than motorized vehicles. Consequently, little driver preparation and instruction are required.

ATVs are capable of speeds up to 70 miles per hour. The instability of ATVs on rough terrain, along with lack of helmet use by the drivers, makes them very unsafe (Runyan and Gerken, 1989). Head injuries are the primary cause of death. The majority of injuries involve the moped and another vehicle, but burn injuries have been reported from contact with the hot muffler, especially when youngsters are riding double (Bantz and Auerbach, 1982). It has been recommended that moped use be regulated, including establishing a minimum age for driving, and making mandatory the use of helmets, riding within prescribed limits (within 3 feet of the right side of the road), and the provision of safety equipment on the moped (e.g., rearview mirror, turning signals).

Firearms

Improper use of firearms continues to be one of the leading causes of death in the adolescent age-group, occurring mainly in or on home premises. The natural interest in gun-related activities is accelerated at this time, when almost half the victims of firearm fatalities are between ages of 15 and 24. Instruction in the use of firearms should be taught at an appropriate age by parents and is probably best accomplished in cooperation with a youth organization or professional association. Most injuries from firearms can be prevented when proper safety precautions are taken in the use and storage of firearms. For example, loaded guns should never be permitted in or around the home, and guns and ammunition must be stored where only appropriate adults have access to them.

Nonpowder firearms. Nonpowder guns (air rifles, BB guns), although viewed as toys by many, account for almost as many injuries as powder guns. Among children ages 5 to 14, the incidence of injury is three times that of powder guns (Christoffel and others, 1984). The regulations regarding nonpowder guns are relaxed; they can be purchased legally by youngsters and are labeled as suitable for children as young as 8 years. Few states regulate their use. As child advocates, nurses can push for legislation to regulate the sale of these potentially dangerous "toys."

Sports and Recreational Injuries

Injuries from sports and recreational activities are the most common nonfatal injuries among adolescents. The leading cause of sports injuries among males is participation in football, whereas females are injured while participating in gymnastics (Goldberg and others, 1988). Poor equipment and inadequate supervision seem to play a role in the cause of injury. Coaching staff need education in injury prevention and the management of acute sports injuries. See Chapter 39 for a discussion of sports injuries.

Occupational Injuries

Occupational injuries have received little attention in health care literature. Depending on the site of employment, youth can be at risk for a variety of injuries. Convenience store and gas station employees are at risk for shootings. The use of hot grease by fast-food restaurants can result in burn injuries, and youths working in agricultural settings are at risk for severe injuries to limbs and crush injuries from operating heavy farm equipment (Runyan and Gerken, 1989).

Nursing Considerations

Because of the magnitude of the problem, greater attention is being given to the science of injury prevention and understanding the theory of risk in adolescents. Prevention can occur on a variety of levels. Safety advocacy, changing public policy, and legislation can curtail injuries. Examples of such approaches are laws that mandate wearing seat belts,

Table 19-2 Injury prevention during adolescence

DEVELOPMENTAL ABILITIES RELATED TO RISK OF INJURY	INJURY PREVENTION
Need for independence and freedom Testing independence Age permitted to drive a motor vehicle (varies) Propensity for risk taking Feeling of indestructibility Need for discharging energy, often at expense of logical thinking and other control mechanisms Strong need for peer approval May attempt hazardous feats Peak incidence for practice and participation in sports Access to more complex tools, objects, and locations Can assume responsibility for own actions	**Motor vehicles** *Pedestrian*—emphasize and encourage safe pedestrian behavior *Passenger*—promote appropriate behavior while riding in a motor vehicle *Driver*—provide competent driver education; encourage judicious use of vehicle, discourage drag racing, "chicken"; maintain vehicle in proper condition (brakes, tires) Teach and promote safety and maintenance of two-wheeled and all-terrain vehicles Promote and encourage wearing of safety apparel such as helmet, long trousers Reinforce the dangers of drugs, including alcohol, when operating a motor vehicle **Drowning** Teach to swim (if adolescent unable to do so) Teach basic rules of water safety: Judicious selection of place to swim Sufficient water depth for diving Swimming with companion **Burns** Reinforce proper behavior in areas involving contact with burn hazards (gasoline, electric wires, fires) Advise regarding excessive exposure to sunlight (ultraviolet burn) Discourage smoking Encourage use of sunscreen **Poisoning** Educate in hazards of drug use, including alcohol **Falls** Teach and encourage general safety measures in all activities **Bodily damage** Promote acquisition of proper instruction in sports and use of sports equipment Promote use of appropriate arena for sports activities Instruct in safe use of and respect for firearms and other devices with potential danger (e.g., power tools, firecrackers) Provide and encourage use of protective equipment when using potentially hazardous devices Promote access to and/or provision of safe sports and recreational facilities Be alert for signs of depression (potential suicide) Discourage use of and/or availability of hazardous sports equipment (trampoline, surfboards) Instruct regarding proper use of corrective devices such as glasses, contact lenses, hearing aids Encourage and foster judicious application of safety principles and prevention

mandatory helmet use while driving moving vehicles other than automobiles, increasing the legal drinking age to 21 years, and instituting curfews for teen drivers.

In addition to improving the environment, health education for teenagers and significant adults is essential. Helping adolescents understand their need for engaging in risk behavior, exploring possible negative outcomes, and weighing possible alternatives are critical components of injury prevention (Vance and others, 1989).

School nurses, in cooperation with other persons involved with youth, such as teachers, activity leaders, and parent groups, can help to evaluate sports and athletic programs, assess environmental conditions, and institute changes that emphasize prevention of injury. They can help to assess the needs for emergency services, institute such services, and provide care and guidance when needed. Developmental characteristics of adolescents that predispose them to injury and suggestions for injury prevention related to these developmental expectations are listed in Table 19-2.

Nurses need to be involved at all levels of intervention, such as through professional organizations that sponsor policy initiatives or health education programs. Participation in local civic organizations or school districts to devise and implement such programs with youths and parents is vital.

Box 19-3 GUIDANCE DURING ADOLESCENCE

Accept adolescent as a human being.
Respect adolescent's ideas, likes and dislikes, wishes.
Provide opportunity for choosing options and accept natural consequences of these choices.
Allow youngster to learn by doing, even when choices and methods differ from those of adults.
Provide adolescent with clear, reasonable limits.
Clarify house rules and consequences for breaking them.
Use family conferences to negotiate house rules.
Allow increasing independence within limitations of safety and well-being.
Be available but avoid pressing youngster too far.
Respect adolescent's privacy.
Try to share adolescent's feelings of joy or sorrow.
Respond to feelings as well as words.
Give space to a teenager who is in a bad mood.
Be available to answer questions, give information, and provide companionship.
Listen and try to be open to youngster's views, even when they disagree with parental views.
Try to make communication clear.
Assist adolescent in selecting appropriate career goals and preparing for adult role.
Provide undemanding love.

Be aware that:
Adolescent is struggling for independence.
Adolescent is extraordinarily sensitive to feelings and behavior that affect him or her.
Message given to adolescent may not be message received.
Friends are extremely important to adolescent.
Adolescent has a strong need "to belong."
Adolescent sees things in black or white, good or bad.

ANTICIPATORY GUIDANCE—CARE OF FAMILIES

The parents of the adolescent are usually as confused and perplexed as the youngster is about the changes and behavior of this stage of development. They also need support and guidance to help them through this trying time. They need to understand the changes taking place and to understand and accept the expected behaviors that accompany the process of detachment, to be prepared to "let go," and to promote the changed relationship from one of dependency to one of mutuality. Suggestions for anticipatory guidance of parents with an adolescent are listed in Box 19-3. Nurses interested in providing family-centered care are referred to the Bibliography for additional information on this expanding topic. (See also Communicating with Children, Chapter 6.)

KEY POINTS

- Adolescence is an important period of development in which significant psychologic, social, and maturation adjustments are made in the move toward adulthood.
- Biologic development during puberty is characterized primarily by hormonal activity in which sexual maturation and skin changes take place.
- According to Erikson, the major developmental crisis of adolescence is establishing a sense of identity.
- In Freudian terms, adolescence marks the beginning of the genital period, in which sexual maturation prepares the individual to satisfy the sex instinct through procreation.
- Cognitive development in adolescence is revealed through thinking beyond the present, logical thought, and a sense of idealism.
- According to Kohlberg's theory of moral development, adolescents begin to question existing moral values and learn to make choices; Gilligan observed differences in the way males and females make moral decisions.
- Spiritual development is characterized by the questioning of family values and ideals, a move to more philosophical thinking, and emphasis on personal religion.
- Adolescent relationships with parents may be strained, whereas the influence of the peer group and heterosexual relationships increases.
- Development of body image is closely tied to sexual awareness, as adolescents cope with sexual maturation.
- Maturation of reproductive organs precipitates sexual feelings in adolescents; heterosexual relationships offer adolescents the opportunity to test new feelings and make decisions regarding sexual activities.
- Homosexual youths have unique issues to cope with in identity formation.
- Emotionality in adolescence fluctuates between periods of stability and periods of instability.

- **Nutritional needs for protein, minerals, and iron may be impaired by adolescents' eating habits of snacking and irregular mealtimes.**
- **Motor vehicle injuries and drowning are the greatest causes of mortality from injuries in this age-group.**

REFERENCES

American Academy of Pediatrics, Committee on Adolescence: Homosexuality and adolescence, Pediatrics 72:249-250, 1983.

Bantz, E., and Auerbach, J.: Leg burns from mopeds, Pediatrics 70:304-305, 1982.

Bidwell, R.J.: The gay and lesbian teen: a case of denied adolescence, J. Pediatr. Health Care 2:3-8, 1988.

Black, J.L.: School-based clinics: filling unmet needs for teens, Compr. Pediatr. 6(3):117-140, 1989.

Blos, P.: The adolescent passage: developmental issues, New York, 1979, International Universities Press, Inc.

Brooks-Gunn, J., and Furstenberg, F.: Adolescent sexual behavior, Am. Psychol. 44:249-257, 1989.

Brown, R.C., Sanders, J.M., and Schonberg, S.K.: Driving safety and adolescent behavior, Pediatrics 77:603-607, 1986.

Christoffel, K.K., and others: Childhood injuries caused by nonpowder firearms, Am. J. Dis. Child. 138:557-561, 1984.

Conger, J.J., and Petersen, A.C.: Adolescence and youth. Psychologic development in a changing world, ed. 3, New York, 1984, Harper & Row, Publishers, Inc.

Dickinson, G.E.: Changing religious behavior of adolescents 1964-1979, Youth Soc. 13:283-288, 1982.

Elkind, D.: All grown up and no place to go: teenagers in crisis, Menlo Park, CA, 1984, Addison-Wesley Publishing Co., Inc.

Erikson, E.H.: Childhood and society, ed. 2, New York, 1963, W.W. Norton & Co., Inc.

Faelten, S.: Rock music: can it hurt your child? Children, pp. 69-73, Aug. 1988.

Fedler, F., Hall, J., and Tanzi, L.: Popular songs emphasize sex, deemphasize romance, Mass. Commun. Rev. 9:10-15, 1982.

Gaddis, A., and Brooks-Gunn, J.: The male experience of puberty, J. Youth Adolesc. 14:61-69, 1985.

Gagnon, J.H.: Human sexuality, Glenview, IL, 1977, Scott, Foresman & Co.

Gagnon, J.H., and Simon, W.: The sexual scripting of oral genital contacts, Arch. Sex Behav. 16:1-25, 1987.

Galanter, M.: Psychological induction into the large group: findings from a contemporary religious sect, Am. J. Psychiatry, 137:154-159, 1980.

Garn, S.M., LaVelle, M., and Pilkington, J.J.: Comparisons of fatness in premenarcheal and postmenarcheal girls of the same age, J. Pediatr. 103:328-331, 1983.

Gilligan, C.: In a different voice: psychological theory and women's development, Cambridge, MA, 1982, Harvard University Press.

Goldberg, B., and others: Injuries in youth football, Pediatrics 81:255-261, 1988.

Gordon, S., and Snyder, C.W.: A guidebook for better sexual health, Boston, 1989, Allyn & Bacon, Inc.

Grant, L.M., and Demetriou, E.: Adolescent sexuality, Pediatr. Clin. North Am. 35:1271-1289, 1988.

Harris, L., and others: American teens speak: sex, myths, TV and birth control, New York, 1986, Planned Parenthood Federation of America.

Harris, L., and others: Sexual material on American network television during the 1987-1988 season, New York, 1988, Planned Parenthood Federation of America.

Hayes, C.D., editor: Risking the future: adolescent sexuality, pregnancy, and childbearing, vol. 1, Washington, DC, 1987, National Academy Press.

Hoelter, J., and Harper, L.: Structural and interpersonal family influences on adolescent self-conception, J. Marriage Fam. 49:129-139, 1987.

Kaluger, G., and Kaluger, M.F.: Human development: the span of life, ed. 4, St. Louis, 1988, Mosby–Year Book, Inc.

Kaplan, S.A.: Clinical pediatric and adolescent endocrinology, Philadelphia, 1982, W.B. Saunders Co.

Katchadourian, H.: Adolescent sexuality, Pediatr. Clin. North Am. 27:17-28, 1980.

Keenan, T.: School-based adolescent health-care programs, Pediatr. Nurs. 12:365-369, 1986.

Kohlberg, L.: The cognitive-developmental approach to moral education, Phi Delta Kappan 56:670-677, 1975.

Marino, D.D., and King, J.C.: Nutritional concerns during adolescence, Pediatr. Clin. North Am. 27:125-140, 1980.

Muuss, R.E.: Theories of adolescence, ed. 5, New York, 1988, Random House.

Nokes, K.M.: Rethinking moral reasoning theory, Image 21:172-175, 1989.

Orr, D.P., and others: Reported sexual behaviors and self-esteem among young adolescents, Am. J. Dis. Child. 143:86-90, 1989.

Peterson, A., and Spiga, R.: Adolescence and stress. In Goldberg, L., and Breznitz, M., editors: Handbook of stress: theoretical and clinical aspects, New York, 1982, Free Press.

Rivara, F.P.: Motor vehicle injuries during adolescence, Pediatr. Ann. 17:107-113, 1988.

Runyan, C.W., and Gerken, E.A.: Epidemiology and prevention of adolescent injury, JAMA 262:2273-2279, 1989.

Sanford, N.D.: Providing sensitive health care to gay and lesbian youth, Nurse Pract. 14(5):30-47, 1989.

Savin-Williams, R.C.: Theoretical perspectives accounting for adolescent homosexuality, J. Adolesc. Health Care 9:95-104, 1988.

Shelly, J.A.: The spiritual needs of children, Downers Grove, IL, 1982, Inter-Varsity Press.

Sherman, B.L., and Dominick, J.R.: Violence and sex in music video: TV and rock 'n' roll, J. Commun. 36:79-93, 1986.

Silverman-Watkins, L.T.: Sex in the contemporary media. In Maddock, J.W., Neubeck, G., and Sussman, M.B., editors: Human sexuality and the family, New York, 1983, The Haworth Press, Inc.

Simmons, R., and others: The impact of cumulative change in early adolescence, Child Devel. 58:1220-1234, 1987.

Soderman, A., as reported in Child. Teens Today 8(5):3, 1988.

Sprafkin, J., and Silverman, L.T.: Physically intimate and sexual behavior on prime-time television, 1978-1979, J. Commun. 31:34-40, 1981.

Strasburger, V.C.: Adolescent sexuality and the media, Pediatr. Clin. North Am. 36:747-773, 1989.

Street, S.: Feedback and self-concept in high school students, Adolescence 23:449-456, 1988.

Sun, S.W., and Lull, J.: The adolescent audience for music videos and why they watch, J. Commun. 36:115-125, 1986.

Thornburg, H.: Adolescent sources of information on sex, J. Sch. Health 51:274-277, 1981.

Troiden, R.R.: Homosexual identity formation, J. Adolesc. Health Care 9:105-113, 1988.

Udry, J.R., and others: Serum androgenic hormones motivate sexual behavior in adolescent boys, Fertil. Steril. 43:90-94, 1985.

Vance, C.J., and others: Preventing adolescent injury: roles for the health professionals, Newton, MA, 1989, Education Development Center, Inc.

Voss, J.R.: A model for helping adolescents make decisions about sex in the age of AIDS: Reported in Child. Teens Today 8(10):5, 1988.

Wattleton, F.: American teens: sexually active, sexually illiterate, J. Sch. Health 57:379-380, 1987.

Westman, J.A., and Morrow, G., III: Moped injuries in children, Pediatrics 74:820-822, 1984.

Woods, N.F.: Toward a holistic perspective of human sexuality: alterations in sexual health and nursing diagnoses, Holistic Nurs. Practice 1(4):1-11, 1987.

BIBLIOGRAPHY

General

American Academy of Pediatrics, Committee on Communications: Impact of rock lyrics and music videos on children and youth, Pediatrics 83:314-315, 1989.

Bane, M.J., and Ellwood, D.T.: One fifth of the nation's children: why are they poor? Science 245:1047-1053, 1989.

Boggs, K.U.: Pubertal status and social support-seeking behavior in early adolescents, J. Pediatr. Nurs. 3:229-236, 1988.

Brooks-Gunn, J., and Petersen, A.C.: Problems in studying and defining pubertal events, J. Youth Adolesc. 13:181-196, 1984.

Brown, E.F., and Hendee, W.R.: Adolescents and their music, JAMA 262:1659-1663, 1989.

Carr, M., and others: Curling-iron cornea (letter), N. Engl. J. Med. 319:1672, 1988.

Dornbusch, S.M., and others: The relation of parenting style to adolescent school performance, Child Dev. 58:1244-1257, 1987.

Duryea, E.J., and Hammes, M.J.: Cognitive development and the dynamics of decision-making among adolescents, J. Sch. Health 56:224-226, 1986.

Erikson, E.H.: Identity: youth and crisis, New York, 1968, W.W. Norton & Co., Inc.

Erikson, E.H.: Dimensions of a new identity, New York, 1974, W.W. Norton & Co., Inc.

Gilligan, C., Ward, J.V., and Taylor, J.M. editors: Mapping the moral domain, Cambridge, MA, 1988, Harvard University Press.

Gillis, C.L., and others: Toward a science of family nursing, Menlo Park, CA, 1989, Addison-Wesley Publishing Co., Inc.

Goldenring, J.M., and Cohen, E.: Getting into adolescent heads, Contemp. Pediatr. 5(7):75-90, 1988.

Grady, K., Gersick, K.E., and Boratynski, M.: Preparing parents for teenagers: a step in the prevention of adolescent substance abuse, Fam. Rel. 34:541-549, 1985.

Hamburg, D., Nightningale, E.O., and Takanishi, R.: Facilitating the transitions of adolescence, JAMA 257:3405-3406, 1987.

Havens, B., and Swenson, I.: Menstrual perceptions and preparation among female adolescents, JOGNN 15:406-411, 1986.

Irwin, C.E., and Millstein, S.G.: Biopsychosocial correlates of risk-taking behaviors during adolescence: can the physician intervene? J. Adolesc. Health Care 7(suppl):82S, 1986.

Kerrins, K.M.: Comparing the self-image of prepubescent girls before and after four sessions on body awareness, J. Sch. Health 53:541-543, 1983.

Koval, J.E.: Violence in dating relationships, J. Pediatr. Nurs. 3:298-304, 1989.

Lerner, R.M., and Foch, T.T.: Biological-psychosocial interactions in early adolescence, Hillside, NJ, 1987, Lawrence Erlbaum Assoc.

Levine, M.D., and McAnarney, E.R., editors: Early adolescent transitions, Lexington, MA, 1988, Lexington Books.

Long, T.J., and others: Basic issues in adolescent medicine, Curr. Probl. Pediatr. 14(10):3-49, 1984.

Lowery, G.H.: Growth and development of children, ed. 8, Chicago, 1986, Mosby–Year Book, Inc.

Morse, I.M., and McKinnon, D.: Adolescents' response to menarche, J. Sch. Health 57:385-388, 1987.

Newman, B., and Newman, P.: The impact of high school on social development, Adolescence 22:525-533, 1987.

Offer, D., Ostrov, E., and Howard, K.I.: Adolescence: what is normal? Am. J. Dis. Child. 143:731-736, 1989.

Orr, D.P., and Ingersoll, G.M.: Adolescent development: a biopsychosocial review, Curr. Probl. Pediatr. 18:443-499, 1988.

Piaget, J.: The theory of stages in cognitive development, New York, 1969, McGraw-Hill, Inc.

Schmitt, B.D.: Dealing with normal adolescent rebellion, Contemp. Pediatr. 7(7):55-60, 1990.

Schwartz, I.D., and Root, A.W.: Puberty in girls: normal or delayed? Contemp. Pediatr. 6(11):83-104, 1989.

Shaffer, D.R.: Developmental psychology: theory, research, and applications, Monterey, CA, 1985, Brooks/Cole Publishing Co.

Slap, G.B.: Normal physiological and psychosocial growth in the adolescent, J. Adolesc. Health Care 7(suppl):13-23, 1986.

Stanwyck, D.J.: Self-esteem through the life span, Fam. Community Health 6(2):11-28, 1983.

Steinberg, L., and Silberberg, S.S.: The vicissitudes of autonomy in early adolescence, Child. Dev. 57:841-851, 1986.

Stone, L.J., and Church, J.: Childhood and adolescence, ed. 5, New York, 1983, Random House, Inc.

Tanner, J.M.: Issues and advances in adolescent growth and development, J. Adolesc. Health Care 8:470-478, 1987.

Thomas, M.A., and Rebar, R.W.: The endocrinology of normal and abnormal puberty, Curr. Opin. Obstet. Gynecol. 1:259-265, 1989.

Vaughn, V.C., and Litt, I.F.: Child and adolescent development: clinical implications, Philadelphia, 1990, W.B. Saunders Co.

Willits, F.K.: Adolescent behavior and adult success and well-being: a 37-year panel study, Youth Society 20:68-87, 1988.

Sexuality and Sex Education

Adger, H., Jr., and DeAngelis, C.: Sexuality education: our schools can do better, Contemp. Pediatr. 6(10):56-65, 1989.

Burke, P.J.: Adolescents' motivation for sexual activity and pregnancy prevention, Issues Compr. Pediatr. Nurs. 10:161-171, 1987.

Calderone, M.S.: Adolescent sexuality: elements and genesis, Pediatrics 76:699-703, 1985.

Committee on Adolescence: Homosexuality and adolescence, Pediatrics 72:249-250, 1983.

Crooks, R., and Baur, K.: Our sexuality, ed. 4, Redwood City, CA, 1990, The Benjamin/Cummings Publishing Co.

Hofferth, S.L., and Hayes, C.D., editors: Risking the future: adolescent sexuality, pregnancy and childbearing, Washington, DC, 1987, National Academy Press.

Kenney, R.D.: A guide to sexual abstinence couseling, Contemp. Pediatr. 6(12):83-95, 1989.

Lowry, L.W., and McGinnis, D.G.: Intergenerational education in human sexuality, MCN 14:341-345, 1989.

Powell, L.H., and Jorgensen, S.R.: Evaluation of church-based sexuality education program for adolescents, Fam. Rel. 34:475-482, 1985.

Remafedi, G.: Adolescent homosexuality: psychosocial and medical implications, Pediatrics 9:331-337, 1987.

Remafedi, G.: Homosexual youth: a challenge to contemporary society, JAMA 258:222-225, 1987.

Remafedi, G.: Male homosexuality: the adolescent's perspective, Pediatrics 79:326-330, 1987.

Sheehan, M.K., Ostwald, S.K., and Rothenberger, J.: Perceptions of sexual responsibility: do young men and women agree? Pediatr. Nurs. 12:17-21, 1986.

Stout, J.W., and Rivara, F.P.: Schools and sex education: does it work? Pediatrics 83:375-379, 1989.

Taylor, M.O.: Teaching parents about their impaired adolescent's sexuality, MCN 14:109-112, 1989.

Wattleton, F.: American teens: sexually active, sexually illiterate, J. Sch. Health 57:379-380, 1987.

Health Promotion During Adolescence

Adams, B.N.: Adolescent health care: needs, priorities and services, Nurs. Clin. North Am. 18:237-248, 1983.

American Medical Association, Council on Scientific Affairs: Harmful effects of ultraviolet radiation, JAMA 262:380-384, 1989.

American Medical Association, Council on Scientific Affairs: Providing medical services through school-based health programs, JAMA 261:1939-1942, 1989.

Barley, Z.B.: Adolescent health: a Colorado experience, Issues Compr. Pediatr. Nurs. 10:315-329, 1987.

Bearinger, L., and Gephardt, J.: Priorities for adolescent health: recommendations of a national conference, MCN 12:161-164, 1987.

Bradley, J.M.: Do adolescents practice what they preach about health? Pediatr. Nurs. 10:285-289, 1984.

Church, J.L., and Baer, K.J.: Examination of the adolescent; a practical guide, J. Pediatr. Health Care 1:65-72, 1987.

Craft, M.J.: Health care preferences of rural adolescents: types of service and companion choices, J. Pediatr. Nurs. 2:3-12, 1987.

Cromer, B.A., and others: Psychosocial determinants of compliance in adolescents with iron deficiency, Am. J. Dis. Child. 143:55-58, 1989.

Elkind, D.: Teenage thinking: implications for health care, Pediatr. Nurs. 10:383-385, 1984.

Ell, K., and Northern, H.: Families and health care: psychosocial practice, New York, 1990, Adline de Gruyter.

Epidemiologic Notes and Reports: Injuries associated with ultraviolet tanning devices—Wisconsin, MMWR 38:333-334, 1989.

Fisher, M., and others: Are adolescents able and willing to pay the fee for confidential health care? J. Pediatr. 170:480-483, 1985.

Food and Nutrition Board, National Research Council: Recommended dietary allowances, ed. 10, Washington, DC, 1989, National Academy of Sciences.

Greene, J.: Making adolescent space in a pediatric office, Pediatr. Nurs. 15:402-403, 1989.

Greene, J.W., and others: Stressful life events and somatic complaints in adolescents, Pediatrics 75:19-22, 1985.

Hoffman, A.D. and Greydanus, D.E., editors: Adolescent medicine, ed. 2, Norwalk, CT, 1989, Appleton & Lange.

Joffe, A., Radius, S., and Gall, M.: Health counseling for adolescents: what they want, what they get, and who gives it, Pediatrics 82:481-485, 1988.

Jordan, D., and Kelfer, L.S.: Adolescent potential for participation in health care, Issues Compr. Pediatr. Nurs. 6:147-156, 1983.

Klerman, L.V.: School absence—a health perspective, Pediatr. Clin. North Am. 35:1253-1269, 1988.

Kulbok, P., Earls, F.J., and Montgomery, A.C.: Life-style and patterns of health and social behavior in high-risk adolescents, Adv. Nurs. Sci. 11:22-35, 1988.

Leiman, A.H., and Strasburger, V.C.: Counseling parents of adolescents, Pediatrics 76:664-667, 1985.

Litt, I.F.: Know thyself—adolescents' self-assessment of compliance behavior, Pediatrics 75:693-696, 1985.

Lyons, J.A.F.: Adolescent health and school-based clinics, Issues Compre. Pediatr. Nurs. 10:303-314, 1987.

Magilvy, J.K.: Health of adolescents: research in school health, Issues Compr. Pediatr. Nurs. 10:291-302, 1987.

Mahan, L.K., and Rees, J.M.: Nutrition in adolescence, St. Louis, 1984, Mosby–Year Book, Inc.

Marks, A., and Fisher, M.: Health assessment and screening during adolescence, Pediatrics 80 (suppl):135-158, 1987.

Millstein, S.G.: Adolescent health: challenges for behavioral scientists, Am. Psychol. 44:837-842, 1989.

Newacheck, P.W.: Improving access to health services for adolescents from economically disadvantaged families, Pediatrics 84:1056-1063, 1989.

Newacheck, P.W.: Adolescents with special health needs: prevalence, severity, and access to health services, Pediatrics 84:872-881, 1989.

Olds, R.S.: Promoting child health through comprehensive school health programs: an investment in America's future, Fam. Community Health 11(4):32-40, 1989.

Panzarine, S., and others: Adolescent health care: a challenge for nursing educators, J. Nurs. Ed. 27:278-280, 1988.

Perry, C.L., and Murray, D.M.: Enhancing the transition years: the challenge of adolescent health promotion, J. Sch. Health 52:307-311, 1982.

Pipes, P.L.: Nutrition in infancy and childhood, ed. 4, St. Louis, 1989, Mosby–Year Book, Inc.

Sachs, B.P: Cognitive screening for adolescent health education, J. Pediatr. Nurs. 2:113-119, 1987.

Smith, K.L., Turner, J.G., and Jacobsen, R.B.: Health concerns of adolescents, Pediatr. Nurs. 13:311-315, 1987.

Sobal, J., and others: Health concerns of high school students and teachers' beliefs about student health concerns, Pediatrics 81:218-223, 1988.

Wildey, L.S., and Barton, A.P.: Training in adolescent health for nurse practitioners, J. Pediatr. Health Care 2:195-199, 1988.

Injury Prevention

American Academy of Pediatrics, Committee on Accident and Poison Prevention: Snowmobile statement, Pediatrics 82:798-799, 1988.

Bass, J.L., Gallagher, S.S., and Mehta, K.A.: Injuries to adolescents and young adults, Pediatr. Clin. North Am. 32:31-39, 1985.

Blocker, S., Coln, D., and Chang, J.H.T.: Serious air rifle injuries in children, Pediatrics 9:751-754, 1982.

Christoffel, K.K., and Christoffel, T.: Handguns: risks versus benefits, Pediatrics 77:781-782, 1986.

Christoffel, K.K., and Tanz, R.: Motor vehicle injury in childhood, Pediatr. Rev. 4:247-250, 1983.

Greensher, J.: Non-automotive vehicle injuries in adolescents, Pediatr. Ann. 17:114-121, 1988.

Jack, M.S.: Personal fable: a potential explanation for risk-taking behavior in adolescents, J. Pediatr. Nurs. 4:334-338, 1989.

Lawrence, H.S.: Fatal nonpowder firearm wounds: case report and review of the literature, Pediatrics 85:177-181, 1990.

Lee, E.J., and Jacobson, J.M.: Accident reports: survey of high school injuries, Pediatr. Nurs. 13:151-154, 1987.

Lee, E.J., Jacobson, J.M., and Levanas, V.: Stressful life events and accidents at school, Pediatr. Nurs. 15:140-142, 1989.

Myre, L.E., and Black, R.E.: Serious air gun injuries in children: update of injury statistics and presentation of five cases, Pediatr. Emerg. Care 3:168-170, 1987.

Orlowski, J.: Adolescent drownings: swimming, boating, diving, and scuba accidents, Pediatr. Ann. 17:125-132, 1987.

Osguthorpe, N.C., and Osguthorpe, J.D.: Scuba diving hazards: emergency management, Am. J. Nurs. 81:1456-1458, 1981.

Paulson, J.A.: The epidemiology of injuries in adolescents, Pediatr. Ann. 17:84-96, 1988.

Sadowski, L.S., Cairns, R.B., and Earp, J.A.: Firearm ownership among nonurban adolescents, Am. J. Dis. Child. 143:1410-1413, 1989.

Schetky, D.H.: Children and handguns, Am. J. Dis. Child. 139:229-231, 1985.

Spivak, H., Prothrow-Stith, D., and Hausman, A.J.: Dying is no accident: adolescents, violence, and intentional injury, Pediatr. Clin. North Am. 35:1339-1347, 1988.

Steinberg, L.: Single parents, stepparents, and the susceptibility of adolescents to antisocial behavior, Child Dev. 58:269-275, 1987.

Tanz, R., Christoffel, K.K., and Sagerman, S.: Are toy guns to dangerous? Pediatrics 75:265-268, 1985.

Tedesco, L.A., and Gaier, E.L.: Friendship bonds in adolescence, Adolescence 23:127-135, 1988.

Thompson, C.E., and Stroud, S.D.: The motorized tricycle: an accident waiting to happen, J. Pediatr. Nurs. 2:120-125, 1987.

Wintemute, G.J., Teret, S.P., and Kraus, J.F.: Plastic handguns that resemble toy guns: new technology creates a uniquely hazardous product, Pediatrics 81:316-317, 1988.

CHAPTER 20

Physical Health Problems of Adolescence

RELATED TOPICS

Behavioral health problems of adolescence, Ch. 21
Disorders affecting the skin, Ch. 18
Genitalia (examination), Ch. 7
Health promotion of the adolescent and family, Ch. 19
Infection control, Ch. 27
Precocious puberty, Ch. 38

GLOSSARY

CDC Centers for Disease Control
IM Infectious mononucleosis
IUD Intrauterine device
IVDU Intravenous drug user
Miscarriage Spontaneous abortion
PID Pelvic inflammatory disease
PIH Pregnancy-induced hypertension
STD Sexually transmitted disease

There are 36 million children in the United States between the ages of 10 and 19 years. More than one fourth of these youth are members of ethnic minorities, including 15% black and 9% Hispanic. Poverty is playing an increasingly important role in determining their quality of life and access to medical care today. It is estimated that one of every five children lives in poverty (Bane and Ellwood, 1989; Wise and Meyers, 1988). Also, an estimated 6.5 million adolescents (ages 10 to 19) live in poverty and 3.3 million of these are minority children (Hamburg, Nightingale, and Takanishi, 1987). This creates a dilemma for health care providers who support access to optimum health care in the face of social forces that impede quality care.

Adolescence is a period of rapid biologic growth and psychosocial transitions and is frequently perceived as a time of optimum wellness. Logically, promotion of optimum wellness, which emphasizes not only absence of disease but a positive sense of well-being and personal achievement, should have its inception during this developmental stage. Examination of information about the health status of adolescents has lead to a growing concern of professionals from many health disciplines (e.g., nursing, medicine, psychology, social work, nutrition, education), many of whom are involved with research or delivery of health services to this group (Millstein, 1989). A noticeable increase in risk-taking behaviors occurs with adolescents, which can lead to either death or disability during this otherwise generally healthy time of life.

Accidental injuries account for 70% of deaths among persons age 10 to 19 years. Adolescents are the only age-group who have not experienced a decline in their death rate since 1950. These injuries are often the result of volitional behaviors, many of which could be prevented or minimized (Irwin and Millstein, 1986). These include drinking and driving, under use of protective devices (e.g., seat belts, helmets), and poor coping and stress management, which result in violent deaths from homicide or suicide (see Chapter 19 for a discussion of injury prevention).

In addition to mortality, behaviors that alter quality of life or life expectancy have their onset during this time. Cigarette smoking provides a classic illustration of a long-term negative health habit that begins during the teenage years. Smoking usually starts at age 12 to 13 years and is established as a lifelong pattern in 95% of all smokers by age 20 (Runyan and Gerkin, 1989). One in four adolescents does not graduate from high school, severely limiting the ability to succeed in the job market. Early onset of sexual activity frequently leads to unintentional pregnancy or sexually transmitted disease (STD), which can have a variety of negative outcomes (Hamburg, Nightingale, and Takanishi, 1987).

Efforts to combat the magnitude of health problems that occur during adolescence have never been sufficient. Surveys reveal that most health care professionals believe they received inadequate educational preparation to deal with the complexity of health and behavioral issues experienced by teenagers. Nurses have not been exempt from this void in professional education (Bearinger and Gephart, 1987; Panzarine and others, 1988). The emphasis of this chapter is on the physical problems of adolescence and the nurse's role in health management.

Jeanette M. Broering, R.N., M.S., C.P.N.P., assisted in the revision of this chapter.

COMMON HEALTH PROBLEMS OF ADOLESCENCE

There are a number of health problems that have their onset in adolescence or are more prominent at this stage of development than at earlier or subsequent ages.

ACNE

Adolescents are subject to the same skin conditions that affect the school-age child, such as bacterial, viral, and fungal infection; contact dermatitis; and drug reactions. However, there is one skin disorder that, although not limited to the adolescent age-group, appears predominantly at this time—*acne vulgaris* (common acne). Acne is an almost universal occurrence during these years and involves anatomic, physiologic, biochemical, genetic, immunologic, and psychologic factors of significant import.

It is estimated that about 70% of the population will have had acne by the end of the teenage years, and as many as 25% to 50% of children before the age of 10 have evidence of the disorder. However, the peak incidence is in late adolescence, at about age 16 to 17 in girls and 17 to 18 years in boys, and the disorder is more common in males than in females (Yonkosky and Pochi, 1986). After this, the disease usually decreases in severity, but it may persist well into adulthood. The degree to which an individual is affected may range from nothing more than a few isolated comedones to a severe inflammatory reaction. Although the disease is self-limited and is not life-threatening, its significance to the affected adolescent is great, and it is a mistake to underestimate the impact that it can have on young persons.

Etiology

The etiology of acne is still unclear, although a number of factors appear to be related to its development. Its distribution in families and a high degree of concordance in identical twins suggest that hereditary factors predispose to susceptibility to acne. Androgens are implicated, since observations indicate a diminished effect on acne during pregnancy, its virtual absence in castrated males and young children, and its higher incidence in adolescent males. The disease seems to be aggravated by emotional stress, hot, humid environment, some stimulant drugs, and the premenstrual period. There is no positive evidence that any specific foods are factors, except perhaps with individual youngsters. Corticosteroids administered systemically over a period of weeks may produce a form of acne with typical lesions that does not appear to be associated with sebaceous hyperplasia and that slowly subsides after the steroids have been discontinued.

Pathophysiology

Acne is a disease that involves the pilosebaceous follicles (the hair follicle and sebaceous gland complex) of the face, neck, shoulders, back, and upper chest—the so-called "flush areas" of the skin. However, there is no abnormality of the gland; it is the glandular secretion, sebum, initiated by androgenic hormones, that is involved in the pathogenesis of this disease. Increased sebum production begins at the time of adrenocortical maturation (adrenarche) and subtly continues to increase until the late teens.

There are two basic types of lesions seen in acne: (1) *noninflamed* lesions called *comedones,* consisting of compact masses of keratin, lipids, fatty acids, and bacteria that dilate the follicular duct, which may be plugged (closed comedones, or whiteheads with no visible opening) or open (blackheads, with visible dilated openings that are discolored as fatty acids are oxidized by air); and (2) *inflamed* lesions that result when the follicular wall ruptures to produce papules, pustules, nodules, and cysts (Fig. 20-1). The inflammatory acne is responsible for the destructiveness and propensity for scarring.

The maturation of the sebaceous glands begins as an early pubertal occurrence, and the development of acne as adolescence progresses appears to be the result of the hormones of puberty. Under the influence of the accelerated androgen secretion from the adrenal glands and gonads, the sebaceous gland increases in size, secretory productivity, and turnover of the follicular epithelium. These changes are accompanied by an alteration in the follicular lining that allows the accumulation and stagnation of sebum and keratinized material derived from the lining cells. Normally the growing hair shaft prevents this accumulation by functioning as a "pipe cleaner" and moving the material out of the follicle. In acne the small, fine, vellus hairs occupying sebaceous follicles are unable to move the fixed material and the acne lesion develops. The noninflammatory comedones may resolve or become infected pustules.

A normally harmless bacterium, *Propionibacterium acnes,* is attracted to the sebum, which it hydrolyzes into fatty acids. These fatty acids are the major tissue irritants in the sebum and initiate the inflammatory response. Inflammation is preceded by rupture of the distended follicles, which allows the follicular contents to leak into the dermis. The resultant damage causes a further wall-rupturing effect from leukocytes that invade the dermis. Those that become cystic are likely to form scars when they heal.

Secondary invasion by *Staphylococcus albus* can complicate the acne lesion, and adolescents' concern about their appearance tempts them to pick, finger, squeeze, and otherwise manipulate the lesions, which plays an important role in the perpetuation of acne. In addition to the precipitating factors mentioned previously, the application of creams, oils, and some cosmetics that add to the plugging of the follicles may aggravate acne; therefore cosmetic agents should be selected to avoid those with greasy or occlusive bases. It has also been shown that iodides markedly increase the cellular phase of inflammation.

Exposure to oily substances, chlorinated hydrocarbons, and coal tar distillates profoundly exaggerates acne, which may influence the choice of occupation among adolescents. Exposure to excessive warmth and humidity may cause marked exacerbations in adolescents with more severe types of acne. It appears that sweating decreases the openings of the pilosebaceous ducts. This may necessitate more aggressive management to enable the adolescent to continue in active sports, such as football or wrestling, or

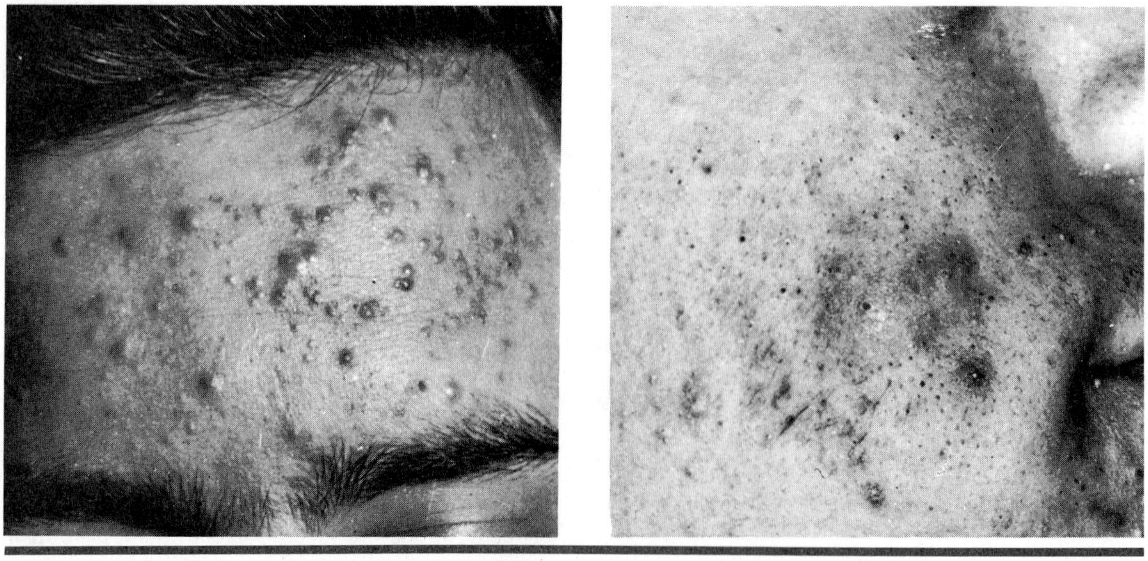

Fig. 20-1. Acne vulgaris. Papular pustules and comedones. (See also Color Plate 18.)
From Stewart, W.D., Danto, J.L., and Maddin, S.: Dermatology: diagnosis and treatment of cutaneous disorders, ed. 4, St. Louis, 1978, Mosby–Year Book, Inc.

employment in a hot, humid environment, for example, working as a cook.

Therapeutic Management

There is little evidence that treatment shortens the duration of the entire course of the disease. However, much can be done to control acne, reduce the inflammatory process and scarring, and improve the appearance. All too often parents and health professionals have a tendency to dismiss acne as a normal part of "growing up."

The treatment of acne requires long-term management with patience and perseverance on the part of patient, family, and health professionals. Unlike many dermatologic conditions the acne lesions resolve slowly, and improvement may not be apparent for many weeks. Also, in early stages of treatment the persistent postinflammatory erythematous macules may lead the patient to believe the therapy has been ineffective.

No single therapeutic agent is effective in the management of acne except in a few mild cases. It is usually more effective to employ a combination of therapies. The treatment most commonly consists of measures directed toward improving the general health of the youngster, removing comedones, preventing their formation, controlling excessive sebaceous gland activity, controlling infection, and preventing scar formation. The treatment consists of some general measures of care and specific treatments largely determined by the type of lesions involved and the preference of the practitioner. Although the combination of therapies and brands selected vary, the objectives are similar.

General measures. A general explanation of the disease process and the plan of care is given to the youngster, with emphasis on compliance to carry out the program faithfully for as long as the process persists. It is also important to obtain the cooperation, understanding, and support of the parents; therefore they should be present at the initial discussion.

Improvement of the adolescent's overall health status is part of the general management. Adequate rest, moderate exercise, a well-balanced diet, reduction of emotional stress, and elimination of any foci of infection are all part of general health promotion. There is no convincing evidence to implicate any single dietary item or combination of foods in the exacerbation of acne, with the possible exception of iodides and bromide in therapeutic amounts. Occasionally a youngster will demonstrate an aggravation of symptoms after each ingestion of a given food. In such instances the food is eliminated for a time to assess its influence on the disease.

Medications. There is a wide range of types and combinations of topical agents for the treatment of acne, with selection depending on the type and severity of the lesions. Tretinoin (retinoic acid) is the only drug that effectively interrupts abnormal follicular keratinization that produces microcomedones, the invisible precursors of the visible comedones. Tretinoin alone is usually sufficient for management of comedonal acne (Shalita, 1986).

Since most patients also have some inflammatory lesions accompanying the comedones, a topical antibacterial agent is prescribed. Benzoyl peroxide, clindamycin, tetracycline, erythromycin, and minocycline are the agents of choice. Benzoyl peroxide also functions as an exfoliant and comedolytic.

The most effective therapy involves the use of benzoyl peroxide, tretinoin, or a combination of these. Both agents can cause redness and peeling early in their use; therefore the treatment usually begins with graded increases in concentration and/or frequency of application according to the patient's tolerance. Both are available in cream or gel preparations. Creams are less irritating, but the gels, which offer more efficient penetration, are favored as the most effective vehicle (Melski and Arndt, 1980; Tunnessen, 1984). The usual regimen is to apply one medication in the morning and the other at night. They should not be applied together, since the benzoyl peroxide may oxidize the retinoic acid and render it impotent (Tunnessen, 1984).

Systemic antibiotic therapy may be needed for some patients who do not respond to topical therapy for inflammatory acne. Isotretinoin, 13-*cis*-retinoic acid (Accutane), a very potent and effective oral agent, is reserved for severe cystic acne. Management of this regimen should be rendered only by a dermatologist. The use of isotretinoin is limited as a universal treatment of inflammatory acne because of its side effects, which include dryness of skin and mucous membranes, musculoskeletal symptoms, and premature epiphyseal closure. The drug has also been found to be teratogenic and therefore unsuitable for pregnant women (Lammer and others, 1987). All sexually active teenagers should be identified before treatment and the drug given only if they use an effective form of contraception during and for 3 to 4 months after completion of treatment (American Academy of Pediatrics, Committee on Drugs, 1983).

Intralesional injections of steroids can hasten the resolution of inflammatory nodules, which decrease in size in about 48 hours (Yonkosky and Pochi, 1986). However, systemic corticosteroids, because of their acneogenic properties, are not used in the treatment of acne. Estrogen-progestin therapy in a cyclic routine has produced good responses in carefully selected older teenage females.

Other topical agents for treatment of acne include sulfur, resorcin, and salicylic acid. Although their beneficial effects have been proved over the years, they now have only a minor place in acne management.

Cleansing. Gentle cleansing with a mild cleanser once or twice daily is usually sufficient. Harsh, rough soaps and excessive scrubbing may irritate the skin and cause rupture of the pilosebaceous ducts, thus enhancing papulopustule formation (Tunnessen, 1984). For some adolescents, hygiene of the hair and scalp appears to be related to the clinical activity of acne. In these persons, acne of the forehead can be improved by brushing the hair away from the forehead and more frequent shampooing.

Nursing Considerations

The nurse may be the initial contact with teenagers for health services in either the school setting or community-based clinics, and it is often the nurse to whom adolescents confide their health concerns.

NURSING CARE PLAN
The Adolescent with Acne

NURSING DIAGNOSIS: Impaired skin integrity related to excretions/secretions

GOAL 1

Reduce lesions

INTERVENTIONS

Teach child and family to:
- *Express comedones periodically as prescribed
  - Blackheads—By direct pressure with comedone extractor
  - Whiteheads—Nick gently and superficially with No. 11 blade before extrusion
- *Apply medication (e.g., retinoic acid) as prescribed

EXPECTED OUTCOME

Lesions are expressed without difficulty

NURSING DIAGNOSIS: Potential impaired skin integrity related to presence of secretions, presence of infective organisms

GOAL 1

Prevent inflammation and scarring

INTERVENTIONS

Carefully cleanse skin with soap and water prior to expression of comedones
Caution against using excessive pressure in comedone expression
Express limited number of comedones each day
*Apply peeling agent(s) as prescribed
Teach correct cleansing techniques and medical asepsis
Caution against too vigorous scrubbing to prevent skin damage
Impress the importance of following instructions, such as using only prescribed preparations and appliances
Instruct about shampooing, hairstyling, and the selection and use of cosmetics
Instruct in proper care of equipment used for therapy
*Administer oral corticosteroids and assist with intralesion injections of the drug
*Administer antibiotics as prescribed
Stress to those on retinoic acid therapy the importance of avoiding exposure to sun; apply sunscreen for protection
Prepare adolescent for surgical procedure(s)
Assist with incision and drainage of cystic or pustular lesions
Prepare adolescent for and assist with x-ray therapy

EXPECTED OUTCOME

Lesions heal with minimum scarring

GOAL 2

Reduce number of lesions

INTERVENTIONS

Avoid oily applications to the skin
Shampoo hair and scalp frequently (if prescribed)
Style hair off the forehead
Avoid use of cosmetic preparations if possible; otherwise avoid oil-base products
Avoid face contact with other areas of the body, for example, chin resting on hands, lying with face on arm
*Administer estrogens (in selected female cases)

EXPECTED OUTCOME

Adolescent uses appropriate precautions

GOAL 3

Promote general health

INTERVENTIONS

Encourage adequate rest and moderate exercise
Help adolescent plan a well-balanced diet
Help adolescent find mechanisms to reduce emotional stress
Implement measures to correct constipation (if it exists)
Assess for any foci of infection and initiate measures to eliminate them
Eliminate any given food the adolescent has found that aggravates the symptoms

EXPECTED OUTCOME

Adolescent complies with general hygiene measures

NURSING DIAGNOSIS: Body image disturbance related to perception of facial lesions

GOAL 1

Educate the adolescent

INTERVENTIONS

Dispel myths regarding the etiology of the condition
Reassure adolescent regarding unfounded fears
Provide accurate information regarding the disease process and the therapy to be implemented

EXPECTED OUTCOME

Adolescent demonstrates an understanding of etiology of lesions

GOAL 2

Obtain medical treatment

INTERVENTIONS

Be alert to cues that the adolescent wants to discuss the skin problem
Broach the subject of therapy for the adolescent with obvious skin lesions
Suggest an understanding dermatologist who is sympathetic to the special need of the adolescent
Discourage self-treatment with over-the-counter preparations

*Dependent nursing action.

NURSING CARE PLAN
The Adolescent with Acne—cont'd

EXPECTED OUTCOMES

Adolescent discusses feelings and concerns
Adolescent complies with suggestions

GOAL 3

Encourage self-care

INTERVENTIONS

Reemphasize importance of cleanliness and medical asepsis
Provide written instructions, including the cause of the lesions and the therapeutic regimen outlined
Motivate the adolescent to assume responsibility for following through on instructions
Instruct in the technique of comedo extraction and other therapeutic and hygienic measures
Discourage mirror gazing and "picking" at lesions

EXPECTED OUTCOME

Adolescent assumes responsibility for care of skin lesions and complies with preventive measures

GOAL 4

Support the adolescent

INTERVENTIONS

Allow the adolescent to express feelings about the disorder, its effect on appearance, and the length of time required for therapy
Provide positive reinforcement for compliance
Encourage maintenance of normal activities and interaction with peers
Explore job opportunities and after-school interests with the adolescent
Explore positive aspects, such as the self-limited nature of the disorder, the efficacy of therapy, and improvement in appearance
Assist adolescent in selection of grooming and other items to enhance appearance

EXPECTED OUTCOME

Adolescent discusses feelings and concerns regarding appearance and identifies positive aspects of appearance

NURSING DIAGNOSIS: Altered family processes related to the child with a troublesome skin problem

GOAL 1

Obtain cooperation and understanding of family

INTERVENTIONS

Explain the disorder and therapy prescribed
Caution the family against nagging about compliance
Teach family the technique of comedo extraction
Explain the nature of the adolescent personality and the effect the disorder has on self-image and identity formation

EXPECTED OUTCOME

Family demonstrates an understanding of the adolescent's skin problem and shows a supportive attitude

Assessment

The health screening interview should contain questions regarding the adolescent's concern about acne. Because acne is so common and its appearance may seem so mild, the adult health provider may underestimate the relative importance of this phenomenon to adolescents. A better approach is to assess the individual adolescent's level of distress, current management, and perceived success of any regimen before initiating a referral. It is estimated that 80% to 90% of all cases of acne can be managed by the primary care provider without referral to a dermatologist (Atton and Tunnessen, 1988).

Nursing Diagnoses

Based on a thorough assessment, several nursing diagnoses are identified. The more common diagnoses for the child with acne are included in the Nursing Care Plan. Others may apply in specific situations.

Planning

Nursing objectives for the adolescent with acne include the following:

1. Reduce the number and extent of lesions.
2. Prevent infection.
3. Promote a positive body image.
4. Provide support and educate the adolescent and family about carrying out therapy properly.

Implementation

Once a treatment regimen has been prescribed, adolescents need ongoing support to comply effectively with management of the disorder and application of medications. Reinforcing and clarifying information are crucial, including causes of acne, rationale for treatment, correct use of medication, and expected side effects of therapy. Teenagers need supportive, caring individuals to help them maintain the persistence required to deal with this chronic condition.

NURSING TIP: OIL-BASE COSMETICS

Oil-base and water-base cosmetics can be differentiated by placing a small amount on the tip of the fingers, rinsing under running water for 10 seconds, then blotting the fingertip with a tissue. Oil-base preparations do not rinse off.

Specific information regarding skin care helps enhance compliance. Teenagers are subject to the influence of commercial advertising from a variety of media; therefore information that dispels myths regarding use of abrasive skin-cleansing products as a means of removing blackheads can prevent unnecessary costs. Washing with a mild, nonabrasive soap is adequate for cleansing.

As noted, use of oil-based cosmetic preparations or moisturizers can aggravate acne because it contributes to plugging of pilosebaceous ducts. Nurses can help females select appropriate water-base cosmetic preparations (see Nursing Tip). Liquid products are best suited to acne but frequently separate into water and flesh-tone cosmetic base when not in use. Shaking the container will reconstitute the water base into a usable suspension for application. Cosmetics should be removed at bedtime and not worn overnight.

Certain acne preparations, such as retinoic acid and tetracycline, have been known to cause photosensitivity; therefore application of a sunscreen with a sun protective factor of at least 15 is strongly recommended. Affected teenagers are also instructed to employ other measures that minimize sun exposure, such as wearing a hat or sun visor to reduce exposure to potentially harmful ultraviolet rays (see Sunburn, Chapter 18).

Teenagers need to be educated about other factors that may aggravate acne and damage skin, such as too vigorous scrubbing. Picking, squeezing, and manual expression with fingernails break down ductal walls and cause acne to worsen. Other factors that exacerbate the lesions include wearing the hair over the face and application of oily hair preparations. Mechanical irritation, such as clothing that rubs over areas predisposed to acne, can cause the development of lesions. Since acne lesions may not be limited to the face, adolescents need to be instructed to apply medication to other affected areas, such as the shoulders and back.

Medications. Because of the complexity of multiple medication regimens, an instruction sheet describing the etiology of acne and the therapy is helpful. Teenagers should be advised not to expect any visible improvement for 4 to 6 weeks after initiation of therapy. Initially the acne may appear worse as the microcomedones, not previously apparent, work their way to the surface of the skin. Also, medications often cause erythema, peeling, itching, burning, and drying when first applied, tempting the youngsters to discontinue their use (see Nursing Tip).

NURSING TIP: APPLICATION OF MEDICATION

The adolescent can be advised that side effects may be minimized by delaying application of medication until the skin is completely dry (20 to 30 minutes after cleansing).

Adolescents are instructed to apply the medication to the entire facial area, not just to the lesions. Furthermore, too heavy application, especially in skin crevices around the nose or chin, can result in redness and cracking of this skin. An innovative unit dose apparatus, which can be screwed to the top of the tube of retinoic acid, helps standardize the amount of medication that is applied daily. This minimizes the possibility of overapplication and increases the length of time between prescription refills, thereby decreasing expense. The nurse needs to be aware of these potential side effects of therapy that may discourage compliance and cause youngsters to discontinue treatment before any measurable success is observed. Appropriate counseling before initiating therapy and return visits to the nurse 2 weeks after initiation may decrease the dropout rate for treatment, and teenagers benefit greatly from the support received at this visit.

Expression of comedones. The nontraumatic removal of comedones serves two purposes. It reduces the risk of future inflammatory lesions and scarring and produces a prompt improvement in the youngster's appearance. Blackheads, which have open communication with the skin surface, can be effectively expressed with a comedo extractor, a small metal scoop with a hole in the center. The hole is placed directly over the blackhead and pressure applied against the skin with a slight sliding movement across the skin. Initially the procedures are carried out in the practitioner's office by the physician or nurse, but the adolescent or the parents can be taught to remove comedones with the extractor. Whiteheads, which do not have open communication with the skin surface, cannot be removed easily with the extractor alone. The epidermal covering of the whitehead must be gently and superficially nicked with a No. 11 Bard-Parker scalpel blade point before extrusion with the comedo extractor. Some extractors are constructed with a blade attached to the end opposite the loop.

The face should be cleansed before and after extraction and the instrument cleaned and cared for in the manner directed by the individual practitioner. The instrument usually is cleaned with soap and water and then either stored in alcohol or wiped with alcohol and stored in a receptacle such as a clean, dry envelope. Handwashing before handling the instrument or touching the skin is emphasized.

The parents and adolescent are cautioned against excessive pressure that might bruise the skin. A blackhead that cannot be removed readily should be left until another time. Some dermatologists limit home treatment to removal of blackheads only. Satisfactory results can be obtained by the removal of a small number (5 or 10) each day on a regular basis. Although the comedones tend to recur in the same follicle, periodic removal properly carried out by this procedure will produce no scarring and will reduce the likelihood of follicular rupture and subsequent inflammation with possible scar formation.

Evaluation

The effectiveness of nursing interventions is determined by continual reassessment and evaluation of care based on the following observational guidelines and expected outcomes:

1. Observe skin for evidence of exacerbation, reduction of lesions, and/or healing.
2. Observe skin for evidence of infection.
3. Interview youngster regarding feelings and concerns.
4. Youngster and family demonstrate the ability to carry out therapy.

Expected outcomes:
See Nursing Care Plan, pp. 910-911.

INFECTIOUS MONONUCLEOSIS

Infectious mononucleosis (IM) is an acute, self-limiting infectious disease that is relatively common among young persons between 12 and 25 years of age. However, recent evidence indicates that the disease is more common in younger children than previously thought (Sumaya, 1989; Sumaya and Ench, 1985). The disease is characterized by an increase in the mononuclear elements of the blood and general symptoms of an infectious process. The course is usually mild but occasionally can be severe or, rarely, accompanied by serious complications.

Pathophysiology

Recent evidence establishes the herpeslike Epstein-Barr virus (EBV) as the principal cause of infectious mononucleosis. The disease appears in both sporadic and epidemic forms, the sporadic cases being more common. The mechanism of spread has not been conclusively established, although the disease is believed to be transmitted by direct intimate contact through saliva, contact with infected objects, or (less commonly) blood transfusions. It also appears to be only mildly contagious, and the period of communicability is unknown. The incubation period after exposure is 4 to 6 weeks. There is enlargement of lymph nodes from mononuclear infiltration and variable infiltration of most body tissues.

Clinical Manifestations

The onset of symptoms of infectious mononucleosis appears anywhere from 10 days to 6 weeks after exposure and may be acute or insidious. The common presenting symptoms vary greatly in type, severity, and duration. The characteristics of the disease are malaise, sore throat, and fever with generalized lymphadenopathy and splenomegaly that may persist for several months. Most often the symptoms appear insidiously with fatigue, lack of energy, and sore throat that may not become prominent. The youngster's chief complaint is difficulty in maintaining the usual level of activity. This is often attributed to lack of sleep, an upper respiratory infection, or both. In many instances the manifestations never arouse enough concern to bring the affected individual to medical attention. Many cases of infectious mononucleosis are no doubt never recognized as such. Many young children do not develop all the expected clinical and laboratory findings; often a complication is the only or presenting symptom (Alpert and Fleisher, 1984).

A skin rash is present in a few cases, most often a discrete macular eruption most prominent over the trunk. More young children have rashes, and older children have abdominal pain. Other symptoms may include headache and epistaxis. The tonsils may be enlarged, reddened, and sometimes covered with a diphtheria-like membrane. Failure to thrive, otitis media, and episodes of recurrent tonsillopharyngitis are more closely associated with childhood disease. Hepatic involvement to some degree is almost always present, often associated with jaundice, which may cause the disease to be confused with infectious hepatitis. The extensive mononuclear infiltration produces symptoms related to any body tissue so that the clinical picture can resemble that of many conditions, including neurologic manifestations and cardiac involvement.

The clinical manifestations of infectious mononucleosis are usually less severe (often subclinical or unapparent) and the convalescent phase is shorter in younger children than in older children and young adults. There is a decided relationship between early-acquired disease and poor economic and hygienic conditions. Children in lower socioeconomic levels acquire the virus at a younger age than middle-class children, who remain susceptible well into adolescence. This probably accounts for the higher incidence of the illness among young people in colleges and universities.

Diagnostic Evaluation

The diagnosis is established on the basis of clinical manifestations, absolute increase in atypical leukocytes in a peripheral blood smear, and a positive heterophil agglutination test. Differential diagnosis depends on the clinical symptoms present. For example, the pharyngitis may simulate symptoms of other diseases such as diphtheria and streptococcal pharyngitis. Lymphadenopathy, fever, and malaise are all characteristic of numerous disorders. Jaundice, nervous system manifestations, and skin eruptions each similarly indicate a variety of conditions. The leukocyte count may be normal or low, but usually lymphocyte leukocytosis develops.

The heterophil antibody test determines the extent to which the patient's serum will agglutinate sheep red blood cells. In infectious mononucleosis a titer of 1:160 is considered diagnostic, although a rising titer during the earlier stages is the best indicator. Because young children have a lower rate of heterophil antibody responses, the diagnosis may be overlooked in this group (Sumaya and Ench, 1985).

The "spot test" (Monospot), a slide test of high specificity, has been developed for the diagnosis of infectious mononucleosis. It is rapid, sensitive, inexpensive, and easy to perform, and it has the advantage that it can detect significant agglutinins at lower levels, thus permitting earlier diagnosis.

Therapeutic Management

The course of infectious mononucleosis is self-limiting and usually uncomplicated. Contrary to popular belief, mononucleosis is not necessarily a difficult, prolonged, disabling disease, and the prognosis is generally good. Acute symptoms usually disappear within 7 to 10 days, and the persistent fatigue subsides within 2 to 4 weeks. A number of affected youngsters may need to restrict activities for 2 to 3 months; the disease rarely extends for longer periods.

There is no specific treatment for infectious mononucleosis. Common symptoms are ordinarily relieved by simple remedies. A mild analgesic is usually sufficient to relieve the bothersome symptoms of headache, fever, and malaise. Bed rest is encouraged for fatigue but is not imposed for any specified period of time. Affected youngsters are instructed to regulate activities according to their own tolerance, unless complicating factors are present. If the spleen is enlarged, for example, activities in which they might receive a blow to the abdomen or chest should be avoided.

A short course of oral penicillin is sometimes prescribed for sore throat, especially if β-hemolytic streptococci are present. Administration of ampicillin frequently precipitates a maculopapular rash in affected persons; therefore its use is contraindicated. Sore throat can be relieved by gargles, hot drinks, analgesic troches, or analgesics. The use of corticosteroids has demonstrated effectiveness in reducing respiratory distress from tonsillar hypertrophy, hemolytic anemia, thrombocytopenia, and neurologic complications. Although steroids can shorten the course of the illness, their use is reserved for complicated cases.

Complications are uncommon but can be serious and require appropriate management. Liver involvement is present to some degree in almost all cases and may become chronic. Neurologic complications are seen in some outbreaks and vary in severity and outcome. Other complications include pneumonitis, myocarditis, hemolytic anemia, thrombocytopenia, and ruptured spleen. There is also some evidence to indicate a depressed cellular immune reactivity during the course of the disease and for some time afterward so that live vaccines are best avoided until several months after recovery.

Nursing Considerations

Nursing responsibilities are directed toward comfort measures to relieve the symptoms and helping affected youngsters and their families determine appropriate activities according to the stage of the disease and their interests. They may need diet counseling to select foods that contain sufficient calories to meet growth and energy needs and yet are easy to swallow. Every effort should be made to prevent a secondary infection; therefore the adolescents are counseled to limit contact with persons outside the family, especially during the acute phase of the illness.

The protracted nature of the illness and its associated weakness and fatigue frequently cause depression and resentment on the part of the usually vigorous, active teenagers. It is important to spend time with youngsters to listen to their concerns and to allow them to express their feelings and vent their anger. Adolescents need to be reassured that the limitations are only temporary and that social activities, so essential at this stage of development, can be resumed after the acute phase and that they will have sufficient autonomy to determine the extent of their capabilities and the rate of resumption of activities.

ALTERATIONS IN GROWTH AND MATURATION

The absence of sexual maturation at a time when other children are experiencing positive evidence of sexual development and its associated spurt in growth and physical strength is a matter of concern to both parents and affected child. In most instances the slow growth is a simple physiologic or constitutional delay that merely represents one end of the normal genetically influenced variation of pubertal growth. These children will go through normal puberty in their late teens and catch up with their more rapidly developing age-mates. However, this becomes a psychosocial problem for some young people.

Less benign is delayed development caused by endocrine disorders or chromosomal aberrations. In other situations delayed development may be a result of malnutrition or chronic diseases that are serious enough to retard the developmental process, such as malabsorption, chronic asthma, and poorly controlled diabetes mellitus.

ASSESSMENT

Serial measurements of growth are plotted periodically on standard growth charts to determine the pattern of growth and to compare the individual child with the norm for that particular age-group. When assessing children in the extremes of height ranges, it is important to compare their height with the height of their parents and siblings. As a whole, children usually can be categorized into one of six groups according to their pattern of maturation (Box 20-1).

Diagnostic Evaluation

Clinical diagnosis of delayed development can usually be determined with relative ease on the basis of the simple criteria outlined in Box 20-2.

SHORT STATURE

Short stature is a nonspecific finding that may be the first manifestation of a serious disorder, or it may be of no consequence medically. It is often the reason an adolescent is brought to the attention of health professionals and is the most common presenting complaint in endocrine clinics. Although it occurs with equal frequency in girls and boys,

Box 20-1 CATEGORIES OF GROWTH ACCORDING TO PATTERN OF MATURATION

Average children—closely approximate the mean for height and weight at all ages
Early-maturing children—tall in childhood but not unusually tall adults
Early-maturing children who are also genetically tall—above the mean at all ages
Late-maturing children—shorter than average in childhood but not necessarily short adults
Late-maturing children who are also genetically short—below the mean at all ages
Children who deviate significantly from the normal growth curve—very rapid- and early-maturing children; much later- and slower-maturing children

the problem is more distressful to boys than to girls. Therefore it is boys who more often seek assistance. Since the psychosocial factors are of importance and there are rare situations in which delayed development is caused by a pathogenic condition, it is important to determine the reason for the short stature.

In most instances the cause of short stature is either *familial short stature* or a simple *constitutional growth delay* in which the child appears to be delayed because development is behind that of age-mates. Familial short stature refers to otherwise healthy children who have ancestors with adult height in the lower percentiles, and whose height during childhood is appropriate for genetic background.

Constitutional growth delay refers to individuals (usually boys) with delayed linear growth, in whom commensurate delays in skeletal and sexual maturation suggest that they will reach normal adult height (Ad Hoc Committee on Growth Hormone Usage, The Lawson Wilkins Pediatric Endocrine Society, and Committee on Drugs, 1983; Lanes and others, 1986). Often there is a history of a similar pattern of growth in one of the parents or other family members of children with constitutional growth delay. The untreated child will proceed through normal changes as expected on the basis of bone age. These changes, although occurring later than in the average child, will appear in normal sequence and manner, and treatment is not usually indicated.

Therapeutic Management

Management consists of continued medical observation, attention to general health and nutrition, and psychologic support. Further assurance can be provided by predicting the youngster's adult height from available tables and other criteria devised from comprehensive studies of child development. Very often the longer a youngster takes to pass through puberty, the better are the prospects for achieving an acceptable adult height, since epiphyseal fusion is more advanced in youngsters who mature earlier.

Most youngsters can be managed with detailed explanation, reassurance, and observation. Unlike growth hormone–deficient children, who do not usually demonstrate maladjustment, children with constitutional delay often display characteristic behavioral difficulties (Gordon and others, 1982). Where the growth delay is accompanied by poor

Box 20-2 DIAGNOSIS OF DELAYED DEVELOPMENT

Family History
History of similar delayed growth and maturation in parents and/or other relatives
Height and weight of siblings at comparable ages and their present measurements are helpful

Child's History
Prenatal—factors that could influence normal growth
Birth—height and weight (usually appropriate for gestational age)
Concurrent chronic diseases
Past illnesses such as head injuries and gastrointestinal, renal, or neurologic disorders
Dietary habits
Strength and stamina
Susceptibility to infection
Attainment of development milestones
School progress
Emotional problems or problems of social adjustment, especially those that may indicate past family instability (prolonged emotional upset has a significant influence on growth)

Previous Growth Pattern
Records available:
- Decrease during any year or period (e.g., second year of life, just before puberty)
- Remained relatively small throughout growth period with a growth curve parallel to or slightly below 3rd percentile

Records not available:
- Determine when first noticed that the child was small compared with other children

Physical Examination
Accurate measurements of height and weight (child stripped to underclothing)
Measurement of body proportions
- Crown to pubis
- Pubis to heel

Signs of sexual development using standard criteria (see Chapter 19)
- Breast budding in girls
- Testicular enlargement (testicular volume greater than 2 ml) in boys
- If present, normal sexual development can be expected to follow in 1 to 2 years

Bone Age
Assessed from wrist x-ray films (always delayed)

Endocrine Studies
Hormonal investigations essentially normal
- Growth hormone (GH) response
- Gonadotropin levels
- Gonadotropin-releasing factor (GnRF) responses

Usually low for the child's chronologic age but consistent with bone age
Plasma testosterone and estrogen levels consistent with bone age
Urinary excretion of 17-ketosteroids consistent with bone age
Corresponding change in endocrine response consistent with normal pubertal changes occurs with maturation

self-esteem and incompetence, the psychosocial situation is such that for the youngster (usually a boy) who is miserable as a result of peer ridicule and indignities, hormonal therapy in addition to psychologic support has proved to be advantageous, and many authorities recommend treatment in these instances. Some success in increasing growth velocity has been reported in prepubertal children with administration of oral clonidine at bedtime (Castro-Magaña and others, 1986). It appears to be less effective in adolescents (Batista and others, 1987).

Often a brief course of androgen therapy induces rapid development of secondary sexual characteristics. Lengthy treatments or large doses affect epiphyseal closure; therefore criteria for selection of candidates must be precise. Treatment usually results in excellent growth, a significant improvement in self-image adjustment, and a dramatic increase in both school-related and extraschool social activity (Rosenfeld, Northcraft, and Hintz, 1982; Wilson and Rosenfeld, 1987; Wilson and others, 1988).

Thyroid hormone is of no value unless hypothyroidism is present; and human growth hormone, although capable of increasing height, is expensive and generally confined to the treatment of growth hormone deficiency (see Chapter 38). With the availability of synthetic growth hormone produced from recombinant DNA technology, the treatment may become commonplace for children of short stature who may require larger amounts of hormone than normally produced or who produce hormone with abnormal structure. The dangers of therapy are a possible diabetogenic effect and overuse in the treatment of short stature. There may be pressures from parents who want their children to be taller than they are genetically constituted. (See Questions and Controversies).

QUESTIONS AND CONTROVERSIES

Should children without growth pathology be given growth hormone in an attempt to increase their eventual height?

The approval and availability of a biologically active human growth hormone produced by recombinant DNA technology has dramatically changed the therapeutic prospects for children with short stature. It has been shown to be effective in facilitating growth in selected cases with no growth hormone failure (Gertner and others, 1984; Van Vliet and others, 1983). It is still not certain precisely which children will benefit from therapy, and the probability of side effects has yet to be thoroughly evaluated.

The Ad Hoc Committee on Growth Hormone Usage, The Lawson Wilkins Pediatric Endocrine Society, and Committee on Drugs (1983) investigated the therapeutic use of growth hormone. Side effects that can occur include formation of antibodies to growth hormone with possible attenuation of growth, hypothyroidism, insulin resistance, hyperinsulinism, and hypertension. Their recommendation is that the only established indication for use of growth hormone is in growth hormone–deficient children. There is still too little experience with the substance to use it indiscriminately. Landos, Siegler, and Cuttler (1989) state that "routine GH therapy for children without documented deficiency of GH secretion (is) outside current pediatric ethical norms."

The multiple questions that arise from the possibilities of accelerating growth will affect health professionals:

1. Should the growth hormone be given to children with familial short stature in the attempt to gain a height in excess of the expected height?
2. Should it be given to young athletes with normal height in whom additional height might be potentially advantageous (e.g., outstanding basketball players)?
3. Should it be routine treatment for constitutional delay?
4. Will treatment produce a better adjusted adult?
5. Should health professionals be swayed by parental pressures to administer growth hormone?

Nursing Considerations

Deviation from the normal course of puberty is always of concern to affected adolescents, and to some it assumes monumental proportions. This distress is often so intense that the youngsters hesitate to voice their concerns for fear that their worries and doubts will be confirmed. Nurses, especially school nurses, working with adolescents encounter young people who are delayed in development or who are destined to be shorter in stature than their average agemates.

Most of the problems of delayed development are those caused by simple constitutional delay of puberty, and in this situation the child can be assured that the normal course of events will eventually take place. This is not always reassuring to such children. They are impatient to grow and are not easily convinced. Even after direct and thorough discussion of growth and the normal variations in rate and timing of maturation, they often doubt that they will grow. It is important to maintain contact with these children, convey to them a concern about their feelings, and let them know that they are accepted as they are.

Those young people who cannot be assured that they will eventually achieve more than a minimum height will need even more acceptance and support. The suffering is especially acute in young boys who may have hoped for success in athletics or those who may have been hurt by thoughtless remarks of their more fortunate associates. They need to know that they have a sympathetic listener who understands their anguish and who can help them develop their potential in areas that do not demand size in order that they will find recognition and acceptance and acquire self-confidence and self-esteem.

One of the difficulties related to a size that is incongruent with chronologic and mental age is the manner in which others, especially adults, relate to the child. People quite naturally respond to children with short stature as though they are younger than their age. Consequently these children often react with babyish or juvenile behavior, thus setting in motion a circular pattern of behavior and response. Conversely, children who are tall or physically advanced for their age are treated as though they are more advanced than their years. They are often considered to be retarded or behaviorally immature when they actually perform according to the normal behavioral expectations for their age.

Listening to distressed adolescents and conveying to them genuine interest and concern are prerequisites to any successful intervention. Counseling and therapy are individualized to meet the needs of each youngster and his or her problems. Encouraging these children to accentuate the positive aspects of their bodies and personalities with sound health practices and good grooming helps foster a more positive self-image. Helpful devices include a padded brassiere and hairstyling for girls and selection of clothing that adds the illusion of height (or diminishes it in the tall girl). In many areas there are special clothing and footwear stores that cater to persons with atypical sizes and where the youngster can find age-appropriate clothing. Children can also be taught to make their own clothing.

Youngsters with permanent short stature need help to redirect their goals from aspirations that are unattainable to those commensurate with their capabilities. Adjustments may be accompanied by psychophysiologic or behavioral manifestations, and health workers need to be alert for signs and prepare the parents for this possibility with anticipatory guidance.

TALL STATURE

Tallness is rarely a problem to boys, but to the girl who is or is likely to be much taller than her age-mates, it can be a source of acute distress. Despite the average height of both boys and girls steadily increasing, there is still a small group of children who are excessively tall when compared with their contemporaries. In almost all cases the tall girl is expressing an expected genetically determined growth pattern. Many girls like the idea of being tall and manage to cope effectively with any height-related problems that may arise. For others, it can be a source of intense anxiety and a severe social handicap.

When the rate of height change before puberty suggests the probability of excessive adult height, treatment with hormones may be considered. Cyclic administration of estrogens has proved effective in controlling height when therapy is initiated prior to menarche and before the end of the adolescent growth spurt that normally precedes menarche. Estrogen therapy is continued over several years until the epiphyses are fused, as determined by periodic wrist x-ray films. If treatment is stopped before that time, growth will continue. Although estrogen treatment has reduced the height from that estimated on prediction tables in a number of cases, there is still a good deal of controversy regarding its use for this purpose.

Before therapy is instituted, a number of factors must be considered: the prediction of future height based on present height and bone age; determination of whether predicted height is really excessive, that is, greater than 178 cm (70 inches); assessment of the child's and parents' attitudes toward the predicted height; and evaluation of the child's capacity to cope with day-to-day problems associated with such height.

Hormonal therapy has also been shown to be effective in reducing the ultimate height of excessively tall teenage boys. Long-acting testosterone esters administered periodically over 1 year have proved effective in a small sample. The testosterone has the effect of accelerating bone maturation and growth with more rapid epiphyseal closure. As with girls, selection of boys for therapy is made by careful evaluation of physical, psychologic, and social factors.

Nursing Considerations

Nursing intervention with a girl of tall stature has much in common with that for children with short stature. It is primarily directed toward support of the child and the family. Sometimes the concern is primarily that of the parent, especially a tall mother who does not wish to have her daughter experience the same distress as the mother did as a child. The child may not view it as a problem. Therefore the initial goal of care is to determine the source and extent of the perceived problem. Some teenage girls are overwhelmed by a height of 170 cm (5 feet 7 inches), whereas most youngsters are well adjusted and happy with a height of 178 cm (5 feet 10 inches). Much depends on the social attitudes that affect what is considered to be a desirable or acceptable body image.

If hormone therapy is elected, the parents and the young girl will need to know the anticipated length of treatment, the probability of success, the side effects associated with estrogen administration, such as menorrhagia (progesterone is usually added on the last 7 days of the ovarian cycle to ensure sloughing of endometrium); dark pigmentation of areolae, nipples, and labia; and in some cases moderate obesity. Both parents and child will need continued support and encouragement during the extent of therapy.

PRECOCIOUS PUBERTY

Precocious puberty is the manifestation of pubertal development that appears before the expected age of onset. Although puberty is gradually appearing earlier in most societies, the appearance of secondary sexual characteristics before 8 years of age is considered precocious. Signs of puberty in girls between ages 8 and 10 indicate "early adolescence" rather than precocious puberty (Schwartz and Root, 1990) (see Chapter 38 for a discussion of precocious puberty).

TURNER SYNDROME

Although Turner syndrome is often recognized at birth, it is diagnosed most frequently at puberty because of three outstanding features: short stature, sexual infantilism, and amenorrhea. The incidence of the condition in the population is considered to be from 1:2500 to 1:8000 live female births (Cohen, 1984).

Etiology

Turner syndrome is caused by absence of one of the X chromosomes; as a result the number of chromosomes in these girls is 45—44 pairs of autosomes and one X chromosome (45,X), sometimes referred to as *monosomy X.*

The disorder is caused by nondisjunction during germ cell formation and, unlike most nondisjunction phenomena, is related to paternal meiotic error. The reason for the growth retardation is unknown. The child's growth is usually normal until 3 years of age then slows, gradually drifting away from the normal growth curve. There is no prepubertal growth spurt.

Clinical Manifestations

A tentative diagnosis can be made on the physical appearance in most instances. Only a few persons with this syndrome manifest all the possible clinical features listed in Box 20-3 (Fig. 20-2). Girls with Turner syndrome have been found to have difficulty with peer relationships and understanding social cues. They exhibit more behavioral problems, especially in relation to immature, socially isolated behavior (McCauley, Ito, and Kay, 1986).

Diagnostic Evaluation

Diagnosis can be suspected in the newborn period by the presence of lymphedema and characteristic hairline, in childhood by short stature, and at puberty by delayed development. Absence of a Barr body, or negative chromatin, is consistent with the disorder. Definitive diagnosis is confirmed by chromosome analysis.

Therapeutic Management

Therapy is always individualized for these girls and consists primarily of hormone treatment and psychologic counseling for both child and parents. When the diagnosis is made early enough, growth is stimulated with administration of androgen therapy with or without growth hormone at about 10 to 11 years of age. Androgen therapy is followed at about age 14 or 15 by estrogen therapy to promote the development of secondary sex characteristics. When linear growth begins to level off, the dosage is increased and combined with progesterone to effect a normal cyclic pattern. Responses to estrogen therapy vary from girl to girl, but gradual feminization is accomplished to some degree in most individuals, accompanied by a positive effect on the young girl's self-image.

Administration of growth hormone results in increased growth velocity and an increase in predicted height (Raiti and others, 1986). The availability of synthetic growth hormone has made possible the treatment that, because of its scarcity, was impossible with growth hormone from human cadavers. The results of studies are encouraging, although the achieved adult height can only be determined by follow-up studies.

Cardiac and other anomalies, if present, require treatment, and surgical correction of the webbed neck may be undertaken if the defect is disfiguring.

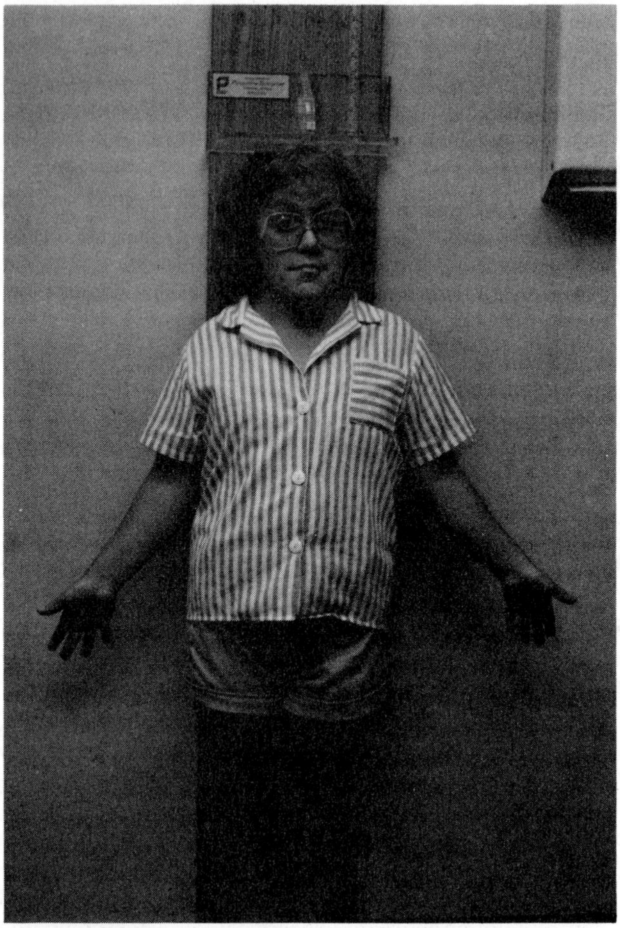

Fig. 20-2. Turner syndrome in 13-year-old girl. Note short stature (126 cm; weight, 37.2 kg), webbed neck, increased carrying angle, and broad chest.

Box 20-3 CHARACTERISTICS OF TURNER SYNDROME

- Significant short stature, which is common to all (many adults are less than 150 cm, or 5 feet, tall) and begins to be apparent at about 4 years, becoming more severe by 8 years of age
- Redundant skinfolds on the neck (webbed neck) with low posterior hairline (present in 40% to 50% of cases)
- Multiple pigmented nevi
- Rather "old" facial appearance with micrognathia and low-set and sometimes malformed ears
- Shield-shaped chest with widely spaced hypoplastic nipples
- Increased carrying angle at the elbow (cubitus valgus)
- Cardiac anomalies, principally coarctation of the aorta or aortic valvular stenosis
- Moderate degrees of learning difficulty (poor spatial perception)
- Abnormal growth patterns: absence of normal growth spurts and sexual development at puberty with primary amenorrhea and sterility; sparse pubic and axillary hair; gonads replaced by fibrous streaks
- In the newborn, lymphedema of hands and feet
- Genitourinary tract anomalies: horseshoe kidney, duplication of collecting system, aberrant renal vasculature, position anomalies

Nursing Considerations

Most of the nursing interventions described for the youngster with short stature apply to the girl with Turner syndrome. The diagnosis should be made as early as possible so that she and her parents can be counseled regarding what to expect. The girl is given some idea of the final height projected in her particular case and the expectations for developing secondary sex characteristics as a result of successful treatment. The girl and parents should understand that the short stature will probably remain despite hormone therapy. It is often reassuring for them to see others who have undergone successful treatment and who are able to adapt to the compromised stature.

It is important that families understand some of the health problems associated with the disorder. The tendency toward obesity may require special attention to diet. The increased tendency for otitis media presents the need for prompt treatment of respiratory infections and regular hearing tests. Other complications commonly associated with Turner syndrome that should be evaluated periodically include hypertension, cardiac anomalies, thyroid disorders, inflammatory bowel disease, and urinary tract anomalies (Cohen, 1984).

The fact or decided probability of sterility should be explained to the child and family. This presents a need for special sex education during adolescence, particularly in relation to fertility and alternative routes to parenthood. However, it should be emphasized at the appropriate age that the girl will be able to marry if she wishes and enjoy sexual relationships (Cohen and Durham, 1986).

Because children with Turner syndrome may have more difficulty in peer relationships and in understanding social cues and have more behavior problems, they often require more structure to socialize and complete tasks. Several national organizations offer information and support to families with congenital disorders. These include **March of Dimes Birth Defects Foundation,*** **National Easter Seal Society,†** and, in Canada, **Turner Syndrome Society.‡**

KLINEFELTER SYNDROME

Young boys with Klinefelter syndrome are seldom seen before puberty, at which time varying degrees of failure of adolescent virilization occur. Some males are not detected until they appear for evaluation for infertility. All have absence of sperm in the semen (azoospermia), small testes, and defective development of secondary sex characteristics. The incidence of the disorder is estimated to be approximately 1:500 live male births.

Etiology

The most common of all chromosomal abnormalities, Klinefelter syndrome is caused by the presence of one or more additional X chromosomes, probably as a result of meiotic nondisjunction. The majority of males with this syndrome have a chromosomal complement of 47,XXY, but there are numerous variants in the number of extra sex chromosomes, and the clinical features are essentially the same in all.

Clinical Manifestations

There are no physical characteristics that are helpful in detecting Klinefelter syndrome before the advent of puberty, with the possible exception of mental retardation. Mental impairment of varying degrees is a frequent finding and appears to have a direct relationship to the number of X chromosomes in the cells. The severity of retardation increases with the number of X chromosomes. Characteristic features of the Klinefelter syndrome are listed in Box 20-4 (Fig. 20-3).

Boys with Klinefelter syndrome have essentially normal intelligence but may have gross motor skill difficulties, developmental language delay, poor verbal skills, and re-

Box 20-4 CHARACTERISTICS OF KLINEFELTER SYNDROME

- Tall, eunuchoid figure with legs disproportionately long in relation to the trunk
- Sparse facial and pubic hair, often with female distribution pattern
- Gynecomastia of some degree (seen in half the cases and often the reason for seeking medical advice)
- Small, firm, and insensitive testes; small penis in childhood (usually normal at adolescence)
- Aspermia or oligospermia

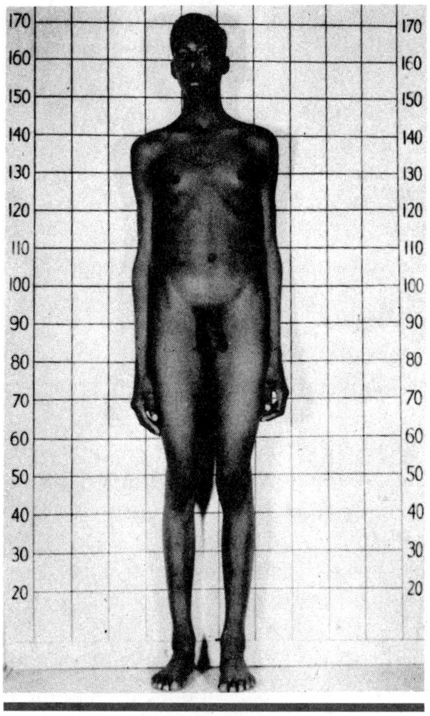

Fig. 20-3. Klinefelter syndrome.
From McKusick, V.A.: J. Chron. Dis. 12:1-202, 1960.

*1275 Mamaroneck Ave., White Plains, NY 10605; (914) 428-7100.
†2023 West Ogden Ave., Chicago, IL 60612; (312) 243-8400 (voice); (312) 243-8880 (TDD).
‡Behavioral Science Building, York University, 4700 Keele St., Downsview, Ontario, Canada M3J 1P3; (416) 736-5023.

duced auditory memory. Shyness, passivity, behavioral problems, and school difficulties are often associated with the disorder, but this may be related to the difference in body build, delayed development, and tendency toward clumsiness (Bender and others, 1983; Walzer and others, 1982).

Diagnostic Evaluation

Diagnosis is suspected on the basis of clinical manifestations, and the extra chromosome is apparent on chromosomal analysis.

Therapeutic Management

The major effort in medical treatment is directed toward enhancing the masculine characteristics through administration of male hormones, principally testosterone. Cosmetic surgery will eliminate embarrassment for a boy with gynecomastia. As with other pubertal development, psychologic counseling and support are considered along with psychologic problems associated with developmental difficulties.

Nursing Considerations

Special nursing considerations in the care of the youngster with Klinefelter syndrome include counseling or referral for problems associated with peer relationships, techniques for handling difficult social situations, and increasing self-esteem (Cohen and Durham, 1986). The child should be informed at the appropriate time that marriage and sexual relationships are possible, even in the absence of fertility, and alternative reproductive options discussed, such as artificial insemination and adoption.

DELAYED DEVELOPMENT CAUSED BY PATHOLOGIC CONDITIONS

A small group of children suffer delay of growth or onset of adolescence because of disorders that may or may not be amenable to treatment. From a worldwide point of view, the most common cause of short stature and/or delayed development is probably inadequate nutrition; however, the major disorders that produce delayed development are most often caused by chronic diseases, endocrine dysfunction, and primary gonadal dysgenesis, usually Turner or Klinefelter syndromes (see previous sections).

Chronic Diseases

Chronic diseases can interfere with growth, but, unless the illness is unduly prolonged, catch-up growth will occur. There are a number of chronic illnesses that fit in this category, and these are discussed where appropriate. Those encountered most frequently are respiratory disorders such as asthma, cystic fibrosis, and recurrent upper respiratory infection; illnesses caused by defective organ or disturbed immune mechanisms; gastrointestinal diseases such as parasitic infestations, cystic fibrosis, and other malabsorption syndromes; cardiac anomalies and blood dyscrasias such as sickle cell anemia; and chronic renal disturbances, especially renal tubular acidosis. It appears that the duration of the illness is more significant than the intensity in its effect on growth, although the precise length of time necessary to affect growth permanently has not been determined.

Skeletal Defects

Skeletal disorders that affect growth in stature are principally those described as dwarfism. Most are caused by a variety of congenital defects and disorders, such as achondroplasia, and some of the inborn errors of metabolism, such as Hurler or Hunter syndrome. Whereas some are readily apparent at or shortly after birth, milder cases may not be recognized until later in life and are diagnosed by x-ray and biochemical examinations.

Endocrine Dysfunction

The major hormones that promote physical growth are thyroid hormone, growth hormone, and sex hormones. Insulin can be said to promote growth by its effect on carbohydrate metabolism, whereas cortisol inhibits growth. Therefore deficiencies of growth-promoting hormones or an excess of cortisol can cause growth retardation in children. Endocrine deficiencies can be the result of abnormal secretory function in the glands responsible for their production, the pituitary hormones that stimulate their secretion, or the releasing factors from the hypothalamus. In some instances growth retardation may be the result of increased production of factors that inhibit hormone secretion. The complex relationships of endocrine function and their disturbances are discussed in Chapter 38.

Sex hormone deficiency. Sex hormone deficiency that causes delayed puberty can occur as a result of either pituitary dysfunction or hypogonadism. A hypofunctioning pituitary gland, as briefly discussed in the preceding segment on endocrine dysfunction, can produce a deficiency in either the gonadotropic hormones, which retards maturation of the gonads, or growth hormone, which will diminish total growth during childhood. In addition, there is a large variety of disorders that cause absence or deficiency of sex hormone secretion by their effect on the gonads directly. These may be genital abnormalities that are related to defective gonadal differentiation or those that are associated with functional abnormalities of the already differentiated fetal gonad. The largest group of disorders in which deficient gonadal development is a prominent feature includes the sex chromosomal aberrations. Two of these, Turner and Klinefelter syndromes, are elaborated in previous sections.

Cortisol Excess

Cortisol excess as a result of organic factors or of prolonged cortisone therapy also has an adverse effect on growth in children. This effect is produced by direct action on growing cartilage, interference with production of growth hormone, or interference with the response to or production of somatomedin. Because of the growth-suppressing effect of cortisone, therapy is limited to short-term administration whenever possible.

PSYCHOSOCIAL DWARFISM

Psychosocial, or deprivation, dwarfism is a term applied to stress-induced growth failure and appears to be more prevalent than previously thought. Psychosocial dwarfism is defined as growth retardation in children over 2 years of age caused by environmental (emotional) stress and is associated with marked delay in physical growth, delayed developmental skills, and immature behavior.

Children from homes in which they receive little, if any, psychosocial stimulation display markedly delayed skeletal development, and various tests in these children for growth hormone release are consistent with those that indicate a pituitary dysfunction. When these children are removed from the deprived environment, their growth proceeds at a normal or accelerated rate. This has been repeatedly demonstrated in infants and very young children (see Failure to Thrive, Chapter 13). Some investigations attribute the growth retardation to malnutrition. This may be a factor in infants and may also be a contributing factor in adolescents with short stature and delayed puberty secondary to psychosocial factors, particularly in the loss of appetite related to the disorder anorexia nervosa.

Although the mechanism is not entirely clear, it is hypothesized that deprivation dwarfism occurs as a response to increased cortisol secretion that results from the prolonged stress of a disturbed environment or unsettled patterns of sleep. Evidence indicates that deprivation dwarfism is also associated with sleep abnormalities. Since growth hormone is secreted in largest amounts during sleep, it follows that anything interfering with normal sleep patterns will interfere with the hormone secretion.

Children with psychosocial dwarfism have a sad look and exhibit infantile behavior. Interpersonal relationships are disturbed, including lack of attachment, poor peer interaction (these children usually prefer adults), and labile age appropriateness. They may display bizarre behaviors such as temper tantrums, increased or decreased motor activity, behaviors related to food (usually increased appetite and thirst), disturbed sleep, and pain insensitivity (may engage in self-injury).

Disturbed environmental clues can include any of numerous observations: maternal depression, marital conflict, an angry and hostile parent (usually the father), emotionally absent father, physical abuse, history of deprivation in a parent's background, poor communication between parents, a power struggle between parent and child, denial of child's size, scapegoating of the child, and symbiotic relationships. Growth measurements confirm growth retardation. Height and growth velocity are below normal, and skeletal maturation and bone age are delayed, although dental age is appropriate to chronologic age.

Therapeutic Management

The objectives of management for children with psychosocial dwarfism are to ensure catch-up growth, return the children to their growth potential, remove the home stress leading to the growth suppression, and maintain normal growth and development. These children are removed from the pathologic environment and placed in a foster home with limited young children—no children younger than the child being placed. Siblings are usually separated unless they thrive when together. There is limited contact with the natural home, and visitation of parents should take place at a neutral site.

Nursing Considerations

Nursing is essentially the same as that for the abused or neglected child (see Chapter 16).

■ HEALTH PROBLEMS OF THE MALE REPRODUCTIVE SYSTEM

It is fortunate for the male that most of the parts of the reproductive system are external and therefore visible and palpable. In most instances obvious anomalies have been identified and corrective measures instituted during childhood. A number of the conditions present in the newborn or young child can affect the development of appropriate sexuality during adolescence. Functional disorders such as enuresis may persist, and gynecomastia, a cause of concern in the pubescent male, may become a problem. Conditions related to urinary function are frequently those that involve the renal system as a whole and are discussed in Chapter 30. Some conditions are related to trauma; others are associated with sexually transmitted diseases.

INFECTIONS

Genitourinary tract infections in general are discussed in Chapter 30; those related to sexually transmitted disease are discussed later in this chapter. The most common infections in adolescent males are urethritis and epididymitis.

Urethritis

Urethritis is the most common genital tract infection occurring among adolescent males. Symptoms of dysuria, penile discharge, and itching on urination are the result of urethral inflammation. Most urethral infections among adolescent males are related to sexual contact. Infections caused by coliform bacteria are usually the result of congenital anomalies in the urogenital tract, most of which are identified in childhood. Therefore among sexually active males, *Neisseria gonorrhoeae, Chlamydia trachomatis,* and *Ureaplasma urealyticum* are the most common etiologic agents. Other less frequently implicated organisms are *Trichomonas vaginalis,* yeast, herpes simplex virus (HSV), *Staphylococcus saprophyticus,* and *Escherichia coli* (Bowie, 1990; Larson and Shapiro, 1988).

Concerns about asymptomatic urethritis among adolescent males have received greater attention. Although men with new gonococcal infections are asymptomatic, some may complain of mild burning and discharge, which are difficult to ignore. Since asymptomatic males remain sexually active, they have the potential for continuing to transmit these bacteria to their female partners. Also, complications such as epididymitis can occur as a result of these sexually transmitted pathogens. Routine urinalysis of the first 10 to 15 ml of voided urine from the sexually active male has been advocated to screen for the presence of asymptomatic urethritis (Shafer and others, 1989).

Diagnosis is usually made through laboratory techniques, such as urethral Gram stain or appropriate cultures. Treatment is administration of a suitable antibiotic (see Sexually Transmitted Diseases, p. 939).

Epididymitis

Epididymitis is an inflammatory reaction of the epididymis of the testicle as a result of either infection or, occasionally, local trauma. The clinical presentation is a sudden onset of unilateral scrotal pain, redness, and swelling. Associated symptoms include urethral discharge, dysuria, fever, and pyuria. The causative factors seem to be related to age, sexual activity, and sexual orientation. In young heterosexual men under 35 years of age the primary cause of epididymitis is infection, primarily from *C. trachomatis* and *N. gonorrhoeae* (Edelsberg and Surh, 1988). The diagnosis is made on the basis of urinalysis, Gram stain, and urethral culture. Mild presentation of symptoms may mimic testicular torsion, which requires immediate surgical intervention. Therefore immediate evaluation by a practitioner is indicated. Treatment consists of analgesics, scrotal support, bed rest, and initiation of appropriate antibiotic therapy. For males with a culture-verified sexually transmitted disease, treatment of their sexual partners is also indicated.

Nursing Considerations

The adolescent male may be self-conscious about his changing body and refuse a genital examination. However, research indicates that few males are uncomfortable with a genital examination (Neinstein and others, 1989). The most successful approach to assessment of the adolescent male is to assume a matter-of-fact attitude to the examination, explain precisely what will take place, and maintain a continuous commentary about what is being done and the findings at each phase of the examination. Experiencing an erection at an inappropriate moment is one of the greatest fears of the adolescent male. If this occurs during examination of the genitalia, he can be assured that it is a normal physiologic response to touch that is essentially no different from a reflex response in other areas of the body, such as the knee jerk or the pupil response to light.

The adolescent male is approached as someone important as a person, with the nurse interested in his concerns. The health assessment during adolescence is no different than the health assessments that have taken place periodically throughout childhood. The nurse should point out normal changes taking place in other areas of the body, such as developing muscles, and assure the youngster that slower developing changes, such as chest and facial hair, will eventually become apparent.

PENILE PROBLEMS

Common congenital anomalies of the penis are almost always detected and corrected in infancy or early childhood, although some boys who need several operative procedures to repair a hypospadias (the most common congenital deformity of the penis) reach adolescence with a penis that looks different from those of their friends. A few who have received no medical care have uncorrected deformities that can cause serious psychologic problems during this sensitive period of development, when being different is intolerable. These young boys need to be identified for surgical repair of the defect.

Uncircumcised males may encounter some problems during adolescence. Some young men have tight foreskins that cannot be retracted over the enlarging glans; some may not cleanse the area properly even though they know that the foreskin should be retracted and the penis bathed regularly. These boys suffer more frequently from infection. *Penile carcinoma* occurs almost exclusively in uncircumcised persons and is more common in those in whom circumcision was delayed until adolescence.

Trauma to the penis may occur in various ways, including burns and accidental injuries. The frenulum (the fold on the lower surface of the glans that connects it with the prepuce) can be torn after retraction of the foreskin, masturbation, or coitus. It can be terrifying to the young boy but usually heals spontaneously with minimum care. However, any extensive bleeding may require suturing of the tissues.

Other problems include an *adherent penis,* a common condition in which the ventral surface of the penis adheres to the scrotum, producing a severe ventral curvature during erection, thus preventing satisfactory coitus; and *priapism,* a rarer disorder consisting of painful, sustained penile erection without sexual desire. The adherent penis can be surgically corrected; treatment of priapism is directed toward treating conditions with which it is often associated, such as sickle cell disease, leukemia, the use of certain medications, and central nervous system lesions.

A frequent concern of adolescent males is *penile size.* Many boys erroneously assume that the size of the penis is directly related to virility and male prowess; the boy with a small penis is often the object of remarks from more amply endowed age-mates. Rarely, micropenis occurs. This condition may improve somewhat with hormonal treatment but seldom to the extent desired. More often the smaller size is related to late maturation, in which case the youngster can be reassured that the problem will resolve in the normal course of maturation. A concerned young man can also be reassured that the size of the flaccid penis is unrelated to the size of the erect penis and that the length is usually adequate for satisfactory coitus. Repeated follow-up visits are employed for reassurance and to reinforce the fact that the examiner views the adolescent's concern with sincerity.

Nursing Considerations

The nursing care of the adolescent male with specific problems is the same as the general approach and management.

TESTICULAR TUMORS

Tumors of the testes are not a common condition, but when manifested in adolescence they are generally malignant. The usual presenting symptom is a heavy, hard, painless mass, palpable on the anterior or lateral aspect of a testis.

The tumor may be smooth or nodular and does not transilluminate unless accompanied by a hydrocele. The involved testicle hangs lower and is therefore more susceptible to trauma. Although not all scrotal masses are malignant, any firm swelling of the testis demands immediate evaluation. If a firm swelling is noted, the youth should be subjected to a minimum of preoperative palpation and referred immediately for surgical exploration. There is seldom delay in seeking medical advice if the mass is painful, but in the absence of pain the condition may go unattended for some time.

Treatment for testicular cancer consists of surgical removal of the affected testicle (orchiectomy) and the adjacent lymph nodes, if affected. If metastases are evident in more distant nodes or organs, chemotherapy and radiation therapy are implemented (see Chapters 23 and 36).

Nursing Considerations

To supplement routine health assessment, every adolescent male should be taught to perform frequent testicular self-examination (TSE) to familiarize him with his own anatomy and to ensure early detection of any abnormality.* Ideally, self-examination should be performed once a month beginning in early adolescence. Each testicle is examined individually, preferably after a warm bath or shower when scrotal skin is more relaxed, using the thumbs and fingers of both hands and applying a small amount of firm, gentle pressure. The normal testicle is a firm organ with a smooth egg-shaped contour. The epididymis can be palpated as a raised swelling on the superior aspect of the testicle and should not be confused with an abnormality. The efficacy of teaching TSE to adolescent males has been tested and found to be successful (Klein, Berry, and Felice, 1990).

VARICOCELE

A varicocele most often appears as a scrotal mass and is characterized by elongation, dilation, and tortuosity of the veins of the spermatic cord superior to the testicle. It is ordinarily small and requires no treatment. Varicoceles are found most often on the left side because of the greater length of the left spermatic vein and its entry into the left renal artery; the right spermatic vein enters the vena cava directly and at a lesser angle, which may be a source of future difficulty. A varicocele can be palpated as a wormlike mass situated above the testicle that decreases in size when the youth is recumbent and becomes distended and tense when he is upright. There may be discomfort during sexual stimulation in some males. The condition frequently improves spontaneously. Surgical ligation of the varicocele is recommended when there is volume loss of the ipsilateral testis; in other cases periodic reexamination is the usual suggested approach (Kass, Chandra, and Belman, 1987).

*To aid in teaching adolescents self-examination, an excellent pamphlet, *What You Need to Know About Cancer of the Testis,* is available from the U.S. Department of Health and Human Services. Material is also available from local branches of the **American Cancer Society,** 1599 Clifton Rd., NE, Atlanta, GA 30329; (404) 329-7617.

TESTICULAR TORSION

Torsion of the testicle is a condition in which the tunica vaginalis, which normally encases the testicle, fails to do so and the testis hangs free from its vascular structures. This condition can result in partial or complete venous occlusion with rotation around this vascular axis. In severe torsion the organ can become swollen and painful; the scrotum becomes red, warm, and edematous and appears to be immobile or fixed as a result of spasm of the cremasteric fibers.

Typically the onset is acute and frequently follows intense activity or trauma. Often the patient has a history of a similar pain that was shorter in duration and less intense. An increased incidence of testicular torsion has also been observed in cold weather, presumably caused by contraction of the cremaster muscle (Williamson, 1983). The cold-related torsion is more common in young than in older children because of the more reactive reflex in young children. Nausea, vomiting, abdominal pain, and a slight fever may accompany the pain. Surgical intervention is mandatory to prevent hemorrhagic necrosis.

Nursing Considerations

Nurses should be alert to the possibility of testicular torsion in children who complain of scrotal pain. Since torsion often results from trauma to the scrotum, school nurses are the persons who are likely to encounter such injuries and should refer the youngster for medical evaluation immediately.

OTHER DISORDERS OF THE SCROTUM AND TESTES

Examination of the scrotal contents is part of the routine health assessment (see Chapter 7). Problems such as cryptorchidism (undescended testes) are usually detected early and corrected in childhood. However, many adolescents have had minimum health care, and the possibility of an imperfectly descended testicle cannot be overlooked in these young men. *Cryptorchid* or *ectopic testes* should be treated as early as possible to reduce the likelihood of malignancy, trauma, or emotional problems resulting from an empty scrotum. A *hydrocele* in the adolescent is most often the result of trauma but rarely may be caused by infection. The fluid generally disappears spontaneously, but aspiration may be required to reduce a large hydrocele or if a hematoma is suspected.

GYNECOMASTIA

Some degree of bilateral or unilateral breast enlargement occurs frequently in young boys during puberty. It is estimated that approximately half of adolescent boys have transient gynecomastia, usually lasting less than 1 year (Biro and others, 1990), that subsides spontaneously with achievement of male development. Occasionally, however, it is associated with abnormalities such as Klinefelter syndrome or endocrine dysfunction; therefore these possibilities are ruled out by appropriate diagnostic examination. Gynecomastia has also been reported in males receiving oral ketoconazole for fungal infection (Pont and others, 1982).

If the condition persists or is extensive enough to cause acute embarrassment or to produce doubts about gender identity in the young boy, plastic surgery is indicated for cosmetic and psychologic considerations. Administration of testosterone has no effect on breast development or regression and may even aggravate the condition.

Nursing Considerations

Treatment usually consists of assurance to the boy and his parents that this is a benign and temporary situation. Since the boy is distressed about his physical integrity and masculinity, he will need reassurance regarding this apparently incongruous development.

HEALTH PROBLEMS OF THE FEMALE REPRODUCTIVE SYSTEM

Unlike the male, the reproductive organs of the female are located internally; therefore, abnormalities are less apparent and more difficult to detect. Infections are a major source of morbidity, especially those described as sexually transmitted diseases. However, the problems most often brought to the attention of health professionals are those related to menstruation—menstrual delay, irregularities, or discomfort. Any concern is worthy of consideration and understanding from health professionals.

THE GYNECOLOGIC EXAMINATION

One of the most difficult experiences facing the adolescent girl is the gynecologic examination. Whether it is her first experience or not, she is most likely filled with apprehension. Almost all adolescent girls are extremely self-conscious about their bodies and the changes taking place. The girl will need continuing support in the form of anticipatory guidance regarding what she can expect and suggestions of what she can do to help herself relax during the procedure.

The ideal time to begin to prepare the youngster for pelvic examination is during childhood as she is maturing. External genitalia examination is always a part of a routine physical assessment; avoiding the genitals reinforces the attitude that sexuality is wrong and should be avoided. During this time the child and parents are informed that a pelvic examination should be performed during adolescence.

The timing of the initial pelvic examination is controversial, but examination in early assessment has several advantages. Criteria listing indications for a pelvic examination during adolescence are listed in Box 20-5. The girl and her parents can be assured that her body is normal, which contributes to a positive body image. It provides an excellent opportunity for health teaching in the areas of hygiene, body functions, and sexuality. The girl should be encouraged to ask questions about her changing body and its implications. For those who object to examination in early adolescence, it can be delayed until middle adolescence, although any genitally related problems that arise before that time can be more stressful if the youngster has not experienced the examination before. The pelvic examination should be made as nonstressful as possible.

Box 20-5 INDICATIONS FOR PELVIC EXAMINATION OF ADOLESCENT FEMALES

- Menstrual disorders:
  - Amenorrhea
  - Irregular uterine/vaginal bleeding
  - Dysmenorrhea unresponsive to therapy
- Undiagnosed abdominal pain
- Any sexually active adolescent
- Request for a prescription method of birth control
- Suspected pelvic mass
- Rape
- Request by patient

The teenager is usually given the option of choosing a supportive person to be present during the pelvic examination. Suggested individuals might include a parent (usually the mother), best friend, boyfriend, or other health professional, such as the nurse or medical assistant. The use of models and drawings and a display of equipment to be used facilitate understanding. The youngster is also given the choice of wearing a gown or her own clothing during the procedure. Description of the examination includes information about the procedure, and words that describe anticipated feelings and sensations experienced during the examination have been demonstrated to reduce anxiety. Of major concern to the adolescent is fear of discovery of pelvic pathology. Reassurance regarding normal physical findings is extremely important (Millstein, Adler, and Irwin, 1988).

Usually the stressful experience of being placed in stirrups in the traditional lithotomy position can be avoided. Most girls favor a semisitting position, which has the additional advantage of allowing eye contact during the procedure. The youngster who is relaxed may be examined in the supine position. Girls experiencing their first pelvic examination have been found to be more relaxed when examined by a female. Those having had a previous examination appear to be equally relaxed with a male examiner (Seymore and others, 1986). Sometimes a pillow will help the patient feel more comfortable and less vulnerable. If a female nurse is not the examiner, it is essential for her to remain with the patient during the examination to offer support and guidance. Most examiners provide a mirror that allows the girl to see what is taking place if she so desires and helps the examiner explain various aspects of anatomy.

Numerous techniques have been described to teach the youngster how to relax, including breathing exercises, imaging, and other stress-reduction strategies (see Chapter 26). However, they are not effective with all individuals. When the examination is over, the findings are discussed with the youngster (and the parents) and necessary referrals made if indicated. Written teaching materials are useful adjuncts to teaching. For diagnosis of menstrual problems, ultrasound is gradually replacing the pelvic examination.

DELAYED MENARCHE/AMENORRHEA

It is not unusual for an adolescent to skip a menstrual period or two when establishing normal menstrual and ovulatory cycles. Two thirds of adolescent females will establish regular menstrual cycles by 2 years after menarche. This is of little concern unless it creates undue anxiety on the part of the girl and her parents, which can ordinarily be allayed by explanation and reassurance. Careful examination will reveal any congenital defects of the genital tract (a rare cause).

Amenorrhea is considered to be *primary* when menarche is delayed beyond age 17, although some prefer the term *delayed menarche. Secondary* or *postmenarchal* amenorrhea is prolonged absence of menstruation for 6 months or more between periods in the first 2 years after menarche or when more than three periods have been missed after menses have become established.

Delayed Menarche

Delayed menarche may be the result of absence or malformation of the female genital structures or the inability of normal structures to respond to hormonal stimulation. This can be of hypothalamic, pituitary, ovarian, or uterine origin and can include hypopituitarism, Turner syndrome, tumors, and infections. Primary amenorrhea resulting from congenital anomalies, which obstruct the outflow of menses, can be caused by imperforate hymen or transverse vaginal septum. Imperforate hymen and transverse vaginal septum are unusual causes of absent menses in a girl who exhibits all the evidences of estrogen production and sexual maturation and who complains of periodic (usually monthly) lower abdominal pain. The treatment is simple surgical perforation and drainage.

A group of systemic disorders that may affect the functions of the reproductive tract are thyroid hypofunction or hyperfunction, prolonged or severe infections, adrenal hyperplasias, diabetes mellitus, and other chronic diseases. Obesity, malnutrition (including protein, vitamin, or iron deficiencies), or any rapid change in weight either up or down can produce amenorrhea. A common cause of delayed menarche is strenuous physical activity sufficient to reduce body fat content (see Injuries and Health Problems Related to Sports Participation, Chapter 39). Management of delayed menarche involves determining and treating the cause or reassurance if the absence of menses is simply delayed normal maturation.

Secondary Amenorrhea

The most common cause of secondary amenorrhea in adolescence is pregnancy. Other factors, which disturb the hypothalamic-pituitary-gonadal axis and cause secondary amenorrhea, include immaturity, extreme physical stress, severe emotional stress, sudden environmental change, hyperthyroidism or hypothyroidism, chronic systemic illness, extreme weight loss or gain, anorexia nervosa (even before marked weight loss), ovarian disturbance, and extrinsic pharmacologic agents (e.g., prescribed medications, abused substances, hormones) (Greydanus and Shearin, 1990).

DYSMENORRHEA

A certain amount of discomfort during the first day or two of the menstrual flow is extremely common. Most girls experience cramping, abdominal pain, backache, and leg ache, but in a few the pain is intolerable and incapacitating. The term *primary dysmenorrhea* is applied to these symptoms when there is no pelvic disease to account for cramping discomfort that is severe enough to interfere with normal activity. Primary dysmenorrhea occurs almost always in ovulatory cycles and commonly appears within 6 to 12 months of the onset of menarche, when ovulatory cycles are usually established. Primary dysmenorrhea is the most common gynecologic complaint, affecting 50% of all female adolescents, and is the leading cause of recurrent school absenteeism among adolescent females in the United States (Alvin and Litt, 1982). Therefore the discussion is primarily concerned with this disorder.

Dysmenorrhea beginning more than 2 years after menarche is more suggestive of *secondary dysmenorrhea,* painful menstruation secondary to pelvic pathology. Endometriosis and pelvic inflammatory disease (PID) are the most frequent causes of secondary dysmenorrhea in adolescents.

Etiology

The etiology of primary dysmenorrhea has been established, and some contributory factors are recognized (Beach, 1988). The factor present in all instances of primary dysmenorrhea is occurrence of prior ovulation. Although it is not invariable, the symptoms do not occur during the first few postmenarchal months or months of irregular anovulatory menses. Estrogen production alone does not appear to be related to uterine discomfort, and progesterone is associated with diminished uterine contractility.

There is a relationship between uterine contractility and the secretion of prostaglandins. Prostaglandins of the F classes cause uterine muscles to contract. The secretion of prostaglandins increases at about the twenty-fifth to the twenty-eighth day of the menstrual cycle and follows the beginning decrease in progesterone secretion. Local discomfort may be related to vascular changes in the endometrial bed during menstruation caused by alternating vasoconstriction and vasodilation of endometrial vessels that induce local ischemia, edema, necrosis, and slough. Nerve terminals also become sensitive to prostaglandins by lowering the threshold of these nerve terminals to the action of chemical and physical stimuli. In some girls the discomfort may be a result of low pain tolerance.

Psychogenic dysmenorrhea. Adolescents who are found to have no demonstrable pelvic pathology through laparoscopy and who do not respond to either prostaglandin inhibitors or oral contraceptives may have a psychogenic etiology for their menstrual cramps. Multiple causes of psychogenic pain have been identified. The most common cause is a prior episode of sexual assault or abuse. Development of abstract thinking allows the adolescent to reflect on any previous episode of sexual abuse in a different perspective. Feelings of shame, guilt, blame, or anger may surface for the first time, and she may need to deal with these feelings within the context of a therapeutic counseling situation.

In the absence of abuse, other causes include familial conditioning, sex-role ambivalence, or a mechanism to avoid stressful situations, such as an unhappy school or family environment. Clinical indexes of psychogenic pain have been described, including onset of pain at menarche, pain that begins with the onset of menses and continues throughout the entire menstrual period, no response to any medication regimens, no evidence of organic pathology by pelvic examination and laparoscopy (if done), and a prior history of sexual abuse. (Beach, 1988).

Clinical Manifestations

Typical complaints of the girl with dysmenorrhea are lower abdominal cramping, pain or discomfort, and nausea (often with vomiting), diarrhea, and fatigue. Sometimes syncope and collapse occur. The pain usually begins some hours before the appearance of visible vaginal bleeding, is most severe on the first day of menstruation, and may last from a few hours to a day but seldom exceeds 2 to 3 days. The symptoms and degree of discomfort vary considerably from one individual to another and from one period to another in the same youngster. The pain may be only a mild fleeting discomfort or so severe as to be incapacitating, requiring absence from school. After adolescence the menstrual discomfort decreases with age (Alvin and Litt, 1982).

Mittelschmerz, a symptom observed in some girls, is a midcycle lower quadrant pain that sometimes occurs in association with ovulation and is believed to be caused by pelvic irritation from discharged ovarian follicular contents. The discomfort is unilateral and on alternate sides each month, often accompanied by mild bleeding or changes in vaginal secretions. The discomfort may last from several hours to 3 to 4 days.

Therapeutic Management

A thorough gynecologic examination is carried out to exclude any pelvic abnormalities, and a careful history is taken regarding the type and duration of pain, its relationship to menstrual flow, and any associated symptoms. These questions not only provide information to the examiner but also serve to provide the girl with evidence that her problem is being taken seriously. An explanation of the physiology of menstruation helps to give reassurance.

The treatment of choice for adolescents is the administration of nonsteroidal antiinflammatory drugs, the drugs that block the formation of prostaglandins (called antiprostaglandins, prostaglandin inhibitors, or prostaglandin synthetase inhibitors). Antiprostaglandins are taken for only 2 to 3 days of the menstrual cycle. Prophylactic aspirin has proved effective when begun a few days before the onset of the menses—approximately 11 days after ovulation. The relief appears to be the result of prostaglandin-inhibitory (rather than analgesic) effect.

A variety of drugs that are taken at the onset of the dysmenorrheic symptoms are available without prescription as over-the-counter medications, such as ibuprofen. The fenamates have the additional benefit of antagonizing the action of already formed prostaglandins. Sometimes cyclic estrogen therapy to prevent ovulation provides dramatic and predictable relief from pain. Oral contraceptives are effective in approximately 90% of cases but are usually reserved for patients who also want contraception control (Dawood, 1983). See Contraception, p. 933, for a discussion of oral contraceptives in adolescence.

Nursing Considerations

The nurse is most frequently the person to whom a young girl turns for advice regarding menstrual problems or problems related to vaginal discharge. Usually all the youngster needs is reassurance about this normal function, but this also provides an opportunity for the nurse to listen to what the adolescent is saying and to engage in health teaching concerning menstrual physiology and hygiene and the importance of a well-balanced diet, exercise, and general health maintenance. It is a time to dispel any myths the girl may have in relation to menstruation and her femininity. When assessment indicates a potential problem and need for evaluation, the girl is referred to a physician, health service, or clinic.

Most of the prostaglandin inhibitors are available without prescription. Whatever drug the girl chooses to use, she needs to be told how the drug produces its effect, how to take the drug for maximum effect, and to try a different drug if one is not effective or if unpleasant side effects are noted. The drug should be taken with food, which is an important aspect of teaching since many teenagers eat no breakfast. Side effects that have been observed are gastrointestinal symptoms (indigestion, heartburn, nausea, vomiting, abdominal pain, diarrhea, and melena), central nervous system manifestations (headache, dizziness, vertigo, visual or hearing disturbances, irritability, depression, drowsiness), or other manifestations, including allergic reactions, skin rash, edema, and bronchospasm. If no satisfactory relief is achieved, the girl is referred for further evaluation. It is especially important if the girl is using oral contraceptive drugs.

Simple exercises similar to those recommended for relief of prenatal discomfort, such as pelvic rocking, assuming the knee-chest position, and breathing exercises, may also be beneficial. The girl is encouraged to practice good hygiene and participate in regular activities.

PREMENSTRUAL TENSION SYNDROME

Premenstrual tension syndrome (PMS) is a loosely defined congestive dysmenorrhea (sometimes called pelvic congestion syndrome) that begins approximately 7 to 10 days before and ends at the onset of menses. The manifestations most frequently cited are headache, backache, increased fatigue, weight gain, irritability, crying spells, depression, bloating, and breast congestion before menstrual flow.

The etiology is unclear, but water and sodium retention as a result of progesterone production after ovulation appear to be factors. Characteristically these symptoms are present several days before the menstrual period and are relieved at the onset of the menstrual flow. The symptoms do not seem to occur before ovulatory cycles begin and are not ordinarily a problem in adolescence but may occur in some older adolescents.

Therapy is controversial, although relief is sometimes achieved by salt restriction or addition of naturally diuretic foods. Sometimes a mild diuretic during the week preceding the onset of menstrual flow is prescribed.

Nursing Considerations

Nursing care is primarily supportive. Adequate rest, good nutrition, and regular exercise are frequently beneficial in lessening unpleasant symptoms.

ENDOMETRIOSIS

Endometriosis is much more common in adolescents than has previously been thought. This painful disorder is caused by the presence of endometrial tissue refluxed from the fallopian tubes during menstruation or developing from embryonic rests that is seeded anywhere in the pelvis. This ectopic tissue forms multiple small cysts on the ovaries, uterine surface, pelvic ligaments, or peritoneum that swell during the menstrual cycle, irritating nerve endings or creating adhesions between pelvic structures. The resulting pain is localized in the lower abdomen, back, groin, thigh, and/or deep pelvis and can be cyclic or acyclic. It is aggravated by coitus but usually relieved by rest.

Laparoscopic examination confirms the diagnosis. Treatment consists of cyclic hormone administration for 3 to 6 months. However, the disorder tends to become a chronic, recurring condition. Continuing management is usually referred to a gynecologist, and surgical intervention may be required.

DYSFUNCTIONAL UTERINE BLEEDING

Dysfunctional uterine bleeding (DUB) is abnormal vaginal bleeding that occurs in the absence of pregnancy, infection, neoplasms, or any other demonstrable pathologic condition or disease (Anderson, Irwin, and Snyder, 1986). During adolescence abnormalities in the timing (intervals of less than 20 days or greater than 40 days), length (greater than 8 days' duration), and amount (more than 80 ml) of menstrual flow can occur frequently. This irregularity is usually attributed to immaturity of the positive feedback mechanism between the hypothalamic-pituitary-gonadal axis and absence of the luteinizing hormone (LH) surge late in the menstrual cycle. This results in anovulatory cycles, which occur at unpredictable intervals ranging from continual spotting to heavy vaginal bleeding.

A comprehensive health history and physical examination, including a pelvic examination, is indicated to ascertain the cause of bleeding. Common causes of vaginal bleeding need to be ruled out before the diagnosis of DUB can be established. The most common reason for vaginal bleeding in adolescence is pregnancy. Bleeding can also represent an impending spontaneous abortion or completed miscarriage. In view of the prevalence of sexual activity among adolescent females, evaluation for pregnancy is always indicated. Other causes of vaginal bleeding can be related to anatomic anomalies, foreign bodies, endocrine disease (e.g., thyroid disease), chronic illness (e.g., renal disease), or previously undetected familial bleeding disorders.

Treatment of vaginal bleeding depends on determination of the underlying mechanism.

In persistent cases hormonal therapy, in the form of oral, cyclic, high-dose estrogen-progesterone combinations available as contraceptive agents, has proved beneficial. The girl needs to know that at the completion of the recommended regimen there will probably be a heavy flow with cramping for 3 to 4 days. If she is not given this information, the youngster may believe that her condition is worse and assume that the treatment was ineffective. This "withdrawal bleeding" requires no additional treatment, but most physicians prescribe a lower-dose cyclic-type combination to begin the fifth day of menstrual bleeding. This medication is continued for 3 weeks and followed a week later by menstruation. The regimen is continued for several months, after which the bleeding irregularities seldom recur.

Dilatation and curettage may be necessary to control hemorrhage in severe cases or in those that do not respond to more conservative management. Supplemental iron is sometimes needed to correct anemia if bleeding has been excessive.

Nursing Considerations

Ordinarily only reassurance and attention to general health status are needed, with emphasis on a well-balanced diet, adequate rest, and moderate exercise. Anticipatory supportive care includes preparation for procedures, if these are a possibility (e.g., dilatation and curettage).

VAGINITIS AND VULVITIS (VULVOVAGINITIS)

A small quantity of vaginal mucus is normal and in adolescent girls usually increases at the time of ovulation and before the onset of menstruation. It is characteristically clear and, except in rare instances when it appears in large amounts, causes no discomfort. However, some teenagers mistakenly believe it to be a sign of vaginal infection. After an examination, the girl can generally be reassured. Since increased secretions may be associated with sexual excitement, this association with lovemaking should be discussed with the girl.

Leukorrhea is the term used to describe a glutinous, gray-white discharge, which can be caused by physical, chemical, or infectious agents. Physical causes include foreign bodies (especially in prepubertal girls), a forgotten tampon, an intrauterine device, or even tight jeans. It can also be caused by irritation from pinworms, bubble bath, feminine hygiene products, or improper wiping after defecation. The resulting discharge is purulent, blood-tinged, or brown, with an offensive odor. Removal of the foreign material and the use of an acidifying vaginal treatment is all that is usually needed.

Medications that the girl is taking may alter the vaginal environment sufficiently to produce an increased secretion of mucus. The girl receiving tetracycline for severe acne is susceptible to secondary candidiasis, which is often more troublesome than the acne. Contraceptive pills, with their high estrogen content, also increase the quantity of the vaginal discharge. Large quantities of cervical mucus cause the normal acidity of the vagina to become alkaline, which can lead to a change in the vaginal flora. Use of an acidifying agent or a change in the type of contraceptive will usually eliminate the problem.

Many of the infectious causes of vaginitis are sexually transmitted; these are discussed in relation to the specific organisms involved (see Sexually Transmitted Disease later in this chapter). However, many cases can and do occur in teenagers who have not experienced coitus. Also, sexual assault is always a possibility (see p. 936). Therapeutic management is directed toward the cause of the inflammation and/or discharge.

Nursing Considerations

Health teaching is important in the prevention and management of vaginitis. Girls should be taught at an early age the proper hygiene after toileting, that is, wiping from front to back. A careful history can often elicit other causes such as use of irritating substances, foreign bodies, or sexual activity that may be divulged to a sensitive and sympathetic examiner. The youngster will need explanations of how the etiologic agent produced the irritation and the principles behind medical management. The discussion might also elicit questions and concerns the adolescent may have regarding other aspects of her developing body and sexuality.

HEALTH PROBLEMS RELATED TO SEXUALITY

The biologic maturation that forms the foundation of adolescent development and the transition to adulthood is accompanied by conflicting feelings, attitudes, and social practices related to the developing sexuality. Adolescents have expressed various reasons for wanting to be sexually active: to promote self-esteem, to care about someone else and to have someone care about them, experimentation, reaction to peer pressure, to feel grown up, to touch and be touched by another, to feel good, and for retaliation (Tauer, 1983).

A number of environmental influences may be operating. Sexual enticements by the mass media to enhance physical attractiveness conflict with traditional religious and societal expectations for chastity (see Questions and Controversies). Easy access to cars, unsupervised after-school activities, removal of other safeguards, and decline of social and religious controls have contributed to the increased vulnerability of youth to environmental forces to which they are exposed. The importance of having "popular" daughters frequently causes parents to push young girls into situations they are not mature enough to handle. Biologic and sociologic patterns are proceeding in opposite directions. Young people are maturing earlier and marrying later, whereas in earlier times they matured later but married earlier.

Some of the problems engendered by the maturation of sexual capacity, experimentation, acting-out, the need to conform, impulsivity, and the search for a sexual identity are teenage pregnancies and sexually transmitted disease.

> **QUESTIONS AND CONTROVERSIES**
>
> **Do the media contribute to the increase in sexual activity among teenagers?**
>
> There are data to indicate that television serves as an important source of information about sex for teenagers (Palumbo and Licamele, 1983). Television movies that show sexually suggestive behaviors have increased sevenfold in a 5-year period (Sprafkin and Silverman, 1981). Many overly dramatize the sexual aspect of adolescence, including sexual affairs, rape, teenage prostitution, and pornography. Many "sexploitive" movies made for theaters are directed toward the teenage moviegoer (Strasburger, 1985), and television soap operas are among the worst offenders of exploitative sex.
>
> What influence will the increase in the number of homes with videocassette players and the availability of sexually suggestive movies have on teenagers? Can teenagers' access to X-rated movies from adult sources be controlled?

ADOLESCENT PREGNANCY

Each year one in 10 adolescent girls in the United States becomes pregnant—approximately 1 million females under the age of 20 years. About 554,000 of these pregnancies result in a birth; more than 400,000 are terminated by abortion (McAnarney and Hendee, 1989a). Today most teenage mothers choose to keep their babies; consequently, there are 1.3 million infants living with teenage mothers, about half of whom are married. Today in most cases teenage pregnancy is no longer considered to be biologically disadvantageous to the conceptus, but it is still regarded as socially, educationally, psychologically, and economically disadvantageous to the mother.

Medical Aspects

With better facilities available for care, the mortality for teenage pregnancies is decreasing, but the morbidity remains high. Teenage girls and their unborn infants are at greater risk for complications of both pregnancy and delivery. The most frequent complications are premature labor and infants of low birth weight, high neonatal mortality, pregnancy-induced hypertension (PIH), iron deficiency anemia, fetopelvic disproportion, and prolonged labor. It now appears that the major obstetric difficulties are related to the smaller maternal size rather than the younger age or developmental immaturity.

Although teenagers have special needs, the obstetric risk should be no greater than for any pregnant patient. When quality prenatal care is available early in the pregnancy, the progress and outcome of teenage pregnancies compare favorably with the obstetric performance of older women (Zuckerman and others, 1984).

Developmental. Previously it was believed that pregnancy interfered with normal development when a fetus competed with the maternal needs for nutrients during the rapid growth of early adolescence. Since pregnancy can take place only after the girl has achieved an advanced state of growth and sexual maturity, interference with growth is less of a concern than the dietary habits and the increased incidence of cigarette smoking, alcohol and drug use, and sexually transmitted diseases in this age-group.

It does not necessarily follow that early biologic development is accompanied by early emotional and psychologic development. The physically mature young girl is still a teenager who must cope with the developmental tasks of adolescence. When the tasks of motherhood or impending motherhood are superimposed on adolescent needs, the girl is ill prepared to deal appropriately with either. Findings of studies indicate that infants born to young mothers have higher infant death rates than do infants born to older women (McAnarney, 1987) and have increased risks of poisonings, burns, and superficial injuries (Taylor, Wadsworth, and Butler, 1983). The hospitalization rate during the first year for infants of teenage mothers is greater than one and one-half times that for children born to women 20 years of age or more (Wilson, Duggan, and Joffe, 1987).

Complications of pregnancy. The most serious complication of teenage pregnancy is PIH. Girls less than 16 years of age have a five times greater chance of developing PIH than older girls and young women, and since there is greater likelihood of repeat pregnancy at an earlier age, the threat is not eliminated with the termination of one pregnancy. Younger women are statistically destined to have more than the average number of additional pregnancies, and these earlier and repeated episodes of PIH are detrimental to the cardiovascular-renal system. Consequently, each subsequent pregnancy bears the risk of increased severity of PIH, and the resulting renal damage can produce chronic renal disease in the young woman by about age 30.

Anemia is not an unusual finding in nonpregnant adolescent girls, but during pregnancy the deficit is increased because of the normal hemodilution associated with pregnancy and the growth demands of the fetus.

There appears to be little difference in the incidence of placental accidents and antepartum and postpartum hemorrhage in teenagers compared with older women, although the findings vary with the observers. Lacerations of the genital tract are more frequent in smaller patients.

Structural. Labor may be prolonged in younger teenagers; this is directly related to fetopelvic incompatibility and is a reflection of teenagers' smaller stature and incomplete growth process. This is particularly true regarding girls 12 to 16 years of age, and the incidence of prolonged labor is highest in girls less than age 14. Girls 12 and 13 years old have the highest rate of cesarean births, primarily necessary because of cephalopelvic disproportion. However, older adolescents, 15 to 21 years of age, often have labors that are shorter than average, especially those girls who have previously delivered a baby. The critical point between pelvic disproportion and adequacy appears to occur around 15 years of age in the average adolescent.

Nutritional. Caloric requirements during adolescence closely parallel the growth curve, and the need for protein, calcium, and iron is increased concomitantly. Young adolescents tolerate caloric restriction poorly, and the anabolic need for calories during pregnancy places an added burden on their bodies. The nutritional status at the time of pregnancy is a reflection of lifetime nutritional practices. Unfortunately, because of an attempt to attain fashionably slim figures, denial of the pregnancy, and zealous restriction of diet to control pregnancy weight gain, many teenagers have been placed at risk.

Since there is marked variation in the dietary needs of individual teenagers, no hard and fast rule can be laid down to describe the adequate diet for all pregnant girls. The diet must provide sufficient nutrients to meet growth needs of both the prospective mother and the unborn child without the threat of obesity and other evidences of malnutrition. The best guide for determining nutritional needs is the Recommended Daily Allowances of the Food and Nutrition Board (1989) for adolescents of the appropriate age and the additional 300 calories per day needed during the second and third trimesters of pregnancy. However, these do not take into consideration deviations and deficiencies.

Adolescent girls often adopt unusual dietary patterns that can seriously compromise the health of themselves and their infants. Adolescents are often unresponsive to suggestions about food choices. Experience also indicates that many teenagers do not understand the basic food groups nor the phrasing used to describe nutrients (e.g., grams of protein per day and servings).

Infants. There is a higher incidence of prematurity and low birth weight in infants born to teenagers. It is difficult to determine if this is a result of the developmental stage of the mother or a reflection of multiple factors associated with teenage pregnancies, including first pregnancy, poor nutrition, lower socioeconomic status, concomitant disease and deleterious habits, and deficiency or lack of prenatal care. Several factors that demonstrate a high degree of association with prematurity, such as first birth, PIH, immaturity, illegitimacy, and the young age of the mother, can create an accumulative effect that places the pregnant teenager in a perilously high-risk situation.

Causal Factors

The causes of teenage pregnancy are complex, and attempts to disentangle the many facets have yet to be fully successful. Several factors have contributed substantially to the rise in premarital births to teenagers. First, the trend to earlier initiation of sexual activity, which started in the

1970s, continues. Second, only about 1 of 3 sexually active adolescents uses a reliable method of contraception consistently. The two most common reasons for their not using contraception are: (1) the youngsters did not believe they could become pregnant, and (2) they did not plan to have intercourse.

The majority of adolescents choose not to marry and to retain custody of their child. When questioned, 92%, or 5 of 6, unmarried pregnant teenagers report that their pregnancy was not intended (Trussell, 1988). Minority youths appear to be most at risk for unintended pregnancy; blacks and Hispanic adolescents experience the highest rates of pregnancy. Understanding the cultural meanings of childbearing and the impact of poverty on these youths is essential before adequate intervention programs can be designed (Children's Defense Fund, 1987). Clearly, it is agreed that youths who delay childbearing until they have completed their own development and education are socially and economically better prepared to become parents.

Social and Economic Aspects

Statistically, teenage marriages are notoriously unstable. The highest divorce rate occurs in couples who are married between ages 15 and 19 and is three to four times higher than that among those married at a later age. Teenagers find themselves still dependent on parents for support or, unskilled and inexperienced, in an unfavorable position to earn enough to support a family adequately. Poverty is often a result of teenage childbearing. Since many of these youths do not complete their education, job opportunities are limited. Frequently they are employed in service-related positions (Children's Defense Fund, 1987).

Poor school performance usually precedes adolescent pregnancy. Unable to achieve academically, the youth views motherhood as a rite of passage into adult status (Davis, 1989). Another significant aspect of school dropout and accelerated maturity is the girl's alienation and isolation from her peers during a stage of development when identity formation is so closely allied with peer identification. She is deprived of the interrelationship with the adolescent social system that is so essential to the development of a sense of identity. The girl believes that she no longer "belongs" to the peer group and does not qualify for membership in the older peer group normally associated with marriage and motherhood. On the other hand, the pregnancy may provide the youngster with an entrance into a peer group.

Today most communities have some arrangement for continuation of the girl's education by allowing her to remain in regular classes or providing a curriculum to meet her special needs either within the school system or through programs associated with other community agencies. Most community programs designed for the assistance of pregnant teenagers involve the cooperative efforts of several organizations. The major service components of the programs provide for early and consistent prenatal care, continuing education on a classroom basis, and individual or group counseling.

Mother-Infant Relationship

Not only are infants of teenage mothers at risk medically, but they are also at risk in other aspects of their existence. Although many adolescent mothers want their babies and are prepared to care for them in a mature manner, many others have unrealistic expectations for the child. The young mother often sees the infant as a plaything or a love object for herself. Children of adolescent mothers experience more developmental problems than children of adult mothers. There are conflicting reports of suboptimum cognitive development in children of teenage mothers, but reports indicate an increased risk of child abuse in these children (Elster, McAnarney, and Lamb, 1983). Many are raised by grandparents, a situation that can be fraught with problems and confused identities for the child.

Mother-infant interaction has been observed by numerous investigators. It has been found that infants of teenage mothers display a slight but consistent developmental advantage during their first year of life, but this is reversed in later years (Camp and others, 1984). Adolescent mothers tend to interact with their infants with relatively more physical than verbal exchanges when compared with adult mothers (Sandler, Vietze, and O'Connor, 1981), and nonverbal interaction is most commonly employed by the younger teenage mothers (Ragozin, 1982). Teenage mothers are also more authoritarian in their relationships with their children (Camp and others, 1984).

Researchers have also investigated the various factors that influence the mother-infant relationship. Maternal stresses, including changes in circumstances, influence her ability to cope and her sensitivity to the needs of the infant. Teenage mothers classify "stressful" as an argument with parent, boyfriend, or husband, whereas adult mothers tend to focus on problems directly involving the infant (Coll and Oh, 1987). The timing of pregnancy is out of phase with the usual course of life events, and role transition and other situational crises of pregnancy all affect the adolescent, who does not have the maturity or the social support to cope adequately (Elster, McAnarney, and Lamb, 1983). Vocational and educational disadvantages of both teenage mothers and fathers further impinge on coping abilities.

There is also a positive correlation between the total amount of social support and the frequency of appropriate maternal behavior (Colletta and Gregg, 1981). The most important source of support is the mother's family of origin, which serves a variety of functions, including cognitive guidance, social reinforcement, tangible assistance, social stimulation, and emotional support (Hirsch, 1980). There is more material support and assistance with child care available to the youngster who lives at home.

The cognitive development of the adolescent influences the development of attitudes and realistic expectations regarding childrearing. To cope effectively and solve situational dilemmas, pregnant teenagers must be able to use the problem-solving approach to assess and evaluate consequences of social interactions. The concrete thought and self-centeredness of early adolescence can influence mothers' attentiveness to and evaluation of their infants' needs

(Lamb and Easterbrooks, 1981). Adolescent mothers lack knowledge of infant behavior and development, and this directly affects their perception, interpretation, and responsiveness to infant cues. The greater the mothers' knowledge, the more likely they are to interpret the infants' cues correctly and to implement appropriate responses (Elster, McAnarney, and Lamb, 1983).

The characteristics of the infants also influence parental behavior. Teenage parents view their children as more temperamentally difficult than do adult parents, no matter what the infants' temperament (Green and others, 1981). Since temperamentally difficult infants have an adverse effect on sensitive responsiveness of parents, a parent-infant interaction that is not mutually satisfying can alter the parents' feelings of effectiveness and self-worth. This can alter their sensitivity and relationships with the infant. An increased incidence of child abuse has been found in adolescent parents (Leventhal, 1981).

Adolescent Fathers

In the past the role of the father of a child born to an unwed teenage mother was almost completely ignored by health professionals. Contrary to prevalent attitudes, the boy is often concerned about the girl he impregnates and wants to act in a responsible way in supporting the girl and sharing with the burden of decisions regarding the new life. With help, the couple can explore all the alternatives available regarding the future of the child, including marriage, adoption, or either the mother or father assuming responsibility to care for and rear the child (Redmond, 1985). Most teenage fathers are willing to accept their obligations and demonstrate strong paternal feelings for the newborn child. They also need to be made aware of their legal rights in relation to the child.

Nursing Considerations

It is evident from the preceding discussion that nurses play a central role in meeting the needs of pregnant teenagers. It is frequently the nurse to whom the young girl turns for help and guidance in her dilemma and on whom she relies for support and reassurance. It has been found that in comparison with their counterparts, young adolescents who were visited by nurses during their pregnancy gave birth to newborns who were heavier and in those who smoked there was a 75% reduction in the incidence of preterm delivery (Olds and others, 1986).

The first goal in nursing care of the pregnant teenager is to obtain medical care for her if she has not already done so whether she elects to continue or terminate the pregnancy. Typically girls in this age-group are reluctant to seek medical help, in part because of anxiety but more often because of a tendency to deny the pregnancy (especially in younger girls) or in an attempt to conceal their condition as long as possible to avoid being dropped from school (older girls). The importance of early prenatal care is essential for the welfare of both mother and infant when the girl chooses to continue the pregnancy and to facilitate a safe abortion when she elects this option. For guidelines, teaching, and general support measures during pregnancy, the reader is directed to the excellent textbooks available on nursing care throughout the maternity cycle.

Basic to the implementation of any program of care is communication and the establishment of a trusting relationship. Initially the adolescent girl frequently appears apathetic and displays little interest in discussing her pregnancy. She may be abrupt, impatient, defensive, hostile, or indifferent. It is important for the nurse to make every effort to put the youngster at ease and avoid undue pressure until a rapport can be developed so that the girl is comfortable in sharing her feelings and concerns. Conveying a nonjudgmental and genuine caring acceptance of the girl and her goals will assist the nurse in gaining her confidence and trust. The girl may have encountered rejection and open criticism from authority figures and peers, depending on the social and cultural attitudes of the school, the community, and her own family structure.

Communication takes time and patience. Asking open-ended questions and listening for cues will help identify physical, emotional, social, and cultural influences that might affect the adolescent's progress through the maternity cycle. For example, various cultural groups have different attitudes toward unsanctioned pregnancies, and it is important to determine other sources of support, such as the family. Factors that might affect her physical status, such as smoking, drug use, and nutritional state and habits, need to be explored and confronted. Each teenager presents a unique situation in relation to background, life-style, support structure, and coping mechanisms.

Nutrition assessment should focus on the dietary adequacy of iron and calcium; multivitamins with folic acid are prescribed. The youngster is referred for food supplement programs (e.g. Women, Infants, and Children food program), and social work referral for thorough psychosocial assessment and planning is initiated. Programs that have been most successful are comprehensive in approach and use an interdisciplinary team concept (i.e., obstetrician, nurse, social worker, nutritionist).

The young girl needs to know what is happening to her, what is expected of her, and how she can help in developing a plan of care. Adolescents have their own ideas of the type of help they need and support that would be beneficial. They should be consulted and provided with the opportunity to share their ideas and to feel that they make an important contribution to planning their care.

The girl will need help to improve her altered self-image, a crucial factor in adolescence. Giving her as much individual attention as possible, being a sympathetic listener, providing the opportunity for her to know, support, and be supported by other girls in the same situation, and helping her to experience success at every opportunity will facilitate progress toward achieving this goal. Individual or group discussions of clothes, hairstyles, makeup, and involvement in creative and self-improvement activities help to enhance her self-concept.

The nurse also involves the family whenever possible. The parents of the girl and the father of the child need to express feelings and attitudes about the situation. Often they must deal with their own feelings before they are able to provide support and help in problem solving for the pregnant girl. The girl may or may not wish to have these persons involved in her decisions and care. The nurse must attempt to determine the teenager's true feelings regarding these relationships.

Education regarding child care begins during pregnancy, and preparations should be made for continued education and assistance after the birth. The information for which teenage mothers consistently expressed a need is (1) medical information, that is, how to care for an ill child, (2) daily physical care, and (3) protection from injury (Howard and Sater, 1985). Education should also include information on child development, diet, and stress management.

Counseling regarding adoption as a viable option is also important. Unfortunately, only 2% to 4% of pregnant teenagers elect this alternative. A variety of agencies (religious and secular) are available to provide counseling and support. Social work referral is usually indicated to assist in planning a course of action. The same prenatal care is required as for the youngster who plans to keep her infant.

The pregnant adolescent, although still ostensibly under parental control, has legal authority over the conduct of her pregnancy and the disposition of the child. Adolescents who are clearly no longer under parental control, for example, those who are living alone, are married, are economically self-sufficient, or otherwise demonstrate the capacity to give informed consent, are considered "emancipated" or "mature" minors and as such are responsible for their actions in seeking and accepting medical care.

ADOLESCENT ABORTION

In 1973 the landmark Supreme Court case of *Roe v. Wade* concluded that the right to an abortion rested within the rights of the individual. This right was not absolute but subject to certain state restrictions. The right to an abortion is also determined by the stage of pregnancy. During the first trimester the woman and her practitioner can arrive at a decision without government interference.

The rights of minors had a historical precedent when the Supreme Court in 1967 ruled that a juvenile had a right to a just trial before any sentencing could take place (otherwise known as the "mature minor" concept). This antecedent ruling allowed the reproductive rights of adults to be extended to minors. Judicial attempts by parents or guardians to overrule the decision of consenting minors have not been successful (Silber, 1989). Several states have enacted legislation that requires parental or guardian consent, consent by another adult family member, or judicial bypass wherein the judge determines the competency of the youth to consent for an abortion (English, 1989). Clearly, the trend is in the direction of each state regulating minors' access to abortion.

Slightly more than 1 million teenage pregnancies were reported in 1985. Of these, 477,710 were live births, 416,170 induced abortions, and the remainder spontaneous abortions or stillbirths. Women younger that 20 years of age accounted for 26% of all abortions (Henshaw and Van Vort, 1989). Although abortion is a controversial and emotional issue, health care professionals involved in delivery of services to pregnant adolescents are confronted with this reality frequently. National opinion surveys of Americans have revealed that the majority of persons support legal abortions without government intervention. However, two restrictions are noted—parental notification for minors under age 18 years and tests for fetal viability (Digest, Family Planning Perspectives, 1989). Since the law in this area is unsettled, changing rapidly, and varies by state, it is essential that nurses stay abreast of legal changes as they relate to reproductive rights of minors in the state in which they practice (Rhodes, 1988a, 1988b).

The medical safety of a legal abortion has been well established. A higher mortality rate has been associated with a full-term pregnancy than with abortion. A variety of surgical procedures are available to the operator but are beyond the scope of this discussion. First-trimester abortions are performed as an outpatient procedure and require local anesthesia or mild sedation only. Complication rates have been reported to be 1% or less. Problems that arise after abortion are endometritis, hemorrhage, Rh sensitization, genital tract injury, retained fetal elements, and (in rare cases) pulmonary embolism or death (Greydanus and Shearin, 1990). Second-trimester abortions usually require hospital admission. The procedure is more complicated and associated with greater risk from hemorrhage.

Counseling the adolescent about pregnancy options in a nonjudgmental way is essential. Counseling criteria suggested in a policy statement by the American Academy of Pediatrics, Committee on Adolescence (1989) include three guiding principles: (1) the counselor should provide information in an unbiased format, (2) none of the options may be universally accepted by either the patient or the health care provider, and (3) the adolescent and other concerned individuals must be given adequate freedom to arrive at a working decision. The counselor must respect the moral decision and legal right of the youth to have an abortion.

Concerns regarding the psychologic impact of the abortion decision have been raised. Studies have revealed that although teenagers may delay a decision and may find it more difficult, they suffer no long-term negative psychologic sequelae (Adler and Dolcini, 1986). Active involvement in the decision-making process and perception of having made the choice personally can contribute to the adolescent's psychologic growth. Teenage females interviewed 2 years following abortion were more likely to have completed their high-school education or had remained in school, were economically more advantaged, and had experienced no more stress or psychologic problems than those who carried their pregnancies to term (Zabin, Hirsch, and Emerson, 1990).

Nursing Considerations

Early identification of pregnancy is essential, and nurses are in an optimum position to provide counseling on pregnancy options. For the adolescent who chooses to continue the pregnancy, prenatal care referral should be initiated as soon as possible. For the youth who elects abortion as an option, referral should be initiated quickly to ensure that the procedure is performed during the first trimester, when complications are reduced. Pelvic ultrasound may be indicated to assess gestational age correctly for those youth who cannot recall the date of their last menstrual period and when a bimanual pelvic examination is inconclusive. Appropriate preprocedure counseling is also indicated.

Patient education regarding the medical aspects of the abortion before the procedure should be conducted verbally and the patient provided with written instructions. Reviewing relaxation strategies to be used during the procedure is helpful. Parents or other significant adults are encouraged to be present during the medical procedure.

Finally, a discussion of future contraceptive needs is important. Many health care providers dispense a method of contraception to the adolescent during this preabortion counseling. Initiation of oral contraceptive medication can be started within a few days after the abortion. Patients should be seen 2 weeks after abortion to receive medical, contraceptive, and psychologic follow-up care.

Since pregnancy during adolescence may not be socially condoned, little has been written on the needs of an adolescent who must mourn the loss of a pregnancy. The sense of loss and bereavement can be significant for adolescents who have experienced a spontaneous abortion or who have been pressured into having a therapeutic abortion against their will. Poor contraceptive compliance following abortion can be linked to the secret desire to be pregnant in an attempt to compensate for this loss. Providing social support and the opportunity to express their grief is an important component of nursing care for these teenagers.

CONTRACEPTION

Family planning services in general have developed and expanded during recent years, and with the increase in sexual activity among the teenage population there is also an increased awareness of the need for contraceptive services as a part of the health care of adolescents. Although all teenagers need sex education, not all of them are candidates for contraception. Among the large adolescent population there are those youngsters whose voluntary sexual restraint eliminates the need for control measures and those who are married and wish to have a child. Since contraceptive advice and management of premarital and married teenagers differ little from fertility control offered to older women, little need be added regarding this group of teenagers.

The group that represents the greatest difficulty is that of the unmarried, dependent, sexually active girl, whether she has been pregnant or not. The predominant feeling among health professionals is that parental notification is important but that the "parents' rights" view is not necessarily sensitive to the health needs and basic rights of youth. There is no evidence to substantiate the belief that providing contraceptive guidance contributes to sexual irresponsibility and promiscuity. Actually, a request for contraceptive information indicates a responsible effort on the part of the teenager to avoid an undesirable pregnancy.

Contraceptive Methods

A contraceptive method, to be safe and effective, must be suited to the individual. The choice is based on the youngster's preference and the practitioner's judgment. Although a girl may prefer to use oral contraceptives, if her menstrual pattern suggests that she is not ovulating normally, she will be guided to another method. The girl must also be motivated to use whatever method is recommended or prescribed. No matter what method is selected, the provision of a birth control device is only part of a comprehensive sex education program. The advantages and disadvantages of various contraceptive methods recommended for use in adolescents are outlined in Table 20-1.

Simple methods. Sometimes, despite the effectiveness of prescription methods, teenagers persist in using less effective methods because of the necessity for medical screening and supervision inherent in the use of superior devices. Commonplace methods such as withdrawal, douches, and reliance on what are hoped to be "safe" periods are often reported in teenage obstetric histories. Factual knowledge about more effective methods such as the condom and chemicals and clarifying some of the myths regarding safe times in the menstrual cycle help to reduce the incidence of unwanted pregnancy. Although they may have some small use for infrequent or short-term exposure to pregnancy, the simple and relatively effective methods are generally unpopular with teenagers. Their use requires considerable consistency and care in following directions and inhibits the spontaneity of the activity.

Prescription methods. Birth control methods that require a medical prescription are considered by many teenagers to be too premeditated; as a result, they are less popular among teenagers. However, prescription methods are now being used by greater numbers as attitudes are changing in a more open and permissive atmosphere. Oral contraceptives appear to be the preferred method and are usually prescribed unless there are contraindications. Some drugs alter the effect of oral contraceptives; therefore a history must include this information. For example, the efficacy can be inhibited by some antibiotics (tetracycline-type and rifampin), the antifungal griseofulvin, or anticonvulsant drugs (phenytoin, primidone, and phenobarbital) (D'Arcy, 1986; Lipman, 1987).

Intrauterine devices (IUDs) and sterilization, common methods of birth control in adults, are not recommended for teenagers. IUDs increase the risk of PID and its consequences, and nulliparous females are more likely to have difficulty during insertion of the device, to suffer cramping and bleeding, and to expel the IUD. Sterilization is contraindicated for adolescents, especially those who have not borne children (Hatcher and others, 1988; Tyrer, Rothbart, and Anderson, 1989). Most adolescents have neither been tested for fertility nor decided on a reproductive life plan.

Use of Contraception

Although teenagers frequently seek contraceptive advice and do not wish for a pregnancy, they are inconsistent users of contraception. Studies indicate that a large number interviewed had used no contraceptive at the preceding act

Table 20-1 Advantages and disadvantages of contraceptive methods in the adolescent

METHOD	ADVANTAGES	DISADVANTAGES
Abstinence	100% effective if carried out Medically ideal contraceptive	Peer pressure to conform Relatively high failure rate from noncompliance
Withdrawal Withdrawal of penis before ejaculation	Reduced risk of pregnancy Popular method with teenagers	High failure rate Some seminal fluid often released before ejaculation Ejaculate at vaginal orifice may enter vagina
Rhythm Refrain from intercourse during fertile period (time of ovulation)	Only method approved by Roman Catholic Church (for family planning) Teaches women about their menstrual cycle Encourages couple participation	High failure rate Requires enormous motivation by the adolescent and partner Requires a regular, predictable menstrual cycle (unusual in early and middle adolescence)
Barrier methods		
Condom Penile covering to trap sperm Spermicidal condoms increase effectiveness for pregnancy and STD prevention	Popular with teenagers Simple to use Available without prescription Provides some protection from sexually transmitted disease No side effects Girl can carry with her for unexpected sexual encounter Male participation	Requires a highly motivated, responsible adolescent male Requires premeditated intent for sexual union High failure rate (unless used properly) Requires consistent use
Diaphragm Cervical covering to prevent sperm from reaching egg For maximum effectiveness, must be used in conjunction with spermicide	Virgins can be fitted May be inserted 4 to 6 hours before intercourse Low failure rate when used correctly Few contraindications	High failure rate in adolescents because of inconvenience of use Requires consistent use Requires fitting and instruction by medical personnel If inserted early, should be checked for placement before coitus Requires premeditated intent for sexual union Requires body awareness for insertion
Sponge Cervical covering Releases a spermicide	As effective as the diaphragm Can be obtained without a prescription	Similar to diaphragm Expensive
Cervical cap	Can remain in place up to 7 days	Relatively high failure rate
Chemicals—spermicidal foam, jelly, cream, and so on Substance injected into vagina to kill sperm	Available without prescription Inexpensive Easy to use Provides some protection against STDs	High failure rate unless combined with mechanical barrier Possible for sperm to be ejaculated directly into uterine os, bypassing spermicide in vagina Must be used shortly before coitus, therefore requires interruption of sexual experience Repeated sexual union requires repeated application Requires premeditated intent for sexual union
Oral contraceptives Estrogen and progesterone-like compounds Inhibit ovulation by blocking release of gonadotropins from anterior pituitary gland	Theoretically 100% effective Exceedingly safe for adolescents Method of choice for most youngsters Administered by mouth Becomes a ritual not associated with sexual activity	Higher failure rate in adolescents than in older women Need to follow precise instructions; require continued motivation Requires prescription Price substantial for teenager No male participation

Box 20-6 REASONS FOR NOT SEEKING OR USING BIRTH CONTROL

Responses of teenagers at initial interview for contraception in order of frequency:
- Didn't get around to it
- Afraid family would find out
- Waiting for closer relationship with partner
- Thought birth control dangerous
- Afraid of examination
- Thought it cost too much
- Didn't think had sex often enough to get pregnant
- Never thought of it
- Didn't know where to get birth control
- Thought had to be older to get birth control
- Didn't expect to have sex
- Thought too young to get pregnant
- Thought birth control wrong
- Partner objected
- Thought wanted pregnancy
- Thought method used good enough

Modified from Tyrer, L.B., Rothbart, B., and Anderson, K.: What every teen should know about contraceptives, Contemp. Pediatr. 6(10):68-94, 1989; with data from Alan Guttmacher Institute: Teenage pregnancy: the problem that hasn't gone away, New York, 1981, Alan Guttmacher Institute.

of intercourse and that only a small number of sexually active youngsters use contraception with regularity. Delay in seeking contraceptive information is commonplace. Compliance is positively correlated with postmenarchal age, frequency of intercourse, autonomy in making and paying for a clinic appointment for the purpose of contraception, and acceptance of a method at the time of the initial clinic visit (Litt, Cuskey, and Rudd, 1980). There are numerous reasons why teenagers are not making better use of contraception (Box 20-6).

Lack of information. Sometimes health professionals have a tendency to confuse a teenager's sophistication with knowledge. Although youngsters are acutely aware of their sexuality, their understanding of reproductive anatomy and physiology is incomplete. If they are using contraception, they often do so with little or no instruction and with only vague understanding. Misinformation is commonplace. Lacking a fundamental understanding of fertility, they often believe that they are too young or have sex too infrequently to become pregnant. A majority of girls mistakenly believe that maximum fertility begins with menses and that the safe period occurs midway between menstrual periods.

Anxiety regarding contraception. Teenagers often express the fear of arguments or threats if they seek assistance via health services. Some are concerned that parents will be notified (see Questions and Controversies). Many have exaggerated ideas about the hazards of oral contraceptives or other methods.

Conflict about sexual activity. Many teenagers feel ambivalent regarding their sexual activity and avoid many contraceptives because their use seems too premeditated and implies that sex is planned rather than a spontaneous activity. Most of these girls believe that sex is all right if one is "swept away" (after all, what can one do about it?) but that planning to do something to prevent pregnancy is wrong.

Desire for pregnancy. There are a few teenagers who deliberately expose themselves to the risk of a pregnancy as a conscious or unconscious act of hostility, response to entrapment, or expression of self-assertion. Even though the youngster has an effective contraceptive, she may fail to use it, use it improperly (conveniently forgetting to take a pill), or use a method not suited to her needs. The girl may know how a contraceptive works but fail to put her knowledge to use. Teenagers are often embarrassed to purchase over-the-counter contraceptives.

QUESTIONS AND CONTROVERSIES

Should adolescents under 18 years of age be permitted to obtain contraceptive services, abortions, and treatment for sexually transmitted diseases without the consent of their parents?

With the increase in sexual activity among adolescents, more of them are in need of health care related to conditions associated with sexuality. Many are reluctant to seek medical care because they are often unable to do so without parental knowledge and permission. Some facilities provide health care to these youngsters without the consent of the parents; however, others deny treatment for fear of legal recriminations. Some minors are able to consent for care legally, that is, those who are married, teenage mothers, and/or self-supporting.

The new regulations governing family planning services under Title X of the Public Health Service Act require that any health care providers receiving government funding notify parents when daughters 17 years of age and under receive prescription contraceptives or contraceptive devices. There are both support for and opposition to this regulation.

Many believe that parents have the right to know what is happening to their children who are under 18 years of age. If parents do not know the medications their daughters are receiving, they are unable to observe for side effects or other associated problems. Also, they will not know what counseling their youngsters might have received relative to the medications or devices.

Others charge that minors will not attend the clinics for needed services for fear that parents will be notified. Thus, this regulation has come to be known as the "squeal rule." Many health professionals insist that young persons have a right to privacy and ownership of their bodies. One of the major reasons youngsters do not seek medical care for sex-related problems is the fear that their parents will find out. Some research indicates that a parental notification policy will not compel all adolescents to inform parents about their contraceptive use; most adolescents will resort to less effective contraceptive methods (Demetriou and Kaplan, 1989).

Would notification of parents penalize those teenagers who are mature and responsible enough to seek contraceptive advice? Will the rule exacerbate the already high incidence of teenage pregnancy and sexually transmitted disease?

Nursing Considerations

Much of contraceptive education and service is assumed by nurses as part of sex education programs, family planning services, or postpartum health services. The introduction of contraceptive methods should ideally be associated with ongoing sex education. When they are included in this education process, the sexually active school-age adolescent will consider contraceptives as a natural and logical part of sex life. It is important that youngsters learn about sexuality, conception, and contraception from someone who can provide them with accurate information in a straightforward, nonjudgmental manner.

Most youngsters select a family planning clinic when seeking contraceptive advice. Many are reluctant to consult a private physician (especially one they know well) because they fear a lecture on morality or a refusal of their request. They may fear that a family physician will inform their parents.

Girls need instruction in correct use of their contraceptive. An effective way to test the teenager's understanding of her particular method is to have her explain to the nurse how the method works. Peer counseling has proved to be successful in gaining compliance, especially in youngsters who engage in more frequent sexual activity, have sex with one partner, and are worried that they might become pregnant (Jay and others, 1984).

An essential part of contraceptive services to teenagers is follow-up. The recipient is expected to return frequently for a checkup on the effectiveness of the method and her general health, sometimes every 2 months, so that the girl must return at regular intervals to maintain her contraceptive.

Nurses are continually on the alert for clues that indicate physical, mental, or emotional problems. Discussions about contraception may provide some insight into disturbed interpersonal relationships and other problems related to the health and well-being of the sexually active adolescent. Participation in regularly scheduled "rap sessions" has proved to be a most important means for exchange between nurses and both male and female adolescents.

An organization that provides education and services for adolescents, including both individual and group counseling, is **Planned Parenthood Federation of America.*** It has branches in most cities in the United States. Many review articles on contraception are available for nurses who wish to counsel teenagers regularly regarding family planning (see Bibliography).

RAPE

The adolescent girl is particularly vulnerable to sexual assault, and it is estimated that more than 50% of rape victims are between 15 and 19 years of age (Koss, Gidycz, and Wisniewski, 1987). In each instance the victim is potentially subject to serious physical or emotional harm or both. Males may also be assaulted and experience the same range of symptoms observed in female victims (Brookman, 1983).

*810 Seventh Ave., New York, NY 10019; (212) 541-7800.

Legal definitions of rape vary from state to state but include the following categories: *completed rape, attempted rape*, and *statutory rape*. Most of the current definitions of rape are expanded to include all forms of sexual victimization, including anal and oral as well as genital penetration. For example, it may include intrusion of any object or body part into the genital or anal area of another person's body.

Sexual assault is not restricted to vaginal or anal penetration but includes every form of sexual activity. To prove power over the victim, the assailant subjects the victim to sodomy and other types of demeaning sexual acts.

Statutory rape may be charged when the victim is unable to give consent legally by virtue of age (age varies from state to state, but is usually less than 16 years of age), mental deficiency, psychosis, or an altered state of consciousness caused by sleep, drugs (including alcohol), or illness. Fitting the penis between the labia without disruption of the hymen or evidence of ejaculation is also considered sufficient penetration to constitute rape.

Assailants

Three relationships are identified for adolescent assault: stranger, nonstranger, and incest. Although all can have serious and long-lasting effects, they are presumed to be different in a number of important ways: in the nature of the dominant, psychologic, and cognitive behavior they provoke; in the issues they raise for service providers and other potential helpers; and in the techniques that may be helpful for treating existing and new cases (Burgess, 1985).

Nonstranger rapist. The majority of rapes are committed by a nonstranger, which is often referred to as *acquaintance* rape. The acquaintance may be a date, someone who lives near the adolescent (e.g., a neighbor), someone who has contact with the victim through recreational activities or sports, or someone in an official association with the teenager (e.g., a teacher). Some assailants wait for an opportunity when the victim is defenseless, such as the teenager at home alone with an uncle or cousin or the baby-sitter being driven home.

The assailant may be another teenager known through a social activity. Research has investigated the relationship of rape-supportive behavior and sex-role learning, dating patterns, and adherence to rape myths (Koss and Oros, 1982). The nature of sex-role learning in most cultures associates females with softness, nonassertiveness, and dependence on men; socializes young women to be alluring yet sexually unavailable; and assigns women the role of pacesetter in sexual situations. Males are conditioned to be strong, powerful, and aggressive—highly valued measures of masculinity—and to be aggressors in sexual situations (Burgess, 1985; Mosher and Anderson, 1986).

Findings of studies also indicate that not only are teenagers at risk for rape by peers but that they often face multiple assailants or "gang rapes." These variations on teenage rape include multiple assailants and a single victim, multiple assailants and multiple victims, multiple assailants and multiple serial victims, and peer rape in tandem (e.g., offenders who group together specifically to rape).

Stranger rapist. It is believed that stranger rapes probably account for 50% of all rapes reported to police. Victims are frequently selected at random because they are apparently helpless and are usually in a vulnerable situation, such as the teenage runaway, the hitchhiker, or the youngster walking alone in an unprotected neighborhood.

Incest. The most commonly reported incestuous relationships are between daughter and a male in a caretaking role (e.g., a father or a stepfather). The average age of onset for an incestuous ongoing relationship is 8 to 9 years, and its duration is approximately 5 years (Kempe and Kempe, 1984). Significantly, a consistent observation is the unusually high incidence of serious illness or disability in mothers of sexually abused daughters, which places greater responsibility for care of the daughter, usually the eldest, in the hands of the father (Herman, 1985). The victim's participation is gained through the application of authority, subtle pressure, persuasion, or misrepresentation of moral standards. For a further discussion of incest, see Chapter 16.

Clinical Manifestations

Adolescents who have been raped arrive at the emergency room or practitioner's office under a variety of circumstances. They are usually brought in by parents, friends, or police, but some girls may seek medical help on their own. They may display a variety of behaviors, such as hysterical crying or giggling, agitation, feelings of degradation, anger and rage, helplessness, nervousness, and rapid mood swings. Adolescents may alternately appear calm and controlled, masking inner turmoil; they may be angry, confused, and filled with self-blame (American Academy of Pediatrics, Committee on Adolescence, 1989b).

The rape victim may present with evidence of physical force, including roughness, nonbrutal beating (slapping), brutal beating (slugging, kicking, beating repeatedly with fists), and choking or gagging. The predominant reaction of the victim is fear—of the rape and of injury. Thus the victim is faced with the dilemma of submission or resistance. Resistance increases the victim's chances of escape but also increases the likelihood of violence against him or her.

Therapeutic Management

It is advisable to obtain parental consent for examination, but the examination may be performed without consent if the adolescent is legally mature and the parents are unavailable. A female nurse should be present during the history and examination of female victims. Whether a parent should be present during the examination is determined on an individual basis. The parent's presence is usually encouraged but only *if the parent is supportive.* Often the presence of a parent or a police officer inhibits the youngster's ability to describe the incident.

Since rape is a legal matter to be determined by the courts, medical examination merely provides evidence of penetration, ejaculation, and, when possible, use of force. The last is difficult to determine, since many young women are left unmarked when forced to comply at the point of a gun or other weapon.

Initial contact. The circumstances of the initial medical evaluation may be frightening and stressful. The initial contact with the rape victim must be supportive, and the fundamental goal (as in any health problem) is to do no further harm. The interrogating and associated activities have the potential to add to the trauma of the sexual assault. First, the victim needs to know that she is (1) all right and (2) not being blamed for the situation. The first approach is not one of repeated interrogation, but an attempt to reduce the youngster's stress.

History. Although it is important to obtain a clear account of the circumstances of an alleged rape, it is equally essential to minimize any further psychologic trauma that might occur if the adolescent is forced to relive a very painful experience. The youngster will in all likelihood have been questioned by family (or whoever brought the victim for care) and the police (if the rape was reported). If the youngster is too upset, the detailed history may be delayed. The youngster should not be further victimized by insensitive care and unnecessary trauma (American Academy of Pediatrics, Committee on Adolescence, 1988).

The history should be as complete as possible and must be taken and presented in the patient's own words, including any account of force or threats. Some youngsters are able to provide detailed descriptions of the event; others are afraid, stammer, cry, and have difficulty in selecting words or are unable to speak at all. The interview can be more effective if a common vocabulary is established so that both the youngster and the interviewer understand the terms used to describe anatomic features.

Information includes date, time, location, and an accurate description of all types of sexual contact. All related activities are included. For example, evidence can be altered if the victim has bathed, urinated, defecated, douched, or changed clothing; therefore these activities should be recorded. Use of a condom by the alleged assailant can alter evidence. For adequate care, other important data include date of last menstrual period, date of last intercourse (where applicable), use of contraception, and any possibility of a preexisting pregnancy or sexually transmitted disease. Behavior and emotional state should also be recorded, since responses range from outward calm and controlled behavior and affect to excessive agitation or hysteria. Some girls are inappropriately giddy or nonchalant.

Examination. The physical examination is carried out as soon as possible, since physical evidence deteriorates rapidly. The youngster is always told in advance in understandable terms exactly what to expect in the way of tests and procedures, and the explanation is accompanied by strong emotional support. The victim is examined thoroughly, including nongenital areas, for evidence of injury that might substantiate the use of force. Sometimes the stress of the incident makes the girl unaware of physical trauma or even serious injury. The degree and type of injury vary greatly in victims of rape. A few are murdered, many suffer physical injury, and practically all are disturbed emotionally. Photographs are taken of bruises, lacerations, or scratches for evidence, and rips or tears in clothing and the presence of dirt or grass stains are noted and recorded. Perineal, vaginal, or rectal lacerations suggest rape.

Specimens are obtained from the vaginal cul-de-sac, and a hang-drop preparation is examined immediately to assess sperm mobility. A cervical smear is prepared and sent to the laboratory. Vaginal secretions are also tested for acid phosphatase, since this enzyme is not normally present in the female genital tract but is found in high concentrations in semen. This is especially important if the assailant has had a vasectomy or is infertile. Prostatic acid phosphatase has been found up to 22 hours after the alleged assault; the Pap smear is the most reliable test for documentation of sexual intercourse from 14 to 26 hours after the event. Forensic materials should be turned over to law enforcement officials promptly after collection (Paradise, 1990).

A baseline serology is drawn, and a gonococcal culture is obtained to prove that the victim did not have any preexisting infection. The child is reexamined at appropriate intervals (4 to 6 weeks for syphilis; 2 to 3 days for gonorrhea) to determine if the child acquired disease from the assailant.

Treatment. Any injuries sustained by the victim that require surgical treatment are repaired. Lacerations of the vagina and/or rectum are not uncommon. Most physicians prescribe, and many of the victims and/or their parents prefer the girl to receive, prophylactic administration of penicillin at the time of initial examination. Pregnancy prophylaxis with high-dose estrogen is offered to the victim who is not using oral contraceptives, pregnant, or menstruating. Follow-up care is needed to observe the youngster for possible development of pelvic inflammatory disease or other sexually transmitted disease.

Rape Trauma Syndrome

Sexual abuse of children, including rape, is being given increasing attention and concern by health professionals, in both the physical aspects and the psychologic reactions to the trauma (see Sexual Abuse, Chapter 16). Burgess and Holmstrom (1975), through their observations, have identified what they describe as the *rape trauma syndrome*. The rape trauma syndrome involves two phases: (1) the acute phase of disorganization of life-style and (2) a long-term process of reorganization. These phases encompass behavioral, somatic, and psychologic reactions to the stressful event. (See also Posttraumatic Stress Disorder, Chapter 18.)

Acute phase of disorganization. During the acute phase, victims exhibit either an expressed style or a controlled style of demonstrating emotional reactions. Those with the expressed style are able to express their feelings of fear, anger, and/or anxiety. Those with the controlled style hide or mask their feelings and display a calm, subdued affect. Since a common emotional response to sexual assault is terror, the psychologic mechanisms evoked in an attempt to cope with the stress are equally powerful. Often the emotional shock creates an exaggerated sense of unreality and dissociation, giving the victim the appearance of indifference (to an untrained observer). The controlled victim is equally as upset as the victim who expresses her feelings.

Other acute reactions include physical reactions such as body soreness, disturbances in sleep patterns, and alterations in eating patterns. In addition to fear responses, the victims demonstrate other emotional responses, including anger, self-blame, guilt, shame, and/or feelings of degradation. Feelings of embarrassment are prominent in adolescents. Mood swings, enhanced mood lability, and increased irritability with others are often observed. Almost all victims spend a good deal of time thinking about how the assault might have been prevented. Many concerns of youngsters focus on how the event will affect them at school.

Long-term reorganization process. Changes in life-style are often observed during the reorganization phase. Victims may continue previous activities such as attending school but achieve only a minimum level of functioning. A teenager may attend school but be apprehensive that other students know about the incident and are talking about her. When an adolescent girl has been raped by a male student or gang of boys from the school, she is afraid to return to school and may beg to move to a different neighborhood. It is not unusual for the attacker to telephone and taunt the victim or for the girl to receive anonymous obscene calls. Most children experience nightmares, phobias about being left alone, and panic reactions on seeing the assailant, the scene of the crime, or a symbolic reminder of the assault. Sexual fears are prominent and difficult for the victim to discuss.

Feelings of helplessness and powerlessness are experienced as the victim feels that events are totally beyond her control. Many demonstrate a marked degree of self-blame because of society's impression that women provoke sexual attacks. Victims are concerned about the potential effects that the assault will have on their relationships with others, particularly regarding the extent to which persons close to them will blame them for the assault. There are concerns about whom to tell about the event and how to go about telling them. Sexual assault produces varied and profound long-term effects on the victims.

Nursing Considerations

Many of the approaches described for the sexually abused child (see Chapter 16) are applicable to the adolescent. Sexual assault is a devastating experience with long-lasting effects. The primary goal of nursing care is not to inflict further stress on the youngster, who is often angry, confused, frightened, embarrassed, and filled with self-blame. Young rape victims fear pregnancy, bodily injury, and the reactions of their parents and peers. Some believe that their bodies are permanently damaged and may even fear death as a consequence of the experience. On the other hand, health professionals are more likely to be angry at the rapist, concerned about sexually transmitted disease, and worried about the youngster's future sexual relations (Mann, 1981).

The nurse must do everything possible to reduce the stress of the interrogation and examination. Application of stress-reduction techniques during the process can help the adolescent manage the immediate experience. Although most health professionals and law enforcement officers are sensitive to the needs of the youngster and attempt to make the process as nonstressful as possible, the nurse should be alert to cues that indicate the victim is being overstressed.

Follow-up care of the rape victim is essential and extends over a long period of time. Consequently, referral to a public health agency, school nurse, and/or mental health agency should be made as soon as possible. Victims who live in areas with established rape crisis centers are fortunate. In areas where they do not exist, nurses can work with communities to establish such a service.

Aside from the universal need for emotional support, there are no firm guidelines for meeting the needs of rape victims. Their needs vary widely and depend on the nature of the incident, when it took place, the physical and emotional injuries sustained by the victim, the actions being considered as a result, the resources available for informal support, and the anticipated reactions of persons in the informal support network (Burgess, 1985). However, the nurse who knows the nature of the rape trauma syndrome and some of the reactions that might be expected is in a better position to assess and meet the needs of the adolescent sexual assault victim.

Family support. In addition to the needs of the adolescent rape victim, the nurse is also sensitive to the needs and reactions of the youngster's parents. Some will be angry and blame the adolescent; others will feel guilty. Many reactions can be expected at the time of the incident, ranging from despair to extreme agitation. Frequently the parents require as much support and reassurance as the victim. Agitated, angry, or incapacitated parents are unable to provide support for their youngster. Meeting their needs can facilitate their ability to support the teenager during the crisis.

Prevention. With the increasing incidence of rape, many professionals are looking to additional means for preventing rape at all ages. Many schools and organizations arrange for classes on how to avoid an attack and how to behave in the event of an attempted rape. Rape trauma centers and most law enforcement agencies provide this service to schools, organizations, or groups of concerned citizens. Every effort should be made to protect children and adolescents from injury and to teach them how to avoid situations that may promote an attack and how to behave in a threatening situation.

Nurses can be advocates for improving the community environment and street lighting, providing safe housing and transportation, and improving the effectiveness of the criminal justice system. They can work toward educating youngsters about the relationship of risk-taking behaviors and sexual attack. These behaviors include drinking, taking drugs, or hitchhiking; a significant number take place after social interactions in unprotected surroundings, such as going to a house or automobile with a relative stranger (known less than 24 hours) (Jenny, 1988).

SEXUALLY TRANSMITTED DISEASES

Sexually transmitted diseases (STDs) represent one of the major causes of morbidity during adolescence and young adulthood and annually afflict approximately 10 million persons under the age of 25 years. Teenagers represent one of the groups at highest risk, since not all of them have initiated sexual activity (Cates, 1987). The area of STD diagnosis and treatment has become exceedingly complex with the expansion from the five traditional venereal diseases (VDs) to the expanded nomenclature of STD in the mid-1970s, which includes more than 20 different infections and associated syndromes.

Several unique characteristics—biologic, developmental, and environmental—place adolescents at risk for acquisition of STDs. Biologically the immature adolescent female undergoes major physiologic transformation in the area of the endocervix. The thin layer of columnar cells appears to favor attachment of infectious agents (e.g., *Chlamydia trachomatis,* wart viruses, papillomavirus), which accounts in part for the increased prevalence of these infections in adolescents. The unchallenged immune system does not provide localized antibody response at the cervical level when exposed repeatedly to infectious agents. During anovulatory cycles, estrogen predominates, as demonstrated by the clear and watery cervical discharge. This may facilitate the transport of pathogens to the upper genital tract (Bell and Hein, 1984).

Developmentally, teenagers experience biologic discontinuities wherein pubertal maturing precedes psychologic and cognitive maturity. For example, the average age of menarche has declined to 12.5 years, and the age of sexual debut has also declined. By age 16 years 25% of females are sexually active; the majority of males and females are sexually active by age 19 years (Hofferth, Kahn, and Baldwin, 1987). The absence of future planning is often evident in their failure to see the implications of current behavior on future outcome, such as condom use to prevent STD or pregnancy or the need to return for follow-up visits for contraceptive refill or STD treatment. During this time of evolving identity and emerging sexuality, the outcome is teenagers who have reproductive capabilities but insufficient maturity and absent social sanctions to be open and responsible about their sexual behavior.

Designing health care systems and providing in-service education for all health care personnel are essential to provision of services that meet the needs of adolescents. Environmental barriers to health care use by teenagers include high cost, lack of insurance, inconvenient timing of appointments, and inconvenient location of health facilities. Services need to be easily accessible and sensitive to the developmental needs and confidentiality of the adolescent.

GONORRHEA

Although gonorrhea as a clinical disease dates from the Old Testament, its differentiation from syphilis (Neisser in 1879) and its linkage to urethral discharge in men and serious pelvic complications in women (twentieth century) are more recent (Sparling, 1990).

Epidemiology

Several demographic factors have been described for persons who are at risk for acquiring gonorrhea. Adolescents

15 to 19 years of age have the highest overall incidence of gonococcal infection compared with any other age-group when rates are adjusted for sexual activity. Gonorrhea among nonwhites is 10 times more frequent than in whites. Part of this discrepancy can be explained by the fact that nonwhites are more likely to attend public health clinics, where reporting of the disease is better than in the private sector. Other known risk factors are low socioeconomic status, urban residence, early onset of sexual activity, single marital status, and previous history of gonorrhea.

✦ **NURSING ALERT** Prior infection is an important marker and should alert the clinician that the individual is at risk for reinfection.

Epidemiologic evidence suggests that there is a core group, or clustering of individuals, who are never treated or inadequately treated and thus serve as a reservoir for reinfection. This emphasizes the need for partner identification and appropriate treatment to interrupt this cycle of reinfection.

Gonorrhea is almost always sexually transmitted, except when it appears in the conjunctiva. Vertical transmission from the maternal cervix to the newborn's conjunctiva is the usual mode of infection. Gonococcal ophthalmia has been eradicated in developed countries by the routine application of prophylactic antibiotics to the eyes of newborn infants (see Chapter 8). Gonococcal infections do not confer lifelong immunity; therefore individuals are subject to repeated reinfection.

Pathophysiology

The causative organism is *Neisseria gonorrhoeae,* a gram-negative diplococcus. The organisms, commonly known as gonococci, have been divided into four types; types 1 and 2 are pathogenic, and types 3 and 4 are considered nonpathogenic. The difference in pathogenicity appears to be the presence of hairlike projections on types 1 and 2 that cause them to adhere to the mucosa, where they remain attached for 36 to 48 hours, the incubation period of the organism. The organisms have very specific survival requirements. They prefer a moist, alkaline environment (pH 7.2 to 7.6) and a temperature of 35° to 36° C (95° to 96.8° F). They quickly die on drying, exposure to the weakest acids, and an increase of 3° C in temperature. The gonococci survive only on the columnar and transitional epithelium; stratified epithelium is resistant to the onslaught. The organisms spread along the mucosa from the point of entry. They penetrate between the epithelial cells and, when they die, liberate an irritant that produces the inflammatory response, characterized by localized capillary dilation, edema, and leukocytosis. This process accounts for the purulent discharge and erosive balanitis and cervicitis observed in affected persons.

Clinical Manifestations

Symptoms can appear as early as 1 day or as late as 2 weeks after sexual contact. Gonococcal infection can occur in many diverse ways with four basic presentations: asymptomatic, uncomplicated symptomatic, complicated symptomatic, and disseminated disease. The infection can involve a number of organs and a wide range of manifestations (see Table 20-2). The pelvic inflammatory disease (PID) in females simulates the inflammatory process caused by other bacterial infections, and differential diagnosis is made for more definitive medical treatment. Since a large percentage of affected persons are asymptomatic, gonorrhea should be considered in the evaluation of all sexually active adolescents. Lack of clinical symptoms is especially characteristic of the rectal and pharyngeal infections.

There is a difference in the way the disease affects children. Whereas uncomplicated urogenital infection in postpubescent girls involves the cervix, in prepubescent girls it is seen as vulvovaginitis. Early complaints of vulvovaginitis include dysuria and perineal or vulvar discomfort, often associated with perianal soreness that is increased during defecation. Examination reveals edematous vaginal mucosa, and a greenish-yellow discharge may be present; the perianal area often appears inflamed and edematous with some discharge from anal crypts.

Diagnostic Evaluation

The diagnosis is established on identification of the organism from direct smear or culture techniques. In males the diagnosis is relatively easy. Since gram-negative diplococci are not normally present in the male genitourinary tract, their intracellular presence in smears is diagnostic. A false-negative result may be seen in the very early course of the disease, in old, untreated cases, and in persons who have taken penicillin or a wide-spectrum antibiotic within a few hours of the examination.

The diagnosis is more difficult in females, which has been a significant obstacle in effective control programs. Although cervical and urethral smears are fairly reliable in the acute phase of the disease, with less acute or asymptomatic cases there is a high yield of both false-positive and false-negative results. Specimens of pus from the urethra or cervix (not the vagina) should be cultured immediately on special media designed for discriminating these organisms. Because of their adverse effects on organisms, surgical jelly or any fatty substance (including some types of swabs) should not be used in securing the specimen. Presence of menses is not a contraindication; the menstrual secretions provide an optimum environment for growth of the organism.

Therapeutic Management

The emergence of gonococcal strains resistant to penicillin has created new recommendations for treatment. A single intramuscular injection of ceftriaxone is the treatment of choice, with intramuscular injection of spectinomycin the preferred alternative for those who are unable to tolerate ceftriaxone (Centers for Disease Control, 1989; Rawstron and others, 1989). Another concern is the high incidence of coexistent chlamydial infection, which has been documented to occur in up to 45% of those individuals who have gonorrhea. Therefore coverage with antibiotics for chlamydia is always recommended to eradicate the coexist-

Table 20-2 Comparison between gonorrhea and chlamydial infection

CHARACTERISTICS	GONORRHEA	CHLAMYDIAL INFECTION
Incubation period	2-6 days; can be as long as 10-16 days in rare cases	8-21 days
Major site of infection	Urethritis (males) Cervicitis (females)	Urethritis (males) Cervicitis (females)
Local complications	Epididymitis, bartholinitis, salpingitis, prostatitis Conjunctivitis Pharyngitis Proctitis common in homosexual individuals	Epididymitis, bartholinitis, salpingitis Conjunctivitis (trachoma) Pharyngitis Proctitis not yet documented
Systemic complications	Well established; septicemia with resulting arthritis, dermatitis, endocarditis; meningitis; perihepatitis and peritonitis also reported	Possible: arthritis, perihepatitis, peritonitis, endocarditis reported
Carrier state	Recognized, especially in women; can last for months; primary reservoir is the cervix, male urethra a minor one	Recognized, especially in women; can last for months; primary reservoir is the cervix, male urethra a minor one
Effects of maternal infection on newborn	Less well established Ophthalmia neonatorum	Well known: inclusion conjunctivitis and pneumonia
Treatment	Ceftriaxone or spectinomycin Probenecid used in conjunction with antibiotics Shorter period of therapy Treatment of sexual contacts	Doxycycline or tetracycline is drug of choice; erythromycin, sulfonamides, streptomycin, trimethoprim-sulfamethoxazole Regimen of 14 days Treatment of sexual contacts

ent infection. Treatment failure with this combination regimen is rare. Test of cure after completion of antibiotics is not indicated. A more cost-effective strategy recommended by the Centers for Disease Control (CDC) is reexamination in 1 to 2 months after infection to detect either treatment failure or, more often, reinfection (Centers for Disease Control, 1989). It is important that all affected youngsters have a serologic test for syphilis (STS), and all their sexual contacts should be traced and treated.

Complicated and disseminated infections may require longer antibiotic therapy, and complications are treated appropriately. In all cases of gonorrhea the long-term genitourinary problems in the male and possible occlusion of the fallopian tubes or tubo-ovarian abscesses in the female from untreated or repeated infections can lead to severe debilitation in later life or even death. Therefore case finding and early treatment are imperative.

Prevention

A genuine prophylaxis against gonorrheal infections is not yet available. There is a protective vaccine in the process of development, but when it is becomes available, the decision must be made concerning who should be vaccinated and when they should be vaccinated. Until such time as protection is in common use, preventive efforts must be directed toward finding and treating affected persons, locating and examining contacts of affected persons, and educating young people regarding the facts of the disease and its spread. The use of spermicide-coated condoms prevents transmission of the infection.

CHLAMYDIAL INFECTION

Recent evidence indicates that chlamydial infection is a major type of STD in adolescents and young adults and is more common than gonorrhea in its incidence, transmission, range of infection sites, and carrier state. Over 4 million infections occur annually. It is estimated that by 1990, 2.8 billion in health care dollars will be spent on direct and indirect cost of chlamydial infections in men and women (Washington, Johnson, and Sanders, 1987). Like gonorrhea, the causative organism is responsible for a variety of disorders, including cervicitis, salpingitis, epididymitis, urethritis, peritonitis, conjunctivitis, pneumonia, and otitis media. However, the main infections are urethritis in males and cervicitis in females.

Pathophysiology

The disease is caused by *Chlamydia trachomatis*, an organism previously thought to be a virus but now known to be bacteria. Like viruses, chlamydiae are intracellular parasites during part of their life cycle. The organisms consist of alternating forms—the extracellular, or elementary, body and the intracellular, or initial, body. The elementary body attaches to the host cell, where it induces active phagocytosis and is ingested in a vesicle that serves as a setting for the next stage of the cycle.

Unlike other phagocytosed organisms, *C. trachomatis* is able to circumvent host cell defenses and become a part of the cell. Within the host cell the elementary body reorganizes into the larger initial body, which uses the cell's synthetic functions and energy sources for its own metabolic needs. It divides to produce microcolonies of chlamydiae. After 18 to 24 hours the initial bodies again reorganize into elementary bodies and exit from the disrupted host cell to infect new cells. The entire process takes about 40 hours, and the result is a slow, steady accumulation of intracellular inclusions that are diagnostic of the infection.

Clinical Manifestations

The signs and symptoms of infection by *C. trachomatis* are similar to those of gonorrhea, which include meatal erythema and tenderness, urethral discharge, dysuria, or urethral itching in males and mucopurulent cervical exudate, usually associated with erythema, edema, congestion, and increased friability of the cervix in females. The symptoms may be mild enough to be ignored or entirely absent (see Table 20-2).

Diagnostic Evaluation

The diagnosis is confirmed by isolation of the organism in a tissue cell culture or serologic evidence of infection. Because the staining techniques are insensitive, smears are not useful in the specific diagnosis of the disease. The complement fixation test is useful in the diagnosis of lymphogranuloma venereum caused by *C. trachomatis,* and the microimmunofluorescent test is often used for other chlamydial infections. Development of a rapid diagnostic test for chlamydia allows for rapid, inexpensive diagnosis of this infection when expensive culture techniques are not available (Stamm and Mardh, 1990). Abnormal Pap smears have been associated with antichlamydial antibodies in cervical secretions.

Therapeutic Management

The treatment of choice is oral doxycycline daily for at least 14 days, with tetracycline as the alternative (Centers for Disease Control, 1989). It is also recommended that all patients receive a course of therapy for gonorrhea because of the high rate of mixed gonococcal and chlamydial infections (see previous section). Treatment of sexual partners is also an important part of therapy.

HUMAN PAPILLOMAVIRUS

Anogenital warts, caused by the human papillomavirus (HPV), have been evident for centuries, but the true incidence is unknown. However, the number of practitioner-patient consultations increased almost sevenfold from 1966 to 1984 (Becker, Stone, and Alexander, 1987). It is the most common sexually transmitted disease in the United States and, in the adolescent, the majority of (if not all) abnormal Pap smears are related to HPV infection (Davis and Emans, 1989).

Three types of genital warts are known to occur in clinical practice—*condyloma acuminatum, condyloma plana,* and *inverted condyloma*—and can be found on any part of the male and female genitalia and may coexist (Steinmiller, 1988). The first two types are discussed further.

The most visible type is condyloma acuminatum, a raised, polypoid mass with an irregular fingerlike surface and fissures, commonly described as a cauliflower appearance. In females these warts are most commonly seen on the external genitals and, less commonly, the vagina, cervix, or rectum. The shaft of the penis is the most common site in males, but warts may also appear on the meatus, anus, and scrotum. Presence of warts on the rectum or anus of males is frequently associated with anal intercourse; anal warts in females can be associated with autoinoculation.

The second and most difficult wart to diagnose is a flat condyloma, also known as subclinical papillomavirus infection (SPI). These warts are easily visualized after the application of acetic acid (vinegar) and by magnification with the colposcope (Moscicki, 1989).

A growing concern has been expressed regarding HPV infection and its relationship to cancer. Newer diagnostic techniques allow researchers to detect infection with HPV using DNA viral typing. Over 50 different viral types have been described; however, the majority of dysplastic lesions will never progress to cancer. Since no easy method is currently available to predict those that will progress, all lesions are treated. It is estimated that an average of 17% of sexually active females have been infected with this virus. The true incidence is not known, because no reporting mechanism now exists (Moscicki, 1989).

Therapeutic Management

Treatment of external warts on females and males consists of topical applications of chemical agents, such as podophyllin or trichloroacetic acid (TCA). Liquid nitrogen can be used to freeze off dysplastic lesions of the cervix. Other therapies include intravaginal and external applications of the antineoplastic drug, 5-fluorouracil; however, its use is limited to extensive and recurrent disease. Laser therapy, used to vaporize extensive lesions, is performed with the patient under general anesthesia and associated with greater risk; thus its use is limited to severe or unrelenting disease (Moscicki, 1989).

Use of chemical agents requires special instruction. For example, the chemical agent podophyllin needs to be washed off 4 to 6 hours after application in order to prevent absorption of the chemical, which can be neurotoxic. Teenagers have many questions regarding warts and their potential for causing cervical cancer; therefore education and reassurance are important. Encouragement of compliance is also important, need for follow-up care is lengthy, and condom use is essential during treatment.

HUMAN IMMUNODEFICIENCY VIRUS INFECTION AND ACQUIRED IMMUNE DEFICIENCY SYNDROME

Health professionals caring for teenagers have expressed growing concern regarding the transmission of human immunodeficiency virus (HIV), which eventually causes acquired immune deficiency syndrome (AIDS) among specific subgroups of adolescents. Presently this virus is considered to be universally fatal. Its ability to overwhelm the individual's immune system causes death through a variety of diseases. Transmission of the virus takes place through sharing body fluids infected with the HIV. Major mechanisms of transmission are through exchange of sexual fluids (semen, vaginal fluid, menstrual fluid, and blood); receiving blood or blood products infected with HIV (intravenous drug users [IVDUs] sharing unclean needles); and passage of the virus from an infected mother to her unborn child. Consequently, HIV has been called the number-one public health problem facing the United States, although the total number of AIDS cases among teenagers is very small (less than 2%) when compared with all other age-groups with the disease.

Reason for concern about AIDS in teenagers is related to several factors. Sexual partners of female adolescents are often several years older and may have been already infected. The known high prevalence rates of other STDs and pregnancy among adolescents document that adolescents are sexually active but do not take precautions to protect themselves against HIV infection. Of particular concern are ethnic minority female youths who may be infected through heterosexual transmission from an intravenous (IV) drug–using partner. Not only are they at risk for developing AIDS, but they can pass the infection to their unborn child if they become pregnant.

A long latency period between infection and the development of clinical AIDS has been demonstrated (average duration, 7 years). Since the greatest number of reported AIDS cases occur among young adults in their twenties, it can be inferred that many of these infections were acquired in adolescence. Transmission of HIV occurs while affected individuals are asymptomatic for AIDS, and those adolescents infected with the virus can continue to spread the infection without ever knowing they have the disease (Hein, 1989; Hein and Hurst, 1988).

Degrees of risk have been identified for adolescents related to AIDS, with specific recommendations for education and intervention (Box 20-7; see also Acquired Immune Deficiency Syndrome, Chapter 35.)

Box 20-7 DEGREES OF HIV RISK AND INTERVENTIONS AMONG ADOLESCENTS

Category 1

Teenagers who are currently not at risk for AIDS because of current life-style or absence of virus within their sphere of activities; very young, virginal; have received no transfusions; are not IV substance abusers

Issues:
- Worried but healthy; need to learn how to live in atmosphere of concern and maintain appropriate level of concern without undue anxiety; need help to differentiate between myths and facts
- Need for information on casual contacts; encourage to engage in activities that do not place them at risk
- Support decision making about sexual activities

Category 2

Sexually active teenagers who have not yet been exposed to HIV

Issues:
- Knowing (or not being able to "know") their partners
- Reconsider patterns of sexual behavior
- Use of contraceptives in general and condoms in particular

Category 3

Teenagers at risk for HIV acquisition because of exposure to infected individuals (IV drug users, sexual partners of IV drug users, homosexuals or bisexuals, sex partners of homosexuals or bisexuals)

Issues:
- Decisions about HIV testing
- Knowledge of serostatus of partner(s)
- Need for barrier methods of contraception
- Reconsideration of patterns of sexual behavior
- Decision about continuing pregnancy
- Need for services geared to adolescent age-group for crisis intervention and follow-up of HIV-infected teenagers and partners

Modified from Hein, K.: Commentary on adolescent acquired immunodeficiency syndrome: the next wave of the human immunodeficiency virus epidemic? J. Pediatr. 114:144-149, 1989.

HEPATITIS B

Hepatitis B virus (HBV) is an infection of the liver, which affects 300,000 persons annually, 10,000 of whom require hospitalization (see Chapter 33). Major concerns have been voiced because of the increased rate of infection, particularly among high-risk populations—IVDUs, heterosexual sex partners of HBV-infected individuals, and homosexual males. Another area of concern is transmission of HBV from pregnant women to their infants. It is estimated that infants whose mothers are positive for HBV will have a 70% to 90% chance of becoming infected, and nearly all these infants will develop chronic HBV carrier status (U.S. Preventive Services Task Force, 1989).

Many potential negative outcomes can be avoided with primary prevention, adequately achieved through immunization. Broader immunization strategies, which target noninfected infants and adolescents before the onset of high-risk behaviors (e.g., sexual activity, IV drug use), may soon be implemented in an attempt to diminish the devastating effects of HBV (Centers for Disease Control, 1988).

VAGINITIS

Seeking gynecologic care for a complaint of vaginal discharge associated with other signs and symptoms (e.g., dysuria, pruritus, foul smell, abnormal bleeding) is common among adolescent females, and among sexually active girls a pelvic examination and collection of cultures for STDs are an important part of health care. Since not all vaginal infections are sexually transmitted, such as candidiasis, adolescent females require considerable health teaching in understanding their bodies.

SEXUALLY TRANSMITTED GENITAL LESIONS

Many sores or lesions that appear on the genitals are the result of STDs. Experienced clinicians can correctly diagnose these lesions by visual examination only 60% of the time; therefore a complete health history, physical examination, and appropriate diagnostic cultures are needed to determine the causative factors. Nurses who interact with adoles-

Table 20-3 Vaginitis and genital lesions in adolescents

DISEASE (AGENT)	MANIFESTATIONS	THERAPY	NURSING CONSIDERATIONS
▪ Vaginitis			
Trichomoniasis *(Trichomonas vaginalis)*—unicellular, anaerobic, flagellated protozoa)	Pruritus and edema of vagina and external genitalia; thin, grayish vaginal discharge; frequency, dysuria; dyspareunia May be asymptomatic, especially in males	Oral metronidazole Clotrimazole vaginal suppository during pregnancy	Nonsexual transmission not well documented Patient should not consume alcohol while taking medication and for at least 3 days following last dose Identify and treat infected partner
Bacterial vaginosis (multiple organisms)	Gray-white, malodorous, nonirritating vaginal discharge; uniformly adherent to vagina	Metronidazole Clindamycin (alternative)	Routine treatment of sexual partner not indicated—no evidence of this entity in males
Candidiasis, or moniliasis *(Candida albicans)*	Edema and erythema of vulva White, cheesy vaginal discharge (less than 50% of cases) May be satellite lesions on groin, thighs, and buttocks Cutaneous lesions on penis May be asymptomatic Usually vulvar pruritus	Miconazole vaginal suppository Butoconazole cream Clotrimazole vaginal tablets Terconazole vaginal suppository	Possibility of predisposing factors such as oral contraceptives, pregnancy, and diabetes mellitus (which alter vaginal environment) or antibiotics Increased risk of neonatal thrush
▪ Genital lesions			
Herpes simplex (Herpesvirus hominis—type II [90%]; type I [10%])	Prodrome: intense burning or itching at site of outbreak First lesions: clear, raised vesicles; rupture in 24 hours; painful Resolving: painful, shallow, white, wet ulcers	Acyclovir (Zovirax) ointment decreases healing time and pain	Immunocompromised patient at risk for overwhelming infection Sex partner not treated unless lesions present Pregnancy should be avoided in sexually active girls Infection can be transmitted to infant during birth
Molluscum (virus)	Solitary clusters of raised, pearly white, firm, nontender papules Umbilicated dimpled lesions	Excision and expression of core material Trichloroacetic acid Cryotherapy	No known complications Sex partner not treated unless lesions present
Primary syphilis *(Treponema pallidum)*	Chancre: a hard, nontender, red, sharply defined lesion with indurated base, raised border, eroded surface, and scanty yellow discharge; usually located on penis, vulva, or cervix	Penicillin Alternative: doxycycline Pregnant women: erythromycin	Viability of organism outside body is short Rapidly killed by oxygen, soap, common bacterial agents, and drying About 95% transmitted sexually; affected person most infectious during first year of disease Transmission from mother to fetus (congenital syphilis)

cents are in a primary position to obtain a health history and refer any sexually active youngster for appropriate evaluation. Follow-up health education regarding any treatment regimen and prevention strategies is a major nursing role. A summary of the most common genital lesions seen in adolescents is outlined in Table 20-3.

PELVIC INFLAMMATORY DISEASE

Pelvic inflammatory disease (PID) is an infection of the upper genital tract (endometrium and fallopian tubes), most commonly caused by sexually transmitted bacteria, such as *N. gonorrhoeae, C. trachomatis,* and a variety of other anaerobic bacteria. PID represents one of the most serious complications of STDs among adolescent females because of the damage that can occur from tubal scarring. It is estimated that each year 1 million females of reproductive age experience an episode of PID with approximately 20% of cases occurring among teenagers. Economic consequences are significant, with estimates of up to $3 billion annually spent on the disease (Sweet, 1987).

Several risk factors associated with PID have been identified. Women under the age of 25 years have a 1 in 8 chance of experiencing PID compared with those over 25 years, whose risk is 1 in 80. Nonwhite females are twice as likely to develop PID as white adolescents. STDs, especially *N. gonorrhoeae* (25% to 50% of cases) and *C. trachomatis* (25% to 43% of cases), have been associated with PID. Contraceptives, such as barrier methods (condoms) or spermicides, which protect against STDs, are used inconsistently by teenagers. Biologically the immature adolescent cervix is in the process of undergoing considerable change, and the area of transformation (ectopy) at the endocervical os seems less resistant to attack by infectious agents (Shafer and Sweet, 1989).

Presenting symptoms in the adolescent may be generalized, with fever, abdominal pain, urinary tract symptoms, and vague influenza-like manifestations, such as malaise, nausea, diarrhea, or constipation. A pelvic examination is indicated for every sexually active female who complains of lower abdominal pain to evaluate the possibility of PID.

PID is of major concern to nurses because of the devastating effects on the reproductve tract of affected adolescents. Approximately 25% of women experiencing PID may have short-term complications, such as acute abscess formation in the fallopian tubes (tubo-ovarian abscess), or long-term complications, such as chronic pelvic pain, dyspareunia (painful coitus), or formation of adhesions. Most significant, however, is the increased risk for ectopic pregnancy and/or infertility, which results from tubal scarring. Outpatient management may be initiated, but hospitalization is preferred to ensure compliance, response to treatment, and preservation of future fertility (Shafer and Sweet, 1989; Washington, Sweet, and Shafer, 1985).

Prevention is the primary concern of health care professionals. Use of barrier contraceptive methods, such as condoms with addition of spermicide, seem to offer the best protection for preventing STDs and this serious complication. Sexually active teenage females should be screened routinely to detect those with asymptomatic STDs, and treatment is needed to prevent PID and all associated complications.

NURSING CONSIDERATIONS IN SEXUALLY TRANSMITTED DISEASE

Nursing responsibilities encompass all aspects of sexually transmissible disease education, prevention, and treatment. The sex education of young people should include information about these diseases, such as their symptoms and treatment, and dispelling the myths associated with their mode of transmission. These diseases are not contracted from toilet seats, drinking glasses, or bath towels. Herpes simplex virus has been shown to remain viable on some surfaces and materials that have been in contact with infected lesions; however, the risk is extremely low (Larson and Bryson, 1985; Nerurkar and others, 1983). Most persons in the vulnerable teenage population are uninformed or misinformed about these diseases. Helping to promote the inclusion of STD information in school sex education programs is an important function of the nurse.

No matter what their area of practice, nurses are in a position to disseminate information, identify probable cases, and refer these cases for treatment. In the hospital, school, clinic, or private practice, nurses who recognize the signs and symptoms of disease can call these to the attention of the attending practitioner. This includes not only nurses working in pediatric practice but those in prenatal and obstetric services as well. A characteristic rash or lesion on a pregnant woman may be evidence of disease and a threat to the unborn child. It is nurses who are most successful in persuading pregnant women to receive early and regular prenatal care. The earlier the mother is treated, the less the hazard to the unborn child, especially in the case of syphilis, which does not affect the fetus during the first 4 months of gestation. Gonorrheal, chlamydial, and herpes infections are most dangerous to the child during delivery and in the postpartum period.

Nurses, too, should not overlook the need for care in handling infected infants and children to prevent cross-contaminating others or contracting the disease themselves. Gloves should be worn when handling secretions and areas most likely to contain the organisms, and any breaks in the skin should receive special protective covering.

The increasing incidence of sexually transmitted diseases in young people is influenced to a great extent by the larger numbers of teenagers who engage in sexual activity, at younger ages, and with more partners. In addition, the changing pattern of contraceptive use is a contributing factor to more promiscuous sexual activity and the concomitant rise in gonorrhea and chlamydial infection. The newer contraceptive methods, oral contraceptives and intrauterine devices, appear to provide no protection against sexually transmitted diseases, and barrier devices, such as the condom, that offer some protection are not well accepted by teenagers. Unfortunately, many girls who take oral contraceptive pills mistakenly believe that they are also effective in preventing sexually transmitted diseases. To decrease the likelihood of infection, sexually active youngsters should be encouraged to use a mechanical barrier (condom).

Essential measures for control of the disease are treating the disease, reporting it *promptly,* and tracing and treating contacts. Very often teenagers who suspect they have a sexually transmitted disease will seek a trusted nurse for help rather than their parents. When dealing with adolescents, nurses need highly developed interviewing skills and a nonjudgmental approach to elicit a history of sexual contacts. The belief that these diseases are "dirty" and that "nice" people from "nice" families do not contract the diseases, and the fear of parental displeasure and of "squealing" on friends, can be deterrents to getting needed information.

Several characteristics of teenagers influence the way health professionals address specific issues related to STDs. Teenagers have cognitive differences, which affect the processing of information, and differences in coping styles. They are "sexual adventurers" and lack availability to services that are convenient, appropriate, and attractive to youth (Hein, 1989). To gain youngsters' cooperation, the nurse conveys acceptance, helps them feel at ease, and assures them that the information they give will be used to help those persons whom they name as contacts. They can be reassured that their identity and the identities of the persons they name as contacts will be kept confidential. The purpose is not to embarrass or punish but to trace and treat affected persons. This is the most effective means presently available for controlling these diseases.

Several resources are available for education, information, and care. *AIDS: Trading Fears for Facts,* a book written especially for youngsters 13 to 18 years of age, describes myths, transmission, and information about testing and treatment and is also a resource guide, with telephone numbers of service agencies.* The national AIDS hotline is available 24 hours a day to answer questions and provide guidance.†

Confidentiality

Providing confidential health services with a mechanism for payment is crucial. Confidentiality implies the notion of a private and personal relationship between the provider and the patient. In most states, adolescents have the ability to consent for their care in a private and confidential manner for health services as they relate to sexuality and, to a limited extent, mental health and substance abuse. Adolescents should also be judged on their own economic status or inability to pay for these services regardless of their parents' health insurance or economic status. Reliance on parental health care benefits for payment may adversely affect confidentiality, since costs generated for the diagnosis and treatment of pregnancy or STD may violate the teenager's right to privacy. Many states have special funds to pay for confidential health services. Laws that protect confidentiality are not intended to exclude parents in the delivery of health care to their children.

Since teenagers may delay seeking services because of fear of disclosure to parents, in some states the law allows them to access care to avoid negative outcomes that might result from no medical care. For example, poor pregnancy outcome may occur when prenatal care is delayed until late (or not at all), or sequelae such as PID may result from untreated STD. Inclusion of a parent can take place, if indicated, after the youth is established in the health care system and a plan negotiated between the youth and the provider regarding the need for parental involvement (Hoffman, 1980; Silber, 1986).

Nurses need to be familiar with state law in their practice settings as it relates to provision of family planning, pregnancy testing and diagnosis, abortion services, obstetric care, and STD diagnosis and treatment. Knowledge of the law allows the nurse to function in the capacity of advocate for the teenage client. Also, youth may seek optional services, such as contraception or abortion, when they have no emergent medical indications. In these situations it is imperative to review risk/benefit ratios and alternative approaches to treatment, provide opportunity for the youth to ask questions, and respect their right to refuse treatment. Delivery of care to adolescents requires a developmental perspective. Understanding of the biologic, psychosocial, and legal issues affects the delivery of health care to adolescent clients and their families.

*Available for $3.95 from Consumer Reports Books, 9180 LeSaint Dr., Fairfield, OH 45014-5452; (513) 860-1178.

†National AIDS hotline: (800) 342-AIDS; in Canada: AIDS Information Line, (800) 972-2437.

KEY POINTS

- Typical adolescent health-seeking behaviors center on skin problems, obesity, headaches, abdominal discomfort, menstrual symptoms, and anxieties about physical development and sexual change.
- Acne is prevalent in the teen years; medication and hygiene are the treatments of choice.
- Alterations in growth and maturation may be manifest in short stature; tall stature; precocious puberty; Turner syndrome; Klinefelter syndrome; pathologic conditions such as chronic disease, skeletal defects, endocrine dysfunction, and cortisol excess; and psychosocial dwarfism.
- Assessment of growth consists of taking a family history, determining previous growth patterns, conducting a physical examination, determining bone age, and conducting endocrine studies.
- The most frequent problems related to the male reproductive system are infections, scrotal conditions, and gynecomastia.
- The most frequent problems of the female reproductive system involve menstruation—delays, irregularities, discomfort—, and infections.
- Adolescent pregnancy has profound social, educational, psychologic, and economic ramifications; physiologically the pregnancy necessities special attention to nutrition and psychologic and emotional support for the mother and father.
- Abortion as an alternative to birth has been determined to have no long-term psychologic sequelae.
- Contraception is often not used because of lack of information, anxiety regarding use, conflict over sexual activity, and desire for pregnancy.
- Rape is a serious problem among adolescent females; common forms are rape by stranger, rape by nonstranger, and incest.
- Sexually transmitted diseases are the most frequently occurring infectious diseases and a major cause of adolescent morbidity.

REFERENCES

Ad Hoc Committee on Growth Hormone Usage, The Lawson Wilkins Pediatric Endocrine Society, and Committee on Drugs: growth hormone in the treatment of children with short stature, Pediatrics 72:891-894, 1983.

Adler, N.E., and Dolcini, P.: Psychological issues in abortion for adolescents. In Melton, G.B., editor: Adolescent abortion: psychological and legal issues, Lincoln, NE, 1986, University of Nebraska Press.

Alpert, G., and Fleisher, G.R.: Complications of infection with Epstein-Barr virus during childhood: a study of children admitted to the hospital, Pediatr. Infect. Dis. 3:304-307, 1984.

Alvin, P.E., and Litt, I.F.: Current status of the etiology and management of dysmenorrhea in adolescence, Pediatrics 70:516-525, 1982.

American Academy of Pediatrics, Committee on Adolescence: Counseling the adolescent about pregnancy options, Pediatrics 83:135-137, 1989.

American Academy of Pediatrics, Committee on Adolescence: Rape and the adolescent, Pediatrics 81:595-597, 1988.

American Academy of Pediatrics, Committee on Drugs: New therapy for severe cystic acne, Pediatrics 72:258-259, 1983.

Anderson, M.M., Irwin, C.E., and Snyder, D.L.: Abnormal vaginal bleeding in adolescents, Pediatr. Ann. 15:697-707, 1986.

Atton, A.V., and Tunnessen, W.W., Jr.: Acne update: help your patients help themselves, Contemp. Pediatr. 5(10):18-50, 1988.

Bane, M.J., and Ellwood, D.T.: One fifth of the nation's children: why are they poor? Science 245:1047-1053, 1989.

Batista, M.C., and others: Low-dose oral clonidine: effective growth hormone releasing agent in children but not in adolescents, J. Pediatr. 111:564-567, 1987.

Beach, R.K.: Menstrual cramps need not be a curse, Contemp. Pediatr. 6(10):41-72, 1988.

Bearinger, L., and Gephart, J.: Priorities for adolescent health: recommendations of a national conference, MCN 12:161-164, 1987.

Becker, T.M., Stone, K.M., and Alexander, E.R.: Genital human papillomavirus infection: a growing concern, Obstet. Gynecol. Clin. North Am. 14:389-397, 1987.

Bell, T.A., and Hein, K.: Adolescents and sexually transmitted diseases. In Holmes, K.K., and others: Sexually transmitted diseases, New York, 1984, McGraw-Hill, Inc.

Bender, B. and others: Speech and language development in 41 children with sex chromosome anomalies, Pediatrics 71:262-267, 1983.

Biro, F.M., and others: Hormonal studies and physical maturation in adolescent gynecomastia, J. Pediatr. 116:450-455, 1990.

Bowie, W.E.: Urethritis in males. In Holmes, K.K., and others: Sexually transmitted diseases, ed. 2, New York, 1990, McGraw-Hill, Inc.

Brookman, R.R.: Adolescent sexuality and related health problems. In Hoffman, A.D., editor: Adolescent medicine, Menlo Park, CA, 1983, Addison-Wesley Publishing Co., Inc.

Burgess, A.W.: The sexual victimization of adolescents, DHHS Pub. No. (ADM) 858-1382, Washington, DC, 1985, U.S. Government Printing Office.

Burgess, A.W., and Holmstrom, L.L.: Sexual trauma of children and adolescents: pressure, sex, and secrecy, Nurs. Clin. North Am. 10:551-563, 1975.

Camp, B.W., and others: Infants of adolescent mothers, Am. J. Dis. Child. 138:243-246, 1984.

Castro-Magaña, M. and others: Effect of prolonged clonidine administration on growth hormone concentrations and rate of linear growth in children with constitutional growth delay, J. Pediatr. 109:784-787, 1986.

Cates, W.: Epidemiology and control of sexually transmitted diseases: strategic evolution, Infect. Dis. Clin. North Am. 1:1-23, 1987.

Centers for Disease Control: Changing patterns of groups at high risk for hepatitis B in the United States, MMWR 37:429-432, 1988.

Centers for Disease Control: Sexually transmitted diseases: treatment guidelines, MMWR 38:S-80, 1989.

Children's Defense Fund: Adolescent pregnancy: an anatomy of a social problem in search of comprehensive solutions, Washington, DC, 1987, Adolescent Pregnancy Prevention Clearinghouse.

Cohen, F.L.: Clinical genetics in nursing practice, Philadelphia, 1984, J.B. Lippincott Co.

Cohen, F.L., and Durham, J.D.: Children with sex chromosome variations: implications for pediatric nursing practice, J. Pediatr. Nurs. 1:12-23, 1986.

Coll, C.T.G., and Oh, W.: The social ecology and early parenting of Caucasian American mothers, Child Dev. 58:955-963, 1987.

Colletta, N.D., and Gregg, C.H.: Adolescent mothers' vulnerability to stress, J. Nerv. Ment. Dis. 169:50-54, 1981.

D'Arcy, P.F.: Drug interactions with oral contraceptives, Drug Intell. Clin. Pharm. 20:353-358, 1986.

Davis, S.: Pregnancy in adolescents, Pediatr. Clin. North Am. 36:665-680, 1989.

Davis, A.J., and Emans, S.J.: Human papilloma virus infection in the pediatric and adolescent patient, J. Pediatr. 115:1-9, 1989.

Dawood, M.Y.: Dysmenorrhea, Clin. Obstet. Gynecol. 27:719-727, 1983.

Demetriou, E., and Kaplan, D.W.: Adolescent contraceptive use and parental notification, Am. J. Dis. Child. 143:1166-1172, 1989.

Digest: Majority of Americans oppose overturning Roe v. Wade and banning abortion outright, polls show, Fam. Plann. Perspect. 18:250-254, 1989.

Edelsberg, J.S., and Surh, Y.S.: The acute scrotum, Emerg. Clin. North Am. 6:521-546, 1988.

Elster, A.B., McAnarney, E.R., and Lamb, M.E.: Parental behaviors of adolescent mothers, Pediatrics 71:494-503, 1983.

English, A.: Minors' consent for abortion: new developments in state law, Youth Law News 10(6):12-15, 1989.

Food and Nutrition Board: Recommended dietary allowances, Washington, DC, 1989, National Academy of Sciences—National Research Council.

Gertner, J.M., and others: Prospective clinical trial of human growth hormone in short children without growth hormone deficiency, J. Pediatr. 104:172-176, 1984.

Gordon, M., and others: Psychosocial aspects of constitutional short stature: social competence, behavior problems, self-esteem, and family functioning, J. Pediatr. 101:477-480, 1982.

Green, J.W., and others: Child rearing attitudes, observed behavior, and perception of infant temperament in adolescent versus older mothers, Pediatr. Res. 15:442, 1981.

Greydanus, D.E., and Shearin, R.B.: Adolescent sexuality and gynecology, Philadelphia, 1990, Lea & Febiger.

Hamburg, D., Nightingale, E.O., and Takanishi, R.: Facilitating the transitions of adolescence: Council on Adolescent Development, JAMA 257:3405-3406, 1987.

Hatcher, R.A., and others: Contraceptive technology, 1988-1989, ed. 14, New York, 1988, Irvington.

Hein, K.: Commentary on adolescent acquired immunodeficiency syndrome; the next wave of the human immunodeficiency virus epidemic? J. Pediatr. 114:144-149, 1989.

Hein, K., and Hurst, M.: Human immunodeficiency virus infection in adolescence: a rationale for action, Adolesc. Pediatr. Gynecol. 1:73-82, 1988.

Henshaw, S.K., and Van Vort, J.: Teenage abortion, birth and pregnancy statistics: an update, Fam. Plann. Perspect. 21(2):85-88, 1989.

Herman, J.: Father-daughter incest. In Burgess, A.W., editor: Handbook on rape research, New York, 1985, Garland Publishing, Inc.

Hirsch, B.J.: Natural support systems and coping with major life changes, Am. J. Community Psychol. 8:159-172, 1980.

Hofferth, S.L., Kahn, J.R., and Baldwin W.: Premarital sexual activity among U.S. teenage women over the past three decades, Fam. Plann. Perspect. 19:46-53, 1987.

Hoffman, A.D.: A rational policy toward consent and confidentiality in adolescent health care, J. Adolesc. Health Care 1:9-17, 1980.

Howard, J.S., and Sater, J.: Adolescent mothers: self-perceived health education needs, JOGNN 14:399-404, 1985.

Irwin, C.E., and Millstein, S.G.: Biopsychosocial correlates of risk-taking behaviors during adolescence: can the physician intervene? J. Adolesc. Health Care 7(suppl.):82S, 1986.

Jay, M.S., and others: Effect of peer counselors on adolescent compliance in use of oral contraceptives, Pediatrics 73:126-131, 1984.

Jenny, C.: Adolescent risk-taking behavior and the occurrence of sexual assault, Am. J. Dis. Child. 142:770-772, 1988.

Kass, E.J., Chandra, R.S., and Belman, A.B.: Testicular histology in the adolescent with a varicocele, Pediatrics 79:996-998, 1987.

Kempe, R.S., and Kempe, C.H.: The common secret: sexual abuse of children and adolescents, New York, 1984, W.H. Freeman & Co., Publishers.

Klein, J.F., Berry, C.C., and Felice, M.: The development of a testicular self-examination instructional booklet, J. Adolesc. Health Care 11:235-239, 1990.

Koss, M.P., Gidycz, C.A., and Wisniewski, N.: The scope of rape: incidence and prevalence of sexual aggression and victimization in a national sample of higher education students, J. Consult. Clin. Psychol. 55:162-170, 1987.

Koss, M.P., and Oros, C.J.: Sexual experience survey: a research instrument investigating sexual aggression and victimization, J. Consult. Clin. Psychol. 50:455-457, 1982.

Lamb, M.E., and Easterbrooks, A.: Individual differences in parental sensitivity: origins, components, and consequences. In Lamb, M.E., and Sherrod, L.R., editors: Infant social cognition: empirical and theoretical considerations, Hillsdale, NJ, 1981, Lawrence Erlbaum Associates, Inc.

Lammer, E.S., and others: Risk for malformations among human fetuses exposed to isotretinoin (13-cis-retinoic acid), Teratology 35:68A, 1987.

Landos, J., Siegler, M., and Cuttler, L.: Ethical issues in growth hormone therapy, JAMA 261:1020-1024, 1989.

Lanes, R., and others: Growth hormone secretion in patients with constitutional delay of growth and pubertal development, J. Pediatr. 109:781-783, 1986.

Larson, R.E., and Shapiro, M.A.: Sexually transmitted urogenital diseases, Emerg. Med. Clin. North Am. 6:487-508, 1988.

Larson, T., and Bryson, Y.J.: Fomites and herpes simplex virus (letter), J. Infect. Dis. 151:746-747, 1985.

Leventhal, J.M.: Risk factors for child abuse: methodologic standards in case-control studies, Pediatrics 68:684-690, 1981.

Lipman, A.G.: Drugs affecting oral contraceptive efficacy, Mod. Med. 55:189-192, 1987.

Litt, I.F., Cuskey, W.R., and Rudd, S.: Identifying adolescents at risk for noncompliance with contraceptive therapy, J. Pediatr. 96:742-745, 1980.

Mann, E.M.: Interviews reveal multifaceted reactions, Am. Fam. Physician 23:219-222, 1981.

McAnarney, E.R.: Young maternal age and adverse neonatal outcome, Am. J. Dis. Child. 141:1053-1059, 1987.

McAnarney, E.R., and Hendee, R.: Adolescent pregnancy and its consequences, JAMA 262:74-77, 1989a.

McAnarney, E.R., and Hendee, R.: The prevention of adolescent pregnancy, JAMA 262:78-82, 1989b.

McCauley, E., Ito, J., and Kay, T.: Psychosocial functioning in girls with Turner syndrome and short stature: social skills, behavior problems, and self-concept, J. Am. Acad. Child Psychiatry 25:105-112, 1986.

Melski, J.W., and Arndt, K.A.: Topical therapy for acne, N. Engl. J. Med. 302:503-506, 1980.

Millstein, S.G.: Adolescent health: challenges for behavioral scientists, Am. Psychol. 4:837-842, 1989.

Millstein, S.G., Adler, N.E., and Irwin, C.E.: Sources of anxiety about pelvic examinations among adolescent females, Sex. Active Teenagers 2(2):66-72, 1988.

Moscicki, A.B.: HPV infection: an old STD revisited, Contemp. Pediatr. 6(4):12-50, 1989.

Mosher, D.L., and Anderson, R.D.: Macho personality, sexual aggression, and reactions to guided imagery or realistic rape, J. Res. Perspect. 20:77-87, 1986.

Neinstein, L.S., and others: Comfort of male adolescents during general and genital examination, J. Pediatr. 115:494-497, 1989.

Nerurkar, L., and others: Survival of herpes simplex virus in water specimens collected from hot tubs in spa facilities and on plastic surfaces, JAMA 250:3081-3083, 1983.

Olds, D.L., and others: Improving the delivery of prenatal care and outcomes of pregnancy: a randomized trial of nurse home visitation, Pediatrics 77:16-28, 1986.

Palumbo, F.M., and Licamele, W.L.: The adolescent and the media. In Shearin, R.B., and Wientzen, R.L., editors: Clinical adolescent medicine—morbidity and mortality, Boston, 1983, G.K. Hall Medical Publishers.

Panzarine, S., and others: Adolescent health care: a challenge for nursing educators, J. Nurs. Educ. 27:278-280, 1988.

Paradise, J.E.: The medical evaluation of the sexually abused child, Pediatr. Clin. North Am. 37:839-862, 1990.

Pont, A., and others: Ketoconazole blocks testosterone synthesis, Arch. Intern. Med. 142:2137-2140, 1982.

Ragozin, A.S., and others: Effects of maternal age on parenting role, Dev. Psychol. 18:627-634, 1982.

Raiti, S., and others: Growth-stimulating effects of human growth hormone therapy in patients with Turner syndrome, J. Pediatr. 109:944-949, 1986.

Rawstron, S.A., and others: Ceftriaxone treatment of penicillinase-producing *Neisseria gonorrhoeae* infections in children, Pediatr. Infect. Dis. 8:445-448, 1989.

Redmond, M.A.: Attitudes of adolescent males toward adolescent pregnancy and fatherhood, Fam. Rel. 34:337-342, 1985.

Rhodes, A.M.: Defining minors' abortion rights, MCN 13:321, 1988a.

Rhodes, A.M.: Options and issues for pregnant adolescents, MCN 13:427, 1988b.

Rosenfeld, R.G., Northcraft, G.B., and Hintz, R.L.: A prospective, randomized study of testosterone treatment of constitutional delay of growth and development in male adolescents, Pediatrics 69:681-687, 1982.

Runyan, C.W., and Gerkin, E.A.: Epidemiology and prevention of adolescent injury: a review and research agenda, JAMA 262:2273-2279, 1989.

Sandler, H.M., Vietze, P.M., and O'Conner, S.: Obstetric and neonatal outcomes following intervention with pregnant teenagers. In Scott, K.G., Field, T., and Robertson, E., editors: Teenage parents and their offspring, New York, 1981, Grune & Stratton, Inc.

Schwartz, I.D., and Root, A.W.: Puberty in girls: early, incomplete, or precocious? Contemp. Pediatr. 7(1):147-156, 1990.

Seymore, C., and others: Influence of position during examination, and sex of examiner on patient anxiety during pelvic examination, J. Pediatr. 108:312-317, 1986.

Shafer, M.A., and Sweet, R.L.: Pelvic inflammatory disease in adolescent females, Pediatr. Clin. North Am. 36:513-533, 1989.

Shafer, M.A., and others: Urinary leukocyte esterase screening test for asymptomatic chlamydial and gonococcal infections in males, JAMA 262:2562-2566, 1989.

Shalita, A.R.: Disorders of sebaceous glands and sweat glands. In Gellis, S.S., and Kagan, B.M.: Current pediatric therapy 12, Philadelphia, 1986, W.B. Saunders Co.

Silber, T.J.: Ethical considerations in the medical care of adolescents consulting for treatment of sexually transmitted diseases, Int. J. Adolesc. Med. Health 2:153-157, 1986.

Silber, T.J.: Ethical and legal issues relating to abortion in adolescence, Pediatr. Ann. 18:231-236, 1989.

Sparling, P.F.: Biology of *Neisseria gonorrhoeae.* In Holmes, K.K., and others, editors: Sexually transmitted diseases, ed. 2, New York, 1990, McGraw-Hill, Inc.

Sprafkin, J.N., and Silverman, L.T.: Uptake: physically intimate and sexual behavior on prime-time television, J. Commun. 31:34-40, 1981.

Stamm, W.E., and Mardh, P.A.: *Chlamydia trachomatis.* In Holmes, K.K., and others, editors: Sexually transmitted diseases, ed. 2, New York, 1990, McGraw-Hill, Inc.

Steinmiller, V.: Chlamydia and condyloma acuminatum, JOGNN 17:86, 1988.

Strasburger, V.C.: Sex, drugs, rock' n' roll: are solutions possible—a commentary, Pediatrics 76:704-712, 1985.

Sumaya, C.V.: New perspectives on infectious mononucleosis, Contemp. Pediatr. 6(11):58-76, 1989.

Sumaya, C.V., and Ench, Y.: Epstein-Barr virus infectious mononucleosis in children. II. Heterophil antibody and viral-specific responses, Pediatrics 75:1011-1019, 1985.

Sweet, R.L.: Pelvic inflammatory disease and infertility in women, Infect. Dis. Clin. North Am. 1:199-215, 1987.

Tauer, K.M.: Promoting effective decision-making in sexually active adolescents, Nurs. Clin. North Am. 18:275-292, 1983.

Taylor, B., Wadsworth, J., and Butler, N.R.: Teenage mothering, admission to hospital, and accidents during the first 5 years, Arch. Dis. Child. 58:6-11, 1983.

Teenage pregnancy: the problem that hasn't gone away, New York, 1981, Alan Guttmacher Institute.

Trussell, J.: Teenage pregnancy in the United States, Fam. Plann. Perspect. 20:262-272, 1988.

Tunnessen, W.W.: Acne: an approach to therapy for the pediatrician, Curr. Probl. Pediatr. 14(5):1-35, 1984.

Tyrer, L.B., Rothbart, B., and Anderson, K.: What every teen should know about contraceptives, Contemp. Pediatr. 6(10):68-94, 1989.

U.S. Preventive Services Task Force: Screening for hepatitis B, Am. Fam. Physician 40(1):131-133, 1989.

Van Vliet, G., and others: Growth hormone treatment for short stature, N. Engl. J. med. 309:1016-1022, 1983.

Walzer, S., and others: Preliminary observations on language and learning in XXY boys, Birth Defects Original Article Series 18(18):185-192, 1982.

Washington, A.E., Johnson, R.E., and Sanders, L.L.: *Chlamydia trachomatis* infections: what are they costing us? JAMA 257:2070-2072, 1987.

Washington, A.E., Sweet, R.L., and Shafer, M.A.: Pelvic inflammatory disease and its sequelae in adolescents, J. Adolesc. Health Care 6:298-310, 1985.

Williamson, R.: Cold weather and testicular torsion, Br. Med. J. 286:1436, 1983.

Wilson, D.M., and Rosenfeld, R.G.: Treatment of short stature and delayed adolescence, Pediatr. Clin. North Am. 34:865-879, 1987.

Wilson, D.M., and others: Effects of testosterone therapy for pubertal delay, Am. J. Dis. Child. 142:96-99, 1988.

Wilson, M., Duggan, A., and Joffe, A.: Correlates of hospitalization in the first year of life of infants born to adolescent mothers (abstract), Am. J. Dis. Child. 141:368, 1987.

Wise, P., and Meyers, A.: Poverty and child health, Pediatr. Clin. North Am. 35:1169-1186, 1988.

Yonkosky, D.M., and Pochi, P.E.: Acne vulgaris in childhood: pathogenesis and management, Dermatol. Clin. 4:127-136, 1986.

Zabin, L.S., Hirsch, M.B., and Boscia, J.A.: Differential characteristics of adolescent pregnancy test patients: abortion, childbearing and negative test groups, J. Adolesc. Health Care 11:107-113, 1990.

BIBLIOGRAPHY

General

American Academy of Pediatrics, Committee on Infectious Disease: Report of the Committee on Infectious Disease, Evanston, IL, 1988, American Academy of Pediatrics.

Bidwell, R.J.: The gay and lesbian teen: a case of denied adolescence, J. Pediatr. Health Care 1:3-8, 1988.

Friedman, I.M.: Promoting adolescents' compliance with therapeutic regimens, Pediatr. Clin. North Am. 33:955-973, 1986.

Hoffman, A.D., and Greydanus, D.E., editors: Adolescent medicine, ed. 2, Norwalk, CT, 1989, Appleton & Lange.

Irwin, C.E., and Millstein, S.G.: Biopsychosocial correlates of risk-taking behaviors during adolescence: can the physician intervene? J. Adolesc. Health Care 7(suppl.):82S, 1986.

Krugman, S., and others: Infectious diseases of children, ed. 8, St. Louis, 1985, Mosby–Year Book, Inc.

Litt, I.F., editor: Symposium on adolescent medicine, Pediatr. Clin. North Am. 27(1): entire issue, 1980.

Muscari, M.E.: Obtaining the adolescent sexual history, Pediatr. Nurs. 13:307-310, 1987.

Neinstein, L.S.: Adolescent health care: a practical guide, Baltimore, 1984, Urban & Schwarzenberg, Inc.

Oski, F.A., chairman: Ethical dilemma: how far can confidentiality stretch? Contemp. Pediatr. 4(1):55-64, 1987.

Robinson, D.P., Greene, J.W., and Walker, L.S.: Functional somatic complaints in adolescence: relationship to negative life events, self-concept, and family characteristics, J. Pediatr. 113:588-593, 1988.

Acne

Acne products: do fewer teens mean lower sales? Am. Druggist 192:117-118, 146, 1985.

Castiglia, P.T.: Acne, J. Pediatr. Health Care 3:259-261, 1989.

De la Cruz, E., and others: Multiple congenital malformations associated with maternal isotretinoin therapy, Pediatrics 74:428-430, 1984.

Lucky, A.W.: Update on acne vulgaris, Pediatr. Ann. 16:29-38, 1978.

Lucky, A.W.: Endocrine aspects of acne, Pediatr. Clin. North Am. 30:495-499, 1983.

Matsuoka, L.Y.: Acne, J. Pediatr. 103:849-854, 1983.

Novotny, J.: Adolescents, acne, and the side-effects of Accutane, Pediatr. Nurs. 15:247-248, 1989.

Rademaker, M., Garioch, J.J., and Simpson, N.B.: Acne in schoolchildren: no longer a concern for dermatologists, Br. Med. J. 298:1217-1219, 1989.

Rasmussen, J.E., and Smith, S.B.: Patient concepts and misconceptions about acne, Arch. Dermatol. 119:570-573, 1983.

Stone, A.C.: Facing up to acne, Pediatr. Nurs. 8:229-234, 1982.

Thomson, E.J., and Cordero, J.F.: The new teratogens: Accutane and other vitamin-A analogs, MCN 14:244-248, 1989.

Infectious Mononucleosis

Feigin, R.D., and Cherry, J.D.: Textbook of pediatric infectious disease, ed. 2, Philadelphia, 1987, W.B. Saunders Co.

McSherry, J.A.: Diagnosing infectious mononucleosis, Am. Fam. Physician 32:129-132, 1985.

Sumaya, C.V., and Ench, Y.: Epstein-Barr virus infectious mononucleosis in children. I. Clinical and general laboratory findings, Pediatrics 75:1003-1010, 1985.

Altered Growth and Maturation

Bercu, B.: Growth hormone treatment and the short child: to treat or not to treat, J. Pediatr. Health Care 110:991-995, 1987.

Cohen, F.L., and Durham, J.D.: Update your knowledge of Klinefelter syndrome, J. Psychosoc. Nurs. 23:19-25, 1985.

Cohen, F.L., and Durham, J.D.: Sex chromosome variations in school-aged children, J. Sch. Health 55:99-102, 1985.

Cuttler, L.: Evaluation of growth disorders in children, Pediatrician 14:109-120, 1987.

Ferholt, J.B., and others: A psychodynamic study of psychosocial dwarfism, J. Am. Acad. Child Psychol. 1:49-53, 1985.

Galatzer, A., and others: Intellectual function of girls with precocious puberty, Pediatrics 74:246-249, 1984.

Graham, J.M., and others: Oral and written language abilities of XXY boys: implications for anticipatory guidance, Pediatrics 81:795-806, 1988.

Green, W.H.: Psychosocial dwarfism: psychological and etiological considerations, Adv. Clin. Child Psychol. 9:245-278, 1986.

Grew, R.S., and others: Facilitating patient understanding in the treatment of growth delay, Clin. Pediatr. 22:685-690, 1983.

Hein, K.: The interface of chronic illness and the hormonal regulation of puberty, J. Adolesc. Health Care 8:530-540, 1987.

Lee, P.D., and Rosenfeld, R.G.: Psychosocial correlates of short stature and delayed puberty, Pediatr. Clin. North Am. 34:851-863, 1987.

Lin, T., Kirkland, J.L., and Kirkland, R.T.: Growth hormone assessment and short-term treatment with growth hormone in Turner syndrome, J. Pediatr. 112:920-922, 1988.
Mahoney, C.P.: Evaluating the child with short stature, Pediatr. Clin. North Am. 34:825-849, 1987.
Ott, M.J., and Jackson, P.L.: Precocious puberty: identifying early sexual development, Nurse Pract. 14(11):21-30, 1986.
Pugliese, M.T., and others: A survey to determine the prevalence of abnormal growth patterns in adolescents from a suburban school district, J. Adolesc. Health Care 9:181-187, 1988.
Richards, G.E., Marshall, R.N., and Kreuser, I.L.: Effect of stature on school performance, J. Pediatr. 106:841-842, 1985.
Rieser, P.: Role of the school nurse in the assessment of linear growth, Community Nurse Forum 4(1):1-10, 1987.
Rosenfeld, R.G., and others: Three-year results of a randomized prospective trial of methionyl human growth hormone and oxandrolone in Turner syndrome, J. Pediatr. 113:393-400, 1988.
Solomon, S.B.: Children with short stature, J. Pediatr. Nurs. 1:80-89, 1986.
Stern, N., and Zaiken, H.: Assessing the child with short stature, Pediatr. Nurs. 11:106-110, 1985.
Underwood, L.E.: Growth hormone treatment for short children, J. Pediatr. 104:237-239, 1984.
Wilson, D.M., and others: Effects of testosterone therapy for pubertal delay, Am. J. Dis. Child. 142:96-99, 1988.

Disorders of the Male Reproductive System

Casey, M.P.: Testicular cancer: the worst disease at the worst time, RN 50(2):36-40, 1987.
Diamond, F., Jr., and others: Effects of drug and alcohol abuse upon pituitary-testicular function in adolescent males, J. Adolesc. Health Care 7:28-33, 1986.
Fonkalsrud, E.W.: Testicular undescent and torsion, Pediatr. Clin. North Am. 34:1305-1317, 1987.
Goldbloom, R.B.: Self-examination by adolescents, Pediatrics 76:126-128, 1985.
Goldenring, J.M., and Purtell, E.: Knowledge of testicular cancer risk and need for self-examination in college students: a call for equal time for men in teaching of early cancer detection techniques, Pediatrics 74:1093-1096, 1984.
Jenkins, B., and Carbaugh, C.: Action stat! Testicular torsion, Nursing '89 19(7):33, 1989.
Likitnukul, S., and others: Epididymitis in children and adolescents: a 20 year retrospective study, Am. J. Dis. Child. 141:41-44, 1987.
Mitchell, J.R.: Male adolescents' concern about a physical examination conducted by a female, Nurs. Res. 29:165-169, 1980.
Moss, J.R.: Teaching adolescents testicular self-examination, Child. Nurse 6(4):4-5, 1988.
Vaz, R.M., Best, D.L., and Davis, S.W.: Testicular cancer: adolescent knowledge and attitudes, J. Adolesc. Health Care 9:474-479, 1988.
Vaz, R.M., and others: Evaluation of a testicular cancer curriculum for adolescents, J. Pediatr. 114:150-153, 1989.
Williams, A.W.: Screening for testicular cancer, Pediatr. Nurs. 7(5):38-40, 1981.

Disorders of the Female Reproductive System

Beach, R.K.: Routine breast exams: a chance to reassure, guide, and protect, Contemp. Pediatr. 4(10):70-100, 1987.
Brown, M.A., and Zimmer P.A.: Personal and family impact of premenstrual symptoms, JOGNN 15:31-38, 1986.
Coupey, S.M., and Ahlstrom, P.: Common menstrual disorders, Pediatr. Clin. North Am. 36:551-571, 1989.
Coyne, C.M., Woods, N.F., and Mitchell, E.S.: Premenstrual tension syndrome, JOGNN 14:446-454, 1985.
Frank, E.P.: What are nurses doing to help PMS patients? Am. J. Nurs. 86:137-140, 1986.
Gemberling, C.L.: The adolescent gynecologic examination: an overview, J. Pediatr. Health Care 1:141-150, 1987.
Gidwani, G.P.: Endometriosis: more common than you think, Contemp. Pediatr. 6(10):99-110, 1989.
Goldstein, D.P.: Acute and chronic pelvic pain, Pediatr. Clin. North Am. 36:573-580, 1989.
Havens, B., and Swenson, I.: Menstrual perceptions and preparation among female adolescents, JOGNN 15:406-411, 1986.
Khoiny, F.W.: Adolescent dysmenorrhea, J. Pediatr. Health Care 2:29-37, 1988.
Lavery, J.P., and Sanfilippo, J.S., editors: Pediatric and adolescent obstetrics and gynecology, New York, 1985, Springer-Verlag New York, Inc.
Lublanezki, N., and Fischer, R.G.: OTC menstrual pain preparations, Pediatr. Nurs. 13:435, 1987.
Murata, J.: Primary amenorrhea, Pediatr. Nurs. 15:125-129, 1989.
Paradise, J., and Willis, E.D.: Probability of vaginal foreign body in girls with genital complaints, Am. J. Dis. Child. 139:472-476, 1985.
Primrose, R.B.: Taking the tension out of pelvic exams, Am. J. Nurs. 84:72-74, 1984.
Rosenfeld, W.D., and Clark J.: Vulvovaginitis and cervicitis, Pediatr. Clin. North Am. 36:489-511, 1989.
Rx drugs switched to OTC, FDA Drug Bull. 13(3):29-30, 1984.
Sasso, S.C.: Prostaglandin inhibitors for primary dysmenorrhea, MCN 9:177, 1984.
Soules, M.R.: Adolescent amenorrhea, Pediatr. Clin. North Am. 34:1083-1103, 1987.
Szydlo, V.L.: Approaching an adolescent about a pelvic exam, Am. J. Nurs. 88:1502-1506, 1988.
Talbot, C.W.: The gynecologic examination of the pediatric patient, Pediatr. Ann. 15:501-508, 1986.
Tunnessen, W.W., Jr.: A teenage girl's abdominal pain: which of many causes? Contemp. Pediatr. 4(6):57-64, 1987.
Wawrzyniak, M.N.: The painless pelvic, MCN 11:78, 1986.

Adolescent Pregnancy

American Academy of Pediatrics, Committee on Adolescence: Adolescent pregnancy, Pediatrics 83:132-133, 1989.
American Academy of Pediatrics, Committee on Adolescence: Care of adolescent parents and their children, Pediatrics 83:138-140, 1989.
Anisfel, E., and Pincus, M.: The post-partum support project: serving young mothers and older women through home visiting, Zero to Three 8(1):13-15, 1987.
Baisch, M.J., and others: Teen pregnancy service: infant outcomes through two years of age, J. Pediatr. Nurs. 3:329-337, 1988.
Barret, R.L., and Robinson, B.E.: Adolescent fathers: other forgotten parents, Pediatr. Nurs. 12:273-277, 1986.
Berland, A.: Young fathers' support group, Pediatr. Nurs. 13:255-256, 276, 1987.
Bobak, I.M., Jensen, M.D., and Zalar, M.K.: Maternity and gynecologic care: the nurse and the family, ed. 4, St. Louis, 1989, Mosby–Year Book, Inc.
Burke, P.J.: A community health model for pregnant teens, MCN 8:340-344, 1983.
Children's Defense Fund: Welfare and teen pregnancy: what we know, what we do, Washington, DC, 1986, Adolescent Pregnancy Prevention Clearinghouse.
Cusson, R.M.: Attitudes toward breast-feeding among female high-school students, Pediatr. Nurs. 11:189-191, 1985.
Daniels, M.B., and Manning, D.: A clinic for pregnant teens, Am. J. Nurs. 83:68-71, 1983.
DeAngelis, C., chairman: Confronting the crisis of teenage pregnancy, Contemp. Pediatr. 4(9):68-90, 1987.
Desrosiers, M.C.: A nursing response to the teen pregnancy epidemic, RN 52(4):22-24, 1989.
Elster, A.B., Lamb, M.E., and Kimmerly, N.: Perceptions of parenthood among adolescent fathers, Pediatrics 83:758-765, 1989.

Elster, A.B., and Panzarine, S.: Teenage fathers, Clin. Pediatr. 22:700-703, 1983.

Fuller, S.A.: Care of postpartum adolescents, MCN 11:398-403, 1986.

Fuller, S.A., and others: A small group can go a long way, MCN 13:414-418, 1988.

Heller, R.G.: School-based clinics: impact on teenage pregnancy prevention, Pediatr. Nurs. 14:103-106, 1988.

Henshaw, S.K.: Induced abortion: a worldwide perspective, Fam. Plann. Perspect. 18:250-254, 1986.

Janowski, M.J.: The road not taken, Am. J. Nurs. 87:334-335, 1987.

Joffe, A., and Radius, S.M.: Breast versus bottle: correlates of adolescent mothers' infant-feeding practices, Pediatrics 79:689-695, 1987.

Levine, L., Coll, C.T.G., and Oh, W.: Determinants of mother-infant interaction in adolescent mothers, Pediatrics 75:23-29, 1985.

McAnarney, E.R., editor: Adolescent pregnancy and parenthood, Early Child. Update 4(3):1-8, 1988.

McAnarney, E.R., and others: Adolescent mothers and their infants, Pediatrics 73:358-362, 1984.

Mecklenburg, M.E., and Thompson, P.G.: The adolescent family life program as a prevention measure, Public Health Rep. 98:21-29, 1983.

Mercer, R.: Assessing and counseling teenage mothers during the perinatal period, Nurs. Clin. North Am. 18:293-301, 1983.

Moore, D.S., Erickson, P.I., and Wurgel, M.: Adolescent pregnancy and parenting: the role of the nurse, Top. Clin. Nurs. 6(3):72-78, 1984.

Moore, M.L.: Recurrent teen pregnancy: making it less desirable, MCN 14:104-108, 1989.

Morgan, B.S., and Barden, M.E.: Unwed and pregnant: nurses' attitudes toward unmarried mothers, MCN 10:114-117, 1985.

Nakashima, I.I., and Camp, B.W.: Fathers of infants born to adolescent mothers: a study of paternal characteristics, Am. J. Dis. Child. 138:452-454, 1984.

Namerow, P.B., Lawton, A.I., and Philliber, S.G.: Teenagers' perceived and actual probabilities of pregnancy, Adolescence 22:475-485, 1987.

Palmore, S.U., and Shannon, M.D.: Risk factors for adolescent pregnancy in students, Pediatr. Nurs. 14:241-245, 1988.

Paperny, D.M., and Starn, J.R.: Adolescent pregnancy prevention by health education computer games: computer-assisted instruction of knowledge and attitudes, Pediatrics 83:742-752, 1989.

Porter, L.S., and Sobong, L.C.: Differences in maternal perception of the newborn among adolescents, Pediatr. Nurs. 16:101-104, 1990.

Proctor, S.E.: A developmental approach to pregnancy prevention with early adolescent females, J. Sch. Health 56:313-316, 1986.

Rivara, F.P., Sweeney, P.J., and Henderson, B.F.: Black teenage fathers: what happens when the child is born? Pediatrics 78:151-158, 1986.

Rivara, F.P., Sweeney, P.J., and Henderson, B.F.: Risk of fatherhood among black teenage males, Am. J. Public Health 77:203-205, 1987.

Rossi, A.S., and Bhavani, S.: Abortion in context: historical trends and future changes, Fam. Plann. Perspect. 20:273-281, 1988.

Ruff, C.C.: How well do adolescents mother? MCN 12:249-253, 1987.

Sachs, B.: Reproductive decisions in adolescence, Image 18(2):69-72, 1986.

Sewall, K.S.: Peer-group reality therapy for the pregnant adolescent, MCN 8:67-69, 1983.

Slager-Earnest, S.E., Hoffman, S.J., and Beckmann, C.J.A.: Effects of a specialized prenatal adolescent program on maternal and infant outcomes, JOGNN 16:422-429, 1987.

Smith, D.L.: Meeting the psychosocial needs of teen-age mothers and fathers, Nurs. Clin. North Am. 19:369-379, 1984.

Smith, K.E., Spires, M.V., and Frese, M.P.: Adolescent mothers' successful participation in a well-baby care program, J. Adolesc. Health Care 8:193-197, 1987.

Smoke, J., and Grace, M.: Effectiveness of prenatal care and education for pregnant adolescents, J. Nurse Midwife 33:178-180, 1988.

Stephenson, J.N.: Pregnancy testing and counseling, Pediatr. Clin. North Am. 36:681-696, 1989.

Story, M., and Alton, I.: Nutrition issues and adolescent pregnancy, Contemp. Nutr. 12(1), 1987.

Tuttle, J.I.: Adolescent pregnancy: factoring in the father of the baby, J. Pediatr. Health Care 2:240-244, 1988.

vonWindeguth, B.J.: Teenagers and the mothering experience, Pediatr. Nurs. 15:517-520, 1989.

Vukelich, C., and Kliman, D.S.: Mature and teenage mothers' infant growth expectations and use of child development information sources, Fam. Rel. 34:189-196, 1985.

Wells, N.: Management of pain during abortion, J. Adv. Nurs. 14:56-62, 1989.

Wildey, L.S.: Diagnosis and initial management of the pregnant adolescent, J. Pediatr. Health Care 1:60-64, 1987.

Yoos, L.: Perspectives on adolescent parenting: effect of adolescent egocentrism on the maternal-child interactions, J. Pediatr. Nurs. 2:193-200, 1987.

Zdanuk, J.M., Harris, C.C., and Wisian, N.L.: Adolescent pregnancy and incest: the nurse's role as counselor, JOGNN 16:99-104, 1987.

Contraception

Babington, M.A.: Adolescent use of oral contraceptives, Pediatr. Nurs. 10:111-114, 1984.

Hewson, P.M.: Research on adolescent male attitudes about contraceptives, Pediatr. Nurs. 12:114-116, 1986.

Jay, M.S., DuRant, R.H., and Litt, I.F.: Female adolescents' compliance with contraceptive regimens, Pediatr. Clin. North Am. 36:731-746, 1989.

Kulig, J.W.: Adolescent contraception: nonhormonal methods, Pediatr. Clin. North Am. 36:717-730, 1989.

Milan, R.J., and Kilmann, P.R.: Interpersonal factors in premarital contraception, J. Sex Res. 23:289-292, 1987.

Panzaarine, S., and Gould, C.L.: Knowledge about contraceptive use and conception among a group of urban, black adolescent mothers, JOGNN 17:279-282, 1988.

Reis, J., and Herz, L.: Young adolescents' contraceptive knowledge and attitudes: implications for anticipatory guidance, J. Pediatr. Health Care 1:247-254, 1987.

Shearin, R.B., and Boehlke, J.R.: Hormonal contraception, Pediatr. Clin. North Am. 36:697-715, 1989.

White, J.E.: Initiating contraceptive use: how do young women decide? Pediatr. Nurs. 10:347-352, 1984.

White, J.E.: Influence of parents, peers, and problem-solving on contraceptive use, Pediatr. Nurs. 13:317-321, 1987.

Yoos, L.: Adolescent cognitive behaviors, Pediatr. Nurs. 13:247-250, 1987.

Rape

Burgess, A.W., and Brodsky, S.L.: Applying flight education principles to rape prevention, Fam. Community Health 4(2):45-51, 1981.

Dennis, L.L.: Adolescent rape: the role of nursing, Issues Compr. Pediatr. Nurs. 11:59-70, 1988.

Foley, T.S. and Davies, M.A.: Rape: nursing care of victims, St. Louis, 1983, Mosby–Year Book, Inc.

Moore, K.A., Nord, C.W., and Peterson, J.L.: Noninvoluntary sexual activity among adolescents, Fam. Plann. Perspect. 21:110-114, 1989.

Muehlenhard, C.L., and Linton, M.A.: Date rape and sexual aggression in dating situations: incidence and risk factors, J. Counsel. Psychol. 34:186-190, 1987.

Platt, C.R., Hicks, D.J., and Mori, D.M.: Medical care for the rape victim. In Reinhardt, A.M., and Quinn, M.D., editors: Family-centered community nursing, vol. 2, St. Louis, 1981, Mosby–Year Book, Inc.

Prentky, R.A., and others: Victim responses by rapist type: an empirical and clinical analysis, J. Interpers. Violence 1(1):73-79, 1986.

Resisting rape without getting killed, Am. J. Nurs. 85:947-948, 1985.

Woodling, B.A., and Kossoris, P.D.: Sexual misuse: rape, molestation, and incest, Pediatr. Clin. North Am. 28:481-499, 1981.

Sexually Transmitted Diseases

AIDS: what shall we teach the children, Contemp. Pediatr. 5(5):58-87, 1988.

Alexander-Rodriguez, T., and Vermund, S.H.: Gonorrhea and syphilis in incarcerated urban adolescents: prevalence and physical signs, Pediatrics 80:561-564, 1987.

American Academy of Pediatrics, Committee on Adolescence: Sexuality, contraception, and the media, Pediatrics 78:535-536, 1986.

American Academy of Pediatrics, Committee on Adolescence: Role of the pediatrician in management of sexually transmitted diseases in children and adolescents, Pediatrics 79:454-456, 1987.

American Academy of Pediatrics, Commmittee on School Health: Acquired immunodeficiency syndrome education in schools, Pediatrics 82:278-279, 1988.

Becker, T.M., Stone, K.M., and Alexander, E.R.: Genital human papillomavirus infection: a growing concern, Obstet. Gynecol. Clin. North Am. 14:387-397, 1987.

Blythe, M.J., and others: Historical and clinical factors associated with *Chlamydia trachomatis* genitourinary infection in female adolescents, J. Pediatr. 112:1000-1004, 1988.

Bourcier, K.M., and Seidler, A.J.: Chlamydia and condylomata acuminata: an update for the nurse practitioner, JOGNN 16(1):17-22, 1987.

Brown, H.P.: Recognizing STDs in adolescents, Contemp. Pediatri. 6(1):17-36, 1989.

Brown, R.T., and others: Pharyngeal gonorrhea screening in adolescents: is it necessary? Pediatrics 84:623-625, 1989.

Bump, R.C., Sachs, L.A., and Buesching, W.J.: Sexually transmissible infectious agents in sexually active and virginal asymptomatic adolescent girls, Pediatrics 77:488-494, 1986.

Centers for Disease Control: Guidelines for effective school health education to prevent spread of AIDS, MMWR 37(suppl.):S-2, 1988.

Centers for Disease Control: Progress toward achieving the 1990 objectives for the nation for sexually transmitted disease, MMWR 39:53-57, 1990.

Chacko, M.R., and Lovchik, J.C.: *Chlamydia trachomatis* infection in sexually active adolescents: prevalence and risk factors, Pediatrics 73:836-840, 1984.

Davidson, J., and Grant, C.: Growing up is hard to do . . . in the AIDS era, MCN 13:352-356, 1988.

DiClemente, R.J., Zorn, J., and Temoshok L: Adolescents and AIDS: a survey of knowledge, attitudes and AIDS in San Francisco, Am. J. Public Health 76:1443-1445, 1986.

DiRubbo, N.C.: The condom barrier, Am. J. Nurs. 87:1306-1309, 1987.

Golden, N., Neuhoff, S., and Cohen, H.: Pelvic inflammatory disease in adolescents, J. Pediatr. 114:138-143, 1989.

Golden, N., and others: The use of pelvic ultrasonography in the evaluation of adolescents with pelvic inflammatory disease, Am. J. Dis. Child. 141:1235-1238, 1987.

Goodman, E., and Cohall, A.T.: Acquired immunodeficiency syndrome and adolescents: knowledge, attitudes, beliefs, and behaviors in the New York City adolescent minority population, Pediatrics 84:36-42, 1989.

Gurevich I.: Counseling the patient with herpes, RN 53(2):22-28, 1990.

Hein, K.: Adolescent acquired immunodeficiency syndrome, Am. J. Dis. Child. 144:46-48, 1990.

Holmes, K.K., and others: Sexually transmitted diseases, ed. 2, New York, 1990, McGraw-Hill, Inc.

Huszti, H.C., Clopton, J.R., and Mason, P.J.: Acquired immunodeficiency syndrome educational program: effects on adolescents' knowledge and attitudes, Pediatrics 84:986-994, 1989.

Kaplan, K.M., and others: Social relevance of genital herpes simplex in children, Am. J. Dis. Child. 138:872-874, 1984.

Kegeles, S.M., Adler, N.E., and Irwin, C.E.: Adolescents and condoms, Am. J. Dis. Child. 143:911-915, 1989.

Khoiny, F.E.: Pelvic inflammatory disease in the adolescent, J. Pediatr. Health Care 3:230-236, 1989.

Loucks, A.: Chlamydia: an unheralded epidemic, Am. J. Nurs. 87:920-922, 1987.

Marvin, C., and Slevin A.: Chlamydia—cause, prevention, and cure, MCN 12:318-321, 1987.

McElhose, P.: The "other" STDs: as dangerous as ever, RN 51(6):51-54, 1988.

McQuiston, C.M.: The relationship of risk factors for cervical cancer and HPV in college women, Nurse Pract. 14(4):22-24, 1989.

Nettina, S.M.: When patients with genital herpes turn to you for answers, Nursing '89 19(8):61-64, 1989.

Nettina, S.M., and Kauffman, F.H.: Diagnosis and management of sexually transmitted genital lesions, Nurse Pract. 15(1):20-39, 1990.

Portnoy, J.: Oral acyclovir for genital herpes: not a cure, but close, Can. Med. Assoc. J. 136:697, 1987.

Richwald, G.A.: Are condom instructions readable? Results of a readability study, Public Health Rep. 103:355-359, 1988.

Rosenfeld, W.D., and Clark, J.: Vulvovaginitis and cervicitis, Pediatr. Clin. North Am. 36:489-512, 1989.

Rosenfeld, W.D., and others: High prevalence rate of human papillovirus infection and association with abnormal Papanicolaou smears in sexual active adolescents, Am. J. Dis. Child. 143:1443-1447, 1989.

Sacks, S.: The role of oral acyclovir in the management of genital herpes simplex, Can. Med. Assoc. J. 136:701-707, 1987.

Spitzer, M., and Krumholz, B.A.: Pap screening for teenagers: a lifesaving precaution, Contemp. Pediatr. 4(5):41-52, 1987.

Steiner, J.D., and others: Are adolescents getting smarter about acquired immunodeficiency syndrome? Am. J. Dis. Child. 144:302-306, 1990.

Strunin, L., and Hingson, R.: Acquired immunodeficiency syndrome and adolescents: knowledge, beliefs, attitudes, and behaviors, Pediatrics 79:825-828, 1987.

Vermund, S.H., and others: Acquired immunodeficiency syndrome among adolescents, Am. J. Dis. Child. 143:1220-1225, 1989.

CHAPTER 21

Behavioral Health Problems of Adolescence

RELATED TOPICS

Childhood depression, Ch. 18
Cocaine exposure, Ch. 10
Communicating with children, Ch. 6
Fetal alcohol syndrome, Ch. 11
Health promotion of the adolescent and family, Ch. 19
Infants of mothers who smoke, Ch. 10
Narcotic-addicted infants, Ch. 10
Nutritional assessment, Ch. 6
Obesity, Ch. 13
Passive smoking, Ch. 32

GLOSSARY

AN Anorexia nervosa

drug abuse The regular use of drugs for other than accepted medical purposes and to the extent that it results in physical or psychologic harm to the user and/or is used in a way that is detrimental to society

drug misuse The overzealous use of drugs or the exercise of bad judgment in their use

drug tolerance The clinical need to increase the dosage of a drug in order to attain the same desired effect, caused by an increased capacity to metabolize and eliminate the drug or the ability of the individual's tissues to adapt to the drug

impulsive act A rage response designed to punish or manipulate a loved person

narcotic addiction Behavioral pattern of overwhelming involvement with obtaining and using a narcotic for its psychic effects rather than for medical reasons, thereby eliciting social disapproval

physical dependence An adaptive physiologic state that occurs when a drug is taken in increasing amounts and that is manifest by the development of physiologic symptoms when the drug is withdrawn

suicidal attempt An act intended to cause injury or death

suicidal gesture An act made without any real attempt to cause serious injury or death

suicidal ideation Thoughts about or plans for suicide

Adolescence is a time of transition, maturational crisis, and adjustment. The transition to adulthood is characterized by change, growth, and stress. Ineffective and unsuccessful accomplishment of the developmental tasks of adolescence produces a sense of diffuse discomfort within some adolescents, who may use faulty problem solving in their search for relief from the discomfort and stress of this transitional period of life.

EATING DISORDERS

Eating disorders are among the most frequently encountered health problems of adolescence. Overeating often begins in infancy and continues throughout childhood; deliberate undereating usually does not become apparent until later childhood or adolescence. Either overeating or undereating can have a detrimental effect on health and well-being and, if extreme, can be a threat to life.

The term *eating disorder* is often applied to the two major eating disorders, anorexia nervosa and bulimia. However, for the purpose of this discussion the two are considered separately because of their age distribution and their characteristics.

ADIPOSE TISSUE

There is wide variation between individuals in the degree of fatness or thinness at all ages because of a multitude of factors. Fat is contained in connective tissue cells that are usually referred to as adipose tissue; this tissue has a distinct lifetime pattern of development and distribution. Fat is characteristically found in subcutaneous tissues (except those of the eyelids, external ear, nose, scrotum, and backs of hands and feet, which contain very little), in the omentum, and in close relation to some viscera, such as the heart and kidneys. Although it contributes substantially to body weight, whether fat "grows" like other tissues is uncertain. The deposits of fat throughout the body function primarily as a means for storing energy. Therefore it is a labile tissue markedly affected by the nutrition of the individual.

Normal fat distribution during childhood follows a definite pattern. Fat first appears in the subcutaneous tissues of the fetus at approximately the sixth month of prenatal life. There is a rapid accumulation from the seventh month through the first 6 postnatal months, and the amount of subcutaneous fat present in the newborn correlates with the weight of the infant. However, at the end of the first year the infant who was lean at birth has approximately the same length and muscle mass as infants who were fatter initially. The significance of subcutaneous fat related to both the specialized "brown fat" and gestational age is discussed in relation to problems of prematurity and temperature regulation in the newborn (see Chapters 8 and 10).

After 6 months of age the rate of fat accumulation declines rapidly and then decreases steadily in both sexes until 6 to 8 years of age. All children begin to slim down soon after the first birthday, but the decrease is somewhat less in girls than in boys; thus at any age girls are slightly fatter than boys. From the ages of 6 to 8 years fat again begins to accumulate slowly. It is during this period that obesity may begin in some children. Many children also put on excess fat just before the adolescent growth spurt.

Up until the onset of puberty there is very little difference in fat accumulation and distribution in boys and girls. During the adolescent growth spurt the amount of fat in boys decreases sharply (especially in the limbs) and is not regained until early adulthood. Their increase in body weight and mass is primarily the result of accelerated bone and muscle growth. In many boys a preadolescent period of fat growth, often a source of social concern to both the child and his parents, precedes the general changes of adolescence. In girls the fat accumulation continues but assumes a typical distribution pattern that produces the feminine curves of the mature female.

The amount and distribution of fat also correlate with a genetically controlled body build that appears to be unrelated to caloric intake. In addition, culturally determined diets, amount of exercise, emotions, and numerous other factors that influence caloric consumption are reflected in increased fat deposits. It is now believed that the number of fat cells is established at an early age and that overfeeding during this time may have a significant influence on development of obesity at a later age.

OBESITY

Probably no problem related to adolescence is so obvious to others, is so difficult to treat, and has such long-term effects on psychologic and physical health status as obesity. It is the most common nutritional disturbance of children and one of the most challenging contemporary health problems at all ages. The prevalence of obesity has been determined to be 25% to 30% of prepubertal children and from 18% to 25% of adolescents. Although the prevalence of obesity has increased 40% during the past 15 years in both children and adolescents, more rapid increases in prevalence have occurred among black children than among whites (Dietz, 1986). Also, in one study 26% of boys and 57% of girls were found to be at risk for compulsive overeating (Marston and others, 1988). Since adult obesity is associated with increased mortality and morbidity from a variety of complications, both physical and psychologic, the presence of adolescent obesity is a serious condition that deserves the interest and attention of health professionals.

The definition of obesity has always led to some confusion and, at best, is very imprecise. Because there is such variability in height and weight among normal healthy children, it is often difficult to determine the presence or extent of obesity by comparing a set of numbers with a standardized table of weights and heights. This is especially true in adolescence, when there is normally a period of rapid weight gain and linear growth together with varying rates of muscular development.

The greatest amount of confusion is related to the distinction between the terms *overweight* and *obesity*. *Obesity* is an increase in body weight resulting from an excessive accumulation of fat or simply the state of being too fat. *Overweight* refers to the state of weighing more than average for height and body build, which may or may not include an increased amount of fat. It is possible for two children to have the same height and weight and for one to be obese whereas the other is not. This is particularly evident during early adolescence when there are considerable differences in the rates of muscular development. Obesity is easily recognized, although it is difficult to assess its severity, especially in children who are overweight to a lesser degree.

Etiology/Pathophysiology

Obesity results from a caloric intake that consistently exceeds caloric requirements and expenditure and may involve a variety of interrelated influences, including metabolic, hypothalamic, hereditary, social, cultural, and psychologic factors. Birth weight offers no clue in detection and prediction of childhood obesity; obese children do not have higher birth weights than nonobese children. However, there is a high correlation of childhood adiposity with both parental adiposity and children's daytime activity levels (Berkowitz and others, 1985). A brief description of some of the major theories regarding childhood obesity is presented here.

Genetic factors. The incidence of obese children born to obese parents is significantly higher than the incidence of obese children born to parents of normal weight: 3% to 7% of children born to parents of normal weight are obese, 40% of obese children have one parent who is obese, and 80% of obese children have two obese parents. Comparison of natural and adopted children shows a positive correlation for weight between children and their natural parents (Strunkard and others, 1986; Van Itallie, 1986). Moreover, studies of identical and fraternal twins reveal an extremely high correlation between identical twins—even identical twins who were reared in different environments—but not fraternal twins.

General body build seems to have some effect on obesity. Children who are inclined toward a rounded body build with soft body contours and larger amounts of subcutaneous fat are somewhat predisposed to the accumulation of fat. Some humans may inherit a metabolic defect that interferes with the breakdown of fat once it has been stored in adipose tissue, which makes maintaining an ideal weight more difficult than it is for others.

It is almost impossible to distinguish between hereditary and environmental factors, since both may be operative in any situation, especially when other family members are also obese. Family eating patterns, ethnic diet, and psychologic factors play an important role; to many persons, fat is still considered to be an indication of good health. The tendency toward obesity is manifest whenever environmental conditions are favorable, such as an abundance of food and reduced or minimal physical activity (from such causes as excessive television viewing and the availability of automobiles).

Diseases. In less than 5% of cases childhood obesity can be attributed to an underlying disease. Such diseases include hypothyroidism, adrenal hypercorticoidism, hyperinsulinism, and dysfunction or damage to the central nervous system as a result of a tumor, injury, infection, or vascular accident. Obesity is a frequent complication of muscular dystrophy and paraplegia as a result of myelomeningocele.

Five recognized congenital syndromes have obesity as a feature (Laurence-Moon-Biedl, Prader-Willi, Vasquez, and Alstrom syndromes and pseudohypoparathyroidism). The most common of these is Prader-Willi syndrome, a disorder characterized by hypogonadism, slow intellectual development, short stature, and dysmorphic facial features, including a narrowed bifrontal diameter, almond-shaped eyes, and triangular-shaped mouth. These children are very hypotonic and will go to great lengths to obtain food.

Metabolic and endocrine factors. The complex interrelationships between hunger, satiety, the central nervous system, and the metabolism of carbohydrates, fats, and protein continue to be investigated in relation to their role in obesity. Theories advanced in an attempt to explain individual variability in energy requirements include increased metabolic efficiency in the obese person that facilitates fat storage, enhanced adipose tissue triglyceride synthesis, and retarded adipocyte lipolysis facilitating fat retention:

- **Brown fat theory**—obese people have less heat-producing brown fat than normal persons, and their brown fat works less efficiently. The body's heat production influences food intake, and this may explain why some individuals are able to overeat and remain slim.
- **Adipose cell theory**—adipose tissue is hyperplastic, hypertrophic, or a combination of the two. *Hyperplastic,* or hypercellular, obesity occurs when the number of cells in adipose tissue is increased, producing lifelong and intractable obesity. Hyperplastic obesity is associated with earlier onset. *Hypertrophic* obesity is associated with an increase in cell size and therefore is more likely to be responsive to treatment. Obese children have larger cells that stay the same size once they reach a maximum, and their fat cells appear to increase in number during childhood.
- **Set point theory**—individuals have a programmed level, or set point, for body weight that remains relatively stable during adulthood. With increased caloric intake the metabolic rate increases to burn the excess; when intake is reduced, metabolism decreases to conserve energy.
- **Sodium (Na)/potassium (K) pump theory**—basal enzyme is used to keep potassium in and sodium out of body cells. Obese persons have less of the required substance and therefore need less energy to maintain equilibrium.
- **Lipoprotein lipase theory**—this enzyme on fat cells is responsible for depositing globules in fat cells. When weight is lost, the body increases production of the enzyme to grasp and store fat. Obese persons are unable to inhibit this process during normal fat intake.

It has also been observed that on the whole, obese children tend to be taller than average with somewhat larger lean body mass. There is some evidence to indicate that growth is accelerated by overnutrition much the same as it is retarded by undernutrition. Consequently, children who are obese in infancy seem to attain relatively greater height than those with later-onset obesity.

Caloric equilibrium. It is consistently observed that obese children are less active than lean children, but it is uncertain whether the inactivity creates the obesity or whether the obesity is responsible for the inactivity. However, it appears that in childhood overeating is the dominant feature, whereas in adult life reduced physical activity with normal intake is more likely to be the rule.

Although the intake of obese persons who are inactive may be lower than that of leaner persons, obese persons eat more at a given sitting and tend to eat more rapidly than nonobese persons. It appears characteristic that obese persons not only exhibit an overwhelming appetite, but also overeat when they are not hungry or have no appetite. They apparently respond to other cues, as well as to the hunger stimulus. It has also been shown that feeding habits and frequency of food ingestion may produce alterations in enzyme activities in both adipose cells and muscle cells. Comparison of individuals who consume similar amounts of calories ingested either as one meal (gorging) or intermittently over a period of time (nibbling) shows an increase of body fat in the "gorgers." It appears that lipogenesis is accelerated following "gorging" patterns of food intake when compared with "nibbling" patterns. Obese adolescents are characteristically night eaters and often skip meals, particularly breakfast.

Sociocultural factors. Patterns of eating are culturally and socially based in most instances, and in some the food preferences of the culture contribute to the development of obesity. Many cultures consider plumpness a sign of health, and some look on obesity as evidence of well-being and foster weight gain as a desirable feature. In others obesity is a status symbol or an indication of affluence. It is not uncommon for obese children to be a product of families in which eating patterns of large meals are emphasized or in which children are admonished for leaving any food on their plates. Parents often have an exaggerated concept of the amount of food children should eat and expect them to eat more than they need.

It has also been observed that in the developed countries, such as the United States and those in Western Europe, there is a marked difference in the prevalence of obesity between upper- and lower-class children and that these differences are frequently apparent before 6 years of age. Lower socioeconomic groups have a greater prevalence of obesity, especially in girls, and this obese state is established earlier and increases at a more rapid rate.

Psychologic factors. Psychologic factors may provide a basis for eating patterns in childhood. In infancy the child first experiences relief from discomfort through feeding and learns to associate eating with feelings of well-being, security, and the comforting presence of the mothering person. Soon eating is deeply associated with the feeling of being loved. To the infant, to be fed is to be loved; satiety is security. In addition, the pleasurable oral sensation of sucking provides an additional connection between emotions and early eating behavior. Many parents use food, such as candy and other "treats," as a positive reinforcer for desired behavior or as a way to compensate for their own feelings of guilt, especially if the child was unwanted or overvalued because of loss of a previous child. This practice soon acquires symbolic significance to the extent that the child continues to use food as a reward, a comfort, and a means by which to deal with feelings of depression or hostility.

In some children overweight may be the normal state and may simply represent the upper end of the normal distribution curve. These children are most comfortable when they are well filled out, and they may or may not have emotional problems. Others may begin overeating and reducing activity in response to a traumatic or upsetting event in their lives, such as the death of a parent or sibling, separation from parents, or social or scholastic failure, or as a response to illness or surgery.

Obesity may be one manifestation of a disturbed way of life. Typically families of obese children are markedly socially introverted and rely on family members for socialization. Television viewing is the primary source of entertainment. Frequently the family is composed of a domineering, ambitious mother and a passive, docile father. Marital disharmony is common. There are usually only one or two children in the family. The obese child assumes the role of active participant, with dependent, submissive, and generally immature behavior. The child follows the family's social pattern of isolation and tends to react to frustration with withdrawal or hostility. On school entrance the child is totally unprepared for experiences outside the shelter of the family group. Consequently, the child turns to food for solace, which has become a means of coping with traumatic experiences, failure, and disappointment. Once obesity has developed, the family patterns of personal and social interaction tend to perpetuate it.

Obesity in Adolescence

Obesity in adolescence may appear simultaneously with the onset of adolescence, or it may have existed before puberty. Although there may be differences in the psychophysiologic dynamics in its development, the effect of the obese condition on the teenager is the same. A great deal has been hypothesized about the psychogenic factors in obesity; however, the psychologic *effects* of being obese are undoubtedly underestimated. Obesity is a serious handicap to the social life of a child and, to an even greater extent, to the life of a teenager. The common emotional sequelae of obesity in adolescence are defective body image, low self-esteem, social isolation, and feelings of rejection and depression.

Adolescent-onset obesity appears to be closely related to an inability to master the developmental tasks of adolescence; as a result children regress to the self-satisfying tactic of overeating to compensate. Unfortunately, this mechanism only creates an additional obstacle to achieving the desired goal. The obesity, however, serves to ward off the pressures engendered by the internal changes of puberty and the outside world. The obesity becomes the safeguard. As long as they remain fat, children do not have to deal with this repressed emotional material. They may come to view the obesity as a handicap responsible for all their disappointments. Consequently, they avoid making the adaptations necessary to growth and maturation. Eating is their means of coping with the normal drives of adolescence and more closely binds them to the family, especially the mother, who provides the food. Thus they become increasingly dependent on food as a means of gratification. This impedes the normal processes of separation and individuation, since they tend to shy away from their peers and become more closely bound to the family.

Vulnerable personality. Obesity is most often a symptom in passive-dependent, compliant youngsters who are readily controlled by guilt and shame. They are easily influenced by outside forces (such as parents, peers, and school) that they consider to be more powerful than themselves. When faced with an internal or external stress, these youngsters react with helplessness, ambivalence, and a tendency to seek support from someone they see as stronger than themselves, either adult or peer.

There are many psychologic implications in the development and perpetuation of obesity. It may represent aggression directed at the self, an attempt (in younger children) to grow bigger in order to physically deal with a hated person, or a means to bring shame and embarrassment to another (often the mother). Many overweight adolescents use obesity as a means of revenge. However, they easily become a scapegoat for the frustrations and anger of parents and others as a source of embarrassment and shame. A common problem is the ambivalence of mothers who like to see their daughters eat but at the same time desire them to have slender figures.

Self-concept and obesity. Obese adolescents score higher on depression-measurement tests than thinner teenagers and significantly lower on body-image tests, indicating a less positive or a more impaired body concept. Unlike many disorders, a youngster's obesity is a matter of general knowledge, continually on display for others to see. Some of the personality characteristics reflecting the psychologic effects of obesity have been likened to those of ethnic and racial minorities who have been subjected to intense discrimination. These include passivity, obsessive concern with the self-image, expectation of rejection, and progressive withdrawal. This sets into motion a cyclic pattern wherein youngsters expect rejection, feel awkward and out of place in social situations, isolate themselves from social contacts, and then experience actual rejection. Decreased opportunity for activity outside the home provides increased exposure to food, leading to an increase in obesity.

Obese adolescents, particularly obese girls, consider obesity undesirable and intensely dislike their figures and physical characteristics. They are concerned about their obesity, are extremely self-deprecating, and judge other people in terms of degree of adiposity. They express contempt for fat persons and admiration for thin ones. They consider their bodies to be grotesque and are certain that others, too, are contemptuous of them. Stylish, age-appropriate clothing is difficult to find and, when available, is restricted to special shops or departments with labels that further emphasize the negative aspects of their appearance. Sexual attractiveness is severely impaired or nonexistent; obese youngsters rarely date.

There are three major factors that contribute to the development of a disturbed body image:

- Age of onset of the obesity. Body-image disturbances are primarily found in persons who were obese as children and adolescents or as adolescents alone.
- Presence of emotional disturbances or neuroses. A stable personality and a secure childhood appear to prevent body-image distortion, whereas emotional disturbances caused by the effects of a disturbed family will invite the development of a distorted body image.
- A negative evaluation of the obesity by others. The child internalizes the attitudes conveyed by significant others.

It appears that there is a critical period for development of a distorted body image that is characteristic of persons who were obese during adolescence. Those who become obese as adults rarely demonstrate this disturbance. During adolescence and when the youngster is establishing a sense of identity, derogatory views by peers and parents are incorporated into enduring views of the self. Fig. 21-1 shows interrelated factors that contribute to adolescent obesity. However, obesity does not necessarily imply a low self-esteem. Results of a recent study show that although obese children have average self-esteem, lean children have high self-esteem (Kaplan and Wadden, 1986).

Complications of Childhood Obesity

The most prevalent complication of childhood obesity is its persistence into adulthood, with remarkable resistance to treatment. With few exceptions, clearly identifiable hazards are rarely present in childhood, but the dangers of obesity increase with its duration. The adult with long-standing obesity is subject to the development of associated medical complications that include hypertension, diabetes, and cardiovascular disease.

The most serious physical effect of severe obesity encountered in childhood is the pickwickian syndrome, named after the Charles Dickens character "Fat Boy Joe," who was continually falling asleep. Although the mechanism is unknown, narcolepsy associated with this obese state is thought to be caused by carbon dioxide narcosis from a decreased ventilatory capacity. There is an increased incidence of certain orthopedic problems in obese children, especially Legg-Perthes disease and genu valgum (knockknee). Probably the most destructive complications

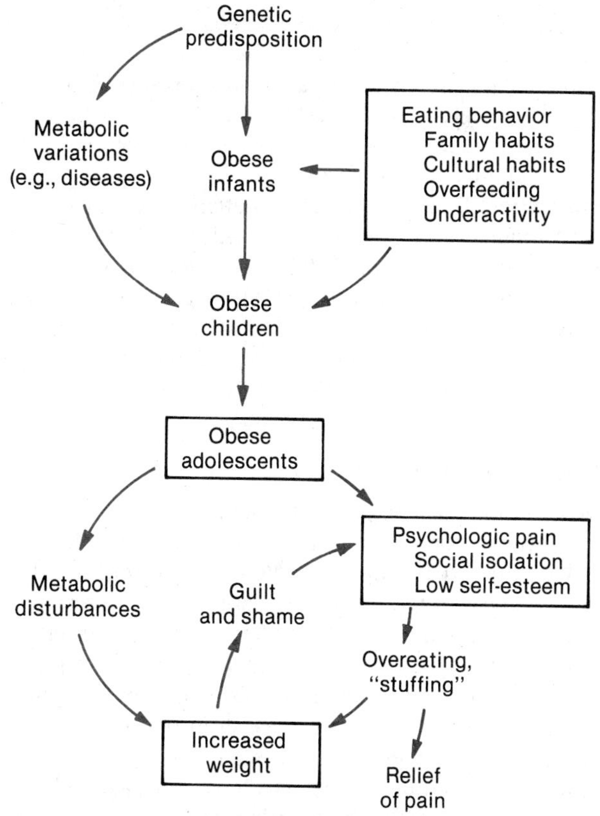

Fig. 21-1. Complex relationships in adolescent obesity.

are the psychosocial problems that affect obese youngsters as a result of teasing, ridicule, and rejection by peers and family.

Diagnostic Evaluation

The presence of obesity is obvious from appearance alone, and a gross determination can be made by a rough comparison of height and weight with standard growth charts. Children who are 20% over normal for their height and weight should undergo further evaluation, including a height and weight history of the child, parents, and siblings, as well as eating habits, appetite and hunger patterns, and physical activities. A careful history is taken regarding the development of the obesity, and a physical examination is carried out to help differentiate simple obesity from increased fat resulting from organic causes. Psychologic assessment, accomplished via interviews with the child and standardized personality tests, provides insight into personality and emotional problems that contribute to obesity and that might interfere with therapy. Appropriate diagnostic tests rule out suspected metabolic and endocrine disorders.

It is useful to have an estimation of the degree of fatness in order to have some idea of the component of body weight that can be modified. Several tests, both scientific and unscientific, can be employed to assess obesity. The most widely used means for determining obesity is measurement of skinfold thickness with special skinfold calipers. This device, calibrated in millimeters, allows the operator to control the pressure on the skinfold and provides a more precise measurement of its thickness. The Committee on Nutritional Anthropometry of the National Research Council recommends use of the triceps and subscapular areas for skinfold measurements (Chapter 7).

More sophisticated techniques have been developed for quantitating body fat and estimating its regional distribution. These include the *bioelectric impedance* method of determining body fat from measures of impedence of electrical current by way of electrodes attached to the arm and leg; *computed tomography (CT),* used to estimate subcutaneous and intraabdominal fat deposition; *magnetic resonance imaging (MRI),* which provides clear images of fat deposits compared with tissues containing water and other components; and total-body *neutron activation,* which provides an estimation of water and fat, as well as calcium, protein, and other components.

Therapeutic Management

Because of the self-perpetuating nature of obesity, efforts to treat the condition have been universally disappointing. A high proportion of obese children become obese adults. Because most of the nonsurgical approaches to weight reduction and maintenance suffer from a lack of lasting success, a more effective and sustained approach is a preventive one—early recognition and establishment of control measures before the child arrives at an obese state. However, varying degrees of success have been achieved in some highly motivated individuals through weight-reduction techniques, including diet, exercise, behavior modification, and psychologic support.

Box 21-1 ESSENTIALS OF A GOOD DIETARY REGIMEN FOR CHILDREN AND ADOLESCENTS

The diet should provide for:
- Rapid weight loss
- Lack of metabolic complications
- Lack of hunger
- Preservation of lean body mass
- Absence of psychiatric reactions
- Normal activity
- Growth

Diet. Diet modification is essential to any weight-reduction program. The ideal diet regimen for children and adolescents should meet the criteria listed in Box 21-1. For extremely obese youngsters the calories are markedly restricted, and the diet management is under the close supervision of health workers with specialized skills and experience.

Formal calorie-limited diets are more difficult to maintain than more flexible methods. Although short-term weight loss is accomplished, long-term maintenance is usually unsuccessful. In mildly obese youngsters with good motivation, correction of undesirable food habits and establishment of sensible eating and exercise behavior are sometimes effective. The dietary management requires nutrition reorientation and education.

Children below 5 years of age will lose weight on 600 to 800 kcal/day without interference with growth or development of ketosis. A diet containing 800 to 1200 kcal/day is usually suggested for children over 5 years of age (Taitz, 1983). The rate of weight loss varies with the level of physical activity and depends on how large the gap is between intake and normal maintenance requirements. An accumulated deficit of 3500 kcal is required to lose 1 pound of fat. The average caloric maintenance requirements for children over 5 years of age are listed in Table 21-1.

Exercise. Some type of regular exercise is incorporated in a weight-reduction program. In the absence of exercise, both fat and lean body mass are generally lost and weight regained is primarily fat (Fox and Mathews, 1981). For the self-conscious, reluctant youngster it is often more effective to begin the program at the time when some loss has been achieved from dieting and the loss has begun to level off somewhat. The youngster is less likely to feel unwilling to engage in the activity. Parents should be reassured that tapering off in the rate of loss is not related to diet failure but to altered metabolism that must be balanced by increasing activity (Taitz, 1983). Significant decreases in percentage of overweight have been observed in children who exercise in conjunction with diet when compared with those on a diet regimen alone (Epstein and others, 1985). Activities should be those that stress self-improvement rather than competition.

Behavior modification. Behavior modification approaches to weight loss are based on the observation that obese individuals have abnormal eating practices that can

Table 21-1 Average calorie requirements for maintenance from age 5 years

AGE	BOYS	GIRLS
5	1350	1300
6	1400	1370
7	1600	1450
8	1650	1500
9	1750	1600
10	1800	1700
11	1900	1800
15	2400	2100
18	2500	2200

Data from Merritt, R.J., and others: Consequences of modified fasting in obese pediatric and adolescent patients. I. Protein-sparing modified fast, J. Pediatr. 96:13-19, 1980.

be altered. The attention is focused not on food but on the social and behavioral aspects surrounding food consumption. The technique has been used primarily with older children and adolescents.

Behavior weight modification programs appear to be more successful when the management includes a problem-solving component. Youngsters who are able to identify problems and determine possible solutions have significantly greater success with weight loss both immediately following the program and at follow-up evaluations (Graves, Meyers, and Clark, 1988).

Drugs. Prescribing appetite-suppressant drugs to children and adolescents is not favored by most practitioners. There is little if any convincing evidence that they are more effective than diet and exercise in maintaining long-term weight loss. Probably more important is a concern regarding habituation to amphetamines and similar drugs. Occasionally some drugs (e.g., fenfluramine) may be desirable for short-term loss but are usually discouraged (Taitz, 1983).

Surgical techniques. Surgical techniques are available that bypass substantial portions of the intestine or occlude a large segment of the stomach to produce a marked diet restriction and hence weight loss. These shunting techniques are hazardous surgical procedures with many metabolic complications, including severe water and electrolyte depletion, persistent diarrhea, vitamin deficiency, internal herniation, and fatty infiltration and degeneration of the liver. Use of such a drastic measure in children and adolescents is still controversial. Most authorities believe that the complex metabolic effects need clarification and that this procedure should be restricted to those massively obese youngsters in whom other therapies have failed and whose obesity is life-threatening in disease states that demand weight loss for effective management. It should not be considered a cosmetic procedure that is available on request.

Nursing Considerations

Many successful weight-reduction programs involve professional nurses. Few physicians are able or inclined to devote time to the long-term supportive care needed to maintain the motivation of obese youngsters. Although therapy involves a team approach that includes the physician, dietitian, family, and the children themselves, nurses play a dominant role in any regulated and promising program of weight reduction. Interested nurse practitioners are able to evaluate, treat, and follow overweight adolescents. They also assume an important position in recognizing potential weight problems and assisting parents and their children in programs of prevention.

There are several factors related to the adolescent that health professionals must keep in mind when planning treatment for youngsters in this age-group. First, weight gain and anabolism are normal and necessary to healthy development during adolescent years, and any weight-reduction program must protect the teenager from prolonged catabolism that may permanently impair growth. Second, energy-absorbing developmental tasks of adolescence are stressful enough in themselves that the psychologic stress of food deprivation may be more than an adolescent can handle.

Assessment

The presence of obesity is obvious from appearance alone, and a gross determination can be made by a rough comparison of height and weight with standard growth charts. Children who are 20% over the normal for their height and weight should be further evaluated. Evaluation includes a height and weight history of the child, parents, and siblings, as well as eating habits, appetite and hunger patterns, and physical activities. It is useful to have an estimation of the degree of fatness in order to have some idea of the component of body weight that can be modified.

Nursing Diagnoses

Based on a thorough assessment, several nursing diagnoses are identified. The more common diagnoses for the obese child are included in the Nursing Care Plan on pp. 960-961. Others may apply in specific situations.

Planning

Nursing objectives for the obese child include the following:

1. Modify diet to provide loss of fat content without interfering with growth, normal activity, and psychologic well-being.
2. Implement a regular exercise program.
3. Modify eating behavior.
4. Provide psychologic support.

Implementation

The reasons behind the desire to lose weight need to be explored with youngsters, but success is rarely achieved unless they are motivated to lose weight and take personal responsibility for dietary habits and exercise programs. Teenagers who are forced by parents to seek help are seldom sufficiently motivated, become rebellious of parental nagging, and are unwilling to control dietary intake. A rigid approach or one based on parental enforcement of the regimen is usually doomed from the start. The strained relation-

NURSING CARE PLAN
The Child Who Is Obese

NURSING DIAGNOSIS: Altered nutrition: more than body requirements related to dysfunctional eating patterns, hereditary factors

GOAL 1

Identify eating patterns and behaviors

INTERVENTIONS

Instruct child and family to:
- Keep a record of everything eaten, including:
  - Time eaten
  - Amount eaten
  - Where food was consumed
  - Activity engaged in while eating
  - With whom the food was eaten or if it was eaten alone
  - Feelings at the time food was eaten, e.g., angry, depressed, lonely, elated
- Identify food stimuli
  - Feelings of hunger
  - Television commercials
  - Smell or sight of food
- Assess eating environments
  - Where food is eaten
  - With whom food is eaten, or eaten alone
  - Feelings at time of food consumption
  - Activity in which engaged while eating
- Analyze preceding data for patterns of eating and relationships of other factors as a basis for making adjustments

EXPECTED OUTCOME

Child's eating patterns become apparent

GOAL 2

Control food stimuli

INTERVENTIONS

Encourage child to:
- Separate eating from other activities
- Minimize food cues
- Get rid of "junk" food
- Prepare and serve only amounts to be eaten
- Put snacks out of sight
- Avoid purchase of problem foods such as fast foods (see Table 21-2)
- Serve food from stove or other place out of reach of the established eating place

EXPECTED OUTCOME

Child demonstrates an understanding of eating patterns and endeavors to alter destructive patterns

GOAL 3

Change eating patterns

INTERVENTIONS

Encourage child to:
- Eat at a specific place reserved just for eating
- Eat orderly meals at regular hours
- Use smaller plates to make amounts of food appear larger
- Eat at slow pace
- Leave a small amount of food on plate
- Eliminate eating during television viewing
- Substitute raw vegetables for "junk" food snacks

EXPECTED OUTCOME

Child alters eating behaviors

GOAL 4

Alter activity patterns

INTERVENTIONS

Encourage child to:
- Use activities other than eating to deal with emotional stress, boredom, and fatigue
- Engage in hobby activity, take a walk, straighten up room
- Become involved in activities away from food

EXPECTED OUTCOME

Child engages in suitable activities according to age and interest

GOAL 5

Eat the prescribed diet

INTERVENTIONS

Assist the child with meal planning
Employ strategies outlined above

EXPECTED OUTCOMES

Child conforms to prescribed diet plan
Child evidences a steady weight loss (or weight maintenance in a growing child)

NURSING DIAGNOSIS: Activity intolerance related to sedentary life-style, physical bulk

GOAL 1

Increase physical activity

INTERVENTIONS

Arrange programmed activity such as running, swimming, cycling
Encourage routine activity such as walking, climbing stairs

NURSING CARE PLAN
The Child Who Is Obese—cont'd

EXPECTED OUTCOME

Child engages in preferred exercise and activities regularly (specify)

NURSING DIAGNOSIS: Ineffective individual coping related to little or no exercise, poor nutrition, personal vulnerability

GOAL 1

Promote goal attainment

INTERVENTIONS

Implement a school weight-loss program
- Employ a buddy system
- Use peers as sponsors and positive reinforcers
- Employ frequent weigh-ins conducted by involved adult, nurse, teacher, physical education instructor
- Provide reinforcement for weight change
  - Social—praise
  - Tangible—contract that earns simple rewards
- Graph positive weight changes and display graph where others in the program can see it
- Provide nutrition education

Have a family member serve as a monitor at home to help in progress toward goals and to encourage child with positive statements daily

EXPECTED OUTCOME

Child engages in school-based program (specify)

NURSING DIAGNOSIS: Self-esteem disturbance related to perception of physical appearance, internalization of negative feedback

GOAL 1

Promote goal attainment

INTERVENTIONS

Encourage child to discuss his or her feelings and concerns
Reinforce accomplishments

EXPECTED OUTCOMES

Child expresses feelings and concerns regarding problems
Child maintains a positive attitude toward the weight-loss program

GOAL 2

Maximize positive aspects of appearance

INTERVENTIONS

Encourage good grooming, hygiene, and posture
Assist with exploring positive aspects of appearance and ways to enhance these aspects

EXPECTED OUTCOME

Child makes measurable efforts to improve appearance (specify)

GOAL 3

Improve self-esteem

INTERVENTIONS

Relate to child as an important, worthwhile individual
Encourage to set small, attainable goals for self
Encourage and support positive thinking (overweight persons are negative thinkers)
Encourage in activities to relieve boredom
Encourage interaction with peers

EXPECTED OUTCOMES

Child sets realistic short-term goals for self-improvement (specify)
Child voices positive attitudes toward self
Child engages in appropriate activities and interactions with peers (specify)

NURSING DIAGNOSIS: Altered family processes related to management of an obese child

GOAL 1

Involve family in child's weight-loss program

INTERVENTIONS

Educate family regarding weight-loss program, including nutrition, relationship of food intake and exercise, psychologic support

Encourage family to:
- Use appropriate reinforcement
- Alter food and eating environment
- Maintain proper attitudes regarding program
- Assist in monitoring eating behavior, food intake, physical activity, weight change
- Eliminate food as a reward
- Encourage youngster with positive statements only

EXPECTED OUTCOME

Family becomes actively involved in child's weight-loss program ships between parents and teenager are intensified by parental coercion, and because adolescents get food outside the home, adults simply cannot control their food intake. The result is an angry, sullen, and rebellious youngster who gains rather than loses weight.

Nutrition counseling. Planning caloric restriction for the adolescent during the rapid growth period requires care. Adolescents are unusually sensitive to caloric restriction, both physically and psychologically. It is extremely difficult to achieve the ideal reduction in body fat without concurrent loss in lean body mass. Sharp restriction in calories may result in relatively large losses of lean body mass and is not recommended for children or adolescents.

Sometimes the most realistic approach, especially during growth, is simply to prevent an increase in body fat. Children who are still growing will, by restricting calories, eventually grow into their weight. This can be accomplished by adjusting three aspects of eating: (1) reducing the *quantity* eaten by purchasing, preparing, and serving smaller portions; (2) altering the *quality* consumed by substituting low-calorie foods for high-calorie foods (especially for snacks); and (3) altering *situations* by severing associations between eating and other stimuli, such as eating while watching television (Copeland and Baucom-Copeland, 1981).

The most successful diets are those that use ordinary foods in controlled portions rather than diets that require the avoidance of any specific food. The youngster and parents are taught how to incorporate favorite foods into the diet and how to select substitutes that are also satisfying. The dieting youngster should eat what the rest of the family eats, but less of it. When parents buy and prepare smaller amounts, tempting second helpings and leftovers are eliminated. For older children exchange diets are useful. There are a multitude of restricted calorie diets available from a number of sources, such as the **American Dietetic Association,*** and the caloric values for a wide variety of commercial foods are available to facilitate meal planning.

For the teenager snacking is an integral part of the daily routine, which makes dieting especially difficult for the obese adolescent. Consequently, the youngster who is serious about dieting should be helped in elimination or judicious selection of snack foods. For example, getting rid of high-calorie junk foods and placing snack foods out of sight help divert attention away from eating. When snacking, several of a particular item are usually eaten; therefore substituting several items with lower caloric value for one item higher in calories is more satisfying. Foods containing complex carbohydrates are more satisfying than those containing simple sugars. The caloric values for common fast foods and snack items are listed in Table 21-2.

No adolescent should be encouraged to initiate a reduction diet without a health assessment, evaluation, and counseling. It is also important to emphasize the undesirable nature of the fad diets and crash programs that continually appear in various publications. Although some success has been achieved with low-carbohydrate, high-fat diets, their unpalatability and dietary boredom contribute to a high failure rate. Exotic diets have not been successful, and their unbalanced nature makes them potentially dangerous for growing children or adolescents. To be successful from all aspects, a dietary program should be nutritionally sound with sufficient satiety value, produce the desired weight loss, and be accompanied by nutrition education and continued support.

Behavior modification. Altering eating behavior has been found essential to weight reduction, especially in maintaining long-term weight control. This approach emphasizes identification and elimination of inappropriate eating habits. Although the long-term effects of this method are still in need of evaluation, it appears to hold promise for the treatment of obesity in adolescents. The behavior modification programs are based on various concepts, primarily those that incorporate the following (Taitz, 1983):

- A description of the behavior to be controlled, such as eating habits
- Attempts to modify and control stimuli governing eating
- Development of eating techniques designed to control speed of eating
- Positive reinforcement for these modifications by a suitable reward system

Some of the techniques used in this approach are listed in the Nursing Care Plan on pp. 960-961.

Group involvement. Some persons on weight-reduction programs find that the support and mutual reinforcement provided by a group of persons with a similar problem help them adjust to the changes needed for successful accomplishment of their goals, including weight loss. Commercial groups or diet workshops composed primarily of adults may be helpful to a few teenagers, but for most teenagers a group composed of other adolescents is more acceptable and usually more successful. Types of teenage groups include summer camps designed for obese youngsters and conducted by health professionals, school groups organized and led by a school nurse, and groups associated with special clinics.

The group not only is concerned with weight loss, but also emphasizes the development of a positive self-image. Nutrition education and diet planning are essential elements of the group function, but equally important are discussions centered around better grooming and improvement of social skills. Improvement is measured by positive changes in all aspects of endeavor. Group support and reinforcement are basic to success.

Family involvement. There is a definite connection between family environment and interaction and obesity (Huse and others, 1982a, 1982b). Involving the family facilitates weight loss, but the nature and extent of the involvement are related to the age of the child. With adolescents parents need education in the purposes of the therapeutic measures and their role in management. The family is given nutrition education and counseled regarding the reinforcement plan, altering the food environment, and maintaining proper attitudes. They assist in monitoring the child's eating behavior, food intake, physical activity, and weight changes.

*216 W. Jackson Blvd., Suite 800, Chicago, IL 60606; (312) 899-0040.

Table 21-2 Caloric values for selected fast food

FOOD	CALORIC VALUE
Burger King	
Cheeseburger	317
Hamburger	275
Whopper, regular	640
w/cheese	723
Double beef, plain	850
w/cheese	950
French fries, regular	227
Onion rings, regular	274
Chocolate shake	320
McDonald's	
Big Mac	570
Hamburger	263
Cheeseburger	328
Chicken McNuggets (6 pieces)	323
Quarter Pounder	427
w/cheese	525
Egg McMuffin	340
French fries, regular	220
Filet-O-Fish	435
Milk shake, vanilla	352
chocolate	383
Wendy's	
Hamburger, single	350
Hamburger, double	570
Chicken sandwich	320
French fries	280
Frosty	400
Long John Silver's	
Fish, 2 pieces and fries	651
3 pieces and fries	853
Fish sandwich	357
Cole slaw	180
Hushpuppies (3)	145
Taco Bell	
Beef Burrito	466
Burrito Supreme	457
Beefy Tostado	291
Dairy Queen	
Super Hot Dog/chili	570
Super Hot Dog w/cheese	580
Fries, small	200
Pizza Hut	
Thin 'n Crispy (¼ medium)	
Standard cheese	340
Superstyle cheese	410
Standard pepperoni	370
Superstyle pepperoni	430
Thick 'n Chewy (¼ medium)	
Standard cheese	390
Superstyle cheese	450
Standard pepperoni	450
Superstyle pepperoni	490
Supreme	480
Super Supreme	590
Fruit	
Apple w/skin, 2½ in. diameter	66
Banana, medium	100
Peach w/skin, 2 in. diameter	38
Cookies and cakes	
Hostess, 1 cup cake	
orange	151
chocolate	166
Hostess Twinkie, 1	147
Oreo, each	50
Chocolate chip	50-80
Cookies and cakes—cont'd	
Brownie	200
Fig Newton, 1	60
Doughnut, regular, 1 oz	113
old fashioned, 1 oz	151
powdered, 1 oz	117
Crackers	
Cheese balls and curls, 1 oz	160
Corn chips, 1 oz	150-160
Graham crackers, 1 piece	30
Pretzels, 1 oz	110-116
Rye Krisp, 1 triple	25
Saltine, 1 piece	12-18
Tortilla chips, 1 oz	130-140
Trisket, 1 piece	20
Wheat Thins, 1 piece	9
Candy	
Heath, 2½ oz	334
Hershey's, 1.2 oz bar	187
Nestle's, 1.1 oz bar	159
Hershey's Kisses, 1 piece	27
Krackle bar, 0.35 oz	52
Life Savers, 1 piece	10
Milk Duds, ¾ oz box	89
1¼ oz box	148
M & Ms, peanut, 1½ oz	219
plain, 1½ oz	202
Mr. Goodbar, 1½ oz	233
Snickers, 1.8 oz	247
Crackerjack, ¾ oz	90
Chewing gum	
Any brand, 1 stick	10
Dentyne, 1 stick	4
Chiclets, Beechies, 1 piece	6
Miscellaneous snacks	
Potato chips, 1 oz	150-160
Pringles, 1 oz	172
Yogurt, plain, 8 oz	150-160
fruit, 8 oz	230-262
Popcorn, plain, 1 cup	54
Nuts	
Almonds, 1 oz	170-178
Peanuts, dry roasted, 1 oz	160-173
oil roasted, 1 oz	179
Pecans, 1 oz	190-220
Pistachios, 1 oz	174
Pumpkin seeds, unshelled, 1 oz	116
Sunflower seeds, shelled, 1 oz	164
unshelled, 1 oz	86
Dessert snacks	
Popsicle, 1 twin pop	70
Turnover	310-340
Pop Tart	200-220
Baskin-Robbins	
Ice cream, 1 scoop	
vanilla	147
French vanilla	181
chocolate	165
chocolate fudge	178
Sherbet, 1 scoop	99-139
Beverages	
Chocolate milk, 8 oz	213
Skim milk, 8 oz	88
Whole milk, 8 oz	159
Coca Cola, 8 oz	96
Sprite, 8 oz	95

Box 21-2 STAGES OF PROBLEM SOLVING RELATED TO WEIGHT CONTROL

Stage 0: Denial. Youngsters have not identified weight control as a personal problem and consider the obesity a result of causes outside themselves. They describe present and future goals that are incompatible with their present weight (e.g., becoming a model).
Objective of counseling: Help youngsters realize their responsibility in weight control.

Stage I: Awareness. Youngsters recognize that they have a weight-control problem; they feel guilty, helpless, and responsible and are able to identify inappropriate habits or behaviors causing the problem.
Objective of counseling: Direct energies into close self-examination of current energy-balance behaviors.

Stage II: Alterable causes. Youngsters recognize that weight control is a personal problem. They can identify inappropriate habits and behaviors but have not considered alternatives.
Objective of counseling: Help youngsters begin to formulate plans of action.

Stage III: Mechanisms. Youngsters understand the relationships of diet, activity, and weight control. They can identify factors in their lives that are responsible for weight gain and could be modified but have not made the behavioral changes needed for weight control.
Objective of counseling: Help youngsters select the most reasonable mechanisms of change in regard to obesity-producing factors identified in stage II and to make only those changes that seem reasonable to them.

Stage IV: Implementation. Youngsters have initiated habit and behavioral changes to control the weight problem. They are able to identify persons or situations that affect their ability to manage weight control. They are able to work through the problem-solving stages and handle new threats.
Objective of counseling: Encourage youngsters to exercise the plan whenever feasible and to remind them that successful adoption will probably create new difficulties for which they must be alert.

More success has been achieved when counselors meet with adolescents and their parents separately (Brownell, Kelman, and Strunkard, 1983). Younger children and parents meet together, and parents are counseled alone when the children are very young.

Prognosis. Lifelong eating habits and psychologic problems make weight reduction extremely difficult and the failure rate very high. Some predictions can be made on the basis of experience. Weight reduction is more successful in obese adolescents who are older, who have lean parents who are married, who have a good academic performance, who have no affective disorder, and who have had no recent stressful life event (such as parents' divorce or a death).

Huse and others (1982a) determined that obese youngsters fit into various attitudinal stages indicating stages of problem solving. These stages of problem solving and their relation to weight control are outlined in Box 21-2.

Prevention. Unfortunately, weight loss programs do not enjoy the successes of therapeutic interventions for most other disorders. The failure rate is dismally high. Consequently, the best approach is to identify the infant and child at risk and attempt to prevent obesity. Gradual accumulation of adipose tissue during childhood establishes a pattern of eating that is virtually irreversible by the time a child reaches adolescence (Taitz, 1983). Children who are at risk of obesity, or those considered likely to become fat, are worthy of attempts at prevention. Risk factors in the development of obesity include familial obesity, severe disabilities leading to immobility (e.g., myelomeningocele), and syndromes associated with obesity (e.g., Prader-Willi syndrome). Cultural and social factors, including the perception of fat as a sign of good health, are deterrents to prevention.

Evaluation

The effectiveness of nursing interventions is determined by continual reassessment and evaluation of care based on the following observational guidelines and expected outcomes:

1. Assess weight at regular intervals (usually weekly); discuss with the youngster his or her feelings, reactions, and concerns; analyze daily recordings (log) of activities (eating, behavior, exercise) and feelings.
2. Review exercise program with the youngster.
3. Review log of eating behaviors; discuss the observations with the youngster.
4. Interview the youngster about the plan of care and progress toward short-term goals.

Expected outcomes:
See Nursing Care Plan, pp. 960-961.

ANOREXIA NERVOSA

Anorexia nervosa (AN) is the term applied to a long-recognized disorder characterized by severe weight loss in the absence of obvious physical cause. The term *anorexia nervosa* inaccurately describes the disorder in which individuals do not lack hunger but deny its existence. Emaciation occurs as a result of self-inflicted starvation. AN occurs predominantly in middle- and upper-class white females between 12 and 35 years of age, and the incidence appears to be increasing significantly. Fewer than 5% of persons with AN are males (Comerci, 1988). However, young school-age children (grades 3 through 9) admit preoccupation with diet and atypical eating habits (Maloney and others, 1989).

Etiology/Pathophysiology

The onset of AN has two peaks: between 12 and 14 and between 16 and 17 years of age (Herzog and Copeland, 1985). Young women who have this disorder are described as "good children," perfectionists, academically high achievers, conforming, and conscientious. Typical patients are female with high energy levels, even with marked emaciation. There is a distinct psychologic component, and the diagnosis is based primarily on psychologic and behavioral criteria. Nevertheless, the physical manifestations of AN lend support to possible organic factors in the etiology. A strong extrinsic motive has, for some reason, suppressed the vital function of eating. Because the disorder predominately involves females, the feminine pronoun is used in the ensuing discussions.

Psychologic aspects. Dominating the psychologic aspects of AN are a relentless pursuit of thinness and a fear of fatness, which are usually preceded by a period of a year or two of mood disturbances and behavior changes. The weight loss is usually triggered by a typical adolescent crisis, such as the onset of menstruation or a traumatic interpersonal incident, that precipitates serious dieting, and this dieting continues out of control. Frequently there is an exaggerated misinterpretation of the normal fat deposition characteristic of the early adolescent period, or someone may comment that the adolescent girl is putting on weight. The weight loss may be a response to teasing, some change in her life (such as changing schools or going to college), or an incident that requires an independent decision that she is unprepared to make (such as a career choice).

The current emphasis on slimness is a significant factor contributing to the increasing incidence in this disorder among young women. The standard for beauty is one exemplified by the models chosen for advertising clothing. Bigness is considered the ideal for men, and smallness is desired for women; and feminine success has long been based on appearance. Consequently, the pressure to diet and be slim continues relentlessly. Youngsters entering the growth phase of puberty when biologic fat accumulation is the normal course of development are particularly vulnerable. However, this standard is not universal. Women in countries where hunger and famine are facts of life do not consider extreme thinness a sign of beauty.

The syndrome of AN consists of three major areas of disordered psychologic functioning (Box 21-3). Some current evidence suggests that AN is a symptom of family psychopathology that is not usually apparent until the child has improved. These girls are usually strongly dependent on their parents, and frequently an ambivalent mother-daughter relationship is present. There is often a history of family strife, with the AN being a symptom of the family's problems. Families are usually rigid, incapable of resolving conflict, overly enmeshed, excessively controlling, and unable to display their feelings (Joffe, 1990).

Affected youngsters are model daughters who are afraid to assume adult responsibilities. They usually find it difficult to formulate an identity and feel ineffective in their personal lives even if they appear successful and capable (Joffe, 1990). They usually feel out of control in all aspects of their lives and choose control of food intake to express their autonomy. Any interventions are viewed as an attempt to remove this control.

Organic etiology. Evidence of organic etiology has been accumulated that may implicate abnormalities of hypothalamic-pituitary and end-organ function in individuals with AN. This is based on the observation that secondary amenorrhea is a common finding and that appetite and satiety are hypothalamic functions. Associated symptoms manifested in AN that relate to hypothalamic dysfunction include abnormalities of thermoregulation, water conservation, and secretion of catecholamines.

Box 21-3 AREAS OF DISORDERED FUNCTIONING IN ANOREXIA NERVOSA

1. **Disturbed body image and body concept of delusional proportions.** The young girl identifies with her emaciation, defending the skeleton-like appearance as normal, actively maintains it, and denies that it is abnormal. She indicates that it is rewarding to achieve and maintain this emaciated state. She is increasingly fearful of weight gain and interprets the concern of others as attempts to make her fat.
2. **Inaccurate and confused perception and interpretation of inner stimuli.** Inaccurate hunger awareness is pronounced. The adolescent does not recognize signs of nutritional need in herself and is unable to assess the amounts of food taken. She may feel "full" after only a few bites and derives pleasure from the refusal of food. A preoccupation and tremendous involvement with food and related activities are associated with this eating behavior; the girl frequently assumes all meal planning and preparation for others. Girls with anorexia nervosa often increase their activity to help counteract the possibility of weight gain. This hyperactivity may continue until emaciation is far advanced.
3. **Paralyzing sense of ineffectiveness that pervades all aspects of daily life.** Youngsters with anorexia nerovsa are overwhelmed by a deep sense of ineffectiveness. They are convinced that they only function in response to demands and wishes of others rather than doing as they want or choose. They have always been compliant children, but careful analysis reveals this to be mechanical obedience and overconformity that is not recognized as a reflection of a serious problem—a self-doubt regarding their ability to stand up for themselves or even the right for self-assertion.

Modified from Bruch, H.: Anorexia nervosa, Nutr. Today 13(5):14-18, 1978.

Clinical Manifestations

The most obvious manifestation of this disorder is the severe and profound weight loss induced by self-imposed starvation. The youngsters identify with this skeleton-like appearance and do not regard it as abnormal or ugly. They attempt to hide their extreme thinness by wearing bulky sweaters and baggy pants. Girls with AN also tend to overestimate the size of others. Patients absolutely refuse to eat and have a repertoire of excuses for not eating. Surprisingly, they display a marked preoccupation with food—preparing meals for others, talking about food, and hoarding food. The youngsters become obsessed with fasting and engage in frequent strenuous exercise, self-induced vomiting, and/or taking laxatives in an attempt to speed up the weight-loss process.

These youngsters tend to withdraw from peer relationships and engage in self-imposed social isolation. They are continually striving for perfection, which may be demonstrated in other compulsive behaviors such as stinginess.

Table 21-3 Some characteristics of eating disorders

FACTORS	ANOREXIA NERVOSA	BULIMIA
Food	Turns away from food to cope	Turns to food to cope
Personality	Introverted Avoids intimacy Negates feminine role	Extroverted Seeks intimacy Aspires to feminine role
Behavior	"Model" child Compulsive/obsessive	Often "acts out" Impulsive
School	High achiever	Variable school performance
Control	Maintains rigid control	Loses control
Body image	Body distortion	Infrequent body distortion
Health	Denies illness	Recognizes illness
Weight	Marked weight loss	Within 5 to 15 lb of normal body weight
Sexuality	Not sexually active	Often sexually active

They are usually overachievers, and their schoolwork is very important to them.

In the wake of the severe weight loss, these young girls exhibit physical signs of altered metabolic activity. They develop secondary amenorrhea, bradycardia, lowered body temperature, decreased blood pressure, and cold intolerance. They have dry skin and brittle nails and develop lanugo hair. The changes are usually reversible with adequate weight gain and improved nutritional status (see Table 21-1). Table 21-3 lists the differences between AN and bulimia.

Diagnostic Evaluation

Diagnosis is made on the basis of clinical manifestations and conformity to the criteria established by the American Psychiatric Association (1987) (Box 21-4).

Therapeutic Management

The treatment and management of AN involve three major thrusts: reinstitution of normal nutrition or reversal of the severe state of malnutrition, resolution of the disturbed patterns of family interaction, and individual psychotherapy to correct deficits and distortions in psychologic functioning. Because of the psychogenic nature of the disorder, treatment is difficult and lengthy. Because most therapeutic interventions require a team approach, the bulk of management is discussed in relation to nursing considerations.

Nutrition. The initial goal is to treat the life-threatening malnutrition with strict adherence to dietary requirements, which sometimes necessitates intravenous and/or tube feedings, although such methods are usually reserved for severe situations. This is combined with resolution of the family interaction and psychotherapy to improve the underlying psychologic misconceptions about the weight loss. Weight gain alone cannot be considered a cure for the disease and is an unreliable sign of progress. Relapses are frequent as the young girl reverts to previous eating patterns when removed from the therapeutic environment.

An adjunct to therapy is deconditioning by producing a mild euphoria that is incompatible with maintaining an anxiety about eating. There is a decided relationship between AN and depression. Decreasing the patient's consciousness of and vigilance about eating makes her less anxious and more amenable to other suggestions. This includes the administration of antidepressant or antianxiety agents. However, these drugs must be carefully monitored because of their cardiovascular side effects.

Some observations indicate that there may be a link between zinc and some aspects of AN. It is unclear whether the reduced serum zinc levels in these patients are secondary to the inadequate dietary intake or whether a premorbid zinc deficiency precipitates the eating behavior (Bryce-Smith and Simpson, 1984).

Psychotherapy. Psychotherapy for the affected youngster is essential. The patient herself needs to be an active participant in the treatment process and to become aware of the impulses, feelings, and needs originating within herself. It is essential that the patient rely on her own thinking, become more realistic in her self-appraisal, and become capable of living as a self-directed, competent individual who can enjoy what life has to offer and no longer needs to manipulate the body and its functions in this bizarre way.

Children whose illness can be clearly related to a dysfunctional family situation respond to therapy best when

Box 21-4 DIAGNOSTIC CRITERIA FOR ANOREXIA NERVOSA

1. Refusal to maintain body weight over a minimal normal weight for age and height, e.g., weight loss leading to maintenance of body weight 15% below that expected; or failure to make expected weight gain during period of growth, leading to body weight 15% below that expected.
2. Intense fear of gaining weight or becoming fat, even though underweight.
3. Disturbance in the way in which one's body weight, size, or shape is experienced, e.g., the person claims to "feel fat" even when emaciated, believes that one area of the body is "too fat" even when obviously underweight.
4. In females, absence of at least three consecutive menstrual cycles when otherwise expected to occur (primary or seconday amenorrhea). (A woman is considered to have amenorrhea if her periods occur only following hormone, e.g., estrogen, administration.)

From American Psychiatric Association: Diagnostic and statistical manual of mental disorders, ed. 3 (DSM-III-R), Washington, DC, 1987, The Association.

separated from the family. Many of those whose therapy plan is implemented in the hospital need a continued behavior modification program after discharge in order to maintain the desired weight. Psychotherapy is aimed at helping the child resolve the adolescent identity crisis, particularly as it relates to a distorted body image.

Prognosis

The complete recovery rate for AN is less than ideal. Only 15% of affected individuals attain full recovery; 50% improve substantially, although they may relapse during times of stress. A few report a more favorable outcome with a small number of patients (Kreipe, Churchill, and Strauss, 1989). The fatality rate for this disorder is approximately 5% and is almost always associated with long-standing symptoms (Comerci, 1988) and such factors as depression, bulimia, and vomiting. Although the changes are often reversible, long-term effects of severe malnutrition may be evident. For many, AN will be a lifelong problem. The prognosis is best for teenagers in whom the disorder is diagnosed at a relatively early age, before abnormal eating patterns and other weight-loss techniques are established and emaciation has set in (Joffe, 1990).

Evidence indicates that patients restored to normal weight still demonstrate a very low self-esteem, are highly sensitive to social interactions, and remain "obsessoid" (Toner, 1986). There is a strong underlying suicidal tendency, and although patients may not be aware of it, the efforts to starve themselves may be a manifestation. This should be explored in psychotherapy.

Nursing Considerations

Management of the youngster with AN is usually difficult and involves long-term commitment to care. Often these patients are relegated to mental health specialists, but the pediatric generalist may also encounter them in day-to-day practice.

Assessment

Because AN is becoming increasingly prevalent in the pediatric age-group, nurses should be alert to the possibility of the disorder when weight loss becomes evident during a routine assessment. The health interview and nutritional assessment often provide clues and guidelines for further investigation.

Nursing Diagnoses

Based on a thorough assessment, several nursing diagnoses are identified. The more common diagnoses for the child with AN are included in the Nursing Care Plan on pp. 968-969. Others may apply in specific situations.

Planning

Nursing objectives for the child with AN include the following:

1. Help the youngster to normalize eating behaviors.
2. Help the youngster develop realistic perceptions of the body and food.
3. Help the youngster develop adaptive ways to cope with the distorted body image and interpersonal relationships.
4. Provide family support and guidance.

Implementation

Nurses need to adopt and maintain a kind, supportive, yet firm manner in managing the care of a child with AN without creating a passive-dependent attitude in the child. The child requires sustained support and reassurance as she copes with ambivalent feelings related to her own body concept and the desire to see herself as cooperative, reliable, and worthy of the kindness she receives. Encouraging the child with education and activities that strengthen her self-esteem facilitates her resocialization process and social acceptance among her peers.

Diet. Rapid weight gain should be avoided. It can be medically unsafe, and it overwhelms the patient, who feels out of control immediately. Many of the deaths associated with AN occur during rehabilitation as a result of cardiovascular overload. A safe and reasonable target weight is calculated by the physician and dietitian—usually 18% fat. Initially the child resists the target weight as "too heavy," but without a target weight she feels out of control and believes people want her to gain weight indefinitely. Establishing a "maintenance weight range" of 1 kg over or under the target weight also helps the youngster feel in control and teaches how weight is maintained through good dietary habits (e.g., uncontrollable weight gain is not inevitable when an individual consumes a normal diet).

It is also important for nurses to be aware of some of the physical side effects of AN. Patients with AN often limit their fluid intake, which can lead to urinary tract problems. Ketones and proteins are frequently detected in the urine as a result of fat and protein breakdown. Vital sign instability can be severe, including orthostatic hypotension; the heartbeat becomes irregular and the pulse rate decreases markedly. The bradycardia and hypothermia can result in cardiac arrest.

Behavior therapy. The behavior modification approach to therapy has both supporters and detractors. Providing privileges or activities for weight gain or positive eating behaviors has had some success, although this approach alone ignores the youngster's individuality and does not address the conflict precipitating the disorder (Pipes, 1989). A clearly defined behavior modification plan is communicated to the child and maintained through a unified team approach by all persons involved in care.

The team responsible for the management of youngsters with AN arranges a carefully structured environment. A number of aspects are essential. First, there must be consistency. The team decides on an approach and adheres to it. The plan is structured with reality testing regarding caloric intake and body-image perception as an essential component. The team members provide a unified front to avoid any possibility of manipulation or inconsistency. Second,

NURSING CARE PLAN
The Child with Anorexia Nervosa

NURSING DIAGNOSIS: Altered nutrition: less than body requirements related to self-starvation

GOAL 1
Restore nutritional status

INTERVENTIONS
Implement high-calorie diet as prescribed
Explain nutritional plan to child and family
With dietitian and patient select balanced diet with the prescribed incremental increase in calories
Help patient prepare a dietary diary

EXPECTED OUTCOME
Child evidences weight gain

GOAL 2
Enforce behavior modification plan (if implemented)

INTERVENTIONS
Make certain all members of the health team determine an approach, understand the plan, and adhere to it consistently
Involve all team members, including the patient
Ensure continuity of caregivers (team members)
Provide for clear communication among team members and with the patient so that patient understands precisely what is expected
Consult with patient regarding progress
Avoid coercive techniques
Support the patient in efforts (e.g., positive feedback for accomplishments)

EXPECTED OUTCOME
Expectations are met consistently (specify)

GOAL 3
Reduce energy expenditure

INTERVENTIONS
Monitor physical activity
Supervise selection and performance of activity
Be alert to evidence of secretive exercising

EXPECTED OUTCOME
Child engages in quiet and specified activities

NURSING DIAGNOSIS: Body image disturbance related to altered perception

GOAL 1
Provide patient with appropriate feeling of control

INTERVENTIONS
Channel need for control and feeling of effectivenes in appropriate directions (rather than control of weight)
Obtain psychiatric referral as indicated
Encourage patient to monitor own care as appropriate

EXPECTED OUTCOME
Child expresses self in acceptable ways

GOAL 2
Support child

INTERVENTIONS
Maintain open communications with child
Convey an attitude of caring and protection to child
Avoid conveying an attitude of intrusion
Encourage participation in own care

EXPECTED OUTCOMES
Child expresses feelings and concerns
Child becomes actively involved in own care and management

GOAL 3
Alter disorted self-image

INTERVENTIONS
Support psychiatric plan of care

EXPECTED OUTCOME
Child displays evidence of developing a positive self-image

NURSING DIAGNOSIS: Ineffective individual coping related to unrealistic perceptions

GOAL 1
Prevent relapse

INTERVENTIONS
Maintain consistency in therapeutic approach selected
Maintain vigilance to detect signs of sabotaging the therapeutic plan, such as self-induced vomiting, hoarding food, disposing of food, placing weighted material in clothing for weigh-in
Provide positive reinforcement for progress
Be alert for signs of depression
Support psychotherapeutic measures
Help arrange for follow-up care

EXPECTED OUTCOME
Child and family conform to therapeutic program (specify behaviors)

NURSING CARE PLAN
The Child with Anorexia Nervosa—cont'd

NURSING DIAGNOSIS: Family coping: potential for growth related to ambivalent family relationships

GOAL 1

Resolve disturbed pattern of family interaction

INTERVENTIONS

Observe family interaction
Explore feelings and attitudes of family members
Support psychotherapeutic measures for redirecting malfunctioning family processes
Help arrange for referral to individuals and groups that further therapeutic goals

EXPECTED OUTCOME

Family patterns of interaction are outlined and evaluated

GOAL 2

Prepare for home care

INTERVENTIONS

Make certain both patient and family understand therapeutic plan
Arrange for follow-up care
Refer to special agencies for additional information and support

EXPECTED OUTCOME

Family demonstrates an understanding of the etiology of the disorder and conforms to therapeutic program

all members of the team must be involved. The responsibility of the program cannot be left to one person. The role and boundaries of each member are clearly spelled out and understood. Third, it is best to have continuity of team members. If possible, it is helpful to have the same staff persons all the time.

Fourth, communication among team members is essential, including clear communication with the patient regarding what is expected from her. Sometimes the limit-setting needed may seem unreasonable, and if the youngster does not know the rationale for the limits, she may sabotage the entire program. It is also important to communicate with the family. Fifth, the plan must provide for support of patient, family, and staff. The patient needs positive feedback for accomplishments made in normalizing eating habits and behaviors. Meetings are held to discuss and process feelings and concerns. This includes group meetings of team members, minimeetings of immediate caregivers and the patient, and structured rounds.

All of those involved in therapy must keep in mind the adolescent's distorted sense of body image and self-awareness and her feelings of self-doubt, ineffectiveness, and helplessness that prompt such bizarre behavior in order to feel in control. The underlying principle in most behavior modification programs is to make conditions extremely uncomfortable and to grant privileges only as a reward for weight gain (Table 21-4). Patients who view the program as coercive and become depressed by this approach seldom maintain weight gain outside the hospital environment.

A *behavioral contract,* an agreement that the patient makes with the others involved to change a maladaptive behavior, has proved to be effective in some cases. The written contract, constructed by the therapeutic team, is approved and signed by the patient. Unless the patient agrees to its terms, the contract can become the source of a power struggle. However, it can be an effective tool by placing the responsibility on the patient for weight gain or other behavior change (Carino and Chmelko, 1983).

Family support. Family therapy seems to be effective when begun soon after the onset of illness, but it is less successful when the condition has existed for some time. Therapy is directed toward disengagement and redirection of malfunctioning processes in the family, but this usually requires individual psychotherapy for family members.

Nurses, patients, and families can find assistance and information from organizations that provide services for young persons suffering from this disorder. The **American Anorexia/Bulimia Association, Inc.,*** also provides information, referrals, counseling, programs, and activities aimed at combating eating disorders. The **National Association of Anorexia Nervosa and Associated Disorders, Inc. (ANAD),†** provides counseling, referral, and self-help programs for young people with AN. The **National Anorectic Aid Society, Inc.,‡** provides information and support services for both patients and families. Others include **Anorexia Nervosa and Related Eating Disorders (ANRED)§** and **Bulimia, Anorexia Self-Help.||**

Prevention. There are no easy ways to prevent AN. However, public and professional awareness of signs and symptoms can help identify patients early so that treatment can be implemented in order to prevent or reduce the long-

*418 E. 76th St., New York, NY 10021; (212) 734-1114.
†P.O. Box 7, Highland Park, IL 60035; (312) 831-3438.
‡5796 Karl Rd., Columbus, OH 43229; (614) 436-1112.
§P.O. Box 5102, Eugene, OR 97405; (503) 344-1144.
||6125 Clayton Ave., Suite 215, St. Louis, MO 63139; (314) 567-4080 or (800) 762-3334 (crisis hotline).

Table 21-4 Behavior modification plan for achieving weight gain in anorexia nervosa

WEIGHT (LB)*	PRIVILEGE LOST OR GAINED
70	Hospitalize
	In room; full bed rest
	No telephone, television, radio, phonograph, and so on
	No books, schoolwork, or craft materials
	No visitors
−3	Tube feeding
+¼	Bathroom privileges
+½	May have books, schoolwork, craft materials
+1	May have radio
+1½	May have television
+2	May have brief visit with parents
+2½	May have telephone
+3	May go out of room
+3½	May have friends visit
+5	May go home
−5	Rehospitalize with all restrictions
−8	Reinstitute tube feedings

From Hofmann, A.D., editor: Adolescent medicine, Menlo Park, CA, 1983, Addison-Wesley Publishing Co., Inc., p. 324.
*Privileges should be accorded at ¼ lb gains in the beginning. Later they may be set at ½ lb intervals. This listing is only an example of one behavior modification approach.

Box 21-5 EARLY SIGNS OF ANOREXIA NERVOSA

The youngster:
- Consumes an inappropriate diet (excessively strict) or may refuse to eat altogether
- Develops peculiar eating habits such as toying with food, food "rituals," preparing and forcing food on family members without eating any herself
- Engages in excessive exercise, such as compulsive jogging, running up and down stairs, rigorous calisthenics to burn off calories—often to the point of exhaustion
- Withdraws from social interaction—starts to spend all her time in her room studying, exercising, or otherwise occupied
- Ceases to have menstrual periods after sudden or excessive weight loss—sometimes almost as soon as dieting begins
- Takes laxatives, diuretics, or enemas to speed intestinal transit time to lose added weight and empty intestines to flatten abdomen
- Vomits deliberately—may go to bathroom after a meal and turn on faucets to avoid being heard
- Denies hunger even after eating practically nothing for days or even weeks
- Develops a distorted body image—states she "feels fat" as she becomes increasingly thinner
- Loses weight—growing girls fail to achieve the 25th percentile on normal growth curves

term adverse consequences. Some of the early signs of AN are outlined in Box 21-5. Education about the disorder may help prevent some cases.

Evaluation

The effectiveness of nursing interventions is determined by continual reassessment and evaluation of care based on the following observational guidelines and expected outcomes:

1. Perform nutritional assessment, measure weight; review diet and nutritional intake (e.g., log); interview child regarding food and eating behaviors; observe eating behaviors.
2. Interview the youngster regarding self-perceptions; observe behavior; confer with psychologist and other members of the health team regarding evidence of progress.
3. Observe child's behavior and interview the youngster regarding attitudes and concerns.
4. Interview family and confer with team members regarding progress; observe interpersonal interactions between child and others, especially family members.

Expected outcomes:
See Nursing care plan, pp. 968-969.

BULIMIA

Bulimia (from the Greek meaning "ox hunger") is the term applied to an eating disorder, similar to AN, that is characterized by binge eating. The binge behavior consists of secretive, frenzied consumption of large amounts of high-calorie (or "forbidden") foods during a brief period of time (usually less than 2 hours). The binge is counteracted by a variety of weight control methods (purging), including self-induced vomiting, diuretic and laxative abuse, and rigorous exercise. These binge/purge cycles are followed by self-deprecating thoughts, a depressed mood, and an awareness that the eating pattern is abnormal.

Clinical Manifestations

Bulimia is observed more frequently in older adolescent girls and young women; male bulimics are uncommon. Dynamically persons with bulimia have many issues in common with other eating disorders—control being a major issue. Many begin with only occasional binges and purges "just for fun," enjoying the control over their weight while eating amounts of food that would normally produce obesity. As the disease progresses, the frequency of binges increases, the amount of food consumed increases, and the bulemic gradually loses control over the binge/purge cycle. The binge/purge cycle provides relief from feelings of guilt resulting from the enormous amounts of costly food consumed. The family becomes angry, and the individual with bulimia becomes frightened, frustrated, and increasingly guilt-ridden, which only increases the symptoms in the self-destructive cycle.

The frequency of binging can be anywhere from once per week to seven or eight times per day. Because persons with bulimia usually binge on high-calorie foods, especially sweets, ice cream, and pastries, insulin production is stimulated to cope with the added carbohydrates. When the food is vomited, the unused insulin stimulates hunger and the desire to eat. An intake of 20,000 to 30,000 calories per day is not unusual. The disorder is almost never seen in lower socioeconomic groups because of the difficulty in obtaining volumes of food.

Characteristically persons with bulimia are those who have been unsuccessful dieters, have low impulse control, and may have been self-conscious about overweight in childhood. They may consciously or unconsciously suppress their feelings and have a strong desire to fit into the group.

Individuals with bulimia appear to fall into two categories: (1) those who consume vast quantities of food followed by purging but who, if unable to purge, still consume large amounts and (2) those who restrict their caloric intake, especially when unable to purge. Some bulimic women are of normal or (more often) slightly above normal weight; others become as underweight as individuals with AN. This latter type with a tendency to restrict intake is also called *bulimarexia*. (See Table 21-3 for a comparison of AN and bulimia.)

Complications. Women with bulimia suffer from several medical complications as a result of the frequent vomiting. Loss of fluids and electrolytes can occur very rapidly as in any other disorder characterized by gastrointestinal losses. Potassium depletion causes diminished reflexes, fatigue, and, if severe, possible cardiac arrhythmias. Potassium losses are more likely to occur with diuretic abuse. Laxative abuse can interfere with absorption of fat, protein, and calcium, as well as produce abdominal complaints, such as cramping, and sluggish bowel function.

Vomiting produces a number of serious complications. Irritation from stomach acid causes erosion of tooth enamel and an increase in dental caries. Chronic esophagitis, chronic sore throat, difficulty swallowing, inflammation, and parotitis are frequent findings. Vomiting may be so severe that the patient suffers esophageal tears, hiatal hernia, and spontaneous bleeding in the eye. Anemia is common.

Diagnostic Evaluation

The diagnosis may be first suspected from the presence of complications. Final diagnosis is made on the basis of criteria established by the American Psychiatric Association (1987) (Box 21-6). Distinctive hand lesions have also been observed in bulimic persons. The backs of the hands are often scarred and cut from repeated abrasion of the skin against the maxillary incisors during self-induced vomiting (Williams, Friedman, and Steiner, 1986).

Box 21-6 DIAGNOSTIC CRITERIA FOR BULIMIA NERVOSA

1. Recurrent episodes of binge eating (rapid consumption of a large amount of food in a discrete period of time)
2. A feeling of lack of control over eating behavior during the eating binges
3. Regularly engages in either self-induced vomiting, use of laxatives or diuretics, strict dieting or fasting, or vigorous exercise in order to prevent weight gain
4. A minimum of two binge eating episodes a week for at least 3 months
5. Persistent overconcern with body shape and weight

Modified from American Psychiatric Association: Diagnostic and statistical manual of mental disorders, ed. 3 (DSM-III-R), Washington, DC, 1987, The Association.

Therapeutic Management

Therapy is similar to the management of AN. Hospitalization may be required, especially for complications, which are treated symptomatically. Intravenous fluids and potassium replacement are the essential elements of care, and cardiac monitoring is indicated.

Two approaches to behavior therapy may be employed. The first advocates eliminating binge/purge opportunity by locking up both food and bathroom. The patient is fed a regular diet. The second approach allows the binge/purge behavior but uses behavior modification to decrease the unwanted behaviors. This approach allows the patient more control as opposed to staff control. (See therapeutic management of AN, p. 966.)

Nursing Considerations

Nursing care is similar to care of the patient with AN. Acute care also involves careful monitoring of fluid and electrolyte alterations and observation for signs of cardiac complications.

"FEAR OF FAT" SYNDROME

A new phenomenon has been identified that affects preteens and teenagers—the fear of becoming fat (Pugliese and others, 1983). In their enthusiasm to avoid becoming overweight, these youngsters restrict their caloric intake to the degree that they stop growing normally and pubertal changes do not take place. The disorder is distinct from AN in which the patients have a distorted body image. Youngsters who are afraid of obesity worry that overweight will make them physically unattractive, jeopardize their health, and shorten their life spans.

The desire for thinness in these youngsters is often triggered by the normal gain in weight and fat accumulation of adolescent growth and development (Attie and Brooks-Gunn, 1989). The dissatisfaction with their appearance often causes young people to resort to fad diets and severely reduce their intake far below the recommended daily allowances for nutrients. As many as 51% of underweight adolescents described themselves as extremely fearful of being overweight, and 36% were preoccupied with body fat (Moses, Banilivy, and Lifshitz, 1989). Unfortunately, to achieve low-calorie, low-fat diets, teenagers eliminate many basic foods such as milk, cheese, eggs, and meat without replacing them with other nutritious items such as cereal and bread. Their diets are lacking in essential minerals as well, especially zinc, a mineral closely tied to growth and onset of puberty (Lifshitz and Moses, 1988).

Many children worry about their weight long before adolescence, even when there is no reason for concern (Feldman, Feldman, and Goodman, 1988). In one study 45% of children (mean age 9.7 years) expressed a desire to be thinner, and 37% reported dieting in an attempt to lose weight; 10% reported binging, and 1% vomited in order to control weight (Maloney and others, 1989). The media emphasis on thinness and the nationwide emphasis on prevention of obesity may be detrimental to this vulnerable age-group.

Nurses who encounter youngsters who impose unwarranted dieting on themselves need to focus on education regarding normal body changes and the hazards of dieting, which are more serious than the risks associated with unwanted weight gain. Although most authorities suggest a weight maintenance program for overweight children during the growth years, there are those who recommend that no child or adolescent in the growth-spurt period be encouraged or counseled to lose weight (Mallick, 1982). Also, investigations of possible eating disorders might well focus on children before adolescence to learn how preoccupation with weight begins and why thinness is thought to be so attractive (Feldman, Feldman, and Goodman, 1988).

DESTRUCTIVE BEHAVIORS

The turmoil and stress associated with the pubertal changes of adolescence, limited problem-solving capacity, and the struggle for independence experienced by many adolescents make them vulnerable to superimposed stresses. Some youngsters who are unable to cope with these complex problems and feelings indulge in behaviors that are life-threatening or physically harmful.

SMOKING

The problem of smoking among teenagers is becoming increasingly serious. The habit appears to be spreading among teenagers even as the evidence of the relationship between smoking and health problems increases. Smoking is considered to be a dependence disorder and is formally included in the diagnostic nomenclature of the American Psychiatric Association (1987). Although the number of smokers has declined in recent years, cigarette smoking is still considered to be the chief avoidable cause of death in the United States (State-specific estimates, 1988).

Findings in one area disclosed that 22% of the girls and 11% of the boys were smoking. In addition, 35% of the boys admitted using smokeless tobacco (Guggenheim and others, 1986); another study reported 37% of males and 2.2% of females using smokeless tobacco (Marty and others, 1986).

The hazards of smoking at any age are undisputed (Surgeon General's report, 1989); however, a preventive approach to teenage smoking is especially important for several reasons. There is high probability that regular smoking in childhood leads to a lifetime habit with concomitant increases in morbidity and mortality.

Etiology

In most instances the smoking habit begins in adolescence, and there are a variety of reasons why teenagers begin smoking. The significant factors related to onset of smoking can be categorized as social, sociodemographic, psychosocial, and biologic. Once smoking behavior is established, smoking itself is thought to produce enough reinforcement to sustain the practice without the initial pressure (Bragg and Hughes, 1984).

Social factors. Social pressures to smoke include imitation of the smoking behavior and attitudes of parents and other adults, the association of smoking with maturity or as representative of "mature" behavior, pressures from peers who view smoking as the popular thing to do, and the use of smoking as an outlet for real or imagined school, social, or home pressures. Other pressures come from advertisers who aim directly at members of this vulnerable age-group.

Parental approval or disapproval of their children's smoking is an important force in predicting teenage smoking. In one study 34% of teenage smokers had smoked at least one cigarette in their homes, implying that smoking was accepted by the parents (Biglan and others, 1984). The social influence of same-sex family members or peers is an important factor, and the number of smokers in the immediate environment increases the probability of subsequent smoking by a youngster. However, researchers have concluded that children are less likely to develop the smoking habit if someone in the family was a model for quitting. Having an ex-smoker model was influential enough to outweigh previous smoking effects on the child (Peterson and Peterson, 1986).

The social nature of smoking is also significant (Flay and others, 1983), as well as anticipation of enjoyment. However, the influence of friends on beliefs and behavior depends in part on the adolescent's tendencies toward rebelliousness and disobedience (McAlister, Krosnick, and Milburn, 1984).

The mass media have contributed to the incidence of smoking in easily influenced adolescents. In advertisements smokers are engaged in activities and dressed in clothes suitable for adolescents, and the ads imply that smoking is associated with fun, risk taking, and sexual adventure, as well as a sign of maturity and autonomy (Davis, 1987). The ads also imply an association between smoking and "youthful vigor, good health, good looks, and personal, social, and professional acceptance and success" (Staff report, 1981).

Sociodemographic factors. Sociodemographic factors include socioeconomic status, sex, and performance in school. A consistent, negative association has been observed between socioeconomic status and smoking (especially among boys), and there is a consistent correlation between low academic goals and performance and smoking (cited in Flay and others, 1983). At least 30% of persons who have not proceeded beyond a high school education are smokers, whereas less than 10% of college graduates smoke (Pierce and others, 1989). Researchers report that students who focus on schoolwork and who have high educational goals for themselves are significantly less likely than their peers to develop a long-term smoking habit (Newcomb, McCarthy, and Bentler, 1989). Smokers have been found to be from families of lower socioeconomic levels (Eckert, 1983) and do not participate in school activities. Adolescents who participate in and dominate school activities tend to come from the upper end of the social continuum (Eckert, 1983).

Psychosocial factors. A primary feature of early adolescence is development of an identity, an autonomous self-concept. During this time the self-conscious young adolescent endeavors to alter the real self-image to approximate the ideal self-image (Chassin and others, 1981). It appears that adolescents who are performing well academically and in school-related activities, especially athletics, derive their status through seniority in the system; the significant minority who are failing place a premium on status that can be achieved through voluntary group associations. Cigarette smoking may be an attempt on the part of these youngsters to emulate the personality traits of toughness, friendliness, confidence, attractiveness, and enthusiasm—traits that are popularly attributed to smokers. They feel a need for social skills that make them appear to be adroit, fluent, authoritative, and worthwhile persons who are sufficiently attractive to warrant inclusion in significant peer groups. Smoking is an easily mastered vehicle with motor activities that convey an air of ease and social adeptness (Wong-McCarthy and Gritz, 1982).

Biologic factors. Biologic factors serve to both encourage and deter further experimentation of would-be smokers. Initial harshness, nausea, and irritation are sufficient to influence many youngsters not to try smoking again; to others it may represent a challenge to overcome. Smoking has been found to lower endurance by decreasing breathing capacity or ventilatory muscle endurance (Dessendorfer, Amsterdam, and Odland, 1983). Dependence is thought to be the result of nicotine, the primary alkaloid in tobacco. Nicotine exerts both stimulating and sedating effects on the central and peripheral nervous systems and several organ systems. Attempts at stopping the smoking habit are accompanied by severe craving and withdrawal symptoms.

Process of Becoming a Smoker

Researchers have identified three stages in the process: trying the first cigarette, experimental smoking (less than weekly), and regular smoking (at least weekly) (Flay and others, 1983). Some recognize a preparation or initiation stage in which psychosocial, environmental, and possibly biologic factors prepare certain youngsters to be smokers (Box 21-7).

Box 21-7 STAGES OF BECOMING A SMOKER

Preparation—early learning experiences provided in the environment (e.g., parent or sibling smokers in the family)
Initiation—trying the first cigarette; peer influences are more important than family influences in determining when cigarettes are first tried
Experimentation—learning to smoke by repeated experimentation: decision to quit or continue
Regular smoking—smoke sufficiently often to be considered a regular smoker

Data from Leventhal, H., and Cleary, P.D.: The smoking problem: a review of the research and theory in behavioral risk modification, J. Personality Soc. Psychol. 88:370-405, 1981.

Smokeless Tobacco

The term *smokeless tobacco* refers to tobacco products that are placed in the mouth but not ignited, for example, snuff and chewing tobacco. This increasingly popular substitute for cigarettes is now posing a serious hazard to children and adolescents, even school-age children, as well as young adults (Goldsmith, 1988). These products have been proved to be carcinogenic, and regular use has been reported to cause dental diseases including foul-smelling breath, periodontal disease, erosion of teeth, and tooth loss (Greer, 1983). The American Academy of Pediatrics, Committee on Environmental Hazards (1985) states that "for the protection of the present and future health of the children of this nation, the selling and advertising of all forms of smokeless tobacco must be controlled without delay."

Nursing Considerations

Prevention of regular smoking in teenagers appears to be the most effective way to reduce the overall incidence of smoking. Obviously, early education is the ideal approach, but most school-based or large-scale public information campaigns have had no significant impact on smoking habits. A variety of methods have been employed to deal with the problem. Posters, charts, displays, statistics, and the use of examples of actual damaged lungs to communicate the hazards of smoking all have their supporters and doubters. While some believe that these are a waste of time, others give evidence that many children are influenced by these "scare tactics." Presentation of films and demonstrations in science classes have proved to be of value in some schools. However, even youngsters who "know better" are not deterred by knowledge of health risks (Marwick, 1988).

For the most part, smoking-prevention programs that focus on negative long-term effects of smoking on health have been uniformly ineffective. Those emphasizing immediate effects and youth-to-youth programs have been somewhat more effective, but primarily in improving the teenagers' attitudes toward smoking (Silvis and Perry, 1987). Because smoking and smoking-related behavior function as a key social symbol, antismoking campaigns must be addressed to the norms of the potential smokers, and anything that ridicules or threatens the social norms of the group can be unproductive or counterproductive (Eckert, 1983). Also, investigators have found that teaching resistance to peer pressure to smoke may be effective in early adolescence but loses effectiveness as adolescents age (Morgan and Grube, 1989). Emphasis on negative consequences of smoking is more likely to be effective with older adolescents.

Two areas of focus are gaining interest among health advocates: peer-led programming and use of media in smoking prevention, that is, videotapes and films. Peer-led programs emphasizing social consequences of not smoking have proved most successful. If a significant number of in-

Box 21-8 RECOMMENDED NONSMOKING STRATEGIES

Provide only a cursory mention of long-term health consequences (e.g., cardiovascular and cancer risks)
Discuss immediate physiologic consequences in some detail (e.g., changes in heart rate and blood pressure, minor respiratory symptoms, and blood carbon monoxide concentrations)
Mention alternatives to smoking for establishing a self-image that appears tough, independent, mature, or sophisticated (e.g., establishing a weight-lifting regimen, jogging and dancing, joining a Boys' Club or a Girls' Club, engaging in volunteer work for a hospital or political or religious group)
Mention the negative effects of smoking (e.g., earlier wrinkling of skin, yellow stains on teeth and fingers, tobacco odor on breath and clothing)
Mention the increasing ostracism of smokers by nonsmokers, both legal and informal, in places of work and public places
Mention the increasing evidence that second-hand smoke is injurious to the health of nonsmokers who are regularly exposed, especially small children
Acknowledge that many adults once believed that important social benefits were associated with smoking; but point out that the vast majority of adult smokers would now quit smoking if they could
Arm the cooperative adolescent with arguments for dealing with peer pressure (e.g., by not smoking, a teenager demonstrates independence and nonconformity, traits normally prized by youth)
Request posters and pamphlets from local voluntary agencies (e.g., American Cancer Society, American Heart Association, and American Lung Association) to display prominently

Modified from Wong-McCarthy, W.J., and Gritz, E.R.: Preventing regular teenage cigarette smoking, Pediatr. Ann. 11:683-689, 1982.

fluential peers can "sell" their classmates on the idea that the habit is not popular, the followers will imitate their behavior. Short-term rather than long-term consequences are emphasized, for example, the effects of smoking on personal appearance, such as the unattractive stains on teeth and hands and the unpleasant odor that smoking gives to the breath and clothing.

Smoking bans in schools also accomplish several goals: (1) they discourage students from starting to smoke; (2) they reinforce knowledge of the health hazards of cigarette smoking and exposure to environmental tobacco smoke; and (3) they promote a smoke-free environment as the norm (School policies, 1989).

Nurses in schools and other agencies of the community are in a position to implement and reinforce teaching, to serve as consultants and counselors to student, teacher, and parent groups, and to be advocates in all areas in which antismoking campaigns might be effective. Several strategies are recommended (Box 21-8). Information can also be obtained from **Stop Teenage Addiction to Tobacco (STAT),** a national organization devoted to educating the public and professionals.*

*121, Lyman St., Suite 210, Springfield, MA 01103; (413) 732-STAT.

SUBSTANCE ABUSE

The use of substances, primarily drugs, by children and adolescents to produce an altered state of consciousness is widespread and is believed to reflect the variety of changes taking place in their lives and the stresses engendered by these changes. The discomfort associated with the growth and changes of this prolonged and intense transitional process encourages the adolescent to search for relief, escape, or self-exploration. To relieve this discomfort, young people often turn to the exhilarating, mind-easing, euphorigenic qualities of drugs.

Most drugs to which young people turn induce changes in perception, a feeling of well-being, and a sense of closeness. To most, they provide a feeling of happiness. With the exception of some stimulant drugs used for practical purposes, such as working better, studying, or increasing cognitive effectiveness, the drugs used are simply pleasure-promoting chemicals used in the hope for altered consciousness or the attainment of a different level of functioning. Most of these drugs have some hallucinogenic properties. Far more frequent is the use of alcohol or marijuana as recreational drugs without significant disruption of behavior or performance (American Academy of Pediatrics, Committee on Adolescence, 1983). Since teenagers and parents do not always consider these to be a health issue, the problem may not be called to the attention of health professionals.

Definitions

The greatest area of misinformation and confusion is related to the terms applied to drug use (see Glossary). The most important differences among these terms is the distinction between voluntary and involuntary behavior and between culturally defined and physiologically identified events. *Drug abuse, misuse,* and *addiction* are culturally defined and are voluntary behaviors. *Drug tolerance* and *physical dependence* are involuntary behaviors based on physiologic changes. Consequently, an individual can be addicted to a narcotic with or without being physically dependent, whereas a person may be physically dependent on a narcotic without being addicted, such as patients who are experiencing pain.

The broad term *drug abuse,* which is often applied to all forms of drug misuse, can be confusing and does not necessarily define the problem related to drug use. Many of the substances are controlled by law and accompanied by severe penalties for their illegal use; others are sanctioned from a legal, social, and medical standpoint. Problems concerning drug use can therefore be defined as legal, social, medical, and individual (Box 21-9).

Patterns of Drug Use

Many factors influence the extent to which drugs are used by teenagers. The type of drug used, mode of administration, duration of use, frequency of use, and single or multiple drug use must be considered in determining the severity of the individual drug problem. Most drug use begins with experimentation. The individual may try a drug only once, it may be used occasionally, or it may become an integral

Box 21-9 PROBLEMS RELATED TO DRUG USE

Legal—the drug being taken is strictly controlled by law and is accompanied by severe penalties for its use or possession.
Social—use of a substance leads to disruptive or bizarre behavior that alienates the user from the rest of society; this results in a social problem.
Medical—current or continued use of a substance may adversely affect the physical or mental health of the youngster.
Individual—focuses on the role that drug use plays in the individual's life and factors that contribute to the individual's need for the drug.

part of a drug-centered life-style. Identification of the pattern of drug use in an individual facilitates the formulation of an approach to the problem. Patterns have been observed based on dose and frequency of use.

There are two broad categories of adolescents who use drugs: the *experimenters* and the *compulsive users.* There is a wide range of use between these groups that represents two ends of a continuum in terms of degree of use. With the exception of a "bad trip" or accidental overdose, the experimenters present few medical problems, although they probably represent the bulk of adolescent drug users. Some of these youngsters with a predisposition to heavy drug use proceed to compulsive use after a time, but by and large they are in the minority.

Between the experimenters and compulsive users is a broad range of *recreational* users of drugs, principally drugs such as marijuana, cocaine, and alcohol. For many the goal is merely relaxation, and these fit more closely with the experimenting, intermittent users. For others the goal is intoxication, and these are more nearly like the compulsive users. The groups of greatest concern to health workers are those whose patterns of use involve high doses with the danger of overdose and those compulsive users with the threat of dependence, withdrawal syndromes, and altered life-style.

Motivation

There are several common motives for drug use. Adolescents try drugs out of curiosity, for kicks. Drugs produce for some persons a dreamy state of altered consciousness and a feeling of power, excitement, heightened acuity, or confidence. Others seek visual hallucinatory experiences and sexual sensation. Many youngsters use drugs not only for the perceptual and sensory experiences, but also for the social aspects.

Teenagers are highly influenced by fads and fashions within their society, and they are, developmentally, sensation-hungry risk takers. It is characteristic that they are eager to test their mental and physical capabilities to the utmost. Adolescents are also trying to find a means to cope with their disenchantment with the adult world and its social and technologic concerns and with their powerlessness to change it. They seek escape from reality and want to achieve a sense of closeness and intimacy with other people, to escape from distress or decision making, and to feel a sense of insight into the mysteries of God, death, and rebirth.

During early and middle teenage years, drug use seems to fall into rather distinct groups in relation to motivation.

Social group. These youngsters are members of the same social group who indulge in occasional use as a social act of sharing. They pass around a bottle so that each youngster can take a drink or a marijuana cigarette so that each member can have a puff. The pleasant act of sharing reinforces membership in the group, sets them apart from adults, and provides them with an atmosphere of doing something against the rules—something that is fun to get away with. With most youths drug use is a passing fancy and after a few times is dispensed with and forgotten.

Escapist group. The majority of youths who experiment with drugs are seeking escape from feelings of anger and depression when they are unable to communicate effectively with their parents concerning their problems or to cope with their emotions. Getting drunk or "freaking out" seems to work for them. Unfortunately, this flight not only leaves the problems unsolved, but also interferes with the satisfactory resolution of the problems. Consequently, the retreat into use of drugs tends to be repeated.

Punitive group. This smaller group of adolescents seem determined to punish the world for making them angry, depressed, or frustrated. Although they use, sell, and/or push drugs, they do so in the hope that they will be discovered and arrested so that their families will suffer the anguish that the youngsters themselves feel.

Self-destructive group. A few youths are openly self-destructive individuals who internalize their anger to the extent that death seems to provide the only relief from their anger. These youngsters often give evidence of suicidal thoughts or demonstrate suicidal behavior.

Types of Drugs Abused

Any drug can be abused, and most are potentially harmful to adolescents still going through formative life experiences. Although rarely considered drugs by society, the chemically active substances most frequently abused are the xanthines and theobromines contained in chocolate and in common beverages such as tea, coffee, and colas. Common analgesics (e.g., Darvon Compound, Fiorinal), ethyl alcohol, and nicotine are others that, although recognized as drugs, are sanctioned by society. Any of these can produce mild to moderate euphoric and/or stimulant effects and can lead to physical and psychic dependence.

A great many factors determine personal preferences for gratification. Many drugs are not harmful for all teenagers, and some, used intermittently, will probably not produce ill effects or result in dependence. Reactions vary according to the drug used and its purity, the expectations of the user, and the context in which the drug is used. These factors determine to a great extent whether the experience is viewed

Table 21-5 Major drugs abused by adolescents

CHEMICAL AGENT/ROUTE	PHYSICAL SIGNS	BEHAVIOR	COMPLICATIONS
Opiates			
Heroin, morphine, methadone—injected subcutaneously or intravenously (IV), intranasal (sniffing), oral	Constricted pupils, respiratory depression, cyanosis Needle marks	Initial euphoria, tranquilization, lethargy, coma	Overdose: coma, respiratory arrest, death Injection site infection, hepatitis, abscesses, septicemia, tetanus, pulmonary complications Withdrawal: muscle cramps, stomach cramps, diarrhea, runny nose and eyes, restlessness, convulsions, death Dental caries
Depressants			
Barbiturates—secobarbital, amobarbital, pentobarbital, amobarbital/secobarbital—oral, IV	Slurred speech, ataxia, slowed reflexes, constricted pupils (barbiturates); dilated pupils (glutethimide)	Short attention span, impaired judgment, combativeness, violence	Overdose: respiratory depression, coma, death Injection site infection, hepatitis, septicemia Withdrawal: hyperreflexia, irritability, convulsions, death
Nonbarbiturates—methaqualone (Quaalude), ethchlorvynol (Placidyl)—oral	Incoordination, tremors, ataxia, confusion, slurred speech, hyperreflexia, diplopia, general muscle weakness	Hyperexcitability; euphoria of methaqualone similar to opiate experience	Overdose: delirium and coma, convulsions, hepatic damage, respiratory arrest, death Withdrawal: similar to barbiturates and alcohol
Alcohol (ethanol)—oral	Incoordination	Impaired judgment and perception, loss of inhibitions, emotional lability, quarrelsomeness, aggressiveness, hostility Lethargy	Hazards related to impaired judgment, e.g., automobile accidents, fights Nutritional deficiencies Gastritis Overdose: coma, death, especially when used in combination with barbiturates Withdrawal: anxiety, tremors, hallucinations, hyperreflexia, convulsions, death
Minor tranquilizers			
Chlordiazepoxide (Librium), diazepam (Valium), meprobamate—oral	Nonspecific	Decreased anxiety and tension Occasional disinhibition	Similar to barbiturates but with reduced intensity
Organic solvents			
Hydrocarbons and fluorocarbons—glue, cleaning fluid, lighter fluid, aerosol sprays, nail polish, gasoline—sniffed	Nonspecific	Euphoria, dysphoria, confusion, impaired perception and coordination Loss of consciousness	Secondary trauma, asphyxia from plastic bags used to inhale fumes Lead poisoning Possible irreversible damage to central nervous system, kidneys, liver, and bone marrow
Stimulants			
Amphetamines—amphetamine sulfate, dextroamphetamine, methamphetamine—oral, subcutaneous, IV	Hypertension, weight loss, dilated pupils Sweating (when injected)	Psychologic and motor stimulation Hyperactivity, false bravado, euphoria, increased alertness, insomnia, anorexia, irritability, personality change	Injection site infection Paranoia, severe depression with suicidal tendency when drug stopped

Table 21-5 Major drugs abused by adolescents—cont'd

CHEMICAL AGENT/ROUTE	PHYSICAL SIGNS	BEHAVIOR	COMPLICATIONS
Cocaine—intranasal, IV, smoke	Hypertension, tachycardia, hyperreflexia	Restlessness, hyperactivity, intense euphoria	Nausea and vomiting, inflammation or perforation of nasal septum
▪ Hallucinogens			
Cannabis—marijuana, hashish—smoke, oral	Occasionally tachycardia, delayed response time, poor coordination	Simple euphoria, mild intoxication, heightened sensory awareness, drowsiness	Occasionally depressive or anxiety reactions
LSD, PCP, DMT, STP, THC, mescaline—oral	Dilated pupils, reddened eyes, occasionally hypertension, hyperthermia, piloerection	Euphoria, heightened sensory awareness, increased appetite, hallucinations, confusion, paranoia	Primarily psychiatric: may intensify latent psychotic tendencies, panic, suicide possible, flashbacks

as pleasant or unpleasant. The type of drugs used also varies according to geographic location, socioeconomic status, urban as opposed to suburban areas, and various times.

A drug that is popular with one "generation" of adolescents may not be attractive to another, and changing trends are influenced by the adolescent's constant search for new and different experiences. The present concern is the use of alcohol, tobacco, and cocaine.

Drugs with mind-altering capacity that are available on the black market and that are of medical and legal concern are the hallucinogenic, narcotic, hypnotic, and stimulant drugs. In addition, health professionals are concerned about use of various volatile substances, such as antifreeze, plastic model airplane cement, organic solvents, and typewriter correction fluid, that are inhaled to achieve altered sensation in the user. Drugs available on the street are often mixed with other compounds and fillers so that the purity of the drug, its strength, and the nature of additives are highly variable. Many of the hazards associated with drug use are related to driving a car or operating equipment that may be harmful when carelessly used while under the influence of the drug. Some of the more commonly abused substances and their general manifestations are outlined in Table 21-5.

Alcohol. Acute or chronic abuse of ethanol, a socially accepted depressant, is responsible for many acts of violence, suicide, and accidental injury and death. Ethanol reduces inhibitions against aggressive and sexual acting out. Abrupt withdrawal is accompanied by severe physical and psychologic symptoms, and long-term use leads to slow tissue destruction, especially of the brain and liver cells.

Teenage drinking is not a new phenomenon, but because of its social acceptance, peer pressure, and easy accessibility, alcohol appears to have become the drug of choice. It is the most widely accepted drug, can be purchased legally by adults, is relatively inexpensive, is often used as part of a meal (wine, beer), and is approved by adults throughout the world when used in moderation. Youngsters may be afraid of hard drugs, but they feel comfortable with alcohol. Most have been exposed to alcohol all their lives.

The pattern of frequent, heavy drinking often begins in the eighth grade, increases with age, and peaks between the ages of 18 and 22 years (O'Malley, Bachman, and Johnston, 1984). Some surveys indicate that 11% of eighth graders report consuming the equivalent of 5.6 oz of absolute alcohol per week, and twelfth grade students admitted to averaging two six-packs of beer per week, often consumed at one or two parties (reported by Schwartz and others, 1986). The majority of youngsters in one study reported high self-esteem, good health, and few psychologic problems, and 63% reported having drunk alcohol at some time. The proportion of youngsters stating that they never drank alcohol becomes progressively smaller with age (Schwartz and others, 1986).

The most noticeable effects of alcohol are on the central nervous system; these include changes in emotional and autonomic functions, such as judgment, memory, learning ability, and other intellectual capacities. Marked mood changes are characteristic of adolescent drinkers, who are described as hard to live with, unable to make up their minds, and acting like persons with split personalities. They can be identified by the way in which they use alcohol. Adolescent alcoholics enjoy the effect of the alcohol and look forward to becoming intoxicated. They drink rapidly to obtain a "high" emotional state, often drink alone, cannot predictably control their use of alcohol, and protect their supply, afraid that they will be caught without anything to drink.

Teenage alcoholics rely on alcohol as a defense against depression, anxiety, fear, and anger. They become increasingly tolerant to the drug, and there is an increased use of sedatives with the alcohol. Some alcoholics have difficulty remembering things done while intoxicated and often intend to swear off the drug or cut down on its use. Not all of these characteristics are observed in the alcoholic, but if several of the signs are evident, the youngster should be considered at risk and detoxification therapy should be initiated to ensure safe and complete withdrawal from the drug. Information about alcohol and answers to questions can be obtained by calling the **Alcohol Hotline.***

Cocaine. Cocaine is the most potent antifatigue agent known, and although it is not a narcotic, it is legally categorized as such. Cocaine is available in two forms: water-soluble cocaine hydrocholoride administered by insufflation or "snorting" and a nonsoluble alkaloid (freebase) used primarily for smoking. "Crack" or "rock" is a newer, purer, and more menacing form of the drug; it can be produced cheaply and smoked in either water pipes or mentholated cigarettes. The increased use of cocaine is related to its availability and affordability, the false perception of safety in its use, its association with persons in glamorous occupations, its snob appeal, its reputation as a sexually enhancing drug, and peer pressure (Tarr and Macklin, 1987).

Cocaine creates a sense of euphoria, or an indefinable high. Withdrawal does not produce the dramatic symptoms observed in withdrawal from other substances. The effects are those more commonly seen in depression, including lack of energy and motivation, irritability, appetite changes, psychomotor retardation, and irregular sleep patterns. More serious symptoms include cardiovascular manifestations and seizures. Withdrawal is not to be confused with the so-called crash after a cocaine high, which consists of a long period of sleep. Answers to questions about health risks of cocaine can be obtained by calling the **National Cocaine Hotline.*** It also provides referrals to support groups and treatment centers.

Narcotics. Narcotic drugs include opiates such as heroin, morphine, meperidine hydrochloride (Demerol), and codeine. They produce a state of euphoria by removing painful feelings and creating a pleasurable experience of a specific quality and a sense of success accompanied by clouding of consciousness and a dreamlike state. Physical signs of narcotic abuse include constricted pupils, respiratory depression, and, often, cyanosis. Needle marks may be visible on arms or legs in chronic users. Withdrawal from opiates is extremely unpleasant unless controlled with supervised substitution of methadone.

Perhaps more important are the indirect consequences related to the illegal status of narcotic use and the problems associated with securing the drug—time-consuming searches and methods used to meet the high cost. Health problems result from self-neglect of physical needs (nutrition, cleanliness, dental care), overdose, contamination, and infection, including acquired immune deficiency syndrome (AIDS) and hepatitis.

Central nervous system depressants. A variety of hypnotic drugs that produce physical dependence and withdrawal symptoms on abrupt discontinuation may be used by adolescents. They create a feeling of relaxation and sleepiness but impair general functioning. Drugs in this category include barbiturates and nonbarbiturates (e.g., methaqualone [Quaalude]), as well as alcohol. Barbiturates combined with alcohol produce a profound depressant effect.

Central nervous system stimulants. Amphetamines and cocaine do not produce strong physical dependence and can be withdrawn without much danger. However, psychologic dependence is strong, and acute intoxication can lead to violent aggressive behavior or psychotic episodes manifest by paranoia, uncontrollable agitation, and restlessness. When combined with barbiturates, the euphoric effects are particularly addictive.

Methamphetamine is gradually assuming an important place in drug abuse. The drug can be snorted, injected, swallowed, or smoked and produces a burst of energy in its users, along with intense, alternating attacks of boldness and paranoia. It provokes excitement far more intense than that caused by crack and cocaine. The drug, with the street names "crank," "meth," and "crystal," is inexpensive and has a longer period of action than cocaine. Instead of a short (few minutes) high, as achieved with crack, a user can remain "up" for hours on a similar dose of crank. Authorities fear that this drug may become the next popular substance of abuse.

Hydrocarbons and fluorocarbons. Glue "sniffing" and the inhalation of plastic cement, typewriter correction fluid, and other volatile substances (e.g., gasoline, gold and silver spray paint) that youngsters breathe directly or place in paper or plastic bags from which they rebreathe the fumes produce an immediate euphoria and altered consciousness. The substances are extremely hazardous to the individual, causing rapid loss of consciousness and respiratory arrest. Many persons taking these drugs do not have time to remove the bag from their heads and quickly become asphyxiated.

Mind-altering drugs. Hallucinogens (psychedelic, psychotomimetic, psychotropic, or illusionogenic) are drugs that produce vivid hallucinations and euphoria. These drugs do not produce physical dependence, since they can be abruptly withdrawn without ill effect. However, acute and long-term effects are variable, and in some individuals the dissociative behavior may be unduly protracted. This category includes cannabis (marijuana, hashish) and lysergic acid diethylamide (LSD).

Terminology. Drug users have developed a specialized vocabulary for the abused substances (Box 21-10). The terminology varies in different localities, and new descriptive terms arise spontaneously wherever drugs are part of the environment.

Therapeutic Management

Adolescents experiencing toxic drug effects or withdrawal symptoms are frequently seen in emergency rooms. Experienced emergency room personnel are familiar with the management of acute drug toxicosis; the signs, symptoms, and behavioral characteristics of a variety of substances; and differences and similarities among them. When the drug is questionable or unknown, knowledge of these factors facilitates handling of the youngster and implementation of a treatment regimen.

The treatment for drug toxicity or withdrawal varies according to the drug and the method used. Every effort should be made to determine the type and amount of drug

*(800) ALCOHOL.

*(800) COCAINE.

Box 21-10 GLOSSARY OF DRUG JARGON

Amphetamines

Bams
Beans
Benn
Bennies
Black beauties
Black cadillacs
Black dex
Bombido (injectable)
Browns
Cartwheels
Chalk
Co-pilots
Cranks
Cross
Crystal
Dexies
Dice
Doe
Drives
Eyeopeners
Fives (5 mg)
Footballs
Goofballs
Green hearts
Greenies
Greens
Heart(s)
Horse hearts
Jolly babies
Leapers
Lid rollers
Lightning
Meth
Orange hearts
Peaches
Pep pills
Rippers
Roses
Speed
Splash
Thrusters
Truck drivers
Wake-up
White crosses
White dexies
Whites
Yellow bams
Zeeters
Zip

Barbiturates (General)

Barbs
Courage pills
Downers
Golf balls
Goofers
Idiot pills
Nimbie
Nimbles
Peanuts
Sleepers

Barbiturates (Specific)

Blue birds (amobarbital)
Blue devils (amobarbital)
Blue heaven (amobarbital)
Canary (pentobarbital)
Christmas trees (mixtures)
Downers (amobarbital)
F-40s (secobarbital)
F-66s (amobarbital sodium and secobarbital sodium) (gorilla pills)
Mexican yellows (pentobarbital)
Nemmies (pentobarbital)
Phennies
Pink ladies (secobarbital)
Pinks (secobarbital)
Rainbow (secobarbital; amobarbital)
Red birds (secobarbital)
Red devils (secobarbital)
Reds (secobarbital)
Seggy, seccy (secobarbital)
Tooies (tuinal)
Yellow jackets (pentobarbital)
Yellows (pentobarbital)

Cocaine

Bernies flake
C
Candy
Cecil
Charlie
Coca-cola
Coke
Cokomo (Kokomo)
Crack
Dust
Flake
Gift of the Sun God
Gold dust
Happy trails
Incentive
Lady snow
Leaf (the)
Movie star drug
Nose
Nose candy
Pimp
Pimp's drug
Rich man's drug
Rock
Schoolboy
Snow
Society high
Star-spangled powder
Stardust
White horse
White stuff

Heroin

Big Harry
Blanco
Boy
Caballo
Chiva
Deuce (a $2 packet)
Doojee
Dust
H
Harry; hairy
Horse
Joy powder
Scag
Scat
Smack
Stuff
Sugar
Ticata
White lady
White stuff

Morphine

Dreamer
Dust
Emma (Miss)
Emsel
Hard stuff
Hocus
M
Monkey
Morf
Morpho
Unkie
White stuff

Marijuana

Acapulco gold (potent)
Bush
Butter
Flower
Grass
Griffo
Hemp
Hooch
Hooter
Indian hay
J
Jive
Joint
Kif
Mary Jane
Mohasky
Mooters
Mu
Mutah
Panama red
Pot
Reefer (cigarette)
Rockets
Smoke
Splimi
Stick (cigarette)
Straw
Superjoint
Texas tea
Tie stick (mixed with opium and tied to a popsicle stick)
Weed

LSD (Lysergic Acid Diethylamide)

Acid
Blotter acid (on paper)
Blue microdot
Cube (the)
D (big)
Heavenly blue
Purple haze
Royal blue
Sugar
Wedding bells
Windowpane

PCP (Phencyclidine)

Angel dust
Busy bee
DOA
Elephant
Goon
Hog (also chloral hydrate)
Horse tranquilizer
Magic mist
Peace pills
Rocket fuel
Sherman's
White horizon
Wobble

Other Hallucinogens

DMT (dimethyltryptamine): businessman's special
DMZ (Benactyzine)
DOM (4-methyl-2,5-dimethoxyamphetamine), STP
Hashish: black hash; black Russian (potent)
STP (dimethoxymethylamphetamine), DOM (syndicate acid, tranquility)
THC (tetrahydrocannabinol): hallucinogen in marijuana and hashish

Mixed Substances

Chicago green (marijuana/opium)
Double trouble (amobarbital/secobarbital)
Fours (acetaminophen with 60 mg codeine)
Fuel (marijuana/insecticide)
Hog (phencyclidine/vegetable material [veterinary drug])
In-betweens (barbiturates/amphetamines)
Mickey Finn (chloral hydrate/alcohol)
Speedball (heroin/cocaine; Percodan/methedrine)
Star-spangled powder (heroin/cocaine)

Miscellaneous

Alcohol: mountain dew, alley juice (methyl alcohol) moonshine (ethyl alcohol), sauce, hootch, booze, juice
Amyl nitrite: aimes, snappers
Chloral hydrate: joy juice
Ethchlorvynol (Placidyl): dyls, plastic red, K-H, K-N
Meperidine hydrochloride: Diane
Mescaline: chief, mesc, mescalito, mescal beans
Methadone: dolls, dollies fizzies (tablets)
Methaqualone (Quaalude): 714, ludes, sopors, westcoast, lemons
Opium for smoking: black stuff
Paregoric: licorice, bitter
Peyote: button, cactus, Hikori, Kikuli, Huatari, Wokouri, seni, tops
Tobacco: coffin, deck (pack), fag

taken, the time it was taken, the mode of administration, and factors related to the onset of presenting symptoms.

It is helpful to know the patient's pattern of use. For example, if two types of drugs are involved, they may require different treatments. Gastric lavage may be employed when the drug has been ingested recently and the cough reflex is intact, but it would be of little value when the drug has been administered by the intravenous ("mainlined") or intranasal ("sniffed") route. Since the actual content of most street drugs is highly questionable, other pharmaceutical agents are administered with caution, except perhaps the narcotic antagonists in cases of suspected opiate overdose. It is necessary to assess for possible trauma sustained while the patient was under the influence of the drug.

Rehabilitation from hard drug use may require withdrawing the youngster from the environment, as well as from the chemical agent. Programs must be suited to the individual and may involve foster home placement or a residential treatment setting, although many youngsters are handled in an ambulatory setting. Programs often include group sessions with other troubled adolescents. Information regarding help can be obtained from the **National Institute on Drug Abuse (NIDA)** hotline.*

Nursing Considerations

Nurses in almost every setting are increasingly likely to have contact with youthful drug abusers or to be in a position to serve as educator and patient advocate. They are often in a position to serve as listener, confidant, and counselor to troubled youngsters. Nurses are essential members of health teams whose efforts are directed toward short-term and long-term therapy for drug abusers.

Often observation or a description of the behavior is more valuable than a report by patients or their friends as to the chemical agent taken (see Box 21-11 for diagnostic criteria). For example, aggressive behavior and disorientation are often seen in barbiturate, alcohol, stimulant, or hallucinogen intoxication but not in opiate intoxication. Overdose from either barbiturates or opiates can result in respiratory failure and coma. Pinpoint pupils are seen only in opiate toxicity. Nurses must be alert for life-threatening consequences of drug toxicity; therefore equipment and personnel should be available or the patient should be transferred to facilities that are prepared to provide supportive measures for physiologic depression and psychogenic phenomena.

Stimulation should be kept to a minimum for agitated, frightened youngsters. Treatment or tests that are not required immediately are best postponed. These youngsters primarily need psychologic support in a nonthreatening environment and close contact with a sympathetic person who can stay with them and help them maintain contact with reality.

Obstetric and nursery personnel sometimes encounter the problem of drug dependence and withdrawal in newborn infants or in a compulsive drug-using mother. Affected infants are at risk and require special surveillance for complications of withdrawal; therefore the nursing staff should be aware of the drug dependence in those mothers who come to the hospital for delivery (see Chapter 10).

Long-term management. A major factor in the treatment and rehabilitation of young drug users is careful assessment, in the nonacute stage, to determine the function that the drug plays in these youngsters' lives. Adolescents need help to identify the problem that motivated them to resort to drugs and to recognize their own role in self-destructive, inappropriate drug-abuse behavior before they can embark on a rehabilitation program.

The motivation phase of treatment is directed toward exploring the factors that influence drug use and establishing in the youngster a feeling of self-worth and a commitment to self-help. It requires a trust relationship between the youngster and the health team and involves a thorough physical examination and assessment of physical, psychologic, educational, and vocational status. A realistic appraisal of the adolescent's potential and efforts aimed at short-term goal satisfaction along with building self-esteem lay the groundwork for a successful rehabilitation program.

Rehabilitation begins when youngsters decide that with the help of concerned and supportive adults, they can and are willing to change. Rehabilitation implies not only environmental manipulation and involvement therapy, but also commitment on the part of the patient to substitute dependency on people for dependency on drugs and to explore alternative mechanisms for problem solving and coping with stress. Persons working with troubled youths must be

*(800) 662-HELP.

Box 21-11 DIAGNOSTIC CRITERIA FOR PSYCHOACTIVE SUBSTANCE DEPENDENCE

Any person with a psychoactive substance abuse disorder will be diagnosed as "dependent" if any three of the following criteria are met:

1. Frequent preoccupation with, seeking, or taking the substance
2. Frequent use in larger amounts or over a longer period than intended
3. Need for increased amounts of the substance to achieve intoxication or desired effect, or diminished effect with continued use of the same amount
4. Display of characteristic withdrawal symptoms
5. Frequent use of the substance to relieve or avoid withdrawal symptoms
6. Persistent desire or repeated efforts to cut down or control substance use
7. Frequent intoxication or impairment from substance use when expected to fulfill social or occupational obligations, or when substance use is hazardous (e.g., driving when drunk)
8. Relinquishment of some important social, occupational, or recreational activity to seek or take the substance
9. Continuation of substance use despite a significant social, occupational, or legal problem, or a physical disorder that the person knows is exacerbated by the use of the substance

Modified from American Psychiatric Association: Diagnostic and statistical manual of mental disorders, ed. 3 (DSM-III-R), Washington, DC, 1987, The Association.

prepared for recidivism, or the tendency to relapse, and maintain a plan for reentry into the treatment process.

Organizations that have achieved success in helping others cope with problems of drug abuse are excellent sources for both youngsters and their families. The **Toughlove*** philosophy first employed by Alcoholics Anonymous and Al-Anon is based on the conviction that parents have the right and the responsibility to be the policymakers in the family, set limits on the behavior of their children, and take control of the household from out-of-control teenagers. The premise is that allowing teenagers to experience the negative consequences of their behavior will bring them closer to accepting help and/or changing their behavior (Newton, 1985). Parents no longer take responsibility for the youngsters' behavior and suffer the negative consequences. Adolescents are offered the choice of (1) getting treatment for mental health or their drug problem or (2) finding another place to live. It is difficult for parents, and some older youngsters do leave home, but most return when they have rethought their decision after experiencing the real world.

Other groups that provide support and counseling for families experiencing crises with their children include **Parents Anonymous†** and **Parental Stress, Inc.,‡** both of which maintain crisis counseling on a 24-hour basis.

Prevention. Drug abuse in adolescence is both an individual and a community problem, and nurses play an important role in education and legislation, as well as in individual observation, assessment, and therapy. In this drug-oriented society patterns of drug use may be established, through parental models and the influence of the media, as an effective means to make the user "feel better." Impressionable youths need to be educated regarding appropriate use of chemicals. More important, those associated with adolescents should listen to what they are saying, determine what is bothering them, and try to help them meet these needs before they resort to drugs.

Researchers have observed that high levels of parental support and nurturance are associated with the lowest average number of alcohol problems, illicit drug use, and deviant acts. Therefore "working with families to develop better parenting skills relevant to nurturance and control can have long-term benefits for adolescents, their families, and society at large" (Barnes and Windle, 1987).

SUICIDE

The problem of suicide is worldwide and increasing in many countries. A striking feature is the rise among persons in the younger age-groups. It is the second leading cause of death among persons ages 15 to 24 years in the United States (Brent and others, 1988), claiming more than 6000 youths annually (National Center for Health Statistics, 1986). There are 50 to 220 suicide attempts for every completion (Shaw, Sheehan, and Fernandez, 1987).

Suicide is defined as the deliberate act of self-injury with the intent that the injury should kill. Most authorities distinguish between a suicidal ideation, gesture, and attempt, and all three must be acknowledged. Suicidal *ideation* is thoughts about or plans for suicide. A *gesture* is made without any real attempt to cause either serious injury or death but rather to send out a signal that something is wrong. An *attempt,* unlike a gesture, is intended to cause injury or death. Teenagers sometimes make a number of gestures to draw attention to the fact that they are unable to cope. If the signals are not detected and responded to promptly, they may escalate in seriousness until they become serious attempts or completed acts. Another category, an *impulsive act,* describes a rage response designed to punish or manipulate a loved person perceived as withdrawing that love (Hofmann, 1983). Moreover, many experts believe that numerous "accidental" deaths are actually suicides (Eisenberg, 1984).

Incidence

The true incidence of suicide in children and adolescents is not known because of general underreporting. Frequently deaths by suicide are reported as accidental because of pressures exerted by family and society to avoid the cultural and religious stigma associated with self-destruction. There also appears to be some degree of certainty that the high accident rate in persons in this age-group may reflect suicides masked by accidental death or homicide.

There are some differences in suicides in relation to ethnic and racial factors. There is a lower incidence of suicide in Asians and Jews, and although older blacks have a lower incidence, the suicide rate for black teenagers is rapidly approaching that for whites (Maris, 1985). Girls make suicidal gestures or attempts four to eight times more often than boys and account for 90% of suicide attempts, whereas boys account for 70% of successful suicides (Raley, 1985). Gestures are made at home when someone else is nearby, usually in the evening or afternoon. Depression is the most frequent diagnosis and occurs in 35% to 79% of all those who attempt suicide (Friedman and others, 1984).

Etiology

The reasons youngsters attempt suicide are numerous and varied. Some contributing factors include the changing times, especially within families. There is an increase in two-career families and more separation and divorce, which make youngsters feel more vulnerable and decrease feelings of stability. The young people of today are faced with an increasingly competitive society that encourages them to have high expectations for themselves and fosters a fear of failure that makes them feel highly pressured.

Developmental factors. Adolescence has always been characterized by turmoil, heightened emotionality, and wide variations in mood. Youngsters display moods

*P.O. Box 1069, Doylestown, PA 18901; (215) 348-7090.

†22330 Hawthorne Blvd., #208, Torrance, CA 90505; (800) 352-0386 (California) and (800) 421-0353 (elsewhere).

‡(617) 742-7535 (Massachusetts) and (800) 632-8188 (elsewhere). Other sources of information include **National Clearinghouse for Alcohol and Drug Abuse Information,** P.O. Box 2345, Rockville, MD 20852, (800) 729-6686; **National Federation of Parents for Drug-Free Youth,** (800) 554-KIDS or (301) 585-5437 (Maryland); and **National Institute on Drug Abuse Prevention Branch,** (800) 638-2045 or (301) 443-2450 (Maryland).

that range from the depths of depression to the heights of elation. It is sometimes difficult to determine whether a youngster is exhibiting a normal mood swing or is at risk for true depression and suicide. No period in life is fraught with such major changes, and teenagers have limited ability to understand these changes. With limited capacities for problem solving and with fewer and less sophisticated resources for resolving difficulties, they may resort to methods of handling problems that were acquired at an earlier age. It often appears to adults that adolescents "overreact" to situations. Actually, they experience emotions and react to events more intensely than adults.

Some teenagers have difficulty coping well with critical events, especially a situation that is forced on them, such as the death of a friend, parent, or sibling. Studies have found that suicidal children experienced increasing and significantly greater amounts of stress as they matured, including a number of specific chaotic and disruptive family events that resulted in losses and separations from important people. Most adolescents can function quite well, but when health professionals see those who do not, further investigation is indicated.

A surprising number of children 5 to 9 years of age commit or attempt to commit suicide. This behavior is often wrongly assumed to be accidental. Children in this age-group are unable to think in abstract terms and therefore do not comprehend the permanence and irreversibility of death. Immature adolescents with poor ego development tend to react impulsively to situations much as they did at a younger age. Turning aggression inward in stressful situations, they seek to avoid discomfort, join a lost object, or gain love.

Family factors. Suicidal youngsters almost invariably come from a disturbed family situation, such as one experiencing economic stress, family disintegration, medical problems, or psychiatric illness. Broken homes, divorce, separation, abandonment, alcoholism, and death are highly significant factors and are frequently noted in the histories of suicidal youth. In instances in which the family is intact, the disorganization is manifested by marital discord, lack of or disturbed communication, abnormal patterns of interaction, physical aggression, and general lack of unity and solidarity within the family system. Often there is a history of a suicide by another family member.

Parents are often inadequate and unable to cope. There is usually a lack or loss of communication links with the parents. Sometimes there is hostility, indifference, or overt rejection by one or both parents. There may be extreme parental control. Younger children who are treated badly at home react with rebellious behavior and may commit suicide for fear of punishment. Parents may set impossibly high expectations for the youngster, or there may be parental indifference with very low expectations. There is often a lack of parental supportive response to the child's problems. Parents have a low understanding of the child and have not noticed the behavior changes displayed by the suicidal youngster. If families seek help immediately after a suicide attempt, there is less possibility of a repeat attempt. If they are negative and apathetic, there is a greater risk of another, more lethal attempt.

Psychoses. When evaluating youngsters for therapy, it is important to rule out those with affective disorders, especially borderline and character disorders. Many of these youngsters exhibit self-destructive behavior, such as scratching at their wrists, that is not likely to succeed as a lethal method. It is manipulative behavior and a bid for attention; although these youngsters may talk about suicide dramatically, they rarely want to kill themselves. Most manipulative behaviors are managed by ignoring the behavior, but these youngsters may inadvertently do severe damage as their manipulative behavior increases. There are also those who are psychotic and who may be hearing voices that tell them to kill themselves.

Suicidal Methods

The outcome of suicidal behavior is influenced to some extent by the method used. Violent methods of destruction, such as jumping from heights or in front of trains, which are used by adults, are less frequently employed by younger persons. Overdose of drugs is the method of choice for most adolescents who attempt suicide, and these are usually medications prescribed for parents, such as barbiturates and antidepressants, those intended for household use (such as aspirin), or solvents. Youngsters do not have the sophistication to know the lethality of most drugs. They tend to use drugs that are available.

Ingesting pills and wrist lacerations are the favored methods of females; males tend to use more lethal methods such as knives, guns, cars, and jumping from heights (Hofmann, 1983). Younger children (under 13½ years) are more likely to resort to hanging (Garfinkel and others, 1982).

Sometimes an adolescent will threaten suicide in order to manipulate the environment. Unfortunately, with no self-destructive intent, a youngster may make a half-hearted attempt that leads to death or permanent injury. A "partial" or chronic suicide is illustrated by the adolescent with a chronic illness, such as diabetes, who refuses to comply with the prescribed medical regimen, the accident-prone adolescent, and the drug-abusing youngster. Risk factors for suicide are outlined in Box 21-12.

Motivation

Suicidal gestures are not uncommon among adolescents, and most are impulsive acts committed to force parents or other significant persons in their lives to pay attention to their need for help. The attempt usually is the culmination of a behavioral pattern. These youngsters often have a history of attention-getting behaviors that range from minor acts to increasingly dramatic ones. With the ultimate act of attempted suicide, the teenagers finally make themselves heard. They seldom actually plan a suicidal act because they really want to die; they want to be free from stress created by an intolerable situation. The attempt is made when there is someone around or when they know someone is coming home. These youngsters need someone to act in a controlling manner.

Box 21-12 RISK FACTORS FOR YOUTH SUICIDE

Past History
History of child abuse or neglect
Death of a parent when child was young (age 3 to 5 years)
Alcohol or substance abuse
Physical/body image problems (delayed puberty, chronic illness, disability)
Thinking disorder (wishes to join a deceased person; hears voices telling to kill self)
Chronic depression; rejects help
Previous suicide attempts
Past psychiatric hospitalization

Family Factors
Previous suicide attempts by family member(s)
Family history of suicide (parent or relative)
Depression
Difficult home situation—long, bitter, parent-child conflict
Hostile parents
Overt rejection by one or both parents; may be thrown out of home
Divorce or separation of parents
Recent or impending move
Exposure to unrealistically high expectations from parents
Parental indifference with very low expectations

Mood Affect
Marked persistent depression
Feelings of hopelessness, helplessness, isolation
Deteriorating schoolwork
Remains distant, sad, remote
Flat affect—has "frozen" facial expression
Persistently looks or sounds sad and unhappy
Describes self as worthless
Feelings of self-hatred or excessive guilt
Feelings of humiliation, often brought on by inadequate performance at school
Sudden cheerfulness following deep depression
Wish to be punished

Behavior
Changes in physical appearance—a child previously neat and well groomed will stop bathing and begin to look slovenly
Loss of function due to illness or trauma
Loss of energy—loss of interest, listlessness, exhaustion without obvious cause
Sleep disturbances—difficulty going to sleep or sleeping excessively; takes voluntary naps during afternoon or evening
Increased irritability, argumentativeness, or stubbornness
Physical complaints—recurrent stomachaches, headaches
Repeated visits to doctor's office or emergency room for treatment of injuries
Antisocial behavior—engages in drinking, uses drugs, fights, commits acts of vandalism, runs away from home, becomes sexually promiscuous
*Preoccupation with death—focuses on morbid thoughts; speaks repeatedly about people getting killed
May begin referring to own death

School and Interpersonal Relationships
Resists or refuses to go to school
May become truant, cut classes, does not complete assignments
Social withdrawal from friends, activities, interests that were previously enjoyed
*Wants to give away cherished possessions
Lacks an effective social support system

Precipitating Factors
Environmental change (friend moved away, relocated to new community or school)
Failure to achieve specific goals in school, job, personal life
Fight with close friend
Breakup of important relationship
Discovery of pregnancy plus family crisis and/or rejection by boyfriend
Death of a close friend, relative, or pet

Coping Skills
Loses reality boundaries
Withdraws and isolates self
No use of support systems
Sees self as totally helpless, a victim of fate

*Absolute red flags.

Suicidal ideation is not uncommon in adolescents. It represents numerous fantasies, such as relief from suffering, a means to gain comfort and sympathy, or a means of revenge against those who have hurt them. The youngsters have the erroneous perception that the act of suicide will evoke remorse and pity and that they will be able to return and witness the grief. They expect people to care and be concerned. A frequent motive for suicide in children and younger adolescents is the desire to punish others who will be grieved by their death. Angry children who are unable to punish directly those who have injured or insulted them will take revenge on those who love them through self-destruction ("They'll be sorry when they find me dead"; "They'll be sorry they were mean to me"). This motive is more common and more likely to persist longer in girls. This, of course, is faulty judgment on the part of those attempting suicide.

Occasionally there are adolescents who are so severely depressed that suicide appears to them to be the only means of release from their despair. These youngsters rarely give evidence of their intent, concealing their suicidal thoughts for fear of outside intervention. Sometimes this self-destructive behavior is a desire to punish themselves for guilt-filled actions, such as masturbation or, more often, thoughts. Peer pressure, too, has convinced many young persons that there is something wrong with them if they feel lonely or depressed; therefore they direct these feelings inward to avoid the risk of rejection.

Adolescents often respond to feelings of anger, failure, or loss with overt flight reactions. Some of these adaptive techniques are rebellion, withdrawal into the self with silence, physical withdrawal, such as running away from home, or, the most drastic of all, suicide. Social isolation is seen in many suicidal adolescents, but it appears to be the most significant factor in distinguishing those who will kill themselves from those who will not. It is more characteristic of those who complete suicides than of those who make attempts or threats.

Although suicide is often linked to a specific event, such as a family fight, an important school examination, the death of a teen idol, or the breakup of a youthful romance, that produced an impulsive response in the child, careful analysis will usually reveal an ongoing depressive process that has been expressed periodically and behaviorally. Teachers often report changes in the behavior of children who previously had not been behavior problems. They may become easily irritated, demonstrate a low frustration point, or exhibit clowning and active, restless behavior. Older children may begin using drugs and alcohol.

A cluster phenomenon, known as "contagion," has also been observed. Sometimes referred to as a teenage "epidemic," this situation occurs when one suicide appears to trigger several other suicides in a group such as a school or community (Davidson and others, 1989). Suicide of a public figure sometimes serves as a role model and prompts a number of suicides. This has also been termed the *Werther effect,* named for the fictional character who, in love with a girl who belonged to another, penned a farewell love note and shot himself (Phillips, 1985). In the story the act generated considerable sympathy and pity from acquaintances, including the lady love.

It has often been a general tendency to dismiss a suicide attempt as an impulsive act resulting from a temporary crisis or depression. If this drastic move fails to draw attention to their problems or makes them worse, adolescents may conclude that taking their lives is their only means to solve these escalating, unsolvable, and unbearable problems.

Depression

Depression is a symptom common to all human beings. It is a normal part of life, and even adolescents who are healthy and happy experience alternating periods of depression and elation as a part of the growth process. Depression is part of the breaking-away process. When adolescents break away from their parents, they need something or someone to belong to; belonging to a peer group is a way of coping. However, this and other coping mechanisms are often stretched to the utmost, and adolescents' heightened vulnerability to added stresses sometimes precipitates maladaptive behavior. The ego is under pressure to adapt to the physical changes and instinctual drives of puberty, whereas at the same time the expectations of the family and the environment for mature, independent, and responsible behavior must be met. Although some suicides occur in conjunction with a psychotic process, most frequently they are a part of the general picture of depression. When depression appears as a predominant mood, persists for a long time, or is so disabling that the adolescent is unable to fulfill the normal tasks of this period of life, the condition is serious and warrants special attention and intervention.

Depression is recognized by both subjective symptoms and objective signs that reflect adolescents' grief. Depressed persons describe feelings of sadness, despair, helplessness, hopelessness, boredom, loss of interest, and isolation. They may also feel self-reproach, self-deprecation, and guilt. These subjective symptoms are evidenced by changes in behavior and attitude.

Therapeutic Management

Suicidal threats should be taken very seriously. Most youngsters respond quickly to intervention. It offers them the opportunity to talk things out. Often the problems are very specific ones that environmental manipulation, such as a change of school or classroom or conferences with parents, can solve. Sometimes simply forming an attachment to a sympathetic, caring adult figure (therapist, nurse, or counselor) is sufficient. This attachment can be highly significant in helping children get through a crisis in the face of fear of rejection or anger from the family and feelings of guilt. They need to be made aware that suicide is a permanent solution to a temporary problem and that the problem will pass if they simply wait it out.

Children need to know that someone cares and must be provided with swift and efficient crisis intervention. Most larger communities have 24-hour service in the form of "hotlines"—telephone communication that is within reach of troubled youngsters or their families where they can make ready contact with someone who will listen to them. The function of the hotline is to help them through the immediate crisis. Through skillful questioning, but without imposing solutions on them, the listener helps callers arrive at a course of action that will contribute to a solution for their problems.

Children should be given no false reassurance, but it is essential to make it clear to them that their lives are considered of great importance and that they will be protected from doing themselves harm. Hospitalization, even if brief, is usually recommended. Youngsters need to be removed from the acute situation that troubles them and given the structure and security they need during the crisis period. They need someone to act in a controlling manner to alleviate the desire to die and encourage the wish to live. Hospitalization provides the surveillance that is impossible to accomplish in the home and reinforces the seriousness of a gesture or attempt. It is especially valuable if youngsters can be placed in a unit where other adolescents can offer warmth, support, and understanding.

Although an acute depressive reaction can be managed without difficulty by ordinary practitioners, the youngster who has made a serious attempt or has a plan for suicide should receive competent psychiatric care. Antidepressant medication is not usually recommended for acute depression but may be indicated for the youngster who is (1) chronically depressed and suicidal and (2) in an acute crisis situation, that is, when the child is admitted to the hospital for 2 to 3 weeks and is still very agitated and/or depressed. The medications take too long to achieve an antidepressant effect to be used for short-term therapy, and the potential for misuse is always a consideration.

Nursing Considerations

Care of the suicidal adolescent includes early recognition, management, and prevention. Probably the most important aspect of management is the recognition of prodromal signs that indicate that a youngster is troubled and might attempt suicide. Health professionals need to be alert to the signs of adolescent depression, and any youngster who exhibits such behavior, subtle or overt, should be referred for thorough psychologic assessment. Depression can be manifested in two different ways: youngsters who feel depressed may talk about suicide and feelings of worthlessness, or they may build themselves a solid defense against such intolerable feelings of depression with behavioral or psychosomatic disturbances.

NURSING ALERT No threat of suicide should be ignored or challenged in any way. It is a symptom that must be taken seriously. Too often suicidal threats or minor attempts are confused with bids for attention. It is also a mistake to be lulled into a false sense of security when the adolescent's depression is apparently relieved. The improvement in attitude may very well mean that the youngster has made the decision to carry out the threat.

Peers or other confidants are excellent sources of information and valuable observers. They may not be able to diagnose depression, but they are able to sense when a friend has undergone a marked personality change. It is important to emphasize that the peer who detects any clues in a friendship is a "potential rescuer" (Allen, 1986) and should not remain quiet about the observations. Friendship does not imply collusion. A peer who believes that a friend may be suicidal should alert someone who is in a position to help—a parent, teacher, guidance counselor, or other person.

As soon as the youngster who attempts suicide is out of danger from medical problems resulting from the attempt, the data-gathering process should begin. It should include information from several sources to help evaluate the extent to which the child is suffering, the direction for therapy, and the probability of a repeated attempt. At least 10% to 15% of those who attempt suicide ultimately *do* commit suicide, and at least 25% of those who commit suicide have made previous attempts (Adolescent in despair, 1985).

The youngster should be questioned directly about the depression or suicidal behavior—it should never be dismissed. Clues to a youngster's feelings may be elicited by questions such as, "You look so sad. What is troubling you?" or "Sometimes people feel life is no longer worth living. Have you had such thoughts?" Sometimes the youngster is relieved to know others have had similar thoughts. The important objective is to get the teenager to talk about thoughts and feelings. "Where do you see yourself 5 years from now?" may offer clues to future plans. "It's too bad you thought about dying. Have you made any plans?" "What did [do] you think would [will] happen to you as a result of taking the medications [or other means]?" and "When something is not going well, is there someone you can go to?" are questions that provide clues regarding the seriousness of the intent (Box 21-13).

Box 21-13 GUIDELINES FOR EVALUATING A SUICIDE GESTURE OR ATTEMPT

Social setting—determine what steps were taken to prevent rescue, if another person was present in the room or the house during the attempt, and if others were aware of the attempt either before or immediately after.
Intent—determine how detailed the suicidal plans were (if a suicide note or letter was written). Such communication often expresses the true depth of a youth's despair.
Method—examine the means selected and the youngster's understanding of the method (e.g., kind, number, and action of pills taken).
History—determine if the attempt was an isolated event and, if not, the number and nature of previous attempts or gestures. A family history of suicide is significant.
Stress—determine the nature of the precipitating event, the alternative courses of action available to the child, and previous methods of coping with stress.
Mental status—assess the present mental status of the youngster and compare it with preattempt status as described by others.
Support—evaluate the type of support that could be expected from the youngster's family, friends, peers, teachers, and others.

Not only is it important to treat the suicidal adolescent, but since the suicide attempt is frequently an outgrowth of family distress, it is essential to deal with the family as well. Ideally the most effective approach is recognition of susceptible youngsters during the early stages of intrafamily distress so that family counseling can be instigated. This emphasizes again the importance of parent-child relationships and the role of the nurse in assessing family interactions and recognizing disturbed relationships. Prevention efforts must be directed toward improving childrearing practices through support and education of parents and changing societal conditions that generate defeat, despair, and maladaptive behavior.

Follow-up care is of utmost importance. Although confidentiality is the usual approach with adolescent counseling, in the case of self-destructive behaviors this cannot be honored. The suicidal behavior is reported to the family and other professionals, and youngsters are informed that this will be done. They are told that the health professional cannot let the youngster do this! Such action conveys an important message to an attempter—that the professionals understand and that they care.

Some schools have instituted suicide-prevention programs. Most are designed for high school–age youth, but many are attempting to reach the younger ages, including elementary school children. Schools with programs in operation offer services such as drop-in counseling services and a peer counseling telephone line. Information can be obtained from the **American Association of Suicidology.*** The **Youth Suicide National Center†** provides information about local 24-hour crisis intervention centers.

*2459 S. Ash, Denver, CO 80222; (303) 692-0985.
†1825 I St., N.W., Washington, DC 20006; (202) 429-0190.

KEY POINTS

- The change, growth, and stress accompanying the transition to adulthood may predispose adolescents to faulty problem solving.
- The major eating disorders of adolescence are obesity, anorexia nervosa, and bulimia.
- Age of onset of obesity, presence of emotional disturbances or neuroses, and negative evaluation of obesity by others may all contribute to the development of a disturbed body image in the adolescent.
- Diet, exercise, and behavior modification are the hallmarks of treatment for obesity.
- The nurse's involvement in obesity control includes nutritional counseling, behavior modification, group programs, and family counseling.
- Anorexia nervosa, a disorder characterized by severe weight loss in the absence of obvious physical cause, consists of three areas of disordered psychologic functioning: disturbed body image and body concept of delusional proportions, inaccurate and confused perception and interpretation of inner stimuli, and paralyzing sense of ineffectiveness that pervades all aspects of daily life.
- Therapeutic management of anorexia involves reinstitution of normal nutrition, resolution of the disturbed patterns of family interaction, and individual psychotherapy to correct deficits and distortions in psychologic functioning.
- Bulimics fall into two categories: those who consume vast quantities of food followed by purging but who, if unable to purge, still consume large amounts and those who restrict their caloric intake, especially when unable to purge.
- Smoking is a widespread problem among teenagers; reasons for smoking include social pressure, mass media influence, and a need to develop a self-concept.
- Substance abuse is a severe problem in adolescence, and abusers include experimenters and compulsive users.
- Common types of drugs abused include alcohol, hydrocarbons and fluorocarbons, mind-altering drugs, narcotics, central nervous sytem depressants, and central nervous system stimulants.
- Suicide, the deliberate act of self-injury with the intent to kill, may occur in adolescents because of difficulties in coping with stress, disturbed family environment, and psychoses.

REFERENCES

The adolescent in despair, Emerg. Med. 17(9):51-66, 1985.

Allen, R.R.: Teen suicide prevention, Washington, DC, 1986, Teen Suicide Task Force.

American Academy of Pediatrics, Committee on Adolescence: The role of the pediatrician in substance abuse counseling, Pediatrics 72:251-252, 1983.

American Academy of Pediatrics, Committee on Environmental Hazards: Smokeless tobacco—a carcinogenic hazard, Pediatrics 76:1009-1011, 1985.

American Psychiatric Association: Diagnostic and statistical manual of mental disorders, ed. 3 (DSM-III-R), Washington, DC, 1987, The Association.

Attie, I., and Brooks-Gunn, J.: Development of eating problems in adolescent girls: a longitudinal study, Dev. Psychol. 25:70-77, 1989.

Barnes, G.M., and Windle, M.: Family factors in adolescent alcohol and drug abuse, Pediatrician 14:13-18, 1987.

Berkowitz, R.I., and others: Physical activity and adiposity: a longitudinal study from birth to childhood, J. Pediatr. 105:734-738, 1985.

Biglan, A., and others: A situational analysis of adolescent smoking, J. Behav. Med. 1:109-114, 1984.

Bragg, C., and Hughes, G.H.: Understanding and managing patients who smoke, Fam. Community Health 7:12-21, 1984.

Brent, D.A., and others: Risk factors for adolescent suicide, Arch. Gen. Psychiatry 45:581-588, 1988.

Brownell, K.D., Kelman, J.H., and Strunkard, A.J.: Treatment of obese children with and without their mothers: changes in weight and blood pressure, Pediatrics 71:515-523, 1983.

Bryce-Smith, D., and Simpson, R.I.D.: Case of anorexia nervosa responding to zinc sulfate (letter), Lancet 2:350, 1984.

Carino, C.M., and Chmelko, P.: Disorders of eating in adolescence: anorexia nervosa and bulimia, Nurs. Clin. North Am. 18:343-352, 1983.

Chassin, L., and others: Self-images and cigarette smoking in adolescence, Perspect. Soc. Psychol. Bull. 7:670-676, 1981.

Comerci, G.D.: Eating disorders in adolescents, Pediatr. Rev. 10:1-6, 1988.

Copeland, E.T., and Baucom-Copeland, S.: Childhood obesity: a family systems view, Am. Fam. Physician 24(8):153-155, 1981.

Davidson, L.E., and others: An epidemiologic study of risk factors in two teenage suicide clusters, JAMA 262:2687-2692, 1989.

Davis, R.M.: Current trends in cigarette advertising and marketing, N. Engl. J. Med. 316:725-732, 1987.

Dessendorfer, E.A., Amsterdam, E.A., and Odland, T.M.: Adolescent smoking and its effect on aerobic exercise tolerance, Phys. Sports Med. 11:109-119, 1983.

Dietz, W.H.: Prevention of childhood obesity, Pediatr. Clin. North Am. 33:823-833, 1986.

Eckert, P.: Beyond the statistics of adolescent smoking, Am. J. Public Health 73:439-441, 1983.

Eisenberg, L.: The epidemiology of suicide in adolescents, Pediatr. Ann. 13:47-54, 1984.

Epstein, L.H., and others: Effect of diet and controlled exercise on weight loss in obese children, J. Pediatr. 107:358-361, 1985.

Feldman, W., Feldman, E., and Goodman, J.T.: Culture versus biology: children's attitudes toward thinness and fatness, Pediatrics 81:190-194, 1988.

Flay, B.R., and others: Cigarette smoking: why young people do it and ways of preventing it. In McGrath, P.J., and Firestone, P.: Pediatric and adolescent behavioral medicine: issues in treatment, New York, 1983, Springer Publishing Co., Inc.

Fox, E.L., and Mathews, D.K.: The physiological basis of physical education and athletics, Philadelphia, 1981, W.B. Saunders Co.

Friedman, R.C., and others: Family history of illness in the seriously suicidal adolescent: a life-cycle approach, Am. J. Orthopsychiatry 54:390-397, 1984.

Garfinkel, B.D., and others: Suicide attempts in children and adolescents, Am. J. Psychiatry 129:1257-1261, 1982.

Goldsmith, M.F.: Increasing use of smokeless tobacco leads to fears of young lives being "snuffed out," JAMA 260:1511-1512, 1988.

Graves, T., Meyers, A.W., and Clark, L.: An evaluation of parental problem-solving training in the behavioral treatment of childhood obesity, J. Consult. Clin. Psychol. 56:245-250, 1988.

Greer, J.E.: Adolescent abuse of typewriter correction fluid, South. Med. J. 77:297-298, 1983.

Guggenheim, J., and others: Changing trends of tobacco use in a teenage population in Western Pennsylvania, Am. J. Publ. Health 76:196-197, 1986.

Herzog, D.B., and Copeland, P.M.: Eating disorders, N. Engl. J. Med. 313:295-299, 1985.

Hofmann, A.D., editor: Adolescent medicine, Menlo Park, CA, 1983, Addison-Wesley Publishing Co., Inc.

Huse, D.M., and others: The challenge of obesity in childhood. I. Incidence, prevalence, and staging, Mayo Clin. Proc. 57:279-284, 1982a.

Huse, D.M., and others: The challenge of obesity in childhood. II. Treatment guidelines by stage, Mayo Clin. Proc. 57:285-288, 1982b.

Joffe, A.: Too little, too much: eating disorders in adolescents, Contemp. Pediatr. 7(3):114-135, 1990.

Kaplan, K.M., and Wadden, T.A.: Childhood obesity and self-esteem, J. Pediatr. 109:367-370, 1986.

Kreipe, R.E., Churchill, B.H., and Strauss, J.: Long-term outcome of adolescents with anorexia nervosa, Am. J. Dis. Child. 143:1322-1327, 1989.

Lifshitz, F., and Moses, N.: Nutritional dwarfing: growth, dieting, and fear of obesity, J. Am. Coll. Nutr. 7:367-370, 1988.

Mallick, M.J.: Health hazards of obesity and weight control in children: a review of the literature, Am. J. Public Health 73:73-78, 1982.

Maloney, M.J., and others: Dieting behavior and eating attitudes in children, Pediatrics 84:482-489, 1989.

Maris, R.: The adolescent suicide problem, Suicide Life Threat. Behav. 15:91-109, 1985.

Marston, A.R., and others: Characteristics of adolescents at risk for compulsive overeating on a brief screening test, Adolescence 23:59-65, 1988.

Marty, P.J., and others: Patterns of smokeless tobacco use in a population of high school students, Am. J. Public Health 76:190-192, 1986.

Marwick, C.: Even "knowing better" about smoking, other health risks, may not deter adolescents, JAMA 260:1512-1513, 1988.

McAlister, A.L., Krosnick, J.A., and Milburn, M.A.: Causes of cigaret smoking: tests of a structural equation model, Soc. Psychol. Q. 47:24-36, 1984.

Morgan, M., and Grube, J.W.: Adolescent cigarette smoking: a developmental analysis of influences, Br. J. Dev. Psychol. 7:179-189, 1989.

Moses, N., Banilivy, M.M., and Lifshitz, F.: Fear of obesity among adolescent girls, Pediatrics 83:393-398, 1989.

National Center for Health Statistics: Annual summary of births, marriages, divorces and deaths: United States, 1985, Washington, DC, 1986, Department of Health, Education, and Welfare, Publication (PHS)86-1120.

Newcomb, M.D., McCarthy, W.J., and Bentler, P.M.: Cigarette smoking, academic lifestyle, and social impact efficacy: an eight year study from adolescence to young adulthood, J. Appl. Soc. Psychol. 19:251-281, 1989.

Newton, B.: Tough love: help for parents with troubled teenagers—reorganizing the hierarchy in disorganized families, Pediatrics 76:691-694, 1985.

O'Malley, P.M., Bachman, J.G., and Johnston, L.D.: Period, age, and cohort effects on substance abuse among American youth, 1976-1982, Am. J. Public Health 74:882-888, 1984.

Peterson, C.C., and Peterson, J.L.: Children and cigarettes: the effect of a model who quits, J. Appl. Dev. Psychol. 7:293-306, 1986.

Phillips, D.P.: The Werther effect, Sciences 25(4):33-39, 1985.

Pierce, J.P., and others: Trends in cigarette smoking in the United States, JAMA 261:61-65, 1989.

Pipes, P.L.: Nutrition in infancy and childhood, ed. 4, St. Louis, 1989, Mosby–Year Book, Inc.

Pugliese, M.T., and others: Fear of obesity: a cause of short stature and delayed puberty, N. Engl. J. Med. 309:513-518, 1983.

Raley, G.: Youth suicide: the federal response, Soc. Legis. Bull. 29:65-68, 1985.

School policies and programs on smoking and health—United States, 1988, MMWR 38:202-203, 1989.

Schwartz, R.H., and others: Drinking patterns and social consequences: a study of middle-class adolescents in two private pediatric practices, Pediatrics 77:139-143, 1986.

Shaw, K.R., Sheehan, K.H., and Fernandez, R.C.: Suicide in children and adolescents, Adv. Pediatr. 34:313-334, 1987.

Silvis, G.L., and Perry, C.L.: Understanding and deterring tobacco use among adolescents, Pediatr. Clin. North Am. 34:363-379, 1987.

Staff report on the cigarette advertising investigation: Federal Trade Commission, 1981.

State-specific estimates of smoking-attributable mortality and years of potential life lost—United States, 1985, MMWR 37:689-692, 1988.

Strunkard, A.J., and others: An adoption study of human obesity, N. Engl. J. Med. 314:193-198, 1986.

The surgeon general's 1989 report on reducing the health consequences of smoking: 25 years of progress, MMWR (suppl)38(S-2):1-30, 1989.

Taitz, L.S.: The obese child, Boston, 1983, Blackwell Scientific Publications, Inc.

Tarr, J.E., and Macklin, M.: Cocaine, Pediatr. Clin. North Am. 34:319-331, 1987.

Toner, B.B.: Long-term follow-up of anorexia nervosa, Psychosom. Med. 48:520-529, 1986.

U.S. Department of Health and Human Services: The health consequences of smoking for women: a report of the surgeon general, Washington, DC, 1980, U.S. Government Printing Office.

U.S. Public Health Service: Smoking and health: a report of the surgeon general, Washington, DC, 1979, Department of Health and Human Services.

Van Itallie, T.B.: Bad news and good news about obesity, N. Engl. J. Med. 314:239-240, 1986.

Williams, J.F., Friedman, I.M., and Steiner, H.: Hand lesions characteristic of bulimia, Am. J. Dis. Child. 140:28-29, 1986

Wong-McCarthy, W.J., and Gritz, E.R.: Preventing regular teenage cigarette smoking, Pediatr. Ann. 11:683-689, 1982.

BIBLIOGRAPHY

Obesity

Becque, M.D., and others: Coronary risk incidence of obese adolescents: reduction by exercise plus diet intervention, Pediatrics 81:605-612, 1988.

Bray, G.A.: Obesity: a blueprint for progress, Contemp. Nutr. 12(7), 1987.

Brownell, K.D., and others: School-based behavior modification, nutrition education and physical education program for obese children, Am. J. Clin. Nutr. 35:277-281, 1982.

Cecere, M.C.: PIP (Positive Image Program): a group approach for obese adolescents, Nurs. Clin. North Am. 18:249-256, 1983.

Castiglia, P.T.: Obesity in adolescence, J. Pediatr. Health Care 3:221-223, 1989.

Dietz, W.H., Jr.: Prevention of childhood obesity, Pediatr. Clin. North Am. 33:823-833, 1986.

Dietz, W.H., Jr.: The overweight child: psychosocial effects and treatment, Feelings 31(1):1-4, 1989.

Dietz, W.H., Jr., and Gortmaker, S.L.: Do we fatten our children at the television set? Obesity and television viewing in children and adolescents, Pediatrics 75:807-812, 1985.

Epstein, L.H., Wing, R.R., and Valoski, A.: Childhood obesity, Pediatr. Clin. North Am. 32:363-379, 1985.

Epstein, L.H., and others: Effects of weight loss on fitness in obese children, Am. J. Dis. Child. 137:654-657, 1983.

Franz, M.J.: Figuring fast food, Diabetes Forecast, pp. 49-54, Nov. 1987.

Hoerr, S.M.: An overlooked factor in adolescent obesity, Food Nutr. News 57:17-19, 1985.

Hoover, M.L.: The self-image of overweight adolescent females: a review of the literature, MCN 13:125-137, 1984.

Kaplan, K.M.: Obesity in children, Child Care Newsletter 5(2):1-3, 1986.

Klesges, R.C., and others: Accuracy of self-reports of food intake in obese and normal-weight individuals: effects of parental obesity on reports of children's dietary intake, Am. J. Clin. Nutr. 48:1252-1256, 1988.

Mahan, L.K.: Family-focused behavioral approach to weight control in children, Pediatr. Clin. North Am. 34:983-996, 1987.

Mellin, L.M.: Adolescent obesity, Contemp. Nutr. 12(8), 1987.

Mendelson, B.K., and White, D.R.: Development of self-body-esteem in overweight youngsters, Dev. Psychol. 21:90-96, 1985.

Mogan, J.: Prevention of childhood obesity, Issues Compr. Pediatr. Nurs. 9:33-38, 1986.

Moore, D.C.: Body image and eating behavior in adolescent boys, Am. J. Dis. Child. 144:475-479, 1990.

Poissonnet, C.M., LaVelle, M., and Burdi, A.R.: Growth and development of adipose tissue, J. Pediatr. 113:1-9, 1988.

Rocchini, A.P., and others: Blood pressure in obese adolescents: effect of weight loss, Pediatrics 82:16-23, 1988.

Rosenbaum, M., and Leibel, R.L.: Pathophysiology of childhood obesity, Adv. Pediatr. 35:73-138, 1988.

Silber, T., Randolph, J., and Robbins, S.: Long-term morbidity and mortality in morbidly obese adolescents after jejunoileal bypass, J. Pediatr. 108:318-322, 1986.

Wadden, T.A., and others: Obesity in black adolescent girls: a controlled clinical trial of treatment by diet, behavior modification, and parental support, Pediatrics 85:345-352, 1990.

Young, E.A., and others: Fast foods update, nutrient analyses, Feelings 29(4):15-26, 1987.

Anorexia Nervosa/Bulimia

Block, P.J.: Working with anorexic and bulimic adolescents, Food Nutr. News 56:33-34, 1984.

Castiglia, P.T.: Anorexia nervosa, J. Pediatr. Health Care 3:105-107, 1989.

Castiglia, P.T.: Bulimia, J. Pediatr. Health Care 3:167-169, 1989.

Danziger, Y., and others: Parental involvement in treatment of patients with anorexia nervosa in a pediatric day-care unit, Pediatrics 81:159-162, 1988.

Drewnowski, A., Hopkins, S., and Kessler, R.: The prevalence of bulimia nervosa in the U.S. college student population, Am. J. Public Health 78:1322-1325, 1988.

Fallon, A: Standards of attractiveness: their relationship toward body image perceptions and eating disorders, Food Nutr. News 59(5):79-80, 1987.

Ferraro, A.R.: Bulimia: a look from within, Pediatr. Nurs. 16:187-191, 1990.

Flood, M.: Addictive eating disorders, Nurs. Clin. North Am. 24:65-69, 1989.

Garner, D.M., and Garfinkel, P.E.: Handbook of psychotherapy for anorexia nervosa, New York, 1985, Guilford Press.

Goodwin, R.A., and Mickalide, A.D.: Parent-to-parent support in anorexia nervosa and bulimia, Child. Health Care 14:32-37, 1985.

Harding, S.E.: Anorexia nervosa, Pediatr. Nurs. 11:275-277, 1985.

Hayes, D., and Ross, C.E.: Concern with appearance, health beliefs, and eating habits, J. Health Soc. Behav. 28:120-130, 1987.

Humphrey, L.L.: Observed family interactions among subtypes of eating disorders using structural analysis of social behavior, J. Consult. Clin. Psychol. 57:206-214, 1989.

Inbody, D.R., and Ellis, J.J.: Group therapy with anorexic and bulimic patients: implications for therapeutic intervention, Am. J. Psychother. 39:411-420, 1985.

Lakin, J.A., and McClelland, E.: Binge eating and bulimic behaviors in a school-age population, J. Community Health Nurs. 4:143-164, 1987.

Litt, I.F., and Glader, L.: Anorexia nervosa, athletics, and amenorrhea, J. Pediatr. 109:150-153, 1986.

Lucas, A.R.: Update and review of anorexia nervosa, Contemp. Nutr. 14(9), 1989.

Mansfield, M.J., and Emans, S.J.: Anorexia nervosa, athletics and amenorrhea, Pediatr. Clin. North Am. 36:533-549, 1989.

Mitchell, J.E.: Bulimia nervosa, Contemp. Nutr. 14(10), 1989.

Muscari, M.E.: Identification and management of the early anorectic child, J. Pediatr. Health Care 1:196-203, 1987.

Muscari, M.E.: Effective nursing strategies for adolescents with anorexia nervosa and bulimia nervosa, Pediatr. Nurs. 14:475-482, 1988.

Palla, B., and Litt, I.F.: Medical complications of eating disorders in adolescents, Pediatrics 81:613-623, 1988.

Potts, N.: The secret pattern of binge/purge, Am. J. Nurs. 84:32-35, 1984.

Rees, J.M.: Eating disorders. In Mahan, L.K., and Rees, J.M.: Nutrition in adolescence, St. Louis, 1984, Mosby–Year Book, Inc.

Sanger, E., and Cassino, T.: Eating disorders—avoiding the power struggle, Am. J. Nurs. 84:31-35, 1984.

Shisslak, C.: Primary prevention of eating disorders, J. Consult. Clin. Psychol. 55:660-667, 1987.

Silber, T.J., and others: Prevalence of PCP use among adolescent marijuana users, J. Pediatr. 112:827-829, 1988.

Twiss, J.J.: The plight of a female adolescent—anorexia or bulimia: an overview, Issues Compr. Pediatr. Nurs. 9:289-298, 1986.

Smoking

Altman, D.G., and others: Reducing the illegal sale of cigarettes to minors, JAMA 261:80-83, 1989.

American Academy of Pediatrics, Committee on Adolescence: Tobacco use by children and adolescents, Pediatrics 79:479-481, 1987.

Coe, R.M., and others: Patterns of change in adolescent smoking behavior and results of a one year follow-up of a smoking prevention program, J. School Health 52:348-353, 1982.

Demuth, P.J.: Clove cigarettes: a hazardous fad, Am. J. Nurs. 85:950-951, 1985.

Goldstein, A.O., and others: Relationship between high school student smoking and recognition of cigarette advertisements, J. Pediatr. 110:488-491, 1987.

Macdonald, D.I.: Prevention of adolescent smoking and drug use, Pediatr. Clin. North Am. 33:995-1005, 1986.

Masironi, R., and Roy, L.: Smoking and youth: a special report, World Smoking and Health 8(1):27-31, 1983.

McCaul, K.D., and others: Predicting adolescent smoking, J. School Health 52:342-346, 1982.

McMahon, A., and Maibusch, R.M.: How to send quit-smoking signals, Am. J. Nurs. 88:1498-1499, 1988.

Murray, M., Kiryluk, S., and Swan, A.V.: School characteristics and adolescent smoking: results from the MRC/Derbyshire smoking study 1974-8 and from a follow-up in 1981, J. Epidemiol. Community Health 38:167-172, 1984.

Perry, C.L., and Silvis, G.L.: Smoking prevention: behavioral prescriptions for the pediatrician, Pediatrics 79:790-799, 1987.

Tonnesen, P., and others: Effect of nicotine chewing gum in combination with group counseling on the cessation of smoking, N. Engl. J. Med. 318:15-18, 1988.

Young, T.L., and Rogers, K.D.: School performance characteristics preceding onset of smoking in high school students, Am. J. Dis. Child. 140:257-259, 1985.

Substance Abuse

American Academy of Pediatrics, Committee on Adolescence, Committee on Bioethics, and Provisional Committee on Substance Abuse: Screening for drugs of abuse in children and adolescents, Pediatrics 84:396-398, 1989.

Anglin, T.M.: Interviewing guidelines for the clinical evaluation of adolescent substance abuse, Pediatr. Clin. North Am. 34:381-398, 1987.

Bertino, J.S., and Reed, M.D.: Barbiturate and nonbarbiturate sedative hypnotic intoxication in children, Pediatr. Clin. North Am. 33:703-722, 1986.

Bloch, J., Bloch, J.H., and Keyes, S.: Longitudinally foretelling drug usage in adolescence: early childhood personality and environmental precursors, Child Dev. 59:336-355, 1988.

Blum, R.W.: Adolescent substance abuse: diagnostic and treatment issues, Pediatr. Clin. North Am. 34:523-537, 1987.

Brown, R.T., and Braden, N.J.: Hallucinogens, Pediatr. Clin. North Am. 34:341-347, 1987.

Burpo, R.H.: A step beyond "just say no," MCN 13:428-431, 1988.

Coulehan, J.L., and others: Gasoline sniffing and lead toxicity in Navajo adolescents, Pediatrics 71:113-117, 1983.

DuPont, R.L.: Teenage drug use: opportunities for the pediatrician, J. Pediatr. 102:1003-1007, 1983.

DuPont, R.L.: Prevention of adolescent chemical dependency, Pediatr. Clin. North Am. 34:495-505, 1987.

Farrow, J.A., Rees, J.M., and Worthington-Roberts, B.S.: Health, developmental, and nutritional status of adolescent alcohol and marijuana abusers, Pediatrics 79:218-223, 1987.

Golb, C.S.: Substance abuse: what turns casual use into chronic dependence? Contemp. Pediatr. 3(10):26-41, 1986.

Hahn, E., and Papazian, K.: Substance abuse prevention with preschool children, J. Community Health Nurs. 4:165-170, 1987.

Hoffmann, N.G., Sonis, W.A., and Halikas, J.A.: Issues in the evaluation of chemical dependency treatment programs for adolescents, Pediatr. Clin. North Am. 34:449-459, 1987.

Huberty, D.J., and others: Family issues in working with chemically dependent adolescents, Pediatr. Clin. North Am. 34:507-521, 1987.

Isralowitz, R., and Singer, M., editors: Adolescent substance abuse: a guide to prevention and treatment, New York, 1983, The Haworth Press.

Joshi, N.P., and Scott, M.: Drug use, depression, and adolescents, Pediatr. Clin. North Am. 34:1349-1364, 1987.

King, N.M.P., and Cross, A.W.: Moral and legal issues in screening for drug use in adolescents, J. Pediatr. 111:249-250, 1987.

Kulberg, A.: Substance abuse: clinical identification and management, Pediatr. Clin. North Am. 33:325-361, 1986.

Lukwikowski, K.L.K.: PPA: an innocent over-the-counter drug? Pediatr. Nurs. 10:387-390, 1984.

Macdonald, D.I.: Drugs, drinking, and adolescence, Am. J. Dis. Child. 138:117-125, 1984.

Macdonald, D.I.: Just say no, J. Pediatr. 114:673-675, 1989.

McHugh, M.J.: The abuse of volatile substances, Pediatr. Clin. North Am. 34:333-340, 1987.

Morrison, M.A., and Smith, Q.T.: Psychiatric issues of adolescent chemical dependence, Pediatr. Clin. North Am. 34:461-480, 1987.

Pallikkathayil, L., and Tweed, S.: Substance abuse: alcohol and drugs during adolescence, Nurs. Clin. North Am. 18:313-321, 1983.

Rice, M.A., and Kibbee, P.E.: Review: identifying the adolescent substance abuser, MCN 8:139-142, 1983.

Richardson, J.L, and others: Substance use among eighth-grade students who take care of themselves after school, Pediatrics 84:556-566, 1989.

Robinson, D.P., and Green, J.W.: The adolescent alcohol and drug problem: a practical approach, Pediatr. Nurs. 14:305-310, 1988.

Rumack, B.H.: Acetaminophen overdose in children and adolescents, Pediatr. Clin. North Am. 33:691-701, 1986.

Sanders, J.M.: Adolescents and substance abuse, Pediatrics 76:630-632, 1985.

Schaffner, A.T., and Dieterich, D.: Streetwise narcotic safety, Am. J. Nurs. 86:707-708, 1986.

Schwartz, R.H.: Are you ready to deal with the pot-smoking patient? Contemp. Pediatr. 4(4):84-106, 1987.

Schwartz, R.H.: Marijuana: an overview, Pediatr. Clin. North Am. 34:305-317, 1987.

Schwartz, R.H., Comerci, G.D., and Meeks, J.E.: LSD: patterns of use by chemically dependent adolescents, J. Pediatr. 111:936-938, 1987.

Schwartz, R.H., and others: Short-term memory impairment in cannabis-dependent adolescents, Am. J. Dis. Child. 143:1214-1219, 1989.

Strasburger, V.C.: Prevention of adolescent drug abuse: why "just say no" just won't work, J. Pediatr. 114:676-681, 1989.

Swaim, R.C., and others: Links from emotional distress to adolescent drug use: a path model, J. Consult. Clin. Psychol. 57:227-231, 1989.

Wheeler, K., and Malmquist, J.: Treatment approaches in adolescent chemical dependency, Pediatr. Clin. North Am. 34:437-447, 1987.

Zarek, D, Hawkins, J.D., and Rogers, P.D.: Risk factors for adolescent substance abuse, Pediatr. Clin. North Am. 34:481-493, 1987.

Alcohol

American Academy of Pediatrics, Committee on Adolescence: Alcohol use and abuse: a pediatric concern, Pediatrics 79:450-453, 1987.

Barnes, G.M., Farrell, M.P., and Cairns, A.: Parental socialization factors and adolescent drinking behaviors, J. Marriage Fam. 8:27-36, 1986.

Casswell, S., and others: What children know about alcohol and how they know it, Br. J. Addict. 3:223-227, 1988.

Castiglia, P.T., and others: Influences on children's attitudes toward alcohol consumption, Pediatr. Nurs. 15:263-266, 1989.

Felter, R., Izsak, E., and Lawrence, H.S.: Emergency department management of the intoxicated adolescent, Pediatr. Clin. North Am. 34:399-421, 1987.

Killen, J.D.: Evidence for an alcohol-stress link among normal weight adolescents reporting purging behavior, Int. J. Eating Disorders 6:349-356, 1987.

Kiltzner, M., and others: Screening for risk factors for adolescent alcohol and drug use, Am. J. Dis. Child. 141:45-49, 1987.

Macdonald, D.I.: How you can help prevent teenage alcoholism, Contemp. Pediatr. 3(11):50-72, 1986.

Macdonald, D.I.: Patterns of alcohol and drug use among adolescents, Pediatr. Clin. North Am. 34:275-288, 1987.

Petchers, M.K., and Singer, M.I.: Perceived-benefit-of-drinking scale: approach to screening for adolescent alcohol abuse, J. Pediatr. 110:977-981, 1987.

Rich, J.: Action stat! Acute alcohol intoxication, Nursing '89 19(9):33, 1989.

Rogers, P.D., Harris, J., and Jarmuskewicz, J.: Alcohol and adolescence, Pediatr. Clin. North Am. 34:289-303, 1987.

Schuckit, M.A.: Genetics and the risk of alcoholism, JAMA 254:2614-2617, 1985.

Cocaine

Acee, A.M., and Smith, D.: Crack, Am. J. Nurs. 87:614-617, 1987.

Bateman, D.A., and Heagarty, M.C.: Passive freebase cocaine ("crack") inhalation by infants and toddlers, Am. J. Dis. Child. 143:25-27, 1989.

Brown, B.S., and others: Kids and cocaine—a treatment dilemma, J. Subst. Abuse Treat. 6:3-8, 1989.

Clouet, D., Asghar, K., and Brown, R., editors: Mechanisms of cocaine abuse and toxicity, NIDA Research Monograph 88, Washington, DC, 1988, U.S. Government Printing Office.

Estroff, T.W., Schwartz, R.H., and Hoffmann, N.G.: Adolescent cocaine abuse, Clin. Pediatr. 28:550-555, 1989.

Farrar, H.C., and Kearns, G.L.: Cocaine: clinical pharmacology and toxicology, J. Pediatr. 115:665-675, 1989.

Heagarty, M.C.: Crack cocaine: a new danger for children, Am. J. Dis. Child. 14:756-757, 1990.

Mofenson, H.C., Copeland, P., and Caraccio, T.R.: Cocaine and crack: the latest menace, Contemp. Pediatr. 3(10):44-50, 1986.

Mofenson, H.C., and Caraccio, T.R.: Cocaine, Pediatr. Ann. 16:864-874, 1987.

Shannon, M., and others: Cocaine exposure among children seen at a pediatric hospital, Pediatrics 83:337-342, 1989.
Smith, D.E., Schwartz, R.H., and Martin, D.M.: Heavy cocaine use by adolescents, Pediatrics 83:539-542, 1989.

Suicide

American Academy of Pediatrics, Committee on Adolescence: Suicide and suicide atttempts in adolescents and young adults, Pediatrics 81:322-324, 1988.
Bakkala, C.F.: The role of the school nurse in suicide prevention, School Nurse 6(1):13-15, 1990.
Baron, P., and Joly, E.: Sex differences in the expression of depression in adolescents, Sex Roles 18:1-7, 1988.
Beardslee, W.R.: Familial influences in childhood depression, Pediatr. Ann. 13:32-36, 1984.
Berman, A.L., and Schwartz, R.H.: Suicide attempts among adolescent drug users, Am. J. Dis. Child. 144:310-314, 1990.
Carmack, B.J.: Suspect a suicide? RN 46(44):43-45, 90, 1983.
Christoffel, K.K., and others: Adolescent suicide and suicide attempts: a population study, Pediatr. Emerg. Care 4:32-40, 1988.
Earls, F.: The epidemiology of depression in children and adolescents, Pediatr. Ann. 13:23-31, 1984.
Faust, J., Forehand, R., and Baum, C.G.: An examination of the association between social relationships and depression in early adolescence, J. Appl. Dev. Psychol. 6:291-297, 1985.
Fazen, L.E., Lovejoy, F.H., and Crone, R.K.: Acute poisoning in a children's hospital: a 2-year experience, Pediatrics 77:144-151, 1986.
Gemma, P.B.: Coping with suicidal behavior, MCN 14:101-103, 1989.
Gould, M.S., and Shaffer, D.: The impact of suicide in television: evidence of imitation, N. Engl. J. Med. 315:690-694, 1986.
Gyulay, J.E.: What suicide leaves behind, Issues Compr. Pediatr. Nurs. 12:103-118, 1989.
Harris, J.C.: Don't overlook depression in children and adolescents, Contemp. Pediatr. 4(3):70-90, 1987.
Hatton, C.L., and Valente, S.M.: Suicide: assessment and intervention, ed. 2, New York, 1984, Appleton-Century-Crofts.
Hergenroeder, A.C., and others: The pediatrician's role in adolescent suicide, Pediatr. Ann. 15:787-798, 1986.
Hoffman, Y.: Surviving a child's suicide, Am. J. Nurs. 87:955-956, 1987.
Kaminer, Y., and Robbins, D.R.: Attempted suicide by insulin overdose in insulin-dependent diabetic adolescents, Pediatrics 81:526-528, 1988.
King, G.S., Smialek, J.E., and Troutman, W.G.: Sudden death in adolescents resulting from the inhalation of typewriter correction fluid, JAMA 253:1604-1606, 1985.
Lamb, J.M.: The suicidal adolescent: how you can help, Nursing '90 20(5):72-76, 1990.
Litt, I.F., Cuskey, W.R., and Rudd, S.: Emergency room evaluation of the adolescent who attempts suicide: compliance with follow-up, J. Adolesc. Health Care 4:106-109, 1983.
Mitchell, K.: Suicide: a preventable tragedy, Pediatr. Nurs. 11:165, 1985.
Muscari, M.E.: Adolescent suicide attempts by acetaminophen ingestion, MCN 12:32-35, 1987.
Ostroff, R.B., and others: Adolescent suicides modeled after television movies, Am. J. Psychiatry 142:989-1004, 1985.
Pfeffer, C.R.: The suicidal child, New York, 1987, Atcom, Inc.
Pfeffer, C.R.: Spotting the red flags for adolescent suicide, Contemp. Pediatr. 6(2):59-70, 1989.
Phillips, D.P., and Carstensen, L.L.: Clustering of teenage suicides after televison news stories about suicide, N. Engl. J. Med. 315:685-689, 1986.
Rankin, W.W.: Teenage suicide, J. Pediatr. Nurs. 4:130-131, 1989.
Raskind, S.M.: Suicide by burning: emotional needs of the suicidal adolescent on the burn unit, Issues Compr. Pediatr. Nurs. 9:369-382, 1986.
Slap, G.B., and others: Risk factors for attempted suicide during adolescence, Pediatrics 84:762-772, 1989.
Stivers, C.: Parent-adolescent communication and its relationship to adolescent depression and suicide proneness, Adolescence 23:291-295, 1988.
Tishler, C.L.: Depression in children and adolescents: identification and intervention, Public Health Curr. 24:1-3, 1984.
Valente, S.: Suicide in school aged children: theory and assessment, Pediatr. Nurs. 9:25-29, 1983.
Valente, S.M.: Assessing suicide risk in the school-age child, J. Pediatr. Health Care 1:14-20, 1987.
Velez, C.N., and Cohen, P.: Suicidal behavior and ideation in a community sample of children: maternal and youth reports, J. Acad. Child. Adolesc. Psychiatry 27:349-356, 1988.
Wright, L.S.: High school polydrug users and abusers, Adolescence 20:853-861, 1985.

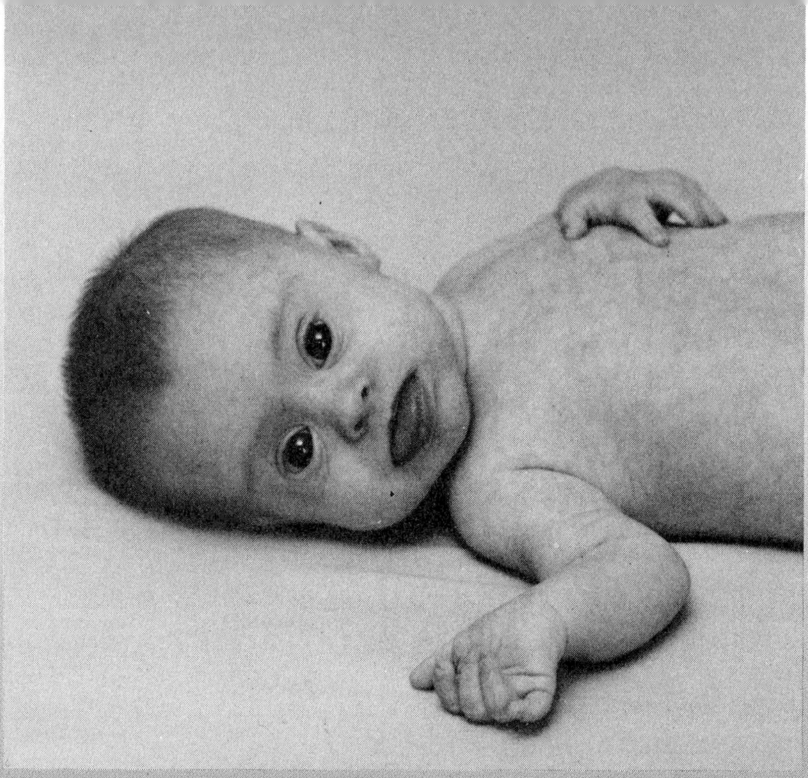

The Child and Family with Special Needs

UNIT VIII

Units III through VII have focused on the growth and development of the well child. Most of the health problems discussed for each age-group were those that temporarily incapacitated the child. Unit VIII is concerned with the child who has special needs imposed by a permanent or chronic physical and/or developmental disability. These children need to master the same developmental achievements as other children, in accordance with their potential abilities and despite the limitations of their condition. Families of these children are faced with exceptional challenges for which there is little guidance and few role models. As a result, the entire family unit is highly vulnerable to psychologic and sometimes physical problems that arise from unsuccessful attempts to deal with the child's special needs.

Chapter 22, *Impact of Chronic Illness or Disability on the Child and Family,* is an overview of the child's and family's reactions to the disorder and nursing interventions that assist each member in adjusting to the condition and developing to the fullest despite the disability. This chapter serves as a basis for understanding the stresses and needs of families when the child is chronically ill, physically disabled, mentally retarded, or sensory impaired. Chapter 23, *Impact of Life-Threatening Illness on the Child and Family,* focuses on the special needs of families when the diagnosis is potentially fatal. Chapter 24, *The Child with Cognitive Impairment,* is primarily concerned with the child who is mentally retarded and the nursing interventions required to help the child develop optimally. Chapter 25, *The Child with Sensory or Communication Impairment,* deals with the child who has a sensory loss or a communication disorder. Emphasis is placed on the effect of the impairment on development, detection of the disorder, and nursing interventions that promote rehabilitation.

CHAPTER 22

Impact of Chronic Illness or Disability on the Child and Family

RELATED TOPICS

Birth of a child with a physical defect, Ch. 11
Childhood morbidity, Ch. 1
Communicating with families, Ch. 6
Developmental assessment, Ch. 7
Discharge planning and home care (high-risk newborn), Ch. 10
Facilitating parent-infant relationships (high-risk newborn), Ch. 10
Family assessment, Ch. 6
Health promotion: infant, Ch. 12; toddler, Ch. 14; preschooler, Ch. 15; school-age child, Ch. 17; and adolescent, Ch. 19
Impact of life-threatening illness on the child and family, Ch. 23
Reaction of the child and family to illness and hospitalization, Ch. 26
Recommendations for health supervision, Ch. 7
School phobia, Ch. 18

GLOSSARY

approach behaviors Coping behaviors that result in movement toward adjustment and resolution of a crisis

avoidance behaviors Coping behaviors that result in movement away from adjustment or maladaptation to a crisis

benevolent overreaction A cycle of overprotective, permissive parent and dependent, demanding child

chronic illness A condition that interferes with daily functioning for more than 3 months in a year, causes hospitalization of more than 1 month in a year, or (at time of diagnosis) is likely to do either of these (Hobbs and Perrin, 1985)

developmental delay A maturational lag—an abnormal, slower rate of development in which a child demonstrates a functioning level below that observed in normal children of the same age (Thompson and Quinn, 1979)

developmental disability Any severe, chronic disability attributable to a mental or physical impairment, or a combination of both, that is manifested before age 22 years, is likely to continue indefinitely, and will result in substantial limitation of function (American Academy of Pediatrics, 1979)

developmental model Focuses on the child's developmental needs rather than on the medical diagnosis

disability The restriction or lack of ability to perform normally as a result of impairment (Jones, 1987)

early intervention Any sustained and systematic effort to assist children who are disabled and developmentally vulnerable from birth to age 3 years and their families

empowerment The interaction of professionals with families in such a way that families maintain or acquire a sense of control over their family lives and attribute positive changes that result from helping behaviors that foster their own strengths, abilities, and actions (Johnson, McGonigel, and Kaufmann, 1989)

enabling families Creating opportunities and means for all family members to display their present abilities and competencies and to acquire new ones that are necessary to meet the needs of the child and family (Johnson, McGonigel, and Kaufmann, 1989)

family-centered care A philosophy of care that recognizes that the family is the constant in a child's life and that service systems and personnel must support, respect, encourage, and enhance the strength and competence of the family (Johnson, McGonigel, and Kaufmann, 1989)

functional burden A factor used in predicting family adjustment that weighs the issues related to caring for and living with a child with special needs against the family's resources and ability to cope

handicap An environmental barrier that prevents or makes it difficult for full participation or integration, such as curbs or steps for a person in a wheelchair (Rush and League of Human Dignity, 1983); individuals with chronic illnesses or disabilities are not necessarily handicapped

home care Parent and/or professionally provided health care and related services delivered in the home environment

IEP Individual Education Program

IFSP Individual Family Service Plan

impairment A loss or abnormality of structure or function

mainstreaming The process of integrating children with special needs into regular classrooms and child care centers

normalization The principle that children and families should have access to services provided in as usual a fashion and environment as possible (Johnson, McGonigel, and Kaufmann, 1989); establishing a normal pattern of living.

parent/professional partnership A relationship between one or more professionals and a family who function collaboratively using agreed-on roles for a common goal

PL 94-142 The Education for All Handicapped Children Act of 1975

PL 99-457 The Education of the Handicapped Act Amendments of 1986

technology-dependent child A child between the ages of birth to 21 years with a chronic disability that requires the routine use of a medical device to compensate for the loss of a life-sustaining body function; daily, ongoing care and/or monitoring is required by trained personnel (Report to Congress, 1988)

In a complex society there are innumerable abilities necessary for functioning. Loss of any physical or cognitive power immediately poses an obstacle to a person's ability to meet societal expectations. With advances in early diagnosis and treatment of many chronic illnesses and with improved technology for people with physical impairments, there is a growing number of children who need care. Because nurses are intimately involved in care for every type of health deviation, it is inevitable that they will be responsible for some phase of care with families who have children with special needs imposed by a physical or mental limitation. This chapter is primarily concerned with families' responses to the disorder, the effects of chronic illness or disability on the child and family unit, and nursing interventions that promote the optimum adjustment of each family member and acceptance of the child as a unique individual with special attributes as well as needs.

Judy Holt Rollins, R.N., M.S., assisted in the revision of this chapter.

PERSPECTIVES IN THE CARE OF CHILDREN WITH SPECIAL NEEDS

Children with special needs comprise an increasingly important group of children who require both routine and specialized health care. The following discussion is an overview of the incidence of chronic illness and disability in children and the current trends in caring for these children.

SCOPE OF THE PROBLEM

Despite the interest and concern for children with special needs, exact definitions and incidence rates of chronic illness and disability do not exist. For the purposes of this chapter, see the definitions listed in the Glossary for the following terms: chronic illness, developmental delay, developmental disability, disability, handicap, impairment, and technology-dependent child.

Statistics regarding chronic illness and disability are at best only estimates of the true incidence of the problem and vary, depending on the definitions used, the methods of study, and the population investigated (Gortmaker and Sappenfield, 1984). Overall rates of children with any chronic disorder range from 10% to 15%; approximately 1% to 2% of the total population (1 to 2 million children) have a severe chronic illness (Hobbs and Perrin, 1985). Two thirds of all cases of chronic illness are attributable to asthma and congenital heart defects; however, in terms of mortality, congenital heart defects, spina bifida, and leukemia are the most lethal (Harkey, 1983). While there has been little change in the survival patterns for asthma, cleft lip/palate, and muscular dystrophy in recent years, there have been improvements in other diseases. For example, 20 years ago children who developed acute lymphocytic leukemia lived an average of 3 to 4 months; today 68% can expect to survive. Children with Hodgkin disease, almost always fatal 20 years ago, can now expect an 88% cure rate (American Cancer Society, 1988). The median life expectancy for a child with cystic fibrosis has increased from 5 years of age in 1955 to 27 years today (Cystic Fibrosis Foundation, 1990). The most dramatic progress, however, has occurred in the treatment of spina bifida. In 1955, 90% of children born with spina bifida died in infancy; today, 90% to 95% survive infancy and have a normal life expectancy if they receive timely and appropriate medical intervention (Spina Bifida Association, 1990).

In addition, technologic advances have increased survival rates of extremely premature infants and full-term low-birth-weight infants (Report to Congress, 1988). In the United States in 1960 only 3 out of 10 very-low-birth-weight newborns survived at least 1 month; by 1980 twice as many survived, with a greater increase expected in the 1990s (Office of Technology, 1987). The resulting progress for these children at risk contributes to the growing number of children with chronic and/or disabling conditions, many of whom remain dependent on technology.

Broadly expanding chronic conditions to include speech, learning, emotional, sensory, and cognitive disorders yields an estimated 40% of children from kindergarten through sixth grade who have a significant long-term condition (Reynolds, 1984). The vast majority of children with chronic illness or disability live at home with their families. Considering that the average American family has between three and four members, the number of individuals intimately affected by these children is staggering.

The numbers alone suggest that comprehensive nursing approaches are required to meet the immense needs of children, youth, and families. Clearly, nurses have a more crucial role than ever before in early screening, case finding, assessment, and diagnostic studies, as well as supportive interventions that minimize the disruptive effects of the condition on the family. Another major responsibility is preventing disabling disorders by eliminating their known causes. Nurses are responsible for ensuring immunization programs, identifying infants and mothers who may be at risk prenatally or postnatally, identifying the disability early, promoting injury prevention policies and programs, and implementing innovative health education programs.

CHANGING TRENDS IN CARE

Several changes have occurred in providing services to children with special needs. Current emphasis is placed on a "noncategoric" approach, which avoids classifying needs and services by medical diagnoses, since most psychosocial and developmental needs of children with chronic conditions are not disease specific (Yoos, 1987). Influenced by technologic advances, economic considerations, and the need for more meaningful models of care, changes not only reflect the kinds of care and services children receive, but also indicate shifts in who provides that care and where services are provided.

Developmental Focus

Using the developmental approach rather than chronologic age emphasizes the child's abilities and strengths rather than disabilities. In the past health professionals have viewed persons with a disability within a pathologic framework, probing for weaknesses and negative features. While much attention has been given to the technologic aspects of the child's care and health needs, less attention has been paid to the child's individuality, personality, or strengths, the family's needs, and the overall concerns of those who interact with these children. Under the developmental model, attention is directed to the child's functional development, changes, and adaptation to the environment. Nurses often are in vital positions to redirect attention from the pathologic to the developmental model to meet the unique needs of the child and family.

Family Development

A developmental focus also considers family development. Duvall (1977) defined a model of family development based on the changing ages and developmental needs of both children and adults, as well as on the changing demands by external forces and crises as the family matures. Families are challenged to achieve specific developmental tasks at various stages in the family life cycle (e.g., leaving one's parents and forming a new relationship during the couple stage; accepting the influence of others on children's behavior during the school-age stage; refocusing on the marital role when children leave home) from the couple's courtship through their parenting years and into retirement (Carney, 1987). A family member's serious illness or disability can cause significant stress or crisis at any stage of the cycle. Just as with individual development, family development may be interrupted or even regress to an earlier, inappropriate level of functioning. Nurses can use the concept of family development to plan meaningful interventions and evaluate care (see Developmental Theory, Chapter 3).

Family-Centered Care

Family-centered care is a philosophy of care that recognizes that the family is the constant in a child's life and that service systems and personnel must support, respect, encourage, and enhance the strength and competence of the family (Johnson, McGonigel, and Kaufmann, 1989). Families are supported in their natural caregiving and decision-making roles by building on their unique strengths as individuals and families. Patterns of living at home and in the community are promoted. The needs of all family members, not just the child's, are considered.

Two basic concepts in this process are enabling and empowerment. Professionals *enable* families by creating opportunities and means for all family members to display their present abilities and competencies and to acquire new ones that are necessary to meet the needs of the child and family. *Empowerment* describes the interaction of professionals with families in such a way that families maintain or acquire a sense of control over their family lives and attribute positive changes that result from helping behaviors that foster their own strengths, abilities, and actions.

A three-level model of empowerment has been described (Fire, 1990). At the first level, parents need information and basic support. Parents develop their competencies in caring and advocating for their child at level two. At the third level, parents develop requisite leadership skills to be effective teachers, advocates, and supporters for other families and professionals. Depending on circumstances, parents can move very rapidly from one level to another. For example, a sudden appearance of new symptoms can send the parent at level three into the level-one stage of gathering and absorbing as much information as possible to understand the new development and its implications.

The *parent-professional partnership* is a powerful mechanism for enabling and empowering families. Parents have moved from feeling "more hostage than partner to a gang of powerful professionals who sustained [my child's] life and taught me the rules of a strange new variety of motherhood" (Oster, 1985), to serving as respected equals with professionals committed to developing optimum quality in the delivery of all levels of health care.* In a parent-professional partnership, parents have the rightful role in deciding what is important for themselves and their family; the professional's role is to support and strengthen the family's ability to nurture and promote its members' development in a way that is both enabling and empowering.

Partnerships imply the belief that partners are capable individuals who become more capable by sharing knowledge, skills, and resources in a manner that benefits all participants (Dunst, Trivette, and Deal, 1988). Collaboration is viewed as a continuum. Families have the option of being anywhere along that continuum, depending on the strengths and needs of the child, the family, and the professionals who are involved (Shelton, Jeppson, and Johnson, 1987). Approximately 10% to 15% of the families of children with special needs will bring a previous history of serious personal and/or family problems and will need special help (Spinetta and Deasy-Spinetta, 1986). However, *every* family has strengths as well as needs. The nurse can help even high-risk families identify their strengths, build on them, and assume a comfortable level of participation. While family-centered care is an important concept in the care of all children, it is crucial to optimum care for children with chronic illnesses or disabilities. (See Box 22-1 for elements of family-centered care.)

*For information about parent-professional partnerships, a free pamphlet, *Equals in This Partnership*, is available from The National Center for Clinical Infant Programs, 2000 14th St. N., Suite 380, Arlington, VA 22201; (703) 528-4300.

Box 22-1 KEY ELEMENTS OF FAMILY-CENTERED CARE

Recognizing that the family is the constant in a child's life, while the service systems and personnel within those systems fluctuate

Facilitating parent/professional collaboration at all levels of health care:
- Care of an individual child
- Program development, implementation, and evaluation
- Policy formation

Honoring the racial, ethnic, cultural, and socioeconomic diversity of families

Recognizing family strengths and individuality and respecting different methods of coping

Sharing with parents, on a continuing basis and in a supportive manner, complete and unbiased information

Encouraging and facilitating family-to-family support and networking

Understanding and incorporating the developmental needs of infants, children, and adolescents and their families into health care systems

Implementing comprehensive policies and programs that provide emotional and financial support to meet the needs of families

Designing accessible health care systems that are flexible, culturally competent, and responsive to family-identified needs

From National Center for Family-Centered Care, Bethesda, MD, 1990, Association for the Care of Children's Health.

Normalization

Normalization refers to establishing a normal pattern of living (see also Box 22-13). It implies child and family access to services in as usual a fashion and environment as possible (Johnson, McGonigel, and Kaufmann, 1989). Normalization permits the child and family to become or remain part of the community. By applying the principles of normalization, the environment for the child is "normalized" and "humanized."

Home Care

Concurrent with the trend toward normalization has been the earlier discharge of children from acute or chronic care facilities to the family and community. *Home care* represents the return to a system and set of priorities in which family values are as important to the care of a child with a chronic health problem as they are in the care of other children. Home care seeks to achieve goals that are consistent with the developmental model (Stein, 1985):

1. Normalize the life of a child with special needs, including those with technologically complex care, in a family and community context and setting.
2. Minimize the disruptive impact of the child's condition on the family.
3. Foster the child's maximum growth and development.

With appropriate training and support, families today provide complex procedures and treatments in the home. Parents are challenged to retain a homelike setting among monitors, ventilators, and other sophisticated equipment. Throughout the text, home care is discussed as appropriate for specific conditions, and the process of transition from hospital to home is elaborated in Chapter 26.

Mainstreaming

Mainstreaming describes the process of integrating children with special needs into regular classrooms and child care centers. Just as the home is the natural environment for children, so school must also be included as an essential component of the children's overall physical, intellectual, and social development. Children who attend school have the advantages of learning and socializing with a wide group of peers. There is an increased focus on individualization as the academic needs of these children are planned along with those of the rest of the students. A variety of supplemental programs have been designed in the school system to accommodate special needs, thus providing these children with an equal educational opportunity. This change has largely been a result of the passage of Public Law 94-142, the Education for All Handicapped Children Act of 1975 (Downey, 1990).

The 1975 law requires states to identify, diagnose, educate, and provide related services for children 5 to 18 years of age. The age range was extended in 1977 to include children between 3 and 21 years, with services for children between the ages of 3 and 5 remaining optional. Under the law, a multidisciplinary team designs an Individual Education Program (IEP), which contains specific educational and therapeutic strategies and goals for each eligible child. Parents may be involved in educational decisions and have the right to a hearing when the team's decision is viewed as inappropriate or harmful (American Academy of Pediatrics, Committee on Children With Disabilities, 1987).

Early Intervention

Early intervention, or early childhood intervention, consists of any sustained and systematic effort to assist children from birth to age 3 years who are young, disabled, and developmentally vulnerable, as well as their families (Meisels, 1989). Over the last 25 years much has been learned about service provision for very young at-risk children and children with disabilities and how special services can support their development. Public Law 99-457, the Education of the Handicapped Act Amendments of 1986, made a giant step toward translating knowledge about early development into public policy. It directs states to develop and implement statewide comprehensive, coordinated, multidisciplinary interagency programs of early intervention services for infants and toddlers with disabilities, as well as their families (Healy, Keesee, and Smith, 1989).

A central component of the law's implementation is its focus on the family as a means of enhancing the child's development through the Individual Family Service Plan (IFSP). Developed jointly by families and professionals, the IFSP includes information about the infant/toddler's present level of development, family strengths and needs relating to enhancing development, major outcomes expected, services needed, identification of a case manager, and transition steps to preschool services.* All services and outcomes relate to the family's, as well as the child's, needs. The IFSP is a commitment to children and families that their strengths will be recognized and built on, that their needs will be met in a way that respects their beliefs and values, and that their hopes and aspirations will be encouraged and enabled (Johnson, McGonigel, and Kaufmann, 1989).

Nurses have much to contribute to providing care for children covered by PL 99-457. Clinical skills and a traditional philosophy of family-focused care earn nurses a valuable place on interdisciplinary assessment and planning teams, often as case managers. Nurses can assess children in preschool settings, provide ongoing family and staff education, coordinate care with health care providers, develop health promotion programs for family and school staffs, and participate in community nursing networks (Hansen, Holaday, and Miles, 1990).

THE CHILD AND FAMILY WITH SPECIAL NEEDS

The family of the child with special needs is faced with the crisis of losing a perfect child and the task of adjusting to and accepting the child and his or her condition. Nurses who understand the responses to the diagnosis and the usual effects the diagnosis has on each family member are able to emotionally support the family, anticipate and prevent potential problems, and foster growth despite the disorder. In addition to the following discussion, the response of parents to a newborn with a physical defect is discussed in Chapter 11, and the family's response to loss, specifically a child with a life-threatening disorder, is presented in Chapter 23.

*The following resource is recommended for developing an IFSP: *Guidelines and Recommended Practices for the Individualized Family Service Plan* by B. Johnson, M. McGonigel, and R. Kaufmann, available from the Association for the Care of Children's Health, 7910 Woodmont Ave., Suite 300, Bethesda, MD 20814; (301) 654-6549.

REACTIONS OF FAMILIES TO A CHRONIC ILLNESS OR DISABILITY

When the diagnosis of a disability or chronic illness is made, the family progresses through a fairly predictable sequence of stages, regardless of the actual nature of the condition. Numerous investigators have studied families' responses and have postulated a number of "stages"; however, no one set of phases is universally accepted (Blacher, 1984). The following discussion focuses on stages that are common to most families, with the exception of out-of-home placement. Not all families experience this process, and each family member varies widely in the time needed to progress through any of the stages.

The nurse is cautioned to explore family reactions for all possible interpretations, not just negative ones. For example, too often a parent's angry reaction has been attributed to a stage of adjustment or a maladaptive reaction, rather than a rational response to, for instance, an insulting remark (Stone, 1989). Professionals are gradually replacing the past emphasis on the negative with a positive, more supportive stance in their interactions with families coping with the birth or diagnosis of a child with special needs.

Shock and Denial

The initial stage is a period of intense emotion and is characterized by shock, disbelief, and sometimes denial, especially if the disorder is not obvious, such as in chronic illness. Denial as a defense mechanism is a necessary cushion to prevent disintegration and is a normal response to grieving any type of loss. Probably all family members experience various degrees of adaptive denial as they learn of the impact that the diagnosis has on their lives. Denial becomes maladaptive when it prevents recognition of treatment or rehabilitative goals necessary for the child's optimum survival or development. For example, protracted denial may be seen in the response of a family to mental retardation; as long as the family can maintain a fiction of normality and handle the deviance within the present familial roles and values, there may exist no recognition of the diagnosis. Instead, the problem is explained as slow maturation or an easily remedied disorder. The denial may be enforced by the child's social development, which belies the degree of motor and speech retardation. Not infrequently this ability to rationalize delayed development is successful until the child enters school and is compared with other children, making his or her differences blatantly evident. At this point the family may begin to recognize the diagnosis as a crisis and react with shock and disbelief.

Shock and denial can last from days to months, sometimes even longer. Examples of denial that may be exhibited at the time of diagnosis include: (1) physician shopping, (2) attributing the symptoms of the actual illness to a minor condition, (3) refusal to believe the diagnostic tests, (4) delay in agreeing to treatment, (5) acting very happy and optimistic despite the revealed diagnosis, (6) refusing to tell or talk to anyone about the condition, (7) insisting that no one is telling the truth, regardless of others' attempts to do so, (8) denying the reason for admission, and (9) asking no questions about the diagnosis, treatment, or prognosis. Each of these mechanisms allows individuals to distance themselves from the onslaught of a tremendous emotional impact and to collect and mobilize their energies toward goal-directed, problem-solving behaviors.

In some instances, various indicators of denial can be viewed as adaptive. Searching for another professional opinion may mean that parents cannot obtain answers to their questions or that they are looking for a different approach to treatment that better meets the needs of their child and family. When parents discuss their strengths and the benefits they derive from caring for their child with special needs, it does not necessarily reflect refusal to accept their difficult circumstances (Stone, 1989). Sometimes delay in making decisions or failure to ask questions simply reflects a lack of information.

Partial denial, such as seeking additional professional consultations or occasionally acting as if nothing were wrong, is common for families with children who have life-threatening conditions. Without such a temporary protective mechanism, few people could survive the constant emotional drain of anticipating their own death or the death of a family member. Partial denial allows the child and family to absorb stressful information—or "dose" themselves—in amounts they can personally manage at the time.

Denial is probably the least understood and most poorly dealt with reaction. Health professionals typically label denial as "maladaptive" and actively attempt to strip it away by repeated and sometimes blunt explanations of prognosis.

Poor communication between parents and professionals can lead to misunderstandings. For example, Mulhern, Crisco, and Camitta (1981) found that physicians had lower prognostic views than parents concerning the child's diagnosis and that neither group displayed an understanding of the disagreement. The physicians studied were largely unaware of parental hopefulness or denial, suggesting that poor communication existed between the groups. In other cases thoughts are communicated but misunderstood. The term *hope,* for example, may translate as "hope for a cure" to one person and "hope for a pain-free death" to another. Nurses must avoid projecting personal interpretations of *hope* or other terms to parents when assessing parental reactions.

In children, the importance of denial has repeatedly been demonstrated as a factor in their positive coping with the diagnosis. O'Malley and others (1979) found that children who used denial to cope with illness were able to deal with anxiety and have a productive attitude about life. Similarly, a study by Zeltzer and others (1980) of the coping styles of ill adolescents found that denial allowed even seriously ill adolescents to function adaptively and with hope.

Probably the crucial word here is *hope.* Denial allows an individual to maintain hope in the face of overwhelming odds. Like hope, denial may be an adaptive mechanism for dealing with loss that persists until a family or patient is ready or needs other responses. Relatives of critically ill patients also identify hope as a universal need (Hickey, 1990) (see Box 22-14).

Adjustment

Adjustment gradually follows shock and is usually characterized by an open admission that the condition exists. This stage is one of "chronic sorrow" and only partial acceptance (Fraley, 1990) and is manifest by several responses, probably the most universal of which are *guilt* and *self-accusation.* Guilt arises from a human need to find rational causes for events. The concept of cause and effect implies an ability to change future events. It is often greatest when the cause of the disorder is directly traceable to the parent, such as in genetic diseases or from accidental injury. However, it occurs even without any scientific or realistic basis for parental responsibility. Frequently the guilt stems from a fallacious assumption that the disability is a result of personal failing or wrongdoing, such as drinking, smoking, not eating correctly, having sex or an affair, exercising, or not doing something correctly during pregnancy or the birth (Childs, 1985). Guilt may be related to thoughts of wishing the child dead, especially when the demands of care seem overwhelming and unrelenting. Guilt may also be associated with religious beliefs. Some parents are convinced that they are being punished for some previous misdeed. Others may see the disorder as a sacrifice sent by God to test their religious strength and faith. It is always advisable to pursue the meaning of each person's religious background to identify hidden sources of guilt and punishment, as well as potential support. The ability to master resentful and self-accusatory feelings of having "caused" the child's disorder is a crucial factor in determining the parents' acceptance of their child.

Children, too, may interpret their serious illness as retribution for past misbehavior. The nurse should be particularly sensitive to the child who passively accepts all painful procedures. This child may believe that such acts are inflicted as deserved punishment. It is always vital to assure children that what happens to them during diagnosis or treatment is to make them better.

Other common reactions are bitterness or anger. Anger directed inward may be evident as self-reproaching or punitive behavior, such as neglecting one's health and verbally degrading oneself. Anger directed outward may be manifest in open arguments or withdrawal from communication and may be evident in the person's relationship with any number of individuals, such as the spouse, the child, and siblings. Passive anger toward the ill child may be evident in decreased visiting, refusal to believe how sick the child is, or inability to provide comfort. One of the most common targets for parental anger is members of the staff. Parents may complain about the nursing care, the insufficient time physicians spend with them, or the lack of skill of those who draw blood or start intravenous infusions.

Children are apt to respond with anger as well, and this includes the affected child, as well as the well siblings. Children are aware of the loss engendered by their illness or disability and may react angrily to the restrictions imposed or the feelings of being different. Siblings may also feel anger and resentment toward the ill child and parents for the loss of routine and parental attention. It is difficult for older children and almost impossible for younger children to comprehend the plight of the affected child. Their perception is of a brother or sister who has the undivided attention of their parents, is showered with cards and gifts, and is the focus of everyone's concern.

Children of various ages manifest anger differently. Young children may demonstrate their uncooperativeness by yelling, screaming, and physically fighting off the adversary. Older children may verbally express anger through abusive language. Passive anger, expressed in statements such as, "I don't know" or "I don't care," usually evokes aggressive anger in others. Such passive anger may be misinterpreted as sullen, obnoxious, or hostile reactions. As a result, these statements are effective in keeping people at a distance, when the hidden message really is, "I need to talk. Please help me understand what is happening."

A number of other reactions among family members, especially parents, are typical and include:

- **Lowered self-esteem,** in which parents perceive a defect in their child as a defect in themselves; their life goals may be abruptly and dramatically altered, and they lose the fantasy of immortality through their child
- **Shame,** in which parents anticipate social rejection, pity, or ridicule and related loss of social prestige and may experience social withdrawal
- **Ambivalence,** in which the simultaneous experience of love and hatred normally experienced by parents toward their children is likely to be greatly intensified
- **Depression,** in which parents experience chronic feelings of sorrow as a reaction to having an affected child; for example, to some parents mental retardation symbolizes the child's death and therefore precipitates a grief reaction
- **Self-sacrifice,** in which parents become acutely sensitive to implied criticism of their child and may react with resentment and belligerence, or they may deny the existence of the problem and seek professional opinions to substantiate their own belief that "there is really nothing wrong with our child"

During the period of adjustment, four types of parental reactions to the child influence the child's eventual response to the disorder (Box 22-2; see also p. 1008). The most common initial response, especially among mothers, is *benevolent overreaction* (Boone and Hartman, 1972). It is usually a consequence of unresolved guilt or fear, such as ambivalent feelings or not wanting the child during pregnancy, feeling responsible for the disorder, believing that

Box 22-2 PARENTAL RESPONSES THAT INFLUENCE CHILD RESPONSE TO DISORDER

Overprotection, in which the parents fear letting the child achieve any new skill, avoid all discipline, and cater to every desire to prevent frustration

Rejection, in which the parents detach themselves emotionally from the child but usually provide adequate physical care or constantly nag and scold the child

Denial, in which parents act is if the disorder does not exist or attempt to have the child overcompensate for it

Gradual acceptance, in which parents place necessary and realistic restrictions on the child, encourage self-care activities, and promote reasonable physical and social abilities

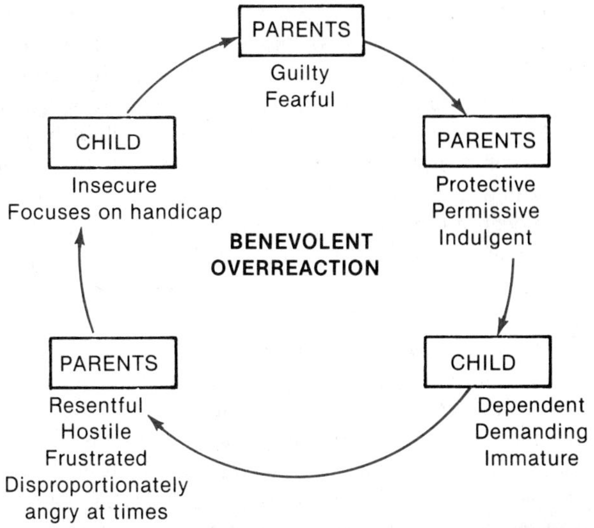

Fig. 22-1. Common cyclical response between parents and child.
From Boone, D.R., and Hartman, B.H.: Clin. Pediatr. 11(5):268-271, 1972.

Box 22-3 CHARACTERISTICS OF PARENTAL OVERPROTECTION

Sacrifices self and rest of family for the child
Continually helps the child, even when the child is capable
Is inconsistent with regard to discipline or employs no discipline; frequently different rules apply to the other siblings
Is dictatorial and arbitrary, making decisions without considering the child's wishes, such as keeping the child from attending school
Hovers and offers suggestions; calls attention to every activity, overdoing praise
Protects the child from every possible discomfort
Restricts play, often because of fear that the child will be injured
Denies the child opportunities for growing up and assuming responsibility, such as learning to give own medications or perform treatments
Does not understand the child's capabilities and sets goals too high or too low
Monopolizes the child's time, such as sleeping with the child, permitting few friends, or refusing participation in social or educational activities

the child would die at the time of birth or diagnosis, or reactivated feelings about a previous death of a loved one. It results in a vicious cycle of overprotective, permissive parent and dependent, demanding child (Fig. 22-1). It prevents the child from developing self-control, independence, initiative, and self-esteem. It is a reaction that responds to early intervention and prevention but is resistant to change once firmly established. Overprotection is so common a parental reaction that it behooves the nurse to assess for its presence and to begin counseling as soon as possible (Box 22-3). Many of these characteristics are also observed in vulnerable child syndrome and could occur or continue should the child recover from illness or injury (see Chapter 10).

Reintegration and Acknowledgment

For many families the last stage is characterized by realistic expectations for the child and reintegration of family life with the illness or disability in proper perspective. Since a large portion of this phase is one of grief for a loss, total resolution is not possible until the child dies or leaves home as an independent adult. Therefore one can regard adjustment to chronic sorrow as "increased comfortableness" with everyday living.

This adjustment phase also involves social reintegration in which the family broadens its activities to include relationships outside of the home, with the child as an acceptable and participating member of the group. This last criterion often differentiates the reaction of gradual acceptance during the adjustment period from total acceptance, or perhaps is more descriptive of the acknowledgment process.

One of the most important aspects of acceptance for health professionals to understand is that it is not an "all-or-none" phenomenon. Rather, it is interspersed with periods of intensified sorrow for the loss. Grieving is most likely seen at each period of the child's development. Parental feelings of recurrent grief resurface when the child experiences a situational or developmental crisis (Fraley, 1990) (Box 22-4). Consequently, even families who have achieved a high level of adjustment and acceptance are at predictable times in need of support from professionals or other families who have coped successfully with similar experiences.

Out-of-Home Placement

If strategies of coping cannot be employed to minimize the stress and disorganization of maintaining the child within the home to tolerable levels, the affected child may be permanently placed outside the home in a residential setting. Evolution of this phase is directly related to the degree of physical and mental disability.

This phase is not necessarily one of maladjustment. Placement may be the only option that will preserve the integrity of the family. Aging parents may be forced to accept this alternative from progressive inability to meet the demands imposed by a severe disability. Relinquishing the role of primary caregiver is followed by an initial sense of loss, relief, guilt, and ambivalence, a pattern of reactions not unlike that seen following the death of a terminally ill child (see Chapter 23).

IMPACT OF THE CHILD'S CHRONIC ILLNESS OR DISABILITY ON FAMILY MEMBERS

Each family who has a child with special needs is affected by the experience. The effects on the parents and their responses are so critical that they directly influence the other members' reactions. In addition, the extended family is affected, and their response, as well as the community's acceptance of the child, can further assist or hinder the fami-

Box 22-4 STRESSES OF FAMILIES WITH A CHILD WITH SPECIAL NEEDS

Day-to-Day Stresses
Constant attention
Reactions of other children and the larger community
Social relations
Effect on siblings
Marital relations

Life Maintenance Stresses
Financial stress, insurance
Housing
Transportation
Clothing and appliances
Need for support

Worries About the Future
Future children
Schooling and vocational training
Residential care

Anticipated Parental Stress Points
Diagnosis of the condition—requires considerable learning, as well as dealing with emotional response
Developmental milestones—times children normally achieve walking, talking, self-care are delayed or impossible for the child
Start of schooling—particularly stressful are situations in which appropriate schooling will not be in a regular class placement
Reaching the ultimate attainment—situations, such as realizing that ambulation will be impossible or that the child will not learn to read, must be handled
Adolescence—issues such as sexuality and independence become prominent
Future placement—decisions about placement must be made when the child becomes an adult or when the parents can no longer care for the child
Death of the child

Anticipated Sibling Stress Points
Birth of another child—may be the affected sibling or the subsequent birth of an unaffected child
Diagnosis of condition—in certain illnesses, times of remission and exacerbations are difficult
Start of schooling—particularly stressful if friends reject the child with special needs
Adolescence—when dating begins, may be embarrassed to bring dates home
Future placement—may worry about responsibility for the affected sibling, especially if the parents are ill or die
Death of the child

ly's coping with the stresses imposed by caring for a child with special needs.

Parents

Besides grieving for the loss of a perfect child, parents may or may not receive positive feedback from transactions with their child. Many parents feel satisfaction and fulfillment from the parenting role. For others, parenting may be a series of unrewarding experiences, which continually support the parents' feelings of inadequacy and failure. These responses may be most evident in parents who are responsible for the child's care. For example, they may become preoccupied with their ability to carry out certain procedures, overlooking the child's personal comfort and satisfaction or failing to offer praise for anything less than perfect cooperation or performance. They may pursue a frustrating activity until they achieve "success"—long after the child has become irritable and uncooperative. As a result, the parent can become caught in a pattern of interaction that is mutually unrewarding and minimally productive. For these parents it may be beneficial to reduce the quantity of time spent with the child to increase the quality of the relationship.

Parental roles. Excessive demands may be placed on parental time, energy, and financial resources. Depending on the roles assumed by each spouse, the wife often receives the brunt of the time and energy demands, and the husband the financial responsibilities. However, with changing sex roles these responsibilities may be shared or shifted more heavily to one member. In a shared approach, parents often divide tasks in a very specific way, according to their skills or level of comfort. For example, the parent with patience for waiting may be the logical person to take the child for tests, examinations, and procedures. The parent who deals best with the sickness and side effects of treatment can ready the environment for the child's return home. It is important for nurses to realize that the absence of one parent from the hospital or clinic does not necessarily indicate that the shared parent pattern is not in effect (Clements, Copeland, and Loftus, 1990).

In other families changing sex roles mean added responsibilities for one parent. For example, the working mother may feel the need to continue employment to help defray the expenses, but she also incurs the added burden of additional child/home responsibilities.

The result can eventually be marital conflicts as one partner views his or her share as unequal (see Questions and Controversies). In addition, the partner who is not included in the caregiving activities may feel neglected, since all the attention is directed toward the child, and resentful that he or she is not sufficiently informed to be competent in the care. Without active participation in the care of the child, the parent has little appreciation of the time and energy involved in performing those activities. When the less competent partner does attempt to participate, the other parent frequently criticizes the less skillful efforts. As a result, communication breaks down and neither is able to support the other. Unfortunately, the problems are seldom recognized until they are well established rather than early, when intervention can be most effective.

Communication tends to be centered on the affected child, with mothers typically assuming the role of interpreter between the child and other family members. This, combined with mothers' heavy investment in the caregiving role, leads to a very close relationship between the child and parent, usually the mother. However, problems frequently arise as the mother interferes with the child's functioning at maximum potential (Cleveland, 1980). Levels of stress appear to be related to the ease with which mothers can relate to their child and the demands their children make on them. Feelings of restriction and social isolation

QUESTIONS AND CONTROVERSIES

What are the effects on the marriage of having a child who is chronically ill or disabled?

Numerous reports in the literature support the finding that having a child with special needs places additional stress on the marriage. Reviews of current research document that increased marital discord is common among the partners and that other negative effects include feelings of low self-esteem, helplessness, and unmet dependency needs among the spouses. However, in a review of 34 published papers on the impact of chronic illness on marital adjustment, Leventhal and Sabbeth (1986) found that divorce rates in families with chronic illness were not substantially higher than those for the general population, even though higher levels of marital distress were reported. Other studies that have examined well-matched groups of families and those that have been careful to include as many eligible families as possible have generally found no differences (Kazak, 1989). The stressors often cited as having an impact on the marriage are (1) the home care program with the burden of care assumed by primarily one parent, (2) the financial burden, (3) the fear of the child dying, (4) pressure from relatives, (5) the hereditary nature of the disease (if applicable), and (6) fear of pregnancy. Other causes of tension often center on the inconveniences associated with care, such as long waiting for appointments, lack of parking near care facilities, or lack of overnight accommodations (Kalnins, 1983). Certainly, these last stressors are within health professionals' domain to minimize, if not eliminate.

Kazak (1989) suggests that families of children with chronic conditions who make poor adjustments to the illness are those that had more problematic levels of adjustment before the illness. A couple's marital functioning before the birth or diagnosis of a child with special needs may well be the best predictor of long-term marital adjustment.

add further stress (Byrne and Cummingham, 1985), thus compounding the negative aspects of an overly close and exclusive relationship with the affected child.

Mother/father differences. Mothers and fathers in the same family appear to experience distinct differences in adjusting and coping as parents of a child with special needs. In a survey of parents of children with Down syndrome, 68% of the mothers reported a peaks-and-valleys periodic crisis pattern, whereas 83% of the fathers depicted their adjustment in terms of steady, gradual recovery (Damrosch and Perry, 1989).

The father of a child with special needs struggles with issues that may be quite distinct from those of the mother (Association for the Care of Children's Health, 1990). He may feel that his role of protector is challenged because he does not know how to help and cannot protect the family from the seemingly overwhelming recurring problems. Dreams of lineage, ego fulfillment, and athletic and vocational achievement are threatened and, in turn, may threaten the father's self-esteem. Because the traditional paternal role, particularly with sons, emphasizes joint recreation over caregiving, fathers seem to have more difficulty adjusting to a son with special needs than to a daughter with special needs. With today's increased emphasis on fathers' involvement in the lives of their children, this loss is felt more profoundly than in the past. The extensive stresses in the family can leave the father feeling depressed, weak, guilty, powerless, isolated, embarrassed, and very angry. Yet, fearful that he will lose control or be viewed as weak or ineffectual, the father will often hide his feelings and display an outward confidence that may lead others to believe that everything is fine. Feelings are further exacerbated by a health care system that frequently excludes and disregards men. Too often the father feels like an afterthought in the care of his child (May, 1990).

Fathers worry about what the future holds for their children, as well as about the ability to manage the increasing financial burden. Some fathers escape in their work as a means for dulling the pain. Others view all of the difficulties of having a child with special needs as challenges to overcome and are not afraid to push limits and be assertive to acquire the needed services for their children (May, 1990).

Single-parent families. Single-parent families are of special concern. The absence of a parent may be due to divorce or death, or the parents may never have married. As the only parent of a child who may require extensive, sophisticated, and lifelong care, the single parent may feel an enormous burden. Nurses must recognize that external sources of support and personal inner strength are particularly crucial for single parents to enable them to care for their child (Clements, Copeland, and Loftus, 1990).

Siblings

Siblings can be deeply affected by the affected child's membership in the family. Younger siblings in particular may be affected because they are uprooted and displaced more than older children. For example, firstborn children with cognitive impairment become the "youngest" by virtue of their developmental age. Conversely, second-born children become the oldest, often shouldering adultlike responsibilities and achieving parental expectations that would have been reserved for the eldest.

Siblings are likely to show symptoms of irritability, social withdrawal, and fear for their own health. Healthy siblings may have a wide variety of physical complaints, such as headache, abdominal pain, or symptoms mimicking those of the sick or disabled child, as a reflection of their anxiety and fear. Their reactions to the child often do not parallel the severity of the condition. The family's financial and social resources available to deal with the implications of the child's condition are believed to be more important factors (Lobato, 1990; Powell and Ogle, 1985).

Most parents can identify specific behaviors in well children that have a negative effect on the family, such as jealousy, increased competition and fighting among siblings, anger, hostility, social withdrawal, attention-seeking behavior, and a decline in school performance. However, positive behaviors are also cited, such as increased nurturing, cooperation, sensitivity, compassion, and mastery of new skills. Sibling constellation variables such as age spacing and birth order appear to play an important role in sibling adjustment. The closer the siblings are in age, the more fertile the ground for competition and rivalry (Wagner, Schubert, and Schubert, 1985). The number of children in the family is also considered a factor. Siblings in families with three or more children are more likely to develop the characteristics of tolerance and understanding (Lobato, 1990). The trend of having only two children 2 to 3 years apart may place many of today's siblings at greater risk for poor adjustment (Rollins, 1990).

Siblings reveal feelings of isolation, deprivation, inferiority, and inadequate knowledge about the child's condition. Their lives are most affected in terms of the parent-child relationship, the medical care and treatment, and play and socialization. For example, the greatest effect of the ill child on the well siblings is a feeling of isolation and of being outside the parent(s)/sick child dyad. This is often increased by social restriction in peer relationships because of additional responsibilities in the home. Many siblings report receiving rewards in terms of "bribes" to overlook shortcomings in their parent-child relationship, but few receive any reward in the form of praise, personal attention, or tangible items. They often feel left out and uninvolved in the child's care, especially when the child is treated away from home. In particular, they report feeling ignored by health care members. One study found that while 89% of siblings interviewed had some information about their brother's or sister's medical condition, the amount of knowledge varied greatly, as did accuracy (Tritt and Esses, 1988). Extent of knowledge and understanding did not differ as a function of age. In some cases there seemed to be an unspoken family rule about not asking questions.

While sibling constellation and characteristics of an illness or disability seem to play a role in sibling adjustment, research suggests that the ways family members feel about one another and cope with stress play the major roles in sibling adjustment (Lobato, 1990). Such findings emphasize that although positive, maturing attitudes can form in these siblings, the responsibility of health professionals is to involve the entire family unit in the adjustment process.

Extended Family Members and Society

Two other groups of people may experience the effects of a child's chronic illness or disability: (1) the significant nonnuclear family members or friends and (2) society as a whole. Although extended family relationships are often helpful to parents in rearing a child with special needs, they may also be sources of stress (Byrne and Cunningham, 1985). Grandparents may have far more difficulty in accepting the diagnosis than the parents themselves do, and parents may have concerns about the best way in which to respond to the grandparents' anger over the diagnosis or criticism regarding parental care. For example, grandparents or other well-meaning relatives may attempt to reassure the parents that the child "will grow out of" his or her slowness at a time when parents are struggling to accept reality.

Nurses need to remember that grandparents often experience a double grief, both for their grandchild and for their child, the parent. The future is now unpredictable not only for the grandchild, but for the child's parents as well. Grandparents do not often acknowledge these emotions, and they are left to adapt on their own (Vadasy, 1987).

Although society's views of individuals with chronic illness or disability are changing toward a more accepting, nonjudgmental, and open attitude, parents, siblings, and the affected child frequently are victims of prejudice, ostracism, or criticism. A great deal of this stems from public ignorance and fear, and this remains a crucial area for intervention by health professionals.

FACTORS AFFECTING THE FAMILY'S ADJUSTMENT

The diagnosis of a child with a serious health problem or disability is a major situational crisis that tremendously affects the entire family system. However, families can experience positive outcomes as they successfully deal with the many challenges that accompany a child with chronic illness or disability (Futcher, 1988). One nursing goal is to assess which families are at greater or lesser risk for succumbing to the effects of the crisis. Six variables—available support system, perception of the event, coping mechanisms, reactions to the child, available resources, and concurrent stresses within the family—influence the resolution of a crisis. Although researchers suggest that approximately 85% of families cope well, the needs of families at risk are great (Schulman, 1983). If they receive emotional support and guidance early, there is an increased likelihood that they will also cope successfully.

Although it is easy to assume that families of children with the most severe illnesses or disabilities would have the poorest adjustment, the severity of the condition reflects only one part of the overall picture. The level of adjustment is significantly influenced by the *functional burden* on the individual family (Stein, 1985). This concept considers the issues related to caring for and living with the child in relation to the family's resources and ability to cope (Box 22-5). Thus, the family of a child with multiple disabilities demanding complex care—yet having many resources and coping skills—may adjust more successfully to his or her situation than the family of a child with a less serious condition and a paucity of resources to counter the balance.

Available Support System

The significant others who are available to individuals for emotional strength during periods of crisis comprise their support system. Support systems may be available through a variety of relationships and may consist of one significant other, such as a marital partner, or a group of significant others, such as the extended family or members of the health team.

Research indicates that the source of support is a determining factor in the effectiveness of certain forms of support, suggesting that professionals should provide different types of support than those provided by family and friends (Woods, Yates, and Primomo, 1989). Lin (1986) proposed that expressive support is best provided by individuals with whom one has strong ties and who are like oneself. On the

Box 22-5 CONCEPT OF FUNCTIONAL BURDEN

Impact of Child with Special Needs
The child's need for medical and nursing care
The child's fixed deficits
The child's age-inappropriate dependency in activities of daily living
The disruptions caused by the care in the family routine
The psychologic burden of the prognosis on the family

Family Resources and Ability to Cope
The family's physical resources
The family's emotional resources
The family's educational resources
The family's social supports and available help
The competing demands for family members' time and energy

Data from Stein, R.E.K.: Home care: a challenging opportunity, Child. Health Care 14(2):90-95, 1985.

other hand, instrumental support can best be provided by those to whom the family has weaker ties and who can link the family to a broader, more diverse social network. Therefore, the most appropriate sources of informational support might include both professionals who have theoretic and practical knowledge and nonprofessionals—parents—whose experience equips them as experts. When professionals develop a strong therapeutic relationship with the family, they, too, can be appropriate sources of emotional support (see discussion on parent-professional partnerships, pp. 995 and 1015).

Although a support system exists, it may not be effective unless the individual is able to use the system through mutual channels of communication.

Status of the marital relationship. The marital relationship is a prime source of potential support and overall is considered the best predictor of coping behavior and adjustment (Kazak, 1989; Trute, 1990). When the spouses can openly discuss their feelings, there tend to be much less guilt, anger, blame, and indecision. Each crisis during the long period of chronic illness is successfully resolved, lessening the accumulation and overlapping of multiple stresses.

Alternate support systems. Support systems may be available with significant others outside the marital relationship. For example, the single-parent family may have the support of extended family, such as that of the parent's own parents. Occasionally parents may be able to communicate with each other but are unable to talk with the child. This is particularly evident with very young children, who communicate least through verbalization, and with adolescents, who may be unwilling to discuss with or listen to adults. In this case the child is left without an available support system.

Ability to communicate. Besides the availability of significant others, family members must have the ability to use the support system. Almost all methods of psychologic intervention, such as support through active listening, counseling, or crisis intervention, require verbal communication between two individuals. The ability to verbalize about feelings such as anger, fear, guilt, or anxiety helps individuals cope with the particular emotion. Verbalization allows for validation of feelings and thoughts.

Not all individuals are able to communicate verbally. Some rely on religious faith and silent prayers for support. Others, such as children, communicate best through nonverbal methods, such as play, drawing, or writing. Some individuals may not be able to communicate with anyone because of their interpersonal withdrawal and social isolation. These individuals are most at risk because, even if a support system is available, they may be unable to share their problems with others.

Perception of the Illness/Disability

The meaning and significance of the child's condition are influenced by the individual's perception of the diagnosis. In particular, the association of guilt may complicate one's ability to realistically view the death and ultimately resolve the grief. Guilt implies a degree of control over one's actions. The more guilt an individual has, the more control that person perceives in the prevention or alteration of the diagnosis. Assessment of specific perceptions concerning the illness or disability aids in evaluating the individual's ability to cope with various aspects of the crisis and identifies possible areas for intervention.

Previous knowledge. Although family members may be shocked to learn that their child has a serious illness or disability, they usually have some knowledge about the disorder from previous associations. It is important to explore the extent of that information, since there is a great tendency to compare the recently disclosed facts with the other knowledge. Because research indicates that people generally act in accordance with their beliefs, it is important to know what parents believe about their child's medical condition and if their beliefs are based on accurate information (Austin, 1990).

Influence of religion. Religious beliefs and spirituality have various meanings for different people. For some, religion comprises the foundation of their support system—all of life revolves around their relationship with God. Healing and faith are synonymous, and any criticism of the family's spirituality can weaken their trust in the medical care. For others, it may intensify feelings of guilt, shame, bitterness, or punishment. For example, some individuals may interpret the illness as a punishment from God. They may exclaim, "What have I done to deserve this?" or "God, why are you punishing me in this way?" It is important to take such statements seriously and to explore reasons why the person believes that this is a punishment.

Imagined cause. Although the cause of many disorders is unknown, parents and children usually supply their own answers. Sometimes this is associated with religious beliefs, but it may also be influenced by previous events. For example, children may interpret the reason for the illness as a punishment for not obeying others. Parents may be convinced that the disease was inherited. Sometimes there is a strong belief in curses, occult witchcraft, or devils as perpetrators of the disorder. Once the fantasied cause is revealed, the person can be helped to deal with the irrationalities of that thinking and, hopefully, will be relieved of feelings of guilt, blame, or anger.

Effects on the family. How the child's illness or disability affects the family reveals how its members perceive the event. For example, the following statements could represent a particular reaction:

- **Denial:** "Everything is the same as it always was."
- **Inability to express feelings:** "We have more *things* to do."
- **Anger, blame, or bitterness:** "We never should have had children."
- **Resentment and hostility:** "My sister gets everything because she is sick."
- **Acceptance and ability to express feelings:** "The perspective of time has changed because we realize how precious and limited it is."

Coping Mechanisms

Coping mechanisms are those behaviors aimed at reducing the tension caused by a crisis. *Approach behaviors* are those coping mechanisms that result in movement toward adjustment and resolution of the crisis. *Avoidance behaviors* result in movement away from adjustment or maladaptation to the crisis. Several approach and avoidance behaviors used in coping with a chronic illness or disability are listed in Box 22-6. None of the indices can be used singly to assess the possible success or failure in resolving the crisis. Each behavior must be viewed in the context of all the variables affecting the family. For example, the observation of several avoidance behaviors in an emotionally healthy family may denote significantly less risk to the successful resolution of the crisis than an equal number of avoidance behaviors in a poorly adjusted family or in an individual who has few available supports.

Two long-term coping strategies of familial adaptation to chronic and severe childhood illness have been significantly associated with a high level of family functioning (Venters, 1981). The first is the parents' ability to endow the illness with meaning within an existing spiritual or medical/scientific philosophy of life. There is an optimistic belief that all things work out for the good and a focus on the positive qualities of the situation. Statements such as "God has chosen our family to care for this special child" are reflective of the religious philosophy.

The second is an ability to share the burdens of the illness with individuals both inside and outside the family constellation. Intrafamilial relationships encourage togetherness of the family members and maintain a mutual acknowledgment that all members are important contributors to the family unit. Extrafamilial supports help preserve meaningful external contacts and provide needed help to the family.

Reactions to previous crises. Exploring the way in which a family dealt with a previous crisis identifies their possible reactions to the present stressful event. The type of family structure frequently offers valuable clues to the general approach the family may use to solve the crisis.

In the authoritarian family one or both parents decide what is best for all its members. As a result, the type of coping behavior demonstrated is usually chosen by a specific individual, regardless of others' needs. In the laissez-faire family new coping mechanisms may be explored, but family members offer little direction, approval, or validation of the effectiveness of the behavior. In the authoritative or democratic family there are flexibility and respect for each other's opinions, although the adults exercise direction and guidance for decision making. This type of family usually

Box 22-6 GUIDELINES FOR ASSESSING COPING BEHAVIORS

Approach Behaviors

Asks for information regarding diagnosis and child's present condition
Seeks help and support from others
Anticipates future problems; actively seeks guidance and answers
Endows the illness or disability with meaning
Shares burden of disorder with others
Plans realistically for the future
Acknowledges and accepts child's awareness of diagnosis and prognosis
Expresses feelings, such as sorrow, depression, and anger, and realizes reason for the emotional reaction
Realistically perceives child's condition; adjusts to changes
Recognizes own growth through passage of time, such as earlier denial and nonacceptance of diagnosis
Verbalizes possible loss of child

Avoidance Behaviors

Fails to recognize seriousness of child's condition despite physical evidence
Refuses to agree to treatment
Intellectualizes about the illness, but in areas unrelated to child's condition
Is angry and hostile to members of the staff, regardless of their attitude or behavior
Avoids staff, family members, or child
Entertains unrealistic future plans for child, with little emphasis on the present
Is unable to adjust to or accept a change in progression of disease
Continually looks for new cures with no perspective toward possible benefit
Refuses to acknowledge child's understanding of disease and prognosis
Uses magical thinking and fantasy, may seek "occult" help
Places complete faith in religion to point of relinquishing own responsibility
Withdraws from outside world; refuses help
Punishes self because of guilt and blame
Makes no change in life-style to meet needs of other family members
Resorts to excessive use of alcohol or drugs to avoid problems
Verbalizes suicidal intents
Is unable to discuss possible loss of child or previous experiences with death

demonstrates the most ability in exploring new coping mechanisms that are aimed at successful resolution of the crisis for the ultimate benefit of the entire family.

Reactions to the Child

An awareness of the family members' reactions to the child is important and can uncover the type of childrearing practices or attitudes that may not only hamper the child's optimum development but also influence the family's adjustment (see Table 22-1 for assessment questions). Parental reactions are driven by feelings such as guilt, love, fear, power, shame, pride, pity, concern, and confusion. These reactions in turn affect attitudes and choice of childrearing practices, which can cause resounding effects throughout the family system.

Available Resources

Resources are the available means that exist or can be developed either within the family members, the family unit, or in the community. For example, nurses can consider family members' age, intelligence, education, willingness and ability to learn the child's care, sense of humor, and sense of optimism as resources they can bring to a situation. Resources within the family unit include cohesion, adaptability, sense of coherence, and hardiness—these are aspects of the family system that can help considerably in the family's adjustment (McCubbin, 1988).

Community resources, such as health care resources, parent support groups, availability of respite care, alternatives for schooling, and educational facilities and recreational programs, are key elements in family adjustment. These kinds of resources are better developed in some areas than in others, meaning that what is available to a family depends largely on where they live. In an urban area, families of children with special needs may find a greater number of programs and services for their children. The rural setting, however, may offer more social support because of a greater sense of community and less anonymity (Patterson, in press). Communities, like families, have different strengths.

How well the community meets the needs of families of children with special needs is influenced not only by the location of the community but by a balanced fit between family and community needs and resources. This fit is best achieved when the attitudes and beliefs shared by professionals in the community create a community climate or atmosphere that is supportive and empowering of families. Nurses who work with families of children with special needs are in unique positions to build professional understanding of family-centered care.

✦ **NURSING ALERT** Be aware that many families—nearly half of the families in a recent survey—do not have a telephone, a service most practitioners consider essential for families of children with special needs (Wissow and Warshow, 1990). Other families may have telephones but are reluctant to reveal the telephone number. To overcome these difficulties, use the following strategies:

Help family identify telephone access close to home (e.g., neighbor's home, nearby store).

Explore methods to obtain telephone service for the family (e.g., social service agencies, charitable organizations).

Be sensitive to family's concern for privacy when asking for a telephone number; explain reason for needing number and to whom it will be given.

Concurrent Stresses Within the Family

The ability to deal with the already overwhelming stresses of a lifelong disability or illness is challenged when additional stresses are present. Ongoing stresses and strains in the family "pile up," increasing the family's vulnerability and reducing its ability to adapt and adjust to a child with special needs. For some family members, non-disease-related stressors are perceived as more stressful than those associated with a child's chronic condition. In a study of siblings of children with cancer, concurrent stressors—such as the pending remarriage of a parent—appeared to be causing some siblings more concern than having a brother or sister with cancer (Rollins, 1990).

Stressors may be situational or developmental. They may be related to marital difficulties, financial pressures, homelessness, or social isolation. With the alarming increase in drug abuse and reports ranging from one household in three to one in five reporting alcohol-related problems (Gallup, 1986; NACOA charts, 1983), it is reasonable to assume that 20% to 33% of the families may be struggling with a family member's alcohol or other drug problem. Even the more minor stresses such as arranging care for siblings, managing the home, and traveling to distant treatment centers can jeopardize the family's ability to cope successfully (see also Box 22-4).

Child or family developmental stressors predictably compound situational stress. For example, a common developmental stressor in the family life cycle is the birth of a first child, an event that requires adaptation by the spouse dyad. The birth of a child with a congenital health problem adds situational stress to the equation (Harber, 1989).

IMPACT OF CHRONIC ILLNESS OR DISABILITY ON THE CHILD

The child's reaction to chronic illness or disability depends to a great extent on his or her developmental level, temperament, and available coping mechanisms; on the reactions of significant others; and to a lesser extent on the condition itself. Knowledge of these variables is essential in providing the kind of support needed by these children to cope with a sometimes overwhelming situation.

Developmental Aspects

The impact of a chronic illness or disability is influenced by the age of onset. Chronic illness affects children of all ages, but the developmental aspects of each age-group dictate particular stresses and risks for the child. The nurse must also recognize that children need to redefine their condition and its implications as they develop and grow. An understanding of these factors facilitates planning care to support the child and minimize the risks (see also Table 22-2).

Infancy. During infancy the child is engaged in the task of developing trust, which necessitates a reciprocal satisfying relationship between child and parent. When illness or disability occurs, this relationship is potentially affected. For example, a visible defect can retard parent bonding as the parent mourns the loss of the perfect child. In addition, prolonged illness may impose separations that prevent the child and parent from normal attachment and deprive the infant of the nurturing relationship.

The illness itself affects the infant, especially since sensorimotor experiences are critical at this age. Illness and/or disability often impairs the child's motor abilities, confining the child to a crib and lessening contact with the environment. Certainly the messages transmitted to infants about their body are influenced by the amount of pain and discomfort they experience. Associating touch with pain can compromise the infant's ability to give and receive affection. Lack of pleasurable sensations can lead to an irritable and unhappy child. Consequently, parents may interpret the behaviors as evidence that they are inadequate in meeting the child's physical and emotional needs, which further affects the parent-child relationship and the acquisition of trust.

To compensate for some of these feelings, parents, especially the mother, may become overly involved with the infant and promote increased dependency. This is significant during infancy when one of the tasks is separation and individuation from the parent. Such a response hinders the child's future self-development and often leads to the pattern of marked dependency, fearfulness, and passivity. One of the critical aspects of this pattern is that it is amenable to change if intervention is begun *early*.

Toddler. The toddler is in the stage of autonomy; the need for mastery of locomotor and language skills is paramount. The child learning to walk and talk progresses toward becoming a separate person, both physically and psychologically. However, illness or disability can hinder mobility and deprive the child of mastery. In addition, the parents' overprotection can magnify the problem by setting limits on the child's exploration and experimentation for fear of injury or exertion. Even the most basic self-help skills, such as feeding and dressing, may be done for the child. Age-appropriate tasks such as toilet training may be delayed. With such limited opportunities for testing mastery, children soon fear to venture on their own and develop little confidence in their abilities. Over time they may feel defeated and become apathetic, passive, and clinging (Perrin and Gerrity, 1984).

Illness can impose separations that are detrimental to the toddler. Like the infant, separation is the most anxiety-producing event for toddlers. A chronic illness or disability can necessitate repeated hospitalizations and painful procedures. If the need to preserve the parent-child relationship is not appreciated, the child may become depressed and eventually detach from the parent. Children seem to have a tremendous capacity to withstand stress, provided their attachment to the parent is preserved.

Preschooler. The preschooler is in the stage of initiative; numerous tasks are achieved during this age that can be severely hampered by chronic illness and disability. Impairment can limit the preschooler's learning about the environment, especially in terms of social development. Rather than being encouraged to play with peers and participate in nursery school activities, the chronically ill preschooler may be confined to the home with socialization limited to the secure and tolerant family. Immature behavior may be tolerated because age-appropriate standards and discipline are not enforced. Consequently, when paired with children the same age or placed in school, the child is deficient in knowing how to act and can easily be criticized by peers who view him or her as a "baby." In fact, the child's illness or disability may provoke much less criticism than his or her inappropriate behavior. Faced with such reactions from others in contrast to the security of the home, the child may gradually choose a life of social isolation and loneliness, especially during the school-age years.

One of the major tasks of this period is establishing sexual identity, and one of the principal methods is through imitation of sex-related activities. However, the sick child may have fewer opportunities to engage in such activity and may view the parent predominantly in the caregiving role, since this may be the focus of their relationship. In some families it is expected that the mother will assume the care of the child while the father provides the financial base by working outside the home. This can limit the child's identification with the male role.

In addition to sexual identity, the child's body image is forming. Children's knowledge of their body image is limited to what they see, feel, and use. If the child is chronically ill, body awareness is focused on the body's causing pain and anxiety. The child with a disability may have difficulty forming a mental image of impaired body parts, such as paralyzed extremities. This poorly developed sense of body integrity makes children especially fearful of intrusive or mutilating experiences, which can be frequent during prolonged illness.

One of the more critical influences of chronic illness or disability on preschoolers is the feeling of guilt that they "caused" the condition by a real or imagined misdeed (Gratz and Piliavin, 1984). This is probably less of a factor if the child is born with the disorder than if it occurs during the preschool years. Such guilt can greatly affect the child's developing but fragile self-esteem. Unlike the child with a temporary physical impairment who has additional opportunities for achieving mastery and thus overcoming feelings of guilt and inferiority, the child with a chronic illness or disability experiences continual insults. Unless situations are structured for success, life can become a series of failures—of never being strong enough or good enough to compete with peers.

School-age child. The child of school age is striving to achieve a sense of accomplishment while overcoming a sense of inferiority. Successful mastery of this task depends on the child's ability to cooperate and to compete with others. Consequently, physical impairments can greatly affect the ability to achieve and compete. For example, physical disability may hinder participation in sports and repeated absences from school caused by illness can place the child at an academic disadvantage. To repeat a grade can saddle the child with feelings of shame, inadequacy, and inferiority. However, the decision to remain in the same grade can also enhance feelings of success because the work requirements may be easier and new classmates provide a second chance for forming friendships.

During this age there is a transition from relationships with family members to strong identification with peers. Peers increasingly influence school-age children's view of themselves and their self-esteem. Anything that labels children as "different" can affect their sense of belonging to the group. Many children cope with their "differentness" by retreating from socialization. As they draw farther from the group, their sense of belonging diminishes, and intense loneliness and isolation dominate. However, if they are helped to deal with their feelings of not being "normal and perfect" and to recognize their unique abilities, these children can cope very well. It is to be expected that all children are unable to master every task and that they will feel some degree of inferiority. If this is stressed to children with physical impairment, the burden to achieve is lessened.

As school-age children identify more with the peer group and authority figures outside the home, there is a concurrent striving for independence from the family. However, the ill child may be forced into an extended period of dependency either from the disorder or from parental overprotectiveness. Attempts to demonstrate independence may be manifest as resentment toward the parents, refusal to comply with treatment, or risk-taking behavior, such as cheating on the special diet. If parents can understand that these behaviors represent a normal phase of development, they may be more tolerant and able to find appropriate outlets for independence (e.g., increasing child's responsibility for home care or increasing child's control in non-disease-related activities).

Adolescence. The impact of illness or disability can be most detrimental during adolescence. Before this age, the child's self-image, self-esteem, and basic adjustment to life were primarily dependent on his or her relationship with the parents. A young child with impaired health reared in a home with loving parents who are sensitive to the child's needs generally copes well with the disorder. However, adolescence is different—even with all the benefits of parental love, the adolescent is striving for an independence away from parents and in many ways must deal with the impact of impairment alone.

The major task of adolescents is to establish an identity of their own. Pubertal changes must be integrated into the self-image while the teenager is gaining control and mastery over increased physical capabilities and sexuality. During early adolescence this takes place primarily within the peer group. Illness or injury at this time interferes with teenagers' sense of mastery and control over a changing body. They are different at a stage of development when being different is unacceptable to the peer group, who may view a disability in one member as a threat to the established uniformity by which all are measured. At no time of life is an individual so vulnerable to the emotional stress of biologic impairment (Hofmann, 1980). Appearance, skills, and abilities are highly valued by peers; a teenager who is limited in any of these qualities is subject to rejection by this important group. This is especially marked when a physical disability interferes with sexual attractiveness.

These teenagers are faced with the task of incorporating their disability into the changing self-concept. The youngster who develops the illness or acquires the disability during the crucial adolescent years has more difficulty accomplishing this task than does the teenager who has been affected since childhood. It appears that the earlier the onset of a limiting condition, the better the individual is able to adapt to it. The youngster with a newly acquired disorder will have the additional task of grieving for a lost "perfection" while adjusting to the changes taking place as a natural course of events. The teenager often feels rejected because of personal appearance or an inability to engage in activities expected of a healthy adolescent (Coupey and Cohen, 1980). The threat is greatest during middle adolescence, when the teenager has less available energy to cope with illness, since emotional resources are being used to meet the normal demands of this developmental phase.

The severity, type, and visibility of the illness also influence the adjustment process and appear to be sex related. Boys seem to be more concerned about diseases or therapies that interfere with their ability to function independently and to achieve vocational and academic goals. Consequently, they may tolerate wearing a visible device or having a somewhat altered appearance as long as their physical and academic goals are not affected; for them confinement and restricted independence are less tolerable. While girls, too, are concerned about issues of independence and vocational and academic goals, they seem more upset by conditions that they perceive to interfere with their ability to attract important others and maintain relationships. Thus they are more likely to tolerate restriction of movement and confinement, provided they continue to look attractive; however, disorders or treatments that affect their appearance are devastating (Coupey and Cohen, 1984).

Adolescence is a time for achieving independence from the family and planning for future goals and responsibilities. Adolescents with long-term chronic illness tend to be less future directed and less independent than well peers (Orr and others, 1984). Enforced dependency from physical impairment can exacerbate the parent-child conflicts surrounding independence. Lack of understanding from both parties can result in bitter feelings and intrafamilial turmoil. The tendency toward rebellion may be directed at the disorder and reflected in decreased compliance with treatment, denying the disorder to preserve a sense of normalcy with peers, and risk-taking behavior that can place the teenager in jeopardy, such as driving a car despite a disorder that increases the chance of an injury. Such behaviors can further strain an already tense parent-child relationship.

Coping Mechanisms

Children's innate and learned coping mechanisms are very important in their ability to deal with their disorder. In a study of well children, their most common response to daily stressors was submission or endurance—quite possibly a fairly accurate view of the children's realization that they have little sense of control over daily life (Sorenson, 1990). Individual characteristics that influence a child's ability to cope with stress are listed in Box 22-7. In addition to these variables, the social support afforded these children is critically important. Therefore the better the family copes, the better the child is able to deal with the stressors imposed by the illness or disability.

Because it is often easier to recognize children who cope poorly with illness or disability, it is helpful to describe those behaviors typical of well-adjusted children. Well-adapted children gradually learn to accept their physical limitations but find achievement in a variety of compensatory motor and intellectual pursuits. They function well at home, at school, and with peers. They have an understanding of their disorder that allows them to accept their limitations, assume responsibility for care, and assist in treatment and rehabilitation regimens.

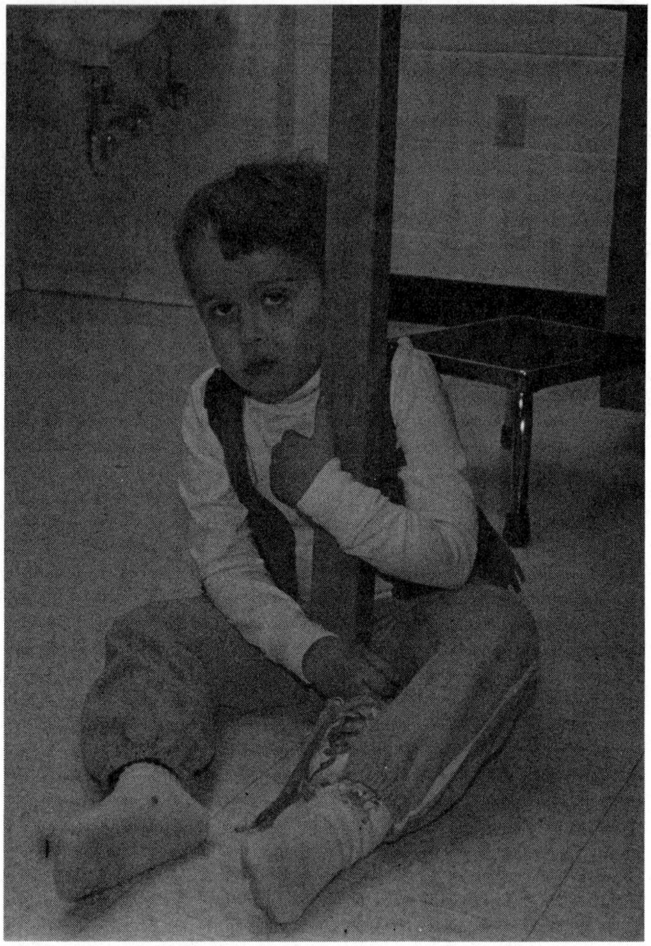

Fig. 22-2. Periods of sadness and anger are appropriate in the child's adjustment to a chronic illness or disability, especially during exacerbations of the disorder.

They express appropriate emotions, such as sadness, anxiety, and anger at times of exacerbations but confidence and guarded optimism during periods of clinical stability (Fig. 22-2). They are able to identify with other similarly affected individuals, promoting positive self-images and displaying pride and self-confidence in their ability to master a productive, successful life despite the disability.

Box 22-7 INDIVIDUAL CHARACTERISTICS THAT AFFECT COPING IN CHILDREN

Gender
Males are more vulnerable to stress than females.
Females are more likely to use emotional sensory and emotional expression responses than boys.
Males are more likely to use physical aggression in coping.

Age
Children between ages 6 months and 4 years are considered most vulnerable.

Temperament
The "difficult child" is considered more vulnerable than the easy child.
The more active, strong-willed child seems to cope better than the passive child.

Preexisting Conditions
The child with preexisting anxiety is considered at greater risk for coping poorly.

Self-Concept
The child with low self-esteem and/or a low sense of self-direction is at greater risk for coping poorly.

Social Skills
The child with few social skills is at greater risk for coping poorly.

Genetic Factors
Inborn traits influence the overall ability to adapt (e.g., vulnerability to alcoholism, sociopathy, mood disorders).

Intelligence
Children with above-average intelligence tend to have fewer psychiatic problems than children with lower intelligence.

References: Adams and Fras, 1988; Rutter, 1983; Sorenson, 1990.

Responses to Parental Behavior

The parents' behavior toward the child, especially in terms of childrearing, is one of the most important influencing factors in the child's adjustment. For example, children whose parents are overprotective tend to have marked dependency, especially on the mother, fearfulness, inactivity, and lack of outside interests. Children who are raised by oversolicitous and guilt-ridden parents are often overly independent, defiant, and high-risk takers. Children who are reared by parents who emphasize their deficits and tend to "hide" or isolate them appear as shy and lonely individuals who harbor resentful and hostile attitudes toward normal persons. In contrast, children who are reared by parents who establish reasonable limits tend to develop independence that is appropriate for their age and achievement commensurate with their limitations. They often display pride and confidence in their ability to cope successfully with the challenges imposed by their disorder.

A common consequence of parental behaviors is progressive control of family functioning by the affected child. Perhaps the most critical factor is the control the child has over the emotional reactions of family members. Many of these children have the ability to cause emotional suffering in their parents and siblings and to ease that suffering by selectively activating parental or sibling feelings of guilt (Cleveland, 1980). Consequently, families with unresolved guilt are most vulnerable to this type of manipulation.

Despite their ability to control members of the family, these children also may feel responsible for much of the stress created by their condition, such as marital discord, financial problems, additional responsibilities on other members, interruption of previous life-style, and interference with future goals. They may also feel insecure in terms of their true worth to the family. For example, it is not unusual for children to wonder if the concern and attention focused on them are the result of their condition. They may question their real worth as a person, especially if their disability has received more emphasis than their abilities.

Type of Illness or Disability

The type of illness or disability also influences the child's emotional response. Interestingly, children with *more severe* disorders often cope better than those with milder conditions (Pless, 1984). Considering children's cognitive ability and their delay in achieving abstract thinking until adolescence, it is likely that an obvious condition is easier to accept because its limitations are concrete. For example, children who are blind or crippled are constantly reminded of their inability to run. However, children with hemophilia not only live by rules they do not understand but also only vaguely and occasionally sense their illness, such as when they run and accidentally initiate a bleeding episode. Therefore some chronic illnesses pose special threats to children.

The onset of a crippling condition may generate a state of confusion for children, who may have trouble differentiating between actual body functions and their image of their bodies. They may also experience problems in identifying themselves and those extensions of self (e.g., wheelchairs, braces, crutches, or other mechanical or prosthetic devices) and may have tremendous difficulty in accepting functional aids.

NURSING CARE OF THE FAMILY AND CHILD WITH SPECIAL NEEDS

The major nursing goal is to help the family remain intact and functioning at maximum levels throughout the child's life. This involves not merely supporting the child and family during the critical period of the newborn phase when the infant is being diagnosed or when the parents encounter problems in the child of preschool or school age. It involves forming parent-professional partnerships that invite the parents' early input, encourage them to be accountable and responsible for the child's care, and do not reinforce the dangerous attitude that the professional will "fix" the child and give him or her back to the parents. It also reinforces the fact that it is not so much the condition itself that affects the child's progress and developmental outcomes but the family's ability to cope successfully with the child's problems. Thus long-term, comprehensive, systematic, family-centered approaches must be applied.

The nurse should strive to understand and accept individual response styles when planning interventions and not assume a common definition for what constitutes a need for help. Families that express no interest in psychosocial interventions are not necessarily resistant (Fritz, Williams, and Amylon, 1988). A "cookbook" approach is ineffective; helpful programs must respond to individual needs.

A Nursing Care Plan for the child with special needs and the family is provided on pp. 1026-1030.

ASSESS THE FAMILY'S STRENGTHS AND LEVEL OF ADJUSTMENT

Since the nurse may meet a family during any phase of the adjustment process, it is essential to assess the family members' individual strengths, coping mechanisms, and reactions to the disorder. Ideally assessment should begin as soon as the family learns the diagnosis. Sample questions designed to elicit information for evaluating the family's adjustment are listed in Table 22-1.

Several instruments can be used to assess the family's overall functioning and support system (see Chapter 6), and specific tools have been developed for these families. For example, the Coping Health Inventory for Parents (CHIPS) is an 80-item checklist providing self-report information about how parents perceive their overall response to the management of family life with a child with a chronic illness. Coping behaviors (e.g., "believing that my child[ren] will get better" or "talking with the medical staff [nurses, social workers, etc.] when we visited the medical center") are listed, and parents are asked to record how "helpful" (0 to 3) the coping items are to them in managing the home illness situation (McCubbin and others, 1983). A number of other instruments can be used to assess various aspects of the family's needs and resources (Bailey and Simeonsson, 1988; Dunst, Trivette, and Deal, 1988; McCubbin and Thompson, 1987).

Regardless of the approach, assessment must be a continuous process because approach behaviors during one phase of the illness do not ensure reciprocal coping mechanisms in subsequent phases. Since support systems may change and perception of events may be altered at any point during the illness, nurses must continually evaluate the effectiveness of their interventions.

The nurse also assesses the parents' reaction to the

Table 22-1 Assessment of factors affecting family adjustment

FACTORS AFFECTING ADJUSTMENT	ASSESSMENT QUESTIONS
Available support system	
Status of marital relationship	Whom do you talk to when you have something on your mind? (If answer is not the spouse, ask for the reason.)
Alternate support systems	When something is worrying you, what do you do? What helps you most when you are upset?
Ability to communicate	Does talking seem to help when you feel upset?
Perception of the illness/disability	
Previous knowledge of disorder	Have you ever heard the word (name of diagnosis) before? Tell me about it (if answer is yes).
Influence of religion	Has your religion or faith been of help to you? Tell me how (if answer is yes).
Imagined cause of disorder	What are your thoughts about the causes of the disorder?
Effects of illness or disability on family	How has your child's illness or disability affected you and your family? How has your life-style changed?
Coping mechanisms	
Reactions to previous crises	Tell me one time you've had another crisis (problem, bad time) in your family. How did you solve that problem?
Reactions to the child Childrearing practices Attitudes	Do you find yourself being a little more cautious with this child than with your other children? Do you feel as comfortable disciplining this child as compared with your other children? How is this child different from the siblings or other children of similar age? Describe your child's personality. Is it easy, difficult, or in-between? When you think of your child's future, what thoughts come to mind?
Available resources	What parts of your child's care are causing the most difficulty for you and/or your family? What services are available to help? What services do you need that presently are not available?
Concurrent stresses	What other problems are you facing now? (Be specific—ask about financial, marital, sibling, and extended family/friends concerns.)

child, using as a guideline the four categories of responses—overprotection, rejection, denial, and acceptance. Observing how parents interact with the child can provide valuable information (Bean, 1987):

- Do the parents cuddle the infant during feeding or maintain distance by positioning the baby on a bed or infant seat?
- Do they touch or stroke an older child who is fed in a high chair other than during actual feeding activities?
- During feeding, dressing, and play, do the parents periodically make direct eye contact with the child?
- Do the parents talk with the child and respond positively to vocalization?

The parents' and child's understanding of the condition is another significant assessment area. Parental knowledge fosters coping and is particularly important since most children seek information from the parents (Nolan and others, 1986). One method of eliciting information is to ask how the person would explain the child's condition to a stranger. This approach frequently eliminates the use of medical jargon that the family has learned to conveniently cover up their true feelings. For example, if a parent explains that mental retardation means an IQ (intelligence quotient) of 75, the nurse can respond that the stranger is unfamiliar with such numbers and needs to know what it means to have an IQ of 75.

While inquiring about the parents' level of understanding, the nurse also focuses on the child's and siblings' knowledge of the condition. It is not unusual for parents who appear well adjusted and knowledgeable to state that they have never told the children the truth. Although this is less of a problem when the condition is visible, it may occur when the disability can be cloaked in terms such as "a little behind" or "slow learner." Conflict arises when the child or siblings learn of the diagnosis from nonparental sources. (See also Informing Children of Life-Threatening Diagnosis, Chapter 23.)

There are special challenges in assessing children's feelings about having a disability. The discussion on communication technique in Chapter 6 focuses on several approaches to encourage children to discuss feelings about their diagnosis and future. For example, using drawing and play as a method of communication is appropriate in the child who may lack verbal skills or for any child dealing with difficult feelings.

Traditionally the mother and child have been active participants and receivers of professional care, whereas fathers and siblings have been excluded. However, to achieve the goal of optimum development for the family unit, each member must be included. This involves scheduling office and/or home visits at times when other family members can be present. Although occasionally this necessitates appointments during evenings or weekends, it can also be done late in the afternoon or early morning. Fathers often will change their work schedule to meet with a health profes-

Box 22-8 GUIDELINES FOR ASSESSING CHILD'S HOME AND SCHOOL ENVIRONMENT

Observe the child's home and classroom behaviors, such as the ability to sit, follow directions, and comply with requests; determine appropriate responses to questions; and determine the child's independence in functioning.
Gather data on reported behavioral problems such as "hyperactivity," "noncompliance," or "stubbornness."
Observe the child's interactions with siblings and peers.
Observe the child's behaviors in structured and nonstructured activities.
Observe the parents' and teacher's appropriate and nonappropriate interactions with the child.
Observe the parents' and teacher's teaching strategies with the child. (Are school strategies consistent with home teaching?)
Observe the child's relationships with adults.
Determine the parents' and teacher's concerns and expectations of the child.
Administer standardized screening tools with the parent or teacher.
Observe the child's behavior before, during, and following a medication regimen.
Observe the child's eating patterns at home and at school.
Collaborate with the parents and teacher in future planning for the child.
Determine the effectiveness of programs of care for the child.
Coordinate parents, teachers, and others' plans for the child.
Assess the teacher's and/or school nurse's understanding of the child's disorder.

sional once an invitation is extended.

The task of including other family members in a visit is approached positively. If they have not been included previously, they may interpret such an invitation as a portent of more bad news or an indication of their own difficulties. One way of welcoming others to join in a visit is to state that after hearing so often about the other siblings and the father, the nurse wishes to meet them. This casual approach is nonthreatening and implies friendly connotations.

Ideally a thorough assessment includes observing the child and family in a variety of settings, including the home and school. Tools that can be used to systematically assess the home environment are the Home Observation for Management of the Environment (HOME) and the Home Screening Questionnaire (see Chapter 6).

The second most important environment for a child is school. Teachers exert a tremendous influence on the child's developmental progress, feelings of self-esteem, learning capacity, and formation of social relationships. Whenever feasible, the nurse should visit the school to observe directly the child's behavior and interaction among teachers and classmates. A summary of objectives for home and school visits is presented in Box 22-8.

PROVIDE SUPPORT AT THE TIME OF DIAGNOSIS

The impact of the crisis usually occurs at the time of diagnosis, which may be at the time of birth, following a long period of physical and/or psychologic testing, or immediately after a tragic injury. It may begin before the diagnosis is made, when parents are aware that something is wrong with their child but before medical confirmation (Clements, Copeland, and Loftus, 1990).

The time of diagnosis is a critical time for parents. Although they may not hear or remember all that is said to them, they frequently sense a certain attitude of acceptance, rejection, hope, or despair that may influence their ability to absorb the shock and to begin adapting to the family's altered future (Halpern, 1984).

Although it is usually the physician's responsibility to inform the family of the diagnosis, nurses are increasingly responsible for acting as a collaborator with the physician, giving follow-up information, and coordinating services with other agencies. Regardless of the exact role nurses assume, they must have guidelines to follow during the informing interview to provide the family with support during this critical time. Such guidelines are presented in Box 22-9.

Parents are encouraged to be together when they are informed of their child's condition, thus avoiding the problem of one parent having to interpret complex findings and deal with the initial emotional reaction of the other (Fig. 22-3). It also provides an opportunity to observe the interaction between the parents as they are confronted with the tragedy of discovering a serious problem in their child. Expressions on their faces, the times they look down, their ability to maintain eye contact with the nurse, their behaviors that show they are avoiding what the nurse is saying, such as turning their heads, looking around, or looking away, or any other activity that shows that they are indeed dealing with a very difficult subject is observed.

The informing session should take place in a private, comfortable setting free of distractions and interruptions. The atmosphere should be one in which parents feel free to express their emotions. If their feelings can be expressed and acknowledged, the parents can be helped to deal openly with them, and their need for further counseling can be determined. Their emotional needs are acknowledged by showing acceptance of such expressions as crying, sadness, anger, and disappointment. Emotional support is offered by having tissues available if a family member cries and demonstrating through facial and bodily language that indeed this is a difficult and painful period. Although touching is a powerful expression of empathy, it must be used wisely. For example, it can prematurely terminate free expression of feelings, especially when combined with statements such as "Everything will be all right." Nurses should also be aware of cultural issues regarding touching (see Chapter 2).

Parents should receive the kind of information they desire. Most parents report wanting a clear, simple explanation of the diagnosis, a prediction of possible futures for the child, advice on what to do next, an opportunity to ask questions, a warm and sympathetic listener, and, most important, time (Halpern, 1984). Clarification of explanations is elicited with such questions as, "Do you see what I mean?" or "Is this clear to you?" Technical terms are used with simple definitions. If the parents are unaware of the

Box 22-9 GUIDELINES FOR INFORMING THE FAMILY OF A SERIOUS CONDITION

Initial Discussion

Discuss suspicions of a problem with parents when waiting for a definite diagnosis to help prepare them for a potentially serious diagnosis.

Have both parents present or have a friend or family member accompany a single parent.

Let the practitioner who knows the family best present the diagnosis with the primary nurse present.

Share information about the child's diagnosis:

- Use the correct terminology for the diagnosis.
- Avoid names of symptoms to define the disorder that immediately have negative connotations. For example, instead of saying "Down syndrome is retardation," say, "Down syndrome is a chromosome abnormality." Once the dialogue has begun, tell parents other characteristics of the condition, for example, "A characteristic of Down syndrome includes mental retardation."
- Mention alternative names for the condition.
- Discuss the possible range of functioning.
- Explain other medical problems and how these are or are not related to the child's diagnosis.

Be willing to repeat information, if necessary.

Convey kindness and understanding by sitting down near the parents, touching the parent's hand or shoulder, calling the child by name, and saying the parent's name during the conversation.

Stress the personhood of the child by showing love, concern, and respect for the child as an individual.

Allow parents to express emotion and to work through feelings naturally.

Encourage parents to ask questions, and provide a telephone number for them to call with questions later or if they just want to talk more.

Be patient if the parents continue to ask the same questions.

Help parents feel competent and in control:

- Assure parents that they will be kept informed to enable them to participate effectively in decision making regarding their child's treatment and care.
- Provide parents with information about parent support groups or family resource centers, as well as knowledge about services and resources and financial assistance programs.
- Ask for permission to call and give their name and phone number to a parent self-help organization, enabling the organization to reach out to them.
- Discuss the siblings and assure parents that siblings tend to do well, especially if kept informed and included in the child's care.

Ongoing Information

Share complete information with parents on an ongoing basis.

Share information in manageable doses. Ask parents what information they want to receive at a given time to determine readiness and to avoid overload.

Be sensitive to parents' reactions.

Listen carefully when parents identify their needs, remembering that they may not always know the label of the service they require (e.g., that respite service is having someone else take over for awhile so they can get some rest).

Provide technical information in understandable terms, yet link these explanations with medical terminology.

Explain why certain questions are being asked.

Offer to share information with the child or with others involved in the child's care (e.g., brothers, sisters, grandparents, other extended family members, teachers, caregivers).

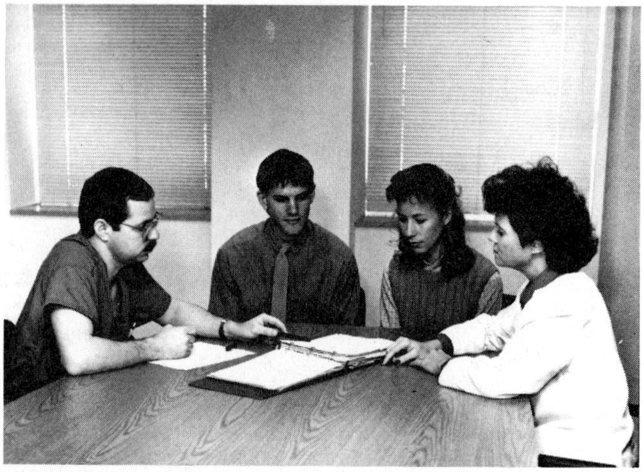

Fig. 22-3. Parents should be together when information about their child is given, especially during the informing conference.

term, they are given written literature or at least a written summary of the diagnosis (see Nursing Tip, p. 1015).

Finally, the informing conference should not end with the presentation of devastating news. Instead, the child's strengths, appealing behaviors, and potential for development are stressed, as well as available rehabilitation efforts or treatment. Parents are encouraged to view life with their child as very similar to life with other children. Their experiences should be thought of as a series of challenges that they are capable of handling, particularly with available professional feedback. The parents are assured that the nurse will be available to answer questions and to provide further assistance as it is needed in the future.

The preceding discussion relates primarily to the initial informing interview. However, because of the need for long-term follow-up, it is only one in a series of continuing discussions. In all interactions the family's input is solicited and incorporated into the plan of care (see also the guidelines in Box 22-11).

ACCEPT THE FAMILY'S EMOTIONAL REACTIONS

One of the most supportive interventions is to accept the family's emotional reactions to the diagnosis in as nonjudgmental a manner as possible. Although all families respond differently and in varying degrees of intensity, three responses are so common and often so poorly handled that they deserve special consideration.

Denial

Nurses' response to denial is a critical component of the individual's continuing need for this defense mechanism. The most effective method of support is active listening. Silence neither reinforces nor rejects denial (or any other emotional reaction) but implies a willingness and acceptance of the person's need for this behavior. However, silence alone can be misinterpreted. For example, if the person demonstrates denial, such as by saying, "I am sure the doctors made a mistake," and the nurse responds silently and leaves, the person may infer disapproval, agreement, avoidance, or rejection from this behavior.

To be effective, silence and listening must be accompanied by physical and mental concentration and use of body language to communicate interest and concern. Direct eye contact, touch, physical closeness, and body posture, such as sitting and leaning slightly forward, demonstrate silent but effective communication. Sometimes accepting people where they are, from their own perspective, is likely to give them the acknowledgment necessary to become more aware of their motives and to consider change.

Guilt

Since guilt is such a common response and can cause family members tremendous anxiety, they should be told directly that there is no known cause of the disorder when appropriate and that they are not to be blamed. Using the third-person technique (see Chapter 6) is valuable in eliciting thoughts of guilt. For example, with children an appropriate statement may be, "When people get sick, they often wonder if they did anything to make themselves sick." This allows children an opportunity to explore any feelings of responsibility they harbor.

If family members are expressing feelings of guilt, it is important to allow them to talk about their feelings rather than quickly trying to dispel them with long "scientific" explanations. Statements such as "If you believe you are responsible for Johnny's condition, then no wonder you feel so bad," acknowledge the family member's feelings. This step is frequently appreciated and necessary before the facts can be presented and absorbed. An effective method in lessening guilt is to *encourage the irrationality of thought.* For example, one mother stated that her son probably developed cancer by sitting too close to the television, which she could have prevented by being more strict. By following her reasoning and talking about how *many* children sit close to the television and how *few* of them ever have cancer, the nurse was able to help the mother realize that this activity was not a cause.

Anger

Anger is one of the more difficult reactions to accept and deal with therapeutically. The responses to anger may be reciprocal anger, fear, acceptance, and/or encouragement. The first two reactions close off communication and express disapproval and rejection of the person. They most commonly occur when the listener views the anger as a personal assault. The last two responses allow the individual to ventilate his or her feelings in an atmosphere of nonjudgmental acceptance. Two basic rules for dealing with the angry person are to avoid losing one's temper and to encourage the person to talk. See Box 22-10 for guidelines to encourage expression of emotions.

One essential element to the successful implementation of this process is to wait for the person to respond to a statement before proceeding to the next step. Since the objective of each statement is for the person to speak freely, the responses should avoid "yes" or "no" types of answers. For example, the behavior can be described (Box 22-10) or the nurse can ask directly, "Are you angry?" The latter question, however, may hinder further expressive communication and places the burden of subsequent conversation on the nurse, who should be the listener (see Therapeutic Dialogue, p. 1014).

Box 22-10 GUIDELINES FOR ENCOURAGING EXPRESSION OF EMOTION

Describe the behavior: "You seem angry at everyone."
Give evidence of understanding: "Being angry is only natural."
Give evidence of caring: "It must be difficult to endure so many painful procedures."
Help focus on feelings: "Maybe you wonder why this happened to your child."

HELP THE FAMILY COPE

In order for the family to meet the stresses of optimally adjusting to the child's condition, each member must be individually supported so that the family system is strong. Although the family unit can indefinitely support a member who is in need of assistance, its greatest strength lies in every member supporting each other. The nurse should bear in mind that the "member in need" is not necessarily the affected child but may be a parent or sibling who is dealing with stresses that require intervention.

Parents

The nurse can provide support by being attentive to families' responses to their children. Mothers and fathers need to experience success, joy, and pride in their children to give the support they need. Children, too, require support for their interactions, adjustments, and efforts. They must be reinforced for attempts to get to know their care providers and to communicate their needs to them.

Nurses must examine their attitudes to determine their ability to engage in parent-professional partnerships. An essential characteristic is the belief that parents are equal to professionals and that parents are experts regarding their child. The partnership is based on trust, which appears to evolve from continuity in the relationship, active participation by professional caregivers, mutual participation of the child and family, advocacy, a focus on coping and competence, a developmental perspective, and a family-centered focus (Drotar, Crawford, and Ganofsky, 1984). See Box 22-11 for guidelines for developing successful partnerships with parents.

Since the majority of mothers and fathers of children with special needs have little or no experience with children who have chronic or disabling conditions, the nurse can role model appropriate interactions with the child. Above all, the nurse should ensure that the parents and sib-

THERAPEUTIC DIALOGUE

Facilitating Emotional Expression

A young school-age child awaiting a lumbar puncture snatches a toy truck from his younger brother. When the sibling protests, a fistfight ensues. The nurse separates the children and begins the conversation as follows with the child awaiting treatment.

NURSE: You really seem angry today.

CHILD: Well, Bobby is playing with my favorite truck.

NURSE: Yes, I thought that was your favorite. I see you playing with it whenever you visit the clinic. But I have also seen you share that truck with Bobby. You really seem to not feel like doing that today.

CHILD: Well, who feels like being nice when somebody's going to stick needles in your back?

NURSE: Sounds like a really good reason to be angry to me. It must be hard to have to go through so many painful things—LPs, bone marrows, even finger sticks.

CHILD: Bobby doesn't have to have all this stuff; just me, always me.

NURSE: Some children tell me that they think it was something they did that made them get sick and have to go through all this.

(PAUSE) after no response

NURSE: Maybe sometimes you wonder why this happened to you.

CHILD: Momma told me that eating cookies before dinner isn't good for you. Bobby doesn't ever do it, but sometimes I do.

NURSE: Eating lots of sweets before dinner isn't good for you, but I've never heard that it can cause cancer. Have you?

SUMMARY

The nurse continues the conversation by clarifying misconceptions, reviewing coping strategies for dealing with painful procedures, and discussing anticipated pleasurable activities after the event. Just before the procedure begins, the child turns to his sibling and offers the truck, asking, "Can I play with it after my test?"

lings learn to perceive the child as a child first, with unique and individual needs. The nurse needs to convey a humanistic, accepting approach of the child so that the parents can observe this acceptance. This attitude of liking, concern for, and acceptance of the child should begin in early infancy and continue throughout the child's life.

Communication among all family members is encouraged. Parent group sessions are helpful in assisting parents to verbalize thoughts and feelings to each other but often do not take into account siblings' or the child's viewpoint. Therefore the nurse may need to set up a family session, such as during a home or clinic visit. Although the ideal situation is to have all the members present at once, this is often not possible within the confines of traditional nursing practice. However, inviting members to participate at various visits is an appropriate alternative.

Parents are encouraged to discuss their feelings toward the child, the impact of this event on their marriage, and associated stresses, such as financial burdens. For most families, regardless of their income or insurance coverage, financial concerns exist. The costs of caring for a child with special needs can be overwhelming. For example, the average yearly cost of care for many chronic illnesses is over $10,000, with additional "hidden" costs in out-of-pocket expenses that may be as much as 25% of the family income (Perrin and Ireys, 1984). Children with functional limitations account for one third of child hospital days; their hospital stays average twice as long and they visit physicians twice as often as children without limitations (Horwitz and Stein, 1990). In addition, the family wage earner may have to sacrifice job opportunities to remain close to a medical facility or to avoid losing insurance benefits.*

Every effort is made to include the father in visits, such as to the nursery, clinic, special school, and stimulation programs. His relationship with the child is observed, noting verbal interactions, tendency to assist the child, ability to give praise or set limits, and sensitivity to the child's needs. He is included in the assessment process, with specific emphasis on having him describe the child's strengths and difficulties (Box 22-12). It is not unusual to find two parents who have opposing views of the child's abilities, especially in the area of developmental disabilities.

Numerous volunteer and community resources are available that provide assistance, rehabilitation, equipment, and funding for a variety of health problems.† National and local disease-oriented organizations may provide needed assistance and support to families that qualify. Many of these are discussed elsewhere in the text under the diagnosis. State and federal departments of health, mental health, social service, and labor may be able to help locate appropri-

*Information regarding financial issues is available from the **Federation for Children with Special Needs,** 95 Berkeley St., Suite 104, Boston, MA 02116; (617) 482-2915.

†General sources of information are **Clearinghouse for Disability Information,** Room 3132, Switzer Building, C St. S.W., Washington, DC 20202-2524, (202) 732-1250; and **National Information Center for Children and Youth with Disabilities,** P.O. Box 1492, Washington, DC 20013, (703) 893-6061 or (800) 999-5599. A comprehensive list of books and pamphlets for parents and teachers is available from the **National Easter Seal Society,** 70 E. Lake St., Chicago, IL 60601; (312) 726-6200. Other sources of information are listed in Appendix E.

Box 22-11 GUIDELINES FOR DEVELOPING SUCCESSFUL PARENT-PROFESSIONAL PARTNERSHIPS

Promote primary nursing; in nonhospital settings designate a case manager.
Acknowledge the parents' overall competence and their unique expertise with their child.
Respect the parents' time as having equal value to that of other members of the child's health care team.
Explain or define any medical, technical, or disciplinary-specific terms (see Nursing Tip).
Tell families, "I am not sure" or "I don't know" when appropriate.
Facilitate the family's effectiveness in team meetings:
- Provide families the opportunity to decide on the appropriate family members and professionals to include in assessment conferences and other meetings.
- Provide information to parents in a face-to-face meeting before convening any formal decision-making meeting about their child.
- Distribute meeting agendas to all participants, including the family, before the date of the meeting. Families, like all other team members, should always be made aware of why a meeting is being held, who will be there, and what to expect.
- Introduce other professionals who may be involved with the child to the parents before any group meeting.
- Provide parents with the same information as other participants so that they can contribute to any decision about their child (e.g., child development checklist, copies of assessment reports).
- Invite parents to speak first and often throughout any information-giving or decision-making meetings, to give their perspectives and describe their observations before professionals give theirs.
- Be open with families and with other professionals when there is disagreement about any aspect of assessment or programming.

References: Bruder, 1989; Johnson, McGonigel, and Kaufmann, 1989; Redburn and others, in press.

NURSING TIP: COMMONLY USED TERMS

Develop a glossary of commonly used terms, acronyms, and "initials" to distribute to parents. The list can stand alone or become a part of patient or parent handbooks.

ate regional resources. For example, state **Programs for Children with Special Health Needs** (formerly Crippled Children's Services) provide financial assistance for children with many disabling conditions. Nurses should become acquainted with those in their communities and with vocational programs for special groups.

Although community resources may exist, it is often very difficult for parents to locate suitable services, and coordination among several agencies may be lacking. Fragmented care is one of the chief complaints from families, with specific problems of delayed referral and negative experiences with agency personnel cited as other concerns (Strauss and

Box 22-12 GUIDELINES FOR WORKING WITH FATHERS*

Regard fathers as able, effective parents, competent and capable of coping with the challenges they face.
Invite the father to family meetings from the very beginning.
Schedule meetings at convenient times, such as weekends; give sufficient notice for fathers to accommodate their work schedule.
Value the problem-solving, pragmatic approach and expertise that many men bring to the difficult challenges their families face (e.g., legislative advocacy, building adaptive devices, making videotapes).
Examine existing programs for families, from policy to implementation.
Design programs in which men support other men and topics are relevant to men, such as financial issues.
Use social situations to introduce fathers to each other, such as family weekends, potluck dinners, and/or sporting events.

Data from May, J.: Fathers of children with special needs: new horizons, Washington, DC, 1990, Association for the Care of Children's Health; and May, J., and Davis, P.: Service delivery issues in working with fathers of children with special needs, ACCH Network 8(2):4, 1990.
*Excellent resources on fathers' issues are presented in a training film, *Special Kids, Special Dads: Fathers of Children with Disabilities,* and a monograph, *Fathers of Children with Special Needs: New Horizons,* which are available from the Association for the Care of Children's Health, 7910 Woodmont Ave., Suite 300, Bethesda, MD 20814, (301) 654-6549.

Munton, 1985). Consequently, community networking for improved services is essential (Johnson and Steele, 1983). Although this topic is beyond the scope of the present discussion, nurses can become key figures in coordinating services. Several excellent resources are available,* and many projects are currently addressing this significant issue (Bock and others, 1983; Case and Matthews, 1983; Pierce and Freedman, 1983; Stein, 1983).

Parent-to-parent support. The support a parent receives from another parent is unique and unobtainable from any other source. A growing number of hospitals and clinics now have a parent on staff. The services these parents provide are particularly valuable for parents of children with special needs who are likely to experience frequent and lengthy hospitalizations, as well as numerous routine clinic visits.

Just being with another parent who has shared similar experiences is helpful. A parent of a child with the same diagnosis is not always necessary, for parents in the process of adjusting to a child with special needs—or finding respite services, educational or rehabilitative services, special equipment vendors, financial counseling—tread a common path. If the agency does not have a parent staff position, the nurse can contact parent groups, who will often send a rep-

Guidelines for Developing Community Networks: Support for Families of Children with Chronic Illness or Handicapping Conditions,* available from the **Association for the Care of Children's Health, 7910 Woodmont Ave., Suite 300, Bethesda, MD 20814, (301) 654-6549; *Workbook Series for Providing Services to Children with Handicaps and Their Families,* available from **Georgetown University Child Development Center,** 3800 Reservoir Rd. N.W., Washington, DC 20007, (202) 687-8635.

resentative. Another strategy is ask another parent to talk to the parents.* The nurse should seek out a parent who is a good listener, has a nonjudgmental approach to differences in families, and possesses good advocacy and problem-solving skills.

The parent self-help group is another way to promote parent-to-parent support.† Group members feel less alone and have the opportunity to observe both coping and mastery role modeling from other members. Parents' groups are rich resources for information. Even if parents are unable to attend meetings, they can still benefit from group newsletters and other literature that often accompany membership. The nurse can foster parent participation in self-help groups by serving as a referral agent, a group advisory board member, a resource person, a group member, or an assistant in founding a group (Rollins, 1987) (see Nursing Tip). Sometimes all that is required in starting a group is identifying one or two parents as leaders, sharing with them the names, telephone numbers, and addresses of other families, and guiding them in how to initiate a first meeting.‡

Advocate for empowerment. Nurses can advocate for methods that foster opportunities for parent empowerment. For example, nurses can suggest reimbursement for travel and child care, plus stipends to enable parents' voices to be heard at meetings and conferences. They can encourage parent membership on staff, committees, and boards. They can help keep parents informed of pending legislation on child health issues or take action when parents inform them.§ Nurses can assess parental level of empowerment and provide the support and resources most needed at each level.

NURSING TIP: SELF-HELP GROUP INFORMATION

Use cards and a file box to store information about parent self-help groups. The system facilitates adding new groups, updating old ones, and keeping cards in easy-to-retrieve alphabetic order.

The Child

Through ongoing contacts with the child, the nurse (1) observes the child's responses to the disorder, ability to function, and adaptive behaviors within the environment and with significant others; (2) explores the child's own understanding of the nature of his or her illness or condition; and (3) provides support while the child learns to cope with his or her feelings. Children are encouraged to express their concerns rather than allowing others to express them for them, since open discussions may reduce anxiety.

Parents sometimes convey concern because the child cannot express the anxieties *he or she feels.* If the child cannot or will not talk, the child may have to play out his or her feelings. He or she can be provided with toys to express threatening or stressful emotions. The nurse may find that the child responds best to drawing pictures or telling stories (see Chapter 6). Puppets can also be used. By demonstrating to parents how useful these techniques are, the nurse also helps them learn new ways of communicating with the child. For youngsters with extremely serious handicaps and/or persistent maladjustment, psychiatric evaluation and management may be needed.

One of the most important interventions is alleviating the child's feeling of being different and normalizing his or her life as much as possible. The principles in Box 22-13 are fundamental in implementing the normalizing process (Bossert and others, 1990; Krulik, 1980). Whenever possible, the nurse should assess the child's daily routine for in-

Box 22-13 GUIDELINES FOR PROMOTING NORMALIZATION

Preparation. Prepare the child in advance for changes that may occur from the illness or disability; for example, the child is told in advance of the possible side effects of drug therapy.

Participation. Include the child in as many decisions as possible, especially those relating to his or her care regimen; for example, the child is responsible for taking medications or scheduling home treatments.

Sharing. Allow both family members and the child's peers to be a part of the care regimen whenever possible; for example, the child is given his or her medication when the other siblings receive their vitamins; the parent cooks the same menu for the whole family; and if the child is invited to another's home, the parent advises the family of the child's dietary restrictions.

Control. Identify areas where the child can be in control so that feelings of uncertainty, passivity, and helplessness are decreased; for example, the child identifies activities that are appropriate to his or her energy level and chooses to rest when fatigued.

Expectation. Apply the same family rules to the child with a chronic illness or disability as to the well siblings or peers; for example, the child is disciplined, expected to fulfill household responsibilities, and attends school in accordance with abilities.

---

*The *Parent Resource Directory* lists over 400 parents of children with chronic illness or disabilities in the United States and Canada, including addresses, phone numbers, the child's condition, and the health facility where the child receives care. It is available from the **Association for the Care of Children's Health,** 7910 Woodmont Ave., Suite 300, Bethesda, MD 20814; (301) 654-6549.

†Information about self-help groups, as well as books and pamphlets, is available from the **National Self-Help Clearinghouse,** CUNY Graduate Center, 33 W. 42nd St., Room 620N, New York, NY 10036, (212) 642-2944; **Saskatchewan Self-Help Developmental Unit,** 410 Cumberland Ave., N., Saskatoon, Saskatchewan S7M1M6, (306) 652-7817.

‡The following resources are recommended: *Organizing and Maintaining Support Groups for Parents of Children with Chronic Illness and Handicapping Conditions* by Minna Newman Nathanson, available from the **Association for the Care of Children's Health,** 7910 Woodmont Ave., Suite 300, Bethesda, MD 20814, (301) 654-6549; and *The Self-Help Sourcebook: Finding and Forming Mutual Aid Self-Help Groups* by E.J. Madara and A. Meese, available from the **New Jersey Self-Help Clearinghouse,** Saint Clares–Riverside Medical Center, Denville, NJ 07834, (201) 625-9565.

§An excellent resource for becoming involved in political action is the *Public Affairs Public Issues Handbook,* available from the **American Cancer Society,** National Public Affairs Office, 316 Pennsylvania Ave., S.E., Suite 200, Washington, DC 20003; (202) 546-4011.

dications of lack of normalizing practices. For example, the child who remains in a bedroom all day is in need of a restructured daily routine to provide activities in different parts of the house, such as eating in the kitchen with the family. Such children may also be deprived of social, recreational, and academic activities that can be recognized by applying normalization practices.

Children who are concerned that their condition detracts from their physical attractiveness need attention focused on the normal aspects of appearance and capabilities. Health professionals must help strengthen and consolidate the self-image by emphasizing the normal, while at the same time allowing children to express anger, isolation, fear of rejection, feelings of sadness, and loneliness (Coupey and Cohen, 1980). They need positive reinforcement for compliance and any evidence of improvement. Anything that might improve attractiveness and contribute to a positive self-image is employed, such as makeup for a teenager with a scar, clothing that disguises a prosthesis, or a hairstyle or wig to cover a deformity or lost hair.

Children, particularly adolescents, are sensitive to the presence or absence of hope. Hopefulness is an internal quality that mobilizes humans into goal-directed action that may be satisfying and life-sustaining. A sense of hopefulness produces increased participation in health-seeking behaviors, improved sense of well-being, lifting of depression, and acceptance of the dying process (Hinds, Martin, and Vogel, 1987). Nurses can influence hopefulness through interpersonal and environmental means (Box 22-14).

Siblings

As pointed out, the presence of a child with special needs in a family may result in parents paying less attention to the other children or expecting older siblings to take on greater responsibility for the care of the child. Siblings may respond by developing negative attitudes toward the child or by expressing anger in different forms. The nurse can help by using "anticipatory guidance," questioning the parents about what they believe is the best way to have siblings respond to the child and about whether they have any concerns about the way in which they are assigning responsibility to older siblings. This questioning should take place before serious negative effects occur.

Siblings may also experience embarrassment associated with the stigma of a disorder such as mental retardation. Parents are then faced with the difficulty of responding to this embarrassment in an understanding and appropriate manner without punishing the siblings for feeling the way they do. Parents should talk with the siblings about how they view their affected sibling. For example, siblings of a child who is retarded may express fears about their ability to bear normal children. Adolescents in particular may not be able to discuss these vital issues with their parents and may prefer to consult with the nurse. Many siblings benefit from sharing their concerns with other young people who are experiencing a similar situation.* Support groups for siblings help decrease isolation, promote expression of negative feelings, and provide an opportunity to learn from each other (Heiney and others, 1990).

Many parents express concern about when and how to inform the other children in the family about the birth or the presence of a child who is disabled. The answer depends on each child's level of sophistication and understanding. However, it is usually best to inform the siblings before a neighbor or other nonfamily member does so. Nurses can show by their behavior that they see the parents as being capable in their own unique style of imparting information about the condition. However, they should make it clear that if the parents postpone informing the siblings, they assume the risk of hindering the siblings' ability to develop a realistic understanding of the problem. Uninformed siblings may fantasize or develop apprehensions that are out of proportion to the child's actual condition. Furthermore, if parents choose to be silent or deceptive about the issue, they are setting a negative precedent for the siblings to follow, rather than encouraging the siblings to cope with the experience in a healthy and nurturing way.

The nurse must be sensitive to the reactions of siblings and whenever possible intervene to promote more positive adjustments. For example, siblings often mention that they are expected to take on additional responsibilities to help the parents care for the child. It is not unusual for them to express a positive reaction to assuming the extra duties but a negative response to feeling unappreciated for doing so. Such feelings can often be minimized by encouraging the siblings to discuss this with the parents and by suggesting to parents ways of showing gratitude, such as an increase in allowance, special privileges, and most significantly verbal praise (see Parent Guidelines, p. 1018.).

Box 22-14 GUIDELINES FOR FACILITATING HOPEFULNESS

- Give honest reports of conditions or events.
- Encourage and participate with the child in physical activities (e.g., arrange activities, play games, or go for walks together).
- Convey a fond, personal interest in the child (give hugs, ask follow-up questions from previous discussions).
- Direct conversations to neutral, non-disease-related or less sensitive topics (discuss child's favorite sports, tell stories).
- Convey competence and gentleness when delivering care.
- Provide information about other children in similar situations who are doing well.
- Encourage the child to think ahead to more comfortable and preferred natural times.
- Be lighthearted and initiate or respond to teasing or other playful interactions with the child.

Modified from Hinds, P., Martin, J., and Vogel, R.J.: Nursing strategies to influence adolescent hopefulness during oncologic illness, J. Assoc. Pediatr. Oncol. Nurses 4(1/2):14-22, 1987.

*For information on the **Sibling Information Network,** contact the Information Network, CUAP, 991 Main St., East Hartford, CT 06108; (203) 282-7050.

PARENT GUIDELINES
Supporting Siblings

Promote healthy sibling relationships

Value each child individually, and avoid comparisons. Remind each child of his or her positive qualities and contribution to other family members.

Help siblings see the differences and similarities between themselves and a child with special needs. Create a climate in which children can achieve successes without feeling guilty.

Teach siblings ways to interact with the child.

Seek to be fair in terms of discipline, attention, and resources; require the affected child to do as much for himself or herself as possible.

Let siblings settle their own differences; intervene only to prevent siblings from hurting one another.

Legitimize reasonable anger. Even children with special needs behave badly sometimes.

Respect a sibling's reluctance to be with or to include the child with special needs in activities.

Help siblings cope

Listen to siblings to let them know that their thoughts and suggestions are valued.

Praise siblings when they have been patient, have sacrificed, or have been particularly helpful. Do not expect siblings to always act in this manner.

Acknowledge the personal strengths siblings have and their ability to cope with stress successfully.

Provide age-appropriate information about the child's condition, and update when appropriate.

Let teachers know what is happening so they can be understanding and helpful.

Recognize special stress times for siblings and plan to minimize negative effects (see Box 22-4).

Schedule special time with siblings; have a friend or family member substitute when parent is unavailable.

Encourage sibling to join or help establish a sibling support group.

Use the services of professionals when needed. If parent feels that such a service is necessary, it should be provided in as vigorous a manner as a service for the child with special needs.

Involve siblings

Seek out ways to realistically include siblings in the care and treatment of the child with special needs.

Limit caregiving responsibilities and give recognition when siblings perform them.

Develop a library of children's books on special needs.

Invite siblings to attend meetings to develop plans for the child with special needs (e.g., IEP, IFSP).

Discuss future plans with them.

Solicit their ideas on treatment and service needs.

Have them visit professionals who work with the child.

Help them develop competencies to teach the child new skills.

Provide opportunities for siblings to advocate for the child.

Allow siblings to set their own pace for learning and involvement.

Modified from Powell, T., and Ogle, P.: Brothers and sisters—a special part of exceptional families, Baltimore, 1985, Paul H. Brooks Publishing Co.; and Spokane Washington Deaconess Medical Center Pediatric Oncology Unit: Tips for dealing with siblings, The Candlelighters Childhood Cancer Foundation Quarterly Newsletter 11(3, 4):7, 1987.

Extended Family Members and Society

The nurse must also be sensitive to family's cues regarding sources of stress from extended members, such as grandparents. For example, the nurse may encourage the parents to invite the grandparents to be present during one of the child's visits to a clinic, during the diagnostic workup, or to a parent conference or to provide appropriate literature. Including grandparents in a discussion in which they can share their concerns may help them deal with their feelings, thus reducing stress on the entire family. Grandparents' feelings of blame and anger as well as any "cure fantasies" they harbor can be brought out in the open and discussed if necessary. Grandparents can be helped to understand the effects of their behavior on the family with an appropriate statement, such as, "Your daughter is currently experiencing a great deal of pain and anguish. We realize that this is difficult for you as well as your daughter; however, you can be of tremendous help by being supportive toward her."

Considerable stress can also arise from nonfamilial sources, such as friends, neighbors, or strangers. Inability to cope with comments about the disorder or curious stares by others may foster the tendency to isolate and protect the child within the home. The family needs guidance in preparing for these inevitable experiences. One approach is encouraging parents to dress the child as much as possible like other children. Good grooming is very important in minimizing differences in appearance. Through role playing parents can practice responses to comments such as, "Is your child retarded?" or "Has he always been crippled?" Through parent groups family members can share experiences and learn from each other how they successfully deal with probing questions or unkind remarks. Such interventions must include the siblings and the affected child, who also must face and deal with these events. Nurses can be instrumental in teaching young children about disabilities to familiarize them with the special needs and abilities of these individuals. For example, school nurses can simulate experiences such as having only one leg by using role playing, can use books or films, or can invite community guests with physical limitations to visit the class (Hedahl, 1981).*

*The President's Committee on Employment of People with Disabilities, 1111 20th St., N.W., Washington, DC 20036, (202) 653-5044, offers a free activity guide, *People Just Like You,* to help children learn about individuals with disabilities.

Special dolls can be used to help children become comfortable and familiar with a variety of disabilities.*

FOSTER REALITY ADJUSTMENT

Fostering a reality adjustment primarily involves family education regarding the disorder, as well as general health care, developmental needs of the child, and realistic goal setting. Ideally education should be aimed at preventing problems, rather than at relearning to change existing dilemmas. Like the interventions previously discussed, this goal requires an ongoing process that is part of assessment and emotional support of the family.

Educate About the Disorder and General Health Care

Educating the family about the disorder is actually an extension of revealing the diagnosis, especially those points listed in Box 22-9.† Education involves not only supplying technical information but also discussing how the condition will affect the child. For example, it is of little benefit to discuss mental retardation in terms of numbers. Rather parents need to understand what the child can do in terms of self-help, academic learning, and independence. Similarly, the child who has lost a limb needs more than an explanation of the prosthetic leg. He or she must know the limitations it places on activity as well as available opportunities.

Parents also need guidance in how the condition may interfere with or alter activities of daily living, such as eating, dressing, sleeping, and toileting. One area frequently affected is nutrition. Common problems are undernutrition as a result of food being inappropriately restricted, loss of appetite, vomiting, or motor deficits that interfere with feeding and overnutrition usually caused by a caloric intake in excess of energy expenditure or boredom and lack of stimulation in other areas. Although the child requires the same basic nutrients as other children, the daily requirements may differ. Special nutritional considerations are discussed as appropriate throughout the text.

In addition to special nutritional needs, another very important area in which modifications may be needed is car safety. Children with conditions such as low birth weight or orthopedic, neuromuscular, or respiratory problems often cannot safely use conventional care restraints. For example, children with hip spica casts cannot sit properly in child safety seats (see Congenital Hip Dysplasia, Chapter 11). Modifications can be made to some commercial models,‡ and for older children a special vest§ is available that secures the child in a lying-down position to the back seat. Children in wheelchairs present special challenges because the wheelchair should be anchored with four points of attachment to the vehicle (two in front and two behind) and should always face forward (Richards, 1989). The family should consult the wheelchair manufacturer for specific instructions regarding safe car transportation.

*Hal's Pals for Challenged Kids are available from Mattel, Inc., 5959 Triumph St., City of Commerce, CA 90040; (800) 824-4000.

†See Wong, D.L., and Whaley, L.F.: Clinical manual of pediatric nursing, ed. 3, St. Louis, 1990, Mosby–Year Book, Inc., for home care instruction sheets, which may be copied and given to families.

‡Information on restraints for children with special needs is available from Automotive Safety for Children Program, Riley Hospital for Children, 702 Barnhill Dr., S-139, Indianapolis, IN 46223; (317) 274-2977 or (800) KID-N-CAR (in Indiana).

§E-Z-On Vest is available from E-Z-On Products, 500 Commerce Way West, Jupiter, FL 33458; (407) 747-6920 or (800) 323-6599 (outside Florida).

Children with special needs require all the usual health care recommended for any child. Attention to injury prevention, immunizations, dental health, and regular physical examinations is essential. Nurses can play an important role in reminding parents of these aspects of care that are so often neglected when the concern is focused on the child's specific illness or disability. See Recommendations for Health Supervision in Chapter 7 for assessing general aspects of health maintenance. Specific discussions of nutrition, sleep and activity, dental health, and injury prevention are presented in the chapters on health promotion for specific age-groups. Immunizations are discussed in Chapter 12.

Parents also need to be aware of the importance of communicating the child's condition in the event of a medical emergency. Young children are unable to give information about their disorder, and although older children may be reliable sources, after an accident they may be physically unable to speak. Therefore all children with any type of chronic condition that may affect medical care should wear some type of identification, such as a Medic-Alert bracelet,* which lists the medical condition and a collect phone number for emergency medical records and other personal information.

Children need information about their condition, the therapeutic plan, and how the disease or the therapy might affect their particular situation. Children nearing puberty also need to understand the maturation process and how their disability may alter this event. For example, the youngster with Crohn disease should understand that this disorder is associated with growth failure and delayed puberty; the child with diabetes needs to know that hormonal changes and increased growth needs will alter food and insulin requirements at this time; and the sexually active girl with sickle cell anemia or systemic lupus erythematosus needs to be aware of the hazards of pregnancy. The information should not be given all at once but timed appropriately to meet the changing needs of the youngsters, and it should be described and repeated as often as the situation demands.

The subject of sexuality related to the effects of the disorder is a prominent concern of adolescents, but they rarely initiate a discussion of this sensitive topic. Any probable interference in sexual function because of the disability should be discussed openly and candidly with the teenager. Unfortunately, many nurses are reticent to discuss sexual issues with adolescents. One study of pediatric nurses caring for adolescent cancer patients revealed that although most of the nurses agreed that sexuality should be a routine component of nursing care, less than half of them had actually

*P.O. Box 1009, Turlock, CA 95380-1009; (800) ID-ALERT.

discussed an alteration in sexuality with an adolescent patient (Williams and Wilson, 1989). Adults often underestimate the degree to which adolescents engage in unrealistic fantasies regarding sexual activities and related matters, or even sexual activity itself. In a study that compared parent and adolescent responses on perceived health care needs, parents were unaware of their teenagers' sexual activity (Dragone, 1990).

Throughout the long process of caring for a child with special needs family members become expert in management of their child's care. Unfortunately, this expertise is often not recognized by health professionals who tend to be directive, rather than collaborative, in their approach to the family. This is particularly common during periods of hospitalization, when parents are placed in a "double-bind"—at home they are expected to care for their child yet in the hospital they are ignored as participants in care, especially treatment regimes (Robinson, 1985). A supportive atmosphere must include coordination of care with family members, respect for their knowledge, and willingness to include their suggestions in the treatment plan.

Promote Normal Development

Aside from knowledge of the condition and its effect on the child's abilities, the family must be guided toward fostering appropriate development in their child. Although each stage may take longer to achieve, parents are guided to helping the child fully realize potential in preparation for the next phase of development. See Table 22-2 for developmental aspects of chronic illness or disability and for supportive interventions.

Early childhood. During infancy the child is achieving basic *trust* through a satisfying, intimate, consistent relationship with his or her parents. However, the affected child's early existence may be stressful, chaotic, and unsatisfying. Consequently he or she may need more parental support and expressions of affection to achieve trust. Likewise the parents require assistance in ways of meeting the infant's needs, such as how to hold a rigid or flaccid infant, how to feed a child with tongue thrust or episodes of dyspnea, and how to stimulate a child who seems incapable of achieving any skills. If hospitalizations are frequent or prolonged, every effort is made to preserve the parent-child relationship (see also Chapter 26).

During early childhood the goal is to achieve separation from mother, autonomy, and initiative. However, the natural parental response to having a sick child is overprotection. Parents need help in realizing the importance of brief separations from the child, including others in the child's care, and providing social experiences outside the home whenever possible. Respite care, which provides temporary relief for family members, is essential in allowing caregivers time away from the daily demands of caring for a child with special needs.* (Warren and Cohen, 1985).

*Information on guidelines to develop a respite care program is available in *Keeping Families Together: Providing Respite and Other Short-Term Care for People with Disabilities,* Alaska Governor's Council for the Handicapped and Gifted, 600 University Ave., University Plaza West, Suite B, Fairbanks, AK 99709; (907) 474-2440.

In spite of need, parents report extreme difficulty finding competent respite care (Palfrey and others, 1989). New respite programs have developed in response to this need. The **National Down Syndrome Society,** for example, designed a program to foster the skills of independence and socialization in children with Down Syndrome, to provide a regular, planned respite for the children's parents, and to educate volunteer host families and communities about the potential of individuals with this genetic disorder* (National Down Syndrome Society, 1988). The National Council on the Aging created **Family Friends,** a unique intergenerational program that uses older adult volunteers to assist and support families who have children with chronic illnesses living at home† (Kuehne, 1989).

Young children also need the opportunity to develop independence. Frequently the child is able to learn self-help skills, such as holding the bottle, finger-feeding, and removing simple articles of clothing, but the parent continues to perform the act. Therefore the nurse must guide parents to the usual milestones expected from the child. Initially this requires developmental assessment of functional age (see Developmental Assessment, Chapter 7). The self-contract is a useful tool for promoting independence and self-care. Although formalized self-contracts are most successful with school-age or older children, a simplified version can be effective with preschoolers (Wesolowski, 1988). For more on self-contracts see Chapter 27 under Compliance.

Periodically the child's developmental progress is evaluated. Since each child develops at his or her own rate, there are no rigid guidelines for expecting when particular skills will be achieved. However, lack of progress in any one area is investigated. For example, sometimes a delay in self-feeding is not caused by lack of motor skill but by the parents' impatience in waiting for the skill to develop. Cleaning up the spilled food may seem like one more unnecessary task unless the importance of using a cup or spoon is stressed. All that may be necessary to encourage parent participation are suggestions to avoid large accidents, such as pouring only a small amount of juice in a cup or having the child feed himself or herself mashed potatoes (a sticky food) rather than gelatin (a slippery food). Placing food on a tray or cookie sheet is also helpful in keeping the food within the child's reach.

Not all children with disabilities are capable of achieving normal developmental milestones. For example, the child with mental impairment may never achieve cognitive skills above a preschool level. The child who is deaf may achieve only rudimentary verbal language. In these situations adjustments must be made to compensate for the lack of or severely delayed achievement in one area. However, such adjustments must be based on an understanding of normal development. Since motor limitations are present in a majority of conditions, this disability is used as an example to

*A "how-to" manual, containing step-by-step information for establishing this program, is available for $5.00 from the National Down Syndrome Society, 666 Broadway, Suite 810, New York, NY 10012; (212) 460-9330 or (800) 221-4602.

†Information is available from Family Friends, Box 1214, Cardinal Station, 620 Michigan Ave., N.E., Washington, DC 20064; (202) 635-5949.

Table 22-2 Developmental aspects of chronic illness or disability on children

AGE/DEVELOPMENTAL TASKS	POTENTIAL EFFECTS OF CHRONIC ILLNESS OR DISABILITY	SUPPORTIVE INTERVENTIONS
▪ Infancy		
Develop a sense of trust	Multiple caregivers and frequent separations, especially if hospitalized Deprived of consistent nurturing	Encourage consistent caregivers in hospital or other care settings Encourage parents to visit frequently or "room in" during hospitalization and to participate in care
Bond/attach to parent	Delayed because of separation, parental grief for loss of "dream" child, parental inability to accept the condition, especially a visible defect	Emphasize healthy, perfect qualities of infant Help parents learn special care needs of infant for them to feel competent
Learn through sensorimotor experiences	Increased exposure to painful experiences over pleasurable ones Limited contact with environment from restricted movement or confinement	Expose infant to pleasurable experiences through all senses (touch, hearing, sight, taste, movement) Encourage age-appropriate developmental skills, e.g., holding bottle, finger feeding, crawling
Begin to develop a sense of separateness from parent	Increased dependency on parent for care Overinvolvement of parent in care	Encourage all family members to participate in care to prevent overinvolvement of one member Encourage periodic respite from demands of care responsibilities
▪ Toddlerhood		
Develop autonomy	Increased dependency on parent	Encourage independence in as many areas as possible, e.g., toileting, dressing, feeding
Master locomotor and language skills	Limited opportunity to test own abilities and limits	Provide gross motor skill activity and modification of toys or equipment, such as modified swing or rocking horse Give choices to allow simple feeling of control, e.g., choice of what book to look at or what kind of sandwich to eat
Learn though sensorimotor experience, beginning preoperational thought	Increased exposure to painful experiences	Institute age-appropriate discipline and limit-setting Recognize that negative and ritualistic behavior are normal Provide sensory experiences, e.g., water play, sandbox, finger paint
▪ Preschool		
Develop initiative and purpose Master self-care skills	Limited opportunities for success in accomplishing simple tasks or mastering self-care skills	Encourage mastery of self-help skills Provide devices that make task easier, e.g., self-dressing
Begin to develop peer relationships	Limited opportunities for socialization with peers; may appear "like a baby" to age-mates Protection within tolerant and secure family may cause child to fear criticism and withdraw	Encourage socialization, such as inviting friends to play, daycare experience, trips to park Provide age-appropriate play, especially associative play opportunities
Develop sense of body image and sexual identification	Awareness of body may center on pain, anxiety, and failure Sex role identification focused primarily on mothering skills	Emphasize child's abilities; dress appropriately to enhance desirable appearance Encourage relationships with same-sex and opposite-sex peers and adults Help child deal with criticisms; realize that too much protection prevents child from realities of world
Learn through preoperational thought (magical thinking)	Guilt (thinking he or she caused the illness/disability or is being punished for wrongdoing)	Clarify that cause of child's illness or disability is not his or her fault or a punishment
▪ School age		
Develop a sense of accomplishment	Limited opportunities to achieve and compete, e.g., many school absences or inability to join regular athletic activities	Encourage school attendance; schedule medical visits at times other than school; encourage to make up missed work Educate teachers and classmates about child's condition, abilities, and special needs
Form peer relationships	Limited opportunities for socialization	Encourage sports activities, e.g., Special Olympics Encourage socialization, e.g., Girl Scouts, Campfire, Boy Scouts, 4-H Clubs, having a best friend or a club
Learn through concrete operations	Incomplete comprehension of the imposed physical limitations or treatment of the disorder	Provide child with knowledge about his or her condition Encourage creative activities, e.g., Very Special Arts

Continued.

Table 22-2 Developmental aspects of chronic illness or disability on children—cont'd

AGE/DEVELOPMENTAL TASKS	POTENTIAL EFFECTS OF CHRONIC ILLNESS OR DISABILITY	SUPPORTIVE INTERVENTIONS
Adolescence		
Develop personal and sexual identity	Increased sense of feeling different from peers and less able to compete with peers in appearance, abilities, special skills	Realize that many of the difficulties the teenager is experiencing are part of normal adolescence (rebelliousness, risk taking, lack of cooperation, hostility toward authority) Provide instruction on interpersonal and coping skills Encourage socialization with peers, including peers with special needs and those without special needs
Achieve independence from family	Increased dependency on family; limited job/career opportunities	Provide instruction on decision making, assertiveness, and other skills necessary to manage personal plans Encourage increased responsibility for care and management of the disease or condition, such as assuming responsibility for making and keeping appointment (ideally alone), sharing assessment and planning stages of health care delivery, contacting resources
Form heterosexual relationships	Limited opportunities for heterosexual friendships; less opportunity to discuss sexual concerns with peers	Encourage activities appropriate for age, such as attending mixed-sex parties, sports activities, driving a car
Learn through abstract thinking	Increased concern with issues such as why did he or she get the disorder, can he or she marry and have a family Decreased opportunity for earlier stages of cognition may impede achieving level of abstract thinking	Be alert to cues that signal readiness for information regarding implications of condition on sexuality and reproduction Emphasize good appearance and wearing stylish clothes, use of makeup Understand that adolescent has same sexual needs and concerns as any other teenager Discuss planning for future and how condition can affect choices

illustrate psychologic implications in making developmental changes.

During early childhood the basic innate drive for movement is dominant. During toddlerhood there is rapid development of motor skills, which eventually becomes the basis for learning and coping with the complex world. Psychologically this period is critical for developing a desire for independence. Language development, bowel control, locomotion, and fine-motor control all converge to produce a feeling of competency. Gradually during the early school years this basic motor urge shifts to a more goal-directed, symbolic expression in which words and thoughts replace actions as a way of problem-solving.

When the young child has a disability that interferes with motor development, there is the potential hazard of shifting to development of compensatory intellectual pursuits before the child is ready. If this occurs, achievement of autonomy and initiative may be severely compromised, setting the stage for emotional problems. Therefore intervention must be based on providing activities that allow maximum motor development. For example, if a child has paraplegia, it is not sufficient to strengthen the upper extremities to compensate for the lower ones. Rather the activity must take into account the child's need for social interaction, sense of control over the body, feeling of competence and achievement, and an outlet for aggression. Suitable activities may include ball throwing, swimming and water activities such as races, bubble blowing, and splashing, building blocks, or pounding with a hammer (Bernard and others, 1981).*

With slight modifications, children with disabilities may be able to ride a tricycle by using self-adhering straps to secure the hands (Fig. 22-4). Wheelchair races are always a popular activity. Programs such as the **Special Olympics**† offer children an opportunity to compete with their peers and to achieve athletic skill. Summer camps‡ also provide

*Information on a toy library system for children with sensory deficits, motor disabilities, and developmental delay is available from the **National Lekotek Center,** 2100 Ridge Ave., Evanston, IL 60201; (708) 328-0001.

†1350 New York Ave., N.W., Suite 500, Washington, DC 20005-1581; (202) 628-3630. Several pamphlets are available from the **National Easter Seal Society,** 70 E. Lake St., Chicago, IL 60601, (312) 726-6200, and the **American Alliance for Health, Physical Education, Recreation and Dance (AAHPERD),** 1900 Association Dr., Reston, VA 22091, (703) 476-3400, on sports and recreation for children with disabilities.

‡A directory of camps for children with a variety of chronic illnesses or general physical disabilities is available for a fee from **American Camping Association,** Publications Service, 100 Bradford Woods, Martinsville, IN 46151; (800) 428-CAMP.

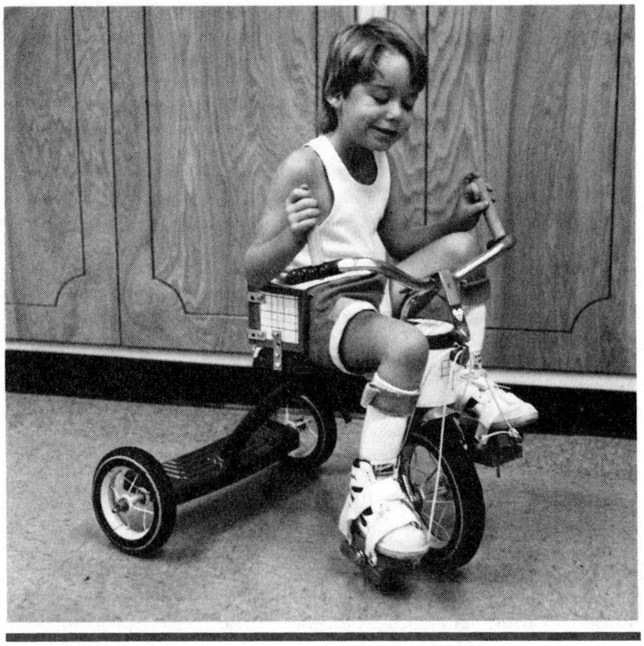

Fig. 22-4. A modified tricycle with block pedals, self-adhering straps for support, and modified seat and handlebars can help a child with disabilities gain mobility.

children with unique opportunities to associate with similarly affected peers and develop a wide variety of skills, including increased independence in activities of daily living and special needs associated with their condition, such as administering medication. With innovation many adaptations can be implemented in children's environment to increase their mobility and independence.* Technologic advances are mushrooming, especially in the application of computers, and parents should be directed to the latest developments that may help their child (Desch, 1986).

Children with special needs derive enormous benefits from expressive activities, such as art, music, poetry, dance, and drama. With adaptive equipment and imagination, children can participate in a variety of activities. Organizations such as **Very Special Arts** offer children an opportunity to celebrate and share their accomplishments.†

Another critical component for normal child development is discipline. Unfortunately this is one of the earliest childrearing practices eliminated when parents react with "over-benevolence." Not only does lack of discipline destroy the child's security because no boundaries exist on which to test behavior, it also fails to teach the child socially acceptable behavior and creates resentment and hostility among the siblings if different standards are applied to each child. The nurse's responsibility is to help parents learn successful methods of controlling behaviors before they become problems (see Chapter 14).

School age. For school-age children, the major tasks are entry into school and achieving a sense of industry. While the importance of school in the life of all children is generally acknowledged, studies indicate that school absences are significantly higher among children with chronic illness, especially if psychosocial problems, such as behavior or family difficulties, coexist, than among their healthy peers (Weitzman, Walker, and Gortmaker, 1986). Some children, especially those with potentially terminal illnesses, may not return to school, despite a long period of remission. The more school absences the child experiences, the more difficult it is to return, and "school phobia" may result. Psychosocial factors that contribute to the risk of school phobia include depression, change in appearance, fear of separation (child and parents), and resistance on the part of school personnel. To prevent school phobia, the child should resume school as quickly as possible following diagnosis (Lansky, List, and Ritter-Sterr, 1988). (See also School Phobia, Chapter 18.)

Preparation for entry or resumption of school is best accomplished through a team approach with the parents, child, school teacher, school nurse, and primary nurse in the hospital. Ideally this planning should begin well before hospital discharge, provided the child is well enough to resume usual activities. A structured plan should be developed, with attention to those aspects of care that must be continued during school hours, such as administration of medication or other treatments (see Chapter 17). Teachers need to be aware of the child's abilities in order to set realistic academic and athletic expectations (Larcombe and others, 1990). Parents' feelings regarding school resumption also need to be considered. Parents, especially mothers, may have difficulty relinquishing the intensive parenting role, particularly if many of their other social attachments have weakened. A successful approach is to plan school attendance concurrently with the parents' recommencement of prediagnosis activities.

Children also need preparation before entering or resuming school. Having a tutor in the hospital or home as soon as children are physically able helps them realize that school will continue and gives them time to consider this prospect (Fig. 22-5). They need to investigate possible answers to the many questions others will ask. One method of anticipatory preparation is to role play, with the child as the "returned pupil" and the nurse as "other schoolmates." The nurse asks questions about the reason for the child's absence, the name of the disease, and so on. The child is thus provided with a safe opportunity to explore possible answers and to experience some of the possible reactions of others. If the child returns to school with some obvious physical change, such as hair loss, amputation, or visible scar, the nurse might also ask questions about these alterations to prompt preparatory responses from the child.

Initially the child may find it easier to attend half-day sessions or to participate in a limited number of activities. It is preferable to plan the school program with as much partic-

*An excellent publication is *The More We Do Together: Adapting the Environment for Children with Disabilities,* Monograph No. 31. Although it is out of print, a photocopy is available for a fee from IEEIR, c/o The Institute on Disability, University of New Hampshire, Durham, NH 03824-3577; (603) 862-4767.

†Very Special Arts has affiliate chapters in all 50 states and in selected sites internationally—yearly festivals are held throughout the world. Information is available from **Very Special Arts,** Education Office, John F. Kennedy Center for the Performing Arts, Washington, DC 20566; (202) 662-8899.

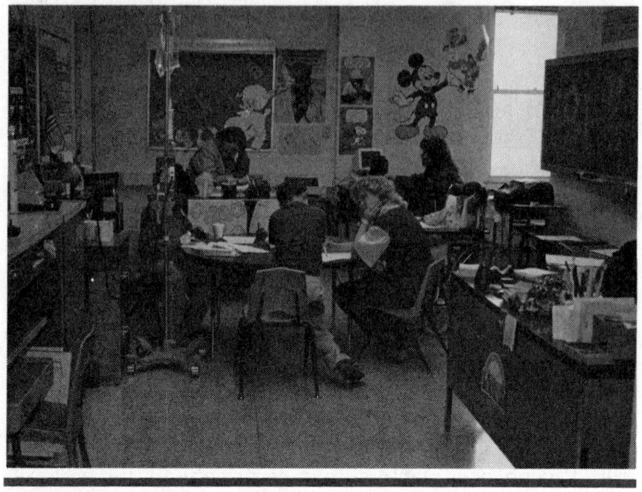

Fig. 22-5. Children with special needs should continue their schooling as soon as their condition permits.

ipation and leadership from the child as possible. Once children return, regular assessments of their progress are essential to assure a satisfactory adjustment. For example, some children appear to be doing well by investing all of their energies in academic endeavors to the detriment of social and/or physical activities. In essence the scholastic achievement may represent a retreat from other areas of school life that are equally important.

Classroom peers also need preparation, and a joint plan between the school teacher, nurse, and child is best. At a minimum the classmates should be given a description of the child's condition, prepared for any visible changes in the child, and allowed an opportunity to ask questions. The child should have the option of attending this session. As the child's condition changes, particularly if the illness is potentially fatal, school personnel, including the students, need periodic appraisal of the child's status and preparation for what to expect (see also Chapter 23).*

Children with special needs are encouraged to maintain or reestablish relationships with peers and to participate according to their capabilities in any age-appropriate activities. Alternative activities may be substituted for those that are impossible or that place a strain on their condition. It is important for these children to have the opportunity to interact with healthy peers, as well as to engage in activities with groups or clubs composed of similarly affected agemates. Such organizations as ostomy clubs, diabetic clubs, and cerebral palsy groups share information and provide support related to the special problems the members face.

Peer interaction is especially important in relation to cognitive development, social development, and maturation. Cognitive development is facilitated by interaction—by exploration of personal, social, and ethical values with peers, parents, and teachers. Youngsters whose isolation hampers their ability to interact with peers miss this opportunity to expand their thinking (Coupey and Cohn, 1980). Too many of these children withdraw to the passive companionship of television.

*Several publications are available to help prepare school personnel, health professionals, and families for the child's return to school and are listed at the end of this chapter.

Adolescence. Adolescence can be a particularly difficult period for the teenager and family. All the needs discussed before apply to this age-group as well. Developing independence or autonomy, however, is a major task for the adolescent as planning for the future becomes a prominent concern. While the emphasis in the past has been on achieving independence from physical assistance, recent developments in the fields of special education, adolescent development, and family systems suggest redefining autonomy in terms of individuals' capacities to take responsibility for their own behavior, to make decisions regarding their own lives, and to maintain supportive social relationships (Crittenden, 1990). With this new definition, even individuals with severe impairment can be viewed as autonomous if they perceive their own needs and take responsibility for meeting them—either directly or by engaging the assistance of others. As adolescents become more autonomous, the nurse can help them discover and articulate how others can be of greatest assistance.

Physical symptoms are high on the teenager's list of health-related concerns (Dragone, 1990). Because adolescence is a time of enormous physical and emotional changes, it is important for the nurse to make a distinction between body changes that are related to disability and those that are a result of normal body development. It is a great comfort for these teenagers to know that many of the changes they experience are normal developmental outcomes.

A sense of feeling different from peers can lead to loneliness, isolation, and depression. Participation in groups of teenagers with chronic conditions or disabilities can alleviate feelings of isolation and smooth the transition to a meaningful relationship with one person in adulthood.*

Establish Realistic Future Goals

One of the most difficult adjustments is setting realistic future goals for the child and for those involved in the child's continued care. Sometimes the impact of this decision does not surface until the child finishes school or the parents near retirement, when a crisis can arise because all the family roles and relationships that maintained stability are now disrupted.

Planning for the future should be a gradual process. All along, the parents should cultivate realistic vocations for the child. For example, children with physical disabilities can be directed to intellectual, artistic, or musical pursuits. Children with developmental disabilities can be taught

*Lasting Impressions, a well-developed psychosocial support program for adolescent cancer patients and their parents, provides an excellent model for supporting adolescents with cancer and other chronic conditions. For information about the program contact Sue P. Heiney, M.N., R.N., C.S., Children's Hospital at Richmond Memorial, 5 Richland Medical Park, Columbia, SC 29203.

skills that can be performed in a special workshop. In this way the child's development proceeds in the direction of self-support through gainful employment.

With prolonged survival for many chronic illnesses, surviving young people must deal with new decisions and problems, such as marriage, employment, and insurance coverage (see Questions and Controversies). With appropriate guidance many of these individuals are capable of gainful employment* and may choose to marry and raise a family. For those whose conditions are genetic, there is the need for counseling regarding future offspring. Prospective spouses often benefit from an opportunity to discuss their feelings regarding marriage to an individual with continued health needs and possibly a limited life span. Health insurance coverage is a critical issue because some private carriers may no longer insure a young person who leaves home or may be unwilling to reinsure the person who is independent. Life insurance is another dilemma, especially when children have serious defects, such as congenital heart anomalies (Truesdell, Skorton, and Lauer, 1986). These issues are only beginning to receive attention but will become increasingly prominent as the number of survivors increases.

One solution that is gaining acceptance is transferring the older adolescent to adult care. The medical and psychosocial needs of adolescents approaching adulthood may be more easily managed by caregivers who are more familiar with adult issues.

Determining readiness for transfer is an important consideration. Arbitrary transfer to adult services based on age criterion alone can compromise both physical and psychosocial care for some young adults. Furthermore, age does not provide any information on how prepared the adolescent may be for transfer. A study using a questionnaire to determine readiness in adolescents with cystic fibrosis revealed that while age is an important criterion for transfer, other indicators (e.g., knowledge of condition and related treatments, medications, and precautions; child initiation; and compliance with regimens) were found to be better predictors (Cappelli, MacDonald, and McGrath, 1989).

Abrupt transfer to adult services can prove difficult for the young adult. Many adolescents have received care in the same medical setting since birth and have established trusting and meaningful relationships with practitioners and staff members. At Temple University Medical School and Hospital children with cystic fibrosis are identified as "in transition" at 16 years of age. To ease the transition, adult care practitioners work with the pediatric team in the pediatric clinic with 16- to 18-year-old adolescents and their families. At 18 approximately 90% of the adolescents move to the adult facility where familiar faces await.†

*Information about employment is available from The President's Committee on Employment of People With Disabilities, 1111 20th St., N.W., Washington, DC 20036; (202) 653-5044.

†For more information about the program contact Stanley B. Fiel, M.D., Chief, Pulmonary Disease Section, and Associate Professor of Medicine, Temple University Medical School and Hospital, 3401 N. Broad St., Philadelphia, PA 19140; (215) 221-3336.

QUESTIONS AND CONTROVERSIES

What ethical issues are young people and families facing as a result of improved survival from chronic illness?

Chronically ill adolescents are faced with a number of serious ethical dilemmas as they enter adulthood. For example, should they share the truth of their condition with dating partners, prospective spouses, or potential employers? Should they seek a job with good health insurance rather than pursue a career with less employee benefits? Should they have the right to refuse further treatment, especially when the prospects for cure or even palliation are minimal? Whose wishes should be upheld when a conflict exists between the parents and young person? Should they transfer to adult care services? Will adult care practitioners be prepared to treat "childhood" diseases or conditions?

Such questions have no clear-cut answers. Rather, adolescents should be encouraged to weigh decisions, investigate alternatives, and choose their own solution (Silber, 1984). For example, in a study of adolescents with disabilities concerning their decision to have surgery, assessment of the teenager's view of surgery as "routine" or "nonroutine," the adolescent's and parents' goals, the alternatives to surgical intervention, how much power the teenager had in making the decision, and the young person's feelings regarding the decision-making process were important factors in arriving at an answer (Deatrick, 1984).

Consent and confidentiality are frequent dilemmas in providing care to any minor adolescent and are often made more complex by the teenager's health problem. For example, do these adolescents have the right to request health care without parents' knowledge or permission? If they are engaging in potentially hazardous activities, such as the teenager with cystic fibrosis who begins to smoke or the young man with hemophilia who engages in contact sports or tests HIV positive and becomes sexually active, should parents be informed? Two principles may be used in resolving such ethical questions: the principle of *autonomy,* which states that a person should have a say in any action that will affect him or her, and the principle of *benevolence,* which states that whenever something beneficial can be done, it should be done. Obviously, autonomy and benevolence support the adolescent's right to health care. However, in the best interests of the teenager, parents may need to be informed of activities that jeopardize one's life (Silber, 1984).

As more is learned about treating the adult phases of childhood conditions, more young adults will likely opt for adult services. In addition to assessing readiness, pediatric nurses can play a significant role in preparing adolescents and adult care providers for this important transition.

Unfortunately, vocational pursuits and independence are not realistic goals for all persons. Persons with multiple or severe disabilities may require lifelong care and assistance. In these situations parents must look to the time when they will no longer be able to care for their child. Residential placement may be very difficult unless the family mutually participates in the decision-making and planning process.

NURSING CARE PLAN
The Child with a Chronic Illness or Disability

NURSING DIAGNOSIS: Altered growth and development related to chronic illness or disability, parental reactions (overbenevolence), repeated hospitalization

GOAL 1
Promote development appropriate to child's age and abilities

INTERVENTIONS

See Table 22-2

EXPECTED OUTCOME

Child achieves appropriate physical, psychosocial, and cognitive development for age and abilities

NURSING DIAGNOSIS: Altered family processes related to situational crisis (child with a chronic disease or disability)

GOAL 1
Help family adjust to the diagnosis

INTERVENTIONS

Provide opportunity for family to adjust to discovery of diagnosis
Anticipate the usual grief reaction to loss of "perfect" child
Explore family's feelings regarding the child and their ability to cope with the disorder
Encourage family to express their concerns
Repeat information as often as necessary
Serve as a role model regarding attitudes and behavior toward the child

EXPECTED OUTCOMES

Parents verbalize feelings and concerns regarding implications of the disease
Family demonstrates an attitude of acceptance and adjustment

GOAL 2
Increase family's understanding of the disorder

INTERVENTIONS

Assist family to understand the disorder, its therapies, and implications
Reinforce information given by others
Clarify misconceptions
Provide accurate information at a rate family can absorb
Discuss advantages and limitations of therapeutic plan
Encourage family to ask questions and express concerns

EXPECTED OUTCOME

Family demonstrates an understanding of the disease (specify)

GOAL 3
Reduce family's fears and anxieties

INTERVENTIONS

Explore family's concerns and feelings of irritation, guilt, anger, disappointment, inadequacy
Help family distinguish between realistic fears and unfounded fears; eliminate unfounded fears
Discuss with parents their fears regarding
- Dealing with the child's anxiety about condition
- Fear of dreadful developments
- Fear of death
- Fear of tests and procedures
- Child's ability to compete with peers

Explore their feelings regarding prescribed therapies

EXPECTED OUTCOME

Family members discuss their fears and concerns

GOAL 4
Promote positive adaptation to the child

INTERVENTIONS

Explore family's reaction to the child and the disorder
Assess family's coping skills, abilities, and resources
Help family to achieve a realistic view of the child and capabilities and limitations
Foster positive family relationships
Assess interpersonal relationships within the family, especially behaviors that reflect family attitudes toward the affected child
Intervene appropriately if there is evidence of maladaptation
Encourage parents in their attempts to promote child's development
Emphasize positive aspects of the child's abilities or attributes
Help family gain confidence in their ability to cope with the child, the disorder, and its impact on other family members

EXPECTED OUTCOMES

Family verbalizes feelings and concerns regarding the special needs of the child and their effect on the family process
Family members demonstrate an attitude of confidence in their ability to cope

GOAL 5
Promote family's ability to provide child's care

INTERVENTIONS

Help family develop a thorough plan of care
Teach skills needed to provide optimum care
Interpret child's behavior to parents (e.g., anger, depression, regression, physical modifications as a result of disorder)
Help family plan for the future

EXPECTED OUTCOME

Family sets realistic goals for selves, child, and others

NURSING CARE PLAN
The Child with a Chronic Illness or Disability—cont'd

GOAL 6
Foster growth-promoting family relationships

INTERVENTIONS

Identify family support systems (immediate family, extended family, friends, health service providers)
Assess systematically the number, affiliation, and interrelationships (if any) of persons the family sees as important
Assist family to assign specific tasks to specific people
Reinforce positive coping mechanisms
Encourage family members to discuss their feelings about each other
Impress upon parents the importance of providing as normal a life as possible for the affected child
Help family feel adequate in their maternal-paternal roles by emphasizing growth and developmental progress of their child
Help family foster child's development by stimulating child to age-appropriate goals consistent with activity tolerance

EXPECTED OUTCOMES

Family demonstrates positive, growth-promoting behaviors
Family avails itself of support

GOAL 7
Provide support

INTERVENTIONS

Be available to the family
Listen to family members—singly or collectively
Allow for expression of feelings, including feelings of guilt, helplessness, and their perception of the impact that the condition may have (or does have) on the family
Refer to community agencies or special organizations providing assistance—financial, social, and support
Refer to genetic counseling if appropriate
Help family learn to expect feelings of frustration and anger toward the child; reassure that it is not a reflection on their parenting
Assist family in problem solving
Encourage interaction with other families who have a similarly affected child
  Introduce to families
  Provide information regarding support groups
Help families learn when to accept and when to "fight"

EXPECTED OUTCOMES

Family maintains contact with health providers
Family demonstrates an understanding of the needs of the child and the impact the condition will have on them
Problems are dealt with early
Family becomes involved with local agencies and support groups

GOAL 8
Prepare family for hospitalized child's discharge

INTERVENTIONS

Teach skills needed for home care
Assess home situation, including family's strengths, weaknesses, and support systems
Help devise an individualized plan of care based on assessment of family's needs and resources
Encourage family involvement in care while still in the hospital
Encourage family to ask questions regarding posthospital care
Explore family's attitudes toward the child's entry (or reentry) into the home
Help family acquire needed drugs, supplies, and equipment
Refer to special agencies based on need assessment
Arrange for regular follow-up care to reassess effectiveness of home management

EXPECTED OUTCOMES

Family demonstrates an understanding of needed skills (specify skills and method of demonstration)
Family members avail themselves of resources within their community (specify)
Family complies with home care program

GOAL 9
Continue ongoing evaluation

INTERVENTIONS

Participate in follow-up care
Coordinate team management of child and family
Be alert to comments by child or family members that indicate possible problems
Assess interpersonal relationships within the family, especially behaviors that reflect family attitudes toward the child
Be alert for cues that signal undue anxiety and guilt; preoccupation with causative factors, constant analysis of effects of therapies, experimentation with diets and folk remedies, seeking magical cures
Be alert for overprotective behaviors such as assuming self-care activities for child, restricting child's activities of interaction with peers
Allow family to express discouragement at interference with activities and what appears to be slow progress

EXPECTED OUTCOMES

Family participates in follow-up care
Family expresses both positive and negative reactions to child's progress
*Signs that may indicate family's difficulty in adjusting to the child's condition are identified early

*Nursing outcome.

Continued.

NURSING CARE PLAN
The Child with a Chronic Illness or Disability—cont'd

GOAL 10

Support siblings of affected child

INTERVENTIONS

Assess siblings to identify areas of concern
Communicate honestly with siblings about the child's disease or disability
Provide opportunity for siblings to ask questions and express feelings but avoid lengthy explanations before they ask
Help parents talk to siblings about the child's condition and interpret the siblings' needs and questions
Encourage parents to spend special time with their child (or children) who are not ill or disabled
Help siblings and family understand that it is normal for them to have negative feelings about the child
Prepare siblings in advance for any household changes
Allow sibling(s) to participate in the child's care and therapy as appropriate
Help siblings learn how to explain the child's condition to their peers and others
Acknowledge siblings' strengths and abilities to cope
Refer to sibling groups and networks composed of siblings of children with the same or similar conditions
Assess siblings periodically to determine their adjustment to the family situation

EXPECTED OUTCOMES

Siblings verbalize or otherwise demonstrate their feelings and concerns
Parents include siblings in discussions of the disabled child
Parents make an effort to spend time with other children
Siblings exhibit an understanding of household changes
Siblings assist with affected child's care (specify)
Siblings become involved in support groups (specify)

NURSING DIAGNOSIS: Anxiety/fear related to tests, procedures, hospitalization, etc. (specify)

GOAL 1

Prepare for tests and procedures, hospitalization, etc. (specify)

INTERVENTIONS

See Preparation for Procedures, Chapter 27
See Preparation for Hospitalization, Chapter 26

EXPECTED OUTCOME

Child copes with stresses of procedures, tests, etc. (specify)

NURSING DIAGNOSIS: Potential for injury (specify)

GOAL 1

Decrease risk of injury

INTERVENTIONS

Assess environment for hazards if indicated
Teach safety precautions
Encourage activities that are compatible with the disease or disability

EXPECTED OUTCOME

Child remains free of injury and complications

GOAL 2

Help child adjust to restricted activities

INTERVENTIONS

Help devise alternatives for restricted activities and help child cope with physical limitations

EXPECTED OUTCOME

Child demonstrates appropriate adaptation to limitations (specify)

GOAL 3

Prevent complications

INTERVENTIONS

Stress importance of sound health practices and frequent health supervision
Make certain child and family understand the therapeutic measures prescribed
Encourage older child to choose activities but take responsibility for own safety
Plan with allied personnel (e.g., teachers, coaches, counselors) appropriate activities
Confer with school nurse (or other person) regarding any special needs of the child
Discuss with parents any indicated limit-setting

EXPECTED OUTCOME

Child maintains optimum health

NURSING DIAGNOSIS: Diversional activity deficit related to environmental lack of diversion, physical limitations (specify), hospitalization

GOAL 1

Provide diversion

INTERVENTIONS

Provide appropriate stimulation
Encourage activities appropriate to age, interests, and capabilities of child
Encourage physical exercise that does not overtax the child (if indicated)
Incorporate therapeutic needs in play activities as appropriate
Supervise and encourage activities of daily living
Encourage child's natural tendency to be active
Encourage interaction with family and peers
Include child in planning and scheduling care

NURSING CARE PLAN
The Child with a Chronic Illness or Disability—cont'd

EXPECTED OUTCOMES

Child engages in age-appropriate activities within the limits of capabilities
Child accepts efforts of family and caregivers

GOAL 2

Discourage sedentary habits

INTERVENTIONS

Encourage child to participate in normal childhood activities commensurate with interests and capabilities
Encourage and reinforce age-appropriate behaviors, experiences, and socialization with peers
Discourage physical inactivity

EXPECTED OUTCOME

Child engages in nonsedentary activities within the limits of disability

NURSING DIAGNOSIS: Impaired social interaction related to hospitalization, confinement to home, frequent illness, activity intolerance, fatigue (specify)

GOAL 1

Promote interpersonal relationships

INTERVENTIONS

Encourage to maintain usual activities
Arrange for continued interpersonal contacts while hospitalized or otherwise confined
Provide opportunities for interaction with others, especially peers
Encourage regular school attendance (including daycare, beginning school, return to school)
Arrange for rest periods at school if needed
Promote peer contact wherever possible
Encourage recreational outlets and after-school activities appropriate to the child's interests and capabilities
Discourage activities that increase isolation from others

EXPECTED OUTCOMES

Child engages in appropriate activities
Child associates with peers and family
Child attends school with reasonable regularity

NURSING DIAGNOSIS: Self-care deficit (specify) related to specific impairment (specify)

GOAL 1

Promote self-help (self-care)

INTERVENTIONS

Teach child about the disease and therapies
Encourage child to assist in own care as age and capabilities permit
Provide and/or help devise methods to facilitate maximum functioning
Incorporate play that encourages desired behavior
Select toys and activities that allow maximum participation by the child
Modify environment if needed (specify)
Assist with self-care activities where needed (specify)
Avoid undue persistence to accomplish a goal
Provide incentives to achieve desired behavior
Instruct when to seek assistance from family or health care providers

EXPECTED OUTCOME

Child engages in self-help activities commensurate with capabilities (specify activities and extent of involvement)

GOAL 2

Enhance child's sense of competence and mastery

INTERVENTIONS

Capitalize on child's assets; help child compensate for liabilities
Praise child for accomplishments and "near" accomplishments, such as partial completion of a task
Ensure adequate rest before attempting energy-expending activities
Emphasize the child's abilities and focus on realistic endeavors
Emphasize positive coping behaviors
Discourage activities that are beyond the child's capabilities; promote and reinforce successful endeavors
Encourage participation in own care to the extent that child is able
Teach and encourage responsibility for use of equipment, appliances, testing, medication (specify)
Help child become adept at self-management to maximum capabilities

EXPECTED OUTCOMES

Child takes responsibility for self-care according to age and capabilities (specify)
Child engages in appropriate activities without undue fatigue

NURSING DIAGNOSIS: Body image disturbance related to perception of disability (self and others), feeling of differentness, inability to participate in specific activities (specify)

GOAL 1

Meet child's emotional needs

INTERVENTIONS

Convey an attitude of understanding, caring, and acceptance
Avoid conveying an attitude of intrusion
Maintain open communications with child
Relate to the child on appropriate cognitive level
Serve as a role model for others

EXPECTED OUTCOME

Child maintains a positive attitude (specify behaviors)

Continued.

NURSING CARE PLAN
The Child with a Chronic Illness or Disability—cont'd

GOAL 2

Determine extent of disturbance

INTERVENTIONS

Encourage verbalization of feelings and perceptions, especially feelings of "differentness"
Explore feelings concerning disease or disability and its implications: stress of being "different," physical limitations, difficulty competing, relationships with peers, self-image
Encourage child to discuss feelings about how he/she thinks others feel about the disorder

EXPECTED OUTCOME

Child openly discusses feelings and concerns about the condition, therapies, and perceived reactions of others

GOAL 3

Help child cope with actual and perceived differentness

INTERVENTIONS

Acknowledge feelings and facilitate sharing feelings with family and other health professionals
Clarify misconceptions child may have acquired
Assist child to identify positive aspects of situation

EXPECTED OUTCOME

Child discusses the disorder and feelings regarding limitations imposed by it

GOAL 4

Assist child in adjusting to the disorder and its effects

INTERVENTIONS

Help child assess own strengths and assets; emphasize strengths
Identify coping behaviors
Support positive coping mechanisms and extinguish negative ones
Help child set realistic goals
Encourage as much independence as condition allows
Introduce child to other children who have adjusted well to this or a similar disorder
Suggest involvement with special groups and facilities for children with similar problems

EXPECTED OUTCOMES

Child identifies own assets and strengths realistically
Child verbalizes positive suggestions for adjusting to the disability
Child becomes involved with special group activities

GOAL 5

Help child build self-esteem and a positive self-concept

INTERVENTIONS

Encourage an appealing physical appearance: good body hygiene, clean straight teeth, good grooming, stylish clothing, makeup for teenage girls
Assist with improving appearance and grooming
Point out positive aspects of own coping, appearance, and other capabilities
Promote constructive thinking in child; encourage to maximize strengths
Reinforce positive behaviors
Assist child to determine and engage in activities that foster self-esteem
Promote independence

EXPECTED OUTCOMES

Child demonstrates a positive appearance and attitude (specify)
Child appears clean, well groomed, and attractively dressed
Child exhibits behaviors that indicate elevated self-esteem (specify)

GOAL 6

Provide child with appropriate feeling of control

INTERVENTIONS

Channel need for control and feeling of effectiveness in appropriate directions
Encourage child to monitor own care as appropriate
Provide opportunities for child to make choices and participate in care when appropriate
Assist the child with vocational planning when appropriate

EXPECTED OUTCOME

Child becomes actively involved in own care and management

GOAL 7

Help prepare hospitalized child for discharge

INTERVENTIONS

Begin early in hospitalization to discuss "going home"
Help child develop independence and self-help capabilities
Encourage visits from friends to help child assess the impact of any change in appearance or behavior that might interfere with returning to previous environments

EXPECTED OUTCOME

Child verbalizes and otherwise demonstrates interest in going home

See also:
Nursing Care Plan: The Child in the Hospital, Chapter 26
Nursing Care Plan: The Family of the Ill or Hospitalized Child, Chapter 26
Nursing Care Plan: The Child Who Is Terminally Ill or Dying, Chapter 23

Institutionalization should not be viewed as abandonment. Not infrequently it is the only way to preserve the family unit. The nurse should help the family investigate suitable placements, discuss their feelings regarding this decision, and explore measures to maintain meaningful communication with the member who has a disability. The nurse can prepare and educate the public to smooth the transition and help normalize the experience for the child, the family, and the community.

KEY POINTS

- Trends in the treatment of children with chronic illness have focused on developmental stages, the child's strengths and uniqueness, family relationships, establishment of normalization, early discharge, home care, mainstreaming, and early intervention.
- Families' reactions to disability or chronic illness are manifested in the following stages: shock and denial, adjustment, reintegration and acknowledgment, and freezing out.
- In response to the child with chronic illness or disability, parents may be affected by feelings of inadequacy and failure; excessive demands on time, energy, and financial resources; and strain on spouse communication.
- Effects of chronic illness on siblings include changes in role status, irritability and physical complaints, jealousy, competition, anger, hostility, attention-seeking behavior, social withdrawal, and decline in school performance.
- Major factors affecting the family's adjustment to a child's chronic illness are the availability of a support system, their perception of the event, their coping mechanisms, reactions to the child, available resources, and concurrent stresses.
- The coping mechanisms parents use in dealing with the child with chronic illness are approach behaviors—movement toward adjustment and resolution of crisis—and avoidance behaviors—maladaptation or movement away from adjustment.
- The child's reaction to illness or disability depends on developmental level, coping mechanisms, others' reactions, and the illness itself.
- A family-centered approach to care that enables and empowers parents offers the greatest opportunity for appropriate interventions that meet the unique needs of all family members.
- Mutual participation in care by child and parent facilitates better communication and alleviates feelings of parental inadequacy and child inferiority.
- Assessment of the family's coping mechanisms and reactions entails understanding the family's functioning and observing the child in home and school.
- To help parents cope with their child's chronic illness, nurses must offer attentiveness, humanistic support, solicitation of suggestions for care, facilitation of communication, verbalization of feelings, and referral to volunteer and community agencies.
- Supporting the child involves encouraging self-expression, alleviating feelings of being different, and strengthening self-image.
- Fostering reality adjustment entails supplying information about the disorder, promoting normal development, and establishing realistic future goals.

REFERENCES

Adams, P., and Fras, I.: Beginning child psychiatry, New York, 1988, Brunner/Mazel, Inc.

American Academy of Pediatrics, Committee on Children With Disabilities: Pediatrician's role in development and implementation of an individual education plan, Pediatrics 80(5):750-751, 1987.

American Academy of Pediatrics: Official statement to the Committee on Children with Handicaps, The Developmental Disability Council, U.S. Department of Health, Education and Welfare, April 1979.

American Cancer Society: Trends in survival of cancer by site of children under 15: 1977-83, CA 30(1):21, 1988.

Association for the Care of Children's Health: Focusing on fathers of children with special needs, ACCH Network 8(2):1, 1990.

Austin, J: Assessment of coping mechanisms used by parents and children with chronic illness, MCN 15(2):98-102, 1990.

Bailey, D., and Simeonsson, R., editors: Family assessment in early intervention, Columbus, OH, 1988, Merrill Publishing Co.

Bean, M.: Assessing families of children with developmental disabilities. In Wright, L., and Leahey, M., editors: Families and chronic illness, Springhouse, PA, 1987, Springhouse Corp.

Bernard, B., and others: Exercise for children with physical disabilities, Issues Compr. Pediatr. Nurs. 5:99-107, 1981.

Blacher, J.: Sequential stages of parental adjustment to the birth of a child with handicaps: fact or artifact? Ment. Retard. 22(2):55-68, 1984.

Bock, R.H., and others: There's no place like home, Child. Health Care 12(2):93-96, 1983.

Boone, D.R., and Hartman, B.H.: The benevolent over-reaction, Clin. Pediatr. 11(5):268-271, 1972.

Bossert, E., and others: Strategies of normalization used by parents of chronically ill school-age children, Child Adolesc. Psychiatr. Mental Health Nurs. 3(2):57-61, 1990.

Bruder, M.: Parent and professional partnerships under PL 99-457, Early Childhood Update 5(2):1-2, 1989.

Byrne, E.A., and Cunningham, C.C.: The effects of mentally handicapped children on families—a conceptual review, J. Child. Psychol. Psychiatry 26(6):847-864, 1985.

Cappelli, M., MacDonald, N., and McGrath, P.: Assessment of readiness to transfer to adult care for adolescents with cystic fibrosis, Child. Health Care 18(4):218-224, 1989.

Carney, I.: Working with families. In Orelove, F., and Sobsey, D., editors: Educating children with multiple disabilities: a transdisciplinary approach, Baltimore, 1987, Paul H. Brookes Publishing Co.

Case, J., and Matthews, S.: CHIP: the Chronic Health Impaired Program of the Baltimore City Public School System, Child. Health Care 12(2):97-99, 1983.

Childs, R.: Maternal psychological conflicts associated with the birth of a retarded child, MCN 14(3):175-182, 1985.

Clements, D., Copeland, L., and Loftus, M.: Critical times for families with a chronically ill child, Pediatr. Nurs. 16(2):157-161, 224, 1990.

Cleveland, M.: Family adaptation to traumatic spinal cord injury: response to crisis, Fam. Relations 29:558-565, 1980.

Coupey, S., and Cohen, M.: A developmental approach to the chronically ill adolescent, Feelings Med. Signif. 22(2):7-10, 1980.

Coupey, S., and Cohen, M.: Special considerations for the health care of adolescents with chronic illnesses, Pediatr. Clin. North Am. 31(1):211-219, 1984.

Crittenden, P.: Toward a concept of autonomy in adolescents with a disability, Child. Health Care 19(3):162-168, 1990.

Cystic Fibrosis Foundation: Personal communication Aug. 13, 1990.

Damrosch, S., and Perry, L.: Self-reported adjustment, chronic sorrow, and coping of parents of children with Down syndrome, Nurs. Res. 38(1):25-30, 1989.

Deatrick, J.A.: It's their decision now: perspectives of chronically disabled adolescents concerning surgery, Issues Compr. Pediatr. Nurs. 7:17-31, 1984.

Desch, L.W.: High technology for handicapped children: a pediatrician's viewpoint, Pediatrics 77(1):71-87, 1986.

Downey, W.: Public Law 99-457 and the clinical pediatrician, Clin. Pediatr. 29(3):158-161, 1990.

Dragone, M.: Perspectives of chronically ill adolescents and parents on health care needs, Pediatr. Nurs. 16(1):45-50, 108, 1990.

Drotar, D., Crawford, P., and Ganofsky, M.: Prevention with chronically ill children. In Roberts, M., and Peterson, I., editors: Prevention of problems in childhood, New York, 1984, John Wiley & Sons, Inc.

Dunst, C., Trivette, C., and Deal, A.: Enabling and empowering families, Cambridge, MA, 1988, Brookline Books.

Duvall, E.: Marriage and family development, ed. 5, New York, 1977, J.B. Lippincott Co.

Fiel, S.B.: Personal communication, Aug. 16, 1990.

Fire, N.: Personal communication, Aug. 26, 1990.

Fraley, A.: Chronic sorrow: a parental response, J. Pediatr. Nurs. 5(4):268-273, 1990.

Fritz, G., Williams, J., and Amylon, M.: After the treatment ends: psychosocial sequelae in pediatric cancer survivors, Am. J. Orthopsychiatry 58(4):552-561, 1988.

Futcher, J.: Chronic illness and family dynamics, Pediatr. Nurs. 14(5):381-385, 1988.

Gallup, G.: An American paradox, Alcoholism & Addiction, July-Aug., 1986.

Gortmaker, S.L., and Sappenfield, W.: Chronic childhood disorders: prevalence and impact, Pediatr. Clin. North Am. 31(1):3-18, 1984.

Gratz, R.R., and Piliavin, J.A.: What makes kids sick: children's beliefs about the causative factors of illness, Child. Health Care 12(4):156-162, 1984.

Halpern, R.: Physician-parent communication in the diagnosis of child handicap: a brief review, Child. Health Care 12(4):170-173, 1984.

Hansen, S., Holaday, B., and Miles, M.: The role of pediatric nurses in a federal program for infants and young children with handicaps, J. Pediatr. Nurs. 5(4):246-251, 1990.

Harber, J.: Response to self-reports of differentiation of self and marital compatibility as related to family functioning in the third and fourth stages of the family life cycle, Scholarly Inquiry Nurs. Pract. 3(3):177-180, 1989.

Harkey, J.: The epidemiology of selected chronic childhood health conditions, Child. Health Care 12(2):62-71, 1983.

Healy, A., Keesee, P., and Smith, B.: Early services for children with special needs, ed. 2, Baltimore, 1989, Paul H. Brookes Publishing Co.

Hedahl, K.J.: Helping children establish positive attitudes towards disabled persons, Pediatr. Nurs. 7(6):11-15, 1981.

Heiney, S.P., and others: The effects of group therapy on siblings of pediatric oncology patients, J. Assoc. Pediatr. Oncol. Nurses 7(3):95-100, 1990.

Hickey, M.: What are the needs of families of critically ill patients? A review of the literature since 1976, Heart Lung 19(4):401-415, 1990.

Hinds, P., Martin, J., and Vogel, R.J.: Nursing strategies to influence adolescent hopefulness during oncologic illness, J. Assoc. Pediatr. Oncol. Nurses 4(1/2):14-22, 1987.

Hobbs, N., and Perrin, J.M., editors: Issues in the care of children with chronic illness, San Francisco, 1985, Jossey-Bass Inc.

Hofmann, A.D.: Managing handicapped adolescents with impaired body image, Feelings Med. Signif. 22(4):13-18, 1980.

Horwitz, S., and Stein, R.: Health maintenance organizations vs indemnity insurance for children with chronic illness, Am. J. Dis. Child. 144:581-586, 1990.

Johnson, B., McGonigel, M., and Kaufmann, R., editors: Guidelines and recommended practices for the Individualized Family Service Plan, Washington, DC, 1989, Association for the Care of Children's Health.

Johnson, B.H., and Steele, B.B.: Community networking for improved services to children with chronic illnesses and their families, Child. Health Care 12(2):100-102, 1983.

Jones, B.: Impairment, disability and handicap (editorial), Child. Care Health Dev. 13:359, 1987.

Kalnins, I.: Cross-illness comparisons of separation and divorce among parents having a child with a life-threatening illness, Child. Health Care 12(2):72-77, 1983.

Kazak, A.: Families of chronically ill children: a systems and social-ecological model of adaptation and challenge, J. Consult. Clin. Psychol. 57(1):25-30, 1989.

Krulik, T.: Successful "normalizing" tactics of parents of chronically ill children, J. Adv. Nurs. 5(6):573-578, 1980.

Kuehne, V.: "Family friends": an innovative example of intergenerational family support services, Child. Health Care, 18(4):237-246, 1989.

Lansky, S.B., List, M.A., and Ritter-Sterr, C.: Psychiatric and psychological support of the child and adolescent with cancer. In Pizzo, P., and Poplack, D., editors: Principles and practice of pediatric oncology, Philadelphia, 1988, J.B. Lippincott Co.

Larcombe, I.J., and others: Impact of childhood cancer on return to normal schooling, Br. Med. J. 301(6744):169-171, 1990.

Leventhal, J., and Sabbeth, F.: In Yogman, M., and Brazelton, T.B., editors: In support of families, Cambridge, MA, 1986, Harvard University Press.

Lin, N.: Conceptualizing social support. In Lin, N., Dean, A., and Ensel, W., editors: Social support, life events and depression, New York, 1986, Academic Press, Inc.

Lobato, D.: Brothers, sisters, and special needs, Baltimore, 1990, Paul H. Brookes Publishing Co.

May, J.: Fathers of children with special needs: new horizons, Washington, DC, 1990, Association for the Care of Children's Health.

McCubbin, H., and Thompson, A.: Family assessment inventories for research and practice, Madison, 1987, The University of Wisconsin—Madison.

McCubbin, H., and others: CHIP—Coping Health Inventory for Parents: an assessment of parental coping patterns in the care of the chronically ill child, J. Marriage Fam. 45:359-370, 1983.

McCubbin, M.: Family stress, resources, and family types: chronic illness in children, Fam. Relations 37:203-210, 1988.

Meisels, S.: Meeting the mandate of Public Law 99-457: early childhood intervention in the nineties, Am. J. Orthopsychiatry 59(3):451-460, 1989.

Mulhern, R.K., Crisco, J.J., and Camitta, B.M.: Patterns of communication among pediatric patients with leukemia, parents, and physicians: prognostic disagreements and misunderstandings, J. Pediatr. 99(3):480-483, 1981.

NACOA charts its course, Alcoholism 3(5):18, 1983.

National Down Syndrome Society: Respite program goes national, Update 4(1):1, 1988.

Nolan, T., and others: Knowledge of cystic fibrosis in patients and their parents, Pediatrics 77(2):229-235, 1986.

Office of Technology Assessment: Technology-dependent children: hospital vs home care, a technical memorandum, Washington, DC, 1987, U.S. Government Printing Office.

O'Malley, J.E., and others: Psychiatric sequelae of surviving childhood cancer, Am. J. Orthopsychiatry 49(4):608-616, 1979.

Orr, D.P., and others: Psychosocial implications of chronic illness in adolescence, J. Pediatr. 104(1):152-157, 1984.

Oster, A.: Keynote address. In Equals in this partnership, Washington, DC, 1985, National Center for Clinical Infant Programs.
Palfrey, J., and others: Patterns of response in families of chronically disabled children: an assessment in five metropolitan school districts, Am. J. Orthopsychiatry 59(1):94-103, 1989.
Patterson, J. Supporting family life. In Fire, N., and others, editors: Coordinate for kids: the family is the reason, Oklahoma City, in press, Oklahoma State Department of Health.
Perrin, E.C., and Gerrity, P.S.: Development of children with a chronic illness, Pediatr. Clin. North Am. 31(1):19-31, 1984.
Perrin, J.M., and Ireys, H.T.: The organization of services for chronically ill children and their families, Pediatr. Clin. North Am. 31(1):235-257, 1984.
Pierce, P.M., and Freedman, S.A.: The REACH project: an innovative health delivery model for medically dependent children, Child. Health Care 12(2):86-89, 1983.
Pless, I.B.: Clinical assessment: physical and psychological functioning, Pediatr. Clin. North Am. 31(1):33-45, 1984.
Powell, T., and Ogle, P.: Brothers and sisters—a special part of exceptional families, Baltimore, 1985, Paul H. Brookes Publishing Co.
Redburn, L., and others: Caring for children and families: guidelines for hospitals, Bethesda, MD, in press, Association for the Care of Children's Health.
Report to Congress and the Secretary by the Task Force on Technology-Dependent Children: Fostering home and community-based care for technology-dependent children, vol. 2, U.S. Department of Health and Human Services, Health Care Financing Administration, HCFA Pub. No. 88-02171, 1988.
Reynolds, M.C.: The educational needs of disabled children and youths. In Blum, R., editor: Chronic illness and disabilities in childhood and adolescence, New York, 1984, Grune & Stratton, Inc.
Richards, D.D.: The challenge of transporting children with special needs, AAP Safe Ride News, pp. 1-4, spring 1989.
Robinson, C.: Double bind: a dilemma for parents of chronically ill children, Pediatr. Nurs. 11(2):112-115, 1985.
Rollins, J.: Self-help groups for parents, Pediatr. Nurs. 13(6):403-409, 1987.
Rollins, J.: Childhood cancer: Siblings draw and tell, Pediatr. Nurs. 16(1):21-27, 1990.
Rush, W.L., and The League of Human Dignity: Write with dignity: reporting on people with disabilities, Lincoln, NB, 1983, Hitchcock Center.
Rutter, M.: Stress, coping, and development: some issues and some questions. In Garmezy, N., and Rutter, M., editors: Stress, coping, and development in children, New York, 1983, McGraw-Hill, Inc.
Schulman, J.: Coping with major disease: child, family, pediatrician, J. Pediatr. 102(6):988-991, 1983.
Shelton, T., Jeppson, E., and Johnson, B.: Family-centered care for children with special health care needs, Washington, DC, 1987, Association for the Care of Children's Health.
Silber, T.J.: Ethical considerations in the care of the chronically ill adolescent. In Blum, R., editor: Chronic illness and disabilities in childhood and adolescence, New York, 1984, Grune & Stratton, Inc.
Sorensen, E.: Children's coping responses, J. Pediatr. Nurs. 5(4):259-267, 1990.
Spina Bifida Association: Personal communication, Aug. 13, 1990.
Spinetta, J., and Deasy-Spinetta, P.: The patient's socialization in the community and school during therapy, Cancer 58(2):512-515, 1986.
Spokane Washington Deaconess Medical Center Pediatric Oncology Unit: Tips for dealing with siblings, The Candlelighters Childhood Cancer Foundation Quarterly Newsletter 11(3/4):7, 1987.
Stein, R.: A home care program for children with chronic illness, Child. Health Care 12(2):90-92, 1983.
Stein, R.E.K.: Home care: a challenging opportunity, Child. Health Care 14(2):90-95, 1985.
Stone, D.: Professional perceptions of parental adaptation to a child with special needs, Child. Health Care 18(3):174-177, 1989.
Strauss, S.S., and Munton, M.: Common concerns of parents with disabled children, Pediatr. Nurs. 11(5):371-375, 1985.
Thompson, R.J., and Quinn, A.N.: Developmental disabilities, New York, 1979, Oxford University Press.
Tritt, S., and Esses, L.: Psychosocial adaptation of siblings of children with chronic medical illnesses, Am. J. Orthopsychiatry 58(2):211-220, 1988.
Truesdell, S.C., Skorton, D.J., and Lauer, R.M.: Life insurance for children with cardiovascular disease, Pediatrics 77(5):687-691, 1986.
Trute, B.: Child and parent predictors of family adjustment in households containing young developmentally disabled children, Fam. Relations 39(3):292-297, 1990.
Vadasy, P.: Grandparents of children with special needs: support especially for grandparents, Child. Health Care 9(4):43-51, 1987.
Venters, M.: Familial coping with chronic and severe childhood illness: the case of cystic fibrosis, Soc. Sci. Med. 15A:289-297, 1981.
Wagner, M., Schubert, H., and Schubert, D.: Effects of sibling spacing on intelligence, interfamilial relations, psychosocial characteristics, and mental and physical health. In Reese, H.W., editor: Advances in child development and behavior, vol. 19, New York, 1985, Academic Press, Inc.
Warren, R., and Cohen, S.: Respite care, Rehab. Lit. 46(3-4):66-71, 1985.
Weitzman, M., Walker, D.K., and Gortmaker, S.: Chronic illness, psychosocial problems, and school absences, Clin. Pediatr. 25(3):137-141, 1986.
Wesolowski, C.: Self-contracts for chronically ill children, MCN 13(1):20-23, 1988.
Williams, H., and Wilson, M.: Sexuality in children and adolescents with cancer: pediatric oncology nurses' attitudes and behaviors, J. Assoc. Pediatr. Oncol. Nurs. 6(4):127-132, 1989.
Wissow, L., and Warshow, M.: Prevalence of home telephone service among families using an inner-city hospital's outpatient services, Am. J. Dis. Child. 144:426, 1990.
Woods, N., Yates, B., and Primomo, J.: Supporting families during chronic illness, IMAGE: J. Nurs. Scholarship 21(1):46-50, 1989.
Yoos, L.: Chronic childhood illnesses: developmental issues, Pediatr. Nurs. 13(1)25-28, 1987.
Zeltzer, L., and others: Psychologic effects of illness in adolescence. II. Impact of illness in adolescents—crucial issues and coping styles, J. Pediatr. 97(1):132-138, 1980.

BIBLIOGRAPHY

Adams, J.A., and Weaver, S.J.: Self-esteem and perceived stress in young adolescents with chronic disease, J. Adolesc. Health Care 7:173-177, 1986.
Ahmann, E.: An annotated bibliography on respite care for children and families, Child. Health Care 14(3):183-186, 1986.
American Academy of Pediatrics, Ad Hoc Task Forces on Home Care of Chronically Ill Infants and Children: Guidelines for home care of infants, children and adolescents with chronic disease, Pediatrics 74(3):434-436, 1984.
American Academy of Pediatrics: Health care financing for the child with catastrophic costs, Pediatrics 80(5):752-757, 1987.
American Academy of Pediatrics, Committee on Child Health Financing: Financing health care for the medically indigent child, Pediatrics 80(6):957-960, 1987.
American Academy of Pediatrics, Committee on Children With Disabilities: Screening for developmental disabilities, Pediatrics 78(3):526-528, 1986.
American Academy of Pediatrics, Committee on Children With Disabilities: Transition of severely disabled children from hospital or chronic care facilities to the community, Pediatrics 78(3):531-534, 1986.
Association for the Care of Children's Health: Family support in the home, Washington, DC, 1988, The Association.

Bean, M.: Assessing families of children with developmental disabilities. In Wright, L., and Leahey, M., editors: Families and chronic illness, Springhouse, PA, 1987, Springhouse Corp.

Bluebond-Langner, M., and others: Children's knowledge of cancer and its treatment: impact of an oncology camp experience, J. Pediatr. 116(2):207-213, 1990.

Blum, R.: Chronic illness and disabilities in childhood and adolescence, New York, 1984, Grune & Stratton, Inc.

Blumberg, B.D., and others: Responding to the information needs of young people whose parents or siblings have cancer: a description of a National Cancer Institute booklet, J. Assoc. Pediatr. Oncol. Nurses 5(1/2):16-19, 1988.

Boren, H.A., and Meell, H.: Adolescent amputee ski rehabilitation program, J. Assoc. Pediatr. Oncol. Nurses 2(1):16-23, 1985.

Brett, K.M.: Sibling response to chronic childhood disorders: research perspectives and practice implications, Issues Compr. Pediatr. Nurs. 11:43-57, 1988.

Brewer, E.J., and others: Family-centered, community-based, coordinated care for children with special health care needs, Pediatrics 83(6):1055-1060, 1989.

Brill, N., and others: Caring for chronically ill children: an innovative approach for care, Child. Health Care 16(2):105-111, 1987.

Butler, J.A., and others: Health insurance coverage and physician use among children with disabilities: findings from probability samples in five metropolitan areas, Pediatrics 79(1):89-98, 1987.

Byme, J., and others: Marriage and divorce after childhood and adolescent cancer, JAMA 262(19):2693-2699, 1989.

Cadman, D., and others: Chronic illness, disability, and mental and social well-being: findings of the Ontario child health study, Pediatrics 79(5):805-813, 1987.

Carraccio, C.L., McCormick, M.C., and Weller, S.C.: Chronic disease: effect on health cognition and health locus of control, J. Pediatr. 110(6):982-987, 1987.

Centers for Disease Control: Chronic disease reports in the Morbidity and Mortality Weekly Report, MMWR 38(suppl. S-1):1-7, 1989.

Chekryn, J., Deegan, M., and Reid, J.: Normalizing the return to school of the child with cancer, J. Assoc. Pediatr. Oncol. Nurses 3(2):20-24, 1986.

Chekryn, J., Deegan, M., and Reid, J.: Impact on teachers when a child with cancer returns to school, Child. Health Care 15(3):161-165, 1987.

Clark, H.B., and others: A social skills development model: coping strategies for children with chronic illness, Child. Health Care 18(1):19-29, 1989.

Clements, D.B., Copeland, L.G., and Loftus, M.: Critical times for families with a chronically ill child, Pediatr. Nurs. 16(2):157-161, 224, 1990.

Cohen, D.S., and others: Instruments to measure parent-child communication regarding pediatric cancer, Child. Health Care 18(3):142-145, 1989.

Cohen, M.H., and Martinson, I.M.: Chronic uncertainty: its effect on parental appraisal of a child's health, J. Pediatr. Nurs. 3(2):89-96, 1988.

Crocker, A.: The care of children with developmental disabilities, Curr. Opin. Pediatr. 1:162-167, 1989.

Crowley, A.: Integrating handicapped and chronically ill children into day care centers, Pediatr. Nurs. 16(1):39-44, 1990.

Crummette, B.: Assessing the impact of illness upon an adolescent and family, MCN 12(3):155-167, 1983.

Deatrick, J.A., and Knafl, K.A.: Management behaviors: day-to-day adjustments to childhood chronic conditions, J. Pediatr. Nurs. 5(1):15-22, 1990.

Decker, V.B.: Counseling approaches to the cancer patient, Issues Oncol. 4(1):4-7, 1987.

Dunst, C.J., and others: Enabling and empowering families of children with health impairments, Child. Health Care 17(2):71-81, 1988.

Eiser, C., and Town, C.: Teachers' concerns about chronically sick children: implications for paediatricians, Dev. Med. Child Neurol. 29(1):56-63, 1987.

Fee, M.A., Charney, E.B., and Robertson, W.W.: Nutritional assessment of the young child with cerebral palsy, Inf. Young Child. 9(1):33-40, 1988.

Feller, N., and others: A multidisciplinary approach to developing safe transportation for children with special needs, Orthopaedic Nurs. 5(5):25-27, 1986.

Ferrari, M.: Perceptions of social support by parents of chronically ill versus healthy children, Child. Health Care 15(1):26-31, 1986.

Fowler, M.G., Johnson, M.P., and Atkinson, S.S.: School achievement and absence in children with chronic health conditions, J. Pediatr. 106(4):683-687, 1985.

Fox, H.B., and Newacheck, P.W.: Private health insurance of chronically ill children, Pediatrics 85(1):50-57, 1990.

Frauman, A.C., and Morton, J.L.: Well child care for the chronically ill child, J. Pediatr. Health Care 2(6):288-294, 1988.

Freedman, S.A., Pierce, P.M., and Reiss, J.G.: REACH: a family-centered community-based case management model for children with special health care needs, Child. Health Care 16(2):114-117, 1987.

Galbehouse, B., and Gitterman, B.: Maternal understanding of commonly used medical terms in a pediatric setting, Am. J. Dis. Child. 144:419, 1990.

Gallo, A.M.: The special sibling relationship in chronic illness and disability: parental communication with well siblings, Holistic Nurs. Pract. 2(2):28-37, 1988.

Goldfarb, L.A., and others: Meeting the challenge of disability or chronic illness—a family guide, Baltimore, 1985, Paul H. Brookes Publishing Co.

Goldfarb, L., and others: Meeting the challenge of disability or chronic illness, Baltimore, 1986, Paul H. Brookes Publishing Co.

Goodell, A.: Peer education in schools for children with cancer, Issues Compr. Pediatr. Nurs. 7:101-106, 1984.

Gortmaker, S.L., and others: Chronic conditions, socioeconomic risks, and behavioral problems in children and adolescents, Pediatrics 85(3):267-276, 1990.

Grindley, J.F.: The handicapped child in school: considerations for health care, Holistic Nurs. Pract. 2(2):11-19, 1988.

Haase, J.E.: Components of courage in chronically ill adolescents: a phenomenological study, Adv. Nurs. Sci. 9(2):64-80, 1987.

Hall, D.M.B.: The child with a handicap, Boston, 1984, Blackwell Scientific Publications, Inc.

Halpern, P.: Respite care and family functioning in families with retarded children, Health Soc. Work 10(2):138-150, 1985.

Healy, A., Keesee, P., and Smith, B.: Early services for children with special needs, ed. 2, Baltimore, 1989, Paul H. Brookes Publishing Co.

Heiney, S.P., and others: The effects of group therapy on parents of children with cancer, J. Assoc. Pediatr. Oncol. Nurses 6(3):63-69, 1989.

Heiney, S.P., and others: Lasting impressions: a psychosocial support program for adolescents with cancer and their parents, Cancer Nurs. 13(1):13-20, 1990.

Hinds, P.S., and Martin, J.: Hopefulness and the self-sustaining process in adolescents with cancer, Nurs. Res. 37(6):336-340, 1988.

Hingsburger, D.: Stranger in a strange bed, Can. Nurse 83(7):21-22, 1987.

Hochstadt, N.J., and Yost, D.M.: The health care–child welfare partnership: transitioning medically complex children to the community, Child. Health Care 18(1):4-11, 1989.

Hockenberry-Eaton, M.J., and Cotanch, P.H.: Evaluation of a child's perceived self-competence during treatment for cancer, J. Pediatr. Oncol. Nurses 6(3):55-62, 1989.

Holaday, B.: Patterns of interaction between mothers and their chronically ill infants, MCN 16(1):29-45, 1987.

Holaday, B., and Turner-Henson, A.: Chronically ill school-age children's use of time, Pediatr. Nurs. 13(6):410-414, 1987.

Horner, M.M., Rawlins, P., and Giles, K.: How parents of children with chronic conditions perceive their own needs, MCN 12(1):40-43, 1987.

Hostler, S.L., and others: Adolescent autonomy project: transition skills for adolescents with physical disability, Child. Health Care 18(1):12-18, 1989.

Jamison, R.N., Lewis, S., and Burish, T.G.: Psychological impact of cancer on adolescents: self-image, locus of control, perception of illness, and knowledge of cancer, J. Chron. Dis. 39(8):609-617, 1986.

Johnson, B.: The changing role of families in health care, Child. Health Care 19(4):234-241, 1990.

Kinrade, L.C.: Preventive group intervention with siblings of oncology patients, Child. Health Care 14(2):110, 1985.

Knafl, K.A., and Deatrick, J.A.: Family management style: concept analysis and development, J. Pediatr. Nurs. 5(1):4-14, 1990.

Knox, J.E., and Hayes, V.E.: Hospitalization of a chronically ill child: a stressful time for parents, Issues Compr. Pediatr. Nurs. 6:217-226, 1983.

Kopala, B.: Mothers with impaired mobility speak out, MCN 14:115-119, 1989.

Kornblatt, E.S., and Heinrich, J.: Needs and coping abilities in families of children with developmental disabilities, Ment. Retard. 23(1):13-19, 1985.

LaMontagne, L.L.: Adopting a process approach to assess children's coping, J. Pediatr. Nurs. 3(3):159-163, 1987.

Levenson, P.M., and Singer, B.: Using computers to help children cope with chronic illness, Child. Health Care 14(2):76, 1985.

Leventhal, J.M.: Psychosocial assessment of children with chronic physical disease, Pediatr. Clin. North Am. 31(1):71-86, 1984.

Lewis, C., and others: Patient, parent, and physician perspectives on pediatric oncology rounds, J. Pediatr. 112(3):378-384, 1988.

Mann, J.R.: Psychosocial aspects of leukemia and other cancers during childhood. In Aaronson, N.K., and Beckmann, J.H.: The quality of life of cancer patients, New York, 1987, Raven Press.

McAnear, S.: Parental reaction to a chronically ill child, Home Healthcare Nurse 8(3):35-40, 1990.

McCormick, D.: School re-entry program for oncology patients, J. Assoc. Pediatr. Oncol. Nurses 3(3):13-17, 25, 1986.

McCubbin, M.A.: Family stress and family strengths: a comparison of single- and two-parent families with handicapped children, Res. Nurs. Health 12:101-110, 1989.

McDonnell, P.M., and others: Do artificial limbs become part of the user? New evidence, J. Rehabil. Res. Dev. 26(2):17-24, 1989.

McElheny, J.E.: Parental adaptation to a child with bronchopulmonary dysplasia, J. Pediatr. Nurs. 4(5):346-352, 1989.

McLane, J.B.: Lekotek: a unique play library for families with handicapped children, Child. Health Care 14(3):178-182, 1986.

Menke, E.M.: The impact of a child's chronic illness on school-aged siblings, Child. Health Care 15(3):132-140, 1987.

Miller, M., and Diao, J.: Family friends: new resources for psychosocial care of chronically ill children in families, Child. Health Care 15(4):259-264, 1987.

Monsen, R.: Phases in the caring relationship: from adversary to ally to coordinator, MCN 11(5):316-318, 1986.

Newacheck, P.W.: Adolescents with special health needs: prevalence, severity, and access to health services, Pediatrics 84(5):872-881, 1989.

Noh, S., and others: Delineating sources of stress in parents of exceptional children, Fam. Relations 38:456-461, 1989.

Ohanian, N.A.: Informational needs of children and adolescents with cancer, J. Assoc. Pediatr. Oncol. Nurses 6(3):94-97, 1989.

Opie, N.D., and Tse, A.M.: Perceptions of factors influencing individualized educational plan conference outcomes: implications for health care, J. Pediatr. Nurs. 3(1):2-10, 1988.

Oremland, E.: Communicating over chronic illness: dilemmas of affected school-aged children, Child. Health Care 14(4):218-223, 1986.

Palfrey, J., and others: Providing therapeutic services to children in special educational placements: an analysis of the related services provisions of Public Law 94-142 in five urban school districts, Pediatrics 85(4):518-526, 1990.

Patton, A.C., Ventura, J.N., and Savedra, M.: Stress and coping responses of adolescents with cystic fibrosis, Child. Health Care 14(3):153-156, 1986.

Perrin, E.C., West, P.D., and Culley, B.S.: Is my child normal yet? Correlates of vulnerability, Pediatrics 83(3):355-363, 1989.

Perrin, J.M., and MacLean, W.E.: Children with chronic illness: the prevention of dysfunction, Pediatr. Clin. North Am. 35(6):1325-1335, 1988.

Phillips, M., and Brostoff, M.: Working collaboratively with parents of disabled children, Pediatr. Nurs. 15(2):180-185, 1989.

Pidgeon, V.: Children's concepts of illness: implications for health teaching, Issues Compr. Pediatr. Nurs. 14(1):23-35, 1985.

Pilon, B.H., and Smith, K.A.: A parent group for the Hispanic parents of children with severe cerebral palsy, Child. Health Care 14(2):96-102, 1985.

Pipes, P.L., and Glass, R.: Nutrition and feeding of children with developmental delays and related problems. In Pipes, P.L., editor: Nutrition in infancy and childhood, ed. 4, St. Louis, 1989, Mosby–Year Book, Inc.

Pittman, J.F., and Lloyd, S.A.: Quality of family life, social support, and stress, J. Marriage Fam. 50(2):53-67, 1988.

Pollard, A., and others: School and the child with cancer: a program to assist school personnel, J. Assoc. Pediatr. Oncol. Nurses 2(3):7-10, 1985.

Poyadue, F.S.: In my opinion . . . parents as teachers of health care professionals, Child. Health Care 17(2):82-84, 1988.

Rawlins, P.S., and Horner, M.M.: Does membership in a support group alter needs of parents of chronically ill children? Pediatrics 14(1):70-72, 1988.

Reynolds, C., and Mann, L.: Encyclopedia of special education, New York, 1987, John Wiley & Sons, Inc.

Riley-Lawless, K.: School re-entry programs, J. Assoc. Pediatr. Oncol. Nurses 6(3)92-93, 1989.

The Robert Wood Johnson Foundation: Serving handicapped children: a special report, Princeton, NJ, 1988, The Foundation.

Rose, M.H.: The concepts of coping and vulnerability as applied to children with chronic conditions, Issues Compr. Pediatr. Nurs. 7:177-186, 1984.

Rose, M.H., and Thomas, R.B., editors: Children with chronic conditions, Orlando, FL, 1987, Grune & Stratton, Inc.

Rosenbaum, P.: Prevention of psychosocial problems in children with chronic illness, Can. Med. Assoc. J. 139(4):293-295, 1988.

Rosenbaum, P.L., Armstrong, R.W., and King, S.M.: Determinants of children's attitudes toward disability: a review of evidence, Child. Health Care 17(1):32-39, 1988.

Rudin, M.M., Martinson, I.M., and Gilliss, C.L.: Measurement of pyschosocial concerns of adoloscents with cancer, Cancer Nurs. 11(3):144-149, 1988.

Sahin, S.: The physically disabled child. In Johnson, S., editor: Nursing assessment and strategies for the family at risk, ed. 2, Philadelphia, 1986, J.B. Lippincott Co.

Sahler, O.J., and Carpenter, P.J.: Evaluation of a camp program for siblings of children with cancer, Am. J. Dis. Child. 143(6):690-696, 1989.

Savage, T.A., and Culbert, C.: Early intervention: the unique role of nursing, J. Pediatr. Nurs. 4(5):339-345, 1989.

Scheiber, K.K.: Developmentally delayed children: effects on the normal sibling, Pediatr. Nurs. 15(1):42-44, 1989.

Schlomann, P.: Developmental gaps of children with a chronic condition and their impact on the family, J. Pediatr. Nurs. 3(3):180-187, 1988.

Selekman, J.: When the nurse knows and the patient does not: waiting for a diagnosis, Holistic Nurs. Pract. 4(1):1-7, 1989.

Seligman, S.: Concepts in infant mental health: implications for work with developmentally disabled infants, Inf. Young Child. 1(1):41-51, 1988.
Silberman, M.A., Fochtman, D., and Baum, E.S.: One step at a time: summer camping for children with cancer, J. Assoc. Pediatr. Oncol. Nurses 2(1):24-30, 1985.
Singer, L., and Farkas, K.J.: The impact of infant disability on maternal perception of stress, Fam. Relations 38:444-449, 1989.
Spinetta, J.J., and others: Long-term adjustment in families of children with cancer, J. Psychosocial Oncol. 6(3,4):179-191, 1988.
Stein, R.E.K., and Jessop, D.J.: General issues in the care of children with chronic physical conditions, Pediatr. Clin. North Am. 31(1):189-198, 1984.
Stern, F.M., and Gorga, D.: Neurodevelopmental treatment (NDT): therapeutic intervention and its efficacy, Inf. Young Child. 1(1):22-32, 1988.
Stutzman, H.: Explaining leukemia to classmates, J. Assoc. Pediatr. Oncol. Nurses 2(1):15, 1985.
Tamlyn, D., and Arklie, M.M.: A theoretical framework for standard care plans: a nursing approach for working with chronically ill children and their families, Issues Compr. Pediatr. Nurs. 9(1):39-45, 1986.
Thomas, R.B.: Nursing assessment of childhood chronic conditions, Issues Compr. Pediatr. Nurs. 7:165-176, 1984.
Tripp-Reimer, T.: Ethnicity and families with chronic illness. In Wright, L.M., and Leahey, M., editors: Families and chronic illness, Springhouse, PA, 1987, Springhouse Corp.
Van Cleve, L.: Parental coping in response to their child's spina bifida, J. Pediatr. Nurs. 4(3):172-176, 1989.
Wacht, M.: The mentally disabled child. In Johnson, S., editor: Nursing assessment and strategies for the family at risk, ed. 2, Philadelphia, 1986, J.B. Lippincott Co.
Walker, C.L.: Stress and coping in siblings of childhood cancer patients, Nurs. Res. 37(4):206-212, 1988.
Walker, D.K.: Care of chronically ill children in schools, Pediatr. Clin. North Am. 31(1):221-233, 1984.
Walker, D.K., and others: Perceived needs of families with children who have chronic health conditions, Child. Health Care 18(4):196-201, 1989.
Wikler, L., Wasow, M., and Hatfield, E.: Seeking strengths in families of developmentally disabled children, Social Work 28(4):313-315, 1983.
Williams, H.A.: Social support and social networks: a review of the literature, J. Am. Pediatr. Nurs. 5(3):6-10, 1988.
Wright, L.M., and Leahey, M.: Families and chronic illness, Springhouse, PA, 1987, Springhouse Corp.
Young, M.H., and others: Use of the health and illness questionnaire with chronically ill and handicapped children, Child. Health Care 16(2):97-104, 1987.
Zeltzer, L.K., and LeBaron, S.: Fantasy in children and adolescents with chronic illness, Dev. Behav. Pediatr. 7(3):195-198, 1986.

Publications for School Attendance

Back to school: a handbook for teachers of children with cancer (also one for parents), Atlanta, 1989, American Cancer Society.
Lorn, A., and Martinez, I.: When you have a visually handicapped child in your classroom: suggestions for teachers, New York, 1985, American Federation for the Blind, Inc.
Morrow, G.: Helping chronically ill children in school, New York, 1985, Parker Publishing Co., Inc.
Students with cancer: a resource for the educator, U.S. Department of Health and Human Services, National Institutes of Health, NIH Pub. No. 87-2086, Washington, DC, 1987. (Order from Office of Cancer Communications, National Cancer Institute, Building 31, Room 10A24, Bethesda, MD 20892).
Suggestions for teachers and school counselors, Oak Brook, IL, 1983, The Compassionate Friends.
When your child is ready to return to school, Chicago, 1982, Association for Brain Tumor Research.

CHAPTER 23

Impact of Life-Threatening Illness on the Child and Family

RELATED TOPICS

The child with cancer, Ch. 36
Communicating with families, Ch. 6
Compliance, Ch. 27
Ethical decision making, Ch. 1
Impact of chronic illness or disability on the child and family, Ch. 22
Long-term sequelae of treatment, Ch. 36
Neonatal loss, Ch. 10
Pain assessment; pain management, Ch. 26
Sudden infant death syndrome, Ch. 13

GLOSSARY

acute grief Somatic symptoms and intense subjective distress that occur within hours or days after a significant loss
anticipatory grief Grieving before an actual loss
bereavement Period of mourning
DNR Do not resuscitate
life-threatening illness Serious disorder with a potentially fatal outcome
mourning Prolonged process of resolving grief
terminal illness A condition wherein a life is near or approaching its end

Although most childhood illnesses respond favorably to treatment, some do not. However, with advances in treatment many invariably fatal illnesses are now amenable to a prolonged period of remission and possibly cure. Despite this, families constantly live under the threat of potential loss of their child. As a result, health professionals are faced with the challenge of providing the best care possible to meet the family's psychologic and emotional needs both during the course of the illness and at the time of death.

There is probably no more difficult death to face than that of a child, because the end of life is premature and parents are robbed of the fulfillment and joy of seeing their child grow. This chapter establishes some theoretic and practical guidelines for helping families cope with the loss of a child. An overview of children's concept of death, the grieving process before and after death, each family member's reaction to a life-threatening illness, and nursing interventions to assist the family through each phase of the illness are presented.

The chapter concludes with a discussion of the impact of caring for dying children on nurses.

CHILDREN AND DEATH

Most children have relatively little experience with death. However, for some the tragedy of death becomes an indelible memory, and the reactions of others to their loss greatly influence how this event affects their lives. The following discussion is concerned with the development of the death concept in children and awareness of fatally ill children of their own death.

CHILDREN'S UNDERSTANDING OF AND REACTIONS TO DYING AND DEATH

The concept of death is acquired through the sequential development of cognitive abilities and follows closely Piaget's stages. Although throughout childhood death is greatly influenced by the child's personal experiences with it and the explanations and attitudes offered by others, the abstract adult meaning of death as irreversible, inevitable, and universal is not understood by most children until preadolescence. Unless nurses understand how children perceive death, the fears associated with death in each age-group, and the personal meanings of death and bereavement during various stages of development, they cannot effectively counsel parents and children through the multiple crises associated with expected or unexpected death.

Knowledge about preschool and older children's concept of death is primarily based on the work of Maria Nagy (1948), who asked several hundred Hungarian children ranging in age from 3 to 10 years to draw pictures and write down (if they were old enough) everything they could think of about death. From analyzing their responses, she concluded that there were three main stages of death interpretation. Although more recent studies have corroborated most of her findings, they have not found evidence of the personification seen in school-age children, but support for a concrete connotation of death, with naturalistic explanations about why people die, such as from old age or a gunshot wound (Table 23-1) (Wass, 1985). These findings may reflect differences in the religious and cultural orientation of the children studied by Nagy and those studied by current investigators.

Table 23-1 Children's concept of death

COGNITIVE STAGE	CONCEPT
Sensorimotor (infancy, toddler)	No concept of death but reacts to loss
Preoperational thought (early childhood)	Death is temporary and reversible Death is seen as a departure or separation
Concrete operations (school age)	Death is irreversible but not necessarily inevitable Death may be personified and viewed as destructive Explanations for death are naturalistic and physiologic
Formal operations (later school age, adolescence)	Death is irreversible, universal, and inevitable Death is still seen as a personal but distant event Explanations for death are physiologic and theologic

Infants and Toddlers

Exactly how preverbal children view death is a mystery because there is no way of reliably assessing their views of death. It is quite likely, on the basis of their cognitive abilities, that they have no concept of death. Toddlers' egocentricity and vague separation of fact and fantasy make it impossible for them to comprehend absence of life. Although they may repeat what initially sounds like a correct definition of death, such as, "Grandpa is dead; he went to heaven," they may later refer to Grandpa as if he still exists. They can only think about events in terms of their own frame of reference—living.

Reactions to dying. Immobilization, regression to less independent levels of behavior, separation, intrusive or painful procedures, and alteration in ritualistic routine represent the greatest threats to children in this age-group. However, they may perceive the seriousness of their illness from the parents' reactions of anxiety, sadness, depression, or anger. Although the children are unaware of the reason for such emotions, they are disturbed and upset by their parents' behavior. Helping parents deal with their feelings allows them more emotional reserve to meet the needs of their children. Encouraging them to stay in the hospital as much as possible and to participate in the child's care promotes the parents' and child's adjustment to a serious, potentially fatal illness.

Reactions to death. To the amazement and dismay of adults, toddlers may persist in wanting to visit the dead person, request that all that person's possessions and living quarters remain unchanged, and talk about the deceased as if nothing has happened. Dealing honestly and openly with such reactions is preferable to admonishing the child or trying to prove what dead means. For example, the parent can restate that the person cannot visit because he or she is dead and in a special place (cemetery, heaven, or other explanation) and can offer to bring the child to visit the burial plot if possible.

Ritualism is extremely important to toddlers, so any change in the home following the death can produce anxiety. There is no harm in allowing the ritualism, such as setting an extra place at the table for the deceased person, because, for the child, imagining the person to be present is almost as real as life. What is important is to stress that, although the place is set at the table, the dead person will return only in thoughts and memories. As children grow older, form new attachments, and develop stronger ego defenses, they will be increasingly able and willing to let go of this fantasy person.

Preschool Children

Several characteristics of preschoolers' cognitive and psychologic development affect their conception of death. Because of their sense of precausality, they are unable to differentiate physical cause from logical or psychologic motivation. In addition, their egocentricity implies a tremendous sense of self-power and omnipotence. Therefore they believe that their thought is sufficient to cause events. The consequence of such magical thinking is the burden of guilt, shame, and punishment.

Concept of death. Children between ages 3 and 5 have usually heard the word "death" and have some connotation of its meaning. They see death as a departure, possibly as a kind of sleep. They may recognize the fact of physical death but do not separate it from living abilities. The dead person in the coffin still breathes, eats, and sleeps. Death is temporary and gradual; life and death can change places with one another. Because of their immature concept of time, there is no real understanding of the universality and inevitability of death. Words such as "forever" and "everyone" have meaning only in the child's egocentric thinking. Waiting until Christmas may be "forever," and anybody the child denotes is "everyone."

Reactions to dying. If preschoolers become seriously ill during this time, they conceive of the illness as a punishment for their thoughts or actions. The usual diagnostic and treatment procedures, combined with enforced hospitalization, only confirm their belief that they are being punished. If the parents do not stay with them during hospitalization or prevent the traumatic procedures, they are convinced that the parents are retaliating for the child's previous misdeeds or bad thoughts.

The same principles of magical thinking and omnipotence affect preschoolers when a sibling becomes critically ill or dies. One of the most significant types of death is sudden infant death syndrome (SIDS). Because it occurs unexpectedly to a healthy infant, who may have been rejected and unwanted by a jealous sibling, preschoolers find no evidence to support a physical cause of death. Indeed, the parents are frequently unaware of the reason for the fatality and may question any possible cause. If preschoolers are in any way accused or suspected of having harmed the infant, they may feel extremely guilty and responsible for the tragedy. On observing their parents' acute grief, they may interpret the anger or depression as a rejection of them.

When a sibling becomes ill, the well siblings experience the loss of routine and parental attention. It is natural for them to resent such disruptions and to blame the changes on the ill child. However, preschoolers have less ability to understand the reasons for the parents' prolonged absence from the home than older children. Even though parents may explain how ill the sibling is, what the hospital is like, and why they must be there, preschoolers only see the special attention and the material rewards that the ill sister or brother receives. Because they are also unable to differentiate causes for separation of the parents and ill child, they fear that the parents may never return. If they should learn that the ill child may not get well or come home, they interpret this to mean that the parents will also never return. Their greatest fear concerning death is separation from parents.

Reactions to death. In relation to death, preschoolers may engage in activities that seem strange or abnormal to adults. For example, if a pet dies, preschoolers usually request a "funeral" or some ceremony to symbolize their loss. Perceptive parents realize that the function of such rites of passage is as important to the preschooler for the loss of a pet as to an adult for the loss of a significant person. After the "funeral" and "burial," preschoolers may dig up the remains. Many parents are confused by this behavior. However, children have no concept of the irreversible nature of death and must continually reassure themselves that the animal has not returned or gone somewhere else. If left alone to satisfy their curiosity, they will see that the dead animal is still in the ground.

Because young children accept the literal meaning of words, it is important for others to examine the implications of possible explanations for death. Those with a religious affiliation may equate death with an afterlife and explain that dead animals or people go to heaven. The act of digging up the dead pet may be a result of trying to ascertain whether the animal did go to heaven. Parents who are aware of the reason for this behavior can explain that the "soul" goes to heaven but the body remains in the earth. If parents dismiss this activity without some clarification, the child may interpret the religious message as a lie.

Another common euphemism for death is "gone to sleep." Again preschoolers attach the literal meaning of sleep to death and may fear going to sleep for fear of dying or never waking up. One 5-year-old child who had been told that her aunt died because she was very tired refused to engage in any strenuous activity and took naps frequently. Her parents became concerned about her sudden lassitude and finally asked her why she was always tired. The child exclaimed that she *was not* tired; she took naps to avoid fatigue because she did not want to die like her aunt. When the parents explained that her aunt was tired from old age and sickness, not from playing too much or sleeping too little, the child immediately resumed her usual behaviors.

Because of their fewer defense mechanisms for dealing with loss, young children may react to a less significant loss with more outward grief than to the loss of a very significant person. This can be extremely disconcerting to parents who view their child's undisturbed behavior as evidence of lack of interest or response to the tragedy. However, the reverse is most likely true. The loss is so deep, painful, and threatening that the child must deny it for the present to survive its overwhelming impact. Behavioral reactions such as giggling, joking, attracting attention, or regressing to earlier developmental skills indicate children's need to distance themselves from the tremendous loss. Understanding the function of such behaviors and supporting children through the reactions until such time as they feel enough self-control to grieve will help them gradually resolve the loss.

School-Age Children

Although school-age children have a better understanding of causality, less egocentricity, and advanced perception of time, they still associate misdeeds or bad thoughts with causing death and feel intense guilt and responsibility for the event. However, because of their higher cognitive abilities, they respond well to logical explanations and comprehend the figurative meaning of words more than children in younger age-groups. Although they are less likely to interpret explanations in a purely literal sense, they are still prone to self-referenced definitions. It is important for adults to clarify the meanings of statements and to repeatedly ask them what they think.

Concept of death. Much of what pertains to the preschool period regarding the understanding of death also relates to school-age children, particularly those near 6 or 7 years of age. However, these children have a deeper understanding of death in the concrete sense. According to Nagy, they attempt to ascribe a more comprehensible meaning to the event by personifying death as a devil, God, ghost, or "bogeyman." According to others, they have naturalistic-physiologic explanations of why death occurs and what happens to the dead body. Factual explanations, such as "When you die, your body decays in the ground," are consistent with their concrete thinking.

By age 9 or 10 years most children have an adult concept of death. They realize that it is inevitable, universal, and irreversible. Their attitudes toward death are greatly influenced by the reactions and attitudes of others, particularly their parents.

Reactions to dying. School-age children's increased ability to comprehend and reason poses additional risks for them. They may fear the reason for the illness, communicability of the disease to themselves or others, consequences of the disease on their functioning and relationships with others, and the process of dying and death itself. They tend to fear the expectation of the event more than its realization. Their fear of the unknown is greater than that of the known; like preschoolers, their fantasy explanations for the unexpected or unknown are usually much more frightening and extreme than the actual situation. For this reason anticipatory preparation is very necessary and effective. These children respond well to explanations of the disease, names of drugs, and so on. Inasmuch as the developmental task of this age is industry, helping children maintain control over their bodies by understanding what is happening to them and participating in what is done to them allows these youngsters to achieve independence, self-worth, and self-esteem and to avoid a sense of inferiority.

Because dying is loss of control over every aspect of living, the realization of impending death or failing to recover is a tremendous threat to their sense of security and ego strength. These children are likely to exhibit their fear more through verbal uncooperativeness than actual physical aggression. Health professionals may erroneously interpret this behavior as rude, impolite, insolent, or stubborn. In reality the words are conveying the same meaning as physical attempts to run away or to fight others off. This verbal "flight or fight" reaction to stress is a plea for some control and power. Encouraging children to talk about their feelings and providing outlets for aggression through play are means of dealing with this type of uncooperativeness.

Reactions to death. School-age children are very interested in postdeath services, such as wakes, funerals, and burials. They may be inquisitive about what happens to the body—who dresses it, how the body feels, or what happens in an autopsy. Adults sometimes find these questions distressing, particularly when they concern the death of a significant person. However, such inquiries are children's way of assimilating all the facts about death into a concrete, logical framework. Avoiding such questions or fabricating euphemistic stories only confuses and frustrates children's attempts at understanding what may happen *to them* if they should die.

Adolescents

By the time most children reach adolescence they have a mature understanding of death, and as abstract thinking develops there is more questioning of death and related topics, such as the religious meaning of afterlife. However, their other developmental needs, especially identity, make this an exceptionally difficult time for these young people to cope with the loss of a loved one or their own impending death.

Concept of death. Although adolescents have a mature understanding of death, they are still very much influenced by "remnants" of magical thinking and are subject to the feelings of guilt and shame. Adolescents are exploring many new areas of interpersonal relationships and are likely to see deviations from accepted behavior as reasons for their illness. It is important to clarify that thoughts and activities, especially sexual experimentation, do not cause diseases, such as cancer.

Reactions to dying. Adolescents have the most difficulty in coping with death. Although they have reached the level of adult comprehension of the concept of death, they are least likely to accept cessation of life, particularly if it is their own. Developmentally the rejection of death is understandable because the adolescents' tasks are to establish an identity by finding out who they are, what their purpose is, and where they belong. Any suggestion of being different or nonbeing is a tremendous threat to the answers to such questions. Adolescents' concern is for the present much more than the past or future.

Adolescents strive for group acceptance and independence from parental constraints. As a result, they rely on peer rules and beliefs for personal direction and reject opposing parental demands. However, when they are faced with the crisis of serious illness, they may consider themselves alienated from peer associations and unable to communicate with their parents for emotional support. Therefore they may be virtually alone in their struggle for survival.

Healthy adolescents must deal with several maturational crises, such as acceptance of bodily changes and socialization of intensifying sexual impulses. Any threat to either task increases the vulnerability of adolescents to the stress of coping with such crises. The ravages of a terminal illness and the deleterious effects of chemotherapy may be greater concerns than the prospect of dying. Adolescents' orientation to the present compels them to worry about physical changes even more than the prognosis for future recovery.

Sometimes parents fail to understand the emotional impact on the adolescent of side effects from chemotherapy, such as hair loss, weight gain, fatigue, or skin eruptions. They wonder why the adolescent cannot accept the temporary altered body image for the possible benefit of the treatment. Intellectually adolescents can understand the necessity of treatment, but emotionally they have great difficulty in overcoming the feelings of being different, unable to equal others, and physically compromised because of the illness.

Nurses are in a most advantageous position in working with terminally ill adolescents; in the hospital setting they spend the greatest amount of time with them. They can structure the hospital admission to allow for maximum self-control and independence, while allowing the adolescent the opportunity to learn to know the nurse. Answering adolescents' questions honestly, treating them as mature individuals, and respecting their needs for privacy, solitude, and personal expressions of emotions such as anger, sadness, or fear convey to adolescents the adult's true concern for their physical and emotional welfare. Nurses can help parents to communicate with their adolescent children by acting as role models, avoiding alliances with either parent or child, and allowing parents the opportunity to ventilate their feelings of frustration, incompetence, or failure in an atmosphere of acceptance and nonjudgment.

Reactions to death. The adolescent's reactions to death straddle the transition from the childhood to adulthood. Although some teenagers are able to cope with death by expressing appropriate emotions, talking about the loss, and resolving the grief, others may appear undisturbed by the event, extremely angry, or unusually silent and withdrawn.

Because of their idealistic view of the world, they may criticize funeral rites as barbaric, money making, and unnecessary. Their fear of the unknown and inability to deal with these thoughts may prevent them from attending funeral services. They are sometimes horrified and angry over adults' concerns for practical matters such as immediate financial arrangements. Statements such as, "Daddy isn't even buried yet and you [mother] are worrying about his money," can cause great conflict and misunderstanding between child and parent. Helping adults understand why teenagers have such thoughts can avert an unnecessary and painful strain among family members.

Nursing Considerations

Nurses in almost any area of pediatrics have an opportunity to help children develop positive attitudes toward death. First, they can counsel parents regarding children's age-specific understanding of death and appropriate ways to handle behaviors, such as digging up the dead pet.

Second, nurses can encourage parents to take advantage of "small deaths" to help children become familiar and more comfortable with loss. The death of a pet, flowers, or a television character may present such an opportunity (Fig. 23-1). Certainly such events should not be covered up, such as replacing a pet with a new one so the child thinks it is the same animal. Many children's books are available that present death in a sensitive and nonthreatening manner and, when read to children, offer opportunities for dialogue. (see also Communication Techniques, Chapter 6; sources of books are listed at the end of the chapter).

Third, nurses may take part in organized programs on death education, especially in the schools, or serve as resources for planning such programs (Wass and others, 1980). Through a formal curriculum devoted to this topic, youngsters are introduced to the many facets of death as a part of life. Such programs can also ease the reentry of children with life-threatening disorders back to school. When

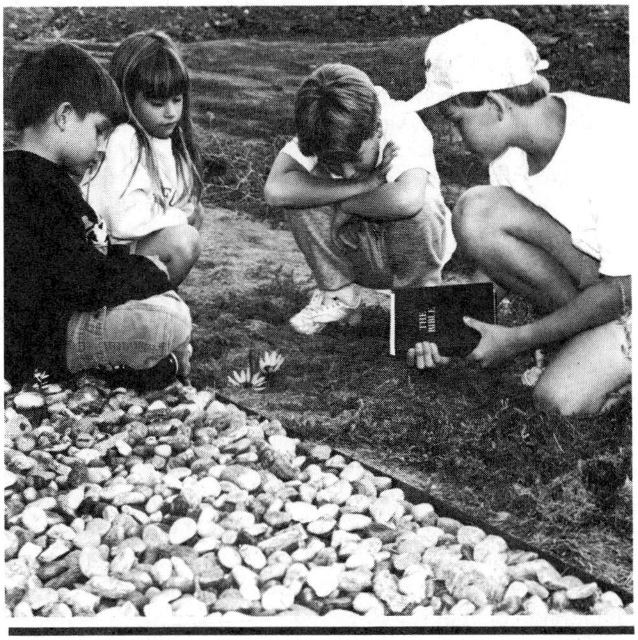

Fig. 23-1. Children learn about death and related rituals, such as burial, through losses, such as death of a pet.

persons die who are known to children, such as classmates or teachers, special bereavement sessions can be instituted to help the students understand and deal with the loss (Schonfeld, 1989).

Finally, nurses can serve as resources to parents and others involved with children in answering questions about children and death. For example, many parents are concerned with how to handle "small deaths" constructively or whether young or school-age children should attend funeral or burial services of loved ones (see p. 1049). Routine inquiry into such topics should be part of well-child care because it can promote healthy attitudes and prepare children to cope with loss when it occurs.

AWARENESS OF DYING IN CHILDREN WITH LIFE-THREATENING ILLNESS

One of the initial reactions of parents (and some health professionals) to the discovery of a life-threatening illness is to protect the child from the impact of the diagnosis. However, terminally ill children develop awareness of the seriousness of their diagnosis, even when protected from the truth (Waechter, 1985). Anxiety may not be attributable to fear of death but may be demonstrated in relationship to separation, pain, intrusive procedures, bodily change or mutilation, loneliness, immobilization, and punishment. Children as young as 2 or 3 years of age perceive their parents' emotions and react accordingly.

Studies of children' experiences with life-threatening illness demonstrate that children learn about their situation through the acquisition of information, at which time they develop different conceptions of themselves. Five stages have been defined (Bluebond-Langner, 1978, 1989):

Stage I: Disease is a serious illness. New identity of "sick" child.

Stage II: Discovery of the relationship of medication and recovery. Learns the taboos of disease and death.

Stage III: Marked understanding of the purposes and implications of special procedures. Sense of well-being begins to fade and perceives self as different from other children.

Stage IV: Illness is viewed as a permanent condition. Sense of always being sick and never getting better.

Stage V: Realization that there is only a finite number of medications. Awareness (directly or indirectly) of their fatal prognosis.

Experience is considered the critical factor in the passage through these various stages. The experience of having a disease allows children to assimilate information by relating what they see and hear to what they feel and think. Experience also explains why age and intellectual ability are not related to the speed or completeness with which children pass through the various stages of awareness. Some 3- and 4-year-olds of average intelligence know more about their prognosis than very intelligent 9-year-olds who are still in their first remission, have had fewer clinical experiences, and are aware only that they have a serious illness (Greenham and Lohmann, 1982).

Time lapse between stages tends to be the same for all children regardless of age. Passage from the first stage to the second stage occurs rapidly on relapse. Passage through the second, third, and fourth stages takes somewhat longer, but passage to the fifth stage may take place as soon as the child learns of the death of another, and all knowledge from previous stages is quickly synthesized into a new self-awareness.

Informing Children of Life-Threatening Diagnosis

All children should be told about the diagnosis by their parents or with the assistance of appropriate practitioners. Children need honest and accurate information about their illness, treatments, and prognosis. Appropriate literature about the disease is helpful.* Providing an atmosphere of open communication early in the course of the illness facilitates answering difficult questions as the child's condition worsens (Lansky, List, and Ritter-Sterr, 1988).

Exactly how and what to tell children about serious illness, dying, and death is a very individual matter. However, guidelines can help in determining how to present facts in a way that fosters trust, enhances meaningful communication, and offers emotional support to the child and parents.

Developmental age. A primary concern in any relationship with children is their age, because the level of comprehension is a function of children's cognitive develpement. As discussed earlier, children at various ages have different understandings and fears of death. The younger child fears separation, which can be imposed by any number of circumstances, only one of which is death or illness. The older child fears the results of illness, particularly pain or bodily injury, as well as death itself. Anyone working with children must be aware of such developmental variations and be sensitive to their verbal and nonverbal language.

Previous knowledge. Besides age, another essential principle is first to find out what the child is thinking. Before any explanations (true or false) are offered to children, they have invented their own. Answers to such questions as "What do you think is wrong with you?" or "What have you heard others say?" provide information on which to structure further explanations. Very often a child will respond with an answer of such detailed, accurate information that the only element lacking is the name of the disease. Other answers may reveal possible areas of misconception, which can then be clarified or refocused.

Sometimes parents and other adults hear the children's words but fail to comprehend their meaning. They erroneously assume that because children recite all the facts they also understand their implications or have dealt with all their fears. This may not be so; intellectualizing about one's condition can be a powerful defense mechanism. For example, an adolescent who was undergoing serious open-heart surgery knew precisely every detail of the operation, preoperative and postoperative care, and involved risks. The med-

*Excellent resources for children with cancer are Baker, L.: You and leukemia: a day at a time, ed. 2, Philadelphia, 1989, W.B. Saunders Co.; Gaes, J.: My book for kids with cansur, Aberdeen, SD, 1987, Melius & Peterson, Publishing, Inc.; and What it is I have, don't want, didn't ask for, can't give back, and how I feel about it, New York, 1983, Leukemia Society of America.

THERAPEUTIC DIALOGUE

Questions on Death

Shortly after learning of the diagnosis of cancer and beginning chemotherapy, a school-age child has the following conversion with the nurse.

CHILD: What is happening to me?
NURSE: What do you mean?
CHILD: I feel so awful. I hate the throwing up after those drugs. Sometimes I think I may die.
NURSE: What do you think about dying?
CHILD: I get very scared. I don't know how it would be or if anyone would be there to help me. (Starts to cry; nurse comforts child in her arms.) Am I going to die?
NURSE: I don't know. You have a serious illness, but we hope these medications will make it go away. But no matter what happens, you won't be alone. People who care for you, like your parents and I, will be here.
CHILD: I'm glad. Being by myself scares me.

SUMMARY

Nurse remains silent to allow the child to continue with the conversation but stays with the child for a short time to reinforce the promise that the child won't be left alone.

ical and nursing staff considered her exceptionally well prepared. However, everyone had failed to ask her about how she felt. When the nurse asked her this before her surgery, the child answered, "I fear that I may die." Once this was verbalized, the child, her parents, and the nurse focused on her fears instead of on the facts of the illness.

Honesty. The last principle in explaining events such as death to children is honesty. Although the truth is usually the most difficult answer to give, in the long run it lessens many of the conflicts or problems that arise from lies, half-truths, or conspiracies. The truth provides answers for future questions. It also fosters trust. Children adeptly perceive the maxim: Do as I say, not as I do. It is very difficult to encourage children to be honest, to confide in others, and to openly discuss their fears if parents refuse to do the same.

Honesty is certainly not the easiest solution; the truth may prompt children to ask other distressing questions. The question many parents and health professionals dread the most is "Am I going to die?" When children have the answer to this question, the next question is "When?" Children need answers that are straightforward, yet caring (see Therapeutic Dialogue). In telling children that a cure is no longer possible, one must also leave room for hope. The hope is redirected from care to comfort (Lansky, List, and Ritter-Sterr, 1988).

If given the opportunity, children will tell others how much they want to know. Asking questions such as, "If the disease came back, would you want to know?" "Do you want others to tell you everything, even if the news isn't good?" or "If someone were not getting better [or more directly, "were dying"], do you think they would want to know?" helps children set the limits for how much truth they can accept and cope with. Children need time to proceed through the stages of denial, shock, and anger before they can assimilate and hopefully accept the inevitable fact of mortality.

SIBLINGS' RESPONSES TO LIFE-THREATENING ILLNESS AND DEATH

The experience of a child with life-threatening illness and/or the child's death has profound effects on the family, including the siblings. Many of the siblings' responses reflect those discussed in Chapter 22 regarding chronic illness or disability in a brother or sister. Predominant feelings of children when the sibling's diagnosis is potentially fatal, such as cancer, include isolation and displacement—the parents devote the majority of their time to care of the ill child, causing the siblings to feel left out of the parent/sick child partnership and regarded as unimportant family members.

Siblings may also express concern for their own health status, recognizing the possibility of death and at times manifesting physical symptoms similar to those of the child. Siblings' knowledge of the diagnosis tends to be inadequate, although many children perceive of cancer as the "scariest disease" (Martinson and others, 1990).

Guilt and shame can surface. Guilt arises when children imagine their own responsibility for the illness. One 5-year-old child stated that her brother got sick when he caught her sore throat. Guilt may also be related to their feeling fortunate about not having the illness, yet jealous of the ill child's lavished attention. Shame may be another source of guilt—shame at having a sibling in the family who is seriously ill, disfigured, or dying (Sourkes, 1986).

When a brother or sister dies, siblings grieve for the loss of the child, must deal with the stress of having grieving parents, and at times may feel like "the replaced child" or the "less special" child. For example, when a parent(s) memorializes the dead child, the surviving siblings are constantly reminded of this child's specialness and may feel that they can never "live up" to the memories or expectations (Davies, 1987).

Some studies have reported a negative impact on children experiencing sibling death. Behavior problems, such as acting out, poorer school performance, and antisocial behavior, have been reported. Whether these are temporary or have a lasting influence on subsequent adjustment is unclear. However, positive benefits are also possible. Bereaved siblings can have higher self-concepts than their nonbereaved peers; they perceive that they have matured and grown psychologically as a result of the experience. Parents also report that the surviving siblings are more compassionate (Martinson, Davis, and McClowry, 1987). Factors influencing positive or negative adjustment are not fully understood, although open communication between the family and siblings and increased involvement with the ill child's care and death are likely to aid in positive adjustment (Birenbaum, 1989; Lauer and others, 1985). (See also Questions and Controversies, p. 1049).

These findings give direction for nursing intervention. Children need information about the sibling's illness and death, especially if the death was unexpected. Children should be told directly that they did not cause the illness or death (except in rare intentional killings) and that it is normal to feel guilty, jealous, or angry. Their fears of becoming ill or dying should be addressed, and, whenever possible, the siblings should be involved in the child's care, praised for their cooperation, and made to feel "special." Parents are encouraged to spend quality time with the well children and to be aware of times they may make the surviving children feel like "replacements," such as inadvertently calling the sibling by the dead child's name. Such interventions have the potential to help the entire family cope successfully with an overwhelming crisis.

GRIEF PROCESS IN EXPECTED AND UNEXPECTED DEATH

In response to any loss there is a grief reaction. *Acute grief* develops within hours to days and is characterized by somatic symptoms and intense subjective distress. *Grief work* or *mourning* refers to the lengthy process that begins with acute grief and extends into a period of reorganization of psychologic life, with attachment to new people and interests. *Bereavement* often refers to the period of mourning, although grief, mourning, and bereavement are used interchangeably.

Numerous investigators have contributed greatly to the present understanding of grief and bereavement, and those whose work is considered classic are presented in the following paragraphs. In expected death the child and family must be involved in the plan for intervention both before and after the death. In unexpected death the survivors face the tremendous task of integrating the loss into their lives, with no opportunity for anticipatory grief. In either situation nurses can facilitate the grief process by being aware of expected psychologic and somatic reactions and supporting the grievers through each stage of the mourning process.

Box 23-1 STAGES OF DYING (KÜBLER-ROSS)

Denial
Person responds with shock and disbelief
"No, not me" reaction occurs regardless of whether the person is explicitly told the diagnosis

Anger
Usually follows denial; may occur and recur at any time during the dying process
"Why me?" reaction; anger, rage, hostility, envy, or resentment may be directed at oneself or at others

Bargaining
Dying person's attempt to postpone the inevitable
Bargaining may be with God, with oneself, or with the most significant other person

Depression
Generally two types: for past losses (loss of hair from therapy, loss of a body part or function, restricted physical ability, and change in life-style) and for anticipated or impending losses (signals the person's preparation for the impending loss of all love objects)

Acceptance
Person is no longer angry or depressed
Not a happy time, but one of inner peace and resolution that death is a certainty

KÜBLER-ROSS: STAGES OF DYING

Although most research on grief has focused on the reactions following a loss, Elisabeth Kübler-Ross (1969) has identified five stages that adults experience in terms of expected death (Box 23-1). That children experience the same set of behaviors is likely but not confirmed. These stages represent a set of *ever-changing behaviors* that surface as the need for them arises within the individual's attempts to cope with expected loss. They are not sequential stages that dying persons progress through. Kübler-Ross maintains that the helping person's role in all stages of dying is to support the person where he or she is, not to maneuver from one stage to another. If support is truly therapeutic, the strength gained from this active intervention will help the person proceed independently to another stage.

LINDEMANN: SYMPTOMATOLOGY OF GRIEF

Lindemann (1944) analyzed and described the reactions of adult survivors following the loss of significant others and found that acute grief has the following characteristics:

1. It is a definite syndrome with psychologic and somatic symptoms (Box 23-2).
2. The syndrome may appear immediately after a crisis, be delayed, be exaggerated, or be apparently absent.
3. In place of the normal syndrome there may appear distorted reactions that represent one special aspect of the syndrome.
4. Through intervention, distorted reactions can be transformed into normal grief work with successful resolution.

Box 23-2 SYMPTOMATOLOGY OF NORMAL GRIEF

Sensations of Somatic Distress
Feeling of tightness in the throat
Choking, with shortness of breath
Marked tendency to sighing
Empty feeling in abdomen
Lack of muscular power
Intense subjective distress described as tension or mental pain

Preoccupation with Image of the Deceased
Hears, sees, or imagines that the dead person is present
Slight sense of unreality
Feeling of emotional distance from others
May believe that he or she is approaching insanity

Feelings of Guilt
Searches for evidence of failure in preventing the death
Accuses self of negligence or exaggerates minor omissions

Feelings of Hostility
Loss of warmth toward others
Tendency to irritability and anger
Wish not be bothered by friends or relatives

Loss of Usual Patterns of Conduct
Restlessness, inability to sit still, aimless moving about
Continual searching for something to do or what he or she thinks should be done
Lack of capacity to initiate and maintain organized patterns of activity

Modified from Lindemann, E.: Symptomatology and management of acute grief, Am. J. Psychiatry 101:141-143, 1944. Copyright 1944 American Psychiatric Association.

The identification of "distorted" reactions is controversial. Lindemann described behaviors such as overactivity without a sense of loss, conspicuous change in social relationships, and acquiring symptoms of the deceased as maladaptive signs. More current research suggests that such behaviors may represent normal, but more variable, grief reactions. Psychosomatic symptoms such as compulsive-obsessive behavior and depression are seen in parents 2 years after the death of a child and do not reflect mental illness (Moore, Gillis, and Martinson, 1988).

Health professionals should emphasize that grief reactions such as hearing the dead person's voice, feeling distant from others, or seeking reassurance that they did everything possible for the lost person are normal, necessary, and expected. They in no way signify insanity or approaching mental breakdown. On the contrary, such behaviors signify that the survivor is working through the acute grief and will probably satisfactorily resolve the loss and resume or restructure a meaningful role in the social environment.

PARKES: MOURNING

Whereas Lindemann's work focused on the symptoms of acute grief, several other researchers have attempted to analyze the behaviors and responses of the bereaved during the long and difficult process of mourning. Although there are numerous commonalities among the stages proposed by these authorities, the work of C. Murray Parkes with widows and widowers is considered classic (Glick, Weiss, and Parkes, 1974); according to Parkes' findings, the grief process consists of at least four phases, which do not necessarily proceed in sequence and may recur at any time. Contrary to the common belief that mourning is completed in a year, data from clinical studies indicate that resolution of grief may take years, and one study reported an *intensification* of grief during the third year (Rando, 1983).

Resolution of grief may not always result in "letting go" of the loved one. Many survivors describe the pressure of an "empty space" in their lives 9 years after the death of a child. Families attempt to fill the emptiness by keeping busy, often through altruistic involvements in self-help groups or by maintaining the connection with the lost child through recalling cherished memories. Feelings of emptiness intensify around holidays and anniversaries and with questions such as "How many children are in the family?" To exclude the dead child in the answer is to ignore his or her significance, but to include the child opens communication that makes many acquaintances uncomfortable. The intensity of both the emptiness and the bereavement responses appears directly related to the closeness of the family members to the deceased (Davies, 1988; McClowry and others, 1987).

Shock and Disbelief

Shock, numbness, and disbelief are seen during the immediate phase of grief. As one parent described, "We were as prepared for our son's death as anyone could be, but it was a shock when in a moment his life was finished. I just can't get over the rapidity with which life ends." This temporary numbness protects the survivors from the overwhelming pain associated with grief. Often decisions are made automatically, and only certain details are remembered.

Expression of Grief

When the numbness fades, there begins a period of intense grief characterized by a yearning and loneliness for the deceased. During this stage many of the signs of acute grief are evident, and physical complaints such as inability to sleep and appetite changes are common. There is a tendency to review the events of the deceased's life and to evaluate the relationship with the loved one. At this time feelings of guilt and anger are common.

Disorganization and Despair

During this stage the pain of the loss is replaced primarily by emptiness, apathy, and deep depression. There is a feeling that life has no meaning and that the pain will never end. This is particularly relevant for parents. For example, mothers often comment that they feel a great emptiness from suffering a double loss—loss of their child and loss of the mothering role (Wong, 1980). Feelings of estrangement from other loved ones are common, and social isolation may foster the depression.

Reorganization

Reorganization refers to recovery from the loss. It is a very gradual process in which the survivors again find meaning in living, readjust to life without the deceased, develop new or renewed relationships, and learn to live with the memory of the deceased with much less pain. It never means that the loved one is forgotten and the pain is gone. There always remains a deep ache that is never totally replaced with happiness and one that returns more intensely, for example, on holidays or anniversaries.

EXPECTED VS UNEXPECTED CHILDHOOD DEATH

Remarkably little research has been conducted comparing grief responses in survivors when the child's death was expected or unexpected. When death is expected, there is time for anticipatory grieving, and it has been suggested that this may favorably affect the grief process. However, a comparison of emotional and physical symptoms of parents whose child died after a chronic illness or an accident found no difference between the two groups (Miles, 1985). However, parents of children who died suddenly did experience more guilt, a prolonged period of numbness and shock, intense loneliness and emptiness, anxious fear that someone else would die, and intense anger at those responsible for the injury (Miles and Perry, 1985). Preliminary findings from a study done with Filipino children suggest that siblings of children who died suddenly may remain in the early stages of grief longer and may experience greater loneliness than siblings of children who died after an extended illness (Atuel, Williams, and Camar, 1988).

Although the grief process may be relatively unaltered by the timing of the child's death, there are differences for the families. In long-term, potentially fatal illnesses the grief for anticipated loss becomes chronic. The parents mourn the loss of their child long before the death. Unlike parents who experience a sudden loss, these family members are unable to resolve their grief until the child is considered cured or is dead. Each time they see the pain the child must endure or anticipate the sudden loss of hope during a relapse, they are reminded of their child's uncertain future.

However, the prolonged period of chronic grief provides families with the precious opportunity to complete all "unfinished business," such as helping the child and siblings understand and cope with a fatal prognosis. Many families reflect on their changed perspective of time after learning of the diagnosis, particularly their heightened awareness of the value and worth of each day. As one father stated, "I used to plan ahead for a better job, more money, and more prestige. But now I find myself wanting to stay home to be with my family. I never before realized how important time really is. Now I only wish we had more of it."

In sudden, unexpected death the family is deprived of any of the advantages of anticipatory grief. There is no opportunity to prepare oneself or others for the death, only the cruel reality that nothing remains of their child except memories. Because of this lack of time to prepare, many families feel great guilt and remorse for not having done something additional or different with the child. For example, they may berate themselves for not having prevented the accident or for depriving the child of some desired material object or privilege.

SPECIAL DECISIONS AT THE TIME OF DYING AND DEATH

Rarely are people prepared to cope with the numerous decisions that must be made when a loved one is dying or dies. When the death is expected, there is the opportunity to make plans in advance, such as where the child should spend the last days or what type of funeral arrangements are desired. When death is unexpected the shock is sufficient to render the survivors incapable of making even simple decisions. Those in attendance at the death and those caring for the dying child can be instrumental in initiating discussions that may facilitate the grief process. The following is a brief review of selected instances when nurses can help parents make decisions related to the expected or unexpected death.

Hospice or Hospital Care

When the child is dying, parents should be given the choice of hospice* or hospital care for the terminal stage of illness. Hospital care refers to the traditional practices of caring for dying patients; hospice is a concept, not necessarily a facility. Hospice is holistic care for the patient and family that is intended to maximize the present quality of life whenever there is no reasonable expectation of cure—Hospice intends for the child to live life to the fullest without pain, with choices and dignity, and with family support (Armstrong-Dailey, 1990; Corr and Corr, 1985). The three basic ways of providing hospice care are in a hospice, in a facility that employs the hospice concept, or in the child's home. If the home is chosen, the child may or may not die in the home. Reasons for final admission to a hospital vary but may be related to the parent's or sibling's wish to have the child die outside the home, exhaustion on the part of the caregivers, physical problems, such as sudden, acute pain or respiratory distress, and insufficient nursing services in the home (Martinson and others, 1986).

Hospice care is based on a number of important concepts that significantly set it apart from hospital care. First, the family are the principal caregivers, supported by a team of professional and volunteer staff. Second, the priority of care is comfort that considers the child's physical, psychologic, social, and spiritual needs. Pain and symptom control are primary concerns, and no extraordinary efforts are used to attempt a cure or prolong life. Third, the needs of the family are considered as important as those of the pa-

*Information on hospice services for children is available from the National Hospice Organization, 1901 N. Moore St., Arlington, VA 22209; (800) 658-8898. A recommended resource is *Home Care: A Manual for Parents* by D. Moldow and I. Martinson, available from Children's Hospice International, 700 Princess St., Suite 3, Alexandria, VA 22314; (800) 24-CHILD.

tient. Fourth, hospice is concerned with the family's post-death adjustment, and care may continue for a year or more.

With children, home care has been the more common environment for implementing the hospice concept and benefits the family in a variety of ways. Children who are dying are allowed the opportunity to remain with those they love and with whom they feel secure. Many children who were thought to be in imminent danger of death have gone home and lived longer than expected. Siblings feel more involved in the care and have more positive perceptions of the death (see Questions and Controversies, p. 1049). Parental adaptation has been more favorable, as shown by their perceptions of how the experience at home affected their marriage, social reorientation, religious beliefs, and views on the meaning of life and death. They also feel significantly less guilt after the child's death than families whose child died in the hospital (Lauer and others, 1983). There is also the economic advantage of home care (Moldow and others, 1982), although private insurance may not cover all outpatient and related services.

Home care may engender stress for the family, particularly anxiety about what to expect at the time of death and how to provide the care. The questions parents most frequently ask are "How long will it be (before the child dies)?" and "How will he die?" (Kohler and Radford, 1985). Parents providing home care may experience more physical fatigue than if the child received hospital care. A potential stress is the lack of support from familiar hospital staff when a new agency provides home assistance (Carlson and others, 1985).

Nurses working in hospice settings and with children dying at home are critical members of the health team. They often prepare the family for the home care experience, provide psychologic support for the family, and teach the physical care, especially comfort measures, such as pain control (see Chapter 26). They need to be available to the family and cognizant of times when the family may need relief from home care. If the child is at home, all families should have the option of admitting their child to the hospital if they feel they are unable to deal with the death. The child who dies at home must be pronounced dead, and hospice programs have provisions so this may proceed smoothly, or the police may be notified with an explanation of the circumstances to prevent unnecessary concern for abuse. Providing the police with the number of the responsible practitioner is usually all that is necessary to confirm the cause of death. Some parents may wish to keep the body at home for the funeral service. Although state laws vary, usually the wake can be held at home, but if the body is not embalmed, it should not remain for any length of time (usually no longer than 24 to 48 hours). Unless the family can also dispose of the body or has special wishes (e.g., tissue donation or autopsy), arrangements need to be made for mortuary services.

Right to Die

One of the benefits of hospice has been the recognition of patients' right to die as they wish, with emphasis on the *quality* of life. Unfortunately, this is not always the focus of care, especially in the traditional hospital setting. Many families are not given the option of terminating treatment when cure is unlikely, and staff may be reluctant to make decisions about "no code" or do not resuscitate (DNR) orders (withholding cardiopulmonary resuscitation in response to cardiac arrest). Some of these situations, such as the dying child's right to refuse additional treatment, often pose difficult ethical questions (see Questions and Controversies). Of even greater complexity is the cessation of life-sustaining measures, such as artificial ventilation or tube feeding, in patients who are in a persistent vegetative state. The legal and ethical questions in these cases remain unanswered and highly controversial (McClung and Kamer, 1990; O'Neil, 1987).

As the group of health professionals who are most involved with families, nurses are in an excellent position to ensure that families are given the options available to them at the time of death. The nurse's first responsibility is to explore the family's wishes. This is best done in concert with the physician, but at times may need to be initiated by the nurse. Statements such as, "Tell me about your thoughts for

QUESTIONS AND CONTROVERSIES

Does the dying child have the right to refuse further treatment?

Traditionally, minor children (age of minority varies with state law) have not had the legal right to give informed consent for treatment or to refuse treatment. However, there is a growing concern for children in the end stage of fatal disease to have a voice in their care during the terminal phase. One of the major issues is the age at which children have the cogniitive ability to understand the medical information, consider and comprehend the consequences of the decision—death, and choose freely among the options (Leikin, 1989). According to children's development of the death concept, a mature understanding of death does not occur until about 9 years of age. However, centers that have developed protocols for allowing informed choice by children document that youngsters as young as 6 years of age understand the implications of their disease as incurable and death as irreversible (Nitschke and others, 1982). These findings are consistent with those of Bluebond-Langner, who found that fatally ill children progress through a series of stages that shape their understanding of their disease and death (see p. 1042).

Other issues raised by opponents include the concern for dispelling hope in the child once death is pronounced imminent, parents' guilt if they later question the decision, and possible conflict between the child's and parents' wishes (Shumway, Grossman, and Sarles, 1983; Stanfill and Strong, 1985). Although there is insufficient research to answer these concerns, it seems unlikely that they will occur if the family is allowed to choose therapeutic alternatives in an atmosphere of professional support and with sufficient information. In addition, staff need to assess each child's capacity to understand the implications of refusing treatment, with documentation of the child's words and actions that support their conclusions (Foley, 1985).

the kind of care you want your child to receive when he is dying" or "Have you considered the kinds of interventions you would like us to use when your child is near death?" can begin discussion of this sensitive but critical aspect of terminal care. If parents choose "DNR," they must be aware of exactly what will and will not be done for the child and assured that this does not mean "no care." For example, the family may wish that oxygen be given to the child for difficult breathing but not want active resuscitation. Once a decision is made, it must be communicated to all members of the health team and include a *written* medical order for the use or withholding of lifesaving measures. An order of "slow" or "delay" code is not legal (Saunders and Valente, 1986). Because the child's condition or the family's wishes may change, DNR orders are reviewed regularly (Olson and Hooke, 1988).

Visualization of the Body

Although most institutions recognize the need for parents to hold and spend time with the dead child, a dilemma may arise when the body is mutilated. Although the memory of the child's disfigurement can be extremely upsetting and generate concern for how much the child suffered, not seeing the body leaves the parents with imagined ideas of how their child looked, which can be worse than the reality and can delay the acceptance of the death (Miles and Perry, 1985). However, family members need preparation for this upsetting experience. They should be told what to expect and why certain parts of the body are covered or bandaged. It is desirable to place the body in a private room, without medical apparatus, and as presentable as the situation allows (Schulman and Rehm, 1983). Some people appreciate the presence of a nurse in the room with them; others desire privacy. Regardless of how badly the body is harmed, parents may want to hold the child. Such options are offered and respected. Family members should be given as much time as they need to say good-bye; for many, viewing the body is a sign of closure to finish their good-byes and leave the hospital (Jost and Haase, 1989).

Tissue Donation/Autopsy

A topic that is rarely considered when a child dies is tissue donation. However, for some families this may be a meaningful act—one that benefits another human being despite the loss of their child. Unfortunately, initiating a discussion about tissue donation is often very stressful for staff, and there may be confusion regarding whose responsibility this is. In centers where transplants are performed, a full-time transplant coordinator is usually available to inform the family about organ donation and to take care of details. If such services are not available, the staff needs to discuss which members should discuss this topic with the family. Ideally this should be the person who knows the family best, knows when the death is expected, or has the opportunity to spend time with the family when the death is unexpected. Often nurses are in an optimum position to suggest tissue donation after consultation with the attending physician (Peele, 1989). The request should be made in a private and quiet area of the hospital and should be simple and direct, with questions such as "Are you a donor family?" or "Have you ever considered organ donation?" (Weber, 1985). Most states have "required request" laws that mandate that the hospital make a request for tissue donation from the family of the deceased, especially if the patient is brain dead. A written consent from the family is required before donation can proceed (Giordano, 1989).

Nurses need to be aware of common questions about organ donation to help families make an informed decision. Healthy children who die unexpectedly are excellent candidates for organ donation, although their age is a determinant of organ suitability. For example, very young donors present technical difficulties in organ removal (Williams, 1985). Children with cancer, chronic disease, or infection or who have suffered prolonged cardiac arrest may not be suitable candidates, although this is individually determined. The nurse should inquire if organ donation was discussed with the child or if the child ever expressed such a wish.* Any number of body tissues or organs can be donated (skin, eyes, bone, kidney, heart, liver, pancreas), and their removal does not mutilate or desecrate the body or cause any suffering. The family may have an open casket, and there is no delay in the funeral. There is no cost to the donor family, but organ donation does not eliminate funeral or cremation responsibilities. Most religions permit organ donation as long as the recipient benefits from the transplant, although Orthodox Judaism forbids it (Carbary, 1985; Gershan, 1985).

In cases of unexplained death, violent death, or suspected suicide, autopsy is required by law. In other instances it may be optional, and parents should be informed of this choice. The procedure, as well as forms that require signing, should be explained. The family should know that the child can be in an open casket following an autopsy (Jost and Haase, 1989).

Siblings' Attendance at Burial Services

One of the most frequent concerns of parents is whether young or school-age children should attend funeral or burial services (see Questions and Controversies). Sharing moments of deep significance with parents helps children understand the experience and deal with their own feelings of shock, sorrow, and grief; depriving them of this opportunity may leave children with lifelong regrets (Fig. 23-2). However, children need preparation for postdeath services. They should be told what to expect, particularly how the deceased person will look if the coffin is open. Ideally the parent should explain the details to the child, but, if the parent's grief prevents this communication, a significant family member or friend should substitute.

It is often helpful to bring children to the funeral service before many visitors arrive. They are allowed private time to say good-bye but are spared some of the unpredictable

*Information about being an organ donor is available from **The Living Bank,** P.O. Box 6725, Houston, TX 77265, (713) 528-2971 (in Texas) or (800) 528-2971; and from **The United Network for Organ Sharing (UNOS),** (800) 24-DONOR.

QUESTIONS AND CONTROVERSIES

Should children attend the funeral or burial services of a loved one?

This question generates much controversy among the general public and professionals. Many lay people feel it is too frightening for children to be exposed to the dead and that it is better for them to remember the loved person as he or she was when alive. There is a general attitude of protecting children from unhappy or distressing events. However, among health professionals involved with children there is a fairly general consensus that children should attend such services (Salladay and Royal, 1981; Schultz, 1980), and some authors suggest that no child is too young merely by virtue of age (Foley, 1986). Others recommend that the parents make the decision regarding attendance until children are 6 or 7 years of age, at which time children should choose (Zelauskas, 1981). Children, like adults, have "unfinished business," and visiting the dead person may represent an opportunity to complete those affairs. For example, the child may wish to say good-bye (verbally or written) or to leave a memento. Kübler-Ross (1983) tells of a 7-year-old child who chose a puzzle that her brother received shortly before he lost sight from a brain tumor. She matter of factly explained that he could finish it "when he arrives in heaven."

Unfortunately, little research has focused on the difference in adjustment between children who do or do not attend postdeath services. However, one study provides substantial evidence of the benefit of involving children in the experience of their dying sibling. Lauer and others (1985) compared children's perceptions of their sibling's death at home vs in the hospital. The home care group (ages 5 to 23 years) reported they were prepared for the impending death, received consistent information and support from their parents, were involved in most activities, found the funeral experience comforting, and viewed their own involvement as the most important aspect of the experience. The non–home care group (ages 2 to 26 years) had opposite perceptions. Another study found that greater participation in the child's care and death, including funeral attendance, was associated with higher self-esteem in the siblings (Michael and Lansdown, 1986). Thus it appears that *increased involvement* with the death rather than isolation and "protection" benefits children.

emotional reactions of others, which can be very distressing to them. Allowing children to stay as long as they wish, but respecting their need to leave, provides maximum control for them over their ability to grieve comfortably.

THE FAMILY OF THE CHILD WITH LIFE-THREATENING ILLNESS

In many respects families who are experiencing life-threatening illness in their child respond to the diagnosis in much the same manner as families whose child has a chronic illness or disability. Because of the advances in medical treatment, many fatal illnesses, such as cancer, are now chronic disorders with a potentially life-threatening outcome.

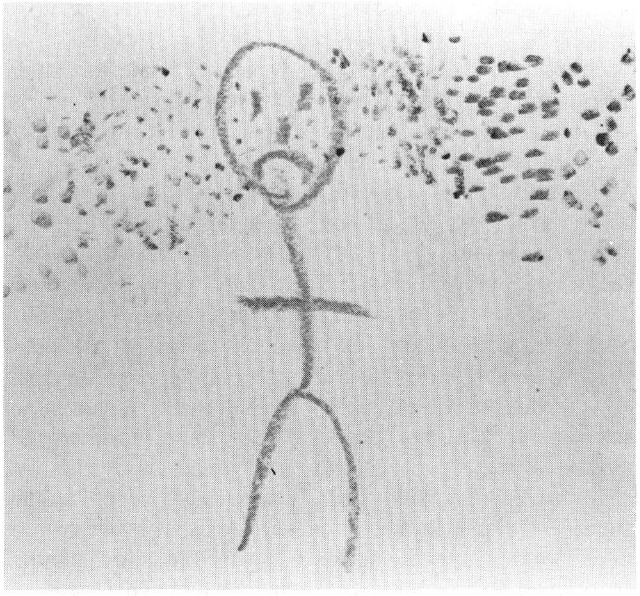

Fig. 23-2. Drawing, made by 7-year-old child whose sister died in a car crash, shows the boy sad and crying (dots are tears) because he was not allowed to see his dead sibling.

REACTIONS OF THE FAMILY TO A LIFE-THREATENING ILLNESS

All families whose child has some type of physical or cognitive disability experience reactions to the loss of the "perfect" child that are similar, despite the diagnosis. The reader is urged to review the concepts in Chapter 22 and apply them to this discussion. The following section focuses on five phases in which there are significant differences in reactions to chronic disease vs life-threatening illness, with cancer used as an example of life-threatening illness. A Nursing Care Plan for the child who is terminally ill or dying is presented on pp. 1057-1059.

Phase I—Revelation and Dawning Reality: Diagnosis and Treatment

When parents first learn of the diagnosis of cancer, their immediate reactions are similar to those of other families whose child has a chronic illness, except that the initial impact can be much more pessimistic and overwhelming because of the generally negative connotation regarding the disease. For children, principal concerns center around the diagnostic tests and treatments and their effects.

Almost immediately after the diagnosis is confirmed, induction therapy aimed at total remission of the disease begins. During this period families commonly react with quiet anger, depression, ambivalence, and bargaining. Much of the psychic energy is directed at waiting for the confirmation of a remission. If that does not occur, all the initial reactions may be repeated again, with increased anticipatory grieving.

Shock and disbelief. Many parents relate that after they heard the diagnosis they were deaf to everything else told to them. As one mother described, "All I heard the doctor say was the word leukemia. I didn't hear anything else. All I could think of was that leukemia was fatal. I was certain my child was going to die. My husband heard the doctor say it was curable, but I didn't. I won't believe that until I see it. Even if my child is 50 years old, I will worry about it coming back." The pessimistic response of this mother is typical of many parents who are afraid to believe that their child will recover despite a favorable prognosis. Anticipatory grieving for the possible loss of the child is common, and if parents are not helped to understand the improved prognosis of these diseases, they may react by psychologically burying the child. This "alarm stage" of emotional chaos and belief in a terminal prognosis typically lasts a week to month after the actual diagnosis, but is highly influenced by the family's personal attitudes and sense of skepticism or faith (Brett and Davies, 1988).

Anger. Children often may feel angry, particularly because of all the traumatic procedures done to them as part of diagnosis and treatment. Once they begin to feel better, they frequently express their anger through uncooperativeness. Parents receive the brunt of much of the child's anger and often find coping with it extremely difficult. A common reaction is to ignore it and try to pacify the child by giving in to requests whenever possible. Overprotectiveness and permissiveness are typical reactions during remission, and helping parents deal with the child's anger constructively during the hospitalization also prevents some of the potential future problems.

Reactions to altered body image. One side effect of chemotherapy or cranial irradiation that has particular psychologic significance for children in different age-groups and for parents is hair loss.

Young children. For young children baldness has little significance. Preschoolers may attach superficial concern to the hair loss, particularly if it affects their sex role image. For example, one 4-year-old girl was disturbed about her baldness because she thought she looked like a boy. Once her parents emphasized her femaleness in dress, she was unconcerned about the temporary change.

Parents of young children may have a difficult adjustment. However, they may be unwilling to admit their concern and lack of acceptance. For example, the mother of a 3-year-old boy refused to openly discuss the hair loss in front of her son. She had decided to hide the change from him until new hair grew in. She had formulated a fantastic conspiracy to maintain the secret. For example, she planned to remove all mirrors in the house, to isolate him from children, to keep his head always covered with hats, and to buy a soft brush and groom the hair as if it were still present. She explained that this was necessary because he was very vain. When asked what she would do if he discovered the baldness, she calmly said, "I'll just tell him what happened." It was not possible for her to see the pitfalls of such a scheme until she verbalized her personal feelings about the hair loss.

School-age children. The reactions of school-age children depend on their preparation for the loss and the type of parental adjustment. Much of their anxiety relates to the anticipation of the loss rather than the actual baldness. Telling children about the chance before it occurs, stressing that it is temporary, and suggesting ways of camouflaging it, such as with a wig, hat, or scarf, fosters better adjustment to the altered body image.

Adolescents. Adolescents have the most difficulty in accepting and adjusting to hair loss because it occurs at a time when peer acceptance and group conformity are essential. They need the opportunity to express their anger and fears of rejection without being judged or reproached. Sometimes parents try to reason with their adolescent child that the hair loss is a small sacrifice for a possible future recovery. Although true, it does little to comfort the adolescent in his or her present struggle.

Involving adolescents in selecting a wig *before* the hair falls out provides them with a feeling of participation and allows them to secure a wig that is most similar to their own hair.

Nursing considerations. The time of diagnosis is a critical period for the development of therapeutic relationships. Ideally, the primary nurse should be present with family members when the diagnosis is given. The same guidelines as discussed in Chapter 22 apply; parents want information that they consider critical—information related to the diagnosis and prognosis, disease process, need for additional diagnostic tests, immediate therapeutic plan, and availability of the physician (Greenberg and others, 1984). They value an open, sympathetic, direct, and uninterrupted discussion, with sufficient time to hear the information and ask questions. Information should be repeated and clarified (Woolley and others, 1989).

In many instances the child's care is so complex that numerous specialists are involved. Consequently the nurse becomes the only consistent person for the family. For example, in the case of a child with Wilms tumor, a pediatrician, urologist, surgeon, radiologist, and hematologist/oncologist participate in the medical/surgical care of the child. Even under the best of circumstances, parents can receive opposing messages from health team members and can become confused about who can answer their questions. The nurse is in an advantageous position to interpret those messages and to direct the parents to the most appropriate source of information.

In many instances care in the hospital is limited to a few days for diagnosis and initiation of treatment. However, in some cases an extended admission may be necessary. Many parents elect to stay with their child and to participate as much as possible in the care. Because the possibility of death in a child is a highly emotional experience, nurses may unknowningly usurp parents' roles or relinquish nursing responsibilities. They need to be aware of their approach toward parents in order to support them in the way most comfortable for the parents. Planning the child's care *with* family members is a most effective way of communicating genuine concern and avoiding either hazard.

During the remission phase, parents, ill children, and siblings need reassurance that their reactions are normal and expected. The interventions discussed in Chapter 22 apply. Because of the shock usually experienced when a catastrophic illness is diagnosed, the needs of well family members, particularly siblings, may be neglected. Siblings can be helped to understand the reason for the abrupt change in family life by keeping them informed of the child's condition and by continuing as much contact as possible with the hospitalized child (and absent parents if necessary) through visiting, telephone contact, letter writing, cards, or photographs.

Parents and children need thorough, detailed, and repeated explanations of the diagnostic tests and plan of therapy. They need reassurance that a change in the child's condition is most likely a result of therapy, not the disease. Decreasing the chance for the unexpected lessens the opportunities for increased anxiety. For example, forewarning the family about the side effects of therapy, such as alopecia, weight gain, constipation, stomatitis, and nausea and vomiting, as well as the necessary laboratory procedures, prepares them for these expected events and increases their sense of security and control.

Phase II—Reprieve: Remission and Maintenance Therapy

Once the child is in remission, there is a long period of hope for an eventual recovery and fear of a possible relapse. Parents commonly react with heightened vigilance by overprotecting the child, encouraging dependency, and liberalizing discipline. These reactions support the child's sick role and hinder optimum physical and emotional development. Family members may attempt to escape or avoid the problems of this period through social isolation.

Overprotectiveness. Although many children return home in relatively stable and much improved physical health, parents frequently treat them as invalids. One of the most common manifestations of overprotectiveness is parents' inability to set appropriate limits. It is understandable that, under the stress of potential loss, parents might respond by overindulging the child, giving in to every desire and wish. Although this is probably part of the grieving process during the initial phase of the illness, persistence of this reaction culminates in special problems during the often long period of remission (see Fig. 22-1).

For ill children, overprotection and "special" treatment increase their fears of serious illness and failure to recover. In addition, if they are given everything during periods of wellness, they will become very frustrated, unhappy, and demanding children during the terminal phase, when it will be impossible to meet all their requests.

Dependency. Closely associated with the overprotectiveness is increased dependency between parents and child. This is often evident in parents' unwillingness to send their child to school. If not helped toward reintegration of usual activities, they may use the hair loss or frequent visits for treatment as excuses for keeping the child home. The same needs and interventions regarding school that are discussed in Chapter 22 apply. However, school personnel may have special concerns.* A common, often unvoiced fear of school personnel is that the child will have some dramatic episode, such as massive hemorrhage, while in the classroom, and die (Klopovich and others, 1981). During the discussion of the disease the nurse should include the usual course of the illness and its specific implications, for example, the child's increased susceptibility to common childhood diseases or unexpected epidemics such as chickenpox. In this case the school nurse should report the instance of prevalent illness to the parent.

Several issues should also be approached with the school teacher and nurse, particularly other parents' questions about the disease, such as the chance of communicability, preparation of the class for expected physical changes, and possible future absences. During the terminal phase the parents should also discuss the likelihood of the child's death and the need for discussing this with the other students. Teachers of siblings who attend the same school should also be included in the discussions. For example, the siblings may be demonstrating in school their difficulties in adjusting to the child's illness. Such behavior may erroneously be interpreted as learning disabilities, behavioral or emotional problems, or delinquency, for example. Unless the teachers are aware of the extenuating circumstances, these children can be saddled with negative labels for the rest of their academic life.

Anxiety. In addition to the concerns discussed in the preceding paragraphs are many other anxiety-provoking stresses. The financial strain of a chronic illness is a constant worry. Job security is always a necessary consideration, because unemployment may jeopardize insurance coverage. There are also costs besides the actual medical care, such as transportation to the hospital, meals away from home, baby-sitting for other siblings, or temporary housing for distant medical care.† The nurse can provide assistance by referring the family to available organizations, such as the **Leukemia Society of America**‡ or the **American Cancer Society,**§ who may be able to provide financial help, and to **The Candlelighters Childhood Cancer Foundation**‖ for information and psychologic support.

Nutrition is also a continuing concern. Many drugs cause severe nausea and vomiting, thereby decreasing the child's appetite. The illness usually results in marked weight loss. Mealtime can become a battleground for family members.

---

*See suggested readings on p. 1036 for information concerning students with serious illness.

†Ronald McDonald Houses provide inexpensive homelike accommodations for families when distance to the hospital is a major factor. They are located in several large cities, and application for lodging is usually made through the social service department of the medical center.

‡733 Third Ave., New York, NY 10017; (212) 573-8484.

§1599 Clifton Rd., NE, Atlanta, GA 30329; (404) 329-7617. Also, Canadian Cancer Society, 77 Bloor St. West, Suite 1702, Toronto, Ontario M55 3A1; (416) 961-7223.

‖1901 Pennsylvania Ave., NW, Washington, DC 20006; (202) 659-5136.

The nurse can prevent some of the problems by forewarning parents of the expected change in appetite and by suggesting ways of encouraging children to eat without causing a power struggle. For example, during the course of steroid therapy, appetite improves dramatically. Parents should be told that the increased hunger is a result of medication, not a change in the child's behavior or attitude. During periods of chemotherapy when the appetite is decreased, providing small, frequent meals of favorite foods often encourages some cooperation. Growth may also be slowed during the treatment phase from the various drugs and use of radiation. If parents are aware of some of these expected changes, they may be more accepting of the child's fluctuating appetite.

Nursing considerations. Often remission and "going home" from the cancer center coincide, and a number of problems can be anticipated and often prevented by a thorough discussion at this time: maintenance of normal family patterns, school attendance, and relationships among family and friends (Lansky, 1985). Because of the usual reaction by parents to overprotect the child, they should be advised to continue appropriate discipline of the child and siblings by resuming preillness rules and limits. The importance of resuming school and other daily activities as soon as possible is stressed, and other family members, particularly mothers, may benefit from resuming their previous functions, including employment. Parents are encouraged to schedule appointments for visits at times that least interfere with the child's daily routine, such as late on Friday, which leaves the weekend for recuperation from any unpleasant side effects (Fig. 23-3).

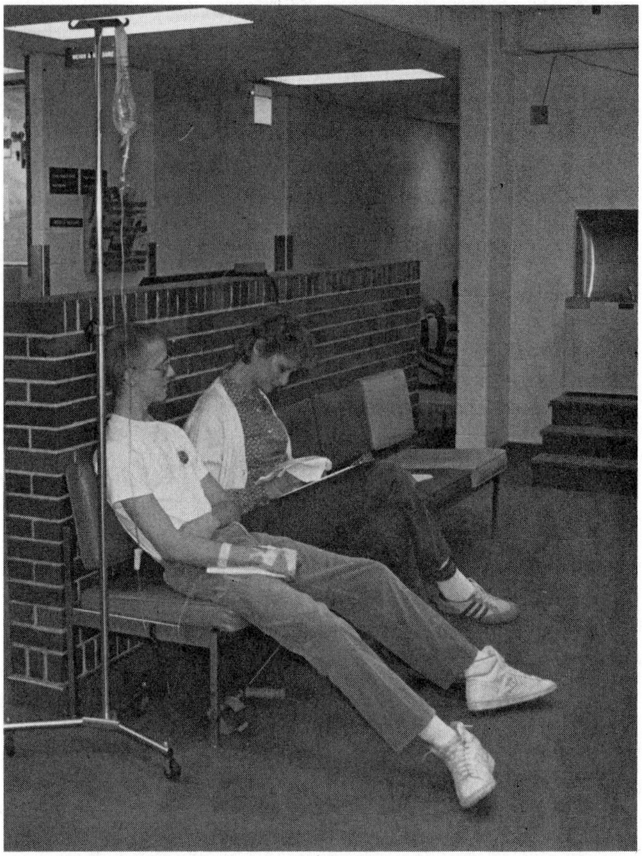

Fig. 23-3. Treatment often involves long periods of outpatient visits that should be scheduled at times that least interfere with the youngster's daily routine.

Ongoing compliance with medical treatment is a very important aspect of care, with prognosis closely related to treatments. However, noncompliance is a serious problem among children with cancer, especially adolescents, who refuse to take the medication at home or keep treatment appointments. Not only can noncompliance affect chance of survival, it can also cause unnecessary diagnostic tests and warranted change in treatment protocols. Strategies for enhancing compliance, especially in teenagers, are to include the youngster in treatment discussions, help the family set clear expectations and clarify roles (for example, who is responsible for administering the drug or supervising the administration), and provide written instructions (Lansky, List, and Ritter-Sterr, 1988). (See also Compliance, Chapter 27.)

To avoid unnecessary social isolation the parents need to be prepared for common responses of friends and relatives, such as staying away from the family, fearing the child's illness, especially concern for contagion, and giving unsolicited advice. Families should take the initiative in informing others about the child's condition and asking directly that they remain in contact with each other. Being the first to express, "I know it's hard to know what to say and do in a situation like this," can put others at ease. A more difficult situation is the offering of unsolicited advice regarding treatment, particularly information about "new" but unproved methods. Parents need to take a firm but tactful approach; they can comment that they will inquire about the method with their health professional but that they feel assured that they are receiving the best care available. Many families benefit from associating with other similarly affected families. There is a special camaraderie between these parents that seems to sustain them through the long ordeal (Lyman, 1987). Once these friendships develop, families often ask staff about other children's status. Staff may be concerned with sharing confidential information, but at least one study found families accepting of the practice (Patno, Young, and Dickerman, 1988). Sources of information about self-help groups are discussed under Help the Family Cope, Chapter 22.

Because many children are treated in tertiary centers located at a distance from their home, there may not be one primary nurse who can act as liaison and coordinator among the nurses in the hospital, school, clinic, practitioner's office, and community. Often this results in a lack of preventive intervention. Nurses who are in a particularly advantageous position to become a primary link with the family are nurse practitioners and community nurses, and a nurse network should be established before discharge to ensure continuity of care.

Phase III—Recovery: Cessation of Therapy and Possible Cure

The maintenance period may be followed by cessation of therapy in the hope of a permanent recovery. Although this is a very happy time, it is mixed with feelings of grief, ambivalence, and concern for the future.

Denial and ambivalence. At the time the decision is made to terminate therapy, many parents deny that treatment is no longer warranted. They may express ambivalence with such questions as, "Are you sure that a longer period of drugs wouldn't guarantee a better chance for a cure?" There is difficulty in giving up the security of the rituals of medication, radiation therapy, and frequent examinations. Occasionally health professionals erroneously label the ambivalence or denial as a psychologic need for the child's sick role.

In general this reaction is characteristic of the grieving for the loss of security afforded by medical intervention and adjustment to the hazards of "waiting it out" again. Parents need almost as much support during this phase as they did when they were told of the diagnosis.

Overprotectiveness. Parents also relate a resurgence of the need to overprotect and isolate their child from any potential physical harm. As one mother stated, "I became fanatical about examining my child for signs of recurring illness when the drugs were stopped. If he had a runny nose or sore throat, I immediately took him to the doctor, requesting a blood count. I was so sure those leukemic cells had returned." She later compared this reaction to the ways in which she treated the child after his first remission. She added, "You would think that after 3 years of living with drugs, side effects, blood tests, and doctors, I would be thrilled to give it all up, but here I am, almost as shaky and nervous as if I had just found out he had the disease."

Concern for the future. When cure is a realistic possibility, the family's concern for the *quantity* of life shifts to the *quality* of life. This is a legitimate concern, because chemotherapy and radiation are not without their immediate and long-term complications. The need for continued medical supervision of these children cannot be overemphasized. (See Long-Term Sequelae of Treatment, Chapter 36.) Survivors worry most about their psychologic normalcy, schooling, and relationships with family and friends. They have concerns about having children, transmitting cancer to their offspring, and recurrence of their disease or another cancer. Some worry about employment discrimination, obtaining insurance, and access to future medical care (Chesler and Lozowski, 1988).

For families who did not have the benefit of anticipatory guidance, the prospect of a cure may represent a rethinking of their childbearing practices. For example, these parents may have indulged the child and tolerated negative or regressive behaviors because of the thought of death. Now that the child's future is much more positive, there may be recognition that changes must occur to reestablish normal behavior. Such families benefit from professional guidance to gradually change behavioral patterns.

Nursing considerations. Probably the most important component of care is acceptance of the family's mixed reactions to cessation of therapy. Parents need to feel comfortable in calling the nurse or clinic about any concern or problem. They also should be encouraged to verbalize their feelings and thoughts of cessation of therapy. It may be helpful for the nurse to acquaint them with another family who has progressed through this transition period.

Nurses working with these families must be aware of the long-term consequences of treatment and be vigilant of signs indicating problems, such as retarded growth or evidence of a second malignancy. Psychosocial problems may surface, and young people are particularly concerned about fertility and sexuality. Adolescents frequently equate the information about impaired fertility with impaired sexual performance, and even when such concerns are not voiced, they need clarification that sexual performance is not physiologically affected.

Phase IV—Recurrence: Relapse and Death

The most dreaded news other than the initial diagnosis is confirmation of a relapse. For many children the first relapse is followed by another remission, but subsequently by future relapses, with the final one followed by death. The family's reactions during the terminal stage are influenced by their previous acceptance or denial of the child's illness. It is a period of intense anticipatory grieving, characterized by the relapse reactions of depression, loss of hope, and possibly acceptance. As the child's condition worsens, there is intensification of numerous fears.

Loss of hope and depression. One of the most difficult realizations for the family is the knowledge that with each relapse the chances for eventual recovery diminish. The reality of possible death looms before them, particularly during the reinduction phase when a recurrent remission may or may not be feasible. Once another remission is attained, reason for hope is again present.

However, many families relate that after termination of the primary remission they never again feel as hopeful or optimistic. Some also discuss their silent preparation and grieving for the child's eventual death. Nurses need to be sensitive to such thoughts and aware of the possible beneficial aspect of this reaction, because repeated relapses are associated with poorer prognoses.

The usual reaction to loss of hope is depression. This may be the type of depression for past losses, but most often is anticipatory grieving for impending losses. Nurses need to carefully assess the reason for the depression and realistically plan intervention. For example, if another remission is likely, the nurse should plan to help the parents work through their depression. However, if this relapse is actually the commencement of the terminal stage, the nurse should plan to support the family in preparing for the death.

Fear of death. The most prevalent fear is of death itself. Parents frequently ask about death through questions such as, "What will he die from?" "How will we know she is dying?" and "What will happen when he dies?" It is important to listen sensitively to such questions because the real concern may be hidden behind the question. For example, when parents ask, "What will he die from?" they may not be so concerned with the medical cause of death, such as hemorrhage or infection, but may really be asking, "What is hemorrhage like?" Most people have a fantasy idea of how death will occur that is much more horrifying than the actual event. For example, parents will relate that their idea of hemorrhage is uncontrollable gushing of blood from every orifice. In reality it is usually internal bleeding and often oozing of blood from the nose. When the nurses are aware of the imagined events, they can clarify the misconceptions and supply the correct information.

Fear of pain. The fear of uncontrollable pain is almost universal. Whatever bargaining occurs during the dying stage is for a peaceful, quiet, and quick death. Often parents will relate that the child has pain even when it appears that the child is comfortable. It is important for nurses to understand that pain is much more than physical. Watching one's child die is a pain that must certainly be immeasurable and that subjectively shadows one's perception of surrounding events.

Fear of loss of control. A fear that is shared by the dying and the survivors is losing emotional and physical control as death approaches. Some parents attempt to cope with this fear by requesting that their child be heavily sedated during the terminal stage. However, the loss of control imposed by medication may make the child very distraught. Inasmuch as nurses usually regulate the administration of drugs, it is important for them to carefully assess the needs of both the child and the parents. Supporting parents at the time of impending death by being physically present, making the child as comfortable as possible, and talking to the awake child helps parents feel in control without the need for sedating the child.

Fear of isolation and loneliness. Parents fear that their child will die when they are not present. Dying children often request that their parents stay with them (Fig. 23-4), and this request should always be respected. Although everyone dies alone, no one need die in lonely isolation.

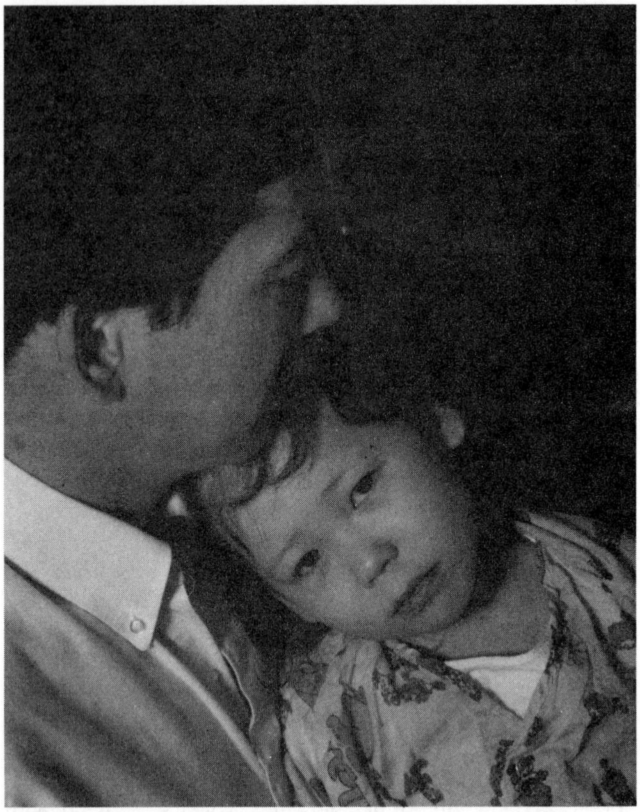

Fig. 23-4. For the dying child there is no greater comfort than the security and closeness of a parent.

Nursing considerations. Relapse is a difficult phase for nurses because it often initiates a loss of hope and their own grieving process. One of the dangers during the phase of relapse is that nurses may transfer their feelings of pessimism or optimism to the parents. It is extremely important to assess one's own personal response to the relapse and to plan the intervention according to the person's needs. This seems to be particularly critical during the final relapse. Nurses can help parents and children formulate realistic short-term goals and establish reasonable priorities of care. It is also the time to discuss with parents their wishes and expectations for the terminal phase. For some families the alternative of hospice or home care is a very significant and fulfilling means of sharing their child's last days (see p. 1046).

During the terminal stage the fears of parents and children form the foundation for nursing care. These fears may be particularly worrisome for those parents who have chosen home care because they must assume primary responsibility for the child. The nurse's role includes preparing them to deal with each fear and providing assistance through home visits, telephone counseling, and the alternative of hospital admission at any time. As death approaches, nurses should recognize the physical signs (Box 23-3) and summon the parents to the child's bedside. If death approaches sooner than expected, families should be prepared. Sometimes health professionals' need to deny death is so strong that parents are continually given messages of false hope that prevent them from preparing themselves for the worst news. Although others may think such false hope is helpful, in reality it may be extremely painful for family members to live in uncertainty.

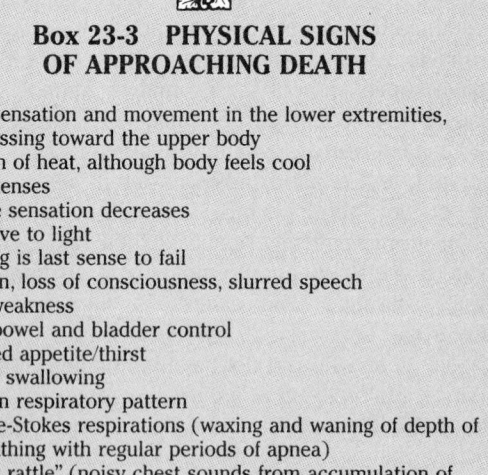

Box 23-3 PHYSICAL SIGNS OF APPROACHING DEATH

- Loss of sensation and movement in the lower extremities, progressing toward the upper body
- Sensation of heat, although body feels cool
- Loss of senses
  - Tactile sensation decreases
  - Sensitive to light
  - Hearing is last sense to fail
- Confusion, loss of consciousness, slurred speech
- Muscle weakness
- Loss of bowel and bladder control
- Decreased appetite/thirst
- Difficulty swallowing
- Change in respiratory pattern
  - Cheyne-Stokes respirations (waxing and waning of depth of breathing with regular periods of apnea)
  - "Death rattle" (noisy chest sounds from accumulation of pulmonary and pharyngeal secretions)
- Weak, slow pulse; decreased blood pressure

The goal in caring for dying children is comfort, and no intervention is more important than control of pain. Analgesics, especially opioids, are administered around the clock to prevent pain, with adjustments made in dosage and schedule as needed to maintain maximum comfort. This often requires increasing dosage of opioids beyond those normally recommended, decreasing the duration between doses, and changing routes of administration to comply with the child's needs and wishes. Whenever possible the oral route is preferred, but when no longer possible, continuous intravenous infusion administration may provide the greatest benefit. Parents and the child need to be reassured that the opioids are needed and that addiction is not a problem. If tolerance and/or physical dependence occur, these normal, involuntary responses to opioids are explained to prevent any misconception that they represent addiction. Any nonpharmacologic measures that may augment pain relief and relaxation are used, such as cutaneous stimulation (for example, rocking, stroking the skin) or diversion (for example, reading to the child or playing music). (See also Chapter 26 for an extensive discussion of pain assessment and management.)

Both the family and the child may have heightened spiritual needs at the time of death. Spiritual support includes respect for the diverse beliefs of families, willingness to discuss matters of spirituality with them, and provision for the rituals and sacraments of organized religion (Conrad, 1985). Many families desire a priest, minister, or rabbi, and the nurse can summon the clergy to be with the family. In those cases in which it may not be possible to reach a member of the clergy, the nurse may have to provide the spiritual needs by praying with the family, reading from the Bible, or listening to the review of their life. (See also Box 23-4 and the Nursing Care Plan on pp. 1057-1059.)

Phase V—The Beginning: Postdeath

The crisis of loss does not end with the child's death. In many ways it only begins. Families can prepare themselves for the expected loss, but when it occurs there is a period of acute grief, followed by an extended phase of mourning (see p. 1045). It is important for families to understand that mourning takes a long time. Whereas acute grief may last only weeks or months, resolving their loss is measured in years. Holidays and anniversaries can be particularly difficult, and people who previously had been supportive may now expect the family to have "adjusted." Consequently, prolonged mourning is often silent and lonely.

Nursing considerations. Part of the difficulty in helping the bereaved family is lack of opportunity for follow-up in the traditional nursing structure. Consequently, many of these families never receive the support and guidance that could help them resolve the loss. Fortunately, hospice programs recognize this need and provide regular follow-up after the death. If only one meeting is arranged, a waiting period of 1 month has been suggested to give the family time to overcome the phase of shock and disbelief (Jankovic and others, 1989). The optimum time and number of visits is not known. Self-help groups, such as **The Com-**

Box 23-4 GUIDELINES FOR SUPPORTING GRIEVING FAMILIES*

General

Stay with the family; sit quietly if they prefer not to talk; cry with them if desired.
Accept the family's grief reactions; avoid judgmental statements, e.g., "You should be feeling better by now."
Avoid offering rationalizations for the child's death, e.g., "You should be glad your child isn't suffering anymore."
Avoid artificial consolation, e.g., "I know how you feel," or "You are still young enough to have another baby."
Deal openly with feelings such as guilt, anger, and loss of self-esteem.
Focus on feelings by using a feeling word in the statement, e.g., "You're still feeling all the pain of losing a child."
Refer the family to an appropriate self-help group or for professional help if needed.

At the Time of Death

Reassure the family that everything possible is being done for the child, if they wish lifesaving interventions.
Do everything possible to ensure the child's comfort, especially relieving pain.
Provide the child and family the opportunity to review special experiences or memories in their lives.
Express personal feelings of loss and/or frustrations, e.g., "We will miss him so much," or "We tried everything; we feel so sorry that we couldn't save him."
Provide information that the family requests and be honest.
Respect the emotional needs of family members, such as siblings, who may need brief respites from the dying child.
Make every effort to arrange for family members, especially parents, to be with the child at the moment of death, if they wish to be present.
Allow the family to stay with the dead child for as long as they wish and to rock, hold, or bathe the child.
Provide practical help when possible, such as collecting the child's belongings.
Arrange for spiritual support, such as clergy; pray with the family if no one else can stay with them.

After the Death

Attend the funeral or visitation if there was a special closeness with the family.
Initiate and maintain contact, e.g., sending cards, telephoning, inviting them back to the unit, or making a home visit.
Refer to the dead child by name; discuss shared memories with the family.
Discourage the use of drugs or alcohol as a method of escaping grief.
Encourage all family members to communicate their feelings rather than to remain silent to avoid upsetting another member.
Emphasize that grieving is a painful process that often takes *years* to resolve.

*The *family* refers to all significant persons involved in the child's life, such as the parents, siblings, grandparents, or other close relatives or friends.

passionate Friends,* an international organization for bereaved parents and siblings, and specialty groups, such as **Parents of Murdered Children,†** also provide informal bereavement help. When such groups are not available, nurses can be instrumental in facilitating parent and sibling groups.

Follow-up can help the family understand the process of mourning, particularly its duration and pain, and can provide assistance in making decisions that involve the loss. One especially difficult dilemma faced by many parents is the decision to have additional children. The advisability of having another child soon after the death is controversial. If the grief is unresolved, there is the danger of the subsequent offspring becoming a "replacement child" (Poznanski, 1972). However, this view is not shared by all professionals or by bereaved families who have successfully conceived another offspring (Glassman-Feibusch 1983; Weiss, 1984). Consequently, the nurse's role cannot be one of giving answers but of assessing readiness for another pregnancy through knowledge of the parents' progress through grief and their motivations in conceiving. (See also Sudden Infant Death Syndrome, Chapter 13.)

At times family members may need assistance in their grieving. Mothers, in particular, often feel a great sense of loneliness and emptiness, and part of their resolving the grief is finding a substitute role that is fulfilling and rewarding. Nurses can be instrumental in this process by (1) preparing the mother for anticipating the *normal* feelings of emptiness, loneliness, and sometimes even failure, (2) helping her reevaluate her role as parent and spouse, stressing that giving up the lost child must occur before she can reestablish emotional relationships, (3) encouraging her to explore fulfilling activities that use her special interests, talents, and qualifications, and (4) supporting her as her role changes, particularly assisting with communication between affected family members (Wong, 1980).

Nurses should also be aware of behaviors that indicate siblings' difficulty with resolving their grief, such as persistent blame and guilt, patterns of overactivity with aggressive and destructive outbursts, compulsive caregiving, persistent anxieties (such as fear of another family death or of their own), excessive clinging to the parent, difficulty with forming new relationships, problems at school (poor concentration, restlessness, preferring to be alone, not being liked by classmates), or delinquency (such as stealing) (Krupnick, 1984; Michael and Lansdown, 1986). In these situations professional assistance may be required, and the nurse can provide appropriate referral.

Communication with the bereaved family is essential, but often there is a feeling of not knowing what to say and of helplessness in offering words of comfort. Regrettably, reports from bereaved families indicate that the majority (80%) consider the information or counseling from professionals to be inadequate and even harmful (Segal, Fletcher, and Meekison, 1986). Harmful comments included:

At stillbirth: "It's horrible; don't look"; "Stop crying."
During hospital stay: "You need to be strong for your wife"; "You shouldn't be so upset. You should have expected it."
After unexpected death: "Why did it take you so long to go to Emergency?"

Harmful behaviors included:

Leaving the parents alone after the child's death
Prescribing tranquilizers in the first 24 hours after the death
Not providing explanations when treating the child

In analyzing the type of "helping" statements frequently made in responding to the bereaved, researchers found that 80% were considered nonhelpful (low facilitative) (Davidowitz and Myrick, 1984). Nonhelpful statements included:

Advice or evaluation—suggests or tells people what they might or ought to do ("You shouldn't question God's will," "You've got to get out more," "Stop feeling sorry for yourself.").
Interpreting or analyzing—attempts to connect events, explain behaviors and causative factors ("It was God's will," "It's better now because she is at peace," "You're acting that way because you choose to suffer.").
Reassurance and support—intend to be encouraging but more often than not also communicate that people need not feel the way they do ("You know, death comes to all of us; it's just a part of life," "At least you still have your father," "Time is a great healer, and you'll be stronger later," "I know how you feel.").

Of the helpful statements (high facilitative), those that conveyed feelings were considered most supportive, but others included questions and clarifying and summarizing statements:

Feeling-focused statements—convey that feelings are understood; require the use of a feeling word in the statement ("You're uncertain about what to do next," "You're feeling confused, and angry, too," "You're still struggling and feeling the pain."); communicate the most understanding, acceptance, and respect.
Questions either open or closed—sometimes have advice implied in them. Behind every question is an assumption ("Can I be of any help?" or "Have you decided who the pallbearers will be?").
Clarifying and summarizing—attempts to seek an understanding of what a person has said or to identify the most salient ideas that seem to be emerging from the conversation ("If I'm following you, you don't want to talk with anyone right now." "Correct me if I'm wrong, but you intend to make all arrangements.").

Guidelines for supporting grieving families are presented in Box 23-4.

THE NURSE AND THE FATALLY ILL CHILD

It would not be complete to discuss the nurse's role in caring for the family and dying child without exploring the effects of this stressful, yet extremely rewarding, area of nurs-

*P.O. Box 3696, Oak Brook, IL 60522-3696; (708) 990-0010.
†100 E. 8th St., Rm. B41, Cincinnati, OH 45202; (513) 721-5683.

NURSING CARE PLAN
The Child Who Is Terminally Ill or Dying

NURSING DIAGNOSIS: Altered growth and development related to terminal illness and/or impending death

GOAL 1

Support child during terminal phase

INTERVENTIONS

Encourage children to talk about their feelings and provide safe, acceptable outlets for aggression
Answer questions as honestly as possible while maintaining a positive, hopeful approach
Explain all procedures and therapies, especially physical effect child will experience
Help child distinguish between consequences of therapies and manifestations of disease process
Structure hospital environment to allow for maximum self-control and independence within the limitations imposed by child's developmental level and physical condition
Respect the child's need for privacy without neglecting the child
Provide for presence of customary support systems
Encourage family to remain near the child as much as possible

EXPECTED OUTCOMES

Child expresses feelings freely
Child demonstrates an understanding of symptoms

GOAL 2

Provide physical comfort and nurturing at time of dying

INTERVENTIONS

Keep bedsheets untucked
Keep child uncovered if sheets are bothersome
Apply loose, cool clothing
Keep fresh air circulating in room (open window, use small fan)
Change child's position only as tolerated
Give cool sponge baths
Use pillows or other supports to prop child in comfortable position
Carry (if possible) to other areas for diversion if desired
Place absorbent pads under hips
Help child to toilet if desired
Limit care to essentials
 May need to forego usual hygienic measures such as bath or clothing change but provide comfort measures (e.g., mouth care, wiping forehead, gentle back rub)
Avoid bright, direct light, but do not keep room too dim
Administer anticholinergic drugs (atropine or scopolamine) to reduce secretions (lessens "death rattle," which can be distressing to family)
Position with head slightly elevated or in well-supported sitting position if tolerated
Provide pain relief as needed (see Nursing Care Plan: The Child in Pain, Chapter 26.)

EXPECTED OUTCOME

Child exhibits minimal or no evidence of physical discomfort

GOAL 3

Provide emotional support at time of dying

INTERVENTIONS

Talk to child even though may not appear awake
Sit at head of bed where child can easily see face
Talk to child in clear, distinct voice, not whispers
Avoid conversation about the child in child's presence
Offer calm reassurance and orient child to surroundings when awake
Phrase questions for yes or no answers
Do not disturb child with repeated measurements of vital signs
Play favorite music (may soothe child)
Preserve physical closeness with family members (e.g., parent may want to rock child in chair or lie next to child in bed)

EXPECTED OUTCOME

Child appears calm and relaxed

NURSING DIAGNOSIS: Altered nutrition: less than body requirements related to loss of appetite, disinterest in food

GOAL 1

Provide nutriments

INTERVENTIONS

Offer any food and fluids child desires
Provide small meals and snacks several times a day
Avoid excess encouragement to eat or drink
Avoid foods with strong odors
Provide pleasant environment for eating
Serve foods that require the least energy to eat (soups, shakes)
Feed slowly
*Administer antiemetic as prescribed if nausea/vomiting is a problem
Provide mouth care before and after eating; lubricate lips with petrolatum

EXPECTED OUTCOME

Child consumes some nutriments

*Dependent nursing action.

Continued.

NURSING CARE PLAN
The Child Who Is Terminally Ill or Dying—cont'd

NURSING DIAGNOSIS: Fear/anxiety related to diagnosis, tests, and therapies and prognosis

GOAL 1
Reduce anxiety

INTERVENTIONS
Limit interventions to palliation only; discuss need for nonpalliative treatment with family and physician
Explain all procedures and other aspects of care to child
Remain with child or provide for constant attendance
Determine what child has been told about prognosis
Determine what the family wishes the child to know about the prognosis
Emphasize importance of honesty
Answer child's questions as openly and honestly as possible
Involve parents in child's care
Remain nonjudgmental regarding child's behavior

EXPECTED OUTCOME
Child discusses fears without evidence of stress

NURSING DIAGNOSIS: Anticipatory grieving related to potential loss of a child

GOAL 1
Support family

INTERVENTIONS
Identify stage of grieving process the family is experiencing
Provide opportunities for family to express emotions
Help parents deal with their feelings, allowing them more emotional reserve to meet the needs of their children
Encourage the parents to remain as near to the child as possible, yet be sensitive to the parents' needs
Provide information regarding child's status, anticipated reactions
Help parents to understand behavioral reactions of their children, especially that concern for present crisis, such as loss of hair, may be much greater than for future ones, including possible death
Facilitate family's assistance with child's care
Provide comfort measures for child and family
Encourage family to maintain own health care needs
Provide as much privacy as possible
Assess family's need for referral services, e.g., hospice services, specific organizations for grieving families
Encourage parents to honestly answer questions about dying rather than avoiding or fabricating euphemisms
Encourage parents to share their moments of sorrow with their children
Provide preparation for postdeath services
Discuss with family their preferences for care if death is imminent
Arrange for appropriate spiritual care in accordance with family's beliefs and/or affiliations
Maintain contact with family
Provide support for families who choose home care for their child
See Guidelines for Supporting Grieving Families, p. 1055

EXPECTED OUTCOMES
Family expresses fear, concerns, and any special desires for terminal child
Family demonstrates an understanding of child and his or her needs (specify)
Family members avail themselves of services
See also:
- Nursing Care Plan: The Child in the Hospital, Chapter 26
- Nursing Care Plan: The Family of the Ill or Hospitalized child, Chapter 26

GOAL 2
Provide interpersonal comfort

INTERVENTIONS
Offer calm reassurance to child
Reassure child of the love of others
Continue to set some limits for the child to provide a sense of security
Spend time with the child when not directly involved in care
Reinforce to the child that what is happening is not the child's fault
Involve child in routine activities as tolerated
Maintain a "normal" atmosphere
Talk to the child even though may not appear to be awake
- Situate self and others where easily visible to child
- Speak to child in clear, distinct voice; avoid whispering
- Avoid conversation about the child's condition in presence of child

Play favorite music and read stories to child
Orient child to surroundings when awake
Phrase questions for "yes" or "no" answers when possible to conserve child's energy

EXPECTED OUTCOME
Child exhibits no evidence of loneliness

NURSING CARE PLAN
The Child Who Is Terminally Ill or Dying—cont'd

NURSING DIAGNOSIS: Anticipatory grief related to imminent death of a child

GOAL 1

Support family

INTERVENTIONS

Be available to the family
Convey an attitude of caring for both child and family
Encourage at least one family member to stay with child
Help family to provide care of the child as they desire without forcing involvement
*Administer medications or other agents as prescribed to reduce unpleasant manifestations
- Oxygen for respiratory distress
- Anticonvulsants for seizures
- Anticholinergic drugs to reduce secretions ("death rattle")
- Analgesics for pain
- Stool softeners/laxatives for constipation
- Antiemetics for nausea/vomiting

Help and encourage family to express feelings appropriately
Encourage family to meet their own physical needs
Provide privacy
Provide for physical comfort of the family
Provide emotional support and comfort to the family
Encourage family to talk to child
Involve family and other children in decision making whenever possible, especially regarding alternatives for terminal care (hospital, home, hospice)
Support and assist family in giving explanations to other family members regarding child's status
Maintain a nonjudgmental attitude toward behavior of family members

EXPECTED OUTCOMES

Family members discuss their feelings
Family members are actively involved in child's care

GOAL 2

Support family's decision to take child home to die, if they wish

INTERVENTIONS

Teach family physical care of the child
Provide family with means for contacting health professionals at any time, e.g., phone numbers
Maintain daily contact with family, e.g., telephone call, home visit
Refer to community agencies as appropriate
Reassure family that they can readmit child to the hospital at any time
Help plan with family what to do when the child dies and what to expect

EXPECTED OUTCOMES

Family demonstrates the ability to provide care for the child
Family contacts appropriate support groups

*Dependent nursing action.

ing practice on the caregiver. Recognition of the potential stresses is essential in coping with the emotional demands imposed by sharing the family's loss and grief.

NURSES' REACTIONS TO CARING FOR FATALLY ILL CHILDREN

Nurses experience reactions to a fatal illness that are very similar to the responses of family members. Some of these help nurses provide care by protecting them from the emotional impact of the event. Others interfere with the establishment of a therapeutic relationship with family members. Analysis and understanding of these reactions are as important in providing effective care to the dying child as is the recognition of specific responses in the family.

Denial

When children are admitted to a pediatric unit with a suspected diagnosis of a serious illness, the initial response from some nurses is shock and denial. However, their behavioral reaction may be withdrawal from the child and family. They choose the "cure" philosophy over the "care" philosophy as a method of distancing themselves from the implications of emotional involvement. Because of their own dependency on denial, nurses may support denial in parents. There are several methods of conveying this message, such as emphasizing only optimistic "survival statistics," negating the seriousness of the illness, focusing on "cheering up" the family, and engaging in casual conversation to avoid meaningful dialogue. Although this increases nurses' comfort in caring for the dying child, it does little to provide family members with an opportunity to progress beyond denial and begin anticipatory grieving.

Some denial is as important for nurses as it is for the child or parents; it protects nurses from the overwhelming reality of death. It would be extremely difficult to participate in the medical treatment plan without some expectation of a cure. Denial is also necessary to prevent feelings of failure. The nursing and medical goal is curing illness and saving lives, not allowing patients to die. However, denial loses its beneficial functions when nurses refuse to admit failure and adhere to the "curing" regimen, regardless of its effectiveness or value.

Anger and Depression

Some nurses may be angry for having been assigned to the "leukemia case," because the very exposure to potential failure in a fatal illness is extremely threatening. Others may feel angry for having to subject the child to painful procedures or for being unable to relieve the child's physical and emotional suffering. Instead of anger, some nurses may feel depression for any of these reasons.

However, without an understanding of the reason for the emotion, nurses may project the anger onto others, particularly family members. They may be unable to tolerate the child's uncooperative behavior or the parents' continual requests for information. Anger fuels more anger, and parents react with hostility and think the members of the nursing staff are rejecting them. A vicious cycle of resentment, mistrust, and frustration results.

Depression also has adverse effects on a therapeutic relationship, because nurses may withdraw from the child and parents as a method of controlling their sadness. Unaware of the reason for the avoidance, family members interpret it as evidence of inadequate care. This reaction also fosters a nonsupportive cycle of avoidance, withdrawal, resentment, and frustration. However, the messages are usually more covert than when the nurses' reaction is anger, and may prevent a climax that could result in a solution to the problem.

Guilt

Nurses who feel unable to deal with fatal illness in a child often experience guilt. Nurses who become angry or depressed when caring for a dying child often reveal that they are very uncomfortable with this response but are unable to choose a more direct, constructive approach. They express guilt for having been intolerant of the child's or parents' behavior and, even more important, realize the missed opportunity to provide these individuals with professional support and guidance.

Nursing staff may experience guilt even when they can deal effectively with the family. There is often a feeling that the family's needs are never completely met. Such nurses tend to set expectations that are beyond anyone's ability to meet, such as the expectation that they are supposed to save lives, not let people die.

The one important difference between a dying child and an ill child is that there may be no second chance to meet the needs of the dying child. This finality is difficult to comprehend but can be a catalyst toward better understanding of one's own responses to dying. For example, when guilt makes one uncomfortable enough to seek alternate behavior patterns, there is an opportunity for change to occur, provided the individual is given some assistance and support.

Ambivalence

One of the most universal reactions of nurses is ambivalence in their feelings toward a dying child. There is the fluctuating adherence to hope for a cure and fear of a relapse. Sometimes the motivations for either are more for personal needs. For example, they may hope that the child recovers to avoid readmissions. Or they may wish for a remission so that discharge is assured. Such thoughts are certainly understandable in light of the emotional toll of nursing a dying child.

Ambivalence may be demonstrated in a particular type of bargaining. Rather than bargaining for extra time, nurses may hope that their colleagues are assigned the patient, or that a death may occur on a shift other than their own. Bargaining for a temporary absence from the dying child is a healthy response, because it denotes nurses' awareness of their own emotional limits. Nurses who are unable to recognize their personal emotional limits are in danger of seeking from the professional relationship their own needs for gratification, achievements, and fulfillment. This results in the loss of an objective evaluation of therapeutic interventions and the increased potential for subjective overinvolvement with the family.

Coping with Stress

One of the hazards of caring for dying children is the risk of *burnout,* a state of physical, emotional, and mental exhaustion (Pines, 1981). It occurs as a result of prolonged involvement with individuals in situations that are emotionally demanding. Nurses working in intensive care units are particularly prone to this occupational hazard, but staff nurses also can experience it when dealing with groups of children such as those who may die. To cope constructively, effectively, and therapeutically with children who are dying in spite of the stress generated, while avoiding burnout, requires deliberate and concerted effort on the part of the nurse.

Self-awareness and consciousness raising. The initial step in effectively caring for a dying child is making a deliberate choice to become involved. Many nurses react negatively to the word "involvement" because they believe that professionals must remain uninvolved in order to maintain objectivity. Involvement does not displace objectivity. On the contrary, allowing oneself to feel with the other person expands one's ability to comprehend the meaning and depth of that emotion. Maslach (1979) suggests that the achievement of *detached concern,* in which the health care practitioner provides sensitive, understanding care by being sufficiently detached to make objective, rational decisions, is the ideal.

Involvement does have the potential risk of clouding objectivity, but awareness of one's reactions and investments in the care of a dying child minimizes this hazard. Developing awareness requires the willingness to investigate one's motivations for choosing to work in such an area and an understanding of the stresses inherent in the role, to review one's resolution of past losses, and to contemplate one's own fears of death. Often nurses realize that their cold, impersonal reaction to dying patients stems from previous unresolved conflicts or losses. Once they are able to talk about such experiences, they are usually able to gain insight into their behavior and begin to form alternative methods of reacting.

Knowledge and practice. Intervening therapeutically with terminally ill children and their families requires more than self-awareness. It also necessitates basing nursing practice on sound theoretic formulations and empiric observations that serve as a general, concise analysis of the typical reactions of families. Although every individual is different and responds to events or crises in a way that is influenced by all of his or her previous life's experiences, there must be some beginning point for understanding the more typical responses of individuals and for making some decision as to their importance in the eventual resolution of the crisis. In this way nurses can plan care that meets the needs of each family member in terms of prevention as well as intervention of problems.

Nurses also must explore ethical issues surrounding the definition of death, the use of extraordinary, lifesaving measures vs passive or active euthanasia, and patients' rights to know and choose their own destiny. Once they have soundly formulated principles by which to practice, they need opportunities for decision making. When a team approach is used, nurses can be valuable members of the group, provided their own values are clarified and they have critically assessed the family's responses. (See Ethical Decision Making, Chapter 1.)

Support sytems. Support systems are essential to continued functioning in a high-stress environment. They allow for regeneration of energies by sharing feelings and concerns with others. Social supports may be personal family members such as parents or spouses, extended relatives, and friends. Professional supports include colleagues, consultants, teachers, and supervisors. Peers may be sources of technical and practical advice and can provide a frame of reference and feedback for the nurse to gauge his or her own work (Cherniss as cited in McElroy, 1982). Professional persons may be of their own field or from related disciplines.

Other strategies. Any number of other strategies may be used to reduce stress. These include maintaining good general health practices, especially regular exercise, and diversionary activities that are of personal interest beyond the workplace (Vachon and Pakes, 1985). Distancing techniques are also effective, such as leaving work at work, informing other staff not to contact them on their days off, periodically assuming less demanding assignments, and taking time off when needed. For caregivers who find the demands of this kind of nursing too emotionally draining, the ultimate distancing strategy is resignation (Munley, 1985).

A final technique is to focus on the positive aspects of the caregiving role. Despite the difficult times in caring for these children and families, there are many rewarding experiences that must be remembered. Dedicated efforts reap numerous rewards, and these must not be forgotten or minimized. Reflection on positive feedback from appreciative families can revitalize self-esteem and job satisfaction. Attending the funeral services can be a supportive act for both the family and the nurse and in no way detracts from the professionalism of care. For the family it conveys a sense of worth and caring by the nurse. For the nurse it provides a sense of "closure" with the family and assists in the resolution of personal grief (Irvine, 1985).

KEY POINTS

- To counsel families and children regarding death, nurses need to understand children's perceptions of death, the fears in each age-group, and personal meanings of death and bereavement during developmental stages.
- Toddlers' egocentricity and separation of fact from fantasy make death incomprehensible; they may still refer to a dead person as if the person exists.
- Because of their sense of precausality and self-power, preschoolers may believe that their thoughts actually cause another person's death.
- With their reasoning power and fear of the unknown, school-age children may feel intense guilt and responsibility about someone's death.
- Adolescents have difficulty accepting death because of their preoccupation with developing a sense of identity.
- Nurses may offer the following assistance in assessment and education about death: counseling parents about children's age-specific understanding of death, encouraging parents to help children become familiar and comfortable with loss, taking part in organized death education in schools, and serving as a resource to answer children's questions.
- What children are told about their serious illness is based on several general principles regarding developmental age, previous knowledge, and honesty.
- Kübler-Ross' stages of dying are denial, anger, bargaining, depression, and acceptance.
- According to Lindemann, acute grief is a syndrome with psychologic and somatic symptomatology that may appear after a crisis or be delayed, exaggerated, or apparently absent. Distorted reactions may represent one aspect of the syndrome and can be transformed into normal grief work.
- Parke's grief process consists of four phases that do not necessarily proceed in sequence and may recur at any time: shock and disbelief, expression of grief, disorganization and despair, and reorganization.
- Special decisions at the time of dying and death may involve hospital or hospice care, the child's right to die, visualization of the body, tissue donation/autopsy, and siblings' attendance at the funeral.
- There are five phases of family reactions to a life-threatening illness: Phase I—shock and disbelief, guilt, anger, anticipatory grieving, depression and ambivalence, bargaining; Phase II—overprotectiveness, dependency, social isolation, hope, fear, and anxiety; Phase III—denial and ambivalence, overprotectiveness, and concern for the future; Phase IV—heightened anticipatory grieving, loss of hope and despair, fear of death, fear of loss of control, and fear of isolation and loneliness; Phase V—acute grief and extended phase of mourning.
- In dealing with stress related to the dying patient, the nurse can cope successfully through self-awareness, consciousness raising, knowledge and practice, available support system, maintaining general good health, and focusing on the positive rewards of involvement with dying children and their families.

REFERENCES

Armstrong-Dailey, A.: Children's hospice care, Pediatr. Nurs. 16(4):337-339, 409, 1990.

Atuel, T.M., Williams, P.D., and Camar, M.T.: Determinants of Filipino children's responses to the death of a sibling, Matern. Child Nurs. J. 17(2):115-134, 1988.

Birenbaum, L.K.: The relationship between parent-sibling communication and coping of siblings with death experience, J. Pediatr. Oncol. Nurs. 6(3):86-91, 1989.

Bluebond-Langner, M.: The private worlds of dying children, Princeton, NJ, 1978, Princeton University Press.

Bluebond-Langner, M.: Worlds of dying children and their well siblings, Death Studies 13:1-16, 1989.

Brett, K.M., and Davies, E.M.B.: "What does it mean?" Sibling and parental appraisals of childhood leukemia, Cancer Nurs. 11(6):329-338, 1988.

Carbary, L.J.: Easing the family's pain: organ donation, Nurs. Life 5(1):26-28, 1985.

Carlson, P., and others: Helping parents cope: a model home-care program for the dying child, Issues Compr. Pediatr. Nurs. 8(1-6):113-128, 1985.

Chesler, M., and Lozowski, S.: Problems and needs of children off treatment, The Candlelighters Childhood Cancer Foundation 12(2/3):2-3, 1988.

Conrad, N.L.: Spiritual support for the dying, Nurs. Clin. North Am. 20(2):415-426, 1985.

Corr, C.A., and Corr, D.M.: Pediatric hospice care, Pediatrics 76(5):774-780, 1985.

Davidowitz, M., and Myrick, R.: Responding to the bereaved: an analysis of "helping" statements, Death Educ. 8:1-10, 1984.

Davies, B.: Family responses to the death of a child: the meaning of memories, J. Palliative Care 3(1):9-15, 1987.

Davies, B.: Shared life space and sibling bereavement responses, Cancer Nurs. 11(6):339-347, 1988.

Foley, G.: Conflicts in practice: the argument for, J. Assoc. Pediatr. Oncol. Nurs. 2(3):22-24, 1985.

Foley, G.V.: Facilitating death discussions with children, Pediatrics: Nursing Update, lesson 19, Princeton, NJ, 1986, Continuing Professional Educational Corp.

Gershan, J.A.: Judaic ethical beliefs and customs regarding death and dying, Crit. Care Nurse 5(1):32-34, 1985.

Giordano, M.S.: What required-request laws mean to you, Am. J. Nurs. 89(10):1296-1297, 1989.

Glassman-Freibusch, B.: Extremely uncaring (letter), MCN 8(6):442, 1983.

Glick, I., Weiss, R., and Parkes, C.: The first year of bereavement, New York, 1974, John Wiley & Sons, Inc.

Greenberg, L.W., and others: Giving information for a life-threatening diagnosis, Am. J. Dis. Child. 138(7):649-653, 1984.

Greenham, D.E., and Lohmann, R.A.: Children facing death: recurring patterns of adaptations, Health Social Work 7:89-94, 1982.

Irvine, P.: The attending at the funeral, N. Engl. J. Med. 312(26):1704-1705, 1985.

Jankovic, M., and others: Meetings with parents after the death of their child from leukemia, Pediatr. Hematol. Oncol. 6:155-160, 1989.

Jost, K.E., and Haase, J.E.: At the time of death: help for the child's parents, Child. Health Care 18(3):146-152, 1989.

Klopovich, P., and others: School phobia, J. Kans. Med. Soc. 82(3):125-127, 1981.

Kohler, J.A., and Radford, M.: Terminal care for children dying of cancer: quantity and quality of life, Br. Med. J. 291:115-116, 1985.

Krupnick, J.: Bereavement during childhood and adolescence. In Osterweis, M., Solomon, F., and Green, M., editors: Bereavement: reactions, consequences, and care, Washington, DC, 1984, National Academy Press.

Kübler-Ross, E: On death and dying, New York, 1969, Macmillan Publishing Co.

Kübler-Ross, E: On children and death, New York, 1983, Macmillan Publishing Co.

Lansky, S.B.: Management of stressful periods in childhood cancer, Pediatr. Clin. North Am. 32(3):625-632, 1985.

Lansky, S.B., List, M.A., and Ritter-Sterr, C.: Psychiatric and psychological support of the child and adolescent with cancer. In Pizzo, P., and Poplack, D., editors: Principles and practice of pediatric oncology, Philadelphia, 1988, J.B. Lippincott Co.

Lauer, M.E., and others: A comparison study of parental adaptation following a child's death at home or in the hospital, Pediatrics 71(1):107-112, 1983.

Lauer, M.E., and others: Children's perceptions of their sibling's death at home or hospital: the precursors of differential adjustment, Cancer Nurs. 8(1):21-27, 1985.

Leikin, S.: A proposal concerning decisions to forego life-sustaining treatment for young people, J. Pediatr. 115(1):17-22, 1989.

Lindemann, E.: Symptomatology and management of acute grief, Am. J. Psychiatry 101:141-148, Sept. 1944.

Lyman, M.J.: The parent network in pediatric oncology: supportive or not? Cancer Nurs. 10(4):207-216, 1987.

Martinson, I.M., Davies, E.B., and McClowry, S.G.: The long-term effects of sibling death on self-concept, J. Pediatr. Nurs. 2(4):227-235, 1987.

Martinson, I.M., and others: Home care for children dying of cancer, Res. Nurs. Health 9(1):11-16, 1986.

Martinson, I.M., and others: Impact of childhood cancer on healthy school-age siblings, Cancer Nurs. 13(3):183-190, 1990.

Maslach, C.: The burn-out syndrome and patient care. In Garfield, C., editor: Stress and survival: the emotional realities of life-threatening illness, St. Louis, 1979, Mosby–Year Book, Inc.

McClowry, S.G., and others: The empty space phenomenon: the process of grief in the bereaved family, Death Studies 11:361-374, 1987.

McClung, J.A., and Kamer, R.S.: Implications of New York's do-not-resuscitate law, N. Engl. J. Med. 323(4):270-272, 1990.

McElroy, A.M.: Burnout—a review of the literature with application to cancer nursing, Cancer Nurs. 5(3):211-217, 1982.

Michael, S., and Lansdown, R.: Adjustment to the death of a sibling, Arch. Dis. Child. 61:278-283, 1986.

Miles, M.S.: Emotional symptoms and physical health in bereaved parents, Nurs. Res. 34(2):76-81, 1985.

Miles, M.S., and Perry, K.: Parental responses to sudden accidental death of a child, Crit. Care Q. 8(1):73-84, 1985.

Moldow, D., and others: The cost of home care for dying children, Med. Care 20(11):1154-1160, 1982.

Moore, I.M., Gilliss, D.L., and Martinson, I.: Psychosomatic symptoms in parents 2 years after the death of a child with cancer, Nurs. Res. 37(2):104-107, 1988.

Munley, S.A.: Sources of hospice staff stress and how to cope with it, Nurs. Clin. North Am. 20(2):343-355, 1985.

Nagy, M.: The child's view of death, J. Genet. Psychol. 73:3-27, 1948.

Nitschke, R., and others: Therapeutic choices made by patients with end-stage cancer, J. Pediatr. 101(3):471-476, 1982.

Olson, V.T., and Hooke, M.M.: The complexities of do not resuscitate orders, MCN 13(3):157-169, 1988.

O'Neil, E.A.: Treatment decisions with the terminally ill incompetent patient, Nurs. Econ. 5(1):32-35, 1987.

Patno, K.M., Young, P.C., and Dickerman, J.D.: Parental attitudes about confidentiality in a pediatric oncology clinic, Pediatrics 81(2):296-300, 1988.

Peele, A.S.: The nurse's role in promoting the rights of donor families, Nurs. Clin. North Am. 24(4):939-949, 1989.

Pines, A.: Burnout: a current problem in pediatrics, Curr. Probl. Pediatr. 11(7):2-32, 1981.

Poznanski, E.: The "replacement child"—a sign of unresolved parental grief, J. Pediatr. 81(6):1190-1193, 1972.

Rando, T.: An investigation of grief and adaptation in parents whose children have died from cancer, J. Pediatr. Psychiatry 8(1):3-20, 1983.

Salladay, S.A., and Royal, M.E.: Children and death: guidelines for grief work, Child Psychiatry Hum. Dev. 11(4):203-212, 1981.

Saunders, J.M., and Valente, S.M.: No code: the question that won't go away, Nursing '86 16(3):60-64, 1986.

Schonfeld, D.J.: Crisis intervention for bereavement support: a model of intervention in the children's school, Clin. Pediatr. 28(1):27-33, 1989.

Schulman, J.L., and Rehm, J.L.: Assisting the bereaved, J. Pediatr. 102(6):992-998, 1983.

Schultz, C.: Grieving children, J. Emerg. Nurs. 6:30-36, 1980.

Segal, S., Fletcher, M., and Meekison, W.: Survey of bereaved parents, Can. Med. Assoc. J. 134(1):38-42, 1986.

Shumway, C.N., Grossman, L.S., and Sarles, R.M.: Therapeutic choices by children with cancer (letter), J. Pediatr. 103(1):168, 1983.

Sourkes, B.M.: Siblings of the child with a life-threatening illness, Feelings Med. Signif. 28(5):19-24, 1986.

Stanfill, P., and Strong, C.: Conflicts in practice: the argument against, J. Assoc. Pediatr. Oncol. Nurs. 2(3):25-26, 1985.

Vachon, M.L.S., and Pakes, E.: Staff stress in the care of the critically ill and dying child, Issues Compr. Pediatr. Nurs. 8(1-6):151-182, 1985.

Waechter, E.: Dying children: patterns of coping, Issues Compr. Pediatr. Nurs. 8(1-6):51-68, 1985.

Wass, H.: Concepts of death: a developmental perspective, Issues Compr. Pediatr. Nurs. 8(1-6):3-24, 1985.

Wass, H., and others: Death education: an annotated resource guide, Washington, DC, 1980, Hemisphere Publishing Corp.

Weber, P.: The human connection: the role of the nurse in organ donation, J. Neurosurg. Nurs. 17(2):119-122, 1985.

Weiss, R.: Reactions to particular types of bereavement. In Osterweis, M., Soloman, F., and Green, M., editors: Bereavement: reactions, consequences, and care, Washington, DC, 1984, National Academy Press.

Williams, L.: Organ procurement: what nurses need to know, Crit. Care Q. 8(1):27-30, 1985.

Wong, D.: Bereavement: the empty-mother syndrome, MCN 5(6):385-389, 1980.

Woolley, H., and others: Imparting the diagnosis of life threatening illness in children, Br. Med. J. 298(6688):1623-1626, 1989.

Zelauskas, B.: Siblings: the forgotten grievers, Issues Compr. Pediatr. Nurs. 5:45-52, 1981.

BIBLIOGRAPHY

Adams, D.W.: Helping the dying child: practical approaches for nonphysicians, Issues Compr. Pediatr. Nurs. 8(1-6):95-112, 1985.

Amenta, M.O.: Hospice in the United States: multiple and varied programs, Nurs. Clin. North Am. 20(2):269-280, 1985.

Antonacci, M.: Sudden death: helping bereaved parents in the PICU, Crit. Care Nurse 10(4):65-70, 1990.

Bachmann, A.T.: Helping the survivors cope with sudden death, Point of View 26(2):6-7, 1989.

Balk, D.: Effects of sibling death on teenagers, J. Sch. Health 53(1):14-18, 1983.

Baskin, C.H., and others: Helping teachers help children with cancer: a workshop for school personnel, Child. Health Care 12(2):78-83, 1983.

Benoliel, J.Q.: Nursing research on death, dying, and terminal illness: development, present state, and prospects. In Werley, H.H., and Fitzpatrick, J.J., editors: Annual review of nursing research, vol. 1, New York, 1983, Springer Publishing Co, Inc.

Blotcky, A.D., and Cohen, D.G.: Psychological assessment of the adolescent with cancer, J. Assoc. Pediatr. Oncol. Nurs. 2(1):8-14, 1985.

Bossert, E., and Martinson, I.: Kinetic family drawings—revised: a method of determining the impact of cancer on the family as perceived by the child with cancer, J. Pediatr. Nurs. 5(3):204-213, 1990.

Bosworth, T.: Leukemia through a teenager's eyes, MCN 14(2):93-94, 1989.

Brunnquell, D., and Hall, M.D.: Issues in the psychological care of pediatric oncology patients, Am. J. Orthopsychiatry 52(1):32-44, 1982.

Castiglia, P.T.: Death of a parent, J. Pediatr. Health Care 2(3):157-159, 1988.

Castiglia, P.T.: Death of a sibling, J. Pediatr. Health Care 2(4):211-213, 1988.

Chase, D.: Dying at home with hospice, St. Louis, 1986, Mosby–Year Book, Inc.

Chee, C.M.: A child's right to die, MCN 7(2):81-88, 1982.

Chekryn, J., Deegan, M., and Reid, J.: Impact on teachers when a child with cancer returns to school, Child. Health Care 15(3):161-165, 1987.

Coleman, F.W., and Coleman, W.S.: Helping siblings and other peers cope with dying, Issues Compr. Pediatr. Nurs. 8(1-6):129-150, 1985.

Coolican, M.B.: Katie's legacy: organ donation helped this family begin to resolve the tragedy, Am. J. Nurs. 87(4):483-485, 1987.

Corr, C.A., and Corr, D.M., editors: Hospice approaches to pediatric care, New York, 1985, Springer Publishing Co, Inc.

Corr, C.A., and Corr, D.M.: In our opinion . . . what is pediatric hospice care? Child. Health Care 17(1):4-11, 1988.

Davies, B.: The family environment in bereaved families and its relationship to surviving sibling behavior, Child. Health Care 17(1):22-31, 1988.

Davis, A.J.: Breaking the news . . . to inform relatives of a family member's death, Am. J. Nurs. 83(10):1457-1478, 1983.

Davis, F.D.: Organ procurement and transplantation, Nurs. Clin. North Am. 24(4):823-836, 1989.

Dufour, D.F.: Home or hospital care for the child with end-stage cancer: effects on the family, Issues Compr. Pediatr. Nurs. 12(5):371-383, 1989.

Edwardson, S.R.: The choice between hospital and home care for terminally ill children, Nurs. Res. 32(1):29-34, 1983.

Erlen, J.A.: The child's choice: an essential component in treatment decisions, Child. Health Care 15(3):156-160, 1987.

Foley, G.V.: Facilitating death discussions with children, Pediatrics: nursing update, lesson 19, Princeton, NJ, 1986, Continuing Professional Educational Corp.

Gaffney, D.A.: Death in the classroom: a lesson in life, Holistic Nurs. Pract. 2(2):20-27, 1988.

Gifford, B.J., and Cleary, B.B.: Supporting the bereaved, Am. J. Nurs. 90(2):48-53, 1990.

Granstrom, S.L.: Spiritual nursing care for oncology patients, Top. Clin. Nurs. 7(1):39-45, 1985.

Grogan, L.B.: Grief of an adolescent when a sibling dies, MCN 15(1):21-24, 1990.

Gyulay, J.: The death of a child, Issues Compr. Pediatr. Nurs. 12(1):1-137, 1989.

Gyulay, J.: The death of a child, part II, Issues Compr. Pediatr. Nurs. 12(2-3):139-260, 1989.

Gyulay, J.: The death of a child, part III, Issues Compr. Pediatr. Nurs. 12(4):261-338, 1989.

Hays, J.C.: Hospice policy and patterns of care, Image 18(3):92-97, 1986.

Hazinski, M.F.: Pediatric organ donation: responsibilities of the critical care nurse, Pediatr. Nurs. 13(5):354-357, 1987.

Henretta, C.B., and Van Brunt, P.F.: Sudden pediatric death: meeting the needs of family and staff, Nurse Educ. 7(6):13-16, 1982.

Hogan, N.S.: The effects of time on the adolescent sibling bereavement process, Pediatr. Nurs. 14(4):333-335, 1988.

Hogan, N.S., and Balk, D.E.: Adolescent reactions to sibling death: perceptions of mothers, fathers, and teenagers, Nurs. Res. 39(2):103-106, 1990.

Homedes, N., and Ahmed, S.M.: In my opinion . . . death education for children, Child. Health Care 15(1):34-36, 1987.

Jacobson, L.A.: When a child's parent dies: the PNP's role, Pediatr. Nurs. 14(5):366-368, 372, 1988.

Johnson, S.E.: After a child dies: counseling bereaved families, New York, 1987, Springer Publishing Co., Inc.

Johnson-Soderberg, S.: The development of a child's concept of death, Oncol. Nurs. Forum 8(1):23-26, 1981.

Kinrade, L.C.: Preventive group intervention with siblings of oncology patients, Child. Health Care 14(2):110, 1985.

Komp, D.M.: Lessons from long-term survivors of childhood cancer, Pediatrics 84(5):910-911, 1989.

Koocher, G.P.: Psychosocial care of the child cured of cancer, Pediatr. Nurs. 11(2):91-93, 1985.

Krulik, T.: Helping parents of children with cancer during the midstage of illness, Cancer Nurs. 5(6):441-445, 1982.

Krulik, T., Holaday, B., and Martinson, I.M.: The child and family facing life-threatening illness, Philadelphia, 1987, J.B. Lippincott Co.

Kübler-Ross, E.: Death: the final stage of growth, Englewood Cliffs, NJ, 1975, Prentice-Hall, Inc.

Kübler-Ross, E.: Living with death and dying, New York, 1981, Macmillan Publishing Co.

Kübler-Ross, E., and Warshaw, M.: To live until we say goodbye, Englewood Cliffs, NJ, 1978, Prentice-Hall, Inc.

Lewandowski, W., and Jones, S.L.: The family with cancer: nursing interventions throughout the course of living with cancer, Cancer Nurs. 11(6):313-321, 1988.

Martinson, I.M.: Impact of childhood cancer on family care in Taiwan, Pediatr. Nurs. 15(6):636-637, 1989.

Martinson, I.M., and others: Home care for children dying of cancer, Res. Nurs. Health 9(1):11-16, 1986.

Martinson, I., Nesbitt, M., and Kersey, J.: Children's adjustment to death of a sibling from cancer, Adv. Thanatol. 6:1-7, 1987.

Martocchio, B.C.: Grief and bereavement: healing through hurt, Nurs. Clin. North Am. 20(2):327-342, 1985.

Martocchio, B.C., and Dufault, K., editors: Symposia on hospice and compassionate care and the dying experience, Nurs. Clin. North Am. 20(2):267-466, 1985.

McCown, D.E.: When children face death in a family, J. Pediatr. Health Care 2(1):14-19, 1988.

McEvoy, M., Duchon, D., and Schaefer, D.S.: Therapeutic play group for patients and siblings in a pediatric oncology ambulatory care unit, Top. Clin. Nurs. 7(1):10-18, 1985.

McNeil, J.N.: Death education in the home: parents talk with their children, Issues Compr. Pediatr. Nurs. 8(1-6):293-313, 1985.

Miles, A.: Caring for families when a child dies, Pediatr. Nurs. 16(4):346-347, 1990.

Miles, M.S.: Helping adults mourn the death of a child, Issues Compr. Pediatr. Nurs. 8(1-6):219-241, 1985.

Miller, J.F.: Hope doesn't necessarily spring eternal—sometimes it has to be carefully mined and channeled, Am. J. Nurs. 85(1):23-25, 1985.

Monaco, G.P.: Resources available to the family of the child with cancer, Cancer 58:516-521, 1986.

Moore, I., Kramer, R., and Perin, G.: Care of the family with a child with cancer: diagnosis and early stages of treatment, Oncol. Nurs. Forum 13(5):60-66, 1986.

Moseley, J.R.: Alterations in comfort, Nurs. Clin. North Am. 20(2):427-438, 1985.

Norris, M.K.G.: How to manage tissue donation, Am. J. Nurs. 89(10):1300-1302, 1989.

Parkes, C., and Weiss, R.: Recovery from bereavement, New York, 1983, Basic Books, Inc.

Pazola, K.J., and Gerberg, A.K.: Privileged communication—talking with a dying adolescent, MCN 15(1):16-21, 1990.

Petix, M.: Explaining death to school-age children, Pediatr. Nurs. 13(6):394-396, 1987.

Pidgeon, V.: Compliance with chronic illness regimens: school-aged children and adolescents. J. Pediatr. Nurs. 4(1):36-47, 1989.

Pitel, A.U., and others: Parent consultants in pediatric oncology, Child. Health Care 14(1):46, 1985.

Rando, T.A., editor: Parental loss of a child, Champaign, IL, 1986, Research Press.

Riley-Lawless, K.: School reentry programs, J. Pediatr. Oncol. Nurs. 6(3):92-93, 1989.

Ross-Alaolmolki, K.: Supportive care for families of dying children, Nurs. Clin. North Am. 20(2):457-466, 1985.

Rudin, M., Martinson, I., and Gilliss, C.: Measurement of psychosocial concerns of adolescents with cancer, Cancer Nurs. 11(3):144-149, 1988.

Snyder, L.A., and Peter, N.K.: How to manage organ donation, Am. J. Nurs. 89(10):1294-1298, 1989.

Sodestrom, K., and Martinson, I.: Patients' spiritual coping strategies: a study of nurse and patient perspectives, Oncol. Nurs. Forum 14(2):41-46, 1987.

Stutzer, C.A.: Work-related stresses of pediatric bone marrow transplant nurses, J. Pediatr. Oncol. Nurs. 6(3):70-78, 1989.

van Eys, J.: In my opinion . . . normalization while dying, Child. Health Care 17(1):18-21, 1988.

van Eys, J., editor: The truly cured child: the new challenge in pediatric cancer care, Baltimore, 1977, University Park Press.

Waechter, E., and others: Concomitants of death imagery in stories told by chronically ill children undergoing intrusive procedures: a comparison of four diagnostic groups, J. Pediatr. Nurs. 1(1):2-11, 1986.

Walker, C.: Siblings of children with cancer, Oncol. Nurs. Forum 17(3):355-360, 1990.

Wass, H., and Corr, L., editors: Special issue on childhood and death, Issues Compr. Pediatr. Nurs. 8(1-6):3-383, 1985.

Wasserman, A.B.: Helping families get through the holidays after the death of a child, Am. J. Dis. Child. 142:1284-1286, 1988.

Weber, J.A., and Fournier, D.G.: Family support and a child's adjustment to death, Fam. Relat. 34(1):43-49, 1985.

Wofford, L.G.: "Cured!" . . . Now what? Pediatr. Nurs. 13(4):252-254, 1987.

Wong, D.: The terminally ill child. In Johnson, S., editor: Nursing assessment and strategies for the family at risk, ed. 2, Philadelphia, 1986, J.B. Lippincott Co.

Yoak, M., Chesney, B.K., and Schwartz, N.H.: Active roles in self-help groups for parents of children with cancer, Child. Health Care 14(1):38-45, 1985.

RESOURCES FOR CHILDREN'S BOOKS ON DEATH*

Aradine, C.: Books for children about death, Pediatrics 57(3):372-378, 1976.

Bernstein, J.: Literature for young people: non-fiction books about death, Death Educ. 3:111-119, 1979.

Delisle, R., and McNamee, A.: Children's perceptions of death: a look at the appropriateness of selected picture books, Death Educ. 5:1-13, 1981.

Fassler, J.: Helping children cope: mastering stress through books and stories, New York, 1978, The Free Press.

McBride, M.: Children's literature on death and dying, Pediatr. Nurs. 5(3):31-33, 1979.

Mills, G.: Books to help children understand death, Am. J. Nurs. 79(2):291-295, 1979.

Wass, H.: Books for children, Issues Compr. Pediatr. Nurs. 8(1-6):373-376, 1985.

Wass, H., and Corr, C., editors: Helping children cope with death: guidelines and resources, ed. 2, Washington, DC, 1984, Hemisphere Publishing Corp.

*Other sources of publications on life-threatening illness and death are **The Compassionate Friends,** P.O. Box 3696, Oak Brook, IL 60522-3696, (708) 990-0010; **Centering Corporation,** P.O. Box 3367, Omaha, NE 68103-0367, (402) 553-1200; **Pediatric Projects, Inc.,** P.O. Box 1880, Santa Monica, CA 90406, (818) 705-3660; **Children's Hospice International,** 700 Princess St., Ste. 3, Alexandria, VA 22314, (703) 684-0330, (800) 24-CHILD; **National Cancer Institute,** Public Inquiries Office, Bldg. 31, Rm. 10A16, Bethesda, MD 20892, (301) 496-5583; **National Childhood Grief Institute,** 6200 Colonial Way, Minneapolis, MN 55436, (616) 920-0737.

CHAPTER 24

The Child with Cognitive Impairment

RELATED TOPICS

The child with sensory or communication impairment, Ch. 25
Dental health, Ch. 14
Developmental assessment, Ch. 7
Fetal alcohol syndrome, Ch. 11
Hereditary influences on health promotion of the child and family, Ch. 5
Impact of chronic illness or disability on the child and family, Ch. 22
Infantile autism, Ch. 13
Limit-setting and discipline, Ch. 14
Play: infant, Ch. 12; toddler, Ch. 14; preschooler, Ch. 15; and school-age child, Ch. 17
Preparation for hospitalization, Ch. 22
Toilet training, Ch. 14
Toy safety, Ch. 4

GLOSSARY*

AAMR American Association on Mental Retardation
CHD Congenital heart disease
cognitive impairment General term for any type of mental deficiency; also refers to MR
DS Down syndrome
EMR Educable MR
IQ Intelligence quotient
MR Mental retardation
TMR Trainable MR

*See also Glossary, Chapter 5.

Cognitive impairment, or mental retardation, is the most common developmental disability in the United States, affecting some 3% of the population. In recent years major changes have occurred in the philosophy of care toward people with cognitive impairment, especially with the trend toward home care. Therefore parents need role models and adequate preparation to effectively teach the child to function at an optimum level within the home and community environment. Nurses are in a strategic position to assume a vital role in assisting these parents with observation, problem solving, and decision making. With expanded roles in nursing, nurses are assuming additional responsibility for the care of these children in schools, sheltered workshops, group homes, residential settings, and ambulatory care centers, as well as in hospitals.

This chapter is concerned with the complex problem of mental retardation—specifically its definition and causes—

and strategies that parents can use to rear these children successfully. In addition, two syndromes associated with cognitive impairment are discussed, Down syndrome and fragile X syndrome. Although the needs and concerns of the family are a primary focus throughout the chapter, the reader is encouraged to review Chapter 22, which details the family's adjustment to disabilities in general.

PERSPECTIVES IN THE CARE OF CHILDREN WITH COGNITIVE IMPAIRMENT

Cognitive impairment is a general term that encompasses any type of mental deficiency. In this chapter the term is used synonymously with *mental retardation (MR).*

MR is a complex disorder, whose very definition has generated considerable controversy throughout the ages. It is caused by numerous factors, many of which leave families with guilt because of the hereditary component. For families, living with a child with cognitive impairment is more than a challenge of childrearing, particularly if other physical disabilities exist. There are educational dilemmas, the need for other special services, decisions regarding future care, and coping with a society that often denigrates those who are retarded. However, for many families the special challenges are more than compensated for from the joy of having this child. Nurses, as part of an interdisciplinary team, can lend support and guidance to help the family cope with the special challenges and concerns associated with the diagnosis of MR, while promoting a healthy, thriving family unit.

GENERAL CONCEPTS

The American Association on Mental Retardation (AAMR) defines MR as "significantly subaverage general intellectual functioning existing concurrently with deficits in adaptive behavior and manifested during the developmental period" (Grossman, 1983). *General intellectual functioning* refers to the results of various individually administered general intelligence tests. *Significantly subaverage intellectual functioning* is defined as an intelligence quotient (IQ) of approximately 70 or below. *Adaptive behavior* is the effectiveness or degree with which individuals meet the standards of personal independence and social responsibility expected for age and cultural group. It is a critical component of the definition, since it implies that IQ alone is not the criterion for mental retardation. For example, individuals with IQ scores near 70 may not be classified as retarded based on their ability to adapt to the environment. *Developmental period* comprises the period between conception and the 18th birthday. Consequently, if cognitive impairment occurs after this time, such as from injury or disease, the person is not considered retarded.

Diagnosis and Classification

The diagnosis of MR is usually made after a period of suspicion by professionals and/or the family that the child's developmental progress is delayed. In some cases it is made at birth because of recognition of distinct syndromes, such as Down syndrome. At the other extreme, it is made after the child begins school, when problems such as speech delays arouse concern when compared to peer achievement. In all cases a high index of suspicion for developmental delay and behavioral signs (Box 24-1) is necessary for early diagnosis, and routine developmental screening (see Chapter 7) can assist in early identification. Delays are commonly seen in gross and fine motor and speech development, although the latter is most predictive. Although gross motor skills such as walking may be delayed, a number of children with even severe retardation may walk at or near the usual age. Thus age of walking is not necessarily a good predictor of intelligence (Hreidarsson, Shapiro, and Capute, 1983). Other common misconceptions that delay early diagnosis include physical stereotyping ("all retarded children are dumb looking") and that children are too young to be tested. In fact, cute children may be retarded, and no child is too young to be evaluated (Coplan, 1982).

Box 24-1 EARLY BEHAVIORAL SIGNS SUGGESTIVE OF COGNITIVE IMPAIRMENT

Nonresponsiveness to contact
Poor eye contact during feeding
Diminished spontaneous activity
Decreased alertness to voice or movement
Irritability
Slow feeding

From Crocker, A., and Nelson, R.: Mental retardation. In Levine, M., and others: Developmental-behavioral pediatrics, Philadelphia, 1983, W.B. Saunders Co., p. 760.

The diagnosis and classification of MR are based on standard IQ tests. Several tests may be employed depending on the child's age. Two of the most commonly used tests are the Stanford-Binet Test and Wechsler Intelligence Scale for Children–Revised (WISC-R). These tests should be administered only under favorable conditions and individually (never as a group test) by specially trained clinicians, such as psychometrists or child development specialists. Tests available for assessing adaptive behaviors include the Vineland Social Maturity Scale and the AAMR Adaptive Behavior Scale. Informal appraisal of adaptive behavior may be made by those fully acquainted with the child (e.g., teachers, parents, or other care providers). Frequently these observations are what lead parents to seek evaluation of the child's development (Grossman, 1983).

The severity of retardation is based on the IQ scores, which represent mild, moderate, severe, and profound levels of deficit. The classification shown in Table 24-1 is based on the AAMR system and uses the same criteria as the American Psychiatric Association (DSM-III-R) (1987). Clinicians are encouraged to use professional judgment in determining adaptive deficit. The revised AAMR system includes a significant change from its previous classification

Table 24-1 Classification of mental retardation

LEVEL (IQ)*	PRESCHOOL (BIRTH-5 YEARS)—MATURATION AND DEVELOPMENT	SCHOOL AGE (6-21 YEARS)—TRAINING AND EDUCATION	ADULT (21 YEARS AND OLDER)—SOCIAL AND VOCATIONAL ADEQUACY
Mild—50-55 to approximately 70	Often not noticed as retarded by casual observer but is slower to walk, feed self, and talk than most children; follows same sequence in development as normal children	Can acquire practical skills and useful reading and arithmetic to a third- to sixth-grade level with special education; can be guided toward social conformity; achieves mental age of 8 to 12 years	Can usually achieve social and vocational skills adequate to self-maintenance; may need occasional guidance and support when under unusual social or economic stress; can adjust to marriage but not childrearing
Moderate—35-40 to 50-55	Noticeable delays in motor development, especially in speech; responds to training in various self-help activities	Can learn simple communication, elementary health and safety habits, and simple manual skills; does not progress in functional reading or arithmetic; achieves mental age of 3 to 7 years	Can perform simple tasks under sheltered condition; participates in simple recreation; travels alone in familiar places; usually incapable of self-maintenance
Severe—20-25 to 35-40	Marked delay in motor development; little or no communication skills; may respond to training in elementary self-help, for example, self-feeding	Usually walks, barring specific disability; has some understanding of speech and some response; can profit from systematic habit training; achieves mental age of toddler	Can conform to daily routines and repetitive activities; needs continuing direction and supervision in protective environment
Profound—below 20-25	Gross retardation; minimum capacity for functioning in sensorimotor areas; needs total care	Obvious delays in all areas of development; shows basic emotional responses; may respond to skillful training in use of legs, hands, and jaws; needs close supervision; achieves mental age of young infant	May walk; needs complete custodial care; has primitive speech; usually benefits from regular physical activity

*Based on classification from American Association on Mental Retardation.

in that *borderline retarded* is eliminated to reflect current thinking in the field and to be consistent with other classification systems (Grossman, 1983).

A more useful approach for clinical application is classification based on educational potential or symptom severity. For educational purposes the terms *educable mentally retarded (EMR)* and *trainable mentally retarded (TMR)* may be used. EMR corresponds to the mildly retarded group, which constitutes about 85% of all people with MR. TMR is generally equivalent to children with moderate levels of cognitive impairment and accounts for about 10% of the MR population (American Psychiatric Association, 1987). Although nurses should be familiar with the approximate range of IQ for classifying severity, they should refrain from using numbers as the criterion for assessing or evaluating the child's abilities, since numbers are of little value in counseling parents or training these children.

Etiology

The causes of severe MR are primarily genetic, biochemical, viral, and developmental. In mild retardation, familial, social, and environmental causes predominate. Associated factors include maternal life-styles, such as poor nutrition, cigarette smoking, and chemical abuse, all of which increase the risk of prematurity and intrauterine growth retardation (Task Force on Joint Assessment, 1985). Among individuals with severe retardation, chromosomal disorders account for 20% to 25% of cases and the majority are Down syndrome. Another 25% are caused by identifiable disorders or syndromes, and about 10% to 20% are associated with severe cerebral palsy, microcephaly, or infantile spasms (Hall, 1984). The prenatal, perinatal, and postnatal causes of MR are listed in Box 24-2 (Grossman, 1983).

Prevention

Currently there is much concern with prevention of MR. The major intervention is improved support for the small premature infant and other high-risk newborns (Crocker, 1982). Other *primary prevention strategies*—those designed to preclude the occurrence of the condition that causes retardation—include rubella immunization; genetic counseling, especially in terms of Down or fragile X syndrome; education regarding the dangers of ingesting alcohol during pregnancy and lead during childhood; adequate prenatal care and childhood nutrition; and reduction of nonintentional and intentional (abuse) cerebral injuries.

Box 24-2 CAUSES OF MENTAL RETARDATION

Infection and intoxication—any agent associated with abnormalities or malformations, such as rubella, syphilis, toxoplasmosis, maternal drug consumption (including alcohol), exposure to industrial chemicals, increased blood levels of lead, Rh incompatibility resulting in kernicterus, or maternal disorders, such as eclampsia

Trauma or physical agent—injury to brain suffered during prenatal, perinatal, or postnatal period, including physical injury, lack of oxygen, or exposure to radiation

Metabolism or nutrition—imbalances in fat, carbohydrates, and amino acids; inadequate nutrition; and metabolic or endocrine disorders, such as phenylketonuria or congenital hypothyroidism

Gross postnatal brain disease—diseases characterized by skin eruptions, lesions, and tumors, such as neurofibromatosis and tuberous sclerosis

Unknown prenatal influence—cerebral, spinal, and craniofacial malformations, such as microcephaly, hydrocephaly, meningomyelocele, and craniostenosis

Chromosomal abnormalities—chromosomal aberrations resulting from radiation, viruses, chemicals, parental age, and genetic mutations, such as Down and fragile X syndromes

Other conditions originating in the perinatal period—prematurity, low birth weight, and postmaturity

Psychiatric disorders with onset during the child's developmental period up to age 18 years—for example, autism

Environmental influences—evidence of a deprived environment associated with a history of mental retardation among parents and siblings

Secondary prevention activities—those designed to identify the condition early and institute treatment to avert cerebral damage—include prenatal diagnosis or carrier detection of disorders, such as Down syndrome, and newborn screening for treatable inborn errors of metabolism, such as congenital hypothyroidism, phenylketonuria, and galactosemia.

Tertiary prevention strategies—those concerned with treatment to minimize long-term consequences—include early identification of conditions and appropriate therapies and rehabilitation services. These include medical treatment of coexisting problems, such as hearing impairment in Down syndrome, and programs for infant stimulation, parent training, preschool education, and counseling services to preserve the integration of the family unit.

NURSING CARE OF CHILDREN WITH COGNITIVE IMPAIRMENT

The goal of caring for children with MR is to promote their optimum development as individuals within a family and community. Since the general guidelines for coping with and adjusting to the child with special needs are discussed extensively in Chapter 22, the following discussion focuses on principles involved in educating these children, specific interventions to teach self-care skills, guidelines for promoting optimum development, helping families adjust to future care, and caring for these children during hospitalization.

THERAPEUTIC DIALOGUE

Developmental Delay

During a well-child visit the nurse performs a Denver Developmental Screening Test on a 13-month-old child. The child has delays in each of the four sectors. However, the mother has not expressed any concern for the child's delayed development.

NURSE: Mrs. M., when I was seeing what Carey is able to do, was his performance typical?

MOTHER: Yes, I would say so.

NURSE: How do you think Carey is developing?

MOTHER: I think he is a little slow, but he was born 2 weeks early and I have read that premature babies can take longer to catch up.

NURSE: Were you told that the baby was premature?

MOTHER: No, but the baby was early and I thought that meant he was premature.

NURSE: Usually, if babies are 2 weeks early or late, they are still considered born at the correct time. I wouldn't expect Carey to have any slower development because of his birth date.

MOTHER: Do you think he is behind? What did that Denver test show?

NURSE: The Denver Developmental Screening Test is only a way to screen children to see how they are developing. It isn't a diagnostic test, but it does show that Carey is behind in these areas. (Nurse explains the results and what delays mean.)

MOTHER: It doesn't seem like very good news. I don't have any other children to compare with Carey, but I thought he should be sitting up by now and talking a little. Anytime I mentioned my concern to my family, they always told me not to worry. They said that Carey is so cute and lovable that he had to be normal.

NURSE: Unfortunately, cute and lovable children can have problems also. At your next visit I will do the Denver again, and I will talk with Carey's doctor. I believe your concerns are correct. Carey should be sitting up by himself and imitating some speech sounds.

MOTHER: I wish what you are saying weren't true, but if it is, I want to find out right away so that we can get the help we need.

NURSE: I can understand that this is difficult news. Once we know more, I can discuss with you what community programs are available. Starting early is very important.

Assessment

Nurses play a major role in identifying children with cognitive impairment. In the newborn and early infancy period few signs are present, with the exception of Down syndrome (see p. 1082). However, after this age delayed developmental milestones are the major clues to MR. In addition, nurses must have a high index of suspicion for early behavioral patterns that may suggest cognitive impairment (see Box 24-1) and be aware of stereotypes that may delay diagnosis, such as "retarded children have to look dumb." Parental concerns, such as delayed development compared to siblings, need to be taken seriously. All children should receive regular developmental assessment, and the nurse is often the person responsible for performing such developmental screening tests (see Chapter 7). When delays are found, the nurse must use sensitivity and discretion in revealing this finding to parents (see Therapeutic Dialogue).

Nursing Diagnoses

A number of nursing diagnoses are prominent in the nursing care of the child with cognitive impairment and the child's family; other diagnoses specific to individual cases become evident. The most common nursing diagnoses are outlined in the Nursing Care Plan on p. 1070.

Planning

The goals of nursing care for the child with MR and family are:

1. Educate the child using effective teaching strategies.
2. Teach the child self-care skills.
3. Promote the child's optimum development.
4. Help the family adjust to future care.
5. Care for the child during hospitalization.
6. Assist in measures to prevent MR.

Implementation

Once the goals are identified, specific interventions are carried out. The following discussion presents general interventions for most children with mental disability. Modifications are needed in specific situations and in accordance with the child's educability.

Educate the child and family. To learn how to teach children with cognitive impairment, it is necessary to investigate their learning abilities and deficits. These children have a marked deficit in their ability to discriminate between two or more stimuli because of difficulty in paying attention to relevant cues. Unfortunately the ability to discriminate between symbols is essential in learning the alphabet for reading or numbers for arithmetic. However, these children can learn to discriminate if the cues are presented in an exaggerated concrete form and all extraneous stimuli are eliminated. For example, the use of colors to exaggerate visual cues or music for auditory cues can help the child learn. The latter is particularly effective for teaching speech by singing the same word rather than only saying it.

These children's deficit in discrimination also implies that concrete ideas are learned much more effectively than abstract concepts. Therefore demonstration is preferable to verbal explanation, and learning is directed toward mastering a skill rather than understanding scientific principles underlying the procedure.

Another deficit is in short-term memory. Whereas children with average intelligence can remember several words, numbers, or directions at one time, children with cognitive impairment are unable to do so. Thus they need simple one-step directions. They respond to learning how to remember, such as by "clustering" pairs or triads together. This approach is helpful when trying to teach them their telephone number. Rather than having them memorize the entire seven-digit number, the teacher breaks it into pairs. After memorizing the pairs, the child puts them together.

Teaching through a step-by-step process requires a task analysis—each task is divided into its necessary components (see Box 24-3). For example, if the child is learning to tie a shoe, the teacher must practice the skill, divide it into steps (task analysis), and teach each step completely before proceeding to the next activity.

One critical area of learning that has had a tremendous impact on education for cognitively impaired individuals is motivation. Programs based on the motivation principles of behavior modification, employing positive reinforcement for specific tasks or behaviors, have demonstrated marked improvement in children's ability to learn. Two techniques are especially important with this group of learners:

Fading—physically taking the child through each sequence of the desired activity and gradually fading out physical assistance so that the child becomes more independent

Shaping—waiting for the child to give a response that approximates the desired behavior, then reinforcing the child by social approval, such as touching or talking to him or her

Such principles can easily be implemented in the home in teaching self-help skills. Maintaining feelings of success in accomplishing specified goals also promotes a feeling of self-esteem in the child.

When behavior modification is employed, it is crucial not only to reinforce desirable behavior but also consistently to ignore undesirable behavior. Ignoring the child is particularly difficult for many parents, because they may equate ignoring their child with being a "bad parent." Therefore the nurse must be especially supportive as the parent attempts negative reinforcement. The parent should realize that repetition plays an important part in the child's learning. As the child gains mastery, the parent is encouraged to decrease the social or physical reinforcement the child has been offered. The parent should understand that if a learning program does not move forward successfully, both parent and nurse will reevaluate the last sequence the child mastered to see if they are expecting too much too soon.

Advances in technology have greatly aided in providing active stimulation,* especially in children who are severely retarded and may have physical disabilities that limit their

*Information on active stimulation is available from Educational Technology Center, Inc., Box 64, Foster, RI 02825.

NURSING CARE PLAN
The Child with Mental Retardation

NURSING DIAGNOSIS: Altered growth and development related to impaired cognitive functioning

GOAL 1
Promote optimum development

INTERVENTIONS
Involve child and family in an early infant stimulation program
Assess child's developmental progress at regular intervals; keep detailed records to distinguish subtle changes in functioning
Help family set realistic goals for child
Encourage learning of self-care skills as soon as child achieves readiness
Reinforce self-care activities (see Tables 24-2 to 24-5)
Encourage family to investigate special daycare programs and educational classes as soon as possible
Emphasize that child has same needs as other children (e.g., play, discipline, social interaction)
Before adolescence, counsel child and parents regarding physical maturation, sexual behavior, marriage, and family
Encourage optimum vocational training

EXPECTED OUTCOMES
Child and family are actively involved in infant stimulation program
Family applies concepts and continues activities in home care of child
Child performs activities of daily living at optimum capacity
Family investigates educational programs
Appropriate limit setting, recreation, and social opportunities are provided
Adolescent issues are explored and implemented as appropriate

NURSING DIAGNOSIS: Altered family processes related to having a child with mental retardation

GOAL 1
Support family at time of diagnosis

INTERVENTIONS
Inform family as soon as possible after birth
Have both parents present at informing conference
Give family written information about the condition, when possible (e.g., a specific syndrome or disease)
Discuss with family members benefits of home care vs institutionalization; allow them opportunities to investigate all residential alternatives before making a decision
Encourage family to meet other families with a similarly affected child
Refrain from giving definitive answers about the degree of retardation; stress the potential learning abilities of retarded children, especially with early stimulation
Demonstrate acceptance of child through own behavior
Emphasize normal characteristics of child
Encourage family members to express their feelings and concerns

EXPECTED OUTCOMES
Family expresses feelings and concerns regarding the birth of a child with MR and its implications
Family members make realistic decisions based on their needs and capabilities
Family members demonstrate acceptance of child

GOAL 2
Help family prepare for future care of child

INTERVENTIONS
As child grows older, discuss with parents options to home care, especially as parents near retirement or old age
Help family investigate residential settings other than institutionalization
Encourage family to include affected member in planning and to continue meaningful relationships after placement
Refer to agencies that provide support and assistance

EXPECTED OUTCOMES
Family identifies realistic goals for future care of child
Family avails themselves of supportive services

See also Nursing Care Plan: The Child with a Chronic Illness or Disability, Chapter 22.

range of capabilities. For example, with the use of specially designed switches, children are given control of some event in the environment, such as turning on the television (Fig. 24-1). The television becomes reinforcement for activating the switch. Repetitive use of these switches provides an early, simplistic association with a technical device that may progress to the child using increasingly complex aids.

Early intervention programs. Early intervention or stimulation programs have been widely promoted for children with developmental disabilities. This group comprises an extensively diverse group of children with MR, cerebral palsy, language and learning disabilities, sensory disorders, autism, and other conditions. Consequently the types of programs vary widely in philosophy and interventions, and the issue of benefit from such programs is often confusing and conflicting.

One analysis of early intervention programs for infants with disabilities found that effectiveness was greatest in centers involving both parents and children in the interventions, in programs having a well-defined curriculum, and in centers that served a heterogenous group of children (possibly because these programs tended to enroll children at a

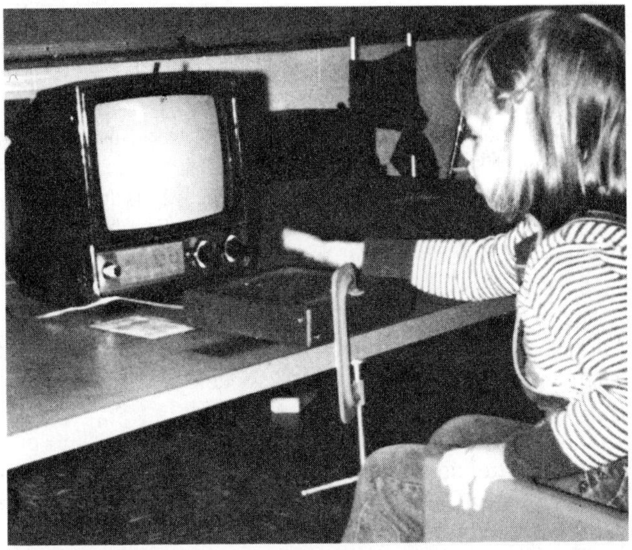

Fig. 24-1. A single push panel allows a child with cognitive impairment to turn a television on and off.

younger age than programs targeted at a specific disability group) (Shonkoff and Hauser-Cram, 1987).

Nurses need to be aware of the types of programs in their community to direct families to groups whose philosophy is best suited to the family's needs. Early intervention programs are provided by a number of organizations. Under Public Law 99-457, the Education for the Handicapped Amendment Act, local departments of education are required to provide education programs for children from 3 years of age, and states are provided incentives for initiating education programs starting at birth. Services may be provided under state **Programs for Children with Special Health Needs** (formerly **Crippled Children's Program**) or by private organizations such as the **National Easter Seal Society*** and the **Association of Retarded Citizens of the United States.†** Parents should inquire about these programs by contacting the appropriate agencies. The child's education should begin as soon as possible, not at 5 or 6 years of age. As children grow older, their education should be directed toward vocational training that prepares them for as independent a life-style as possible within their scope of abilities (American Academy of Pediatrics, Committee on Children with Disabilities, 1986).

Promote independent self-help skills. When a child with cognitive impairment is born, parents need assistance in promoting normal developmental skills that are almost automatically learned by other children. There is no way to predict when a child should be able to master self-help skills, and studies demonstrate that wide variability exists in the ages at which these children accomplish such functions (see Table 24-6). For the nurse to be successful in meeting this goal, the parents must be supported, included as the primary rehabilitators with the child, and provided with detailed written descriptions of the stimulation program. The following discussion is concerned with activities of daily living; promoting gross motor development is outlined in Table 24-7. Parents also need to be aware that numerous devices are commercially available that can aid in achievement of independence.*

Feeding. Self-feeding is recognized as the first major self-help skill that children learn. It involves the integration of fine and gross motor skills and visual perception. Most parents take for granted that they will be successful in teaching their children to feed themselves. Therefore the nurse must also be especially sensitive to the needs of the parent as well as of the child when assistance is offered.

Before beginning a self-feeding program, the nurse should do a task analysis, breaking the process of feeding into its smallest components (Box 24-3). It is important to observe the child in an eating situation to determine whether any of these small steps that make up the entire task of self-feeding have been mastered. If so, the nurse should comment about them positively to the parent and child.

In addition to a task analysis, a number of other factors are assessed, such as the shape of the child's mouth and control of mouth, lips, and tongue movements (whether the tongue moves forward and backward or from side to side, whether there are rotary movements). The presence of teeth determines the textures and consistencies of food that may be offered to the child. The child's developmental readiness for self-feeding, such as the ability to maintain head and trunk support and to sit without support, eye-hand coordination, the firmness of the grasp, and ability to reach for an

Box 24-3 SAMPLE TASK ANALYSIS: SPOON FEEDING

1. Orients to the food by looking at it
2. Looks at the spoon
3. Reaches for it
4. Touches it
5. Grasps it
6. Lifts it
7. Delivers the spoon to the bowl
8. Lowers it into the food
9. Scoops food onto the spoon
10. Lifts it
11. Delivers the spoon to the mouth
12. Opens the mouth
13. Inserts the spoon into the mouth
14. Moves the tongue and mouth to receive the food
15. Closes the lips
16. Swallows the food
17. Returns the spoon to the bowl

*70 E. Lake St., Chicago, IL 60601; (312) 726-6200 or (800) 221-6827.

†P.O. Box 6109, Arlington, TX 76005; (817) 640-0204.

Information on early intervention programs in each state is available from the **National Down Syndrome Society,** 666 Broadway, Suite 810, New York, NY 10012; (212) 460-9330 or (800) 221-4602.

*A resource for a wide variety of equipment, including self-help devices, is available from J.A. Preston, *Catalog: Materials for Exceptional Children,* 60 Page Rd., Clifton, NJ 07012; (201) 777-2700 or (800) 631-7277.

object, hold it, and release it, are examined. If the child has any physical impairments that interfere with holding or grasping the utensil, specially designed utensils can be substituted (Fig. 24-2) or homemade modifications can be used, such as building the handle up with a sponge or piece of wood or bending it to accommodate arm movement.

Further data are obtained from the parent by asking specifically about the family's approach to feeding. For example, who feeds the child regularly? Is the child fed when hungry or according to a prescribed schedule? What are the child's appetite patterns? Does the parent know when the child is full? What foods does the child like? How long does feeding take? A short feeding time, such as 10 or 20 minutes, might indicate that the child is being deprived of sensory experiences or appropriate interactions; a long time might indicate frustration and fatigue on the parent's part. Is the feeding environment described as quiet and nondistracting? What is the best time to begin teaching this new task? If the family is going on vacation, if someone is visiting, or if there has been a major stress in the family, this may not be the ideal time to begin a teaching program.

Preparation for the feeding activity is also discussed, such as proper placement of the child at the table and protection of the area against spills. The principle of normalization (see Box 22-13) is employed to make feeding a family activity. For example, the child is fed in the kitchen, at the table, or in a high chair in a sitting position, and with other family members whenever possible. Food should be served in attractive receptacles; offered in separate servings, not pureed or mixed together; served at the appropriate temperature, not routinely lukewarm; and of sufficient variety and texture from each of the basic four food groups.

Once the feeding program is begun, the nurse is in an important position to give parents supportive feedback. The parents' observational skills, their ability to share observations, keep records of the child's progress, and establish a goal that is appropriate and realistic for both the child and the parents are praised. By acknowledging these aspects, the nurse promotes mastery of a task that is extremely important to the child who is mentally retarded. Table 24-2 lists activities to help the child learn self-feeding.

Toileting. Independent toileting is another major self-help skill that can be taught using behavior modification principles. It should be started after self-feeding, since this is the normal sequence of development. Plans for a toileting program begin by assessing the child's physical and psychologic readiness (Table 24-3; see also Box 14-1). Because of physical or developmental limitations, certain signs may not be possible. For example, children who cannot walk can be trained once they are able to sit with good balance, and children with poor speech may need to rely on gesturing to signal their toileting needs.

Parents are interviewed regarding their readiness to pursue a toilet-training program that is characterized by a positive, consistent, individualized, nonpunitive, nonpressured style of teaching. It is important to explore the parents' willingness to participate, the time they have to invest in the program, the advantages they see, the inconveniences that toilet training may cause them, the reason they wish to start, and whether this is the best time for both the parents and the child to begin.

Any past attempts at toilet training the child are reviewed: When and why did the parents start training? What methods did they use? Did they experience feelings of frustration, indifference, or discomfort? How long did they attempt training, and what were their reasons for discontinuing training efforts? Looking back, how did they view the experience for themselves and the child? Were their efforts consistent? What did they do most consistently? Do they think it is important to try again? If the parents admit to using punishment in any form, including spanking, scolding, withholding privileges, using suppositories, withholding fluid, or getting the child up in middle of the night, the nurse appeals to them to discontinue these unnecessary, ineffective methods.

As part of the procedure for determining the readiness of both parents and child to become involved in a successful

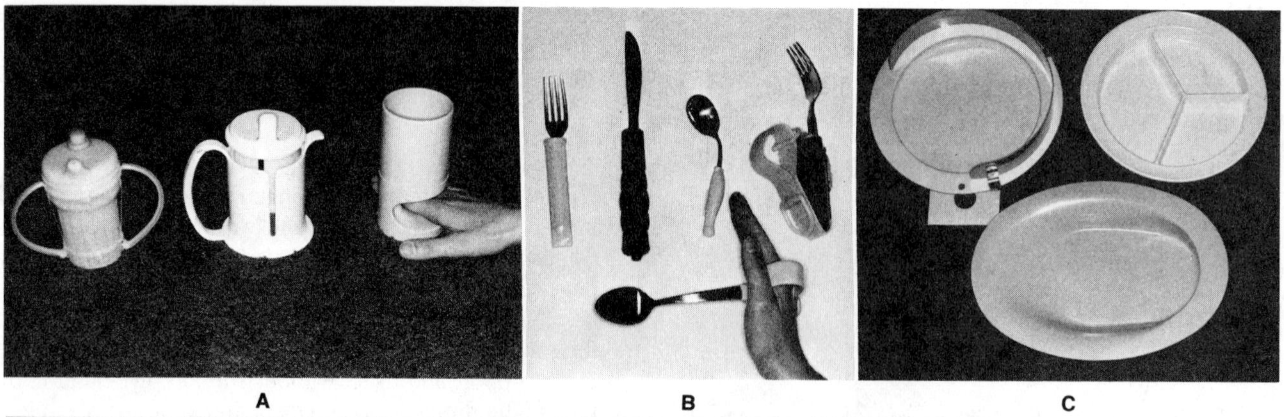

Fig. 24-2. Self-help aids for feeding. **A,** *Left to right,* Modified drinking cup, glass with holder and lid, pedestal cup. **B,** *Left to right,* Soft built-up handle utensil, weighted knife, child's bent spoon, Quad-Quip utensil holder (holds most household utensils); *bottom,* vertical palm self-handle utensil. **C,** *Left to right, top,* Plastic plate with suction feet and optional metal food guard, partitioned scoop dish, *bottom,* scoop dish.

Table 24-2 Infant stimulation program for self-feeding

USUAL AGE OF ACHIEVEMENT (MONTHS)	BEHAVIOR	ACTIVITY
Birth	Has sucking, rooting, and swallowing reflexes	Gently stroke around child's lips and mouth to stimulate puckering in order to strengthen lip muscles if sucking is weak Maintain in midline and slightly flexed
1	Is able to take food from a spoon	Press spoon on the tongue to stimulate jaw closure; press gently above the thyroid cartilage to stimulate swallowing; after spoon is withdrawn, close the mouth by pushing up on the mandible; wipe excess food from the lips in one stroke to prevent disrupting the normal closing and swallowing sequence Introduce pureed foods of different tastes and textures
4-5	Can approximate cup to lips	Offer small amounts of formula from a cup Place hands on lower jaw to provide better lip closure
5-6	Can use fingers to bring food to mouth	Give child dry toast, zwieback, pretzel, or cracker Dip fingers into food and bring hand to child's lips Place food in child's hand and gradually make child reach for it if child is not used to voluntarily grasping objects
6-7	Is able to chew solids	Introduce soft foods that require some chewing (cooked carrots, baked meats, baked potato, cheese, and so on) Place a small piece of food on the back molar area to stimulate chewing
8-9	Holds a spoon and plays with it during feeding	Give child a small spoon at feeding time Reinforce any attempts at self-feeding (putting spoon in mouth, in food, and so on) Improvise appropriate utensil if child has difficulty in holding spoon
9	Holds own bottle Finger feeds	Place the bottle in child's hands and bring it to the mouth; gradually release your hand Fill it only partway with milk or use a small (4-ounce) bottle Purchase a special nipple with a straw attached that draws milk from the bottom of the bottle if child is unable to tilt the bottle Give firmly cooked food cut into small pieces
12	Drinks from a cup with much spilling	Give child a cup, beginning with the same procedure as for a bottle
15	Drinks from a cup with less spilling	Use a wide, unbreakable cup with two handles Introduce a straw if child is unable to lift a cup; to initiate sucking liquid up the straw, fill the straw with juice, cover the top end with your finger, place the bottom end in child's mouth, and gradually release your finger to let the fluid in when child makes sucking movements Wean child gradually from one bottle at a time, eliminating the nighttime one last
18	Uses a spoon with much spilling	Give child a spoon, a bowl, and "sticky" food (applesauce or mashed potatoes) Guide child's hand toward the bowl and then into mouth if child is unwilling to feed self; gradually fade out the assistance Anchor the bowl to the table if child has poor motor coordination
24	Holds cup in one hand Uses spoon with little spilling	Give a small-diameter cup that is easily grasped with one hand; add small amount of liquid
36	Begins to use fork; holds it in fist	Give a small-handled and short-pronged fork Guide the hand to pierce the food if child is reluctant
48	Eats with fork held with fingers	Continue encouraging use of fork
72-84	Uses knife	Encourage "spreading" with knife, followed by cutting tender foods Introduce knife and fork cutting

Table 24-3 Child stimulation program for self-toileting

USUAL AGE OF ACHIEVEMENT (YEARS)	BEHAVIOR	ACTIVITY
1-2½	Is able to Sit unsupported Walk and stand alone Walk alone backward/forward Balance well Climb onto a chair Retain urine for at least 2 hours	Assess physical behaviors that indicate readiness for training; begin after most signs are evident Begin bowel training before bladder training Record approximate schedule of evacuation Place on potty-chair at regular intervals (on awakening, after meals, before bedtime) Stay with child while on potty-chair (usually 5-20 minutes) Keep potty-chair in bathroom Use training pants rather than diapers; whenever possible, leave diapers off child to experience feeling of voiding without clothing
	Recognizes urge to let go and hold on Is able to communicate this sensation to parent Has desire to please parent by voluntarily controlling elimination	Assess psychologic readiness for toileting Point out when diapers are wet or dry Use consistent words or gestures to indicate need for elimination Praise for success Avoid punishment or excessive pressure
3 (may be as long as 5 years)	Stays dry during night	Take to toilet just before bedtime Do not offer excessive fluids before bedtime
	Seats self on toilet	When child is trained, gradually reduce use of potty-chair for regular toilet If needed, keep small stool by toilet for climbing onto seat (sitting with legs facing tank reduces feeling of "falling in")
3-3½	Voids standing up (male)	Use imitation of watching father (or other male) Provide small stool for easy access to toilet May need to direct stream initially
	Washes/dries hands with supervision	Turn on faucets for child; provide small stool Make hygiene routine part of toileting
3½-4	Attempts to wipe self but is unsuccessful	Offer toilet paper Teach correct procedure from front to back
	Undresses/dresses self	Use clothing that is easy to manage (elastic waist pants, dress)
	Flushes toilet	Remind to flush toilet after elimination
	Completely cares for self at toilet, including wiping and handwashing	Encourage independence

toilet-training program, parents are asked to keep detailed records for 7 days. They should be cautioned to discontinue record keeping if the child becomes ill or if fluid intake is changed. Record keeping includes the following events:

1. The child ate or drank, no matter how little was consumed.
2. The child's behavior was suddenly distinctly different, for example, when the child was noticeably more quiet or louder, started fussing or tugging at clothes, pointed toward the bathroom, cried, or squirmed.
3. Parents gave the child positive attention related to toileting behaviors only, in the form of praise, concrete rewards, affection, or approval.
4. Parents gave attention in the form of scolding, threatening, or spanking if the child had wet or soiled the underclothes or did not tell them before eliminating.
5. The child indicated the need to go to the toilet by either gestures or words.
6. The child was noted to have dry underclothes.
7. The child was noted to have wet underclothes.

It is crucial to refrain from beginning any toilet-training program until such records are completed, because they show how parents are responding to the child's behaviors and at what times the child is most likely to eliminate.

The goal of any toilet-training program is to help the child achieve small goals and experience comfort and success and to help the parents simultaneously experience feelings of adequacy, minimum tension, and success. Parents should understand that they will be capitalizing on the times the child is most likely to eliminate and that they should respond immediately to any cues indicating this need.

A task analysis of toileting includes the same discrete steps as outlined for feeding (see Box 24-3). A positive and relaxed attitude toward toilet training is important and differs little from the approach used with other children (see Chapter 14). Activities to help the child learn independent toileting are presented in Table 24-3.

Dressing. Dressing skills develop without special training in most children, usually as a consequence of autonomy and imitation. For children who are retarded, special training is necessary to promote this skill. Factors that interfere with spontaneous learning include immature motor skills, lack of motivation, physical impairments, or lack of opportunity. The last variable should always be considered when assessing delayed development of independent dressing.

The level of independence in dressing varies according to the degree of retardation. Children with mild and moderate retardation and no accompanying physical limitations can become independent in all dressing skills, except for more complex tasks such as color coordination. Those who are severely retarded can achieve most dressing skills, except the ability to fasten complicated closures such as buttons or ties. Those who are profoundly retarded are usually able to assist in undressing and dressing but achieve no independent skills.

Children are considered mentally ready for dressing training if they can sit quietly for 3 to 5 minutes while working on a task, can watch what they are doing while working on a task, can follow physical gestures or cues, can follow verbal commands, and can relate clothing to the appropriate body part, such as socks with feet. As with other self-help skills, the child may not be able to master every task but should be evaluated for evidence of willingness to participate at his or her level of readiness. The use of teaching devices such as dolls with mock closures and reinforcement for success in managing the fasteners can increase the child's manipulative skills, which may be transferred to ready-to-wear clothing.

After the assessment of the child's readiness, a detailed record is kept of what the child can do in dressing, what is being taught, and how well the child is progressing with the new skill. The program for self-dressing follows the same sequence as normal development, as outlined in Table 24-4.

Choice of clothing is an important aspect of the training program. Clothes should be clean, up-to-date, and well fitted. They should be easy to put on and take off, easy to fasten, comfortable and nonrestricting, capable of disguising a physical disability, and easy to maintain. Minimizing the abnormal appearance of a "retarded" child is a major goal in promoting acceptance from others and self-esteem in the child.

Grooming. Self-grooming is usually learned along with other independent skills, such as washing hands during toilet training. The same principles are followed in teaching grooming procedures as have already been discussed: assess the child's readiness and present level of competency, proceed with skills in the normal sequence of development, analyze the task into its component parts, and set up an individualized teaching program. As with self-dressing, a major factor in learning independent grooming is the opportunity to practice the skills. Table 24-5 suggests activities for promoting self-grooming. Complete independence for bathing and hair washing is learned during the school years; these are therefore late skills for these children.

Special mention must be made of dental hygiene. An odor-free mouth and a white set of teeth are essential in promoting a positive image. In addition, healthy teeth are necessary for proper mastication and speech. Diseased teeth and gums increase drooling and prevent proper preparation of food for subsequent digestion. Missing teeth interfere with proper tongue positioning for clear speech.

Most causes of dental problems in these children are a result of neglected dental hygiene and excessive quantities of carbohydrates, including the use of candy to reward behavior. Most dental problems are preventable with the same dental hygiene practices discussed in Chapter 14.

If the child has physical impairments that limit the ability to brush, special devices may be necessary, such as a larger handle or a curved toothbrush, to reach all surfaces of the teeth. Electric toothbrushes may be a worthwhile investment for some children. The use of dental disclosing tablets is an excellent aid in visually showing the child (and parent) the thoroughness (or lack) of cleaning. Any devices that help motivate the child to brush should be used. For example, the parent can place a special "tooth calendar" on the wall and mark each date with stars to represent the number of brushings per day. At the end of a specified number of stars the child can receive a special reward.

The child should be routinely taken to a dentist. It is important to prepare the child for such visits, since it is much more difficult to change an unsatisfactory experience than to prevent one. Once the child is traumatized by the experience, parents may be less inclined to take the child back for fear of temper tantrums or other resisting behavior. The nurse can assist families by locating dentists who are familiar with treating these children and discussing with parents preparatory procedures for the visit.

Promote optimum development. Optimum development involves more than achieving independence. It requires appropriate guidance for establishing acceptable social behavior and personal feelings of self-esteem, worth, and security. These attributes are not simply learned through a stimulation program. Rather they must arise from the genuine love and caring that exists among family members. However, families need guidance in providing an environment that fosters optimum development. Often it is the nurse who can provide continuing assistance in these areas of childrearing.

Play. Children who are retarded have the same need for play as any other children. However, because of the child's slower development, parents may be less aware of the need to continue appropriate stimulation. They may also feel inadequate in playing with the child, since the usual reciprocal satisfaction between child and parent may be slower in developing. Therefore the nurse guides parents toward selection of suitable toys and interactive activities. Since play has been discussed for children in each age-group in earlier

Table 24-4 Stimulation program for self-dressing

USUAL AGE OF ACHIEVEMENT (MONTHS)	BEHAVIOR	ACTIVITY
15	Cooperates by extending arm or leg	Give child verbal directions ("Put your hands over your head") and assist child in procedure; gradually give only verbal command
18	Takes off mittens, hat, or socks	Demonstrate taking off article of clothing; then give only verbal command Use loose-fitting socks
	Unzips	Place child's finger on zipper head; assist to pull it down; gradually reduce assistance until child can do it on verbal command
	Tries to put on shoes	Begin with having child extend foot, put open shoe or slipper in child's hand, and demonstrate getting it over toes; demonstrate how to push foot into shoe and hit the sole with the hand to make sure heel is inside; demonstrate "stepping into" shoes Use oversized shoes at first
21	Undresses	Demonstrate step-by-step procedure, for example, pants: pull down pants to child's ankles, have child pull them off, then pull down to knees, then hips, and last, have child pull them from waist For shirt: unbutton shirt, pull off shoulders and one arm, have child pull off other arm, then pull off shoulders only and have child do both arms
24	Removes shoes	Loosen shoes completely; demonstrate taking them off by pushing from heel; take them off partway, have child do rest; gradually have child do it by self Demonstrate untying shoe by placing two beads or bells at the ends of the laces, grasping each, and pulling the bow out; have child first pull one string with parent until gradually can do both unaided
	Helps in dressing	Use same technique as for learning to cooperate with undressing (15 months) and self-undressing (21 months) Concentrate on putting the clothes on first and fastening them later Sew tabs or colorful appliques on shirts and pants to indicate front or back Practice buttoning with large buttons; use front-fastening clothes Use apparel that is easy to put on and take off*

*Suggested clothing for use in a training program: undershirts with large neck openings; brassieres that have elastic straps and front fasteners; half-slips with flared design; underpants with elastic waists; boxer shorts for boys; slip-on polo shirts with large armholes and wide neck openings (not tight turtleneck sweaters); front-buttoning shirts or dresses; pants with elastic waistbands or large, side hook fasteners; wool or cotton ankle socks (not tight nylon knee socks); panty hose with sewn-in panty for girls; slip-on shoes; and apparel with self-adhering (Velcro) closures.

chapters, only the exceptions for these children are discussed.

The type of play is based on the child's developmental age, although the need for sensorimotor play may be prolonged for several years. Parents should use every opportunity to expose the child to as many different sounds, sights, and sensations as possible. Appropriate play includes musical mobiles, stuffed toys, water play, floating toys, rocking chair or horse, swing, bells, and rattles. The child should be taken on outings, such as trips to the grocery store or shopping center; other people should be encouraged to visit in the home; and the child should be related to directly, such as cuddling, holding, rocking, talking to the child in the *en face* position, and giving "rides" on the parents' shoulders.

Toys are selected for their recreational and educational value. For example, a large inflatable beach ball is a good water toy, encourages interactive play, and can be used to learn motor skills, such as balance, rocking, kicking, and throwing. Attractive toys encourage a child to reach, thus assisting in the development of motor skills (Fig. 24-3). A doll with removable clothes and different types of closures can help the child learn dressing skills. Musical toys that mimic animal sounds or respond with social phrases are excellent ways of encouraging speech. Toys should be simple in design so that the child can learn to manipulate them without help. For children with severe cognitive and physical impairment, electronic switches can be used to allow them to operate toys (Fig. 24-4).

Safety is a major consideration in selection of toys. Toys that may be appropriate developmentally may present dangers to a child who is strong enough to break them. Even if more advanced toys are suitable for the child's developmental skills, the parent must keep in mind the child's level of responsibility in using them properly. For example, the child may be physically able to use a bow and arrow but may lack the judgment in using it to shoot only at a target.

Supervision during play and other activities is stressed,

Table 24-5 Stimulation program for self-grooming

USUAL AGE OF ACHIEVEMENT (MONTHS)	BEHAVIOR	ACTIVITY
14	Brushes teeth mainly with help	Establish a routine (after each meal and before bedtime) Demonstrate toothbrushing to child on yourself Use small toothbrush with minute amount of pleasant-tasting toothpaste (preferably containing fluoride) Use a mirror for child to observe procedure Place toothbrush in child's hand and assist in brushing Teach child how to rinse toothbrush and mouth
18	Helps with bath	Explain to child what you are doing ("I am washing my face") Give child washcloth and soap, guide hand to imitate your action; gradually reduce assistance
24	Washes hands with help	Demonstrate procedure Place child by sink with a stool so bowl can be reached easily Regulate water, give child soap, help rub soap on hands, rinse, and dry; gradually reduce assistance
	Helps with washing hair	Place child's hands in hair while lathering scalp; show child the bubbles on hands and use a mirror for child to observe shampooing; as child learns to rub scalp, gradually reduce assistance During rinse, give child a towel to hold over the eyes Give child a large-toothed comb for hair; guide child's hand in learning to comb own hair
30-36	Brushes teeth alone (but with parents' assistance and supervision)	Demonstrate placing paste on toothbrush Encourage child to brush own teeth using "any direction" method Reinforce any previously learned skills Remind child to brush according to set routine Begin visits to the dentist (if not begun sooner)
36	Washes hands alone	Place all utensils within easy reach Regulate water for child (safety measure against burning) Teach child to turn off faucets Reinforce all previously learned skills When child has sense of responsibility concerning danger (hot), teach how to regulate water and check the temperature each time

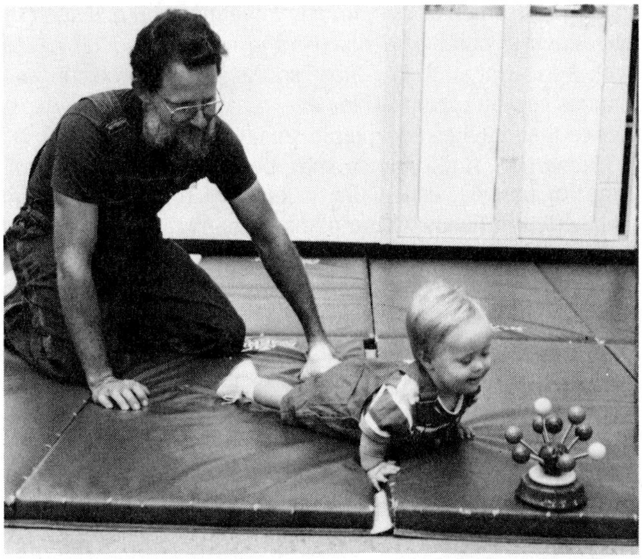

Fig. 24-3. Placing an attractive object out of child's reach encourages crawling movements.

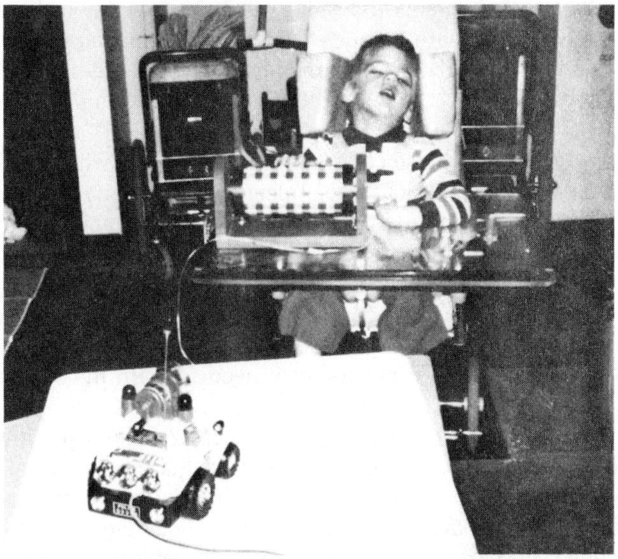

Fig. 24-4. A barrel switch allows a child with cognitive impairment to play with a battery-operated truck.

since these children are slow to learn inherent dangers. Parents may need to place reminders around the house to prevent injuries, such as signs to keep the yard gate locked.

These children often lack the motivation to institute appropriate play activities on their own. As a result of boredom, they may resort to self-stimulatory behavior, such as rocking, twirling, masturbating, or finger sucking, and self-injurious behaviors, such as head banging, biting, head hitting, body hitting, and scratching (Hyman and others, 1990). Such behaviors limit developmental progress and impede social acceptance. If such behaviors exist, appropriate play activities, especially as a method of distraction from self-stimulation, are discussed with the parents. Behavior techniques, such as ignoring children when they engage in such behavior and attending to them when they are behaving acceptably, should also be used.

Communication. Verbal skills are often delayed more than other physical skills and are frequently the first clues of cognitive deficits. Since suggestions for promoting speech development are discussed in Chapter 25, only brief comments are included here.

Speech requires hearing and interpretation (receptive skills) and facial muscle coordination (expressive skills). Both may be impaired in these children. For example, in children with Down syndrome the large protruding tongue often interferes with speech. These children may need tongue exercises to correct the tongue thrust or gentle reminders to keep the lips closed. Deficits in discrimination impede learning of different sounds. Often it helps to associate the sound with other stimuli, such as singing, which attracts and sustains the child's attention. Parents also must remember that since learning is slower, their teaching must continue longer. The nurse encourages them not to give up or believe that speech is hopeless.

Shaping techniques are useful in fostering meaningful vocalization. Every time the child vocalizes a sound that represents either a letter of the alphabet or an intelligible syllable, the parent responds with praise and social approval. Parents are instructed to record all meaningful vocalizations the child has learned in the past in order to continue reinforcing them. A written record also helps parents monitor evidence of progress in this area.

For some of these children, especially those with severe cognitive and physical impairments, speech acquisition is not possible and nonverbal methods of communication should be employed, such as sign language. Several nonverbal systems are available, but the clinician must be knowledgeable of the cognitive level required to learn and use the method. In order for these children to communicate, others in their environment need to learn the system as well.

Discipline. As discussed in Chapter 22, one of the first childrearing practices eliminated when the parents have a child with a disability is discipline. This not only can result in serious behavior problems, but also interferes with the child's developing a sense of security and self-control. It may also foster resentment from siblings who are forced to abide by a double standard.

Discipline must begin early. For children with cognitive impairment, limit-setting measures must be simple, consistent, and appropriate for their mental age. Control measures are based on teaching a specific behavior, not on having the child understand the reasons behind it. Stressing moral lessons is of little value to a child who cannot learn from self-criticism. Behavior modification, especially reinforcement of desired actions, and time-out are appropriate forms of behavior control (see Chapter 14).

Socialization. Acquiring social skills is a complex task, as is learning self-care procedures. Active rehearsal with role playing and practice sessions and positive reinforcement for desired behavior have been the most successful approaches (Davies and Rogers, 1985). Parents are encouraged early to teach their child socially acceptable behavior, such as waving good-bye, saying hello and thank you, responding to his or her name, greeting visitors but not being overly affectionate, and sitting modestly. The teaching of socially acceptable sexual behavior is especially important to minimize sexual exploitation (Williams, 1983). Parents also need to expose the child to strangers so he or she can practice manners, since there is not automatic transfer of learning from one situation to another.

Before preschool age the parents should contact the nearest day-training center or special school. Not only do these centers provide appropriate education and training, they also offer an opportunity for social experiences among the children. As children grow older, they should have peer experiences similar to those of other children, including group outings, sports, and organized activity, such as Boy Scouts, Girl Scouts, or **Special Olympics.*** These children often experience greater success in individual and dual sports than in team sports and enjoy themselves with children of the same developmental age (American Academy of Pediatrics, Committee on Sports Medicine, 1987).

Adolescents who are retarded also need social outlets for heterosexual experiences. Unfortunately, few schools or communities provide for this recreational need. The nurse can be instrumental in indirectly initiating such activities by encouraging parents to discuss these unmet social needs with educational staff. Clubs, sports, hobby projects, and dances can be organized for the teenagers to provide experience that teaches acceptable social behavior.

Sexuality. Adolescence may be a particularly difficult time for parents, especially in terms of the child's sexual behavior and needs, future plans to marry, and ability to be independent. Frequently little anticipatory guidance has been offered parents to prepare the child for physical and sexual maturation, and the degree of the adolescent's interest in sex has been underestimated. Studies have found that as many as half of the youngsters with mild retardation (a proportion comparable to the general adolescent population), a third of the moderately retarded, and 9% of the severely retarded have had sexual intercourse, and less than one half of the total group used contraception. In addition, these young people have increased rates of sexual abuse or

*1350 New York Ave., N.W., Suite 500, Washington, DC 20005-4709; (202) 628-3630. In Canada, **Canadian Special Olympics, Inc.,** 40 St. Clair Ave. West, Suite 209, Toronto, Ontario M4V 1M6.

QUESTIONS AND CONTROVERSIES

What are the issues surrounding the question of sterilization of individuals who are mentally retarded?

Although parents may ordinarily consent to any necessary medical or surgical treatment for their minor children, consent for sterilization is an exception (Williams, 1983). Currently the decision regarding sterilization of minors and incompetent adults, in particular those who are mentally retarded, is a moral and legal one. State laws vary; some allow no sterilization, and others permit review of sterilization requests. Basically, two opposing viewpoints dominate the controversy: those who feel that the *right to procreate* is fundamental and those who maintain that the *right not to procreate* is equally important. Proponents of the latter view consider laws preventing sterilization to be in violation of human rights (Passer and others, 1984).

In allowing the young person who is mentally retarded to make an informed consent, a basic issue is the individual's level of competency. Assessing competency is a complex process. Silva (1984) presents a detailed review of elements and tests of competency and proposes that the main elements of decision-making competency are (1) internalization of a set of goals and values, (2) ability to comprehend and communicate information, and (3) ability to reason and make choices. Tests of competency must be employed on an individual basis, and nurses may be instrumental in presenting information in a simple and concrete manner that increases the person's understanding and level of competence. When a person is considered mentally incompetent, four areas need to be addressed: (1) identification of an appropriate decision maker, (2) alternatives to sterilization, (3) the person's best interests, and (4) current understanding of applicable laws (American Academy of Pediatrics, Committee on Bioethics, 1990).

rape, with one third of adolescents who are mildly retarded and one fourth of those who are moderately retarded having been victims (Chamberlain and others, 1984).

Nurses can help in this area by providing parents with information about sex education that is geared to the child's developmental level. For example, the adolescent female needs a *simple* explanation of menstruation and instructions on personal hygiene during the menstrual cycle.*

These adolescents need also practical sexual information regarding anatomy, physical development, and conception. Because of their easy persuasion and lack of judgment, they need a well-defined, concrete code of conduct. The subtleties of social sexual behavior are less beneficial than specific instructions for handling certain situations. For example, a girl should be firmly told never to go alone anywhere with any person she does not know well. A boy should be warned of intimate advances from other males. To protect him or her from abusive sexual activities, parents must closely observe their teenager's activities and associates.

The question of contraceptive protection for female retarded adolescents is often a parental concern. Permanent contraception through sterilization is a special dilemma because of moral and ethical questions as well as psychologic effects on the adolescent (see Questions and Controversies). Parents seem to be most interested in sterilization of daughters who are more severely retarded and for elimination of menses to avoid the problems of hygiene (Passer and others, 1984).

Parents of these adolescents are often very concerned about the advisability of marriage between two individuals with significant cognitive impairment. There is no conclusive answer; each situation must be judged individually. In many instances marriage would help the couple achieve a mutually satisfying and supportive relationship, meaningful companionship, and a more normal social sexual adjustment. However, parenthood is usually not desirable because of the complexity of childrearing and the problem of perpetuating mental deficiency. The nurse should discuss this topic with parents and with the prospective couple, stressing suitable living accommodations and contraceptive methods to prevent pregnancy.

Help families adjust to future care. Not all families are able to cope with home care of these children, especially those who are severely or profoundly retarded and/or multiply disabled. Parents who do choose home care may not be able to continue with care responsibilities once they reach retirement or old age. The decision regarding residential placement is difficult for families. The nurse's role is to assist parents in exploring the reasons for desiring placement, especially of adolescents; investigating alternatives to home care before they become necessary; and establishing ways in which to maintain contact and communication with the family member. Guidelines for assessing out-of-home care facilities are listed in Box 24-4.

A number of alternatives exist regarding out-of-home care, but the availability of these facilities varies widely depending on the community's resources. Basically, care options range from the least to the most restrictive types of environments—foster homes, group residences, semi-independent living programs, and state institutions (Sirrocco, 1987). The current trend is toward noninstitutional care settings. Some communities have special vocational or day programs, which allow the individual an opportunity for some measure of gainful employment and the family temporary respite from care.

Care for the child during hospitalization. Caring for children with MR during hospitalization is a special challenge to nurses. Frequently nurses are unfamiliar with these children; nurses may cope with their feelings of insecurity and fear by ignoring or isolating the child. Not only is this approach nonsupportive, it may also be destructive for the child's sense of self-esteem and optimum development and may impair the parents' ability to cope with the stress of the experience. To prevent use of this nontherapeutic approach, nurses can use the mutual participation model in

*Sources of information on sexuality and conception are the **Association for Retarded Citizens of the United States,** P.O. Box 6109, Arlington, TX 76005, (817) 640-0204; and **Planned Parenthood Federation of America,** 810 Seventh Ave., New York, NY 10019, (212) 541-7800.

Box 24-4 GUIDELINES FOR ASSESSING OUT-OF-HOME CARE FACILITIES

1. Clarify the facility's philosophy of care.
2. Assess the environment for adequacy of inanimate and animate stimuli for the residents.
3. Determine the appropriateness of amounts of stimuli in the environment.
4. Observe care provider-to-resident ratios.
5. Observe care personnel interacting with residents in a variety of teaching and learning experiences.
6. Determine the appropriateness of the setting for the person being considered for placement.
7. Observe the quality of physical care administered.
8. See if the residents are attended to regularly and consistently, instead of when inappropriate behaviors occur.
9. Determine if activities are age appropriate for the residents.
10. Determine the existence of structured and nonstructured activities.
11. Determine if individual plans of care are available and implemented.
12. Determine the functional levels of those who reside in settings, for example, are they ambulatory and is speech encouraged?
13. Determine if speech, physical, and occupational therapies are available.
14. Determine if each person is perceived as unique and distinct and if care is given to residents according to their needs.
15. Determine if and to what degree official standards of care are met.
16. Meet with parents of those who reside in special settings to hear their comments, both positive and negative.

planning the child's care. Parents are encouraged to room with their child but should not be made to feel as if the responsibility is totally theirs.

Assessment of the child's abilities, special needs, and the family's or other caregiver's successful management techniques is essential. Ideally a hospital staff should make a prehospital visit to the home or care facility. This not only provides information about the child's usual environment, but also minimizes the unfamiliarity of the hospital setting, since one staff person will be recognized on admission (Wasch, 1981). When the child is admitted, a detailed history (see Chapter 26) is taken, especially in terms of all self-help activity. During the interview the child's developmental age is assessed. Although it is not unreasonable to ask about IQ level, such questioning must be done sensitively. Also, the information often tells little about the child's actual abilities.

Questions about the child's abilities are approached positively. For example, rather than asking, "Is your child toilet trained yet?" the nurse may state, "Tell me about your child's toileting habits." The assessment should also focus on any special devices the child uses, effective measures of limit-setting, unusual or favorite routines, and any behaviors that may require intervention. For example, if the parent states that the child engages in self-stimulatory or self-injurious activities, the events that precipitate them and techniques the parents use to manage them are assessed. Once the functional level is known, the child is encouraged to be as independent as possible in the hospital setting.

Procedures are explained to the child using methods of communication that are at the appropriate cognitive level. Generally, explanations should be simple, short, and concrete, emphasizing what the child will *physically* experience. Demonstration either through actual practice or with visual aids is preferable to verbal explanation. The nurse repeats instructions often and evaluates the child's understanding by asking questions—"What did I say it will feel like?" "What will the doctor look like?" "Show me how you must lie," or "Where will the dressing be?" Parents are included in preprocedural teaching for their learning and to help the nurse learn effective methods of communicating with the child.

During hospitalization the nurse should also focus on growth-promoting experiences for the child. For example, hospitalization may be an excellent opportunity to emphasize to parents abilities the child does have but has not had the opportunity to practice, such as self-dressing. It may also be an opportunity for social experiences with peers, group play, or new educational/recreational activities. For example, one child who had had the habit of screaming and kicking demonstrated a definite decrease in these behaviors after learning to pound pegs and use a punching bag. Through social services the parents may become aware of specialized programs for the child. Nutritional counseling is available if the child is overweight or has evidence of specific deficiencies, such as iron deficiency. Hospitalization may also offer parents a respite from everyday care responsibilities and an opportunity to discuss their feelings with a concerned professional.

Assist in measures to prevent retardation. Besides having a responsibility to families of a child with MR, nurses also need to be involved in programs aimed at preventing MR. Many of the familial, social, and environmental factors known to cause mild retardation are preventable. Counseling and education can reduce or eliminate such factors, for example, poor nutrition, cigarette smoking, and chemical abuse, which also increase the risk of prematurity and intrauterine growth retardation. Consequently, the major interventions are directed at improving maternal health and educating women regarding the dangers of chemicals, including alcohol, during pregnancy.

Other preventive strategies include taking part in immunization programs, especially for rubella; ensuring that neonatal screening is done on all newborns in the nurse's care; and helping identify families who may benefit from prenatal testing and genetic counseling.

5 Evaluation

The effectiveness of nursing interventions is determined by continual reassessment and evaluation of care based on the following observational guidelines and expected outcomes:

1. Observe the techniques used to teach the child and their success in accomplishing education; inquire if child is enrolled in early stimulation program.
2. Observe those activities of daily living that the child can completely or partially perform.

3. Interview the family regarding the provision of appropriate play, socialization, and discipline for the child; observe the child's ability to communicate with others; if possible, interview the child regarding feelings of self-worth.
4. Interview the family regarding any plans for future care and their awareness of community services.
5. Check medical record or Kardex for evidence of nursing admission history, especially for self-help activities; observe parent's involvement in child's care; observe social interaction of child and family with other patients.
6. Investigate community programs aimed at preventing retardation and inquire as to nursing involvement in these efforts.

Expected outcomes:
See Nursing Care Plan, p. 1070.

SYNDROMES ASSOCIATED WITH COGNITIVE IMPAIRMENT

Numerous chromosomal syndromes are associated with varying degrees of cognitive impairment. Two of them, Down syndrome and fragile X syndrome, are particularly important because of their relative frequency in the general population. The following discussion is concerned with specific aspects of each syndrome. The reader is encouraged to apply the concepts discussed earlier in this chapter and those in Chapter 22 regarding the family's response to the diagnosis and nursing interventions to promote adjustment and acceptance of the child.

DOWN SYNDROME

Down syndrome (DS), also known by the unacceptable name *mongolism* because of the particular facial characteristics that resemble those of the Mongol race, is the most common chromosomal abnormality of a generalized syndrome, occurring in 1:800 to 1000 live births. It occurs in slightly more whites than blacks, although the incidence is unchanged in various socioeconomic classes (Pueschel, 1983).

Etiology

The cause of DS is not known. A number of theories, including genetic predisposition to nondisjunction, radiation prior to conception, and infection, have been proposed, but none of the hypotheses has been substantiated. Recent reports in cytogenetic and epidemiologic studies support the concept of multiple causality.

Although the etiology is unclear, the cytogenetics of the disorder are well established. Approximately 92% to 95% of all cases of DS are attributable to an extra chromosome 21 (group G), hence the name *trisomy 21.* Although children with trisomy 21 are born to parents of all ages, there is a statistically greater risk in older women, particularly those over 35 years of age (see Table 5-2). However, the majority (about 80%) of infants with DS are born to women under age 35. This trend toward younger families may be caused by the availability of amniocentesis to older women, desire for smaller families, or some unidentified environmental or constitutional factor. Paternal age is also a factor and may account for 20% to 30% of cases resulting from trisomy 21 in DS. The risk appears significant only in males 55 years and over (Cohen, 1984).

About 4% to 6% of the cases may be caused by *translocation* of chromosomes 15 and 21 or 22. This type of genetic aberration is usually hereditary and is not associated with advanced parental age. From 1% to 3% of affected persons demonstrate *mosaicism,* which refers to cells with both normal and abnormal chromosomes. The degree of physical and cognitive impairment is related to the percentage of cells with the abnormal chromosome makeup. (For a discussion of the genetics involved in DS, see Maldistribution of Chromosomes, Chapter 5.)

Except for mosaicism, the mechanism by which the syndrome occurs has little effect on the characteristics displayed by the affected child and the management of the disorder. However, it is significant for purposes of genetic counseling. Whereas nondisjunction is usually a sporadic event associated with a low risk of recurrence (0.5% to 1%), a translocation is more often hereditary with a recurrence risk that depends on the type of translocation and the sex of the parent (Smith, 1982). In DS caused by translocation, testing of the parents is necessary to identify the carrier and offer genetic counseling.

Clinical Manifestations

DS can usually be diagnosed by the clinical manifestations alone, although no one physical feature is diagnostic (Box 24-5 and Fig. 24-5), and there is considerable variation in phenotypic expression. In addition, some infants may have characteristics of DS, such as epicanthal folds, narrow palate, short broad hands, and a simian crease, but may be cytologically normal. Therefore, a chromosomal analysis is done to confirm the genetic abnormality. The following are other outstanding features of the syndrome:

Intelligence—varies from severely retarded to low-normal intelligence but is generally within the moderate range and may be related to parental intelligence (Sharav, Collins, and Shlomo, 1985). Initial development may appear near normal, although slow development, especially in speech, is characteristic and highly variable (see Table 24-6). Although some reports suggest a relative decline in IQ scores during early childhood, followed by a slight increase during adolescence (Carr, 1988), this needs further investigation, with the present emphasis on early stimulation.

Social development—may be 2 to 3 years beyond the mental age, especially during early childhood. Temperamental characteristics show the same range as those found in normal peers, although there is a trend toward the easy child pattern (Gunn and Perry, 1985).

Congenital anomalies—about 30% to 40% have a congenital heart disease (CHD), especially septal defects. Other structural defects include renal agenesis, duodenal atresia, Hirschsprung disease, and tracheoesophageal fistula. Skeletal defects include patella dislocation, hip subluxation, and atlantoaxial instability (instability of the first and second cervical vertebrae).

Sensory problems—ocular problems include strabismus, nystagmus, astigmatism, myopia, hyperopia, head tilt, excessive tearing, and cataracts (Caputo and others, 1989). Con-

Box 24-5 CLINICAL MANIFESTATIONS OF DOWN SYNDROME

Head
*Separated sagittal suture
Brachycephalic
Skull rounded and small
Flat occiput
Sparse hair (variable)

Face
Flat profile

Eyes
*Oblique palpebral fissures (upward, outward slant)
Inner epicanthal folds
Speckling of iris (Brushfield's spots)
Short, sparse eyelashes
Blepharitis

Nose
*Small
*Depressed nasal bridge (saddle nose)

Ears
Small
Short pinna (vertical ear length)
Overlapping upper helices
Sometimes low set

Mouth
*High-arched palate
Small osseous orbit
Protruding tongue, may be fissured at lip and furrowed on the surface
Hypoplastic mandible
Downward curve (especially noted when crying)

Teeth
Delayed eruption
Alignment abnormalities common

Neck
*Skin excess and laxity, lateral aspects
Short and broad

Abdomen
Protruding
Muscles lax and flabby
- Diastasis recti
- Umbilical hernia

Genitalia
Small penis
Cryptorchidism
Bulbous vulva

Hands
Broad, short
Stubby fingers
Incurved little finger (clinodactyly)
Transverse palmar crease (simian line)
Characteristic dermal ridge patterns
- Distally located axial triradius
- Increased ulnar loops on fingers

Feet
*Wide space between big and second toes
*Plantar crease between big and second toes
Broad, stubby

Musculoskeleton
*Hyperextensible and lax joints
*Muscle weakness
Hypotonic
Atlantoaxial instability

Skin
Dry, cracked, and frequent fissuring
Cutis marmorata (mottling)

*Most common findings (Pueschel, 1983).

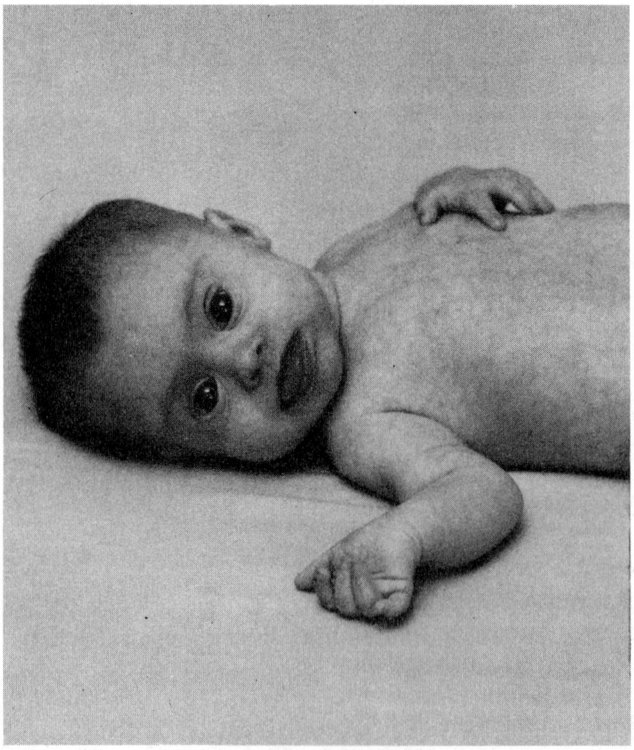

Fig. 24-5. Down syndrome in infant. Note small square head with upward slant to eyes, flat nasal bridge, protruding tongue, mottled skin, and hypotonia.

ductive hearing loss occurs in a large percentage (up to 80%), probably secondary to otitis media and impacted cerumen in the small ear canals, and is mainly in the mild to moderate range; significantly, binaural loss may be present in more than 60% of these children (Balkany and others, 1979).

Other physical disorders—respiratory infections are very prevalent; when combined with cardiac anomalies, they are the chief cause of death, particularly during the first year (Declining mortality, 1990). The incidence of leukemia is 10 to 30 times more frequent than expected in the general population (cited in Arenson and Forde, 1989) and is thought to be related to immunologic defects. Thyroid dysfunction, including hypothyroidism and hyperthyroidism, is common; the incidence of persistent primary congenital hypothyroidism has been reported as 28 times more frequent than in the general population (Fort and others, 1984).

Growth—growth in both height and weight is reduced, but weight gain is more rapid than growth in stature, often resulting in overweight by 36 months of age. Deficient growth rate is most marked during infancy and adolescence. Growth of children with a moderate or severe CHD is more affected than those with a mild or no CHD (Cronk and others, 1988).

Sexual development—may be delayed, incomplete, or both. Male genitalia may be underdeveloped, as well as secondary sex characteristics such as facial hair. The breast development of females is mild to moderate. Menstruation usually occurs at the average age, and postpubertal women can be fertile; a small number have had offspring, the majority of whom were born with some type of abnormality. Men with Down syndrome are infertile.

Therapeutic Management

Although there is no cure for DS, a number of controversial therapies are advocated, such as megadoses of vitamins and minerals (orthomolecular therapy), sicca cell therapy (injection of lyophilized material prepared from fetal animal tissue), surgery to correct the physical stigmata, and administration of drugs, such as thyroid hormone, dimethyl sulfoxide (DMSO), and 5-hydroxytryptophan (Golden, 1984; Pueschel, 1985). Controlled studies have failed to document the effectiveness of any of these treatments, especially the popular orthomolecular therapy (Bennett and others, 1983; Smith and others, 1984) or cell therapy (Van Dyke and others, 1990).

Children with DS may require surgery to correct serious congenital anomalies and benefit from regular medical care. Evaluation of sight and hearing is essential, and treatment of otitis media is required to prevent auditory loss, which can influence cognitive function (Libb and others, 1985). Neonatal and subsequent periodic testing of thyroid function is recommended. Special growth charts are available to monitor nutrition, thyroid function, weight control, and general aspects of well-child care (Cronk and others, 1988).

Children participating in sports that may involve stress on the head and neck, such as gymnastics, diving, butterfly stroke in swimming, high jump, and soccer, should be evaluated for atlantoaxial instability; if they have this skeletal abnormality, they should not engage in these activities (American Academy of Pediatrics, Committee on Sports Medicine, 1984). Symptoms of the disorder, such as neck pain, weakness, and torticollis, require prompt attention. Some authorities recommend routine radiologic examination of all children with DS to identify the problem (Msall and others, 1990; Pueschel, 1988).

Prognosis. Life expectancy has improved in recent years but remains significantly lower than that for the general population. Survival at 1 year of age is 76% for children with a CHD and 91% for those without a CHD; at age 20 years the rates are 53% and 82%, respectively. There is a dramatic increase in mortality after age 44 years, and virtually all these deceased individuals have neurologic changes associated with Alzheimer disease (Baird and Sadovnick, 1987, 1988).

Nursing Considerations

Caring for the child with DS involves several short- and long-term goals. Support for parents from health professionals, especially nurses, is increasingly important with the present trend to rear these children at home. This discussion focuses on supporting parents at the time of diagnosis and preventing physical problems in the child. Long-term psychologic interventions for the child and family are discussed in Chapter 22, and decisions for the future are explored earlier in this chapter.

Assessment

Assessment of the child with DS usually presents little difficulty because of the obvious physical characteristics (see Box 24-5). However, the nurse needs to be aware of newborns who manifest these stigmata in order to ensure early diagnosis and support for the family.

Nursing Diagnoses

A number of nursing diagnoses are prominent in the nursing care of the child with DS and the child's family; other diagnoses specific to individual cases become evident. The most common nursing diagnoses are outlined in the Nursing Care Plan on p. 1084.

Planning

The goals of nursing care for the child with DS and family are:

1. Support the family at time of diagnosis.
2. Assist the family in preventing physical problems.
3. Promote child's developmental progress.
4. Assist in prenatal diagnosis and genetic counseling.

Implementation

Once the goals are identified, specific interventions are carried out. The following discussion presents general interventions for most children with DS. Long-term interventions for the child with MR are discussed earlier in this chapter.

NURSING CARE PLAN
The Child with Down Syndrome

NURSING DIAGNOSIS: Potential for infection related to hypotonia, increased susceptibility to respiratory infection

GOAL 1

Prevent respiratory infection

INTERVENTIONS

- Teach family good handwashing
- Stress importance of changing child's position frequently, especially sitting posture
- Encourage use of cool-mist vaporizer
- Teach suctioning of nares
- Stress importance of good mouth care (follow feedings with clear water)

EXPECTED OUTCOME

Child exhibits no evidence of infection or respiratory distress

NURSING DIAGNOSIS: Impaired swallowing related to hypotonia, large tongue, cognitive impairment

GOAL 1

Minimize feeding difficulties in infancy

INTERVENTIONS

- Suction nares before each feeding
- Schedule small frequent feedings; allow child to rest during feedings
- Feed solid food by pushing it to back and side of mouth; use long, straight-handled infant spoon
- Point out to family that tongue thrust does not indicate refusal of food
- Calculate caloric needs to meet energy requirements; base intake on height and weight, not chronologic age
- Monitor height and weight at regular intervals
- Provide sufficient fiber and fluids to prevent constipation
- Refer to specialists for specific feeding problems

EXPECTED OUTCOMES

- Infant consumes an adequate amount of food for age and size (specify)
- Family reports satisfactory feeding
- Infant gains weight in accordance with standard weight tables
- Family avails themselves of specialist services.

NURSING DIAGNOSIS: Altered family processes related to having a child with Down syndrome

See Nursing Care Plan: The Child with Mental Retardation, p. 1070

See Nursing Care Plan: The Child with a Chronic Illness or Disability, Chapter 22

GOAL 1

Prepare family for care of associated defect(s) (specify)

INTERVENTIONS

See Nursing Care Plan: The Child with Congenital Heart Disease, Chapter 34

See Nursing Care Plan: The Child with Acute Respiratory Infection, Chapter 32

Refer family to community agencies and support groups

EXPECTED OUTCOME

Family is able to cope with the care needed by the specific health problem (specify)

GOAL 2

Provide support

INTERVENTIONS

- Refer to genetic counseling services if indicated and/or desired
- Refer to organizations and parent groups designed for families with a child with DS
- Emphasize positive aspects of rearing child at home

EXPECTED OUTCOMES

- Family avails themselves of support groups
- Family demonstrates positive attitude

NURSING DIAGNOSIS: Altered growth and development related to impaired cognitive functioning

GOAL 1

Promote optimum development

INTERVENTIONS AND EXPECTED OUTCOMES

See Nursing Care Plan: The Child with Mental Retardation, p. 1070.

NURSING DIAGNOSIS: Potential for injury (physical) related to parental age factors

GOAL 1

Prevent DS

INTERVENTIONS

- Discuss with high-risk women risks of giving birth to child with DS
- Encourage all pregnant women at risk (over age 35, family history of DS, or previous birth of child with DS) to consider amniocentesis during twelfth to sixteenth week of pregnancy to rule out DS in fetus
- Discuss option of elective abortion with women who are carrying an affected fetus
- Discuss with parents of adolescent children with DS the possibility of conception in a female and the need for contraceptive methods

EXPECTED OUTCOMES

- Pregnant women at risk seek evaluation for DS
- Families demonstrate an understanding of options available to them
- Families of an affected female child seek contraceptive advice

Support family at time of diagnosis. Because of the characteristic facies and other physical characteristics, the infant with DS is usually diagnosed at birth. Generally, parents wish to know the diagnosis as soon as possible. This approach prevents such dilemmas as experiencing unconfirmed doubt over the child's development and telling others that the child has DS after indicating that the infant is fine. Most parents prefer that both of them be present during the informing interview because it is a problem that both will have to face; they can emotionally support each other, and it eliminates the difficult task of revealing the diagnosis to the other partner.

The parents' responses to the child may greatly influence decisions regarding future care. Whereas some families willingly plan to take the child home, others consider foster care or adoption. The nurse must carefully answer questions regarding developmental potential, since the responses may influence the parents' decision. It is obvious from ranges such as those in Table 24-6 that these children's potential for developmental achievement varies greatly. Therefore it would be inaccurate and unfair to predict the child's intellectual capacity at birth. It is important to stress that a decision regarding placement will affect all of their lives and need not be made at the time of diagnosis. The nurse should emphasize every available source of assistance, such as parent groups, professional guidance, and literature, to help the family learn to live with the child and deal with childrearing problems.*

It may also be helpful for parents to know that studies of families who chose to rear the child at home report many favorable responses. Parental feelings toward the child usually are very positive; parents believe the experience of having this special child makes them stronger and more accepting of others. Behavioral problems among the siblings are similar to those found among families without children with DS, and divorce rates in the DS families are less than those in the general population (Carr, 1988; Cooper, 1989).

Assist family in preventing physical problems. Many of the physical characteristics of DS present nursing problems. The hypotonicity of muscles and hyperextensibility of joints complicate positioning. The limp, flaccid extremities resemble the posture of a rag doll; as a result, holding the infant is difficult and cumbersome. Sometimes parents perceive this lack of molding to their bodies as evidence of inadequate parenting. The extended body position promotes heat loss because more surface area is exposed to the environment. Parents are encouraged to swaddle or wrap the infant tightly in a blanket before picking up the infant to provide security and warmth. The nurse also discusses with parents their feelings concerning attachment to the child, emphasizing that the child's lack of clinging or molding is a physical characteristic, not a sign of detachment or rejection.

Table 24-6 Developmental milestones in children with Down syndrome

	AVERAGE (MONTHS)	RANGE (MONTHS)
Smiling	2	1.5 to 4
Rolling over	8	4 to 22
Sitting alone	10	6 to 28
Crawling	12	7 to 21
Creeping	15	9 to 27
Standing	20	11 to 42
Walking	24	12 to 65
Talking, words	16	9 to 31
Talking, sentences	28	18 to 96
Eating		
Finger feeding	12	8 to 28
Using spoon and fork	20	12 to 40
Toilet training		
Bladder	48	20 to 95
Bowel	42	28 to 90
Dressing		
Undressing	40	29 to 72
Putting clothes on	58	38 to 98

Modified from Pueschel, S.M.: The child with Down syndrome. In Levine, M.D., and others, editors: Developmental-behavioral pediatrics, Philadelphia, 1983, W.B. Saunders Co., p. 359.

Decreased muscle tone compromises respiratory expansion. In addition, the underdeveloped nasal bone causes a chronic problem of inadequate drainage of mucus. The constant stuffy nose forces the child to breathe by mouth, which dries the oropharyngeal membranes, increasing the susceptibility to upper respiratory infections. Measures to lessen infection including clearing the nose with a bulb-type syringe,* rinsing the mouth with water after feedings, increasing fluid intake and using a cool-mist vaporizer to keep the mucous membranes moist and the secretions liquefied, changing the child's position frequently, performing postural drainage and percussion if necessary, practicing good handwashing, and properly disposing of soiled articles, such as tissues (Steele and others, 1989). If antibiotics are ordered, the importance of completing the full course of therapy for successful eradication of the infection and prevention of growth of resistant organisms is stressed.

The large, protruding tongue and hypotonia also interfere with feeding, including breast-feeding, bottle-feeding, and introduction of solid foods. Parents need to know that the tongue thrust does not indicate refusal to feed but is a physiologic response. Parents are advised to use a small but long, straight-handled spoon to push the food toward the

*Sources of information are: **Association for Retarded Citizens of the United States,** P.O. Box 6109, Arlington, TX 76005, (817) 640-0204; **American Association on Mental Retardation,** 1719 Kalorama Rd., N.W., Washington, DC 20009, (202) 387-1968 or (800) 424-3688; **National Down Syndrome Society,** 666 Broadway, Suite 810, New York, NY 10012, (212) 460-9330 or (800) 221-4602; **National Down Syndrome Congress,** 1800 Dempster St., Park Ridge, IL 60068, (708) 823-7550 or (800) 232-6372; **Parents of Down Syndrome Children,** 11600 Nebel St., Rockville, MD 20852, (301) 984-5792; **National Association for Down Syndrome,** P.O. Box 4542, Oak Brook, IL 60522, (708) 325-9112; and **Association for Children with Down Syndrome, Inc.,** 2616 Martin Ave., Bellmore, NY 11710, (516) 221-4700.

*Home care instructions for using a bulb syringe are available in Wong, D.L., and Whaley, L.F.: Clinical manual of pediatric nursing, ed. 3, St. Louis, 1990, Mosby–Year Book, Inc.

back and side of the mouth. If food is thrust out, it is refed. At times the family may require the assistance of a specially trained individual, such as a lactation expert or speech pathologist, to guide them in dealing with feeding problems.

Dietary intake needs supervision. Decreased muscle tone affects gastric motility, predisposing the child to constipation. Dietary measures such as increased fiber and fluid promote evacuation. The child's eating habits need careful monitoring to prevent obesity. Height and weight measurements should be obtained on a serial basis, especially during infancy, since excessive weight gain can impede motor development. The child receives calories in accordance with height and weight, not chronologic age.

During infancy the child's skin is pliable and soft. However, it gradually becomes rough and dry and is prone to cracking and infection. Skin care involves the use of minimum soap and application of lubricants. Lip balm is applied to the lips, especially when the child is outdoors, to prevent excessive chapping.

Promote child's developmental progress. The hypotonicity affects muscular development. Supporting skills such as rolling over, sitting up, standing, or pulling oneself to a sitting or standing position may be delayed. These children should be involved in an early stimulation program. If a formally organized program is not available, the nurse can individualize one by assessing the infant's present abilities and selecting appropriate activities. Table 24-7 lists several exercises to help a child learn gross motor skills. Suggestions for teaching independent self-help behaviors are discussed earlier in this chapter and are summarized in Tables 24-2 to 24-5.

At regular intervals the child's developmental progress is assessed to ensure compliance with a stimulation program. Developmental screening tests are not sufficiently detailed to evaluate indices of progress such as increased strength, balance, coordination, or muscle tone. Therefore, detailed written records of the child's motor abilities can be kept in order to distinguish subtle changes in functioning, as well as periodic formal testing.

The parents are encouraged to investigate special daycare programs for the child as soon as possible. They should also investigate the public school system for special education classes, including infant stimulation programs and preschools. In essence, the same childrearing goals established for normal children are pursued for these children, with attention to preventing the problems of overprotection and including family members, especially the father and siblings, in the caring role.

Assist in prenatal diagnosis and genetic counseling. Prenatal diagnosis of DS is possible through amniocentesis, since chromosomal analysis of fetal cells can detect the presence of trisomy or translocation. However, analysis will not identify sporadic cases in young women when there is no indication for amniocentesis. However, testing for low maternal-serum α-fetoprotein levels may identify affected young women, who can then undergo amniocentesis (American Academy of Pediatrics, Committee on Genetics, 1989). There is also evidence that ultrasonography can detect anatomic peculiarities of DS (thickened nuchal fold and short femur length) with subsequent amniocentesis to confirm the diagnosis (Benzcerraf, Gelman, and Frigoletto, 1987).

The nurse has a role in genetic counseling of women who are of advanced maternal age or who have a family history of the disorder to discuss the possibility of amniocentesis. If the fetus is affected, the nurse must allow the parents to express their feelings concerning elective abortion and support their decision to terminate or proceed with the pregnancy.

Evaluation

The effectiveness of nursing interventions is determined by continual reassessment and evaluation of care based on the following observational guidelines:

1. Observe the parents' response to the newborn; interview family regarding plans for home care or residential placement.
2. Observe the parents' ability to care for child; monitor weight and height; observe condition of the skin.
3. Observe the child's gross motor abilities; compare with expected developmental milestones.
4. Interview parents regarding their beliefs on abortion if result of amniocentesis is positive; check follow-up if family is referred for genetic counseling.

Expected outcomes:
See Nursing Care Plan, p. 1084.

FRAGILE X SYNDROME

The fragile X syndrome is thought to be the most common inherited cause of MR and the second most common chromosomal cause of MR after DS. It has been described in all ethnic groups and races; the incidence of the disorder is 1 in 1000 males, although the incidence of carriers is higher.

The syndrome is caused by an abnormal gene(s) on the lower end of the long arm of the X chromosome. Chromosomal analysis demonstrates a fragile site (a region that fails to condense during mitosis and is characterized by a nonstaining gap or narrowing) in some cells of all affected males and in most carrier females. The syndrome does not uniformly follow the pattern of X-linked recessive disorders. For example, mental impairment is present in about one third of the carrier females and in about three fourths of affected males; the remaining one fourth of males are carriers. This is in contrast to the classic X-linked recessive pattern where all carrier females are normal, all affected males have symptoms of the disorder, and no males are carriers. Another peculiarity in fragile X syndrome is that daughters of carrier males are more likely to have affected sons than are mothers of carrier males (Chudley and Hagerman, 1987). Consequently, genetic counseling of affected families is more complex than that for families with a classic X-linked recessive disorder, such as hemophilia.

Prenatal techniques can detect the fragile X chromosome but are not widely available. Amniocentesis is the most widely used procedure; chorionic villus sampling and percutaneous umbilical blood sampling are also under investi-

Table 24-7 Infant stimulation program for gross motor development

USUAL AGE OF ACHIEVEMENT (MONTHS)	BEHAVIOR	ACTIVITY*
Birth	Assumes flexed position, kicks, has dance reflex	Exercise limbs several times each day Place child in flexed position; encourage movement such as kicking Hold child upright with feet touching a flat surface to stimulate dance reflex
3-4	Holds head erect	Hold child prone; encourage to raise head Place child supine and pull up by arms; encourage to raise head forward Place child in sitting position, hold head erect, gradually release support on sides of head to learn muscle control If child holds head erect, tilt child to one side to learn balance Support child in sitting position with head erect; if head falls forward, attract child's attention to encourage to look up
4-5	Rolls over—prone to supine	Place child prone but slightly lying on one side; place hand on hip and push down while pulling up on the ipsilateral arm; encourage child to push with arm underneath body; gradually encourage child to use free arm to push self over completely
5-6	Rolls over—supine to prone	Place child supine, cross one leg over the other, and gently push child to one side; reduce assistance as child learns to roll alone Roll child over and over
8	Sits up unsupported	Place child in sitting position but supported several times each day Support child in sitting position; gently tilt to one side to learn balance Place child in sitting position with the back against a wall; kneel in front of child and encourage leaning away from the wall to learn balance Sit child on floor with knees in an Indian position; place child's hands on floor to balance self Use same Indian position, kneel down in front of child, and gently push child to one side to practice righting self Sit child on large beach ball with feet flat on the floor; sway child from side to side to regain balance
9-10	Goes from sitting to standing position	Sit child on a low stool or chair with feet firmly placed on floor; place a towel around the chest and gently pull up to standing position; help child sit down again; gradually reduce assistance Place child in crib or playpen and in sitting position; encourage to get up to reach an object
10	Crawls	Place child on abdomen; encourage child to come forward by moving an object away Place child over a large, rolled towel that is high enough to allow hands to rest on the floor; encourage bearing weight on hands; straighten arms to increase weight bearing Use same position but with small towel so that elbows and lower arms rest on floor; encourage to lift up or come forward slightly; press down on child's shoulders to stimulate effort to maintain this position When bearing weight on hands, place rolled towel or beach ball under child's chest to stimulate getting on all fours; gently support around the waist and pull child up; release assistance as bears more weight Lay child across beach ball; roll forward, backward, and to each side to stimulate balance in either direction Play wheelbarrow; hold at hips and let child walk forward on hands; as child bears more weight, hold by feet and let child move forward Encourage "walking like a bear" (last step before walking); stand child upright, support at the hips, and have child lean forward or gently push over to bear weight on hands; encourage to walk in this position and to straighten up

Modified from Gregory, P.: Pediatr. Nurs. 1(4):23-29, 1975.
*With each activity the parent continues the actual behavior with a verbal command and praises the child for each increment in motor development, as well as for cooperation and/or signs of enjoyment.

Continued.

Table 24-7 Infant stimulation program for gross motor development—cont'd

USUAL AGE OF ACHIEVEMENT (MONTHS)	BEHAVIOR	ACTIVITY*
	Stands with support	If child resists standing, place child upright with back against the wall, grasp the knees, and manually straighten the legs; as child controls legs, reduce the amount of assistance While child is in crib or playpen, place in standing position and holding onto railing While child is in standing position, holding your hands, encourage to bear weight and "jump" up and down
10-12	Stands alone for short periods	With child in standing position, release support for a moment to encourage standing alone
12-14	Walks with support	Hold both of child's hands in front of you and guide in walking; gradually hold only one hand Encourage child to cruise around furniture and push a chair or carriage
14	Walks alone	Place child in standing position in front of you; reach out to child but do not provide support; encourage to walk forward Hold by one hand; release your grasp while child is walking

gation as reliable prenatal tests for the disorder. DNA testing for carrier detection is offered on an experimental basis at a limited number of centers (Cronister and Hagerman, 1989).

Clinical Manifestations

The classic trend of physical findings in adult males with fragile X syndrome consists of a long face with a prominent jaw (prognathism); large, protruding ears; and large testes (macro-orchidism). However, in prepubertal children these features may be less obvious, and behavioral manifestations may initially suggest the diagnosis (Box 24-6). In one study developmental delay was noted in all the children, with language delay seen in 95% of the subjects (Simko and others, 1989). The syndrome is strongly associated with autism; autistic behavior (e.g., rocking, talking to self, spinning, hand flapping, hand biting, poor eye contact, social unresponsiveness, echolalia) is seen in many affected males, and males with autism may be positive for the fragile X chromosome (Chudley and Hagerman, 1987).

In carrier females the clinical manifestations are extremely varied. Both affected sexes are fertile and therefore capable of transmitting the fragile X disorder.

Therapeutic Management

There is no cure for fragile X syndrome. Medical treatment may include the use of phenothiazines to control violent temper outbursts and central nervous system (CNS) stimulants to improve attention span and decrease hyperactivity. The use of folic acid, which affects the metabolism of CNS transmitters, is controversial.

All affected children require early speech and language therapy, occupational therapy, and special education assistance. Without appropriate intervention, progressive decline in IQ can occur (Chudley and Hagerman, 1987).

Box 24-6 CLINICAL MANIFESTATIONS OF FRAGILE X SYNDROME

Physical Features
Long, wide, and/or protruding ears
Long face, prominent jaw
High, arched palate
Flattened nasal bridge
Macrocephaly with apparent hypertelorism
Epicanthal folds
Simian creases (palms), vertical creases (soles)

Behavioral Features
Mild to profound MR (occasional normal IQ with learning disabilities)
Speech delay; speech may be rapid, with stuttering and repetition of words
Short attention span, hyperactivity
Mouthing beyond expected age for behavior
Temper tantrum
Autistic-like behaviors

Nursing Considerations

Since cognitive impairment is a fairly consistent finding in individuals with fragile X syndrome, the care afforded to these families is the same as for any child with MR. Because the disorder is hereditary, genetic counseling is necessary to inform parents and siblings of the risks of transmission. In addition, any male or female with unexplained or nonspecific mental impairment should be referred for chromosomal analysis and appropriate genetic counseling. Families with a member affected by the disorder should be referred to the **National Fragile X Foundation.***

*1441 York St., Suite 215, Denver, CO 80206; (800) 688-8765 or (303) 333-6155

KEY POINTS

- Mental retardation is the most common developmental disability in the United States, affecting about 3% of the population.
- According to the American Association of Mental Retardation, mental retardation is a "significantly subaverage general intellectual functioning existing concurrently with deficits in adaptive behavior and manifested during the developmental period."
- Diagnosis of cognitive impairment is based on standard intelligence tests, and no child is too young to be assessed.
- Causes of severe mental retardation are primarily genetic, biochemical, viral, and developmental. Mild retardation is associated primarily with familial, social, and environmental causes, whereas severe retardation is more likely associated with specific syndromes.
- Primary prevention efforts focus on support for the premature neonate and other high-risk newborns, rubella immunization, genetic counseling, education regarding alcohol, adequate prenatal nutrition, and reduction of nonintentional and intentional cerebral injuries.
- Secondary prevention activities include prenatal diagnosis or carrier detection.
- Tertiary prevention is aimed at minimizing long-term consequences through medical treatment.
- Education of children with cognitive impairment emphasizes sensory and verbal discrimination, improvement of short-term memory, motivation, and technologic support.
- Promotion of independent self-help skills is aimed at feeding, toileting, dressing, and grooming.
- Promoting optimum development may be achieved through family guidance regarding play, communication, discipline, socialization, and sexuality.
- For the hospitalized child, nurses must be aware of the child's abilities and needs, provide a familiar setting, and support families.
- Down syndrome, a chromosomal abnormality, is characterized by subnormal intelligence, slowed social development, congenital anomalies, sensory problems, diminished growth and sexual development, and reduced life expectancy.
- Fragile X syndrome is characterized by mental retardation and phenotypic findings in affected males. It is considered the most common hereditary form of mental retardation and the second most common chromosomal cause after Down syndrome.

REFERENCES

American Academy of Pediatrics, Committee on Bioethics: Sterilization of women who are mentally handicapped, Pediatrics 85(5):868-871, 1990.

American Academy of Pediatrics, Committee on Children with Disabilities: Role of the pediatrician in prevocational and vocational education of children and adolescents with developmental disabilities, Pediatrics 78(3):529-530, 1986.

American Academy of Pediatrics, Committee on Genetics: Prenatal diagnosis for pediatricians, Pediatrics 84(4):741-744, 1989.

American Academy of Pediatrics, Committee on Sports Medicine: Atlantoaxial instability in Down syndrome, Pediatrics 74(1):152-154, 1984.

American Academy of Pediatrics, Committee on Sports Medicine, Committee on Children with Disabilities: Exercise for children who are mentally retarded, Pediatrics 80(3):447-448, 1987.

American Psychiatric Association: Diagnostic and statistical manual of mental disorders, ed 3, revised, (DMS-III-R), Washington, DC, 1987, The Association.

Arenson, E.B., and Forde, M.D.: Bone marrow transplantation for acute leukemia and Down syndrome: report of a successful case and results of a national survey, J. Pediatr. 114:69-72, 1989.

Baird, P.A., and Sadovnick, A.D.: Life expectancy in Down syndrome, J. Pediatr. 110:849-854, 1987.

Baird, P.A., and Sadovnick, A.D.: Life expectancy in Down syndrome adults, Lancet 2(8624):1354-1356, 1988.

Balkany, T.J., and others: Hearing loss in Down's syndrome: a treatable handicap more common than generally recognized, Clin. Pediatr. 18(2):116-118, 1979.

Bennett, F.C., and others: Vitamin and mineral supplementation in Down's syndrome, Pediatrics 72(5):707-713, 1983.

Benzcerraf, B., Gelman, R., and Frigoletto, F.: Sonographic identification of second-trimester fetuses with Down's syndrome, N. Engl. J. Med. 317(22):1371-1376, 1987.

Caputo, A.R., and others: Down syndrome: clinical review of ocular features, Clin. Pediatr. 28(8):355-358, 1989.

Carr, J.: Six weeks to twenty-one years old: a longitudinal study of children with Down's syndrome and their families, J. Child. Psychol. Psychiatry 29(4):407-431, 1988.

Chamberlain, A., and others: Issues in fertility control for mentally retarded female adolescents. I. Sexual activity, sexual abuse, and contraception, Pediatrics 73(4):445-450, 1984.

Chudley, A.E., and Hagerman, R.J.: Fragile X syndrome, J. Pediatr. 110(6):821-831, 1987.

Cohen, F.: Clinical genetics in nursing practice, Philadelphia, 1984, J.B. Lippincott Co.

Cooper, E.: Nurses' and parents' views of parents' adjustment to having a child with Down's syndrome, unpublished master's thesis, Halifax, Nova Scotia, Canada, 1989, Dalhousie University.

Coplan, J.: Three pitfalls in the early diagnosis of mental retardation, Clin. Pediatr. 21(5):308-310, 1982.

Crocker, A.C.: Current strategies in prevention of mental retardation, Pediatr. Ann. 11(5):450-457, 1982.

Cronister, A.E., and Hagerman, R.J.: Fragile X syndrome, J. Pediatr. Health Care 3(1):9-19, 1989.

Cronk, C., and others: Growth charts for children with Down syndrome: 1 month to 18 years of age, Pediatrics 81(1):102-110, 1988.

Davies, R.R., and Rogers, E.S.: Social skills training with persons who are mentally retarded, Ment. Retard. 23(4):186-196, 1985.

Declining mortality from Down syndrome—no cause for complacency, Lancet 335(8694):888-889, 1990.

Fort, P., and others: Abnormalities of thyroid function in infants with Down syndrome, J. Pediatr. 104(4):545-549, 1984.

Golden, G.S.: Controversies in the therapies for children with Down syndrome, Pediatr. Rev. 6(4):116-120, 1984.

Grossman, H.J., editor: Manual on terminology and classification in mental retardation, American Association on Mental Deficiency, Baltimore, 1983, Garamond Pridemark Press.

Gunn, P., and Perry, P.: The temperament of Down's syndrome toddlers and their siblings, J. Child Psychol. Psychiatry 26(6):973-979, 1985.

Hall, D.M.B.: The child with a handicap, Boston, 1984, Blackwell Scientific Publications, Inc.

Hreidarsson, S.J., Shapiro, B.K., and Capute, A.J.: Age of walking in the cognitively impaired, Clin. Pediatr. 22(4):248-250, 1983.

Hyman, S.L., and others: Children with self-injurious behavior, Pediatrics 85:437-441, 1990.

Libb, J.W., and others: Hearing disorder and cognitive function of individuals with Down syndrome, Am. J. Ment. Defic. 90(3):353-356, 1985.

Msall, M.E., and others: Symptomatic atlantoaxial instability associated with medical and rehabilitative procedures in children with Down syndrome, Pediatrics 85:447-449, 1990.

Passer, A., and others: Issues in fertility control for mentally retarded female adolescents. II. Parental attitudes toward sterilization, Pediatrics 73(4):451-454, 1984.

Pueschel, S.M.: The child with Down syndrome. In Levine, M.D., and others, editors: Developmental-behavioral pediatrics, Philadelphia, 1983, W.B. Saunders Co.

Pueschel, S.M.: Down syndrome: defining problems and exposing useless 'therapy,' Consultant 25(11):77-84, 1985.

Pueschel, S.M.: Atlantoaxial instability and Down syndrome, Pediatrics 81(6):879-880, 1988.

Sharav, T., Collins, R., and Shlomo, L.: Effect of maternal education on prognosis of development in children with Down syndrome, Pediatrics 76(3):387-391, 1985.

Shonkoff, J.P., and Hauser-Cram, P.: Early intervention for disabled infants and their families: a quantitative analysis, Pediatrics 80(5):650-657, 1987.

Silva, M.C.: Assessing competency for informed consent with mentally retarded minors, Pediatr. Nurs. 10(4):261-265, 306, 1984.

Simko, A., and others: Fragile X syndrome: recognition in young children, Pediatrics 83(4):547-552, 1989.

Sirrocco, A.: The 1986 inventory of long-term care places: an overview of facilities for the mentally retarded. Advance data from Vital and Health Statistics, No. 143, DHHS Pub. No. (PHS) 87-1250, Public Health Service, Hyattsville, MD, 1987.

Smith, D.W.: Recognizable patterns of human malformation: genetic, embryologic and clinical aspects, ed. 3, Philadelphia, 1982, W.B. Saunders Co.

Smith, G.F., and others: Use of megadoses of vitamins with minerals in Down syndrome, J. Pediatr. 105(2):228-234, 1984.

Steele, S., and others: Home management of URI in children with Down syndrome, Pediatr. Nurs. 15(5):484-488, 1989.

Task Force on Joint Assessment of Prenatal and Perinatal Factors Associated with Brain Disorders: National Institutes of Health report on causes of mental retardation and cerebral palsy, Pediatrics 76(3):457-458, 1985.

Van Dyke, D.C., and others: Cell therapy in children with Down syndrome: a retrospective study, Pediatrics 85(1):79-84, 1990.

Wasch, S.W.: Hospitalization of profoundly and severely mentally retarded children, Child. Health Care 9(4):126-131, 1981.

Williams, J.K.: Reproductive decisions: adolescents with Down syndrome, Pediatr. Nurs. 9(1):43-44+, 1983.

BIBLIOGRAPHY

Mental Retardation

American Academy of Pediatrics, Committee on Drugs: Medroxyprogesterone acetate (Depo-Provera), Pediatrics 65(3):648, 1980.

Bernardo, M.L.: Premarital counseling and the couple with disabilities: a review and recommendations, Rehabil. Lit. 42(7-8):213-216, 1981.

Blum, R.W.: Sexual health needs of physically and intellectually impaired adolescents. In Blum, R., editor: Chronic illness and disabilities in childhood and adolescence, New York, 1984, Grune & Stratton, Inc.

Brizee, L., Sophos, C., and McLaughlin, J.: Nutrition issues in developmental disabilities, Inf. Young Child. 2(3):10-21, 1990.

Bromley, B., and Blacher, J.: Factors delaying out of home placement of children with severe handicaps, Am. J. Ment. Retard. 94(3):284-291, 1989.

Colwell, S.O.: The adolescent with developmental disorders. In Blum, R., editor: Chronic illness and disabilities in childhood and adolescence, New York, 1984, Grune & Stratton, Inc.

Crocker, A.C., and Nelson, R.P.: Mental retardation. In Levine, M.D., and others, editors: Developmental-behavioral pediatrics, Philadelphia, 1983, W.B. Saunders Co.

Diamond, D.L.: Medical care of the mentally retarded, Pediatr. Ann. 11(5):445-449, 1982.

Doernberg, N.L.: Issues in communication between pediatricians and parents of young mentally retarded children, Pediatr. Ann. 11(5):438-444, 1982.

Fagan, J.F., and others: Selective screening device for the early detection of normal or delayed cognitive development in infants at risk for later mental retardation, Pediatrics 78(6):1021-1026, 1986.

Forness, S.R., and Hecht, B.: Special education for handicapped and disabled children: classification, programs, and trends, J. Pediatr. Nurs. 3(2):75-88, 1988.

Friedrich, W.N., Cohen, D.S., and Wilturner, L.T.: Specific beliefs as moderator variables in maternal coping with mental retardation, Child. Health Care 17(1):40-44, 1988.

Johnson, D.M., and Johnson, W.R.: Sexuality and the mentally retarded adolescent, Pediatr. Ann. 11(10):847-853, 1982.

Krywanio, M.L., and Jones, L.C.: Developing an early intervention program for infants at risk, J. Pediatr. Nurs. 3(6):375-382, 1988.

Lynch, E.C., and Staloch, N.H.: Parental perception of physicians' communication in the informing process, Ment. Retard. 26(2):77-81, 1988.

Mahoney, G., Finger, I., and Powell, A.: Relationship of maternal behavioral style to the development of organically impaired mentally retarded infants, Am. J. Ment. Defic. 90(3):296-302, 1985.

Morgan, C.D., and Elias, S.: Prenatal diagnosis of genetic disorders, J. Perinat. Neonatal Nurs. 2(4):1-12, 1989.

Pipes, P.L., and Glass, R.: Nutrition and feeding of children with developmental delays and related problems. In Pipes, P.L., editor: Nutrition in infancy and childhood, ed. 4, St. Louis, 1989, Mosby–Year Book, Inc.

Sameroff, A.J., and others: Intelligence quotient scores of 4-year-old children: social-environmental risk factors, Pediatrics 79(3):343-350, 1987.

Steele, S.: Assessment of functional wellness behaviors in adolescents who are mentally retarded, Issues Compr. Pediatr. Nurs. 9:331-340, 1986.

Steele, S.: Deinstitutionalization of persons with mental retardation/developmental disabilities, Issues Compr. Pediatr. Nurs. 10:235-250, 1987.

Steele, S.: Fostering potentiality in persons with mental retardation, Issues Compr. Pediatr. Nurs. 11:283-290, 1988.

Steele, S.: Preschool children with developmental delays: nursing intervention, J. Pediatr. Health Care 2(5):245-252, 1988.

Steele, S.M.: Assessing developmental delays in preschool children, J. Pediatr. Health Care 2(3):141-145, 1988.

Stern, F., and Gorga, D.: Neurodevelopmental treatment (NDT): therapeutic intervention and its efficacy, Inf. Young Child. 1(1):22-32, 1988.

Sullivan-Volyai, S.: Practical aspects of toilet training the child with a physical disability, Issues Compr. Pediatr. Nurs. 9(2):79-96, 1986.

Taylor, M.O.: Teaching parents about their impaired adolescent's sexuality, MCN 14:109-112, 1989.

Ulvund, S.E.: Predictive validity of assessments of early cognitive competence in light of some current issues in developmental psychology, Hum. Dev. 27(2):76-83, 1984.

Varley, C.K., and Fururkawa, M.J.: Psychopathology in young children with developmental disabilities, Child. Health Care 19(2):86-92, 1990.

Vessey, J.A.: Care of the hospitalized child with a cognitive developmental delay, Holistic Nurs. Pract. 2:48-54, 1988.

Wolraich, M.L., Siperstein, G.N., and O'Keefe, P.: Pediatricians' perceptions of mentally retarded individuals, Pediatrics 80(5):643-649, 1987.

Down Syndrome

Atlantoaxial instability in Down syndrome, Lancet 1(8628):24, 1989.

Bovicelli, L., and others: Reproduction in Down's syndrome, Obstet. Gynecol. 59(6)(suppl.):135-175, 1982.

Brinkworth, R.: Helping the child with Down's syndrome, Midwife Health Visitor Community Nurse 19:93-96, 1983.

Brown, F.R., and others: Intellectual and adaptive functioning in individuals with Down syndrome in relation to age and environmental placement, Pediatrics 85:450-452, 1990.

Chatterjee, M.S.: Paternal age and Down's syndrome, Contemp. OB/GYN 21(5):171-174, 1983.

Churchill, L.R.: Bone marrow transplantation, physician bias, and Down syndrome: ethical reflections, J. Pediatr. 114(1):87-88, 1989.

Cutler, A.T., Benezra-Obeiter, R., and Brink, S.J.: Thyroid function in young children with Down syndrome, Am. J. Dis. Child. 14:479-483, 1986.

Davidson, R.G.: Atlantoaxial instability in individuals with Down syndrome: a fresh look at the evidence, Pediatrics 81(6):857-865, 1988.

Goodwin, B.A., and Huether, C.A.: Revised estimates and projections of Down syndrome births in the United States and the effects of prenatal diagnosis utilization, 1970-2002, Prenat. Diagn. 7(4):261-271, 1987.

International Commission for Protection Against Environmental Mutagens and Carcinogens: ICPEMC Meeting Report No. 3: Is the incidence of Down syndrome increasing? Mutat. Res. 175:263-266, 1986.

Kerr, R., and Blais, C.: Motor skill acquisition by individuals with Down syndrome, Am. J. Ment. Defic. 90(3):313-318, 1985.

Lockitch, G., and others: Infection and immunity in Down syndrome: a trial of long-term low oral doses of zinc, J. Pediatr. 114:781-787, 1989.

Marino, B., and others: Ventricular septal defect in Down syndrome, Am. J. Dis. Child. 144:544-545, 1990.

Miola, E.S.: Down syndrome: update for practitioners, Pediatr. Nurs. 13(4):233-237, 1987.

Pueschel, S.M., editor: New perspectives on Down syndrome, Baltimore, 1987, Paul H. Brookes Publishing Co.

Pueschel, S.M., editor: The young person with Down syndrome: transition from adolescence to adulthood, Baltimore, 1988, Paul H. Brookes Publishing Co.

Pueschel, S.M.: Atlantoaxial instability, sport, and Down syndrome, Lancet 1(8635):438-439, 1989.

Pueschel, S.M., and Scola, F.H.: Atlantoaxial instability in individuals with Down syndrome: epidemiologic, radiographic, and clinical studies, Pediatrics 80(4):555-560, 1987.

Pueschel, S.M., and others: Atlantoaxial instability in Down syndrome: roentgenographic, neurologic, and somatosensory evoked potential studies, J. Pediatr. 110:515-521, 1987.

Schneider, D.S., and others: Patterns of cardiac care in infants with Down syndrome, Am. J. Dis. Child. 143:363-365, 1989.

Sharav, T., Collins, R.M., Jr., and Baab, P.J.: Growth studies in infants and children with Down's syndrome and elevated level of thyrotropin, Am. J. Dis. Child. 142:1302-1306, 1988.

Shepperdson, B.: Changes in the characteristics of families with Down's syndrome children, J. Epidemiol. Community Health 39(4):320-324, 1985.

Spencer, K., and Carpenter, P.: Screening for Down syndrome using serum alpha-fetoprotein: a retrospective study indicating caution, Br. Med. J. 290(6486):1940-1943, 1985.

Uchida, I.A., and Freeman, V.C.P.: Trisomy 21 Down syndrome. II. Structural chromosome rearrangements in the parents, Hum. Genet. 72(2):118-122, 1986.

Walden, B.J.: The newborn infant with Down syndrome: realities and possibilities, J. Perinat. Neonatal Nurs. 2(4):72-82, 1989.

Fragile X Syndrome

Brown, W.T.: The fragile X syndrome, Neurol. Clin. 7(1):107-121, 1989.

Hagerman, R.J., Murphy, M.A., and Wittenberger, M.D.: A controlled trial of stimulant medication in children with the fragile X syndrome, Am. J. Med. Genet. 30(1-2):377-392, 1988.

Hagerman, R.J., and Sobesky, W.E.: Psychopathology in fragile X syndrome, Am. J. Orthopsychiatry 59(1):142-152, 1989.

Reiss, A.L., and Freund, L.: Fragile X syndrome, Biol. Psychiatry 27(2):223-240, 1990.

Simensen, R.J., and Rogers, R.C.: Fragile-X syndrome, Am. Fam. Physician 39(5):185-193, 1989.

Sutherland, G.R., and Mulley, J.C.: Diagnostic molecular genetics of the fragile X, Clin. Genet. 37(1):2-11, 1990.

Webb, T., Crawley, P., and Bundey, S.: Folate treatment of a boy with fragile-X syndrome, J. Ment. Defic. Res. 34(pt. 1):67-73, 1990.

CHAPTER 25

The Child with Sensory or Communication Impairment

RELATED TOPICS

Auditory testing, Ch. 7
The child with cognitive impairment, Ch. 24
Denver II, Ch. 7
Impact of chronic illness or disability on the child and family, Ch. 22
Language development, Ch. 4; infant, Ch. 12; toddler, Ch. 14; preschooler, Ch. 15
Optic, otic, and nasal administration (of medication), Ch. 27
Otitis media, Ch. 32
Vision testing, Ch. 7

GLOSSARY

agnosia Inability to interpret sound correctly
amblyopia Reduced visual acuity in one eye despite appropriate optical correction, in the absence of any pathologic defect
anisometropia Difference of refractive strength in each eye
aphasia Inability to express ideas in any form, either written or verbally
ASL American Sign Language
astigmatism Unequal curvatures in the cornea or lens
blindisms Self-stimulatory habits
block Absence of sound when person who stutters tries to speak
BSL British Sign Language
cataract Opacity of the crystalline lens
central auditory imperception Hearing loss that is not from defects in the conductive or sensorineural structures
communication impairment Inability to receive and/or process a symbol system, represent concepts or symbol systems, and/or transmit and use symbol systems
conductive hearing loss Loss from interference of transmission of sound to the middle ear
DASE Denver Articulation Screening Examination
dB decibel; unit of loudness
deaf Refers to a person whose hearing disability precludes successful processing of linguistic information through audition, with or without a hearing aid
dysacusis Difficulty in processing details or discriminating among sounds
ELM Early Language Milestone Scale
emmetropia Absence of refractive errors
expressive language Formulation of verbal symbols
glaucoma Condition in which intraocular pressure is increased, causing pressure on the optic nerve and eventually atrophy and blindness

hard-of-hearing Refers to a person who, generally with the use of a hearing aid, has residual hearing sufficient to enable successful processing of linguistic information through audition
hearing aid Device that amplifies all incoming sound
hearing impairment Generic term indicating disability that may range in severity from mild to profound and includes the subsets of deaf and hard-of-hearing
hearing-threshold level Measurement of an individual's hearing threshold by means of an audiometer
hyperopia Farsightedness; ability to see objects clearly at a distance but not at close range
language Symbol system used to convey thoughts and feelings
legal blindness Visual acuity of 20/200 or less and/or a visual field of 20 degrees or less in the better eye
light perception Vision limited to recognizing shades of light
lipreading Understanding what is being said by watching movements of speaker's mouth and facial expressions
mixed conductive-sensorineural hearing loss Loss from interference with transmission of sound in the middle ear and along neural pathways
myopia Nearsightedness; ability to see objects clearly at close range but not at a distance
receptive language Comprehension of spoken word
school vision Visual acuity between 20/70 and 20/200 (also known as partially sighted)
sensorineural hearing loss Nerve deafness from damage to the inner ear structures and/or the auditory nerve
sign language Visual-gestural language that uses hand signals to represent words and concepts
speech Oral production of language, including articulation of sounds, rhythm, and tone
stuttering Dysfluent speech characterized by tense repetition of sounds or complete blockages of sound
TDD Telecommunication devices for the deaf
tinnitus Ringing in the ears
travel vision Visual acuity of 20/400
TTY Teletypewriters
vision impairment General term referring to visual loss that cannot be corrected with regular prescriptive lenses

Sensory impairments pose special threats to a child's developmental potential. Deprived of visual or auditory cues, the child must rely more heavily on other sensory experiences to learn about and relate to the environment. The child with a communication disorder may function well during early childhood but be unable to achieve in an academic setting. Without assistance and rehabilitation, these children are vulnerable to the lifelong disadvantages of being an individual with a disability.

Parents are the major rehabilitators of the child. However, they need guidance and support from specially trained professionals to help the child learn. The nurse is often in a strategic position to prevent and identify sensory or communication disorders, support the family in adjusting to the disorder, and assist them in learning methods of overcoming or compensating for the impairment. This chapter is primarily concerned with prevention, identification, and rehabilitation. Psychosocial interventions to assist the family in coping with the impairment are discussed in Chapter 22, and the reader is encouraged to review those concepts.

HEARING IMPAIRMENT

Hearing impairment is one of the most common disabilities in the United States. An estimated 1 in 750 infants in the low-risk newborn population is born with some degree of bilateral sensorineural hearing impairment. In high-risk neonates the incidence rises sharply to approximately 1 in 25 to 50 infants (Roush, 1990). There are about 1 million hearing-impaired children ranging in age from birth to 21 years of age in the United States. Of these children 47,000 require specialized educational settings (Jackson, 1989). Approximately 30% of hearing-impaired children have associated disabilities, such as visual problems or cognitive deficits (Hall, 1984).

DEFINITION AND CLASSIFICATION

A number of definitions exist regarding categories of hearing impairment, including such terms as *deaf and dumb, mute,* or *deaf-mute.* However, these terms are unacceptable; hearing-impaired persons are not dumb and, if mute, have no physical speech defect other than that caused by the inability to hear. Acceptable definitions focus on the child's educational and psychologic potential (see *hearing impairment, deaf,* and *hard-of-hearing* in Glossary) (Davis and Silverman, 1978).

Hearing defects may also be classified according to etiology, pathology, or symptom severity. Each is important in terms of treatment, possible prevention, and rehabilitation.

Etiology

Hearing loss may be caused by various prenatal and postnatal conditions. These include a family history of childhood hearing impairment, anatomic malformations of the head or neck, low birth weight, severe perinatal asphyxia, perinatal infection (cytomegalovirus, rubella, herpes, syphilis, toxoplasmosis, bacterial meningitis), chronic ear infection, cerebral palsy, Down syndrome, or administration of ototoxic drugs (see also Assessment, p. 1095).

In addition, high-risk neonates surviving formerly fatal prenatal or perinatal conditions may be susceptible to hearing loss from the disorder or its treatment. For example, sensorineural hearing loss may be the result of continuous humming noises or high noise levels associated with incubators, oxygen hoods, or intensive care units, especially when combined with the use of potentially ototoxic antibiotics.

In very-low-birth-weight infants, risk factors for sensorineural hearing loss may include ototoxic drugs (e.g., aminoglycosides), low pH, hypoxemia, high bilirubin levels, and poorer overall medical status (Salamy, Eldredge, and Tooley, 1989).

Environmental noise is a special concern. Sounds loud enough to damage sensitive hair cells of the inner ear can produce irreversible hearing loss. Very loud, brief noise, such as gunfire, can cause immediate, severe, and permanent loss of hearing. Longer exposure to less intense but still hazardous sounds can also produce hearing loss (Consensus Conference, 1990). In addition to hearing loss, noise can also interfere with learning, increase stress, and provoke aggression (Bronzaft, 1989).

The exact sound level that produces hearing loss is unknown; duration of exposure and individual susceptibility to the sound influence the degree of risk. As a general rule, sound appreciably louder than conversational speech is potentially harmful if the sound persists for a sufficient time.

✦ **NURSING ALERT** Suspect hazardous noise if the listener experiences (1) difficulty in communication while hearing the sound, (2) ringing in the ears (tinnitus) after exposure to the sound, or (3) muffled hearing after leaving the sound (Consensus Conference, 1990).

Pathology

Disorders of hearing are divided according to location of the defect. *Conductive* or middle-ear hearing loss results from interference of transmission of sound to the middle ear. It is the most common of all types of hearing loss and most frequently is a result of recurrent serous otitis media. Conductive hearing impairment mainly involves interference with loudness of sound.

Sensorineural hearing loss, also called perceptive or nerve deafness, involves damage to the inner ear structures and/or the auditory nerve. The most common causes are congenital defects of inner ear structures or consequences of acquired conditions, such as kernicterus, infection, administration of ototoxic drugs, or exposure to excessive noise. Sensorineural hearing loss results in distortion of sound and problems in discrimination. Although children hear some of everything going on around them, the sounds are distorted, severely affecting discrimination and comprehension.

Mixed conductive-sensorineural hearing loss results from interference with transmission of sound in the middle ear and along neural pathways. It frequently results from recurrent otitis media and its complications.

Central auditory imperception includes all hearing losses that do not demonstrate defects in the conductive or sensorineural structures. They are usually divided into organic or functional losses. In the *organic type* of central auditory imperception, the defect involves the reception of auditory stimuli along the central pathways and the expression of the message into meaningful communication. Examples are *aphasia,* an inability to express ideas in any form, either written or verbally; *agnosia,* the inability to interpret sound correctly; and *dysacusis,* difficulty in processing details or discrimination among sounds.

In the *functional type* there is no organic lesion to explain a central auditory loss. Examples of functional hearing loss are conversion hysteria (an unconscious withdrawal from hearing to block remembrance of a traumatic event), infantile autism, and childhood schizophrenia.

Symptom Severity

For clinical purposes, hearing impairment is described according to the degree or severity of loss. Hearing is expressed in decibels (dB), which are units of loudness (Table 25-1); it is measured at various frequencies, such as 500, 1000, and 2000 cycles per second, the critical listening speech range. Calculation of the relationship between decibels and intensity of a noise involves logarithmic formulas, the discussion of which is beyond the scope of this book. An example is that the loudness of a noise at 40 dB is 31 times that of the noise at 10 dB. The same relationship applies to the loudness of noise for any fourfold change in decibels. For example, the loudness of a noise at 160 dB is also 31 times that of a noise at 40 dB.

The term *hearing-threshold level* refers to the measurement of an individual's hearing threshold by means of an audiometer (see Auditory Testing, Chapter 7). Hearing impairment can be classified according to hearing-threshold level and the degree of symptom severity as it affects speech (Table 25-2). These classifications offer only general guidelines regarding the effect of the impairment on any individual child, since children differ greatly in their ability to use residual hearing.

Most deaf children have some perception of loud sounds but no usable hearing. Their primary mode of communication is visual (lipreading or sign language). Children who

Table 25-1 Intensity of sounds expressed in decibels

DECIBELS (dB)	REPRESENTATIVE SOUND
0	Softest sound normal ear can hear
10	Heartbeat, rustling of leaves
20	Whisper at 1.8 m (5 feet)
40-50	Normal conversation
60	Noise in average restaurant
70-80	Street noises
80	Loud radio in home
90-100	Train
120	Thunder, rock music
140	Jet airplane during departure
>140	Pain threshold

Table 25-2 Classification of hearing loss based on symptom severity

CLASS	EFFECT ON SPEECH	EDUCATIONAL RECOMMENDATIONS
Slight (hard-of-hearing)—30 dB or better	Difficulty in hearing faint or distant speech Likely to "get along" in school and to have normal speech	Should be given benefit of favorable seating in regular classrooms May be assisted by special instruction in lipreading
Mild to moderate (hard-of-hearing)—30-55 dB	Usually understand conversational speech at a distance of 3 to 5 feet without great difficulty May have some defects in articulation of their own speech May have difficulty in hearing adequately in school if talker's voice is faint or if face is not visible	Should wear hearing aids and be trained in their use Should be taught lipreading, receive benefit of speech correction, and learn conservational speech Should have advantage of favorable seating in classrooms
Marked (hard-of-hearing)—55-70 dB	Understand conversational speech only if it is loud Have considerable difficulty in group and classroom discussions Language and especially vocabularies may be limited Abnormalities of articulation and voice production are obvious	Hearing aids and auditory training, special training in speech, and special language work are all essential May be able to continue in regular classes; may derive more benefit from special classes
Severe (deaf)—70-90 dB	May hear sound of loud voice about 1 foot from ear May identify some environmental noises and may distinguish vowels but have difficulty with consonants Must be taught both speech and language	Should be taught by means of educational procedures for deaf child, with special emphasis on speech, auditory training, and language
Extreme (deaf)—90 dB or worse	Are deaf, even though may hear some very loud sounds Speech and language must be developed through careful and extensive training	Require special educational procedures

Modified from Davis, H., and Silverman, S.R.: Hearing and deafness, ed. 4, New York, 1978, Holt, Rinehart & Winston, p. 436.

are hard-of-hearing use auditory cues together with visual cues to communicate. Educational recommendations based on the severity of hearing are also presented in Table 25-2.

THERAPEUTIC MANAGEMENT

Treatment of hearing loss depends on the cause and type of hearing impairment. Many conductive hearing defects are amenable to medical or surgical treatment, such as antibiotic therapy for acute otitis media or insertion of tympanostomy tubes for chronic otitis media. When the conductive loss is permanent, hearing can be improved with the use of a hearing aid to amplify sound.

Treatment for sensorineural hearing loss is much less satisfactory. Since the defect is not one of intensity of sound, hearing aids are of less value in this type of defect. The use of cochlear implants (a surgically implanted prosthetic device) is providing hope for some affected children (Miyamoto and others, 1987).

Disorders of central auditory imperception depend on the cause. Functional types, such as conversion hysteria, may require psychologic intervention, but others, such as autism, may not respond to any therapy.

NURSING CARE OF THE CHILD WITH HEARING IMPAIRMENT

Nursing care of hearing-impaired children is often a specialized area, requiring additional training in auditory testing and rehabilitation. However, general nursing goals that focus on assessment, prevention, and rehabilitation are every nurse's responsibility. In addition, nurses may have to care for a hearing-impaired child who is hospitalized and must know how to best meet the child's and family's special needs.

Assessment

Assessment of children for hearing impairment is a critical nursing responsibility. Discovery of a hearing impairment within the first 6 to 12 months of life is essential to prevent social, physical, and psychologic damage to the child. Assessment involves (1) identifying those children whose history places them at risk (Box 25-1; see also Box 8-2), (2) observing for behaviors that indicate a hearing loss, and (3) screening all children for auditory function. This discussion focuses on developmental/behavioral indices associated with hearing impairment.

Auditory testing is presented in Chapter 7. Since hearing-

Box 25-1 GUIDELINES FOR ASSESSING A CHILD FOR IMPAIRED HEARING

Family History
Genetic disorders associated with hearing impairment
Family members, especially siblings, with hearing disorders

Prenatal History
Miscarriages
Illnesses during pregnancy (rubella, syphilis, diabetes)
Drugs taken
Exposure to childhood diseases
Eclampsia

Delivery
Duration of labor, type of delivery
Fetal distress
Presentation (especially breech)
Drugs used
Blood incompatibility

Birth History
Apgar score
Weight
Associated anomalies
Cyanosis, oxygen therapy
Jaundice, transfusions

Past Health History
Immunizations
Serious illness (e.g., bacterial meningitis)
Convulsions
High unexplained fevers
Ototoxic drugs
No history (adopted child)
Colds, ear infections, allergies
Treatment of ear problems
Visual difficulties

Hearing
Parental concerns regarding hearing loss (what cues, at what age)
Response to name calling, loud noises, sounds of different frequencies (crinkling paper, whisper, bell, rattle)
Results of previous audiometric testing

Speech Development
Age of babbling, first meaningful words, phrases
Intelligibility of speech
Present vocabulary

Motor Development
Age of sitting, standing, walking
Level of independence in self-care, feeding, toileting, grooming

Adaptive Behavior
Play activities
Socialization with other children
Behaviors: temper tantrums, stubbornness, self-vexation, vibratory stimulus
Educational achievement
Recent behavioral/personality changes

Box 25-2 CLINICAL MANIFESTATIONS OF HEARING IMPAIRMENT

Infants
Lack of startle or blink reflex to a loud sound
Failure to be awakened by loud environmental noises
Failure to localize a source of sound by 6 months of age
Absence of babble or inflections in voice by age 7 months
General indifference to sound
Lack of response to the spoken word; failure to follow verbal directions
Response to loud noises as opposed to the voice

Children
Use of gestures rather than verbalization to express desires, especially after age 15 months
Failure to develop intelligible speech by age 24 months
Monotone quality, unintelligible speech, lessened laughter
Vocal play, head banging, or foot stamping for vibratory sensation
Yelling or screeching to express pleasure, annoyance (tantrums), or need
Asking to have statements repeated or answering them incorrectly
Responding more to facial expression and gestures than verbal explanation
Avoidance of social interaction; often puzzled and unhappy in such situations, prefers to play alone
Inquiring, sometimes confused facial expression
Suspicious alertness, sometimes interpreted as paranoia, alternating with cooperation
Frequently stubborn because of lack of comprehension
Irritable at not making themselves understood
Shy, timid, and withdrawn
Often appear "dreamy," "in a world of their own," or markedly inattentive

impaired children rely on vision to supplement communication skills and since many have associated visual defects, a careful assessment of ocular impairments is also needed (see Assessment, p. 1106).

Infancy. At birth the nurse can observe the neonate's response to auditory stimuli, as evidenced by the startle reflex, head turning, eye blinking, and cessation of body movement. The infant may vary in the intensity of the response, depending on the state of alertness. However, a consistent absence of a reaction should lead to suspicion of hearing loss. Other clinical manifestations of hearing impairment in the infant are summarized in Box 25-2.

Childhood. The profoundly deaf child is much more likely to be diagnosed during infancy than the less severely affected one. If the defect is not detected during early childhood, it probably will surface during entry to school, when the child has difficulty in learning. Unfortunately, some of these children are erroneously placed in special classes for students with learning disabilities or mental retardation. Therefore it is essential that the nurse suspect a hearing impairment in any child who demonstrates the behaviors listed in Box 25-2.

Of primary importance is the effect of hearing impairment on speech development. A child with a mild conductive hearing loss may speak fairly clearly but in a loud, monotone voice. A child with a sensorineural defect usually has difficulty in articulation. For example, inability to hear higher frequencies may result in the word *spoon* being pronounced *poon.* Children with articulation problems need to have their hearing tested.

✦ **NURSING ALERT** When parents express concern about their child's hearing and speech development, refer the child for a hearing evaluation.

Nursing Diagnoses

A number of nursing diagnoses are prominent in the nursing care of the child with hearing impairment and the child's family; other diagnoses specific to individual cases become evident. The most common nursing diagnoses are outlined in the Nursing Care Plan on pp 1098-1099.

Planning

The goals of nursing care for the child with hearing impairment and family are as follows:

1. Promote the child's optimum development through enhancing the communication process and socialization.
2. Support the child and family.
3. Care for the child during hospitalization.
4. Assist in measures to prevent hearing impairment.

Implementation

Once the goals are identified, specific interventions are carried out. The following discussion presents general interventions for most children with hearing impairment. Modifications are needed in specific situations, particularly if other physical or mental disabilities coexist.

Promote the communication process. The nurse's initial role in rehabilitation is to encourage the family to participate in an auditory training program.* Rehabilitation training consists of using a hearing aid and learning lipreading (speech reading), sign language, and verbal communication.

Hearing aids. The nurse should be familiar with the types, basic care, and handling of hearing aids, especially when the child is hospitalized.† Types of aids include those worn in or behind the ear, models incorporated into an eyeglass frame, or types worn on the body with a wire connection to the ear (Fig. 25-1).

Another option for sound amplification is the radio frequency (FM) system, which combines binaural ear-level instruments with an additional receiver worn on the child's body and an FM transmitter used by the speaker. With this system the speaker can talk directly into the transmitter from a greater distance, and the background noise is minimized. When the FM transmitter is turned off, the device functions as a standard hearing aid (Roush, 1990).

*Home training correspondence programs are sponsored by the **John T. Tracy Clinic,** 806 West Adams Blvd., Los Angeles, CA 90007; (213) 748-5481. Other sources of information on several aspects of hearing loss and on the International Parents' Organization are the **Alexander Graham Bell Association for the Deaf,** 3417 Volta Place, N.W., Washington, DC 20007, (202) 337-5220; and **Canadian Hearing Society,** 271 Spadina Rd., Toronto, Ontario M5R 2V3, (416) 964-9595.

†Information about hearing aids is available from the **National Hearing Aid Society,** 20361 Middlebelt Rd., Livonia, MI 48152; (800) 521-5247 or (313) 478-2610 (in Michigan).

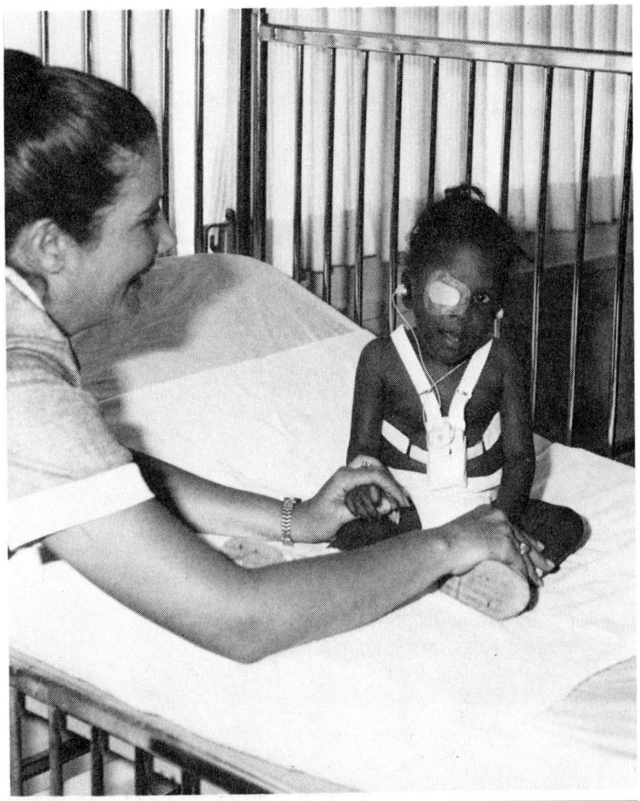

Fig. 25-1. On-the-body hearing aids are convenient for young children, such as this child with severe bilateral hearing loss. Note the eye patching for strabismus.

NURSING TIP: HEARING AID

To reduce or eliminate whistling from a hearing aid, try reinserting the aid, making certain that no hair is caught between the ear mold and canal, cleaning the ear mold or ear, or lowering the volume of the aid.

One of the most common problems with a hearing aid, especially an ear-level device, is *acoustic feedback,* an annoying whistling sound usually caused by improper fit of the ear mold. Sometimes the whistling may be at a frequency that the child cannot hear but that is annoying to others. In this case, if children are old enough, they are told of the noise and asked to readjust the aid (see Nursing Tip).

As children grow older, they may be self-conscious about the device. Every effort is made to make the aid inconspicuous, such as an appropriate hairstyle to cover behind-the-ear or in-the-ear models, attractive frames for glasses, and placement of the on-the-body type where it is not seen, such as under a blouse or sweater. Children are given responsibility for the care of the device as soon as they are able, since fostering independence is a primary goal of rehabilitation.

Lipreading. Even though the child may become expert

NURSING CARE PLAN
The Child with Hearing Impairment

NURSING DIAGNOSIS: Sensory/perceptual alterations (auditory) related to hearing impairment

GOAL 1

Maximize residual hearing

INTERVENTIONS

Help family investigate reliable hearing aid dealers
Discuss types of hearing aids and their proper care
Teach child how to regulate hearing aid for maximum benefit
Help child focus on all sounds in the environment and talk about them
For older child, discuss methods of camouflaging the aid to make it less conspicuous

EXPECTED OUTCOME

Child acquires and uses hearing aid

NURSING DIAGNOSIS: Impaired verbal communication related to inability to hear auditory cues

GOAL 1

Promote communication process

INTERVENTIONS

Encourage family to attend the rehabilitation program in order to continue learning in the home; encourage them to learn sign language
Teach language that serves a useful purpose
Encourage use of language and books in the home
Encourage spontaneous language but correct speech impairments

EXPECTED OUTCOMES

Family continues communication practices in the home environment
Family provides stimulation to the child

GOAL 2

Facilitate lipreading

INTERVENTIONS

Test child for visual problems that may interfere with learning to lipread or use sign language
Teach family and others involved with child (e.g., teacher) behaviors that facilitate lipreading (see Box 25-3)

EXPECTED OUTCOMES

Child communicates with others in manner taught (specify)
Persons communicating with child use good communication techniques

NURSING DIAGNOSIS: Altered growth and development related to defective communication

GOAL 1

Promote independence and development

INTERVENTIONS

Help family transfer normal childrearing practices to this child
Emphasize importance of attaining independence in self-care
Provide child with devices that foster independence (hearing ear dog, special signaling aids for telephone or doorbell)
Discuss importance of discipline and limit setting

EXPECTED OUTCOME

Child performs activities of daily living appropriate to level of development

GOAL 2

Provide opportunities for play and socialization

INTERVENTIONS

Guide family in selection of toys that maximize visual and tactile senses, as well as residual hearing
Encourage child to participate in group activities
Help child follow group discussion by pointing out the speaker and arranging the group in a semicircle
Help child develop friendships among hearing and deaf peers
Help child achieve a sense of security in ability to compete with peers

EXPECTED OUTCOME

Child engages in activities appropriate to developmental level

GOAL 3

Encourage education within a regular classroom

INTERVENTIONS

Discuss with teacher ways of communicating effectively with child (e.g., through facilitating lipreading)
Promote socialization with classmates

EXPECTED OUTCOME

Child attends school regularly

NURSING CARE PLAN
The Child with Hearing Impairment—cont'd

NURSING DIAGNOSIS: Potential for injury related to environmental hazards, infection

GOAL 1
Prevent hearing loss

INTERVENTIONS
Infancy
- Encourage immunization at appropriate age
- Minimize noise levels in intensive care unit
- Prevent ear infection; detect early

Childhood
- Assess hearing ability of infants and children receiving ototoxic antibiotics
- Promote compliance with treatment regimens for otitis media
- Discuss with parents measures to prevent otitis media
- Evaluate auditory ability of children prone to chronic ear or respiratory problems
- Assess sources of excessive noise in child's environment; institute appropriate measures to decrease sound levels (turn music lower, use ear protection)
- Participate in immunization program for children

EXPECTED OUTCOMES
Infant or child does not develop hearing loss
Child is not exposed to excess noise levels
Child is properly immunized

NURSING DIAGNOSIS: Altered family processes related to diagnosis of deafness of a child

GOAL 1
Assist the family in adjusting to child's loss of hearing

INTERVENTIONS
Anticipate the usual grief reaction to loss
Help family deal with any guilt feelings regarding previous responses to child when true nature of the problem was unknown
Help family realize extent of child's disability and its tremendous influence on speech and language development
Discuss advantages and limitations of amplifying devices with different types of hearing loss
Encourage formal rehabilitation as soon as possible

EXPECTED OUTCOMES
Family expresses feelings and concerns regarding the child's loss of hearing
Family demonstrates an understanding of the implications of hearing loss
Family becomes involved in programs

GOAL 2
Provide emotional support

INTERVENTIONS
Be available to the family for assistance
Encourage family members to discuss their feelings regarding the disability
Stress child's abilities rather than disability
Become familiar with techniques used for communication if following the family on a long-term basis
Refer family to appropriate community agencies for medical, psychiatric, educational, vocational, or financial assistance
Involve parents in local parent groups for deaf children

EXPECTED OUTCOMES
Family expresses feelings and concerns about the disability and its ramifications
Family members avail themselves of available resources

GOAL 3
Promote parent-child attachment

INTERVENTIONS
Help family identify clues other than verbal ones that signify infant's communication with them
Encourage family to stimulate child with visual and tactile cues
Stress importance of continuing to talk to child even though child may not hear their voices

EXPECTED OUTCOME
Parents and child demonstrate a positive relationship

See also Nursing Care Plan: The Child with a Chronic Illness or Disability, Chapter 22

Box 25-3 GUIDELINES FOR FACILITATING LIPREADING

Attract child's attention before speaking; use light touch to signal speaker's presence.
Stand close to child.
Face child directly or move to a 45-degree angle.
Stand still; do not walk back and forth or turn away to point or look elsewhere.
Establish eye contact and show interest.
Speak at eye level and with good lighting on speaker's face.
Be certain nothing interferes with speech patterns, such as chewing food or gum.
Speak clearly and with a slow and even rate.
Use facial expression to assist in conveying messages.
Keep sentences short.
Do not repeat if child does not understand the words; rephrase message.

at lipreading, only about 40% of the spoken word is understood, and less if the speaker has an accent, mustache, or beard. Exaggerating pronunciation or speaking in an altered rhythm further lessens comprehension. Parents can help the child understand the spoken word by using the suggestions in Box 25-3. The child learns to supplement the spoken word with sensitivity to visual cues, primarily body language and facial expression (e.g., tightening the lips, muscle tension, and eye contact).

Sign language. Sign language, such as the American Sign Language (ASL) or British Sign Language (BSL), is a visual-gestural language that uses hand signals that roughly correspond to specific words and concepts in the English language. Family members are encouraged to learn signing because using or watching hands requires much less concentration than lipreading or talking. Also, a symbol method enables some deaf children to learn more and to learn faster.

Speech therapy. The most formidable task in the education of a deaf child is learning to speak. Speech is learned through a multisensory approach, using visual, tactile, kinesthetic, and auditory stimulation. Since the usual mechanism for learning language (imitation and reinforcement) is not available to the deaf child, systematic formal education is required. Parents are encouraged to participate fully in the learning process.

Additional aids. Everyday activities present problems to the older child. For example, the child may not be able to hear the telephone, doorbell, or alarm clock. Several commercial devices are available to help the deaf person adjust to these dilemmas. Flashing lights can be attached to a telephone or doorbell to signal its ringing. Trained hearing-ear dogs can provide great assistance to deaf individuals because they alert the person to sounds, such as someone approaching, a moving car, a signal to wake up, and a child's cry. Special teletypewriters (TTY) or telecommunications devices for the deaf (TDD) help deaf people communicate with each other over the telephone; the typed message is conveyed via the telephone lines and displayed on a small screen.*

Any audiovisual medium presents dilemmas to children because, although they can see the picture, they cannot hear the message. However, *closed captioning* offers a solution. Through a special decoding device attached to a television, the audio portion of a program is translated into subtitles that appear on the screen.†

For a limited number of older children, vibrotactile devices (tactual vocoders) may be useful. The device presents amplified speech signals through vibrating stimulators worn on the body, such as the forearm.

As deaf children learn to compensate for their lack of hearing, they become extremely perceptive to visual and vibratory changes. They often know when another person wishes to talk to them because the person will walk close by but not pass. They learn to be alert to other people approaching them by seeing their shadows or feeling the vibrations of their footsteps. They are acutely aware of facial expressions and may comprehend the unspoken word more quickly than the spoken word.

Socialization. Since socialization is extremely important to the child's development, the nurse discusses with the family methods of fostering social contact. If children attend a special school for the deaf, they are able to socialize with peers in that setting. Classmates become a potential source of close friendships because they communicate more easily among themselves. Parents are encouraged to promote these relationships whenever possible.

Children with a hearing impairment may need special help in school or social activities. For those children wearing hearing aids, background noise should be kept to a minimum. Since many of these children are able to attend regular classes, the teacher may need assistance in adapting methods of teaching for the child's benefit. The school nurse is often in an optimum position to emphasize methods of facilitated communication, such as lipreading (see Box 25-3). Since group projects and audiovisual teaching aids may hinder the deaf child's learning, these educational methods should be carefully evaluated.

In a group setting, it is helpful for the other members to sit in a semicircle in front of the child. Since one of the difficulties in following a group discussion is that the deaf child is unaware of who will speak next, it helps to have someone point out each speaker. This can be accomplished by giving speakers numbers or using their names and marking this down as that person talks. If one person writes down the main topic of the discussion, the child is able to follow lipreading more closely. Such suggestions can increase the child's ability to participate in sports, clubs such as Boy Scouts or Girl Scouts, and group projects.

---

*Directory listings stating "TDD only" before a phone number indicate that regular telephone use is not possible; "TDD and voice" indicates that both TDD users and speaking/hearing people can use the telephone number.

†Additional information is available from the **National Captioning Institute,** Inc., 5203 Leesburg Pike, Falls Church, VA 22041; (703) 845-1992 or (703) 998-2400 (TDD Voice).

Support the family. Once the diagnosis of hearing impairment is made, parents need extensive support to adjust to the shock of learning about their child's disability. This may be the first time they learn that the child's poor speech development and behavior problems are the result of a hearing deficit, not because of difficulty with the tongue, refusal to talk, or disobedience. Parents may need time to deal with guilt feelings over previous attempts to teach the child to talk or past punishment for the child's misbehavior.

Parents also need an opportunity to realize the extent of the hearing loss. Sometimes parents benefit from a demonstration of what it is like to be deaf or hard-of-hearing. For example, showing them a moving film without sound helps them appreciate the profound effect of living in a world devoid of hearing and the great difficulty in comprehending the spoken word. If the child has a selective hearing loss, the parents can better understand the distortion of sound and difficulty with discrimination if they are placed in a soundproof room and allowed to hear only the frequencies the child hears. Central auditory imperception is similar to hearing a foreign language with no understanding of the meaning of the words.

The parents gradually need to adjust to the idea that the child's major obstacle will be the development and use of language. The parents may benefit from being told that with appropriate teaching the child can learn receptive language skills. This step will precede attempts to use expressive language, because children need to know and understand what is being communicated to them before they can be expected to communicate expressively to others.

After the parents have been able to assimilate the magnitude of their child's loss, they may benefit from encouragement and support to set realistic goals for themselves and for their child. A hearing-impaired child's education cannot wait until the child is 6 years of age. It must begin as early as possible and be continued in the home, where the parents play a significant role in teaching and reinforcing language skills.

Parents need to know how impaired hearing affects a child's normal development. For example, infants with a hearing loss, especially in the moderate or greater range, are unaware of parental verbal cues. Consequently they are less likely to demonstrate the same degree of reciprocity in relating to the parents as a hearing child. However, they do acknowledge significant others by looking at them, nestling in their arms during holding, or quieting when their needs are met. These behaviors are stressed to help parents establish meaningful contact with the infant. Although the child is unable to hear, parents are encouraged to talk as they would to a hearing child, supplement stimulation needs with visual and tactile cues, and relate in the en face (face-to-face) position to help the child learn facial expressions.

Care for the child during hospitalization. The needs of hospitalized deaf children are the same as those of other hospitalized children, but the disability presents special challenges to the nurse. For example, verbal explanations as the primary method of preparation for admission or procedures must be supplemented with tactile and visual aids, such as books or actual demonstration and practice. When written materials are used, the reading level must be appropriate for the child. Although the acquired reading skill depends on the child's age and individual abilities, the average reading comprehension of deaf adults is fourth-grade level because sign language, not English, is their primary language (Harrison, 1990).

Children's understanding of the explanation needs to be constantly reassessed. If their verbal skills are poorly developed, they can answer questions through drawing, writing, or gesturing. When explaining procedures or conditions related to the body, the nurse needs to be very specific. Deaf children's perception of internal body parts is less clearly developed than hearing children's perception (Gibbons, 1985). For example, if the nurse is attempting to clarify where a spinal tap is done, the child is asked to point to where the needle is placed. Since deaf children often need more time to grasp the full meaning of an explanation, the nurse is careful not to judge the slowness as a sign of retardation and to allow ample time for understanding.

When communicating with the child, the nurse should use the same principles as those outlined for facilitating lip-reading. Ideally, nurses without foreign accents should be assigned to the child. The child's hearing aid is checked to ensure that it is working properly. If it is necessary to awaken the child at night, the nurse gently shakes the child to signal the nurse's presence or turns on the hearing aid before arousing the child. The nurse always makes sure that the child can see him or her before any procedures are performed, even routine ones such as changing a diaper or regulating an infusion. It is important to remember that the child may not be aware of one's presence until alerted through visual or tactile cues.

Ideally, parents are encouraged to room with the child. However, it must be conveyed to them that this is not to serve as a convenience to the nurse but as a benefit to the child. Although the parents' aid can be enlisted in familiarizing the child with the hospital and explaining procedures, the nurse also talks directly to the child, encouraging expression of feelings about the experience. If there is difficulty in understanding the child's speech, an effort is made to become familiar with the child's pronunciation of words. Parents often can be helpful by explaining the child's usual speech habits.

Nonvocal communication devices that employ pictures or words that the child can point to are also available (see p. 1115). Such boards can also be made up by drawing pictures or writing the words of common needs on cardboard, such as parent, food, water, or toilet.

The nurse has a special role as child advocate with deaf children and is in a strategic position to alert other health team members and other patients to the child's special needs regarding communication. For example, the nurse should accompany other practitioners on visits to the child's room to ensure that they speak to the child and that the child understands what is said. Caregivers sometimes forget that the child has the abilities to perceive and learn despite a hearing loss and consequently communicate only with the parents. As a result, the child's needs and feelings remain unrecognized and unmet.

Since deaf children often have difficulty in forming social relationships with other children, the child is introduced to roommates and encouraged to engage in play activities. The hospital setting can provide growth-promoting opportunities for social relationships. With the assistance of a child-life specialist, the child can learn new recreational activities, experiment with group games, and engage in therapeutic play. The use of puppets, dollhouses, role playing with dress-up clothes, building with a hammer and nails, finger painting, needle play, and water play can help the child express feelings that previously were suppressed.

Assist in measures to prevent hearing impairment. A primary nursing role is prevention of hearing loss. Since the most common cause of impaired hearing is chronic otitis media, it is essential that appropriate measures be instituted to treat existing infections and prevent recurrences (see Chapter 32). Children with histories of ear or respiratory infections or any other condition known to increase the risk of hearing impairment should receive periodic auditory testing.

To prevent the causes of hearing loss that begin prenatally and perinatally, pregnant women need counseling regarding the necessity of early prenatal care, including genetic counseling for known familial disorders; avoidance of all ototoxic drugs, especially during the first trimester; tests to rule out syphilis, rubella, or blood incompatibility; medical management of maternal diabetes; control of alcoholism; and adequate dietary intake. During childhood the necessity of routine immunization to eliminate the possibility of acquired sensorineural loss from rubella, mumps, and measles (encephalitis) is stressed.

Exposure to excessive noise pollution is a well-established cause of sensorineural hearing loss. The nurse should routinely assess the possibility of environmental noise pollution and advise children and parents of the potential danger. When individuals engage in activities associated with high-intensity noise, such as flying model airplanes, target shooting, or snowmobiling, they should wear ear protection such as earmuffs or earplugs (not ordinary dry cotton). Even common household equipment can be hazardous, such as lawn mowers, power vacuum cleaners, and cordless telephones.

Evaluation

The effectiveness of nursing interventions for hearing impairment is determined by continual reassessment and evaluation of care based on the following observational guidelines and expected outcomes:

1. Observe the techniques used to communicate with the child. Inquire if child is enrolled in auditory training program. Inquire about socialization opportunities for the child (i.e., who are child's friends, what are child's extracurricular activities).
2. Interview the family regarding their adjustment to the sensory impairment. Observe the family members' relationship with the child. Interview the child regarding feelings about the sensory impairment and its effect on activities of daily living (especially important if a recent impairment).
3. Observe types of preparation/communication used to prepare child for hospitalization or procedures. Observe parents' involvement in child's care. Observe interaction of child and family with other patients.
4. Investigate community programs aimed at preventing or detecting hearing loss and inquire about nursing involvement in these efforts.

Expected outcomes:
See Nursing Care Plan, pp. 1098-1099.

VISION IMPAIRMENT

Visual impairments are a common problem during childhood; prevalence rates for some degree of visual impairment even with corrective glasses is approximately 20 to 35 per 1000 children. Of this group, 0.5 to 1.0 per 1000 are considered legally blind (Gortmaker and Sappenfield, 1984). Almost 50% of blind children under 5 years of age have no useful vision, and for the remainder the visual acuity is unknown (Vision problems, 1980). The nurse's role is clearly one of detection, referral, and in some instances rehabilitation.

DEFINITION AND CLASSIFICATION

Vision impairment is a general term referring to visual loss that cannot be corrected with regular prescriptive lenses. However, a more useful system for classifying visual impairments is based on the type of activity in which the child can be expected to engage, which may include the following categories (Helveston and Ellis, 1984):

School vision—visual acuity between 20/70 and 20/200 (also known as partially sighted). The child should be able to obtain an education in the usual public school system with the use of normal-sized print. Near vision is almost always better than distance vision.

Legal blindness—visual acuity of 20/200 or less and/or a visual field of 20 degrees or less in the better eye. This is useful only as a legal definition, not as a medical diagnosis. It allows special considerations with regard to taxes, entrance into special schools, eligibility for aid, and other benefits.

Travel vision—visual acuity of 20/400. This vision allows the child to travel in unfamiliar surroundings provided the child is otherwise healthy. The use of print may be possible but difficult. Learning braille may be required.

Light perception—this is primarily important for the child's sense of well-being and may be an aid in mobility, but it is not useful for other educational purposes.

ETIOLOGY

The etiology of visual impairment can be classified according to several divisions. In addition, diseases such as cataracts, optic atrophy, or glaucoma may cause any number of visual defects. Factors causing vision impairment include:

Familial factors—genetic diseases associated with visual defects, such as Tay-Sachs disease, albinism, galactosemia, or retinoblastoma

Prenatal/intrauterine factors—especially maternal infections, such as rubella, syphilis, herpes simplex, or toxoplasmosis

Perinatal factors—prematurity, maternal infection (ophthalmia neonatorum), and oxygen toxicity (retinopathy of prematurity)

Postnatal factors—primarily trauma, infections (mumps, measles, rubella, poliomyelitis, chickenpox), and disorders such as juvenile rheumatoid arthritis, leukemia, and myasthenia gravis

Refractive errors are the most common types of visual disorders in children. The term *refraction* means bending and refers to the bending of light rays as they pass through the lens of the eye. Normally, light rays enter the lens and fall directly on the retina *(emmetropia)*. However, in refractive disorders the light rays either fall in front of the retina *(myopia)* or beyond it *(hyperopia)* (Fig. 25-2). Other eye problems, such as strabismus, may or may not include refractive errors but are important because, if untreated, they may result in blindness from amblyopia (Table 25-3).

Amblyopia, or "lazy eye," is a reduced visual acuity in one eye despite appropriate optical correction and can occur in the absence of any pathologic defect (e.g., cataract, scarred cornea) in the affected eye. Amblyopia develops when one eye does not receive sufficient visual stimulation during the critical period of cortical development. Misplaced, blurred, or absent retinal images during early childhood cause loss of vision in the visually deprived eye. It does not occur after 9 years of age, when the retinal system is mature. The most common types of amblyopia are secondary to strabismus and to unequal refractive errors *(anisometropia)*. Other causes include cataracts, corneal opacities, or prolonged occlusion of one or both eyes (a condition that can occur from prolonged therapeutic patching for strabismus) (Friendly, 1987).

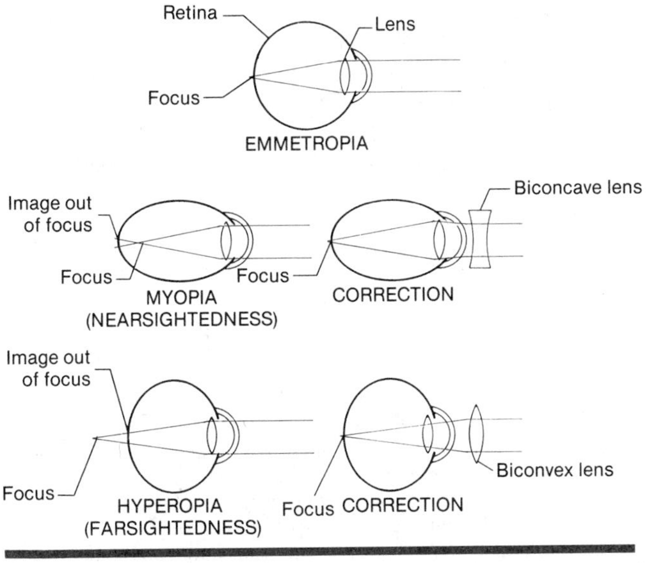

Fig. 25-2. Comparison of normal vision and refractive errors. **A,** Emmetropia (normal vision). **B,** Myopia (nearsightedness). **C,** Hyperopia (farsightedness).

Box 25-4 MOST COMMON CAUSES OF OCULAR INJURY

Balls	Assorted toys
Sticks	Guns, BBs
Fists, fingers	Hangers
Falls	Belts, buckles
Rocks, stones	Fireworks
Metal foreign bodies	Auto accidents
Glass	Kicking
Animal bites	Knives, scissors
Projectiles (nonspecific)	

Data from DeRespinis, P.A., and others: A survey of severe eye injuries in children, Am. J. Dis. Child. 143:711-716, 1989.

Trauma is a common cause of blindness in children. The most common sources are balls, especially baseballs, fists, and sticks (Box 25-4). Injuries to the eyeball and adnexa (supporting or accessory structures; e.g., eyelids, conjunctiva, lacrimal glands) can be classified as penetrating or nonpenetrating. *Penetrating wounds* damage tissue in the outer coat of the eye, cornea, and sclera and may perforate through the entire thickness of the structures. Penetrating wounds are most often the result of sharp instruments, such as knives or scissors; propulsive objects, such as firecrackers, guns, bows and arrows, slingshots, or twist-off bottle caps; and a powerful contusion by a blunt object, which may occur during a fight, with racquet sports, or from a serious car injury. *Nonpenetrating injuries* damage the outermost surface of the eye and may be the result of foreign objects in the eyes, lacerations, a blow from a blunt object such as a fist, and thermal or chemical burns. Although most instances of eye trauma are unintentional, the possibility of child abuse should be considered, especially when marked facial trauma, bilateral corneal abrasions, unexplained hyphemas, and cigarette burns are present (Frey, 1983).

Infections of the adnexa and the structures of the eyeball or globe also may occur in children. The most common eye infection is conjunctivitis (see Chapter 16). Keratitis (inflammation and infection of the cornea) has become more common among wearers of contact lenses who use homemade saline solutions, wear lenses (even the extended-wear type) for prolonged periods, and swim with the lenses (Stehr-Green and others, 1987).

THERAPEUTIC MANAGEMENT

Treatment of eye disorders depends on the specific problem and is outlined for several ocular defects in Table 25-3. In all instances the goal is preservation of vision. Treatment in early childhood is necessary to prevent vision loss from amblyopia, especially resulting from strabismus; treatment must be instituted as soon as possible after serious trauma.

Treatment of strabismus may involve surgery of affected muscles, prescription lenses to correct refractive errors, and

Table 25-3 Types of visual impairment

DEFECT/DESCRIPTION	PATHOPHYSIOLOGY	CLINICAL MANIFESTATIONS	TREATMENT
Refractive errors			
Myopia (nearsightedness)—ability to see objects clearly at close range but not at a distance	Results from eyeball that is too long, causing image to fall in front of retina	*Behavioral manifestations:* Rubs eyes excessively Tilts head or thrusts head forward Has difficulty in reading or other close work Holds books close to eyes Writes or colors with head close to table Clumsy; walks into objects Blinks more than usual or is irritable when doing close work Is unable to see objects clearly Does poorly in school, especially in subjects that require demonstration, such as arithmetic *Signs/symptoms:* Dizziness Headache Nausea following close work	Corrected with biconcave lenses that focus rays on retina
Hyperopia (hypermetropia or farsightedness)—ability to see objects clearly at a distance	Results from eyeball that is too short, causing image to focus beyond retina	Because of accommodative ability, child can usually see objects at all ranges Most children normally hyperopic until about 7 years of age	If correction is required, use convex lenses to focus rays on retina
Astigmatism—unequal curvatures in refractive apparatus	Results from unequal curvatures in cornea or lens that cause light rays to bend in different directions	Depends on severity of refractive error in each eye May have clinical manifestations of myopia	Corrected with special lenses that compensate for refractive errors
Anisometropia—different refractive strengths in each eye	May develop amblyopia as weaker eye is used less	Depends on severity of refractive error in each eye May have clinical manifestations of myopia	Treated with corrective lenses, preferably contact lenses, to improve vision in each eye so they work as a unit
Amblyopia ("lazy eye")—reduced visual acuity in one eye	Results when one eye does not receive sufficient stimulation Each retina receives different images, resulting in diplopia (double vision) Brain accommodates by suppressing less intense image Visual cortex eventually does not respond to visual stimulation with loss of vision in that eye	Poor vision in affected eye	Preventable if treatment of primary visual defect, such as anisometropia or strabismus, begins before 6 years of age
Strabismus ("squint" or "cross-eye")—malalignment of eyes Esotropia—inward deviation of eye (Fig. 25-3) Exotropia—outward deviation of eye	May result from muscle imbalance or paralysis, poor vision, or as congenital defect Since visual axes not parallel, brain receives two images, and amblyopia can result	*Behavioral manifestations:* Squints eyelids together or frowns Has difficulty in focusing from one distance to another Inaccurate judgment in picking up objects	Treatment depends on cause of strabismus May involve occlusion therapy (patching stronger eye) to increase visual stimulation to weaker eye Early diagnosis essential to prevent vision loss

Table 25-3 Types of visual impairment—cont'd

DEFECT/DESCRIPTION	PATHOPHYSIOLOGY	CLINICAL MANIFESTATIONS	TREATMENT
Strabismus—cont'd		Unable to see print or moving objects clearly Closes one eye to see Tilts head to one side If combined with refractive errors, may see any of the manifestations listed for refractive errors *Signs/symptoms:* Diplopia Photophobia Dizziness Headache Cross-eye	
Cataracts—opacity of crystalline lens	Prevents light rays from entering eye and refracting them on retina	*Behavioral manifestations:* Gradually less able to see objects clearly May lose peripheral vision *Signs/symptoms:* Nystagmus (with complete blindness) Gray opacities of lens Strabismus Absence of red reflex	Requires surgery to remove cloudy lens and replacement of lens (intraocular lens implant, removable contact lens, prescription glasses) Must be treated early to prevent blindness from amblyopia
Glaucoma—increased intraocular pressure	Congenital type results from defective development of some component related to flow of aqueous humor Increased pressure on optic nerve causes eventual atrophy and blindness	*Behavioral manifestations:* Mostly seen in acquired types—loses peripheral vision May bump into objects not directly in front Sees halos around objects May complain of mild pain or discomfort (severe pain, nausea, vomiting if sudden rise in pressure) *Signs/symptoms:* Redness Excessive tearing (epiphora) Photophobia Spasmodic winking (blepharospasm) Corneal haziness Enlargement of eyeball (buphthalmos)	Requires surgical treatment (goniotomy) to open outflow tracts May require more than one procedure

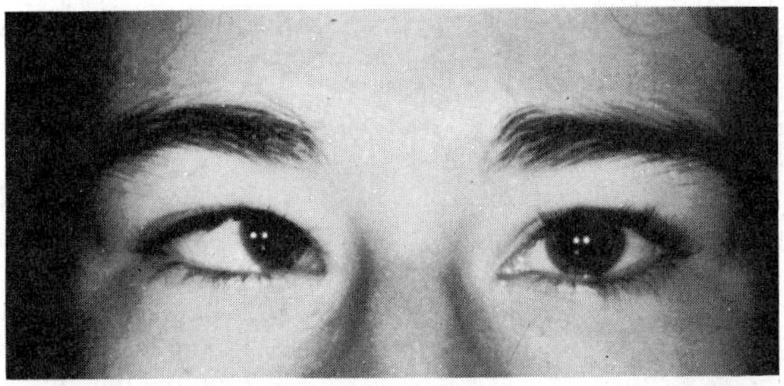

Fig. 25-3. Strabismus. Note obvious malalignment of eyes. Light reflections are centered in left cornea and to side of right cornea.

From Havener, W.H., and others: Nursing care in eye, ear, nose, and throat disorders, ed. 3, St. Louis, 1976, Mosby–Year Book, Inc.

occlusion therapy. Sometimes anticholinesterase agents are administered to reduce the accommodative effort in an attempt to bring the image into clearer focus. Occlusion therapy is a common procedure and involves patching the stronger eye to increase the visual stimulation to the weaker eye to prevent amblyopia. A careful schedule of patching must be followed to avoid occlusion amblyopia. Some practitioners prescribe 1 week of patching for every year of the child's age, followed by an examination to assess visual acuity in the occluded eye. Other authorities recommend alternative patching and uncovering each day to provide periodic stimulation to the covered eye (Kovalesky, 1985).

The goal in treating strabismus is preservation of vision, binocularity, and improvement in cosmetic appearance. However, all of these goals may not be achieved. Vision loss is always a concern, and some children may require low-vision aids to compensate for the impairment. Fortunately, lack of binocularity is not a serious handicap for most children. However, it does result in failure to develop stereopsis, or depth perception, the ability to locate an object in spatial relationship to another object. The individual has difficulty in judging distances, such as when driving a car or reaching for a close object, and when using binocular instruments, such as a microscope or field glasses. Certain vocations, such as aviation, may not be available for these people, and appropriate counseling should begin early.

Treatment of ocular injury involves adequate examination of the injured eye (with the child sedated or anesthetized in severe injuries), appropriate immediate intervention such as removal of the foreign body or suturing of the laceration (see Emergency Treatment), and prevention of complications, such as administration of antibiotics or steroids and complete bed rest to allow the eye to heal and blood to reabsorb. Prognosis varies according to the type of injury. It is usually guarded in all cases of penetrating wounds because of the high risk of serious complications, especially retinal detachment, panophthalmitis (infection of uvea, retina, vitreous body, and sclera), and sympathetic ophthalmia (autoimmune disease of the uveal tract occurring in the uninjured eye). Treatment of infections is usually ophthalmic antibiotics. Severe infections may require systemic antibiotic therapy. Steroids are used cautiously because they exacerbate viral infections such as herpes simplex, increasing the risk of damage to the involved structures.

NURSING CARE OF THE CHILD WITH VISION IMPAIRMENT

Nursing care of visually impaired children is often a specialized area, requiring additional training in vision testing and rehabilitation. However, general nursing goals that focus on assessment, prevention, and rehabilitation are every nurse's responsibility. In addition, nurses may have to care for a vision-impaired child who is hospitalized and must know how to best meet the child's and family's special needs.

Assessment

Assessment of children for vision impairment is a critical nursing responsibility. Discovery of a vision impairment as early as possible is essential to prevent social, physical, and psychologic damage to the child. Assessment involves (1) identifying those children whose history places them at risk, (2) observing for behaviors that indicate a vision loss, and (3) screening all children for visual acuity and signs of other ocular disorders, such as strabismus. The clinical manifestations of various types of visual problems are presented in Table 25-3. Vision testing is discussed in Chapter 7.

Infancy. At birth the nurse should observe the neonate's response to visual stimuli, such as following a light or object and cessation of body movement. The infant may vary in the intensity of the response, depending on the state of alertness.

NURSING ALERT Suspect blindness if the newborn fails to react to light and if parents express concern.

Of special importance in detecting visual impairment during infancy are the parents' concerns regarding visual responsiveness in their child. Their concerns must be taken seriously, such as lack of eye-to-eye contact from the infant. During infancy the child should be tested for strabismus. Lack of binocularity after 4 months of age is considered abnormal and must be treated to prevent amblyopia.

Childhood. Since the most common visual impairments during childhood are refractive errors, testing for visual acuity is essential. The school nurse usually assumes major responsibility for vision testing in school children. Besides refractive errors, the nurse should be aware of signs and symptoms that indicate other ocular problems. If a referral is made to the family requesting further eye testing, the nurse is responsible for follow-up concerning the recommendation.

Nursing Diagnoses

A number of nursing diagnoses are prominent in the nursing care of the child with visual impairment and the child's family; other diagnoses specific to individual cases become evident. The most common nursing diagnoses are outlined in the Nursing Care Plan on pp. 1108-1109.

Planning

The goals of nursing care for the child with visual impairment and family are as follows:

1. Support the child and family.
2. Promote parent-child attachment.
3. Promote the child's optimum development.
4. Care for the child during hospitalization.
5. Assist in measures to prevent vision impairment.

Implementation

Once the goals are identified, specific interventions are carried out. The following discussion presents general interventions for most children with vision impairment, especially blindness. Modifications are needed in specific situations, particularly if other physical or mental disabilities coexist.

Support the child and family. The shock of learning that their child is blind or partially sighted is an immense crisis for families. Of all types of disabilities, many people fear loss of sight the most. Vision is involved in almost every activity of daily living. Parents need support during the initial phase of learning about the diagnosis and help to gain a realistic understanding of their child's abilities. The family is encouraged to investigate appropriate stimulation and educational programs for their child as soon as possible. Sources of information include state **Commissions for the Blind,** local schools for the blind, the **American Foundation for the Blind,* National Federation of the Blind,† National Association for Parents of the Visually Impaired, Inc.,‡ National Association for Visually Handicapped,§** and **American Council of the Blind.**‖¶

When blindness is not congenital but acquired, newly blind children need much support to help them adjust to the disability. They are usually frightened and confused by the sudden or progressive loss of sight and benefit from an environment that provides security and familiarity.

Promote parent-child attachment. A crucial time in the life of blind infants is when they and their parents are getting acquainted with each other. Pleasurable patterns of interaction between the infant and parents may be lacking if there is not enough reciprocity. For example, if the parent gazes fondly at the infant's face and seeks eye contact but the infant fails to respond because he or she cannot see the parent, a troubled cycle of responses may occur. The nurse can help parents learn to look for other cues that indicate the infant is responding to them, such as whether the eyelids blink; whether the activity level accelerates or slows; whether respiratory patterns change, such as faster or slower breathing when they come near; and whether the infant makes throaty sounds when they speak to the infant. In time parents learn that the infant has unique ways of relating to them. They are encouraged to show affection using nonvisual methods, such as talking or reading, cuddling, and walking the child.

Promote the child's optimum development. Promoting the child's optimum development requires rehabilitation in a number of important areas. These include learning self-help skills and appropriate communication techniques to become independent. Although nurses may not be directly involved in such programs, they can provide direction and guidance to families regarding the availability of programs and the need to promote these activities in their child.

EMERGENCY TREATMENT
Eye Injuries

Foreign object

Examine eye for presence of a foreign body (evert upper lid to examine upper eye).
Remove a freely movable object with pointed corner of gauze pad lightly moistened with water.
Do not irrigate eye or attempt to remove a penetrating object (see below).
Caution child against rubbing eye.

Chemical burns

Irrigate eye copiously with tap water for 20 minutes.
Evert upper lid to flush thoroughly.
Hold child's head with eye under tap of running lukewarm water.
Take to emergency room.
Have child rest with eyes closed.
Keep room darkened.

Ultraviolet burns

If skin is burned, patch both eyes (make sure lids are completely closed); secure dressing with Kling bandages wrapped around head rather than tape.
Have child rest with eyes closed.
Refer to an ophthalmologist.

Hematoma ("black eye")

Use a flashlight to check for gross hyphema (hemorrhage into anterior chamber; visible fluid meniscus across iris; more easily seen in light-colored than in brown eyes).
Apply ice for first 24 hours to reduce swelling if no hyphema is present.
Refer to an ophthalmologist immediately if hyphema is present.
Have child rest with eyes closed.

Penetrating injuries

Take child to emergency room.
Never remove an object that has penetrated eye.
Follow strict aseptic technique in examining eye.
Observe for:
- Aqueous or vitreous leaks (fluid leaking from point of penetration)
- Hyphema
- Shape and equality of pupils, reaction to light
- Prolapsed iris (not perfectly circular)

Apply a Fox shield if available (not a regular eye patch).
Maintain bed rest with child in 30-degree Fowler position.
Apply patch over unaffected eye to prevent bilateral movement.
Caution child against rubbing eye.

EMERGENCY TREATMENT

---

*15 W. 16th St., New York, NY 10011.
†1800 Johnson St., Baltimore, MD 21230.
‡2180 Linway Dr., Beloit, WI 53511; (800) 562-6265.
§22 W. 21th St., New York, NY 10010.
‖1010 Vermont Ave., N.W., Washington, DC 20005.
¶Sources of information in Canada include the **Canadian National Institute for the Blind,** 1931 Bayview Ave., Toronto, Ontario M4G 4C8; **Low Vision Association of Canada,** 145 Adelaide St. West, Toronto, Ontario M5H 3H4; and **Blind Organization of Ontario,** 597 Parliament St., Suite B-3, Toronto, Ontario M4X 1W3.

NURSING CARE PLAN
The Child with Vision Impairment

NURSING DIAGNOSIS: Altered growth and development related to sensory/perceptual alterations (visual)

GOAL 1
Promote development and independence

INTERVENTIONS

Provide visual-motor activities for infant (sitting in chair or swing, holding head up, standing, crawling, grasping for objects)
Provide an environment that fosters familiarity and security; arrange furniture to allow safe ambulation; place identifying markers to denote steps or other dangerous areas
Enroll child in special programs for the blind as soon as possible to learn independent skills, braille reading and writing, and navigational skills (cane method, sighted guide, guide dog)
Encourage participation in active play
Discuss need for experimenting with active play in safe environment and with other children

EXPECTED OUTCOMES

Infant or child engages in appropriate activities for level of development (specify)
Child demonstrates an attitude of security in the environment

GOAL 2
Provide opportunities for play/socialization

INTERVENTIONS

Talk to child about the environment
Guide family to selection of play material that encourages motor development and stimulates the sense of hearing and touch
Discuss with family how play for blind children differs from that of sighted children
Encourage family to initiate play activities and teach child how to use toys
Assess adequacy of environmental stimulation if blindisms are present
Use behavior modification to discourage blindisms
Discuss importance of consistent limit setting in helping child learn acceptable behavior and tolerate frustration
Discuss with child's family possible opportunities for socialization

EXPECTED OUTCOME

Parents engage in appropriate activities with the blind child and have realistic expectations for the child

NURSING DIAGNOSIS: Altered family processes related to diagnosis of blindness in a child

GOAL 1
Assist family in adjusting to child's loss of sight

INTERVENTIONS

Anticipate the usual grief reactions to loss
Stress to family (and older child) that such feelings are normal and that grief takes time to resolve
Help family gain a realistic concept of child's disability and abilities
Encourage formal rehabilitation as soon as realistically feasible
Assist family in orienting newly blind child to environment and in making immediate surroundings safe to encourage ambulation
Listen to family's concerns regarding the child's visual loss
Refer to community agencies and support groups

EXPECTED OUTCOMES

Parents express their feelings and concerns regarding loss of sight
Parents demonstrate an understanding of the child's disability and its implications

GOAL 2
Promote parent-child attachment

INTERVENTIONS

Help parents identify clues other than eye contact from the infant that signify communication with them
Encourage parents to discuss their feelings regarding lack of visual contact or smiling from the child
Stress that lack of such responses is not an indication of child's rejection or dislike of parents
Demonstrate by own example acceptance of the child
Emphasize positive abilities or attributes
Encourage parents in their attempts to promote child's development

EXPECTED OUTCOME

Parents and child exhibit a positive relationship

NURSING DIAGNOSIS: Potential for injury related to environmental hazards, noncompliance with therapeutic plan

GOAL 1
Prevent defects of vision

INTERVENTIONS

Provide prophylactic eye care at birth
Administer oxygen cautiously to premature infant
Periodically screen all children from birth through adolescence for visual impairment
Participate in immunization programs for children
Teach safety regarding common causes of eye injuries
Stress importance of good eye care—use of proper lighting, avoidance of excessive close work, proper rest and nutrition, and yearly eye examinations
See Guidelines for Preventing Eye Injuries, Box 25-5

NURSING CARE PLAN
The Child with Vision Impairment—cont'd

EXPECTED OUTCOME

Healthy child does not acquire visual defect

GOAL 2

Prevent complications from eye trauma

INTERVENTIONS

Prevent further injury by instituting appropriate emergency care (see Emergency Treatment, p. 1107)
Avoid any implication of guilt
Reassure parent and child; avoid giving false reassurance; apprise them of each step of treatment, especially if therapy interferes with vision (patching eyes)

EXPECTED OUTCOME

Child exhibits no evidence of complications

GOAL 3

Prevent complications from infection

INTERVENTIONS

Teach family correct procedure for instilling ophthalmic preparations (always in conjunctival cul-de-sac)
Ensure proper dosage by holding dropper vertically, slowly closing the lids, and having child rotate the eyeball for even distribution
Wipe excess medication from inner canthus outward to prevent contamination of contralateral eye
Emphasize regular administration of drug for entire term of therapy to eradicate infection completely

EXPECTED OUTCOME

Family complies with instructions and performs procedures correctly (specify)

GOAL 4

Prevent complications of eye defects

INTERVENTIONS

Encourage compliance with corrective therapies
Strabismus:
- Discuss with school-age child necessity of patch in preserving vision; allow child to verbalize feelings regarding altered facial appearance; help overcome visual difficulties imposed by seeing with weaker eye (favorable seating in school, large-print books, additional time to complete assignments)
- Teach parents correct procedures for instilling anticholinesterase drugs

Refractive errors:
- For secure fit of glasses, use ones with rounded temporal pieces or attach elastic strap to handles and around back of head
- Include older child in selection of frames
- Encourage parents to compare value of more expensive attractive frames and inducement for wearing them against cost
- If glasses are recommended for continuous wearing, discuss possibility of temporary removal for special occasions
- Encourage use of protective shields during contact sports
- Stress improvement in visual acuity as reason for wearing glasses
- Discuss feasibility of contact lenses with selected families
- Know procedures for care, insertion, and removal of lens; teach these to parents and older children

EXPECTED OUTCOMES

Child and family comply with therapy and perform procedures correctly
Child wears corrective lenses and cares for equipment correctly

See also Nursing Care Plan: The Child with a Chronic Illness or Disability, Chapter 22

Development and independence. Motor development is almost as dependent on sight as verbal communication is on hearing. From earliest infancy parents are encouraged to expose infants to as many visual-motor experiences as possible, such as sitting supported in an infant seat or swing and being given opportunities for holding up the head, sitting unsupported, reaching for objects, and crawling.*

Despite visual impairment the child can become independent in all aspects of self-care. The same principles used for promoting independence in sighted children apply, with additional emphasis on nonvisual cues. For example, the child may need help in dressing, such as special arrangement of clothing for style coordination and braille tags to distinguish colors and prints.

The blind child also must learn to become independent in navigational skills. The two main techniques are the *tapping method* (use of a cane to survey the environment for direction and to avoid obstacles) and *guides,* such as a human sighted guide or a dog guide, such as a Seeing Eye dog. Partially sighted children may benefit from ocular aids, such as a monocular telescope.

Play and socialization. Blind children do not learn to play automatically. Because they cannot imitate others or actively explore the environment as sighted children do, they depend much more on others to stimulate and teach them how to play. Parents need help in selecting appropriate play material, especially those that encourage fine and

*Suggested references are *Move with Me* and *Learning to Play: Common Concerns for the Visually Impaired Preschool Child,* available at no charge from Blind Children's Center, 4120 Marathon St., P.O. Box 29159, Los Angeles, CA 90029-0159; (213) 664-2153.

NURSING TIP: HELPING CHILDREN LEARN BODY PARTS

To help the young child learn body parts and enjoy music, use the tune to "This Is the Way We Wash Our Clothes" and change the words to "This is the way we touch our head [or other part], touch our head, touch our head. This is the way we touch our head, so early in the morning [or other times of day, week, month]."

From National Association for Parents of the Visually Impaired, Inc.: Awareness, p. 11, 4th quarter, 1987.

gross motor development and stimulate the senses of hearing, touch, and smell.* Toys with educational value are especially useful, such as dolls with various clothing closures. (See also Nursing Tip.)

Blind children have the same needs for socialization as sighted children. Since they have little difficulty in learning verbal skills, they are able to communicate with age-mates and participate in suitable activities. The nurse discusses with parents opportunities for socialization outside of the home, especially regular nursery schools. The trend is to include these children with sighted children to help them adjust to the outside world for eventual independence.

To compensate for inadequate stimulation, these children may develop *blindisms,* such as body rocking, finger flicking, or arm twirling. Such habits retard the child's social acceptance and should be discouraged. Behavior modification is often successful in reducing or eliminating blindisms.

Education. The main obstacle to learning in blind children is their total dependence on nonvisual cues. Although they can learn via verbal lecturing, they are unable to read the written word or to write without special education. Therefore they must rely on *braille,* a system that uses raised dots to represent letters and numbers. The child can then read the braille with the fingers and can write a message using a braille writer. However, unless others read braille, this is not useful for communicating with others. A more portable system for written communication is the use of a braille slate and stylus (Fig. 25-4) or a microcassette tape recorder. A recorder is especially helpful for leaving messages for others and for taking notes during classroom lecturing. Both the braille slate and stylus and the tape recorder are as important to a blind person as paper and pencil are to a sighted individual. For mathematical calculations portable calculators with voice synthesizers are available.†

Records and tapes are significant sources of reading material other than braille books, which are large and cumbersome. The **Library of Congress*** has talking books, braille books, and a special records program, which are available at many local libraries, state libraries, and directly from the Library of Congress. The talking book machine and tape player are provided at no cost to families, and there is no postage fee for returning the materials. **Recording for the Blind, Inc.†** also provides texts and tapes of books, which are very helpful for secondary and college students who are blind.

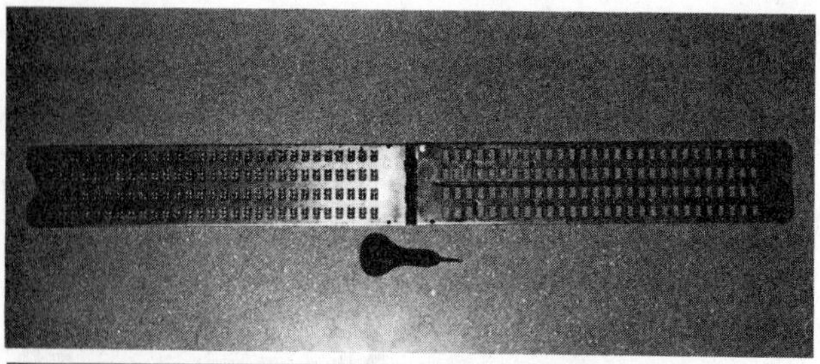

Fig. 25-4. Braille slate and stylus. The hinged slate consists of a series of open rectangles on one side and standard braille cells on the other. The paper is clamped or sandwiched between these two metal bars, and the appropriate dots are punched with the stylus.

Learning to use a regular typewriter is another form of writing but has the disadvantage of the blind person being unable to check the accuracy of the typing. Recent developments with computers have eliminated this drawback. A home computer with a voice synthesizer can be adapted to speak each letter or word that has been typed.

The partially sighted child benefits from specialized visual aids, which produce a magnified retinal image. The basic devices are accommodation, such as bringing the object closer, special plus lenses, hand-held and stand magnifiers, telescopes, video projection systems, and large print. Special equipment is available to enlarge print. Information about services for the partially sighted is available from the **National Association for Visually Handicapped** and **American Foundation for the Blind.** An excellent newsletter is published by the **National Association for Parents of the Visually Impaired.** Children with diminished vision often prefer to do close work without their glasses and compensate by bringing the object very near to their eyes. This should be allowed. The exception is the child with vision in only one eye, who should always wear glasses for protection.

Care for the child during hospitalization. Because nurses are more likely to care for children who are hospitalized for procedures that involve temporary loss of vision than for children who are blind, the following discussion concentrates primarily on the needs of such children. The nursing care objectives in either situation are to (1) reassure the child and family throughout every phase of treatment, (2) orient the child to his or her surroundings, (3)

*Suggested references are *Move with Me* and *Learning to Play: Common Concerns for the Visually Impaired Preschool Child,* available at no charge from Blind Children's Center, 4120 Marathon St., P.O. Box 29159, Los Angeles, CA 90029-0159; (213) 664-2153.

†A catalog of numerous products for people with vision problems is available from the American Foundation for the Blind.

***Division for the Blind and Visually Handicapped,** 1291 Taylor St., N.W., Washington, DC 20542; (202) 707-5100 or (800) 424-8567.

†20 Roszel Rd., Princeton, NJ 08540; (609) 452-0606.

provide a safe environment, and (4) encourage independence. Whenever possible the same nurse should care for the child to ensure consistency in the approach. These same principles also apply to a blind child who requires hospitalization.

When sighted children temporarily lose their vision, almost every aspect of the environment becomes bewildering and frightening. They are forced to rely on nonvisual senses for help in adjusting to the blindness without the benefit of any special training. Nurses have a major role in minimizing the effects of temporary loss of vision. They need to talk to the child about everything that is occurring, emphasizing aspects of procedures that are felt or heard. They should approach the child by always identifying themselves as soon as they enter the room. Since unfamiliar sounds are especially frightening, these are explained. Parents are encouraged to room with their child and participate in the care. Familiar objects, such as a teddy bear or doll, should be brought from home to help lessen the strangeness of the hospital. As soon as the child is able to be out of bed, he or she is oriented to the immediate surroundings. If the child is able to see on admission, this opportunity is taken to point out significant aspects of the room. The child is encouraged to practice ambulating with the eyes closed to become accustomed to this experience.

The room is arranged with safety in mind. For example, a stool or chair is placed next to the bed to help the child climb in and out of bed. The furniture is always placed in the same position to prevent collisions. Cleaning personnel are reminded of the need to keep the room in order. If the child has difficulty navigating by feeling the walls, a rope can be attached from the bed to the point of destination, such as the bathroom. Attention to details such as well-fitting slippers or robes that do not hang on the floor is important in preventing tripping. Unlike the child who is blind, these children are not familiar with navigating with a cane.

The child is encouraged to be independent in self-care activities, especially if the visual loss may be prolonged or potentially permanent. For example, during bathing the nurse sets up all the equipment and encourages the child to participate. At mealtime the nurse explains where each food item is on the tray, opens any special containers, prepares cereal or toast, but encourages the child in self-feeding. Favorite finger foods, such as sandwiches, hamburgers, hot dogs, or pizza, may be good selections. The child is praised for efforts at being cooperative and independent. Any improvements made in self-care, no matter how small, are stressed.

Appropriate recreational activities are provided, and if a child life specialist is available, such planning is done jointly. Since children with temporary blindness have a wide variety of play experiences to draw on, they are encouraged to select activities. For example, if they like to read, they may enjoy being read to. If they prefer manual activity, they may appreciate playing with clay or building blocks or feeling different textures and naming them. If they need an outlet for aggression, activities such as pounding or banging on a drum can be helpful. Simple board and card games can be played with a "seeing partner" or if the opponent helps with the game. They should have familiar toys from home to play with, since familiar items are more easily manipulated than new ones. If parents wish to bring presents, they should be objects that stimulate hearing and touch, such as a radio, music box, or stuffed animal.

Occasionally children who are blind come to the hospital for procedures to restore their vision. Although this is an extremely happy time, it also requires intervention to help them adjust to sight. They need an opportunity to take in all that they see. They should not be bombarded with visual stimuli. They may need to concentrate on people's faces or their own to become accustomed to this experience. They often need to talk about what they see and to compare the visual images with their mental ones. The child may also go through a period of depression, which must be respected and supported. The nurse or parents should refrain from statements such as, "How can you be so sad when you can see again?" Instead the child should be encouraged to discuss how it feels to see, especially in terms of seeing himself or herself.

Newly sighted children also need time to adjust to the ability to engage in activities that were impossible before. For example, they may prefer to use braille to read, rather than learning a new "visual approach," because of familiarity with the touch system. Eventually, as they learn to recognize letters and numbers, they will integrate these new skills into reading and writing. However, parents and teachers must be careful not to push them before they are ready. This applies to social relationships and physical activities as well as learning situations.

Assist in measures to prevent vision impairment. An essential nursing goal is to prevent visual impairment. This involves many of the same interventions discussed under hearing impairments, namely (1) prenatal screening for pregnant women at risk, such as those with rubella or syphilis infection and family histories of genetic disorders associated with visual loss; (2) adequate prenatal and perinatal care to prevent prematurity and iatrogenic damage from excessive administration of oxygen; (3) periodic screening of all children, especially newborns through preschoolers, for congenital blindness and visual impairments caused by refractive errors, strabismus, and so on; (4) rubella immunization of all children; and (5) safety counseling regarding the common causes of ocular trauma (Box 25-5).

Following detection of eye problems, the nurse has a responsibility to prevent further ocular damage by ensuring that corrective treatment is employed. For the child with strabismus, this often necessitates occlusion patching of the stronger eye. Compliance with the procedure is greatest during the early preschool years. It is more difficult to encourage school-age children to wear the occlusive patch because the poor visual acuity of the uncovered weaker eye interferes with schoolwork and the patch sets them apart from their peers. In school they benefit from being positioned favorably (closer to the blackboard) and allowed extra time to read or complete an assignment. If treatment of the eye disorder requires instillation of ophthalmic medica-

Box 25-5 GUIDELINES FOR PREVENTING EYE INJURIES

Infants and Toddlers

Avoid any toys with long pointed handles, such as a pinwheel on a stick.
Keep pointed instruments and tools out of reach (e.g., scissors, knives, screwdrivers, rulers, pencils, sticks).
Do not allow child to *walk* or *run* with any pointed object in the hand (e.g., spoon, lollipop, toothbrush).
Keep child away from play of older children and adults that involves projectile activities (throwing a ball, golf, target shooting, swings).
Stress importance of fire safety and poison protection in preventing thermal/chemical burns to eye.
Shield child's eyes when in direct sunlight.

Preschoolers

Supervise use of sharp or pointed objects, especially scissors.
Teach proper use of pointed objects, such as toy guns or scissors, namely, to always point them *away* from the face or from anyone else at close range.
Teach child to walk carefully (never run) while carrying any sharp or pointed object.
Keep child away from projectile activities.
Begin teaching respect for firearms.

School-Age Children and Adolescents

Teach proper use and respect for potentially dangerous equipment such as power tools (flying objects from them), firearms, firecrackers where legally permitted, and racquet sports.
Stress use of eye protection when playing ball (baseball, racquetball, tennis), shooting, practicing archery, gardening with power tools, riding motorcycles, or using equipment such as power saws or chemistry sets.
Teach child to open soda bottles with screw cap pointing away from face.
Encourage safe use of curling iron.
Advise child of danger of excessive sunlight (ultraviolet burns).
Warn child to never look directly at the sun even with sunglasses.
Monitor duration of wear of contact lens to prevent corneal scratching and possible scarring.
Store nail glue away from eye drop containers to avoid mistaking the glue for the medication.

tion, the family is taught the correct procedure (see Chapter 27).*

The nurse helps children with reflective errors adjust to wearing glasses. Young children who often pull glasses off benefit from temporal pieces that wrap around the ears or an elastic strap attached to the frames and around the back of the head to hold them on securely. Once children appreciate the value of clear vision, they are more likely to wear the corrective lenses.

Glasses should not interfere with any activity. Special protective guards are available during contact sports to prevent accidental injury, and all corrective lenses should be made from safety glass, which is shatterproof. Often corrective lenses improve visual acuity so dramatically that children are able to compete more effectively in sports. This in itself is a tremendous inducement to continue wearing glasses.

Contact lenses are a popular alternative, especially for adolescents. Several types are available, such as hard lenses, including gas-permeable ones, and soft lenses, which may be designed for daily or extended wear. Contact lenses offer several advantages over glasses, such as greater visual acuity, total corrected field of vision, convenience (especially with the extended-wear type), and optimum cosmetic benefit. However, they require much more care than glasses, including considerable practice to learn techniques for insertion and removal. If they are prescribed, the nurse can be very helpful in teaching parents or older children how to care for the lenses. General guidelines for care include regular removal and cleaning (daily for both hard and soft lenses or every 7 days or less for the extended-wear type), thorough handwashing before handling lenses, and only use of commercially prepared saline solutions—not tap water or homemade saline solutions—for soft lenses. In addition, soft lenses require periodic disinfection.

Since trauma is the leading cause of blindness, the nurse has the major responsibility of preventing further eye injury until the specific treatment is instituted (see Emergency Treatment, p. 1107). Patients with a serious eye injury fear blindness, so the nurse should stay with the child and family to provide support and reassurance.

Evaluation

The effectiveness of nursing interventions for vision impairment is determined by continual reassessment and evaluation of care based on the following observational guidelines and expected outcomes:

1. Interview the family regarding their adjustment to the sensory impairment. Observe the family members' relationship with the child. Interview the child regarding feelings about the sensory impairment and its effect on activities of daily living (especially important if a visual loss).
2. Have parents identify cues that indicate the infant is responding to them. Observe nonvisual behaviors of parents as they respond to their infant.
3. Observe the techniques the child uses to read and navigate. Inquire if the child is enrolled in a visual training program. Inquire about socialization opportunities for the child (i.e., who are child's friends, what are child's extracurricular activities).
4. Observe preparation of room and self-care activities that provide for the child's safety and independence during hospitalization.
5. Investigate community programs aimed at preventing or detecting vision loss and inquire about nursing involvement in these efforts.

Expected outcomes:
See Nursing Care Plan, pp. 1108-1109.

*Home care instructions for giving eye medication are available in Wong, D.L., and Whaley, L.F.: Clinical manual of pediatric nursing, ed. 3, St. Louis, 1990, Mosby–Year Book, Inc.

THE DEAF-BLIND CHILD

The most traumatic sensory impairment is loss of sight and hearing. One of the chief causes of deaf blindness was congenital rubella syndrome, but immunization has decreased its incidence. Other causes are usually the result of one congenital sensory impairment combined with an acquired impairment, such as congenital blindness and acquired deafness from meningitis. Most children with multisensory impairments have some residual hearing and vision to supplement the senses of touch, smell, and taste.

Auditory and visual impairments have profound effects on the child's development. They interfere with the normal sequence of physical, intellectual, and psychosocial growth. Although the child often achieves the usual motor milestones, they are delayed. Children only learn communication with specialized training. Finger spelling is one desirable method often taught to these children. The letters are spelled into the deaf-blind child's hand, and the child spells out ideas to the other person. Another type of tactile communication, the Tadoma method, involves the child placing the hand over the speaker's face and neck to monitor facial movements associated with speech production (Reed and others, 1989). Children with residual hearing can learn to speak. Whenever possible, speech is encouraged, since it allows communication with individuals not familiar with the preceding approaches.

Programs for these children vary. The John T. Tracy Clinic offers a home correspondence course for parents, and the **American Foundation for the Blind,** the **Helen Keller National Center,*** the **Perkins School for the Blind,†** and the **Foundation for the Junior Blind‡** provide special services; the last two organizations have residential educational programs.

NURSING CONSIDERATIONS

Caring for children with multisensory impairments is an area in which few nurses have much experience. It involves an overwhelming adjustment for families, and the child's educational needs cannot be met in most public school programs. Most of the interventions discussed for the hearing or visually impaired child are applicable to the care of these children, such as activities to facilitate learning self-care and increased stimulation for motor development. The following discusses some of the special problems encountered by these families and constructive interventions.

One of the major concerns of families with deaf-blind children is helping them establish communication. The nurse is in a vital position to help parents with this goal. Since infants cannot coo, laugh, or make eye movements, they are limited in the cues they can send and receive. Therefore initiating and maintaining communication is the caregiver's responsibility. The nurse discusses with parents behaviors that signal the infant's recognition of them, such as quieting behavior, blinking, and change in respiration. The parents are encouraged to find ways of increasing stimulation for the child, especially cues that help the child identify each parent. For example, each person involved with the child should choose something that he or she, and only he or she, does, such as a kiss on the forehead or a stroke on the cheek. In this way the infant learns to discriminate among people in the environment.

The infant should be held close to the adult with the child's hands placed on the face while the person talks or changes facial expression. Eventually this technique becomes structured to associate a certain facial vibration with a word. However, such associations take time, patience, and effort from both the child and the parents.

As many sensory experiences as possible are provided, such as placing children in different positions during the day in relation to light and providing variation in stimuli so that they will be motivated to move toward, reach, touch, and explore the environment. Changing position also encourages muscle development and movement patterns. Sounds should be brought near and made interesting to these children. For example, they can participate in hearing by placing the hand on a radio or on a person's throat. Consistent tactile cues should be associated with a change of position and activities so that the movement is experienced as a positive, nonthreatening experience. The nurse encourages family members to urge the child to participate in games that require repositioning and body action, such as peekaboo and pat-a-cake.

Deaf-blind children need secure, safe experiences while learning to walk and gaining confidence. Once ambulatory, they need help in exploring the environment on a gradual *planned* basis. The environment should not be haphazard, since children may become fearful and avoid growth-producing experiences. After they succeed in becoming well oriented to the environment and can overcome any abnormal movement patterns, they are ready for a plan of locomotion. Sighted guide, trailing (movement directed by touching objects, such as the wall), and cane walking are three methods. An individually planned mobility program is based on the child's age, needs, and functional status and is shared with the child's therapist, teachers, parents, and siblings.

The future prospects for deaf-blind children are at best unpredictable. Sometimes congenital blindness and/or deafness is accompanied by other physical or neurologic handicaps, which further lessen the child's learning potential. The most favorable prognosis is often for children who have acquired deaf blindness and have few, if any, associated disabilities. Their learning capacity is greatly potentiated by their developmental progress before the sensory impairments. Although total independence, including gainful vocational training, is the goal, some deaf-blind children are unable to develop to this level. They may require lifelong parental or residential care. The nurse working with

*Middle Neck Rd., Sands Point, NY 11050; (516) 944-8900 (voice/TDD).
†175 N. Beacon St., Watertown, MA 02172; (617) 924-3434.
‡5300 Angeles Vista Blvd., Los Angeles, CA 90043; (213) 295-4555.

such families helps them deal with future goals for the child, including possible alternatives to home care during the parents' advancing years. In this respect much of the nurse's role is similar to that discussed in Chapter 24 for the child with cognitive impairment.

■ COMMUNICATION IMPAIRMENT

One of the most outstanding differences between human beings and lower animals is the human ability to communicate by using verbal language. The profound effect of hearing loss on speech development, discussed earlier in this chapter, laid a foundation for understanding how inability to communicate impacts a child's life. However, hearing impairment is only one of several reasons for communication disorders. Often the child has language and speech but is still unable to communicate effectively. This discussion focuses on types of communication disorders, guidelines for detecting children who require referral, and techniques to promote language/speech development and prevent problems.

GENERAL CONCEPTS

Communication impairment is a broad term that refers to the inability to (1) receive and/or process a symbol system, (2) represent concepts or symbol systems, and/or (3) transmit and use symbol systems (Definitions, 1982). Although communication disorders are concerned with verbal symbols of the spoken word, other symbol systems include nonverbal methods, such as gestures, sign language, and braille. With severe communication impairment, these methods may be needed to substitute for the spoken word.

Because of the complexity of communication, various classification systems are available and there is no universal agreement on one system. Basically, a communication impairment may occur in language, speech, or hearing or any combination of these. The problems encountered when hearing is affected are discussed earlier in this chapter. *Language* primarily refers to the symbol system used to convey thoughts or feelings to others. The two major types are *receptive* language, or understanding the spoken word, and *expressive* language, or speaking verbal symbols. *Speech* is the oral production of language, including articulation of sounds, rhythm, and tone.

Delayed development of language and speech is the most common symptom of developmental disability in children and affects from 5% to 10% of all children (Coplan, 1985). Speech problems are more prevalent than language disorders, and both impairments decline as children grow older. Males are affected three to four times more often than females (U.S. Department of Health and Human Services, 1988).

Etiology

The most common cause of communication impairment is mental retardation, followed by hearing impairment. Other causes include (1) central nervous system dysfunction, such as attention deficit disorders or learning disabilities; (2) severe emotional disturbance, such as autism and schizophrenia; (3) organic problems, such as cerebral palsy, cleft palate, vocal cord injury, and paralysis or foreshortening of the soft palate and uvula; and (4) some genetic disorders, such as cri-du-chat syndrome and Gilles de la Tourette syndrome. In some instances, such as in stuttering, the cause is unknown or speculative. Although the exact influence of environmental factors is controversial, the current thinking deemphasizes the importance of laziness, birth order, or bilingualism on delayed language development (Coplan, 1985).

Language Impairment

Language disorders include an inability to:

1. Assign meaning to words (vocabulary)
2. Organize words into sentences
3. Alter word forms to indicate tense, possession, and plurality

Examples of language disorders are failure to develop vocabulary at the expected age, a reduced vocabulary for age, poor sentence structure, such as "Me see dog," or omitting words from the sentence, such as "Me fun." Such short or "telegraphic" phrases are normal during the first 2 years but should be replaced by more complete statements during the preschool years.

Clinical manifestations of language disorders are presented in Box 25-6.

Speech Impairment

Speech impairments include differences from normal in articulation, fluency, and voice production. *Articulation* errors

Box 25-6 CLINICAL MANIFESTATIONS OF LANGUAGE DISORDERS

Assigning Meaning to Words
First words not uttered before second birthday
Vocabulary size reduced for age or fails to show steady increase
Difficulty in describing characteristics of objects, although may be able to name them
Infrequent use of modifier words (adjectives or adverbs)
Excessive use of jargon past 18 months

Organizing Words into Sentences
First sentences not uttered before third birthday
Short and incomplete sentences
Tendency to omit words (articles, prepositions)
Misuse of the "be," "do," and "can" verb forms
Difficulty understanding and producing questions
Plateaus at an early developmental level; uses easy speech patterns

Altering Word Forms
Omission of endings for plurals and tenses
Inappropriate use of plurals and tense endings
Inaccurate use of possession words

Box 25-7 CLINICAL MANIFESTATIONS OF SPEECH DISORDERS

Dysfluency (Stuttering)

Noticeable repetition of sounds, words, or phrases after age 4 years
Obvious frustration with attempts to communicate
Demonstration of struggling behavior while talking (head jerks, eye blinks, retrials, circumlocution)
Embarrassment about own speech

Articulation Deficiency

Intelligibility of conversational speech absent by age 3 years
Omission of consonants at beginning of words by age 3 and at end of words by age 4
Persisting articulation faults after age 7
Omission of a sound where one should occur
Distortion of a sound
Substitution of an incorrect sound for a correct one

Voice Disorders

Deviations in pitch (too high or too low, especially for age and sex); monotone
Deviations in loudness
Deviations in quality (hypernasality or hyponasality)

refer to those sounds that a child makes incorrectly or inappropriately. For example, the child tends to distort or substitute a few consonants or blends, especially those that are learned last—*s, l, r,* and *th*—or child omits many consonants, usually at the end of words, and substitutes the letters *t, d, k,* or *y* for them.

Dysfluencies, or rhythm disorders, usually consist of repetitions of sounds, words, or phrases. One of the most common and potentially serious dysfluencies is stuttering. *Stuttering,* or the less frequently used term *stammering,* describes dysfluent speech characterized by tense repetition of sounds or complete blockages of sounds or words. A stutter is sometimes referred to as a *block* when no sound comes out when the person tries to speak (Guitar, 1989).

Voice disorders are characterized by differences in pitch, loudness, and/or quality. Clinical manifestations of speech disorders are presented in Box 25-7.

NONSPEECH COMMUNICATION

Another category receiving increased attention is concerned with individuals who have severe disabilities, such as cerebral palsy, mental retardation, or multiple physical impairments, that prevent acquisition of meaningful verbal speech. Many of these people comprehend language but are unable to speak. Consequently, they benefit from communication methods that employ nonverbal symbols such as sign language. Besides the use of hand or body gestures, numerous other communication systems exist. For example, *Blissymbols* are a highly stylized system of graphic symbols that represent words, ideas, and concepts (Murray, 1984). Although Blissymbols require education for their use, no reading skill is needed. These symbols or other self-

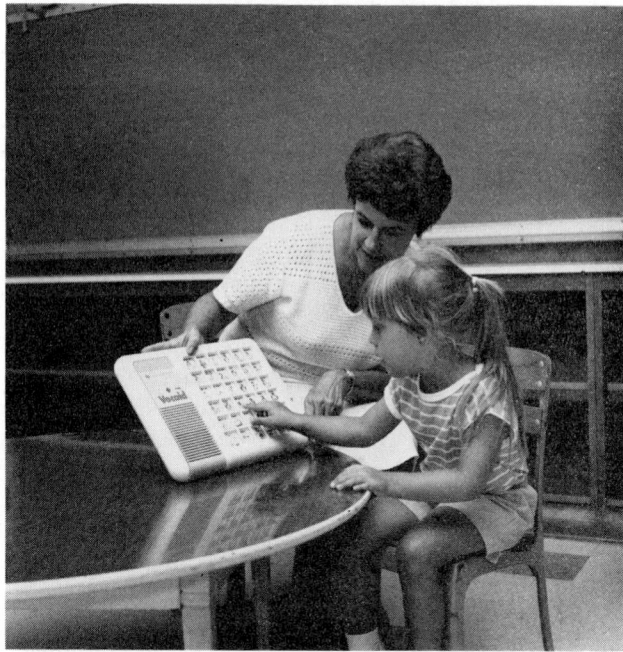

Fig. 25-5. The Vocaid is a communication board with a voice synthesizer. The child pushes the picture she wants, and that word or phrase is spoken.
(Manufactured by Texas Instruments, Dallas, TX.)

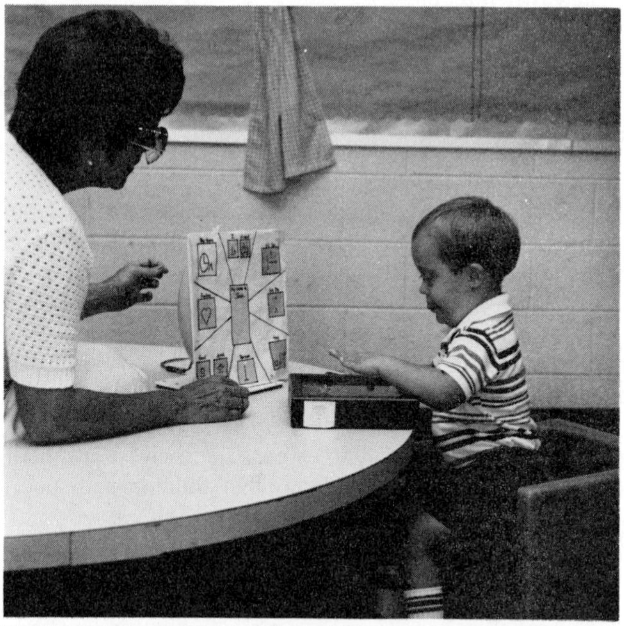

Fig. 25-6. Blissymbols can help a young child communicate nonverbally. This device uses a light behind each symbol; the light is rotated around the board by pressing the push panel.

explanatory graphics are usually arranged on a board, and the person points to the symbol(s) to convey a message; more sophisticated devices employ voice synthesizers that "speak" the symbol's meaning (Fig. 25-5). For children with physical limitations that prevent fine hand movements, numerous devices are available that facilitate isolating a symbol (Fig. 25-6). Noncommunication systems are allowing severely disabled individuals a much more meaningful life; many children are able to learn more and faster because of the advances in augmentative communication (Lloyd and Karlan, 1984).*

NURSING CARE OF THE CHILD WITH COMMUNICATION IMPAIRMENT

Nursing goals focus primarily on assessment of communication disorders and prevention of primary problems or development of further difficulties, especially through parent education. Since nurses are frequently involved in preventive health maintenance of well preschool children and care of ill or hospitalized youngsters, they are in an optimum position to assess children for adequate communication development, detect deviations, and begin counseling.

Prevention

The primary intervention for communication disorders is prevention. Much of prevention directly relates to factors that predispose to causes of language/speech impairment, namely, mental retardation and hearing loss. Infants at risk for either condition (see Boxes 8-2 and 24-2) should be referred for audiologic evaluation before 6 months of age so that audiologic and speech therapy can be initiated immediately, when required.

Prevention also involves early recognition of children at risk for language delays and involves timely intervention to promote adequate language development. Nurses are often able to provide education for families that foster the child's communication skills. Specific interventions are presented in the Parent Guidelines.

One area that is particularly important in terms of preventing communication impairment through appropriate parental guidance is stuttering. This hesitancy or dysfluency in speech pattern is a *normal* characteristic of language development during the preschool years. It occurs because children's advancing mental ability and level of comprehension exceed vocabulary acquisition. Children know what they want to say but hesitate or repeat words or sounds as they try to find the vocabulary to express themselves. Eventually their language skills parallel the other abilities, and speech becomes fluent.

However, when parents or other significant persons place undue emphasis or stress on this pattern of dysfluency, an abnormal speech pattern may result. Chances for reversal of stuttering are good until about 5 years of age. Therefore prevention must begin early. The nurse discusses with parents the normal dysfluencies in children's speech. When stuttering does occur, parents are advised to use the suggestions listed under Parent Guidelines to prevent inadvertently reinforcing the dysfluent pattern. If excessive concern of the parent or frustration and struggling behavior from the child are noted, the child is referred for language and speech evaluation.*

PARENT GUIDELINES
Stuttering in Young Children

To be encouraged

- Viewing hesitancy and dysfluency as a normal part of speech development
- Giving the child plenty of time and the impression that you are not rushed or in a hurry
- Looking directly at the child while he or she is talking; being patient and never ridiculing or criticizing
- Setting a good example by speaking clearly and articulating well
- Identifying situations when stuttering increases, and avoiding them or ignoring the hesitancy
- Minimizing stress, such as talking at the child's eye level; avoiding frequent questioning; and preventing interruptions while the child is speaking
- Capitalizing on periods of fluent speech with positive reinforcement, such as singing songs or repeating nursery rhymes

To be avoided

- Practicing the natural tendency to "help" or finish the sentence for the child by supplying the word when the child has a block
- Telling the child to stop and start over, to think before speaking, or to take it easy and go slowly
- Showing great concern, embarrassment, or disapproval for hesitancy
- Doing *anything* that emphasizes stuttering and calls the child's attention to speech skills
- Promising a reward for proper speech

NURSING ALERT The critical point to remember is that the dysfluency must be arrested before the child develops an awareness or anticipation of the difficulty and begins to mistrust his or her speech skills.

Assessment

Communication disorders can occur at any age but are most often found during childhood. The preschool period is considered critical to language development and therefore is a prime age for assessment and intervention. Failure to detect communication disorders during early childhood affects the development of social relationships and emotional interactions, increases difficulty in developing academic skills, and lessens the chances for successful correction of deficit skills.

Assessment of abnormalities requires knowledge of normal language and speech development. Awareness of when

*Information about communication aids for children is available from the Crestwood Company, 6625 North Sidney Pl., Milwaukee, WI 53209; (414) 352-5678.

*Information about sources of assistance is available from the **Stuttering Resource Foundation,** 123 Oxford Rd., New Rochelle, NY 10804; (914) 632-3925 (Westchester) or (800) 232-4773 (outside local calling areas).

Table 25-4 Normal language/speech development during early childhood

AGE (YEARS)	DEVELOPMENT	INTELLIGIBILITY
1	Says two to three words with meaning Imitates sounds of animals Omits most final and some initial consonants	Usually no more than 25% intelligible to unfamiliar listener Height of unintelligible jargon at age 18 months
2	Uses two- to three-word phrases Has vocabulary of about 300 words Uses "I," "me," and "you" Articulation lags behind vocabulary	50% intelligible in context
3	Says four- to five-word sentences Has vocabulary of about 900 words Uses "who," "what," and "where" in asking questions Uses plurals, pronouns, and prepositions Often repeats and hesitates	75% intelligible
4-5	Has vocabulary of 1500 to 2100 words Able to use most grammatical forms correctly, such as past tense of verb with "yesterday" Uses complete sentences with nouns, verbs, prepositions, adjectives, adverbs, and conjunctions	At age 4 years, speech is 100% intelligible, although some sounds are still imperfect
5-6	Has vocabulary of 3000 words Comprehends "if," "because," and "why" Masters most sounds; still distorts *s, z, sh, ch,* and *j*	

children achieve such milestones enables nurses to distinguish when specific communication characteristics are expected and when they are considered deviations (Table 25-4). Nurses must also be aware of clinical manifestations of language and speech impairment (see Boxes 25-6 and 25-7), as well as hearing or cognitive deficits (see Box 25-2 and Chapter 24).

Three methods are available for assessing speech and language development:

1. Direct observation of the child's verbal skills
2. Questioning of the parents
3. Testing

Direct observation necessitates spontaneous language interaction between the child and the nurse. Suggestions for initiating conversation include showing children an object and asking them to describe it (asking children to name the object often results in one-word responses that are too limited for evaluation of speech, although appropriate for evaluation of language) or posing questions such as, "If you could have three wishes, what would you want?" The word-imitative procedure may also be used by having children repeat sentences or words. This approach is valid because children are not able to reproduce statements using correct grammatical forms that they have not previously learned to use. Whenever possible, the child's conversation should be tape-recorded for serial documentation of progressive language/speech development and further evaluation by or consultation with a language or speech therapist.

Indirect assessment relies on parental information obtained through a history. Key questions that reflect problems in language or speech are listed in Box 25-8. Information obtained from the history is critically important, and parental comments such as, "He doesn't say much" or "Her use of words is so much slower than her older brother's was" must be taken seriously. However, caution must also be exercised in evaluating parental comments. Parents may be unaware of the child's difficulties because of lack of comparison with normal language development. Also, they may not realize the degree of unintelligible speech because of familiarity with the child's approximation of words. Conversely, parents may have unrealistic expectations regarding verbal development and may exaggerate the degree of dysfluency, misarticulation, or word usage. Consequently, screening tests are a very important component of objective measurement of speech development.

Denver Articulation Screening Examination. The Denver Articulation Screening Examination (DASE) (see Appendix B) employs the word-imitative procedure and is one of the most frequently used tests. The child repeats 22 words but pronounces 30 different sound elements. The raw score, or the number of correctly pronounced sounds, is then compared with the percentile rank for children in that age-group. The examiner must be careful to evaluate the specific sound rather than the quality of the entire word. For beginning examiners it is helpful to validate the final score by comparing the results with a different examiner, ideally a speech therapist. The child is also scored on intelligibility, by selection of one of four possible categories: (1) easy to understand, (2) understandable half of the time, (3) not understandable, or (4) cannot evaluate. The DASE is a reliable, effective screening tool because it requires only 10

Box 25-8 GUIDELINES FOR ASSESSING COMMUNICATION IMPAIRMENT

Key Questions for Language Disorders

1. How old was your child when he (or she) began to speak his (or her) first words?
2. How old was your child when he (or she) began to put words into sentences?
3. Does your child have difficulty in learning new vocabulary words?
4. Does your child omit words from sentences (i.e., do sentences sound telegraphic?) or use short or incomplete sentences?
5. Does your child have trouble with grammar, such as the verbs "is," "am," "are," "was," and "were"?
6. Can your child follow two to three directions given at once?
7. Do you have to repeat directions or questions?
8. Does your child respond appropriately to questions?
9. Does your child ask questions beginning with "who," "what," "where," and "why"?
10. Does it seem that your child has made little or no progress in speech and language in the last 6 to 12 months?

Key Questions for Speech Impairment

1. Does your child ever stammer or repeat sounds or words?
2. Does your child seem anxious or frustrated when trying to express an idea?
3. Have you noticed certain behaviors, such as blinking the eyes, jerking the head, or attempting to rephrase thoughts with different words, when your child stammers?
4. What do you do when any of these occur?
5. Does your child omit sounds from words?
6. Does it seem like your child uses *t, d, k,* or *g* in place of most other consonants when speaking?
7. Does your child omit sounds from words or substitute the correct consonant with another one (such as "rabbit" with "wabbit")?
8. Do you have any difficulty in understanding your child's speech? How much of it is intelligible?
9. Has anyone else ever remarked about having difficulty in understanding your child?
10. Has there been any recent change in the sound of your child's voice?

Box 25-9 GUIDELINES FOR REFERRAL REGARDING COMMUNICATION IMPAIRMENT

Age 2 Years

Failure to speak any meaningful words spontaneously
Consistent use of gestures rather than vocalizations
Difficulty in following verbal directions
Failure to respond consistently to sound

Age 3 Years

Speech largely unintelligible
Failure to use sentences of three or more words
Omission of initial consonants
Frequent omission of final consonants
Use of vowels rather than consonants

Age 5 Years

Stutters or has any other type of dysfluency
Sentence structure noticeably impaired
Substitutes easily produced sounds for more difficult ones
Omits word endings (plurals, tenses of verbs, etc.)

School Age

Poor voice quality (monotonous, loud, or barely audible)
Vocal pitch inappropriate for age
Any distortions, omissions, or substitutions of sounds after age 7 years
Connected speech characterized by use of unusual confusions or reversals

General

Any child with signs suggesting a hearing impairment (see p. 1096)
Any child who is embarrassed or disturbed by his or her speech
Parents who are excessively concerned or who pressure the child to speak at a level above that appropriate for the child's age

minutes for the examiner to perform and is designed to discriminate between significant speech delay and normal variations in the acquisition of speech sounds. It also detects common abnormal physical conditions such as hyponasality, hypernasality, tongue thrust, and lateral lisp.

Early Language Milestone Scale. The Early Language Milestone Scale (ELM)* is a standardized screening instrument for assessing language development in children less than 3 years of age. The test focuses on expressive, receptive, and visual language, and the revised form includes intelligibility (Coplan and Gleason, 1988; Coplan and others, 1982). The ELM relies primarily on the parent's report, with occasional direct testing of the child, and takes 1 to 4 minutes to administer. The best age range for the ELM is 25 to 36 months (Walker and others, 1989).

Other tests. A number of other tests are available to screen children for impaired language development. The Denver II, a revision of the Denver Developmental Screening Test, includes an expanded section on language items, and delays in that area provide an early indication for those children who require further evaluation (see Chapter 7). For children 2½ to 18 years the *Peabody Picture Vocabulary Test–Revised* is a useful screening instrument for word comprehension (Dunn and Dunn, 1981).

Referral. Following assessment and detection of language or speech problems, the nurse must make a decision regarding appropriate referral. The all-too-frequent advice of "let's wait and see what happens" or "your child will grow out of it" is often to the detriment of the child's future development. Since children normally vary greatly in their development of verbal skills, the nurse needs some guidelines for determining which child's development is abnormal. Box 25-9 lists general recommendations for referring children for specialized audiologic and language evaluations. Information regarding available services for language,

*The complete testing kit can be purchased from Pro-Ed, Inc., (512) 451-3246 (call collect).

PARENT GUIDELINES
Helping a Child Learn Language

Provide listening opportunities:
- Select a small group of words connected to a specific activity (e.g., say "open" each time a door is opened).
- Repeat the word with the activity several times, then repeat the word but wait for the child to initiate the activity.

Choose vocabulary that is useful, easy to pronounce, and understandable to the child.

Encourage vocabulary by having the child say the word rather than gesture before fulfilling a request (e.g., expect the child to say all or part of the word "drink" before giving a beverage).

Speak at a level slightly above the child's level (e.g., if the child speaks two words, use three- or four-word phrases).

Expand the statement, preserving the child's intent.*
- Expand the statement using the same noun.
  - CHILD: Kitty jump
  - ADULT: The kitty is on the chair.
- Replace the noun with a pronoun.
  - CHILD: Kitty jump
  - ADULT: She is jumping.
- Expand the statement adding new information.
  - CHILD: Kitty jump
  - ADULT: The dog is jumping, too.

Respond by indicating the meaning of the child's utterance, rather than its linguistic accuracy (or inaccuracy).*
- CHILD: Kitty jump
- ADULT: Yes, the kitty is jumping.

Substitute questions with statements about an observed activity (e.g., rather than asking, "What's that?" say, "Look at the kitten").

Reinforce the child's attempt to use language with verbal praise and affection.

*Data from U.S. Department of Health and Human Services: Developmental speech and language disorders: hope through research, Pub. No. 188-2757, Bethesda, MD, 1988, Public Health Service, National Institutes of Health.

speech, and hearing can be obtained from the **American Speech-Language-Hearing Association*** and the **Council for Exceptional Children†** (see also p. 1097 for organizations devoted to hearing impairment).

Education

When a child is delayed in language development, it becomes very important to try to structure the parents' communication to expand the child's language, including new words, new sentence construction, and rules of grammar. The underlying principle is not to bombard children with words so that they learn more language, but to plan what will be said to them, what responses will be expected, and how they will be reinforced. Suggestions to help parents foster their child's attainment of language skills are presented in the Parent Guidelines.

Parents should also be aware that children learn language through imitation. Therefore serving as role models by speaking clearly, fluently, and with proper grammar is essential to children's mastery of language and speech. Parents need guidance regarding normal language and speech development so that they expect neither too little nor too much from their child.

*10801 Rockville Pike, Rockville, MD 20852.

†Division for Children with Communication Disorders, 1920 Association Dr., Reston, VA 22091.

KEY POINTS

- Hearing defects may be categorized according to etiology, pathology, or symptom severity; treatment, prevention, and rehabilitation are based on these factors.
- Hearing disorders may be classified according to the location of the defect: conductive, sensorineural, mixed conductive-sensorineural, and auditory imperception.
- Some of the effects of hearing loss on growth and development are impaired knowledge of objects, emotional behavior, poor motor development, impaired academic learning, and decreased socialization.
- Prevention of hearing loss is the nurse's major responsibility. Efforts include treatment of infection, auditory testing, immunization, pregnancy and genetic counseling, and reduction of excessive noise.
- Rehabilitation for hearing loss involves parent education and support, hearing aids, lipreading, sign language, speech therapy, and promotion of socialization.
- Visual impairments are often classified, for convenience, by activity: school vision, legal blindness, travel vision, and light perception.
- Visual impairment may result from familial factors, prenatal/intrauterine factors, perinatal factors, and postnatal factors.
- Common visual impairments in childhood are refractive errors, amblyopia, strabismus, cataracts, glaucoma, trauma, and infections.
- Effects of visual impairment on development include impaired motor function, lack of stimulation, and diminished academic learning.
- Prevention of visual impairment focuses on prenatal screening, prenatal and perinatal care, periodic vision screening of all children, immunization, and safety counseling.
- Nursing goals in visual rehabilitation are helping the family and child adjust to the child's visual impairment, promoting parent-child attachment, fostering optimum development and independence, providing for play and socialization, and being aware of educational facilities.
- For the child undergoing ocular surgery, nursing care is aimed at reassuring the child and family throughout treatment, orienting the child to the surroundings, providing a safe environment, and encouraging independence.

- Nursing interventions for the deaf-blind child are helping the family adjust to the child's impairment, choosing appropriate educational channels, facilitating self-care, promoting communication, and assisting with ambulation.
- Communication impairment broadly refers to the inability to receive and/or process a symbol system, to represent concepts or symbol systems, and to transmit and use symbol systems.
- Causes of impaired communication include mental retardation, hearing impairment, central nervous system dysfunction, severe emotional disturbances, and organic problems.
- Assessing speech and language development is accomplished by direct observation of verbal skills, questioning of parents, and testing.
- Dysfluency in speech is normal during the preschool years and can become problematic stuttering if the child becomes anxious over the speech pattern.

REFERENCES

Bronzaft, A.L.: Noise is hazardous to child's health and well-being, Child Behav. Dev. Lett. 5(10):1-4, 1989.

Consensus Conference: Noise and hearing loss, JAMA 263(23):3185-3190, 1990.

Coplan, J.: Evaluation of the child with delayed speech or language, Pediatr. Ann. 14(3):202-208, 1985.

Coplan, J., and Gleason, J.: Unclear speech: recognition and significance of unintelligible speech in preschool children, Pediatrics 82(3, pt. 2):447-452, 1988.

Coplan, J., and others: Validation of an early language milestone scale in a high-risk population, Pediatrics 70(5):677-683, 1982.

Davis, H., and Silverman, S.R.: Hearing and deafness, ed. 4, New York, 1978, Holt, Rinehart & Winston, Inc.

Definitions: Communicative disorders and variations, Am. Speech Lang. Hear. Assoc. J. 24:949-950, 1982.

Dunn, L., and Dunn, L.: The Peabody Picture Vocabulary Test–Revised, Circle Pines, MN, 1981, American Guidance Service.

Frey, T.: Pediatric eye trauma, Pediatr. Ann. 12(7):487-497, 1983.

Friendly, D.S.: Amblyopia: definition, classification, diagnosis, and management considerations for pediatricians, family physicians, and general practitioners, Pediatr. Clin. North Am. 34(6):1389-1401, 1987.

Gibbons, C.L.: Deaf children's perception of internal body parts, Matern. Child Nurs. J. 4(1):37-46, 1985.

Gortmaker, S.L., and Sappenfield, W.: Chronic childhood disorders: prevalence and impact, Pediatr. Clin. North Am. 31(1):3-18, 1984.

Guitar, B.: Stuttering, Feelings Med. Signif. 31(3):9-12, 1989.

Hall, D.M.B.: The child with a handicap, Boston, 1984, Blackwell Scientific Publications.

Harrison, L.L.: Minimizing barriers when teaching hearing-impaired clients, MCN 15(2):113, 1990.

Helveston, E., and Ellis, F.: Pediatric ophthalmology practice, ed. 2, St. Louis, 1984, Mosby–Year Book, Inc.

Jackson, C.B.: Primary health care for deaf children, part I, J. Pediatr. Health Care 3(6):316-318, 1989.

Kovalesky, A.: Nurses' guide to children's eyes, New York, 1985, Grune & Stratton, Inc.

Lloyd, L.L., and Karlan, G.R.: Non-speech communication symbols and systems: where have we been and where are we going? J. Ment. Defic. Res. 28:3-20, 1984.

Miyamoto, R.T., and others: Cochlear implants in children, Insights Otolaryngol. 2(5):1-8, 1987.

Murray, F.: Language for the handicapped, Point of View 21(3):8-9, 1984.

Reed, C., and others: Analytic study of the Tadoma method: effects of hand position on segmental speech production, J. Speech Hear. Res. 32:921-929, 1989.

Roush, J.: Acoustic amplification for hearing-impaired infants and young children, Inf. Young Child. 2(4):59-71, 1990.

Salamy, A., Eldredge, L., and Tooley, W.H.: Neonatal status and hearing loss in high-risk infants, J. Pediatr. 114(5):847-852, 1989.

Stehr-Green, J., and others: *Acanthamoeba* keratitis in soft contact lenses wearers, JAMA 258(1):57-60, 1987.

U.S. Department of Health and Human Services: Developmental speech and language disorders: hope through research, Pub. No. 1 88-2757, Bethesda, MD, 1988, Public Health Service, National Institutes of Health.

Vision problems in the United States, New York, 1980, National Society to Prevent Blindness.

Walker, D., and others: Early Language Milestone Scale and language screening of young children, Pediatrics 83(2):284-288, 1989.

BIBLIOGRAPHY

Hearing Impairment

Boothroyd, A., and Hnath-Chisolm, T.: Spatial, tactile presentation of voice fundamental frequency as a supplement to lipreading: results of extended training with a single subject, J. Rehabil. Res. Dev. 25(3):51-56, 1988.

Church, M.W., and Gerkin, K.P.: Hearing disorders in children with fetal alcohol syndrome: findings from case reports, Pediatrics 82(2):147-154, 1988.

Coplan, J.: Deafness: ever heard of it? Delayed recognition of permanent hearing loss, Pediatrics 79(2):206-213, 1987.

Epstein, S., and Reilly, J.S.: Sensorineural hearing loss, Pediatr. Clin. North Am. 36(6):1501-1520, 1989.

Hanawalt, A., and Troutman, K.: If your patient has a hearing aid, Am. J. Nurs. 84(7):900-901, 1984.

Holder, L.: Hearing aids: handle with care, Nursing '82 12(4):64-67, 1982.

Jackson, C.B.: Primary health care for deaf children, part II, J. Pediatr. Health Care 4(1):39-41, 1990.

Kaplan, S.L., and others: Onset of hearing loss in children with bacterial meningitis, Pediatrics 73(5):575-578, 1984.

Kaufman, D.H., Grothe, G., and Brasser, B.: Early identification and ear infection and hearing loss in an early childhood population, School Nurse, pp. 18-21, Jan./Feb. 1987.

Lynch, M., Eilers, R., and Oller, D.: Profoundly hearing impaired subjects: use of tactile aids in speech perception tasks, Volta Rev. 91(5):113-126, 1989.

Lynch, M.P., and others: Speech perception by congenitally deaf subjects using an electrocutaneous vocoder, J. Rehabil. Res. Dev. 25(3):41-50, 1988.

Matkin, N.D.: Early recognition and referral of hearing-impaired children, Pediatr. Rev. 6(5):151-156, 1984.

Matkin, N.: Key considerations in counseling parents of hearing impaired children, Semin. Speech Lang. 9:209-222, 1988.

McGarr, N.: Research on the use of sensory aids for hearing-impaired people, Volta Rev. 91(5):1-138, 1989.

McKerrow, K.: Minimal hearing loss may not be benign, Am. J. Nurs. 87(7):904-905, 1987.

Northern, J., and Downs, M.: Hearing in children, ed. 4, Baltimore, 1984, Williams & Wilkins.

Oberklaid, F., Harris, C., and Keir, E.: Auditory dysfunction in children with school problems, Clin. Pediatr. 28(9):397-403, 1989.

Robinson, T.: Early identification of vision and hearing problems. In Pediatrics: nursing update, vol. 1, no. 12, Princeton, NJ, 1986, Continuing Professional Education Center, Inc.

Shimizu, Y.: Microprocessor-based hearing aid for the deaf, J. Rehabil. Res. Dev. 26(2):25-36, 1989.
Thomas, K.A.: How the NICU environment sounds to a preterm infant, MCN 14:249-251, 1989.
Weibley, T.: Inside the incubator, MCN 14(2):96-100, 1989.

Vision Impairment

Bateman, J.B.: Genetics in pediatric ophthalmology, Pediatr. Clin. North Am. 30(6):1015-1031, 1983.
Blinding missiles: soft drink twist-off bottle caps, Sightsaving 53(1):2-7, 1984.
Borders, C.R.: Strabismus/amblyopia: when to refer, Patient Care 18(17):21-52, 1984.
Buncic, J.R.: The blind infant, Pediatr. Clin. North Am. 34(6):1403-1413, 1987.
Carr, M., and others: Curling-iron cornea (letter), N. Engl. J. Med. 319:1672, 1988.
Chew, E., and Morin, J.D.: Glaucoma in children, Pediatr. Clin. North Am. 30(6):1043-1060, 1983.
Cromie, B.W.: Superglue inadvertently used as eyedrops, Br. Med. J. 300(6725):680, 1990.
DeRespinis, P.A.: Cyanoacrylage nail glue mistaken for eye drops, JAMA 263(17):2301, 1990.
DeRespinis, P.A., and others: A survey of severe eye injuries in children, Am. J. Dis. Child. 143:711-716, 1989.
Fiore, P.M., and Wagner, R.S.: Halloween hazards: ocular injury from flying eggs, N. Engl. J. Med. 319(7):1159, 1988.
Fulton, A.B., and Robb, R.M.: Special diagnostic and therapeutic modalities in pediatric ophthalmology, Pediatr. Clin. North Am. 34(6):1543-1556, 1987.
Gray, R., and others: Pecking injury of the eye, N. Engl. J. Med. 319(15):1021-1022, 1988.
Grin, T.R., Nelson, L.B., and Jeffers, J.B.: Eye injuries in childhood, Pediatrics 80(1):13-17, 1987.
Grosvenor, T.: Myopia: what can we do about it clinically? Optom. Vision Sci. 66:415-419, 1989.
Holds, J.B., and others: Water balloon orbitopathy, JAMA 260(13):1884, 1988.
Ingram, R.M.: Amblyopia, Br. Med. J. 298(6668):204, 1989.
Jan, J.E., and others: Eye-pressing by visually impaired children, Dev. Med. Child. Neurol. 25(6):755-762, 1983.
Kodadek, S.M., and Haylor, M.J.: Using interpretive methods to understand family caregiving when a child is blind, J. Pediatr. Nurs. 5(1):42-49, 1990.
Lubniewski, A., and others: Ocular dangers in the garden, Ophthalmology 95(7):906-910, 1988.
Lyons, C., Stevens, J., and Bloom, J.: Superglue inadvertently used as eyedrops, Br. Med. J. 300:328, 1990.
Martyn, L.J., and DiGeorge, A.T.: Selected eye defects of special importance in pediatrics, Pediatr. Clin. North Am. 34(6):1517-1542, 1987.
Melamed, M.: Complications of contact lenses, Emerg. Med. 14(4):218-224, 1982.
Nelson, L.B.: The visually handicapped child, Pediatr. Rev. 6(6):173-182, 1984.
Nelson, L.B., Wilson, T.W., and Jeffers, J.B.: Eye injuries in childhood: demography, etiology, and prevention, Pediatrics 84(3):438-441, 1989.
Nelson, L.B., and others: Developmental aspects in the assessment of visual function in young children, Pediatrics 73(3):375-381, 1984.
Norris, R.M.: Commonsense tips for working with blind patients, Am. J. Nurs., pp. 360-361, March 1989.
Osguthorpe, N.C.: If your patient has contact lenses, Am. J. Nurs. 84(10):1255-1256, 1984.
Phillips, S., and Hartley, J.T.: Developmental differences and interventions for blind children, Pediatr. Nurs. 14(3):201-204, 1988.
Questions and answers about strabismus, Patient Care 18(17):184, 1984.
Randall, K.: Contact lenses for infants after congenital cataract surgery, Sightsaving 53(1):8-13, 1984.
Rollins, J.A.: National Library Service for the Blind and Physically Handicapped, Pediatr. Nurs. 14(6):522, 1988.
Ruttum, M.S., and others: Detection of congenital cataracts and other ocular media opacities, Pediatrics 79(5):814, 1987.
Scheiner, A.P., and Moomaw, M.: Care of the visually handicapped child, Pediatr. Rev. 4(3):74-81, 1982.
Simmons, J.N.: Mediating the environment: a case study approach, Child Care Health Dev. 11(4):195-207, 1985.
Tongue, A.C.: Refractive errors in children, Pediatr. Clin. North Am. 34(6):1425-1437, 1987.
Tumulty, G., and Resler, M.M.: Eye trauma, Am. J. Nurs. 84(6):740-744, 1984.

Communication Impairment

Accardo, P., and Whitman, B.: Toe walking: a marker of language disorders, Clin. Pediatr. 28(8):347-350, 1989.
Blamey, P., and others: Speech perception using combinations of auditory, visual, and tactile information, Vet. Admin. J. Rehabil. Res. Dev. 26(1):15-24, 1989.
Casper, J.: Disorders of speech and voice, Pediatr. Ann. 14(3):220-229, 1985.
Choi, S., and Cotton, R.: Surgical management of voice disorders, Pediatr. Clin. North Am. 36(6):1535-1549, 1989.
Cohen, C.: Augmentative communication: a perspective for pediatricians, Pediatr. Ann. 14(3):232-240, 1985.
Fischel, J., and others: Language growth in children with expressive language delay, Pediatrics 82(2):218-227, 1989.
Fuller, C.W.: Speech and hearing problems. In Green, M., and Haggerty, R.J., editors: Ambulatory pediatrics, III, Philadelphia, 1984, W.B. Saunders Co.
Goldberg, R.: Identifying speech and language delays in children, Pediatr. Nurs. 15(4):252-259, 1984.
Graham, J.M., Jr., Bashir, A.S., and Stark, R.E.: Communicative disorders. In Levine, M.D., and others, editors: Developmental-behavioral pediatrics, Philadelphia, 1983, W.B. Saunders Co.
Hall, D.: Delayed speech in children, Br. Med. J. 297(6659):1281-1282, 1988.
Lombardino, L., Stapell, J., and Gerhardt, K.: Evaluating communicative behaviors in infancy, J. Pediatr. Health Care 1(5):240-246, 1987.
Menyuk, P.: Language development in a social context, J. Pediatr. 109(1):217-224, 1986.
Resnick, T.J., Allen, D.A., and Rapin, I.: Disorders of language development diagnosis and intervention, Pediatr. Rev. 6(3):85-92, 1984.
Smith, R., and others: Effectiveness of a writing system using a computerized long-range optical pointer and 10-branch abbreviation expansion, Vet. Admin. J. Rehabil. Res. Dev. 26(1):51-62, 1989.
Speech dysfluency, Lancet 8637(1):530-532, 1989.

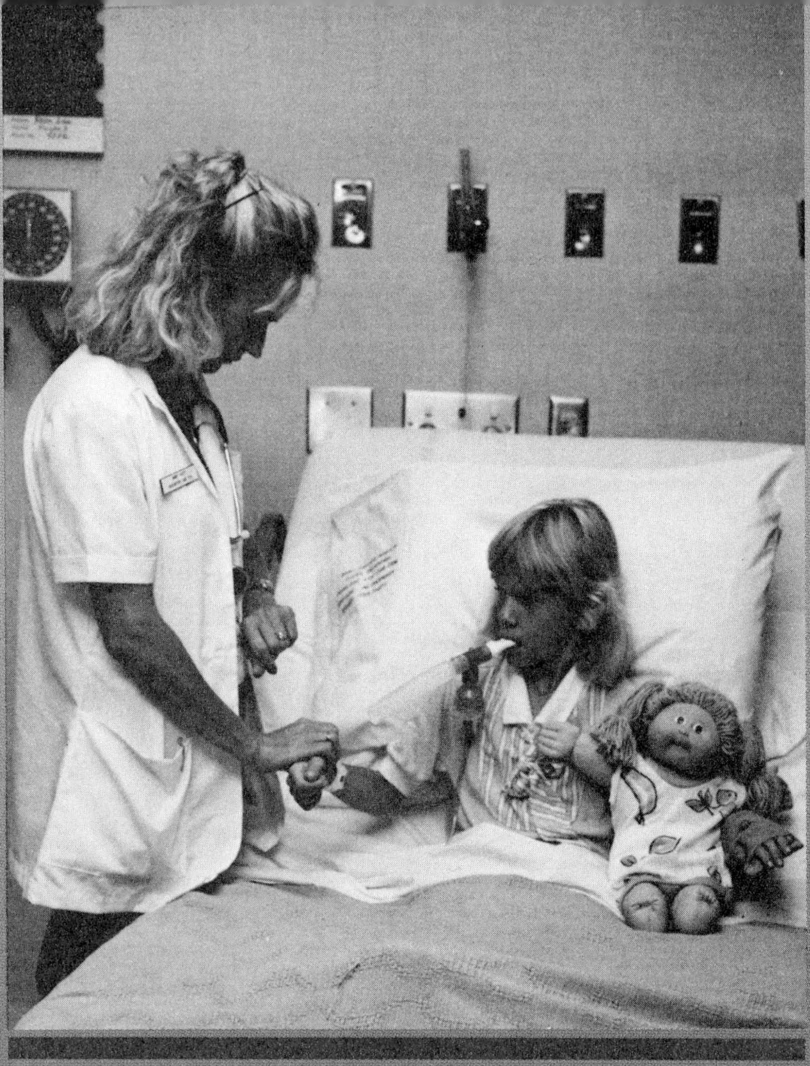

NURSING CARE OF THE ILL OR HOSPITALIZED CHILD

PART

II

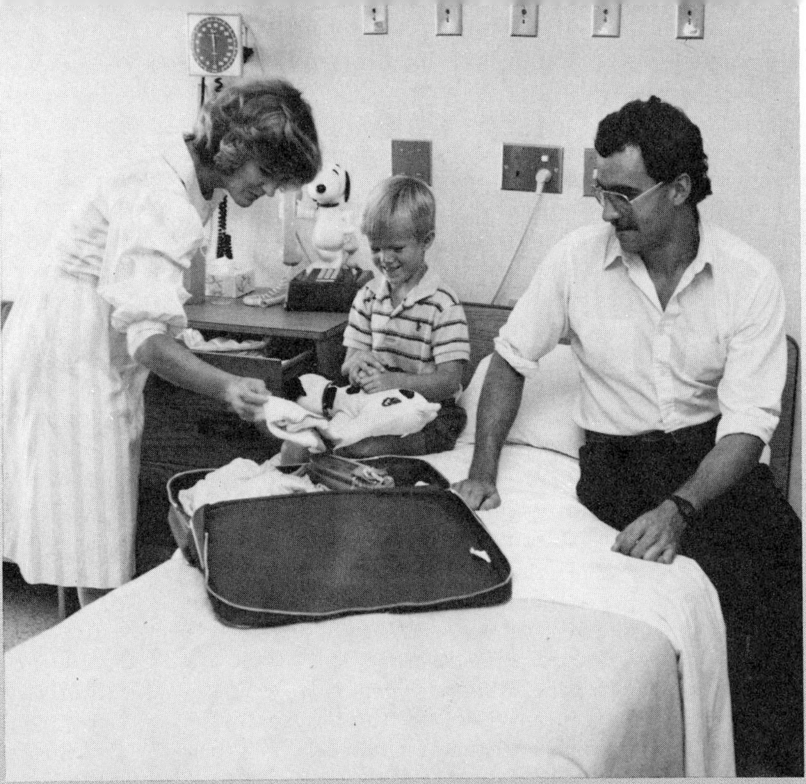

Impact of Hospitalization on the Child and Family

UNIT IX

When illness requires hospitalization, it creates a crisis for the child and family. Depending on their age, children must deal with separation from familiar caregivers and environment, exposure to painful experiences, loss of independence, and disruption of nearly every aspect of their usual lifestyle. Often the reason for the hospitalization is of much less concern to the child than the consequences of confinement. Emergency and intensive care admissions pose an even greater threat because of the lack of time to prepare the child and the seriousness of the child's condition. In addition, treatments are often painful and frightening.

Chapter 26, *Reaction of the Child and Family to Illness and Hospitalization,* is concerned with the child's age-related reactions to illness and hospitalization. It discusses interventions that lessen the psychologic trauma of the experience, particularly parent participation and preparation for hospital admission. The effects of the child's hospitalization on the family are considered, since care is extended to these important individuals as well. The needs of the child and family during special hospital situations also are explored. The chapter concludes with a discussion of discharge planning and home care.

Chapter 27, *Pediatric Variations of Nursing Interventions,* deals with pediatric variations of nursing procedures and psychologic and physical preparation of the child for various procedures. It is not designed to present a detailed description of how to perform specific procedures, but rather how to implement them safely with children.

CHAPTER 26

Reaction of the Child and Family to Illness and Hospitalization

RELATED TOPICS

Administration of medication, Ch. 27
Communication and health assessment of the child and family, Ch. 6
Compliance, Ch. 27
Cultural/religious influences on health care, Ch. 2
Impact of chronic illness or disability on the child and family, Ch. 22
Impact of life-threatening illness on the child and family, Ch. 23
Neonatal pain, Ch. 11
Nursing care of the surgical neonate, Ch. 11
Physical and developmental assessment of the child, Ch. 7
Preparation for procedures, Ch. 27
Surgical procedures, Ch. 27

GLOSSARY

analgesia Absence of pain without loss of consciousness
ATC Around the clock
drug tolerance Clinical need to increase the drug dosage in order to attain the same desired effect
ICU Intensive care unit
IM Intramuscular
IV Intravenous
narcotic Legal term for any substance causing psychologic dependence
narcotic addiction Behavioral pattern of overwhelming involvement with obtaining and using a narcotic for its psychic effects rather than for medical reasons
NSAID Nonsteroidal antiinflammatory drug
opioid Natural or synthetic analgesic with morphinelike actions
physical dependence Adaptive physiologic state that occurs when a drug is taken in increasing amounts and that is manifest by development of withdrawal symptoms
PO Oral
PRN Administer as needed
SC Subcutaneous

For children and their families, illness and hospitalization constitute a stressful experience. It is often the first crisis children must confront. Children, especially during the early years, are particularly vulnerable to the crises of illness and hospitalization because (1) stress represents a change from the usual state of health and environmental routine, and (2) children have a limited number of coping mechanisms to resolve the stressful events. Children's reactions to these crises are influenced by their developmental age; previous experience with illness, separation, or hospitalization; available support system; their innate and acquired coping skills; and the seriousness of the diagnosis.

This chapter focuses on the various aspects of illness and hospitalization in children to assist nurses in providing the quality of care that promotes optimum resolution of the crisis and positive growth from the experience for the entire family unit.

STRESSORS AND REACTIONS RELATED TO DEVELOPMENTAL STAGE

Children's understanding of, reaction to, and method of coping with illness or hospitalization are influenced by the significance of individual *stressors* (those events that produce stress) during each developmental phase. The major stressors of separation, loss of control, bodily injury, and pain and children's behavioral reactions are discussed in this section. However, a review of the previous chapters on normal growth and development will facilitate a more thorough understanding of children's physical, psychosocial, and cognitive abilities and limitations. In addition, Chapters 22 and 23 present an in-depth discussion of children's and family members' reactions to a disability and chronic or life-threatening illness.

SEPARATION ANXIETY

The major stress from middle infancy throughout the preschool years, especially for children ages 15 to 30 months, is separation anxiety, also called *anaclitic depression.* The principal behavioral responses of these children to the three phases of separation anxiety are summarized in Box 26-1.

During the phase of *protest,* children cry loudly, scream for the parent, refuse the attention of anyone else, and are inconsolable in their grief (Fig. 26-1). They may continue this behavior for a few hours to several days. Some children may protest continuously, ceasing only from physical exhaustion. If a stranger approaches them, children will initially protest even louder.

During the phase of *despair,* the crying stops. The child is much less active, is disinterested in play or food, and withdraws from others. The child looks sad, lonely, isolated, and apathetic (Fig. 26-2). The major behavior characteristic is depression, a result of increasing hopelessness, grief, and mourning.

The third phase is *detachment,* sometimes also called *denial.* Superficially the child appears to have finally adjusted to the loss. The child becomes more interested in the surroundings, plays with others, and seems to form new relationships. However, this behavior is the result of resignation and is not a sign of contentment. The child detaches from the parent in an effort to escape the emotional pain of desiring the parent's presence. The child copes by forming shallow relationships with others, becoming increasingly self-centered, and attaching primary importance to material objects. This is the most serious phase, since reversal of the potential adverse effects is less likely to occur once detachment is established. However, in most situations the temporary separations imposed by hospitalization do not cause such prolonged parental absences that the child enters into detachment. In addition, considerable evidence suggests that, even with stresses such as separation, children are re-

Box 26-1 MANIFESTATIONS OF SEPARATION ANXIETY IN YOUNG CHILDREN

Phase of Protest

Observed behaviors during later infancy
- Cries
- Screams
- Searches for parent with eyes
- Clings to parent
- Avoids and rejects contact with strangers

Additional behaviors observed during toddlerhood
- Verbally attacks strangers (e.g., "Go away")
- Physically attacks strangers (e.g., kicks, bites, hits, pinches)
- Attempts to escape to find parent
- Attempts to physically force parent to stay

Behaviors may last from hours to days

Protest, such as crying, may be continuous, ceasing only with physical exhaustion

Approach of stranger may precipitate increased protest

Phase of Despair

Observed behaviors
- Inactive
- Withdraws from others
- Depressed, sad
- Uninterested in environment
- Uncommunicative
- Regresses to earlier behavior (e.g., thumb-sucking, bed-wetting, use of pacifier, use of bottle)

Behaviors may last for variable length of time

Child's physical condition may deteriorate from refusal to eat, drink, or move

Phase of Detachment

Observed behaviors
- Shows increased interest in surroundings
- Interacts with strangers or familiar caregivers
- Forms new but superficial relationships
- Appears happy

Detachment usually occurs after prolonged separation from parent; rarely seen in hospitalized children

Behaviors represent a superficial adjustment to loss

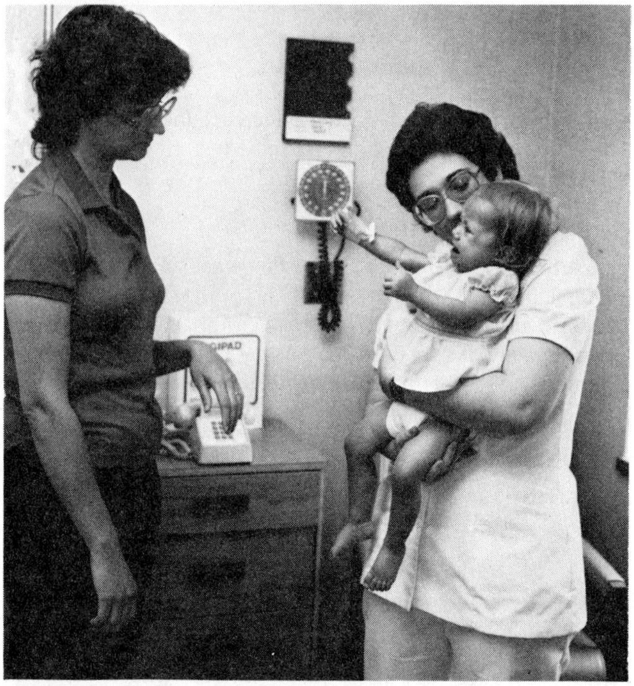

Fig. 26-1. In the protest phase of separation anxiety, children cry loudly and are inconsolable in their grief for the parent.

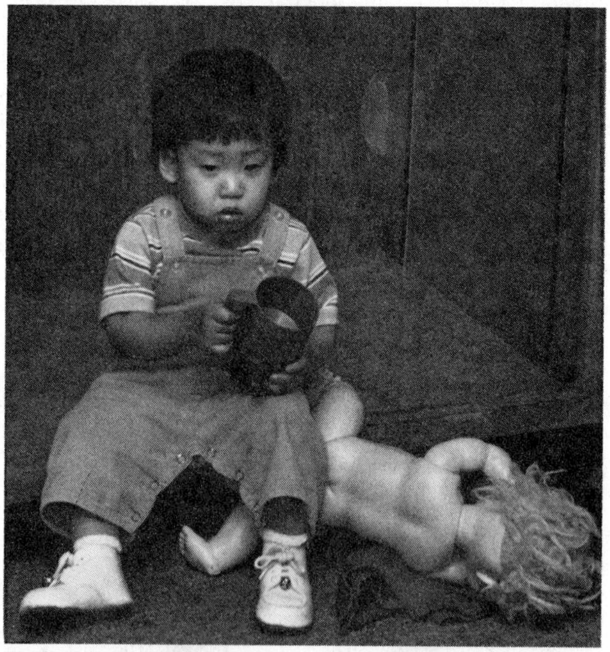

Fig. 26-2. During the despair phase of separation anxiety, children are sad, lonely, and disinterested in play or food.

markably resilient, and permanent ill effects are rare (see Questions and Controversies, p. 549).

While progression to detachment is uncommon, the initial phases are frequently observed even with very brief separations from either parent. Without an understanding of the meaning of each stage of behavior, health team members may erroneously label the behaviors as positive or negative. In the phase of protest, they may view the loud crying as "bad" behavior. Since the protesting increases if a stranger approaches, staff may interpret the reaction as evidence of their need to stay away. During the quiet, withdrawn phase of despair, they regard the child as finally "settling in" to the new surroundings and see the detachment behaviors as proof of a "good adjustment." The faster a child reaches this stage, the more likely the child will be regarded as the "ideal patient."

Since children seem to react "negatively" to visits by their parents, uninformed observers feel justified in restricting parental visiting privileges. For example, during the protest phase, children outwardly do not appear happy to see their parents. Instead, they may cry louder than before the parents' visit. If children are depressed, they may reject their parents or begin to protest once more. Often they cling to their parents in an effort to ensure their continued presence. Consequently, such behavior reactions may be regarded as "disturbing" the child's adjustment to the surroundings. If the separation has progressed to the phase of detachment, children will respond no differently to their parents than to any other strange or familiar person.

Such reactions are equally distressing to parents, who may be unaware of their meaning. If they are regarded as intruders, parents will view their absence as "beneficial" to the child's adjustment and recovery. They may respond to the child's behavior by staying for short periods, decreasing the frequency of visits, or deceiving the child when it is time to leave. Consequently a *destructive* cycle of misunderstanding and unmet needs results.

Early Childhood

Separation anxiety is most evident during the ages of 6 to 30 months and is the greatest stress imposed by hospitalization. If separation is avoided, young children have a tremendous capacity to withstand any other stress. During this time the typical reactions just described are seen. However, children in the toddler stage demonstrate more goal-directed behaviors. For example, they may verbally plea for their parents to stay and physically attempt to secure or find them. They may demonstrate displeasure on the parents' return or departure by having temper tantrums; refusing to comply to the usual routines of mealtime, bedtime, or toileting; or regressing to more primitive levels of development.

Since preschoolers are much more secure interpersonally than toddlers, they can tolerate brief periods of separation from their parents and are more inclined to develop substitute trust in other significant adults. However, the stress of illness usually renders them less able to cope with separation; as a result they manifest many of the stage behaviors of separation anxiety. In general the protest behaviors are more subtle and passive than those seen in younger children. Preschoolers may demonstrate separation anxiety through refusing to eat, difficulty in sleeping, crying quietly for their parents, continually asking when they will visit, or withdrawing from others. They may express anger indirectly by breaking their toys, hitting other children, or refusing to cooperate during usual self-care activities. Nurses need to be sensitive to these less obvious signs of separation anxiety to intervene appropriately.

Later Childhood

Although school-age children are better able to cope with separation in general, the stress imposed by illness or hospitalization may increase their need for parental security and guidance. This is particularly true for young school-age children who have only recently left the safety of the home and are struggling with the crisis of school adjustment. Middle and late school-age children may react more to the separation from their usual activities and peers than to absence of their parents. Their high level of physical and mental activity frequently finds no suitable outlets in the hospital environment. Even when they dislike school, they admit to missing its routine and associated activities and worry that they will not be able to compete or "fit in" with their classmates on returning to school. Feelings of loneliness, boredom, isolation, and depression are common. It is important to recognize that such reactions may occur more as a result of separation than from concern over the illness, treatment, or hospital setting.

School-age children may need and desire parental guidance or support from other adult figures but be unable or unwilling to ask for it. Because the goal of attaining independence is so important to them, they are reluctant to seek help directly for fear that they will appear weak, childish, or dependent. Cultural expectations to "act like a man" or to "be brave and strong" bear heavily on these children, especially males, who tend to react to stress with stoicism, withdrawal, or passive acceptance. Often the need to express hostile, angry, or other negative feelings finds alternate outlets, such as irritability and aggression toward parents, withdrawal from hospital personnel, inability to relate to peers, rejection of siblings, or subsequent problems in school.

For adolescents, separation from home and parents may be a welcomed and appreciated event. However, loss of peer-group contact may be a severe emotional threat because of loss of group status, inability to exert group control or leadership, and loss of group acceptance. Deviations within peer groups are poorly tolerated, and, although members may express concern for the adolescent's illness or need for hospitalization, they continue their group activities, quickly filling the gap of the absent member. During the temporary separation from their usual group, ill adolescents may benefit from group associations with other hospitalized age-mates.

LOSS OF CONTROL

One of the factors influencing the amount of stress imposed by hospitalization is the amount of control that persons perceive themselves as having. Lack of control increases the perception of threat and can affect children's coping skills (LaMontagne, 1984). Many hospital situations decrease the amount of control a child feels. Although the usual sensory stimulations are lacking, the additional hospital stimuli of sight, sound, and smell may be overwhelming. Without an insight into the type of environment conducive to children's optimum growth, the hospital experience can at best temporarily slow development and at worst permanently retard it. Because the needs of children vary greatly depending on their age, the major areas of loss of control in terms of physical restriction, altered routine or rituals, and dependency are discussed for each age-group.

Toddlers

Toddlers are striving for autonomy, and this goal is evident in most of their behaviors—motor skills, play, interpersonal relationships, activities of daily living, and communication. When their egocentric pleasures meet with obstacles, toddlers react with negativism, especially temper tantrums. Any restriction or limitation of movement, such as the simple act of laying toddlers on their back, can cause forceful resistance and noncompliance.

Loss of control also results from altered routines and rituals. Toddlers rely on the consistency and familiarity of daily rituals to provide a measure of stability and control in their complex world of growing and developing. The hospitalization or illness severely limits their sense of expectation and predictability, since most details of the hospital environment differ from those of the home.

Toddlers' main areas for rituals include eating, sleeping, bathing, toileting, and play. When the routines are disrupted, difficulties can occur in any or all of these areas. The principal reaction to such change is regression. For example, when mealtime and food choices differ from those at home, toddlers often refuse to eat, demand a bottle, or request others to feed them. Although regression to earlier forms of behavior may seem to increase toddlers' security and comfort, in reality it is very threatening for them to relinquish their most recently acquired achievements.

Enforced dependency is a chief characteristic of the sick role and accounts for the numerous instances of toddler negativism. For example, rigid schedules, altered caregiving activities, unfamiliar surroundings, separation from parents, and medical procedures usurp toddlers' control over their world. Although most toddlers initially react negatively and aggressively to such dependency, prolonged loss of autonomy may result in passive withdrawal from interpersonal relationships and regression in all areas of development. Therefore the effects of the sick role are most severe in instances of chronic, long-term illnesses or in those families who foster the sick role despite the child's improved state of health.

Preschoolers

Preschoolers also suffer from loss of control caused by physical restriction, altered routines, and enforced dependency. However, their specific cognitive abilities, which make them feel omnipotent and all-powerful, also make them feel out of control. This loss of control in the context of their sense of self-power is a critical influencing factor in their perception of and reaction to separation, pain, illness, and hospitalization.

Preschoolers' egocentric and magical thinking limits their ability to understand events because they view all experiences from their own self-referenced perspective. Without adequate preparation for unfamiliar settings or experiences, preschoolers' fantasy explanations for such events are usually more exaggerated, bizarre, and frightening than the facts. One typical fantasy to explain the reason for illness or hospitalization is that it represents punishment for real or imagined misdeeds. The response to such thinking is usually feelings of shame, guilt, and fear.

Preschoolers' cognitive ability is also concrete. Explanations are understood only in terms of real events. Purely verbal instructions are often inadequate for them because of their inability to abstract and synthesize beyond what their senses tell them. When combined with their egocentric and magical powers, they can interpret any message according to their particular past experiences. Even with the best preparation for a procedure, they may misconstrue the details.

Transductive reasoning implies that preschoolers deduct from the particular to the particular, rather than from the specific to general, or vice versa. For example, if preschoolers' concept of nurses is that they inflict pain, preschoolers will think that every nurse (or everyone wearing a similar uniform) will also inflict pain.

School-Age Children

Because of their striving for independence and productivity, school-age children are particularly vulnerable to events that may lessen their feeling of control and power. In particular, altered family roles; physical disability; fears of death, abandonment, or permanent injury; loss of peer acceptance; lack of productivity; and inability to cope with stress according to perceived cultural expectation may result in loss of control.

Because of the nature of the patient role, many routine hospital activities usurp individual power and identity. For these children, dependent activities such as enforced bed rest, use of a bedpan, inability to choose a menu, lack of privacy, help with a bed bath, or transport by a wheelchair or stretcher can be a direct threat to their security. Although all of these procedures seem routine and inconsequential, they allow no freedom of choice to children who want to "act grown-up." However, when children are allowed to exert a measure of control, regardless of how limited it may be, they generally respond very well to any procedure. For example, some of the most cooperative, satisfied, and contented patients are school-age children who help make their beds, choose their schedule of activities, assist in procedures, and help the nurses care for the younger children. An increased sense of control usually results from a feeling of usefulness and productivity.

In addition to the hospital environment, illness may also cause a feeling of loss of control. One of the most significant problems of children in this age-group centers on boredom. When physical or enforced limitations curtail their usual abilities to care for themselves or to engage in favorite activities, school-age children generally respond with depression, hostility, or frustration. Keeping a normally active child on bed rest is no small challenge. However, emphasizing areas of control and capitalizing on quiet activities, particularly hobbies such as building models or collecting specific objects, promote their adjustment to physical restriction. Nursing judgment regarding selection of a roommate is one of the most important contributing factors to their overall adjustment to illness and hospitalization.

Adolescents

Adolescents' struggle for independence, self-assertion, and liberation centers on the quest for personal identity. Anything that interferes with this poses a threat to their sense of identity and results in a loss of control. Illness, which limits their physical abilities, and hospitalization, which separates them from usual support systems, constitute major situational crises.

The patient role fosters dependency and depersonalization. Adolescents may react to dependency with rejection, uncooperativeness, or withdrawal. They may respond to depersonalization with self-assertion, anger, or frustration. Regardless of which response they manifest, hospital personnel generally tend to regard them as difficult, unmanageable patients. Parents may not be a source of help because these behaviors serve to further isolate them from understanding the adolescent. Although peers may visit, they may not be able to offer the type of support and guidance needed. Sick adolescents often voluntarily isolate themselves from age-mates until they feel they can compete on an equal basis and meet group expectations. As a result, ill adolescents may be left with virtually no support systems.

Loss of control also occurs for many of the reasons discussed for school-age children. However, adolescents are more sensitive to potential instances of loss of control and dependency than younger children. For example, both groups seek information about their physical status and rely heavily on anticipatory preparation to decrease fear and anxiety. However, adolescents react not only to what information is supplied, but also to how it is conveyed. They may feel very threatened by others who relate facts in a derogatory manner. Adolescents want to know that others can relate to them on their own level. This necessitates a careful assessment of their intellectual abilities, previous knowledge, and present needs. It may also require the nurse's willingness to learn the adolescent's language.

BODILY INJURY AND PAIN

Fears of bodily injury and pain are prevalent among children. Recent research documents that young children, including newborns, react to painful stimuli. In caring for children, nurses must appreciate the concerns related to bodily harm and children's reactions to pain at different developmental periods. Developmental considerations related to children's understanding of illness and pain are summarized in Table 26-1. Developmental characteristics of children's reactions to pain are also important (see Box 26-4).

Infants

Of the research exploring children's development of illness concepts and how their understanding of illness relates to fears of bodily injury, no findings are available for preverbal children. Consequently, the following discussion is limited to infants' reactions to pain. Neonatal pain is discussed in Chapter 11.

Infants' response to pain after the neonatal period is quite similar to earlier reactions, although there is marked variability in measures of distress, especially initial cry and heart rate, which may decrease in some infants (Dale, 1986). The most consistent indicator of distress is a facial expression of discomfort (Fig. 26-3). Body movements include squirming, writhing, jerking, and flailing (Mills, 1989). The individual differences may be the result of temperamental characteristics, which require further research and

Table 26-1 Children's developmental concepts of illness and pain

COGNITIVE STAGE (AGE)	CONCEPT OF ILLNESS*	CONCEPT OF PAIN†
Preoperational thought (2 to 7 years)	*Phenomenism:* Perceives an external, unrelated, concrete phenomenon as the cause of illness; e.g., "being sick because you don't feel well" *Contagion:* Perceives cause of illness as proximity between two events that occurs by "magic"; e.g., "getting a cold because you are near someone who has a cold"	Conceives of pain primarily as physical, concrete experience Thinks in terms of magical disappearance of pain May view pain as punishment for wrongdoing Tends to hold someone accountable for own pain and may strike out at person
Concrete operational thought (7 to 10+ years)	*Contamination:* Perceives cause as a person, object, or action external to the child that is "bad" or "harmful" to the body; e.g., "getting a cold because you didn't wear a hat" *Internalization:* Perceives illness as having an external cause but as being located inside the body; e.g., "getting a cold by breathing in air and bacteria"	Conceives of pain physically; e.g., headache, stomach-ache Able to perceive psychologic pain; e.g., someone dying Fears bodily harm and annihilation (body destruction and death) May view pain as punishment for wrongdoing
Formal operational thought (13 years and older)	*Physiologic:* Perceives cause as malfunctioning or nonfunctioning organ or process; can explain illness in sequence of events *Psychophysiologic:* Realizes that psychologic actions and attitudes affect health and illness	Able to give reason for pain; e.g., fell and hit nerve Perceives several types of psychologic pain Has limited life experiences to cope with pain as adult might cope despite mature understanding of pain Fears losing control during painful experience

*Data from Bibace, R., and Walsh, M.E.: Development of children's concepts of illness, Pediatrics 66(6):912-917, 1980.
†Data from Hurley, A., and Whelan, E.G.: Cognitive development and children's perception of pain, Pediatr. Nurs. 14(1):21-24, 1988.

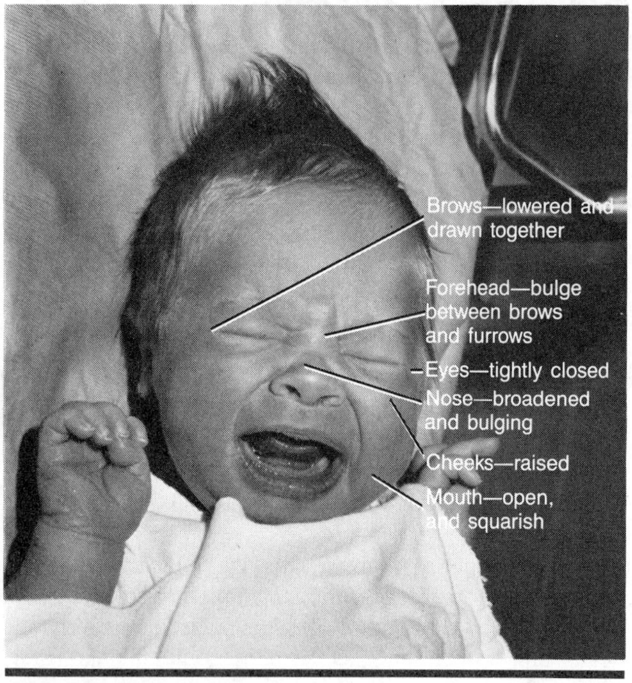

Fig. 26-3. Facial expression of physical distress is the most consistent behavioral indicator of pain in infants.

study. Some infants may cry loudly following the procedure, whereas others are easily calmed by a gentle hug. It is important to recognize and respect such early signs of individuality and to realize that children who react less intensely may still be experiencing significant discomfort (Broome and others, 1990).

Infants less than 6 months of age seem to have no memory of previous painful experiences and react to a potentially stressful situation with less apprehension and fear than older children. However, after this time, children's response to pain is influenced by their recall of prior painful experiences and the emotional reaction of parents during the procedure. Older infants react intensely with physical resistance and uncooperativeness. They may refuse to lie still, attempt to push the person away, or try to escape with whatever motor activity they have achieved. Distraction does little to lessen their immediate reaction to pain, and anticipatory preparation, such as showing them the equipment, tends to increase their fear and resistance.

Toddlers

Toddlers' concept of body image, particularly the definition of body boundaries, is very poorly developed. Intrusive experiences, such as examining the ears or mouth or taking a rectal temperature, are very anxiety producing. Toddlers may react to such painless procedures as intensely as they do to painful ones.

Toddlers' reactions to pain are similar to those seen during infancy, except that the number of variables influencing the individual response is highly complex and varied. Memory, physical restraint, parent separation, emotional reactions of others, and lack of preparation partially determine the intensity of the behavioral response. In general, children in this age-group continue to react with intense emotional upset and physical resistance to any actual or perceived painful experience. Behaviors indicating pain include grimacing, clenching their teeth/lips, opening their eyes wide, rocking, rubbing, and aggressiveness, such as biting, kicking, hitting, or running away. Unlike adults, who usually decrease their activity when in pain, young children typically become restless and overly active; frequently this response is not recognized as a consequence of pain.

By the end of this age period, toddlers usually are able to communicate about their pain. Although they have not developed the ability to describe the type or intensity of the pain, they usually are able to localize it by pointing to a specific area.

Preschoolers

Concepts of illness begin during the preschool period and are influenced by the cognitive abilities of the preoperational stage. Preschoolers differentiate poorly between themselves and the external world. Their thinking is focused on externally perceived events, and causality is based on the proximity of two events. Consequently, children define illness according to what they are told or are given external evidence of, such as, "You are sick because you have a fever." The cause of illness is seen as a concrete action the child does or fails to do, such as, "Catching a cold because you go out into cold weather" (Perrin and Gerrity, 1981); consequently, it implies a degree of responsibility and self-blame. Another explanation may be based on contagion, that the proximity of two objects or persons causes the illness; for example, "A person gets a cold when someone else with a cold gets near him" (Bibace and Walsh, 1980).

The psychosexual conflicts of children in this age-group make them very vulnerable to threats of bodily injury. Intrusive procedures, whether painful or painless, are threatening to preschoolers, whose concept of body integrity is still poorly developed. Preschoolers may react to an injection with as much concern for withdrawal of the needle as for the actual pain. They fear that the intrusion or puncture will not reclose and that their "insides" will leak out.

Concerns of mutilation are paramount during this age period. Loss of any body part is threatening, but preschool boys' fears of castration complicate their understanding of surgical or medical procedures associated with the genital area, such as circumcision, repair of hypospadias or epispadias, cystoscopy, or catheterization. Their limited comprehension of body functioning also increases their difficulty in understanding how or why body parts are "fixed." For example, telling preschoolers that their tonsils are to be removed may be interpreted as "taking out their voice," or having the penis "fixed" may be understood as cutting it off. Words such as "dye," "cut off," "take out," or "draw" (e.g., "draw some blood") are understood literally and can lead to confusion and fear.

Reactions to pain tend to be similar to those seen during toddlerhood, although some differences become apparent. For example, preschoolers respond more favorably to preparatory interventions, such as explanation and distraction, than younger children. Physical and verbal aggression are more specific and goal directed. Instead of showing total body resistance, preschoolers may push the offending person away, try to secure the equipment, or attempt to lock themselves in a safe place. Much more thought is evident in their plan of attack or escape.

Verbal expression in particular demonstrates their advanced development in response to stress. They may verbally abuse the attacker by stating, "Get out of here" or "I hate you." They may also use the more cunning approach of trying to persuade the person to give up the intended activity. A common plea is, "Please don't give me a shot; I'll be good." Some statements are not only attempts to avoid the event but also evidence of children's perceptions about the experience.

Attempts to be comforted may also be evident through behaviors such as clinging to a parent, wanting to be held, or refusing to be left alone. A typical expression denoting the need for dependency is, "Help me." It is important to recognize such requests as the need for support from others during a time of stress. Admonishing children to act grown-up or encouraging them to do things by stating, "I know you can do it yourself," deprives them of the support they are requesting and increases their own feelings of guilt and shame.

School-Age Children

Fears of the physical nature of the illness surface at this time. School-age children may be less concerned with pain than with disability, uncertain recovery, or possible death. Girls tend to express more and stronger fears than boys, and previous hospitalizations may have no effect on the frequency or intensity of these fears (Aho and Erickson, 1985). Because of their developing cognitive abilities, school-age children are aware of the significance of different illnesses, the indispensability of certain body parts, potential hazards in treatments, lifelong consequences of permanent injury or loss of function, and the meaning of death. A major concern of hospitalized school-age children is their fear of not being well again (May and Sparks, 1983). They generally take a very active interest in their health or illness. Even those children who rarely ask questions usually reveal detailed knowledge of their condition by attentively listening to all that is said around them. They request factual information and quickly perceive lies or half-truths. Seeking information tends to be one way of their maintaining a sense of control despite the stress and uncertainty of illness.

The school-age child defines illness by a set of multiple concrete symptoms, such as signs of a cold, and views the cause as primarily germs or bacteria. The germs have a powerful, almost magical quality, so that in the child's mind, illness can be prevented by avoiding people with the germs (Perrin and Gerrity, 1981). There is also the idea of contamination, which is similar to that seen in the younger age-group; for example, the illness occurs because of physical contact or because the child engaged in a harmful action and became contaminated (Bibace and Walsh, 1980). Consequently, feelings of self-blame and guilt may be associated with the reason for becoming ill (Wood, 1983).

School-age children begin to show concern for the potential beneficial and hazardous effects of procedures. Besides wanting to know if a procedure will hurt, they want to know what it is for, how it will make them better, and what injury or harm could result. For example, these children fear the actual procedure of anesthesia. Unlike preschoolers who fear the mask and the strange surroundings, school-age children fear what may happen while they are asleep, whether they will wake up, and if they may die. Preadolescents also worry about the procedure itself, particularly one that will result in visible changes in body appearance.

Intrusive procedures of a nonsexual nature, such as routine physical examination of the ears, nose, mouth, and throat, are generally well tolerated. However, concerns for privacy become evident and increasingly significant. Although school-age children may be cooperative during examination of, or procedures performed on, the genital area, it is usually very stressful for them, especially for preadolescents who are beginning pubertal changes. Nurses who respect children's need for privacy can provide them with much assurance and support.

By the age of 9 or 10, most school-age children show less fright or overt resistance to pain than younger children. They generally have learned passive methods of dealing with discomfort, such as holding rigidly still, clenching their fists or teeth, or trying to act brave by the "grin-and-bear-it" routine. If they do display signs of overt resistance, such as biting, kicking, pulling away, trying to escape, crying, or plea bargaining, they may deny such reactions later, especially to their peers for fear of embarrassment.

School-age children verbally communicate about their pain in respect to its location, intensity, and description. Unlike younger children, who may have difficulty choosing words to describe pain, children 8 years and older use a wide variety of words and phrases, such as hurting, sore, burning, stinging, aching, and "like a sharp knife" (Tesler and others, 1989).

School-age children also use words as a means of controlling their reactions to pain. For example, these children may ask the nurse to talk to them during a procedure. Some prefer to participate in a procedure, whereas others choose to distance themselves by not looking at what is happening. Most appreciate an explanation of the procedure and seem less fearful when they know what to expect. Others try to gain control by attempting to postpone the event. A typical request is, "Give me the shot when I am finished with this." Although the ability to make decisions does increase their sense of control, unlimited procrastination results in heightened anxiety. When choices are allowed, such as selection of the injection site, it is best to structure the number of possible sites and to limit the number of "procrastination" techniques.

Similar to their more passive acceptance of pain is their nondirective request for support or help. School-age children will rarely initiate a conversation about their feelings or request someone to stay with them during a lonely or stressful period. Their visible composure, calmness, and acceptance often mask their inner longing for support. It is especially important to be aware of nonverbal clues, such as a serious facial expression, a halfhearted reply of "I am fine," silence, lack of activity, or social isolation, as signs of the need for help. Usually when someone identifies the unspoken messages and offers support, they readily accept it.

Adolescents

Although the development of body image begins at birth, its relevance is paramount during adolescence. Injury, pain, disability, and death are viewed primarily in terms of how each affects adolescents' views of themselves in the present. Any change that differentiates the adolescent from peers is regarded as a major tragedy. For example, diseases such as diabetes mellitus often present a more difficult adjustment period for children in this age-group than for younger children because of the necessary changes in the adolescent's life-style. Conversely, serious, even life-threatening illnesses that entail no visible body changes or physical restrictions may have less immediate significance for the adolescent. Therefore the nature of bodily injury may be more important in terms of adolescents' perception of the illness than its actual degree of severity.

Adolescents' rapidly changing body image during pubertal development often makes them feel insecure about their bodies. Illness, medical or surgical intervention, and hospitalization increase their existing concerns for normalcy. They may respond to such events by asking numerous questions, withdrawing, rejecting others, or questioning the adequacy of care. Frequently their fear for loss of control and body image change is demonstrated as overconfidence, conceit, or a "know-it-all" attitude.

Because of sexual changes, adolescents are very concerned about privacy. Lack of respect for this need can cause greater stress than physical pain. In addition, adolescents look for signs that indicate that they are developing normally and according to acceptable standards. When illness occurs, they fear that growth may be retarded, leaving them behind their peers. Although they may not voice this concern, they may demonstrate it by carefully observing others' reactions to them.

Adolescents react to pain with much self-control. Physical resistance and aggression are unusual at this age, unless the adolescents are totally unprepared for a procedure. As with older school-age children, they are very concerned with remaining composed and feel embarrassed and ashamed of losing control. They are able to describe their pain experience and to use any of the pain assessment tools developed for adults. However, they may be reluctant to disclose their pain unless the nurse is willing to listen closely and observe physical indications, such as limited movement, excessive quiet, or irritability. They may also believe that the nurse knows how they feel; thus they may see no need to ask for analgesia (Favaloro and Touzel, 1990).

SUBSEQUENT EFFECTS OF HOSPITALIZATION

Children not only react to the stresses of illness and hospitalization during admission but may demonstrate temporary behavioral changes following discharge, especially children under 4 years of age (Box 26-2). These effects result from (1) separation from significant people, (2) a lack of opportunity to form new attachments, and (3) a strange environment.

Box 26-2 POSTHOSPITAL BEHAVIORS IN CHILDREN

Young Children

Some initial aloofness toward parents; may last from a few minutes (most common) to a few days

Frequently followed by dependency behaviors:
- Tendency to cling to parents
- Demand parents' attention
- Vigorously oppose any separation (e.g., staying at nursery school or with a baby-sitter)

Other negative behaviors include:
- New fears (e.g., nightmares)
- Resistance to going to bed, night waking
- Withdrawal and shyness
- Hyperactivity
- Temper tantrums
- Food finickiness
- Attachment to blanket or toy
- Regression in newly learned skills (e.g., self-toileting)

Older Children

Negative behaviors include:
- Emotional coldness, followed by intense, demanding dependence on parents
- Anger toward parents
- Jealousy toward others (e.g., siblings)

Previous studies done on hospitalization and development of subsequent long-term emotional disturbance have found that *repeated* hospital admissions and a single hospitalization of *4 weeks or more* were significantly associated with later disturbances. Children from disadvantaged homes were more at risk for developing emotional problems than children from nondisadvantaged homes. However, more recent reviews of the relationship between duration of hospital stay in preschool years and behavior at age 6 years does not completely support these findings. Shannon, Fergusson, and Dimond (1984) found no significant association between duration of hospitalization and children's behavior problems when family and social factors were controlled. The authors propose that the changes in pediatric hospital care currently, as compared to the stricter practices in the 1940s and 1950s, may account for the differences in subsequent behavior of children who are hospitalized during their preschool years.

■ STRESSORS AND REACTIONS OF THE FAMILY OF THE HOSPITALIZED CHILD

The crisis of childhood illness and hospitalization affects every member of the nuclear family and, to varying degrees, members of the extended family. The stressors and reactions of families have been discussed in detail in Chapter

22 in relation to chronic illness and in Chapter 23 in relation to life-threatening illness. In many respects they differ little regardless of the diagnosis except for their intensity and persistence, which are proportional to the degree of severity of the illness. Consequently, when a child is admitted to an intensive care facility, the family members' reactions and needs are typically greater than when a child is admitted with a less serious condition to the regular pediatric unit. The following discussion briefly reviews the common reactions of the family; specific reactions during intensive care admissions are discussed on p. 1174.

PARENTAL REACTIONS

Parents' reactions to illness in their child depend on a variety of influencing factors. Although one cannot predict which factors are most likely to influence their response, a number of variables have been identified (Box 26-3).

Almost all parents respond to their child's illness and hospitalization with remarkably consistent reactions. Initially parents may react with *disbelief*, especially if the illness is sudden and serious. Following the realization of illness, parents react with *anger, guilt*, or both. They tend to search for self-blame regarding why the child became ill or to project anger at others for some wrongdoing. Even in the mildest of illnesses, parents question their adequacy as caregivers and review any actions or omissions that could have prevented or caused the illness. When hospitalization is indicated, parental guilt is intensified because they feel helpless in alleviating the child's physical and emotional pain.

Fear, anxiety, and *frustration* are common feelings expressed by parents. Fear and anxiety may be related to the seriousness of the illness and the type of medical procedures involved. Often a great deal of anxiety is related to the trauma and pain inflicted on the child because of the various procedures. Feelings of frustration are often related to lack of information about procedures and treatments, unfamiliarity with hospital rules and regulations, a sense of unwelcomeness from the staff, or fear of asking questions. Much frustration can be alleviated in a pediatric unit where parents participate in their child's care and are regarded as the most significant contributors to the child's total health.

Parents eventually may react with some degree of *depression*. The depression usually occurs when the acute crisis is over, such as following hospital discharge or complete recovery. Mothers often comment on their feeling of physical and mental exhaustion after all the other family members have adapted to the crisis. Other reasons for anxiety and depression are related to concerns for the child's future well-being, including negative effects produced by the hospitalization and any subsequent financial burden incurred from the hospitalization.

Box 26-3 FACTORS AFFECTING PARENTS' REACTIONS TO THEIR CHILD'S ILLNESS

Seriousness of the threat to the child
Previous experience with illness or hospitalization
Medical procedures involved in diagnosis and treatment
Available support systems
Personal ego strengths
Previous coping abilities
Additional stresses on the family system
Cultural and religious beliefs
Communication patterns among family members

SIBLING REACTIONS

Siblings' reactions to a sister's or brother's illness or hospitalization are discussed in Chapters 22 and 23 and differ little when a child becomes temporarily ill. Their main reactions are anger, resentment, jealousy, and guilt. Various factors have been identified that influence the effects of the child's hospitalization on siblings. Although these factors are similar to those seen when a child has a chronic illness, the following are related specifically to the hospital experience and were found to *increase* the effects on the siblings (Craft, Wyatt, and Sandell, 1985):

- Fear of contracting the illness
- Younger age
- Close relationship to sick sibling
- Out-of-home residence during period of hospitalization
- Minimum explanation of the sick child's illness
- Perceived changes in parenting, such as increased parental anger

Parents are often unaware of the number of effects that siblings experience during the sick child's hospitalization and of the benefit of simple interventions to minimize such effects, such as explicit explanations about the illness and provisions for the siblings to remain at home. Although sibling visitation is advocated and is probably advantageous, effects on siblings who do visit the sick child are still evident but may be different. Those who do not visit may experience more difficulty concentrating in school, feelings of being less healthy, and nail biting, while those who visit are more likely to become angry (Craft and Wyatt, 1986).

NURSING CARE OF THE HOSPITALIZED CHILD AND THE FAMILY

Children and their families require competent and sensitive care to minimize the potential negative effects of hospitalization and also to promote positive benefits from the experience. Interventions should focus on (1) eliminating or minimizing the stressors of separation, loss of control, and bodily injury and pain for children (see Nursing Care Plan: The Child in the Hospital, pp. 1136 to 1140); and (2) providing specific supportive strategies for family members, such as fostering family relationships and providing information (see Nursing Care Plan: The Family of the Ill or Hospitalized Child, pp. 1163 to 1166).

NURSING CARE PLAN
The Child in the Hospital

NURSING DIAGNOSIS: Anxiety/fear related to separation from accustomed routine and support system; unfamiliar surroundings

GOAL 1
Prevent or minimize separation

INTERVENTIONS
Provide consistency of nursing personnel as much as possible; assign a primary nurse
Arrange workload and schedule to allow personal contact with the child
Encourage parents to room-in whenever possible
Provide an atmosphere of warmth and acceptance for both child and parents
Encourage parents and others to cuddle, fondle, and otherwise demonstrate affection for the child
Recognize the child's separation behaviors as normal
- Allow the child to cry
- Provide support through physical presence

Maintain the child's contact with parents and siblings
- Talk about the child's parents frequently
- Encourage the child to talk about and remember parents
- Stress the significance of the parents' visits, telephone calls, or letters

Help the parents understand the behaviors of separation anxiety and suggest ways of supporting the child
- Explain to the child when they leave and when they will return
- Tell the hospitalized child the reason for leaving
- Convey the expected time of return in terms of anticipated events. For example, if the parents will return in the morning, they can say they will see the child, "After the sun comes up," or, "When (a favorite program) is on television"
- Use a clock or calendar for an older child
- Visit for short but frequent times rather than one long time; encourage parents and relatives to take turns visiting
- Allow siblings to visit
- Leave favorite home articles, such as a blanket, toy, bottle, feeding utensil, or article of clothing, with the child
- Respect treasured objects or older objects of older children, such as a stuffed animal
- Encourage the family to provide photographs of family members and tape recordings of the parents' voices, such as reading a story, singing a song, saying prayers before bedtime, or relating events at home

Play family tape recordings at lonely times, such as before sleep
Encourage the child to talk about family members
Suggest that the family leave small gifts for the child to open each day; if the parents know when their next visit will be, have them leave the number of packages that correspond to the days between visits
Assign a "foster grandparent" or consistent volunteer to be with the child if available

EXPECTED OUTCOMES
Child has consistent caregivers
Parents visit as much as possible
Parents cooperate in care (specify)
Child accepts and responds positively to comforting measures
Child discusses the family, including pets
Parents demonstrate an understanding of separation behaviors
Siblings visit as much as possible
Family provides the child with familiar and/or cherished articles from home
Assigned person spends time with the child (specify amount)

GOAL 2
Allow expression of feelings

INTERVENTIONS
Accept expression of feelings
Provide an atmosphere that encourages free expression of feelings
Provide opportunities for the child to verbalize, "play out," or otherwise express feelings without fear of punishment

EXPECTED OUTCOME
Child verbalizes or plays out feelings or concerns

GOAL 3
Keep the child calm

INTERVENTIONS
Do nothing to make the child more anxious
Maintain calm, relaxed, and reassuring manner
Establish rapport with the child and parents
Instill confidence in both parents and child
Try to avoid intrusive procedures

EXPECTED OUTCOMES
Child exhibits no signs of apprehension
Parents relate readily with personnel and calmly with child
Child rests quietly and calmly

GOAL 4
Establish a trusting relationship with the child

INTERVENTIONS
Be positive in approach to the child
Be honest with the child
Convey to the child the behaviors expected
Be consistent in expectations and relationships with the child
Treat the child fairly and help the child to feel this
Encourage parents to maintain a truthful relationship with the child
Make certain the child has call light or other signal device within reach

EXPECTED OUTCOMES
Child develops rapport with primary nurse
Child maintains trust of family

GOAL 5
Help the child to feel cared for as a person

INTERVENTIONS

Maintain the child's identity
- Address the child by name or usual nickname
- Avoid assigning a nickname to the child or converting a given name to its counterpart in another language (e.g., using Joe instead of José)

Avoid communicating any signals of rejection, distaste, or other negative feelings to the child
Criticize or communicate disapproval of unacceptable *behavior,* not disapproval of the *child*
Communicate (verbally and nonverbally) that the child is a valued person

EXPECTED OUTCOMES

Child interacts with staff
*Staff demonstrates respect for the child

GOAL 6

Reduce or alleviate fear of the unknown

INTERVENTIONS

Explain routines, items, procedures, and events in a language appropriate to the child's developmental level; use simple language
Reassure the child and repeat reassurance as necessary
Absolve the child from any guilt about being hospitalized
Allow the parent(s) to participate in the child's care
Allow the child to handle items that may seem strange or threatening
Give encouragement and positive feedback for cooperation in care

EXPECTED OUTCOMES

Child exhibits understanding of information presented (specify information and means of demonstration)
Child discusses procedures and activities without evidence of anxiety

GOAL 7

Allow for regression during periods of illness

INTERVENTIONS

Recognize that regressive behavior is a feature of illness
Accept regressive behavior and help the child with dependency
Assist the child in reconquering the negative counterpart of the psychosocial stage to which child has regressed (e.g., overcome mistrust; facilitate development of trust)

EXPECTED OUTCOME

*Staff and parents exhibit an attitude of acceptance of regressive behaviors

GOAL 8

Provide comfort measures

INTERVENTIONS

Provide pacifier to meet oral needs, if appropriate
Hold infant or young child when this does not interfere with therapy
Touch, talk, and otherwise comfort child who cannot be held
Provide sensory stimulation and diversion appropriate to child's level of development
Encourage family members to visit and allow them to comfort and care for child to the extent possible

EXPECTED OUTCOMES

Child engages in nonnutritive sucking
Child exhibits no signs of distress
Family is involved in care

NURSING DIAGNOSIS: Anxiety/fear related to distressing procedures, events

GOAL 1

Prepare for hospitalization

INTERVENTIONS

Prepare the child as needed
Select appropriate preparatory materials
Involve the parents
Modify preparation in special situations (e.g., day hospital, emergency admission, ICU)

EXPECTED OUTCOME

Child is prepared for hospital experience

GOAL 2

Decrease fear of bodily injury

INTERVENTIONS

Recognize developmental fears associated with illness and procedures
Provide age-appropriate explanations for procedures, especially those that are intrusive or involve the genitals
Reassure the child that certain body parts can be removed without producing harm (e.g., blood, tonsils, appendix)
Provide privacy for any procedure that exposes the body
Protect the child from seeing unclothed patients
Use interventions that preserve the child's concept of body integrity (e.g., bandages over puncture sites)

EXPECTED OUTCOME

Child displays minimum fear of bodily injury

GOAL 3

Support the child during tests and procedures

INTERVENTIONS

Prepare the child for procedures according to age and level of understanding (see Chapter 27)
Remain with the child
Prepare the child and family for surgery if prescribed
Answer questions and explain purposes of activities
Keep informed of progress

EXPECTED OUTCOME

Child remains calm and cooperative during procedures

*Nursing outcome.

Continued.

NURSING CARE PLAN
The Child in the Hospital—cont'd

NURSING DIAGNOSIS: Powerlessness related to the health care environment

GOAL 1
Modify the hospital environment to resemble home

INTERVENTIONS
Determine from the parents or other caregiver the child's customary routine and manner of handling (see Box 26-15)
Maintain a routine similar to the one the child is accustomed to at home
Minimize a hospital-like environment as much as possible; allow the child to sit at table to eat meals, wear own pajamas or street clothes
Use terms familiar to the child, such as those for body functions

EXPECTED OUTCOME
Child's routines and environment are similar to those at home (specify)

GOAL 2
Provide opportunities for acceptable control

INTERVENTIONS
Allow the child choices whenever possible, such as food selection, clothing, options for time of basic care (bath, play, bedtime), selection of television channels
Use time structuring with an older child, a jointly planned and written schedule of daily activities
Permit freedom on the unit within defined and enforced limitations
Limit use of restraints
Encourage self-care according to the child's abilities
Assign tasks to an older child, especially in extended hospitalization (e.g., making the bed, supervising younger children, distributing menus, collating charts)
Respect the child's need for privacy

EXPECTED OUTCOMES
Child participates in planning care (specify)
Child moves about the unit but respects limits
Child participates in care activities (specify activities)
Child assumes responsibility for tasks (specify)
*Child's need for privacy is maintained

NURSING DIAGNOSIS: Diversional activity deficit related to impaired mobility, musculoskeletal impairment, confinement to hospital or home, effects of illness

GOAL 1
Provide opportunity for activities

INTERVENTIONS
Schedule therapies and periods of rest to allow for activities
Involve the child in planning care to the extent of capabilities
Arrange for and encourage interaction with others as feasible
Encourage visits from family and friends
Provide opportunity to socialize with noninfectious children

EXPECTED OUTCOMES
Child helps plan care and schedule
Child interacts with family and other children

GOAL 2
Provide diversion

INTERVENTIONS
Spend time with the child
Change position of bed in room periodically to alter sensory stimuli, if the child is confined to bed
Provide activities appropriate to the child's condition, physical limitations, and developmental level
Encourage family to fondle and hold infant or child
Maintain accustomed routine at home and, when possible, if hospitalized
Provide diversional activities or consult with a child-life specialist
Encourage interaction with other children
Choose a roommate compatible in age, sex, and physical abilities
Monitor time spent watching television vs interactive or creative activities
Allow ample time for play
Make play materials available to the child
Encourage play activities and diversions appropriate to the child's age, condition, and capabilities
Use play as a teaching strategy and an anxiety-reducing technique

EXPECTED OUTCOMES
Child engages in activities appropriate for age, interests, and physical limitations (specify activities)
Child receives attention and comfort
Child engages in age-appropriate play (specify)

*Nursing outcome.

NURSING CARE PLAN
The Child in the Hospital—cont'd

NURSING DIAGNOSIS: Activity intolerance related to generalized weakness, fatigue, imbalance between oxygen supply and demand

GOAL 1
Conserve energy

INTERVENTIONS
Assess the child's level of physical tolerance
Anticipate the child's need, as evidenced by irritability, short attention span, and fretfulness; assist the child in those activities of daily living that may be beyond tolerance
Provide entertainment and quiet diversional activities appropriate to the child's age and interest
Provide diversional play activities that promote rest and quiet but prevent boredom and withdrawal
Choose an appropriate roommate of similar age and interests and one who requires restricted activity
Instruct child to rest when feeling tired
Balance rest and activity when ambulatory

EXPECTED OUTCOMES
Child plays and rests quietly and engages in activities appropriate to age and capabilities (specify)
Child exhibits no evidence of intolerance
Child tolerates increasingly more activity

GOAL 2
Promote rest

INTERVENTIONS
Provide quiet environment
Organize activities for maximum sleep time
Schedule visiting to allow for sufficient rest
Keep visiting periods with friends and family short
Encourage parents to remain with child
*Administer sedatives and analgesics as indicated if ordered for restlessness and pain
Encourage frequent rest periods
Enforce regular sleep times
Implement measures to ensure sleep, such as quiet, darkened room

EXPECTED OUTCOMES
Child remains calm, quiet, and relaxed
Child gets a sufficient amount of rest (specify)

*Dependent nursing activity.

NURSING DIAGNOSIS: Potential for injury/trauma related to unfamiliar environment, therapies, hazardous equipment

GOAL 1
Promote safety

INTERVENTIONS
Employ environmental safety measures
Report any potential hazards (e.g., slippery floors, poor illumination, electrical hazards, damaged or malfunctioning furniture or equipment, unprotected windows, stairwells)
Dispose of small breakable items appropriately (thermometers, bottles)
Keep potentially hazardous articles out of the child's reach
Check bath water for temperature before bathing infant or child
Maintain surveillance of children in bathtubs
Keep crib sides up and securely fastened, siderails on children who may fall out of bed; use safety restraints when applicable
Maintain hand contact while caring for a child in a crib with siderails down
Transport infants and children appropriately
  Held with proper support
  Fasten safety belt on gurney, wheelchair
Alert ancillary hospital personnel regarding the child's physical tolerance and need for assistance during activity

EXPECTED OUTCOME
Child remains free of injury

GOAL 2
Prevent complications from restraining devices, if used

INTERVENTIONS
Remove restraints from extremities as often as possible
Change position at least every 2 hours
Frequently observe circulation, position, and pressure points

EXPECTED OUTCOME
Extremities remain free of constriction and pressure

Continued.

NURSING CARE PLAN
The Child in the Hospital—cont'd

NURSING DIAGNOSIS: Bathing/hygiene and dressing/grooming self-care deficit related to physical or cognitive disability, mechanical restrictions

GOAL 1

Promote self-help

INTERVENTIONS

Assist with bathing
Allow the child to help plan own daily routine and choose from alternatives when appropriate
Encourage participation in self-care activities according to developmental level and capabilities
Provide devices, equipment, and methods to assist the child in self-care
Assist with dressing, grooming

EXPECTED OUTCOME

Child engages in self-help activities to maximum capabilities

NURSING DIAGNOSIS: Toileting self-care deficit related to physical or cognitive disability, mechanical restrictions

GOAL 1

Facilitate elimination

INTERVENTIONS

Sit in upright position when possible
Employ special devices where appropriate (e.g., fracture pan, commode, elevated toilet seat); modify utensils when indicated
Carry out bowel training program with hydration, high-fiber diet, stool softeners, and mild laxatives if needed
Provide privacy

EXPECTED OUTCOME

Child has daily bowel movement

NURSING DIAGNOSIS: Altered patterns of urinary elimination related to discomfort, positioning

GOAL 1

Stimulate voiding

INTERVENTIONS

Position as upright as possible to void
Hydrate to adequate urinary output for age
Stimulate bladder emptying with warm water, running water, stroking suprapubic area
Catheterize as indicated

EXPECTED OUTCOME

Child voids without difficulty

See also:
Nursing Care Plan: The Child with a Chronic Illness or Disability, Chapter 22
Nursing Care Plan: The Child Undergoing Surgery, Chapter 27
Nursing Care Plan: The Child in Pain, p. 1158
Nursing Care Plan: The Child Who Is Terminally Ill or Dying, Chapter 23
Nursing Care Plan for specific health problem(s)

PREVENTING OR MINIMIZING SEPARATION

The primary nursing goal is to prevent separation, particularly in children under 5 years of age. However, this is not always possible, and measures to minimize the effects of separation must be implemented. The importance of a primary nurse for the child cannot be overemphasized. There is no substitute for the consistency provided by primary nursing and its advantages for the child and family.

Parent Participation and "Rooming-In"

Prevention of separation requires rooming-in facilities in pediatric hospital settings. Although some health facilities provide special accommodations for parents, the concept of "rooming-in" can be instituted anywhere. The first requirement is the staff's positive attitude toward parents. When hospital staff genuinely appreciate the importance of continued parent-child attachment, they foster an environment that encourages parents to stay. When parents are included in the care planning and made to feel as if they are a contributing factor to the child's recovery, they are more inclined to remain with their child and have more emotional reserves to support themselves and the child through the crisis.

Since the mother tends to be the usual family caregiver, she spends more time in the hospital than the father. However, not all mothers feel equally comfortable in assuming responsibility for their child's care. Some may be under such great emotional stress that they need a temporary reprieve from total participation in caregiving activities. Others may feel insecure in participating in specialized areas of care, such as bathing the child after surgery. Individual assessment of each parent's preferred involvement is necessary to prevent the effects of separation while supporting parents in their needs as well (Stull and Deatrick, 1986).

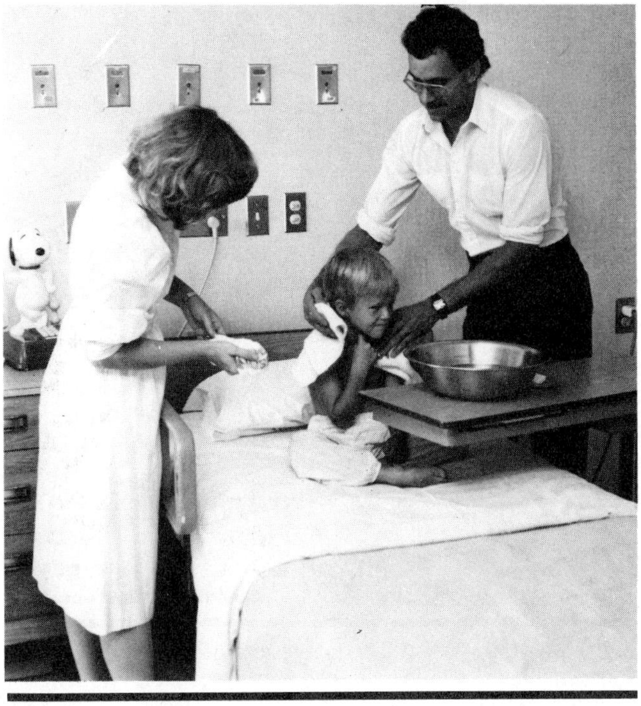

Fig. 26-4. Parents are encouraged to participate in their child's care to the extent that they feel comfortable.

Both underinvolvement and overinvolvement of parents in the child's care can be detrimental; therefore every effort is extended to help parents identify moderate amounts of visiting and participation (O'Donnell as cited in Thompson, 1985) (Fig. 26-4).

With life-styles and sexual roles changing, some fathers may assume all or some of the usual mothering roles in the household. In this case it may be the father-child relationship that requires preservation. Fathers need to be included in the plan of care and respected for their parental role. For some fathers the child's hospitalization may represent an opportunity to alter their usual caregiving role and increase their involvement (Knafl and Dixon, 1984). It is equally important to support the mother's role as family provider or parttime housekeeper in order to meet each parent's needs. In single-parent families the caregiver may not be a parent but an extended family member, such as a grandparent or aunt.

One of the potential problems with continuous parent visiting is neglect of the parent's need for sleep, nutrition, and relaxation. Often the sleeping accommodations are limited to a chair and sleep is disrupted by nursing procedures. After a few days parents can become exhausted but feel obligated to stay. Encouraging them to leave for brief periods, arranging for sleeping quarters on the unit but outside the child's room, and planning a schedule of alternating visiting with the other parent or with a family member can minimize the stresses for the parent (see Nursing Tip).

All too often nurses respond to parental participation by abandoning their patient responsibilities. Nurses need to restructure their roles to complement and augment the caregiving functions of parents. Even in units structured to provide care by parents, parents frequently feel anxiety in their caregiving responsibilities; those more involved in direct care may feel more anxiety than those less involved in direct care. Therefore 24-hour responsibility may be too much for some parents (Monahan and Schkade, 1985). Assistance and relief by nursing personnel should always be available to these families.

NURSING TIP: PARENT "BEEPERS"

If parents are reluctant to leave the hospital (usually for fear of not being there when the child awakens or the physician visits), try to arrange for them to have a remote "beeper" that can provide immediate communication regardless of their location.

Strategies to Minimize the Effects of Separation

When separation cannot be prevented, numerous strategies can be employed to minimize the effects of temporary separation on children. Ideally a primary nurse is assigned to meet the child's needs. Becoming a surrogate parent requires a thorough, detailed nursing history that specifically identifies the child's established daily routine. Usual daily activities such as food preparation and method of feeding help establish a complementary schedule of caregiving practices. It also helps the parent feel as if he or she is participating in the child's care but through another person. A nursing admission history for children is outlined in Box 26-15.

The nurse caring for the child must have an appreciation of the child's separation behaviors. As discussed earlier, the phases of protest and despair are normal. The child is allowed to cry. Even if the child rejects strangers, the nurse provides support through physical presence in the room. The nurse may say, "I know you are unhappy because you miss your mommy and daddy. It's all right to cry. I will sit here for awhile so you are not alone." This reinforces for children the nurse's awareness of their feelings without abandoning them. If detachment behaviors are evident, the nurse maintains the child's contact with the parents by frequently talking about them, encouraging the child to remember them, and stressing the significance of their visits, telephone calls, or letters.

Separation may be equally as difficult for parents, especially when they do not understand the behaviors of separation anxiety. To avoid the immediate protest, parents may sneak out or lie to the child about leaving. As a result, the child does not learn that absence is associated with a guaranteed return but that absence means loss of parents. Helping parents recognize that separation behaviors are normal and expected can decrease their anxiety and may ease their fears about leaving without telling the child. Explaining to parents how the child reacts after they leave may also be helpful. Many parents think the child cries for hours after they leave, whereas in reality the child may cry for a few minutes but settle down when comforted by someone else.

Toddlers and preschoolers have a very limited concept of time. The young child's question, "Will my mommy come yesterday?" symbolizes a lack of understanding for usual measurements of time, such as days, hours, and weeks. Time is measured in associations, such as, "Eating dinner when daddy comes home." Therefore, when helping parents with their fears of separation, nurses need to suggest ways of explaining leaving and returning. For example, if parents must leave to go to work or to make meals for the other family members, they should tell the hospitalized child the reason for leaving. They also need to convey the expected time of return in terms of anticipated events. For example, if the parents return in the morning, they can tell the child that they will see him or her "After the sun comes up" or "When [a favorite program] is on television."

The young child's ability to tolerate parental absence is very limited. Therefore parental visits should be frequent. For example, it is better for parents to visit three times a day for short periods than once a day for an extended time. This may necessitate that each parent visit at different times to lessen the length of separation. When parents cannot visit, the presence of other significant people can be comforting for the child (Fig. 26-5).

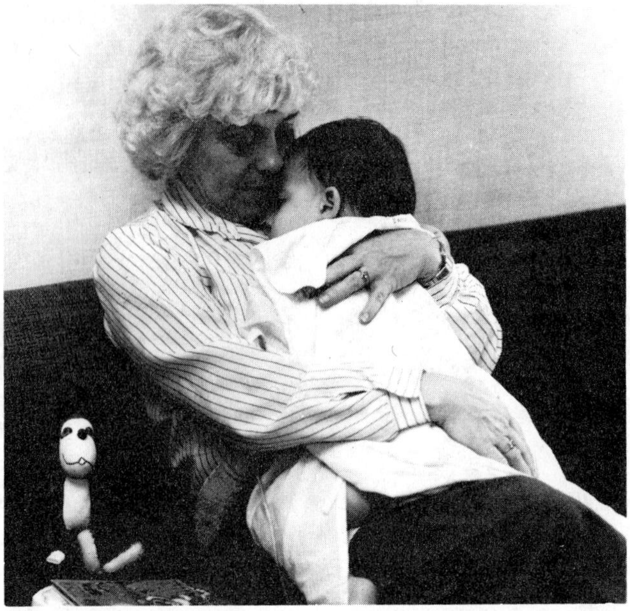

Fig. 26-5. When parents cannot visit, other significant persons, such as a grandparent, can provide comfort to the hospitalized child.

If parents leave after the child is asleep, they still need to communicate their absence. The parents of a 5-year-old boy solved this problem by devising a sign; on one side they drew a picture of a telephone and on the other a hamburger. Before they left, they turned the sign to the appropriate side to tell the child when he awoke that they were out using the telephone or eating.

For older children who know how to tell time, it is helpful to give them a clock or watch. However, these children have the same needs for honesty from their parents regarding visiting schedules. Because peer groups are also important, adolescents often appreciate planning visiting hours with their parents to provide them with some private time for friends.

Familiar surroundings also increase the child's adjustment to separation. If parents cannot room-in, they should leave favorite home articles with the child, such as a blanket, toy, bottle, feeding utensil, or article of clothing. Since young children associate such inanimate objects with significant people, they gain comfort and reassurance from such possessions. They make the association that if the parent left this, the parent will surely return. Placing an identification band on the toy lessens the chances of its being misplaced and provides a symbol that the toy is experiencing the same needs as the child. Other momentos of home include photographs and tape recordings of family members' reading a story, singing a song, saying prayers before bedtime, relating events at home, or taking a "talking walk" through the home. The tapes can be played at lonely times, such as on awakening or before sleeping (McCain, 1982). Some units allow pets to visit, which can be a special event for a child and can have therapeutic benefits (Davis, 1985).

Older children also appreciate familiar articles from home, particularly photographs, a radio, a favorite toy or game, and the usual pajamas. Often the importance of treasured objects for school-age children is overlooked or criticized. However, it is reported that about half of school-age children have a special object to which they formed an attachment in early childhood and that this is a normal and healthy phenomenon (Sherman and others, 1981). Therefore such treasured or transitional objects can help even older children feel more comfortable in a strange environment.

Helping children maintain their usual nonhome contacts also minimizes the effects of separation imposed by hospitalization. This includes continuing school lessons during the illness and confinement, visiting with friends either directly or through letter writing or telephone calls, and participating in extracurricular projects whenever possible.

For extended hospitalizations, youngsters enjoy personalizing the hospital room to make it "home" by decorating the walls with posters and cards, rearranging the furniture (when possible), and displaying a collection or hobby. Growing plants can also be a constructive activity because it gives the child something to care for (Fig. 26-6). Hardy and fast-growing plants are best, such as beans, sunflowers, and marigolds. A terrarium is useful for a child in an oxygen tent because it can be used to explain the oxygen cycle. When considering plants, the nurse needs to be aware that certain circumstances may preclude this activity, such as children with specific allergies or those who are susceptible to infections (Gough, 1986).

MINIMIZING LOSS OF CONTROL

Feelings of loss of control result from separation, physical restriction, changed routines, enforced dependency, magical thinking, and altered roles within the family or peer

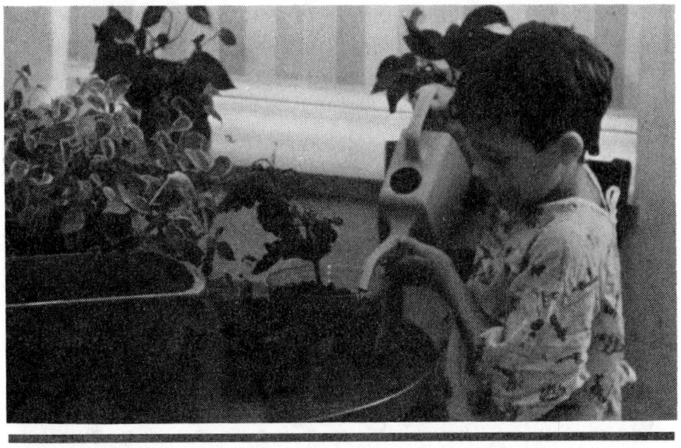

Fig. 26-6. For extended hospitalizations, school-age children enjoy having projects to occupy their time, such as caring for plants.

group. Although some of these cannot be prevented, most of them can be minimized through individualized planning of nursing care.

Physical Restriction

Younger children react most strenuously to any type of physical restriction or immobilization. Although some restraint, such as immobilizing an extremity for maintenance of an intravenous line, is frequently necessary, most physical restriction can be prevented if the nurse gains the child's cooperation.

For young children, particularly infants and toddlers, preserving parent-child contact is the best means of decreasing the need for or stress of restraint. For example, almost the entire physical examination can be done in a parent's lap, with the parent hugging the child for procedures such as otoscopy. For painful procedures the parents' preferences for assisting, observing, or waiting outside the room are assessed (see also Questions and Controversies, p. 1191).

Environmental factors also influence the need for physical restraint. Keeping children in cribs or playpens may not represent immobilization in a concrete sense, but it certainly limits sensory stimulation. Increasing mobility by transporting children in carriages, wheelchairs, carts, wagons, or on stretchers or beds provides them with mechanical freedom.

In some cases physical restraint or isolation is necessary for recovery. Whenever possible, restraints should be removed to allow the child some period of supervised freedom, such as during the bath or when parents visit. When restraints or isolation cannot be discontinued, such as in severe burns, the environment can be manipulated to increase sensory freedom. For example, moving the bed toward the door or window; opening window shades; providing musical, visual, or tactile toys; and increasing interpersonal contact can substitute mental mobility for the limitations of physical movement.

Altered Routines

Altered daily schedules and loss of rituals are particularly stressful for toddlers and early preschoolers and may increase the stress of separation. As stated previously, the nursing admission history provides a baseline for planning care around the child's usual home activities.

Children's response to loss of routine and ritualism is often demonstrated in problems with activities such as feeding, sleeping, dressing, bathing, toileting, and social interaction. Although some regression is to be expected in all these areas, sensitivity to the special needs of children can minimize the negative effects. For example, loss of appetite and marked food preferences are common in ill or hospitalized children. In addition, the food selections on hospital menus may differ greatly from preferred cultural or ethnic food preparation. Encouraging the child to eat while avoiding a battle is often a challenge, yet it is an essential nursing responsibility. Suggestions for feeding sick children are discussed in Chapter 27.

Although regression is expected and normal, nurses also have the responsibility of fostering children's optimum growth and development. Hospitalization can become a significant opportunity for learning and advancing. For example, extended hospitalization for long-term chronic illness or situations of failure to thrive, abuse, or neglect represent instances in which regression must be seen as an adjustment period, to be followed by plans for promoting appropriate developmental skills.

A frequently neglected aspect of altered routines is the change in the child's daily activities. A nonhospitalized child's day, especially during the school years, is structured with specific times for eating, dressing, going to school, playing, and sleeping. However, this time structure vanishes when the child is hospitalized. Although the nurses have a set schedule, the child is frequently unaware of it; new schedules are imposed that may be rigid or flexible. For example, some units have uniform nap and bedtimes for all children while others allow children to stay up very late. Many children obtain significantly less sleep in the hospital than at home; the primary causes are delay in sleep onset and early termination of sleep because of hospital routines (Hagemann, 1981a, 1981b). Not only are hours of sleep disrupted, but waking hours are spent in passive activities. For example, few institutions impose any regulation on the amount of time the child spends watching television. Studies show that children spend an average of 8 hours a day watching television in the hospital, which is considerably more time than that spent at home (McCain and Bies, 1983).

One technique that can minimize the disruption in the child's routine is *time structuring* (Volz, 1981). This approach is most suitable for the noncritically ill school-age and adolescent child who has mastered the concept of time. It involves scheduling the child's day to include all those activities that are important to the nurse and child, such as treatment procedures, schoolwork, exercise, television, playroom, and hobbies. Together, the nurse, parent, and child then plan a daily schedule with time and activity written down (Fig. 26-7). This is left in the child's room, and a clock or watch is available for the child's use. Whenever possible, a calendar is also constructed with special events marked, such as favorite television programs, visits by

ERIC'S DAILY SCHEDULE:

7:00 AM	Breakfast, Watch TV, Brush Teeth, Wash up	3:00 PM	Tutor (M,W,F) Study Time (T,Th)
9:00	Tub Room, Dressing Change	4:00	Physical Therapy
		5:00	Dinner
10:00	Rest, TV, Snack	6:30	Dressing Change
11:00	Physical Therapy	7:00 to 9:00	TV, Reading, Snack, Friends Visit
12:00 PM	Lunch		
1:00	Playroom, Quiet Play, Rest, Friends Visit	9:00	Brush Teeth, Wash up
		9:15	Bedtime

Fig. 26-7. Time structuring is an effective strategy for normalizing the hospital environment and increasing the child's sense of control.

friends or relatives, events in the playroom, and holidays or birthdays. If specific changes in treatment are expected (e.g., "beginning physical therapy in 2 days"), these are added.

Enforced Dependency

The dependent role of the hospitalized patient imposes tremendous feelings of loss on older children. Principal interventions should focus on respect for individuality and the opportunity for decision making. Although these sound simple, their efficacy lies with nurses who are flexible, tolerant, and personally secure. The last is particularly important because when decision making is geared toward the patient, nurses can feel threatened by a sense of lessened control.

Promoting children's control involves maintaining independence, and the concept of *self-care* can be most beneficial. Self-care refers to the practice of activities that individuals personally initiate and perform on their own behalf in maintaining life, health, and well-being (Orem, 1985). Although self-care is limited by the child's age and physical condition, most children beyond infancy can perform some activities with little or no help. Whenever possible, these activities are encouraged in the hospital. Other approaches include jointly planning care; time structuring; wearing street clothes; making choices in food selections, bedtime, and so on; continuing school activities; and rooming with an appropriate age-mate. For example, although school-age children may enjoy the responsibility of caring for a toddler or preschooler in their room, adolescents generally prefer quarters separate from the pediatric unit (see p. 1172).

Lack of Understanding

Loss of control can occur from feelings of having too little influence on one's destiny as well as from sensing overwhelming control or power over fate. Although preschoolers' cognitive abilities predispose them most to magical thinking and self-power, all children are vulnerable to misinterpreting causes for stresses such as illness and hospitalization.

Most children feel more in control when they know what to expect, because the element of fear is reduced. Anticipatory preparation and providing information help greatly to lessen stress and prevent lack of understanding (see Preparation for Procedures, Chapter 27).

Altered Family and Social Roles

In addition to the effects of separation on family roles, loss of parenting, sibling, and offspring roles may affect each family member differently. One of the most common reactions of parents is specialized and intensified attention toward the sick child. The other siblings usually regard this as unfair and interpret the parents' attitude toward them as rejection. Although such responses are usually unconscious and unintended, they place unique burdens on ill children. For example, the ill child may feel obligated to play the sick role in order to meet parents' expectations, especially children who have had limited physical ability and regain normal health status, such as following corrective heart surgery. Parents, as well, may be unable to perceive the child's recovery and therefore need to continue the pattern of overprotection and indulgent attention.

Ill children may also feel jealousy and resentment from other siblings. Because of their singular position in the family, they may be denied the companionship of their brothers and sisters. Rivalry between siblings tends to be greatest in the sibling who is nearest the ill child's age. Without an understanding of the interpersonal dynamics between siblings, parents are likely to blame the well children for antisocial behavior.

Illness may also result in children's loss of status within either their family or social group. For example, illness in the oldest child may temporarily terminate special privileges as "big" brother or sister. The hospitalized adolescent loses rank within the peer group. The effects of such losses have already been discussed.

MINIMIZING BODILY INJURY

Beyond early infancy all children fear bodily injury either from mutilation, bodily intrusion, body image change, disability, or death. In general, preparation of children for painful procedures decreases their fears. Manipulating procedural techniques for children in each age-group also minimizes fear of bodily injury. For example, since toddlers and young preschoolers are traumatized by insertion of a rectal thermometer, axillary temperatures or electronic temperature probes can effectively be substituted. Whenever procedures are performed on young children, the most supportive intervention is to do them as quickly as possible and maintain parent-child contact.

Because of young children's poorly defined body boundaries, the use of bandages may be particularly helpful. For example, telling them that the bleeding will stop after the needle is removed does little to relieve their fears, whereas applying a small Band-Aid usually provides much reassurance. The size of bandages is also significant to children in this age-group. The larger the bandage, the more importance is attached to the wound. Using successively smaller surgical dressings is one way of their measuring healing and improvement. Prematurely removing a dressing may cause them considerable concern for their well-being.

In children who fear mutilation of body parts, repeatedly stressing the reason for a procedure and evaluating their understanding is essential to minimize fear. For example, explaining cast removal to preschoolers may seem simple enough, but the child's comprehension of the details may vary considerably from the explanation. Asking them to draw a picture of what they think will happen provides substantial evidence of how they perceive events.

Children may fear bodily injury from a great variety of sources. X-ray machines, use of strange equipment for examination, unfamiliar rooms, or awkward positions can be perceived as potentially hazardous. In addition, thoughts and actions can be imagined sources of bodily damage. For older children, masturbation or sex play may be perceived as powerful weapons of potential destruction. Therefore it is important to investigate imagined reasons, particularly of a sexual nature, for illness. Since children may fear revealing such thoughts, using projective techniques such as drawing or doll play may demonstrate previously undisclosed misconceptions.

Older children fear bodily injury of both internal and external origins. For example, school-age children are aware of the heart's significance and may fear the actual procedure as much as the pain, the stitches, and the possible scar. Adolescents may express concern for the surgery but be much more anxious over the resulting scar. An appreciation of each child's special concerns helps nurses focus on critical areas during preparation for procedures or when explaining the disease processes.

Children can grasp information only if it is presented according to their cognitive development. This necessitates an awareness of the words used to describe events or processes. The example of a 7-year-old who interpreted the physician's statement of "there's edema in your belly" as "there's a demon in your belly" is proof of the necessity of choosing words carefully and reevaluating the child's understanding of the message (Perrin and Gerrity, 1981).

When children are upset about their illness, their perception can be changed by (1) providing a somewhat different and less negative account of the disease or (2) offering an explanation that is characteristic of the next stage of cognitive development (Bibace and Walsh, 1980). An example of the first strategy is reassuring a preschool child who fears that after a tonsillectomy, another sore throat means a second operation. Explaining that once tonsils are "fixed" they do not need fixing again can help relieve the fear. An example of the second strategy is to explain that germs made the tonsils sick and even though germs can cause another sore throat, they cannot cause the tonsils to ever be sick again. This higher level explanation is based on the school-age child's concept of germs as a cause of disease.

QUESTIONS AND CONTROVERSIES

Are hospitalized children under medicated for pain?

Several studies have examined the pattern of pain medication for children as compared to adults and have found remarkably consistent findings—that children are grossly undermedicated for pain. Eland and Anderson (1977) investigated the incidence of administration of analgesics to 25 hospitalized children for postoperative pain. Twelve of the children received a total of 24 doses of analgesics; the remaining 13 children were never given any medication for pain relief. In contrast, 18 adults with identical diagnoses received 372 narcotic analgesic doses and 299 nonnarcotic analgesic doses for a total of 671 doses. One of the saddest findings was that more than twice as many children had pain medication ordered as received it. This lack of response to the need for pain medication directly relates to the nurses who failed to administer the analgesic.

Another study investigating analgesic prescriptions given to children and adults after open heart surgery found that all of the adults received medication for a total of 564 doses but only three fourths of the children were given medication for a total of 237 doses during the first 3 postoperative days. This difference was even greater on the fifth postoperative day, when 83% of the adults continued to receive analgesics (a total of 136 doses) but only 12% of the children were medicated (a total of 10 doses) (Beyer and others, 1983). Another study on postoperative pain found that 75% of the children reported pain on the day of surgery and if orders for narcotic or nonnarcotic analgesics were written, the nonnarcotic was given exclusively. In addition, the doses ordered were usually too small and/or too infrequent to be maximally effective. Most orders were written "PRN," which was often interpreted by nursing staff as "as little as possible" (Mather and Mackie, 1983). Younger children are less likely to have narcotics offered, and "PRN" orders may place these children at a further disadvantage because of their inability to communicate their discomfort (Schechter, Allen, and Hanson, 1986).

The situation is even more serious with infants. One analysis of anesthetic practices with newborns undergoing surgical ligation of patent ductus arteriosus found that 76% of the infants received only a muscle relaxant and nitrous oxide (Anand and Aynsley-Green, 1985). In a survey of nurses working in neonatal intensive care units, 79% believed that infants were undermedicated for pain. The same study found that more than half of the medications used for pain relief had no analgesic properties (Franck, 1987).

Practices such as these have prompted the American Academy of Pediatrics (1987) and the American Society of Anesthesiologists to publish jointly a statement on neonatal anesthesia that encourages the use of local or systemic pharmacologic agents "according to the usual guidelines for the administration of anesthesia to high-risk, potentially unstable patients." If medication is withheld, the decision should be based on the same medical criteria used for older patients, not on the infant's age or perceived degree of cortical maturity.

PAIN ASSESSMENT

Pain assessment is a critical component of the nursing process. Unfortunately, health professionals, including nurses, tend to underestimate the existence of pain in children. Several studies have documented the enormous disparity between medication practices with children and adults (see Questions and Controversies). One of the reasons for inad-

Table 26-2 Fallacies and facts about children and pain

FALLACIES	FACTS
Infants and children do not feel pain or feel pain less than adults do.	Neonates and infants demonstrate physiologic, behavioral, and biochemical indicators of pain (Anand, Phil, and Hickey, 1987; Marshall, 1989; Shapiro, 1989). (See also Neonatal Pain, Chapter 11.) Children's sensitivity to pain actually *decreases* with age (Haslam, 1969). Younger children tend to rate procedure-related pain higher than older children do (Wong and Baker, 1988).
Children cannot tell where they hurt.	Children beyond infancy can accurately point to the body area or mark the site on a drawing. By age 3 years, they can use simple pain scales (e.g., faces) (Beyer, 1988; Savedra and others, 1989; Wong and Baker, 1988).
Children always tell the truth about their pain.	Children may be frightened by an injection and not admit having pain to avoid one. Because of constant pain, they may not realize how much they are hurting. Because of egocentric thinking, children and adolescents may believe that others know how they are feeling and not ask for analgesia. (Eland, 1985; Favaloro and Touzel, 1990; Hester, 1989).
Children tolerate pain better than adults and become accustomed to pain or painful procedures.	Children may not demonstrate decreased behavioral signs of discomfort with repeated painful procedures (Dolgin and others, 1989; Fitzgerald, Millard, and MacIntosh, 1988; Katz, Kellerman, and Siegel, 1980).
Behavioral manifestations of pain reflect pain intensity.	Behavioral manifestations do not necessarily correlate with pain intensity. Developmental level, coping skills, and temperament influence children's behavioral responses to pain (Broome and others, 1990; Wallace, 1989; Young, 1988).
Narcotics are dangerous drugs for children. They cause addiction and respiratory depression.	Narcotics (opioids) are no more dangerous for children than they are for adults. Addiction from narcotics (opioids) used to treat pain is extremely rare in adults, and no reports substantiate this fear in children. Reports of respiratory depression in children are rare. (See text.)

equate management of pain is a lack of understanding of what pain is—a personal phenomenon that *cannot* be experienced by any other individual. Therefore defining pain in terms of another's perceptions is inappropriate and inaccurate. An operational definition that is useful in clinical practice is: *pain is whatever the experiencing person says it is, existing whenever the person says it does* (McCaffery and Beebe, 1989). This definition implies a very important attitude toward patients—*that they are believed.* It includes both verbal and nonverbal expressions of pain.

Fallacies and Facts

Children are undertreated for pain for a number of complex and interrelated reasons, including professionals' misconceptions about pain; the complexities of pain assessment, particularly in nonverbal children; and the lack of information regarding currently available pain reduction techniques. A number of fallacies continue to flourish because of incorrect knowledge about pain in infants and children, despite these fallacies having been disproved by current research on pediatric pain (Table 26-2). Two fallacies that probably promote undertreatment of pain the most are unrealistic fears about respiratory depression and addiction from opioids.*

Fear of addiction. A major concern that prevents health professionals from adequately using opioids to relieve pain is an unwarranted fear of addiction. Studies on addiction rates in patients treated with opioids have found an incidence of 0.03%, and all the patients who developed addiction following their hospitalization had a prior history of substance abuse (Porter and Jick, 1980). Reports of addiction in children receiving opioids for pain management are virtually nonexistent. There are, however, anecdotal reports of children receiving opioids for severe pain, such as sickle cell crisis, who have not become addicted (Morrison and Vedro, 1989). The American Pain Society (1989) has made the following statement regarding addiction from opioid use in pain management for children: "There is no evidence that preadolescent or adolescent children are at higher risk for developing psychologic dependence (addiction) than the general population when given opioids for the management of pain."

One of the reasons for the unfounded and prevalent fear regarding addiction is confusion between three terms: narcotic addiction, drug tolerance, and physical dependency. Health professionals erroneously equate all three terms with addiction, when in reality these terms reflect completely different behavioral and physiologic actions (Jaffe, 1985):

Narcotic addiction—*behavioral* pattern of overwhelming involvement with obtaining and using a narcotic for its psychic effects rather than for medical reasons

Drug tolerance—*clinical* need to increase the dosage of a drug

*The term *opioid* refers to natural or synthetic analgesics with morphinelike actions. It is preferred to the term *narcotic,* which in a legal context refers to any substance that causes psychologic dependence, such as cocaine, which is not an opioid. The word "narcotic" also engenders fears of addiction in older children and parents that are unwarranted when opioids are used for pain control.

to attain the same desired effect, either because of increased metabolism of the drug or body tissues adapting to the drug

Physical dependence—adaptive *physiologic* state that occurs when the drug is taken in increasing amounts and that is manifest by the development of withdrawal symptoms when the drug is abruptly discontinued

Fear of respiratory depression. Respiratory depression is the most serious side effect of opioids; however, it is a rare occurrence in children. Several studies document the safety of appropriately dosed opioids in infants and children (Beasley and Tibballs, 1987; Billmire, Neale, and Gregory, 1985; Dilworth and MacKellar, 1987). Evidence suggests that in children over 3 months of age (and possibly younger) opioids cause no greater respiratory depression than in adults (Hertzka and others, 1989; Olkkola and others, 1988). Respiratory depression is most likely to occur when the opioid is administered with other drugs, such as sedatives, that also depress respirations (Yaster and others, 1990). Unlike sedatives, opioids have the advantage of an antidote, naloxone (Narcan), that rapidly reverses the respiratory depression. In addition, as tolerance to the analgesic effect of opiates occurs, tolerance to the respiratory depressant effect also occurs. Pain acts as a natural antagonist to the action of opioids. With increased pain, a patient can receive increased opioids and, except for constipation, will not experience increased side effects.

Principles of Pain Assessment in Children

Since pain is both a sensory and an emotional experience, using several assessment strategies provides qualitative and quantitative information about pain. One approach to pain assessment in children is QUESTT (Baker and Wong, 1987):

Question the child.
Use pain rating scales.
Evaluate behavior and physiologic changes.
Secure parents' involvement.
Take cause of pain into account.
Take action and evaluate results.

Question the child. Children's verbal statements and descriptions of pain are the most important factors in assessing pain. However, young children may not know what the word "pain" means and may need help in describing it using familiar language. Therefore, using a variety of words to describe pain, such as "owie," boo-boo," "feel funny," or "hurt," is necessary. Older children also benefit from using simple words to describe pain. Suggested questions for obtaining information about children's experiences with pain are presented in Box 26-4. Asking children to locate the pain is also helpful, and play can provide other means for helping children to reveal discomfort (see Nursing Tips).

When asking children about pain, the nurse must remember that they may deny pain because they fear receiving an injectable analgesic or because they believe they deserve to suffer as punishment for some misdeed. They may also deny pain to a stranger but readily admit it to a parent. This behavior should not be interpreted as seeking attention from the parent, but as a valid indication of pain.

Use a pain rating scale. Pain rating scales provide a subjective quantitative measure of pain. Although various pain scales exist (Table 26-3), not all of them are appropriate for young children. For the most valid and reliable pain intensity rating, a scale is selected that is suitable to the child's age, abilities, and preference. Scales using facial expressions are readily accepted by children and can be used by very young children better than other scales (Wong and Baker, 1988).

It is best to use the same scale with children to avoid confusing them with different instructions. Ideally, children should be taught to use the scale before pain is expected, such as preoperatively. Familiarizing children with the scale facilitates its use when children are actually in pain.

Evaluate behavior and physiologic changes. Behavioral changes are common indicators of pain and are especially valuable in assessing pain in nonverbal children. Children's behavioral responses to pain change with age and follow a developmental trend (Box 26-5). However, children vary widely in their responses and may exhibit behaviors at one age that are more typically seen at a different

Box 26-4 PAIN EXPERIENCE INVENTORY

Questions for Parents

Describe any pain your child has had before.
How does your child usually react to pain?
Does your child tell you or others when he or she is hurting?
How do you know when your child is in pain?
What do you do to ease discomfort for your child when your child is hurting?
What does your child do to get relief when hurting?
Which of these actions work best to decrease or take away your child's pain?
Is there anything special that you would like me to know about your child and pain? (If yes, have parent[s] describe.)

Questions for Child

Tell me what pain is.
Tell me about the hurt you have had before.
What do you do when you hurt?
Do you tell others when you hurt?
What do you want others to do for you when you hurt?
What don't you want others to do for you when you hurt?
What helps the most to take away your hurt?
Is there anything special that you want me to know about you when you hurt? (If yes, have child describe.)

From Hester, N., and Barcus, C.: Assessment and management of pain in children. In Pediatrics: nursing update 1(14):3, Princeton, NJ, 1986, Continuing Professional Education Center, Inc.

NURSING TIPS: HELPING CHILDREN LOCATE PAIN

Ask child to point to where it hurts or to "where Mommy or Daddy would put a Band-Aid."
Have child mark or color the painful area on a drawing of a human figure (see Fig. 27-1).
Ask child to tell how a puppet, doll, or stuffed animal is feeling or to point out areas on these models that "hurt" or "don't feel good."

Table 26-3 Pain rating scales for children

PAIN SCALE/DESCRIPTION	INSTRUCTIONS	RECOMMENDED AGE
Faces Scale* (Wong and Baker, 1988) Consists of six cartoon faces ranging from very happy, smiling face for "no pain" to increasingly less happy faces to final sad, tearful face for "worst pain"	Explain to child that each face is for a person who feels happy because there is no pain (hurt) or sad because there is some or a lot of pain. Face 0 is very happy because there is no hurt. Face 1 hurts just a little bit. Face 2 hurts a little more. Face 3 hurts even more. Face 4 hurts a whole lot, but Face 5 hurts as much as you can imagine, although you don't have to be crying to feel this bad. Ask child to choose face that best describes own pain.	Children as young as 3 years

PAIN SCALE/DESCRIPTION	INSTRUCTIONS	RECOMMENDED AGE
Oucher† (Beyer, 1988) Consists of six photographs of child's face representing "no hurt" to "biggest hurt you could ever have"; also includes a vertical scale with numbers from 0 to 100	*Photographs:* Explain to child that face at bottom has "no hurt, no hurt at all"; second picture, "just a little bit of hurt"; third picture, a "little bit more"; fourth picture, "even more hurt"; fifth picture, "*pretty* much hurt"; and last picture, "biggest hurt you could ever have." Ask child to choose face that best describes own pain. *Numbers:* Explain to child that 0 means you have "no hurt"; 0 to 29, "little hurts"; 30 to 69, "middle hurts"; 70 to 99, "big hurts"; and 100, "biggest hurt you could ever have." Ask child to choose any number between 0 and 100, not just numbers pictured on Oucher, that best describes own pain.	Children as young as 3 years; use numeric scale if child can count to 100; otherwise use photographic scale
Numeric Scale Uses straight line with end points identified as "no pain" and "worst pain"; divisions along line are marked in units from 0 to 10 (high number may vary)	Explain to child that at one end of the line is a 0, which means that a person feels no pain (hurt). At the other end is a 10, which means the person feels the worst pain imaginable. The numbers 1 to 9 are for a very little pain to a whole lot of pain. Ask child to choose number that best describes own pain.	Children as young as 5 years, provided they can count and have some concept of numbers

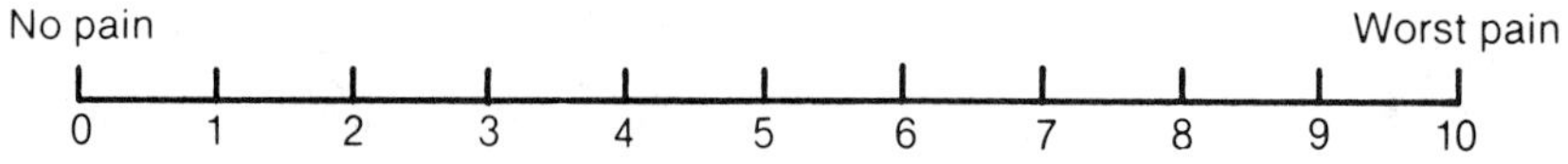

PAIN SCALE/DESCRIPTION	INSTRUCTIONS	RECOMMENDED AGE
Poker Chip (Hester, 1979, 1989) Uses plastic (poker) chips; several variations in color and number of chips have been described; original used four white chips	Explain to child that these are "pieces of hurt." One piece is a "little bit of hurt," and four pieces is the "most hurt." Ask child to choose number of pieces that describes own pain. If child replies "no pain," record a 0.	Children as young as 4 to 4½ years, provided they can count and have some concept of numbers
Color Tool (Eland, 1985) Uses crayons or markers for child to construct own scale	Ask child to identify things that have hurt in the past and what has hurt the worst. Give child eight crayons or markers (yellow, orange, red, green, blue, purple, brown, and black) in a random order. Ask child which color is like the worst pain experienced. Place that crayon or marker aside and ask child to identify crayon that is like a hurt not quite as bad as the worst hurt. Place that crayon aside and ask which other crayon is like something that hurts just a little. Place that crayon with the others and ask child which crayon is like no hurt at all. Show four crayon choices to child in order from worst-hurt color to no-hurt color. Ask child to show on body outline where it hurts using crayon of color that most nearly is like own pain. When colors are ranked, assign them a numeric value of 0 to 3.	Children as young as 4 years, provided they know their colors and are not color blind

*Several variations of faces scales exist (Bieri and others, 1990; Kuttner and LePage, 1989; McGrath, de Veber, and Hearn, 1985). Wong/Baker Faces Scale is available from Purdue Frederick Co., 100 Connecticut Ave., Norwalk, CT 06856; (800) 243-5667, ext. 4010.

†Oucher is available from Judith E. Beyer, Ph.D., R.N., Associate Professor, University of Colorado Health Sciences Center, School of Nursing, Campus Box C288, 4200 E. Ninth Ave., Denver, CO 80262; (303) 270-4317.

Table 26-3 Pain rating scales for children—cont'd

PAIN SCALE/DESCRIPTION	INSTRUCTIONS	RECOMMENDED AGE
Simple Descriptive Scale Uses descriptive words (may vary according to scale) to denote varying intensities of pain	Explain to child that at one end of line is *no pain* because person feels no hurt. At the other end is *worst pain* because person feels the worst pain imaginable. The words in between are *mild* for just a little pain, *moderate* for a little more, *quite a lot* for even more, and *very bad* for a whole lot of pain. Ask child to choose word that best describes own pain.	Children as young as 5 years, although words may need explanation
	No pain 0 — Mild 1 — Moderate 2 — Quite a lot 3 — Very bad 4 — Worst pain 5	
Visual Analogue Scale Uses 10 cm horizontal line with end points marked "no pain" and "worst pain"	Ask child to place a mark on line that best describes amount of own pain. With a centimeter ruler, measure from the "no pain" end to the mark and record this measurement as the pain score.	Young school-age children; may understand concept better if presented as vertical line with anchor phrases such as "no hurt" and "biggest hurt you could ever have" (Beyer and Aradine, 1987) and described as thermometer

Box 26-5 DEVELOPMENTAL CHARACTERISTICS OF CHILDREN'S RESPONSES TO PAIN

Young Infants
Generalized body response of rigidity or thrashing, possibly with local reflex withdrawal of stimulated area
Loud crying
Facial expression of pain (brows lowered and drawn together, eyes tightly closed, mouth open and squarish) (see Fig. 26-3)
Demonstrates no association between approaching stimulus and subsequent pain

Older Infants
Localized body response with deliberate withdrawal of stimulated area
Loud crying
Facial expression of pain and/or anger (same facial characteristics as pain but eyes may be open)
Physical resistance, especially pushing the stimulus away *after* it is applied

Young Children
Loud crying, screaming
Verbal expressions of "Ow," "Ouch," or "It hurts"
Thrashing of arms and legs
Attempts to push stimulus away *before* it is applied
Uncooperative; needs physical restraint
Requests termination of procedure
Clings to parent, nurse, or other significant person
Requests emotional support, such as hugs or other forms of physical comfort
May become restless and irritable with continuing pain
All these behaviors may be seen in anticipation of actual painful procedure

School-Age Children
May see all behaviors of young child, especially *during* painful procedure but less in anticipatory period
Stalling behavior, such as "Wait a minute" or "I'm not ready"
Muscular rigidity, such as clenched fists, white knuckles, gritted teeth, contracted limbs, body stiffness, closed eyes, wrinkled forehead

Adolescents
Less vocal protest
Less motor activity
More verbal expressions, such as "It hurts" or "You're hurting me"
Increased muscle tension and body control

Data from Craig, K.D., and others: Developmental changes in infant pain expression during immunization injections, Soc. Sci. Med. 19(12):1331-1337, 1984; and Katz, E., Kellerman, J., and Siegel, S.: Behavioral distress in children with cancer undergoing medical procedures: developmental considerations, J. Consult. Clin. Psychol. 48(3):356-365, 1980.

age. In addition, temperament affects coping style, and children with more positive moods may appear to be in less pain than they actually are. Children who use passive coping behaviors (offering no resistance, cooperating) may rate pain as more intense than children who use active coping behaviors (resisting, attacking) (Broome and others, 1990). Cultural background may also play a role in children's pain responses, although the influence appears slight (Abu-Saad, 1984). Unfortunately, nurses often make judgments about pain based on behavior, which results in some children receiving inadequate pain medication (Wallace, 1989).

Depending on the type and location of pain, children may display behaviors that indicate local body pain, such as pulling the ears for ear pain; rolling the head from side to side for head and ear pain; lying on the side with legs flexed for abdominal pain; limping for leg or foot pain; and refusing to move a body part. Children who experience chronic or repeated pain often develop effective behavioral coping strategies, such as squeezing a hand, talking, counting, relaxing, or thinking about pleasant events. Once these coping skills are identified, the child can be encouraged to use them in future experiences with pain.

Physiologic responses indicating pain include flushing of the skin; increases in sweating, blood pressure, pulse, and respiration; restlessness; and dilation of the pupils. However, these signs vary considerably—for example, heart rate may actually decrease (Dale, 1986)—and they may be produced by emotions such as fear, anger, or anxiety. They occur primarily in acute pain from stimulation of the sympathetic nervous system. If pain persists, the body begins to adapt and these responses decrease or stabilize. Consequently, if nurses rely primarily on observing these physiologic indications before believing that pain exists, many instances of pain will go unrecognized.

One of the most valuable clues to pain is a change in behavior and vital signs after administration of an analgesic. Improved behavior (e.g., less irritability, cessation of crying) and decreased pulse, respirations, and blood pressure provide important evidence for pain. Often the change in vital signs is attributed to the depressant effect of opioids, when in reality the return to more normal physiologic functioning is due to pain relief.

Secure parents' involvement. Parents know their child and are sensitive to changes in behavior. However, little documentation exists on parents' ability to recognize pain in their children. Some parents may never have seen their child in severe pain and may equate certain responses, such as irritability or withdrawal, with discomfort. However, others are aware that certain behaviors signal pain because the child has acted similarly during previous painful events. In addition, parents usually know what comforts their child, such as rocking, stroking, or talking.

To better assess the child's pain, the nurse can interview the parents about their child's previous pain experiences (see Box 26-4). Ideally this questioning should occur before the child is in pain, such as on admission to the hospital. Parents need to realize that their knowledge of their child is important in providing care. Parents sometimes leave the assessment of pain up to the nurse because "nurses are more experienced," and consequently parents do not report pain (Mills, 1989). Parents need to be taught nonverbal pain behaviors in children and encouraged to inform the staff when they occur.

Take cause of pain into account. When children exhibit behaviors or other clues that suggest pain, reasons for discomfort should be investigated. Pathology may give clues to expected intensity and type of pain. For example, pain associated with vaso-occlusive crises in sickle cell disease is severe. Pain caused by bone marrow puncture is typically greater than the discomfort associated with a venipuncture.

✦ **NURSING ALERT** A golden rule to follow in pain assessment is: Whatever is painful to an adult is painful to an infant or child until proved otherwise (Franck, 1989).

Take action and evaluate results. The reason for assessing pain is to relieve it. Total pain relief should be the goal, with the combined use of pharmacologic and nonpharmacologic interventions (see following discussion). Regardless of the type of pain intervention, evaluation of the results is essential. No one pain reduction technique is effective for all children. Therefore, a pain assessment record is used to monitor the effectiveness of the interventions (Fig. 26-8). With nonverbal children, behavioral and physiologic signs are evaluated for evidence of pain relief. With verbal children, their statements about pain relief and pain ratings are also recorded. Changes in the medication regimen are made as needed to provide the maximum pain relief with the minimum side effects. Family members are often excellent allies for keeping a pain assessment record for the nurse.

PAIN MANAGEMENT

Relief of pain is a basic need and right of all children, yet physicians and nurses are often reluctant to order and administer analgesics and lack knowledge of well-documented approaches to pharmacologic pain control.*

Effective pain management requires that health professionals be willing to try a number of interventions to achieve optimum results. Basically, pain-reducing methods can be grouped into two categories: nonpharmacologic and pharmacologic. Whenever possible, both should be used; however, nonpharmacologic measures should not be considered substitutes for analgesics.

Nonpharmacologic Management

A number of nonpharmacologic techniques exist for lessening the perception of pain and, when used with analgesics, can enhance these drugs' effectiveness. However, nonpharmacologic strategies can also produce a cooperative child who continues to suffer "in silence" (Zeltzer, Jay, and Fisher, 1989). Therefore, nurses must carefully evaluate the

*An excellent resource is *Principles of Analgesic Use in the Treatment of Acute Pain and Chronic Cancer Pain,* available from the American Pain Society, 5700 Old Orchard Rd., Skokie, IL 60077-1024; (708) 966-5595.

PAIN ASSESSMENT RECORD

Directions:
1. Record time of administering drug and assess analgesic effect 30 minutes later and then hourly.
2. State "Reason for drug administration" in behavioral terms, e.g., "child says he hurts" or "child crying and irritable."
3. Use column "Reason for drug administration" to record behavior during reassessment, e.g., "child says he feels better" or "child playing."
4. Use pain rating scale if child understands its use and only when child is awake. Name of scale: ________________; Rating: No pain = ________ and Worst pain = ________.
5. Suggested guidelines for safe minimum respiratory rates for children receiving opioids are 10 to 16 breaths/minute. Consider child's age (with age, respiratory rate decreases) and physiologic status (shallow respiration, decreased oxygen saturation, decreased consciousness) when evaluating respirations.

Date	Time	Drug administered	Reason for drug administration	Pain rating	Respirations	Signature

Fig. 26-8. Pain assessment record.

effectiveness of the intervention in truly reducing pain and avoid setting an expectation of passive acceptance. Aside from this risk, nonpharmacologic methods are extremely safe and most are independent nursing functions.

Nonpharmacologic interventions include *general strategies* that are effective with most children, especially those who can benefit from explanations. However, *specific nonpharmacologic strategies* are more effective with certain children than with others (Box 26-6). Experimentation with several strategies that are suitable to child's age, pain intensity, and abilities is often necessary to determine the most effective approach.

✦ **NURSING ALERT** Most specific nonpharmacologic strategies require children's understanding and cooperation. Therefore, try to match the strategy with the pain severity. Children in severe pain may not be able to expend the effort necessary to learn the technique, and those with very mild symptoms may not be motivated to learn. Therefore, these strategies may be most useful with mid-range pain (Cleeland, 1986).

In the selection of a pain reducer, it is best to use a strategy familiar to the child or to describe several strategies and let the child select the most appealing one. Parents should be involved in the selection process; they may be familiar with the child's usual coping skills and can help identify potentially successful strategies. Involving parents also encourages their participation in learning the skill with the child and acting as coach. If the parent cannot assist the child, other appropriate persons may include a grandparent, older sibling, nurse, or child-life specialist.

Children should learn a specific strategy *before* pain occurs or before it becomes severe. To reduce the child's effort, instructions for a strategy, such as distraction or relaxation, can be audiotaped and played during a period of discomfort.

Pharmacologic Management

Using pharmacologic methods to control pain requires attention to four "rights": right drug, right dose, right route, and right time. Although nurses may not prescribe the medication, knowledge of these essential principles assists in optimally implementing analgesic orders and discussing with other practitioners possible strategies to improve pain control. In addition, observing for side effects of the drugs and using supportive approaches with children when administering the drug are important nursing interventions.

Right drug. Nonopioids, collectively referred to as nonsteroidal antiinflammatory drugs (NSAIDs), are sometimes suitable for mild to moderate pain; opioids are needed for moderate to severe pain. A combination of the two analgesics attacks pain on two levels: nonopioids at the peripheral nervous system and opioids at the central nervous system. This approach provides increased analgesia without increased side effects. Several commercially available combinations, such as Tylenol with Codeine, may have increasing doses of the opioid but a constant dose of the nonopioid (Box 26-7). Therefore, before increasing the opioid, it may be preferable to increase the nonopioid component, for example, adding one plain Tylenol (300 mg) to Tylenol with Codeine No. 3 before advancing to Tylenol with Codeine No. 4.

The safety of various opioids differs. Morphine is considered the drug of choice. When morphine is not a suitable opioid, drugs such as hydromorphone (Dilaudid) and fentanyl (Sublimaze) are effective substitutes. Meperidine (Demerol, pethidine) is not recommended for chronic use be-

Box 26-6 GUIDELINES FOR NONPHARMACOLOGIC PAIN MANAGEMENT

General Strategies

Form a trusting relationship with child and family.
- Express concern regarding their reports of pain.
- Take an active role in seeking effective pain management strategies.

Use general strategies to prepare child for painful procedure (see Chapter 27).

Prepare child before potentially painful procedures but avoid "planting" the idea of pain. For example, instead of saying: "This is going to (or may) hurt," say "Sometimes this feels like pushing, sticking, or pinching and sometimes it doesn't bother people. You tell me what it feels like to you."
- Use "nonpain" descriptors when possible (e.g., "It feels like intense heat" rather than "It's a burning pain").
- This allows for variation in sensory perception, avoids suggesting pain, and gives child control in describing reactions.

Avoid evaluative statements or descriptions (e.g., "This is a terrible procedure" or "It really will hurt a lot").

Stay with child during a painful procedure.
- Encourage parents to stay with child if child and parent desire; encourage parent to talk softly to child and to remain near child's head.
- Involve parents in learning specific nonpharmacologic strategies and assisting child in their use.

Educate child about the pain, especially when explanation may lessen anxiety (e.g., that child's pain is expected after surgery and does not indicate something is wrong; reassure that child is not responsible for the pain).

For long-term pain control give child a doll, which becomes "the patient," and allow child to do everything to the doll that is done to the child; pain control can be emphasized through the doll by stating, "Dolly feels better after the medicine."

Specific Strategies

Distraction

Involve parent and child in identifying strong distractors.

Involve child in play; use radio, tape recorder, record player; have child sing or use rhythmic breathing.

Have child concentrate on yelling or saying "ouch" by focusing on "yelling loud or soft as you feel it hurt; that way I know what's happening."

Use humor, such as watching cartoons, telling jokes or funny stories, or acting silly with child.

Relaxation

With an infant or young child:
- Hold in a comfortable, well-supported position, such as vertically against the chest and shoulder.
- Rock in a wide, rhythmic arc in a rocking chair or sway back and forth, rather than bouncing child.
- Repeat one or two words softly, such as "Mommy's here."

With a slightly older child:
- Ask child to take a deep breath and "go limp as a rag doll" while exhaling slowly, then ask child to yawn (demonstrate if needed).
- Help child assume a comfortable position (e.g., pillow under neck and knees).
- Begin progressive relaxation: starting with the toes, systematically instruct child to let each body part "go limp" or "feel heavy"; if child has difficulty with relaxing, instruct child to tense or tighten each body part and then relax it.
- Allow child to keep eyes open, since children may respond better if eyes are open rather than closed during relaxation.

Guided imagery

Have child identify some highly pleasurable real or pretend experience.

Have child describe details of the event, including as many senses as possible (e.g., "feel the cool breezes," "see the beautiful colors," "hear the pleasant music").

Have child write down or record script.

Encourage child to concentrate only on the pleasurable event during the painful time; enhance the image by recalling specific details, such as reading the script or playing the record.

Combine with relaxation.

Positive self-talk

Teach child positive statements to say when in pain (e.g., "I will be feeling better soon," "When I go home, I will feel better," "Relaxing will make me hurt less").

Thought-stopping

Identify positive facts about the painful event (e.g., "It does not last long").

Identify reassuring information (e.g., "If I think about something else, it does not hurt as much").

Condense positive and reassuring facts into a set of brief statements, and have child memorize them (e.g.: "Short procedure, good veins, little hurt, nice nurse, go home").

Have child repeat the memorized statements whenever thinking about or experiencing the painful event.

Cutaneous stimulation

Includes simple rhythmic rubbing; use of pressure, electric vibrator; massage with hand lotion, powder, or menthol cream; application of heat or cold, such as an ice cube on the site before giving injection or application of ice to the site opposite the painful area (e.g., if right knee hurts, place ice on left knee).

A more sophisticated method is transcutaneous electrical nerve stimulation (TENS) (use of controlled low-voltage electricity to the body via electrodes placed on the skin).

Behavioral contracting

Informal—may be used with children as young as 4 or 5 years:
- Use stars or tokens as rewards.
- Give uncooperative or procrastinating children (during a procedure) a limited time (measured by a visible timer) to complete the procedure.
- Proceed as needed if child is unable to comply.
- Reinforce cooperation with a reward if the procedure is accomplished within specified time.

Formal—use written contract, which includes the following:
- Realistic (seems possible) goal or desired behavior
- Measurable behavior (e.g., agrees not to hit anyone during procedures)
- Contract written, dated, and signed by all persons involved in any of the agreements
- Identified rewards or consequences are reinforcing
- Goal can be evaluated

Box 26-7 SELECTED COMBINATION OPIOID AND NONOPIOID ORAL ANALGESICS WITH INGREDIENTS

Non-Aspirin Products	
Darvocet-N 50	50 mg propoxyphene napsylate 325 mg acetaminophen
Darvocet-N 100	100 mg propoxyphene napsylate 650 mg acetaminophen
Percocet-5	5 mg oxycodone HCl 325 mg acetaminophen
Tylenol with Codeine No. 1	7.5 mg codeine 300 mg acetaminophen
Tylenol with Codeine No. 2	15 mg codeine 300 mg acetaminophen
Tylenol with Codeine No. 3	30 mg codeine 300 mg acetaminophen
Tylenol with Codeine No. 4	60 mg codeine 300 mg acetaminophen
Tylenol and Codeine Elixir (each 5 ml)	12 mg codeine 120 mg acetaminophen 7% alcohol
Tylox	5 mg oxycodone HCl 500 mg acetaminophen
Vicodin	5 mg hydrocodone 500 mg acetaminophen
Aspirin Products*	
Darvon Compound	32 mg propoxyphene HCl 389 mg aspirin 32.4 mg caffeine
Darvon Compound-65	65 mg propoxyphene HCl 389 mg aspirin 32.4 mg caffeine
Darvon with A.S.A.	65 mg propoxyphene HCl 325 mg aspirin
Darvon-N with A.S.A.	100 mg propoxyphene napsylate 325 mg aspirin
Percodan	4.5 mg oxycodone HCl 0.38 mg oxycodone terephthalate 325 mg aspirin
Percodan-Demi	2.25 mg oxycodone HCl 0.19 mg oxycodone terephthalate 325 mg aspirin

*Aspirin is not recommended for children because of its possible association with Reye syndrome.

cause of the accumulation of the metabolite, normeperidine, a central nervous system stimulant that can produce anxiety, tremors, myoclonus, and generalized seizures that are not reversed with naloxone (American Pain Society, 1989; Kaiko and others, 1983).

Opioids are frequently combined with other drugs that are considered "potentiators." One common mixture is the "DPT," or "lytic" cocktail—Demerol, Phenergan, and Thorazine (see Physical Preparation for Procedures, Chapter 27). However, there is little evidence that any drug potentiates the analgesic effect of opioids; rather, drugs such as promethazine (Phenergan) produce sedation, which is erroneously equated with analgesia. Several drugs, known as *adjuvant analgesics,* may be used alone or with opioids to control pain symptoms, although they may or may not have analgesic properties. They may be given for depression, anxiety, sleeplessness, or agitation. Frequently used drugs to relieve anxiety, cause sedation, and provide amnesia are diazepam (Valium) and midazolam (Versed); however, they are not analgesics.

At times health professionals question whether pain really exists and administer placebos to "see if the pain is real." This practice is unjustified; a positive response to a placebo, such as a saline injection, is common in patients who have a documented organic basis for pain. Therefore, the deceptive use of placebos does not provide useful information about the presence or severity of pain (Goodwin, Goodwin, and Vogel, 1979). In addition, the use of placebos can cause side effects similar to those of opioids, can destroy the client's trust in the health care staff, and raises serious ethical and legal questions (Perry and Heidrich, 1981). Therefore the use of placebos should be avoided (American Pain Society, 1989).

Right dosage. The optimum dosage is one that controls pain without causing severe side effects. This usually requires *titration,* the gradual adjustment of drug dosage (usually by increasing the dose) until optimum pain relief without excessive sedation is achieved. Dosage recommendations, such as those in Tables 26-4 and 26-5, are only safe initial dosages, not optimum dosages. Children (except infants younger than about 3 months of age) metabolize drugs more rapidly than adults; younger children may require higher doses of opioids to achieve the same analgesic effect (Hertzka and others, 1989; Olkkola and others, 1988). Therefore, the therapeutic effect and duration of analgesia vary. Children's dosages are usually calculated according to body weight, body surface area, or, less precisely, as a percentage of the recommended starting adult dose (Box 26-8).

If pain relief is inadequate, the initial dosage can be increased (usually by 50% if pain is moderate or by 100% if pain is severe) to provide greater analgesic effectiveness. Decreasing the interval between doses may also provide more continuous pain relief. A major difference between opioids and nonopioids is that nonopioids have a *ceiling effect,* which means that doses higher than the recommended dose will not produce greater pain relief. Opioids do not have a ceiling effect other than that imposed by side effects; therefore, larger dosages can be given safely for increasing severity of pain.

Parenteral and oral dosages of opioids are not the same. Because of the *first-pass effect,* an oral drug is rapidly absorbed from the gastrointestinal tract and enters the portal circulation, where it is partially metabolized before reaching the central circulation. Therefore, oral dosages must be

Table 26-4 Nonsteroidal antiinflammatory drugs (NSAIDs) approved for children*

DRUG (TRADE NAME)	DOSE	COMMENTS
Acetaminophen (Tylenol and other brands)	10-20 mg/kg/dose every 4-6 hours not to exceed 5 doses in 24 hours	Available in drops (80 mg/0.8 ml), elixir (160 mg/5 ml), tablets (80 mg), swallowable caplets (160 mg), and rectal suppositories (several dosages) Nonprescription Higher dosage range may provide increased analgesia
Choline magnesium trisalicylate (Trilisate)	Children 37 kg or less: 50 mg/kg/day divided into 2 doses Children over 37 kg: 2250 mg/day divided into 2 doses	Available in elixir 500 mg/5 ml Prescription
Ibuprofen		
PediaProfen	Children 6 months to 12 years: 5-10 mg/kg/dose every 6-8 hours not to exceed 40 mg/kg/day for fever Children over 12 years: 200-400 mg/dose every 6-8 hours	Available in suspension 100 mg/5 ml Prescription Recommended for fever reduction in children 6 months to 12 years, but also indicated for juvenile rheumatoid arthritis and mild to moderate pain in children over 12 years
Children's Advil	Children 12 months and older: 5-10 mg/kg/dose every 6-8 hours not to exceed 40 mg/kg/day for fever	Available in suspension 100 mg/5 ml Prescription Dosage recommendation is for juvenile rheumatoid arthritis and fever
Naproxen (Naprosyn)	Children over 2 years: 10 mg/kg/day divided in 2 doses	Available in elixir 125 mg/5 ml Prescription
Tolmetin (Tolectin)	Children over 2 years: 20 mg/kg/day divided in 3 or 4 doses	Available in scored 200 mg tablets Prescription

All product information approved by U.S. Food and Drug Administration (FDA) as of September 1990.
*All NSAIDs in the table except acetaminophen have significant antiinflammatory, antipyretic, and analgesic actions. Acetaminophen has a weak antiinflammatory action, and its classification as an NSAID is controversial. Patients respond differently to various NSAIDs; therefore, changing from one drug to another may be necessary for maximum benefit.
Acetylsalicylic acid (aspirin) is also an NSAID but is not recommended for children because of its possible association with Reye syndrome. The NSAIDs in the table have no known association with Reye syndrome. However, caution should be exercised in prescribing any salicylate-containing drug (e.g., Trilisate) for children with known or suspected viral infection.
Side effects of ibuprofen, naproxen, and tolmetin include nausea, vomiting, diarrhea, constipation, gastric ulceration, bleeding nephritis, and fluid retention.
Acetaminophen and choline magnesium trisalicylate are well tolerated in the gastrointestinal tract and do not interfere with platelet function. NSAIDs except acetaminophen should not be given to patients with allergic reactions to salicylates. All the NSAIDs should be used cautiously in patients with renal impairment.

Box 26-8 GUIDELINES FOR CALCULATING CHILDREN'S INITIAL ANALGESIC DOSAGE*

Children 2 to 6 years: 20% to 25% of starting adult dose
Children 7 to 12 years: 50% of starting adult dose
Children 12 years and older: full starting adult dose

Data from American Pain Society: Principles of analgesic use in the treatment of acute pain or chronic cancer pain, Skokie, IL, 1989, The Society.
*These guidelines are used only when pediatric dosage recommendations are not available.

larger to compensate for the partial loss of analgesic potency. Conversion factors for selected opioids, when a change is made from IM or IV to oral, are listed in Table 26-5.

Right route. Several routes of administration exist (Box 26-9). Children should not have to endure pain, such as from intramuscular (IM) injections, to achieve pain relief. Therefore, the most effective and least traumatic route of administration should be selected. When parenteral routes are used, changing to the oral route requires appropriate dosage conversion to achieve *equianalgesia* (equal analgesic effect) because of the first-pass effect. Parenteral to oral conversion can be immediate or gradual (Box 26-10). *Immediate conversion* is usually successful if the child does not associate the parenteral form with superior pain relief. *Gradual conversion* may be used when the child associates the parenteral form with superior pain relief and doubts the effectiveness of the oral preparation. Gradual conversion should also be used when large parenteral doses have been given for severe pain, since immediate conversion to an equianalgesic oral dose may be excessive. Equianalgesic charts are merely a guideline for initial doses. Immediate conversion from IM or intravenous (IV) to the suggested equianalgesic oral dose may result in a substantial error in the individual child. For example, the dose may be significantly more or less than what that child requires. Small changes ensure small errors.

Right time. The right timing for administering analgesics depends on the type of pain. For continuous pain con-

Table 26-5 Dosage and therapeutic activity of selected opioids for children

DRUG (ROUTE)*	INITIAL DOSE†	CONVERSION FACTOR IM TO PO‡	ADULT INITIAL IM DOSE (mg) EQUIVALENT TO EACH OTHER§	THERAPEUTIC ACTIVITY FOR IM ROUTE EXCEPT AS NOTED‖
Morphine (IV, IM, SC, PO)	0.1-0.2 mg/kg IM	3-6	10	O = 15-60 minutes P = 0.5-1 hour D = 3-7 hours
Fentanyl (Sublimaze) (IV, transdermal)	2-3 μg/kg IV	—	0.1	IV route: O = 7-8 minutes P = No data D = 1-2 hours
Codeine (IM, PO)	0.5-1 mg/kg PO	1.5	130	O = 15-30 minutes P = 0.5-1 hour D = 4-6 hours
Methadone (Dolophine) (IM, PO)	0.1-0.2 mg/kg PO	2	10	O = 30-60 minutes P = 0.5-1 hour D = 4-6 hours‖
Hydromorphone (Dilaudid) (IV, SC, PO)	0.015-0.03 mg/kg IM	5	1.5	O = 15-30 minutes P = 0.5-1 hour D = 4-5 hours
Levorphanol (Levo-Dromoran) (SC, IV, PO)	0.02-0.04 mg/kg IM	2	2	O = 30-60 minutes P = 0.5-1 hour D = 4-8 hours
Meperidine (¶) (Demerol) (IV, IM, PO)	1 to 2 mg/kg IV or IM	4	75	O = 10-45 minutes P = 0.5-1 hour D = 2-4 hours

Data from American Pain Society: Principles of analgesic use in the treatment of acute pain or chronic cancer pain, Skokie, IL, 1989, The Society.
*IV, Intravenous; IM, intramuscular; SC, subcutaneous; PO, oral.
†These dosages are considered *initial (starting) doses* for moderate to severe pain in children who have not developed tolerance to the drug. The *optimum dose* is determined by titration: increasing or decreasing the dose according to the child's response. Dosages for hydromorphone and levorphanol are based on the equianalgesic dose of parenteral morphine.
To calculate hourly infusion rate, divide child's IM dose by drug's expected duration. For example, divide morphine 2 mg (dose for 20 kg child) by duration of 4 hours for initial starting dose of 0.5 mg/hour/IV.
‡To convert an IM dose to a PO dose, multiply the IM dose by the conversion factor. Based on clinical experience, IM and IV doses are considered equianalgesic. However, some clinicians suggest that ½ the IM dose equals the IV dose, especially for an initial IV bolus dose. For morphine a conversion factor of 3 is recommended for repetitive dosing.
§When converting from one drug to another drug, be certain that the dosages of the drugs are equivalent. For example, 5 mg of IV morphine is equal to 0.75 mg of IV or 4 mg of PO hydromorphone.
‖O = onset; P = peak; D = duration. With IV administration, times may be shorter, and with PO administration, times may be longer. Times for all drugs are approximate and may be shorter in children due to their more rapid metabolism of the drug. With repeated dosing, duration of methadone and levorphanol increases. Sustained-release preparations of oral morphine are available (MS Contin, 8-12 hours: Roxanol-SR, 8 hours).
¶Should not be used chronically, particularly in patients with compromised renal function or for treatment of sickle cell crisis pain, because of accumulation of the metabolite, normeperidine, which causes central nervous system irritability (anxiety, tremors, myoclonus, generalized seizures).

trol, such as for postoperative or cancer pain, a preventive schedule of medication around the clock (ATC) is effective. The ATC schedule avoids the low plasma concentrations that permit "breakthrough" pain. If analgesics are administered only when pain returns (a typical use of the PRN, or "as needed," order), pain relief may take several hours. This may require higher doses, leading to a cycle of undermedication of pain alternating with periods of overmedication and drug toxicity. This cycle of erratic pain control also promotes "clock watching," which may be erroneously equated with "addiction." Nurses can effectively use PRN orders by giving the drug at regular intervals, since "as needed" can be interpreted to mean "as needed to prevent pain."

Preventive pain control is best provided through continuous IV infusion rather than intermittent boluses. If intermittent boluses are given, the intervals between doses should not exceed the drug's expected duration of effectiveness. For extended pain control with fewer administration times, drugs that provide longer duration of action (e.g., some NSAIDs, time-released morphine, methadone, levorphanol) can be used.

NURSING ALERT Since "breakthrough" pain can occur even with optimum ATC scheduling, there should be an order for PRN "rescue" doses of an analgesic.

Continuous analgesia is not always appropriate, because not all pain is continuous. Frequently, temporary pain control is needed to provide analgesia before a scheduled pro-

Box 26-9 ROUTES AND METHODS OF ANALGESIC DRUG ADMINISTRATION

Oral

Preferred because of convenience, cost, and relatively steady blood levels

Higher dosages of oral form of opioids required for equivalent parenteral analgesia

Peak drug effect occurs after 1½ to 2 hours for most analgesics

- Delay in onset a disadvantage when rapid control of severe pain or fluctuating pain is desired

Sublingual/Buccal

Tablet or liquid placed between cheek and gum (buccal) or under tongue (sublingual)

Highly desirable because more rapid onset than oral

- Avoids first-pass effect through liver, which normally reduces analgesia from oral opioids (unless sublingual/buccal form swallowed, which occurs often in children)

Few drugs commercially available in this form

- Many drugs can be compounded into a sublingual troche or lozenge (Wong and Redding, 1987)*

Few published data on effectiveness and safety

Intravenous (IV) (Bolus)

Preferred for rapid control of severe pain

Provides most rapid onset of effect, usually in about 5 minutes

- Advantage for acute pain, procedural pain, and breakthrough pain

Initial bolus dose is controversial; one recommendation is one-half IM dose

Needs to be repeated hourly for continuous pain control

- Drugs with short half-life (morphine, fentanyl, hydromorphone) are preferred to avoid toxic accumulation of drug

Intravenous (Continuous)

Preferred over bolus and IM for maintaining control of pain

Provides steady blood levels

Easy to titrate dosage

Suggested initial dose is controversial; one approach to calculating hourly infusion rate is to divide IM dose by drug's expected duration for IM route

Full peak effect is delayed; best if combined with initial IV bolus dose

Subcutaneous (SC) (Continuous)

Used when oral and IV routes not available

Provides equivalent blood levels to continuous IV infusion

Suggested initial bolus dose to equal 2-hour IV dose; total 24-hour dose usually equal to total IV or IM 24-hour dose

Patient-Controlled Analgesia (PCA)

Generally refers to self-administration of drugs, regardless of route

Typically uses programmable infusion pump (IV or SC) that permits self-administration of boluses of medication at preset dose and time interval (*lockout interval* is time between doses)

Best pain control achieved with initial bolus and continuous (basal or background) infusion of opioid

Optimum lockout interval not known, but must be at least as long as time needed for onset of drug

- Should effectively control pain during movement or procedures
- Longer lockout requires larger dose

Used successfully with children as young as 2 years of age who can understand concept of "pushing button when in pain"

- Parent may assist younger child (Gaukroger, Tomkins, and van der Walt, 1989; Gureno and Reisinger, in press)

May be used as a convenient analgesic delivery system for neonates; nurse pushes button for increased pain control

Intramuscular (IM)

Available in many opioid preparations

Painful administration (hated by children)

Some drugs (e.g., meperidine) can cause tissue damage

Wide fluctuation in absorption of drug from muscle

Faster absorption from deltoid than gluteal sites

Shorter duration and more expensive than oral drugs

Time consuming for staff

Intradermal

Used primarily for skin anesthesia (e.g., for lumbar puncture, bone marrow aspiration, arterial puncture, skin biopsy)

Local anesthetics (lidocaine) cause stinging, burning sensation

- Duration of stinging may depend on type of "caine" used

To avoid stinging sensation associated with lidocaine:

- Buffer the solution by adding 1 part of sodium bicarbonate (1 mEq/ml) to 10 parts of 1% lidocaine (McKay, Morris, and Mushlin, 1987)

Topical/Transdermal

Limited number of applications

EMLA (eutectic [easily melted] mixture of local anesthetics [lidocaine/prilocaine]) cream† (Juhlin and Evers, 1990)

- Provides skin anesthesia for up to 4 hours
- Eliminates or reduces pain from most procedures involving skin puncture
- Must be placed over puncture site under occlusive dressing for 1 hour before procedure

TAC (tetracaine/adrenalin/cocaine) liquid (Engebo, 1990)

- Provides skin anesthesia about 5 to 15 minutes after application
- Used primarily for suturing lacerations
- Allowed to drip or soak into wound
- Must not be used on mucous membranes and denuded areas because of the risk of systemic absorption and toxicity

Transdermal fentanyl (Duragesic)

- Available as "patch" for continuous cancer pain control (Miser and others, 1989)
- Safety and efficacy not established in children under 12 years

Transmucosal fentanyl ("lollipop")†

- Used for preoperative medication (Streisand and others, 1989)

Data primarily from American Pain Society: Principles of analgesic use in the treatment of acute pain or chronic cancer pain, Skokie, IL, 1989, The Society; and McCaffery, M., and Beebe, A.: Pain: clinical manual for nursing practice, St. Louis, 1989, Mosby–Year Book, Inc.

*For further information about compounding drugs in troches or suppositories, contact Technical Staff, Professional Compounding Centers of America, P.O. Box 368, Sugarland, TX 77487; (800) 331-2498.

†Under investigation as of this writing.

Box 26-9 ROUTES AND METHODS OF ANALGESIC DRUG ADMINISTRATION—cont'd

Rectal
Alternative to oral or parenteral routes
Variable absorption rate
Generally disliked by children, but often preferred over IM injection
Acceptance may be culturally influenced
Many drugs can be compounded into rectal suppositories*

Regional Nerve Block
Use of long-acting anesthetic (bupivacaine) injected into site, usually at end of surgery
Provides prolonged analgesia postoperatively, such as following inguinal herniorrhaphy (Hinkle, 1987)
May be used to provide local anesthesia for surgery, such as dorsal penile nerve block for circumcision (Stang and others, 1988)

Inhalation
Use of anesthetics, such as nitrous oxide or halothane
Used to produce partial or complete analgesia for painful procedures (Griffin, Campbell, and Jones, 1981; Perin and Frase, 1985)

Epidural/Intrathecal
Used postoperatively or in selected terminal care (Krane and others, 1987)
Involves catheter placed into epidural or intrathecal space for continuous drip or intermittent administration of opioid (with or without a long-acting anesthetic, e.g., bupivacaine)
Analgesia primarily from drug's direct effect on opiate receptors in spinal cord
Provides steady drug levels and long-lasting analgesia
No less risk of respiratory depression and urinary retention when compared to continuous IV or SC infusion
Uncertainty about optimum drug choice and indications for choosing this route over other routes

Box 26-10 GUIDELINES FOR CONVERTING FROM IV OR IM TO PO ANALGESICS

Convert directly by giving next dose of analgesic orally (PO) in equivalent dosage without any parenteral form of the same drug.

or

Convert gradually to PO form using the following steps:
- Convert half the parenteral dose to a PO dose.
- Administer half the parenteral dose and the PO dose.
- Assess pain relief.
- If pain relief is inadequate, increase the PO dose as needed.
- If sedation occurs, decrease the PO dose as needed.
- When the parenteral and PO doses are effective, discontinue the parenteral dose and give twice the PO dose.

Box 26-11 SIDE EFFECTS OF OPIOIDS

General
Respiratory depression
Sedation
Constipation (possibly severe)
Nausea and vomiting
Agitation, euphoria
Mental clouding
Hallucinations
Orthostatic hypotension
Pruritus
Urticaria
Sweating
Miosis (sign of toxicity)
Anaphylaxis (rare)

Signs of Tolerance
Decreasing pain relief
Decreasing duration of pain relief

Signs of Physical Dependence
Initial signs of withdrawal:
- Lacrimation
- Rhinorrhea
- Yawning
- Sweating

Later signs:
- Restlessness
- Irritability
- Tremors
- Anorexia
- Dilated pupils
- Gooseflesh

cedure. When pain can be predicted, the drug's peak effect should be timed to coincide with the painful event. For example, with opioids the peak effect is approximately ½ to 1 hour for the IM or subcutaneous (SC) route (considerably less for the IV route); with nonopioids the peak effect occurs about 2 hours after oral administration. For rapid onset and peak of action, opioids that quickly penetrate the blood-brain barrier (e.g., IV fentanyl) provide excellent pain control. (See also Physical Preparation for Procedures, Chapter 27.)

Observe for side effects. Both NSAIDs and opioids have side effects, although the major concern is with those from opioids (Box 26-11). Respiratory depression is the most serious complication and is most likely to occur in sedated patients. The respiratory rate may decrease gradually or may cease abruptly; lower limits of normal are not established for children, but any significant change from a previous rate calls for increased vigilance. A slower respiratory rate does not necessarily reflect decreased arterial oxygenation; an increased depth of ventilation may compensate for the altered rate (Rowbotham and others, 1989).

If respirations slow, most children respond to verbal reminders to breathe and to use of a manual resuscitation bag. Decreasing the dosage may also prevent a slower rate, but analgesia may be compromised. When these measures are not adequate, immediate intervention with IV naloxone (Narcan), an opioid antagonist that rapidly reverses analgesia, is required. The recommended dose is 0.1 mg/kg for infants and children from birth to 5 years of age or 20 kg of body weight; children older than 5 years of age or weighing

NURSING CARE PLAN
The Child in Pain

NURSING DIAGNOSIS: Pain related to (specify)

GOAL 1

Promote coping strategies; reduce perception of pain

INTERVENTIONS

Employ nonpharmacologic strategies to help child manage pain
Select appropriate strategy (see Box 26-6)
Use strategy familiar to child or describe several strategies and let child select one
Involve parent in selection of strategy
Select appropriate person(s) to assist child with strategy
Develop individualized child and family goals for decreasing pain and increasing coping strategies
Teach child to use specific nonpharmacologic strategies before pain occurs or before it becomes severe
Assist or have parent assist child with using strategy during actual pain

EXPECTED OUTCOMES

Child exhibits reduced or tolerable pain level
Child learns and implements effective coping strategies
Parent learns coping skills and is effective in assisting child to cope

GOAL 2

Relieve pain

INTERVENTIONS

Plan to administer prescribed analgesic before procedure so that its peak effect coincides with inducement of pain (see Table 26-5)
Plan preventive schedule of medication around the clock, not as needed, when pain is continuous and predictable (e.g., postoperatively)
Administer analgesia by mouth or into intravenous line whenever possible (avoid injection)
Prepare child for administration of analgesia
Use supportive statements
- Reinforce effect of the analgesic by stating that child will begin to feel better in X amount of time (according to drug use); use a clock or timer to measure onset of relief with child; reinforce the cause and effect of pain and the analgesic, so child becomes conditioned to *expecting* relief
- Avoid saying, "I am going to give you an injection for pain," since this is another pain in addition to the existing pain; if child refuses an injection, explain that the "little hurt from the needle will take away the bigger hurt for a long time"
- Avoid statements such as, "This is enough medicine to take away anyone's pain," or "By now you shouldn't need so much pain medicine"
- Give child control whenever possible (e.g., choosing which leg for an injection, taking bandages off, holding the tape or other equipment)

*Administer prescribed analgesic
- Titrate dosage for maximum pain relief
- Begin with recommended dosage for age and weight (see Tables 26-4 and 26-5)
- Increase dosage and/or decrease dose interval between dosages if pain relief is inadequate

If using parenteral route, change to oral route as soon as possible using equianalgesic dosages (see Box 26-10)
Combine nonopioids with opioids
Avoid combining opioids with so-called potentiators
Avoid using placebos to verify "if pain is real"

EXPECTED OUTCOMES

Child exhibits absence of or minimum evidence of pain
Child accepts administration of analgesia with minimum distress

NURSING DIAGNOSIS: Potential for poisoning or injury related to sensitivity, overuse, decreased gastrointestinal motility

GOAL 1

Prevent respiratory distress

INTERVENTIONS

Have emergency drugs and equipment in case of respiratory depression from narcotics
Decrease drug dosage if excessive sedation or decreased respiratory rate occurs
Have emergency drugs and equipment available
*Administer naloxone (Narcan) for respiratory depression

EXPECTED OUTCOME

Child's respirations remain within acceptable limits (see inside front cover for normal variations)

GOAL 2

Prevent minor side effects from becoming serious

INTERVENTIONS

*Administer stool softener or laxative to prevent constipation
Stop or decrease medication if evidence of rash or other reaction

EXPECTED OUTCOMES

Child has regular bowel movements
Child exhibits no evidence of reaction

GOAL 3

Manage tolerance and physical dependency

INTERVENTIONS

Recognize signs of tolerance and withdrawal (physical dependence) (see Box 26-11)
*Help treat tolerance and physical dependence appropriately
Never refer to child who is tolerant or physically dependent as addicted

EXPECTED OUTCOME

Child receives appropriate therapy for tolerance or dependency

*Dependent nursing action.

more than 20 kg are given 2.0 mg (American Academy of Pediatrics, Committee on Drugs, 1990).

✦ **NURSING ALERT** Since naloxone's duration of action (about 1 to 4 hours) may be shorter than the duration of the narcotic, repeated doses may be required to prevent recurrence of respiratory depression. Respiratory depression from morphine is most likely to occur 7 minutes after IV infusion, 30 minutes after IM administration, and 90 minutes after oral ingestion.

Constipation is a common and sometimes troublesome side effect of opioids. Prevention with stool softeners and laxatives, especially senna, is more effective than treatment once constipation occurs. Pruritus from epidural or intrathecal infusion can be treated with low doses of naloxone infused slowly or with IV nalbuphine. Pruritus from IV infusion usually responds to oral antihistamines. Nausea, vomiting, and sedation usually subside after 2 days of opioid administration, although oral or rectal antiemetics may be necessary.

Both tolerance and physical dependence can occur with prolonged use of opioids. Treatment of tolerance involves increasing the dose or decreasing the duration between doses. Treatment of physical dependence involves gradually reducing the dose over 7 to 10 days to prevent occurrence of withdrawal symptoms (similar to tapering of steroid dosages after chronic steroid therapy); the use of methadone in tapering doses over 5 days is effective in reducing symptoms of withdrawal (Miser and others, 1986).

Use supportive statements when administering analgesics. The effectiveness of analgesics can be enhanced by a supportive attitude toward the child. By reinforcing the cause and effect of the medication and analgesia, child can become conditioned to expect pain relief, provided the regimen is likely to be effective. Ideally, injections should not be given, but when they are, children need to understand that the "little hurt from the needle will take away the bigger hurt for a long time."

Parents and older children may have concerns about the use of opioids because of fear of addiction. These concerns should be addressed with assurance that any such risk is extremely low. It may be helpful to ask the question, "If you did not have this pain, would you want to take this medicine?" (McCaffery and Beebe, 1989). The answer is invariably no, which reinforces the solely therapeutic nature of the drug.

Other supportive interventions, as well as a review of pain management interventions, are described in the Nursing Care Plan on p. 1158.

USE OF PLAY TO MINIMIZE STRESS

Play is one of the most important aspects of a child's life and one of the most effective tools for managing stress. Since illness and hospitalization constitute crises in the child's life and often involve overwhelming stresses, playing out fears and anxieties gives the child a means to cope with these stresses.

Box 26-12 FUNCTIONS OF PLAY IN THE HOSPITAL

- Provides diversion and brings about relaxation
- Helps the child feel more secure in a strange environment
- Helps to lessen stress of separation and the feelings of homesickness
- Provides a means for release of tension and expression of feelings
- Encourages interaction and development of positive attitudes toward others
- Provides an expressive outlet for creative ideas and interests
- Provides a means for accomplishing therapeutic goals (see Box 27-5)
- Places child in active role and provides opportunity to make choices and be in control

Play is the "work" of children. It is essential to their mental, emotional, and social well-being. As with their developmental needs, the need for play does not stop when children are ill or when they enter the hospital. On the contrary, play in the hospital serves many functions (Box 26-12). Of all hospital facilities, no room probably does more to alleviate the stressors of hospitalization than the playroom. In this room children temporarily distance themselves from the fears of separation, loss of control, and bodily injury. They can work through their feelings in a nonthreatening, comfortable atmosphere and in the manner most natural for them. They also know that the boundaries of this room are safe from intrusive or painful procedures, strange faces, and probing questions. The playroom becomes a sanctuary of peace and safety in an otherwise frightening environment.

Children in various age-groups require different types of play facilities. Infants and toddlers need maximum safety, whereas school-age children and adolescents benefit most from group recreation. Providing space for special needs of children in each age-group can be difficult in overcrowded institutions, but innovative solutions can ensure practical answers. Playroom schedules can accommodate children in one age-group at one session and another group at a later time; for example, adolescents can use the facility in the evening when younger children are asleep. Older children can also congregate in one patient's room and listen to music, play games, or just talk about their experiences. If the location of the recreational session is rotated each evening, older children can look forward to arranging or setting up for the activities.

Diversional Activities

Almost any form of play can be used for diversion and recreation, but the activity should be selected on the basis of the child's age, interests, and limitations (Fig. 26-9). Children do not necessarily need special direction for using play materials. All they require is the raw materials with which to work and adult approval and supervision to help keep their natural enthusiasm or expression of feelings from getting out of control. Small children enjoy a variety of small, colorful toys they can play with in bed or in their

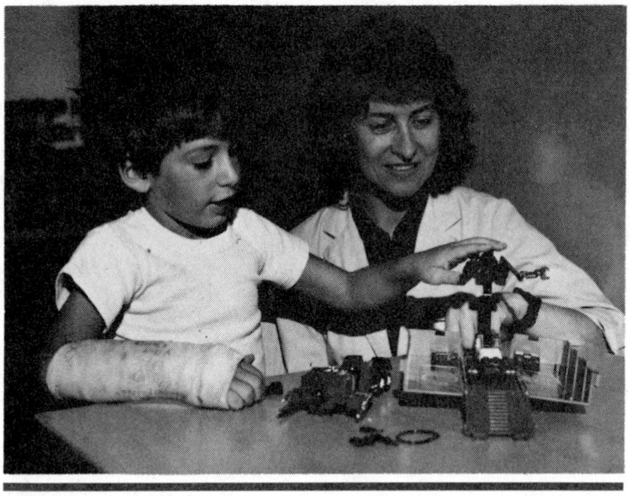

Fig. 26-9. Play materials for hospitalized children need to be appropriate for their age, interests, and limitations.

room or more elaborate play equipment, such as playhouses, sandboxes, rhythm instruments, and large boxes and blocks, that may be a part of the hospital playroom.

Games that can be played alone or with another child or an adult are popular with older children, as are puzzles; reading material; quiet individual activities such as sewing, stringing beads, and weaving; and Tinker-Toys, Lego blocks, and other building materials. Assembling models is an excellent pastime, but one should make certain that all pieces and necessary materials are included in the package so that the child is not disappointed.

Well-selected books are of infinite value to the child. Children never tire of stories. To have someone read aloud provides endless hours of pleasure and is of special value to the child who has limited energy to expend in play. A radio or television, part of most hospital room equipment, is a useful tool for entertaining a child, but parents and nurses should monitor program selection. Also, it should not be used as a substitute for social interaction or therapeutic play.

When supervising play for ill or convalescent children, it is best to select activities that are simpler than would normally be chosen according to the child's developmental level. These children usually do not have the energy to cope with more challenging activities. Other limitations also influence the type of activities. Special consideration must be given to the child who has limited movement, has a restricted extremity, or is isolated. Toys for isolated children must be capable of being disposed of or disinfected after use.

Toys. Parents of hospitalized children often ask nurses about the types of toys that would be best to bring for their child. Most want to bring new ones to cheer and comfort the child and assuage their own guilt feelings regarding the child's need for hospitalization. The nurse should tell the parents that, although wanting to provide these things for their child is natural, it is often better to wait awhile to bring new things, especially for younger children. Small children need the comfort and reassurance of familiar things, such as the stuffed animal the child hugs for comfort and takes to bed at night. These are a link with home and the world outside the hospital.

Large numbers of toys often confuse and frustrate a small child. A few small, well-chosen toys are usually preferred to one large, expensive one. Children who are hospitalized for an extended time benefit from changes. Rather than a confusing accumulation of toys, older toys should be replaced periodically as interest wanes. A helpful suggestion is to have parents provide the child with a shoe box, a child's small suitcase, or knapsack to attach to the bed for an easy storage receptacle to prevent small items from becoming lost in the sheets or under the bed. Children love putting things in and taking things out of a larger container. Many simple items, such as a small magnifying glass, a magnet, grooming aids, a small mirror, crayons and coloring books, colorful paper with scissors and paste, a magic slate, small dolls or toy soldiers, small cars, and beads to string, provide endless hours of amusement. The nurse is responsible for assessing the safety of the toys brought to the child.

A highly successful diversion for a child who is hospitalized for a length of time and whose parents are unable to visit frequently is for them to bring a box with seven small, inexpensive, and brightly wrapped items with a different day of the week printed on the outside. The child will eagerly anticipate the time for opening each one. When the parents know when their next visit will be, they can provide the number of packages that corresponds to the days between visits. In this way the child knows that the diminishing packages also represent the anticipated visit from the parent.

Expressive Activities

Play provides one of the best opportunities for encouraging emotional expression, including the safe release of anger and hostility. Nondirective play that allows children freedom for expression can be very therapeutic. Therapeutic play, however, should not be confused with the psychologic technique of play therapy. *Play therapy* is reserved for use by trained and qualified therapists who use the technique as an interpretative method with emotionally disturbed children. *Therapeutic play,* on the other hand, is a very effective nondirective modality for helping children deal with their concerns and fears; at the same time it often helps the nurse to gain insights into their needs and feelings (Clatworthy, 1981).

Tension release can be facilitated through almost any activity. With younger ambulatory children, large-muscle activity such as use of tricycles and wagons is especially beneficial. Much aggression can be safely directed into games and activities that involve pounding and throwing. Bean bags are often thrown at a target or open receptable with surprising vigor and hostility. A pounding board is employed with enthusiasm by young children; clay and Play-Doh are beneficial at any age. An angry child of 9 or 10 years of age may attack a mound of clay with the same intensity as a 3- or 4-year-old.

Creative expression. Drawing and painting are excellent media for expression. The child needs only to be supplied with the raw materials, such as crayons and paper; pots of bright poster color, large brushes, and an ample supply of newsprint supported on easels; or materials for finger painting. Children usually require little direction for self-expression; however, older children may be given some direction in what to paint or draw. For example, they may be asked to draw the hospital room or draw what they like or do not like about the hospital. Groups of children can enjoy this creative activity either working individually or, with older children, collaborating on a group project such as a mural painted on a long piece of paper. For children confined to bed, an old sheet (acquired from the laundry) spread over the bed and a large gown that extends down over the bedclothes to cover their own gown provide protection for clean linen.

Holidays provide stimulus and direction for unlimited creative projects. The children can participate in decorating the pediatric unit, and making pictures and decorations for their rooms gives the children a sense of pride and accomplishment. This is especially beneficial for immobilized and isolated children. Making gifts for someone at home helps to maintain interpersonal ties.

Dramatic play. Dramatic play is a well-recognized technique for emotional release, allowing children to reenact frightening or puzzling hospital experiences. Through use of puppets, replicas of hospital equipment, or some actual hospital equipment, children can play out the situations that are a part of their hospital experience. Dramatic play enables children to learn about procedures and events that will concern them and to assume the roles of the adults in the hospital environment.

Puppets are universally effective for communicating with children. Most children view them as peers and readily communicate with them. Children will tell the puppet feelings that they hesitate to express to adults. Puppets can share children's own experiences and help them to find solutions to their problems. Puppets dressed to represent figures in the child's environment—for example, a physician, nurse, child patient, therapist, and members of the child's own family—are especially useful (Fig. 26-10). Small, appropriately attired dolls are equally effective in encouraging the child to play out situations, although puppets are usually best for direct conversation.

In planning any play activities, the nurse must not forget that the reason for the child's hospitalization always takes precedence over other considerations, including the need for play. Play must be scheduled around medical needs and any limitations imposed by the child's condition. For example, small children may eat paste and other creative media; therefore a child who is allergic to wheat should not be given finger paint made from wallpaper paste or play dough made with flour. A child on a restricted salt intake should not play with modeling dough, since salt is one of its major constituents.* Treatment schedules and the institution's rules and policies must also be considered. At home the play program should be planned around the therapy regimen. However, play can be satisfactorily incorporated into the child's care if the nurse and others involved allow some flexibility and use creativity in planning for play.

*A national clearinghouse for research and education in visual and performing arts can be contacted at the **Center for Safety in the Arts,** 5 Beckman St., Suite 1030, New York, NY 10038; (212) 227-6220.

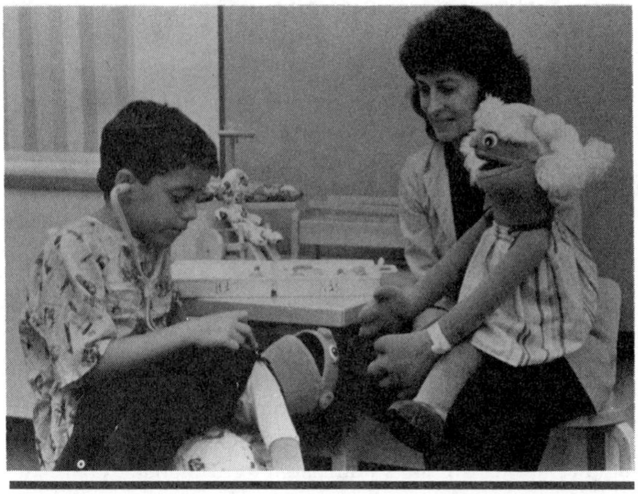

Fig. 26-10. Playing with miniature hospital equipment and puppets allows children to explore feelings and concerns safely.

MAXIMIZING POTENTIAL BENEFITS OF HOSPITALIZATION

While hospitalization generally represents a stressful time for children and families, it also presents an opportunity for facilitating positive change within the child and among family members. Therefore nursing interventions must also focus on maximizing the potential benefits of the experience.

Fostering Parent-Child Relationships

The crisis of illness or hospitalization can mobilize parents into more acute awareness of their children's needs. For example, one school-age child who was diagnosed with a serious physical condition commented to the nurse that he "enjoyed" the hospital because it was the first time that he had seen so much of his parents. He expressed concern over discharge because he anticipated the loss of the intensified love and attention. The nurse was able to discuss these feelings with the parents and to increase their awareness of their child's need for them.

Hospitalization provides opportunities for parents to learn more about their children's growth and development. When parents are helped to understand children's usual reactions to stress, such as regression or aggression, they are not only better able to support the child through the hospital experience but also may extend their insights into childrearing practices following discharge.

Difficulties in parent-child relationships that may result in feeding problems, negative behavior, and enuresis may decrease during hospitalization. The temporary cessation of such problems sometimes alerts parents to the role they may be playing in propagating the negative behavior. With assistance from health professionals, parents can restructure ways of relating to their children to foster more positive behavior.

Hospitalization may also represent a temporary reprieve or refuge from a disturbed home. Typically abused or neglected children's dramatic physical and social improvement during hospitalization is proof of the growth potential of this experience. Hospitalized children temporarily are able to seek support, reassurance, and security from new relationships, particularly with nurses, hospitalized peers, and others.

Providing Educational Opportunities

Illness and hospitalization represent excellent opportunities for children and other family members to learn more about their bodies, each other, and the health professions. For example, during a child's admission for a diabetic crisis, the child may learn about the disease; the parents may learn about the child's needs for independence, normalcy, and appropriate limits; and each of them may find a new support system in the hospital staff.

During extended hospitalization, special tutoring can help children advance their studies and concentrate on difficult subjects. The child's relationship with a tutor can foster a more positive attitude toward school and learning.

Illness or hospitalization can also help older children in choosing a vocational career. Frequently children have impressions of physicians or nurses that are disproportionately glorified or horrified. However, experience with different health professionals can influence their decision for or against a health career.

Promoting Self-Mastery

The experience of facing a crisis such as illness or hospitalization, coping successfully with it, and maturing as a result of it constitutes an opportunity for self-mastery. Younger children have the chance to test out fantasy vs reality fears. They realize that they were not abandoned, mutilated, castrated, or punished. In fact, they were loved, cared for, and treated with respect for their individual concerns. It is not unusual to hear children who have undergone hospitalization or surgery tell others of how "it was nothing" or proudly display their scars or bandages. For older children, hospitalization may represent an opportunity for decision making, independence, and self-reliance. They are proud of having survived the experience and may feel a genuine self-respect for their achievements. Nurses can facilitate such feelings of self-mastery by emphasizing aspects of personal competence in the child and not acknowledging uncooperative or negative behavior.

Providing Socialization

Hospitalization may offer children a special opportunity for social acceptance. Lonely, asocial, sometimes delinquent children find a sympathetic environment in the hospital. Children who are physically deformed or in some other way "different" from their age-mates may find an accepting social peer group. Although this does not always spontaneously occur, nurses can structure the environment to foster a supportive child group. For example, judicious selection of a roommate can help children gain a new friend and learn more about themselves. Forming relationships with significant members of the health care team, such as the physician, nurse, child-life specialist, or minister, can greatly enhance the child's adjustment in many areas of life.

Parents may also encounter a new social group in other parents who have similar problems. The waiting room or hallway "self-help" groups are part of every institution. Nurses can capitalize on this informal gathering by encouraging parents to discuss collectively their concerns and feelings. They can also refer parents to organized parent groups or can use the help and support of recovered hospitalized patients.

SUPPORTING FAMILY MEMBERS

The term *family-centered care* defines the focus of pediatric care because nursing of children cannot be optimally performed unless each family member is designated the "patient" or "client" (see Family-Centered Care, Chapter 22; also Box 22-1). Support involves the willingness to stay and listen to parents' verbal and nonverbal messages. Sometimes the support is not given directly by the nurse. For example, the nurse may offer to stay with the child to allow the parents time alone or may discuss with other family members the parents' need for extra relief. Often extended relatives and friends want to help but do not know how. The nurse can suggest baby-sitting, preparing meals, tending the garden or home, doing laundry, or transporting the siblings to school as ways to lessen the parents' responsibilities.

Support may also be provided through the clergy. Parents with deep religious beliefs may appreciate the counsel of a clergy member, but because of their stress they may not have sufficient energy to initiate the contact. Nurses can be supportive by arranging for clergy to visit and by respecting and upholding parents' religious beliefs.

Support involves an acceptance of cultural, socioeconomic, and ethnic values. For example, health and illness are defined differently by various ethnic groups. For some, disorders that have few outward manifestations of illness, such as diabetes, hypertension, or cardiac problems, are not viewed as a sickness. Consequently, following a prescribed treatment may be seen as unnecessary. Nurses who appreciate the influences of culture are more likely to intervene therapeutically (see also Chapter 2 for an extensive discussion of cultural/religious influences on health care).

Parents need help in accepting their own feelings toward the ill child. If given the opportunity, parents often disclose their feelings of loss of control, anger, and guilt. They often resist admitting to such feelings because they expect others to disapprove of behavior that is less than perfect. Unfortunately, health personnel, including nurses, sometimes show little tolerance for deviation from the expected norm. This only increases the psychologic impact of a child's illness on family members. Helping parents identify the specific reason for such feelings and emphasizing that each is a normal, expected, and healthy response to stress provides them with an opportunity to lessen their emotional burden.

NURSING CARE PLAN
The Family of the Ill or Hospitalized Child

NURSING DIAGNOSIS: Anxiety/fear related to situational crisis, threat to role functioning, change in environment

GOAL 1

Help family adjust to the hospital

INTERVENTIONS

Introduce family to significant staff members
Describe hospital routine that affects the child
Acclimate family to the new and strange surroundings
  Physical layout of unit, including playroom, unit kitchen, toilet, telephone, where they can stay
Direct family to areas they may need to use outside the unit (e.g., dining room, chapel)
Provide an atmosphere that promotes questioning, expression of doubts and feelings
Be available to family
Be alert to signs of tension in family members
Provide for privacy

EXPECTED OUTCOMES

Family demonstrates familiarity with hospital environment
Family members ask questions

GOAL 2

Make family feel important as members of the health team

INTERVENTIONS

Employ a polite approach and demeanor
Greet family by name when they arrive on the unit
Encourage frequent visiting
Include family in planning patient care
Encourage family to select and assume specific roles in the child's care
Offer encouragement for their efforts
Ask family to share with the staff what they know about the child's care and needs
Convey an attitude of collegiality with family, not competition

EXPECTED OUTCOME

Family becomes involved in planning and carrying out care for the child

GOAL 3

Reduce apprehension

INTERVENTIONS

Allow for expression of feelings about the child's hospitalization and illness
Provide needed information
Prepare family for what to expect (e.g., procedures, behaviors)
Explore family's concerns and feelings of irritation, guilt, anger, disappointment, inadequacy
Explore family's fears and anxieties regarding the child's status and expectations of results of procedures or therapy
Introduce parents to other families who have a child in the hospital, especially a child who is similarly affected
Provide something constructive for family to focus on (e.g., keeping record of intake and output, pain relief record, ensuring a specified amount of fluid intake, collecting a specimen)

EXPECTED OUTCOMES

Family members verbalize feelings and concerns
Family demonstrates an understanding of procedures and behaviors (specify manner of demonstration and learning)
Family interacts with other families
Family complies with directions (specify)

GOAL 4

Prepare family for special procedures (radiology, diagnostic tests, surgery)

INTERVENTIONS

Assess family's understanding of the procedure and its purpose
Provide needed information; clarify misconceptions
Explain special preparation needed (e.g., nothing by mouth [NPO], shaving, preprocedure medication or equipment)
Describe
  Where the child will be during the procedure
  Whether the family can be with the child
  Where the family can wait
  Approximate length of time procedure requires
Reassure family that they will be notified regarding progress of the procedure

EXPECTED OUTCOME

Family demonstrates an understanding of procedures and tests (specify)

GOAL 5

Support the family during child's absence

INTERVENTIONS

Provide a comfortable place for the family to wait
Suggest activities to help reduce anxiety (e.g., go to the coffee shop or dining room, take a short walk [specify activity])
Be available to family
Make contact with family at frequent intervals to relay information, provide comfort

EXPECTED OUTCOME

Family takes advantage of suggestions (specify)

GOAL 6

Help family adjust to the child's appearance and behavior following procedure(s) or in special care unit

INTERVENTIONS

Remain calm
Describe the environment, if appropriate (e.g., ICU)
Apply principles of learning to explanations
  Begin with small amounts of information
  Begin with very general information
  Allow ample time for family to absorb information and to ask questions

Continued.

Explain how the child will look and the reasons for the child's appearance and equipment
Explain what the child is experiencing
Prepare the child and surroundings to lessen the impact of first impression
- Tidy the bed
- Personalize the bed and bedside with a toy or other item(s)
- Provide chairs for the family
- Be prepared for possible adverse reaction (e.g., fainting)

Convey an attitude of caring *about* as well as *for* the child
Accompany the family to the child's bedside

EXPECTED OUTCOME

Family comes to child's bedside without evidence of distress

GOAL 7

Alleviate fears

INTERVENTIONS

Help family distinguish between realistic and unfounded fears
Help eliminate unfounded fears
Discuss with family their fears regarding
- Child's signs and symptoms
- Child's anxiety
- Dire consequences of disease or therapy
- Deterioration of child's condition
- Tests and procedures
- Death

Answer questions honestly and compassionately

EXPECTED OUTCOME

Family members verbalize fears and explore nature and ramifications of these fears

NURSING DIAGNOSIS: Powerlessness related to health care environment

GOAL 1

Provide a sense of control

INTERVENTIONS

Encourage family visiting at times convenient for them (there will be cultural variations in the amount and type of visiting)
Allow expression of concerns regarding the child's care and progress
Explore the family's feelings regarding prescribed therapies
Permit the family as much control as possible in the child's management
- Encourage participation in the child's care
- Include family in setting goals for care
- Involve family in scheduling and other aspects of care
- Explain what family can do for the child and how to handle the child to maintain therapy (e.g., how to pick up the child who has an intravenous line)
- Employ family's suggestions regarding the child's care whenever possible

EXPECTED OUTCOMES

Family schedules visiting times
Family readily discusses feelings and concerns
Family contributes to care and management of the child
*Family's suggestions are incorporated into plan of care

NURSING DIAGNOSIS: Altered family processes related to situational crisis (threat to role functioning, hospitalization of a child)

GOAL 1

Help family understand the child's illness

INTERVENTIONS

Recognize family's concern and need for information, support
Assess family's understanding of diagnosis and plan of care
Reinforce and clarify health professional's explanation of the child's condition, suggested procedures and therapies, and the prognosis
Use every opportunity to increase the family's understanding of the disease and its therapies
Repeat information as often as necessary
Interpret technical information
Help family interpret the infant's or child's behaviors and responses
Do not appear rushed; if time is inappropriate, set a date for discussion as soon as feasible
- Keep appointment faithfully

EXPECTED OUTCOME

Family demonstrates an understanding of the disease and its therapies (specify knowledge)

GOAL 2

Help alleviate guilt feelings

INTERVENTIONS

Provide accurate and specific information regarding the causes of the illness
Clarify misconceptions and false assumptions

EXPECTED OUTCOME

Family verbalizes their understanding of the cause of the illness (specify)

GOAL 3

Support family

INTERVENTIONS

Respect parental rights
Convey an attitude of respectful caring for both child and family
Support and emphasize the family's strengths and abilities
Provide feedback and praise for compliance

*Nursing outcome.

Refer to other professionals for additional interpersonal and concrete support (e.g., social service, clergy)

EXPECTED OUTCOMES

Family exhibits behaviors that indicate a feeling of self-respect
Family uses supportive services

GOAL 4

Help family cope with the child's behavior

INTERVENTIONS

Determine family's understanding of the normal childhood responses to the stress of illness and hospitalization
Explain child's regression, magical thinking, egocentricity, separation anxiety, fears
Explain behavioral reactions generally expected of the child (specify according to age and developmental level)
Explain what the child is (family are) permitted to do in coping with the child's behavior
Reinforce family's endeavors

EXPECTED OUTCOME

Family demonstrates an understanding of the child's unfamiliar behaviors (specify manner of demonstration—verbalization, physical attitude, behaviors with child)

GOAL 5

Help family assist the child to cope with hospitalization

INTERVENTIONS

Help parents determine the best way to prepare the child for hospitalization, procedures
Provide family with precise information about what will take place so they know what the child is likely to experience
Encourage family to trust the child's capacity to cope
Impress on family the need for honesty in relating to the child
Encourage family to use play as a coping strategy
Suggest appropriate items to bring to the child (e.g., pajamas, favorite toys)
See also Nursing Care Plan: The Child in the Hospital, p. 1136

EXPECTED OUTCOMES

Family helps in planning strategies
Family is honest with the child and staff
Family uses play as a tool for relating with the child

GOAL 6

Promote and foster positive family relationships

INTERVENTIONS

Recognize that family members know the child best and are "cued in" to the child's needs
Allow unlimited visiting times
Encourage family to bring other significant family members to visit (e.g., siblings, grandparents, and [where permitted] pets)
Encourage family to provide the child with significant, but manageable, items from home

EXPECTED OUTCOMES

Child and family exhibit behaviors that indicate positive coping
Family visits the child at appropriate times and in appropriate numbers
Child demonstrates an attitude of security with familiar persons and things

GOAL 7

Promote family health

INTERVENTIONS

Stress the importance of maintaining family members' health during the child's illness and hospitalization
Encourage adequate rest
- Provide sleeping facilities where possible
- Encourage members to alternate visiting with the child to allow some time at home
- Explore means for respite care of dependent family members

Convey to family the assurance that the child will receive optimum care in their absence
Provide relief for family from direct care of child as needed
Promote adequate nutrition
- Provide meals for parents if possible
- Direct family to nutritious resources for meals
- Encourage regular mealtimes away from unit

EXPECTED OUTCOMES

Family shows no evidence of illness
Family members appear well rested
Family members eat regularly

GOAL 8

Promote a smooth transition from hospital to home

INTERVENTIONS

Assess the family's learning needs
Outline and carry out a teaching plan
Determine services needed and make necessary referrals
Include family in planning and problem solving
Maintain open communication between family and health care providers

EXPECTED OUTCOME

Child and family demonstrate the ability to provide needed care in the home

GOAL 9

Prepare for discharge

INTERVENTIONS

Assess the family's knowledge
Teach family the skills needed to carry out the therapeutic program (specify)
- Allow ample time for preparation
- Teach necessary techniques and observations
- Help family by demonstration
- Distribute appropriate home care instructions or other educational materials or both
- Encourage questions and expression of feelings and concerns

Continued.

NURSING CARE PLAN
The Family of the Ill or Hospitalized Child—cont'd

- Allow sufficient time for family to perform procedures under supervision
- Inform parents of
  - Signs of progress to observe for
  - Any unfavorable signs to be alert for
  - Problems that can be anticipated (e.g., care of equipment or devices)
  - Behaviors that indicate special needs (e.g., pain medication, imminent seizures)
  - A course of action to follow (e.g., seizure care)
- Make certain family knows how to contact appropriate persons if or when needed
- Prepare family for possible posthospital behaviors of the child (see Box 26-2)
- Ensure family's comprehension of the child's needs before discharge

EXPECTED OUTCOMES

Family demonstrates the procedures needed to care for the child in the home (specify learning and method of demonstration)
Family is aware of how to seek help

GOAL 10

Maintain continuity of care

INTERVENTIONS

Inform family of community resources available
Refer to agencies as appropriate (specify)
Help identify support group(s) for family
Be available to family by telephone or other means
Schedule follow-up appointments as needed

EXPECTED OUTCOMES

Family seeks appropriate assistance
Family keeps appointments

See also:
Nursing Care Plan: The Child in the Hospital, p. 1136
Nursing Care Plan: The Child with a Chronic Illness or Disability, Chapter 22
Nursing Care Plan: The Child Who Is Terminally Ill or Dying, Chapter 23

Providing Information

One of the most important nursing interventions is to provide information regarding (1) the disease, its treatment, and prognosis; (2) the child's emotional, as well as physical, reaction to illness and hospitalization; and (3) the probable emotional reactions of family members to the crisis.

For many families the child's illness is their first contact with the hospital experience. Often parents are not prepared for the child's behavioral reactions to hospitalization, such as separation behaviors, regression, aggression, and hostility. Providing the parents with information about these normal and expected behavioral responses can lessen the parents' anxiety during the hospital admission (Vulcan and Nikulich-Barrett, 1988). The family is equally unfamiliar with hospital rules, which often adds to feelings of confusion and anxiety. Therefore the family needs clear explanations about what to expect and what is expected of them. Nurses can also help family members become more adept at seeking information about their child's condition by asking questions that elicit meaningful information (Box 26-13). In giving information, nurses need to be alert to information overload (see Box 6-2).

Box 26-13 GUIDELINES FOR HELPING FAMILIES ELICIT INFORMATION

- Find out what the family wants to know.
- Teach them to avoid general questions, such as, "Why is my child sick?"
- Help them prepare specific questions, such as, "What is causing my child's pain?" or "What does this drug do?"
- Encourage the use of short and open-ended questions.
- Have the family write down the questions, preferably in a diary or journal that is kept in an accessible area, such as a pocket, to have available when needed.
- Encourage the family to speak up when they do not understand an answer and to have it explained in clearer or easier language.
- Have the family repeat the information to be certain they understand it and to record unfamiliar terms.

Modified from Norris, L.: Coaching the question, Nursing 86 16(5):100, 1986.

Parents also need to be aware of the effects of illness on the family and strategies that prevent negative changes. Specifically, parents should keep the family well informed and communicating as much as possible. They should treat all the children as equally and as normally as before the illness occurred. Discipline, which initially may be lessened for the ill child, should be continued to provide a measure of security and predictability. When ill children know that their parents expect certain standards of conduct from them, they feel certain that they will recover. When all limits are removed, they fear that something catastrophic will happen.

Helping parents understand and accept the meaning of posthospitalization behaviors in the sick child is necessary for them to tolerate and support such behaviors. Consequently, they should be forewarned of the usual continuance of such reactions following discharge. Parents who do not expect such reactions may misinterpret them as evidence of the child's "being spoiled" and demand perfect behavior at a time when the child is still reacting to the stress of illness and hospitalization. If the behaviors, especially the demand for attention, are dealt with in a supportive manner, most children are able to relinquish them and assume precrisis levels of functioning.

Nurses should also forewarn parents of the reactions of siblings to the ill child—particularly anger, jealousy, and resentment. Older siblings may deny such reactions because they provoke feelings of guilt. However, everyone needs outlets for emotions, and the repressed feelings may surface as problems in school, with age-mates, as psychosomatic illnesses, or in delinquent behavior.

Probably one of the most neglected areas involves giving information to siblings. Age frequently becomes the only factor that leads to an awareness of this problem, since older children may begin to ask questions or request explanations. However, even in this situation the information may be seriously inadequate. Children in every age-group deserve some explanation of the child's illness or hospitalization, preferably appropriate written information for children. Although the exact wording may differ, the answer should focus on the following concerns: (1) "Will I get sick and have to go to the hospital?" (2) "Did I cause the illness?" (for actual or imagined reasons), and (3) "Will my parents abandon me if my brother or sister doesn't recover?" If parents or nurses address the explanations to these three questions, the siblings' own fears of illness, guilt, and abandonment are minimized.

Nursing approaches with siblings can be direct or indirect. Direct services might include (1) incorporating siblings into hospital admission programs; (2) liberalizing visiting regulations; (3) extending parent participation programs to include sibling involvement, such as through family dining or group play sessions; and (4) developing programs designed specifically for siblings, such as group sessions to discuss their concerns or posthospital discharge visits to evaluate the siblings' adjustment. Older siblings may not wish to attend a group; the nurse can be available for casual talks or for a tour, which may encourage the youngster to talk.

Indirect services, which can be influenced by any existing nursing role, involve helping parents understand, cope with, and support the siblings' reactions to the experience. Measures, such as ensuring siblings understand what is happening and providing for them to remain at home rather than with a neighbor or relative, can help minimize some of the negative effects (Craft, Wyatt, and Sandell, 1985; Knafl and Dixon, 1983). Other interventions include helping the sick and well siblings maintain contact through telephone calls or sending tape recordings, letters, or postcards (see also Parent Guidelines: Supporting Siblings, Chapter 22).

■ PREPARATION FOR HOSPITALIZATION

The rationale for preparing children for the hospital experience and related procedures is based on the principle that fear of the unknown (fantasy) exceeds fear of the known. Therefore, decreasing the elements of the unknown results in less fear. When children do not have paralyzing fear to cope with, they can then direct their energies toward dealing with the other unavoidable stresses of hospitalization and benefit optimally from the growth potential of the experience.

For children past infancy and early toddlerhood, in-hospital and/or home preparation for hospitalization reduces children's stress (Bates and Broomes, 1986). Even when children are too young to benefit from direct preparation, parents need prehospital counseling to lessen their fears and thus increase their ability to support the child psychologically. Prehospital counseling has two major goals:

1. To make the hospital less strange and frightening to parents and children
2. To establish a positive atmosphere and trusting relationship with hospital staff and family members

GUIDELINES IN PREPARING FOR HOSPITALIZATION

While preparation for hospitalization is a common practice, there is no universal standard or program that is advocated in both general and children's hospitals. Some hospital admission programs focus on group preparation before actual admission, whereas others prepare each child either before or on the day of admission. There is also a trend to prepare well children for future hospitalizations, although the benefits and disadvantages are controversial (Azarnoff, 1985). The primary audience of most hospital preparation programs is children who are experiencing an initial hospitalization. However, readmission is also stressful; children's fear and fantasies may not subside with repeated hospital stays but may intensify. These children need preparation as well, although the type of program needs to be individualized and may differ from the following guidelines for planning prehospital tours for groups or individual families who have not yet experienced hospital admission.

Ideally, preparatory procedures should be:

- Planned by the hospital staff before any child's admission to the hospital
- Appropriately designed for each child's developmental age
- Sufficiently individualized to account for different children's previous experience with hospitalization, present reason for admission, and available support system

In addition to the following discussion, the reader is also encouraged to review Preparation for Procedures, Chapter 27.

Group Size and Timing of Preparation

Group size should be small (about 10 children to a group) to provide individualized attention and facilitate discussion

(Huth, 1983). If tours are arranged for each child, the parents should be included and possibly the well siblings, although the actual benefit to these children has not been researched.

Prehospital admission programs should be scheduled for the time of day when staff members are most available and most treatment procedures are completed. They should occur before actual admission. However, no firm consensus exists on the timing of the event. Some authorities recommend preparing children 4 to 7 years of age about 1 week in advance so they can assimilate the information and ask questions. For older children the time may be longer. However, for young children, who may begin to fantasize about what they observed, 1 or 2 days before admission is sufficient time for anticipatory preparation (Petrillo and Sanger, 1980). Other research has found that children ages 5 to 12 years prefer to know about impending hospitalization from several weeks to a few minutes before the event, suggesting that the optimum approach is one that is individualized for each child (Ross and Ross, 1984). The length of the session should be suited to the children's attention span—the younger the child, the shorter the program.

Setting of the Tour

The setting of the tour should avoid any frightening aspects of the hospital environment and should typically include an inpatient room, the playroom (a highlight of the tour), the parents' waiting room, the nurses' station, and other special areas, such as the group dining room. Other areas that may be visited are the radiology department and laboratory area, the slumber or induction room, and the recovery room. Different hospitals may tailor this tour to include special rooms, such as the "OR playroom," where children and parents first go before any induction is administered. Children who are undergoing serious surgery requiring special postoperative care may be taken to visit the intensive care unit. Children scheduled for special tests, such as cardiac catheterization or cystoscopy, are sometimes shown these areas. Young children may respond better to shorter tours that concentrate on the areas of most concern, such as the pediatric unit, playroom, and recovery room. In any case, throughout the tour, the nurse (or other guide) must be alert to signs of concern or fear in the children. Strange noises, sights, sounds, and smells that are routine to hospital personnel can be frightening to children.

Preparatory Materials

The most suitable type of presentation for children includes a variety of preparatory materials, including films, lecture, demonstration, and play. The following discussion explores some of the typical methods that may be used in preparing children for elective surgery.

A puppet show may reenact the basic steps of hospitalization—admission procedures; preparation for surgery, the operating room, and the recovery room; and postsurgical treatment. The main focus of each scene is the use of concrete actions and models to familiarize the family members with what will occur. The puppets talk about children's common fears—pain, anesthesia, and parent separation. Although the sophistication of the materials varies, the basic characters should include a puppet family (mother, father, child) and hospital staff (physician, nurse) that are racially representative of the patient and hospital population. For example, both black and white dolls are required in many urban areas. Hospital equipment includes mask, cap, gloves, gown, intravenous bottle, stand, tubing, syringes, thermometer, blood pressure machine, stethoscope, scale, oxygen mask, suture removal set, bandages, bed, and sheets. If children are routinely admitted for diagnostic evaluations, miniature replicas of machinery (e.g., x-ray equipment) or the use of slides as visual aids may be used. The use of scaled-down models is especially beneficial for young children, who may be frightened by the actual proportions of some equipment. However, the *intent* of what is conveyed greatly surpasses the sophistication of the materials used.

Opportunity for Discussion

Any type of preparatory program needs to provide ample opportunity for discussion both before and after the tour. During the tour family members are encouraged to ask questions and to familiarize themselves with the environment by sitting on a bed, using the electric bed controls, riding in a wheelchair, or handling the equipment in the special rooms. Ideally the tour should also be an opportunity for meeting the child's primary nurse. Although this is not always possible because of staffing schedules, the nursing staff should be introduced to the children by name. Introducing them to one specific nurse, such as the head nurse or clinical specialist, helps them feel more comfortable in knowing who is available for questions or concerns during the hospital stay.

Following the tour there should be a question-and-answer period, monitored by a nurse. Sometimes the group is reticent about asking questions. In this case the nurse can stimulate discussion by posing a question to the audience or inviting the children to see and touch the puppets and equipment. Allowing children to play with the equipment and draw pictures about what they observed are excellent methods of evaluating the learning process and clarifying any misconceptions.

The tour may conclude with serving refreshments, which helps people relax, gather their thoughts, and ask a last-minute question. By informally visiting each table, the nurse has an excellent opportunity to discuss individual concerns. At this time the parents can also be invited to call the pediatric unit for any reason before admission, since questions may arise during this interval.

Prehospital Counseling by Parents

In many situations the preparation of children for hospitalization is left up to parents. Parents may abdicate this responsibility for a variety of reasons. For example, they sometimes think the child is too young to understand or is better off not knowing beforehand; often they are unable to prepare the child because of their own lack of knowledge and understanding.

Professionals can help parents prepare their children by

adequately informing them of the specific details of hospitalization and related procedures, through both direct discussion and written material. Responsibility for such guidance often rests with office and clinic nurses. They can discuss with parents the appropriate timing of the preparation and the methods, such as picture books about going to the hospital (see p. 1183). Many hospitals develop their own books and photograph albums for this purpose. Nurses working with these parents should also assess their level of anxiety regarding the impending hospitalization to prevent emotional contagion to the child.

HOSPITAL ADMISSION

The preparation that children require on the day of admission depends on their prehospital counseling. If they have been prepared in a formalized program, they will usually know what to expect in terms of initial medical procedures, inpatient facilities, and nursing staff. However, prehospital counseling does not preclude the need for support during procedures such as drawing blood, x-ray tests, or physical examination. For example, undressing young children before they feel comfortable in their new surroundings can be very upsetting. Causing needless anxiety and fear during admission may adversely affect the nurse's establishment of trust with these children. Therefore nursing assistance during the admission procedure is vital, regardless of how well prepared any child is for the hospitalization. In addition, spending this time with the child gives the nurse an opportunity to evaluate understanding of subsequent procedures, such as surgery (Fig. 26-11). The usual admission procedures for children are outlined in Box 26-14.

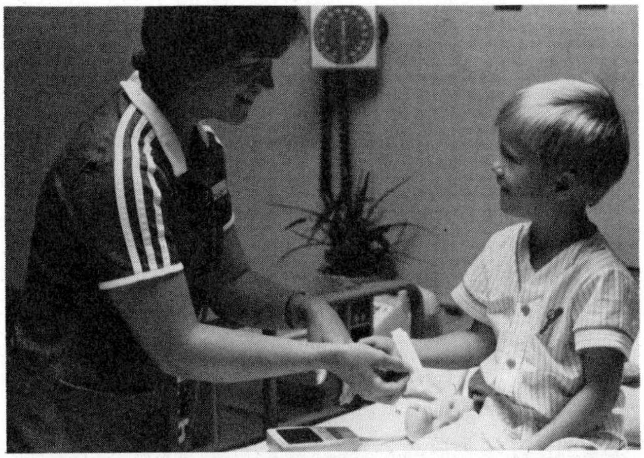

Fig. 26-11. The initial admission procedures allow the nurse to begin knowing the child and assessing his or her understanding of the hospital experience.

Box 26-14 GUIDELINES FOR ADMISSION

Preadmission

Assign a room based on developmental age, seriousness of diagnosis, communicability of illness, and projected length of stay.
Prepare roommate(s) for the arrival of a new patient; when children are too young to benefit from this consideration, prepare parents.
Prepare room for child and family, with admission forms and equipment nearby to eliminate need to leave child.

Admission

Introduce primary nurse to child and family.
Orient child and family to inpatient facilities, especially to assigned room and unit; emphasize positive areas of pediatric unit.
  Room: explain call light, bed controls, television, etc.; direct to bathroom, telephone, etc.
  Unit: Direct to playroom, desk, dining area, or other areas
Introduce family to roommate and his or her parents.
Apply identification band to child's wrist, ankle, or both (if not done).
Explain hospital regulations and schedules (e.g., visiting hours, mealtimes, bedtime, limitations [give written information if available]).
Perform nursing admission history (see Box 26-15).
Take vital signs, blood pressure, height, and weight.
Obtain specimens as needed and order needed laboratory work.
Support child and perform or assist practitioner with physical examination (for purposes of nursing assessment).

Guidelines for Emergency Admission

Lengthy preparatory admission procedures are often impossible and inappropriate for emergency situations.
Unless an emergency is life-threatening, children need to participate in their care to maintain a sense of control.
Focus on essential components of admission counseling, including:
  Appropriate introduction to the family
  Use of child's name, not terms such as "honey" or "dear"
  Determination of child's age and some judgment about developmental age (if the child is of school age, asking about the grade level will offer some evidence for concurrent intellectual ability)
  Information about child's general state of health, any problems that may interfere with medical treatment (e.g., sensitivity to medication), and previous experience with hospital facilities
  Information about the chief complaint from both the parents and the child

Guidelines for Admission to Intensive Care Unit

Prepare child and parents for elective ICU admission, such as for postoperative care after cardiac surgery.
Prepare child and parents for unanticipated ICU admission by focusing primarily on the sensory aspects of the experience and on usual family concerns (e.g., persons in charge of child's care, schedule for visiting, area where family can wait).
Prepare parents regarding child's appearance and behavior when they first visit child in ICU.
Accompany family to bedside to provide emotional support and answer questions.
Prepare siblings for their visit; plan length of time for sibling visitation; monitor siblings' reactions during visit to prevent them from becoming overwhelmed.

Nursing Admission History

The nursing admission history refers to a systematic collection of data about the child and family that allows the nurse to plan individualized care. The nursing admission history presented in Box 26-15 is organized according to the Functional Health Patterns outlined by Gordon (1987) (see Nursing Diagnosis, Chapter 1), which facilitates the formulation of nursing diagnoses. One of the main purposes of the history is to assess the child's usual health habits at home to promote a more normal environment in the hospital. Therefore questions related to activities of daily living are a major part of the assessment. The questions found under the health perception–health management pattern are directed toward evaluation of the child's preparation for hospitalization and are key factors in determining if additional preparation is needed.

As with any history form, the questions are only guidelines; for maximum communication, nurses should ask

Box 26-15 NURSING ADMISSION HISTORY ACCORDING TO FUNCTIONAL HEALTH PATTERNS*

Health Perception–Health Management Pattern

Why has your child been admitted?
How has your child's general health been?
What does your child know about this hospitalization?
- Ask the child why he or she came to the hospital.
- If answer is "For an operation or for tests," ask the child to tell you about what will happen before, during, and after the operation or tests.

Has your child ever been in the hospital before?
- How was that hospital experience?
- What things were important to you and your child during that hospitalization? How can we be most helpful now?

What medications does your child take at home?
- Why are they given?
- When are they given?
- How are they given (if a liquid, with a spoon; if a tablet, swallowed with water; or other)?
- Does your child have any trouble taking medication? If so, what helps?
- Is your child allergic to any medications?

Nutrition-Metabolic Pattern

What are the family's usual mealtimes?
Do family members eat together or at separate times?
What are your child's favorite foods, beverages, and snacks?
- Average amounts consumed or usual size portions
- Special cultural practices, such as family eats only ethnic food

What foods and beverages does your child dislike?
What are your child's feeding habits (bottle, cup, spoon, eats by self, needs assistance, any special devices)?
How does your child like the food served (warmed, cold, one item at a time)?
How would you describe your child's usual appetite (hearty eater, picky eater)?
- Has being sick affected your child's appetite?

Are there any known or suspected food allergies? Is your child on a special diet?
Are there any feeding problems (excessive fussiness, spitting up, colic); any dental or gum problems that affect feeding?
What do you do for these problems?

Elimination Pattern

What are your child's toilet habits (diaper, toilet trained–day only or day and night, use of word to communicate urination or defecation, potty chair, regular toilet, other routines)?
What is your child's usual pattern of elimination (bowel movements)?
Do you have any concerns about elimination (bed-wetting, constipation, diarrhea)?
What do you do for these problems?
Have you ever noticed that your child sweats a lot?

Sleep-Rest Pattern

What is your child's usual hour of sleep and awakening?
What is your child's schedule for naps; length of naps?
Is there a special routine before sleeping (bottle, drink of water, bedtime story, nightlight, favorite blanket or toy, prayers)?
Is there a special routine during sleep time, such as waking to go to the bathroom?
What type of bed does your child sleep in?
Does your child have a separate room or share a room; if shares, with whom?
What are the home sleeping arrangements (alone or with others, e.g., sibling, parent, other person)?
What is your child's favorite sleeping position?
Are there any sleeping problems (falling asleep, waking during night, nightmares, sleep walking)?
Are there any problems awakening and getting ready in the morning?
What do you do for these problems?

Activity-Exercise Pattern

What is your child's schedule during the day (nursery school, daycare center, regular school, extracurricular activities)?
What are your child's favorite activities or toys (both active and quiet interests)?
What is your child's usual television viewing schedule at home?
- What are your child's favorite programs?
- Are there any TV restrictions?

Does your child have any illness or disabilities that limit activity? If so, how?
What are your child's usual habits and schedule for bathing (bath in tub or shower, sponge bath, shampoo)?
What are your child's dental habits (brushing, flossing, fluoride supplements or rinses, favorite toothpaste); schedule of daily dental care?
Does your child need help with dressing or grooming, such as hair combing?
Are there any problems with the above (dislike of or refusal to bathe, shampoo hair, or brush teeth)?
What do you do for these problems?
Are there special devices that your child requires help in managing (eyeglasses, contact lenses, hearing aid, orthodontic appliances, artificial elimination appliances, orthopedic devices)?

NOTE: Use the following code to assess functional self-care level for feeding, bathing/hygiene, dressing/grooming, toileting:
- **0:** Full self-care
- **I:** Requires use of equipment or device
- **II:** Requires assistance or supervision from another person
- **III:** Requires assistance or supervision from another person and equipment or device
- **IV:** Is dependent and does not participate

*The focus of the admission history is the child's psychosocial environment. Most of the questions are worded in terms of parental responses. Depending on the child's age, they should be addressed directly to the child when appropriate.

Box 26-15 NURSING ADMISSION HISTORY ACCORDING TO FUNCTIONAL HEALTH PATTERNS—cont'd

Cognitive-Perceptual Pattern
Does your child have any hearing difficulty?
Does the child use a hearing aid?
Have "tubes" been placed in your child's ears?
Does your child have any vision problems?
Does the child wear glasses or contact lenses?
Does your child have any learning difficulties?
What is the child's grade in school?
For information on pain, see Box 26-4

Self-Perception–Self-Concept Pattern
How would you describe your child (e.g., takes time to adjust, settles in easily, shy, friendly, quiet, talkative, serious, playful, stubborn, easygoing)?
What makes your child angry, annoyed, anxious, or sad? What helps?
How does your child act when annoyed or upset?
What have been your child's experiences with and reactions to temporary separation from you (parent)?
Does your child have any fears (places, objects, animals, people, situations)? How do you handle them?
Do you think your child's illness has changed the way he or she thinks about self (e.g., more shy, embarrassed about appearance, less competitive with friends, stays at home more)?

Role-Relationship Pattern
Does your child have a favorite nickname?
What are the names of other family members or others who live in the home (relatives, friends, pets)?
Who usually takes care of your child during the day/night (especially if other than parent, such as baby-sitter, relative)?
What are the parents' occupation and work schedules?
Are there any special family considerations (adoption, foster child, stepparent, divorce, single parent)?
Have any major changes in the family occurred lately (death, divorce, separation, birth of a sibling, loss of a job, financial strain, mother beginning a career, other)? Describe child's reaction.
Who are your child's play companions or social groups (peers, younger or older children, adults, prefers to be alone)?
Do things generally go well for your child in school or with friends?
Does your child have "security" objects at home (pacifier, thumb, bottle, blanket, stuffed animal or doll)? Did you bring any of these to the hospital?
How do you handle discipline problems at home? Are these methods always effective?
Does your child have any condition that interferes with communication? If so, what are your suggestions for communicating with your child?
Will your child's hospitalization affect the family's financial support or care of other family members, (e.g., other children)?
What concerns do you have about your child's illness and hospitalization?
Who will be staying with your child while hospitalized?
How can we contact you or another close family member outside of the hospital?

Sexuality-Reproductive Pattern
(Answer questions that apply to your child's age-group.)
Has your child begun puberty (developing physical sexual characteristics, menstruation)? Have you or your child had any concerns?
Does your daughter know how to do breast self-examination?
Does your son know how to do testicular self-examination?
How have you approached topics of sexuality with your child?
Do you feel you might need some help with some topics?
Has your child's illness affected the way he or she feels about being a boy or a girl? If so, how?
Do you have any concerns with behaviors in your child, such as masturbation, asking many questions or talking about sex, not respecting others' privacy, or wanting too much privacy?
Initiate a conversation about an adolescent's sexual concerns with open-ended to more direct questions and using the terms "friends" or "partners" rather than "girlfriend" or "boyfriend":
Tell me about your social life.
Who are your closest friends? (If one friend is identified, could ask more about that relationship, such as how much time they spend together, how serious they are about each other, if the relationship is going the way the teenager hoped.)
Might ask about dating and sexual issues, such as the teenager's views on sex education, "going steady," "living together," or premarital sex.
Which friends would you like to have visit in the hospital?

Coping–Stress Tolerance Pattern
(Answer questions that apply to your child's age-group.)
What does your child do when tired or upset?
If upset, does your child want a special person or object?
If so, explain.
If your child has temper tantrums, what causes them and how do you handle them?
Whom does your child talk to when worried about something?
How does your child usually handle problems or disappointments?
Have there been any big changes or problems in your family recently?
How did you handle them?
Has your child ever had a problem with drugs or alcohol or tried suicide?
Do you think your child is "accident prone"? If so, explain.

Value-Belief Pattern
What is your religion?
How is religion or faith important in your child's life?
What religious practices would you like continued in the hospital (e.g., prayers before meals/bedtime; visit by minister, priest, or rabbi; prayer group)?

these questions as a part of conversation, not as a direct questionnaire. Answers to questions, such as, "What does your child know about this hospitalization?" that are broad and nonspecific, need to be followed by more directive questions, such as, "Tell me what you told him." Children may respond to questions regarding their knowledge of hospitalization with statements such as, "I don't know why I am here." Although this may be correct, frequently they have been given some explanation concerning the reason for hospitalization. Such an answer may mean that the explanation was inadequate, their anxiety blocked the recall, or they are testing out the explanation by prompting the nurse to supply additional information.

Once the data are collected, they must be applied to the nursing process and communicated to other staff. It makes little sense to assess a child's home routine if none of this knowledge is integrated into the plan of care. Most nursing units have provisions for care plans in which specific information about the child's habits and needs are recorded.

Physical Assessment

Although physical examinations by practitioners are a required part of the admission procedure, nurses should also use the valuable information gained from physical assessments in their planning of care (see Chapter 7). Subjecting children to two separate examinations is unnecessary if the nurse and other practitioners cooperate during the procedure. For example, when the nurse is present to support the child psychologically, the opportunity can also be used to observe the child's body for any bruises, rash, signs of neglect, deformities, or physical limitations.

The nurse should also listen to the heart and lungs to assess overall physical status. For example, it is impossible to evaluate improvement in respiratory function in a child admitted with pulmonary disease unless there are baseline data with which to compare subsequent findings. Collaboration also prevents the often frustrating and needless waste of the family's time in repeating histories and examinations, especially when the child has a chronic condition that requires many hospitalizations.

Placing the Child

Room assignments are usually made before the child is admitted to the pediatric unit. The minimum considerations for room assignment are age, sex, and nature of the illness. Ideally, however, room selection should be based on a variety of developmental and psychobiologic needs. Determining compatible roommates, both for the children and for rooming-in parents, greatly influences the growth potential from the hospital experience.

Although there are no absolute rules to govern room selection, in general placing children of the same age-group and with similar types of illness in the same room is both psychologically and medically advantageous. However, there are many exceptions. For example, a school-age child may thrive on the responsibility of caring for a younger child. A child in traction may be very therapeutic for another child confined to bed because of a serious illness. A child who is very independent despite physical disabilities may help another child with similar or different limitations and the parents achieve deeper insight and acceptance of the disorder.

NURSING CARE DURING SPECIAL HOSPITAL SITUATIONS

In addition to a general pediatric unit, children may be admitted to special facilities, such as a day hospital, an adolescent unit, an isolation room, or an intensive care unit. Some admissions are unexpected and frequently constitute medical emergencies. Such situations require special preparation of the child and family and nursing care interventions based on an awareness of the child's needs and the unique stressors associated with these hospital facilities.

Day Hospital

The concept of a day hospital is to provide needed medical services for the child while eliminating the necessity of overnight admission. Among the benefits of a day hospital are (1) minimization of the stressors of hospitalization, especially separation from the family; (2) reduced chance of infection; and (3) economic saving. Admission to the day hospital usually is for surgical or diagnostic procedures, such as insertion of tympanostomy tubes, hernia repair, adenoidectomy, tonsillectomy, cystoscopy, or bronchoscopy.

Because of the limited contact with the child, nursing admission procedures are extremely important. Ideally, each child and family should receive preadmission counseling, including a tour of the facility and a review of the expected day's procedures. However, when this is not possible, surgery should be scheduled to allow some time for children to become acquainted with their surroundings and for nurses to assess, plan, and complement appropriate teaching.

Discharge instructions must also be explicit (see Discharge Planning and Home Care, p. 1176). Parents need guidelines on when to call their practitioner regarding a change in the child's condition. It is helpful for the nurse to make a follow-up telephone call or to specify a time for the family to report on the child's progress. Even hints for taking the child home in the car are appreciated (see Nursing Tips).

Adolescent Unit

In recent years there has been increased awareness of children's needs based on developmental considerations. To meet the unique needs of adolescents, special units have been developed that provide privacy, increased socialization, and appropriate activities for these young people. Typically these units are set apart from the general pediatric facility so that the teenagers do not share space with younger children, who are often perceived as a threat to their maturity. These units also provide more flexible routines and activities, such as more group activity, wearing of street clothes, provisions to leave the adolescent unit temporarily, and access to the items so critical to teenagers—tele-

NURSING TIPS: DISCHARGE FROM THE DAY HOSPITAL

Help the family prepare for the car ride with the discharged child by offering these suggestions:

- Have a blanket and pillow in the car.
- Take a basin or plastic bag in case of vomiting.
- Use a cup with a cap and straw for the child to drink fluids.
- Give any prescribed pain medication before leaving the facility.

phones, record and tape players, video recorders, and televisions. Because adolescents' food habits are rarely limited to the three traditional meals a day, a ready supply of snacks should be available. However, the most important benefit of these units is increased socialization with peers. In addition, staff members usually enjoy working with this age-group and are well suited to establishing the trust so essential for communication.

Despite the advantages of adolescent units, all young people require preparation for the experience. They need orientation to the unit, introduction to staff and other patients, and an atmosphere of warmth and welcome. Just as teenagers form "cliques" in normal social relationships, this same tendency occurs in the hospital. Staff must be aware of exclusiveness of group membership, especially when new patients are admitted. Scheduled and supervised group meetings are effective in preventing feelings of "nonbelonging" and in facilitating introductions and new friendships. They also provide an excellent opportunity for discussions about typical adolescent concerns (e.g., sexuality, drugs, drinking, parental relations) and special concerns of ill adolescents (e.g., peer rejection for being different) (Pazola and Gerberg, 1985).

Isolation

Admission to an isolation room increases all the stressors typically associated with hospitalization. There is further separation from familiar persons, additional loss of control, and added environmental changes, such as sensory deprivation and the strange appearance of visitors. These stressors are compounded by children's limited understanding of isolation. Preschool children have difficulty understanding the rationale for isolation because they cannot comprehend the cause-and-effect relationship between germs and illness. They are likely to view isolation as punishment. Older children understand the causality better but still require information to decrease fantasizing or misinterpretation (Broeder, 1985).

When a child is placed in isolation, preparation is essential for the child to feel in control. With young children the best approach is a simple explanation, such as, "You need to be in this room to help you get better. This is a special place to make all the germs go away. The germs made you sick and you could not help that."

All children, but especially younger ones, need preparation in terms of what they will see, hear, or feel in isolation. Therefore they are shown the mask, gloves, and gown and are encouraged to "dress up" in them. Playing with the strange apparel lessens the fear of seeing "ghostlike" people walk into the room. Before entering the room, nurses and other health personnel should introduce themselves and let the child see their face before donning a mask. In this way the child associates them with significant experiences and gains a sense of familiarity in an otherwise strange and lonely environment.

When the child's condition improves, appropriate play activities are provided to minimize boredom. Rather than dwelling on the negative aspects of isolation, the child can be encouraged to view this experience as challenging and positive. For example, the nurse can help the child look at isolation as a method of keeping others out and letting only special people in. Children often think of intriguing signs for their doors, such as "Enter at your own risk" or "Many have entered but few have left." These posterlike signs also encourage people "on the outside" to talk with the child about the ominous greetings.

Emergency Admission

One of the most traumatic hospital experiences for the child and parents is an emergency admission. The sudden onset of an illness or the occurrence of an injury leaves little time for preparation and explanation. Sometimes the emergency admission is compounded by admission to an intensive care unit or the need for immediate surgery. However, even in those instances requiring outpatient treatment, the child is exposed to a strange, frightening environment and to people who often inflict pain. Thus every medical emergency requires psychologic intervention to reduce the fear and anxiety frequently associated with the experience.

There is a wide discrepancy between what constitutes a medically defined emergency and a client-defined emergency. Studies show that acute life-threatening emergencies account for less than 1% of all emergency visits and that acute non-life-threatening emergencies account for approximately 6%. In pediatric populations most visits are for respiratory infections, with skin conditions, gastrointestinal disorders, and trauma such as poisoning accounting for the remainder of the cases. The most common reason parents give for bringing the child to the emergency room is concern about the illness worsening. However, practitioners generally do not consider the progressive symptoms as necessitating emergency care. Therefore the word "emergency" is perceived differently by various people. One of nursing's primary goals is to assess the parents' perception of the events and their reason for considering it serious or life-threatening.

Lengthy preparatory admission procedures are often inappropriate for emergency situations. In such instances nurses must focus their nursing interventions on the essential components of admission counseling (see Box 26-14) and complete the process as soon as the child's condition is stabilized.

THERAPEUTIC DIALOGUE

"Postvention" Counseling

A child admitted to the hospital for an emergency appendectomy described the usual admission and preoperative procedures correctly but had no understanding of why they were done. His most prominent recollection focused on all the "shots" he had received (blood tests, intravenous fluid, sedation).

NURSE: Tell me about all these shots.
CHILD: I got millions of shots!
NURSE: Tell me what they were for.
CHILD: To make me better.
NURSE: Why wouldn't one shot have been enough?
CHILD: I guess because I didn't tell my mommy about my stomachache soon enough.
NURSE: I'm not sure about that. Let's count how many shots you got and why you got them. (The nurse reviewed with the child the entire admission, preoperative procedure, and postoperative care and the reason for each injection and venipuncture.) Now, how many shots did we count?
CHILD: Six.
NURSE: Is that a little less than a million?
CHILD: Yes, but they still feel like a million shots when you get them!
NURSE: I can understand that, but do you understand why you got them?
CHILD: I guess so.
NURSE: Do you still think you got extra shots because you didn't tell your mom about your stomachache?
CHILD: Well, you told me everybody gets these same shots when they have their appendix taken out, so I don't think so. My stomach didn't hurt that bad in the beginning, so I didn't say anything until it hurt a lot.
NURSE: That's right. There were reasons for all the shots, and you didn't do anything wrong. In fact, you should feel proud of yourself for having the operation and doing so well.
CHILD: Thanks. I'm going to tell my friends about my operation and how brave I was to get so many shots.

Unless an emergency is life-threatening, children need to participate in their care to maintain a sense of control. Because emergency rooms are frequently hectic, there is a tendency to rush through procedures in order to save time. However, the extra few minutes needed to allow children to participate may save many more minutes of useless resistance and uncooperativeness during subsequent procedures. Other supportive measures include ensuring privacy, accepting various emotional responses to fear or pain, preserving parent-child contact, explaining all events before or as they occur, and personally remaining calm.

At times, because of the child's physical condition, little or no preparatory counseling for emergency hospitalization can be done. In such situations the implementation of *postvention,* or counseling subsequent to the event, has therapeutic value. The process of postvention involves evaluating children's thoughts regarding admission and related procedures. It is similar to precounseling techniques; however, instead of supplying information, the nurse listens to the explanations offered by the child. Projective techniques such as drawing, doll play, or storytelling are especially effective. The nurse then bases additional information on what has already been revealed (see Therapeutic Dialogue).

Intensive Care Unit

Admission to an intensive care unit (ICU) can be a particularly traumatic event for both the child and the parents. The nature and severity of the illness and the circumstances surrounding the admission are major factors, especially for parents. Parents experience significantly more stress when the admission is unexpected rather than expected (Eberly and others, 1985). Stressors for the child and family are described in Box 26-16.

The family's emotional needs are important when a child is admitted to an ICU. While the same interventions that were discussed earlier for the stressors of separation, loss of control, and bodily injury and pain apply here, frequently they are not implemented or adjustments need to be made to accommodate the family's needs despite the often hectic and stressful atmosphere.

When an ICU admission is expected, such as for postoperative care after cardiac surgery, the child and parents should be prepared for the event. Some units advocate a tour, whereas others use picture books of the unit to familiarize the family with the environment and usual equipment. Dolls can be used to demonstrate the types of tubes that the child may have. Special care or effects of the tubes are discussed, such as the need to move despite the presence of chest tubes and inability to talk with an endotracheal tube. As much reassurance as possible should accompany the introduction of stressful information. For example, children should be reassured that they can talk when the tube is removed and that in the meantime they can use a communication board to convey their needs.

When parents first visit the child in the ICU, they need preparation for how the child will look and what the child is experiencing if awake. Ideally the nurse should accompany the family to the bedside to provide emotional support and answer any questions. If siblings visit, they need the same preparation as parents. Whether they should visit soon after the child is admitted or after the child's condition has stabilized is controversial. Early visiting minimizes the opportunity for siblings to fantasize about the experience and imagine fears that are probably greater than the actual situation (Shonkwiler, 1985). However, visiting early may be frightening, especially when the child is in pain or unresponsive

Box 26-16 NEONATAL/PEDIATRIC ICU STRESSORS FOR THE CHILD AND FAMILY

Physical Stressors
Pain and discomfort (e.g., injections, intubation, suctioning, dressing changes, other invasive procedures)
Immobility (e.g., use of restraints, bed rest)
Sleep deprivation
Inability to eat or drink
Changes in elimination habits

Environmental Stressors
Unfamiliar surroundings (e.g., crowding)
Unfamiliar sounds
- Equipment noise (e.g., monitors, telephone, suctioning, computer printout)
- Human sounds (e.g., talking, laughing, crying, coughing, moaning, retching, walking)

Unfamiliar people (e.g., health care professionals, patients, visitors)
Unfamiliar and unpleasant smells (e.g., alcohol, adhesive remover, body odors)
Constant lights
Activity related to other patients
Sense of urgency among staff

Psychologic Stressors
Lack of privacy
Inability to communicate (if intubated)
Inadequate knowledge and understanding of situation
Severity of illness
Parental behavior (expression of concern)

Social Stressors
Disrupted relationships (especially with family and friends)
Concern with missing school/work
Play deprivation

Data primarily from Tichy, A.M., and others: Stressors in pediatric intensive care units, Pediatr. Nurs. 14(1):40-42, 1988.

and attached to numerous tubes and machinery. The length of time for sibling visitation should be planned ahead and monitored during the visit to prevent the well child from becoming overwhelmed.

Children admitted to the ICU need their parents' comfort and security, and parents are encouraged to stay with their child. If visiting hours are limited, the schedule should be flexible to accommodate parental needs. Family members should be given a written schedule of the times permitted and assured that they can call the unit at any time. With liberalization of visiting hours, many parents think they must stay; nurses need to be sensitive to their needs, suggesting periodic respites from the tense, stressful ICU environment.

Since altered parental roles are a major stress for parents, nurses need to implement interventions to minimize this concern, such as (1) educating and preparing parents for the expected role changes; (2) identifying ways in which parents can continue to fulfill parenting functions, such as helping with the bath or feeding and touching and talking to the child; and (3) determining new roles, such as helping with procedures (Miles and others, 1984; Rennick, 1986). Information sharing can increase parents' sense of control and responsibility, but facts must be conveyed simply, repeated often, and monitored to prevent overwhelming family members. Since medical jargon abounds in a complex environment such as the ICU, unfamiliar terms need to be clarified and simpler terms substituted (see Box 27-4).

As in emergency admissions, there is a tendency in the ICU to perform procedures quickly and without attention to the child's preparational needs. Therefore nurses need to remember the special concerns of children in each age-group about bodily injury. Explaining each procedure, altering it whenever possible to decrease the child's fears, and supporting the child are essential. Giving children an object that symbolizes their courage, such as a "hero badge" or an "ICU diploma," helps them face their fears and anxiety. It is a positive memento of an otherwise stressful experience. Because of the numerous procedures performed on the child and the nature of the illness, pain management needs to receive a high priority.

Of particular importance in decreasing fear is ensuring that discussions that do not directly include the family are held where the child and family cannot overhear them. Casual conversation in the nursing station or in the halls can often be overheard and taken out of context. When discussions are held at the bedside, it is very easy to forget the patient and make remarks that are misunderstood. Usually a quiet reminder of how frightened the child can become from listening to these discussions is sufficient. If bedside conferences are necessary, the nurse interprets them for family members in language they can comprehend or if appropriate, asks the family to leave the area during report.

Extensive monitoring makes a usual day-night cycle difficult in an ICU. However, some schedule should be established that maintains a similarity to daily events in the child's life. These include organizing care during normal waking hours, keeping regular bedtime schedules, including quiet times when televisions and radios are lowered or turned off, closing and opening drapes as appropriate, dimming lights, placing a curtain around the bed for privacy and decreased stimulation, and having clocks or calendars in easy view for older children. In particular, staff members must realize the need for quiet and refrain from loud talking or laughing. Equipment noise should be kept to a minimum by turning alarms as low as safely possible, performing treatments requiring equipment at one time, turning off bedside equipment not in use (e.g., suction, oxygen), and avoiding loud, abrupt noises (e.g., clattering bedpans, toilet flushing) (Snyder-Halpern, 1985). Such measures can reduce the sensory overload and the sleep deprivation commonly associated with ICU admissions.

Despite the stresses normally associated with ICU admission, a special security develops from being carefully monitored and receiving individualized care. Therefore planning for transition to the regular unit is essential and should include (1) assignment of a primary nurse on the regular unit who visits before the transfer, (2) continued visits by the ICU staff to assess the child's and parents' adjustment and to act as a temporary liaison with the nursing staff, (3) explanation of the differences between the two units and the rationale for the change to less intense monitoring of the child's physical condition, and (4) selection of an appropriate room, such as one close to the nursing station, and a compatible roommate.

DISCHARGE PLANNING AND HOME CARE

Most hospitalizations necessitate some type of discharge planning. Often this involves education of the family for continued care and follow-up in the home. Depending on the diagnosis, this may be relatively simple or considerably complex. With the current concern for cost containment and recognition of children's emotional needs, home care for children with technologically complex care, such as youngsters on ventilators, has become increasingly common. Preparing the family for home care demands a high degree of competence in planning and implementing discharge instruction. Although this is usually a team effort, nurses are often key individuals in initiating the process and collaborating with others in the planning and implementing stages. While it is not possible to discuss all the details needed for effective discharge planning and home care, this section presents a brief overview of the more critical aspects. More specific details are discussed throughout the text for conditions such as home apnea monitoring, tracheostomy care, or hyperalimentation, and numerous sources of information exist in the literature (Steele and Harrison, 1986).

Assessment

Discharge planning for home care must begin with an assessment of the family's desire and capability in assuming care responsibilities. Ideally, at least two individuals should be committed to learning the skills needed for home care. A thorough assessment of the family and home environment should be done to ensure that the family's emotional and physical resources are sufficient to manage the tasks of home care (for a discussion of family and home assessment strategies, see Chapter 6). In addition to adequate family resources, an investigation of community services, including respite care, is needed to ensure that appropriate support agencies are available, such as emergency facilities, home health agencies, and equipment vendors. To coordinate the immense task of assessment and to plan implementation, a case coordinator should be appointed early in the discharge program (Stein, 1985).

Planning

Ideally, preparation for hospital discharge and home care begins during the admission assessment with the establishment of short- and long-term goals. These goals are concerned with the child's physical needs as well as the psychologic needs of the child and family. For children who require complex care, discharge planning focuses on those skills that parents or children are expected to continue at home. In planning appropriate teaching, nurses need to assess (1) the actual and perceived complexity of the skill, (2) the parents' or child's ability to learn the skill, and (3) the parents' or child's previous or present experience with such procedures. (See Compliance, Chapter 27, for guidelines for effective teaching.)

The teaching plan should incorporate levels of learning, such as observing, participating with assistance, and finally acting without help or guidance. The skill should be divided into discrete steps, and each step taught to the family member until it is learned. Return demonstration of the skill should be requested before new skills are introduced. A record of teaching and performance provides an efficient checklist for evaluation. All families should receive detailed *written* instructions about home care before they leave the hospital, as well as telephone numbers for assistance.*

Transitional Care

Once the family is competent in performing the skill, they should be given responsibility for the care. Whenever possible, the family should have a transition or trial period to assume care with minimum supervision. This may be arranged on the unit, during a home pass, or in a facility (e.g., a motel) near the hospital. Some programs incorporate a hospital trial into their discharge criteria, necessitating that the family successfully manage this phase before discharge to home (Steele and Harrison, 1986). Such transitions provide a safe practice period for the family, with assistance readily available when needed, and are especially valuable when the family lives at a distance to the treating center.

Evaluation and Continuing Support

Evaluation is a critical part of any discharge plan and assumes even more importance in home care of children with complex needs. Factors to consider in home care programs are need for subsequent hospitalization, child's developmental and physical progress, effects of home care on the family, actual vs expected use of resources by the family and home care team, financial costs and savings, and improved survival (American Academy of Pediatrics, Ad Hoc Task Forces on Home Care of Chronically Ill Infants and Children, 1984).

In most instances parents need only simple instructions and understanding of follow-up care. However, the often overwhelming care assumed by some families necessitates continued professional support after discharge. Appropriate referrals and resources may include visiting nurse or home health agencies, private nurse services, the school system, physical therapist, mental health counselor, social worker, or various community agencies, including special organizations. Sharing the important issues surrounding the child's and family's needs is essential. Referral summaries should be concise, specific, and factual. When numerous support services are involved, periodic collaboration among the professionals involved and the family is an excellent strategy to ensure efficient implementation and comprehensive delivery of services.

---

*Home care instructions for a wide variety of technical skills are available in Wong, D.L., and Whaley, L.F.: Clinical manual of pediatric nursing, ed. 3, St. Louis, 1990, Mosby–Year Book, Inc.

KEY POINTS

- Children are particularly vulnerable to the stresses of illness and hospitalization because stress represents a change from the usual state of health and routine and because they possess limited coping mechanisms.
- The three phases of separation anxiety are protest, despair, and detachment.
- Feelings of loss of control are caused by unfamiliar environmental stimuli, physical restriction, altered routine, and dependency.
- Fear of bodily pain may be manifested in the following ways: infants—expressions, body movements; toddlers—intense emotional upset, physical resistance; preschoolers—aggression, verbal expression, dependency; school-age children—precise verbalization of pain, passive requests for support or help, procrastination technique; adolescents—self-control, irritability, limited movement.
- Because of their separation from significant people, hospitalized children may lack the opportunity to form new attachments in the strange environment and may exhibit negative behaviors after discharge.
- Family reactions are influenced by the seriousness of illness, experience with illness or hospitalization, diagnostic or therapeutic procedures, available support systems, personal ego strengths, coping abilities, additional stresses, cultural and religious beliefs, and family communication patterns.
- The following increase the negative effects of a brother's or sister's illness/hospitalization on siblings: fear of contracting illness, their younger age, a close relationship with the ill sibling, substitute child care, minimum explanation of the illness, and perceived changes in parenting.
- Nursing care of the hospitalized child and family is aimed at preventing or minimizing separation, decreasing loss of control, minimizing bodily injury and pain, using play to lessen stress, maximizing potential benefits of hospitalization, and supporting family members.
- Pain assessment includes questioning the child, using pain rating scales, evaluating behavior and physiologic changes, securing parents' involvement, taking the cause of pain into account, and taking action.
- Pain management should incorporate both pharmacologic and nonpharmacologic methods. Pharmacologic methods focus on four rights: right drug, right dose, right route, and right time.
- Diversional or expressive play is an effective tool in minimizing stress.
- The nurse can maximize potential benefits of hospitalization by fostering parent-child relations, providing educational opportunities, promoting self-mastery, and encouraging socialization.
- Supporting family members involves listening to parents' verbal and nonverbal messages; providing clergy support; accepting cultural, socioeconomic, and ethnic values; and giving information to families and siblings.
- The major goals of prehospital counseling are to make the hospital less strange and frightening to parents and children and to establish a positive atmosphere and trusting relationships with staff and family members.
- In preparing families for hospitalization, the nurse should consider small group size and timing of the event, setting of the tour, inclusion of preparatory materials, time for discussion, and prehospital counseling for parents.
- Emergency admission or admission to a day hospital, isolation room, or intensive care unit requires additional intervention strategies to meet the child's and family's needs.

REFERENCES

Abu-Saad, H.: Cultural group indicators of pain in children, Matern. Child Nurs. J. 13(3):187-196, 1984.

Aho, A.C., and Erickson, M.T.: Effects of grade, gender, and hospitalization on children's medical fears, Dev. Behav. Pediatr. 6(3):146-153, 1985.

American Academy of Pediatrics: Neonatal anesthesia, Pediatrics 80(3):446, 1987.

American Academy of Pediatrics, Ad Hoc Task Forces on Home Care of Chronically Ill Infants and Children: Guidelines for home care of infants, children, and adolescents with chronic disease, Pediatrics 74(3):434-436, 1984.

American Academy of Pediatrics, Committee on Drugs: Naloxone dosage and route of administration for infants and children: addendum to emergency drug doses for infants and children, Pediatrics 86(3):484-485, 1990.

American Pain Society: Principles of analgesic use in the treatment of acute pain or chronic cancer pain, Skokie, IL, 1989, The Society.

Anand, K., and Aynsley-Green, A.: Metabolic and endocrine effects of surgical ligation of patent ductus arteriosus in the human preterm neonate: are there implications for further improvement of postoperative outcome? Mod. Probl. Paediatr. 23:143-157, 1985.

Anand, K.J.S., Phil, D., and Hickey, P.: Pain and its effects in the human neonate and fetus, N. Engl. J. Med. 317(21):1321-1329, 1987.

Azarnoff, P.: Preparing well children for possible hospitalization, Pediatr. Nurs. 11(1):53-56, 1985.

Baker, C., and Wong, D.: Q.U.E.S.T.: a process of pain assessment in children, Orthopaed. Nurs. 6(1):11-21, 1987.

Bates, T.A., and Broome, M.: Preparation of children for hospitalization and surgery: a review of the literature, J. Pediatr. Nurs. 1(4):230-239, 1986.

Beasley, S.W., and Tibballs, J.: Efficacy and safety of continuous morphine infusion for postoperative analgesia in the paediatric surgical ward, Aust. N.Z. J. Surg. 57:233-237, 1987.

Beyer, J.E.: The Oucher: a user's manual and technical report, Denver, CO, 1988, University of Colorado.

Beyer, J.E., and Aradine, C.R.: Patterns of pediatric pain intensity: a methodological investigation of a self-report scale, Clin. J. Pain 3:130-141, 1987.

Beyer, J., and others: Patterns of postoperative analgesic use with adults and children following cardiac surgery, Pain 17:71-81, 1983.

Bibace, R., and Walsh, M.E.: Development of children's concepts of illness, Pediatrics 66(6):912-918, 1980.

Bieri, D., and others: The Faces Pain Scale for the self-assessment of the severity of pain experienced by children: development, initial validation, and preliminary investigation for ratio scale properties, Pain 41(2):139-150, 1990.

Billmire, D.A., Neale, H.W., and Gregory, R.O.: Use of IV fentanyl in the outpatient treatment of pediatric facial trauma, J. Trauma 25(11):1079-1080, 1985.

Broeder, J.L.: School-age children's perceptions of isolation after hospital discharge, Matern. Child Nurs. J. 14(3):153-174, 1985.

Broome, M., and others: Children's medical fears, coping behaviors, and pain perceptions during a lumbar puncture, Oncol. Nurs. Forum 17(3):361-367, 1990.

Clatworthy, S.: Therapeutic play: effects on hospitalized children, Child. Health Care 9(4):108-113, 1981.

Cleeland, C.: Behavioral control of symptoms, J. Pain Symptom Manag. 1(1):36-38, 1986.

Craft, M.J., and Wyatt, N.: Effect of visitation upon siblings of hospitalized children, Matern. Child Nurs. J. 15(1):47-59, 1986.

Craft, M.J., Wyatt, N., and Sandell, B.: Behavior and feeling changes in siblings of hospitalized children, Clin. Pediatr. 24(7):374-378, 1985.

Craig, K.D., and others: Developmental changes in infant pain expression during immunization injections, Soc. Sci. Med. 19(12):1331-1337, 1984.

Dale, J.C.: A multidimensional study of infants' responses to painful stimuli, Pediatr. Nurs. 12(1):27-31, 1986.

Davis, J.H.: Children and pets: a therapeutic connection, Pediatr. Nurs. 11(5):377-379, 1985.

Dilworth, N.M., and MacKellar, A.: Pain relief for the pediatric surgical patient, J. Pediatr. Surg. 22:264-266, 1987.

Dolgin, M., and others: Behavioral distress in pediatric patients with cancer receiving chemotherapy, Pediatrics 84(1):103-110, 1989.

Eberly, T.W., and others: Parental stress after the unexpected admission of a child to the intensive care unit, Crit. Care Q. 8(1):57-65, 1985.

Eland, J.M.: The child who is hurting, Semin. Oncol. Nurs. 1(2):116-122, 1985.

Eland, J.M., and Anderson, J.E.: The experience of pain in children. In Jacox, A., editor: Pain: a source book for nurses and other health professionals, Boston, 1977, Little, Brown & Co., Inc.

Engebo, D.: Safe and effective use of tetracaine, adrenaline, and cocaine (TAC) solution anesthetic for anesthetizing of lacerations, J. Emerg. Nurs. 16(2):100-101, 1990.

Favaloro, R., and Touzel, B.: A comparison of adolescents' and nurses' postoperative pain ratings and perceptions, Pediatr. Nurs. 16(4):414-417, 424, 1990.

Fitzgerald, M., Millard, C., and MacIntosh, N.: Hyperalgesia in premature infants, Lancet 6(8580):292, 1988.

Franck, L.: A national survey of the assessment and treatment of pain and agitation in the neonatal intensive care unit, JOGNN 16:387-393, 1987.

Franck, L.S.: Pain in the nonverbal patient: advocating for the critically ill neonate, Pediatr. Nurs. 15(1):65, 1989.

Gaukroger, P., Tomkins, D.P., and van der Walt, J.: Patient-controlled analgesia in children, Anaesth. Intensive Care 17(3):264-268, 1989.

Goodwin, J.S., Goodwin, J.M., and Vogel, A.V.: Knowledge and use of placebos by house officers and nurses, Ann. Intern. Med. 91:106-110, 1979.

Gordon, M.: Nursing diagnosis: process and application, ed. 2, New York, 1987, McGraw-Hill, Inc.

Gough, W.C.: A growing interest, Am. J. Nurs. 86(2):165-166, 1986.

Griffin, G.C., Campbell, V.D., and Jones, R.: Nitrous oxide–oxygen sedation for minor surgery: experience in a pediatric setting, JAMA 245(23):2411-2413, 1981.

Gureno, M.A., and Reisinger, C.L.: Patient controlled analgesia for the young pediatric patient, Pediatr. Nurs. (in press).

Hagemann, V.: Night sleep of children in a hospital. Part 1. Sleep duration, Matern. Child Nurs. J. 10:1-13, 1981a.

Hagemann, V.: Night sleep of children in a hospital. Part 2. Sleep disruption, Matern. Child Nurs. J. 10:127-142, 1981b.

Haslam, D.R.: Age and the perception of pain, Psychosom. Sci. 15:86, 1969.

Hertzka, R., and others: Fentanyl-induced ventilatory depression: effects of age, Anesthesiology 70:213-218, 1989.

Hester, N.: The preoperational child's reaction to immunization, Nurs. Res. 28(4):250-255, 1979.

Hester, N.O.: Comforting the child in pain. In Funk, S.G., and others, editors: Key aspects of comfort, New York, 1989, Springer Publishing Co., Inc.

Hinkle, A.J.: Percutaneous inguinal block for the outpatient management of post-herniorrhaphy pain in children, Anesthesiology 67:411-413, 1987.

Huth, M.M.: Guidelines for conducting hospital tours with early school-age children, Pediatr. Nurs. 9(6):414-415, 1983.

Jaffe, J.: Drug addiction and drug abuse. In Gilman, A., and others, editors: Goodman and Gilman's the pharmacological basis of therapeutics, ed. 7, New York, 1985, Macmillan Publishing Co.

Juhlin, L., and Evers, H.: EMLA: a new topical anesthetic, Adv. Dermatol. 5:75-92, 1990.

Kaiko, R.F., and others: CNS excitatory effects of meperidine in cancer patients, Ann. Neurol. 13(2):180-185, 1983.

Katz, E., Kellerman, J., and Siegel, S.: Behavioral distress in children with cancer undergoing medical procedures: developmental considerations, J. Consult. Clin. Psychol. 48(3):356-365, 1980.

Knafl, K.A., and Dixon, D.M.: The role of siblings during pediatric hospitalization, Issues Compr. Pediatr. Nurs. 6:13-22, 1983.

Knafl, K.A., and Dixon, D.M.: The participation of fathers in their children's hospitalization, Issues Compr. Pediatr. Nurs. 7(4-5):269-281, 1984.

Krane, E.J., and others: Caudal morphine for postoperative analgesia in children: a comparison with caudal bupivacaine and intravenous morphine, Anesth. Analg. 66:647-653, 1987.

Kuttner, L., and LePage, T.: Face scales for the assessment of pediatric pain: a critical review, Can. J. Behav. Sci. 21(2):198-209, 1989.

LaMontagne, L.L.: Children's locus of control beliefs as predictors of preoperative coping behavior, Nurs. Res. 33(2):76-79, 1984.

Marshall, R.E.: Neonatal pain associated with caregiving procedures, Pediatr. Clin. North Am. 36(4):885-903, 1989.

Mather, L., and Mackie, J.: The incidence of postoperative pain in children, Pain 15:271-282, 1983.

May, B.K., and Sparks, M.: School-age children: are their needs recognized and met in the hospital setting? Child. Health Care 11(3):118-121, 1983.

McCaffery, M., and Beebe, A.: Pain: clinical manual for nursing practice, St. Louis, 1989, Mosby–Year Book, Inc.

McCain, G.C.: Parent-created tape recordings for hospitalized children, Child. Health Care 10(3):104-105, 1982.

McCain, G.C., and Bies, D.C.: Television viewing and the hospitalized child, Pediatr. Nurs. 9(1):33-35, 1983.

McGrath, P., de Veber, L., and Hearn, M.: Multidimensional pain assessment in children. In Fields, H., Dubner, R., and Cervero, F., editors: Advances in pain research and therapy, vol. 9, New York, 1985, Raven Press.

McKay, W., Morris, R., and Mushlin, P.: Sodium bicarbonate attenuates pain on skin infiltration with lidocaine, with or without epinephrine, Anesth. Analg. 66:572-574, 1987.

Miles, M.S., and others: Maternal and paternal stress reactions when a child is hospitalized in a pediatric care unit, Issues Compr. Pediatr. Nurs. 7:333-342, 1984.

Mills, N.M.: Acute pain behavior in infants and toddlers. In Funk, S.G., and others, editors: Key aspects of comfort: management of pain, fatigue, and nausea, New York, 1989, Springer Publishing Co., Inc.

Miser, A.W., and others: Narcotic withdrawal syndrome in young adults after the therapeutic use of opiates, Am. J. Dis. Child. 140:603-604, 1986.

Miser, A., and others: Transdermal fentanyl for pain control in patients with cancer, Pain 37:15-21, 1989.

Monahan, G.H., and Schkade, J.K.: Comparing care by parent and traditional nursing units, Pediatr. Nurs. 11:463-468, 1985.

Morrison, R., and Vedro, D.: Pain management in the child with sickle cell disease, Pediatr. Nurs. 15(6):595-599, 613, 1989.
Olkkola, K., and others: Kinetics and dynamics of postoperative intravenous morphine in children, Clin. Pharmacol. Ther. 44:128-136, 1988.
Orem, D.: Nursing: concepts of practice, ed. 3, New York, 1985, McGraw-Hill, Inc.
Pazola, K.J., and Gerberg, A.K.: Teen group: a forum for the hospitalized adolescent, MCN 10(4):265-269, 1985.
Perin, G., and Frase, D.: Development of a program using general anesthesia for invasive procedures in a pediatric outpatient setting, J. Assoc. Pediatr. Oncol. Nurs. 3(4):8-10, 1985.
Perrin, E.C., and Gerrity, P.S.: There's a demon in your belly: children's understanding of illness, Pediatrics 67(6):841-849, 1981.
Perry, S.W., and Heidrich, G.: Placebo response: myth and matter, Am. J. Nurs. 81(4):720-725, 1981.
Petrillo, M., and Sanger, S.: Emotional care of hospitalized children, ed. 2, Philadelphia, 1980, J.B. Lippincott Co.
Porter, J., and Jick, H.: Addiction rare in patients treated with narcotics, N. Engl. J. Med. 302(2):123, 1980.
Rennick, J.: Reestablishing the parental role in a pediatric intensive care unit, J. Pediatr. Nurs. 1(1):40-44, 1986.
Rowbotham, D., and others: Transdermal fentanyl for the relief of pain after upper abdominal surgery, Br. J. Anaesth. 63:56-59, 1989.
Ross, D.M., and Ross, S.A.: Childhood pain: the school-age child's viewpoint, Pain 20(2):179-191, 1984.
Savedra, M., and others: Pain location: validity and reliability of body outline markings by hospitalized children and adolescents, Res. Nurs. Health 12:307-314, 1989.
Schechter, N.L., Allen, D.A., and Hanson, K.: Status of pediatric pain control: a comparison of hospital analgesic usage in children and adults, Pediatrics 77(1):11-15, 1986.
Shannon, F.T., Fergusson, D.M., and Dimond, M.E.: Early hospital admissions and subsequent behavior problems in 6-year olds, Arch. Dis. Child. 59:815-819, 1984.
Shapiro, C.: Pain in the neonate: assessment and intervention, Neonatal Network 8(1):7-21, 1989.
Sherman, M., and others: Treasured objects in school-aged children, Pediatrics 68(3):379-386, 1981.
Shonkwiler, M.A.: Sibling visits in the pediatric intensive care unit, Crit. Care Q. 8(1):67-72, 1985.
Snyder-Halpern, R.: The effect of critical care unit noise on patient sleep cycles, Crit. Care Q. 7(4):41-50, 1985.
Stang, H.J., and others: Local anesthesia for neonatal circumcision: effects on distress and cortisol response, JAMA 259(10):1507-1511, 1988.
Steele, N., and Harrison, B.: Technology-assisted children: assessing discharge preparation, J. Pediatr. Nurs. 1(3):150-158, 1986.
Stein, R.: Home care: a challenging opportunity, Child. Health Care 14(2):90-95, 1985.
Streisand, J.B., and others: Oral transmucosal fentanyl citrate premedication in children, Anesth. Analg. 69:28-34, 1989.
Stull, M.K., and Deatrick, J.A.: Measuring parental participation. Part I. Issues Compr. Pediatr. Nurs. 9(3):157-165, 1986.
Tesler, M.D., and others: Children's words for pain. In Funk, S.G., and others, editors: Key aspects of comfort: management of pain, fatigue, and nausea, New York, 1989, Springer Publishing Co., Inc.
Thompson, R.H.: Psychosocial research on pediatric hospitalization and health care: a review of the literature, Springfield, IL, 1985, Charles C Thomas, Publisher.
Tichy, A.M., and others: Stressors in pediatric intensive care units, Pediatr. Nurs. 14(1):40-42, 1988.
Volz, D.D.: Time structuring for hospitalized school-aged children, Issues Compr. Pediatr. Nurs. 5:205-210, 1981.
Vulcan, B., and Nikulich-Barrett, M.: The effect of selected information on mothers' anxiety levels during their children's hospitalizations, J. Pediatr. Nurs. 3(2):97-102, 1988.
Wallace, M.: Temperament: a variable in children's pain management, Pediatr. Nurs. 15(2):118-121, 1989.
Wong, D., and Baker, C.: Pain in children: comparison of assessment scales, Pediatr. Nurs. 14(1):9-17, 1988.
Wong, D., and Redding, B.: Lozenges can be "lifesavers," Am. J. Nurs. 87(9):1129-1130, 1987.
Wood, S.P.: School-aged children's perceptions of the causes of illness, Pediatr. Nurs. 9(2):101-104, 1983.
Yaster, M., and others: Midazolam-fentanyl intravenous sedation in children: case report of respiratory arrest, Pediatrics 86(3):463-467, 1990.
Young, M., and Fu, V.: Influence of play and temperament on the young child's response to pain, Child. Health Care 16(3):209-215, 1988.
Zeltzer, L.K., Jay, S.M., and Fisher, D.M.: The management of pain associated with pediatric procedures, Pediatr. Clin. North Am. 36(4):941-964, 1989.

BIBLIOGRAPHY

Hospitalization: The Child and Family

Alexander, D., White, M., and Powell, G.: Anxiety of non-rooming-in parents of hospitalized children, Child. Health Care 15(1):14-20, 1986.
Alexander, D., and others: Anxiety levels of rooming-in and non-rooming-in parents of young hospitalized children, Matern. Child Nurs. J. 17(2):79-99, 1988.
Algren, C.L.: Role perception of mothers who have hospitalized children, Child. Health Care 14(1):6-9, 1985.
American Academy of Pediatrics, Committee on Hospital Care: Hospital care of children and youth, Elk Grove Village, IL, 1986, The Academy.
Banks, E.: Concepts of health and sickness of preschool- and school-aged children, Child. Health Care 19(1):43-48, 1990.
Betz, C.L., and Poster, E.C.: Incorporating play into the care of the hospitalized child, Issues Compr. Pediatr. Nurs. 7:343-355, 1984.
Bolig, R., and Weedle, K.D.: Resiliency and hospitalization of children, Child. Health Care 16(4):255-260, 1988.
Bordeaux, B.R.: Television viewing patterns of hospitalized school-aged children and adolescents, Child. Health Care 15(2):70-75, 1986.
Brown, J., and Ritchie, J.A.: Nurses' perceptions of parent and nurse roles in caring for hospitalized children, Child. Health Care 19(1):28-36, 1990.
Burke, S.O., Costello, E.A., and Handley-Derry, M.H.: Maternal stress and repeated hospitalizations of children who are physically disabled, Child. Health Care 18(2):82-90, 1989.
Caty, S., Ritchie, J.A., and Ellerton, M.: Helping hospitalized preschoolers manage stressful situations: the mother's role, Child. Health Care 18(4):202-209, 1989.
Caty, S., Ritchie, J.A., and Ellerton, M.L.: Mothers' perception of coping behaviors in hospitalized preschool children, J. Pediatr. Nurs. 4(6):403-410, 1989.
Clements, D.B.: Reminiscence: a tool for aiding families under stress, MCN 11(2):114-117, 1986.
Coucouvanis, J.A., and Solomons, H.C.: Handling complicated visitation problems of hospitalized children, MCN Child Nurs. 8(2):131, 1983.
Cozad, J.: Children, hospitalization and stress, Point View 27(2):7-11, 1990.
Craft, M.J.: Validation of responses reported by school-aged siblings of hospitalized children, Child. Health Care 15(1):6-13, 1986.
Craft, M.J., and Craft, J.L.: Perceived changes in siblings of hospitalized children: a comparison of sibling and parent reports, Child. Health Care 18(1):42-48, 1989.
Crocker, E.: In my opinion . . . television for hospitalized children: the issue of control, Child. Health Care 15(2):76-78, 1986.

Curry, N.E.: Enhancing dramatic play potential in hospitalized children, Child. Health Care 16(3):142-149, 1988.

DelPo, E.G., and Frick, S.B.: Directed and nondirected play as therapeutic modalities, Child. Health Care 16(4):261-267, 1988.

Denholm, C.J.: Hospitalization and the adolescent patient: a review and some critical questions, Child. Health Care 13(3):109-116, 1985.

Denholm, C.J.: The adolescent patient at discharge and in the post-hospitalization environment: a review, Matern. Child Nurs. J. 16(2):95-102, 1987.

Denholm, C.J.: Reactions of adolescents following hospitalization for acute conditions, Child. Health Care 18(4):210-217, 1989.

Denholm, C.J.: Memories of adolescent hospitalization: results from a 4-year follow-up study, Child. Health Care 19(2):101-105, 1990.

Denholm, C.J., and Ferguson, R.V.: Strategies to promote the developmental needs of hospitalized adolescents, Child. Health Care 15(3):183-187, 1987.

Elfert, H., and Anderson, J.M.: More than just luck, Can. Nurse 83(4):14-17, 1987.

Ellerton, M., Ritchie, J.A., and Caty, S.: Nurses' perceptions of coping behaviors in hospitalized preschool children, J. Pediatr. Nurs. 4(3):197-205, 1989.

Faller, H.S.: A child's perception of the hospital, MCN 13:38, 1988.

Flint, N.S., and Walsh, M.: Visiting policies in pediatrics: parents' perceptions and preferences, J. Pediatr. Nurs. 3(4):237-246, 1988.

Fosarelli, P.: In my opinion . . . advocacy for children's appropriate viewing of television: what can we do? Child. Health Care 15(2):79-81, 1986.

Garot, P.A.: Therapeutic play: work of both child and nurse, J. Pediatr. Nurs. 1(2):111-116, 1986.

Goldberger, J.: Issue-specific play with infants and toddlers in hospitals: rationale and intervention, Child. Health Care 16(3):134-141, 1988.

Gratz, R.R., and Piliavin, J.A.: What makes kids sick: children's beliefs about the causative factors of illness, Child. Health Care 12(4):156-162, 1984.

Graves, J.K., and Ware, M.E.: Parents' and health professionals' perceptions concerning parental stress during a child's hospitalization, Child. Health Care 19(10):37-42, 1990.

Grimm, D.L., and Pefley, P.T.: Opening doors for the child "inside," Pediatr. Nurs. 16(4):368-369, 1990.

Harris, C.: Programming for special groups through closed-circuit television, Child. Health Care 15(2):91-94, 1986.

Hester, N.O.: Health perceptions of school-age children, Issues Compr. Pediatr. Nurs. 10:137-147, 1987.

Hudson, C., and others: Storytelling: a measure of anxiety in hospitalized children, Child. Health Care 16(2):118-122, 1987.

Jessee, P., and others: Nature experiences for hospitalized children, Child. Health Care 15(1):55-57, 1986.

Knafl, K.A., Cavallari, K.A., and Dixon, D.M.: Pediatric hospitalization: family and nurse perspectives, Boston, 1988, Scott, Foresman & Co.

Kreger, B.E., and Restuccia, J.D.: Assessing the need to hospitalize children: pediatric appropriateness evaluation protocol, Pediatrics 84(2):242-247, 1989.

Lamb, J.M., and Rodgers, D.R.: Assisting the hostile, hospitalized child, MCN 8(5):336-339, 1983.

LaMontagne, L.L.: Three coping strategies used by school-age children, Pediatr. Nurs. 10(1):25-28, 1984.

LaMontagne, L.L.: Children's preoperative coping: replication and extension, Nurs. Res. 36(3):163-167, 1987.

Lynn, M.R.: Siblings' responses in illness situations, J. Pediatr. Nurs. 4(2):127-129, 1989.

Maheady, D.C.: Health concepts of preschool children, Pediatr. Nurs. 12(3):195-197, 1986.

Marchant, R.: Caring for hospitalized inner-city children, Pediatr. Nurs. 11(2):129-131, 1985.

McCain, G.C.: Family functioning 2 to 4 years after preterm birth, J. Pediatr. Nurs. 5(2):97-104, 1990.

McClowry, S.G.: A review of the literature pertaining to the psychosocial responses of school-aged children to hospitalization, J. Pediatr. Nurs. 3(5):296-311, 1988.

McClowry, S.G.: The relationship of temperament to pre- and posthospitalization behavioral responses of school-age children, Nurs. Res. 39(1):30-35, 1990.

McClowry, S.G., and McLeod, S.M.: The psychosocial responses of school-age children to hospitalization, Child. Health Care 19(3):155-161, 1990.

McCue, K.: Medical play: an expanded perspective, Child. Health Care 16(3):157-161, 1988.

McLeod, S.M., and McClowry, S.G.: Using temperament theory to individualize the psychosocial care of hospitalized children, Child. Health Care 19(2):79-85, 1990.

Meer, P.A.: Using play therapy in outpatient settings, MCN 10(6):378-380, 1985.

Merkens, M.J.: A pediatric chronic illness transition unit, Child. Health Care 19(1):4-9, 1990.

Miller, S.A.: Promoting self-esteem in the hospitalized adolescent: clinical interventions, Issues Compr. Pediatr. Nurs. 10:187-194, 1987.

Miron, J.: What children think about hospitals, Can. Nurs. 86(3):23-25, 1990.

Nugent, K.E.: Routine care: promoting development in hospitalized infants, MCN 14:318-321, 1989.

Oremland, E.K.: Mastering developmental and critical experiences through play and other expressive behaviors in childhood, Child. Health Care 16(3):150-156, 1988.

Pass, M.D., and Pass, C.M.: Anticipatory guidance for parents of hospitalized children, J. Pediatr. Nurs. 2(4):250-258, 1987.

Poster, E.C., and Betz, C.L.: Survey of sibling and peer visitation policies in Southern California hospitals, Child. Health Care 15(3):166-171, 1987.

Powell, G.M., and others: Maternal anxiety and the nature of sleep onset latency in hospitalized children, Pediatr. Nurs. 13(6):397-401, 1987.

Reynolds, E.A., and Ramenofsky, M.L.: The emotional impact of trauma on toddlers, MCN 13(2):106-109, 1988.

Robinson, C.A.: Preschool children's conceptualizations of health and illness, Child. Health Care 16(2):89-95, 1987.

Robinson, C.A.: Roadblocks to family centered care when a chronically ill child is hospitalized, Matern. Child Nurs. J. 16(3):181-193, 1987.

Ruddy-Wallace, M.: Temperament: assessing individual differences in hospitalized children, J. Pediatr. Nurs. 2(1):30-36, 1987.

Saunders, R.B., Miller, B.B., and Cates, K.M.: Pediatric family care: an interdisciplinary team approach, Child. Health Care 18(1):53-58, 1989.

Savedra, M., Tesler, M., and Ritchie, J.: Parents' waiting: is it an inevitable part of the hospital experience? J. Pediatr. Nurs. 2(5):328-332, 1987.

Schum, T.T.: Effects of hospitalization derived from a family diary: review of the literature, Clin. Pediatr. 28(8):366-370, 1989.

Stevens, M.: Adolescents' perception of stressful events during hospitalization, J. Pediatr. Nurs. 1(5):303-313, 1986.

Stevens, M.S.: Which adolescents breeze through surgery? Am. J. Nurs. 87(12):1564-1565, 1987.

Stevens, M.S.: Application of a stress and coping framework to one adolescent's experience with hospitalization, Matern. Child Nurs. J. 17(1):51-61, 1988.

Stevens, M.S.: Benefits of hospitalization: the adolescent's perspective, Issues Compr. Pediatr. Nurs. 11(4):197-212, 1988.

Stevens, M.: Coping strategies of hospitalized adolescents, Child. Health Care 18(3):163-169, 1989.

Strickland, M.P.: Children's adjustment to the hospital: a rural/urban comparison, Matern. Child. Nurs. J. 16(3):251-260, 1987.

Terry, D.G.: The needs of parents of hospitalized children, Child. Health Care 16(1):18-20, 1987.

Vessey, J.A., Braithwaite, K.B., and Weidmann, M.: Teaching children about their internal bodies, Pediatr. Nurs. 16(1):29-33, 1990.

White, J.E.: Special nursing needs of hospitalized children with learning disabilities, MCN 8:209-212, 1983.
White, M.A., and others: Distress and self-soothing bedtime behaviors in hospitalized children with non-rooming-in parents, Matern. Child Nurs. J. 17(2):67-77, 1988.
White, M.A., and others: Sleep onset latency and distress in hospitalized children, Nurs. Res. 39(3):134-139, 1990.
Wilson, C.J.: Comparison of two methods of preparation for hospitalization, Child. Health Care 16(1):24-27, 1987.
Winch, A.E., and Christoph, J.M.: Parent-to-parent links: building networks for parents of hospitalized children, Child. Health Care 17(2):93-97, 1988.
Winkelstein, M.L., and Carson, V.J.: Adolescents and rooming-in, Matern. Child Nurs. J. 16(1):75-88, 1987.
Yap, J.N.: The effects of hospitalization and surgery on children: a critical review, J. Appl. Dev. Psychol. 9:349-358, 1988.

Pain Assessment

Aradine, C.R., Beyer, J.E., and Tompkins, J.M.: Children's pain perception before and after analgesia: a study of instrument construct validity and related issues, J. Pediatr. Nurs. 3(1):11-23, 1988.
Beyer, J.E., and Aradine, C.R.: Content validity of an instrument to measure young children's perceptions of the intensity of their pain, J. Pediatr. Nurs. 1(6):386-395, 1986.
Beyer, J.E., and Byers, M.L.: Knowledge of pediatric pain: the state of the art, Child. Health Care 13(4):150-159, 1985.
Beyer, J.E., and Knapp, T.R.: Methodologic issues in the measurement of children's pain, Child. Health Care 14(4):233-241, 1986.
Beyer, J.E., and Levin, C.R.: Issues and advances in pain control in children, Nurs. Clin. North Am. 22(3):661-676, 1987.
Beyer, J.E., and Wells, N.: The assessment of pain in children, Pediatr. Clin. North Am. 36(4):837-854, 1989.
Bradshaw, C., and Zeanah, P.D.: Pediatric nurses' assessments of pain in children, J. Pediatr. Nurs. 1(5):314-322, 1986.
Broome, M.E.: The child in pain: a model for assessment and intervention, Crit. Care Q. 8(1):47-56, 1985.
Carpenter, P.J.: New method for measuring young children's self-report of fear and pain, J. Pain Symptom Manag. 5(4):233-240, 1990.
Chapman, C.R., and others: Pain measurement: an overview, Pain 22:1-31, 1985.
Dale, J.C.: A multidimensional study of infants' behaviors associated with assumed painful stimuli: phase II, J. Pediatr. Health Care 3(1):34-38, 1989.
Gaffney, A., and Dunne, E.A.: Developmental aspects of children's definitions of pain, Pain 26:105-117, 1986.
Hawley, D.D.: Postoperative pain in children: misconceptions, descriptions, and interventions, Pediatr. Nurs. 10(1):20-23, 1984.
Hurley, A., and Whelan, E.G.: Cognitive development and children's perception of pain, Pediatr. Nurs. 14(1):21-24, 1988.
International Association for the Study of Pain: Pain terms: a current list with definitions and notes on usage, Pain 3:S216-S221, 1986.
Lynn, M.R.: Pain in the pediatric patient: a review of research, J. Pediatr. Nurs. 1(3):198-201, 1986.
McGrath, P.A.: Evaluating a child's pain, J. Pain Symptom Manag. 4(4):198-214, 1989.
McGrath, P.J., and Craig, K.D.: Developmental and psychological factors in children's pain, Pediatr. Clin. North Am. 36(4):823-836, 1989.
McGrath, P.J., and Unruh, A.: Pain in children and adolescents, New York, 1988, Elsevier Science Publishing Co., Inc.
Ross, D.M., and Ross, S.A.: Childhood pain: current issues, research, and management, Baltimore, 1988, Urban & Schwarzenberg, Inc.
Schechter, N.L.: The undertreatment of pain in children: an overview, Pediatr. Clin. North Am. 36(4):781-794, 1989.
Thorpe, D.M.: Pain assessment. I. Matching the tool to patient needs, Dimens. Oncol. Nurs. 3(2):19-25, 1989.
Wilkie, D.J., and others: Measuring pain quality: validity and reliability of children's and adolescents' pain language, Pain 41:151-159, 1990.
Wofford, L.G.: Pain in children with cancer: an assessment, J. Assoc. Pediatr. Oncol. Nurs. 2(2):34-37, 1985.

Pain Management

Beasley, S.W., and Tibballs, J.: Efficacy and safety of continuous morphine infusion for postoperative analgesia in the paediatric surgical ward, Aust. N.Z. J. Surg. 57:233-237, 1987.
Bell, S.G., and Ellis, L.J.: Use of fentanyl for sedation of mechanically ventilated neonates, Neonatal Network 6:27-31, 1987.
Bonadio, W.A., and Wagner, V.: Efficacy of TAC topical anesthetic for repair of pediatric lacerations, Am. J. Dis. Child. 142(2):203-205, 1988.
Broadman, L.M.: Patient-controlled analgesia in children and adults. In Ferante, F.M., Ostheimer, G.W., and Covino, B.G., editors: Patient-controlled analgesia, Boston, 1990, Blackwell Scientific Publications, Inc.
Bucknell, S., and Sikorski, K.: Putting patient-controlled analgesia to the test, MCN 14(1):37-40, 1989.
Christoph, R., and others: Pain reduction in local anesthetic administration through pH buffering, Ann. Emerg. Med. 17(2):117-120, 1988.
Cole, T., and others: Intravenous narcotic therapy for children with severe sickle cell crisis pain, Am. J. Dis. Child. 140:1255-1259, 1986.
Crockett, R.K.: Pain management in the pediatric emergency department, Int. Pediatr. 4(1):14-18, 1989.
Dalens, B.: Regional anesthesia in children, Anesth. Analg. 68:654-672, 1989.
Davies, G.G., and From, R.: A blinded study using nalbuphine for prevention of pruritus induced by epidural fentanyl, Anesthesiology 69:763-765, 1988.
Dothage, J., Arndt, C., and Miser, A.: Use of a continuous intravenous morphine infusion for pain control in an infant with terminal malignancy, J. Assoc. Pediatr. Oncol. Nurs. 3(4):22-24, 1986.
Eland, J.M.: The effectiveness of transcutaneous electrical nerve stimulation (TENS) with children experiencing cancer pain. In Funk, S.G., and others, editors: Key aspects of comfort, New York, 1989, Springer Publishing Co., Inc.
Frayling, I.M., and others: Methaemoglobinaemia in children treated with prilocaine-lignocaine cream, Br. Med. J. 301(6744):153-154, 1990.
Gilman, A., and others, editors: Goodman and Gilman's the pharmacological basis of therapeutics, ed. 7, New York, 1985, Macmillan Publishing Co.
Halperin, D.L., and others: Topical skin anesthesia for venous, subcutaneous drug reservoir and lumbar punctures in children, Pediatrics 84(2):281-284, 1989.
Hegenbath, M.A., and others: Comparison of topical tetracaine, adrenaline, and cocaine anesthesia with lidocaine infiltration for repair of lacerations in children, Ann. Emerg. Med. 19:63-67, 1990.
Koren, G., and Maurice, L.: Pediatric uses of opioids, Pediatr. Clin. North Am. 36(5):1141-1156, 1989.
Lacouture, P.G., Gaudreault, P., and Lovejoy, F.H., Jr.: Chronic pain of childhood: a pharmacologic approach, Pediatr. Clin. North Am. 31(5):1133-1151, 1984.
Lindsley, C.B., and Warady, B.A.: Nonsteroidal antiinflammatory drugs: renal toxicity, a review of pediatric issues, Clin. Pediatr. 29(1):10-13, 1990.
Maguire, D.P., and Maloney, P.: A comparison of fentanyl and morphine use in neonates, Neonatal Network 7(1):27-32, 1988.
McManus, M., and Panzarella, C.: The use of dextroamphetamine to counteract sedation for patients on a morphine drip, J. Assoc. Pediatr. Oncol. Nurs. 3(1):28-29, 1986.
Miser, A.W., Dothage, J.A., and Miser, J.S.: Continuous intravenous fentanyl for pain control in children and young adults with cancer, Clin. J. Pain 3:152-157, 1987.
Miser, A.W., and Miser, J.S.: The use of oral methadone to control moderate and severe pain in children and young adults with malignancy, Clin. J. Pain 1:243-248, 1985.

Mofenson, H., and Caraccio, T.: Tack up a warning on TAC, Am. J. Dis. Child. 143(5):519, 1989.
Nelson, P.S., and others: Comparison of oral transmucosal fentanyl citrate and an oral solution of meperidine, diazepam, and atropine for premedication in children, Anesthesiology 70:616-621, 1989.
Norton, S.J.: After effects of morphine and fentanyl analgesia: a retrospective study, Neonatal Network 7(3):25-28, 1988.
Rodgers, B.M., and others: Patient-controlled analgesia in pediatric surgery, J. Pediatr. Surg. 23(3):259-262, 1988.
Rogers, A.G.: The use and availability of rectal narcotics, J. Pain Symptom Manag. 1(4):229-230, 1986.
Ryan, E.A.: The effect of musical distraction of pain in hospitalized school-aged children. In Funk, S.G., and others: Key aspects of comfort, New York, 1989, Springer Publishing Co., Inc.
Schechter, N.L., Altman, A., and Weisman, S.: Report of the Consensus Conference on the Management of Pain in Childhood Cancer, Pediatrics 86(5, suppl.): 813-834, 1990.
Shannon, M., and Berde, C.B.: Pharmacologic management of pain in children and adolescents, Pediatr. Clin. North Am. 36(4):855-871, 1989.
Tipton, G., DeWitt, G., and Eisenstein, S.: Topical TAC (tetracaine, adrenaline, cocaine) solution for local anesthesia in children: prescribing inconsistency and acute toxicity, South. Med. J. 82(11):1344-1346, 1989.
Whitman, H.H.: Sublingual morphine: a novel route of narcotic administration, Am. J. Nurs. 84(7):939, 1984.
Yaster, M., and Deshpande, J.K.: Management of pediatric pain with opioid analgesics, J. Pediatr. 113(3):421-429, 1988.

Hospital Preparation and Special Admissions

Alcock, D., and others: Environment and waiting behaviors in emergency waiting areas, Child. Health Care 13(4):174-180, 1985.
Bernardo, L.M., Conway, K., and Bove, M.: The ABC method of emotional assessment and intervention: a new approach in pediatric emergency care, J. Emerg. Nurs. 16(2):70-76, 1990.
Broome, M.E.: Working with the family of a critically ill child, Heart Lung 14(4):368-372, 1985.
Byers, M.L.: Same day surgery: a preschooler's experience, Matern. Child Nurs. J. 16(3):277-282, 1987.
Cagan, J.: Weaning parents from intensive care unit care, MCN 13:275-277, 1988.
Caine, R.M.: Families in crisis: making the critical difference, Focus Crit. Care 16(3):184-189, 1989.
Curley, M.A.: Effects of the nursing mutual participation model of care on parental stress in the pediatric intensive care unit, Heart Lung 17(6, pt. 1):682-688, 1988.
Deatrick, J.A., and Knafl, K.A.: Developing programs for hospitalized children: clinical significance of qualitative research, J. Pediatr. Nurs. 3(2):123-126, 1988.
deChesnay, M.: Promoting healthy family functioning in acute care units, J. Pediatr. Nurs. 1(2):96-101, 1986.
Dracup, K.: Are critical care units hazardous to health? Appl. Nurs. Res. 1(1):14-21, 1988.
Edwinson, M., Arnbjornsson, E., and Ekman, R: Psychologic preparation program for children undergoing acute appendectomy, Pediatrics 81(1):30-36, 1988.
Epsersen, S., and Hardy, C.D.: Pediatric care plan for adult ICU nurses, Crit. Care Nurse 5(2):14-18, 1985.
Etzler, C.A.: Parents' reaction to pediatric critical care settings: a review of the literature, Issues Compr. Pediatr. Nurs. 7:319-331, 1984.
Ferguson, C.K.: Childhood coping: adaptive behavior during intensive care hospitalization, Crit. Care Q. 6(4):81-93, 1984.
Gillis, A.J.: Hospital preparation: the children's story, Child. Health Care 19(1):19-27, 1990.
Goldbloom, R.B., and Macleod, M.U.: Impact of preadmission evaluations on elective hospitalization of children, Pediatrics 73(5):656-660, 1984.
Gross, S.: Pediatric tours of hospitals—positive or negative? MCN 11:336-338, 1986.
Hansen, M., Young, D.A., and Carden, F.E.: Psychological evaluation and support in the pediatric intensive care unit, Pediatr. Ann. 15(1):60-69, 1986.
Hazinski, M.F.: Nursing care of the critically ill child: a seven-point check, Pediatr. Nurs. 11(6):453-461, 1985.
Hickey, M.: What are the needs of families of critically ill patients? A review of the literature since 1976, Heart Lung 19(4):401-415, 1990.
Jansen, M.T., and others: Meeting psychosocial and developmental needs of children during prolonged intensive care unit hospitalization, Child. Health Care 18(2):91-95, 1989.
Johnson, P.A., Nelson, G.L., and Brunnquell, D.J.: Parent and nurse perceptions of parent stressors in the pediatric intensive care unit, Child. Health Care 17(2):98-105, 1988.
Kasper, J.W., and Nyamathi, A.M.: Parents of children in the pediatric intensive care unit: what are their needs? Heart Lung 17(5):574-581, 1988.
Kidder, C.: Reestablishing health: factors influencing the child's recovery in pediatric intensive care, J. Pediatr. Nurs. 4(2):96-103, 1989.
King, S.L., and Gregor, F.M.: Stress and coping in families of the critically ill, Crit. Care Nurse 5(4):48-51, 1985.
LaMontagne, L.L., and Pawlak, R.: Stress and coping of parents of children in a pediatric intensive care unit, Heart Lung 19(4):416-421, 1990.
Miles, M.S., and Carter, M.C.: Sources of parental stress in pediatric intensive care units, Child. Health Care 11(2):65-69, 1982.
Miles, M.S., and Carter, M.C.: Assessing parental stress in intensive care units, MCN 8(5):354-359, 1983.
Miles, M.S., and Carter, M.C.: Coping strategies used by parents during their child's hospitalization in an intensive care unit, Child. Health Care 14(1):14-21, 1985.
Moore, A.C.: Crisis intervention: a care plan for families of hospitalized children, Pediatr. Nurs. 15(3):234-236, 1989.
Munn, V.A., and Tichy, A.M.: Nurses' perceptions of stressors in pediatric intensive care, J. Pediatr. Nurs. 2(6):405-411, 1987.
O'Mears, K., and others: Preadmission programs: development, implementation, and evaluation, Child. Health Care 11(4):137-141, 1983.
Orsuto, J., Sr., and Corbo, B.H.: Approaches of health caregivers to young children in a pediatric intensive care unit, Matern. Child Nurs. J. 16(2):157-175, 1987.
Philichi, L.M.: Family adaptation during a pediatric intensive care hospitalization, J. Pediatr. Nurs. 4(4):268-276, 1989.
Proctor, D.L.: Relationship between visitation policy in a pediatric intensive care unit and parental anxiety, Child. Health Care 16(1):13-17, 1987.
Rushton, C.H.: Family-centered care in the critical care setting: myth or reality? Child. Health Care 19(2):68-78, 1990.
Rushton, C.H.: Strategies for family-centered care in the critical care setting, Pediatr. Nurs. 16(2):195-199, 1990.
Terry, D.G.: The needs of parents of hospitalized children, Child. Health Care 16(1):18-20, 1987.
Tichy, A.M., and others: Stressors in pediatric intensive care units, Pediatr. Nurs. 14(1):40-42, 1988.
Titus, S., and Porter, P.: Orem's theory applied to pediatric residential treatment, Pediatr. Nurs. 15(5):465-468, 556, 1989.
Tompkins, J.M.: Intrahospital transport of seriously ill or injured children, Pediatr. Nurs. 16(1):51-53, 1990.
Tse, A.M., Perez-Woods, R.C., and Opie, N.D.: Children's admissions to the intensive care unit: parents' attitudes and expectations of outcome, Child. Health Care 16(2):68-75, 1987.
Welch, T.C.: Ambulatory surgery centers: an aspect of surgical patient care, Point View 27(2):14-18, 1990.
Wilson, C.J.: Comparison of two methods of preparation for hospitalization, Child. Health Care 16(1):24-27, 1987.
Wilson, T., and Broome, M.E.: Promoting the young child's development in the intensive care unit, Heart Lung 18(3):274-281, 1989.

Wyckoff, P.M., and Erickson, M.T.: Mediating factors of stress on mothers of seriously ill, hospitalized children, Child. Health Care 16(1):4-12, 1987.

Discharge Planning and Home Care

Bass, L.W.: The neglected discharge instruction, Pediatrics 78(2):362-364, 1986.
Foster, S.D.: The role of education in discharge planning, MCN 13:403, 1988.
Giesy, J.: Teaching discharge management, J. Pediatr. Nurs. 2(5):353-354, 1987.
Jones, M.: Home care for the chronically ill or disabled child: a manual and sourcebook for parents and professionals, New York, 1985, Harper & Row, Publishers, Inc.
Kasprisin, C.: Home care instructions. In Wong, D.L., and Whaley, L.F.: Clinical manual of pediatric nursing, ed. 3, St. Louis, 1990, Mosby–Year Book, Inc.
Kruger, S.F., and Rawlins, P.: Pediatric dismissal protocol to aid the transition from hospital care to home care, Image 16(4):120-125, 1984.
McHatton, M.: A theory for timely teaching, Am. J. Nurs. 85(7):798-800, 1985.
Miller, A.: When is the time ripe for teaching? Am. J. Nurs. 85(7):801-804, 1985.
Sanborn, C.W., and Blount, M.: Standard plans for care and discharge, Am. J. Nurs. 84(11):1394-1396, 1984.
Steele, B.: Home care for children: an annotated bibliography, Washington, DC, 1984, Association for the Care of Children's Health.
Wong, D.L.: Transition from hospital to home for children with complex medical care, J. Pediatr. Oncol. Nurs. 8(1):3-9, 1991.

SELECTED BOOKS FOR CHILDREN

Chase, F., and Coleman, L.: A visit to the hospital, New York, 1974, Grosset & Dunlap, Inc.
Clark B.: Pop-up going to the hospital, New York, 1970, Random House, Inc.
Collier, J.: Danny goes to the hospital, New York, 1970, W.W. Norton & Co., Inc.
Howe, J.: The hospital book, New York, 1981, Crown Publishers, Inc.
Rey, M., and Rey, H.: Curious George goes to the hospital, New York, 1966, Houghton Mifflin Co.
Stein, S.: A hospital story, New York, 1974, Walker & Co.
Weber, A.: Elizabeth gets well, New York, 1970, Thomas Y. Crowell Co.

OTHER RESOURCES

Association for Care of Children's Health, 7910 Woodmont Ave., Suite 300, Bethesda, MD 20814; (301) 654-6549.

Talks About the Hospital, a series written by Fred Rogers, is available from Family Communications, Inc., 4802 Fifth Ave., Pittsburgh, PA 15213; (412) 687-2990.

See also Bibliography in Chapter 6, Box 6-3.

CHAPTER 27

Pediatric Variations of Nursing Interventions

RELATED TOPICS

Communicating with families, Ch. 6
Dental health: infant, Ch. 12; toddler, Ch. 14; preschooler, Ch. 15; school-age child, Ch. 17; and adolescent, Ch. 19
Feeding resistance, Ch. 10
Injury prevention: infant, Ch. 12; toddler, Ch. 14; preschooler, Ch. 15; school-age child, Ch. 17; and adolescent, Ch. 19
Limit-setting and discipline, Ch. 14
Long-term venous access, Ch. 28
Neonatal pain, Ch. 11
Nursing care of the surgical neonate, Ch. 11
Nutritional assessment, Ch. 6
Pain management, Ch. 26
Parenteral fluid therapy, Ch. 28
Preparation for hospitalization, Ch. 26
Preparation for procedures, Ch. 36
Temperature (measurement), Ch. 7
Use of play to minimize stress, Ch. 26

GLOSSARY

antipyretic An agent that relieves or reduces fever
BSI Body substance isolation
CDC Centers for Disease Control
emancipated minor One who is legally under the age of majority (age at which child becomes an adult) but is recognized as having the legal capacity of an adult, as prescribed by law

febrile Pertaining to fever
fever Elevation in set point such that body temperature is regulated at a higher level
HIV Human immunodeficiency virus
hyperthermia Body temperature exceeds the set point
IM Intramuscular
informed consent Legal and ethical requirement that patients/parents must completely understand proposed treatments, including risks and benefits
IV Intravenous
NSAID Nonsteroidal antiinflammatory drug
PACU Postanesthesia care unit
set point Temperature around which body temperature is regulated by a thermostat-like mechanism in the hypothalamus
UP Universal precautions

Children are not simply small adults. They differ from their older counterparts in the areas of biologic, cognitive, and emotional function and response. Consequently many standard interventions employed in nursing practice must be altered to meet the special needs of children at various developmental stages. The chapter presents an overview of psychologic preparation of children for procedures; strategies to enhance compliance; application of principles of growth and development in planning, implementing, and evaluating nursing procedures; and selected aspects of skills that require modification in caring for infants and children.

GENERAL CONCEPTS RELATED TO PEDIATRIC PROCEDURES

Children, regardless of their age, require preparation for procedures. Family members, especially parents, also need adequate preparation and, for some procedures, are required to give informed consent. This section discusses informed consent, general aspects of preparation for procedures, and preparation for a specific procedure, surgery. Preparation of the child for hospitalization is presented in Chapter 26. Because play is such an integral part of children's lives, a discussion on the use of play in procedures is included. The section concludes with a discussion of compliance, an essential aspect of continued care.

INFORMED CONSENT*

Informed consent refers to the legal and ethical requirement that patients must completely understand proposed treatments, including significant risks associated with treatment. Patients must also be informed of possible benefits of the proposed treatment, possible alternative treatments, and risks of nontreatment before giving informed consent. To obtain valid informed consent, three conditions must be met (Hogue, 1988):

1. The person must be capable of giving consent; he or she must be over the *age of majority* (age at which a child becomes an adult) and must be considered competent, that is, possess the mental capacity to make choices and understand their consequences.
2. The person must receive the information needed to make an intelligent decision.
3. The person must act voluntarily when exercising freedom of choice without force, fraud, deceit, duress, or other forms of constraint or coercion.

Many state legislatures have adopted laws (statutes) that address issues of informed consent. Nurses must understand what is required in their practices by reviewing applicable statutes in each jurisdiction in which they practice. There are, however, some general principles associated with informed consent that are generally applicable in all states. The following discussion of informed consent is presented in general terms and is not to be interpreted as legal advice. Although informing patients or parents of the risks, benefits, and alternatives of procedures is physicians' responsibility, nurses frequently are asked to secure patients' signatures on consent forms (Cushing, 1984). In caring for children, special dilemmas may arise regarding who may sign consent forms when a parent is unavailable. The age of majority is especially important when caring for adolescents, and competence is a key issue in decisions involving minors who are retarded or otherwise mentally incapacitated (see Questions and Controversies, p. 1079). Consequently, nurses need to be familiar with this highly significant and complex subject and must keep current on legal aspects of practice within their communities.

Requirements for Obtaining Informed Consent

Informed consent from a parent or legal guardian is usually required for medical or surgical treatment of children, including many diagnostic procedures. Informed consent must be obtained for each surgical or invasive diagnostic procedure and for certain situations that are not directly related to medical treatment (Box 27-1).

Assent for proposed treatments should also be obtained from the child age 7 years or older who is at least in the concrete operations period. Assent requires that the child be informed about the proposed treatment or plan of care

Donna Phillips Smith, R.N., M.S., assisted in the revision of this chapter.
*Elizabeth E. Hogue, J.D., assisted in the revision of this section.

Box 27-1 PROCEDURES AND SITUATIONS REQUIRING INFORMED CONSENT

Major surgery
Minor surgery—cutdown, biopsy, dental extraction, suturing a laceration (especially one that may have a cosmetic effect), removal of a cyst, closed reduction of a fracture
Diagnostic tests with an element of risk—bronchoscopy, needle biopsy, angiography, electroencephalogram, lumbar puncture, cardiac catheterization, ventriculography, bone marrow aspiration
Medical treatments with an element of risk—blood transfusions, thoracentesis or paracentesis, radiation therapy, shock therapies
Taking photographs for medical, educational, or other public use
Removal of children from health care institutions against medical advice
Postmortem examinations, except in unexplained deaths, such as sudden infant death, violent death, or suspected suicide
Release of medical information

and agree or concur with the decisions made by the person(s) who can give informed consent. By including children in the decision-making process and gaining their acceptance, children are treated with respect (Erlen, 1987). Assent must also be obtained in research involving children. Considerable controversy surrounds the use of children as research subjects, and nurses involved in research must be aware of the legal and ethical guidelines and requirements before initiating pediatric research (Rae and Fournier, 1986).

Eligibility for Giving Informed Consent

In most situations either a parent or legal guardian gives informed consent. However, problems may arise when parents are not available to give consent, the child seeks certain treatments, the child is a so-called emancipated minor, or parents neglect or refuse treatment for their minor child. The judicial system may intervene in cases where the parents' views and the child's best interests conflict (Nix, 1991). However, laws significantly favor parental authority, and clear and convincing evidence must be presented before the court will intervene (Rhodes, 1988).

Problems may also occur when the child's parents are divorced. Generally speaking, both custodial and noncustodial parents may consent to treatment for their minor children. Consent from either divorced parent is sufficient; the consent of both parents is generally not required (Hogue, 1988).

Informed consent of parents or legal guardians. Parents have full responsibility for the care and rearing of their minor children, including legal control over them. Therefore, as long as children are minors, parents or persons designated as legal guardians for the child are required to give informed consent before medical treatment is rendered or any procedure is performed on the child. Parents also have a right to withdraw consent later.

Evidence of consent. A signed consent form is only evidence that the process of informed consent has occurred; it is not legally required, although it may be an institutional policy. Verbal consent is also evidence of the process. For example, when parents are unavailable to sign consent forms, verbal consent may be obtained via telephone. Verbal consent may also be obtained from parents who are unable to sign, for example, because of injury. It is good risk management to have a witness to a parent's or guardian's verbal consent. Another nurse may be present or listening on a telephone extension. Both nurses record that informed consent was given and the name, address, and relationship of the person giving consent, together with their signatures indicating that they witnessed the consent.

Informed consent of mature and emancipated minors. State laws differ with regard to the so-called age of majority. Although some variation still exists, children become adults on their eighteenth birthdays in most states. Competent adults can give informed consent on their own behalf. Nonetheless, some courts have permitted minors to consent to their treatment based on the *mature minors doctrine.* This doctrine permits minors to give consent even though they are not technically adults as long as they understand the consequences of their decisions.

Statutes in many states permit minors to give consent on their own behalf to certain treatments, such as for:

- Sexually transmitted diseases
- Contraceptive services
- Pregnancy
- Drug or alcohol abuse

Pediatric nurses should carefully review laws in the states in which they practice to determine when minors may consent to treatment on their own behalf.

An *emancipated minor* is one who is legally under the age of majority but is recognized as having the legal capacity of an adult under circumstances prescribed by state law. Minors may become emancipated by the following (Selbst, 1985):

- Pregnancy
- Marriage
- High school graduation
- Living independently
- Military service

Some states require emancipated minors to appear in court to prove their status. Such hearings usually result in court orders that are useful to nurses as proof of emancipation and the ability to consent to treatment. In other states one or more of the events just listed triggers emancipation without the need for any proof in court. Nurses who practice in such states are not necessarily required to seek proof of emancipation in order to accept consent from emancipated minors.

Consent to abortion is more complex. The U.S. Supreme Court has decided that parental consent is not required before performing abortions. The issue of parental notification before or after an abortion is still undecided.

Treatment without parental consent. Exceptions to

requiring parental consent before treating minor children occur when children need prompt medical or surgical treatment and a parent is not readily available to give consent or refuses to give consent. In the absence of parents or legal guardians, some providers permit persons in charge of the child to give informed consent for treatment. In emergencies, consent is not needed; it is implied according to the law (Hogue, 1988). Emergencies include danger to life or possibility of permanent injury.

Refusal to give consent can occur when the treatment, such as blood transfusions, conflicts with the parents' religious beliefs. All states recognize such exceptions and have statutory procedures to permit treatment if the life or health of such a minor is in jeopardy or if delayed treatment would create a risk to the health of the minor. The state is also able to intervene in situations that jeopardize the health and welfare of children, as in cases in which parents neglect or impose excessive or improper punishment on a child. In most communities there are procedures by which custody of the child can be transferred to a governmental or a private agency when parental neglect or abuse can be proved.

PREPARATION FOR PROCEDURES

Psychologic Preparation*

Preparing children for procedures decreases their anxiety, promotes their cooperation, supports their coping skills and may teach them new ones, and facilitates a feeling of mastery in experiencing a potentially stressful event. Preparatory methods may be formal, such as group preparation for hospitalization (see Chapter 26). Most preparation strategies used by nurses are informal, focus on providing information about the experience, and are directed at stressful and/or painful procedures. Although research has been conducted on many types of preparation (e.g., using dolls, puppets, plays, books, videotapes, or slides), no one method is universally more effective than another. However, young children respond better to play materials, and older youngsters benefit more from viewing peer-modeling films (Bates and Broome, 1986). Preparatory interventions are most effective in reducing behavioral distress (crying, resisting), followed by decreasing children's rating of pain, and last, by reducing signs of physiologic distress (heart rate, blood pressure, oxygen saturation) (Broome and Lillis, 1989; Broome, Lillis, and Smith, 1989).

General guidelines for preparing children for procedures are described in Box 27-2, and age-specific guidelines that consider children's developmental needs and cognitive abilities are presented in Box 27-3. In addition to these suggestions, nurses should consider the child's temperament, existing coping strategies, and previous experiences in individualizing the preparatory process. Children who are distractible and highly active, as well as those who are "slow to warm up," may need individualized sessions that are shorter for the active child but more slowly paced for the shy child (McLeod and McClowry, 1990). Youngsters who tend to cope well may need more emphasis on using their present skills, whereas those who appear to cope less adequately can benefit from more time devoted to simple coping strategies, such as relaxing, breathing, counting, squeezing a hand, or singing (Patterson and Ware, 1988). Children with previous health-related experiences still need preparation for repeat or new procedures, but the nurse must assess what they know, correct misconceptions, supply new information, and introduce new coping skills as indicated by their previous reactions (Bates and Broome, 1986).

Children also are different in their "information-seeking dimension"; some want and actively solicit information about the intended procedure, whereas others characteristi-

Box 27-2 GENERAL GUIDELINES FOR PREPARING CHILDREN FOR PROCEDURES

- Determine the details of the exact procedure to be performed.
- Review the parents' and child's present level of understanding.
- Plan the actual teaching based on the child's developmental age and existing level of knowledge.
- Incorporate parents in the teaching if they desire, and especially if they plan to participate in the care.
- Inform parents of their role during procedure, such as stand near child's head or in line of vision and talk softly to child.
- While preparing the child and family, allow for ample discussion to prevent information overload and ensure adequate feedback.
- Use concrete, not abstract, terms and visual aids to describe the procedure. For example, use a simple line drawing of a boy or girl (Fig. 27-1), and mark the body part that will be involved in the procedure.
- Emphasize that no other body part will be involved.
- If the body part is associated with a specific function, stress the change or noninvolvement of that ability (e.g., following tonsillectomy, the child can still speak).
- Use words appropriate to the child's level of understanding (a rule of thumb for number of words is the age in years plus 1).
- Avoid words/phrases with dual meanings (see Box 27-4) unless the child understands such words.
- Clarify all unfamiliar words (e.g., "Anesthesia is a *special* sleep").
- Emphasize the sensory aspects of the procedure—what the child will feel, see, smell, and touch and what the child can do during the procedure (e.g., lie still, count out loud, squeeze a hand, hug a doll).
- Allow the child to practice those procedures that will require cooperation (e.g., turning, deep breathing, using an incentive spirometer or mask).
- Introduce anxiety-laden information last (e.g., the preoperative injection).
- Be honest with the child about the unpleasant aspects of a procedure but avoid creating undue concern. When discussing that a procedure may be uncomfortable, state that it feels differently to different people and have the child describe how it felt.
- Emphasize the end of the procedure and any pleasurable events afterward (e.g., going home, seeing the parent).
- Stress the positive benefits of the procedure (e.g., "After your tonsils are fixed, you won't have as many sore throats").

*Marion E. Broome, R.N., Ph.D., assisted in the revision of this section.

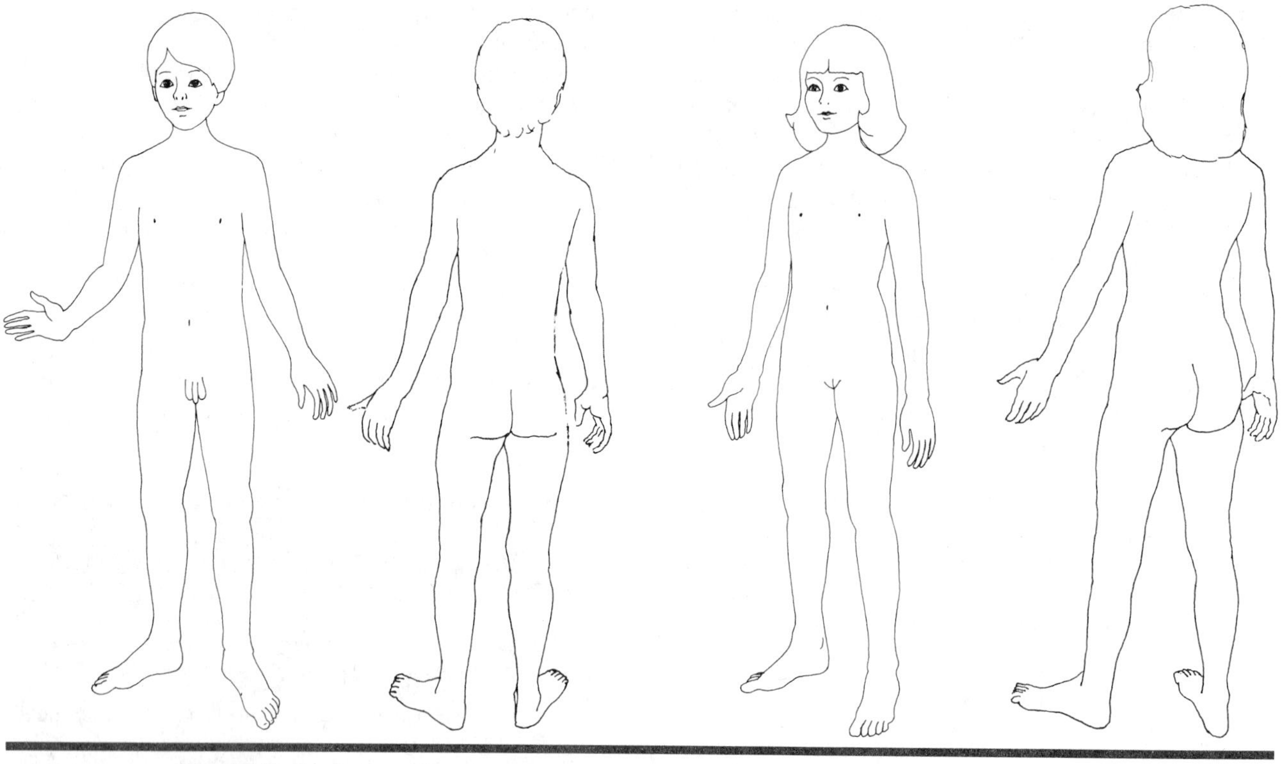

Fig. 27-1. Examples of line drawings to be used in preparing child for procedures.

cally avoid information (Peterson and Toler, 1986). Parents can often guide nurses in deciding how much information is enough for the child, since parents know if the child is typically inquisitive or satisfied with short answers. Asking older children their preferences about the amount of explanation is also important. Questions such as, "Do you like to know everything about new experiences or just the basic facts?" or "How much of an explanation do you want—just what you will experience or why things are done?" are also helpful in tailoring information to avoid overpreparation or underpreparation (see also Box 6-2 for signs of information overload).

The exact timing of the preparation for a procedure varies with the child's age and the type of procedure. There are no exact guidelines to govern timing, but in general the younger the child, the closer the explanation should be to the actual procedure to prevent undue fantasizing and worrying. With complex procedures more time may be needed for assimilation of information, especially with older children. For example, the explanation for an injection can immediately precede the procedure for all ages, but preparation for surgery may begin the day before for young children and a few days before for older children, although older children's preferences should be elicited (see Preparation for Hospitalization, Chapter 26).

Establish trust and provide support. The nurse who has spent time with and who has established a positive relationship with a child will usually find it easier to gain cooperation. If the relationship is based on trust, the child will associate the nurse with caregiving activities that give comfort and pleasure most of the time and not as someone who brings discomfort and stress. If the nurse does not know the child, it is best if the nurse is introduced by another staff person whom the child trusts. The first visit with the child ideally focuses on the child first and then on explanation of the procedure only; performing the procedure should be avoided. When talking with the child, the nurse uses the same guidelines for communicating with children that are discussed in Chapter 6.

Children need support during procedures, and for young children the greatest source of support is the parents. However, controversy exists regarding the role parents should assume during the procedure, especially if discomfort is involved (see Questions and Controversies). Nurses need to consider the issues in deciding whether parental presence is beneficial. The parents' preferences for assisting, observing, or waiting outside the room should be assessed, as well as the child's preference for parental presence. The child's choice should be respected (Rollins and Brantly, 1991). Parents who wish to stay need preparation for what will occur and how they can help. Simple instructions such as clarifying where parents can stay in the room and positioning them where they have eye contact with the child provide support and lessen anxiety. Parents who do not wish to be present or participate are supported in their decision and encouraged to remain close by so that they can be available to console the child immediately following the procedure. Parents should also know that someone will be

Box 27-3 AGE-SPECIFIC GUIDELINES FOR PREPARING CHILDREN FOR PROCEDURES BASED ON DEVELOPMENTAL CHARACTERISTICS

Infancy: Developing a Sense of Trust

Attachment to parent	*Involve parent in procedure if desired. Keep parent in infant's line of vision. If patient is unable to be with infant, place familiar object with infant (e.g., stuffed toy).
Stranger anxiety	*Have usual caregivers perform or assist with procedure. Make advances slowly and in nonthreatening manner. *Limit number of strangers entering room during procedure.
Sensorimotor phase of learning	During procedure use sensory soothing measures (e.g., stroking skin, talking softly, giving pacifier). *Use analgesics (e.g., local anesthetic, intravenous opioid) to control discomfort. Cuddle and hug child after stressful procedure; encourage parent to comfort child.
Increased muscle control	Expect older infants to resist. Restrain adequately. Keep harmful objects out of reach.
Memory for past experiences	Realize that older infants may associate objects or persons with prior painful experiences and will cry and resist at sight of them. *Keep frightening objects out of view. *Perform painful procedures in a separate room, not in crib (or bed).
Imitation of gestures	Model desired behavior (e.g., opening mouth).

Toddler: Developing a Sense of Autonomy

	Use same approaches as for infant in addition to following:
Egocentric	Explain procedure in relation to what child will see, hear, taste, smell, and feel. Emphasize those aspects of procedure that require cooperation (e.g., lying still). Tell child it's okay to cry, yell, or use other means to express discomfort verbally.
Negative behavior	Expect treatments to be resisted; child may try to run away. Use firm, direct approach. Ignore temper tantrums. Use distraction techniques (e.g., singing a song *with* a child). Restrain adequately.
Limited language skills	Communicate using behaviors. Use a few, simple terms familiar to child. Give one direction at a time (e.g., "Lie down," then "Hold my hand"). Use small replicas of equipment; allow child to handle equipment. Use play; demonstrate on doll but avoid child's favorite doll since child may think doll is really "feeling" procedure. Prepare parents separately to avoid child's misinterpreting words.
Limited concept of time	Prepare child shortly or immediately before procedure. Keeping teaching sessions short (about 5 to 10 minutes). Have preparations completed before involving child in procedure. Have extra equipment nearby (e.g., alcohol swabs, new needle, Band-Aids) to avoid delays. Tell child when procedure is completed.
Striving for independence	Allow choices whenever possible but realize that child may still be resistant and negative. Allow child to participate in care and to help whenever possible (e.g., drink medicine from a cup, hold a dressing).

Preschooler: Developing a Sense of Initiative

Preoperational thought: egocentric	Explain procedure in simple terms and in relation to how it affects child (as with toddler, stress sensory aspects). Demonstrate use of equipment. Allow child to play with miniature or actual equipment. Encourage "playing out" experience on a doll both before and after procedure to clarify misconceptions. Use neutral words to describe the procedure (see Box 27-4).
Increased language skills	Use verbal explanation but avoid overestimating child's comprehension of words. Encourage child to verbalize ideas and feelings.
Concept of time and frustration tolerance still limited	Implement same approaches as for toddler but may plan longer teaching session (10 to 15 minutes); may divide information into more than one session.
Illness and hospitalization often viewed as punishment	Clarify why each procedure is performed; a child will find it difficult to understand how medicine can make him or her feel better and can taste bad at the same time. Ask child thoughts regarding why a procedure is performed. State directly that procedures are never a form of punishment.

*Applies to any age.

Continued.

Box 27-3 AGE-SPECIFIC GUIDELINES FOR PREPARING CHILDREN FOR PROCEDURES BASED ON DEVELOPMENTAL CHARACTERISTICS—cont'd

Preschooler: Developing a Sense of Initiative—cont'd	
Fears of bodily harm, intrusion, and castration	Point out on drawing, doll, or child where procedure is performed. Emphasize that no other body part will be involved. Use nonintrusive procedures whenever possible (e.g., axillary temperatures, oral medication). Apply a Band-Aid over puncture site. Encourage parental presence. Realize that procedures involving genitals provoke anxiety. Allow child to wear underpants with gown. Explain unfamiliar situations, especially noises or lights.
Striving for initiative	Involve child in care whenever possible (e.g., hold equipment, remove dressing). Give choices whenever possible but avoid excessive delays. Praise child for helping and attempting to cooperate; never shame child for lack of cooperation.
School-Age Child: Developing a Sense of Industry	
Increased language skills; interest in acquiring knowledge	Explain procedures using correct scientific/medical terminology. Explain reason for procedure using simple diagrams of anatomy and physiology. Explain function and operation of equipment in concrete terms. Allow child to manipulate equipment; use doll or another person as model to practice using equipment whenever possible (doll play may be considered "childish" by older school-age child). Allow time before and after procedure for questions and discussion.
Improved concept of time	Plan for longer teaching sessions (about 20 minutes). Prepare in advance of procedure.
Increased self-control	Gain child's cooperation. Tell child what is expected. Suggest ways of maintaining control (e.g., deep breathing, relaxation, counting).
Striving for industry	Allow responsibility for simple tasks (e.g., collecting specimens). Include in decision making (e.g., time of day to perform procedure, preferred site). Encourage active participation (e.g., removing dressings, handling equipment, opening packages).
Developing relationships with peers	May prepare two or more children for same procedure or encourage one to help prepare another peer. Provide privacy from peers during procedure to maintain self-esteem.
Adolescent: Developing a Sense of Identity	
Increasingly capable of abstract thought and reasoning	Supplement explanations with reasons why procedure is necessary or beneficial. Explain long-term consequences of procedures. Realize that adolescent may fear death, disability, or other potential risks. Encourage questioning regarding fears, options, and alternatives.
Conscious of appearance	Provide privacy. Discuss how procedure may affect appearance (e.g., scar) and what can be done to minimize it. Emphasize any physical benefits of procedure.
Concerned more with present than future	Realize that immediate effects of procedure are more significant than future benefits.
Striving for independence	Involve in decision making and planning (e.g., choice of time; place; individuals present during procedure, such as parents; clothing to wear). Impose as few restrictions as possible. Suggest methods of maintaining control. Accept regression to more childish methods of coping. Realize that adolescent may have difficulty in accepting new authority figures and may resist complying with procedures.
Developing peer relationships and group identity	Same as for school-age child but assumes even greater significance.

Continued.

with their child to provide support. Ideally this person should inform the parents after the procedure about how the child did.

Provide an explanation. Children need an explanation for anything that involves them directly. Before performing a procedure, the nurse explains to children what is to be done and what is expected of them. The explanation should be short, simple, and appropriate to the child's level of comprehension. Long explanations are not necessary and may only increase anxiety in a small child. This is especially true regarding painful procedures. When explaining the procedure to parents with the child present, the nurse uses language appropriate to the child because unfamiliar words can be misunderstood (Box 27-4). If the parents need

QUESTIONS AND CONTROVERSIES

Should parents be allowed to stay with their children during stressful procedures?

Health professionals have basically adopted two opposing philosophies in relation to parental presence during procedures. One view purports that parents should not be present, since the child may view the parent's presence and/or participation as complicity and then blame the parent for allowing such indignities to be inflicted on the child. Since children normally associate parents with a comforting, "make it better" role, these professionals believe that parents should be a source of comfort and security to the child, which is best served by reuniting the child and parents after the procedure. The opposite view holds that not allowing the parents to be present inflicts the additional stress of separation and deprives the child of the parent's support. No consensus exists on whether parents who are present with the child should participate in the procedure, such as assisting in restraint.

Although relatively little research has focused on this important issue, most of the available research finds that parental presence is supportive. Vernon, Foley, and Schulman (1967) compared preschoolers' responses to stress during admission and anesthesia induction with the parent present or absent. They found no differences in the preschoolers' behavior during admission procedures but considerably more distress in children whose parent was not present during induction, especially at the final phase after the mask was placed on the face. Several more recent studies found similar results when parents were permitted to stay with unpremedicated children during induction anesthesia in an outpatient setting (Gauderer, Lorig, and Eastman, 1989; Hannallah and Rosales, 1983; Schofield and White, 1989).

Shaw and Routh (1982) assessed the effect of parental presence on young children during an injection and found that the children separated from the parent cried less and for less time. They concluded that the increased negative behavior in the children when the parent was present did not necessarily indicate greater upset; rather, it showed the children's greater expression of emotion in a supportive atmosphere. Another study on parental presence during dental treatment did not find a statistically significant difference between children's stress levels and parental presence or absence. However, it did find that when the parents were with them, children were more relaxed (Venham, Bengston, and Cipes, 1978). While some health professionals maintain that parents are disruptive during a procedure, studies have found that most parents choose to participate, are not disruptive of the procedure, and even when they find the experience difficult and stressful, are able to support their children (Bauchner, Vinci, and Waring, 1989; Merritt, Sargent, and Osborn, 1990; Savedra, 1981). Parents can become stressed by the experience, and parents with high anxiety tend to cause more anxiety in the child, although the child may not behave any differently during the actual procedure (Broome and Endsley, 1989; Johnston and others, 1988).

Some of the most significant evidence in favor of parental presence during stressful procedures comes from children. When children are asked for their preference, the response is overwhelmingly in favor of having their parents stay with them. All children ages 4 to 18 years wanted their parents to accompany them during a bone marrow test (Hamner and Miles, 1988). More than 80% of children ages 5 to 11 years wanted parents at the time of anesthesia induction, and more than 90% wanted them to be in the postanesthesia care unit (Hanna and Sherlock, 1983). Seventy percent of adolescents ages 14 to 19 years preferred their parents to be present during cancer-related procedures (Weekes and Savedra, 1988). When school-age children were asked what would help most if they were in pain, 99.2% of them answered having their parents present, even though most realized that the parent could do nothing but be there (Ross and Ross, 1984).

additional preparation, this is done in an area away from the child. Teaching sessions are planned at times most conducive to the child's learning (e.g., after a rest period) and usual span of attention.

Special equipment is not necessary for preparing a child, but for young children who cannot yet think in concepts, using objects to supplement verbal explanation is important. Allowing children to handle actual items that will be used in their care, such as a stethoscope, sphygmomanometer, or oxygen mask, helps them to develop familiarity with these items and to reduce the threat often associated with their use. Miniature versions of hospital items such as gurneys and x-ray and intravenous equipment can be used to explain what the children can expect and permit them to safely experience situations that are unfamiliar and potentially frightening. Written and illustrated materials are also valuable aids to preparation.*

Physical Preparation

For most procedures no special physical preparation is needed. However, some do require physical preparation, such as cleansing and shaving of the skin before surgery.

*Sources of preparatory materials are the *You're Gonna Do What?* series of diagnosis and treatment procedures, available from Arkansas Children's Hospital, Attn: Barbara Widell, 800 Marshall St., Little Rock, AR 72202, (501) 320-1199; *Talks About the Hospital Series* by Fred Rogers, available from Family Communications, Inc., 4802 Fifth Ave., Pittsburgh, PA 15213, (412) 687-2990; and *Child Care Series—Patient Education for Children,* available from the Centering Corp., P.O. Box 3367, Omaha, NE 68103-0367, (402) 553-1200.

Box 27-4 GUIDELINES FOR SELECTING NONTHREATENING WORDS OR PHRASES

Words/Phrases to Avoid	Suggested Substitutions
Shot, bee sting, stick	Medicine under the skin
Organ	Special place in body
Test	See how [specify body part] is working
Incision	Special opening
Edema	Puffiness
Stretcher, gurney	Rolling bed
Stool	Child's usual term
Dye	Special medicine
Pain	Hurt, discomfort, "owie," "boo-boo"
Deaden	Numb, make sleepy
Cut, fix	Make better
Take (as in "take your temperature")	See how warm you are
Put to sleep, anesthesia	Special sleep
Catheter	Tube
Monitor	TV screen
Electrodes	Stickers, ticklers
Specimen	Sample

One area of special concern is the administration of appropriate sedation and/or analgesia before stressful procedures. The drug is given before the procedure to allow time for the medication to reach its peak effect. Whenever possible, the intravenous (through an existing infusion), oral, transdermal, or rectal route is used rather than the intramuscular route because children dislike injections. Some institutions are using short-acting anesthetics (e.g., ketamine), general anesthetics, or potent analgesics (e.g., fentanyl) to eliminate the pain and trauma associated with treatments, such as bone marrow tests, lumbar punctures, burn debridement, and suturing (Billmire, Neale, and Gregory, 1985; Forlini, Morin, and Treacy, 1987; Maunuksela, Rajantie, and Simes, 1986; Perin and Frase, 1985). (See also Pain Management, Chapter 26.)

Performance of Procedure

Supportive care continues during the procedure and can be a major factor in a child's ability to cooperate and achieve mastery. Ideally the same nurse who explains the procedure should perform it or assist. Before beginning, all equipment is assembled and the room is readied to prevent unnecessary delays and interruptions that only serve to increase the child's anxiety. If at all possible, procedures are performed in a special treatment room rather than the child's hospital room. Traumatic procedures should never be performed in "safe" areas, such as the playroom. If the procedure is lengthy, conversation that could be misinterpreted by the child is avoided. As the procedure is nearing completion, the nurse should inform the child that it is almost over.

Expect success. Nurses who approach children with confidence and who convey the impression that they expect to be successful are less likely to encounter difficulty. It is best to approach a child as though cooperation is expected. Children sense anxiety in an adult and will respond to a perceived threat by striking out or actively resisting. Although it is not possible to eliminate such behavior in every child, a firm approach with a positive attitude from the nurse tends to convey a feeling of security to most children.

Involve the child. As in any other aspect of care, involving children helps to gain their cooperation. Permitting them to make choices gives them some measure of control. However, a choice is given only in situations in which one is available. To ask children, "Do you want to take your medicine now?" or "I'm going to give you a shot now, okay?" leads them to believe that there is an option and provides them with the opportunity to legitimately refuse or delay the medication. This places the nurse in an awkward, if not impossible, position. It is much better to state firmly, "It's time to drink your medicine now." Children usually like to make choices, but the choice must be one that they do indeed have, for example, "It's time for your medicine. Do you want to drink it plain or with a little juice?"

Many children respond to tactics that appeal to their maturity or courage. This also gives them a sense of participation and achievement. For example, preschool children will be proud that they can hold the dressing during the procedure or remove the tape. The same is true for the school-age child who often cooperates with minimum resistance.

Provide distraction. A child who is occupied with an interesting activity is less likely to focus on the procedure. For example, when an injection is given, it is helpful to give the child something to do or something on which to focus attention. For example, asking the child to point the toes inward and wiggle them not only helps relax the gluteal muscles but provides a diversion. Other strategies for diverting attention are to have the child tightly squeeze the hands of a parent or an assistant, count aloud, sing a familiar song such as a nursery rhyme, or verbally express discomfort (see Nursing Tip). (For other interventions that may lessen discomfort, see Nonpharmacologic Pain Management, Chapter 26.)

Allow expression of feelings. The child should be allowed to express feelings of anger, anxiety, fear, frustration, or any other emotion. It is natural for children to strike out in frustration or to try to avoid stress-provoking situations. The child needs to know that it is all right to cry. Whatever the response, the nurse must accept the behavior for what it is. Telling a child with limited verbal skills, such as a toddler, to stop kicking, biting, or otherwise expressing frustration conveys to the child that he or she is not being understood. Behavior is children's primary means of communication and coping and should be permitted unless it inflicts harm on them or those caring for them.

NURSING TIP: COPING

Help the child to select and practice a coping technique before the procedure.

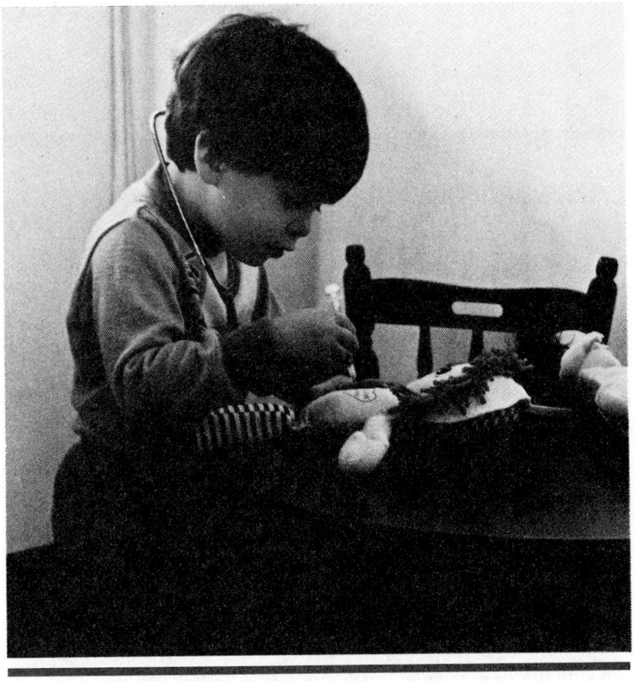

Fig. 27-2. Needle play provides child an opportunity to play out fears and concerns.

Postprocedural Support

After the procedure the child continues to need reassurance that he or she performed well and is accepted and loved. If the parents did not participate, the child is united with them as soon as possible so that they can provide comfort.

Encourage expression of feelings. Planned activity after the procedure is helpful in encouraging constructive expression of feelings. For verbal children reviewing the details of the procedure can clarify misconceptions and provide feedback for improving the nurse's preparatory strategies. Play is an excellent activity for all children. Infants and young children are given the opportunity for gross motor movement. Even older children are able to vent their anger and frustration in acceptable pounding or throwing activities. Play-Doh is a remarkably versatile medium for pounding and shaping. Dramatic play provides an outlet for anger and places the child in a position of control, in contrast to the position of helplessness in the real situation. One of the most effective interventions is therapeutic play, which includes well-supervised activities such as permitting the child to give a "shot" to a doll or stuffed toy to reduce the stress of injections (Fig. 27-2). (See next section and also Use of Play to Minimize Stress, Chapter 26.)

Praise the child. Children need to hear from adults that the youngsters did the best they could in the situation—no matter how they behaved. It is important for children to know that their worth is not being judged on the basis of behavior in a stressful situation. Reward systems, such as earning stars or tokens or saving the empty medicine cup as evidence of achievement, are often helpful. Children who require distasteful medications or injections over time can look with pride on a series of stars or stickers on a calendar, especially if an accumulated number represents a special privilege or reward.

Returning to the child a short while after the procedure helps the nurse to strengthen a supportive relationship. Relating with the child in a relaxed and nonstressful period allows him or her to see the nurse not only as someone associated with stressful situations but as someone with whom to share pleasurable experiences as well.

Use of Play in Procedures

The use of play is an integral part of relationships with children. As such, its value in specific situations is discussed throughout this book, such as in Chapter 26 in relation to hospitalization. Many institutions have very elaborate and well-organized play areas and programs under the direction of child life specialists; other institutions have limited facilities. However, no matter what the institution provides for children, nurses can still include play activities as part of nursing care. Play can be used to teach, for expression of feelings, or as a method to achieve a therapeutic goal. Consequently, it should be included in preparing children for and encouraging their cooperation during procedures. Play sessions after procedures can be structured, such as directed toward needle play, or general, with a wide variety of equipment available for children to play with. Even "routine" procedures such as temperature taking and oral administration of medication may be of concern to children (Ellerton, Caty, and Ritchie, 1985). Suggestions for incorporating play into nursing procedures and activities for the hospitalized child that facilitate learning and adjustment to a new situation are described in Box 27-5.

Surgical Procedures

Some of the most traumatic procedures for children involve surgery. Both the psychologic and physical aspects of care are significant in the child's adjustment and recovery. Although procedures related to type of surgery differ, the following is an overview of general nursing interventions.

Preoperative care. Children experiencing surgical procedures require both psychologic and physical preparation. In general, psychologic preparation is similar to that discussed earlier for any procedure and employs many of the same techniques used in preparing a child for hospitalization, such as films, books, play, and tours (see Chapter 26). However, some important differences exist. Even though children are asleep for the actual surgical intervention, they are subjected to numerous preoperative and postoperative procedures, which require a series of preparatory sessions to prevent overstressing the child with too much information. Six stress points before and after surgery have been identified as being significant in terms of causing anxiety (Visintainer and Wolfer, 1975):

1. Admission
2. The blood test
3. The afternoon of the day before surgery
4. Injection of preoperative medication
5. Before and during transport to the operating room
6. Return from the postanesthesia care unit (PACU)

Box 27-5 PLAY ACTIVITIES FOR SPECIFIC PROCEDURES

Fluid Intake

Make freezer pops using child's favorite juice.
Cut Jell-O into fun shapes.
Makes game of taking sip when turning page of book or in games such as "Simon Says."
Use small medicine cups; decorate the cups.
Color water with food coloring or Kool-Aid.
Have tea party; pour at small table.
Let child fill a syringe and squirt it into mouth or use it to fill small decorated cups.
Cut straws in half and place in small container (much easier for child to suck liquid).
Decorate straw: cut out small design with two holes and pass straw through; place small sticker on straw.
Use a "crazy" straw.
Make a "progress poster"; give rewards for drinking a predetermined quantity.

Deep Breathing

Blow bubbles with bubble blower.
Blow bubbles with straw (no soap).
Blow on pinwheel, feathers, whistle, harmonica, balloons, toy horns.
Practice band instruments.
Draw face on rubber glove to expand when blown up.
Have blowing contest using balloons, boats, cotton balls, feathers, marbles, Ping-Pong balls, pieces of paper; blow such objects on a tabletop over a goal line, over water, through an obstacle course, up in the air, against an opponent, or up and down a string.
Suck paper or cloth from one container to another using a straw.
Use blow bottles with colored water to transfer water from one side to the other.
Dramatize stories, such as "I'll huff and puff and blow your house down" from the Three Little Pigs.
Do straw-blowing painting.
Take a deep breath and "blow out the candles" on a birthday cake.
Use a little paint brush to "paint" nails with water and blow nails dry.

Range of Motion and Use of Extremities

Throw bean bags at fixed or movable target, wadded paper into wastebasket.
Touch or kick Mylar balloons held or hung in different positions (if child is in traction, hang balloon from trapeze).
Play "tickle toes"; wiggle them on request.
Play Twister game or "Simon Says."
Play pretend and guess games (e.g., imitate a bird, butterfly, horse).
Have tricycle or wheelchair races in safe area.
Play kick or throw ball with soft foam ball in safe area.
Position bed so that child must turn to view television or doorway.
Climb wall like a "spider."
Pretend to teach "aerobic" dancing or exercises; encourage parents to participate.
Encourage swimming, if feasible.
Play video games or pinball (fine motor movement).
Play "hide and seek" game: hide toy somewhere in bed (or room, if ambulatory) and have child find it using specified hand or foot.
Provide clay to mold with fingers.
Paint or draw on large sheets of paper placed on floor or wall.
Encourage combing own hair; play "beauty shop" with "customer" in different positions.

Soaks

Play with small toys or objects (cups, syringes, soap dishes) in water.
Wash dolls or toys.
Bubbles may be added to bath water if permissible; move bubbles to create shapes or "monsters."
Pick up marbles, pennies* from bottom of bath container.
Make designs with coins on bottom of container.
Pretend a boat is a submarine by keeping it immersed.
Have Instant Products† (a capsule filled with a design that when immersed in warm water dissolves and foam rubber animals or other surprises appear) for child over age 3 years.
Read to child during soaks, sing with child, or play game, such as cards, checkers, or other board game (if both hands are immersed, move the board pieces for the child).
Sitz bath: give child something to listen to (music, stories) or look at (Viewmaster, book).
Punch holes in bottom of plastic cup, fill with water, and let it "rain" on child.

Injections

Let child handle syringe, vial, alcohol swab and give an injection to doll or stuffed animal.
Use syringes to decorate cookies with frosting, squirt paint, or target shoot into a container.
Draw a "magic circle" on area before injection; draw smiling face in circle after injection.
Allow child to have a "collection" of syringes (without needles); make "wild" creative objects with syringes.
If multiple injections or venipunctures, make a "progress poster"; give rewards for predetermined number of injections.

Ambulation

Give child something to push.
- Toddler: push-pull toy
- School-age child: wagon or decorated IV stand
- Adolescent: a baby in a stroller or wheelchair

Have a parade; make hats, drums, etc.

Extending Environment (Patients in Traction, etc.)

Make bed into a pirate ship or airplane with decorations.
Put up mirrors so patient can see around room.
Move patient's bed frequently, especially to playroom, hallway, or outside.

*Small objects such as marbles or coins are unsafe for young children.
†Instant Products, Inc., P.O. Box 33068, Louisville, KY 40232.

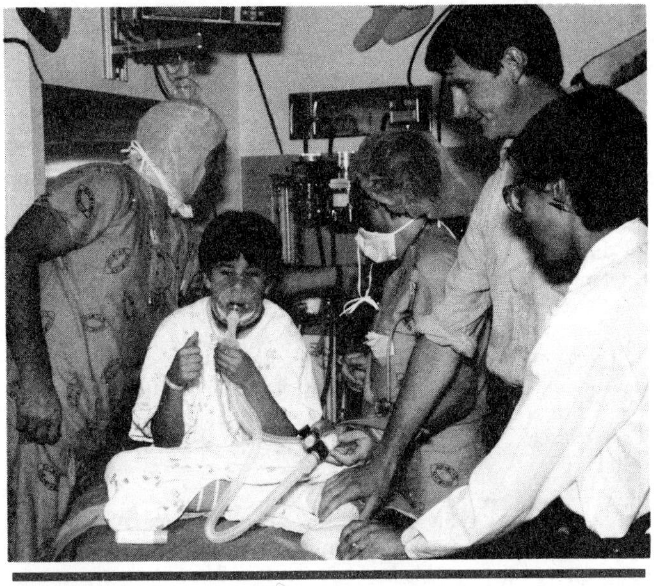

Fig. 27-3. Parental presence during induction of anesthesia can minimize the child's and parents' anxiety during the preoperative period.

Psychologic intervention consisting of systematic preparation, rehearsal of the forthcoming events, and supportive care at each of these points has been shown to be more effective than a single session preparation (which is a common method of preoperative preparation) or consistent supportive care without systematic preparation and rehearsal. Play is always an effective strategy in preparing children, and increased familiarity with medical procedures decreases anxiety (Siaw, Stephens, and Holmes, 1986).

Surprisingly little research has been conducted on children's perception of the surgical experience and their fears of the event. Although fear of anesthesia is thought to be a major concern among children, little evidence for this exists. One study of school-age children reported few remembered events and even fewer fears. Those events recalled more often were the ride to and arriving in the operating room, the preoperative or induction injection, waking up in pain, and not being allowed to eat or drink. The most feared events were the injection and the mask on the face. Although parents were not allowed to be with the children, more than 80% of the children wanted them during induction of anesthesia and in the PACU (Hanna and Sherlock, 1983).

Parental presence during induction is becoming a more common practice, although few institutions endorse the policy (Fig. 27-3). Reports from parents who attend the induction are very favorable. Even though some may become anxious, most parents can control their anxiety, do not disrupt the induction, and support the child (Gauderer, Lorig, and Eastwood, 1989; Hanallah and Rosales, 1983; Schofield and White, 1989).

There is some concern regarding the appropriateness of this practice for all parents. A few parents are visibly upset by the rapid succession of induction events, observing their child becoming limp, and leaving the child in the care of strangers (Vessey, Caserza, and Bogetz, 1990). Parents who are very anxious before surgery tend to become even more anxious after the induction, while the reverse is true of parents with little anxiety (Johnston and others, 1988).

However, based on the parents' favorable response to the practice and most children's desire to have parents with them during any stressful procedure (see Questions and Controversies, p. 1191), a policy of offering parents the option of attending the induction, combined with a program that prepares them for what to expect and what is expected of them, seems justified. When parents choose not to or are not allowed to attend this induction, leaving a favorite possession with the child and uniting the child and parents as soon as possible after surgery (preferably in the PACU) are important interventions. During surgery the family should have a designated place to wait and needs to be kept informed of the child's progress. They also should know where and when they can visit the child after surgery.

Aside from possibly being separated from the parents before and after surgery, children also may be cared for by a number of unfamiliar practitioners. Although the same supportive nurse should remain with the child through as many of the procedures as possible, the child may have other nurses, especially if the patient returns to a special care unit postoperatively. However, joint planning of care between the various nursing staffs, such as in pediatrics and the PACU, can overcome some of the disadvantages of unfamiliar nurses caring for the child. Many hospitals have surgical tours for children and parents to familiarize them with the strange environment and to introduce them to other individuals who will be involved in their care.

Besides psychologic preparation, children usually require various types of physical care before surgery, such as those listed in the Nursing Care Plan on pp. 1196-1199. Infants require special attention to fluid needs. They should not be without oral fluids for an extended period preoperatively to avoid glycogen depletion and dehydration. Current recommendations for food or fluids prior to anesthesia induction are (1) no milk or solids after midnight before scheduled procedures and (2) the following guidelines for clear liquids: birth to 3 years of age, up to 4 hours before the procedure; 3 to 6 years, up to 6 hours before the procedure; and 7 years or older, up to 8 hours before the procedure (American Academy of Pediatrics, Committee on Drugs, 1985). New research, however, indicates that clear liquids up to 2 hours before surgery for children at any age do not pose additional risk for pulmonary aspiration in those undergoing elective surgery (Schreiner and others, 1990).

Although most preoperative care procedures are routine, nurses should keep in mind that they can be anxiety provoking for children and parents. For example, for young children, having to wear a loose-fitting hospital gown without the security of underpants or pajama bottoms can be traumatic.

The most upsetting event for children is generally the preoperative injection. Unfortunately, little research has been done on the value of this practice, but evidence in adults suggests that the injection does little to relieve anxi-

NURSING CARE PLAN
The Child Undergoing Surgery

Preoperative care

NURSING DIAGNOSIS: Potential for injury related to surgical procedure, anesthesia

GOAL 1

Ensure legal authorization

INTERVENTIONS

Check chart for signed informed consent form or obtain informed consent
- Contact physician to determine if parents have been informed of procedure (informed consent is physician's responsibility)

Obtain and/or witness signature if not obtained earlier

EXPECTED OUTCOME

*Appropriate permissions are obtained

GOAL 2

Provide hygienic preparation

INTERVENTIONS

Bathe child, groom hair
Provide mouth care
Check for loose teeth
- Inform anesthesiologist if detected

Cleanse operative site according to prescribed method, if ordered

EXPECTED OUTCOME

Child is cleansed and prepared appropriately (specify)

GOAL 3

Provide physical preparation

INTERVENTIONS

Carry out special procedures as prescribed (e.g., colonic enemas)
Administer antibiotics as ordered, observing for known side effects
Order and/or assist with special tests such as radiographs
Consult with physician for appropriate change in schedule or route of administration of any medication child ordinarily receives
Attire child appropriately (e.g., special operating room gown)
- Allow child to wear underwear or pajama bottoms, if possible
- Label personal articles and clothing

Remove any makeup and/or nail polish (to observe for cyanosis)
Remove jewelry and/or prosthetic devices (e.g., mouth retainers)

EXPECTED OUTCOME

Child is prepared appropriately (specify)

*Nursing outcome

GOAL 4

Prevent complications

INTERVENTIONS

Maintain child NPO (nothing by mouth) as ordered
Be sure child is well hydrated before NPO begins, especially infants
Take and record vital signs
- Report any deviations from admission readings, especially elevated temperature, which may indicate infection

Have child void before preoperative medication is administered to prevent bladder distention or incontinence during anesthesia
- Record time of last voiding if unable to void

Be certain allergies are clearly indicated on chart
Check laboratory values for any sign of systemic abnormality, such as infection (increased white blood cells), anemia (decreased hemoglobin and/or hematocrit), or bleeding tendencies (reduced platelets or prolonged bleeding or clotting time)

EXPECTED OUTCOMES

Child is NPO for designated time preoperatively
Child voids
*Pertinent information about child is visible

GOAL 5

Ensure safety

INTERVENTIONS

Ascertain that identification band is securely fastened
Check identification band with surgical personnel
Fasten siderails of bed or crib
Use restraints during transport by use of stretcher (or other conveyance)
Do not leave child unattended

EXPECTED OUTCOME

Child is safe from immediate harm

GOAL 6

Prepare to receive child on return from surgery

INTERVENTIONS

Collect needed equipment for assessment and recording (e.g., record sheets, IV pump, restraints, thermometer, blood pressure apparatus)
Turn down covers or prepare surgical bed as appropriate

EXPECTED OUTCOME

*Room is prepared for child's return from surgery

NURSING DIAGNOSIS: Anxiety/fear related to separation from support system, unfamiliar environment, knowledge deficit

GOAL 1
Increase child's sense of security

INTERVENTIONS
Institute preoperative teaching
Orient child to strange surroundings
Explain where parents will be while child is in operating room

EXPECTED OUTCOME
Child demonstrates minimum insecurity or anxiety

GOAL 2
Prepare child and family for expected surgical procedure and postoperative care

INTERVENTIONS
Prepare for postoperative procedures, as indicated (e.g., nasogastric tube, IV fluids, nothing by mouth, dressing changes, wound drains if necessary)
Explain reason for surgery; if special operative procedure is to be performed, explain basic principles and briefly outline care needed
Explain all preoperative procedures (e.g., blood work, any other laboratory test)
In emergency situation, explain most essential components of surgery (e.g., where child will be before and after surgery, anesthesia, dressing)
Accept behavioral reactions of parents and child

EXPECTED OUTCOMES
Child and family demonstrate an understanding of forthcoming events (specify methods of learning and evaluation)
*Family's behavioral reactions are accepted and supported

GOAL 3
Achieve optimum relaxation and sedation before child arrives in operating room

INTERVENTIONS
Administer preoperative sedation (preferably oral), if ordered
Place unfamiliar equipment out of child's view
Place child in quiet room with minimum distraction
Do not leave child unattended
Explain what is happening, unless child is asleep
Encourage parents to stay with child as long as permitted
Permit parent to hold child until child falls asleep, if desired
Encourage parents to accompany child as far as possible, preferably through induction of anesthesia
Allow significant objects to accompany child (e.g., a favorite toy)

EXPECTED OUTCOMES
Child falls asleep or lies quietly
Child is not left alone

*Nursing outcome.

NURSING DIAGNOSIS: Altered family processes related to a surgical procedure

GOAL 1
Support and reassure family

INTERVENTIONS
Reinforce and clarify information given by practitioner
Explain associated diagnostic tests and procedures (e.g., x-ray examinations)
Explain child's schedule
- When child will receive premedication
- Time child will leave for surgery
- Where parents can wait for child to return
- Room to which child will return
- Postprocedural care and routines

Explore family's feelings regarding the procedure and its implications
Include parents in preparation of child
Be available to family
See also Nursing Care Plan: The Family of the Ill or Hospitalized Child, Chapter 26

EXPECTED OUTCOMES
Family demonstrates an understanding of procedure (specify demonstration) and related information (specify)
Family complies with directives (specify)

Postoperative care

NURSING DIAGNOSIS: Potential for injury related to surgical procedure, anesthesia

GOAL 1
Receive child on return from surgery

INTERVENTIONS
Place child in bed (unless transported in own bed or crib) using techniques appropriate to type of surgery
Hang IV apparatus, and connect any needed equipment (e.g., suction apparatus, traction)
Place in position of comfort and safety in accordance with surgeon's orders
Perform stat (immediate) activities

EXPECTED OUTCOME
Child is transferred to bed without injury and with minimum stress

GOAL 2
Promote wound healing and prevent wound infection

Continued.

NURSING CARE PLAN
The Child Undergoing Surgery—cont'd

INTERVENTIONS

Use proper handwashing techniques, especially if wound drainage is present
Employ careful wound care
- Keep wound clean and dry
- Change dressings if indicated, whenever soiled; carefully dispose of soiled dressings
- Carry out special wound care as prescribed: irrigation, drain care, etc.
- Cleanse with prescribed preparation (if ordered)
- Apply antibacterial solutions and/or ointments as ordered
- Report any unusual appearance or drainage

Place diapers below abdominal dressing to prevent contamination, if appropriate
When child begins oral feedings, provide nutritious diet as ordered

EXPECTED OUTCOME

Child exhibits no evidence of wound infection

GOAL 3

Prevent other complications

INTERVENTIONS

Ambulate as prescribed
Maintain child NPO until fully awake
Encourage to void when awake
- Offer bedpan
- Boys may be allowed to stand at bedside

Notify practitioner if unable to void
Maintain abdominal decompression, chest tubes, or other equipment, if prescribed
Provide diet as prescribed; advance as appropriate

EXPECTED OUTCOME

Child exhibits no evidence of complications

NURSING DIAGNOSIS: Anxiety/fear related to surgery, unfamiliar environment, separation from support systems, discomfort

GOAL 1

Relieve anxiety

INTERVENTIONS

Maintain calm, reassuring manner
Encourage expression of feelings
Explain procedures and other activities before initiating
Answer questions and explain purposes of activities
Keep informed of progress
Remain with child as much as possible
Give encouragement and positive feedback for cooperation in care
Encourage parental presence as soon as permitted
If emergency procedure, review child's memory of previous events

EXPECTED OUTCOMES

Child rests quietly and calmly
Child discusses procedures and activities without evidence of anxiety

NURSING DIAGNOSIS: Pain related to surgical incision

GOAL 1

Relieve pain

INTERVENTIONS

See Pain Assessment; Pain Management, Chapter 26
Do not wait until child experiences severe pain to intervene
Avoid palpating the operative area unless necessary
Insert rectal tube, if indicated
Encourage to void, if appropriate
Administer mouth care
Lubricate nostril to decrease irritation from nasogastric tube, if present
Allow the child position of comfort if not contraindicated
Perform nursing activities and procedures (e.g., dressing change, deep breathing) after analgesia
*Administer analgesics prescribed
*Administer antiemetics as ordered
Monitor effectiveness of analgesics

EXPECTED OUTCOME

Child rests quietly and exhibits minimum or no evidence of pain (specify)

NURSING DIAGNOSIS: Potential fluid volume deficit related to NPO before and/or after surgery, loss of appetite, vomiting

GOAL 1

Promote adequate hydration

INTERVENTIONS

Monitor IV infusion at prescribed rate
- Attach pediatric IV apparatus if not done in operating room

Offer fluids as soon as ordered or child tolerates
- Start with small sips of water and advance as tolerated

Encourage to drink
- Tempt with favorite fluids, ice chips, or popsicles

EXPECTED OUTCOMES

Child exhibits no evidence of dehydration
Child takes and retains fluid when allowed (specify)

*Dependent nursing action.

NURSING CARE PLAN
The Child Undergoing Surgery—cont'd

NURSING DIAGNOSIS: Potential for infection related to weakened condition, presence of infective organisms

GOAL 1
Prevent respiratory complications

INTERVENTIONS

Assess need for pain medication before respiratory hygiene
Assist to turn, deep breathe
- Splint operative site with hand or pillow if possible before coughing (if coughing prescribed)
- Stimulate infant to cry

Assist with use of incentive spirometer or blow bottle
Perform percussion and vibration, if indicated
Suction secretions if needed

EXPECTED OUTCOME

Lungs remain clear

NURSING DIAGNOSIS: Altered family processes related to situational crisis (emergency hospitalization of child), knowledge deficit

GOAL 1
Support and reassure child and family

INTERVENTIONS

Explain all procedures
Prepare child and family for surgery
Keep family informed of child's progress
Encourage expression of feelings
Review child's memory of events if an emergency procedure
Refer to public health nurse if indicated
Refer to appropriate agency or persons for specific help (e.g., social service, clergy)
See also Nursing Care Plan: The Child in the Hospital, Chapter 26
See also Nursing Care Plan: The Family of the Ill or Hospitalized Child, Chapter 26

EXPECTED OUTCOMES

Family discusses child's condition and therapies comfortably
Family demonstrates an awareness of child's progress (specify method of evaluation)
Family members avail themselves of appropriate assistance

GOAL 2
Instruct family regarding needed knowledge for home care

INTERVENTIONS

If dressing changes are required at home, teach parents sterile or aseptic procedures; provide written list of necessary equipment and instructions
Instruct parents regarding administration of medications (if ordered), including possible side effects and untoward reactions
Instruct parents in care and management of special procedures (e.g., ostomy care, irrigations)

EXPECTED OUTCOME

Family demonstrates an understanding of instructions (specify methods of learning and evaluation)

ety (Catchpole, 1984). If children have no preoperative pain, are well prepared psychologically for surgery, and have their parents nearby, preanesthetic medication may be unnecessary. When drugs are used, they should be "atraumatic" by using oral, existing intravenous, or rectal routes. Several drug options exist, such as morphine, midazolam, diazepam, methohexital (Brevital), and fentanyl. Fentanyl "lollipops," currently under investigation, have been found to be an effective preoperative medication (Feld and others, 1989; Nelson and others, 1989).

Research on children who received no premedication, an oral sedative, or an opioid and an anticholinergic drug and whose parents accompanied them during induction found no difference in the ease of induction. The group receiving the opioid had better postoperative pain control but more nausea and vomiting (Schofield and White, 1989).

Numerous preanesthetic drug regimens are used with children, and there is no consensus on the optimum method. Drugs used should achieve three goals: (1) decrease anxiety and facilitate induction of anesthesia, (2) provide amnesia of the perioperative period, and (3) relieve preoperative and postoperative pain. At least one popular drug combination—meperidine (pethidine [Demerol]), promethazine (Phenergan), and chlorpromazine (Thorazine), known as DPT or lytic cocktail—falls short of these goals.

Meperidine, a short-acting analgesic, provides pain relief for only 2 to 3 hours, can cause orthostatic hypotension and respiratory depression, and is irritating to the tissues. Promethazine has antianalgesic properties, produces excessive sedation, and can cause extrapyramidal reactions (spasms of neck, face, tongue, and back; fixed eyeballs). All these drugs lower the seizure threshold, a particular risk to those with a convulsive disorder. In addition, the "cocktail" is usually administered intramuscularly, causing additional pain (Howland and Goldfrank, 1986; Ros, 1987; Snodgrass and Dodge, 1989).

Children may also be fearful of the induction of anesthesia by mask. Practices that can minimize anxiety related to inhalation anesthesia are (1) disguising the unpleasant odor of anesthetic gases by applying a pleasant-smelling substance on the mask; (2) using a transparent plastic mask rather than an opaque black mask and gradually bringing it toward the face; (3) directing a stream of gas toward the child's face from the bare tube until the child becomes drowsy, then using the mask; and (4) allowing the child to sit up rather than lie down for anesthesia induction (Jones, 1985).

Postoperative care. After surgical procedures, various physical interventions and observations are required to prevent or minimize possible untoward effects (see Nursing Care Plan, pp. 1196-1199). Although most of these interventions are prescribed by physicians, it is the nurse's responsibility to exercise judgment in their implementation. For example, vital signs are taken as frequently as necessary until they are stable. Simply recording temperature, pulse, respiration, and blood pressure without comparing the present readings with previous ones is a useless technical

Table 27-1 Potential causes of postoperative vital sign alterations in children

ALTERATION	POTENTIAL CAUSE	COMMENTS
▪ Heart rate		
Increase	Decreased perfusion (shock) Elevated temperature Pain Respiratory distress (early) Medications (atropine, morphine, epinephrine)	Heart rate may increase to maintain cardiac output
Decrease	Hypoxia Vagal stimulation Increased intracranial pressure Respiratory distress (late) Medications (prostigmine)	Bradycardia is of more concern in the young child than tachycardia
▪ Respiratory rate		
Increase	Respiratory distress Fluid volume excess Hypothermia Elevated temperature Pain	Body responds to respiratory distress primarily by increasing rate
Decrease	Anesthetics, opioids Pain	Decreased respiratory rate from opioids may be compensated by increased depth of respiration
▪ Blood pressure		
Increase	Excess intravascular volume Increased intracranial pressure Carbon dioxide retention Pain Medications (ketamine, epinephrine)	Serious in premature infants because it increases risk of intraventricular hemorrhage
Decrease	Vasodilating anesthetic agents (halothane, isoflurane, enflurane) Opioids (morphine) Shock (late sign)	Decreased blood pressure is late sign of shock due to elasticity and constriction of vessels to maintain cardiac output
▪ Temperature		
Increase	Infection Environmental causes (warm room, excess coverings) Malignant hyperthermia	Fever associated with infection usually occurs later than fever of noninfectious origin Absence of fever does not rule out infection, especially in infants Malignant hyperthermia requires immediate treatment
Decrease	Vasodilating anesthetic agents (halothane, isoflurane, enflurane) Muscle relaxants Environmental causes (cool room) Infusion of cool fluids/blood	Neonates are especially susceptible to hypothermia with serious or fatal consequences

From Smith, D.P., and others, editors: Comprehensive child and family nursing skills, St. Louis, 1991, Mosby–Year Book, Inc.

function. Each vital sign is evaluated in terms of side effects from anesthesia and signs of impending shock or respiratory compromise (Table 27-1).

A change in vital signs that demands immediate attention is elevated temperature due to malignant hyperthermia, a potentially lethal genetic myopathy. In susceptible children certain anesthetic agents trigger the disorder, producing elevated temperature, muscle rigidity, hypermetabolism, and muscle cell destruction. The symptoms may or may not occur during surgery; therefore, alert observation in the PACU and regular care unit is essential. Treatment includes immediate discontinuation of triggering agents, hyperventilation with 100% oxygen, and intravenous dantrolene (Sessler, 1986).

NURSING ALERT When taking the preoperative history, ask the family if any relatives have had anesthetic difficulties suggesting malignant hyperthermia; report findings immediately. Observe for early signs of the disorder:

- Tachycardia
- Rising blood pressure
- Tachypnea
- Mottled skin
- Muscle rigidity

Pain is assessed and the child given analgesics as needed to provide comfort and facilitate cooperation in postoperative procedures, such as ambulating and deep breathing. Routinely scheduled analgesics, rather than PRN (as necessary) orders, afford more satisfactory pain control (see Pain Management, Chapter 26).

During the recovery period, some time should be spent with children to assess their perception of surgery. Play, drawing, and storytelling are excellent methods of discovering their thoughts. With such information the nurse can support or correct their perceptions and assist children in achieving mastery for having endured a stressful procedure.

COMPLIANCE

One of the most significant nursing interventions concerning procedures that must be repeated in the hospital and/or continued at home is related to compliance. Compliance, also termed adherence (Bishop, 1987), refers to the extent to which the patient's behavior in terms of taking medication, following diets, or executing other life-style changes coincides with the prescribed regimen (Blum, 1984). Reviews of compliance rates in children and adolescents with chronic diseases estimate that the rate of noncompliance ranges from 36% to more than 80% (Pidgeon, 1989). Since nurses are frequently responsible for teaching families about treatment protocols, they must have knowledge of factors that influence compliance, methods to measure compliance, and strategies to enhance adherence to prescribed treatment.

Assessment

In developing strategies to improve compliance, the nurse must first assess the patient's level of compliance. Since many children are too young to assume partial or total responsibility for their care, parents are usually the primary caregivers in terms of home management. Consequently the nurse needs to assess their ability to carry out instructions. The first approach to assessment is knowledge of those factors that influence compliance. The second is to apply methods to assess more objectively the child's and parents' levels of compliance.

Box 27-6 FACTORS THAT POSITIVELY INFLUENCE COMPLIANCE

Individual/Family Factors
High self-esteem
Positive body image
High degree of autonomy (increased locus of control)
Supportive and well-adjusted family
Effective family communication
Family expectation for successful completion of therapy

Care Setting Factors
Perceived satisfaction with care
Positive interactions with practitioners
Continuity of care
Individualized care
Minimum waiting time for appointments
Convenient care setting

Treatment Factors
Simple regimen
Minimum disruption in usual life-style
Short duration
Inexpensive
Visible benefits
Tolerable side effects

Factors that influence compliance. Research on compliance has identified several factors that influence compliance (Box 27-6). The first area relates to factors about the patient. Contrary to what might be expected, no typical characteristics of noncompliers exist, and even education is not correlated with compliance (Rosenstock, 1988). Some evidence suggests that higher levels of self-esteem and increased autonomy favorably affect adolescent compliance (Pidgeon, 1989). However, family factors are important, and characteristics associated with good compliance include family support, family reminders, good communication, and expectations for successful completion of therapeutic regimen (Cromer and others, 1989; Meichenbaum, 1989; Pidgeon, 1989).

Factors relating to the care setting are very important in determining compliance and provide useful guidelines in planning strategies to improve compliance. Basically, any aspect of the health care setting that increases the family's satisfaction with the physical setting and the relationship with the practitioner positively influences adherence to the treatment regimen. In addition, the type of care required to manage the disorder is important. The more complex, expensive, inconvenient, longer, and disruptive the treatment protocol, the less likely the family is to comply. During long-term conditions that involve multiple treatments and considerable rearrangement of life-style, compliance is most severely affected.

Measurement of compliance. While it is helpful to know those factors that influence compliance, especially in assessing the likelihood of compliance in a family, assessment must include more direct measurement techniques. A number of methods exist, each with their advantages and disadvantages. The most successful approach includes a combination of at least two of the following methods:

Clinical judgment—the nurse judges family compliance. This is a very poor method that is subject to bias and inaccuracy unless the nurse carefully evaluates the criteria used in evaluation.

Self-reporting—the family is asked about their ability to carry out the prescribed treatments. Although a simple method, most people overestimate their compliance by about 20%, even when they admit to lapses in treatment.

Direct observation—the nurse directly observes the patient or family perform the treatment. Although this approach is very effective in identifying errors related to the correct procedure, it is difficult to employ outside the health care setting. Also, the family's awareness of being observed frequently affects their performance.

Monitoring appointments—the family's attendance at scheduled appointments is recorded. Keeping appointments indicates general levels of compliance but only indirectly indicates compliance with the prescribed care.

Monitoring therapeutic response—the child's response in terms of benefit from treatment is monitored, preferably recorded on a graph or chart. Unfortunately, few treatments yield directly measurable results (e.g., decreased blood pressure, weight loss), making this a less satisfactory method for most types of therapies. Also, adherence does not ensure clinical improvement, and less than 100% may *achieve therapeutic results,* reinforcing partial compliance (Meichenbaum, 1989).

Pill counts—the nurse counts the number of pills remaining in the original container and compares the amount missing with the number of days the medication should have been taken. Although this is a simple method, families may forget to bring the container or deliberately alter the number of pills to avoid detection. This method is also poorly suited to liquid medication, which is so often prescribed in pediatrics. A new technique is the use of pill container caps that record every opening as a presumptive dose (Cramer and others, 1989).

Chemical assay—for certain drugs, such as digoxin and phenytoin, measurement of plasma drug levels provides information on the amount of drug recently ingested. However, this method is expensive, indicates only short-term compliance, and requires precise timing of the assay for accurate results.

Compliance Strategies

Strategies to improve compliance are concerned with those interventions that encourage families to follow the prescribed treatment regimen. Ideally such strategies should be implemented before or concurrent with the initiation of therapy to avoid compliance problems. A number of strategies have been identified as effective, but, as with measurement methods, no one approach is always successful, and the best results occur when at least two strategies are employed. The following is an overview of compliance strategies.

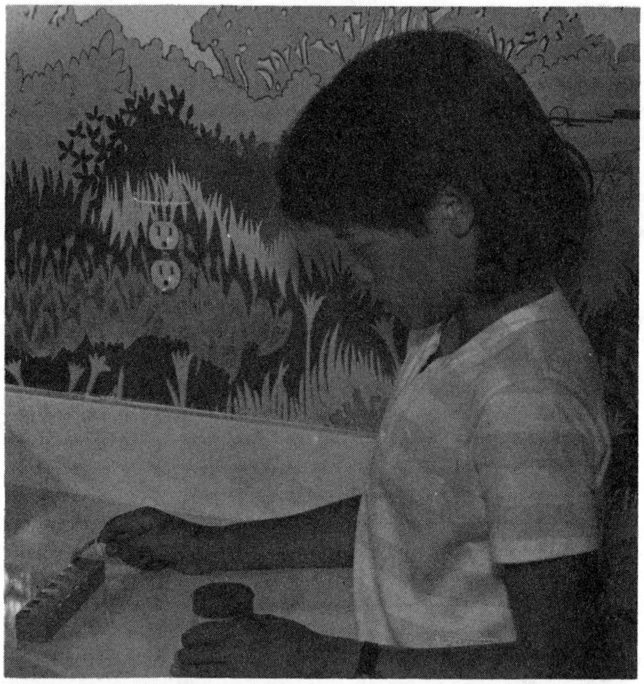

Fig. 27-4. Pill dispensers can help children assume responsibility for their care at home, serve as reminders that medication needs to be taken, and facilitate checking compliance.

Organizational strategies. Organizational strategies refer to those interventions concerned with the care setting and the therapeutic plan. They include manipulating the factors listed in Box 27-6, which are known to positively affect compliance (Young, 1986). Depending on the individual situation, this may involve increasing the frequency of appointments, designating a primary practitioner, reducing the cost of medication by purchasing generic brands, reducing the disruption of the treatment on the family's lifestyle, and the use of "cues" to minimize forgetting. Numerous devices are available commercially or can be improvised for cueing, such as pill dispensers; watches with alarms; charts to record completed therapy; reminders, such as messages on the refrigerator or morning coffeepot; and treatment schedules that incorporate the treatment plan into the daily routine, such as physical therapy after the evening bath (Fig. 27-4).

Educational strategies. Educational strategies are concerned with instructing the family about the treatment plan. Although education is an important component in enhancing compliance and patients who are more knowledgeable about their condition are more likely to comply, education alone does not ensure compliant behavior. Also, for education to be effective, it must incorporate teaching principles known to enhance understanding and retention of material (Box 27-7). Written materials are essential, especially in any regimen requiring multiple or complex treatments, and need to be readable by the average individual, which appears to be at the fourth grade level (50% of health care clients have difficulty or are unable to read at a fifth

Box 27-7 GUIDELINES FOR EFFECTIVE TEACHING OF FAMILY MEMBERS

Establish rapport; reduce anxiety and fear.
Assess what family knows and expects to learn, especially if they have concerns, and address their concerns before beginning teaching.
Assess family's learning style; ask if they prefer having everything explained in detail or knowing only the major facts.
Direct teaching to family decision maker.
Use a variety of teaching materials (lecture, demonstration, video or slide presentation, written material).
Speak family's language, avoid jargon, and clarify all terms.
Be specific when giving information; divide information into small steps.
Keep information short, simple, and concrete.
Introduce most important information first.
Use "verbal" headings to organize information, such as, "There are two things you need to learn: how to give the medicine and what side effects to look for. First, how to give. . . . Second, what side effects. . . ."
Stress importance of instructions and expected benefits; explain detrimental effects of inadequate treatment but avoid fear tactics.
Evaluate teaching by eliciting feedback to ensure that family understands information.
Repeat information as needed.
Reward family for learning through verbal praise.
Use "teachable" moments—times when family is most likely to accept new information (e.g., when symptoms are present).

grade level) (Streiff, 1986). Including the culturally significant decision maker (e.g., maternal grandmother) in teaching sessions will help improve compliance (Faber, 1986).

Behavioral strategies. Behavioral strategies encompass those interventions designed to modify behavior directly. Several strategies are effective in encouraging the desired behavior and are very useful with children. Ideally, positive reinforcement should be employed to strengthen the behavior and may consist of earning stars or tokens, which gains the child a special privilege or gift. A more formal method is the use of contracting (see following discussion). However, at times disciplinary techniques, such as time-out for young children (see p. 619) or withholding privileges for older children, may be needed to reduce noncompliance (Rapoff, 1986).

Contracting. Contracting is a process in which the exact elements of desired behavior are explicitly outlined in the form of a written contract (Steckel, 1982). Based on behavior modification, it is a very effective method of shaping behavior, especially with older children who are involved in the process of defining the rules of the agreement. Ideally it should involve tangible rewards but may include negative consequences, such as demerits or "checks" for failing to comply. In deciding whether to use positive or negative reinforcers, the nurse should question parents about their opinion regarding powerful motivators for the child. Often the contract includes a commitment from the parent, such as agreeing to stop nagging about taking medication.

Box 27-8 COMPONENTS OF A CONTRACT

The goal or desired behavior is realistic and seems possible.
The behavior is measurable (e.g., agreeing to take the drug before leaving for school without reminding).
The contract is written and signed by all those involved in any of the agreements.
The contract is dated, and if appropriate, a date is specified when a goal should be reached (e.g., number of pounds of weight loss in 2 weeks).
The identified rewards or consequences are reinforcing.
The goal can be evaluated (e.g., counting the number of tablets, using a scale for weight measurement).

An effective contract includes components listed in Box 27-8, although more informal arrangements can be used with young children, such as awarding desired behavior with stars, stickers, or other small novelties. Once the contract is implemented, it is evaluated at the end of the time specified in the agreement and revisions are made, such as extending the time or terminating the contract. If the contract has not been successful, every effort is made to ascertain if the goals were realistic, the time period was sufficient for accomplishing the goal, and the rewards or consequences were motivating.

GENERAL HYGIENE AND CARE

Hygienic care is continued throughout the child's hospital stay and is essentially no different from that provided to persons of any age. The primary differences are those related to the patient's size. Grooming aids and attractive attire are important adjuncts to hygienic care. Older children are delighted with anything that makes them feel more attractive.

Certain caregiving activities present special challenges, especially feeding the sick child. In addition, children often have high fevers that require attention. Any of these activities presents excellent opportunities for family health teaching.

BATHING

Unless contraindicated, most infants and children can be bathed in a tub at the bedside, on the bed, or in a standard bathtub located on the unit, which is often conveniently adapted for pediatric use. For infants and young children confined to bed, the towel method can be used. Two towels are immersed in a dilute soap solution and wrung damp. With the child lying supine on a dry towel, one damp towel is placed on top of the child and used to gently clean the body. This towel is discarded, then the child is dried and turned prone. The procedure is repeated using the second damp towel.

Infants and small children are *never* left unattended in a bathtub, and infants who are unable to sit alone are se-

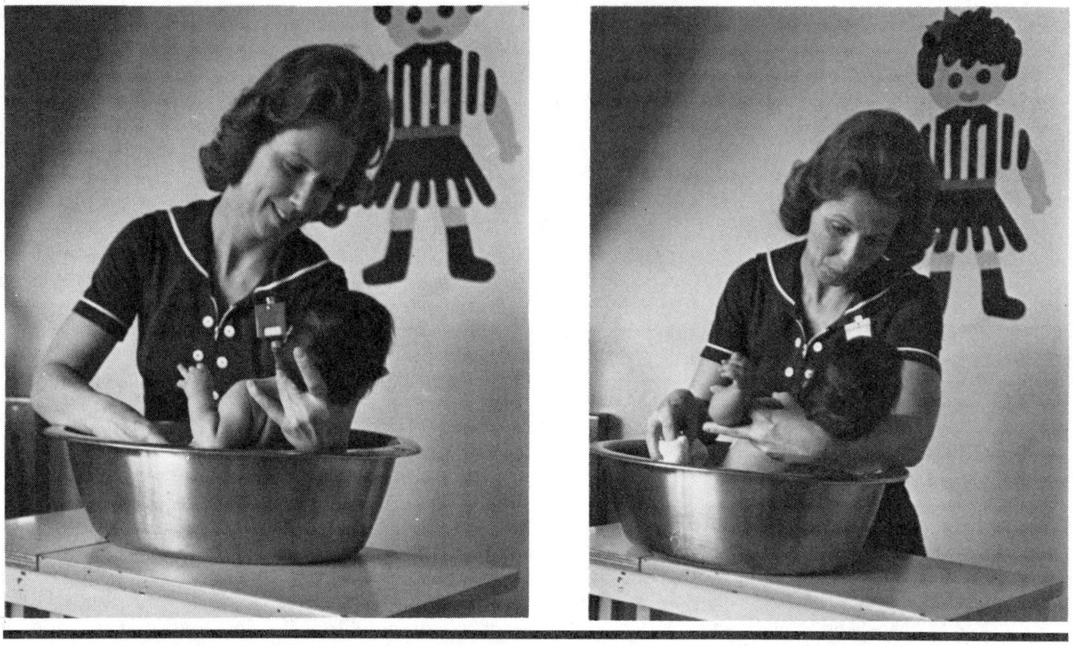

Fig. 27-5. Proper method for holding infant for tub bath. **A,** Supporting neck. **B,** Neck supported on wrist.

curely held with one hand during the bath. The infant's head is supported securely with one hand or the farther arm is firmly grasped in the nurse's hand while the head rests comfortably on the wrist. This provides secure control of the infant while the other hand is free to wash the infant's body (Fig. 27-5). Infants or children who are able to sit without assistance need only close supervision and a pad placed in the bottom of the tub to prevent slipping and loss of balance, which could result in a bumped head or submersion of the face.

Older children may enjoy a shower if it is available. School-age children may be reluctant to bathe, and many are not accustomed to a daily bath. However, most children who feel well require little encouragement to participate in their daily care. Nurses will need to use judgment regarding the amount of supervision the child requires. Some can be trusted to assume this responsibility unaided, whereas others will need someone in constant attendance. Children with cognitive impairments, physical limitations such as severe anemia or leg deformities, or suicidal or psychotic problems (who may commit bodily harm) require close supervision.

Areas that require special attention during bed baths and for children performing their own care are the ears, between skinfolds, the neck, the back, and the genital area. The genital area should be carefully cleansed and dried with particular care to skinfolds, and in uncircumcised boys the foreskin should be gently retracted and the exposed surfaces cleansed and then the foreskin replaced. If the condition of the glans indicates inadequate cleaning, such as accumulated smegma, inflammation, phimosis, or foreskin adhesions, teaching proper hygiene is indicated. In the Vietnamese and Cambodian cultures the foreskin is traditionally not retracted until adulthood (Krueger and Osborn, 1986). Older children have the tendency to avoid the genitalia; therefore they may need a gentle reminder.

Children who are ill or debilitated will need more extensive assistance with bathing and other aspects of hygienic care, but they should be encouraged to perform as much as they are capable without overtaxing their energies. Increasing involvement can be expected with improved strength and endurance. Children with limited capacity for self-help but no other contraindications benefit greatly from tub baths. They can be transported to the tub and, with the aid of lifting devices and/or an appropriate number of persons to assist, gain the advantages of a tub bath.

ORAL HYGIENE

Mouth care is an integral part of daily hygiene and should be continued in the hospital. Infants and debilitated children will require the nurse or a family member to perform mouth care. Although small children can manage a toothbrush and are encouraged to use it, most will need assistance to perform a satisfactory job. Older children, although capable of brushing without assistance, sometimes need to be reminded that this is a part of their hygienic care. Most hospitals have equipment available for those children who do not have toothbrush or toothpaste of their own. (See Dental Health, Chapters 12, 14, 15, 17, and 19; and Chapter 36 for mouth care of children with mucosal ulcers.)

HAIR CARE

Brushing and combing hair are a part of the daily care for all persons in the hospital, including infants and children. If the child does not have a brush or comb, many hospitals provide one as part of the usual admission kit. If not, the parents should be asked to bring hair care equipment for the child's use. Both boys and girls are helped to comb or brush their hair, or it is done for them, at least once daily. The hair is styled for comfort and in a manner pleasing to the child and parents. A satisfactory style for girls with longer hair is French braiding, which is created by starting with three equal portions of hair from the top of the scalp; as the hair is braided, segments of hair are added at successive intervals until all the hair has been incorporated into one or more neat, head-hugging braids. The ends are firmly anchored with a malleable holder or barrette. The hair should not be cut without parental permission, although shaving hair to provide access to a scalp vein for intravenous needle insertion may be necessary.

If children are hospitalized for more than a few days, the hair may need shampooing. With infants, the hair may be washed during the daily bath or less frequently. For most children washing the hair and scalp once or twice weekly is sufficient, unless there is an indication to wash it more frequently, such as following a high fever and profuse sweating. Some hospitals have shampoo basins, but almost any child can be conveniently transported by a gurney to an accessible sink or washbasin for shampooing. Those who are unable to be transported can receive a shampoo in their beds with adequate protection and/or specially adapted equipment or positioning. A convenient method involves positioning the child near the edge of the bed, placing towels under the shoulders, and draping a large plastic garbage bag at the edge of the bed with one open side under the shoulders and the other side opened away from the head so that the hair is inside the opening. Water can be transported in a basin or placed in an empty enema bag (see Nursing Tip).

Teenagers, with their normally increased oily sebaceous secretions, are particularly in need of frequent hair care and usually require more frequent shampoos. Commercial "dry shampoo" products also may prove useful on a short-term basis.

Black children require special hair care, and this need is frequently neglected or inadequately managed. For the black child with kinky hair, most standard combs are inadequate and may cause hair breakage and discomfort to the child. If a special comb with widely spaced teeth is not available on the unit, the parent can be reminded to bring a comb, if possible, for the child's use. It is also much easier to comb the hair after shampooing, when it is wet (Joyner, 1988). This type of hair requires a special hair dressing or pomade, which usually has a coconut oil base. The preparation is rubbed on the hands and then transferred to the hair to make it more pliable and manageable. The child's parents should be consulted regarding the preparation they wish to be used on their child's hair and asked if they can provide some for use during the child's hospitalization. Petroleum jelly should *not* be used. If braiding or plaiting the hair is desired, the hair should be damp and loosely woven. The hair tightens as it dries, which could result in tension folliculitis (Joyner, 1988).

NURSING TIP: SHAMPOOING HAIR IN BED

For a convenient source of water, fill an empty enema bag with warm water and hang the bag from an intravenous pole; use the clamp on the bag's tubing to adjust the flow of water (Bourgault, 1985).

FEEDING THE SICK CHILD

Loss of appetite is a symptom common to most childhood illnesses and is frequently the initial evidence of illness, preceding fever and other overt signs of infection. In most cases children can be permitted to determine their own need for food. Since an acute illness is usually short, the nutritional state is seldom compromised. In fact, urging foods on the sick child may precipitate nausea and vomiting and in some cases even cause an aversion to the feeding situation that can extend into the convalescent period and beyond.

Refusing to eat may also be one way children can exert power and control in an otherwise helpless situation. For young children, loss of appetite may be related to the depression of separation from their parents and their natural tendency toward negativism. Parents' concern with eating can intensify the problem. Forcing a child to eat only meets with rebellion and reinforces the behavior as a control mechanism. Parents are encouraged to relax any pressure during an acute illness. Although it is best to encourage high-quality nutritious foods, the child may desire foods and liquids that contain mostly calories. Some well-tolerated foods include gelatin, diluted clear soups, carbonated drinks, popsicles, dry toast, crackers, and hard candy. Even though these substances are not nutritious, they can provide necessary fluid and calories.

Dehydration is always a hazard when children are febrile or anorexic, especially when this is accompanied by vomiting or diarrhea. An adequate fluid intake is encouraged by offering small amounts of favored fluids at frequent intervals and by providing salty foods if allowed. If diarrhea is present, high-carbohydrate liquids (e.g., carbonated beverages, gelatin, popsicles) are avoided because they may aggravate the diarrhea by an osmotic effect (Ghishan, 1988). Also, replacing abnormal losses with plain water or undiluted broth, which may worsen the electrolyte imbalance, is not advocated. Fluids should not be forced, and the child is not wakened from rest to take fluids. Forcing fluids may create the same difficulties as urging unwanted food. Gentle persuasion with preferred beverages will usually meet with success. Using play techniques can also be very effective (see Box 27-5).

In general, hot dogs, hamburgers, peanut butter and jelly sandwiches, fruit yogurt, milkshakes, spaghetti, tacos, macaroni and cheese, and pizza are favorite foods of most children. Although alone they may not typify well-balanced di-

Box 27-9 GUIDELINES FOR FEEDING THE SICK CHILD

Take a dietary history (see Chapter 6) and use information to make eating time as much like home as possible.
Encourage parents or other family members to feed child or to be present at mealtimes.
Have children eat at tables in groups; bring nonambulatory children to eating area in wheelchairs, beds, strollers, gurneys, or wagons.
Use familiar eating utensils, such as a favorite plate, cup, or bottle for small children.
Make mealtimes pleasant; avoid any procedures immediately before or after eating; make sure child is rested and pain free.
Have a nurse present at mealtimes to offer assistance, prevent disruptions, and praise children for their eating.
Serve small, frequent meals rather than three large meals or serve three meals and nutritious between-meal snacks.
Bring in foods from home, especially if food preparation is very different from hospital's; consider cultural differences.
Provide finger foods for young children.
Involve children in food selection and preparation whenever possible.
Serve small portions, and serve each course separately, such as soup first, followed by meat, potatoes, and vegetables, and ending with dessert; with young children camouflage size of food by cutting meat thicker so less appears on plate or by folding a cheese slice in half; offer second helpings; ensure a variety of foods, textures, and colors.
Provide food selections that are favorites of most children, such as peanut butter and jelly sandwiches, hot dogs, hamburgers, macaroni and cheese, pizza, spaghetti, tacos, fried chicken, corn on the cob, and fruit yogurt.
Avoid foods that are highly seasoned, have strong odors, are served hot, or are all mixed together, unless typical of cultural practices.
Provide fluid selections that are favorites of most children, such as fruit punch, cola, ginger ale, sweetened tea, ice pops, sherbet, ice cream, milk and milkshakes, eggnog, pudding, gelatin, clear broth, or creamed soups. (See also Box 27-5.)
Offer nutritious snacks, such as frozen yogurt or pudding, ice cream, oatmeal or peanut butter cookies, hot cocoa, cheese slices or "kisses," pieces of raw vegetable or fruit, and dried fruit or cereal.
Make food attractive and different, for example:
- Serve a "picnic lunch" in a paper bag.
- Pack food in a Chinese-food container; decorate container.
- Put a "face" or a "flower" on a hamburger or sandwich with pieces of vegetable.
- Use a cookie-cutter to shape a sandwich.
- Serve pudding, yogurt, or juice frozen as a popsicle.
- Make slurpies or snowcones by pouring flavored syrup on crushed ice.
- Add vegetable coloring to water or milk.
- Serve fluids through brightly colored or unusually shaped straws.
- Make "bowtie" sandwiches by cutting them in triangles and placing two points together.
- Slice sandwiches into "fingers."
- Grate mounds of cheese.
- Cut apples horizontally to make circles.
- Put a banana on a hot dog bun and spread with peanut butter.
- Break uncooked spaghetti into toothpick lengths and skewer cheese, cold meat, vegetables, or fruit chunks.

Praise children for what they do eat.
Do *not* punish children for not eating by removing their dessert or putting them to bed.

ets, they can be adjusted to include sufficient amounts from the basic four food groups. It is better to work with preferred food choices than with selections that children rarely eat. Approaches to food preparation that can increase the child's interest in eating are presented in Box 27-9.

An understanding of children's feeding habits can also increase food consumption. For example, if children are given all their food at one time, they will generally eat the dessert first. Likewise, if they are presented with large portions, they often push the food away because the amount overwhelms them. If young children are not supervised during mealtime, they tend to play with the food rather than eat it. Therefore nurses should present food in the usual order, such as soup first, followed by small portions of meat, potatoes, and vegetables, and ending with dessert. The principles of conservation (see Cognitive Development, Chapter 15) can also be used to increase food consumption.

Once the child is feeling better, appetite usually begins to improve. It is best to take advantage of any hungry period by serving high-quality foods and snacks. If the child still refuses to eat, nutritious fluids, such as prepared breakfast drinks, should be encouraged. Parents can be very helpful by bringing in these food items from home. This is especially important if the family's cultural eating habits differ from the hospital's food services.

When children are placed on special diets, such as clear liquids after surgery or during episodes of diarrhea, assessment of their intake and readiness to advance to more complex foods is essential.

NURSING ALERT Evidence of lack of readiness to advance the diet:
- Vomiting or diarrhea
- Decrease in appetite
- Abdominal cramping or distention
- Absence of bowel sounds
- Dehydration or weight loss

Regardless of the type of diet, charting the amount consumed is an important nursing responsibility. Descriptions need to be detailed and accurate, such as "4 ounces of orange juice, one pancake, no bacon, and 8 ounces of milk." Comments such as "ate well" or "ate poorly" are inadequate. Percentage of meal eaten is also inadequate unless food is measured before serving. If parents are involved in the child's care, they are encouraged to keep a list of everything eaten. Using a premeasured cup for fluids ensures a more accurate estimate of intake. A comparison of the intake at each meal can isolate food deficiencies, such as insufficient intake of meat or vegetables. Behaviors associated with mealtime also identify possible factors influencing appetite. For example, the observation, "Child eats well when with other children but plays with food if left alone in room," helps the nurse plan mealtime activities that stimulate the appetite.

CONTROLLING ELEVATED TEMPERATURES

An elevated temperature, most frequently from fever but occasionally caused by hyperthermia, is one of the most common symptoms of illness in children. This manifestation is frequently misunderstood and of great, but often unnecessary, concern to parents. To facilitate an understanding of fever, the following terms are defined (McCarthy, 1985):

Set point—the temperature around which body temperature is regulated by a thermostat-like mechanism in the hypothalamus

Fever—an elevation in set point such that body temperature is regulated at a higher level; may be arbitrarily defined as temperature above 38° C (100° F)

Hyperthermia—a situation in which body temperature exceeds the set point, which usually results from the body or external conditions creating more heat than the body can eliminate, such as in heat stroke, aspirin toxicity, or hyperthyroidism

Body temperature is regulated by a thermostat-like mechanism in the hypothalamus. This mechanism receives input from centrally and peripherally located receptors. When temperature changes occur, these receptors relay the information to the thermostat, which either increases or decreases heat production to maintain a constant set point temperature. However, during an infection, pyrogenic substances cause an increase in the body's normal set point, a process that is mediated by prostaglandins. Consequently the hypothalamus increases heat production until the core temperature reaches the new set point.

Most fevers in children are of viral origin, are of relatively brief duration, and have limited consequences. In addition, there is mounting evidence that fever plays a role in enhancing the development of both specific and nonspecific immunity and aiding recovery and survival from infection (Reeves-Swift, 1990). Contrary to popular belief, neither the rise in temperature nor its response to antipyretics indicates the severity or etiology of infection, which casts doubt on the value of using fever as a diagnostic or prognostic indicator (Baker, Fosarelli, and Carpenter, 1987; Weisse, Miller, and Brien, 1987).

Therapeutic Management

Treatment of elevated temperature depends on whether it is due to a fever or hyperthermia. Because the set point is normal in hyperthermia, but increased in fever, different approaches must be used to lower body temperature successfully. An unusual presentation of elevated temperature is malignant hyperthermia; management of this emergency condition differs from the usual measures for fever or hyperthermia (see p. 1201).

Fever. The principal reason for treating fever is the relief of discomfort; no specific degree of fever requires treatment. Relief measures include pharmacologic and/or environmental intervention. The most effective intervention is the use of antipyretics to lower the set point.

Antipyretic drugs include acetaminophen, aspirin, and nonsteroidal antiinflammatory drugs (NSAIDs). Acetaminophen is the preferred drug; aspirin should not be given to children because of the possible association between aspirin use in children with influenza virus or chickenpox and Reye syndrome. One prescription NSAID, ibuprofen, is approved for fever reduction in children as young as 6 months of age (see Table 26-4). Dosage is based on the initial temperature level: 5 mg/kg of body weight for temperatures less than 39.1° C (102.5° F) or 10 mg/kg for temperatures greater than 39.1° C (102.5° F). The duration of fever reduction is generally 6 to 8 hours and is longer with the higher dose (Watson and others, 1989). Nonprescription ibuprofen (Advil, Nuprin, Motrin IB, Medipren) is not approved for use in children under 12 years of age.

The recommended dosages of acetaminophen are listed in Table 27-2. It should be given every 4 hours, but no more than five times in 24 hours. Since body temperature normally decreases at night, three to four doses in 24 hours are usually sufficient to control most fevers. The temperature is usually retaken 30 minutes after the antipyretic is given to assess its effect but should not be repeatedly measured. The child's level of discomfort is the best indication for continued treatment.

Table 27-2 Dosage recommendations for acetaminophen (Tylenol)*

AGE	WEIGHT (POUNDS)	DOSE (mg)	FORM†
Under 3 months	6-11	40	½ dropper
4-11 months	12-17	80	1 dropper or ½ tsp elixir
12-23 months	18-23	120	1½ droppers or ¾ tsp elixir or 1½ chewable tablets
2-3 years	24-35	160	2 droppers or 1 tsp elixir or 2 chewable tablets
4-5 years	36-47	240	1½ tsp elixir or 3 chewable tablets
6-8 years	48-59	320	2 tsp elixir or 4 chewable tablets or 2 swallowable tablets
9-10 years	60-71	400	2½ tsp elixir or 5 chewable tablets or 2½ swallowable tablets
11 years	72-95	480	3 tsp elixir or 6 chewable tablets or 3 swallowable tablets
12-14 years	96+	640	4 swallowable tablets

*Doses should be administered four or five times daily, but not to exceed five doses in 24 hours.
†1 dropper = 80 mg/0.8 ml; elixir = 160 mg/5 ml; chewable tablet = 80 mg each; junior-strength swallowable tablets = 160 mg each.

Environmental measures to reduce fever may be used if tolerated by the child and if they do not induce shivering. Shivering is the body's way of maintaining the elevated set point by producing heat. Compensatory shivering greatly increases metabolic requirements above those already caused by the fever.

> ✦ **NURSING ALERT** Treatment of shivering is directed at modifying or interfering with the rate of heat loss by warming the body with increased clothing (especially on the extremities), higher environmental temperature, and warm baths (Holtzclaw, 1990).

Traditional cooling measures, such as minimum clothing, exposing the skin to the air, reducing room temperature, increasing air circulation, and cool moist compresses to the skin (e.g., the forehead), are effective if employed approximately 1 hour *after* an antipyretic is given so that the set point is lowered. Cooling procedures such as sponging or tepid baths are ineffective in treating febrile children either when used alone or in combination with antipyretics, and they cause considerable discomfort (Newman, 1985).

Seizures associated with a fever occur in 3% to 4% of all children, usually in those between 3 months and 5 years of age. Although most children never have febrile seizures after the first occurrence, a younger age at onset and a family history of febrile seizures are associated with recurring episodes (Berg and others, 1990). For children who have febrile seizures, administration of antipyretics does not prevent recurrences. Prophylactic therapy with anticonvulsants is controversial but seems to be more effective with fewer side effects when administered intermittently, at the onset of a febrile illness (Rosman, 1989).

Hyperthermia. Unlike in fever, antipyretics are of no value in hyperthermia, because the set point is already normal. Consequently, cooling measures are used. Cool applications to the skin help to reduce the core temperature. Cooled blood from the skin surface is conducted to inner organs and tissues, and warm blood is circulated to the surface, where it is cooled and recirculated. The surface blood vessels dilate as the body attempts to dissipate heat to the environment and facilitate this cooling process.

Commercial cooling devices, such as cooling blankets or mattresses, are available to reduce body temperature. They are placed on the bed and covered with a sheet or lightweight blanket. Frequent temperature monitoring is essential to prevent excessive cooling of the body.

Cool applications can also be given in a tub or in the bed or crib. For tepid tub baths, it is usually best to start with warm water and gradually add cool water until the desired water temperature of 37° C (98.6° F) is reached to accustom the child to the lower water temperature. Place the child directly into the tub of tepid water for 20 to 30 minutes while gently squeezing water from a washcloth over the back and chest or gently spraying it over the body from a sprayer. In the bed or crib, use cool washcloths or towels, exposing only one area of the body at a time. Continue the sponging for approximately 30 minutes.

> ✦ **NURSING ALERT** Isopropyl alcohol should never be used for sponging; neurotoxic effects such as stupor, coma, and even death have been reported (Arditi and Killner, 1987).

After the tub or sponge bath, the child is dried and dressed in lightweight pajamas, nightgown, or diaper and placed in a dry bed. The temperature is retaken 30 minutes after the tub bath or sponge bath. The child is dried by gently rubbing the skin surface with a towel to stimulate circulation. The bath or sponge should not be continued or restarted until the skin surface is warm or if the child feels chilled. Chilling causes vasoconstriction, which defeats the purpose of the cool applications. In this condition little blood is carried to the skin surface; the blood remains primarily in the viscera to become heated.

Whether a temperature elevation in the critically ill child is caused by fever or hyperthermia, it should be treated more aggressively. The metabolic rate increases 10% for every 1° C increase in temperature and three to five times during shivering, increasing oxygen, fluid, and caloric requirements. If the child's cardiovascular or neurologic system is already compromised, these increased needs are especially taxing (Holtzclaw, 1990; Reeves-Swift, 1990). In all children with elevated temperature, attention to adequate hydration is essential. Most children's needs can be met through additional oral fluids.

FAMILY TEACHING AND HOME CARE

Nurses have a unique opportunity for teaching the family about health care practices while the child is hospitalized. Although most children have learned self-care and hygiene in the home or at school, many have not. For some young children this is their first introduction to the use of a toothbrush. Much health teaching can be accomplished even when the child is hospitalized for only a short time. The daily bath, handwashing before meals and after bowel and bladder evacuation, and conscientious dental hygiene are taught by example during routine care. Clean hair, nails, and clothing, as well as good grooming, are emphasized as essential to a pleasing appearance. Positive reinforcement of good hygiene practices helps to create a positive body image, promote the development of self-esteem, and prevent health problems (e.g., teaching girls to wipe the genital area from front to back after toileting).

While sick children's appetites may be poor and not characteristic of their home eating habits, the hospital stay provides numerous opportunities for nurses to assess the family's knowledge of good nutrition and to implement teaching as needed to improve nutritional intake. Creative games can be employed that not only teach but provide diversion as well (Dininny, 1977; Mandelbaum, 1983).

Parental education about elevated temperatures is essential, since many parents are unaware of what constitutes a fever, have unrealistic fears about the dangers of fever, and are apt to over- or undermedicate the febrile child (Gribetz and Cronley, 1987; Kilman, 1987). Parents also need to

Box 27-10 GUIDELINES FOR PARENTS OF CHILD WITH FEVER

Call immediately if:
- Child is <2 months of age.
- Fever is >40.5° C (105° F).
- Child is crying inconsolably.
- Child is difficult to awaken.
- Child is confused or delirious.
- Child has had a seizure.
- Child has a stiff neck.
- Child has purple spots on the skin.
- Breathing is difficult, and child does not feel better after nose is cleared.
- Child is acting very sick.
- Child has an underlying risk factor for serious infection (e.g., sickle cell disease).

Call during office hours if:
- Child is 2 to 4 months old (unless fever is due to a diphtheria-pertussis-tetanus [DPT] vaccination).
- Fever is 40° to 40.5° C (104° to 105° F), especially if child is <2 years old.
- Burning or pain occurs with urination.
- Fever has been present for >72 hours.
- Fever has been present for >24 hours without an obvious cause or location of infection.
- Fever disappeared for >24 hours and then returned.
- Child has a history of febrile seizures.
- Parents have other questions.

Modified from Schmitt, B.D.: Fever in childhood, Pediatrics 74(5, suppl.):934, 1984.

know that sponging is indicated for elevated temperatures from hyperthermia rather than fever and that ice water and alcohol are inappropriate, potentially dangerous, solutions. Parents should know how to take the child's temperature, read the thermometer accurately, and have guidelines for seeking professional care (Box 27-10). Some of the newer temperature-measuring devices, such as plastic strip or digital thermometers, may be better suited for home use (see Temperature, Chapter 7). Many parents are unable to read a mercury thermometer or calculate the correct decimal point (Banco and Jayashekaramurthy, 1990). If the use of acetaminophen is indicated, the parents need instruction in administering the drug.* It is important to emphasize accuracy in both the amount of drug given and the time intervals at which the drug is administered. Since many forms of acetaminophen are available, the nurse must be certain of the type being used in the home when discussing dosage. For example, the specially coated swallowable tablets for older children contain *twice* the amount of drug of the chewable tablets. If parents switch from the infant drops to the elixir, they are cautioned against using the dropper to measure the elixir, which is much less concentrated than the drops. Also, as children grow, the dosage needs to be recalculated. To ensure the correct dose, it is recommended that a dose for a small child be calculated on the basis of 15 mg/kg/dose rather than 10 mg/kg/dose (Gribetz and Cronley, 1987).

*Home care instructions on measuring temperature and giving medications are available in Wong, D.L., and Whaley, L.F.: Clinical manual of pediatric nursing, ed. 3, St. Louis, 1990, Mosby–Year Book, Inc.

SAFETY

Safety is an essential component of any patient's care, but children have special characteristics that require an even greater concern for safety. Since small children are separated from their usual environment and do not possess the capacity for abstract thinking and reasoning, it is the responsibility of everyone who comes in contact with them to maintain protective measures throughout their hospital stay. Nurses need a good understanding of the age level at which each child is operating and plan for safety accordingly.

Name bands, a part of hospital safety practices, are particularly important for children in the pediatric age-group. Infants and unconscious patients are unable to tell or respond to their names. Toddlers may answer to any name or to a nickname only. Older children may exchange places, give an erroneous name, or choose not to respond to their own names as a form of joke, unaware of the hazards of such practices.

INFECTION CONTROL

The need for medical asepsis and appropriate barrier precautions to reduce the risk of nosocomial (hospital-associated) infections is essential in caring for children. Children are frequently infected with organisms, such as varicella (chickenpox), that are transmissible and may be dangerous to others, especially immunocompromised patients. In addition, children may not have developed good hygiene habits, such as handwashing after toileting. Young children are especially at risk for infection because of their high oral activity. Children in diapers present infection risks if caregivers do not practice meticulous cleaning techniques. Because of the importance of reducing the risk of nosocomial infection in children, a brief overview of the traditional and current trends in isolation practices is presented.

Although institutions can design their own system, most hospitals have adopted one of the following two basic systems for isolation precautions recommended by the Centers for Disease Control (CDC) (1983):

Category-specific isolation precautions—isolation categories group diseases for which similar isolation precautions are indicated. Instructions for each category include taking all the precautions necessary to prevent transmission of the most infectious disease in each category. Seven categories are used: strict isolation, contact isolation, respiratory isolation, tuberculosis isolation, enteric precautions, drainage/secretion precautions, and blood/body fluid precautions (replaced in 1987/1988 by Universal Blood and Body Fluid Precautions ["Universal Precautions"]).

Disease-specific isolation precautions—each disease is listed with only the precautions needed to prevent transmission of that disease. Consequently, there is more variability in instructions with this system.

Table 27-3 Comparison of body substance isolation and universal precautions

	BODY SUBSTANCE ISOLATION (BSI)*	CENTERS FOR DISEASE CONTROL (CDC) UNIVERSAL PRECAUTIONS (UP)†	COMMENTS
Purpose	Reduces risk of cross-transmission of organisms, including human immunodeficiency virus (HIV), between patients and from patients to personnel Depends on the interaction between the caregiver and patient, regardless of diagnosis	Minimizes risk of blood-borne infection (HIV, hepatitis B virus [HBV]) Must also use category- or disease-specific isolation precautions for diagnosed infections Depends on type of patient contact and diagnosis	Major difference between BSI and UP: BSI system considers all patients potentially infectious for all pathogens (interaction driven); UP system considers all patients potentially infectious only for blood-borne infections and requires additional protections once diagnosis is made (diagnosis driven)
Body substances considered potentially infectious	All, including: Blood Feces Urine Vomitus Wound and other drainage Oral secretions	Blood Semen Vaginal secretions Cerebrospinal fluid Synovial fluid Pleural fluid Peritoneal fluid Pericardial fluid Amniotic fluid Fluids *not* included unless they contain visible blood: Feces Nasal secretions Sputum Sweat Tears Urine and vomitus	UP do not apply to human breast milk or saliva except in special situations: Frequent exposure to breast milk (i.e., in breast milk banking) During dental procedures where saliva may be contaminated with blood
Handwashing	Performed for 10 seconds with soap, running water, and friction any time the hands are visibly soiled and between most patient contacts even if gloves are worn Not necessary between sequential low-risk patient contacts involving intact skin, such as taking vital signs or administering medications	Immediately and thoroughly wash hands and other skin surfaces that are contaminated with body fluids to which UP apply	Handwashing is the single most important strategy for preventing infection transmission
Gloves	Must be used when contact with mucous membranes, nonintact skin, or moist body substances is likely to occur; changed between patient contacts	Must be worn when touching fluids to which UP apply Use during phlebotomy depends on risk of exposure to blood and prevalence of blood-borne pathogens. General guidelines include: If operator has breaks in skin If operator is receiving training in phlebotomy If hand contamination with blood is likely (e.g., performing phlebotomy on uncooperative patient) Finger and/or heel sticks on infants and children	Washing or disinfecting gloves for reuse is not recommended Washing with surfactants may cause "wicking"; i.e., the enhanced penetration of liquids through undetected holes in the glove Disinfecting agents can deteriorate the glove General CDC control practices for saliva include use of gloves for digital examination of mucous membranes and endotracheal suctioning

*Data from Lynch, P., and others: Rethinking the role of isolation practices in the prevention of nosocomial infections, Ann. Intern. Med. 107:243-246, 1987.

†Data from Centers for Disease Control: Update: Universal precautions for prevention of transmission of human immunodeficiency virus, hepatitis B virus, and other bloodborne pathogens in healthcare settings, MMWR 37(24):377-387, 1988.

NOTE: The American Academy of Pediatrics has published guidelines on infection control, but because they are limited only to HIV infection and depend on the prevalence of HIV infection in an area, which is rarely known, they are not included (Task Force on Pediatric AIDS, 1988).

Table 27-3 Comparison of body substance isolation and universal precautions—cont'd

	BODY SUBSTANCE ISOLATION (BSI)*	CENTERS FOR DISEASE CONTROL (CDC) UNIVERSAL PRECAUTIONS (UP)†	COMMENTS
Gowns or plastic aprons	Worn when it is likely that body substances will soil the clothing; changed between patient contacts	Same as BSI	With young children, use of a gown or plastic apron with adequate shoulder and chest protection may be needed during feeding and bubbling
Masks and/or eye protection	Worn when likely that the eyes and/or nose and mouth will be splashed with body substances or when personnel are working directly over large, open skin lesions	Same as BSI except only for substances considered infectious and as recommended by CDC guidelines (1983)	Benefit of masks in preventing transmission of airborne infection is questionable BSI system does not recommend masks for protection from airborne infections CDC guidelines (1983) recommend masks for protection from airborne infection UP system does not address masks except for protection from splashes, since HIV and HBV are not airborne Eyeglasses generally adequate to provide eye protection
Needle/syringe units and other sharp instruments	Used needles not generally removed from disposable syringes, recapped or broken; all sharp instruments are disposed of in a rigid, puncture-resistant container located preferably near the site of use (e.g., patient's room, treatment rooms)	Same as BSI	Needle punctures are a leading cause of nosocomial (hospital-associated) transmission of blood-borne pathogens Gloves cannot prevent penetrating injuries caused by needles or other sharp instruments Adherence to proper handling of sharp instruments is essential If recapping is necessary, a one-handed scoop technique should be used
Trash and linen	Bagged securely in leakproof containers and disposed of or cleaned according to institutional policy	Same as BSI	CDC recommendations include extensive discussions of environmental considerations for HIV transmission, although there is no evidence of casual or environmental transmission of HIV
Private rooms	Desirable for children who soil the environment with body substances; required for children with airborne, communicable diseases unless they can share a room with roommate(s) known to be immune to the disease	Not addressed other than to use disease- or category-specific isolation precautions	According to CDC, diseases affecting children that require use of a private room for strict or respiratory isolation precautions are varicella (chickenpox), diphtheria, mumps, pertussis, measles, erythema infectiosum, epiglottitis, meningitis (*Haemophilus influenzae*, meningococcal), pneumonia (*H. influenzae*, meningococcal), and meningococcemia

Both these systems are *diagnosis driven;* that is, the patient's diagnosis determines the type of precautions needed to interrupt the transmission of the infectious agent. However, these systems are not designed to provide protection when the infected person is undiagnosed. A problem with any diagnosis-driven approach to isolation precautions is that most communicable diseases are infectious before the diagnosis is made (Lynch and others, 1987).

Recent concern for possible transmission of infection such as hepatitis B and human immunodeficiency virus (HIV) from undiagnosed patients to other patients and health care workers prompted the CDC (1988) to issue guidelines for treating all patients as potentially infectious. This system developed by the CDC is known as *universal precautions* (UP). One type of universal precautions is the *body substance isolation* (BSI) system. Important differences exist between these two systems (Table 27-3).

Nurses caring for young children are frequently in contact with body substances, especially urine, feces, and vomitus. In using BSI, nurses need to exercise judgment for those situations when gloves, gowns, or masks are necessary. For example, gloves and possibly gowns should be worn for changing diapers when there are loose or explosive stools. Otherwise, the plastic lining of disposable diapers provides a sufficient barrier between the hands and body substances. During feedings, gowns should be worn if

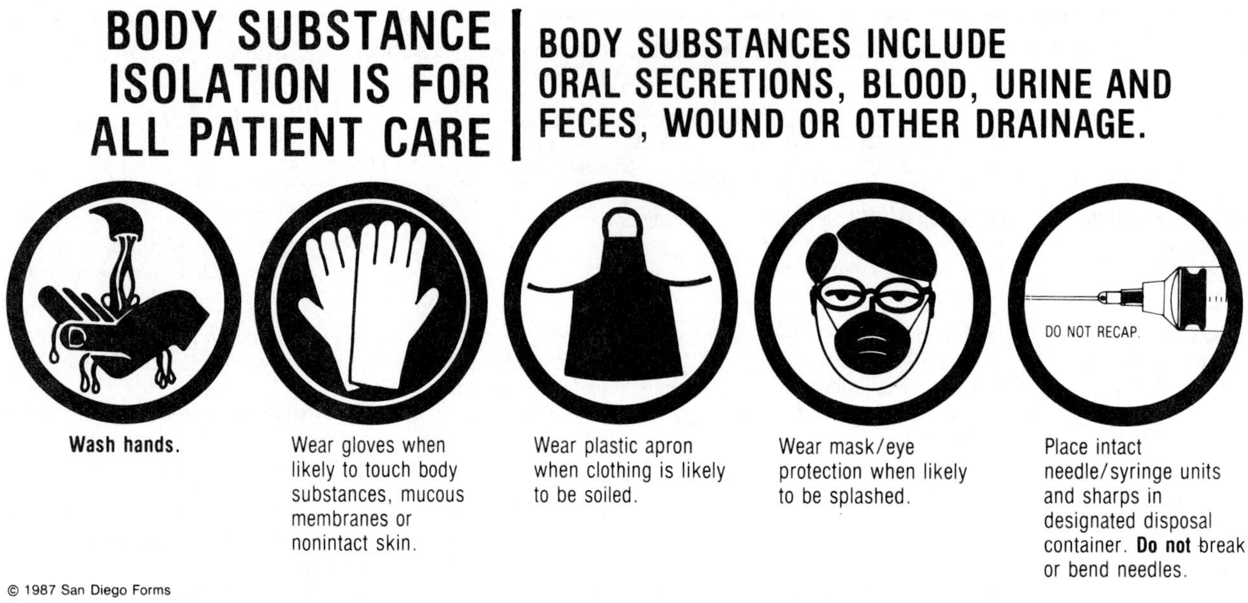
BODY SUBSTANCE ISOLATION IS FOR ALL PATIENT CARE
BODY SUBSTANCES INCLUDE ORAL SECRETIONS, BLOOD, URINE AND FECES, WOUND OR OTHER DRAINAGE.
DO NOT RECAP.
Wash hands.
Wear gloves when likely to touch body substances, mucous membranes or nonintact skin.
Wear plastic apron when clothing is likely to be soiled.
Wear mask/eye protection when likely to be splashed.
Place intact needle/syringe units and sharps in designated disposal container. Do not break or bend needles.
© 1987 San Diego Forms

Fig. 27-6. decal can be displayed in a prominent location, such as on a towel dispenser, to remind personnel to use precautions with all body substances.

the child is likely to vomit or spit up, which often occurs during burping. If aprons with minimum shoulder protection are worn, the child should be sitting on the nurse's lap, not upright against the shoulder, when the child is bubbled. Even when gloves are worn, the hands are washed thoroughly after removing the gloves, since studies have found both latex and vinyl gloves fail to provide consistent protection (Korniewicz, Laughon, and Butz, 1989; Larson, 1989).

Another essential practice of UP and BSI is that all needles (uncapped and unbroken) should be disposed of in a rigid, puncture-resistant container located near the site of use. Consequently, these containers are installed in patients' rooms. Since children are naturally curious, extra attention is needed in selecting a suitable container and a location that discourage access to the disposed needles. To encourage staff to practice BSI, reminders can be placed in strategic areas (Fig. 27-6).

ENVIRONMENTAL FACTORS

All the environmental safety measures for the protection of adults apply to children as well, such as good illumination, floors clear of fluid or other objects that might contribute to falls, and nonskid surfaces in showers and tubs. Electrical equipment is maintained in good working order, is used only by personnel familiar with its use, and is not in contact with moisture or near tubs, where it could prove to be a shock hazard. Beds of ambulatory patients are locked in place and at a height that allows easy access to the floor. Staff members practice proper care and disposal of small breakable items, such as thermometers and bottles, and know a well-organized fire plan. A special hazard for children is the danger of entrapment under an electronically controlled bed when it is activated to descend (Merz, 1983).

All windows should be securely screened and elevators and stairways made safe. Ideally, electrical outlets should be provided with covers to prevent burns in small children, whose exploratory activities may extend to inserting objects into the small openings. Bath water is carefully checked before placing the child in it, and children must never be left alone in a bathtub. Infants are helpless in water, and small children (and some older ones) may turn on the hot water faucet and be severely burned.

Furniture is safest when it is scaled to the child's proportions, is sturdy, and is well balanced to prevent its being easily tipped over. Infants and small children must be securely strapped into infant seats, feeding chairs, and strollers. Baby walkers should be discouraged because they provide access to hazards, resulting in burns, falls, and poisonings. Infants, young children, and those who are weak, paralyzed, agitated, confused, sedated, or cognitively impaired are never left unattended on treatment tables, on scales, or in treatment areas. Even premature infants are capable of surprising mobility; therefore portable incubators must be securely fastened when not in use.

Crib sides are kept up and fastened securely unless an adult is at the bedside. It is safer to leave crib sides up, even when the crib is unoccupied, to remove the temptation to climb in. Anyone attending an infant or small child in a crib with the sides down should never turn away without maintaining hand contact with the child; that is, one hand is kept on the child's back or abdomen to prevent rolling, crawling, or jumping from the open crib (Fig. 27-7). Banco and Powers (1988) reported that falls from cribs by infants tended to occur when siderails had carelessly been left down. Children in beds, however, tended to fall despite

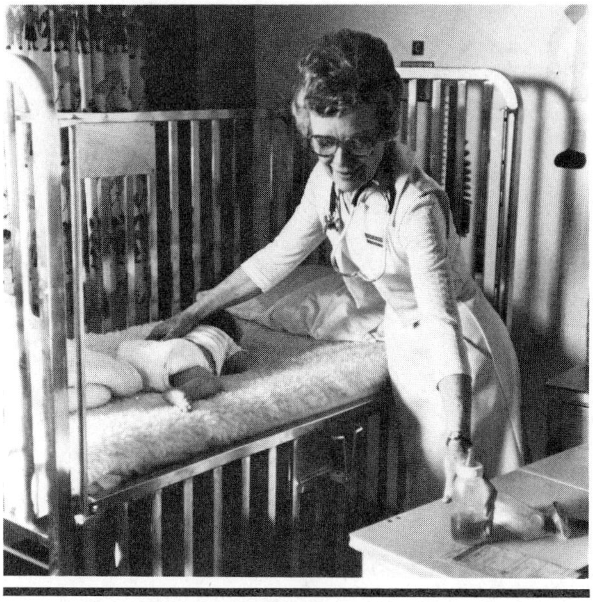

Fig. 27-7. Nurse maintains hand contact when back is turned.

raised siderails by climbing over them. A child who tends or seems inclined to climb over the sides of the crib is safest when placed in a specially constructed crib with a cover or a safety net over the top. If the net is used, it must be tied to the frame so that there is ready access to the child in case of emergency. Nets are never tied to the movable crib sides, and the knots are tied in a manner that permits quick release. (See also Injury Prevention, Chapter 12.)

TOYS

Toys play a vital role in the everyday life of children, and they are no less important in the hospital setting. However, nurses are responsible for assessing the safety of toys brought to the hospital by well-meaning parents and friends. Toys should be appropriate to the child's age, condition, and treatment. For example, if the child is in an oxygen tent, electrical or friction toys or equipment cannot be placed in the tent, because sparks can cause oxygen to ignite. Toys are inspected to make certain that they are nonallergenic, washable, and unbreakable and that they have no small, removable parts that can be aspirated or swallowed or that can otherwise inflict injury to a child.

LIMIT-SETTING

Setting limits is essential to a child's safety. Children must understand where they are permitted to go and what they are permitted to do in the hospital. These limitations are made clear to them, consistently enforced, and repeated as frequently as necessary to make certain that they are understood. The nurse is responsible for where children are at all times. Children can easily wander off unnoticed. Normally active older children often become restless when their activity is restricted and may resort to pillow fights, water fights, and other rough play that might endanger the safety of other children, staff, or visitors. Children in the hospital require surveillance, and appropriate tension-reducing activities can be planned and supervised by nurses and/or by the play therapist. A useful discipline technique is time-out (see Limit-Setting and Discipline, Chapter 14).

TRANSPORTING INFANTS AND CHILDREN

In the course of a hospital stay, infants and children usually need to be transported within the unit and to areas outside the pediatric unit. It is ordinarily safe to carry infants and small children for short distances within the unit, but for more extended trips the child should be securely transported in a suitable conveyance.

Small infants can be held or carried in the horizontal position with the back supported and the thigh grasped firmly by the carrying arm (Fig. 27-8, *A*). In the football hold the infant is carried on the nurse's arm with the head supported by the hand and the body held securely between the nurse's body and elbow (Fig. 27-8, *B*). Both these holds leave the nurse's other arm free for activity. The infant can be held in the upright position with the buttocks on the nurse's forearm and the front of the body resting against the nurse's chest. The infant's head and shoulders are supported by the nurse's other arm to allow for any sudden movement by the infant (Fig. 27-8, *C*). Older infants are able to hold their heads erect but are still subject to sudden movements.

Infants can be transported to other areas, such as the radiology department, in their bassinet or crib. Baby carriages are sometimes used for infants who are not likely to stand up. Strollers and wheeled feeding chairs or tables are also convenient transporters in some situations, such as trips to the playroom, nurse's station, or sun porch.

The method of transporting children is determined by their age, condition, and destination. Most older children are safe in wheelchairs or in gurneys. Younger children can be transported in their crib, on a gurney, in a wagon with raised sides, or in a wheelchair with a safety belt. Gurneys should be equipped with high sides and a safety belt, both of which are kept in place during transport.

RESTRAINTS

Some method of restraint frequently is needed to ensure a child's safety or comfort, to facilitate examination, or to carry out procedures. Restraint can be accomplished with the hand or with physical devices. Restraining the child with the hand provides an element of human contact that is lacking in restraint by mechanical means. The use of physical devices may require a physician's order, although it is the nurse's responsibility to decide when mechanical restraints are needed. Restraints can often be avoided with adequate preparation of the child, parental or staff supervision of the child, and adequate protection of a vulnerable site, such as an infusion device.

Mechanical restraints are never used as a punishment or as a substitute for observation. When a child must be re-

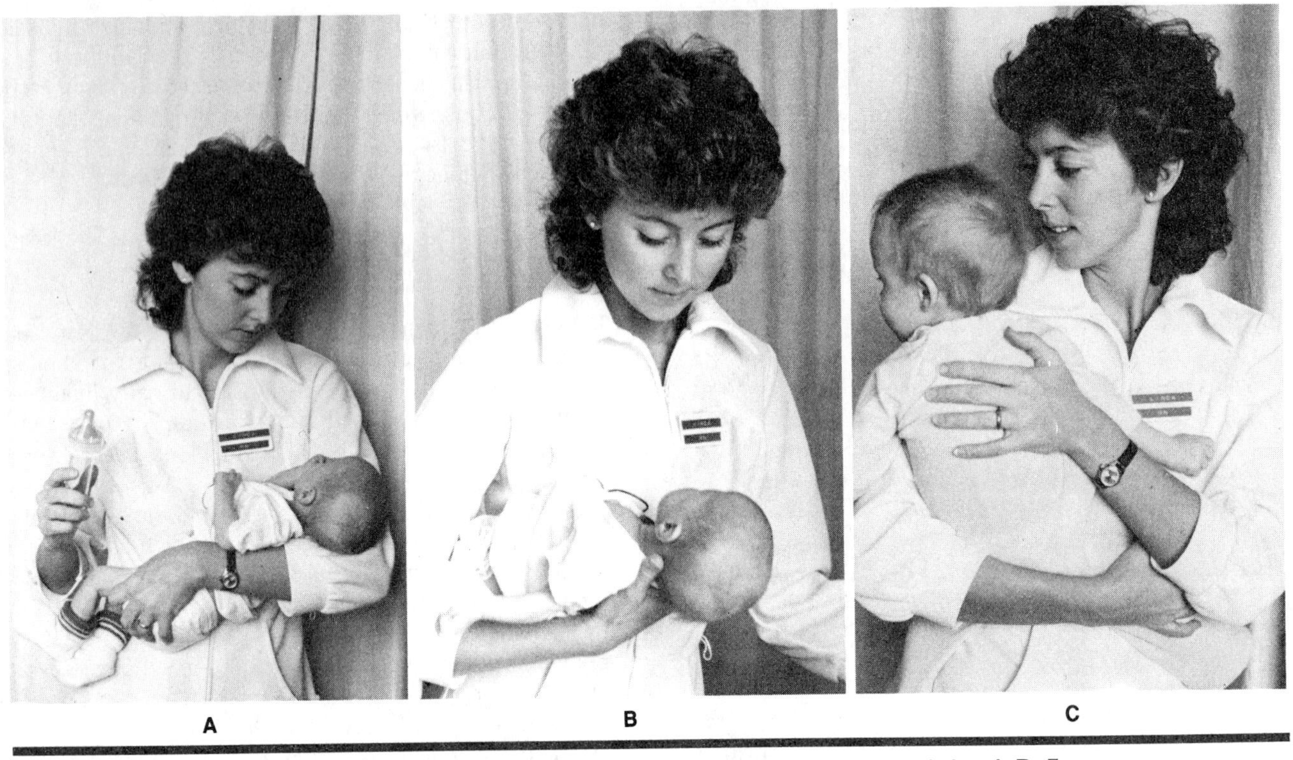

Fig. 27-8. Transporting infants. **A,** Infant's thigh firmly grasped in nurse's hand. **B,** Football hold. **C,** Back supported.

strained, the child and parents need a simple explanation. If the restraint is applied for an extended time, the explanation must be repeated often to gain cooperation and to help the child understand that it is not a punishment. Restraining devices are not without risk and must be checked every 1 to 2 hours. This ensures that restraints are accomplishing their purpose, that they are applied correctly, and that they do not impair circulation, sensation, or skin integrity.

Parents need to know the purpose of restraints, how to remove and reapply them, and the signs of complications from their use. Parents are sometimes upset when their child must be restrained and need to understand how they can help to ensure the maximum benefit and minimize the stress related to restraints. Children, too, should be prepared for the procedure or the circumstance for which the restraint is required.

Removing restraints whenever possible (at least every 2 hours when children are awake) is an essential part of nursing care of children who are restrained for treatments or other purposes. Alternate methods may be devised to replace the need for passive restraints. Holding children for periods is a pleasant alternative, as is restraining them in a highchair, where they can observe nearby activities. If feasible, distraction techniques such as play and reading are employed to gain the child's cooperation without resorting to restraints. Parental participation is always encouraged.

Mummy Restraint

When an infant or small child requires short-term restraint for examination or treatment that involves the head and neck (e.g., venipuncture, throat examination, gavage feeding), the mummy device effectively controls the child's movements. A blanket or sheet is opened on the bed or crib with one corner folded to the center. The infant is placed on the blanket with shoulders at the fold and feet toward the opposite corner (Fig. 27-9, *A*). With the infant's right arm straight down against the body, the right side of the blanket is pulled firmly across the infant's right shoulder and chest and secured beneath the left side of the body (Fig. 27-9, *B*). The left arm is placed straight against the infant's side, and the left side of the blanket is brought across the shoulder and chest and locked beneath the infant's body on the right side (Fig. 27-9, *C*). The lower corner is folded and brought over the body and tucked or fastened securely with safety pins (Fig. 27-9, *D*). Safety pins can be used to fasten the blanket in place at any step in the process.

To modify the mummy restraint for chest examination, the folded edge of the blanket is brought over each arm and under the back, after which the loose edge is folded over and secured at a point below the chest to allow visualization and access to the chest.

Jacket Restraint

A jacket restraint is sometimes used as an alternative to the crib net to prevent the child from climbing out of the crib or to keep the child safe in various chairs. The jacket is put on the child with the ties in back so that the child is unable to manipulate them. The long tapes, secured to the understructure of the crib, keep the child inside the crib (Fig. 27-

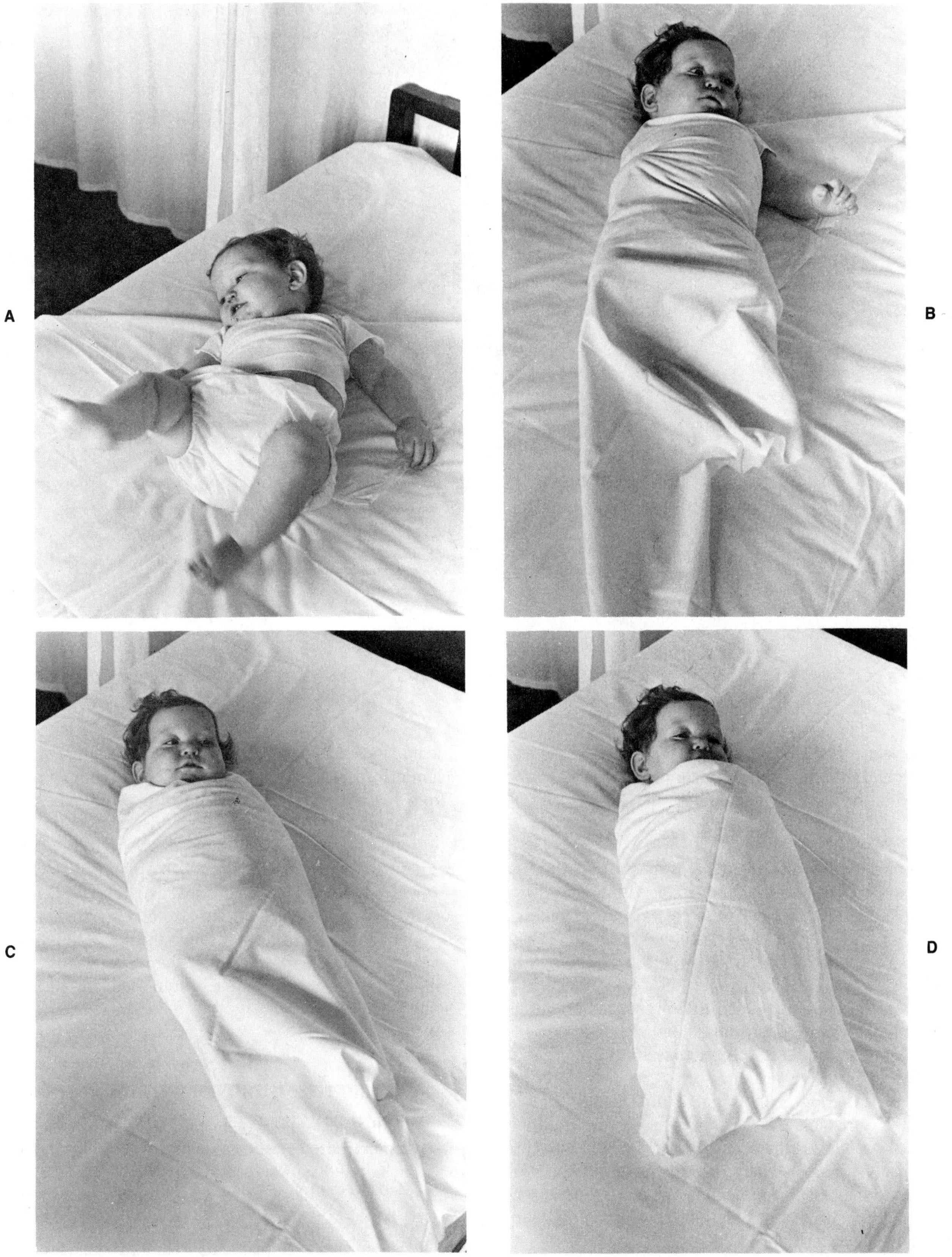

Fig. 27-9. Application of mummy restraint. **A,** Infant placed on folded corner of blanket. **B,** One corner of blanket brought across body and secured beneath body. **C,** Second corner brought across body and secured. **D,** Lower corner folded and tucked or pinned in place.

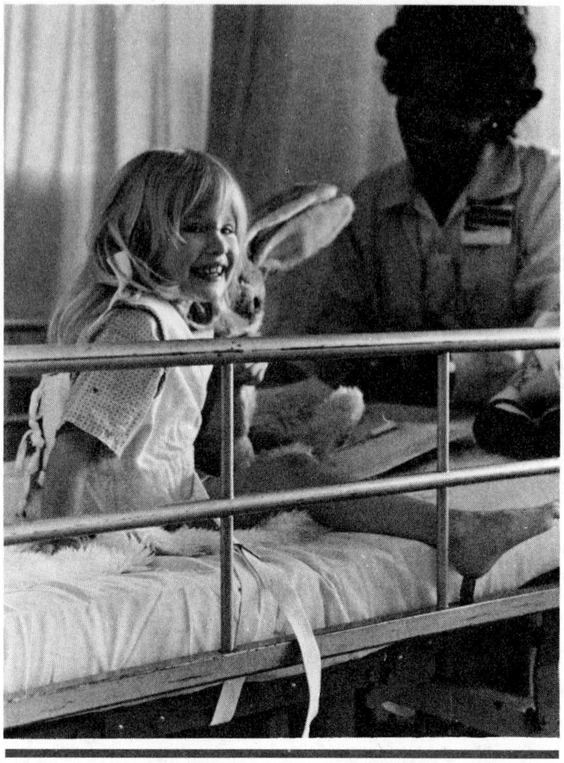

Fig. 27-10. Jacket restraint.

10). The jacket restraint is also useful as a means to maintain the child in a desired horizontal position. A Posey belt scaled to fit the child is an alternative device.

Arm and Leg Restraints

Occasionally one or more extremities must be restrained or limited in motion. Several commercial restraining devices are available, including disposable wrist and ankle restraints, or a restraint can be fashioned from gauze tape, muslin strips, or a length of narrow stockinette. When this type of restraint is used, it must be appropriate to the child's size; it must be padded to prevent undue pressure, constriction, or tissue injury; and the extremity must be observed frequently for signs of irritation or impaired circulation. The ends of the restraints are never tied to the crib rails, since lowering of the rail will disturb the extremity, frequently with a jerk that may hurt or injure the child.

The *clove hitch* restraint is fashioned from a length of gauze or muslin tape. When properly applied, the restraint provides a snug fit with minimum danger of pulling too tightly. Fig. 27-11 illustrates the method of tying and applying a clove hitch restraint.

Elbow Restraint

Sometimes it is important to prevent the child from reaching the head or face, for example, after lip surgery, when a scalp vein infusion is in place, or to prevent scratching in skin disorders. For this purpose, elbow restraints fashioned from a variety of materials function very well. The most common form of elbow restraint consists of a piece of muslin long enough to reach comfortably from just below the axilla to the wrist, with a number of vertical pockets into which tongue depressors are inserted (Fig. 27-12). The restraint is wrapped around the arm and secured with tapes or pins. It may be necessary to pin the top of the restraint to the undershirt sleeve to prevent the restraint from slipping. Similar restraints can be made from readily available items (see Nursing Tips).

NURSING TIPS: IMPROVISED ELBOW RESTRAINTS

Pad the ends of large-diameter towel rollers or appropriately sized plastic containers from which the tops and bottoms have been removed. Apply adhesive tabs to the top end and pin the tabs to the child's sleeves to prevent the restraint from slipping from the extremity.

Fashion adjustable restraints from tongue blades placed vertically against strips of adhesive and then covered with adhesive; secure with adhesive tabs as just described.

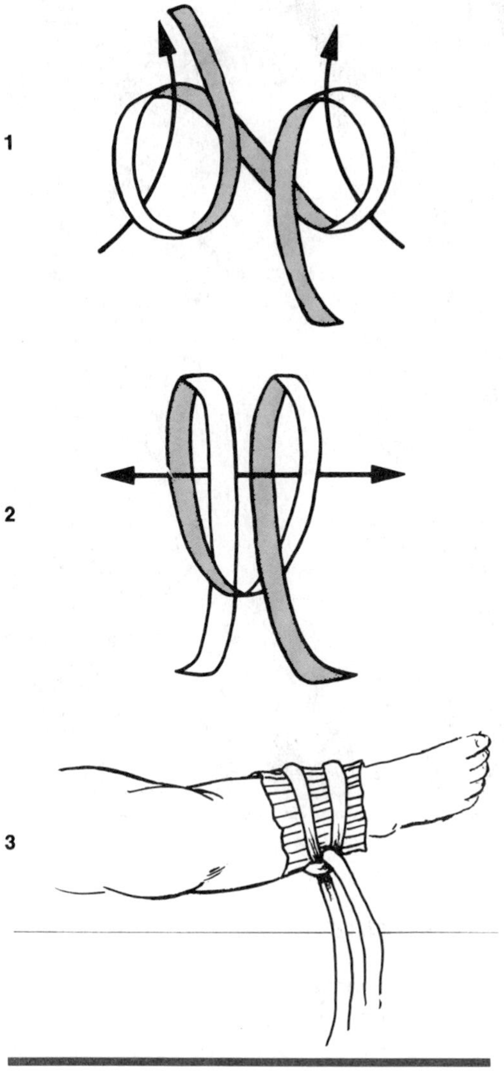

Fig. 27-11. Clove hitch restraint.

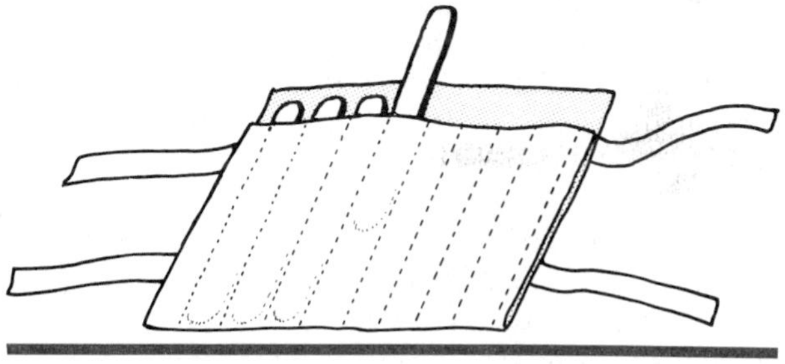

Fig. 27-12. Elbow restraint.

■ POSITIONING FOR PROCEDURES

Infants and small children are unable to cooperate for many procedures; therefore the nurse is responsible for minimizing their movement and discomfort with proper positioning. Older children usually need only minimum, if any, restraint. Careful explanation and preparation beforehand and support and simple guidance during the procedure are usually sufficient.

JUGULAR VENIPUNCTURE

The large, superficial external jugular vein is frequently used to obtain blood specimens from infants and young children. For easy access to the vein, the child is first placed in a mummy restraint in which the top edge of the restraint is low enough to permit access to the vein. The child is placed so that the head and shoulders extend over the edge of a table or a small pillow with the neck extended and the head turned sharply to the side (Fig. 27-13). One alternate method for restraining arms and legs is with the nurse holding the child's arms and legs at the same time that the child's head is restrained and positioned. It is important for the nurse holding the infant to maintain control of the infant's head without interfering with the operator's approach to the vein. The infant's crying during the procedure increases intravenous pressure, which facilitates visualization of the vein. Following venipuncture, digital pressure is applied to the site with a dry gauze square for 3 to 5 minutes or until bleeding stops. Care must be taken not to apply excessive pressure that might compromise circulation or breathing during or following the procedure.

FEMORAL VENIPUNCTURE

Other frequently used sites for venipuncture are the large femoral veins. The nurse restrains the infant by placing the child supine with the legs in a frog position to provide extensive exposure of the groin area. Both the arms and the legs of the infant can be effectively controlled by the nurse's forearms and hands (Fig. 27-14). Only the side used for the venipuncture is uncovered so that the operator is protected should the child urinate during the procedure. Pressure is applied to the site after the withdrawal of blood to prevent oozing from the site.

EXTREMITY VENIPUNCTURE

The most common sites of venipuncture are the veins of the extremities, especially the arm and hand. A convenient position for restraint is having one person on either side of the bed. The child's outstretched arm is partially stabilized by the technician drawing the blood. The other person leans across the child's upper body, preventing movement, and uses an arm to immobilize the venipuncture site. This type of restraint also comforts the child because of the close body contact and allows each person to maintain eye contact (Fig. 27-15).

LUMBAR PUNCTURE

The technique for lumbar puncture in infants and children is similar to that in the adult, although modifications are

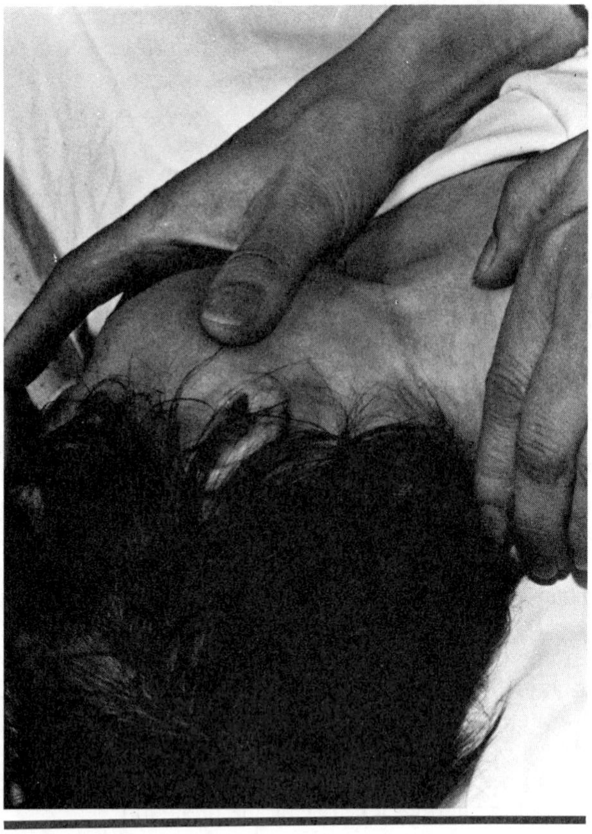

Fig. 27-13. Restraining child for jugular vein puncture.

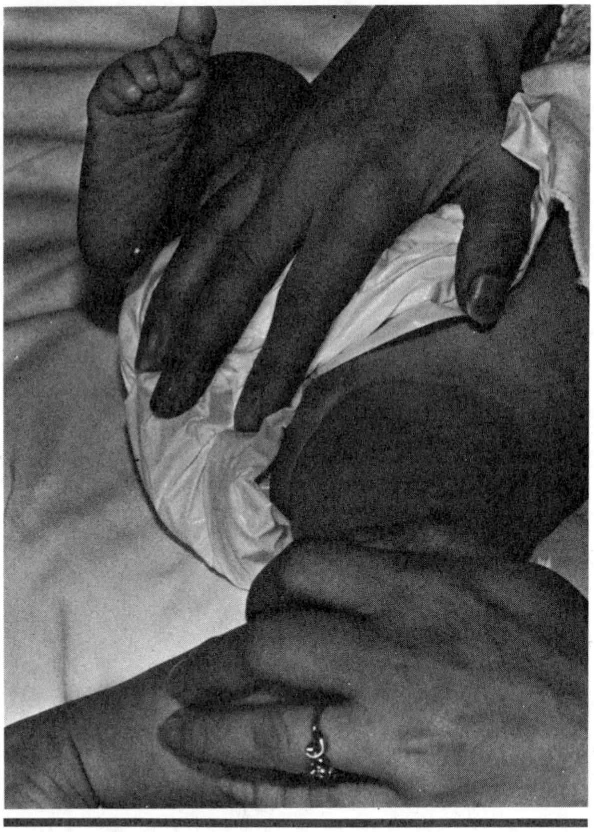

Fig. 27-14. Restraining infant for femoral vein puncture.

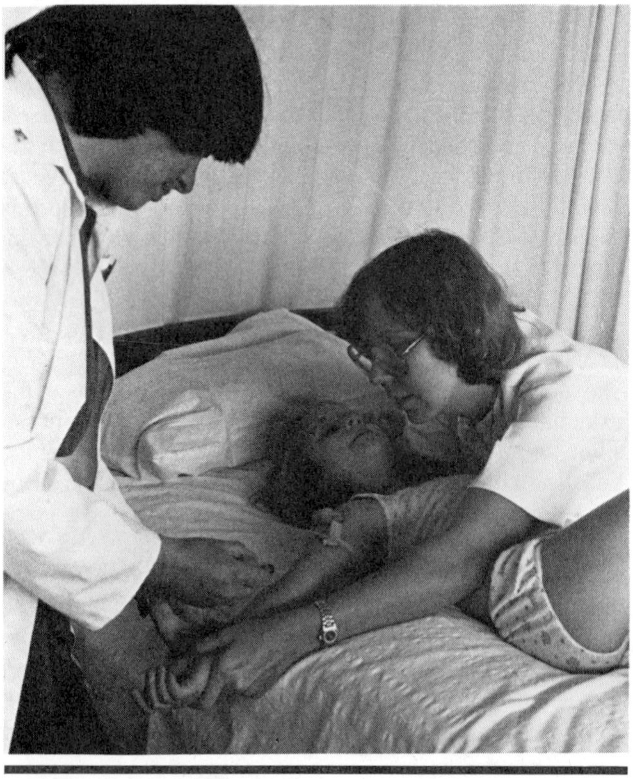

Fig. 27-15. Restraining child for extremity venipuncture. NOTE: Procedure is being performed in emergency department, not in child's hospital room.

suggested in premature infants (see p. 429). Pediatric lumbar puncture sets contain smaller spinal needles, but sometimes the practitioner will specify a particular size or type of needle that the nurse should make certain is placed on the tray.

Children are usually controlled best in the side-lying position, with the head flexed and the knees drawn up toward the chest. Even cooperative children need to be restrained to prevent possible trauma from unexpected, involuntary movement. They can be reassured that, although they are trusted, the restraint will serve as a reminder to maintain the desired position. It also provides a measure of support and reassurance to them.

The child is placed on the side with the back close to the edge of the examining table on the side from which the practitioner is working. The nurse maintains the child's spine in a flexed position by holding the child with one arm behind the neck and the other behind the thighs. The position can be effectively stabilized if the nurse's hands are clasped in front of the child's abdomen (Fig. 27-16, *A*). The flexed position enlarges the spaces between the lumbar vertebral spines, which facilitates access to the spinal fluid space. It is helpful to wrap the legs before positioning to decrease leg movement.

An alternate position used with small infants and some older children is the sitting position. The child is placed with the buttocks at the edge of the table and with the neck flexed so that the chin rests on the chest. The infant's arms

A

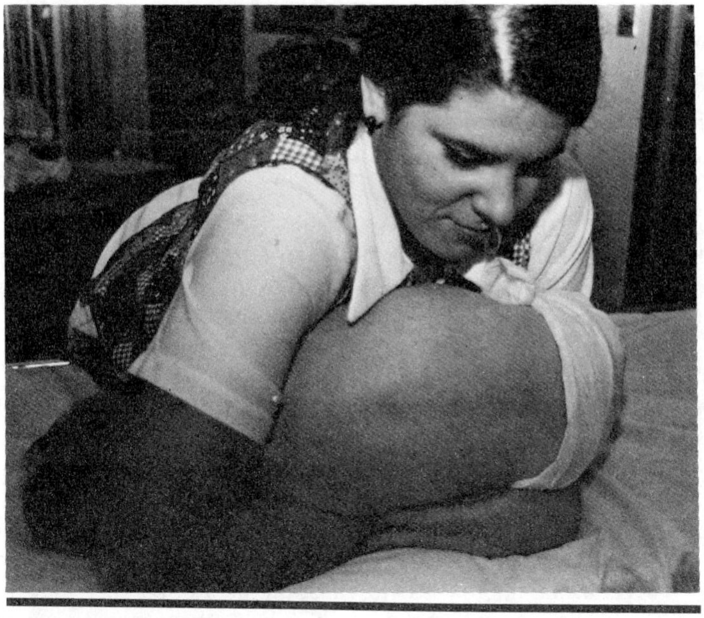

B

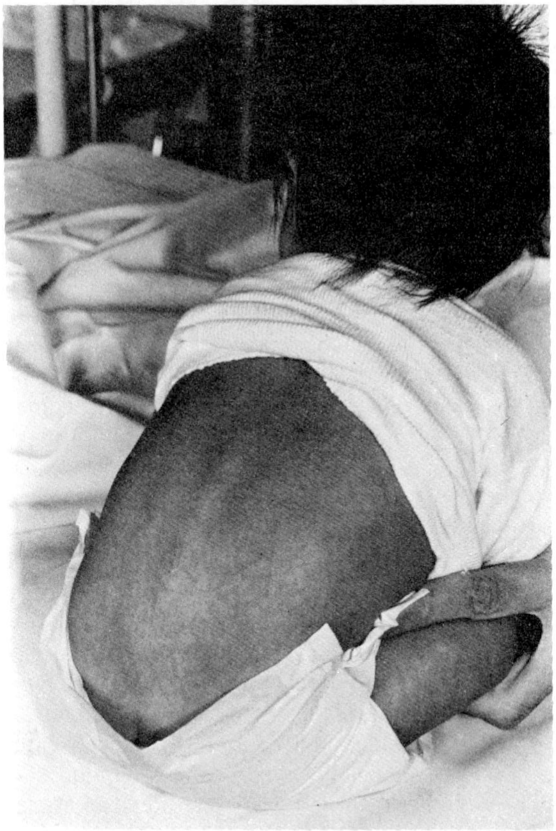

Fig. 27-16. Position for lumbar puncture. **A,** Lying on side. **B,** Sitting.

and legs are immobilized by the nurse's hands (Fig. 27-16, *B*).

✦ **NURSING ALERT** The sitting position may interfere with chest expansion and diaphragm excursion, and in infants the soft, pliable trachea may collapse. Therefore observe the child for difficulty with breathing.

Another position that employs close and comforting contact for the child involves holding the child upright against the nurse's (or parent's) chest with the child's legs wrapped around the adult's waist. The adult's arms are used to hug and restrain the child. For ease of the examiner, the adult should be standing. A small pillow is placed between the child's abdomen and the adult to help arch the child's back. If the pillow proves unsuccessful, a third person can place an arm in this space to achieve the desired position (Brown, 1984).

Specimens and spinal fluid pressure are obtained, measured, and sent for analysis in the same manner as for the adult patient. Vital signs are taken as ordered, and the child is observed for any changes in level of consciousness, motor activity, or other neurologic signs. Postlumbar puncture headache may occur and is related to postural changes; this is less severe when the child lies flat. Headache is seen much less frequently in young children than adolescents (Boulder, 1986).

BONE MARROW ASPIRATION/BIOPSY

Position for a bone marrow aspiration or biopsy depends on the location of the chosen site. In children the posterior or anterior iliac crest is most frequently used, although in infants the tibia may be selected because of easy access to the site and restraint of the child. The sternum, which is the most frequent site in adults, is generally avoided in children because the bone is more fragile and adjacent to vital organs.

If the posterior iliac crest is used, the child is positioned prone. Sometimes a small pillow or folded blanket is placed under the hips to facilitate obtaining the bone marrow specimen. In children who have not received adequate analgesia or anesthesia, restraint is needed and is best applied with two people—one person to immobilize the upper body and a second person to immobilize the lower extremities. If the other sites are used, the child is placed supine and restraint is applied in a similar manner, with modifications for access to the tibia or anterior iliac crest.

OTHER PROCEDURES

For subdural puncture through a fontanel or burr hole, the infant is wrapped in a mummy restraint and placed in the supine position with the head accessible to the examiner. To control the head, the nurse uses a firm hold on each side of it. Procedures for immobilizing the head are discussed in Chapter 7 under Ears; Nose; Mouth and Throat.

■ COLLECTION OF SPECIMENS

Many of the specimens needed for diagnostic examination of children are collected in much the same way as they are for adults. Older children are able to cooperate if given proper instruction regarding what is expected from them. Infants and small children, however, are unable to follow directions or control body functions sufficiently to help in collecting some specimens.

URINE SPECIMENS

Children admitted to the hospital or seen in a clinic or office may require a urine specimen as a routine diagnostic procedure. Older children and adolescents will readily use the bedpan or urinal or can be trusted to follow directions for collection in the bathroom. However, they may have special needs. School-age children are cooperative but curious. They are concerned about the reasons behind things and are likely to ask questions regarding the disposition of their specimen and what one expects to discover from it. Self-conscious adolescents may be reluctant to carry a specimen bottle through a hallway or waiting room and appreciate a paper bag or other means for disguising the container. The presence of menses may be an embarrassment or a concern to teenage girls; therefore it is a good idea to ask them about this and make adjustments as necessary. The specimen can be delayed or a notation made on the laboratory slip to explain the presence of red blood cells.

Preschoolers and toddlers are less cooperative, primarily because they are usually unable to void on request. It is often best to offer them water or other liquids that they enjoy and wait about 30 minutes until they are ready to void voluntarily or set a timer to alert them to void shortly (see also Nursing Tips). Children will better understand what is expected if the nurse uses familiar terms for the function, such as "pee-pee" or "tinkle." Some will have difficulty voiding in an unfamiliar receptacle. Potty-chairs or a bedpan placed on the toilet are usually satisfactory. Toddlers who have recently acquired bladder control may be especially reluctant, since they undoubtedly have been admonished for "going" in places other than those approved by parents. A useful approach is to enlist the help of parents; they are likely to be successful, and this helps them to feel a part of the child's care.

For infants and toddlers who are not toilet trained, special urine collection devices are used. These devices are clear plastic, single-use bags with self-adhering material around the opening at the point of attachment. To prepare the infant, the genitalia, perineum, and surrounding skin are washed and dried thoroughly, since the adhesive will not stick to a moist, powdered, or oily skin surface. The collection bag is easiest to apply if attached first to the perineum, progressing to the symphysis (Fig. 27-17). With little

NURSING TIPS: ENCOURAGING INFANTS TO VOID

Wipe abdomen with alcohol pad and fan it dry; cooling effect often causes voiding within 2 minutes (Ellis, 1989).

Apply pressure over suprapubic area or stroke paraspinal muscles (along spine) to elicit Perez reflex; in infants 4 to 6 months of age, reflex causes crying, extension of back, flexion of extremities, and urination.

A

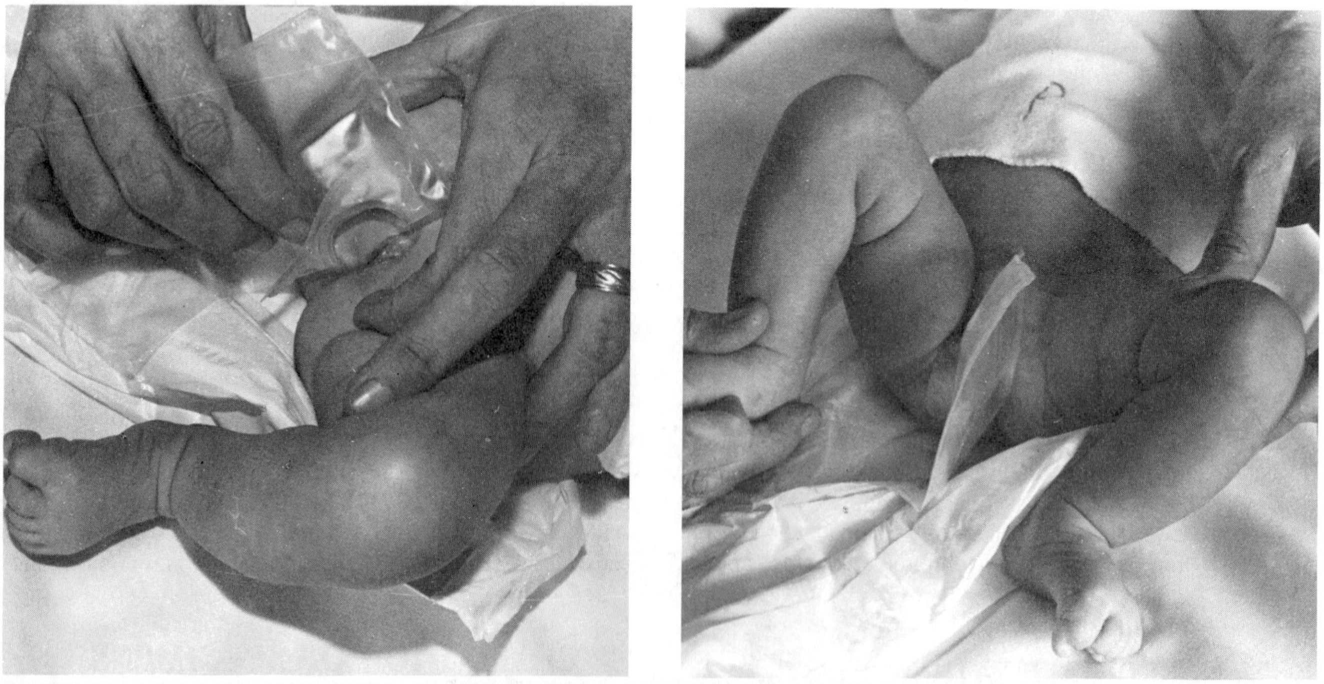

B

Fig. 27-17. Application of urine collection bag. **A,** For female infants, adhesive portion is applied to exposed and dried perineum first. **B,** Bag adheres firmly around perineal area to prevent urine leakage.

NURSING TIPS: URINE COLLECTION

When using a urine collection bag, cut a small slit in the diaper and pull the bag through to allow room for urine to collect and to facilitate checking on the contents.
To obtain small amounts of urine, use a syringe without needle to aspirate urine directly from the diaper; if diapers with absorbent gelling material that trap urine are used, place a small gauze dressing or some cotton balls inside the diaper to collect urine and aspirate the urine with a syringe.

girls the perineum is stretched taut during application to that area to ensure a leak-proof fit. With small boys the penis and scrotum are placed inside the bag. The adhesive portion of the bag must be firmly applied to the skin all around the genital area to avoid possible leakage. The diaper is carefully replaced (see Nursing Tips). The bag is checked frequently and removed as soon as the specimen is available, since the moist bag may become loosened on an active child. For some types of urine testing, such as checking specific gravity, ketones, sugar, and protein, urine can be aspirated directly from the diaper (Suri, 1988) (see Nursing Tips).

Immediate determination of urine specific gravity from a diaper sample is not essential. Studies report no significant change in specific gravities taken from diaper samples up to 4 hours after urination, provided that the diaper is folded closed and taped and is not exposed to air, heat, or light (Lybrand, Medoff-Cooper, and Monro, 1990; Stebor, 1989). Diapers exposed to the environment, especially when radiant heat is used, may lose moisture through evaporation, which may affect the accuracy of specific gravity measurement (Cooke, Werkman, and Watson, 1989). When urine is collected for culture, the bag is removed immediately. If the urine is not tested within 30 minutes, the specimen is refrigerated or placed in a sterile container with a preservative (Goodman and others, 1985; Lewis and Alexander, 1980). Leaving the bag on the perineum for up to 30 minutes has been shown not to affect culture results (Schlager and others, 1990).

At times parents may be requested to bring a urine sample to a health care facility for examination, especially when infants are unable to void during an outpatient visit. In this instance parents need instruction on applying the collection device and storage of the specimen.* Ideally the specimen should be brought to the designated place as soon as possible; if there is a delay, the sample should be refrigerated and the lapsed time reported to the examiner.

*Home care instructions on obtaining a urine sample are available in Wong, D.L., and Whaley, L.F.: Clinical manual of pediatric nursing, ed. 3, St. Louis, 1990, Mosby–Year Book, Inc.

Clean-Catch Specimens

Clean-catch specimens traditionally refer to urine samples obtained for culture after the urethral meatus is cleaned and the first few milliliters of urine are voided before the urine is collected (midstream specimen). The procedure consists of cleaning the perineum or tip of the penis with a soap- or antiseptic-soaked sterile pad, and in females wiping from front to back only once with each pad. This is repeated at least two times. The area may be wiped with sterile water to prevent accidental contamination of the urine with a solution that may destroy the pathogens, although minute amounts of antiseptic such as iodine do not alter bacterial counts. Although this traditional cleansing procedure is often practiced, studies have found that it does not significantly reduce contamination rates in infants, circumcised or uncircumcised males, or toilet-trained prepubertal children. Also, midstream collection does not significantly reduce contamination rates over nonmidstream specimens (Lohr, Donowitz, and Dudley, 1989; McDonald and others, 1985; Saez-Llorens and others, 1989).

Twenty-Four-Hour Collection

The need to collect urine voided over a 24-hour period creates a special challenge in infants and children. Collection bags and sometimes restraining methods are required in infants and small children. Older children require special instruction about notifying someone when they need to void or have a bowel movement so that urine can be collected separately and not discarded. Some older school-age children and adolescents can be trusted to take responsibility for collection of their own 24-hour specimens. These children can keep output records and transfer each voiding to the 24-hour collection container if this is permitted.

As in any 24-hour urine collection, the collection period always starts and ends with an empty bladder. At the time the collection begins the child is instructed to void and the specimen is discarded. All urine voided in the subsequent 24 hours is saved in a container with a preservative or is placed on ice. Twenty-four hours from the time the precollection specimen was discarded, the child is again instructed to void, the specimen is added to the container, and the entire collection is taken to the laboratory for examination.

Infants and small children who are bagged for 24-hour urine collection require a special collection bag; frequent removal and replacement of adhesive collection devices can produce skin irritation. A thin coating of sealant, such as Skin-Prep, applied to the skin helps to protect it and aids adhesion. Plastic collection bags with collection tubes attached are ideal when the container must be left in place for a time. These can be connected to a collecting device or emptied periodically by aspiration with a syringe. When such devices are not available, a regular bag with a feeding tube inserted through a puncture hole at the top of the bag serves as a satisfactory substitute. However, care is taken to empty the bag as soon as the infant urinates to prevent leakage and loss of contents.

Special Techniques

Catheterization or *suprapubic aspiration* is employed when a specimen is urgently needed or when the child is unable to void or otherwise provide an adequate specimen. Catheterization is most often used when urethral obstruction or anuria caused by renal failure is believed to be the cause of the child's failure to void. Suprapubic aspiration is useful in clarifying the diagnosis of suspected urinary tract infection in acutely ill infants.

Catheterizing a child requires aseptic technique, good light, and gentle, thorough cleansing of the vulva or glans penis. Most children, including female infants, accommodate a size 8 or 10 French catheter, but in male infants or when the larger catheters cannot be passed, a smaller, soft plastic feeding tube may be needed. Most children are frightened of this procedure, and few small children are entirely cooperative; therefore even when the procedure is adequately explained, an assistant is needed to help restrain and reassure the child. Special care must be exercised when catheterizing young males to avoid trauma to the ductal and glandular openings into the urethra, which might result in sterility.

Suprapubic aspiration, which is performed by a practitioner skilled in the procedure, involves aspirating bladder contents by inserting a 20- or 21-gauge needle in the midline approximately 1 cm above the symphysis and directed vertically downward. The skin is prepared as for any needle insertion, but the bladder should contain an adequate volume of urine. This can be assumed if the infant has not voided for at least 1 hour or the bladder can be palpated above the symphysis. This technique is especially useful for obtaining sterile specimens from young infants. The bladder is an abdominal organ at this time and is easily accessible.

STOOL SPECIMENS

Stool specimens are frequently collected in children to identify parasites and other organisms that cause diarrhea, to assess gastrointestinal function, and to check for occult (hidden) blood. Ideally, stool should be collected without contamination with urine, but in children wearing diapers this is difficult unless a urine bag is applied. Children who are toilet trained should urinate first, flush the toilet, then defecate in the toilet or in a bedpan (preferably one that is placed on the toilet to avoid embarrassment). An ample amount of stool is collected using a tongue blade and placed in the appropriate container, which is covered and labeled. If several specimens are needed, the containers are marked with the date and time and kept in a specimen refrigerator. Special care is exercised in handling the specimen because of the risk of contamination.

BLOOD SPECIMENS

Although most blood specimens are obtained by the laboratory staff or physicians, nurses are increasingly responsible for specimen collection, especially if the child has an arterial or venous access device. However, whether the specimen is collected by the nurse or others, the nurse is responsible for making certain that specimens, such as serial examinations and fasting specimens, are collected on time and that the proper equipment is available, such as correct collection tubes and ice for blood gas samples.

Venous blood samples can be obtained by venipuncture or by aspiration from a peripheral or central access device. Withdrawing blood specimens through heparin lock devices in small peripheral veins has met with varying degrees of success. Although it avoids an additional venipuncture for the child, attempting to aspirate blood from the heparin lock may shorten the life of the device. When using an intravenous infusion site for specimen collection, it is important to consider the type of fluid being infused. For example, a specimen collected for glucose determination would be inaccurate if removed from a catheter through which glucose-containing solution is being administered (see Nursing Tips).

Arterial blood samples are sometimes needed for blood gas measurement, although noninvasive techniques, such as transcutaneous oxygen monitoring and pulse oximetry, are being used more frequently. Arterial samples may be obtained by arteriopuncture using the radial, brachial, or femoral arteries; by deep heel puncture; or from indwelling arterial catheters. Adequate circulation should be assessed prior to arterial puncture by observing capillary refill or performing the Allen test, a procedure that assesses the circulation of the radial, ulnar, or brachial arteries (Millam, 1988; see also Blood Gas Determination, Chapter 31). Since unclotted blood is required, only heparinized collection tubes are used. In addition, no air bubbles should enter the tube, since they can alter blood gas concentration. Crying, fear, and agitation also affect blood gas values; therefore every effort is used to comfort the child. The blood samples are packed in ice to reduce blood cell metabolism and are taken to the laboratory for immediate analysis.

Capillary blood samples are taken from children by finger or earlobe stick methods, just as in the adult patient. The best method for taking peripheral blood samples from infants is by a heel stick. Before the blood sample is taken, the heel is warmed with warm, moist compresses for 5 to 10 minutes to dilate the vessels in the area. The area is cleansed with alcohol, and with the infant's foot firmly restrained with the free hand, the heel is punctured with a Bard-Parker no. 11 or Redi-Lance blade.

The most serious complication of infant heel puncture is

NURSING TIPS: BLOOD SPECIMENS

To obtain a blood specimen from a central venous line or heparin lock when the infusion solution may interfere with the test results, first aspirate a minimum quantity of blood equal to the volume of fluid in the catheter and discard; then aspirate the blood sample.

For a blood culture, use the first sample of blood, since organisms are most likely to collect within the catheter itself (Schreiner, 1987).

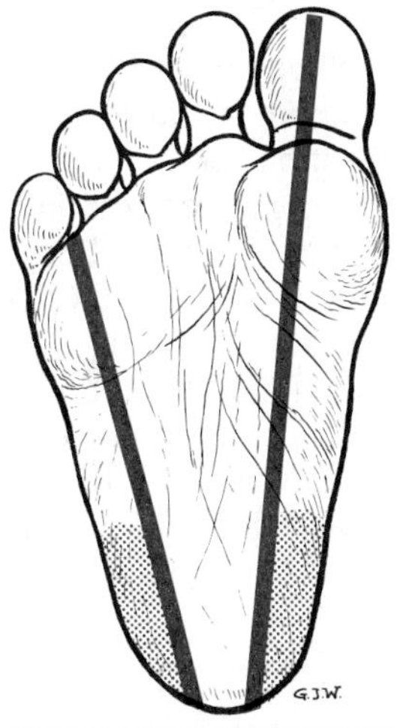

Fig. 27-18. Puncture site *(red stippled area)* on sole of infant's foot.

NURSING TIP: VENIPUNCTURE

Keep arm extended, not flexed, while applying pressure for a few minutes after venipuncture in the antecubital fossa to reduce bruising (Dyson and Bogod, 1987).

necrotizing osteochondritis from lancet penetration of the underlying calcaneus bone. To avoid this, the puncture should be no deeper than 2.4 mm and should be made at the outer aspect of the heel. The boundaries of the calcaneus can be marked by an imaginary line extending posteriorly from a point between the fourth and fifth toes and running parallel to the lateral aspect of the heel and another line extending posteriorly from the middle of the great toe and running parallel to the medial aspect of the heel (Fig. 27-18). In addition, repeated trauma to the walking surface of the heel can cause fibrosis and scarring that may interfere with locomotion. Frequent heel punctures have been associated with development of plantar warts at a later age.

The needed specimens are quickly collected, and pressure is applied to the puncture site with a dry gauze square until bleeding stops (see Nursing Tip). The site is then covered with a Band-Aid. In young children, "spot" Band-Aids pose an aspiration hazard; their use should be avoided, or the Band-Aid should be removed as soon as the bleeding stops. Applying warm compresses to ecchymotic areas increases circulation, helps remove extravasated blood, and decreases pain.

No matter how or by whom the specimen is collected, children, even some older ones, fear the loss of their blood. This is particularly true for children whose condition requires frequent blood specimens. Ignorant about the process of hemopoiesis, they mistakenly believe that blood removed from their bodies is a threat to their lives. Explaining to them that their blood is continually being produced by their bodies provides them with a measure of reassurance regarding this aspect of the stress-provoking procedure. When the blood is drawn, a simple comment such as, "Just look how red it is. You're really making a lot of nice red blood," confirms this information and affords them an opportunity to express their concern. A Band-Aid gives them added assurance that the vital fluids will not leak out through the puncture site.

Children also dislike the discomfort associated with venous, arterial, or capillary punctures. In fact, children have identified these procedures as the ones most frequently causing pain during hospitalization and arterial punctures as being one of the most painful of all procedures experienced (Wong and Baker, 1988). Younger children are more distressed by venipuncture than older children (Fradet and others, 1990). Consequently, nurses need to institute pain reduction techniques to lessen the discomfort of these procedures. The use of topical and intradermal anesthetics significantly reduces the pain, and nonpharmacologic strategies, such as distraction and relaxation, may also be effective (see Pain Management, Chapter 26).

RESPIRATORY SECRETION SPECIMENS

Collection of sputum or nasal discharge is sometimes required for diagnosis of respiratory infections, especially tuberculosis and respiratory syncytial viruses. Older children and adolescents are able to cough as directed and supply sputum specimens when given proper directions. It must be made clear to them that a coughed specimen, not mucus cleared from the throat, is needed. It is helpful to demonstrate a deep cough so that communication is clear. Infants and small children are unable to follow directions to cough and will swallow any sputum produced when they do; therefore gastric washings (lavage) may be used to collect a specimen. Sometimes a satisfactory specimen can be obtained by using a suction device such as a mucous trap if the catheter is inserted into the trachea and the cough reflex elicited. A catheter inserted into the back of the throat is not sufficient. For children with a tracheostomy, a specimen is easily aspirated from the trachea or major bronchi by attaching a collecting device to the suction apparatus.

Nasal washings are usually obtained to diagnose an infection of respiratory syncytial virus (RSV) (Nederhand and others, 1989). The child is placed supine, and 1 to 3 ml of sterile normal saline is instilled with a sterile syringe (without needle) into one nostril. The contents are aspirated using a small, sterile bulb syringe and are placed in a sterile container. To prevent any additional discomfort to the child, all the equipment should be ready before beginning the procedure. Other respiratory secretion collection methods include nasopharyngeal swabs to diagnose *Bordetella pertussis* and throat cultures.

✦ **NURSING ALERT** Do not attempt to obtain a throat culture if acute epiglottitis is suspected. The trauma from the swab may increase edema, possibly occluding the airway (Battaglia, 1986).

ADMINISTRATION OF MEDICATION

The administration of medications to children presents problems that are not encountered when giving medication to adult patients. Children vary widely in age, weight, surface area, and the ability to absorb, metabolize, and excrete medications. Nurses must be particularly alert when computing and administering drugs to infants and children.

DETERMINATION OF DRUG DOSAGE

It is the physician's responsibility to prescribe drugs in the correct dosage to achieve the desired effect without endangering the child's health. However, nurses must have an understanding of the safe dosage of medications they administer to children as well as the expected action, possible side effects, and signs of toxicity. Unlike adult medications, there are few standardized dosage ranges for children in the pediatric age-groups, and with a few exceptions, drugs are prepared and packaged in average adult-dosage strengths.

Factors related to growth and maturation significantly alter an individual's capacity to metabolize and excrete drugs, and deficiencies associated with immaturity become more important with decreasing age. Immaturity or defects in any or all of the important processes of absorption, distribution, biotransformation, or excretion can significantly alter the effects of a drug. Newborn and premature infants with immature enzyme systems in the liver (where most drugs are broken down and detoxified), lower plasma concentrations of protein for binding with drugs, and immaturely functioning kidneys (where most drugs are excreted) are particularly vulnerable to the harmful effects of drugs. Beyond the newborn period, many drugs are metabolized more rapidly by the liver, necessitating larger doses or more frequent administration. This is particularly important in pain control, when the dosage may need to be increased or the interval between administering analgesics may need to be decreased (Singleton, Rosen, and Fisher, 1987).

Other factors that create problems in drug dosages in children include the difficulty in evaluating drug response. For example, how is a toxic manifestation such as ringing in the ears assessed in a preverbal child? In disease states, particularly in children, water losses and water requirements are both increased, whereas the fluid intake decreases. Since water is required to excrete the drug, dehydration poses the danger of toxic accumulation.

Various formulas involving age, weight, and body surface area (BSA) as the basis for calculations have been devised to determine children's drug dosage from a standard adult dose. Since the administration of medication is a nursing responsibility, nurses need not only a knowledge of drug action and patient responses, but also some resources for estimating safe dosages for children. The method most often used to determine children's dosage is based on surface area.

Body Surface Area

The most reliable method for determining children's dosage is to calculate the proportional amount of body surface area to body weight. The ratio of body surface area to weight varies inversely to length; therefore the infant who is shorter and weighs less than an older child or adult has relatively more surface area than would be expected from the weight.

The usual determination of surface area requires the use of the West nomogram (Fig. 27-19). Body surface area is estimated from the child's height and weight. Then this information is applied to a formula for dosage, such as either of the following formulas, which require different types of information:

$$\frac{\text{Body surface area of child}}{\text{Body surface area of adult}} \times \text{Adult dose} = \text{Estimated child's dose}$$

$$\text{Surface area of child (m}^2\text{)} \times \text{Dose/m}^2 = \text{Estimated child's dose}$$

PREPARATION FOR SAFE ADMINISTRATION

Unit dose packaging, which is gaining wide usage in hospital pharmacies, frequently does not extend to pediatric medications. Therefore the ability to calculate fractional doses from larger dosages is absolutely essential. In addition, measuring doses, identifying patients, and gaining cooperation create problems not usually encountered in giving medications to adults.

Checking Dosage

Administering the correct dosage of a drug is a shared responsibility between the physician who orders the drug and the nurse who carries out that order. Children react with unexpected severity to some drugs, and ill children may be especially sensitive to drugs. Therefore checking the dose if there is any doubt about its accuracy is a professional duty. When a dose is ordered that is outside the usual range or if there is some question regarding the preparation or the route of administration, the nurse should always check with the physician before proceeding with the administration, since the nurse is legally liable for any drug administered.

Administering some medications requires added safeguards. Even when it has been determined that the dosage is correct for a particular child, many drugs are potentially hazardous or lethal. Most hospital units or other facilities where medications are given to children have regulations requiring that specified drugs be double-checked by another nurse before they are given to the child. Among those drugs that require such safeguards are digoxin, heparin, and insulin. Others that are frequently included are epinephrine, opioids, and sedatives. Even if this precaution is not mandatory, nurses would be wise to take such precautions for their own sense of security. Errors in decimal point placement may easily occur and may result in a tenfold or more dosage error (Koren, Barzilay, and Greenwald, 1986).

Identification

Before the administration of any medication, the child must be correctly identified, since children are not totally reliable

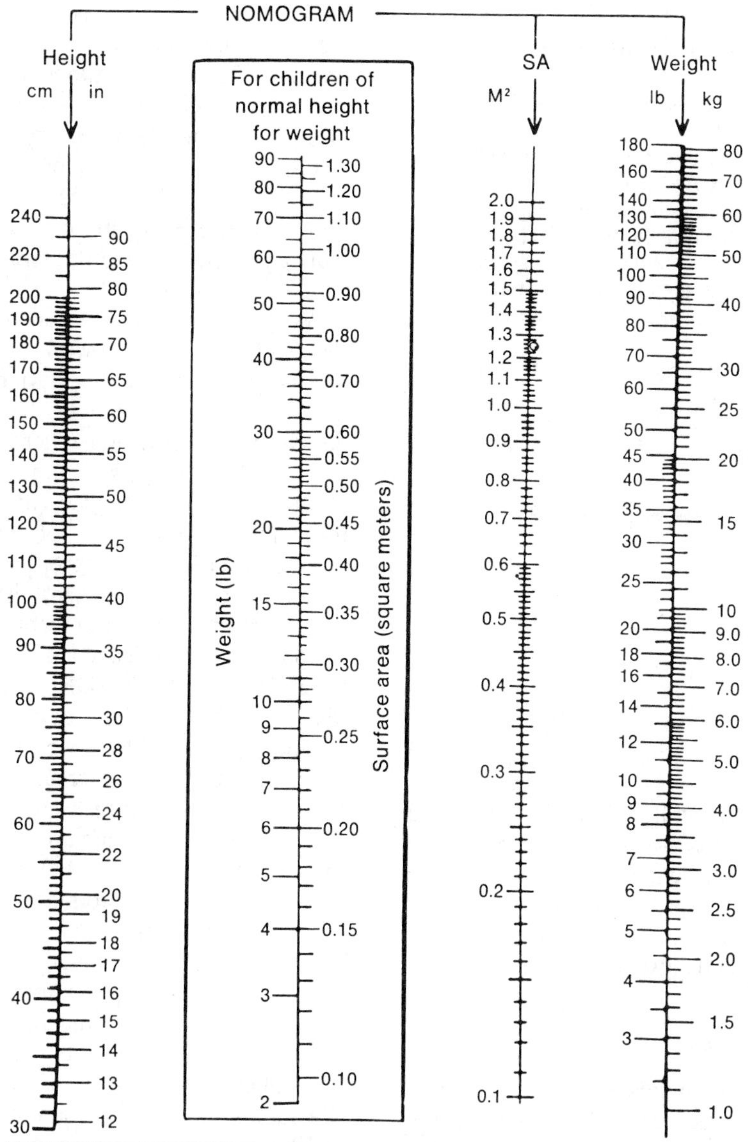

Fig. 27-19. West nomogram (for estimation of surface areas). Surface area is indicated where a straight line connecting height and weight intersects surface area (SA) column, or if patient is approximately of normal proportion, from weight alone (enclosed area).
Nomogram modified from data of E. Boyd by C.D. West; from Behrman, R.E., and Vaughan, V.C., editors: Nelson textbook of pediatrics, ed. 13, Philadelphia, 1987, W.B. Saunders Co., p. 1521.

in giving correct names on request. Infants are unable to give their name, toddlers or preschoolers may admit to any name, and school-age children may deny their identity in an attempt to avoid the medication. Children sometimes exchange beds during play. Parents may be present to identify their child, but the only safe method for identifying children is to check their hospital identification bands with the medication card.

Parents

Parents can be useful sources of information regarding the child and his or her capabilities. Nearly all parents have given some type of medication to their child and can describe the approaches that they have found to be successful. They can also provide information regarding the child's reaction to similar experiences if the child has been hospitalized before or has been given medication in a practitioner's office or clinic. In some cases it is less traumatic for the child if a parent gives the medication, provided the nurse prepares the medication and supervises its administration and the practice is consistent with hospital or ward policy. Children being given daily medications at home are accustomed to the parent's functioning in this capacity and are less apt to fuss than they would if the medication were administered by a stranger. Individual decisions need to be made regarding parental presence and participation, such

NURSING TIPS: ORAL MEDICATION

To encourage the child's acceptance of oral medications:

- Give the child a popsicle or small ice cube to suck to numb the tongue before giving the drug.
- Mix the drug with a small amount (about 1 tsp) of sweet-tasting substance, such as honey (except in infants because of the risk of botulism), flavored syrups, jam, fruit purees, or ice cream; avoid essential food items, since the child may later refuse to eat them.
- Give a "chaser" of water, juice, a soft drink, or a popsicle or frozen juice bar after the drug.
- If nausea is a problem, give a carbonated beverage poured over finely crushed ice before or immediately after the medication.

as in helping with restraint, during injections (see Questions and Controversies, p. 1191).

Child

Every child requires psychologic preparation for parenteral administration of medication and supportive care during the procedure (see p. 1187). Even if children have received several injections, they rarely become accustomed to the discomfort and have as much right to understanding and patience from those involved in giving the injection as any other child. Safe administration of any drug requires meticulous attention to the safeguards discussed here.

ORAL ADMINISTRATION

The oral route is preferred for administering medications to children whenever possible. Because of the ease of administration of oral medications, most are dissolved or suspended in liquid preparations. Although some children are able to swallow or chew solid medications at an early age, solid preparations are not recommended for young children. There is danger of aspiration in any oral preparation, but solid forms (pills, tablets, capsules) are especially hazardous if their administration causes extreme resistance or crying.

Most pediatric medications come in palatable and colorful preparations for added ease of administration. Some have a slightly unpleasant aftertaste, but the majority of children will swallow these liquids with little if any resistance. The nurse should taste a minute amount of an oral preparation to ascertain if it is palatable or bitter. In this way legitimate complaints of dislike from the child can be accepted and the taste camouflaged whenever possible. Most pediatric units have preparations available for this purpose (see Nursing Tips).

Preparation

Selecting a vehicle to measure and administer a medication requires careful consideration. The devices available to measure medicines are not always sufficiently accurate for measuring the small amounts needed in pediatric nursing practice (Fig. 27-20). Although molded plastic cups offer reasonable accuracy in measuring moderate or large doses of liquids, paper cups are likely to have irregularly shaped or crumpled bottoms. Calibrations on the cups (especially the teaspoon mark) and the personal equation or interpretation of a given measure are highly variable. Measures less than a teaspoon are impossible to determine accurately with a medicine cup.

Many liquid preparations are prescribed in measurements of teaspoons. However, teaspoons and soup spoons are inaccurate measuring devices and are subject to error from a number of variables. For example, teaspoons vary greatly in capacity, and different persons using the same spoon will pour different amounts. This variability is also influenced by the adequacy of available light, the color of the liquid, and the size of the bottle from which it is poured. Therefore a drug ordered in teaspoons should be measured in milliliters—the established standard is 5 ml per teaspoon. A convenient hollow-handled medicine spoon is available to accurately measure and administer the drug* (see Fig. 27-20, *A*). Household *measuring* spoons can also be used when other devices are not available.

Another unreliable device for measuring liquids is the drop, which varies to a greater extent than the teaspoon or measuring cup. Droppers are available in numerous sizes but, even with the standard USP dropper, the volume of a drop will vary according to the viscosity of the liquid measured. Viscid fluids produce much larger drops than thin liquids. Many medications are supplied with caps or droppers designed for measuring each specific preparation. These are accurate when used to measure that specific medication but are not reliable for measuring other liquids. Emptying dropper contents into a medicine cup invites additional error. Since some of the liquid clings to the sides of the cup, a significant amount of the drug can be lost.

The most accurate means for measuring small amounts of medication is the plastic disposable (never glass) syringe, especially the tuberculin syringe for volumes less than 1 ml. Not only does the syringe provide a reliable measure, but it also serves as a convenient means for transporting and administering the medication. The medication can be placed directly into the child's mouth from the syringe. For added safety, a short length of flexible tubing can be placed on the tip of the syringe to prevent injury to the mouth, although the tubing must be completely emptied of medication.

Young children and some older children have difficulty in swallowing tablets or pills. Since a number of drugs are not available in pediatric preparations, the tablet will need to be crushed before it can be given to these children. Commercial devices† are available or simple methods can be

*Manufactured by Apex Medical Corp., P.O. Box 1235, Sioux Falls, SD 57101-1235; (800) 328-2935.

†Trademark Medical manufactures a pill crusher and has compiled a list of more than 190 medications that should not be crushed or chewed. Both are available from Trademark Medical, 1053 Headquarters Park, Fenton, MO 63026-2033; (314) 349-3265.

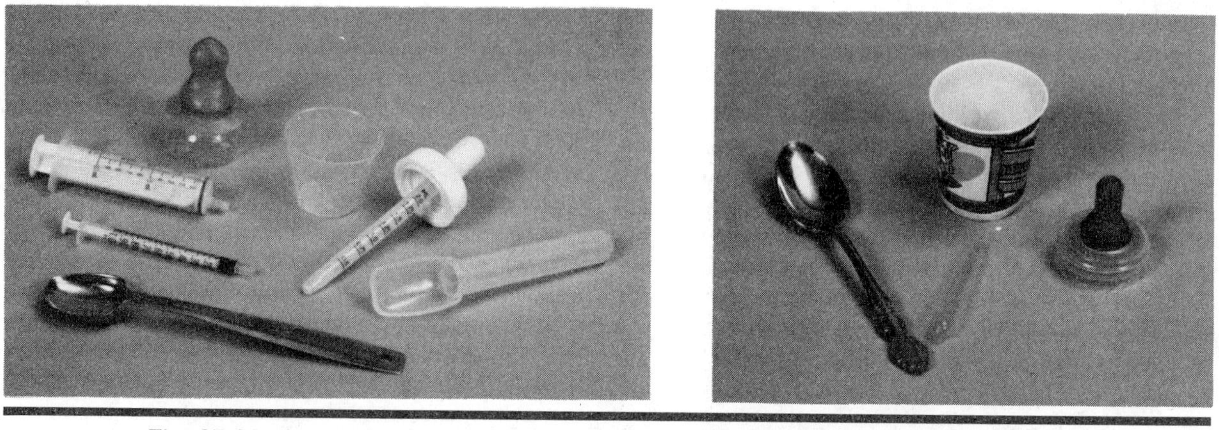

A B

Fig. 27-20. A, Acceptable devices for measuring and administering oral medication to children *(clockwise):* measuring spoon, plastic syringes, calibrated nipple, plastic medicine cup, calibrated dropper, hollow-handled medicine spoon. **B,** Acceptable devices only for administering premeasured oral medication *(clockwise):* household teaspoon, paper cup, nipple, uncalibrated dropper.

NURSING TIP: CRUSHING TABLETS

To minimize loss of the drug, crush the tablet between two spoons or place the tablet either in a medicine cup or between two small paper soufflé cups and use a pestle for crushing; collect the bits of pulverized medication that tend to cling to the sides of the cup or spoon and mix the crushed tablet with a palatable substance.

NURSING TIP: ENCOURAGING SWALLOWING

In infants up to 11 months of age and children with neurologic impairments, blowing a small puff of air in the face frequently elicits a swallow reflex (Orenstein and others, 1988).

employed for crushing tablets (see Nursing Tip). Another alternative is to have the pharmacist prepare the drug in a flavored, chewable troche or lozenge (Wong and Redding, 1987).

Not all drugs can be crushed, for example, medication with an enteric or protective coating or formulated for slow release.† For some children it may be possible to encourage swallowing the tablet or capsule by using a special glass designed with a shelf that holds the drug (manufactured by Apex Medical Corp.). The child drinks normally, and the tablet is carried to the back of the throat. For children who must take solid oral medication for an extended period, training sessions using progressively larger candy to teach the child to swallow can be beneficial (Funk, Mullins, and Olson, 1984).

Since pediatric doses often require dividing adult preparations of medication, the nurse may be faced with the dilemma of accurate dosage. With tablets, only those that are scored can be halved or quartered accurately. If the medication is soluble, the tablet or contents of a capsule can be mixed in a small, premeasured amount of liquid and the appropriate portion given. If half a dose is required, the tablet is dissolved in 5 ml of water and 2.5 ml is given.

Administration

While administering liquids to infants is relatively easy, care must be observed to prevent aspiration. With the infant held in a semireclining position, the medication is placed in the mouth from a spoon, plastic cup, plastic dropper, or plastic syringe (without needle). The dropper or syringe is best placed along the side of the infant's tongue and administered slowly in small amounts, waiting for the child to swallow between deposits. To encourage swallowing, see Nursing Tip.

Medicine cups can be used effectively for older infants who are able to drink from a cup. Because of the natural outward tongue thrust in infancy, medications may need to be retrieved from lips or chin and refed. Allowing the infant to suck the medication that has been placed in an empty nipple or inserting the syringe or dropper into the side of the mouth, parallel to the nipple, while the infant nurses are other convenient methods for giving liquid medications to infants. Medication is not added to the infant's formula feeding.

The young child who refuses to cooperate or resists consistently despite explanation and encouragement may require mild physical coercion. If so, it is carried out quickly and carefully. Every effort is made to determine why the child resists, and the reasons for this alternative are explained in such a way that the child will know that it is being carried out for his or her well-being and is not a form of punishment. There is always a risk in using even mild forceful techniques. A crying child can aspirate a medication, particularly when lying on the back. If the nurse holds the

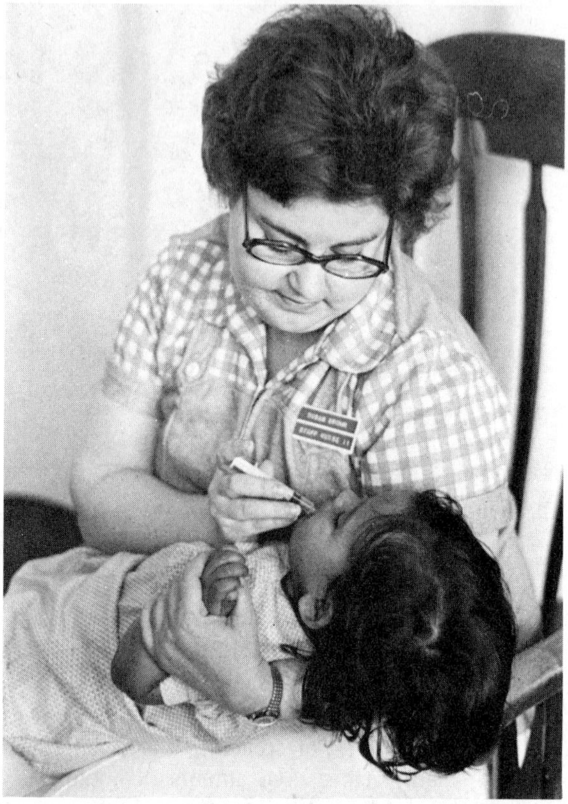

Fig. 27-21. Nurse partially restrains child for easy and comfortable administration of oral medication.

child in the lap with the child's right arm behind the nurse, the left hand firmly grasped by the nurse's left hand, and the head securely restrained between the nurse's arm and body, the medication can be slowly poured into the mouth (Fig. 27-21).

INTRAMUSCULAR ADMINISTRATION

Injections, including intramuscular (IM), intradermal, subcutaneous, and intravenous (IV), constitute some of the most traumatic health-related experiences for children. No one likes an injection, especially young children, who may associate the procedure with other meanings such as fear of body mutilation and punishment. At times it can be no less stressful to the nurse who must inflict the distress. Consequently, injections are given only when the drug cannot be given by any other route. Because many drugs are given intramuscularly, this section is devoted to IM injections.

Selecting Syringe and Needle

The volume of medication prescribed for small children and the small amount of tissue for injection require that a syringe be selected that can measure very small amounts of solution. For volumes less than 1 ml, the tuberculin syringe, calibrated in one-hundredth increments, is appropriate. Very minute doses may require the use of a 0.5 ml, low-dose syringe. These syringes with specially constructed needles minimize the possibility of inadvertently administering incorrect amounts of a drug because of dead space, which allows fluid to remain in the syringe and needle after the plunger is pushed completely forward. A minimum of 0.2 ml of solution remains in a standard needle hub; therefore when very small amounts of two drugs are combined in the syringe, such as mixtures of insulin, the ratio of the two drugs can be altered significantly (Wong, 1982).

Dead space is also an important factor to consider when injecting medication, since flushing the syringe with an air bubble or parenteral fluid adds an additional amount of medication to the prescribed dose. This can be hazardous when very small amounts of a drug are given. For example, a tuberculin syringe filled to the 0.05 ml mark can deliver *more than twice* the calculated dose of medication when it is flushed with parenteral fluid from an IV line. This has resulted in overadministration of digoxin, a drug with a narrow margin of safety between therapeutic and toxic dose (Berman and others, 1978).

Consequently flushing is not recommended, especially when less than 1 ml of medication is given. Syringes are calibrated to deliver a prescribed drug dose, and the amount of medication left in the hub and needle is not part of the syringe barrel calibrations. However, the air-bubble technique (drawing up about 0.2 ml of air into the syringe after withdrawing the medication) may be beneficial with certain drugs, such as iron dextran and diphtheria and tetanus toxoid, to avoid tracking the drug through the tissue (Chaplin, Shull, and Welk, 1985). Other techniques to minimize tracking include changing the needle after withdrawing the fluid from the vial and using the Z track method.

The needle length must be sufficient to penetrate the subcutaneous tissue and deposit the medication into the body of the muscle. Limited research is available on adequate needle length for children. One study found that a 1-inch needle is necessary to adequately penetrate the vastus lateralis muscle in 4-month-old infants and probably is needed for 2-month-old infants (Hicks and others, 1989). Some suggestions for estimating needle length are provided in the Nursing Tips. Needle gauge should be as small as possible to deliver the fluid safely. Small gauges (25 to 30) cause the least discomfort, but larger sizes are needed for viscous medication and when longer length needles are used (to prevent accidental bending).

NURSING TIPS: NEEDLE LENGTH

To estimate needle length for IM injection, first grasp lateralis or deltoid muscle and choose needle length that is approximately half the distance between thumb and index finger.

With ventrogluteal or dorsogluteal site, only subcutaneous tissue is grasped, so choose needle length that is slightly more than half the distance.

Choose a final needle length that allows for small portion of needle to be exposed at skin surface as precaution if needle should break off from hub (Lenz, 1983).

Determining Site

Factors that are considered when selecting a site for an IM injection on an infant or child include:

- The amount and character of the medication to be injected
- The amount and general condition of the muscle mass
- The frequency or number of injections to be given during the course of treatment
- The type of medication being given
- Factors that may impede access to or cause contamination of the site
- The ability of the child to assume the required position safely

Older children and adolescents usually pose few problems in selecting a suitable site for IM injections, but infants, with their small and underdeveloped muscles, have fewer available sites. It is sometimes difficult to assess the amount of fluid that can be safely injected into a single site. Usually 1 ml is the maximum volume that should be administered in a single site to small children and older infants. The muscles of small infants may not tolerate more than 0.5 ml. As the child approaches adult size, volumes approaching those given to adults may be used. However, the larger the amount of solution, the larger must be the muscle into which it is injected.

Injections must be placed in muscles large enough to accommodate the medication, but major nerves and blood vessels must be avoided. There is no universal agreement regarding the best IM injection site for children. The preferred site for infants is the vastus lateralis. General recommendations for using the gluteal sites are after children have been walking (length of suggested time varies but is usually a minimum of 1 year after walking), since the muscle develops with locomotion. Unfortunately, this recommendation is often applied to the ventrogluteal muscle site as well as the dorsogluteal site. However, there are significant differences between these two sites that warrant recognition. The ventrogluteal site is relatively free of major nerves and blood vessels, is a relatively large muscle with less subcutaneous tissue than the dorsal site, has well-defined landmarks for safe site location, and is easily accessible in several positions (Beecroft and Redick, 1990; Intramuscular injections, 1985). These advantages make it a preferred site over the dorsogluteal muscle and challenge the recommendation that the ventrogluteal site not be used until children have been walking. The deltoid muscle, a small muscle near the axillary and radial nerves, can be used for small volumes of fluid in children as young as 18 months of age. Its advantages are less pain and fewer side effects from the injectate (as observed with immunizations) as compared with the vastus lateralis (Ipp and others, 1989). Table 27-4 summarizes the four major injection sites and illustrates the location of the preferred IM injection sites for children.

Administration

Although injections that are executed with care seldom produce trauma to the child, there have been reports of serious disability related to IM injections in children. Repeated use of a single site has been associated with fibrosis of the muscle with subsequent muscle contracture. Injections close to large nerves, such as the sciatic nerve, have been responsible for permanent disability, especially when potentially neurotoxic drugs are administered. There are several reports of tissue damage from penicillin; one of the difficulties in administering the opaque preparations, such as Bicillin, is that aspirated blood cannot be detected at the bottom of the syringe, thus increasing the risk of injecting into a blood vessel. When such drugs are injected, great care must be used in locating the correct site. When aspirating, the nurse should look for blood at the *top* of the syringe near the plunger, since blood may be drawn up through the column of penicillin (Stoller and Losey, 1985).

A reported potential hazard with medication in glass ampules is the presence of glass particles in the ampule after the container is broken. When the medication is withdrawn into the syringe, the glass particles are also withdrawn and are subsequently injected into the patient. As a precaution, medication from glass ampules should only be drawn up through a needle with a filter or injected intravenously through a site in the tubing that is distal to an IV filter (Shaw and Lyall, 1985). Other precautions related to proper disposal of the needle are on p. 1211. Safety precautions for administering chemotherapeutic drugs are discussed in Chapter 36.

Most children are unpredictable and few are totally cooperative when receiving an injection. Even children who appear to be relaxed and constrained can lose control under the stress of the procedure. It is advisable to have someone available to help restrain the child if needed. Since children often jerk or pull away unexpectedly, it is a good idea to carry an extra capped needle to exchange for a contaminated one so that delay is minimized. The child, even a small one, is told that he or she is receiving an injection, and then the procedure is carried out as quickly and skillfully as possible to avoid prolonging the stressful experience. Delay caused by lengthy explanations, attempts to hide the syringe from sight, or efforts to soothe the child will only serve to increase anxiety. It must be kept in mind that intrusive procedures such as injections are especially anxiety provoking in preschool children and that small children usually associate any assault to the "behind" area with punishment.

Small infants offer little resistance to injections. Although they squirm and may be difficult to hold in position, they can usually be restrained without assistance. The muscle mass of the thigh to be injected is firmly grasped in one hand to stabilize the limb and compress the muscle mass for injection with the other hand. The body of a larger infant can be securely restrained between the nurse's arm and body (Fig. 27-22).

If medication is given around the clock, the nurse must be careful to wake the child before giving the injection. Although it may seem easier to surprise the sleeping child and do it as quickly as possible, performing the procedure in this way can cause the child to fear going back to sleep. If awakened first, children will know that nothing will be done to them unless forewarned. Box 27-11 summarizes ad-

Table 27-4 Intramuscular injection sites in children

SITE | **DISCUSSION**

VASTUS LATERALIS

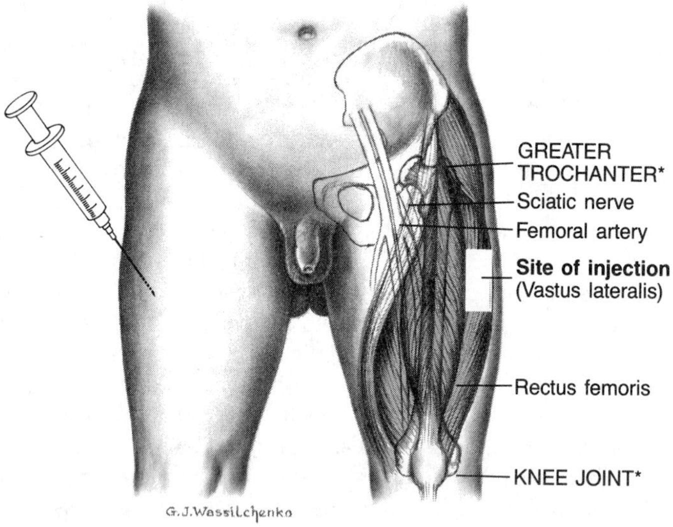

Location*

Palpate to find greater trochanter and knee joints; divide vertical distance between these two landmarks into quadrants; inject into middle of upper quadrant.

Needle insertion and size

Insert needle at 45-degree angle toward knee in infants and in young children or needle perpendicular to thigh or slightly angled toward anterior thigh.

22 to 25 gauge, ⅝ to 1 inch†

Advantages

Large, well-developed muscle that can tolerate larger quantities of fluid (0.5 ml [infant] to 2.0 ml [child])

No important nerves or blood vessels in this location

Easily accessible if child is supine, side lying, or sitting

A tourniquet can be applied above injection site to delay drug hypersensitivity reaction if necessary

Disadvantages

Thrombosis of femoral artery from injection in midthigh area

Sciatic nerve damage from long needle injected posteriorly and medially into small extremity

VENTROGLUTEAL

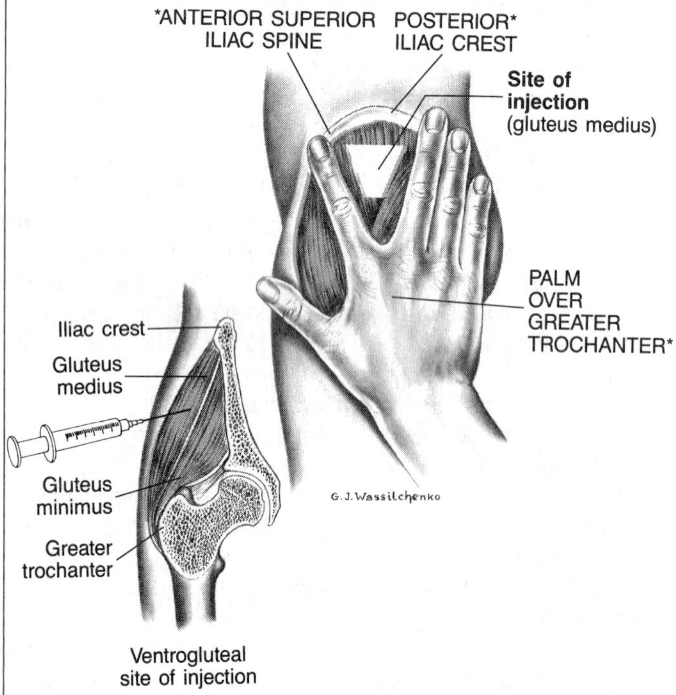

Location*

Palpate to locate greater trochanter, anterior superior iliac tubercle (found by flexing thigh at hip and measuring up to 1 to 2 cm above crease formed in groin), and posterior iliac crest; place palm of hand over greater trochanter, index finger over anterior superior iliac tubercle, and middle finger along crest of ilium posteriorly as far as possible; inject into center of V formed by fingers.

Needle insertion and size

Insert needle perpendicular to site but angled slightly toward iliac crest.

22 to 25 gauge, ½ to 1 inch

Advantages

Free of important nerves and vascular structures

Easily identified by prominent bony landmarks

Thinner layer of subcutaneous tissue than in dorsogluteal site, thus less chance of depositing drug subcutaneously rather than intramuscularly

Can accommodate larger quantities of fluid (0.5 ml [infant] to 2.0 ml [child])

Easily accessible if child is supine, prone, or side lying

Less painful than vastus lateralis

Disadvantages

Health professionals' unfamiliarity with site

Not suitable for use of a tourniquet

*Locations are indicated by asterisks on illustrations.

†Research has shown that a 1-inch needle is needed for adequate muscle penetration in infants 4 months old and possibly in infants as young as 2 months (Hicks, and others, 1989). Other recommendations for needle size and volume of fluid are based on traditional practice and have not been verified by research.

Table 27-4 Intramuscular injection sites in children—cont'd

SITE | **DISCUSSION**

DORSOGLUTEAL

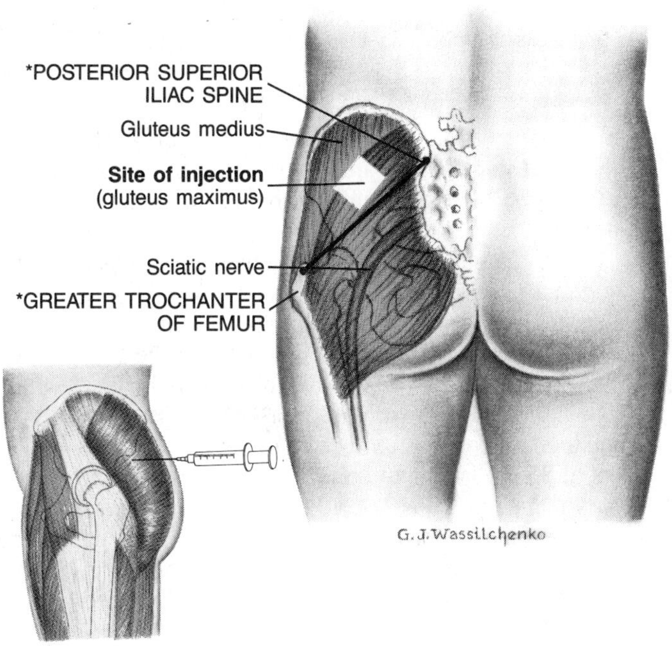

Location*
Locate greater trochanter and posterior superior iliac spine; draw imaginary line between these two points and inject lateral and superior to line into gluteus maximus or medius muscle.

Needle insertion and size
Insert needle perpendicular to surface on which child is lying when prone.
20 to 25 gauge, ½ to 1½ inches

Advantages
In older child, large muscle mass; well-developed muscle can tolerate greater volume of fluid (up to 2.0 ml)
Child does not see needle and syringe
Easily accessible if child is prone or side lying

Disadvantages
Contraindicated in children who have not been walking for at least 1 year
Danger of injury to sciatic nerve
Thick, subcutaneous fat, predisposing to deposition of drug subcutaneously rather than intramuscularly
Not suitable for use of a tourniquet
Inaccessible if child is supine
Exposure of site may cause embarrassment in older child

DELTOID

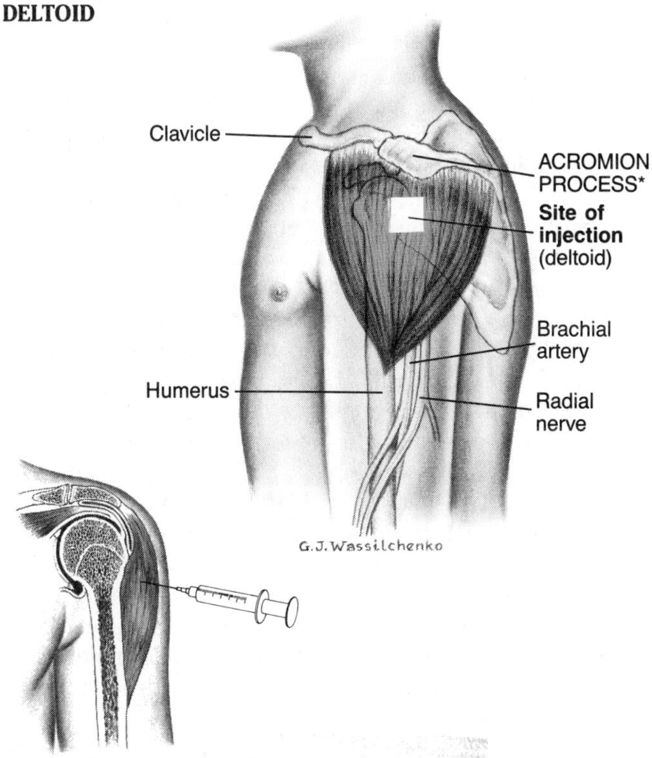

Location*
Locate acromion process; inject only into upper third of muscle that begins about 2 fingerbreadths below acromion.

Needle insertion and size
Insert needle perpendicular to site but angled slightly toward shoulder.
22 to 25 gauge, ½ to 1 inch

Advantages
Faster absorption rates than gluteal sites
Tourniquet can be applied above injection site
Easily accessible with minimum removal of clothing
Less pain and fewer local side effects from vaccines as compared with vastus lateralis

Disadvantages
Small muscle mass; only limited amounts of drug can be injected (0.5 to 1.0 ml)
Small margins of safety with possible damage to radial nerve and axillary nerve (not shown, lies under deltoid at head of humerus)

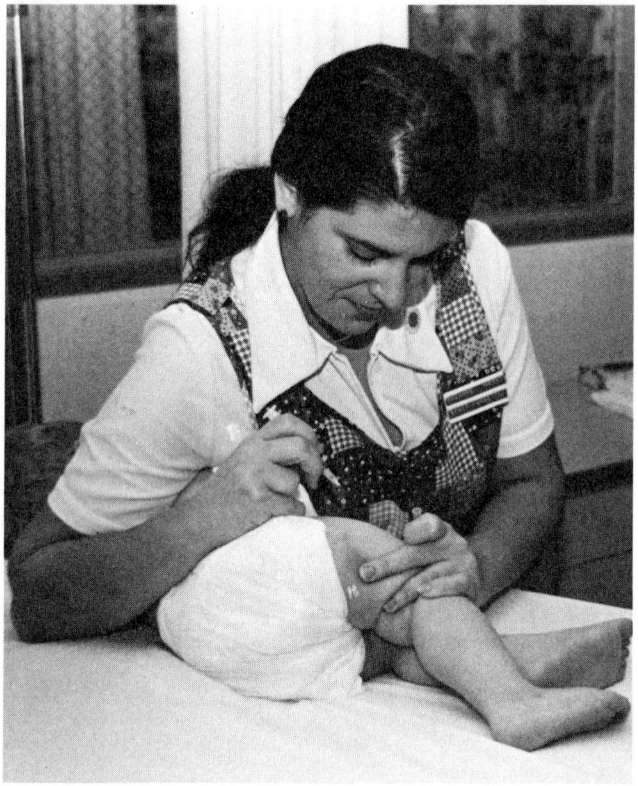

Fig. 27-22. Restraining small child for intramuscular injection. Note how nurse isolates and stabilizes muscle.

ministration techniques that maximize safety and minimize the discomfort often associated with injections.

INTRAVENOUS ADMINISTRATION*

The IV route for administering medications is frequently used in pediatric therapy. For some important drugs it is the only effective route of administration. This method is used for giving drugs to children who have poor absorption as a result of diarrhea, dehydration, or peripheral vascular collapse; children who need a high serum concentration of a drug; children who have resistant infections that require parenteral medication over an extended time; children who need continuous pain relief; and children who require emergency treatment.

Insertion sites and observation of the IV infusion are discussed in Chapter 28 under Parenteral Fluid Therapy and Long-Term Venous Access. However, several factors need to be considered in relation to IV medication. When a drug is administered intravenously, the effect is almost instantaneous and further control is limited. Most drugs for IV administration require a specified minimum dilution and/or rate of flow, and many are highly irritating or toxic to tissues outside the vascular system. In addition to the precautions and nursing observations related to IV therapy, factors to consider when preparing and administering drugs to infants and children by the IV route include:

- Amount of drug to be administered
- Minimum dilution of drug and if child is fluid restricted
- Type of solution in which drug can be diluted
- Length of time over which drug can be safely administered
- Rate of infusion that child and vessels can tolerate
- IV tubing volume capacity
- Time that this or another drug is to be administered
- Compatibility of all drugs that child is receiving intravenously and compatibility with infusion fluids

Before any IV infusion, the site of insertion is checked for patency. Medications are never administered with blood products. Only one antibiotic should be administered at a time.

When a drug is to be administered within a specific time, such as 1 hour, the infusion rate should take into account the volume of fluid in the tubing from the injection point that must infuse before the drug reaches the bloodstream. For example, if a drug is added to 10 ml in the gravity drainage apparatus (e.g., Volutrol, Burette, Soluset, Metriset) and the tubing contains 10 ml of fluid, the infusion rate must be set at 20 drops/minute (microdropper) or 20 ml/hour (infusion pump) (to infuse the 10 ml in the tubing and the 10 ml in the Volutrol) for all the medication to enter the bloodstream in 1 hour. Therefore the rate must always be considered to ensure that the entire dose is administered over the desired time.

For accuracy, the nurse must verify the correct tubing volume for the manufacturer brand and the types of tubing used for the infusion. For example, an extension tubing added to a primary line may have a tubing volume of 3 ml, which must be added to the total tubing volume. Guidelines for calculating the IV rate to infuse medications are presented in Box 27-12.

The method in Box 27-12 is suitable for children who can tolerate the necessary infusion rate and the extra fluid needed to administer the medication. For the very small infant or fluid-restricted child who is not able to tolerate the increased rate or fluids, other IV methods available are the direct technique and the retrograde technique. Although the medication must still be minimally diluted as recommended, the dose is administered closer to the child's vein, avoiding the need to also infuse the tubing volume.

For the *direct technique,* appropriately diluted medication is injected into the tubing at the site of the Y connection or through a stopcock in the direction of the child. A syringe pump may be used for a controlled rate. As syringe pumps become increasingly available, this method is being used more often for pediatric patients because of convenience, greater control over administration time, and the need to flush with less fluid when administering medications.

For the *retrograde technique,* appropriately diluted medication is injected into the IV tubing at the site of the Y connection or a stopcock, in the direction away from (retrograde) the child. The tubing is clamped, or the stopcock to the child is turned off. After the medication is injected, the

*Dorothy C. Blome, R.N.,C., M.N., assisted in the revision of this section.

Box 27-11 GUIDELINES FOR INTRAMUSCULAR ADMINISTRATION OF MEDICATION

Use safety precautions in administering medication (e.g., check child's identification).
Prepare medication.
- Select needle and syringe appropriate to the following:
  - Amount of fluid to be administered (syringe size)
  - Viscosity of fluid to be administered (needle gauge)
  - Amount of tissue to be penetrated (needle length)
- Maximum volume to be administered in a single site is 1 ml for older infants and small children.

Determine the site of injection (see Table 27-4); make certain muscle is large enough to accommodate volume and type of medication.
- Older children: select site as with adult patient; allow child some choice of site, if feasible.
- Following are acceptable sites for infants and small or debilitated children:
  - Vastus lateralis muscle
  - Ventrogluteal muscle
- Dorsogluteal muscle is insufficiently developed to be a safe site for infants and small children.

Administer medication.
- Provide for sufficient help in restraining child; children are often uncooperative, and their behavior is usually unpredictable.
- Explain briefly what is to be done and, if appropriate, what child can do to help.
- Expose injection area for unobstructed view of landmarks.
- Select a site where skin is free of irritation and danger of infection; palpate for and avoid sensitive or hardened areas. With multiple injections, rotate sites.
- Place child in a lying or sitting position; child is not allowed to stand because:
  - Landmarks are more difficult to assess.
  - Restraint is more difficult.
  - Child may faint and fall.
- Use a new, sharp needle with smallest diameter that permits free flow of the medication.
- Grasp muscle firmly between thumb and fingers to isolate and stabilize muscle for deposition of drug in its deepest part; in obese children, spread skin with thumb and index finger to displace subcutaneous tissue and grasp muscle deeply on each side.
- Allow skin preparation to dry completely before skin is penetrated.
- Have medication at room temperature.
- Decrease perception of pain:
  - Distract child with conversation.
  - Give child something on which to concentrate (e.g., squeezing a hand or bed rail, pinching own nose, humming, counting, yelling "Ouch!").
  - Place a cold compress or wrapped ice cube on site about a minute before injection, or apply cold to contralateral site.
  - Say to child, "If you feel this, tell me to take it out, please."
  - Have child hold a small Band-Aid and place it on puncture site after IM injection is given.
- Insert needle quickly, using a dartlike motion.
- Avoid tracking any medication through superficial tissues:
  - Replace needle after withdrawing medication, or wipe medication from needle with sterile gauze.
  - If withdrawing medication from an ampule, use a needle equipped with a filter that removes glass particles; then use a new, nonfilter needle for injection.
  - Use the Z track and/or air-bubble technique as indicated.
  - Avoid any depression of the plunger during insertion of the needle.
- Aspirate for blood.
  - If blood is found, remove syringe from site, change needle, and reinsert into new location.
  - If no blood is found, inject into a relaxed muscle:
    - Dorsogluteal—place child on abdomen with legs and toes rotated inward.
    - Ventrogluteal—place child on side with upper leg flexed and placed in front of lower leg.
- Inject medication slowly (over 20 seconds).
- Remove needle quickly; hold gauze sponge firmly against skin near needle when removing it to avoid pulling on tissue.
- Apply firm pressure to site after injection; massage site to hasten absorption unless contraindicated, as with irritating drugs and heparin.
- Place a small Band-Aid on puncture site; with young children decorate Band-Aid by drawing a smiling face or other symbol of acceptance.
- Hold and cuddle young child and encourage parents to comfort child; praise older child.
- Allow expression of feelings.

Discard syringe and uncapped, uncut needle in puncture-resistant container located near site of use.
Record time of injection, drug, dose, and injection site.

tubing is unclamped or the stopcock opened, and the infusion resumes, with subsequent administration of the medication. The rate may still need to be adjusted using the formula in Box 27-12 to deliver the medication in the specified time. This method does result in displacement of the fluid in the IV tubing, since the diluted medication is injected retrogradely. This fluid can be accommodated by an empty drip chamber (but not more than 3 ml), or by an empty syringe connected to an upper Y site or stopcock, which will accept the displaced fluid for discard. If the empty syringe method is used, the tubing volume between the two Y sites or stopcocks must be greater than the amount of diluted medication volume injected to avoid the medication reaching the discard syringe.

NURSING ALERT An often unrecognized source of contamination for vascular access lines (peripheral and central) is stopcock ports. Unaccessed ports should be covered at all times with a sterile cap or syringe, which is changed if contaminated during access for medication administration or blood collection (Brosnan and others, 1988).

Regardless of the technique used, the nurse must know the minimum dilutions for safe administration of IV medications to infants and children. In the example in Box 27-12 of ampicillin 500 mg, the recommended minimum dilution is 50 mg/1 ml. Therefore, for a 500 mg dose, the ratio would be:

Box 27-12 GUIDELINES FOR CALCULATING IV INFUSION RATE FOR MEDICATION ADMINISTRATION IN CHILDREN

General Formula

$$\text{Rate} = \text{Volume to be infused} \times \frac{\text{Drop factor of administration set}}{\text{Desired time to infuse in minutes}}$$

Volume to be infused includes diluted medication volume added to the volume control chamber *plus* tubing volume (e.g., 12 ml)

Drop factor of administration set (e.g., 60 drops/minute) for a microdrop (pediatric) set

Desired time to infuse in minutes (e.g., 15, 30, or 60 minutes)

Example

Determine the rate to administer ampicillin 500 mg IV over 30 minutes. The medication is diluted as recommended in 10 ml in the volume control chamber of a set that has a tubing volume of 12 ml.

Volume to be infused = 10 ml (diluted ampicillin) + 12 ml (tubing volume) = 22

Drop factor of administration set = 60

Desired time to infuse in minutes = 30

$$\text{Rate of infusion} = 22 \times \frac{60}{30} = 44 \text{ ml/hour}$$

Adjust the IV infusion rate to 44 ml/hour to deliver the tubing volume, medication volume, and the "flush" volume (an amount equal to the tubing volume added after the medication volume empties from the volume control chamber) until the flush reaches the child, clearing the tubing of medication.

After a total time of 30 minutes, the dose is completed; readjust the IV rate to the originally ordered rate.

$$\frac{50 \text{ mg}}{1 \text{ ml}} = \frac{500 \text{ mg}}{x}$$

After solving the equation, the acceptable minimum dilution is 10 ml.

Several other methods of long-term venous access are available and include the heparin lock device, central venous catheters, and implanted infusion ports (see Chapter 28, Long-Term Venous Access).

NASOGASTRIC, OROGASTRIC, OR GASTROSTOMY ADMINISTRATION

When a child has an indwelling feeding tube or a gastrostomy, oral medications are usually given via that route. An advantage of this method is the ability to administer oral medications around the clock without disturbing the child. A disadvantage is the risk of occluding or "clogging" the tube, especially when giving viscous solutions through small-bore feeding tubes. The most important preventive measure is adequate flushing after the medication is instilled (Leff and Roberts, 1988; Williams, 1989). See Box 27-13 for guidelines for administration.

Box 27-13 GUIDELINES FOR NASOGASTRIC, OROGASTRIC, OR GASTROSTOMY MEDICATION ADMINISTRATION IN CHILDREN

Use elixir or suspension (rather than syrup) preparations of medication whenever possible.

If administering tablets, crush tablet to a very fine powder and dissolve drug in a small amount of warm water.
- Never crush enteric-coated or sustained-release tablets or capsules.

Avoid oily medications because they tend to cling to side of tube.

Dilute viscous medication if possible.

Do not mix medication with enteral formula unless fluid is restricted. If adding a drug:
- Check with pharmacist for compatibility.
- Shake formula well and observe for any physical reaction (e.g., separation, precipitation).
- Label formula container with name of medication, dosage, date, and time infusion started.

Have medication at room temperature.

Measure medication in calibrated cup.

Check for correct placement of nasogastric or orogastric tube.

Attach syringe (with adaptable tip but without plunger) to tube.

Pour medication into syringe.

Unclamp tube and allow medication to flow by gravity.

Adjust height of container to achieve desired flow rate (e.g., increase height for faster flow).

As soon as syringe is empty, pour in water to flush tubing.
- Amount of water depends on length and gauge of tubing.
- Determine amount before administering any medication by using a syringe to completely fill an unused nasogastric or orogastric tube with water. The amount of flush solution is usually $1\frac{1}{2}$ times this volume.
- With certain drug preparations (e.g., suspensions) more fluid may be needed.

If administering more than one drug at the same time, flush the tube between each medication with clear water.

Clamp tube after flushing, unless tube is left open.

RECTAL ADMINISTRATION

The rectal route for administration is less reliable but sometimes used when the oral route is difficult or contraindicated. Some of the drugs available in suppository form are aspirin, sedatives, analgesics (morphine), and antiemetics. The difficulty in using the rectal route is that, unless the rectal ampulla is empty at the time of insertion, the absorption of the drug may be delayed, diminished, or prevented by the presence of feces. Sometimes the drug is later evacuated, securely surrounded by stool. However, the rectal route is used most frequently in children who are unable to take anything by mouth and are unlikely to have large amounts of stool. It is also used when oral preparations are unsuitable to control vomiting.

The wrapping on the suppository is removed, and the suppository is lubricated with water-soluble jelly or warm water. Using a glove or finger cot, the suppository is quickly but gently inserted into the rectum, making certain that it is placed beyond both the rectal sphincters. The buttocks are then held or taped together firmly to relieve pressure on the anal sphincter until the urge to expel the suppository has passed—5 to 10 minutes. Sometimes the amount of drug ordered is less than the dosage available. The irregular shape of most suppositories makes the process of dividing them into a desired dose difficult if not dangerous. If it must be halved, it should be cut lengthwise. However, there is no guarantee that the drug is evenly dispersed throughout the petrolatum base.

If medication is administered via a retention enema, the same procedure is used. Drugs given by enema are diluted in the smallest amount of solution possible to minimize the likelihood of being evacuated.

OPTIC, OTIC, AND NASAL ADMINISTRATION

There are few differences in administering eye, ear, and nose medication to children and to adults. The major difficulty is in gaining children's cooperation or employing restraining techniques. The infant's or young child's head is immobilized in the same manner as described in Fig. 7-33. Older children need only explanation and direction. Although the administration of optic, otic, and nasal medication is not painful, these drugs can cause unpleasant sensations, which can be eliminated with various techniques (see Nursing Tips).

To instill eye medication, the child is placed supine or sitting with the head extended and is asked to look up. One hand is used to pull the lower lid downward; the hand that holds the dropper rests on the head so that it may move synchronously with the child's head, thus reducing the possibility of trauma to a struggling child or dropping medication on the face (Fig. 27-23). As the lower lid is pulled down, a small conjunctival sac is formed; the solution or ointment is applied to this area, never directly on the eyeball. Another effective technique is to pull the lower lid down and out to form a cup effect, into which the medication is dropped.

NURSING TIPS: EYE/EAR/NOSE DROPS

To reduce unpleasant sensations:

- **Eye:** Apply finger pressure to the lacrimal punctum at the inner aspect of the lid for 1 minute to prevent drainage of medication to the nasopharynx and the unpleasant "tasting" of the drug.
- **Ear:** Allow medications stored in the refrigerator to warm to room temperature before instillation.
- **Nose:** Position the child with the head hyperextended to prevent strangling sensations caused by medication trickling into the throat rather than up into the nasal passages.

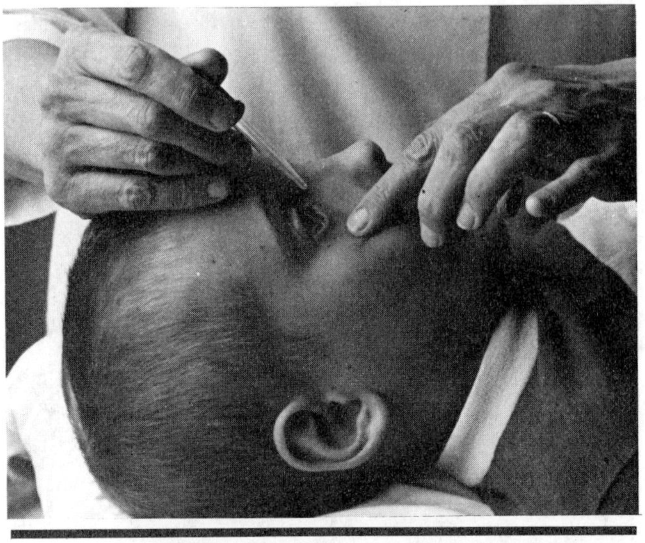

Fig. 27-23. Administering eye drops.

The lids are gently closed to prevent expression of the medication, and the child is asked to look in all directions to enhance even distribution of the preparation. Excess medication is wiped from the inner canthus outward to prevent contamination to the contralateral eye.

Instilling eye drops in infants can be difficult because they often clench the lids tightly closed. One approach is to place the drops in the nasal corner where the lids meet. The medication pools in this area, and when the child opens the lids, the medication flows onto the conjunctiva. For young children, playing a game can be helpful, such as instructing the child to keep the eyes closed until the count of 3, then to open them, at which time the drops are quickly instilled. Ointment can be applied when the child is sleeping by gently pulling down the lower lid and placing the ointment in the lower conjunctival sac.

✦ **NURSING ALERT** If both eye ointment and drops are ordered, give drops first, wait 3 minutes, then apply the ointment to allow each drug to work. When possible, administer eye ointments before bedtime or naptime, since the child's vision will be blurred for a while.

Ear drops are instilled with the child restrained in the supine position and the head turned to the appropriate side. For children younger than 3 years of age, the external auditory canal is straightened by gently pulling the pinna downward and straight back. The pinna is pulled upward and back in children older than 3 years of age (see Fig. 7-28). To advance the drops into the ear canal without contaminating the tip of the dropper, place a disposable ear speculum in the canal and administer the drops through the speculum. After instillation, the child should remain lying on the opposite side for a few minutes. Gentle massage of the area immediately anterior to the ear facilitates the entry of drops into the ear canal. The use of cotton pledgets pre-

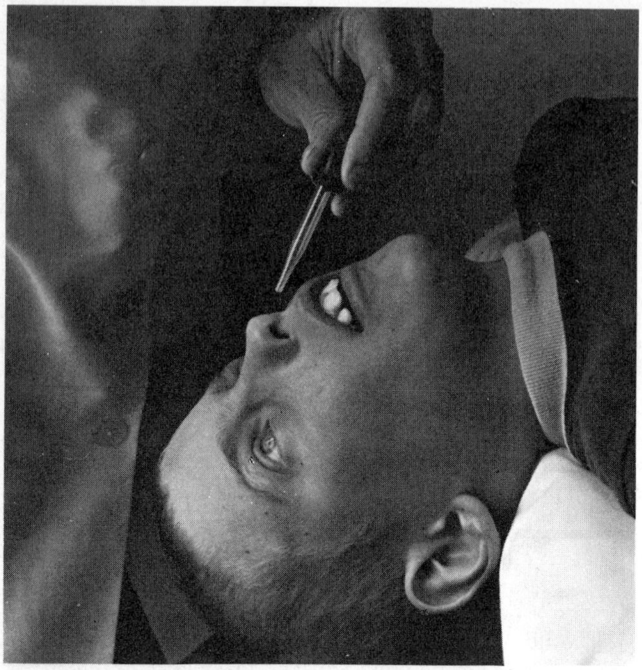

Fig. 27-24. Proper position for instilling nose drops.

vents medication from flowing out of the external canal. However, they should be loose enough to allow any discharge to exit from the ear. Premoistening the cotton with a few drops of medication prevents the wicking action from absorbing the medication instilled in the ear.

Nose drops are instilled in the same manner as in the adult patient. Unpleasant sensations associated with medicated nose drops are minimized when care is taken to position the child with the head extended well over the edge of the bed or a pillow (Fig. 27-24). Depending on their size, infants can be positioned in the football hold (see Fig. 27-8), in the nurse's arm with the head extended and stabilized between the nurse's body and elbow and the arms and hands immobilized with the nurse's hands, or with the head extended over the edge of the bed or a pillow. Following instillation of the drops, the child should remain in position for 1 minute to allow the drops to come in contact with the nasal surfaces.

FAMILY TEACHING AND HOME CARE

The nurse usually assumes the responsibility for preparing families to administer medications at home. The family should have an understanding of why the child is receiving the medication and the effects that might be expected, as well as the amount, frequency, and length of time the drug is to be administered. Instruction should be carried out in an unhurried, relaxed manner, preferably in an area away from busy ward or office routine, following the same guidelines for teaching outlined in Box 27-7.

The caregiver is carefully instructed regarding the correct dosage, and the nurse is responsible for preparing parents for the specifics of the task. Some persons have difficulty in understanding or interpreting terminology from the pharmacy, and just because they nod or otherwise indicate an understanding, it cannot be assumed that the message is clear. It is important to ascertain their interpretation of a teaspoon, for example, and to be certain they have acceptable devices for measuring the drug. If the drug is packaged with a dropper, syringe, or plastic cup, the nurse should show the point on the device that indicates the prescribed dose and demonstrate how the dose is drawn up into a dropper or syringe and measured and the bubbles eliminated. If the nurse has any doubts about the parent's ability to administer the correct dose, the parent should give a return demonstration. This is especially important when the drug has potentially serious consequences from incorrect dosage, such as insulin or digoxin, or when more complex administration is required, such as parenteral injections. When teaching a parent to give an injection, adequate time for instruction and practice must be allotted.

Home modifications are often necessary because the availability of equipment or assistance can differ from the hospital setting. For example, restraint is often required when giving medications to children, and the parent may need guidance in devising methods that allow for one person to restrain the child and safely give the drug. One successful method is described in the Nursing Tip on one-person restraint.

The time that the drug is to be administered is clarified with the parent. For instance, when a drug is prescribed in

NURSING TIP: ONE-PERSON RESTRAINT

To administer oral, nasal, or optic medication when only one person is available to restrain the child, use the following procedure:

- Place child supine on flat surface (bed, couch, floor).
- Sit facing child so that child's head is between operator's thighs and child's arms are under operator's legs.
- Place lower legs over child's legs to restrain lower body, if necessary.
- To administer oral medication, place small pillow under child's head to reduce risk of aspiration.
- To administer nasal medication, place small pillow under child's shoulders to aid flow of liquid through nasal passages.

NURSING TIP: COLOR-CODED MEDICATION INSTRUCTIONS

If parents have difficulty reading or understanding English, use colors to convey instructions. For example, mark each drug with a color and place the appropriate color on a calendar chart or on a drawing of a clock to identify when the drug needs to be given.

association with meals, the number of meals that the family is accustomed to eat influences the amount of drug the child receives. Do they have meals twice a day or five times a day? When a drug is to be given several times during the day, together the nurse and parents can work out a schedule that accommodates the family routine. This is particularly significant if the drug must be given at equal intervals throughout a 24-hour period. For example, telling them that the child needs 1 teaspoon of medicine four times a day is subject to misinterpretation, since parents may routinely schedule the doses at incorrect times. Instead, a preplanned schedule based on 6-hour intervals should be set up with the number of days required for therapeutic dosage listed. Written instruction should accompany all drug prescriptions* (see Nursing Tip on instructions).

GASTRIC FEEDING TECHNIQUES

Some children are unable to take nourishment by mouth because of conditions such as anomalies of the throat, esophagus, or bowel; impaired swallowing capacity; severe debilitation; respiratory distress; or unconsciousness. These children are frequently fed by way of a tube inserted orally or nasally to the stomach (orogastric or nasogastric gavage) or duodenum/jejunum (enteral gavage) or by a tube inserted directly into the stomach (gastrostomy) or jejunum (jejunostomy). Such feedings may be intermittent or by continuous drip. Although the newer small-bore tubes may be used for enteral feedings, the following discussion is limited to gastric gavage and gastrostomy. Feeding resistance, a problem that may result from any long-term feeding method that bypasses the mouth, is discussed in Chapter 10. During nonoral feedings, infants are given a pacifier. Nonnutritive sucking has been shown to have several advantages, such as increased weight gain and decreased crying (Anderson, 1986). However, only pacifiers with a safe design must be used to prevent the possibility of aspiration. Using improvised pacifiers made from bottle nipples is not a safe practice.

When a child is concurrently receiving continuous-drip gastric or enteral feedings and parenteral (intravenous) therapy, the potential exists for inadvertent administration of the enteral formula through the circulatory system. The possibility for error increases when the parenteral solution is a fat emulsion, a milky appearing substance. Safeguards to prevent this potentially serious error include (Garvin and Franck, 1989):

- Use a separate, specifically designed enteral feeding pump mounted on a separate pole for continuous-feeding solutions.
- Label all tubing for continuous enteral feeding with brightly colored tape or labels.
- Use specifically designed continuous-feeding bags to contain the solutions instead of parenteral equipment, such as a burette.

*Home care instructions on giving medications are available in Wong, D.L., and Whaley, L.F.: Clinical manual of pediatric nursing, ed. 3, St. Louis, 1990, Mosby–Year Book, Inc.

GAVAGE FEEDING

Infants and children can be fed simply and safely by a tube passed into the stomach through either the nares or the mouth. The tube can be left in place or inserted and removed with each feeding. In older children it is usually less traumatic to tape the tube securely in place between feedings. When this alternative is used, the tube should be removed and replaced with a new tube according to hospital policy, specific orders, and the type of tube used. Meticulous handwashing is practiced during the procedure to prevent bacterial contamination of the feeding, especially during continuous-drip feedings.

Preparation

The equipment needed for gavage feeding includes:

- A suitable tube selected according to the size of the child and the viscosity of the solution being fed. Feeding tubes are available in silicone rubber, polyurethane, polyethylene, or polyvinylchloride. Polyurethane and silicone rubber tubes are smaller in diameter and more flexible than the others and are often referred to as small-bore tubes.
- A receptacle for the fluid; for small amounts a 10 to 30 ml syringe barrel or Asepto syringe is satisfactory; for larger amounts a 50 ml syringe with a catheter tip is more convenient.
- A syringe to aspirate stomach contents and/or to inject air after the tube has been placed.
- Water or water-soluble lubricant to lubricate the tube; sterile water is used for infants.
- Paper or nonallergenic tape to mark the tube and to attach the tube to the infant's or child's cheek.
- A stethoscope to determine the correct placement in the stomach.
- The solution for feeding.

Not all feeding tubes are the same. Polyethylene and polyvinylchloride types lose their flexibility and need to be replaced frequently, usually every 3 to 4 days. The polyurethane and silicone rubber tubes are indwelling and remain flexible so that they can remain in place longer and afford more patient comfort. Use of these small-bore tubes for continuous feeding has greatly reduced the incidence of complications, such as pharyngitis, otitis media, and incompetence of the lower esophageal sphincter (Wesley, 1988). While the increased softness and flexibility of the tubes are advantages, they also cause disadvantages, such as difficult insertion (may require a stylet, or metal guide wire), collapse of the tube during aspiration of gastric contents to test for correct placement, dislodgment during forceful coughing, and unsuitability for thick feedings (Moore and Green, 1985). Traditional methods for verifying placement are less reliable with the small-bore tubes (Metheny, 1988).

Procedure

Infants will be easier to control if they are first wrapped in a mummy restraint (see Fig. 27-10). Even tiny infants with random movements can grasp and dislodge the tube. Premature infants do not ordinarily require restraint, but if they do, a small towel folded across the chest and secured be-

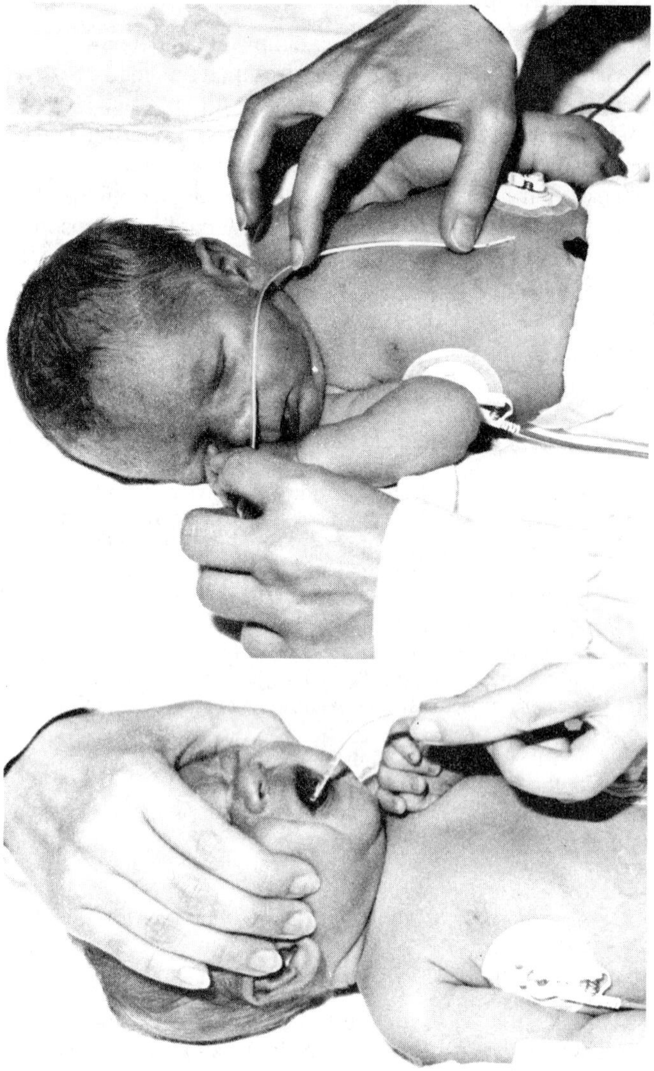

A

B

Fig. 27-25. Gavage feeding. **A,** Measuring tube for orogastric feeding from tip of nose to earlobe and to midpoint between end of xiphoid process and umbilicus. **B,** Inserting the tube.

neath the shoulders is usually sufficient. Care must be taken so that breathing is not compromised.

Whenever possible, the infant should be held during the procedure to associate the comfort of physical contact with the feeding. When this is not possible, gavage feeding is carried out with the infant or child on the back or toward the right side and the head and chest elevated. Feeding the child in a sitting position helps maintain the placement of the tube in the lowest position, thus increasing the likelihood of correct placement in the stomach.

The feeding tube can be passed through either the nose or the mouth. Since most young infants are obligatory nose breathers, insertion through the mouth causes less distress and helps to stimulate sucking. A tube passed through one of the nares in older infants and children is satisfactory once the tube is in place. An indwelling tube is almost always placed through the nose; the tube is alternated between nares with each insertion to minimize irritation, chance of infection, and possible breakdown of mucous membranes from pressure that occurs over time.

Two important issues remain unresolved regarding gavage feeding: measuring the insertion distance and checking the tube placement. Two standard methods of measuring tube length for insertion are (1) measuring from the nose to the bottom of the earlobe and then to the end of the xiphoid process or (2) measuring from the nose to the earlobe and then to a point midway between the xiphoid process and umbilicus (Fig. 27-25, *A*). However, research on using these methods in premature infants has found both placements to be too high (in the esophagus), although the second method provided better placement (Weibley and others, 1987). In a study on children 1 month to 18 years of age, the first method resulted in the *tip* of the tube, but not necessarily the side holes, being in the stomach 90% of the time. In the other 10% of the cases the tip was above the esophageal sphincter (Welch and others, 1990). Until more definitive data are available, no method that results in a shorter distance than these methods should be used.

Unfortunately, "bedside" methods used to verify the placement of the tube have serious shortcomings (Box 27-14). The only accurate method for testing tube placement is radiography, but this practice is not feasible before each feeding (Metheny, 1988). One method that appears promising is pH testing of aspirated fluid, since respiratory, gastric, and intestinal fluid have different pH (Metheny and others, 1989). Until pH is studied further, especially in children, nurses need to use the traditional methods with an awareness of their limitations. If doubt exists regarding correct placement, the physician should be consulted. The procedure for gavage feeding is described in Box 27-14.

GASTROSTOMY FEEDING

Feeding by way of gastrostomy tube is a variation of tube feeding often used for children in whom passage of a tube through the mouth, pharynx, esophagus, and cardiac sphincter of the stomach is contraindicated or impossible. It is also used to avoid the constant irritation of a nasogastric tube in children who require tube feeding over an extended period. Placement of a gastrostomy tube may be performed with the child under general anesthesia or percutaneously using an endoscope and local anesthesia (Nelson and Hallgren, 1989). The tube is inserted through the abdominal wall into the stomach about midway along the greater curvature and secured by a purse-string suture. The stomach is anchored to the peritoneum at the operative site. The tube used can be a Foley, wing-tip, or mushroom catheter. Immediately after surgery the catheter is left open and attached to gravity drainage for 24 hours or more.

Postoperative care of the wound site is directed toward

Box 27-14 GUIDELINES FOR NASOGASTRIC TUBE FEEDINGS IN CHILDREN

Place the child supine with head slightly hyperflexed or in a sniffing position (nose pointed toward ceiling).

Measure the tube for approximate length of insertion, and mark the point with a small piece of tape.

Insert the tube that has been lubricated with sterile water or water-soluble lubricant through either the mouth or one of the nares to the predetermined mark. Since most young infants are obligatory nose breathers, insertion through the mouth causes less distress and helps to stimulate sucking. In older infants and children the tube is passed through the nose and alternated between nostrils. An indwelling tube is almost always placed through the nose.

- When using the nose, slip the tube along the base of the nose and direct it straight back toward the occiput.
- When entering through the mouth, direct the tube toward the back of the throat (Fig. 27-25, *B*).
- If the child is able to swallow on command, synchronize passing the tube with swallowing. (See Nursing Tip: Encouraging Swallowing, p. 1227).

Check the position of the tube by using *both* of the following:

- Attach the syringe to the feeding tube and apply negative pressure. Aspiration of stomach contents indicates proper placement, but aspiration of respiratory secretions may be mistaken for stomach contents. However, absence of fluid is not necessarily evidence of improper placement. The stomach may be empty, or the tube may not be in contact with stomach contents. Note the amount and character of any fluid aspirated and return the fluid to the stomach.
- With the syringe, inject a small amount of air (0.5 to 1 ml in premature or very small infants to 5 ml in larger children) into the tube while simultaneously listening with a stethoscope over the stomach area. Sounds of gurgling or growling will be heard if the tube is properly situated in the stomach, although it is possible to hear the air entering the stomach even when the tube is positioned above the gastroesophageal sphincter.

Stabilize the tube by holding or taping it to the cheek, not to the forehead, because of possible damage to the nostril. To maintain correct placement, measure and record the amount of tubing extending from the nose or mouth to the distal port when the tube is first positioned. Recheck this measurement before each feeding.

Warm the formula to room temperature. Pour formula into the barrel of the syringe attached to the feeding tube. To start the flow, give a gentle push with the plunger, but then remove the plunger and allow the fluid to flow into the stomach by gravity. The rate of flow should not exceed 5 ml every 5 to 10 minutes in premature and very small infants and 10 ml/minute in older infants and children to prevent nausea and regurgitation. The rate is determined by the diameter of the tubing and the height of the reservoir containing the feeding and is regulated by adjusting the height of the syringe. A usual feeding may take from 15 to 30 minutes to complete.

Flush the tube with sterile water (1 or 2 ml for small tubes to 5 ml or more for large ones, or see discussion of flushing for administering medication through nasogastric tubes in Box 27-13 to clear it of formula.

Cap or clamp indwelling tubes to prevent loss of feeding.

- If the tube is to be removed, first pinch it firmly to prevent escape of fluid as the tube is withdrawn. Withdraw the tube quickly.

Position the child on the right side or abdomen for at least 1 hour in the same manner as following any infant feeding to minimize the possibility of regurgitation and aspiration. If the child's condition permits, bubble the youngster after the feeding.

Record the feeding, including the type and amount of residual, the type and amount of formula, and how it was tolerated. For most infant feedings, any amount of residual fluid aspirated from the stomach is refed to prevent electrolyte imbalance, and the amount is subtracted from the prescribed amount of feeding. For example, if the infant is to receive 30 ml and 10 ml is aspirated from the stomach before the feeding, the 10 ml of aspirated stomach contents is refed plus 20 ml of feeding.

prevention of infection and irritation. The area is cleansed and covered with a sterile dressing daily or as often as needed to keep the area dry. After healing occurs, meticulous care is needed to keep the area surrounding the tube clean and dry to prevent excoriation and infection. Daily applications of antibiotic ointment or other preparations may be prescribed to aid in healing and prevention of irritation. Care is exercised to prevent excessive pull on the catheter that might cause widening of the opening and subsequent leakage of highly irritating gastric juices. Sliding the tube through a sterile disposable nipple whose tip is cut off and whose base is then taped to the abdomen keeps the tube from rotating and causing erosion and enlargement of the skin opening (Perez and others, 1984).

For children on long-term gastrostomy feeding, the recently developed skin level device (Button, Gastroport) offers several advantages. The small, flexible silicone device protrudes slightly from the abdomen, is cosmetically pleasing in appearance, affords increased comfort and mobility to the child, is easy to care for, and is fully immersible in water. The one-way valve at the proximal end minimizes reflux and eliminates the need for clamping. However, the skin level device requires a well-established gastrostomy site and is more expensive than the conventional tube. In addition, the valve may become clogged and, when functioning, prevents air from escaping. Therefore the child requires frequent bubbling. During feeding the child must remain fairly still, since the tubing easily disconnects from the device if the child moves (Huth and O'Brien, 1987). Also, residual is not checked with these devices, because it may disrupt the function of the one-way valve.

Positioning and feeding of water, formula, or pureed foods are done in the same manner and rate as for gavage feeding. However, residual may not be aspirated. After feedings the infant or child is positioned on the right side or in Fowler position, and the tube may be left open and sus-

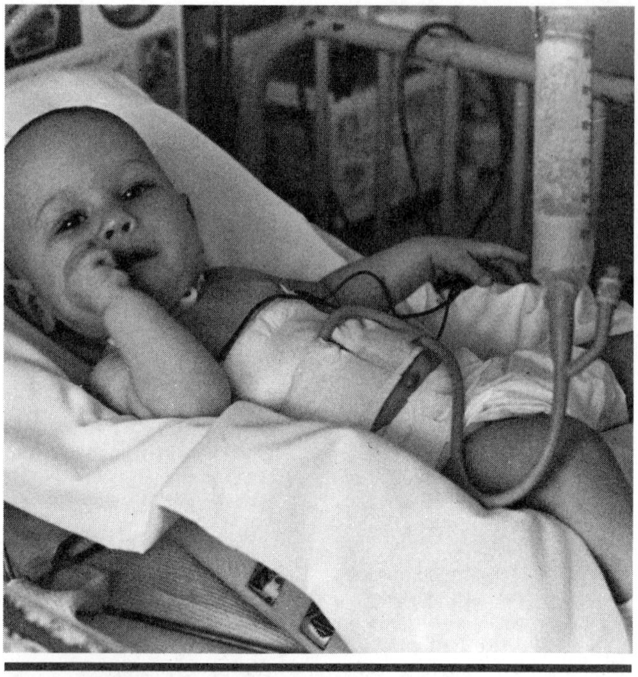

Fig. 27-26. Gastrostomy feeding. Syringe barrel suspended to allow thick formula to enter stomach by gravity. Note child sucking on thumb for oral gratification.

pended or clamped between feedings, depending on the child's condition (Fig. 27-26). A clamped tube allows more mobility but is only appropriate if the child can tolerate intermittent feedings without vomiting or prolonged backup of feeding into the tube. Sometimes a Y tube is used to allow for simultaneous decompression during feeding. If a Foley catheter is used as the gastrostomy tube, very slight tension is applied and the tube is securely taped to maintain the balloon at the gastrostomy opening and prevent its progression toward the pyloric sphincter, where it may occlude the stomach outlet. As a precaution, the length of the tube is measured postoperatively and then remeasured each shift to be sure it has not slipped. When the gastrostomy tube is no longer needed, it is removed; the skin opening usually closes spontaneously by contracture.

FAMILY TEACHING AND HOME CARE

When gastric tube feedings are needed for an extended period, the child may be discharged home before the tube is removed. The family will require appropriate instruction and preparation for performing the skill. The same principles are applied as discussed earlier in this chapter for compliance, especially in terms of education (see Box 27-7). and in Chapter 26 for discharge planning and home care.*

*Home care instructions for gavage and gastrostomy feeding are available in Wong, D.L., and Whaley, L.F.: Clinical manual of pediatric nursing, ed. 3, St. Louis, 1990, Mosby–Year Book, Inc.

PROCEDURES RELATED TO ELIMINATION

Children seldom have problems with elimination, but in cases of severe constipation or when an empty rectum is needed before surgery or diagnostic procedures, an enema may be administered to stimulate rectal emptying. Various conditions in the newborn and childhood period also require formation of an ostomy for purposes of elimination.

ENEMA

The procedure for giving an enema to an infant or child does not differ essentially from that for an adult, except for the type and amount of fluid administered and the distance for inserting the tube into the rectum (Box 27-15).

NURSING ALERT Proper insertion of the catheter tip, especially in infants, is essential to prevent rectal damage and perforation (see Fig. 7-10, *B*). If insertion of the enema tip causes discomfort, remove the tip and notify the physician.

An isotonic solution is used in children (see Nursing Tip). Plain water is not used because, being hypotonic, it can cause rapid fluid shift and fluid overload. The Fleet enema (pediatric or adult sized) is not advised for children because of the harsh action of its ingredients (sodium biphosphate and sodium phosphate). Commercial enemas can be dangerous to patients with megacolon and to dehydrated or azotemic children. The osmotic effect of the Fleet enema may produce diarrhea, which can lead to metabolic acidosis. Other potential complications are extreme hyperphosphatemia, hypernatremia, and hypocalcemia, which may lead to neuromuscular irritability and coma (Martin and others, 1987).

Since infants and young children are unable to retain the solution after it is administered, the buttocks must be held together for a short time to retain the fluid. The enema is administered and expelled while the child is lying with the buttocks over the bedpan and with the head and back supported by pillows. Older children are ordinarily able to hold the solution if they understand what to do and if they are not expected to hold it for too long. The nurse should have the bedpan handy or, for the ambulatory child, ensure that the bathroom is readily available before beginning the pro-

Box 27-15 GUIDELINES FOR ADMINISTRATION OF ENEMAS TO CHILDREN

Age	Amount (ml)	Insertion Distance (cm/inches)
Infant	120-240	2.5 (1 inch)
2-4 years	240-360	5.0 (2 inches)
4-10 years	360-480	7.5 (3 inches)
11 years	480-720	10.0 (4 inches)

NURSING TIP: HOMEMADE SALINE

If prepared saline is not available, it can be made by adding 1 tsp table salt to 500 ml (1 pint) tap water.

cedure. An enema is an intrusive procedure and thus threatening to the preschool child; therefore a careful explanation is especially important to ease possible fear.

A preoperative bowel preparation solution given orally or through a nasogastric tube is increasingly being used instead of an enema. The polyethylene glycol–electrolyte lavage solution (Golytely) mechanically flushes the bowel without significant absorption, thereby avoiding potential fluid and electrolyte imbalances (Konings, 1989).

OSTOMIES

Children may require stomas for various health problems. The most frequent causes are necrotizing enterocolitis and imperforate anus in the infant, less often Hirschsprung disease. In the older child the most frequent causes are inflammatory bowel disease, especially Crohn disease (regional enteritis), and ureterostomies for distal ureter or bladder defects.

Care and management of ostomies in the older child differ little from the care of ostomies in the adult patient. The major emphasis in pediatric care is the preparation of the child for the procedure and teaching care of the ostomy to the child and family. The basic principles of preparation are the same as for any procedure (see p. 1187). Simple, straightforward language is most effective, together with the use of illustrations and a replica model; for example, drawing a picture of a child with a stoma on the abdomen and explaining it as "another opening where bowel movements [or any other term the child uses] will come out." At another time the nurse can draw a pouch over the opening to demonstrate how the contents are collected. Using a doll to demonstrate the process is an excellent teaching strategy and special books are available.*

Except in infants, an appliance is usually fitted immediately after surgery. Once an appliance is in place, drainage is directly measured from the collecting pouch. To measure colostomy drainage accurately before a collecting appliance is in place, the nurse weighs the dry dressing and reweighs it when wet. The difference in weight is calculated as fluid because 1 g equals 1 ml. If formed stool is passed, it is not weighed and calculated as part of fluid loss.

Ostomies performed on infants create special problems. The fragile nature of the skin increases the risk of breakdown, and the small surface area of the abdomen is ill suited to the standard appliances. Regardless of the type of stoma (ileostomy or colostomy), initially most infants are left with a gauze dressing over the stoma. The dressing may

Chris Has an Ostomy, available from United Ostomy Association, Inc., 36 Executive Park, Suite 120, Irvine, CA 92714-6744; (714) 660-8624.

NURSING TIPS: COLOSTOMY DRESSING

To secure a dressing over the colostomy site:

- Use a self-adhering wrap (Coban) or an expansible wrap (Kerlix, Ace) around the abdomen, and secure the end of the wrap with tape or a safety pin.
- Use a diaper (may be applied alone or with a dressing over the site).
- Use Montgomery straps: on either side of the dressing, apply one or more strips of nonirritating tape to the skin and attach cloth ties to the end of the tapes; lace the ties across the dressing.

or may not be saturated with petroleum jelly or other protective material. The skin is cleansed well after each bowel movement, and a nonporous substance (e.g., zinc oxide ointment [Desitin], karaya products, or a mixture of the zinc oxide ointment and karaya powder) is applied.

Various inexpensive techniques have been devised to absorb drainage around the stoma. Squares of paper towel, disposable diaper, or gauze with openings cut to fit the stoma are gently pressed against the layer of protective substance on the area around the stoma. They can be kept in place with a variety of methods that avoid repeated use of tape on the skin (see Nursing Tips). As a rule, if a sigmoid colostomy is to be performed on an infant, a colostomy appliance is usually not used because the stools are formed and less likely to irritate the skin. Usually only diapers and a nonporous ointment (e.g., zinc oxide) around the stoma are used.

When the stoma has healed and the infant has grown to a size that permits its use, an appropriate-sized infant pouch with skin barrier water is introduced. Before the pouch is applied, the skin is prepared with a skin sealant that is allowed to dry. Then stoma paste is applied around the base of the stoma. The sealant and paste work together to prevent peristomal breakdown.

FAMILY TEACHING AND HOME CARE

Since these children are almost always discharged with a functioning colostomy, preparation of the family should begin as early as possible in the hospital. The family is instructed in the application of the device (if used), care of the skin, and instructions regarding appropriate action in case skin problems develop. Early evidence of skin breakdown or stomal complications, such as ribbonlike stools, excessive diarrhea, bleeding, prolapse, or failure to pass flatus or stool, is brought to the attention of the physician, the nurse, or the stoma specialist. The same principles are applied as discussed earlier in this chapter for compliance, especially in terms of education (see p. 1202), and in Chapter 26 for discharge planning and home care.*

*Home care instructions on caring for a colostomy are available in Wong, D.L., and Whaley, L.F.: Clinical manual of pediatric nursing, ed. 3, St. Louis, 1990, Mosby–Year Book, Inc.

KEY POINTS

- Informed consent is valid when the person is capable of giving consent (is over the age of majority and is competent), the person is supplied with information needed to make an intelligent decision, and the person acts voluntarily when exercising freedom of choice.
- Informed consent is needed for major surgery, minor surgery, and diagnostic tests and medical treatments with an element of risk.
- The major principles in psychologic preparation of the child for surgery are to establish trust, provide support, and give an explanation in easy-to-understand terms.
- Most parents and children want to be together during stressful procedures and should be offered this opportunity, with guidance on how the parent can comfort the child.
- In the performance of a procedure the nurse should expect success, involve the child when possible in the procedure, provide distraction, and allow for expression of feelings.
- In giving postprocedural support, the nurse should encourage children to express their feelings and praise them for completion of the procedure.
- Six stressful times before and after surgery that produce anxiety in children are the day of admission, blood tests, the afternoon of the day before surgery, injection of preoperative medication, transportation to the operating room, and return from the postanesthesia care unit.
- Assessment of compliance entails measuring factors that affect compliance (through clinical judgment, self-reporting, and direct observation), monitoring therapeutic response, taking pill counts, and performing chemical assay.
- Compliance strategies may be classified as organizational, educational, and behavioral.
- Knowledge of the sick child's eating habits and favorite foods can help in maintaining adequate nutrition.
- Control of elevated temperatures may be accomplished, depending on cause, by pharmacologic means (administration of antipyretics) and environmental means (minimum clothing, increased air circulation, cool compresses).
- Ensuring safety in the hospital setting is a major concern and can be achieved through environmental measures, infection control measures, limit-setting, and safe transportation.
- Common types of physical restraints for children are jacket, mummy, arm and leg, and elbow.
- Factors that affect drug dosage determination are growth and maturation, difficulty in evaluating drug response, and body surface area.
- Family teaching regarding medication administration includes telling parents why the child is receiving the drug, its possible effects, and the amount, frequency, and length of time the drug is to be administered.
- The major forms of gastric feeding for children are gavage feeding and gastrostomy feeding.
- In the care of children with ostomies, nurses play an important role in family support and instruction in care of the stoma site.

REFERENCES

American Academy of Pediatrics, Committee on Drugs, Section on Anesthesiology: Guidelines for the elective use of conscious sedation, deep sedation, and general anesthesia in pediatric patients, Pediatrics 76(2):317-321, 1985.

Anderson, G.C.: Pacifiers: the positive side, MCN 11(2):122-124, 1986.

Arditi, M., and Killner, M.: Coma following use of rubbing alcohol for fever control, Am. J. Dis. Child. 141(3):237-238, 1987.

Baker, M., Fosarelli, P., and Carpenter, R.: Childhood fever: correlation of diagnosis with temperature response to acetaminophen, Pediatrics 80(3):315-318, 1987.

Banco, L., and Jayashekaramurthy, S.: The ability of mothers to read a thermometer, Clin. Pediatr. 29(6):343-345, 1990.

Banco, L., and Powers, A.: Hospitals: unsafe environments for children, Pediatrics 82(5):794-797, 1988.

Bates, T., and Broome, M.: Preparation of children for hospitalization and surgery: a review of the literature, J. Pediatr. Nurs. 1(4):230-234, 1986.

Battaglia, J.D.: Severe croup: the child with fever and upper airway obstruction, Pediatr. Rev. 7(8):227-233, 1986.

Bauchner, H., Vinci, R., and Waring, C.: Pediatric procedures: do parents want to watch? Pediatrics 84(5):907-909, 1989.

Beecroft, P., and Redick, S.: Intramuscular injection practices of pediatric nurses: site selection, Nurse Educ. 15(4):23-28, 1990.

Berg, A.T., and others: Predictors of recurrent febrile seizures: a metaanalytic review, J. Pediatr. 116(3):329-337, 1990.

Berman, W., and others: Inadvertent overadministration of digoxin to low-birth weight infants, J. Pediatr. 92(6):1024-1025, 1978.

Billmire, D., Neale, H., and Gregory, R.: Use of IV fentanyl in the outpatient treatment of pediatric facial trauma, J. Trauma 25(11):1079-1080, 1985.

Bishop, B.E.: Compliant: isn't it time to retire this word? (editorial), MCN 12:381, 1987.

Blum, R.W.: Compliance with therapeutic regimens among children and youths. In Blum, R., editor: Chronic illness and disabilities in childhood and adolescence, New York, 1984, Grune & Stratton, Inc.

Boulder, P.M.: Postlumbar puncture headache in pediatric oncology patients, Anesthesiology 65(6):696-698, 1986.

Bourgault, A.: A hair piece, Nursing '85 15(9):80, 1985.

Broome, M., and Endsley, R.: Maternal presence, childrearing practices, and children's response to an injection, Res. Nurs. Health 12:229-235, 1989.

Broome, M., and Lillis, P.: A descriptive analysis of pediatric pain management research, J. Appl. Nurs. Res. 2(2):74-81, 1989.

Broome, M., Lillis, P., and Smith, M.: Pain interventions in children: a meta-analysis of the research, Nurs. Res. 38(3):154-158, 1989.

Brosnan, K.M., and others: Contamination stopcock, Am. J. Nurs. 88(3):320-323, 1988.

Brown, S.R.: An anxiety reduction technique during lumbar punctures in infants and toddlers, J. Assoc. Pediatr. Oncol. Nurs. 1(3):24-25, 1984.

Catchpole, M.: Does preop medication promote stress? Am. J. Nurs. 84(10):1202, 1984.

Centers for Disease Control: Guidelines for the prevention and control of nosocomial infections, Atlanta, 1983, CDC.

Centers for Disease Control: Update: universal precautions for prevention of transmission of human immunodeficiency virus, hepatitis B virus, and other bloodborne pathogens in health care settings, MMWR 37(24):377-387, 1988.

Chaplin, G., Shull, H., and Welk, P.C., III: How safe is the air-bubble technique for I.M. injections? Nursing '85 15(9):59, 1985.
Cooke, R., Werkman, S., and Watson, D.: Urine output measurements in premature infants, Pediatrics 83(1):116-118, 1989.
Cramer, J.A., and others: How often is medication taken as prescribed? A novel assessment technique, JAMA 261(22):3273-3277, 1989.
Cromer, B.A., and others: Psychosocial determinants of compliance in adolescents with iron deficiency, Am. J. Dis. Child. 143(1):55-58, 1989.
Cushing, M.: Informed consent: an MD responsibility? Am. J. Nurs. 84(4):437-440, 1984.
Dininny, J.B.: Food rummy, the game of nutrition, MCN 2(2):90-91, 1977.
Dyson, A., and Bogod, D.: Minimizing bruising in the antecubital fossa after venipuncture, Br. Med. J. 294(6588):1659, 1987.
Ellerton, M.L., Caty, S., and Ritchie, J.A.: Helping young children master intrusive procedures through play, Child. Health Care 13(4):167-173, 1985.
Ellis, R.: Once more into the void, Contemp. Pediatr. 6(8):164, 1989.
Erlen, J.A.: The child's choice: an essential component in treatment decisions, Child. Health Care 15(3):156-160, 1987.
Faber, M.M.: A review of efforts to protect children from injury in crashes, Fam. Community Health 4(3):25-41, 1986.
Feld, L.H., and others: Preanesthetic medication in children: a comparison of oral transmucosal fentanyl citrate versus placebo, Anesthesiology 71(3):374-377, 1989.
Forlini, J., Morin, D.M., and Treacy, S.: Painless peds procedures, Am. J. Nurs. 87(3):321-323, 1987.
Fradet, C., and others: A prospective survey of reactions to blood tests by children and adolescents, Pain 49(1):53-60, 1990.
Funk, M.J., Mullins, L.L., and Olson, R.A.: Teaching children to swallow pills: a case study, Child. Health Care 13(1):20-23, 1984.
Garvin, G., and Franck, L.: Preventing delivery of enteral formula via parenteral route, Pediatr. Nurs. 15(1):17-18, 1990.
Gauderer, M., Lorig, J., and Eastwood, D.: Is there a place for parents in the operating room? J. Pediatr. Surg. 24(7):705-707, 1989.
Ghishan, F.K.: The transport of electrolytes in the gut and the use of oral rehydrating solutions, Pediatr. Clin. North Am. 35(1):35-51, 1988.
Goodman, L.J., and others: A urine preservative system to maintain bacterial counts, Clin. Pediatr. 24(7):383-386, 1985.
Gribetz, B., and Cronley, S.: Underdosing of acetaminophen by parents, Pediatrics 80(5):630-633, 1987.
Hamner, S.B., and Miles, M.S.: Coping strategies in children with cancer undergoing bone marrow aspirations, J. Assoc. Pediatr. Oncol. Nurs. 5(3):11-15, 1988.
Hanna, W.J., and Sherlock, H.: Recall and fears of anaesthesia and surgery in 50 Jamaican paediatric patients, West Indian Med. J. 32:75-82, 1983.
Hannallah, R., and Rosales, J.: Experience with parents' presence during anaesthesia induction in children, Can. Anaesth. Soc. J. 30(3):287-290, 1983.
Hicks, J.F., and others: Optimum needle length for diphtheria-tetanus-pertussis inoculation of infants, Pediatrics 84(1):136-137, 1989.
Hogue, E.E.: Informed consent: implications for critical care nurses, Pediatr. Nurs. 14(4):315-316, 1988.
Holtzclaw, B.J.: Control of febrile shivering during amphotericin B therapy, Oncol. Nurs. Forum 17(4):521-524, 1990.
Howland, M., and Goldfrank, L: Meperidine usage in patients with sickle cell crisis, Ann. Emerg. Med. 15(12):1506-1507, 1986.
Huth, M.M., and O'Brien, M.E.: The gastrostomy feeding button, Pediatr. Nurs. 13(4):241-245, 1987.
Intramuscular injections: a guide to sites and techniques, Philadelphia, 1985, Wyeth Laboratories.
Ipp, M.M., and others: Adverse reactions to diphtheria, tetanus, pertussis-polio vaccination at 18 months of age: effect of injection site and needle length, Pediatrics 83(5):679-682, 1989.
Johnston, C.C., and others: Parental presence during anesthesia induction, AORN J. 47(1):187-194, 1988.
Jones, S.T.: Reducing children's psychological stress in the operating suite, Ophthalmic Plast. Reconstr. Surg. 1:199-203, 1985.
Joyner, M.: Hair care in the black patient, J. Pediatr. Health Care 2(6):281-287, 1988.
Kilman, C.: Parents' knowledge and practices related to fever management, Pediatr. Health Care 1(4):173-179, 1987.
Konings, K.: Preop use of Golytely in pediatrics, Pediatr. Nurs. 15(5):473-474, 1989.
Koren, G., Barzilay, Z., and Greenwald, M.: Tenfold errors in administration of drug doses: a neglected iatrogenic disease in pediatrics, Pediatrics 77(6):848-849, 1986.
Korniewicz, D., Laughon, B., and Butz, A.: Integrity of vinyl and latex procedure gloves, Nurs. Res. 38:144-146, 1989.
Krueger, H., and Osborn, L.: Effects of hygiene among the uncircumcised, J. Fam. Pract. 22(4):353-355, 1986.
Larson, E.: Handwashing: it's essential—even when you use gloves, Am. J. Nurs. 89(7):934-939, 1989.
Leff, R., and Roberts, R.: Enteral drug administration practices: report of a preliminary survey, Pediatrics 81(4):549-551, 1988.
Lenz, C.L.: Make your needle selection right to the point, Nursing '83 13(2):50-51, 1983.
Lewis, J.F., and Alexander, J.J.: Overnight refrigeration of urine specimens for culture, South. Med. J. 73(3):351-352, 1980.
Lohr, J., Donowitz, L., and Dudley, S.: Bacterial contamination rates in voided urine collections in girls, J. Pediatr. 114(1):91-93, 1989.
Lybrand, M., Medoff-Cooper, B., and Monro, B.: Periodic comparisons of specific gravity using urine from a diaper and collecting bag, MCN 15(4):238-239, 1990.
Lynch, P., and others: Rethinking the role of isolation practices in the prevention of nosocomial infections, Ann. Intern. Med. 107:243-246, 1987.
Mandelbaum, J.: The food square: helping people of different cultures understand balanced diets, Pediatr. Nurs. 9(1):20-21, 1983.
Martin, R., and others: Fatal poisoning from sodium phosphate enema: case report and experimental study, JAMA 257:2190-2192, 1987.
Maunuksela, E., Rajantie, J., and Simes, M.: Flunitrazepam-fentanyl-induced sedation and analgesia for bone marrow aspiration and needle biopsy in children, Acta Anaesthesiol. Scand. 30:409-411, 1986.
McCarthy, D.O.: The adaptive value of fever during infection, Diet. Curr. 12(3):13-18, 1985.
McDonald, N., and others: Efficacy of chlorhexidine cleansing in reducing contamination of bagged urine specimens, Can. Med. Assoc. J. 133:1211-1213, 1985.
McLeod, S.M., and McClowry, S.G.: Using temperament theory to individualize the psychosocial care of hospitalized children, Child. Health Care 19(2):79-85, 1990.
Meichenbaum, D.: Noncompliance, Feelings Med. Signif. 31(2):5-8, 1989.
Merritt, K., Sargent, J., and Osborn, L.: Attitudes regarding parental presence during medical procedures, Am. J. Dis. Child. 144(3):270-271, 1990.
Merz, B.: Hospital-bed deaths, injuries force downswitch modifications, JAMA 250(7):871-872, 1983.
Metheny, N.: Measures to test placement of nasogastric and nasointestinal feeding tubes: a review, Nurs. Res. 37(6):324-329, 1988.
Metheny, N., and others: Effectiveness of pH measurements in predicting feeding tube placement, Nurs. Res. 38(5):280-285, 1989.
Millam, D.A.: Getting into an artery, Am. J. Nurs. 88(9):1214-1217, 1988.
Moore, M.C., and Green, H.L.: Tube feedings of infants and children, Pediatr. Clin. North Am. 32(2):401-417, 1985.
Nederhand, K., and others: Respiratory syncytial virus: a nursing perspective, Pediatr. Nurs. 15(4):342-345, 1989.
Nelson, C., and Hallgren, R.: Gastrostomies: indications, management, and weaning, Inf. Young Child. 2(1):66-74, 1989.

Nelson, P.S., and others: Comparison of oral transmucosal fentanyl citrate and an oral solution of meperidine, diazepam, and atropine for premedication in children, Anesthesiology 70(4):616-621, 1989.
Newman, J.: Evaluation of sponging to reduce body temperature in febrile children, Can. Med. Assoc. J. 132:641-642, 1985.
Nix, K.S.: Obtaining informed consent. In Smith, D.P., and others, editors: Comprehensive child and family nursing skills, St. Louis, 1991, Mosby–Year Book, Inc.
Orenstein, S., and others: The Santmyer swallow: a new and useful infant reflex, Lancet 1(8581):345-346, 1988.
Patterson, K.L., and Ware, L.L.: Coping skills for children undergoing painful medical procedures, Issues Compr. Pediatr. Nurs. 11:113-143, 1988.
Perez, R.C., and others: Care of the child with a gastrostomy tube: common and practical concerns, Issues Compr. Pediatr. Nurs. 7(2-3):107-119, 1984.
Perin, G., and Frase, D.: Development of a program using general anesthesia for invasive procedures in a pediatric outpatient setting, J. Pediatr. Oncol. Nurs. 3(4):8-10, 1985.
Peterson, L., and Toler, S.: An information seeking disposition in child surgery patients, Health Psychol. 5(4):343-358, 1986.
Pidgeon, V.: Compliance with chronic illness regimens: school-aged children and adolescents, J. Pediatr. Nurs. 4(1):36-47, 1989.
Rae, W.A., and Fournier, C.J.: Ethical issues in pediatric research: preserving psychosocial care in scientific inquiry, Child. Health Care 14(4):242-248, 1986.
Rapoff, M.A.: Helping parents to help their children comply with treatment regimens for chronic diseases, Issues Compr. Pediatr. Nurs. 9(3):147-156, 1986.
Reeves-Swift, R.: Rational management of a child's acute fever, MCN 15(2):82-85, 1990.
Rhodes, A.M.: Children and the law, MCN 13:171, 1988.
Rollins, J., and Brantly, D.: Preparing the child for procedures. In Smith, D.P., and others, editors: Comprehensive child and family nursing skills, St. Louis, 1991, Mosby–Year Book, Inc.
Ros, S.: Outpatient pediatric analgesia—a tale of two regimens, Pediatr. Emerg. Care 3(4):228-230, 1987.
Rosenstock, I.M.: Enhancing patient compliance with health recommendations, J. Pediatr. Health Care 2(2):67-72, 1988.
Rosman, N.P.: Evaluation and management of febrile seizures, Curr. Opin. Pediatr. 1:318-323, 1989.
Ross, D.M., and Ross, S.A.: Childhood pain: the school-aged child's viewpoint, Pain 29(2):179-191, 1984.
Saez-Llorens, X., and others: Bacterial contamination rates for non-clean catch and clean catch midstream urine collections in uncircumcised boys, J. Pediatr. 114(1):93-95, 1989.
Savedra, M.: Parental responses to a painful procedure performed on their child. In Azarnoff, P., and Hardgrove, C., editors: The family in child health care, New York, 1981, John Wiley & Sons, Inc.
Schlager, T.A., and others: Bacterial contamination rate of urine collected in a urine bag from healthy non-toilet-trained male infants, J. Pediatr. 116(5):738-739, 1990.
Schofield, N.M., and White, J.B.: Interrelations among children, parents, premedication, and anaesthetists in paediatric day stay surgery, Br. Med. J. 299(6712):1371-1375, 1989.
Schreiner, M.S., and others: Ingestion of liquids compared with preoperative fasting in pediatric outpatients, Anesthesiology 72(4):593-597, 1990.
Schreiner, V.: Don't discard this specimen, Nursing '87 17(10):5, 1987.
Selbst, S.M.: Treating minors without their parents, Pediatr. Emerg. Care 1:168-173, 1985.
Sessler, D.I.: Malignant hyperthermia, J. Pediatr. 109(1):9-14, 1986.
Shaw, E.G., and Routh, D.K.: Effect of mother presence on children's reaction to aversive procedures, J. Pediatr. Psychol. 7(1):33-42, 1982.
Shaw, N., and Lyall, E.: Hazards of glass ampoules, Br. Med. J. 291(6506):1390, 1985.
Siaw, S.N., Stephens, L.R., and Holmes, S.S.: Knowledge about medical instruments and reported anxiety in pediatric surgery patients, Child. Health Care 14(3):134-141, 1986.
Singleton, M.A., Rosen, J.I., and Fisher, D.M.: Plasma concentrations of fentanyl in infants, children and adults, Can. J. Anaesth. 34(2):152-155, 1987.
Snodgrass, W.R., and Dodge, W.F.: Lytic/"DPT" cocktail: time for rational and safe alternatives, Pediatr. Clin. North Am. 36(5):1285-1291, 1989.
Stebor, A.: Posturination time and specific gravity in infant's diapers, Nurs. Res. 38(4):244-245, 1989.
Steckel, S.: Patient contracting, New York, 1982, Appleton-Century-Crofts.
Stoller, K.P., and Losey, R.: Inadvertent intra-arterial injection of penicillin: an unseen danger, Pediatrics 75(4):785-786, 1985.
Streiff, L.D.: Can clients understand our instructions, Image 18(2):48-52, 1986.
Suri, S.: Simplifying urine collection from infants and children without losing accuracy, MCN 13(12):438-441, 1988.
Task Force on Pediatric AIDS: Pediatric guidelines for infection control of human immunodeficiency virus (acquired immunodeficiency virus) in hospitals, medical offices, schools, and other settings, Pediatrics 82(5):801-807, 1988.
Venham, L.L., Bengston, D., and Cipes, M.: Parent's presence and the child's response to dental stress, J. Dent. Child. 45(3):213-217, 1978.
Vernon, D.T.A., Foley, J.M., and Schulman, J.L.: Effect of mother-child separation and birth order on young children's responses to two potentially stressful experiences, J. Pers. Soc. Psychol. 5(2):162-174, 1967.
Vessey, J., Caserza, L., and Bogetz, M.: In my opinion . . . another Pandora's box? Parental participation in anesthetic induction, Child. Health Care 19(2):116-118, 1990.
Visintainer, M.A., and Wolfer, J.A.: Psychological preparation for surgical pediatric patients: the effect of children's and parents' stress responses and adjustment, Pediatrics 56(2):187-202, 1975.
Watson, P.D., and others: Ibuprofen, acetaminophen, and placebo treatment of febrile children, Clin. Pharmacol. Ther. 46(1):9-17, 1989.
Weekes, D.P., and Savedra, M.C.: Adolescent cancer: coping with treatment-related pain, J. Pediatr. Nurs. 3(5):318-328, 1988.
Weibley, T.T., and others: Gavage tube insertion in the premature infant, MCN 12:24-27, 1987.
Weisse, M.E., Miller, G., and Brien, J.: Fever response to acetaminophen in viral vs. bacterial infections, Pediatr. Infect. Dis. J. 6:1091-1094, 1987.
Welch, J.A., and others: Staff nurses' experiences as co-investigators in a clinical research project, Pediatr. Nurs. 16(4):364-367, 396, 1990.
Wesley, J.R.: Special access to the intestinal tract. In Enteral feeding: scientific basis and clinical application, Report of the 94th Ross Conference on Pediatric Research, Columbus, OH, 1988, Ross Laboratories.
Williams, P.J.: How do you keep medicines from clogging feeding tubes? Am. J. Nurs. 89(2):181-182, 1989.
Wong, D.L.: Significance of dead space in syringes, Am. J. Nurs. 82(8):1237, 1982.
Wong, D.L., and Redding, B.: Lozenges can be "lifesavers," Am. J. Nurs. 87(9):1129-1130, 1987.
Wong, D.L., and Baker, C.M.: Pain in children: comparison of assessment scales, Pediatr. Nurs. 14(1):9-17, 1988.
Young, M.S.: Strategies for improving compliance, Top. Clin. Nurs. 7(4):31-38, 1986.

BIBLIOGRAPHY

Informed Consent

Appelbaum, P.S., and Grisson, T.: Assessing patients' capacities to consent to treatment, N. Engl. J. Med. 319(25):1635-1638, 1988.

Davis, A.J.: Clinical nurses' ethical decision making in situations of informed consent, Adv. Nurs. Sci. 11(3):63-69, 1989.

Erickson, S., and others: Gray areas: informed consent in pediatric and comatose adult patients, Heart Lung 16(3):323-325, 1987.

Erlen, J.A.: The child's choice: an essential component in treatment decisions, Child. Health Care 15(3):156-160, 1987.

Hogue, E.E.: Consent for minors, Pediatr. Nurs. 15(4):404, 1989.

Holder, A.R.: Parents, courts, and refusal of treatment, J. Pediatr. 104(4):515-520, 1983.

Leikin, S.: A proposal concerning decisions to forgo life-sustaining treatment for young people, J. Pediatr. 115(1):17-22, 1989.

Northrop, C.E., and Kelly, M.E.: Legal issues in nursing, St. Louis, 1987, Mosby–Year Book, Inc.

Rhodes, A.M.: Consent for medical treatment, MCN 12(2):133, 1987.

Rhodes, A.M.: Obtaining consent to treat minors, MCN 12(3):209, 1987.

Rhodes, A.M.: When parents refuse to consent, MCN 12(4):289, 1987.

Rhodes, A.M.: The rights of minors, MCN 13(4):281, 1988.

Rhodes, A.M.: A minor's refusal of treatment, MCN 15(4):261, 1990.

Siantz, M.L.D.: Defining informed consent, MCN 13(2):94, 1988.

Silva, M., and Zeccolo, R.: Informed consent: the right to know and the right to choose, Nurs. Manage. 17(8):18-19, 1986.

Preparing for Procedures/Use of Play

Bates, T.A., and Broome, M.: Preparation of children for hospitalization and surgery: a review of the literature, J. Pediatr. Nurs. 1(4):230-239, 1986.

Broome, M.E.: The relationship between children's fears and behavior during a painful event, Child. Health Care 14(3):142-145, 1986.

Goldberger, J., and Wolfer, J.: Helping children cope with health-care procedures, Contemp. Pediatr. 7(3):141-162, 1990.

Perry, S.E.: Teaching tools made by peers: a novel approach to medical preparation, Child. Health Care 15(1):21-25, 1986.

Petrillo, M., and Sanger, S.: Emotional care of hospitalized children, ed. 2, Philadelphia, 1980, J.B. Lippincott Co.

Pridham, K.F., Adelson, F., and Hansen, M.F.: Helping children deal with procedures in a clinic setting: a developmental approach, J. Pediatr. Nurs. 2(1):13-22, 1987.

Streiff, L.D.: Can clients understand our instructions? Image 18(2):48-52, 1986.

Waidley, E.K.: Show and tell: preparing children for invasive procedures, Am. J. Nurs. 85(7):811-812, 1985.

Surgical Procedures

Addleman, C.D.: What do you look for in the pediatric postanesthesia patient? J. Post Anesth. Nurs. 3(1):3-10, 1988.

Atsberger, D.B., and Shrewsbury, P.: Postoperative pain management: the PACU nurse's challenge, J. Post Anesth. Nurs. 3(6):399-403, 1988.

Berde, C.B.: Pediatric postoperative pain management, Pediatr. Clin. North Am. 36(4):921-940, 1989.

Carter, J.H., and Hancock, J.: Caring for children: how to ease them through surgery, Nursing '88 18(10):46-50, 1988.

Cote, C.J.: NPO after midnight for children—a reappraisal, Anesthesiology 72(4):589-592, 1990.

Demarest, D.S., Hooke, J.F., and Erickson, M.T.: Preoperative intervention for the reduction of anxiety in pediatric surgery patients, Child. Health Care 12(4):179-183, 1984.

Feychting, H.: Premedication and psychological preparation, Clin. Anaesthesiol. 3(3):505-514, 1985.

Johnson, J.E.: Coping with elective surgery. In Werley, H.H., and Fitzpatrick, J.J., editors: Annual review of nursing research, vol. 2, New York, 1984, Springer Publishing Co., Inc.

Krane, E.J., and others: Caudal morphine for postoperative analgesia in children: a comparison with caudal bupivacaine and intravenous morphine, Anesth. Analg. 66:647-653, 1987.

Litwack, K.: Practical points in the use of midazolam, J. Post Anesth. Nurs. 3(6):408-410, 1988.

McIlvaine, W.B.: Perioperative pain management in children: a review, J. Pain Symptom Manage. 4(4):215-229, 1989.

Mendelson, L.S.: Pain management for ambulatory surgery, J. Post Anesth. Nurs. 3(2):109-113, 1988.

Moushey, R., Sinacore, M., and Diomede, B.: A perioperative teaching program: a collaborative process, J. Pediatr. Nurs. 3(1):40-45, 1988.

Ogilvie, L.: Hospitalization of children for surgery: the parents' view, Child. Health Care 19(1):49-56, 1990.

Olkkola, K.T., and others: Kinetics and dynamics of postoperative intravenous morphine in children, Clin. Pharmacol. Ther. 44(2):128-136, 1988.

Rowland, M.A.: Myths—and facts—about postop discomfort, Am. J. Nurs. 90(5):60-64, 1990.

Rushton, C.H.: The surgical neonate: principles of nursing management, Pediatr. Nurs. 14(2):141-151, 1988.

Taylor, M.B., Vine, P.R., and Hatch, D.J.: Intramuscular midazolam premedication in small children, Anaesthesia 41:21-26, 1986.

Thomas, S.D.: Malignant hyperthermia, Crit. Care Nurse 9(6):58-68, 1989.

Tobias, J.D., and others: Postoperative analgesia: use of intrathecal morphine in children, Clin. Pediatr. 29:44-48, 1990.

Vogelsang, J., and Hayes, S.R.: Stadol attenuates postanesthesia shivering, J. Post Anesth. Nurs. 14(4):222-227, 1989.

Wilmore, D.W., and others: American College of Surgeons care of the surgical patient, vol. 2, New York, 1989, Scientific American, Inc.

Zeltzer, L.K., Jay, S.M., and Fisher, D.M.: The management of pain associated with pediatric procedures, Pediatr. Clin. North Am. 36(4):941-964, 1989.

Compliance

Austin, J.K.: Predicting parental anticonvulsant medication compliance using the theory of reasoned action, J. Pediatr. Nurs. 4(2):88-95, 1989.

Baer, C.L.: Compliance: the challenge for the future, Top. Clin. Nurs. 7(4):77-85, 1986.

Burckhardt, C.S.: Ethical issues in compliance, Top. Clin. Nurs. 7(4):9-16, 1986.

Clark, S.R.: Compliance and health behaviors, Top. Clin. Nurs. 7(4):39-46, 1986.

Connaway, N.: My patient won't follow the medical plan treatment. What should I do to protect myself—legally? . . . home health care, Home Healthcare Nurse 3(4):6-8, 1985.

DiFlorio, I.A., and Duncan, P.A.: Design for successful patient teaching, MCN 11:246-249, 1986.

Friedman, I.M., and Litt, I.F.: Promoting adolescents' compliance with therapeutic regimens, Pediatr. Clin. North Am. 33(4):955-973, 1986.

Korsch, B.M.: What do patients and parents want to know? What do they need to know? Pediatrics 74(5, suppl.):917-920, 1984.

Littlefield, L.C.: Therapeutic drug monitoring in ambulatory pediatrics, J. Pediatr. Health Care 1(2):113-116, 1987.

Lucas, C.M.: Compliance and illness responses, Top. Clin. Nurs. 7(4):47-56, 1986.

McCord, M.A.: Compliance: self-care or compromise? Top. Clin. Nurs. 7(4):1-8, 1986.

McHatton, M.: A theory for timely teaching, Am. J. Nurs. 85(7):798-800, 1985.

Melnyk, K.: Barriers to care: operationalizing the variable, Nurs. Res. 39(2):108-112, 1990.

Miller, A.: When is the time ripe for teaching? Am. J. Nurs. 85(7):801-804, 1985.

Padrick, K.P.: Compliance: myths and motivators, Top. Clin. Nurs. 7(4):17-22, 1986.

Russell, F.F., Mills, B.C., and Zucconi, T.: Relationship of parental attitudes and knowledge to treatment adherence in children with PKU, Pediatr. Nurs. 14(6):514-516, 523, 1988.

Sallis, J.F.: Improving adherence to pediatric therapeutic regimens, Pediatr. Nurs. 11(2):118-120, 1985.

Spicher, C.M., and Yund, C.: Effects of preadmission preparation on compliance with home care instructions, J. Pediatr. Nurs. 4(4):255-262, 1989.

Stang, H.: Compliance: get parents in on the diagnosis, Contemp. Pediatr. 7(3):170, 1990.

Williams, R.L., and others: Educational strategies to improve compliance with an antibiotic regimen, Am. J. Dis. Child. 140(3):216-220, 1986.

Wysocki, T., and others: Behavior modification in pediatric hemodialysis, ANNA J. 17(3):250-254, 1990.

Yoos, L.: Factors influencing maternal compliance to antibiotic regimens, Pediatr. Nurs. 10(2):141-147, 1984.

General Care and Hygiene/Fever

Baker, R.C., and others: Severity of disease correlated with fever reduction in febrile infants, Pediatrics 83(6):1016-1019, 1989.

Burson, J.Z., and Brannigan, C.N.: The use of play in the nutritional support of hospitalized children, Issues Compr. Pediatr. Nurs. 7(4-5):283-289, 1984.

Ibuprofen vs acetaminophen in children, Med. Lett. 31(807):109-110, 1989.

Irwin, M.: Encourage oral intake—yes, but how? Am. J. Nurs. 87(1):100-106, 1989.

Kilmon, C.A.: Home management of children's fevers, J. Pediatr. Nurs. 2(6):400-404, 1987.

Kleiman, M.B.: Feverish children, frightened parents, Contemp. Pediatr. 6(3):161-167, 1989.

McCarthy, P.L., and others: Observation, history, and physical examination in diagnosis of serious illnesses in febrile children <24 months, J. Pediatr. 110(1):26-30, 1987.

Perry, A.G., and Potter, P.A.: Clinical nursing skills and techniques, ed. 2, St. Louis, 1990, Mosby–Year Book, Inc.

Younger, J.B., and Brown, B.S.: Fever management: rational or ritual? Pediatr. Nurs. 11(1):26-28, 1985.

Safety/Collection of Specimens

DeGroot-Kosolcharoen, J., and Jones, J.J.: Permeability of latex and vinyl gloves to water and blood, Am. J. Infect. Control 17:196-201, 1989.

Jackson, M.M.: Implementing universal body substance precautions, Occup. Med. 4:39-44, 1989.

Jackson, M.M.: Infection prevention and control for HIV and other infectious agents in obstetric, gynecologic and neonatal settings, Clin. Issues Perinat. Women's Health Nurs. 1(1):115-121, 1990.

Jackson, M.M., and Lynch, P.: The epidemiology of HIV infection, AIDS, and health care worker risk issues, Fam. Community Health 12(2):34-42, 1989.

Jackson, M.M., and others: Why not treat all body substances as infectious? Am. J. Nurs. 87(9):1137-1139, 1987.

Kelly, P.M.: Are you ready to perform arterial punctures? Nursing '87 17(5):39-43, 1987.

Klein, B.S., Perloff, W.H., and Maki, D.G.: Reduction of nosocomial infection during pediatric intensive care by protective isolation, N. Engl. J. Med. 320:1714-1721, 1989.

Lynch, P., and others: Implementing and evaluating a system of generic infection precautions: body substance isolation, Am. J. Infect. Control 18(1):1-11, 1990.

Millam, D.A.: Venous blood samples: sharpen your drawing skills, Nursing '87 17(12):56-61, 1987.

Preusser, B.A., and others: Quantifying the minimum discard sample required for accurate arterial blood gases, Nurs. Res. 38:276-279, 1989.

Rutledge, J.C.: Pediatric specimen collection for chemical analysis, Pediatr. Clin. North Am. 36(1):37-47, 1989.

Administration of Medication

Beecroft, P.C., and Redick, S.: Possible complications of intramuscular injections on the pediatric unit, Pediatr. Nurs. 15(4):333-376, 1989.

Bergeson, P.S.: Immunizations to the deltoid region (letter), Pediatrics 85(1):134, 1990.

Bergeson, P.S., Singer, S.A., and Kaplan, A.M.: Intramuscular injections in children, Pediatrics 70(6):944-948, 1982.

Birdsall, C., and Uretsky, S.: How do I administer medication by NG? Am. J. Nurs. 84(10):1259-1260, 1984.

Faller, H.S.: Calculating pediatric I.V. dosages, Nursing '88 18(9):67-68, 1988.

Ford, D.C., Leist, E.R., and Phelps, S.T.: Guidelines for administration of intravenous therapy to pediatric patients, ed. 6, Bethesda, MD, 1988, American Society of Hospital Pharmacists.

Frank, T., and Fischer, R.G.,: What are some of the most common reasons for medication errors? Pediatr. Nurs. 10(4):294, 1984.

Gahart, B.L.: Intravenous medications: a handbook for nurses and other allied health personnel, ed. 6, St. Louis, 1990, Mosby–Year Book, Inc.

Glassman, S.K., and Measel, C.P.: A makeshift mini-bottle: accurate small volume fluid or oral medication administration to infants, Neonatal Network 7(4):29-31, 1989.

Knight, M.M., and others: Medication education for children: is it worthwhile? Child Adolesc. Psychiatr. Ment. Health Nurs. 3(1):25-28, 1990.

McConnell,E.A.: The subtle art of really good injections, RN 45(2):24-34, 1982.

Nahata, M.C.: Methods of intravenous drug infusion in pediatric patients, Am. J. Intraven. Ther. Clin. Nutr. 11(5):6-7, 1984.

Nelson, J.D.: Pocketbook of pediatric antimicrobial therapy, Baltimore, 1989, Williams & Wilkins.

Penatzer, M., and others: Common pediatric IV meds at a glance, Pediatr. Nurs. 14(1):56-58, 1988.

Raju, T.N., and others: Medication errors in neonatal and paediatric intensive-care units, Lancet 2(8659):374-376, 1989.

Rettig, F.M., and Southby, J.R.: Using different body positions to reduce discomfort during dorsogluteal injection, Nurs. Res. 31(4):219-221, 1982.

Weir, M.R.: Intravascular injuries from intramuscular penicillin, Clin. Pediatr. 27(2):85-90, 1988.

Wolf, Z.R.: Medication errors and nursing responsibility, Holistic Nurs. Pract. 4(1):8-17, 1989.

Wooldridge, J.B., and Jackson, J.G.: Evaluation of bruises and areas of induration after two techniques of subcutaneous heparin injection, Heart Lung 17:476-482, 1988.

Wordell, D.C.: Should you crush that tablet? Nursing '88 18(1):48-49, 1988.

Gastric Feeding Techniques/Elimination

Guiness, R.: How to use the new small-bore feeding tubes, Nursing '86 16(4):51-56, 1986.

Huddleston, K., and others: MIC or Foley: comparing gastrostomy tubes, MCN 14(1):20-23, 1989.

Metheny, N.A., Spies, M.A., and Eisenberg, P.: Measures to test placement of nasoenteral feeding tubes, West. J. Nurs. Res. 10:367-383, 1988.

Metheny, N.M.: 20 ways to prevent tube-feeding complications, Nursing '85 15(1):47-50, 1985.

Paarlberg, J., and Balint, J.P.: Gastrostomy tubes: practical guidelines for home care, Pediatr. Nurs. 11(2):99-102, 1985.

Saltzstein, R., and others: Anorectal injuries incident to enema administration: a recurring avoidable problem, Am. J. Phys. Med. Rehabil. 67:186-188, 1988.

Smith, D.B.: The ostomy: how is it managed? Am. J. Nurs. 85(11):1246-1249, 1985.

Wink, D.M.: The physical and emotional care of infants with gastrostomy tubes, Compr. Pediatr. Nurs. 6:195-203, 1983.

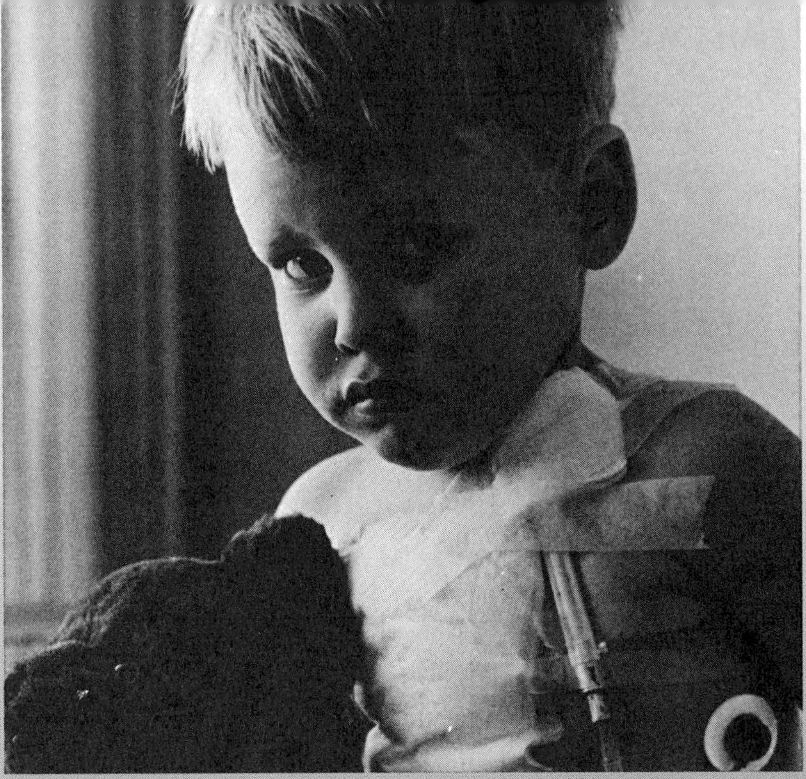

The Child with Disturbance of Fluid and Electrolytes

UNIT X

Some of the most common problems associated with the care of infants and children are related to the assessment and maintenance of fluid balance. The physiologic characteristics of young children render them more susceptible to fluid imbalances, and almost any early childhood illness is complicated by fluid disturbances. These differences are particularly noted in the infant, whose proportion of total body water is considerably greater than that of the adult or older child. In addition, the usual childhood responses to illness, such as fever and loss of appetite, further contribute to water depletion and dehydration.

It is essential that nurses who work with children have an understanding of the basic principles underlying the pathologic processes that produce fluid and electrolyte disturbances, the rationale behind fluid therapy, and the role of the nurse in maintaining or restoring fluid balance. Chapter 28, *Balance and Imbalance of Body Fluids,* provides a brief review of the basic concepts of fluid and electrolyte balance and imbalance and the nurse's role in fluid administration. Chapter 29, *Conditions That Produce Fluid and Electrolyte Imbalance,* discusses some of the major causes of fluid disturbance, and Chapter 30, *The Child with Genitourinary Dysfunction,* deals with the more specific fluid problems of genitourinary dysfunction.

CHAPTER 28

Balance and Imbalance of Body Fluids

RELATED TOPICS

Acute infectious gastroenteritis, Ch. 29
Burns, Ch. 29
The child with gastrointestinal dysfunction, Ch. 33
The child with genitourinary dysfunction, Ch. 30
Collection of specimens, Ch. 27
Diarrhea, Ch. 29
Gastric feeding techniques, Ch. 27
Intravenous administration of medication, Ch. 27
Oral hygiene, Ch. 27
Pain management, Ch. 26
Preparation for procedures, Ch. 27
Shock states, Ch. 29
Vomiting, Ch. 29

GLOSSARY

acidosis pH equal to or less than 7.35
ADH Antidiuretic hormone
alkalosis pH equal to or greater than 7.45
azotemia Accumulation of excessive amounts of nitrogenous products in the blood
BMR Basal metabolic rate
BUN Blood urea nitrogen
COP Colloidal osmotic pressure
ECF Extracellular fluid
electrolyte An element or compound that, when dissolved in a liquid (e.g., water), dissociates into ions and is able to conduct an electric current
H^+ Hydrogen ion
HCO_3 Base bicarbonate
H_2CO_3 Carbonic acid
HTPN Home total parenteral nutrition
hypertonic Having a greater osmotic pressure than a reference solution
hypotonic Having a lesser osmotic pressure than a reference solution
ICF Intracellular fluid
insensible Loss of fluid from the body by evaporation and/or respiration
isotonic Having the same osmotic pressure as a reference solution
K^+ Potassium ion

mEq Milliequivalent
Na⁺ Sodium ion
NaCl Sodium chloride
NPO Nothing by mouth
osmolality Number of particles (proteins or electrolytes) suspended in fluid
pH Expression of hydrogen ion concentration
SIADH Syndrome of inappropriate antidiuretic hormone
solute A substance dissolved in a solution
TBW Total body water
TPN Total parenteral nutrition
VAD Venous access device

The basic elements related to fluid and electrolyte balance—body water, electrolytes, and pH—are so closely interrelated that they rarely can be separated in clinical disorders; however, for simplicity they will be reviewed separately. An understanding of the basic principles of fluid dynamics and acid-base balance is essential for the nurse to be able to interpret observations, correlate these findings with the course of the disease process, and comprehend the rationale behind therapy in order to participate intelligently in a treatment regimen.

DISTRIBUTION OF BODY FLUIDS

Water is the major constituent of body tissues, and the total body water (TBW) in an individual ranges from 45% to 75% of total body weight. Its importance to body function is related not only to its abundance but also to the fact that it is the medium in which body solutes are dissolved and all metabolic reactions take place. Since these metabolic processes are affected by even small alterations in fluid composition, precise regulation of the volume and composition of the fluid is essential. In healthy individuals body water remains singularly constant, but marked alterations in either its volume or distribution that occur in many disease states can produce severely damaging physiologic consequences.

WATER BALANCE

Under normal conditions the amount of water ingested closely approximates the amount of urine excreted in a 24-hour period, and the water in food and from oxidation balances that lost in feces and through evaporation. In this way equilibrium is maintained.

Mechanisms of Fluid Movement

Water is retained in the body in a relatively constant amount and, with few exceptions, is freely exchangeable between all body fluid compartments. The proximity of the extravascular compartment to the cells allows for continual change in volume and distribution of fluids, largely determined by solutes (especially sodium) and physical forces (Box 28-1). Transport mechanisms are the basis for all activity within the cells and, since they have limited ability to store materials, movement in and out of cells must be

Box 28-1 PHYSICAL FORCES INFLUENCING FLUID BALANCE

Hydrostatic pressure—the pumping action of the heart increases fluid pressure in the arterial portion of the circulatory system, forcing fluid through the capillary walls into the interstitial spaces and from glomerular capillaries into the collecting tubules of the kidneys.
Osmotic pressure—the physical force, or "pull," created by a solution of higher concentration across a semipermeable membrane. Fluid in the solution of lesser concentration moves to the solution of greater concentration to equalize the concentration on each side of the membrane. Major osmotic forces in body fluids are sodium and intravascular proteins.
Diffusion—random movement of molecules from a region of greater concentration to regions of lesser concentration. Rate of diffusion is influenced by the size (small particles move more rapidly than large ones), temperature (heat increases the rate of movement), and agitation (stirring hastens movement). *Facilitated diffusion* employs a carrier substance to assist solute movement across a membrane.
Active transport—a substance is transported by way of a carrier substance *against* a pressure gradient.
Vesicular transport—a portion of a membrane engulfs a large molecule and releases it on the other side of the membrane. Substances move into cells by *pinocytosis* and out of cells by *exocytosis.*

Box 28-2 INTERNAL CONTROL MECHANISMS INFLUENCING FLUID BALANCE

Thirst—the impetus to ingest water is stimulated by increased solute concentration (osmolality) of extracellular fluid and/or diminished intravascular volume.
Antidiuretic hormone (ADH)—released from the posterior pituitary gland in response to increased osmolality and decreased volume of intravascular fluid; promotes water retention in the renal system by increasing the permeability of renal tubules to water.
Aldosterone—secreted by the adrenal cortex; enhances sodium reabsorption in renal tubules, thus promoting osmotic reabsorption of water.
Renin-angiotensin system—diminished blood flow to the kidneys stimulates renin secretion, which reacts with plasma globulin to generate angiotensin, a powerful vasoconstrictor. Angiotensin also stimulates the release of aldosterone.

rapid. Internal control mechanisms are responsible for distribution and maintenance of fluid balance (Box 28-2).

Table 28-1 shows electrolyte concentrations of various body fluids.

Maintaining water balance. Maintenance water requirement is the volume of water needed to replace insensible water loss (through the skin and respiratory tract) and losses through urine and stool formation. The amount and type of these losses may be altered by disease states such as fever (with increased sweating), diarrhea, gastric suction, and sequestration of body fluids in a body space.

Basal maintenance calculations are used for conditions in which a child is in a normal state of hydration, for example, preoperative preparation or in a coma. Requirements for a 24-hour period are: 100 ml/kg of body weight for the first 10 kg plus 50 ml/kg for next 10 kg plus 20 ml/kg for greater than 20 kg, or 1500 ml/m^2 (Abelson and Smith, 1987).

Maintenance fluids contain both water and electrolytes and can be estimated from the child's age, body weight, degree of activity, and body temperature. *Basal metabolic rate (BMR)* is derived from standard tables and adjusted for the child's activity, temperature, and disease state. For example, for afebrile patients at rest the maintenance water requirement is approximately 100 ml for each kilocalorie expended (Barness, 1986). Children with fluid losses or other alterations require adjustment of these basic needs to accommodate abnormal losses of both water and electrolytes as a result of a disease state. For example, insensible losses are increased when basal expenditure is increased by unusual activity in bed, fever, and hypermetabolic states. Hypometabolic states, such as hypothyroidism and hypothermia, decrease the BMR.

Table 28-1 Electrolyte concentration of body fluids (mEq/L)

SOURCE	Na^+	K^+	Cl^-
Stomach	20-80	5-20	100-150
Ileostomy	45-135	3-156	20-115
Diarrhea	10-90	10-80	10-110
Sweat	10-30	3-10	10-35
Burn	140-145	4-5	110

NURSING ALERT Nurses need to be alert for altered fluid requirements in various conditions:

- Increased requirements:
  - Fever (add 12% per rise of 1° C)
  - Vomiting, diarrhea
  - High-output renal failure
  - Diabetes insipidus
  - Tachypnea
- Decreased requirements:
  - Congestive heart failure
  - Meningitis (syndrome of inappropriate antidiuretic hormone [SIADH])
  - Mechanical ventilation
  - Postoperatively
  - Oliguric renal failure

Changes in Fluid Volume Related to Growth

The percentage of total body water varies among individuals and in adults and older children is related primarily to the amount of body fat. Consequently females, who have significantly more body fat than males, and obese persons have less water content in relation to weight.

The embryo is composed primarily of water with little tis-

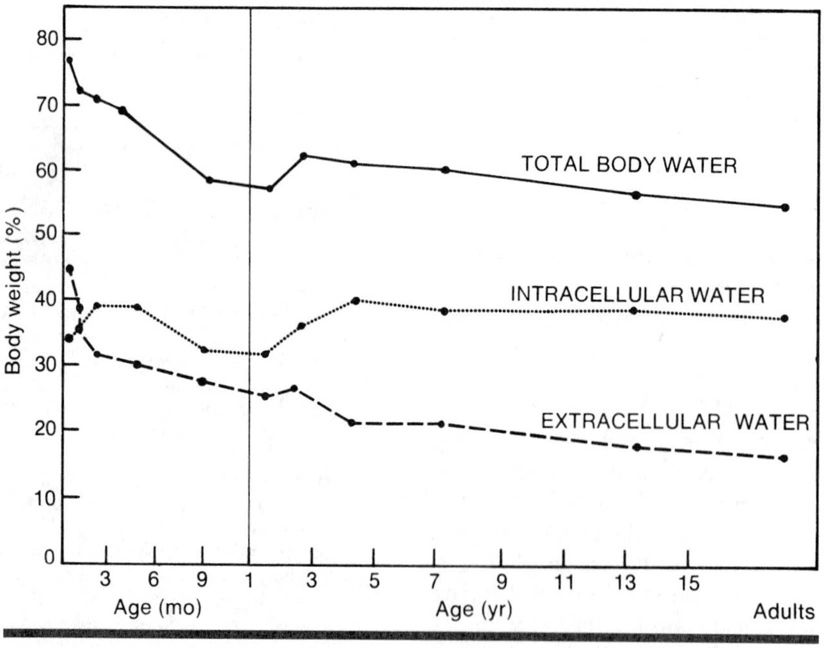

Fig. 28-1. Changes in total body water, extracellular water, and intracellular water in percentages of body weight.
After Fris-Hansen, B.: Pediatrics 28:169, 1961.

sue substance. As the organism grows and develops, there is a progressive decrease in total body water, with the fastest rate of decline taking place during fetal life. The changes in water content and distribution that occur with age reflect the changes that take place in the relative amounts of bone, muscle, and fat comprising the body. The percentage of total body water falls from 90% in the 1-month-old embryo to 75% or 80% of total body weight at birth. In a child 3 years of age total body water comprises 63% of body weight and decreases slowly until age 12, when it reaches approximately 58%. At maturity the percentage of total body water is somewhat higher in the male than in the female and is probably a result of the differences in body composition, particularly fat and muscle content (Fig. 28-1).

Another important aspect of growth change as it corresponds to water distribution is related to the intracellular fluid (ICF) and extracellular fluid (ECF) compartments. In the fetus and prematurely born infant, the largest proportion of body water is contained in the ECF compartment. As growth and development proceed, the proportion within this fluid compartment decreases as the ICF and cell solids increase. The ECF diminishes rapidly from approximately 40% of body weight at birth to 25% at 2 years of age and 20% at maturity. The different effects on males and females become apparent at puberty.

Water Balance in Infants

Because of several characteristics, infants and young children have a greater need for water and are more vulnerable to alterations in fluid and electrolyte balance. Newborns have an appreciably larger water content than older infants and children. This is partially because the newborn has less fat and a greater proportion of body mass, especially the larger percentage of mass composed of the visceral organs. Compared to older children and adults, infants have a greater fluid intake and output relative to size, water and electrolyte disturbances occur more frequently and more rapidly, and infants adjust less promptly to these alterations. The ECF compartment comprises over half of the total body water at birth and contains a greater relative content of extracellular sodium and chloride. Most of this neonatal "excess" ECF is lost in the first 10 days of life through insensible perspiration, which can amount to 5% to 10% of the infant's birth weight.

Until about 2 years of age, the infant maintains a larger amount of ECF than the adult, and this fluid volume, together with other anatomic and physiologic differences, contributes to greater and more rapid water loss and poorer adjustment during this age period. Infants are subject to rapid and profound water depletion in dehydration states as a result of intake restriction or excessive losses from disease. Similarly, overhydration from excessive intake, especially in intravenous (IV) fluid administration, is more serious in infants.

During the first year there is a sharp decrease in total body water when expressed as a percentage of body weight. The percentage of ECF also decreases from approximately 45% to 27%. The gradual alteration in water distribution that accompanies growth and maturation is a result of several changes that occur from infancy to childhood. Muscle growth associated with expanding size of individual cells increases the actual and relative ICF volume and decreases the relative volume of ECF. In addition to muscle growth, other organs also increase in size; for example, the size of nerve cells grows with a corresponding decrease in ECF volume, and the fraction of total body water contained in the skin diminishes during growth. Furthermore, the daily volume of secretions into the gastrointestinal tract is relatively much higher in infants than in children. The net result of these changes is a decrease in the proportion of ECF as the infant grows older.

Surface area. The infant's relatively greater surface area allows larger quantities of fluid to be lost in insensible perspiration through the skin. It is estimated that the body surface area of the premature neonate is proportionately five times as great, and that of the newborn is two to three times as great, as that of the older child or adult. The gastrointestinal tract, sometimes considered to be an extension of the body surface area, is also relatively larger in infancy and is a source of proportionately greater fluid loss, especially from diarrhea. The large surface area is an important factor in metabolism and heat production, which also influence fluid loss.

Metabolic rate. The rate of metabolism in infancy is significantly higher than in adulthood because of the larger surface area in relation to the mass of active tissue. Consequently there is a greater production of metabolic wastes that must be excreted by the kidneys. Any condition that increases metabolism causes a rise in heat production, with its concomitant insensible fluid loss and growing need for water for excretion.

Kidney function. The kidneys of the infant are functionally immature at birth and are therefore inefficient in excreting waste products of metabolism. Of particular importance for fluid balance is the inability of the infant's kidneys to concentrate or dilute urine, to conserve or excrete sodium, and to acidify urine. Therefore the infant is less able to handle large quantities of solute-free water than the older child and is more apt to become dehydrated when given concentrated formulas.

Fluid requirements. As a result of these characteristics, infants ingest and excrete a greater amount of fluid per kilogram of body weight than older children. Since electrolytes are excreted with water and the infant has limited ability for conservation, maintenance requirements include both water and electrolytes. The daily exchange of ECF in the infant is much greater than that in older children, which leaves little fluid volume reserve in dehydration states. Water requirements for infants and children at various ages are listed in Table 28-2.

DISTURBANCES OF FLUID AND ELECTROLYTE BALANCE

Disturbances of fluids and their solute concentration are closely interrelated. Alterations in fluid volume affect the

Table 28-2 Maintenance requirements

WEIGHT (kg)	SURFACE AREA (m^2)	WATER (ml/kg)	Cal/kg	Na^+/kg (mEq)	K^+/kg (mEq)
3	0.20	100	40-50	3-4	3-4
5	0.27	90	50-70	3-4	3-4
10	0.45	75	40-60	2-3	2-3
15	0.64	65	40-50	2-3	2-3
30	1.10	55	35-45	2-3	1-2
50	1.50	45	25-40	1-2	1-2
70	1.75	40	15-20	1-2	1-2

From Barness, L.A.: Fluid and electrolyte therapy. In Gillis, S.S. and Kagan, B.M., editors: Current pediatric therapy 12, Philadelphia, 1986, W.B. Saunders Co., p. 762.
Requirements/m^2: water 1500 ml, Na^+ 60 mEq, K^+ 45 mEq.

electrolyte component, and changes in electrolyte concentration influence fluid movement. Since intracellular water and electrolytes move to and from the ECF compartment, any imbalance in the ICF is reflected by an imbalance in the ECF. Disturbances in the ECF involve either an excess or a deficit of fluid and/or electrolytes; of these, fluid loss occurs more frequently.

Depletion of ECF, usually caused by gastroenteritis, is one of the most common problems encountered in infants and children (see Chapter 29). Until modern techniques for fluid replacement were perfected, it was one of the chief causes of infant mortality. Fluid and electrolyte problems related to specific diseases and their management are discussed throughout the book where appropriate. The major fluid disturbances, their usual causes, and clinical manifestations are outlined in Table 28-3; the most common distur-

Table 28-3 Disturbances of fluid and electrolyte balance

MECHANISMS/SITUATIONS	MANIFESTATIONS	MANAGEMENT/NURSING CARE
▪ Water depletion		
Failure to absorb or reabsorb water Complete sudden cessation of intake or prolonged diminished intake: Neglect of intake by self or caregiver—confused, psychotic, unconscious, or helpless Loss from gastrointestinal tract—vomiting, diarrhea, nasogastric suction, fistula Disturbed body fluid chemistry: inappropriate ADH secretion Excessive renal excretion: glycosuria (diabetes) Loss through skin or lungs: Excessive perspiration or vaporization—febrile states, hyperventilation, increased ambient temperature Impaired skin integrity—transudate from injuries Hemorrhage Iatrogenic: Overzealous use of diuretics Improper postoperative fluid replacement	General symptoms: Thirst Variable temperature—increased (infection) Dry skin and mucous membranes Poor skin turgor Poor perfusion (decreased pulse, slowed capillary refill time) Weight loss Fatigue Diminished urine output Irritability and lethargy Tachycardia Tachypnea Altered level of consciousness Symptoms depend to some extent on proportion of electrolytes lost with water Laboratory findings: High urine specific gravity Increased hematocrit Variable serum electrolytes Variable urine volume Increased blood urea nitrogen (BUN) Increased osmolality	Provide replacement of fluid losses commensurate with volume depletion Provide maintenance fluids Determine and correct cause of water depletion Measure intake and output Monitor vital signs
▪ Water excess		
Water intake in excess of output: Excessive oral intake Excessive intravenous infusion Hypertonic fluid overload Plain water enemas Failure to excrete water in presence of normal intake: Kidney disease Congestive heart failure Malnutrition	Edema: Generalized Pulmonary (moist rales) Intracutaneous (noted especially in loose areolar tissue) Elevated venous pressure Hepatomegaly Slow, bounding pulse Weight gain Lethargy Increased spinal fluid pressure Central nervous system manifestations (seizures, coma) Laboratory findings: Low urine specific gravity Decreased serum electrolytes Decreased hematocrit Variable urine volume	Limit fluid intake Administer diuretics Monitor vital signs Determine and treat cause of water excess Analyze laboratory electrolyte measurements frequently

Table 28-3 Disturbances of fluid balance—cont'd

MECHANISMS/SITUATIONS	MANIFESTATIONS	MANAGEMENT/NURSING CARE
▪ Sodium depletion (hyponatremia)		
Prolonged low-sodium diet Fever Excess sweating Tachypnea (infants) Cystic fibrosis Burns and wounds Vomiting, diarrhea, nasogastric suction, fistulas Adrenal insufficiency Renal disease Diabetic acidosis	Associated with water loss: Same as with water loss—dehydration, weakness, dizziness, nausea, abdominal cramps, apprehension Mild—apathy, weakness, nausea, soft pulse Moderate—decreased blood pressure Laboratory findings: Sodium concentration <130 mEq/L (may be normal if volume low) Specific gravity depends on water deficit or excess	Determine and treat cause Administer IV fluids with appropriate saline concentration
▪ Sodium excess (hypernatremia)		
High salt intake—nasogastric or IV Renal disease	Intense thirst Dry, sticky mucous membranes Flushed skin Temperature may be increased Hoarseness Oliguria Nausea and vomiting Irritability and possible progression to disorientation, convulsions Laboratory findings: Serum sodium concentration ≥ 150 mEq/L High plasma volume Alkalosis	Determine and treat cause Administer fluids as prescribed Measure intake and output Monitor laboratory data
▪ Potassium depletion (hypokalemia)		
Starvation Clinical conditions associated with poor food intake Malabsorption IV fluid without added potassium Diarrhea, vomiting, fistulas, nasogastric suction Diuresis Administration of diuretics Administration of corticosteroids Diuretic phase of nephrotic syndrome Healing stage of burns Potassium-losing nephritis Hyperglycemic diuresis (e.g., diabetes mellitus) Familial periodic paralysis IV administration of insulin in ketoacidosis Alkalosis	Muscle weakness, cramping, stiffness, paralysis, hyporeflexia Hypotension Cardiac arrhythmias, gallop rhythm Tachycardia or bradycardia Ileus Apathy, drowsiness Irritability Fatigue Laboratory findings: Decreased serum potassium concentration ≤ 3.5 mEq/L Abnormal ECG—flat, notched, or inverted T waves, prolonged ST segment	Determine and treat cause Monitor vital signs, including ECG Administer supplemental potassium Assess for adequate renal output before administration IV: administer slowly Oral: offer high-potassium fluids and foods
▪ Potassium excess (hyperkalemia)		
Renal disease Renal shutdown Adrenal insufficiency (Addison disease) Associated with metabolic acidosis Too rapid administration of IV potassium chloride Transfusion with old donor blood Severe dehydration Crushing injuries Burns Hemolysis from sudden massive water intake Dehydration	Muscle weakness, flaccid paralysis Twitching Hyperreflexia Bradycardia Ventricular fibrillation and cardiac arrest Oliguria Apnea—respiratory arrest Laboratory findings: High serum potassium concentration ≥ 5.5 mEq/L Variable urine volume Flat P wave on ECG, peaked T waves	Determine and treat cause Monitor vital signs, including ECG Administer exchange resin, if prescribed Administer IV fluids as prescribed Administer insulin (if ordered) to facilitate movement of potassium into cells Monitor serum potassium levels

Continued.

Table 28-3 Disturbances of fluid balance—cont'd

MECHANISMS/SITUATIONS	MANIFESTATIONS	MANAGEMENT/NURSING CARE
▪ Calcium depletion (hypocalcemia)		
Inadequate dietary calcium Vitamin D deficiency Rapid transit through gastointestinal tract Advanced renal insufficiency Administration of diuretics Hypoparathyroidism Alkalosis Trapped in diseased tissues Increased serum protein (albumin) Cow's milk formula—tetany of the newborn Exchange transfusion with citrated blood	Neuromuscular irritability Tingling of nose, ears, fingertips, toes Tetany Laryngospasm Generalized convulsions May be changes in clotting Positive Chvostek sign Hypotension Cardiac arrest Laboratory findings: Decreased serum calcium concentration (N = 8.8 − 10.8 mEq/L) or Increased serum protein	Determine and treat cause Administer calcium supplements as prescribed; administer slowly Monitor IV site; calcium may cause vascular irritation Monitor serum calcium levles Monitor serum protein levels
▪ Calcium excess (hypercalcemia)		
Acidosis Prolonged immobilization Conditions associated with increased bone catabolism Hypoproteinemia Kidney disease Hypervitaminosis D Hyperparathyroidism	Few problems (ordinarily) Constipation Anorexia Dryness of mouth (thirst) Muscle hypotonicity Bradycardia/cardiac arrest Increased calcium concentration in urine may cause formation of kidney stones Laboratory findings: Increased serum calcium levels or Decreased serum protein levels	Determine and treat cause Monitor serum calcium levels Monitor ECG

Box 28-3 AREAS OF CONCERN IN PLANNING MANAGEMENT OF FLUID PROBLEMS

- Volume of the body fluids (i.e., the water content of the patient)
- Osmolality of the body fluids, a factor that has an effect on the distribution of body water among the various compartments
- Hydrogen ion status (i.e., whether or not there has been a disturbance in the pH of body fluids or a disturbance in the homeostatic mechanisms that maintain the pH)
- Electrolyte deficits from cells as well as extracellular water
- Disturbances in the equilibrium between the mineral skeleton and body fluids

bances—dehydration and edema—are elaborated further. Problems of fluid and electrolyte disturbance always involve both water and electrolytes; therefore replacement includes administration of both, calculated on the basis of ongoing processes and laboratory serum electrolyte values.

In problems that involve alterations in the amount and composition of body fluid compartments, five areas are considered when planning management (Box 28-3). The following discussion is concerned with the general concepts of two common fluid volume disturbances, dehydration and edema, that are features of a variety of conditions. Specific disorders are discussed in Chapters 29 and 30 and elsewhere in the book when appropriate.

DEHYDRATION

Dehydration is a common body fluid disturbance encountered in the nursing of infants and children; it occurs whenever the total output of fluid exceeds the total intake, regardless of the underlying cause. Although dehydration can result from lack of oral intake (especially in elevated environmental temperatures), more often it is a result of abnormal losses, such as those that occur in vomiting or diarrhea, when oral intake only partially compensates for the abnormal losses. Other significant causes of dehydration are diabetic ketoacidosis and extensive burns.

In early dehydration (during the first 2 days) fluid loss is derived from both the ECF and the ICF, since the increased osmolality of the diminished ECF volume causes fluid from the ICF compartment to move into the ECF compartment. As dehydration becomes chronic, the cellular losses predominate.

Types of Dehydration

Sodium is the primary osmotic force that controls fluid movement between the major fluid compartments; therefore describing dehydration according to plasma sodium concentrations (i.e., isonatremic, hyponatremic, or hypernatremic) would be more descriptive. However, other osmotic forces may play the dominant role in dehydration, such as glucose in diabetic dehydration and protein in nephrotic syndrome. Consequently dehydration is conventionally classified as (1) isotonic, (2) hypotonic, and (3) hypertonic.

Isotonic dehydration. Isotonic (isosmotic or isonatremic) dehydration occurs in conditions in which electrolyte and water deficits are present in approximately balanced proportion. The observable fluid losses are not necessarily isotonic, but losses from other avenues make adjustments so that the sum of all losses, or the net loss, is isotonic. Since there is no osmotic force present to cause a redistribution of water between the ICF and ECF, the major loss is sustained from the ECF compartments. This significantly reduces the plasma volume and hence the circulating blood volume with its effect on skin, muscle, and kidneys. Shock is the greatest threat to life in isotonic dehydration, and the child with isotonic dehydration displays symptoms characteristic of hypovolemic shock. Plasma sodium remains within normal limits, between 130 and 150 mEq/L.

Hypotonic dehydration. Hypotonic (hyposmotic or hyponatremic) dehydration occurs when the electrolyte deficit exceeds the water deficit. Since ICF is more concentrated than ECF in hypotonic dehydration, water transfers from the ECF to the ICF to establish osmotic equilibrium. This movement further increases the ECF volume loss, and shock is a frequent result. Because there is a greater proportional loss of ECF in hypotonic dehydration, the physical signs tend to be more severe with smaller fluid losses than isotonic or hypertonic dehydration. Plasma sodium concentration is less than 130 mEq/L.

Hypertonic dehydration. Hypertonic (hyperosmotic or hypernatremic) dehydration results from water loss in excess of electrolyte loss and is usually caused by a proportionately larger loss of water and/or a larger intake of electrolytes. This sometimes occurs in infants with diarrhea who are given fluids by mouth that contain large amounts of solute or in children receiving high-protein nasogastric tube feedings that place an excessive solute load on the kidneys. In hypertonic dehydration, fluid shifts from the lesser concentration of the ICF to the ECF. Plasma sodium concentration is greater than 150 mEq/L.

Since the ECF volume is proportionately larger, hypertonic dehydration consists of a greater degree of water loss for the same intensity of physical signs. Shock is less apparent in hypertonic dehydration. However, neurologic disturbances, such as seizures, are more likely to occur. Cerebral changes are serious and may result in permanent damage. These include disturbance of consciousness, poor ability to focus attention, lethargy, increased muscle tone with hyperreflexia, and hyperirritability to stimuli (tactile, auditory, bright light).

Degree of Dehydration

Traditionally the magnitude of fluid loss has been described as a percentage (5%, 10%, 15%) and ascertained by a comparison of preillness weight and current weight, since any weight loss is substantially equivalent to the amount of water lost. However, water constitutes only 60% to 70% of infant weight, and adipose tissue, which contains little water, is highly variable in individual infants and children. Rather than percentage, a more accurate means of describing dehydration is to reflect acute loss (over 48 hours or less) in milliliters per kilogram of body weight (Finberg, 1990). For example, a 50 ml/kg loss is considered to be a mild fluid loss, whereas 100 ml/kg produces severe dehydration.

Clinical signs provide clues to the extent of dehydration (Table 28-4). The earliest detectable sign is usually tachycardia, followed by dry skin and mucous membranes, sunken fontanel, signs of circulatory failure (coolness and mottling of extremities), loss of skin elasticity, and delayed capillary filling time.

Compensatory mechanisms attempt to maintain fluid volume by adjusting to these losses. Interstitial fluid moves into the vascular compartment to defend the blood volume in response to hemoconcentration and hypovolemia, and vasoconstriction of peripheral arterioles helps maintain pumping pressure. When fluid losses exceed the body's ability to sustain blood volume and blood pressure, circulation is seriously compromised and the blood pressure falls. This results in tissue hypoxia with accumulation of lactic

Table 28-4 Intensity of clinical signs associated with varying degrees of isotonic dehydration in infants

	DEGREE OF DEHYDRATION		
	MILD	MODERATE	SEVERE
Fluid volume loss	<50 ml/kg	50-90 ml/kg	≥100 ml/kg
Skin color	Pale	Gray	Mottled
Skin elasticity	Decreased	Poor	Very poor
Mucous membranes	Dry	Very dry	Parched
Urine output	Decreased	Oliguria	Marked oliguria and azotemia
Blood pressure	Normal	Normal or lowered	Lowered
Pulse	Normal or increased	Increased	Rapid and thready
Capillary filling time	<2 seconds	2-3 seconds	>3 seconds

acid, pyruvate, and other acid metabolites, which contributes to the development of metabolic acidosis.

Renal compensation is impaired by reduced blood flow through the kidneys, and little urine is formed. Increased serum osmolality stimulates the secretion of antidiuretic hormone to conserve fluid and initiates the renin-angiotensin mechanisms in the kidney, causing further vasoconstriction. Aldosterone is released to promote sodium retention and conserve water in the kidneys. If dehydration increases in severity, urine formation is markedly diminished and metabolites and hydrogen ions that are normally excreted by this route are retained.

Shock is a common manifestation of severe depletion of ECF volume accompanied by tachycardia and signs of poor perfusion. Peripheral circulation is poor as a result of reduced blood volume; therefore the skin is cool and mottled, with poor capillary filling after blanching. Impaired kidney circulation often leads to oliguria and azotemia. While low blood pressure may accompany other symptoms of shock, in infants and young children it is usually a late sign and may herald the onset of cardiovascular collapse.

Diagnostic Evaluation

To initiate a therapeutic plan, several factors must be determined: the degree of dehydration based on physical assessment; the type of dehydration based on the pathophysiology of the specific illness responsible for the dehydrated state; specific physical signs other than general signs; initial plasma sodium concentrations; and associated electrolyte (especially serum potassium) and acid-base imbalances. Initial and regular ongoing evaluations are carried out to assess the patient's progress toward equilibrium and the effectiveness of therapy.

Therapeutic Management

Medical management is directed at correcting the fluid imbalance and treating the underlying cause. When the child is alert, awake, and not in shock, correction of dehydration may be attempted with oral fluid administration. Most dehydration is mild and can be managed at home by this method. Several commercial rehydration fluids are available for use (see Table 29-1). Oral rehydration management consists of rapid replacement of fluid loss over 4 to 6 hours, replacement of continuing losses, and providing for maintenance fluid requirements. Amounts and rates are determined from body weight and are increased if rehydration is incomplete or if excess losses continue. Full diet is usually withheld until the child is well hydrated and the basic problem is under control (see Diarrhea, Chapter 29).

Parenteral fluid therapy. Parenteral fluid therapy is instigated whenever the child is unable to ingest sufficient amounts of fluid and electrolytes to (1) meet ongoing daily physiologic losses, (2) replace previous deficits, and (3) replace ongoing abnormal losses. Patients who usually require IV fluids are those with severe dehydration, those with uncontrollable vomiting, those who are unable to drink for any reason (e.g., extreme fatigue, coma), and those with severe gastric distention (Barness, 1986).

Since dehydration constitutes the greatest threat to life, the first priority is the restoration of circulation by rapid expansion of the ECF volume in order to treat shock or prevent its occurrence. IV administration of fluid is begun immediately, even though the exact nature of the dehydration and the serum electrolyte values are not known. The solution selected is based on what is known regarding the probable type and cause of the dehydration—usually a saline solution.

A suggested formula is to replace one half the estimated deficit over the first 8 to 16 hours and one half over the next 16 to 24 hours, depending on the type of dehydration; thus the deficit is recovered within 24 to 48 hours. Maintenance fluid volumes are calculated and added to the infusion therapy during replacement therapy.

Sodium bicarbonate may be added, since acidosis is usually associated with severe dehydration, but potassium is not administered until kidney function is restored, unless the child is known to be hypokalemic (as in diabetic ketoacidosis). As the circulation improves, the glomerular filtration pressure increases to improve renal function, which is essential to electrolyte readjustments.

The goal of the next phase is the restoration of ECF volume. With improved circulation, water and electrolyte deficits can be evaluated and acid-base status corrected either directly through the administration of fluids or indirectly through improved renal function. Next, potassium lost in ICF must be replaced slowly by way of the ECF. Finally, the body fat and protein stores are replaced through diet. If the child is unable to eat or if feeding aggravates the condition (e.g., diarrhea), IV alimentation is provided to prevent serious malnourishment.

Although the initial phase of fluid replacement is rapid in both isotonic and hypotonic dehydration, it is contraindicated in hypertonic dehydration because of the risk of water intoxication, especially in the brain cells. There is an apparent physiologic difference in the manner and length of time for diffusion of sodium into and out of brain cells. There is a significant time lag for sodium to reach a steady state in these cells, whereas water diffuses almost instantaneously. Consequently, rapid administration of fluid will cause equally rapid diffusion of water into the dehydrated brain cells, causing marked cerebral edema. Since ECF volume is maintained relatively well in hypertonic as opposed to the other types of dehydration, shock is not a usual manifestation.

WATER INTOXICATION

Water intoxication, or water overload, is observed less often than dehydration. However, it is important that nurses and others who care for children are aware that this can occur and be alert to the possibility in certain situations. Patients who ingest excessive amounts of fluid develop a concurrent decrease in serum sodium and central nervous system symptoms. There is a large urine output and, because water moves into the brain more rapidly than sodium moves out, the child also exhibits irritability, somnolence, headache, vomiting, diarrhea, and generalized seizures. The affected child usually appears well hydrated but may be edematous or even dehydrated.

Fluid intoxication can occur during acute IV water overloading, too rapid dialysis, tap water enemas, or with too rapid reduction of glucose levels in diabetic ketoacidosis. Patients with central nervous system infections occasionally retain excessive amounts of water. Administration of inappropriate hypotonic solutions (e.g., 5% dextrose in water) may cause a rapid reduction in sodium and result in symptoms of water overload.

Infants are especially vulnerable to fluid overload. Their thirst mechanism is not well developed; therefore they are unable to "turn off" fluid intake appropriately. A decreased glomerular filtration rate does not allow for repeated excretion of a water load, and ADH levels may not be maximally reduced. Consequently infants are unable to excrete a water overload effectively.

Administration of inappropriately prepared formula is one of the more common causes of water intoxication, often related to feeding mismanagement (Schulman, 1980). Families who cannot afford to buy enough expensive formula may dilute the formula to increase the volume or even substitute water for the formula. A family may run out of formula and dilute the remaining amount to make it last until they are able to purchase replacement formula. In addition, water is sometimes used for pacification. Water intoxication can also occur in infants who receive overly vigorous hydration during a febrile illness.

A number of clinicians have reported water intoxication in infants following swimming lessons (Bennett, Wagner, and Fields, 1983; Goldberg and others, 1982; Kropp and Schwartz, 1982). Although they hold their breath, some infants apparently swallow a large amount of water during repeated submersion. This is probably not a common occurrence, since parents who observe their infants swallowing water tend to keep the infant's head above water (Phillips, 1987). Anticipatory guidance to parents should include a discussion of swimming instruction and advice to stop a lesson if the child is observed to swallow unusual amounts of water or exhibit any symptoms of hyponatremia.

EDEMA

Edema is the presence of excess fluid in the interstitial spaces as a result of some defect in the normal circulation of body fluids that causes increased pressure in the interstitial spaces. Fluid removal from the interstitial spaces depends on venous hydrostatic pressure, oncotic pressure of intravascular and interstitial spaces, an intact semipermeable capillary wall, tissue tension, and lymphatic flow.

Mechanisms of Edema Formation

A defect in any of the homeostatic mechanisms maintaining fluid balance can cause accumulation of interstitial fluid. Disequilibrium results from anything that (1) alters the retention of sodium, such as renal disease or hormonal influences; (2) affects the formation or destruction of plasma proteins, such as starvation or liver disease; or (3) alters membrane permeability, such as nephrotic syndrome or trauma.

Edema may be localized to a small or large area, such as that occurring in urticaria, infection, and pulmonary congestion, or it can be generalized, as in the hypoproteinemia of the nephrotic syndrome and starvation. A severe, generalized accumulation of great amounts of fluid in all body tissues is termed *anasarca.*

Increased venous pressure. The colloidal osmotic pressure (COP) of the plasma proteins draws fluid back into the vascular system as long as this force is greater than the venous hydrostatic pressure. However, when the venous pressure is increased, fluid tends to be retained in the interstitial spaces. This can occur when an individual remains in the same position for a long time, such as swollen ankles and feet after standing or sitting for long periods. Constrictive dressings or restraints applied too tightly to extremities will obstruct venous return, increase venous and capillary pressure, and cause edema. The most graphic pathologic illustrations are pulmonary edema caused by pulmonary circulation overload in cardiac defects with a left-to-right shunt and ascites caused by portal hypertension. Edema from any cause is increased in dependent areas because of this added factor of increased venous hydrostatic pressure and the gravitational effects in these areas.

Capillary permeability. Damage to capillary walls or alteration in their permeability permits exudation of plasma protein into the interstitial space. Most often this occurs as local edema, such as manifested in inflammatory and hypersensitivity reactions. Capillary damage from burns allows extensive exudation of protein-rich fluid into the interstitial spaces to compound edema formation.

Diminished plasma proteins. A fall in plasma protein levels hampers the osmotic pull back into the vessels. Consequently fluid remains in the interstitial spaces. Although other factors play a role, such as hydrostatic pressure of both the arterial vascular system and the tissues and Na^+ concentration, significantly low protein levels (below 4.5 mg/dl) are associated with edema. Examples of this are the massive albumin losses of the nephrotic syndrome, diminished serum protein from insufficient dietary protein, and (sometimes) hemodilution of plasma proteins from IV fluid administration in chronic dehydration.

Lymphatic obstruction. Obstruction of lymph flow creates edema high in protein content. This is uncommon in childhood but can result from trauma to the lymphatic glands or removal of lymph nodes.

Tissue tension. Tissue hydrostatic pressure is ordinarily of little consequence. However, it plays a significant role in determining distribution of edema fluid in certain pathologic conditions. Loose tissues allow a greater amount of fluid accumulation than tissues that are tightly bound by dense fibrous bands in which tissue pressure rapidly increases to limit further extravasation of fluid. Edema appears earlier and more readily in loose structures such as those in the periorbital and genital tissues. The areolar structure of lung tissue is probably a contributing factor in pulmonary edema as well as in increased hydrostatic pressure in the pulmonary vessels.

Other factors in edema formation. Any factor that causes Na^+ retention by the kidneys will produce or augment edema formation. This includes stimulation of the renin-angiotensin-aldosterone mechanisms for Na^+ reabsorption created by the diminished plasma volume in edema, which resulted from primary causes. The salt-retaining property of steroids is responsible for the edema associated with their administration.

A particularly threatening form of edema is cerebral edema caused by trauma, infection, or other etiologic factors, including vascular overload or injudicious IV administration of hypotonic solutions. The problems and assessment of cerebral edema are always nursing considerations in fluid administration.

Therapeutic Management

The primary goal in the management of edema is treatment of the basic disease process, which is discussed in relation to the specific disorders. However, an essential aspect in the management of any fluid overload is early recognition, in which nurses play a vital role.

DISTURBANCES OF ACID-BASE BALANCE

The ability of the body to regulate the acid-base status is one of its most crucial physiologic functions. Many disease states, such as diarrhea, vomiting, or febrile conditions, are complicated by disturbances in the acid-base balance, which are often more hazardous to the child's survival than the primary disease process. Sometimes simply providing adequate hydration, replacing electrolytes, and correcting acid-base disturbances are all that is needed to sustain an infant or child until the primary disorder has run its course.

ACID-BASE IMBALANCE

A disturbance of acid-base equilibrium in the direction of acidosis or alkalosis may come about in a variety of ways. However, very simply stated, *acidosis (acidemia)* results from either accumulation of acid or loss of base, and *alkalosis (alkalemia)* results from either accumulation of base or loss of acid.

Hydrogen Ion Concentration

The pH represents the concentration of H^+ in solution and only indicates whether the imbalance is more acidic or more alkaline. It does not reflect the nature of the imbalance, that is, whether it is of metabolic or respiratory origin. Body metabolism affects primarily the base bicarbonate (HCO_3); therefore alterations in the concentration of HCO_3 are termed *metabolic* disturbances of acid-base balance. Also, since the amount of CO_2 exhaled through the lungs affects the carbonic acid (H_2CO_3), changes in H_2CO_3 concentration are referred to as *respiratory* disturbances. Consequently the simple disturbances (those with a single primary cause) are categorized as metabolic acidosis or alkalosis and respiratory acidosis or alkalosis.

It is also significant that the major signs and symptoms of hydrogen ion imbalances, acidosis and alkalosis, reflect central nervous system involvement. Depression of the central nervous system, manifested by lethargy, diminished mental capacity, delirium, stupor, and coma, is observed in acidosis of either metabolic or respiratory origin. On the other hand, alkalosis produces clinical manifestations of nervous system stimulation and excitement, including overexcitability, nervousness, tingling sensations, and tetany that may progress to convulsions. Persons with epilepsy are particularly susceptible to seizures, which can be precipitated by hyperventilation.

It is also important to note that eventually all body systems will become dysfunctional if the "normal" limits of pH are violated for very long. The extent and severity of signs and symptoms depend on the length of time the imbalance has existed and the magnitude or degree of the deviation from normal. A rapid, severe imbalance will seriously compromise the compensatory mechanisms to the point where it is incompatible with life, whereas the body will be able to compensate adequately for a mild, gradual distortion and produce few if any observable signs or symptoms.

Compensatory Mechanisms

When the fundamental acid-base ratio is altered for any reason, the body attempts to correct the deviation. In a simple disturbance there is a single *primary* factor that affects one component of the acid-base pair and is usually accompanied by a *compensatory* or *secondary* change in the component that is not primarily affected. For example, increased formation of metabolic acid rapidly reduces the HCO_3 in the formation of H_2CO_3. The respiratory mechanism immediately attempts to compensate for the imbalance by eliminating the H_2CO_3 through exhaled CO_2 and water. The imbalance is corrected when the kidneys excrete hydrogen and ammonium ions in exchange for reabsorbed sodium bicarbonate.

When the secondary changes (the hyperventilation and renal excretion of H^+ in the preceding example) succeed in preventing a distortion of the acid-base ratio and the pH is restored to normal, the disturbance is described as *compensated.* The *uncompensated* state exists when there is no compensatory effect and the pH remains uncorrected. The imbalance is said to be *corrected* when physiologic mechanisms fully correct the primary abnormality.

Laboratory Measurements

Several laboratory tests are employed to assess the nature and extent of acid-base disturbances. The importance of these data is readily apparent when a clinical observation such as hyperventilation can represent either the primary factor in respiratory alkalosis or a secondary or compensatory factor in metabolic acidosis. The laboratory tests of value in the assessment of acid-base status are outlined in Table 28-5. To determine the acid-base status, three variables—the respiratory component (P_{CO_2}), the metabolic component (arterial HCO_3, or serum CO_2), and the serum

Table 28-5 Laboratory tests employed in assessment of acid-base status

ABBREVIATION	TEST	NORMAL VALUES*	DESCRIPTION
pH	Partial pressure of hydrogen	Birth: 7.11-7.36 1 day: 7.29-7.45 Child: 7.35-7.45	Expression of hydrogen ion concentration
P_{CO_2}	Partial pressure of carbon dioxide or carbon dioxide tension	Newborn: 27-40 Infant: 27-41 Girls: 32-45 Boys: 35-48	Measure of carbon dioxide tension; reflects carbonic acid (H_2CO_3) concentration of plasma
HCO_3 (serum) arterial	Carbon dioxide content or carbon dioxide combining power	Infant: 21-28 mEq/L	Concentration of base bicarbonate
BE	Base excess (whole blood)	Newborn: −2 to −10 Infant: −1 to −7 Child: +2 to −4 Thereafter: +3 to −3	Used to express extent of deviation from normal buffer base concentration; indicates quantity of blood buffers remaining after hydrogen ion is buffered

*Data from Behrman, R.E., and Vaughan, V.C., III, editors: Nelson textbook of pediatrics, ed. 13, Philadelphia, 1987, W.B. Saunders Co.

Table 28-6 Summary of simple acid-base disturbances (partially compensated)

DISTURBANCE	PLASMA pH	PLASMA P_{CO_2}	PLASMA HCO_3
Respiratory acidosis	↓	↑	↑
Respiratory alkalosis	↑	↓	↓
Metabolic acidosis	↓	↓	↓
Metabolic alkalosis	↑	↑	↑

pH—must be determined. Measurement of any two will allow computation of the third. A summary of relationships between these and other variables is outlined in Table 28-6.

Associated Disturbances in Acid-Base Balance

Physiologic functions of the body take place optimally when the pH is maintained within a normal range. The disequilibrium created by moderately altered pH can produce disordered function of physiologic and enzyme systems, but great divergences are incompatible with life. In addition, electrolyte shifts that take place in response to changes in pH alter the electrolyte concentration in the fluid compartments to disturb the normal concentrations. For example, cell membrane permeability is affected by changes in pH. A lowered pH allows K^+ to move from the ICF to the ECF. Serum K^+ levels increase with acidosis and decrease with alkalosis.

Serum potassium. One of the disturbances that complicates both fluid losses and acid-base imbalance is an alteration in K^+ levels. During dehydration, fluid moves out of the ICF compartment into the ECF compartment in an attempt to balance the fluid losses. In doing so, K^+ also moves out, creating a total body K^+ depletion. Since renal function is drastically reduced in dehydration, normal excretion of K^+ does not take place. This causes elevated serum levels that can produce all the signs and symptoms of hyperkalemia. During rapid rehydration therapy for gastrointestinal losses and diabetic ketoacidosis, the ECF K^+ moves back into the ICF compartment, thereby posing the risk of hypokalemia unless there is an anticipated replacement. However, K^+ is not replaced until the ICF is sufficient to restore adequate renal function.

Serum calcium. Disturbed ECF calcium (Ca^+) levels may occur in various types of dehydration. Usually the disturbance is in the form of reduced serum Ca^+ levels, especially where there is a concomitant potassium loss. Although hypocalcemia is a common finding, it rarely reaches a point of tetany in current practice, which includes adequate replacement of potassium losses. Immediate effects of Ca^+ imbalance associated with acidosis or alkalosis are tetany of metabolic alkalosis; long-term effects of chronic acidosis are related to bone resorption from renal disturbances.

Oxygen combination. The capacity of oxygen (O_2) to combine with hemoglobin is also affected by changes in pH. The affinity of hemoglobin for O_2 decreases with a decrease in pH so that, in a state of acidosis, less O_2 will be picked up by the hemoglobin as blood travels through the lungs. However, O_2 is more easily released to the tissues when the pH is lowered. The opposite effects operate during an increase in pH.

Blood flow. Blood flow in various areas is altered by changes in pH. Pulmonary circulation constricts in acidosis, whereas decreased pH (acidosis) causes vasodilation in systemic vessels.

RESPIRATORY ACIDOSIS

Respiratory acidosis results from diminished or inadequate pulmonary ventilation that causes an elevation in plasma P_{CO_2} and thus an increased concentration of dissolved H_2CO_3, which leads to elevated carbonic acid and H^+ concentration. Conditions that produce respiratory acidosis can

Box 28-4 ORIGINS OF INADEQUATE GAS EXCHANGE

Factors that depress the respiratory center, such as head injury, depressant or narcotizing drugs, and infections of the central nervous system
Factors that affect the lung proper, such as obstructive pulmonary disease, pneumonia, cystic fibrosis, acute pulmonary edema, atelectasis, and occlusion of respiratory passages
Factors that interfere with the bellows action of the chest wall, including trauma to the chest wall, skeletal diseases or deformities, and diseases of the thoracic muscles or their innervation (e.g., muscular dystrophy or muscular atrophy)

originate at three levels in the respiratory system and result in inadequate gas exchange (Box 28-4).

Compensation is mediated through the kidneys, which are stimulated to conserve and thus increase the plasma HCO_3 concentration and to excrete hydrogen ions. Laboratory findings in respiratory acidosis include elevated plasma HCO_3 concentration (over 29 mEq/L in older children, over 28 mEq/L in young children) and elevated Pco_2 (above 38 mm Hg, arterial).

The treatment of respiratory acidosis is aimed at correcting the primary defect and improving gas exchange at the alveolar level to provide more efficient removal of CO_2. Administration of buffers such as bicarbonate to reduce H^+ concentration remains controversial, since their addition *without* adequate ventilatory control providing ongoing elimination of CO_2 may only serve to aggravate acidosis.

RESPIRATORY ALKALOSIS

Conversely, respiratory alkalosis is caused by a primary increase in the rate and depth of pulmonary ventilation, resulting in unusually large amounts of CO_2 being exhaled or "blown off." This reduces the plasma Pco_2, H_2CO_3, and H^+ concentration and leaves an excess of HCO_3. Conditions that cause stimulation of the respiratory center to produce hyperventilation are listed in Box 28-5.

A frequent cause of hyperventilation in children is voluntary hyperventilation before underwater swimming. It is also a consideration in the care of persons having assisted ventilation. Incorrectly set mechanical ventilators can cause respiratory rates and tidal volumes in excess of physiologic needs.

Compensation of respiratory alkalosis takes place in the kidneys and consists of excretion of H_2CO_3 in association with Na^+ and K^+ to conserve H^+. Laboratory findings include elevated plasma pH (over 7.43), depressed plasma H_2CO_3 concentration (less than 23 mEq/L in older children, less than 20 mEq/L in young children), and lowered Pco_2 (less than 35 mm Hg).

Treatment of respiratory alkalosis consists of correction of the primary defect and prevention of lost anions and the associated K^+ deficit. CO_2 administered by mask slows respirations and provides rapid relief.

Box 28-5 CONDITIONS THAT PRODUCE HYPERVENTILATION

Primary central nervous system stimulation resulting from emotions, including hysteria, fear, or apprehensions; central nervous system infection (encephalitis); and certain drug reactions, such as early salicylate intoxication (a primary respiratory stimulant)
Reflex central nervous system stimulation from peripheral chemoreceptors as a result of hypoxia, which provides the stimulus for hyperventilation at high altitudes, fever or high environmental temperatures, and cardiac conditions
Reflex central nervous system stimulation from intrathoracic stretch receptors, which is believed to be the cause of hyperventilation in localized pulmonary disease

Box 28-6 METABOLIC ACIDOSIS

Strong acid is gained by:
- Gain of exogenous acid (e.g., ammonium chloride) by ingestion or infusion
- Incomplete oxidation of fatty acids, which occurs in conditions such as diabetic ketoacidosis, starvation (including patients receiving nothing by mouth for therapeutic purposes), and salicylate poisoning
- Incomplete oxidation of carbohydrate that produces large amounts of lactic acid as a result of primary lactic acidosis (rare) or secondary to tissue hypoxia from excessive exercise, serious trauma, and severe infection
- Inability of the renal system to excrete the normal, ongoing volume of inorganic acid metabolites, which results from the azotemic acidosis of advanced renal failure

Base bicarbonate is lost by:
- Losses from the gastrointestinal tract—secretions distal to the pyloric sphincter contain large amounts of bicarbonate, which may be lost during conditions that produce diarrhea or vomiting, including fistula drainage and suction
- Losses as a result of inappropriate bicarbonate excretion in the kidneys because of renal tubular acidosis

METABOLIC ACIDOSIS

Metabolic acidosis is a lowered plasma pH caused by any process that reduces the HCO_3 concentration. Metabolic acidosis can be produced by the gain of nonvolatile acids or the loss of HCO_3. Strong acid is gained, and HCO_3 is lost by several specific mechanisms and routes (Box 28-6).

Compensation of metabolic acidosis is respiratory. Strong acids are immediately buffered to generate the weaker H_2CO_3, which the respiratory system attempts to eliminate through increased alveolar ventilation. In this respiratory effort the breathing is deep and rapid—the Kussmaul or air-hunger type of respirations. HCO_3 conservation and excretion by the kidneys is a slower mechanism. Laboratory findings of uncompensated metabolic acidosis include lowered plasma pH (below 7.33), diminished plasma HCO_3 concentration (below 23 mEq/L in older children, be-

Box 28-7 METABOLIC ALKALOSIS

Loss of acid can result from the following:
- In children the most common cause of hydrogen ion depletion is loss of hydrochloric acid (HCl) incident to hypertrophic pyloric stenosis. The infant produces large amounts of HCl, which is vomited with repeated feedings.
- Less often, hydrogen ions are lost through the kidneys in diuretic therapy, potassium depletion, or administration of adrenocortical hormones.

A gain in base is usually iatrogenic and relatively uncommon in children but can result from the following:
- Gain of exogeneous bicarbonate from ingestion or infusion
- Oxidation of salts or organic acid from infusion or ingestion of lactate, citrate, or acetate

low 20 mEq/L in young children), and CO_2 combining power that is lowered and approximately equivalent to the plasma HCO_3 in concentration.

Treatment is directed at correcting the basic defect and replacing the excessive losses of HCO_3 with sodium or potassium bicarbonate or sodium lactate.

METABOLIC ALKALOSIS

Metabolic alkalosis is an elevated plasma pH that occurs when there is a reduction in H^+ concentration and an excess of HCO_3. This can be caused by a gain in base or a loss of acid, which is almost the same as base gain (Box 28-7).

Compensation in metabolic alkalosis theoretically should be respiratory; however, such compensation is irregular and unpredictable. In addition, renal correction is complicated by losses of Na^+, K^+, and Cl^-, which are lost in pyloric stenosis through vomiting. The kidneys will attempt to conserve the Na^+ and K^+ concentration at the expense of H^+ concentration and acid-base balance. Laboratory findings include elevated urine pH (often above 7; may be lowered if associated with K^+ depletion), elevated plasma pH (above 7.43), elevated plasma HCO_3 (above 29 mEq/L in older children, above 28 mEq/L in young children), and, if in conjunction with chloride deficit, reduced Cl^- concentration (below 98 mEq/L).

Treatment of metabolic alkalosis is aimed at preventing further losses of acid and replacement of lost electrolytes.

NURSING RESPONSIBILITIES IN FLUID AND ELECTROLYTE DISTURBANCES

Nursing observation and intervention are essential to the detection and therapeutic management of disturbances in fluid and electrolyte balance. There are a wide variety of circumstances in which imbalances may be precipitated, and the balance is so precarious, especially in infants, that changes can take place in a very short time. Therefore an important nursing responsibility is perceptive observation for any signs of imbalance, particularly in those situations and conditions in which imbalance is likely to occur. Conditions in which changes can develop with surprising rapidity in young children include diarrhea; vomiting; sweating; fever; disorders such as diabetes, renal disease, and cardiac anomalies; administration of certain drugs such as diuretics and steroids; and trauma, such as major surgery, burns, and other extensive injury.

Nurses need to be comfortable with equipment used to deliver fluids to infants and children and be familiar with the knowledge and techniques for assessment. An understanding of normal serum levels provides additional data on which to base assessments and interventions and to validate observations. Data that are helpful in assessment related to fluid and electrolyte balance are the medical diagnosis, the treatment that the child is receiving (especially medications and fluid therapies), laboratory reports, history, and records of intake and output. An important nursing role in child care is teaching parents to recognize early signs of dehydration.

ASSESSMENT

Whether the child is at home, in the practitioner's office or clinic, or in the hospital, nursing assessment is an essential part of the nursing care plan. The assessment of suspected or potential fluid and electrolyte disturbance begins with the observation of general appearance. Ill children usually have drawn, flaccid expressions, and their eyes lack luster. Loss of appetite is one of the first behaviors observed in the majority of childhood illnesses, and the infant's or child's activity level is diminished. The cry of an ill infant is less vigorous, often whining, and higher pitched than usual. The child is irritable, seeks the comfort and attention of the parent, and displays purposeless movements and inappropriate responses to people and familiar things. As the child's illness becomes more severe, the irritability progresses to lethargy and even unconsciousness.

History

Much of the information regarding the child's behavior can be elicited from the parent. In addition to initial observations, a good history is extremely valuable to the assessment. The amount and type of intake and output (especially abnormal output) are important. An accurate estimate of fluid losses is beyond the capacity of history givers, but rough estimates of excessive fluid losses or diminished output can usually be obtained from information such as the number and consistency of stools the child has passed in the past 24 hours, the number of times the child voided, and the type and amount of food and fluid ingested or vomited. Parents frequently omit this information from their discussion with the health professional. They tell how much has been taken but not how much was excreted unless asked specifically for this information.

Both the type and the amount of intake provide valuable information. The quality and quantity can be determined—if intake is sustained, excessive, or curtailed. Loss early in diarrheal illness progresses rapidly, and the water losses can exceed sodium losses leading to hypernatremia. Hypernatremic dehydration indicates a significant interference with water intake. Also important is a history of normal or increased intake of an unusual fluid such as one containing sugar, tea, athletic hydration fluid (e.g., Gatorade), or other solute-containing fluids, which can contribute to hyponatremic dehydration in the face of abnormal losses (Finberg, 1990).

History of gradual weight gain and observations of any puffiness, especially in areas with less dense tissues (periorbital, scrotal), or "clothes fitting tighter" offer early clues to edema. History of excessive intake, especially when associated with diminished output, is important in assessing edema and water intoxication.

Clinical Observations

Tachycardia, the earliest manifestation of dehydration, can also be produced by fever and infection; therefore these are considered in the assessment of dehydration. Dry skin and mucous membranes usually appear early. A sunken fontanel is a useful observation if the configuration of the fontanel is known when the child is healthy. Signs of circulatory failure usually indicate severe dehydration, since compensatory mechanisms are able to sustain blood pressure in the low normal range for some time. Loss of skin elasticity, generally manifest in children less than 2 years of age, is measured by the length of time it takes for pinched abdominal skin to recoil. This sign is also observed in undernourished children. Also, in hypertonic dehydration the skin has a smooth, velvety feel before it develops disturbed elasticity.

Capillary filling time is assessed by pinching the abdominal skin, a toe, or a thumb and estimating the time that blood is observed to return. Capillary filling time in mild dehydration is less than 2 seconds, increasing to over 3 seconds in severe dehydration. The technique is effective in children of all ages. However, it can be altered in the presence of heart failure, which affects circulation time, and hypertonic dehydration, in which fluid loss is primarily intracellular.

The observations outlined in Table 28-7 are also used to arrive at a meaningful assessment. When caring for the ill child, vital signs are assessed as often as every 15 to 30 minutes, and weight is recorded frequently during the initial phase of therapy. It is important to use the same scale each time the child is weighed and to predetermine the weight of any equipment or devices that must remain attached during the weighing process, including arm boards and sandbags. Routine weights should be taken at the same time each day.

Table 28-7 Significance of observations and probable problem

OBSERVATION	SIGNIFICANT VARIATION	PROBABLE IMBALANCE	COMMENTS
Temperature	Elevated	Early water depletion Sodium excess	Elevated temperature will increase rate of water loss
	Lowered	Fluid volume deficit	Caused by reduced energy output Shock is outcome of severe fluid deficit
Pulse	Rapid, weak, thready, easily obliterated	Circulatory collapse may result from fluid deficit, hemorrhage, plasma-to-interstitial fluid shift	Pulse rate should include assessment of volume and quality as well as rate
	Bounding, easily obliterated	Impending circulatory collapse Sodium deficit	Pulse may be influenced by activity or emotions
	Bounding, not easily obliterated	Fluid volume excess Interstitial fluid-to-plasma shift	
	Weak, irregular, rapid	Severe potassium deficit	
	Weak, irregular, slowing	Severe potassium excess	
	Increased	Sodium excess Magnesium deficit	
	Decreased	Magnesium excess	
Respiration	Slow, shallow	Respiratory alkalosis	Rapid respirations increase water loss
	Rapid, deep	Metabolic acidosis	Not a reliable sign of respiratory alkalosis in infants
	Dyspnea	Fluid volume excess either general or pulmonary	
	Moist rales	Fluid volume excess Pulmonary edema	
	Shallow	Potassium excess or deficit	
	Stridor	Severe calcium deficit	
Blood pressure	Increased	Fluid volume excess	Blood pressure not a reliable sign in young children
	Decreased	Sodium deficit	

Table 28-7 Significance of observations and probable problem—cont'd

OBSERVATION	SIGNIFICANT VARIATION	PROBABLE IMBALANCE	COMMENTS
		Diminished vascular volume (loss of plasma-to-interstitial fluid shift) Severe potassium excess or deficit	Elasticity of blood vessels may keep blood pressure stable
Skin			
Color	Pallor	Protein deficit Fluid deficit Fluid compartment shifts	
	Flushed	Sodium excess	
Temperature	Cold mottled extremities	Severe fluid volume deficit, even with fever Severe sodium depletion	Caused by decreased peripheral blood flow
Feel	Dry	Fluid depletion Sodium excess	
	Clammy, cold	Sodium deficit Plasma-to-interstitial fluid shift Hypotonic dehydration	
	Poor capillary filling	Fluid volume deficit	
Elasticity (turgor)	Poor to very poor	Fluid depletion	Pinch of skin from abdomen or inner thigh is lifted and remains raised for several seconds
Edema	Slight to severe	Fluid volume excess Plasma-to-interstitial fluid shift	Obese infants may appear normal
Mucous membranes	Dry Longitudinal wrinkles on tongue	Fluid volume depletion	
	Sticky; rough, red, dry tongue	Sodium excess Hypertonic dehydration	
Salivation and tearing	Absent	Fluid volume deficit	
Fontanel	Sunken Bulging	Fluid volume deficit Fluid volume excess	
Eyeballs	Sunken Soft	Fluid volume deficit	
Sensory alterations	Tingling in fingers and toes	Calcium deficit Alkalosis	Sensory alterations unreliable in infants and young children who are unable to communicate symptoms
	Abdominal cramps	Sodium deficit Potassium excess	
	Muscle cramps	Calcium deficit Potassium deficit	
	Lightheadedness	Respiratory alkalosis	
	Nausea	Calcium excess Potassium excess Potassium deficit	
	Thirst	Fluid deficit Sodium excess Calcium excess	May be difficult to assess in infants May be masked by nausea Any condition that reduces intravascular volume will stimulate thirst receptors

Continued.

Table 28-7 Significance of observations and probable problem—cont'd

OBSERVATION	SIGNIFICANT VARIATION	PROBABLE IMBALANCE	COMMENTS
Neurologic signs	Hypotonia	Potassium deficit Calcium excess	
	Flaccid paralysis	Severe potassium deficit Severe potassium excess	
	Weakness	Metabolic acidosis	
	Hypertonia		
	Positive Chvostek sign	Calcium deficit	Children may suffer calcium deficit easily, since growing bones do not readily relinquish calcium to circulation
	Tremors, cramps, tetany	Alkalosis with diminished calcium ionization Calcium deficit	
	Twitching	Magnesium deficit	
Behavior	Lethargy	Fluid volume deficit overload	Behavioral changes are among the first indications of dehydration as reported by parents
	Irritability	Fluid volume deficit	
	Comatose condition	Hypotonic fluid deficit Profound acidosis of alkalosis	
	Lethargy with hyperirritability on stimulation	Hypertonic fluid deficit	
	Extreme restlessness	Potassium excess	
Weight	Loss	Fluid deficit	See Tables 28-2 and 28-3
	Up to 5%	Mild	
	5% to 9%	Moderate	
	10% or higher	Severe Protein or calorie deficiency	
	Gain	Edema—general or pulmonary Ascites	Check for hepatomegaly; children sequester excess fluid in the liver
Urine			
Volume	Increased (polyuria)	Interstitial fluid-to-plasma shift Increased renal solute load	Normal range Infant: 2 ml/kg/hr Child: 1-2 ml/kg/hr Adolescent: 0.5-1 ml/kg/hr (varies with intake and other factors)
	Diminished	Mild fluid deficit	
	Oliguria	Moderate to severe fluid deficit Plasma-to-interstitial fluid shift Sodium deficit Potassium excess Severe sodium excess Renal insufficiency	
Specific gravity	Low (≤1.010)	Adequate hydration Fluid excess Renal disease Sodium deficit	Used to monitor hydration status in infants Fixed low reading occurs in renal disease
	High (≥1.030)	Fluid deficit Sodium excess Glycosuria Proteinuria	
pH	Acid	Acidosis—metabolic or respiratory Alkalosis accompanied by severe potassium deficit Fluid deficit	
	Alkaline	Alkalosis, metabolic or respiratory Hyperaldosteronism Acidosis accompanied by chronic renal infection and renal tubular dysfunction Diuretic therapy with carbonic anhydrase inhibitors	

Intake and Output Measurement

One of the most important roles of the nurse in fluid and electrolyte disturbance is related to intake and output (I & O). Accurate measurements are essential to the assessment of fluid balance. Measurements from all sources—including both gastrointestinal and parenteral intake and output from urine, stools, vomitus, fistulas, nasogastric suction, sweat, and drainage from wounds—must be taken and considered. Although the physician usually indicates when I & O are to be recorded, it is a nursing responsibility to keep an accurate I & O record on certain patients:

- Receiving intravenous therapy
- After major surgery
- Severe thermal burns or injuries
- Renal disease or damage
- Congestive heart failure
- Dehydration
- Diabetes mellitus
- Oliguria
- Receiving diuretic therapy
- Receiving corticosteroid therapy

Infants or small children who are unable to use a bedpan or those who have bowel movements with every voiding will require the application of a collecting device (see Urine Specimens, Chapter 27). Collecting bags may not be suitable for all infants, for example, preterm and other infants whose fragile skin does not tolerate self-adhesive appliances. If collecting bags are not used, wet diapers or pads are carefully weighed to ascertain the amount of fluid lost. This includes liquid stool, vomitus, and other losses. The volume of fluid in milliliters is approximately equivalent to the weight of the fluid measured in grams. The specific gravity as a measure of osmolality is determined with a urinometer or a refractometer and assists in assessing the degree of hydration.

Disadvantages of the weighed diaper method of fluid measurement include (1) inability to differentiate one type of loss from another because of admixture; (2) loss of urine or liquid stool from leakage or evaporation, especially if the infant is under a radiant warmer; and (3) additional fluid in diaper (superabsorbent disposable type) from absorption of atmospheric moisture (high-humidity incubators) (Hermansen and Buches, 1987 and 1988). Evaporative losses render measurements inaccurate unless the diaper is weighed and measured for specific gravity at least every 30 minutes when critical values are needed. Evaporative losses are greater in infants under radiant warmers or being treated with phototherapy. However, research indicates that accurate specific gravity measurements can be made for up to 2 hours on urine obtained from a diaper that has been removed from an infant, folded, and stored in a utility room (Lybrand, Medoff-Cooper, and Munro, 1990).

It is important to measure and record all intake, oral and parenteral, and output from all sources, including urine, stool, emesis, drainage tubes, fistulas, and wounds from which appreciable amounts of fluid are lost.

At home parents are advised to observe the number of times and how much the child voids. Infants younger than 1 year of age normally void every 1 to 2 hours; toddlers urinate approximately every 3 hours. As children get older, they void less frequently. The parents are instructed to notify the nurse or clinician if the child appears to be voiding an insufficient amount or persistently losing fluid through vomiting or diarrhea (see Nursing Tip, p. 332).

ORAL FLUID INTAKE

Under ordinary circumstances an adequate oral intake is no problem in children who are able to respond to thirst cues. Hydration becomes a nursing problem when infants or children are unable to respond to the thirst mechanism and when fatigue or discomfort makes them reluctant to swallow. Children with elevated temperatures, those with continued gastrointestinal losses, and those with labile diabetes are especially prone to dehydration. Occasionally dehydration caused by inadequate intake has been observed in breast-fed infants (Rowland and others, 1982).

A number of common fluids found in hospitals and in the home are acceptable for encouraging fluid intake and preventing dehydration, including diluted fruit juice, liquid or solid gelatin, sweetened tea, Popsicles, and decarbonated cola or ginger ale. When teaching parents about fluid management, it is always wise to determine whether or not they understand the concept of clear liquids. It is important to emphasize that milk is not a liquid, since it forms curds when it comes in contact with stomach renin.

When an electrolyte formula is prescribed, it is advisable to have the parents demonstrate their ability to prepare it, because a mistake or misunderstanding of measurements (e.g., substitution of a tablespoon for the teaspoon measure, using heaping rather than level measurements, or adding other ingredients, such as milk) can significantly alter the electrolyte concentration. Parents are cautioned about including broth as fluid intake. When prepared as directed on the labels, most commercial broths contain unusually high sodium concentrations. Parents should consult with a dietitian or the health practitioner for proper dilution of these fluids before offering them to a child who is suffering from large fluid losses. The calorie content and electrolyte composition of some common fluids are listed in Table 28-8.

NURSING TIP: CLEAR LIQUIDS

Any liquid through which newsprint can be read is considered to be clear.

NURSING TIP: DECARBONATING BEVERAGES

To decarbonate beverages, pour the beverage into a cup and place in a microwave oven for 15 seconds. Allow the beverage to cool before serving it.

Table 28-8 Sodium, potassium, and caloric content of commonly administered oral fluids

FLUID	NA+* (mEq/L)	K+* (mEq/L)	CALORIES (kcal/L)
Water	0	0	0
Sugar water (5%)	0	0	200
Lytren	25	25	280
Pedialyte	30	20	280
Coca-Cola	3.6	0	435
Pepsi Cola	0	0	480
Ginger ale	4.5	0.1	300
7-Up	0.5	0	420
Sprite	7.6	0	400
Orange juice (unsweetened)	2	48.5	410
Apple juice	0.43	25	483
Gatorade	23.5	2.5	170
Grape juice	0.8	29.6	660
Jello (half strength)	5.5-16.5†	0.1-0.2	404

*Varies according to mineral content of water used for bottling.
†Varies according to flavor (Na^+ highest in wild cherry, lowest in grape and black raspberry).

Persuading a reluctant child to drink fluids can be a nursing challenge and is not uncommon in the care of infants and children. Older children will often respond to the challenge of meeting a specific goal for fluid intake (or deprivation) and can be active participants in planning an intake schedule. Contracts and rewards are effective strategies. However, young children require more creative tactics. A number of suggestions for encouraging children to drink fluids are discussed in Chapter 27. See Chapter 27 for a discussion of nasogastric alimentation.

The Child Who Is NPO

Infants or children who are unable or not permitted to take fluids by mouth (NPO) have special needs. To ensure that they do not receive fluids, a sign can be placed in some obvious place, such as over their beds or pinned to their shirts, to alert others to the NPO status. Fluids are removed from the bedside to reduce the temptation. Drinking fountains and wash basins are monitored.

Oral hygiene, a part of routine hygienic care, is especially important when fluids are restricted or withheld (see Chapter 27). For young children who cannot brush the teeth or rinse the mouth without swallowing fluid, the mouth and teeth can be cleaned and kept moist by swabbing with saline-moistened gauze or other appliance. Judicious administration of ice chips provides moist, cool relief (if permitted by the practitioner). A thin layer of petrolatum (Vaseline) or other commercial lip aid helps to keep lips soft and prevents cracking and caking.

NURSING TIP: MOUTH MOISTENING

Water sprayed into the mouth from an atomizer is refreshing and relieves a dry mouth.

To meet the need to suck, infants should be provided with a pacifier, preferably an acceptable commercial variety. Aspiration of a nipple used to construct a pacifier has been reported (Millunchick and McArtor, 1986).

The child on restricted fluids provides an equal challenge. Limiting fluids is often more difficult for the child than NPO, especially when IV fluids are also eliminated. To make certain the child does not drink the entire amount allowed early in the day, the daily allotment is calculated to provide fluids at periodic intervals throughout the child's waking hours. Serving the fluids in small containers gives the illusion of larger servings. No extra liquid is left at the bedside if compliance is a problem.

PARENTERAL FLUID THERAPY

Since most hospitalized infants and children with serious disturbance of fluid and electrolyte balance are maintained with IV fluids, monitoring IV fluid replacement is a major nursing responsibility. Most of the general principles of IV therapy apply to infants and children, but with a number of important variations.

Intravenous Infusion

Before an IV infusion is started, several preparatory activities must take place. All needed equipment is gathered so that the operator can proceed without interruption. More importantly, the child and the family must be prepared for this universally stressful procedure.

Solution. The composition of IV solution is selected on the basis of tonicity (osmolality) and electrolyte content. A solution that is *isotonic* has the same osmolality, or tonicity, as body fluids such as plasma. A *hypertonic* solution is one that has a greater concentration of solutes than plasma; a *hypotonic* solution has a lower concentration. Examples of isotonic solutions are 0.9% saline solutions and 5% dextrose in water; 10% glucose in water is a hypertonic solution; plain water and 0.2% sodium are hypotonic solutions. Although it is larger, one molecule of glucose has only half the osmolality of one molecule of NaCl because the NaCl ionizes in solution into two particles, the Na^+ and the Cl^- ions. Thus one molecule of NaCl exerts twice the osmotic pressure of one molecule of glucose.

Most common pediatric maintenance solutions include a combination of dextrose (usually 5% or 10%) and NaCl (usually 0.22% to 0.3%). The hypotonic solution is necessary for children, since their daily turnover of "free" water exceeds that of adults. Because infants and young children are subject to rapid fluid shifts, any IV solution given to them contains at least 0.2% NaCl to prevent brain edema, a disorder to which they are susceptible if given plain water. Glucose is rapidly metabolized; therefore the osmolality of 5% glucose is further diminished.

Equipment. For IV infusions in most children, a 22- or 24-gauge over-the-needle catheter is preferred. For small scalp veins a butterfly needle may be used, and in situations in which fluids are urgently needed and there is difficulty in entering a vein, a polyethylene tube inserted by the surgical cutdown procedure may be necessary. The vein of choice for this alternative is the internal saphenous vein located just anterior to the medial malleolus of the tibia or the external saphenous vein on the lateral side.

Other equipment needed includes alcohol and povidone-iodine swabs to clean the site, a tourniquet, an appropriate-sized padded armboard (when an extremity is used), sandbags, rolled towels or small blankets for maintaining position of head or extremity, tape (or dressing and bacteriostatic ointment if hospital dictates), and a device to protect the IV site after insertion. The prescribed solution, tubing, filter, and infusion pump are prepared in advance, ready to connect to the needle after insertion.

Infusion pumps. There are several modifications in equipment used for IV infusion for children. A gravity drainage apparatus used for children is much the same as that for adults except that it is designed to deliver a reduced drop size (60 drops/ml) and contains a calibrated volume control chamber (e.g., a Buretrol or Solu-set) that regulates the amount of fluid that can be infused. A microdropper greatly facilitates calculation of flow rate because a prescribed number of milliliters per hour equals the number of drops per minute. For example, if the solution is to infuse at a rate of 30 ml per hour, the infusion is regulated to deliver 30 drops per minute.

A variety of infusion pumps are available, but all have a limited capacity, refillable from the bottle above or contained in syringe pumps, to minimize the possibility of overloading the circulation. It is an important nursing responsibility to calculate the amount to be infused in a given length of time, set the infusion rate, and monitor the apparatus frequently (at least every 1 to 2 hours) to make certain that the desired rate is maintained, the integrity of the system remains intact, the site remains intact (free of infiltration or irritation), and the infusion does not stop.

Continuous infusion pumps, although convenient and efficient, are not without attendant risks. Overreliance on the accuracy of the machine can cause either too much or too little fluid to be infused; therefore its use does not obviate careful periodic assessment by the nurse. Excess pressure can build up if the machine is set at a rate faster than the vein is able to accommodate (or continues to pump when the needle is out of the lumen). This is especially true in very small infants and when circumstances necessitate the use of a capillary. No matter what device is used, a thorough understanding of the apparatus is essential for safe fluid administration.

Preparing the Child and Parents

Children of any age are anxious and fearful of injections, and unless the IV infusion is implemented as an emergency procedure, there will be time to prepare them (see Preparation for Procedures, Chapter 27). Many children have never undergone the procedure, and those who have will retain memories of the experience. It is useful to ask them what they think about the procedure and why it is needed for them specifically. Children's perceptions of the anticipated experience furnish information on misconceptions that need to be clarified and help the nurse prepare children for what they can expect. In addition, children's observations provide some insight into how to cope with a child's reactions during the insertion procedure and throughout the course of the IV therapy.

Play, always an excellent stress-reducing technique, can be employed during the preparation process. Allowing children to handle the equipment and to "start" an IV infusion on a toy animal or doll helps familiarize them with the frightening aspects of the procedure. In some instances it may be helpful to introduce a child to another child who is coping well in the same situation (Piercy, 1981).

It is best to arrange for a quiet, private setting for the child during the insertion. The assurance of privacy relieves the child of some anxieties concerning loss of control in front of others. It also avoids subjecting other children to the potentially stress-provoking scene. The child should be provided with some distracting activity, such as those described for injections, and perhaps be allowed to "help" by holding supplies such as a gauze square, helping to clean the site with alcohol, and assisting in taping the site after the procedure.

Children will usually cooperate better and feel more in command if they are allowed to sit up during the process, although this may not be possible even in some older, normally cooperative children. It is a mistake to assume that children will not lose control even after they promise to cooperate. It is wise to have ample assistance available in the event a child cannot control anxiety. The child need not be restrained until necessary, but the assisting nurse should be prepared to grasp a child gently but firmly during the insertion. Explaining to children what is being done during each step of the procedure and how they can participate helps to obtain their cooperation and reduce their stress.

Since the procedure is painful and anxiety producing, the child should also be prepared for these aspects of the procedure. Although the anticipation of pain may increase the child's anxiety initially, it allows the child to mobilize any coping strategies and thus ultimately promotes a sense of trust in the nurse. Application of a topical anesthetic to the injection site before needle insertion should be considered as a means of reducing the pain of injection (see Chapter 27). See Chapter 26 for a discussion of nonpharmacologic pain reduction techniques.

Parents should be told about the procedure, including the reason for the procedure, how long the needle must remain in place, and what they can expect during and after the insertion. They should be offered the option of remaining with their child or leaving (see Questions and Controversies p. 1191).

The Procedure

The site selected for IV infusion depends on accessibility and convenience. In older children any accessible vein may be used. Whenever possible, it is best to avoid the child's favored hand in order to reduce the disability related to the procedure. A site is chosen that restricts the child's movements as little as possible—a site over a joint in an extremity is avoided. An older child can help to select the site and thereby maintain some measure of control. In small infants a scalp vein or a superficial vein of the wrist, hand, foot, or

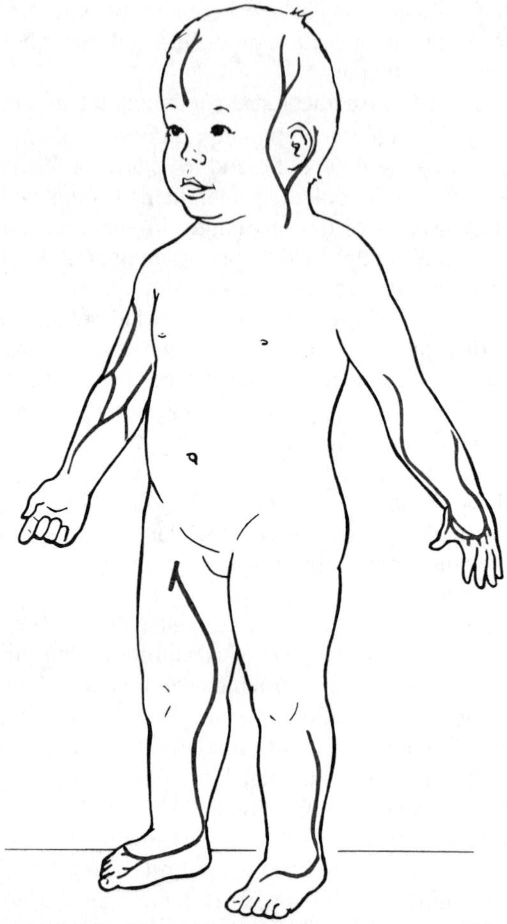

Fig. 28-2. Superficial veins used most often for intravenous infusion in infants and very young children.
From Kempe, C.H., Silver, H.K. and O'Brien, D.: Current pediatric diagnosis and treatment, ed. 9, Los Altos, Calif., 1986, Lange Medical Publications.

arm is usually convenient and most easily stabilized (Fig. 28-2).

Most children have one or two possible IV sites on each arm and foot and four to eight sites on the scalp. Since superficial veins of the scalp have no valves, they can be infused in either direction and are frequently used for IV therapy in infants less than 9 months of age. The temporal and forehead areas are suitable and do not interfere with side-to-side head movements. Scalp veins have little subcutaneous tissue to obscure visualization of the vein, and there are no joints to interfere with movement. However, the use of a scalp vein site requires shaving the area around the site to better visualize the vein and provide a smooth surface on which to tape the tubing (Fig. 28-3). Shaving off a portion of the infant's hair is very upsetting to parents; therefore they should *always* be told what to expect and reassured that the hair will grow in again rapidly (save the hair because parents often wish to keep it). As little as possible is removed directly over the insertion site. A rubber band slipped onto the head from brow to occiput will usually suffice as a tourniquet.

NURSING TIP: TOURNIQUET

A small adhesive tape tab slipped over the rubber band tourniquet provides a convenient way to grasp and remove the band.

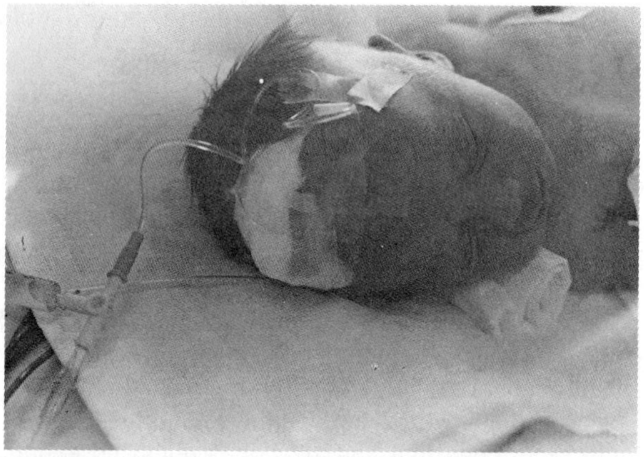

Fig. 28-3. Scalp vein infusion.

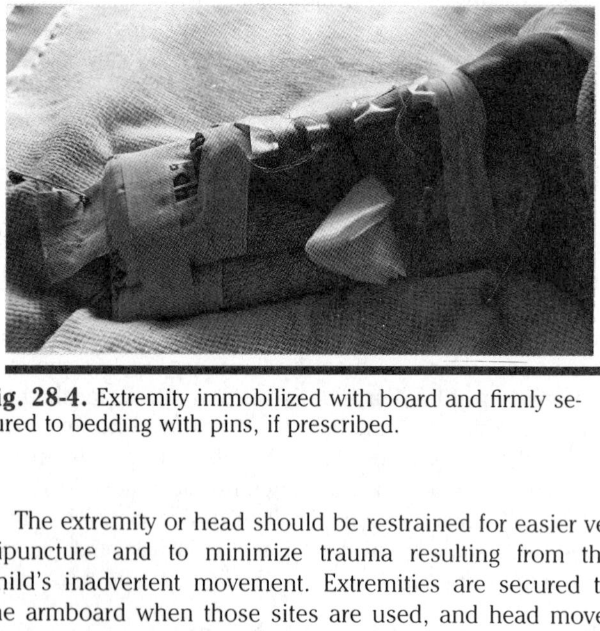

Fig. 28-4. Extremity immobilized with board and firmly secured to bedding with pins, if prescribed.

The extremity or head should be restrained for easier venipuncture and to minimize trauma resulting from the child's inadvertent movement. Extremities are secured to the armboard when those sites are used, and head movements are restrained for scalp venipuncture. (See also Chapter 27 for additional restraining methods.) For a scalp site it is helpful to visualize the way in which the needle will be secured following insertion (Arthur, 1984).

Locating a vein may be difficult because the veins are smaller and children have a significant amount of subcutaneous fat. When veins are not readily visible, applying a warm compress to the site or, when using an extremity, holding the limb in a dependent position below body level will help fill the veins for better visualization. Gentle tapping sometimes causes the veins to stand out. A flashlight held against the skin below the intended site sometimes assists in locating vessels. If these measures do not help, a tourniquet applied with light pressure medially to the site may be needed. Although the tourniquet makes the veins more visible and provides a more rapid blood return, the added venous pressure may cause fragile veins to "blow" when punctured, producing a hematoma.

The needle must be placed in the direction of the blood flow, which creates no problem when an extremity is used. Scalp veins are more difficult to assess. In general, the venous blood flows from the top of the head toward the neck. To test the direction before insertion, the forefinger is placed on the vein at the site chosen for venipuncture. While the finger gently presses the vein, a second finger is used to "strip" the vein in the direction of the top of the head. The pressure from the second finger is released. If the vein fills distal to the compressing finger, the direction of flow is toward the stationary finger (Arthur, 1984).

To maintain the integrity of the IV site, adequate protection of the site will be required for the child. An attempt is made to position the extremity in a natural anatomic position with the use of gauze pads or rolls as needed. A sandbag or a small board, well padded with plastic foam and a cloth or stockinette cover, provides a suitable means for immobilization (Fig. 28-4). Some form of resilient padding is required to prevent areas of pressure necrosis over bony prominences such as the ankle or pressure on the peroneal nerve on the lateral aspect of the knees. The head can be immobilized with covered sandbags. To prevent trauma to the skin from removal of tape, gauze can be placed between the skin and the adhesive.

Following insertion, the needle is firmly secured at the puncture site with nonallergenic tape and protected from becoming dislodged by immobilization of the extremity. The insertion site and about 1 inch of skin beyond the site are left uncovered for early detection of infiltration. Clear plastic dressings are ideal because they allow ready visualization of the insertion site. Some finger or toe areas are left unoccluded by dressings or tape to allow for assessment of circulation. The thumb is never immobilized because of the danger of contractures with limited movement later on. A plastic or wax paper cup that is cut in half (with the rigid edges covered with tape) and applied directly over the needle site will further protect the infusion. Some needle containers make excellent protective covers. A colorful and interesting sticker can be applied to the armboard or protecting device to add a positive note to the procedure.

Older children who are alert and cooperative can usually be trusted to protect the IV site. An IV infusion is not always a deterrent to mobility. When the child is feeling well and the insertion site is well secured, the child can be held or be walked, but precautions must be observed to preserve the integrity of the IV system.

Infants, small children, and uncooperative children require varying degrees of immobilization, and on rare occasions, complete restriction of movement may be needed to prevent removal of the IV infusion. The board is secured to the bed, and the remaining extremities that might be used to dislodge the needle are restrained. This includes feet as well as hands, since most infants will attempt to brush away the offending attachment by rubbing it against another extremity or body part.

Immobilization is intolerable to the naturally active child, and every effort should be extended to relieve the stress of immobilization (see Chapter 39). Frequent removal of the restraints provides the child with the opportunity to move the extremities. Whenever possible, the infant or child should be held and cuddled to help meet emotional needs during this trying time (Fig. 28-5). Range of motion exer-

QUESTIONS AND CONTROVERSIES

Should a nurse irrigate an intravenous catheter that is not running and may be clotted?

Considerable controversy has been generated by the question of whether or not an intravenous catheter can be safely irrigated to reestablish flow. The problem is rarely addressed in textbooks, and no controlled scientific studies have been conducted to confirm or refute the practice. All agree that the standard practice of aspirating should precede other alternative actions. Although most hospital policies discourage irrigating, the practice is widespread and supports the justification for irrigating. No confirmed pulmonary embolism from irrigating a peripheral or central catheter has been reported (Feldstein, 1985).

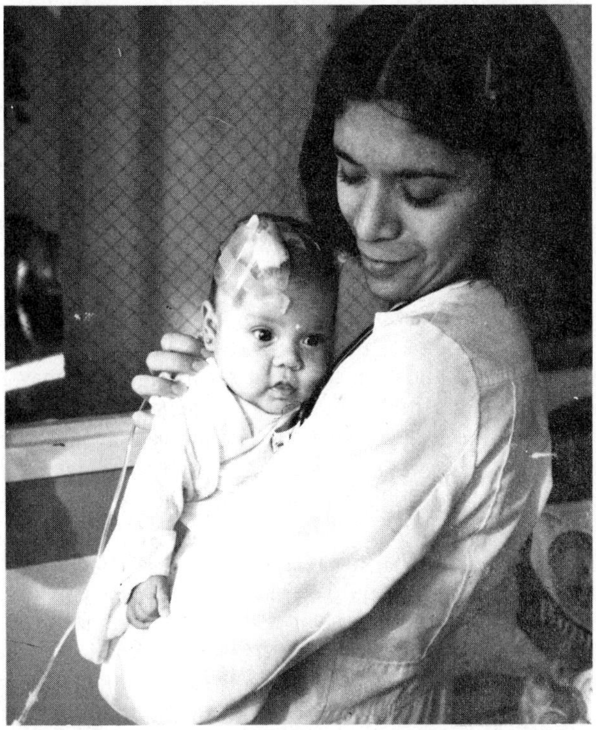

Fig. 28-5. Intravenous infusion does not prevent infant from being picked up and cuddled.

cises are employed on infants and children who are too ill or unable to move their extremities, but others should be encouraged to move their arms and legs in response to a natural stimulus. Most infants or small children will instinctively move their extremities when released. If not, a toy or other stimulus can provide incentive.

When it comes time to discontinue an IV infusion, many children are distressed by the thought of needle removal. Therefore, they need a careful explanation of the process and suggestions for helping. One way is to allow children to remove or help remove the tape from the site. It provides them with a measure of control and often encourages their cooperation. The procedure consists of turning off any pump apparatus, occluding the IV tubing, removing the tape, and pulling out the needle or catheter in the direction of insertion, while exerting firm pressure at the site. A dry dressing (adhesive bandage strip) is placed over the puncture site. If a catheter was used for the IV infusion, the tip is inspected to make certain the catheter is intact and no portion remains in the vein.

Complications. The same precautions regarding maintenance of asepsis, prevention of infection, and observation for infiltration are carried out with patients of any age. However, infiltration is more difficult to detect in infants and small children than it is in adults. The increased amount of subcutaneous fat and the amount of tape used to secure the needle often obscure the signs of early infiltration. When the fluid appears to be infusing too slowly or ceases, the usual assessment for obstruction within the apparatus, that is, kinks, screw clamps, shutoff valve, and positioning interference (e.g., a bent elbow), often locates the difficulty. When these actions fail to detect the problem, it may be necessary to carefully remove some of the tape and other material that obscure a clear view of the venipuncture site. Dependent areas, such as the palm and undersides of the extremity or the occiput and behind the ears, are examined.

Whenever possible, the IV infusion should be placed in an extremity to which the identification band (or bracelet) is not attached. Serious circulatory impairment can result from infiltrated solution distal to the band, which acts as a tourniquet preventing adequate venous return. To check for return blood flow through the needle, the bottle is lowered below the level of the infusion site. If the tubing is connected to an infusion pump, it must be removed from the pump before lowering.

Since IV therapy is often used in pediatrics and tends to be difficult to maintain, extravasation injuries are reported with relative frequency. A number of drugs are toxic to subcutaneous tissues and can result in varying degrees of damage with extended hospitalization and treatment. Hyaluronidase has been used effectively to diffuse extravasated fluids rapidly through the tissue and increase its absorption rate (Laurie and others, 1984). The IV infusion is discontinued and the needle removed as soon as extravasation is recognized, and hyaluronidase is injected (as prescribed) into the area surrounding the site. The affected limb is elevated to promote venous return, and the area is assessed every 15 minutes for approximately 2 hours. No heat is applied to the area.

Prevention of infection is a major nursing function during IV therapy. The infusion site is protected from trauma and entry of bacteria. When an IV infusion continues for several days or longer, the tubing and bottle are changed at regular intervals according to hospital policy. Frequency ranges from every 24 to every 72 hours—most often every 48 hours. To ensure that the equipment is changed regularly, it is labeled with the date and time that the new bottle and tubing are attached. Any signs of inflammation such as redness or pain should be reported immediately. This usually requires removal of the infusion and restarting it at another site.

Intraosseous Infusion

Situations may occur in which rapid establishment of a systemic access is vital and venous access may be hampered by peripheral circulatory collapse, cardiopulmonary arrest, burns, or other conditions. Intraosseous infusion provides an alternate route for administration of fluids and medications until intravascular access can be attained. The technique has been used satisfactorily by paramedics, emergency nurses, and physicians (Peck and Altieri, 1988). A needle is inserted into the medullary cavity of a long bone, most often the distal femur, proximal tibia, and distal tibia (Spivey, 1987). Although a variety of needles can be used, the task has proved to be easier and faster with a bone marrow needle (Wagner and McCabe, 1988).

LONG-TERM VENOUS ACCESS

Even greater mobility is possible with the use of some form of venous access device (VAD). The heparin lock is used as an alternative for a keep-open infusion when extended access to a vein is required without the need for fluid. It is most frequently employed for intermittent infusion of medication into a peripheral venous route. A short, flexible catheter (occasionally a butterfly needle) is used for the heparin lock device, and a site is selected where there will be minimum movement, such as the forearm. The needle is inserted and secured in the same manner as any IV infusion device, but the needle hub is occluded with a stopper.

The type of device used may vary among medical establishments, and the care and use of the heparin lock are carried out according to the specific protocol of the institution or unit. However, the general concept is the same. The needle or catheter remains in place and is flushed with heparin following infusion of the medication. The heparin solution prevents blood from clotting in the device between infusions. Children may be discharged with a heparin lock in place in order that they can continue receiving medications without hospitalization. Heparin locks are usually reserved for children who require medications on a short-term basis. Those who require long-term chemotherapy are best managed with a central VAD.

The children and parents are taught the procedure before discharge from the hospital, including preparation and injection of the prescribed medication, the heparin flush, and dressing changes. A protective device may be recommended for some active children to prevent their accidentally dislodging the needle. An eye bubble shield taped over the needle provides excellent protection. Many children take responsibility for preparing and administering medications. The procedure is explained and demonstrated. Both verbal and written step-by-step instructions are provided for the learners, as are ample opportunities for questions and practice (see Home Care Instructions: Caring for a Heparin Lock*).

*In Wong, D.L., and Whaley, L.F.: Clinical manual of pediatric nursing, ed. 3, St. Louis, 1990, Mosby–Year Book, Inc.

Central Venous Catheters

Other alternatives for long-term venous access include the indwelling central venous catheters (Broviac or Hickman catheters) and implanted infusion ports (Infus-A-Port, Medi-Port, Port-a-cath). See Table 28-9 for a comparison of catheters and infusion ports.

With the patient under local or general anesthesia, the central venous catheter of choice is placed with aseptic technique. A vein, such as the jugular or subclavian, is entered through a small cutdown site, and the catheter is threaded to the junction of the superior vena cava and right atrium, confirmed by fluoroscopic dye injection, and then

Table 28-9 Comparison of long-term venous access devices

DEVICE	DESCRIPTION	ADVANTAGES	DISADVANTAGES
Hickman/Broviac catheter (includes several other trade names)	Silicone, radiopaque, flexible catheter with open ends One or two Dacron cuffs on catheter(s) enhance tissue ingrowth	Reduced risk of bacterial migration after tissue adheres to Dacron cuff Easy to use for self-administered infusions	Requires daily heparin flushes Must be clamped or have clamp nearby at all times Must keep exit site dry Heavy activity restricted until tissue adheres to cuff Risk of infection still present Protrudes outside body; susceptible to damage from sharp instruments and may be pulled out; may affect body image More difficult to repair Patient/family must learn catheter care
Groshong catheter	Clear, flexible, silicone, radiopaque catheter with closed tip and two-way valve at proximal end Dacron cuff on catheter enhances tissue ingrowth	Reduced time and cost for maintenance care; no heparin flushes needed Reduced catheter damage—no clamping needed because of three-way valve Increased patient safety because of minimum potential for blood backflow or air embolism Reduced risk of bacterial migration after tissue adheres to Dacron cuff Easily repaired Easy to use for self-administered infusions	Requires weekly irrigation with normal saline Must keep exit site dry Heavy activity restricted until tissue adheres to cuff Risk of infection still present Protrudes outside body; susceptible to damage from sharp instruments and may be pulled out; can affect body image Patient/family must learn catheter care
Implanted ports (Port-a-cath, Infus-A-Port, MediPort)	Totally implantable metal or plastic device that consists of self-sealing injection port with preconnected or attachable silicon catheter that is placed in large blood vessel	Reduced risk of infection Placed completely under the skin; therefore cannot be pulled out or damaged No home maintenance care and reduced cost for family Heparinized monthly and after each infusion to maintain patency No limitations on regular physical activity, including swimming No dressing needed No or only slight change in body appearance (slight bulge on chest)	Must pierce skin for access; pain with insertion of needle; can use local anesthetic before accessing port Special needle (Huber) with angled tip must be used to inject into port Skin preparation needed before injection Hard to manipulate for self-administered infusions Catheter may dislodge from port, especially if child "plays" with port site ("twiddler syndrome") Vigorous contact sports (football, soccer, hockey) generally not allowed

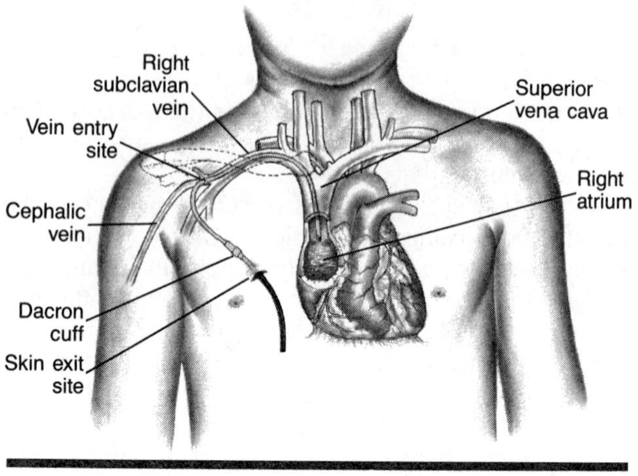

Fig. 28-6. Central venous catheter insertion and exit site.

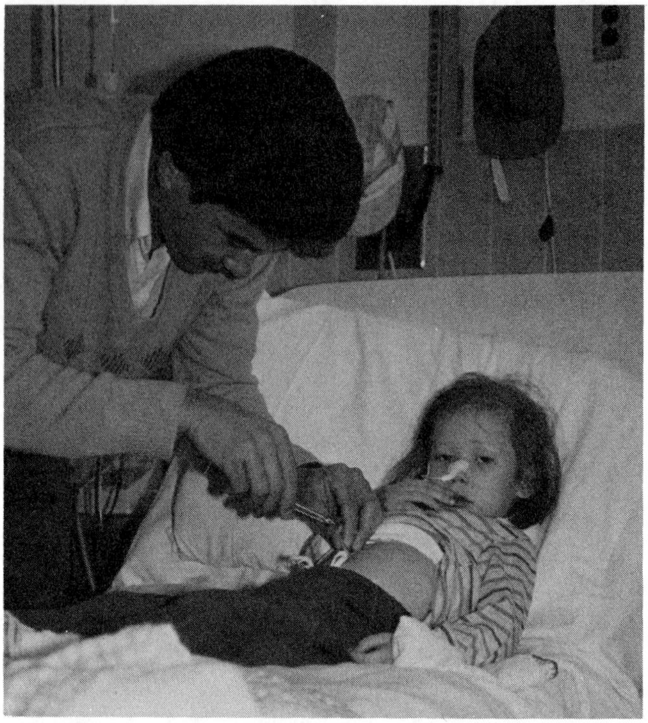

Fig. 28-7. A parent flushing a central venous catheter.

sutured in place. To stabilize the catheter and reduce the risk of infection, the remainder is tunneled beneath the skin to exit through a small incision at a convenient location on the anterior aspect of the chest or upper abdomen (Fig. 28-6). One or two Dacron cuffs on the catheter remain in the subcutaneous tunnel; as tissue adheres to the cuff, the cuff provides a barrier to infection. The cutdown site is surgically closed, the catheter is sutured to the skin at the exit site, and a sterile dressing is applied.

The smaller Broviac catheter is most appropriate for children. Regardless of which catheter is used, the child and family are taught the care and management of the device with provision for practice under supervision (Fig. 28-7). It can be frightening to both child and parents to know that the catheter tip is situated near the heart. They need reassurance that with reasonable care they will do no harm to the apparatus. It is often useful to introduce the family to other children and families who are using central venous catheters successfully and with whom they can share concerns and helpful tips regarding care and management. This sharing is especially valuable for teenage patients. Because teenagers usually have a positive attitude toward the catheter, it is beneficial for them to share their experiences with adolescents who face the prospects of catheter placement (Bergman, 1985).

Parents of children who engage in outside activities, go to school, or are otherwise under the supervision of another adult should inform the teacher, school nurse, coach, and baby-sitter about the presence of the central venous catheter. A written information sheet concerning the VAD, including its purpose, pertinent facts about any restrictions for the child, and directions related to management of the device, should be provided for their reference. Grandparents and other family members who care for the child are taught the care and management of the catheter by the nurse or the parents.

Procedures and published standards for catheter care vary widely among organizations, and there is no evidence that one method is superior over another. For example, some advocate covering the healed catheter site with a dressing; others do not. All companies that manufacture central catheters have patient and professional teaching kits. The user should become thoroughly familiar with the specific device selected for use. (See also Home Care Instructions: Caring for a Central Venous Catheter.*)

The catheter is not a deterrent to most activities, including showers or tub bathing. However, the practitioner is consulted before activities such as swimming or physical contact sports are attempted. Swimming is usually prohibited, but may be allowed in certain situations. If the exit site is healed and the cuff adheres to the tissue, a transparent dressing can be placed over the catheter and exit site and swimming may be permitted for a limited time such as 1 hour or less in a chlorinated pool. Most contact sports are prohibited because of the possibility of the catheter being hit or pulled.

Infection and a clotted catheter are possible complications of central venous catheters. Although neither is an emergency, both require treatment—antibiotics for infection and streptokinase or urokinase for clots. Uncapping can be prevented by taping the cap securely to the catheter and the clamped line to the dressing. Leaks can be prevented by using a smooth-edged clamp only. Parents are cautioned to keep scissors away from the child to prevent accidental cutting of the catheter. If the catheter leaks, they are instructed to tape it above the leak and then clamp the catheter at the taped site. The child should be taken to the practitioner as soon as possible to prevent infection or clotting following a cathteter leak.

*In Wong, D.L., and Whaley, L.F.: Clinical manual of pediatric nursing, ed. 3, St. Louis, 1990, Mosby–Year Book, Inc.

NURSING TIP: VAD AND ACTIVITY

A pocket sewn on the inside of a T-shirt provides a place in which to coil the catheter line while the child is at play if a dressing is not used.

✦ **NURSING ALERT** If a central venous catheter is accidentally removed, apply pressure to the *entry* site to the vein, not the exit site on the skin (Marcoux, Fisher, and Wong, 1990).

Implanted Ports

Adolescents may benefit from the implanted ports, which consist of a small, circular "port of entry" that is placed under the skin (while the patient is under local or general anesthesia) over a bony prominence to provide a stable surface—usually under the distal third of the clavicle. A tunnel is created from the port to the point where the catheter enters a central vein leading to the entrance to the right atrium. Medication or other solution is injected with a special needle through the skin into the port. The device can remain situated indefinitely. Adolescents who are highly concerned about body image and may be troubled by the visible central venous catheter often prefer this method of venous access. One disadvantage of an infusion port is that it requires repeated skin punctures, which may make it less acceptable to children. The use of a topical anesthetic, eutectic mixture of local anesthetics (EMLA), can make the puncture painless. (See also Pain Management, Chapter 26, and Box 26-9.)

INTRAVENOUS ALIMENTATION

Total parenteral nutrition (TPN), also known as intravenous alimentation or hyperalimentation, provides for the total nutritional needs of infants or children whose lives are threatened because feeding by way of the gastrointestinal tract is impossible, inadequate, or hazardous. Common conditions for which TPN is used therapeutically include chronic intestinal obstruction from peritoneal sepsis or adhesions, bowel fistulas, inadequate intestinal length, chronic nonremitting severe diarrhea, extensive body burns, abdominal tumors treated by surgery, irradiation, and chemotherapy. TPN may also be initiated prophylactically when prolonged starvation is expected.

Hyperalimentation therapy involves IV infusion of highly concentrated solutions of protein, glucose, and other nutrients. The hyperalimentation solution is infused through conventional tubing with a special filter attached to remove particulate matter or microorganisms that may have contaminated the solution. The highly concentrated solutions require infusion into a vessel with sufficient volume and turbulence to allow for rapid dilution. The wide-diameter vessels selected are the superior vena cava and innominate or intrathoracic subclavian veins approached by way of the external or internal jugular veins. In some situations the inferior vena cava from a femoral vein serves as an alternative route. Central VADs are ideal for long-term and home TPN.

The highly irritating nature of concentrated glucose precludes the use of the small peripheral veins in most instances. However, dilute glucose-protein hydrolysates that are appropriate for infusing into peripheral veins are being used with increasing frequency. When peripheral veins are used, intralipids become the major calorie source. This fat solution cannot be mixed with the glucose solutions; it requires administration through a multilumen catheter or a separate bottle and tubing that enters the circuit near the venous entry site through a type of injection adapter.

The major nursing responsibilities are the same as for any IV therapy: control of sepsis, monitoring of infusion rate, and continuous observations. The TPN solution must be prepared under rigid aseptic conditions best accomplished by specially trained technicians. In some institutions the solution and tubing are changed and the infusion site is redressed by specially trained nurses, using meticulous aseptic precautions.

The infusion is maintained at a uniform rate by means of a constant infusion pump to ensure proper concentrations of glucose and amino acids. This requires accurate calculation of the rate required to deliver a measured amount in a given length of time. Since alterations in flow rate are relatively common, the drip should be checked frequently to ensure an even, continuous infusion. If for some reason the infusion rate slows, the rate should not be increased to compensate for the uninfused amount.

General assessments such as vital signs, intake and output measurements, and checking results of laboratory tests facilitate early detection of infection or fluid and electrolyte imbalance. Additional amounts of K^+ and Na^+ are often required in hyperalimentation; therefore observation for signs of K^+ or Na^+ deficit or excess is part of nursing care. This is rarely a problem except in children with reduced renal function or metabolic defects.

Hyperglycemia may occur during the first day or two as the child adapts to the high-glucose load of the hyperalimentation solution. Addition of insulin may be required to assist the body's adjustment to the hyperglycemia. Nursing responsibilities include blood glucose testing to monitor the effectiveness of insulin therapy. To prevent hypoglycemia at the time hyperalimentation is discontinued, the rate of infusion and the amount of insulin are decreased gradually. The high concentration of glucose may produce an osmotic diuresis with the risk of hypertonic dehydration.

Because many children are treated with hyperalimentation regimens for long periods of time, it is especially important to be attuned to developmental needs. An infant stimulation program is initiated as early as feasible to prevent developmental delays (see Developmental Intervention, Chapter 10). Delays in the areas of gross motor and language skills are observed most frequently in infants receiving long-term TPN (greater than 3 months) (Allen and Harper, 1983). The program is maintained throughout the hospital stay and extended into the home, where home hyperalimentation is implemented. In most instances children achieve a satisfactory developmental level by 2 years of age (Ralston and others, 1984).

Complications

Complications from TPN are numerous, and a major nursing responsibility is to prevent these when possible and to be alert to signs of their development. Complications either (1) are related to the infusate (metabolic complications) or (2) result from the presence of the indwelling catheter.

Metabolic complications are associated with the infant's or child's capacity for the various components of the hyperalimentation solution. Excessive intake of any of the components will create an imbalance, such as hyperglycemia, azotemia, acid-base disorders, anemia, bone demineralization, vitamin and mineral deficiencies, hyperosmotic dehydration and coma, fluid overload, and a variety of electrolyte imbalances.

Liver disease is the most important gastrointestinal complication in pediatric populations. The cause is obscure, but liver disease appears to be more prevalent in preterm infants who have minimum enteral feedings and who were begun on TPN at an early age (Ament, 1986). Affected children develop cholestasis, hepatocellular necrosis, and, in advanced disease, cirrhosis or hepatic failure. Manifestations include hepatomegaly, jaundice, and elevated serum transaminase, bilirubin, and alkaline phosphatase levels, which become evident approximately 2 weeks after initiation of TPN. Cholelithiasis is an uncommon but possible occurrence in pediatric patients. Therefore children on TPN should be assessed periodically for signs and symptoms of cholelithiasis and/or cholecystitis (Roslyn and others, 1983).

Catheter-related complications include those involving catheter placement, such as pneumothorax, hemothorax, perforation, and catheter dislodgement. However, the major complication associated with the catheter is infection: infection at catheter entrance site, catheter "seeding" sepsis, venous thrombosis with infection and embolization, and endocarditis. In addition to the many problems associated with TPN, delays have been noted in various aspects of development, especially in feeding (see Feeding Resistance, Chapter 10).

Home Total Parenteral Nutrition

Some children require total parenteral nutrition over an extended period, often weeks or months. For many children home total parenteral nutrition (HTPN) is an alternative for long-term hospitalization. The child must be one who is unable to maintain adequate enteral alimentation, has no medical problems requiring hospitalization, has a parent who is able to manage the home care (or is an older child who can participate in his or her own care), and has the potential to benefit from the treatment.

Before a home care program can be implemented, a thorough assessment is made of the family and the home situation. The parents must be capable of performing the technical aspects of the procedure and be able to adapt to the changes inherent in the home program. Psychosocial readiness of the family, family support systems, and practical considerations are investigated, including availability of a pharmacy to prepare the hyperalimentation solution, a physician to handle day-to-day emergency needs, and a cooperating insurance company or agency (because of the exorbitant cost of maintaining long-term parenteral feeding). In most areas home health care agencies are able to assume the major management of HTPN for families.

The needs of the particular child and the family situation are the basis for development and implementation of a care plan. The parent (or parents) and child learn to carry out the procedure under the supervision of a specially trained nurse; detailed, step-by-step instructions are written out. Before discharge the parent (or parents) is prepared for taking over the child's total care. A room is provided at the hospital or the parent and child are housed at a nearby motel for 3 to 4 days. The parent assumes full responsibility for the child's total care, with help readily available if needed.

The emotional and economic benefits of this approach are readily apparent. The familiar environment and the atmosphere of normality are enormously therapeutic, and the stress of separation is avoided. With support from health professionals, a home care program can be the ideal alternative to hospitalization for a capable, motivated family of a child who requires total parenteral nutrition.

The family is encouraged to make the home life as normal as possible for the child within the limits imposed by the therapy. For example, having the infant or child at the table during mealtimes and including the child in family activities contribute to a normal family atmosphere. Quiet play should be encouraged during the HTPN, and it may be helpful to have a potty-chair available at the bedside. Toddlers who may crawl out of a crib may need to be protected from becoming tangled or catching IV tubing on the rail. It is also important to make certain the child's dental care is not neglected.

The family is referred to community agencies that provide support and practical assistance. The **Oley Foundation,*** a nonprofit research and education organization, maintains a national registry of persons receiving HTPN and publishes a bimonthly newsletter for consumers, families, clinicians, and home care services.

*214 Hun Memorial, Albany Medical Center, Albany, NY 12208; (518) 445-5079.

KEY POINTS

- Water distribution and maintenance are determined by solutes, physical forces, internal control mechanisms, and boundary organs through which external exchanges occur.
- Infants are subject to fluid depletion because of their relatively greater surface area, their high rate of metabolism, and their immature kidney function.
- Management of fluid volume disturbances focuses on the following areas: volume of body fluids, osmolality, hydrogen ion status, electrolyte deficits, and disturbances in mineral skeleton and body fluid equilibrium.
- Fluid disturbances experienced by childeren are dehydration, water intoxication, and edema.

- Dehydration may be classified as isotonic, hypotonic, and hypertonic.
- Parenteral fluid therapy is initiated to meet ongoing daily physiologic losses, restore previous deficits, and replace ongoing abnormal losses.
- Fluid gains or losses from the interstitial spaces depend on the following factors: venous hydrostatic pressure, colloidal osmotic pressure, semipermeable capillary wall, tissue tension, and lymphatic flow.
- Edema formation is caused by increased venous pressure, capillary permeability, diminished plasma proteins, lymphatic obstruction, or decreased tissue tension.
- Disturbances in acid-base balance are respiratory acidosis, respiratory alkalosis, metabolic acidosis, and metabolic alkalosis.
- Respiratory acidosis may result from factors that depress the respiratory center, factors that affect the lung, and factors that interfere with the bellows action of the chest wall.
- Respiratory alkalosis results primarily from central nervous system stimulation.
- Metabolic acidosis is a lowered plasma pH caused by any process that reduces base bicarbonate concentration or increases metabolic acid formation.
- Metabolic alkalosis is an elevated plasma pH that occurs when there is a reduction of hydrogen ion concentration or an excess of base bicarbonate.
- Nursing assessment of fluid and electrolyte disturbances entails observation of general appearance, vital signs, intake and output measurement, and review of relevant laboratory results.
- Long-term venous access is accomplished by heparin lock, indwelling central venous catheters, or implanted ports.
- Intravenous alimentation provides total nutritional needs when feeding via the gastrointestinal tract is impossible, inadequate, or hazardous.
- Before initiating home total parenteral nutrition, the following factors are assessed: parents' ability to perform the procedure, existence of family support systems, availability of nearby pharmacies, and insurance coverage.

REFERENCES

Ableson, W.H., and Smith, R.G.: Residents handbook of pediatrics, ed. 7, Toronto, 1987, B.C. Decker, Inc.

Allen, S.S., and Harper, K.L.: Developmental delays in infants on long-term TPN, Nutr. Support Serv. 3:42-43, 1983.

Ament, M.E.: Home parenteral nutrition in infants and children. In Rombeau, J.L., and Caldwell, M.D., editors: Parenteral nutrition, Philadelphia, 1986, W.B. Saunders Co.

Arthur, G.M.: When you littlest patients need IVs, RN 47(4):30-35, 1984.

Bennett, H.J., Wagner, T., and Fields, A.: Acute hyponatremia and seizures in an infant after a swimming lesson, Pediatrics 72:125-127, 1983.

Bergman, T.: Verbal responses of adolescents to right atrial catheters, J. Assoc. Pediatr. Oncol. Nurses 3:31-36, 1985.

Feldstein, A.G.: Consultation: irrigating question, Nursing '85 15(8):22, 1985.

Finberg, L.: Assessing the clinical clues to dehydration, Contemp. Pediatr. 7(4):45-57, 1990.

Goldberg, G.N., and others: Infantile water intoxication after a swimming lesson, Pediatrics 70:599-600, 1982.

Hermansen, M.C., and Buches, M.: Super diapers and premature infants, Pediatrics 79:1056-1057, 1987.

Hermansen, M.C., and Buches, M.: Urine output determination from superabsorbent and regular diapers under radiant heat, Pediatrics 81:428-431, 1988.

Kropp, R.M., and Schwartz, J.F.: Water intoxication from swimming, J. Pediatr. 101:947-948, 1982.

Laurie, S.W., and others: Intravenous extravasation injuries: the effectiveness of hyaluronidase in their treatment, Ann. Plast. Surg. 13:191-194, 1984.

Lybrand, M., Medoff-Cooper, B., and Munro, B.H.: Periodic comparisons of specific gravity using urine from a diaper and collecting bag, MCN 15:238-239, 1990.

Marcoux, C., Fisher, S., and Wong, D.: Central venous access devices in children, Pediatr. Nurs. 16:123-133, 1990.

Millunchick, E.W., and McArtor, R.D.: Fatal aspiration of a makeshift pacifier, Pediatrics 77:369-370, 1986.

Peck, K.R., and Altieri, M.: Intraosseous infusions: an old technique with modern applications, Pediatr. Nurs. 14:296-298, 1988.

Phillips, K.G.: Swimming and water intoxication in infants (letter), Can. Med. J. 1136:1147, 1987.

Ralston, C.W., and others: Somatic growth and developmental functioning in children receiving prolonged home total parenteral nutrition, J. Pediatr. 105:842-846, 1984.

Roslyn, J.J., and others: Increased risk of gallstones in children receiving total parenteral nutrition, Pediatrics 71:784-789, 1983.

Schulman, J.: Infantile water intoxication at home, Pediatrics 66:119-122, 1980.

Spivey, W.H.: Intraosseous infusions, J. Pediatr. 111:639-643, 1987.

Wagner, M.B., and McCabe, J.B.: A comparison of four techniques to establish intraosseous infusion, Pediatr. Emerg. Care 4:87-91, 1988.

BIBLIOGRAPHY

General

Baliga, R., and Lewy, J.E.: Pathogenesis and treatment of edema, Pediatr. Clin. North Am. 34:639-648, 1987.

Barta, M.A.: Correcting electrolyte imbalances, RN 50(2):30-33, 1987.

Carroll, P.F.: Aspirated feeding solution, Nursing '86 16(1):33, 1986.

Chenevey, B.: Overview of fluid and electrolytes, Nurs. Clin. North Am. 22:749-759, 1987.

Folk-Lighty, M.: Solving the puzzles of patients' fluid imbalances, Nursing '84 14(2):34-41, 1984.

Hazinski, M.F.: Understanding fluid balance in the seriously ill child, Pediatr. Nurs. 14:231-236, 1988.

Lancaster, L.E.: Renal and endocrine regulation of water and electrolyte balance, Nurs. Clin. North Am. 22:761-772, 1987.

Lattanzi, W.E.: Simplifying the approach to fluid therapy, Contemp. Pediatr. 6(2):72-88, 1989.

Lowrey, S.J.: Diminishing the risks of I.V. potassium chloride, Nursing '88 18(6):64, 1988.

O'Rourke, M.E.: Reducing the risk of venous air embolism, Am. J. Nurs. 88:886-890, 1988.

Poyss, A.S.: Assessment and nursing diagnosis in fluid and electrolyte disorders, Nurs. Clin. North Am. 22:773-783, 1987.

Reams, P.K., and Deane, D.M.: Bagged versus diaper urine specimens and laboratory values, Neonatal Network 6(6):17-20, 1988.

Romanski, S.O.: Interpreting ABGs in four easy steps, Nursing '86 16(9):58-63, 1986.

Schwartz, M.W.: Potassium imbalances, Am. J. Nurs. 87:1292-1299, 1987.

Siegel, N.J., and Lattanzi, W.E.: Fluid and electrolyte therapy in children. In Arieff, A.L., and DeFronzo, R.A., editors: Fluid, electrolyte and acid-base disorders, vol. 2, New York, 1985, Churchill Livingstone, Inc.

Toto, K.H.: When the patient has hyperkalemia, RN 50(4):34-37, 1987.

Toto, K.H.: When the patient has hypokalemia, RN 50(3):38-41, 1987.

Young, M.E., and Flynn, K.T.: Third-spacing: when the body conceals fluid loss, RN 51(8):46-48, 1988.

Parenteral Therapy

Abrams, L., and others: Effect of peripheral IV infusion on neonatal axillary temperature measurement, Pediatr. Nurs. 15:630-632, 1989.

Axton, S.E., and Fugate, T.: A protocol for pediatric IV meds, Am. J. Nurs. 87:943-945, 1987.

Barrus, D.H., and Danek, G.: Should you irrigate an occluded I.V. line? Nursing '87 17(3):63-64, 1987.

Boykoff, S.L., Boxwell, A.O., and Boxwell, J.J.: 6 ways to clear the air from an I.V. line, Nursing '88 18(2):46-48, 1988.

Bosque, E., and Weaver, L.: Continuous versus intermittent heparin infusion of umbilical artery catheters in the newborn infant, J. Pediatr. 108:141-143, 1986.

Dyson, A., and Bogod, D.: Minimizing bruising in the antecubital fossa after venipuncture, Br. Med. J. 294:1659, 1987.

Ellerhorst-Ryan, J.M.: Troubleshooting the venous access system, Am. J. Nurs. 85:795, 1985.

Fay, M.J.: The special challenges of pediatric IVs, Dimens. Crit. Care Nurs. 2:23-29, 1983.

Few, B.J.: Hyaluronidase for treating intravenous extravasations, MCN 12:23, 1987.

Holder, C., and Alexander, J.: A new and improved guide to IV therapy, Am. J. Nurs. 90:43-47, 1990.

Koszuta, L.E.: Choosing the right infusion control device for your patient, Nursing '84 14(3):55-57, 1984.

Lenox, A.C.: IV therapy: reducing the risk of infection, Nursing '90 20(3):60-61, 1990.

Maki, D.G., and others: Prospective study of replacing administration sets for intravenous therapy at 48- vs 72-hour intervals, JAMA 258:1777-1781, 1987.

Millam, D.A.: Managing complications of I.V. therapy, Nursing '88 18(3):34-42, 1988.

Millam, D.A.: Are nurses prepared to perform I.V. therapy? Nursing '88 18(8):43, 1988.

Moriarty-Sheehan, M.: Clearing up infusion pump problems, RN 49(7):40-41, 1986.

Neish, S.R., and others: Intraosseous infusion of hypertonic glucose and dopamine, Am. J. Dis. Child. 142:878-880, 1988.

Nelson, R., and Miller, H.: Keeping air out of I.V. lines, Nursing '86 16(3):57-59, 1986.

Seigler, R.S., Tecklenburg, F.W., and Shealy, R.: Prehospital intraosseous infusion by emergency medical services personnel: a prospective study, Pediatrics 84:173-177, 1989.

Sherman, J.E., and Sherman, R.H.: I.V. therapy that clicks, Nursing '89 19(5):50-51, 1989.

Tietjen, S.D.: Starting an infant's IV, Am. J. Nurs. 90:44-47, 1990.

Viall, C.D.: Your complete guide to central venous catheters, Nursing '90 20(2):34-41, 1990.

Long-Term Venous Access

Birdsall, C.: What are dos and don'ts for Hickman/Broviac catheters? Am. J. Nurs. 86:385, 1986.

Brosnan, K.M., and others: Stopcock contamination, Am. J. Nurs. 88:320-323, 1988.

Cosentino, F.: Preparing your patient for home I.V. therapy, Nursing '88 18(11):87-88, 1988.

Cyganski, J.M., Donahue, J.M., and Heaton, J.S.: The case for the heparin flush, Am. J. Nurs. 87:796-799, 1987.

Dunn, D.L., and Lenihan, S.F.: The case for the saline flush, Am. J. Nurs. 87:798-799, 1987.

Favazza P., Brennan, M., and Carney, K.: The pediatric approach to home IV therapy: a case study, Rx Home Care, pp. 51-57, June 1987.

Goodman, M.S., and Wickham, R.: Venous access devices: an overview, Oncol. Nurs. Forum 11(5):16-23, 1984.

Gullatte, M.M.: Managing an implanted infusion device, RN 52(1):45-49, 1989.

Harris, L.C., Rushton, C.H., and Hale, S.J.: Implantable infusion devices in the pediatric patient: a viable alternative, J. Pediatr. Nurs. 2:174-183, 1987.

Hook, M.L., and others: Arterial line patency maintained with nonheparinized flush solution, Heart Lung 16:693-699, 1987.

Knox, L.S.: Implantable venous access devices, Crit. Care Nurse 7(1):70-73, 1987.

Meeske, K., and Davidson, L.T.: Teacher's reference on right atrial catheters, J. Pediatr. Nurs. 3:351-353, 1988.

Miller, D.: Tips on drawing blood through a heparin lock, RN 49(7):22-23, 1986.

Wildblood, R.A., and Strezo, P.L.: The how-to's of home IV therapy, Pediatr. Nurs. 13:42-46, 68, 1987.

Wilkes, G., Vannicola, P., and Starck, P.: Long-term venous access, Am. J. Nurs. 85:793-796, 1985.

Wurzel, C.L., and others: Infection rates of Broviac-Hickman catheters and implantable venous devices, Am. J. Dis. Child. 142:536-540, 1988.

Intravenous Alimentation

Atkins, J.M., and Oakley, C.W.: A nurse's guide to TPN, RN 49(6):20-24, 1986.

Berry, R.K., and Jorgensen, S.: Growing with home parenteral nutrition: adjusting to family life and child development, Pediatr. Nurs. 14:43-45, 1988.

Berry, R.K., and Jorgensen, S.: Growing with home parenteral nutrition: maintaining a safe environment, Pediatr. Nurs. 14:155-157, 1988.

Birdsall, C.: When is TPN safe? Am. J. Nurs. 85:73, 1985.

Carr, P.: When the patient needs TPN at home, RN 49(6):25-27, 1986.

Committee on Nutrition: Commentary on parenteral nutrition, Pediatrics 71:547-552, 1983.

Dahlstrom, K.A., and others: Nutritional status in children receiving home parenteral nutrition, J. Pediatr. 107:219-224, 1985.

Fox, B., and Stegall, B.: TPN: take precautions now, Nursing '85 15(5):48-49, 1985.

Garvin, G., and Franck, L.S.: Preventing delivery of enteral formula via parenteral route, Pediatr. Nurs. 15:17-18, 1989.

Geertsma, M.A., and others: Feeding resistance after parenteral hyperalimentation, Am. J. Dis. Child. 139:255-256, 1985.

Greene, H.L., and others: Guidelines for the use of vitamins, trace elements, calcium, magnesium, and phosphorus in infants and children receiving total parenteral nutrition: report of the Subcommittee on Pediatric Parenteral Nutrient Requirements from the Committee on Clinical Practice Issues of The American Society of Clinical Nutrition, Am. J. Clin. Nutr. 48:1324-1342, 1988.

Johndrow, P.D.: Making your patient and his family feel at home with T.P.N., Nursing '88 18(10):65-69, 1988.

Ramos, L.: Care and management of long-term right atrial catheters, Crit. Care Nurse 7:66-69, 1987.

Munro-Black, J.: The ABCs of total parenteral nutrition, Nursing '84 14(2):50-56, 1984.

O'Connor, M.J., Ralston, C.W., and Ament, M.E.: Intellectual and perceptual-motor performance of children receiving prolonged home total parenteral nutrition, Pediatrics 81:231-236, 1988.

Orr, M.J., and Allen, S.S.: Optimal oral experiences for infants on long-term total parenteral nutrition, Nutr. Clin. Pract., pp. 288-295, 1986.

Ward, J.: Evaluation of enteral feeding pumps for pediatric use, J. Pediatr. Nurs. 1:133-136, 1986.

Wesley, J.: Home parenteral nutrition: indications, principles and cost-effectiveness, Compr. Ther. 9:29-36, 1983.

Wilhelm, L.: Helping your patient "settle in" with TPN, Nursing '85 15(4):60-64, 1985.

Zlotkin, S.H., Stallings, V.A., and Pencharz, P.B.: Total parenteral nutrition in children, Pediatr. Clin. North Am. 32:381-400, 1985.

CHAPTER 29

Conditions That Produce Fluid and Electrolyte Imbalance

RELATED TOPICS

The child with cardiovascular dysfunction, Ch. 34
The child with gastrointestinal dysfunction, Ch. 33
Disorders affecting the skin, Ch. 18
Injury prevention: infant, Ch. 12; toddler, Ch. 14; and school-age child, Ch. 17
Pain assessment; pain management, Ch. 26

GLOSSARY

acidosis Serum pH equal to or less than 7.35
alkalosis Serum pH equal to or greater than 7.45
ARDS Adult respiratory distress syndrome
CNS Central nervous system
CNSD Chronic nonspecific diarrhea
colitis Inflammation of the colon
CVP Central venous pressure
diarrhea Increase in number and/or consistency of stools based on the individual's normal stool pattern
dysentery Intestinal inflammation accompanied by cramping, abdominal pain, tenesmus, and watery stools containing blood and mucus
electrolyte An element or compound that, when dissolved in a liquid (e.g., water), dissociates into ions and is able to conduct an electric current
enteral By way of the alimentary tract
enteritis Inflammation of the intestine
gastritis Inflammation of stomach
gastroenteritis Inflammation of stomach and intestines
GI Gastrointestinal
hypertonic Having a greater osmotic pressure than a reference solution
hypotonic Having a lesser osmotic pressure than a reference solution
ICP Intracranial pressure
insensible Loss of fluid from the body by evaporation and/or respiration
isotonic Having the same osmotic pressure as a reference solution
ORS Oral rehydration solution
osmolality Number of particles (proteins or electrolytes) suspended in fluid
parenteral By some means other than through the digestive tract
regurgitation Return of undigested food from the stomach
septic Relating to or caused by sepsis
solute a substance dissolved in a solution
TSS Toxic shock syndrome

Fluid and electrolyte disturbances are common in the pediatric age-group. Acute attacks of vomiting and diarrhea are so common in this group that they can almost be regarded as part of the normal way of life. However, the nature of the anatomic and physiologic structure of the infant and small child renders them particularly vulnerable to imbalances when pathologic changes affect the fluid compartments. The most serious disturbances are those involving the gastrointestinal tract or the cardiovascular system, and losses resulting from massive burn injury.

■ GASTROINTESTINAL DISORDERS

The numerous secretions of the gastrointestinal (GI) tract are produced in large amounts, but under ordinary conditions most fluid is reabsorbed in the lower bowel. Except for saliva, which is hypotonic, the total solute concentration in most of the GI secretions is similar to that of interstitial fluid, but there are marked differences in electrolyte composition among the secretions. Consequently, fluid lost from the GI tract depends largely on the composition of the fluid that is lost. Fluid losses from the GI tract in vomiting, diarrhea, or other routes (fistula, nasogastric tube) not only produce rapid and profound depletion of extracellular volume but can cause marked distortion in the electrolyte composition as well. Most illnesses create some disturbance in body fluids or electrolytes, and in many children these disturbances are more threatening than the primary disorder. Replacement requires careful attention to both volume and solute composition.

DIARRHEA

Diarrhea is a symptom that can result from disorders involving digestive, absorptive, and secretory functions. It is usually defined as an increase in the number of stools or a decrease in their consistency. However, there are wide variations in colonic function between individuals. For example, normally one infant may have one firm stool every second or third day, whereas another normally passes from five to eight small, soft stools daily. More important are (1) a noticeable or sudden increase in number of stools, (2) a reduction in their consistency with an increase in fluid content, and (3) a tendency for the stools to be greenish in color.

Diarrhea may be acute or chronic, inflammatory or noninflammatory, and the physiologic consequences vary considerably in relation to its severity, duration, associated symptoms, age of the child, and the child's nutritional status before the onset of diarrhea. Diarrhea related to inflammatory processes is usually described as *gastroenteritis,* and the terms are often used interchangeably.

Etiology

Diarrhea can be attributed to a large number of specific causes, mechanisms, and predisposing factors (Box 29-1).

Box 29-1 FACTORS THAT PREDISPOSE TO DIARRHEA

Age. As a rule, the younger the child, the greater is the susceptibility and the more severe the diarrhea. Diarrhea occurs more frequently in infancy, is a lesser threat in early childhood, and usually constitutes only a minor problem in older children.

Impaired health. Malnourished or debilitated children are more susceptible and tend to have more severe diarrhea.

Climate. Saprophytic organisms (organisms that grow more readily in warmer weather) are more prevalent in warm weather and are more apt to proliferate in areas in which sanitation and refrigeration are a problem. Dehydration that accompanies diarrhea is also aggravated by hot weather.

Environment. Diarrhea occurs with greater frequency where there is crowding, substandard sanitation, poor facilities for preparation and refrigeration of food, and generally inadequate health care and education. The frequency of diarrhea in infancy is closely related to the ingestion of contaminated milk; there is a lower incidence of diarrhea in breast-fed infants.

Box 29-2 MECHANISMS KNOWN TO PRODUCE DIARRHEA

Osmotic factors. Osmotic gradients cause water to passively cross intestinal mucosa in isotonic proportions. Unabsorbed solutes create an osmotic gradient that results in movement of sodium and water in the intestinal lumen (e.g., ingestion of nonabsorbable solutes and malabsorption of water-soluble nutrients).

Diminished absorption or increased secretion of water and electrolytes. Diminished absorption of solutes causes decreased absorption of water and electrolytes (e.g., mucosal disease). Increased secretion can result from passive secretion secondary to inflammation or active secretion secondary to stimulation of mucosal cells (e.g., toxin-producing bacteria).

Reduction in anatomic or functional surface area. The anatomically short bowel has reduced absorptive surfaces to absorb all ingested substances.

Altered motility. Both hypermotility and hypomotility reduce the amount of substance absorbed by the intestinal mucosa.

Data from Silverman, A., and Roy, C.C.: Pediatric clinical gastroenterology, ed. 3, St. Louis, 1983, Mosby–Year Book, Inc.

Several major mechanisms produce diarrhea in infants or children who are susceptible or exposed to a causative agent, and more than one mechanism may be operative (Box 29-2). Some agents create their effect by direct invasion of the intestinal tract; others exert their effect through parenteral means.

A variety of factors can produce diarrhea in the infant or child either as the initial symptom or an associated symptom. Often a specific etiologic diagnosis is lacking. Diarrheal disturbances can involve any portion of the GI tract. Enteropathologic organisms are frequent causes of diarrhea

Box 29-3 CAUSES OF ACUTE DIARRHEA

Dietary
Overfeeding
Introduction of new foods
Unripe fruit
Reinstituting milk too soon after diarrheal episode
Osmotic diarrhea from excess sugar or fat in formula

Toxic
Ingestion of
- Heavy metals (arsenic, lead, mercury)
- Organic phosphates
- Ferrous sulfate
- Antibiotics

Enteropathologic
Bacteria: *Escherichia coli, Shigella, Salmonella, Yersinia enterocolitica, Campylobacter, Staphylococcus aureus, Clostridium perfringens, Vibro cholerae, Vibro parahaemolyticus,* tuberculosis
Viruses: Adenoviruses, rotavirus, parvovirus-like organisms
Infestations: Amebiasis, giardiasis, ascariasis, coccidioidosis

Parenteral Infection
Communicable diseases
Upper respiratory tract infections
Urinary tract infections
Otitis media

Inflammatory Bowel Disease
Necrotizing enterocolitis of the newborn
Enterocolitis secondary to Hirschsprung disease

Emotional
Episodes of nervous excitement
Periods of emotional tension
Fatigue
Psychogenic "irritable colon syndrome" in hyperactive children

in infancy and childhood and are further discussed in relation to gastroenteritis p. 1284.

Acute diarrhea. Acute diarrhea, a sudden change in frequency and consistency of stools, is often caused by an inflammatory process of infectious origin but may also be the result of toxic reaction to ingestion of poisons, dietary indiscretions, or infection outside the alimentary tract (Box 29-3). Most are self-limited and will ultimately subside without specific treatment if consequent dehydration does not create a serious complication.

Antibiotic therapy is a common cause of diarrhea in children. Antibiotics such as ampicillin, neomycin, and tetracyclines cause a decrease in glucose absorption and disaccharidase activity. They should be discontinued and a lactose-free diet implemented if diarrhea occurs. Antibiotics can also cause diarrhea by allowing an overgrowth of a bacterium responsible for pseudomembranous colitis.

Dietary indiscretions and sensitivities are observed at any age. However, the most common causes, especially in infancy, are high-osmolar formulas and food sensitivities, discussed in Chapter 13. Children can have an innate sensitivity to certain foods, but more often the sensitivity develops from repeated exposure to specific antigenic substances. Sorbitol, the sweetener in some "sugar-free" gum, dietetic candies, and other products, is poorly absorbed in the GI tract and may produce osmotic diarrhea if ingested in large amounts.

Chronic diarrhea. Chronic diarrhea, the passage of loose stools with increased frequency of more than 2 weeks' duration, is likely to be associated with disorders of malabsorption, anatomic defects, abnormal bowel motility, hypersensitivity (allergic) reaction, or a long-term inflammatory response (Box 29-4). The remainder of this discussion is restricted to acute diarrhea.

Intractable diarrhea of infancy. Intractable diarrhea of infancy is a syndrome defined as diarrhea occurring in the first 3 months of life that persists for longer than 2 weeks with no recognized pathogens and is refractory to treatment. It is classified as either primary, which is identified as nonspecific enterocolitis, or secondary, which is associated with disease entities such as allergy, bowel anomalies, or a variety of congenital diseases. The age of onset ranges from 4 days to 3 months.

The primary form, although the triggering factor is not well defined, may be secondary to such trivial causes as an infection or feeding difficulties, but in most cases no predisposing cause can be identified. The immediate concerns are dehydration and electrolyte imbalances, but these children universally suffer from malnutrition and its consequences. Because the diarrhea occurs during a period of high caloric need, affected infants can quickly become severely ill.

The diarrhea rapidly becomes self-perpetuating through a combination of secondary consequences: malnutrition deprives the infant of the elements protein, vitamins, calcium, and magnesium needed for mucosal regeneration; the villi of the small intestine atrophy; the bowel wall becomes inflamed and irritated by undigested foodstuffs or microorganisms; and secondary digestive and absorptive disorders develop as a result of malnutrition, various patterns of motility, and overgrowth of bacteria caused by the infant's debilitated state (Fig. 29-1).

Clinical Manifestations

The most serious and immediate physiologic disturbances associated with severe diarrheal disease are (1) dehydration, (2) acid-base derangements with acidosis, and (3) shock that occurs when dehydration progresses to the point that circulatory status is seriously disturbed (see Dehydration, Chapter 28). Mild diarrhea is described as a few loose stools each day without other evidence of illness that terminates in a few days. With moderate diarrhea the child is sicker, may have a fever, vomits, appears fretful and irritable, and passes several loose or watery stools daily. Although the child may not gain weight or may even show a slight loss, signs of dehydration are usually absent.

In severe diarrhea the child has numerous to continuous stools and evidence of moderate to severe diarrhea; the child is drawn, flaccid, and expressionless; the eyes lack luster; and the cry lacks vigor and is often whining and

Box 29-4 CAUSES OF CHRONIC DIARRHEA*

Anatomic or Mechanical
Small bowel syndrome
Hirschsprung disease
Partial small bowel obstruction (stenosis)
Malrotation
Fistula
Intestinal lymphangiectasis
Chronic idiopathic intestinal pseudo-obstruction

Biochemical Causes
Celiac disease
Specific carbohydrate or fat malabsorption syndromes caused by enzyme deficiencies such as lactase deficiency, bile-salt deficiency

Endocrinopathies
Hyperthyroidism
Congenital adrenal hyperplasia
Addison disease

Hepatic and Pancreatic Disorders
Cystic fibrosis
Cirrhosis
Hepatitis
Chronic pancreatitis
Pancreatic exocrine deficiency
Pancreatic hypoplasia
Nonspecific enterocolitis of infancy

Neoplastic Disorders
Lymphoma
Neuroblastoma
Polyposis
Adenocarcinoma
Pancreatic islet cell tumor
Ganglioneuroma
Medullary thyroid carcinoma

Immune Deficiencies
Acquired hypoglobulinemia
Wiskott-Aldrich syndrome
Agammaglobulinemia
Severe combined immune deficiency disease
Thymic hypoplasia
Selective IgA deficiency
Acquired immune deficiency syndrome

Food Allergy
Milk allergy
Allergic gastroenteropathy

Inflammatory Bowel Disease
Ulcerative colitis
Regional enteritis (Crohn disease)
Nonspecific enterocolitis of infancy
Pseudomembranous enterocolitis

Malnutrition
Protein malnutrition (kwashiorkor)
Protein-calorie malnutrition (marasmus)

*See Chapter 33 for discussion of chronic gastrointestinal disorders.

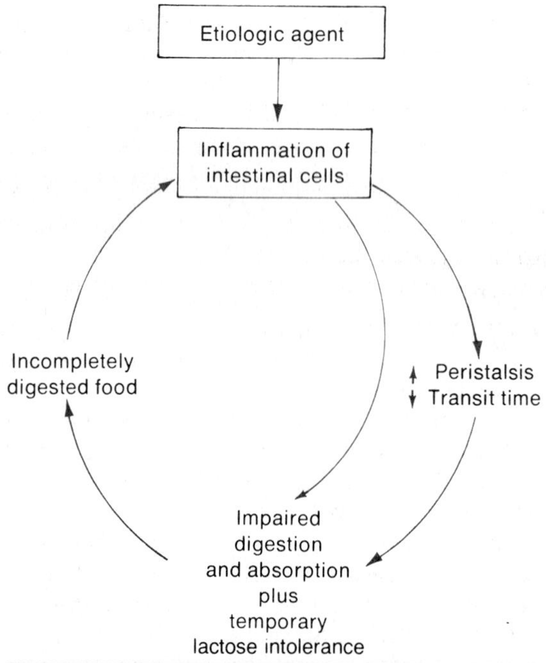

Fig. 29-1. Vicious pathologic cycle in diarrhea with temporary lactose intolerance.

higher pitched than usual. The child is irritable, seeks the comfort and attention of the parents, and displays purposeless movements and inappropriate responses to people and familiar things. The child may become lethargic, moribund, or comatose.

Fluid losses and metabolic acidosis in severe diarrhea contribute to rapid deterioration in diarrheal disease in infancy (Box 29-5), and although the fluid deficit cannot be stated precisely, it can be estimated from changes in body weight and objective clinical signs.

Alterations in body potassium occur in association with both fluid losses and acidosis. Potassium is continually lost in stools, cellular potassium leaves the cells in exchange for sodium and hydrogen ions entering the cells, and potassium is lost from cells damaged by hypoxia. Thus the cellular potassium is seriously depleted. However, because renal excretion is impaired as a result of the circulatory adjustments, the serum levels of potassium are normal or even elevated. When circulatory volume and renal function are restored, potassium redistribution and excretion may produce a potassium deficit unless adequate amounts are restored during rehydration.

Box 29-5 CONSEQUENCES OF DIARRHEA

Dehydration

Voluminous losses of fluid and electrolytes in frequent watery stools
Losses when there is frequent vomiting
Reduced fluid intake resulting from nausea or anorexia
Increased insensible losses from fever, hyperpnea, and sometimes, high environmental temperature
Continued (although diminished) obligatory renal losses

Metabolic Acidosis

Losses of bicarbonate, sodium, and potassium in diarrheal stools
Impaired renal function
Accumulation of lactic acid from tissue hypoxia secondary to hypovolemia
Ketosis from fat metabolism when glycogen stores are depleted in untreated diarrheal dehydration or inadequate carbohydrate intake

Diagnostic Evaluation

The history provides valuable information regarding exposure to infectious agents, personal contact, travel, or probable contact with contaminated foods. Allergic and dietary history may indicate food sensitivities or allergies. Crowding and close person-to-person contact, as in institutions, make epidemics with any enteric pathogen more likely.

The age of the child provides clues to the cause of diarrheal disturbances. For example, milk sensitivity or intolerance of formula constituents is suspected in early infancy. In later infancy new foods added to the diet are frequent offenders. Parenteral infections, especially viral, are very common causes of diarrhea in infancy. Most acute, inflammatory diarrheas are infectious, and the type of stools and symptoms associated with diarrhea provide clues to the organism. For example, fever is not a symptom of *Escherichia coli* disease until late, whereas it is a common early feature even in mild cases of shigellosis. Abdominal cramps are also common in shigellosis. Explosive onset of diarrhea accompanied by or preceded by vomiting suggests food poisoning. Although vomiting may occur in all infectious diarrheas, it is not a major feature.

Laboratory examination. The specimen obtained from evacuated stool should include mucus or tissue shreds, if present. The specimen is examined with indicator paper for pH, and a Clinitest tablet will detect the acid stool containing sugar that is characteristic of disaccharide intolerance. Bulky stools containing fat suggest malabsorption diarrhea.

The breath hydrogen test for carbohydrate malabsorption (lactose, sucrose) provides a simple, rapid, and noninvasive method to detect a variety of GI disorders. The end products of many metabolic processes, carbon dioxide and hydrogen, are normally absorbed, transported by the bloodstream, and eliminated by the lungs. In children with carbohydrate malabsorption the breath hydrogen excretion rate is two to eight times greater than normal after ingestion of the specific testing carbohydrate. The test has also been perfected to detect bacterial overgrowth (Davidson, Robb, and Kirubakaran, 1984).

The specimen is also examined for the presence of red blood cells. Rectal swabs for culture are indicated for a rotazyme test or whenever a bacterial agent is suspected. Serum electrolyte values are obtained in the young infant who is hospitalized with diarrhea because of the likelihood of complicating dehydration and associated electrolyte imbalances, particularly in relation to sodium and potassium alterations. Dehydrated infants will have an elevated hematocrit as a result of volume loss, and elevated blood urea nitrogen will be found in the presence of reduced renal circulation.

Therapeutic Management

Mild or moderate diarrhea is usually managed by simple measures, and the child seldom requires hospitalization. The extent to which the child should be examined and observed by a nurse or a practitioner depends a great deal on the intelligence and cooperation of the caregiver in following instructions and assessing the progress of treatment. When the competency of the caregiver is questionable in regard to estimating the child's condition, the child should be seen daily by a health worker. If the diarrhea persists, if the child loses weight, if there is blood in the stools, or if associated signs develop, such as deep breathing, listlessness, or reduced urinary output, that may signal complications, the child should be seen by the practitioner. When the moderate diarrhea becomes worse or does not respond to simple measures, hospitalization is indicated. This provides the opportunity for closer observation and examination and for a brief course of parenteral fluid therapy, which usually results in rapid improvement.

Rehydration. Orally administered rehydration solutions (ORS) are currently the therapy of choice in treatment of diarrhea of any cause and in a wide range of age-groups except in severe dehydration or other complicating circumstances. The ORS recommended by the Diarrheal Disease Control Program of the World Health Organization is used successfully throughout the world, but seldom in the United States. The Committee on Nutrition of the American Academy of Pediatrics (1985) states that it is appropriate for rapid rehydration but is not suitable for maintaining fluid balance in infants with ongoing losses. The large amount of sodium in the solution contributes to the risk of hyperelectrolytemia. In addition, it is typically prepared in powder form, which must be mixed with water for administration; thus the chance of inaccurate measurement increases the likelihood of error in preparation. In the United States commercially prepared formulas are available (Table 29-1) and used almost exclusively for oral rehydration.

The usual approach is to administer ORS with initial fluid provided within 4 hours to 6 hours for mild or moderate dehydration. The amounts and rates are increased if the patient does not appear fully hydrated or continues to have

Table 29-1 Composition of oral rehydration solutions

FORMULA	Na^+ (mEq/L)	K^+ (mEq/L)	CL^- (mEq/L)	BASE (mEq/L)	CARBOHYDRATE (g/L)
Lytren (Mead-Johnson)	50	25	45	30 (citrate)	20 (dextrose, corn syrup, solids)
Pedialyte (Ross)	45	20	35	30 (citrate)	25 (dextrose)
Rehydralyte (Ross)	75	20	65	30 (citrate)	25 (dextrose)
Gastrolyte	50	20	52	18	20
Infalyte powder (Pennwalt)	50	20	40	30 (bicarbonate)	20 (glucose)
WHO (World Health Organization)	90	20	80	30 (bicarbonate)	18 (dextrose)

diarrhea. The amounts are decreased if the patient appears to be fully hydrated earlier than expected or signs of overhydration (e.g., periorbital edema) develop. Infants can be allowed to continue breast-feeding as desired after treatment has been started.

When oral rehydration is complete, maintenance therapy is begun. Most mild to moderate acute diarrhea can be managed at home under careful health supervision. The volume of ORS ingested should equal the volume of stool losses. Some authorities advocate ad libitum intake of ORS with an additional one bottle of plain or flavored water for every two bottles of ORS (Bass and Walker, 1986).

The issue of continued or delayed feedings has not been resolved. Some advocate continuing the child's regular diet; others advise removing all milk for 24 to 36 hours. Research has indicated that infants recover from mild disease regardless of the carbohydrate ingested (Groothuis, Berman, and Chapman, 1986), and unrestricted diet does not appear to affect the course or symptoms in mild diarrhea (Conway and others, 1989; Margolis and others, 1990). Breast milk is generally well tolerated by infants. The current trend is toward rapid resumption of the previous diet after oral or intravenous (IV) hydration.

Hypernatremic diarrheal dehydration is usually managed by *slow* oral rehydration (over 12 hours) to avoid cerebral edema with accompanying seizures (Pizarro, Posada, and Levine, 1984).

Diluted fruit juices and soft drinks are not recommended for rehydration, especially in infants. The high carbohydrate content of these fluids aggravates the diarrhea by an osmotic effect produced by nonabsorbable carbohydrate (Ghishan, 1988). Some antibiotics (such as ampicillin, which destroy bacteria that normally break down and ferment carbohydrate) may increase the carbohydrate load in the colon. Cola soft drinks are deficient in electrolyte replacement, especially sodium and potassium (Ghishan, 1988; Weizman, 1986). Recently observers have advocated cereals or rice as a source of glucose to reduce the osmolality of rehydration solution (Carpenter, Greenough, and Pierce, 1988).

Lactose-free formulas are often substituted (Brown and MacLean, 1984), and investigators have found that introduction of a soy-based, lactose-free formula (usually diluted 50%) after the initial 4 hours of rehydration reduced stool output and duration of diarrhea in most infants (Santosham and others, 1985). In some children a secondary lactase deficiency may cause a temporary intolerance to milk and exacerbation of diarrhea; therefore, reintroduction of lactose is attempted progressively. Milk is usually withheld until at least a week after the disappearance of symptoms, and the feeding consists of some type of hydrolyzed lactose-free formula. Feeding lactose-containing formulas as a sole nutrient source can cause diarrhea sufficient to increase the risk of dehydration in these children (Penny, Paredes, and Brown, 1989).

Medications. Antimicrobial therapy is instituted in some types of diarrhea. It significantly shortens the course of shigellosis and appears to be beneficial in *E. coli* infections but does not affect the course of *Salmonella* disease. It is always indicated in bacteremia, and parenteral infections are treated with appropriate drugs.

Antidiarrheal medications such as opiates (paregoric), which inhibit peristaltic action, are seldom employed in treatment of diarrhea in the pediatric age-group. They have little or no effect on the course of infantile diarrhea and are more likely to cause toxicity. Diphenoxylate hydrochloride with atropine sulfate (Lomotil) is sometimes prescribed for older children, but is contraindicated in infants and children younger than 2 years of age because of its narrow margin of safety.

Adsorbents, such as kaolin and pectin, alter consistency and cosmetic appearance of stools and decrease the frequency of evacuation but do not reduce the amount of fluid loss and may actually mask significant fluid losses. Although of questionable value, they are sometimes prescribed to provide parents with a sense that something is being done for the child. Antidiarrheal agents are not administered to infants, but may be of limited value in older children.

Severe diarrhea. Severe diarrhea is largely a problem of infants and very young children, and regardless of the cause, successful management relies primarily on appropriate treatment of physiologic disturbances and is only secondarily concerned with specific treatment of the etiologic agent. Severe diarrhea warrants hospitalization, comprehensive evaluation, and parenteral fluid therapy. Intravenous fluid therapy is directed toward rapid replacement of (1) the fluid deficit, (2) ongoing normal losses, and (3) abnormal ongoing losses. The magnitude of the deficit is determined from loss of body weight and ongoing losses by calculating the energy requirements of the child. The energy requirements include not only predicted caloric expenditure for age and size but other factors that increase the use of energy, such as elevated temperature (metabolism increases by about 12% for each 1° C) and hyperventilation. Additional replacement covers abnormal losses as determined by output measurement, weight, and electrolyte determinations.

Once the severe effects of dehydration are under control, specific diagnostic and therapeutic measures are instigated to detect and treat the cause of the diarrhea. This includes mild sedation, antimicrobial therapy when indicated, and treatment of secondary effects of the illness or its therapy. For example, secondary bacterial growth may be countered with a short course of nonabsorbable antibiotics or oral administration of lactobacilli to recolonize the normal flora of the GI tract.

Typically the frequency and volume of stools will subside within 48 hours in fasted patients receiving intravenous fluids. If the child is alert and no intervening complications arise, such as persistent vomiting or distention, an ORS is generally initiated. The caloric intake is increased gradually until the usual dietary intake is reestablished, usually within 7 to 8 days.

Intractable diarrhea. The initial concern in the first 24 to 48 hours is correction of acidosis, dehydration, and electrolyte disturbances, with nothing by mouth, to place the bowel at rest. Infants who have difficulty adjusting to oral feedings require peripheral alimentation with dextrose and amino acids to supplement enteral feedings. Intralipid may be given slowly to provide additional calories. The orally administered formula is usually increased in concentration while the infant is receiving peripheral alimentation. When full-strength formula is tolerated, the volume is gradually increased and the intravenously administered fluids are decreased accordingly (Bass and Walker, 1986).

Severely ill infants who are unable to tolerate continuous enteral feedings are usually provided with peripheral alimentation with lipids. If sufficient caloric intake is not achieved by this route, a central venous catheter is required. Central alimentation may be needed for several weeks before the infant is able to tolerate enteral feedings. When an elemental diet is established and weight gain is satisfactory, the infant is discharged with careful follow-up care and observation. Milk protein and lactose are usually avoided for at least 6 months (Bass and Walker, 1986).

Nursing Considerations

The observation of children who receive treatment at home is often the responsibility of a nurse. Management involves assessment, therapy, and education. The status of the child must be evaluated to determine the extent of disease—the nature and frequency of stools, associated signs (e.g., tenesmus, cramping, vomiting, fever), and assessment of the state of hydration. When the diarrhea consists of a few loose stools each day without evidence of illness, it is managed with continued observation and diet management.

The duration of time before initial feedings and the amount and type of fluids suggested depend on the philosophy of the health practitioner, and the parent should be cautioned against giving fluids other than those prescribed. The ORS is usually well tolerated by infants, but older children find it unpalatable. Some type of flavoring may improve the taste, but many flavorings contain glucose; therefore caution should be observed in their selection. The fluids recommended for dehydration (see Chapter 28) are well tolerated by children, but caution must be observed to avoid aggravating the diarrhea or depleting essential electrolytes.

The parent is encouraged to give fluids to the child. Fluids are usually tolerated best at room temperature, and it is best to begin with small, frequent feedings. Parents are instructed to maintain a record of the fluids taken and the child's output, both stool and urine. The health practitioner should be notified if the child refuses to take fluids, there is an increase in stooling or persistent vomiting, or the child exhibits any evidence of dehydration (see Chapter 28) or overhydration (e.g., periorbital edema).

Soft foods are gradually added when liquids are well tolerated, as evidenced by no vomiting and an increased consistency and decrease in number of stools. Appropriate soft foods include gelatin desserts, soups (not creamed), bananas, applesauce, strained carrots, crackers (including pretzels), rice, and toast with jelly.

Part of the home assessment includes a history to help elicit probable etiologic agents, such as introduction of a new food, travel to an area of high susceptibility, contact with foods that might be contaminated, and contact with pets that are known to be sources of enteric infections. Unrefrigerated milk and egg products provide excellent media for growth of *Staphylococcus,* and fowl, both wild and domestic, is a well-known source of *Salmonella.* Animals of all varieties can be infected by other animals and birds. Pet chickens, mammals (e.g., dogs, cats, mice), and reptiles, especially small turtles, have been implicated as sources of infection in children.

Home assessment should include detection of such sources of contamination as well as observation of general cleanliness and sanitation in preparation and storage of food. It is especially important to emphasize the need for handwashing before food preparation, feeding, or otherwise handling the infant or child and after elimination or diapering.

Severe diarrhea. The infant or child admitted to the hospital with diarrhea is always isolated from other children, and appropriate precautions are implemented to prevent possible spread to other children and personnel. Each hospital has a policy regarding enteric precautions (see Infection Control, Chapter 27).

The child is weighed on admission and frequently during the emergency phase of rapid hydration. Accurate intake and output measurement is imperative, and a urine collection (see Chapter 27) is placed to determine the volume of output, measure specific gravity, and ascertain that renal blood flow is sufficient to permit administration of potassium. Unless urine is separated from stool, this essential information cannot be obtained.

Children who are sufficiently ill to require hospitalization are almost always given parenteral fluid therapy with nothing by mouth for 12 to 48 hours. Monitoring the intravenous infusion is a primary nursing function, with careful attention to ascertain that the correct fluid and electrolyte concentration is infused, the flow rate is adjusted to deliver the desired volume over a given period, and the intravenous site is maintained. Restraint of some type is needed with infants and small children, whose purposeful or random movements might disturb the catheter placement (see Chapter 28). Frequent assessment of the intravenous site for infiltration and of the restrained limbs for circulation and pressure areas is necessary. Restraints should be released as frequently as possible to allow the child to move the extremities. Children are sufficiently active that range of motion exercises are seldom necessary when they are unconstrained and not in severe pain.

The nurse is responsible for examination of stools and the collection of specimens for laboratory examination. Care is exerted in obtaining and transporting stools to prevent possible spread of infection. Specimens are manipulated and transported to the laboratory in appropriate media and containers and in accordance with hospital policy. Tests for pH, blood, and sugar can be done without removing the stool from the diaper. A clean tongue depressor can be used to obtain specimens for laboratory examination when a larger volume is needed or as an applicator for transfer to a culture medium.

Because diarrheal stools are highly irritating to the skin, extra care is needed to protect the skin of the diaper region from becoming excoriated. Exposing the reddened areas to air and light is an effective method to facilitate healing. Active children may require restraint to maintain proper exposure, prevent any possibility of injury, and minimize possible spread of any feces that may be expelled. Contamination is especially likely in children with explosive bowel movements. Holding an infant or small child in the lap, protected with blankets or diapers, during exposure serves as an excellent means for observing and restraining the child as well as providing tactile stimulation.

NURSING TIP: DRYING THE BUTTOCKS

Using a hair dryer on a low or cool setting is helpful for drying the skin of the diaper area.

NURSING TIP: COMMERCIAL WIPES

Many commercial baby wipes contain alcohol, which can sting. Therefore nurses and families should be cautioned against their use on excoriated or denuded areas of skin.

Oral feedings are begun according to the philosophy of the attending practitioner, and resumption of feedings is usually begun with a diluted soy formula (e.g., Isomil or ProSoBee), which is gradually strengthened as tolerated until the full-strength formula is taken without exacerbation of the diarrhea. Milk and lactose-containing formulas are usually withheld for at least a week in children with severe diarrhea. Hydrolyzed protein formulas with nonlactose sugar (e.g., Nutramigen or Pregestimil) are often substituted until the GI tract is again able to tolerate milk and milk products.

ACUTE INFECTIOUS GASTROENTERITIS

When diarrhea is presumed or established to be caused by a microorganism, the term *infectious gastroenteritis* or *bacterial gastroenteritis* is applied. In the pediatric age-group infectious gastroenteritis is second only to upper respiratory tract infections as a cause of illness (Silverman and Roy, 1983). Although ordinarily benign and self-limited, they are a major pediatric problem and account for a significant number of hospital admissions.

Epidemiology

A variety of organisms are responsible for GI tract disorders in infants and children, and most are spread by the fecal-oral route. Organisms can be transmitted by direct person-to-person contact (especially where sizable groups are in direct contact, such as in daycare centers), animals (primarily family pets), foods (especially raw milk and poultry), and water (including swimming water). Most of the illnesses show seasonal variations. Viral gastroenteritis is seen more frequently in winter months; most bacterial disorders are more prevalent during the summer and fall.

Although acute gastroenteritis affects all age-groups, certain patterns are discernible. There is a greater frequency of diarrheal disease in younger children, and specific organisms are more prominent at different ages, for example, *E. coli* in the newborn, rotaviruses in children younger than 2 years of age, and *Giardia, Shigella, Yersinia,* and *Campylobacter* in toddlers. The relative chance of a given illness being associated with *C. jejuni* is greater in older children, and the Norwalk-like viruses are a frequent cause of epidemics in school-age children (Guerrant, Lohr, and Williams, 1986). Adolescents who are sexually active are subject to enteric pathogens that are transmitted by sexual contact as well as the traditional sexually transmitted organisms that present with diarrhea or proctitis (e.g., *Neisseria gonorrhoeae,* syphilis, *Chlamydia,* and herpes simplex).

Traveler's diarrhea is a common problem for some persons traveling to other countries, especially developing countries. Daycare centers are a prime source of infection in younger children, especially in centers that care for children in diapers. Toddlers not only explore their environment with their mouths, but many are not toilet trained and engage in direct contact with other children and caregivers (see the discussion of infections in daycare centers in Chapter 15). Other persons at risk are children with immune system disorders.

Etiology/Pathophysiology

Many organisms can cause diarrheal disturbances in children, especially in infants. These can be enteric pathogens primarily, such as the *Shigella* and *Salmonella* groups of bacteria, or other organisms that have the potential to produce diarrhea under favorable circumstances, such as *Staphylococcus aureus.* Most infectious organisms are transmitted through unwashed hands, contaminated feedings, or infected "carriers," including animal reservoirs such as dogs, cats, hamsters, birds, and turtles.

Bacterial invasion of the GI tract produces diarrhea and related symptoms by interaction with intestinal mucosa (Box 29-6). Organisms that are considered "normal flora" in most situations are enteropathic under certain conditions and in susceptible children, particularly newborn and young infants.

S. aureus produces an enterotoxin that can cause diarrhea by (1) food poisoning from contamination (especially milk or egg products) with exotoxin production, (2) enteritis as a result of prolonged broad-spectrum antibiotic therapy that destroys and eliminates enteric organisms that normally control staphylococcal invasion, (3) enteritis as a complication of staphylococcal infection elsewhere (skin or lungs), and (4) primary staphylococcal infection in newborns who have not yet established competing enteric flora.

Clinical Manifestations

Infectious diarrheas have some features in common, such as vomiting, and there is frequently abdominal discomfort. Bacterial infections and some viral infections are accompanied by fever. The severity is variable among the various forms (Table 29-2).

Diagnostic Evaluation

Laboratory confirmation of the specific organism confirms the diagnosis and serves as a guideline for appropriate medical therapy.

Therapeutic Management

The primary concern in infectious gastroenteritis, as in all conditions in which fluid is lost in large amounts, is dehydration and the attendant deterioration. Fluid replacement and monitoring of electrolyte status with replacement are the same as for any diarrheal disorder. When the organism is identified, appropriate antibiotics are prescribed for those diarrheas for which specific therapy has been found to be effective.

Box 29-6 MECHANISMS OF DIARRHEA PRODUCTION BY ORGANISMS

Enterotoxin production. Organisms produce their effect by multiplication in the GI tract, followed by adhesion to the mucosa, where they release an exotoxin that binds to the small bowel villi. Interaction of this toxin and mucosa stimulates profuse secretion of water and electrolytes. Examples include *Shigella, E. coli,* and *Vibrio cholerae.*

Invasion and destruction of epithelial cells. Organisms invade intestinal epithelium directly, where they multiply and destroy cells, causing superficial ulcerations of the mucosa. Infection proceeds from the upper to the lower intestines, producing bloody mucoid stools. Organisms also produce a powerful endotoxin that promotes loss of fluids and electrolytes into the intestine. Examples include *Shigella* and *E. coli.*

Penetration and systemic invasion. Organisms invade the thin layer of connective tissue (lamina propria) lying directly beneath the epithelium of the mucosal membrane in the distal small bowel and colon, causing local inflammation and stimulating the excretion of intestinal fluids. The mucosa becomes hyperemic and edematous. From this point the organism has access to the systemic circulation, in which it can produce foci of infection elsewhere in the body. An example is *Salmonella.*

Adherence without destruction of mucosa and without enterotoxin production (unconfirmed mechanism). Enteropathic organisms (e.g., *E. coli*) penetrate the covering (glycocalyx) of some cells and adhere to the enterocyte surface, where they disrupt the microvilli and have a blunting effect on the villi, interfering with villi functioning.

Data from Silverman, A., and Roy, C.C.: Pediatric clinical gastroenterology, ed. 3, St. Louis, 1983, Mosby–Year Book, Inc.

Nursing Considerations

Basic nursing care for the infant or child with infectious gastroenteritis is the same as for any diarrheal disease. However, appropriate precautions are carried out to prevent the spread of the infection to others (see Infection Control, Chapter 27). Assessment of stooling and history of the symptoms and circumstances surrounding the onset are important to identification of the causative organisms.

✦ **NURSING ALERT** Children with a cluster of three characteristics—abrupt onset, more than four stools per day, and absence of vomiting before onset of diarrhea—have been found to have a high incidence of positive stool cultures for bacterial diarrhea (DeWitt, Humphrey, and McCarthy, 1985).

It may be necessary to obtain stool specimens from the child and other family members who are affected or suspected to be carriers of infectious organisms. The parents

Table 29-2 Enteropathologic causes of acute gastroenteritis

ORGANISM	PATHOLOGY	CHARACTERISTICS	COMMENTS
Viral agents			
Rotavirus Incubation period: 1-3 days	Remains unexplained Severely distorted mucosal architecture with atrophic mucosa and severe inflammatory changes	Abrupt onset Fever (38° C or above) lasting approximately 48 hours Associated upper respiratory tract infection Diarrhea may persist for more than a week	Incidence higher in cool weather (80% in winter) Affects all age-groups; 6- to 24-month-old infants more vulnerable Usually mild and self-limited Important cause of nosocomial infections in hospitals and gastroenteritis in children attending daycare centers
Norwalk-like organisms Incubation period: 1-3 days	Mechanism of effect unknown Blunting of villi and inflammatory changes in lamina propria Reduced enzymes	Fever Loss of appetite Nausea/vomiting Abdominal pain Diarrhea Malaise	Source of infection: drinking water, recreation water, food (including shellfish) Affects all ages Benign; seldom lasts more than 3 days Self-limited (2-3 days)
Bacterial agents			
Pathogenic *Escherichia coli* Incubation period: highly variable; depends on strain	Usually caused by enterotoxin production (small bowel) Reduces absorption and increases secretion of fluids and electrolytes	Onset gradual or abrupt Variable clinical manifestations Most—green, watery diarrhea with mucus; becomes explosive Vomiting may be present from onset Abdominal distention Diarrhea Fever; appears toxic	Incidence higher in summer Usually interpersonal transmission but may transmit via inanimate objects A cause of nursery epidemics With symptomatic treatment only, may continue for weeks Full breast-feeding has a protective effect Symptoms generally subside in 3-7 days Relapse rate approximately 20%
Salmonella groups (nontyphoidal)—gram negative, nonencapsulated, nonsporulating Incubation period: 6-72 hours for gastroenteritis (usually less than 24); 3-60 days for enteric fever (usually 7-14)	Penetration of lamina propria (small bowel and colon) Local inflammation—no extensive destruction Stimulation of intestinal fluid excretion Systemic invasion of other sites	Rapid onset Variable symptoms—mild to severe Nausea, vomiting, and colicky abdominal pain followed by diarrhea, occasionally with blood and mucus Chills may occur Hyperactive peristalsis and mild abdominal tenderness Symptoms usually subside within 5 days May have fever, headache, and cerebral manifestations, e.g., drowsiness, confusion, meningismus, or seizures Infants may be afebrile and nontoxic May result in life-threatening septicemia and meningitis	Two thirds of patients are younger than 20 years of age; highest incidence in children younger than age 9 years, especially infants Highest incidence occurs July through October, lowest from January through April Transmission primarily via contaminated food and drink—most from animal sources, including fowl, mammals, reptiles, and insects Most common sources are poultry and eggs In children—pets, e.g., dogs, cats, hamsters, and especially pet turtles Communicable as long as organisms are excreted
S. typhi	Rapid invasion of bloodstream from minor sites of inflammation Marked inflammation and necrosis of intestinal mucosa and lymphatics	Variable in infants Older children—irregular fever, headache, malaise, lethargy Diarrhea occurs in 50% at early stage Cough is common In a few days, fever rises and is consistent; fatigue, cough, abdominal pain, anorexia, and weight loss develop; diarrhea begins	Decreased incidence in last decade Acute symptoms may persist for a week or more Transmitted by contaminated food or water (primary), infected animals (e.g., pet turtles)

Table 29-2 Enteropathologic causes of acute gastroenteritis—cont'd

ORGANISM	PATHOLOGY	CHARACTERISTICS	COMMENTS
Shigella groups—gram negative, nonmotile, anaerobic bacilli Incubation period: 1-7 days, usually 2-4	Enterotoxin Stimulates loss of fluids and electrolytes Invasion of epithelium with superficial mucosal ulcerations *S. dysenteriae* forms exotoxin	Onset variable but usually abrupt Fever and cramping abdominal pain initially Fever—may reach 40.5° C Convulsions in about 10%—usually associated with fever Patient appears sick Headache, nuchal rigidity, delirium Watery diarrhea with mucus and pus starts about 12-48 hours after onset Stools preceded by abdominal cramps; tenesmus and straining follow Symptoms usually subside in 5-10 days	Approximately 60% of cases in children younger than age 9 years with more than one third between ages 1 and 4 years Peak incidence late summer Transmitted directly or indirectly from infected persons Communicable for 1-4 weeks Self-limited disease Treat with antibiotics Severe dehydration and collapse can affect all patients Acute symptoms may persist for a week or more
Yersinia enterocolitica Incubation period: dose dependent; 1-3 weeks		Diarrhea—may be bloody Fever (>38.7° C) Abdominal pain right lower quadrant (RLQ) Vomiting, diarrhea	Seen more frequently in winter Majority in first 3 years of life Transmitted by food and pets Can resemble appendicitis May be relapsing and last for months
Campylobacter jejuni Incubation period: 1-7 days or longer	Precise mechanism unclear Jejunum and ileum involvement Extensive ulceration with hemorrhagic ileitis Broadening and flattening of mucosa	Fever Abdominal pain—often severe, cramping, periumbilical Watery, profuse, foul-smelling diarrhea Vomiting	Person-to-person transmission May be transmitted by pets (e.g., cat, dog, hamster) Food (especially chicken) and water-borne transmission Relapse possible Most patients recover spontaneously Antibiotics advocated to speed recovery Peak incidence in summer
Vibrio cholerae (cholera) groups Incubation period: usually 2-3 days; range from few hours to 5 days	Enterotoxin causes increased secretion of chloride and possibly bicarbonate Intestinal mucosa congested with enlarged lymph follicles Intact mucosal surface	Sudden onset of profuse, watery diarrhea without cramping, tenesmus, or anal irritation, although children may complain of cramping Stools are intermittent at first, then almost continuous Stools are whitish, almost clear, with flecks of mucus—"rice water stools"	Rare in infants younger than 1 year old Mortality high in both treated and untreated infants and small children Transmitted via contaminated food and water Endemic in Bengal Attack confers immunity
▪ Food poisoning			
Staphylococcus Incubation period: 4-6 hours	Produce heat-stable enterotoxin	Nausea, vomiting Severe abdominal cramps Profuse diarrhea Shock may occur in severe cases May be a mild fever	Transferred via contaminated food—inadequately cooked or refrigerated, e.g., custards, mayonnaise, cream-filled or -topped desserts Self-limited; improvement apparent within 24 hours Excellent prognosis
Clostridium perfringens Incubation period: 8-24 hours, usually 8-12	Produces heat-resistant and heat-sensitive toxins	Moderate to severe crampy, midepigastric pain	Self-limited illness Transmission by commercial food products, most often meat and poultry
Clostridium botulinum Incubation period: 12-26 hours (range, 6 hours to 8 days)	Highly potent neurotoxin	Nausea, vomiting Diarrhea Central nervous system (CNS) symptoms with curare-like effect Dry mouth, dysphagia	Transmitted by contaminated food products Variable severity—mild symptoms to rapidly fatal within a few hours Antitoxin administration

are provided with specimen containers and instructed in collection and disposition of stool samples.

Reports suggest that traveler's diarrhea can be prevented by prophylactic administration of trimethoprim/sulfamethoxazole (Bactrim, Septra) (Freeman and others, 1983), doxycycline (Vibramycin, Vibra-Tabs) (Dupont and others, 1983), or subsalicylate bismuth suspension (Pepto-Bismol) (Dupont and others, 1980; Graham and others, 1983). Although the medications appear to be safe for adults, parents should be cautioned against giving any of the drugs to children. The drugs may be inappropriate or untested for use in children. For example, the large doses of Pepto-Bismol recommended for adults may contain toxic amounts of salicylates when given to children, and the bismuth may cause neurologic deficits.

Until vaccines or other prophylactic measures are proved safe for children, the best prevention is to allow children to drink only bottled water and carbonated beverages (from the container through a straw supply brought from home). Tap water, ice, unpasteurized dairy products, raw vegetables, and unpeeled fruits should be avoided. Meats and seafoods may be risky as well.

CHRONIC NONSPECIFIC DIARRHEA

Chronic nonspecific diarrhea (CNSD) (sometimes called protracted diarrhea or irritable bowel syndrome) is the most common cause of prolonged diarrhea in young children between 6 and 36 months of age and appears to be caused by decreased transit time in the alimentary tract. Characteristically there is diarrhea for at least 3 weeks, normal growth, and no evidence of enteric pathogens.

A number of mechanisms have been suggested for CNSD, including abnormal GI motility, food intolerances, dietary fat restriction, excessive fluid intake, and carbohydrate malabsorption associated with fruit juice intake, especially those containing sorbitol (Hyams and others, 1988). Intake of fluid appears to have been associated with the development of CNSD in some children. The incidence has increased significantly since the implementation of oral rehydration therapy, and affected children developed normal stool patterns following fluid restriction (Greene and Ghishan, 1983).

CNSD is most common in the toddler age-group. Some instances of CNSD have been attributed to specific causes such as laxative abuse (Munchausen syndrome by proxy), bacterial overgrowth, allergic gastroenteropathy, postgastroenteritis syndrome, transient protein intolerance, and iatrogenic diarrhea (from administration of some drugs) (Andres, 1988).

It has also been observed that persistent diarrhea is an important side effect of exogenous prostaglandins administered to pregnant women to initiate labor. Prostaglandins have also been implicated as a cause of diarrhea associated with some tumors. Increased circulating prostaglandin levels have been found in some children with CNSD. These children respond well to administration of prostaglandin synthetase inhibitors such as aspirin or indomethacin (Dodge and others, 1981).

Nursing Considerations

A careful history is important in assessment and management of CNSD, since causation is basic to therapy and nursing care. The most common cause in infancy is postinfectious lactose intolerance, which is managed with lactose-free formula. Teaching parents about diet modification, stool specimen collection, and record-keeping is a major nursing responsibility (see previous discussions for nursing care).

VOMITING

Vomiting, a very common symptom in childhood, is usually of little concern. Often it is of a minor and temporary nature, but when vomiting is persistent and prolonged, the consequences to the infant or child can be rapid and serious. An associated hazard, especially in very young and debilitated infants and children, is the risk of aspiration with the possibility of asphyxiation, atelectasis, or pneumonia.

The amount and character of the vomiting are important observations, and nurses should be able to distinguish between and describe the various forms this behavior takes. *Vomiting* is the forcible ejection of stomach contents and is usually accompanied by nausea. In *projectile vomiting* vomitus is forcefully ejected as far as 2 to 4 feet (0.6 to 1.2 m) from the child. Projectile vomiting is not associated with nausea. Spitting up and regurgitation, characteristic of infants, are described in Chapter 13.

Vomiting in childhood can be caused by numerous intrinsic and extrinsic factors, but is usually caused by readily detected infections or psychologic causes. Vomiting and diarrhea are common manifestations of a variety of infectious disorders, responses to an allergen or ingestion of drugs or other toxic substances, and symptoms associated with appendicitis or GI tract obstruction. Recurrent, prolonged, or persistent vomiting is also associated with encephalographic variations and results from increased intracranial pressure (ICP).

Many children are prone to motion sickness when riding in an automobile or airplane or even when swinging in a swing. Some children, especially overly dependent children, maladjusted children, or children who react to environmental stress (e.g., a high-anxiety home environment) with somatic symptoms, respond to tension or stress with stomach upset and vomiting. (See also Rumination, Chapter 13.)

Occasionally children will vomit as an oral defense mechanism, such as when children resist feedings they do not want. They may think eating is an obligation they are powerless to resist. Other children resort to contentious vomiting when they become angry with someone they know loves and cares for them. For example, struggles over independence in 2-year-old children can trigger intense emotions. A child who vomits during a conflict with parents soon realizes that this inadvertent occurrence causes concern in the parents, who view kicking and screaming as behavior but vomiting as illness. Consequently, the reflexive vomiting may become conditioned and reinforced by the parents' response to it (Fleisher, 1986).

The *cyclic vomiting syndrome* usually begins between 2 and 9 years of age with episodes that tend to be stereotypic and self-limited. Typically they begin at night or on rising and last 12 to 48 hours, although some children may have symptoms for as little as a few hours, and others for as long as 10 days. Attacks occur fairly regularly in most patients and may occur weekly or several months apart. In the majority of cases specific events trigger an attack, such as vacations or other nonnoxious excitement, noxious emotional experiences, and colds or flu. There is no cure, but in most children the disorder remits during adolescence (Fleisher, 1986).

Older children may practice vomiting as an act of malingering, deceiving parents or others in order to gain something or to be relieved of some obligation. This manipulative behavior stops as soon as it ceases to work. Bulimia, practiced by some adolescents, is described in Chapter 21.

Pathophysiology

Vomiting, one of the most primitive protective functions with which animals are endowed, is controlled through the vomiting center located in the reticular core of the medulla. The vomiting center receives stimuli from three sources (Box 29-7).

Vomiting involves a complex reflex that is associated with widespread autonomic discharge that causes salivation, pallor, sweating, and tachycardia. Motor reaction, transmitted to the upper GI tract, causes the vomiting act. The stomach antrum and duodenum contract; the remainder of the stomach, the esophagus, and its sphincters relax; the glottis closes to occlude the pulmonary airway; and the soft palate closes the nasopharynx. Then the diaphragm and abdominal muscles contract sharply, raising intraabdominal pressure, which compresses abdominal contents and propels them into the esophagus and out through the mouth. Actual vomiting is usually preceded by severe cycles of reflux into the esophagus.

Assessment

Vomiting is the first symptom of a variety of common infections as well as a manifestation of more serious conditions.

Box 29-7 SOURCES OF VOMITING STIMULI

Higher cortical centers—either deep-seated or superficial psychologic disturbances. Stimuli include those associated with unpleasant sights, repugnant odors, and fright.

Chemosensitive trigger zone—transmits impulses to cortical center; located on the floor of the fourth ventricle. Stimuli include chemical stimulation by drugs (e.g., apomorphine, morphine, ipecac, and some digitalis derivatives), toxins (e.g., from uremia, infections, or radiation), cerebral hypoxia, increased ICP, and disturbances of the semicircular canals of the inner ear.

Reflex excitement (vagal and sympathetic afferent nerves)—results from disturbed GI and other viscera. Stimuli include irritation, inflammation, or mechanical disturbance in GI tract (e.g., distention or obstruction); irritation of other viscera (e.g., heart, renal pelvis, bladder); and pain.

It is a relatively frequent symptom during the neonatal period, usually caused by simple regurgitation from overfeeding or insufficient bubbling, and has little clinical significance. However, it can indicate the presence of GI tract disorders or increased ICP. The following nursing observations can provide valuable information for evaluating the nature and importance of vomiting.

Character of vomitus. Esophageal vomitus contains unchanged food and no gastric juice. A relaxed cardiac sphincter or rumination (habitual regurgitation) will produce frequent small amounts of vomitus emitted with little force. The presence of sour milk curds with no green or brown color indicates vomitus from the stomach and excludes an esophageal cause. Uncurdled milk may also be vomited during or shortly after feedings. Vomitus containing greenish material indicating the presence of bile pigment is most likely to occur when an obstruction is situated below the ampulla of Vater; bile in the vomitus almost always excludes pyloric stenosis. Vomitus with a fecal odor suggests a lower intestinal obstruction or peritonitis.

Blood in the vomitus may appear as bright red, bloody streaks or brown coffee grounds emesis and may be insignificant or of major importance. Hematemesis is sometimes observed in the immediate neonatal period in infants who have swallowed maternal blood during delivery or occasionally from a cracked nipple. Other causes of hematemesis in early infancy include hemorrhagic disease of the newborn or other defects of coagulation and early esophageal erosion associated with regurgitation of gastric juice related to reflux (see Chapter 33). Trauma from nasogastric tubes or tracheal catheters may cause bleeding followed by vomiting of swallowed blood.

In older children hematemesis may be caused by swallowed blood from epistaxis or after nose or throat surgery. Rupture of esophageal varices and peptic ulcer can cause profuse hematemesis. Coagulation defects or vascular damage may cause bloody vomiting in many diseases.

Frequency and persistence. Frequent or persistent vomiting indicates that the causative factor is still operating. The primary danger is loss of fluids and electrolytes, which increases with the frequency and duration of vomiting. In early infancy the most frequent causes of persistent vomiting are pylorospasm, pyloric stenosis, adrenocortical insufficiency, and urinary tract infections. Recurrent vomiting suggests GI allergy, an epileptic equivalent ("abdominal epilepsy"), a childhood form of migraine, or intermittent intestinal obstruction, as might occur with malrotation of the colon. It is frequently associated with the onset of a febrile illness or a period of increased emotional tension.

Amount. The amount of the emesis should be measured and recorded because it often furnishes information regarding the amount of fluid lost in relation to intake. This provides a clue to the extent of dehydration. Overfeeding or too rapid feeding may cause the child to vomit part of the feeding.

Force of vomiting. Repeated regurgitation is most often related to rumination or gastroesophageal reflux. Forceful vomiting during or after a meal is usually caused by overdistention with milk and air. Repeated forceful vomiting of a projectile nature is one of the cardinal signs of pyloric stenosis in early infancy and can be a result of increased ICP at any age. When combined with abdominal distention, it suggests intestinal obstruction.

Relationship to feeding. Emesis in infants may be related to the nature of their formula. Highly diluted formula may cause hungry infants to consume so much that they vomit from overdistention. High-fat or acidified formulas may cause others to vomit. Food that is contaminated by bacteria or food that is inappropriate for the child, such as unripe fruits or rich, highly seasoned foods, may cause a child to vomit.

Vomiting soon after eating may be a symptom of food allergy or acute, febrile illness. More often vomiting is initiated by gastric distention by milk and air, which is caused by such feeding practices as failure to bubble the infant during and immediately after feedings, feeding formula through nipples with holes so small that the infant takes in air while sucking for milk, improper positioning of the bottle so that air instead of milk enters the nipple, feeding too rapidly, and swallowing air from prolonged sucking on an empty breast. Underfeeding leads to hunger, causing the infant to swallow air while sucking on fingers or fists. Cold formula may cause a few infants to vomit, and hurried eating at any age may precipitate vomiting, particularly when the child is excited or overly tired.

History. Sometimes the cause of vomiting is readily apparent from the history. Vomiting associated with diarrhea is usually caused by gastroenteritis; vomiting that occurs suddenly in a previously healthy child suggests the early stages of an infection. When several children or members of a family who have eaten together vomit, food poisoning is the most likely possibility. Vomiting accompanied by fever, abdominal pain, and tenderness is a common symptom of appendicitis or other abdominal conditions requiring surgical repair. Vomiting is not an uncommon reaction to toxins or drugs taken as prescribed or ingested accidentally.

Diagnostic Evaluation

When vomiting is persistent and cannot be attributed to an obvious and temporary condition, a more comprehensive evaluation is warranted. It may be the child's only symptom or, more often, only one clinical feature of a variety of disorders. The importance of vomiting also varies. It may be a minor manifestation or the dominant feature of a serious illness. Vomiting that is not associated with feeding may be an indication of increased ICP.

Diagnostic tests. Physical examination and routine tests of blood and urine are performed, but special laboratory tests are seldom employed. Radiographic studies can detect anomalies of the alimentary tract. If vomiting has persisted to the degree that dehydration and electrolyte imbalance are present, the child's weight and serum electrolyte, blood urea nitrogen, and carbon dioxide content of the blood are determined to assess the state of hydration and to serve as the basis for therapy.

Therapeutic Management

Management is directed toward detection and treatment of the cause of the vomiting and prevention of complications of the vomiting. Vomiting that results in fluid loss of considerable degree may require parenteral fluid therapy. Fluids are administered in the same manner and in a similar electrolyte composition to those administered in diarrhea. This includes both parenteral and oral fluids.

Although most children respond well to these measures, centrally acting antiemetic drugs may be prescribed when the cause of the vomiting is known and the vomiting is predictable and of limited duration. Antiemetics can exert their effect on neural labyrinth pathways, depress the chemoreceptor trigger zone and the vomiting center, or act on the aural vestibular apparatus.

Nursing Considerations

The major emphasis of nursing care of the vomiting infant or child is on observation and reporting of vomiting behavior and associated symptoms and the implementation of measures to reduce the vomiting. Accurate assessment of the type of vomiting, the appearance of the vomitus, and the child's behavior associated with the vomiting greatly aids in establishing a diagnosis of disorders that have vomiting as a clinical manifestation.

Nursing interventions will be determined by the cause of the vomiting. When the vomiting is identified as a manifestation of improper feeding methods, establishing proper techniques through teaching and example will usually correct the problem. If vomiting is determined to be a manifestation of probable GI obstruction, food is usually withheld or special feeding techniques are implemented. In situations in which vomiting is related to concurrent infection, dietary indiscretion, or emotional factors, efforts are directed toward maintaining hydration or preventing dehydration by offering small amounts of palatable fluids, much the same as the oral intake described for dehydration (see Oral Fluid Intake, Chapter 28).

The thirst mechanism is the most sensitive guide to fluid needs, and ad libitum administration of a glucose-electrolyte solution to an alert child will restore water and electrolytes satisfactorily. It is important to include carbohydrate to spare body protein and to avoid ketosis resulting from exhaustion of glycogen reserves. Once vomiting has abated, more liberal amounts can be offered, followed by simple foods such as gelatin, crackers, clear broth, and buttered toast in small amounts, when the child desires, followed by gradual resumption of the regular diet. Some health practitioners believe that small, frequent feedings actually induce further losses through activation of the gastrocolic reflex, and they prescribe large volumes initially at less frequent intervals.

The vomiting infant or child is positioned to prevent aspiration and observed for evidence of dehydration (see Chapter 28). It is important to emphasize the need for the child to brush the teeth or rinse the mouth after vomiting to dilute hydrochloric acid that comes in contact with the teeth. A flavored mouthwash or brushing also helps freshen the mouth. Careful monitoring of fluid and electrolyte status must be exercised to avoid the possibility of hyperelectrolytemia.

SHOCK STATES

A number of conditions constitute medical and nursing emergencies; severe shock is one of these conditions. Nurses should be prepared for this possibility and intervene early and appropriately when patients display signs that indicate circulatory impairment.

SHOCK

Shock, or circulatory failure, is a clinical syndrome characterized by prostration and tissue perfusion that is inadequate to meet the metabolic demands of the body, resulting in depressed vital cell function. Although the causes are different, the physiologic consequences are the same: hypotension, tissue hypoxia, and metabolic acidosis.

Etiology

Circulatory failure in children is the result of hypovolemia, altered peripheral vascular resistance, pump failure, or obstruction (Fig. 29-2). The most common type of circulatory failure in children is hypovolemia, or *hypovolemic shock,* which follows a reduction in circulating blood volume related to blood, plasma, or extracellular fluid losses beyond the child's physical ability to compensate (Crone, 1980). *Cardiogenic shock* resulting from decreased output is not common in children. The types of shock and their most frequent causes are listed in Box 29-8.

Pathophysiology

The circulatory system of the healthy child is able to transport oxygen and metabolic substrates to meet the essential needs of body tissues, which demand varying amounts of nutrients in relation to one another and relative to alterations in conditions such as exercise and disease states. The cardiac output and distribution to the various body tissues can change very rapidly in response to intrinsic (myocardial and intravascular) or extrinsic (neuronal) control mechanisms. In shock states these mechanisms are altered or challenged.

Reduced blood flow, as in hypovolemic shock, causes diminished venous return to the heart, low central venous pressure (CVP), low cardiac output, and hypotension. The reduced intravascular volume triggers a chain of compensatory mechanisms. Fluid is mobilized from the extracellular compartment. Vasomotor centers in the medulla are signaled, causing depressed vagal activity and increased sympathetic activity that increase the force and rate of cardiac contraction and constrict the arterioles and veins, thereby increasing peripheral vascular resistance.

Simultaneously the lowered blood volume also leads to the release of large amounts of catecholamines, antidiuretic hormone, adrenocorticosteroids, and aldosterone in an effort to conserve body fluids. The catecholamines augment the vasomotor activity to produce vasoconstriction and reduce blood flow to the skin, kidneys, muscles, and splanchnic viscera in order to shunt the available blood to the brain and heart. Consequently the skin feels cold and clammy, there is poor capillary filling, and glomerular filtration and urine output are significantly reduced.

Impaired perfusion to peripheral tissues also produces metabolic alterations. Oxygen depletion causes the cells to revert to anaerobic glycolytic metabolism, forming pyruvic

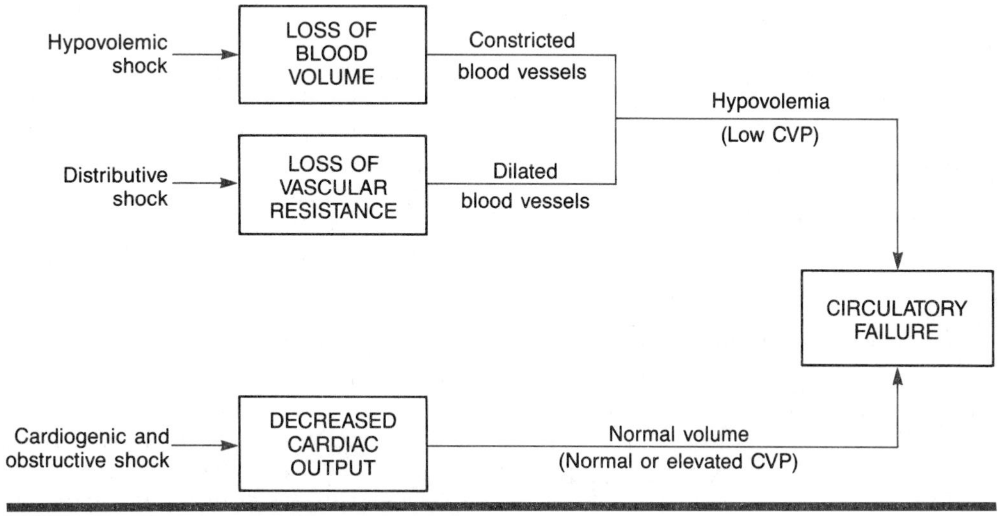

Fig. 29-2. Causes of circulatory failure in children.
Modified from Crone, R.K.: Pediatr. Clin. North Am. 27:525-538, 1980.

Box 29-8 TYPES OF SHOCK

Hypovolemic Shock

Characteristics
Reduction in size of vascular compartment
Falling blood pressure
Poor capillary filling
Low central venous pressure (CVP)

Most frequent causes
Blood loss (hemorrhagic shock)—trauma, GI bleeding, intracranial hemorrhage
Plasma loss—increased capillary permeability associated with sepsis and acidosis, hypoproteinemia, burns, peritonitis
Extracellular fluid loss—vomiting, diarrhea, glycosuric diuresis, sunstroke

Distributive Shock

Characteristics
Reduction in peripheral vascular resistance
Profound inadequacies in tissue perfusion
Increased venous capacity and pooling
Acute reduction in return blood flow to the heart
Diminished cardiac output

Most frequent causes
Anaphylaxis (anaphylactic shock)—extreme allergy or hypersensitivity to a foreign substance
Sepsis (septic shock, bacteremic shock, endotoxic shock)—overwhelming sepsis and circulating bacterial toxins
Loss of neuronal control (neurogenic shock)—interruption of neuronal transmission (spinal cord injury)
Myocardial depression and peripheral dilation—exposure to anesthesia or ingestion of barbiturates, tranquilizers, narcotics, antihypertensive agents, or ganglionic blocking agents

Obstructive Shock

Characteristic
Inflow or outflow obstruction of main bloodstream

Most frequent sites of obstruction and probable causes
Vena cava—compression
Pericardium—tamponade, pneumopericardium
Cardiac chambers—ball-valve thrombus, anatomic obstruction (atresia)
Pulmonary circuit—embolism, pulmonic stenosis, tension pneumothorax, pleural effusion
Aorta—coarctation

Cardiogenic Shock

Characteristic
Decreased cadiac output

Most frequent causes
Congenital heart disease in infancy—usually systemic-to-pulmonary shunting
Primary pump failure—myocarditis, myocardial trauma, biochemical derangements
Dysrhythmias—paroxysmal atrial tachycardia, atrioventricular block, and ventricular dysrhythmias; secondary to myocarditis or biochemical abnormalities (occasionally)

acid, which is then converted to lactic acid, thus producing lactic acidosis. The acidosis places an extra burden on the lungs as they attempt to compensate for the metabolic acidosis by increased rate. Impaired cellular uptake and metabolism of glucose create hyperglycemia. When plasma fluid is lost, hemoconcentration and diminished blood flow increase the viscosity of the blood and further impair perfusion.

Prolonged vasoconstriction results in fatigue and atony of the resisting peripheral arterioles and, augmented by the release of vasodilator substances such as histamine, leads to vasodilation. Venules, less sensitive to vasodilator substances, remain constricted for a time, causing massive pooling in the capillary and venular beds and transudation of plasma fluid into the tissues to further deplete blood volume. In all types of shock these circulatory alterations take place, but in neurogenic, septic, and anaphylactic shock there are some variations.

In neurogenic shock control mechanisms that maintain vascular tone are interrupted, causing reduced vascular resistance and peripheral pooling of blood; with this increased vascular capacity, there is loss of effective circulating blood volume. Septic shock produces a hyperdynamic state in which there is often an elevated plasma volume and reduced peripheral resistance that leads to widespread vasodilation. In many cases there is a high cardiac output caused by the vasodilation in infected tissues and elsewhere plus a high metabolic rate resulting from the elevated body temperature. Degenerating tissues cause aggregation of red blood cells and sludging of the blood. Development of disseminated intravascular coagulation, triggered by either the degenerating tissue or bacterial toxins, consumes the clotting factors, which produces widespread hemorrhages. (See discussion in Chapter 35.)

Complications of shock create further hazards. Central nervous system (CNS) hypoperfusion may eventually lead to cerebral edema, cortical infarction, or intraventricular hemorrhage. Renal hypoperfusion causes renal ischemia with possible tubular or glomerular necrosis and renal vein thrombosis. Reduced blood flow to the lungs can interfere with surfactant secretion and result in "shock lung," which is characterized by sudden pulmonary congestion and atelectasis with formation of a hyaline membrane. Gastrointestinal tract bleeding and perforation are always a possibility following splanchnic ischemia and necrosis of intestinal mucosa. Metabolic complications of shock may include hypoglycemia, hypocalcemia, and other electrolyte disturbances.

Clinical Manifestations

Shock can be regarded as a form of compensation for circulatory failure and, because of its progressive nature, can be divided into three stages or phases: *compensated, uncompensated,* and *irreversible.* At all stages the principal differentiating signs are observed in degree of (1) tachycardia and perfusion to extremities, (2) level of consciousness, and (3) blood pressure. Additional signs or modifications of these more universal signs may be present depending on the type and cause of the shock.

Compensated shock. When vital organ function is maintained by intrinsic mechanisms and the child's ability to compensate is effective, cardiac output and systemic arterial blood pressure are usually normal or increased, but blood flow is generally uneven or maldistributed in the microcirculation. Early clinical signs are subtle, including apprehension, irritability, normal blood pressure, narrowing pulse pressure, thirst, pallor, and diminished urinary output.

✦ **NURSING ALERT** Unexplained mild tachycardia and a decrease in perfusion of the hands and feet are differentiating features of compensated shock.

Decompensated shock. As shock progresses, perfusion in the microcirculation becomes marginal despite compensatory adjustments, and signs are more obvious and indicate early decompensation. These signs are tachypnea, moderate metabolic acidosis, oliguria, and cool, pale extremities with decreased skin turgor and poor capillary filling. The outcomes of circulatory failure that progress beyond the limits of compensation are tissue hypoxia, metabolic acidosis, and eventual dysfunction of all organ systems.

✦ **NURSING ALERT** Tachycardia is pronounced, blood pressure is still maintained, but pulse pressure becomes narrowed, there is poor capillary filling, and the child in decompensated shock exhibits decreased responsiveness, confusion, and sleepiness.

Irreversible shock. Irreversible, or terminal, shock implies damage to vital organs such as the heart or brain of such magnitude that the entire organism will be disrupted regardless of therapeutic intervention. There is pronounced systemic vasoconstriction and hypoxia of visceral and cutaneous circulations with hypotension, acidosis, lethargy or coma, and oliguria or anuria. The child is totally obtunded. Thready, weak pulse; hypotension; periodic breathing or apnea; anuria; and stupor or coma are signs of impending cardiopulmonary arrest. Death occurs even if cardiovascular measurements return to normal levels with therapy (Perkin and Levin, 1982a).

Diagnostic Evaluation

The cause of shock can be discerned from the history and the physical examination. The extent of the shock is determined by measurement of vital signs, including CVP and capillary filling. Laboratory tests that assist in assessment are blood gas measurements, pH, and sometimes various liver function tests such as serum glutamic oxaloacetic transaminase (SGOT), bilirubin, and total serum protein (TSP). Coagulation status (prothrombin time [PT], partial thromboplastin time [PTT], platelet count, fibrinogen, fibrin) is evaluated when there is evidence of bleeding, such as oozing from a venipuncture site, bleeding from any orifice, or petechiae. Cultures of blood and other sites are indicated when there is a high suspicion of sepsis. Renal function tests are performed when impaired renal function is evident.

Therapeutic Management

Treatment of shock consists of three major thrusts: (1) ventilation, (2) fluid administration, and (3) improvement of the pumping action of the heart (vasopressor support). The first priority is to establish an airway and administer oxygen. Once the airway is assured, circulatory stabilization is the major concern. Placement of an intravenous catheter for rapid volume replacement is the most important action for reestablishment of circulation. Where individuals are familiar with and skilled in the technique, percutaneous cannulation of the internal jugular or subclavian veins is preferred. An alternative is rapid surgical cutdown cannulation of the saphenous vein. The vein is anatomically accessible, can accommodate the volumes of fluid needed, and is situated where it does not interfere with any resuscitation procedures that might be necessary. Another effective emergency method is intraosseous administration of fluids (see Chapter 28).

Ventilatory support. The lung is the organ most sensitive to shock. The decreased or redistribution of blood flow to respiratory muscles plus the increased work of breathing can rapidly lead to respiratory failure. Critically ill patients are unable to maintain an adequate airway. To place the lung at rest and improve ventilation, tracheal intubation is initiated early with positive-pressure ventilation and supplemental oxygen. Blood gases and pH are monitored frequently.

Increased extravascular lung water caused by edema—both hydrostatic and permeable—contributes to the development of respiratory complications. Hydrostatic edema occurs from elevation of pulmonary microvascular pressure as a result of left ventricular dysfunction; permeable edema occurs when damage to alveolar cell and pulmonary capillary epithelium causes fluid to leak into the interstitial space resulting in the so-called adult respiratory distress syndrome (ARDS) or shock lung (see Chapter 32). Therapy is directed toward maintaining normal arterial blood gas measurements, normal acid-base balance, and circulation. Efforts are made to remove fluid and prevent its accumulation by increasing oncotic pressure and decreasing microvascular hydrostatic pressure. Elevated oncotic pressure is promoted by diuresis with furosemide or mannitol, colloid administration, or both (Perkin and Levin, 1982b).

Cardiovascular support. In the majority of cases rapid restoration of blood volume is all that is needed for resuscitation of the child in shock. The nature of the fluid depends primarily on the availability of the appropriate fluid and the kind of fluid loss incurred. It may be a crystalloid solution such as lactated Ringer's solution, a colloid in the form of fresh frozen plasma, or blood. Successful resuscitation will be reflected by an increase in blood pressure and a reduction in heart rate. An increased cardiac output will result in improved capillary circulation and skin color. For these children effective monitoring includes accurate measurements and recording of vital signs and objective observations. Urinary output measurement is an important indicator of adequacy of circulation.

For the critically ill child with shock and multisystem dysfunction more aggressive monitoring is needed. Central venous measurements of right atrial pressure or pulmonary wedge pressure help guide fluid therapy. In children with persistent shock a Swan-Ganz catheter should be placed for more accurate monitoring. Determination of arterial blood gases, hematocrit, serum electrolytes, glucose, and calcium concentrations provides additional information concerning composition of circulating blood. Correction of acidosis, hypoxemia, and any metabolic derangements is mandatory.

Vasopressor support. Temporary pharmacologic support may be required to enhance myocardial contractility, to reverse metabolic or respiratory acidosis, and to maintain arterial pressure. The principal agents used to improve cardiac output and circulation are the sympathetic amines administered by constant infusion pump. Dopamine is the preferred drug in most situations because it also improves renal perfusion. Other agents used to improve cardiac output (e.g., dobutamine, isoproterenol, epinephrine) may be used as appropriate depending on the situation. Digitalis may be given to augment myocardial contractility in a failing heart, thereby increasing cardiac output.

Other drugs with vasopressor action may be used in specific situations, including phenylephrine and methoxamine. Vasodilators that are sometimes employed include nitroprusside (Nipride) and hydralazine (Apresoline). Nitroprusside is both a venous and an arteriolar vasodilator with immediate action, but it can be toxic to CNS tissues and therefore is reserved for short-term treatment. Hydralazine, a relatively pure arteriolar dilator, is difficult to titrate but may be used for more extended treatment.

Metabolic acidosis is usually corrected with adequate tissue perfusion and improved renal function. This is accomplished with adequate ventilatory support, including oxygen, and restoration of blood volume and peripheral circulation. The administration of sodium bicarbonate may be associated with complications; therefore it is used only to partially correct the pH to levels that do not pose a threat to life (Perkin and Levin, 1982b).

Calcium chloride may be administered to improve cardiac function and to offset the reduced ionized calcium associated with large amounts of albumin, whole blood, or fresh-frozen plasma. Diuretics, such as furosemide (Lasix), cause a reduction in the ventricular filling pressures without changing cardiac output or heart rate and promote sodium and water excretion by the kidney in cases where pulmonary congestion is a problem.

Other therapies. Peritoneal dialysis may be necessary if hyperkalemia, acidosis, hypervolemia, or altered mental status occurs. Nutritional support is provided by both enteral and parenteral routes. Prevention of infection is a primary concern because host resistance is depressed in patients in shock. Other complicating disorders, for example, disseminated intravascular coagulation and gastrointestinal problems (e.g., paralytic ileus, stress ulceration), are managed appropriately.

Corticosteroids are controversial in the treatment of shock. When used, they are given in massive doses on a short-term basis. They may be administered for anaphylactic shock, but time is required for their effects to develop. The intraaortic balloon pump (IABP) may be employed for the child with low cardiac output who is refractory to conventional medical management (Webster and Veasy, 1985). Extracorporeal membrane oxygenation (ECMO) is used occasionally as a last resort where this therapy is available.

Nursing Considerations

The child in shock requires intensive observation and care. When shock is a likely complication, the child should be observed carefully for any early signs such as irritability, unexplained increase in heart rate, thirst, pallor, or diminished urinary output. Appearance of any of these signs requires further evaluation and initiation of therapy.

The initial action in care of the child in shock is assuring adequate tissue oxygenation. The nurse should be prepared to administer oxygen by the appropriate route and to assist with any intubation and ventilatory procedures indicated. Other procedures and activities that require immediate attention are establishing an intravenous line, weighing the child, obtaining baseline vital signs, placing an indwelling catheter, obtaining blood gas and other measurements, and administering medications as indicated.

The child is best positioned flat with legs elevated. Hypotensive patients show no benefit from the traditional Trendelenburg position. Head-down positioning tends to increase intracranial pressure, decrease diaphragmatic excursion and lung volume, and decrease venous return to the heart because of the altered thoracic pressure. Elevating the lower extremities decreases pooling in the extremities, thereby returning blood supply to the heart.

The nurse's responsibilities are to monitor the intravenous infusion, intake and output, vital signs (including CVP), and general systems assessments on a routine basis. Intravenous medications are titrated according to patient responses, and vital signs are taken every 15 minutes during the critical periods and thereafter as needed. Urine output is measured hourly, and blood gases, hematocrit, pH, and electrolytes are monitored frequently to assess the status of the child and the efficacy of therapy. Apnea and cardiac monitors are attached and monitored continuously. In the initial stages of acute shock the care of the child often requires the attendance of more than one nurse in order to manage all the necessary activities that must be carried out simultaneously.

Throughout the intense activity the parents must not be overlooked. Someone should contact them at frequent intervals to inform them about what is being done and if there is any progress. Ideally, someone should remain with the parents to serve as liaison between them and the intensive care team. However, this is not always feasible in such a critical situation. As soon as possible they should be allowed to see the child. A member of the clergy may be called to help provide comfort and support.

Because assessment and management of shock are so complex and require intensive nursing care, a detailed, comprehensive discussion is beyond the scope of this book. Therefore the reader is directed to the many resources on the topic that provide a more detailed discussion.

SEPTIC SHOCK

Septic shock occurs frequently and is associated with high mortality rates in children and differs in pathology from other forms of shock (Perkin and Anas, 1986). The mechanisms producing septic (bacteremic) shock are not clear but appear to be the result of many interrelated factors. Multiple vasoactive substances, released in response to endotoxin exposure, produce a marked reduction in systemic vascular resistance (Zimmerman and Dietrich, 1987). Uneven blood flow and inadequate tissue oxygenation result in progressive decompensation of the capillary circulation and tissue cells.

Three stages have been identified in septic shock (Lamb, 1982; Perkin and Levin, 1982a) (Box 29-9). In early septic shock there are chills, fever, and vasodilation with increased cardiac output that results in the warm, flushed skin reflecting vascular tone abnormalities and *hyperdynamic,* or hyperdynamic-compensated, responses. The patient has the best chance for survival from this stage. The *normodynamic,* cool, or hyperdynamic-uncompensated stage lasts for only a few hours. With advancing disease, signs progress through decompensatory manifestations, which deteriorate to signs of circulatory collapse indistinguishable from late shock of any cause. In *hypodynamic* shock cardiovascular function progressively deteriorates even with aggressive therapy. This is the most dangerous stage of shock. A later and ominous development is disseminated intravascular coagulation (the major hematologic complication of septic shock), which is evidenced by petechiae or purpura fulminans, a severe form of subcutaneous hemorrhage (Lamb, 1982; Perkin and Levin, 1982a) (see Chapter 35).

Nursing Considerations

Nursing observations and care follow medical management as in all types of shock. Because many deaths from septic shock occur as a result of the pathophysiologic responses to the endotoxin and cardiac function is compromised early, the immediate concern is recognizing and treating the shock (Zimmerman and Dietrich, 1987). Broad-spectrum antibiotics are administered and the underlying source is identified as soon as possible to guide specific therapy.

As in any case of shock pulmonary support is a major concern, but is especially important since the most common cause of death in septic shock is ARDS. In addition to multiple factors that increase vascular permeability in ARDS, endotoxin action causes direct damage to lung endothelium, resulting in noncompliant and atelectatic lungs. To optimize and maintain oxygen delivery, early institution of mechanical ventilation is often recommended (Zimmerman and Dietrich, 1987).

✚ **NURSING ALERT** To aid in early identification and management, nurses caring for children at risk for septic shock should be alert to early evidence of dysfunction—fever, tachycardia, and tachypnea.

ANAPHYLAXIS

Anaphylaxis is the acute clinical syndrome resulting from the interaction of an allergen and a patient who is hypersensitive (Zimmerman, 1985). Severe reactions are immediate in onset, are often life threatening, and frequently involve multiple systems, primarily the cardiovascular, respiratory, gastrointestinal, and integumentary. Exposure to the antigen can be by ingestion, inhalation, or injection. The most common allergens are listed in Box 29-10.

Prevention of a reaction is the primary goal of anaphylaxis. Preventing exposure is more easily accomplished in children known to be at risk, including those with (1) a history of previous allergic reaction to specific antigen, (2) a

Box 29-9 STAGES OF SEPTIC SHOCK

Hyperdynamic Stage (Warm Shock, Pink Shock)	Normodynamic Stage (Cool Shock)	Hypodynamic Stage (Cold Shock)
Tachycardia	Tachycardia	Tachycardia
Tachypnea	Hyperventilation	Respiratory distress
Chills and fever	Normal temperature	Profound hypothermia
Skin flushed, warm	Skin cool	Skin cold, clammy
Warm extremities	Cool extremities	Cold, pale extremities
Bounding pulses	Normal pulses	Weak, thready pulses
Normal or elevated systemic blood pressure	Normal or slightly elevated systemic blood pressure	Severe hypotension
Wide pulse pressure	Normal to slightly narrow pulse pressure	Narrow pulse pressure
Normal urine output or polyuria	Oliguria	Severe oliguria or anuria
Mental confusion	Depressed sensorium	Lethargy or coma

Box 29-10 COMMON ALLERGENS ASSOCIATED WITH ANAPHYLAXIS

Drugs
Antibiotics (penicillin, cephalosporins, tetracycline, aminoglycosides, streptomycin, amphotericin B)
Analgesics (aspirin, indomethacin, codeine, phenylbutazone)
Local anesthetics (lidocaine, procaine, bupivacaine, tetracaine)
Chemotherapeutic agents (adriamycin, bleomycin, cisplatin, cyclophosphamide, L-asparaginase, melphalan)
Diagnostic contrast media (sulfobromophthalein sodium [BSP] dye, dehydrocholic acid [Decholin], iodinated contrast media, iopanoic acid [Telepaque])

Foods
Eggs
Seafood (fish, shellfish)
Milk and milk products
Chocolate
Nuts and seeds
Berries
Legumes (soybeans, beans, lentils, peanuts)
Wheat
Citrus fruits

Venoms
Hymenoptera (bee, yellow jacket, hornet, wasp, fire ant)
Snake
Jellyfish
Spider

Biologic agents
Allergen extracts
Antisera (snake, tetanus, diphtheria)
Enzymes
Hormones
Immune globulin (gammaglobulin, cryoprecipitate, blood, plasma)

history of atopy, (3) a history of severe reactions in immediate family members, and (4) a reaction to a skin test, although skin tests are not available for all allergens.

Pathophysiology

An anaphylactic reaction occurs as a result of interaction between an allergen and preexisting specific immunoglobulin E (IgE). When the antigen enters the circulatory system, a generalized reaction rapidly takes place. Vasoactive amines (principally histamine or histamine-like substance) are released and cause vasodilation, bronchoconstriction, and increased capillary permeability. Consequently there is increased venous capacity and pooling, reduced arterial pressure, and rapid loss of fluid into interstitial spaces, causing a marked decrease in venous return to the heart.

Clinical Manifestations

The onset of clinical symptoms usually occurs within seconds or minutes of exposure to the antigen, and the rapidity of the reaction is directly related to its intensity—the sooner the onset, the more severe the reaction. Typically the reaction is preceded by one or more prodromal signs and symptoms, including vague complaints of uneasiness or impending doom, restlessness, irritability, severe anxiety, headache, dizziness, paresthesia, and disorientation. The patient may lose consciousness. Cutaneous signs are the most common initial sign, and the child may complain of feeling warm. Angioedema is most noticeable in the eyelids, lips, tongue, hands, feet, and genitalia. Any or all of several reactions may affect one or more organ systems, as outlined in Box 29-11.

Box 29-11 POSSIBLE MANIFESTATIONS OF ANAPHYLACTIC REACTION

Cardiovascular
Tachycardia
Dysrhythmia
Hypotension
Relative hypovolemia

Respiratory
Rhinitis—sneezing, nasal itching, rhinorrhea
Laryngeal edema—stridor
Bronchospasm—cough, wheezing

Gastrointestinal
Nausea and vomiting
Abdominal pain
Diarrhea

Skin
Diffuse flushing
Urticaria
Angioedema—periorbital, perioral

Central Nervous System
Seizures
Loss of consciousness

Cutaneous manifestations are often followed by bronchiolar constriction. Bronchiolar constriction causes a narrowing of the airway, dilated pulmonary circulation produces pulmonary edema and hemorrhages, and there is often life-threatening laryngeal edema. Shock occurs as a result of mediator-induced vasodilation and sudden inadequacy of the circulation. The hypovolemia is further enhanced by increased capillary permeability and loss of intravascular fluid into the interstitial space. Laryngeal edema with its acute upper airway obstruction and related hypovolemic shock carry a more ominous prognosis.

Therapeutic Management

Successful outcome of anaphylactic reactions depends on rapid recognition and institution of treatment. The goals of treatment are to provide ventilation, restore adequate circulation, and prevent further exposure by identifying and removing the cause when possible.

A mild reaction with no evidence of respiratory distress or cardiovascular compromise can be managed with antihistamines, such as diphenhydramine (Benadryl) and epinephrine. Moderate or severe distress presents a potentially life-threatening emergency and requires immediate intervention. Severely unresponsive patients are transferred to hospital intensive care units when possible.

As in any shock state, the airway is the first concern. The most important drug is aqueous epinephrine 1:1000 (0.1 to 0.5 ml [0.01 mg/kg]) administered subcutaneously for mild reactions and intramuscularly for moderate reactions. The dose may be repeated three times at 15- to 20-minute intervals. When cardiovascular collapse is present or imminent, the drug may be diluted in 10 ml saline solution and administered slowly over several minutes by the intravenous route (Bailit, 1986). If the site of the antigen injection is known (e.g., drug, sting), the site is isolated by application of a tourniquet proximal to the site and then epinephrine injected directly to the area (Morriss, 1984).

Other drugs that may be used but are not universally applied are aminophylline and diphenhydramine (Benadryl). Vasopressors may be required for severe shock from any cause. Corticosteroids are controversial, but some authorities advocate their use for control of persistent or recurrent symptoms. The time required for them to achieve their effect diminishes their value for emergency therapy.

The child is positioned and monitored the same as any shock patient. If this is the initial anaphylactic reaction, it is especially important to identify the allergen and implement measures to prevent any future reaction. A Medic-Alert bracelet, tag, or other identification should be carried by the patient at all times. Desensitization may be recommended in certain cases.

Nursing Considerations

The major nursing responsibility in anaphylaxis is anticipating which children are likely to develop a reaction, recognizing the early signs, and intervening appropriately. When an anaphylactic reaction is suspected, both immediate intervention and preparation for medical therapy are nursing responsibilities. Help will be needed and the practitioner notified, but the nurse must not leave the patient. Ventilation is assured by placing the child in a head-elevated position, unless contraindicated by hypotension, to facilitate breathing and administer oxygen. If the child is not breathing, cardiopulmonary resuscitation is initiated.

If the cause can be determined, measures are implemented to slow the spread of the offending substance. For example, a tourniquet is applied above the point of entry (e.g., sting, injection) or intravenous medication or dye infusion is discontinued. If an intravenous infusion line is not in place, one is established immediately and the flow rate monitored carefully. Vital signs are monitored every 15 minutes, and urine output is measured at regular intervals. Medications are administered as prescribed with regular assessment to monitor effectiveness and to detect signs of side effects of medication and fluid overload.

To prevent an anaphylactic reaction, parents are always asked about possible allergic responses to foods, medications, and environmental conditions. (See Guidelines for Taking a Drug Allergy History, Box 6-13.) These are displayed prominently on the patient's chart. The specific allergen is noted, as well as the type and severity of the reaction. Parents are excellent historians, especially when the child has displayed a pronounced reaction to a substance. Drugs, including related drugs (e.g., penicillin, nafcillin), that have produced a reaction previously are *never* given.

The child and the parents need as much reassurance as can be provided without giving false hope. They are kept informed of the child's progress, the reasons for the therapies, and what they can reasonably expect. It is a frightening experience and one which the family will remember and will make every effort to prevent recurring. The idea of medical information in a convenient and visible form, such as the Medic-Alert items, is reinforced. For the child who is allergic to insect venom, the family is instructed to purchase an emergency kit to be kept with the child at all times (e.g., Ana-Kit,* EpiPen Auto-Injector, or EpiPen Jr. Auto-Injector†). Both the family and the child, if the child is old enough and is likely to be away from the family (e.g., at school), are taught how to use the equipment (see also Chapter 27).

TOXIC SHOCK SYNDROME

Toxic shock syndrome (TSS) is a relatively rare disease that occurs predominantly (but not exclusively) in previously healthy young women during their menstrual periods. Studies have shown a striking relationship between the disease and the use of tampons (Centers for Disease Control, 1980), although other foci have been identified, including contraceptive sponges, nasal packing, and wounds. Some cases reported in children were unrelated to any identifiable foci (Surh and Read, 1984; Wiesenthal and Todd, 1984).

Pathophysiology

Evidence from several sources suggests that TSS occurs secondary to infection with phage group-1 *Staphylococcus aureus*. The organism is believed to produce an epidermal toxin, but the precise mode of transmission is not known. The disease has been observed primarily in women who use tampons during a menstrual period. The tampons may carry the organism from the fingers or the vulva into the vagina during insertion, the tampon might traumatize the vaginal wall and provide a focus of infection, or the tampon itself may provide a favorable environment for growth of the organism or elaboration of its toxin. The superabsorbent tampons appear to be more likely to contribute to development of the disease. Persistent use throughout the menstrual cycle also alters the vaginal mucosa by absorbing protective secretions and subjects it to greater mechanical trauma and microulcerations.

Clinical Manifestations

The sudden development of high fever, vomiting and diarrhea, profound hypotension, shock, oliguria, and an erythe-

---

*Hollister-Stier Laboratories, 400 Morgan Lane, West Haven, CT 06516; (203) 773-2123.

†Center Labs, 35 Channel Dr., Port Washington, NY 11050; (516) 767-1800.

matous macular rash with subsequent desquamation are characteristic manifestations of TSS. Other manifestations might include headache, blurred vision, purulent conjunctivitis, abdominal guarding, and purulent vaginal discharge. Inasmuch as various signs and symptoms are associated with the disease and affected individuals seldom exhibit all of them, the Centers for Disease Control has published a case definition of TSS (Box 29-12).

Complications include respiratory distress, cardiac dysfunction, hematologic changes (particularly disseminated intravascular coagulation), and abnormal liver function. Impaired perfusion to extremities may become severe, with eventual necrosis and loss of extremities.

Diagnostic Evaluation

Diagnosis is established on the basis of the criteria of the Centers for Disease Control's toxic case definition. A history of tampon use contributes to the diagnosis. Additional laboratory tests include cultures from blood, vagina, cervix, and discharge from any suspected source of infection. Other laboratory tests are those that facilitate the management of shock.

Therapeutic Management

The management of TSS is the same as management of shock of any cause. Because the disease is highly varied in intensity, therapy is directed toward supportive care in mild cases to hospitalization and intensive care in severe cases. Appropriate parenteral antibiotics are usually administered after cultures are obtained. Preventing complications of impaired circulation demands constant observation and immediate therapeutic intervention for hypotension, pulmonary dysfunction, acidosis, hematologic changes, and renal impairment.

Box 29-12 CASE DEFINITION OF TOXIC SHOCK SYNDROME

1. Fever (temperature at or above 38.9° C, or 102° F)
2. Rash (diffuse macular erythroderma)
3. Desquamation 1 to 2 weeks after onset of illness, particularly of the palms and soles
4. Hypotension (systolic blood pressure at or below 90 mm Hg for adults or below the fifth percentile for age for children younger than 16 years of age, or orthostatic syncope)
5. Involvement of three or more of the following organ systems:
   a. Gastrointestinal (vomiting or diarrhea at onset of illness)
   b. Muscular (severe myalgia or creatine phosphokinase level above two times the upper limits of normal)
   c. Mucous membrane (vaginal, oropharyngeal, or conjunctival hyperemia)
   d. Renal (blood urea nitrogen or creatinine levels above two times the upper limits of normal or above five white blood cells per high-power field—in the absence of a urinary tract infection)
   e. Hepatic (total bilirubin, SGOT [serum glutamic oxaloacetic transaminase], or SGPT [serum glutamic pyruvic transaminase] above two times the upper limits of normal)
   f. Hematologic (platelets below 100,000/mm^3)
   g. Central nervous system (disorientation or alterations in consciousness without focal neurologic signs when fever and hypotension are absent)
6. Negative results on the following tests, if obtained:
   a. Blood, throat, or cerebrospinal fluid cultures
   b. Serologic tests for Rocky Mountain spotted fever, leptospirosis, or measles

From Centers for Disease Control: MMWR 29:442, 1980.

Nursing Considerations

Nursing care and observation of the acutely ill patient are the same as those described for shock of any cause. Because the disease is relatively rare, the major efforts of nursing are directed toward prevention. The association between the disease and the use of tampons provides some direction for education. Avoiding the use of tampons offers the most certain preventive measure, although this approach is probably unacceptable to most adolescent girls. Most young women prefer the freedom, comfort, and inconspicuousness that tampons afford, and are unlikely to comply with this advice.

Adolescent girls who use tampons can be taught general hygiene measures, such as handwashing before insertion of the tampon and not to use a tampon that has been dropped or otherwise soiled. Tampons should be inserted carefully to avoid vaginal abrasion. Also, it is wise to modify their use. For example, tampons may be used intermittently during the menstrual cycle, alternating with sanitary napkins—perhaps using the napkins during the night, when at home during the day, and when flow is slight. Young girls are advised not to use superabsorbent tampons and not to leave any tampon in the body for more than 12 hours (3 to 6 hours is preferable). A strong association has been found between absorbency and risk of illness.

Patients who use tampons need to understand that they should remove the tampon and consult their health professional if they develop a sudden high fever, vomiting, diarrhea, muscle pain, dizziness, fainting or near fainting when standing up, or rash that resembles a sunburn. Excellent posters and handout materials for use as teaching aids are available from the **Food and Drug Administration.***

■ BURNS

Minor thermal injuries are experienced by everyone in day-to-day living and are relatively commonplace in nursing practice. Extensive burns, on the other hand, are relatively uncommon; however, they account for some of the most difficult nursing problems encountered in the pediatric age-group. Serious burn injury accounts for a very large number of children who must undergo prolonged, painful, and restrictive hospitalization, many of whom emerge from the experience with scars to both body and personality that profoundly affect their social and emotional development. It is

*FDA, HFE-88 (or HFW-40 for multiple copies), Rockville, MD 20857; (301) 443-3170.

tragic, too, that the great majority (75%) of burn injuries are preventable.

OVERVIEW

Although severe burns are manifest primarily in damage to the skin, they produce a complex illness that requires the utmost in nursing skill and care. Every organ system becomes involved, and sometimes the treatment even creates additional problems. Nursing care of patients with extensive burns involves an understanding of a variety of specialized areas, including surgical principles and techniques, respiratory physiology, fluid and electrolyte physiology, nutrition, bacteriology, growth and development, occupational therapy, physical therapy, and principles of psychiatric nursing.

Epidemiology

More than 2 million persons each year in the United States sustain significant burns. At least half of these injuries occur in the pediatric age-group (Dyer, 1980) and account for approximately 3000 deaths from burn injury in persons younger than 15 years of age (Harmel, Vane, and King, 1986). The second most important cause of death from *trauma* in childhood, burns are outranked only by motor vehicle casualties. Figures contributed from major burn centers that specialize in the care of children reveal that children under 4 years of age are at greatest risk of hospitalization for burn injury and that burns occur most frequently at home and between the hours of 6 PM and midnight (Robinson and Seward, 1987). Males outnumber females 2 to 1 (Coren, 1987). Table 29-3 describes the types of burn that are most often associated with children at different developmental levels.

House fires cause three fourths of all fire deaths, especially of young children and elderly persons. Cigarettes used by adults are the leading cause of ignition of fatal house fires—from 30% to 45% of deaths. Approximately 2% of residential fire deaths are attributed to children playing with matches or other ignition sources (Baker, O'Neill, and Karpf, 1984).

Age. Children younger than age 5 years sustain 70% of burn injuries, and the incidence is often related to the quality and quantity of adult supervision. Very young children have an innate curiosity to learn about their environment, limited perception of danger, less control of elements in their environment, and limited ability to react promptly and properly to a fire or burn situation (McLoughlin and Crawford, 1985). Burns in children in this age-group occur more often in large than in small families.

Whereas young children receive more scalds, older children are likely to be burned severely by flaming clothing from open flames, heaters, and explosions—very often in an unsupervised play situation in which combustible materials, such as gasoline and matches or cigarette lighters, are present. Fascination with fire seems to be a normal trait, and natural curiosity will lead young children who have access to matches or cigarette lighters to experiment with them (McLoughlin and Crawford, 1985). Match play generally occurs in the bedroom, where the child goes to be alone. Somewhat older children (especially boys) playing with matches or gasoline tend to be with friends, out of sight of adults (Libber and Slayton, 1984).

Table 29-3 Burn hazards of children

AGE-GROUP	TYPE OF BURN	HAZARD	TIME/PLACE
Toddler (6-24 months)	Scalds	Playing underfoot in kitchen, overturning cups, pulling electric cords off coffeepots or frying pans; bath water too hot; parental neglect/abuse	Daytime/home
	Electric burns	Chewing extension cords	
	Contact burns	Curling irons, heaters, oven doors	
Young children (2-6 years)	Flame burns	Playing with matches, climbing on stove, warming with heating source	Early morning/kitchen, bedroom, etc.
	Scalds	Overturning containers of hot liquids; bath water	
6- to 14-year-old children	Scalds	Water too hot	
Boys	Flame burns	Playing/working with gasoline, campfires, barbecues, chemistry sets, firecrackers, rockets, matches, etc.	After school, holidays/outdoors, indoors
	Electric burns	Climbing around high-tension wires	
Girls	Flame burns	Reaching over stove, candles, making candles, "innocent bystander" (observing others play with fire or gasoline)	Morning, evening/kitchen; after school/yard
All children	Flame burns	House fires; gas tank explosion during automobile accident	Usually night, anytime

Modified from Northern California Burn Council, San Francisco, and Elizabeth McLoughlin, Director of Burn Injury Project, Shriners Burns Institute, Boston, Mass.

Electric burns of the mouth from chewing on an electric cord are more typical of children in the crawling or toddler stage of development. Younger children are more likely to be burned by poking metal objects into electric outlets, whereas burns from tension wires occur in older children. Many children die or are seriously injured in burning buildings, especially when left unattended. A significant number of burns occur in garages and basements in which there is an open gas heating unit or pilot light.

Seasonal incidence. Burns also have a seasonal incidence. Inasmuch as furnaces and other heating devices are used most extensively during cold weather, burns from heaters, wood stoves, and house fires are more frequent in the winter months. Flash burns from explosive ignition of outdoor barbecues with volatile liquids increase in summer months. Burns caused by clothing catching fire from campfires occur in summer, and from burning leaves in autumn. Some types of burns occur on specific dates, for example, sunburns on Memorial Day weekend and blast and burn injuries from Independence Day firecrackers (McLoughlin and Crawford, 1985). In all seasons young girls sustain burn injuries to the chest and arms when loose, frilly clothes (especially nightwear) are ignited by an open fire, gas ranges or heaters, and candelabra. Fortunately these burns have decreased significantly since regulation of inflammable clothing has been established.

Psychologic factors. Psychologic factors are often related to burn injury in children. For example, burns inflicted as punishment are a common form of child abuse, and it is the unwanted or least desirable child who is the last to be rescued from a burning building. Burns are a significant mechanism of child abuse—as common as CNS injury, and two to three times as frequent as skeletal injury, soft tissue injury, abdominal injury, or sexual abuse (Caniano, Beaver, and Boles, 1986; Guzzetta and Holihan, 1988). Therefore, when abuse is suspected, it is important to look for associated injuries.

The frequency of burn injury, as well as other accidental injuries, is increased in families in which there is emotional disturbance, such as marital discord, a disturbed parent, or a disturbed or retarded child. Setting fires by small boys and burns of either boys or girls can often be interpreted as a signal of distress related to loss of a parent to whom the child had a strong attachment. In many children difficult behavior for varying periods of time precedes the burn injury. Not only do these psychologic and behavioral problems contribute to the injury, but they also influence the child's hospitalization and convalescence.

Etiology

Burns can be caused by thermal, chemical, electric, or radioactive agents. Most burn injuries are caused by thermal agents, principally flame, direct contact (stove, heater), and hot water (scalding water, steam), and to a lesser extent by friction and frostbite. Chemical burns can be caused by either acids or alkalis, and radiation burns by either x-rays or ultraviolet radiation. The extent of tissue destruction is determined by the intensity of the heat source, the duration of contact or exposure, and the speed with which the heat energy is dissipated by the burned surface. For example, a brief exposure to high-intensity heat, such as a flame, or a longer exposure to low-intensity heat, such as hot water, can produce similar burn injuries. Burns caused by boiling oil or liquid fat tend to cause deep partial-thickness burns. Prolonged exposure to the sun's rays or to a heated object, such as a sidewalk, is also capable of producing significant burns.

Full-thickness destruction frequently occurs when clothing is ignited. Cotton and nylon clothing burns most easily, whereas clothing made from wool or other animal fibers burns less readily. Synthetic fabrics melt and stick to the skin surface. Contact burns from heated metal or liquids (e.g., tar) at extreme temperatures, prolonged immersion in hot water, chemical burns without rinsing with water, and electric burns are all significant in the cause of severe burn trauma. Chemical agents continue to cauterize the tissues until the injurious agent is chemically united with tissue elements, neutralized, or removed by washing with running water.

Electric burns are especially deceptive, because they are characterized by more extensive thrombosis that is not evident until 24 to 36 hours after injury. Electricity is converted to thermal energy as it encounters resistance. Inasmuch as body tissues vary in the degree of resistance they offer, the type of tissue through which an electric current passes plays a role in the extent of the burn injury. Bone offers the greatest amount of resistance. Other tissues in descending order of resistance are fat, tendon, skin, muscle, blood, and nerves. Although blood offers less resistance than most tissues, it is an extremely good conductor of electric current. All other things being equal, the greater the skin resistance, the more severe is the local burn; the less the skin resistance, the greater are the systemic effects. The extensive destruction of an electric burn has been described as resembling a crush injury.

BURN WOUND CHARACTERISTICS

The physiologic responses, therapy, prognosis, and disposition of the injured child are all directly related to the *amount of tissue destroyed;* therefore the severity of the burn injury is assessed on the basis of percentage of body surface burned, depth of the burn, and location of the burn(s).

Also important in determining the seriousness of the injury are age of the child, etiologic agent, extent of respiratory tract involvement, general health of the child, and presence of any associated injury or condition. Suspected or confirmed child abuse is significant because of the associated impact on long-term progress and additional risk.

Extent of Injury

The extent of a burn is usually expressed as a percentage of total body surface area, which is most accurately estimated by using specially designed age-related charts (Fig. 29-3). Because of the body proportions, especially the head and lower extremities, the standard "rule of nines" charts used for adults are not applicable to small children.

A

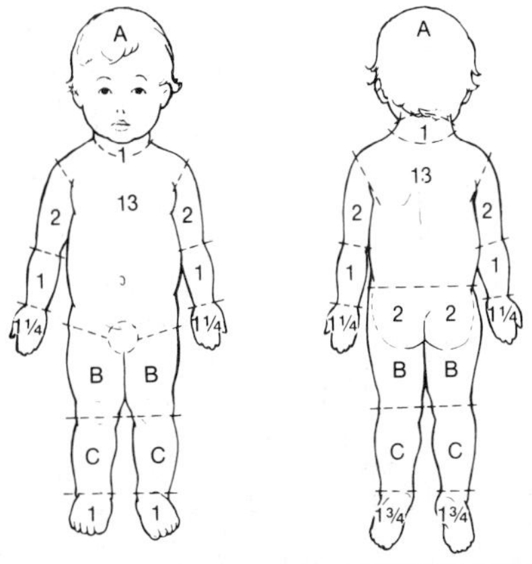

RELATIVE PERCENTAGES OF AREAS AFFECTED BY GROWTH

AREA	BIRTH	AGE 1 YR	AGE 5 YR
A = 1/2 of head	9 1/2	8 1/2	6 1/2
B = 1/2 of one thigh	2 3/4	3 1/4	4
C = 1/2 of one leg	2 1/2	2 1/2	2 3/4

B

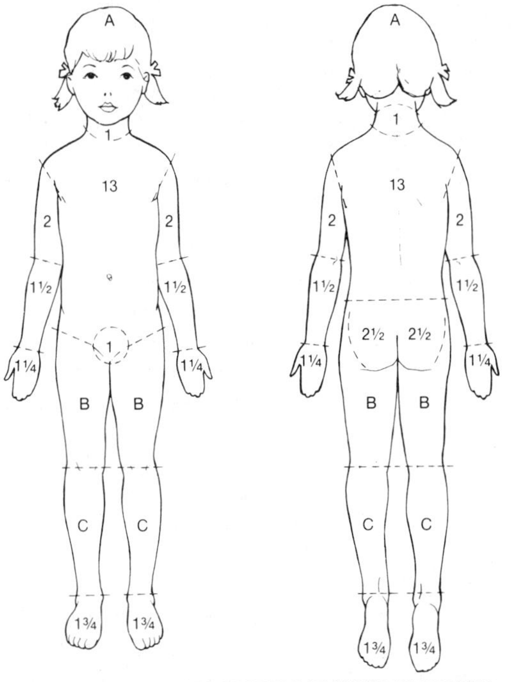

RELATIVE PERCENTAGES OF AREAS AFFECTED BY GROWTH

AREA	AGE 10 YR	AGE 15 YR	ADULT
A = 1/2 of head	5 1/2	4 1/2	3 1/2
B = 1/2 of one thigh	4 1/2	4 1/2	4 3/4
C = 1/2 of one leg	3	3 1/4	3 1/2

Fig. 29-3. Estimation of distribution of burns in children. **A,** Children from birth to age 5 years. **B,** Older children.

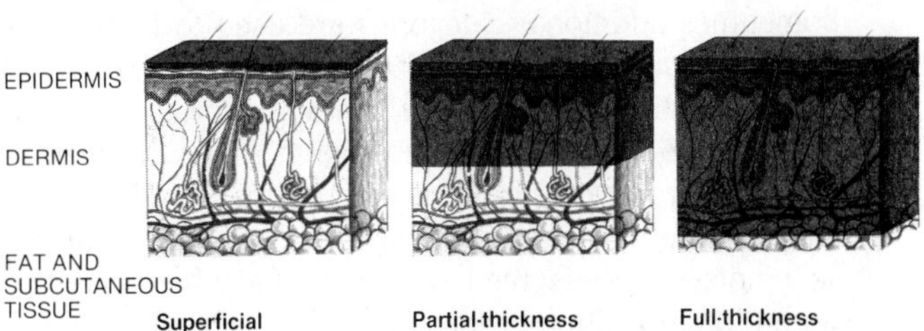

	Superficial (first degree)	Partial-thickness (second degree)	Full-thickness (third degree)
Type of burn	Sunburn; low-intensity flash; brief scald	Scalds; flash flame	Fire; contact with hot objects
Appearance	Dry surface; red; blanches on pressure and refills	Blistered; moist; mottled pink or red, reddened; blanches on pressure and refills	Tough, leathery; brown, tan, black, or red; does not blanch on pressure; dull, dry
Sensation	Painful	Very painful	Little pain

Fig. 29-4. Classification of burn depth. (See also Color Plates 21 to 24.)

Depth of Injury

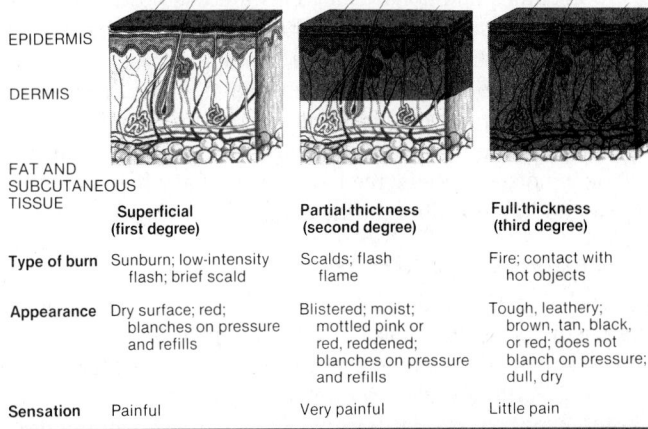

A thermal injury is a three-dimensional wound and therefore is also assessed in relation to depth of injury. Traditionally the terms *first-*, *second-*, and *third-degree* have been used to describe the depth of tissue injury. However, with the current emphasis on burn healing, these are gradually being replaced by more descriptive terms based on the extent of destruction to the epithelializing elements of the skin. Partial-thickness burns heal in time; full-thickness burns require skin grafting for closure. Partial-thickness injury is further categorized by many as superficial or deep dermal burns, depending on how rapidly they heal. Because both terminologies are used, often interchangeably, both are presented in describing the characteristics of burn wounds (Fig. 29-4).

Superficial (first-degree) burns are usually of minor significance. There is frequently a latent period followed by erythema. Tissue damage is minimal, protective functions remain intact, and systemic effects are rare. Pain is the predominant symptom.

Partial-thickness (second-degree) burns are deeper and involve not only the epithelium but also a minimal to substantial portion of the corium. The severity of the injury and the rate of healing are directly related to the amount of undamaged corium from which new tissue can regenerate. Superficial burns are often classified with first-degree burns and heal uneventfully. Deep dermal burns, although classified as second-degree or partial-thickness burns, in many respects resemble third-degree burns. There is hyperemia in areas with less heat, and leakage of protein in areas with the most heat. Systemic effects are similar to those that occur with deeper burns. Whereas first-degree and superficial partial-thickness burns are painful, deep dermal burns are often anesthetic for the first 1 or 2 days after injury.

Full-thickness (third-degree) burns are serious injuries in which all layers of the skin are destroyed, may involve underlying tissues as well, and are usually combined with extensive partial-thickness damage. Presence of visible thrombosed veins in the burn wound is pathognomonic of a full-thickness burn. Systemic effects can be life threatening and involve every organ system in the body. Although a notable characteristic of third-degree burns is lack of sensation at the wound surface, this is misleading. Superficial nerve endings are destroyed in the full-thickness areas, but nerve endings are hypersensitive on wound edges (described by Kibbee, 1984). In addition, deep somatic pain is present in the full-thickness area as a result of inflammation and ischemia (LaMotte and Thalhammer, 1982).

Sometimes additional categories are used to further describe full-thickness burns. Fourth-degree burns involve fat and are difficult to prepare for grafting. Burns involving muscle may be designated as fifth-degree burns. Because of the myoglobin released from muscle destruction, burns involving muscle may lead to kidney damage. Burns that destroy bone are sixth-degree burns, are usually hard and dry, and lead to amputation of the affected part (Jacoby, 1984).

Severity of Injury

Burns are also appraised on the basis of their severity. This is useful in determining the disposition of the patient for treatment. Burned patients can usually be distinguished as (1) those with a critical burn who require the services and equipment of a special burn facility, (2) those with moderate burns who may be treated in any hospital unit, and (3) those with minor burns who are able to be treated on an outpatient basis. Although each burn unit and specialist in the field of burn management has criteria for admission to special units, there are a number of factors that influence the effects of the injury, the probability of recovery, and response to therapy.

Initial assessment to estimate the extent of skin destruction is made on the basis of observation and simple diagnostic techniques. The extent of surface involvement is readily calculated, and the surface appearance of the wound provides clues to whether the injury involves the full thickness of the skin or only a portion of the skin layers. The extent to which the wound is capable of regeneration depends on the areas destroyed. Epithelial regeneration can take place from residual basilar cells and from the epithelial lining of sweat glands and hair follicles.

Blisters do not occur in full-thickness burns, but with superficial burns in general, the deeper the burn, the more common is blister formation. Blisters increase in size in the hours immediately after the burn occurs, and usually the larger the blister, the deeper the burn. Touching injured surfaces gives more additional information. Testing for capillary filling by blanching and refilling indicates whether circulation in the area is intact. Because the sensory end organs are concentrated in the deep dermal areas, presence of sensation indicates tissue viability; absence of sensation suggests full skin thickness destruction. This is easily determined by pulling out a hair, which lifts out readily in a full-thickness injury.

The burn source can help to estimate and classify the extent of the injury. Hot liquids may result in partial-thickness injury, whereas full-thickness injury is associated with flame burns. This can vary with the age of the child, however. Because infants' skin is so thin, it is readily destroyed by thermal agents. This makes estimation of depth difficult in children in this age-group, especially in scalds. Electric burns appear to be less serious than they actually are, because they often involve deep structures. Electric current follows nerves and blood vessels and may cause thrombosis with subsequent severe tissue destruction. Severe burns of hands and/or feet can interfere with normal growth and development. Children with facial burns or burns acquired in an enclosed area or those in whom inhalation injury is suspected for other reasons are at risk for developing airway obstruction or severe hypoxia during the hours after inhalation.

Children younger than 2 years of age have a significantly higher mortality than older children with burns of similar magnitude. They are subject to rapid fluid shifts, which places them in jeopardy in the early hours, and their immune competence is not well developed; therefore, sepsis is a frequent complication. The classification of burns according to severity is outlined in Box 29-13.

Box 29-13 BURN SEVERITY CRITERIA

Minor Burns

Partial-thickness burns of less than 10% of body surface area (BSA)
Full-thickness burns of less than 2% of BSA

Moderate Burns

Partial-thickness burns of 15% to 25% of BSA (age related; see Major or Critical Burns)
Full-thickness burns of less than 10% of BSA, except in small children and when the burns involve critical areas, such as the face, hands, feet, or genitalia

Major or Critical Burns

Burns complicated by respiratory tract injury
Partial-thickness burns of 25% of BSA or greater
Burns of face, hands, feet, or genitalia, even if they appear to be partial thickness
Full-thickness burns of 10% of BSA or greater
Any child younger than 2 years of age, unless the burn is very small and very superficial (20% of BSA or greater considered critical in child less than 2 years of age)
Electric burns that penetrate
Deep chemical burns
Respiratory tract damage
Burns complicated by fractures or soft tissue injury
Burns complicated by concurrent illness, such as obesity, diabetes, epilepsy, and cardiac and renal diseases

Local Responses

Local changes at the site of the burn injury begin to occur at approximately 45° C (113° F); tissues die at 65° C (149° F) and higher because of coagulation necrosis. The tissue coagulates, desiccates, or becomes carbonized, depending on the extent of exposure to the source of heat. At the same time, changes in the intercellular cement that binds the epidermis to the dermis cause the epidermis to detach and either peel away or form a blister between the two layers. In infants and young children the skin is so thin and contains such shallow dermal appendages that full-thickness loss occurs easily on exposure to heat. There are also fewer skin appendages in prepubescent children than in adolescents.

The burn wound consists basically of three distinct layers (Fig. 29-5), as described in Box 29-14. It is within the two outer zones that significant changes take place, and these zones are involved in the pathophysiology of the burn wound and the systemic responses to the initial burn injury.

Edema formation. Thermal injury to the vessels in the two outer zones causes increased capillary permeability. At

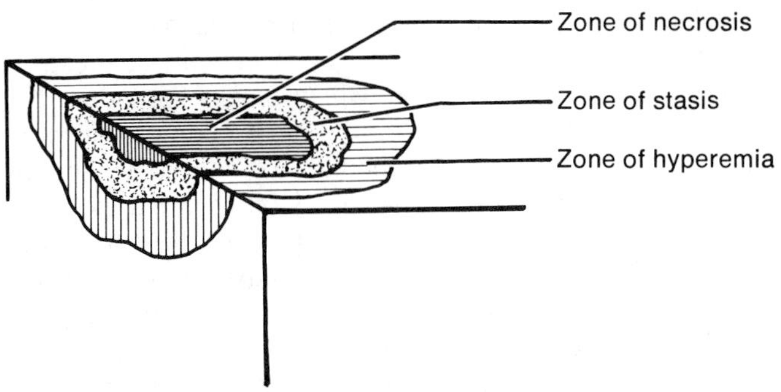

Fig. 29-5. Zones of injury in burn.
After Zawacki, B.: Ann. Surg. 180:98-102, 1974.

Box 29-14 ZONES OF BURN INJURY

Zone of coagulation (necrosis)—area beneath obviously destroyed tissue; capillary flow has ceased and tissue destruction is irreversible; tissue is dead.
Zone of stasis—area beneath and surrounding zone of coagulation; markedly reduced capillary flow; tissue severely damaged from heat but not coagulated. Tissue in this zone can be saved with prevention of further injury and adequate perfusion.
Zone of hyperemia—area metabolically active; displays usual response to tissue injury.

the same time vasodilation results in increased hydrostatic pressure within the capillaries. The increased hydrostatic pressure plus the increased capillary permeability cause loss of water, protein, and electrolytes from the intravascular compartment into the interstitial spaces. This shift is further enhanced by a diminishing intravascular oncotic pressure, as protein and sodium are lost to the interstitial spaces. Although the edema involves both burned and nonburned areas, at the site of injury the accumulation of edema fluid beneath and around the burn can reach tremendous proportions until the extravasation of fluid is limited by tissue tension.

In addition, there are also changes in the permeability of tissue cells in and around the burned area that allow an abnormal exchange of electrolytes between the cells and the interstitial fluid; that is, sodium enters the cells in exchange for potassium, causing further depletion of intravascular sodium.

Fluid loss. Without the protective skin, fluid loss at the air-wound interface can be extremely high. These losses reach a maximum about the fourth day after the burn occurs but continue to pose problems until the denuded surfaces are debrided and grafted.

Circulatory stasis. Significant circulatory alterations take place in the zone of stasis located around the coagulated dead tissue. Heated red blood cells become spherical in shape when heated. These heat-damaged cells, together with hemoconcentration from fluid loss, depressed cardiac output, and tissue edema, reduce the blood flow in the burn area, causing capillary stasis. Thrombi develop that further impede circulation, producing tissue ischemia and eventual necrosis, which may also prolong the edema phase. Further hyperviscosity and impaired blood flow are attributed to the release of substances from damaged cells, such as thromboplastin and clot-activating factors, that cause the production of microthrombi, platelet adhesiveness and aggregation, and increased pain and swelling.

Circulation in the area around partial-thickness burns ceases immediately after injury but is rapidly restored within 24 to 48 hours. In full-thickness burns, however, the vascular supply is completely occluded, and no appreciable circulation is reestablished until granulation takes place at the interface between burned and unburned tissue.

Burn wound. In first-degree destruction of the vascular epithelium, tissue damage is minimal. Protein loss is insignificant and edema barely perceptible. The burning sensation and pain resolve in 48 to 72 hours, and in 5 to 10 days the damaged epithelium peels off in small scales or sheets, leaving no scar.

Considerable edema and more severe capillary damage occurs in second-degree, partial-thickness burns. In 3 to 5 days a crust of dried exudate and injured tissue covers the wound to form a protective seal while healing takes place from underneath. With reasonable care superficial burns heal spontaneously and uneventfully through the generative capacity of the stratum germinativum and epithelial cells of the lining of skin appendages. The crust separates in 10 to 14 days with minimum or no scarring.

Deep dermal burns heal more slowly by regeneration from the epithelial lining of skin appendages, sweat glands, and hair follicles. A thin epithelial covering develops in 25 to 35 days, but this type of burn may require several months to heal. Scarring is common, and trauma or infection can easily convert a partial-thickness burn to a full-thickness injury, especially in young children with their normally thinner skin. Fluid loss and metabolic effects may be considerable.

Cell destruction by coagulation necrosis takes place in third-degree, full-thickness burns. Dead tissue and exudate convert to a thick, leathery eschar in 48 to 72 hours, which liquefies and begins to separate in 12 to 21 days as a result of autolysis, leukemic digestion, and disintegration of collagen fibers. New granulation tissue forms on the wound bed, which, if not grafted, heals by slow proliferation from the edges with high risk of infection and severe scarring. Full-thickness burns cause severe edema with fluid and electrolyte shifts and extensive metabolic changes.

Systemic Responses

Along with and subsequent to the pathophysiologic response at the site of thermal injury, a number of systemic responses occur.

Circulation. The immediate postburn period is marked by dramatic alterations in circulation, known as *burn shock*. There is a precipitous drop in cardiac output (about 50% of normal resting values) that precedes any changes in circulating blood or plasma volume. With the large fluid losses through denuded skin, vasodilation, and edema formation, the blood volume decreases rapidly and cardiac output is reduced even further, usually leveling off at 20% of normal resting values. Cardiac output returns to normal spontaneously in 24 to 36 hours, although the plasma volume lags far behind.

The initial decrease in cardiac output is attributed to a circulating myocardial depressant factor, associated with severe burn injury, that affects the contractility of heart muscle directly. The blood volume deficit, although slower in onset, can be profound and appears to be directly proportional to the extent and depth of the burn.

Capillary permeability with leakage of fluid takes place in noninjured areas including bowels, brain, and other organs, as well as in the outer zones of the burn wound. Edema fluid accumulates rapidly in the first 18 hours after injury to reach a maximum in about 48 hours. Capillary permeability returns to normal and fluid is reabsorbed, chiefly by way of the lymphatics. Reabsorption usually proceeds at the rate of fluid accumulation, although it may persist longer. Redistribution of fluid is often complex and unpredictable. After a time the lymphatics become incompetent, and inapparent lymph accumulation may take place in compartments within the trunk or extremities.

In most children the cardiovascular system is able to withstand the demands placed on it, although shock is a prominent feature of large thermal injuries and many children are prone to congestive heart failure and pulmonary edema. In addition, peripheral circulation in the infant is less efficient and more labile, which complicates burn response and therapy in children in this age-group.

Anemia. Initially red blood cell destruction is reflected by an increased hematocrit. A significant loss of circulating red cell mass is associated predominantly with deep burns. The anemia characteristic of thermal injury is attributed to several factors—red blood cells are damaged or destroyed by heat; circulating red blood cells are lost in the zone of stasis; hemolysis from circulating plasma and from *Pseudomonas* invasion occurs; there is direct bleeding from the wound; bone marrow is depressed as a result of sepsis; and (later) loss from bleeding during repeated debridement of the wound surface occurs.

Renal. Loss of fluid from the intravascular compartment causes renal vasoconstriction that in turn leads to reduced renal plasma flow and depressed glomerular filtration. When adequate fluids are provided, the glomerular filtration rate returns to normal, and by the third or fourth day of fluid therapy, urine output increases as edema fluid is mobilized and eliminated. In the first few days oliguria is more commonly the result of inadequate fluid replacement than of acute renal failure. If the patient does not respond to treatment or if there is inadequate fluid resuscitation, acute renal failure may develop with permanent kidney damage. Children with a history of a prior kidney disorder are at increased risk.

Blood urea nitrogen and creatinine levels are elevated from tissue breakdown and oliguria. Hematuria may also be evident from hemolysis of red blood cells, and oliguria may develop as a consequence of the increased pigment load the kidneys must handle, especially myoglobin from extensive electric burn destruction, which blocks the kidney tubules. Except for electrical burns, renal failure is uncommon in burns involving less than 20% of the body surface. Cell destruction following electrical burns releases large amounts of myoglobin, which places the victim at high risk for renal failure. Renal failure also occurs more frequently following flame burns sustained indoors than after scalds.

Metabolism. The metabolic rate in burned patients is greatly accelerated, and the nitrogen losses are far in excess of those seen in other types of injuries. The magnitude of energy requirements of a burned child frequently exceeds the requirements of a normal active child, and when the burned area is extensive, may approach twice the normal requirements.

The stress of injury places high demands on the body. Stress-invoked glycogen breakdown depletes the energy stores in 12 to 24 hours, after which the body resorts to glyconeogenesis for high energy needs. Blood glucose levels are elevated and, inasmuch as insulin resistance is evident, remain elevated for some time. Protein breakdown is rapid, as reflected in blood urea nitrogen and urine urea nitrogen levels. Each gram of urinary urea nitrogen represents a loss of 30 g of lean body mass.

Many of the metabolic consequences of extensive burn injuries are attributed to the amount of energy needed for the energy-consuming process of evaporation of water from the damaged skin surface. Infants or young children are especially vulnerable because of the large surface area relative to metabolically active tissue. Burning destroys a lipid layer and converts skin that is normally virtually impermeable to water to a freely water-permeable state that transmits water vapor at least four times as rapidly as normal skin. In partial-thickness burns this loss is greatest the day of injury; in full-thickness areas it rises slowly at first and then rapidly increases to reach a peak about the fourth day after the burn occurs. Evaporative losses are maintained until partial-thickness burns are healed and full-thickness injuries are grafted. Thus body stores of energy are rapidly depleted unless sufficient replacement is provided or losses are reduced.

Neuroendocrine system. As a response to stress of any origin, the hypothalamic-hypophyseal mechanism restores equilibrium by secreting tropic hormones, which stimulate various target organs of the neuroendocrine system. Adrenal activity is stimulated maximally. The medulla responds by secreting increased amounts of the catecholamines epinephrine and norepinephrine, which appear to have a sustained elevation. Adrenocortical hormones are elevated and reach a peak immediately after injury but remain high for some time. Aldosterone secretion is elevated and sustained at a high level throughout hospitalization, and there is release of antidiuretic hormone. Despite this increased adrenal activity, adrenal insufficiency is a rare complication.

Acidosis. Most burned patients exhibit some degree of metabolic acidosis. Reduced blood volume and cardiac output result in diminished tissue perfusion with resultant tissue hypoxia, which causes a shift to anaerobic metabolism with formation of metabolic acids. However, this is usually sufficiently compensated by increased ventilation as a result of pulmonary irritation or an independent respiratory alkalosis. Renal compensatory mechanisms are impaired by the decreased blood flow.

Growth changes. Changes in the growth pattern are frequently observed, particularly in older children who have burns covering large areas of their body. As in any severely burned individual, nail and hair growth essentially cease during the catabolic phase of burn response. It is believed that bone growth is also affected; weight loss is marked. During convalescence following full recovery, there is a catch-up spurt in bone growth and weight recovery. Prepubertal children who suffer thermal injury frequently experience a rapid acceleration of pubertal changes, with development of secondary sex characteristics, which may occur 2 to 3 years before usual. It is believed that these changes are probably caused by a prolonged and heavy production of growth hormone.

Complications

Thermally injured children are subject to a number of serious complications, both from the wound and from systemic alterations resulting from the wound. The immediate threat to life is asphyxia resulting from irritation and edema of the lungs and respiratory passages. In the first 48 to 72 hours the greatest hazard is unremitting shock with its associated complications. During healing, infection—both local and generalized sepsis—is the primary complication. Mortality associated with thermal injury in children decreases with the age of the child and increases with the extent of the burn. In children older than age 3 years the fatality rate is similar to that in adults, but below this age resistance to the burn or its complications is considerably lessened. Although the cause for this is unknown, it may be a function of physiologic immaturity.

Pulmonary. Pulmonary problems persist as the major cause of fatality in patients with thermal burns or a result of injury to or complications in the respiratory tract. A full range of respiratory insufficiency can occur, including inhalation injury, aspiration in unconscious patients, bacterial pneumonia, pulmonary edema, pulmonary embolus, and posttraumatic pulmonary insufficiency.

Inhalation injury may be caused by heat injury to the tissues of the airway or inhalation of carbon monoxide or other noxious gases. Although direct thermal injury to the upper airway may occur, heat damage below the vocal cords is rare. Above the glottis the damage is thermal (laryngeal edema); below the glottis damage is chemical. Inspired heated air is cooled in the upper airway before reaching the trachea, and reflex closure of the cords and laryngeal spasm prevent full inhalation. Evidence of direct thermal injury to the upper airway includes burns of the face, lips, and nasal hairs and signs of pharyngeal swelling or necrosis. Acute edema formation may lead to airway obstruction and asphyxiation. Symptoms may not develop for as long as 24 hours. Wheezing, prolonged expiratory phase, wet rales, and sooty secretions are signs of respiratory tract involvement. In such situations tracheal intubation with gentle suction is indicated to clear the bronchial tree.

Inhalation of carbon monoxide is suspected when the injury occurs in a closed space (see Smoke Inhalation Chapter 32, for a discussion of carbon monoxide inhalation). Inhalation of other by-products of combustion, that is, smoke and toxic chemicals, can produce varying degrees of lung damage, depending on the type of burning material. Burning wood smoke is extremely irritating, and smoke from burning plastic material, especially polyvinyl chloride, is the most irritating. Poisonous gases such as chlorine, sulfuric acid, or cyanide can be lethal if absorbed into the bloodstream. Respiratory injury is manifest as severe mucosal edema followed by sloughing of the mucosa and replacement by a mucopurulent membrane. This purulent material together with edema seriously compromises respiration. Acute bronchitis and bronchopneumonia commonly develop within a few days of injury.

The most common etiologic factor in respiratory failure in the pediatric age-group is bacterial pneumonia, which may be secondary to airway injury, contamination from intubation, or acquired through hematogenous spread of bacteria, usually from the burn wound. However, the largest percentage (65%) is caused by airborne infection, which occurs early in the postburn period and is associated with poor mentation, abdominal distention, and immobilization. The hematogenous variety occurs later from either the septic burn wound or other foci, such as phlebitis at a previous cutdown site.

Less common pulmonary complications are pulmonary emboli and pulmonary edema resulting from fluid overload during early fluid replacement. Sometimes deep burns of the chest may cause restriction of chest movement secondary to the effect of the binding, inelastic eschar formation. This is relieved by longitudinal incision of the eschar to prevent fatal hypoxia. Posttraumatic pulmonary insufficiency, which is difficult to distinguish from bacterial pneumonia, is sometimes a consequence of severe burns and is associated with sepsis and intravascular coagulation. It is the result of pulmonary capillary damage and leaking of fluid and protein into interstitial spaces of the lung, which causes loss of compliance and interference with oxygenation.

Wound sepsis. Sepsis is the most critical problem in treatment of burns and is an ever-present threat after the shock phase. Initially burns are relatively pathogen free, unless the wound is contaminated with potentially infectious material (e.g., dirt, polluted water). However, dead tissue and exudate provide a fertile field for bacterial growth. Early colonization of the wound surface by a preponderance of gram-positive organisms (primarily staphylococci) changes, on about the third postburn day, to predominantly gram-negative organisms, particularly *Pesudomonas aeruginosa* organisms. By the fifth postburn day the bacterial invasion is well underway beneath the surface of the wound.

Characteristics of the burn wound contribute to the proliferation of pathogenic organisms. Vascular supply to full-thickness burns is occluded immediately, and no appreciable blood is supplied to the area for approximately 3 weeks after the injury. In partial-thickness burns the circulation to the burn area stops immediately, but returns in about 24 to 48 hours, unless infection supervenes. Thrombosis from bacterial invasion will impair circulation sufficiently to convert partial-thickness injury to full-thickness destruction. These large amounts of nonviable tissue also provide an excellent medium for the growth of microorganisms.

Occlusion of the local blood supply is believed to impair the delivery of both humoral and cellular defense mechanisms to the burn area. Initially there is a decrease in inflammatory and phagocytic cells to the area, but the number of phagocytes gradually increases until they are present in abundance by the third postburn week, when good granulation tissue is forming. Granulating tissue, with its rich blood supply, affords increasing resistance to infection. Inasmuch as organisms are normally a part of skin flora, cultures that reveal an organism concentration of 10^5/g of tissue have been arbitrarily set as the level at which burn wound invasion occurs.

Normally there is a cyclic variation in the ability of phagocytes to kill ingested bacteria, and it appears that burn injury accentuates this process markedly. Burn wound sepsis occurs most often during the periods when this phagocytic killing power is depressed. Although the amount of complement (the system of plasma enzymes that mediate the antigen-antibody response) is also depressed, it is still present in sufficient quantities. This has led to development of a specific antibody against *P. aeruginosa*, the primary organism involved in burn wound sepsis. The success of this approach is presently being evaluated.

✦ **NURSING ALERT** Disorientation in the burned patient is one of the first signs of overwhelming sepsis. A spiking fever and usually paralytic ileus develop and progressively increase in severity over 2 to 3 days, after which the temperature falls to below normal. At this time the wound deteriorates, the white blood cell count is depressed, and septic shock becomes manifest.

Gastrointestinal. Recurrent or intermittent bleeding resulting from Curling, or stress, ulceration is a major noninfectious complication of burns. Routine antacid administration has reduced the incidence of this complication in recent years, but these superficial erosive lesions still occur in a number of burn injuries. The cause is obscure, and although gastric ulcers are more common in the total burn population, duodenal ulcers occur twice as frequently in children as in adults. Whereas gastric ulcers are observed in persons in all age-groups during the first postburn month, the peak occurrence of duodenal lesions is in the first week in adults but not until the third or fourth week in children. Children with significant (greater than 50% total body surface area) burn injury may be given cimetidine intravenously.

Children with burns covering more than 20% of body surface usually develop a partial paralytic ileus in the early postburn period that lasts for 2 to 3 days. Gastric decompression and parenteral nutrition are needed until bowel motility is reestablished and oral feedings are started.

Central nervous system. In children a frequent complication of both large and small burn injuries is CNS dysfunction. The manifestations range from hallucinations, personality change, and delirium to seizures and coma. Postburn seizures seem to be unique to children. In most cases the cause of this burn encephalopathy can be attributed to hypoxemia, electrolyte imbalance (hyponatremia), hypovolemia, septicemia, and drug administration. When the cause is determined, appropriate treatment can be initiated. Although the cause is unknown in one third of cases, full neurologic recovery is usual, even with prolonged and serious manifestations.

Hypertension. Approximately one third of children with severe thermal injuries develop arterial hypertension. The cause is unclear but may be related to the increased secretion of catecholamines or high plasma renin levels. Hypercalcemia caused by immobilization is occasionally a factor. It may appear at any time during the burn course and may persist for a few days or several months. Control is achieved by administration of diuretic and antihypertensive drugs. Mild hypertension is managed with administration of morphine sulfate or furosemide (Lasix); hydralazine may be required for more refractory problems (Harmel, Vane, and King, 1986).

THERAPEUTIC MANAGEMENT

The treatment of burns is commonly divided into phases because of the nature of the pathologic processes. The phases are described and titled differently by various authorities. However, for the purpose of this discussion, the emergency care is discussed first, followed by the medical management for minor and major burns. No phases are delineated.

Emergency Care

The aims of immediate treatment of thermal injury are to stop the burning process, cover the burn, transport the child to medical aid, and provide reassurance.

Stop burning process. The chief aim of rescue in flame burns is to smother the fire, not to fan it. Children tend to panic and run, which only serves to fan the flames and make assistance more difficult. The victim should not run and should not remain standing. The injured child should be placed in a horizontal position and rolled in a blanket, rug, or similar article, being careful not to cover the head and face because of the danger that the child might inhale the toxic fumes. If no article is available, the victim should be made to lie down and roll over slowly. Remaining in a vertical position may cause the hair to ignite or it may cause the child to inhale flames, heat, or smoke.

Spontaneous cooling of burns by slow immersion in cool water or any nonflammable liquid helps to relieve the pain, inhibit edema formation, and slow the process of heat damage, especially in the zone of stasis. However, if a large amount of skin surface is denuded, immersion may precipitate hypothermia. Ice water or ice packs are contraindicated because the resulting vasoconstriction interferes with capillary perfusion and carries the risk of further damage from cold burn. Unless there is nothing else available, no dirt or sand should be thrown on the burn. In chemical burns it is particularly important to wash the burn with copious amounts of cool running water. The exception to this rule is when the chemical irritant is a powder; addition of water will spread the caustic agent.

Burned clothing is removed gently to prevent further damage from smoldering fabric or hot beads of melted synthetic material. This also provides better access to the wound and precludes more painful removal later on. Special care must be exerted in removing any clothing that adheres to the skin.

Emergency procedures. As soon as the flames are extinguished, the condition of the victim is assessed. Airway, breathing, and circulation are the priority concerns. Cardiopulmonary or cerebral emergencies are always a possibility following a severe injury. Cardiopulmonary resuscitation is begun if indicated from the assessment. Cardiopulmonary complications may result from hypovolemic (or electric) shock and seizures may be caused by lack of oxygen to the brain, inhalation of noxious fumes, or aggravation of a preexisting tendency to convulsions by stress of the injury.

Cover burn. The burn wound should be covered with a clean cloth to prevent contamination and to alleviate pain by avoiding air contact. The child with extensive burns is covered to prevent hypothermia and help ease pain from contact with the air. No attempt should be made to treat the burn. Application of topical ointments, oils, or other home remedies is avoided.

Transport child to medical aid. The child with an extensive burn should not be given anything by mouth because of the risk of aspiration and water intoxication. The child is transported to the nearest place where medical aid is available. If this cannot be accomplished within a relatively short time and if facilities for intravenous fluid therapy and oxygen administration are available, they should be instigated to prevent burn shock. IV access is established with a large-bore catheter, preferably in an unburned area, and oxygen is administered at 5 liters per minute. A report of the initial assessment is given to the person assuming charge of the child's care.

Provide reassurance. Providing reassurance and psychologic support to both the parents and the child helps immeasurably during postinjury crisis. Reducing anxiety helps to conserve energy needed to cope with the physiologic and emotional stress of a traumatic injury.

Management of Minor Burns

Treatment of burns classified as minor usually can be managed adequately on an outpatient basis when it is determined that the *caregivers can be relied on to carry out instructions for care and observation.* Children with burns of the hands and most children with burns of the feet are admitted to the hospital so that they can receive careful local wound care and proper splinting to prevent deformity. In addition, children with burns of the face should be observed for airway obstruction and cosmetic reasons.

The wound is cleansed and debrided (all foreign material and devitalized tissue removed) with a tepid (approximately 32° C [90° F]), dilute, nonirritating, nonalkaline soap solution and rinsed with sterile saline solution. In minor injury coolness reduces pain and probably reduces edema, which can interfere with capillary flow in the zone of stasis. Blisters may or may not be debrided. Removal of the dead skin makes a cleaner wound and reduces the chance of infection in the blister fluid, but it is more painful and the intact blister skin provides a biologic dressing. When there is any doubt regarding intactness of the blister it is debrided and appropriately covered.

Most practitioners favor covering the wound with a dry dressing or fine-mesh gauze lightly lubricated with water-soluble antiseptic or antimicrobial cream and then wrapping it with bulky, dry, gauze dressings. This helps to keep the wound clean and to protect it from trauma. The caregivers are instructed to cleanse the wound with mild soap and tepid water, change the dressings once or twice daily, and return to the office or clinic as directed for wound observation. Occasionally the practitioner prefers to leave an occlusive dressing in place for several days if it remains clean and the child afebrile.

If there is a high probability of infection or other complications or if there is doubt about their ability to carry out

EMERGENCY TREATMENT
Burns

Minor burns

Stop burning process:
- Apply cool water to burn or hold burned area under cool running water.

Do not disturb any blisters that form.
Do not apply anything to wound.
Leave small burns exposed to air.
Apply dry, nonstick dressing if risk of damage or contamination.
Observe for signs of infection.

Major burns

Stop burning process:
- Flame burns—smother fire.
- Place victim in horizontal position.
- Roll victim in blanket or similar object; avoid covering head.
- Immerse in cool water or any nonflammable liquid.

Remove burned clothing.
Assess for adequate airway and breathing.
- If not breathing, begin mouth-to-mouth resuscitation.

Cover wound with clean cloth.
Transport to medical aid.

the directions, parents may be directed to return daily for dressing change and inspection or a nurse may be assigned to make a home visit for that purpose. Frequent removal of dressings is an effective mode of debridement. Soaking the dressing in tepid water before removal will help loosen the dressings and debris and reduce the discomfort. Superficial burns about the face are usually treated by exposure; a protective crust will form in 24 to 36 hours if the atmosphere is cool and dry. Partial-thickness burns are covered as a protection against infection.

A tetanus history is obtained on admission. When there is no history of immunization, human tetanus antitoxin should be administered. Administration of antibiotics for minor burns is controversial. Most mild burns heal with little difficulty, but if the wound margin becomes erythematous, gross purulence is noted, or the child develops evidence of systemic reaction, such as fever or tachycardia, hospitalization is indicated. A mild analgesic such as acetaminophen is usually sufficient to relieve any discomfort, and the antipyretic effect of the drug helps alleviate the sensation of heat.

Management of Major Burns

When a child with serious burns is admitted to the hospital for treatment, a variety of assessments are made and therapies initiated. Of these, the priority concerns are to (1) establish and maintain an adequate airway, (2) establish a lifeline for fluid resuscitation, and (3) care for the burn wound. Although the order of implementation may vary from institution to institution and from patient to patient, a number of procedures and activities generally are initiated on admission. Some are carried out simultaneously (Box 29-15).

Box 29-15 OUTLINE OF MAJOR BURN WOUND MANAGEMENT

Ascertain the adequacy of the airway and provide oxygen, intubation, and ventilatory assistance as indicated.
Insert an intravenous line in an unburned area (if possible) that is sufficiently ample to deliver fluids at a rapid rate and, in patients with extensive injury, to accommodate a central venous pressure line.
Remove clothes and examine for trauma to head, skeleton, or nervous system.
Weigh the child.
Control pain with appropriate analgesics.
Provide intravenous sedation only after adequate oxygenation is ensured, fluid resuscitation is established, and comfort measures have not calmed the child.
Insert an indwelling Foley catheter to obtain specimens and measure hourly output.
Empty stomach through nasogastric tube.
Obtain blood sample for baseline laboratory studies.
Examine the burn wound and evaluate the extent and depth of injury.
Carry out an escharotomy (incision through the eschar) for constricting circumferential eschar of chest or extremities, if necessary (usually not an emergency procedure).
Cover flame or contact burns and apply topical medication and gauze dressings.
Calculate fluid requirements and establish appropriate regimen.
Administer appropriate protection against tetanus.
Obtain history regarding the injury and other pertinent data.

Other needs and therapies, including nutritional support, splinting to prevent contractures, treatment of anemia and hypoproteinemia, psychologic support, and rehabilitative aspects of burn management, are initiated as appropriate throughout the course of treatment.

Establishment of adequate airway. The first priority of care is airway maintenance. Thermal injuries to the face, nares, or upper torso; history of fire in an enclosed area; or examination of the oral and nasal membranes that reveals edema of these membranes, hyperemia, burns of mucous membranes, or evidence of trauma to upper respiratory passages all suggest inhalation of noxious agents or presence of respiratory burn. Oxygen is administered and blood gases, including carbon monoxide, are quickly determined. If the child exhibits changes in sensorium, air hunger, or otherwise appears in critical condition, an endotracheal tube is inserted to maintain the airway. The usual practice is to place a tube if there is any question regarding the possibility of respiratory problems. Pharyngeal edema may make delayed intubation difficult, and the child will become restless from hypoxia.

Tracheostomy is rarely employed, because it has been associated with serious complications and significant mortality in childhood burn injuries, such as a high incidence of infection, tracheobronchitis, delayed hemorrhage, and cannula obstruction from secretions and granulations. Inasmuch as early edema subsides within 24 to 48 hours and many have been managed successfully for longer periods without significant damage, nasotracheal intubation is the safer and preferred approach. It allows for the delivery of humidified air with oxygen, the easy removal of secretions from respiratory passages, and the use of a pressure ventilator if needed.

Frequently placing the child in semi-Fowler position inside a tent or under an oxygen hood with a high flow of oxygen and maximum humidity is sufficient to reduce reflex bronchospasm produced by trauma to the bronchial mucosa. To combat continued respiratory distress, sometimes a large dose of antiinflammatory corticosteroid compound is given rapidly by the intravenous route to augment the already elevated blood level of circulating steroids. This therapy still remains very controversial, however, because of the effect of corticosteroids on the immune response and the high risk of infection with major burns.

Fluid replacement therapy. The objectives of fluid therapy are to (1) compensate for water and sodium lost to traumatized areas and interstitial spaces, (2) replenish sodium deficits, (3) restore plasma volume, (4) obtain adequate perfusion, (5) correct acidosis, and (6) improve renal function.

Fluid and electrolyte therapy for children in the first 24 hours after a burn is still controversial. This controversy is centered primarily around whether colloid solution, usually albumin, dextran, Plasmanate, or plasma, should be part of the resuscitation phase of fluid therapy. Those who favor crystalloid solutions believe that during this time the altered capillary membrane is unable to provide a structural barrier and that, therefore, colloid solutions are of questionable value in restoring the plasma oncotic pressure. Instead, the colloid crosses the membrane and becomes trapped in the interstitial spaces as capillary permeability is restored during the next 24 hours, augmenting the extravascular fluid retention. This has serious implications for fluid accumulation in the lungs and brain.

The composition of the fluid selected varies with the philosophy of the individual practitioner or the burn unit and may consist of isotonic saline solution, a near-isotonic solution (e.g., Ringer's lactate), or even a hypertonic saline solution. Needs are determined by several parameters, such as vital signs, including blood pressure, urine volume and character, pulse, adequacy of capillary filling, and state of sensorium. In complicated cases arterial, central venous, and pulmonary artery pressures are monitored. These criteria, based on individual needs, are more effective for fluid resuscitation. Periodic monitoring of potassium, chloride, carbon dioxide, blood urea nitrogen, and osmolality helps determine the adequacy of fluid therapy and evidence of acidosis (Herndon and others, 1985).

✦ **NURSING ALERT** Capillary refill, alterations in sensorium, and urine output are the most reliable indicators for assessing adequacy of fluid resuscitation in burned children. Blood pressure can remain normotensive even in a state of hypovolemia.

After diuresis, in 48 to 72 hours when capillary permeability is restored, fluid requirements decrease to a constant that remains so long as the burn wound is open. Sometimes colloid solutions such as albumin or plasma are used in maintaining plasma volume. During this phase interstitial fluid is returning rapidly to the vascular compartment, and increasing intake to match urine output may cause circulatory overload. Early enteral feeding is the rule and may begin within the first 24 hours postburn (Guzzetta and Holihan, 1988). Fluid balance may continue to be a problem throughout the course of treatment, especially during the periods in which there may be considerable evaporative loss from the wound.

Nutrition. The high metabolic requirements and catabolism in severe burns make nutritional needs of paramount importance and often difficult to provide. Hypermetabolism, increased glucose flow, and severe protein and fat wasting are characteristic of the response to major trauma and infection. Children with multiple trauma and who are respiratory dependent can have metabolic requirements 30% to 75% above normal. The metabolic rate of those with burns greater than 40% total body surface is 100% greater than normal (Herndon and others, 1985) and may reach 200% of normal resting energy expenditure (Harmel, Vane, and King, 1986).

The diet must provide sufficient protein to prevent negative nitrogen balance and extra calories to utilize the proteins, sustain the adaptive hypermetabolism, and spare protein breakdown. Normal protein requirements may be three times the standard adult intake and increase proportionately as a result of trauma and stress. The child's proportionately less body fat and substantially smaller muscle mass predispose to the rapid development of protein-calorie malnutrition (Harmel, Vane, and King, 1986). Extra calories should be derived from carbohydrates, because fat, although higher in total calories, will not spare protein. The normal energy stores of glycogen are depleted; therefore exogenous glucose must be provided early. Intravenous 5% glucose can supply minimum requirements, but these are inadequate to meet added needs.

Most burn patients are able to eat, and the child is given oral feedings as soon as possible. A liquid diet is instituted and gradually advanced to a regular diet. Because burned children have poor appetites and the caloric requirements may be as much as two to three times their usual requirements for size and age, the diet is high in calories and protein, supplemented with high doses of vitamins B and C and iron. An adequate anabolic state is reached when the blood urea nitrogen level begins to fall.

Nasogastric feedings may be needed to supplement oral intake, and peripheral parenteral alimentation has been used to provide a large amount of concentrated glucose and amino acids, especially in infants. The anorexia, delayed gastric emptying, and osmotic diarrhea secondary to high-solute tube feedings lead to this mode of nutrition despite difficulties encountered in placement of the catheter and the increased risk of sepsis.

To facilitate growth and proliferation of epithelial cells, administration of vitamin A is begun early in the postburn period. Zinc sulfate is also administered by some practitioners, because zinc stores are depleted during catabolism and it appears to facilitate wound healing and epithelialization.

Medication. Controversy also exists regarding the use of antibiotics during the first few days after injury. Some authorities believe that low doses of penicillin should be given prophylactically to all children with serious burns because of (1) their susceptibility to rapidly spreading cellulitis as a result of streptococcal infection, and (2) lowered immunoglobulin levels. Others prefer to treat the streptococci only when they become a problem. Fevers are evaluated and antibiotics administered if no immediate source of the elevation can be identified. The use of topical antibacterial creams, which are effective against both gram-negative and gram-positive organisms, also renders prophylactic antibiotics unnecessary. Broad-spectrum antibiotics are avoided to prevent the possibility of a superimposed infection. In addition, impaired circulation in the wound area prevents their access to the site.

Some form of sedation and analgesia is required in the care of burned children. During the first 12 to 24 hours sedation is kept at a minimum to allow for observation of sensorium, to assess brain perfusion, and to evaluate cerebral status when head trauma is established or suspected. Also, there is increased risk of respiratory distress in some patients. Suitable opioids such as morphine sulfate or fentanyl are administered intravenously and titrated as needed. The unstable circulatory status precludes the use of intramuscular injections. Beyond 24 hours the amount and type of sedation are determined on an individual basis based on the needs of the child. General anesthesia is required for extensive debridement, but during dressing changes and debridement a number of methods are available.

Management of Burn Wound

After the initial period of shock and restoration of fluid balance, the primary concern is the burn wound. The objectives of management for epidermal and superficial (first- and second-degree) burns is to prevent infection by providing an environment as aseptic as possible. Occlusive dressings help to reduce pain by minimizing exposure to air. The exposure method allows the wound to dry and is used primarily for mild to moderate face wounds. All methods employ topical antibacterial applications, or daily hydrotherapy, or both, to remove loose tissue and debris and to allow inspection of the wound. The objectives for management of full-thickness wounds are prevention of invasive infection, removal of dead tissue, protection from mechanical trauma, and closure of the wound.

Debridement. The use of hydrotherapy has reduced the need for surgical debridement under general anesthesia. Debridement is painful and requires some type of analgesic before the procedure (Fig. 29-6). Morphine and fentanyl are drugs of choice in most units. Ketamine hydrochloride in subanesthetic doses has proved highly effective in children, and nitrous oxide inhalation is employed in a number of burn units. The child will require instruction in how to breathe the gas at the appropriate time and coaching during its use.

Soaking in the Hubbard tank for 20 to 30 minutes once or twice daily facilitates the loosening and removal of sloughing tissue, eschar, exudate, and topical medications. Mesh gauze serves to entrap exudative slough and is readily removed during hydrotherapy (Fig. 29-7). Any loose tissue or eschar is carefully trimmed away before redressing (Fig. 29-8). However, hosing is rapidly replacing tubbing as a

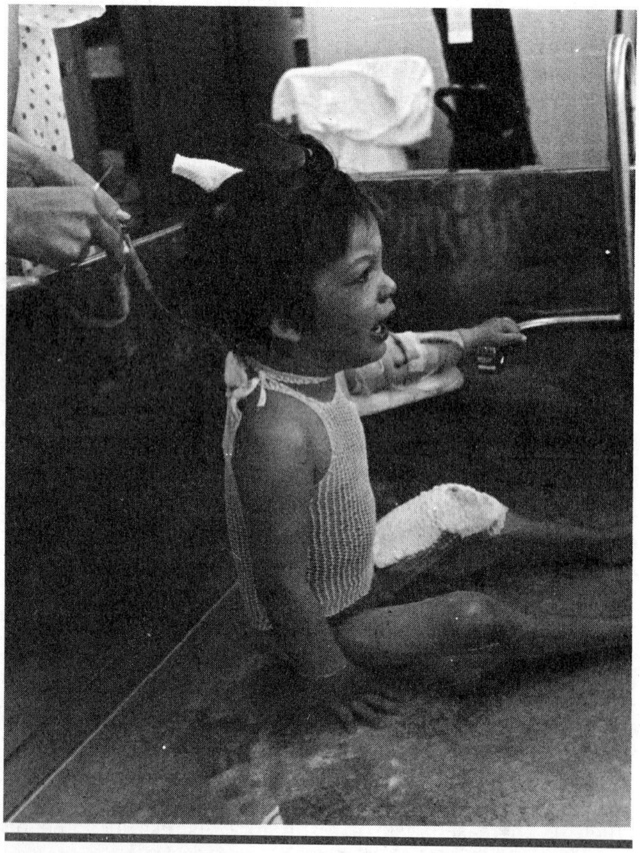

Fig. 29-6. An analgesic is administered before removal of dressings and debridement. In this instance analgesic is injected directly into intravenous line at time of hydrotherapy.

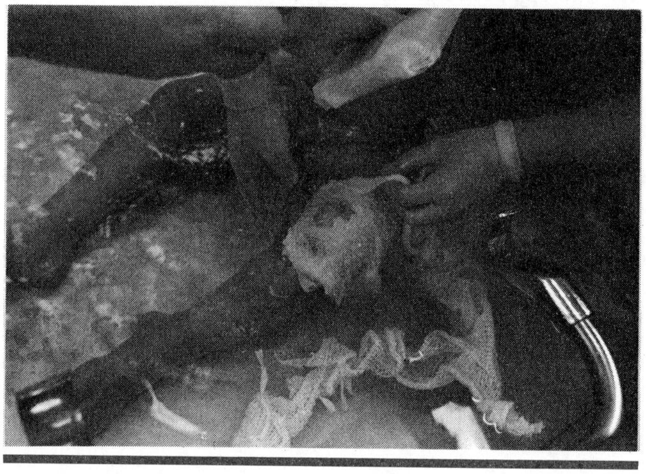

Fig. 29-7. Removal of dressing during hydrotherapy.

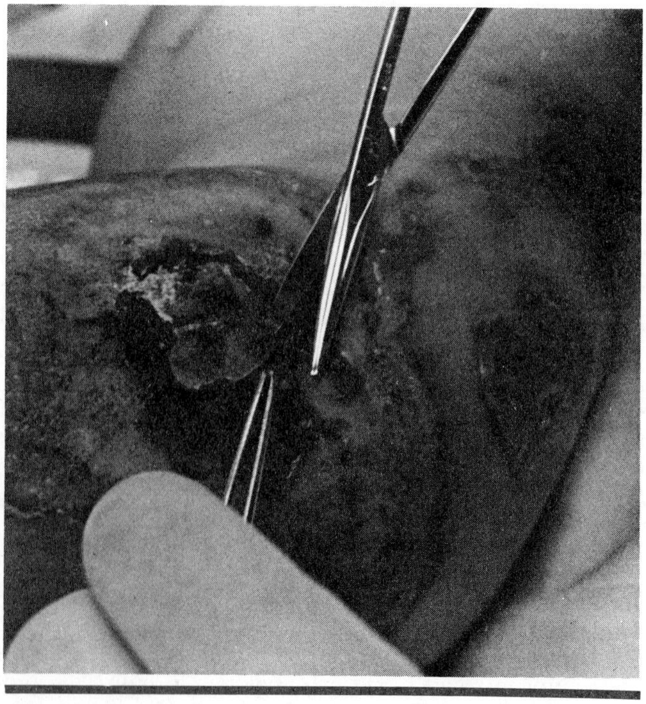

Fig. 29-8. Dead skin and debris are carefully trimmed away before dressing is applied.

method of hydrotherapeutic debridement because there is less risk of infection.

Topical antimicrobial agents. Several methods are used for covering the burn wound (Box 29-16). All meet the objective of preparation for permanent wound coverage and all employ some type of topical agent. Before the development of effective topical agents for reducing the incidence of invasive organisms, wound sepsis was the major cause of mortality from burn injury. Systemic administration cannot reach the area because of thrombosed vessels. Topical agents do not eliminate organisms from the burn wound, but they can effectively inhibit or delay bacterial growth. Successful burn therapy relies on both topical antibacterial applications and thorough cleansing and debridement to reduce the amounts of necrotic material on which the bacteria grow. To be effective, a topical application must be nontoxic, capable of diffusing through eschar, harmless to viable tissue, inexpensive, and easy to apply. It should not cause an increase in resistant strains and should produce minimum electrolyte derangements (Fig. 29-9).

Box 29-16 METHODS OF BURN WOUND MANAGEMENT

Exposure—wounds are left open to the air; crust forms on partial-thickness wounds, and eschar forms on full-thickness wounds.
Open—topical antimicrobial ointment is applied directly to wound surface, but wound is left uncovered.
Modified—ointment is applied directly to wound or impregnated into thin gauze and applied to wound; a stretched gauze or net covering secures the area (Fig. 29-10).
Occlusive—ointment-impregnated gauze or ointment covered with gauze layer is placed on the burn wound; multiple layers of bulky gauze are placed over the primary layer and secured with stretched gauze or net.

A number of topical agents are employed, but those used most frequently are 0.5% silver nitrate solution, 10% mafenide acetate (Sulfamylon), and 1% silver sulfadiazine (Silvadene). All three are effective bacteriostatic agents, but each has advantages and disadvantages. Less frequently used are 0.1% gentamicin sulfate (Garamycin) and povidone-iodine (Betadine) ointment. Furacin-saturated gauze dressings have been used by some burn units, but renal impairment has been observed in some patients, caused by the polyethylene glycol base in which it is prepared (Food and Drug Administration, 1982). The significant aspects of each are summarized in Table 29-4.

Biologic skin coverings. Biologic dressings are used during the acute phase of therapy to cover wound surfaces, protect the wound from bacterial invasion, limit fluid and protein loss, reduce pain, and increase rate of epithelialization (Herndon and others, 1985) (Box 29-17).

The type of graft particularly suitable and used most frequently for temporary covering in children is the porcine xenograft (Fig. 29-11). The split-thickness pigskin is available commercially and is an effective covering agent after eschar separation. Changed regularly, it reduces evaporative loss, protects the wound bed, and is believed to protect the wound from infection and trauma. The grafts usually adhere within a few hours, and dressings are not needed. They are particularly effective in children with second-degree scald burns of hands and face, because they allow relatively pain-free movement, which reduces contracture and has the added benefit of improved appetite and morale. Pigskin dressings are replaced daily or at least every 3 to 4 days; as a result acceptance of the graft is minimal. When left in

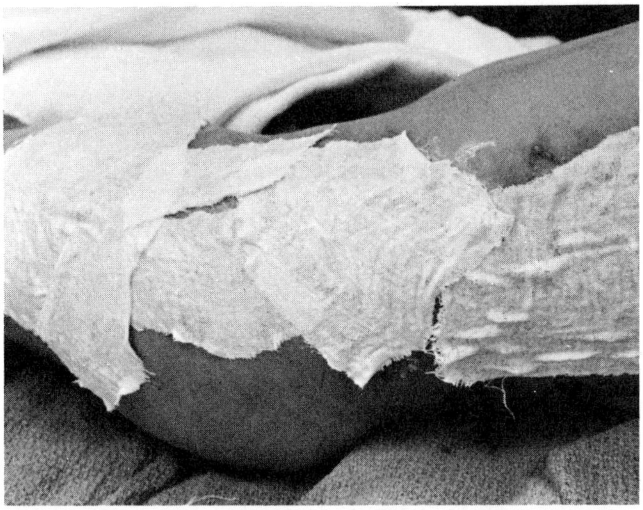

Fig. 29-9. Gauze impregnated with ointment applied to burn wound.

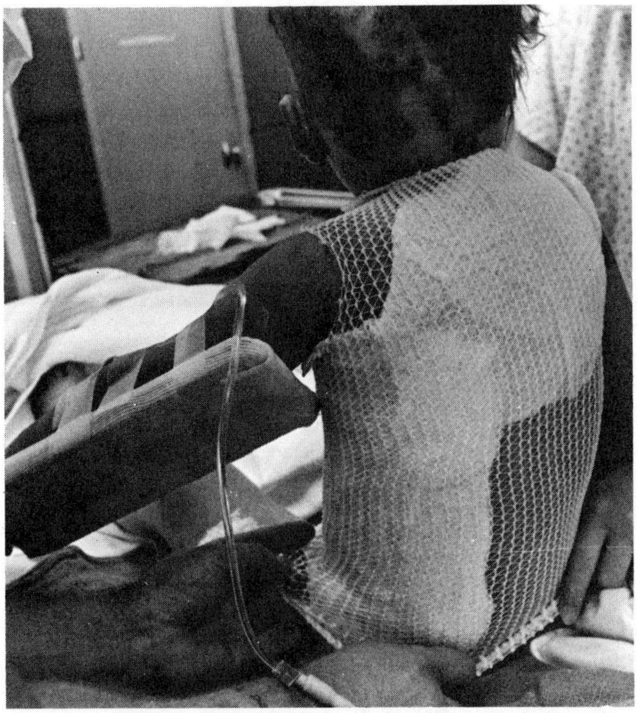

Fig. 29-10. Burn wound covered with gauze dressings and secured with tabular elastic netting.

Table 29-4 Comparison of common topical preparations

AGENT	DRESSINGS	ADVANTAGES	DISADVANTAGES
Silver nitrate, 0.5% ($AgNO_3$)	Exposure, modified or occlusive Impedes joint movement Dressings changed twice daily	Greatly reduces evaporative losses, thus lower metabolic rate and lower weight loss Does not interfere with wound healing Nonallergenic Inexpensive Effective against major burn flora, including *Pseudomonas* and *Staphylococcus*	Cannot allow dressings to become dry; requires frequent wetting (at least every 2 hours) Difficult to use Ineffective on established burn wound infections Does not penetrate eschar; therefore, should be applied before bacterial growth established Hypotonicity pulls electrolytes from wound, causing depletion of sodium, chloride, potassium, and magnesium that necessitates continuous monitoring and replacement Little effect on *Klebsiella* and *Aerobacter* groups Stains skin, linens, clothes
Mafenide acetate (Sulfamylon), 10%	Usually exposure Occasionally with dressings Reapplied twice daily	Diffuses rapidly into burn wound and underlying tissues Rapidly excreted Easily applied Penetrates through eschar and deeply into burn wound; therefore, effective in deep flame, electric, and older wounds Effective against many gram-positive and gram-negative organisms, including *Pseudomonas* and *Clostridium*	Mild acidosis caused by inhibition of carbonic anhydrase in kidney Hypersensitivity reaction in many children Causes discomfort during application Inhibits wound healing
Silver sulfadiazine (Silvadene), 1% (AgSD)	Occlusive Motion of joints maintained Applied once or twice daily	Nontoxic Combines advantages of silver nitrate and mafenide acetate Painless (relatively) Easy to apply Absorbs slowly Bactericidal for up to 48 hours Effective against gram-positive and gram-negative bacteria and *Candida albicans*	Does not penetrate eschar as well as mafenide acetate or gentamicin sulfate Children complain that the application feels "cold"; may be interpreted as pain May cause neutropenia; usually reverses in 48 hours
Gentamicin sulfate (Garamycin), 0.1%	Exposure, modified or occlusive	No pain associated with use Relatively nontoxic Penetrates burn wound quickly Especially effective against *Klebsiella* and *Enterobacter*	40% of pseudomonal organisms have become resistant Occasionally nephrotoxicity and ototoxicity
Povidone-iodine (Betadine) ointment	Exposure, modified or occlusive Impedes joint movement	Apparently nontoxic Effective against broad spectrum of organisms	Elevation of protein-bound iodine (PBI) Use associated with considerable pain Causes eschar to "tan" and become very stiff, making debridement and evaluation of burn wound difficult May cause acidosis

place for longer periods, antibody development causes increasingly rapid rejection.

Other allografts that are used are from human cadavers, when available. Rejection of these grafts occurs in about 14 days. Skin allografts from closely histocompatible living related donors, used in conjunction with immunosuppression therapy, maintain wound coverage continuously over a longer period of time. Short-term coverage can be accomplished with human amnion (obtained by stripping the amniotic membrane from the placenta).

Synthetic skin coverings. A number of satisfactory biologic dressings and skin substitutes are available for

Box 29-17 TYPES OF SKIN GRAFTS

Temporary Grafts

Allografts (homografts)—skin is obtained from genetically different members of the same species, living or dead, usually cadavers, that are free from disease.

Xenografts (heterografts)—skin is obtained from members of a different species, primarily pigskin, either fresh or frozen.

Permanent Grafts

Autografts—tissues are obtained from undamaged areas of the patient's own body.

Isografts—histocompatible tissue is obtained from genetically identical individuals, that is, the patient's identical twin.

Methods of Applying Split-Thickness Grafts

Full-cover graft—a sheet of skin, removed from the donor site, is placed intact over the recipient site and sutured in place or maintained in place by pressure dressings.

Postage-stamp graft—a sheet of skin from the donor site is cut into postage-stamp pieces and placed on the recipient bed; may be covered with a dressing or left exposed for inspection and rolling serum from beneath the graft.

Mesh, lace, or slit graft—a sheet of skin is removed from donor site with multiple slits so that, when stretched, it expands to cover from one and one-half to nine times (usually three times) the area of a full-cover graft; requires suturing to maintain tension; may be exposed or covered with occlusive dressing for about 48 hours; effective for large areas (Fig. 29-12).

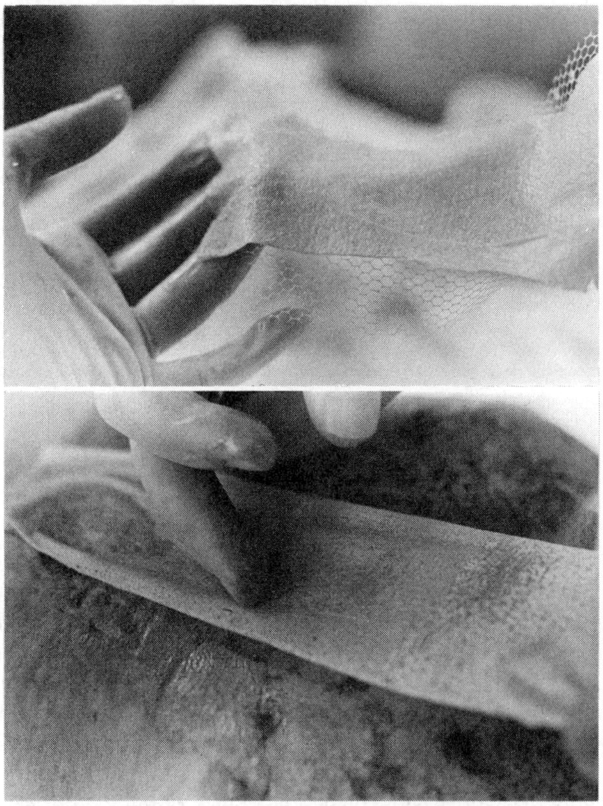
A

B

Fig. 29-11. Porcine dressing. **A,** Removed from net backing. **B,** Applied to wound.

burn wound management. Ideally the dressing should provide many of the properties of human skin—adherent, elastic, durable, and hemostatic—and be inexpensive and available.

Synthetic skin substitutes are available in several forms. Examples include dressings consisting of a layer of polyurethane foam laminated to outer sheets of microporous polypropylene film, a silicone polymer membrane, a semisynthetic membrane composed of Silastic nylon and collagen (Biobrane), and a mixture of polymer powder and polyethylene glycol liquid that forms a flexible, adherent, transparent, water-soluble dressing (Hydron). Synthetic adhesive, vapor-permeable polyurethane film dressings (Op-Site, Clingfilm, Via-film, and Tegaderm) are also available and especially valuable for fresh, small partial-thickness wounds treated on an outpatient basis. All synthetic dressings are reputed to hasten the healing of some partial-thickness burns and donor sites and to reduce wound discomfort.

Combined biologic and synthetic skin substitutes have been developed for covering burns and skin graft sites. This is the collagen wound dressing and contains a porous collagen fibrillous "dermal" layer combined with an impermeable "epidermal" layer of Silastic. The synthetic skin is gradually replaced with normal vascularized connective tissue elements as it is slowly biodegraded. This new tissue is then ready to support a standard split-thickness skin graft, which is placed as the Silastic is removed (Burke and others, 1981).

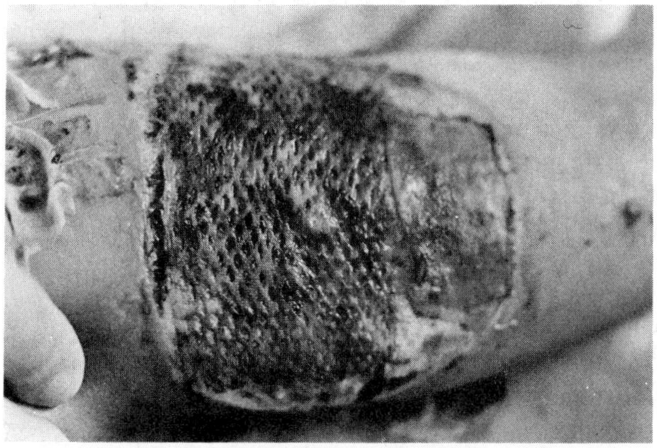

Fig. 29-12. Mesh graft.

Permanent skin covering. Permanent skin grafting is part of the rehabilitative stage to restore cosmetic appearance and to achieve maximum functional capacity. Permanent grafting of full-thickness burns is usually accomplished with a split-thickness skin graft, which can be obtained from only two sources: autograft from the patient's own tissue or isografts from an identical twin.

A permanent skin graft consists of the epidermis and part

Box 29-18 REQUIREMENTS FOR A SUCCESSFUL GRAFT

Sufficient nourishment until new blood supply grows in from the base of the recipient bed
Primary tissue contact, that is, actual contact between cut surface of the graft and the recipient bed
Avoidance of bleeding; the possibility of even the slightest bleeding must be controlled with light pressure
Prevention of infection, especially in full-cover grafts; postage-stamp grafts will often "take" in contaminated areas

of the dermis being removed from an undamaged area by a special instrument, the dermatome, which is designed to excise split-thickness skin. The priority areas for coverage are the face, neck, and areas around joints, especially the hands. With extensive burns it is often difficult to find enough viable skin to cover the wounds; therefore, available donor sites are used to the best advantage by special techniques. The various methods of applying split-thickness grafts are described in Box 29-17. Full-sheet grafts are used in areas in which a cosmetic effect is desired. Patch and mesh grafts result in a less desirable appearance. Requirements of a successful "take," regardless of the type of graft used, are listed in Box 29-18.

Until blood supply is established, the grafted skin is nourished by osmotic interchange with the recipient bed. Wound healing takes place as the recipient area throws out fibrin that attaches the graft to the new bed. The fibrin is infiltrated by leukocytes and fibroblasts, and the capillary buds of the granulation tissue spread through the fibrin. Within 3 days there is vascularization of the graft; after 2 weeks the graft is attached to the base by connective tissue.

The donor site is dressed with either a xenograft or fine-mesh gauze and left exposed until the dressing falls off in about 10 to 14 days. Dressings are not changed on donor sites to prevent tearing the new, delicate epithelium.

An important nursing role in management of permanent skin grafts is facilitating adhesion between surfaces by removal of serum accumulated beneath the graft. The graft area is carefully rolled with a sterile applicator to move the serum from beneath the graft to its edge. This process is especially important with mesh and postage-stamp grafts.

When burns are extensive and donor sites for split-thickness grafts are inadequate for coverage, it is possible to culture epidermal cells from a small skin biopsy and produce coherent epithelial sheets that can be grafted to generate a permanent epidermal surface. Some children have been successfully treated with this autologous cultured epithelium method (Gallico and others, 1984; O'Conner and others, 1982).

Primary excision. Excision and immediate grafting of small full-thickness and deep partial-thickness burns hastens recovery in selected cases. In many areas this method is replacing standard topical therapy. Primary excision should take place as early as possible after restoration of physical balance.

NURSING CONSIDERATIONS

Nursing care is the most important aspect of burn therapy. Because the care of severely burned children encompasses such a broad range of skills and foci, it is divided into segments that correspond with the major phases of burn treatment: the *acute phase* (also referred to as the resuscitative, emergent, or metabolic phase), which involves the first 24 to 48 hours; the *management phase,* which extends from the time a child has been adequately resuscitated until the major rehabilitative aspects of care are initiated; and the *rehabilitative phase,* which begins with permanent grafting. This phase continues until all full-thickness injuries are covered and reconstructive procedures and corrective measures have been accomplished. This often extends over a period of months or years.

Acute Phase

The primary emphasis during the initial phases of burn care is prevention of burn shock. Checking vital signs, monitoring the intravenous infusion line, and measuring urinary output are ongoing nursing activities in the hours immediately after injury. The intravenous infusion is started immediately by intracatheter or cutdown and is regulated according to urine output and specific gravity, laboratory data, and objective signs of adequate hydration. Urine volume, measured at least every hour, should be 1 to 2 ml/kg of body weight/hour.

✦ **NURSING ALERT** Assessment of sensorium is an important indicator of adequacy of hydration.

Children are observed for all parameters. They require constant observation and assessment with special attention to signs of complications. Respiratory, cardiac, and renal complications may appear early in the postburn period.

Care of the burn wound is secondary to the more critical problems of circulatory or respiratory failure. When a special burn facility is available, the child is wrapped in a sterile sheet and covered with a blanket for warmth during transfer, and the burn wound is attended to after arrival at the unit. If no burn unit is available, the wound is cleansed and dressed in the emergency department. Many units take photographs of the burn wound initially and periodically as a record of wound progress and for legal purposes, if needed—especially in cases of suspected child abuse. Usually the child with a major burn and unstable condition is given a bed bath with warm saline. Evaluation of the wound is more accurately accomplished during or after cleansing.

The burn wound is treated according to the protocol of the specific burn facility. Extensive wounds may require the use of special beds, such as CircOlectric beds, flotation beds, and alternating pressure mattresses, and many other devices, depending on the extent and location of the wound. When inhalation injury is suspected, the nurse observes the child for evidence of pulmonary involvement. Activities include listening for inspiratory wheezing and detecting increasing hoarseness.

Throughout the acute phase of care children's emotional needs must not be overlooked. They are frightened, uncomfortable, and often confused. Children are isolated from familiar persons and surroundings, and the often overwhelming physical needs at this time are the primary focus of staff and parents. Children need to be reassured that they are all right and that they will get better.

Management and Rehabilitative Phases

After the patient's condition is stabilized, the lengthy management phase begins. During this phase the major goal is care of the wound to facilitate healing and prepare for permanent closure. The rehabilitative phase begins when permanent closure of the wound begins, although rehabilitation essentially begins with initiation of care.

Assessment

Wound assessment continues to be a major observation as well as comprehensive assessment of the child's general condition and behaviors. Observation for signs of complications, especially infection, and assessing the need for and effectiveness of pain management are important nursing functions.

Nursing Diagnoses

Based on a thorough assessment, several nursing diagnoses are identified. The more common diagnoses for the child with burns are included in the Nursing Care Plan on pp. 1316-1318. Others may apply in specific situations.

Planning

Nursing objectives for the child with burns include:

1. Relieve pain.
2. Facilitate wound healing and permanent closure.
3. Provide nutrition and reduce metabolic losses.
4. Prevent acute complications (management phase).
5. Prevent long-term complications (rehabilitative phase).
6. Support child and family.

Implementation

The management phase of burn care involves intensive nursing care, which can be arduous for patient, family, and nursing staff. Except for minor burns, care usually takes place in a burn unit.

Relieve pain. The severe pain of the wound and the therapies, the anxiety generated by these experiences, and the conscious and unconscious interpretations of traumatic events contribute to the psychologic reactions frequently observed in burned children. Much of the difficulty encountered in managing burned children is related to these factors. Soon after hospitalization many burned children become irritable, depressed, hostile, and aggressive toward the members of the health team. When pain is not a factor, as in the case of burns to a paralyzed area, this behavior has not been observed. In their helplessness, children often resort to angry outbursts against anything and anybody.

The burn pain is overwhelming, engulfing, and irrepressible. Consequently the pain causes anxiety and a feeling of profound helplessness in a child and can produce reactions of confusion, fear, and panic. Compounding the pain is a child's interpretation of it and of the procedures; this is closely related to the developmental level of a child. Many burned children believe their pain is punishment for past misdeeds and therefore deserved. There are often feelings of anger, guilt, and depression, and, as in all illness, regressive behavior. When children appear to accept their pain and show little or no aggressive behavior, psychologic consultation is usually in order.

It is always difficult to deal with children in pain, and to inflict pain on helpless children is contrary to the empathetic nature of nursing. Adequate management of pain is essential to reduce discomfort of the burn and the necessary therapeutic procedures. Management of pain consists of choosing the (1) correct analgesic (opioids are needed for severe pain), (2) adequate dosage, and (3) appropriate timing. For example, to relieve pain adequately, the *onset* of action of the drug must be considered in order that the peak effect occurs when the treatment is performed. An analgesic administered shortly before the procedure will exert its effect *after* the procedure is completed.

Management of pain follows the principles described in Chapter 26.

Care of burn wound. The nurse has the major responsibility for cleansing, debriding, and applying topical medication and dressings to the burn wound. Because dressing removal is a painful procedure, children should receive adequate analgesia before the scheduled tubbing. It should be administered so that the peak effect of the drug coincides with the procedure. Both nurses and children must recognize it for exactly what it is—a dreadful but absolutely necessary procedure. Because it is painful, children should know that it is all right to cry when the treatment hurts, but only *when it hurts.* An effective approach is to conduct the procedure as a team with one nurse to perform the painful activities while the other provides support and comfort to the child. In the process of supporting, the comforting nurse also prevents injury by holding the child firmly during the procedure.

Because it is easy for children to give way to emotional excesses they cannot control, they need the firm control and guidance of a caring adult. This includes both actual and anticipated hurt. Children need help to gain and maintain control of their emotions. They benefit from knowing why things are being done to them, how these things will help them get better, and how they can contribute.

Research has demonstrated that children are more cooperative and demonstrate less anxiety and depression when they are allowed to be active participants in their care (Kavanagh and Freeman, 1984). Predictability and controllabil-

NURSING CARE PLAN
The Child with Burns: Management and Rehabilitative Stages

NURSING DIAGNOSIS: Impaired skin integrity related to thermal injury

GOAL 1

Facilitate wound healing

INTERVENTIONS

Shave hair from wound and area immediately surrounding burn, if needed
Thoroughly cleanse wound and surrounding skin; debride of devitalized tissues
Keep child from scratching and picking at wound
  Provide distraction
  Older child: explain reasons
  Young child: apply restraining devices as needed
Maintain care in handling wound to avoid damaging epithelializing and granulating tissues
Offer high-calorie, high-protein meals and snacks
Prevent infection
*Administer supplementary vitamins and minerals—vitamins A, B, and C and zinc sulfate

EXPECTED OUTCOME

Wound heals without evidence of damage or inflammation

GOAL 2

Protect graft area

INTERVENTIONS

Position for minimum disturbance of graft site
Restrain if necessary

EXPECTED OUTCOME

Skin graft remains intact

NURSING DIAGNOSIS: Pain related to skin trauma, therapies

GOAL 1

Relieve pain

INTERVENTIONS

Assess need for pain medication (see Chapter 26)
Position for comfort
Employ appropriate nonpharmacologic pain-reduction techniques (see Chapter 26)
*Administer analgesics as needed

EXPECTED OUTCOME

Child exhibits only minimum evidence of pain

GOAL 2

Prevent pain

INTERVENTIONS

Avoid touching or moving painful areas
Reduce irritation; for example, avoid drafts, movement
Anticipate need for pain medication and administer before onset of pain

*Dependent nursing action

EXPECTED OUTCOME

Child exhibits only minimum evidence of pain

NURSING DIAGNOSIS: Potential for infection related to denuded skin, presence of pathogenic organisms

GOAL 1

Control bacterial growth on wound

INTERVENTIONS

Implement and maintain infection control precautions according to unit policy
Maintain careful handwashing by members of staff and visitors
Wear clean or sterilized gown, cap, mask, and sterile gloves when handling wound area
Avoid injury to crust and eschar
Avoid patient contact with persons who have upper respiratory or skin infection
Cover wound and/or patient according to protocol of unit
Administer good oral hygiene
*Apply prescribed topical antimicrobial preparation and dressings (if ordered) to wound
Obtain wound cultures three times per week to ascertain any increase in wound flora

EXPECTED OUTCOMES

Possible sources of infection are eliminated
Wound displays minimum or no evidence of infection

NURSING DIAGNOSIS: Altered nutrition: less than body requirements related to increased catabolism, loss of appetite

GOAL 1

Maintain adequate nutrition and prevent nitrogen loss

INTERVENTIONS

Provide high-calorie, high-protein meals and snacks

EXPECTED OUTCOME

Child maintains a positive nitrogen balance—no weight loss

GOAL 2

Stimulate appetite

INTERVENTIONS

Encourage oral feeding (see Feeding the Sick Child, Chapter 27)
Provide foods child likes
Allow self-help
Provide meals when child is most likely to eat well
Provide attractive meals and surroundings
Provide companionship at meals
Employ "contract" with older children

EXPECTED OUTCOMES

Child consumes a sufficient amount of nutrients (specify)
Child interacts with older child

NURSING CARE PLAN
The Child with Burns: Management and Rehabilitative Stages—cont'd

NURSING DIAGNOSIS: Impaired physical mobility (specify level) related to pain, impaired joint movement

GOAL 1

Promote optimum functioning (physical)

INTERVENTIONS

Carry out range of motion exercises
Encourage mobility if child is unable to move extremities
Ambulate as soon as feasible
Splint involved joints at night and rest periods
Encourage and promote self-help activities
Administer analgesia before painful activity (e.g., physical therapy)

EXPECTED OUTCOME

Joints remain flexible with maximum functional capacity

GOAL 2

Minimize scar formation

INTERVENTIONS

Position in functional attitude for minimum deformity and optimum function
Apply splints as ordered and designed
Wrap healing tissue with elastic bandage or dress in elastic garments as ordered
Carry out physical therapy

EXPECTED OUTCOME

Wound heals with minimum scar formation; joints remain flexible and functional

NURSING DIAGNOSIS: Body image disturbance related to perception of appearance and mobility

GOAL 1

Meet emotional needs

INTERVENTIONS

Convey positive attitude toward child
Encourage parents to visit
Encourage as much independence as condition allows
Arrange for continued schooling
Promote peer contact where possible

EXPECTED OUTCOMES

Child accepts efforts of family and caregivers
Child engages in activities with others according to age and capabilities

GOAL 2

Help build positive body image

INTERVENTIONS

Explore feelings concerning physical appearance
Discuss feelings about returning to home and family, school, and friends
Provide reinforcement of positive aspects of appearance and capabilities
Point out evidence of healing
Discuss aids that camouflage disfigurement
- Wigs
- Clothing, for example, turtleneck sweaters
- Makeup

Provide recreational and diversional activities
Promote constructive thinking in child

EXPECTED OUTCOMES

Child discusses feelings and concerns regarding appearance and perceived reactions of others
Child verbalizes positive suggestions for adjusting to appearance

GOAL 3

Promote self-care

INTERVENTIONS

Assist with self-care activities as needed
Encourage self-care according to capabilities
Begin early in hospitalization to discuss "going home"
Accept regressive behavior where appropriate
Help child develop independence and self-help capabilities

EXPECTED OUTCOMES

Child verbalizes and otherwise demonstrates interest in going home
Child engages in self-help activities

NURSING DIAGNOSIS: Altered family processes related to situational crisis (child with a serious injury)

GOAL 1

Prepare family for discharge

INTERVENTIONS

Teach wound care to caregiver
Discuss diet, rest, and activity
Explore attitudes toward child's reentry into the family
Explore family's concept regarding child's capabilities and the possible restrictions and freedom they will allow
Help family set realistic goals for themselves, child, and other family members
Help family acquire needed equipment and supplies

EXPECTED OUTCOMES

Family demonstrates an understanding of the needs of the child and the impact child's condition will have on them
Family sets realistic goals for selves, child, and others

Continued.

NURSING CARE PLAN
The Child with Burns: Management and Rehabilitative Stages—cont'd

GOAL 2

Participate in follow-up care

INTERVENTIONS

Coordinate team management of child and family
Arrange for return visits
Assess needs of family
Arrange for referral to agencies based on needs assessment
Collaborate with school nurse to help with child's reintegration into school and the world of peers
Visit school to prepare teacher and peers, if possible

EXPECTED OUTCOMES

Family maintains contact with health providers
Child attends school regularly and interacts with age-mates

See also:
Nursing Care Plan: The Child in the Hospital, Chapter 26
Nursing Care Plan: The Family of the Ill or Hospitalized Child, Chapter 26

ity are promoted during dressing changes. Predictability is increased by providing cues (nurses wearing specific clothing for dressing changes), focusing the patient on the procedure, and providing children with information about physical sensations they are likely to experience (e.g., pulling, stinging, pressure) before they experience them. Controllability is enhanced by providing the children with as many choices as possible during the burn care and encouraging active participation. These strategies are unlike the traditional approaches of distraction and passivity. "Learned helplessness" is most intense when the outcomes are unpleasant and the situation is perceived to be unchangeable (Murphy, 1982). See suggestions for reducing the stress of burn wound management outlined in Box 29-19.

New procedures or changes in routine need to be explained. When possible, there should be consistency in members of the staff who care for the children and the routine for procedures and activities. Providing some order in their world reduces the anxieties related to apprehension about the unknown. Children feel comfortable with the known, the routine.

Outer dressings (if any) are removed before placing a child in the tub, but adherent dressings are more easily removed after soaking in the water. Loose or easily detached tissue is also removed during hydrotherapy, and children are encouraged to move about as much as possible to exercise muscles and reduce contracture formation. They need encouragement and every little bit of healing pointed out as evidence that they are getting better. Merely saying that they are better is insufficient as they gaze at unsightly wounds. Providing something constructive to do helps the child to focus on something other than the procedure. In dressing the wound, it is important that all areas be clean, that medication be amply applied, and that no two burned surfaces touch each other, such as fingers or toes, or the ears touching the head.

Ointments are applied directly to the burn wound surface with sterile tongue blades or the sterile gloved hand. The layer of cream or ointment should be applied ⅛ inch thick. It can be left uncovered or covered with a layer of fine-mesh gauze and secured with stretch gauze or elastic tubular netting. For areas that are small or difficult to cover, strips of fine-mesh gauze are impregnated with the medication and then applied to the wound.

There are some psychologic implications that may influence a child's reaction to the hydrotherapy and application of medication. Children who acquired the burn from hot water are particularly fearful, especially if the injury was inflicted as a punishment (battered child). Application of the medication also can be a painful experience, when mafenide (Sulfamylon) cream is the agent employed. Both the nurse and the children must understand that there is a painful sensation often described as "burning" that may have special significance for these children, who must be reassured that the medication is not inflicting further injury.

When occlusive dressings are applied, elastic bandages are worn over dressings to prevent epithelial breakdown, to

Box 29-19 GUIDELINES FOR EASING DISTRESS OF DRESSING CHANGES IN BURN MANAGEMENT

Have all materials ready before beginning.
Administer appropriate analgesics
Remind child of impending procedure to provide sufficient time for child to prepare for the ordeal.
Allow child to test and approve the temperature of the water for hydrotherapy.
Allow child to state on which area of the body to begin.
Allow child to request *one* short rest period during procedure.
Allow child to remove dressings if desired.
Provide something constructive for child to do during procedure (e.g., holding a package of dressings or roll of Kerlix, holding someone's hand).
Inform child when the procedure is near completion.
Praise child for cooperation.

stimulate circulation, and to make mobility easier. The bandage is applied in a figure eight to promote optimum circulation. A stable dressing is especially important when the children are ambulatory.

There are other aspects of burn care of which nurses should be aware. Many children are placed in protective isolation, which severely limits their contact with others. Complete coverings on all who enter their presence, including most of the face, serve to further isolate these children. Children who are accustomed to having someone nearby continuously, as in the intensive care burn unit, may become anxious and uneasy when transferred to a transitional unit or a regular unit where staff members are available only intermittently or when summoned.

Nutrition. After the initial phase of care, children are usually allowed oral feedings (unless paralytic ileus persists). If they will not eat, tube feeding is necessary, but every effort should be made to encourage oral intake without a power struggle. Food is often the one area in which the child can exert considerable control. Serving regular meals even though a child may take only a small amount helps to maintain the habit of eating by mouth. For older children, forming a contract with them (with suitable reward) can encourage oral intake and avoid the need for supplemental tube feeding.

Because children frequently lack appetite and their caloric needs and protein needs are markedly increased, a great deal of encouragement, help, and patience is required on the part of the nursing staff. Consultation with the parents and the dietitian is arranged to determine the best way to provide needed nutrients in foods the child will be more likely to eat. Children who are old enough to participate should be included in the planning. Nourishing snacks are provided between regularly scheduled mealtimes, and if children eat better at times other than scheduled mealtimes, that is when they should be fed. Most important, meals should not be scheduled immediately after a dressing change. Most children are too physically exhausted and too emotionally upset to eat at this time.

Many children eat better when they can feed themselves and when they can eat in an atmosphere more nearly like what they are accustomed to at home. Even if they are unable to feed themselves (e.g., if their arms are bandaged), they do better if they can sit up or at least see the tray of food so that they can instruct the person feeding them how they prefer their food and what they want to be fed next. When their condition allows, children enjoy sitting at a table for their meals, especially with other children. Parents are encouraged to bring a child's favorite dish from home.

Prevent complications: acute care. Attempts should be made to decrease the excess metabolic expenditures of burned children. This means avoiding overheating and underheating. The hypermetabolic response is temperature sensitive but not temperature dependent. Environmental temperatures greater than skin temperature cause the metabolic rate of patients with burns in excess of 40% to increase twice the normal rate. Therefore the environmental temperature in the child's room should be maintained between 28° and 33° C (82.4° to 91.4° F) to minimize metabolic expenditure and maximize comfort (Herndon and others, 1985).

Hypothermia is also a threat, and a means must be provided to prevent heat loss, such as expeditious dressing changes to avoid prolonged exposure and intermittent hypothermia that result in "cold stress." An overhead warming unit may be provided to maintain body heat. Although evaporative heat loss is unchanged, the warmer air reduces the conductive, convective, and radiant heat losses from the denuded areas. Heat is often provided by means of a heat cradle over the child, but, if employed, the heat source should be situated well away from the child's body. Other methods include electric heaters, which should be situated 4 to 5 feet (1.2 to 1.5 m) away to avoid overheating, and maintaining room temperature sufficiently elevated to reduce evaporative loss. This can be extremely uncomfortable for persons attending the child, however.

The chief danger in this phase of burn care is infection—wound infection, generalized sepsis, and bacterial pneumonia. All burn patients are treated in a protected environment. Staff and visitors change into "scrub" clothing when entering the burn unit (Fig. 29-13). Children on open units are placed in protective isolation. It is important to make accurate ongoing assessments of all parameters that provide clues for diagnosis. For example, wound cultures are done at least three times weekly, and a blood culture is indicated in any child with a rectal temperature of 39.5° C (103° F) or higher.

Antacids are usually administered prophylactically to prevent or minimize the effect of Curling ulcer, but nurses must be alert for any signs of bleeding.

Continued observations are made to detect any indica-

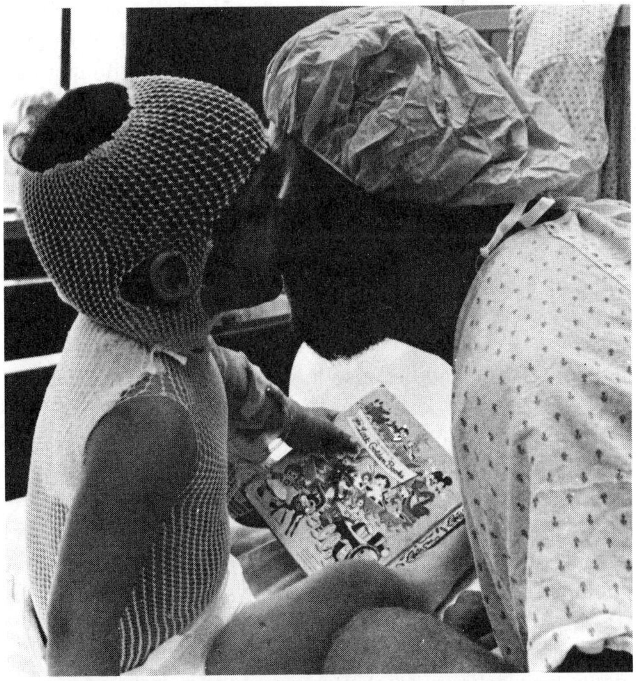

Fig. 29-13. Visitors wear cover gowns and hair coverings while child is in a protected environment.

tion of other complications associated with burns and their management. Rashes are not uncommon in children and may be of viral origin or a reaction to medications. They should be evaluated. The nurse must be alert to the possibility of any of the complications described previously—hypertension, renal disorders, and convulsion disorders.

Because children are reluctant to move because doing so causes pain or discomfort, stiffness and joint contracture develop easily. In an effort to prevent this complication, they are encouraged to move whenever feasible and active physiotherapy is included as an essential aspect of burn care. When children are resting or sleeping, contracture is prevented by proper splinting. Children's natural tendency is to be active, and they will usually move spontaneously unless the pain is severe.

Prevent complications: long-term care. The rehabilitative phase of burn care begins when permanent closure of the wound is implemented. The primary focus of this phase is to obtain functional use of burned areas and cosmetic results as nearly normal as possible. Efforts in the care of children with skin grafts are directed toward facilitating a "take." Trauma, infection, and bleeding must be avoided for a successful transplantation to occur. When the grafted area is left exposed, children must be immobilized to prevent the graft from becoming dislodged. Flat surfaces usually pose few problems, but grafts over irregular or mobile areas may require special techniques such as splints or skeletal traction. Small children usually need to be restrained, and sedation is sometimes needed for very restless or uncooperative children for the first 2 or 3 days after surgery.

The exposed method allows for easier inspection of the grafts, and collection of fluid under the graft can be removed by gently rolling the fluid out with a sterile applicator. This should be attempted with collections of fluid 1.25 cm (½ inch) or less from the edge of the graft. For those further toward the middle, a tiny slit is made in the graft tissue through which the fluid can be rolled. The less disturbance to any fibrous attachments, the better.

Some plastic surgeons prefer to use occlusive pressure dressings over the grafted tissue or secured with sutures attached to normal surrounding skin and tied over the grafted skin to hold it in place. Wet dressings are occasionally applied over lace grafts and kept moist with antimicrobial agents, silver nitrate, or normal saline solution. Moist dressings are covered with dry absorbent gauze. Plastic wraps are contraindicated because they cause buildup of heat and moisture that may cause maceration of the graft.

Wound contraction and scar tissue formation are normal parts of wound healing (Fig. 29-14). Scar tissue is metabolically active tissue that continually rearranges itself; as a result, disabling contractures, deformity, and disfigurement are ever-present possibilities. Part of home care frequently includes continuation of regular physical therapy (Fig. 29-15). Splints and other methods are employed to minimize these long-term effects. Pressure splints and elastic bandages or elasticized (Jobst) garments help reduce scar hypertrophy and are sometimes worn for months after hospitalization (Fig. 29-16). Parents should be advised that these garments are expensive and need to be replaced frequently. It is also advisable to have two garments if the child wears it 24 hours a day, to allow for laundering and care.

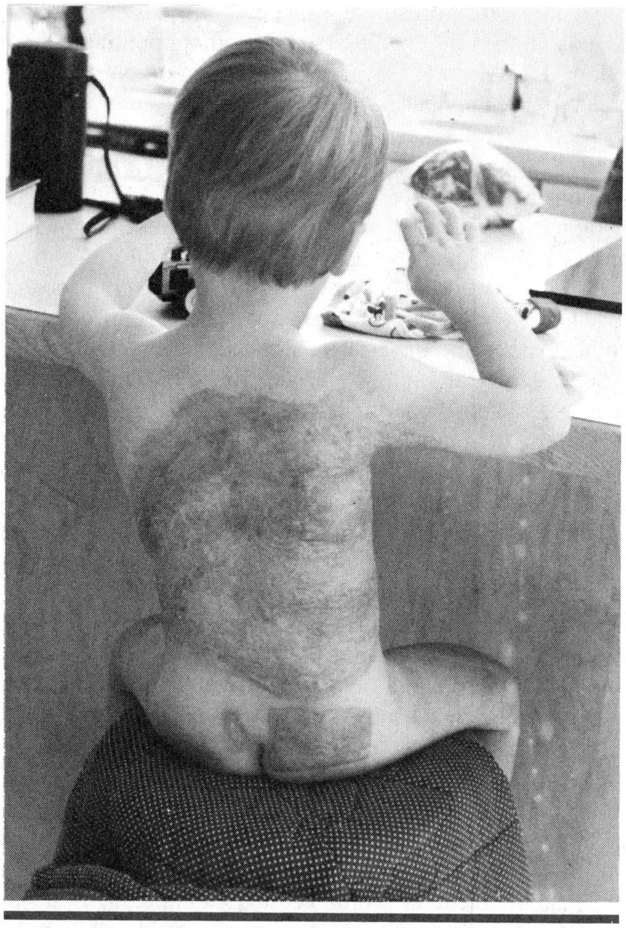

Fig. 29-14. Extensive scars from flame burn. Note donor graft site on right buttock.

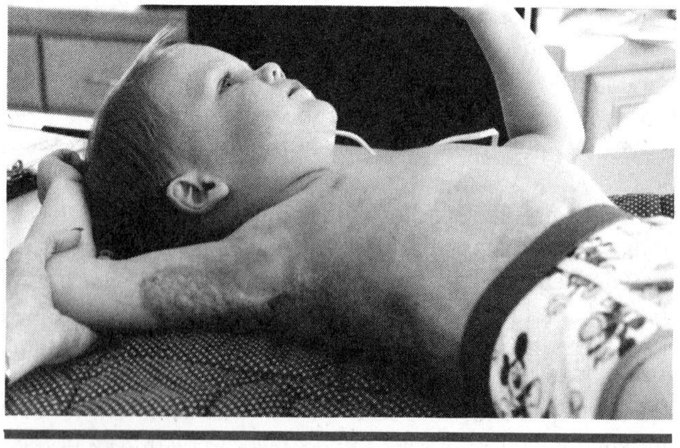

Fig. 29-15. Daily physical therapy to prevent contracture deformity is continued at home.

Scar tissue has some properties that are significant, particularly for growing children. Intense itching occurs in healing burn wounds and scar tissue until the scar is no

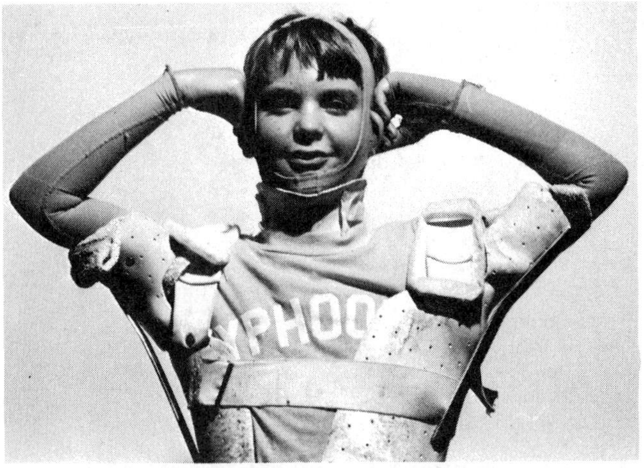

Fig. 29-16. Child in elasticized (Jobst) garment and "airplane" splints.

longer edematous and raised. It is usually treated with administration of diphenhydramine (Benadryl) or hydroxyzine (Atarax) and frequent application of a moisturizer such as Eucerin cream, cocoa butter, or vitamin E lotion along with massage therapy. Scar tissue does not grow as do normal tissues, which may create difficulties, especially in areas such as hands. Additional surgery is sometimes needed to maintain function in contracted areas. Because scar tissue has no sweat glands, children with extensive scarring may have difficulty during hot weather or when they develop a fever. Parents need to be informed of this characteristic so that they can be prepared to find alternative cooling methods when indicated.

Severely burned children must return to the hospital periodically for additional skin grafts and scar revisions, especially to release contractures over joint spaces and for cosmetic considerations. Achievement of optimum results frequently requires years. In the meantime, burn scars are unsightly, and although improvements can be made, hope should not be extended to the parents and child for complete cosmetic and functional repair.

The psychologic pain and sequelae of severe burn trauma are as intense as the physical trauma. All burned children have a tremendous amount of pain, often continuous for varying periods, and are separated from the family for extended periods. During the painful ordeal of hospitalization, children develop coping mechanisms for dealing with the acute and ever-present pain. Self-induced hypnosis is not uncommon. In addition, a continual barrage of painful therapeutic and diagnostic procedures is inflicted by others. This pain, however, is usually psychologically repressed as children attempt to forget these painful incidents.

Life becomes a struggle for children after burn trauma. They are puzzled, confused, and bombarded by a new way of life in a frightening world of strange people, things, and language. They wonder why this has happened to *them*—what they have done that they should be punished so. Past experiences cannot serve them in this crisis. They do not understand the "ugliness" and disfigurement they see as their bodies. They wonder, "Am I going to die?"

Preparation for facing friends and classmates may be more than they are able to cope with; some severely burned children are ashamed to show their bodies in the hospital. In addition, pressure garments and other therapeutic measures greatly intensify the feeling of being different. It is not difficult to imagine how children dread facing a world of stares or imagined stares. Undressing at school can be a painful experience. It is not surprising that many children withdraw from contacts with others, even at a very early age. In time, as understanding and acceptance increase, they may feel more comfortable with themselves, and the emotional scars may fade somewhat.

The impact of such severe injury taxes the capabilities of children at all ages, but young children, who suffer acutely from separation anxiety, and adolescents, who are developing an identity, are probably most affected psychologically. Toddlers cannot begin to comprehend why the parents whom they love and who have protected them from hurt can leave them in such a dreadful place and allow others to inflict such painful indignities on them. Adolescents, in the process of achieving independence from families and seeking to find out who they are in the world, find themselves in a dependent position with a damaged body. Being different from others at a time when conformity and being like their peers are so important is difficult to accept. These children need understanding adults to help them deal with the struggles concerning resentment and other feelings generated by such a catastrophe. A psychiatric nurse is often an integral member of the burn team and is invaluable to the total management of the children and their families.

Child support. One of the most difficult aspects of burn care, especially in children, is the impact it has on nurses. The appearance and smell of the burn and the necessary discomfort that must be inflicted on the child as a part of the therapy are often beyond the nurse's ability to cope and remain therapeutic. Throughout the entire process of burn management, nurses must deal with their own feelings and anxieties regarding their therapeutic role in burn care.

Children should begin early to do as much for themselves as possible and to be active participants in their care. It takes a great deal of warm firmness and fortitude on the part of the nurse to force these children to do this. Moving hurts. Many children are able to move and help themselves. Others need considerable help and encouragement. If children are unable to move, they should be told firmly but gently that it must be done, that the nurses will help them, and that it will be done as quickly as possible. They should be told how they can help to make it easier.

It is difficult to handle children with extensive burns. It is almost impossible to move and turn them without touching a burned area. Fortunately the discomfort lasts only for the short time they are being handled; once they are repositioned, it hurts no longer. Children may cry, but they usually stop once the procedure is over. Some children cry in anticipation of the move and may continue to cry afterward, but

THERAPEUTIC DIALOGUE

Burns

A 9-year-old child who has sustained 60% partial- and full-thickness burns from a barbecue fire is talking to the nurse.

CHILD: Why did God punish me like this?
NURSE: What do you mean?
CHILD: Why did God let me get burned when my grandpa was the one who started the grill?
NURSE: Your grandpa wasn't burned?
CHILD: No, only me. And it isn't fair. I was just sitting a little way from the grill.
NURSE: It sounds like you're wondering what you did to deserve this.
CHILD: That's right. God must hate me for letting me get burned.
NURSE: What could you have done to make God hate you?
CHILD: I don't know.
NURSE: Do you think that sometimes things just happen to people, and maybe nobody meant to hurt them?
CHILD: Yes, like in car accidents or plane acccidents.
NURSE: So why do you think your accident is any different?
CHILD: I don't know. Do you think it was just bad luck for me but not for my grandpa?
NURSE: Yes, I do. I don't believe anyone is punishing you. These unhappy things just happen, and nobody is to blame.

SUMMARY

This conversation helped the child deal with his guilt and also his resentment toward the grandfather, whom he had refused to see.

even small children learn that the hurt stops when the moving is over. Special frames and beds can be used to facilitate the process and to keep children positioned in an attitude that prevents contracture deformity. Fowler position is comfortable but may produce hip and knee contractures that take months to correct.

Children should be encouraged to participate in as many aspects of their care as possible. With illness, children always regress to the developmental level that allows them to deal with the stress. However, there are limits to how long they should be permitted to remain at a lower level of functioning. To lie passively while others tend to their needs is not "normal" and may be detrimental. As their condition permits, children can be expected to do things that they were capable of doing for themselves before they were burned, such as oral hygiene, face washing, feeding themselves, and playing. Allowing children to make choices and to help make decisions about the time of their care and recreational activities makes them feel a part of the team and provides them a small measure of control. They will probably require assistance; however, as children see themselves contributing to their care, they gain confidence and self-esteem. Fears and anxieties diminish with accomplishment and self-confidence.

Activities are selected and encouraged according to each child's level of development and interest, but, as with any ill child, they should be somewhat simpler and less challenging than would be expected in a state of health. Otherwise their already taxed energies may be further depleted and self-esteem threatened. Quiet games and activities such as reading, coloring, drawing, games, and puzzles are always appropriate. Television is a satisfactory diversion but should not replace active participation and should not substitute for contacts with others. Play that encourages the expression of feelings of guilt, frustration, and anger is especially therapeutic. Contacts should also include those that help children to understand what can be expected, their role, and what the nurse will do. During the acute, resuscitative phase, children are frequently isolated, but they should be moved to where they have contact with others, especially other children, as soon as their physical condition allows. School-age children should continue with schoolwork.

Children need to be bolstered in other ways. They like to look and smell nice, and the unattractive burns, dressings, and assorted paraphernalia do little to foster a positive self-image. They know how they appear to others, and small things such as careful hair combing and a bright ribbon, colorful nightgown or pajamas (when possible), slippers, or any decoration (a flower, pin, necklace, badge) will help make them feel that they look better and are worthwhile to others.

All hospitalized children, especially those who must undergo painful procedures, must be allowed to express their anger and frustration appropriately through verbalization or play. They need to know that their injury and the treatments are not punishment for specific or general, real or imagined transgressions and to know that nurses understand their fears, anger, and discomfort. They also need body contact. This is often difficult to arrange for the child with massive injury. The discomfort associated with moving and the bulky, messy dressings or the bare open wound are deterrents and frequently provide justification for the nurse to avoid such action because of fear or repulsion. Even older children enjoy sitting on the nurse's or parent's lap and being cuddled and hugged. This can be a comfort in times of stress or used as a reward, but most of all it should be kept in mind that it is a natural part of childhood.

Family support. Members of the family as well as the child feel the impact of severe burn injury. They are concerned about the child's survival, recovery, and future appearance. Because they, too, have overwhelming anxieties, fears, frustrations, and feelings of guilt, their needs must be met in order that they, in turn, can provide the support and encouragement so desperately needed by the child. It is the family, particularly the parents, who are the most significant persons in the child's life.

As in any emergency situation, all attention is focused on the child, and the parents are forced to abandon their child to others. Often they do not know what is happening, how their child is doing, or if their child is even alive. They feel powerless and ineffectual. Nurses can alleviate parents' anxiety simply by acknowledging that they appreciate their concern, explain what is being done, explain why the child is crying, and offer whatever physical comfort is available.

Most parents feel overwhelming guilt about their child's illness. Whether justified or not, they feel responsible for the accident or injury—as if in some way they should have been able to prevent it. These feelings sometimes impede the child's rehabilitation. Parents may indulge the child and give in to every whim. Some are unable to look at or touch the child who is edematous, lethargic, and covered with unsightly eschar. Parents need to be told what to expect in the child, concerning both appearance and behavior. The burn wound will look worse before it looks better, and the child may exhibit unpredictable behavior when the parents are present. Ill children often cry when the parents are around, almost certainly when they prepare to leave; at other times they may reject the parents.

Nurses are in the most opportune position to assist parents to cope with the stresses of the child's illness and their own feelings of guilt and helplessness. The parents need to be informed of the child's progress and helped in their efforts to cope with their feelings while providing support to the child. The nurse is the person who can help them understand that it is not selfish to look after themselves and their own needs in order that they can better meet the needs of the child. For parents whose response to the illness is too severe or whose response to stress is manifest in destructive behavior, professional help may be needed.

Evaluation

The effectiveness of nursing interventions is determined by continual reassessment and evaluation of care based on the following observational guidelines and expected outcomes:

1. Observe child's behavior during all aspects of care; listen for verbal cues; use pain assessment record to evaluate effectiveness of analgesia.
2. Observe the burn wound and the patient's general condition.
3. Observe child's eating behavior and amount of food consumed; weigh daily or as indicated.
4. Inspect burn wound for signs of infection; take vital signs; observe for evidence of gastric bleeding, respiratory complications, weight loss, altered hemoglobin level, and neurologic signs.
5. Observe for evidence of healing and scar formation; assess effectiveness of physical therapy and appliances (splints, pressure garments).
6. Observe the child's and family's behaviors; interview the child and family regarding their feelings and concerns.

Expected outcomes:
See Nursing Care Plan, pp. 1316-1318.

Prevention of Burn Injury

Nurses have an obligation to be active in educating parents, children, and others in prevention of burn injuries. Children can be taught the hazards of flame and what to do in case of fire. They should be taught respect for matches, lighters, and other items, such as firecrackers and torches, that might cause fires or catch clothing afire. Items that create a flame, such as cigarette lighters, should not be used to entertain children as toys or thrown away where children have access to them. Any heating unit, flame heater, or fire is a potentially lethal device, and children must learn to maintain a safe distance from the heat source. They can learn to be "fire marshals" and inspect their homes and neighborhood for fire hazards.

Children can also be taught how to behave in case of fire. Every family should practice fire drills and designate specific responsibilities for the child in getting himself to safety from any location. Special decals are available that can be placed in windows to help firemen identify children's rooms in burning buildings. Older children should know how to report a fire and the location of the nearest fire alarm box. All children should be taught to crawl to safety. Children have a tendency to crawl under beds or into cupboards, where they are difficult to locate. Children need an explanation regarding the appearance of firemen, whose protective clothing and masks may be misinterpreted as "monsters" coming to get them. Children should also be taught how to behave if their clothing becomes ignited. For example, a child who calmly walked to the kitchen where her mother was working and reported that her nightgown was afire received much less severe burns than a child in a similar situation who ran around in a panic.

Parent education should be aimed at prevention and emergency care for burns. Hot water heaters should be set at a safe temperature, and infant formulas do not need to be warmed and should not be heated in a microwave oven (see also Chapter 12). See Fig. 29-17 for temperatures related to common household activities. Parents can be taught commonsense safety precautions. Many persons are not aware that simple acts can prevent tragedy. Small or helpless children should not be left alone in the kitchen or bathroom. Children can turn on a gas range, especially where the knobs are situated at the front of the stove; run hot water; and pull hot items onto themselves, including

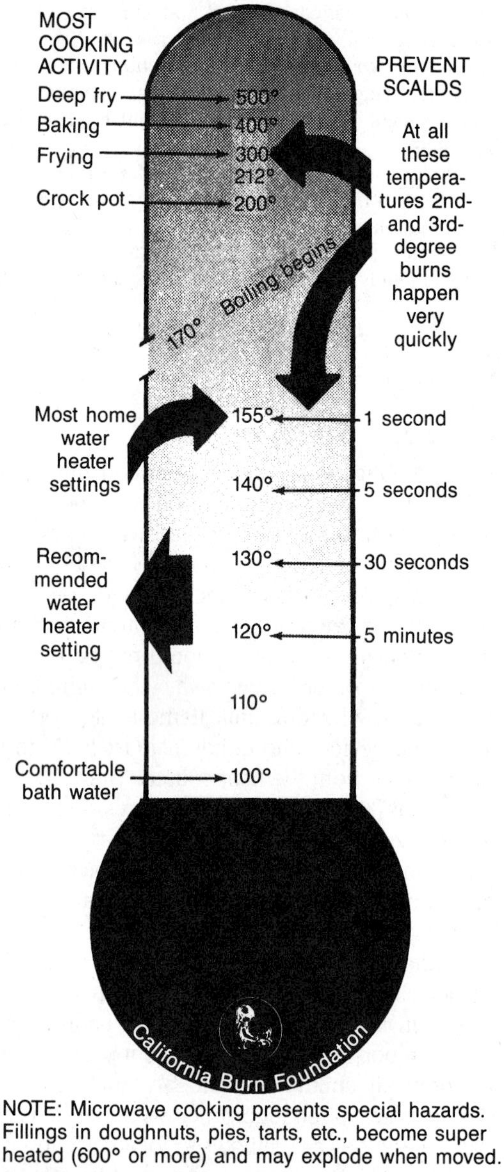

Fig. 29-17. Temperatures associated with common burn injuries in the home. NOTE: Most authorities recommend that water heaters be kept at the lowest safe setting of 120° F.
Reproduced with permission of the California Burn Foundation, Canoga Park, CA.

small children in walkers, who can also back into a fire or a heater.

It is also characteristic of small children in a bathtub of hot water to remain still or even to squat down rather than to climb out. Crawling infants or toddlers should be kept away from electric cords on which they might chew. Parents should recognize that children's thin skin is sensitive to direct sunlight and limit the time the child is exposed to the sun (see Chapter 18). Preventive measures regarding burns are discussed in Chapters 12 and 14. A handy resource for parents, the *Fire Safety Book,** outlines activities for presenting safety messages appropriate for preschoolers.

Instruction in emergency first-aid measures should be part of parent education. Most lay persons still treat burns with application of butter or petroleum jelly. They need to be aware that current treatment is cooling the area with cool water. It is important that they have some criteria for determining when the injury can be treated with a simple dressing and when to seek medical aid.

Public education through community groups, the communication media, and offices, clinics, and homes is part of nurses' responsibility in preventive care. Information regarding safety devices for the home, such as sprinkling systems, smoke detectors, and fire extinguishers, can be disseminated to a large audience. Nurses can be effective campaigners for safety legislation, such as fireproofing children's clothing and for improvement of substandard housing. As health professionals, their voices can and should be heard.

Additional information on burn care and prevention can be obtained from the **American Burn Association*** and the **National Safety Council.†** The **Alisa Ann Ruch Burn Foundation‡** provides assistance to burn victims and burn centers, supports research to improve burn care and treatment, and promotes public education in fire and burn prevention. The *Shriners Burns Institutes* are staffed to treat patients with acute burns, needing plastic or reconstructive surgery as a result of healed burns, with severe scarring resulting in contractures or interference of proper limb mobility, or with scarring and deformity of the face. Applications can be obtained through the Shrine Temple, Shrine Club, or Shriners Hospitals or by contacting the **International Shrine Headquarters.§**

*Available for $2.00 from The Children's Television Workshop, Community Education Service Division, Dept. FS, 1 Lincoln Plaza, New York, NY 10023.

*New York–Cornell Medical Center, 525 E. 68th St., Rm. F758, New York, NY 10021; (212) 746-5454.
†444 North Michigan Ave., Chicago, IL 60611; (800) 621-7615.
‡20944 Sherman Way, Suite 115, Canoga Park, CA 91303; (818) 883-7700.
§2900 Rocky Point Dr., Tampa, FL 33607; (800) 237-5055; in Florida (800) 282-9161.

KEY POINTS

- Acute gastrointestinal disorders of childhood that cause fluid depletion are diarrhea and vomiting.
- Mechanisms known to produce diarrhea are osmotic factors, diminished absorption or increased secretion of water and electrolytes, reduction in anatomic or functional surface area, and altered bowel motility.
- Acute infectious gastroenteritis is caused by enterotoxin production, invasion and destruction of epithelial cells, penetration and system invasion, or adherence without destruction of mucosa and without enterotoxin production.

- Vomiting may result from infectious disorders, responses to an allergen or ingestion of drugs or other toxic substances, symptoms associated with appendicitis or gastrointestinal obstruction, motion sickness, environmental stress, and oral-defense mechanisms.
- Nurses should observe character, frequency, amount, and force of vomitus.
- Shock is divided into three stages: compensated, uncompensated, and irreversible.
- Types of shock are hypovolemic, including hemorrhagic, plasma loss, and extracellular fluid loss; distributive, including anaphylactic, septic, and neurogenic; cardiogenic, resulting from congenital heart disease, primary pulmonary failure, and dysrhythmias; and obstructive, from inflow or outflow obstruction.
- Persons at risk for anaphylaxis may be identified by a history of previous allergic reaction, history of atopy, history of severe reactions in family, and positive skin test to the allergen.
- Nursing management of the patient with toxic shock syndrome focuses on prevention and education.
- Burns are caused by thermal, chemical, electric, or radioactive agents.
- Burns are assessed on the basis of percentage of body surface burned, depth, location, age, etiologic agent, respiratory involvement, general health, and presence of associated injury or condition.
- Emergency measures for severe burns include stopping the burning process; assessing for airway, breathing, and circulation; covering the burn; transporting the child to medical aid; and providing reassurance to child and family.
- Management of minor burns is facilitating wound healing, relieving discomfort, and preventing complications.
- Management of major burns is facilitating wound healing, relieving discomfort, replacing destroyed skin, preventing and/or treating complications, and providing rehabilitation.

REFERENCES

American Academy of Pediatrics, Committee on Nutrition: Use of oral fluid therapy and posttreatment feeding following enteritis in children in a developed country, Pediatrics 75:358-361, 1985.

Andres, J.M.: Advances in understanding the pathogenesis of persistent diarrhea in young children, Adv. Pediatr. 35:483-498, 1988.

Bailit, I.W.: Anaphylaxis. In Gellis, S.S., and Kagan, B.M., editors: Current pediatric therapy 12, Philadelphia, 1986, W.B. Saunders Co.

Baker, S.P., O'Neill, B., and Karpf, R.: The injury fact book, Lexington, MA, 1984, Lexington Books.

Bass, D.M., and Walker, W.A.: Acute and chronic nonspecific diarrhea syndromes. In Gellis, S.S., and Kagan, B.M., editors: Current pediatric therapy 12, Philadelphia, 1986, W.B. Saunders Co.

Brown, K.H., and MacLean, W.C., Jr.: Nutritional management of acute diarrhea: an appraisal of the alternatives, Pediatrics 73:119-125, 1984.

Burke, J.F., and others: Successful use of a physiologicallly acceptable artificial skin in the treatment of extensive burn injury, Ann. Surg. 194:413-428, 1981.

Caniano, D.A., Beaver, B.L., and Boles, E.T.: Child abuse: an update on surgical management in 256 cases, Ann. Surg. 203:219-224, 1986.

Carpenter, C.C., Greenough, W.B., and Pierce, N.E.: Oral-rehydration therapy—the role of polymeric substrates, N. Engl. J. Med. 319:1346-1348, 1988.

Centers for Disease Control: Follow-up on toxic-shock syndrome, MMWR 29:441-445, 1980.

Coren, C.V.: Burn injuries in children, Pediatr. Ann. 16:328-339, 1987.

Crone, R.K.: Acute circulatory failure in children, Pediatr. Clin. North Am. 27:525-538, 1980.

Davidson, G.P., Robb, T.A., and Kirubakaran, C.P.: Bacterial contamination of the small intestine as an important cause of chronic diarrhea and abdominal pain: diagnosis by breath hydrogen test, Pediatrics 74:229-235, 1984.

DeWitt, T.G., Humphrey, K.F., and McCarthy, P.: Clinical predictors of acute bacterial diarrhea in young children, Pediatrics 76:551-556, 1985.

Dodge, J.A., and others: Toddler diarrhea and prostaglandins, Arch. Dis. Child. 56:705-707, 1981.

Dupont, H., and others: Prevention of traveler's diarrhea (emporiatic enteritis): prophylactic administration of subsalicylate bismuth, JAMA 243:237-241, 1980.

Dupont, H., and others: Prevention of traveler's diarrhea with trimethoprim-sulfamethoxazole and trimethoprim alone, Gastroenterology 84:75-80, 1983.

Dyer, C.: Burn care in the emergent period, J. Emerg. Nurs. 6:9-16, 1980.

Fleisher, D.R.: Nausea and vomiting. In Gellis, S.S., and Kagan, B.M., editors: Current pediatric therapy 12, Philadelphia, 1986, W.B. Saunders Co.

Food and Drug Administration: Topical PEG in burn ointments, FDA Drug Bull. 12(3):25-26, 1982.

Freeman, L., and others: Brief prophylaxis with doxycycline for the prevention of traveler's diarrhea, Gastroenterology 84:276-280, 1983.

Gallico, G.G., and others: Permanent coverage of large burn wounds with autologous-cultured human epithelium, N. Engl. J. Med. 311:448-451, 1984.

Ghishan, F.K.: The transport of electrolytes in the gut and the use of oral rehydration solutions, Pediatr. Clin. North Am. 35:35-51, 1988.

Graham, D.Y., and others: Double-bind comparison of bismuth subsalicylate and placebo in the prevention and treatment of enterotoxigenic *Escherichia coli*–induced diarrhea in volunteers, Gastroenterology 85:1017-1022, 1983.

Greene, H.L., and Ghishan, F.K.: Excessive fluid intake as a cause of chronic diarrhea in young children, J. Pediatr. 102:836-840, 1983.

Groothuis, J.R., Berman, S., and Chapman, J.: Effect of carbohydrate ingested on outcome in infants with mild gastroenteritis, J. Pediatr. 108:903-906, 1986.

Guerrant, R.L., Lohr, J.A., and Williams, E.K.: Acute infectious diarrhea. I. Epidemiology, etiology and pathogenesis, Pediatr. Infect. Dis. 5:353-359, 1986.

Guzzetta, P., and Holihan, J.: Burns. In Eichelberger, M., and Pratsch, G., editors: Pediatric trauma care, Rockville, MD, 1988, Aspen Systems Corp.

Harmel, R.P., Vane, D.W., and King, D.R.: Burn care in childen: special considerations, Clin. Plast. Surg. 13:95-105, 1986.

Herndon, D.N., and others: Treatment of burns in children, Pediatr. Clin. North Am. 32:1311-1332, 1985.

Hyams, J.S., and others: Carbohydrate malabsorption following fruit juice ingestion in young children, Pediatrics 82:64-68, 1988.

Jacoby, F.: Care of the massive burn wound, Crit. Care Q. 7(3):44-53, 1984.

Kavanagh, C.K., and Freeman, R.: Burn care and the pediatric patient: a preliminary report, PRN Forum 3(2):1-3, 1984.

Kibbee, E.: Burn pain management, Crit. Care Q. 7(3):54-62, 1984.

Lamb, L.S.: Think you know septic shock? Nursing '82 12(1):34-43, 1982.

LaMotte, R., and Thalhammer, J.: Peripheral neural mechanisms of cutaneous hyperalgesia following mild injury by heat, Neuroscience 2:765-781, 1982.

Libber, S.M, and Slayton, D.J.: Childhood burns reconsidered: the child, the family, and the burn injury, J. Trauma 24:245-252, 1984.

Margolis, P.A., and others: Effects of unrestricted diet on mild infantile diarrhea, Am. J. Dis. Child. 144:162-164, 1990.

McLoughlin, E., and Crawford, J.D.: Burns, Pediatr. Clin. North Am. 32:61-75, 1985.

Morriss, F.C.: Analphylaxis. In Levin, D.L., Morriss, F.C., and Moore, G.C., editors: A practical guide to pediatric intensive care, ed. 2, St. Louis, 1984, Mosby–Year Book, Inc.

Murphy, S.A.: Learned helplessness: from concept to comprehension, Perspect. Psychiatr. Care 20(2):27-32, 1982.

O'Conner, N.E., and others: Grafting of burns with cultured epithelium prepared from autologous epidermal cells, Lancet 1:75-78, 1982.

Penny, M.E., Paredes, P., and Brown, K.H.: Clinical and nutritional consequences of lactose feeding during persistent postenteritis diarrhea, Pediatrics 84:835-844, 1989.

Perkin, R.M., and Anas, N.G.: Cardiovascular evaluation and support in the critically ill child, Pediatr. Ann. 15(1):30-41, 1986.

Perkin, R.M., and Levin, D.L.: Shock in the pediatric patient, part I, J. Pediatr. 101:163-169, 1982a.

Perkin, R.M., and Levin, D.L.: Shock in the pediatric patient. II. Therapy, J. Pediatr. 101:319-323, 1982b.

Pizarro, D., Posada, G., and Levine, M.M.: Hypernatremic diarrheal dehydration treated with "slow" (12-hour) oral rehydration therapy: a preliminary report, J. Pediatr. 104:316-319, 1984.

Robinson, M.D., and Seward, P.N.: Thermal injury in children, Pediatr. Emerg. Care 3(4):266-270, 1987.

Santosham, M., and others: Role of soy-based, lactose-free formula during treatment of acute diarrhea, Pediatrics 76:292-298, 1985.

Silverman, A., and Roy, C.C.: Pediatric clinical gastroenterology, ed. 3, St. Louis, 1983, Mosby–Year Book, Inc.

Surh, L., and Read, S.E.: Staphylococcal tracheitis and toxic shock syndrome in a young child, J. Pediatr. 105:585-587, 1984.

Vesikari, T., and others: Protection of infants against rotovirus diarrhoea by RIT 4237 attenuated bovine rotovirus strain bacteria, Lancet 1:977-981, 1984.

Webster, H., and Veasy, L.G.: Intra-aortic balloon pumping in children, Heart Lung J. Crit. Care 14:548-555, 1985.

Weizman, Z.: Cola drinks and rehydration in acute diarrhea (letter), N. Engl. J. Med. 315:768, 1986.

Wiesenthal, A.M., and Todd, J.K.: Toxic shock syndrome in children aged 10 years or less, Pediatrics 74:112-117, 1984.

Zimmerman, J.J., and Dietrich, K.A.: Current perspectives on septic shock, Pediatr. Clin. North Am. 34:131-163, 1987.

Zimmerman, S.S.: Anaphylaxis. In Zimmerman, S.S., and Gildea, J.H.: Critical care pediatrics, Philadelphia, 1985, W.B. Saunders Co.

BIBLIOGRAPHY

Diarrhea

Anderson, B.J.: Tube feeding: is diarrhea inevitable, Am. J. Nurs. 86:705-706, 1986.

Boyne, L.J., Kerzner, B., and McClung, H.J.: Chronic nonspecific diarrhea: the value of a preliminary observation period to assess diet therapy, Pediatrics 76:557-561, 1985.

Brown, K.H., and others: Effect of continued oral feeding on clinical and nutritional outcomes of acute diarrhea in children, J. Pediatr. 112:191-200, 1988.

Buzby, M.: Chronic diarrhea: management in pediatrics, J. Pediatr. Health Care 3(3):163-165, 1989.

DeBenham, J.J., and others: Initial assessment and management of chronic diarrhea in toddlers, Pediatr. Nurs. 11(4):281-285, 1985.

DeSantis, L.: Cultural factors affecting newborn and infant diarrhea, J. Pediatr. Nurs. 3:391-398, 1988.

Farrell, M.K.: The diagnosis and treatment of diarrhea in children, Pediatr. Consult. 5(1):1-8, 1986.

Finberg, L.: Oral rehydration: finding the right solution, Contemp. Pediatr. 4(2):61-67, 1987.

Fitzgerald, J.F.: Management of the infant with persistent diarrhea, Pediatr. Infect. Dis. 4:6-9, 1985.

Grill, B.: Oral rehydration, food allergy, and specialized nutrition, Curr. Opin. Pediatr. 1:384-393, 1989.

Hamilton, J.R.: Treatment of acute diarrhea, Pediatr. Clin. North Am. 32:419-427, 1985.

Lifschitz, C.H., and others: Carbohydrate malabsorption in infants with diarrhea studied with the breath hydrogen test, J. Pediatr. 102:371-375, 1983.

Morgan, S.R., and Parks, B.: What is the role of oral electrolyte solution in diarrheal dehydration in children? Pediatr. Nurs. 11(3):215, 227, 1985.

Orenstein, S.R.: Enteral versus parenteral therapy for intractable diarrhea of infancy: a prospective, randomized trial, J. Pediatr. 109:277-286, 1986.

Pickering, L.K.: Antimicrobial therapy of gastrointestinal infections, Pediatr. Clin. North Am. 30:373-388, 1983.

Pizarro, D., and others: Oral rehydration in hypernatremic and hyponatremic diarrheal dehydration: treatment with oral glucose/electrolyte solution, Am. J. Dis. Child. 137:730-734, 1983.

Santosham, M., and others: Oral rehydration therapy for acute diarrhea in ambulatory children in the United States: a double-blind comparison of four different solutions, Pediatrics 76:159-166, 1985.

Sharifi, J., and Ghavami, F.: Oral rehydration therapy of severe diarrheal dehydration, Clin. Pediatr. 23:87-90, 1984.

Tucker, J.A., and Sussman-Karten, K.: Treating acute diarrhea and dehydration with an oral rehydration solution, Pediatr. Nurs. 13:169-174, 1987.

Infectious Gastroenteritis

Bartlett, A.V., and others: Diarrheal illness among infants and toddlers in day care centers. I. Epidemiology and pathogens, J. Pediatr. 107:495-502, 1985.

Bartlett, A.V., and others: Diarrheal illness among infants and toddlers in day care centers. II. Comparison with day care homes and households, J. Pediatr. 107:503-509, 1985.

Bartlett, A.V., III, Reves, R.R., and Pickering, L.K.: Rotavirus in infant-toddler day care centers: epidemiology relevant to disease control strategies, J. Pediatr. 113:435-441, 1988.

Cohen, M., and Balistreri, W.F.: Diagnosing and treating diarrhea, Contemp. Pediatr. 6(3):89-114, 1989.

Goodman, R.A., and others: Infectious diseases and child day care, Pediatrics 74:134-139, 1984.

Hamilton, J.R.: Viral enteritis, Pediatr. Clin. North Am. 35:89-101, 1988.

Hoffman, R.E., and Shillam, P.J.: The use of hygiene, cohorting, and antimicrobial therapy to control an outbreak of shigellosis, Am. J. Dis. Child. 144:219-221, 1990.

Kovacs, A., and others: Rotavirus gastroenteritis, Am. J. Dis. Child. 141:161-166, 1987.

Pickering, L.K, and others: Asymptomatic excretion of rotavirus before and after rotavirus diarrhea in children in day care centers, J. Pediatr. 112:361-365, 1988.

Radetsky, M.: Laboratory evaluation of acute diarrhea, Pediatr. Infect. Dis. 5:230-238, 1986.

Riesenberg, D.E.: How to protect day-care center children from infectious disease? JAMA 255:1245-1251, 1986.

St. Louis, M., and others: The emergence of grade A eggs as a major source of *Salmonella enteritidis* infections, JAMA 259:2103-2107, 1988.

Thompson, C.M., Jr., and others: *Clostridium difficile* in a pediatric population, Am. J. Dis. Child. 137:271-274, 1983.

Zedd, A.J., and others: Nosocomial *Clostridium difficile* reservoir in a neonatal intensive care unit, Pediatr. Infect. Dis. 3:429-432, 1984.

Shock

Briening, E.P.: Septic shock: tough cases that teach the most, RN 51:36-39, 1988.

Cohen, M.R.: Action stat! Drug-induced anaphylaxis, Nursing '85 15(2):43, 1985.

Corse, K.M., and Lambert, L.E.: Multisystem disorders: shock and trauma. In Smith, J.B., editor: Pediatric critical care, New York, 1983, John Wiley & Sons, Inc.

Hackleman, N.: The unwritten rules that saved Katie, RN 47(1):52-53, 1984.

Holt, M., McKenny, S., and Pribyl, C.: Shock—detecting it soon enough to save your patient: seven fast refreshers, part I, Nurs. Life 4(6):33-40, 1984.

Holt, M., McKenny, S., and Pribyl, C.: Shock—detecting it soon enough to save your patient: nine more fast refreshers, part II, Nurs. Life 5(1):33-40, 1985.

Kaplan, S.L., and Vargo, T.A.: Endotoxin shock in children. In Dickerman, J.D., and Lucey, J.F., editors: The critically ill child: diagnosis and medical management, ed. 3, Philadelphia, 1985, W.B. Saunders Co.

Keely, B.R.: Septic shock, Crit. Care Q. 7(4):59-67, 1985.

Morse, T.S.: Shock in infants and children. In Pierog, J.E., and Pierog, L.J., editors: Pediatric critical illness and injury, Rockville, MD, 1984, Aspen Systems Corp.

Randall, B.J.: Reacting to anaphylaxis, Nursing '85 16(3):34-40, 1986.

Rice, V.: Shock management. Part I. Fluid volume replacement, Crit. Care Nurse 4(6):69-82, 1984.

Rice, V.: Shock management. Part II. Pharmacologic intervention, Crit. Care Nurse 5(1):42-46, 48-49, 51-57, 1985.

Rimar, J.M.: Recognizing shock syndromes in infants and children, MCN 13:32-37, 1988.

Rimar, J.M.: Shock in infants and children: assessment and treatement, MCN 13:98-105, 1988.

Wahl, S.C.: Shock: how to detect it early, Nursing '89 19(1):53-59, 1989.

Toxic Shock Syndrome

Barbour, S.D., Shlaes, D.M., and Guertin, S.R.: Toxic-shock syndrome associated with nasal packing: analogy to tampon-associated illness, Pediatrics 73:163-165, 1984.

Buchdahl, R., and others: Toxic shock syndrome, Arch. Dis. Child. 60:563-567, 1985.

Dart, R., and Levitt, A.: Toxic shock syndrome associated with the use of the vaginal contraceptive sponge, JAMA 253:1877, 1985.

Faich, G., and others: Toxic shock syndrome in the vaginal contraceptive sponge, JAMA 255:216-218, 1986.

Resnick, S.D.: Toxic shock syndrome: recent developments in pathogenesis, J. Pediatr. 116:321-328, 1990.

Toxic shock syndrome: an update on symptoms and treatment, Nursing '85 15(9):74, 1985.

Whettam, J.: Update on toxic shock: how to spot it and treat it, RN 47(2):55-56, 58, 60, 1984.

Burns

Acres, C., and Kraft, E.R.: Skin transplantation, Am. J. Nurs. 81:1466-1467, 1981.

Arneson, S.W., and Triplett, J.L.: How children cope with disfiguring changes in their appearance. In Fore, C., and Poster, E.C., editors: Meeting psychosocial needs of children and families in health care, Washington, DC, 1985, Association for the Care of Children's Health.

Atchison, N., Guercio, P., and Monaco, C.: Pain in the pediatric burn patient: nursing assessment and perception, Issues Compr. Pediatr. Nurs. 9:399-409, 1986.

Baker, M.D., and Chiaviello, C.: Household electrical injuries in children, Am. J. Dis. Child. 143:59-62, 1989.

Bayley, E.W., and Smith, G.A.: The three degrees of burn care, Nursing '87 17(3):34-41, 1987.

Berkner, P., Kastner, T., and Skolnick, L.: Palatal burn due to bottle warming in a microwave oven, Pediatrics 82:382-385, 1988.

Bingham, H.: Electrical burns, Clin. Plast. Surg. 13:75-85, 1986.

Brown, A.S., and Barot, L.R.: Biologic dressings and skin substitutes, Clin. Plast. Surg. 13:69-74, 1986.

Bush, A.: What to look for when the patient suffers an electrical injury, RN 50(9):39-43, 1987.

Cameron, C.O., Juszczak, L., and Wallace, N.: Using creative arts to help children cope with altered body image, Child. Health Care 12:108-112, 1984.

Cockington, R.A.: Ambulatory management of burns in children, Burns 15:271-273, 1989.

Donovan, M.K.: Do nurses know and teach burn prevention and safety in practice? Issues Compr. Pediatr. Nurs. 10:13-32, 1987.

Grossman, E.R.: Floor furnace burns (letter), Pediatrics 73:568-569, 1984.

Harris, J.R., Kobayashi, J.M., and Frost, F.: Injuries from fireworks, JAMA 249:2460, 1983.

Hurt, R.A.: More than skin deep: guidelines on caring for the burn patient, Nursing '85 15(6):52-57, 1985.

Kavanagh, C.: Psychological intervention with the severly burned child: report of an experimental comparison of two approaches and their effects on psychological sequelae, J. Am. Acad. Child Psychiatry 22:145-156, 1983.

Kinner, M.A.: Relationship between knowledge of burn prevention and emergency treatment and risk-taking attitudes in 11-15 year olds, Issues Compr. Pediatr. Nurs. 9:353-367, 1986.

Langley, J.: Description and classification of childhood burns, Burns 10:231, 1984.

Lasoff, E.M., and McEttrick, M.A.: Participation versus diversion during dressing change: can nurses' attitudes change? Issues Compr. Pediatr. Nurs. 9:391-398, 1986.

Luterman, A., Adams, M., and Curreri, P.W.: Nutritional management of the burn patient, Crit. Care Q. 7(3):34-43, 1984.

Marvin, J.A.: Planning home care for burn patients, Nursing '83 13(8):65-67, 1983.

Mikhail, J.N.: Acute burn care: an update, J. Emerg. Nurs. 14(1):9-18, 1988.

Moylan, K.: Amnion dressing—a natural for wounds, Nursing '86 16:68, 1986.

Osgood, P.F., and Szyfelbein, S.K.: Management of burn pain in children, Pediatr. Clin. North Am. 36:1001-1013, 1989.

Poteet, G.W., Hilld, A.S., and Roberson, V.S.: Care of the burned patient with herpes simplex, J. Pediatr. Nurs. 1:376-385, 1986.

Puczynski, M., Rademaker, D., and Gatson, R.L.: Burn injury related to the improper use of a microwave oven, Pediatrics 72:714-715, 1983.

Ressijac, R.H.: High voltage electrical injuries, Issues Compr. Pediatr. Nurs. 9:383-389, 1986.

Robertson, K.E., Cross, P.J., and Terry, J.C.: Burn care: the crucial first days, Am. J. Nurs. 85:30-50, 1985.

Smith, G.A., and Savinski-Bozinko, G.: Giving emergency care for burns, Nursing '89 19(9):55-62, 1989.

Stoddard, F.J.: Coping with pain: a developmental approach to treatment of burned children, Am. J. Psychiatry 139:736-740, 1982.

Surveyer, J.A., and Clougherty, D.M.: Burn scars: fighting the effects, Am. J. Nurs. 83:746-751, 1983.

Thomas, K.A., Hassanein, R.S., and Christophersen, E.R.: Evaluation of group well-child care for improving burn prevention practices in the home, Pediatrics 74:879-882, 1984.

Thompson, J.C., and Ashwal, S.: Electrical injuries in children, Am. J. Dis. Child. 137:231-235, 1983.

Tobiasen, J., Hiebert, J.M., and Edlich, R.F.: The abbreviated burn severity index, Ann. Emerg. Med. 11:260-262, 1982.

Wagner, M.M., editor: Care of the burn-injured patient, Littleton, MA, 1981, PSG Publications Co., Inc.

Yanofsky, N.N., and Morain, W.D.: Upper extremity burns from woodstoves, Pediatrics 73:722-726, 1984.

CHAPTER 30

The Child with Genitourinary Dysfunction

RELATED TOPICS

Administration of medication, Ch. 27
Collection of specimens, Ch. 27
Defects of the genitourinary tract, Ch. 11
Physical examination: genitalia, Ch. 7

GLOSSARY

acidosis Lowered blood pH
AGN Acute glomerulonephritis
anuria Absence of urine formation
APSGN Acute poststreptococcal glomerulonephritis
ARF Acute renal failure
ASO Antistreptolysin O
azotemia Excessive amounts of nitrogenous compounds in the blood
bacteriuria Growth of bacteria in uncontaminated urine
CAPD Continuous ambulatory peritoneal dialysis
CAVH Continuous arteriovenous hemofiltration
CCPD Continuous cycling peritoneal dialysis
CGN Chronic glomerulonephritis
COP Colloidal osmotic pressure
CRF Chronic renal failure
CRP C-reactive protein
cystitis Inflammation of the bladder
dialysis Process of separating colloids and crystalline substances in solution by the difference in their rate of diffusion through a semipermeable membrane
ESR Erythrocyte sedimentation rate
ESRD End-stage renal disease
hemodialysis Dialysis in which blood is circulated outside the body through artificial membranes
HUS Hemolytic uremic syndrome
hyperkalemia Abnormal potassium concentration in the blood
IVP Intravenous pyelogram
MCNS Minimal change nephrotic syndrome
NDI Nephrogenic diabetes insipidus
oliguria Diminished output of urine
osteodystrophy Defective bone formation
peritoneal dialysis Dialysis in which the peritoneum serves as a semipermeable membrane
RTA Renal tubular acidosis
tubular Involving renal tubules
uremia Presence of excessive amounts of urea and other nitrogenous waste in the blood
urethritis Inflammation of the urethra
UTI Urinary tract infection
VUR Vesicoureteral reflux

Diseases involving the kidneys are relatively common in childhood and are caused by a variety of etiologic factors. To better understand the way in which the pathologic processes produce an effect, the basic kidney structure and function are briefly reviewed, and the most frequently used tests of renal function are outlined to help the reader understand the relationship of these studies to renal physiology and pathology. Discussion of the more common disorders of renal function is followed by discussion of the critical therapies of dialysis and renal transplant.

RENAL STRUCTURE AND FUNCTION

The primary responsibility of the kidney is to maintain the composition and volume of the body fluids in equilibrium. To maintain this constant internal environment, the kidney must respond appropriately to alterations in the internal environment caused by variations in dietary intake and extrarenal losses of water and solutes. This is accomplished by the formation of urine (the product of glomerular filtration), tubular reabsorption, and tubular secretion. *Reabsorption* is the transport of a substance from the tubular lumen to the blood in surrounding vessels. *Secretion* is transport in the opposite direction, that is, from the blood to the lumen. These processes can be active or passive. *Excretion* is the elimination of a substance from the body, in this case urine.

A secondary function of the kidney is the production of certain humoral substances. One such substance is an enzyme, *erythropoietin stimulating factor (ESF,* or *erythrogenin),* which acts on a plasma globulin to form erythropoietin, which in turn stimulates erythropoiesis in the bone marrow. Its production is increased in the presence of hypoxia and androgens. Few red blood cells are formed in the absence of erythropoietin, which accounts in some measure for the anemia associated with advanced renal disease. Another enzyme, *renin,* is also secreted by the kidney in response to reduced blood volume, decreased blood pressure, or increased secretion of catecholamines. Renin stimulates the production of the angiotensins, which produce arteriolar constriction and an elevation in blood pressure and stimulate the production of aldosterone by the adrenal cortex.

RENAL PHYSIOLOGY

The structural and functional unit of the kidney is the nephron, which is composed of a complex system of tubules, arterioles, venules, and capillaries (Fig. 30-1). The nephron consists of the *Bowman capsule,* enclosing a tuft of capillaries, which is joined successively to the *proximal convoluted tubule, the loop of Henle,* the *distal convoluted tubule,* and the *straight,* or *collecting duct.* Collecting tubules join larger ducts, and all of the larger collecting ducts of one renal pyramid join to form a single duct that opens into a *minor calyx.* A number of calyces empty into one of several *major calyces* that converge into the *renal pelvis.* The renal pelvis narrows after it leaves the kidney and forms what then becomes a *ureter,* through which urine drains into the *urinary bladder.*

The blood supply to the kidneys constitutes about one fifth of the total cardiac output; therefore profuse bleeding can accompany renal trauma. Because interstitial tissue is sparse, individual nephrons with their blood vessel component are closely packed together. Each nephron is supplied by a sizable *afferent arteriole,* which separates into capillary loops that comprise the glomerular tuft. Blood leaves by a smaller *efferent arteriole.* From there the efferent arterioles branch into a *peritubular capillary* network and hairpin loops called the *vasa recta,* which parallel the Henle loops and the collecting ducts. The total surface area of the renal capillaries is approximately equal to the total surface of the tubules.

The Bowman capsule is composed of two cellular layers that separate the blood from the glomerular filtrate—the capillary endothelium and a layer of tubular epithelial lining cells. Situated between these layers is the basal lamina, or basement membrane. The permeability of this glomerular membrane is a result of its structure; the capillary endothelium is fenestrated with pores or *fenestrae,* and the outer surface of the glomerular epithelium consists of fingerlike projections *(pseudopodia,* or *podocytes),* which cover the entire surface to form slits called *slit pores.* The basement membrane has no visible openings but behaves as if it contains pores or channels. Consequently the glomerular filtrate, which has essentially the same composition as plasma except for the large protein molecules and cellular elements, passes through these three layers and does so at a very rapid rate. The structure of these layers becomes altered in kidney disease.

Glomerular Filtration

Filtration through the glomerular capillaries is governed by the same mechanism as filtration across other capillaries in the body, that is, the size of the capillary bed, the permeability of the capillaries, and the hydrostatic and osmotic pressure gradients across the capillaries. The filtration capacity of the glomerulus is the product of three pressure forces— glomerular hydrostatic pressure, colloidal osmotic (oncotic) pressure (COP), and intracapsular pressure—and permeability of the glomerular capillaries.

Blood enters the nephron at a substantial pressure. This hydrostatic pressure forces plasma fluid and solutes through the capillary membrane into the collecting apparatus of the unit. As this filtrate travels through the renal tubules, water and solutes are selectively reabsorbed back into the vascular compartment. That which is not reabsorbed is excreted as urine. Filtration takes place as long as hydrostatic pressure within the glomerular capillaries exceeds the opposing COP of the plasma proteins. If the pres-

---

Elizabeth J. Heywood, R.N., M.S.N., P.N.P., assisted in the revision of this chapter.

STRUCTURE	GLOMERULUS WITHIN BOWMAN CAPSULE	PROXIMAL TUBULE	LOOP OF HENLE	DISTAL TUBULE	CONNECTING DUCT
FUNCTION	Filtration	Reabsorption of Na^+ (majority) Glucose K^+ Amino acids HCO_3^- PO_4^- Urea H_2O (ADH not required) Secretion of H^+ Foreign substances	Concentration of urine (countercurrent mechanism) Descending loop Water reabsorption Na^+ diffuses in Ascending loop Na^+ reabsorbed (active transport) Water stays in	Reabsorption of Na^+ H_2O (ADH required) HCO_3^- Secretion of K^+ Urea H^+ NH_3^+ Some drugs	Reabsorption of H_2O (ADH required) Reabsorption or secretion of Na^+ K^+ H^+ NH_3^+
TONICITY OF FLUID (WITHIN DUCTS)		Isotonic	Isotonic → Hypertonic → Hypotonic	Isotonic or hypotonic	Final concentration

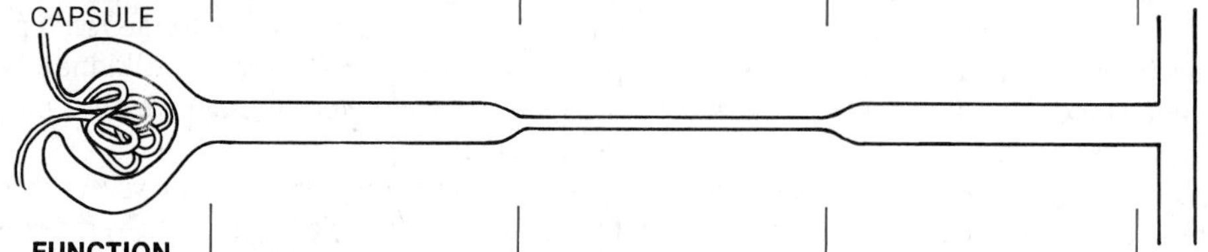

Fig. 30-1. Major functions of nephron components.

sure becomes equal through decreased hydrostatic pressure or decreased COP, no further filtration takes place. In a state of dehydration, more water is reabsorbed; when water intake is increased, more is excreted as urine. In conditions that produce osmotic diuresis (i.e., when large solutes, such as glucose, are filtered through the capillaries in such excessive amounts that they cannot be reabsorbed), the osmotic attraction of the solute causes less water to be reabsorbed, resulting in water being excreted in the urine with the solute.

Tubular Function

The function of the renal tubules is to modify the glomerular filtrate. Tubular cells may add more of a substance to the filtrate (tubular secretion), remove some or all of a substance from the filtrate (tubular reabsorption), or both. The reabsorption is selective and discriminating for substances essential to body processes and equilibrium, whereas nonessential substances are eliminated as waste. The substances are secreted or reabsorbed in the tubules by osmosis, passive diffusion down a chemical or electric gradient, or actively transported against these gradients. These processes operate throughout the length of the tubules, but there are variations in the types, amounts, and mechanisms by which substances are secreted or reabsorbed in the different tubular segments, caused in large part by the cellular characteristics of each segment.

Active transport mechanisms move vital substances both inward and outward from the tubular filtrate. For example, essential items such as glucose, amino acids, and sodium ions are reabsorbed in the proximal tubule and returned directly to the blood. Active transport mechanisms, as elsewhere, have a limited capacity, or threshold, for moving the solute. When the maximum of the transport mechanism is reached, no more of the substance is reabsorbed, and the remainder is excreted in the urine. For example, when blood glucose concentrations exceed their transport capacity, the surplus remains in the filtrate to be excreted in the urine (glycosuria). When two substances share a common transport mechanism, the first substance may be blocked by the addition of a second substance (selective inhibition). The effect of many therapeutic agents, for example, diuretics, depends on this process.

Electrolytes are moved by both active transport and diffusion, and the transport of some, particularly sodium, has important effects on other substances. For example, sodium is actively transported from all parts of the nephron. The movement of sodium ions produces both an electric and an osmotic gradient, which causes chloride ions and water to diffuse from the tubules in an effort to establish equilibrium. This is the obligatory water reabsorption in the kidneys. There is a limit to the concentration gradient against which sodium can be transported out; therefore when larger than normal amounts of sodium ions remain in the tubules, water is obliged to remain with the sodium.

Under normal conditions the kidneys are able to adjust the urine and solute excretion in response to the requirements for body water and electrolyte balance. They are able to excrete or conserve both water and most electrolytes in addition to excreting end products of protein metabolism, principally urea. The volume of urine excreted by the kidneys in a given period of time depends on the water balance (including intravascular filtration pressure), the quantity of solutes presented to the kidneys, and the capacity of the kidneys to dilute or concentrate the filtrate.

Renal Development and Function in Early Infancy

Development of the kidney begins within the first weeks of embryonic life but is not completed until about the end of the first year after birth. The nephrons increase in number throughout gestation and reach their full complement by birth. However, they are immature and less efficient than at later ages. Many of the tubular sections are not fully formed, and the glomeruli enlarge considerably after birth.

Glomerular filtration and absorption are relatively low and do not reach adult values until the child is between 1 and 2 years of age. This appears to be related to a barrier imposed by more cuboidal-shaped glomerular epithelial cells and higher afferent arteriole resistance. Consequently, the newborn is unable to dispose of excess water and solute rapidly or efficiently.

Tubular length of nephrons is highly variable; glomerular size is less variable. The juxtaglomerular nephrons show more advanced development than cortical nephrons. The loop of Henle (the site of the urine-concentrating mechanism) is short in the newborn, which reduces the ability to reabsorb sodium and water, producing a very dilute urine, although adequate amounts of antidiuretic hormone are secreted by the newborn pituitary gland. The length of tubules gradually increases until concentrating ability reaches adult levels about the third month of life. Urea synthesis and excretion are slower during this time, and the newborn retains large quantities of nitrogen and essential electrolytes in order to meet needs for growth in the first weeks of life. Consequently the excretory burden is minimized. The lower concentration of urea, the principal end product of nitrogen metabolism, also reduces concentrating capacity, since it also contributes to the concentration mechanism.

Other characteristics of the newborn's kidneys create differences in renal function from that of older children and adults. Because of some as yet undetermined cause, newborn infants are unable to excrete a water load at rates similar to those of older persons. Hydrogen ion excretion is reduced, acid secretion is lower for the first year of life, and plasma bicarbonate levels are low. As a result of these inadequacies of the kidney along with less efficient blood buffers, the newborn is more liable to develop severe metabolic acidosis. Sodium excretion is reduced in the immediate newborn period, and the kidneys are less able to adapt to deficiencies and excesses of sodium. For example, an isotonic saline infusion may produce edema because of impaired ability to eliminate excess. Conversely, inadequate reabsorption of sodium from tubules may increase sodium losses in disorders such as vomiting or diarrhea. Moreover, infants have a diminished capacity to reabsorb glucose and, during the first few days, to produce ammonium ions.

Because of the small, conical pelvis, the urinary bladder is an abdominal organ in infancy, but, as the pelvis expands with growth, the bladder settles into it to become a pelvic organ. The kidney functions during fetal life and produces urine that contributes to the amniotic fluid volume. The 24-hour urine volume is low at birth, rapidly increases in the neonatal period, and steadily increases with normal growth (see Appendix D).

ASSESSMENT OF RENAL FUNCTION

Assessment of kidney and urinary tract integrity and the diagnosis of renal or urinary tract disease are based on several evaluative tools. Physical examination, history, and observation of symptoms are the initial procedures. In suspected urinary tract diseases or disorders, further assessment by laboratory, radiologic, and other evaluative methods is carried out.

Clinical Manifestations

As in most disorders of childhood, the incidence and type of kidney or urinary tract dysfunction change with the age and maturation of the child. In addition, the presenting complaints and the significance of these complaints vary with maturation. For example, a complaint of enuresis has greater significance at age 8 years than at age 4. In the newborn, urinary tract disorders are associated with a number of obvious malformations of other body systems, including the curious and unexplained but frequent association between malformed or low-set ears and urinary tract anomalies. Important signs and symptoms that suggest possible renal or genitourinary tract disease in children at different ages are outlined in Box 30-1.

Many of the clinical manifestations are common to a variety of childhood disorders, but their presence is an indication to obtain further information from past history, family history, and laboratory studies as part of a complete physical examination. Suspected renal disease can be further evaluated by means of radiographic studies and renal biopsy.

Laboratory Tests

Both urine and blood studies contribute vital information for detection of renal problems. The single most important test is probably the routine urinalysis. Specific urine and blood tests provide additional information. Since nurses are usually the persons who collect the specimens for examination and who often perform many of the screening tests, they should be familiar with the test, its function, and factors that can alter or distort the results of the test (see Collection of Specimens, Chapter 27).

Glomerular filtration rate is a measure of the amount of plasma from which a given substance is totally cleared in 1 minute. Clearance is calculated from the ratio of substance

Box 30-1 SIGNS AND SYMPTOMS OF URINARY TRACT DISORDERS OR DISEASE AT DIFFERENT AGES

Neonatal Period (Birth to 1 Month)
Poor feeding
Vomiting
Failure to gain weight
Rapid respiration (acidosis)
Respiratory distress
Spontaneous pneumothorax or pneumomediastinum
Frequent urination
Screaming on urination
Poor urinary stream
Jaundice
Convulsions
Dehydration
Other anomalies or stigmata
Enlarged kidneys or bladder

Infancy (1 to 24 Months)
Poor feeding
Vomiting
Failure to gain weight
Excessive thirst
Frequent urination
Straining or screaming on urination
Foul-smelling urine
Pallor
Fever
Persistent diaper rash
Convulsions (with or without fever)
Dehydration
Enlarged kidney or bladder

Childhood (2 to 14 Years)
Poor appetite
Vomiting
Growth failure
Excessive thirst
Enuresis, incontinence, frequent urination
Painful urination
Swelling of face
Convulsions
Pallor
Fatigue
Blood in urine
Abdominal or back pain
Edema
Hypertension
Tetany

excreted to the concentration of that substance in the plasma. A number of substances can be used, but the most useful clinical estimation of glomerular filtration is the clearance of creatinine, an end product of protein metabolism in muscle and a substance that is freely filtered by the glomerulus and secreted by renal tubular cells. The production and secretion of creatinine remain relatively constant from day to day, and its appearance in the urine is determined by the serum level. When the collection is complete and accurately timed, the results are fairly reliable and compare favorably with clearance of other substances, such as inulin, that require special equipment to evaluate and long immobilization of the child.

Any significant degree of renal disease can diminish the glomerular filtration rate, but diseases of the glomerulus and renal vascular disease have the most immediate effect. The nurse's responsibility in this test is collection of urine, usually a 12- or 24-hour specimen.

The major urine and blood tests are outlined in Tables 30-1 and 30-2. Special tests and nursing responsibilities are briefly described in Table 30-3.

Nursing Considerations

Nursing responsibilities in assessment of genitourinary disorders and/or diseases begins with observation of the child for any manifestations that might indicate dysfunction. In addition to the general manifestations (Box 30-1), many conditions have specific characteristics that distinguish them from other disorders. These are discussed as appropriate throughout the chapter.

The nurse is generally the one who is responsible for preparing infants, children, and parents for tests and collection of urine and (sometimes) blood specimens (see Preparation for Procedures, Chapter 27, and Collection of Specimens, Chapter 27, for observation and laboratory analysis). Nurses maintain careful intake and output measurements on most children with genitourinary dysfunction and those who might be at risk to develop renal complications (e.g., children in shock, postoperative patients). Nurses observe the characteristics of urine collected, often perform any of a number of tests on urine specimens (e.g., urine specific gravity, protein, blood, glucose, ketones), and assist with more complex diagnostic tests (e.g., radiography, cystoscopy). Nurses must be familiar with significant laboratory tests and their implications.

GENITOURINARY TRACT DISORDERS

Urinary tract anomalies and disorders may adversely affect urinary excretion by producing inflammation, tissue damage, and scarring of tissue components. Infection of the genitourinary tract is one of the most common conditions in childhood, and in many instances the predisposing cause is obstruction within the kidneys and urinary drainage and storage structures. Obstructive uropathy has been discussed in relation to congenital anomalies. This section is devoted to infections in the genitourinary tract and a common etiologic condition, vesicoureteral reflux.

URINARY TRACT INFECTION

Urinary tract infection (UTI) is the term used to describe a clinical condition that may involve the urethra, bladder (lower urinary tract), and/or the ureters, renal pelvis, calyces, and renal parenchyma (upper urinary tract). Because it is often impossible to localize the infection, the broad designation UTI is applied to the presence of significant num-

Table 30-1 Urine tests of renal function

TEST	NORMAL RANGE	DEVIATIONS	SIGNIFICANCE OF DEVIATIONS
▪ Physical tests			
Volume	Age related	Polyuria	Osmotic factors (urinary glucose level in diabetes mellitus)
		Oliguria	Retention caused by obstructive disease Inadequate bladder emptying caused by neurogenic bladder or obstructive disorder
		Anuria	Obstruction of urinary tract; acute renal failure
Specific gravity	With normal fluid intake: 1.016-1.022 Newborn: 1.001-1.020	High	Dehydration Presence of protein or glucose Presence of radiopaque contrast medium after radiologic examinations
	Others: 1.001-1.030	Low	Excessive fluid intake Distal tubular dysfunction Insufficient antidiuretic hormone Diuresis
		Fixed at 1.010	Chronic glomerular disease
Osmolality	Newborn: 50-600 mOsm/L Thereafter: 50-1400 mOsm/L	High or low	Same as for specific gravity More sensitive index than specific gravity
Appearance	Clear pale yellow to deep gold	Cloudy	Contains sediment
		Cloudy reddish pink to reddish brown	Blood from trauma or disease Myoglobin following severe muscle destruction
		Light	Dilute
		Dark	Concentrated
		Red	Trauma
▪ Chemical tests			
pH	Newborn: 5-7 Thereafter: 4.8-7.8 Average: 6	Weak acid or neutral	If associated with metabolic acidosis, suggests tubular acidosis If associated with metabolic alkalosis, suggests potassium deficiency Urinary infection Metabolic alkalosis
		Alkaline	Metabolic alkalosis
Protein level	Absent	Present	Abnormal glomerular permeability, for example, glomerular disease, changes in blood pressure Most kidney disease Orthostatic in some individuals
Glucose level	Absent	Present	Diabetes mellitus Infusion of concentrated glucose-containing fluids Glomerulonephritis Impaired tubular reabsorption
Ketone levels	Absent	Present	Conditions of acute metabolic demand (stress) Diabetic ketoacidosis
▪ Microscopic tests			
White blood cell count	Less than 1 or 2	More than 5 polymorphonuclear leukocytes/field	Urinary tract inflammatory process
		Lymphocytes	Allograft rejection Malignancy
Red blood cell count	Less than 1 or 2	4-6/field in centrifuged specimen	Trauma Stones Glomerular injury Infection Neoplasms

Continued.

Table 30-1 Urine tests of renal function—cont'd

TEST	NORMAL RANGE	DEVIATIONS	SIGNIFICANCE OF DEVIATIONS
Presence of bacteria	Absent to a few	More than 100,000 organisms/ml in centrifuged specimen	Urinary tract infection
Presence of casts	Occasional	Granular casts	Tubular or glomerular disorders Degenerative process in advanced renal disease
		Cellular casts	
		White blood cell	Pyelonephritis
		Red blood cell	Glomerulonephritis
		Hyaline casts	Proteinuria; usually transient

Table 30-2 Blood tests of renal function

TEST	NORMAL RANGE (mg/dl)	DEVIATIONS	SIGNIFICANCE OF DEVIATIONS
Blood urea nitrogen (BUN)	Newborn: 4-18 Infant, child: 5-18	Elevated	Renal disease—acute or chronic (the higher the BUN, the more severe the disease) Increased protein catabolism Dehydration Hemorrhage High protein intake Corticosteroid therapy
Uric acid	Child: 2.0-5.5	Increased	Severe renal disease
Creatinine	Infant: 0.2-0.4 Child: 0.3-0.7 Adolescent: 0.5-1.0	Increased	Severe renal impairment

Table 30-3 Radiologic and other tests of renal function

TEST	PROCEDURE	PURPOSE	COMMENTS AND NURSING RESPONSIBILITIES
Intravenous pyelography (IVP) (intravenous urogram; excretory urogram)	Intravenous injection of a contrast medium Medium secreted and concentrated by tubules X-ray films made 5, 10, and 15 minutes after injection	Defines urinary tract Provides information about integrity of kidneys, ureters, and bladder Retroperitoneal masses visualized when they shift position of ureters	Preparation for test: Infants less than 2 years of age—no solid food, omit one bottle on morning of examination, studies should be done early to avoid withholding of fluids Children aged 2-14 years—give cathartic evening before examination, nothing orally after midnight, enema (Fleet or soapsuds) morning of examination

Table 30-3 Radiologic and other tests of renal function—cont'd

TEST	PROCEDURE	PURPOSE	COMMENTS AND NURSING RESPONSIBILITIES
Time-sequence IVP	Modification of those for IVP Films made every 5 minutes after injection of contrast medium	More accurately distinguishes differences between kidneys Differences in times of excretion indicate unilateral disease	Support during procedure Normal kidneys show dye before abnormal ones
Retrograde pyelography	Contrast medium injected through catheter inserted into kidney pelvis via urethra, bladder, and ureter	Visualizes pelvic calyces, ureters, and bladder	Rarely necessary during childhood
Renal angiography	Contrast medium injected directly into renal artery via catheter placed in femoral artery (or umbilical artery in newborn) and advanced to renal artery	Visualizes renal vascular system, especially for renal arterial stenosis	Give cathartic if ordered Give preoperative medication if ordered Observe for reaction to contrast medium Monitor vital signs following procedure
Radioisotope renography and renal scanning	Radioisotopes injected intravenously and recorded with special camera and computer analysis	Measures renal function and renal blood flow by recording appearance and disappearance of radioactivity in each kidney Gives detailed picture of excretory performance Helps define intrarenal masses Delineates nonfunctioning kidney	Insert or assist insertion of intravenous infusion Monitor intravenous infusion
Voiding cystourethrography	Contrast medium injected into bladder through urethral catheter until bladder is full; films taken before, during, and after voiding	Visualizes bladder outline and urethra, reveals reflux or urine into ureters, and shows complications of bladder emptying	Prepare child for catheterization
Scout film (KUB)	Flat plate roentgenogram of abdomen and pelvis	Detects and establishes renal outlines, presence of calculi, or opaque foreign bodies in bladder	Prepare as for routine x-ray film
Cystoscopy	Direct visualization of bladder and lower urinary tract through small scope inserted via urethra	Investigation of bladder and lower tract lesions; visualizes urethral openings, bladder wall, trigone, and urethra	Give nothing orally after midnight Carry out preoperative preparations
Renal biopsy	Removal of kidney tissue by open or percutaneous technique for study by light, electron, or immunofluorescent microscopy	Yields histologic and microscopic information about glomeruli and tubules; helps to distinguish between types of nephrotic syndromes Distinguishes other renal disorders	Give nothing orally 4-6 hours before test Premedicate as ordered Prepare setup for procedure Assist with procedure Take vital signs Apply pressure to area with pressure dressing and, if feasible, a sandbag Bed rest for 24 hours Observe for abdominal pain, tenderness Monitor input and output; surgical incision may be required in infants

Continued.

Table 30-3 Radiologic and other tests of renal function—cont'd

TEST	PROCEDURE	PURPOSE	COMMENTS AND NURSING RESPONSIBILITIES
Nephrosonography	Transmission of ultrasonic sound waves through kidney areas to outline kidney mass	Distinguishes between cystic and solid masses and renal and nonrenal masses, localizes kidneys, and delineates nonfunctional kidney	Administer sedation if needed
Computed tomography	Narrow-beam x-rays and computer analysis provide precise reconstruction of area	Visualizes vertical or horizontal cross section of kidney Especially valuable to distinguish tumors and cysts	Noninvasive Similar to preparation for pyelography
Urine culture and sensitivity	Collection of sterile specimen	Determines presence of pathogens and the drugs to which they are sensitive	Does not require specific parental permission Send specimen to laboratory immediately after collection Catheterization, clean-catch, or suprapubic specimen

Box 30-2 CLASSIFICATION OF URINARY TRACT INFECTION OR INFLAMMATION

Bacteriuria—growth of bacteria in uncontaminated urine (greater than 100,000 colonies/ml)
Asymptomatic bacteriuria—significant bacteriuria with no clinical evidence of active infection
Symptomatic bacteriuria—significant bacteriuria accompanied by physical symptoms
Recurrent UTI—repeated symptomatic episodes, usually caused by entry of new organisms from the perineal-fecal flora (sometimes termed *reinfection)*
Relapse of UTI—persistence of the same organism despite appropriate antibiotic therapy
Urethritis—inflammation of the urethra
Cystitis—inflammation of the bladder
Ureteritis—inflammation of the ureters
Pyelonephritis—inflammation of the kidney and upper tract (may be acute or chronic)

bers of microorganisms anywhere within the urinary tract (except the distal one third of the urethra, which is usually colonized with bacteria).

Infection of the urinary tract may be present with or without clinical symptoms. As a result, the site of infection is often difficult to pinpoint with accuracy. Various terms used to describe urinary tract disorders are listed in Box 30-2.

The peak incidence of UTI not caused by structural anomalies occurs between 2 and 6 years of age. Except for the neonatal period, females have a 10 to 30 times greater risk for developing UTI than males. Approximately 3% to 5% of girls will have one or more episodes of UTI prior to puberty (Jodal and Winberg, 1987). The likelihood of recurrence is 50% or greater in girls; the recurrence rate is lower in boys (Edelmann, 1988).

UTI in newborns differs in some respects from infections occurring in older children. In this group males outnumber females. At all ages asymptomatic bacteriuria is more common than symptomatic disease, and recurrence is not uncommon, especially in girls. An increased incidence of UTI is observed in adolescents, especially those with evidence of sexual activity (Weir and Lampe, 1984).

Etiology

A variety of organisms can be responsible for UTI. *Escherichia coli* (80% of cases) and other gram-negative enteric organisms are most frequently implicated; all are common to the anal, perineal, and perianal region. Other organisms associated with UTI include *Proteus, Pseudomonas, Klebsiella, Staphylococcus aureus, Haemophilus,* and coagulase-negative *Staphylococcus* (Ogra and Faden, 1985). A number of factors contribute to the development of UTI. These include anatomic, physical, and chemical conditions or properties of the host urinary tract.

Anatomic and physical factors. The structure of the lower urinary tract is believed to account for the increased incidence of bacteriuria in females. The short urethra, which measures about 2 cm (¾ inch) in young females and 4 cm (1½ inches) in mature women, provides a ready pathway for invasion of organisms. In addition, the closure of the urethra at the end of micturition may return contaminated bacteria to the bladder.

The longer male urethra (as long as 20 cm [8 inches] in an adult) and the antibacterial properties of prostatic secretions inhibit the entry and growth of pathogens. Reports indicate an increased incidence of UTI in infants less than 1 year of age who are not circumcised when compared to infants who are circumcised (Herzog, 1989; Roberts, 1988; Wiswell and Geschke, 1989; Wiswell and Roscelli, 1986). The presence of a foreskin is associated with a greater quantity of periurethral bacteria that can ascend the urethra easily (Wiswell and others, 1988; Fussell and others, 1988). The incidence of renal scarring is greatest in patients whose first infection occurs during infancy.

The single most important host factor influencing the occurrence of UTI is urinary stasis. Ordinarily urine is sterile, but at 37° C (98.6° F) it provides an excellent culture medium. Under normal conditions the act of completely and repeatedly emptying the bladder flushes away any organisms before they have an opportunity to multiply and invade surrounding tissue. However, urine that remains in the bladder allows bacteria from the urethra to rapidly become established in the rich medium.

Incomplete bladder emptying (stasis) may result from reflux (see p. 1340 for a discussion of reflux), anatomic abnormalities (especially those involving the ureters), dysfunction of the voiding mechanism, or extrinsic ureteral or bladder compression. Pressure of overdistention within the bladder may increase the risk of infection by decreasing host resistance, probably as a result of lessened blood flow to the mucosa. This frequently occurs in neurogenic bladder or as a consequence of voluntarily holding back urine despite the urge to void.

Extrinsic factors that may be responsible for *functional* bladder neck obstruction are chronic and intermittent constipation and pregnancy. In both conditions, the full rectum or uterus displaces the bladder and posterior urethra in the fixed and limited space of the bony pelvis, causing obstruction, incomplete micturition, and urinary stasis. Treating constipation along with antibiotic therapy for UTI reduces the recurrence of infection, whereas failure to relieve the fecal retention in spite of adequate treatment of the UTI may result in recurrence.

Other extrinsic factors that can contribute to UTI include catheters, especially short-term indwelling catheters, and administration of antimicrobial agents. Antimicrobials alter the host's normal perineal flora, allowing easier colonization with uropathogens. Tight clothing or diapers, poor hygiene, and local inflammation, such as from vaginitis, masturbation, or pinworm infestation, may also increase the risk of ascending infection. The essential oils in bubble baths and shampoos have been found to irritate the urethra of both boys and girls, causing painful and frequent urination (Rogers, 1985). Consequently, bubble baths are discouraged. There is no evidence that plain tub baths increase the risk of UTI, but infections have been related to the use of hot tub or whirlpool baths (Salmen and others, 1983). Sexual intercourse may produce transient bacteriuria in females and is associated with an increased risk of UTI.

Altered urine and bladder chemistry. Several chemical characteristics of the urine and bladder mucosa help maintain urinary sterility. An increased fluid intake promotes flushing of the normal bladder and lowers the concentration of organisms in the infected bladder. Water diuresis also seems to enhance the antibacterial properties of the renal medulla. One effect of water diuresis is increased blood flow to the medulla (where it is normally low), thereby increasing the availability of white cells at the site of inflammation.

Most pathogens favor an alkaline medium. Normally urine is slightly acidic, but it can be made more acidic by diet (apple or cranberry juices, large amounts of ascorbic acid, animal protein) or acid-forming drugs. When the urine pH is about 5, bacterial multiplication is hampered, although the acidification rarely eliminates the bacteriuria. However, it may enhance the therapeutic effectiveness of drugs and of the natural defense mechanisms, as well as help relieve some of the symptoms. Infection by some organisms, such as *Proteus*, increases the pH by decomposing urea to ammonia, thereby increasing the favorable conditions for the continued growth of the organism.

The bladder mucosa seems to have bactericidal effectiveness by destroying the bacteria in the very thin layer of urine left on the walls after complete voiding. Since close contact of the bacteria with the mucosa is essential for lysis to occur, any residual urine prevents the mechanism from functioning.

Pathophysiology

Inflammatory changes are usually confined to the bladder (cystitis) in uncomplicated infection. However, recurrent infection of the bladder may produce changes that distort the normal anatomic relationships of the ureter as it traverses the bladder wall, causing incompetence of the vesicoureteral valve. This may permit reflux of urine during voiding, which can allow access of organisms to the upper urinary tract.

Infection of the upper collecting system (pyelitis) and kidney (pyelonephritis), although much less common than cystitis, is usually acquired through an ascending infection from the lower tract. Infection of the renal parenchyma may also be introduced hematogenously, especially in infants in whom this is the more common route. Infection causes acute and chronic inflammatory changes in the pelvis and medulla with resulting scarring and loss of renal tissue, usually symmetric. Recurrent or chronic episodes cause an increase in fibrotic tissue and kidney contraction. In acute pyelonephritis the kidney is swollen and edematous with diffuse infiltration of polymorphonuclear cells. The scarring in relation to reflux appears to occur mainly in children under 5 years of age (Kroovand and Perlmutter, 1983).

Clinical Manifestations

The clinical manifestations of UTIs depend on the age of the child. In newborn infants and children less than 2 years of age the signs are characteristically nonspecific. They more nearly resemble gastrointestinal tract disorders: failure to thrive, feeding problems, vomiting, diarrhea, abdominal distention, and jaundice. Newborns may have fever or hypothermia and/or sepsis. Other evidence that may be observed includes frequent or infrequent voiding, constant squirming and irritability, strong-smelling urine, and abnormal stream. A persistent diaper rash may also be a helpful clue.

The classic symptoms of UTI are often observed in children over 2 years of age. These include enuresis or daytime incontinence in the child who has been been toilet trained, fever, strong or foul-smelling urine, increased frequency of urination, dysuria, or urgency. They may also complain of abdominal pain or costovertebral angle tenderness (flank pain). Some will present with hematuria; preschoolers may vomit. There is a high frequency of obstructive uropathy in young infants and boys that is characterized by dribbling of urine, straining with urination, or a decrease in the force and size of the urinary stream. High fever and chills accompanied by flank pain, severe abdominal pain, and leukocytosis suggest pyelonephritis. However, flank pain and tenderness may be the only indication of pyelonephritis on physical examination.

Manifestations in adolescents are more specific. Symptoms of lower tract infections include frequency and painful urination of a small amount of turbulent urine that may be grossly bloody. Fever is usually absent. Upper tract infection is characterized by fever, chills, flank pain, and lower tract symptoms, which may appear 1 or 2 days after the upper tract symptoms.

A large proportion (40%) of UTIs in children are asymptomatic or atypical in clinical presentation, and many complaints may be unrelated to the urinary tract (Hellerstein and others, 1984). Many are treated as respiratory or gastrointestinal infections. It is important that these children be identified so that treatment can be initiated. Significant scarring can take place, especially in infants and very young children.

Diagnostic Evaluation

The diagnosis of UTI depends on a high degree of suspicion, evaluation of history and physical examination, and urinalysis and culture. Urine characteristic of possible infection appears cloudy, hazy, or thick with noticeable strands of mucus and pus; it also smells fishy and unpleasant even when fresh. Presumptive UTI diagnosis can be made on the basis of microscopic examination of the urine, which often reveals pyuria (5 to 8 white blood cells/ml of uncentrifuged urine) and the presence of at least one bacterium in a Gram stain. However, a normal urinalysis may also be present in conditions of asymptomatic bacteriuria.

Diagnosis of UTI is confirmed by detection of bacteriuria in urine culture, but urine collection is often difficult, especially in infants and very small children (see Collection of Specimens, Chapter 27). Several factors may alter a urine specimen. Contamination of a specimen by organisms from sources other than the urine is the most frequent cause of false-positive results. Bag urine specimens are frequently contaminated by perineal and perianal flora and are usually considered inadequate for a definitive diagnosis. Clean-catch urine specimens have been determined to be no better than a regular midstream specimen. Unless the specimen is a first morning sample, a recent high fluid intake may indicate a falsely low organism count. Therefore children should not be encouraged to drink large volumes of water in an attempt to obtain a specimen quickly.

More accurate estimates of bacterial content are obtained from suprapubic aspiration (children less than 2 years of age) and properly performed bladder catheterization (as long as the first few milliliters are excluded from collection). Care of a urine specimen obtained for culture is an important nursing aspect related to diagnosis. The specimen should be taken to the laboratory for culture immediately. If culture is delayed, the sample can be placed in a refrigerator for up to 24 hours, but storage can result in loss of formed elements such as blood cells and casts (Bailie, 1986).

Recently developed tests to detect bacteriuria are being used with increased frequency in screening for UTI. The plastic dipstick, Chemstrip, and the agar-coated slide tests are quick and inexpensive methods for detecting infection prior to obtaining final culture results.

Localization of the infection site may involve more specific tests, including ureteral catheterization and bladder washout procedures. Other tests, such as ultrasonography, voiding cystourethrogram (VCUG), intravenous pyelogram (IVP), and DSMA (dimercaptosuccinic acid) scan may be performed after the infection subsides to identify anatomic abnormalities contributing to the development of infection and existing kidney changes from recurrent infection.

Therapeutic Management

The objectives of treatment of children with UTI are (1) to eliminate the infection, (2) to detect and correct functional or anatomic abnormalities, (3) to prevent recurrences, and (4) to preserve renal function (Krugman and others, 1985). Antibiotic therapy should be initiated based on identification of the pathogen, the child's history of antibiotic use, and the location of the infection. A variety of antimicrobial drugs are available for treating UTI, but all of them can occasionally be ineffective because of resistance of organisms. Antibacterial compounds used in the management of UTI include (1) systemic penicillins and sulfonamides, which are used for a short, intensive course of therapy; and (2) antiseptic preparations, which are often continued over longer periods to maintain urinary sterility, especially in children with long-term susceptibility to infection, such as those with neurogenic bladder.

The optimum length of therapy for UTI in children is not well established. Conventional therapy for uncomplicated infection, a single oral antibiotic (e.g., ampicillin, a sulfonamide, or nitrofurantoin) that the patient has not taken recently, can be administered for 10 to 14 days. Short-course and single-dose antibiotic therapies are controversial and not universally accepted but may be employed in special situations. In all cases follow-up laboratory evaluation is needed.

Children with suspected pyelonephritis and fever are admitted to the hospital and given appropriate antibiotics intravenously for a minimum of 48 hours. Blood and urine cultures are obtained on admission and following therapy. Urine cultures are usually repeated at monthly intervals for 3 months and at 3-month intervals for 6 months (Smith, 1986).

Newborn infants with documented UTI, UTI in boys of any age, and females 2 to 3 years of age with a second or subsequent UTI infection warrant somatographic or radiographic evaluation (Hellerstein and others, 1984). If anatomic defects such as primary reflux or bladder neck obstruction are present, surgical correction of these abnormalities may be necessary to prevent recurrent infection.

Follow-up study is an important component of medical management, since the relapse rate is high and recurrent infection tends to occur 1 to 2 months after termination of treatment. Even with recurrent infections, renal damage is rare if no anatomic abnormalities complicate the condition. The aim of therapy and careful follow-up in such cases is to prevent morbidity rather than reduce the chance of renal failure.

Prognosis. With prompt and adequate treatment at the time of diagnosis, the long-term prognosis for UTIs is usually excellent. However, the hazard of progressive renal injury is greatest when infection occurs in young children (es pecially under 2 years of age) and is associated with congenital renal malformations and reflux. Therefore early diagnosis of children at risk is particularly important during infancy and toddlerhood.

Nursing Considerations

Objectives of nursing care include identification of children with UTI and education of parents and child regarding prevention and treatment of infection. Aside from the influence of renal abnormalities, females between the ages of 2 and 6 years are in general a high-risk group. Since they are not a captive population, mass screening is difficult. However, the annual health examinations should include a routine urinalysis. In addition, nurses should instruct parents to observe regularly for clues suggesting UTI. Unfortunately the signs of UTI are not as evident as those of upper respiratory infection. Therefore many cases go undetected because no one thought to investigate this very common problem.

NURSING ALERT A child who exhibits the following should be evaluated for urinary tract infection:
- Incontinence in a toilet-trained child
- Strong-smelling urine
- Frequency and/or urgency

Since infants and young children are unable to express their feelings and sensations verbally, it is difficult to detect discomfort they may be experiencing from dysuria. A careful history regarding voiding habits and episodes of unexplained irritability may assist in detecting less obvious cases of UTI. Consequently parents should be encouraged to observe for specific clues of UTI in suspected cases (see Nursing Tip).

NURSING TIP: CLUES FOR DETECTING UTI IN INFANTS AND TODDLERS

Check the diaper every ½ hour (increases the opportunity for observing the stream for such findings as straining or fretting before voiding begins, signs of discomfort before and during urinating, starting and stopping the stream intermittently, and frequent dripping of small amounts of urine).

When infection is suspected, collecting an appropriate specimen is essential. It is the nurse's responsibility to take every precaution to obtain acceptable clean-voided specimens in order to avoid the use of other collecting procedures except when absolutely indicated.

Frequently other tests are performed to detect anatomic defects. Children are prepared for these tests as appropriate for their age. Children who are old enough to understand need an explanation of the procedure, its purpose, and what they will experience (see Preparation for Procedures, Chapter 27). Sometimes a simple description of the urinary system is helpful. Especially for preschool children, the nurse must clarify that the urinary tract is separate from any sexual function and that the test is for a problem that they did not cause. It is not uncommon for children to associate blame for perceived wrongdoing (e.g., masturbation) or unacceptable thoughts with the reason for the illness or the tests. For young children under 3 to 4 years of age, the procedure can be explained on a doll. For those who are older, a simple drawing of the bladder, urethra, ureters, and kidneys makes the explanation more understandable.

Children may be treated as outpatients to avoid overnight separation from home for such procedures. In such cases nurses must be careful not to overlook the need for adequate preparation, since, if surgery is subsequently indicated, the child will be able to encounter the impending operation with facts and understanding from these procedures, which will help to decrease his fear and anxiety of more extensive medical-surgical intervention.

Since antibacterial drugs are indicated in UTI, the nurse advises parents of proper dosage and administration. Ampicillin is frequently the drug of choice, but it must be given every 6 hours to maintain high blood levels. This generally requires waking the child during sleep for one dose. Amoxicillin allows for 8-hour intervals, which is more convenient, but the drug is more expensive than ampicillin. When antiseptics such as nitrofurantoin are used for prolonged therapy to maintain urine sterility, parents need an explanation of their continued necessity when no signs of infection are present. For all children an adequate or increased fluid intake is encouraged.*

*For home care instructions for giving medications to children and a nursing care plan for the child with urinary tract infection, see Wong, D.L, and Whaley, L.F.: Clinical manual of pediatric nursing, ed. 3, St. Louis, 1990, Mosby–Year Book, Inc.

Box 30-3 GUIDELINES FOR PREVENTION OF URINARY TRACT INFECTION

Factors Predisposing to Development	Measures of Prevention
Short female urethra close to vagina and anus	Perineal hygiene—wipe from front to back Avoid tight clothing or diapers; wear cotton panties rather than nylon Check for vaginitis or pinworms, especially if child scratches between legs
Incomplete emptying (reflux) and overdistention of bladder	Avoid "holding" urine; encourage child to void frequently, especially before a long trip or other circumstances where toilet facilities are not available Empty bladder completely with each void Avoid straining at stool
Concentrated and alkaline urine	Encourage generous fluid intake Acidify urine with juices such as apple and a diet high in animal protein

Box 30-4 VESICOURETERAL REFLUX GRADING SYSTEM

Grade I: VUR into the lower ureter only
Grade II: Ureteral and pelvic filling without calyceal dilation
Grade III: Ureteral and pelvic filling with mild calyceal blunting
Grade IV: Marked distention of pelvis, calyces, and ureter
Grade V: Massive VUR associated with severe hydronephrosis

Prevention. Prevention is the most important goal in both primary and recurrent infection, and most preventive measures are simple to very simple, ordinary hygienic habits that should be a routine part of daily care. Any signs of intestinal parasites (e.g., scratching between the legs and around anal area) should be investigated and treated appropriately. Sexually active adolescent females are advised to urinate as soon as possible after intercourse to flush out bacteria introduced during sex play. Parents and older children are taught health practices that prevent UTI (Box 30-3).

Children with disabilities involving the bladder are frequently on a prophylactic regimen, such as acidifying agents and prescribed fluid intake. The importance of compliance should be reinforced on parents and responsible children.

VESICOURETERAL REFLUX

Vesicoureteral reflux (VUR) refers to the retrograde flow of bladder urine into the ureters. Reflux increases the chance for and perpetuates infection, since with each void urine is swept up the ureters and then allowed to empty after voiding. Therefore the residual urine from the ureters remains in the bladder until the next void (Fig. 30-2). The International Classification System describes the degree of reflux from the bladder into upper genitourinary tract structures (Box 30-4).

Primary reflux results from the congenitally abnormal insertion of the ureters into the bladder and predisposes to development of infection. A familial incidence of VUR is sometimes observed. *Secondary reflux* occurs as a result of infection. Normally the ureters enter the bladder wall in such a manner that the accumulating urine compresses the submucosal segment of the ureter, preventing reflux. However, the edema caused by bladder infection renders this mechanism at the ureterovesicular junction incompetent. In

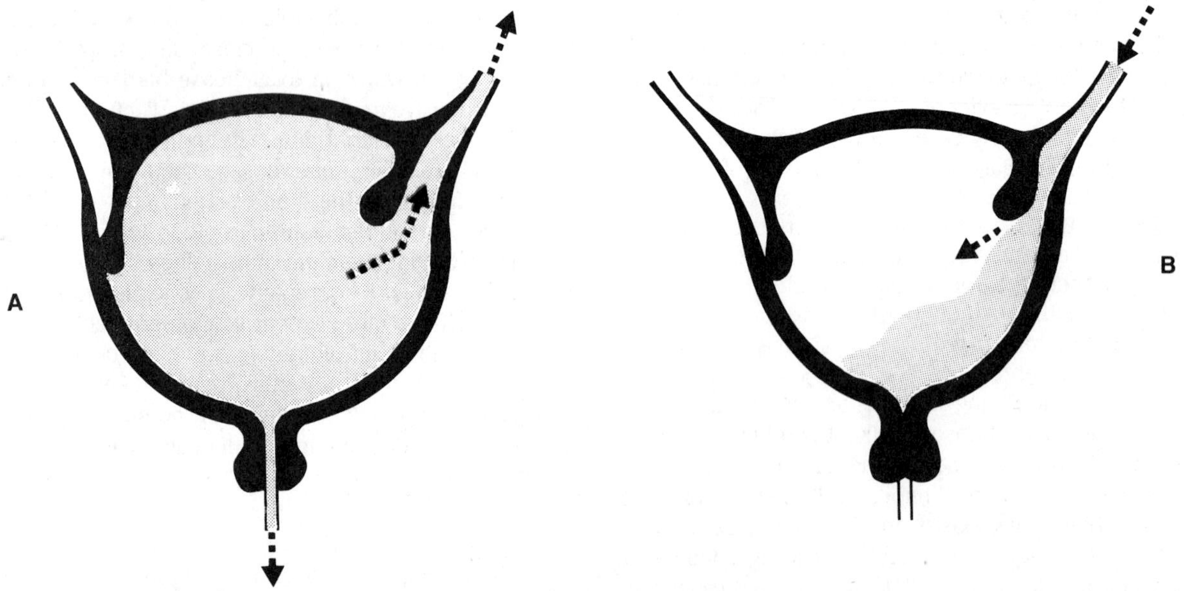

Fig. 30-2. Mechanisms of vesicoureteral reflux. **A,** During voiding, urine refluxes into ureter. **B,** After voiding, residual urine from ureter remains in bladder.

addition, in infants and young children the shortness of the submucosal portion of the ureter decreases the effectiveness of this antireflux mechanism. Other causes of secondary reflux are neurogenic bladder from either chronic obstruction or neural dysfunction or as an iatrogenic result from progressive dilation of the ureters following surgical urinary diversion.

Reflux with infection can lead to kidney damage, since refluxed urine ascending into the collecting tubules of the nephrons allows the microorganisms to gain access to the renal parenchyma, initiating renal scarring. The shape of renal papillae and the angle of entry of collecting ducts change with advancing age, making intrarenal reflux difficult (Edelmann, 1988). Therefore, most renal scars associated with reflux occur at a very young age and are present at the time of diagnosis; few develop after 5 years of age. However, between 30% and 60% of children with VUR have evidence of renal scarring, and scarring is almost always found in association with reflux (Ehrlich, 1982). Therefore UVR is an important cause of renal damage, and careful examination for its presence is indicated. Careful routine follow-up is a critical part of management of children with urinary tract infection (UTI), and children with reflux, documented by voiding cystoureterography, are assessed repeatedly during ensuing years (Hellerstein, 1984).

Therapeutic Management

Conservative, nonoperative therapy is effective in controlling infection in most cases of VUR. There is a high incidence of spontaneous resolution over time—approximately 20% to 30% for each 2-year period throughout childhood (Ehrlich, 1982). An 80% probability of remission may occur in Grades I and II reflux when managed medically (Hensle and Burbige, 1986). Therapy consists of continuous low-dose antibacterial therapy with frequent urine cultures, which can usually be done at home by the dip slide or Chemstrip methods. This long-term therapy requires medical supervision and reliable, cooperative parents. Surgical correction of reflux may be required for Grades IV and V reflux. Grade III is managed conservatively unless complications interfere.

The major indications for surgical intervention include significant anatomic abnormality at the ureterovesical junction, recurrent UTI, high grades of VUR, noncompliance with medical therapy, intolerance to antibiotics, and VUR after puberty in females (Hensle and Burbige, 1986). Antireflux surgery consists of reimplantation of the ureters. Postsurgical antibiotic therapy is continued until a voiding cystourethrogram demonstrates no further VUR. Postoperative excretory urograms are performed before discharge, at 3 months, and at 1 year and 3 years after surgery to assess renal growth. Accelerated renal growth is observed in some children after surgery.

Nursing Considerations

The primary nursing goal in children on medical therapy is encouraging compliance. The importance of maintaining the medical regimen should be emphasized to parents and older children. The medications prescribed are usually well tolerated by children, but parents may need help in encouraging children to take the medication. The methods described in Chapter 27 provide some guidelines for administration and encouraging compliance. The importance of hygiene and a frequent voiding schedule are also discussed. (See Nursing Care Plan: The Child with Urinary Tract Infection.*)

GLOMERULAR DISEASE

The glomerulus is responsible for the initial step in formation of urine by separating a fraction of the water and disolved solutes from the formed elements and macromolecules of the blood flowing through the glomerular capillaries. The rate of filtration is determined by physical forces previously described; the efficiency of filtration depends on an intact glomerular membrane. The permeability of the membrane far exceeds that of capillaries in skeletal muscle due to the increased number of pores through which filtration takes place. Anything that alters the rate of flow or the filtrating capacity can disturb the body equilibrium.

ACUTE GLOMERULONEPHRITIS

Acute glomerulonephritis (AGN) as a classification includes a number of distinct entities. It may be a primary event or a manifestation of a systemic disorder (Table 30-4), and the disease can range from minimal to severe. The common features include oliguria, edema, hypertension and circulatory congestion, hematuria, and proteinuria. Most are postinfectious and have been associated with pneumococcal, streptococcal, and viral infections. All postinfectious diseases are presumed to result from immune complex formation and glomerular deposition, and the clinical presentations may be indistinguishable.

Acute poststreptococcal glomerulonephritis (APSGN) is the most common of the noninfectious renal diseases in childhood and the one for which a cause can be established in the majority of cases. APSGN can occur at any age but affects primarily early school-age children with a peak age of onset of 6 to 7 years. It is uncommon in children younger than 2 years of age, and males outnumber females 2:1 (Jordan and Lemire, 1982).

Etiology

It is now generally accepted that APSGN is an immune-complex disease, that is, a reaction that occurs as a by-product of an antecedent streptococcal infection with certain strains of the group A β-hemolytic streptococcus. Most streptococcal infections do not cause APSGN. A latent period of 10 to 14 days occurs between the streptococcal infection and the onset of clinical manifestations. The peak incidence of disease corresponds to the incidence of streptococcal infections. Disease secondary to streptococcal pharyngitis is

*In Wong, D.L., and Whaley, L.F.: Clinical manual of pediatric nursing, ed. 3, St. Louis, 1990, Mosby–Year Book, Inc.

Table 30-4 Renal involvement associated with a systemic disease process

DISEASE	MECHANISM	RENAL MANIFESTATION	COMMENTS
Systemic lupus erythematosus (SLE)	Deposition of autoantibody-antigen complexes in kidney	Variable degrees of hematuria and proteinuria More severe—nephrotic syndrome, hypertension, renal insufficiency	Responsive to corticosteroid and antimetabolite therapy Renal failure most common cause of death from SLE Rare before adolescence but may occur in school-age children
Anaphylactoid (Henoch-Schönlein) purpura	Unknown	Hematuria (gross or microscopic) Less common—edema, hypertension Nephrotic syndrome with oliguria and hypertension indicates severe involvement Rarely—acute renal failure	Incidence from 20% to 70% of cases Renal involvement most serious manifestation of the disease More common in children over age 6 years Responsive to corticosteroid therapy Management similar to that for persistent glomerulonephritis
Sickle cell disease	Infarction of renal vessels by sickled cells (especially medullary) Results in decreased circulation in vasa recta and impaired sodium and chloride ion reabsorption in collecting ducts	Hematuria Nephrotic syndrome Defective urine collection Progressive glomerulonephritis	Irreversible with increasing age Severe urinary tract infections with bacteremia not uncommon
Polyarteritis nodosa	Fibroid necrosis of arterial walls Large vessels—patchy renal infarction Microscopic vessels—necrotizing glomerulitis	Proteinuria Hematuria Severe hypertension	Kidney involvement of secondary importance in infancy Variable course Long-term prognosis guarded
Bacterial endocarditis	Focal or diffuse, immune-complex deposition related to chronic bacteremia Some embolization of glomeruli by bacteria and fibrin from endocardial vegetations	Proteinuria Hematuria	Seen in about 50% of cases Renal involvement seldom of major significance
Prolonged bacteremia (infected atrioventricular shunts)	Immune-complex deposition with exudation and cellular proliferation	Variable degrees of persistent nephrotic syndrome	Vigorous antibiotic therapy and/or removal of infected shunt required

more common in the winter or spring, but, when associated with pyoderma (principally impetigo), it may be more prevalent in later summer or early fall, especially in warmer climates. Multiple cases tend to occur in families. Second attacks are rare.

Pathophysiology

The mechanism by which the reaction takes place is still speculative. The most popular proposal to explain the pathologic process is that the streptococcal infection is followed by the release of a membranelike material from the specific organism into the circulation. Because it is antigenic, antibody is formed, and, after the appropriate period of time, an immune-complex reaction occurs. These immune complexes become trapped in the glomerular capillary loop, much the same as experimental serum sickness.

The kidney itself appears normal or moderately enlarged, but microscopic examination reveals a diffuse proliferative and exudative process. Glomerular capillary loops are almost obliterated by swelling, and infiltration with polymorphonuclear leukocytes adds to the appearance of increased cellularity. Consequently, the glomeruli appear dense and bloodless. Further examination reveals discrete nodules or "humps" on the basement membrane, which are identified as deposits of immune complexes. These deposits are not evident after about 6 weeks.

Endothelial cell proliferation and edema occlude the capillary lumen of affected glomeruli, and the afferent arteriole is probably constricted by vasospasm, both of which significantly reduce the glomerular filtration rate. This occurs without a proportional decrease in renal blood flow and results in a reduced capacity to form filtrate from the glomerular plasma flow. Vascular and tubular changes are mild and nonspecific; therefore, tubular function is less severely impaired.

The decreased filtration of plasma results in an excessive accumulation of water and an avid retention of sodium. These cause expanded plasma and interstitial fluid volumes that lead to circulatory congestion and edema. It is unclear whether the decreased glomerular filtration rate, increased capillary permeability, or vascular spasm is responsible for these various manifestations. The cause of the hypertension associated with acute glomerulonephritis is also unexplained. Plasma renin activity is low during the acute phase, but the hypervolemia may be a factor.

Clinical Manifestations

Typically, affected children are in good health until they experience the antecedent infection. In some instances there is no history of an infection, or it is only described as a mild cold. The onset of nephritis appears after an average latent period of about 10 days. Since the child appears well during this time, the association is not recognized by parents.

Initial signs of nephrotic reaction include puffiness of the face, especially around the eyes (periorbital edema), anorexia, and passage of dark-colored urine. The edema is more prominent in the face in the morning but spreads during the day to involve the extremities and abdomen. The edema is only moderate and may not be appreciated by someone unfamiliar with the child's normal appearance. The urine is cloudy, smoky brown, or what parents describe as resembling tea or cola, and severely reduced in volume.

✦ **NURSING ALERT** A child who exhibits the following should be evaluated for possible acute glomerulonephritis:

- Orbital edema, which parents report is worse in the morning
- Loss of appetite
- Decreased output
- Dark-colored urine revealed by examination
- Antecedent streptococcal infection

The child is pale, irritable, and lethargic. He appears unwell but seldom expresses specific complaints. Older children may complain of headaches, abdominal discomfort, and dysuria. Vomiting is not uncommon. On examination there is usually a mild-to-moderate elevation in blood pressure (diastolic, 80 to 120 mm Hg; systolic, 120 to 180 mm Hg). Occasionally a child will have an atypical mode of onset with severe symptoms such as convulsions (secondary to cerebral ischemia and/or hypertension), pulmonary and circulatory congestion, minimal urine findings, or hematuria in the absence of hypertension and edema. For a comparison between APSGN and minimal change nephrotic syndrome (see Table 30-5).

Clinical course. The acute edematous phase of glomerulonephritis usually persists from 4 to 10 days but may persist for 2 or 3 weeks, during which time the child remains listless, anorexic, and apathetic. The weight fluctuates, the urine remains thick and smoky brown in color, and the blood pressure may suddenly reach dangerously high levels at any time during this phase.

The first sign of improvement is a small increase in urine output with a corresponding decrease in body weight, followed in 1 or 2 days by copious diuresis. With diuresis the child begins to feel better, the appetite improves, and the

Table 30-5 Comparison of poststreptococcal glomerulonephritis and nephrotic syndrome

MANIFESTATIONS	ACUTE POSTSTREPTOCOCCAL GLOMERULONEPHRITIS	MINIMAL CHANGE NEPHROTIC SYNDROME
Streptococcal antibody titers	Present	Absent
Blood pressure	Elevated	Normal or decreased
Edema	Primarily periorbital and peripheral	Generalized severe
Circulatory congestion	Common	Absent
Proteinuria	Moderate	Massive
Hematuria	Gross or microscopic	Microscopic or none
Casts	Present	Present
Azotemia	Present	Absent
Serum potassium levels	Increased	Normal
Serum protein levels	Minimum reduction	Markedly decreased
Serum lipid levels	Normal	Elevated
Fatigue	Present	Present
Age at onset (years)	5-7	2-3

blood pressure decreases to normal with the reduction of edema. Gross hematuria diminishes, in part because of dilution of the red blood cells in the more dilute urine, but microscopic hematuria may persist for weeks or months. The blood urea nitrogen level decreases during diuresis, but it, along with a slight to moderate proteinuria, may persist for several weeks.

Prognosis. Almost all children correctly diagnosed as having APSGN recover completely, and specific immunity is conferred so that subsequent recurrences are uncommon. Deaths from complications still occur but are, fortunately, rare. A few of these children may develop chronic disease, but many of these cases are believed to be (probably) different glomerular diseases misdiagnosed as poststreptococcal disease.

Complications. The major complications that may develop during the acute phase of glomerulonephritis are hypertensive encephalopathy, acute cardiac decompensation, and acute renal failure. Normally cerebral blood flow responds to acute arterial hypertension by vasoconstriction. However, acute and severe hypertension may cause this protective autoregulation of cerebral blood flow to fail, leading to hyperperfusion of the brain and cerebral edema. The premonitory signs of encephalopathy are headache, dizziness, abdominal discomfort, and vomiting. If the condition progresses there may be transient loss of vision and/or hemiparesis, disorientation, and generalized convulsions of the grand mal type.

Cardiac decompensation during the acute edematous phase of nephritis is caused by hypervolemia and not by cardiac failure. Signs of circulatory congestion are evident, however. The heart is enlarged, and increased pulmonary vascular markings are evident on roentgenographic examination. Increased pulmonary capillary permeability is also believed to be an important factor in the development of pulmonary edema.

Acute renal failure with persistent oliguria or anuria is an uncommon complication but one that requires an appropriate treatment regimen.

Diagnostic Evaluation

Urinalysis during the acute phase characteristically shows hematuria, proteinuria, and increased specific gravity. The specific gravity is moderately elevated and seldom exceeds 1.020. Proteinuria generally parallels the hematuria, and the content usually shows 3+ or 4+ but is not the massive proteinuria seen in nephrotic syndrome. Gross discoloration of urine reflects its red blood cell and hemoglobin content. Microscopic examination of the sediment shows many red blood cells, leukocytes, epithelial cells, and granular and red blood cell casts. Bacteria are not seen, and urine cultures are negative.

Blood examination reveals normal electrolytes (sodium, potassium, and chloride ions) and carbon dioxide levels, unless the disease has progressed to renal failure. Azotemia resulting from impaired glomerular filtration is reflected in elevated blood urea nitrogen and creatinine levels in at least 50% of cases. When proteinuria is heavy, there may be changes associated with nephrotic syndrome, that is, transient hypoproteinemia and hyperlipidemia.

Cultures of the pharynx are positive for streptococci in only a few cases, and the numbers are not significantly greater than the normal carrier incidence in many communities. Positive cultures help to establish a diagnosis. Cultures should be obtained from other household members, and persons positive for group A streptococci should receive a course of antistreptococcal therapy.

Some serologic tests may help in diagnosis. Antibody responses to the extracellular products of the streptococci provide indirect evidence of previous streptococcal infection. These include antistreptolysin O (ASO), antistreptokinase (ASKase), antihyaluronidase (AHase), antideoxyribonuclease-B (ADNase-B), and antinicotyladenine dinucleotidase (ANADase). The ASO titer is the most familiar and readily available test for streptococcal antibodies. ASO appears in the serum about 10 days after the initial infection and persists for 4 to 6 weeks; however, there is no correlation between the degree of elevation and its duration and the severity or prognosis of the glomerulonephritis. It is a useful diagnostic tool when nephritis follows a pharyngeal infection but is of less value after pyoderma. An ASO titer of 250 Todd units or higher is of diagnostic significance, as is a rising titer in two samples taken a week apart. More consistent and reliable antibody tests following streptococcal skin infections are elevated AHase and ADNase-B titers.

Nonspecific acute-phase reactants that reflect acute inflammatory processes, such as the erythrocyte sedimentation rate (ESR), C-reactive protein (CRP), and serum mucoprotein tests are elevated during the early stages of acute disease and then gradually return to normal as healing takes place. The ESR is sometimes used as a guide to the progress of the nephritis.

Since glomerulonephritis is an immune-complex disease, there is reduced total serum complement activity in the early stages of acute disease. The simpler measurements of the C3 complement component (beta$_1$ C globulin) are used as an index of total complement activity. The test is most useful in children with no edema or minimal urine findings.

Other studies that are employed include a chest x-ray examination, which shows characteristic generalized cardiac enlargement, pulmonary congestion, and pleural effusion during the edematous phase of acute disease. Electrocardiography reveals elevation or depression of the ST segment, prolonged QRS and ST segments, lengthening of the P-R interval, and flattened or inverted T waves. Renal biopsy for diagnostic purposes is seldom required but may be useful in the diagnosis of atypical cases.

Correlations between laboratory and morphologic findings indicate a significant relationship between creatinine clearance and severity of glomerular damage. Greater damage is reflected in a reduced creatinine clearance and is also associated with a higher blood urea nitrogen level. An increased excretion of cellular protein is associated with increasing glomerular capillary obliteration. There appears to be no correlation between the extent of glomerular damage and ASO titer, oliguria, or blood pressure.

Therapeutic Management

No specific treatment is available for acute glomerulonephritis, but recovery is spontaneous and uneventful in most cases. Management consists of general supportive measures and early recognition and treatment of complications. Children who have normal blood pressure and a satisfactory urine output can generally be treated at home. Those with substantial edema, hypertension, gross hematuria, and/or significant oliguria should be hospitalized because of the unpredictability of complications. Short hospitalization is the rule in uncomplicated cases; prolonged hospitalization is required only for children with severely impaired renal function.

General measures. Bed rest may be recommended during the acute phase, but ambulation does not seem to have an adverse effect on the course of the disease once the gross hematuria, edema, hypertension, and azotemia have abated. Since they are generally listless and experience fatigue and malaise, most children voluntarily restrict their activities during the most active phase of the disease.

Fluid balance. Regular measurement of vital signs, body weight, and intake and output is essential in order to monitor the progress of the disease and to detect complications that may appear at any time during the course of the disease. A record of daily weight is the most useful means to assess fluid balance and should be kept for children treated at home as well as for those who are hospitalized. Water restriction is seldom necessary unless the output is significantly reduced (less than 2 to 3 dl/24 hours). In these children the water allowed is equivalent to the calculated insensible loss plus the volume of urine excreted. Children on restricted fluids, especially those who are severely edematous or those who have lost weight, should be observed for signs of dehydration.

Diuretics are usually of limited value, since very little sodium reaches the distal tubules as a result of the reduced filtration rate. However, diuretic therapy, usually furosemide, is helpful if significant edema and fluid overload are present. Digitalis may be employed sometimes, although there is question regarding its effectiveness in acute nephritis. Rarely children with acute glomerulonephritis develop acute renal failure with oliguria that significantly alters the fluid and electrolyte balance. These children require careful management that may include peritoneal dialysis or hemodialysis.

Loss of glomerular filtration may produce electrolyte imbalances in children with severe forms of APSGN, especially hyperkalemia, acidosis, hypocalcemia, and hyperphosphatemia. Management of these electrolyte disturbances is described under acute renal failure.

Hypertension. Acute hypertension must be anticipated and identified early. Blood pressure measurements are taken every 4 to 6 hours. Significant but not severe hypertension is controlled with hydralazine (Apresoline), usually in conjunction with a diuretic. Oral hydrochlorothiazide is used to control mild hypertension. Seizure activity associated with hypertensive encephalopathy requires anticonvulsant therapy as well as antihypertensive agents (see Renal Failure, p. 1357 for management of severe hypertension).

Nutrition. Dietary restrictions depend on the stage and severity of the disease, especially the extent of edema. Regular diet is permitted in uncomplicated cases, but the intake of sodium is usually limited (no salt is added to foods). Moderate sodium restriction is usually instituted for children with hypertension or edema. Foods with substantial amounts of potassium are generally restricted during the period of oliguria. Protein restriction is reserved only for children with severe azotemia resulting from prolonged oliguria. The loss of appetite associated with the disease usually limits the protein intake sufficiently. During the acute stage calories may be restricted to carbohydrates and fats.

Antibiotics. Antibiotic therapy is indicated only for those children with evidence of persistent streptococcal infections. The antibiotics do not alter the course of the disease but are often recommended to prevent transmission of nephritogenic streptococci to other family members (Fish and Fouser, 1986). Authorities are divided in their use of prophylactic antimicrobials for other family members.

Nursing Considerations

Nursing care of the child with glomerulonephritis involves careful assessment of the disease status, with regular monitoring of vital signs (including frequent measurement of blood pressure), fluid balance, and behavior. Vital signs provide clues to the severity of the disease and early signs of complications. They are carefully measured, and any abnormalities reported and recorded. The volume and character of urine are noted, and the child is weighed daily. Assessment of the child's appearance for signs of cerebral complications is an important nursing function, since the severity of the acute phase is variable and unpredictable. The child with edema, hypertension, and gross hematuria may be subject to complications, and anticipatory preparations such as seizure precautions and intravenous equipment are included in the nursing care plan.

For most children a regular diet is allowed, but it should contain no added salt. Foods high in sodium and salted treats are eliminated, and parents and friends should be advised not to bring items such as potato chips or pretzels. However, the total amount of salt ingested is usually less than prescribed because of poor appetite. Fluid restriction, if prescribed, is more difficult, and the amount permitted should be evenly divided throughout the waking hours and served in small cups to give the illusion of larger servings. Meal preparation and service require special attention, since the child has a poor appetite and is indifferent to meals during the acute phase. Again, collaboration with parents and the dietitian and special consideration for food preferences facilitate meal planning.

During the acute phase children are generally quite content to lie in bed, but activities should be those that require little expenditure of energy. As they begin to feel better and their symptoms subside, activities should be planned to allow for frequent rest periods and avoidance of fatigue.

Children with mild edema and no hypertension, as well as convalescent children being treated at home, need follow-up care. Parents are instructed regarding general measures, including activity, diet, and prevention of infection. Strenuous activity is usually restricted until there is no evidence of proteinuria or macroscopic hematuria.

Health supervision is continued with weekly, followed by monthly, visits for evaluation and urinalysis. Parent education and support in preparation for discharge and home care include education in home management and the need for follow-up care and health supervision. (See Nursing Care Plan: The Child with Acute Poststreptococcal Glomerulonephritis.*)

CHRONIC OR PROGRESSIVE GLOMERULONEPHRITIS

The majority of cases of renal glomerular disease are acute glomerulonephritis, minimal change nephrotic syndrome, and glomerulonephritis associated with systemic diseases. These pose relatively few problems of diagnosis, and their natural course is fairly predictable. A few cases present a prolonged course and a poor ultimate prognosis. They are a rather heterogeneous group, defined by correlating the clinical manifestations, pathologic conditions, and natural course of the individual diseases.

Persistent glomerulonephritis is used to describe those cases of glomerulonephritis that have no specific histologic picture but that fail to show the rapid recovery expected in acute nephritis. *Chronic glomerulonephritis (CGN)* describes advanced glomerular disease, which includes a variety of different disease processes. *Rapidly progressive glomerulonephritis* is used to describe an acute illness with severe, acute onset resembling acute poststreptococcal glomerulonephritis but that causes rapidly progressive deterioration of renal function in weeks to months.

Pathophysiology

In most cases of CGN immunologic mechanisms can be implicated either through direct attack on the kidney or secondary to the accumulation of immune complexes in the glomerular filter or fibrin deposition from previously damaged glomeruli. Either can contribute to further glomerular damage and can initiate chronic changes in the glomerular structure. In many cases there is no history of an attack of acute glomerular disease. In other cases it may represent one of a succession of exacerbations of a preexisting disease. CGN that is not associated with other diseases may go undetected for years and be relatively asymptomatic until kidney destruction produces marked reduction in renal function. Consequently, the disease is more common in adolescents than in younger children. Renal insufficiency with all its manifestations occurs as the ultimate event.

Clinical Manifestations

The varied clinical manifestations and laboratory findings generally reflect deteriorating renal function. Nephrotic syndrome, with its usual manifestations, frequently develops. Hypertension, edema, proteinuria, cardiac failure, dyspnea, osteodystrophy, and anemia are common manifestations of progressive disease.

Diagnostic Evaluation

Laboratory findings may include proteinuria, with casts and red and white blood cells. Failing renal function is evidenced by elevated blood urea nitrogen, creatinine, and uric acid levels. Electrolyte alterations include metabolic acidosis, decreased sodium from the chronic salt-losing state, elevated potassium, elevated phosphorus, and decreased calcium levels. As the disease progresses, urine specific gravity eventually stabilizes at an isotonic state (about 1.012) as a result of the inability of the kidney to reabsorb solutes or respond to antidiuretic hormone. The renal insufficiency may extend from 5 to 15 years and even longer, or rapid deterioration may progress to end-stage renal disease (ESRD) in 1 to 2 years.

Therapeutic Management

Early in the course of the disease, treatment is appropriate to the underlying disease and is largely symptomatic in most cases. Efforts are directed toward providing optimal conditions for the child's physical, psychologic, and social development. As few restrictions as feasible are imposed, and the child is allowed to live as normal a life as possible for as long as possible. Drug treatment offers little lasting benefit, although diuretic therapy may be helpful occasionally for edema or hypertension. Marked hypertension is controlled with antihypertensive agents, and anemia may require periodic transfusion with fresh packed cells. Salt is only moderately restricted. Ultimately dialysis and transplantation may restore relatively good health; however, these are usually not available alternatives until renal failure is far advanced. (See Chronic Renal Failure, p. 1363, for more detailed management of specific problems.) Children with rapidly progressive glomerulonephritis are usually referred to a center specializing in renal disease.

Nursing Considerations

The problems of CGN and those encountered in chronic renal insufficiency from any cause are discussed in association with chronic renal failure.

NEPHROTIC SYNDROME

Nephrotic syndrome is the most common presentation of glomerular injury in children. It is defined as massive proteinuria, hypoalbuminemia, hyperlipemia, and edema, but the disorder is a clinical manifestation of a large number of distinct glomerular disorders in which increased glomerular permeability to plasma protein results in massive urinary protein loss. Following a description of the three major

*In Wong, D.L., and Whaley, L.F.: Clinical manual of pediatric nursing, ed. 3, St. Louis, 1990, Mosby–Year Book, Inc.

forms of nephrotic syndrome, the remainder of the discussion is devoted to minimal change disease.

Types of Nephrotic Syndrome

Nephrotic syndrome can be classified as *primary,* when the syndrome is restricted to glomerular injury, or *secondary,* when it develops as part of a systemic illness. Although it may have several different histologic variations, the most common form of the primary disease is *minimal change nephrotic syndrome.* A congenital form is also recognized.

Minimal change nephrotic syndrome (MCNS). Approximately 80% of cases of nephrotic syndrome in children occur in the absence of recognizable systemic disease or preexisting renal disease and are categorized as idiopathic. MCNS can present at any age but is predominantly a disease of the preschool child. In 74% of children, the onset of the disease occurs between the ages of 2 and 7 years (McEnery and Strife, 1982). The disease is rare in children younger than 6 months of age, uncommon in infants younger than 1 year of age, and unusual after the age of 8. The incidence of the disease in North America is approximately 2:100,000 children per year, and males outnumber females 2:1 (Drummond, 1983). In adolescence the ratio is 1:1.

The cause of MCNS (also known as idiopathic nephrosis, "minimal lesion" nephrosis, childhood nephrosis, lipoid nephrosis, or uncomplicated nephrosis) remains obscure. Often a nonspecific illness, usually a viral upper respiratory infection, precedes the manifestations by 4 to 8 days but is considered to be a precipitating factor rather than a cause.

Secondary nephrotic syndrome. Nephrotic syndrome may occur after or in association with glomerular damage of known or presumed etiology. Prominent among causes of glomerular damage is acute or chronic glomerulonephritis. Less commonly, secondary nephrotic syndrome occurs during the course of collagen diseases (such as disseminated lupus erythematosus and anaphylactoid purpura) or as the result of toxicity to drugs (such as trimethadione and heavy metals), stings, or venom. Nephrotic syndrome is the major presenting symptom of renal disease in pediatric patients with acquired immune deficiency syndrome (AIDS). Diverse, rare causes are sickle cell disease, hepatitis, malaria, cyanotic heart disease, diabetes mellitus, amyloidosis, tuberculosis, infected ventriculojugular shunts, renal vein thrombosis, or malignancies.

Congenital nephrotic syndrome. The hereditary form of nephrotic syndrome is caused by a recessive gene on an autosome. Infants who have nephrotic syndrome are small for gestational age, and proteinuria and edema are manifest early. The disease does not respond to the usual therapy, and death in the first year or two of life is the rule if the infant does not receive a successful renal transplant.

Pathophysiology

The pathogenesis of MCNS is not understood. There may be a metabolic, biochemical, or physiochemical disturbance in the basement membrane of the glomeruli that leads to increased permeability to protein, but the causes and mechanisms are only speculative.

The glomerular membrane, which is normally impermeable to albumin and other large proteins, becomes permeable to proteins, especially albumin, which leak through the membrane and are lost in urine (hyperalbuminuria). This reduces the serum albumin level (hypoalbuminemia), which decreases the colloidal osmotic pressure in the capillaries. As a result, the hydrostatic pressure exceeds the pull of the colloidal osmotic pressure, and fluid accumulates in the interstitial spaces and body cavities, particularly the abdominal cavity (ascites). The shift of fluid from the plasma to the interstitial spaces reduces the vascular fluid volume (hypovolemia), which in turn stimulates the renin-angiotensin system and the secretion of antidiuretic hormone and aldosterone. Tubular reabsorption of sodium and water is increased in an attempt to increase intravascular volume. The elevation of serum cholesterol, phospholipids, and triglycerides is unexplained. The sequence of events in nephrotic syndrome is diagrammed in Fig. 30-3.

Clinical Manifestations

A previously well child begins to gain weight, which progresses insidiously over a period of days or weeks. Puffiness of the face, especially around the eyes, is apparent on arising in the morning but subsides during the day, when swelling of the abdomen and lower extremities is more prominent. The generalized edema develops so slowly that parents may consider it to be a sign of healthy growth. Although an acute infection may precipitate severe generalized edema (*anasarca*), the usual course is one of progressive weight gain until either rapid or gradual increase in edema prompts the family to seek medical evaluation. Usually present are periorbital edema, abdominal swelling from ascites, and labial or scrotal swelling (Fig. 30-4). Edema of the intestinal mucosa may cause diarrhea, loss of appetite, and poor intestinal absorption. The volume of urine is decreased, and it appears darkly opalescent and frothy.

Extreme skin pallor is often present, and the child has a tendency toward skin breakdown during periods of edema. The child is irritable and may be easily fatigued or lethargic but does not appear seriously ill. Weight loss from poor appetite and loss of protein is not uncommon, although it is frequently obscured by edema. Changes in the nails appear as white (Muercke) lines parallel to the lanula, which are caused by prolonged hypoalbuminemia. The blood pressure is usually normal or slightly decreased. The child is more susceptible to infection, especially cellulitis, pneumonia, peritonitis, or septicemia.

✦**NURSING ALERT** A child who exhibits the following should be be evaluated for the possibility of nephrotic syndrome:

- Weight gain over that expected based on previous pattern
- Parent observation that the child's clothes fit tightly
- Decreased urine output
- Pallor, fatigue

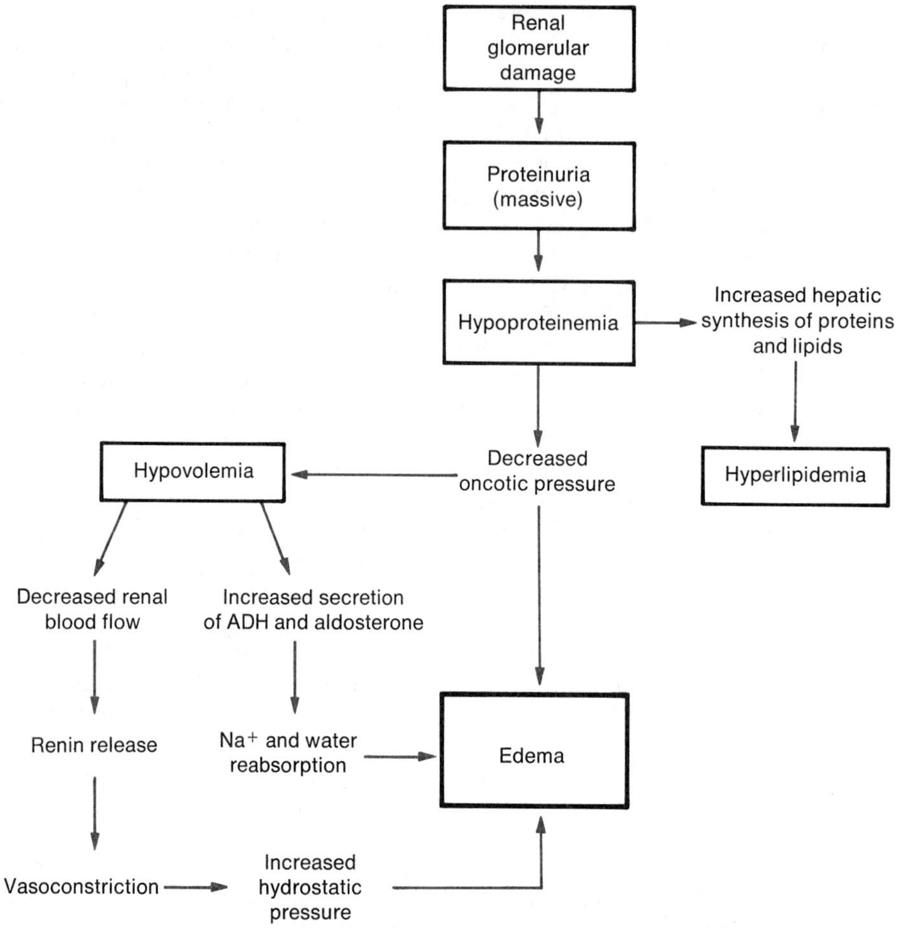

Fig. 30-3. Sequence of events in nephrotic syndrome.

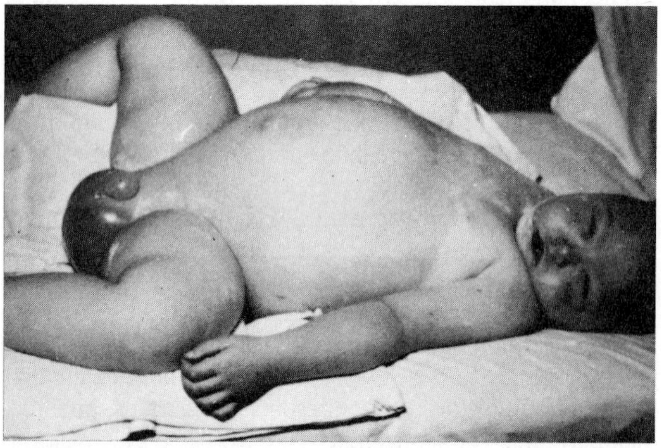

Fig. 30-4. Two-year-old child with nephrosis.
From Shirkey, H.C., editor: Pediatric therapy, ed. 6, St. Louis, 1980, Mosby–Year Book, Inc.

In children with MCNS, in rare instances there is significant or persistent hypertension, gross or persistent hematuria, significant or persistent azotemia (presence of increased nitrogenous products in the blood), or depression of serum $\beta 1_c$ globulin.

Diagnostic Evaluation

The diagnosis of MCNS is made on the basis of history and clinical manifestations (edema, proteinuria, hypoalbuminemia, and hypercholesterolemia in the absence of hematuria and hypertension) in children presenting between the ages of 2 and 4 years. Massive proteinuria is reflected in urine excretion of protein that frequently reaches levels in excess of 2 g/m^2/day of body surface with relatively greater clearance of low-molecular-weight proteins. Hyaline casts from high protein and sluggish flow and oval fat bodies, as well as a few red blood cells, can be found in the urine of most affected children, although there is seldom gross hematuria. Specific gravity is high and proportionate to the amount of protein concentration. If hypovolemia is not significant and the child is well hydrated, the glomerular filtration rate is usually normal.

Total serum protein concentrations are reduced, with the albumin fractions significantly reduced (less than 2 g/dl) and plasma lipids elevated. Serum cholesterol may be as high as 450 to 1500 mg/dl. Hemoglobin and hematocrit are usually normal or elevated, and the platelet count is high (500,000 to 1,000,000) as a result of hemoconcentration. Serum sodium concentration is usually low, about 130 to 135 mEq/L.

If renal biopsy is performed, it provides information regarding the glomerular status and type of nephrotic syndrome, response to drugs, and probable course of the disease. Under the microscope the foot processes of the basement membrane appear fused. The major focuses in differential diagnosis are to establish the edema as renal in origin and to distinguish minimum change nephrotic syndrome from other glomerulopathies with nephrotic syndrome as a manifestation.

Therapeutic Management

The medical management consists of both general and specific measures. The primary objective is to reduce the excretion of urinary protein and maintain a protein-free urine. Additional objectives include prevention or treatment of acute infection, control of edema, establishment of good nutrition, and readjustment of any disturbed metabolic processes. Children with severe symptoms or whose disease is newly recognized are hospitalized for assessment and observation for evidence of infection, response to therapy, and parental education.

General measures. General treatment is principally supportive. During the edema phase the child is often placed on bed rest, but activity is not restricted during remission. Children can be remarkably active with no evidence that restriction affects the ultimate outcome. Acute and intercurrent infections are treated with appropriate antibiotics, and efforts are made to eliminate possible infection.

Diet. The child who is in remission is allowed a regular diet; however, during periods of massive edema, salt is restricted in the form of no added salt at the table and excluding foods with very high salt content. This is usually tolerated by the child for a time, but it should be adjusted to the child's appetite and must not interfere with nutrient intake. Although edema cannot be removed by a low-sodium diet, its rate of increase may be reduced. Water is seldom restricted. A diet generous in protein is logical, but there is no evidence that it is beneficial or alters the outcome of the disease (Kim and Grupe, 1986). The presence of azotemia and renal failure is a contraindication for high-protein intake.

Corticosteroid therapy. The response of most affected children to corticosteroids has established these drugs as prime therapeutic agents in management of nephrotic syndrome. Corticosteroid therapy is begun as soon as the diagnosis has been determined and administered orally in a dosage of 2 mg/kg of body weight or 60 mg/m^2/day in evenly divided doses. Prednisone, the safest and least expensive drug, is the steroid of choice. The drug is continued until the urine is free from protein and remains normal for 10 days to 2 weeks (Drummond, 1983).

The course of the disease is fairly predictable. There is little change during the first few days of therapy. In most patients diuresis occurs as the urine protein excretion diminishes within 7 to 21 days after the initiation of steroid therapy. Other clinical manifestations stabilize or return to normal shortly thereafter. Almost 95% of patients between 1 and 10 years of age with no hypertension, hematuria, or renal insufficiency and who have satisfactory laboratory measurements of C3 complement and a renal clearance of IgG will have complete resolution of proteinuria with therapy (Kim and Grupe, 1986).

If the child has not responded to therapy in 28 days of daily steroid administration, the likelihood of subsequent response diminishes rapidly. When the child is free of proteinuria and edema, the total daily dose of prednisone is usually given for a time as a single daily dose every 48 hours. The dose is gradually tapered to discontinuation over a variable period, from several weeks to months, depending on the medical philosophy. Once a satisfactory response is achieved, steroid therapy is reduced to every other day (q.o.d.). This dosage is less likely to depress pituitary-adrenal function and produces fewer side effects during prolonged therapy. If a tendency to relapse is demonstrated, the number of relapses can be reduced with administration of a low-dose, q.o.d. schedule of prednisone therapy that continues for 6 months to 1 year (provided remission is achieved and successful tapering to low-dose q.o.d. therapy occurs).

Children with MCNS are often described according to their response to corticosteroid therapy (Box 30-5). Children with MCNS typically relapse one to three times per year. Children who are steroid-dependent tend to have frequent relapses over many years and receive large amounts of steroids, which results in cushingoid features and growth retardation. They also require supportive treatment (diuretics, diet). The prognosis for children who are steroid-unresponsive is less predictable than for those who are steroid-responsive (McEnery and Strife, 1982).

Children who require frequent courses of steroid therapy are highly susceptible to complications of steroids, such as growth retardation, cataracts, obesity, hypertension, gastrointestinal bleeding, bone demineralization, infections, and hyperglycemia. Children who do not respond to steroid therapy, those who have frequent relapses, and those in whom the side effects threaten their growth and general health may be considered for a course of therapy using other immunosuppressant medications.

Box 30-5 CLASSIFICATION OF NEPHROTIC SYNDROME ACCORDING TO STEROID RESPONSE

1. "Steroid-sensitive" (20% to 40%)—response to a single short course of steroids without evidence of relapse after cessation of therapy.
2. "Frequent relapsers" or "steroid-dependent" (60% to 80%)—respond to steroids and can be tapered off completely; have three or more relapses in a 6- to 12-month period; remit when placed on steroids but tend to relapse on lowered dosage.
3. "Steroid-unresponsive" or "steroid-resistant"—never respond to steroids or become resistant to steroids at some point during the course of disease.

Modified from McEnery, P.T., and Strife, C.F.: Nephrotic syndrome in childhood, Pediatr. Clin. North Am. 89:875-894, 1982.

Immunosuppressant therapy. It is often possible to reduce the relapse rate and induce long-term remission with administration of an oral alkylating agent, usually cyclophosphamide (Cytoxan), alternating with prednisone. Both drugs are administered for up to 2 to 3 months, after which cyclophosphamide is discontinued abruptly, and the prednisone is decreased by decrements. Chlorambucil has also proven effective when given with corticosteroids. The two drugs share many characteristics, and response to both appears to depend on dose, duration of therapy, age, and the duration of the disease.

Significant side effects of cyclophosphamide must be considered and discussed with parents of children for whom this drug is contemplated. Leukopenia must be anticipated, and evidence suggests that cyclophosphamide may cause azoospermia with potential sterility in males treated for more than 2 to 3 months and variable effects on gonadal function in females.

Diuretics. One characteristic of the edema of nephrotic syndrome is its usual lack of responsiveness to diuretic agents. However, in cases in which edema interferes with respiration or there is hypotension, hyponatremia, or evidence of skin breakdown, loop diuretics are sometimes useful, usually furosemide in combination with metolazone. In addition, plasma expanders such as salt-poor human albumin may be administered to severely edematous children requiring prompt control; however, they must be administered frequently, since the glomeruli are readily permeable to albumin in the acute stage.

Prognosis. The prognosis for ultimate recovery in most cases is good. It is a self-limiting disease, and in children who respond to steroid therapy the tendency to relapse decreases with time. With early detection and prompt implementation of therapy to eradicate proteinuria, progressive basement membrane damage is minimized, so that when the tendency to exacerbations is past, renal function is usually normal or near normal. It is estimated that approximately 80% of nephrotic children have this favorable prognosis, although half the children have relapses even after 5 years, and 20% after 10 years (Kim and Grupe, 1986).

Nursing Considerations

Whether nephrotic syndrome occurs as an initial disorder, a recurrent health problem, or a complication of another disorder, the affected child presents a nursing challenge.

Assessment

Continuous monitoring of fluid retention or excretion is an important nursing function. Strict and accurate records of intake and output are essential but may be difficult in very young children. Application of collection bags is highly irritating to edematous, sensitive skin, already subject to breakdown. Other methods of monitoring progress include urine examination for specific gravity and albumin, daily weight, and measurement of abdominal girth. Assessment of edema such as increased or decreased swelling around eyes and dependent areas, degree of pitting (if noted), and color and texture of skin are part of nursing care. Vital signs are monitored to detect any early signs of complications such as shock or an infective process.

Nursing Diagnoses

Constant reassessment and evaluation reveal a number of nursing diagnoses that are relevant to the care of these children and their families (see Nursing Care Plan, pp. 1351-1352). Others will be apparent in specific situations.

Planning

The goals of nursing care for the child with nephrotic syndrome are as follows:

1. Reduce the excretion of urinary protein and maintain a protein-free urine.
2. Prevent skin breakdown and infection.
3. Establish and maintain good nutrition.
4. Support and educate child and family.

Implementation

Children hospitalized with MCNS may be placed on bed rest during the edema phase of the disease. They seldom offer resistance, since they are usually lethargic and easily fatigued, and their cumbersome edematous bulk is not conducive to movement. Most are content to lie in the prone position. These children must be encouraged and helped to turn regularly to prevent tissue breakdown. Areas that are particularly edematous, such as the scrotum, abdomen, and legs, may require support, and skin surfaces should be cleaned and separated with clothing, cotton, or antiseptic powder to prevent intertrigo.

Infection is a constant source of danger to edematous children and those on corticosteroid therapy. These children are particularly vulnerable to upper respiratory infection; therefore, they must be kept warm and dry, turned frequently, and protected from contact with infected roommates, visitors, and personnel. Vital signs are monitored to detect any early signs of an infective process.

Loss of appetite that accompanies active nephrosis creates a perplexing problem for nurses. During this time the combined efforts of nurse, dietitian, parents, and the child himself are needed to formulate a nutritionally adequate and attractive diet. Salt is usually restricted, but not eliminated, during the edema phase. Every effort should be made to serve attractive meals with a minimum of fuss, but it usually requires a considerable amount of ingenuity and enticement to get the child to eat. Games, rewards, and special treats often help, but each child is unique, and it may require considerable trial and error to arrive at a successful strategy. Also, the same strategy may not work consistently (see Feeding the Sick Child, Chapter 27).

As the edema subsides, children are allowed increased activity. Although they are easily fatigued, they are usually able to adjust activities according to their individual tolerance but may require guidance in selection of play activities. Suitable recreational and diversional activities are an important part of their care. Once edema fluid has been

NURSING CARE PLAN
The Child with Nephrotic Syndrome

NURSING DIAGNOSIS: Fluid volume excess (total body) related to fluid accumulation in tissues and third spaces

GOAL 1
Detect evidence of fluid retention

INTERVENTIONS
Assess intake relative to output
- Measure and record intake and output accurately
- Weigh daily (or more often, if indicated)

Assess changes in edema
- Measure abdominal girth at umbilicus
- Test urine for specific gravity, albumin
- Collect specimens for laboratory examination

EXPECTED OUTCOME
Measurements reveal desired information

GOAL 2
Prevent fluid retention

INTERVENTIONS
*Administer corticosteroids as prescribed
*Administer diuretics if ordered
Limit fluids as indicated

EXPECTED OUTCOME
Child exhibits no evidence of fluid accumulation (specify parameters)

GOAL 3
Prevent increased fluid intake

INTERVENTIONS
Regulate fluid intake carefully
Monitor intravenous infusion to maintain prescribed intake
Employ strategies to prevent undesired intake
- Use small containers for fluid intake
- Divide allowed intake into small volumes spread over entire day
- Spray mouth with atomizer (mist) to prevent feeling of dryness

Keep lips lubricated

EXPECTED OUTCOME
Child receives no more fluid than prescribed

*Dependent nursing action.

NURSING DIAGNOSIS: Potential (intravascular) fluid volume deficit related to protein (reduced COP) and fluid loss, edema

GOAL 1
Detect evidence of intravascular fluid loss

INTERVENTIONS
Monitor vital signs to detect physical evidence of fluid depletion
Assess pulse quality and rate
Measure blood pressure
Report any deviations from normal

EXPECTED OUTCOME
Child displays no evidence of hypovolemia

GOAL 2
Assist in raising COP

INTERVENTION
*Administer salt-poor albumin if prescribed

EXPECTED OUTCOME
Child exhibits no evidence of intravascular fluid loss or hypovolemic shock

NURSING DIAGNOSIS: Potential for infection related to lowered body defenses, fluid overload

GOAL 1
Prevent infection

INTERVENTIONS
Protect child from contact with infected persons
- Place in room with noninfectious children
- Restrict contact with persons who have infections, including family, other children, friends, and staff members
- Observe medical asepsis
  - Practice good handwashing
- Teach visitors appropriate preventive behaviors

Keep child warm and dry
Monitor vital signs for early evidence of infection

EXPECTED OUTCOMES
Child and family apply good health practices
Child exhibits no evidence of infection

Continued.

NURSING CARE PLAN
The Child with Nephrotic Syndrome—cont'd

NURSING DIAGNOSIS: Potential impaired skin integrity related to edema, lowered body defenses

GOAL 1
Prevent skin breakdown

INTERVENTIONS

Provide meticulous skin care
Cleanse and powder opposing skin surfaces several times per day
Separate opposing skin surfaces with soft cotton
Support edematous organs, such as scrotum
Cleanse edematous eyelids with warm saline wipes
Change position frequently; maintain good body alignment

EXPECTED OUTCOME

Child's skin displays no evidence of redness or irritation

NURSING DIAGNOSIS: Altered nutrition: less than body requirements related to loss of appetite

GOAL 1
Provide good nutrition

INTERVENTIONS

Offer nutritious diet
Restrict sodium during edema and steroid therapy
*Administer supplementary vitamins and iron as ordered
Enlist aid of child, parents, and dietitian in formulation of diet

EXPECTED OUTCOME

Child consumes an adequate diet (specify)

GOAL 2
Stimulate appetite

INTERVENTIONS

Provide cheerful, clean, relaxed atmosphere during meals
Serve small quantities initially to stimulate appetite; encourage seconds
Provide special and preferred foods
Serve foods in an attractive manner
See also Feeding the Sick Child, Chapter 27

EXPECTED OUTCOME

Child consumes an adequate amount of food

NURSING DIAGNOSIS: Body image disturbance related to change in appearance

GOAL 1
Establish good mental hygiene

INTERVENTIONS

Explore feelings and concerns regarding appearance
Point out positive aspects of appearance and evidence of diminished edema
Encourage activity within limits of tolerance
Encourage socialization with persons without active infection
Provide positive feedback
Explore areas of interest and encourage their pursuit

EXPECTED OUTCOMES

Child discusses feelings and concerns
Child engages in activities appropriate to interests and abilities

NURSING DIAGNOSIS: Activity intolerance related to fatigue

GOAL 1
Conserve energy

INTERVENTIONS

Maintain bed rest initially if severely edematous
Balance rest and activity when ambulatory
Plan and provide quiet activities
Instruct child to rest when begins to feel tired

EXPECTED OUTCOME

Child engages in activities appropriate to capabilities

NURSING DIAGNOSIS: Altered family processes related to a child with a serious disease

GOAL 1
Support family

INTERVENTIONS AND EXPECTED OUTCOMES

See Nursing Care Plan: The Family of the Ill or Hospitalized Child, Chapter 26

See also Nursing Care Plan: The Child in the Hospital, Chapter 26

*Dependent nursing action.

lost, children are allowed to resume their usual activities with discretion. Irritability and mood swings accompanying the inactivity, disease process, and steroid therapy are not unusual manifestations in these children, which create an additional challenge to the nurse and the family.

Family support and home care. Many children are treated at home during exacerbations. Parents are taught to detect signs of relapse and to bring the child for treatment at the earliest indications. Unless the edema and proteinuria are severe or the parents, for some reason, are unable to care for the ill child, home care is preferred. Parents are instructed in testing urine for albumin, administration of medications, and general care. Salt is restricted to no additional salt during relapse and steroid therapy, but a regular diet is suitable for the child in remission. Parents are instructed regarding avoiding contact with infected playmates, but the child is permitted to attend school. It is important for parents of children on corticosteroid therapy to be aware of the common side effects of steroid therapy, such as rounding of the face, increased appetite, abdominal distention, and hirsutism, and to distinguish some of these from the edema formation of the disease. They should be reassured that the symptoms will disappear gradually after discontinuation of the drug. The child should receive close medical and/or nursing observation to detect unusual but more serious side effects.

The prolonged course of the relapsing form of nephrotic syndrome is taxing to both the child and the family. The up-and-down course of remissions and exacerbations with periodic disruption of family life by hospitalization places a severe strain on the child and the family, both psychologically and financially. Parents and children over 5 or 6 years of age need reassurance regarding this characteristic of the course of the disease so that they will not become discouraged with the frequent relapses. At the same time it is important to impress on them the importance of long-term care to gain their cooperation. A satisfactory response is more likely when relapses are detected and therapy is instituted early, and remissions are prolonged when instructions are carried out faithfully. For example, one child had an exacerbation when his mother reduced the dosage of his drug because it was so expensive.

Social isolation is a concomitant problem for these children. Isolation is related to frequent hospitalization or confinement during relapse, the risk of infection that may precipitate an exacerbation, lack of energy, and the child's reluctance to face friends at home or school because of the changes in appearance resulting from the disease or the medication. Both parents and child need someone to listen to their complaints, to assist them to cope with both short-term and long-term problems associated with the disease, and to find solutions to their problems. Continuous support of the child and family is one of the major nursing considerations.

5 Evaluation

The effectiveness of nursing interventions is determined by continual reassessment and evaluation of care based on the following observational guidelines and expected outcomes:

1. Measure intake and output and examine urine for albumin.
2. Monitor vital signs and assess skin for evidence of breakdown or infection.
3. Assess appetite and eating behaviors.
4. Observe and interview child and family regarding their understanding of the disease, therapies, and compliance with prescribed regimen.

Expected outcomes:
See Nursing Care Plan, pp. 1351-1352.

RENAL TUBULAR DISORDERS

Disorders of renal tubular function include a variety of conditions in which there are one or more abnormalities in specific mechanisms of tubular transport or reabsorption, whereas initially glomerular function is normal or comparatively less impaired. Eventually there may be more widespread kidney destruction with renal failure. In some cases the dysfunction has little, if any, effect on renal function. These disorders may be permanent or transient and may originate as primary defects or arise as a secondary effect of metabolic disease or exogenous toxins. Renal tubular disorders may be congenital (usually displaying characteristic patterns of genetic transmission), appear without evidence of hereditary transmission, or be acquired as a result of known or unknown causes.

Unlike the classic manifestations of glomerular diseases, edema and hypertension are absent and the blood urea nitrogen level and routine urinalysis are usually normal. Proteinuria may be demonstrated but only by elaborate tests. Manifestations of tubular disorders are primarily metabolic disturbances or deficiencies, such as failure to thrive, metabolic bone disease, or persistent acidosis. The variety of these disorders is extensive and the incidence rare.

TUBULAR FUNCTION

The function of the proximal tubules is the reabsorption of substances from the glomerular filtrate, including sodium, potassium, chloride, bicarbonate, glucose, phosphate, and amino acids. A number of disorders feature impairment of reabsorption of one or more filtrate constituents and most involve defects in the transport mechanisms for these substances. Impaired tubular reabsorption of any specific substance will cause that substance to appear in the urine, usually with reduced levels in the blood.

The primary functions of the distal renal tubules are acidification of urine, potassium secretion, and the selective and differential reabsorption of sodium, chloride, and water, which determines the final urinary concentration. Since the contribution of the distal tubule to urine composition depends in part on the volume and composition of the filtrate from the proximal tubule, the net contribution of the distal tubule is related to proximal tubular function and glomerular filtration.

RENAL TUBULAR ACIDOSIS

Renal tubular acidosis (RTA) is a syndrome of sustained metabolic acidosis in which there is impaired reabsorption of bicarbonate and/or excretion of net hydrogen ion, but in which glomerular function is normal or comparatively less impaired. On the basis of underlying pathophysiology, renal tubular acidosis is divided into *proximal renal tubular acidosis,* which results from a defect in bicarbonate absorption, and *distal renal tubular acidosis,* which results from inability to establish an adequate gradient of pH between blood and tubular fluid (Behrman and Vaughan, 1987).

Proximal Tubular Acidosis (Type II)

Proximal tubular acidosis is caused by impaired bicarbonate reabsorption in the proximal tubule. It may occur as an isolated defect (primary); however, more often it appears in association with other proximal tubular disorders (secondary). As a result of a depressed renal threshold, bicarbonate reabsorption in the proximal tubule is incomplete, causing the plasma concentration of bicarbonate to stabilize at a lower level than normal. This results in a hyperchloremic metabolic acidosis. There is no impairment of distal tubular integrity or, in most cases, of the distal acidifying mechanism. A more complex abnormality in the proximal tubules is the *Fanconi syndrome* in which transport mechanisms are damaged by the accumulation of toxic metabolites or the tubular epithelium is damaged by heavy metals such as lead or arsenic.

The cause of the primary disorder is unknown, but it appears to be almost entirely restricted to male infants. The major clinical manifestation and presenting symptom is growth failure. Tachypnea from hyperchloremic metabolic acidosis is also evident. Dehydration, vomiting, episodic fever, nephrolithiasis secondary to hypercalciuria, muscle weakness or paralysis as a result of hypokalemia, and episodes of severe, life-threatening acidemia (sometimes triggered by a concurrent infection) may be seen also.

Complications are rare. The disorder appears to be transient and resolves spontaneously in time.

Distal Tubular Acidosis (Type I)

Distal tubular acidosis is caused by the inability of the kidney to establish a normal pH gradient between tubular cells and tubular contents. Its most characteristic feature is the inability to produce a urinary pH below 6.0 despite the presence of severe metabolic acidosis.

Distal renal tubular acidosis may occur as a primary, isolated defect or in association with other diseases or disorders. Most secondary causes are rare. The primary disorder is usually considered to be a hereditary defect with a variable degree of expression and a greater penetrance in females. After the age of 2 years the child usually has growth failure, although there is often a history of vomiting, polyuria, dehydration, anorexia, and failure to thrive. Evidence of bone demineralization (see hypophosphatemic rickets) may be present along with, occasionally, the formation of urinary calculi (urolithiasis) in older children.

The inability to secrete hydrogen ion causes an accumulation of the ion in the body, which soon depletes the available hydrogen buffer, producing a sustained acidosis. Acidosis retards normal somatic growth, and demineralization of bone occurs as bone salts are mobilized to buffer the excessive hydrogen ions. Increased serum levels of both calcium and phosphorus contribute to the development of stones within the renal system. Both sodium and potassium are secreted in larger amounts. Serum potassium levels are depleted as the distal tubules excrete large amounts of potassium ions in an attempt to conserve sodium, since hydrogen ions are unable to participate in the exchange. Hyponatremia stimulates increased aldosterone secretion, which further aggravates the hypokalemia. With the depletion of bicarbonate ions, more chloride is reabsorbed in the proximal tubule to create a hyperchloremia.

Prognosis. The primary disorder is usually permanent, but with early diagnosis and therapy secondary effects on growth and stone formation can be avoided. When it occurs as a secondary complication and renal damage is prevented, the prognosis is good.

Therapeutic Management

Treatment of both proximal and distal disorders consists of administration of sufficient bicarbonate or citrate to balance metabolically produced hydrogen ions and maintain the plasma bicarbonate level within normal range and to correct associated electrolyte disorders, especially hypokalemia. Proximal disorders require large volumes of bicarbonate to compensate for urinary losses; in distal disorders the alkali required to maintain a normal plasma concentration is low. Most authorities favor a mixture of sodium and potassium bicarbonate (or citrate) in order to prevent deficiencies of either cation. The citrate solutions (Bicitra, Polycitra, or Shohl solution) are usually more easily tolerated than bicarbonate solutions. Shohl solution is very effective but has the disadvantage of requiring preparation by a pharmacist.

Nursing Considerations

Nursing goals include recognizing the possibility of RTA in children who fail to thrive or display other symptoms suggestive of the disorders and referring these children for medical evaluation. Helping parents understand the importance of compliance in administration of medications on a long-term basis is a primary goal of nursing management (see Compliance, Chapter 27, and Administration of Medication, Chapter 27). Children who must continue the medication indefinitely are taught the importance of taking the medications as soon as they are old enough to assume responsibility for their own care.

NEPHROGENIC DIABETES INSIPIDUS

Nephrogenic diabetes insipidus (NDI) is the major disorder associated with a defect in the ability to concentrate urine. In this disorder the distal tubules and collecting ducts are insensitive to the action of antidiuretic hormone or its exogenous counterpart, vasopressin. The nature of the defect is unknown but it occurs primarily in males, which supports

X-linked recessive inheritance. The disease is more variable in female carriers of the defective gene who may exhibit only a mild defect in urine-concentrating ability. The differential diagnosis for NDI should include chronic obstructive renal disorders, sickle cell disease, renal tuberculosis, and other renal disorders, which may cause high urine output with failure of the kidney to respond to vasopressin.

Clinical Manifestations

The disease is manifest in the newborn period by vomiting, unexplained fever, failure to thrive, and severe recurrent dehydration with hypernatremia. The passage of copious amounts of dilute urine, which produces severe dehydration and hypoelectrolytemia, is a serious threat to life during this period and may be responsible for the high incidence of mental and motor retardation found in affected persons. Growth retardation is probably related to diminished food intake and poor general health because of uncontrolled polydipsia. Diagnosis is suspected on the basis of patient and family history and confirmed by a urine osmolality value consistently below that of plasma. Lack of response to vasopressin administration rules out other causes.

Therapeutic Management

Therapy involves provision of adequate volumes of water to compensate for urinary losses. As a result of an insatiable thirst, most of the child's time is spent drinking and voiding, with little time for activity and stimulation. These children may go to great lengths to satisfy their thirst. A low-sodium/low-solute diet and the use of chlorothiazide or ethacrynic acid diuretics to increase the reabsorption of sodium and water in the proximal tubule help to reduce the amount of tubular fluid delivered to the distal tubules and diminish the volume of water excreted. Urine output has been reported to be reduced when prostaglandin inhibitors such as tolmetin sodium, indomethacin, ibuprofen, and aspirin are administered in conjunction with chlorothiazide (Garin and Richard, 1983; Libber, Harrison, and Spector, 1986). Supplemental potassium may be required to prevent hypokalemia as a result of thiazide therapy. If the disease is recognized early and treatment instituted and maintained, normal growth can be expected, and a normal life span anticipated.

Nursing Considerations

Nursing goals for children and families with NDI are to recognize signs of the disorder early and assist them in coping with the long-term inconvenience of the continual thirst and elimination problems. Families need to be taught to administer medications and help with diet planning for those on sodium restriction and who need supplemental potassium. The problem of ensuring adequate hydration is lifelong, and families need to adapt to away-from-home fluid needs and to avoid activities that contribute to dehydration when fluids may not be available. Genetic counseling is recommended.

MISCELLANEOUS RENAL DISORDERS

Renal damage occurs as a major or minor complication in many systemic diseases and with varying degrees of severity. In some cases the renal complication may be the principal cause of death or one of several complications with fatal consequences. In other cases it may be only a source of discomfort but no direct threat to life. Sometimes renal complications provide a clue to diagnosis of the underlying disease; at other times renal involvement confuses the diagnosis.

There are a wide variety of hereditary disorders of renal function. It is estimated that 15% of renal diseases are genetically determined. These may be glomerular function disorders, tubular defects, metabolic disorders that may lead to renal damage, disorders involving more than one system, or structural abnormalities and tumors. In addition, there are a number of miscellaneous renal conditions for which a cause is unknown.

HEMOLYTIC-UREMIC SYNDROME

Hemolytic-uremic syndrome (HUS) is an uncommon acute renal disease that is characterized by a triad of manifestations: acute renal failure, hemolytic anemia, and thrombocytopenia. HUS occurs primarily in infants and small children between the ages of 6 months and 3 years. It has been recognized predominantly in whites and, although it occurs worldwide, is more prevalent in South Africa, Argentina, and the West coasts of North and South America. There have also been reports of increased incidence in families (Fong, de Chadarevian, and Kaplan, 1982). HUS represents one of the main causes of acute renal failure in early childhood (Rizzoni and others, 1988).

Etiology

In the majority of cases no causative agents have been identified, although recent theories implicate genetic factors, prostacyclin deficiency, neuraminidase and agglutination, endotoxins (especially *Shigella* endotoxin), antithrombin-III deficiency, deficiency of antioxidants, and reduced platelet aggregation. The appearance of the disease has been associated with *Rickettsia,* viruses (especially *Escherichia coli,* Coxsackie, ECHO, and adenovirus), pneumococci, *Shigella,* and *Salmonella* and may represent an unusual response to these infections. A strong association has been found between HUS and enteric infection with verocytotoxin-producing *E. coli,* specifically the O157:H7 serotype (Karmali and others, 1985; Neill and others, 1987).

The disease usually follows an acute gastrointestinal or upper respiratory infection and tends to occur in scattered outbreaks in small geographic areas. HUS is clinically and pathologically similar to thrombocytopenic purpura, except for the hypertension that is associated with HUS. Some have speculated that thrombocytopenic purpura may be the adult version of the hemolytic-uremic syndrome of infancy and early childhood.

Pathophysiology

The primary site of injury appears to be the endothelial lining of the small glomerular arterioles, although other organs and tissues may be involved (e.g., the liver, brain, heart, pancreatic islet cells, and muscles). The endothelium becomes swollen and occluded with deposition of platelets and fibrin clots (intravascular coagulation). Red blood cells are damaged as they move through the partially occluded blood vessels. These fragmented red blood cells are removed by the spleen, causing acute hemolytic anemia. Fibrinolytic action on the precipitated fibrin causes these fibrin-split products to appear in the serum and urine. The platelet aggregation within damaged blood vessels or the damage and removal of platelets produce the characteristic thrombocytopenia.

Clinical Manifestations

The disease is preceded by a prodromal period during which there is an episode of diarrhea and vomiting. Less often the illness is an upper respiratory infection and occasionally varicella, measles, or urinary tract infection.

The hemolytic process persists for several days to 2 weeks. During this time the child is anorectic, irritable, and lethargic. There is marked and rapid onset of pallor, accompanied by hemorrhagic manifestations such as bruising, purpura, or rectal bleeding. Severely affected patients are anuric and are frequently hypertensive. Convulsions and stupor suggest central nervous system involvement, and there may be signs of acute heart failure. Mild cases demonstrate anemia, thrombocytopenia, and azotemia; urine output may be reduced or increased.

Diagnostic Evaluation

The triad of anemia, thrombocytopenia, and renal failure is sufficient for diagnosis. Renal involvement is evidenced by proteinuria, hematuria, and presence of urinary casts; blood urea nitrogen and serum creatinine levels are elevated. A low hemoglobin and hematocrit and a high reticulocyte count confirm the hemolytic nature of the anemia.

Therapeutic Management

In general, treatment is directed toward control of the complications and hematologic manifestations of renal failure. The initial supportive measures for most children are those used in managing renal failure—fluid replacement (calculated with great care), treatment of hypertension, and correction of acidosis and electrolyte disorders. The most consistently effective treatment is early and repeated hemodialysis or peritoneal dialysis, which is instituted in any child who has been anuric for 24 hours or who demonstrates oliguria with uremia or hypertension and seizures. Blood transfusions with fresh, washed packed cells are administered for severe anemia but are used with caution to prevent circulatory overload from added volume.

Once vomiting and diarrhea have resolved, the child is restarted on enteral nutrition. Sometimes parenteral nutrition is required for children with severe persistent colitis and in those in whom tissue catabolism is marked. There is no substantial evidence that heparin, corticosteroids, or fibrinolytic agents are beneficial, and in some instances they may aggravate the condition. The usefulness of plasma infusion for treatment of HUS is currently being studied.

Prognosis. With prompt treatment the recovery rate is about 95%, but residual renal impairment ranges from 10% to 50% in various areas. Death is usually caused by residual renal impairment or central nervous system injury.

Nursing Considerations

Nursing care is the same as that provided in acute renal failure and, for children with continued impairment, includes management of chronic disease. Because of the sudden and life-threatening nature of the disorder in a previously well child, parents are often ill-prepared for impact of hospitalization and treatment. Therefore support and understanding are especially important aspects of care.

FAMILIAL GLOMERULOPATHY (ALPORT SYNDROME)

The syndrome of chronic hereditary nephritis consists of hematuria, high-frequency sensorineural deafness, ocular disorders, and chronic renal failure. The disease appears to be inherited as an autosomal-dominant trait, which suggests a possible X-linked dominant trait, although rare male-to-male transmission occurs. It is uncommon but not rare and accounts for a significant percentage of persistent glomerular disease in childhood.

The clinical manifestations are indistinguishable from mild acute nephritis. Initial symptoms include hematuria, proteinuria, malaise, and mild edema. Onset of gross hematuria may be associated with an acute respiratory infection. The average age of onset is 6 years, but the condition may be noted in infancy. It begins slowly and progresses until uncontrollable renal failure develops in adolescence or early adulthood. There is usually a positive family history. Most untreated boys develop severe symptoms, whereas affected girls generally have a milder disease and a normal life expectancy.

Treatment is symptomatic and supportive. Dialysis and renal transplantation are ultimate therapeutic measures for renal involvement. Hearing loss and ocular disorders should receive appropriate attention, and families should be counseled regarding the genetic implications of the disease.

UNEXPLAINED PROTEINURIA

Often apparently healthy children with no suggestion of renal disease will demonstrate proteinuria on routine urinalysis. The percentage of children with unexplained proteinuria ranges from 1% at 6 years of age to 11% at puberty, reaching a maximum prevalence at age 13 in girls and age 16 in boys.

Unexplained proteinuria can be categorized as (1) *transient (inconstant),* (2) *persistent,* or (3) *orthostatic,* or *postural.* Transient proteinuria is a common finding with no known cause, but it sometimes increases with febrile illness, exercise, cold, or emotions.

Persistent proteinuria usually signifies renal disease. Orthostatic proteinuria is seen in 3% to 5% of adolescents and young adults, and, although proteinuria is evident in the recumbent as well as the erect position, it is readily detected by qualitative tests. Reactions of 2+ or 3+ are frequently encountered. The cause is unknown, but minor glomerular changes occur in many instances. The condition is benign and generally resolves over a period of time.

In cases of unexplained proteinuria, it is important to confirm or exclude renal disease with appropriate diagnostic tests. Repeated examination for proteinuria, an orthostatic test, urine culture, and (if proteinuria is persistent) more definitive tests, including 24-hour protein excretion, renal ultrasound, and renal scan, are indicated.

RENAL TRAUMA

Serious injuries of the genitourinary tract are not uncommon in the pediatric age-group, the peak incidence occurring between the ages of 10 and 20 years. The kidneys are among the organs most often injured in children, despite their relatively protected location. However, the kidneys in children are more mobile than they are in the adult, and the outer borders are less well protected. They are separated from the skin surface by only 2 to 3 cm (¾ to 1¼ inches) in young children. Most injuries are of the nonpenetrating or "blunt" type, usually involving falls, athletic injuries, and motor vehicle accidents. Penetrating trauma (e.g., gunshot or stab wound) occurs much less frequently in children. In many children preexisting renal abnormalities, particularly congenital anomalies associated with mild to moderate hydronephrosis, are found that were unrecognized before the accident.

Renal injury can be suspected in children who complain of flank pain, and frequently there are abrasions or contusions on the overlying skin. Hematuria is consistently present, but the amount of blood in the urine is not a reliable indicator of the seriousness of the injury. Many relatively insignificant injuries are associated with grossly bloody urine, whereas some of the most severe injuries are found in children with only microscopic hematuria (Box 30-6).

Box 30-6 CLASSIFICATION ACCORDING TO EXTENT OF RENAL INJURY

Type I: A relatively mild renal contusion in which the capsule, parenchyma, and collecting system are usually intact but subcapsular bleeding frequently occurs into the parenchyma and appears in the urine. Renal contusion is an important cause of gross hematuria in active children.

Type II: Laceration of the kidney, injury to a major renal vessel, or injury to the collecting system with intracapsular extravasation of urine.

Type III: Multiple renal lacerations or injury to the main renal artery.

Renal rupture involves the actual splitting open of the kidney capsule, causing extravasation of blood or a mixture of blood and urine into the surrounding retroperitoneal space. Renal vascular injury, although unusual, requires immediate recognition and surgical intervention. Since the volume per minute blood flow through the kidney is greater (25% of cardiac output) than to any other abdominal organ, injury to the kidney may result in a rapid loss of blood (Hoover, 1984).

In active children there may or may not be history of unusual trauma. Abdominal or flank pain and tenderness are caused by bleeding around the kidney and may or may not be associated with fever. Clots passing down the ureter may cause pain similar to that of renal colic, and dysuria is common. Patients with more severe injuries may complain of nausea or abdominal pain. There may be a palpable abdominal mass caused by loss of blood and/or urine loss into the retroperitoneum. The fibrous capsule enclosing the kidney prevents expansion of a hematoma; therefore exsanguination and shock are seldom observed even in severe renal trauma.

Diagnosis is made on the basis of intravenous pyelography, angiography, and/or retrograde pyelography. Unsuspected hydronephrosis often is first detected as a result of traumatic injury.

Therapeutic Management

Severe injury requires close observation in the hospital intensive care unit, as well as blood replacement if there is severe internal or external bleeding. In most cases bleeding subsides spontaneously. Surgical exploration is indicated in multiple injuries, extravasation of blood around the kidneys, or disruption of the major vessels or the collecting system. Children with less severe injury, such as contusions only, are placed on bed rest. They should remain on bed rest for 3 days after cessation of gross bleeding, since the substance released from injured renal tissue (urinary urokinase) has strongly fibrinolytic properties that may precipitate serious bleeding. Prognosis depends on the nature and extent of the injury.

Nursing Considerations

Nursing management is directed toward recognizing and assisting in the diagnosis of renal injury. Care of both child and family is primarily supportive. All the concepts related to emergency hospitalization and care are implemented (see Chapter 26). Postsurgical care, if indicated, is the same as for any other surgical patient.

RENAL FAILURE

Renal failure is the inability of the kidneys to excrete waste material, concentrate urine, and conserve electrolytes. The disorder can be acute or chronic and affects most of the systems in the body. Two terms that are often used in relation to renal failure need some clarification: *azotemia* is the accumulation of nitrogenous waste within the blood; *ure-*

mia is a more advanced condition in which retention of nitrogenous products produces toxic symptoms. Azotemia is not life threatening, whereas uremia is a serious condition that often involves other body systems.

ACUTE RENAL FAILURE

Acute renal failure (ARF) is said to exist when the kidneys suddenly are unable to regulate the volume and composition of urine appropriately in response to food and fluid intake and the needs of the organism. The principal feature is oligoanuria* associated with azotemia, acidosis, and diverse electrolyte disturbances. ARF is not common in childhood, but the outcome depends on the cause, associated findings, and prompt recognition and treatment.

Etiology

ARF can develop as a result of a large number of related or unrelated clinical conditions—poor renal perfusion, acute renal injury, or the final expression of chronic, irreversible renal disease. The most common cause in children is transient renal failure resulting from dehydration or other causes of poor perfusion that respond to restoration of fluid volume. Causes of ARF are usually classified as to *prerenal, intrinsic renal,* and *postrenal* causes. This implies that only renal causes are characterized by damage to the renal parenchyma, whereas prerenal and postrenal causes can be more easily remedied. However, severe or long-standing prerenal or postrenal etiologies can produce severe secondary renal damage.

Prerenal causes. Prerenal causes of ARF are most common in children and are always related to reduction of renal perfusion in an anatomically and physiologically normal kidney and collecting system. Dehydration secondary to diarrheal disease or persistent vomiting is the most frequent cause of prerenal failure in infants and children. Surgical shock and trauma (including burns) are also common causes. Hypovolemia and decreased renal perfusion cause a decreased glomerular filtration rate and stimulate the secretion of renin, aldosterone, and antidiuretic hormone, which further diminish urine flow. Extended and severe hypoperfusion (secondary to such procedures as cardiac surgery) can produce cortical or tubular necrosis; however, when medical care is available, this is seldom allowed to occur. Azotemia that accompanies this type of renal failure generally is rapidly reversible with prompt attention to expansion of the extracellular fluid volume. Prerenal failure is often difficult to distinguish from tubular or cortical necrosis.

Intrinsic renal causes. Intrinsic renal causes of ARF comprise the largest group that requires extended management. These include diseases and nephrotoxic agents that damage the glomeruli, tubules, or renal vasculature. Glomerular disease is the most common cause of glomerular damage, whereas tubular destruction is more often caused by ischemia or nephrotoxins. Vascular damage is an uncommon cause of renal failure in childhood. The type and extent of damage determine the degree and duration of renal insufficiency, and it is difficult to predict in any given case whether or not acute necrosis will develop.

Postrenal causes. ARF resulting from obstructive uropathy is uncommon in children except during the first year of life. However, renal function can be restored by relief of the obstruction. The degree of recovery depends on the duration of the renal failure.

Pathophysiology

ARF is usually reversible, but the deviations of physiologic function can be extreme, and mortality in the pediatric age-group is still high. There is severe reduction in glomerular filtration rate, an elevated blood urea nitrogen level, and decreased tubular reabsorption of sodium from the proximal tubule. Consequently, there is increased concentration of sodium in the distal tubule, which causes stimulation of the renin mechanism. The local action of angiotensin causes vasoconstriction of the afferent arteriole, which further reduces glomerular filtration and prevents urinary losses of sodium. There is a significant reduction in renal blood flow.

The pathologic conditions that produce acute renal failure caused by glomerulonephritis, hemolytic-uremic syndrome, and other renal disorders have been discussed in relation to those disease processes. The necrotic processes within the nephron can be cortical, tubular, or both.

Cortical necrosis. Complete cortical necrosis usually results from severe ischemia, infection, or intravascular coagulation and represents a severe irreversible cause of acute renal failure. In the pediatric age-group this occurs as a fatal event most frequently during the neonatal period as a result of hypoxia and shock. When cortical destruction is incomplete, some recovery of renal function may occur. Intravascular coagulation is believed to play a significant role as an intermediate factor in the development of ARF, especially in cases related to sepsis.

Tubular necrosis. Damage to the renal tubules can be broadly classified as (1) secondary to renal ischemia and (2) associated with the ingestion or inhalation of substances toxic to the kidneys. Renal tubules are particularly vulnerable to a wide variety of toxic agents that produce vasoconstriction and to focal patches of ischemia that cause a uniform necrosis of the tubular epithelium down to, but not including, the basement membrane. A lesion produced by sustained reduction in renal blood flow involves the basement membrane as well, which may become fragmented and ruptured to the extent that the continuity of tubular structure is disrupted. The lesions may affect any segment of the tubules, appearing at irregular intervals along with normal segments throughout the kidney.

Healing of tubular lesions is accomplished by reepithelialization in the areas with intact basement membrane. In those areas in which the basement membrane has been disrupted, such healing is unable to take place, and connective tissue grows through the ruptured membrane, thus preventing reestablishment of tubular integrity. Individual cells

*The definition of oligoanuria varies extensively, from 1.8 to 4 dl/m^2/24 hours, in the literature.

within the nephron are capable of regeneration, but the entire nephron is not capable of this.

Clinical course. The clinical course of the child with ARF is variable and depends on the cause. In reversible ARF there is a period of severe oliguria, or the low-output phase, followed by an abrupt onset of diuresis, or a high-output phase, followed by a gradual return to, or toward, normal urine volumes. The length of the oliguric phase in older children and adolescents is 10 to 14 days, although it is highly variable at all ages. It tends to be shorter (3 to 5 days) in infants, children, and milder cases. The onset of the diuretic phase appears unexpectedly and over several days proceeds in stepwise fashion from very low to above normal urine volumes. During the oliguric phase manifestations of uremia are present but may also be accompanied by other clinical disorders that make assessment difficult, such as infection, anoxia, and shock.

Clinical Manifestations

In many instances of ARF the infant or child is already critically ill with the precipitating disorder, and the explanation for development of oliguria may or may not be readily apparent. Often the underlying illness overshadows the renal failure and frequently assumes the priority of care—for example, the patient who is in shock from endotoxemia, the infant who is severely dehydrated from gastroenteritis, or a child who is subject to seizures as a result of hypertensive encephalopathy associated with acute glomerulonephritis.

The prime manifestation of ARF is oliguria, generally a urine output less than 50 ml/24 hours. Anuria is uncommon except in obstructive disorders. Other symptoms related to ARF include edema, drowsiness, circulatory congestion, and cardiac arrhythmia from hyperkalemia. Seizures may be caused by hyponatremia or hypocalcemia and tachypnea from metabolic acidosis. With continued oliguria, biochemical abnormalities can develop rapidly, and circulatory and central nervous system manifestations appear.

Diagnostic Evaluation

When a previously well child develops ARF without obvious cause, a careful history is taken to reveal symptoms that may be related to glomerulonephritis, to obstructive uropathy, or regarding exposure to nephrotoxic chemicals, such as ingestion of heavy metals or inhalation of carbon tetrachloride or other organic solvents or drugs, such as methicillin, sulfonamides, neomycin, polymyxin, and kanamycin. Laboratory data reflect the kidney dysfunction—hyperkalemia, hyponatremia, metabolic acidosis, hypocalcemia, anemia, or azotemia (Table 30-6).

Therapeutic Management

The most effective management of ARF is prevention. The development of ARF is a known risk in certain situations. This should be anticipated and recognized, and adequate therapy should be implemented—for example, fluid therapy for children with hypovolemia in such conditions as dehydration, burns, and hemorrhage. Nephrotoxic drugs should be used with caution or avoided in children with renal disease, and all personnel should be knowledgeable about precautions related to their administration. For example, a generous fluid intake is needed for children receiving antimetabolite drugs and after radiotherapy.

Table 30-6 Laboratory findings associated with acute renal failure

CLINICAL PROBLEM	MECHANISM	CLINICAL CONSIDERATIONS
Azotemia Elevated BUN levels	Ongoing protein catabolism Significantly decreased excretion	Lower rate of production in neonates and persons with depleted protein stores Increased in situations involving large amounts of necrotic tissue or extravasated blood
Elevated plasma creatinine levels	Continued production Significantly decreased excretion	Production less affected by other factors More sensitive measure of intensity of azotemia Low in neonate because of small muscle mass relative to size
Metabolic acidosis	Continued endogenous acid production Significantly decreased excretion Depletion of extracellular and intracellular fluid buffers	Compensatory hyperventilation Opisthotonos Major threat to life
Hyponatremia	Dilution of extracellular fluid Decreased excretion of water	May develop cerebral signs
Hyperkalemia	Ongoing protein catabolism Decreased excretion compounded by metabolic acidosis	Most important electrolyte to be considered in acute renal failure May contribute to cardiac arrhythmia With ECG changes, major threat to life May be lost from gastrointestinal tract
Hypocalcemia	Associated with metabolic acidosis and hyperphosphatemia	During alkali therapy, may cause tetany

The treatment of ARF is directed toward (1) treatment of the underlying cause, (2) management of the complications of renal failure, and (3) provision of supportive therapy within the constraints imposed by the renal failure. Treatment of poor perfusion resulting from dehydration consists of volume restoration, as described in the treatment of dehydration (see Chapter 28). If oliguria persists after restoration of fluid volume or if the renal failure is caused by intrinsic renal damage, the physiologic and biochemical abnormalities that have resulted from kidney dysfunction must be corrected or controlled. Central venous pressure monitoring is usually implemented.

Initially a Foley catheter is inserted to rule out urine retention, to collect available urine for electrolytes and analysis, and to monitor results of diuretic administration. The catheter may or may not be removed. Many authorities who believe that it serves little purpose during the oliguric phase and predisposes to bladder infection prefer collection bags for measuring urine output. Others maintain a catheter for hourly urine measurements.

Oliguria. When there is persistent oliguria in the presence of adequate hydration and no lower tract obstruction, mannitol, furosemide, or both may be administered rapidly as a test to provoke a flow of urine. When glomerular function is intact, the administration of these substances will behave as nonreabsorbable solute in the tubular fluid to evoke an osmotic diuresis. The presence of mannitol in tubular fluid and the obligatory water that follows it also serve to dilute the concentration of any nephrotoxin that may be present in the tubules below toxic levels. The furosemide blocks reabsorption of tubular filtrate. If urine flow is generated to the extent of 6 to 10 ml/kg of body weight in 1 to 3 hours, the initial dosage is reduced and continued, if needed, to sustain the flow. If no urine is produced within 2 hours after the single dose, the drugs are not repeated, and an oliguric regimen is instituted to control water balance and other abnormalities.

Fluid and calories. The amount of exogenous water provided should not exceed the amount needed to maintain zero water balance. It is calculated on the basis of estimated endogenous water formation and losses from sensible (primarily gastrointestinal) and insensible sources. No allotment is calculated for urine as long as oliguria persists.

The child with ARF has a tendency to develop water intoxication and hyponatremia, which make it difficult to provide calories in sufficient amounts to meet the needs of the child and reduce the tissue catabolism, metabolic acidosis, hyperkalemia, and uremia. If the child is able to tolerate oral foods, concentrated food sources high in carbohydrate and fat but low in protein, potassium, and sodium may be provided. However, many children have functional disturbances of the gastrointestinal tract, such as nausea and vomiting; therefore the intravenous route is generally preferred and usually consists of essential amino acids or a combination of essential and nonessential amino acids administered by the central venous route.

Control of water balance in these patients requires careful monitoring of feedback information, such as accurate intake and output, body weight, and electrolyte measurements. In general during the oliguric phase no sodium, chloride, or potassium is given unless there are other large ongoing losses. Regular measurement of plasma electrolyte, pH, blood urea nitrogen, and creatinine levels is required to assess the adequacy of fluid therapy and to anticipate complications that require specific treatment.

Hyperkalemia. Elevated serum potassium is the most immediate threat to the life of the child with ARF. Potassium ions are not being excreted, whereas at the same time release of potassium from cells is accelerated by acidosis, stress, and tissue breakdown in cases associated with internal bleeding or trauma. Since cardiac arrhythmia and cardiac arrest may result, electrocardiograms as well as serum potassium ion levels are monitored regularly. Hyperkalemia can be minimized and sometimes avoided by eliminating potassium from all food and fluid, by reducing tissue catabolism, and by correcting acidosis.

✦ **NURSING ALERT** Any of the following signs of hyperkalemia constitute an emergency situation and should be reported immediately:

- Serum potassium concentrations in excess of 7 mEq/L
- Presence of ECG abnormalities, such as prolonged QRS complex, depressed ST segment, high peaked T waves, bradycardia, or heart block

Several measures are available to reduce the serum potassium concentration, and the priority of implementation is usually based on the rapidity with which the measures are effective. Temporary measures that produce a rapid but transient effect are:

1. Calcium gluconate, 0.5 ml/kg, administered intravenously over 2 to 4 minutes, with continuous ECG monitoring, exerts a protective effect on cardiac conduction.
2. Sodium bicarbonate, 2 to 3 mEq/kg, administered intravenously over 30 to 60 minutes, elevates the serum pH to cause a transient shift of extracellular fluid potassium into the intracellular fluid. However, there is risk of hypocalcemia, tetany, and fluid overload.
3. Glucose, 50%, and insulin, 1 U/kg, administered intravenously, accelerate glycogen synthesis, causing glucose and potassium to move into the cells. Insulin facilitates the entry of glucose into cells.

These effects produce only transient protection by redistributing existing potassium stores; they do not remove potassium from the body. However, they provide relief while more definitive but slower-acting measures are being implemented. Potassium can be removed by:

1. Administration of an ion-exchange resin such as polystyrene sodium sulfonate (Kayexalate), 1 g/kg, administered orally or rectally, to bind potassium and remove it from the body. This requires time to be effective, and a sodium ion is exchanged for each potassium ion. This increased sodium concentration adds to the body fluids, which may contribute to fluid overload, hypertension, and cardiac failure.
2. Dialysis (discussed on p. 1368). Hemodialysis is efficient but requires specialized facilities. Peritoneal dialysis is simpler and can be carried out in almost any hospital setting. Indications for dialysis in ARF are continued oliguria associated with any of the following:

Severe, persistent acidosis
Inability to reduce serum potassium levels to a safe range with other methods
Clinical uremic syndrome, consisting of nausea and vomiting, drowsiness, and progression to coma
Circulatory overload, hypertension, and evidence of cardiac failure

A popular philosophy is to institute dialysis after 24 to 48 hours of oliguria, regardless of other symptoms. Supporters of this approach believe that early and frequent dialysis is associated with reduced morbidity and mortality and that it permits improved nutrition with relaxed diet restrictions. The combination of dialysis and nutrition tends to reduce the complications of ARF.

Hypertension. Hypertension is a frequent and serious complication of ARF, and, to detect it early, blood pressure determinations are taken every 4 to 6 hours. The most common cause of hypertension in ARF is overexpansion of the extracellular fluid and plasma volume together with activation of the renin-angiotensin system. The goal of therapy is to prevent hypertensive encephalopathy and avoid overtaxing the cardiovascular system.

When there is a threat of encephalopathy, labetalol (a β and α blocker) may be administered intravenously as bolus infusions or a continuous drip. Sodium nitroprusside may be given but requires close monitoring. For less urgent situations, hydralazine, clonidine, or verapamil may be given intravenously. Oral drugs used for acute hypertension include captopril, minoxidil, hydralazine, propranolol, or furosemide (Lasix) (Dillon, 1987).

Other complications. Other complications that may occur with ARF are anemia, convulsions and coma, cardiac failure, and pulmonary edema. *Anemia* is frequently associated with ARF, but transfusion is not recommended unless the hemoglobin level drops below 6 g/dl. Transfusions consist of fresh, packed red blood cells given slowly to reduce the likelihood of increasing blood volume, hypertension, and hyperkalemia.

Seizures occur rather often when renal failure progresses to uremia and are also related to hypertension, hyponatremia, and hypocalcemia. Treatment is directed to the specific cause when known. More obscure etiologies are managed with anticonvulsant drugs.

Cardiac failure with pulmonary edema is almost always associated with hypervolemia. Treatment is directed toward reduction of fluid volume, with water and sodium restriction and administration of diuretics. Digitalis is ineffective and can be hazardous.

Diuretic, or high-output, phase. When the output begins to increase, either spontaneously or in response to diuretic therapy, the intake of fluid, potassium, and sodium must be monitored, and adequate replacement provided to prevent depletion and its consequences. In some cases the high-output phase is mild and lasts only a few days; in others enormous amounts of electrolyte-rich urine are passed.

Prognosis. The prognosis of ARF depends largely on the nature and severity of the causative factor or precipitating event and the promptness and competence of management. The mortality rate is less than 20%. The outcome is least favorable in children with rapidly progressive nephritis and cortical necrosis. Children in whom ARF is a result of hemolytic-uremic syndrome or acute glomerulitis may recover completely, but residual renal impairment or hypertension is more often the rule. Complete recovery is usually expected in children whose renal failure is a result of dehydration, nephrotoxins, or ischemia. ARF following cardiac surgery is less favorable. It is often impossible to assess the extent of recovery for several months.

Nursing Considerations

Nursing care of the infant or child with ARF involves care of the underlying cause plus careful observation and management of the renal status. The major goal is reestablishment of renal function, with emphasis on providing an adequate caloric intake to minimize reduction of protein stores, prevention of complications, and monitoring of fluid balance, laboratory data, and physical manifestations. The probability of dialysis must be considered, and the necessary equipment made available in anticipation of such an eventuality. Because the child requires intensive observation and often specialized equipment, admission to an intensive care unit where equipment and personnel trained in its use are available is the usual disposition.

Assessment

Meticulous attention to the fluid intake and output is mandatory, including all the physical measurements discussed previously in relation to problems of fluid balance. Monitoring of fluid balance and vital signs is continuous, and observers are constantly on the alert for signs of complications so that appropropriate interventions can be implemented.

NURSING ALERT Diminished urinary output and lethargy in a child who is dehydrated, in shock, or recently postoperative should be evaluated for possible acute kidney failure.

Nursing Diagnoses

A number of diagnoses are evident following a thorough assessment of the child with ARF (see Nursing Care Plan, p. 1362. Others will be noted, depending on the age of the child, the cause of the renal failure, and any concomitant complications.

Planning

Major goals in the care of the child with ARF are as follows:

1. Monitor laboratory data and physical manifestations.
2. Provide an adequate caloric intake to minimize reduction of protein stores.
3. Prevent and/or manage complications.
4. Support and educate child and family.

Implementation

The major nursing task in the care of the infant or child with ARF is monitoring and assessing fluid and electrolyte bal-

NURSING CARE PLAN
The Child with Acute Renal Failure

NURSING DIAGNOSIS: Fluid volume excess related to failure or compromised renal regulatory mechanisms

GOAL 1

Help remove excess fluid

INTERVENTIONS

Perform or assist with dialysis
Monitor progress

EXPECTED OUTCOME

Child exhibits no evidence of accumulated fluid and waste products

GOAL 2

Regulate fluid intake

INTERVENTIONS

*Administer intravenous or oral fluids as prescribed
Monitor intravenous infusion to maintain prescribed intake
Employ strategies to prevent undesired intake
- Remove fluids from access by child
- Divide allowed intake into small volumes spread over entire day
- Keep mouth moist with atomizer (avoid excess use which would increase intake)

EXPECTED OUTCOME

Child exhibits no evidence of fluid gain

NURSING DIAGNOSIS Potential for injury related to accumulated electrolytes and waste products

GOAL 1

Help remove excess levels of electrolytes and nitrogenous waste

INTERVENTIONS

*Assist with dialysis
*Administer Kayexalate as prescribed
*Provide diet low in protein, potassium, and sodium, if prescribed
Observe for evidence of accumulated waste products (hyperkalemia, hypernatremia, uremia)

EXPECTED OUTCOME

Child exhibits no evidence of waste product accumulation

GOAL 2

Reduce blood pressure

INTERVENTIONS

*Administer antihypertensives as prescribed
Avoid situations that increase child's anxiety and apprehension
Provide quiet, calm environment

EXPECTED OUTCOME

Child's blood pressure remains within acceptable limits (specify)

NURSING DIAGNOSIS: Potential for infection related to lowered body defenses, fluid overload

GOAL 1

Prevent infection

INTERVENTIONS

Protect child from contact with infected persons
- Place in room with noninfectious children
- Restrict contact with persons who have infections, including family, other children, friends, and staff members
- Observe medical asepsis
  - Practice good handwashing
- Teach visitors appropriate preventive behaviors

Keep child warm and dry
Monitor vital signs for early evidence of infection

EXPECTED OUTCOMES

Child and family apply good health practices
Child exhibits no evidence of infection

NURSING DIAGNOSIS: Altered family processes related to a child with a serious disease

GOAL 1

Support family

INTERVENTIONS AND EXPECTED OUTCOMES

See Nursing Care Plan: The Family of the Ill or Hospitalized Child, Chapter 26

See also Nursing Care Plan: The Child in the Hospital, Chapter 26

*Dependent nursing action.

ance. Limiting fluid intake requires ingenuity on the part of caregivers to cope with the child who is thirsty. Rationing the daily intake in small amounts of fluid served in containers that give the impression of larger volumes is one strategy. Older children who understand the rationale of fluid limits can help determine how their daily ration should be distributed.

Meeting nutritional needs is sometimes a problem, since

the child may be nauseated and encouraging concentrated foods without fluids may be difficult. When nourishment is provided by the IV route, careful monitoring is essential to prevent fluid overload. In addition, nursing measures, such as maintaining an optimum thermal environment, reducing any elevation of body temperature, and reducing restlessness and anxiety, are employed to decrease the rate of tissue catabolism.

The nurse must be continually alert for changes in behavior that indicate the onset of complications. Infection from reduced resistance, anemia, and general morbidity is a constant threat. Fluid overload and electrolyte disturbances can precipitate cardiovascular complications such as hypertension and cardiac failure. Fluid and electrolyte imbalances, acidosis, and accumulation of nitrogenous waste products can produce neurologic involvement manifest by coma, convulsions, or alterations in sensorium.

Although children with ARF are usually quite ill and voluntarily diminish their activity, infants may become restless and irritable, and children are often anxious and frightened. Frequent, painful, and stress-producing treatments and tests must be performed. The presence of a supportive, empathetic nurse can provide comfort and stability in a threatening and unnatural environment.

Family support. Providing support and reassurance to parents is among the major nursing responsibilities. The seriousness and emergency nature of ARF are stressful to parents, and most feel some degree of guilt regarding the child's condition, especially when the illness is the result of ingestion of a toxic substance, dehydration, or a genetic disease. They need reassurance and a sympathetic listener. They also need to be kept informed of the child's progress and provided explanations regarding the therapeutic regimen. The equipment and the child's behavior are sometimes frightening and anxiety provoking. Nurses can do much to help parents comprehend and deal with the stresses of the situation.

Evaluation

The effectiveness of nursing interventions is determined by continual reassessment and evaluation of care based on the following observational guidelines and expected outcomes:

1. Carry out frequent assessment of vital signs and behaviors.
2. Observe eating behaviors and energy expenditure; monitor intake of protein and calories; carefully monitor intake and output, weigh daily or more often as prescribed.
3. Monitor vital signs, sensorium and other neurologic signs; evaluate laboratory results and observe for signs of electrolyte imbalance.
4. Observe and interview child and family regarding their understanding of the disease and therapies; encourage child and family to express their feelings and concerns.

Expected outcomes:
See Nursing Care Plan, p. 1362.

CHRONIC RENAL FAILURE

The kidneys are able to maintain the chemical composition of fluids within normal limits until more than 50% of functional renal capacity is destroyed by disease or injury. Chronic renal failure (CRF) or insufficiency begins when the diseased kidneys can no longer maintain normal chemical structure of body fluids under normal conditions. Progressive deterioration over months or years produces a variety of clinical and biochemical disturbances that eventually culminate in the clinical syndrome known as *uremia*. When the kidneys can no longer function, even with medical intervention, and the patient must resort to dialysis for clearing wastes, the term *end-stage renal disease (ESRD)* is applied. The pattern of renal dysfunction is remarkably uniform no matter what disease process initiates the advanced disease.

Etiology

A variety of diseases and disorders can result in CRF. The most frequent causes of CRF before age 5 years are congenital renal and urinary tract malformations (particularly renal hypoplasia and dysplasia) and vesicoureteral reflux. Glomerular and hereditary renal disease predominate in children 5 to 15 years of age. Glomerular diseases that most frequently lead to CRF are chronic pyelonephritis, chronic glomerulonephritis, and glomerulonephropathy associated with systemic diseases such as anaphylactoid purpura and lupus erythematosus. Hereditary nephritis, congenital nephrotic syndrome, Alport syndrome, polycystic kidney, and several other hereditary disorders result in renal failure in childhood. Renal vascular disorders such as hemolytic-uremic syndrome, vascular thrombosis, or cortical necrosis are less frequent causes.

Pathophysiology

Early in the course of progressive nephron destruction, the child remains asymptomatic with only minimal biochemical abnormalities. Unless its presence is detected in the process of routine assessment, signs and symptoms that indicate advanced renal damage frequently emerge only late in the course of the disease. Midway in the disease process, as increasing numbers of nephrons are totally destroyed and most others are damaged in varying degree, the few that remain intact are hypertrophied but functional. These few normal nephrons are able to make sufficient adjustments to stresses to maintain reasonable degrees of fluid and electrolyte balance. Definitive biochemical examination at this time will reveal restricted tolerance to excesses or restrictions. As the disease progresses to the terminal stage, because of severe reduction in the number of functioning nephrons, the kidneys are no longer able to maintain fluid and electrolyte balance, and the features of the uremic syndrome appear.

The pathophysiology of specific biochemical abnormalities is briefly summarized in the following sections.

Retention of waste products. Moderate decrease in renal function is not associated with a rise in fasting blood urea nitrogen concentration. With progressive nephron destruction and diminished function, the serum level of these end products of protein metabolism increases. However, the blood urea nitrogen level is affected by protein intake, whereas the creatinine concentration is not; therefore creatinine is a more reliable index of renal failure.

Water and sodium retention. The damaged kidneys are able to maintain sodium and water balance under normal circumstances, although the few remaining functional nephrons are required to increase their rate of filtration and reabsorption in proportion to their numbers. The limitations of this capacity become apparent under stress. The nature of abnormalities in adjustment depends on the underlying renal disease: infants and small children with kidney dysplasia or urinary obstructive disease tend to excrete large volumes of dilute urine low in sodium content, children with glomerular disease tend to retain both sodium and water as a result of a greater reduction in glomerular filtration than of tubular reabsorption, and children with defective sodium reabsorption from tubular disease tend to lose sodium with a corresponding osmotic water loss. Consequently, sodium excesses may cause edema and hypertension, whereas sodium deprivation can result in hypovolemia and circulatory failure. Only in end-stage renal disease is markedly reduced glomerular filtration inadequate to handle normal amounts of sodium and water. Retention of these substances leads to edema and vascular congestion.

Hyperkalemia. Dangerous hyperkalemia is an infrequent occurrence in CRF until the terminal stages. However, the kidneys are unable to adjust readily to increased ingestion of potassium, and they require a longer period of time to rid the body of this excess.

Acidosis. A sustained metabolic acidosis is characteristic of CRF; it results from the inability of the damaged kidney to excrete a normal load of metabolic acids generated by normal metabolic processes. There is reduced capacity of the distal tubules to produce ammonia and impaired reabsorption of bicarbonate. Although there is continual hydrogen ion retention and bicarbonate loss, the plasma pH is maintained at a level compatible with life by other buffering mechanisms, particularly the bone salt (see following sections).

Box 30-7 FACTORS RELATED TO BONE DEMINERALIZATION IN CHRONIC RENAL FAILURE

1. In a state of acidosis there is dissolution of the alkaline salts of bone, which serve as buffers, and the release of phosphorus and calcium into the bloodstream.
2. Reduced glomerular filtration and excretion of inorganic phosphate lead to an elevation of plasma phosphate with a concomitant decrease in serum calcium.
3. Decreased serum calcium concentration stimulates the secretion of parathyroid hormone (PTH), which results in resorption of calcium from bones. Under normal circumstances parathyroid hormone inhibits the tubular reabsorption of phosphates.
4. Diseased kidneys are unable to complete the synthesis of vitamin D to its most active form, 1,25-dihydroxycholecalciferol, which is necessary for the absorption of calcium from the gastrointestinal tract and deposition of calcium in bone. This acquired resistance to vitamin D decreases calcium absorption, permits retention of phosphorus, and contributes to secondary hyperparathyroidism.

Box 30-8 CAUSES OF ANEMIA IN CHRONIC RENAL FAILURE

1. Shortened life span of red blood cells caused by some extracorpuscular factor associated with the uremic state
2. Impaired red blood cell production resulting from decreased production of erythropoietin
3. Increased tendency to bleed, associated with a prolonged bleeding time, probably related to impaired platelet function
4. Superimposed nutritional anemia

Box 30-9 PROBABLE CAUSES OF GROWTH FAILURE IN CHRONIC RENAL FAILURE

1. Renal osteodystrophy
2. Poor nutrition associated with dietary restrictions (especially protein) and loss of appetite
3. Biochemical abnormalities associated with renal failure, such as sustained acidosis, hyperkalemia, chronic hyposmolarity secondary to hyposthenuria (secretion of urine with low specific gravity), and phosphorus depletion

Calcium and phosphorus disturbances. One of the distressing features of CRF is its effect on calcium and phosphorus homeostasis. Profound and complex disturbances in the metabolism of these substances result in significant bone demineralization and impaired growth. This appears to be related to several factors (Box 30-7). The result of these complex disturbances in calcium, phosphorus, and bone metabolism produces growth arrest or retardation, bone pain, and deformities known as *renal osteodystrophy,* sometimes called *renal rickets,* since the disorganization of bone growth and demineralization is similar to that caused by vitamin D–resistant rickets.

Anemia. A consistent feature of chronic renal insufficiency is anemia that appears to result from several factors (Box 30-8).

Growth disturbance. One of the most striking effects of CRF in childhood, and one that can have profound psychologic and social consequences for the developing child, is retarded growth. The cause is poorly understood but may be related to nutritional and biochemical factors (Box 30-9).

Sexual maturation may be delayed or may not occur in children with CRF, and secondary amenorrhea frequently develops in girls past puberty. CRF can also cause sexual dysfunction by creating imbalances in gonadal hormone levels. Decreased testosterone levels impair spermatogenesis in males; decreased estrogen, luteinizing hormone, and progesterone cause anovulation and menstrual irregularities (usually amenorrhea) in females. Autonomic neuropathy and anemia are also factors that can alter sexual function.

Other disturbances. Children with CRF are more susceptible to infection, especially pneumonia, urinary tract infection, and septicemia, although the reason for this is not entirely clear. Hyperventilation, a manifestation of the respiratory compensatory mechanism for metabolic acidosis, and pulmonary edema may contribute to upper respiratory infection. These children become extraordinarily sensitive to changes in vascular volume that may cause, in addition to pulmonary overload, cerebral symptoms and circulatory manifestations such as hypertension and cardiac failure.

Numerous neurologic manifestations appear with advanced renal failure, although no specific toxin or biochemical defect has been identified. However, disturbances in enzyme function, disturbances in water and electrolyte balance, altered calcium ion concentration, hypertension, and accumulation of various "uremic toxins" have been implicated.

Clinical Manifestations

The first evidence of difficulty is usually loss of normal energy and increased fatigue on exertion. For example, the child may prefer quiet, passive activities rather than participation in more active games and outdoor play. The child is usually somewhat pale, but it is often so inconspicuous that the change may not be evident to parents or others. Sometimes the blood pressure is elevated.

As the disease progresses, other manifestations may appear. The child eats less well (especially breakfast), shows less interest in normal activities, such as schoolwork or play, and has a decreased or increased urinary output and a compensatory intake of fluid. For example, a child who has achieved bladder control may wet the bed at night. Pallor becomes more evident as the skin develops a characteristic sallow, muddy appearance as the result of anemia and deposition of urochrome pigment in the skin. The child may complain of headache, muscle cramps, and nausea. Other signs and symptoms include weight loss, facial puffiness, malaise, bone or joint pain, growth retardation, dryness or itching of the skin, bruised skin, and sometimes sensory or motor loss. Amenorrhea is common in adolescent girls.

Therapy is generally instigated before the appearance of the *uremic syndrome,* although there are occasions in which the symptoms may be observed. Manifestations of untreated uremia reflect the progressive nature of the homeostatic disturbances and general toxicity. Gastrointestinal symptoms include loss of appetite, and nausea and vomiting. Bleeding tendencies are apparent in bruises, bloody diarrheal stools, stomatitis, and bleeding from lips and mouth. There is intractable itching, probably related to hyperparathyroidism, and deposits of urea crystals appear on the skin as "uremic frost." There may be an unpleasant "uremic" odor to the breath. Respirations become deeper as a result of metabolic acidosis, and circulatory overload is manifest by hypertension, congestive heart failure, and pulmonary edema. Neurologic involvement is reflected by progressive confusion, dulling of sensorium, and, ultimately, coma. Other signs may include tremors, muscular twitching, and seizures.

Diagnostic Evaluation

The diagnosis of CRF is usually suspected on the basis of any of a number of clinical manifestations, history of prior renal disease, and/or biochemical findings. The onset is usually gradual, and the initial signs and symptoms are vague and nonspecific. Laboratory and other diagnostic tools and tests are of value in assessing the extent of renal damage, biochemical disturbances, and related physical dysfunction. Often they can help establish the nature of the underlying disease and differentiate between other disease processes and the pathologic consequences of renal dysfunction.

Therapeutic Management

In irreversible renal failure the goals of medical management are to promote effective renal function, to maintain body fluid and electrolyte balance within acceptable limits, to treat systemic complications, and to promote as active and normal a life as possible for the child for as long as possible. This becomes increasingly difficult as the disease progresses toward its inevitable end. Even therapeutic measures designed to relieve one manifestation may prove detrimental to another. For example, antihypertensive agents may further impair renal function.

Activity. Children are allowed unrestricted activity and to set their own limits regarding rest and extent of exertion. They are encouraged to attend school. When the effort is too great, home tutoring is arranged.

Diet. Regulation of diet is the most effective means, short of dialysis, for reducing the quantity of materials that require renal excretion. The goal of the diet in renal failure is to provide sufficient calories and protein for growth while limiting the excretory demands made on the kidney, to minimize metabolic bone disease (osteodystrophy), and to minimize fluid and electrolyte disturbances. Dietary phosphorus, principally the intake of cow's milk, is restricted. This reduces the protein load on the kidneys, the phosphorus content in the diet, and one of the principal sources of metabolic acids.

Limited protein in the diet should include foods high in essential amino acids; those foods with protein of lesser value can be omitted. Bottle-fed infants are placed on a low-protein, low-electrolyte formula with additional caloric supplements. When given with meals, substances that bind phosphorus in the intestines prevent its absorption and allow a more liberal intake of phosphorus-containing protein. Sodium and water are not usually limited, unless there is evidence of edema or hypertension.

Potassium is not restricted as long as creatinine clearance remains at acceptable limits (greater than or equal to 30 to 35 ml/min). Restrictions are instituted for patients with oliguria or anuria, however. Restrictions of any or all these minerals may be imposed in later stages or at any time in which factors cause abnormal serum concentrations.

Because of modified dietary intake, altered metabolism, and poor appetite, some dietary supplementation is usually needed. Because fat-soluble vitamins can accumulate in patients with CRF, vitamins A, E, and K are not supplemented beyond normal dietary intake. Vitamin D is prescribed, and water-soluble vitamin supplementation may be required if diet is inadequate. Other dietary needs are discussed in relation to osteodystrophy and anemia.

Osteodystrophy. Measures directed at prevention or correction of the calcium/phosphorus imbalance are reduction of dietary phosphorus, administration of a phosphorus-binding agent, provision of supplemental calcium, control of acidosis, and administration of vitamin D.

Dietary phosphorus is controlled by the reduction of protein and milk. Phosphorus levels can be further reduced by the oral administration of aluminum hydroxide gel (Amphojel) or tablets that combine with the phosphorus to decrease gastrointestinal absorption and thus the serum levels of phosphate. However, aluminum phosphate binders have been shown to cause aluminum loading when used on a continuous basis in children; therefore, these substances are used only for very short periods to treat hyperphosphatemia (Sedman, 1986a; Griswold and others, 1983). These children should be monitored for aluminum accumulation and evidence of aluminum intoxication, such as altered sensorium, inability to talk, ataxia, or seizures.

To avoid aluminum exposure in children (especially infants) calcium carbonate preparations can be used. These medications act as (1) phosphate binders, (2) calcium supplements, and (3) alkalizing agents. Calcium carbonate preparations can be given with meals to bind phosphorus if the child is hyperphosphatemic or mildly hypocalcemic. If given 1 to 2 hours after meals, they act as calcium supplements for children with stable phosphorus but low calcium levels.

When serum phosphate levels are within a normal range, appropriate vitamin D therapy is instituted. The drugs that are administered to increase the absorption of calcium through the gastrointestinal tract include dehydrotachysterol (Hytakerol) or 1,25-dihydroxyvitamin D_3 (Rocaltrol). The serum calcium level is monitored weekly during periods when the drugs are being changed or regulated. Parathyroid hormone levels are measured every 2 to 3 months.

Osseous deformities that result from renal osteodystrophy, especially those related to ambulation, are troublesome and require correction as soon as feasible. It has been found that noticeable deformities develop in one third of patients with osteodystrophy despite medical therapy (Hsu and others, 1982). Deformities are particularly frequent and severe in children whose renal failure develops in infancy. However, until the osteodystrophy is healed and under control, the deformities will recur.

Acidosis. Pharmacologic treatment of acidosis is initiated early in children who have chronic renal insufficiency. In addition to reducing the formation of metabolic acids by decreasing the dietary intake of protein, acidosis is alleviated by alkalizing agents such as sodium bicarbonate or a combination of sodium and potassium citrate (Bicitra, Polycitra, or Shohl solution*). Correction of acidosis is best attempted after calcium levels are elevated, since rapid correction may precipitate tetany in a hypocalcemic child.

Anemia. Because the anemia associated with renal failure is related to decreased production of erythropoietin, it usually cannot be successfully managed with hematinic agents. However, sufficient sources of folic acid and iron should be provided in the diet, although this is difficult when protein sources are restricted. Inadequate intake and iron losses that may occur are managed by supplemental iron, usually ferrous sulfate. Providing adequate sources of ascorbic acid at the same time that iron-rich foods or supplement are given enhances the absorption.

Blood transfusions are used to treat symptomatic anemia. Children with chronic renal failure may require a transfusion of packed red blood cells as often as every 6 weeks to maintain their hematocrit and hemoglobin. A new medication, recombinant human erythropoietin (rHuEPO), corrects anemia (improving energy level and general well-being) and eliminates the need for frequent blood transfusions in patients with CRF (Eschbach and Adamson, 1989).

Hypertension. Hypertension of advanced renal disease may be managed initially by cautious use of a low-sodium diet, fluid restriction, and perhaps diuretics such as thiazides or furosemide. Strict restriction of sodium intake may be necessary in oliguric patients. Severe hypertension may require the use of a combination of a beta blocker and a vasodilator (propranolol and hydralazine). Other drugs that may be used include nifedipine, atenolol, minoxidil, prazosin, captopril, or labetalol singly or in combinations.

Growth retardation. One major consequence of CRF is growth retardation, especially in the preadolescent. These children grow poorly both before and after initiation of hemodialysis. Depletion of body protein is characteristic of children with CRF, in addition to a number of metabolic abnormalities. Studies are now being conducted in various pediatric centers to evaluate the use of recombinant human growth hormone to accelerate growth in children with growth retardation secondary to CRF or following renal transplant. Evidence indicates marked acceleration in growth velocity in children treated with growth hormone (Koch and others, 1989).

Miscellaneous complications. Intercurrent infections are treated with appropriate antimicrobials at the first sign of infection. Most of these drugs are excreted through the kidneys; therefore, the dosage is usually reduced in proportion to the decrease in renal function and the interval between doses extended in these children to avoid possible toxic effects from accumulation. Any drug eliminated through the kidneys is administered with caution. Serum levels of ototoxic and/or nephrotoxic drugs (e.g., gentamycin or kanamycin) are assessed regularly to assure a safe nontoxic level.

Dental defects are common in children with chronic kidney disease, and the earlier the onset of the disease the more severe are the dental manifestations. These include hypoplasia, hypomineralization, tooth discoloration, alteration in size and shape of teeth, malocclusion (secondary to deficient skeletal growth), ulcerative stomatitis, occa-

*Each milliliter of Shohl solution contains 1 mEq of citrate ion, which metabolizes to yield 1 mEq of bicarbonate. Citric acid exerts no effect on acid-base balance but enhances the palatability of the mixture.

sional oral hematomas, and an increase in calcific deposits around the teeth (Cooley and Sobel, 1982). Regular dental care is especially important in these children. Other nondental complications are treated symptomatically, for example, chlorpromazine (Thorazine) or prochlorperazine (Compazine) are given for nausea, anticonvulsants for seizures, and diphenhydramine (Benadryl) for pruritus. Once evidence of ESRD appears in a child, the disease runs its relentless course and terminates in death in a few weeks, unless waste products and toxins are removed from body fluids by dialysis and/or kidney transplantation. Since these techniques have been adapted for infants and small children, the outlook for them has improved remarkably. These alternatives are implemented in most cases of renal failure once palliative management is no longer effective.

Nursing Considerations

The child with CRF is a prime example of an individual whose life is maintained by drugs and artificial means, and the multiple stresses placed on these children and their families are often overwhelming. The unrelenting course of the disease process is one of progressive deterioration. There is no means to prevent the irreversible progress of renal insufficiency, nor is there any known cure. As the affected child progresses from renal insufficiency to uremia and then to hemodialysis and transplantation with a need for intensity of therapy, the need for supportive nursing care is also intensified. Team effort is more important than ever and involves coordination of personnel from medicine, nursing, social services, physical/ocupational therapy, dietetics, and psychologic or psychiatric specialties.

Progressive disease places a number of stresses on the child and his family. There is continuing need for repeated examinations that often entail painful procedures, side effects, and frequent hospitalizations. Diet therapy becomes progressively more restricted and intense, and parents may need help in learning to select appropriate foods, reading labels carefully for sodium and potassium content, and modifying meals to accommodate the special needs of the child. The child is required to take a variety of medications. Compliance is difficult when long-term therapies are involved. Ever present in all aspects of the treatment regimen is the agonizing realization that without treatment death is the inevitable outcome.

ESRD presents the same nonspecific stresses on child and family as any other chronic (Chapter 22) or life-threatening (Chapter 23) illness. The reactions and adaptation of the child and family depend on the age and developmental stage of the child, the cultural and socioeconomic background of the family, the quality of the interpersonal relationships of family members, and the communication patterns within the family. In general the problems observed and emotional responses to the stress of the illness are influenced less by the nature of the illness than by the family relationships and the personalities of its members.

One of the first and most noticeable changes is the alteration in physical appearance—fluctuations in weight, anemia, and failure to grow. Children must adjust to the fact that they will always be different from their peers in some ways. They will be shorter, often more tired, and unable to participate in all the activities that are attractive to young people. Children who have had diversion procedures, dialysis shunts, and other surgeries or who urinate into a bag must learn to adjust to these differences. Children must educate their friends to accept them as they are or learn to bear the teasing if they are unable to adjust. Such difficulties can lead to behavior problems in these children.

School is often difficult for these children. Frequent absences for illnesses, evaluations, or treatments disrupt the educational process and socialization. Teachers and school systems are not always sympathetic to the rights and needs of a child with a chronic illness—e.g., the right to equal education and the need for flexibility and special help at times, which places an additional burden on the parents. Sometimes a teacher will pass a failing child because of pity (Dracopoulos and Weatherly, 1983).

In some families illness and stressful experiences act as a unifying force; in others stress aggravates preexisting problems and contributes to family disharmony. The relentless nature of the disease and its therapies not only place physical and emotional stresses on the family but are also a chronic drain on the family finances. Insurance rarely covers the full cost of the multiple hospitalizations and outpatient expenses. Hidden costs abound, such as transportation to special treatment centers, meals, and sometimes lodging away from home. Some temporary assistance may be provided by private foundations, churches, and community groups, and nurses should become familiar with those in the area of their practice that can be of financial and educational service to these families. For example, the **National Kidney Foundation*** and numerous other agencies provide services and information for families, including pamphlets and descriptive literature. Particularly useful are booklets written for children with renal disease.†

Some specific stresses related to ESRD and its treatment are predictable. When it first becomes apparent that kidney failure is inevitable, both parents and child experience great depression and anxiety. Acceptance is particularly difficult if renal failure progresses rapidly after diagnosis. Denial and disbelief are usually pronounced, especially among parents. Once the kidney failure is established and symptoms become progressively more distressing, the initiation of hemodialysis is usually perceived as a positive experience, and, after the initial concerns of implementing the treatment, the child begins to feel better, and parental anxiety is relieved for a time. (See Nursing Care Plan: The Child with Chronic Renal Failure.‡)

*National Kidney Foundation, 30 E. 33rd St., New York, NY 10016, (212) 889-2210 or (800) 622-9010.

†Recommended is Pamplin, H.H., Light, J.A., and Hyman, L.R.: Sidney kidney, Washington, D.C., 1974, Walter Reed Army Medical Center; and Orrbine, E. and Wolfish, N.N.: Understanding kidney failure: a handbook for parents (available for $2.00 from Children's Hospital of Eastern Ontario Foundation, 385 Smyth Road, Ottawa, Ontario, Canada K1H 8L2).

‡In Wong, D.L., and Whaley, L.F.: Clinical manual of pediatric nursing, ed. 3, St. Louis, 1990, Mosby–Year Book, Inc.

Box 30-10 PROCESSES OF FLUID AND ELECTROLYTE MOVEMENT

Osmosis—passive movement of water from a solution of lower concentration to a solution of higher concentration of particles
Diffusion—random movement of particles from an area of greater concentration to an area of lower concentration
Ultrafiltration—movement of fluid, under pressure, through filtering material with minute pores

TECHNOLOGIC MANAGEMENT OF RENAL FAILURE

Technologic advances in the care of children with acute and chronic renal failure have provided a means for maintaining excretory function in acute disease and for prolonging life in those with ESRD. The primary modalities are hemodialysis, peritoneal dialysis, hemofiltration, and transplantation.

Dialysis is the process of separating colloids and crystalline substances in solution by the difference in their rate of diffusion through a semipermeable membrane. This movement across the membrane is accomplished by three processes: osmosis, diffusion, and utrafiltration (Box 30-10).

Methods of dialysis currently available for clinical management of renal failure are:

1. **Hemodialysis,** in which blood is circulated outside the body through artificial cellophane membranes that permit a similar passage of water and solutes
2. **Peritoneal dialysis,** wherein the abdominal cavity acts as a semipermeable membrane through which water and solutes of small molecular size move by osmosis and diffusion according to their respective concentrations on either side of the membrane
3. **Hemofiltration,** in which blood filtrate is circulated outside the body by hydrostatic pressure exerted across a semipermeable membrane and replaced (simultaneously) by electrolyte solution

The choice of whether to use hemodialyis, peritoneal dialysis, or hemofiltration is determined by the nature of the renal failure (acute vs chronic), the cause of renal failure, and patient/parent preference. Hemodialyis is more efficient than peritoneal dialysis, but is technically more difficult in infants and very young children. Hemofiltration may be a viable substitute for dialysis in these children. As a rule, dialysis is reserved for children who are in end-stage renal failure, since it requires creation of a venous access and special equipment. It may be used acutely for such conditions as severe metabolic acidosis, accidental poisoning, intractable heart failure, hypernatremia, hyperkalemia, and hepatic coma.

The absolute indications for dialysis are life-threatening electrolyte abnormalities, severe volume overload, and children with bilateral neoplastic disease or bilateral nephrectomies performed for various reasons, including intractable hypertension. Although each child is assessed on an individual basis, indications for instituting dialysis in CRF are biochemical abnormalities including elevated BUN, acidosis, severe hyperphosphatemia, elevated potassium, and anemia requiring transfusion (placing child at risk for fluid overload). Other indications include deteriorating CNS function or congestive heart failure that is unresponsive to other therapy. Growth failure, severe osteodystrophy, insufficient caloric intake, and inability to carry out normal activities are sometimes criteria for dialysis.

Most children show rapid clinical improvement with the implementation of dialysis, although it is directly related to the duration of uremia before dialysis and the extent to which dietary regulations are followed. Growth rate and skeletal maturation improve, but recovery of normal growth is uncommon. In many cases sexual development, although delayed, has progressed to completion. Females generally remain amenorrheic while on dialysis.

HEMODIALYSIS

Hemodialysis is the preferred dialytic method for children with *acute* conditions such as life-threatening hyperkalemia or poisoning with dialyzable compounds. Protein loss is less extensive than with peritoneal dialysis. However, it is not recommended for small children whose delicately balanced cardiovascular dynamics may be upset by the rapid changes in blood volume and systemic blood pressure that may occur with hemodialysis. In addition, it may be difficult to place vascular access for hemodialysis in small children.

Hemodialyis is the preferred form of dialysis for children who need *chronic* treatment and for certain family situations in which any one person is unable to take time and responsibility to perform the procedures at home. It is best suited to children who live close to the dialysis center, since they must come to the center as often as three times per week for treatments. Children who are not good candidates for peritoneal dialysis because of family noncompliance, recurrent peritoneal infections, or unstable living conditions must elect hemodialysis.

Procedure

Hemodialysis requires the use of special dialysis equipment—the hemodialyzer, or so-called artificial kidney. Hemodialyzers are available in three forms—coil, parallel flow (plate), and hollow fiber—but not all are suited to pediatric patients. Hollow fiber dialyzers are preferable for children because their blood compartment is relatively small and rigid (Novello, 1986a). Pediatric dialysis can be safely carried out when the fluid volume required to fill both hemodialyzer and blood tubing does not exceed 10% of the child's calculated blood volume.

Hemodialysis also requires blood access by three types of means: grafts, fistulas, and temporary access. An *atriovenous fistula* is an access in which a vein and artery are connected surgically. The preferred site is the radial artery and a forearm vein. Sometimes alternate vessels are used, including the tibial artery and the long saphenous vein, especially for home dialysis. An alternative to the external Teflon shunt is the creation of a subcutaneous (internal) arteriovenous fistula by anastomosing a segment of a saphenous vein autograft or a bovine arterial xenograft to the brachial artery and brachiocephalic vein, which produces dilation and thickening of the superficial vessels of the forearm to provide easy access for repeated venipuncture. Fewer complications and less restriction of activity are observed with this approach. Both the graft and fistula require needle insertion at each dialysis. For *temporary vascular access,* percutaneous catheters are inserted in the femoral, subclavian, or internal jugular veins, even in very small children.

Various hemodialysis schedules are employed, but most centers recommend dialysis three times a week for 4 to 6 hours, depending on the size of the child. For a complete description of the highly specialized process of hemodialysis, the reader is directed to the numerous references available on this topic.

Dietary limitations are necessary in chronic dialysis to avoid biochemical complications and to facilitate adequate dialysis. Fluid and sodium are restricted to prevent fluid overload with its associated symptoms of hypertension, cerebral manifestations, and congestive heart failure. Potassium is restricted to prevent complications related to hyperkalemia; phosphorus restriction helps to prevent parathyroid hyperactivity and its attendant risk of abnormal calcification in soft tissues. Limited protein intake reduces high levels of blood urea nitrogen. Fluid is usually limited to 5 $dl/m^2/day$ plus an amount equal to daily urine output.

Seizures during or after hemodialysis are not uncommon. The cause is uncertain, but they probably result from cerebral edema caused by alterations in osmolality in the brain when the blood urea nitrogen level is lowered rapidly. Hyponatremia may be a factor as well. Seizures are most likely to occur at the time dialysis is first initiated, when large changes in serum osmolality may occur.

Home Hemodialysis

With appropriate cannulization and proper training and education of both the child and parents, hemodialysis can be performed at home. Time spent in transportation is eliminated, the environment is more pleasant and secure, and the child is able to assume a more active role in the treatment program. Home dialysis is especially advantageous for children waiting for a transplant who live a great distance from the dialysis center or for children who have had one or more kidney transplant failures.

Home hemodialysis units are available to some children, and the preparation and management are similar to that required for hemodialysis in the hospital. The patient is equipped with a dialysis unit that is used with the vascular access established for outpatient dialysis. Parents of children on home hemodialysis must know how to operate the equipment, connect the unit to the vascular access, and assess the status of the child. They must palpate an internal

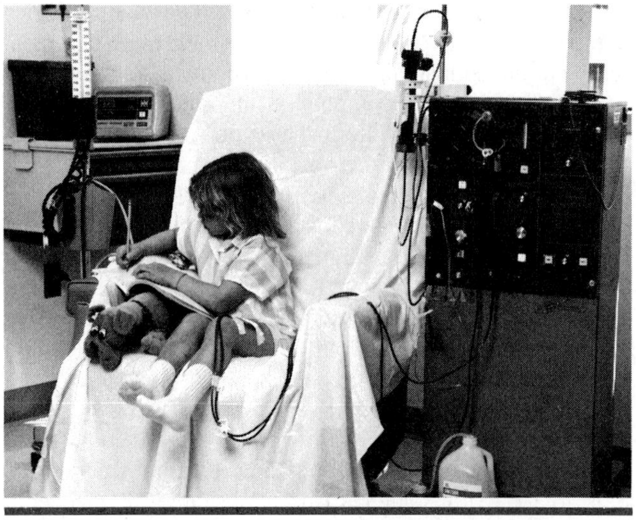

Fig. 30-5. Child undergoing hemodialysis.

shunt for evidence of patency and auscultate it for a bruit sound.

Nursing Considerations

Initiating a hemodialysis regimen is a traumatic and anxiety-provoking experience for most children. It involves surgery for implantation of the graft or fistula, and the initial experience with the hemodialysis machine and its implication are frightening to most children. They need reassurance about the nature of the preparations for dialysis and conduct of the treatment. They are anxious concerning repeated venipunctures (with implanted shunts and for blood chemistries) and the sight of their blood leaving their body and entering the machine. Once the initial fear of the machine has been resolved, younger children adjust fairly well to maintenance hemodialysis (Fig. 30-5).

Adolescents, with their increased need for independence and their urge for rebellion, may adapt less well. They resent the control and enforced dependence imposed by the rigorous and unrelenting therapy program. They resent dependency on a machine, parents, and professional staff. Depression, hostility, or both are common in adolescents undergoing hemodialysis. The adverse consequences of the disease include the need for diet restrictions, limitations to physical activity (resulting from lack of energy, frequent illnesses, and specific restrictions related to access), and the sense of being different from other children. Withdrawal from peers and social isolation are the rule, and noncompliance with the therapeutic regimen is not uncommon.

Body changes related to the disease process, such as growth retardation, skin color, and lack of sexual maturation, are stress provoking. Dietary restrictions are particularly burdensome for both children and parents. Children feel deprived when unable to eat foods previously enjoyed and unrestricted for other family members. Consequently, failure to cooperate is not uncommon. Diet restrictions are interpreted as punishment and, since they may not be able to fully understand the purpose of the restrictions, some will sneak forbidden food items at every opportunity. Allowing children, especially adolescents, maximum participation in and responsibility for their own treatment program is helpful. The extent of compliance and adjustment depends on the personalities of the involved persons, the quality of their relationships, and their coping mechanisms.

After weeks or months of hemodialysis, parents and child feel anxiety associated with the prognosis and continued pressures of the treatment. The relentless need for treatment interferes with family plans. Transportation to and from the dialysis unit and the time spent on the machine restrict the time available for outside activities, including school. Graft and fistula problems are not uncommon and present a common source of aggravation. The occurrence of seizures during dialysis is highly stressful to both child and family. Most families and children on hemodialysis look to renal transplanation as a desirable alternative to long-term treatment.

PERITONEAL DIALYSIS

For *acute* conditions peritoneal dialysis (PD) is quick, relatively easy to learn, safe to perform, and requires a minimum amount of equipment and specially trained nurses. PD is a slow gentle process, which decreases the stress on body organs that can occur with the rapid chemical and volume changes of hemodialysis. The procedure is indicated for neonates, children with severe cardiovascular disease, or those with bleeding abnormalities who are poor risks for vascular access and heparinization.

Chronic PD is the preferred form of dialysis for children/parents who are independent, families who live a long distance from the medical center, infants, school-age children, and children who prefer fewer dietary restrictions and a gentler form of dialysis. Chronic peritoneal dialysis is most often performed at home.

Contraindications for use of PD include recent abdominal surgery, peritoneal adhesions and scarring, or paralytic ileus. A higher rate of infection (peritonitis and pneumonia) is observed with this modality, as well as a lower rate of efficiency in children with hypotension and reduced visceral blood flow when compared with hemodialysis.

Procedure

In acute situations PD catheter insertion may be accomplished at the bedside; catheters for long-term use are placed surgically in the operating room under anesthesia. A catheter is inserted through the anterior abdominal wall, and the catheter cuff sutured into place. At the time of dialysis, a commercially prepared dialysis solution (dialysate) is allowed to flow by gravity through the catheter into the peritoneal cavity, where it remains while equilibrium between plasma and dialysis fluid takes place. Approximately 30 to 50 ml/kg of dialysate is instilled at each treatment. The fluid is then allowed to flow by gravity drainage into a receptacle, and fresh dialysate is again instilled.

In acute PD, each pass generally takes about 30 minutes: 5 minutes for the fluid to flow into the peritoneal cavity, 20 minutes for equilibration, and 5 to 10 minutes for removal (Sedman, 1986b). The procedure is usually continued until renal funcion is restored, poisons are reduced, or (in prolonged need) the patient is placed on a form of chronic PD—*continuous ambulatory peritoneal dialysis (CAPD)* or *continuous cycling peritoneal dialysis (CCPD)*. If placed aseptically, catheters may be used to treat ARF for several weeks provided the aseptic exit site, bag exchanges, and tubing changes are performed by the dialysis or intensive care nursing staff.

Home Dialysis

The development of satisfactory methods for CAPD and its alternative, CCPD, has provided additional means for managing ESRD at home. In both methods commercially available sterile dialysate solution is instilled into the peritoneal cavity through the surgically implanted indwelling catheter. The warmed solution is allowed to enter the peritoneal cavity by gravity and remains a variable length of time according to the procedure used.

In CAPD the dialysate is instilled, the line clamped off, and the empty solution bag is rolled up and worn attached to the abdomen or thigh or even placed in a pocket. The solution is allowed to remain in the peritoneum for 4 to 6 hours. The bag is then unrolled and placed on the floor, the line is unclamped, and the fluid is drained into the bag by gravity. Another heated bag is hung, and the process is repeated so that there is fluid in the abdomen continuously. The procedure is performed three times during the day and once at night. For an active child CAPD has proved to be a satisfactory alternative to hemodialysis that can be continued for an indefinite time.

CCPD is a modification of CAPD and intermittent peritoneal dialysis. The dialysis exchange is performed only at night using an automatic dialysis machine, which controls the timed cycles of inflow and outflow of dialysate. The catheter is opened only at night rather than four times per day, although an additional exchange may be prescribed during the day. The nighttime dialysis allows the child more freedom during the day and relieves parents from having to perform multiple exchanges (Alliapoulos and others, 1984).

The care and management of the procedure are the responsibility of the parents of young children. School nurses can perform the procedure for younger school-age children. Older children and adolescents are able to carry out the procedure themselves, thus providing them with some control and less dependency. This is especially important for adolescents.

Complications. CAPD and CCPD are presently considered to be the methods of choice for most children who require dialysis because they are easier to initiate and maintain than hemodialysis. Peritonitis is the major complication of home peritoneal dialysis, but no differences in the incidence of infection have been found between the two methods (Warady and others, 1984; Alliapoulos and others, 1984). The patients are treated intraperitoneally with antibiotics, and some may require catheter replacement. Although the risk of infection is continuously present, most practitioners believe that it is not great enough to discourage the use of these methods (Fine and others, 1983).

However, other complications have been noted in patients on home peritoneal dialysis. Tunnel infections are evidenced by swelling, warmth, and tenderness along the subcutaneous catheter tract; however, they can be managed with administration of antibiotics. Peritoneal leaks and ventral hernias caused by the sustained hydraulic pressure that develops within the peritoneum have also been found in a significant number of children. Most of these patients respond to reduction in dialysate volume.

Nursing Considerations

The availability of home dialysis has offered a greater degree of freedom for persons undergoing long-term dialysis. The need for a residence convenient to a dialysis unit and the necessity for frequent trips to the unit are eliminated except for monthly evaluations. The nurse is responsible for teaching the family. Education focuses on (1) the disease, its implications, and the therapeutic plan; (2) the possible psychologic effects of the disease and the treatment; and (3) the technical aspects of the procedure.

The family must learn how to take vital signs before and after the dialysis and how to interpret the significance of blood pressure and temperature variations. They need to know how to vary the composition of the dialysate to compensate for variations in the vital signs and to maintain an accurate record of all aspects of the treatment.

Parents of the young child using CAPD are taught how to exchange bags and manage the procedure at home. Even newborn infants are able to benefit from peritoneal dialysis. Older children can be taught to take responsibility for their own treatments as much as possible. The family is encouraged to ask questions throughout the preparation time, including those that clarify anatomy and physiology, mechanical functioning, and side effects of the disease and the treatment. The peritoneal dialysis schedule is outlined to meet the individual needs of the patient and the family. Most schedules are arranged for uninterrupted sleep at night and to coordinate the dialysis with school and other activities. The diet, medication, and activity are discussed, and feelings about the entire therapeutic program are explored with the child and the family.

Infection is the greatest hazard of peritoneal dialysis; therefore the family is instructed to contact the appropriate persons at the earliest evidence of peritonitis. In most instances of peritonitis the infection can be controlled with administration of antibiotics. Unfortunately there is a high incidence of peritonitis; episodes occur approximately 6 months to a year apart (Sedman, 1986b). Repeated infections may necessitate replacement of the catheter or its removal and abandonment of the peritoneum as an access route.

The importance of emotional, as well as material, support cannot be overemphasized. The National Kidney Foundation, mentioned previously, provides a number of services and information for families of children with renal disease. A relatively new organization, the **American Association of Kidney Patients (AAKP),*** has been organized to promote the interest and welfare of kidney patients. It provides education and support for patients and public education regarding all areas of kidney disease.

*Suite LL1, 1 Davis Blvd., Tampa, FL 33606; (813) 254-2558.

CONTINUOUS ARTERIOVENOUS HEMOFILTRATION

A third type of dialysis used primarily in acute care settings is continuous arteriovenous hemofiltration (CAVH), a gentle form of dialysis that employs specialized equipment (filter, pump, tubing connected to a vascular access) to ultrafiltrate blood continuously at a very slow rate. With this procedure, fluid balance may be achieved within 24 to 48 hours after initiation. CAVH is a procedure used to remove excess fluid from patients with severe oliguric fluid overload.

CAVH is an ideal form of dialysis for childen with fluid overload from surgical procedures (such as cardiovascular surgery) who do not have severe biochemical abnormalities. It is frequently used for critically ill children who require volume-expanding fluids such as hyperalimentation solution, albumin, or packed red cells. It creates space for the infusion of these replacement solutions in fluid-sensitive patients. CAVH has proven to be a highly successful alternative form of dialysis for critically ill children who might not survive the rapid volume changes that occur with hemodialysis and peritoneal dialysis.

TRANSPLANTATION

Renal transplantation is now an acceptable and effective means of therapy in the pediatric age-group. Although peritoneal dialysis and hemodialysis are life-preserving and are able to be carried out in the home in a large number of cases, neither method is compatible with a normal lifestyle. Transplantation, on the other hand, offers the opportunity for a relatively normal life. It is presently regarded as the preferred form of treatment for many children with chronic renal failure.

Kidneys for transplant are available from two sources: a living related donor (LRD), usually a parent or sibling, and cadaver donor (CD), wherein the family of a dead or brain-dead patient consent to donation of a healthy kidney. The criteria for selection of kidney recipients are quite liberal, but uniform criteria have not been established among the various centers that specialize in the procedure. In general there is no limit to age. In some cases, a person's mental status (e.g., mental retardation, emotional instability, or noncompliant behavior) may be reason to defer transplantation until the recipient's psychoemotional status improves and it is reasonable to assume that the posttransplant regimen will be carried out (Novello, 1986b).

Generalized infection must be eradicated before attempted transplantation, and the recipient should have adequate bladder capacity, although this is not considered to be a contraindication. Children with abnormal bladders may be subject to more posttransplant urologic complications and infection than they would otherwise be. Nevertheless, many children with systemic disease and tumors have

QUESTIONS AND CONTROVERSIES

Who should be denied renal transplantation?

The criteria for selection of renal transplant recipients sometimes create dilemmas for professionals. In most cases the decision is simply a matter for the transplant team and the family to resolve for the benefit of the child involved. However, in some situations, especially in view of the scarcity of donor kidneys and the expense of the procedure, the solution is less clear. The matter creates more questions than answers.

For example, should a child with a severe mental or physical disability take priority over one without these disabilities? Should financial responsibility be a consideration? Some youngsters with renal transplants have discontinued taking their medications, thereby either causing damage to their kidney or losing the graft (Korsch, 1981). Should these youngsters receive a second transplant? Should very young children whose families have proven too unreliable in complying with a therapeutic regimen be given a transplant when the success of the graft depends on following a prescribed therapeutic plan? Are very young, unwed adolescent mothers likely to be less compliant in following the prescribed medical regimen? Can persons on limited incomes manage to acquire the costly medications? If not, should the government subsidize payment?

What solutions to these dilemmas are available and how are decisions justified? Who should make the decisions?

had successful transplants. On the other hand, there is a high incidence of recurrent disease in the donor kidney in children who receive a transplant for rapidly progressive glomerulonephritis, hemolytic-uremic syndrome, or focal segmental glomerulonephritis.

Procedure

The kidney graft is placed in the extraperitoneal space, usually the anterior iliac fossa, the renal artery is anastomosed to the internal iliac or hypogastric artery, the renal vein is anastomosed to the hypogastric vein, and the ureter is implanted into the bladder or anastomosed to the recipient's ureter. Small children receiving a large donor kidney may require placement within the abdomen with vessel anastomoses to the aorta and inferior vena cava. Unless there is medical contraindication, the recipient's failed kidneys are left in place. Severe hypertension, neoplasm, and obstructive uropathy are the usual causes for nephrectomy.

The primary goal in transplantation is the long-term survival of the grafted tissue. The means by which this is attempted is (1) securing tissues that are antigenically similar to that of the recipient and (2) suppressing the recipient's immune mechanism.

Selection of Donor Tissue

The source of a donor kidney is either a live person or a cadaver soon after death. The closer the genetic relationship between the donor and recipient, the better the possibility of long-term survival. The only truly compatible tissue match is that between identical twin siblings. The next best possible match is a sibling, then a parent, and finally an uncle or aunt. In some states use of siblings is impossible until the possible donor is of age to give consent for removal of a kidney. Unrelated donors are least likely to be compatible. Careful immunologic studies are carried out to determine the donor whose kidney is least likely to be rejected by the recipient.

Suppression of the Immune Response

After the best possible tissue match is obtained for a transplant, the survival time can be significantly lengthened by suppressing the immune response of the recipient. The immunosuppressant therapy of choice in kidney transplantation is corticosteroids (prednisone) in conjunction with cyclosporine and azathioprine. Other therapies include antilymphoblast globulin or monoclonal antibodies, administered intravenously for 14 days after transplant.

The administration of these drugs is not without hazard. The major problem encountered with nonspecific immunosuppression is that it not only suppresses the immune response to the grafted tissue but also suppresses the body's capacity to respond to other antigenic stimuli. Consequently, the child is vulnerable to overwhelming infections.

Prednisone is a powerful immunosuppressant and antiinflammatory agent that acts to stabilize cell walls, reduce migration of white blood cells into the inflamed area, and inhibit deposition of fibrin and collagen. It also depresses T-cells, B-cells, and phagocytes. A number of complications that are directly attributable to corticosteroid therapy are cause for concern for children on steroid therapy. Interference with calcium absorption retards linear growth, and in most centers alternate-day administration is being used in an effort to improve growth rates and to decrease other long-term side effects. Other corticosteroid-induced side effects may include the characteristic cushingoid facies, cataracts, fluid and sodium retention, gastric ulcer, and obesity.

Cyclosporine is a powerful immunosuppressant that acts to decrease production of T-cells. Side effects of this drug are arterial hypertension, which may appear within 3 weeks of transplant; hirsutism; and nephrotoxicity, a major concern in renal transplantation. Maintenance doses of cyclosporine are determined by serum blood levels. Low therapeutic cyclosporine levels usually prevent untoward side effects, as well as rejection. After the initial intravenous therapy immediately following transplant, the drug is administered orally. It has a rather unpleasant taste; however, this can be satisfactorily disguised by the addition of chocolate milk or juices.

Azathioprine is a powerful immunosuppressant that interferes with cellular protein synthesis. The problem related to the toxic effect of azathioprine is mainly neutropenia, which is usually managed by reduced dosage. (See Chapter 36 for a discussion of immunosuppressant therapy and related nursing care.)

Rejection

Rejection of a transplanted kidney is the most frequent cause of transplant failure. Rejection can be one of three types—hyperacute, acute, or chronic. Hyperacute rejection is irreversible, develops immediately or within a few hours after revascularization, and is related to circulating antibodies preformed in the recipient against the donor tissue antigens. These are seen in second transplants or in persons sensitized from blood transfusions.

Acute rejection usually occurs between the first few days and 6 months after transplantation but may occur as late as 1 or 2 years later. Rejection is evidenced by both biochemical and clinical abnormalities. The most frequent finding is fever, which is usually accompanied by swelling and tenderness over the graft, hypertension, and diminished urine output. A severe reaction may cause oliguria. Increases in serum blood urea nitrogen and creatinine levels are laboratory evidence of decreased transplant function. Most acute rejection episodes respond to intravenous administration of methylprednisolone sodium succinate (Solu-Medrol), antilymphoblast globulin, or monoclonal antibodies.

NURSING ALERT The child with a recent kidney transplant (a few days) or one who was grafted approximately 6 months previously who exhibits any of the following should be evaluated immediately for possible rejection:
Fever
Swelling and tenderness over graft area
Diminished urine output
Elevated blood pressure

Chronic rejection is characterized by slow, gradual deterioration of renal function that typically begins 6 months or more after transplantation. Evidence of rejection may be heralded by proteinuria and/or hematuria, and the rejection may have symptomatology indistinguishable from the original kidney disease. No present therapy can halt the progressive process, which inevitably leads to loss of the implanted kidney.

Prognosis

The 2-year survival rate of transplants varies from 65% to 95% for relative donors and 42% to 80% for cadaver grafts. Posttransplant complications include infection, hypertension, steroid toxicity, hyperlipidemia, aseptic necrosis, malignancy, and growth retardation (Ettenger and Fine, 1987). Long-term graft survival is not guaranteed, and many children require a second or third transplant. Successful renal transplantation does improve rehabilitation of children with CRF, both educationally and psychologically.

Nursing Considerations

The possibility of renal transplantation often comes as a hope for relief from the rigors of hemodialysis and the hated diet restrictions. Except for children with preexisting personality problems or residual physical disabilities, most children and families respond well to kidney transplant, and the majority return to normal life within a year after surgery. The dynamics related to accepting and donating kidneys are fraught with emotional overtones, caused in part by the issues related to the child's receiving an organ from another person.

A variety of serious emotional and psychologic conflicts may arise as a consequence of donor selection, including ambivalence of donors faced with surgery and relinquishing a kidney, feelings of guilt if one should prove to be unacceptable as a donor, and the emotional impact of having a live-relative donated kidney rejected by the recipient. This is especially guilt-producing when a parent is the donor.

The child recipient responds in various ways to kidney transplant. The concept of having a foreign body, especially a cadaver kidney, inside their own body is sometimes disturbing to children. They often speculate about the age, sex, personality, and physical characteristics of the donor. They may fear that the kidney will wear out if it came from an older person. Some children are distressed to find that their donor kidney came from a person of the opposite sex. Corticosteroid therapy, necessary in kidney transplants, creates undesirable side effects—for example, growth failure, obesity, characteristics of Cushing syndrome (see Fig. 38-3), acne, and hirsutism—that are frequently a source of emotional and social problems for older children. Characteristic facial changes (coarseness, thickened nares, puffy cheeks, prominent supraorbital ridges, and mandibular prognathism) have also been reported in children on cyclosporine (Reznik and others, 1987).

The most frequent reason for noncompliance in childhood renal transplant recipients is dislike of undesirable side effects. The cosmetic implications of the side effects can be overwhelming, especially to adolescent girls. Deliberate discontinuation of the drugs is most commonly observed in teenage girls. Noncompliance is also seen frequently in children from poorly communicating families who are not very supportive (see Compliance, Chapter 27).

Working with children and their families during the various stages of renal failure, dialysis, and transplantation is a difficult and challenging experience. Nurses must become familiar with the family; assess family strengths, weaknesses, and coping mechanisms; and be prepared to provide intensive support and guidance during the prolonged experience. The child and family need help in accepting what is happening to them, learning anticipatory guidance regarding predictable stresses, and dealing constructively with the physical, emotional, and financial burdens that are an ongoing part of this prolonged disability.

KEY POINTS

- The main function of the kidney is to maintain the composition and volume of body fluids in equilibrium.
- Common inflammatory disorders of the genitourinary tract include urinary tract infection, nephrotic syndrome, and acute glomerulonephritis.
- Management of UTIs is directed at eliminating infection, detecting and correcting functional or anatomic abnormalities, preventing recurrences, and preserving renal function.

- Vesicoureteral reflux is the retrograde flow of bladder urine into the ureters.
- Common features of acute glomerulonephritis are oliguria, edema, hypertension, circulatory congestion, hematuria, and proteinuria.
- Therapeutic management of acute glomerulonephritis is maintenance of fluid balance, treatment of hypertension, and antibiotic therapy.
- Nephrotic syndrome is characterized by increased glomerular permeability to protein.
- Management of nephrotic syndrome is aimed at reducing excretion or protein, reducing or preventing fluid retention by tissues, and preventing infection and other complications, dietary control, corticosteroid therapy, immunosuppressant therapy, use of diuretics, and use of antimicrobials.
- Primary functions of the distal renal tubules are acidification of urine, potassium secretion, and selective and differential reabsorption of sodium, chloride, and water.
- The most common renal tubular disorders are renal tubular acidosis and nephrogenic diabetes insipidus.
- Management of hemolytic-uremic syndrome is aimed at control of complications and hematologic manifestations of renal failure.
- In acute renal failure, management is directed at determining treatment of underlying cause, management of complications of renal failure, and supportive therapy.
- Abnormalities in chronic renal failure are waste product retention, water and sodium retention, hyperkalemia, acidosis, calcium and phosphorus disturbance, anemia, and growth disturbances.
- When the child will need home dialysis, the nurse educates the family on the disease, its implications, the therapeutic plan, possible psychologic effects of the disease, and the treatment and technical aspects of the procedure.
- The major concerns in renal transplantation are tissue matching and prevention of rejection; psychologic concerns involve self-image as related to possible body changes as a result of the effects of corticosteroid therapy.

REFERENCES

Alliapoulos, J.C., and others: Comparison of continuous cycling peritoneal dialysis with continuous ambulatory peritoneal dialysis in children, J. Pediatr. 105:721-725, 1984.

Bailie, M.D.: Rapid screening and diagnosis of UTI, Contemp. Pediatr. 3:33-41, 1986.

Behrman, R.E., and Vaughan, V.C., III: Tubular disorders. In Behrman, R.E., and Vaughan, V.C., III, editors: Nelson's textbook of pediatrics, ed. 13, Philadelphia, 1987, W.B. Saunders Co.

Cooley, R.O., and Sobel, R.S.: Dental treatment considerations for the medically compromised child, Pediatr. Clin. North Am. 29:613-629, 1982.

Dillon, M.J.: Drug treatment of hypertension. In Holiday, M.A., Barratt, T.M., and Vernmier, R.L., editors: Pediatric nephrology, Baltimore, 1987, Williams & Wilkins.

Dracopoulos, D.T., and Weatherly, J.B.: Chronic renal failure: the effects on the entire family, Issues Compr. Pediatr. Nurs. 6:141-146, 1983.

Edelmann, C.M., Jr.: Urinary tract infection and vesicoureteral reflux, Pediatr. Ann. 17:568-582, 1988.

Ehrlich, R.M.: Vesicoureteral reflux: a surgeon's perspective, Pediatr. Clin. North Am. 29:827-834, 1982.

Eschbach, J.W., and Adamson, J.W.: Guidelines for recombinant human erythropoietin therapy, J. Kidney Dis. 14:2-8, 1989.

Ettenger, R.B., and Fine, R.N.: Renal transplantation. In Holiday, M.A., Barratt, T.M., and Vernmier, R.L., editors: Pediatric nephrology, Baltimore, 1987, Williams & Wilkins.

Fine, R.N., and others: Peritonitis in children undergoing continuous ambulatory peritoneal dialysis, Pediatrics 71:806-809, 1983.

Fish, A.J., and Fouser, L.S.: Glomerulonephritis. In Gellis, S.S., and Kagan, B.M., editors: Current pediatric therapy 12, Philadelphia, 1986, W.B. Saunders Co.

Fong, J.S.C., de Chadarevian, J., and Kaplan, B.S.: Hemolytic-uremic syndrome, Pediatr. Clin. North Am. 29:835-856, 1982.

Fussell, E.N., and others: Adherence of bacteria to human foreskins, J. Urol. 140:997-1001, 1988.

Garin, E.H., and Richard, G.A.: Prostaglandin inhibitors in treatment of nephrogenic diabetes insipidus, J. Pediatr. 104:174, 1983.

Griswold, W.R., and others: Accumulation of aluminum in a nondialyzed uremic child receiving aluminum hydroxide, Pediatrics 71:56-58, 1983.

Hellerstein, S., and others: Consensus: roentgenographic evaluation of children with urinary tract infection, Pediatr. Infect. Dis. 3:291-293, 1984.

Hensle, T.W., and Burbige, K.A.: Vesicoureteral reflux. In Gellis, S.S., and Kagan, B.M., editors: Current pediatric therapy 12, Philadelphia, 1986, W.B. Saunders Co.

Herzog, L.W.: Urinary tract infections and circumcision: a case-control study, Am. J. Dis. Child. 143:348-350, 1989.

Hoover, D.L.: Genitourinary trauma. In Pierog, J.E., and Pierog, L.J., editors: Pediatric critical illness and injury, Rockville, MD, 1984, Aspen Systems Corp.

Hsu, A.C., and others: Renal osteodystrophy in children with chronic renal failure: an unexpectedly common and incapacitating complication, Pediatrics 70:742-750, 1982.

Jodal, I.U., and Winberg, J.: Management of children with unobstructed urinary tract infection, Pediatr. Nephrol. 1:647-650, 1987.

Jordan, S.C., and Lemire, J.M.: Acute glomerulonephritis, Pediatr. Clin. North Am. 29:857-873, 1982.

Karmali, M.A., and others: The association between idiopathic hemolytic uremic syndrome and infection by verotoxin-producing *Escherichia coli*, J. Infect. Dis. 151:775-782, 1985.

Kim, M.S., and Grupe, W.E.: The nephrotic syndrome. In Gellis, S.S., and Kagan, B.M., editors: Current pediatric therapy 12, Philadelphia, 1986, W.B. Saunders Co.

Koch, V.H., and others: Accelerated growth after recombinant human growth hormone treatment of children with chronic renal failure, J. Pediatr. 115:365-371, 1989.

Korsch, B.: The impact of end-stage renal disease. In Azarnoff, P., and Hardgrove, C., editors: The family in child health care, New York, 1981, John Wiley & Sons, Inc.

Kroovand, R.L., and Perlmutter, A.D.: The genitourinary system. In Behrman, R.E., and Vaughan, V.C., III, editors: Textbook of pediatrics, ed. 12, Philadelphia, 1983, W.B. Saunders Co.

Libber, S., Harrison, H., and Spector, D.: Treatment of nephrogenic diabetes insipidus with prostaglandin synthesis inhibitors, J. Pediatr. 108:305-311, 1986.

McEnery, P.T., and Strife, C.F.: Nephrotic syndrome in childhood, Pediatr. Clin. North Am. 89:875-894, 1982.

Neill, M.A., and others: *Escherichia coli* O157:H7 as the predominant pathogen associated with the hemolytic uremic syndrome: a prospective study in the Pacific Northwest, Pediatrics 80:37-40, 1987.

Novello, A.C.: Hemodialysis. In Gellis, S.S., and Kagan, B.M., editors: Current pediatric therapy 12, Philadelphia, 1986a, W.B. Saunders Co.

Novello, A.C.: Renal transplantation. In Gellis, S.S., and Kagan, B.M., editors: Current pediatric therapy 12, Philadelphia, 1986b, W.B. Saunders Co.

Ogra, P.L., and Faden, H.S.: Urinary tract infections in childhood: an update, J. Pediatr. 106:1023-1028, 1985.

Reznik, V.M., and others: Changes in facial appearance during cyclosporin treatment, Lancet 1:1405-1406, 1987.

Rizzoni, G., and others: Plasma infusion for hemolytic-uremic syndrome in children: results of a multicenter controlled trial, J. Pediatr. 112:284-290, 1988.

Roberts, J.A.: URI: an argument for circumcision, Contemp. Pediatr. 5(8):42-54, 1988.

Rogers, W.B.: Shampoo urethritis, Am. J. Dis. Child. 139:748-749, 1985.

Salmen, P., and others: Whirlpool-associated *Pseudomonas aeruginosa* urinary tract infection, JAMA 250:2025-2026, 1983.

Sedman, A.B.: Chronic renal failure. In Gellis, S.S., and Kagan, B.M., editors: Current pediatric therapy 12, Philadelphia, 1986a, W.B. Saunders Co.

Sedman, A.B.: Peritoneal dialysis. In Gellis, S.S., and Kagan, B.M., editors: Current pediatric therapy 12, Philadelphia, 1986b, W.B. Saunders Co.

Smith, F.G.: Urinary tract infections. In Gellis, S.S., and Kagan, B.M., editors: Current pediatric therapy 12, Philadelphia, 1986, W.B. Saunders Co.

Warady, B.A., and others: Peritonitis with continuous ambulatory peritoneal dialysis and continuous cycling peritoneal dialysis, J. Pediatr. 726-730, 1984.

Wiswell, T.E., and Geschke, D.W.: Risks from circumcision during the first month of life compared with those for uncircumcised boys, Pediatrics 83:1011-1015, 1989.

Wiswell, T.E., and Roscelli, J.D.: Corroborative evidence for the decreased incidence of urinary tract infections in circumcised male infants, Pediatrics 78:96-99, 1986.

Wiswell, T.E., and others: Effect of circumcision status on periurethral bacterial flora during the first year of life, J. Pediatr. 113:442-446, 1988.

BIBLIOGRAPHY

General

Alon, U., and Pery, M.: Percutaneous kidney needle biopsy in children is less traumatic than in adults, Nephrology 50:57-60, 1988.

Anderson, G.F., and Smey, P.: Current concepts in the management of common urologic problems in infants and children, Pediatr. Clin. North Am. 32:1133-1149, 1985.

Benitez, O.A., and others: Inaccuracy in neonatal measurement of urine concentration with a refractometer, J. Pediatr. 108:613-616, 1986.

Chambers, J.K.: Fluid and electrolyte problems in renal and urologic disorders, Nurs. Clin. North Am. 22:815-826, 1987.

Frank, A., and Murray, S.M.: A no-guess guide for urinary color assessment, RN 51(6):46-47, 49, 51, 1988.

Guarda, N.P.: If your patient must undergo fine-needle biopsy, RN 49(10):34-35, 1986.

Hogg, R.J.: Recent advances in the diagnosis of hematuria in children, Pediatr. Ann. 17:560-567, 1988.

Kallen, R.J.: What's causing the hematuria? Contemp. Pediatr. 8:55-71, June 1986.

Krugman, S., and others: Infectious diseases of children, ed. 8, St. Louis, 1985, Mosby–Year Book, Inc.

Norman, M.E.,: An office approach to hermaturia and proteinuria, Pediatr. Clin. North Am. 34:545-560, 1987.

Oliphant, M.: Ultrasound: a primary screening tool for GU disorders, Contemp. Pediatr. 3:71-78, 1986.

Silva, F., and others: Overview of pediatric nephrology, Kidney Int. 33:1016-1032, 1988.

Urinary Tract Infection/Reflux

Alon, U., and others: Ultrasonography in the radiologic evaluation of children with urinary tract infection, Pediatrics 78:58-64, 1986.

Bergstein, J.M.: Hematuria, proteinuria, and urinary tract infections, Pediatr. Clin. North Am. 20:55-66, 1982.

Brogna, L., and Lakaszawski, M.L.: The continent urostomy, Am. J. Nurs. 86:160-163, 1986.

Burns, M.W.: Pediatric urinary tract infection: diagnosis, classification and significance, Pediatr. Clin. North Am. 34:1111-1120, 1987.

Conti, M.T., and Euthropius, L.: Preventing UTI's: What works? Am. J. Nurs. 87:307-309, 1987.

Edelmann, C.M., Jr.: Urinary tract infection and vesicoureteral reflux, Pediatr. Ann. 17:568-582, 1988.

Heldrich, F.J.: Pinning down the diagnosis of UTI, Contemp. Pediatr. 5:52-78, 1988.

Johnson, C.E., and others: Renal ultrasound evaluation of urinary tract infections in children, Pediatrics 78:871-878, 1986.

Lerner, G.R., Fleischmann, L.E., and Perlmutter, A.D.: Reflux nephropathy, Pediatr. Clin. North Am. 34:747-770, 1987.

Winberg, J.: Urinary tract infections in infants and children. In Walsh, P.C., and others, editors: Campbell's urology, ed. 5, Philadelphia, 1986, W.B. Saunders Co.

Woodward, J.R., and Rushton, H.G.: Reflux uropathy, Pediatr. Clin. North Am. 34:1349-1364, 1987.

Glomerular Diseases

Berns, J.S., and others: Steroid responsive nephrotic syndrome of childhood: a long-term study of clinical course, histopathology, efficacy of cyclophosphamide therapy, and effects of growth, Am. J. Kidney Dis. 9:108-114, 1987.

Brodehl, J., and Ehrich, J.H.H.: Short versus standard prednisone therapy for initial treatment of idiopathic nephrotic syndrome in children, Lancet 1:380-383, 1988.

Earle, D.P.: Poststreptococcal acute glomerulonephritis, Hosp. Pract. 20(7):48E-48J, 48O-P, 48U, 48Z, 48AA-BB, 1985.

MacDonald, N.E., and others: Role of respiratory viruses in exacerbations of primary nephrotic syndrome, J. Pediatr. 108:378-382, 1986.

Mahan, J.D., and others: Congenital nephrotic syndrome: evolution of medical management and results of renal transplantation, J. Pediatr. 105:549-553, 1984.

McVicar, M., and Chandra, M.: Pathogenic mechanisms in the nephrotic syndrome of childhood, Adv. Pediatr. 32:269-286, 1985.

Schnaper, H.W.: The immune system in minimal change nephrotic syndrome, Pediatr. Nephrol. 3:101-110, 1989.

Srivastava, R.N., and others: Later resistance to corticosteroids in nephrotic syndrome, J. Pediatr. 107:66-70, 1985.

Tejani, A., and others: Cyclosporin A–induced remission in relapsing nephrotic syndrome in children, Kidney Int. 33:729-734, 1988.

Ueda, N., and others: Intermittent versus long-term tapering prednisolone for initial therapy in children with idiopathic nephrotic syndrome, J. Pediatr. 112:122-126, 1988.

Vernier, R.L., and Chavers, B.: Glomerular permeability: new concepts, Pediatr. Ann. 17:590-600, 1988.

Warshaw, B.L., and Hymes, L.C.: Daily single-dose and daily reduced-dose prednisone therapy for children with the nephrotic syndrome, Pediatrics 83:694-699, 1989.

Wynn, S.R., and others: Long-term prognosis for children with nephrotic syndrome, Clin. Pediatr. 27:63-68, 1988.

Hemolytic-Uremic Syndrome

Cleary, T.G.: Cytotoxin-producing *Escherichia coli* and the hemolytic uremic syndrome, Pediatr. Clin. North Am. 35:485-501, 1988.

Havens, P.L., and others: Laboratory and clinical variables to predict outcome in hemolytic-uremic syndrome, Am. J. Dis. Child. 142:961-964, 1988.

Kavi, J., and Wise, R.: Causes of the haemolytic uraemic syndrome, Br. Med. J. 298:65-67, 1989.

Novillo, A.A., and others: Haemolytic uremic syndrome associated with faecal cytotoxin and verotoxin neutralizing antibodies, Pediatr. Nephrol. 2:288-290, 1988.

Siegler, R.L.: Management of hemolytic-uremic syndrome, J. Pediatr. 112:1014-1020, 1988.

Acute Renal Failure

Coleman, E.: When the kidneys fail, RN 49:28-38, 1986.

Engle, W.D.: Evaluation of renal function and acute renal failure in the neonate, Pediatr. Clin. North Am. 33:129-151, 1986.

Fildes, R.D., Springate, J.E., and Feld, L.G.: Acute renal failure. II. Management of suspected and established disease, J. Pediatr. 109:567-571, 1986.

Gaudio, K.M., and Siegel, N.J.: Pathogenesis and treatment of acute renal failure, Pediatr. Clin. North Am. 34:771-787, 1987.

Hahn, K.: The many signs of renal failure, Nursing '87 17:34-41, 1987.

Kon, V., and Ichikawa, I.: Research seminar: physiology of acute renal failure, J. Pediatr. 105:351-357, 1984.

Nace, G.: Preventing adverse drug reactions in patients with renal failure, J. Nephrol. Nurs. 2:30-32, 1985.

Ruley, E.J., and Bock, G.H.: Acute renal failure in infants and children. In Shoemaker, W.C., and others, editors: Textbook of critical care, ed. 2, Philadelphia, 1989, W.B. Saunders Co.

Chronic Renal Failure

Bock, G.H., and others: Disturbances of brain maturation and neurodevelopment during chronic renal failure in infancy, J. Pediatr. 114:231-238, 1989.

Crittenden, M.R., and Holaday, B.: Physical growth and behavioral adaptations of children with renal insufficiency, ANNA J 16:87-92+, 1989.

Fennell, R.S., and others: Growth in children with various therapies for end-stage renal disease, Am. J. Dis. Child. 138:28-31, 1984.

Fine, R.N., Salusky, I.B., and Ettenger, R.B.: The therapeutic approach to the infant, child, and adolescent with end-stage renal disease, Pediatr. Clin. North Am. 34:789-801, 1987.

Foreman, J.W., and Chan, J.C.M.: Chronic renal failure in infants and children, J. Pediatr. 113:793-800, 1988.

Frauman, A.C., and Gilman, C.: "Normal" life—a goal for the child with chronic renal failure, ANNA J 12:252-254, 1985.

Gertner, J.M.: Phosphorus metabolism and its disorders in childhood, Pediatr. Ann. 16:957-965, 1987.

Langman, C.: Childhood uremic bone disease, Pediatr. Ann. 16:974-978, 1987.

Lierance, C.: Adolescents with end stage renal disease, J. Nephrol. Nurs. 2:34-35, 1985.

McCrory, W.W., and others: Effects of dietary phosphate restriction in children with chronic renal failure, J. Pediatr. 111:410-412, 1987.

Quinlan, M.: Nursing assessment and management of malnutrition in uremic infants, ANNA J 15:19-22, 1988.

Ray, P.E., and Holliday, M.A.: Growth rates in infants with impaired renal function, J. Pediatr. 113:594-600, 1988.

Trachtman, H., and Gauthier, B.: Parenteral calcitriol for treatment of severe renal osteodystrophy in children with chronic renal insufficiency, J. Pediatr. 110:966-970, 1987.

Weiss, R.: Management of chronic renal failure, Pediatr. Ann. 17:584-589, 1988.

Dialysis

Bell, S.: CAVH in pediatrics: Meeting the challenge, ANNA J 15:25-26, 1988.

Dirkes, S.M.: Making a critical difference with C.A.V.H., Nursing '89 19(11):57-60, 1989.

Gharbieh, P.A.: Renal transplant: surgical and psychologic hazards, Crit. Care Nurse 8(6):58-70, 1988.

Gold, L.M., and others: Psychosocial issues in pediatric organ transplantation: the parents' perspective, Pediatrics 77:738-743, 1986.

Harmon, W.E., and Ingelfinger, J.R.: Dialytic management of end stage renal disease. In Tune, B.M., and others, editors: Contemporary issues in nephrology: pediatric nephrology, ed. 12, New York, 1984, Churchill Livingstone, Inc.

House, R.M., and Thompson, T.L., II: Psychiatric aspects of organ transplantation, JAMA 260:535-539, 1988.

Kadas, N.: Reducing fluid overload without hemodialysis, RN 49(5):27-31, 1986.

Kennedy, J.M.: The development of CAPD dialyzable dolls, J. Nephrol. Nurs. 2:46-47, 1985.

Malti, J., and Wellons, D.: CAPD: a dialysis breakthrough with its own burdens, RN 51:46-52, 1988.

McFarland, K.: Pediatric peritoneal dialysis, Pediatr. Nurs. 14:426-429, 1988.

Moskop, J.C.: Organ transplantation in children: ethical issues, J. Pediatr. 110:175-179, 1987.

Neff, E.J.: Nursing the child undergoing dialysis, Issues Compr. Pediatr. Nurs. 10:173-185, 1987.

Nova, G.: Dialyzable drugs, Am. J. Nurs. 87:933-942, 1987.

Pascual, J.F., Lopez, J.D., and Molina, M.: Hemofiltration in children with renal failure, Pediatr. Clin. North Am. 34:803-818, 1987.

Sander, V., Murray, C., and Robertson, P.: School and the in-center pediatric hemodialysis patient, ANNA J 16:72-74, 1989.

Sheldon, C.A., McLorie G.A., and Churchill, B.M.: Renal transplantation in children, Pediatr. Clin. North Am. 34:1209-1232, 1987.

Sheldon, C.A, and others: Surgical considerations in childhood end-stage renal disease, Pediatr. Clin. North Am. 34:1187-1208, 1987.

Sinai-Trieman, L., Salusky, I.B., and Fine, R.N.: Use of subcutaneous recombinant human erythropoietin in children undergoing continuous cycling peritoneal dialysis, J. Pediatr. 114:550-554, 1989.

Stephenson, T., and Jakubawski, J.A.: Kidney camp, J. Nephrol. Nurs. 2:46-47, 1985.

Suddaby, E.C., Bell, S.B., and Murphy, K.J.: Continuous hemofiltration in infants and children, Pediatr. Nurs. 16:79-82, 1990.

Tank, E.S., and Hatch, D.A.: Hernias complicating chronic ambulatory peritoneal dialysis in chidlren, J. Pediatr. Surg. 21:41-42, 1986.

Walker, L.: Adolescent dialysands in group therapy, Soc. Casework 66:21-29, 1985.

Transplantation

Conley, S.B., and others: Use of cyclosporine in pediatric renal transplant recipients, J. Pediatr. 106:45-49, 1985.

Frauman, A.C., and Miles, M.S.: Parental willingness to donate the organs of a child, ANNA J 14:401-404, 1987.

Funnell, B.: Orthoclone OKT #3 sterile solution in the treatment of acute allograft rejection: relevant nursing issues, CAANT 2:11-13, 1987.

Hollander, L.A.: Renal transplantation in schoolage children: beyond physiologic care, ANNA J 12:252-254, 1985.

Hudson, K., and Hiott, K.: Coping with pediatric transplant rejection, ANNA J 13:261-263, 1985.

Kegg, D.L.: My kidney transplant—a preoperative teaching tool, J. Nephrol. Nurs. 2:267-270, 1985.

Morris, P.J.: Therapeutic strategies in immunosuppression after transplantation, J. Pediatr. 111(6):1004-1007, 1987.

Oyler-Mooney, J., Taylore, S., and Ulrich, B.: Care of the renal transplant patient receiving cyclosporin, J. Nephrol. Nurs. 2:274-276, 1985.

Rimar, J.M.: Cyclosporine for organ transplantation, MCN 10:237, 1985.

Sheldon, C.A., McLorie, G.A, and Churchill, B.M.: Renal transplantation in children, Pediatr. Clin. North Am. 34:1209-1232, 1987.

van Diemen-Steenvoorde, R., and others: Growth and sexual maturation in children after kidney transplantation, 110:351-356, 1987.

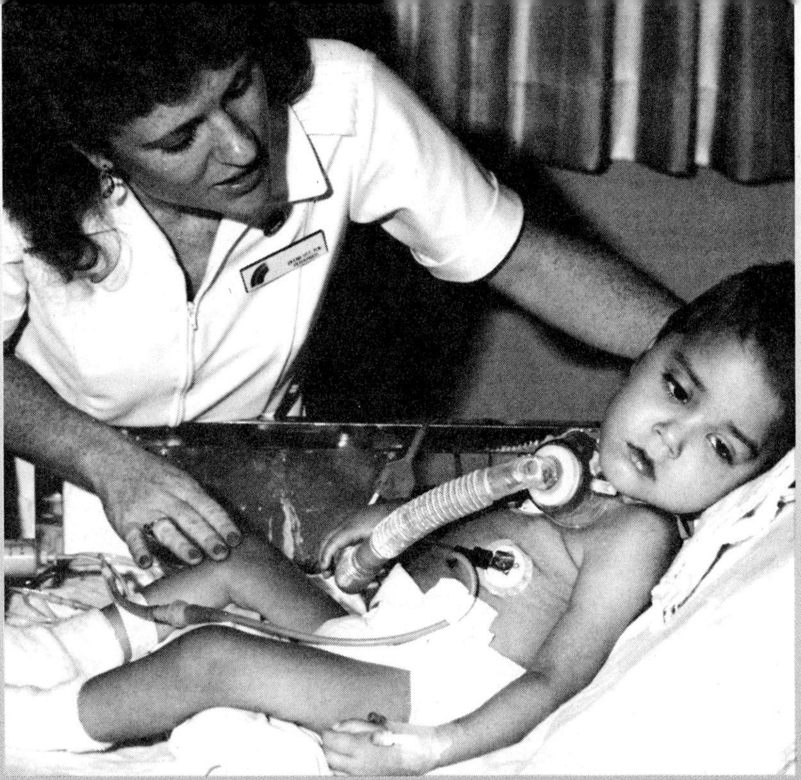

The Child with Problems Related to Transfer of Oxygen and Nutrients

UNIT XI

The survival of an individual depends on a continuous supply of energy for maintaining the function of all the cells in the body. This energy is obtained through oxygen and nutrients incorporated by the body and converted to energy by the process of oxygenation-reduction. Any circumstance or condition that requires an increase in energy requires a concomitant increase in the materials that the body converts into energy.

The need for oxygen is acute. Without this vital substance, the body is unable to survive more than a few minutes without permanent damage to vital structures or death. Therefore oxygen must be supplied constantly. Nutrients and water, on the other hand, can be stored within the body for use at times of increased need or diminished supply.

Alterations in the ability to supply oxygen or nutrients are some of the most common health problems of childhood. Interference with respiratory and gastrointestinal function is encountered at all ages, but very young children are especially vulnerable to dysfunctions in these systems. Respiratory and gastrointestinal disorders are encountered more frequently and the effects are more serious in children in the younger age-groups. Chapter 31, *The Child with Disturbance of Oxygen and Carbon Dioxide Exchange,* and Chapter 32, *The Child with Respiratory Dysfunction,* describe the more common conditions that impair the exchange of oxygen and carbon dioxide. Chapter 33, *The Child with Gastrointestinal Dysfunction,* is concerned with factors that interfere with digestion or absorption of body nutrients. There are other situations in which there are disturbances in the availability of oxygen and nutrients for energy, for example, diabetes mellitus and disorders of fluid and electrolyte balance, but these are more appropriately discussed elsewhere.

CHAPTER 31

The Child with Disturbance of Oxygen and Carbon Dioxide Exchange

RELATED TOPICS

The child with respiratory dysfunction, Ch. 32
High risk related to disturbed respiratory function, Ch. 10
Discharge planning and home care, Ch. 26
Physical examination: chest, lungs, Ch. 7
Shock, Ch. 29

GLOSSARY

ABG Arterial blood gas
ALS Advanced life support
apnea Absence of airflow (breathing)
BLS Basic life support
CO_2 Carbon dioxide
CPAP Continuous positive airway pressure
CPR Cardiopulmonary resuscitation
dyspnea Difficulty breathing
EMS Emergency medical services
ET Endotracheal
FIO_2 Fraction of inspired oxygen
hyperpnea Deep, rapid, or labored respiration
hypopnea Slow or shallow respirations
hypoxemia Deficiency of oxygen in the arterial blood
hypoxia Inadequate, reduced tension of cellular oxygen
MV Minute volume (total volume per minute measured by collection of expired gas)
O_2 Oxygen
Pa Pressure of gas in arteries
$Paco_2$ Partial pressure (tension) of carbon dioxide in arteries
Pao_2 Partial pressure (tension) of oxygen in arteries
PAo_2 Partial pressure (tension) of oxygen in alveoli
P_B Barometric pressure
Pco_2 Partial pressure (tension) of carbon dioxide
pH Expression of hydrogen ion concentration
PIo_2 Pressure of inspired oxygen
Po_2 Partial pressure (tension) of oxygen
respiration Process of oxygen and carbon dioxide exchange within the body tissues from the lungs to cellular oxidation processes
respiratory arrest Cessation of respiration
respiratory failure Inability of the respiratory apparatus to maintain adequate oxygenation
respiratory insufficiency Increased work of breathing or inability to maintain normal blood gas tensions
Sao_2 Oxygen saturation
tachypnea Abnormally rapid rate of breathing
TCM Transcutaneous monitoring
TV Tidal volume (amount of air inhaled and exhaled during normal ventilation)
ventilation Process by which gases are moved into and out of the lungs

Disorders involving the respiratory tract, many of which can be life-threatening, occur frequently in infancy and childhood. Various factors influence the development of respiratory disease during these periods. To enhance understanding of how pathologic processes produce an effect, the basic anatomy and physiology of the respiratory tract are reviewed. The physiologic responses are no different in the child than in the adult; for example, gas exchange, oxygen (O_2) and carbon dioxide (CO_2) tension, and the activity of chemoreceptors are much the same in children and in adults. Anatomically, however, there are a number of differences that influence the way in which children, particularly infants, respond to respiratory disturbances.

RESPIRATORY TRACT STRUCTURE AND FUNCTION

The respiratory tract consists of a complex of structures that function under neural and hormonal control. The primary responsibility of these structures is to distribute air and exchange gases so that cells are supplied with O_2 for body metabolism and CO_2, the volatile product of metabolism, is removed. The organs of the respiratory system—nose, pharynx, larynx, trachea, bronchi, and lungs—provide the means whereby gases enter the body; the circulatory system distributes gases to and from the millions of cells throughout the body. All the structures of the respiratory system, except the minute air sacs (alveoli) of the lung tissue, function in air distribution. It is within the alveoli that the gas exchange takes place.

STRUCTURE

The thoracic cavity, which is encased in the bony framework provided by the ribs, vertebrae, and sternum, consists of three major partitions: the three-lobed lung on the right, the two-lobed lung on the left, and the space between them—the mediastinum—which contains the esophagus, trachea, large blood vessels, and heart. The entire thoracic cavity is lined by the smooth parietal pleura, which adheres to the ribs and superior surface of the diaphragm. Each lung is encased in a separate visceral pleural sac that, when inflated, lies against the parietal pleura. Normally the two pleural membranes are separated by only enough fluid to lubricate the surface for painless movement during filling and emptying of the lungs. In disease states this space may contain air *(pneumothorax)* or fluid *(pleural effusion)*, more specifically serum *(hydrothorax)*, blood *(hemothorax)*, or pus (*pyothorax*, also known as *empyema*). Inflammation of the pleura causes the painful friction of pleurisy during respiratory movements.

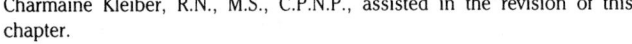

Charmaine Kleiber, R.N., M.S., C.P.N.P., assisted in the revision of this chapter.

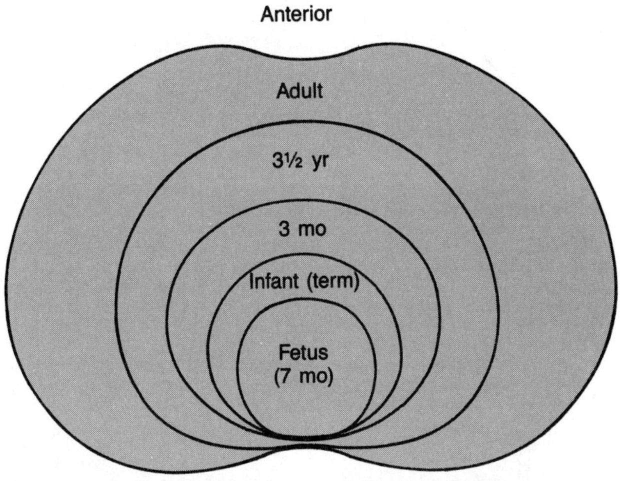

Fig. 31-1. Changes in chest shape with age.

Chest

The chest has a relatively round configuration at birth but changes gradually to one that is more or less flattened in the anteroposterior diameter in adulthood (Fig. 31-1). In certain lung diseases chronic overinflation causes changes in these measurements. For example, in severe obstructive lung disease (e.g., asthma, cystic fibrosis) the anteroposterior measurement approaches the transverse measurement to produce the so-called barrel chest. Periodic measurements provide clues to the course of lung disease or the efficacy of therapy.

The elliptic shape of the ribs and the angle at which they are attached to the spine allow the thorax to change size during respiration. Contraction of the intercostal muscles lifts the ribs from a downward angle to a more horizontal angle, which increases both the anteroposterior and the lateral dimensions of the chest. This also changes the diameter of the bronchi. The diameter increases during inspiration and decreases during expiration, an important factor when the bronchi are narrowed as a result of obstruction or inflammation. Contraction and relaxation of the diaphragm cause the chest cavity to lengthen and shorten, which also increases the volume of the chest cavity during inspiration. Normal expiration is passive, although contraction of the internal intercostal muscles pulls the rib cage downward, and contraction of the abdominal muscles forces the diaphragm upward to decrease the chest size actively.

An adult's ribs articulate with the vertebrae and sternum from a downward and lateral angle. Contraction of the intercostal muscles raises the ribs to a horizontal position in a "bucket-handle" type of respiratory motion, causing the chest cavity to enlarge. In the newborn infant the ribs articulate with the spine at a horizontal rather than a downward slope and, if raised further, decrease the diameter of the chest (Fig. 31-2). Therefore the infant relies almost entirely on diaphragmatic-abdominal breathing. During inspiration the diaphragm is forced downward, increasing the available

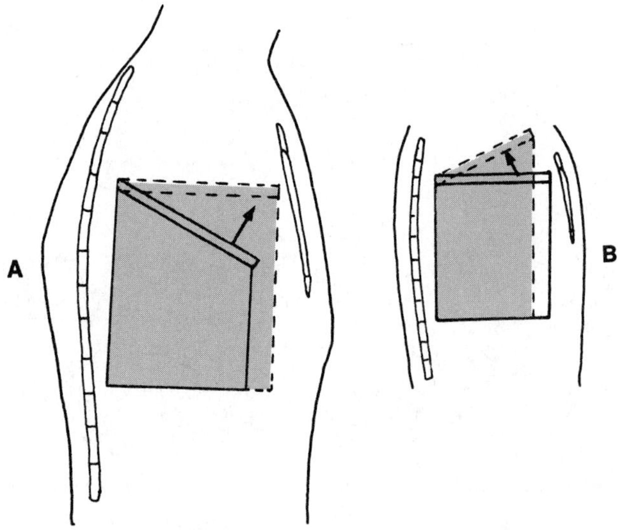

Fig. 31-2. Mechanisms of respiratory excursion. **A,** Downward and lateral position of rib in adult and expansion of lung capacity on thoracic inspiration. **B,** More horizontal position of rib in infant and decreased expansion of lung capacity of thoracic inspiration.

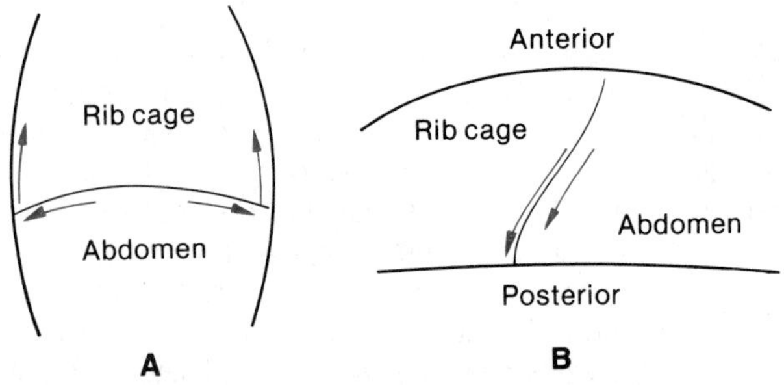

Fig. 31-3. Relationship of diaphragm and abdominal contents in, **A,** upright, and **B,** supine positions.

space for lung expansion. The intercostal muscles serve primarily as stabilizing forces.

Also facilitating respiration are (1) the elastic properties of lung tissue, which allow them to expand with increasing volume (compliance) and to collapse away from the pleural wall with decreased volume (elastic recoil), and (2) the presence of a lipoprotein (surfactant) layer at the air-fluid interface, which allows even alveolar expansion and prevents alveolar collapse.

Compliance also changes with age. It is very high in the newborn, facilitated in part by a more pliant rib cage. This increased compliance in the newborn causes the rib cage to be easily distorted with increased negative pressure in the pleural cavity or when factors inhibit the stabilizing action of the intercostal muscles. This can be observed in the infant with lung disease. Inspiration causes an inward movement of the rib cage as the abdomen moves outward, because the greater negative pleural pressure required to move the lungs pulls in the soft, compliant, and easily distorted rib cage. Factors that interfere with compliance and recoil increase the work of respiration. Examples include a deficiency of surfactant in respiratory distress syndrome or reduced compliance from fibrotic changes resulting from chronic lung disorders such as cystic fibrosis and chronic asthma.

Variations also occur in lung volume relative to posture. In the upright position the evenly distributed weight of the abdominal contents contributes to uniform application of negative intrathoracic pressure. However, in the supine position the abdominal contents apply weight caudally to create a nonuniform distribution of positive pressure to the diaphragm. Consequently, lung volume is increased in the upright position and decreased in the supine position. In addition, the mechanical attachment of the diaphragm to the rib cage is such that contraction will elevate the rib cage in the upright position but in the supine position tends to pull in the rib cage (Fig. 31-3).

In the newborn the diaphragm is attached higher in front and consequently is longer. Therefore this already stretched diaphragm is unable to contract as far or as forcefully as that of the older infant or child. Also, young infants are less able to withstand diaphragmatic fatigue because of fewer energy-producing components. Abdominal distention from gas or fluid can impede diaphragmatic excursion significantly.

Airways

The rigid nasal structures, which are lined with ciliated mucous membranes, serve as passageways for air, warming and moistening air and filtering it of impurities. In infancy the nasal passages are narrow, and infants are primarily nose-breathers, which substantially increases airway resistance. Any factor that decreases the size of the passages and further increases airway resistance, such as nasal mucosal swelling and mucous accumulation, hampers infants' breathing and feeding.

The upper airway is shared by both the respiratory and the alimentary tracts, and many of the muscles in this area participate in several complex acts. However, the sequence of airway muscle activation is different in breathing and swallowing. The upper airway dilates during inspiration and constricts during exhalation. During certain activities these dimensions are modified; for example, inspiration is short during crying, coughing, and sneezing, but with crying the larynx and pharynx dilate. The net result of swallowing is closure of the upper airway with interruption of airflow. Consequently the timing and magnitude of muscle activation have important implications for airway dimension and patency.

The pharynx is also a passageway for the entry and exit of air, and it plays a role in phonation by helping produce vowel sounds. The pharynx contains the palatine and lingual tonsils, which are involved in infection control.

The larynx, situated at the upper end of the trachea, is constructed of a rigid circular framework of cartilage and contains the epiglottis and the glottis (vocal cords). These structures prevent solids or liquids from entering the airway during swallowing, and the vibrations of the vocal cords produce voice sounds. In infancy the glottis is located more cephalad than in later childhood, and the laryngeal reflexes are very active. The epiglottis is longer and projects further posteriorly in infants. The narrowest portion of the larynx is at the level of the cricoid cartilage. In the infant and young child the ciliated columnar epithelium below the vocal cords is loosely bound with areolar tissue and is therefore more susceptible to edema formation. Swelling of the glottis and epiglottis produces hoarseness and often life-threatening obstruction of this narrow portion of the airway (croup).

The trachea, which is composed of smooth muscle supported by C-shaped rings of cartilage, ensures an open airway to the bronchi and lungs. The trachea divides into two primary bronchi. The right one is situated slightly more vertical than the left, which causes aspirated objects to lodge more frequently in the right bronchus. Each bronchus enters the lung on its respective side, where it divides into secondary bronchi that continue to branch and divide into progressively smaller bronchioles. The entire bronchial tree is lined with mucous membrane and is composed of spiral smooth muscle supported by rings of cartilage. As the bronchioles become smaller, the cartilaginous rings become increasingly irregular and then disappear completely in the smallest bronchioles, the walls of which consist of only a single layer of cells (Fig. 31-4).

All the structures are subject to obstruction from edema or foreign objects, but the degree of obstruction from constriction of smooth muscle differs. The diameter of the relatively rigid upper airway is less subject to constriction than the lower airways, which contain very little cartilaginous support. The highly reactive bronchiolar smooth muscle of the lower airways can cause life-threatening obstruction during bronchoconstriction. The airway cartilage in young infants is very soft and compressible; therefore the intrathoracic airways are highly reactive to stimuli, such as vagal stimulation.

The airways of the newborn have very little smooth muscle, but in children 4 to 5 months of age they contain sufficient muscle to cause narrowing in response to irritating stimuli. By 1 year of age, smooth muscle development and reactivity are comparable to those in the adult. Growth of the respiratory system follows the general growth curve during the early weeks of life, but the airways grow faster than the thoracic and cervical portions of the vertebral column. Consequently, the larynx and trachea descend in relation to the upper spine. For example, the bifurcation of the trachea that lies opposite the third thoracic vertebra in the infant descends to a position opposite the fourth in adulthood (Fig. 31-5). Likewise, the cricoid cartilage descends from a position opposite the fourth cervical vertebra in the infant to opposite the sixth cervical vertebra in the adult. These anatomic changes produce differences in the angle of access to the trachea at various ages and must be considered when the infant or child is to be positioned for resuscitation and airway clearance.

The function of the tracheobronchial tree is to distribute air to the alveoli of the lung. A variety of diseases and conditions, such as mucosal swelling, muscular contraction, and mechanical obstruction by mucus or a foreign body, can cause localized or generalized airway occlusion.

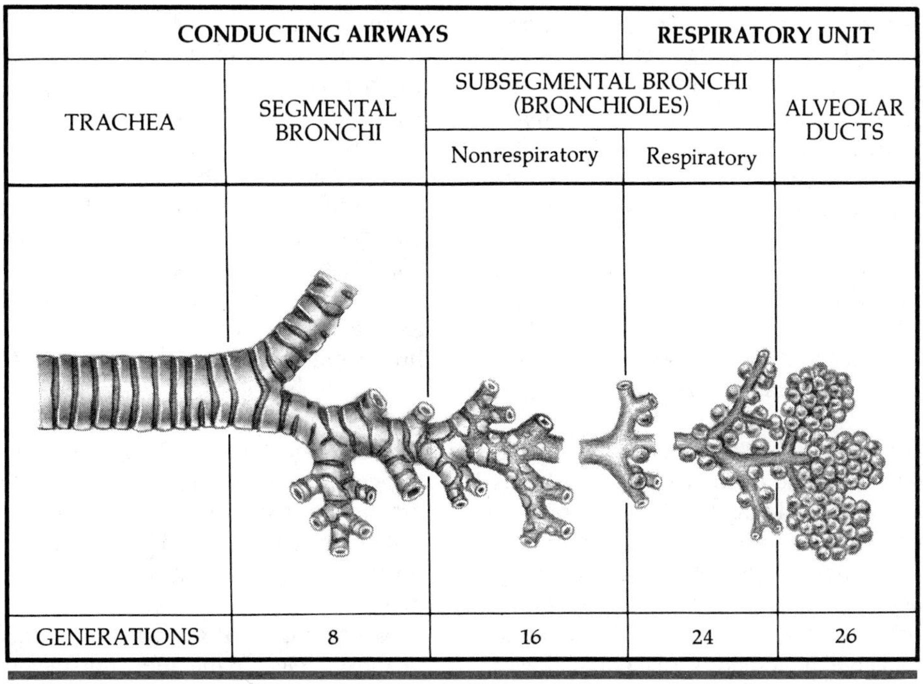

Fig. 31-4. Structures of the lower airway.
From Thompson, J.M., and others: Mosby's manual of clinical nursing, ed. 2, St. Louis, 1989, Mosby–Year Book, Inc.

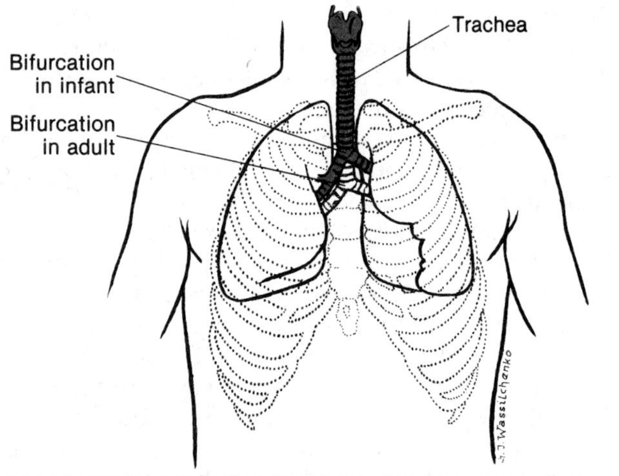

Fig. 31-5. Difference in level of bifurcation of trachea in infant and adult.

Respiratory Units

The two cone-shaped lungs consist of the bronchi, bronchioles, and innumerable small air sacs, or alveoli. Through these thin-walled structures, gas exchange occurs between the inspired air and the bloodstream. The amount of gas exchanged depends on many factors, including the amount and composition of air inhaled, thickness of the alveolar wall, adequacy of circulation to the alveoli, and substances within the alveoli that either prevent their inflation (e.g., surface-active substance surfactant) or prevent gas exchange (e.g., fluids).

With age, changes take place in the air passages that increase respiratory surface area. The major changes are in the number and size of alveoli and in the increased branching of terminal bronchioles. Whereas the number of conducting airways is complete early in fetal life, the air sacs are shallow with wide necks but have few septa at birth. This promotes patency but limits surface area for gas exchange. The alveoli are large with thick septa that have little elastic recoil (not unlike the emphysemic lung). During the first year bronchioles continue to branch, and the globular alveoli formed earlier in the terminal units rapidly increase in number with each generation. These alveoli partition and divide existing alveoli to form smaller lobular units separated by thinner septa, thus enlarging the area available for gas exchange.

Alveoli increase steadily in number, but it is unclear when septal division ceases and an increase in size begins. It appears to occur sometime during middle childhood, although evidence indicates that an increase in number of alveoli for each terminal airway takes place at puberty. Approximately nine times as many alveoli are present at age 12 years than at birth. In later stages of growth the structures lengthen and enlarge. In addition, collateral pathways of ventilation develop, including pores through alveolar walls and possibly pathways between bronchioles.

All of these factors are significant to respiratory disorders in young children. Infants and young children have less alveolar surface area for gas exchange, the narrowly branching peripheral airways become easily obstructed, and lack of collateral pathways inhibits ventilation beyond obstructed units. Consequently, young children are more readily subject to obstruction and atelectasis, especially as a result of repeated infection.

A variety of pathologic conditions can affect lung growth. A postural defect such as kyphoscoliosis reduces the number of alveoli. Rare infections of the respiratory tract (e.g., coxsackievirus) can permanently alter lung development, resulting in decreased numbers of small airways. Replication of alveoli is inhibited, so the remaining alveoli are large but decreased in number. Lung growth can also be enhanced by changes in hormone levels. Glucocorticosteroids promote lung maturation, and prenatal administration of corticosteroids has reduced the incidence of neonatal respiratory distress syndrome. Thyroxine and prolactin also enhance lung development, and lack of thyroid hormone results in immature lungs. Biochemical substances that enhance lung growth are theophylline, estrogen, isoxsuprine, epidermal growth factor, and heroin injected during pregnancy. Lung growth is inhibited by phenobarbital or excess insulin (Inselman and Mellins, 1981).

FUNCTION

Respiratory movements are first evident at approximately 20 weeks of gestation, and throughout fetal life amniotic fluid is exchanged in the alveoli. In the neonate the respiratory rate is rapid to meet the needs of a high metabolism. During growth the rate steadily decreases until it levels off at maturity (see inside front cover). The volume of air inhaled increases with the growth of the lungs and is closely related to body size. In addition, a qualitative difference exists in expired air at different ages. The amount of O_2 in the expired air gradually decreases and the amount of CO_2 increases during growth.

Ventilation occurs as air moves in and out of the lungs. This results from changes in pressure gradients created by changes in the size of the thoracic cavity. Contraction of the diaphragm and external intercostal muscles increases the size of the thorax and decreases the intrathoracic pressure. As a result, air moves from the atmosphere, which has a higher pressure, into the lungs, which have a lower pressure. The principles of artificial ventilation are based on this concept. Artificial respiratory devices increase the pressure entering the air passages (positive-pressure breathing devices), lower the pressure around the body (negative-pressure ventilator), or increase the negative pressure within the thoracic cavity (rocking bed). The shorter abdominal length of infants makes this last method ineffectual.

The alveoli are surrounded by pulmonary capillaries, and in most areas of the lung the membranes that separate these structures are exceedingly thin. The gas exchange takes place by simple diffusion in the alveoli; gas in other parts of the respiratory tract is unavailable for exchange with capillary blood.

The diameter of the airways and thus the airflow are determined by the balance of forces that tend to widen or narrow the airways. One of these is neural regulation of bronchial smooth muscles mediated through autonomic nerves. Sympathetic impulses relax the airways; parasympathetic impulses constrict them. Reflex constriction occurs in response to irritating inhalants such as dust, smoke, or sulfur dioxide; arterial hypoxemia and hypercapnia; cold air; and some drugs, such as acetylcholine and histamine. Other factors that alter airway size are peribronchial pressure, which tends to narrow the airways, and intraluminal pressure, which tends to keep airways open. For example, forced expiration causes increased peribronchial pressure and hence narrowing of the airways; a positive-pressure breathing apparatus increases intraluminal pressure, keeping the airways open.

Gas Exchange*

Gases in the blood are measured by the partial pressures (tensions) of the individual gases and are expressed in millimeters of mercury, also called *torr.* With O_2 therapy it is important to understand the relationship between the concentration of the inspired gas and the partial pressure of that gas in the arteries (PaO_2). Inspired O_2 is expressed as the fraction of inspired O_2 (FIO_2), with 1.0 meaning 100% O_2, 0.5 meaning 50% O_2, and so on. Patients breathing room air would have an FIO_2 of 0.21, since ambient air contains 21% O_2. Understanding the relationship between inspired gases and their partial pressures in the blood begins with a knowledge of gases in ambient air and how the pressure they exert creates a gradient between the alveoli and capillary blood.

Ambient air is composed of 21% O_2, trace amounts of CO_2, and 79% nitrogen (N). Water vapor (H_2O) also exerts a pressure. The water vapor does not change with the barometric pressure (PB), but exerts a constant pressure of 47 mm Hg when the gas is fully saturated at body temperature. Each contributes to the total PB as follows:

$$PB = PO_2 + PCO_2 + PN_2 + PH_2O$$

The significance of inspired gases lies in the FIO_2 and the pressure it exerts (PIO_2). At sea level this can be calculated as follows:

$$PIO_2 = FIO_2 \times (PB - PH_2O)$$
$$PIO_2 = 0.21 \times (760 - 47)$$
$$PIO_2 = 0.21 \times 713$$
$$PIO_2 = 150 \text{ mm Hg}$$

When the FIO_2 is increased, the pressure exerted also increases:

$$PIO_2 = 0.50 \times (760 - 47)$$
$$PIO_2 = 0.50 \times 713$$
$$PIO_2 = 356.5 \text{ mm Hg}$$

*This section was written by Kathleen Rossman, R.R.T.

As the inspired gas travels down the airway and reaches the alveoli, the pressure drops as CO_2 is added to the mixture. Ambient air contains only traces of CO_2. As the gas diffuses from the capillary blood to the alveoli, however, the amount and pressure of CO_2 in the alveoli increase to the CO_2 levels in the venous blood. By subtracting the PCO_2 from the PIO_2, the alveolar O_2 pressure (PAO_2) can be determined. The $PACO_2$ is first divided by 0.8. This correlation factor, or respiratory quotient (RQ), is used to calculate the ratio of O_2 absorbed to CO_2 eliminated. The alveolar pressure can then be expressed as:

$$PAO_2 = PIO_2 - (PACO_2 \div 0.8)$$
$$PAO_2 = 150 - (40 \div 0.8)$$
$$PAO_2 = 150 - 50$$
$$PAO_2 = 100 \text{ mm Hg}$$

Since normal venous PO_2 is approximately 40 mm Hg, a gradient is created when the PAO_2 is 100 mm Hg and diffusion occurs between the alveoli and capillary blood. When the patient's PaO_2 decreases, the FIO_2 can be raised to increase the PAO_2, thereby increasing the gradient for diffusion.

Because CO_2 is more soluble than O_2, it diffuses 21 times faster; therefore diffusion of CO_2 from the blood to the alveoli is not impaired. The amount of O_2 that diffuses into the blood and the amount of CO_2 removed by the lungs depend on several factors (Box 31-1).

Oxygen transport. Once O_2 has diffused from the alveolus to the pulmonary capillary, it is transported throughout the body in two ways. A small amount (PaO_2) is transported as a solute dissolved in the plasma and the water of red blood cells. A larger portion (40 to 70 times as much) is carried by hemoglobin as oxyhemoglobin. Since each gram of hemoglobin can combine with 1.34 ml of oxygen, the transport capacity is largely determined by the amount of hemoglobin present. For example, children with severe ane-

Box 31-1 FACTORS AFFECTING GAS DIFFUSION IN ALVEOLI

Pressure gradient between alveolar air and capillary blood—in order for gases to diffuse across this gradient, the gas molecules must pass through the barrier of liquid surfactant lining the alveolus. Disease can greatly increase this barrier, thus interfering with the diffusion process.

Alveolar ventilation, or amount of air that reaches the alveoli—any obstruction to air passing from the upper airways through the bronchi to the alveoli decreases the volume of air available for diffusion. *Minute ventilation* (MV) is the amount of air inhaled in a normal breath (*tidal volume* [TV]) multiplied by the respiratory rate. Factors affecting the respiratory rate or TV may decrease the amount of air available for diffusion.

Relationship between amount of alveolar air and alveolar perfusion—factors that decrease the amount of alveolar perfusion increase the ventilation/perfusion ratio. Factors or disease states that increase or decrease the amount of alveolar air also create a ventilation/perfusion mismatch and abnormal levels of PO_2 or PCO_2 in the blood.

mia tend to be fatigued, be somewhat cyanotic, and breathe more rapidly. In addition, increasing the amount of oxygen delivered to the alveoli can increase the amount carried by the blood only in relation to the amount of hemoglobin present. For example, at a Pao_2 of 100 mm Hg, hemoglobin is 97.5% saturated.

It is important to understand the relationship between the Pao_2 and the O_2 saturation (Sao_2) of the hemoglobin. This relationship is described by the oxyhemoglobin dissociation curve (Fig. 31-6). The degree to which O_2 combines with hemoglobin is affected by several factors. A shift of the curve to the left causes an increased affinity of hemoglobin for O_2. This represents an increase in the Sao_2 if measured against the same Pao_2 of the normal oxyhemoblobin dissociation curve. This left shift can be caused by an increase in blood pH, a decrease in arterial carbon dioxide pressure ($Paco_2$), or a decrease in body temperature.

A shift of the curve to the right causes a decreased affinity of hemoglobin for O_2. This represents a lower Sao_2 if measured against the same Pao_2 of the normal oxyhemoglobin dissociation curve. This right shift can be caused by a decrease in blood pH, an increase in $Paco_2$, or an increase in body temperature.

CO_2 is carried in the blood in a number of ways. A small amount ($Paco_2$) is transported dissolved in the plasma and the water of red blood cells. A large amount, more than half, hydrates to form carbonic acid, which dissociates and is carried as bicarbonate and hydrogen ions. The remaining CO_2 combines with certain plasma proteins and hemoglobin. The association of CO_2 with hemoglobin is accelerated by an increasing $Paco_2$ and a decreasing Pao_2 and is decreased by the opposite conditions. The diffusion of CO_2 into the alveoli is very rapid. Thus the equilibrium between the $Paco_2$ of the pulmonary capillaries and the alveoli is achieved promptly.

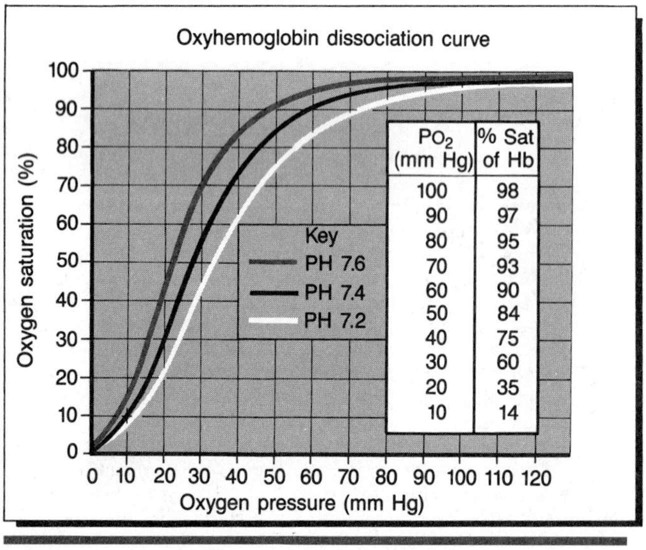

Fig. 31-6. Oxyhemoglobin dissociation curve. Changes in the affinity of hemoglobin for oxygen shift the position of the oxyhemoglobin dissociation curve. Shift to the left *(red line)* indicates increased affinity of hemoglobin for oxygen. Shift to the right *(white line)* indicates decreased affinity of hemoglobin for oxygen.

Transport between blood and tissue cells is accomplished down a diffusion gradient, just as it is between the blood and the alveoli.

Regulation of respiration. The mechanisms that control respiration can be divided into two large categories: (1) a neural system that maintains a coordinated, rhythmic respiratory cycle and regulates the depth of respiration and (2) a chemical (neurohumoral) system that regulates alveolar ventilation and maintains normal blood gas pressures.

Neural control in the respiratory center is located in three areas:

1. **A pneumotaxic center,** which modulates respiratory frequency and depth
2. **An apneustic center** which produces an inspiratory spasm and is modulated by the pneumotaxic and medullary centers and by vagal afferent impulses
3. **Medullary respiratory centers,** both inspiratory and expiratory, which regulate the rhythmicity of respirations

Impulses from other areas also affect the respiratory centers. *Proprioceptive vagal* impulses in the lung parenchyma are sensitive to stretching. When lungs become stretched, impulses are transmitted by the vagus nerve to the respiratory center, which inhibits further inflation and prevents overdistention—the *Hering-Breuer reflex.* The cerebral cortex also helps to control respirations by voluntary inhibition or acceleration of rate and depth of respirations. Reflex apnea can result from sudden painful stimulation, sudden cold stimulation, and stimulation to the larynx or pharynx (the choking reflex, which serves to prevent aspiration).

Chemical, or neurohumoral, control is mediated by specialized structures that respond to changes in pH, Pco_2, and Po_2—central chemoreceptors, probably located in the medulla, and peripheral chemoreceptors, located in the great vessels. Peripheral chemoreceptors of greatest physiologic importance are the carotid bodies, located at the division of the common carotid artery into its external and internal branches, and the aortic bodies that lie between the ascending aorta and the pulmonary artery. CO_2 and hydrogen ions control respiration by acting directly on the respiratory center; the peripheral chemoreceptors respond to changes in Po_2. Thus an increase in ventilation can result from either (1) stimulation of the respiratory center by an increased $Paco_2$ or pH or (2) a decreased Pao_2, which stimulates the carotid and aortic bodies. These bodies then transmit signals to the brain to excite the respiratory center.

The lungs also have an important role in acid-base balance. Less rapid than the chemical buffers, the respiratory mechanism begins to act within 1 to 3 minutes to make adjustments in pH by eliminating or retaining CO_2. When the levels of CO_2 are altered sufficiently, the respiratory centers in the brain respond by either increasing or decreasing the rate and depth of respirations. For example, when the pH of the blood drops, as from increased exercise, a compensatory increase in respirations rids the body of the CO_2 derived from carbonic acid, which is formed from buffered acid metabolites. CO_2 buildup from breath-holding produces the same response, again increasing the carbonic acid and reducing the serum pH. Therefore the lungs are the compensatory organs in metabolic disturbances and respond quite rapidly.

Defenses of the Respiratory Tract

The respiratory tract has several anatomic and biochemical characteristics that provide natural defenses against the many biologic and inanimate agents that can damage respiratory tissues. Intact defenses help to repel and resist the impact of injurious agents; factors that reduce the integrity of these mechanisms increase the vulnerability of these tissues to invasion and disease. Respiratory tract defenses include:

Lymphoid tissues—faucial, lingual, and pharyngeal tonsils (adenoids) and other pharyngeal lymphoid tissues form a protective circle around the entrance to the respiratory tract. These help to localize and contain invading organisms so that they can be destroyed by the body's humoral defense mechanisms.

Viscid secretions—the epithelium of the respiratory tract secretes a sticky mucus to which airborne organisms adhere.

Ciliary action—the mucus secreted by the columnar epithelium of the respiratory tract is kept flowing, carrying microorganisms and other hostile agents away from the lungs to be coughed or swallowed.

Epiglottis—the epiglottis and the epiglottis reflex protect the respiratory tract from invading material, including infectious exudate from the upper tract, and prevent such material from being aspirated into the lower tract.

Cough—the expulsive force of the cough reflex propels foreign material out of the lower tract.

Tracheobronchial dynamics—the tracheobronchial tree elongates and dilates on inspiration and shortens and narrows on expiration.

Position changes—changes in body position encourage drainage of tracheobronchial passages.

Lymphatics—lymphatics draining the terminal bronchi and bronchioles remove invading organisms, which are filtered and destroyed in the regional lymph nodes.

Humoral defenses—organisms and other foreign material are removed and/or destroyed by phagocytes, enzymes, and immunoglobulins, especially immunoglobulin A (IgA).

Although effective, these natural barriers are frequently breached. For example, some children have conditions that predispose to infection as a result of interference with the efficiency of these mechanisms, such as chronic asthma, cystic fibrosis, and the various immunodeficiency disorders. Frequent, intense exposure to organisms that accompanies conditions of crowding or continual exposure to irritating substances in the air results in breakdown of healthy defenses. Concurrent illness, malnutrition, or fatigue reduces the efficiency of natural defenses. Also, drying of the mucous membranes inhibits the activity of immunoglobulins.

ASSESSMENT OF RESPIRATORY FUNCTION

A variety of procedures relating to respiratory function can assist in diagnosis and therapy. Some can be performed by most health professionals; others require specialized skills or equipment. This section discusses only the ones used more frequently.

PHYSICAL ASSESSMENT

The nurse can obtain much information about the child's respiratory status from simple observations of physical signs and behavior. However, to make a useful assessment, the nurse needs to know what to look for and what it means (see Physical Examination: Chest, Chapter 7). *Auscultation* of the lung fields is helpful in identifying specific pathologies and in assessing the child's responses to treatment. Also, auscultation is essential to determine airway patency. *Palpation* and *percussion* provide information regarding areas of pain and tissue density. Breath sounds and their terminology are also described in Chapter 7.

Respiration

Much can be determined from the configuration of the chest and the pattern of respiratory movement, including rate, regularity, symmetry of movements, depth, effort expended in respiration, and use of accessory muscles of respiration. To assess deviations from the usual, the observer must know the normal type and rate of respiration in relation to the child's size and age (see inside front cover). Respirations are best determined when the child is sleeping or quietly awake.

Tachypnea is observed with anxiety, with elevated temperature, with severe anemia, and as the result of metabolic acidosis. Sometimes it is associated with respiratory alkalosis caused by psychoneurosis and with central nervous system disturbances. The progress of disorders that contribute to low compliance, such as the pneumonias, pulmonary edema, and pleural effusion, can be followed and evaluated by observing changes in respiratory rate.

Alterations in the depth of respirations—too deep *(hyperpnea)* or too shallow *(hypopnea)*—are recognized as abnormal only in the extremes. Hyperpnea is noted with fever, severe anemia, respiratory alkalosis associated with psychosis, central nervous system disturbances, and respiratory acidosis that accompanies disorders such as diabetes mellitus or diarrhea. Hypoventilation is less easily detected and occurs with metabolic alkalosis in conditions such as pyloric stenosis and respiratory acidosis that accompanies diaphragmatic paralysis or central nervous system depression.

Associated Observations

Associated observations also contribute to assessment. *Retractions,* or a sinking in of soft tissues relative to the cartilaginous and bony thorax, may be noted in some pulmonary disorders. Although slight intercostal retractions are normal, in disease states (particularly in severe airway obstruction) retraction becomes extreme. Subcostal retraction, observed anteriorly at the lower costal margins, indicates a flattened diaphragm, since it not only lowers the floor of the thorax but also pulls on the rib cage in response to a greater than normal decrease in intrathoracic pressure. In

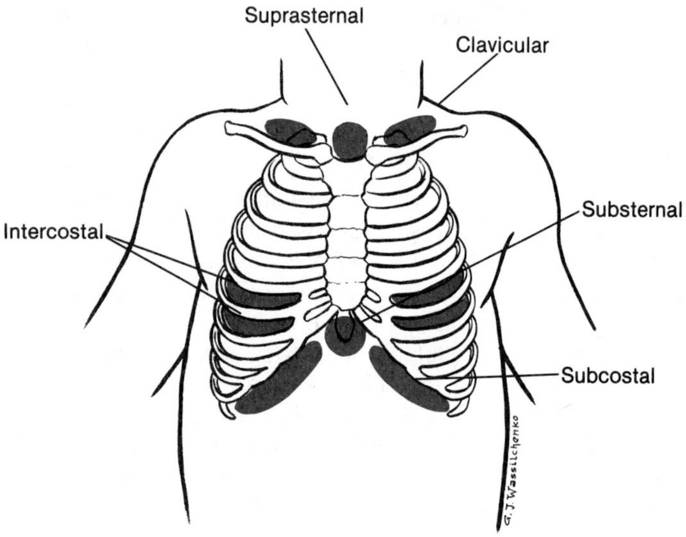

Fig. 31-7. Location of retractions.

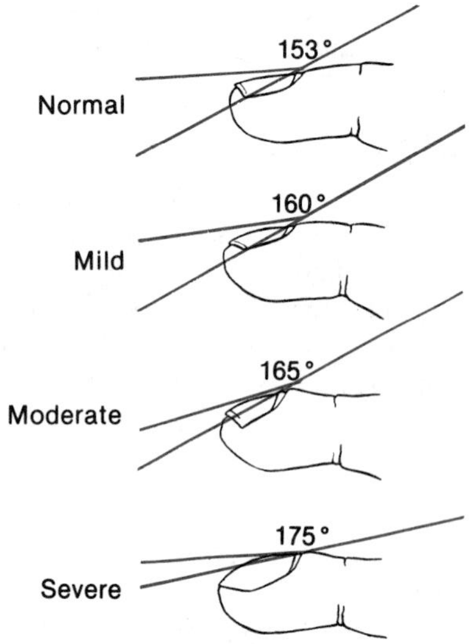

Fig. 31-8. Stages of clubbing. Degree of angle formed above finger at skin-nail junction indicates extent of clubbing. Angle greater than 160 degrees and decided curvature of nail are good criteria for presence of clubbing.

Modified from Waring, W.W.: The history and physical examination. In Kendig, E.L., Jr., and Chernick, V., editors: Disorders of the respiratory tract in children, ed. 4, Philadelphia, 1983, W.B. Saunders Co.

severe obstruction, retractions extend to the supraclavicular areas and the suprasternal notch. (See Fig. 31-7 for location of retractions.)

Nasal flaring is a sign of increased work of breathing. The enlargement of the nostrils helps reduce nasal resistance and maintain airway patency. Nasal flaring may be intermittent or continuous and should be described as minimal or marked.

Head bobbing in a sleeping or exhausted infant is a sign of dyspnea. The head, supported on the caregiver's arm only at the suboccipital area, will bob forward with each inspiration. This is caused by neck flexion resulting from contraction of the scalene and sternocleidomastoid muscles. Noisy breathing such as "snoring" is frequently associated with hypertrophied adenoidal tissue, choanal obstruction, polyps, or a foreign body in the nasal passages.

Grunting is frequently a sign of chest pain, suggesting acute pneumonia or pleural involvement. It is also observed in pulmonary edema and is a characteristic of respiratory distress syndrome. It serves to increase end-expiratory pressure and thus prolong the period of O_2 and CO_2 exchange across the alveolocapillary membrane.

Color changes of the skin, especially the distribution, degree, and duration of *cyanosis,* are noted. Except for the peripheral bluish discoloration resulting from circulatory stasis in the newborn, cyanosis is significant and usually indicates cardiopulmonary disease. The most common causes of cyanosis in children are listed in Box 31-2.

Chest pain may be a complaint of older children and may have a variety of causes, both pulmonary and nonpulmonary. It may be caused by disease of any of the chest structures—esophagus, pericardium, diaphragm, pleura, or chest wall. Parietal pleural pain is usually localized over the affected area and is aggravated by respiratory movements. The pain of diaphragmatic pleural irritation may be referred to the base of the neck posteriorly and anteriorly or to the abdomen. Most pleural pain is related to respiration; therefore respiratory movements are shallow and rapid.

Clubbing, or proliferation of tissue about the terminal phalanges, accompanies a variety of conditions, frequently those associated with chronic hypoxia, primarily cardiac defects and chronic pulmonary disease. Although clubbing often worsens with lung disease, it does not reflect disease progression accurately (Orenstein, 1989). The degree of clubbing is determined by the extent to which the nail base is lifted on the dorsal surface of the phalanx by the tissue proliferation. The greater the angle formed above the finger at the skin-nail junction, the more pronounced the clubbing, especially when there is a decided curvature to the nail (Fig. 31-8).

Box 31-2 COMMON CAUSES OF CYANOSIS IN CHILDREN

Acute or chronic alveolar hypoventilation, as seen in airway obstruction, weakness of the respiratory muscles, or a depressed respiratory center

Uneven distribution of gas and blood throughout the lungs, as might occur in bronchopneumonia

Anatomic right-to-left shunts of blood that occur in some forms of congenital heart disease or congenital arteriovenous aneurysms of the lung

Disturbances of alveolocapillary diffusion, a rare cause of cyanosis as a result of interstitial pneumonia or pulmonary fibrosis

Box 31-3 COUGH ASSESSMENT

Onset and duration
Type—dry, hacking, moist, barking, brassy, paroxysmal (a sudden attack, outburst, or intensification of symptoms)
Progress—better, worse, unchanged, persistent
Pattern—daytime, nighttime, both, different intensity with time or activity
Associated symptoms—sore throat, dyspnea, pain and its location
Secretions—sputum presence, consistency, color, frequency, evidence of swallowing sputum, postnasal drip

Cough is often associated with respiratory disease. A cough can be initiated voluntarily, although it is usually a result of a complex reflex consisting of three components: afferent nerve fibers, the cough center, and efferent nerve fibers. Much of the respiratory epithelium contains afferent receptors that are sensitive to mechanical or chemical stimuli. These receptors are concentrated in the areas of the larynx, the carina, and the bifurcations of the large and medium-sized bronchi. When a stimulus is applied to these areas, impulses are transmitted via the vagus nerve to the cough center in the brainstem. Efferent impulses travel via the vagus, phrenic, and spinal motor nerves to the larynx, intercostal muscles, diaphragm, abdominal muscles, and pelvic floor. An inspiratory gasp and closure of the glottis are followed by contraction of muscles in the chest wall, diaphragm, abdomen, and pelvic floor. The resulting compression and increase in pleural, alveolar, and subglottic pressure cause a sudden opening of the glottis and immediate release of trapped air at extremely rapid expiratory flow rates, which forces undesirable material from the respiratory tract.

Inflammation or infection almost anywhere in the upper or lower respiratory tract may produce coughing. Some types of cough are characteristic of specific diseases. For example, severe cough is associated with measles and cystic fibrosis, and the paroxysmal cough accompanied by an inspiratory "whoop" is pathognomonic of pertussis. A brassy cough is part of the symptomatology of croup and foreign body aspiration. Because there are no cough receptors in the alveoli, a cough may be absent in a child with lobar pneumonia in the early stages of the disease. Cough is assessed according to the features listed in Box 31-3.

DIAGNOSTIC PROCEDURES

Various procedures are available for assessing respiratory function and diagnosing respiratory disease. For nurses caring for the child with respiratory disorders, understanding how the tests are carried out helps them to devise the best strategies for preparing children for the tests, gaining their cooperation, and supporting them during the procedure. Moreover, this knowledge provides nurses with information on which to base nursing interventions, such as positioning, use of supplemental O_2, and assistance with coughing or deep breathing.

Pulmonary Function Tests

Noninvasive pulmonary mechanics can easily be measured with new technology at the bedside of infants and children with the use of pneumotachography. This information is sometimes limited in diagnosis, since the same functional abnormality may occur in different diseases. These tests are useful to evaluate the severity and course of a disease and to study the effects of treatment. A listing of the measured parameters is provided in Table 31-1.

Radiology and Other Diagnostic Procedures

Radiography is used frequently in diagnostic evaluation of children. Although no definitive information exists on the effects of low-dose radiation, measures are carried out to protect vulnerable areas from possible damage. When possible, technicians and others try to prevent unnecessary exposure of the child (and personnel), and the more radiosensitive areas should be protected. Careful protection of the immature gonads of the infant or child with lead shields is essential. Other sensitive areas are the thyroid gland, ocular lens, and bone marrow.

Although nurses have limited control over the length, frequency, and correct application of the x-ray beam, they can make certain that the infant or child receives proper protection from possible hazards. Lead shields, correctly placed and consistently applied to areas not needed for diagnostic purposes, are essential. Play and modification of methodology can be used effectively to reduce the trauma sometimes associated with the procedure and to gain the child's cooperation. Special radiologic examinations used in respiratory diagnosis are outlined in Table 31-2.

Several other procedures are employed in diagnosing lung disorders (Table 31-3). Most require specialized equipment and skills. All require some type of preparation of the child.

Blood Gas Determination

Blood gas measurements are sensitive indicators of change in respiratory status in acutely ill patients. They provide valuable information regarding lung function, lung adequacy, and tissue perfusion and are essential for monitoring conditions involving hypoxemia, CO_2 retention, and pH. For the nurse who cares for the acutely ill respiratory patient, this information provides cues for decision making regarding therapeutic interventions, such as adjusting the ventilator, increasing chest physiotherapy, administering O_2, or positioning the child for maximum ventilation.

Noninvasive monitoring. For continuous monitoring of blood gases, noninvasive measurements are used whenever possible. Electronic equipment has proved to be valuable in the treatment of both hospitalized and ambulatory patients.

Transcutaneous monitoring (TCM) provides continual monitoring of both transcutaneous Po_2 ($tcPo_2$) and transcu-

Table 31-1 Pulmonary function tests used in children

TEST	MEASUREMENT	SIGNIFICANCE
Vital capacity (VC) (peak flow)	Maximum amount of air that can be expelled from the lungs after maximum inspiration	Reduced in obesity Reduced in obstructive airway disease Normal in restrictive disease
Forced expiratory volume in 1 (FEV_1) or 3 (FEV_3) seconds	Amount of air that can be forced from the lungs after maximum inspiration in 1 and 3 seconds	Normally 80% of VC is exhaled in 1 second Reduced in obstructive disease
Tidal volume (TV or V_T)	Amount of air inhaled and exhaled during any respiratory cycle	Multiplied by respiratory rate to provide minute volume Information needed to determine rate and depth of artificial ventilation
Functional residual volume (FRV); functional residual capacity (FRC)	Volume of air remaining in the lungs after passive expiration	Allows for aeration of alveoli Increased in hyperinflated lungs of obstructive lung disease
Minute ventilation	Amount of air exchanged over 1 minute	See Tidal Volume
Dynamic compliance	Relationship between change in volume and pressure difference	Reflects elastic recoil of lung Normal volume but decreased airflow in obstructive disease (e.g., asthma) Normal flow but decreased volume in restrictive disease (e.g., pulmonary fibrosis)
Pulmonary resistance	Changes in pressure with changes in flow on inspiration and expiration	
Work of breathing	Total work expended moving lung and chest	
Respiratory time constancy	Time for proximal and alveolar airway pressure to equilibrate	
Blood oxygenation		
Transcutaneous O_2/CO_2 monitoring (TCM)	Skin surface electrodes heated and applied to well-perfused areas of the trunk; measurements in mm Hg	Provides continuous and reliable trends of arterial O_2 and CO_2 Noninvasive
Oximetry	Photometric measurement of O_2 saturation Measurements in percentages	Provides continuous noninvasive measurements of hemoglobin saturation
Capnography	Measures CO_2 during inhalation and exhalation cycle and produces a graph of CO_2 concentration over time	Provides end-tidal CO_2 levels to determine trends and identify shunts

NURSING TIP: APPLYING THE OXIMETER SENSOR

Infant: Tape the sensor securely to the great toe and tape the wire to the sole of the foot (or use a commercial holder that fastens with self-adhering closure). Place a snugly fitting sock over the foot.

Child: Tape the sensor securely to the index finger and tape the wire to the back of the hand. Place a finger cot or a finger cut from a latex glove over the sensor.

taneous Pco_2 ($tcPco_2$). An electrode is attached to the warmed skin to facilitate arterialization of cutaneous capillaries. The site of the electrode must be changed every 3 to 4 hours to prevent burning the skin, and the machine must be calibrated with every site change. This monitoring is used frequently in neonatal intensive care units, but it may not reflect Pao_2 in infants with impaired local circulation or in older infants whose skin is thicker.

Pulse oximetry measures the amount of light absorbed by oxyhemoglobin and uses this information to calculate the Sao_2. A sensor with a bright light is taped to a finger or toe. The sensor must identify every pulse beat to calculate an accurate Sao_2. Since movement can interfere with sens-

Table 31-2 Radiologic examinations

TEST	DESCRIPTION	PURPOSE	COMMENT
Radiography	Pictures obtained by passing x-rays through body and recording them on sensitized film	Produces images of internal structures of chest, including air-filled lungs, airways, vascular markings, heart, and great vessels	Requires preparation, cooperation, and immobilization of child
Fluoroscopy	Electronically intensified image to allow its projection on viewing screen	Used primarily to study diaphragmatic excursion and respiratory motion of the lungs Examination of barium-filled esophagus to outline mediastinal abnormalities	Requires preparation and immobilization of child
Bronchography	Contrast medium is instilled directly into bronchial tree through opaque catheter inserted via orotracheal tube	Most valuable to demonstrate and inspect bronchiectasis Detects distal bronchial obstruction Detects malformations	Carried out under general anesthesia or sedation Used less frequently than other examinations Prepare child for anesthesia
Barium swallow	Esophagus is outlined when barium solution or colloid is swallowed	Esophageal displacement defines mediastinal masses Detects swallowing disorders and malformations (e.g., tracheoesophageal fistula)	Valuable adjunct for diagnosis Performed under fluoroscope Prepare child for procedure
Angiography	Injection of dye to produce image of pulmonary vasculature	Investigation of pulmonary vascular anomalies and pulmonary hypertension	Performed under general anesthesia Prepare child for anesthesia
Computed tomography (CT)	Sequence of x-rays, each representing a cross section or "cut" through lung tissue at different depth	Useful in identifying presence of calcium or a cavity within a lesion, hilar adenopathy, mediastinal masses, or abnormalities	Usually reserved for children old enough to be able to suspend respiration voluntarily Prepare child for procedure
Magnetic resonance imaging (MRI)	Use of large magnet and radio waves to produce two- or three-dimensional image	Clearly identifies soft tissues	Requires cooperation and usually sedation of child Prepare child for procedure or anesthesia
Radioisotope scanning	Intravenous injection of albumin labeled with radioisotopes or inhalation of radioactive aerosols or xenon gas followed by radiation scanning	Delineates defects in pulmonary arterial perfusion and diseased areas of lung Detects location of aspirated foreign body	Requires cooperation of child or sedation Prepare child for procedure
Ultrasonography	Transmission of sound waves through chest	Identifies opacification	Limited use in diagnosis of respiratory disorders Prepare child for procedure

Table 31-3 Diagnostic procedures used in respiratory disorders

PROCEDURE	DESCRIPTION	PURPOSE
Tracheal aspiration	Sputum obtained by direct aspiration from trachea	Obtains secretions for examination, culture
Bronchoscopy	Direct observation of tracheobronchial tree via bronchoscope	Localizes abnormalities in major airways Provides access to (1) remove aspirated foreign bodies from major airways, (2) remove obstructive mucous plugs, and (3) perform bronchial lavage
Lung puncture	Needle aspiration of lung fluid via syringe and needle through intercostal space	Obtains lung aspirate for histologic study or culture
Lung biopsy	Removal of lung tissue via open thoracotomy or closed-needle procedures	Diagnosis of protracted pulmonary disease unexplained by other means
Brush biopsy	Material for biopsy obtained with nylon brush on end of wire passed through tube placed via nose, pharynx, trachea, and airways (via fluoroscope) to involved lung segment	Obtains material for culture and histologic examination
Percutaneous transtracheal aspiration	Needle and catheter aspiration of tracheal secretions through thyroid cartilage	Obtains secretions for laboratory examination and culture
Arterial puncture	Arterial blood obtained from temporal (neonates), brachial, radial, posterior tibial, and femoral arteries	Obtains blood for gas analysis (Po_2, Pco_2, pH)

ing, false alarms occur when the patient is active. However, some devices synchronize the arterial saturation reading with the heartbeat, thereby reducing the interference caused by motion.

✦ **NURSING ALERT** It is important to make certain that sensory connectors and oximeters are compatible. Some companies make connectors for their sensors that can be inserted into oximeters from other companies. However, the wiring is incompatible and can generate considerable heat at the tip of the sensor. Second- and third-degree burns have been reported in a neonate when sensors from one company were inadvertently used on oximeters from another firm (Murphy, 1990).

Oximetry offers several advantages over TCM. Oximetry (1) does not require heating the skin, thus reducing the risk of burns; (2) eliminates a delay period for transducer equilibration; and (3) maintains an accurate measurement regardless of the patient's age or skin characteristics or the presence of lung disease. However, oximetry is insensitive to hyperoxia because hemoglobin approaches 100% saturation for all Pao_2 readings above approximately 100 mm Hg (Lough and Carlo, 1988). This can be dangerous for the premature infant at risk for developing retinopathy of prematurity (see Chapter 10). Therefore, the premature infant being monitored with oximetry should have upper limits identified and a protocol established for decreasing O_2 when saturations are high (Harbold, 1989).

The Pao_2 can be related to the Sao_2 by means of the oxyhemoglobin dissociation curve (see Fig. 31-6). In the steep portion of the curve, small changes in Pao_2 result in large changes in Sao_2; therefore the oximeter reflects hypoxemia and O_2 availability to tissue better than transcutaneous measurements. In the flat portion of the curve, large changes in Pao_2 result in only small changes in Sao_2. Consequently, hyperoxia cannot be detected reliably when Sao_2 is 95% to 100%.

NURSING TIP: CALCULATION

A quick formula for calculating correlation of Pao_2 to Sao_2 is the 30-60, 60-90 rule. Assuming a normal pH, $Paco_2$, and body temperature, this rule can apply: when Pao_2 = 30, Sao_2 = 60; when Pao_2 = 60, Sao_2 = 90.

Arterial blood sampling. Some controversy surrounds the collection of "arterialized" capillary blood for blood gas measurements; however, many believe it to be a safe, convenient, and relatively accurate method. The blood samples are obtained by taking a deep heel stick after dilatation of the vascular bed by warming (see Fig. 27-18). The first drop of blood is discarded, and subsequent blood is collected directly into heparinized capillary tubes held in a horizontal position. The tube is delivered to the laboratory as soon as possible.

Arterial blood samples are obtained through an indwelling catheter or by arteriopuncture. The artery most frequently used is the radial artery, since there are no nearby veins. The temporal, posterior tibial, and umbilical arteries can be used effectively in the newborn. The femoral and brachial arteries may also be used. The radial and posterior tibial arteries are the first choice for intermittent arterial blood sampling because of the collateral circulation present.

Adequacy of collateral circulation can be determined by the *Allen test,* which should be performed before arterial puncture is attempted. To perform the test, the extremity distal to the puncture site is blanched by squeezing gently. The two arteries supplying blood flow to the extremity are then occluded and pressure is removed from one artery. Color return to the blanched extremity indicates collateral circulation. The procedure is repeated with the other artery.

✦ **NURSING ALERT** Nurses should perform the Allen test as a precautionary measure regardless of whether or not they perform the arterial puncture.

Normal arterial blood gas (ABG) values are much the same for all ages and depend on the concentration of O_2 the child is breathing. The arterial Po_2 should rise in proportion to the O_2 concentration being inhaled. Therefore when one is assessing the significance of ABG values, the data should include the percentage of O_2 administered (if any); the child's body temperature, since as little as 1° F can alter the blood gas values 5% to 8%; and the presence of anxiety, which causes many children to hyperventilate and blow off extra CO_2. Crying can cause breath-holding and apnea, which can decrease Pao_2.

Unclotted blood is required; therefore a syringe rinsed with heparinized solution is used to draw blood samples, and no air bubbles should enter the syringe to alter the blood gas concentration. Many institutions use prepackaged ABG sampling kits. These kits allow air-free samples to be drawn without the need for heparin dilutions. The amount collected depends on the child's size. Depending on the laboratory facilities, as little as 0.1 ml may be sufficient in small infants. Table 31-4 lists normal ABG and pH measurements in patients breathing room air at sea level.

The significance of ABG determination is related primarily to the relationships among these three determinations: pH, Po_2, and Pco_2. Much of this is discussed in relation to acid-base imbalance in Chapter 28. Sometimes a specified schedule is ordered; at other times the sample is to be drawn as indicated by clinical observations. Any change in a blood gas value must be compared with the other values and with previous readings as well as with the child's clinical appearance and behavior, medical history, and associated physiologic factors. Other factors that influence blood gas levels include the amount and method of O_2 administration, the assessment of the child, and the nature of the respiratory disorder.

Signs that indicate the need for blood examination include a change in color, depth or rate of respirations, behavior or sensorium, and sometimes other vital signs. The nurse may or may not be able to obtain the blood sample by arteriopuncture, depending on the institution's policies. Nurses are usually able to withdraw the sample from an arterial catheter, and they should become skilled in the techniques of drawing blood and flushing the line. No matter who obtains the sample, the nurse is responsible for its speedy transport for analysis.

Table 31-4 Blood gas analysis

COMPONENT	DEFINITION	NORMAL VALUE	ACIDOSIS	ALKALOSIS
pH	Indicates acid-base status of body	7.40	Less than 7.40 indicates an excess of acid	Greater than 7.40 indicates an excess of base
Pco_2	Pressure exerted by dissolved CO_2 in blood Under control of lungs Respiratory component	40 mm Hg	Greater than 40 mm Hg Causes: obstructive lung disease, hypoventilation of any cause	Less than 40 mm Hg Causes: hypoxia, pulmonary embolism, hyperventilation of any cause
HCO_3	Buffers effect of acid in blood Under control of kidneys Metabolic component	24 mEq/L	Less than 24 mEq/L Causes: diarrhea, lactic acidosis, renal failure, shock, therapy with acetazolamide, diabetic ketoacidosis, drainage of pancreatic juice	Greater than 24 mEq/L Causes: fluid loss from upper gastrointestinal tract, diuretics, corticosteroid therapy
Base excess (BE)	Reflects status of all bases in the blood	0	Negative	Positive
Po_2	Pressure exerted by dissolved O_2 in blood Indicates effectiveness of oxygenation by the lungs	80-100 mm Hg	Less than 80 mm Hg hypoxia Causes: obstructive lung disease, high CO_2 levels, low FIo_2, hypoventilation	Greater than 100 mm Hg hyperoxygenation Causes: high FIo_2, hyperventilation

Reprinted from Quick Reference to Pediatric Intensive Care Nursing by P.A. Brown et al., p. 92, with permission of Aspen Publishers, Inc. © 1989.

NOTE: The Sao_2 printed with blood gas reports cannot be used as a standard to confirm oximetry readings. Blood gas analyzers provide only approximate blood O_2 saturations based on calculations using measured blood gases, pH, and Pao_2.

The results of the gas analysis provide the nurse with information on which to base further nursing action. Nurses must be able to understand the report's significance and to implement nursing activities, for example, adjusting the concentration of O_2 the patient is receiving, changing the position, performing suction, administering prescribed drugs, or notifying the attending physician, according to the interpretation of the gas analysis. Because of increased use of continuous monitoring, painful arterial punctures can be minimized.

RESPIRATORY THERAPY

Procedures to improve ventilation are employed with increasing frequency in the prevention and management of pulmonary dysfunction. Most of these involve the nurse in the hospital or the home situation.

Respiratory care is an all-inclusive term that encompasses a variety of therapies that involve changing the composition, volume, or pressure of inspired gases. This includes primarily increasing the O_2 concentration of inspired gas *(oxygen therapy)*, increasing the water vapor content of inspired gas *(humidification)*, adding airborne particles with beneficial properties *(aerosol therapy)*, and employing various means for controlling or assisting respiration *(artificial ventilation*, or *continuous positive airway pressure)*.

Although the major responsibility for providing therapies is assumed by the respiratory care practitioner, in most institutions nurses take a prominent role in observation and ongoing management. Chest physiotherapy and suctioning are often nursing responsibilities.

OXYGEN THERAPY

The indication for administration of O_2 is *hypoxemia*, as evidenced by reduced Pa_{O_2} and cyanosis. O_2 is administered by mask, hood, nasal cannula, face tent, O_2 tent, or ventilator. The mode of delivery is selected on the basis of the concentration needed and the child's ability to cooperate in its use. The concentration of O_2 delivered should be regulated according to the individual child's needs. There are hazards related to its use; therefore O_2 should not be continued after the indication for its use is no longer present. Since O_2 is dry, it is always humidified in some manner.

O_2 therapy is primarily carried out in the hospital, although increasing numbers of children are receiving O_2 in the home. It is the responsibility of the nurse or respiratory care practitioner to ensure uninterrupted delivery of the appropriate O_2 concentration and monitoring of the child's response to the therapy.

✦ **NURSING ALERT** Oxygen is a drug and is prescribed by dose.

Oxygen Administration

Oxygen delivered to infants is best tolerated by plastic hood (Fig. 31-9). Low and high concentrations of O_2 can be easily

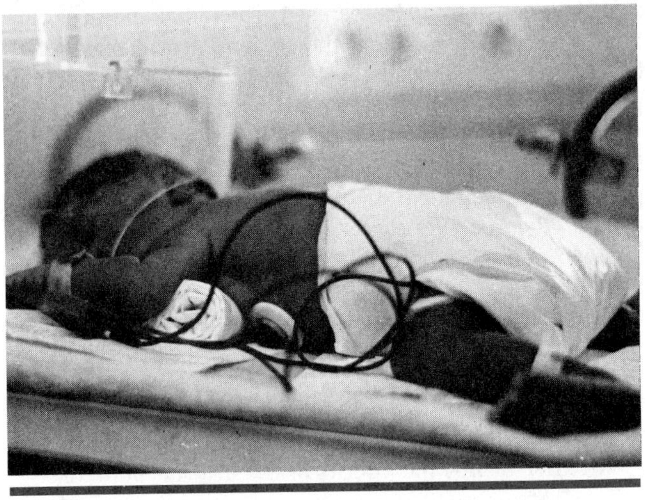

Fig. 31-9. Oxygen administered to infant by plastic hood.

maintained in this head hood, and most nursing procedures can be continued without interrupting the O_2 delivery. This is not possible when delivering O_2 directly into the incubator. At least 4 to 5 L/minute of flow is needed to maintain O_2 concentrations and remove the exhaled CO_2.

The gas should not be allowed to blow directly into the face of an infant in a hood. Cold fluid or air applied to the face stimulates receptors that trigger the diving reflex, which causes bradycardia and shunting of blood from peripheral to central circulation. The O_2 hood should not rub against the infant's neck, chin, or shoulder. Older infants and children can use a nasal cannula or prongs, which can supply a concentration of about 50%. Nasal catheters or masks are not well tolerated by children. A nasal cannula, designed especially for infants and young children, allows for more freedom for infant and caregiver and facilitates breast-feeding because the upper lip is not restricted.*

Oxygen Toxicity

Oxygen is essential to life and a valuable therapeutic aid. However, prolonged exposure to high O_2 tensions can be damaging to lung tissue. Although the exact pathogenesis of the pulmonary changes is unclear, evidence indicates damage to lung capillaries, which causes diffuse microhemorrhagic changes, diminished mucus flow, inactivation of surfactant, and altered ciliary function. The total effect appears to be the direct result of "lung burn" and is therefore a result of the PA_{O_2} and not the Pa_{O_2}. The result of these changes is a gradual impairment of alveolar ventilation.

Atelectasis may occur as the result of the "washing out" of nitrogen from the alveoli by the high concentrations of O_2. This is more likely to occur in persons with low tidal volume and retention of mucus or other secretions.

Oxygen-induced CO_2 narcosis is a physiologic hazard of O_2 therapy that may occur in persons with chronic pulmo-

*For information contact John Timmons, ESP, Inc., 2929 Tallevast Rd., Sarasota, FL 34243; (813) 351-3698.

nary disease. It is seldom encountered in children except those with cystic fibrosis. These children have chronic alveolar hypoventilation with a concomitant chronic CO_2 retention and hypoxemia. In these patients the respiratory center has adapted to the continuously higher $Paco_2$ levels, and therefore hypoxia becomes the more powerful stimulus to respiration. When the Pao_2 is elevated during O_2 administration, the hypoxic drive is removed, causing progressive hypoventilation and increased $Paco_2$ levels, and the child rapidly becomes unconscious. CO_2 narcosis can also be induced by the administration of sedation in these patients.

Other suspected toxic effects of O_2 include changes in the renal tubules, sympathoadrenal medullary stimulation precipitating neurogenic seizures, and an increased rate of destruction of red blood cells. In preterm infants the risk of retinopathy of prematurity is a major concern in O_2 administration (see Chapter 10).

ADJUNCTIVE THERAPIES

Several therapies are carried out in a management of respiratory dysfunction. Same are administered as an isolated therapy; others are performed in conjunction with O_2 administration.

Aerosol Therapy

Aerosol therapy can be effective in depositing medication directly into the airway. This can be used to avoid systemic side effects of certain drugs and reduce the amount of drug necessary to achieve the desired effect. Bronchodilators, steroids, and antibiotics, suspended in particulate form, can be inhaled so that the medication reaches the small airways. Aerosol therapy is particularly challenging in children who are too young to cooperate in controlling rate and depth of breathing. Administration of medications by this route requires skill, patience, and creativity on the part of the respiratory care practitioner.

Medications can be aerosolized with air or with O_2-enriched gas. Hand-held nebulizers are the most frequently used equipment. The medicated mist is discharged into a small plastic mask, which the child holds over the nose and mouth. To avoid particle deposition in the nose and pharynx, the child is instructed to take slow, deep breaths through an open mouth during treatment. For home use, an air compressor is necessary to force air through the liquid medication to form the aerosol. Relatively compact, portable units can be rented from health equipment companies.

The metered dose inhaler (MDI) is a self-contained, hand-held device that allows for intermittent delivery of a specified amount of medication. Many bronchodilators are available in this form and are used successfully by children with asthma (see Chapter 32). For children less than 5 or 6 years of age, a "spacer" device attached to the MDI can help coordinate breathing and aerosol delivery and allows the aerosolized particles to remain in suspension for a longer time.

A major nursing responsibility during aerosol therapy is to assess the effectiveness of the treatment and the patient's tolerance of the procedure. Assessment of breath sounds and work of breathing should be performed before and after treatments. Small children who become upset with a mask held close to the face may become fatigued from fighting the procedure and may appear worse during and immediately after the therapy. Careful assessment is needed by the nurse and practitioner to determine if the treatment is of value. It may be necessary to take time to calm the child after the therapy, allowing vital signs to return to baseline levels, in order to assess accurately changes in breath sound and work of breathing.

Continuous administration of mist, or aerosolized water, for the treatment of inflammatory conditions of the airways has no proven benefit (Alderson and Warren, 1984), but improvement has been noted in some cases. For example, the use of a mist tent or a very humid environment (e.g., a steamy bathroom) for treatment of croup is a common practice. For other pathologies, mist therapy can be detrimental. For example, bronchoconstriction in children with asthma can be exacerbated by mist therapy. Contrary to popular beliefs, inhaled mist does not affect the water content of expectorated mucus. Oral or parenteral rehydration normalizes water content of respiratory mucus effectively.

Mist Therapy

For most children beyond early infancy the mist tent, or canopy, is a satisfactory means for providing a high-humidity atmosphere, sometimes in conjunction with O_2 (Fig. 31-10). A tent does not require any device to come into direct contact with the face, but the concentration of O_2 within the tent is difficult to control and to maintain above about 40%.

The enclosed tent becomes very warm; therefore some

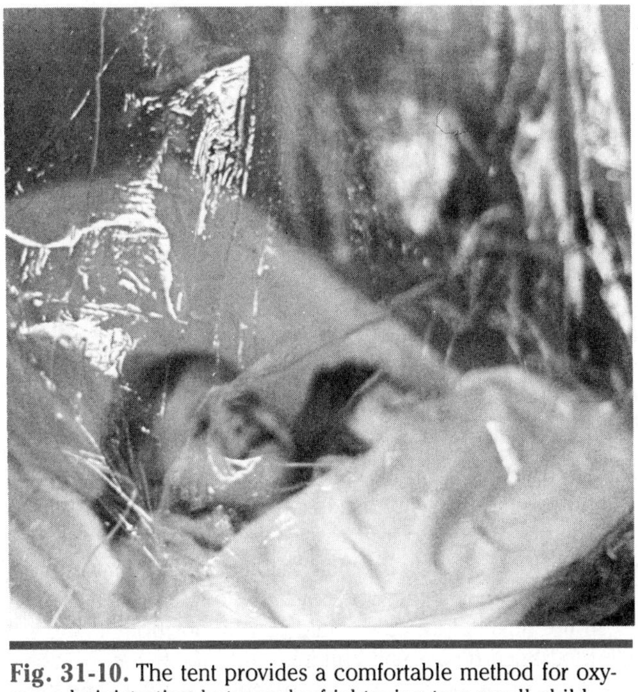

Fig. 31-10. The tent provides a comfortable method for oxygen administration but may be frightening to a small child, even when shared by a familiar "friend."

type of refrigeration unit is provided. The temperature inside the tent must be checked periodically to be certain that it is maintained at the desired level. It is important to make certain that the child is kept warm and dry. Moisture condenses on tent walls and bedding. Therefore the child's bedding and clothing are examined periodically and changed as needed to prevent chilling.

The reactions of children to the mist tent vary. Some, especially older children, feel comfortable in the tent and like the cozy, close privacy it affords. Others, more often younger children, may be frightened by the forced enclosure. The plastic walls distort their view of the world and constitute a barrier between them and their source of comfort, the parents. Their distress can be minimized if they are able to see someone nearby and are reassured that they will not be left alone. A favorite toy or object can accompany the child inside the tent. However, if O_2 is administered in conjunction with mist, toys should be inspected for safety and suitability. The high oxygen environment makes any source of sparks (e.g., metal toys, some mechanical toys) a potential fire hazard. Other familiar items can be placed at the foot of the bed or otherwise in view.

The child can be removed from the tent for activities such as feeding and bathing, whereas in other cases the child is placed in the tent only during periods of rest. Increased respiratory effort or restlessness is an indication to return the child to the oxygen tent. The equipment is changed and/or cleaned at regular intervals (at least once weekly) to prevent bacterial growth when the child requires O_2 over an extended period.

Bronchial (Postural) Drainage

Bronchial drainage is indicated whenever excessive fluid or mucus in the bronchi is not being removed by normal ciliary activity and cough. The techniques of segmental drainage, percussion, and vibration assist the normal cleansing mechanisms of the lung. Positioning the child to take maximum advantage of gravity further facilitates removal of secretions. The effect is sometimes dramatic in children with chronic lung disease (e.g., asthma, cystic fibrosis) characterized by thick mucous secretions.

Postural drainage is carried out three to four times daily and is more effective when it follows other respiratory therapy, such as bronchodilator and/or nebulization medication. Bronchial drainage is generally performed before meals (or 1 to 1½ hours after meals) to minimize the chance of vomiting and is repeated at bedtime. The length and duration of treatment depend on the child's tolerance level—usually 20 to 30 minutes. There are positions to facilitate drainage from all major lung segments (Fig. 31-11), but all positions are not used at each session. Children will usually cooperate for four to six positions, but more than six tend to exceed their limits of tolerance. Older children can be expected to tolerate longer periods.

In the hospital an older child can be positioned over an elevated knee rest. Small children and infants can be positioned with pillows or on the practitioner's lap and legs (Fig. 31-12). Infants should not be placed in the Trendelenburg position because they do not have autonomic regulation of blood flow to the head. Special modifications of the techniques are required in children whose conditions contraindicate the standard positioning, such as head injuries, some types of surgical incisions or burns, and casts or traction. At home, small children can be positioned on a padded ironing board. Children who require postural drainage over months or years may benefit from specially constructed tables padded and adjusted to their individual needs. The positions used and the frequency and duration of treatment are individualized.

Chest Physiotherapy

Chest physiotherapy usually means the use of postural drainage in combination with adjunctive techniques that are thought to enhance the clearance of mucus from the airway. These techniques include manual percussion, vibration, and squeezing of the chest; cough; forceful expiration; and breathing exercises. However, the efficacies of techniques, both individually and combined, are controversial (Kyff, 1987). Postural drainage in combination with forced expiration has been shown to be beneficial, but the benefit of other techniques has yet to be demonstrated.

The most common technique used in association with postural drainage is manual *percussion* of the chest wall and is carried out frequently in the United States despite controversy over its effectiveness. Nurses are often responsible for this maneuver if respiratory care coverage is not available; therefore they should become skilled in the technique. The patient is dressed in a light shirt and placed in a postural drainage position. The practitioner then gently but firmly strikes the chest wall with a cupped hand. A "popping," hollow sound should be the result, not a slapping sound. Percussion should be done over the rib cage only and should be painless. Percussion can be performed with a soft circular mask (adapted to maintain air trapping) or a percussion cup marketed especially for the purpose of aiding the loosening of secretions.

Vibration can be used to help move secretions cephalad during exhalations. Hand-held vibrators should be approved for use in an O_2-enriched environment (tent, head hood). Larger children may benefit from a more powerful vibrator. This therapy is subject to patient tolerance, and oximetry is an excellent monitoring tool for therapy tolerance.

Chest physiotherapy is contraindicated when patients have pulmonary hemorrhage, pulmonary embolism, end-stage renal disease, increased intracranial pressure, osteogenesis imperfecta, or minimum cardiac reserves. Chest physiotherapy is a time-consuming procedure and effective for only certain patients. After an exhaustive review of the literature, Sutton (1988) has offered the guidelines for performing chest physiotherapy (see Box 31-4).*

Squeezing is sometimes a useful maneuver while the child is in the drainage position. The child is directed to

*Home care instructions are available in Wong, D.L., and Whaley, L.F.: Clinical manual of pediatric nursing, ed. 3, St. Louis, 1990, Mosby–Year Book, Inc.

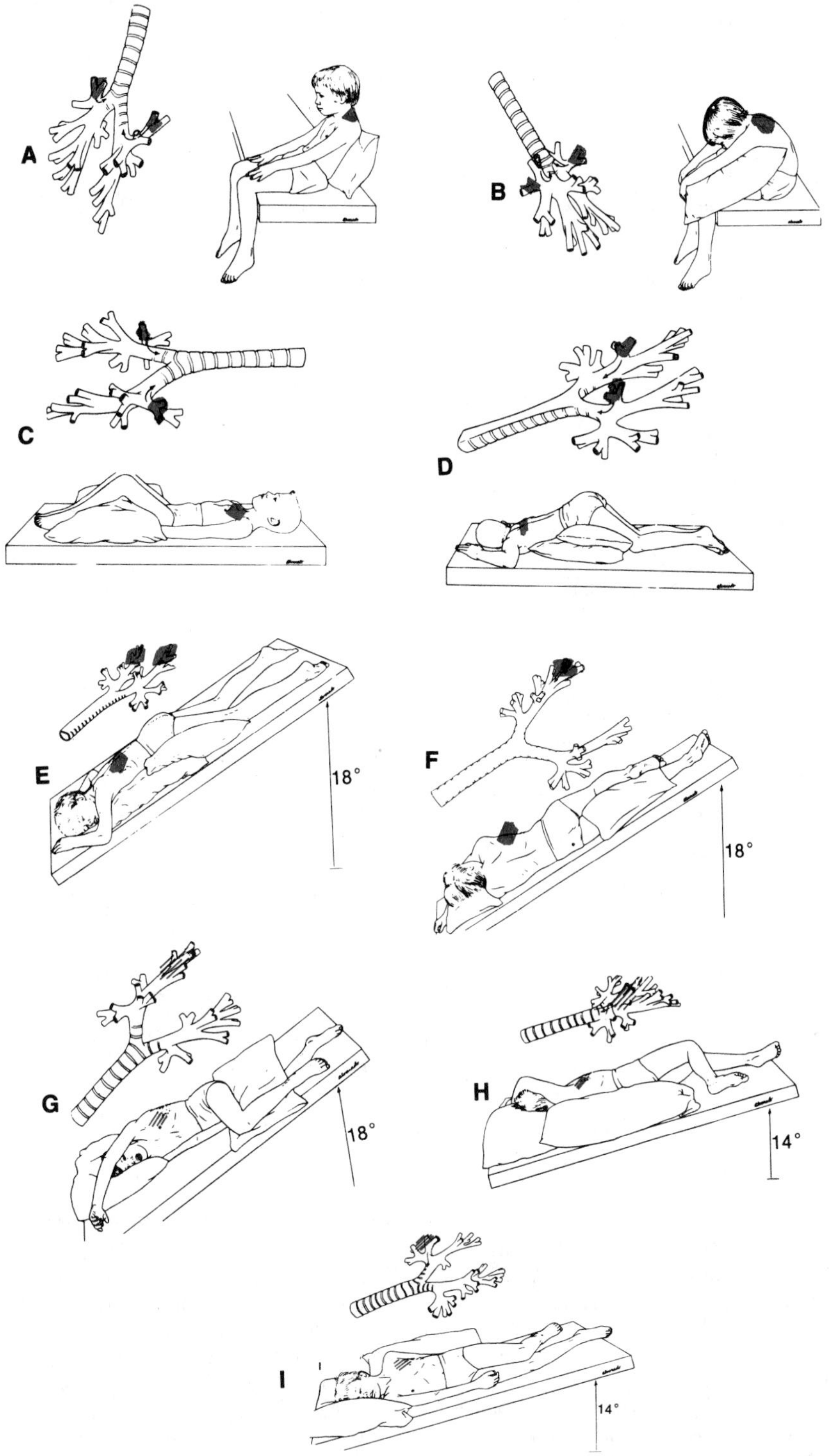

Fig. 31-11. Bronchial drainage positions for all major lung segments of child. For each position, model of tracheobronchial tree is projected beside child to show segmental bronchus *(striped)* being drained and pathway *(arrow)* of secretions out of bronchus. Drainage platform is horizontal unless otherwise noted. Striped area on child's chest indicates area to be cupped or vibrated by therapist. **A,** Apical segment of right upper lobe and apical subsegment of apical-posterior segment of left upper lobe. **B,** Posterior segment of right upper lobe and posterior subsegment of apical-posterior segment of upper left lobe. **C,** Anterior segments of both upper lobes; child should be rotated slightly away from side being drained. **D,** Superior segments of both lower lobes. **E,** Posterior basal segments of both lower lobes. **F,** Lateral basal segments of right lower lobe; left lateral basal segment would be drained by mirror image of this position (right side down). **G,** Anterior basal segment of left lower lobe; right anterior basal segment would be drained by mirror image of this position (left side down). **H,** Medial and lateral segments of right middle lobe. **I,** Lingular segments (superior and inferior) of left upper lobe (homologue of right middle lobe).

From Kendig, E.L., Jr., editor: Disorders of the respiratory tract of children, ed. 4, Philadelphia, 1983, W.B. Saunders Co.

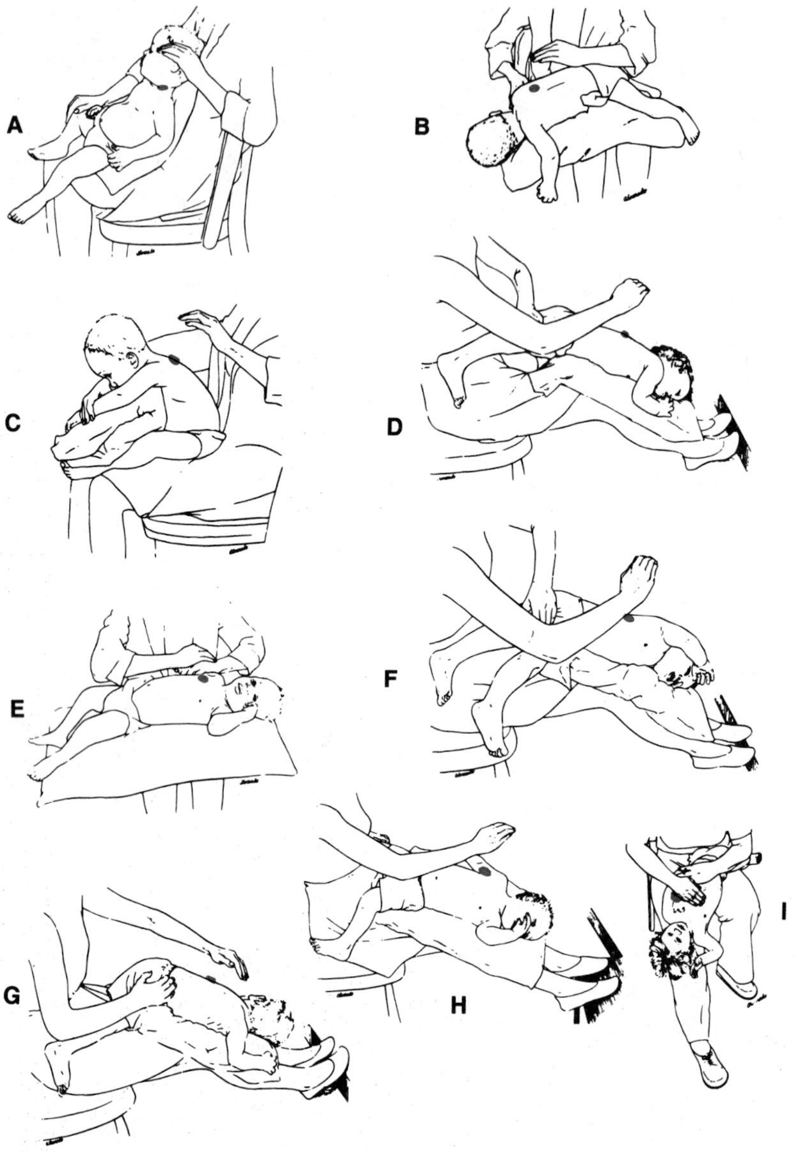

Fig 31-12. Bronchial drainage positions for major segments of all lobes in infant. Procedure is most easily carried out in therapist's lap. Therapist's hand on chest indicates area to be cupped or vibrated. **A,** Apical segment of left upper lobe. **B,** Posterior segment of left upper lobe. **C,** Anterior segment of left upper lobe. **D,** Superior segment of right lower lobe. **E,** Posterior basal segment of right lower lobe. **F,** Lateral basal segment of right lower lobe. **G,** Anterior basal segment of right lower lobe. **H,** Medial and lateral segments of right middle lobe. **I,** Lingular segments (superior and inferior) of left upper lobe.

Modified from Infant segmental bronchial drainage. Reprinted with permission of Cystic Fibrosis Foundation, Rockville, MD.

take a deep breath and then to exhale through the mouth rapidly and as completely as possible. The depth of the expiratory effort is increased by brief, firm pressure from the practitioner's hands compressing the sides of the chest. This decreases the volume of the tracheobronchial tree and facilitates the expression of secretions. The inspiration after the activity often stimulates a deep, productive cough (reinforced by the operator).

Deep breathing is often encouraged when the child is relaxed in the desired position for drainage. The child is directed to take several deep breaths using diaphragmatic breathing. The use of deep breathing enlarges the tracheobronchial tree, enabling air to circulate around and through secretions that are not affected by usual tidal volumes. Expirations after these deep breaths often carry secretions and may stimulate a cough. Other methods that can be employed to stimulate deep breathing are blow bottles of various types, incentive spirometers, and incorporation of play that extends the expiratory time and increases expiratory pressure. For example, such play may include using items

Box 31-4 GUIDELINES FOR PERFORMING CHEST PHYSIOTHERAPY

Chest physiotherapy should be used for patients who have increased sputum production. It is probably of no value to the uncomplicated postoperative patient or the patient with pneumonia.
Forced expiration combined with postural drainage is more effective than cough alone.
Percussion and vibration have no proven value.
Appropriate use of bronchodilators before chest physiotherapy will enhance mucus clearance.

such as pinwheel toys, moving small items by blowing through a straw, blowing cotton balls or a Ping-Pong ball on a table, preventing a tissue from falling by blowing it against a wall, blowing up balloons (under supervision), and singing loudly (especially songs with a lot of words between breaths).

With or without stimulation, children are encouraged to *cough,* not to suppress a cough, and not to waste strength and energy with repeated weak and ineffective coughs. One or two hard coughs after a deep breath are more efficient. Since many children have difficulty in coughing when in a dependent position, they should be encouraged to sit up while they cough. Having the child hug a stuffed toy or a small pillow offers comfort, as well as physical support, during coughing. As an alternative, the practitioner can reinforce the child's efforts by encircling the chest with the practitioner's hands and compressing the sides of the lower chest in synchrony with the cough. This is less fatiguing and increases the effectiveness of the cough efforts.

Breathing and *postural exercises* have not been widely applied to children but are useful techniques with older, motivated children. They are especially of value to children with kyphoscoliosis, cystic fibrosis, asthma, and bronchiectasis. Breathing exercises are employed as part of a total therapy program and are more convenient when performed in association with bronchial drainage.

The goals of breathing exercises are to (1) develop more effective diaphragmatic and lower intercostal breathing; (2) relax all muscles, especially those of the upper chest, shoulder girdle, and neck; and (3) attain a good easy posture. The number and type of exercises depend on the child's age, motivation, and strength, as well as the type and extent of the physiologic disturbance. Breathing exercises are selected to meet the specific child's needs or are alternated in their use. The most important exercises are diaphragmatic breathing and side bending, concentrating on both abdominal expansion and lateral expansion.

ARTIFICIAL VENTILATION

A variety of methods are available for controlling or assisting ventilation. Temporary assistance can be provided by a hand-operated self-inflating ventilation bag with a mask and a nonreturnable valve to prevent rebreathing. With the mask placed on the nose and mouth, the bag is rhythmically compressed, forcing gas from the bag into the patient's airways. The bag should be supplied with 100% O_2 and should have a reservoir so that 100% O_2 is delivered to the patient. An open airway is established by correct positioning with the patient's chin directed forward and the neck extended to the "sniffing" position. It is important not to hyperextend an infant's neck, because this can occlude the airway.

For more prolonged assistance, mechanical ventilation is used to replace the function of the diaphragm and thoracic chest wall muscles. The lungs are inflated by application of either positive or negative pressure. A positive-pressure machine inflates the lung by increasing airway pressure above atmospheric pressure, and a negative-pressure ventilator creates a subatmospheric pressure around the chest wall and inside the chest, thus allowing air to move into the chest. Application of positive pressure by mechanical means usually improves gas distribution within the lung and often reinflates partially collapsed lung segments. The overall effect is improvement of gas exchange.

Ventilators are usually classified according to the factors that regulate cycling. The method by which inspiration is terminated can be categorized as pressure cycled, volume cycled, and time cycled (Box 31-5). Ventilators are attached to the patient by endotracheal (ET) tube or tracheostomy.

Box 31-5 TYPES OF VENTILATORS

Pressure-cycled ventilator—terminates the respiratory cycle when a preset inspiratory pressure is reached. Volume will differ greatly depending on the preset inspiratory time and the flow rate of the delivery gas. The compliance of the lung will affect the tidal volume even though the pressure will remain constant.
Volume-cycled ventilator—terminates respiration when a preset volume (tidal volume) is delivered. The compliance and resistance of the lung will change the pressure needed to deliver the preset volume.
Time-cycled ventilator—terminates inspiration when a preset time is reached. Tidal volume is greatly affected by the compliance of the ventilator tubing, compliance and resistance of the lung, and flow rate of the delivered gas. The duration of the inspiratory pressure will be affected by the preset inspiratory time and the flow rate of the delivered gas.

✦ **NURSING ALERT** Patients requiring mechanical ventilation should always have a self-inflating ventilation bag at the bedside. When the patient's condition or the ventilator's operation is in doubt, the ventilation bag should be used.

Care of the Patient

The regulation and maintenance of mechanical ventilators are the responsibility of respiratory care practitioners. However, nurses should understand the function of the ventilator being used and be able to detect signs of malfunction and deviations from the desired settings. The nurse also promotes the effectiveness of ventilation by suctioning, positioning, and providing support and reassurance to the child receiving mechanical ventilation. (See Chapter 10 for assisted and controlled ventilation in the neonate.)

Weaning the patient from a ventilator involves gradual physical and psychologic withdrawal from dependence on the mechanical device. Criteria for beginning the weaning process varies with the primary disease and the practitioner's preference.

The child who is to be extubated is deprived of oral intake. In some regions of the United States, steroids are administered before the extubation to control laryngeal edema. Sedation or other respiratory depressants are contraindicated so that the child can be observed for respiratory activity. The child is placed on a cardiac and apnea monitor if one is not already attached. Resuscitation and reintubation equipment is available at the bedside. Vigorous chest physiotherapy and suctioning are ordinarily performed just before tube removal, and cool mist is begun immediately after extubation. The child is monitored for respiratory distress, and ABG measurements are observed. The most common complications are airway edema, fatigue, and atelectasis. Airway edema often responds to nebulized racemic epinephrine, which can be given several times to prevent reintubation.

Endotracheal Airways

An artificial airway is usually used in association with artificial ventilation and in children with upper airway obstruction. Endotracheal intubation can be accomplished by the nasal (nasotracheal), oral (orotracheal), or direct tracheal (tracheostomy) routes. Oral intubation is usually the method of choice for emergency situations, but for prolonged intubation a nasotracheal tube is more often used. Although it is more difficult to place technically, nasotracheal intubation is preferred to orotracheal intubation because it facilitates oral hygiene and provides more stable fixation, which reduces the complication of tracheal erosion and the danger of accidental extubation.

Although newborn infants have been successfully maintained on ET tubes for longer periods, in older children who require intubation beyond a week, tracheostomy is usually performed. The decision to change from ET tube to tracheostomy is made on an individual basis. The tracheostomy allows the child to speak (by temporarily occluding the opening with a clean fingertip) and eat and also facilitates clearing of secretions. Suctioning an ET tube is carried out with the same care as suctioning a tracheostomy (see Tracheostomy at right).

Complications. The most severe complication related to immediate intubation is hypoxia with accompanying bradycardia. Patients must be closely monitored during intubation attempts and, if hypoxia occurs, the procedure is discontinued until vital signs are stable. Ventilation with bag-valve-mask and O_2 is reinstituted. Other complications include trauma to mouth and teeth, epistaxis, creation of air leaks, and vagal-mediated changes in vital signs. The most common sequela of intubation is sore throat, which is benign and disappears within 48 to 72 hours without therapy, although humidified atmosphere is beneficial. Other complications include traumatic laryngitis, infection, glottic edema, and mucosal lesions of the larynx secondary to pressure exerted by the rigid ET tube. The most severe sequela of intubation is laryngeal stenosis secondary to fibrosis.

TRACHEOSTOMY

Tracheostomy consists of a surgical opening in the trachea between the second and fourth tracheal rings (Fig. 31-13). It is usually performed in children to (1) bypass upper airway obstruction caused by conditions (e.g., congenital or acquired subglottic stenosis, paralysis of vocal cords) or infectious processes (e.g., croup, epiglottitis) or (2) provide access to the airway for long-term ventilatory support.

Pediatric tracheostomy tubes are usually made of plastic or Silastic (Fig. 31-14). These tubes are constructed with a more acute angle than adult tubes, and they soften at body temperature, conforming to the contours of the trachea. Since these materials resist the formation of crusted respiratory secretions, they are made without an inner cannula. However, some children require a metal tracheostomy tube, which contains an inner cannula.

Tracheostomy Care

Before the tracheostomy is performed, it is important to prepare the child and family. Preoperative teaching should include communication methods that will be used with that

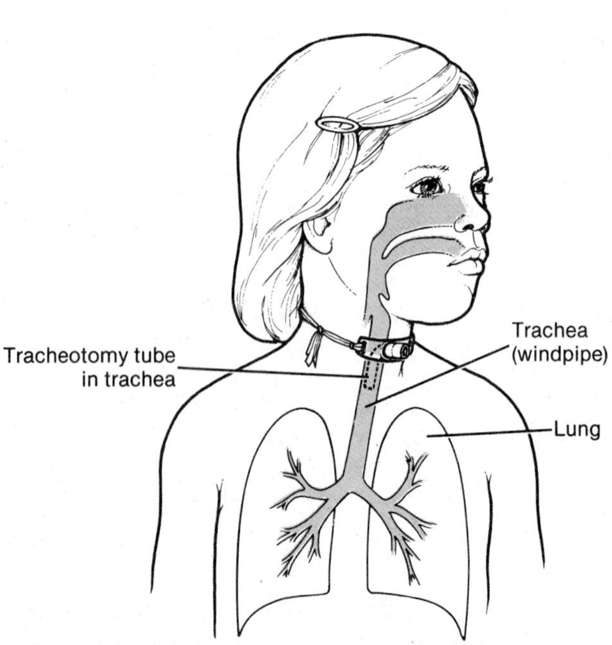

Fig. 31-13. Tracheostomy tube in trachea and securely tied with tape.

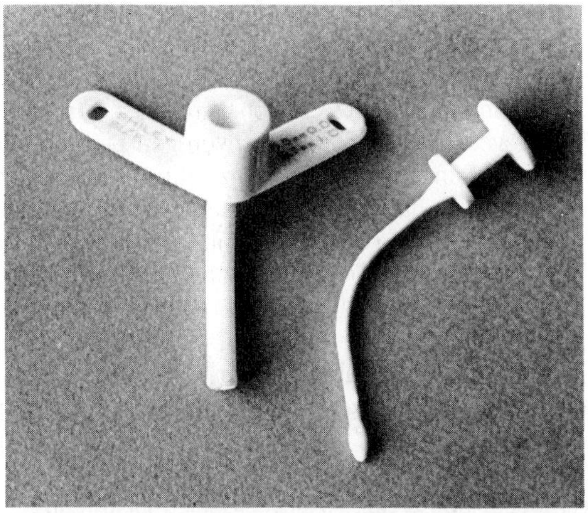

Fig. 31-14. Silastic pediatric tracheostomy tube and obturator for insertion of tube.

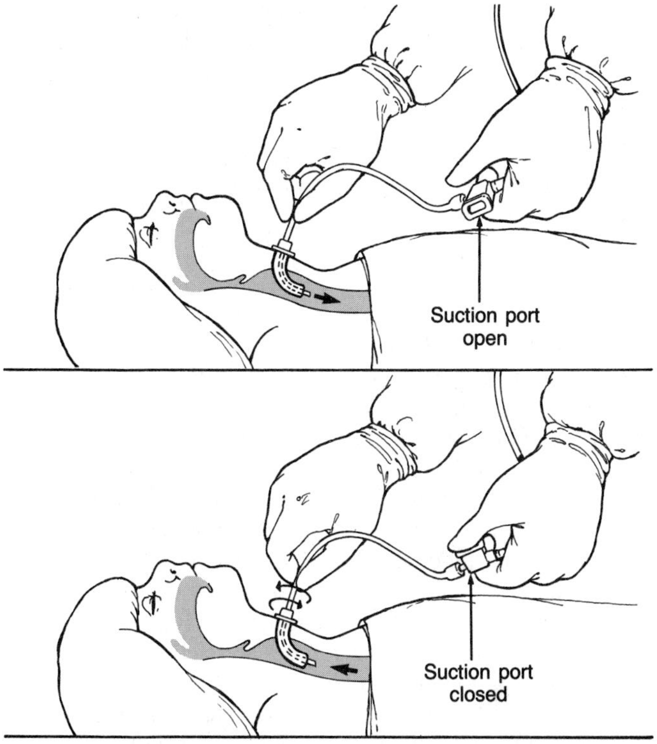

Fig. 31-15. Tracheostomy suctioning. **A,** Insertion, port open. **B,** Withdrawal, port occluded.

particular child, preparation for the appearance of the stoma, and routine postoperative management.

Children who have undergone tracheostomy must be monitored continually for the first few days after surgery. The focus of postoperative nursing care is maintaining a patent airway, facilitating removal of pulmonary secretions, and preventing complications.

Since the child may be unable to signal for help, direct observation and use of respiratory and cardiac monitors is essential. Respiratory assessments (including breath sounds and work of breathing, vital signs, and tightness of the tracheostomy ties) are performed every 15 minutes until the patient is stable and then every 1 to 2 hours for the first 24 hours. Assessments thereafter are every 2 to 4 hours or more frequently if needed. Some bleeding from the surgical site can be expected, but profuse bleeding is unusual and the practitioner should be notified immediately if this occurs.

The child is positioned with the head of the bed raised, or in the position most comfortable to the child, with the call bell easily available. Suction catheters, suction source, gloves, sterile saline, sterile gauze for wiping away secretions, scissors, an extra tracheostomy tube of the same size with ties already attached, and another tracheostomy tube (one size smaller) are kept at the bedside. A source of humidification is provided to the tracheostomy, since the normal humidification and filtering functions of the airway have been bypassed. Intravenous fluids ensure adequate hydration until the child is able to swallow sufficient amounts of fluids.

The child returns from the operating room with the tracheostomy tube in place and long sutures taped to the chest. These sutures are attached to the tracheal rings and can be used to hold the tracheostomy stoma open in the event of accidental decannulation. In approximately 5 days a tract is formed in the trachea, subcutaneous tissue, and skin, at which time the stay sutures are no longer required.

Suctioning. The airway must remain patent and requires frequent suctioning during the first few hours after tracheostomy to remove mucous plugs and excessive secretions. Proper vacuum pressure and suction catheter size are important to prevent atelectasis and decrease hypoxia from the suctioning procedure. Vacuum pressure should range from 80 to 100 mm Hg. Unless secretions are thick and tenacious, the lower range of negative pressure is recommended. Tracheal suction catheters are available in a variety of sizes. The catheter selected should have a diameter one half the diameter of the tracheostomy tube. If the catheter is too large, it can obliterate the airway. The catheter is constructed with a side port so that the catheter is introduced without suction and removed while simultaneous intermittent suction is applied by obliterating the port with the thumb (Fig. 31-15). The catheter is inserted to 0.5 cm beyond the end of the tracheostomy tube (see Nursing Tip). A

NURSING TIP: CATHETER INSERTION

To measure the length for catheter insertion, place the catheter near a sample tracheostomy tube (same size as child's tube) with the end of the catheter 0.5 cm beyond the end of the tube; grasp catheter with sterile-gloved hand to mark the length and insert catheter until hand reaches stoma.

small amount of sterile isotonic saline (a few drops to 0.5 to 2 ml, depending on the child's size) injected into the tube helps loosen secretions and crusts for easier aspiration.

✦ **NURSING ALERT** Suctioning should require no more than 3 to 4 seconds (American Heart Association, 1987).

Counting 1–one thousand, 2–one thousand, 3–one thousand, and so on while suctioning is a simple means for monitoring the time. Without a safeguard the airway may be obstructed for too long a period. Hyperventilating the child with 100% O_2 before and after suctioning should also be performed to prevent hypoxia.

Suctioning is carried out at frequent intervals to prevent buildup of crusts and as often as needed for signs of mucus in the airway, such as bubbling, noisy breathing, or coughing. The cough, although noisy, is ineffectual because the glottis, which normally closes and releases suddenly to effect a cough, is bypassed by the tracheostomy. The child is allowed to rest for 30 to 60 seconds after each aspiration to allow O_2 tension to return to normal; then the process is repeated until the trachea is clear. Suctioning should be limited to about three aspirations in one period. Oximetry is an effective feedback tool to monitor suctioning and prevent hypoxia.

Aseptic technique is essential during care of the tracheostomy. Secondary infection is a major concern, since the air entering the lower airway bypasses the natural defenses of the upper airway. Two gloves are worn during the aspiration procedure, although a sterile glove is needed only on the hand touching the catheter. A new tube, gloves, and sterile saline solution are used each time.

Routine care. The tracheostomy stoma requires daily care. Assessments of the stoma area include observations for signs of infection and breakdown of the skin. The skin is kept clean and dry, and secretions around the stoma are gently removed with half-strength hydrogen peroxide. Special sterile dressings made of nonshredding material can be placed under the flanges of the tracheostomy tube if desired. These should be changed frequently, however, since a soiled dressing may be a reservoir for bacteria (Sigler, 1985).

The tracheostomy tube is held in place with tracheostomy ties made of a durable, nonfraying material. The ties are changed daily and when soiled. New ties are looped through the flanges (Fig. 31-16) and tied snugly in a triple knot at the side of the neck *before* the soiled ties are cut and removed. Some nurses have found that threading the ties through a piece of ¼-inch surgical tubing cushions the ties; others have found the tubing to be irritating to the skin. The ties should be tight enough to allow just a fingertip to be inserted between the ties and the neck (Fig. 31-17). It is easier to ensure a snug fit if the child's head is flexed rather than extended while ties are being secured. Ties fastened with self-adhering closure are also available but are used only on children who are unlikely to pull and undo the fastening.

Routine tracheostomy tube changes are carried out at least weekly after a tract has been formed to minimize formation of granulation tissue (Sigler, 1985). The first change is usually performed by the surgeon; subsequent changes are performed by the nurse. Ideally two caregivers participate in the procedure to assist with positioning the child.

Changing the tracheostomy tube is accomplished using sterile technique. The new, sterile tube is prepared by inserting the obturator and attaching new ties. The child is suctioned before the procedure to minimize secretions,

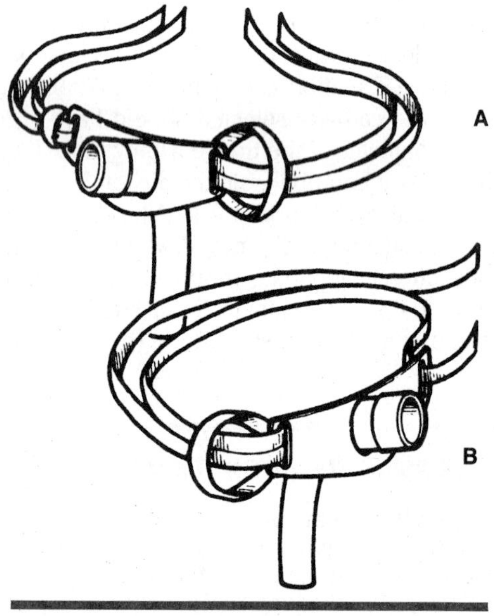

Fig. 31-16. Pediatric tracheostomy tube. **A,** Tape secured at both sides to be tied in back. **B,** Tape secured on one side and looped through other side to be tied at side.

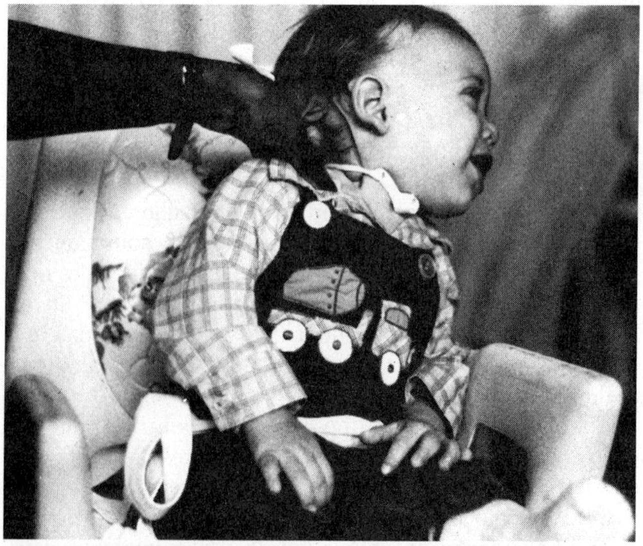

Fig. 31-17. Securing tracheostomy tube. A snug fit, but finger can be inserted beneath ties.

then restrained and positioned with the neck slightly extended. One caregiver cuts the old ties and removes the tube from the stoma. The new tube is inserted gently into the stoma (using a downward and forward motion that follows the curve of the trachea), the obturator is removed, and ties are secured. The adequacy of ventilation must be assessed after a tube change because the tube can be inserted into the soft tissue surrounding the trachea. Therefore breath sounds and respiratory effort should be carefully monitored.

Supplemental O_2 is always delivered with a humidification system to prevent drying of the respiratory mucosa (Fig. 31-18). Humidification of room air for an established tracheostomy can be intermittent if secretions remain thin enough to be coughed or suctioned from the tracheostomy. Direct humidification via tracheostomy mask can be provided during naps and at night so the child is able to be up and around unencumbered during much of the day. Room humidifiers are also used successfully (Lichtenstein, 1986). The system chosen depends on the viscosity of the secretions and the practitioner's preference.

The inner cannula, if used, should be removed with each suctioning, cleaned with sterile saline and pipe cleaners to remove crusted material, and reinserted.

Emergency care: tube occlusion and accidental decannulation. Occlusion of the tracheostomy tube is life-threatening, and infants and children are at greater risk than adults because of the smaller diameter of the tube. Maintaining patency of the tube is accomplished by frequent suctioning and routine tube changes to prevent formation of crusts that can occlude the tube.

✦ **NURSING ALERT** Life-threatening occlusion is apparent when the child displays signs of respiratory distress and a suction catheter cannot be passed to the end of the tube, despite several attempts and instillation of saline. This situation requires an immediate tube change.

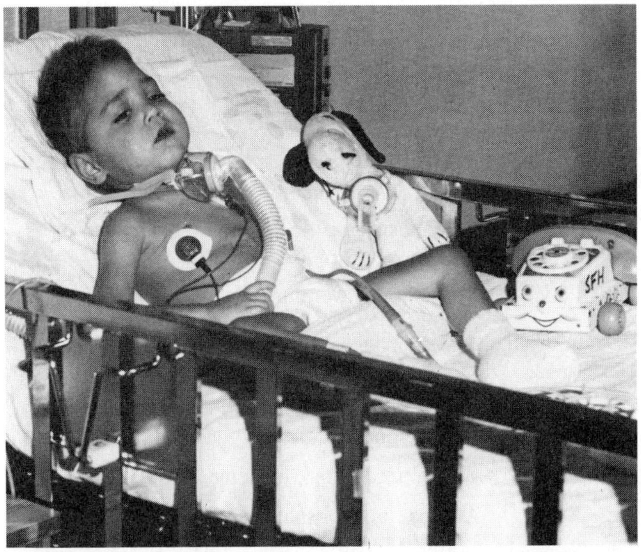

Fig. 31-18. Child with a tracheostomy and a mist collar.

Accidental decannulation also requires immediate tube replacement. Some children have a fairly rigid trachea, so that the airway remains partially open when the tube is removed. However, others have malformed or flexible tracheal cartilage, which causes the airway to collapse when the tube is removed or dislodged. Since many infants and children with upper airway problems have little airway reserve, if replacement of the dislodged tube is impossible, a smaller-sized tube should be inserted. If the stoma cannot be cannulated with another tracheostomy tube, oral intubation should be performed.

Decannulation

The tracheostomy tube is removed as soon as it is no longer needed. Diseases of short duration (e.g., croup) usually allow early removal, but some conditions (e.g., tracheomalacia, tracheal stenosis, paralysis) may require that the tube remain in place indefinitely. Opinions differ regarding the best means for removing the tube, especially after lengthy intubation. Usually the child is weaned to the smallest possible tracheostomy tube. When the tube has been in place for 24 hours and the child's respiratory status is unimpaired, the tube is occluded. After another 24 hours the tube is removed. The procedure is carried out in a hospital setting where continuous observation is available and emergency reintubation can be accomplished without delay, if necessary. Following successful decannulation, the child remains under close observation in the hospital for an additional 48 hours (Johnson, Reilly, and Mallory, 1985).

■ RESPIRATORY DYSFUNCTION

Disorders of respiratory structure and function that may result in ventilatory failure are a significant cause of childhood illness. They may have a variety of causes, both pulmonary and nonpulmonary, and the pulmonary dysfunction can result in disturbances in other organs and systems. The primary function of the lungs is to provide sufficient O_2 for metabolic needs and to remove the CO_2 produced. Inadequacy of the O_2-supplying role results in *hypoxemia* and tissue *hypoxia;* inadequate CO_2 removal causes *hypercapnia.* Often both gases may be insufficiently exchanged.

RESPIRATORY FAILURE

In general, the term *respiratory insufficiency* is applied to two conditions: (1) children with increased work of breathing while preserving gas exchange function near normal and (2) children who are unable to maintain normal blood gas tensions and develop hypoxemia and acidosis secondary to CO_2 retention.

Respiratory failure is defined as the inability of the respiratory apparatus to maintain adequate oxygenation of the blood, with or without CO_2 retention.

Respiratory arrest is the cessation of respiration.

Apnea is absence of airflow (breathing). Apnea can be (1) central, in which respiratory efforts are absent; (2) obstructive, in which respiratory efforts are present; and (3) mixed, in which both central and obstructive components are present.

Effective pulmonary gas exchange requires clear airways, normal lungs and chest wall, and adequate pulmonary circulation. This functional pulmonary unit plus normal respiratory control mechanisms ensures adequate total alveolar ventilation and perfusion, which are reflected in O_2 and CO_2 tensions in arterial blood leaving the lung. Anything that affects these functions or their relationships can compromise respiration.

Respiratory dysfunction may have an abrupt or an insidious onset. Respiratory failure therefore can occur as an emergency situation or may be preceded by gradual and progressive deterioration of respiratory function. Most clinical manifestations are nonspecific and are affected by variations among individual patients and differences in the severity and duration of inadequate gas exchange.

The diagnosis of respiratory failure is determined by the combined application of three sources of information (Wade, 1982):

1. Presence or history of a condition that might predispose to respiratory failure
2. Observation of respiratory failure
3. Measurement of ABGs and pH

Conditions That Predispose to Respiratory Failure

Respiratory disorders are more conveniently classified according to three dominant functional abnormalities, although all three types may be present in the disease. The three primary types of functional disorders and examples of each are:

1. *Obstructive lung disease,* in which there is increased resistance to airflow in either the upper or the lower respiratory tract (Table 31-5)
2. *Restrictive lung disease,* in which there is impaired lung expansion resulting from loss of lung volume, decreased distensibility, or chest wall disturbance (Table 31-6)
3. *Primary inefficient gas transfer,* in which there is insufficient alveolar ventilation for CO_2 removal or impaired oxygenation of pulmonary capillary blood as a result of dysfunction of the respiratory control mechanism or a diffusion defect (Table 31-7)

Table 31-5 Causes of obstructive respiratory disease

SITE OF DISTURBANCE	NEWBORN AND EARLY INFANCY	LATE INFANCY AND CHILDHOOD
Upper airway		
Anomalies	Choanal atresia, Pierre-Robin syndrome, flabby epiglottis, laryngeal web, tracheal stenosis, vocal cord paralysis, tracheomalacia, vascular ring	Tracheal stenosis, vocal cord paralysis, vascular ring, laryngotracheomalacia
Aspiration	Meconium, mucus, vomitus	Foreign body, vomitus
Infection	Pneumonia, pertussis	Laryngotracheitis, diphtheria, epiglottitis, peritonsillar or retropharyngeal abscess
Tumors	Hemangioma, cystic hygroma, teratoma	Papilloma, hemangioma, lymphangioma, teratoma, hypertrophy of tonsils and adenoids
Allergic or reflex	Laryngospasm from local irritation (intubation) or tetany	Laryngospasm from local irritation (aspiration, intubation, drowning) or tetany, allergy, smoke inhalation
Lower airway		
Anomalies	Bronchostenosis, bronchomalacia, lobar emphysema, aberrant vessels	Bronchostenosis, lobar emphysema, aberrant vessels
Aspiration	Amniotic contents, tracheoesophageal fistula, pharyngeal incoordination, gastroesophageal reflux	Foreign body, vomitus, pharyngeal incoordination (Riley-Day syndrome), drowning, gastroesophageal reflux
Infection	Pneumonia, pertussis	Bronchiolitis, pneumonia, tuberculosis (endobronchial, hilar adenopathy), cystic fibrosis, bronchiectasis
Tumors		Bronchogenic cyst, teratoma
Allergic or reflex		Asthma, bronchospasm secondary to inhalation of noxious gases

From Pagtakhan, R.D., and Chernick, V.: Intensive care for respiratory disorders. In Kendig, E.L., and Chernick, V., editors: Disorders of the respiratory tract in children, ed. 4, Philadelphia, 1983, W.B. Saunders Co.

Table 31-6 Causes of restrictive respiratory disease

SITE OF DISTURBANCE	NEWBORN AND EARLY INFANCY	LATE INFANCY AND CHILDHOOD
Parenchymal		
Anomalies	Agenesis, hypoplasia, lobar emphysema, congenital cyst, pulmonary sequestration	Hypoplasia, congenital cyst, pulmonary sequestration
Atelectasis	Hyaline membrane disease	Thick secretions, foreign body
Infection	Pneumonia	Pneumonia, cystic fibrosis, bronchiectasis, pneumatocele
Alveolar rupture	Pneumothorax (spontaneous or iatrogenic), intestinal emphysema	Pneumothorax (trauma, asthma)
Others	Pulmonary hemorrhage, pulmonary edema, Wilson-Mikity syndrome, sudden infant death syndrome	Pulmonary edema, lobectomy, chemical pneumonitis, pleural effusion, near-drowning
Chest wall		
Muscular	Diaphragmatic hernia, eventration, edema	Amyotonia congenita, poliomyelitis, diaphragmatic hernia, eventration, myasthenia gravis, muscular dystrophy, botulism
Skeletal malformations	Hemivertebrae, absence of ribs, thoracic dystrophy	Kyphoscoliosis, hemivertebrae, absence of ribs
Others	Abdominal distention	Obesity, flail chest

From Pagtakhan, R.D., and Chernick, V.: Intensive care for respiratory disorders. In Kendig, E.L., and Chernick, V., editors: Disorders of the respiratory tract in children, ed 4, Philadelphia, 1983, W.B. Saunders Co.

Table 31-7 Causes of primary inefficient gas transfer

SITE OF DISTURBANCE	SPECIFIC DISEASE CONDITIONS
Pulmonary diffusion defect	
Increased diffusion path between alveoli and capillaries	Pulmonary edema, pulmonary fibrosis, collagen disorders, *Pneumocystis carinii* infection, sarcoidosis
Decreased alveolocapillary surface area	Pulmonary embolism, sarcoidosis, pulmonary hypertension, mitral stenosis, fibrosing alveolitis
Inadequate erythrocytes and hemoglobin	Anemia, hemorrhage
Respiratory center depression	
Increased cerebrospinal fluid pressure	Cerebral trauma (birth injuries), intracranial tumors, central nervous system infection (meningitis, encephalitis, sepsis)
Excessive central nervous system depressant drugs	Maternal oversedation; overdose with barbiturates, opioids, or diazepam
Excessive chemical changes in arterial blood	Severe asphyxia (hypercapnia, hypoxemia)
Toxic	Tetanus

From Pagtakhan, R.D., and Chernick, V.: Intensive care for respiratory disorders. In Kendig, E.L., and Chernick, V., editors: Disorders of the respiratory tract in children, ed. 4, Philadelphia, 1983, W.B. Saunders. Co.

Recognition of Respiratory Failure

Respiratory failure that occurs as a result of acute obstruction of a major airway or cardiac arrest is sudden and readily apparent. Gradual and more covert development of signs and symptoms is less easily recognized. Insufficient alveolar ventilation from any cause ultimately leads to hypoxemia and hypercapnia. However, situations occur in which severe respiratory distress may be present without significant CO_2 retention, and hypoxemia may occur without clinically detectable cyanosis. Therefore evaluation of respiratory adequacy is based on both clinical assessment and laboratory studies. Nursing observation and judgment are vital to successful management of respiratory failure. Nurses must be able to assess a situation and initiate appropriate action within moments.

Unless respiratory arrest occurs suddenly, signs of hypoxemia and hypercapnia are usually subtle in their development and become more obvious as respiratory failure progresses. The unknowing observer may attribute early signs such as mood changes and restlessness to other causes, and some signs can be altered by other factors, for example, anemia. Hemoglobin is needed to show some cyanosis; therefore it may not be observed in the child with a hemoglobin of less than 6 g/dl. Cyanosis is usually apparent at a Pao_2 of 40 to 50 mm Hg. The signs of respiratory failure are outlined in Box 31-6.

In clinical situations in which impaired ventilation can be anticipated or clinical manifestations indicate impending hypoxemia, serial measurements of blood gases should be obtained and monitored to detect impending respiratory failure and implement therapy before respiratory acidosis becomes extreme.

Box 31-6 SIGNS OF RESPIRATORY FAILURE

Cardinal Signs
Restlessness
Tachypnea
Tachycardia
Diaphoresis

Early but Less Obvious Signs
Mood changes, such as euphoria or depression
Headache
Altered depth and pattern of respirations
Hypertension
Exertional dyspnea
Anorexia
Increased cardiac output and renal output
Central nervous system symptoms (decreased efficiency, impaired judgment, anxiety, confusion, restlessness, irritability)
Flaring nares
Chest wall retractions
Expiratory grunt
Wheezing and/or prolonged expiration

Signs of More Severe Hypoxia

Hypotension or hypertension	Dyspnea
Dimness of vision	Depressed respirations
Somnolence	Bradycardia
Stupor	Cyanosis, peripheral or central
Coma	

MANAGEMENT AND RELATED NURSING CONSIDERATIONS

The interventions used in the management of respiratory failure are often dramatic, requiring special skills, and are frequently emergency procedures. If respiratory arrest occurs, the primary objectives are to recognize the situation and initiate resuscitative measures within moments. When the situation is not an arrest, the suspicion of respiratory failure is confirmed by assessment and the severity defined by ABG analysis. When severity is established, an attempt is made to determine the underlying cause by thorough evaluation.

Treatment of respiratory dysfunction involves both specific and nonspecific therapy. Specific therapies are directed toward reversal of the causative factors. However, sometimes nonspecific measures are needed to maintain oxygenation and enhance CO_2 removal until specific methods take effect. The major reasons for implementing nonspecific treatments are (1) unknown etiology, (2) lack of specific treatment for a known cause, (3) lack of time for a specific treatment to take effect, and (4) need for specialized personnel or equipment for specific treatment.

The principles of management are to (1) maintain oxygenation, (2) maintain ventilation, (3) apply specific and nonspecific therapy, and (4) anticipate complications. Monitoring the patient's condition is critical, and some of the techniques employed to maintain oxygenation and assist ventilation are described in the previous section.

Observation and Monitoring

The child is monitored to evaluate the cause of the failure, help determine a course of action, and assess the patient's response to treatment. If close continuous monitoring is required, the child is transferred to an intensive care unit. Ap-

Box 31-7 NURSING OBSERVATIONS FOR THE CHILD WITH RESPIRATORY FAILURE

Visual inspection of skin color to estimate level of arterial O_2 saturation
Observation of respiratory effort or distress—nasal flaring, grunting, gasping, retraction
Observation of diaphragmatic movement, lung expansion, and use of accessory muscles—depth, symmetry, inspiration/expiration ratio
Auscultation of thorax to assess:
- Breath sounds—presence, intensity, quality, symmetry
- Abnormal sounds—stridor, wheezes, crackles, rubs, crepitation, increase or decrease in sounds
- Tube placement and need for endotracheal suction when child is intubated

propriate treatment modalities are applied according to the specific functional disturbance and the underlying etiology.

The child's cardiac and respiratory status are monitored by observation and by electronic means. However, no monitoring equipment can replace conscientious nursing observations (Box 31-7).

Hourly temperature assessments are needed, and assessments should be performed more often if the child, usually an infant, requires a thermally controlled environment. Optimum temperature is maintained, since fever increases the need for O_2 and increases respiratory efforts. Blood gases are usually monitored continuously via electronic devices or regular measurements by laboratory analysis, as described previously.

Family Support

Children who are fatigued and in distress before a procedure will probably fall into a restful sleep after establishment of an airway. However, unless they remain unconscious or semiconscious, they will probably be anxious and frightened when they are unable to communicate. Children who are old enough to write and not too fatigued can use a pad of paper and a pencil or spelling board to express their needs and concerns. Other alternative means for communication are pictures illustrating various items and activities. Simple sign language has proved to be an effective and easily learned communication medium.

It is often a terrifying experience for young children to discover that they are unable to make vocal sounds, including crying. It is also stressful to parents to watch their children plead with frightened eyes and cry noiselessly. It is important to talk to children and reassure them that their voices will return when they are able to breathe again. Children whose tracheostomies are more or less permanent but needed to facilitate pulmonary toilet are taught to occlude the opening with a clean finger so that they can use the vocal cords to communicate.

Parents have numerous concerns relative to tracheostomies, ET tubes, and ventilators. If time allows before a tracheostomy, the reasons for the decision to implement the therapy, the expected results, and the approximate length of time it will remain in place should be discussed with them. Parental concern is centered around the (often) life-threatening implications generated by the need for the procedure and the possible long-term effects on the child, both physiologic and psychologic. Parents are concerned about the visible wound and the scar. Parents who must face the possibility of caring for the child with a tracheostomy at home have additional worries regarding their ability to assume this responsibility.

Some children may be discharged from the hospital with tracheostomy tubes. Before discharge, the parents will need careful instruction and practice in the care and management of the tracheostomy,* including basic life support (BLS) (cardiopulmonary resuscitation [CPR]). Some institutions provide BLS classes especially for families; others refer the families to the classes offered by the **American Red Cross.*** During hospitalization the parents should be involved in the child's care as soon as possible in anticipation of home care. The more comfortable they are with all aspects of tracheostomy care, the more confident and less anxious they will be when faced with total care of the child at home. It sometimes requires weeks before they feel comfortable with suctioning, cleaning, and changing the tube. Instructions should be detailed and explicit. To facilitate their adjustment, supplies identical to the ones they are accustomed to should be available to the parents. Parents often become anxious when they encounter even small differences from the familiar. In the event of substitution, they need to be reassured that the unfamiliar equipment is safe to use on their child.

A nurse from the public health department or other service should be available to the family and should periodically assess the family's ability to carry out the activities needed in care of the child. The parents may find it helpful to talk to other parents of children with tracheostomies. They also need to know whom to call and where they can obtain help and support in times of uncertainty or in an emergency.

Parents are encouraged to provide as normal a life as possible for their child and other family members (Fig. 31-19). The child who is physically able (e.g., a child with a tracheostomy without respiratory disability such as recurrent laryngeal polyps) can usually be allowed to engage in most activities appropriate for the child's age. The child may even play outdoors with a scarf or other protection to cover the tracheostomy stoma. Both child and parents must be cautioned regarding play near any body of water, such

*Home care instructions on caring for a child with a tracheostomy and cardiopulmonary resuscitation are available in Wong, D.L., and Whaley, L.F.: Clinical manual of pediatric nursing, ed. 3, St. Louis, 1990, Mosby–Year Book, Inc.

*Make referrals to classes available through the local chapter of the American Red Cross. Most units keep a list of dates and times of classes in their areas.

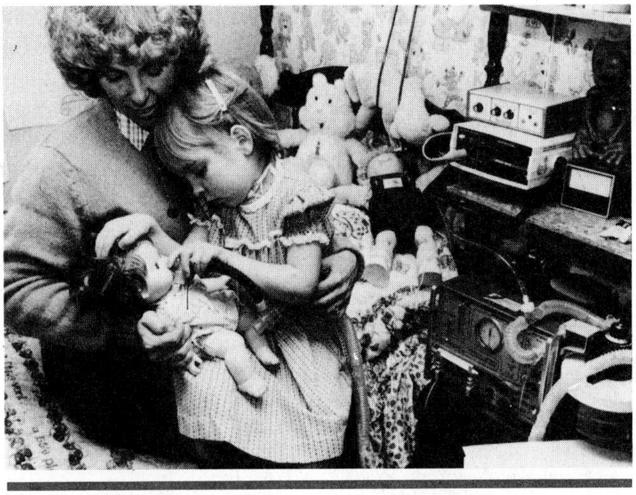

Fig. 31-19. Child with tracheostomy being managed at home.

as a swimming pool or stream, and informed about safety precautions in the bathtub. The child should not be exposed to noxious fumes (e.g., paint, varnish, hair spray) and baby powder. Young children who may spill food near the stoma should wear a fabric bib (without plastic lining) or other device to prevent dribbled food or crumbs from being aspirated.

Home Care of the Technology-Assisted Child

Advanced technology and medical knowledge have improved the survival of children with a number of respiratory problems formerly considered fatal. Children have been sent home on low or intermittent O_2 therapy for quite some time. However, the ventilator-dependent child is now able to be managed at home with proper equipment and a dedicated family. This has created a new category of children with disabilities—one created by technology.

Discharge planning begins in the hospital, when it is determined that the child can be managed at home and the family can assume the needed care. All family members who might be involved in the child's care should be included in the teaching sessions. Equipment and means of replacement are sought and families learn how to maintain the equipment and ensure an adequate supply for daily use. Backup equipment, such as a mouth suction apparatus that can be used when a mechanical suction machine malfunctions and as an alternative when the child is away from the machine for a short period (e.g., in another room, in the yard), should be at hand. See also Discharge Planning and Home Care, Chapter 26.

The length and intensity of preparation vary among families and according to the child's condition. Complex procedures, such as changing the tracheostomy tube, that are frightening tasks are usually left until the family is comfortable with other aspects of care (Calvi, 1985).

The child is protected from infection, and visitors are kept to a minimum to avoid inadvertent exposure to infections. As the child grows and develops, many of the problems of rearing a child are altered (see Impact of Chronic Illness or Disability on the Child and Family, Chapter 22). The multiple problems that might be encountered by the child with a respiratory disability and the family are beyond the scope of this discussion. A beginning list of references dealing with both general and specific aspects of home care is provided in the bibliography at the end of this chapter and Chapter 22. Organizations such as the **American Lung Association,*** those providing services for children with disabilities in general (see list of resources in Appendix E), and those devoted to special health problems (see the specific disease) offer education and support to families. Of particular interest are organizations such as **SKIP (Sick Kids Need Involved People, Inc.),†** an organization that provides information, planning, education, and referral services for families of children receiving home care.

*1740 Broadway, New York, NY 10019; (212) 315-8700.
In Canada: **Canadian Lung Association,** 75 Albert St., Suite 908, Ottawa, Ontario K1P 5E7; **The Lung Association,** 1573 King St. East, Suite 201, Toronto, Ontario M5A 1M5.
†990 2nd Ave., New York, NY 10022; (212) 421-9161.

CARDIOPULMONARY RESUSCITATION*

Cardiac arrest in the pediatric population is less often of cardiac origin than from prolonged hypoxemia secondary to inadequate oxygenation, ventilation, and circulation (shock). Some causes include injuries, suffocation (e.g., foreign body aspiration), smoke inhalation, sudden infant death syndrome (SIDS), or infection. Respiratory arrest has been associated with a better survival than cardiac arrest. Once cardiac arrest occurs, the outcome of resuscitative efforts is poor (American Heart Association, 1987).

Complete apnea signals the need for rapid and vigorous action to prevent cardiac arrest. In such situations nurses must be prepared to initiate action immediately. Neurologically intact survival has been only in those children who receive immediate resuscitation and respond promptly (Torphy, Minter, and Thompson, 1984). In the hospital, emergency equipment should be readily available in areas in which respiratory arrest might take place, and the status of this resuscitation equipment should be checked at least once daily. Regardless of the cause of the arrest, some very basic procedures are carried out, modified somewhat according to the child's size.

✦ **NURSING ALERT** Rescuers who have infections (regardless of type) that may be transmitted by blood or saliva or who believe they have been exposed to such an infection should not perform mouth-to-mouth resuscitation if the circumstances allow other immediate or effective methods of ventilation (e.g., use of a bag-valve-mask) (Special Communications, 1989).

Outside the hospital situation, the first action in an emergency is to assess quickly the extent of any injury and determine whether the child is unconscious. A child who is struggling to breathe but conscious should be transported immediately to an advanced life support (ALS) facility, allowing the child to maintain whatever position affords the most comfort. However, attempting to transport a child by automobile wastes valuable time in obtaining help. Transport by an emergency medical service (EMS) is recommended or preferable. Services in larger communities can institute ALS immediately or en route to a medical facility.

An unconscious child is managed with care to prevent additional trauma if a head or spinal cord injury has been sustained. The circumstances in which the child is found offer some clues to a possible injury. For example, a child

*Home care instructions for CPR in infants, children 1 to 8 years of age, and children over 8 years are available in Wong, D.L., and Whaley, L.F.: Clinical manual of pediatric nursing, ed. 3, St. Louis, 1990, Mosby–Year Book, Inc.

who has been thrown from a bicycle or fallen from a tree is more likely to sustain trauma than a child who is discovered in bed. The child should be turned as a unit with firm support to the head and neck to prevent rolling, twisting, or tilting backward or forward.

Resuscitation Procedure

For effective CPR the victim is placed on the back on a firm flat surface, employing appropriate precautions (Figs. 31-20 and 31-21).

With loss of consciousness the tongue, which is attached to the lower jaw, relaxes and falls back, obstructing the airway. To open the airway, the head is positioned with either head tilt/chin lift or jaw thrust. Health professionals should be able to use both maneuvers. *Head tilt* is accomplished by placing one hand on the victim's forehead and applying firm, backward pressure with the palm to tilt the head back. The fingers of the free hand are placed under the bony portion of the lower jaw near the chin to lift and bring the chin forward *(chin lift)*. This supports the jaw and helps tilt the head back (Fig. 31-22, *A*).

The *jaw thrust* is accomplished by grasping the angles of the victim's lower jaw and lifting with both hands, one on each side, displacing the mandible forward while tilting the head backward (Fig. 31-22, *B*). After restoration of a patent airway by removal of foreign material and secretions (if indicated) and if the child is not breathing, continuation of the airway is maintained and rescue breathing is initiated. To ventilate the lungs in the infant (age birth to 1 year of age), the operator's mouth is placed in such a way that both the mouth and the nostrils are included (Fig. 31-22, *C*). Children (over 1 year of age) are ventilated through the mouth while the nostrils are firmly pinched for airtight contact (Fig. 31-22, *D*).

✦ **NURSING ALERT** The volume of air in an infant's lungs is small and the air passages are considerably smaller, with resistance to flow potentially higher than in adults. Therefore small puffs of air are delivered.

Since the differences are relative and vary according to the child's size, the correct volume of air and force of the rescue breaths cannot be stated with certainty. If air enters freely and the chest rises, the airway is assumed to be clear. Breaths should be given slowly with sufficient volume to make the chest rise. Volume must be provided without causing abdominal distention. Gastric distention, which interferes with diaphragmatic excursion, frequently occurs when more volume than necessary is delivered and the breaths are delivered too rapidly.

After an initial two breaths, a peripheral pulse is palpated to ascertain the presence of a heartbeat. The carotid is the most central and accessible artery (Fig. 31-22, *E*). However, the very short and often fat neck of the infant renders the carotid pulse (ordinarily used in adults and in children over 1 year of age) difficult to palpate. Therefore it is preferable to use the brachial pulse, located on the inner side of the upper arm midway between the elbow and shoulder (Fig. 31-22, *F*). Absence of carotid or brachial pulse is considered sufficient indication to begin external cardiac massage.

Chest compression. External chest compression consists of serial, rhythmic compressions of the chest to maintain circulation to vital organs until the child achieves spontaneous vital signs or ALS can be provided. Chest compressions are always accompanied by simultaneous ventilation of the lungs. For optimum compressions, it is essential that the child's spine is supported on a firm surface during compressions of the sternum, and sternal pressure must be forceful but not traumatic. The child's head is positioned for optimum airway opening using the head tilt/chin lift maneuver. It is essential to prevent overextension of the head of small infants, since this tends to close the flexible trachea.

The placement of the fingers for compression in infants is now determined to be lower than previously thought, that is, at a point on the lower rather than the middle sternum (Orlowski, 1984). The site is one fingerbreadth below the intersection of the sternum and an imaginary line drawn between the nipples (Fig. 31-22, *G*). Compressions on the child 1 to 8 years of age are applied to the lower sternum two fingerbreadths above the sternal notch (Fig. 31-22, *H*). Sternal compression to infants is applied with two or three fingers on the sternum exerting a firm downward thrust; for children, pressure is applied with the heel of one hand. The depth of compression is also adapted to the child's size. The location, rate, and depth for children over 8 years are the same as for adults. Previously there was concern regarding the possibility of rib fractures during CPR; this has been found to be a rare occurrence (Feldman and Brewer, 1984).

Ventilation and compression are continued by the mouth-to-mouth method or bag-valve-mask, at a ratio of one breath for five compressions (for two-person CPR) until signs of recovery appear. These are evidenced by palpable peripheral pulses, return of pupils to normal size, the disappearance of mottling and cyanosis, and possibly return of spontaneous respiration.

Medications. Medications are an important adjunct to resuscitation, especially cardiac arrest, and are used during and following resuscitation. Medications are employed to (Chameides, 1988):

Correct hyoxemia.
Increase perfusion pressure during chest compression.
Stimulate spontaneous or more forceful myocardial contraction.
Accelerate cardiac rate.
Correct metabolic acidosis.
Suppress ventricular ectopy.

Appropriate fluid therapy is initiated immediately to children in the hospital or by EMS personnel during transport (see Parenteral Fluid Therapy, Chapter 28, and Shock, Chapter 29). A complete supply of emergency medications is kept and maintained in all EMS vehicles and on all hos-

One-rescuer CPR

	Objectives	Actions: Adult (over 8 yr)	Child (1 to 8 yr)	Infant (under 1 yr)
A. AIRWAY	**1.** Assessment: Determine unresponsiveness.	Tap or gently shake shoulder.		
		Say, "Are you okay?"		Observe
	2. Get help.	Call out "Help!"		
	3. Position the victim.	Turn on back as a unit, supporting head and neck if necessary. (4-10 seconds)		
	4. Open the airway.	Head-tilt/chin-lift		
B. BREATHING	**5.** Assessment: Determine breathlessness.	Maintain open airway. Place ear over mouth, observing chest. Look, listen, feel for breathing. (3-5 seconds)		
	6. Give 2 rescue breaths.	Maintain open airway.		
		Seal mouth to mouth		Mouth to nose/mouth
		Give 2 rescue breaths, 1 to 1½ seconds each. Observe chest rise. Allow lung deflation between breaths.		
	7. Option for obstructed airway	**a.** Reposition victim's head. Try again to give rescue breaths.		
		b. Activate the EMS system.		
		c. Give 6-10 subdiaphragmatic abdominal thrusts (the Heimlich maneuver).		Give 4 back blows.
				Give 4 chest thrusts.
		d. Tongue-jaw lift and finger sweep	Tongue-jaw lift, but finger sweep only if you see a foreign object.	
		If unsuccessful, repeat a, c, and d until successful.		
C. CIRCULATION	**8.** Assessment: Determine pulselessness.	Feel for carotid pulse with one hand; maintain head-tilt with the other. (5-10 seconds)		Feel for brachial pulse; keep head-tilt.
	9. Activate EMS system.	If someone responded to call for help, send them to activate the EMS system.		
	Begin chest compressions: **10.** Landmark check	Run middle finger along bottom edge of rib cage to notch at center (tip of sternum).		Imagine a line drawn between the nipples.
	11. Hand position	Place index finger next to finger on notch:		Place 2-3 fingers on sternum, 1 finger's width below line. Depress ½-1 in.
		Two hands next to index finger. Depress 1½-2 in.	Heel of one hand next to index finger. Depress 1-1½ in.	
	12. Compression rate	80-100 per minute		At least 100 per minute
CPR CYCLES	**13.** Compressions to breaths.	2 breaths to every 15 compressions.	1 breath to every 5 compressions.	
	14. Number of cycles.	4 (52-73 seconds)	10 (60-87 seconds)	10 (45 seconds or less)
	15. Reassessment.	Feel for carotid pulse. (5 seconds)		Feel for brachial pulse.
		If no pulse, resume CPR, starting with 2 breaths.	If no pulse, resume CPR, starting with 1 breath.	
OPTION FOR ENTRANCE OF 2ND RESCUER: "I KNOW CPR. CAN I HELP?"	1st rescuer ends CPR.	End cycle with 2 rescue breaths.	End cycle with 1 rescue breath.	
	2nd rescuer checks pulse (5 seconds).	Feel for carotid pulse.		Feel for brachial pulse.
	If no pulse, 2nd rescuer begins CPR.	Begin one-rescuer CPR, starting with 2 breaths.	Begin one-rescuer CPR, starting with 1 breath.	
	1st rescuer monitors 2nd rescuer.	Watch for chest rise and fall during rescue breathing; check pulse during chest compressions.		
OPTION FOR PULSE RETURN	If no breathing, give rescue breaths.	1 breath every 5 seconds	1 breath every 4 seconds	1 breath every 3 seconds

Fig. 31-20. One-rescuer CPR.

Two-rescuer CPR

Step	Objective	Critical performance
1. AIRWAY	**One rescuer (ventilator):** Assessment: Determine unresponsiveness.	Tap or gently shake shoulder.
		Shout "Are you OK?"
	Position the victim.	Turn on back if necessary (4-10 sec).
	Open the airway.	Use a proper technique to open airway.
2. BREATHING	Assessment: Determine breathlessness.	Look, listen, and feel (3-5 sec).
	Ventilate twice.	Observe chest rise: 1-1.5 sec/inspiration.
3. CIRCULATION	Assessment: Determine pulselessness.	Feel for carotid pulse (5-10 sec).
	State assessment results.	Say "No pulse."
	Other rescuer (compressor): Get into position for compressions.	Hand, shoulders in correct position.
	Locate landmark notch.	Landmark check.
4. COMPRESSION/ VENTILATION CYCLES	**Compressor:** Begin chest compressions.	Correct ratio compressions/ventilations: 5/1
		Compression rate: 80-100/min (5 compressions/3-4 sec).
		Say any helpful mnemonic.
		Stop compressing for each ventilation.
	Ventilator: Ventilate after every 5th compression and check compression effectiveness.	Ventilate 1 time (1-1.5 sec/inspiration).
		Check pulse occasionally to assess compressions.
	(Minimum of 10 cycles.)	Time for 10 cycles: 40-53 sec.
5. CALL FOR SWITCH	**Compressor:** Call for switch when fatigued.	Give clear signal to change.
		Compressor completes 5th compression.
		Ventilator completes ventilation after 5th compression.
6. SWITCH	Simultaneously switch:	
	Ventilator: Move to chest.	Move to chest.
		Become compressor.
		Get into position for compressions.
		Locate landmark notch.
	Compressor: Move to head.	Move to head.
		Become ventilator.
		Check carotid pulse (5 sec).
		Say "No pulse."
		Ventilate once (1-1.5 sec/inspiration)
7. CONTINUE CPR	Resume compression/ventilation cycles.	Resume Step 4.

Fig. 31-21. Two-rescuer CPR. NOTE: If CPR is in progress with one rescuer (layperson), the entrance of the two rescuers occurs after the completion of one rescuer's cycle of five compressions and one ventilation. The EMS should be activated first. The two new rescuers start with Step 6. If CPR is in progress with one health care provider, the entrance of a second health care provider is at the end of a cycle after check for pulse by the first rescuer. The new cycle starts with one ventilation by the first rescuer, and the second rescuer becomes the compressor. Applies to children 1 year and older.

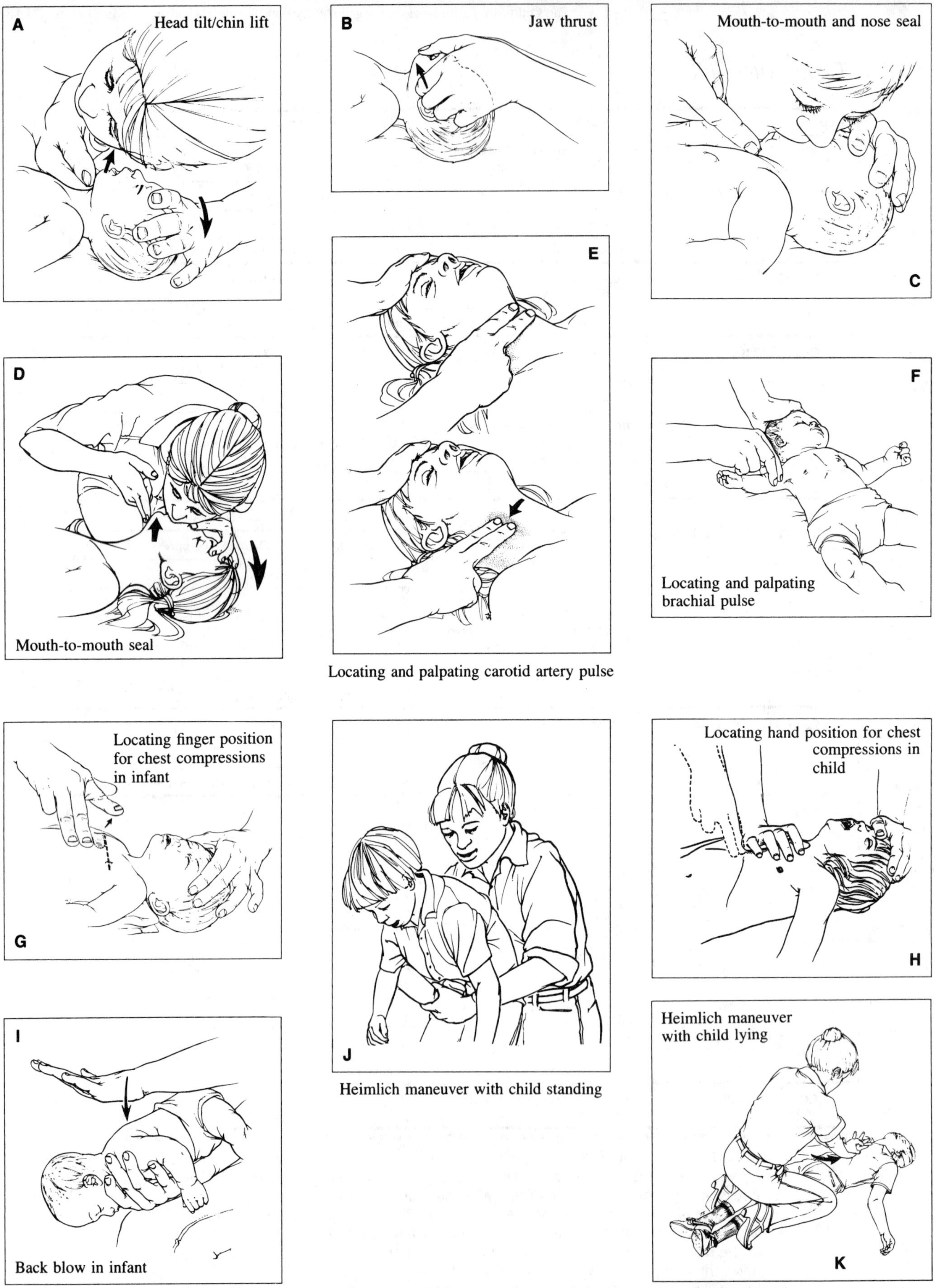

Fig. 31-22. Procedures for cardiopulmonary resuscitation, **A** to **H,** and airway obstruction, **I** to **K.**

Modified from Standards for Cardiopulmonary Resuscitation (CPR) and Emergency Cardiac Care (ECC). Part IV. Pediatric basic life support, JAMA 225(21):2954-2960, 1986.

Foreign body airway obstruction management

Signs of life-threatening obstruction

The truly choking child *cannot speak, becomes cyanotic,* and *collapses.*

	Objectives	Actions: Adult (over 8 yr)	Actions: Child (1 to 8 yr)	Actions: Infant (under 1 yr)
CONSCIOUS VICTIM	**1.** Assessment: Determine airway obstruction.	Ask, "Are you choking?" Determine if victim can cough or speak.		Observe breathing difficulty.
	2. Act to relieve obstruction.	Perform subdiaphragmatic abdominal thrusts (Heimlich maneuver).		Give 4 back blows. Give 4 chest thrusts.
	Be persistent.	Repeat Step 2 until obstruction is relieved or victim becomes unconscious.		
VICTIM WHO BECOMES UNCONSCIOUS	**3.** Position the victim; call for help.	Turn on back as a unit, supporting head and neck, face up, arms by sides. Call out, "Help!" If others come, activate EMS.		
	4. Check for foreign body.	Perform tongue-jaw lift and finger sweep.	Perform tongue-jaw lift. Remove foreign object only if you actually see it.	
	5. Give rescue breaths.	Open the airway with head-tilt/chin-lift. Try to give rescue breaths.		
	6. Act to relieve obstruction.	Perform subdiaphragmatic abdominal thrusts (Heimlich maneuver).		Give 4 back blows. Give 4 chest thrusts.
	7. Check for foreign body.	Perform tongue-jaw lift and finger sweep.	Perform tongue-jaw lift. Remove foreign object only if you actually see it.	
	8. Try again to give rescue breaths.	Open the airway with head-tilt/chin-lift. Try to give rescue breaths.		
	9. Be persistent.	Repeat Steps 6-8 until obstruction is relieved.		
UNCONSCIOUS VICTIM	**1.** Assessment: Determine unresponsiveness.	Tap or gently shake shoulder. Shout, "Are you okay?"		Tap or gently shake shoulder.
	2. Call for help; position the victim.	Turn on back as a unit, supporting head and neck, face up, arms by sides. Call out, "Help!" If others come, activate EMS.		
	3. Open the airway.	Head-tilt/chin-lift		Head-tilt/chin-lift, but do not tilt too far.
	4. Assessment: Determine breathlessness	Maintain an open airway. Ear over mouth; observe chest. Look, listen, feel for breathing. (3-5 seconds)		
	5. Give rescue breaths.	Make mouth-to-mouth seal.		Make mouth-to-nose-and-mouth seal.
		Try to give rescue breaths.		
	6. Try again to give rescue breaths.	Reposition head. Try rescue breaths again.		
	7. Activate the EMS system.	If someone responded to the call for help, that person should activate the EMS system.		
	8. Act to relieve obstruction.	Perform subdiaphragmatic abdominal thrusts (Heimlich maneuver).		Give 4 back blows. Give 4 chest thrusts.
	9. Check for foreign body.	Perform tongue-jaw lift and finger sweep.	Perform tongue-jaw lift. Remove foreign object only if you actually see it.	
	10. Rescue breaths.	Open the airway with head-tilt/chin-lift. Try again to give rescue breaths.		
	11. Be persistent.	Repeat Steps 8-10 until obstruction is relieved.		

Fig. 31-23. Foreign body airway obstruction management.

Table 31-8 Drugs for pediatric cardiopulmonary resuscitation

DRUG/DOSE	ACTION	IMPLICATIONS
Epinephrine HCl 0.01 mg/kg	Adrenergic Acts on both alpha- and beta-receptor sites, especially heart and vascular and other smooth muscle	Most useful drug in cardiac arrest Disappears rapidly from bloodstream after injection May produce renal vessel constriction and decreased urine formation
Sodium bicarbonate 1 mEq/kg	Alkalinizer Buffers pH	Infuse slowly and only when ventilation is adequate
Atropine sulfate 0.02 mg/kg	Anticholinergic-parasympatholytic Increases cardiac output, heart rate by blocking vagal stimulation in heart	Used to treat bradycardia after ventilatory assessment Maximum dose: infants and children, 1.0 mg; adolescents, 2.0 mg
Calcium chloride 20 mg/kg	Electrolyte replacement Needed for maintenance of normal cardiac contractility	Used only for hypocalcemia, calcium blocker overdose, hyperkalemia, or hypermagnesemia Administer slowly
Lidocaine HCl 1 mg/kg	Antidysrhythmic Inhibits nerve impulses from sensory nerves	Used for ventricular dysrhythmias only
Bretylium tosylate 5 mg/kg	Antidysrhythmic Inhibits release of norepinephrine in postganglionic nerve endings that control ventricular tachycardia	Used if lidocaine not effective
■ **Infusions**		
Epinephrine HCl infusion 0.1-1.0 μg/kg/min	Adrenergic See above	Titrated to desired hemodynamic effect
Dopamine HCl infusion 2-20 μg/kg/min	Agonist Acts on alpha receptors, causing vasoconstriction Increases cardiac output	Titrated to desired hemodynamic response
Dobutamine HCl infusion 5-20 μg/kg/min	Adrenergic direct-acting $beta_1$-agonist Increases contractility and rate of heart	Titrated to desired hymodynamic response Little vasconstriction, even at high rates
Isoproterenol HCl infusion 0.1-1.0 μg/kg/min	Adrenergic Increases contractility of heart by acting on beta-receptors Vasoconstriction	Titrated to desired hemodynamic effect
Lidocaine HCl infusion 20-50 μg/kg/min	Antidysrhythmic Increases electrical stimulation threshold of ventricle	See above Lower infusion dose used in shock Used for ventricular tachycardia

pital units. The supply is checked on a regular basis (usually once on each 8-hour shift). Resuscitation medications are listed in Table 31-8.

AIRWAY OBSTRUCTION*

Attempts at clearing the airway should be considered for (1) children in whom aspiration is witnessed or strongly suspected and (2) unconscious, nonbreathing children whose airways remain obstructed despite the usual maneuvers to open them.

NURSING ALERT In a conscious choking child attempt at relieving the obstruction only if:
- The child is unable to make any sounds.
- The cough becomes ineffective.
- There is increasing respiratory difficulty with stridor.

When a child is obviously choking, the initial step is to open the mouth and attempt to visualize and dislodge the object. Although strong controversy surrounds the optimum method for relieving foreign body obstruction in children, the methods currently recommended are a combination of *back blows* and *chest thrusts* for infants less than 1 year of age and the *Heimlich maneuver* for children over 1 year of age. Because of the risk of injury to abdominal organs, abdominal thrusts are not recommended for infants 1 year of age or less.

Infants

A choking infant is placed face down over the rescuer's arm with the head lower than the trunk and the head supported (Fig. 31-22, *I*). Additional support can be achieved if the rescuer supports the arm firmly against the thigh. Four quick, sharp, back blows are delivered between the infant's shoulder blades with the heel of the rescuer's hand. Less force is required than would be applied to an adult. After delivery of the back blows, the rescuer's free hand is placed flat on the infant's back so that the infant is "sandwiched" between the two hands, making certain the neck and chin are well supported. While the rescuer maintains support with the infant's head lower than the trunk, the infant is turned and placed supine on the rescuer's thigh, where four chest thrusts are applied in rapid succession in the same manner as external chest compressions described for CPR. Four back blows and four chest thrusts are continued until the object is removed or the infant becomes unconscious.

Children

The Heimlich maneuver, a series of subdiaphragmatic abdominal thrusts, is recommended for children over 1 year of age. The maneuver creates an artificial cough that forces air, and with it the foreign body, out of the airway. The procedure is carried out with the child in a standing, sitting, or lying position (Fig. 31-22, *J* and *K*). In the conscious choking child, upward thrusts are delivered to the upper abdomen with the fisted hand at a point just below the rib cage (see Fig. 31-23). To prevent damage to the internal organs, the rescuer's hands should not touch the xiphoid process of the sternum or the lower margins of the ribs. Six to 10 thrusts are repeated in rapid succession until the foreign body is expelled.

It is neither necessary nor desirable to squeeze or compress the arms during the procedure. It is not a punch or a bear hug. The child may vomit after relief of the obstruction and should be positioned to prevent aspiration. After breathing is restored, the child should receive medical attention and be assessed for complications.

The success of the technique is primarily a result of the obstruction occurring at the end of a maximum respiration. The victim is most likely to choke on food during inspiration; therefore the tidal volume plus expiratory reserve volume is present in the lungs. When pressure is exerted on the diaphragm by the maneuver, the food bolus is ejected with considerable force by this trapped air.

*Home care instructions for managing obstructed airway (choking) in infants and children are available in Wong, D.L., and Whaley, L.F.: Clinical manual of pediatric nursing, ed. 3, St. Louis, 1990, Mosby–Year Book, Inc.

KEY POINTS

- The major functions of the respiratory tract are to distribute air and exchange gases to supply cells with oxygen (O_2) and to remove carbon dioxide (CO_2).
- Several anatomic features predispose infants and young children to airway obstruction and atelectasis: there is less alveolar surface for gas exchange, narrowly branching peripheral airways become easily obstructed, and lack of collateral pathways inhibits ventilation beyond obstructed units.
- Gas exchange depends on the amount and composition of gases inhaled, thickness of the alveolar wall, adequacy of circulation to the alveoli, and substances within the alveoli that prevent their inflation or gas exchange.
- The amount of O_2 that diffuses into the blood depends on a pressure gradient between alveolar air and capillary blood, total functional surface area of the alveolocapillary membrane, minute volume, and alveolar ventilation.
- Defense mechanisms of the respiratory tract include the lymphatic system, viscid secretions, ciliary action, epiglottis, cough reflex, tracheobronchial dynamics, body position changes, and humoral defenses.
- Complete assessment of respiratory function involves a detailed history, physical examination, pulmonary function tests, radiography, and blood gas determination.
- Pulse oximetry is a noninvasive method of determining the O_2 saturation in the blood. One limitation of the technology is that it does not identify dangerously high O_2 levels.

- Improvement in respiratory function may be accomplished with measures such as O_2 therapy, positioning, humidification, aerosol therapy, and artificial ventilation.
- O_2 for administration must always be humidified in some manner.
- Chest physiotherapy is useful for patients with increased sputum production but is contraindicated for some.
- Respiratory failure is defined as the inability of the respiratory system to maintain adequate oxygenation of the blood, with or without CO_2 retention.
- Management of respiratory failure is to provide O_2, maintain ventilation, apply appropriate therapy, and anticipate complications.
- Indications for tracheostomy in children include upper airway obstruction, central nervous system dysfunction, neuromuscular disease, obstruction from secretions, and disturbances of gas diffusion or distribution.
- Occlusion of the tracheostomy tube is life-threatening; therefore equipment for replacing a tube must always be at hand.
- Two essentials of cardiopulmonary resuscitation are to support the patient's spine and to apply forceful, but not traumatic, sternal pressure.
- The Heimlich maneuver is reserved for children for whom aspiration is witnessed or strongly suspected. A combination of back blows and chest thrusts is used for infants with obstructed airways.

REFERENCES

Alderson, S.H., and Warren, R.H.: Pediatric aerosol therapy guidelines, Clin. Pediatr. 23:553-557, 1984.

American Heart Association: Instructor's manual for basic life support, Dallas, TX, 1987, American Heart Association.

Calvi, A.: Care of the child requiring long-term mechanical ventilation, Pediatr. Nurs. Update 1(6):1-8, 1985.

Chameides, L., editor: Textbook of pediatric advanced life support, Dallas, TX, 1988, American Heart Association.

Feldman, K.W., and Brewer, D.K.: Child abuse, cardiopulmonary resuscitation and rib fractures, Pediatrics 73:339-342, 1984.

Harbold, L.A.: A protocol for neonatal use of pulse oximetry, Neonatal Network 8(1):41-42, 55-57, 1989.

Inselman, L.S., and Mellins, R.B.: Growth and development of the lung, J. Pediatr. 98:1-15, 1981.

Johnson, J.T., Reilly, J.S., and Mallory, G.B.: Decannulation. In Myers, E.N., Stool, S.E., and Johnson, J.T., editors: Tracheostomy, New York, 1985, Churchill Livingston, Inc.

Kyff, J.V.: Current thoughts on chest physical therapy, Respir. Manage. 17(6):70-73, 1987.

Lichtenstein, M.A.: Pediatric home tracheostomy care: a parent's guide, Pediatr. Nurs. 12:41-48, 69, 1986.

Lough, and Carlo, W.A.: In Carlo, W.A., and Chatburn, R.L.: Neonatal respiratory care, ed. 2, St. Louis, 1988, Mosby–Year Book, Inc.

Murphy, K.G., and others: Severe burns from a pulse oximeter anesthesiol. 73:350, 1990.

Orenstein, D.M.: Cystic fibrosis: a guide for patient and family, New York, 1989, Raven Press.

Orlowski, J.P.: Optimal position for external cardiac massage in infants and children, Crit. Care Med. 12:224-229, 1984.

Sigler, B.A., and Wills, J.M.: Nursing care of the patient with a tracheostomy. In Meyers, E.N., Stool, S.E., and Johnson, J.T., editors: Tracheostomy, New York, 1985, Churchill Livingston, Inc.

Special Communications: Risk of infection during CPR training and rescue: supplemental guidelines, JAMA 262:2714-2715, 1989.

Sutton, P.P.: Chest physiotherapy: time for reappraisal, Br. J. Dis. Chest 82:127-137, 1988.

Torphy, D.E., Minter, M.G., and Thompson, B.M.: Cardiorespiratory arrest and resuscitation in children, Am. J. Dis. Child. 138:1099-1102, 1984.

Wade, J.F.: Respiratory nursing care: physiology and technique, ed. 3, St. Louis, 1982, Mosby–Year Book, Inc.

BIBLIOGRAPHY

General

Ahrens, T.S., and Rutherford, K.A.: The new pulmonary math. Applying the a/A ratio, Am. J. Nurs. 87:337-340, 1987.

Dudell, G., Cornish, J.D., and Bartlett, R.H.: What constitutes adequate oxygenation? Pediatrics 85:39-41, 1990.

Lareau, S., and Larson, J.L.: Ineffective breathing pattern related to airflow limitation, Nurs. Clin. North Am. 22:179-191, 1987.

Mathew, O.P.: Maintenance of upper airway patency, J. Pediatr. 106:863-869, 1985.

Wilmott, R.W.: Pursuing the cause of persistent cough, Contemp. Pediatr. 4(10):26-43, 1987.

Wolff, P.S.: An ingenious way to treat psychogenic cough, MCN 13:118-120, 1988.

Pulmonary Assessment

Birdsell, C.: How do you measure transcutaneous oxygen? Am. J. Nurs. 87:1273-1274, 1987.

Birdsell, C.: How and when do you use pulse oximetry? Am. J. Nurs. 87:158-165, 1989.

Chatburn, R.L.: Evaluation of pediatric pulmonary function: theory and application, Respir. Care 34:597-608, 1989.

Ehrhardt, B.S., and Graham, M.: Pulse oximetry: an easy way to check oxygen saturation, Nursing '90 20:50-54, 1990.

Fanconi, S., and others: Pulse oximetry in pediatric intensive care: comparison with measured saturations and transcutaneous oxygen tension, J. Pediatr. 107:362-366, 1985.

Fruthaler, G.J.: Snurgles and gurgles: respiratory sounds that worry parents, Comtemp. Pediatr. 5(7):42-46, 1988.

Hader, C.F., and Sorensen, E.R.: The effects of body position on transcutaneous oxygen tension, Pediatr. Nurs. 14:469-473, 1988.

Hartsell, M.B.: Noninvasive oxygen monitoring, J. Pediatr. Nurs. 2:64-65, 1987.

Hickenlooper, G.B., and Sowan, N.A.: Comparison of cardiorespiratory fitness tests for children, Pediatr. Nurs. 14:485-487, 491, 1988.

Kulick, R.M.: Pulse oximetry, Pediatr. Emerg. Care 3:127-130, 1987.

Nielsen, L.: Assessing patients' respiratory problems, Am. J. Nurs. 80:2192-2196, 1980.

Praud, J.P., and others: Accuracy of two wavelength pulse oximetry in neonate and infants, Pediatr. Pulmonol. 6:180-182, 1989.

Rooth, G., Huch, A., and Huch, R.: Transcutaneous oxygen monitors are reliable indicators of arterial oxygen tension (if used correctly), Pediatrics 9:283-286, 1987.

Salyer, J.W., Chatburn, R.L., and Dolcini, D.M.: Measured vs calculated oxygen saturation in a population of pediatric intensive care patients, Respir. Care 34:342-348, 1989.

Schroeder, C.H.: Pulse oximetry: a nursing care plan, Crit. Care Nurse 8(8):50-66, 1988.

Sherman, J.M.: New options for examining children's airways, Contemp. Pediatr. 6(1):30-44, 1989.

Ward, J.J.: Lung sounds: easy to hear, hard to describe, Respir. Care 34:17-19, 1989.

Wimsatt, R.: Unlocking the mysteries behind the chest wall, Nursing '85 15(11):58-64, 1985.

Therapeutic Procedures

Alderson, S.H., and Warren, R.H.: Pediatric aerosol therapy guidelines, Clin. Pediatr. 23:553-557, 1984.

Bailey, C., and others: Shallow versus deep endotracheal suctioning in young rabbits: pathologic effects on the tracheobronchial wall, Pediatrics 82:746-751, 1988.

Clarke, P.H.: The child in a mist tent, Pediatr. Nurs. 14:446-450, 1988.

Hartsell, M.B.: Chest physiotherapy and mechanical vibration, J. Pediatr. Nurs. 2:135-137, 1987.

Hoffman, L.A., Mazzocco, M.C., and Roth, J.E.: Fine tuning your chest PT, Am. J. Nurs, 87:1566-1572, 1987.

Kleiber, C., Krutzfield, N., and Rose, E.F.: Acute histologic changes in tracheobronchial tree associated with different suction catheter insertion techniques, Heart Lung 17:10-14, 1988.

Artificial Ventilation

Birdsall, C.: How do you use a closed suction adapter, Am. J. Nurse. 86:1222-1223, 1987.

Chulay, M.: Arterial blood gas changes with a hyperinflation and hyperoxygenation suctioning intervention in critically ill patients, Heart Lung 17:654-661, 1989.

Dixon, M., and Holmes, R.B.: The care of a ventilator-dependent child on a general pediatric unit, J. Pediatr. Nurs. 2:184-192, 1987.

Dougherty, J.M.: Negative pressure devices in pediatric practice, Pediatr. Nurs. 16:135-138, 1990.

Fuller, R.A.: Optimizing care for the infant with a tracheostomy, Neonatal Network 5(2):55-61, 1986.

Gordin, P.: High-frequency jet venilation for severe respiratory failure, Pediatr. Nurs. 15:625-629, 1989.

Hall, S.S., and Weatherly, K.S.: Using sign language with tracheostomized infants and children, Pediatr. Nurs. 15:362-267, 1989.

Hess, D.: Bedside monitoring of the patient on a ventilator, Crit. Care Q. 6(2):23-31, 1983.

Janowsky, M.J.: Accidental disconnections from breathing systems, Am. J. Nurs. 84:241-244, 1984.

Landis, K., and Smith, S.: The mechanically ventilated patient: a comprehensive nursing care plan, Crit. Care Q. 6(2):43-52, 1983.

Ritz, R., and others: Contamination of a multiple-use suction catheter in a closed-circuit system compared to contamination of a disposable, single-use suction catheter, Resp. Care 31:1086-1091, 1986.

Runton, N., and Zazal, G.H.: The decannulation process in children, J. Pediatr. Nurs. 4:370-373, 1989.

Simon, B.M., and McGowan, J.S.: Tracheostomy in young children: implications for assessment and treatment of communication and feeding disorders, Inf. Young Child. 1(3):1-9, 1989.

Walsh, C.M., and others: Controlled supplemental oxygenation during tracheobronchial hygiene, Nurs. Res. 36:211-215, 1987.

Whitford, K.M.: Health care needs of ventilator-dependent children, Pediatr. Nurs. 14:216-219, 1988.

Wolford, R.W.: Management of the pediatric airway, Emerg. Care Q. 3(3):52-62, 1987.

Endotracheal Airways

Blatzheim, L., Lipsey, A., and Warburton, D.: Pediatr. Pulm. 2:108-109, 1986.

Browning, D.H., and Graves, S.A.: Incidence of aspiration with endotracheal tubes in children, J. Pediatr. 102:582-584, 1983.

Corbo, B.H.: Endotracheal intubation: adolescent ICU experiences, Crit. Care Q. 8(1):35-46, 1985.

Feaster, S.C., West, C., and Ferketich, S.: Hyperinflation, hyperventilation, and hyperoxygenation before tracheal suctioning in children requiring long-term respiratory care, Heart Lung 14:379-384, 1985.

Finer, N.N., and others: Limitations of self-inflating resuscitators, Pediatrics 77:417-420, 1986.

Fuller, R.A.: Optimizing care for the infant with a tracheostomy, Neonatal Network 5(2):55-61, 1986.

Harris, R., and Hyman, R.: Clean vs. sterile tracheostomy care and level of pulmonary infection, Nurs. Res. 33:80-85, 1984.

Nieves, J.: Avoiding spontaneous extubation of nasotracheal or oral tracheal tubes, Pediatr. Nurs. 12:215-218, 1986.

Riegel, B., and Forshee, T.: A review and critique of the literature on preoxygenation for endotracheal suctioning, Heart Lung 14:507-518, 1985.

Runton, N., and Zazal, G.H.: The decannulation process in children, J. Pediatr. Nurs. 4:370-373, 1989.

Scott, P.H., and others: Predictability and consequences of spontaneous extubation in a pediatric ICU, Crit. Care Med. 13:228-232, 1985.

Shekleton, M.E., and Nield, M.: Ineffective airway clearance related to artificial airway, Nurs. Clin. North Am. 22:167-178, 1987.

Home Care

Aday, L.A., and Wegner, D.H.: Home care for ventilator-assisted children: implications for the children, their families, and health policy, Child. Health Care 17:112-120, 1988.

Anderson, K.L.: Long-term oxygen therapy: indications and guidelines for use,Home Healthcare Nurse 7(3):40-48, 1989.

Andrews, M.M., and Nielson, D.W.: Technology dependent children in the home, Pediatr. Nurs. 14:111-114, 151, 1988.

Bendell, D., and others: Behavioral treatment of CPR anxiety: a case study, Child. Health Care 13:77-81, 1984.

Briggs, N.J.: Selecting a pediatric home care program, Pediatr. Nurs. 13:191, 1987.

Czarniecki, L.: Caring for a young child with a tracheostomy, Caring 4(5):30-32, 1985.

Fanconi, S.: Outcome of home mechanical ventilation (letter), J. Pediatr. 108:791, 1986.

Frates, R.C., and others: Outcome of home mechanical ventilation in children, J. Pediatr. 106:850-856, 1985.

Giovannoni, R.: Chronic ventilator care: from hospital to home, Rx Home Care 7(1):51-52, 54, 56-57, 1985.

Goldberg, A.I., and others: Home care for life-supported persons: an approach to program development, J. Pediatr. 104:785-795, 1984.

Graber, H.P., and Balas-Stevens, S.: A discharge tool for teaching parents to monitor infant apnea at home, MCN 9:178-180, 1984.

Grammatica, G.: Developing a quality home care program for children, Pediatr. Nurs. 15:33-35, 1989.

Groeneveld, M.: Sending infants home on low-flow oxygen, JOGNN 15:237-241, 1986.

Harris, P.J.: Sometimes pediatric home care doesn't work, Am. J. Nurs. 88:81-854, 1988.

Harrison, L.L.: Teaching parents to provide home-care for ventilator-dependent children, MCN 14:281, 1989.

Hazinski, M.F.: Pediatric home tracheostomy care: a parent's guide, Pediatr. Nurs. 12:41-48, 69, 1986.

Hazlett, D.E.: A study of pediatric home ventilator management: medical, psychosocial, and financial aspects, J. Pediatr. Nurs. 4:284-294, 1989.

Kaufman, J., and Hardy-Ribakow, D.: Home care: a model of a comprehensive approach for technology-assisted chronically ill children, J. Pediatr. Nurs. 2:244-249, 1987.

Kaufman, J., and Hardy-Ribakow, D.: What parents need to know about trach care, RN 51:99-104, 1988.

Kenney, M.M.: Hospital to home: care of the child with a tracheostomy, Neonatal Network 6(1):21-24, 1987.

Kennelly, C.: Tracheostomy care: parents as learners, MCN 12:264-267, 1987.

Kirkhart, K.A., and others: Louisiana's ventilator assisted care program: case management services to link tertiary with community-based care, Child. Health Care 17:106-111, 1988.

Kopacz, M.A., and Moriarty-Wright, R.: Multidisciplinary approach for the patient on a home ventilator, Heart Lung 13:255-262, 1984.

Kruger, S., and Rawlins, P.: Pediatric dismissal protocol to aid the transition from hospital to home care, Image 16:120-125, 1984.

Leighton, E.M., Davis, R.H., and Anderson, L.J.W.: An orientation program for high-technology home care nursing, Pediatr. Nurs. 16:182-185, 1990.

McCarthy, M.F.: A home discharge program for ventilator-assisted children, Pediatr. Nurs. 12:331-335, 380, 1986.

McCrory, L.: Pediatric home tracheostomy care alternatives (letter), Pediatr. Nurs. 12:223, 1986.

Mizuki, J.A.: There's no place like home, Am. J. Nurs. 84:646-648, 1984.

O'Pray, M.: Working with families with infants with respiratory equipment in the home, Issues Compr. Pediatr. Nurs. 10:113-121, 1987.

Scharer, K., and Dixon, D.M.: Managing chronic illness: parents with a ventilator-dependent child, J. Pediatr. Nurs. 4:236-247, 1989.

Schreiner, M.S., Donar, M.E., and Kettrick, R.G.: Pediatric home mechanical ventilation, Pediatr. Clin. North Am. 34:47-60, 1987.

Steele, N.F., and Harrison, B.: Technology-assisted children: assessing discharge preparation, J. Pediatr. Nurs. 1(3):150-158, 1986.

Steele, N.F., and Morgan, J.: Emergency planning for technology-assisted children, J. Pediatr. Nurs. 4:81-87, 1989.

Stroup, K.B., Wylie, P., and Bull, M.J.: Car seats for children with mechanically assisted ventilation, Pediatrics 80:290-292, 1987.

Thilo, E.H., Comito, J., and McCulliss, D.M.: Home oxygen therapy in the newborn, Am. J. Dis. Child. 141:766-768, 1987.

Wasserman, A.L.: A prospective study of the impact of home monitoring on the family, Pediatrics 74:323-329, 1984.

Wegener, D.H., and Aday, L.A.: Home care for ventilator-assisted children: predicting family stress, Pediatr. Nurs. 15:371-376, 1989.

Wessel, G.L., Prumo, M.O., and Harrison, P.: School placement and the oxygen-dependent child, J. Pediatr. Nurs. 6:435-436, 1989.

Respiratory Failure

Carter, J.H.: Pediatric cardiopulmonary resuscitation, Child Care Newsletter 6(1):6-5, 1987.

Curley, M.A.Q., and Vaughan, S.M.: Assessment and resuscitation of the pediatric patient, Crit. Care Nurse 7(3):26-42, 1987.

Curley, M.A.Q., and Vaughan, S.M.: Pediatric resuscitation: mock code, MCN 12:277-280, 1987.

Escher-Neidig, J.R.: Pediatric respiratory arrest: emergency airway management in the critical care setting, Crit. Care Nurse 8(8):22-33, 1988.

Raphaely, R.C.: Acute respiratory failure in infants and children, Pediatr. Ann. 15:315-321, 1986.

Rimar, J.M.: Sodium bicarbonate during CPR, MCN 11:245, 1986.

Wright, S., Norton, C., and Kesten, K.: Retention of infant CPR instruction by parents, Pediatr.Nurs. 15:37-41, 1989.

Cardiopulmonary Resuscitation

Bardossi, K.: Newest guidelines on pediatric CPR and first aid, Contemp. Pediatr. 4(6):47-56, 1987.

Brill, J.E.: Cardiopulmonary resuscitation, Pediatr. Ann. 15:24-29, 1986.

Fiser, D.H., and Wrape, V.: Outcome of cardiopulmonary resuscitation in children, Pediatr. Emerg. Care 3:235-238, 1988.

Goetting, M.G., and Sowa, B.: Retinal hemorrhage after cardiopulmonary resuscitation in children: an etiologic reevaluatiion, Pediatrics 85:585-588, 1990.

Phillips, G.W.L., and Zideman, D.A.: Relation of infant heart to sternum: its significance in cardiopulmonary resuscitation, Lancet 1:1024-1025, 1986.

Schuman, A.J.: Pediatric advanced life support: an update and review, Contemp. Pediatr. 6(5):26-50, 1989.

Scientific Board, California Medical Association: Transmission of disease via mouth-to-mouth resuscitation, West. J. Med. 143:468, 1985.

Airway Obstruction

American Academy of Pediatrics, Committee on Accident and Injury Prevention: First aid for the choking child, 1988, Pediatrics 81:740-743, 1988.

Day, R.L.: Differing opinions on the emergency treatment of choking, Pediatrics 71:976-977, 1983.

Kilhman, H., Gillis, J., and Benjamin, B.: Severe upper airway obstruction, Pediatr. Clin. North Am. 34:1-14, 1987.

Mofenson, H.C., and Greensher, J.: Management of the choking child, Pediatr. Clin. North Am. 32:183-192, 1985.

CHAPTER 32

The Child with Respiratory Dysfunction

RELATED TOPICS

Administration of medication, Ch. 27
The child with disturbance of oxygen and carbon dioxide exchange, Ch. 31
Compliance, Ch. 27
Controlling elevated temperatures, Ch. 27
High risk related to disturbed respiratory function, Ch. 10
Immunizations, Ch. 12
Infection control, Ch. 27
Pain assessment; pain management, Ch. 26
Physical examination: ears, nose, mouth and throat, chest, lungs, Ch. 7
Smoking, Ch. 21
Surgical procedures, Ch. 27

GLOSSARY

AOM Acute otitis media
ARDS Adult respiratory distress syndrome
bronchiolitis Inflammation of the bronchioles
bronchitis Inflammation of the bronchi
CF Cystic fibrosis
CNS Central nervous system
COHb Carboxyhemoglobin
COPD Chronic obstructive pulmonary disease
Coryza Acute nasal congestion
CPT Chest physiotherapy
EIA Exercise-induced asthma
epiglottitis Inflammation of the epiglottis
ET Endotracheal
GABHS Group A β-hemolytic streptococci
GI Gastrointestinal
IgE Immunoglobulin E
INH Isoniazid
laryngitis Inflammation of the larynx
LTB Laryngotracheobronchitis
MDI Metered-dose inhaler
OM Otitis media
OME Otitis media with effusion
Pa_{O_2} Arterial oxygen
PA_{O_2} Alveolar oxygen
P_{CO_2} Partial pressure of carbon dioxide
PE Pressure equalizing

PFT Pulmonary function tests
PPD Purified protein derivative (tuberculin)
RAST Radioallergosorbent test
RMP Rifampin
RSV Respiratory syncytial virus
stridor (laryngeal) A shrill, harsh respiratory sound, often described as a "crowing" sound, which is particularly marked during inspiration
T & A Tonsillectomy and adenoidectomy
TB Tuberculosis
URI Upper respiratory infection

Some of the most common problems in the pediatric age-group are related to disturbed respiratory function, and respiratory failure is the chief cause of morbidity in the newborn period. Respiratory illness can be caused by disease, trauma, or physical anomalies or can be seen as a manifestation of a disturbance in another organ or system, such as neurologic disorders involving the respiratory center or innervation to the respiratory musculature. Most communicable diseases have respiratory symptoms.

The type and pattern of respiratory disturbances also vary tremendously according to the age of the child. There are differences in susceptibility to infections and in response to different organisms and conditions at various ages. Moreover, manifestations of illness vary according to the age of the child and may involve different organ systems. For example, diarrhea is often the manifestation of a viral infection in infancy that produces a pharyngoconjunctivitis in the older child. This chapter is primarily concerned with infections, allergic responses, and mechanical disturbances.

RESPIRATORY INFECTION

Acute infection of the respiratory tract is the most common cause of illness in infancy and childhood. Young children ordinarily have four or five such infections each year, which manifest a wide range of severity from trivial to severe or even fatal illness. The type of illness and the physical response are also related to a variety of factors, including the type of infectious agent, the age of the child, and the integrity of the child's defense mechanisms. Despite the effectiveness of the natural defense mechanisms in the respiratory tract, circumstances alter their ability to repel invading organisms.

GENERAL ASPECTS OF RESPIRATORY INFECTIONS

Infections of the respiratory tract are described in a number of different ways according to the general areas of involvement in the more common infections. The upper respiratory tract, or upper airway, consists primarily of the nose and pharynx. The lower respiratory tract consists of the bronchi and bronchioles (which constitute the reactive portion of the airway because of their smooth muscle content and ability to constrict) and the alveoli. Authorities disagree about the designation for the structurally stable portion of the airway (including the epiglottis, larynx, and trachea). Some consider these structures to be part of the lower airway, whereas others categorize them as upper airway structures. For this discussion, the trachea is considered with lower tract disorders, and infections of the epiglottis and larynx are categorized as croup syndromes.

Respiratory infections seldom fall neatly into discrete anatomic areas. Infections tend to spread from one structure to another because of the contiguous nature of the mucous membrane lining the entire tract. Consequently, infections of the respiratory tract involve several areas rather than a single structure, although the effect on one may predominate in any given illness.

Etiology and Characteristics

Respiratory infections account for a large majority of acute illnesses in children. The etiology and course of these infections are influenced by a number of factors, including the age of the child, season, living conditions, and preexisting medical problems.

Infectious agents. The respiratory tract is subject to a wide variety of infective organisms, but the largest percentage of infections are caused by viruses, particularly in the upper respiratory passages. These infections account for a large majority of acute illnesses in children. Other agents that may be involved in primary or secondary invasion include group A β-hemolytic streptococci, staphylococci, *Haemophilus influenzae, Chlamydia trachomatis, Mycoplasma,* and pneumococci.

Age. The pattern of respiratory infection varies considerably with the age of the child. Infants under the age of 3 months have a lower infection rate, presumably because of the protective function of maternal antibodies. The infection rate soars from age 3 to 6 months, the time between the disappearance of maternal antibodies and the infant's own antibody production. The viral infection rate continues to be high during the toddler and preschool years but drops steadily. By the time the child reaches 5 years of age, viral respiratory infections are much less frequent, but the incidence of *Mycoplasma pneumoniae* and group A β-streptococcal infections increases.

Some of the viral agents produce a mild illness in older children but cause severe lower respiratory tract illness and croup in infants. The amount of lymphoid tissue increases

Charmaine Kleiber, R.N., M.S., C.P.N.P., assisted in the revision of this chapter.

throughout middle childhood, and repeated exposure to organisms confers increasing immunity as the child grows older; thus older children have a greater resistance to most organisms. Whooping cough is a relatively harmless tracheobronchitis in childhood but a serious disease in infancy.

Risk of aspiration is increased during the first year, partially related to the feeding and postfeeding positions. During feeding, the infant is in a recumbent position that facilitates entry of fluids into the airway, which can cause upper lobe changes. In children beyond infancy, most aspiration occurs when they are in the upright position.

Size. Anatomic differences influence the degree to which children respond to respiratory tract infections. The diameter of the airways is smaller in young children than in older children and is therefore subject to considerable narrowing from edematous mucous membranes and increased production of secretions. In addition, the distance between structures within the tract is shorter anatomically in the young child; therefore organisms move more rapidly down the respiratory tract for more extensive involvement. Also, the relatively short and open eustachian tube in infants and young children allows pathogens easy access to the middle ear.

Resistance. The ability to resist invading organisms depends on several factors. Deficiencies of the immune system place the child at risk for any infectious process. The general conditions that appear to decrease resistance to infection are malnutrition, anemia, fatigue, and chilling of the body. Conditions affecting the respiratory tract that weaken its defenses and predispose to infection include allergies such as allergic rhinitis and asthma, cardiac anomalies that have the tendency to develop pulmonary congestion, and cystic fibrosis of the pancreas.

Seasonal variations. The most common respiratory

Box 32-1 SIGNS AND SYMPTOMS ASSOCIATED WITH RESPIRATORY INFECTIONS IN INFANTS AND SMALL CHILDREN

Fever

- May be absent in newborn infants
- Greatest at ages 6 months to 3 years
  - Temperature may reach 39.5° to 40.5° C (103° to 105° F) even with mild infections
- Often appears as first sign of infection
- May be listless and irritable or somewhat euphoric and more active than normal, temporarily; some children talk with unaccustomed rapidity
- Tendency to develop high temperatures with infection in certain families
  - May precipitate febrile seizures (sudden temperature rise to 40° C [104° F])
  - More gradual temperature rise will not elicit a seizure
  - Febrile seizures uncommon after 3 or 4 years of age

Meningismus

- Meningeal signs without infection of the meninges
- Occurs with abrupt onset of fever
- Accompanied by:
  - Headache
  - Pain and stiffness in the back and neck
  - Presence of Kernig and Brudzinski signs
- Subsides as the temperature drops

Anorexia

- Common to most childhood illnesses
- Almost invariably accompanies acute infections in small children
- Frequently the initial evidence of illness
- Persists to a greater or lesser degree throughout febrile stage of illness; often extends into convalescence

Vomiting

- Small children vomit readily with illness
- A clue to the onset of infection
- May precede other signs by several hours
- Usually short lived, but may persist during the illness

Diarrhea

- Mild transient diarrhea
- Often accompanies respiratory infections, especially viral infections
- May be severe

Abdominal Pain

- Common complaint
- Sometimes indistinguishable from pain of appendicitis
- Mesenteric lymphadenitis may be cause
- Muscle spasms from vomiting may be a factor, especially in nervous, tense children

Nasal Blockage

- Small nasal passages of infants easily blocked by mucosal swelling and exudation
- Can interfere with respiration and feeding in infants
- Contributes to the development of otitis media and sinusitis

Nasal Discharge

- Frequently accompanies respiratory infections
- May be thin and watery (rhinorrhea) or thick and purulent
  - Depends on the type and/or stage of infection
- Associated with itching
- May irritate upper lip and skin surrounding the nose

Cough

- Common feature of respiratory disease
- May be evident only during the acute phase
- May persist several months after a disease

Respiratory Sounds

- Sounds associated with respiratory disease:
  - Cough
  - Hoarseness
  - Stridor
  - Wheezing
- Auscultation:
  - Wheezing
  - Crackles
  - Hyperresonance
  - Absence of sound

Sore Throat

- Frequent complaint of older children
- Young children (unable to describe symptoms) may not complain even when highly inflamed
  - Elastic nature of the tissues in young children may cause less pressure on nerve endings

tract pathogens appear in epidemics during the winter and spring months, but mycoplasma infections occur more often in autumn and early winter. Infection-related asthma (e.g., asthmatic bronchitis) occurs more frequently during cold weather.

Clinical Manifestations

Infants and young children, especially those between 6 months and 3 years of age, react more severely to acute respiratory tract infection than older children, and they appear to be much more ill than their local manifestations would indicate. Young children display a number of generalized signs and symptoms, as well as local manifestations, that differ from those seen in older children and adults. An infant or child may display any or all of the signs and symptoms listed in Box 32-1.

Nursing Considerations

Because respiratory infections are common in children, they are the illnesses most frequently observed by nurses.

Assessment

The general assessment of the respiratory system follows the guidelines described in Chapter 7 (for nose, mouth and throat, chest, and lungs), and normal vital signs can be found on the inside front cover. In addition, special attention is given to the specific observations outlined in Box 32-1 using the guidelines in Box 32-2.

Nursing Diagnoses

After a thorough assessment, a number of nursing diagnoses may be identified. The most likely diagnoses are outlined and discussed in the Nursing Care Plan on pp. 1421-1422. Others may be apparent in individual cases.

Planning

The nursing goals for care of the child with an acute respiratory infection are as follows:

1. Facilitate respiratory efforts.
2. Promote rest.
3. Promote comfort.
4. Prevent spread of primary infection to others.
5. Reduce temperature (if significantly elevated).
6. Prevent dehydration and provide nourishment.
7. Prevent complications.
8. Educate and support family.

Implementation

Since the majority of children with upper respiratory tract infections are treated at home, most of the nursing care is directed toward education and guidance of parents in caring for their child and serving as resources for problem solving. If the practitioner has given the parents written instructions, these are explained and reinforced as appropriate. If written instructions have not been furnished, the nurse should provide the parents with written guidelines and, in some cases, outlines of procedures to be carried out.

Ease respiratory efforts. Most acute respiratory infections are mild and cause few distressing symptoms. Although children may feel uncomfortable and suffer from a "stuffy" nose and some mucosal swelling, respiratory distress is uncommon. The interventions described in the remainder of the discussion are usually sufficient to relieve most minor discomfort and ease respiratory efforts. However, children with croup or epiglottitis may develop suffi-

Box 32-2 GUIDELINES FOR ASSESSMENT OF RESPIRATORY FUNCTION

Respirations

The pattern of respirations is observed for rate, depth, ease, and rhythm of breathing:

Rate—rapid (tachypnea), normal, or slow for the particular child

Depth—normal depth, too shallow (hypopnea), too deep (hyperpnea); usually estimated from the amplitude of thoracic and abdominal excursion

Ease—effortless, labored (dyspnea), orthopnea, associated with intercostal and/or substernal retractions (inspiratory "sinking in" of soft tissues in relation to the cartilaginous and bony thorax), pulsus paradoxus (blood pressure falls with inspiration and rises with expiration), flaring nares, head bobbing (head of sleeping child with suboccipital area supported on mother's forearm bobs forward in synchrony with each inspiration), grunting, or wheezing

Labored breathing—continuous, intermittent, becoming steadily worsening, sudden onset, at rest or on exertion, associated with wheezing, grunting, associated with pain

Rhythm—variation in rate and depth of respirations

Other Observations

In addition to respirations, particular attention is addressed to the following:

Evidence of infection—check for elevated temperature, enlarged cervical lymph nodes, inflamed mucous membranes, and purulent discharges from the nose, ears, or lungs (sputum)

Cough—observe the characteristics of the cough (if present); for example, under what circumstances the cough is heard (e.g., night only, on arising), the nature of the cough (paroxysmal with or without wheeze, "croupy" or "brassy"), frequency of cough, associated with swallowing or other activity

Wheeze—expiratory or inspiratory, high-pitched or musical, prolonged, slowly progressive or sudden, associated with labored breathing

Cyanosis—note distribution (peripheral, perioral, facial, trunk as well as face), degree, duration, associated with activity

Chest pain—may be a complaint of older children. Note location and circumstances: localized or generalized, referred to base of neck or abdomen, dull or sharp, deep or superficial, associated with rapid, shallow respirations or grunting

Sputum—supervised older children may provide sputum sample. Note volume, color, viscosity, and odor

Bad breath—may be associated with some lung infections

NURSING CARE PLAN

The Child with Acute Respiratory Infection

NURSING DIAGNOSIS: Ineffective breathing pattern related to inflammatory process, pain

GOAL 1

Ease respiratory efforts

INTERVENTIONS

Allow position of comfort
Promote rest
Maintain patent airway
Provide high-humidity atmosphere
Position for comfort and maximum lung expansion
Implement measures to reduce anxiety and apprehension
Organize activities to allow for minimal expenditure of energy

EXPECTED OUTCOMES

Child rests and sleeps quietly
Respirations are unlabored
Respirations remain within normal limits (see inside front cover for normal variations)

GOAL 2

Increase oxygen supply to lungs

INTERVENTIONS

Position for maximum ventilatory efficiency such as high-Fowler position or sitting, leaning forward
Avoid constricting clothing, linens, restraints
Place in Croupette with cool vapor, if prescribed
*Provide oxygen as prescribed and/or needed
*Provide nebulization, if prescribed

EXPECTED OUTCOMES

Child breathes easily
Respirations remain within normal limits (see inside front cover for normal variations)

GOAL 3

Reduce anxiety and apprehension

INTERVENTIONS

Provide constant attendance during acute phase of illness
Encourage presence of parents
Provide comfort and cuddling when possible
Remove restraining devices when and as often as possible
Provide quiet diversion appropriate to child's age and condition
*Administer medications that promote breathing (bronchodilators, expectorants)

EXPECTED OUTCOMES

Child exhibits no signs of distress
Parents remain with child and provide comfort
Child engages in quiet activities appropriate for age, interest, and condition

NURSING DIAGNOSIS: Ineffective airway clearance related to mechanical obstruction, inflammation, increased secretions, pain

GOAL 1

Maintain patent airway

INTERVENTIONS

Aspirate (suction) secretions from airway as needed
Avoid neck hyperextension
Position to prevent aspiration of secretions
- Semiprone position
- Side-lying position

Assist child to expectorate sputum
- Provide nebulization with appropriate solution and equipment as prescribed

Give nothing by mouth to prevent aspiration of fluids (severe tachypnea)

EXPECTED OUTCOMES

Airways remain clear
Child breathes easily; respirations are within normal limits (see inside front cover)

GOAL 2

Promote expectoration of mucous secretions

INTERVENTIONS

Ensure adequate fluid intake
Provide humidified atmosphere
Assist child to cough effectively; provide tissues
Remove accumulated mucus; suction, if needed

EXPECTED OUTCOME

Older child expectorates secretions appropriately and without undue stress and fatigue

*Dependent nursing action.

Continued.

NURSING CARE PLAN
The Child with Acute Respiratory Infection—cont'd

NURSING DIAGNOSIS: Fear/anxiety related to hospitalization, difficulty breathing

GOAL 1
Keep child calm

INTERVENTIONS
Explain unfamiliar procedures and equipment to the child
Remain with child during procedures
Employ calm, reassuring manner
Provide constant attendance
Hold and cuddle child whenever possible—preferably by parent or other familiar person
Be aware of child's sleep/rest cycle or pattern in planning nursing activities
Provide security devices such as familiar toy, blanket
Encourage parental attendance and, when possible, involvement in child's care
Do nothing to make the child more anxious than already is
Maintain a relaxed manner
Establish rapport with the child and parents
Instill confidence in both parents and child
Try to avoid any intrusive procedures
*Administer sedatives as indicated if ordered for restlessness and pain

EXPECTED OUTCOMES
Child responds positively to comforting measures
Parents relate readily with personnel and calmly with child
Child remains calm and cooperative

NURSING DIAGNOSIS: Pain related to inflammatory process, surgical incision

GOAL 1
Relieve pain

INTERVENTIONS AND EXPECTED OUTCOMES
See Nursing Care Plan: The Child in Pain, Chapter 26

NURSING DIAGNOSIS: Potential for injury related to presence of infective organisms

GOAL 1
Help eradicate infective organisms

INTERVENTIONS
*Administer antibiotics as prescribed
Provide nutritious diet according to child's preferences and ability to consume nourishment

EXPECTED OUTCOME
Child exhibits evidence of diminishing symptoms

GOAL 2
Prevent spread of infection to others

INTERVENTIONS
Employ appropriate infection control (see Chapter 27)
Instruct others (parents, members of staff) in appropriate precautions
Teach affected children protective methods to prevent spread of infection, e.g., hand washing, handling genital area, care after using bedpan or toilet
Endeavor to keep infants and small children from placing hand and objects in contaminated areas
Assess home situation and implement protective measures as feasible in individual circumstances
*Administer antimicrobial medications if prescribed
Support body's natural defenses, e.g., good nutrition

EXPECTED OUTCOME
Others remain free from infection

NURSING DIAGNOSIS: Altered family processes related to illness and/or hospitalization of a child

GOAL 1
Reduce parental anxiety

INTERVENTIONS
Recognize parental concern and need for information and support
Explain therapy and child's behavior
Provide support as needed
Encourage family to become involved in child's care

EXPECTED OUTCOME
Parents ask appropriate questions, discuss the child's condition and care calmly, and become involved positively in child's care

See also:
Nursing Care Plan: The Family of the Ill or Hospitalized Child, Chapter 26
Nursing Care Plan: The Child in the Hospital, Chapter 26

*Dependent nursing action.

cient swelling to obstruct the airway. These children are hospitalized for observation and therapy (see discussions of specific disorders). Positioning for optimum respiration and observation for signs of respiratory distress are primary nursing functions.

The atmosphere in homes heated during the winter months is often very dry. Warm or cool mist has been a common therapeutic measure for symptomatic relief of respiratory discomfort. The moisture soothes inflamed membranes and seems to be especially beneficial when there is

> **NURSING TIP: HUMIDIFICATION**
>
> A large, wet beach towel hung with one end in shallow water in the bathtub will increase humidity if the bathroom door remains open.

hoarseness or any laryngeal involvement. Mist tents are frequently used in the hospital for humidifying the air and relieving discomfort. However, use of steam vaporizers in the home should be discouraged because of the hazards related to their use and the little evidence to support their efficacy (Colombo, Hopkins, and Waring, 1981). Alternate suggestions are available, such as humidification systems. Shallow pans with wide surface areas for evaporation increase humidity but should be placed where they do not pose a safety hazard.

A time-honored method of producing steam is the shower. Running a shower of hot water into the empty bathtub or open shower stall with the bathroom door closed produces a quick source of steam. Keeping a child in this environment for 10 to 15 minutes offers the same advantages as the mist tent without the fear and restraint often associated with the confines of a tent. A small child can be held on the lap of a parent or other adult. Older children can sit in the bathroom under the supervision of an adult.

Promote rest. Children who have an acute febrile illness should be placed on bed rest. This is usually not difficult while the temperature is elevated but may be difficult when children, particularly young children, feel fairly well. When parents take the advice seriously and consistently keep them in bed, most children learn to cooperate during illness. Often children are more apt to comply if they are allowed to lie quietly on a couch where they can watch television or participate in an alternate quiet activity. If children are unreasoning and expend an inordinate amount of energy in protest, allowing them to play quietly on the floor serves the purpose of rest better than allowing them to cry excessively in bed. A number of entertainment devices, based on individual interests, can be used to keep children quiet.

Promote comfort. Older children are usually able to manage nasal secretions with little difficulty. Parents are instructed about the correct administration of nose drops and throat irrigations, if ordered. For very young infants, who normally breathe through their noses, an infant nasal aspirator or a rubber ear syringe is helpful in removing nasal secretions before feeding. This practice, followed by instillation of saline nose drops, may be all that is necessary to clear nasal passages and promote feeding. Saline nose drops can be prepared at home by dissolving ¾ teaspoon of salt in 1 pint of warm water.*

*Home care instructions for administration of nose drops and nasal aspiration are available in Wong, D.L., and Whaley, L.F.: Clinical manual of pediatric nursing, ed. 3, St. Louis, 1990, Mosby–Year Book, Inc.

For older infants and children who can better tolerate decongestants, vasoconstrictive nose drops may be administered 15 to 20 minutes before feeding and at bedtime. Two drops are instilled, and since this shrinks only the anterior mucous membranes, 2 more drops are instilled 5 to 10 minutes later. Phenylephrine (Neo-Synephrine) 0.25% is the usual choice of decongestant nose drops, although others, such as ephedrine 1%, may be prescribed. Older cooperative children often prefer nasal sprays. They are taught to compress the plastic container at the moment of inspiration to gain relief. Spray bottles and bottles of nose drops should be used for one child only and only for one illness, since they become easily contaminated with bacteria. Nose drops or sprays should not be administered for more than 3 days to avoid rebound congestion.

Hot or cold applications sometimes provide relief for older children with painful cervical adenitis. An ice bag or heating pad applied to the neck may decrease the discomfort, but safety precautions must be observed to prevent burns. The ice bag or heating device must be covered, and the heating pad should not be set at high ranges.

Prevent spread of infection. Careful handwashing should be carried out when caring for children with respiratory infections. Children and families are taught the correct disposal of respiratory secretions and proper behavior related to airborne droplets (coughing and sneezing). They are taught to use a tissue or their hand to cover their nose and mouth when they cough or sneeze and to dispose of the tissues properly.

Every endeavor should be made to remove affected children from contact with other children. Ideally, ill children should be isolated in a separate bedroom at the first sign of illness. This is seldom a problem with only children but is often difficult when living arrangements are crowded and there are several children in the family. If children have no separate bedroom, sometimes another child can sleep on a couch or cot, or with relatives or friends. An effort should be made to teach well children to stay away from ill children if the living conditions allow for segregation, although this may be difficult or impossible to enforce.

Reduce temperature. If the child has a significantly elevated temperature, controlling the fever becomes a major nursing task. The parent should know how to take a child's temperature and read the thermometer accurately. Most parents are able to do this, but nurses cannot make this assumption. Those who cannot will require instruction in use of the thermometer.*

If the practitioner has prescribed acetaminophen, parents may need help administering the drug. Most parents can read the label and calculate the desired dose, but some have difficulty and will require careful instruction or precise direction.* It is important to emphasize accuracy in both the amount of drug given and the time intervals at which the drug is administered in order to avoid accumulation ef-

*Home care instructions for measuring temperature and administration of medication are available in Wong, D.L., and Whaley, L.F.: Clinical manual of pediatric nursing, ed. 3, St. Louis, 1990, Mosby–Year Book, Inc.

fects. Cool liquids are encouraged to help reduce the temperature and to minimize the chances of dehydration. (See Controlling Elevated Temperatures, Chapter 27.)

Promote hydration. Dehydration is always a hazard when children are febrile or anorexic, especially when vomiting or diarrhea is also present. Adequate fluid intake should be encouraged by offering small amounts of favorite fluids at frequent intervals. High-calorie liquids, such as colas, fruit juices, water-flavored and sweetened with corn syrup, or similar drinks, help prevent catabolism and dehydration. Fluids should not be forced, and children should not be awakened to take fluids. Forcing fluids may create the same difficulties as urging unwanted food. Gentle persuasion with preferred beverages will usually be successful.

Parents should know how to assess their child's level of hydration (see Chapter 28) (see Nursing Tip). They are advised to observe the frequency of voiding and notify the nurse or practitioner if there appears to be insufficient voiding.

Provide nutrition. Loss of appetite is characteristic of children with acute infections, and in most cases, children can be permitted to determine their own need for food. Many children show no decrease in appetite, and others respond well to certain foods such as gelatin, soup, and puddings (see also Feeding the Sick Child, Chapter 27). Since the illness is relatively short, the nutritional state is seldom compromised. In fact, urging foods on anorexic children may precipitate nausea and vomiting and in some cases even cause an aversion to the feeding situation that can extend into the convalescent period and beyond.

Family support and home care. Small children with respiratory infections are irritable and often difficult to comfort. Therefore the family needs support, encouragement, and practical suggestions for care. Since most care involves comfort measures and administration of medication, a primary goal of education is related to these activities.

In addition to antipyretics and nose drops, the child may require antibiotic therapy. It is usually the nurse who instructs the parents about continuing medication begun in the hospital or initiating medications at home, especially antibiotics. Parents of children who are sent home with oral antibiotics need to understand the importance of regular administration and continuing the drug for the prescribed length of time, regardless of whether the child appears to be ill.

Parents are also cautioned against giving the child any medications that are not approved by the health practitioner. Adverse effects have been noted in children who have received some preparation intended for adults, for example, some long-acting nose drops (Neo-Synephrine II) and dextromethorphan cough squares (mistaken for candy). They are also cautioned about giving the child unprescribed antibiotics left over from a previous illness. Self-medication with unprescribed antibiotics is a significant problem (Cunningham and others, 1983). It should be emphasized that some drugs interact with others to produce serious side effects, and such a likelihood is increased when medications are administered to children without consultation with the practitioner. The nurse is in an excellent position to provide drug information to families. It has been found that patients who have questions about medications are more likely to ask a nurse than a physician (Morris and others, 1984). (See Chapter 27 for administration of medications and teaching parents.)

NURSING TIP: ASSESSING VOIDING

Counting the number of wet diapers in a 24-hour period is a satisfactory method of assessing output in infants and toddlers.

5 Evaluation

The effectiveness of nursing interventions is determined by continual reassessment and evaluation of care based on the following observational guidelines and expected outcomes:

1. Observe individual child's respiratory behavior and movement.
2. Observe signs and symptoms for progress toward preillness status.
3. Observe child's behavior and activity.
4. Observe other family members and contacts for evidence of infection.
5. Take temperature.
6. Observe for signs of adequate hydration.
7. Observe eating behavior.
8. Assess child for evidence of complications, such as dehydration, weight loss, or spread of infection to other areas of the body.
9. Observe family's behavior and interview members regarding their feelings and concerns.

Expected outcomes:
See Nursing Care Plan, pp. 1421-1422.

UPPER RESPIRATORY TRACT INFECTIONS

Upper respiratory infections (URIs) include infectious processes involving any or all of the structures in the upper respiratory tract. Most are caused by viruses and are self-limited. The average North American preschooler or young school-age child has five or six minor respiratory infections per year (Goldbloom, 1986). Most URIs have a viral etiology and need only symptomatic treatment and support. However, secondary infection or extension of URIs can cause serious or long-lasting effects, especially in infants and very young children. A primary site for extension is the middle ear.

ACUTE VIRAL NASOPHARYNGITIS

Acute nasopharyngitis (the equivalent of the "common cold" in adults) is caused by any of a number of different viruses, usually rhinoviruses, respiratory syncytial virus (RSV), adenovirus, influenza virus, or parainfluenza virus.

Clinical Manifestations

Symptoms of nasopharyngitis are more severe in infants and children than in adults. Fever is common, especially in young children. Older children have low-grade fevers, which appear early and suddenly in children 3 months to 3 years of age and are associated with irritability, restlessness, and decreased appetite and activity. Nasal inflammation may lead to obstruction of passages, producing open-mouth breathing. Other symptoms (e.g., vomiting and diarrhea) may be evident in some children.

The initial symptoms in older children are dryness and irritation of nasal passages and sometimes the pharynx, followed in a few hours by sneezing, chilly sensations, muscular aches, an irritating nasal discharge, and sometimes cough. Nasal inflammation may lead to obstruction, and continual wiping away of secretions causes skin irritation to nares.

The disease is self-limited and usually resolves within 4 to 10 days without complications. The most common complication is otitis media, especially in infants, and this should be suspected if fever recurs. It may occur early or after the initial phase of nasopharyngitis is past. Pneumonia is a less frequent complication and observed more often in infants.

Therapeutic Management

Children with nasopharyngitis are managed at home. There is no specific treatment, and effective vaccines are not yet available. Antipyretics are usually prescribed for mild fever and discomfort (see Chapter 27 for management of fever). Decongestants may be prescribed for children and infants over 6 months of age in an effort to shrink swollen nasal passages. The decongestants that exert their effect by vasoconstriction are usually less effective when taken orally than when applied topically as nose drops. Since these drugs affect *all* vascular beds they should be given with caution to children with diabetes.

Cough suppressants containing dextromethorphan may be prescribed for a dry, hacking cough. Some preparations contain up to 22% alcohol; they should not be administered to young children continuously and must be stored out of reach of children.

Antihistamines are largely ineffective in treatment of nasopharyngitis. The drugs have a weak atropine-like effect that tends to dry secretions, but they can cause drowsiness and, paradoxically, have a stimulatory effect on children. There is no support for the usefulness of expectorants, and antibiotics are usually contraindicated because they can sensitize a child who may need the drugs in a severe illness. Administration of vitamin C has not been shown to have significant therapeutic or prophylactic value (Goldbloom, 1986).

Reports indicate some success with the intranasal administration of interferon (from human white blood cells) or alpha-2-interferon (from recombinant DNA) in preventing nasopharyngitis caused by rhinovirus and coronavirus infections (Douglas and others, 1986; Hayden and others, 1985). Virucidal-treated paper tissues have been reported and are presumed to reduce the spread of infection from person to person (Dick and others, 1986; Hayden and others, 1985). However, since children are the major source of spread, the logistics of effective use are apparent and positive results questionable.

Prevention. Nasopharyngitis is so widespread in the general population that it is impossible to prevent. In addition, children are more susceptible to colds because they have not yet developed resistance to many types of viruses. Very young infants are subject to relatively serious complications; therefore some attempt should be made to protect them from exposure. Bed rest is recommended until the child is free of fever for at least 1 day.

Nursing Considerations

A cold is often the parents' first introduction to an illness in their infants. Parents are assisted in managing the infant or child as described for general care. Most of the distress of nasopharyngitis is related to the nasal obstruction, especially in small infants. Placing the child in a prone position (unless respirations are compromised), suctioning, and vaporization may help provide relief. Saline nose drops and gentle suction with an ear syringe, particularly before feeding, are sometimes useful.

Maintaining adequate fluid intake is essential during any infectious process. Although a child's appetite for solid foods is usually diminished for several days, it is important to offer favorite fluids to prevent dehydration. Fluids can be cool or warm, depending on individual preference. See Nursing Considerations, p. 1420, for other interventions.

Because nasopharyngitis is spread from secretions, the best means for prevention is avoiding contact with affected persons. This goal is difficult in places where large numbers of people are confined in a small area for a long time, such as classrooms. Family members with a cold should try to "keep it to themselves" by carefully disposing of tissues; not sharing towels, glasses, or eating utensils; covering the mouth and nose with tissues when coughing or sneezing; and washing the hands thoroughly after nose blowing or sneezing. The most frequent carriers of infection are the human hands, which deposit viruses on doorknobs, faucets, and other everyday objects. Therefore children should be taught to wash their hands thoroughly before putting them near nose, mouth, or eyes.

Family support. Support and reassurance are important elements of care for families of young children with recurrent URIs. Because URIs are so frequent in children less than 3 years of age, families may feel they are on an endless roller-coaster of illness. They can be reassured that frequent colds are a normal part of childhood and that by 5 years of age their children will have developed immunity to many viruses. Parents who work outside the home should expect to have to take time off to care for ill children during the fall and winter months. If the children are cared for routinely in daycare centers, the infection rate will be higher than if they

Box 32-3 EARLY EVIDENCE OF RESPIRATORY COMPLICATIONS

Parents are instructed to notify the health professional if any of the following are noted:
- Evidence of earache (see p. 1433)
- Respirations faster than 50 to 60 per minute
- Fever over 101° F
- Listlessness
- Increasing irritability with or without fever
- Persistent cough 2 days or more
- Wheezing
- Crying
- Refusal to eat

Modified from National Association of Pediatric Nurse Associates and Practitioners (NAPNAP): Baby's first cold, New York, 1989, Winthrop Consumer Products. Copies available from NaSal Nasal Moisturizing drops, c/o Winthrop Consumer Products, 90 Park Ave., 7th Floor, New York, NY 10016.

were being cared for in the home. Parents should know the signs of respiratory complications and be counseled to notify a health professional if any signs of complications appear or if the child does not improve within 2 or 3 days (Box 32-3).

ACUTE STREPTOCOCCAL PHARYNGITIS

Group A β-hemolytic streptococci (GABHS) infection of the upper airway (strep throat) is not in itself a serious disease, but affected children are at risk for serious sequelae—acute rheumatic fever (ARF), an inflammatory disease of heart, joints, and central nervous system (see Chapter 34), and acute glomerulonephritis, an acute kidney infection (see Chapter 30). Permanent damage can result from these sequelae, especially ARF, which has demonstrated a recent resurgence in the United States. However, only 21% to 50% of children with streptococcal infections have a history of pharyngitis (Ferrieri, 1987), and by 15 years of age the likelihood that group A is responsible is only about 15% (McMillan, 1988).

Clinical Manifestations

GABHS is generally a relatively brief illness that varies markedly in severity from subclinical (no symptoms) to comparatively severe toxicity. The onset is generally abrupt and characterized by pharyngitis, headache, fever, and (especially in small children) abdominal pain. The tonsils and pharynx may be inflamed and covered with exudate (50% to 80% of cases) (see Color Plate 19), which usually appears by the second day of illness. Anterior cervical lymphadenopathy (30% to 50% of cases) usually occurs early, and the nodes are often tender. Pain can be relatively mild to severe enough to make swallowing difficult. Clinical manifestations usually subside in 3 to 5 days unless complicated by sinusitis or parapharyngeal, peritonsillar, or retropharyngeal abscess. Nonsuppurative complications may appear after the onset of GABHS—acute nephritis in about 10 days and rheumatic fever in an average of 18 days (Feigin, 1990).

Diagnostic Evaluation

Clinical diagnosis of GABHS infection can present difficulties. Although 80% to 90% of all cases of acute pharyngitis are viral, a throat culture should be performed to rule out GABHS and (in some cases) *Corynebacterium diphtheriae.* Because some children normally harbor streptococci in their throats, a positive culture is not always conclusive evidence of active disease. Since most streptococcal infections are short-term illnesses, antibody (antistreptolysin O) responses do not appear until relatively late and are useful only for retrospective diagnosis.

Rapid identification of GABHS is possible with diagnostic test kits that can be used in the office or clinic setting. However, because of their questionable sensitivity, they are not yet considered to be a substitute for culture, especially if the organism is endemic in the community.

Therapeutic Management

If streptococcal sore throat infection is present, oral penicillin G is prescribed in a dose sufficient to control the acute local manifestations and to maintain an adequate level for at least 10 days to eliminate any organisms that might remain to initiate rheumatic fever symptoms. Penicillin does not appear to prevent the development of acute glomerulonephritis in susceptible children; however, it may prevent the spread of a nephrogenic strain of GABHS to others in the family (Gerber and Markowitz, 1985). Penicillin usually produces a prompt response within 24 hours. Occasionally patients require retreatment if the organism is not eradicated.

A combination of penicillin and rifampin is more effective in eradicating GABHS than penicillin alone and is recommended for carriers and persons resistant to penicillin (Chaudhary and others, 1985; Tanz and others, 1985). Erythromycin is the alternative medication most often used for children who are sensitive to penicillin. Manifestations are treated symptomatically.

Nursing Considerations

The nurse is often the person who performs a throat smear for culture and instructs the parents about administering penicillin and analgesics as prescribed. Most children prefer to remain in bed during the acute phase of the illness. Cold or warm compresses to the neck may provide relief. In children old enough to cooperate, warm saline gargles offer some relief of throat discomfort. Pain may interfere with oral intake, and the child should not be forced to eat. Cool liquids or ice chips are usually more acceptable than solids and are encouraged.

Special emphasis is placed on correct administration of oral medication and completing the course of penicillin (see Administration of Medication, Chapter 27, and Compliance, Chapter 27). If injections are required, they must be administered deep into a large muscle mass (e.g., the vastus lateralis or gluteus muscle). Parents need to be aware of the residual tenderness, which may cause the child to limp for a day or two. Local applications of heat are helpful in relieving some of the discomfort.

Prevention. No satisfactory method of immunization is available for prevention of streptococcal disease. The organism is spread by close contact with affected persons—direct projection of large droplets or physical transfer of respiratory secretions containing the organism. As a result, spread of infection is common in families, classrooms, and daycare centers. Children with streptococcal infection are noninfectious to others within a few hours after initiation of penicillin therapy. The streptococcus is not virulent when dried but is acquired from close droplet transmission; therefore fomites are not usually a hazard.

It is important to know when the organism is epidemic in the community so that families can be on the alert for symptoms. Directors of daycare centers and school officials should share infectious disease information with parents. Obtaining throat cultures from children who are close family contacts of patients with streptococcal infection is advised. It is even proposed that in populations where streptococcal infection is occurring at an epidemic level over an extended period of time, mass prophylaxis may be advised. Penicillin administration before the onset of symptoms prevents most cases of streptococcal disease.

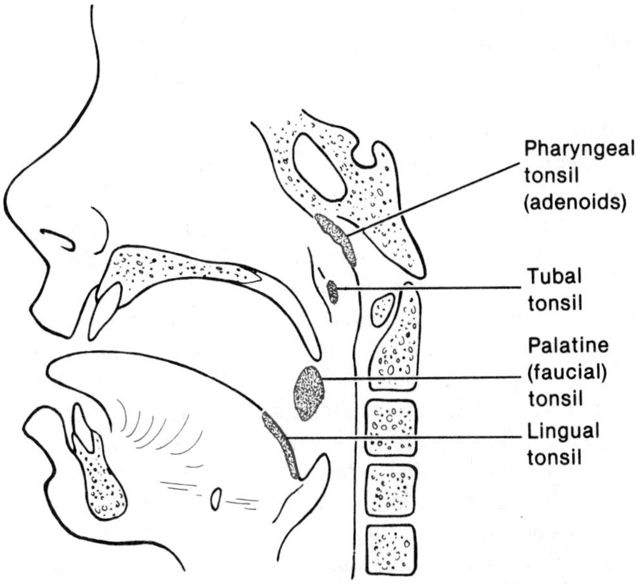

Fig. 32-1. Location of various tonsillar masses.

TONSILLITIS

The tonsils are masses of lymphoid tissue located in the pharyngeal cavity. Their function is to filter and protect the respiratory and alimentary tracts from invasion by pathogenic organisms. They also may have a role in antibody formation. Although the size of tonsils varies, children generally have much larger tonsils than adolescents or adults. This difference is thought to be a protective mechanism at a time when young children are especially susceptible to upper respiratory infection.

Pathophysiology

Several pairs of tonsils are part of a mass of lymphoid tissue encircling the nasal and oral pharynx, known as Waldeyer tonsillar ring (Fig. 32-1). The *palatine,* or *faucial,* tonsils are located on either side of the oropharynx, behind and below the pillars of the fauces (opening from the mouth). A free surface of the palatine tonsils is usually visible during oral examination. The palatine tonsils are those removed during tonsillectomy. The *pharyngeal* tonsils, also known as the *adenoids,* are located above the palatine tonsils on the posterior wall of the nasopharynx. Their proximity to the nares and eustachian tubes causes difficulties in instances of inflammation. The *lingual* tonsils are located at the base of the tongue and only rarely are removed. The *tubal* tonsils, found near the posterior nasopharyngeal opening of the eustachian tubes, are not part of the Waldeyer tonsillar ring.

Etiology

Tonsillitis usually occurs in association with pharyngitis. Because of the abundant lymphoid tissue and the frequency of URIs, tonsillitis is a very common cause of morbidity in young children. The causative agent may be viral or bacterial.

Clinical Manifestations

The manifestations of tonsillitis are chiefly caused by inflammation. As the palatine tonsils enlarge from edema, they may meet in the midline (kissing tonsils), obstructing the passage of air or food. The child has difficulty swallowing and breathing. Enlargement of the adenoids blocks the space behind the posterior nares, making it difficult or impossible for air to pass from the nose to the throat. As a result, the child breathes through the mouth.

If mouth breathing is continuous, the mucous membranes of the oropharynx become dry and irritated. There may be an offensive mouth odor and impaired senses of taste and smell. Because air cannot be trapped for proper speech sounds, the voice has a nasal and muffled quality. A persistent, harassing cough is also common. Because of the proximity of the adenoids to the eustachian tubes, this passageway is frequently blocked by swollen adenoids, interfering with normal drainage and frequently resulting in otitis media and/or difficulty hearing.

Therapeutic Management

The diagnosis is established from visual examination of the throat. The majority of children with tonsillitis respond to medical treatment. However, a significant number undergo surgical intervention, although the exact criteria for this common procedure are controversial.

Medical. Since the illness is self-limiting, treatment of viral pharyngitis is symptomatic. Throat cultures positive for GABHS infection warrant antibiotic treatment. It is important to differentiate between viral and streptococcal infection in febrile exudative tonsillitis. Since the majority of infections are of viral origin, early rapid tests can eliminate unnecessary antibiotic administration. In general, viral tonsillitis has been found to be more common in children younger than 3 years of age and GABHS more common in children 6 years or older (Putto, 1987).

Surgical. Surgical treatment of chronic tonsillitis is a very controversial subject. Tonsillectomy is the pediatric surgical procedure most frequently performed beyond the newborn period, but many authorities believe that the majority of these surgeries are unwarranted. Others, who have seen children improve measurably after tonsillectomy and adenoidectomy, continue to recommend it for selected patients (Paradise and others, 1984). There are a small number of severely affected children for whom surgery is clearly indicated, a larger number for whom it is not indicated, and a considerable number who fall between these two extremes. It is these children over whom most of the controversy occurs.

Tonsillectomy (removal of the palatine tonsils) is indicated for massive hypertrophy that results in difficulty breathing or eating. Absolute indications are malignancy and obstruction of the airway that result in cor pulmonale. *Adenoidectomy* (removal of the adenoids) is recommended for children with recurrent otitis media, especially when associated with hearing loss, and in those children where hypertrophied adenoids obstruct nasal breathing. Their removal may be warranted in the child under 3 years of age and should be performed without a tonsillectomy. Follow-up after adenoidectomy should include assessment of hearing, smell, and taste for expected improvement. Contraindications to either tonsillectomy or adenoidectomy are (1) cleft palate, since both tonsils help minimize escape of air during speech; (2) acute infections at the time of surgery, since the locally inflamed tissues increase the risk of bleeding; and (3) uncontrolled systemic diseases or blood dyscrasias.

Generally, removal of the tonsils should occur after 3 or 4 years of age because of the problem of excessive blood loss in small children and the possibility of regrowth or hypertrophy of lymphoid tissue. The tubal and lingual tonsils often enlarge to compensate for the lost lymphoid tissue, resulting in continued pharyngeal and eustachian tube obstruction.

Nursing Considerations

Nursing care of the child with tonsillitis mainly involves providing comfort. A soft to liquid diet is generally preferred. A cool-mist vaporizer helps keep the mucous membranes moist during periods of mouth breathing. Warm saltwater gargles, throat lozenges, and analgesic/antipyretic drugs such as acetaminophen (Tylenol) are useful to promote comfort.

If surgery is needed, the child requires the same psychologic preparation and physical care as for any other operation (see Chapters 26 and 27). The following discussion focuses on specific nursing care for tonsillectomy and adenoidectomy (T & A).

Assessment

A complete history is taken, with special notation of any bleeding tendencies, since the operative site is highly vascular. Baseline vital signs are important for postoperative monitoring and observation. Signs of any URI are noted and reported, and bleeding and clotting times are included in the usual laboratory work requests. During physical assessment the presence of any loose teeth is noted. (See also Surgical Procedures, Chapter 27.)

Nursing Diagnoses

Based on a careful assessment, a number of nursing diagnoses become apparent. Some are common to all children; others are not. The usual diagnoses are outlined and discussed in the Nursing Care Plan on pp. 1429-1430. Others may be apparent in individual cases.

Planning

The nursing goals for postoperative care of the child with a T & A are as follows:

1. Facilitate drainage of secretions.
2. Promote comfort and relieve pain.
3. Observe for evidence of bleeding.
4. Prevent complications.
5. Provide fluids and nutrition.
6. Instruct family for home care.
7. Support child and family.

Implementation

Until they are fully awake, children are placed on the abdomen or side to facilitate drainage of secretions, and any needed suctioning is performed carefully to avoid trauma to the oropharynx. When alert, children may prefer sitting up, although they should remain in bed for the remainder of the day. They are discouraged from coughing frequently or clearing the throat, which may aggravate the operative site.

Some secretions are common, particularly dried blood from surgery. All secretions and vomitus are inspected for evidence of fresh bleeding (some blood-tinged mucus is expected). Dark brown (old) blood is usually present in the emesis, as well as in the nose and between the teeth. If parents do not expect this, they may be frightened at a time when they need to be calm and reassuring for their children.

The throat is very sore after surgery. An ice collar may provide relief, but many children find it bothersome and prefer not to have it. Most children experience moderate pain after a T & A and should receive pain medication for at least the first 24 hours (Rauen and Holman, 1989). Analgesics are ordered but may need to be given rectally or intravenously to avoid the oral route. Since pain is continuous, ideally pain control should be continuous (see Pain Management, Chapter 26). If children are comfortable, they seldom require sedation. Irritable children may require mild

NURSING CARE PLAN
The Child with Tonsillectomy

NURSING DIAGNOSIS: Altered oral mucous membranes related to raw, denuded surfaces of tonsil sockets

GOAL 1

Prevent bleeding

INTERVENTIONS

Discourage child from coughing frequently or clearing the throat
Avoid use of gargles or hard objects (such as toothbrush) in the mouth
Avoid foods that are irritating (e.g., high acid fruit juices, raw vegetables) or highly seasoned
Encourage cool liquid or semisoft foods

EXPECTED OUTCOMES

Child does not aggravate the operative site
There is no evidence of bleeding

NURSING DIAGNOSIS: Ineffective airway clearance related to discomfort

GOAL 1

Facilitate drainage

INTERVENTIONS

Position on side or stomach while sleeping
Discourage swallowing mucous secretions; provide tissues

EXPECTED OUTCOMES

Breathing remains unlabored
Child disposes of mucus appropriately

NURSING DIAGNOSIS: Impaired swallowing related to inflammation and pain

GOAL 1

Prevent dehydration

INTERVENTIONS

Offer cool, bland liquids; soft, bland foods
Provide pain relief
Position for optimal swallowing

EXPECTED OUTCOME

Child consumes an adequate amount of nourishment

GOAL 2

Prevent aspiration of secretions

INTERVENTIONS

Assist child to expectorate
Position on side or stomach while sleeping

EXPECTED OUTCOME

Child disposes of mucus and drainage appropriately

NURSING DIAGNOSIS: Pain related to surgical site

GOAL 1

Relieve pain

INTERVENTIONS

Avoid offering irritating liquid and solid foods
Employ nonpharmacologic pain reduction techniques (see Chapter 26)
*Administer analgesics as prescribed

EXPECTED OUTCOME

Child rests quietly and exhibits no evidence of pain
See also Nursing Care Plan: The Child in Pain, Chapter 26

GOAL 2

Prevent irritation to operative site

INTERVENTIONS

Offer diet as tolerated
  Cool liquid diet for 12-24 hours
  Soft diet thereafter
  Advance to regular diet as recommended
Avoid substances that irritate denuded areas, e.g.,
  Acid juices
  Rough foods
  Highly seasoned foods
Avoid placing hard objects in mouth

EXPECTED OUTCOME

Child exhibits no evidence of discomfort

*Dependent nursing action.

Continued.

NURSING CARE PLAN
The Child with Tonsillectomy—cont'd

NURSING DIAGNOSIS: Anxiety/fear related to unfamiliar event, discomfort

GOAL 1

Reduce anxiety

INTERVENTIONS

Explain source of discomfort
Anticipate needs
Keep child and bed free from any blood-tinged excretions
Reassure child regarding any blood-tinged drainage
Keep emesis basin within easy reach

EXPECTED OUTCOMES

Child rests quietly and readily attends to verbal and nonverbal communication
Child communicates needs and wants in a calm manner

NURSING DIAGNOSIS: Potential fluid volume deficit related to nothing by mouth, prior to surgery, reluctance to swallow

GOAL 1

Promote adequate hydration

INTERVENTIONS

Administer fluids as ordered
- Intravenous
  - *Administer fluid as prescribed
  - Maintain desired drip rate
  - *Add appropriate electrolytes as prescribed
  - Maintain integrity of infusion site
- Oral
  - Employ play for promoting fluid intake see Box 27-5

EXPECTED OUTCOMES

Child drinks a sufficient amount of fluid (specify type and amount)
Child exhibits evidence of adequate hydration, e.g., moist mucous membranes, good skin turgor, adequate urinary output for age

See also:
Nursing Care Plan: The Family of the Ill or Hospitalized Child, Chapter 26
Nursing Care Plan: The Child in the Hospital, Chapter 26
Nursing Care Plan: The Child Undergoing Surgery, Chapter 27

*Dependent nursing action.

sedation to lessen crying, which irritates the operative site, increasing the chance of bleeding.

Food and fluid are restricted until children are fully alert and there are no signs of hemorrhage. Cool water, crushed ice, popsicles, or dilute fruit juice is given first, although fluids with a red or brown color are avoided to distinguish fresh or old blood in emesis from the ingested liquid. Citrus juice may cause discomfort and is usually poorly tolerated. Milk, ice cream, or pudding is not offered until clear fluids are retained, because milk products coat the mouth and throat, causing the child to clear the throat more often, which may initiate bleeding. Soft foods, particularly gelatin, cooked fruits, sherbet, soup, and mashed potatoes, are started on the first or second postoperative day or as the child tolerates feeding. The pain from surgery often inhibits intake, reinforcing the need for adequate pain control.

Postoperative hemorrhage is unusual but can occur. Therefore the nurse observes the throat directly for evidence of bleeding, using a good source of light and, if necessary, carefully inserting a tongue depressor. Other signs of hemorrhage are increased pulse (above 120 beats per minute), pallor, frequent clearing of the throat, and vomiting of bright red blood. Restlessness, an indication of hemorrhage, may be difficult to differentiate from general discomfort after surgery. Decreasing blood pressure is a later sign and signals impending shock.

✦ **NURSING ALERT** The most obvious early sign is the child's continuous swallowing of the trickling blood. While the child is sleeping, the frequency of swallowing is noted.

If continuous bleeding is suspected, the physician is notified immediately, since a child can lose a considerable amount of blood before overt signs of blood loss are observed. Surgery may be required to ligate a bleeding vessel. Airway obstruction may occur as a result of edema or accumulated secretions and is indicated by progressive cyanosis. Suction equipment should be available after tonsillectomy.

Family support and home care. Discharge instructions include (1) avoiding foods that are irritating or highly seasoned, (2) avoiding the use of gargles or vigorous toothbrushing, (3) discouraging the child from coughing or clearing the throat or putting objects in the mouth, and (4) using mild analgesics or an ice collar for pain. Hemorrhage may occur 5 to 10 days after surgery as a result of tissue sloughing from the healing process. Any sign of bleeding warrants immediate medical attention. Objectionable mouth odor and slight ear pain with a low-grade fever are common for a few days postoperatively. However, persistent severe earache, fever, or cough requires medical evaluation. Most children are ready to resume normal activity within 1 to 2 weeks after the operation.

A T & A often represents the first hospitalization experience for the child and family. Since the surgery is usually an elective procedure, there is ample opportunity to prepare both children and parents for this event. Both need reassurance about what to expect at the time of admission, before and after surgery, and at discharge. Parents are encouraged to visit often or room-in if possible and participate in their child's care if they wish. Children are honestly apprised of postoperative discomfort and reassured that they will be able to talk. Sometimes children believe that the operation will immediately "make the throat all better" and are dismayed to find that it still hurts after the surgery. Ideally, children should have an opportunity to discuss the experiences to gain a feeling of mastery and to overcome any fears or misconceptions.

Evaluation

The effectiveness of nursing interventions is determined by continual reassessment and evaluation of care based on the following observational guidelines and expected outcomes:

1. Monitor the child's vital signs and behavior.
2. Observe for evidence of bleeding.
3. Observe and interview family about their understanding of the child's condition.
4. Have family demonstrate an understanding of home care.
5. Encourage family to discuss concerns that provide some insight into their ability to comply with instructions.

Expected outcomes:
See Nursing Care Plan, pp. 1429-1430.

INFLUENZA

Influenza, or "flu," one of the most common disorders, has been overused in diagnosis of relatively nondescript respiratory infections. Influenza is caused by three of the orthomyxoviruses, which are antigenically distinct: types A and B, which cause epidemic disease, and type C, which is unimportant epidemiologically. The viruses may undergo significant changes from time to time. Major changes that occur at intervals of years (usually 5 to 10) are called *antigenic shift;* minor variations within the same subtypes, *antigenic drift,* occur almost annually. Consequently, antigenic drift that takes place over several years can alter the virus sufficiently to result in susceptibility of individuals to a type for which they were previously immunized or infected.

The disease is spread from one individual to another by direct contact (large-droplet infection) or by articles recently contaminated by nasopharyngeal secretions. There is no predilection for a specific age-group, but attack rates are highest in young children who have not had previous contact with a strain. It is frequently most severe in infants. During epidemics, infection among school-age children is believed to be a major source of transmission in a community. Influenza is more common during the winter months.

The disease has a 1- to 3-day incubation period, and affected persons are most infectious for 24 hours before and after onset of symptoms. The virus has a peculiar affinity for epithelial cells of the respiratory tract mucosa, where it destroys ciliated epithelium with metaplastic hyperplasia of the tracheal and bronchial epithelium with associated edema. The alveoli may also become distended with a hyaline-like material. The viruses can be isolated from nasopharyngeal secretions early after onset of the infection, and serologic tests identify the type by complement fixation or the subgroups by hemagglutination inhibition.

Clinical Manifestations

The manifestations of influenza may be subclinical, mild, moderate, or severe. In most cases of overt illness, the throat and nasal mucosa are dry, there is a dry cough, and there is a tendency toward hoarseness. There is a sudden onset of fever and chills accompanied by flushed face, photophobia, myalgia, hyperesthesia, and sometimes prostration. Subglottal croup is common, especially in infants. The symptoms last for 4 to 5 days. Complications include severe viral pneumonia (often hemorrhagic), encephalitis, and secondary bacterial infections, such as otitis media, sinusitis, or pneumonia. Reye syndrome can be a serious complication of influenza A or B at any age but occurs most often in school-age children. Therefore children with influenza should not receive aspirin.

Therapeutic Management

Uncomplicated influenza in children usually requires only symptomatic treatment—acetaminophen for fever, dextromethorphan for cough (if needed), and sufficient fluids to maintain hydration. Amantadine hydrochloride (Symmetrel) has been effective in reducing symptoms associated with type A disease if administered within 24 to 48 hours after onset. It is ineffective against type B or C influenza or other viral diseases. It should not be given to children under 1 year of age but is recommended for unvaccinated high-risk children, as is late immunization.

Prevention. Inactivated influenza viral vaccines are safe and effective for prevention of influenza provided the antigens in the vaccine correlate with circulating influenza viruses. The Committee on Infectious Diseases recommends that all children receive a single dose of *Haemophilus influenzae* type b conjugate vaccine at 18 months of age (American Academy of Pediatrics, Committee on Infectious Diseases, 1989). For information on immunization see Chapter 12.

Nursing Considerations

Nursing care is the same as for any child with a URI, including helping the family to implement measures to relieve symptoms. The greatest danger to affected children is development of a secondary infection.

NURSING ALERT Prolonged fever or appearance of fever during early convalescence is a sign of secondary bacterial infection and should be reported to the practitioner for antibiotic therapy.

OTITIS MEDIA

Otitis media (OM) is one of the most prevalent diseases of early childhood. It has been determined that approximately 70% of children have had at least one episode and 33% have had three or more episodes by 3 years of age. The incidence is highest in children age 6 months to 2 years; then it gradually decreases with age, except for a small increase at age 5 and 6 years, the time of school entry. OM is uncommon in children over 7 years of age. Boys are affected more frequently than girls in children less than school age; later the sexes are affected equally. The incidence of acute otitis media (AOM) is highest in the winter months. Children living in households with many members (especially smokers) are more likely to have OM than those living with fewer persons, and children with siblings or parents who had a history of chronic OM have a higher incidence than those who do not (McFadden and others, 1985).

OM has been defined in a variety of ways. The acute disease has been known as "suppurative," "purulent," or "bacterial" OM and OM with effusion as "serous," "secretory," "nonsuppurative," and "glue ear." The standard terminology that has been established to describe OM is outlined in Box 32-4.

Etiology

AOM is most frequently caused by *Streptococcus pneumoniae* and *H. influenzae.* The etiology of the noninfectious type is unknown, although it is a frequent result of blocked eustachian tubes from the edema of allergic rhinitis or hypertrophic adenoids. Chronic OM is frequently an extension of an acute episode.

By 1 year of age 65% of children in a Boston study had experienced one or more episodes of AOM; by age 3, 83% had experienced at least one episode. The peak incidence occurred at age 6 months to 1 year of age; a second peak was observed at ages 4 and 5 years. Boys with a sibling history of recurrent AOM and early occurrence of a first episode are at highest risk for recurrent AOM (Teele and others, 1989). Passive smoking has been established as a significant factor in development of OM (see p. 1455). It has been suggested that smoke inhalation increases the risk of a blocked eustachian tube by impairing mucociliary function, causing congestion of soft nasopharyngeal tissues, or predisposing patients to upper respiratory infection (Strachan, Jarvis, and Feyerabend, 1989).

A relationship has been observed between the incidence of OM and the feeding methods in early infancy. Infants fed breast milk have a lower incidence of OM compared with formula-fed infants (Cunningham, 1984; Paradise and Elster, 1984; Teele and others, 1989). Breast-feeding may protect infants against respiratory viruses and allergy and limits the exposure of the eustachian tube and middle ear mucosa to microbial pathogens and foreign proteins (Saarinen, 1982). Also, reflux of milk up the eustachian tubes is less likely in breast-fed infants because of the semivertical positioning during breast-feeding as compared with bottle-feeding. The admonition is to "prop the baby, not the bottle."

Box 32-4 STANDARD TERMINOLOGY FOR OTITIS MEDIA

Otitis media—an inflammation of the middle ear without reference to etiology or pathogenesis
Acute otitis media (AOM)—a rapid and short onset of signs and symptoms lasting approximately 3 weeks
Otitis media with effusion (OME)—an inflammation of the middle ear in which a collection of fluid is present in the middle ear space
Subacute otitis media—middle ear effusion lasting from 3 weeks to 3 months
Chronic otitis media with effusion—middle ear effusion that persists beyond 3 months

Pathophysiology

OM is primarily the result of dysfunctioning eustachian tubes. The eustachian tubes are part of a contiguous system composed of the nares, nasopharynx, eustachian tube, middle ear, and mastoid antrum and air cells (see Fig. 7-29). Eustachian tubes have three important functions relative to the middle ear: (1) protection of the middle ear from nasopharyngeal secretions, (2) drainage of secretions produced in the middle ear into the nasopharynx, (3) and ventilation of the middle ear to equalize air pressure within the middle ear with atmospheric pressure in the external ear canal and replenishment of oxygen that has been absorbed.

Mechanical or functional obstruction of the eustachian tube causes accumulation of secretions in the middle ear. Intrinsic obstruction can be caused by infection or allergy; extrinsic obstruction is usually the result of adenoids or nasopharyngeal tumors. Persistent collapse of the tube during swallowing can cause functional obstruction associated with decreased stiffness or an inefficient opening mechanism. Eustachian tube obstruction results in negative middle ear pressure and, if persistent, produces a transudative middle ear effusion. Drainage is inhibited by sustained negative pressure and impaired ciliary transport within the tube. When the passage is not totally obstructed, contamination of the middle ear can take place by reflux, aspiration, or insufflation during crying, sneezing, nose blowing, and swallowing when the nose is obstructed.

Several factors predispose infants and young children to development of otitis media (Box 32-5).

Complications. The consequences of prolonged middle ear disorders can be either functional or structural. The principal functional consequence is *hearing loss,* although loss in the majority of cases is conductive in nature and mild in severity. The causes of hearing loss are negative middle ear pressure, the presence of effusion in the middle ear, or structural damage to the tympanic membrane. How-

Box 32-5 FACTORS PREDISPOSING TO DEVELOPMENT OF OTITIS MEDIA

The eustachian tubes are short, wide, and straight and lie in a relatively horizontal plane (Fig. 32-2).
The cartilage lining is undeveloped, making the tubes more distensible and therefore more likely to open inappropriately.
The normally abundant pharyngeal lymphoid tissue readily obstructs the eustachian tube openings in the nasopharynx.
Immature humoral defense mechanisms increase the risk of infection.
The usual lying-down position of infants favors the pooling of fluid, such as formula, in the pharyngeal cavity.

ever, the most feared consequence of hearing loss is its adverse effect on development of speech, language, and cognition. It was observed that children who had spent prolonged periods of time with middle ear effusion performed less well on speech and language tests that those who had had few if any middle ear diseases. The association was strongest when the effusion occurred during the first 6 to 12 months of life (Teele and others, 1984).

Structural complications or sequelae involve primarily the tympanic membrane. *Tympanic membrane retraction* or *retraction pocket* occurs when continued negative middle ear pressure draws the tympanic membrane inward, and in areas of low-tensile strength or atrophic segments of the drum head, retraction pockets appear. This retraction may result in impaired sound transmission, perforation of the thinned-out areas, or infection in the pockets and, later, cholesteatoma.

Tympanosclerosis (eardrum scarring) is the deposition of hyaline material into the fibrous layer of tympanic membrane. It is commonly seen in children with inflammatory middle ear disease or those with repeated tympanoplasty tube placement. Eardrum *perforation* is a common complication in AOM and often accompanies chronic disease. Persistent perforation is a complication of tympanostomy tube placement. Surgery is required to close some perforations.

Adhesive otitis media (glue ear) is a thickening of the mucous membrane by proliferation of fibrous tissue that can cause fixation of the ossicles with a resultant hearing loss. *Chronic suppurative otitis media,* an inflammation of the middle ear and mastoid, is evidenced by perforation and discharge (otorrhea). *Labyrinthitis,* infection of the inner ear, and *mastoiditis,* infection of the mastoid sinus, are rare since the advent of antibiotic therapy. *Meningitis* and other suppurative intracranial complications are possible complications of extension of infection from the middle ear or mastoid. However, these complications are uncommon when adequate antibiotic therapy is implemented.

Cholesteatoma is one of the least common but most potentially dangerous sequelae of otitis media with effusion (OME). A cholesteatoma is formed when the keratinizing stratified squamous epithelial cell lining desquamates to form scales that accumulate within the middle ear space.

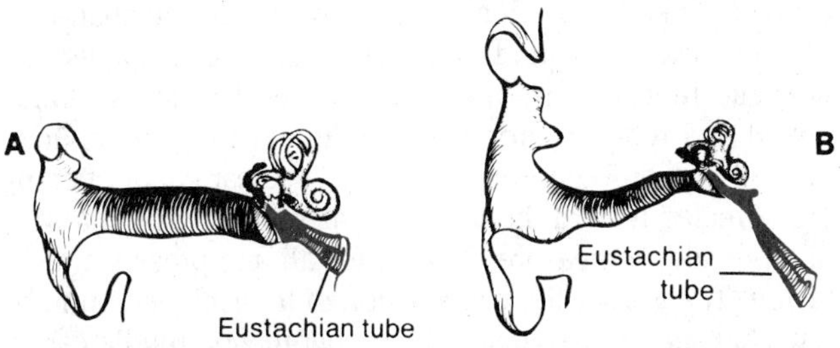

Fig. 32-2. Comparison of anatomic position of eustachian tube in, **A,** child and, **B,** adult.

As it enlarges, the cholesteatoma erodes all the structures it encounters, especially bone, destroying the ossicles and gaining entry to the inner ear and meninges. Clinical signs are a foul-smelling, grayish-yellow discharge, sometimes pain, and permanent progressive hearing loss. Treatment is surgical excision of the entire cholesteatoma.

Clinical Manifestations

As purulent fluid accumulates in the small space of the middle ear chamber, pain results from the pressure on surrounding structures. Infants become irritable and indicate their discomfort by holding or pulling at their ears and rolling their head from side to side. Young children will usually verbally complain of the pain. A temperature as high as 40° C (104° F) is common, and postauricular and cervical lymph glands may be enlarged. Rhinorrhea, vomiting, and diarrhea, as well as signs of concurrent respiratory or pharyngeal infection, may also be present. Loss of appetite is common, and sucking or chewing tends to aggravate the pain. As the exudate accumulates and pressure increases, the tympanic membrane may rupture spontaneously.

✦ **NURSING ALERT** As a result, there is immediate relief of pain, a gradual decrease in temperature, and the presence of purulent discharge in the external auditory canal.

Severe pain or fever is usually absent in OME, and the child may not appear ill. Instead there is a feeling of "fullness" in the ear, a popping sensation during swallowing, and a feeling of "motion" in the ear if air is present above the level of fluid. Since chronic serous otitis media is the most frequent cause of conductive hearing loss in young children, audiometry may reveal deficient hearing.

Diagnostic Evaluation

In AOM otoscopy reveals an intact membrane that appears bright red and bulging, with no visible landmarks or light reflex. The usual landmarks of the bony prominence from the long and the short process of the malleus are obscured by the outwardly bulging membrane. In OME otoscopic findings may include a slightly injected, dull gray membrane, obscured landmarks, and a visible fluid level or meniscus behind the eardrum if air is present above the fluid.

Several tests provide an assessment of mobility of the

tympanic membrane. Pneumatic otoscopy and tympanometry are discussed under Auditory Testing (Chapter 7). Acoustic reflectometry measures the level of sound transmitted and reflected from the middle ear to a microphone located in a probe tip placed against the ear canal opening and directed toward the tympanic membrane. The information provides a measure of canal length and presence of effusion. The greater the cancellation of transmitted sound by reflected sound, the greater the probability of middle ear effusion (Lampe and others, 1985).

Diagnosis is usually based on clinical manifestations, but if purulent discharge is present, it should be cultured and a specific antibiotic chosen for that organism.

Therapeutic Management: Acute Otitis Media

Treatment of AOM is administration of antibiotics, especially ampicillin or amoxicillin. A variety of other antibiotics may be prescribed individually or in combination. With appropriate therapy most children improve within 48 to 72 hours. If not, the child is reexamined and medication altered if indicated.

The usual length of therapy is 10 to 14 days. However, compliance with the recommended schedule is a serious problem. Other measures include the use of analgesic/antipyretic drugs such as acetaminophen (Tylenol) to reduce the pain and/or fever. Oral decongestants, such as pseudoephedrine hydrochloride, may relieve nasal congestion, and antihistamines may provide relief from known or suspected nasal allergy. The efficacy of these drugs in treatment of OM is questioned, but they may provide relief from symptoms of associated upper respiratory infection or allergy. Although they may promote comfort, ear drops are not recommended because they obscure a clear view of the tympanic membrane. Myringotomy (incision of the eardrum) may be required to relieve the symptoms in some children, especially those with acute suppuration who are in severe pain.

Children with AOM should be seen following antibiotic therapy to evaluate the effectiveness of the treatment and to identify potential complications, such as effusion or hearing impairment. Hearing loss may not be noticed by parents but should be determined by audiometric testing. (Screening tests for hearing are discussed in Chapter 7.)

Recurrent otitis media. Children who have recurrent episodes of AOM may require preventive therapy during periods of greatest susceptibility—either immunoprophylaxis with pneumococcal vaccine or chemoprophylaxis with a modified course of an antibiotic agent or combination of antibiotics. Antibacterial prophylaxis has reduced ear infection in children at high risk but can cause toxicity and resistance. The pneumococcal vaccine can reduce the incidence by 50% but currently is not recommended for infants or children under 2 years of age (Klein, 1986).

Children on antibiotic prophylaxis are evaluated once a month to detect any evidence of effusion. Any acute infection during prophylaxis is treated with an alternate antibiotic regimen. If acute episodes are frequent, additional treatment similar to that for OME may be indicated, including myringotomy with insertion of typanostomy tubes to improve middle ear ventilation. The efficacy of these therapies as prophylaxis continues to be a subject of debate.

Therapeutic Management: Otitis Media with Effusion

Many children have fluid that persists in the middle ear for weeks or months, and most have some impairment of hearing. The major goal of therapy is to establish and maintain an aerated middle ear that is free of fluid with a normal mucosa and to achieve normal hearing. The medical management of OME is uncertain and controversial. The widespread use of decongestants and antihistamines to shrink the mucous membranes and increase eustachian tube function is of unproven benefit. Corticosteroids have proved to be of limited value. Occasionally attempts at middle ear inflation by the Valsalva maneuver are successful. Because of the spontaneous improvement in a large percentage of children, one simple method is observation, especially if the child speaks well and has only unilateral involvement.

Surgical management. When medical intervention is unsuccessful in achieving the goals of therapy, surgical intervention may be required. Myringotomy and needle aspiration have been tried with variable degrees of success. Some children benefit from adenoidectomy alone or in combination with tonsillectomy. More often the surgical treatment involves tympanostomy or insertion of ventilating tubes. Mechanical drainage promotes better healing of the membrane and prevents scar formation and loss of elasticity. Tympanostomy tubes (pressure-equalizer [PE] tubes, grommets, or dottles) facilitate continued drainage of fluid and allow ventilation of the middle ear. The objective is to allow the eustachian tube a period of recovery while the tubes perform its functions.

Tympanostomy tubes are usually inserted while the child is under general anesthesia in an outpatient surgical department. The tubes remain in the ear an average of 6 months before being spontaneously rejected. Although an extremely common practice in the United States, the insertion of PE tubes is not without complications and therefore is controversial (Paradise and Rogers, 1986). Some argue that there are no solid data to support the efficacy of the procedure and that the risk of eardrum complications is greater with tubes (Stickler, 1984). Others cite the loss of hearing and risk of delayed speech and language development as sufficient justification for use of tubes (Teele and others, 1984). Additional disadvantages relative to the surgery include the psychologic trauma of surgery, anesthetic risks, and secondary infection (Paradise, 1981). The controversy remains unresolved.

Tubes also tend to become plugged and often require reinsertion. The complications of repeated or long-term tube placement are tympanosclerosis, localized or diffuse atrophy of the membrane, persistent perforation, or, rarely, cholesteatoma.

Nursing Considerations

Since OM is such a common aftermath of URIs, nurses are continually alert to this possibility when caring for a child with such infections.

Assessment

Examination of the external auditory canal is an integral part of the physical assessment (see discussion in Chapter 7). In some instances, nurses perform audiometry and other tests for hearing. Nurses are always alert to any evidence of ear involvement, including detecting manifestations that indicate possible middle ear infection or dysfunction.

Nursing Diagnoses

Based on a thorough assessment, several nursing diagnoses are identified. The more common diagnoses for the child with AOM are included in the Nursing Care Plan on p. 1436. Others may apply in specific situations and in the case of chronic OM or OME.

Planning

Nursing objectives for the child with AOM include the following:

1. Relieve pain.
2. Facilitate drainage when possible.
3. Prevent complications or recurrence.
4. Educate family in care of the child.
5. Provide emotional support to child and family.

Implementation

Analgesics are often very helpful to reduce severe earache. High fever, particularly in infants, should be reduced with antipyretic drugs to avoid febrile convulsions. The application of heat may reduce pain in some children but may aggravate discomfort in others. Local heat should be placed over the ear while the child lies on the affected side. This position also facilitates drainage of the exudate if the eardrum has ruptured or if myringotomy was performed. An ice compress placed over the affected ear may also provide comfort, since it reduces edema and pressure. If the child is cooperative, either procedure can be tried to determine which offers maximum relief.

If the ear is draining, the external canal may be cleansed with sterile cotton swabs or pledgets soaked in hydrogen peroxide. If ear wicks or lightly rolled sterile gauze packs are placed in the ear after surgical treatment, they should be loose enough to allow accumulated drainage to flow out of the ear; otherwise the infection may be transferred to the mastoid process. Parents should be told to keep these wicks dry during shampoos or baths. Occasionally drainage is so profuse that the auricle and skin surrounding the ear become excoriated from exudate. This is prevented by frequent cleansing and application of petrolatum or zinc oxide to the area.

Parents require some anticipatory guidance regarding temporary hearing loss that accompanies OM. For example, they may need to speak louder, at closer proximity, and while facing the child. They are reminded that the child is not ignoring them but is unaware of being spoken to. Persistent difficulty in hearing beyond the acute stage should be evaluated.

Preventing recurrence requires adequate parent education regarding antibiotic therapy. Antibiotics are frequently considered "miracle" drugs or a "one-dose" cure for everything. Since the symptoms of pain and fever usually subside within 24 to 48 hours, the rapid outward signs of recovery support such thinking. Nurses must emphasize that although the child looks well in a couple of days, the infection is not completely eradicated until all of the prescribed medication is taken. At the risk of alarming parents, it is important to stress the potential complications of OM, especially hearing loss, which can be prevented with adequate treatment and follow-up care (see Administration of Medication, Chapter 27, and Compliance, Chapter 27). See also Home Care Instructions: Administration of Medications.*

A concern presented by the use of tympanostomy tubes is the possibility of water entering the middle ear. Several studies indicate that small amounts of water pose little hazard and that even swimming without earplugs or occlusive bathing caps carries no higher risk for an increased incidence of OM (Lounsbury, 1985). However, diving, jumping, and submerging may be forbidden by some physicians. Bath and shampoo water should be kept out of the ear, if possible, since soap reduces the surface tension of water, facilitating entry through the tube. Lake water, as well as bath water, is contaminated; therefore wearing earplugs, although not watertight, prevents total flooding of the external canal and provides sufficient protection. Parents should be aware of the appearance of a grommet (usually a tiny, white plastic, spool-shaped tube) so that they can observe if it falls out. They are reassured that this is normal and requires no immediate intervention.

Parents sometimes ask about preventing ear discomfort in their infants during ascent or descent of an airplane. During ascent, air in the middle ear expands, but decompression takes place through a normal eustachian tube. If the tissues are congested with a URI, the passage of air may be blocked. A nasal-mucosa shrinking spray or oral decongestant before the trip may be helpful. During descent, the air within the middle ear decreases as atmospheric pressure increases. Swallowing is the simplest and most effective method for inflating the middle ear on descent; therefore feeding or offering a pacifier to infants during descent is beneficial.

Reducing the chances of otitis media is possible with some simple measures, such as sitting or holding an infant upright for feedings. Forceful nose blowing during a URI is discouraged. Any evidence of hearing impairment should be investigated. Early detection of possible middle ear effusion is a primary nursing goal in prevention of complications. Infants and preschool children should be screened for effusion, and all school children, especially those with learning disabilities, should be tested for middle ear effusion. Frequent audiologic evaluations, medical consulta-

*In Wong, D.L., and Whaley, L.F.: Clinical manual of pediatric nursing, ed. 3, St. Louis, 1990, Mosby–Year Book, Inc.

NURSING CARE PLAN
The Child with Acute Otitis Media

NURSING DIAGNOSIS: Pain related to pressure caused by inflammatory process

GOAL 1
Relieve pain

INTERVENTIONS
Position for comfort according to needs of individual child
Apply external heat (with heating pad on low setting) or cool compresses
Avoid chewing by offering liquid or soft foods
Position with affected ear in dependent position; have child lie on affected side
*Administer analgesics

EXPECTED OUTCOME
Child sleeps and rests quietly and exhibits no signs of discomfort

NURSING DIAGNOSIS: Potential for infection/injury related to inadequate treatment, presence of infective organisms

GOAL 1
Prevent reinfection

INTERVENTIONS
Emphasize the importance of following instructions, especially regarding administration of antibiotics
- Maintain regularity of administration
- Complete the course of therapy

Employ simple preventive practices such as
- Sit or hold child upright for feedings
- Promote aeration of middle ear
  - Encourage gentle nose blowing
  - Employ the modified Valsalva maneuver, i.e., pinch the nose, close the lips, and force air up the eustachian tube
  - Use blowing games
  - Chew gum
- Eliminate tobacco smoke and known allergens from child's environment

EXPECTED OUTCOMES
Child remains free of infection
Family complies with directives (specify)

GOAL 2
Prevent complications (especially hearing loss)

INTERVENTIONS
See above
Stress importance of follow-up care
Stress importance of regular hearing tests to assess early signs of impairment
Teach parents to recognize signs of hearing impairment in the infant or child (see Chapter 25)
Avoid excessive water in ear if polyethylene tubes or myringotomy was part of the therapy

EXPECTED OUTCOME
Child remains free of complications

NURSING DIAGNOSIS: Altered family processes related to a child with an infection

GOAL 1
Support family

INTERVENTION
Prepare family for surgical procedure, if appropriate (insertion of pressure equalizer tubes)

EXPECTED OUTCOME
Family demonstrates an understanding of procedure

GOAL 2
Prepare family for discharge and home care

INTERVENTIONS
Cleanse external meatus of draining ear with sterile cotton swabs or pledgets soaked in sterile normal saline
Avoid water from baths or shampoo from dampening wicks, if inserted to facilitate drainage after surgery
Prevent contaminated water (from baths, swimming pools, fresh-water lakes) from entering the external ear
- Suggest use of a good earplug

Notify health professional if grommet (tiny, white plastic spool-shaped tube) falls out of the ear canal
- No immediate intervention needed

EXPECTED OUTCOME
Child recovers from infection and/or surgery without complications

See also:
Nursing Care Plan: The Child in the Hospital, Chapter 26
Nursing Care Plan: The Family of the Ill or Hospitalized Child, Chapter 26

*Dependent or independent nursing function.

tion, and education of parents and children are advised when middle ear effusion is detected.

Evaluation

The effectiveness of nursing interventions is determined by continual reassessment and evaluation of care based on the following observational guidelines and expected outcomes:

1. Observe behaviors that indicate pain relief (see Chapter 26); seek verbal confirmation.
2. Observe skin in and around external auditory canal.
3. Interview family regarding practices that prevent recurrence of infection, especially instructions regarding administration of prescribed medications.
4. Observe and interview family regarding their understanding of OM and therapies.
5. Interview family regarding their feelings and concerns.

Expected outcomes:
See Nursing Care Plan, p. 1436.

OTITIS EXTERNA

Infections of the external ear may result from normal ear flora (*Staphylococcus epidermidis* and *Corynebacterium,* primarily) that assume pathogenic characteristics under conditions of excessive wetness or dryness. Ordinarily the external ear canal is protected by a waxy, water-repellent coating composed of highly viscid secretions of the sebaceous glands and the watery, pigmented secretions of apocrine glands in combination with exfoliated surface cells. Inflammation occurs when this environment is altered by swimming, bathing, or increased environmental humidity *(swimmer's ear);* by infection, dermatoses, or insufficient cerumen; or by trauma from a foreign body or a finger.

Secondary invasion of foreign pathogens also occurs. In addition to the resident flora, the offending agents can be *Pseudomonas aeruginosa* (most commonly), *Enterobacter aerogenes, Proteus mirabilis, Klebsiella pneumoniae,* streptococci, and fungi such as *Candida* and *Aspergillus.* The ear canal becomes irritated, and maceration takes place.

The predominant symptom of external ear infection is ear pain accentuated by manipulation of the pinna, especially pressure on the tragus. The pain often appears to be out of proportion to the degree of inflammation. Conductive hearing loss may be present as a result of the edema, secretions, and accumulation of debris within the canal. Edema, erythema, and a cheesy green-blue-gray discharge and tenderness appear as the infection progresses. The external canal may be so tender and swollen that visualization is difficult. There may be fever. In advanced cases the pain is intense, constant, and aggravated by jaw motion or ear manipulation.

Therapeutic objectives include relief of pain, edema, and itching and restoration of normal flora, cerumen, and canal epithelium. Analgesics are prescribed for pain. Debris is removed with gentle suction and wisps of cotton on metal cotton carriers. Otic preparations containing neomycin with either colistin or polymyxin and corticosteroids are instilled in the canal. A gauze wick is usually inserted to facilitate the medication reaching the site of inflammation. The wick is removed after swelling and pain have subsided, but the drops are continued for at least 3 days after relief of pain. The best management for external ear inflammation is prevention.

> **NURSING TIP: KEEPING THE EAR DRY**
>
> Pull the auricle up and out to straighten the canal, then use a conventional hair dryer, held at a distance of 18 to 24 inches for 30 seconds, three times a day (Hands, 1987).

Nursing Considerations

Nurses can teach parents or patients to apply simple measures to prevent recurrent infections. Children are advised to limit their stay in the water to less than an hour, if possible, and ears should dry completely (1 to 2 hours) before children enter the water again. Shaking the head and judicious use of the corner of a towel can remove most excess water. The ear canal can also be dried with a small tuft of cotton (not a swab). Placing a combination of white vinegar and rubbing alcohol (50/50) in both ear canals upon arising, at bedtime, and at the end of each swim (the most common cause of otitis externa) is effective in preventing recurrence. The solution must remain in the canal for 5 minutes (Marcy, 1989). Youngsters are cautioned not to pick at the ears with a pencil, cotton swab, bobby pin, or other object, which can injure or infect the ear canal.

CROUP SYNDROMES

Croup is a general term applied to a symptom complex characterized by hoarseness, a resonant cough described as "barking" or "brassy" (croupy), varying degrees of inspiratory stridor, and varying degrees of respiratory distress resulting from swelling or obstruction in the region of the larynx. Acute infections of the larynx are of greater importance in infants and small children than they are in older children, in part because of the increased incidence in children in this age-group and the smaller diameter of the airway, which renders it subject to significantly greater narrowing with the same degree of inflammation (Fig. 32-3).

Acute respiratory infections of the nonreactive airway involve all areas to some extent and are seldom restricted to one area. Croup syndromes affect to varying degrees the larynx, trachea, and bronchi. However, laryngeal involvement often dominates the clinical picture because of the severe effects on the voice and breathing. Croup syndromes are usually described according to the primary anatomic area affected, that is, epiglottitis (or supraglottitis), laryngitis, laryngotracheobronchitis (LTB), and tracheitis. In general, LTB tends to occur in very young children, whereas epiglot-

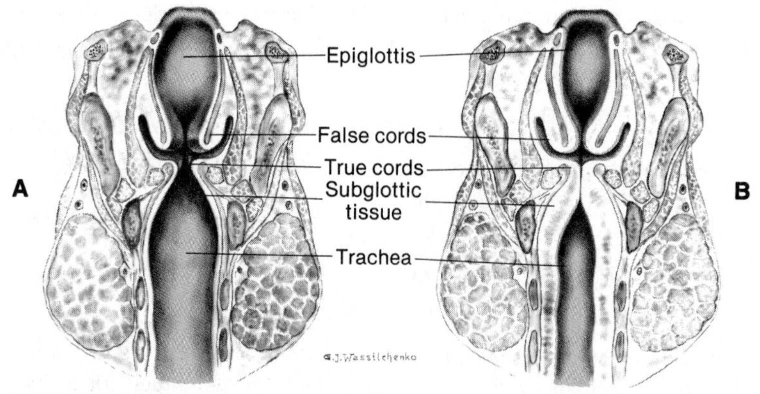

Fig. 32-3. **A,** Normal larynx. **B,** Obstruction and narrowing resulting from edema of croup.

Table 32-1 Comparison of croup syndromes

	ACUTE EPIGLOTTITIS (SUPRAGLOTTITIS)	ACUTE LARYNGO-TRACHEOBRONCHITIS	ACUTE SPASMODIC LARYNGITIS (SPASMODIC CROUP)	ACUTE TRACHEITIS
Age-group affected	1-8 years	3 months–8 years	3 months–3 years	1 month–6 years
Etiologic agent	Bacterial, usually *H. influenzae*	Viral	Viral with allergic component	Bacterial, usually *S. aureus*
Onset	Rapidly progressive	Slowly progressive	Sudden; at night	Moderately progressive
Major symptoms	Dysphagia Stridor aggravated when supine Drooling High fever Toxic Rapid pulse and respirations	URI Stridor Brassy cough Hoarseness Dyspnea Restlessness Irritability Low-grade fever Nontoxic	URI Croupy cough Stridor Hoarseness Dyspnea Restlessness Symptoms waken child Symptoms disappear during day Tends to recur	URI Croupy cough Stridor Purulent secretions High fever No response to LTB therapy
Treatment	Antibiotics Airway protection	Humidity Racemic epinephrine	Humidity	Antibiotics

titis is more characteristic of older children (see Table 32-1 for a comparison of croup syndromes).

ACUTE EPIGLOTTITIS

Acute epiglottitis, or acute supraglottitis, is a serious obstructive inflammatory process that occurs principally in children between 3 and 7 years of age, but can occur from infancy to adulthood. The disorder requires immediate attention. The obstruction is supraglottic as opposed to the subglottic obstruction of laryngitis. The responsible organism is usually *H. influenzae;* LTB and epiglottitis do not occur together.

Clinical Manifestations

The onset of epiglottitis is abrupt and rapidly progressive to severe respiratory distress. The child usually goes to bed asymptomatic to awaken later complaining of sore throat and pain on swallowing. The child has a fever, appears toxic out of proportion to the clinical findings, and presents a classic picture; the child generally insists on sitting upright, leaning forward, with chin thrust out, mouth open, and tongue protruding (tripod position). Drooling of saliva is common because of the difficulty or pain on swallowing and excessive secretions.

✦ **NURSING ALERT** Three clinical observations that have been found to be predictive of epiglottitis are absence of spontaneous cough, presence of drooling, and agitation (Mauro and others, 1988).

The child is irritable and markedly restless, and has an anxious, apprehensive, and frightened expression. The voice is thick and muffled, with a froglike croaking sound on inspiration. The child is not hoarse. Suprasternal and substernal retractions may be visible. The child seldom struggles to breathe, and slow quiet breathing provides better air exchange. The sallow color of mild hypoxia may progress to frank cyanosis. The throat is red and inflamed, and a distinctive large, cherry-red, edematous epiglottis is visible on careful throat inspection. *Throat inspection should be attempted only when immediate intubation can be performed if needed.*

Therapeutic Management

The course of epiglottitis may be fulminant, with respiratory obstruction appearing suddenly. Progressive obstruction leads to hypoxia, hypercapnia, and acidosis followed by decreased muscular tone, reduced level of consciousness, and, when obstruction becomes more or less complete, a rather sudden death. A presumptive diagnosis of epiglottitis constitutes an emergency.

The child suspected of epiglottitis should be examined where facilities are available for coping with this type of emergency. The child is best transported while sitting in a parent's lap to reduce distress. Examination of the throat with a tongue depressor is contraindicated until properly experienced personnel and equipment are at hand to proceed with immediate intubation or tracheostomy in the event that the examination precipitates further or complete obstruction.

If a lateral neck film is indicated, the same experienced personnel should accompany the child to the radiology department. However, most practitioners prefer that the child not be transported but remain on the parent's lap in the examination area during portable radiology.

Endotracheal intubation or tracheostomy is usually considered for *H. influenzae* epiglottitis with severe respiratory distress. It is recommended that the intubation or tracheostomy and any invasive procedure, such as starting an intravenous infusion, be performed in the operating room. Whether or not there is an artificial airway, the child requires intensive observation by experienced personnel. The epiglottal swelling usually decreases after 24 hours of antibiotic therapy, and the epiglottis is near normal by the third day. Intubated children are generally extubated at this time.

Children with suspected bacterial epiglottitis are given antibiotics intravenously, followed by oral administration to complete a 7- to 10-day course. The use of corticosteroids for reducing edema is controversial but may be beneficial during the early hours of treatment. Most intubated children will have had a course of corticosteroids for 24 hours before extubation.

Prevention. The American Academy of Pediatrics, Committee on Infectious Diseases (1990) recommends that all children beginning at 2 months of age receive the *Haemophilus influenzae* type B conjugate vaccine. As administration of the vaccine becomes a routine part of the regular immunization schedule, a decline in the incidence of epiglottitis can be anticipated. (See also Immunizations, Chapter 12.)

Nursing Considerations

Epiglottitis is a serious and frightening disease for child, family, and health professionals. It is important to act quickly but calmly and provide support without unduly increasing anxiety. The child is allowed to remain in the position that provides the most comfort and security, and parents are reassured that everything possible is being done to obtain relief for their child.

✦ **NURSING ALERT** Nurses who suspect epiglottitis should not attempt to visualize the epiglottis directly with a tongue depressor or take a throat culture but should refer the child to a physician immediately.

Acute care of the child is that described for the child with acute respiratory distress and artificial airways in Chapter 31. Continuous monitoring of respiratory status, including blood gases, is part of nursing observations, and the intravenous infusion is maintained as described in Chapter 28.

ACUTE LARYNGITIS

Acute infectious laryngitis is a common illness in older children and adolescents. Infants and smaller children experience more generalized involvement (see following section on laryngotracheobronchitis). Viruses are the usual causative agents and the principal complaint is hoarseness, which may be accompanied by other upper respiratory symptoms (e.g., coryza, sore throat, nasal congestion) and systemic manifestations (e.g., fever, headache, myalgia, malaise). Associated complaints vary with the infecting virus. For example, adenoviruses and influenza viruses are responsible for more systemic involvement; parainfluenza viruses, rhinoviruses, and respiratory syncytial virus (RSV) cause more mild illness (Wald, 1990).

Therapeutic Management and Nursing Considerations

The disease is almost always self-limited without long-term sequelae. Treatment is symptomatic with fluids and humidified air (see Nursing Care Plan on p. 1421).

ACUTE LARYNGOTRACHEOBRONCHITIS

Viral laryngotracheobronchitis (LTB) (viral croup) is the most common of the croup syndromes and primarily affects children less than 5 years of age. Organisms usually responsible for LTB are the parainfluenza viruses. The disease is usually preceded by an upper respiratory infection, which gradually descends to adjacent structures. It is characterized by gradual onset of low-grade fever.

Inflammation of the mucosa lining the larynx and trachea causes a narrowing of the airway. When the airway is

Box 32-6 PROGRESSION OF SYMPTOMS IN LARYNGOTRACHEOBRONCHITIS

Stage I
Fear
Hoarseness
Croupy cough
Inspiratory stridor when disturbed

Stage II
Continuous respiratory stridor
Lower rib retraction
Retraction of soft tissue of neck
Use of accessory muscles of respiration
Labored respiration

Stage III
Signs of anoxia and carbon dioxide retention
Restlessness
Anxiety
Pallor
Sweating
Rapid respiration

Stage IV
Intermittent cyanosis
Permanent cyanosis
Cessation of breathing

As described by Forbes from Krugman, S., and others: Infectious diseases of children, St. Louis, 1985, Mosby–Year Book, Inc., p. 275.

significantly narrowed, the child struggles to inhale air past the obstruction and into the lungs, producing the characteristic inspiratory stridor and suprasternal retractions. When the child is unable to inhale a sufficient volume of air, symptoms of hypoxia become evident. As the work of forcing air past the obstruction increases, negative pressure generated in the thoracic cavity also increases, leading to leakage of pulmonary vascular fluid into interstitial spaces and causing uneven ventilation and hypoxia (Battaglia, 1986). Obstruction severe enough to prevent adequate exhalation of carbon dioxide causes respiratory acidosis, and, eventually, the child experiences respiratory failure. (See progression of symptoms outlined in Box 32-6.)

Therapeutic Management

The major objective in medical management of infectious LTB is maintaining an airway and providing for adequate respiratory exchange. Children with mild croup (no stridor at rest) are managed at home. Parents are taught the signs of respiratory distress so that professional help can be summoned early if needed. Children who progress to stage II respiratory symptoms should receive medical attention, usually with hospitalization.

High humidity with cool mist provides relief for most children. A cool air vaporizer or a steamy bathroom can be used at home. In the hospital setting, huts for infants or mist tents for toddlers are sometimes used to provide increased humidity and supplemental oxygen.

For moderately severe croup aerosolized racemic epinephrine causes vasoconstriction and reduces swelling of the airway. Because the effects of epinephrine are temporary, airway obstruction can return to its original severity in a few hours (Battaglia, 1986). For this reason, the drug should not be used for outpatient therapy, and children receiving it are monitored continuously. With widespread use of the medication, the incidence of intubation and tracheostomy has decreased markedly. Intubation of the airway is performed only if no other method of preventing respiratory collapse is available.

If intubation is required, the procedure should be performed in a controlled environment (preferably the operating room), and the swollen airway necessitates a smaller than normal endotracheal (ET) tube. When the swelling begins to subside, an air leak usually forms around the ET tube, indicating that the obstruction has reversed and extubation can be attempted.

The use of corticosteroids for acute LTB is still controversial, but several research studies support the practice (Kairys, Olmstead, and O'Connor, 1989; Super and others, 1989). Antibiotics are not indicated unless a bacterial infection is detected.

Maintaining hydration may require intravenous fluid therapy. Distressed children may not take a sufficient amount of fluid. Children with severe respiratory distress should be kept NPO to prevent aspiration in the event that intubation becomes necessary. Also, very rapid respiration predisposes to aspiration.

Nursing Considerations

The most important nursing function in the care of children with croup is continuous, vigilant observation and accurate assessment of respiratory status. Cardiac, respiratory, and noninvasive blood gas monitoring equipment supplement visual observations. Changes in therapy are frequently based on nurses' observations and assessment of a child's status, response to therapy, and tolerance of procedures. The trend away from early intubation of children with LTB emphasizes the importance of nursing observation and the ability to recognize impending respiratory failure so that intubation can be implemented without delay. Intubation equipment should be readily accessible and taken with the child during transport to other areas (e.g., radiology, operating room).

NURSING ALERT Early signs of impending airway obstruction include increased pulse and respiratory rate; substernal, suprasternal, and intercostal retractions; flaring nares; and increased restlessness.

To conserve energy, children are given every opportunity to rest. Infants or small children find that being enclosed within a mist tent, coughing, laryngeal spasms, and restraint for intravenous therapy are additional sources of distress. Infants and small children prefer sitting upright, and most want to be held. Children need the security of the parent's presence. Since crying increases respiratory distress and hypoxia, a child's individual tolerance for these therapies must be assessed. An extremely fussy child may do better when held in the parent's lap with cool mist directed toward the child's face.

The rapid progression of croup, the alarming sound of the cough and stridor, and the child's apprehensive behavior and ill appearance combine to create a very frightening experience for the parents. They need reassurance regarding the child's progress and an explanation of treatments. They may feel guilty for not having suspected the seriousness of the condition sooner. The family should be allowed to remain with their child as much as possible, especially when this decreases the child's distress.

The nurse can provide them with an opportunity to express their feelings, thus minimizing any blame or guilt. They need frequent reassurance provided in a calm, quiet manner and education regarding what they can do to make their child more comfortable. Fortunately, as the crisis subsides and the child responds to therapy, breathing becomes easier and recovery is generally prompt. Home care after discharge includes continued humidity, adequate hydration, and nourishment. Parents are encouraged to ask questions about home care and preparation for discharge. Referral to a public health agency for follow-up care may be advisable.

ACUTE SPASMODIC LARYNGITIS

Acute spasmodic laryngitis (spasmodic croup) is distinct from laryngitis and LTB and characterized by paroxysmal attacks of laryngeal obstruction that occur chiefly at night. Signs of inflammation are absent or mild, and there is frequently a history of previous attacks lasting for 2 to 5 days followed by uneventful recovery. It usually affects children ages 1 to 3 years. Some children appear to be predisposed to the condition; allergy and psychogenic factors are implicated in some cases.

The child goes to bed well or with some very mild respiratory symptoms but awakes suddenly with characteristic barking, metallic cough, hoarseness, noisy inspirations, and restlessness. The child appears anxious, frightened, and prostrated. Dyspnea is aggravated by excitement; but there is no fever, the attack subsides in a few hours, and the child appears well the next day.

Therapeutic Management and Nursing Considerations

Children with spasmodic croup are managed at home. Cool mist is recommended for the child's room. Warm mist provided by steam from hot running water in a closed bathroom may be helpful. Sometimes the spasm is relieved by sudden exposure to cold air (as when the child is taken out into the night air to see the physician). Parents are usually advised to have the child sleep in humidified air until the cough has subsided so that subsequent episodes may be prevented. Children with moderately severe symptoms may be hospitalized for observation and therapy with cool mist and racemic epinephrine as for LTB. Patients may respond to corticosteroid therapy. The disease is usually self-limited.

BACTERIAL TRACHEITIS

Bacterial tracheitis, an infection of the mucosa of the upper trachea, is a distinct entity with features of both croup and epiglottitis. The disease is seen in children ages 1 month to 6 years and may be a serious cause of airway obstruction—severe enough to cause respiratory arrest. It is believed to be a complication of LTB, and although *Staphylococcus aureus* is the most frequent organism responsible, group A β-hemolytic streptococci and *H. influenzae* have also been implicated.

Many of the manifestations of bacterial tracheitis are similar to those of LTB but are unresponsive to LTB therapy. There is a history of previous upper respiratory infection with croupy cough, stridor unaffected by position, toxicity, and high fever. A prominent manifestation is the production of thick, purulent tracheal secretions. Respiratory difficulties are secondary to these copious secretions.

Therapeutic Management and Nursing Considerations

Bacterial tracheitis requires vigorous management. Humidified oxygen, antipyretics, and antibiotics are prescribed. Most children require endotracheal intubation and frequent tracheal suctioning to prevent airway obstruction. The emphasis in this disorder is early recognition in order to prevent catastrophic airway obstruction.

■ INFECTIONS OF THE LOWER AIRWAYS

The reactive portion of the lower respiratory tract includes the bronchi and bronchioles in children. Cartilaginous support of the large airway is not fully developed until adolescence. Consequently, the smooth muscle in these structures represents a major factor in the constriction of the airway, particularly in the bronchioles, that portion that extends from the bronchi to the alveoli.

The infectious disorders involving the reactive portion of the airway are diverse in nature and etiology. Inflammation of the bronchi (bronchitis) as an isolated clinical entity is uncommon in childhood, if it exists at all. Bronchial inflammation is usually seen as tracheobronchitis or laryngotracheobronchitis. Infection of the bronchioles (bronchiolitis, or capillary bronchitis) is an entirely different illness that is more closely related to interstitial pneumonia. Table 32-2 compares some of the major features of bronchial and bronchiolar infections. The major portion of the following discussion is focused on bronchiolitis.

BRONCHITIS

Bronchitis (sometimes referred to as tracheobronchitis) describes inflammation of large airways (trachea and bron-

Table 32-2 Comparison of conditions affecting the bronchi

	VIRAL-INDUCED ASTHMA*	BRONCHITIS	BRONCHIOLITIS
Description	Exaggerated response of bronchi to infection Bronchospasm, exudation, and edema of bronchi	Usually occurs in association with URI Seldom an isolated entity	A more common infectious disease of lower airways Maximum obstructive impact at bronchiolar level
Age-group affected	Late infancy and early childhood	Affects children in first 4 years of life	Usually children 2-12 months; rare after age 2 Peak incidence approximately age 6 months
Etiologic agents	Most commonly viruses but may be any of a variety of URI pathogens	Usually viral Other agents (e.g., bacteria, fungi, allergic disorders, airborne irritants) can trigger symptoms	Viruses, predominantly respiratory syncytial viruses; also adenoviruses, parainfluenza viruses, and *M. pneumoniae*
Predominant characteristics	Wheezing, productive cough	Persistent dry, hacking cough (worse at night) becoming productive in 2-3 days	Dyspnea, paroxysmal nonproductive cough, tachypnea with retractions and flaring nares, emphysema, may be wheezing
Treatment	Bronchodilators	Cough suppressants if needed	Oxygen mist Ribavirin if severe

*See Bronchial Asthma, p. 1458.

chi), which is almost invariably associated with an upper respiratory infection. Viral agents are the primary cause of the disease, although *M. pneumoniae* is a common cause in children older than 6 years of age. The condition is characterized by a dry, hacking, and nonproductive cough that is worse at night and becomes productive in 2 to 3 days.

Bronchitis is a mild self-limiting disease that requires only symptomatic treatment, including analgesics, antipyretics, and humidity. Cough suppressants may be useful to allow rest but can interfere with cough clearance of secretions (Neddenriep, Taussig, and Mietens, 1989). Most patients recover uneventfully in 5 to 10 days.

BRONCHIOLITIS

Bronchiolitis is an acute viral infection with maximum effect at the bronchiolar level. The infection occurs primarily in winter and spring and is rare in children over 2 years of age. Although few children with bronchiolitis require hospitalization, it can be a serious disease (McIntosh, 1987). Respiratory syncytial virus (RSV) is responsible for over half of all episodes of bronchiolitis (80% during epidemics) (Guerra, Kemp, and Shearer, 1990; Neddenriep, Taussig, and Mietens, 1989). Adenoviruses and parainfluenza viruses may also cause acute bronchiolitis. The virus becomes epidemic in communities during the late fall and winter months and is easily spread by hand-to-nose transmission.

Pathophysiology

Bronchiole mucosa is swollen, and lumina are filled with mucus and exudate; the walls of the bronchi and bronchioles are infiltrated with inflammatory cells; and peribronchiolar interstitial pneumonitis is usually present. The variable degrees of obstruction produced in small air passages by these changes lead to hyperinflation, obstructive emphysema resulting from partial obstruction, and patchy areas of atelectasis. Dilation of bronchial passages on inspiration allows sufficient space for intake of air, but narrowing of the passages on expiration prevents air from leaving the lungs. Thus air is trapped distal to the obstruction and causes progressive overinflation *(emphysema)*.

Clinical Manifestations

Bronchiolitis begins as a simple upper respiratory infection with serous nasal discharge that may be accompanied by mild fever. The child gradually develops increasing respiratory distress with tachypnea, paroxysmal cough, and irritability. There may be wheezing. Chest radiographs show hyperaeration and areas of consolidation that are difficult to differentiate from bacterial pneumonia. Children may have considerable dyspnea, but do not have the toxic appearance of children with bacterial infections (McIntosh, 1987).

The chest may appear barrel shaped from overinflation, and respiratory excursions are usually shallow and rapid, with flaring nares and suprasternal and subcostal retractions. This in turn causes increased alveolar oxygen tension (PA_{O_2}). Apnea may be the first recognized indicator of RSV infection in very young infants.

Severe disease may be followed by a rise in arterial carbon dioxide tension (Pa_{CO_2}) (hypercapnia), leading to respiratory acidosis. Hypoxemia may persist for 4 to 6 weeks after the peak of the illness, during which time auscultation reveals fine rales, diminished breath sounds, hyperresonance, scattered consolidation, and a prolonged expiratory phase. There may be wheezing.

Diagnostic Evaluation

Diagnosis of bronchiolitis is made on the basis of clinical findings, child's age, season, and epidemiology of the community. Positive identification of RSV is accomplished by enzyme-linked immunosorbent assay (ELISA) from direct aspiration of nasal secretions or nasopharyngeal washings.

The most difficult distinction to make in infants is between bronchiolitis and intrinsic reactive airway disease or asthma. Diagnosis of asthma is favored in repeat attacks, where there is a history of atopy, and if the child responds favorably to administration of bronchodilators. Cystic fibrosis often manifests as repeated bouts of bronchiolitis (see p. 1470). Chest radiotherapy helps rule out pneumonia.

Therapeutic Management

Bronchiolitis is treated symptomatically with high humidity, adequate fluid intake, and rest. The majority of children with bronchiolitis can be managed at home; but hospitalization is usually recommended for children with complicating conditions, such as underlying lung or heart disease, associated debilitated states, or questionable adequacy of caregiver. The child should also be admitted who is tachypneic, has marked retractions, seems listless, or has a history of poor fluid intake (Guerra, Kemp, and Shearer, 1990). Mist therapy is generally combined with oxygen by hood or tent in concentrations sufficient to alleviate dyspnea and hypoxia, after which mist alone is continued for mild dyspnea. Fluids by mouth may be contraindicated because of tachypnea, weakness, and fatigue; therefore intravenous fluids are preferred until the crisis of the disease has passed.

Clinical assessments, noninvasive oxygen monitoring, and blood gas values guide therapy. Medical therapy for bronchiolitis is controversial. Bronchodilators, corticosteroids, cough suppressants, and antibiotics have not proved to be effective in uncomplicated disease and are not recommended for routine use. Corticosteroids, theophylline, and furosemide have all been used for intubated and ventilated infants and children.

Ribavirin, an antiviral agent recently approved for aerosol, is the first specific therapy available for RSV infection. The drug is delivered via hood, tent, or mask; and children receiving the drug for lower respiratory tract involvement have demonstrated improvement (Conrad and others, 1987; Rodriguez and others, 1987). Other investigators question the unclear evidence of benefit from the drug (Ray, 1988; Wald, Dashefsky, and Green, 1988) and cite potential toxic effects to health care workers from its use (Guglielmo, Jacobs, and Locksley, 1989). Teratogenic effects have been reported in laboratory animals. The Committee on Infectious Diseases of the American Academy of Pediatrics (1987) recommends that ribavirin aerosol be administered to:

1. Infants at high risk for severe or complicated RSV infection (i.e., infants with congenital heart disease, bronchopulmonary dysplasia and other chronic lung disease, some premature infants, children with immunodeficiency, recent transplant recipients, and those undergoing chemotherapy for malignancy)
2. Infants hospitalized with RSV lower respiratory tract disease who are severely ill
3. Infants hospitalized with lower respiratory tract disease that is not initially severe, but who may be at some increased risk of progressing to a more complicated course (e.g., less than 6 months of age or those in whom prolonged illness might be particularly detrimental, such as multiple congenital anomalies, neurologic or metabolic disease)

Prognosis. The disease lasts about 3 to 10 days, and the prognosis is generally good. Although most infants with RSV bronchiolitis appear to recover completely, severe disease is associated with recurrent pulmonary infection and bronchospasm. Infants with preexisting cardiopulmonary disease have an increased incidence of death related to RSV infection.

Nursing Considerations

The child is placed in a bed away from others, frequently in a small, segregated area used only for children with respiratory infections. Ideally, a cohort system of nurses should be assigned to these children with responsibility for no other children. Because RSV has been found to be readily transmitted by close contact with hospital personnel, families, and other children by both direct contact (especially cuddling) and fomites (particularly hard, smooth surfaces), precautions against cross-infection are especially important. Up to 50% of family contacts acquire the infection (Wright, 1986). The primary routes of inoculation for the organisms are the nose and eyes; therefore infection control should stress handwashing of all persons caring for affected children and keeping their hands away from faces (see Infection Control, Chapter 27). Disposable plastic goggles are suggested for personnel caring for these children (Agah and others, 1987; Gala and others, 1986). Because of the potential teratogenicity, pregnant female personnel or visitors should be advised of this risk (Centers for Disease Control, 1988).

PNEUMONIA

Pneumonia, inflammation of the pulmonary parenchyma, is common in childhood but occurs more frequently in infancy and early childhood. Pneumonias can be classified according to morphology, etiologic agent, and clinical forms. Clinically pneumonia may occur either as a primary disease or as a complication of some other illness. Morphologically pneumonias are recognized as lobar pneumonia, bronchopneumonia, and interstitial pneumonia (Box 32-7). Other terms that describe pneumonias are hemorrhagic, fibrinous, and necrotizing. *Pneumonitis* is a localized acute inflammation of the lung without the toxemia associated with lobar pneumonia.

The most useful classification of pneumonia is based on the etiologic agent. In general, pneumonia is caused by four etiologic processes: viruses, bacteria, mycoplasmas, and aspiration of foreign substances. Less often pneumonia may be caused by histomycosis, coccidioidomycosis, and other fungi. The clinical manifestations of pneumonia vary greatly

Box 32-7 TYPES OF PNEUMONIA

Lobar pneumonia—all or a large segment of one or more pulmonary lobes is involved. When both lungs are affected, it is known as bilateral or "double" pneumonia.

Bronchopneumonia—begins in the terminal bronchioles, which become clogged with mucopurulent exudate to form consolidated patches in nearby lobules; also called lobular pneumonia.

Interstitial pneumonia—the inflammatory process is more or less confined within the alveolar walls (interstitium) and the peribronchial and interlobular tissues.

depending on the etiologic agent, the age of the child, the child's systemic reaction to the infection, the extent of the lesions, and the degree of bronchial and bronchiolar obstruction. The etiologic agent is identified largely from the clinical history, the child's age, the general health history, the physical examination, radiography, and the laboratory examination.

VIRAL PNEUMONIA

Viral pneumonias occur more frequently than bacterial pneumonia and are seen in children in all age-groups. They are often associated with viral upper respiratory infections, and the pathologic changes involve interstitial pneumonitis with inflammation of the mucosa and the walls of bronchi and bronchioles. Of the many viruses that produce pneumonia in children, RSV accounts for the largest percentage. Others are the influenza virus, parainfluenza virus, psittacosis, rhinovirus, and adenovirus. There are few clinical symptoms to distinguish between the responsible organisms, and differentiations between viruses can be made only by laboratory examination.

Clinical Manifestations

The onset may be acute or insidious, and symptoms are variable, ranging from mild fever, slight cough, and malaise to high fever, severe cough, and prostration. Early in the course of the illness the cough is likely to be unproductive or productive of small amounts of whitish sputum. Breath sounds may include a few rhonchi or fine crackles. Radiography reveals diffuse or patchy infiltration with a peribronchial distribution.

Therapeutic Management and Nursing Considerations

The prognosis is generally good, although viral infections of the respiratory tract render the affected child more susceptible to secondary bacterial invasion. Treatment is usually symptomatic. Although some authorities recommend antimicrobial therapy in hope of reducing or preventing secondary bacterial infection, it is usually reserved for cases in which the presence of such infection is demonstrated by appropriate cultures.

PRIMARY ATYPICAL PNEUMONIA

M. pneumoniae is the most common cause of pneumonia in children between the ages of 5 and 12 years of age (Moffet, 1989). It occurs principally in fall and winter months and is more prevalent in crowded living conditions.

Clinical Manifestations

The onset may be sudden or insidious and is usually manifest first by general systemic symptoms, including fever, chills (in older children), headache, malaise, anorexia, and muscle pain (myalgia). These symptoms are followed by rhinitis, sore throat, and a dry, hacking cough. The cough, initially nonproductive, produces seromucoid sputum that later becomes mucopurulent or blood streaked. The duration and degree of fever vary widely and may last from several days to 2 weeks. Dyspnea is uncommon.

Radiographic examination reveals evidence of pneumonia before physical signs are apparent. There may be fine crepitant crackles over various areas of the lung fields, but consolidation is usually not demonstrated. The pathologic process consists of interstitial round cell infiltration and edema of alveolar septa and varying distribution of areas of inflammation, necrosis, and ulceration of the mucosal lining of bronchi and bronchioles. Areas of consolidation and emphysema are present.

Therapeutic Management and Nursing Considerations

Most affected persons recover from acute illness in 7 to 10 days with symptomatic treatment, followed by a week of convalescence. Hospitalization is rarely necessary.

BACTERIAL PNEUMONIA

Virtually every type of microorganism produces pneumonia. In all age-groups viruses represent the single most frequent cause—RSV in infants and parainfluenza viruses, influenza viruses, and adenoviruses in older children (Eichenwald and Mietens, 1989).

Etiology and Epidemiology

Etiology of pneumonia varies with the age of the child. *S. pneumoniae* (pneumococcus), group A streptococcus, staphylococcus, or enteric bacilli are the most likely agents in infants under 3 months of age. Chlamydial infection is also a cause of pneumonia in this age-group. In the 3-month to 5-year age-group, pneumococcal infection and *H. influenzae* type b are common causes. Pneumococcus accounts for 90% of all bacterial infections in children over age 5 years (Rao, 1988).

Clinical Manifestations

Clinical manifestations of bacterial pneumonia in normal children usually appear acutely with fever and toxic appearance. Older children may complain of headache, abdominal pain, or chest pain. Respiratory distress may or may not be present. Initially cough is usually hacking and nonproductive, and breath sounds are diminished or heard as scattered crackles. When consolidation is present, breath sounds may be tubular in quality with no adventitious noises. As the infection resolves, coarse crackles and rhonchi are heard and the cough becomes productive with purulent sputum.

Lack of specific signs indicating infection makes diagnosis in infancy particularly difficult. First evidence of infection is often irritability or lethargy and poor feeding. Abrupt fever may be accompanied by seizures. Respiratory distress is evident with air hunger, tachypnea, and circumoral cyanosis. Because pneumonia in newborns carry a high morbidity and mortality, bacterial infection should be suspected in those with respiratory symptoms and therapy initiated (Rao, 1988).

Staphylococcal pneumonia is rare but particularly progressive and must be treated aggressively. The onset is rapid, with rapid deterioration. Conjunctivitis and furuncles are signs of a probable staphylococcal infection (Rao, 1988).

Diagnostic Evaluation

Radiographic examination reveals the characteristic pictures described earlier. Laboratory examination shows elevated white blood cell counts (may be normal in infants with staphylococcal disease) and positive blood cultures in a number of patients. Children with streptococcal disease have an elevated antistreptolysin O titer.

Therapeutic Management

Antimicrobial therapy has significantly reduced the morbidity and mortality from bacterial pneumonia. Penicillin G is effective in treatment of pneumococcal and streptococcal pneumonia and is implemented as soon as the diagnosis is suspected. Other antibiotics may be used, however. Because staphylococcal infections are caused by penicillinase-producing (penicillin G–resistant) staphylococci, semisynthetic penicillins are administered. In the hospital, medications are given parenterally for rapid action and maximum effect. Sometimes a single daily dose of procaine penicillin G or oral pencillin every 6 to 8 hours for 7 to 10 days may be given for pneumococcal pneumonia.

The majority of older children with pneumococcal pneumonia can be treated at home, especially if the condition is recognized and treatment initiated early. Antibiotic therapy, bed rest, liberal oral intake of fluid, and administration of antipyretics for fever constitute the principal therapeutic measures. Hospitalization is indicated when pleural effusion or empyema accompanies the disease and is mandatory for children with staphylococcal pneumonia. Pneumonia in the infant or young child is best treated in the hospital, since the course of illness is more variable and complications are more common in very young patients. In addition, intravenous fluid administration is frequently necessary, and oxygen may be required if the child is in respiratory distress.

Prognosis. The prognosis for pneumococcal infections is generally good, with rapid recovery when they are recognized and treated early. The course of staphylococcal pneumonia is generally prolonged. The prognosis varies with the length of the illness before treatment, although early recognition and treatment are usually beneficial.

Use of pneumococcal polysaccharide vaccine is recommended for use in selected individuals such as children over age 2 years who are at risk of acquiring pneumococcal infection or are at risk of serious disease. (See Immunizations, Chapter 12.)

Complications. At present, the classic features and clinical course of pneumonia are rarely seen because of early and vigorous antibiotic and supportive therapy. However, a large number of children, especially infants, with staphylococcal pneumonia develop empyema, pyopneumothorax, or tension pneumothorax. Pneumococci are the most common cause of acute otitis media and a frequent complication of pneumococcal infection. Pleural effusion is not uncommon in children with lobar (pneumococcal) pneumonia. A diagnostic thoracentesis is performed if fluid is suspected to be in the pleural cavity. Nonpurulent effusions, such as occur in pneumococcal pneumonia, do not require surgical drainage.

Continuous closed chest drainage is instituted when purulent fluid is aspirated, a frequent finding in staphylococcal infections. If a large amount of purulent drainage is obtained, an appropriate antibiotic is instilled into the cavity and the suction is discontinued for approximately 1 hour after the instillation. Closed drainage is continued until drainage fluid is free of pathogens—rarely more than 5 to 7 days. Sometimes repeated pleural taps are sufficient to remove fluid; however, the purulent drainage accumulates so rapidly and is so highly viscous that continuous drainage is preferred. In addition, continuous drainage is less traumatic to the child than repeated thoracentesis.

Thoracentesis. Dyspnea resulting from pressure from fluid accumulation in the pleural cavity requires removal by thoracentesis. Thoracentesis is also performed to obtain fluid for culture or to instill antibiotics directly into the pleural cavity. Equipment and preparation for the procedure are the same as for an adult. Nursing responsibilities include obtaining and setting up equipment, preparing the child physically and psychologically, and assisting the practitioner with the procedure. If continuous closed chest drainage is anticipated, this equipment should also be available. Thoracentesis is performed with the child in a sitting position, preferably with arms and trunk bent forward over pillows or over an overbed table with a pillow. Infants are positioned in a semirecumbent position on the unaffected side. The child will need to be physically restrained in the desired position by the nurse. The nurse provides explanation, offers emotional support during the procedure, and observes the child for any changes in color, respiration, and pulse and any alterations in behavior (such as coughing) and sensorium.

After the procedure the child is made comfortable, and observations and recording of physical and emotional responses are continued. The amount and description of the fluid obtained and any medication instilled are recorded, and specimens are sent to the laboratory for culture. Continuous closed chest drainage is managed according to the same protocol as for the child with a thoracotomy.

Nursing Considerations

Nursing care of the child with a lower respiratory tract infection is primarily supportive and symptomatic to meet the needs of each child. Isolation procedures are instituted according to hospital policy. Rest and conservation of energy are encouraged by relief of physical and psychologic stress. The child is disturbed as little as possible by clustering care to encourage the child's regular sleep cycle. If the cough is disturbing, judicious use of antitussives, especially before rest times and meals, is often helpful. To prevent dehydration, fluids are frequently administered intravenously during the acute phase. Oral fluids, if allowed, are given cautiously to avoid aspiration and to decrease the possibility of aggravating a fatiguing cough.

Children may be placed in a mist tent with oxygen. Cool mist moistens the airways and provides a cool atmosphere that aids in temperature reduction. Children often require frequent clothing and linen changes to prevent chilling in the damp atmosphere. They are usually more comfortable in a semierect position but should be allowed to determine the position of comfort. Lying on the affected side (if pneumonia is unilateral) splints the chest on that side and reduces the pleural rubbing that often causes discomfort. Fever is usually controlled by the cool environment and administration of antipyretic drugs as prescribed. Temperature is monitored regularly to detect a rapid rise that might trigger a febrile seizure.

Vital signs and chest sounds are monitored to assess the progress of the disease and to detect early signs of complications. Children with ineffectual cough or those with difficulty handling secretions, especially infants, will require suctioning to maintain a patent airway. A simple bulb syringe is usually sufficient for clearing the nares and nasopharynx of infants, but mechanical suction should be readily available if needed. Older children can usually handle secretions without assistance. Postural drainage and chest physiotherapy are generally prescribed every 4 hours or more often, depending on the child's condition.

The hospitalized child is apprehensive, and many of the treatments and tests are frightening and stress producing. Reducing anxiety and apprehension reduces psychologic distress in the child and, when the child is more relaxed, the respiratory efforts are lessened. Easing respiratory efforts makes the child less apprehensive, and encouraging the presence of the caregiver provides the child with a customary source of comfort and support.

CHLAMYDIAL PNEUMONIA

C. trachomatis is an intracellular microorganism that has a number of properties similar to gram-negative bacteria. It is currently classified as a specialized bacterium. The organism is responsible for one of the most common sexually transmitted diseases, and newborn infants acquire pulmonary infection from their mothers via ascending infection just before or in the process of birth.

Chlamydial pneumonia is a severe, diffuse disease; its onset is in children between 1 and 3 months, and it is characterized by a persistent cough and tachypnea, but minimum or absent fever. Radiographs show nonspecific abnormalities. Treatment with erythromycin and sulfa drugs shortens the course of the illness. Nursing care is the same as for any infant with pneumonia.

■ OTHER INFECTIONS OF THE RESPIRATORY TRACT

Although less common than the previously described illnesses, several infectious disorders are capable of causing significant morbidity, especially in the infant and very young child.

PERTUSSIS (WHOOPING COUGH)

Pertussis, or whooping cough, is an acute respiratory infection caused by *Bordetella pertussis* that occurs chiefly in children younger than 4 years of age who have not been immunized. It is highly contagious and is particularly threatening in young infants, in whom there is a higher morbidity and mortality rate. (See Table 16-1 for signs, symptoms, and management of pertussis.) The incidence is highest in the spring and summer months, and a single attack confers lifetime immunity. Pertussis vaccine is effective, but the immunity diminishes with time after the initial infection or immunization. A small number of asymptomatic adults and immunized children have been shown to be carriers of organisms and transmit the infection to susceptible contacts (Mertsola and others, 1983).

TUBERCULOSIS

Tuberculosis (TB) is an ancient disease and, although controlled in most developed countries, still remains a health hazard and a leading cause of death throughout many parts of the world. TB in children is still a problem. In many areas of the United States the incidence has increased, especially in large cities. This is attributed, in part, to the influx of foreign-born persons and recognition of the disease in the native-born population (Inselman, 1986).

Etiology

TB is caused by *Mycobacterium tuberculosis,* an acid-fast bacillus (i.e., the organism is not readily decolorized by acids after staining). The main types of tubercle bacilli that cause disease in humans are the human *(M. tuberculosis)* and the bovine *(M. bovis).* Children are susceptible to both varieties, and in parts of the world where TB in cattle is not controlled or pasteurization of milk is not practiced, the bovine type is a common source of infection in children.

Although the causative agent is the tubercle bacillus,

Box 32-8 FACTORS AFFECTING RESISTANCE TO TUBERCULOSIS

Heredity
No positive evidence to indicate hereditary tendency
Evidence that resistance to infection may be genetically transmitted

Sex
Early years: no sex differences in incidence
Later childhood and adolescence: morbidity and mortality higher in girls than in boys

Age
Diminished resistance to infection in infancy
- Delay in development of acquired immunity
- Diminished capacity to resist extension of infective process

Increased tendency to develop disease during puberty and adolescence
- New infection superimposed on an old one
- Increased contacts
- Indigenous reinfection stimulated by metabolic changes or suboptimal diets during a period of rapid growth

Stress States
Temporary stressful circumstances (e.g., injury or illness, undernutrition, emotional distress, or chronic fatigue) may increase susceptibility to infection
Increased secretion of adrenal steroids suppresses protective inflammatory response and permits infection to spread
Therapeutic administration of corticosteroids (similar effect)

Nutrition
Active disease inversely proportional to state of nutrition
Excellent nutrition is essential to young children's recovery from disease

Intercurrent Infection
Infectious diseases (especially measles and pertussis) may activate latent tuberculosis

other factors influence the degree to which the organism is able to produce an altered state in the host. Resistance to the bacillus can be modified by several factors (Box 32-8).

Pathophysiology

The source of infection in children is in most situations an infected adult or a teenager, usually a member of the household. It can also be a baby-sitter, domestic worker, or a frequent visitor to the household. The tubercle bacillus from a lung lesion is expelled in microdroplets from the respiratory tract during a cough or a sneeze where they disperse into the air; therefore the lung is the most frequent portal of entry in human beings. Less often the organism gains entrance to the body by ingestion. At the focal site there is first an inflammatory reaction with accumulation of polymorphonuclear leukocytes and then localized acute bronchopneumonia.

There is a proliferation of epithelial cells that surround and encapsulate the multiplying bacilli in an attempt to wall off the invading organisms, thus forming the typical tubercle. During the inflammatory process some of the bacilli leave the focal area and are carried to the regional lymph nodes that drain the anatomic area of the organism; as a result the child develops a fever. Radiographic examinations may be positive if such tests are made, as in cases in which the child is known to have been exposed. The tuberculin test is positive. Outcomes of pulmonary TB can vary.

Extension of the primary lesion at the original site causes progressive tissue destruction as it spreads within the lung, discharges material from foci to other areas of the lungs (e.g., bronchi or pleura), or produces pneumonia. Erosion of blood vessels by the primary lesion can cause widespread dissemination of the tubercle bacillus to near and distant sites (miliary TB). Frequently affected areas include lymph nodes, meninges, and bone.

Clinical Manifestations

Clinical manifestations of TB in children are extremely variable. The disease may be asymptomatic or produce a broad range of symptoms, including general responses such as fever, malaise, anorexia, and weight loss or more specific symptoms related to the site of infection (e.g., lungs, bone, brain, kidneys). Lung disease may or may not include cough (which progresses slowly over weeks to months), aching pain and tightness in the chest, and (rarely) hemoptysis.

As increasing amounts of lung tissue become involved, the respiratory rate increases, the lung on the affected side does not expand as well as the other, auscultation reveals diminished breath sounds and crackles, and there is dullness to percussion. In children (usually infants) who are unable to contain the spread of infection, the fever persists; the generalized symptoms are manifest; and they develop pallor, anemia, weakness, and weight loss.

Diagnostic Evaluation

Several tests and procedures are used to establish a diagnosis. Diagnosis is based on information derived from physical examination, history, reaction to tuberculin tests, radiographic examinations, and organism cultures. In addition, it must be determined whether or not the lesion is in the active, quiescent, or healed stage.

History. Symptoms generally do not contribute significantly to a diagnosis. History of possible contact with a person known to be infected or subsequently found to be infected is helpful. All contacts of an affected child are examined for the disease.

Tuberculin test. The tuberculin test is the single most important test to determine whether a child has been infected with the tubercle bacillus. A primary infection initiates a hypersensitivity reaction to the protein fraction of the tubercle bacillus, which can be detected 2 to 10 weeks after the infection.

Two types of tuberculin preparations are used for skin tests: *old tuberculin (OT)* and *purified protein derivative (PPD)* of tuberculin. The PPD is used most widely, and the standard dose is 5 tuberculin units (TU) in 0.1 ml of solution, injected intradermally *(Mantoux test)*. Also commonly used are the *multiple-puncture tests (Tine, Heaf, ScaloTest, Sternnedle, Mono-Vac)*, which may contain OT or PPD.

Box 32-9 CIRCUMSTANCES PRODUCING FALSE REACTIONS TO TUBERCULIN TESTS

Tuberculin reaction suppressed by:
- Intercurrent diseases, e.g., viral diseases such as measles, rubella, influenza, mumps, varicella, and probably others (about 4 weeks)
- Viral vaccines, e.g., measles, mumps, and rubella vaccines (about 4 weeks)
- Corticosteroids and other immunosuppressive agents

Cellular immune deficiency disease

Severe malnutrition

Too early testing before the body develops a sensitivity to the protein fraction of the tubercle bacillus

Use of impotent, outdated testing material—mixture that has been prepared for too long or has been exposed to sunlight

Faulty technique—e.g., deep injection, no wheal formed, improper measurement of solution, or leaking of solution from a defective or loosely fitting syringe

Overwhelming tuberculosis infections—end-stage and terminal miliary disease; may cause allergy to disappear

Test results are determined according to instructions provided by the manufacturer. A positive reaction indicates that the person has been infected and has developed a sensitivity to the protein of the tubercle bacillus; it does not confirm the presence of active disease. Once individuals react positively, they will continue to do so. A positive reaction in a previously negative reactor indicates the person has been infected since the last test.

In theory, tuberculin testing should not be carried out before or at the same time as measles immunization. Exacerbation of TB is known to occur with natural measles infection and could result from the live attenuated measles virus vaccine. Furthermore, viral interference from the vaccine may cause a false-negative reaction. However, in actual practice neither of these possibilities is considered a contraindication to measles immunization, especially in the event of an epidemic.

Various factors can affect the response to the test and produce false reactions. A negative reaction will usually mean that the child has never been infected with the organism. However, circumstances may produce a false-negative reaction (Box 32-9).

Bacteriologic examination. A definitive diagnosis is made by demonstrating the presence of mycobacteria in culture. The organism is identified from microscopic examination of properly prepared and stained smears from a lesion, sputum, gastric washings, spinal fluid, draining lymph nodes, and so on. Serodiagnosis and biochemical markers (DNA probes) are now available and may improve diagnostic accuracy, especially for extrapulmonary TB (Starke, 1988).

Radiographic studies. Radiographic examinations are usually carried out, but numerous chronic intrathoracic diseases may simulate tuberculous lesions; therefore the use of x-ray examinations is chiefly supplementary to other diagnostic methods.

Therapeutic Management

Medical management of tuberculous lesions in children consists of adequate nutrition, chemotherapy, general supportive measures, unnecessary exposure to other infections that further compromise the body's defenses, prevention of reinfection, and sometimes surgical procedures. The child is placed on bed rest to conserve energy, avoid fatigue, and decrease metabolic demands. Bed rest is continued until the child is free of fever, exhibits evidence of returning strength, has no manifestations that limit ambulation, and desires to be up and about. Since metabolic deficits, particularly negative calcium and nitrogen levels, occur easily in infected children, special attention is given to planning an adequate intake of the necessary nutritional elements.

The need for hospitalization varies. If possible, children with recent PPD conversions or active disease should be hospitalized to obtain culture material, ascertain tolerance and compliance with medication, investigate household contacts for exposure, identify and initiate treatment for the index case, and remove active sources from the environment before returning the child to the home. It also serves as an excellent opportunity for family education regarding the importance of medication and follow-up care.

Chemotherapy. Chemotherapy is the single most important therapeutic modality available for management of TB. A variety of chemical agents can be used, and a regimen involving two or more drugs simultaneously has been found to be effective and is usually the mode of choice. The drugs most commonly used in children are a combination of isoniazid (INH) and rifampin. INH with ethambutol (EMB) or another combination of drugs is used if the child cannot tolerate the other drug(s). Streptomycin (STM) is used less frequently but is important for drug-resistant disease. Pyrazinamide (PZA) and ethambutol are prescribed less often for children.

The rationale for multiple drug therapy is based on three characteristics of the bacillus. Metabolic rates of bacilli vary in different lesions. For example, bacilli in well-oxygenated lesions (e.g., open cavities) replicate rapidly; the organism in a low-oxygen environment can remain dormant for extended periods of time (Starke, 1988). Also, *M. tuberculosis* is particularly prone to mutation to drug-resistant strains, and drugs vary in their ability to penetrate the blood-brain barrier (Engel, 1989). Sometimes a short course of corticosteroids may be used (in conjunction with antituberculosis drugs) to diminish the inflammatory response, especially in meningitis.

The optimum duration of therapy is unknown, but it is important to treat patients for the shortest period of time. This practice reduces the cost of treatment, diminishes the exposure to toxic effects from the drugs, and increases the likelihood of compliance. Nine months of treatment with INH and rifampin will cure 98% of cases when given daily for the first 1 to 2 months then daily or twice weekly thereafter (Starke, 1990).

Surgical procedures. Surgical procedures may be required to remove the source of infection in tissues that are inaccessible to chemotherapy or that are destroyed by the disease. Orthopedic operations for correction of bone deformities, bronchoscopy for removal of a tuberculous granulomatous polyp, or resection of a portion of a diseased lung may also be performed.

Prognosis. Most children recover from primary tuberculosis infection and are often unaware of its presence. However, very young children have a higher incidence of disseminated disease. It is a serious disease during the first 2 years of life and during adolescence. Except in cases of tuberculous meningitis, death seldom occurs in treated children. Antibiotic therapy has decreased the death rate and the hematogenous spread from primary lesions.

Prevention. The only certain means to prevent TB is to avoid contact with the tubercle bacillus. Maintaining an optimum state of health with adequate nutrition and avoidance of fatigue and debilitating infections promotes natural resistance but does not prevent infection. There is no means to induce reliable immunity.

Pasteurization of milk and routine testing and elimination of diseased cattle have helped reduce the incidence of bovine tuberculosis. Infants and children should be given only pasteurized milk from TB-free cattle.

In general, primary pulmonary tuberculosis in young children is noninfectious for older children or adults (Krugman and others, 1985). The contagiosity of chronic pulmonary TB in older children and adolescents is comparable to that of similar disease in adults. Of concern to hospital personnel is that infected family members may spread the disease when visiting a child in the hospital. Therefore the child and all visitors may be restricted to the child's room until the family can be screened for evidence of the disease.

Limited immunity can be produced by administration of the only successful vaccine to date, BCG (bacillus Calmette-Guérin) vaccine containing bovine bacilli with reduced virulence. The freshly prepared vaccine, injected intradermally, produces definite although incomplete protection against tuberculosis. In most instances, positive tuberculin reactions develop after inoculation. The distribution of BCG vaccine is controlled by local or state health departments, but the vaccine is not used extensively, even in areas with a high prevalence of disease.

Greater protection is afforded by daily prophylactic administration of INH. The drug is given to children with a high probability of exposure to TB despite the disadvantage of the need for continuous therapy. A 1-year course has proved to be effective, but most clinicians prescribe preventive therapy for 9 months to coincide with the length of treatment for disease. The drug has no effect on the child's reaction to tuberculin; therefore the test continues to be useful in detecting acquired infection.

Nursing Considerations

Most children with pulmonary tuberculosis are almost always noninfectious; therefore they seldom need to be isolated. There are few bacilli in the sputum, the amount of sputum produced is quite small, and it is swallowed rather than expectorated. Exceptions are children with draining fistulas from cervical adenitis or other infectious lesions and the rare child with cavitating tuberculosis.

Hospitalization is seldom necessary except for needed diagnostic tests. Only those children with the more serious forms are placed in the hospital for therapy; others are managed satisfactorily at home. Therefore, the major nursing care of children with tuberculosis involves nurses in ambulatory settings—outpatient departments, schools, and especially public health agencies.

Asymptomatic children are able to lead an essentially unrestricted life. They can and should attend school (or nursery school), but older children are restricted from vigorous activities such as competitive games and contact sports during the active stage of primary TB. They should be protected from stresses, including parental anxieties, overprotection, and pressures regarding nutritional intake. The regular immunization schedule should be continued. Care should be exerted to maintain an optimum health status with proper diet, adequate rest, and avoidance of infection.

Diagnosis. Nurses assume several important roles in management of the disease, including assisting with radiographic examinations, performing skin tests, and obtaining specimens for laboratory examination. Skin tests, whether used as screening tools or diagnostic aids, must be carried out correctly in order for the results to be accurate. A wheal 6 to 10 mm in diameter is formed in the skin when the solution is injected. If a wheal is not formed, the procedure is repeated.

Sputum specimens are difficult or impossible to obtain in an infant or young child, since they swallow any mucus coughed from the lower respiratory tract. Therefore the best means for obtaining material for smears or culture is by gastric washing, that is, aspiration of lavaged contents from the fasting stomach. The procedure is carried out and the specimen obtained early in the morning before the customary breakfast time.

Ambulatory care. Nursing supervision of the child at home involves teaching parents and child about the disease and its ramifications. Since children usually acquire the disease from an adult in the home, parents often feel guilty. Historically the disease has been regarded with fear, and numerous misconceptions need to be clarified. Reducing parental anxieties helps them to deal with the illness more constructively and to collaborate more effectively in planning for the child's continued care. The success of therapy depends on the acceptance and cooperation of the family. The nurse can help the family to understand the rationale of diagnostic procedures and therapy and the importance of maintaining the therapeutic plan over the extended period needed for recovery. Promoting optimum general health and preventing intercurrent infections and reinfections with the tubercle bacillus are also of primary importance. Excellent patient education materials can be obtained from the **American Lung Association.***

Case finding. Case finding and follow-up of known contacts are important nursing responsibilities. Every case of tuberculosis identified in the community involves nurses in follow-up of known contacts—contacts from which the

*1740 Broadway, New York, NY 10019-4374; (212) 315-8700.

affected person may have acquired the disease and persons who may have been exposed to the diseased individual. Early diagnosis affords a means for early protection or treatment and prevents further spread of the disease.

Periodic skin testing of all school children and adults could serve to identify positive reactors, particularly in populations in which there is a high incidence of the disease. Annual skin tests are recommended for high-risk children such as Native American children and children of parents who have immigrated from Asia, Africa, the Middle East, Latin America, and the Caribbean. Annual testing is not recommended for children from areas where there is a low prevalence of the disease. For these children testing is recommended at three stages: (1) at 12 to 15 months, (2) before school entry, and (3) during adolescence (American Academy of Pediatrics, Committee on Infectious Diseases, 1988).

PULMONARY DISTURBANCE CAUSED BY NONINFECTIOUS IRRITANTS

Inflammation of lung tissue can occur occasionally as the result of irritation from foreign material. Aspiration of food, oral secretions, or other substances by otherwise normal infants or children can set up an inflammatory response or chemical pneumonia. Young children are especially prone to aspiration of foreign substances, and weak and debilitated children are subject to aspiration of food or secretions. Infants may aspirate talcum powder, especially during diaper changes (see Injury Prevention, Chapter 12). The major problems associated with aspiration in children are asphyxia and respiratory tract inflammation as the result of inhaling foreign material. Medical and nursing care of a subsequent pneumonitis and/or bronchitis is similar to that for lower respiratory tract inflammation resulting from infectious agents.

FOREIGN BODY ASPIRATION

Small children characteristically explore matter with their mouths and are therefore particularly prone to aspirate foreign bodies into the air passages. Aspiration of foreign bodies can occur at any age but is most commonly seen in children ages 1 to 3 years. The signs and changes produced depend on the degree of obstruction and the nature of the foreign body. For example, dry vegetable matter, such as a seed, nut, or piece of carrot or popcorn, that does not dissolve and that may swell when wet creates a particularly difficult problem. The high fat content of potato chips and peanuts may cause the added risk of lipoid pneumonia. "Fun foods" of any kind are among the worst offenders.

The types of food items are significant. In a study by Harris and others (1984), over 90% of deaths from food-related asphyxiation occurred in children less than 5 years of age and 65% in infants. Offending foods in the order of frequency of aspiration are hot dog, round candy, peanut or other nut, grape, cooky or biscuit, other meat, carrot, apple, and peanut butter. Round foods are the most frequent offenders. The first four items together comprise more than 40% of all aspirated food items.

A sharp or irritating object produces irritation and edema. A round, pliable object that does not readily break apart is more likely to occlude an airway than an object with a different shape. Balloons are especially hazardous. A small object may cause little if any pathologic change, whereas an object of sufficient size to obstruct a passage can produce various changes, including atelectasis, emphysema, inflammation, and abscess.

Pathophysiology

A foreign body may be arrested in any portion of the air passages from the larynx to the bronchi. The site is usually determined by the size, weight, and configuration of the object. For example, heavy objects such as bullets, coins, and nails are more likely to drop into the most dependent portions of the tracheobronchial tree. The object may remain in the same location or change its situation in the airway. It can be coughed from a smaller to a larger airway and re-aspirated in a different passage—or it might be ejected forcefully into the mouth and subsequently swallowed.

Signs characteristic of obstruction caused by a foreign body in a bronchus can be explained by the same mechanisms that control the flow of fluids in pipes (Fig. 32-4). During normal respiration the caliber of bronchi and bronchioles becomes larger during inspiration and smaller during expiration. When a small object partially obstructs a passage, air passes around the obstruction during both inspiration and expiration (bypass valve). In this type of obstruction a wheeze is heard. A somewhat larger obstruction will allow air to enter the distal portion when bronchioles enlarge during inspiration, but when they diminish in caliber during expiration, the lumen becomes occluded and air becomes trapped distal to the obstruction (check valve). This type of obstruction produces obstructive emphysema. When there is complete blockage of the bronchus by a foreign body or by the foreign body and swollen mucosa, air is unable to move in either direction (stop valve), and the air distal to the obstruction is soon absorbed, leaving an area of obstruction atelectasis. The right bronchus, with its shorter length and straighter angle, is the usual site of bronchial obstruction.

Clinical Manifestations

Initially a foreign body in the air passages produces choking, gagging, wheezing, or cough. The child's face may become livid and sometimes the child falls unconscious and dies of asphyxiation if the object is not removed. If obstruction is partial, there is often an interval of hours, days, or even weeks without symptoms after the initial period. Secondary symptoms are related to the anatomic area in which the foreign body is lodged and are usually caused by a persistent respiratory infection focused distally to the obstruction. A history of recurrent intractable pneumonia is reason to consider a foreign body in an airway. Often, by the time secondary symptoms appear, the parents have forgotten the initial episode of coughing and gagging. The most common

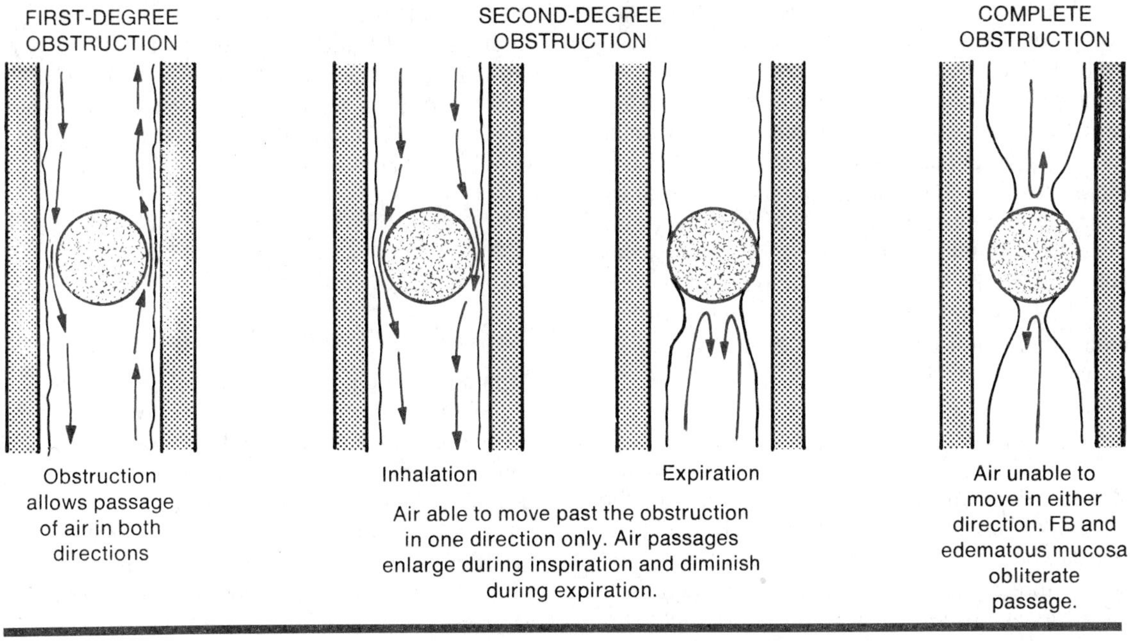
FIRST-DEGREE OBSTRUCTION
SECOND-DEGREE OBSTRUCTION
COMPLETE OBSTRUCTION
Obstruction allows passage of air in both directions
Inhalation
Expiration
Air able to move past the obstruction in one direction only. Air passages enlarge during inspiration and diminish during expiration.
Air unable to move in either direction. FB and edematous mucosa obliterate passage.

Fig. 32-4. Mechanisms of airway obstruction by foreign body *(FB)*.

symptoms observed in children brought to medical attention are stridor, wheezing, sternal retraction, and cough (Esclamado and Richardson, 1987).

Diagnostic Evaluation

The diagnosis of a foreign body is usually suspected on the basis of history and physical signs. Radiographic examination reveals opaque foreign bodies but may be of limited use in localizing vegetable matter. Bronchoscopy is usually required for a definitive diagnosis of foreign bodies in the larynx and trachea. Fluoroscopic examination is a valuable aid in detecting and localizing foreign bodies in the bronchi.

On fluoroscopy a check-valve–obstructed lung will remain expanded, the diaphragm will remain low and fixed on the obstructed side, and the heart and mediastinum will shift to the unobstructed side during expiration. In a stop-valve obstruction the heart and mediastinum are drawn to the obstructed side and remain there during both inspiration and expiration. The diaphragm on the obstructed side remains high, whereas that on the unobstructed side moves normally.

Therapeutic Management

Foreign bodies rarely are coughed up spontaneously; therefore they must be removed instrumentally by direct laryngoscopy or bronchoscopy. This should be carried out as soon as possible, since the progressive local inflammatory process triggered by the foreign material hampers removal, a chemical pneumonia soon develops, and vegetable matter begins to macerate within a few days, causing it to be even more difficult to remove. After removal of the foreign body, the child is placed in a high-humidity atmosphere, and any secondary infection is treated with appropriate antibiotics.

Nursing Considerations

A major role of nurses caring for a child who has aspirated a foreign body is to keep the child as quiet as possible while waiting for surgical removal of the object. The child and the family are naturally upset and frightened, but an agitated child can cause a foreign body to descend and lodge further down in the respiratory tree (e.g., from the larynx or trachea into the right stem bronchus).

All persons working with children should be prepared to deal effectively with aspiration of a foreign body. Choking on food or other material should not be fatal. Two very simple procedures, back blows and the Heimlich maneuver, which can be used by both health professionals and lay persons, can save lives. It is the obligation of nurses to learn the techniques and teach them to parents and other groups. (See Figs. 31-22 and 31-23.)

To aid a child who is choking, nurses need to recognize the signs of distress. Not every child who gags or coughs while eating is truly choking.

✦ **NURSING ALERT** The child in distress (1) *cannot speak,* (2) *becomes cyanotic,* and (3) *collapses.* These three signs indicate that the child is truly choking and requires immediate and quick action. The child can die within 4 minutes.

Prevention. Small children should not be allowed access to enticing small objects that they might place in their mouth. Rubber balloons are high-risk items for children; Mylar balloons are the only safe variety for children. Unlikely items (foil tabs from soft drink containers, Band-Aids applied to fingers of infants or very small children, and plastic tabs from price tags on clothing) can be hazardous. Peanut butter, a staple in the diet of children, should never be given to a child unless it is spread on bread or a cracker.

A spoonful of peanut butter can obstruct the airway and stick to mucous membranes, becoming difficult or impossible for the child to dislodge.

Nurses, as child advocates, are in a position to teach prevention in a variety of settings. They can educate parents singly or in groups about hazards of aspiration in relation to the developmental level of their children and encourage them to teach their children safety. Parents teach by example; therefore they should be cautioned about behaviors that their children might imitate, for example, holding foreign objects, such as pins, nails, and toothpicks, in their lips or mouth. Prevention based on the child's age is discussed in Chapters 12 and 14.

FOREIGN BODY IN THE NOSE

Children will sometimes introduce a foreign object into the nose. This includes such items as food, crayons, small toys, pieces of plastic, beans, beads, erasers, wads of paper, and small stones. A foreign body can be suspected when there is evidence of local obstruction with sneezing, mild discomfort, and (rarely) pain. The irritation produces local mucosal swelling and, with items that increase in size as they absorb moisture (hygroscopic), the signs of obstruction and discomfort increase with time. Infection usually follows as evidenced by foul breath and a purulent or bloody discharge from one nostril.

Although the object is usually situated anteriorly, unskilled attempts at removal may move it further posteriorly. Removal is carried out as soon as possible to prevent the risk of aspiration and to prevent local tissue necrosis. Removal can usually be accomplished with topical anesthesia and either forceps or suction. Sometimes phenylephrine added to the topical anesthesia will help shrink swollen membranes (Templer, 1982). Infection and irritation usually disappear promptly after removal.

FOREIGN BODY IN THE EAR

A variety of objects can be inserted in the external ear canal by children. Such foreign bodies are common in childhood. First an attempt should be made to remove the object by straightening the ear canal by pulling on the pinna and gently shaking the child's head. Many objects can be removed by emergency room personnel with simple tools (Baker, 1987).

A smooth object (such as a bead) can often be removed by applying a cotton-tipped applicator with warmed dental wax or collodion against the object for 1 to 2 minutes, then withdrawing the applicator. The object remains attached to the wax or collodion. Irregularly shaped objects might be removed with bayonet forceps, and steel objects (e.g., a ball bearing) can sometimes be removed with a magnetic probe. A right-angle hook or ear curette can be inserted behind the object and the hook withdrawn, pushing the object ahead of it. A simple suction catheter can remove objects that are not firmly imbedded.

Other options include irrigation by placing the tip of the irrigation tube past the object and directing the flow toward the tympanic membrane to flush the object out of the canal. In this case 70% alcohol is substituted. Using a suction machine is another alternative. However, if the object is large or wedged in place, the child is referred to an otolaryngologist for removal to avoid the risk of damage to the tympanic membrane or ossicles.

✦ **NURSING ALERT** Irrigating is contraindicated for attempted removal of vegetable matter that may swell on contact with water.

ASPIRATION PNEUMONIA

Aspiration of fluid or food substances is a particular hazard in the child who has difficulty with swallowing or is unable to swallow because of paralysis, weakness, debility, congenital anomalies such as cleft palate or tracheoesophageal fistula, or absent cough reflex (unconscious) or who is force fed, especially while crying or breathing rapidly. The newborn may develop a severe pneumonia from aspirating amniotic fluid and debris during the process of birth. Rarely aspiration causes immediate death from asphyxia; more often the irritated mucous membrane becomes a site for secondary bacterial infection. In addition to fluids, food, vomitus, and nasopharyngeal secretions, other substances that cause pneumonia are hydrocarbons, lipids, or powder.

Hydrocarbon Pneumonia

Children frequently develop pneumonia secondary to the ingestion of various forms of hydrocarbons, such as kerosene, gasoline, solvents, and lighter fluid. Petroleum distillates are generally impure substances and contaminated with heavy metals or other toxic chemicals that can cause systemic as well as local effects. Many, but not all, hydrocarbons are made from petroleum (e.g., turpentine is made from pine oil), and many are found in the home or garage.

Hydrocarbons are usually packaged in attractive containers and many have a pleasant aroma. Therefore they are frequently ingested accidentally by young children. They are not often swallowed with the intent of committing suicide, however. On the average, children will swallow less than 30 ml (often about 3 to 4 ml). They begin coughing severely and swallow no more. Although central nervous system abnormalities, gastrointestinal irritation, myocardiopathy, and renal toxicity can all occur, the most serious complication is pneumonitis.

On the whole, distillates that have high volatility, decreased viscosity, and low surface tension are more likely to be aspirated and produce respiratory complications. Lower viscosity enhances penetration into more distal airways; lower surface tension facilitates spread over a larger area of lung surface. Consequently, ingestion of lighter fluid or gasoline frequently causes a pathologic condition, whereas petroleum jelly or tar rarely does.

The pathogenesis of the pulmonary involvement is the subject of conflicting interpretations, but the most generally accepted explanation is irritation from aspiration during swallowing, vomiting, or gastric lavage. Reactions include bronchospasm, atelectasis, and emphysema. Pathologic changes consist of signs of inflammation (edema, hyperemia, and infiltration of polymorphonuclear cells), vascular thrombosis and hemorrhage, and necrosis of bronchial, bronchiolar, and alveolar tissues. Even in small amounts, the hydrocarbon spreads over the surface of tissues. In the lungs it interferes with gas exchange. Coughing and vomiting occur almost immediately after ingestion and probably contribute to aspiration. Central nervous system symptoms may consist of agitation and restlessness, confusion, drowsiness, or coma. The temperature is elevated (37.8° C to 40° C or [100° F to 104° F]).

After swallowing, coughing, and choking, the child becomes short of breath, and older children complain of dyspnea. There are varying degrees of cyanosis, tachycardia, tachypnea, nasal flaring, and retractions. Intercostal retractions, grunting, cough, and fever may appear within 30 minutes or be delayed for a few hours. Localized areas of dullness are felt on percussion and moderately intense rhonchi, wheezes, and crackles are usually heard. Severe injury causes hemoptysis and pulmonary edema that develop rapidly, more severe cyanosis, and death within 24 hours of aspiration.

Inducing the child to vomit is contraindicated because of the renewed danger of aspiration. Hydrocarbons are readily absorbed by the gastrointestinal tract and excreted by the lungs. Bronchitis or pneumonia usually develops early (within the first 24 hours) but may be delayed. Recovery from pulmonary involvement occurs in most instances despite a severe clinical course. Death, if it occurs, is generally the result of hepatic failure complicated by pulmonary factors. Treatment is the same as for any lower respiratory tract inflammation and consists of high humidity, oxygen, hydration, and treatment of any secondary infection.

Lipoid Pneumonia

Oily substances aspirated into the respiratory passages cause progressive changes in lung tissues. First, an interstitial proliferative inflammation occurs that may include an exudative pneumonia. The next stage involves a diffuse, chronic, proliferative fibrosis that is often complicated by acute bronchopneumonia. The final stage features multiple localized nodules or tumorlike paraffinomas. There are no characteristic manifestations. Cough is usually present, and dyspnea is seen in severe cases. Secondary bronchopneumonia infections are common. The outcome depends on the extent of pulmonary damage, the general condition of the infant, and discontinuing the oily inhalation. There is no specific treatment.

Powder

The use of powder has been discouraged for infants; however, although the incidence has decreased, a significant number of infants suffer talcum powder aspiration. Commercial talcum powder is predominantly a mixture of talc (hydrous magnesium silicate) and other silicates. The true incidence of powder inhalation is unknown, but of those with respiratory distress serious enough to be brought to medical attention, the mortality is high (Mofenson and others, 1981). Severe respiratory distress occurs immediately as a result of an inflammatory reaction in small bronchioles initiated by deep inhalation of the extremely light powder. (See Chapter 12 for further discussion of powder inhalation.)

Nursing Considerations

Care of the child with aspiration is the same as that described for the child with pneumonia from other causes. However, the major thrust of nursing care is aimed at prevention of aspiration. Proper feeding techniques should be carried out for weak, debilitated, and uncooperative children; and preventive measures are used to prevent aspiration of any material that might enter the nasopharynx.

Oily nose drops and oil-based vitamin preparations are not appropriate for infants and small children. Solvents, lighter fluid, and other hydrocarbon substances should be kept away from older infants and small children who are apt to put anything in their mouths and who may be attracted by the slightly sweet smell.

Infants and debilitated children should be positioned on the abdomen or the right side after feedings to minimize the possibility of aspirating vomitus or regurgitated feeding. Nurses play a major role in education for injury prevention (see Injury Prevention, Chapters 12 and 14).

ADULT RESPIRATORY DISTRESS SYNDROME

Adult respiratory distress syndrome (ARDS) is now recognized in children, as well as in adults, and poses a major threat to a child recovering from a primary insult. It is characterized by respiratory distress and hypoxemia that occur within 72 hours of a serious injury or surgery in a person with previously normal lungs. It is a syndrome and not a disease and has been variously described as *shock lung, wet lung, stiff lung, congestive atelectasis,* and *posttraumatic lung,* among others. Shock is the most common event associated with the onset of the syndrome.

The hallmark of ARDS is increased permeability of the alveolar-capillary membrane that results in pulmonary edema (Royall and Levin, 1988). The lungs become stiff, gas diffusion is impaired, and eventually there is bronchiolar mucosal swelling and congestive atelectasis. The net effect is decreased functional residual capacity and increased intrapulmonary right-to-left shunting of pulmonary circulation. Surfactant secretion is reduced, and the atelectasis and fluid-filled alveoli provide an excellent medium for bacterial growth. The criteria for diagnosis of ARDS in children are an acute antecedent illness or injury, acute respiratory distress or failure, no evidence of prior cardiopulmonary disease, and diffuse bilateral infiltrates evidenced on chest radiography.

Treatment involves general supportive measures such as prevention of infection, maintenance of vascular pressure, adequate nutrition, comfort measures, positioning to improve functional residual capacity, and psychologic support. Definitive therapy is primarily directed toward improvement of oxygenation. Surfactant therapy that has been successful in infant respiratory distress syndrome (see Chapter 31) may be a definitive therapy for ARDS.

Nursing care involves careful monitoring of pulse, heart rate, perfusion, capillary filling, and urine output, as well as assessment of respiratory status. Blood gas analysis is an important evaluation tool. Respiratory distress is a frightening situation for both the child and the parents, and attention to their psychologic needs is a major element in the care of these children.

SMOKE INHALATION INJURY

A number of noxious substances that may be inhaled are toxic to humans. They are primarily products of incomplete combustion and are believed to cause more deaths from fires than flame injuries. The severity of the injury depends on the nature of the substances generated by the material being burned and whether the victim is confined in a closed space.

General Aspects

Possible inhalation injury is suspected when there is a history of flames in a closed space whether or not burns are present. Sooty material around the nose or in the sputum, singed nasal hairs, or mucosal burns of the nose, lips, mouth, or throat are all signs that the affected person demands observation for possible pulmonary injury from inhalants. A hoarse voice and cough are further evidence of airway involvement, and increased inspiratory and expiratory stridor indicates severe damage to the upper passages. Signs of respiratory distress are also indicated by tachypnea, tachycardia, and diminished or abnormal breath sounds, including crackles, rhonchi, and wheezes. Smoke inhalation causes three different types of injury: heat, local chemical, and systemic.

Heat injury. Heat causes thermal injury to the upper airways, but since air has low specific heat, the injury goes no further than the upper airway. Reflex closure of the glottis prevents injury to lower airways. Heat may reach the middle airway occasionally but it rarely penetrates to the lungs.

Chemical injury. A wide variety of gases may be generated during the combustion of materials such as clothing, furniture, and floor coverings. Acids, alkalis, and their precursors in smoke can produce chemical burns. These substances can be carried deep into the respiratory tract, including the lower respiratory tract, in the form of insoluble gases. Soluble gases tend to dissolve in the upper respiratory tract.

Synthetic materials are especially toxic, producing gases such as oxides of sulfur and nitrogen, acetaldehyde, formaldehyde, hydrocyanic acid, and chlorine. Heated plastics are the source of extremely toxic vapors, including chlorine and hydrochloric acid from polyvinylchloride and hydrocarbons, aldehydes, ketones, and acids from polyethylene. Irritant gases such as nitrous oxide or CO_2 combine with water in the lungs to form corrosive acids; aldehydes cause denaturation of proteins, cellular damage, and edema of pulmonary tissues. Chemical burns to the airways are similar to burns on the skin except they are painless because the tracheobronchial tree is relatively insensitive to pain.

Inhalation of small amounts of noxious irritants produces alveolar and bronchiolar damage that can lead to obstructive bronchiolitis. Severe exposure causes further injury, including alveolar-capillary damage with hemorrhage, necrotizing bronchiolitis, inhibited secretion of surfactant, and formation of hyaline membranes—manifestations of ARDS described in the previous section.

Systemic injury. Gases that are nontoxic to the airways (e.g., carbon monoxide [CO] and hydrogen cyanide) can cause injury and death by interfering with or inhibiting cellular respiration. CO is a colorless, odorless gas with an affinity for hemoglobin 230 times greater than that of oxygen. CO combines at the same point on the hemoglobin molecule as does oxygen; therefore when it enters the bloodstream, CO readily binds reversibly with hemoglobin to form carboxyhemoglobin (COHb). Because it combines more readily and is released less readily, very low levels of tissue oxygen levels must be reached before appreciable amounts of oxygen are released from the hemoglobin. Therefore tissue hypoxia reaches dangerous levels before oxygen is available to meet tissue needs.

Accidental poisoning is most often the result of exposure to fumes from heaters or smoke from structural fires, although poorly ventilated recreational vehicles with improperly operated or maintained gas lamps or stoves and cooking in underventilated areas with charcoal grills or hibachis are also frequent causes. CO is produced by incomplete combustion of carbon or carbonaceous material such as wool or charcoal.

The signs and symptoms of CO poisoning are secondary to tissue hypoxia and vary with the level of COHb. Mild manifestations include headache, visual disturbances, irritability, and nausea, whereas more severe intoxication causes confusion, hallucinations, ataxia, and coma (Box 32-10). CO may increase cerebral blood flow, increase cerebral capillary permeability, and increase cerebrospinal fluid pressure, all of which contribute to the central nervous system (CNS) signs observed. The bright, cherry-red lips and skin often described are less often observed; more frequently pallor and cyanosis are seen.

Therapeutic Management

When inhalation injury is suspected, the patient is given humidified 100% oxygen by mask, and blood is drawn to determine baseline arterial blood gases and COHb levels. Surprisingly, arterial oxygen partial pressure may be within normal limits unless there is marked respiratory depression. If CO poisoning is confirmed, 100% oxygen is continued until COHb levels fall to the nontoxic range of about 10%, and artificial ventilation may be implemented in selected cases. Where a hyperbaric oxygen chamber is available, the breakdown of the CO-hemoglobin bond is greatly accelerated. Other therapies that may be used but that remain controversial are the administration of 5% to 7% CO to stimulate the respiratory center, transfusion with washed red blood cells to increase the oxygen carried to tissues, and hypothermia to reduce the tissue demand for oxygen and to prevent CNS complications.

Respiratory distress may occur early in the course of

Box 32-10 INHALATION INJURY RELATED TO CARBOXYHEMOGLOBIN CONCENTRATION

Signs and Symptoms	Percent of COHb Concentration
Usually none (often questioned)	0-5
Tightness across forehead, may or may not be headache, cutaneous blood vessel dilation	5-15
Throbbing headache plus above	15-30
Severe headache, weakness, dizziness, dimmed vision, nausea, vomiting, cardiovascular collapse (especially infants, anemic children, and those with pulmonary disease)	30-40
Same as above but worse, with greater possibility of cardiovascular collapse, syncope, coma, and lactic acidemia	40-50
Syncope, tachycardia, poor cardiac output, seizures, Cheyne-Stokes respirations, death	50-60
Coma, seizures, decreased cardiac output, respiratory depression, death if not treated*	60-80

*Death can occur with lower concentrations in infants and in children with pulmonary disease or anemia.

smoke inhalation as a result of hypoxia, or patients who are breathing well on admission may later develop sudden respiratory distress. Therefore intubation and/or tracheostomy equipment should be available at the bedside. More often distress is related to transient edema of the airways, which can occur at any level in the tracheobronchial tree. Assessment and localization of the obstruction should be accomplished before severe swelling of head, neck, or oropharynx occurs. Intubation is often necessary when (1) severe burns in the area of the nose, mouth, and face increase the likelihood of developing oropharyngeal edema and obstruction; (2) vocal cord edema causes obstruction; (3) the patient has difficulty handling secretions; and (4) progressive respiratory distress requires artificial ventilation. There is a good deal of controversy regarding tracheostomy, but many prefer this procedure when the obstruction is proximal to the larynx and reserve nasotracheal intubation for lower tract involvement.

Use of corticosteroids, although controversial, may be of value in reducing edema, and bronchodilators (usually isoproterenol) are often given intravenously or by nebulizer. A broad-spectrum antibiotic is sometimes administered prophylactically but this too is controversial.

Nursing Considerations

Nursing care of the child with inhalation injury is the same as that for any child with respiratory distress. Vital signs and other respiratory assessments are performed frequently, and the pulmonary status is carefully observed and maintained. Pulmonary physiotherapy is usually part of the therapeutic program, as well as mechanical ventilation if needed.

In addition to the observation and management of the physical aspects of inhalation injury, the nurse also deals with the psychologic needs of a frightened child and distraught parents. As with any accidental injury, the parents feel overwhelming guilt, even when the injury occurred through no fault of their own. More often, however, the injury could have been prevented, which compounds their guilt feelings. They need a great deal of support and reassurance, as well as information about the child's condition, treatment, and progress.

The increased use of wood-burning stoves as a primary or supplementary source of heat has produced additional air-pollutant particles in residential air. Investigators have noted an increase in respiratory illness in infants and children from households heating with wood-burning stoves (Honicky, Osborne, and Akpom, 1985). A family assessment that reveals frequent respiratory infections in children during the cold winter months should alert the nurse to this possibility.

PASSIVE SMOKING

Numerous researchers have investigated the effects of environmental pollution on children's health and have determined that the worst pollutant is parental smoking, especially maternal smoking. It has been found that children in passive smoking situations have an increased number of respiratory illnesses when compared with children of nonsmoking parents and that the number of illnesses is positively correlated with the number of cigarettes smoked (Chen, Li, and Yu, 1986; Neuspiel and others, 1989; Ogston, 1985; Pattishall and others, 1985; Pedreira and others, 1985).

The incidence of respiratory disease related to passive smoking also correlates with the smoking members of the family. Maternal cigarette smoking is associated with increases of 20% to 35% in the rates of respiratory illnesses and respiratory symptoms. Paternal smoking is associated with smaller but still substantial increases (Ware and others, 1984). Other researchers have found that children of smoking parents have reduced performance on pulmonary function tests. Parental smoking may have a deleterious effect on children's growth (Rona and others, 1981).

Nursing Considerations

Passive smoking during childhood may well be the most important precursor of chronic lung disease in the adult. Nurses and other health care professionals need to be aware of this problem and include this information in all health assessments of children, especially those with respiratory illnesses. In families where smokers refuse to quit, house rules should be established for reducing smoke in the child's environment (Box 32-11). The American Academy of Pediatrics has renewed its statement on hazards of passive smoking (American Academy of Pediatrics, Committee on Environmental Hazards, 1986). Armed with this knowledge, nurses should play a stronger role in ridding

Box 32-11 HOUSE RULES FOR SMOKING HOUSEHOLDS

Do not smoke in same room with children.
Restrict smoking to an isolated area.
Do not smoke in automobile with children.
Do not smoke in rooms children use.

children's environments of tobacco smoke by informing parents; setting an example for children and families; and becoming advocates for "no smoking" ordinances in public places, prohibition of advertising tobacco products in the media, and inclusion of health warnings of sidestream smoke on tobacco products.

LONG-TERM RESPIRATORY DYSFUNCTION

Respiratory disorders that assume a long-term aspect are not uncommon in childhood. They are responsible for significant morbidity and school absenteeism, as well as altering the quality of life and physical and social development of children. Bronchial asthma is prominent among these, and cystic fibrosis is the most common inherited disease of children.

ALLERGIC RHINITIS

Allergic rhinitis is the most common of all allergic disorders and, although not life-threatening, is a significant cause of morbidity in all age-groups. The manifestations may be episodic or perennial. Seasonal allergic rhinitis, also known as "hay fever" or "summer cold," occurs during certain months of the year and does not develop until the individual has been sensitized by two or more pollen seasons. Although the peak incidence is in the postadolescent teenage group, younger children are also affected.

Pathophysiology

The development of allergic rhinitis requires two conditions: a familial predisposition to develop allergy and exposure of a sensitized person to the allergen. Inhalants in the form of microscopic airborne particles, including pollens, mold, animal danders, and environmental dusts, are the principal allergens. It is thought that water-soluble allergens diffuse into the respiratory epithelium from airborne foreign particles that enter the upper respiratory tract with each inhalation. After diffusion, immunoglobulin E antibody production is stimulated in the genetically susceptible child and subsequent sensitization of respiratory tissues takes place. Repeated exposure of these sensitized membranes to specific aeroallergens results in antigen-antibody interactions with the release of mast cell mediators, inflammation, and clinical allergic disease (Mathews, 1982). In exercise-induced bronchospasm, cold, dry air triggers a release of bronchoactive substances in mast cells and epithelial cells of the respiratory tract, which opposes the bronchodilation that normally accompanies exercise (Bar-Yishay and Godfrey, 1985).

Clinical Manifestations

Symptoms of allergic rhinitis may include paroxysms of sneezing; itching of the nose, eyes, palate, pharynx, and conjunctiva; nasal stuffiness progressing to partial or total obstruction of air flow; and mucus secretion, frequently accompanied by postnasal drainage. Nasal itching is troublesome, and the affected child attempts to alleviate the symptoms by rubbing and dorsal manipulation of the nose—the "allergic salute" (Fig. 32-5). The child may develop facial tics and mannerisms in an attempt to avoid scratching the nose (Simons, 1988). Classic facial features often exhibited by affected children include an open mouth caused by chronic nasal obstruction ("allergic gape"), discoloration and edema around the eyes from chronic nasal obstruction ("allergic shiner"), transverse nasal crease from the "allergic salute," and radiating lines in the lower orbitopalpebral grooves (*Dennies lines*).

Other symptoms may appear during peak symptom periods, including tearing and soreness of the eyes and gelatinous conjunctival discharge in the morning, irritability, fatigue, depression, and loss of appetite. Symptoms related to an accompanying otitis media with effusion and eustachian

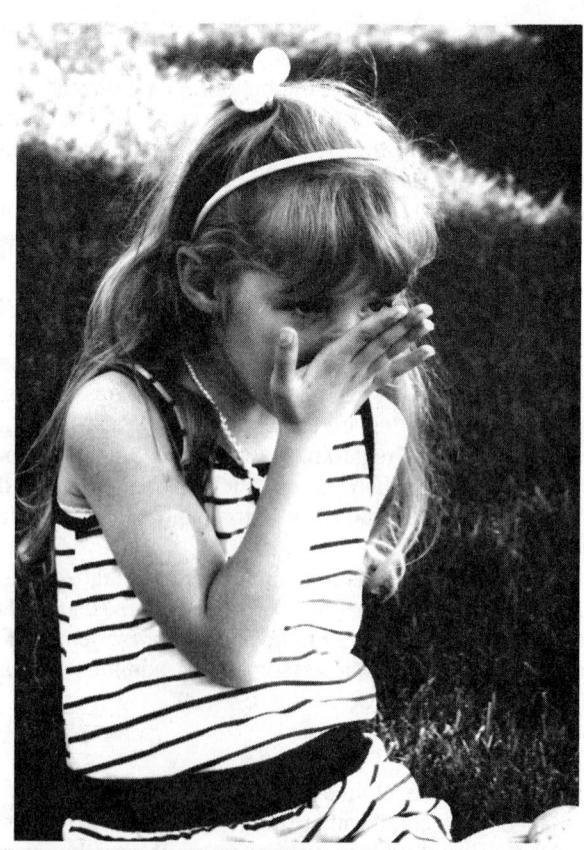

Fig. 32-5. "Allergic salute."

tube dysfunction may be present. Chronic rhinitis leading to significant nasal obstruction can lead to various abnormalities in growth and development and in psychosocial and intellectual development (Pearlman, 1988).

Diagnostic Evaluation

Diagnosis of allergic rhinitis is based on a thorough history and physical examination. Since allergic rhinitis is often associated with atopic dermatitis or asthma, examination of the skin and chest is indicated (Simons, 1988). Other tests that may be used include mucus examination for eosinophils, superficial biopsy of nasal mucosa, fiberoptic rhinoscopy, blood examination for elevated eosinophils, and various challenge tests. Nasal blood flow and nasal air flow measurements are sometimes used.

Sensitization testing. Tests for sensitization to specific allergens include skin tests and the radioallergosorbent test (RAST) and related tests. Skin testing involves injection of specific allergens and remains the most commonly used diagnostic test for allergy. The allergenic extract is introduced into the epidermis by (1) scratch, prick, or puncture; (2) a single intracutaneous injection of a dilute concentration of specific allergen; or (3) serial dilution (threefold or tenfold) injections to determine the end point of reactivity. After a suitable time period (10 to 30 seconds) the size of the resultant wheal and flare reaction is measured to assess the patient's sensitivity (Nalebuff and Fadal, 1986). The magnitude of the wheal and flare response correlates roughly with the severity of symptoms produced by natural exposure to the same allergen; however, a positive skin test does not always indicate the presence of clinical reactivity (Wood and Sampson, 1987).

Skin testing and immunotherapy are generally safe procedures, but they are not without risk. Severe and even fatal reactions can occur within a short period of time, depending on the type of extract used and sensitivity of the individual. To minimize the risk of severe reactions the American Academy of Allergy and Immunology (1990) recommends the patient remain under observation for at least 20 minutes after injection and longer for high-risk patients. In other countries (such as the United Kingdom), in which extracts unapproved in the United States are used, the recommended waiting period is 2 hours.

✦ **NURSING ALERT** Onset of a reaction is often insidious. Mild initial symptoms may include local pruritus, pallor, flushing, cyanosis, shortness of breath, dyspnea, cough, malaise, or abdominal pain. Later developments include hypotension, airway obstruction, chest pain, ventricular fibrillation, and loss of consciousness (Lockey and others, 1987).

The RAST test, which measures the specific immunoglobulin E (IgE), requires only one serum sample. Allergists are divided in their preferences between skin and RAST tests. All agree that the tests should be used as supplemental procedures for history and physical examination and not as screening tools.

Therapeutic Management

Therapy is directed toward avoidance of offending allergens, medication, and immunotherapy (hyposensitization or desensitization). Avoidance measures involve removing allergens from the environment and are usually effective for allergy to foods, drugs, and animals (see Box 32-15).

If a patient is unable to avoid the allergens, symptoms can be controlled with drugs in many cases. However, treatment should be highly individualized. Four main classes of drugs are used: H_1-receptor antagonists (antihistamines), adrenergic and anticholinergic drugs, disodium cromoglycate (cromolyn), and topical corticosteroids (Simon, 1988).

Antihistamines are the preferred medications, and any of a variety of these drugs are effective. If nasal obstruction is a prominent feature, relief can often be obtained from an α-adrenergic decongestant given singly or in combination with an antihistamine. Topical nasal applications of β-adrenergic vasoconstrictors often provide symptomatic relief but should not be used for any length of time. Cromolyn is used prophylactically on a regular basis and is effective in preventing both the early and late responses to antigen. For cases that cannot be controlled with the previous therapies, some suggest the use of topical (nasal) corticosteroids.

Immunotherapy may be necessary if drug therapy and avoidance of allergens are ineffective in controlling symptoms or if drugs evoke undesirable side effects. Skin tests are performed to determine the offending antigens and desensitization injections are carried out. About 80% to 90% of patients achieve significant clinical improvement, but the duration of immunotherapy injections depends on the patient's overall clinical response (Fagin, Friedman, and Fireman, 1981). If improvement is not obtained after a 2-year trial, the child is reevaluated and therapy usually discontinued. With clinical improvement, patients are given the opportunity to stop the immunotherapy after approximately 5 years of injections.

Nursing Considerations

Nurses can help affected children by recognizing the existence of rhinitis and referring them for diagnosis and therapy. Since it is sometimes difficult to distinguish between allergic rhinitis and viral nasopharyngitis, some helpful hints are outlined in the Nursing Tips.

NURSING TIPS: DISTINGUISHING ALLERGIES FROM COLDS

Allergies are seldom accompanied by fever; colds are.
Allergies tend to cause itching in the child's eyes and nose; colds do not.
Allergies usually trigger constant and consistent bouts of sneezing; colds are characterized by sporadic sneezing.

From Judith Acciani, R.N., Director, Nasalcrom and Opticrom Allergy Information Center.
For other tips and information about children's allergy, call the toll-free hotline: (800) 727-5400.

The major nursing goal in care of the child with allergic rhinitis is preparation for skin tests and desensitization injections, which are the source of greatest stress to children. It is difficult to make them understand how inflicting discomfort regularly over a long time is going to make them better. Adolescents can intellectualize the rationale behind the procedures and tolerate the discomfort but still need the support that is provided by sympathetic nursing.

To help allay children's fears of skin tests, they need a careful and thorough explanation of what is to be done and how many shots are involved (usually series of eight on each site, for a total of 30 tests). Very young, anxious patients may benefit from one prick on the arm to demonstrate how it feels. The skin is pricked with a stylet rather than a regular needle and syringe, then a drop of allergen is placed on the pierced skin. A helpful strategy is to have the child count off the number of pricks with the nurse as a distraction.

BRONCHIAL ASTHMA

Asthma is an obstructive disease of the airways characterized by reversible hyperreactivity of the bronchi and trachea to a variety of stimuli. All triggers produce the same response in the airways—constriction of the smooth muscles of the airway, inflammation and edema of the bronchial mucosa, and increased production of bronchial mucus. Manifestations most frequently associated with asthma are coughing and wheezing.

The incidence, severity, and mortality associated with asthma have risen steadily throughout the world (Williams, 1989). Asthma is the most common cause of school absences and is responsible for a major proportion of pediatric admissions to emergency rooms and hospitals (Eggleston, 1990). Although the onset of asthma may be at any age, 80% to 90% of children have their first symptoms before 4 or 5 years of age, and it is estimated that 5% to 10% of children in the United States have manifestations of asthma at some time during childhood (Ellis, 1987). Boys are affected more frequently than girls until adolescence when the incidence is approximately equal (Avery and First, 1989). The severity of the disease varies markedly among children and is not influenced by sex.

Asthma can be classified as *intermittent,* in which the child is symptom-free for extended periods without medication, and *chronic,* which describes the child who requires frequent or continuous medical therapy. Both intermittent and chronic disease are variable in intensity, and the choice of therapy depends on both the classification and the severity.

Etiology

Manifestations of asthma appear to be the result of allergic hypersensitivity to foreign substances, usually those carried in the air, such as plant pollens. However, in some instances no allergic process can be detected. Theories that attempt to explain the hyperresponsiveness of airways include (1) a basic defect in the β-adrenergic receptors on leukocytes and (2) increased cholinergic activity in the airways. Asthma is a complex disorder involving biochemical, immunologic, infectious, endocrine, and psychologic factors to varying degrees in different persons (Ellis, 1987).

There is a family predisposition toward hyperactivity of the airways, and a relationship between asthma and IgE-mediated diseases (especially allergic rhinitis) is established. Frequently, the child has other manifestations of allergy such as nasal allergy, eczema, or urticaria. Although many children with asthma exhibit an allergic component, asthma is not always an inherently allergic disease (Weinberger, 1989); the onset of asthma in childhood generally precedes the presence of identifiable allergens.

Numerous stimuli have been found to provoke an asthma attack, including viruses, allergens, smoking (both active and passive), cold air, exercise, and inhaled irritants. Of these, viral infection of the airways is the most common trigger of asthma in children, with RSV and parainfluenza viruses the most frequent offenders. Bacterial infection is rarely associated with triggering a hyperreactive airway response. Psychologic stress has been named as a trigger in the past, but there is no evidence to indicate that this contributes to asthma in early childhood (Weinberger, 1989). Less frequently, sulfites in food and nonsteroidal antiinflammatory drugs are the responsible triggers.

Pathophysiology

There is general agreement that heightened airway reactivity is characteristic of children with asthma. The reasons for this are less clear, and most theories do not explain all types and causes of asthma. Some of the theories attribute the hyperreactivity to (1) an exaggeration of the normal defenses of the respiratory tract, (2) abnormal tissue reactions in the bronchioles, possibly immunologically induced, or (3) an imbalance of normally balanced responses. However, the mechanisms responsible for the obstructive symptoms of asthma are (Fig. 32-6):

1. Edema of the mucous membranes
2. Accumulation of tenacious secretions from mucous glands
3. Spasm of the smooth muscle of the bronchi and bronchioles, which decreases the caliber of the bronchioles

The role that each of these mechanisms plays varies from patient to patient and during the course of the disease. In some patients, smooth muscle contraction is the major factor early in the episode, followed by mucosal edema and increased mucus secretion, which are predominant in contributing to the obstruction. In others the sequence of the responses is reversed.

Immunologic factors. Many children with asthma exhibit an allergic component. A vast number of substances in the environment are capable of inducing an asthmatic response, but the most significant are those that are antigenic, that is, that evoke the immune response. The antigen (or foreign substance) is deposited on the respiratory mucosa, where lysozymes immediately digest its outer coating,

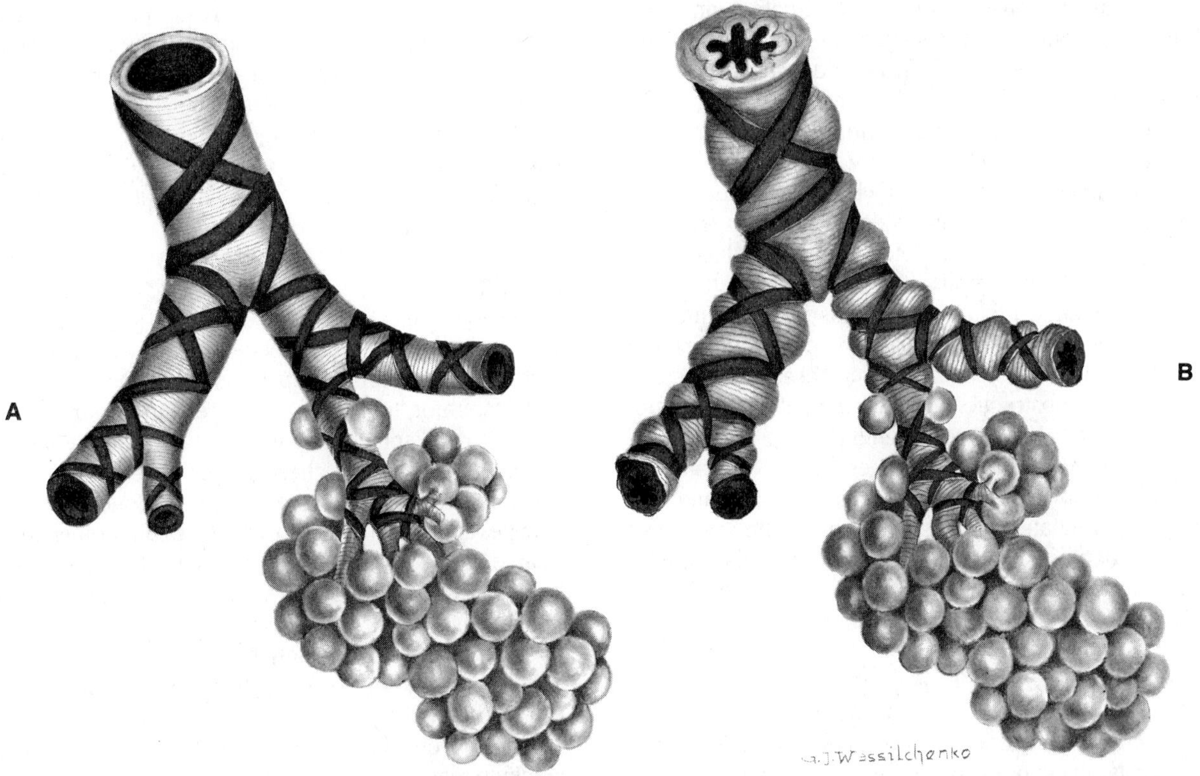

Fig. 32-6. Mechanisms of obstruction in asthma. **A,** Normal bronchus. **B,** Asthmatic bronchus.

releasing fragments of foreign protein that initiate the immune sequence. The antibodies (immunoglobulins) most active in allergic disorders, including asthma, are immunoglobulin E (IgE), located primarily in skin and mucous membranes.

IgE mediates the immediate hypersensitive reaction in the bronchial mucosa that leads to *specific tissue binding.* IgE attachs to surfaces of mast cells and basophils, where it reacts with the specific antigen to which they have developed a bonding capacity. Antigenic substances trigger an immediate hypersensitivity reaction with subsequent release of chemical mediators from mast cells and basophils—histamine, leukotrienes, platelet-activating factor, and other substances including prostaglandins, serotonin, and various kinins. The major effects of the mediators in the airways are increased permeability of the blood vessels, contraction of smooth muscle, and stimulation of mucus secretion.

Vagal stimulation. Normally the balance of vagal and sympathetic nerve influences maintains the tone of bronchial smooth muscle. Irritant receptors on the bronchial mucosa stimulated by various antigenic (pollens, dust) or nonantigenic (smoke, fumes, cold) stimuli trigger a reflex bronchospasm that narrows the airway. This normal reflex mechanism is designed to protect the alveoli from harmful stimuli in the bronchi; however, in the person with asthma the bronchial constriction is abnormally severe. Acetylcholine, a neurotransmitter, mediates the vagal response.

Ventilation. The rigid cartilaginous rings of the upper airways act to modify the constrictive forces, but in the smaller bronchi and the bronchioles the cartilage has been replaced by membranous tissue. The smooth muscle, arranged in spiral bundles around the airway, causes narrowing and shortening of the airway, which significantly increases airway resistance to airflow. Since the bronchi normally dilate and elongate during inspiration and contract and shorten on expiration, the respiratory difficulty is more pronounced during the expiratory phase of respiration.

Increased resistance in the airway causes forced expiration through the narrowed lumen. The volume of air trapped in the lungs increases as airways are functionally closed at a point between the alveoli and the lobar bronchi by the combined mechanisms just described. As the severity of the asthma increases, the airways close at higher residual volume. This gas trapping is the central physiologic feature in the clinical manifestations of asthma, as it forces the individual to breathe at a higher and higher lung volume. This in turn increases the elastic work of breathing and decreases the mechanical efficiency of respiratory muscles. Consequently the person with asthma fights to inspire sufficient air, and hyperinflation of alveoli increases the diameter of the airways by exerting lateral traction on bronchiolar walls. Gas exchange is facilitated, but more energy is required during inspiration to overcome the tension of already stretched elastic lung tissues. The expenditure of effort for breathing causes fatigue, decreased respiratory effectiveness, and increased oxygen consumption and cardiac output at a time when gas exchange and cardiac output are already compromised. In addition, the inspiration occurring at higher lung volumes reduces the effectiveness of the cough. The child becomes progressively dyspneic, cyanotic, and tachypneic.

Gas exchange. The degree to which impaired respiration interferes with gas exchanges depends to a large measure on the ratio of poorly ventilated and hyperextended alveoli to well-ventilated alveoli. Other factors that reduce the ventilatory efficiency include atelectasis and pneumonia. When the number of poorly ventilated alveoli increases, the degree of arterial hypoxemia also increases; in cases of complete airway obstruction there is a right-to-left pulmonary shunt with total absence of ventilation.

While there are a sufficient number of well-ventilated alveolar-capillary units, perfusion remains adequate and carbon dioxide elimination is not impaired. As the severity of obstruction increases, there is a reduced alveolar ventilation with carbon dioxide retention, hypoxemia, respiratory acidosis, and eventually respiratory failure.

Clinical Manifestations

Timing of symptoms varies markedly among patients. Bronchoconstriction in response to an allergen can have an immediate, histamine-type pattern or a late response with airway hypersensitivity lasting for days, weeks, or months (Dolovich and others, 1988). Since a second wave of symptoms sometimes appears 6 to 8 hours after the initial antigen exposure, patients should have sufficient medicine to control late response symptoms if they occur.

It has been observed that children may experience a prodromal itching localized at the front of the neck or over the upper part of the back (David and others, 1984). An asthmatic episode begins with a hacking, paroxysmal, irritative, and nonproductive cough caused by bronchial edema. Accumulated secretions, acting as a foreign body, stimulate the cough. As the secretions become more profuse, the cough becomes rattling and productive of frothy, clear, gelatinous sputum. Bronchial spasm and mucosal edema reduce the size of the bronchial lumen, which is, as a result, more easily occluded by mucous plugs.

A common symptom of asthma is coughing in the absence of respiratory infection, especially at night. This may disrupt sleep, leading to excessive fatigue during the day and poor school performance. Wheezing may be mild or discernible only on auscultation at the end of expiration, or severe enough to be audible. The child is frequently short of breath.

The child with a more severe attack is short of breath and tries to breathe more deeply; the expiratory phase becomes prolonged and is accompanied by an audible wheezing. The child often appears pale but may have a malar flush and red ears. The lips assume a deep, dark red color that may progress to cyanosis observed in the nail beds and skin, especially around the mouth. The child is restless and apprehensive with an anxious facial expression. Sweating may be prominent as the attack progresses. Older children have a tendency to sit upright with shoulders in a hunched-over position, hands on the bed or chair, and arms braced to facilitate the use of accessory muscles of respiration. The child speaks with short, panting, broken phrases. Infants and small children are restless, irritable, and difficult to make comfortable. The severity of the attack can be evaluated on the basis of sweating and the child's refusal to lie down. A nonsweating child who remains upright is moderately ill; one who remains recumbent is the least ill.

The prolonged expiratory phase is less apparent in infants and young children because of a more pliable chest and the normal rapid respiratory rate. Therefore expiratory and inspiratory dyspnea are more difficult to differentiate. Infants may display intercostal and suprasternal retractions.

Examination of the chest reveals hyperresonance on percussion. Breath sounds are coarse and loud, with sonorous crackles throughout the lung fields. Expiration is prolonged. Coarse rhonchi can be heard, as well as generalized inspiratory and expiratory wheezing that becomes more high pitched as obstruction progresses. With minimal obstruction, wheezing may be only mild (discernible only on auscultation at the end of expiration) or even absent, but can be accentuated by rapid, deep breathing.

With severe spasm or obstruction, breath sounds and crackles may become audible. Cough is ineffective despite repeated, hacking maneuvers. This represents lack of air movement and may be misinterpreted as improvement by unknowing examiners.

✦ **NURSING ALERT** Shortness of breath with air movement in the chest restricted to the point of absent breath sounds accompanied by a sudden rise in respiratory rate is an ominous sign indicating ventilatory failure and imminent asphyxia.

Children with chronic asthma develop generalized vascularization, mucosal thickening, and hypertrophy of the mucous glands and fibers of the bronchial musculature. With repeated episodes the thoracic cavity becomes fixed in a hyperventilated state (barrel chest) with depressed diaphragm, elevated shoulders, and use of accessory muscles of respiration. The child's face takes on a typical appearance with flattened malar bones, circles beneath the eyes, narrow nose, and prominent upper teeth.

Diagnostic Evaluation

Asthma is underdiagnosed in childhood and is often mislabeled as "wheezy bronchitis" (König, 1985). This can result in the misuse of cough suppressants, antihistamines, and antibiotics (which are not indicated in the treatment of asthma) and ineffective use of bronchodilators (Neddenriep, Schumacher, and Lemen, 1989). A diagnosis of asthma is most often made on the basis of history of symptoms and physical examination.

Generally, chronic cough in the absence of infection or diffuse wheezing during the expiratory phase of respiration is sufficient to establish a diagnosis. Several observations

Box 32-12 CONDITIONS THAT MAY MIMIC ASTHMA

Foreign body in airway
Cystic fibrosis
Congestive heart failure
Intrathoracic tumors
Vascular rings
Tracheomalacia or laryngomalacia
Tracheoesophageal fistula
Acute inflammation of the airway
Vocal cord paralysis
Cysts or hemangiomas

provide assistance in differential diagnosis of other conditions (Box 32-12). Localized, monophonic wheezing may indicate the obstruction of a single bronchus, caused by foreign body aspiration, bronchial stenosis, or intrathoracic tumor. Stridor, heard primarily on inspiration, usually indicates an extrathoracic obstruction such as laryngotracheomalacia, croup, or epiglottitis. Coarse crackles due to increased mucus secretion are often heard in conjunction with reactive airways, but fine crackles, characteristic of congestive heart failure or pneumonia, are absent. Most children with asthma are well nourished and do not display signs of chronic hypoxia. Poor growth, digital clubbing, or chronic bacterial infection is more likely to be caused by cystic fibrosis, heart disease, or cancer.

Diagnostic tests. The anteroposterior (AP) diameter may be increased (barrel chest), and chest radiographs show hyperexpansion of airways. Pulmonary function tests reveal air trapping and decreased expiratory flow and are helpful in diagnosis and follow-up of patients with asthma. Measurements of forced expiratory volume at 1 second (FEV_1), forced respiratory capacity (FRC), respiratory volume (RV), and total lung capacity (TLC) provide some indication of the degree of obstruction and are used for both diagnosis and as guidelines for management. A simple mechanical spirometer is available for use in offices and clinics as well as a pediatric flowmeter for measurements in young children at home. The children are taught the necessary maneuver by practice on a party favor.

Because allergic rhinitis and eczema often accompany symptoms of allergic asthma, methacholine or histamine challenges are performed occasionally to assess airway responsiveness to an allergen. Skin testing is useful in identifying specific allergens, and those obtained by the puncture technique correlate better than intracutaneous tests with symptoms and measurements of specific IgE antibody. Provocative testing, direct exposure of the mucous membranes to a suspected antigen in increasing concentrations, helps to identify inhaled allergens. The RAST test helps identify antigens against various foods and is often useful in determining appropriate therapy.

Therapeutic Management: General

The overall goal of asthma management is to prevent disability and to minimize physical and psychologic morbidity—to assist the child in living as normal and happy a life as possible (Box 32-13). This includes facilitating the child's social adjustments in the family, school, and community and normal participation in recreational activities and sports. To accomplish these goals, efforts are directed toward recognizing acute episodes early and implementing appropriate therapy, identifying and eliminating irritant and allergic factors from the child's environment, educating parents to the long-term nature of the disease and how to manage exacerbations, and helping the child to deal constructively with the disease. Adherence to the prescribed regimen is essential to successful management.

Allergen control. Basic to any therapeutic plan is an evaluation of the child's general health and an assessment of the specific allergenic factors and the nonspecific factors that precipitate symptoms. House dust mites and other components of house dust are the agents identified most often in children allergic to inhalants. Other causes are animal dander (especially cats and dogs), fungi, and allergenic pollens. Irritants that can cause bronchoconstriction in individuals with asthma, whether or not there is allergy, are cigarette smoking—especially parental smoking (the most common source of local air pollution)—wood-burning stoves, kerosene heaters, and fireplaces.

Specific allergens are identified by skin testing, and steps are taken to eliminate or avoid the offending allergens. Often simply removing the offending environmental factors will decrease the frequency of attacks, for example, removal of a dog or cat from the home of a child sensitive to animal dander. Nonspecific factors that may trigger an attack, such as extremes of temperature, are sometimes controlled by humidifiers or air conditioners.

Drug therapy. Most children do not require continuous medication. The goal is to control the acute attack; therefore early recognition and treatment at the onset are most

Box 32-13 GOALS OF ASTHMA THERAPY

1. Control symptoms to the maximum possible with a minimum number of the safest medications.
2. Relieve airway obstruction and normalize pulmonary function.
3. Prevent acute episodes that require emergency treatment.
4. Reduce the number and frequency of hospitalizations.
5. Educate the patient and family to understand, accept, and manage asthma within the context of the family's life-style.
6. Participate in normal daily activities and sports without restrictions or with minimum and specific restrictions.
7. Improve the long-term prognosis.
8. Achieve normal growth and development.
9. Minimize school absenteeism.

Modified from Hen, J., Jr.: An overview of pediatric asthma, Pediatr. Ann. 15:92-96, 1985.

important. Providing rapid relief of the bronchospasm reduces the need for drastic measures and increases the likelihood that relief will be complete. Medical management of asthma varies considerably among practitioners. Several drugs are prescribed, often in combination, to reverse or prevent bronchospasm.

β-Adrenergic agents. β-Adrenergic agonists (primarily albuterol, metaproterenol, and terbutaline) are the most frequently prescribed as first-line drugs for treating asthma. These drugs bind with the beta receptors on the smooth muscle of airways where they activate adenylate cyclase and convert adenosine monophosphate (AMP) to cyclic AMP (cAMP). It is believed that the increased cAMP enhances binding of intracellular calcium (Ca) to the cell membrane, reducing the availability of Ca and thus allowing smooth muscle to relax. Other effects of the drug help stabilization of mast cells to prevent release of mediators. Most β-adrenergics used in asthma therapy affect only beta-2 receptors, which help eliminate bronchospasm. Beta-1 effects, which are reflected in increased heart rate and gastrointestinal disturbances, have been minimized.

β-Adrenergic agonists can be given via inhalation or as oral or parenteral preparations. The inhaled drug, administered by metered-dose inhaler (MDI) or nebulizer, has a more rapid onset of action than the oral form but is more costly. The MDI may have a spacing unit or reservoir attached, which makes it easier for small children to use. Inhalation also reduces troublesome systemic side effects—irritability, tremor, nervousness, and insomnia.

Inhaled β-adrenergics can be taken two to four times daily for acute symptoms. Children with exercise-induced bronchospasm are advised to use the drug prophylactically 10 to 15 minutes before exercise. Small children who have difficulty using the MDI can get effective relief with nebulization. The medication is mixed with saline or cromolyn and then nebulized with compressed air. Children are instructed to breathe normally with the mouth open to provide a direct route to the trachea.

Methylxanthines. The methylxanthine drugs, principally theophylline, have been used for decades to relieve symptoms and prevent asthma attacks and are prepared for intravenous, intramuscular, oral, or rectal administration. The drug is available in sustained-release form so it can be taken once or twice daily. The rectal form is rarely used because of its variable and unpredictable absorption.

The precise mechanism of action in preventing smooth muscle contraction in the airway is unclear, but the drug is believed to inhibit the effect of phosphodiesterase to prevent the breakdown and thus prolong the action of cAMP, the adrenergic activator. In addition to its potent bronchodilator effect, theophylline is also a central respiratory stimulant and increases respiratory muscle contractility (Galant, 1987).

The dose of theophylline varies with age. Children over 12 months of age metabolize the drug faster than adults, so the dose per kilogram must be higher. Because absorption also varies among individuals, it is important to follow serum levels of the drug until a therapeutic dose is achieved.

Box 32-14 FACTORS AFFECTING THEOPHYLLINE CLEARANCE

Substances That Accelerate Clearance
Phenytoin
Rifampin
Phenobarbital
Valproic acid
Cigarette and marijuana smoke

Factors That Delay Clearance
Erythromycin
Troleandomycin
Cimetidine
Neonatal age
Fever

Serum concentrations of 10 to 20 μg/ml is considered therapeutic. Symptoms of toxicity, which can appear when levels exceed 20 μg/ml, include nausea, tachycardia, and irritability; seizures and dysrhythmias occur at blood levels greater than 30 μg/ml.

Several drugs commonly prescribed in the pediatric population interact with theophylline to affect the rate of clearance (Neddenriep, Schumacher, and Lemen, 1989). These and other conditions influencing blood levels of the drug are listed in Box 32-14.

Recent reports suggest that theophylline causes behavior problems and poor school performance in children (Gutstadt and others, 1989; Rachelefsky and others, 1986) and depression and anxiety (Furukawa and others, 1988). Other researchers challenge these findings (Rappaport and others, 1989; Weinberger and others, 1987). Further and more definitive studies need to be carried out to confirm or deny these observations.

Cromolyn sodium. Cromolyn sodium is neither a bronchodilator nor an antiinflammatory agent, but acts superficially to inhibit mast cell degranulation in both early and late phases of asthma. The action is essentially prophylactic and is of no value when administered after the allergic reaction; it cannot reverse bronchospasm. Systemic absorption is poor, and clearance from the body is rapid. Cromolyn is administered via nebulizer or MDI, and a single dose inhibits allergen–, exercise–, and sulfur dioxide–induced asthma. It has virtually no toxicity and few side effects (Eggleston, 1990), although it may produce airway irritation and aggravation of cough in some patients.

Anticholinergics. The anticholinergic agents, or cholinergic antagonists, which specifically block the effects of acetylcholine at the vagal postganglionic synapse, are potent bronchodilators effective in preventing reflex-mediated constriction (e.g., from irritants) but less effective in exercise-induced (EIA) and allergen-induced asthma (Egglestson, 1990). The principal anticholinergics used occasionally are atropine or its derivative ipratropium. The drug does not cross the blood-brain barrier so there are no CNS effects. Adverse effects include dry mouth, cough, and blurred vision; anticholinergics are not well accepted.

Corticosteroids. Corticosteroids are the most potent drugs available for treatment of asthma. They diminish the inflammatory cell responses and restore β-adrenergic sensitivity and are used to treat asthma that is resistant to bronchodilator therapy. The drugs can be given intravenously, orally, or topically by aerosol. Metabolism is slow; therefore results are delayed for up to 6 hours, and one daily dose is usually sufficient. Inhaled corticosteroids result in fewer side effects but are less effective for acute attacks. Intravenous administration is warranted during acute, severe exacerbations. Oral steroids can be taken without risk of adrenal suppression if given every other day or daily administration is limited to 7 days (Goldenhersh and Rachelefsky, 1989). Tapering must be planned if the hormone is prescribed for an extended period. Authorities differ on the length of time corticosteroids can be given without initiating a tapering schedule. Patients who are steroid dependent may require increased dosage for periods of stress or exacerbation of respiratory illness. Corticosteroids are lifesaving in status asthmaticus.

Chest physiotherapy. Chest physiotherapy (CPT) is a standard adjunct to treatment of chronic asthma. This includes breathing exercises, physical training, and inhalation therapy. These therapies help produce physical and mental relaxation, improve posture, strengthen respiratory musculature, and develop more efficient patterns of breathing. For the motivated child, breathing exercises and controlled breathing are of value in preventing overinflation and improving the strength of respiratory muscles and the efficiency of the cough. Stretch exercises sometimes help increase the flexibility of the ribs. Sit-ups and leg exercises strengthen abdominal muscles and aid expiration.

Hyposensitization. The role of hyposensitization in childhood asthma has not been clarified. In many cases the child demonstrates multiple sensitivities, which makes such therapy impractical. Moreover, the injections can be expensive and uncomfortable. When the allergen can be defined and cannot be avoided or controlled satisfactorily by drugs, specific hyposensitization is seriously considered. Immune therapy is not recommended for allergens that can be eliminated effectively, for example, food sensitivities, drugs, and animal dander. Inhalant allergens such as house dust, pollens, and molds are most often the allergens considered for immune therapy.

Injection therapy is usually limited to clinically significant allergens. The initial dose of the offending allergen(s), based on the size of the skin reaction, is injected subcutaneously. The amount is increased at weekly intervals until a maximum tolerance is reached, after which a maintenance dose is given at 4-week intervals. This may be extended to 5- or 6-week intervals during the off-season for seasonal allergens. Successful treatment is continued for a minimum of 3 years and then stopped. If no symptoms appear, acquired immunity is said to be retained; if symptoms recur, treatment is reinstituted.

Exercise. Airway obstruction often develops in children with asthma. *Exercise-induced bronchospasm*, or *exercise-induced asthma (EIA)*, does not represent a unique syndrome but rather an example of the airway hyperactivity common to all persons with asthma (Wood and Eggleston, 1986). This bronchoconstriction is not limited to children with asthma but also occurs in children with allergic rhinitis. EIA is defined as an acute, reversible, usually self-terminating airway obstruction that develops 5 to 15 minutes after strenuous exercise and lasts 15 to 60 minutes after the onset (Pierson, 1988). Usually, the episode subsides spontaneously in ½ to 1 hour. The severity of an attack increases as the exercise becomes increasingly strenuous. Patients with a history of EIA often have normal pulmonary function tests and are only symptomatic with exercise (American Academy of Pediatrics, Section on Allergy and Immunology, 1989).

The problem is rare in activities that require only short bursts of energy (such as baseball, sprints, gymnastics, skiing) rather than those that involve endurance exercise (e.g., soccer, basketball, distance running). Swimming, even long-distance swimminng, is well tolerated by children with EIA, partly because they are breathing air fully saturated with moisture, but the type of breathing required may also play a role. Exhaling under water prolongs each expiration and increases the end-expiratory pressure within the respiratory tree (essentially pursed-lip breathing).

Pretreatment with a bronchodilator provides relief through the exercise period. Inhaled β-adrenergic agonists or cromolyn sodium provide protection in the majority of cases (American Academy of Pediatrics, Section on Allergy and Immunology, 1989).

Children with asthma are often excluded from exercise by parents, teachers, and physicians, as well as by the children themselves because they are reluctant to provoke an attack. This can seriously hamper peer interaction. It has been found that moderate or even strenuous exercise is advantageous for children with asthma. In fact, some investigators have found significant improvement in work tolerance and cardiopulmonary fitness (Nickerson and others, 1983; Orenstein and others, 1985).

The American Academy of Pediatrics, Committee on Children with Disabilities and Committee on Sports Medicine (1984) agrees that physical activities are useful to these children and that the majority can participate in activities at school and in sports with minimum difficulty, provided the asthma is under control. Participation is encouraged but should be evaluated on an individual basis in terms of tolerance for duration and intensity of effort. Appropriate prophylactic treatment with β-adrenergic agents or cromolyn sodium before exercise will usually permit full participation in strenuous exertion. Restrictions are invoked only when the child's condition makes it necessary.

Prognosis. The outlook for children with asthma varies widely. An impressive number of children become asymptomatic at puberty, but there is no factor that can predict which children will "outgrow" their asthma. Some develop other forms of allergy in adulthood. It has been postulated that just as the skin manifestations of infancy (eczema) shift to the bronchi in childhood, there may be another shift in the susceptible tissues (shock organ) at adulthood—most frequently to the nose.

The prognosis for control or disappearance of symptoms will differ from children who have rare and infrequent attacks to those who are constantly wheezing or are subject to status asthmaticus. In general, the more severe and numerous the symptoms, the longer they have been present, and a family history of allergy increases the likelihood of a poor prognosis. Many who outgrow their attacks are subject to exercise-induced asthma as adults, and the associated disorders such as growth impairment, chest deformity, and airway obstruction are maintained throughout life.

The relationship between childhood asthma and the development of chronic obstructive pulmonary disease (COPD) in adulthood has not been determined satisfactorily. Smoking is the major risk factor for development of COPD, although numerous persons who had asthma have developed COPD without smoking (Coultas and Samet, 1987).

Deaths from asthma have been relatively uncommon, especially in young age-groups (Evans and others, 1987), but increases have been reported from various regions worldwide. The adolescent age-group appears to be the most vulnerable, with the greatest increase occurring in the ages between 10 and 14 years. No reliable data exist to explain this increase. Factors that have been postulated include exposure of atopic persons to more allergens, change in severity of the disease, abuse of drug therapy (toxicity), failure of families and practitioners to recognize severity of asthma, and psychologic factors, such as denial or refusal to accept the disease (Friday and Fireman, 1988). Risk factors for asthma deaths appear to be onset at an early age, frequent attacks, difficult-to-manage disease, adolescence, history of respiratory failure, psychologic problems (refusal to take medications), dependency on or misuse of drugs (high use), presence of physical stigmata (barrel chest, intercostal contractions), and deranged pulmonary function tests. Psychologic differences have also been found between children who died during an attack and similarly ill children who did not. Those who died had many of the risk factors but also had significant psychologic problems, such as extreme reactions to separation or loss, history of family turmoil, and expressed hopelessness or despair (Miller and Strunk, 1989).

Therapeutic Management: Specific

Children are subject to asthmatic attacks at varying intervals, with severity ranging from wheezing to life-threatening status asthmaticus. The modes of management vary according to the frequency and severity of the disease.

Intermittent (mild) asthma. Children with intermittent asthma have extended symptom-free periods, and their symptoms are usually relieved promptly with medical intervention. A variety of drug therapies are available for management, most commonly a short course of inhaled or oral bronchodilators. When symptoms have disappeared for several days, the drugs are discontinued. Occasionally, children with intermittent asthma have severe episodes requiring a short course of corticosteroids for control.

Status asthmaticus. Children who continue to display respiratory distress despite vigorous therapeutic measures, especially injections of epinephrine, are considered to be in *status asthmaticus*. The condition may develop gradually or rapidly, often coincident with complicating conditions such as pneumonia that can influence the duration and treatment of the attack. Status asthmaticus is a medical emergency that can result in respiratory failure and death if untreated.

Persistent hypoventilation leads to accumulation of carbon dioxide, with a decrease in arterial pH and respiratory acidosis. As a result, compensatory buffering mechanisms become overtaxed and the pH may drop to dangerous levels. Vomiting and dehydration cause further reduction of arterial pH by promoting retention of metabolic acids. Therapy of status asthmaticus is directed toward correction of dehydration and acidosis, improvement of ventilation, and treatment of any concurrent infection.

Several scoring systems have been devised for assessing the severity of bronchial obstruction, and most involve blood gas and pH measurements, presence of cyanosis, use of accessory muscles, breath sounds, and mental alertness. A child suspected of status asthmaticus is usually admitted to a pediatric intensive care unit for close observation and continuous cardiorespiratory monitoring.

The child is given intravenous fluids and nothing by mouth except liquids if the condition permits. Intravenous infusion provides a means for hydration and administering medications. Correction of dehydration, acidosis, hypoxia, and electrolyte derangements is guided by frequent determination of arterial pH, blood gases, and serum electrolytes.

Bronchospasm is relieved by constant intravenous infusion of theophylline sufficient to maintain serum levels at 10 to 20 $\mu g/ml$ and β-adrenergic agents via nebulizer, regulated by continual monitoring. Corticosteroids are given for any child with severe asthma who does not improve immediately, who has been taking steroids chronically, or who does not respond to other therapy (Eggleston, 1990). Occasionally, intravenous isoproterenol is administered for recalcitrant bronchospasm.

Humidified oxygen is administered by nasal prongs, hood, or face mask to maintain an arterial Po_2 greater than 65 torr but less than 100 torr to avoid the danger of oxygen narcosis. Mist tents do not allow for the close observation needed for the severely affected child. Since oxygen is a stimulus for respiration, high levels may significantly depress respirations. Controlled ventilation with endotracheal intubation may be needed when the condition progresses to respiratory failure, but it is rarely needed for more than 12 hours.

Sodium bicarbonate is administered to correct acidosis, since pH less than 7.25 impairs systemic, pulmonary, and coronary blood flow; normal pH enhances the response of bronchial smooth muscle to bronchodilator therapy (Galant, 1987). Antibiotics are frequently prescribed, since infection may be masked or may not always be evident and is always a threatening complication. As the attack subsides, fluids and medication are given orally (adrenergic agonists may be administered by MDI) and discharge plans are begun, especially follow-up care. Administration of steroids is withdrawn as rapidly as possible.

Nursing Considerations: Acute Care

Children who are admitted to the hospital with acute asthma are ill, anxious, and uncomfortable. In most instances, children are admitted as an emergency with status asthmaticus and are in acute distress. The importance of continual observation and assessment cannot be overemphasized.

✦ **NURSING ALERT** The child who sweats profusely and remains sitting upright and refuses to lie down is in severe distress. Also, the child who suddenly becomes agitated, or the agitated child who suddenly becomes quiet, may be seriously hypoxic and requires immediate intervention.

An intravenous infusion is begun immediately, and medication, usually corticosteroids and theophylline, is administered to relieve bronchospasm. The child is monitored closely and continuously during theophylline administration for relief of respiratory distress and signs of side effects or toxicity. Pulse, respiration, and blood pressure are taken and recorded every 5 minutes during rapid infusion and every 15 minutes for at least an hour after the drug has been absorbed. Toxicity can ocur with serum levels greater than 20 μg/ml.

✦ **NURSING ALERT** Side effects from theophylline include nausea, headache, irritability, and insomnia. Early signs of toxicity are nausea, tachycardia, and irritability; seizures and dysrhythmias occur at blood theophylline levels over 30 μg/ml.

Some practitioners prefer to administer aerosol β_2-adrenergics and corticosteroids. If aerosol medications are administered, the β-adrenergics are administered first to open the airways before administration of antiinflammatory agents.

It is especially important that the child receive sufficient fluid either orally or intravenously to replace losses through diaphoresis and hyperventilation. Liquids are best tolerated if they are warm or at room temperature. Cold liquids can trigger reflex bronchospasm and should be avoided (Seaman-Bates, 1980). Nourishment is provided in small, frequent feedings to avoid abdominal distention that might interfere with diaphragm excursion.

✦ **NURSING ALERT** Dehydration should be corrected slowly; overhydration can increase the accumulation of interstitial pulmonary fluid to exacerbate small airway obstruction.

Children usually prefer the high-Fowler position, although they may be more comfortable sitting upright or leaning slightly forward. When possible, the nurse communicates in such a way that a child need only reply in a few words to avoid fatigue. Shortness of breath makes talking difficult. Oxygen is indicated for relief of dyspnea and cyanosis; however, it is not administered indiscriminately but regulated according to the blood gas analysis and objective observation of color, respiratory effort, and sensorium. Associated treatments such as intermittent positive-pressure breathing or postural drainage and tests (such as blood gases or pulmonary function tests) may be performed by specialized personnel or may be the nurse's responsibility.

Children in status asthmaticus are apprehensive and anxious. Moreover, they are usually tired from respiratory efforts and loss of sleep. The calm, efficient presence of a nurse helps to reassure them that they are safe and will be cared for during this stressful period. It is important to assure children that they will not be left alone and that their parents are allowed to be near and available when needed.

Parents need reassurance, too. They want to be informed of their child's condition and therapies. They are upset, apprehensive about the child's condition, and feeling guilty. Often they feel that they may have in some way contributed to the child's condition or could have prevented the attack. They may even feel, consciously or unconsciously, anger toward the child for continuing to display symptoms despite their efforts to prevent or control the attack. Reassurance about their efforts expended on the child's behalf and their parenting capabilities can help alleviate their stress. All efforts to reduce parental apprehension will, in turn, help reduce the child's distress. Anxiety is easily communicated to the child from parents and members of the staff.

Nursing Considerations: General Care

Nursing care of children with asthma involves both acute and long-term care and includes therapies and observations described in previous discussions of respiratory disturbances. Nurses who are involved with children in the home, clinic, or practitioner's office play an important role in helping the children and their families learn to live with the condition. The disease can be tolerated if it does not interfere with family life, physical activity, or school attendance or if it does not require hospitalization.

Assessment

Nurses are involved in the initial assessment and workup to determine the cause and extent of the asthma. Physical assessment of asthma involves the same observations and techniques described in Chapters 7 and 31. In addition, some physical characteristics of chronic respiratory involvement are noted and evaluated, including chest configuration (such as barrel chest), posturing, and type of breathing. A history of the current and previous attacks and likely precipitating factors or events provides important information.

Nurses assist with various diagnostic tests, pulmonary function tests, and skin testing as well as a general health assessment. Also the child and family are assessed as to the degree to which the disorder (if previously diagnosed) interferes with everyday activities, the disorder alters the child's self-concept, and the child and family comply with the prescribed therapy.

Nursing Diagnoses

Based on a thorough assessment, several nursing diagnoses are identified. The more common diagnoses for the child with asthma are included in the Nursing Care Plan on p. 1467. Others may apply in specific situations.

Planning

The plan of care for a child with asthma includes the following:

1. Eliminate or avoid proven or suspicious irritants and allergens.
2. Relieve bronchospasm.
3. Maintain optimum health.
4. Prevent complications.
5. Promote normal activities.
6. Support and educate child and family regarding the disease and its management.

Implementation

The major emphasis of nursing care is directed toward outpatient management by the family. Parents are even able to manage acute attacks if they maintain contact with the practitioner and know how to observe for the expected response and signs of probable toxicity.

Allergen avoidance. The primary goal of asthma management is avoidance of an attack. Parents need to know the nature of the disease and, when the allergens are determined, how they can avoid and/or relieve asthmatic attacks. The nurse assists the parent in modifying the environment to reduce contact with the offending allergen(s) (Box 32-15). The parents are cautioned to avoid exposing a sensitive child to excessive cold, wind, or other extremes of weather, smoke, sprays, or other irritants. Passive smoking has been associated with exacerbation of symptoms in children with hyperresponsive airways, especially in boys and older children (Murray and Morrison, 1989).

Although foods are an unusual cause of asthma, foods known to provoke symptoms should be eliminated from the diet. Food additives (especially monosodium glutamate [MSG]), sulfites, and dyes) have been reported to produce allergic responses in sensitive persons. Families are taught to read labels carefully for the presence of these substances.

Since approximately 2% to 6% of children with asthma are sensitive to aspirin, nurses caution the parents to use other analgesic/antipyretic drugs for discomfort or fever. Acetaminophen appears to be a safe drug for these children and is recommended as the analgesic of choice (Fischer and others, 1983). Those children with aspirin-induced asthma may also be sensitive to nonsteroidal antiinflammatory drugs and tartrazine (yellow dye number 5, a common food coloring) (Tan and Collins-Williams, 1982). Other drugs that should be avoided by children with asthma are antihistamines (dry airway secretions, making expectoration difficult), cough suppressants (impair clearance of secretions), and sedatives (depress respirations and aggravate hypoventilation).

Box 32-15 "ALLERGY PROOFING" THE HOME

Reduce House Dust

Child's bedroom should be for sleeping, not playing.
Dust room daily and clean thoroughly weekly; child should not be in house during housecleaning activities.
Floors should be bare and damp mopped several times per week.
Remove from room unnecessary furniture, rugs, stuffed animals, upholstered furniture, etc.
Walls should be covered with washable paint or wallpaper.
Hot-air heating vents should be covered to prevent circulation of dust (e.g., when heat is turned on after summer accumulation of dust); substitute electric heater (properly protected) if possible.
Bedcovers, curtains, and scatter rugs should be made of smooth cotton or synthetic fabric and laundered frequently.
Closets should be free of stored articles, especially woolens.

Reduce Pollen and Other Allergens

Bedding should be free of allergens:
Use foam rubber or Dacron pillows, synthetic blankets.
Wool or feather items should be encased in nonallergenic coverings.
Use foam mattress or cover mattress and box springs with nonallergenic covers.
Windows and doors should remain closed during pollen season.
Pets, furry or feathered, should be excluded from home.

Reduce Exposure to Molds and Mildew

Avoid cellars as play area.
Clean showers and tile areas; spray with antimold agent (e.g., Lysol).
Keep vaporizers, air conditioners (including automobile) clean and free of mold.
Keep plants and aquariums out of a child's room.

Relieve bronchospasm. The parents and older children need to learn how to use the medications prescribed to relieve bronchospasm. They are taught to recognize early signs and symptoms of an impending attack so that it can be controlled before symptoms become distressing. Most children can recognize prodromal symptoms well before an attack (about 6 hours) so that preventive therapy can be implemented. Some objective signs that parents may observe include rhinorrhea, cough, low-grade fever, irritability, itching (especially in front of neck and chest), apathy, anxiety, sleep disturbance, abdominal discomfort, and loss of appetite. A simple, inexpensive peak flowmeter is available for use in the home to help parents assess the extent of the child's symptoms.*

Older children who use a nebulizer or aerosol device to deliver adrenergic drugs need to learn how to use the device correctly. The MDI (Fig. 32-7) combines portability with a rapid and reliable dose for patients managed at home. The objective of the device is to distribute the prescribed medication directly to the narrowed airways. It is important that the child learns to breathe slowly and deeply for better

*HealthScan Products Inc., 882 Pompton Ave., Cedar Grove, NJ 07009.

NURSING CARE PLAN
The Child with Bronchial Asthma

NURSING DIAGNOSIS: Potential for suffocation related to interaction between individual and allergen(s)

GOAL 1

Prevent asthmatic attack

INTERVENTIONS

Use prophylactic medication(s) according to instructions
Teach child and family correct use of bronchodilators, corticosteroids
Teach child and family how to avoid conditions or circumstances that precipitate asthmatic attack
Avoid contact with offending allergens
Assist parents in eliminating allergens that trigger attack
- Meal planning to eliminate allergenic foods
- Removal of pets
- Modification of environment; "allergy proof" home

Assist parents in obtaining and/or installing device to control environment (humidifier, air conditioner, electronic air filter)
Avoid extremes of environmental temperature
Avoid undue excitement and/or physical exertion
Teach child and family to recognize early signs and symptoms so that an impending attack can be controlled before it becomes distressful
Teach child to understand how equipment works
Teach child correct use of inhalers and peak flow meters

EXPECTED OUTCOMES

Family makes every effort to remove or avoid possible allergens or precipitating events
Family is able to detect signs of an impending attack early and implement appropriate actions

GOAL 2

Maintain optimum health

INTERVENTIONS

Encourage sound health practices
- Balanced, nutritious diet
- Adequate rest
- Hygiene
- Appropriate exercise

Prevent infection
- Avoid exposure to infection
- Employ meticulous care of equipment to avoid bacterial and/or fungal growth
- Employ good handwashing

EXPECTED OUTCOMES

Child and parents conform to sound health practices
Child exhibits no evidence of infection

NURSING DIAGNOSIS: Ineffective breathing pattern related to allergenic response in bronchial tree

GOAL 1

Improve ventilatory capacity

INTERVENTIONS

Instruct and/or supervise
- Breathing exercises
- Controlled breathing

Teach correct use of prescribed medication
Assist child and family in selecting activities appropriate to the child's capabilities and preferences
Encourage regular exercise
Encourage good posture
Encourage physical exercise involving stop-and-start activity that does not overtax the respiratory mechanism
Discourage physical inactivity

EXPECTED OUTCOMES

Child breathes easily and without dyspnea
Child engages in activities according to abilities and interest (specify)

NURSING DIAGNOSIS: Activity intolerance related to imbalance between oxygen supply and demand

GOAL 1

Promote rest

INTERVENTIONS

Encourage activities appropriate to the child's capabilities (specify)
Provide ample opportunities for rest and quiet activities

EXPECTED OUTCOMES

Child engages in appropriate activities (specify)
Child appears rested

NURSING DIAGNOSIS: Altered family processes related to having a child with a chronic illness

GOAL 1

Promote positive adaptation to the disorder

INTERVENTIONS

Foster positive family relationships
Be alert to signs of parental rejection or overprotection
Intervene appropriately if there is evidence of maladaptation
Use every opportunity to increase the parents' and child's understanding of the disease and its therapies
Be alert to signs that the child may be using symptoms to manipulate interpersonal relationships
Refer family to appropriate support groups and community agencies

EXPECTED OUTCOMES

Family copes with symptoms and effects of the disease and provides a normal environment for the child

See also Nursing Care Plan: The Child with a Chronic Illness or Disability, Chapter 22

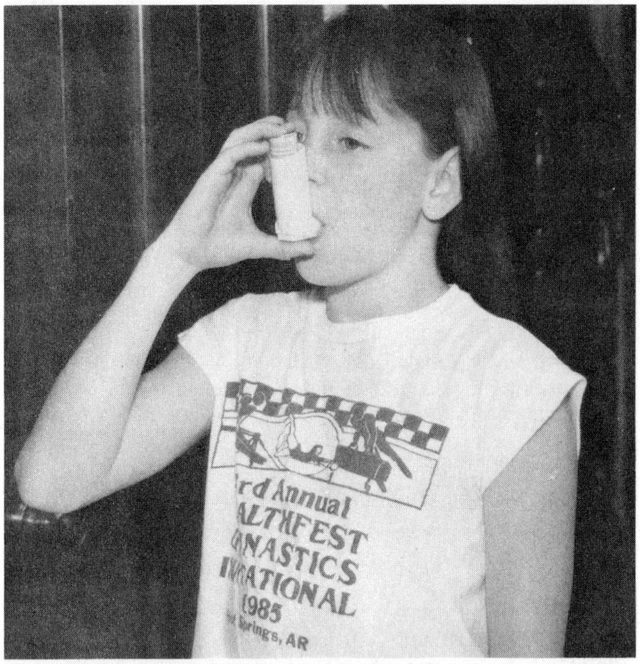

Fig. 32-7. Child using metered-dose inhaler.

Box 32-16 GUIDELINES FOR CORRECT USE OF METERED-DOSE INHALER

1. Shake the inhaler immediately before use with the cap on the mouthpiece.
2. Hold inhaler ready to use and remove cap.
3. Breathe out fully.
4. With the inhaler in an upright position, insert the mouthpiece into the mouth to form an airtight seal between the lips and the inhaler mouthpiece.
5. At the end of a normal expiration, breathe in slowly and deeply, while simultaneously depressing the top of the inhaler canister firmly to release drug mist.
6. Relax the pressure on the top of the canister.
7. Hold the breath for 10 seconds or as long as possible.
8. Remove inhaler and breathe out slowly through the nose.
9. Repeat in 2 to 5 minutes or as instructed by the practitioner.

Modified from Nemec, M.A.: Inhalational medications for chronic asthma, J. Pediatr. Nurs. 1:223-227, 1987.

NURSING TIP: PROPER USE OF INHALER

To determine if children are using an inhaler properly, have them use the device in front of a mirror. If vapor appears on the mirror, the inhaler is being used incorrectly. Children can check their effectiveness daily by this method (Barrow, 1987).

distribution to narrowed airways (Box 32-16). Rapid inspiration causes the drugs to move through unobstructed bronchioles to patent airways where they are less needed. Controversy exists regarding the amount of time to wait between puffs; the recommendations range is from 2 to 10 minutes.

Young children and those who are otherwise unable to manipulate the device or coordinate breathing with activation of the MDI are able to use special chambers called add-on devices, spacers, or extension tubes. These permit an operator to deliver the medication from the MDI into the spacer from which the child inhales.

The child and parents also need to be cautioned about the adverse effects of prescribed drugs and the dangers of overuse. They should know that it is important to use them when needed but not indiscriminately or as a substitute for avoiding the symptom-provoking allergen. Parents and child are taught to report any changing reaction to a drug or if the drug appears to be losing its effectiveness, as evidenced by more frequent need for the drug. Parents are also cautioned against purchasing generic substitutions for prescribed theophylline, since dosage varies considerably. Also, over-the-counter preparations may contain duplicate medications that increase the dosage of a prescribed drug (e.g., Bronkaid R, which contains theophylline). Toxicity has been reported from this practice (Keyes, 1987).

Maintain health and prevent complications. The child should be protected from a respiratory infection that can trigger an attack or aggravate the asthmatic state, especially in young children. Their airways are mechanically smaller and more reactive; therefore edema from infection causes wheezing and other signs of respiratory obstruction. Also, the equipment used for the child, such as nebulizers, must be kept absolutely clean to decrease the chances of contamination with bacteria and fungi. Oral candidiasis is a major complication of aerosolized steroids; therefore children with severe asthma who are taking steroids by this route are taught to rinse the mouth thoroughly with water after each treatment to minimize the risk of infection.

Breathing exercises and controlled breathing are taught and encouraged for the motivated youngster, and the nurse can help to select activities suitable to the child's capacity. Anything that promotes proper diaphragmatic breathing, side expansion, and generally improved mobility of the chest wall is encouraged by many practitioners.

Asthma camps have become popular in recent years as a means of encouraging physical activity in a more homogeneous, controlled, and less competitive environment. Not all persons subscribe to this practice; some support the positive benefits, which are primarily that the denominator of asthma is removed as a factor. Everyone at the camp has asthma; therefore no child is different from the others.

Promote normal activities. Self-care is the hallmark of effective asthma management, and self-management programs are important in helping the child and family to learn as much as possible about the factors that precipitate an

NURSING TIP: BREATHING COLD AIR

To reduce the probability of an attack triggered by cold air, teach the child to breathe through the nose (not the mouth). Also, a reservoir of warm air can be created by having the child wear a mask or swaddling the nose and mouth in a scarf when in cold air.

NURSING TIP: BREATHING EXERCISES

Play techniques that can be used for younger children to extend their expiratory time and increase expiratory pressure include blowing cotton balls or a Ping-Pong ball on a table, blowing a pinwheel, or preventing a tissue from falling by blowing it against the wall.

Box 32-17 OBJECTIVES OF SELF-MANAGEMENT PROGRAMS

To remove the stigma of self-fault for the condition
To integrate the reality of asthma into the life-style of the individual's choice
To learn management skills to avoid or minimize conditions that cause asthma attacks

asthma attack and the most effective means of bringing the disease under control (Box 32-17).

Most self-management programs convey four principles to the child and family regarding the disease and its management. First, asthma is a very common disease, and to have asthma is annoying but not disgraceful. Even though emotions have been implicated in asthma, psychologic aspects are primarily a response to it rather than a cause. Emotions and stress can be major triggers, but the disease, not the individual, is responsible for the symptoms. Absolution of the individual from the responsibility for the etiology makes the concept of a therapeutic plan more sensible and acceptable.

Second, persons with asthma are able to live full and active lives. Learning about others who have accomplished their goals (e.g., Theodore Roosevelt) and meeting children of the same age who are dealing effectively with their disease, including engaging in age-related activities, such as sports, provide positive examples of what is possible.

Third, it is much easier to prevent than to treat an asthmatic attack. The importance of compliance to a therapeutic program and learning the activities or factors that trigger an attack are emphasized. Sustained-release medications and appropriate drug administration before exercise or with a respiratory infection have made it possible for children with asthma to avoid an attack.

Fourth, individuals do not become addicted to asthma medication, but they do prefer to breathe more freely whenever possible. Emphasis is on management rather than cure. The cost/benefit of each medication is explained, and attempts are made to assess the "wheezogenic" potential by tapering the medication periodically to demonstrate that the management process is a dynamic one in which the child and the parent are active participants (Lewiston, 1986).

Several approaches are used to facilitate self-management. Self-contained programs and brochures for patient education are available through the national office of the **Asthma and Allergy Foundation of America (AAFA).*** The **American Lung Association†** also has brochures about asthma available through the local offices. One that is highly recommended is *Superstuff,* a workbook for elementary and junior high school children that includes self-management techniques using a variety of educational aids. An excellent and highly recommended publication is *Children with Asthma: A Manual for Parents.‡* Self-management instruction in group settings (e.g., camps for children with asthma) are a very popular means for education and training. Three such packaged programs are available that have proved successful. Many are funded by organizations with support from local health professionals, institutions, and interested families. One, *ACT (Asthma Care Training),* a five-session program with the theme "You're in the Driver's Seat," using driving and traffic analogies, is available without charge through the **Asthma and Allergy Foundation of America.** *WOW (Winning Over Wheezing)* is a cassette-workbook developed for group instruction.§

Asthma education and awareness are an important aspect of asthma management. Although the principles of self-management are very general and the programs designed for general use, each child and family have their own special needs that require individualized care and attention.

Child and family support. The nurse working with children with asthma can provide them with support in a number of ways. Many asthmatic children voice frustration about the ways their attacks interfere with their goal achievements and social lives. They need education about their disease, and they need to realize that it is not as bad as they might think. Children, their families, and their peers need to know what to do to prevent an attack and what to do during an attack. These children need reassurance from the health team and reinforcement of their coping mechanisms. Last of all, they need "grit"—the courage to help them live and cope with their condition one day at a time.

Both short- and long-term adaptation of affected children to the disease depends to a great extent on the family's ac-

*1717 Massachusetts Ave., Suite 305, Washington, DC 20036; (202) 265-0265.

†National office: 1740 Broadway, New York, NY 10019; (212) 315-8700.

‡Available from Pedipress, Inc., 125 Red Gate Lane, Amherst, MA 01002; (413) 549-7798.

§Winning Over Wheezing, Rhône-Poulenc-Rorer, Inc., 500 Virginia Dr., Fort Washington, PA 19304.

ceptance of the disorder. The task of living day-to-day with affected children involves the family continually. There are periodic crises and the ever-present threat of a crisis, requiring parental vigilance, sleepless nights, frequent emergency trips to the hospital, and often overwhelming medical expenses. Throughout these stresses, parents are expected and encouraged to promote as normal a life as possible for their children without neglecting the needs of siblings.

Evaluation

The effectiveness of nursing interventions is determined by continual reassessment and evaluation of care based on the following observational guidelines and expected outcomes:

1. Interview family about removal or avoidance of known allergens.
2. Observe child for evidence of respiratory symptoms.
3. Assess child's general health.
4. Observe child and interview family about any infections or other complications.
5. Interview child about daily activities.
6. Determine the degree to which the family and child understand the child's condition and the extent to which the therapies are carried out.

Expected outcomes:
See Nursing Care Plan, p. 1467.

CYSTIC FIBROSIS

Cystic fibrosis (CF) is the most common serious pulmonary and genetic disease of children. CF, a multisymptom disorder, primarily affects the exocrine (mucus-producing) glands of white children. In the early 1950s, life expectancy for children with CF was very short. Currently with early diagnosis and treatment more than half of patients survive into adulthood.

Etiology

CF is inherited as an autosomal-recessive trait; therefore the affected child inherits the defective genes from both parents with an overall incidence of 1:4 (see Chapter 5). The incidence of the disease is estimated at approximately 1:1600 births in predominantly white populations, with a carrier prevalence of 1:20 (Nora and Fraser, 1989) and an equal sex distribution. Although the disease is found in all racial and socioeconomic groups, it is almost nonexistent in Asians and is far less prevalent in blacks, occurring primarily in areas in which there is likely to be mixed ancestry.

It has been determined that the gene responsible for CF is located on chromosome 7 and is believed to code for production of a regulator protein that may be a membrane channel for chloride ions.

Pathophysiology

The disease is characterized by several apparently unrelated clinical features—increased viscosity of mucous gland secretions, a striking elevation of sweat electrolytes, an increase in several organic and enzymatic constituents of saliva, and abnormalities in autonomic nervous system function. There is some evidence for overactivity of the autonomic nervous system, which stimulates the cholinergic glands. This theory is plausible, since this system innervates all exocrine glands, but findings are not conclusive. Patients with CF demonstrate decreased pancreatic secretion of bicarbonate and chloride (Kopelman and others, 1988), and the primary transport abnormality in CF involves an electrogenic chloride channel or its regulation (Orlando and others, 1989). An increase in sodium and chloride in both saliva and sweat is characteristic of children with CF and forms the basis for one of the most reliable diagnostic procedures, the sweat chloride test.

The sweat electrolyte abnormality is present from birth throughout life and is unrelated to the severity of the disease or the extent to which other organs are involved. The sodium and chloride content of sweat in children with CF is two to five times greater than that of the controls in 98% to 99% of affected children. It has been demonstrated that a decrease in cellular permeability to chloride may explain the observation of electrolyte alterations in CF and might be the basic generalized biochemical abnormality in this disorder (Quinton and Bijman, 1983).

The primary factor, and the one that is responsible for the multiple clinical manifestations of the disease, is mechanical obstruction caused by the increased viscosity of mucous gland secretions (Fig. 32-8). Instead of forming a thin, freely flowing secretion, the mucous glands produce a thick, inspissated mucoprotein that accumulates and dilates them. Small passages in organs such as the pancreas and bronchioles become obstructed as secretions precipitate or coagulate to form concretions in glands and ducts.

Respiratory tract. Because of the increased viscosity of bronchial mucus, there is greater resistance to ciliary action (probably secondary to infection and ciliary destruction), a slower flow rate of mucus, and incomplete expectoration, which also contributes to the mucous obstruction. This retained mucus serves as an excellent medium for any bacterial growth. Reduced oxygen–carbon dioxide exchange causes variable degrees of hypoxia, hypercapnia, and acidosis. In severe, progressive lung involvement, compression of pulmonary blood vessels and progressive lung dysfunction frequently lead to pulmonary hypertension, cor pulmonale, respiratory failure, and death.

Pulmonary complications are present in almost all children with CF, but the onset and extent of involvement are variable. Symptoms are produced by stagnation of mucus in the airways with eventual bacterial colonization leading to destruction of lung tissue. The abnormally viscous and tenacious secretions are difficult to expectorate and gradually obstruct the bronchi and bronchioles, causing scattered areas of atelectasis and emphysema. The stagnant mucus offers a favorable environment for bacterial growth. Infection usually begins in the early years with *S. aureus* and *H. influenzae; P. aeruginosa* predominates in later years. *P. aeruginosa* infection is highly specific to CF, is confined to the lungs, and does not appear to threaten immunocompetent persons. The bacteria develop resistance to multiple drugs and are almost impossible to eradicate. Multiple antibodies developed by the patient to the bacteria are ineffective in

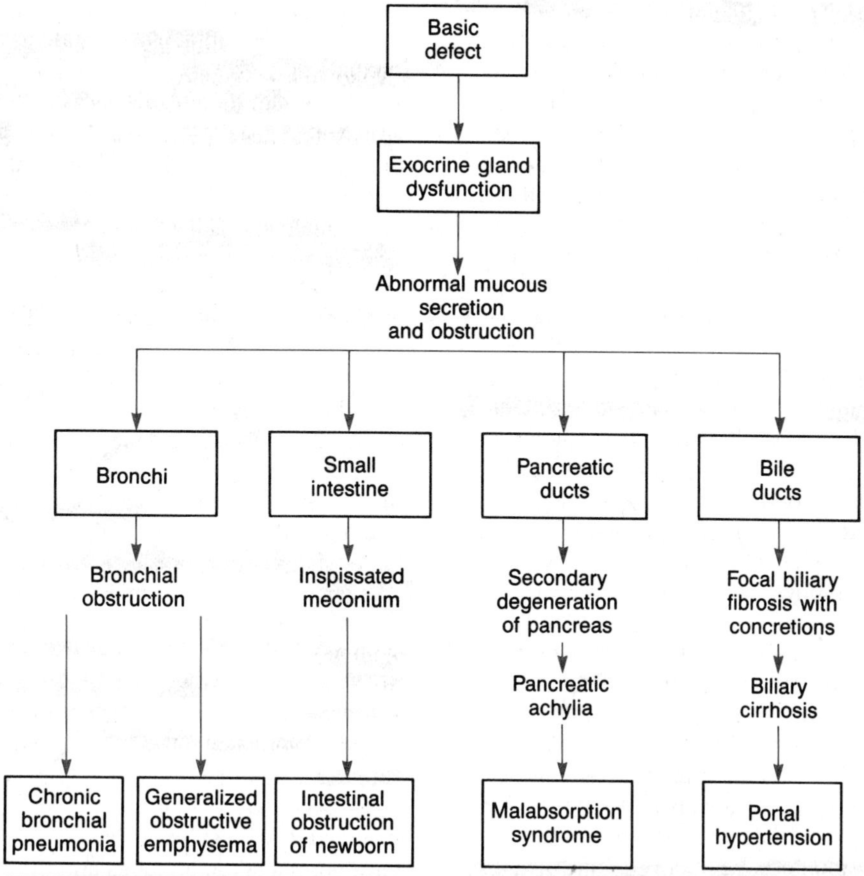

Fig. 32-8. Various effects of exocrine gland dysfunction in cystic fibrosis.

controlling infection, and the host is able to tolerate large concentrations of bacteria without overt evidence of worsening.

Gradual progression of pulmonary disease follows chronic infection, bronchial epithelium is destroyed, and infection spreads to peribronchial tissues, resulting in weakening of bronchial walls and peribronchial fibrosis. The pattern is chronic, progressive fibrosis with decreased O_2 and CO_2 exchange and a concurrent alteration in pulmonary vasculature. Chronic hypoxemia causes contraction and hypertrophy of medial muscle fibers in pulmonary arteries and arterioles, leading to pulmonary hypertension and eventual cor pulmonale. Pneumothorax may occur when peripheral bullae rupture; hemoptysis can occur when the bronchial wall is eroded through to an artery.

Gastrointestinal tract. The extent of gastrointestinal (GI) involvement varies from patient to patient. In the pancreas of many patients, the thick secretions block the ducts, leading to cystic dilations of the acini (small lobes of the gland), which then undergo degeneration and progressive diffuse fibrosis. This event prevents essential pancreatic enzymes from reaching the duodenum, which causes marked impairment in the digestion and absorption of nutrients—particularly fats, proteins, and, to a lesser degree, carbohydrates. Disturbed absorption is reflected in excessive stool fat (steatorrhea) and protein (azotorrhea).

The endocrine function of the pancreas often remains unchanged, since the islets of Langerhans are normal but may decrease in number as pancreatic fibrosis progresses. However, the incidence of diabetes mellitus is greater in these children than in the general population, which may be caused by changes in pancreatic architecture and diminished blood supply over time (Goodchild and Dodge, 1985). Consequently, with increased survival insulin-dependent diabetes is becoming a more frequent finding in the CF population. There is no relationship between the progression of pulmonary disease and the development of diabetes mellitus in CF (Wheeler and Colten, 1988). Diabetic ketoacidosis is rare.

In the liver focal biliary obstruction and fibrosis are common and become more extensive with time, eventually giving rise to a distinctive type of multilobular biliary cirrhosis. A few children develop extensive liver involvement. The gallbladder is small and contains a firm, gelatinous material that also fills the cystic duct. Findings similar to those in the pancreas are found in the salivary glands and contribute to a dry mouth and susceptibility to infection as a result of interference with salivation.

Clinical Manifestations

The clinical manifestations vary widely among children with CF and change as the disease progresses. The usual pattern is one of failure to thrive and gradual deterioration of the respiratory system. The diagnosis is not readily apparent in most cases, especially when there is no familial evidence of disease. Some children display symptoms at birth; others may not develop symptoms for weeks, months, or years. Some show only mild forms of the disease with limited impairment of digestion and respiratory problems, whereas others have severe malabsorption and life-threatening pulmonary complications. Although most affected children display both pulmonary and GI symptoms, a few have only enzyme deficiency without pulmonary disease; a few have only pulmonary disease without pancreatic insufficiency.

Respiratory tract. Initial pulmonary manifestations are often wheezing respirations and a dry, nonproductive cough. Eventually diffuse bronchial and bronchiolar obstruction leads to irregular aeration with progressive pulmonary disturbance and secondary infection. Dyspnea increases, the cough often becomes paroxysmal, and the mucoid impactions within the small air passages cause a generalized obstructive emphysema and patchy areas of atelectasis.

Progressive pulmonary involvement with hyperaeration of functioning alveoli produces the overinflated, barrel-shaped chest in which the anteroposterior diameter approaches the lateral diameter. When ventilation is significantly impaired, cyanosis and clubbing of fingers and toes occur. The child suffers repeated episodes of bronchitis and bronchopneumonia and is subject to chronic sinusitis and nasal polyps. Respiratory symptoms mimic diseases such as pneumonia, bronchitis, asthma, whooping cough, tuberculosis, and bronchiectasis. The incidence of ear, nose, and throat surgeries is higher in this group of children when compared to the general population.

Gastrointestinal tract. The earliest postnatal manifestation of CF is *meconium ileus*, which occurs in 10% to 15% of newborns with the disease (Goodchild and Dodge, 1985). Thick, puttylike, tenacious, mucilaginous meconium blocks the lumen of the small intestine usually at or near the ileocecal valve, which gives rise to signs of intestinal obstruction, including abdominal distention, vomiting, failure to pass stools, and rapid development of dehydration with associated electrolyte imbalance. Thick intestinal secretions continue to be problematic for many people with CF throughout life. Gumlike masses in the cecum can obstruct the bowel, causing pain, nausea, and vomiting. This is referred to as "meconium ileus equivalent."

As the disease progresses, obstruction of pancreatic ducts prevents digestive enzymes (trypsin, chymotrypsin, amylase, lipase) from being released into the duodenum, which prevents conversion of ingested food into compounds that can be absorbed by the intestinal mucosa. Consequently, the nondigested food is excreted (chiefly unabsorbed fats and proteins), increasing the bulk of feces to two or three times the normal amount. The bulky nature of the stools may go unnoticed at first, but usually by 6 months of age the child passes large, loose stools with normal frequency or a chronic diarrhea of unformed stools. As solid foods are added to the diet, the excessively large stools become frothy and extremely foul smelling.

Because so little is absorbed from the intestine, affected children have difficulty maintaining weight despite a healthy appetite and diet. Unable to compensate for the fecal losses, children lose weight and exhibit marked wasting of tissues and failure to grow. The abdomen is distended, the extremities are thin, and the sallow skin droops from wasted buttocks. The impaired ability to absorb fats results in a deficiency of the fat-soluble vitamins A, D, E, and K (which causes easy bruising); and anemia is a common complication. These GI symptoms are similar to those seen in children with celiac disease, and failure to thrive is a frequent initial diagnosis in young children with CF. When the child is ill with an infection, especially *Pseudomonas*, the appetite usually decreases with subsequent weight loss. Sometimes hospitalization is necessary.

The most common GI complication associated with CF in untreated children is *prolapse of the rectum*, which occurs most often in infancy and childhood and is related to large, bulky stools and lack of supportive fat pads around the rectum. The problem is seldom encountered in well-treated patients. Affected children of all ages are subject to peptic ulcers, pancreatic insufficiency, and intestinal obstruction from inspissated or impacted feces. Abdominal distention is common, abdominal cramps may be excessive, and foul-smelling flatus is a common complaint. Malnutrition is another commonly associated problem.

Reproductive system. Reproductive systems of both males and females with CF are affected. Females with CF have normal fallopian tubes and ovaries, but fertility can be inhibited by highly viscous cervical secretions, which act as a plug, blocking sperm entry. With few exceptions males are sterile, which may be caused by blockage of the vas deferens with abnormal secretions or by failure of normal development of the wolffian duct structures (vas deferens, epididymis, and seminal vesicles), resulting in decreased or absent sperm production.

Integumentary system. The consistent finding of abnormally high sodium and chloride concentrations in the sweat is a unique characteristic of CF. Parents frequently observe that their infants taste "salty" when they kiss them. The chloride channel defect in sweat glands prevents reabsorption of sodium and chloride, which leaves the affected person at risk for abnormal salt loss, dehydration, and hypochloremic and hyponatremic alkalosis during hyperthermic conditions. This is especially important to the infant because of limited fluid stores and the potential for inadequate sodium intake with most commercially prepared infant formulas.

The disease is sometimes expressed in other ways, for example, hypoelectrolytemia caused by massive losses through the sweat, especially in high environmental temperatures or febrile episodes. Infants with CF who fail to thrive frequently demonstrate hypoalbuminemia resulting from diminished absorption of protein, which in severe cases causes generalized edema.

Diagnostic Evaluation

An initial evaluation is conducted with general appraisal in the areas of general activity, physical findings, nutritional status, and findings on chest radiographs. The diagnosis of CF is suspected in the child who fails to thrive and/or suffers frequent upper respiratory infections and is established on the basis of duplicate sweat chloride tests. A positive family history aids in diagnosis.

The quantitative sweat chloride test (pilocarpine iontophoresis) involves stimulating the production of sweat, collecting the sweat, and measuring the sweat electrolytes. The quantitative analysis requires a minimum of 50 mg of sweat; 75 to 100 mg is preferable. Two separate samples are collected to assure the reliability of the test for any individual. Because newborns do not have active sweat glands, it is often difficult to obtain an adequate sample for analysis. Therefore if results are questionable, the test is repeated at a later date. The test should be performed only by personnel skilled in the procedure.

Normally sweat chloride content is less than 40 mEq/L, with a mean of 18 mEq/L. A chloride concentration greater than 60 mEq/L is diagnostic of CF; levels of 40 to 60 mEq/L are highly suggestive of the disease. Children with questionable results are followed carefully for any evidence of pulmonary system symptoms so that treatment can be implemented immediately.

Chest radiography reveals characteristic patchy atelectasis and obstructive emphysema. Pulmonary function tests are sensitive indexes of lung function, providing evidence of abnormal small airway function in CF. Other diagnostic tools that may aid in diagnosis include stool fat and/or enzyme analysis. Stool analysis requires a 72-hour sample with accurate recording of food intake during that time. Radiographs, including barium enema, are used for diagnosis of meconium ileus.

Development of DNA probes has enabled the identification of the disease in families in which there is an individual affected with CF. They are used successfully to identify heterozygotes and for prenatal diagnosis in families at risk. The tests detect only the gene defect presently known, which occurs in 70% of all CF carriers. The other 30% of cases are caused by different mutations of the gene (Roberts, 1990). Heterozygote screening and prenatal testing will not be available until the genes are identified.

Therapeutic Management

The goals of therapy are to assure adequate nutrition for growth, prevent or minimize pulmonary complications, and assist the child and family in adapting to a chronic disorder. Normal development should be expected, and life goals for fulfillment and happiness should be encouraged.

Management of pulmonary problems. Management of pulmonary problems is directed toward prevention and treatment of pulmonary infection by improving aeration, removing mucopurulent secretions, and administering antimicrobial agents. Most children will develop respiratory symptoms by 3 years of age. Young children normally have small airways and are predisposed to frequent viral infections. The large amounts and viscosity of respiratory secretions in children with CF contribute to the likelihood of infection. Once infection becomes established in relatively defenseless lungs, it is difficult to eradicate.

Prevention of infection involves a daily routine of chest physiotherapy to maintain pulmonary hygiene (see Chapter 31). In theory, postural drainage and percussion of the lungs loosen and move secretions toward the glottis to facilitate expectoration. Numerous studies have been conducted to evaluate the efficacy of the procedure. Several researchers have pursued the concept that exercise, deep breathing, and directed coughing are just as effective in preventing pulmonary deterioration. However, patients have been found to regress when conventional chest physiotherapy (CPT) is discontinued (Reisman and others, 1988). Therefore, although it is time-consuming for the child and family, CPT remains the cornerstone of pulmonary therapy.

CPT is usually performed twice daily (on rising and in the evening) and more frequently if needed, especially during pulmonary infection. Bronchodilator medication delivered in an aerosol helps open bronchi for easier expectoration and is administered before CPT when the patient exhibits evidence of reactive airway disease. No effective agents are available to decrease viscosity of secretions or break up mucus secretions. Mist therapy is of little proven value.

Forced expiration, or "huffing," with the glottis partially closed helps move secretions from small airways so that subsequent coughing can move secretions forcefully from large airways (Sutton, 1988). Several studies indicate this maneuver enhances the pulmonary function of patients with CF (Bain, Bishop, and Olinsky, 1988).

Physical exercise is an important adjunct to daily CPT. Exercise not only stimulates mucus secretion, it also provides a sense of well-being and increased self-esteem. In some instances exercise can be substituted for CPT. Any aerobic exercise that is enjoyed by the patient should be heartily encouraged. The ultimate aim of exercise is to establish a good habitual breathing pattern.

Pulmonary infections are treated as soon as they are recognized. Some practitioners prefer to prescribe oral antistaphylococcal drugs prophylactically at the time of diagnosis; others begin therapy when pulmonary symptoms arise. Sputum culture and sensitivity guide the choice of antibiotic. The trend is toward aggressive therapy even for milder disease.

Colonization with *P. aeruginosa* signals progressive involvement. Although the bacteria are impossible to eradicate, they can be successfully controlled for many years. Inhaled antibiotics are administered as a prophylactic measure in some centers, but once the organism has become established, antibiotic therapy is most effective given intravenously. Patients with CF metabolize antibiotics more rapidly than normal; therefore drug dosage is often higher than would be expected. The antibiotic selected (usually aminoglycosides, cephalosporins, or semisynthetic penicillins) depends on sensitivity of the organism. Duration of therapy depends on the patient's response, measured with clinical indicators including cough, fatigue, and exercise intolerance in addition to tests such as pulmonary function tests (PFTs), chest radiography, and O_2 and CO_2 measurements.

Intravenous antibiotics can be administered at home as an alternative to hospitalization as long as the family agrees and regular monitoring for toxicity can be accomplished.

Home care has become widely accepted as both medically safe and less costly. Studies indicate that home therapy for CF with pulmonary exacerbations is as effective as in-hospital therapy (Donati, Guenette, and Auerbach, 1987). Most children have central venous access devices for home administration of intravenous medications. When pulmonary function does not improve with outpatient management, hospitalization may be recommended for continued antibiotic therapy and vigorous CPT.

Oxygen administration is usually recommended for children with acute episodes, but since many of these children have chronic CO_2 retention, the unsupervised use of oxygen can be harmful (see Oxygen Toxicity, Chapter 31).

Pneumothorax, which may occur in patients with more advanced disease, may resolve spontaneously or require placement of a chest tube. Aggressive management is more common since recurrence rates have been shown to be 70% to 100% if untreated. Surgical treatment with pleurectomy or pleurodesis is indicated if respiration is impaired (Seddon, 1988).

Hemoptysis occurs frequently in older children with CF but is usually mild and often associated with exacerbation of bacterial infection of the airway. Hemoptysis greater than 300 cc in 24 hours is considered to be life threatening and must be treated (Wheeler and Colten, 1988). Vitamin K is administered and intravenous antibiotics are started. Bronchoscopy may be performed to determine the bleeding site, and bronchial artery embolization or lobectomy may be necessary.

Nasal polyps are removed surgically to relieve blockage of nasal passages. Sinusitis is treated symptomatically with appropriate antibiotic therapy.

Cor pulmonale is right ventricle hypertrophy in response to increased resistance in the pulmonary vascular bed. Low-flow O_2 therapy can reverse some of the pulmonary hypertension induced by alveolar hypoxia. O_2 is usually begun when arterial saturation is below 90% for extended periods and is often administered at nighttime only, so that the patient can be up and about unhindered during the daytime (Wheeler and Colton, 1988). Diuretics, digitalis, and salt restriction can be helpful in decreasing the vascular load on the right heart. In advanced disease, the right heart decompensates and congestive heart failure becomes evident.

A few heart-lung transplants have been successfully performed on children with CF with advanced pulmonary vascular disease and severely disabled by dyspnea and hypoxia. Long-term survival has yet to be evaluated, but improved quality of life in these children is encouraging.

Management of gastrointestinal problems. The principal treatment for pancreatic insufficiency is replacement pancreatic enzymes, which are administered with meals and snacks to ensure that digestive enzymes are mixed with food in the duodenum. Enteric-coated products prevent the neutralization of enzymes by gastric acids, thus allowing activation to occur in the alkaline environment of the small bowel. The amount of enzymes depends on the severity of the insufficiency, the response of the child to enzyme replacement, and the philosophy of the practitioner. Usually 1 to 5 capsules are administered with a meal, and a smaller amount is taken with snacks. Capsules can be swallowed whole or taken apart and the contents sprinkled on a small amount of food to be taken at the beginning of the meal. The amount of enzyme is adjusted to achieve normal growth and a decrease in the number of stools to two or three per day.

The diet for children with CF should be well balanced, and impaired intestinal absorption necessitates a diet significantly higher in calories than is normally required in a child of similar size. Children with CF often need 150% of the recommended daily allowance to meet their needs for growth. Restriction of fat is not necessary (Luder and others, 1989). The uptake of fat-soluble vitamins is decreased in these children because of impaired digestion and absorption of fat in the intestine. Multivitamin preparations are prescribed and vitamin K is administered to infants under 1 year of age and to patients with liver involvement.

Infants with pancreatic insufficiency have special problems in the first months of life. Cow's milk formulas are usually adequate and breast-feeding can be sustained if the infant is given supplemental enzymes before each feeding. A small amount of enzyme is mixed into cereal or fruit. If a child fails to gain weight or becomes hypoproteinemic, an elemental or predigested formula may be prescribed. However, the infant still requires enzyme replacement, and parents are cautioned to be aware of the sodium content of the formula. Very low sodium can lead to hyponatremia in infants with CF.

Children with CF should thrive with adequate replacement therapy and calorie intake. Failure to thrive despite adequate nutritional support usually indicates deterioration of pulmonary status. Occasionally, patients will be placed on supplemental tube feedings of parenteral alimentation in an effort to build up nutritional reserves if there has been a history of inability to maintain weight. This therapy may result in short-term improvement; however, long-term benefits have not been demonstrated (Stern, 1986).

Meconium ileus and meconium ileus equivalent usually improve with rectal administration of diatrizoate methylglucamine (Gastrografin) or acetylcysteine (Mucomyst). Laxatives, stool softeners, and a low-fat diet may also help to relieve the obstruction. Rectal prolapse is managed by simply guiding the rectum back into place with a gloved, lubricated finger and attempting to decrease the bulk of daily stools through enzyme replacement.

Salt depletion through sweating can be a problem during hot weather or physical exertion. Most children are able to adjust salt to their needs, and older children often exhibit a preference for salty foods. Salt supplementation is often needed during hot weather or febrile periods.

Some experimentation is being conducted to evaluate the use of recombinant human growth hormone, much the same as in children with growth hormone deficiency (see Chapter 38). The objective of growth stimulation is to improve physical strength and endurance, thereby promoting activity (e.g., exercise) and, ultimately, respiratory function.

Prognosis. It is the pulmonary involvement that determines the ultimate outcome of the disease. Pancreatic enzyme deficiency is less of a problem if adequate nutrition is ensured. Hemorrhage from liver cirrhosis and massive salt depletion in hot weather are occasional hazards. With early diagnosis and improved therapeutic measures, the life expectancy has improved. Many more children are reaching adulthood; however, the variation in severity of the disease is an important factor in determining the ultimate outcome. Children whose presenting symptoms were gastrointestinal at diagnosis have a good clinical course; those whose initial symptoms at diagnosis were pulmonary frequently demonstrate subsequent clinical deterioration (Katz and others, 1986).

No exact figures are available regarding the life expectancy of a child with CF. Many still die in infancy and early childhood, but increasing numbers are living into the third and fourth decades and even beyond. More than 50% of the patients now live into adulthood. With increasing survival, the incidence of insulin-dependent diabetes mellitus is also increasing, providing an additional management problem.

Nursing Considerations

Nursing care of infants and children with CF involves both acute and chronic management. These children require regular observation and medical supervision, including ongoing assessment of general health and nutritional and pulmonary status.

The nurse's contact with an affected child usually begins when the child is brought to the hospital or clinic for confirmation of the diagnosis. Perhaps the reason for hospitalization is failure to thrive or recurrent respiratory infections. Later, during recurrent admission to the hospital or during ongoing follow-up in the clinic or at home, the nurse and the child develop a sustained relationship.

Assessment

Assessment of the child with CF involves both pulmonary and GI observations. Pulmonary assessment is the same as that described for bronchial asthma (see p. 1465), with special attention to lung sounds, observation of cough, and evidence or degree of finger clubbing. GI assessment primarily involves observing the frequency and nature of the stools and abdominal distention. The observer is also alert to evidence of failure to thrive (e.g., weight loss, wasting, pallor, and fatigue). Family members are interviewed to determine the child's eating and eliminating habits, to observe salty perspiration, and to confirm a history of frequent respiratory infections or bowel obstruction in infancy.

Nursing Diagnoses

Based on a thorough assessment, several nursing diagnoses are identified. The more common diagnoses for the child with CF are included in the Nursing Care Plan on pp. 1476-1477. Others may apply in specific situations.

Planning

Nursing objectives for the child with CF include the following:

1. Promote pulmonary function, especially improve aeration and facilitate lung clearance.
2. Promote intake and absorption of nutrients.
3. Prevent or manage complications.
4. Facilitate growth and maintain optimum health.
5. Promote normal activities.
6. Support and educate child and family.

Implementation

On the initial contact, frequently in the hospital setting, nurses are involved in performing or assisting with diagnostic tests, primarily sweat for laboratory analysis of chloride content and, less often, stool specimens for trypsin and fat. The child, usually an infant, needs comfort during the procedures; young children need distraction while they are confined during iontophoresis. Even short periods of inactivity seem long to an active child. Children beyond very early childhood need an explanation of the strange, and sometimes painful, procedures and the equipment used for tests and treatments.

At first the respiratory equipment is frightening, especially to infants and very young children. The child needs patient support and guidance in using the equipment. Accepting uncharacteristic behavior and explaining this normal stress response to parents are important nursing functions.

Parents are anxious and puzzled. Few of them have any understanding of the disease process and the long-term implications it has for their family. They need patient and careful explanations of the disease, how it might affect their family, and what they can do to provide the best possible care for their child.

The shock associated with the diagnosis is overwhelming to parents. They must face the impact of the chronic, life-threatening nature of the disease and the prospect of intensive treatment, for which they must assume a major part of the responsibility and for which they are ill prepared. They often fear that they will be unable to provide the care the child needs. One of the most difficult aspects of the diagnosis is the implications inherent in its etiology, that is, the recognition that each parent contributed the gene responsible for the defect in their child.

Hospital care. When the child is hospitalized for confirmation of the diagnosis or for pulmonary complications, aerosol therapy is instituted or continued. Respiratory therapy is usually initiated and supervised by a trained respiratory therapist or physiotherapist. In institutions with large support staffs, they may provide all treatments. Otherwise, it becomes the responsibility of the nurse to perform the prescribed aerosol therapy and CPT and to teach supervised breathing exercises. CPT should not be performed before or immediately after meals. Planning the activity so that it does not coincide with meals is difficult in the hospital situation. However, it is very important and is often overlooked by nursing personnel.

Oxygen is cautiously administered to children in respiratory distress, but the child requires frequent assessment. The hazard of oxygen narcosis is a constant threat in chil-

NURSING CARE PLAN
The Child with Cystic Fibrosis

NURSING DIAGNOSIS: Ineffective airway clearance related to secretion of thick, tenacious mucus

GOAL 1
Expectorate mucus

INTERVENTIONS
Assist child to expectorate sputum
Provide nebulization with appropriate solution and equipment as prescribed
Perform chest physiotherapy

EXPECTED OUTCOMES
Child expectorates mucus
Airways are clear

NURSING DIAGNOSIS: Ineffective breathing pattern related to mechanical airway obstruction caused by thick mucus

GOAL 1
Ease respiratory efforts

INTERVENTIONS
Allow position of comfort
Promote rest
Maintain patent airway
Encourage child to engage in appropriate exercise
Implement measures to reduce anxiety and apprehension
Organize activities to allow for minimal expenditure of energy

EXPECTED OUTCOMES
Child rests and sleeps quietly
Respirations are unlabored
Respirations remain within normal limits (see inside front cover for normal variations)

GOAL 2
Increase oxygen supply to lungs

INTERVENTIONS
Position for maximum ventilatory efficiency such as high-Fowler position or sitting, leaning forward
*Provide oxygen as prescribed and/or needed
*Provide nebulization, if prescribed

EXPECTED OUTCOMES
Child breathes easily
Respirations remain within normal limits (see inside front cover for normal variations)

GOAL 3
Promote expectoration of mucous secretions

INTERVENTIONS
Ensure adequate fluid intake
Provide humidified atmosphere
Assist child to cough effectively

EXPECTED OUTCOME
Older child expectorates secretions appropriately and without undue stress and fatigue

GOAL 4
Reduce anxiety and apprehension

INTERVENTIONS
Provide constant attendance during acute phase of illness
Encourage presence of parents
Provide comfort and cuddling when possible
Provide quiet diversion appropriate to child's age and condition
*Administer medications that promote breathing (bronchodilators)

EXPECTED OUTCOMES
Child exhibits no signs of distress
Parents remain with child and provide comfort
Child engages in quiet activities appropriate for age, interest, and condition

NURSING DIAGNOSIS: Altered nutrition: less than body requirements related to inability to digest nutrients, loss of appetite (advanced disease)

GOAL 1
Promote digestion

INTERVENTIONS
*Administer pancreatic enzymes, with meals and snacks as prescribed

EXPECTED OUTCOME
Child takes medication

GOAL 2
Prevent malnutrition

INTERVENTIONS
Provide healthful diet with any modifications that may be prescribed
Provide adequate salt, especially when sweating (e.g., fever, hot weather)
*Administer multiple vitamins, iron as prescribed

EXPECTED OUTCOME
Child eats a balanced diet and exhibits a satisfactory weight gain

*Dependent nursing action.

NURSING CARE PLAN
The Child with Cystic Fibrosis—cont'd

NURSING DIAGNOSIS: Potential for infection related to impaired body defenses, presence of mucus as medium for growth of organisms

GOAL 1

Prevent infection

INTERVENTIONS

Promote good health practices
- Maintain adequate nutrition
- Maintain good hygienic habits

Observe good hand washing

Restrict contact with persons who have infections, including family, other children, friends, and members of staff

Observe medical asepsis, especially respiratory equipment

Keep child dry and warm

Instruct family, and child if old enough, in administration of prophylactic antibiotics

Instruct family to have child immunized yearly against influenza

EXPECTED OUTCOMES

Child and family apply good health practices

Child exhibits no evidence of infection

NURSING DIAGNOSIS: Activity intolerance related to imbalance between oxygen supply and demand

GOAL 1

Conserve energy

INTERVENTIONS

Promote effective breathing

Promote rest

Implement measures to reduce apprehension

Encourage child to engage in activities commensurate with interest and capabilities

EXPECTED OUTCOME

Child rests quietly and engages in activities suitable to energy level

NURSING DIAGNOSIS: Altered growth and development related to inadequate digestion of nutrients, chronic illness

GOAL 1

Promote nutrition

INTERVENTIONS

See Altered nutrition above

EXPECTED OUTCOME

Child exhibits normal growth

GOAL 2

Promote normal development

INTERVENTIONS AND EXPECTED OUTCOMES

See Nursing Care Plan: The Child with a Chronic Illness or Disability, Chapter 22

NURSING DIAGNOSIS: Altered family processes related to a child with a chronic and potentially fatal illness

GOAL 1

Support family

INTERVENTIONS

Refer to appropriate support groups and agencies

EXPECTED OUTCOMES

Family demonstrates the ability to cope with child's illness (specify behaviors)

Family contacts and becomes involved with appropriate agencies

See also:

Nursing Care Plan: The Child with a Chronic Illness or Disability, Chapter 22

Nursing Care Plan: The Child Who Is Terminally Ill or Dying, Chapter 23

dren with long-standing disease who receive oxygen (see Chapter 31). The child requires close observation to assist with cough and expectoration.

The diet is implemented for the newly diagnosed child or continued for the child who is hospitalized for pulmonary disease. Children in the early stages of the disease maintain a good appetite, and some will eat excessively. With infection and increased lung involvement, the appetite diminishes, however. Eventually it becomes a challenge to tempt failing appetites (see Feeding the Sick Child, Chapter 27). Some younger children may object to the extra fluids that are encouraged to prevent dehydration. Food is considered therapy for these patients. The caloric intake should be increased significantly. Pancreatic enzymes are supplied for each meal or snack, and adequate salt is provided, especially for febrile children.

Frequent skin care is carried out to prevent irritation and skin breakdown over bony prominences. Particular attention is necessary after use of the bedpan or when the diaper is changed. Careful cleansing helps to reduce irritation and odor from offensive stools.

The child will need support for the many treatments and tests that are a necessary part of the hospital therapy. Intravenous fluids and blood tests are almost always a part of the treatment, and the child soon associates hospitalization with these stress-provoking procedures. Because these children are usually quite thin with little muscle mass, careful selection of injection sites is required.

Support to both child and family is a vital part of nursing care. The progressive nature of the disease makes each illness requiring hospitalization a potentially life-threatening event. Skilled nursing care and sympathetic attention to the emotional needs of the child and family help them cope with the stresses associated with repeated respiratory infections and hospitalization.

When discussing the nature of the illness and the genetic etiology, families should be informed of services in the community that provide genetic counseling. The inheritance of CF is straightforward and offers little confusion if explained in the context of flipping two coins. It is important that the family fully understands the 1:4 likelihood of an affected child with each pregnancy (see Chapter 5).

Home care. After the diagnosis is confirmed and a treatment program determined, preparation for home care is implemented. A plan of care should be flexible enough so that family activities are disrupted as infrequently as possible. Parents will need help in finding inhalation equipment available for home use that best meets their needs. They will need opportunities to learn about and practice the use of the equipment, as well as some of the problems they may encounter.

They need to learn about the preferred diet of nutritious meals with tolerated fat and ample protein and carbohydrate, and the administration of pancreatic enzymes. Children usually adjust well to taking pancreatic enzymes. For infants and young children, the enzymes can be mixed with pureed fruit, such as applesauce, and fed with a spoon. Capsules are suitable for older children. It is important to stress to parents that the enzymes, in the amount regulated to the child's needs, should be administered with all meals and snacks. They are cautioned about not restricting salt, especially during hot weather, and ensuring an adequate fluid intake, since dehydration aggravates the thick mucus secretions. Oral hygiene is important because of interference with salivation and the increased susceptibility to oral infections.

One of the most important aspects of educating parents for home care is teaching chest physiotherapy and breathing exercises. The success of a therapy program depends on conscientious performance of these treatments regularly as prescribed. The number of times these therapies are performed each day is determined on an individual basis, and often parents readily learn to adjust the number and intensity of the treatments to the child's needs. Although it is usually the physiotherapist who instructs the parents, nurses frequently follow up the care in the home and assist the family with innovative approaches to therapy. For example, using games and normal childhood activities to achieve the desired end reduces the likelihood that treatment will meet with resistance from the child. When additional respiratory exercises are introduced to established routines, the family will need to be reeducated in new techniques, such as "huffing."

Postural drainage can be achieved with simple activities that are fun, such as hanging by the knees from a bar or low-hanging trapeze that can be easily built in the backyard (or indoors), turning somersaults, or playing "wheelbarrow" with the child suspended head down and propelling with the hands while the adult holds on to the feet. Most children respond to a challenge, such as, "How long can you stand on your head?" Small children can "stand on their heads" with their heads on the cushion of a large chair with or without an adult holding on to their feet. Parents soon learn to respond to cues from their children and incorporate spontaneous activities into the treatment regimen.

For pulmonary infection, home intravenous antibiotics may be prescribed. Home intravenous care is preferred for willing and competent families. It reduces tension and usually brings a sense of belonging to the family members. With the use of the venous access devices, the parents and child are taught the technique of direct administration into the intravenous line.* Unfortunately, around-the-clock administration may be difficult for families because it requires waking at least once during the night to give the drug.

The nurse can assist the family in contacting resources that provide help to families with affected children. The various special child health services, many local clinics, private agencies, service clubs, and other community groups often offer equipment and medications either free or at reduced rates. The **Cystic Fibrosis Foundation†** has chapters throughout the United States to provide education and services to families and professionals.

Family support. One of the most important and difficult aspects of providing care for the family of a child with CF is coping with the emotional needs of the child and family. The diagnosis, treatment, and prognosis are fraught with many problems, frustrations, and feelings. The diagnosis with all its implications evokes feelings of guilt and self-recrimination in parents. These feelings may be particularly marked if the newly diagnosed child is the second affected child in the family, and the parents had been counseled about the 1:4 risk of such an event occurring.

The long-range problems are those encountered in the care of a child with a chronic illness (see Chapter 22). Both the child and the family must make many adjustments, the

---

*Home care instructions for giving medications to children are available in Wong, D.L., and Whaley, L.F.: Clinical manual of pediatric nursing, ed. 3, St. Louis, 1990, Mosby–Year Book, Inc.

†6931 Arlington Road, Bethesda, MD 20814-3205; (800) FIGHT CF or (301) 951-4422. In Canada: **Canadian Cystic Fibrosis Foundation,** 586 Eglinton Ave. East, Suite 204, Toronto, Ontario M4P 1P2. Two excellent publications available from the Cystic Fibrosis Foundation are *What Everyone Should Know About Cystic Fibrosis* and *Cystic Fibrosis: A Summary of Symptoms, Diagnosis, and Treatment.*

success of which depends on their ability to cope and also on the quality and quantity of support they receive from outside sources. Combined efforts of a variety of health professionals offer the most comprehensive services to families. It is often the responsibility of the nurse to organize and coordinate these services, to assess the home situation, and to collect the data needed to evaluate the effectiveness of the services in meeting the family's needs.

For the family, the illness means modification of numerous family activities. Meals require planning in order not to place too many restrictions on the affected child or deprive the other members of the family. Limits on mobility restrict family recreational activities, especially when the child's therapy includes respiratory equipment that is not transportable. CPT must be continued wherever the child may be. In addition, members of the family hesitate to take the child too far from familiar and trusted medical care. The illness even determines the family's place of residence and employment, as the child's condition dictates that the family live near medical care facilities that offer the specialized care the child needs.

The persistent need for treatment several times daily also places a strain on the family. Someone must perform the procedures, such as percussion and vibration, even on older children who are able to assume responsibility for their own exercises and respiratory therapy. Children often balk at the treatments, and the parents are placed in the position of insisting on compliance. Sometimes the stress and anxiety related to this continual routine generate feelings of resentment, which are frequently focused on one aspect of the regimen, such as the diet or equipment. When possible, occasional trusted respite care should be made available to the parent or parents to allow them the opportunity to leave the situation for short periods without undue anxiety about the child's welfare.

The affected child also may become resentful about the disease, its relentless routine of therapy, and the necessary curtailment it places on activities and relationships. The child's activities are interrupted or built around treatment, medications, and diet that impose hardships (such as carrying medication to school and other places where the child may eat away from home), and growth retardation associated with most chronic illness may be trying. Any of these aspects of the disease may be the cause of ridicule from other children. However, the child should be encouraged to attend school and join age-appropriate groups, such as scouting, to foster a life that is as normal and productive as possible.

Families afflicted with CF have psychologic hurdles similar to those of all families coping with a child with a chronic illness (see Chapter 22), and a constant source of anxiety for both parents and child is the ever-present fear of death. However, despite the prognosis of a shortened life span, numerous hospitalizations and unpleasant complications, children with CF have been found to be amazingly well adjusted (Cowen, 1986). Patients and their siblings show generally healthy self-esteem, and family functioning is normal.

As the disease progresses, however, family stress should be expected, and the patient may become angry and noncompliant. It is important for the nurse to recognize the changing needs of the family. Families should be made aware of sources for counseling as stressful setbacks occur. Patients need to be guided into activities that enable them to express anger, sorrow, and fear without guilt.

As life expectancy continues to rise for children with CF, issues related to marriage, childbearing, and career choice become more pressing. Men must be informed at some point that they will be unable to produce offspring. It is important that the distinction be made between sterility and impotence. Normal sexual relationships can be expected. Female patients may be able to bear children, but must be made aware of the possible deleterious effects on the respiratory system created by the burden of pregnancy. They need to know that their children will be carriers of the CF gene.

Life as an independent adult, the goal that most families have for their children, should be encouraged for children with CF. From the time that children can take partial responsibility for their own care (e.g., CPT and taking enzymes), independence and accountability should be fostered. Although the prognosis for these children has improved, many do not survive through the second decade. Anticipatory grieving and other aspects related to care of a child with a terminal illness are part of nursing care (see Chapter 23).

Evaluation

The effectiveness of nursing interventions is determined by continual reassessment and evaluation of care based on the following observational guidelines and expected outcomes:

1. Monitor vital signs (especially respiratory parameters), chest physiotherapy, and exercise to assess the expected outcomes (e.g., expectoration of secretions, increased lung expansion).
2. Observe nutritional intake and enzyme administration. For the child at home, interview family about child's intake or have the child maintain a log of nutritional intake. Obtain regular measurements of growth.
3. Monitor child for evidence of respiratory infection, GI dysfunction, and other complications. Interview family about prophylactic medications, procedures, and activities.
4. Perform regular physical assessments. Interview family about the child's health status and maintenance (e.g., dental care).
5. Observe child and activities selected for participation. Interview child and family about school attendance, interaction with peers, and participation in sports and other activities.
6. Explore family's understanding of the disease and its therapies and their ability to carry out the treatment plan. Maintain contact with family (if feasible) at follow-up evaluations and home care. Observe for readmissions. Interview child and family about involvement with agencies and services for children with CF.

Expected outcomes:

See Nursing Care Plan, pp. 1476-1477.

KEY POINTS

- Acute infection of the respiratory tract is the most common cause of illness in infancy and childhood.
- The incidence and severity of respiratory tract infections are influenced by the infectious agent involved, the child's age, and the child's natural defenses.
- Symptoms of respiratory tract infections include fever, febrile convulsions, meningismus, anorexia, vomiting, diarrhea, abdominal pain, nasal blockage and discharge, cough, respiratory sounds, and presence or absence of sore throat.
- Common respiratory tract infections of childhood include acute nasopharyngitis, acute pharyngitis, influenza, tonsillitis, and otitis media.
- Streptococcal infection of the throat is not always associated with pharyngitis.
- Severe bleeding from the tonsil site can occur within 6 hours after surgery or 5 to 10 days after tonsillectomy.
- Factors that predispose children to otitis media are the shape and position of eustachian tubes, undeveloped cartilage lining, abundant pharyngeal lymphoid tissue, immature humoral defense mechanisms, and the recumbent position (in infants).
- Croup syndromes include acute laryngotracheobronchitis, acute spasmodic laryngitis, and acute epiglottitis.
- Epiglottitis is a medical emergency and is characterized by high fever, toxic appearance, and difficulty swallowing.
- The primary nursing function in the care of children with croup is observation for signs of respiratory embarrassment and relief of laryngeal obstruction.
- Common infections of the lower airway include bacterial tracheitis, asthmatic bronchitis, bronchitis, and bronchiolitis.
- Pneumonias are generally classified either by site (lobar, bronchial, or interstitial) or by etiologic agent (viruses, bacteria, mycoplasmas, or associated with foreign bodies).
- Management of uncomplicated bronchiolitis and viral pneumonia is symptomatic in otherwise healthy infants.
- In tuberculosis, resistance to the bacillus can be altered by heredity, sex, age, stress states, poor nutrition, and intercurrent infection.
- Signs of choking include inability to speak, cyanosis, and collapse.
- Inhaled objects are rarely coughed up spontaneously; they must be removed by direct laryngoscopy or bronchoscopy.
- Inducing a child to vomit is contraindicated in the event of hydrocarbon ingestion because of the danger of hydrocarbon aspiration.
- In asthma, hyperreactivity of airways is thought to be attributed to exaggeration of normal defenses of the respiratory tract, abnormal tissue reactions, or imbalance of normally balanced responses.
- Bronchial asthma can be triggered by a variety of agents and is characterized by bronchospasm, edema of the bronchial mucosa, and increased bronchial mucus secretion.
- Cystic fibrosis is the most frequently occurring inherited disease of white children and is transmitted by an autosomal-recessive gene.
- Diagnosis of cystic fibrosis is based on family history, absence of pancreatic enzymes, chronic pulmonary involvement, and an abnormally high sweat chloride concentration.

REFERENCES

Agah, R., and others: Respiratory syncytial virus (RSV) infection rate in personnel caring for children with RSV infections, Am. J. Dis. Child. 141:695-697, 1987.

American Academy of Allergy and Immunology, Executive Committee: The waiting period after allergen skin testing and immunotherapy 85:526-527, 1990.

American Academy of Pediatrics, Committee on Children with Disabilities and Committee on Sports Medicine: The asthmatic child's participation in sports and physical education, Pediatrics 74:155-156, 1984.

American Academy of Pediatrics, Committee on Environmental Hazards: Involuntary smoking—a hazard to children, Pediatrics 77:755-757, 1986.

American Academy of Pediatrics, Committee on Infectious Diseases: Report of the committee on infectious diseases, ed. 21, Elk Grove Village, IL, 1988, American Academy of Pediatrics.

American Academy of Pediatrics, Committee on Infectious Diseases: Ribavirin therapy of respiratory syncytial virus, Pediatrics 79:475-478, 1987.

American Academy of Pediatrics, Committee on Infectious Diseases: *Haemophilus influenzae* type b conjugate vaccine: immunization of children 2 to 15 months of age, AAP News 6(11):19 and 23, 1990.

American Academy of Pediatrics, Section on Allergy and Immunology and Section on Diseases of the Chest: Exercise and the asthmatic child, Pediatrics 84:392-393, 1989.

Avery, M.E., and First, L.R., editors: Pediatric medicine, Baltimore, 1989, Williams & Wilkins.

Bain, J., Bishop, J., and Olinsky, A.: Evaluation of directed coughing in cystic fibrosis, Br. J. Dis. Chest 82:138-148, 1988.

Baker, M.D.: Foreign bodies of the ears and nose in childhood, Pediatr. Emerg. Care 3(2):67-70, 1987.

Barrow, E.N.: Proper technique for using inhaler in asthma (letter), N. Engl. J. Med. 316:951-952, 1987.

Bar-Yishay, E., and Godfrey, S.: Exercise and hyperventilation induced asthma, Clin. Rev. Allergy 3:441-461, 1985.

Battaglia, J.D.: Severe croup: the child with fever and upper airway obstruction, Pediatr. Rev. 7:227-233, 1986.

Centers for Disease Control: Assessing exposures of health care personnel to aerosols of ribavirin—California, MMWR 37:560-563, 1988.

Chaudhary, S., and others: Penicillin V and rifampin for the treatment of group A streptococcal pharyngitis: a randomized trial of 10 days penicillin vs 10 days penicillin with rifampin during the final 4 days of therapy, J. Pediatr. 106:481-486, 1985.

Chen, Y., Li, W., and Yu, S.: Influence of passive smoking on admissions for respiratory illness in early childhood, Br. Med. J. 293:303-305, 1986.

Colombo, J.L., Hopkins, R.L., and Waring, W.W.: Steam vaporizer injuries, Pediatrics 67:661-663, 1981.

Conrad, D.A., and others: Aerosolized ribovarin treatment of respiratory syncytial virus infection in infants hospitalized during an epidemic, Pediatr. Infect. Dis. 6:152-157, 1987.

Coultas, D.B., and Samet, J.M.: Epidemiology and natural history of childhood asthma. In Tinkelman, D.G., Falliers, C.J., and Naspitz, C.K., editors: Childhood asthma pathophysiology and treatment, New York, 1987, Marcel Dekker, Inc.

Cowen, L., and others: Psychologic adjustment of the family with a member who has cystic fibrosis, Pediatrics 77:745-752, 1986.

Cunningham, A.S.: Morbidity in breast-fed and artificially fed infants, part II, J. Pediatr. 95:685, 1984.

Cunningham, D.G., and others: Unprescribed use of antibiotics in common childhood infections, J. Pediatr. 103:747-749, 1983.

David, T.J., and others: Prodromal itching in childhood asthma, Lancet 2:154-155, 1984.

Dick, E.C., and others: Interruption of transmission of rhinovirus colds among human volunteers using virucidal paper handkerchiefs, J. Infect. Dis. 153:352-356, 1986.

Dolovich, J., and others: Early/late response model: implications for control of asthma and chronic cough in children, Pediatr. Clin. North Am. 35:969-979, 1988.

Donati, M.A., Guenette, G., and Auerbach, H.: Prospective controlled study of home and hospital therapy of cystic fibrosis pulmonary disease, J. Pediatr. 111:28-33, 1987.

Douglas, R.M., and others: Prophylactic efficacy of intranasal alpha$_2$-interferon against rhinovirus infections in the family setting, N. Engl. J. Med. 314:65-70, 1986.

Eggleston, P.A.: Asthma. In Oski, F.A., and others, editors: Principles and practice of pediatrics, Philadelphia, 1990, J.B. Lippincott Co.

Eichenwald, H.F., and Mietens, C.: Pneumonias, lung abscess, and empyema. In Eichenwald, H.F., and Ströder, J., editors: Current therapy in pediatrics–2, Philadelphia, 1989, B.C. Decker, Inc.

Ellis, E.F.: Allergic disorders. In Behrman, R.E., and Vaughan, V.C., III: Nelson textbook of pediatrics, ed. 13, Philadelphia, 1987, W.B. Saunders Co.

Engel, N.S.: Multiple drug therapy for pediatric tuberculosis, MCN 14:169, 1989.

Esclamado, R.M., and Richardson, M.A.: Laryngotracheal foreign bodies in children, Am. J. Dis. Child. 141:259-262, 1987.

Evans, and others: The impact of passive smoking on emergency room visits of urban children with asthma, Am. Rev. Respir. Dis. 135:567-572, 1987.

Fagin, J., Friedman, R., and Fireman, P.: Allergic rhinitis, Pediatr. Clin. North Am. 28:797-806, 1981.

Feigin, R.D.: Group A streptococcal infections. In Oski, F.A., and others, editors: Principles and practice of pediatrics, Philadelphia, 1990, J.B. Lippincott Co.

Fischer, T., and others: Adverse pulmonary responses to aspirin and acetaminophen in chronic childhood asthma, Pediatrics 71:313-318, 1983.

Friday, G.A., and Fireman, P.: Morbidity and mortality of asthma, Pediatr. Clin. North Am. 35:1149-1162, 1988.

Furukawa, C.T., and others: Cognitive and behavioral findings in children taking theophylline, J. Allergy Clin. Immunol. 81:83-89, 1988.

Gala, C.L., and others: The use of nose goggles to control nosocomal respiratory syncytial virus infection, JAMA 256:2706-2711, 1986.

Galant, S.P.: Therapeutic approach to acute asthma in children. In Tinkelman, D.G., Falliers, C.J., and Naspitz, C.K., editors: Childhood asthma pathophysiology and treatment, New York, 1987, Marcel Dekker, Inc.

Gerber, M.A., and Markowitz, M.: Management of streptococcal pharyngitis reconsidered, Pediatr. Infect. Dis. 4:518-526, 1985.

Goldbloom, R.B.: Nasopharyngitis. In Gellis, S.S., and Kagan, B.M., editors: Current pediatric therapy 12, Philadelphia, 1986, W.B. Saunders Co.

Goldenhersh, M.J., and Rachelefsky, G.S: Childhood asthma: management, Pediatr. Rev. 10:259-265, 1989.

Goodchild, M., and Dodge, J.: Cystic fibrosis manual of diagnosis and management, ed. 2, Philadelphia, 1985, W.B. Saunders Co.

Guerra, I.C., Kemp, J.S., and Shearer, W.T.: Bronchiolitis. In Oski, F.A., and others, editors: Principles and practice of pediatrics, Philadelphia, 1990, J.B. Lippincott Co.

Guglielmo, B.J., Jacobs, R.A, and Locksley, R.M.: The exposure of health care workers to ribavirin aerosol (letter), JAMA 261:1880-1881, 1989.

Gutstadt, L.B., and others: Determinants of school performance in children with chronic asthma, Am. J. Dis. Child. 143:471-475, 1989.

Hands, B.: Blow-drying for otitis externa, Can. Med. Assoc. J. 137:1077, 1987.

Harris, C.S., and others: Childhood asphyxiation by food: a national analysis and overview, JAMA 251:2231-2235, 1984.

Hayden, G.F., and others: The effect of placebo and virucidal paper handkerchiefs on viral contamination of the hand and transmission of experimental rhinovirus infection, J. Infect. Dis. 152:403-407, 1985.

Honicky, R.E., Osborne, J.S., III, and Akpom, C.A.: Symptoms of respiratory illness in young children and the use of wood-burning stoves for indoor heating, Pediatrics 75:587-593, 1985.

Inselman, L.S.: Tuberculosis. In Gellis, S.S., and Kagan, B.M., editors: Current pediatric therapy 12, Philadelphia, 1986, W.B. Saunders Co.

Kairys, S.W., Olmstead, E.M., and O'Connor, G.T.: Steroid treatment of laryngotracheobronchitis: a meta-analysis of the evidence from randomized trials, Pediatrics 83:683-693, 1989.

Katz, J.N., and others: Clinical features as predictors of functional status in children with cystic fibrosis, J. Pediatr. 108:352-358, 1986.

Keyes, W.G.: Theophylline toxicity caused by an over-the-counter antiasthmatic preparation, Clin. Pediatr. 26:630-633, 1987.

Klein, J.O.: Otitis media. In Gellis, S.S., and Kagan, B.M., editors: Current pediatric therapy 12, Philadelphia, 1986, W.B. Saunders Co.

König, P.: Diagnostic problems in asthma, Ann. Allergy 55:95-101, 1985.

Kopelman, H., and others: Impaired chloride secretion, as well as bicarbonate secretion, underlies the fluid secretory defect in the cystic fibrosis pancreas, Gastroenterology 95:349-355, 1988.

Krugman, S., and others: Infectious diseases of children, ed. 8, St. Louis, 1985, Mosby–Year Book, Inc.

Lampe, R.M., and others: Acoustic reflectometry in the detection of middle ear effusion, Pediatrics 76:75-79, 1985.

Lewiston, N.J.: Asthma self-management programs and education, Pediatr. Ann. 15:127-136, 1986.

Lockey, R., and others: Fatalities from immunotherapy (IT) and skin testing (ST), J. Allergy Clin. Immunol. 79:660-677, 1987.

Lounsbury, B.F.: Swimming unprotected with long-shafted middle ear ventilation tubes, Laryngoscope 95:340-343, 1985.

Luder, E., and others: Efficacy of a nonrestricted fat diet in patients with cystic fibrosis, Am. J. Dis. Child. 143:458-464, 1989.

Marcy, S.M.: A summer refresher: swimmer's ear, Contemp. Pediatr. 6(5):90-91, 1989.

Mathews, K.P.: Respiratory atopic disease, JAMA 248:2587-2610, 1982.

Mauro, R.D., and others: Differentiation of epiglottitis and laryngotracheobronchitis in the child with stridor, Am. J. Dis. Child. 142:679-682, 1988.

McFadden, D.M., and others: Age-specific patterns of diagnosis of acute otitis media, Clin. Pediatr. 24:571-575, 1985.

McIntosh, K.: Respiratory syncytial virus infections in infants and children: diagnosis and treatment, Pediatr. Rev. 9:191-196, 1987.

McMillan, J.A.: Sore throats in teens: strep and beyond, Contemp. Pediatr. 5(3):20-30, 1988.

Mertsola, J., and others: Intrafamilial spread of pertussis, J. Pediatr. 103:359-363, 1983.

Miller, B.D., and Strunk, R.C.: Circumstances surrounding the deaths of children due to asthma, Am. J. Dis. Child. 143:1294-1299, 1989.

Mofenson, H.C., and others: Baby powder—a hazard! Pediatrics 68:265-266, 1981.
Moffet, H.: Pediatric infectious disease, ed. 3, Philadelphia, 1989, J.B. Lippincott Co.
Morris, L., and others: A survey of patient sources of prescription drug information, Am. J. Public Health 74:1161, 1984.
Murray, A.B., and Morrision, B.J.: Passive smoking by asthmatics: its greater effect on boys than on girls and on older than on younger children, Pediatrics 84:451-459, 1989.
Nalebuff, D.J., and Fadal, R.G.: Allergy diagnosis and treatment, Portland, ME, 1986, Ventrex Laboratories, Inc.
Neddenriep, D., Schumacher, M.J., and Lemen, R.J.: Asthma in childhood, Curr. Probl. Pediatr. 19:331-385, 1989.
Neddenriep, D., Taussig, L.M., and Mietens, C.: Infections of the lower respiratory tract. In Eichenwald, H.F., and Ströder, J., editors: Current therapy in pediatrics–2, Philadelphia, 1989, B.C. Decker Inc.
Neuspiel, D.R., and others: Parental smoking and post-infancy wheezing in children: a prospective cohort study, Am. J. Publ. Health 79:168-171, 1989.
Nickerson, B., and others: Distance running improves fitness in asthmatic children without pulmonary complications or changes in exercise-induced bronchospasm, Pediatrics 71:147-152, 1983.
Nora, J.J., and Fraser, F.C.: Medical genetics, ed. 3, Philadelphia, 1989, Lea & Febiger.
Ogston, S.A.: The Tayside infant morbidity and mortality study: effect on health of using gas for cooking, Br. Med. J. 290:957-960, 1985.
Orenstein, D.M., and others: Exercise conditioning in children with asthma, J. Pediatr. 106:556-560, 1985.
Orlando, R.C., and others: Colonic and esophageal transepithelial potential difference in cystic fibrosis, Gastroenterology 96:1041-1048, 1989.
Paradise, J.L.: Otitis media during early life: how hazardous to development? A critical review of the evidence, Pediatrics 68:869-873, 1981.
Paradise, J.L., and Elster, B.A.: Evidence that breast milk protects against otitis media with effusion in infants with cleft palate, Pediatr. Res. 18:283A, 1984.
Paradise, J.L., and Rogers, K.D.: On otitis media, child development, and tympanostomy tubes: new answers or old questions? Pediatrics 77:88-92, 1986.
Paradise, J.L., and others: Efficacy of tonsillectomy for recurrent throat infection in severely affected children: results of parallel randomized and nonrandomized clinical trials, N. Engl. J. Med. 310:674-683, 1984.
Pattishall, E.N., and others: Serum cotinine as a measure of tobacco smoke exposure in children, Am. J. Dis. Child. 139:1101-1104, 1985.
Pearlman, D.: Chronic rhinitis in children, J. Allergy Clin. Immunol. 81:962-966, 1988.
Pedreira, F.A., and others: Involuntary smoking and incidence of respiratory illness during the first year of life, Pediatrics 75:594-597, 1985.
Pierson, W.E.: Exercise-induced bronchospasm in children and adolescents, Pediatr. Clin. North Am. 35:1031-1040, 1988.
Putto, A.: Febrile exudative tonsillitis: viral or streptococcal? Pediatrics 80:6-11, 1987.
Quinton, P.M., and Bijman, J.: Higher bioelectric potentials due to decreased chloride absorption in the sweat glands of patients with cystic fibrosis, N. Engl. J. Med. 308:1185-1189, 1983.
Rachelefsky, G.S., and others: Behavior abnormalities and poor school performance due to oral theophylline use, Pediatrics 78:1133-1138, 1986.
Rao, M.: Chest diseases. In Rajkumar, S., and Toback, C., editors: Principles and practice of ambulatory pediatrics, New York, 1988, Plenum Medical Book Co.
Rappaport, L., and others: Effects of theophylline on behavior and learning in children with asthma, Am. J. Dis. Child. 143:368-372, 1989.
Rauen, K.K., and Holman, J.B.: Pain control in children following tonsillectomies: a retrospective study, J. Nurs. Qual. Assur. 3(3):45-53, 1989.
Ray, C.G.: Ribavirin: ambivalence about an antiviral agent (editorial), Am. J. Dis. Child. 142:488-489, 1988.
Reisman, J., and others: Role of conventional physiotherapy in cystic fibrosis, J. Pediatr. 113:632-636, 1988.
Roberts, N.A., and others: Rational design of peptide-based HIV proteinase inhibitors, Science 248:358-360, 1990.
Rodriguez, W.J., and others: Aerosolized ribavirin in the treatment of patients with respiratory syncytial virus disease, Pediatr. Infect. Dis. 6:159-163, 1987.
Rona, R.J., and others: Parental smoking at home and the height of children, Br. Med. J. 283:1363, 1981.
Royall, J.A., and Levin, D.L.: Adult respiratory distress syndrome in pediatric patients. I. Clinical aspects, pathophysiology, pathology, and mechanisms of lung injury, J. Pediatr. 112:169-173, 1988.
Saarinen, U.M.: Prolonged breast-feeding as prophylaxis for recurrent otitis media, Acta Paediatr. Scand. 71:567, 1982.
Seaman-Bates, N.J.: Emergency management of status asthmaticus, J. Emerg. Nurs. 6(5):9, 1980.
Seddon, D.J., and Hodson, M.E.: Surgical management of pneumothorax in cystic fibrosis, Thorax 43:739-740, 1988.
Simon, P., and others: Carrier prediction of cystic fibrosis in families in 36 families by means of restriction fragment length polymorphism, Eur. J. Pediatr. 147:199-201, 1988.
Simons, F.E.R.: Allergic rhinitis: recent advances, Pediatr. Clin. North Am. 35:1053-1074, 1988.
Starke, J.R.: Modern approach to the diagnosis and treatment of tuberculosis in children, Pediatr. Clin. North Am. 35:441-464, 1988.
Starke, J.R.: Tuberculosis. In Oski, F.A., and others, editors: Principles and practice of pediatrics, Philadelphia, 1990, J.B. Lippincott Co.
Stern, R.: Cystic fibrosis: recent development in diagnosis and treatment, Pediatr. Rev. 7:276-286, 1986.
Stickler, G.B.: The attack on the tympanic membrane, Pediatrics 74:291-292, 1984.
Strachan, D.P., Jarvis, M.J., and Feyerabend, B.T.: Passive smoking, salivary cotinine concentrations and middle ear effusion in 7 year old children, Br. Med. J. 298:1549-1552, 1989.
Super, D.M., and others: A prospective randomized double-blind study to evaluate the effect of dexamethasone in acute laryngotracheitis, J. Pediatr. 115:323-329, 1989.
Sutton, P.: Chest physiotherapy: time for reappraisal, Br. J. Dis. Chest 82:127-137, 1988.
Tan, Y., and Collins-Williams, C.: Aspirin-induced asthma in children, Ann. Allergy 48:1-5, 1982.
Tanz, R.R., and others: Penicillin plus rifampin eradicates pharyngeal carriage of group A streptococci, J. Pediatr. 106:876-880, 1985.
Teele, D.W., and others: Otitis media with effusion during the first three years of life and development of speech and language, Pediatrics 74:282-287, 1984.
Teele, D.W., and others: Epidemiology of otitis media during the first seven years of life in children in Greater Boston: a prospective cohort study, J. Infect. Dis. 160:83-94, 1989.
Templer, J.: Removal of foreign body from the nose, Hosp. Med. 18:77, 1982.
Wald, E.R.: Croup. In Oski, F.A., and others, editors: Principles and practice of pediatrics, Philadelphia, 1990, J.B. Lippincott Co.
Wald, E.R., Dashefsky, B., and Green, M.: In re Ribavirin: a case of premature adjudication? J. Pediatr. 112:154, 1988.
Ware, J.H., and others: Passive smoking, gas cooking, and respiratory health of children living in six cities, Am. Rev. Respir. Dis. 129:366-374, 1984.
Weinberger, M.: Managing asthma, Baltimore, 1989, Williams & Wilkins.

Weinberger, M., and others: Effects of theophylline on learning and behavior: reason for concern or concern without reason? J. Pediatr. 111:471-474, 1987.

Wheeler, W.B., and Colten, H.R.: Cystic fibrosis: current approach to diagnosis and management, Pediatr. Rev. 9:241-248, 1988.

Williams, M.H.: Increasing severity of asthma from 1960 to 1987 (letter), N. Engl. J. Med. 320:1015-1016, 1989.

Wood, R.A., and Eggleston, P.A.: Help your patients prevent exercise-induced asthma, Contemp. Pediatr. 3(12):61-67, 1986.

Wood, R.A., and Sampson, H.A.: A practical guide to allergy testing, Contemp. Pediatr. 4(special issue):8-20, 1987.

Wright, P.F.: Bronchiolitis, Pediatr. Rev. 7:219-222, 1986.

BIBLIOGRAPHY

Respiratory Infection

Bass, J.W.: Pertussis: current status of prevention and treatment, Pediatr. Infect. Dis. 4:614-619, 1985.

Bass, J.W., and others: Sudden death due to acute epiglottitis, Pediatr. Infect. Dis. 4:447-449, 1985.

Baugh, R., and Gilmore, B.B.: Infectious croup: a critical review, Otolaryngol. Head Neck Surg. 95:40-46, 1986.

Breese, B.B., and others: Consensus: difficult management problems in children with streptococcal pharyngitis, Pediatr. Infect. Dis. 4:10-13, 1985.

Cohen, G.J.: Management of infections of the lower respiratory tract in children, Pediatr. Infect. Dis. J. 6:317-323, 1987.

Conrad, D.A., and others: Aerosolized ribavirin in treatment of respiratory syncytial virus infections in infants hospitalized during an epidemic, Pediatr. Infect. Dis. J. 6:159-163, 1987.

Denny, F.W.: Acute respiratory infections in children: etiology and epidemiology, Pediatr. Rev. 9:135-146, 1987.

Denny, F.W.: Current problems in managing streptococcal pharyngitis, J. Pediatr. 111:797-805, 1987.

Eavey, R.D.: A sound workup for evaluating airway obstruction, Contemp. Pediatr. 3:78-83, 1986.

Everett, D.: For a child with pneumonia, there's no place like home, RN 53(3):85-88, 1990.

Fulginiti, V.A.: The current state of pertussis and pertussis vaccines, Am. J. Dis. Child. 143:532-533, 1989.

Gerber, M.A., Randolph, M.F., and Tilton, R.C.: Enzyme fluorescence procedure for rapid diagnosis of streptococcal pharyngitis, J. Pediatr. 108:421-423, 1986.

Gladu, J.M., and Ecobichon, D.J.: Evaluation of exposure of health care personnel to ribavirin, J. Toxicol. Environ. Health 28:1-12, 1989.

Grossman, M., and others: Consensus: management of presumed bacterial pneumonia in ambulatory children, Pediatr. Infect. Dis. 3:497-500, 1984.

Hammerschlag, M.R.: Infections due to *Chlamydia trachomatis*, Pediatr. Ann. 13:673-681, 1984.

Hayden, F.G., and others: Prevention of natural colds by contact prophylaxis with intranasal alpha$_2$-interferon, N. Engl. J. Med. 314:71-75, 1986.

Huston, C.J.: Epiglottitis, Nursing '88 18(4):59, 1988.

Kerfoot, F.E.: The perils of pertussis, J. Pediatr. Nurs. 4:277-283, 1989.

Kim, K.S., and Kaplan, E.L.: Association of penicillin tolerance with failure to eradicate group A streptococci from patients with pharyngitis, J. Pediatr. 107:681-684, 1985.

Ledbetter, E.O.: The many faces of pneumococcal pneumonia, Contemp. Pediatr. 5(11):50-72, 1988.

Longini, I.M., and Monto, A.S.: Efficacy of virucidal nasal tissues in interrupting familial transmission of respiratory agents, Am. J. Epidemiol. 128:639-644, 1988.

Mack, J.E.: Ribavirin: an antiviral agent with promise, Pediatr. Nurs. 14:220-221, 1988.

Mauro, R.D., and Poole, S.R.: Is it croup? A guide to diagnosis and treatment, Contemp. Pediatr. 5(10):51-70, 1988.

McConnochie, R.M., and Roghmann, K.J.: Parental smoking, presence of older siblings, and family history of asthma increase risk of bronchiolitis, Am. J. Dis. Child. 140:806-812, 1986.

Meltzer, E.O., and others: Chronic rhinitis in infants and children: etiologic, diagnostic, and therapeutic considerations, Pediatr. Clin. North Am. 30:847-871, 1983.

Nederhand, K.C, and others: Respiratory syncytial virus: a nursing perspective, Pediatr. Nurs. 15:342-345, 1989.

Ophir, D., and Elad, Y.: Effects of steam inhalation on nasal patency and nasal symptoms in patients with common cold, Am. J. Otolaryngol. 3:149-153, 1987.

Pionteck-Lentz, T.C.: Ribavirin: ready for RSV season, Neonatal Network 7(2):29-35, 1988.

Radetsky, M., and others: Comparative evaluation of kits for rapid diagnosis of group A streptococcal disease, Pediatr. Infect. Dis. 4:274-281, 1985.

Randolph, M.F., and others: Effect of antibiotic therapy on the clinical course of streptococcal pharyngitis, J. Pediatr. 106:870-875, 1985.

Roddey, O.F., and others: Comparison of a latex agglutination test and four culture methods for identification of group A streptococci in a pediatric office laboratory, J. Pediatr. 108:347-351, 1986.

Rubin, B.K.: The evaluation of the child with recurrent chest infections, Pediatr. Infect. Dis. 4:88-98, 1985.

Sheahan, S.L., and Seabolt, J.P.: *Chlamydia trachomatis* infections: a health problem of infants, J. Pediatr. Health Care 3:144-149, 1989.

Skoner, D., and Caliguiri, L.: The wheezing infant, Pediatr. Clin. North Am. 35:1011-1030, 1988.

Smith, T.D., Wilkinson, V., and Kaplan, E.L.: Group A *Streptococcus*-associated upper respiratory tract infections in a day-care center, Pediatrics 83:380-384, 1989.

Spicer, C.M., and Yund, C.: Effects of preadmission preparation on compliance with home care instructions, J. Pediatr. Nurs. 4:255-262, 1989.

Szilagyi, P.G.: What can we do about the common cold? Contemp. Pediatr. 7(2):23-49, 1990.

Todisco, T., de Benedictis, F.M., and Dottorini, M.: Viral and *Mycoplasma pneumoniae* pneumonias in school-age children: three-year follow-up of respiratory function, Pediatr. Pulmonol. 6:232-236, 1989.

Turner, R.B., and others: Pneumonia in pediatric outpatients: cause and clinical manifestations, J. Pediatr. 111:194-200, 1987.

Walson, P.D.: Coughs and colds, Pediatrics 74(suppl.):937-940, 1984.

Otitis Media

Adams, J.L., Evans, G.A., and Roberts, J.E.: Diagnosing and treating otitis media with effusion, MCN 9:22-28, 1984.

American Academy of Pediatrics, Committee on School Health: Impedance bridge (tympanometer) as a screening device in schools, Pediatrics 79:472, 1987.

Bluestone, C.D.: Modern management of otitis media, Pediatr. Clin. North Am. 36:1371-1387, 1989.

Bluestone, C.D., and others: Controversies in screening for middle ear disease and hearing loss in children, Pediatrics 77:57-70, 1986.

Breitzer, G.M.: Practical approach to the treatment of otitis media in infants and children, Pediatr. Basics 51:11-16, 1989.

Bresolin, D., and others: Facial characteristics of children who breathe through the mouth, Pediatrics 73:622-625, 1984.

Castiglia, P.T., Aquilina, S.S., and Kemsley, M.: Focus: nonsuppurative otitis media, Pediatr. Nurs. 9:427-430, 1983.

Dyson, A.T., Holmes, A.E., and Duffitt, D.V.: Speech characteristics of children after otitis media, J. Pediatr. Health Care 1:261-265, 1987.

Fireman, P.: Otitis media and nasal disease: a role for allergy, J. Allergy Clin. Immunol. 82:917-926, 1988.

Fireman, P.: Otitis media and its relationship to allergy, Pediatr. Clin. North Am. 35:1075, 1090, 1988.

Gates, G.A., and others: Effectiveness of adenoidectomy and tympanostomy tubes in the treatment of chronic otitis media with effusion, N. Engl. J. Med. 317:1444-1451, 1987.

Hayden, G.F., and Schwartz, R.H.: Characteristics of earache among children with acute otitis media, Am. J. Dis. Child. 139:721-723, 1985.

Jefferson County Public Schools, School Nurse Practitioner Committee: Protocol ear problems, School Nurse, pp. 22-27, Jan./Feb. 1987.

Kaufman, D.H., Grothe, G., and Brasser, B.: Early identification of ear infection and hearing loss in an early childhood population, School Nurse, pp. 18-21, Jan./Feb. 1987.

Le, C.: Otitis revisited: are ear tubes the answer? Contemp. Pediatr. 9(9):24-45, 1988.

Marchant, C.D., and others: Objective diagnosis of otitis media in early infancy by tympanoplasty and ipsilateral acoustic thresholds, J. Pediatr. 109:590-595, 1986.

Roberts, J.E., and others: Otitis media in early childhood and cognitive, academic, and classroom performance of the school-age child, Pediatrics 83:477-485, 1989.

Schwartz, R.H.: A practical approach to the otitis-prone child, Contemp. Pediatr. 4(1):30-54, 1987.

Smelt, G.J.C., and Yeoh, L.H.: Swimming and grommets, J. Laryngol. Otol. 98:243-245, 1984.

Teele, D.W., and Teele, J.: Detection of middle ear effusion by acoustic reflectometry, J. Pediatr. 104:832-836, 1984.

Wright, P.F., and others: Impact of recurrent otitis media on middle ear function, hearing, and language, J. Pediatr. 113:581-587, 1988.

Tuberculosis

Abernathy, R.S., and others: Short-course chemotherapy for tuberculosis in children, Pediatrics 72:801-806, 1983.

Chest x-ray screening statements, FDA Drug Bull. 13(2):13-14, 1983.

Coleman, D.A.: TB: the disease that's not dead yet, RN 47(9):49-59, 1984.

Hauser, M., and Baier, H.: Interactions of isoniazid with foods, Drug Intell. Clin. Pharm. 16:617-618, 1982.

Jacobs, R.F., and Abernathy, R.S.: The treatment of tuberculosis in children, Pediatr. Infect. Dis. 4:513-517, 1985.

Lorin, M.I., Hsu, K.H.K., and Jacob, S.C.: Treatment of tuberculosis in children, Pediatr. Clin. North Am. 30:333-348, 1983.

Madsen, L.A.: Tuberculosis today, RN 53(3):44-50, 1990.

MMWR: A strategic plan for the elimination of tuberculosis in the United States, MMWR 38(suppl.):S-3, 1989.

Nemir, R.L.: Perspectives in adolescent tuberculosis; three decades of experience, Pediatrics 78:399-405, 1986.

Nemir, R.L., and Krasinski, K.: Tuberculosis in children and adolescents in the 1980s, Pediatr. Infect. Dis. J. 7:441-464, 1988.

Perez-Stable, E.J., and others: Tuberculin skin test reactivity and conversions in United States– and foreign-born Latino children, Pediatr. Infect. Dis. 4:476-479, 1985.

Snider, D.E., Jr., and others: Tuberculosis in children, Pediatr. Infect. Dis. J. 7:271-278, 1988.

Starke, J.R., and Taylor-Watts, K.T.: Tuberculosis in the pediatric population of Houston, Texas, Pediatrics 84:28-35, 1989.

Noninfectious Irritants

Barker-Stotis, K.: CO poisoning, Nursing '87 17(12):33, 1987.

Burchfiel, C., and others: Passive smoking in childhood, Am. Rev. Respir. Dis. 133:966-973, 1986.

Cahan, W.G.: Abusing children by smoking (opinion), CA 37:3132, 1987.

Cotton, E., and Yasuda, K.: Foreign body aspiration, Pediatr. Clin. North Am. 31:937-941, 1984.

Crawford, W.A.: On the health effects of environmental tobacco smoke, Arch. Environ. Health 43:34-37, 1988.

Desai, M.H.: Inhalation injuries in burn victims, Crit. Care Q. 7(3):1-7, 1984.

Evans, D., and others: The impact of passive smoking and effects on emergency room visits of urban children with asthma, Am. Rev. Respir. Dis. 135:567-572, 1987.

Feyerabend, C., and others: Nicotine concentration in urine and saliva of smokers and non-smokers, Br. Med. J. 284:1002-1004, 1982.

Frankowski, B.L., and Secker-Walker, R.H.: Advising parents to stop smoking, Am. J. Dis. Child. 143:1091-1094, 1989.

Friedman, E.M.: Foreign bodies in the pediatric aerodigestive tract, Pediatr. Ann. 17:640-647, 1988.

Friedman, G.D., Petitti, D.B., and Bawol, R.D.: Prevalence and correlates of passive smoking, Am. J. Public Health 73:401-405, 1983.

Gozal, D., and others: Accidental carbon monoxide poisoning: emphasis on hyperbaric oxygen treatment, Clin. Pediatr. 24:132-135, 1985.

Greenberg, R.A., and others: Ecology of passive smoking by young infants, J. Pediatr. 114:774-780, 1989.

Holroyd, H.J.: Foreign body aspiration: potential cause of coughing and wheezing, Pediatr. Rev. 10:59-63, 1988.

Irons, T.G., and Kenney, R.D.: Let's get parents to stop smoking, Contemp. Pediatr. 5(3):107-118, 1988.

Kenna, M.A.: Foreign bodies in the air and food passages, Pediatr. Rev. 10:25-31, 1988.

Kent, J.M.: How serious is that smoke inhalation? Patient Care 18(13):172-176, 179-180, 185-186, 1984.

Klein, B.L, and Simon, J.E.: Hydrocarbon poisonings, Pediatr. Clin. North Am. 33:411-419, 1986.

Laks, Y., and Barzilay, Z.: Foreign body aspiration in childhood, Pediatr. Emerg. Care 4:102-106, 1988.

Lavengood, T.D.W.: Involuntary smoking—children in crisis, Pediatr. Nurs. 14:93-95, 1988.

Lybarger, P.M.: Inhalation injury in children: nursing care, Issues Compr. Pediatr. Nurs. 10:33-50, 1987.

Mohler, S.E.: Passive smoking: a danger to children's health, J. Pediatr. Nurs. 1:298-304, 1987.

Pierson, W.E., Koenig, J.Q., and Bardana, E.J., Jr.: Potential adverse health effects of wood smoke, West. J. Med. 151:339-342, 1989.

Rona, R., Chinn, S., and DuVe Florey, C.: Exposure to cigarette smoking and children's growth, Int. J. Epidemiol. 14:402-429, 1985.

Miscellaneous Respiratory Conditions

A.R.D.S.: Nursing '88 18(9):74-75, 1988.

Dickinson, S.P., and Bury, G.M.: Pulmonary embolism, Nursing '89 19(4):34-41, 1989.

Fanconi, S., and others: Long-term sequelae in children surviving adult respiratory distress syndrome, J. Pediatr. 106:218, 1985.

Gerdes, L.: Recognizing the multisystemic effects of embolism, Nursing '87 17(12):34-41, 1987.

Karnes, N.: Don't let ARDS catch you off guard, Nursing '87 17(5):34-38, 1987.

McConnell, E.A.: Giving intradermal injections, Nursing '90 20(3):70, 1990.

Royall, J.A., and Levin, D.L.: Adult respiratory distress syndrome in pediatric patients. I. Clinical aspects, pathophysiology, pathology, and mechanisms of lung injury, J. Pediatr. 112:169-180, 1988.

Royall, J., and Levin, D.L.: Adult respiratory distress syndrome in pediatric patients. II. Management, J. Pediatr. 112:335-347, 1988.

Bronchial Asthma

Albert, S.: Aminophylline toxicity, Pediatr. Clin. North Am. 34:61-73, 1987.

Alexander, J.S., and others: Effectiveness of a nurse-managed program for children with chronic asthma, J. Pediatr. Nurs. 3:312-316, 1988.

Baker, M.D.: Pitfalls in the use of clinical asthma scoring, Am. J. Dis. Child. 142:183-185, 1988.

Blessing-Moore, J., Fritz, G., and Lewiston, N.J.: Self-management programs for childhood asthma, Chest 87:1-5, 1985.

Blue, C.L.: Exercise-induced asthma: the "silent asthma," J. Pediatr. Nurs. 2:167-174, 1988.

Bowers, K., and Koviach, J.: Self-care management of asthma, Child. Nurse 5(1):1-4, 1987.

Brunette, M.G., Lands, L., and Thibodeau, L.: Childhood asthma: prevention of attacks with short-term corticosteroid treatment of upper respiratory tract infection, Pediatrics 81:624-629, 1988.

Burr, M.L.: Is asthma increasing? J. Epidemiol. Commun. Health 41:185-192, 1987.

Chryssanthopoulos, C., and others: Cardiopulmonary responses of asthmatic children to strenuous exercise, Clin. Pediatr. 23:384-387, 1984.

Conboy, K.: Nursing care plan for the child with status asthmaticus, Crit. Care Nurse 5(2):8-9, 12, 1985.

Donnelly, J.E., Donnelly, W.J., and Thong, Y.H.: Inadequate parental understanding of asthma medications, Ann. Allergy 62:337-341, 1989.

Duffy, D.M., and Halloran, M.C.: Effect of an educational program on parents of children with asthma, Child. Health Care 16:76-81, 1987.

Dworkin, G., and Kattan, M.: Mechanical ventilation for status asthmaticus in children, J. Pediatr. Nurs. 114:545-549, 1989.

Ellis, E.F.: A 15-minute test for theophylline levels, Contemp. Pediatr. 3(special issue):87, 1986.

Ellis, E.F.: Adverse effects of corticosteroid therapy (editorial), J. Allergy Clin. Immunol. 80:515-517, 1987.

Ellis, E.F.: Asthma: current therapeutic approach, Pediatr. Clin. North Am. 35:1041-1052, 1988.

Fischer, T.J., and others: Adverse pulmonary responses to aspirin and acetaminophen in chronic childhood asthma, Pediatrics 71:313-318, 1983.

Frost, L., Kieckhefer, G.M., and Rubino, C.: Incorporating research into a community asthma program, Pediatr. Nurs. 14:197-200, 1988.

Galdès-Sebaldt, M., McLaughlin, F.J., and Levison, H.: Comparison of cold air, ultrasonic mist, and methacholine inhalations as tests of bronchial reactivity in normal and asthmatic children, J. Pediatr. 107:526-530, 1985.

Gurwitz, D.: Family education: effective treatment for asthma, Contemp. Pediatr. 4(3):55-64, 1987.

Haltom, J.R., and Szefler, S.J.: Theophylline absorption in young asthmatic children receiving sustained-release formulations, J. Pediatr. 107:805-810, 1985.

Hen, J.: An overview of pediatric asthma, Pediatr. Ann. 15:92-94, 96, 1986.

Joad, J.P., and others: Extrapulmonary effects of maintenance therapy with theophylline and inhaled albuterol in patients with chronic asthma, J. Allergy Clin. Immunol., 78:1147-1153, 1986.

Kattan, M.: Managing and preventing asthma emergencies, Contemp. Pediatr. 5(11):22-32, 1988.

Kay, A.B., editor: Asthma. Clinical pharmacology and therapeutic progress, Boston, 1986, Blackwell Scientific Publications, Inc.

Kieckhefer, G.M.: Testing self-perception of health theory to predict health promotion and illness management, J. Pediatr. Nurs. 2:381-391, 1987.

König, P., and others: A trial of metaproterenol by metered-dose dose inhaler and two spacers in preschool asthmatics, Pediatr. Pulmonol. 5:247-251, 1988.

Kubly, L.S., and McClellan, M.S.: Effects of self-care instruction on asthmatic children, Issues Compr. Pediatr. Nurs. 7:121-130, 1984.

Lanes, S., and Walker, A.: Do pressurized bronchodilator aerosols cause death among asthmatics? Am. J. Epidemiol. 125:755-760, 1987.

Lee, H., and Evans, H.E.: Aerosol inhalation teaching device, J. Pediatr. 110:249-252, 1987.

Lewis, C.E., and others: A randomized trial of A.C.T. (asthma care training) for kids, Pediatrics 74:478-486, 1984.

Mallol, J., and others: Use of nebulized bronchodilators in infants under 1 year of age: analysis of four forms of therapy, Pediatr. Pulmonol. 3:298-303, 1987.

Mendlowitz, D.R., and others: Understanding respiration and digestion: a developmental comparison of healthy and asthmatic children, Child. Health Care 17:45-49, 1988.

Murray, A.B., and Ferguson, A.C.: Dust-free bedrooms in the treatment of asthmatic children with house dust or house dust mite allergy: a controlled trial, Pediatrics 71:418-422, 1983.

Neild, J.E., and Cameron, I.R.: Bronchoconstriction in response to suggestion: its prevention by an inhaled anticholinergic agent, Br. Med. J. 290:674, 1985.

Nickerson, B.G.: Approach to the wheezing infant, Pediatr. Ann. 15:99-104, 1986.

Nickerson, B.G., and others: Distance running improves fitness in asthmatic children without pulmonary complications or changes in exercise-induced bronchospasm, Pediatrics 71:147-152, 1983.

Odom, J.D., and Taylor, R.W.: Environmental variables and acute asthmatic attacks in children, J. Pediatr. Nurs. 1:335-341, 1986.

O'Neil, S.L., Barysh, N., and Setear, S.J.: Determining school programming needs of special population groups: a study of asthmatic children, J. School Health 55:237, 1985.

Petosa, R: Enhancing the health competence of school-age children through behavioral self-management skills, J. School Health 56:211-214, 1986.

Plaut, T.F.: Helping asthma patients breathe easier, Contemp. Pediatr. 6(special issue):59-76, 1989.

Plaut, T.F.: What a peak flow meter can do for children with asthma, Contemp. Pediatr. 6(special issue):33-52, 1989.

Rachelefsky, G.S.: Asthma self-management programs for children, Child Care Newsletter 3(2):5-8, 1984.

Rachelefsky, G.S., and others: ACT for kids, Chest 87(suppl.):98S-100S, 1985.

Ramsey, A.M., and Siroky, A.S.: The use of puppets to teach school-age children with asthma, Pediatr. Nurs. 14:187-190, 1988.

Rew, L.: The relationship between self-care behaviors and selected psychosocial variables in childen with asthma, J. Pediatr. Nurs. 2:333-341, 1987.

Rimar, J.M.: Albuterol: a selective $beta_2$ bronchodilator, MCN 11:169, 1986.

Rolnick, S.J.: Self-management of pediatric asthma: four programs being studied, J. Pediatr. Nurs. 2:264-266, 1988.

Rubin, D.H., and others: Educational intervention by computer in childhood asthma: a randomized clinical trial testing the use of a new teaching intervention in childhood asthma, Pediatrics 77:1-10, 1986.

Sedlacek, K.K.: Asthma in children: facilitating self-care, Pediatr. Nurs. Update 1(1):1-8, 1985.

Shultz, D.M.: Sulfite sensitivity, Am. J. Nurs. 86:914, 1986.

Skoner, D., and Caliguiri, L.: The wheezing infant, Pediatr. Clin. North Am. 35:1011-1031, 1988.

Stein, R., and others: Severe acute asthma in a pediatric intensive care unit: six year's experience, Pediatrics 83:1023-1028, 1989.

Strunk, R.C.: Asthma deaths in childhood: identification of patients at risk and intervention, J. Allergy Clin. Immunol. 80(suppl.):472-477, 1987.

Tashkin, D.P., and Jenne, J.W.: Alpha and beta adrenergic agents. In Weiss, E.B., Segal, M.S., and Stein, M., editors: Bronchial asthma, Boston, 1985, Little, Brown & Co., Inc.

Taylor, S.L., and Bush, R.K.: Sulfites as food ingredients, Contemp. Nutr. 11(10), 1986.

Towns, S.J., and Mellis, C.M.: Role of acetyl salicylic acid and sodium metabisulfite in chronic childhood asthma, Pediatrics 73:631-637, 1984.

Traver, G.A., and Martinez, M.: Asthma update. I. Mechanisms, pathophysiology, and diagnosis, J. Pediatr. Health Care 2:221-226, 1988.

Traver, G.A., and Martinez, M.: Asthma update. II. Treatment, J. Pediatr. Health Care 2:227-233, 1988.

Weinberger, M.: Antiasthmatic therapy in children, Pediatr. Clin. North Am. 316:1251-1284, 1989.

Zahr, L.K., Connolly, M., and Page, D.R.: Assessment and management of the child with asthma, Pediatr. Nurs. 15:109-114, 1989.

Zimo, D.A., Gaspar, M., and Akhter, J.: The efficacy and safety of home nebulizer therapy for children with asthma, Am. J. Dis. Child. 143:208-211, 1989.

Zwerdling, R.G.: Status asthmaticus, Pediatr. Ann. 15:105-109, 1986.

Cystic Fibrosis

Brissette, S., and others: Nursing care plan for adolescents and young adults with advanced cystic fibrosis, Issues Compr. Pediatr. Nurs. 10:87-97, 1987.

Canam, C.: Talking about cystic fibrosis within the family—what parents need to know, Issues Compr. Pediatr. Nurs. 9:167-178, 1986.

Cassey, J., and others: Totally implantable system for venous access in children with cystic fibrosis, Clin. Pediatr. 27:91-95, 1988.

Cowen, L., and others: Psychologic adjustment of the family with a member who has cystic fibrosis, Pediatrics 77:745-753, 1986.

Dibble, S.L., and Savedra, M.C.: Cystic fibrosis in adolescence: a new challenge, Pediatr. Nurs. 14:299-303, 1988.

Dolan, T.F.: Update: cystic fibrosis, Pediatr. Ann. 15:296-304, 1986.

Gibson, C.: Perspective in parental coping with a chronically ill child: the case of cystic fibrosis, Issues Compr. Pediatr. Nurs. 11:33-41, 1988.

Hymovich, D.P., and Baker, C.D.: The needs, concerns and coping of parents of children with cystic fibrosis, Fam. Rel. 34:91-97, 1985.

Johnson, J.P.: Genetic counseling using linked DNA probes: cystic fibrosis as a prototype, J. Pediatr. 113:957-964, 1988.

Loftus, T.: Helping cystic fibrosis patients with high-tech home care, Caring 6(6):22-27, 1988.

Moore, M.C.: Taurine supplementation: theoretical and practical considerations, Pediatr. Nurs. 14:489-491, 1988.

Myer, P.A.: Parental adaptation to cystic fibrosis, J. Pediatr. Health Care 2:20-28, 1988.

Nolan, T., and others: Knowledge of cystic fibrosis in patients and their parents, Pediatrics 77:229-235, 1986.

Orenstein, D.M.: Exercise tolerance and exercise conditioning in children with chronic lung disease, J. Pediatr. 118:1043-1047, 1988.

Patterson, J.M.: Critical factors affecting family compliance with home treatment for children with cystic fibrosis, Fam. Rel. 34:79-89, 1985.

Patton, A.C., Ventura, J.N., and Savedra, M.: Stress and coping responses of adolescents with cystic fibrosis, Child. Health Care 14:153-156, 1986.

Rose, J., and Jay, S.: A comprehensive exercise program for persons with cystic fibrosis, J. Pediatr. Nurs. 1:323-334, 1986.

Rosenstein, B.J.: A clearer—and somewhat brighter—picture of cystic fibrosis, Contemp. Pediatr. 4(7):71-91, 1987.

Rubenstein, S., Moss, R., and Lewiston, N.: Constipation and meconium ileus equivalent in patients with cystic fibrosis, Pediatrics 78:473-479, 1986.

Stewart, A.: Care in the hospital: cystic fibrosis, part 3, Nurs. Times 80(22):44-45, 1984.

Stullengarger, B., and others: Family adaptation to cystic fibrosis, Pediatr. Nurs. 13:29-31, 1987.

Walker, L.S., Ford, M.B., and Donald, W.D.: Cystic fibrosis and family stress: effects of age and severity of illness, Pediatrics 79:239-246, 1987.

Wells, P.W., and Meghdadpour, S.: Research yields new clues to cystic fibrosis, MCN 13:187-190, 1988.

CHAPTER 33

The Child with Gastrointestinal Dysfunction

RELATED TOPICS

Cystic fibrosis, Ch. 32
Disorders of the gastrointestinal tract, Ch. 11
Encopresis, Ch. 18
Gastric feeding techniques, Ch. 27
Gastrointestinal disorders, Ch. 29
Intestinal parasitic diseases, Ch. 16
Nursing care of high-risk newborns, Ch. 10
Ostomies, Ch. 27
Pain assessment; pain management, Ch. 26
Preparation for procedures, Ch. 27
Procedures related to elimination, Ch. 27
Surgical procedures, Ch. 27

GLOSSARY

CD Celiac disease; Crohn disease
CND Chronic nonspecific diarrhea
diarrhea Increased frequency or decreased consistency of stools
GER Gastroesophageal reflux
GI Gastrointestinal
HAV Hepatitis A virus
HBV Hepatitis B virus
HPS Hypertrophic pyloric stenosis
IBD Inflammatory bowel disease
IBS Irritable bowel syndrome
jaundice Yellowish discoloration of the skin and sclera
NANB non-A, non-B virus
NG Nasogastric
PUD Peptic ulcer disease
SBS Short bowel syndrome
UC Ulcerative colitis

Disorders of the gastrointestinal tract are very common and constitute one of the largest categories of illnesses that occur in infancy and childhood. Structural and obstructive defects interfere with the ingestion and transport of foodstuffs, and inflammatory, malabsorptive, and maldigestive disturbances impair the functional integrity of the gastrointestinal tract. Furthermore, in most of the disorders the primary defect can produce additional complications. For example, obstructive or inflammatory conditions affect digestion and absorption because bowel motility, mucosal functioning, enzymatic activity, and bacterial flora are altered. This chapter is concerned with those conditions that in some way interfere with normal digestion and absorption of nutrients.

Box 33-1 FUNCTIONS OF THE GASTROINTESTINAL TRACT

Process and absorb nutrients necessary to maintain metabolic processes and to support growth and development

Perform an excretory function for both digestive residue and other waste products that pour into the intestine from the blood or are excreted in the bile

Provide detoxification while other routes of elimination (kidneys, liver, skin) are still immature

Participate in maintaining fluid and electrolyte balance in infancy

GASTROINTESTINAL STRUCTURE AND FUNCTION

Knowledge of the basic structure and physiology of digestion and absorption is foundational to the understanding of gastrointestinal (GI) disorders. The following discussion is an overview of the development of the GI tract during early childhood and of the basic physiology of digestion and absorption. For a review of the major anatomic structures within the abdominal cavity, the reader is referred to Fig. 7-44.

GASTROINTESTINAL DEVELOPMENT AND FUNCTION IN EARLY CHILDHOOD

The GI system serves several essential functions (Box 33-1), and all actions are subject to a variety of outside influences at all ages. At all ages children are sensitive to tensions and anxieties, and many diseases and disorders are reflected in altered GI function.

Development of the Gastrointestinal Tract

The primitive digestive system forms during the fourth week of gestation, but the most rapid and extensive development occurs just before birth. As a result, most biochemical and physiologic functions are established at the time of birth. Before birth the exchange of nutrients and waste is assumed by the placenta; therefore the demands on the alimentary tract are minimal. However, the presence in the intestine of a thick, sticky, greenish black material *(meconium)* composed of cast-off epithelial cells, digestive tract secretions (e.g., mucus and bile), and residue from swallowed amniotic fluid attests to prenatal activity. The passage of this meconium after birth provides evidence of the patency of the tract.

The mechanical functions of digestion are relatively immature at birth. Sucking and swallowing are established prenatally but do not become fully developed until after birth. Swallowing is an automatic reflex action for the first 3 months, and the infant has no voluntary control of swallowing until the striated muscles in the throat establish their cerebral connections. This begins at approximately 6 weeks of age. By 6 months the infant is capable of swallowing, holding food in the mouth, or spitting it out at will. The mechanism of sucking is also a reflexive activity in the newborn, and the muscular action of the tongue has a typical forward thrust. With neural and muscular development, the infant gradually acquires the ability to perform the coordinated muscular action typical of the adult type of swallowing (see Chapter 12). The chewing function is facilitated by eruption of the primary teeth. The timing of dietary changes closely parallels these progressive capabilities. First to develop are those that require merely swallowing, then those that need no mastication, and finally those that require biting and chewing.

The stomach, which lies horizontally, is round until the child is approximately 2 years of age. It then gradually elongates until at about 7 years of age it assumes the shape and anatomic position of the adult. This anatomic placement of the stomach in infancy influences positioning practices during and after feeding (see Chapter 8). At birth the capacity of the stomach is only about 10 to 20 ml, but the stomach, a distensible organ, rapidly expands to triple its capacity in 3 weeks and to reach 5 to 10 times its original birth capacity at the age of 1 month (Table 33-1).

The immaturity of the digestive system in the infant is demonstrated by the rapidity with which swallowed food is propelled through the entire tract. The frequency and character of stools are affected by the rate of peristalsis and the nature of ingested food. For example, the frequent, yellow stools of the neonate gradually assume a more adult regularity and character in the infant. The emptying time of the stomach increases from 2½ to 3 hours in the newborn to 3 to 6 hours in older infants and children. The small stomach capacity has implications for determining the amount and frequency of feedings during this period of growth. In addition, in infancy it is not uncommon for peristaltic waves to reverse and cause spitting up or, if vigorous, vomiting of stomach contents. An immature, relaxed cardiac sphincter in infancy and early childhood contributes to this ease of regurgitation.

During the prenatal period the large intestine grows more rapidly than the small intestine, but after birth this rate is reversed. The length of the intestine in infants is 6 times the

Table 33-1 Stomach Capacity (Approximate) at Various Stages of Development

AGE	CAPACITY(ML)
Newborn	10-20
1 week	30-90
2-3 weeks	75-100
1 month	90-150
3 months	150-200
1 year	210-360
2 years	500
10 years	750-900
16 years	1500
Adult	2000-3000

body length and is proportionately greater than that of the full-grown individual, which is 4 to 5 times the body length. There are two periods of accelerated growth of the intestine that correlate with nutritional and physiologic changes taking place: (1) between 1 and 3 years of age, during a period of diet transition, and (2) between 10 and 15 years of age, a period that coincides with the adolescent growth spurt.

The secretory cells of the GI tract are believed to be functional at birth. However, since most of the digestive enzymes depend on a specific pH relationship that is gradually acquired with age, their efficiency may be impaired. The newborn produces only small amounts of saliva, which contains some of the starch-splitting enzyme ptyalin; therefore its primary purpose at this time is to moisten the mouth and throat. It has little time to act on starches in the rapidly swallowed food. By the end of the second year the salivary glands have increased in size about 5 times to reach their full size and function.

Gastric acidity varies during childhood. The acidity of gastric juice is low during infancy and rises during childhood to level off at approximately 10 years of age. At the time of the adolescent growth spurt there is an increase in free hydrochloric acid. It is particularly marked in males, which probably contributes to the simultaneous increase in consumption of food. Most of the chemical activity is functional within these limitations and to the extent that it is dependent on the development of hormonal and neurologic maturation.

Digestion

Digestion refers to the catabolism of foodstuffs from an original complex form to simple, assimilable nutrients. Foodstuffs are composed of six substances: water, vitamins, mineral salts, carbohydrates, proteins, and fats. The processes of digestion are mainly *mechanical* (mixing and propulsion of food along the alimentary tract) and *chemical* (conversion of carbohydrates, proteins, and fats into assimilable forms—simple sugars, amino acids, and fatty acids and glycerol, respectively).

Mechanical digestion begins in the mouth. Chewing movements of teeth and tongue mix food with saliva and reduce the size of particles into a *bolus*. Saliva, in addition to moistening the food sufficiently to aid in swallowing, initiates digestion. The enzyme ptyalin (amylase) catalyzes the more complex carbohydrates or starches into simpler forms, such as maltose. Once the bolus is swallowed, the remainder of mechanical digestion is involuntary.

The pharynx and esophagus are primarily concerned with deglutition, or swallowing. As the tongue pushes food backward into the pharynx, the food is propelled into the esophagus by two mechanisms, which prevent its entry up into the nasal cavity or respiratory tract. First, the soft palate and uvula elevate to block off the nasopharynx. Second, the epiglottis closes over the larynx to prevent food from passing into the airway. As food enters the esophagus, it is propelled forward into the stomach by movements called *peristalsis*, wavelike movements that squeeze food along the entire length of the alimentary tract. The passage of stomach contents is controlled by the cardiac sphincter between the esophagus and stomach and by the pyloric sphincter between the stomach and duodenum, the beginning of the small intestine.

As the bolus passes into the stomach, gastric movements churn the particles, mixing them with gastric juice composed of water, pepsin, hydrochloric acid, rennin, lipase, and mucin. Pepsin (protease), hydrochloric acid, and rennin partially digest proteins; lipase initiates the digestion of fats. Mucin serves primarily to buffer the strong acid and forms a protective barrier between the acid and the stomach. The entire alimentary tract is protected from digestive action of its various secretions by production of mucus and rapid replacement of mucosal cells.

Partially digested food (*chyme*) passes from the stomach into the small intestine, where churning movements mix it thoroughly with intestinal juices and cause it to come in contact with the mucosal lining for absorption. Intestinal epithelial cells contain large quantities of digestive enzymes, which appear to complete digestion while substances are being absorbed into the cells. *Peptidases* split peptides into amino acids; *sucrase, maltase, isomaltase,* and *lactase* convert disaccharides into the monosaccharides glucose, galactose, and fructose; and *lipase* splits fats into fatty acids and glycerol.

Secretions from the liver and pancreas complete digestion in the small intestine. Bile, formed in the liver, contains no enzymes but is important for digestion because it (1) lowers the surface tension of fat, forming an emulsion that allows the water-soluble lipase to exert its enzymatic effect on the fat globules, and (2) increases the absorption of the end products of fat digestion by the intestinal wall. Absence of bile causes about half of ingested fat to appear in the feces *(steatorrhea)* and impairs absorption of fat-soluble vitamins A, D, E, and K.

Pancreatic juice contains three important digestive enzymes: (1) *trypsin* (protease) converts partially digested proteins (proteoses and peptones) and intact proteins into the final end product, amino acids; (2) *lipase* catalyzes bile-emulsified fats into their final end products, fatty acids and glycerol; and (3) *amylase* hydrolyzes most starches and carbohydrates to the disaccharides maltose, sucrose, and lactose. Each of these three enzymes becomes active only after the inactive forms are secreted into the small intestine. For example, enterokinase is necessary for trypsinogen to be converted into trypsin. Otherwise activated enzymes would digest the pancreas and pancreatic duct.

After digestion and absorption of nutritional end products in the small intestine, the remainder of intestinal contents (nondigestible residue and a small amount of undigested fat and protein) pass through the ileocecal valve into the large intestine. Here the contents are prepared for excretion as *feces.* Most of the remaining water and electrolytes are absorbed from the proximal colon. Bacterial flora form vitamin K, vitamin B_{12}, thiamine, riboflavin, and various gases. The odor of feces is primarily caused by products of bacterial action and depends on the type of colonic flora and ingested food. Defects in digestion or absorption notably alter the odor, as well as the appearance, of feces. Color is the result of bilirubin end products converted by bacteria to urobilinogen and then oxidized to urobilin.

As the rectum becomes distended with feces, powerful peristaltic waves are stimulated, propelling colonic contents toward the anus. At the same time, the internal anal sphincter relaxes, and if the external sphincter voluntarily or involuntarily relaxes, defecation occurs.

Absorption

The principal absorbing site in the GI system is the small intestine, the inner lining of which contains many folds. The entire surface of these folds is covered with small, fingerlike projections called *villi.* Millions of *microvilli* make up the luminal surface of intestinal epithelial cells covering each villus, forming the *brush border* of the villi. These structures or coats have been estimated to increase the surface area of the intestine by 600 to 700 times (Klish and Putnam, 1981). In each villus are *crypts of Lieberkühn,* whose main purpose is to replace absorptive cells that are constantly being extruded at each villus tip. This process of regeneration is so effective that normally the intestinal epithelium replaces itself every 5 days.

Unlike this type of surface, the stomach and large intestine are devoid of villi. Most of the absorption that takes place there is by *diffusion* (movement of substances from an area of higher concentration to one of lower concentration). Absorption in the small intestine may be by simple diffusion or *active transport,* which requires energy to transport a substance across an opposing pressure gradient or against an electric potential. The mechanisms of active transport are not completely understood but are thought to be carried on by epithelial cells of intestinal mucosa.

End products of carbohydrate and protein digestion (monosaccharides and amino acids) are absorbed into intestinal capillaries and circulated to the liver by the portal vein. Here they are metabolized and either used for energy or stored as the body's reserves. End products of fat digestion (fatty acids and glycerol) are absorbed by epithelial cells of the villi. Here they are reconverted to triglyceride fat molecules, which then move out of the cells into lymph capillaries (lacteals) of the villi. Lymphatics carry them to the venous circulation by the thoracic duct to the left subclavian vein, superior vena cava, heart, and general circulation. Some undigested emulsified fats directly enter the circulation by intestinal capillaries.

All of the vitamins are believed to be absorbed in the small intestine. Fat-soluble vitamins are absorbed along with digested fats in the presence of bile. Water-soluble vitamins, vitamin B complex and C, are quickly absorbed, although absorption of vitamin B_{12} takes place only in the ileum. Water and electrolytes are also absorbed primarily in the small intestine, although some absorption also takes place in the large intestine.

ASSESSMENT OF GASTROINTESTINAL FUNCTION

Some GI disorders (e.g., vomiting and/or diarrhea) occur as primary and isolated disturbances but are also among the manifestations often associated with a variety of childhood illnesses. Structural and obstructive defects interfere with the ingestion and transport of ingested foodstuffs, and inflammatory, malabsorptive, and maldigestive disturbances impair the functional integrity of the GI tract. Furthermore, in most of the disorders the primary defect can produce additional complications. For example, loss of GI contents causes significant alterations in fluid and electrolytes, and obstructive or inflammatory conditions affect digestion and absorption because bowel motility, mucosal functioning, enzymatic activity, and bacterial flora are altered.

Numerous general observations provide possible clues to specific GI problems (Box 33-2). In some cases only one manifestation may be observed; others may involve several signs and symptoms as part of the disease complex. In many disorders that involve GI losses, particularly large amounts of fluid, dehydration poses a serious threat to life and often dominates the clinical picture (see Dehydration, Chapter 28, and Acute Infectious Gastroenteritis, Chapter 29).

A number of tests may be employed to assess GI function (Table 33-2), and nurses are responsible for collecting specimens (see Collection of Specimens, Chapter 27). Since children may not like to drink contrast media, generally dislike enemas, and are frightened of unfamiliar equipment, they need preparation for procedures and collection of specimens (see Preparation for Procedures, Chapter 27).

■ INGESTION OF FOREIGN SUBSTANCES

Children are prone to ingesting foreign substances as they place their hands and any attractive object or substance into their mouths. Infants and small children in particular explore items with their mouths instinctively. Older children often place items in their mouths and accidentally swallow them. Rarely, a child deliberately swallows unusual objects

Box 33-2 CLINICAL MANIFESTATIONS OF GASTROINTESTINAL DYSFUNCTION IN CHILDREN

Failure to thrive, as evidenced by deceleration from established growth pattern or consistently below the 5th percentile for height and weight on standard growth charts.

Spitting up and/or regurgitation, characteristic of infants, are discussed in Chapter 13.

Vomiting, the forceful ejection of stomach contents, involves a complex reflex that is associated with widespread autonomic discharge that causes salivation, pallor, sweating, and tachycardia. Vomiting is ordinarily accompanied by nausea.

Projectile vomiting, in which the vomitus is forcefully ejected as far as 2 to 4 feet (0.6 to 1.2 m) from the child, is not associated with nausea.

Hematemesis, the vomiting of blood, may result from swallowing blood from the oropharynx or from bleeding in the upper GI tract.

Nausea is an unpleasant sensation vaguely referred to the epigastrium, with an inclination to vomit.

Stools, the number, type, consistency, presence or absence of blood, and associated signs and symptoms provide clues to the etiology of gastrointestinal dysfunction.

Constipation is the regular passage of firm or hard stools or of small, hard masses with associated symptoms such as difficulty expelling the stools, blood-streaked bowel movements, and abdominal discomfort. Suggested lower limit of frequency is six movements per week in children less than 3 years and four per week in older children. The apparent difficulty in passing stools is not a reliable sign, especially in infancy.

Diarrhea is an increase in the number of stools or a decrease in their consistency as a result of alterations of water and electrolyte transport by the alimentary tract. Diarrhea may be acute or chronic.

Abdominal pain, specific or nonspecific, is associated with a number of GI disorders.

Abdominal enlargement or distention is a common observation in a child with GI dysfunction.

Dysphagia, difficulty in swallowing, can be the result of structural abnormalities or neurologic or neuromuscular impairment.

Bowel sounds, or their absence, can provide information about some GI disorders.

Jaundice is the yellow discoloration of the skin associated with liver dysfunction.

Disability in sucking and swallowing is a manifestation often observed in infants.

Fever is a common manifestation of illness in children. In GI disorders it is usually associated with dehydration or infection.

or substances. Hands come into contact with dirt and contaminated objects that contain ova or larvae of a variety of parasites. The following is an overview of ingestion of foreign objects; ingestion of specific substances, such as lead or parasites, is presented in Chapter 16.

PICA

Pica is the Latin word for magpie, a bird of voracious and indiscriminate appetite. The use of the term today refers to the habitual, purposeful, and compulsive ingestion of nonfood substances in the environment. The list of ingested substances is practically endless but most commonly includes clay, dirt, ashes, paint chips, laundry starch, cornstarch, paper, pencils, erasers, crayons, cigarette butts, and matches. Most children have a particular craving for a few items, which is largely determined by the availability of the substance.

It is believed by some that certain forms of pica are manifestations of a deficiency in the diet, especially of minerals. For example, eating clay has been related to zinc deficiency, and eating chalk to calcium deficiency. In most instances pica is relatively harmless, but if the substance ingested contains a harmful ingredient (e.g., lead in paint), the practice becomes a serious matter. If eating of a specific substance persists, it should probably be evaluated. Certainly, if a potentially harmful substance is involved, it should be removed from the environment or the child denied access to it.

EMERGENCY TREATMENT
Foreign Body Ingestion

1. Seek medical treatment *immediately* if:
   a. Any sharp or large object or a battery was ingested.
   b. There are signs that the object may have been aspirated (i.e., coughing, choking, inability to speak, or difficulty in breathing) (see Chapter 31 for emergency treatment of airway obstruction).
   c. There are signs that the object may be lodged in the esophagus (i.e., increased salivation, drooling, gagging, or difficulty with swallowing).
   d. There are signs that the object may be lodged in the pharynx (i.e., discomfort in the throat or chest [more likely with a fish or chicken bone]).
2. Seek medical advice if the object is smooth and small (usually less than the size of a nickel).
3. If no treatment is required, check the stool for passage of the object; do not give laxatives.

FOREIGN BODIES

Children ingest a variety of foreign objects. Most ingested foreign bodies, such as marbles, coins, beads, and small safety pins, pass through the alimentary tract without difficulty once they reach the stomach. Larger items and straight or sharp objects, such as bobby pins, hairpins, pull tabs on beverage cans, needles, tacks, and large safety pins, may become lodged in the esophagus or duodenal loop.

Once an ingested object passes the pylorus, its progress may be followed by radiographs, and the stools are examined for its presence. The child is fed the customary diet. If serial radiographs indicate that the object remains stationary, it is removed by an endoscope or in rare cases by laparotomy. Surgical removal is indicated in instances of perforation, bleeding, or obstruction and when large or long ob-

Table 33-2 Diagnostic procedures

TEST	DESCRIPTION	PURPOSE	COMMENTS
Stool examination	Gross, microscopic, and chemical examination of stool specimen	To detect presence of normal and abnormal constituents	Most tests demand a fresh specimen Provide samples from several areas of the stool
Ova and parasites	Examination of lumen contents for presence of organisms	To aid in diagnosis of parasites or their eggs	Requires a fresh, warm specimen
Fat	Examination for presence of fat	To aid in diagnosis of pancreatic insufficiency	Requires a 72-hour cumulative specimen
Culture and sensitivity	Sample contents grown on culture media and tested with appropriate antimicrobials	To detect presence of bacterial overgrowth, abnormal motility To confirm diagnosis of bacterial gastroenteritis To assess sensitivity to specific antimicrobials	Avoid external contamination of stool Deliver specimen to laboratory promptly Collect a sufficient amount Provide laboratory with necessary clinical information to select suitable media and techniques
Reducing substances (sugars)	Clinitest tablets added to small amount of stool suspended in 15 gtt of water; color change indicates amount of substance present	To detect presence of reducing substances in stool Sucrose not considered a reducing substance	Easily and quickly administered Test should be carried out as soon as possible after collection Test modified for detection of sucrose Test can be performed on unit
Occult blood Guaiac test	Guaiac chemicals added to stool smeared on filter paper reveals blue color in presence of blood	To detect presence of blood in stool	Easily and quickly administered screening test Small amounts of blood (e.g., from bleeding mouth, gums, and nose) may give false-positive results Test can be performed on unit
Hematest	Hematest tablet and water added to stool smeared on filter paper turns blue in presence of blood	To detect presence of blood in stools	
Gastric acidity	Stomach emptied of secretions; removed by suction via NG tube; serial specimens needed; samples measured for amount and acid content	To measure gastric acidity	Requires fast before test: Children: nothing after midnight Infant less than 1 year: 4 to 6 hours before test NG tube placed so that tip lies in most dependent area of stomach
Pancreatic enzymes	Duodenal secretions collected via double-lumen duodenal tube following pancreatic stimulation with IV secretion and pancreazymin Serial samples collected	To determine functional capacity of pancreas	Requires preprocedure fast Requires sedation Child needs preparation for NG tube insertion
Radiography Flat plate	Anterior/posterior and lateral radiographs of abdomen and pelvis	To detect presence of air in gut lumen or peritoneum To detect foreign body and follow progress, if needed	Requires no special preparation Child needs preparation for the procedure
Contrast studies Upper GI series Lower GI series	Radiopaque media (barium or Gastrografin) is swallowed or administered as an enema	To outline lumen of GI tract—esophagus, stomach, bowel, rectum To detect abnormalities in bowel lumen	Children need preprocedure preparation for both barium swallow and enema Barium enema requires cleansing enemas before procedure Encourage fluids following procedure

Table 33-2 Diagnostic procedures—cont'd

TEST	DESCRIPTION	PURPOSE	COMMENTS
Ultrasonography (sonography)	Measures and records reflection of pulsed or continuous high-frequency sound waves	To locate, measure, and delineate deep structures, e.g., the pyloric musculature	Noninvasive technique No radiation involved Child needs preparation for procedure
Computed tomography (CT)	Pinpoint x-ray beam is directed on horizontal or vertical plane to provide series of "cuts" or "slices" that are fed into computer and assembled in image displayed on video screen and transferred to permanent record	To visualize horizontal and vertical cross section of abdomen at any axis To distinguish density of various tissues	Noninvasive procedure Requires sedation Can be performed on outpatient basis Rapid, relatively safe, and accurate
Magnetic resonance imaging (MRI)	Produces radiofrequency emissions from elements (hydrogen, phosphorus), which are converted to visual images by computer	Permits visualization of morphologic features of target structures Permits tissue discrimination unavailable with many techniques	Noninvasive Requires heavy sedation for lengthy immobilization No exposure to radiation No metal can be present in scanner
Manometry			
Esophagus	Measures progressive contractions of esophagus	Useful for evaluation of dysphagia, esophageal spasm, acholasia, dysmotility	Child needs preparation for procedure
Rectal	Records reflex responses of anal sphincter to transient rectal balloon distention	To measure anal sphincter function, especially for screening for constipation, diagnosis of Hirschsprung disease	Child requires preparation for procedure
Biopsy	Removal of small piece of living tissue from an organ for microscopic examination	To confirm or establish a diagnosis, estimate prognosis, or follow course of a disease	Prepare child for procedure
Endoscopy Panendoscopy (esophagus, stomach, duodenum) Esophagoscopy Colonoscopy Rectosigmoidoscopy Anoscopy	Endoscope introduced into area to be examined Fiberoptic endoscopy—light transmitted down flexible tube containing thin, transparent fibers and reflected back to produce an image Endoscope equipped with channels through which instruments can be passed	Direct visualization of lumen of GI tract to evaluate appearance and integrity of mucosa, detect lesions, and provide access for biopsy Allows for instrumental removal of foreign objects or specimens for biopsy	Requires bowel cleansing before procedure Clear liquid diet 48 hours before procedure For lower bowel (colon, rectum) colonic lavage before procedure—Golytely (colonic lavage solution) or magnesium citrate
Breath test	Hydrogen generated in colon by bacterial action on carbohydrate fermentation is excreted as flatus (79%) or absorbed into blood (21%) where it diffuses into alveoli and is excreted via lungs	Useful in detection of conditions that interfere with digestion or absorption of carbohydrate (lactose, sucrose) in gut—primary lactose intolerance, secondary lactose intolerance related to mucosal injury (e.g., enteropathy), bacterial overgrowth	Noninvasive Hydrogen not a product of any known metabolic reaction in humans Amount of hydrogen expelled in each breath is directly related to amount of carbohydrate presented to colonic bacteria
D-Xylose absorption test	10% D-xylose solution administered orally Serum xylose is measured exactly 1 hour later	To evaluate absorptive qualities of small intestine Diagnosis of small bowel malabsorption caused by celiac disease	Requires 8-hour fast before administration of D-xylose Requires venipuncture Child requires preparation for all aspects of procedure

jects have not cleared the stomach within 3 to 5 days (Webb, McDaniel, and Jones, 1984).

Foreign bodies that become lodged in the esophagus require immediate attention, since they may adhere to the esophageal wall, where they cause erosion of the epithelium. Of particular concern is the increasing incidence of ingestion of "button" batteries commonly found in watches, hearing aids, cameras, and calculators. Some have been found to leak their alkaline electrolytes and other corrosive substances or have been acted on by stomach and intestinal secretions. While most button battery ingestions are benign, the most difficulty arises from the larger-diameter batteries, which become impacted in the esophagus. Recommendations for treating battery ingestions include (1) confirming the location by radiographic examination, (2) removing immediately those lodged in the esophagus, (3) observing those beyond the esophagus on an outpatient basis, (4) repeating radiography after 48 hours if the ingested battery is larger than button size and removing those that still remain in the stomach, and (5) repeating radiography if a small battery has not passed in the stool by 4 to 7 days (Litovitz, 1985).

Coins are the most frequently swallowed items and account for most esophageal foreign bodies. If a coin passes into the stomach, it generally passes through the remainder of the GI tract without problems. If it remains in the esophagus, it can be symptomatic or asymptomatic. Usual symptoms are refusal to take foods, increased salivation, pain or discomfort on swallowing, or vomiting. Symptomatic esophageal coin ingestion is managed the same as battery ingestion. Therapeutic management of asymptomatic coin ingestion is controversial. Some advocate immediate radiographic evaluation to determine placement regardless of symptoms (Gracia, Frey, and Balaz, 1984; Schunk, Corneli, and Bolte, 1989). Others recommend that asymptomatic patients be allowed a 24-hour period in which to pass the coin without radiography or intervention (Caravati, Bennett, and MeElwee, 1989; Joseph, 1990). Alternative to removal involves advancing the coin carefully into the stomach for continued travel through the GI tract (Bonadio and others, 1988)

Nursing Considerations

The primary nursing intervention is prevention of foreign body ingestion through preventive family teaching. All children who are old enough to understand should be taught not to put anything in their mouths before asking permission. Infants and young children who cannot follow such advice must have their environment protected for them. Small objects are placed out of their reach or properly discarded. The best suggestion is to search the floor carefully on hands and knees and remove small objects that are accessible to inquisitive young children.

Once an object is swallowed, parents need guidelines on seeking treatment (see Emergency Treatment p. 1491). When no treatment is instituted, parents should examine the stool for verification that the object has passed safely through the GI tract, usually in 3 to 4 days. For children in diapers this is easily accomplished by squeezing the stool between the diaper to locate the object, but in toilet-trained children it requires more effort. A piece of plastic wrap placed across the toilet bowl to collect the stool makes it easier to examine the feces, although a tongue blade or some other disposable object may be needed to break up the stool.

■ DISORDERS OF MOTILITY

A number of GI disorders are caused by disturbance in motility. Some, such as Hirschsprung disease and gastroesophageal reflux, are seen primarily in infancy and cause problems in elimination or feeding. Others, such as constipation, can occur at any age and produce few serious effects, unless the primary disorder can lead to obstruction. The common problems of diarrhea and vomiting are discussed in Chapter 29 because of the importance of the fluid and electrolyte changes they can produce.

CONSTIPATION

Constipation is the regular passage of firm or hard stools or of small, hard masses with associated symptoms such as difficulty in expulsion of the stools, blood-streaked bowel movements, and abdominal discomfort. The frequency of bowel movements is not considered a diagnostic criterion because it varies widely among children. General guidelines for stool frequency suggest a lower limit of six per week in children younger than 3 years and four per week in older children (Corazziari and others, 1985). However, less frequent bowel movements may be normal. Having extremely long intervals between defecation is termed *obstipation.* Constipation with fecal soiling is *encopresis.* The following discussion is concerned primarily with causes of constipation in different age-groups and the treatment of simple constipation during childhood. For a discussion of encopresis, see Chapter 18.

Constipation can be a symptom of a number of abdominal disorders, primarily those that cause an obstruction in the lower intestinal tract, such as Hirschsprung disease or imperforate anus. Physical and mental disorders are often associated with defecation problems, for example, neurologic disorders, mental retardation, hypothyroidism, and hypercalcemia. However, the development and course of constipation can be influenced by a number of familial, cultural, and social factors. Psychologic factors play an important role in bowel habits, as well as toilet-training techniques, diet, overuse of laxatives, and enemas. The most common cause of constipation in children is environmental change, such as change in feeding habits, using a new toilet, birth of a sibling, and relocation of housing or school (Johns, 1985).

Newborn

Normally the newborn passes a first meconium stool within 24 to 36 hours of birth. Any infant who does not do so should be assessed for evidence of intestinal atresia or stenosis, congenital aganglionic megacolon (50% of cases), hypothyroidism, meconium plugs, or meconium ileus. Meconium plugs are caused by meconium that has reduced water content and are usually evacuated following digital examination, but they may require irrigations of normal saline or the iodinated contrast medium *diatrizoate meglumine (Gastrografin).*

Meconium ileus, the initial manifestation of cystic fibrosis, is the presence of thick, mucilaginous meconium that clings to the abdominal wall, making it difficult, if not impossible, to pass. Treatment is the same as for a meconium plug. Rarely, surgical intervention may be necessary.

Infancy

True constipation is relatively rare in infants, but normal stool patterns can vary markedly from infant to infant. Hard, painful bowel movements are mild to moderate problems, but distention associated with constipation requires further evaluation (Rappaport and Levine, 1986). Medical causes such as Hirschsprung disease, hypothyroidism, and strictures must be ruled out in chronic cases of constipation. The assessment history should always include frequency of bowel movements, the composition of the diet, and whether the constipation is recent or has been present since birth.

The most frequent cause of constipation in infancy is dietary mismanagement. It is almost unknown in breast-fed infants, who typically have more stools than bottle-fed infants. Constipation may accompany the change from human milk or modified cow's milk formula to whole cow's milk, presumably because of the greater protein-to-carbohydrate ratio of whole cow's milk. Some bottle-fed infants pass hard stools and develop anal fissures. To avoid the pain in defecation, these infants voluntarily withhold stool. The infant's behavior during withholding of stools is often misinterpreted by parents as constipation. The infant grunts and appears to be straining, displaying a red face and with legs drawn up on the abdomen. However, a red face and straining are normal behavior in infancy.

Simple measures ordinarily correct the problem, such as increasing the amount of fluid or sugar in the formula in the very young infant or adding or increasing the amount of cereal, vegetables, and fruit in the diet of the older infant. If the child has anal fissures, the temporary use of stool softeners, glycerine suppositories, or mineral oil is usually sufficient to break the painful defecation cycle.

Early Childhood

Children between 1 and 3 years of age are most likely to have constipation (Abrahamian and Lloyd-Still, 1984). Most constipation is due to environmental changes or is related to normal development when a child begins to attain control over bodily functions. A child who has experienced discomfort during bowel movements may deliberately try to avoid them. "Stool withholding" behavior is often misinterpreted by parents as extreme straining to pass stool. The child will be observed to hide in the corner of a room or to grip a piece of furniture, assume a longitudinal posture (standing or lying supine) with buttocks squeezed together, and turn red with or without crying. The rectum accommodates the stool accumulation, and the urge to defecate passes. When bowel contents are ultimately evacuated, the result is that accumulated feces are passed with even greater pain, reinforcing the desire to withhold. This generates a self-perpetuating cycle of further retention and discomfort (Pettei, 1987; Rappaport and Levine, 1986).

School-Age Children

School entrance often exacerbates bowel difficulties that were experienced earlier in life, and some children who never had constipation develop retentive tendencies at this time (Rappaport and Levine, 1986). Before school entry children have ample opportunity for toileting in the home setting. Early and hurried departure for school immediately after breakfast is not conducive to leisurely bathroom use. Also school and after-school activities are often rigidly scheduled and regimented. The most common cause of new-onset constipation at school entry is fear of using school bathrooms, which are noted for their lack of privacy. Most schools will liberalize bathroom rules for individual children who have been identified and have a parent or health professional intervene on their behalf.

Therapeutic Management

If constipation is associated with manifestations such as vomiting, abdominal distention or pain, and evidence of growth failure, the condition merits further investigation. Constipation may result from some medications, such as iron preparations, diuretics, antacids, and anticonvulsant agents. Constipation frequently accompanies enuresis, and treatment of the constipation often results in resolution of the enuresis (O'Regan and others, 1986).

The management of simple constipation is based on a plan to keep the bowel relatively empty of stool and dietary management to prevent further constipation. Although authorities differ on the methods to clean out the bowel, all agree that use of laxatives is not usually recommended because of their tendency to produce dependency. Some regimens employ the use of enemas to initially rid the bowel of stool and additional enemas if voluntary evacuation does not occur within 48 hours. During this time a high-fiber diet is instituted, and any foods known to be constipating are eliminated, such as all milk and milk products, apples, apple juice, carrots, bananas, rice, and gelatin. Supplemental bran may be given also (Olness, 1984). When high-fiber foods are added, additional sources of fluid must be given to the child to prevent the fiber from having a binding effect. One of the major functions of fiber is to absorb water to soften the stool. Other regimens may include a stool softener to keep the stool of a consistency that is more easily evacuated.

Nursing Considerations

Constipation, unfortunately, tends to be self-perpetuating. A child who has difficulty or discomfort when attempting to evacuate the bowels has a tendency to retain the bowel contents and thus begins a vicious cycle. Nursing assessment begins with an accurate history of bowel habits, diet, events that may be associated with the onset of constipation, drugs or other substances that the child may be taking, and the consistency, color, frequency, and other characteristics of the stool. If there is no evidence of a pathologic condition that requires further investigation, the major task of the nurse is to educate the parents regarding normal stool patterns and to relieve the cause of the constipation.

Dietary modifications are usually essential in preventing constipation. During infancy simply increasing the carbohydrate (sugar or corn syrup) in an infant formula will often relieve the problem. During childhood the diet should contain increased amounts of fiber and fluid. Parents will benefit from guidance in dietary planning, especially regarding foods that facilitate bowel movements (Table 33-3). If bran is added to the diet, creative ways to disguise the consistency are needed. For example, it can be added to cereal, peanut butter, mashed potatoes, fruit shakes, and baked goods.

An excellent food for providing a high-fiber intake is popcorn. It is readily accepted by children, inexpensive and easy to prepare, and safe for children beyond the age when foreign body aspiration is a hazard. Popcorn has sufficient bulk and can be purchased in a variety of different tastes and forms. The recommended "dose" is 1 to 2 quarts of popcorn per day for several months until regular bowel habits are established (Chen and Sullivan, 1986). Compliance is rarely a problem.

Parents also need reassurance concerning the benign nature of the condition. It is important to discuss with them their attitudes and expectations regarding toilet habits and to discourage the use of stool softeners, laxatives, and enemas. If such measures have been prescribed by a physician, parents should understand that these are merely temporary and not to be continued beyond the current need.

Table 33-3 High-fiber foods

FOOD GROUP	SELECTIONS
Bread, grains	Whole-grain bread or rolls Whole-grain cereals Bran Pancakes, waffles, and muffins with fruit or bran Unrefined (brown) rice
Vegetables	Raw vegetables, especially broccoli, cabbage, carrots, cauliflower, celery, lettuce, and spinach Cooked vegetables, such as those listed above and asparagus, beans, brussels sprouts, corn, potatoes, rhubarb, squash, string beans, turnips
Fruits	Raw fruits, especially those with skins or seeds, other than ripe bananas or avocado Raisins, prunes, or other dried fruits
Miscellaneous	Nuts, seeds, legumes, popcorn

HIRSCHSPRUNG DISEASE (CONGENITAL AGANGLIONIC MEGACOLON)

Hirschsprung disease is a congenital anomaly that results in mechanical obstruction from inadequate motility in part of the intestine. It accounts for about one fourth of all cases of neonatal obstruction, although it may not be diagnosed until later in infancy or childhood. It is four times more common in males than females, follows a familial pattern in a small number of cases, and has a higher incidence in children with Down syndrome. Depending on its presentation, it may be an acute, life-threatening condition or a chronic disorder.

Pathophysiology

The term *congenital (aganglionic) megacolon* describes the primary defect, an absence of autonomic parasympathetic ganglion cells of the submucosal (Meissner) and myenteric (Auerbach) plexuses in one or more segments of colon (*aganglionic*). The defect is probably the result of defective migration of parasympathetic ganglion cell precursors during embryonic development. Lack of innervation produces the functional defect, that is, absence of propulsive movements (peristalsis), which causes accumulation of intestinal contents and bowel distention proximal to the defect (*megacolon* or large colon). In addition, failure of the internal rectal sphincter to relax contributes to clinical manifestations because it prevents evacuation of solids, liquids, and gas.

The length of aganglionic bowel varies greatly, from involving only the internal sphincter to the entire colon. The latter condition is rare (about 12% of all cases) and influences prognosis and mortality significantly (about 54%), although newer surgical techniques have dramatically improved the outlook for these children (Jordan, Coran, and Wesley, 1981). The most commonly affected site is the rectosigmoid colon (Fig. 33-1).

Clinical Manifestations

Clinical manifestations vary according to the age when symptoms are recognized and according to the occurrence of complications, such as enterocolitis. In the newborn the chief signs and symptoms are failure to pass meconium within 24 to 48 hours after birth, reluctance to ingest fluids, bile-stained vomitus, and abdominal distention. If the disorder is allowed to progress, other signs of intestinal obstruction develop, such as respiratory distress and shock.

During infancy the child does not thrive and has constipation, abdominal distention, and episodes of diarrhea and vomiting. Explosive, watery diarrhea, fever, and severe prostration are ominous signs because they often signify the presence of enterocolitis (inflammation of the small bowel and colon), which greatly increases the risk of fatality. Enterocolitis may also be present without diarrhea and is first evidenced with unexplained fever and poor feeding.

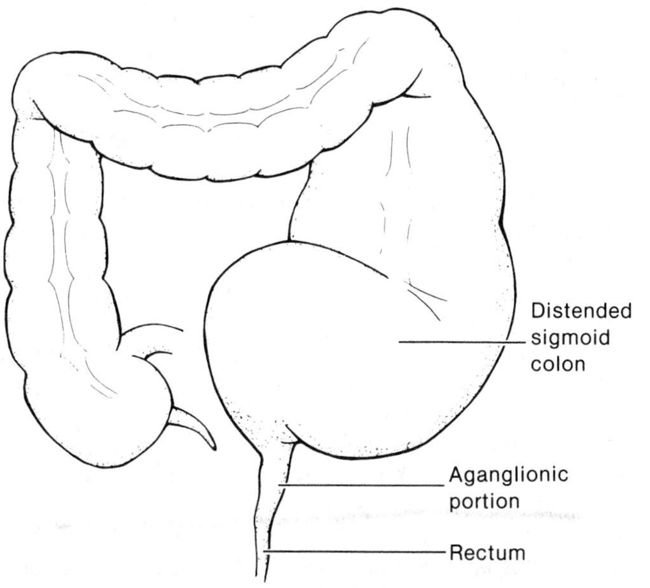

Fig. 33-1. Hirschsprung disease.

During childhood the symptoms become chronic and include constipation, passage of ribbonlike, foul-smelling stools, abdominal distention, and visible peristalsis. Fecal masses are easily palpable. The child is usually poorly nourished, anemic, and hypoproteinemic from malabsorption of nutrients.

Diagnostic Evaluation

In the neonate diagnosis is suspected on clinical signs of intestinal obstruction and failure to pass meconium. In infants and children the history is an important part of diagnosis and typically details a chronic pattern of constipation. On examination the rectum is empty of feces, the internal sphincter is tight, and there is leakage of liquid, offensive, pale stool and accumulated gas. Radiographic studies using a barium enema often demonstrate the transition zone between the dilated proximal colon (megacolon) and the aganglionic distal segment. However, this typical megacolon and narrow distal segment may not develop until 3 to 4 weeks or even months after birth in some children.

To confirm the diagnosis, rectal biopsy is performed either surgically to obtain a full-thickness biopsy for histologic evidence of aganglionic cells or by suction biopsy, performed without anesthesia, to detect the presence of ganglia in the submucosa and increased amounts of the enzyme acetylcholinesterase in a biopsy specimen. Another noninvasive procedure that may be used is anorectal manometry, in which a cylinder with three balloons attached to it is inserted partway into the rectum. Two balloons are positioned at the internal sphincter, and the third at the external sphincter. The test records the reflex response of the sphincters to distention of the balloons. A normal response is relaxation of the internal sphincter followed by contraction of the external sphincter. In Hirschsprung disease the external sphincter contracts normally, but the internal sphincter fails to relax or contract.

Therapeutic Management

Treatment is primarily surgical removal of the aganglionic bowel to ensure continence. A very small number of children with chronic, but not severe, symptoms of megacolon are treated conservatively with occasional enemas to establish a regular pattern of defecation. However, these children represent a distinct exception and may be at continued risk for the development of fatal enterocolitis (Martin and Torres, 1985).

Surgical correction usually involves a two- or three-stage approach. In most cases a temporary colostomy is created in part of the bowel with normal innervation (usually the sigmoid or transverse colon) and at a site that permits the corrective operation to be performed. The colostomy allows the bowel a period of rest in order to resume its normal caliber and tonicity and provides an opportunity for the child to gain weight before the more extensive repair is undertaken.

Definitive correction is usually performed when the child is 8 months to 1 year of age or has reached approximately 20 pounds (Polley, Coran, and Wesley, 1985). The type of surgical procedure for reanastomosis involves "pulling" the end of the intact bowel down to a point near the rectum. The most common surgical techniques are the Swenson, the Soave (endorectal pull-through), and the Duhamel operations, which usually require both an abdominal and a perineal incision.

The third stage (if required) is closure of the colostomy, normally performed within a few (usually 3) months of the definitive repair. Prognosis after complete surgical repair depends on the child's ability to adjust to a normal diet and to learn bowel control and varies depending on the type of surgery. However, most children are able to attain satisfactory defecatory function (Martin and Torres, 1985; Polley, Coran, and Wesley, 1985).

Nursing Considerations

Many of the nursing concerns depend on the child's age and the type of treatment. Nursing observation in the neonatal period is most important as a factor in early diagnosis. In a retrospective study all infants who were diagnosed by biopsy at a later date had onset of constipation in the neonatal period (Landman, 1987). If the disorder is diagnosed during the neonatal period, the main objectives are helping the parents adjust to a congenital defect in their child, fostering infant-parent bonding, preparing them for the medical/surgical intervention, and assisting them in caring for the colostomy after discharge.

When the disorder is not discovered during this period, the nurse can facilitate establishing a diagnosis by carefully listening to the parents' history, with special emphasis on bowel habits. In Hirschsprung disease several areas must be investigated: (1) onset of constipation, especially if present since birth; (2) character of stools, particularly ribbonlike and foul smelling; and (3) frequency of bowel movements. Other clues in the history and physical examination include poor feeding habits, fussiness and irritability, a distended abdomen, and signs of undernutrition, such as thin extremities, pallor, muscle weakness, and fatigue.

The following discussion is limited to the care of the child undergoing surgical correction. For the rare child who is managed with occasional enemas, the nurse needs to teach the parents the correct procedure, as well as inform them of the dangers of using tap water, concentrated salt solutions, soap solutions, or phosphate preparations. Normal saline solution can be purchased without a prescription from a pharmacy or can be prepared at home by adding 1 level measuring teaspoon of noniodized salt to 1 pint of tap water. Since the instructions for preparing the solution and administering the enema require several steps, all the directions should be written down as well as verbally explained.* See Chapter 27 for suggested amounts of solution according to the child's age.

Preoperative care. Much of the child's preoperative care depends on the age and clinical condition. Physical preoperative preparation entails the same measures that are common to any surgery (see Chapter 27). In the newborn, whose bowel is sterile, no additional preparation is required. However, children beyond the newborn period need bowel emptying with repeated saline enemas and reduction of bacterial flora with systemic antibiotics and colonic irrigations using antibiotic solution. A nasogastric (NG) tube may be inserted to prevent abdominal distention, and antibiotic solution instilled through the tube to further prepare the GI tract. All intake and output of irrigant and drainage are noted, particularly a marked discrepancy in retention or loss of fluid. A rectal tube may also be inserted to allow for escape of accumulated fluid and gas. Because of the rectal tube and to prevent damage to the mucosa, only axillary temperatures are taken.

In children with enterocolitis, emergency preoperative care includes frequent monitoring of vital signs and blood pressure for signs of shock; monitoring fluid replacement with electrolytes, plasma, or other blood derivatives; and observing for symptoms of bowel perforation, such as increasing abdominal distention, vomiting, increased tenderness, irritability, dyspnea, and cyanosis.

Since progressive distention of the abdomen is a serious sign, abdominal circumference is measured at the largest diameter, usually at the level of the umbilicus. The point of measurement is marked with a pen to ensure reliability. To lessen any stress to the acutely ill child, the tape measure should be left under the child, rather than removed each time. As a rule of thumb, abdominal measurement can be performed at the same time that vital signs are taken. It is best to record the measurement in serial order so that a change will be readily apparent.

Children need to be prepared for an ostomy (see Ostomies, Chapter 27). Parents also need preparation before surgery. Since a colostomy represents a change in body function and appearance, the nurse should investigate parents' previous knowledge of this procedure. It is not uncommon for parents to have some knowledge about a colostomy. For example, one mother related that a friend's father had a permanent colostomy because of cancer. As soon as the mother heard that her child needed this procedure, she was convinced that the mass in her child's abdomen was a cancerous tumor.

It is best not to assume that parents understand a verbal explanation of a colostomy. Drawing a picture or using the doll is excellent for parents, as well as children. During this teaching session, the nurse should briefly mention methods of care, since presenting too much information can overwhelm the parents.

It is important to stress to parents and older children that the colostomy for Hirschsprung disease is temporary. The nurse should also keep in mind that although a temporary colostomy is favorable in terms of future health and adjustment, it also necessitates additional surgery, which may be very stressful to parents and children.

Since feeding and associated behavioral problems are frequently associated with a chronic pattern of megacolon, the nurse should inform parents that although the defect can be corrected, it will take some time for the child's physical status and feeding practices to improve. Although the benefit of surgery should not be minimized, it is necessary to avoid implying that surgical correction is a panacea to all physical and behavioral complaints.

Postoperative care. Physical postoperative care usually includes (1) nothing by mouth until bowel sounds return and the colostomy and/or anastomosed bowel are ready for feedings, (2) intravenous fluid to maintain hydration and replace lost electrolytes, (3) NG suctioning to prevent abdominal distention, (4) frequent abdominal dressing changes, and (5) perineal dressing changes.

To prevent contamination of the abdominal wound with urine, the diaper should be placed below the dressing. Sometimes a Foley catheter is used in the immediate postoperative period to divert the flow of urine away from the abdomen. Drainage from the NG tube and the colostomy is measured, since fluid and electrolyte replacement is partially calculated on these losses.

For young children who cannot brush their teeth or rinse out their mouths without swallowing fluid, the nurse can institute oral hygiene by wiping the teeth, gums, and tongue with a cloth moistened with saline. It is best to avoid using toothpaste because the foam is difficult to remove without liberally flushing the mouth, in which case the child may ingest or aspirate fluid. Sometimes physicians allow crushed ice after the child is fully alert from anesthesia. If permitted, the crushed ice can be offered on a spoon, or frozen ice in the form of a popsicle can be given. If colored ice is used, the colors red and green are avoided, since they can be confused with blood or bile.

When parents initially visit their child postoperatively, they are frequently unprepared for the numerous tubes and intravenous lines attached to various body parts. Even when

*Home care instructions on giving an enema are available in Wong, D.L., and Whaley, L.F.: Clinical manual of pediatric nursing, ed. 3, St. Louis, 1990, Mosby–Year Book, Inc.

all the procedures are explained beforehand, the actual visual shock can be great. The nurse should explain the function of each piece of equipment, stressing safety features that permit the child to be safely moved and handled, such as length of tubing, use of armboards at intravenous sites, and tape to secure the NG tube to the nose. In this way parents are encouraged and assisted in holding and stimulating their child.

The nurse emphasizes the expected changes in the appearance of the stoma, which initially is large, protruding, red, and raw looking. Since the stomal site appears painful, it is also important to stress that bowel mucosa is nonsensitive but that the surrounding abdominal skin must be protected.

Home care. Postoperatively, parents need instruction concerning colostomy care at home* (see Ostomies, Chapter 27). During the early postoperative period, including parents and the older child in dressing changes can enhance teaching of colostomy care when an appliance is fitted and promote gradual acceptance of the body change. Even a preschooler can be included in the care by handing articles to the parent, rolling up the colostomy bag after emptying, or applying cream to the surrounding skin. Since these children may have had difficulties with bowel training before surgery because of constipation and erratic stool patterns, the period during the temporary colostomy can relieve the pressures previously associated with bowel control. Older children should be involved in colostomy care to the point of total responsibility. A helpful book for families is *The Special Children: The Ostomy Book for Parents of Children with Colostomies, Ileostomies and Urostomies* by K.F. Jeter.† Also, a complete line of pediatric ostomy products is available.‡

In some institutions an enterostomal therapist is available to provide expert assistance in planning procedures for home care, such as preparation of skin, application of the collecting appliance, care of the appliance, control of odor, and signs of stomal complications, such as ribbonlike stools, excessive diarrhea, bleeding, prolapse, or failure to pass flatus or stool. Whenever possible, this person should be used in preparing for colostomy care.

In those children with delayed correction of Hirschsprung disease, feeding problems may be present, including the discomfort from abdominal distention after eating and the likelihood of parental pressure to eat. Hospitalization provides an excellent assessment period for the nurse to observe parent-child interaction during mealtime. Once specific problems are discovered, the nurse can initiate steps to reverse the pattern. It is important to remember that relearning must take place because the behavior has probably been reinforced for a long time.

*Home care instructions on caring for the child with a colostomy are available in Wong, D.L., and Whaley, L.F.: Clinical manual of pediatric nursing, ed. 3, St. Louis, 1990, Mosby–Year Book, Inc.

†Bull Publishing Co., 1982, Palo Alto, CA.

‡Little Ones Ostomy Products, ConvaTec, Dept. MCN, CN 5254, Princeton, NJ 08543-5254; (609) 924-6315.

Behavior modification techniques tend to be especially effective in changing eating patterns but require a thorough assessment and identification of reinforcement factors. Other helpful suggestions include establishing regular frequent mealtimes with small servings, avoiding an argument or any type of parental pressure at mealtime, and serving as many of the child's favorite foods as possible.

Referral to a public health nurse establishes continuity of care, especially in relation to colostomy care and dietary management. The community nurse can also assist parents and children in anticipating subsequent surgery. Sometimes families require financial assistance and additional psychologic support. Therefore a referral to a social worker or other service agency may be necessary.*

GASTROESOPHAGEAL REFLUX

Gastroesophageal reflux (GER, chalasia, cardiochalasia) is relaxation or incompetence of the lower esophageal sphincter, causing frequent return of stomach contents into the esophagus. In newborns this is considered a normal phenomenon because of immature neuromuscular control of the gastroesophageal sphincter. However, in a small percentage of infants reflux continues, producing symptoms that warrant investigation. The exact cause is not known, although it is thought to result from delayed maturation of lower esophageal neuromuscular function or impaired local hormonal control mechanisms. GER is also more common in premature infants, childen with neurologic impairment (such as cerebral palsy or head injury), and children following some kinds of esophageal surgery. With improved diagnosis GER is rapidly becoming one of the more common diagnoses in young children.

Clinical Manifestations

The most common symptoms of GER are vomiting, weight loss, increased appetite, respiratory problems, and bleeding. Vomiting is the most common symptom and in infants is quite forceful. It is frequently so severe that there is a loss of calories sufficient to cause weight loss and failure to thrive.

Reflux of stomach contents to the pharynx predisposes to aspiration and the development of respiratory symptoms, especially pneumonia, cyanotic episodes, reactive airway disease, and apnea. Repeated irritation of the esophageal lining with gastric acid can lead to esophagitis and consequently bleeding. Blood loss in turn causes anemia and is seen as hematemesis or melena (blood in stools). Heartburn is also a frequent symptom in older children, who can describe it, but may go unrecognized in infants.

Diagnostic Evaluation

The history is an important part of the diagnostic evaluation, including observation of the child's feeding habits.

*See Nursing Care Plan: The Child with Hirschsprung Disease (Megacolon) in Wong, D.L., and Whaley, L.F.: Clinical manual of pediatric nursing, ed. 3, St. Louis, 1990, Mosby–Year Book, Inc.

Several tests are available to evaluate the presence of reflux. Generally, the initial test is the barium esophagram. Reflux of barium from the stomach to the esophagus can be seen by fluoroscopy, although it may be missed because of the intermittent nature of the disorder. Other tests include manometry to measure esophageal sphincter pressure; 24-hour intraesophageal pH monitoring, which uses a probe to directly measure the pH of the distal esophagus; and gastroesophageal scintigraphy, which scans the esophagus after a feeding of a radioactive compound to detect reflux or aspiration. Each of these diagnostic tests must be performed accurately to ensure a correct diagnosis.

Therapeutic Management

Therapeutic management of GER depends on its severity. Infants who are thriving ordinarily require no therapy other than parental reassurance that the child will outgrow the condition, although most infants benefit from appropriate positioning during and after feedings. For the symptomatic child, modification of feeding with small, frequent feedings of thickened formula and positioning may be helpful to minimize the symptoms of the reflux until the child grows and a normal physiologic barrier to reflux develops.

There is considerable controversy regarding the most advantageous position. Traditionally, the upright position (usually in an infant seat) has been recommended, but this position has been shown to increase intraabdominal pressure and may cause the reflux to become worse. Research in infants less than 6 months of age demonstrated that positioning the child prone with the body inclined at about a 30-degree angle for 24 hours a day was more effective (Orenstein and Whitington, 1983). This position is easily maintained by use of an upper body harness (Fig. 33-2) or a reflux board. Length of time to recovery is variable.

Drugs that promote gastric emptying and/or relax the pyloric sphincter have been used with some success, including bethanechol (a cholinergic agent), metoclopramide (a dopamine blocker), and domperidone (a benzimidazole derivative with peripheral dopamine antagonist properties). In some cases antacids and H_2 blocking agents, such as cimetidine, have been used to reduce gastric acidity, although there is no evidence to support their value (Carcassonne and others, 1985).

Surgical intervention is selected for those children with severe complications, such as respiratory distress (choking, aspiration, recurrent apnea, severe asthma), esophagitis, esophageal stricture, or failure to thrive. However, a trial of medical management generally precedes surgical intervention. A commonly used surgical procedure is the Nissen fundoplication, which creates a valve mechanism by wrapping the greater curvature of the stomach (fundus) around the distal esophagus. The procedure involves an abdominal incision and generally insertion of a gastrostomy tube. Other antireflux procedures may be used in some centers.

Prognosis. Most infants achieve normal function by 6 to 7 weeks of age and will achieve complete functional maturity without therapy. Infants with continued reflux will exhibit improvement or resolution by 6 months of age; 90% will have complete resolution by 18 months of age (Belknap, 1990).

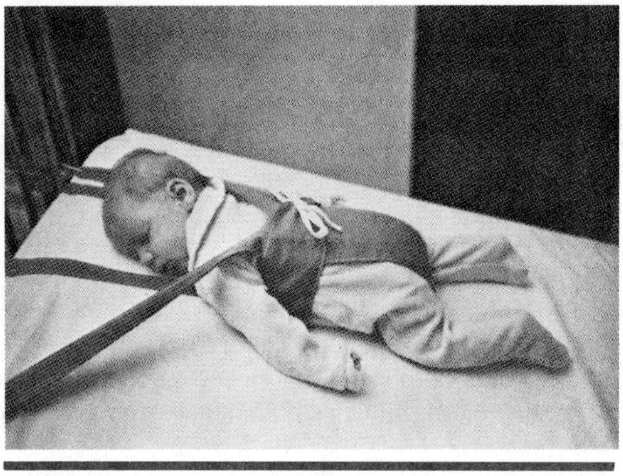

Fig. 33-2. Five-week-old infant positioned in harness.
From Orenstein, S.R., and Whitington, P.F.: Positioning for prevention of infant gastroesophageal reflux, J. Pediatr. 103:534-537, 1983.

Nursing Considerations

Nursing care is directed at (1) identifying children with symptoms suggestive of GER, (2) helping parents with home care of feeding and positioning when indicated, and (3) if appropriate, caring for the child undergoing surgical intervention. For the majority of infants parental reassurance of the benign nature of the condition and its relationship to physiologic maturity is the most important intervention. To help parents cope with the inconvenience of vomiting, simple measures such as using bibs and protective cloths during feeding and upright positioning after feeding are beneficial.

Feeding modification may require some rescheduling of the family's routine to accommodate more frequent feeding times. Formula is thickened with cereal, and the nipple opening may need to be enlarged for easier sucking. If the mother is breast-feeding her infant, a decision regarding the benefit of feeding modification must be made; she can express the milk or change to commercial formula if thickening is recommended. Alternatively, a more concentrated formula may be given to reduce volume or, in severe cases, NG or nasojejunal feedings may be necessary.

Nonnutritive sucking tends to hasten clearance of refluxed material from the esophagus. In infants with GER, nonnutritive sucking was found to affect the frequency of reflux episodes—increasing reflux in prone infants and decreasing it in seated infants (Orenstein, 1988). Nonnutritive sucking also reduces crying behavior.

Infants receiving antacids should be given the medication at the same time as the feeding to improve its buffering (Sutphen, Dillard, and Pipan, 1986). The older child should avoid caffeine-containing foods and beverages (e.g., cola drinks) to reduce gastric acid production. A low-fat diet, avoiding eating 2 to 4 hours before bedtime, and sleeping on a wedge are often beneficial.

For the very young infant, positioning can be accomplished by raising the mattress at the head end and using a harness. When the infant is older and more mobile, positioning becomes increasingly difficult; a special procedure has been described for constructing a bed that comfortably maintains the child's position. It consists of a cradle bed or bassinet that incorporates a wooden base with a wooden spindle under the mattress. The padded spindle protrudes through a hole cut in the mattress. The infant is positioned prone with legs straddling the spindle, and the head end of the bassinet is raised at a 30-degree angle.

Postoperative nursing care is similar to other types of abdominal surgery (see Chapter 27). Gastric decompression by NG tube or gastrostomy must be maintained to avoid distention. When postoperative ileus resolves, the NG tube is removed, or the gastrostomy tube is elevated in preparation for feeding. When feedings are initiated through the gastrostomy, the tube should remain vented for several days or longer to avoid gastric distention from swallowed air. Edema surrounding the surgical site and compression of gastric wrap may prohibit the infant from expelling air through the esophagus. Some infants benefit from clamping of the tube for increasingly longer intervals until they are able to tolerate continuous clamping between feedings. During this time, if the infant displays increasing irritability and evidence of cramping, some relief may be provided by venting the tube. Unvented continuous feeding directly into the gastrostomy is not recommended immediately following surgery.

Preparation for home care. If medication is prescribed or surgery performed, the same nursing responsibilities for helping parents administer the drug at home,* and provide special feeding regimens or formula preparation, gastrostomy care, and postoperative care (see Chapter 27) are instituted. After surgery, symptoms are completely controlled in most cases, with these children attaining normal health and growth. If a gastrostomy tube is inserted during surgery, it may be removed after several weeks unless nutritional supplementation is needed. Problems that may occur following surgery are gas bloat, delayed gastric emptying, inability to vomit, slow eating habits, and choking on solids. Families should be aware of such subsequent changes in order to take appropriate actions, such as increased precaution with foods that can be aspirated and allowing children longer time at the table.

IRRITABLE BOWEL SYNDROME

Irritable bowel syndrome (IBS), abnormally increased motility of the small and large intestines, is a very common condition in childhood, most often observed in children between 8 months and 3 years of age (Klish, 1990). In early childhood the condition is variously known as toddler diarrhea, chronic nonspecific diarrhea (CND), and the IBS of childhood (see Recurrent Abdominal Pain, Chapter 18). Affected children are more likely to have a history of colic with feeding difficulties and a family history of bowel problems.

Typically, the onset of symptoms occurs in children between 16 and 20 months of age who begin having three to six loose stools per day (Levine, 1987). The child is active, appears healthy, has a good appetite, and exhibits normal growth. Most of the stools are passed during waking hours, are loose, and contain undigested foods and mucus. The condition is self-limiting, and symptoms usually clear gradually and spontaneously until most patients are asymptomatic by 40 months. The condition is not associated with pain, malabsorption, or growth retardation.

Therapeutic Management

The long-range goal of treatment is development of regular bowel habits, although therapy fails in 10% to 20% of children (Klish, 1990). Conditioning is of little value in infants and toddlers, but plays a role in bowel training for older children. Despite differences in techniques, common features include enemas to eliminate unusually large fecal accumulations and stimulant or lubricant laxatives individualized to ensure regular and easy passage of one or two stools per day (Davidson, 1987). Diet generally does not play a significant role in therapy. A normal balanced diet is prescribed, sometimes with additional fiber. Psyllium bulk agents are effective in eliminating symptoms in some children but are usually discontinued if no response is observed in 7 to 10 days. Occasionally children respond to administration of cholestyramine or metronidazole.

Nursing Considerations

The primary nursing goal is family support. The disorder is very stressful to parents, whose anxiety may disturb parent-child relationships. Parents need support and reassurance that although the symptoms of the disorder are difficult to deal with, the disorder is not a threat to the child's well-being. Nurses can help the family plan an age-appropriate, balanced diet and support parents and older children with a conditioning regimen.

INFLAMMATORY CONDITIONS

Inflammatory conditions involving large or small segments of the gastrointestinal tract are not uncommon in childhood. They may be acute or chronic, and some are more likely to affect one age-group more than another. For example, necrotizing enterocolitis is seen in the newborn, Meckel diverticulum primarily affects children under age 2 years, ulcerative colitis occurs most frequently in the prepubescent and adolescent child, and acute appendicitis appears at any age.

ACUTE APPENDICITIS

Appendicitis, inflammation of the vermiform appendix, or blind sac, at the end of the cecum, is the most common

*Home care instructions for administration of medications and nasogastric and gastrostomy feedings are available in Wong, D.L., and Whaley, L.F.: Clinical manual of pediatric nursing, ed. 3, St. Louis, 1990, Mosby–Year Book, Inc.

reason for abdominal surgery during childhood. Although rare in children younger than 2 years of age, it is associated with increased complications and mortality in this age-group. Primarily an acute disorder, appendicitis rapidly progresses to perforation and peritonitis if it remains undiagnosed. It is a significant problem, because early diagnosis is frequently delayed as a result of children's inability to verbalize symptoms and failure of health professionals (not parents) to interpret behavioral cues correctly.

While mortality has decreased greatly since the advent of antibiotics, the incidence of appendiceal rupture has still remained high, occurring in about 28% of patients (Berry and Malt, 1984). Other contributing factors are young age, lower social class, presence of fecaliths, absence of family history, and advice given by the first health professional the family contacted, especially the advice to observe the child at home (Brender and others, 1985a).

Etiology

The exact cause of appendicitis is poorly understood, but it is almost always a result of obstruction of the lumen of the appendix, usually by a fecalith (a hard fecal concretion). Sometimes a fold of peritoneum causes the appendix to adhere to the cecum, resulting in an obstructive kink. Other causes include lymphoid hyperplasia, fibrous stenosis from an earlier inflammation, and tumors. Although worms are frequently found in the appendix, their role in the pathophysiology is unclear. There is mounting evidence that dietary habits play a role. Children with diets high in fiber foods have a lower incidence of appendicitis than those whose fiber intake is low (Barker, Morris, and Nelson, 1986; Brender and others, 1985b). Fiber increases the bulk and softness of the stool—a factor that minimizes the chance of obstruction and promotes evacuation.

Pathophysiology

With acute obstruction the outflow of mucus secretions is blocked, and pressure builds within the lumen, resulting in compression of blood vessels. Resulting ischemia is followed by ulceration of the epithelial lining and bacterial invasion. Subsequent necrosis causes perforation or rupture with fecal and bacterial contamination of the peritoneal cavity. The resulting inflammation spreads rapidly throughout the abdomen (*peritonitis*)—especially in young children, who are unable to localize infection and who have a thinner appendiceal wall. The omentum, which is not fully developed, is less efficient in walling off the inflammation, sealing perforated viscera, and confining an intraperitoneal disease process. The proximity of all abdominal and pelvic organs favors the spread of peritonitis to accessory digestive and reproductive organs. Progressive peritoneal inflammation results in functional intestinal obstruction of the small bowel (*ileus*), since intense gastrointestinal reflexes severely inhibit bowel motility. Since the peritoneum represents a major portion of total body surface, the loss of extracellular fluid to the peritoneal cavity leads to electrolyte imbalance and hypovolemic shock.

Clinical Manifestations

The most common signs and symptoms of appendicitis are colicky abdominal pain, tenderness, and fever. Initially the pain is generalized or periumbilical; however, it usually descends to the lower right quadrant. The most intense site of pain may be at the McBurney point, located midway between the anterior superior iliac crest and the umbilicus. Other important signs are a rigid abdomen, decreased or absent bowel sounds, and rebound tenderness (the sudden pain at the point of tenderness elicited by pressing firmly over a part of the abdomen distal to the area of tenderness). Jumping or riding over bumps in an automobile or gurney aggravates the pain.

Vomiting commonly follows the onset of pain, especially in younger children, and constipation or diarrhea may be present. Anorexia is a constant feature. Low-grade fever is typically seen early in the disease but can rise sharply once peritonitis has begun. Probably the most significant clinical manifestation is a change in the child's behavior. The younger, nonverbal child will assume a rigid, motionless, side-lying posture with the knees flexed on the abdomen. The older child may exhibit all of these behaviors while complaining of abdominal pain. The child walks very carefully with decreased range of motion in the right hip and usually lies with the hip flexed.

✦ **NURSING ALERT** Signs of peritonitis in addition to fever include sudden relief from pain after perforation, subsequent increase in pain, which is usually diffuse and accompanied by rigid guarding of the abdomen, progressive abdominal distention, tachycardia, rapid shallow breathing as the child refrains from using abdominal muscles, pallor, chills, irritability, and restlessness.

Diagnostic Evaluation

Diagnosis is based primarily on history and examination. The chief clues that should alert the practitioner to appendicitis are the progression of abdominal pain, location of abdominal tenderness, decreased peristalsis, pain on rectal examination, and absence of any other symptoms or findings suggesting another disorder, such as pneumonia.

Laboratory evaluation includes a white blood cell count, which is usually elevated but is seldom higher than 15,000 to 20,000/mm^3. Radiographic studies of the abdomen are not very helpful but may reveal possible contributing causes of appendicitis, such as fecaliths or a foreign body in the appendix. Ultrasound may be used to locate an abscess before surgery.

Diagnosis is not always straightforward. Numerous infectious processes have features in common. For example, fever, vomiting, abdominal pain, and elevated blood count are associated with inflammatory bowel disease, gastroenteritis, pelvic inflammatory disease, urinary tract infection, right lower lobe pneumonia, constipation, mesenteric adenitis, Meckel diverticulum, and intussusception. Also, diagnosis may be delayed in infants and small children because they do not localize infections well and can become sick more rapidly than older children. Consequently, the risk of perforation is greater. Therefore practitioners must have a high degree of suspicion for appendicitis in the differential diagnosis.

Therapeutic Management

Treatment of appendicitis before perforation is surgical removal of the appendix (appendectomy). Recovery is rapid and generally uneventful unless peritonitis has occurred. The following discussion is concerned with the special care of the child with a ruptured appendix.

Ruptured appendix. Management of the child diagnosed with peritonitis caused by a ruptured appendix often begins preoperatively with intravenous administration of fluid and electrolytes, systemic antibiotics, and NG suction. Postoperative management includes fluid and electrolyte balance maintenance, continued administration of antibiotics, and NG suction for abdominal decompression until intestinal activity returns.

Most surgeons provide for external drainage when abscess formation has occurred, when there is necrotic or severely damaged tissue, or when there are purulent collections within the peritoneum. This is accomplished by sump drainage or a Penrose drain and wound irrigations. The child is maintained in semi-Fowler position to reduce spread of the infection to other parts of the peritoneum, one of the most common of which is the subdiaphragmatic area.

Nursing Considerations

Because successful treatment of appendicitis is based on prompt recognition of the disorder, a primary nursing objective is assisting in establishing a diagnosis. Since the treatment is universally surgical, preoperative and postoperative care are major nursing functions. Although in many instances nurses may not perform the complete history and examination, they are often in a strategic position to make judgments regarding the child's care. For example, nurses in private physicians' offices, ambulatory settings, or emergency units often have the responsibility of counseling parents or triaging patients regarding additional treatment.

When the child with an *acute abdomen* (a general term used to describe conditions associated with acute abdominal pain) is admitted to the pediatric unit, staff nurses usually decide where to place the child, how quickly to arrange for laboratory evaluation, and how much observation and assessment of the child are required and by whom. Even outside the strictly professional relationship, parents may ask nurse friends for advice regarding abdominal pain. Without an appreciation of the signs and symptoms suggestive of appendicitis, these nurses may not make decisions that facilitate rapid diagnosis.

Assessment

Since abdominal pain is the most common childhood complaint, the nurse needs to make some preliminary assessment of the severity of pain (see Chapter 26). One of the most reliable estimates is the degree of change in behavior. A child who stays home from school and voluntarily lies down or refuses to play is much more likely to have considerable pain than the child who is absent from school but plays contentedly at home. For those nurses involved in primary ambulatory care, the responsibility of recognizing a possible instance of appendicitis and prompt medical/surgical referral is particularly great. A detailed history and careful abdominal examination cannot be overstressed. Palpating the abdomen should be delayed until all other assessments have been made. The child is instructed to point with one finger to the "place where it hurts." Rebound tenderness is not a sufficiently reliable test to justify subjecting the child to the exquisite pain. Light percussion (it "shakes" the ilia) will satisfactorily elicit referred pain (see Nursing Tips). Techniques for assessment of the abdomen are discussed in Chapter 7.

NURSING TIPS: PALPATING THE ABDOMEN AND ELICITING ABDOMINAL PAIN

Because children associate the stethoscope with "listening," the bell of the instrument can be used to palpate the abdomen for tenderness. Children usually endure pressure from the stethoscope that they would not tolerate from a probing hand.

Asking the child to lift the heels and drop them to the floor two or three times or hop on one foot will evoke discomfort without more painful probing.

Nursing Diagnoses

Based on a thorough assessment, several nursing diagnoses are identified. The more common diagnoses for the child with acute appendicitis are included in the Nursing Care Plan on p. 1504. Others may apply in specific situations.

Planning

Nursing objectives for the child with acute appendicitis include the following:

1. Prepare the child and family for surgical removal of appendix.
2. Provide competent postoperative care as described for the child undergoing surgery in Chapter 27.

Goals for the child with peritonitis include the above plus:

1. Prevent dehydration.
2. Prevent spread of infection.
3. Provide support to child and family.

Implementation

Physical preparation of the child with appendicitis is the same as that for any child undergoing surgery (see Chapter

NURSING CARE PLAN
The Child with Appendicitis

Preoperative care

NURSING DIAGNOSIS: Pain related to inflamed appendix

GOAL 1
Relieve discomfort

INTERVENTIONS
See Nursing Care Plan: The Child in Pain, Chapter 26
Allow position of comfort
*Administer analgesia, if prescribed

EXPECTED OUTCOME
Child rests quietly

NURSING DIAGNOSIS: Potential for injury related to possibility of rupture

GOAL 1
Prevent rupture

INTERVENTIONS
Avoid application of heat or cold to abdomen
Apply ice pack to abdomen if it provides relief
Avoid palpating the abdomen unless necessary

EXPECTED OUTCOME
Status remains unchanged

NURSING DIAGNOSIS: Potential fluid volume deficit related to decreased intake secondary to loss of appetite, vomiting

GOAL 1
Prevent fluid losses

INTERVENTIONS
Administer fluids as ordered
- Intravenous
  - *Administer fluid as prescribed
  - Maintain desired drip rate
  - *Add appropriate electrolytes as prescribed
  - Maintain integrity of infusion site

EXPECTED OUTCOMES
Child receives sufficient fluids to replace losses
Child exhibits signs of adequate hydration (specify)

Postoperative care
See Postoperative Care: The Child Undergoing Surgery, Chapter 27

*Dependent nursing action.

Ruptured appendix

NURSING DIAGNOSIS: Potential for infection related to presence of infective organisms in abdomen

GOAL 1
Prevent spread of infection

INTERVENTIONS
Position in low Fowler position to localize and prevent upward spread of infection
Implement appropriate isolation precautions
- Careful wound care and disposal of wound dressings

*Administer antibiotics as prescribed

EXPECTED OUTCOME
Infection remains confined to lower right quadrant of abdomen

NURSING DIAGNOSIS: Potential for injury related to absence of bowel activity

GOAL 1
Prevent abdominal distention

INTERVENTIONS
Allow nothing by mouth
Insert rectal tube if indicated
Maintain NG decompression if ordered

EXPECTED OUTCOME
Child does not exhibit signs of discomfort; abdomen remains soft

NURSING DIAGNOSIS: Altered family processes related to a child with a serious illness

GOAL 1
Support family

INTERVENTIONS AND EXPECTED OUTCOME
See Nursing Care Plan: The Family of the Ill or Hospitalized Child, Chapter 26

See also Nursing Care Plan: The Child in the Hospital, Chapter 26

27). In situations in which medical treatment is required to correct problems associated with peritonitis, the nurse must anticipate expected procedures and set up equipment as quickly as possible to prevent any delay in preparing the child for surgery.

NURSING ALERT In any instance in which severe abdominal pain is expected, the nurse must be aware of the danger of administering laxatives or enemas or applying heat to the area. Such measures stimulate bowel motility and increase the risk of perforation.

Psychologic preparation of the child and parents is similar to that used in other emergency situations (see Chapter 27).

Postoperative care. Postoperative care for the nonperforated appendix is the same as for most abdominal operations. Care of the child with a ruptured appendix and peritonitis involves more complex care. The course of recovery is considerably longer and may require up to 2 weeks of hospitalization, in contrast to 1 to 4 days for an uncomplicated appendectomy.

The child is maintained on intravenous fluids, is allowed nothing by mouth, and remains on low intermittent gastric decompression until there is evidence of intestinal activity. Listening for bowel sounds and observing for other signs of bowel activity (such as passage of stool) are part of the routine assessment. Management of intravenous therapy is the same as for any child receiving fluids and parenteral antibiotics.

Positioning the child in semi-Fowler position or lying on the right side after surgery for a ruptured appendix facilitates drainage from the peritoneal cavity and prevents the formation of a subdiaphragmatic abscess. A Penrose drain is often placed in the wound during surgery, and frequent dressing changes with meticulous skin care are essential to prevent excoriation of the surgical area. Sometimes the abdominal wound is irrigated with antibacterial solution.

Psychologic care after surgery is also important. Parents and older children need an opportunity to express their feelings regarding the events surrounding the hospitalization. It is especially important for the nurse to encourage the child to relate all the events he or she remembers concerning admission and treatment in order to clarify misconceptions.

Evaluation

The effectiveness of nursing interventions is determined by continual reassessment and evaluation of care based on the following observational guidelines and expected outcomes:

1. Observe the child preoperatively for reaction to situation and compliance with care.
2. Monitor child's physical and emotional reaction to hospitalization and surgery.
3. Observe child's physical indications of good hydration.
4. Observe child for evidence of infection.
5. Interview and observe child and family for evidence of understanding the illness.

Expected outcomes:
See Nursing Care Plan, p. 1504.

MECKEL DIVERTICULUM

Meckel diverticulum results when the omphalomesenteric or vitelline duct, which connects the midgut to the yolk sac during embryonic development, fails to completely obliterate. Although several different types of malformations can result, such as cysts, fistulas, or fibrotic cords, Meckel diverticulum consists of an outpouching of the ileum, most commonly in proximity to the ileocecal valve. It may vary in size from a small appendiceal process to a segment of bowel several inches long and wide. At times it may be connected to the umbilicus by a cord.

It is the most common congenital malformation of the GI tract and is present in 1% to 2% of the population. It is more common in males than in females, and complications are several times more frequent in males. Often it exists without causing symptoms. Most symptomatic cases are seen in the first 2 years of life.

Pathophysiology

Meckel diverticulum is a sac subject to inflammation (diverticulitis) in the same manner as appendicitis. In over half the cases the diverticulum contains gastric mucosa, which produces hydrochloric acid and pepsin. The acid continually irritates the bowel and erodes the surface, which results in bleeding and, in some instances, may lead to perforation. Mechanical obstruction can occur as a result of volvulus, or twisting of the bowel around the fibrotic Meckel cord. Intussusception can occur if the diverticulum acts as a lead point for invagination.

Clinical Manifestations

Signs and symptoms are based on the specific pathologic process, such as diverticulitis or intestinal obstruction. Rectal bleeding, however, is the chief presenting sign in more than half of the cases. Bright red or dark red rectal bleeding is much more common than black tarry stools and represents acute hemorrhage. Usually there is no evidence of abdominal pain. Severe anemia and shock are consequences of the hemorrhage.

Diagnostic Evaluation

Diagnosis is usually based on the history. Barium enema and radionucleotide scintigraphy confirm the diagnoses. Radiologic studies are not helpful in confirming the diagnosis, because the diverticulum may be too small to be visualized or may fail to fill with barium. Blood studies are usually part of the general laboratory workup to rule out any bleeding disorder and to evaluate the severity of the anemia.

Therapeutic Management

Treatment is surgical removal of the diverticulum. In instances in which severe hemorrhage increases the surgical risk, medical intervention to correct hypovolemic shock (e.g., blood replacement, intravenous fluids, and oxygen) may be necessary. In diverticulitis antibiotics may be used preoperatively to control infection. If intestinal obstruction has occurred, appropriate preoperative measures are used to reverse electrolyte imbalances and prevent abdominal distention.

Nursing Considerations

Nursing objectives are the same as for any child undergoing surgery (see Chapter 27). Since the onset is usually rapid, psychologic support parallels that for other conditions, such as appendicitis. It is important to remember that massive rectal bleeding is most often traumatic to both the child and the parents and may significantly affect their emotional reaction to hospitalization and surgery.

Specific preoperative considerations when rectal bleeding is present include (1) frequent monitoring of vital signs and blood pressure for shock, (2) keeping the child on bed rest, and (3) recording the approximate amount of blood lost in stools. In the absence of rectal hemorrhage, the nurse tests the stools for occult blood.

INFLAMMATORY BOWEL DISEASE

Inflammatory bowel disease (IBD) is a general term used to designate two chronic intestinal disorders—*ulcerative colitis (UC)* and *Crohn disease (CD)*. The term should not be confused with *irritable bowel syndrome (IBS),* which refers to a functional disorder (see p. 1501). Although these two diseases are grouped under the classification of IBD because they have similar epidemiologic, immunologic, and clinical features, they are two distinct conditions with very significant differences, primarily in the intestinal features. The most important reason for differentiating between the two is prognosis. CD is considered the more serious and disabling disorder, and medical/surgical treatment is much less effective than in UC. Unfortunately, the incidence of CD is increasing in the population, although the reason for this change is not known.

Etiology

The cause of IBD is unknown, although infectious, nutritional, immunologic, and psychogenic etiologies have been proposed. It is proposed that IBD is the result of an inappropriate activation of the mechanisms of the immune response in genetically susceptible individuals (Kirschner, 1988). Psychologic factors such as stress or personality characteristics do not play a role in the pathogenesis of the disease but may accentuate symptoms and the severity of a relapse (Silverman and Roy, 1983).

Several genetic and environmental factors influence the incidence of IBD: (1) there is a familial tendency in about 22% to 25% of the cases (Kirschner, 1988), (2) individuals from higher socioeconomic levels and more whites than nonwhites are affected, (3) the incidence is several times greater in Jews living in Europe and North America than in the general population, and (4) there is a higher occurrence of the disease in children living in urban settings than rural areas. A recent report found lack of breast-feeding to be associated with later development of CD (Koletzko and others, 1989).

Pathophysiology: Ulcerative Colitis

UC is a disease characterized by a chronic inflammatory reaction involving the mucosa and submucosa of the large intestine. It occurs in both sexes and in all age-groups. It is basically a disease of young adults, although close to 15% of the cases begin in children younger than 16 years. The mean age of onset in children is around 11.

The inflammatory changes in UC are primarily limited to the mucosa of the colon and rectum. The mucous membranes become hyperemic and edematous with the formation of patchy granulations over the intestinal surface that bleed easily and eventually develop irregular areas of superficial ulcerations. The ulcerated and damaged mucosa is ineffective in reabsorbing nutrients, fluid, and electrolytes. The more extensive the involvement, the more severe is the diarrhea and resulting growth retardation. In long-standing disease the bowel becomes narrowed, smooth, and inflexible, with thin or absent mucosa heavily infiltrated by scar tissue. The greatly reduced absorptive surface results in loose, watery, and sometimes bloody stools.

The *acute remitting* type is more common and follows a pattern of remissions and exacerbations. During the period of remission, the child is usually well, with few or no symptoms of the disease. Periods of exacerbation are severe and acute, although these children usually respond well to medical treatment. The disease may terminate in a permanent remission or ultimately follow the course of chronic colitis.

In *chronic continuous colitis* there are no definitive periods of severe disease with intermittent good health. Intestinal symptoms tend to be less severe, but chronic malnutrition and anemia are common. These children often respond poorly to medical therapy and are more likely to suffer from complications, especially carcinoma of the colon.

Pathophysiology: Crohn Disease

CD may involve any part of the GI tract but most commonly affects the terminal ileum. The disease characteristically involves all layers of the bowel wall (transmural). Acute edema and inflammation eventually progress to deep transverse or longitudinal ulcerations often associated with fissure formation. The thickened bowel wall may lead to obstruction. The asymmetric and patchy distribution of the lesions helps to differentiate CD from the contiguous and symmetric lesions of UC. Local lymph nodes are enlarged.

Clinical Manifestations

Clinical features are similar in both UC and CD, especially systemic and extraintestinal manifestations. Clinical presentations of intestinal signs and symptoms are different (Table 33-4). The diseases occur in both sexes with equal frequency, and both are primarily diseases of adolescence and young adulthood.

Intestinal manifestations. The most common feature of UC is persistent or recurring diarrhea. In the acute, fulmi-

Table 33-4 Comparison of inflammatory bowel diseases—ulcerative colitis and Crohn disease

CHARACTERISTICS	ULCERATIVE COLITIS	CROHN DISEASE
Pathologic changes		
Extent of involvement	Diffuse, mucosal	Focal, transmural (entire wall)
Ulceration	Superficial, extensive	Deep
Distribution of lesions	Contiguous, symmetric	Segmental, asymmetric with "skip" areas
Lymph nodes	Normal	Affected
Primary areas of involvement	Colon, rectum	Ileum, colon, rectum (10%-20%)
Clinical features		
Rectal bleeding	Common	Uncommon
Diarrhea	Often severe	Moderate to absent
Pain	Less frequent	Common
Anorexia	Mild or moderate	Can be severe
Weight loss	Moderate	Severe
Growth retardation	Usually mild	Often marked
Anal and perianal lesions	Rare	Common
Fistulas and strictures	Rare	Common
Surgical resection of affected bowel	Curative	Unsatisfactory because of frequent recurrence
Risk of carcinoma	Related to duration of disease Prevented by surgery	Occurs less frequently Not prevented by surgery

nating disease there is bloody diarrhea preceded by cramping abdominal pain and followed by abdominal distention. Diarrhea may be severe with marked urgency and frequency (20 to 30 stools daily). Radiography reveals characteristic pouches that give the normal colon a scalloped appearance, shortening of its length, and uniform reduction in diameter, all of which give the picture of the *lead-pipe colon.* Nocturnal diarrhea is common and associated with more extensive involvement. Children are usually healthy before the onset of the disease. See Fig. 33-3 for effects of UC.

The onset of CD is usually insidious. Diarrhea and intermittent, cramping pain often resemble that of acute appendicitis. The pain is often triggered by eating. As the disease progresses, however, the abdominal pain becomes a constant aching or soreness. The diarrhea may contain blood, but it is a less frequent finding in children. Malabsorption is more common in CD.

Systemic and extraintestinal manifestations. A number of other symptoms unrelated to the GI manifestations may be seen, including low-grade fever, anorexia, and fatigue. Weight loss occurs more frequently (87% of patients) and to a greater degree (5.7 kg) in CD than in UC (68% and 4.1 kg) (Bouchier, 1984). Arthralgia and arthritis are not uncommmon extraintestinal manifestations of IBD in children. Large joints (especially knees, ankles, and hips) are usually affected and may require antiinflammatory therapy. Pallor and anemia may result from bleeding and reduced dietary intake, and the numerous watery bowel movements often cause depletion of water and electrolytes.

Delayed growth and sexual maturation are prominent features of IBD and manifested as either a change in height percentile or decreased growth velocity. Bone age is usually delayed by at least 2 years in these circumstances (Kirschner, 1988). Although numerous studies have investigated the cause of growth failure, the most consistent explanation is chronic caloric insufficiency.

Oral ulcers and skin lesions may appear during periods of active disease. Some children develop complications involving the urinary tract (renal calculi and hematuria) and eye (conjunctivitis, iritis, and episcleritis).

Diagnostic Evaluation

Diagnosis is usually based on a combination of findings from history, physical examination, and laboratory testing. Specific diagnostic tests to confirm the diagnosis and rule out other possibilities such as anal fissures, GI infections, and diverticulitis include: (1) radiographic studies of the colon, especially barium enema, (2) endoscopy, and (3) mucosal biopsy for histologic evidence of the inflammatory process (especially in CD). Stool samples may be obtained to rule out the presence of pathologic organisms and malabsorptive defects. Blood studies are done to determine severity of anemia, extent of albumin loss, and immunoglobulin levels. Erythrocyte sedimentation rate and C-reactive protein are more likely to be elevated in CD. Diagnosis is established by endoscopy examination and, in CD, biopsy. Endoscopic features considered most useful in discriminating CD and UC include intermittent colonic involvement, perianal lesions, and cobblestoning of mucosa with CD, whereas erosions and mucosal granularity are more suggestive of UC (Bines and Walker, 1989).

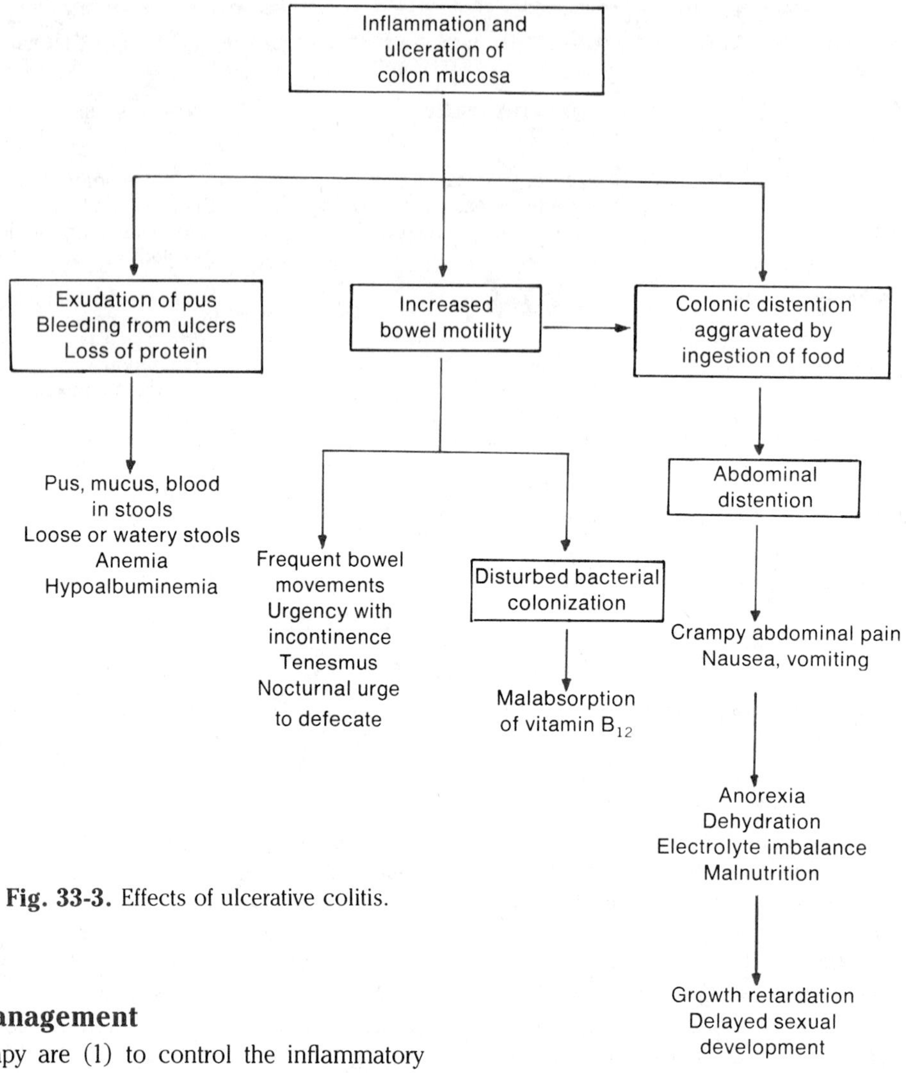

Fig. 33-3. Effects of ulcerative colitis.

Therapeutic Management

The goals of therapy are (1) to control the inflammatory process in order to reduce or eliminate the symptoms, (2) to maintain long-term remission, and (3) to allow as normal a life-style as possible. Treatment must be individualized and managed according to the severity of the disease, location of lesions, and response to therapy.

Medical treatment. The drug sulfasalazine has proved useful in decreasing the frequency of recurrences in patients with mild cases of IBD. Because it interferes with the absorption and utilization of folic acid, daily supplements of folic acid are prescribed.

Corticosteroids are the most important and effective drugs for treating moderate and severe IBD. High doses are administered for acute episodes, then tapered according to the clinical response. Although high doses of corticosteroids interfere with growth, significant growth can be achieved with judicious management and maintenance of optimum nutrition. Sometimes steroid enemas are helpful in reducing the need for systemic administration for children with rectosigmoid involvement.

Other drugs include metronidazole for treatment of perianal CD, antispasmodic agents, which sometimes help relieve the discomfort of diarrhea and cramping, and immunosuppressive agents, which are efficacious in patients on high-dose corticosteroids.

Dietary treatment. Dietary management is often vigorous because of the child's poorly nourished state. The goals are (1) to replace nutrient losses associated with the inflammatory processes, (2) to correct body deficits, and (3) to provide sufficient nutrients to promote energy and nitrogen balance for normal metabolic function (Motil and Grand, 1985). These goals can be accomplished by enteral and/or parenteral routes. The therapeutic diet consists of high protein, high calorie, normal to low fat, and low fiber. Vitamin and mineral supplements are usually provided to correct anemia and other deficiencies.

During the acute stage supplemental nutrition by way of intermittent or continuous drip gastric feedings, intravenous fluids to correct dehydration and associated electrolyte imbalances, and/or parenteral alimentation may be required.

Surgical treatment. In some instances elective surgery is required. A temporary colostomy may be performed to allow the bowel a period of rest. To arrest the disease process, the entire section of ulcerated bowel is removed, in which case total colectomy and ileostomy are usually required. Advances in surgical techniques over the incontinent abdominal stoma now provide options for some children. Surgical alternatives include a *continent (Koch) ileostomy* in which an intraabdominal pouch or reservoir is created to allow continence, or an *ileoanal anastomosis,* which preserves the normal pathway for defecation and eliminates the abdominal stoma.

Removal of the diseased bowel is a permanent remedy for UC and prevents possible development of carcinoma. However, in CD surgical removal of the affected bowel is not curative. The disease tends to recur, and the risk of cancer of the bowel is not affected and requires appropriate screening for early detection.

Nursing Considerations

Many of the nursing considerations relate directly to the therapeutic management in treating colitis. However, the scope of nursing responsibilities extends beyond the immediate period of hospitalization and involves (1) continued guidance of families in terms of dietary management and drug compliance, (2) adjusting to a disease of remissions and exacerbations or one of chronic ill health, and (3) when indicated, preparing the child and parents for the possibility of diversionary bowel surgery.

Since diet therapy is a very important component of therapy, encouraging the anorexic child to consume sufficient quantities of this diet is of primary importance and is frequently a nursing challenge. An approach that is more likely to meet with success involves including the child in meal planning; encouraging small, frequent meals or snacks rather than three large meals a day; serving meals around medication schedules when diarrhea, mouth pain, and intestinal spasm are controlled; and preparing high-protein, high-calorie foods, such as eggnog, milk shakes, cream soups, puddings, or custard (if lactose is tolerated) (see also Feeding the Sick Child, Chapter 27).

Foods that are known to aggravate the condition are avoided, as are high-fiber foods (see Table 33-3). Since the best sources of folic acid and iron are found in high-fiber foods, such as fresh fruits and vegetables, the child is at risk for vitamin deficiency. Also, sulfasalazine inhibits folate absorption. It is important to emphasize the need to make up for these deficiencies with supplements. Occasionally stomatitis further complicates adherence to dietary management. Good mouth care before eating and the selection of bland foods help relieve the discomfort of mouth sores (see Stomatitis, Chapter 16).

The importance of continued drug therapy despite remission of symptoms must be stressed to the parents and child. Failure to adhere to the pharmacologic regimen can result in exacerbation of the disease process (see Chapter 27 for a discussion of compliance).

Attending to the emotional components of a chronic disease requires a thorough assessment of those stress factors that are disease related. Frequently the nurse can be instrumental in helping these children adjust to the problems of growth retardation, delayed sexual maturation, dietary restrictions, feelings of being "different" or "sickly," inability to compete with peers, and necessary absence from school during exacerbations of the illness (see Chapter 22).

In the event that a permanent colectomy/ileostomy is required, the nurse can assist the child and family in accepting and adjusting to the change by teaching them how to care for the ileostomy, by emphasizing the positive aspects of surgery (particularly accelerated growth and sexual development, permanent recovery, and eliminated risk of colonic cancer), and by stressing the normality of life despite bowel diversion. Introducing the child and parents to other ostomy patients, especially those of the child's age, can be the greatest therapeutic measure in fostering eventual acceptance. Whenever possible, the newer continent ostomies should be offered as options to the child, although they are not performed in all centers throughout the United States.

Because of the chronic and often lifelong nature of the disease, families benefit from many of the services provided by organizations such as the **Colitis and Ileitis Foundation,*** which has branches in many major communities and provides education regarding the management of inflammatory bowel disease. If diversionary bowel surgery is indicated, the **United Ostomy Association†** and the **International Association for Enterostomal Therapy‡** are available to assist the ileostomy care and provide important psychologic support through their self-help groups.§||

PEPTIC ULCER

Peptic ulcer disease (PUD) is an ulcerative condition defined as circumscribed loss of tissue lining the stomach or duodenum. A *gastric ulcer* affects the lining of the stomach, whereas a *duodenal ulcer* involves the pylorus or duodenum. PUD is classified as *primary* (idiopathic) when it occurs in otherwise healthy children and *secondary* (stress) when associated with underlying disorders involving injury (e.g., severe burns), illness (e.g., sepsis, acute respiratory disease, collagen vascular disease), or drug therapy (e.g., salicylates, corticosteroids, ferrous sulfate).

Although peptic ulcers are more common in adults, they are also a significant pediatric problem, occurring at any age but primarily in children from 3 months to 17 years of age, with a mean age of 10 years. The male-female ratio for PUD is 1.5:1. Most ulcers are solitary lesions located in the duodenum and less often in the stomach.

Etiology

The etiology of PUD in children is unknown. Both genetic and environmental factors appear to be important in the etiology of PUD. There is an increased frequency among relatives and a positive relationship to blood group O. How-

---

*444 Park Ave., South, New York, NY 10016; (212) 679-1570.

†36 Executive Park, Suite 120, Irvine, CA 92714-6744; (714) 660-8624.

‡2081 Business Center Drive, Suite 290, Irvine, CA 92715; (714) 476-0268.

§In Canada: **Canadian Foundation for Ileitis and Colitis,** 21 St. Clair Ave, East, Suite 301, Toronto, Ontario M4TL 1L9, (416) 920-5035; **United Ostomy Association, Canada,** 5 Hamilton Ave., Hamilton, Ontario L8V 2L3, (416) 389-8822.

||See Nursing Care Plan: The Child with Inflammatory Bowel Disease in Wong, D.L., and Whaley, L.F.: Clinical manual of pediatric nursing, ed. 3, St. Louis, 1990, Mosby–Year Book, Inc.

ever, emotional stress has been implicated as an important contributing factor toward the development, severity, and prognosis of peptic ulcers. Affected children tend to be of above-average intelligence, are overachievers, do not handle anger and frustration well, and internalize their aggressive feelings (Nord, 1988). Association between bereavement or separation and PUD has also been noted (Ackerman, Manaker, and Cohen, 1981; Wessel and McCullough, 1982).

Diet does not appear to influence the development of PUD, but exogenous factors such as alcohol use, cigarette smoking, and caffeine increase the incidence. Alcohol and caffeine stimulate acid production; cigarette smoking decreases pancreatic secretions and alkalinity in the duodenum (Motil, 1990).

Recent reports have demonstrated a strong association between *Helicobacter pylori* (formerly called *Campylobacter pylori*) gastritis and development of peptic ulcers in persons who do not suppress the organism by usual immune mechanisms (Drumm and others, 1987; Kilbridge, Dahms, and Czinn, 1988). The organism infects the antral tissue of the duodenum, rendering the damaged tissue susceptible to the effects of acid and pepsin.

Pathophysiology

The precise mechanism is not understood, but the pathogenesis is thought to be an imbalance between destructive and defensive factors in the GI tract. Destructive elements include endogenous (hydrochloric acid, pepsin, and bile salts) and exogenous (alcohol, drugs, stress) factors. Defensive factors are endogenous and consist of an undisturbed mucous layer, an alkaline (bicarbonate) mucus secretion, prostaglandins, and rapid epithelial cell renewal. Anything that interferes with the protective functions or increases the destructive elements contribute to ulcer formation. Unprotected gastric mucosa is highly vulnerable to the digestive effects of gastric juice. Prolonged contact with the highly acidic contents of the stomach and duodenum causes an erosion of the mucosal wall, especially in those areas least protected, such as the cardia and lesser curve of the stomach and the area immediately beyond the pylorus. Factors that can result in hypersecretion or decreased protection are outlined in Fig. 33-4.

Clinical Manifestations

Signs and symptoms of PUD vary according to the age of the child and the location of the ulcer (Table 33-5). The typical pain-food-relief syndrome seen in adults with peptic ulcer is often absent in young children. Suggestive symptoms of peptic ulcer include chronic abdominal pain, especially when the stomach is empty, such as during the night or early morning, recurrent vomiting after meals, chronic anemia with occult blood in the stools, and vague gastrointestinal complaints with a positive family history for PUD.

Diagnostic Evaluation

Diagnosis is based on the history (pattern of pain), physical examination (pain in the epigastric area), and diagnostic testing such as radiologic studies, barium swallow (identify

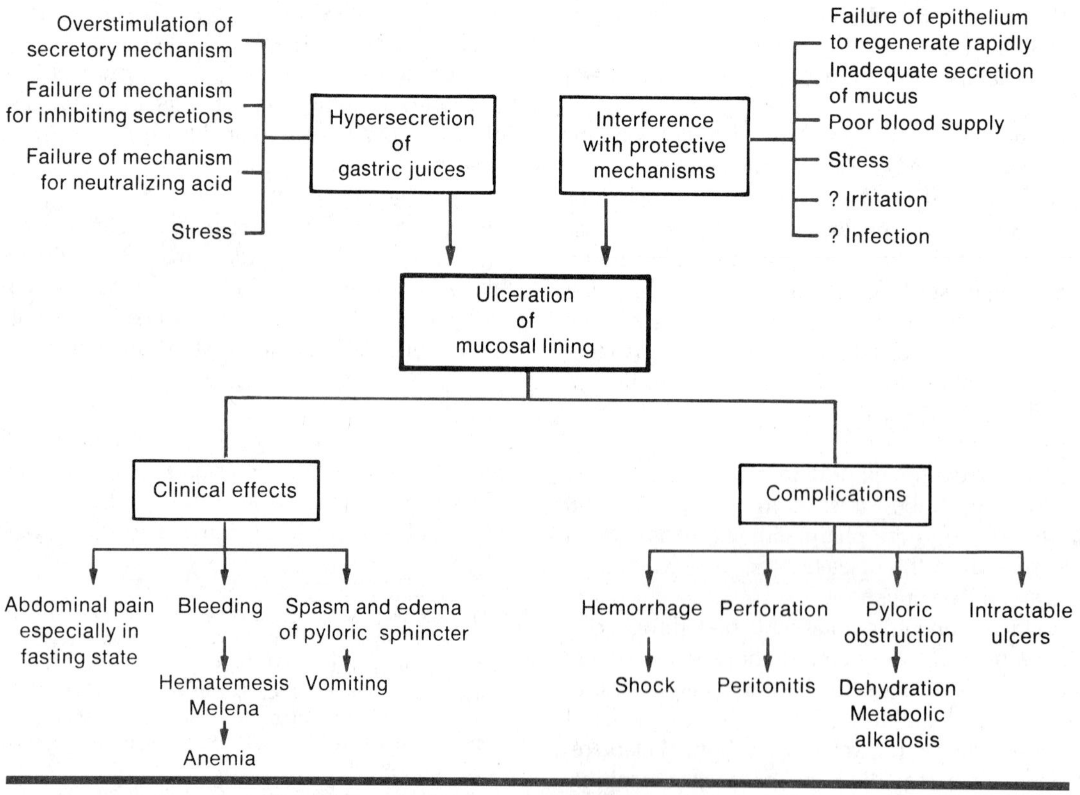

Fig. 33-4. Possible causes and effects of peptic ulcer.

Table 33-5 Clinical manifestations of peptic ulcers

AGE-GROUP	TYPE OF ULCER	MANIFESTATIONS	COMMENTS
Neonates	Usually gastric	Usually perforation Often massive hemorrhage Almost the same as seen in stress ulcers	Usually catastrophic More likely in infants with hypoxia, sepsis, difficult labor/delivery, or nasogastric feeding Prognosis often poor
Infants to 2-year-old children	Gastric or duodenal, primary or secondary	Poor eating, vomiting, crying spells after feeding, abdominal distention, tarry stools, melena Vague discomfort Irritability	Primary ulcers more likely to be gastric with slow onset Usually bleed rather than perforate
2- to 6-year-old children	Gastric or duodenal	No really positive physical findings May have vomiting related to eating, generalized or periumbilical pain, melena, hematemesis Wake at night crying with pain	Diagnosis often made on basis of social history Duodenal ulcers 5:1 over gastric Perforation more likely in secondary ulcers
6- to 9-year-old children	Usually duodenal and primary Often with obstruction	Pain—burning or gnawing sensation in epigastrium related to fasting state, melena, hematemesis, vomiting	Often related to school achievement, change, relationship with peers and/or teachers
Children over 9 years	Usually duodenal	Same as above	More typical of adult type Chances of recurrence greater than 50%

ulcers), and endoscopy. Other tests include blood studies (anemia), stool samples (occult blood), and, occasionally, gastric acid measurements (to isolate hypersecretors). Upper GI series are followed through to rule out CD, a great imitator; endoscopy may be performed for the same reason.

Therapeutic Management

The major objectives of therapy for children with PUD are to relieve discomfort, promote healing, and prevent complications and recurrence. The management of ulcers is primarily medical and consists of administration of medications that reduce or neutralize gastric acid secretion and, when possible, measures to eliminate or reduce stresses.

The child is provided with a nutritious diet but advised to avoid foods that are associated with aggravation of symptoms (see discussion under Nursing Considerations). Milk and other dairy products at frequent intervals are no longer recommended for treatment of ulcers. Milk contains protein and calcium, both of which stimulate gastric acid production. Milk also distends the stomach, further stimulating acid secretion, and exits from the stomach rapidly, thereby negating any prolonged buffering (Mathewson and Farnham, 1984).

Antacids are the preferred agents in the initial treatment of peptic ulcers. The antacid of choice, usually a liquid magnesium preparation, is administered 1 and 3 hours after each meal and before bedtime. The dosage is determined by the size of the child. Sodium bicarbonate (baking soda) is contraindicated because of the danger of metabolic alkalosis. As healing progresses, the frequency is gradually reduced, although the antacids are usually prescribed for several weeks.

H_2-receptor antagonists, potent inhibitors of basal and food-stimulated acid and pepsinogen secretion, are prescribed for most patients. The drugs most commonly used are ranitidine, cimetidine, and famotidine. These drugs offer greater compliance because of decreased frequency of administration, but are much more costly than antacids. Their use in children is not approved; therefore they need to be prescribed with careful consideration given to the risks and benefits.

Sucralfate and anticholinergic agents are useful adjuncts to antacid and H_2-blockers in some patients but are not given as single-agent therapy. Anticholinergic agents are rarely prescribed for children. Most children are treated with antibiotics and a bismuth compound.

A child with an acute ulcer who has developed complications, such as massive hemorrhage, requires emergency care. An NG tube is inserted to remove the blood, prevent abdominal distention, and provide a means of calculating blood loss. Blood replacement, intravenous fluids, and oxygen are usually necessary. Surgical closure of the perforation or bleeding point may be required to stop the hemorrhage.

Surgical management is rarely used in children, except for patients with complications of intractable pain, perforation, hemorrhage, and obstruction. Vagotomy with pyloroplasty is the preferred technique. Gastric resection is rarely performed.

Nursing Considerations

The main nursing objective is to promote healing of the ulcer through compliance with the dietary and medication regimen. The diet is generally not restricted. Foods known to cause symptoms are eliminated, and cola drinks are limited to one can per day. Smoking and alcohol are forbidden. If an analgesic/antipyretic is needed during the course of therapy, acetaminophen is substituted for aspirin.

Drug compliance is essential and can be a problem with frequent administration of antacids. Therefore strategies to improve compliance are instituted early in the course of therapy (see Chapter 27). For traveling and during school the use of antacid tablets rather than liquid is more convenient.

Although the exact role stress plays in the pathogenesis of ulcers in children is unclear, especially since many ulcers occur secondary to other conditions, the nurse should be aware of those family and environmental conditions that may have precipitated or may aggravate the condition. Children may benefit from psychologic counseling and from learning how to cope more constructively with stresses in their lives, such as school, family, and friends (Sibinga, 1983). The adaptive management of stress during childhood is an important area that has yet to be fully explored or researched.*

■ OBSTRUCTIVE DISORDERS

Obstruction of the bowel occurs when the passage of intestinal contents is mechanically impeded by a constricted or occluded lumen or when there is interference with normal muscular contraction. Intestinal obstruction from any cause is characterized by similar signs and symptoms, although the progression may vary greatly.

Classically, acute mechanical intestinal obstruction is characterized by colicky abdominal pain, nausea and vomiting, abdominal distention, and constipation. *Pain* is caused by severe, intermittent muscular contractions proximal to the obstruction as the bowel attempts to move luminal contents along the normal path. *Abdominal distention* is the result of accumulation of gas and fluid above the level of the obstruction. As these secretions continue to accumulate, the gut becomes excessively irritated and stimulates the vomiting center in the medulla to rid itself of the irritants with or without nausea. *Vomiting* is often the earliest sign of a high obstruction and a later sign in lower obstructions. Conversely, *constipation* and *obstipation* are early signs of low obstructions and later signs of higher obstructions. For example, a child with a high obstruction can have normal stools for 1 or 2 days as the bowel evacuates itself distal to the defect.

In acute conditions such as intussusception, the clinical manifestations are apparent within a few hours of the onset of the disorder. In other conditions such as pyloric stenosis, the signs and symptoms may be more gradual and may be missed during early stages of the disorder. If the obstruction is below the stomach, reflux from the small intestine causes intestinal secretions to flow back into the stomach, where they are vomited along with stomach contents. As this progresses, large quantities of fluid and electrolytes are lost, causing *dehydration.*

As distention progresses, the abdomen may be rigid and boardlike, with moderate to severe *tenderness. Bowel sounds* gradually diminish and cease. *Respiratory distress* occurs as the diaphragm is pushed up into the pleural cavity. As proteins are lost from the bloodstream into the intestinal lumen, the plasma volume diminishes and *shock* may occur.

HYPERTROPHIC PYLORIC STENOSIS

Obstruction at the pyloric sphincter by hypertrophy of the circular muscle of the pylorus is one of the most common surgical disorders of early infancy. This functional anomaly is seen soon after birth, with vomiting that becomes progressively more severe and projectile. It is five times more common in male than in female infants, affecting approximately 5 of 1000 males and only 1 of 1000 females (Cohen, 1984). Hypertrophic pyloric stenosis (HPS) is seen less frequently in black and Oriental than in white infants. It is more likely to affect a full-term than a premature infant.

The cause of the increased size of the pyloric musculature is unknown. A higher incidence in first-degree relatives and in monozygotic as opposed to dizygotic twins implicates heredity in the etiology, although the nature of the hereditary factors is only speculative.

Pathophysiology

The circular muscle of the pylorus is grossly enlarged as a result of both hypertrophy and hyperplasia. This produces severe narrowing of the pyloric canal between the stomach and the duodenum. Consequently, the lumen at this point is partially obstructed. Over a period of time inflammation and edema further reduce the size of the opening until the partial obstruction may progress to complete obstruction. The muscle is thickened to as much as twice its usual size—2 to 3 cm (¾ to 1¼ inches) long—and is almost cartilaginous in consistency. The distal portion ends abruptly and is externally distinct and easily palpated, but the proximal end

*See Nursing Care Plan: The Child with Peptic Ulcer Disease in Wong, D.L., and Whaley, L.F.: Clinical manual of pediatric nursing, ed. 3, St. Louis, 1990, Mosby–Year Book, Inc.

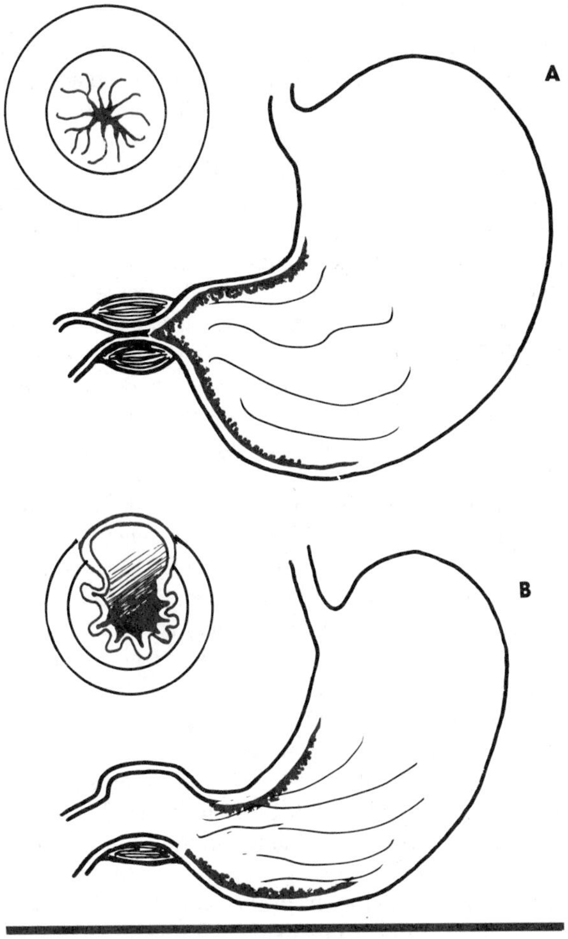

Fig. 33-5. Hypertrophic pyloric stenosis. **A,** Enlarged muscular tumor nearly obliterates pyloric channel. **B,** Longitudinal surgical division of muscle down to submucosa establishes adequate passageway.

merges into the gastric antrum. The stomach is usually dilated (Fig. 33-5, *A*).

Clinical Manifestations

The age of onset and pattern of vomiting are variable. Typically infants with pyloric hypertrophy are well during the first weeks of life. Initially there is only regurgitation or occasional nonprojectile vomiting that begins about the second to the fourth week after birth, although in a few infants symptoms begin at birth. Others do well for the first few weeks and then suddenly develop projectile vomiting that rapidly leads to dehydration. The projectile vomiting usually develops within a week and may lead to complete obstruction by 4 to 6 weeks. The vomitus may be ejected 2 to 4 feet (0.6 to 1.2 m) from the child in a side-lying position, and 1 foot (0.3 m) or more when the infant is lying on the back.

Vomiting occurs most often shortly after a feeding, although it may occur as long as several hours later. In some instances the vomiting may follow each feeding; in others it appears intermittently. The infant is hungry and an avid nurser who eagerly accepts a second feeding after a vomiting episode. The vomitus is nonbilious, containing only gastric contents, but may be blood tinged. The infant does not appear to be in pain other than the discomfort of chronic hunger.

The infant fails to gain weight or may lose weight, the stools diminish in number and size from the reduced intake, and evidence of dehydration becomes increasingly obvious. There is decreased elasticity of the skin, loss of subcutaneous tissue, and sunken eyeballs. The upper abdomen is distended, and diagnosis can be established on the basis of (1) a readily palpable olive-shaped tumor in the epigastrium just to the right of the umbilicus and (2) visible gastric peristaltic waves that move from left to right across the epigastrium. The pyloric tumor is most easily felt when the abdominal muscles are relaxed during a feeding or immediately after vomiting. Positive identification of these physical signs is sufficient evidence to establish a diagnosis.

Difficulty in diagnosis is related to children with feeding difficulties associated with disturbed parent-child relationships or hyperkinetic infants, who are exceptionally reactive to external stimuli and vomit more frequently than usual in the early weeks of life.

Diagnostic Evaluation

If diagnosis is inconclusive from the history and physical signs, upper GI radiographic studies will reveal delayed gastric emptying and an elongated, threadlike pyloric channel. Ultrasound evaluation is as accurate as radiography, is less traumatic, and there is less risk of aspiration of contrast medium. The hazard of aspiration is increased with gastric outlet obstruction. If ultrasound is unavailable, barium ingested for GI radiography should be evacuated from the stomach following evaluation. A palpable "olive" mass can usually be felt in the right upper quadrant.

Laboratory findings reflect the metabolic alterations created by severe depletion of both water and electrolytes from extensive and prolonged vomiting. There are decreased serum levels of both sodium and potassium, although these may be masked by the hemoconcentration from extracellular fluid depletion. Of greater diagnostic value are a decrease in serum chloride levels and increases in pH and bicarbonate (carbon dioxide content) characteristics of metabolic alkalosis. Hemoconcentration is evidenced by elevated hematocrit and hemoglobin values.

Therapeutic Management

Surgical relief of the pyloric obstruction by pyloromyotomy is simple, safe, and effective and is, with very few exceptions, the standard treatment for this disorder. Inasmuch as the surgery is not an emergency procedure, the initial efforts are directed toward rehydration of the infant, replenishment of body potassium stores, and correction of alkalosis with parenteral fluid and electrolyte administration. In well-hydrated infants with no evidence of electrolyte imbalance, surgery is performed without delay. Replacement fluid therapy usually delays surgery for 24 to 48 hours. Most surgeons prefer the stomach to be empty during surgery to diminish postoperative vomiting from gastric irritation. The stomach is decompressed with an NG tube. The tube is often left in place during the surgical procedure to keep the stomach empty of fluid, air, or barium from radiographic procedures.

The surgical procedure is performed through a right upper quadrant incision and consists of a longitudinal incision through the circular muscle fibers of the pylorus down to, but not including, the submucosa (Fredet-Ramstedt operation) (Fig. 33-5, *B*). The procedure has a very high success rate when infants receive careful preoperative preparation to correct fluid and electrolyte imbalances. It may take up to 12 weeks for the pylorus to return to normal size (Okorie and others, 1988).

Feedings are usually begun 4 to 6 hours postoperatively, beginning with small, frequent feedings of glucose in water or electrolyte solution. If clear fluids are retained, about 24 hours after surgery formula is started in the same stepwise increments, gradually increasing the amount and the interval between feedings until a full feeding schedule is reinstated, which usually takes about 48 hours. The infant is ready to be discharged from the hospital by about the second to sixth postoperative day. The prognosis is excellent, and the mortality is low.

Nursing Considerations

Nursing care of the infant with HPS involves primarily observation for physical signs and behaviors that help establish the diagnosis, careful regulation of fluid therapy, and reestablishment of normal feeding behaviors. Nurses are in a position to recognize signs of the disorder in infants and to refer them for medical evaluation.

Assessment

HPS should be considered as a possibility in the very young infant who appears alert but fails to gain weight and has a history of vomiting after meals. Assessment is based on observation of eating behaviors and evidence of characteristic clinical manifestations.

Nursing Diagnoses

Based on a thorough assessment, several nursing diagnoses are identified. The more common diagnoses for the child with HPS are included in the Nursing Care Plan on p. 1515. Others may apply in specific situations.

Planning

Nursing objectives for the child with HPS include the following:

1. Provide nutrition.
2. Prevent vomiting.
3. Prevent complications.
4. Support and educate family.

Implementation

Preoperatively the emphasis is placed on restoring hydration and electrolyte balance and beginning replacement of depleted body fat and protein stores. Many infants need several days or weeks of nutritional support to replace stores and improve surgical risk. These infants are allowed nothing by mouth and given intravenous fluids of glucose and electrolytes based on laboratory serum electrolyte values, usually sodium chloride solution with added potassium (when there is adequate urine output). Depleted calcium must also be replaced. Careful monitoring of the intravenous infusion and assiduous attention to intake, output, and urine specific gravity measurements are important to the success of fluid replacement. Accurate description of any vomiting, as well as the number and character of stools, is recorded.

Observations include assessment of vital signs, particularly those that might indicate fluid or electrolyte imbalances, including glucose levels because glycogen stores may be depleted from prolonged vomiting. These infants are especially prone to metabolic alkalosis from loss of hydrogen ions and to potassium, sodium, and chloride depletion, all of which are contained in gastric secretions. The skin and mucous membranes are assessed for alterations in hydration status, and daily weight measurement provides added clues to water gain or loss (see Chapter 28 for manifestations of fluid and electrolyte disturbances).

It is the responsibility of the nurse to ensure that the NG tube is patent and functioning properly and to measure and record the type and amount of drainage. The infant is usually positioned with the head slightly elevated.

General hygienic care, with particular attention to skin and mouth in dehydrated infants, is an important part of care. Protection from infection is also important, because infants with impaired nutritional status are even more susceptible than normal newborn infants. As with any child in the hospital, parents are encouraged to visit and become involved in the child's care. Vomiting of a projectile nature is frightening to parents, and they often believe that they may have done something wrong. Most parents need support and reassurance that the condition is caused by a structural problem and is in no way a reflection of their parenting skills and capacities.

Postoperative care. Postoperative vomiting is not uncommon, and most infants, even with successful surgery, exhibit some vomiting during the first 24 to 48 hours. Intravenous fluids are administered until the infant is taking and retaining adequate amounts by mouth. Therefore much of the same care that was instituted before surgery is continued postoperatively, that is, observation of physical signs, monitoring of intravenous fluids, careful observation and recording of intake and output, and observation for signs of hypoglycemia (see Chapter 9), including monitoring blood glucose levels. In addition, the infant is observed for responses to the stress of surgery.

The NG tube may be maintained after surgery for a variable length of time. Feedings are usually instituted relatively

NURSING CARE PLAN
The Child with Hypertrophic Pyloric Stenosis

NURSING DIAGNOSIS: Fluid volume deficit related to vomiting

GOAL 1
Prevent dehydration

INTERVENTIONS
*Maintain intravenous fluids as prescribed
Monitor laboratory data

EXPECTED OUTCOME
Child exhibits no evidence of dehydration

GOAL 2
Prevent interference with therapeutic regimen

INTERVENTIONS
Apply appropriate restraining methods where indicated
Provide pacifier for infants who are receiving nothing by mouth

EXPECTED OUTCOMES
Infant does not interfere with fluid therapy
Infant engages in nonnutritive sucking

NURSING DIAGNOSIS: Altered nutrition: less than body requirements related to persistent vomiting

*Dependent nursing action.

GOAL 1
Provide nutrition

INTERVENTIONS
Feed diet for age
Begin with small feeding at frequent intervals to prevent overdistention if vomits, reduce volume and progress slowly
Bubble before and frequently during feedings
Position in high Fowler position and slightly on right side after feeding
Handle minimally and gently after feeding
Reestablish breast-feeding

EXPECTED OUTCOME
Infant consumes and retains a sufficient amount of nourishment

NURSING DIAGNOSIS: Altered family processes related to a child with a life-threatening condition

GOAL 1
Support family

INTERVENTIONS AND EXPECTED OUTCOMES
See Nursing Care Plan: The Family of the Ill or Hospitalized Child, Chapter 26

See also:
Nursing Care Plan: The Child Undergoing Surgery, Chapter 27
Nursing Care Plan: The Child in Pain, Chapter 26.

soon, beginning with clear liquids containing glucose and electrolytes. They are offered slowly and at frequent intervals as ordered by the physician. If the infant has been breast-fed, breast milk, expressed by the mother, may be given by bottle when the infant is able to tolerate feedings, or the mother is instructed to limit nursing to 5 to 8 minutes and gradually increase to previous nursing pattern. Observation and recording of feedings and the infant's responses to feedings and feeding techniques are a vital part of postoperative care. Positioning with the head elevated is usually continued postoperatively. Care of the operative site consists of observation for any drainage or signs of inflammation and care of the incision as directed by the surgeon. Poorly nourished infants may have problems with wound healing.

Developmental intervention (see Chapter 10) is incorporated into the infant's care, parental involvement is encouraged and promoted, and parents require support and reassurance. Illness and surgery in an infant are frightening events for families, especially following a frustrating preoperative experience. Parents are involved in the infant's care as soon as possible after surgery and encouraged to provide comfort and stimulation appropriate to the needs of the infant.

Evaluation

The effectiveness of nursing interventions is determined by continual reassessment and evaluation of care based on the following observational guidelines and expected outcomes:

1. Observe feeding behavior, especially vomiting episodes.
2. Weigh infant daily.
3. Observe for evidence of complications.
4. Observe and interview family regarding feelings, understanding, and concerns.

Expected outcomes:
See Nursing Care Plan, p. 1515.

INTUSSUSCEPTION

Intussusception is one of the most frequent causes of intestinal obstruction during infancy. Half of the cases occur in children younger than 1 year, more commonly between 3 and 12 months of age, and most of the others occur in children during the second year. However, a number of cases have been reported in infants under 4 months of age and children 5 to 15 years of age (Newman and Schuh, 1987; Reijnin, 1987). Intussusception is three times more common in males than in females. Although specific intestinal lesions can be found in a small percentage of the children, generally the cause is not known. The occurrence of intussusception is increased in children with cystic fibrosis and celiac disease.

Pathophysiology

Intussusception is an invagination or telescoping of one portion of the intestine into another. The most common site is the ileocecal valve (*ileocolic*), in which the ileum invaginates into the cecum and then further into the colon (Fig. 33-6). Other forms include *ileoileal* (one part of the ileum invaginates into another section of the ileum) and *colocolic* (one part of the colon telescopes into another area of the colon), usually in the area of the hepatic or splenic flexure or at some point along the transverse colon.

As a result of the invagination, there is obstruction to the passage of intestinal contents beyond the defect. In addition, the two walls of the intestine press against each other, causing inflammation, edema, and eventually decreased blood flow. As incarceration continues, necrosis results with hemorrhage, perforation, and peritonitis. If untreated, this condition is incompatible with life.

Clinical Manifestations

Classic presentation of intussusception is a healthy, thriving child, usually between 3 and 12 months of age, who suddenly has an episode of acute abdominal pain. Typical behavior includes screaming and drawing the knees up to the chest. These episodes of severe pain are characterized by intervals in which the child appears normal and comfortable.

During this initial period vomiting usually occurs, and the child passes one normal brown stool. However, as the condition worsens, the vomiting increases, the child becomes apathetic, and subsequent stools are red and currant jelly–like from the passage of stool mixed with blood and mucus.

The abdomen becomes tender and distended. A sausage-shaped mass may be felt in the upper right quadrant. In contrast, the lower right quadrant usually feels empty (Dance sign) as the bowel distal to the obstruction is less involved and free of contents. If treatment is not sought, the child becomes acutely ill with fever, prostration, and signs of peritonitis (see p. 1502).

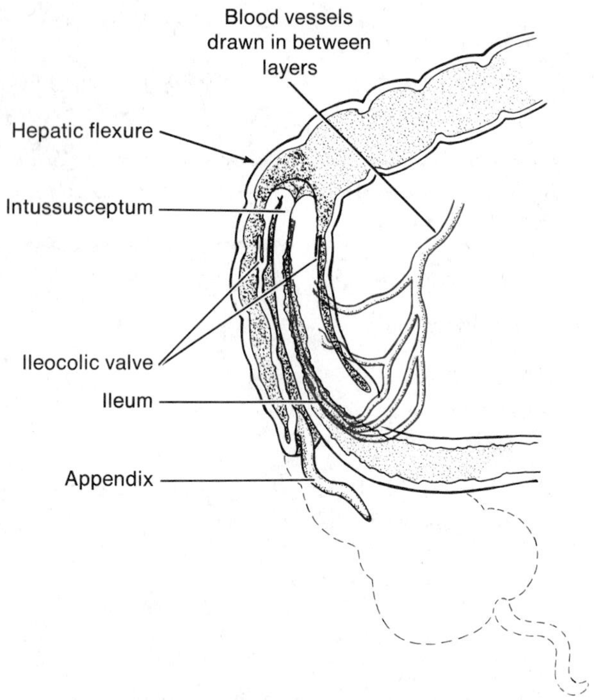

Fig. 33-6. Ileocolic intussusception.

Manifestations in older children. Although the classic signs and symptoms of intussusception are paroxysmal abdominal pain, vomiting, palpable abdominal mass, and currant jelly stools, a more chronic picture may occur, characterized by diarrhea, constipation, occasional vomiting, and periodic colic. Since this condition is potentially life-threatening, the nurse must recognize such signs and closely observe and refer these children for further medical investigation.

Diagnostic Evaluation

Frequently the diagnosis can be made on subjective findings alone. However, definitive diagnosis is based on a barium enema, which clearly demonstrates the obstruction to the flow of barium. A rectal examination reveals mucus, blood, and occasionally a low intussusception itself.

Therapeutic Management

In most cases the initial treatment of choice is nonsurgical hydrostatic reduction by barium enema. Usually correction of the invagination is carried out at the same time as the diagnostic testing. The principle behind this procedure is that the force exerted by the flowing barium will be sufficient to push the invaginated portion of the bowel into its original position, similar to pushing an inverted "finger" out of a glove.

Alternative pressure reduction techniques involve the use of saline for hydrostatic pressure under ultrasound, which reduces the risk of radiographic exposure and spilling of barium into the peritoneal cavity (Wang and Liu, 1988). Pneumonic insufflation with air or oxygen has also been successfully used in reduction (Guo and others, 1986; Tamanaha and others, 1987). It can be accomplished more rapidly than barium and appears to be equally effective.

Since this procedure is not always successful (about 75% in uncomplicated cases) and is not recommended if there are clinical signs of shock or perforation, the child is also prepared for surgery before the attempted reduction. Surgical intervention involves manually reducing the invagination and, where indicated, resecting any nonviable intestine.

Nursing Considerations

The nurse can assist in establishing a diagnosis by carefully listening to the parents' history of the child's physical and behavioral symptoms relating to the complaint. Although parents may not know the medical problem, they are astute diagnosticians in detecting that something is wrong.

✦ **NURSING ALERT** Report of severe colicky abdominal pain in a child combined with vomiting is a significant clue to intussusception.

As soon as a possible diagnosis of intussusception is made, the nurse begins to prepare the parents for the immediate need for hospitalization, the usual nonsurgical techniques, and the possibility of surgery. It is important at this time to explain the basic defect of intussusception, which can be easily demonstrated by pushing the end of a finger on a rubber glove back into itself or using the example of a telescoping rod. The principle of reduction by hydrostatic pressure can be simulated by filling the glove with water, which pushes the "finger" into a fully extended position. By using such demonstrations, the parents are aware of why surgery is sometimes necessary. Without this preparation, they may be left with the feeling that the physician "failed" or that their child had "complications."

Physical care of the child with intussusception differs little from that for any child undergoing abdominal surgery (see Chapter 27). Even though nonsurgical intervention may be successful, usual preoperative procedures are performed. For the child with signs of electrolyte imbalance, hemorrhage, or peritonitis, additional medical preparation such as replacement fluids, whole blood or plasma, and NG suctioning may be included. All stools are monitored before surgery.

✦ **NURSING ALERT** Passage of a normal brown stool usually indicates that the intussusception has reduced itself. This is immediately reported to the physician, who may choose to alter the diagnostic/therapeutic plan of care.

Postprocedural care includes the usual postoperative observations (see Surgical Procedures: Postoperative Care, Chapter 27) with special observation of stool passage and return of bowel sounds. In the case of hydrostatic reduction or autoreduction, the nurse observes for passage of barium and the stool patterns, since recurrences of the intussusception are most likely to occur within the first 36 hours after reduction. For this reason the child is kept in the hospital for 2 to 3 days. Overall recurrence of intussusception after nonsurgical or operative reduction is between 4% and 10% (Silverman and Roy, 1983).

■ MALABSORPTION SYNDROMES

The term *malabsorption syndrome* is applied to a long list of disorders associated with some degree of impaired digestion and/or absorption. Most are classified according to the locations of the supposed anatomic and/or biochemical defect.

CLASSIFICATION AND MANIFESTATIONS

Malabsorption can be classified as (1) failure of digestion (intraluminal), (2) failure of absorption (mucosal), and (3) lymphatic obstruction. Only digestive and absorptive dysfunctions are discussed.

Classification

Digestive failure mainly includes those conditions in which the enzymes necessary for digestion are diminished or absent, such as (1) absence of pancreatic enzymes (cystic fibrosis) or when there is inadequate mixing of enzymes and food (rapid transit), (2) inadequate bile salt concentration (biliary or liver disease), or (3) lactase deficiency (congenital or secondary lactose intolerance).

Absorptive failure includes those conditions in which the intestinal mucosa is impaired. It may be caused by (1) inadequate absorptive surface (short gut syndrome) or (2) mucosal disease (celiac disease), or it may be secondary to inflammatory disease (damaged mucosa and accelerated motility of IBD or viral gastroenteritis).

Obstructive disorders, such as Hirschsprung disease, can also cause secondary malabsorption from enterocolitis, chronic inflammation of the distended small and large bowel. There are also some disorders that result in malabsorption but for which no specific organic cause can be found. One of the classic examples is nonorganic failure to thrive, in which malnutrition results despite adequately functioning body systems and is reversed by a program of emotional stimulation rather than medical intervention. See Box 29-4 for causes of chronic diarrhea.

Manifestations

A number of manifestations are common to chronic malabsorption/maldigestion. Nutritional state is the most important aspect of assessment of chronic diarrhea (see Nutritional Assessment, Chapter 6). Wasting of subcutaneous fat (especially noticeable in the gluteal area) is characteristic of failure to thrive. Edema is observed in children with protein deficiency, and easy bruising often results from inadequate absorption of vitamin C and fat-soluble vitamin K. Celiac syndrome is a major manifestation of some major malabsorption diseases.

Celiac syndrome. *Celiac syndrome* and *malabsorption syndrome* are terms used to describe a symptom complex associated with several different diseases that have four characteristics in common: (1) steatorrhea (fat, foul, frothy, bulky stools), (2) general malnutrition, (3) abdominal distention, and (4) secondary vitamin deficiencies. Two diseases with celiac syndrome as manifestations are celiac disease and cystic fibrosis. Celiac disease, which in adults is often referred to as nontropical sprue, is discussed in the next section. Cystic fibrosis is the most common genetic disorder with celiac syndrome as a feature. Because the pulmonary complications of the disease are the most life-threatening, cystic fibrosis is discussed in Chapter 32.

CELIAC DISEASE (GLUTEN ENTEROPATHY)

Celiac disease (CD), also known as *gluten enteropathy (GE), gluten-sensitive enteropathy (GSE),* and *celiac sprue,* is infrequent in the pediatric population in the continental United States (Whittington, 1990). Although the exact reason is not known, there is an association between changes in feeding practices—specifically, delayed introduction of solid foods and encouragement of breast-feeding—and the declining incidence of celiac disease.

Evidence of a link between the disease and genetic factors is the incidence of histocompatibility antigen HLA-B8 in 60% to 90% of affected individuals, which is a fourfold increase over that found in the general population (Savilahi and others, 1986; Silverman and Roy, 1983).

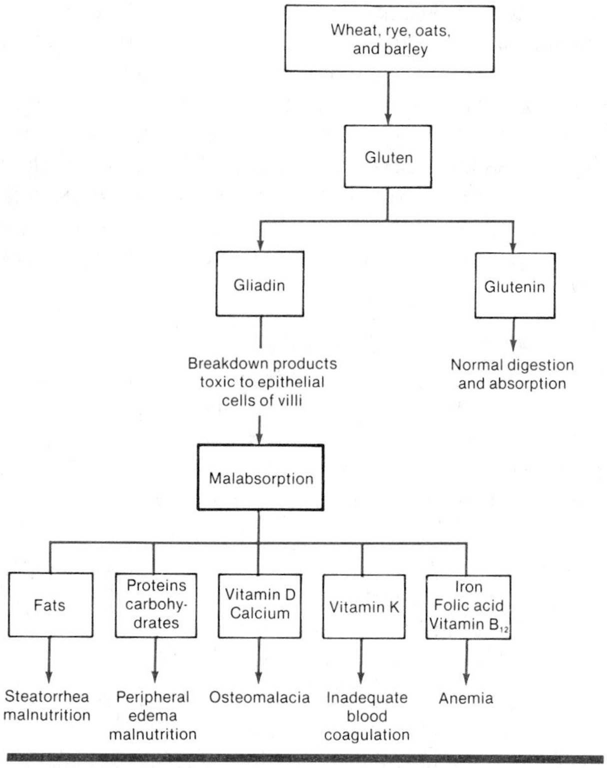

Fig. 33-7. Malabsorptive defect in celiac disease.

Pathophysiology

The disease is characterized by an intolerance for the gliadin faction of gluten, a protein component of wheat, barley, rye, and oats. Although the precise mechanism by which gliadin produces cell damage is not known, inability to fully digest gliadin results in accumulation of the amino acid glutamine, which is toxic to the mucosal cells. Damaged villi eventually atrophy, greatly reducing the absorptive surface and impairing various absorptive processes.

In the early stages of celiac disease fat absorption is primarily affected, resulting in elimination of large quantities of digested fat (soaps and fatty acids) in the stool. The frothy appearance, foul odor, and excessive quantity of stool are the result of altered bacterial flora on the digested, but unabsorbed, fats and proteins. As the pathologic processes in the villi continue, the absorption of protein, carbohydrates, calcium, iron, folic acid, and vitamins D, K, and B_{12} is greatly impaired and contributes to the typical clinical picture seen in the child (Fig. 33-7). Growth failure, muscle wasting (especially in extremities and buttocks), distended abdomen, and anemia are also observed in untreated children.

Clinical Manifestations

Symptoms of celiac disease (described in the preceding paragraph) are first noted about 3 to 6 months following introduction of gluten-containing grains into the diet, typically at 9 to 12 months of age, although it may not be evident until early childhood. Symptoms are usually insidious and chronic. The first evidence of the disease may be failure to regain weight or appetite after a bout of diarrhea. Constipation, vomiting, and abdominal pain may also be initial presenting signs. Behavioral changes, such as irritability, fretfulness, uncooperativeness, or apathy, are common. As the disease progresses, signs of general wasting become evident.

Diagnostic Evaluation

A definitive diagnosis is based on a peroral jejunal biopsy, which demonstrates the atrophic changes in the architecture of the mucosal wall. This procedure is performed by passing a polyethylene tube through the mouth along the alimentary tract to the jejunum of the small bowel. Measuring serum antigliadin and antireticulin antibodies aids in diagnosis.

The other essential criterion of diagnosis is dramatic clinical improvement after adherence to a gluten-restricted diet. Within a day or two after instituting the diet, most children with CD demonstrate a favorable personality change. Weight gain, improved appetite, and disappearance of diarrhea and steatorrhea usually do not occur for several days. Return of symptoms after reintroduction of gluten is positive evidence of gluten sensitivity.

Therapeutic Management

Treatment of chronic celiac disease is primarily dietary management. Although the prescribed diet is called "gluten free," it is in reality low in gluten, since it is impossible to remove every source of this protein. Also, most patients are able to tolerate restricted amounts of gluten. Since gluten is found mainly in the grains of wheat and rye, but also in smaller quantities in barley and oats, these four foods are eliminated. Corn, rice, and millet are substitute grain foods.

In children with severe malnutrition, specific deficiencies are treated with supplemental vitamins, iron, and calories. Because absorption of fat-soluble vitamins is impaired, these are supplied in a water-miscible form.

Most patients with CD have a permanent sensitivity to gluten, which requires lifelong maintenance of a gluten-free diet. A small group of infants exhibit transient gluten sensitivity and are able to digest gluten safely after a period of time.

Celiac crisis, a rare event, requires prompt medical intervention to correct the dehydration and metabolic acidosis. Treatment involves intermittent NG decompression, intravenous fluids with appropriate electrolyte replacement, and intravenous steroid administration to decrease bowel inflammation. The prompt improvement in response to steroids is believed to support the immunologic theory that gluten acts as an antigen to the mucosal cells.

Nursing Considerations

The main nursing consideration is helping the parents and child adhere to diet therapy. This involves considerable time in explaining the disease process to the parents, the specific role of gluten in aggravating the disorder, and those foods that must be restricted. It is especially difficult to maintain a diet indefinitely when the child has no symptoms and temporary transgressions result in no difficulties. Although the chief source of grain is cereal and baked goods, grains are frequently added to processed foods as thickeners or fillers. To compound the difficulty, gluten is added to many foods but obscurely listed on the label as "hydrolyzed vegetable protein." The nurse must advise parents of the necessity of reading all label ingredients carefully to avoid hidden sources of gluten.

Some of children's favorite foods contain these ingredients, including bread, cake, cookies, crackers, doughnuts, pies, spaghetti, pizza, prepared soups, some processed ice cream, many types of chocolate candy, milk preparations such as malts, hot dogs, luncheon meats, meat gravy, some prepared hamburgers, and many soups. Many of these products can be eliminated from the infant's or young child's diet fairly easily, but monitoring the diet of a school-age child or adolescent is a much more difficult situation. Luncheon preparation away from home is particularly difficult, since bread, luncheon meats, and instant soups are not allowed. For families on restricted food budgets, adhering to the diet adds an additional financial burden, since many inexpensive or convenience foods cannot be used. It may be more economical for these families to buy rice or corn flour directly from the milling company. Because the flour is a dietary prescription, the cost is a tax-deductible medical expense (Hartwig, 1983).

Another deterrent to adherence is the recommendation that the child continue the diet indefinitely. This is especially difficult for parents and children to understand when there have been no symptoms of the disease for an extended time and occasional dietary indiscretions have not caused untoward effects. However, evidence demonstrates that the majority of individuals who relax their diet experience a relapse. There is also evidence that terminating the diet predisposes to development of malignant lymphoma of the small intestine, esophageal cancer, and other gastrointestinal cancers in adulthood.

It is important to stress long-range complications, as well as to remind parents of the child's physical status before dietary treatment and dramatic improvement after it was begun. For the child, however, these arguments may not be as convincing, because the future is less significant than the present and the past has little meaning. The nurse can be instrumental in allowing the child to express these feelings, while focusing on ways in which the child can still be "normal." For example, the usual prepared foods, such as hot dogs and hamburgers, may be restricted, but tacos and other Mexican dishes made with corn tortillas are acceptable. Many children complain that the diet is boring because the parent prepares the same food all the time. The child can be encouraged to find new recipes using suitable ingredients. With the present emphasis on natural health foods, the nurse can encourage the child to investigate new foods, such as sesame seeds and rice flour, to enhance their choices, while still being in vogue with peer interests. In some children permanent growth retardation is another emotional crisis.

Several resources are available to assist parents in all aspects of coping with CD. The **American Celiac Society*** and the **Celiac Sprue Association/United States of America**† are organizations that provide support and guidance to families and supply educational materials concerning gluten-free diet, food sources, and recipes, and travel information.‡ A booklet, *Pointers for Parents: Coping with Celiac Sprue,*§ which provides information on shopping, cooking, and otherwise living with an affected child, is available.

SHORT BOWEL SYNDROME

The short bowel syndrome (SBS) refers to a condition in which loss of intestine results in diminished ability to normally digest and absorb a regular diet. It occurs most often in infants or children following intestinal resection for inflammatory conditions such as necrotizing enterocolitis or IBD or congenital bowel anomalies such as small intestine atresias, gastroschisis, or volvulus (twisting of a large section of bowel).

---

*Dept. N83, 45 Gifford Ave., Jersey City, NJ 07304; (201) 432-1207.

†3213 Rocklyn Dr., Des Moines, IA 50322; (515) 270-9689.

‡In Canada: **Canadian Celiac Association, Inc.,** 1087 Meyerside Dr., Suite 5, Mississauga, Ontario L5T 1M5; (416) 673-8200.

§Available from Clinical Dietetics Dept., Children's Memorial Hospital, 2300 Children's Plaza, Chicago, IL 60614; (312) 880-4000.

Both the extent and location of the loss, especially the ileum, are important factors in determining the severity of the condition. As much as 50% of the intestine can be lost without affecting the health of the child, unless it includes the distal ileum. A loss of greater than 75% of the small bowel results in malabsorption. However, the remaining intestine and stomach can adapt to the loss provided the child is kept alive through nutritional support. Adaptation occurs in a compensatory growth of all coats of the bowel wall with increased length and diameter of the remaining gut (Klish and Putnam, 1981).

Therapeutic Management

The goals of treatment are (1) to preserve as much length of bowel surgically as possible and (2) to maintain the child's nutritional status until adaptation of the bowel occurs. Small amounts of dilute formula should be started as soon as possible, since the bowel must be challenged with formula for it to develop enzymes to tolerate feedings. This necessitates a planned schedule of gradually increased concentration of formula; enteral feedings may be prescribed, and severely affected children require total parenteral nutrition to provide sufficient nutrition.

Nursing Considerations

Nursing care is directed toward maintaining the child's nutritional state, and prescribed orders for oral or enteral feedings must be followed exactly. If parenteral alimentation is required, every effort is made to preserve the intravenous line and to prevent complications such as infection. When long-term parenteral nutrition is required, preparing the family for home care of the child is a major nursing responsibility (see Chapter 28). Since hospitalization may be prolonged, the child's developmental and emotional needs must be attended to as well.

HEPATIC DISORDERS

The liver is the largest internal organ in the body and one of the most vital. It performs over 400 functions that broadly include (1) blood storage and filtration; (2) secretion of bile and bilirubin; (3) metabolism of fat, protein, and carbohydrate and synthesis of blood-clotting components; (4) detoxification of hormones, drugs, and other substances; and (5) storage for glycogen, iron, and vitamins A, D, E, and B_{12}. Inflammatory, obstructive, or degenerative disorders that affect the liver will affect all or some of these functions. The following discussion is concerned with two disorders that affect the liver during childhood—hepatitis and cirrhosis. Biliary atresia, a congenital anomaly, is discussed in Chapter 11.

ACUTE HEPATITIS

Hepatitis, or inflammation of the liver, is rapidly emerging as one of the major causes of morbidity and a significant cause of mortality in children. The discussion that follows is primarily concerned with acute hepatitis, although the chronic form of the disease may involve many of the same mechanisms.

Etiology

Hepatitis of viral origin is caused by at least four types of virus: *hepatitis A virus* (HAV), formerly referred to as "infectious" hepatitis; *hepatitis B virus* (HBV), formerly referred to as "serum" hepatitis; *hepatitis D* (HDV); and *non-A, non-B virus* (NANB). HDV is a unique viral agent in that it replicates only in the presence of HBV. NANB agents have not been identified; they refer to instances of hepatitis when other viral agents are excluded (Krugman, 1985). The following discussion is concerned with HAV and HBV. Although these viruses produce the same pathologic changes in the liver and similar clinical manifestations, they are distinct in their epidemiologic and immunologic characteristics. Table 33-6 compares the various features of HAV and HBV.

Hepatitis A. Hepatitis A is a relatively benign, self-limiting, but highly contagious disease that is spread by the fecal-oral route. The most common method is by person-to-person contact (American Academy of Pediatrics, 1988). Frequently reported are cases caused from ingestion of contaminated food or water, including eating shellfish caught in contaminated water, and from swimming in such water. HAV can affect individuals at any age but is seen at a younger age in children in lower socioeconomic groups, where housing conditions are crowded. The disease is endemic in developing countries. Spread occurs readily in households and daycare centers that care for children in diapers. An estimated 30% of HAV outbreaks in the United States have started in daycare centers (Marwick and Simmons, 1984). Because most of the infected children may have only mild symptoms or be asymptomatic, the disease is usually spread long before it is recognized.

Hepatitis B. Hepatitis B is a more insidious and serious form of the disease. HBV is most commonly transmitted by direct (needles) or indirect (cuts, burns, abrasions) parenteral means, although it can be spread to mucous surfaces (intimate contact, contaminated secretions splashed into mouth or eyes during irrigations) and by certain fomites (contaminated equipment, gloves). The virus can be found in almost all body fluids and secretions (except perhaps feces)—saliva, tears, sweat, urine, genital secretions, nasopharyngeal secretions, and possibly mother's milk, although these fluids probably are not sources of transmittable HBV. Persons at risk include close family contacts, clients and staff of custodial institutions for children who are retarded, those requiring frequent blood transfusions and hemodialysis, and health workers—especially those in operating rooms, emergency rooms, dialysis units, intensive care units, laboratories, and dental care units.

The incidence of HBV is significant in adolescent parenteral drug users and their contacts, but most HBV in children is acquired by the nonparenteral route. Newborn infants are also at risk for neonatal hepatitis, especially if the mother is infected with HBV or was a carrier of HBV during

Table 33-6 Comparison of types A and B hepatitis

CHARACTERISTICS	TYPE A	TYPE B
Incubation period	15-45 days, average 25 days	50-180 days, average 120 days
Period of communicability	Unknown Virus in blood and feces 2 to 3 weeks before onset of jaundice and for at least 1 week after onset of jaundice	Variable Virus in blood (probably in stool but no direct proof) during late incubation period and acute stage of disease; may persist in carrier state for years
Mode of transmission	Principal route—oral-fecal Less frequent route—parenteral	Principal route—parenteral Less frequent route—oral, sexual Fetal transfer—transplacental blood (last trimester), at delivery
Clinical features		
Onset	Usually rapid, acute	More insidious
Fever	Common and early	Less frequent
Anorexia	Extreme	Mild to moderate
Nausea and vomiting	Common	Less common
Rash	Rare	Common
Arthralgia	Rare	Common
Pruritus	Rare	Sometimes present
Jaundice	Present	Present
Immunity	Present after one attack; no crossover to type B	Present after one attack; no crossover to type A
Carrier state	None	Yes
Prophylaxis		
Immune serum globulin (ISG)	Passive immunity Successful, especially in early incubation period and preexposure prophylaxis	Passive immunity Inconsistent benefits; probably of no use
Hepatitis B immune globulin (HBIG)	No benefit	Postexposure protection possible if given immediately after definite exposure
Hepatitis B vaccine (See Table 12-11)	Not indicated	Provides active immunity Recommended for those persons at high risk of exposure

pregnancy. Possible routes of maternal-fetal (infant) transmission include (1) leakage of virus across the placenta late in pregnancy or during labor, (2) ingestion of amniotic fluid or maternal blood, and (3) breast-feeding, especially if the mother has cracked nipples (Krugman and others, 1985). The infectivity of colostrum and breast milk is controversial. The severity of hepatitis in the infant varies from no liver disease to a fulminant or chronic, active type.

Chronic carriers of HBV provide a reservoir of virus and are infectious for the duration of their carrier state. Of recent concern is the increased incidence of HBV in refugees from Southeast Asia. Most refugees do not know they are carriers.

Non-A, non-B hepatitis. NANB is now believed to be caused by two distinct viruses. The first is the most common cause of posttransfusion hepatitis in the United States, with a marked propensity to progress to chronic liver disease. The second, transmitted by the fecal-oral route via contaminated water or person-to-person, has caused large outbreaks in Asia, Africa, and the Soviet Union. NANB hepatitis is largely limited to the adult population.

Pathophysiology

The pathologic changes occur primarily in the parenchymal cells of the liver and result in variable degrees of swelling, infiltration of liver cells by mononuclear cells, subsequent degeneration, necrosis, and autolysis. Structural changes within the hepatocyte are thought to account for altered liver functions, such as impaired bile excretion, elevated transaminase and alkaline phosphatase levels, and decreased albumin synthesis.

The disorder is usually self-limiting, with complete regeneration of liver cells without scarring occurring within 2 to 3 months. There are, however, forms of hepatitis that do not result in complete return of liver function. These include *fulminant hepatitis*, which is characterized by a severe, acute course with death frequently occurring within 1 to 2 weeks, and *subacute* or *chronic active hepatitis*, characterized by progressive liver destruction and uncertain regeneration with the possibility of scarring.

Clinical Manifestations

The clinical manifestations for HAV and HBV viral hepatitis are similar, except for a more rapid, acute onset in type A and a slower, more insidious onset in type B. Both types may have flulike symptoms and may never be recognized as actual cases of hepatitis.

The initial anicteric (absence of jaundice)–phase symptoms include nausea and vomiting, extreme anorexia, malaise, easy fatigability, and slight to moderate fever. The child may have abdominal pain (especially epigastric or upper right quadrant), usually acts ill, preferring to rest in bed, and is fretful or irritable. The most significant finding on physical examination is liver tenderness with or without enlargement. This phase usually lasts 5 to 7 days.

The icteric (jaundice) phase begins with darkening of the urine and the presence of light-colored stools, followed by yellowing of the sclera and skin. As jaundice worsens, the child usually begins to feel better, with improved appetite and behavior and the absence of nausea, vomiting, and fever. This opposing course of rising bilirubin and improved clinical signs is regarded as a significant diagnostic and prognostic sign of benign viral hepatitis.

The appearance of jaundice with worsening constitutional symptoms is regarded as a poorer prognostic sign. A majority of these children develop fulminant, subacute, or chronic active hepatitis. Some children never develop jaundice; however, although their course is usually milder, they are still infectious.

The icteric phase commonly lasts less than 4 weeks. Complete recovery with return of normal liver function and a feeling of well-being with absence of fatigue or malaise may take 1 to 3 months. Generally, children recover promptly. However, it is not unusual for the child to experience a short relapse of slight jaundice and clinical symptoms 10 to 12 weeks after the illness. Unless the symptoms persist and continue to worsen, this relapse is considered benign.

Not all affected children exhibit signs of disease. Because the manifestations of hepatitis are the body's response to the viral antigen, individuals who are unable to muster an adequate defense will develop few if any symptoms. However, they may still harbor the virus as carriers. Newborn infants of mothers with HBV who have been exposed to the virus during prenatal life do not recognize the virus as a foreign protein and thus become chronic carriers.

Diagnostic Evaluation

Diagnosis is based on history, physical examination, laboratory evidence of the virus, and liver function tests (Table 33-7). Other assessment factors include evidence of (1) contact with a person known to have hepatitis, especially a family member; (2) questionable sanitation practices, such as impure drinking water; (3) eating certain foods, such as clams or oysters (especially from polluted water;) (4) recent immunizations or blood transfusions; (5) ingestion of hepatotoxic drugs, such as salicylates, sulfonamides, several antineoplastic agents, and many other medications; and (6) parenteral administration of illicit drugs or sexual contact with a person who uses these drugs. The last event is especially important when hepatitis is suspected in an adolescent and should be coupled with a careful examination for signs of needle marks, especially in the antecubital fossa.

Diagnosis is confirmed by detection of antibodies or antigens produced in response to the specific virus, such as HBsAg (hepatitis B surface antigen). Clinical improvement is usually associated with a decrease and disappearance of antigens, followed by the appearance of their antibodies. Since the antibodies persist indefinitely, they are used to identify the carrier state (individuals with the HBV who have no clinical disease but are able to transmit the organism).

Therapeutic Management

There is no specific treatment for hepatitis. Management is primarily treatment of symptoms. For example, antiemetics may be helpful to reduce the nausea or vomiting. The value of bed rest in promoting overall recovery is controversial. The child who feels ill and tired in the anicteric phase usually chooses to stay in bed. However, once improvement of physical complaints begins, the child prefers to resume normal activity gradually. The best approach is probably to allow the child to regulate his or her own pace. Hospitalization is rarely necessary, although proper isolation precautions at home are imperative.

The child is allowed preferred foods, especially during the initial stage when anorexia is severe. Generally low-fat foods cause less stomach distention and are better tolerated than foods high in fat content. Carbohydrates should be encouraged to ensure an adequate caloric intake to spare proteins for cell growth. Vitamin K is administered if prothrombin time is prolonged.

Prevention. Isolation or quarantine of the infected child is not necessary as long as measures are employed to prevent spread of the virus. An attack of either virus confers long-lasting immunity to that virus; however, there is no crossover protection to the other virus. Prophylactic use of immune serum globulin (ISG) is effective in preventing hepatitis virus A in situations of preexposure (such as anticipated travel to areas where HAV is prevalent) or in situations of postexposure during the early part of the incubation period and, to a lesser extent, before the onset of the disease. It is of inconsistent benefit in preventing type B virus.

Passive immunity to HBV can be achieved with hyperimmune gamma globulin (hepatitis B immune serum globulin, HBIG), but it is very expensive. However, it is used for postexposure prophylaxis in the following situations: (1) newborn infants born to HBsAg-positive mothers, (2) accidental needle stick or mucosal exposure to HBsAg-positive blood, or (3) sexual contact with an HBsAg-positive person. The hepatitis B vaccine is highly effective in providing protection against HBV and may be used alone or with HBIG. At present the vaccine is recommended for persons at risk, including hemodialysis patients, recipients of certain blood products (e.g., persons with hemophilia or thalassemia),

Table 33-7 Liver function tests

TEST	NORMAL FUNCTION OF LIVER	ABNORMAL FINDING AND SIGNIFICANCE
▪ Blood		
Serum bilirubin level	Conversion of indirect (unconjugated) bilirubin to direct (conjugated) bilirubin for excretion in bile	Increased indirect bilirubin level denotes damage to hepatic cells Increased direct bilirubin level denotes some blockage of bile duct
Thymol turbidity or cephalin flocculation	Globulins produced by liver	Abnormal globulins produced, especially in acute liver disease
Bromsulphalein (BSP) excretion	Filtration and excretion	Removal of this dye is similar to mechanisms used in excreting bilirubin; therefore excess dye in bloodstream can indicate problems in hepatic blood flow, liver cells, or bile ducts
Blood ammonia level	Detoxification of ammonia to urea	Increased level reflects poorly functioning hepatic cells and impaired hepatic blood flow
Prothrombin time	Prothrombin manufactured by liver	Prothrombin time increased but usually only reflected in severe liver disease
Serum protein levels	Albumin manufactured chiefly by liver; globulins manufactured by liver, spleen, lymphatics, and bone marrow	Albumin usually decreased, whereas globulins increased
Aklaline phosphatase level	Enzyme produced by liver and excreted with bile	Increased level reflects *acute* liver cell disease or bile duct obstruction
Serum glutamic oxaloacetic transaminase (SGOT) level, serum glutamic pyruvic transaminase (SGPT) level, and lactic dehydrogenase (LDH) level	Metabolic enzymes produced by liver	All elevated in *acute* liver destructions as the damaged cells release their enzymes SGOT—found also in heart tissue SGPT—found mostly in liver but a less sensitive indicator than SGOT LDH—found in several organ tissues, therefore not specific for liver disease
▪ Urine		
Urine bilirubin level	Normally bilirubin excreted in bile, broken down to urobilinogen in stool and therefore not excreted in urine	Present in urine, produces deep yellow to brown color Reflects direct bilirubin level because only this form is water soluble
Urine urobilinogen level	Normally contains only small amounts from filtration of blood	Increased
▪ Stool		
Stool sample	Urobilinogen oxidized to pigment urobilin (stercobilin), which gives stool its characteristic color	If bile is not being produced or if its flow is obstructed, stool will be white or clay-colored from lack of bile pigments

and health care workers with frequent exposure to blood.

Transmission from hepatitis Be antigen (HBeAg) can be reduced by passive immunization with hepatitis B immunoglobulin within 48 hours of birth, followed by active immunization at birth, and at 1, 6, and 12 months of age (or other schedule as determined by individual practitioners) (Mowat, 1989). With the increased incidence of HBV infection in families who adopt Asian children, it is recommended that all Asian adoptees be screened for HBV and appropriate members of adopting families (especially parents) be vaccinated (Friede and others, 1988).

Nursing Considerations

Nursing objectives depend largely on the severity of the hepatitis, the rigidity of medical treatment, and factors influencing the control and transmission of the disease. Since children with benign viral hepatitis are frequently cared for at home, the responsibility of explaining any medical therapies and control measures is frequently left to the clinic or office nurse. In instances in which further assistance is needed for parents to comply with such instructions, a public health nursing referral may be necessary.

The emphasis is on encouraging a well-balanced diet

and a realistic schedule of rest and activity adjusted to the child's condition. Since hepatitis type A is not infectious within a week or so after onset of jaundice, the child may feel well enough to resume school shortly thereafter. The parents are also cautioned about administering any medication to the child without the practitioner's knowledge, since normal doses of many drugs may become dangerous because of the liver's inability to detoxify and excrete them. Common drugs that are affected by hepatic failure include acetaminophen (Tylenol), ferrous sulfate (oral iron), and propoxyphene hydrochloride (Darvon).

Handwashing is the single most effective measure in prevention and control of hepatitis in any setting (for a discussion of preventive measures in the daycare center, see Chapter 15). Parents and children need an explanation of the usual ways in which hepatitis virus A (oral-fecal route) and hepatitis virus B (parenteral route) are spread; they may benefit from receiving written instructions.*

Hospitalized children are not usually isolated in a separate room unless they are fecally unreliable or incontinent or if their toys and other items might become contaminated with feces. They are discouraged from sharing their toys. For further discussion of infection control see Chapter 27.

For those children with type B virus who have a known or suspected history of illicit drug use, the nurse has the additional responsibility of helping them realize the associated dangers of drug abuse, stressing the parenteral mode of transmission, and encouraging them to seek counseling from a drug program.†

CIRRHOSIS

Cirrhosis, which means "yellow" and refers to the typical orange-colored nodules of a fibrotic liver, is a result (not a primary cause) of liver destruction. It represents the end stage of chronic disease in which there is generalized destruction of hepatic cells. Cirrhosis is not a common cause of morbidity or mortality in children; therefore the diagnosis may be easily missed. With the alarming escalation in the number of adolescents who are at risk for contracting hepatitis type B from illicit parenteral drug use, it is likely that the occurrence of cirrhosis in early adulthood will also increase. Likewise, improved treatment of genetic diseases, such as cystic fibrosis or sickle cell anemia, will also affect the number of children who are at risk for developing this complication.

Pathophysiology

Cirrhosis is believed to be the result of some type of injury or insult to the liver. The hepatocellular injury (with or without inflammation) activates fibroblasts that respond by synthesizing collagen, thus forming fibrous connective tissue. The balance among fibrogenesis, the mechanisms for fibrous tissue removal, and hepatocyte regeneration appear to determine the degree of permanent hepatic fibrosis.

Once mature fibrous tissue is formed, a vicious cycle ensues. Vascular pathways form within the fibrotic tissues, depriving hepatocytes of their blood supply. The consequent cellular hypoxia, inflammation, and necrosis stimulate further fibroblastic activity. As a result, normal hepatic architecture is sufficiently distorted to affect both hepatocellular function and hepatic blood circulation.

The consequences of liver malfunction are evident in the various processes that depend on the products of liver function. For example, diminished formation of blood proteins results in hypoproteinemia and impaired coagulation, inability to conjugate bilirubin produces jaundice, reduced bile causes malabsorption of fats, and depressed detoxification and destruction result in accumulation of toxic substances. Interference with liver circulation causes hypertension in the portal circulation. This, together with the decreased protein in the blood, leads to fluid accumulation in the abdomen (ascites).

Clinical Manifestations

Clinical manifestations depend on the etiology. In cirrhosis from congenital biliary atresia, jaundice is usually the first sign. In cirrhosis from other causes, the symptoms are usually vague and the onset is insidious. Not infrequently, the first evidence of severe liver failure is a complication such as failure to thrive, ascites, or bleeding esophageal varices. The three major complications of chronic liver disease are (1) bleeding from esophageal varices, (2) ascites, and (3) hepatic encephalopathy (hepatic coma).

Diagnostic Evaluation

Diagnosis rests on (1) the history, especially evidence of prior liver disease, such as hepatitis; (2) physical examination, particularly hepatosplenomegaly, and the cutaneous changes from hemodynamic alterations and increasing hormone levels; and (3) laboratory evaluation, especially liver function tests (see Table 33-7). Definitive diagnosis is based on liver biopsy evidence of histologic changes.

Therapeutic Management

There is no specific treatment for cirrhosis, except in those cases in which a treatable cause, such as an infection, exists. Therapy is directed primarily toward (1) frequent assessment of liver status with physical examination and liver function tests and (2) management of pathologic changes based on these findings. Liver transplant is becoming a more viable option for some children. Most of the liver transplant recipients are children with extrahepatic biliary atresia and biliary hypoplasia and those with metabolic disorders, such as glycogen storage disease (Gartner and others, 1984).

For cirrhosis uncomplicated by ascites or encephalopathy, the diet is one that provides sufficient calories and essential nutrients to maintain growth and prevent specific de-

*Home care instructions for preventing AIDS and hepatitis infection are available in Wong, D.L., and Whaley, L.F.: Clinical manual of pediatric nursing, ed. 3, St. Louis, 1990, Mosby–Year Book, Inc.

†See Nursing Care Plan: The Child with Acute Hepatitis in Wong, D.L., and Whaley, L.F.: Clinical manual of pediatric nursing, ed. 3, St. Louis, 1990, Mosby–Year Book, Inc.

ficiencies. A high-calorie diet with low or moderate fats, moderate high-quality protein, and high carbohydrates is recommended. In addition, supplements of water-soluble preparations of vitamins A, D, E, and K are given. In children with vitamin B_{12} deficiency, injectable supplements are necessary.

The child and parents are advised against strenuous physical exercise and cautioned about the role of trauma, infection, and hepatotoxic drugs as factors that can aggravate the condition.

Complications. The complications of cirrhosis require special treatment:

Hemorrhage from esophageal varices is managed, as in adults, with blood transfusions, fluid and electrolyte replacement, administration of vitamin B complex and vitamin K, and, in life-threatening bleeding, with a Sengstaken-Blakemore balloon tube and oxygen.

Ascites is managed with diuretics and restriction of dietary sodium, limitation of protein, and sometimes intravenous administration of albumin. Fluid restriction may be necessary, but drainage by paracentesis is rarely needed unless abdominal pain or respiratory distress is present.

Hepatic encephalopathy is related to the harmful effects of ammonia; therefore much of the management is aimed at reducing ammonia formation. Treatment attempts to (1) reduce dietary protein, (2) inhibit the growth of organisms active in the formation of ammonia by administration of lactulose, (3) reduce the bacterial flora by administration of antibiotics, and (4) correct any other causes that might precipitate coma, such as infections or fluid and electrolyte imbalances.

Nursing Considerations

Nursing objectives in caring for the child with cirrhosis depend on several factors, including the precipitating cause of the cirrhosis, the severity of complications, and the prognosis. Overall, the last factor has the greatest impact because the prognosis for life is poor. Since treatment of cirrhosis ideally is treatment of the cause, in many instances a fatal outcome is determined by the inability to surgically correct or reverse the underlying problem. Therefore nursing care of this child is the same as that for any ill child with a life-threatening illness (Chapter 23). Hospitalization is usually required when complications such as ascites, bleeding esophageal varices, or hepatic coma occur.

Prevention, however, is an important nursing responsibility in terms of those diseases that may ultimately lead to cirrhosis. For example, genetic counseling would reduce the number of children afflicted with many genetic-metabolic disorders, such as galactosemia, sickle cell disease, or cystic fibrosis. Proper prenatal care and immunization can lessen the possibility of neonatal hepatitis. Public health education regarding the dangers of hepatitis and in particular the usual modes of transmission of hepatitis B virus may eventually decrease the human reservoir.

KEY POINTS

- The essential functions of the GI system are to process and absorb nutrients necessary to maintain metabolic processes and support growth and development, to perform excretory functions, to provide detoxification, and to maintain fluid and electrolyte balance, especially in infancy.
- Digestion is the catabolism of foodstuffs (water, vitamins, mineral salts, carbohydrates, proteins, and fats) from their original complex form to simple, assimilable nutrients.
- The small intestine is the principal absorbing site in the GI system.
- Most ingested foreign bodies pass through the alimentary tract without difficulty. Those lodged in the esophagus require further evaluation.
- Constipation is usually managed by diet management and bowel training.
- Hirschsprung disease requires surgical removal of aganglionic segments of bowel.
- Nursing care of gastroesophageal reflux is aimed at identifying children with suggestive symptoms, helping parents with home care feeding and positioning, and caring for the child undergoing surgical intervention.
- Although the cause of appendicitis is poorly understood, it is commonly a result of obstruction of the lumen, usually by a fecalith. Common signs and symptoms are colicky abdominal pain, tenderness, and fever.
- Meckel diverticulum is a congenital malformation of the GI tract characterized by rectal bleeding.
- Inflammatory bowel disease refers to ulcerative colitis and Crohn disease. Persistent and recurring diarrhea is the most common feature.
- Management of IBD includes high-protein diet, vitamin/mineral supplements, sufasalazine and/or corticosteroids, antibiotics, and general supportive therapy. Surgical removal of inflamed bowel may be necessary.
- Peptic ulcers are poorly understood, but one of two mechanisms probably reflects the basic defect: an increase in the rate of production of gastric juice, or interference with the normal protective mechanisms of the mucosal lining.
- General signs of obstruction include colicky abdominal pain, nausea and vomiting, abdominal distention, and constipation.
- Hypertrophic pyloric stenosis is detected by observation of projectile vomiting without loss of appetite. Therapy is surgical pyloromyotomy.
- Intussusception is a cause of intestinal obstruction during infancy. Treatment is either nonsurgical hydrostatic reduction or surgical reduction.
- Malabsorption syndromes are disorders associated with some degree of impaired digestion and/or absorption. They include digestive defects, absorptive defects, and anatomic defects.

- Celiac disease, the second leading cause of malabsorption in children, is characterized by an intolerance for gluten. The major role of the nurse in the management of celiac disease is helping parents and child adhere to diet therapy and preventing infections.
- Viral hepatitis is caused by at least four types of virus—hepatitis A virus, hepatitis B virus, hepatitis D virus, and non-A, non-B virus.
- Hepatitis A virus is spread by the fecal-oral route, whereas hepatitis B virus is transmitted primarily by the parenteral route. The single most effective measure in prevention and control of hepatitis in any setting is handwashing.

REFERENCES

Abrahamian, F.P., and Lloyd-Still, J.D.: Chronic constipation in childhood: longitudinal study of 186 patients, J. Pediatr. Gastroenterol. Nutr. 3:460-467, 1984.

Ackerman, S.H., Manaker, S., and Cohen, M.I.: Recent separation and the onset of peptic ulcer disease in older children and adolescents, Psychosom. Med. 43:305-310, 1981.

American Academy of Pediatrics: Report of the Committee on Infectious Diseases, Elk Grove, IL, 1988, The Academy.

Barker, D.J.P., Morris, J., and Nelson, M.: Vegetable consumption and acute appendicitis in 59 areas in England and Wales, Br. Med. J. 292:927-930, 1986.

Belknap, W.M.: Sucking and swallowing disorders and gastroesophageal reflux. In Aski, F.A., and others, editors: Principles and Practice of Pediatrics, Philadelphia, 1990, J.B. Lippincott Co.

Berry, J., Jr., and Malt, R.A.: Appendicitis near its centenary, Ann. Surg. 200:567-575, 1984.

Bines, J.E., and Walker, W.A.: Advances in inflammatory bowel disease, Curr. Opin. Pediatr. 1:48-56, 1989.

Bonadio, W.A., and others: Esophageal bougienage technique for coin ingestion in children, J. Pediatr. Surg. 23:917-918, 1988.

Bouchier, I.A.D.: Textbook of gastroenterology, London, 1984, W.B. Saunders Co.

Brender, J.D., and others: Childhood appendicitis: factors associated with perforation, Pediatrics 76(2):301-306, 1985a.

Brender, J.D., and others: Fiber intake and childhood appendicitis, Am. J. Public Health 75(4):399-400, 1985b.

Caravati, E.M., Bennett, D.L., and McElwee, N.E.: Pediatric coin ingestion: a prospective study on the utility of routine roentgenograms, Am. J. Dis. Child. 143:549-551, 1989.

Carcassonne, M., and others: Surgery of gastroesophageal reflux, World J. Surg. 9:269-276, 1985.

Cassell, B.L.: The new trend in ileostomy surgery, RN 47(1):48-51, 1984.

Chen, D., and Sullivan, B.: Constipation, Pediatrics 77:933, 1986.

Cohen, F.L.: Clinical genetics in nursing practice, Philadelphia, 1984, J.B. Lippincott Co.

Corazziari, E., and others: Gastrointestinal transit time, frequency of defecation, and anorectal manometry in healthy and constipated children, J. Pediatr. 106(3):379-382, 1985.

Davidson, M.: Overview of therapy for irritable bowel syndrome, Pediatr. Ann. 116:831-833, 1987.

Drumm, B., and others: *Campylobacter pyloridis*–associated primary gastritis in children, Pediatrics 80:192-195, 1987.

Friede, A., and others: Transmission of hepatitis b virus from adopted Asian children to their American families, Am. J. Public Health 78:26-29, 1988.

Gartner, J.C., and others: Orthotopic liver transplantation in children: two-year experience with 47 patients, Pediatrics 74(1):140-145, 1984.

Gracia, C., Frey, C.F., and Balaz, I.B.: Diagnosis and management of ingested foreign bodies: a ten-year experience, Ann. Emerg. Med. 13:30-34, 1984.

Guo, J., and others: Results of air pressure enema reduction of intussusception: 6,396 cases in 13 years, J. Pediatr. Surg. 21:1201-1203, 1986.

Hartwig, M.S.: Sticking to a gluten-free diet, Am. J. Nurs. 83(9):1308-1310, 1983.

Johns, C.: Encopresis, Am. J. Nurs. 85(2):153-156, 1985.

Jordan, F.T., Coran, A.G., and Wesley, J.R.: Modified endorectal procedure for management of long-segment aganglionosis, Ann. Surg. 194(1):70-75, 1981.

Joseph, P.R.: Management of coin ingestion, Am. J. Dis. Child. 143:449-450, 1990.

Kilbridge, P.M., Dahms, B.B., and Czinn, S.J.: *Campylobacter pylori*–associated gastritis and peptic ulcer disease in children, Am. J. Dis. Child. 142:1149-1152, 1988.

Kirschner, B.S.: Inflammatory bowel disease in children, Pediatr. Clin. North Am. 35:189-208, 1988.

Klish, W.J.: Chronic nonspecific diarrhea of childhood. In Oski, F.A., and others, editors: Principles and practice of pediatrics, Philadelphia, 1990, J.B. Lippincott Co.

Klish, W.J., and Putnam, T.C.: The short gut, Am. J. Dis. Child. 135:1056-1061, 1981.

Koletzko, S., and others: Role of infant feeding practices in development of Crohn's disease in childhood, Br. Med. J. 298:1617-1618, 1989.

Krugman, S.: Viral hepatitis: 1985 update, Pediatr. Rev. 7(1):3-11, 1985.

Krugman, S., and others: Infectious diseases of children, ed. 8, St. Louis, 1985, Mosby–Year Book, Inc.

Landman, G.B.: A five-year chart review of children biopsied to rule out Hirschsprung's disease, Clin. Pediatr. 26:288-291, 1987.

Levine, J.J.: Chronic nonspecific diarrhea, Pediatr. Ann. 16:821-829, 1987.

Litovitz, T.L.: Battery ingestions: product accessibility and clinical course, Pediatrics 75(3):469-476, 1985.

Martin, L.W., and Torres, A.M.: Hirschsprung's disease, Surg. Clin. North Am. 65(5):1171-1180, 1985.

Marwick, C., and Simmons, K.: Changing childhood disease pattern linked with day-care boom, JAMA 251:1245-1251, 1984.

Mathewson, M., and Farnham, C.: Milk therapy in ulcer disease: yes or no? Home Healthc. Nurse 2(4):8, 1984.

Motil, K.J.: Peptic ulcer disease. In Oski, F.A., and others, editors: Principles and practice of pediatrics, Philadelphia, 1990, J.B. Lippincott Co.

Motil, K.J., and Grand, R.J.: Nutritional management of inflammatory bowel disease, Pediatr. Clin. North Am. 32 (2):447-469, 1985.

Mowat, A.P.: Selected developments in pediatric hepatology, Curr. Opin. Pediatr. 1:369-379, 1989.

Newman, J., and Schuh, S.: Intussusception in babies under 4 months of age, Can. Med. Assoc. J. 136:266-269, 1987.

Nord, K.S.: Peptic ulcer disease in the pediatric population, Pediatr. Clin. North Am. 35:117-140, 1988.

Okorie, N.M., and others: What happens to the pylorus after pyloromyotomy? Arch. Dis. Child. 63:1339-1340, 1988.

Olness, K.: Constipation and soiling, Pediatr. Basics 38:4-7, 1984.

O'Regan, S., and others: Constipation a commonly unrecognized cause of enuresis, Am. J. Dis. Child. 140(3):260-261, 1986.

Orenstein, S.R.: Effect of nonnutritive sucking on infant gastresophageal reflux, Pediatr. Res. 24:38-40, 1988.

Orenstein, S.R., and Whitington, P.F.: Positioning for prevention of infant gastroesophageal reflux, J. Pediatr. 103(4):534-537, 1983.

Pettei, M.J.: Chronic constipation, Pediatr. Ann. 16:796-813, 1987.

Polley, T.Z., Jr., Coran, A.G., and Wesley, J.R.: A ten-year experience with ninety-two cases of Hirschsprung's disease, Ann. Surg. 202(3):349-354, 1985.

Rappaport, L.A., and Levine, M.D.: The prevention of constipation and encopresis: a developmental model approach, Pediatr. Clin. North Am. 33:859-869, 1986.
Reijnin, J.A.M., and others: Intussusception in older children, Br. J. Surg. 74:692-693, 1987.
Savilahti, E., and others: Celiac disease in insulin-dependent diabetes mellitus, J. Pediatr. 108(1):690-693, 1986.
Schunk, J.E., Corneli, H., and Bolte, R.: Pediatric coin ingestions: a prospective study of coin location and symptoms, Am. J. Dis. Child. 143:546-548, 1989.
Sibinga, M.S.: The gastrointestinal tract. In Levine, M.D., and others, editors: Developmental-behavioral pediatrics, Philadelphia, 1983, W.B. Saunders Co.
Silverman, A., and Roy, C.C.: Pediatric clinical gastroenterology, ed. 3, St. Louis, 1983, Mosby–Year Book, Inc.
Sutphen, J.L., Dillard, V.L., and Pipan, M.E.: Antacid and formula effects on gastric acidity in infants with gastroesophagal reflux, Pediatrics 78:55-57, 1986.
Tamanaha, K., and others: Air reduction of intussusception in infants and children, J. Pediatr. 111:733-736, 1987.
Wang, G., and Liu, S.: Enema reduction of intussusception by hydrostatic pressure under ultrasound guidance: a report of 377 cases, J. Pediatr. Surg. 23:814-818, 1988.
Webb, W.A., McDaniel, L., and Jones, L.: Foreign bodies of the upper gastrointestinal tract: current management, South. Med. J. 77:1083-1086, 1984.
Wessel, M.A., and McCullough, W.B.: Bereavement—an etiologic factor in peptic ulcer in childhood and adolescence, J. Adolesc. Health Care 2:287-288, 1982.
Whittington, P.F.: Digestive system. In Summitt, R.L., editor: Comprehensive pediatrics, St. Louis, 1990, Mosby–Year Book, Inc.

BIBLIOGRAPHY

General

Adams, D.A., and Selekof, J.L.: Children with ostomies: comprehensive care planning, Pediatr. Nurs. 12:429-433, 1986.
Alterescu, K.B.: The ostomy: what about special procedures? Am. J. Nurs. 85(12):1363-1367, 1985.
American Academy of Pediatrics, Committee on Infectious Diseases, Committee on Drugs, and Section on Surgery: Antimicrobial prophylaxis for pediatric surgical patients, Pediatrics 74:437-439, 1984.
Boarini, J.: The ostomy: what can go wrong? Am. J. Nurs. 85(12):1358-1362, 1985.
Boyle, J.T.: Upper gastrointestinal tract, Curr. Opin. Pediatr. 1:350-357, 1989.
Broadwell, D.C.: Continent ileostomy and ileoanal reservoir: two surgical alternatives for patients once requiring conventional ileostomies, Point of View 23(3):12-15, 1986.
Dalton-Loehner, D., and Connor, P.A.: Beyond ileostomy: surgery for a normal life, RN 52(7):29-33, 1989.
Friedman, E.M.: Caustic ingestions and foreign bodies in the aerodigestive tract of children, Pediatr. Clin. North Am. 36:1403-1410, 1989.
Konings, K.: Preop use of Golytely in pediatrics, Pediatr. Nurs. 15:473-474, 1989.
Lenaerts, C., and others: High incidence of upper gastrointestinal tract involvement in childen with Crohn disease, Pediatrics 83:777-781, 1989.
Milla, P.J.: Small intestine and colon: pathophysiology and therapeutics, Curr. Opin. Pediatr. 1:358-362, 1989.
Milov, D.E., and Andres, J.M.: Sorting out the causes of rectal bleeding, Contemp. Pediatr. 5(10):80-104, 1988.
Neufeldt, J.: Helping the I.B.D. patient cope with the unpredictable, Nursing '87 17(8):47-49, 1987.
Ross, A.J.: The delicate matter of the damaged spleen, Contemp. Pediatr. 6(8):111-122, 1989.
Tranes, S.: Ileal pull-through surgery, Nursing '87 17(11):92, 1987.

Assessment of Gastrointestinal Function

Ament, M.E., and others: Fiberoptic upper intestinal endoscopy in infants and children, Pediatr. Clin. North Am. 35:141-155, 1988.
Bagnell, P.C.: Evaluation and examination of the gastrointestinal tract in children, Curr. Opin. Pediatr. 1:339-344, 1989.
Caulfield, M., and others: Upper gastrointestinal tract endoscopy in the pediatric patient, J. Pediatr. 115:339-3445, 1989.
Harris, J.A.: Pediatric abdominal assessment, Pediatr. Nurs. 12:355-362, 1986.
Jonas, M.M.: Gastrointestinal disease symptoms, Curr. Opin. Pediatr. 1:345-349, 1989.
Kane, N.M., and others: Pediatric abdominal trauma: evaluation by computed tomography, Pediatrics 82:11-15, 1988.
Levine, J.J., Seidman, E., and Walker, W.A.: Screening tests for enteropathy in children, Am. J. Dis. Child. 141:435-438, 1987.
Riddlesberger, M.M., Jr.: Evaluation of the gastrointestinal tract in the child: CT, MRI, and isotopic studies, Pediatr. Clin. North Am. 35:281-310, 1988.
Rossi, T.: Endoscopic examination of the colon in infancy and childhood, Pediatr. Clin. North Am. 35:331-356, 1988.
Smith, C.E.: Assessing bowel sounds, Nursing '88 18(2):42-43, 1988.
Steffen, R.M., and others: Colonoscopy in the pediatric patient, J. Pediatr. 115:507-514, 1989.
Tollison, A.A.: Danger signs: rebound tenderness, Nursing '88 18(2):78-79, 1988.
Winter, H.S.: Breath tests as a diagnostic technique for malabsorption, Pediatr. Ann. 16:258-262, 1987.

Disorders of Motility

Aquilina, S.S.: Gastroesophageal reflux: problem or nuisance? J. Pediatr. Health Care 1:233-239, 1987.
Bailey, D.J., and others: Lack of efficacy of thickened feedings as treatment for gastroesophageal reflux, J. Pediatr. 110:187-189, 1987.
Blount, W.: Gastroesophageal reflux in children, Am. Family Physician 37:201-216, 1988.
Boarini, J.: The ostomy: what can go wrong? Am. J. Nurs. 85(12):1358-1362, 1985.
Cerrato, P.L.: What to tell your patients about dietary fiber, RN 50(1):63-64, 1987.
Grill, B.B., and others: Effects of domperidone therapy on symptoms and upper gastrointestinal motility in infants with gastroesophageal reflux, J. Pediatr. 106(2):311-316, 1985.
Kurer, M., Lowson, J., and Pambakian, H.: Techniques for diagnosing suction biopsy of Hirschsprung's disease, Arch. Dis. Child. 61(1):83-84, 1986.
Levine, J.J.: Chronic nonspecific diarrhea, Pediatr. Ann. 16:821-829, 1987.
Lynn, M.R.: Use of infant seats for gastroesophageal reflux, J. Pediatr. Nurs. 1(2):127-129, 1986.
Milla, P.J.: Gastrointestinal motility disorders in children, Pediatr. Clin. North Am. 35:311-330, 1988.
Opie, J.C., Chaye, H., and Fraser, G.C.: Fundoplication and pediatric esophageal manometry: actuarial analysis over 7 years, J. Pediatr. Surg. 22:935-938, 1987.
Orenstein, S.R., Magill, H.L., and Brooks, P.: Thickening of infant feedings for therapy of gastroesophageal reflux, J. Pediatr. 110:181-186, 1987.
Orenstein, S.R., and Orenstein, D.M.: Gastroesophageal reflux and respiratory disease in children, J. Pediatr. 112:847-858, 1988.
Petersen, M.: Esophageal pH monitoring, J. Pediatr. Nurs. 1:354-357, 1986.
Scallen, C., Puri, P., and Reen, D.: Identification of rectal ganglion cells using monoclonal antibodies, J. Pediatr. Surg. 20(1):37-40, 1985.
Shepherd, R.W., and others: Gastroesophageal reflux in children, Clin. Pediatr. 26:55-59, 1987.

Sondheimer, J.M.: Gastroesophageal reflux: update on pathogenesis and diagnosis, Pediatr. Clin. North Am. 35:103-116, 1988.

Trowell, H., and Burkitt, D.: Physiological role of dietary fiber: a ten-year review, Contemp. Nutr. 11:1-2, 1986.

Tunell, W.P.: Gastroesophageal reflux in childhood: implications for surgical treatment, Pediatr. Ann. 18:192-196, 1989.

Zahr, L.K., and Trentini, P.: Gastroesophageal reflux, fundoplication, and dumping: literature review and case study, Issues Compr. Pediatr. Nurs. 12:385-393, 1989.

Inflammatory Conditions

Adkins, R.B., Jr., and others: The management of gastric ulcers: a current review, Ann. Surg. 201(6):741-750, 1985.

Brender, J.D., and others: Fiber intake and childhood appendicitis, Am. J. Public Health 75:399-400, 1985.

Blumer, J.L., and others: Pharmacokinetic determination of ranitidine pharmacodynamics in pediatric ulcer disease, J. Pediatr. 107(2):301-306, 1985.

Dickson, A.P., and MacKinlay, G.A.: Rectal examination and acute appendicitis, Arch. Dis. Child. 60(7):666-676, 1985.

Edwinson, M., Arnbjórnsson, E., and Ekman, R.: Psychologic preparation program for children undergoing acute appendectomy, Pediatrics 82:30-36, 1988.

Ellett, M.L., and Schibler, K.: Adolescent psychosocial adaptation to inflammatory bowel disease, J. Pediatr. Health Care 2:57-66, 1988.

Farley, J.: Facts and myths about gastrointestinal bleeding, Nursing 88 18(3):25, 1988.

Galladay, E.S., and others: Delayed diagnosis in pediatric appendicitis, South. Med. J. 81:38-42, 1988.

Lessman, M.: Painful chronicle, Am. J. Nurs. 85(5):551-552, 1985.

Lewicki, L.J., and Leeson, M.J.: The multisystem impact on physiologic processes of inflammatory bowel disease, Nurs. Clin. North Am. 19(1):71-80, 1984.

Meyers, S., and others: Fecal alpha-1-antitrypsin measurement: an indicator of Crohn's disease activity, Gastroenterology 89(1):13-18, 1985.

Mezoff, A., and Balistreri, W.F.: New GI therapies: any better than antacids? Contemp. Pediatr. 7(4):101-123, 1990.

Motil, K.J., Altchuler, S.I., and Grand, R.J.: Mineral balance during nutritional supplementation in adolescents with Crohn disease and growth failure, J. Pediatr. 107(3):473-479, 1985.

Postuma, R., and Moroz, S.P.: Pediatric Crohn's disease, J. Pediatr. Surg. 20(5):478-482, 1985.

Soll, A.H.: Pathogenesis of peptic ulcer and implications for therapy, N. Engl. J. Med. 322:909-916, 1990.

Stotts, N.A., Fitzgerald, K.A., and Williams, K.R.: Care of the patient critically ill with inflammatory bowel disease, Nurs. Clin. North Am. 19(1):61-70, 1984.

Wormsley, K.G.: Maintenance treatment with H_2 receptor antagonists in patients with peptic ulcer disease: reduces morbidity in a significant minority of patients, Br. J. Med. 297:1392-1394, 1988.

Obstruction

Breaux, C.W., Jr., and others: Changing patterns in the diagnosis of hypertrophic pyloric stenosis, Pediatrics 81:213-217, 1988.

Breaux, C.W., Jr., and others: The significance of alkalosis and hypochloremia in hypertrophic pyloric stenosis, J. Pediatr. Surg. 24:1250-1252, 1989.

Cargile, N.D.: Buying time when you face a bowel obstruction, RN 48(8):40-46, 1985.

Foley, L.C., and others: Evaluation of the vomiting infant, Am. J. Dis. Child. 143:660-661, 1989.

Jedd, M.B., and others: Factors associated with infantile hypertrophic pyloric stenosis, Am. J. Dis. Child. 142:334-337, 1988.

McConnell, E.A.: Meeting the challenge of intestinal obstruction, Nursing '87 17(7):34-41, 1987.

Puri, P., and Guiney, E.J.: Small bowel tumours causing intussusception in childhood, Br. J. Surg. 72(6):493-494, 1985.

Rollins, M.D., and others: Pyloric stenosis: congenital or acquired? Arch. Dis. Child. 64:138-147, 1989.

Touloukian, R.J., and others: Analgesic premedication in the management of ileocolic intussusception, Pediatrics 79:432-434, 1987.

Malabsorption Syndromes

Anson, O., Weizman, Z., and Zeevi, N.: Celiac disease: parental knowledge and attitudes of dietary compliance, Pediatrics 85:98-103, 1990.

Auricchio, S, Greco, L., and Troncone, R.: Gluten-sensitive enteropathy in childhood, Pediatr. Clin. North Am. 35:157-187, 1988.

Cacciari, E., and others: Can antigliadin antibody detect symptomless celiac disease in children with short stature? Lancet 1(8444):1469-1471, 1985.

Chuan-Hao, L., and others: Nutritional assessment of children with short-bowel syndrome receiving home parenteral nutrition, Am. J. Dis. Child. 141:1093-1098, 1987.

Gantt, L., and Thompson, C.: Short gut syndrome in the infant, Am. J. Nurs. 85(11):1263-1266, 1985.

Thompson, J.S.: The current status of surgical therapy for the short bowel syndrome, Contemp. Surg. 33(12):27-32, 1988.

Tucker, N.T., and others: Antigliadin antibodies detected by enzyme-linked immunosorbent assay as a marker of childhood celiac disease, J. Pediatr. 113:286-289, 1988.

Hepatic Disorders

Balisteri, W.F.: Viral hepatitis, Pediatr. Clin. North Am. 35:637-669, 1988.

Brady, M.: Preventing the perinatal spread of hepatitis, Br. J. Pediatr. Health Care 3:49-51, 1989.

Brainerd, E.: Nursing management of chronic infectious diseases in children, Pediatr. Nurs. Update 1(17):2-7, 1986.

Chin, J.: Prevention of chronic hepatitis B virus infection from mothers to infants in the United States, Pediatrics 71(2):289-292, 1983.

Crawford, F., and Vermund, S.H.: Hepatitis A in day care centers, J. Sch. Health 55:378-380, 1985.

Edwards, M.S.: Hepatitis B serology—help in interpretation, Pediatr. Clin. North Am. 35:503-515, 1988.

Fredette, S.L.: When the liver fails, Am. J. Nurs. 84(1):64-67, 1984.

Genesca, J., Esteban, J.I., and Esteban, R.: Hepatitis B immunoprophylaxis of low-birth-weight infants, Pediatrics 76(6):1020, 1985.

Guenter, P.: Hepatic disease: nutritional implications, Nurs. Clin. North Am. 18:71-80, 1983.

Gurevich, I.: Viral hepatitis, Am. J. Nurs. 83:572-586, 1983.

Keith, J.S.: Hepatic failure: etiologies, manifestations, and management, Crit. Care Nurse 5(1):60-86, 1985.

Kirkman-Liff, B., and Dandoy, S.: Hepatitis B: what price exposure? Am. J. Nurs. 84(4):988-990, 1984.

Pachter, A.: Should nurses receive the hepatitis B vaccination? Nursing '88 18(6):51, 1988.

Poss, J.E.: Hepatitis B virus infection in Southeast Asian children, J. Pediatr. Health Care 3:311-315, 1989.

West, D.J., Calandra, G.B., and Ellis, R.W.: Vaccination of infants and children against hepatitis B, Pediatr. Clin. North Am. 37:585-601, 1990.

Wimpsett, J.: Trace your patient's liver dysfunction, Nursing '84 14(8):56-57, 1984.

Withers, J., and Bradshaw, E.: Preventing neonatal hepatitis-B infection, MCN 11:270-272, 1986.

Xu, Z., and others: Prevention of perinatal acquisition of hepatitis B virus carriage using vaccine: preliminary report of a randomized, double-blind placebo-controlled and comparative trial, Pediatrics 76(5):713-718, 1985.

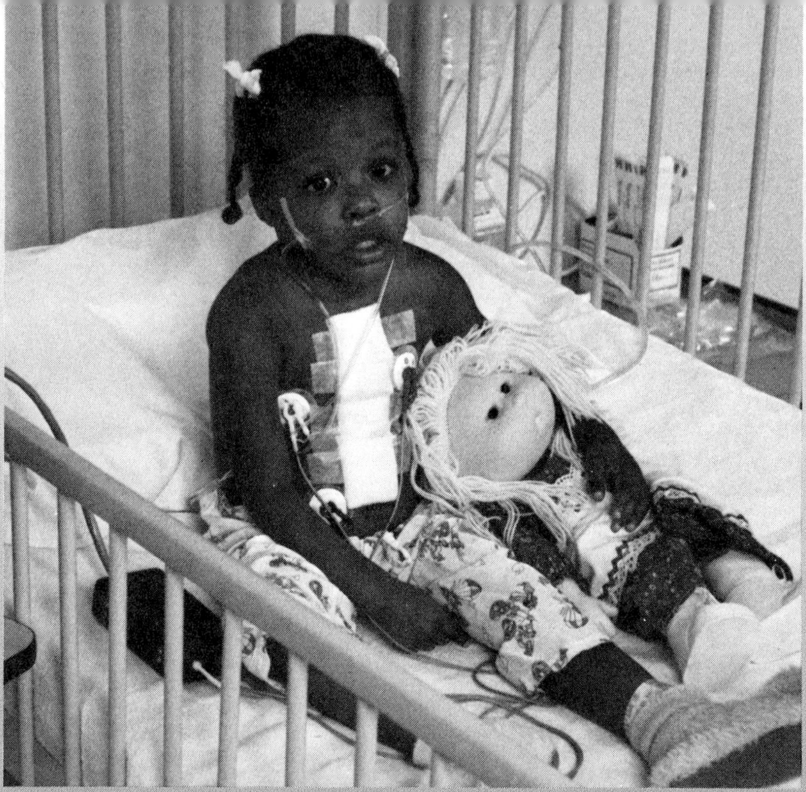

The Child with Problems Related to Production and Circulation of Blood

UNIT XII

Some of the most common and serious childhood conditions are related to the heart and formed elements of the blood. Many of these disorders, especially those of the blood, are inherited and present at birth, whereas others are acquired. Most of them necessitate medical and/or surgical intervention to prevent complications, some of which can be life-threatening. Nursing care at the time of diagnosis, before and during corrective/palliative procedures, and after treatment is essential to promote physical and emotional recovery.

Chapter 34, *The Child with Cardiovascular Dysfunction,* discusses the types of congenital and acquired cardiac disorders and the physical consequences of impaired functioning. It focuses on caring for the child with heart disease, preparation of the family for diagnostic procedures and surgery, and postoperative nursing interventions, including discharge planning for home care. Chapter 35, *The Child with Hematologic or Immunologic Dysfunction,* deals with several disorders related to the formed elements of the blood. Since many of these conditions are inherited and chronic, nursing interventions stress helping the family adjust to the disorder and cope with and prevent its complications.

CHAPTER 34

The Child with Cardiovascular Dysfunction

RELATED TOPICS

Birth of a child with a physical defect, Ch. 11
Compliance, Ch. 27
Controlling elevated temperatures, Ch. 27
Heart (physical assessment), Ch. 7
High risk related to cardiovascular complications, Ch. 10
Impact of chronic illness or disability on the child and family, Ch. 22
Impact of life-threatening illness on the child and family, Ch. 23
Neonatal loss, Ch. 10
Neonatal pain, Ch. 11
Nursing care of the surgical neonate, Ch. 11
Pain assessment; pain management, Ch. 26
Physiologic measurements, Ch. 7
Preparation for procedures, Ch. 27
Skin (physical assessment), Ch. 7
Surgical procedures, Ch. 27
Tissue donation/autopsy, Ch. 23
Transplantation, Ch. 30
Vulnerable child syndrome, p. 411

GLOSSARY

ACE Angiotensin-converting enzyme
afterload Pressure that heart must pump against
AS Aortic stenosis
ASD Atrial septal defect
A-V Atrioventricular
AVC Atrioventricular canal
BE Bacterial endocarditis
bradycardia Abnormally slow heart rate
bradydysrhythmia Abnormally slow heart rate: may have irregular rhythm
cardiac cycle Sequential contraction (systole) and dilatation (diastole) of heart chambers

cardiac output Blood volume ejected by heart in 1 minute
cardiomegaly Enlargement of heart muscle
CHD Congenital heart disease
CHF Congestive heart failure
COA Coarctation of aorta
contractility Ability of heart muscle to pump
corrective procedure Surgical intervention that restores normal circulatory patterns, but does not necessarily create a normal heart
CVA Cerebrovascular accident
CVP Central venous pressure
cyanosis Bluish color in skin from reduced oxygen saturation
diastole Period of dilatation of heart, especially of ventricles
dysrhythmia Abnormal heart rhythm
ECG, EKG Electrocardiogram
ET tube Endotracheal tube
HDL High-density lipoprotein
hemodynamic Pertaining to movements involved in circulation of blood
HLHS Hypoplastic left heart syndrome
HR Heart rate
hypercholesterolemia Elevated level of serum cholesterol
hypercyanotic spells Presence of acute cyanosis and hyperpnea (also called "tet" or "blue" spells)
hyperlipidemia Elevated level of serum lipids
hypoxemia Arterial oxygen tension less than normal
hypoxic Reduction in tissue oxygenation
IVC Inferior vena cava
KD Kawasaki disease
LA Left atrium
LDL Low-density lipoprotein
LV Left ventricle
PA Pulmonary artery
palliative procedure Intervention, such as creating a shunt, that temporarily improves hemodynamic functioning until corrective repair can be performed
Pao_2 Arterial oxygen pressure
PDA Patent ductus arteriosus
polycythemia Increased number of red blood cells
preload Circulating blood volume returning to heart
PS Pulmonic stenosis
pulmonary hypertension Increased arterial pressure in pulmonary vessels
pulmonary vascular resistance (PVR) Pressure exerted by blood vessels in lungs
PV Pulmonary valve
RA Right atrium
RF Rheumatic fever
RV Right ventricle
stroke volume Volume of blood ejected by heart during one contraction
SVC Superior vena cava
SVT Supraventricular tachycardia
systemic perfusion Circulation of blood to tissues throughout body
systemic vascular resistance (SVR) Pressure exerted by arteries and veins in systemic (body) circulation
systole Period of contraction of heart, especially of ventricles
tachycardia Abnormally rapid heart rate
tachydysrhythmia Abnormally rapid heart rate
TAPVC Total anomalous pulmonary venous connection
TC Total cholesterol
TGA Transposition of great arteries
TOF Tetralogy of Fallot
VLDL Very-low-density lipoprotein
VSD Ventricular septal defect

Cardiovascular disorders in children are divided into two major groups, congenital cardiac defects and acquired heart disorders. *Congenital heart defects* are anatomic abnormalities present at birth that result in abnormal cardiac function. The clinical consequences of congenital heart defects fall into two broad categories, congestive heart failure and hypoxemia. *Acquired cardiac disorders* refer to disease processes or abnormalities that occur after birth and can be seen in the normal heart or in the presence of congenital heart defects. They result from various factors, including infection, autoimmune responses, environmental factors, and familial tendencies.

Any disorder that affects the heart provokes anxiety in the family. To help the child and family adjust to a heart condition and to prepare them for the medical and/or surgical management require guidance and support from many health professionals, particularly nurses.

Patricia O'Brien, R.N.,C., M.S.N., P.N.P. (section editor); Annette L. Baker, R.N., M.S.N.; Jeanne T. Boisvert, R.N., B.S.N.; Ann Burns Gerraughty, R.N., M.S.; Lindyce A. Kulik, R.N., B.S.N.; Paula Moynihan, R.N., B.S.N.; Patricia A. O'Hara, R.N., B.S.N.; Suzanne J. Reidy, R.N., B.S.N.; Carole T. Roberts, R.N., M.S., P.N.P.; Patricia Rotondi, R.N., M.S.; and Allison T. Weber, R.N., B.S.N., assisted in the revision of this chapter.

CARDIAC STRUCTURE AND FUNCTION

Understanding the effects of congenital and acquired heart defects requires knowledge of the normal heart's structure and function, including embryologic development, fetal circulation, and the changes that occur with postnatal growth. Basic cardiac physiology is presented in this section; Altered hemodynamics are discussed on p. 1541.

CARDIAC DEVELOPMENT AND FUNCTION

The heart is a muscular four-chambered organ whose primary purpose is to pump blood throughout the body. It is located slightly to the left of the sternum in the space between the two pleural cavities, called the *mediastinum.* The main mass of the heart is formed by the muscular tissue, the *myocardium.* Lining the inner surface of the myocardium is the *endocardium,* a thin layer of endothelial tissue. The heart also has its own special covering, a double-walled membrane called the *pericardium.* Between the two layers is a slight space *(pericardial space),* which is filled with a few drops of serous fluid *(pericardial fluid).* These layers provide for frictionless movement of the heart muscle.

The interior of the heart is divided into four chambers. The two upper chambers are called *atria* and include a right atrium (RA) and a left atrium (LA). The two bottom chambers are *ventricles,* a right ventricle (RV) and a left ventricle (LV). The chambers are separated by walls called the atrial septum and ventricular septum. Located within the heart chambers are four *valves,* whose main function is to prevent the backflow of blood. The valves are attached to the heart muscle by several cordlike structures called *chordae tendineae.* The *tricuspid* valve, so named because it has three flaps or cusps of endocardial tissue projecting into the ventricles, is located between the RA and RV. The *bicuspid,* or *mitral,* valve has two flaps and is located between the LA and LV. Together these two valves are often termed *atrioventricular* (A-V) valves. The *semilunar* valves are located in the pulmonary artery (PA) (*pulmonic* valve) and the aorta (*aortic* valve). Heart sounds (S_1 and S_2) are thought to be related to the vibrations that result during closing of these valves (see Chapter 7).

Embryologic Development

The heart and other components of the circulatory system (blood, blood vessels, lymph) develop from the mesoderm beginning during the fourth week of gestation and are completed by the eighth week. Cardiac development parallels the embryo's increasing nutritional needs.

During the third week, two endocardial tubes fuse to become the heart tube. As the tube elongates, it begins to coil to the right (dextra or D-looping). This looping occurs by approximately the twenty-eighth day, when the heart begins to beat. Concentrations of mesenchymal cells enlarge and cause their lining (endocardium) to bulge into the heart lumen. These internal bulges are called *endocardial cushions* and eventually merge to divide the heart chambers.

The developing heart tube bulges until it finally lies in the pericardial cavity. The tube remains attached to the pericardium at its cephalic and caudal ends but is free at the midsection. During the fifth week the midcardiac tube grows rapidly and assumes a characteristic convoluted shape with identifiable structures. These structures ultimately give rise to the heart chambers and vessels and include (1) a *common atrium;* (2) a *common ventricle;* (3) the *bulbus cordis,* which eventually helps form the outflow tracts of the ventricles; (4) the *sinus venosus,* which develops into the *inferior* and *superior vena cava* and *coronary sinus;* and (5) the *truncus arteriosus,* which divides into the PA and aorta and also gives rise to the aortic arch.

The formation of the heart's internal structures, particularly the cardiac septa (partitions), takes place almost simultaneously. The *atrial septum* is formed by the growth of both the *septum primum* and the *septum secundum* at about the fourth week of fetal growth. Overlapping of the septum primum and septum secundum before fusion results in a temporary flap opening known as the *foramen ovale.*

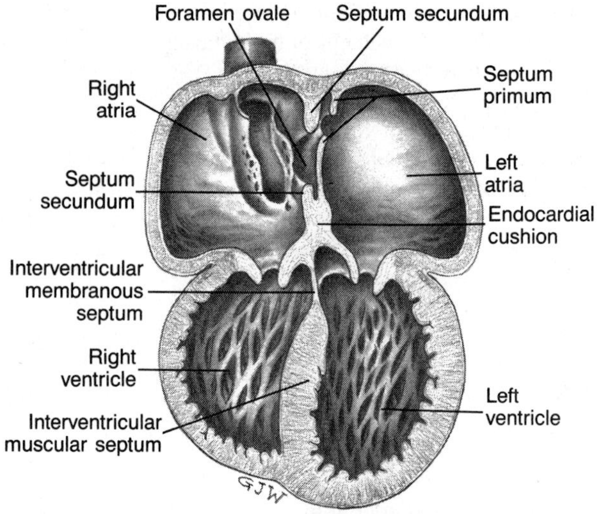

Fig. 34-1. Septal development of the heart.

The *ventricular septum* develops from the joining of the muscular and membranous ventricular septa during the fourth to eighth weeks of growth. The *muscular septum* develops when the right and left ventricular chambers fuse, whereas the *membranous septum* develops out of an intricate growth of the endocardial cushions, conal cushions, and conotruncal septum (Fig. 34-1). During this partitioning process, congenital defects may result if the formation of various structures is disturbed. The structure of the fetal heart provides for a pattern of circulation that is very different from that required during postnatal life. During prenatal life the heart distributes oxygen and nutrients, supplied via the placenta, to the developing fetus through an efficient system of shunts that partially bypass the nonfunctioning lungs.

Fetal circulation. The normal growth and development of the fetus rely on an active, independent metabolism but also require an efficient circulation. During fetal life the lungs are essentially nonfunctional and the liver is only partially functional; therefore less blood is needed in these organs than is required after birth. The fetal brain requires the highest oxygen concentration, and the heart must pump a large amount of blood through the placenta. The characteristics of fetal circulation ensure that the most vital organs and tissues receive the maximum concentration of vital materials for growth.

Blood carrying oxygen and nutritive materials from the placenta enters the fetal system through the umbilicus via the large umbilical vein (Fig. 34-2, *A*). The blood then travels upward to the underside of the liver, where it separates; part of the blood enters the portal and hepatic circulation of the liver, and the remainder travels directly to the inferior

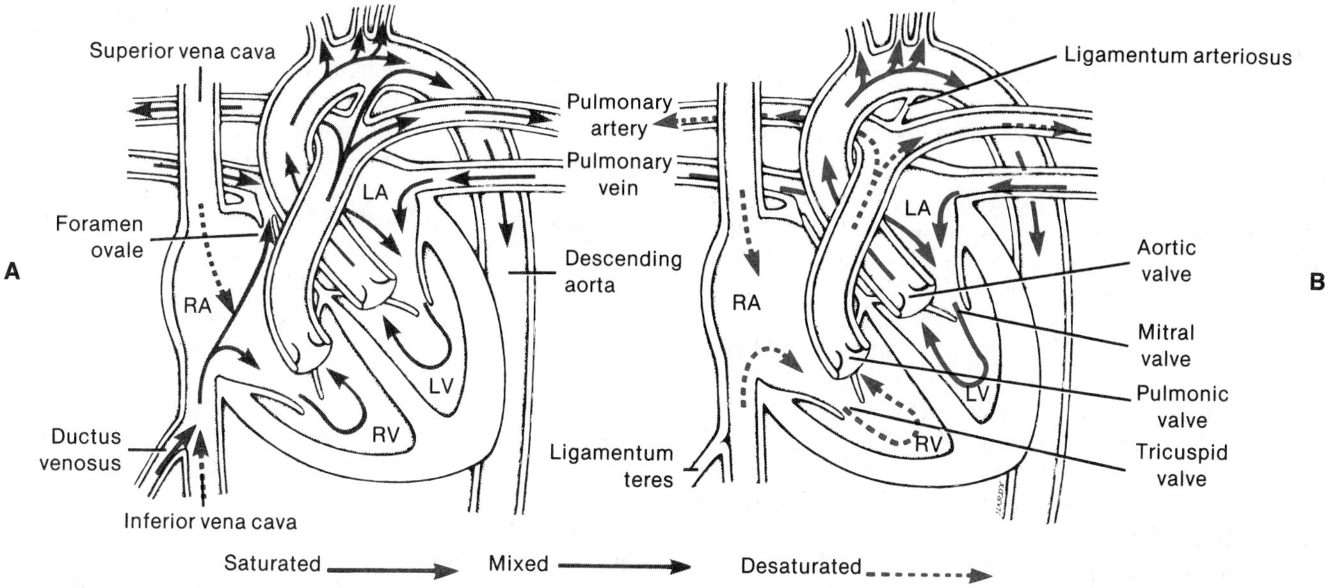

Fig. 34-2. Changes in circulation at birth. **A,** Prenatal circulation. **B,** Postnatal circulation. Arrows indicate direction of blood flow. Although four pulmonary veins enter the LA, for simplicity this diagram shows only two. See Glossary (p. 1530) for abbreviations.

vena cava (IVC) by way of the *ductus venosus.* Because of the higher pressure of blood entering the RA from the IVC, it is directed posteriorly in a straight pathway across the RA and through the foramen ovale to the LA. In this way the better-oxygenated blood enters the LA and LV to be pumped through the aorta to the head and upper extremities. Blood from the head and upper extremities entering the RA from the superior vena cava (SVC) is directed downward through the tricuspid valve into the RV. From here it is pumped through the PA, where the major portion is shunted to the descending aorta via the *ductus arteriosus.* A small amount flows to and from the nonfunctioning fetal lungs. Blood is returned to the placenta from the descending aorta through the two umbilical arteries.

Before birth the high pulmonary vascular resistance created by the collapsed fetal lung causes greater pressures in the right side of the heart and the PAs. At the same time the free-flowing placental circulation and the ductus arteriosus produce a low systemic vascular resistance in the remainder of the fetal vascular system. With the clamping of the umbilical cord and the expansion of the lungs at birth, the hemodynamics of the fetal vascular system undergo pronounced and abrupt changes. These changes are the direct result of cessation of the placental blood flow and the beginning of lung respiration. The changes occurring at birth are discussed in Chapter 8, and the circulatory changes in the heart are shown in Fig. 34-2, *B.*

Postnatal Development

In infancy the size of the heart in relation to total body size is larger, and it occupies a larger space within the lung enclosure. It lies at a transverse angle, but with growth and the enlarging lungs it comes to lie lower and more obliquely at maturity. The ventricle walls are more or less equal in thickness at birth (some believe that the RV may be somewhat larger). With the increased demand of the postnatal peripheral circulation, the left side becomes thicker than the right. During the first years the weight of the heart is doubled; by 5 years, it is increased fourfold, and by 9 years, sixfold (Lowrey, 1986). An increase in heart size accompanies the adolescent growth spurt, with a resulting increase in blood pressure and decrease in heart rate. The heart rate at any age shows an inverse relationship to body size (see inside front cover).

The arteries and veins elongate to keep pace with expanding body dimensions, and the vessel walls thicken to cope with the increased pressure. The systolic blood pressure after birth is low, reflecting the weaker LV of the neonate. With the developing strength and power of the left side of the heart, the systolic pressure rises rather sharply during the first 6 weeks and continues to rise but at a much slower rate until shortly before puberty, at which point it rises rapidly to adult levels (see inside front cover).

Postnatal circulation. Once the cardiorespiratory system adjusts to the changes necessary to support extrauterine life, the circulation through the heart assumes a pathway that allows for oxygenation of venous blood by the lungs and delivery of saturated blood to the systemic circulation. Blood returning from the body via the SVC and IVC is received in the RA. It is then pumped to the RV through the tricuspid valve. The RV pumps the blood through the pulmonic valve into the PA and then to the lungs, where the blood becomes saturated with oxygen. The blood is then returned from the lungs via the pulmonary veins into the LA, where it is pumped through the bicuspid valve to the LV, and finally through the aortic valve to the aorta into the systemic circulation (Fig. 34-2, *B*).

Arteries are blood vessels that carry blood away from the heart and serve primarily the function of distributing highly oxygenated blood to the capillaries. Veins are blood vessels that carry poorly oxygenated blood to the heart and function as both collectors and reservoirs. Their function as a reservoir helps maintain normal circulation. For example, if there is increased resistance to blood flow through the right side of the heart (e.g., as the result of severe pulmonary valvular stenosis), RV end-diastolic and RA pressures may rise. As a result, central venous pressure rises and hepatomegaly may occur. The function of the arterioles is mainly to provide resistance to blood flow to maintain blood pressure and circulation.

Although major blood vessels enter and leave the heart, the heart muscle receives its own coronary blood supply. The *right* and *left coronary arteries,* which arise above the aortic valve, supply all the myocardium. *Coronary veins* collect the blood and return it directly to the RA or through a common venous channel called the *coronary sinus,* which drains into the RA.

Conduction system. To maintain an orderly and effective pumping action, the heart has a specialized electrical conduction system—electrical impulses generated within the heart initiate the mechanical contraction leading to circulation of blood. Although all myocardial cells are capable of developing an action potential and depolarizing without external stimulation, certain specialized cells make up the heart's normal pacemaker. These structures include (Fig. 34-3) (Anthony and Thibodeau, 1983):

1. The *sinoatrial (SA) node,* located within the RA wall near the opening of the SVC
2. The *atrioventricular (A-V) node,* also located within the RA but near the lower end of the septum
3. The *atrioventricular bundle (bundle of His),* which extends from the A-V node along each side of the interventricular septum and then divides into right and left bundle branches
4. *Purkinje fibers,* which extend from the A-V bundle into the walls of the ventricles

The SA node initiates the heart's conduction system and normally is the heart's pacemaker. The impulse spreads from the SA node throughout the atria to cause depolarization. As the atria depolarize, impulses spread to the A-V node to stimulate the ventricles. The A-V node is the major pathway by which the impulses from the atria can be transmitted to the ventricles. The impulses then spread to the A-V bundle and Purkinje fibers to cause simultaneous depolarization of the ventricles.

A *cardiac cycle* is composed of sequential contraction (systole) and relaxation (diastole) of both the atria and the ventricles. First, the atria contract, ejecting blood into the relaxed ventricles. Then, as the atria relax, the ventricles contract to eject blood into the PA and aorta. During atrial diastole, blood enters the atria from the systemic and pulmonary veins, thus completing one cardiac cycle.

Basic Cardiac Physiology

The heart is basically a complex pump, ejecting blood throughout the body. The heart and lungs function together to deliver oxygen to the tissues and remove waste products such as carbon dioxide. The primary function of the cardiopulmonary system is to provide effective oxygen transport to meet the body's metabolic needs. To perform this function, the heart must maintain an adequate cardiac output. By definition, *cardiac output* is the volume of blood ejected by the heart in 1 minute. It is derived by multiplying the heart rate (HR) by the stroke volume. *Stroke volume* is the amount of blood ejected by the heart in any one contraction. Stroke volume is influenced by three factors: preload, afterload, and contractility.

Cardiac output = HR × Stroke volume
↑
Preload
Afterload
Contractility

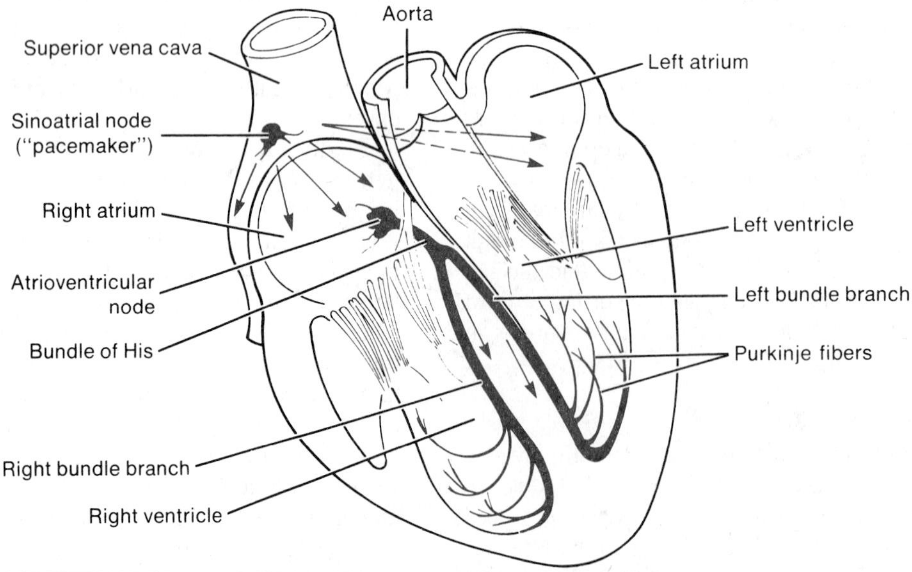

Fig. 34-3. Conduction system of heart.

Heart rate. HR, the number of beats per minute, is influenced by the autonomic nervous system. The sympathetic fibers increase HR, and the parasympathetic fibers, acting through the vagus nerve, decrease HR. Levels of circulating catecholamines and other hormones also influence HR. Generally an increase in HR will increase cardiac output, and a decrease or irregularity in HR (bradycardia, dysrhythmia) will impair cardiac output. However, a very fast HR shortens diastole and impairs coronary artery perfusion, causing eventual impairment of cardiac muscle function.

Preload. In physiologic terms, preload refers to myocardial fiber length. If the amount of blood delivered to the heart increases, then the myocardial fibers lengthen, and a greater amount of blood is pumped out of the heart. In simpler terms the preload is the volume of blood returning to the heart, or the circulating blood volume. The circulating blood volume is most easily assessed clinically using the central venous pressure (CVP).

Afterload. Afterload refers to the resistance against which the ventricles must pump when ejecting blood (ventricular ejection). Conditions that make it more difficult for the heart to pump blood forward into the circulation increase the afterload. It is determined by several complex factors, primarily the relative resistances of the systemic circulation *(systemic vascular resistance)* and the pulmonary circulation *(pulmonary vascular resistance).* Clinically, without the aid of hemodynamic monitoring, measurement of arterial blood pressure gives some indication of afterload—higher blood pressure, greater afterload.

Contractility. Contractility refers to the efficiency of myocardial fiber shortening, or the ability of the cardiac muscle to act as an efficient pump. There is no simple bedside technique to assess contractility, although an echocardiogram may be useful. Contractility is often inferred in clinical practice. Certain states are known to depress contractility (e.g., hypoxia, acidosis). It is often decreased following cardiac surgery in the early postoperative period.

Adequate systemic perfusion depends on an appropriate HR, adequate circulating blood volume, efficient pump function, appropriate systemic and pulmonary vascular resistances, capillary permeability, and tissue utilization of oxygen. The body makes frequent adjustments in the various determinants of cardiac output to maintain a steady state.

Several clinical examples are useful to illustrate these principles. The *Starling law (Frank-Starling curve)* demonstrates that an increase in ventricular end-diastolic volume (caused by an increased preload) somewhat increases stroke volume. Since the myocardial fibers can only stretch to a certain point and still function effectively, any increase in volume beyond this point impairs cardiac output. When decreased cardiac output results from decreased preload (e.g., in hypovolemia due to blood loss), treatment involves providing volume, either with intravenous fluids or blood products. If decreased cardiac output results from a dramatic increase in afterload (e.g., severe hypertension) that increases the myocardial workload, treatment involves reducing afterload with vasodilating drugs. Contractility can be enhanced by medications such as digoxin or intravenous inotropic medications such as dopamine or dobutamine. Adjustments in HR are the most common response to changes in cardiac output; HR is slowest during sleep and can more than double with strenuous physical exercise.

ASSESSMENT OF CARDIAC FUNCTION

As with most other health conditions, assessment of congenital or acquired heart disease is aided by a comprehensive history and physical examination. Understanding of heart physiology helps guide assessment and consequent determination of cardiac output status. Specialized procedures are available to help establish a diagnosis or determine heart function at any given time.

History

Assessment of all functional health patterns helps to establish a thorough history from the family. In taking a history, the nurse should elicit the parents' concerns. Often they have vague, nonspecific complaints, such as "Baby doesn't feed well" or "Baby is too quiet," that offer clues to a less obvious cardiac defect. Parents of children with congenital or acquired heart disease will often report one or more of the following:

- Poor weight gain, poor feeding habits, and fatigue during feeding
- Frequent respiratory infections and difficulties (tachypnea, dyspnea, shortness of breath)
- Cyanosis
- Evidence of exercise intolerance

A history of previous cardiac defects in a sibling, maternal rubella infection during pregnancy, the use of medications or chemicals during pregnancy, or chronic illness in the mother can be important clues to the diagnosis of congenital heart disease. Children with chromosomal abnormalities, such as Turner, Down, or Holt-Oram syndromes, are likely to have associated congenital heart defects, and the history is essential in evaluating their overall health.

In evaluating acquired heart disease, a history of a viral infection or toxic exposure is important if myocarditis is suspected. A history of a previous streptococcal infection is essential in rheumatic fever.

Physical Examination

Several specific areas of physical examination may yield evidence of heart disease (see Chapter 7 for a general discussion of physical assessment of the heart). During inspection, a general examination of overall nutritional status, skin color, particularly the presence of cyanosis with or without clubbing, and position of comfort is performed. During palpation and percussion, the quality of chest activity ("active precordium"), quality and symmetry of all pulses, warmth of extremities, and presence or absence of edema are assessed. Locating the hepatic and splenic borders for evidence of organ enlargement is also important. An essential aspect of heart auscultation is recognition of the heart's position within the chest cavity. The point of maximum intensity and apical impulse should be established, since they may offer clues to the heart's position.

Thorough assessment of aortic, pulmonic, tricuspid, and mitral areas helps determine the overall flow of blood through the heart. A murmur may be audible in one of these areas if either shunting of blood or turbulent flow within the heart is present. Noting the presence or absence of splitting of the second heart sound can also be valuable in assessing valve function. A splitting of the second heart sound is normal; the first component is aortic valve closure, and the second is pulmonic valve closure. Auscultation also includes heart rate and rhythm and determination of blood pressures in the four extremities.

✦ **NURSING ALERT** Unequal blood pressures between upper and lower extremities is a cardinal sign of coarctation of the aorta (see p. 1560).

Auscultation of lung sounds and respiratory rate also provides valuable clues to heart function. Lung sounds may appear coarse from excess fluid within the interstitial spaces. This fluid may remain within the lungs because of the heart's inability to circulate blood adequately. An elevated respiratory rate may also indicate difficulty in circulating blood from the lungs into the heart (see Congestive Heart Failure, p. 1543).

Murmurs. Although many murmurs are benign, they can also be an important sign of cardiac defects. Auscultation of murmurs is discussed in Chapter 7. The following discussion is an overview of the types of murmurs heard in heart defects.

The most frequent cause of murmurs is an abnormal shunting of blood between two heart chambers or between vessels. However, murmurs can also be produced by disturbing the flow of fluid through a vessel as a result of (1) increasing the rate of flow, (2) constricting or dilating the lumen, and (3) creating some type of irregularity on the vessel wall, such as an aneurysm, which vibrates as fluid flows past. Murmurs are classified according to their timing within the cardiac cycle (Box 34-1).

Murmurs caused by congenital defects involving the septum or great vessels are usually heard best near the sternal borders or over the base of the heart. Those of valvular origin are typically loudest over the respective auscultating valvular area, in the direction of blood flow. Murmurs that originate on the right side of the heart are subject to change during respiration as a result of intrathoracic pressure that prolongs right ventricular filling. Thus murmurs originating on the right side of the heart increase during inspiration.

Although the determination of murmurs' significance is generally a medical decision, nurses should be aware of those murmurs most likely associated with cardiac defects. Pathologic murmurs generally include those that are diastolic, pansystolic, systolic, continuous, or very loud (Rosenthal, 1984).

TESTS OF CARDIAC FUNCTION

A variety of invasive and noninvasive tests may be employed in the diagnosis of heart disease. Table 34-1 briefly

Box 34-1 CLASSIFICATION OF MURMURS ACCORDING TO TIMING WITHIN CARDIAC CYCLE

Systolic—between S_1 and S_2 heart sounds
Diastolic—between S_2 and S_1
Systolic ejection—begin after the S_1, attain a peak during midsystole, and terminate before the S_2
Pansystolic or **holosystolic**—during all of systole
Pandiastolic or **holodiastolic**—during all of diastole
Prediastolic—early diastolic
Presystolic—late diastolic
Continuous—continue through all of systole and all or part of diastole

Table 34-1 Procedures for cardiac diagnosis

PROCEDURE	DESCRIPTION
Electrocardiography	Measures electrical potential generated from heart muscle
Echocardiography	Short pulses of ultrasound transmitted through the heart bounce off heart structures; reflected on a screen
Ultrasonography	Similar to echocardiography; it is synchronized with ECG to provide a three-dimensional recording of heart structures
Roentgenography	
Fluoroscopy	Provides direct observation of heart size, position, contour, and relationships
Radiography	Provides permanent record of heart size and configuration
Angiocardiography	Opaque medium injected into circulatory system outlines blood flow through the heart and vessels; performed in conjunction with cardiac catheterization
Cardiac catheterization	Opaque catheter introduced into the heart chambers via large peripheral vessels is observed by fluoroscopy or image intensification; pressure measurements and blood samples provide additional source of information
Digital subtraction angiography (DSA)	Opaque media injected into circulatory system Provides computed images of vessels and tissues containing dye—"subtracts" all tissues not containing dye

outlines cardiac diagnostic procedures. The more frequently conducted tests are described here. Cardiac catheterization, which generates more anxiety than any other cardiac test, is discussed in detail; it may be used for diagnostic and interventional purposes.

Radiography

A chest x-ray examination is the most frequently ordered radiographic test for children with suspected cardiac problems. A chest film provides a permanent record of (1) the heart's size and configuration, its chambers, and the great vessels and (2) the pattern of blood flow, especially in the pulmonary vessels. Fluoroscopy is used mainly in conjunction with cardiac catheterization.

Electrocardiography

An electrocardiogram (ECG or EKG) measures the electrical activity of the heart and records it on graph paper. This allows the evaluation of the sequence and magnitude of the electrical impulses generated by the heart (Fig. 34-4). The normal ECG consists of the P wave, P-R interval, QRS complex, T wave, Q-T interval, and ST segment:

P-wave—represents the spread of the impulse over the atria (atrial depolarization). The sinus node's electrical activity is not represented in the ECG.

P-R interval—represents the time that elapses from the beginning of atrial depolarization to the beginning of ventricular depolarization. It is termed P-R instead of P-Q because the Q wave is frequently absent.

QRS complex—represents ventricular depolarization. It is actually composed of three separate waves—the Q, the R, and the S—that result from the currents generated when the ventricles depolarize before their contraction.

T wave—represents ventricular repolarization.

Q-T interval—represents ventricular depolarization and repolarization. This interval varies with heart rate—the faster the rate, the shorter the Q-T interval. Therefore in children this interval is normally shorter than in adults.

ST segment—represents the time that the ventricles are in absolute refractory period, the period between ventricular depolarization and repolarization.

Information supplied by an ECG includes heart rate and rhythm, abnormalities of conduction, muscular damage (ischemia), hypertrophy, effects of electrolyte imbalance, influence of various drugs, and pericardial disease. The ECG gives no direct information about the mechanical performance of the heart as a pump (Berne and Levy, 1986).

Special uses of the ECG include (1) continuous ambulatory monitoring, which employs a Holter monitor, a transistorized tape recorder attached to chest leads, and (2) exercise stress assessment, in which the ECG is monitored during controlled exercise, usually on a treadmill.

An ECG is taken by placing leads or electrodes on the skin to transmit electrical impulses back to a recording machine. Usually the electrodes are attached to the extremities with a rubber strap or to the chest with adhesive. An electrolyte lubricant is placed between the skin and the lead to increase conductivity. Chest leads must be positioned correctly because even minor misplacement can cause considerable inaccuracy in the recording. One common chest lead placement is illustrated in Fig. 34-5 (see also Nursing Tip, p. 1358). Although all these tests are painless, the leads can be frightening. Children old enough to understand can benefit from an explanation of the procedure. The child must remain still for the standard ECG; infants and young chil-

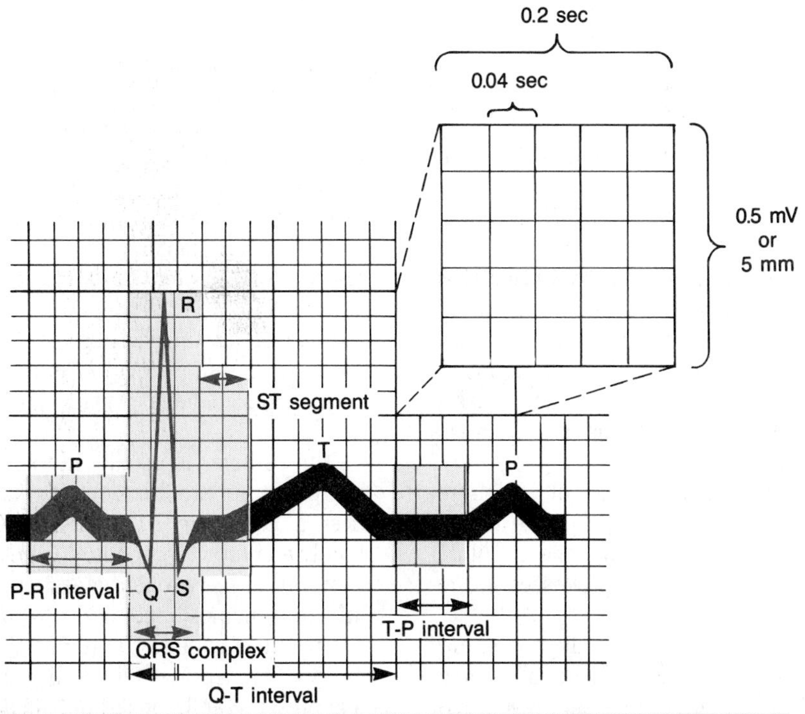

Fig. 34-4. Normal electrocardiogram pattern. Inset *(upper right)* shows conventional time and voltage or amplitude (height) calibrations.

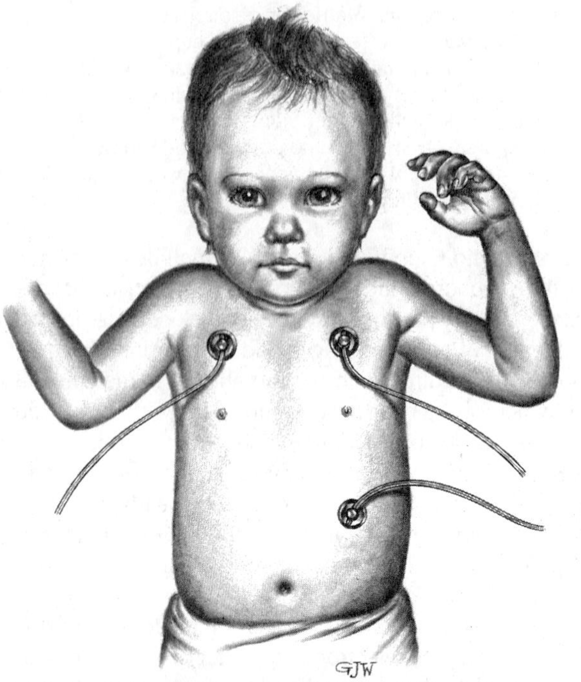

Fig. 34-5. Electrode placement for standard chest lead 1 in ECG monitoring.

NURSING TIP: ELECTRODE PLACEMENT

Electrodes for wires attached to the body are often color coded:
- White for right
- Green (or red) for ground
- Black for left

Always check to ensure these colors are placed correctly.

dren may be more cooperative if held in the parent's lap during the procedure.

Echocardiography

Echocardiography is one of the most frequently used tests for detecting cardiac dysfunction in children. Recent improvements in echocardiographic techniques have made it increasingly possible to confirm the diagnosis without resorting to cardiac catheterization. In selected instances a prenatal diagnosis of congenital heart disease can be made by fetal echocardiography.

Echocardiography involves the use of ultra-high-frequency sound waves to produce an image of the heart's structure. A transducer placed directly on the chest wall delivers repetitive pulses of ultrasound and processes the returned signals (echoes).

There are basically two types of echocardiograms. *Motion mode (M-mode)* provides a one-dimensional view of the heart and is useful in determining its size, presence or absence of structures, and their relationship to one another. A *two-dimensional (2-D),* or *cross-sectional,* echocardiogram provides information about spatial relationships between structures. A *pulse,* or *continuous Doppler,* echocardiogram is primarily a velocity-sensing system and is generally used with 2-D "echo" to provide information about volume flow rate. Depending on the type of test, information can be obtained regarding integrity of septa; chamber size; position and contractility; presence, position, size, and function of the valves; velocity of blood flow; and the relationship between and size of the great vessels.

Although the test is noninvasive, painless, and associated with no known side effects, it can be traumatic for children. The child must lie quietly in the standard echocardiographic positions; crying, nursing, or sitting up often leads to diagnostic errors or omissions (Snider, 1984). Therefore infants and young children may need a mild sedative; older children benefit from psychologic preparation for the test.

CARDIAC CATHETERIZATION

The most diagnostic invasive procedure is cardiac catheterization, in which a radiopaque catheter is inserted through a peripheral blood vessel into the heart. It is usually combined with angiography (angiocardiography), in which a radiopaque contrast material is injected through the catheter into the circulation. Cardiac catheterization provides information regarding:

- Oxygen saturation of blood within the chambers and great vessels
- Pressure changes within these structures
- Changes in cardiac output or stroke volume (the amount of blood pumped out of the LV into the aorta with each contraction)
- Anatomic abnormalities, such as septal defects or obstruction to flow

Cardiac catheterization may be *diagnostic, interventional,* or *electrophysiologic.* Until recently, diagnostic catheterization was the only option. The two main types of diagnostic cardiac catheterizations are (1) *right-sided* or *venous catheterization,* in which the catheter is introduced from a vein into the RA, and (2) *left-sided* or *arterial catheterization,* in which the catheter is threaded by way of a systemic artery retrograde into the aorta and LV or from a right-sided approach to the LA by means of a septal puncture or through an existing abnormal septal opening. In children the most common method is a right-sided catheterization, since septal defects permit entry into the left side of the heart.

The catheter is usually introduced through a percutaneous puncture into the femoral vein (the catheter is threaded over a guidewire inserted through a large-bore needle). Rarely a cutdown procedure is needed to gain access to the vein, but this approach is associated with increased risk of infection, hemorrhage, and obstruction. Once the vessel is entered, the catheter is guided through the heart with the aid of fluoroscopy. As the tubing is advanced, the child may feel pressure at the insertion site and vasospasm (fluttering) of the small vessels. Once the catheter is within the heart,

Table 34-2 Current interventional cardiac catheterization procedures for children

DIAGNOSIS	INTERVENTION/STATUS
Transposition of the great arteries	Balloon atrioseptostomy Well established
Valvular pulmonary stenosis Distal pulmonary artery stenosis Recurrent coarctation of aorta Rheumatic mitral valve	Balloon dilatation Accepted alternative to surgery
Patent ductus arteriosus	Transcatheter closure Routine in some institutions; requires further follow-up
Atrial septal defect	Transcatheter closure Clinical trials
Valvular aortic stenosis	Balloon dilatation Routine in some institutions; requires further follow-up

blood samples and pressure readings are taken for analysis. Then the contrast material may be injected and films taken of the dilution and circulation of the material. As the contrast medium is administered, the child may experience warmth, nausea, vomiting, restlessness, or headache.

Interventional, or therapeutic, cardiac catheterization has become an alternative to surgery in some congenital heart defects, such as isolated valvular pulmonic stenosis and patent ductus arteriosus (Table 34-2).

Electrophysiologic studies are increasingly being used to evaluate dysrhythmias. These diagnostic catheterizations employ catheters with tiny electrodes that record the heart's electrical impulses directly from the conduction system.

Nursing Considerations

Cardiac catheterization has become a routine diagnostic procedure and may be done on an outpatient basis. Catheterization is not, however, without risks, especially in neonates and seriously ill infants and children. Typical reactions include acute hemorrhage from the entry site (more likely with interventional procedures because larger catheters are used), low-grade fever, nausea, vomiting, loss of pulse in the catheterized extremity (usually transient, resulting from a clot, hematoma, or intimal tear), and transient dysrhythmias (generally catheter induced). Rare risks include stroke, seizures, tamponade from myocardial perforation, and death (Roberts, 1989). Therefore good nursing judgment and physical assessment before and after the procedure are essential. A Nursing Care Plan for the child undergoing cardiac catheterization is on p. 1540.

Preprocedural care. A complete nursing assessment is necessary to ensure a safe procedure with minimum complications. This assessment should include an accurate height (essential to correct catheter selection) and weight. Specific attention to signs and symptoms of infection is crucial. Severe diaper rash may be a reason to cancel the procedure if femoral access is required. Since assessment of pedal pulses is important after catheterization, the nurse should assess and mark pulses (dorsalis pedis, posterior tibial) before the child goes to the catheterization room. The presence and quality of pulses in both feet are clearly documented. If pulse oximetry is available, baseline oxygen saturation in children with cyanosis is also recorded. Preparing the child and family for the procedure is the joint responsibility of physician, nurse, and parents. The cardiologist usually explains the procedure to the parents, but nurses can reinforce and clarify the information. Many parents and older children who undergo both cardiac catheterization and cardiac surgery say, in retrospect, that they were more anxious about cardiac catheterization than about the surgery. Preparation for cardiac catheterization requires the same attention to the principles of preparation for procedures described in Chapter 27.

It is important to describe the catheterization ("cath") room because the x-ray machinery can appear frightening. Some institutions routinely take children on a brief tour of the area before the test. Although this is a controversial practice, it has been shown to help decrease children's anxiety (Naylor, Coates, and Kan, 1984). If this is not permitted, the child can be shown a picture (Fig. 34-6).

Other aspects of the procedure that should be explained (using words the child understands) include, specifically, that (1) the groin (or sometimes the antecubital fossa) is cleansed with a special brown solution; (2) the child will receive some medicine (lidocaine) in that area so that the skin will go to sleep; (3) a tube will be placed in a blood vessel, and the child may feel a little pushing at times; (4) when a special "medicine" (referring to the contrast material) is put into the tubing, the child may feel warm for a few seconds; and (5) as soon as the medicine is put in, the lights will go off and a machine will begin to take pictures. The last point is important to stress because younger children may associate the lights going off with "causing" the warm feeling from the contrast agent. As a result, they may become fearful of the dark and the noise from the machines.

Before the test the child may be sedated with several different drugs. A frequently prescribed regimen is meperidine (pethidine [Demerol]) with or without promethazine (Phenergan) and/or chlorpromazine (Thorazine); however, the use of these drugs is questionable (see discussion on p. 1199). Chloral hydrate is often used in infants and morphine sulfate in children with unrepaired tetralogy of Fallot. General anesthesia is usually unnecessary except in selected interventional procedures. The child is allowed nothing by mouth 4 to 6 hours before catheterization, although polycythemic infants and children may require intravenous fluids to prevent dehydration, and neonates may need dextrose solution up to 2 to 3 hours before the procedure to prevent hypoglycemia. Usually the morning dose of all oral

NURSING CARE PLAN
The Child Undergoing Cardiac Catheterization

Preprocedural care

NURSING DIAGNOSIS: Anxiety and fear related to diagnostic procedure, unfamiliar environment

GOAL 1
Relieve anxiety

INTERVENTIONS
See Preparation for Procedures, Chapter 27
See Surgical Procedures: Preoperative Care, Chapter 27
Take to cardiac catheterization room
- Transport infants in bassinet, crib, or Isolette with extra diapers, blanket, and pacifier
- Transport older children on gurney with comfort object (doll, toy, blanket)
- Distract child during procedure by playing tapes of favorite stories or songs; talk to child

EXPECTED OUTCOME
Child is transported to cardiac catheterization room with minimum distress to child and family

Postprocedural care

NURSING DIAGNOSIS: Potential for injury related to operative procedure, blood loss during catheterization, contrast medium

GOAL 1
Prevent complications

INTERVENTIONS
Keep leg on operative side as straight as possible
Avoid hip flexion
Keep incision and dressing clean and dry
Apply pressure if oozing or bleeding is noted
Carry out routine physical assessments
Keep child relatively quiet
Avoid undue excitement

EXPECTED OUTCOME
Child exhibits no evidence of vein obstruction or bleeding

GOAL 2
Prevent dehydration

INTERVENTIONS
Assess skin turgor and oral mucosa for signs of dehydration
Assess for nausea (intravenous hydration and/or antiemetics may be necessary in older child if emesis persists)
Maintain accurate record of intake and output

EXPECTED OUTCOME
Child exhibits no signs of dehydration

GOAL 3
Observe for complications

INTERVENTIONS
Assess physiologic status
- Pulses, especially below the catheterization site, for equality and symmetry
- Temperature and color of the affected extremity
- Respirations (respiratory rate and effort, breath sounds)
- Blood pressure, especially for hypotension

Assess general color and oxygenation by oximetry as prescribed
Check dressing for evidence of bleeding or hematoma formation in the femoral or antecubital area

EXPECTED OUTCOME
*Signs of complications are detected early

GOAL 4
Maintain optimum body temperature

INTERVENTIONS
Provide warmth if child is chilled from exposure during procedure
Avoid either overheating or chilling

EXPECTED OUTCOMES
Child's temperature remains within normal range (see inside front cover)
*Withheld digitalis and other medications are administered if ordered

NURSING DIAGNOSIS: Altered family processes related to child undergoing diagnostic procedure

GOAL 1
Support family

INTERVENTIONS
Keep family informed of child's progress during procedure
Be with family when results of procedure are given
Answer any questions regarding child's care or diagnosis

EXPECTED OUTCOME
Family members demonstrate an understanding of the procedural care and diagnosis

GOAL 2
Prepare for home care

INTERVENTIONS
Teach family signs of complications
- Altered perfusion in the catheterized extremity (cold, pale leg or foot)
- Infection (redness, swelling, or drainage from catheterization site)

Stress need to report these signs to practitioner

EXPECTED OUTCOME
Family demonstrates understanding of signs of complications

See also:
Nursing Care Plan: The Family of the Ill or Hospitalized Child, Chapter 26
Nursing Care Plan: The Child in the Hospital, Chapter 26

*Nursing outcome.

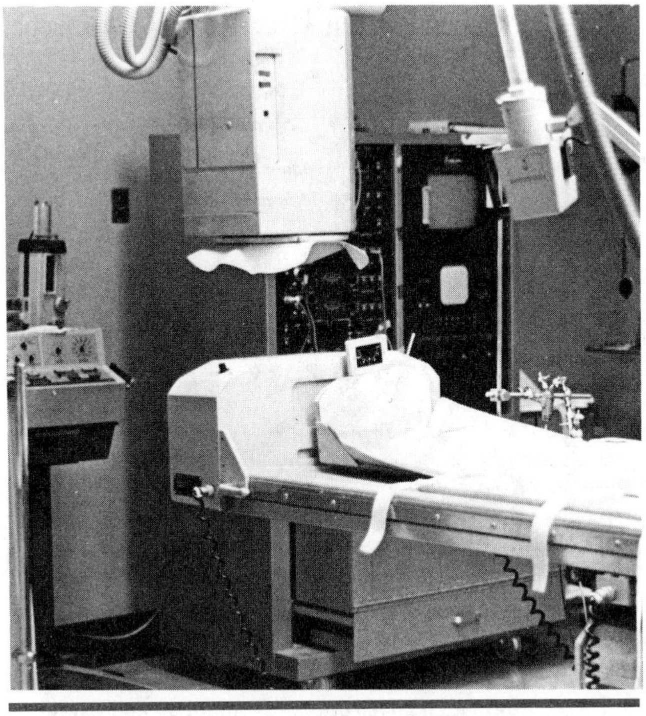

Fig. 34-6. Cardiac catheterization room.

medications is withheld, although this is clarified beforehand with the practitioner.

Postprocedural care. Essentially the care following cardiac catheterization is the same as general postoperative care. However, since children are not anesthetized during the procedure, they usually return directly to their room. The most important nursing responsibility is observation of the following for signs of complications:

- Pulses, especially below the catheterization site, for equality and symmetry (pulse distal to the site may be weaker for the first few hours after catheterization but should gradually increase in strength)
- Temperature and color of the affected extremity, since coolness or blanching may indicate arterial obstruction
- Vital signs, which are taken as frequently as every 15 minutes, with special emphasis on heart rate, which is counted for 1 full minute for evidence of dysrhythmias or bradycardia
- Blood pressure, especially for hypotension, which may indicate hemorrhage from cardiac perforation or bleeding at the site of initial catheterization
- Dressing, for evidence of bleeding or hematoma formation in the femoral or antecubital area

NURSING ALERT If bleeding occurs, direct continuous pressure is applied 2.5 cm (1 inch) *above* the percutaneous skin site to localize pressure over the vessel puncture (Agamalian, 1986).

Depending on hospital policy the child may be kept in bed with the affected extremity maintained straight for 4 to 6 hours after venous catheterization and 6 to 8 hours after arterial catheterization to facilitate healing of the cannulated vessel. If younger children have difficulty complying, they can be held in the parent's lap with the leg maintained in the correct position. The child's usual diet can be resumed as soon as tolerated, beginning with sips of water and advancing as the condition allows. The child is encouraged to void to clear the contrast material from the blood. Generally there is only slight discomfort at the percutaneous site. To prevent infection, the catheterization area is protected from possible contamination. If the child wears diapers, the dressing can be kept dry by covering it with a piece of plastic film and sealing the edges of the film to the skin with tape. The nurse must be careful, however, to continue to observe the site for any evidence of bleeding.

CONGENITAL HEART DISEASE

The incidence of congenital heart disease (CHD) in children is generally reported to be 4 to 10:1000 live births (Hoffman, 1990). CHD is the major cause of death (other than prematurity) in the first year of life. Although there are more than 35 well-recognized defects, the most common heart anomaly is ventricular septal defect (VSD) (Table 34-3). Reports on its incidence indicate that VSD is increasing in frequency in the United States. Although the reason for this is not known, at least part of it probably results from improved detection of small, isolated VSDs, primarily with echocardiography (Martin, Perry, and Ferencz, 1989).

The etiologic factor in CHD is not known in more than 90% of cases. However, several factors are associated with a higher-than-expected incidence of the defect. These include prenatal factors such as (1) maternal rubella during pregnancy, (2) maternal alcoholism, (3) maternal age over 40 years, and (4) maternal insulin-dependent diabetes. Heart defects are found in a much higher percentage of stillbirths, spontaneous abortions, and low-birth-weight infants, especially those small for age (Hoffman, 1990). Children with CHD are also more likely to have extracardiac defects, such as tracheoesophageal fistula, renal agenesis, and diaphragmatic hernias.

Several genetic factors are also implicated in CHD, although the influence is multifactorial. The risk of recurrence in families with an affected parent is variously reported in the literature but may be as high as 16% (Whittemore, Hobbins, and Engle, 1982), especially if the mother has the defect (Rose and others, 1985). The rising recurrence rates may be the result of more children with previously fatal heart defects surviving to adulthood and having offspring. Certain chromosomal aberrations, such as Down and Holt-Oram syndromes, are associated with increased risk of cardiac defects.

ALTERED HEMODYNAMICS

To understand the physiology of heart defects, it is necessary to review the role of pressure gradients, flow, and resistance within the circulation. Blood flows because of pressure gradients in different parts of the body and because of the heart's pumping action. As with any fluid, blood flows from an area of high pressure to one of low pressure and toward the path of least resistance. The rate of flow is directly proportional to the pressure gradient (i.e., the higher

Table 34-3 Percentage distribution of selected congenital heart defects and association with other conditions

DEFECT	PERCENTAGE OF SPECIFIC DEFECTS*	DISORDERS ASSOCIATED WITH INCREASED INCIDENCE OF DEFECT†
Ventricular septal defect	32.1%	Down syndrome Holt-Oram syndrome Fetal alcohol syndrome
Transposition of great arteries	2.6%	Diabetes or prediabetes in mother
Tetralogy of Fallot	3.8%	Down syndrome Fetal alcohol syndrome
Coarctation of aorta	6.7%	Turner syndrome Apert syndrome
Patent ductus arteriosus	8.3%	Rubella syndrome Down syndrome
Hypoplastic left heart syndrome	3.1%	—
Atrioventricular valve defect	3.6%	Down syndrome
Pulmonic stenosis	8.6%	Rubella syndrome Noonan syndrome
Atrial septal defect	7.4%	Noonan syndrome Holt-Oram syndrome Down syndrome Fetal alcohol syndrome
Aortic stenosis	3.8%	Turner syndrome
Truncus arteriosus	1.7%	—

*U.S. multicenter data. From Hoffman, J.I.: Congenital heart disease: incidence and inheritance, Pediatr. Clin. North Am. 37(1):31, 1990.
†Data from Noonan, J.A.: Association of congenital heart disease with syndromes or other defects, Pediatr. Clin. North Am. 25(4):797-816, 1978.

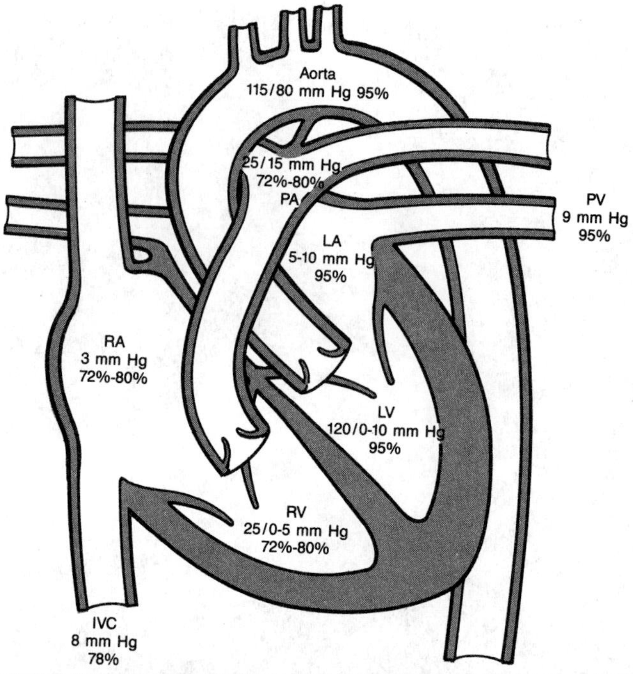

Fig. 34-7. Normal chamber pressures (mm Hg) and oxygen saturations (Sa_{O_2}) in cardiac chambers and great arteries. *PV*, Pulmonary vein; see Glossary (p. 1530) for other abbreviations.

the pressure gradient, the greater the rate of flow) and inversely proportional to the resistance (i.e., the higher the resistance, the less the rate of flow). However, increased resistance does not always decrease flow. If the proximal cardiac chamber can increase the driving pressure proportionately, flow can remain unchanged.

Normally the pressure on the right side of the heart is lower than that on the left side, and the resistance in the pulmonary circulation is less than that in the systemic circulation. Likewise, vessels entering or exiting from these chambers have corresponding pressures (e.g., lower pressure in the PA and higher pressure in the aorta). Therefore, if an abnormal connection exists between the heart chambers, such as a septal defect, blood flows from an area of higher pressure (left side) to one of lower pressure (right side). This directional flow of blood is termed a *left-to-right shunt.* If the opening is small, the amount of blood shunted to the atrium or ventricle may be minimal.

An understanding of saturations within the heart is also helpful in understanding CHD. The blood returning to the heart via the great veins, the SVC, and the IVC should have the lowest oxygen saturation because the tissues should have extracted oxygen, leaving the venous blood desaturated. Saturations in the RA, RV, and PA should be equal. Blood returning from the lungs to the heart through the PVs should be fully saturated, the most oxygen-rich blood in the body. Saturations on the left side of the heart should all be equal, with fully saturated blood entering the aorta and first supplying the heart muscle through the coronary arteries and then supplying the brain (Fig. 34-7). Normally, saturated blood circulates separately from desaturated blood. Depending on the type of defect, mixing of saturated and desaturated blood may occur. The amount of mixed blood that reaches the systemic circulation is a significant feature of several cardiac anomalies and results in varying degrees of hypoxemia and cyanosis.

CLASSIFICATION AND CLINICAL CONSEQUENCES

Congenital heart defects have been divided into two categories. Traditionally, a physical characteristic, cyanosis, has been used as the distinguishing feature, dividing the anom-

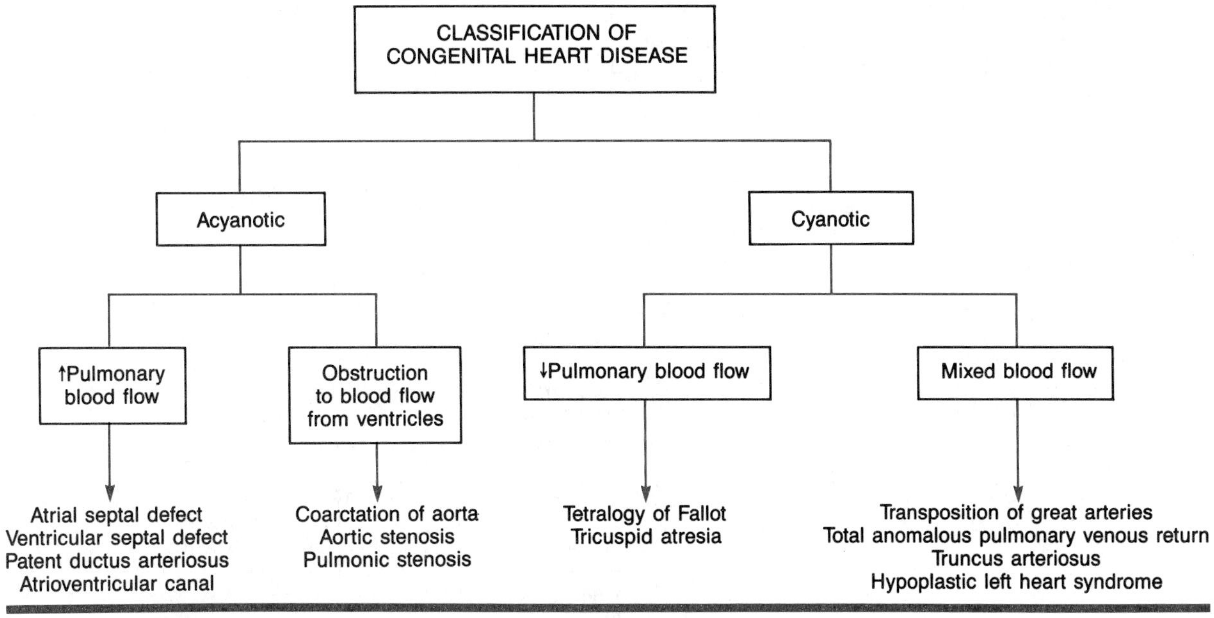

Fig. 34-8. Comparison of acyanotic-cyanotic and hemodynamic classification systems of congenital heart disease.

alies into *acyanotic* and *cyanotic defects.* In clinical practice this system is problematic because children with acyanotic defects may develop cyanosis. Also, more often, those with cyanotic defects may be pink and have more clinical signs of congestive heart failure (CHF). Because of the complexity of many defects and the variability of their clinical manifestations, the cyanotic-acyanotic classification system has proved inadequate and misleading.

Another classification system, based on *hemodynamic characteristics,* or movements involved in circulation of blood, is more frequently used. The defining characteristic is blood flow patterns: (1) increased pulmonary blood flow, (2) decreased pulmonary blood flow, (3) obstruction to blood flow out of the heart, and (4) mixed blood flow, in which saturated and desaturated blood mix within the heart or great arteries. As a comparison, both classification systems are outlined in Fig. 34-8.

With the hemodynamic classification system, the clinical manifestations of each group are more uniform and predictable. Defects that allow blood flow from the high-pressure left side of the heart to the lower-pressure right side (left-to-right shunt) result in increased pulmonary blood flow and cause CHF. Obstructive defects impede blood flow out of the ventricles; obstruction on the left side of the heart results in CHF, whereas severe obstruction on the right side causes cyanosis. Defects that cause decreased pulmonary blood flow result in cyanosis. Mixed lesions present a variable clinical picture based on degree of mixing and amount of pulmonary blood flow; hypoxemia (with or without cyanosis) and CHF usually occur together. (For more detailed explanations, see specific defects later in this chapter.)

Depending on the severity of the cardiac defect and the altered hemodynamics, two principal clinical consequences can occur: CHF and hypoxemia. The conditions can occur alone or together. Nursing care plays a critical role in the early identification and supportive management of these conditions.

CONGESTIVE HEART FAILURE

Congestive heart failure is inability of the heart to pump an adequate amount of blood to the systemic circulation to meet the body's metabolic demands. Causes of CHF can be classified according to the following changes:

Volume overload, especially with left-to-right shunts that may cause the RV to hypertrophy in order to compensate for the additional blood volume

Pressure overload, primarily resulting from obstructive lesions, such as valvular stenosis or coarctation of the aorta

Decreased contractility, primarily factors that affect the contractility of the myocardium, such as cardiomyopathy or myocardial ischemia from severe anemia or asphyxia, heart block, acidemia, and low levels of potassium, glucose, calcium, or magnesium

High cardiac output demands, in which the body's need for oxygenated blood exceeds the heart's cardiac output (even though the volume may be normal), such as in sepsis, hyperthyroidism, and severe anemia

In children, CHF occurs most frequently secondary to congenital heart defects in which structural abnormalities result in an increased volume load or increased pressure load on the ventricles. For example, septal defects can cause large left-to-right shunts, resulting in a volume load on the RV. Obstruction to flow out of the LV, such as narrowing of the aorta (coarctation of the aorta), can cause increased pressure inside the ventricle. CHF can also be the result of an excessive workload on a normal myocardium. Myocardial failure, in which the contractility of the heart muscle is impaired, can result from cardiomyopathy, drugs, electrolyte imbalances, dysrhythmias, and other causes.

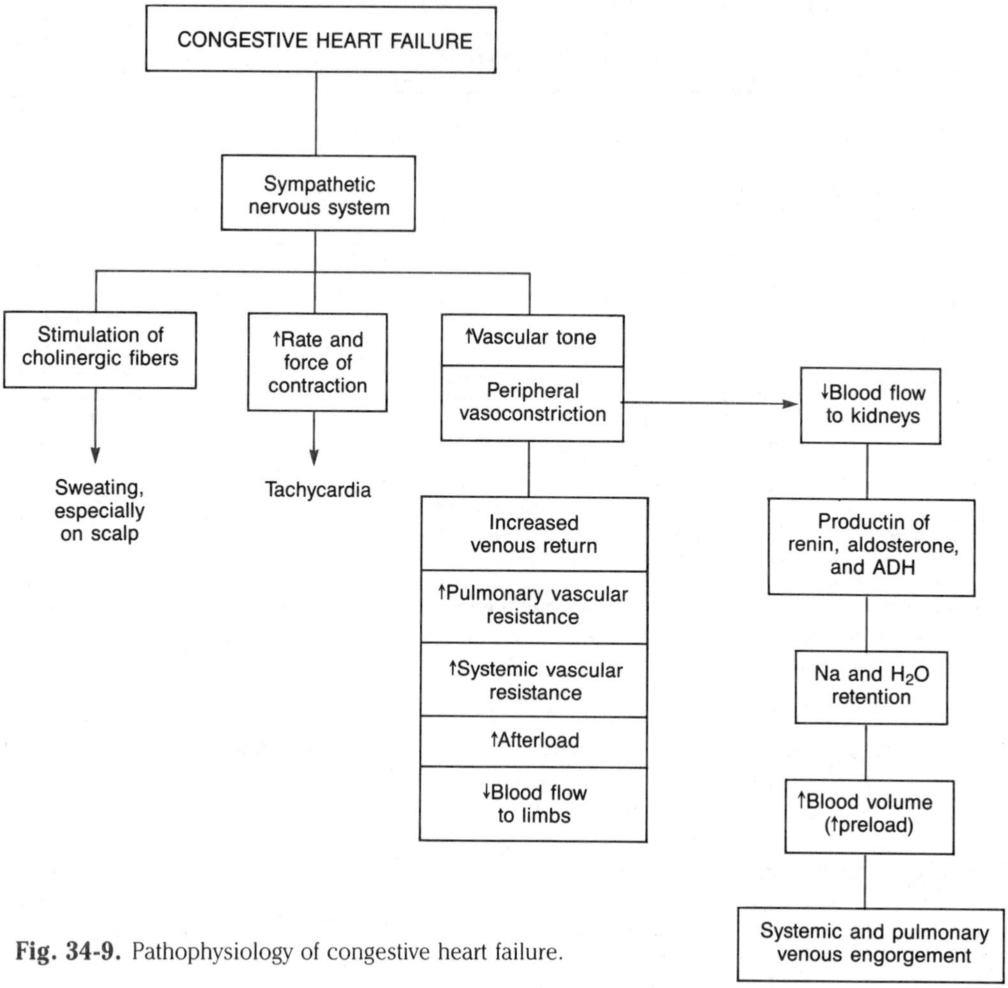

Fig. 34-9. Pathophysiology of congestive heart failure.

Diseases in other organ systems, particularly the lungs, also can cause CHF. Obstructive changes in the lungs result in increased pulmonary vascular resistance, which increases the right ventricular workload. In time the right side of the heart has difficulty pumping blood forward to the lungs, becomes dilated, and hypertrophies; then signs and symptoms of right-sided heart failure are seen. *Cor pulmonale* is the term for CHF resulting from obstructive lung diseases such as cystic fibrosis or bronchopulmonary dysplasia.

Pathophysiology

Heart failure may be theoretically divided into two classifications: right-sided or left-sided failure. In *right-sided failure* right ventricular function is suboptimal. RV end-diastolic pressure rises, causing increased central venous pressure and systemic venous engorgement. Systemic venous hypertension causes hepatomegaly and may cause edema in the extremities. In *left-sided failure* left ventricular dysfunction occurs and LV end-diastolic pressure rises, resulting in increased pressure in the LA and also in the pulmonary veins. The lungs become congested with blood, causing elevated pulmonary pressures and pulmonary edema.

Although each type of heart failure produces different signs and symptoms, clinically it is unusual to observe solely right- or left-sided failure in children. Since both sides of the heart depend on adequate function of the other side, failure of one chamber causes a reciprocal change in the opposite chamber.

Compensatory mechanisms. The heart initially tries to meet the body's demand for increased cardiac output through several compensatory mechanisms called the *cardiac reserve.* These include hypertrophy and dilatation of the cardiac muscle and stimulation of the sympathetic nervous system (Fig. 34-9).

Hypertrophy and dilatation of cardiac muscle. In response to the need to increase cardiac output, the cardiac muscle hypertrophies, developing greater tension. It is able to generate increased pressure within the ventricle, pumping blood out of the heart at a higher pressure. Also, the cardiac muscle can dilate and increase the stretch of its fibers, which increases the force of contraction. However, both hypertrophy and dilatation have potentially negative effects. Hypertrophy may result in decreased ventricular compliance over time. Decreased compliance requires a higher filling pressure to produce the same stroke volume. The increased muscle mass impairs oxygenation to the heart muscle. Beyond a certain amount of dilatation, the force of contraction decreases and the heart fails. (See discussion of Starling law, p. 1535.)

Stimulation of the sympathetic nervous system. When the cardiac output begins to fall, stretch receptors and baroreceptors in the blood vessels stimulate the sympathetic nervous system, releasing catecholamines. Catecholamines increase the force and rate of myocardial contraction, as manifested by tachycardia. They cause peripheral vasoconstriction, resulting in increased systemic vascular resistance, increased venous return, and reduced blood flow to the limbs, viscera, and kidneys. Sympathetic cholinergic fibers cause sweating.

While initially successful in increasing cardiac output, prolonged sympathetic stimulation also has negative effects. By shortening the diastolic period, tachycardia increases oxygen consumption by the heart muscle, eliminates the heart's resting phase, and impairs coronary artery perfusion. A continued increase in systemic vascular resistance increases the afterload on the heart muscle, which requires extra work by the heart muscle and reduces systemic blood flow.

The renal system is particularly sensitive to reductions in blood flow and renal perfusion, activating the renin-angiotensin-aldosterone mechanism. Renin-angiotensin secretion causes vasoconstriction and leads to an increase in aldosterone secretion, which causes retention of salt and water. Retention of salt and water causes an increase in preload. Although at first helpful to the failing heart, the sodium and water retention becomes excessive, resulting in signs of systemic venous congestion and fluid overload.

Clinical Manifestations

As the compensatory mechanisms are exceeded, the child will exhibit signs of CHF because of decreased myocardial contraction, increased preload, and increased afterload. The signs and symptoms of CHF can be divided into three groups: (1) impaired myocardial function, (2) pulmonary congestion, and (3) systemic venous congestion (Box 34-2). Because these hemodynamic changes occur from different causes and at differing times, the clinical presentation may vary among children.

Impaired myocardial function. One of the earliest signs of CHF is *tachycardia* (sleeping heart rate greater than 160 beats/minute in infants), as a direct result of sympathetic stimulation. It is elevated even during rest but becomes extremely rapid with the slightest exertion. Ventricular dilatation and excess preload result in extra heart sounds S_3 and S_4, referred to as *gallop rhythm. Diaphoresis* is often seen, especially on the head during exertion. Children are easily fatigued, have poor exercise tolerance, and are often irritable. Decreased cardiac output results in *poor perfusion,* manifested by cold extremities, weak pulses, low blood pressure, and mottled skin. Extreme pallor or duskiness are ominous signs.

Pulmonary congestion. *Tachypnea* (respiratory rate greater than 60 breaths/minute in infants) occurs in response to decreased lung compliance. Tachypnea can lead to hypoxemia because oxygen does not reach the alveoli for gas exchange in adequate amounts with fast breathing rates. *Mild cyanosis* results from impaired gas exchange and is relieved with oxygen administration. *Dyspnea* is caused by a decrease in the distensibility of the lungs. Inability to feed with resultant poor weight gain is primarily a result of tachypnea and dyspnea on exertion. *Costal retractions* occur as the pliable chest wall in the infant is drawn inward during attempts to ventilate the noncompliant lungs. Initially, dyspnea may only be evident on exertion, but it may progress to the point that even slight activity results in labored breathing. In infants dyspnea at rest is a prominent sign and may be accompanied by flaring nares.

Box 34-2 CLINICAL MANIFESTATIONS OF CONGESTIVE HEART FAILURE

Impaired Myocardial Function
Tachycardia
Sweating (inappropriate)
Decreased urine output
Fatigue
Weakness
Restlessness
Anorexia
Pale, cool extremities
Weak peripheral pulses
Decreased blood pressure
Gallop rhythm
Cardiomegaly

Pulmonary Congestion
Tachypnea
Dyspnea
Retractions (infants)
Flaring nares
Exercise intolerance
Orthopnea
Cough, hoarseness
Cyanosis
Wheezing
Grunting

Systemic Venous Congestion
Weight gain
Hepatomegaly
Peripheral edema, especially periorbital
Ascites
Neck vein distention (children)

As the LV fails, blood volume and pressure increase in the LA, pulmonary veins, and lungs. Eventually the pulmonary capillary pressure exceeds the plasma osmotic pressure, forcing fluid into the interstitial space and finally causing *pulmonary edema.* Increased interstitial lung water also decreases compliance (ability to expand) of the lungs and increases the work of breathing.

Orthopnea (dyspnea in the recumbent position) is caused by increased blood flow to the heart and lungs from the extremities. It is relieved by sitting up because blood pools in the lower extremities, decreasing venous return. In addition, this position decreases pressure from the abdominal organs on the diaphragm. In infants orthopnea may be evident in their inability to lie supine and their desire to be held upright.

Edema of the bronchial mucosa may produce *cardiac wheezing* from obstruction to airflow. Mucosal swelling and irritation result in a persistent, dry, hacking *cough.* As pulmonary edema increases, the cough may be productive from increased secretions. Pressure on the laryngeal nerve results in *hoarseness.* A late sign of heart failure is *gasping* and *grunting respirations.*

Infants with CHF have an increased metabolic rate and require additional caloric intake to grow. The work of the heart and breathing demands all the infant's energy, leaving little for normal activity. As a result of poor weight gain and activity intolerance, infants with CHF demonstrate *developmental delays.* Because of the physical energy and strength needed to sit up, pull to stand, and walk, these infants are delayed most in gross motor activities. The fine motor, social, and cognitive aspects of development seem less impaired. Following surgical correction, most children will catch up to their peers with time. Older children with severe CHF will have decreased exercise tolerance and persistent developmental delays.

Systemic venous congestion. Systemic venous congestion from right-sided failure results in increased pressure and pooling of blood in the venous circulation. *Hepatomegaly* occurs from pooling of blood in the portal circulation and transudation of fluid into the hepatic tissues. The liver may be tender on palpation, and its size is an indication of the course of heart failure.

Edema forms as the sodium and water retention causes systemic vascular pressure to rise. The earliest sign is *weight gain.* However, as additional fluid accumulates, it leads to swelling of soft tissue that is dependent and favors the flow of gravity, such as the sacrum and scrotum (when recumbent) and loose periorbital tissues. In infants edema is usually generalized and difficult to detect. Gross fluid accumulation may produce *ascites* and *pleural effusions.*

Distended neck and *peripheral veins* result from a consistently elevated central venous pressure. Normally neck and hand veins collapse when the head or hands are raised above the level of the heart, since the blood drains by gravity back to the heart. However, when the venous pressure is high, it slows venous return, causing the veins to remain distended. Distended neck veins are difficult to detect in the short, fat neck of infants and are usually observed only in older children.

Diagnostic Evaluation

Diagnosis is made on the basis of clinical symptoms such as tachypnea and tachycardia at rest, dyspnea, retractions, activity intolerance (especially during feeding in infants), weight gain caused by fluid retention, and hepatomegaly. Cardiomegaly resulting from dilatation and hypertrophy is seen on chest radiography. Ventricular hypertrophy appears on the ECG.

Therapeutic Management

The goals of treatment are to (1) improve cardiac function (increase contractility and decrease afterload), (2) remove accumulated fluid and sodium (decrease preload), (3) decrease cardiac demands, and (4) improve tissue oxygenation and decrease oxygen consumption.

Improve cardiac function. Two groups of drugs are used to enhance myocardial performance in CHF: (1) digitalis glycosides, which improve contractility, and (2) angiotensin-converting enzyme inhibitors, which reduce the afterload on the heart, making it easier for the heart to pump. Digitalis has three major actions:

1. Increases the force of contraction (positive inotropic)
2. Decreases the heart rate (negative chronotropic) and slows the conduction of impulses through the A-V node (negative dromotropic)
3. Indirectly enhances diuresis by increased renal perfusion

The beneficial effects are increased cardiac output, decreased heart size, decreased venous pressure, and relief of edema.

In pediatrics digoxin (Lanoxin) is used because of its rapid onset and decreased risk of toxicity as a result of a short half-life. It is available as an elixir (50 μg/ml) for oral administration or in a parenteral preparation (0.1 mg/ml). For infants the dose is often calculated in micrograms (1000 μg = 1 mg). Because digoxin has a very narrow margin of safety, the dosage must be calculated exactly; premature infants are more sensitive to digoxin and require smaller doses because the drug accumulates in the blood faster than in infants and children (Hastreiter and others, 1985).

Treatment is based on a digitalizing dose, given intravenously or orally, in divided doses over a short time span to bring the child's serum digoxin level into the therapeutic range. A maintenance dose, usually one eighth of the digitalizing dose, is given orally twice a day to maintain blood levels (Table 34-4). During digitalization the child is monitored with an ECG to observe for the desired effects (prolonged P-R interval and reduced ventricular rate) and detect side effects, especially dysrhythmias.

✦ **NURSING ALERT** Therapeutic serum digoxin levels range from 0.8 to 2.0 μg/L.

A newer group of drugs that has proved beneficial in the treatment of CHF are the angiotensin-converting enzyme (ACE) inhibitors. As their name implies, these drugs inhibit the normal function of the renin-angiotensin system in the kidney. The production of renin triggers the production of angiotensin I and angiotensin II, which cause vasoconstriction and aldosterone secretion. The ACE inhibitors block the conversion of angiotensin I to angiotensin II so that in-

Table 34-4 Oral digoxin dosage in infants and children

AGE	DIGITALIZING DOSE*	MAINTENANCE DOSE*
Premature infant	20	5
Full-term infant	30	8-10
<2 years	40-50	10-12
2-10 years	30-40	8-10
>10 years	0.75-1.25 mg	0.125-0.25 mg

*Dosage in μg/kg of body weight except as indicated.

Table 34-5 Diuretics used in congestive heart failure

DRUG	ACTION	COMMENTS	NURSING CONSIDERATIONS
Furosemide (Lasix)	Blocks reabsorption of sodium and water in proximal renal tubule and interferes with reabsorption of sodium in loop of Henle and in most proximal portion of distal tubule	Drug of choice in severe CHF Causes excretion of chloride and potassium (hypokalemia may precipitate digitalis toxicity)	Begin to record output as soon as drug is given Observe for dehydration caused by profound diuresis Observe for side effects (nausea and vomiting, diarrhea, ototoxicity, hypokalemia, dermatitis, postural hypotension) Encourage foods high in potassium and/or give potassium supplements Monitor chloride and acid-base balance with long-term therapy Observe for signs of digitalis toxicity
Bumetanide (Bumex)	Loop diuretic similar to furosemide Much more potent than furosemide (1 mg = 40 mg furosemide)	May be used for severe CHF when furosemide is less effective Use cautiously (once a day or several times weekly) because of profound diuresis and electrolyte imbalances	Monitor for dehydration and electrolyte imbalances Observe for side effects (similar to those for furosemide) Observe for renal toxicity and electrolyte disturbances
Chlorothiazide (Diuril)	Acts directly on distal tubules and possibly proximal tubules to decrease sodium, water, potassium, chloride, and bicarbonate absorption Decreases urinary diluting capacity	Most frequently used drug Inexpensive Causes hypokalemia, acidosis from large doses May be given on alternate days or for 4 or 5 days and stopped for 2 days to allow for reabsorption of potassium	Observe for side effects (nausea, weakness, dizziness, paresthesia, muscle cramps, skin eruptions, hypokalemia, acidosis) Encourage foods high in potassium and/or give potassium supplements
Metolazone (Zaroxolyn)	Unique thiazide diuretic Appears effective in patients with reduced renal function	Chronic diuretic; useful in long-term therapy, not for acute diuresis Duration of action: 24 hours Use cautiously (once a day or several times weekly) because of profound diuresis and electrolyte imbalances	Observe for side effects, especially dehydration, nausea, vomiting, electrolyte imbalances Provide foods high in potassium and/or administer potassium supplements
Spironolactone (Aldactone)	Blocks action of aldosterone, which promotes retention of sodium and excretion of potassium	Has potassium-sparing effect; frequently used with thiazides, furosemide Poorly absorbed from gastrointestinal tract Expensive Beneficial for children resistant to other diuretics	Observe for side effects (skin rash, drowsiness, ataxia, hyperkalemia) Do not administer potassium supplements

stead of vasoconstriction, vasodilatation occurs. Vasodilatation results in decreased pulmonary and systemic vascular resistance, decreased blood pressure, a reduction in afterload, and decreased right and left atrial pressures. It also reduces the secretion of aldosterone, which reduces preload by preventing volume expansion from fluid retention and decreases the risk of hypokalemia. Renal blood flow is improved, which enhances diuresis.

Two ACE inhibitors are currently used in pediatrics: captopril (Capoten), given three times a day, and enalapril (Vasotec), given twice a day. Captopril is used in infants and young children because it can be given in smaller doses; its principal side effects are hypotension, renal dysfunction, and cough. Captopril also may have some immune-based side effects, including fever and allergic reactions. Since enalapril has the same principal side effects but fewer immune-based side effects, patients may be switched from one preparation to the other (see Box 34-9) (Opie, 1987).

Remove accumulated fluid and sodium. Treatment consists of diuretics, possible fluid restriction, and possible sodium restriction. Diuretics are the mainstay of therapy to eliminate excess water and salt to prevent reaccumulation. The most commonly used agents are listed in Table 34-5.

Since furosemide and the thiazides cause loss of potassium, potassium supplements and rich dietary sources of the electrolyte are given.

NURSING ALERT A fall in the serum potassium level enhances the effects of digitalis, increasing the risk of digitalis toxicity. Therefore serum potassium levels must be carefully monitored.

Fluid restriction may be required in the acute states of CHF and must be carefully calculated to avoid dehydrating the child, especially if cyanotic CHD and significant polycythemia are present. Infants rarely need fluid restrictions because CHF makes feeding so difficult that they struggle to take maintenance fluids.

Sodium-restricted diets are used less often in children than in adults to control CHF because of their potential negative effects on the child's appetite and ultimate growth. If salt intake is restricted, the diet usually consists of avoiding additional table salt and highly salted foods. Low-salt formulas are available but used infrequently because infants need a normal sodium source to offset the sodium depletion of chronic diuretic therapy. Most infant formulas have slightly more sodium than breast milk.

Decrease cardiac demands. To lessen the workload on the heart, metabolic needs are minimized by (1) providing a neutral thermal environment to prevent cold stress in infants, (2) treating any existing infections, (3) reducing the effort of breathing (semi-Fowler position), and (4) using medication to sedate an irritable child.

Improve tissue oxygenation. All the preceding measures serve to increase tissue oxygenation either by improving myocardial function or by lessening tissue oxygen demands. However, supplemental cool humidified oxygen may also be administered to increase the amount of available oxygen during inspiration. Oxygen administration is especially helpful in patients with pulmonary edema, intercurrent respiratory infections, and increased pulmonary vascular resistance (oxygen is a vasodilator that decreases pulmonary vascular resistance). An oxygen hood is preferred with young infants to provide increased concentration of the gas. A nasal cannula or face tent may be useful with older infants and children. Nasal cannulas are ideal for long-term oxygen administration because the child can be ambulatory and can easily eat and drink. Cool humidification is necessary to counteract the drying effect of oxygen. The amount of cool humidity is carefully regulated to prevent chilling.

Nursing Considerations

The infant or child with CHF is usually quite ill and may be admitted to an intensive care unit. Expert nursing care is essential to reduce the cardiac demands that strain the failing heart muscle. During this time the child and family require emotional support; for some children, severe CHF represents end-stage cardiac disease.

Assessment

Nurses need to be alert to signs of CHF in children with CHD and in infants with suspected CHD (see Box 34-2). Signs of CHF indicate a worsening clinical condition; the earlier they are detected, the sooner treatment can be begun.

NURSING ALERT The early signs of CHF are:
- Tachycardia, especially during rest and slight exertion
- Tachypnea
- Profuse scalp sweating, especially in infants
- Fatigue and irritability
- Sudden weight gain
- Respiratory distress

Nursing Diagnoses

Following a thorough assessment, several nursing diagnoses are evident (see Nursing Care Plan, pp. 1550-1551). Others may become apparent in special circumstances and with children in different age-groups.

Planning

The objectives of nursing care of the infant or child with CHF include:

1. Assist in measures to improve cardiac function.
2. Decrease cardiac demands.
3. Reduce respiratory distress.
4. Maintain nutritional status.
5. Assist in measures to promote fluid loss.
6. Support child and family.

Implementation

Although the objectives of nursing care are the same, the interventions differ depending on the child's age; interventions for infants are quite different from those for older children.

Assist in measures to improve cardiac function. The nurse's responsibility in administering digoxin includes observing for signs of toxicity, calculating and administering the correct dosage, and instituting parental teaching regarding drug administration at home. The child's apical pulse is always checked before administering digoxin. As a general rule the drug is not given if the pulse is below 90 to 110 beats/minute in infants and young children or below 70 beats/minute in older children (the cutoff point for adults is 60). However, since the pulse rate varies in children in different age-groups, the written drug order should specify at what heart rate the drug is withheld. The nurse should also use judgment in evaluating the pulse rate. If it is significantly lower than the previous recording, the dose should be withheld until the practitioner is notified.

The apical rate is taken because a pulse deficit (radial pulse rate lower than apical) may be present with decreased cardiac output. It is auscultated for 1 full minute to evaluate alterations in rhythm. If the child is monitored by means of an ECG, a rhythm strip is obtained and attached to the chart for rate and rhythm analysis, such as abnormal lengthening of the P-R interval (more than a 50% increase over predigitalization interval) and dysrhythmias.

Box 34-3 COMMON SIGNS OF DIGOXIN TOXICITY IN CHILDREN

Gastrointestinal	Cardiac
Nausea	Bradycardia
Vomiting	Dysrhythmias
Anorexia	

Digoxin is a potentially dangerous drug because the margin of safety of therapeutic, toxic, and lethal doses is very narrow. Many toxic responses are extensions of its therapeutic effects. Therefore the nurse must maintain a high index of suspicion for signs of toxicity when administering digoxin (see Box 34-3).

Digoxin: cardiac toxicity. The principal manifestations of cardiac toxicity are abnormalities in heart rate, rhythm, and conduction. An early sign is bradycardia.

Digoxin toxicity can occur from accidental overdose. Since margins of safety between therapeutic and toxic doses are narrow, great care must be taken in properly calculating and measuring the dosage. When converting milligrams to micrograms to milliliters, the nurse carefully checks the placement of the decimal point, since an error causes a significant change in dosage. For example, 0.1 mg is 10 times the dosage of 0.01 mg.

NURSING ALERT No infant should ever receive more than 1 ml (50 μg, or 0.05 mg) in one dose; a higher dose is an immediate warning of a dosage error. To ensure safety, compare the calculation with another staff member before giving the drug.

These same principles are taught to parents in preparation for discharge, although the correct dose in milliliters is usually specified on the container, thus reducing potential errors in calculation. The nurse observes the parent measure the elixir in the dropper and stresses the level mark as the meniscus of the fluid that is observed at eye level. Other instructions for administering digoxin are listed in the Parent Guidelines.

Parents are also advised of the signs of toxicity. According to the practitioner's preference, they may be taught to take the pulse before giving the drug. A return demonstration of the procedure from both parents or other principal caregiver is included as part of the teaching plan. Their level of anxiety in counting the pulse is assessed, since overconcern about the heart rate may result in excessive withholding of the drug.

Digoxin: extracardiac toxicity. The earliest manifestation of toxicity is vomiting, usually with anorexia and nausea, caused by stimulation of the emetic control center in the medulla. Although vomiting should alert the nurse to observe for other evidence of cardiac toxicity, one episode of vomiting does not warrant cessation of the drug because vomiting from other causes frequently occurs, especially in infants. Vomiting associated with digoxin toxicity is often unrelated to feedings, and infants are usually less interested in feeding with a recent decrease in oral intake. When in doubt regarding the cause of the vomiting and if another dose of digoxin should be given, the nurse should seek the practitioner's advice before administering the next dose. Other extracardiac signs of toxicity are neurologic or visual disturbances, which are extremely difficult to identify in children and consequently are of little value in assessing toxicity in infants.

If digoxin toxicity occurs, especially as a result of a drug overdose, all subsequent doses are held. The child is closely monitored for dysrhythmias, which are treated appropriately if they occur. An antidote for digoxin is Digibind, but it has had little use in children (Few, 1987). Because of the long half-life of digoxin (1.5 days), it may be several days before the blood level returns to normal (Opie, 1987).

Afterload reduction. For patients receiving ACE inhibitors for afterload reduction, the nurse should carefully monitor blood pressure before and after dose administration, observe for symptoms of hypotension, and notify the practitioner if blood pressure is low. Serum electrolytes should be monitored. Because ACE inhibitors also block the action

PARENT GUIDELINES
Administering Digoxin

Give digoxin at regular intervals, usually every 12 hours, such as 8 AM and 8 PM.
Plan the times so that the drug is given *1 hour before* or *2 hours after* feedings.
Use a calendar to mark off each dose that is given or post a reminder, such as a sign on the refrigerator.
Have the prescription refilled *before* the medication is completely used.
Administer the drug carefully by slowly directing it on the side and back of the mouth.
Do not mix it with other foods or fluids, since refusal to consume these results in inaccurate intake of the drug.
If the child has teeth, give water after administering the drug; whenever possible, brush the teeth to prevent tooth decay from the sweetened liquid.
If a dose is missed and more than 4 hours has elapsed, withhold the dose and give the next dose at the regular time; if less than 4 hours has elapsed, give the missed dose.
If the child vomits, do not give a second dose.
If more than two consecutive doses have been missed, notify the physician or other designated practitioner.
Do not increase or double the dose for missed doses.
If the child becomes ill, notify the physician or other designated practitioner immediately.
Keep digoxin in a safe place, preferably a locked cabinet.
In case of accidental overdose of digoxin, call the nearest poison control center immediately; the number is usually listed in the front of the telephone directory.

Modified from Jackson, P.L.: Digoxin therapy at home: keeping the child safe, MCN 4(2):105-109, 1979.

NURSING CARE PLAN
The Child with Congestive Heart Failure

NURSING DIAGNOSIS: Decreased cardiac output related to structural defect, myocardial dysfunction

GOAL 1

Improve cardiac output

INTERVENTIONS

*Administer digoxin (Lanoxin, digitalis) as ordered, using established precautions to prevent toxicity
- Make certain dosage is within safe limits
- Ascertain correct preparation for route
- Check dosage with another nurse
- Count apical pulse for 1 full minute before giving drug
  - Withhold medication and notify practitioner if pulse rate is less than 90 to 110 beats/minute (infants) or 70 to 85 (older children), depending on previous pulse readings
- Often an ECG rhythm strip is taken to assess cardiac status before administration
- Ensure adequate intake of potassium
- Monitor serum potassium levels (decrease enhances digitalis toxicity)

*Administer medications to decrease afterload, as ordered
- Check blood pressure
  - Observe for signs of hypotension
- Monitor electrolyte levels

Attach cardiac monitor if ordered

EXPECTED OUTCOMES

Heartbeat is strong, regular, and within normal limits for age (see inside front cover)

Peripheral perfusion is adequate

NURSING DIAGNOSIS: Ineffective breathing pattern related to pulmonary congestion

GOAL 1

Improve ventilation and oxygen supply

INTERVENTIONS

Place in inclined posture of 30 to 45 degrees, tilt mattress support of incubator; place older infant in infant seat

Avoid any constricting clothing or restraints around abdomen and chest

*Administer humidified oxygen as prescribed

EXPECTED OUTCOME

Respirations remain within normal limits, color is good, and infant rests quietly (see inside front cover for normal variations in respirations)

GOAL 2

Reduce anxiety

INTERVENTIONS

Employ flexible feeding schedule that reduces fretfulness associated with hunger

Handle child gently

Hold and comfort infant

Employ comfort measures found to be effective in individual cases

Encourage family to provide comfort and solace

*Administer morphine sulfate as prescribed

EXPECTED OUTCOME

Infant rests quietly and breathes easily

NURSING DIAGNOSIS: Fluid volume excess related to fluid accumulation (edema)

GOAL 1

Help eliminate excess fluid and prevent fluid accumulation

INTERVENTIONS

*Administer diuretics as prescribed

Maintain fluid restriction, if ordered

Provide skin care for children with edema

Change position frequently
- Use resilient mattress or mattress cover (Egg-crate, sheepskin)

EXPECTED OUTCOME

Infant exhibits evidence of fluid loss (frequent urination, weight loss)

NURSING DIAGNOSIS: Activity intolerance related to imbalance between oxygen supply and demand

GOAL 1

Reduce cardiac demands and oxygen consumption

INTERVENTIONS

Maintain neutral thermal environment
- Place newborn in incubator or under warmer
- Keep infant warm
- Treat fever promptly

Feed small volumes at frequent intervals (every 2 to 3 hours) using soft nipple with moderately large opening

Implement gavage feeding if infant becomes fatigued before taking an adequate amount

Time nursing activities to disturb infant as little as possible

Implement measures to reduce anxiety

Respond promptly to crying or other expressions of distress

EXPECTED OUTCOME

Infant rests quietly

*Dependent nursing action.

NURSING CARE PLAN
The Child with Congestive Heart Failure—cont'd

NURSING DIAGNOSIS: Potential for infection related to reduced body defenses, pulmonary congestion

See Infection Control, Chapter 27
See Nursing Care Plan: The Child with Congenital Heart Disease, p. 1572

NURSING DIAGNOSIS: Altered family processes related to a child with a life-threatening illness

GOAL 1
Support family

INTERVENTIONS AND EXPECTED OUTCOMES
See Nursing Care Plan: The Family of the Ill or Hospitalized Child, Chapter 26

GOAL 2
Prepare for home care

INTERVENTIONS
Teach family:
- Medication administration and side effects
- Signs and symptoms of CHF and to report them to designated practitioner
- Feeding techniques and nutritional requirements
- Positioning
- Need for rest
- Growth and developmental considerations
- Growth is slowed
- Gross motor skills may be delayed more than fine motor skills

EXPECTED OUTCOME
Family demonstrates an understanding of the condition and required care at home

of aldosterone, they act as potassium-sparing agents. Most patients do not need potassium supplements or spironolactone (Aldactone) while receiving these medications. Numerous medications affecting the kidney can potentiate renal dysfunction, so children taking multiple diuretics along with an ACE inhibitor require careful assessment.

Decrease cardiac demands. The infant requires rest and conservation of energy for feeding. Every effort is made to organize nursing activities to allow for uninterrupted periods of sleep. Whenever possible, parents are encouraged to stay with their infant to provide the holding, rocking, and cuddling that help children sleep more soundly. To minimize disturbing the infant, changing bed linen and complete bathing are done only when necessary. Feeding is planned to accommodate the infant's sleep and wake patterns. The child is fed when hungry, such as when sucking on fists rather than when crying for a bottle, since the stress of crying exhausts the limited energy supply. Since infants with CHF tire easily and may sleep through feedings, smaller feedings every 3 hours may be helpful. Gavage feedings may be instituted to provide adequate nutrition and allow the infant to rest.

Every effort is made to minimize unnecessary stress. With infants this primarily involves preserving the parent-child relationship and meeting their needs to reduce frustration. Older children need an explanation of what is happening to them to decrease anxiety over their deteriorating physical status. For example, if they are monitored by an ECG or placed in an oxygen tent, the nurse first explains the procedure. The few minutes it takes to reassure a child that ECG leads do not hurt help to lessen physiologic responses to stress.

Temperature is carefully monitored for hyperthermia (a sign of infection) or hypothermia (loss of heat to ambient air). Fever is reported, since infection must be promptly treated. If body temperature is low, the child is kept warm with additional blankets or the use of a radiant heater. Fever increases oxygen demands and is poorly tolerated. Maintaining body temperature is very important for the child who is receiving cool, humidified oxygen and for one who tends to be diaphoretic, losing heat via evaporation.

Skin breakdown from edema is minimized or prevented if possible. The child is placed on sheepskin, Egg-crate pad, or alternating pressure mattress and turned every 2 hours (from side to side while in semi-Fowler position). The skin, especially over the sacrum, is checked for evidence of redness from pressure. Respiratory infections can exacerbate CHF and should be appropriately treated and prevented if possible. The child is protected from persons with respiratory infections and has a noninfectious roommate. With an older child, it is advantageous to choose a roommate who is also confined to bed and relatively quiet in order to promote a restful environment. Good handwashing is practiced before and after caring for any hospitalized child. Antibiotics may be given to combat respiratory infection. The nurse ensures that the drug is given at equally divided times over a 24-hour schedule to maintain high blood levels of the antibiotic.

Reduce respiratory distress. Careful assessment, positioning, and oxygen administration can reduce respiratory distress. Respirations are counted for 1 full minute during a resting state. Any evidence of increased respiratory distress is reported, since this may indicate worsening heart failure.

Infants should be positioned to encourage maximum chest expansion, with the head of the bed elevated; they should sit up in an infant seat or be held at a 45-degree angle. Children prefer to sleep on several pillows and remain in a semi-Fowler or high Fowler position during waking hours. Shirts and diapers are pinned loosely to allow maximum chest expansion. Safety restraints, such as those used with the infant seats, are applied low on the abdomen and loosely enough to provide safety and maximum expansion.

The infant or child is often given humidified supplemental oxygen via oxygen hood or tent, nasal cannula, or mask. The child's response to oxygen therapy is carefully evaluated by noting respiratory rate, ease of respiration, color, and especially oxygen saturations, as measured by oximetry.

Maintain nutritional status. The same interventions discussed on p. 1574 (under Help Family Cope with Effects of the Disorder) apply here. Attention to nutrition is essential and is a nursing challenge because of the fatigue associated with CHF. If the child is hospitalized, parents are encouraged to feed the infant and employ whatever strategies have been successful at home. If such measures are still exhausting, the infant may be fed by gavage. Some infants with severe CHF, neurologic deficits, or significant gastroesophageal reflux may need placement of a gastrostomy tube to allow adequate nutrition.

Assist in measures to promote fluid loss. When diuretics are given, the nurse records fluid intake and output and monitors body weight at the same time each day to evaluate benefit from the drug. Since profound diuresis may cause dehydration and electrolyte imbalance (loss of sodium, potassium, chloride, bicarbonate), the nurse observes for signs indicating either complication, as well as signs and symptoms suggesting reactions to the drugs. Diuretics should be given early in the day to children who are toilet trained to avoid the need to urinate at night. If potassium-losing diuretics are given, the nurse encourages foods high in potassium, such as bananas, oranges, whole grains, legumes, and leafy vegetables, and administers prescribed supplements (see Nursing Tip).

✦ NURSING ALERT Observe for signs of hypokalemia (muscle weakness, hypotension, dysrhythmias, tachycardia or bradycardia, irritability, drowsiness) or hyperkalemia (muscle weakness, twitching, bradycardia, ventricular fibrillation, oliguria, apnea) from supplemental overdose.

Fluid restriction is rarely necessary in infants because of their difficulty in feeding. However, if fluids are restricted, the nurse plans fluid intake schedules for a 24-hour period, allowing for most fluids during waking hours. With toddlers and preschoolers it is psychologically advantageous to give small amounts of liquid in small cups so the containers appear full. Suitable utensils are decorated medicine cups, paper Dixie cups, doll-sized teacups, or measuring cups. It is also important to avoid leaving extra fluids at the bedside, since older children may help themselves to additional servings. Older children's cooperation is gained by placing them in charge of recording fluid intake.

NURSING TIP: POTASSIUM SUPPLEMENTS

Mix the elixir with fruit juice (red punch or grape juice works well) to disguise the bitter taste and to prevent intestinal irritation from a concentrated solution.

If salt is limited, the nurse discusses food sources of sodium with the family and discourages their bringing salt-containing treats to the child. At mealtime the child's tray is checked to make sure the appropriate diet is given.

Support child and family. CHF is a serious complication of heart disease. Parents and older children are usually acutely aware of the critical nature of the condition. Since stress places additional demands on cardiac function, the nurse should focus on reducing anxiety through anticipatory preparation, frequent communication with the parent regarding the child's progress, and constant reassurance that everything possible is being done.

Home care involves many of the same interventions discussed under Plan for Discharge and Home Care (see p. 1580). The nurse teaches the family about the medications that need to be administered and alerts them to the signs of worsening CHF that require medical attention, such as increased sweating, decreased urine output (noted in fewer wet diapers or infrequent use of the toilet), or poor feeding. Compliance is a major issue, and every effort is extended to improve the family's adherence to the medication schedule (see Chapter 27). Written instructions regarding correct administration of digitalis (digoxin) are essential (see Parent Guidelines, p. 1549), including an explanation regarding signs of toxicity.

If CHF is the end stage of a severe heart defect, the nurse cares for this child as for any child who is terminally ill, using the principles discussed in Chapter 23.

Evaluation

The effectiveness of nursing interventions for the family and the child with CHF is determined by continual reassessment and evaluation of care based on the following observational guidelines and expected outcomes:

1. Monitor heart rate and quality, respiratory rate and efforts, and color, and observe behaviors that provide clues to expended effort.
2. Observe nutritional intake, feeding behaviors, and weight.
3. Monitor intake, output, and weight.
4. Interview and observe behaviors of family.

Expected outcomes:
See Nursing Care Plan, pp. 1550-1551.

HYPOXEMIA

Hypoxemia refers to an arterial oxygen tension (or pressure, Pa_{O_2}) that is less than normal and can be identified by a decreased arterial saturation or a decreased Pa_{O_2}. *Hypoxia* is a reduction in tissue oxygenation that results from low oxygen saturations and PaO_2 and results in impaired cellular processes. *Cyanosis* is a blue discoloration in the mucous membranes, skin, and nail beds of the child with reduced oxygen saturation. It results from the presence of deoxygenated hemoglobin (hemoglobin not bound to oxygen) in a concentration of 5 g/dl of blood or more. Cyanosis is usually apparent when arterial oxygen saturations are 75% to 85% (Hazinski, 1984). Determination of cyanosis is subjective. It can vary depending on skin pigment, quality of light, color of the room, or clothing worn by the child. The presence of cyanosis may not accurately reflect arterial hypoxemia because both oxygen saturation and amount of circulating hemoglobin are involved. Children with severe anemia may not be cyanotic despite severe hypoxemia because the hemoglobin level may be too low to produce the characteristic blue color. Conversely, patients with polycythemia may appear cyanotic despite a near normal PaO_2.

Altered Hemodynamics

Heart defects that cause hypoxemia and cyanosis result from desaturated venous blood (blue blood) entering the systemic circulation without passing through the lungs. Three types of defects cause cyanosis in the infant. The first results from severe obstruction to pulmonary blood flow and blood shunting from the right side to the left side of the heart, or *right-to-left shunting.* Tetralogy of Fallot is the most common example. The second is mixing of arterial and venous blood within the chambers of the heart itself; a single ventricle is an example. The third defect, transposition of the great arteries, presents a unique situation in which the pulmonary and systemic circulations are parallel rather than in sequence. Fully oxygenated blood returns to the lungs, and desaturated blood returns to the body. Newborns with transposition of the great arteries depend on intracardiac mixing from a patent foramen ovale, septal defect, or ductus arteriosus to allow oxygenation.

Infants and children with some complex cardiac anomalies can be both hypoxemic and cyanotic and have symptoms of CHF. Defects resulting in one functional ventricle, hypoplastic left heart syndrome, and transposition of the great arteries with a ventricular septal defect are examples.

Adolescents and young adults may become cyanotic because of unrepaired septal defects in which the increased pulmonary blood flow over many years results in pulmonary vascular changes. *Eisenmenger complex (syndrome)* refers to the clinical situation in which a left-to-right shunt becomes a right-to-left shunt because of progressive increase in pulmonary vascular resistance. With increasing pulmonary vascular thickening the resistance in the pulmonary circulation can exceed or equal that in the systemic circulation, causing a reversal of blood flow from the right to the left ventricle.

Clinical Manifestations

Over time, two physiologic changes occur in the body in response to chronic hypoxemia: polycythemia and clubbing. Persistent hypoxemia stimulates erythropoiesis, resulting in *polycythemia,* an increased number of red blood cells. Theoretically a greater number of red blood cells increases the oxygen-carrying capacity of the blood. However, this increased red blood cell formation may result in anemia if iron is not readily available for the formation of hemoglobin. In addition, polycythemia increases the viscosity of the blood and tends to crowd out platelets and other coagulation factors. *Clubbing,* a thickening and flattening of the tips of the fingers and toes, is thought to occur because of chronic tissue hypoxemia and polycythemia (Fig. 34-10).

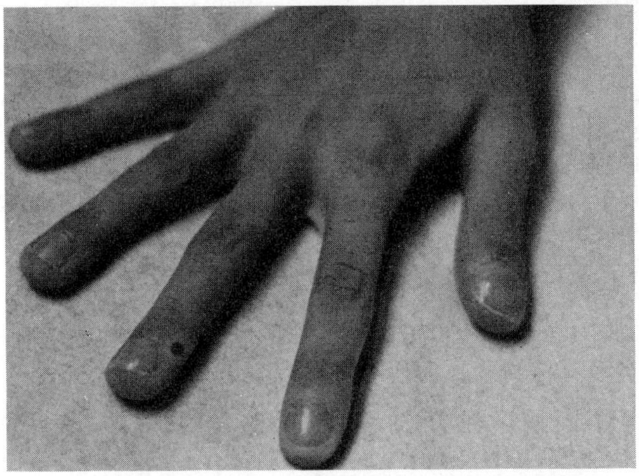

Fig. 34-10. Clubbing of the fingers.

Infants with mild hypoxemia may be asymptomatic except for cyanosis and exhibit near-normal growth and development. Those with more severe hypoxemia may exhibit fatigue with feeding, poor weight gain, tachypnea, and dyspnea. The position of comfort for these infants is either flaccid with extremities extended (in contrast to the normal flexed position) or side-lying with the knees toward the chest. Both positions are thought to be a response to tissue hypoxia and an attempt to reduce oxygen demands. Flaccidity is usually a sign of severe cardiovascular compromise.

Squatting, most characteristic of children with tetralogy of Fallot, is seen in toddlers and older children as an unconscious attempt to relieve chronic hypoxia, especially during exercise. The squatting position is helpful because flexing the legs (1) reduces the return of venous blood from the lower extremities, which is very desaturated; and (2) increases systemic vascular resistance, which diverts more blood flow into the pulmonary artery. Because of early surgical intervention before walking, squatting is rarely seen.

Severe hypoxemia resulting in tissue hypoxia is manifested by clinical deterioration and signs of poor perfusion. The infant is pale and dusky with increased cyanosis, cool to touch with diminished pulses, and lethargic with signs of respiratory distress, including hyperpnea and gasping respirations. Tissue hypoxia causes metabolic acidosis, leading to hyperventilation and a rapidly worsening clinical course unless prompt treatment is instituted.

Hypercyanotic spells, also referred to as blue spells or "tet" spells because they are often seen in infants with tetralogy of Fallot, may occur in any child whose heart defect includes obstruction to pulmonary blood flow and communication between the ventricles. The infant becomes acutely cyanotic and hyperpneic because sudden infundibular spasm decreases pulmonary blood flow and increases right-to-left shunting (the proposed mechanism in tetralogy of Fallot). With other anomalies an increase in oxygen requirements, which the infant is unable to meet, may cause a spell. Hypoxia causes acidosis, which further increases pulmonary vascular resistance, which further decreases pulmonary blood flow; thus a vicious cycle ensues. Spells, rarely seen before 2 months of age, occur most frequently in the first year of life. They occur more often in the morning and may be preceded by feeding, crying, or defecation. Because profound hypoxemia causes cerebral hypoxia, hypercyanotic spells require prompt assessment and treatment to prevent brain damage or possibly death.

Persistent cyanosis as a result of cyanotic cardiac defects places the child at risk for significant neurologic complications. Polycythemia and the resultant increased viscosity of the blood increase the risk of thromboembolic events. Cerebrovascular accidents (CVAs, strokes) may occur in about 2% of patients; infants with severe cyanosis and iron deficiency anemia are at greatest risk (Rosenthal, 1989). They may occur spontaneously but often follow an acute febrile illness, an hypoxic spell, or cardiac catheterization. Signs and symptoms of CVA include sudden paralysis, altered speech, extreme irritability or fatigue, and seizures. There is a 2% incidence of brain abscess in this patient population (Hazinski, 1984). Right-to-left shunting of blood in cyanotic heart defects allows bacteria to colonize the brain, which is vulnerable because of hypoxemia and poor perfusion of the cerebral microcirculation. Rarely seen in children under age 2 years, it should be suspected in older children with fever, headaches, focal neurologic signs, or seizures. Prompt treatment with antibiotics and surgical drainage is critical because death or significant neurologic impairment may result. Also, children who are cyanotic, especially those with systemic-to-pulmonary shunts, are at increased risk of bacterial endocarditis.

Several studies have highlighted the negative developmental consequences, particularly in the area of motor and cognitive development, that result from chronic hypoxemia (Aisenberg and others, 1982; Newburger and others, 1984; O'Dougherty and others, 1983). Fifty percent of postnatal brain growth occurs in the first year of life, so chronic hypoxemia, poor growth, and nutrition during this period can have significant adverse effects. If the risks of CVA, brain abscess, periods of profound cyanosis and hypoxia during hypercyanotic spells, and multiple surgeries, hospitalizations, and cardiac catheterizations are added, the possibility of neurologic insult resulting in developmental delays becomes significant and increases with each year of life. Minimizing these risks is an important factor in the trend toward early corrective surgical repair of cyanotic defects in infancy.

Children who are cyanotic from birth are generally smaller than their peers, exhibit poor weight gain, have dyspnea on exertion, fatigue easily, and have poor exercise tolerance. Hematologic abnormalities are also seen, such as thrombocytopenia, abnormal platelet function, fewer coagulation factors, and prolonged clotting time. These hematologic changes increase the likelihood of postoperative bleeding.

Diagnostic Evaluation

Cyanosis in the newborn can be the result of cardiac, pulmonary, metabolic, or hematologic disease, although cardiac and pulmonary causes occur most often. To distinguish between the two, a hyperoxia test may be helpful. The infant is placed in a 100% oxygen environment, and blood gases are monitored. A Pao_2 of 150 mm Hg or more suggests lung disease (increase in ventilation causes increased oxygenation), and a Pao_2 less than 100 mm Hg suggests cardiac disease (problem is related to inadequate perfusion of the pulmonary bed) (Driscoll, 1990). An accurate history, chest radiograph (demonstrating reduced pulmonary blood flow), and especially an echocardiogram contribute to the diagnosis of cyanotic heart disease.

Therapeutic Management

Newborns generally exhibit cyanosis within the first few days of life as the ductus arteriosus, which provided pulmonary blood flow, begins to close. Prostaglandin E_1, which causes vasodilation and smooth muscle relaxation, thus increasing dilatation and patency of the ductus arteriosus, is administered intravenously to reestablish pulmonary blood flow. The use of prostaglandins has been life-saving for infants with ductus-dependent cardiac defects. The increase in oxygenation allows the infant to be stabilized and a complete diagnostic evaluation to be performed before further treatment is needed.

Hypercyanotic spells occur suddenly, and prompt recognition and treatment are essential. In the hospital setting, spells are often seen during blood drawing or intravenous insertion, when the child is highly agitated, or following cardiac catheterization. Treatment of a hypercyanotic spell is outlined in Box 34-4. Morphine, administered subcutaneously or through an existing intravenous line, is helpful in reducing infundibular spasm. Generally a spell indicates prompt surgical treatment, if possible (Driscoll, 1990). In

Box 34-4 GUIDELINES FOR TREATING HYPERCYANOTIC SPELLS

Place infant in knee-chest position.
Employ calm, comforting approach.
Administer 100% oxygen by face mask.
Give morphine subcutaneously or through existing intravenous line.
Begin intravenous fluid replacement and volume expansion, if needed.
Repeat morphine administration.

some instances propranolol (Inderal) may be given in the interim to prevent infundibular spasm.

The cyanotic infant and child are well hydrated to keep the hematocrit and blood viscosity within acceptable limits to reduce the risk of CVA. Fevers are carefully evaluated because bacteremia can result in bacterial endocarditis. The infant is monitored closely for anemia because of the risk of CVAs and the reduced arterial oxygen-carrying capacity that occurs. Iron supplementation and possibly blood transfusion are used as needed. Older children and adolescents may require serial phlebotomy to reduce blood viscosity and minimize the risk of CVA. The goal is to reduce the hematocrit to approximately 60% by removing small aliquots of blood and replacing blood with normal saline or other intravenous solutions to maintain intravascular volume. This procedure is a temporary measure but may relieve symptoms of dyspnea, headache, and malaise for short periods and can be repeated every 1 or 2 months if polycythemia is severe.

Respiratory infections or reduced pulmonary function from any cause can worsen hypoxemia in the cyanotic child. Aggressive pulmonary hygiene, chest physiotherapy, administration of antibiotics, and use of oxygen to improve arterial saturations are important interventions.

Palliative surgery. Severely hypoxemic newborns with cardiac defects not amenable to corrective repair may have a palliative surgical procedure called a *shunt.* The shunt serves the same purpose as the ductus arteriosus: to increase blood flow to the lungs through a systemic artery–to–pulmonary artery connection. Currently a *modified Blalock-Taussig shunt* using a Gore-Tex or Impra tube graft to create a communication between the right or left subclavian artery and the pulmonary artery on the same side is the preferred procedure. Because of the higher resistance in the systemic circulation, blood flows from the subclavian artery to the pulmonary artery and to the lungs for oxygenation. The small diameter of the subclavian artery (as opposed to the aorta) automatically restricts the volume of blood flow to the pulmonary artery. This procedure sacrifices the brachial and radial pulse on the affected side, and the hand initially may be slightly cooler and paler until collateral circulation develops. Table 34-6 outlines the different shunt procedures, including past ones rarely performed today and those used in specific clinical situations. Corrective surgical repair is always preferred to a palliative shunt procedure if it can be performed at low risk. Corrective techniques are described with the cardiac defect.

Following a shunt procedure, the infant must be as-

Table 34-6 Shunt procedures for children with cardiac defects

TYPE OF SHUNT/LOCATION	COMMENTS
Potts Descending aorta to left pulmonary artery	Rarely performed Shunt often excessive, causing CHF May be difficult to take down at time of definitive repair
Waterston Ascending aorta to right pulmonary artery	Rarely performed Shunt often excessive, causing CHF Kinking at anastomosis can cause obstruction of right pulmonary artery, requiring reconstruction at time of definitive repair
Blalock-Taussig (BT) Subclavian artery to pulmonary artery	Replaced by modified version More difficult to perform in small infants because of small subclavian artery Ligation of subclavian artery may cause growth retardation of affected arm
Modified Blalock-Taussig Subclavian artery to pulmonary artery using Gore-Tex graft	Shunt flow sometimes excessive, requiring use of diuretics Possibility of thrombosis; antiplatelet therapy may be used postoperatively Easy to ligate at time of definitive correction Shunt size fixed and may become too small as child grows
Central Ascending aorta to main pulmonary aorta using Gore-Tex graft	Length of shunt acts to restrict blood flow, limiting symptoms of CHF; may require diuretics Uncommon; used when BT shunt or modified BT shunt cannot be done Easy to perform and remove at time of repair
Glenn Superior vena cava to side of right pulmonary artery, which is ligated from main pulmonary artery Blood flow to right lung only	Used as a second shunt procedure if complete repair not possible High mortality in infants under age 6 months Superior vena cava syndrome may occur Pulmonary arteriovenous fistulas may occur many years later Difficult to take down at time of definitive repair
Bidirectional Glenn Superior vena cava to side of right pulmonary artery Blood flow to both lungs	Done as a second shunt; often as a staging step to a Fontan procedure Can be incorporated into eventual modified Fontan procedure Relieves cyanosis and decreases volume overload on ventricle

Adapted from O'Brien, P.: Surgical repair of cyanotic cardiac defects in young adults, Nurs. Clin. North Am. 19(3):524, 1984.

sessed for signs of increased or decreased pulmonary blood flow. If the shunt is too small or narrowed, the newborn may remain severely hypoxemic, with oxygen saturations below 70%. Surgically revising the shunt or placement of an additional shunt may be needed. More often the shunt is too large and the pulmonary blood flow may be excessive, resulting in signs and symptoms of CHF and oxygen saturations above 85%. The infant may require digoxin and diuretic therapy (see discussion of CHF). Some surgeons place infants on low-dose aspirin therapy for several months to prevent platelet aggregation and subsequent narrowing of the shunt. Acute cyanosis and signs of tissue hypoxia may occur if the shunt is occluded and pulmonary blood flow is severely limited; shunt occlusion is a medical emergency.

Nursing Considerations

The general appearance of infants and children with significant cyanosis poses unique concerns. Blue lips and fingernails are obvious signs of their hidden cardiac defect. Clubbing and small, thin stature in older children further indicate severe heart disease. Body image concerns are important; these children are often teased about their appearance and singled out as different. Adolescents are especially concerned about their body image, and cyanosis can become a particular issue for them. Many children, when asked what surgery will do, reply, "Make me pink." Their joy and excitement following surgery are evident when they see their pink fingers. Accentuating the normal and positive and being careful not to call attention to their cyanosis are helpful interventions. Meeting other children who are cyanotic in the clinic or hospital reassures them that they are not the only ones who are blue.

Parents are often fearful of their child's bluish color, since cyanosis is usually associated with lack of oxygen and severe illness. They also must deal with comments from relatives, friends, and strangers in the community about their child's abnormal color. They need a simple explanation of hypoxemia and cyanosis and reassurance that cyanosis does not imply a lack of oxygen to the brain. Their questions and fears need to be addressed in a calm, supportive manner, and positive aspects of their child's growth and development are emphasized. They are taught the treatment for hypercyanotic spells (see Box 34-4).

Dehydration must be prevented in hypoxemic children because it potentiates the risk of CVAs. Fluid status is carefully monitored, with accurate intake and output and daily weight measurements. Maintenance fluid therapy is the minimum requirement, supplemental fluids should be readily available, and gavage feeding or intravenous hydration is given to children unable to take adequate oral fluids. Fever, vomiting, and diarrhea can cause dehydration and require prompt treatment. Parents are instructed in the importance of adequate fluid intake and measures to prevent dehydration. An oral electrolyte solution such as Pedialyte should be available at home in the event the infant is unable to tolerate the usual formula. The practitioner should be notified of fever, vomiting, diarrhea, or other problems.

Preventive measures and accurate assessment of respiratory infection are important nursing considerations. Any compromise in pulmonary function will increase the infant's hypoxemia. Good handwashing and protection from individuals with an obvious respiratory infection are important. Aggressive pulmonary hygiene, treatment with antibiotics or antiviral agents as indicated, and supplemental oxygen to decrease hypoxemia are necessary measures. Infants may need to be gavage-fed or given parenteral hydration if respiratory distress prevents oral feeding.

✦ **NURSING ALERT** Intracardiac shunting of blood from the right side (desaturated) to the left side of the heart allows air in the venous system to go directly to the brain, resulting in an air embolism. Therefore all intravenous lines should have filters in place to prevent air entering the system, the entire tubing is checked for air, all connections are taped securely, and any air is removed.

■ DEFECTS WITH INCREASED PULMONARY BLOOD FLOW

In this group of cardiac defects, intracardiac communications along the septum or an abnormal connection between the great arteries allows blood to flow from the high-pressure left side of the heart to the lower-pressure right side of the heart (Fig. 34-11). Increased blood volume on the right side of the heart increases pulmonary blood flow at the expense of systemic blood flow. Clinically, patients demonstrate signs and symptoms of CHF. Atrial and ventricular septal defects and patent ductus arteriosus are typical anomalies in this group.

ATRIAL SEPTAL DEFECT

An atrial septal defect (ASD) is an abnormal communication between the two atria resulting from incomplete septation (Fig. 34-12; see also Fig. 34-1). The defect may be one of three major types:

Ostium primum (ASD 1)—opening at the lower end of the septum; may be associated with mitral valve abnormalities
Ostium secundum (ASD 2)—opening near center of septum
Sinus venosus defect—opening near junction of superior vena cava and right atrium; may be associated with partial anomalous pulmonary venous connection

Altered Hemodynamics

Because left atrial pressure slightly exceeds right atrial pressure, blood flows from the left to the right atrium, causing an increased flow of oxygenated blood into the right side of the heart. Despite the low pressure difference, a high rate of flow can still occur because of low pulmonary vascular resistance and the greater distensibility of the right atrium, which further reduces flow resistance. This volume is well tolerated by the right ventricle because it is delivered under much lower pressure than in a ventricular septal defect. Although there is right atrial and ventricular enlargement, cardiac failure is unusual in an uncomplicated atrial septal de-

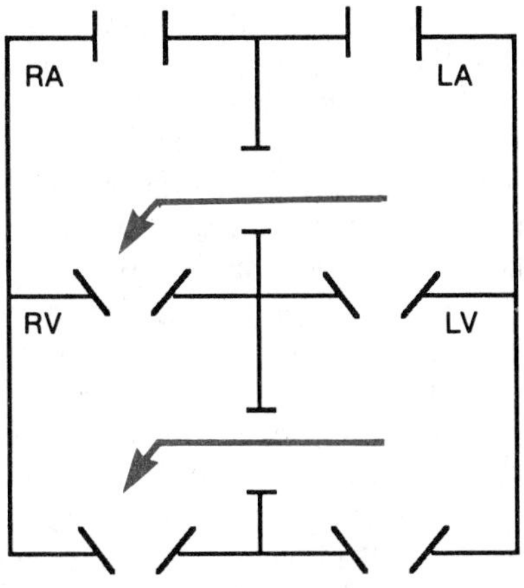

Fig. 34-11. Hemodynamics in defects with increased pulmonary blood flow.

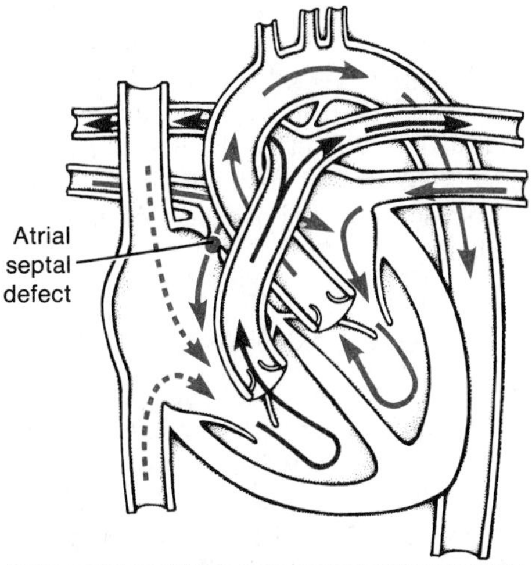

Fig. 34-12. Atrial septal defect. *Red arrows,* Saturated blood; *broken red arrows,* desaturated blood; *black arrows,* mixed blood.

fect. Pulmonary vascular changes usually occur only after several decades if the defect is unrepaired.

Clinical Manifestations

Most children with ASD are asymptomatic. Diagnosis is usually made after discovery of a murmur during routine physical examination. An ASD produces a characteristic crescendo-decrescendo type of systolic ejection murmur over the second to third interspace along the left sternal border. The murmur is not produced by blood flow across the defect, as in ventricular septal defect, but represents increased blood flow through the normal pulmonic valve.

Although the heart sounds are normal in intensity, there is a wide fixed splitting of the second sound. Normally the splitting between the two components of the second sound occurs because closure of the aortic valve precedes closure of the pulmonic valve during inspiration. The split normally widens because the increased venous return prolongs right ventricular emptying, causing a delay in pulmonic valve closure. When an ASD is present, the fixed overload of the right ventricle further prolongs its ejection time, thus widening the delay in closure of the pulmonic valve.

If an ASD remains unrepaired into adulthood, right and left ventricular hypertrophy will be significant. This may produce atrial dysrhythmias, CHF, or emboli formation. These symptoms are usually not apparent until age 20 to 30 years.

Diagnostic Evaluation

The most suggestive signs of ASD are its characteristic murmur and fixed splitting of the second heart sound. Unless clinical signs suggest pulmonary hypertension, clinical examination combined with echocardiography is sufficient to establish diagnosis (Adams, Emmanouilides, and Riemenschneider, 1989).

Therapeutic Management

Because of the risk of CHF and pulmonary vascular obstructive disease later in life, closure of ASD is recommended before school age. Surgical closure is similar to the corrective procedures employed in ventricular septal defect closures. In addition, the sinus venosus defect requires patch placement, so the anomalous right pulmonary venous return is directed to the left atrium with a baffle. The ASD 1 may require repair or, rarely, replacement of the bicuspid (mitral) valve. Surgical closure of all types of ASD is associated with essentially no operative mortality, and postoperative complications are unusual (Adams, Emmanouilides, and Riemenschneider, 1989). Another approach to ASD repair is accomplished in the cardiac catheterization laboratory using a "clamshell" device. This technique is in clinical trials and appears to have promise (Lock, Keane, and Fellows, 1987).

VENTRICULAR SEPTAL DEFECT

A ventricular septal defect (VSD) is an abnormal communication between the right and left ventricles resulting from incomplete septation (Fig. 34-13; see also Fig. 34-1). VSDs may be classified according to location: membranous (accounting for 80%) or muscular. They are frequently associated with other defects, such as pulmonary stenosis, transposition of the great vessels, patent ductus arteriosus, atrial defects, and coarctation of the aorta. Many VSDs (20%-60%) are thought to close spontaneously. Spontaneous closure is most likely to occur during the first year of life in children having small or moderate defects. Closure is a result of growth and proliferation of the muscular septum, apposition of a cusp of the tricuspid valve against the defect, or formation of a membranous diaphragm across the opening (Moller and Neal, 1990).

Altered Hemodynamics

Because of the higher pressure within the left ventricle and because the systemic arterial circulation offers more resistance than the pulmonary circulation, blood flows through the defect into the pulmonary artery. The increased blood

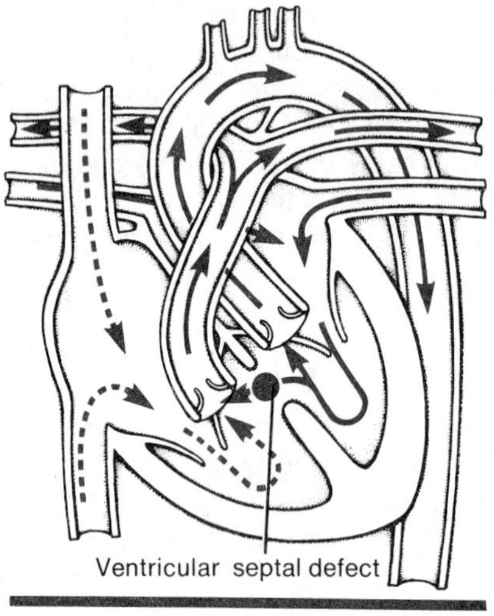

Fig. 34-13. Ventricular septal defect. *Red arrow,* Saturated blood; *broken red arrows,* desaturated blood; *black arrows,* mixed blood.

volume is pumped into the lungs, which may eventually result in increased pulmonary vascular resistance. Increased pressure in the right ventricle as a result of left-to-right shunting and pulmonary resistance causes the muscle to hypertrophy. If the right ventricle is unable to accommodate the increased workload, the right atrium may also enlarge as it attempts to overcome the resistance offered by incomplete right ventricular emptying. In severe defects Eisenmenger syndrome may develop (see p. 1553).

Clinical Manifestations

The infant with VSD has varying symptoms, depending on age, weight, and size of the defect. Failure to thrive and frequent respiratory infections resulting from increased pulmonary blood flow are the typical course.

One of the characteristic signs of VSD is a loud, harsh, pansystolic murmur generally heard best at the left lower sternal border and radiating throughout the precordium. The intensity of the murmur is not necessarily an indication of the defect's size. In neonates the murmur may be absent because of the normally high pulmonary vascular resistance, which tends to equalize the pressure between the two ventricles. A systolic thrill is associated with loud murmurs.

Severe overloading of the right ventricle and occasionally the right atrium causes hypertrophy and an obvious cardiac enlargement. Development of CHF typically occurs.

Diagnostic Evaluation

The ECG and echocardiographic findings of right ventricular hypertrophy and cardiomegaly, and prominent pulmonary markings on chest radiograph usually confirm the diagnosis of VSD. Cardiac catheterization and cineangiography are necessary to measure pulmonary vascular resistance and precisely define the location and number of VSDs.

Therapeutic Management

Preventing the development of pulmonary vascular obstructive disease demands closure of large VSDs within the first year of life. Early repair prevents progressive respiratory disease. Although palliation using a pulmonary artery band is used in some institutions, data suggest that complete primary repair can be performed without an increased risk during the first year of life. Age alone has little influence on the outcome of the repair, although younger infants are frequently sicker in the postoperative period.

Surgical closure is accomplished through a sternotomy and using cardiopulmonary bypass. A patch closure is usually performed, but a stitch closure may be used for smaller defects. The repair is generally approached through an atriotomy and the tricuspid valve. It may be necessary to use a right ventriculotomy approach. Subpulmonic VSDs carry a higher operative risk than other VSDs. Multiple VSDs carry a higher mortality rate, possibly because of longer circulatory arrest time, and more often require a ventriculotomy (Yeager and others, 1984). Muscular VSDs located in the apex may be hard to visualize surgically and may result in a residual VSD. Surgical closure of membranous VSDs, regardless of age and weight, can now be done with a low operative risk in infants, but muscular VSDs continue to have a mortality as high as 30% (Hazinski, 1984). Postoperative complications include residual VSD and conduction disturbances. Advanced pulmonary vascular obstructive disease (Eisenmenger syndrome) contraindicates VSD closure. These patients should be considered for an eventual heart-lung transplant.

ATRIOVENTRICULAR CANAL DEFECT

Atrioventricular canal (AVC) defect, one anomaly in the group of endocardial cushion defects, results from incomplete fusion of the endocardial cushions during fetal life. The incomplete fusion produces abnormalities in both the atrial and the ventricular septa as well as in the atrioventricular valve(s) (Fig. 34-14). Defects are generally classified as transitional (TAVC), partial (PAVC), or complete (CAVC). The most severe form, CAVC, consists of a single atrioventricular valve common to both right and left atrioventricular chambers. The central communication usually involves an ASD 1 above and a large defect in the inlet of the ventricular septum below. It is the most common cardiac defect in children with Down syndrome (Hoffman, 1990).

Altered Hemodynamics

The alterations in the hemodynamics depend on the defect's severity and the child's pulmonary vascular resistance. Immediately after birth, while the newborn's pulmonary vascular resistance is high, there is minimum shunting of blood through the defect. Once this resistance falls, left-to-right shunting occurs and pulmonary blood flow increases. The resultant pulmonary vascular engorgement predisposes to development of CHF.

Clinical Manifestations

At birth, signs and symptoms may be minimal except during crying or on exertion, when cyanosis occurs. If the defect consists of an ASD 1 and mild mitral valve insufficiency, the child is usually asymptomatic. If a complete

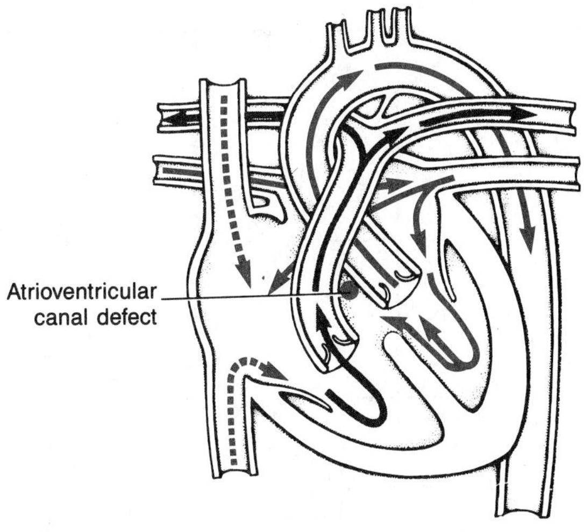

Fig. 34-14. Atrioventricular canal defect. *Red arrows,* Saturated blood; *broken red arrows,* desaturated blood; *black arrows,* mixed blood.

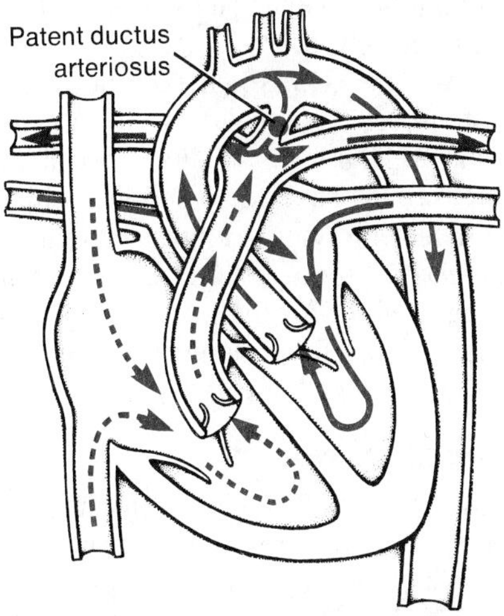

Fig. 34-15. Patent ductus arteriosus. *Red arrows,* Saturated blood; *broken red arrows,* desaturated blood; *black arrows,* mixed blood.

atrioventricular canal is present, cyanosis is more severe. Murmurs characteristic of an ASD or VSD may be found.

Diagnostic Evaluation

The ECG may demonstrate biventricular hypertrophy and a left axis deviation. Echocardiography may reveal separate mitral and tricuspid valves with an ASD 1 and continuity between these valves with a complete atrioventricular canal. Cardiac catheterization findings are characteristic of a left-to-right shunt and indicate the presence and location of septal defects.

Therapeutic Management

Surgical repair consists of patch closure of the septal defect(s) while reconstructing the valves. If the mitral (bicuspid) valve defect is severe, a valve replacement may be needed. Repair of CAVC in infants has improved in the last decade and now has a hospital mortality of less than 10% (Pacifico, 1989). Postoperative complications include bleeding, heart block, dysrhythmias, and CHF. A significant long-term problem is mitral valve regurgitation.

PATENT DUCTUS ARTERIOSUS

A patent ductus arteriosus (PDA) is present when the normal fetal structure fails to close completely after birth (Fig. 34-15). In the fetus, most blood entering the pulmonary artery from the right ventricle escapes to the systemic circulation through the normally present ductus arteriosus. This shunt allows more blood to go to the actively growing fetus and less to the virtually nonfunctioning pulmonary system. During fetal life, patency of the ductus arteriosus appears to be maintained by the combined relaxant effects of low oxygen tension and locally synthesized prostaglandins of the E type. At birth, functional closure of the ductus arteriosus normally occurs within hours from exposure of smooth muscle in its vessel wall to increased oxygen tension and less response to the relaxant effect of prostaglandins (Gersony, 1986). Permanent anatomic closure is usually complete toward the end of the first postnatal month. In some infants this does not occur, and the ductus arteriosus remains patent.

Altered Hemodynamics

The hemodynamic consequences of PDA depend on the size of the ductus and the pulmonary vascular resistance. At birth the resistance in the pulmonary and systemic circulations is almost identical, thus equalizing the resistance in the aorta and pulmonary artery. As the systemic pressure exceeds the pulmonary pressure, blood begins to shunt from the aorta, across the duct, to the pulmonary artery (left-to-right shunt).

The additional blood is recirculated through the lungs and returned to the left atrium and left ventricle. The effect of this altered circulation is increased workload on the left side of the heart, increased pulmonary vascular congestion and possibly resistance, and potentially increased right ventricular pressure and hypertrophy.

Clinical Manifestations

The turbulent flow of blood from the aorta through the PDA to the pulmonary artery results in a characteristic machinery-like murmur, which is auscultated best at the middle to upper left sternal border. Since there is a continuous flow of blood across the shunt, the murmur is heard during all of systole and most of diastole beyond the neonatal period. It is usually associated with a thrill. Another common feature is a widened pulse pressure. Some children have no detectable abnormality except for a murmur; others have frequent respiratory infections, signs of CHF, and failure to thrive.

Diagnostic Evaluation

The machinery-type murmur is almost diagnostic of PDA, but it may be absent in neonates or premature infants because of the normally high pulmonary resistance that tends to equalize the pressure between the two vessels. Radiographic examinations usually demonstrate left atrial and ventricular enlargement and evidence of increased pulmonary blood flow. The ECG is generally normal, although it may demonstrate left ventricular or biventricular enlargement. An echocardiogram is useful, since it may demonstrate an increased left atrial to aortic ratio, which is characteristic of a defect producing increased pulmonary blood flow and increased venous return, as is seen in PDA. Patients of any age with PDA can undergo surgery without cardiac catheterization if all the noninvasive findings are typical (Lock, Keane, and Fellows, 1987).

Therapeutic Management

CHF is an indication for PDA closure in infancy. In asymptomatic patients, PDA closure can be planned electively and is recommended before age 2 years. Because of low surgical risk and possible bacterial endocarditis, correction is recommended for all affected children. Surgical intervention involves surgical division or ligation of the patent vessel. Since the defect is outside the heart, cardiopulmonary bypass is not necessary. However, it is still a major procedure because the thoracic cavity must be entered. The risk of surgical PDA closure, excluding premature infants with respiratory distress syndrome, should approach 0% (Adams, Emmanouilides, and Riemenschneider, 1989).

In the premature infant with respiratory distress syndrome, indomethacin (a prostaglandin inhibitor) has been used to encourage ductal closure. If this is ineffective, operative closure is suggested and is well tolerated (see Persistent Patent Ductus Arteriosus, Chapter 10).

In older infants and children, PDA may also be obliterated with an "umbrella" apparatus placed during cardiac catheterization (Roberts, 1989). A double-umbrella device at the tip of the catheter is passed through the PDA to the descending aorta for opening of the distal arms of half the umbrella. The catheter is pulled back through the PDA for opening of the umbrella's proximal arms against the left pulmonary artery side. The entire unit is then released, thus occluding the opening.

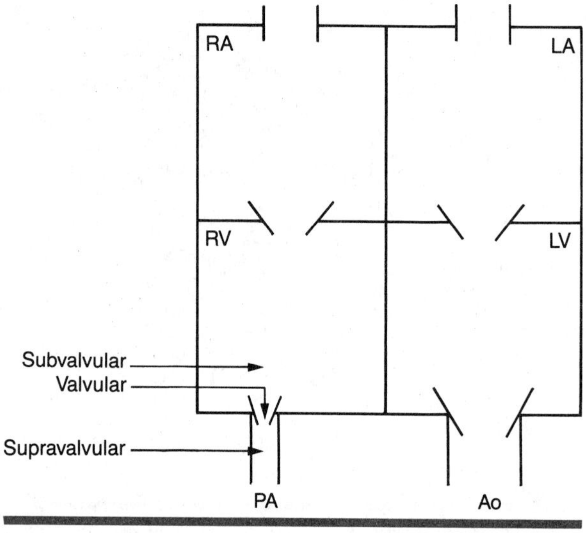

Fig. 34-16. Obstruction to ventricular ejection can occur at the valvular level (shown), below the valve (subvalvular), or above the valve (supravalvular). Pulmonary stenosis is shown here.

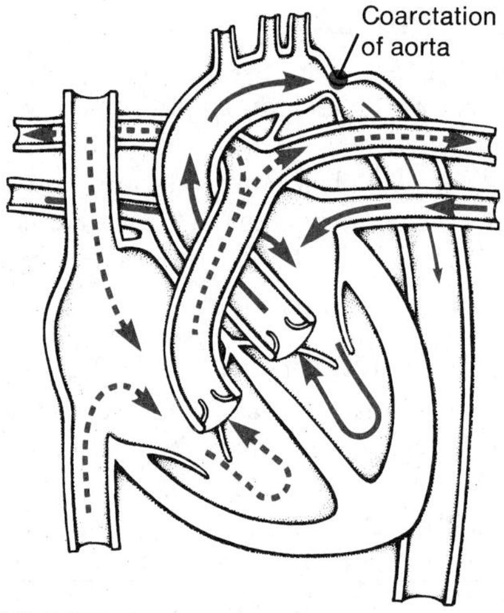

Fig. 34-17. Coarctation of aorta (postductal). *Red arrows,* Saturated blood; *broken red arrows,* desaturated blood.

OBSTRUCTIVE DEFECTS

Obstructive defects are those in which blood exiting the heart meets an area of anatomic narrowing (stenosis), causing obstruction to blood flow. The pressure in the ventricle and in the great artery before the obstruction is increased, and the pressure in the area beyond the obstruction is decreased. The location of the narrowing is usually near the valve (Fig. 34-16):

Valvular—at the site of the valve itself
Subvalvular—narrowing in the ventricle below the valve (also referred to as the *ventricular outflow tract*)
Supravalvular—narrowing in the great artery above the valve

Aortic stenosis, pulmonic stenosis, and coarctation of the aorta (narrowing of the aortic arch) are typical defects in this group. Hemodynamically, there is a pressure load on the ventricle and decreased cardiac output. Clinically, infants and children exhibit signs of CHF. Children with mild obstruction may be asymptomatic. Rarely, as in severe pulmonic stenosis, hypoxemia may be seen.

COARCTATION OF THE AORTA

Coarctation of the aorta (COA) is a narrowing of the aorta. The position of the narrowing is described as follows:

Preductal—proximal to the insertion of the ductus arteriosus usually between that vessel and the left subclavian artery
Postductal—distal to the ductus arteriosus (Fig. 34-17)
Juxtaductal—at the level of the ductus arteriosus

A coexisting bicuspid aortic valve is found in about 50% of patients.

Altered Hemodynamics

The effect of a narrowing within the aorta is increased pressure proximal to the defect and decreased pressure distal to it. In the preductal type of COA the lower half of the body is supplied with blood by the right ventricle through the ductus arteriosus. In the postductal type, right ventricular outflow cannot maintain blood flow to the descending aorta. Therefore collateral circulation develops during fetal life to maintain flow from the ascending to the descending aorta.

Clinical Manifestations

Patients with COA include the symptomatic neonate or infant and the asymptomatic older child. The neonate or young infant frequently has CHF when admitted to the hospital. Often these patients' hemodynamic condition deteriorates rapidly, and they are admitted to the intensive care unit near death, usually severely acidotic and hypotensive. In most older children, COA is first recognized at routine physical examination when upper extremity systemic hypertension, weak or absent femoral pulses, and a heart murmur are found. In those body areas that receive blood from vessels proximal to the defect, blood pressure is high and the pulses are bounding. With postductal COA, hypertension is present in both upper extremities and the head. However, if the constriction is between the insertion of the innominate and left subclavian arteries, only the right arm will have bounding radial pulses and elevated blood pressure. Because of hypertension, the child may experience occasional dizziness, headaches, fainting, and epistaxis. In those body areas distal to the defect, the blood pressure is decreased. The femoral pulses are weak or absent, the lower extremities may be cooler than the upper ones, and muscle cramps may result during increased exercise from tissue anoxia (a condition called *claudication*). A heart murmur is usually heard high on the sternal border because of rapid blood flow through the narrowed area.

Diagnostic Evaluation

In the neonate and young infant the chest radiograph usually shows a greatly enlarged heart and congested lung fields. An echocardiogram and Doppler examination confirm the diagnosis. If the two-dimensional echocardiogram rules out associated intracardiac anomalies, no further studies are needed. However, if a question exists about additional intracardiac pathology, a cardiac catheterization is performed.

In older children the ECG may be either normal or show some degree of left ventricular hypertrophy. The classic radiologic finding of rib notching, caused by erosion of the ribs' underside from enlarged collateral vessels, is rarely seen in a child before age 10 years.

Therapeutic Management

In the sick neonate or infant with COA, mechanical ventilation and inotropic support are often necessary before surgery. Surgical treatment is indicated in all symptomatic infants as soon as they are clinically stable and also in those patients who continue to deteriorate clinically, despite maximum medical management.

Surgical treatment consists of either resection of the coarcted portion with an end-to-end anastomosis of the aorta or enlargement of the constricted section using a graft of prosthetic material or a portion of the left subclavian artery. Because this defect is outside the heart and pericardium, cardiopulmonary bypass is not required and a thoracotomy incision is used.

In neonates and infants with isolated COA, hospital mortality is less than 5%, whereas in patients with COA that coexists with complex congenital heart disease, mortality increases significantly. Beyond early infancy, mortality is less than 1% (Moller and Neal, 1990). Balloon angioplasty as a primary intervention for COA is experimental (Rocchini and others, 1986). Recurrent COA more frequently affects the neonate. In infants beyond the neonatal period the incidence of recoarctation is less than 5% (Zeimer, 1986). Percutaneous balloon angioplasty techniques have proved very effective in relieving residual postoperative coarctation gradients.

Postoperative hypertension (greater than 160 mm Hg) is treated with intravenous sodium nitroprusside, followed by oral medications, such as captopril, hydralazine, and/or propranolol. Residual permanent hypertension after repair of COA seems to be related to age and time of repair. To prevent both hypertension at rest and exercise-provoked systemic hypertension after repair, elective surgery for COA is advised within the first 2 years of life.

AORTIC STENOSIS

Aortic stenosis (AS) is a narrowing or stricture of the aortic outflow tract. *Valvular* stenosis, the most common type, is usually caused by malformed cusps resulting in a bicuspid rather than tricuspid valve or fusion of the cusps (Fig. 34-18). *Subvalvular* stenosis is a stricture caused by a fibrous ring below a normal valve; *supravalvular* stenosis occurs infrequently.

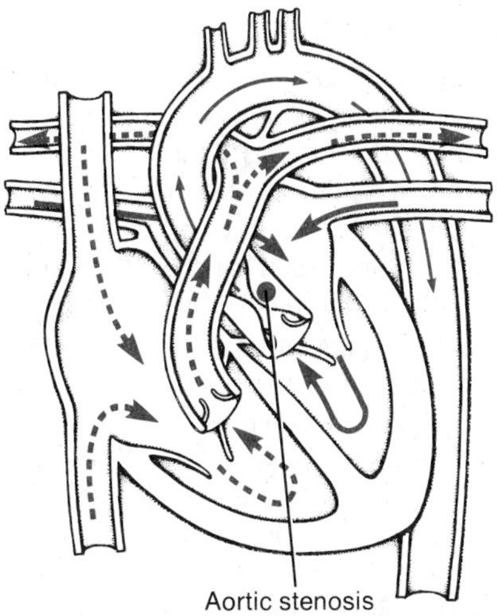

Fig. 34-18. Aortic stenosis. *Red arrows,* Saturated blood; *broken red arrows,* desaturated blood.

Valvular AS is a serious defect for the following reasons: (1) the obstruction tends to be progressive, (2) sudden episodes of myocardial ischemia or low cardiac output can result in sudden death, and (3) surgical repair rarely results in a normal valve. This is one of the rare instances in which strenuous physical activity may be curtailed because of the cardiac condition (Adams, Emmanouilides, and Riemenschneider, 1989).

Altered Hemodynamics

A stricture in the aortic outflow tract causes resistance to ejection of blood from the left ventricle. The extra workload on the left ventricle causes hypertrophy. If left ventricular failure develops, left atrial pressure will increase; this causes increased pressure in the pulmonary veins, resulting in pulmonary vascular congestion (pulmonary edema).

Clinical Manifestations

A serious form of critical AS may occur during the neonatal period. Symptoms of left ventricular failure and low cardiac output (respiratory distress, faint peripheral pulses, decreased urine output, poor feeding) occur during the first 2 weeks of life. Children with less severe AS may not show signs of the defect until preadolescence. Clinical manifestations such as fainting, epigastric or anginal pain, exercise intolerance, and dizziness after prolonged standing may occur. Sudden death after exertion has been reported among children with AS and is thought to result from the development of acute dysrhythmias.

A murmur is typically produced by blood flow through the stenotic area. It is heard best at the upper right sternal border at the second interspace (aortic space).

The prominent anatomic consequence of AS is the hypertrophy of the left ventricular wall, which eventually will lead to increased end-diastolic pressure, resulting in pulmonary venous and pulmonary arterial hypertension. Left ventricular hypertrophy also interferes with coronary artery perfusion and may result in myocardial infarction or scarring of the papillary muscles of the left ventricle, causing mitral insufficiency.

Diagnostic Evaluation

Diagnosis may be made on the basis of the history and physical findings alone. Cardiac catheterization is necessary to determine the location and severity of the stenosis, especially in those children with few symptoms who are at risk for acute dysrhythmias. The catheterization is also diagnostic in terms of the surgical approach; if a thin membrane is present, this is easily removed with excellent results.

Radiographic studies may confirm left ventricular enlargement and a dilated aorta in the poststenotic area; increased pulmonary vascular markings and cardiomegaly may be noted if CHF is present. An ECG may show left ventricular hypertrophy in mild defects. Depression of the ST segment indicates myocardial ischemia and is a very important finding in determining the need for immediate surgery. Echocardiography may show a thick, poorly contractile left ventricular wall and an abnormal aortic valve.

Therapeutic Management

Severe CHF is the main indication for surgical treatment of AS in infancy. In older children a systolic gradient across the obstruction of more than 50 mm Hg on the echocardiogram or angiographic evidence of a discrete subvalvular, valvular, or supravalvular stenosis is the main indication for surgery. All types of AS require open-heart surgery, which is performed through a median sternotomy.

Valvular aortic stenosis. The management of infants and children with congenital AS has changed significantly over the last few years. The neonate with critical AS requires urgent treatment. Although the procedure can be done with cardiopulmonary bypass, many institutions prefer an aortic valvotomy under inflow occlusion. Aortic valvotomy in critically ill neonates and infants still carries a mortality of 10% to 20% in major medical centers (Jonas and others, 1985). Results of aortic valvotomy in older children are very good, with mortality close to 0%. However, aortic valvotomy remains a palliative procedure, and approximately 25% of patients require second surgery within 10 years for recurrent stenosis. A valve replacement may be required at the second procedure.

In recent years, percutaneous balloon aortic valvotomy, performed in the cardiac catheterization laboratory, has become an alternative to surgery in some large centers. This technique has proved effective in the critically ill neonate and also in the older child with congenital AS. Aortic balloon valvotomy is a relatively new procedure without long-term follow-up. The incidence of side effects and complications, including aortic insufficiency or valvular regurgitation, tearing of the valve leaflets, loss of pulse in the catheterized limb, or serious dysrhythmias, is about 40%. In critically ill neonates the mortality rate is similar to that of surgery, approximately 15% to 30% (Perry and others, 1989).

Subvalvular aortic stenosis. Surgical repair of subvalvular AS may involve incising a membrane if one exists or cutting the fibromuscular ring. If the obstruction results from narrowing of the left ventricular outflow tract and a small aortic valve annulus, a patch may be required to enlarge the entire left ventricular outflow tract and annulus, an approach known as the *Konno* procedure. Supravalvular AS may also involve incising a membrane if present; however, an extensive area of narrowing requires enlargement with a patch graft.

Mortality from surgical repair of subvalvular AS is less than 2% in major centers; however, about 10% of these patients develop recurrent subaortic stenosis and require second surgery (Jonas and others, 1985). The Konno procedure is performed infrequently and needs further evaluation.

PULMONIC STENOSIS

Pulmonic stenosis (PS) is a narrowing at the entrance to the pulmonary artery (see Fig. 34-19). The valve may be normal, but the raphae (divisions between the cusps) are fused so that blood flow through the valve is restricted or the valve

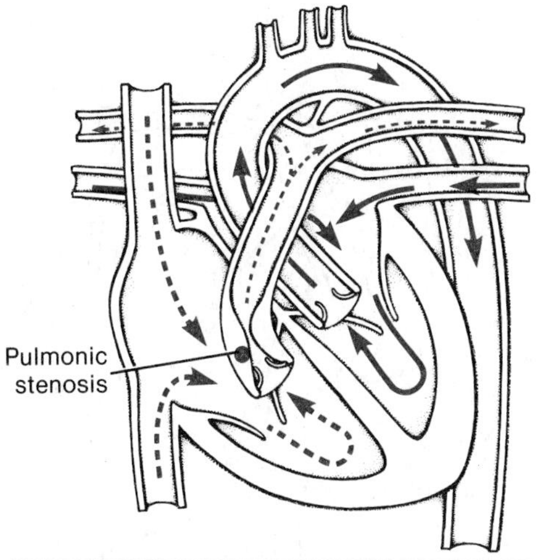

Fig. 34-19. Pulmonic stenosis. *Red arrows,* Saturated blood; *broken red arrows,* desaturated blood.

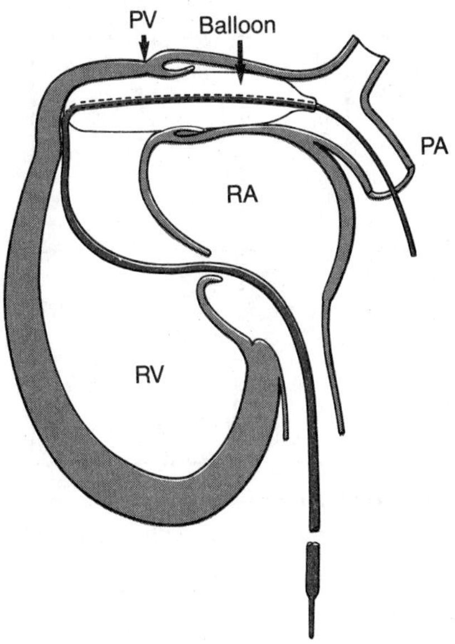

Fig. 34-20. Balloon dilatation of pulmonic valve *(PV).*

may be malformed. Stenosis may also occur from narrowing in the ventricular outflow tract. Pulmonary atresia is the extreme form of PS in that there is total fusion of the commissures and no blood flows to the lungs.

Altered Hemodynamics

When PS is present, resistance to blood flow causes right ventricular hypertrophy. If right ventricular failure develops, right atrial pressure will increase and this may result in reopening of the foramen ovale, shunting of unoxygenated blood into the left atrium, and systemic cyanosis. If PS is severe, CHF occurs, and systemic venous engorgement will be noted. An associated defect such as a PDA partially compensates for the obstruction by shunting blood from the aorta to the pulmonary artery and into the lungs.

Clinical Manifestations

Symptoms depend on the degree of PS and can range from only a murmur to cyanosis and CHF. A systolic ejection murmur is heard best at the upper left sternal border and may be accompanied by a thrill.

Children with moderate defects generally experience dyspnea and fatigue, especially on exertion, since blood flow to the lungs is insufficient to accommodate demands for increased cardiac output. Occasionally, severe PS is associated with a small right ventricle and an intact ventricular septum. These infants develop a large right-to-left shunt through a foramen ovale; pulmonary blood flow is greatly reduced and acute CHF ensues. Without immediate surgical intervention to increase pulmonary blood flow and relieve right ventricular obstruction, death will occur.

Diagnostic Evaluation

An echocardiogram demonstrates the obstruction to the pulmonary artery and any associated defects such as ASD. Cardiac catheterization documents increased pressure in the right side of the heart, and decreased oxygenation in the left side will be noted if a right-to-left shunt is present. Radiographic studies show a normal size heart, usually with normal or decreased pulmonary vascular markings and poststenotic dilatation of the pulmonary artery. An ECG may show several changes, including right atrial and ventricular hypertrophy.

Therapeutic Management

Children with mild degrees of PS may not require invasive intervention but are followed medically with appropriate antibiotic administration to prevent bacterial endocarditis. Treatment is recommended whenever the child demonstrates a significant pressure gradient across the pulmonic valve, since continued right ventricular hypertension contributes to the development of right ventricular fibrosis.

Critical PS in the infant often requires emergency surgery and carries a higher risk of complications. Although children with severe stenosis may require surgery, many pulmonic defects are being successfully treated with balloon angioplasty. Through a percutaneous puncture (similar to cardiac catheterization) a catheter is inserted across the stenotic pulmonic valve into the pulmonary artery, and a balloon at the end of the catheter is inflated and rapidly passed through the narrowed opening (Fig. 34-20). The procedure is associated with few complications and has proved highly effective, with a 50% to 75% reduction in pressure gradient across the pulmonic valve and a low rate of complications (Radtke and Lock, 1990). It is the treatment of choice for discrete PS in most centers and can be done safely in neonates.

In patients requiring surgery, a pulmonary valvotomy is performed. In a very brief procedure the surgeon works through a small incision in the pulmonary artery. The fused commissures are incised, and the pulmonary artery incision

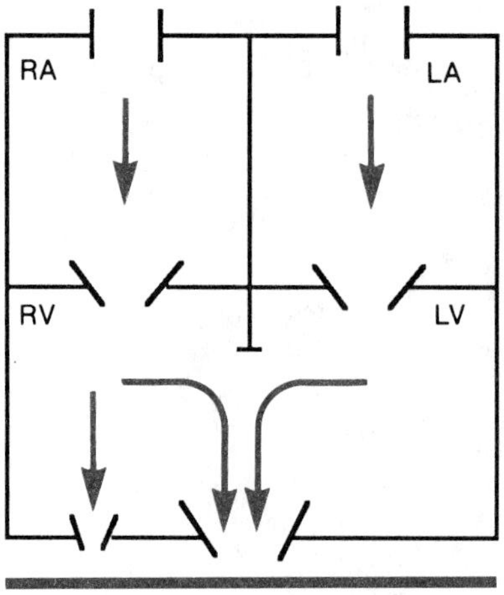

Fig. 34-21. Hemodynamic defects with decreased pulmonary blood flow.

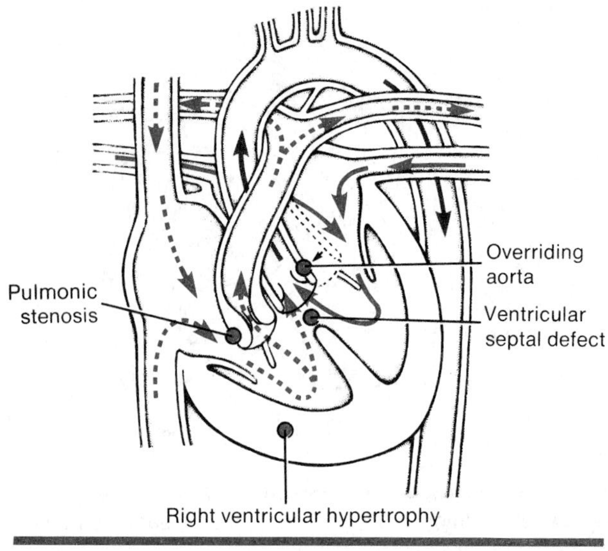

Fig. 34-22. Tetralogy of Fallot. *Red arrows,* Saturated blood; *broken red arrows,* desaturated blood; *black arrows,* mixed blood.

is closed. The surgical risks are very low (mortality less than 1%), and the hemodynamic results are excellent (Adams, Emmanouilides, and Riemenschneider, 1989). Both balloon dilatation and surgical valvotomy leave the pulmonic valve incompetent because they involve opening the fused valve leaflets; however, these patients are clinically asymptomatic. Long-term problems with restenosis or valve incompetence may occur.

DEFECTS WITH DECREASED PULMONARY BLOOD FLOW

In this group of defects, there is obstruction to pulmonary blood flow and an anatomic defect (ASD or VSD) between the right and left sides of the heart (Fig. 34-21). Because blood has difficulty exiting the right side of the heart via the pulmonary artery, pressure on the right side increases, exceeding left-sided pressures. This allows desaturated blood to shunt right to left, causing desaturation in the left side of the heart and in the systemic circulation. Clinically, these patients are hypoxemic and usually appear cyanotic. Tetralogy of Fallot and tricuspid atresia are the more common defects in this group.

TETRALOGY OF FALLOT

Tetralogy of Fallot (TOF) is the most common cyanotic heart defect. The anatomic definition includes four defects: (1) VSD; (2) PS, always subvalvular and often valvular; more accurately called right ventricular outflow tract obstruction; (3) an aorta that overrides the VSD; and (4) right ventricular hypertrophy, which occurs from pulmonary artery obstruction (Fig. 34-22). Wide variation exists in the severity of this defect. Some infants with mild obstruction to pulmonary blood flow have little or no right-to-left shunting and appear pink. They are often referred to as "pink tets." The more typical presentation is mild cyanosis at birth, which worsens with age because the PS is progressive, pulmonary blood flow is reduced, and the degree of right-to-left shunting increases with time.

Some infants with TOF are extremely cyanotic at birth because of severe obstruction and require immediate intervention to provide pulmonary blood flow. The most severely affected infants are those with complete pulmonary atresia (no anatomic connection between right ventricle and pulmonary artery), a rare defect. The following discussion focuses on the most common type of TOF, which manifests as progressive PS and increasing cyanosis with age.

Clinical Manifestations

The infant initially may not be cyanotic because the PDA shunts blood to the lungs, bypassing the PS. When the PDA has closed, hypoxemia and cyanosis become apparent. Cyanosis becomes more severe over time because increasing right ventricular outflow tract obstruction results in decreased pulmonary blood flow and increased right-to-left shunting. Rising hemoglobin and hematocrit concentrations are seen. Hypercyanotic ("tet") spells may occur with increasing obstruction and infundibular spasm. Squatting is rarely seen because children are usually repaired before age 2 years. (See Hypoxemia, p. 1552, for a discussion of cyanosis.) A pansystolic murmur is usually heard at the middle to lower left sternal border. Typically the second heart sound is single rather than split, as normal.

Diagnostic Evaluation

A diagnosis is usually made on the history and physical findings alone. However, a cardiac catheterization and/or echocardiogram is performed to evaluate the severity of the anatomic defects and cardiac changes. Laboratory tests determine the degree of polycythemia and arterial oxygen saturation. Right ventricular hypertrophy is noted on chest radiograph and ECG. The pulmonary arteries vary in size.

Therapeutic Management

The current trend is to repair TOF in infancy; the exact timing depends on the child's overall clinical status and the condition of the pulmonary arteries, but elective repair is usually performed in the first year of life. Indications for repair include increasing cyanosis and the development of hypercyanotic spells. Complete repair involves closure of the VSD and resection of the infundibular stenosis, with a pericardial patch to enlarge the right ventricular outflow tract. The procedure requires a median sternotomy and the use of cardiopulmonary bypass.

In infants who cannot undergo primary repair, a palliative procedure to increase pulmonary blood flow and increase oxygen saturation may be performed. The preferred procedure is the *Blalock-Taussig* or *modified Blalock-Taussig shunt,* which provides blood flow to the pulmonary arteries from the left or right subclavian artery (see Table 34-6). In general, however, shunts are avoided because they may result in pulmonary artery distortion.

The operative mortality for total correction of TOF is less than 5%. With improved surgical techniques there is a lower incidence of dysrhythmias and sudden death; surgical heart block is rare even in severely affected infants (Jonas and Lang, 1988).

TRICUSPID ATRESIA

Tricuspid atresia is failure of the tricuspid valve to develop; consequently there is no communication between the right atrium and right ventricle (Fig. 34-23). Tricuspid atresia is also associated with right ventricular hypoplasia and defects, such as septal defects, that allow some shunting of blood to the left side of the heart, then back to the right ventricle or pulmonary artery. Approximately 25% of these children also have transposition of the great arteries, and as many as 50% have PS. Anatomic variations of tricuspid atresia may produce decreased, normal, or increased pulmonary blood flow, varying the clinical presentation and treatment required.

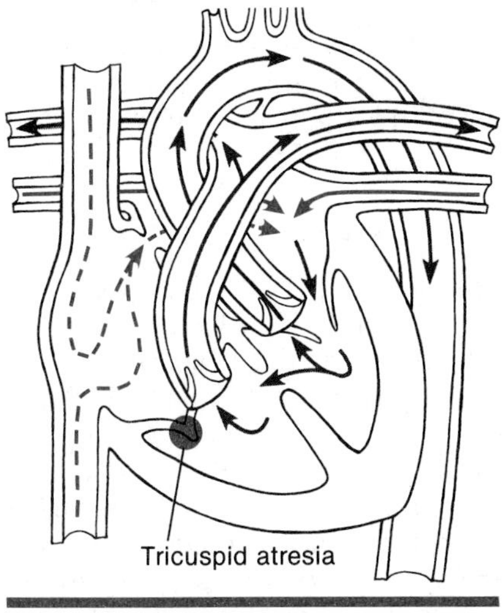

Fig. 34-23. Tricuspid atresia. *Red arrows,* Saturated blood; *broken red arrows,* desaturated blood; *black arrows,* mixed blood.

Altered Hemodynamics

At birth the presence of a patent foramen ovale (or other atrial septal opening) is required to permit blood flow across the septum into the left atrium; the PDA allows blood flow to the pulmonary artery into the lungs for oxygenation. A VSD allows a modest amount of blood to enter the right ventricle and pulmonary artery for oxygenation. Pulmonary blood flow usually is diminished.

Clinical Manifestations

Cyanosis, often evident within the first day of life, is the most consistent clinical sign of tricuspid atresia. The degree of cyanosis depends on the amount of pulmonary blood flow. Tachypnea and dyspnea are often present. Severe cyanosis and hypoxemia may be delayed until the ductus arteriosus closes. If the neonate survives later into infancy, systemic consequences of cyanosis and polycythemia may develop. Hypercyanotic episodes may also occur.

No murmur is characteristic of tricuspid atresia; auscultatory findings are determined by the presence of associated defects. A harsh pansystolic murmur usually indicates a VSD. The second heart sound may be narrowly split because of decreased blood flow to the pulmonary artery, or the pulmonic component may be absent when no VSD is present. Pulmonary findings of CHF occur early if increased pulmonary blood flow is present.

Diagnostic Evaluation

Laboratory findings are those associated with any cyanotic defect (hypoxemia and acidosis). The chest radiograph findings are variable; the heart is often normal or slightly increased in size, and pulmonary vascular markings are normal or decreased. Echocardiography is helpful in confirming the presence of tricuspid atresia. An ECG shows significant right and left atrial and ventricular enlargement. Confirmation of the diagnosis is made by cardiac catheterization, which reveals flow of right atrial blood to the left atrium, inability to enter the right ventricle, and presence of associated defects, such as transposition of the great arteries, VSD, and PS.

Therapeutic Management

For the neonate whose pulmonary blood flow depends on the patency of the ductus arteriosus, a continuous infusion of prostaglandin E_1 is started at 0.1 mg/kg of body weight/minute until surgical intervention can be arranged. Palliative treatment is the placement of a shunt (pulmonary-to-systemic artery anastomosis) to increase blood flow to the lungs. If the ASD is small, an atrial septostomy is done during cardiac catheterization. Some children have increased pulmonary blood flow and require pulmonary artery banding to lessen the volume of blood to the lungs.

The corrective procedure for tricuspid atresia and a variety of other defects in which there is only one functional ventricle is called the *Fontan procedure.* The Fontan procedure has undergone many modifications since it was first described in 1971 and continues to evolve. The principle behind the procedure is that there is sufficient energy in the systemic venous system to propel blood through the lungs without a ventricular pump, as long as pulmonary vascular resistance and left atrial pressure are relatively low. The goals of the Fontan procedure are (1) to separate the systemic and pulmonary circulations by closing any septal defects and previous shunts and (2) to connect the systemic venous structures (venae cavae, right atrium) with the pulmonary arteries (Sade and Fyfe, 1990). This procedure is most effective in children with normal left ventricular function, pulmonary artery anatomy, and pulmonary vascular resistance. Postoperative complications include dysrhythmias, systemic venous hypertension, pleural and pericardial effusions, elevated pulmonary vascular resistance, and ventricular dysfunction. While initial results have been encouraging, long-term survival and morbidity must await future studies.

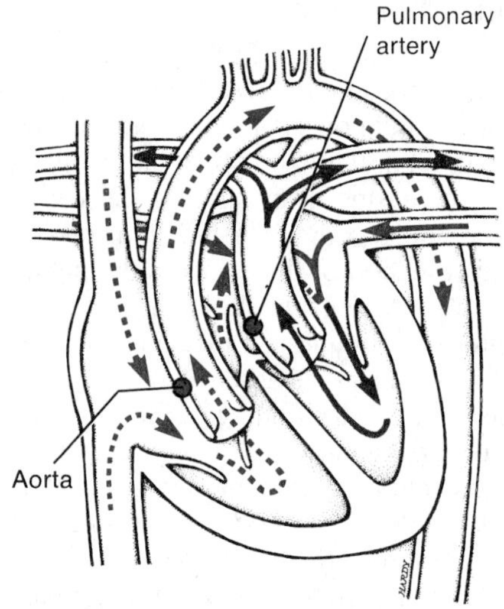

Fig. 34-24. Transposition of the great arteries. *Red arrows,* Saturated blood; *broken red arrows,* desaturated blood; *black arrows,* mixed blood.

MIXED DEFECTS

Many complex cardiac anomalies are classified together in the *mixed* category because survival in the postnatal period depends on mixing of blood from the pulmonary and systemic circulations within the heart chambers. Hemodynamically, fully saturated systemic blood flow mixes with the desaturated pulmonary blood flow, causing a relative desaturation of the systemic blood flow. Pulmonary congestion occurs because the differences in pulmonary artery pressure and aortic pressure favor pulmonary blood flow. Cardiac output decreases because of a volume load on the ventricle. Clinically, these patients have a variable picture that combines some degree of desaturation (although cyanosis is not always visible) and signs of CHF. Some defects, such as transposition of the great arteries, cause severe cyanosis in the first days of life and later cause CHF. Others, such as truncus arteriosus, cause severe CHF in the first weeks of life and mild desaturation.

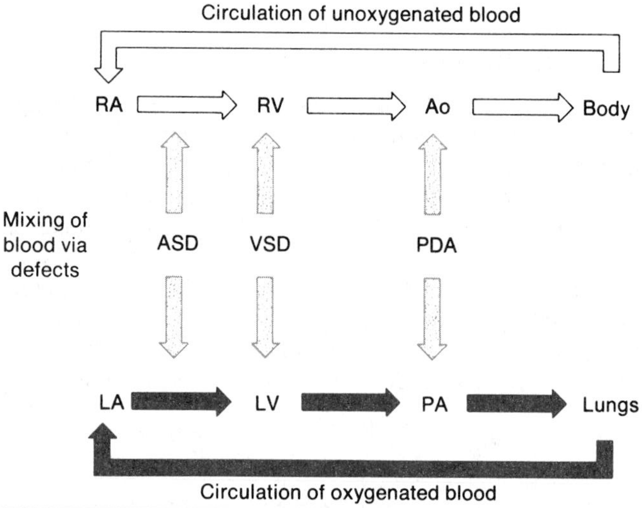

Fig. 34-25. Hemodynamics in transposition of great arteries. *Ao,* Aorta. See Glossary (p. 1530) for other abbreviations.

TRANSPOSITION OF THE GREAT ARTERIES

By definition, transposition of the great arteries (TGA) refers to a condition in which the pulmonary artery leaves the left ventricle and the aorta exits from the right ventricle (Fig. 34-24). This type of circulation is incompatible with extrauterine life because the body receives only desaturated blood and progressive hypoxemia will develop. For survival the parallel circuits must communicate to allow adequate mixing of saturated blood in the pulmonary circulation and desaturated blood in the systemic circulation. This is accomplished through associated defects such as septal defects or a PDA (Fig. 34-25).

Associated Defects and Hemodynamics

The most common defect associated with TGA is a patent foramen ovale. At birth there is also a PDA, although in most instances this closes after the neonatal period. Another associated anomaly may be VSD. Presence of these defects increases the risk of CHF, since they often produce high pulmonary blood flow under high pressure. For example, a large VSD permits blood to flow from the right to the left ventricle, into the pulmonary artery, and finally to the lungs. However, it also produces high pulmonary blood flow under high pressure, which can result in pulmonary vascular resistance. The same series of events occurs with a large PDA, since blood directly from the aorta flows under high pressure into the pulmonary artery and lungs.

Clinical Manifestations

The severity of the child's condition depends on the amount of blood mixing. Neonates with minimum mixing of systemic and pulmonary venous blood or obstruction to pulmonary blood flow are severely cyanotic at birth. Those with large septal defects or a PDA may be less severely cyanotic but develop symptoms of CHF during the first weeks of life. In these infants the only signs at birth may be cyanosis after crying or feeding and progressive hyperpnea. However, hypercyanotic episodes can occur and are thought to result from increased oxygen demand that the cardiovascular system cannot meet.

There is no murmur associated with simple TGA, and if one is present, it is characteristic of the associated defects. Cardiomegaly from right and left ventricular hypertrophy may be evident a few weeks after birth. The infant with a large VSD will have symptoms of CHF in the first weeks to month of life.

Diagnostic Evaluation

Definitive diagnosis of TGA is made on the findings of two-dimensional echocardiography. Radiologic findings may reveal an egg-shaped heart with a narrowed mediastinum as well as some increased pulmonary markings. Cardiac catheterization is indicated to define coronary artery anatomy and measure left-to-right ventricular ratios to determine the left ventricle's ability to assume the work of the systemic circulation.

Therapeutic Management

Both palliative and corrective surgical procedures can be performed for TGA. Whenever possible, however, primary repair is recommended. The administration of prostaglandin E_1 may be initiated to increase blood mixing if systemic and pulmonary mixing is inadequate to provide an oxygen saturation of 75% or to maintain cardiac output. During cardiac catheterization a balloon atrial septostomy (Rashkind procedure) may also be performed to increase mixing and maintain cardiac output over a longer period.

Several surgical approaches are available for correction of TGA. The choice of the reparative procedure depends on the anatomic defects, the surgeon's preference, and the availability of comprehensive postoperative management. The procedure of choice is the *Jatene operation,* or *arterial switch,* which involves transposing the great arteries and mobilizing and reimplanting the coronary arteries. It is a technically challenging procedure because the coronary arteries must be removed from the aorta before the switch is performed, and then they must be reimplanted into the aorta at its new location. Reimplantation of the coronary arteries is critical to the infant's survival, and they must be reattached without torsion or kinking to provide the heart with its supply of oxygen. The advantage of the arterial switch procedure is the reestablishment of normal circulation, with the left ventricle acting as the systemic pump.

The *Mustard* or *Senning operation* involves the creation of an intraatrial baffle to tunnel or divert systemic venous blood to the mitral valve (and the left ventricle and pulmonary artery) and divert pulmonary venous blood to the tricuspid valve (and the right ventricle and aorta). Therefore the procedure does not attempt to transplant the transposed arterial vessels but reverses the function of the atria. An advantage of the Senning operation is the use of the patient's own atrial septum to create the baffle rather than pericardium or prosthetic material, which is used in the Mustard operation. The use of little or no foreign material allows for growth of the biologic baffle.

Another surgical option is the *Rastelli procedure,* which is the operative choice in infants with TGA, VSD, and severe PS. It involves closure of the VSD with a baffle, directing left ventricular blood through the VSD into the aorta. The pulmonic valve is then closed and a conduit placed from the right ventricle to the pulmonary artery, creating a physiologically normal circulation. Unfortunately, this procedure requires multiple conduit replacements as the child grows.

The optimum time for repair depends on the procedure. The Jatene operation can usually be performed safely in the first 3 weeks to 1 month of life. The other surgeries are usually performed within the first year of life. Mortality following repair is influenced by the type of procedure, complexity of the lesion, maturity of the infant, and other complicating factors. Mortality for both the arterial and the atrial switch procedures is less than 5%. However, significant problems occur with late complications following atrial baffle surgery. For example, right ventricular failure, baffle obstructions, and rhythm disturbances occur most often. Only 50% of patients have normal sinus rhythm 10 years after atrial baffle procedures (Castaneda, 1989). Potential complications of the Jatene arterial switch include narrowing at the great artery anastomoses or coronary artery insufficiency.

TOTAL ANOMALOUS PULMONARY VENOUS CONNECTION

Total anomalous pulmonary venous connection (TAPVC), also called total anomalous pulmonary venous return (TAPVR) or total anomalous pulmonary venous drainage (TAPVD), is a rare defect characterized by failure of the pulmonary veins to join the left atrium. Instead, the pulmonary veins are abnormally connected to the systemic venous circuit via the right atrium or various veins draining toward the right atrium, such as the superior vena cava. The abnormal attachment results in mixed blood being returned to the right atrium and shunted from the right to the left through an ASD. The type of TAPVC is classified according to the pulmonary venous point of attachment as:

Supracardiac—attachment above the diaphragm, such as to the superior vena cava (most common form) (Fig. 34-26)
Cardiac—direct attachment to the heart, such as to the right atrium or coronary sinus
Infracardiac—attachment below the diaphragm, such as to the inferior vena cava (most severe form)

Altered Hemodynamics

The right atrium receives all the blood that normally would flow into the left atrium. As a result, the right side of the heart hypertrophies, whereas the left side, especially the left

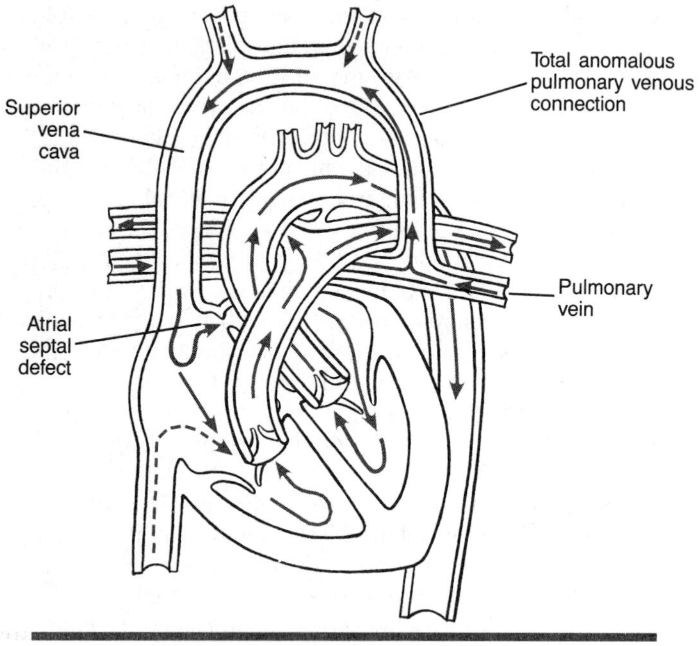

Fig. 34-26. Supracardiac total anomalous pulmonary venous connection. *Red arrows,* Saturated blood; *broken red arrows,* desaturated blood; *black arrows,* mixed blood.

atrium, may remain small. An associated ASD or patent foramen ovale allows systemic venous blood to shunt from the higher-pressure right atrium to the left atrium and into the left side of the heart. As a result, the oxygen saturation of the blood in both sides of the heart (and ultimately, in the systemic arterial circulation) is the same. If the pulmonary blood flow is large, pulmonary venous return is also large and the amount of saturated blood is relatively high. However, if there is obstruction to pulmonary venous drainage, pulmonary venous return is impeded, pulmonary venous pressure rises, and pulmonary interstitial edema develops and eventually contributes to CHF. Infracardiac TAPVC is often associated with obstruction to pulmonary venous drainage and is a surgical emergency.

Clinical Manifestations

Most infants with TAPVC develop cyanosis early in life. The degree of cyanosis is inversely related to the amount of pulmonary blood flow—the more pulmonary blood, the less cyanosis. Children with unobstructed TAPVC may be asymptomatic until pulmonary vascular resistance decreases during infancy, increasing pulmonary blood flow, with resulting tachypnea, feeding difficulties, repeated upper respiratory infections, and other signs of CHF. On physical examination the infants look thin and malnourished. Conversely, cyanosis becomes worse with pulmonary obstruction; once obstruction occurs, the infant's condition usually deteriorates rapidly. Without intervention, cardiac failure will progress to death.

Auscultatory findings depend on the hemodynamics. A blowing systolic murmur from tricuspid regurgitation may be heard at the lower left sternal border. A continuous murmur or venous hum may be present from blood flow through the anomalous venous channels. Because the right side of the heart is hyperdynamic, a gallop rhythm is common.

Diagnostic Evaluation

The chest radiograph reveals increased pulmonary vascular markings and cardiomegaly with right atrial and ventricular enlargement. If pulmonary venous obstruction is present, the heart size is usually normal with a pattern of diffuse pulmonary congestion. The ECG shows right ventricular hypertrophy, and the echocardiogram demonstrates the abnormal connections. The cardiac catheterization reveals the changes in oxygen saturation of the blood within various chambers and vessels. Angiography identifies the site of the pulmonary venous connection.

Therapeutic Management

The current trend is toward corrective repair of TAPVC during early infancy (Jonas and Lang, 1988). In unobstructed veins, cardiac failure is medically managed until surgical correction is performed. If the pulmonary veins are obstructed, a surgical emergency exists. The surgical approach varies with the anatomic defect. In general, however, the common pulmonary vein is anastomosed to the left atrium, the ASD is closed, and the anomalous pulmonary venous connection is ligated. Any other defects, such as PDA, are also repaired.

The success of corrective surgery depends on the location of the defect, absence or presence of pulmonary venous obstruction, and left ventricular function. The cardiac type is most successfully repaired because of ease in restructuring the channels and less chance of pulmonary vein obstruction. The infracardiac type has the greatest incidence of morbidity and mortality. Potential postoperative complications include reobstruction; bleeding; dysrhythmias, particularly heart block; pulmonary artery hypertension; and persistent heart failure.

TRUNCUS ARTERIOSUS

Truncus arteriosus results from failure of normal septation and division of the common trunk into the pulmonary artery and aorta. As a result, a single vessel arises from both ventricles, straddling a VSD and providing blood flow for the pulmonary, systemic, and coronary circulations. The common trunk has a single valve, which may possess two to six cusps. This valve is often malformed, stenosed, or incompetent. There are three major types of truncus arteriosus:

Type I—a single pulmonary trunk arises near the base of the truncus and divides into the left and right pulmonary arteries.
Type II—the left and right pulmonary arteries arise separately from the posterior aspect of the truncus.
Type III—the pulmonary arteries arise independently and from the lateral aspect of the truncus (Fig. 34-27).

Altered Hemodynamics

Blood ejected from the left and right ventricles enters the common trunk, mixing pulmonary and systemic circula-

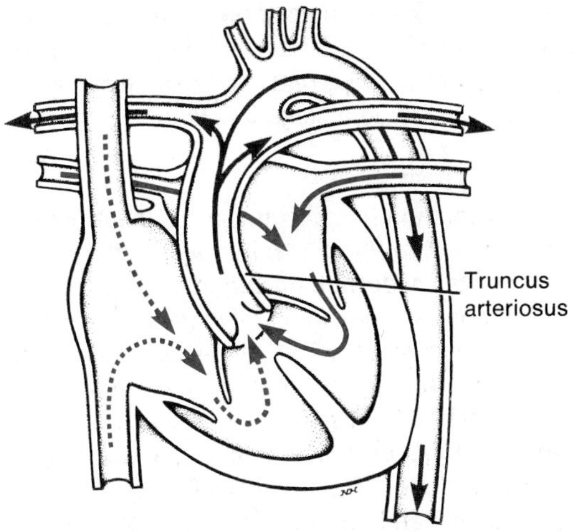

Fig. 34-27. Truncus arteriosus. *Red arrows,* Saturated blood; *broken red arrows,* desaturated blood; *black arrows,* mixed blood.

tions. Blood flow is distributed to the pulmonary and systemic circulations according to the relative resistances of each system. The amount of pulmonary blood flow depends on the size of the pulmonary arteries and the pulmonary vascular resistance. Generally, resistance to pulmonary blood flow is less than systemic vascular resistance, resulting in preferential blood flow to the lungs. Pulmonary vascular disease develops at an early age in patients with truncus arteriosus.

Clinical Manifestations

Clinical manifestations depend on the source and volume of the infant's pulmonary blood flow and the presence of other intracardiac anomalies. The infant without PS often demonstrates mild or moderate cyanosis within the first days of life, which worsens with crying or exertion. However, as pulmonary vascular resistance falls, the lungs receive an increased volume of blood and signs of severe CHF develop. If PS is present, the cyanosis is severe, particularly once the PDA begins to close. However, these infants are less likely to develop CHF.

A harsh systolic ejection murmur is heard along the left sternal border as a result of the VSD and is usually accompanied by a thrill. Opening of the truncal valve may produce a click immediately after the first heart sound. If pulmonary blood flow is increased, the child may demonstrate bounding pulses and a widened pulse pressure.

Diagnostic Evaluation

Diagnostic findings depend largely on the presence of CHF because of the large pulmonary blood flow with or without truncal valve regurgitation. The chest radiograph will show increased pulmonary vascular markings and cardiomegaly. If significant PS is present, pulmonary vascular markings will be decreased and cardiomegaly may not be present. Echocardiography and cardiac catheterization are done to confirm the diagnosis and determine the type of defect.

Therapeutic Management

Most children with truncus arteriosus can be medically managed through the first month of life with aggressive treatment of CHF. Corrective treatment is a modification of the Rastelli procedure. It involves closing the VSD so that the truncus arteriosus receives the outflow from the left ventricle, excising the pulmonary arteries from the aorta, and attaching them to the right ventricle by means of a homograft. Currently, homografts (segments of cadaver aorta and pulmonary artery that are treated with antibiotics and cryopreserved) are preferred over synthetic conduits to establish continuity between the right ventricle and pulmonary artery. The synthetic conduits have been associated with calcification and accumulation of an obstructive pseudointima, leading to obstruction and need for early replacement (Jonas and Lang, 1988). Homografts are more flexible and easier to use during the procedure and appear less prone to obstruction.

The success of corrective surgery depends on the child's age and the severity of existing pulmonary vascular disease. Early elective repair is recommended to prevent severe CHF, severe growth failure, or worsening pulmonary vascular disease. Postoperative complications include persistent heart failure, bleeding, pulmonary artery hypertension, dysrhythmias, and residual VSD. These children require additional procedures to replace the conduit as its size becomes inadequate in relation to the children's growth.

HYPOPLASTIC LEFT HEART SYNDROME

Hypoplastic left heart syndrome (HLHS) refers to a collection of complex congenital heart lesions characterized by abnormal development of the left-sided cardiac structures. A lesion obstructs blood flow to the body, and the left ventricle, aorta, and aortic arch are underdeveloped (Fig. 34-28). A uniformly fatal defect without intervention, infants

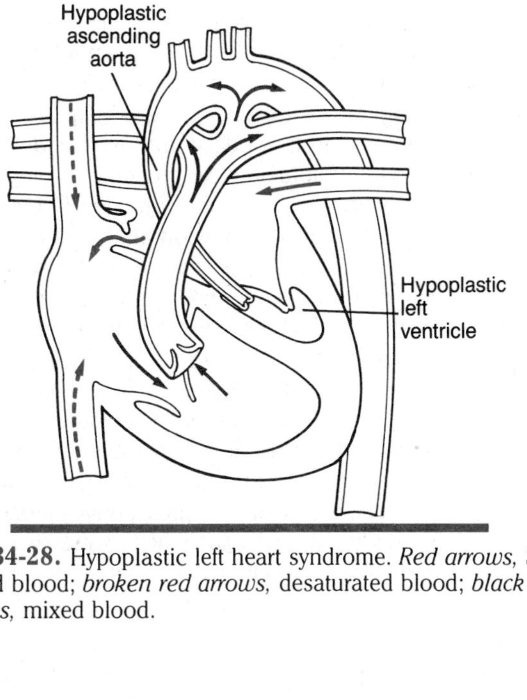

Fig. 34-28. Hypoplastic left heart syndrome. *Red arrows,* Saturated blood; *broken red arrows,* desaturated blood; *black arrows,* mixed blood.

with HLHS have one effective ventricle and depend on the PDA for survival.

Altered Hemodynamics

An ASD or patent foramen ovale allows saturated blood from the left atrium to mix with desaturated blood from the right atrium and to flow through the right ventricle and out into the pulmonary artery. From the pulmonary artery the blood flows to the lungs, then through the ductus arteriosus into the aorta and out to the body. The amount of blood flow to the pulmonary and systemic circulations depends on the relationship between the pulmonary and systemic vascular resistances. The coronary and cerebral vessels receive blood by retrograde flow through the hypoplastic ascending aorta.

Clinical Manifestations

Infants born with HLHS usually appear well developed and normal at birth. Most infants develop mild cyanosis, tachypnea, and progressive dyspnea within the first week of life. As the ductus arteriosus starts to close, systemic perfusion progressively deteriorates, leading to hypoxemia and acidosis. Signs of CHF develop as pulmonary blood flow increases. Generally, acute deterioration and cardiovascular collapse occur with ductal closure.

Diagnostic Evaluation

The chest radiograph demonstrates cardiomegaly and increased pulmonary vascular markings. The ECG reflects underdevelopment of the left side of the heart and prominence of right-sided forces, with right axis deviation, right ventricular hypertrophy, and diminished left ventricular forces. Diagnosis often is made by echocardiography without the need for cardiac catheterization.

Therapeutic Management

Survival depends on prompt recognition and treatment of HLHS. The administration of prostaglandin E_1 to reopen the ductus arteriosus is essential for these infants' survival. Aggressive medical management is required to correct acidosis, control heart failure, and balance systemic and pulmonary blood flow to stabilize these infants until surgical intervention is arranged.

Surgical intervention is a staged approach, requiring the infant to undergo multiple surgical procedures. Stage I palliation begins with the *Norwood procedure* (Norwood, 1989). The surgical goals of palliation are to (1) establish a permanent communication between the right ventricle and aorta, (2) establish pulmonary blood flow and maintain at near-normal levels, and (3) establish a large interatrial communication. Postoperative complications include imbalance of systemic and pulmonary blood flow, bleeding, low cardiac output, and persistent heart failure. Ventricular function, normal pulmonary artery anatomy, and low PVR must be preserved for the child to be a good candidate for the stage II corrective repair (modified Fontan procedures, see p. 1565). Early surgical experiences were disappointing, but with continued modification, successes have been reported (de Leval and others, 1988).

Cardiac transplantation may be another surgical option for infants with HLHS, either as the initial surgical approach (Bailey and Gundry, 1990) or as an alternative therapy if the child is not considered a stage II candidate.

Heart Transplantation

Heart transplantation has become a treatment option for infants and children with worsening heart failure and a limited life expectancy despite maximum medical and surgical management. Indications for cardiac transplantation in children are cardiomyopathy and end-stage congenital heart disease. An important and controversial group of patients with congenital heart disease are infants with HLHS who undergo heart transplantation as their initial treatment (Bailey and others, 1986). The number of heart transplants performed in infants and children has increased tenfold in the last decade, from fewer than 20 transplants in 1983 to more than 200 in 1989. Survival for children over 1 year of age is 76% at 1 year and 62% at 5 years after transplant; infants under 1 year of age have a higher operative mortality and a 1-year survival of 66% (Kriett and Kaye, 1990). Although the outlook for infants and children undergoing heart transplantation has greatly improved in the last decade with improved techniques and treatments and increased clinical experience, it is still considered a palliative procedure, not a cure (Parness and Nadas, 1988).

The heart transplant procedure may be orthotopic or heterotopic. *Orthotopic* heart transplantation refers to removing the recipient's own heart and implanting a new heart from a donor who has had brain death but a healthy heart. The donor and recipient are matched by weight and blood type. *Heterotopic* heart transplantation refers to leaving the recipient's own heart in place and implanting a new heart to act as an additional pump or "piggyback" heart; this type of transplant is rarely done in children.

Before transplantation, potential recipients are carefully evaluated to identify problems in other organ systems that might preclude or increase the risks of transplantation. A psychosocial evaluation of patient and family is done to identify possible problems in complying with the complex medical regimen following transplantation and in providing needed support systems. Patients are listed on a national computer network organized by the **United Network for Organ Sharing (UNOS)** to match donors and recipients. Because of the limited donor supply, increasing numbers of children waiting for heart transplants, and the uncertain medical course of patients with end-stage heart disease, some patients will die waiting for a donor heart (see also Tissue Donation/Autopsy, Chapter 23).

The posttransplant course is complex. Although heart function is greatly improved or normal following transplantation, the risk of rejection is serious. Rejection of the heart is diagnosed primarily by endomyocardial biopsy and several noninvasive tests. Immunosuppressants must be taken for life and have many systemic side effects. Infection is always a risk. Potential long-term problems that may limit survival include chronic rejection, causing coronary artery disease; renal dysfunction and hypertension resulting from cyclosporine administration; lymphoma; and infection (Zuberbuhler, Fricker, and Griffith, 1989). In the short term, following successful transplantation, children are able to return to full participation in age-appropriate activities and appear to adapt well to their new life-style (Parness and Nadas, 1988; Starnes and others, 1987; Trento and others, 1989). The long-term prognosis is unknown.

Nursing considerations. Nursing care following transplantation is demanding and complex, with careful attention to both the physical needs of the child and the emotional needs of the child and family. Immunosuppressants and nursing implications are discussed in Chapter 30 in relation to renal transplantation. Care of the immunosuppressed child is reviewed in Chapter 36. Psychosocial concerns and appropriate interventions for the child with a life-threatening disorder are presented in Chapter 23. Successfully caring for a child following a heart transplant requires the expertise and dedication of many members of the health care team. Nurses play vital roles in assessment, coordination of care, psychosocial support, and patient and family education.

Transplantation raises a number of ethical issues, including the use of anencephalic infants as organ donors (see Questions and Controversies, p. 472), use of animal hearts in human transplantation, scarcity of donors, and donor allocation issues. Other factors, often unique to pediatrics, involve the patient's status as a minor, specifically issues of informed consent and parental responsibility and authority.

NURSING CARE OF THE FAMILY AND CHILD WITH CONGENITAL HEART DISEASE

When a child is born with a severe cardiac anomaly, the parents are faced with the immense psychologic and physical tasks of adjusting to the birth of a child with special needs. The reactions and nursing interventions required to support the family differ little from those discussed in Chapters 11 and 22. Since corrective surgery is being performed at an earlier age, this discussion is primarily directed (1) toward the family of an infant who has a serious heart defect and requires home care before definitive repair and (2) toward preparation and care of the child and family when heart surgery is performed.

Assessment

Nursing care of the child with a congenital heart defect begins as soon as the diagnosis is suspected. However, in many instances symptoms that suggest a cardiac anomaly are not present at birth or, if manifest, are so subtle that they are easily overlooked.

Many heart defects are not evident until the child's growth and/or energy expenditure exceeds the heart's ability to supply oxygenated blood to the tissues. Since the onset of symptoms may be gradual, the child may curtail activity so that the signs of exercise intolerance are less obvious. However, a careful history yields important clues to this change. For example, infants are normally extremely mobile and their energies are directed toward learning gross motor skills. Most infants suck vigorously and fall asleep after finishing a feeding. It is very unusual to hear of a child who prefers to sit rather than crawl or walk or who falls asleep shortly after beginning a feeding. Likewise, a child who needs frequent rests or naps after limited play periods may also be exhibiting exercise intolerance. Such histories should alert the nurse to assess cardiac function.

Other clues are a history of poor weight gain; poor feeding habits, especially the need to pause during feeding; poor suck; difficulty in coordinating sucking, swallowing, and breathing; frequent respiratory infections; cyanosis; and squatting. Since parents may not view any of these findings as abnormal, the nurse must specifically ask about them during a health assessment.

Another indication of heart defects is murmurs. Chapter 7 discusses the usual distinguishing characteristics between innocent and organic murmurs. Nurses who perform primary health assessments must be knowledgeable of the differences in order to correctly refer children with heart murmurs of possible organic origin to a cardiologist. There has been controversy over informing parents of innocent murmurs, since some practitioners believe that the parent may be unduly worried and transfer that concern to overprotectiveness of the child. However, this problem can be avoided by stressing to parents that although a murmur was heard, no heart disease is present, no further cardiac study is needed, and the heart is normal.

Nursing Diagnoses

Many nursing diagnoses are apparent following a thorough assessment of the child and family. Some of these are developed in the Nursing Care Plan on pp. 1572-1573. Others will be evident based on assessment of individual cases.

Planning

The overall plan of care for the infant or child with CHD includes those listed here. The nursing care consists of providing not only direct care to the infant or child, but also indirect care through family members.

1. Help parents and child adjust to the diagnosis.
2. Educate family regarding symptoms of the disease and their management.
3. Help family cope with effects of the disorder.
4. Foster growth-promoting family relationships.
5. Prepare child and family for surgical repair of a defect.
6. Provide care to the child undergoing cardiac surgery.
7. Provide emotional support.
8. Prepare child and family for home care.

Implementation

Many problems face nurses and families when a child is born with a congenital abnormality. Cardiac defects are especially frightening to families because of the serious con-

NURSING CARE PLAN
The Child with Congenital Heart Disease

NURSING DIAGNOSIS: Decreased cardiac output related to structural defect

GOAL 1
Improve cardiac output

INTERVENTIONS
*Administer digoxin as ordered (see Parent Guidelines, p. 1549)
*Administer afterload reduction agents as ordered

EXPECTED OUTCOME
Heart rate and volume indicate satisfactory cardiac output

NURSING DIAGNOSIS: Activity intolerance related to imbalance between oxygen supply and demand

GOAL 1
Reduce energy expenditure

INTERVENTIONS
Allow for frequent rest periods
Encourage quiet games and activities
Help the child select activities appropriate to age, condition, and capabilities
Avoid extremes of environmental temperature

EXPECTED OUTCOME
Child determines and engages in activities commensurate with capabilities

NURSING DIAGNOSIS: Altered growth and development related to inadequate oxygen and nutrients to tissues; social isolation

GOAL 1
Promote physical growth

INTERVENTIONS
Provide well-balanced, highly nutritious diet

EXPECTED OUTCOME
Child achieves normal growth (specify)

GOAL 2
Improve iron-carrying capacity of blood (for children with hypoxemia)

INTERVENTIONS
*Administer iron preparations as prescribed
Encourage iron-rich foods in the diet

EXPECTED OUTCOME
Child assimilates sufficient iron

GOAL 3
Avoid social isolation

INTERVENTIONS
Encourage age-appropriate activities

EXPECTED OUTCOME
Child engages in age-appropriate activities

NURSING DIAGNOSIS: Potential for infection related to debilitated physical status

GOAL 1
Prevent infection

INTERVENTIONS
Avoid contact with infected persons
Provide for adequate rest
Provide optimum nutrition

EXPECTED OUTCOME
Child remains free of infection

*Dependent nursing action.

NURSING CARE PLAN
The Child with Congenital Heart Disease—cont'd

NURSING DIAGNOSIS: Altered family processes related to having a child with a heart condition

See Nursing Care Plan: The Child with a Chronic Illness or Disability, Chapter 22

GOAL 1
Reduce family's fears and anxieties

INTERVENTIONS
Discuss with parents their fears regarding child's symptoms, such as pounding heart, hypercyanotic spells, irritability

EXPECTED OUTCOME
Family discusses their fears and anxieties

GOAL 2
Help family cope with symptoms of disease

INTERVENTIONS
Encourage family to participate in care of the child while hospitalized
Encourage family to include others in child's care to prevent their own exhaustion
Assist family in determining appropriate physical activity and disciplining methods for child

EXPECTED OUTCOME
Family copes with child's symptoms in a positive way

GOAL 3
Prepare family for home care of the infant or child

INTERVENTIONS
Teach skills needed for home care
- Administration of medications
- Feeding techniques
- Interventions for conserving energy and those directed toward relief of frightening symptoms
- Signs that indicate complications
- Where and whom to contact for help and guidance

Anticipate need for further information and support
Refer family to local chapter of the American Red Cross for instruction in cardiopulmonary resuscitation

EXPECTED OUTCOMES
Family demonstrates the ability and motivation for home care of the infant
Family members learn cardiopulmonary resuscitation technique

NURSING DIAGNOSIS: Potential for injury (complications) related to cardiac condition and therapies

GOAL 1
Recognize signs of complications early

INTERVENTIONS
Teach family to recognize signs of complications
- Congestive heart failure (CHF) (see Box 34-2)
- Digoxin toxicity
  - Vomiting (earliest sign)
  - Bradycardia
  - Dysrhythmias
- Increased respiratory effort—tachycardia, retraction, grunting, cough, cyanosis
- Hypoxemia—cyanosis, restlessness, tachycardia
- Cerebral thrombosis—compensatory polycythemia (in cyanotic heart disease) is particularly hazardous when child is dehydrated
- Cardiovascular collapse—pallor, cyanosis, hypotonia

Teach family to intervene during hypercyanotic spells
- Place child in knee-chest position with head and chest elevated
- Remain calm
- Call practitioner

EXPECTED OUTCOMES
Family recognizes signs of complications and institutes appropriate action

GOAL 2
Prepare for diagnostic tests and surgery

INTERVENTIONS
Explain or clarify information presented to family by the practitioner and surgeon
Prepare child and parents for the procedure
Assist with family's decision regarding surgery
Explore feelings regarding surgical options

EXPECTED OUTCOME
Family demonstrates an understanding of tests, surgery, etc. (specify learning and manner of demonstration)

See also:
- Nursing Care Plan: The Child in the Hospital, Chapter 26
- Nursing Care Plan: The Family of the Ill or Hospitalized Child, Chapter 26
- Nursing Care Plan: The Child Undergoing Surgery, Chapter 27
- Nursing Care Plan: The Child in Pain, Chapter 26

notations. The specific interventions for a child with CHD are discussed here and outlined in the Nursing Care Plan on pp. 1572-1573). The care of the infant with CHF and hypoxemia and major physiologic consequences of CHD are presented earlier in the chapter.

Help Family Adjust to the Disorder

Once parents learn of the heart defect, they are initially in a period of shock, followed by high anxiety, especially fear of the child's death. This reaction may occur soon after the child's birth or at a later period in life. Whatever its timing, the family needs a period of grief before assimilating the meaning of the defect. Unfortunately the demands for medical treatment may not allow this, necessitating that the parents be informed of the condition in order to give informed consent for diagnostic/therapeutic procedures. The nurse can be instrumental in supporting parents in their loss, assessing their level of understanding, supplying information as needed, and helping other members of the health team to understand the parents' reactions.

Severely distressed newborns usually remain in the hospital. This can seriously affect parent-infant attachment unless parents are encouraged to hold, touch, and look at their child. Every effort must be made by health personnel to foster attachment. (See Chapter 10 for suggestions in promoting attachment between parents and their hospitalized newborn.)

A child with CHD may constitute a long-term family crisis. Frequently the continuing unremitting stresses of care—physical exhaustion, financial costs, emotional upset, fear of death, and concern for the child's future—are not fully appreciated by those caring for the family. Even when the child's condition is stabilized or corrected, the family may need to make new adjustments in their life-style. Introducing them to other families with similarly affected children can help them adjust to the daily stresses.*

Educate Family About the Disorder

Once parents are ready to hear about the heart condition, it is essential that they be given a clear explanation based on their level of understanding. Lack of familiarity with the cardiovascular system may be a major reason for lack of parental understanding, and it is usually helpful to review the basic structure and function of the heart before describing the defect (Kaden and others, 1985). A simple diagram, pictures, or a model of the heart can be most helpful in visualizing the heart and the congenital defect. Parents appreciate receiving written information about the specific condition.†

Another fact to remember is that different health personnel may convey the same information using different diagrams and medical terms. To prevent this from becoming a problem, which often happens when several health team members work with a family, the same type of diagram should be used, and the parents should write down any unclear terms or ask for clarification. Sometimes it is helpful to provide the family with a glossary of frequently used words for reference.

Parents are primarily interested in two types of information—prognosis and surgery. They are frequently upset about indefinite answers to either. The family should be assured that the health care team will be honest in keeping them informed of the child's condition and of decisions regarding future procedures and treatments. The nurse needs to be aware of alterations in the plan of therapy in order to convey similar messages to the family.

Children of various ages have different ideas about their heart (Reif, 1972). Children between ages 4 and 6 years have heard about the heart, know its approximate anatomic location in the chest or back, illustrate it as valentine shaped, and characterize it by the sounds *tick-tock, thump,* and so on. Children ages 7 to 10 have a clearer concept of the heart, realizing that it is not shaped like a valentine and that it has vital functions, such as, "It makes you live." However, their knowledge of its integrated functions to pump blood through a system of vessels to all parts of the body is still hazy. By the age of 10 or 11 children have a much more involved concept of the heart, with knowledge of veins, valves, pumping action, and circulation. They are beginning to appreciate why death occurs when the heart stops.

Information given to the child must be tailored to the child's developmental age. As the child matures, the level of information is revised to meet the child's new cognitive level. Preschoolers need basic information about what they will experience more than what is actually occurring physiologically. School-age children benefit from a concrete explanation of the defect. Preadolescents and adolescents often appreciate a more detailed description of how the defect affects their heart. Children of all ages need to express their feelings concerning the diagnosis.

Help Family Cope with Effects of the Disorder

Parents also need an explanation regarding the symptoms of the disease. Many children have few symptoms but may develop CHF. Therefore parents should be aware of early signs of worsening physical status, such as sweating, sudden weight gain, decreased exercise tolerance, poor feeding, and increased breathing effort. These symptoms need medical evaluation, but the family is assured the symptoms usually respond quickly to therapeutic intervention.

Another area of parental concern is the child's level of physical activity. Children do not need to restrict activity, and the best approach is to treat the child normally and allow self-limited activity. Deliberately attempting to prevent crying should be avoided because it can establish a maladaptive parental pattern of relating to the infant. Exceptions to self-determined activity primarily involve strenuous recreational and competitive sports.

NURSING ALERT Although decisions regarding activity restrictions are made on an individual basis on the cardiologist's advice, children with aortic stenosis or insufficiency are usually not permitted to engage in strenuous activity (Freed, 1984).

*Some local American Heart Associations have organized parent groups.
†A booklet that can be given to parents is *If Your Child Has a Congenital Heart Defect: A Guide for Parents,* available from the American Heart Association, 7320 Greenville Ave., Dallas, TX 75231; (214) 373-6300.

Children with CHD require good nutrition. The infant may need to be fed small amounts of formula every 2 to 3 hours to ensure adequate nutrition. If several nighttime feedings are required, the nurse should discuss with parents the need to share the responsibility and enlist the help of others whenever possible.

The infant who has more difficulty feeding because of a congenital heart defect should be well supported and in a semiupright position when fed. This ensures a comfortable position for the infant attempting to coordinate the suck/swallow and breathing process and also decreases the risk of aspiration. Caregivers are encouraged not to interrupt infants who suck vigorously. The infants will pause and pace themselves during the feeding, but they should be stimulated to suck in an attempt to complete the feeding. The environment should be conducive to concentration on the feeding by both infant and parent. Eye contact and conversation between the parent and infant can make the experience more enjoyable for both.

The infant with CHD frequently requires caloric supplements because of the inefficient functioning of the heart and lungs. A diet plan specific to the individual infant's needs is calculated and prescribed by the nutritionist in collaboration with the other health personnel. The nurse needs to reinforce this information with the parents as necessary.

Children with severe cardiac defects are often anorexic. Encouraging them to eat can be a tremendous challenge. Because of the parents' concern over eating, children learn early to manipulate parents through eating, such as making unrealistic demands for foods that are not available. The nurse advises parents of this potential problem, since prevention yields greater success than intervention. For example, the child should be given a choice of available high-quality foods. Suggestions for encouraging sick children to eat are discussed in Chapter 27.

The family also needs to be knowledgeable regarding the therapeutic management of the disorder, especially in terms of the medications that the child is receiving. Parents are taught the correct procedure for giving drugs* and cautioned to keep them in a safe area to prevent accidental ingestion (see Parent Guidelines, p. 1549).

Foster Growth-Promoting Family Relationships

The effect of a child with a serious heart defect on the family is complex. No member, regardless of the degree of positive adjustment, is unaffected. Mothers frequently feel inadequate in their mothering ability because they gave birth to a child with a defect and are unable to keep their child well. Mothers often feel constantly exhausted from the pressures of caring for these children and the other family members. Likewise, fathers and siblings may feel neglected and resentful, a reaction similar to the feelings of family members toward other chronic conditions (see Chapter 22). Often parents do not feel confident leaving the child in another's care because they believe that the child will be upset by a change in routine and that the baby-sitter will be unable to cope with the cyanosis and dyspnea. This often sets up a trap for parents, especially mothers, who become locked into the child's care with no relief. Although the parents' fears are justified, they can be minimized by gradually teaching someone (a reliable relative or neighbor) how to care for the child.

The need to maintain discipline and set consistent limits cannot be overemphasized. Using behavior modification techniques, either in the form of concrete awards (e.g., a favorite food) or social reinforcement (e.g., approval), can be effective. However, it is most beneficial if employed *before* the child learns to control the family. Therefore guiding parents toward the need for discipline while the child is in infancy is necessary to prevent later problems. It also teaches these children how to tolerate frustration and delayed gratification, which often are lacking because of immediate satisfaction of all their needs.

Another problem that may develop within family relationships is the child's overdependency. This is often the result of parental fear that the child may die and overcompensation through what has been termed the benevolent overreaction (see Chapter 22). The best approach to dealing with this dilemma is prevention. Parents need guidance to recognize the eventual hazards of continuing dependency and protectiveness as the child grows older, and the nurse can assist parents in learning ways to foster optimum development. Unless parents are helped to see what activities the child can do, they may focus on physical limitations and encourage dependency.

The child also needs opportunities for social development. These children do not need to be isolated from known sources of infection or prevented from playing with other children because of concern regarding overexertion. Such practices only add to the dangers of increased dependency in the home environment. Parents need to be encouraged to seek appropriate social activity, especially before kindergarten.

Prepare Child and Family for Surgery

Few surgical procedures demand as much planning for preoperative preparation and postoperative care as heart surgery. The general principles for preparing children for procedures, such as surgery, are discussed in Chapter 27, and the reader is urged to review them. This discussion focuses on those measures specific to the cardiovascular procedure. Technical differences exist between closed- and open-heart surgery, since the latter involves the use of cardiopulmonary bypass (extracorporeal circulation). Consequently there are some additions to physical care postoperatively in open-heart surgery. However, in general the term *heart surgery* is used regardless of the actual procedures, and the same nursing interventions apply.

The child is usually admitted to the hospital 1 to 2 days before surgery for diagnostic tests. This interval allows time to prepare the child and parents for surgery, although with the present concern on health care costs, less time may be appropriated for admission procedures. With infants the fo-

*Home care instructions on giving medications to children are available in Wong, D.L., and Whaley, L.F.: Clinical manual of pediatric nursing, ed. 3, St. Louis, 1990, Mosby–Year Book, Inc.

cus of preoperative teaching is directed to the parents. Since much information is conveyed, it is important to schedule teaching to prevent information overload and to be alert to signs of overload (see Box 6-2). No well-documented research exists on how extensive preoperative preparation should be, and the nurse must use considerable judgment in planning the aspects of teaching. Preparation can be divided into three categories: equipment, environment, and procedures. The following discussion assumes that the child and/or parents have an understanding of the defect.

Introduce child and family to the environment. Ideally, when the child is admitted, a primary nurse and associate nurses to cover all shifts should be assigned. In some institutions the nurse who will care for the child postoperatively in the intensive care unit is also assigned to the child at admission to facilitate forming a relationship with the family and to share preoperative teaching, such as introduction to the recovery room and intensive care unit. To increase familiarity, all nurses should call the child and parents by name and refer to themselves by name. Wearing a name tag reinforces this point. Postoperatively the family will feel more at ease recognizing familiar names, faces, and voices.

If a visit to the recovery room and/or intensive care unit is planned, it should take place when there is least activity in the area, the parents can accompany the child, and the child is well rested. Usually the day before surgery is ample time to allow the child to ask questions and to prevent undue fantasizing about the experience. If a visit is not included in the teaching plan, the nurse can use a book, preferably with pictures or photographs of the actual rooms, to explain the environment to the child.

During the visit to the intensive care unit, the child and parents should experience everything that directly affects the child's care, such as the sounds of ECG monitors, oxygen tents, and placement of the bed. All positive, nonfrightening aspects of the environment are emphasized, such as the play area, visitors' section, pictures or mobiles in the room, or television. If it is a pediatric intensive care unit, the nurse can introduce the family to other children who may be recovering from surgery. The child should be protected from the frightening sights in the unit, and equipment not in view postoperatively, such as equipment located behind or below the bed, needs less attention. The child and parents are encouraged to ask questions or to explore further any equipment in the room, but they should not be pushed to assimilate more information than they appear to be tolerating.

Familiarize child and family with equipment. Some of the equipment, such as the stethoscope, blood pressure apparatus, and thermometer, will already be familiar to the child and parents. However, the nurse emphasizes that procedures involving such equipment will be done more frequently. If monitoring devices, such as blood pressure or oximetry, are used, the child is told about the placement of the sensor on the skin.

Types of equipment new to many families are the oxygen mask, suction, chest tubes, endotracheal tubes, incentive spirometers, nasogastric tube, and intravenous tubing. Each of these is shown and demonstrated either on the child or on a doll, if he or she appears ready. With a younger child, miniaturized equipment suitable for use with a doll or puppet is often less anxiety producing than the actual samples. If other children in the unit have an intravenous infusion or are in oxygen tents, the older child may benefit from seeing them, but this must be planned carefully to avoid frightening the child.

Several intravenous lines are inserted perioperatively: (1) an ordinary line for infusion of fluids, inserted in a peripheral vein; (2) a venous pressure line, inserted into the right subclavian or jugular vein; and (3) an arterial line for direct measurement of arterial pressure. Younger children need only know the location of each tubing and that both arms may be restrained to prevent dislodging the tubing. Older children may appreciate knowing the reason for each infusion, especially when venous and arterial measurements are taken. Since the lines are inserted during surgery, they are not painful, only uncomfortable because of the restricted movement.

The type and size of dressing the child will have after surgery are discussed and can be shown on a doll. Usually one of two types of incisions is made: a *median sternotomy,* which splits the sternum, or a *lateral thoracotomy,* which extends from the midaxillary line to the scapula. Frequently no sutures are visible because subcuticular, absorbable sutures may be used. If this is done, it should be pointed out to the child and parents, who may fear the incision will open. Sometimes a butterfly incision is used for cosmetic reasons in girls instead of the regular median sternotomy.

The child may be told about chest tubes and their purpose in draining fluid from around the heart and lungs. A picture of the equipment used for drainage can be shown to the child, or the setup can be simulated by attaching one end of the tubes to a doll with a chest dressing and the other end to small bottles (e.g., empty medicine vials). The nurse stresses that the child must move even though the tubes are in place. It can be demonstrated on the doll that the tubing is long enough to permit turning. Since this information may be anxiety producing, it is best left to the end of teaching or eliminated if the child appears too anxious.

An endotracheal (ET) tube is inserted during surgery and may be left in place for ventilatory assistance and tracheobronchial suctioning. However, it may be best to prepare older children for the ET tube only if *prolonged* ventilatory support is planned. The ET tube can be presented as a "breathing tube" that is placed in the nose or mouth (Rushton, 1983). The nurse explains that while the tube is in, the child will feel it in the throat and will not be able to talk, but nothing is wrong. The child can express desires by pointing or using a picture communication board. The nurse stresses that the tube will be removed as soon as possible, often during the first postoperative day.

Preoperative physical care differs little, if any, from that for any other surgery and is discussed in Chapter 27. The child should be assured that the parents will be there when the child wakes up; they should be allowed to accompany their child as far as possible to the operating suite (see Questions and Controversies, p. 1191). After all the equipment and procedures have been explained, it is important to talk about "getting well" and going home. If a doll was used during the preparatory session, the tubes can be removed and the doll can be dressed in regular clothes in anticipation of discharge.

Provide Postoperative Care

Immediate postoperative care is usually provided by specially trained nurses in intensive care units. Many of the procedures, such as arterial pressure and central venous pressure (CVP) monitoring and the observations related to vital functions, require advanced educational training (the reader should refer to critical care texts for further information). However, nurses caring for the child before surgery and during the convalescent period need to be familiar with the major principles of care.

Observe vital signs and arterial/venous pressures. Vital signs and blood pressure are recorded frequently until stable. Heart rate and respirations are counted for 1 full minute, compared with the ECG monitor, and recorded with activity. The heart rate is normally increased after surgery. The nurse observes cardiac rhythm and notifies the practitioner of any changes in regularity. Dysrhythmias may occur postoperatively secondary to anesthetics, acid-base and electrolyte imbalance, hypoxia, surgical intervention, or trauma to conduction pathways.

At least hourly the lungs are auscultated for breath sounds. Diminished or absent sounds most likely indicate an area of atelectasis, which necessitates further medical assessment. Auscultation guides the nurse's selective use of postural drainage and percussion to those pulmonary lobes most in need. It also allows a more objective evaluation of effective ventilation.

Temperature changes are typical during the early postoperative period. Hypothermia is expected immediately after surgery from hypothermia procedures, effects of anesthesia, and loss of body heat to the cool environment. During this period the child is kept warm to prevent additional heat loss. Infants may be placed under radiant heat warmers. During the next 24 to 48 hours the body temperature may rise to 37.7° C (100° F) or slightly higher as part of the inflammatory response to tissue trauma. After this period an elevated temperature is most likely a sign of infection and warrants immediate investigation for probable cause.

Intraarterial monitoring of blood pressure is almost always used following open-heart surgery. Residual vasoconstriction after cardiopulmonary bypass makes indirect blood pressure readings less reliable, and intraarterial monitoring permits continuous rather than intermittent observation. A catheter is passed into the radial artery or the dorsalis pedis or posterior tibial artery, and the other end is attached to an electronic monitoring system, which provides a continuous recording of the blood pressure. Continuous blood pressure readings are compared with those taken indirectly with a sphygmomanometer or oscillometry (Dinamap). A discrepancy between the two may indicate a change in peripheral vascular resistance, a malfunction in the electronic device, or human error in using the wrong-size blood pressure cuff. The nurse also observes for potential complications of intraarterial monitoring, such as arterial thrombosis, infection, air emboli, or blood loss through the catheter. Prevention of each of these hazards is similar to care for any other type of infusion.

The intraarterial line is maintained with a low-rate constant infusion of heparinized saline to prevent clotting. The amount of irrigant is recorded as intake fluid. The dressing at the site is changed daily.

Intracardiac monitoring lines provide data on cardiac function and output. They are placed intraoperatively and may be present in the left atrium, pulmonary artery, or right atrium. Placement of a catheter in the right atrium allows for measurement of the pressure in the right side of the heart. Therefore it indicates right atrial filling pressure, right ventricular function, the relationship between blood volume (venous return) and cardiac output, and early signs of right-sided CHF. The CVP catheter is inserted into the superior vena cava or inferior vena cava, and the other end is attached to a monitor.

CVP continually changes according to blood volume, heart rate, and myocardial function. If the blood volume decreases, such as in shock, the CVP falls. If the efficiency of the left side of the heart decreases, the resistance to right ventricular ejection will ultimately result in an elevated CVP but decreased intraarterial pressure. CHF and/or hypervolemia raise the CVP.

The complications of CVP lines are similar to other infusions, with the addition of atrial dysrhythmias from irritation of the atrial wall; hemothorax, pneumothorax, or hydrothorax from accidental puncture as the catheter enters the thorax; and fluid overload, since the intravenous line is kept patent by a continuous drip. The nurse observes for signs and symptoms indicative of each of these risks.

Maintain respiratory status. The child is generally maintained on mechanical ventilation in the immediate postoperative period. When weaning and extubation are completed, humidified oxygen is delivered by mask or hood to liquefy secretions. The child is kept warm and dry, since excessive chilling from wet linens causes an increased metabolic need and consequent increased cardiac demand. The child is encouraged to cough, turn, and deep breathe at least hourly. Every measure is employed to enhance ventilation and decrease pain, such as splinting of the operative site and judicious use of analgesics. Although crying increases heart rate, it is beneficial in promoting deep respirations.

Postural drainage is done frequently, usually every 2 to 4 hours. It is helpful to have two nurses work together, one to position the child while the other percusses and vibrates. Since the procedure is uncomfortable, it is important to emphasize to the child the necessity of performing it and to clarify that the percussion, sometimes mistakenly viewed as hitting, is done to loosen secretions in the lungs and is not a punishment. The child is usually comforted by the parents, and if they wish to participate, they can be very helpful in positioning the child.

Suctioning is performed as needed. Deep suctioning is performed carefully to avoid vagal stimulation (cardiac dysrhythmias) and laryngospasm, especially in infants. Suctioning is intermittent and maintained for no more than 5 seconds to prevent depleting the oxygen supply. Supplemental oxygen is administered with a manual resuscitation Ambu bag before and after the procedure to prevent hypoxia. Heart rate is monitored after suctioning to detect changes in rhythm or rate, especially bradycardia. The child should always be positioned facing the nurse to permit assessment of the child's color and tolerance to the procedure.

✦ **NURSING ALERT** During suctioning, observe for signs and symptoms of respiratory distress, such as tachypnea, use of accessory muscles for breathing, and restlessness.

Chest tubes are inserted into the pleural and/or mediastinal space during surgery or in the immediate postoperative period to remove secretions and air in order to allow reexpansion of the lung. The chest tube is attached to a water-seal drainage system, usually a disposable type such as Pleur-Evac. The purpose of the underwater drainage is to prevent air from traveling up the tube into the pleural space, causing a pneumothorax. The nursing considerations include (1) do not interrupt water-seal drainage unless the chest tube is clamped, (2) check for tube patency (fluctuation in the water-seal chamber), and (3) maintain sterility.

Drainage is checked hourly for color and quantity. Immediately postoperatively the drainage may be bright red, but afterward it should be serous. The largest volume of drainage occurs in the first 12 to 24 hours and is more copious in extensive heart surgery.

✦ **NURSING ALERT** Chest tube drainage greater than 3 ml/kg/hour for more than 3 consecutive hours is excessive and may indicate postoperative hemorrhage (Mills and others, 1984). The surgeon is notified immediately, since cardiac tamponade can develop rapidly and is life-threatening.

Chest radiographs are taken when the tubes are inserted to check their location and after they are removed to evaluate the inflation of the lungs. Chest tubes are usually removed on the second to third postoperative day. Lung expansion is evidenced by decreased fluctuation in the tube and absence of drainage.

Removal of chest tubes is a painful, frightening experience. Analgesics such as morphine sulfate (0.1 mg/kg), preferably with a local anesthetic, should be given before the procedure. Children are forewarned that they will feel a sharp, momentary pain. After the suture is cut, the tubes are quickly pulled out at the end of full inspiration to prevent intake of air into the pleural cavity. A purse-string suture (placed when the tubes were inserted) is pulled tight to close the opening. A petrolatum-covered gauze dressing is immediately applied over the wound and securely taped on all four sides to the skin so that an airtight seal is formed. The dressing is checked for signs of drainage and any evidence of infection.

Provide maximum rest. After heart surgery, maximum rest should be provided to decrease the workload of the heart and promote healing. Nursing care is planned according to the child's usual activity and sleep patterns. The simplest way to ensure individualized, efficient, high-quality care is to plan at the beginning of the shift the nursing procedures to be done. Periods of rest are identified. The schedule should be shared with parents to allow them to visit at the most advantageous times, such as after a rest period when no special treatments are anticipated.

Provide comfort. Heart surgery is both painful and frightening for children, and comfort should be a primary nursing concern. Unfortunately, children are often poorly medicated for pain after surgery (see Questions and Controversies, p. 1145), especially children who are unable to verbally communicate discomfort (see Pain Assessment, Chapter 26). Recent improvements have been made in the management of pain following cardiac surgery. The increasing clinical experience with continuous intravenous opioid infusions, particularly morphine and fentanyl, has demonstrated the safety and effectiveness of this method of pain control (Maguire and Maloney, 1988). Patient-controlled analgesia may be used with children old enough to understand the concept, and epidural morphine may be another option (Rosen and Rosen, 1989). Paralyzing agents such as pancuronium (Pavulon) or metocurine (Metubine) may also be used with the analgesics for children who are very agitated or hemodynamically unstable. Children receiving opioid infusions for a prolonged period should be weaned slowly from the medication to prevent withdrawal symptoms (Norton, 1988).

Most patients need intravenous analgesics for pain control during the immediate postoperative period. Following extubation and removal of lines and tubes, pain can be satisfactorily controlled with oral medications such as codeine with acetaminophen (Tylenol) or oxycodone and acetaminophen (Tylox). Acetaminophen alone provides adequate pain relief for most children at discharge. Sternotomy incisions are usually well tolerated, with some discomfort when walking and coughing. Thoracotomy incisions are usually more painful because the incision is through muscle; a more aggressive pain management plan with round-the-clock medications for several days is often necessary to allow for adequate rest, ambulation, and pulmonary hygiene.

In addition to pharmacologic pain control, every effort is made to minimize the discomfort of procedures, such as using a firm pillow or favorite stuffed animal placed against the chest incision during coughing, and performing treatments *after* pain medication is given, preferably at a time that coincides with the drug's peak effect. Nonpharmacologic measures are employed to lessen the perception of pain, and parents are encouraged to comfort their child as much as possible. (See also Pain Assessment; Pain Management, Chapter 26.)

Monitor fluids. Intake and output of all fluids must be accurately calculated. Intake is primarily intravenous fluids; however, a record of fluid used to flush the arterial and CVP lines or to dilute medications is also kept. Output includes hourly recordings of urine (usually a Foley catheter is inserted and attached to a closed collecting device), drainage from chest and nasogastric tubes, and blood drawn for analysis. Urine is analyzed for specific gravity to assess the kidneys' concentrating ability and to assess approximately the body's degree of hydration. Renal failure is a potential risk from a transient period of low cardiac output.

✦ **NURSING ALERT** The signs of renal failure are decreased urine output (less than 1 ml/kg/hour) and elevated levels of blood urea nitrogen and serum creatinine (van Breda, 1985).

Fluids are restricted during the immediate postoperative period to prevent hypervolemia, which places additional demands on the myocardium, predisposing to cardiac failure. Two factors influence increased blood volume. In open-heart surgery the cardiopulmonary pump is primed with a large volume of fluid (usually electrolyte solution), which may greatly dilute the patient's blood. During circulation through the body, some of this priming fluid diffuses into the interstitial spaces but postoperatively diffuses back into the systemic circulation.

In addition, the physiologic changes of open- or closed-heart surgery stimulate the adrenal cortex to secrete aldosterone, which increases renal reabsorption of sodium. This results in water retention but increased excretion of potassium. Concurrently the hypothalamus secretes additional antidiuretic hormone (ADH), which causes the distal and collecting tubules to reabsorb more water. Not only can this process result in hypervolemia, but it also may cause electrolyte imbalances, principally hypokalemia. Decreased potassium affects myocardial function and may increase the risk of dysrhythmias. The nurse assesses electrolyte imbalances by observing for signs of hypokalemia (see Nursing Alert, p. 1552) and checking all blood electrolyte analysis reports.

Fluid requirements are based on the child's weight and body surface area. The child is weighed daily, and the same scale is used at approximately the same time each day to avoid errors in measurement. The child is usually given nothing by mouth for the first 24 hours. If an ET tube is inserted, oral fluids are usually withheld until the child is extubated. Fluid restriction may be imposed even when oral fluids are given. The nurse calculates the distribution over a 24-hour period based on the child's preoperative weight and drinking habits. The distribution should allow for the majority of fluid to be given during the child's most wakeful and active periods.

Plan for progressive activity. Fatigue and weakness are common after heart surgery, as a result of both the surgical trauma to the heart and sleep deprivation during the immediate postoperative period. However, moderate activity is essential to prevent pulmonary and vascular complications. Initially, turning, coughing, and deep breathing are sufficient to promote respiratory expansion. However, passive range of motion exercises, especially to the lower extremities, are instituted to prevent venous stasis. All infusion sites are inspected for evidence of thrombophlebitis and emboli. The areas are passively exercised to promote circulation.

A progressive schedule of ambulation and activity is planned, based on the child's preoperative activity patterns and postoperative cardiovascular and pulmonary function. Toys that were enjoyed before surgery are provided to encourage movement. It is important to plan the activity at times when the child is well rested, is comfortable (usually has had analgesic medication), and is not scheduled for any strenuous procedure or treatment immediately afterward.

Ambulation is initiated early, usually by the second postoperative day, when chest tubes, arterial lines, and assisted ventilatory equipment may be removed. The nurse begins ambulation for this child as for a child who had undergone any other postsurgical procedure, progressing from sitting on the edge of the bed and dangling the legs to standing up and to sitting in a chair. Heart rate and respirations are carefully monitored to assess the degree of cardiac demand imposed by each activity. Tachycardia, dyspnea, cyanosis, desaturation, progressive fatigue, or dysrhythmias indicate the need to limit further energy expenditure. Even if the child is able to ambulate to a chair with a moderate increase in heart rate, the effort required to return to bed must be considered. After ambulation a rest period is scheduled.

Observe for complications of heart surgery. Several complications can occur after heart surgery, most of which are related to open-heart surgery and use of cardiopulmonary bypass. Many of the procedures discussed in the preceding paragraphs are aimed at preventing these problems. Only those that have not already been discussed are included here. A serious complication, bacterial endocarditis, is discussed on p. 1581.

Hematologic changes. While passing through the heart-lung machine, blood is exposed to substantial trauma by direct contact with oxygen, mechanical action, foreign substances, and massive doses of anticoagulants. The result of this injury is red blood cell hemolysis and potential renal tubular necrosis, clotting abnormalities from decreased thrombin and prothrombin, heparinization of the blood during extracorporeal circulation, decreased platelets, and altered platelet aggregation.

Hemolysis of red blood cells results in blood loss and anemia, which may require packed red blood cell transfusion. The nurse monitors results of complete blood counts to identify the severity of the hemolysis. All urine is tested for the presence of blood. If transfusions are required, the child is closely observed for signs of reaction (see Table 35-2) and fluid overload. The necessity of measuring urine output hourly has already been discussed.

Since blood clotting mechanisms are affected, signs of hemorrhage are watched for, especially bleeding from the chest tubes and a fall in arterial/venous pressures. Hemorrhage is more likely to occur in patients who have repair of cyanotic heart defects because of the associated physiologic thrombocytopenia.

Normally the filter and bubble trap on the heart-lung machine remove air emboli, tiny clots, fat debris, and organisms from the arterialized (oxygenated) blood before its return to the body. However, impure blood entering the systemic circulation can cause fat emboli, thromboemboli, and infection anywhere in the body, but most importantly in the brain.

Cardiac changes. Cardiac failure may result from increased workload on ventricles that have been hypertrophied before surgery. Consequently, signs of heart failure are watched for, including elevation of the CVP.

Low cardiac output syndrome and decreased peripheral perfusion can occur from hypothermia or inability of the left ventricle to maintain systemic circulation. The most important signs of adequate peripheral perfusion are rapid capillary refill, good skin color, warm extremities, and strong pulses. Evidence of low cardiac output is similar to signs of shock, that is, decreased blood pressure, decreased pulse pressure, cool extremities, metabolic acidosis, and oliguria.

Dysrhythmias can result from electrolyte imbalance, especially hypokalemia, and surgical intervention of the septum or myocardium. The heart rate and rhythm are carefully monitored by observing the ECG pattern and by counting the *apical pulse* for 1 full minute. Dysrhythmias that impair cardiac performance are bradycardias (heart rate less than 80 beats/minute), tachycardia (ventricular rate greater than 180 to 200 beats/minute), extrasystole, or heart block. Epicardial pacing wires may be inserted during surgery for managing cardiac dysrhythmias postoperatively.

Cardiac tamponade is compression of the heart by blood and other effusion (clots) in the pericardial sac, which severely restricts the normal heart movement. A characteristic sign is *paradoxic pulse pressure,* in which the systolic pressure drops during inspiration because accumulated blood compresses the heart, resulting in a drop in cardiac output. Other signs include a rising venous pressure, falling arterial pressure, narrowing pulse pressure, tachycardia, dyspnea, cyanosis, apprehension, and a compensatory posture of sitting and leaning forward. Any evidence of this potentially fatal complication is immediately reported. Treatment consists of prompt pericardiocentesis to remove the blood or fluid. If active hemorrhage and coagulopathy are present, steps are taken to enhance blood clotting.

Pulmonary changes. Areas of atelectasis are common immediately after surgery as a result of deflation of the lung during cardiopulmonary bypass. Other pulmonary complications include pneumothorax, especially caused by faulty chest tubes; pulmonary edema from increased pulmonary blood flow or heart failure; and pleural effusion caused by persistent venous congestion. Signs of pneumothorax are persistent decreased breath sounds, sudden dyspnea, tachycardia, rapid shallow respirations, cyanosis, and sometimes sharp chest pain. Signs of pulmonary edema are rales, wheezing, moist dyspneic respirations, tachycardia, cyanosis, and restlessness. Signs and symptoms of pleural effusions include increased respiratory rate, vomiting, decreased breath sounds, fatigue, and irritability.

Neurologic changes. Cerebral edema and brain damage may occur during open-heart surgery. Although the exact cause is unknown, it is thought to be a result of tissue ischemia or emboli. The nurse checks the equality of strength and reflexes in both extremities for evidence of paralysis; assesses the pupil size, equality, and reaction to light and accommodation; and assesses the child's orientation to the environment. Any evidence of cerebral damage is immediately reported. The nurse also observes for focal or generalized seizure activity, which may be secondary to electrolyte imbalance.

Postpericardiotomy syndrome. This syndrome of fever, leukocytosis, pericardial friction rub, and/or pericardial and pleural effusion can occur anytime the pericardium is opened, either in the immediate postoperative period or after surgery, typically around day 7 to 21. The cause is unknown, although etiologic theories include a viral infection, autoimmune response to myocardial tissue, or a reaction to blood in the pericardium. It is self-limited and is treated with rest, salicylates, and sometimes steroids.

Provide Emotional Support

Children may become depressed after surgery. This is thought to be caused by preoperative anxiety, postoperative psychologic and physiologic stress, and sensory overstimulation. Typically the child's disposition improves on leaving the intensive care unit (see Chapter 26).

Children may also be angry and uncooperative after surgery as a response to the physical pain and to the loss of control imposed by the surgery and treatments. They need an opportunity to express feelings, either orally or through activity. The nurse can be supportive by reassuring children that the procedures that require cooperation, such as coughing and deep breathing, are difficult to perform; by praising them for efforts to cooperate; and by refraining from expecting too much "courage" or "bravery." This approach allows children to express feelings with the nurse's acceptance, regardless of their emotional response. Children also may express feelings of anger or rejection toward parents. The nurse must reassure parents that this is normal and that with continued support the anger will subside.

The nurse can support the parents by being available for information and explaining all the procedures to them. The first few postoperative days are particularly difficult because parents see their child in pain and realize the potential risks from surgery. They often are overwhelmed by the physical environment of the intensive care unit and feel useless because they can do so little for their child. The nurse can minimize such feelings by including parents in caregiving activities if they wish, such as a partial bath, turning, or positioning for postural drainage; by providing information about the child's condition; and by being sensitive to their emotional and physical needs. The importance of their presence in making the child feel more secure is stressed, even if they do not provide physical care.

Plan for Discharge and Home Care

Ideally, discharge planning begins on admission for cardiac surgery and includes an assessment of the parents' adjustment to the child's altered state of health. As mentioned earlier, one of the most common parental reactions is overprotection, and the nurse needs to be aware of times when the family may need help in recognizing the child's improved health status. With surgical correction of heart anomalies occurring during infancy, there is less likelihood of this pattern of overdependency developing. Many of these children are at risk for the vulnerable child syndrome (see p. 411).

The family will need verbal as well as written instructions on medication, nutrition, activity restrictions, subacute bacterial endocarditis, return to school, wound care, and signs and symptoms of infection or complications. Referrals to community agencies may be warranted to assist parents in the transition from hospital to home and to reinforce the teaching.

The parents will also need clear instructions on when to seek medical care, such as for a change in the child's behavior or an unexplained fever. Follow-up with the cardiologist is also arranged before discharge. Appropriate identification, such as a Medic-Alert bracelet, is indicated for children with a pacemaker or a heart transplant and for those receiving anticoagulation therapy or antidysrhythmic medication.

The nurse also discusses common behavior disturbances that may occur after discharge, such as nightmares, sleep disturbances, separation anxiety, and overdependence. A supportive, consistent response is essential to allow the child to overcome the surgical experience. The child may work out feelings and fears through therapeutic play, and this should be encouraged.

Although surgical correction of heart defects has improved dramatically, it is still not possible to totally reverse many of the complex anomalies. For many children repeat procedures are required to replace conduits or grafts or to manage complications, such as restenosis. Consequently the long-term prognosis is uncertain, and full recovery is not always possible. For these families medical follow-up and continued emotional support are essential. The nurse can often serve as an important primary health professional and as a resource for referrals when needed.

Evaluation

The effectiveness of nursing interventions for the family and the child with CHD is determined by continual reassessment and evaluation of care based on the following observational guidelines and expected outcomes:

1. Interview families and observe their behavior with the infant or child.
2. Encourage family to discuss their feelings and concerns; observe their response to education.
3. Interview the child and observe his or her behavior and concerns; encourage the verbal child to express feelings.
4. Interview family and observe family interactions and relationships.
5. Interview family regarding their understanding of the condition and the proposed surgery.
6. Monitor and observe the infant or child and family preoperatively and postoperatively.
7. Interview child and family regarding response to cardiac surgery.
8. Observe and interview child and family regarding their understanding of home care needs, ability to carry out care, and compliance with the plan of care.

Expected outcomes:
See Nursing Care Plan, pp. 1572-1573.

ACQUIRED CARDIOVASCULAR DISORDERS

Acquired cardiac disorders refer to disease processes or abnormalities that occur after birth and can be seen in the normal heart or in the presence of congenital heart defects. They occur for a variety of reasons, including infection, autoimmune responses, environmental factors, and familial tendencies. Nursing care often plays a critical role in the identification and supportive management of these cardiovascular disorders.

BACTERIAL (INFECTIVE) ENDOCARDITIS

Bacterial endocarditis (BE) or infective endocarditis (IE), also referred to as subacute bacterial endocarditis (SBE), is an infection of the valves and inner lining of the heart. Although it can occur without underlying heart disease, it most often is a sequela of bacteremia in the child with acquired or congenital anomalies of the heart or great vessels. It especially affects children with valvular abnormalities, prosthetic valves, recent cardiac surgery with invasive lines, and rheumatic heart disease with valve involvement. In addition, a growing problem is endocarditis associated with drug abuse (Kaplan and Shulman, 1989). The most common causative agent is *Streptococcus viridans;* other causative agents are *Staphylococcus aureus,* gram-negative bacteria, and fungi, such as *Candida albicans.* Endocarditis associated with open-heart surgery is most often caused by *S. aureus,* coagulase-negative staphylococci, or diphtheroids (Kaplan, 1990).

Pathophysiology

The microorganisms usually grow on a section of the endocardium that has been subjected to abnormal blood streaming and turbulence, such as occurs when the flow of blood is restricted by an anatomic narrowing or forced through an abnormal opening. Growth may also begin where the abnormal jet of blood strikes the opposing endocardium, causing a thickening of the lining. Changes in the endocardium predispose it to the growth of invading organisms.

Organisms may enter the bloodstream from any site of localized infection. The most common portals of entry are oral from dental work *(S. viridans);* urinary tract, such as from urinary tract infection after catheterization (gram-negative bacilli); heart, from cardiac surgery, especially if synthetic material is used (valves, patches, conduits); and the bloodstream from long-term indwelling catheters. The microorganisms grow on the endocardium, forming vegetations (verrucae), deposits of fibrin, and platelet thrombi. The lesion may grow to invade adjacent tissues, such as aortic and mitral valves and myocardium, and may break off and embolize elsewhere, especially in the spleen, kidney, central nervous system, lung, skin, and mucous membranes.

Clinical Manifestations

The onset of symptoms is usually insidious, with unexplained low-grade, intermittent fever. Other common nonspecific symptoms are anorexia, malaise, myalgias, arthralgias, headache, and weight loss. A new murmur or a change in a previously existing one is frequently found as a result of damage to valves or perforation of the myocardium. Another finding, especially in those with prolonged illness, is splenomegaly. Other signs that result from emboli formation elsewhere in the body include splinter hemorrhages (thin black lines) under the nails, Osler nodes (red, painful intradermal nodes with white centers found on the pads of the phalanges), Janeway spots (painless hemorrhagic areas on the palms and soles), and petechiae on the oral mucous membranes.

Diagnostic Evaluation

Several laboratory findings may indicate BE, such as ECG changes (prolonged P-R interval), radiographic evidence of cardiomegaly, anemia, elevated erythrocyte sedimentation rate, leukocytosis, and microscopic hematuria. Definitive diagnosis can be made after growth of the organism and identification of the causative agent in the blood and visualization of the vegetations on two-dimensional echocardiography. Usually several blood specimens are drawn for culturing to rule out contamination during venipuncture and dilution technique. As soon as an organism is isolated, sensitivity studies are done to determine appropriate antibiotic therapy.

Therapeutic Management

Treatment is administration of high-dose antibiotics (usually penicillin, ampicillin, methicillin, cloxacillin, streptomycin, and/or gentamicin for specific bacteria or amphotericin B and/or flucytosine for fungi) given intravenously for at least 4 to 6 weeks. Blood cultures are taken periodically to evaluate response to antibiotic therapy. In instances when antibiotic therapy is unsuccessful, CHF develops, or recurrent systemic emboli are present, surgical intervention is warranted. This may include replacing damaged valves with prostheses, debriding and draining myocardial abscesses, excising areas of infection, and removing vegetations (Kaplan and Shulman, 1989).

Successful early medical treatment, especially with BE, occurs in approximately 80% of affected patients. However, cases diagnosed late, those caused by antibiotic-resistant organisms or fungi, or those occurring in infants or patients without preexisting heart disease carry a higher mortality and may necessitate surgical intervention. Death is most often caused by CHF, myocardial infarction from coronary emboli, or cardiac perforation. Nonfatal complications result from embolism to other organs, especially to the central nervous system (causing hemiplegia, aphasia, meningitis, convulsions), kidney (resulting in hematuria, proteinuria), spleen, and bowel.

Prevention of BE in susceptible children is of utmost importance and includes all children with CHD *except* those with (1) isolated ASD 1 and (2) surgical repair of ASD 1, VSD, and PDA without residual effects after 6 months (Dajani and others, 1990). Prevention involves administration of prophylactic antibiotic therapy shortly before and briefly after procedures known to increase the risk of entry of organisms (Box 34-5). Published recommendations provide guidelines for antibiotic prophylaxis, but they are complex and must be individualized for the child (Dajani and others, 1990). Drugs of choice are amoxicillin, penicillin, ampicillin, erythromycin, clindamycin, and vancomycin. The drugs may be given orally or parenterally depending on the procedure to be performed.

Nursing Considerations

Ideally the objective of nursing care is counseling parents of high-risk children concerning the need for prophylactic antibiotic therapy before procedures such as dental work. The family's regular dentist should be advised of existing cardiac problems in the child as an added precaution to ensuring preventive treatment. These children should also maintain the highest level of oral health to reduce the chance of bacteremia from oral infections. (See also discussion on dental care in Chapter 14.)

Parents should also have a high index of suspicion regarding potential infections. Without unduly alarming them, the nurse stresses that any unexplained fever, weight loss,

Box 34-5 PROCEDURES REQUIRING PROPHYLAXIS FOR BACTERIAL ENDOCARDITIS

All dental procedures likely to induce gingival or mucosal bleeding, including professional teeth cleaning (not simple adjustment of orthodontic appliances or shedding of deciduous teeth)
Tonsillectomy and/or adenoidectomy
Surgical procedures or biopsy involving respiratory or intestinal mucosa
Bronchoscopy with a rigid bronchoscope
Incision and drainage of infected tissue
Genitourinary and gastrointestinal procedures, including most diagnostic and therapeutic procedures that are invasive (sclerotherapy for esophageal varices, esophageal dilatation, cystoscopy, urethral dilatation, urethral catheterization or surgery if urinary tract infection is present, prostatic surgery, vaginal hysterectomy and vaginal delivery in presence of infection)

Data from Dajani, A.S., and others: Prevention of bacterial endocarditis: recommendations by the American Heart Association, JAMA 264(22): 2919-2922, 1990.

and change in behavior (lethargy, malaise, anorexia) must be brought to the practitioner's attention. Such symptoms should not be self-diagnosed as a cold or flu. Early treatment is important in preventing further cardiac damage, embolic complications, and growth of resistant organisms.

Treatment of endocarditis requires long-term hospitalization for the duration of parenteral drug therapy. In some cases intravenous antibiotics may be administered at home with nursing supervision for part of the treatment course. Nursing goals during this period are (1) preparation of the child for intravenous infusion, usually a heparin-lock device and several venipunctures for blood cultures; (2) prevention of boredom and depression, especially from restricted mobility caused by hospitalization and need for partial bed rest (if required); (3) observation for side effects of antibiotics, especially inflammation along venipuncture sites; and (4) observation for complications, including embolism and CHF. Follow-up after treatment is also important, and the nurse can be instrumental in arranging for convenient appointments.

RHEUMATIC FEVER

Rheumatic fever (RF) is a poorly understood autoimmune reaction to group A, beta-hemolytic, streptococcal pharyngitis. It is a self-limited disease that involves the joints, skin, brain, serous surfaces, and the heart. If not for cardiac valve damage (referred to as *rheumatic heart disease*), RF would be of little consequence (Fyler, 1990). In the 1920s, however, rheumatic heart disease was the leading cause of death in individuals between 5 and 20 years of age (Bland, 1987).

Recently, in developed countries, RF and rheumatic heart disease have become uncommon, probably as a result of antibacterial control of streptococcal infection, successful treatment of rheumatic heart disease, and a change in the organism itself. However, RF remains a devastating problem in developing (third-world) countries. An estimated 15 to 20 million new cases of RF occur in the world each year, and this number is probably an underestimate (Zabriskie, 1985). There is evidence, however, that RF is increasing in the United States and is reappearing in some areas and affecting enough persons to warrant concern (Kaplan, 1987).

Etiology

Strong evidence supports a relationship between upper respiratory infection with group A streptococci and subsequent development of RF (usually within 2 to 6 weeks). In almost all cases of RF a previous infection with group A streptococci can be documented by laboratory evidence of rising antibody titers. Prevention or treatment of group A streptococcal infection prevents RF.

Pathophysiology/Clinical Manifestations

The principal manifestions of RF are observed in the heart, joints, skin, and central nervous system. In the heart inflammatory hemorrhagic bullous lesions, called *Aschoff bodies,* are formed that cause swelling, fragmentation, and alterations in the connective tissue. Subsequent endocarditis produces vegetations, which when healed become fibrous, scarred areas. The structures of the heart most affected are the mitral and aortic valves. With progressive involvement of the valves, signs of mitral and aortic valve stenosis are evident, especially murmurs. Other signs of carditis are tachycardia that is out of proportion to the degree of fever, especially during rest or sleep; precordial pain from pericarditis; pericardial friction rub; muffled heart sound from pericardial effusion; and an accentuated third sound (prediastolic gallop).

Pathologic changes in the joints are mainly caused by edema, inflammation, and effusion in joint tissue. They are reversible and migratory, favoring large joints such as the knees, elbows, hips, shoulders, and wrists. The affected joint is swollen, hot, red, and exquisitely painful for 1 to 2 days, after which a different joint is affected. The manifestations usually accompany the acute febrile period, most often the first 1 to 2 weeks.

The skin manifestation is an erythematous macule with a clear center and wavy, well-demarcated border. The transitory, nonpruritic rash is most often found on the trunk and proximal portion of extremities. Subcutaneous nodules are small (0.5 to 1 cm), nontender swellings that persist indefinitely after onset of the disease and gradually resolve with no resulting damage. They are rare but may be found in crops over bony prominences, such as feet, hands, elbows, scalp, scapulae, and vertebrae.

Central nervous system involvement is characterized by chorea, which is referred to as *St. Vitus dance* or *Sydenham chorea.* Chorea is characterized by sudden, aimless, irregular movements of the extremities, involuntary facial grimaces, speech disturbances, emotional lability, and muscle weakness that can be profound. It is usually exaggerated by anxiety and attempts at deliberate fine motor activity and is relieved by rest, especially sleep.

In addition to these major manifestations, other vague signs and symptoms include low-grade fever, usually spiking in the late afternoon, unexplained epistaxis, abdominal pain that may be severe enough to simulate appendicitis, arthralgia without arthritic changes, weakness, fatigue, pallor, anorexia, and weight loss.

Diagnostic Evaluation

Diagnosis is based on a set of guidelines recommended by the American Heart Association. These guidelines, known as modifications of the Jones criteria, are listed in Box 34-6.

Streptolysin-O (O because it is oxygen labile) is a streptococcal extracellular product that produces lysis of the red blood cell. Antistreptolysin-O titers measure the concentration of antibodies formed in the blood against this product. Normally the titers begin to rise about 7 days after onset of the infection and reach maximum levels in 4 to 6 weeks. Therefore a rising titer demonstrated by at least two antistreptolysin-O tests is the most reliable evidence of recent streptococcal infection. Normal values are between 0 and 120 Todd units. Elevations over 333 Todd units indicate recent streptococcal infection in children.

Box 34-6 JONES' CRITERIA (REVISED) FOR GUIDANCE IN THE DIAGNOSIS OF RHEUMATIC FEVER

Major Manifestations	Minor Manifestations
Carditis	Clinical
Polyarthritis	Fever
Chorea	Arthralgia
Erythema marginatum	History of previous RF or rheumatic heart disease
Subcutaneous nodules	Laboratory
	Increased erythrocyte sedimentation rate
	C-reactive protein
	Leukocytosis
	Anemia
	Prolonged P-R interval on ECG

Supportive evidence of preceding streptococcal infection:
- Recent scarlet fever
- Positive throat culture for group A β-hemolytic streptococci
- Increased antistreptolysin-O or other streptococcal antibodies

Presence of two major manifestations or one major and two minor manifestations with supportive evidence of recent streptococcal infection indicates a high probability of rheumatic fever.

Therapeutic Management

The goals of medical management are (1) eradication of hemolytic streptococci, (2) prevention of permanent cardiac damage, (3) palliation of the other symptoms, and (4) prevention of recurrences of RF. Penicillin is the drug of choice, with erythromycin as a substitute in penicillin-sensitive children. Salicylates are used to control the inflammatory process, especially in the joints, and reduce the fever and discomfort. Bed rest is recommended during the acute febrile phase but need not be strict. In patients with carditis physical exercise should be limited, at least until the pulse rate returns to normal (Kashani, 1981).

Prophylactic treatment against recurrence of RF is started after the acute therapy and involves monthly intramuscular injections of benzathine penicillin G (1.2 million U), two daily oral doses of penicillin (200,000 U), or one daily dose of sulfadiazine (1 g). The duration of long-term prophylaxis is uncertain. Because of the risk of BE, in rheumatic heart disease the same prophylaxis discussed earlier is implemented. The antibiotic regimens used to prevent recurrences of RF are inadequate for the prevention of BE.

Children who have had acute RF are susceptible to recurrent RF for the rest of their lives and should be followed medically for at least 5 years. As Fyler (1990) states, "Once a rheumatic, always a rheumatic." Therefore medical considerations for these patients continue. Children and families must be aware of the need for continuing antibiotic prophylaxis for dental work, infection, and invasive procedures.

Nursing Considerations

The objectives of nursing care for the child with RF are to (1) encourage compliance with drug regimens, (2) facilitate recovery from the illness, (3) provide emotional support, and (4) prevent the disease. Since compliance is a major concern in long-term drug therapy, every effort is made to encourage adherence to the therapeutic plan (see Compliance, Chapter 27). When compliance is poor, monthly injections may be substituted for daily oral administration of antibiotics, and children need preparation for this often dreaded procedure.

Interventions during home care are primarily concerned with providing rest and adequate nutrition. Usually, once the febrile stage is over, children can resume moderate activity and their appetite improves. If carditis is present, the family must be aware of any activity restrictions and may need help in choosing less strenuous activities for the child.

One of the most disturbing and frustrating manifestations of the disease is chorea. The onset is gradual and may occur weeks to months after the illness, sometimes even occurring in children who have not been diagnosed with RF. It may be mistaken for nervousness, clumsiness, behavioral changes, inattentiveness, and learning disability. It is usually a source of great frustration to the child because the movements, incoordination, and weakness severely limit physical ability. The child needs an opportunity to verbalize feelings. Of utmost importance is stressing to parents and schoolteachers the involuntary, sudden nature of the movements, that the chorea is transitory, and that all manifestations eventually disappear.

Nurses also have a role in prevention, primarily in screening school-age children for sore throats caused by group A streptococci. This may involve actively participating in throat culture screening programs or in referring children with a possible streptococcal infection for testing.

KAWASAKI DISEASE (MUCOCUTANEOUS LYMPH NODE SYNDROME)

Kawasaki disease (KD) is an acute systemic vasculitis of unknown cause. Approximately 80% of the cases occur in children under the age of 5 years, with peak incidence in the toddler age-group. The acute disease is self-limited. Without treatment, however, approximately 1 in 5 children develop cardiac sequelae. Damage to the blood vessels that supply the heart muscle (the coronary arteries) and damage to the heart muscle itself can occur. The most common sequela is dilatation of the coronary arteries, resulting in *ectasia* or aneurysm formation. Infants less than 1 year of age are most seriously affected by KD and are at the greatest risk for heart involvement. KD is the leading cause of acquired heart disease in children in the United States.

KD is seen in every racial group. However, it occurs most

frequently in Japan and in children of Japanese heritage. Blacks are affected slightly more than whites, and males are affected more than females, with approximately a 1.6:1 ratio (Rauch, 1987). The reported incidence is greater in children of higher socioeconomic backgrounds.

The etiology of KD remains a mystery. Although KD is not spread by person-to-person contact, several factors support infectious etiologic factors. It is often seen in geographical and seasonal outbreaks, with the most cases reported in the late winter and early spring. It rarely occurs in the adult population.

Pathophysiology

Although KD is best known for damage to the cardiovascular system, it involves all the small and medium-sized blood vessels (Newburger and Burns, 1989). During the acute stage of the illness there is progressive inflammation of the small vessels (capillaries, venules, arterioles) along with pancarditis. This progresses to the medium-sized muscular arteries (12 to 25 days) and possible formation of coronary artery aneurysms. In addition, aneurysms of the peripheral cervical, axillary, brachial, iliac, and renal arteries can occur, although this is rare. Once damaged, ectatic vessels respond by myointimal proliferation. The walls of the vessel heal inward and may eventually return to normal in one half to two thirds of patients (Takahashi and others, 1987). The vessel, however, is never completely normal again. The affected vessel walls thicken and are subject to scarring, calcification, and stenosis, especially at the distal ends of the aneurysm. Inflammation gradually subsides and eventually ceases in 6 to 8 weeks. Long-term stenosis and scarring may form in affected vessels. In chronic disease, clot formation usually occurs at the site of stenosis and can lead to myocardial ischemia and an acute myocardial infarction. At greatest risk for development of cardiac sequelae are infants and those children with prolonged fever (Koren and others, 1986).

Clinical Manifestations

KD manifests in three phases: acute, subacute, and convalescent. The *acute phase* begins with the abrupt onset of high fever that is unresponsive to antibiotics and antipyretics. The child then develops the remaining diagnostic symptoms. The bulbar conjunctivae of the eyes become reddened, with clearing around the iris (limbal sparing). The eyes are generally dry, without drainage. Inflammation of the pharynx and the oral mucosa develops, with red, cracked lips and the characteristic "strawberry tongue" (the normal coating of the tongue sloughs off, leaving the large papillae exposed, resembling a strawberry). The rash of KD differs from child to child but is never vesicular. It is most often accentuated in the perineum. Often the area affected by the rash may desquamate. In addition, the child's hands and feet become edematous, and the palms and soles become erythematous. The child may have cervical lymphadenopathy (at least a single node 1.5 cm or larger). During this stage the child is typically *very* irritable and inconsolable. Complications during this period include myocarditis with resultant ECG changes, decreased left ventricular function, and occasional symptoms of CHF. Approximately one third of patients will develop a temporary arthritis beginning in the small joints.

The *subacute phase* begins with resolution of the fever and lasts until all clinical signs of KD have disappeared. During this phase the child is at greatest risk for the development of coronary artery aneurysms. If changes in the arteries occur, they can start as early as day 7 and generally peak at 3 to 4 weeks. Thrombocytosis and hypercoagulability place the child at risk for coronary thrombosis. During this period the child often has the characteristic periungual desquamation of the hands and feet. Arthritis that develops during the subacute phase affects mainly the larger weight-bearing joints. Irritability persists during this phase.

In the *convalescent phase* all the clinical signs of KD have resolved. The laboratory values, however, have not yet returned to normal. The erythrocyte sedimentation rate may remain elevated, reflecting lingering inflammation. Thrombocytosis may still be present. Arthritis may continue into this stage, and coronary complications may remain a concern. This phase is complete when all blood values return to normal (6 to 8 weeks after onset). At the end of this stage parents report that the child appears to have returned to normal in terms of temperament, energy, and appetite.

Cardiac involvement. The most serious complication of KD is the potential for myocardial infarction, which generally results from thrombotic occlusion of a coronary aneurysm. The group at highest risk for thrombus formation are children with "giant" aneurysms (greater than 8 mm in diameter). The main symptoms of acute myocardial infarction in children are abdominal pain, vomiting, restlessness, and shock. Complaints of chest pain are more typical in older children (Kato, Ichinose, and Kawasaki, 1986).

Diagnostic Evaluation

Since no specific diagnostic test exists for KD, the diagnosis is established on the basis of clinical findings and associated laboratory results (Box 34-7).

Box 34-7 DIAGNOSTIC CRITERIA FOR KAWASAKI DISEASE

The child must exhibit five of the following six criteria, including fever:

1. Fever for 5 or more days (often diagnosed with shorter duration of fever if other symptoms are present)
2. Bilateral conjunctival infection without exudation
3. Changes in the oral mucous membranes, such as erythema, dryness, and fissuring of the lips; oropharyngeal reddening; or "strawberry tongue"
4. Changes in the extremities, such as peripheral edema, peripheral erythema, and desquamation of palms and soles, particularly periungual peeling
5. Polymorphous rash, often accentuated in the perineal area
6. Cervical lymphadenopathy

These criteria should be used only as guidelines. Many children with KD do not fulfill standard diagnostic criteria, and infants often have an atypical presentation. It is therefore important to consider KD as a possible diagnosis in any infant or child with prolonged elevated temperature that is unresponsive to antibiotics and is not attributable to another cause.

Several associated laboratory findings, when combined with clinical data, can be helpful in making the diagnosis. The typical child with KD is anemic and has a leukocytosis with a "shift to the left" (increased immature white blood cells) during the acute phase. An elevated erythrocyte sedimentation rate reflects ongoing inflammation and generally persists for 6 to 8 weeks. Urinalysis reveals a sterile pyuria with mononuclear cells. This will not be evident with a regular dipstick and white blood count because the white blood cells are not polymorphonuclear neutrophils. A transient elevation of liver enzymes typically occurs. Thrombocytosis with hypercoagulability becomes evident in the subacute phase and peaks in 3 to 4 weeks.

Echocardiograms are used to monitor myocardial and coronary artery status. A baseline echocardiogram should be obtained at the time of diagnosis for comparison with future studies. In addition, follow-up echocardiograms should be performed at approximately 2 weeks after onset and again at 6 to 8 weeks to determine the diameter of the coronary arteries, as well as left ventricular contractility and valvular function. If cardiac involvement is evident, more frequent studies may be necessary.

Therapeutic Management

Therapeutic management of KD has evolved significantly over the past 5 years. The use of gamma globulin has greatly altered the course of this disease; before its use, fever and symptoms usually lasted several weeks. With administration of intravenous gamma globulin, symptoms generally resolve rapidly. The current treatment of KD includes high-dose intravenous gamma globulin along with traditional salicylate therapy. Aspirin is given initially in an antiinflammatory dose (80 to 100 mg/kg/day in divided doses every 6 hours) to control fever and symptoms of inflammation. Once fever has subsided, aspirin is continued at an antiplatelet dose (3 to 5 mg/kg/day). Low-dose aspirin is continued in patients without echocardiographic evidence of coronary abnormalities until the platelet count has returned to normal (6 to 8 weeks). If the child develops coronary abnormalities, salicylate therapy is continued indefinitely.

Gamma globulin has been demonstrated to be effective at reducing the incidence of coronary artery abnormalities when given within the first 10 days of the illness (Newburger and others, 1986). Gamma globulin has traditionally been given in four consecutive daily infusions (400 mg/kg/dose). In a recent multicenter randomized trial the 4-day infusion was compared with a single large infusion of 2 g/kg over 8 to 10 hours. The single infusion was found to be as safe and more effective in reducing fever and aneurysm formation in up to 85% of cases (Newburger and others, 1990). The exact mechanism by which gamma globulin works is unknown.

Prognosis

Most children with KD recover fully following treatment. However, when cardiovascular complications occur, serious morbidity may result. The long-term cardiac effects are not known because the disease is relatively recent, preventing longitudinal data analysis. Death occurs in approximately 0.3% of children and almost always results from coronary thrombosis.

Nursing Considerations

The nursing care of children with KD is challenging. Inpatient care focuses on symptomatic relief, emotional support, medication administration, diagnostic assistance, and education of the child and family.

In the initial phase the nurse must monitor the child's cardiac status carefully. Intake and output and daily weight measurements are recorded. Although the child may be reluctant to eat and therefore may be partially dehydrated, fluids need to be administered with care because of the usual finding of myocarditis. The child should be assessed frequently for signs of CHF, including decreased urinary output, gallop rhythm, tachycardia, and respiratory distress. Cardiac monitoring is suggested in the following cases: before the initial ECG and echocardiogram are completed and shown to be normal, during the infusion of intravenous gamma globulin (because of the large fluid load), for children less than 1 year of age, and for any child with cardiac symptoms. Sedation is generally required before echocardiography in children under 3 years of age, since the child needs to remain completely still for up to an hour.

Most nursing care focuses on symptomatic relief. To minimize skin discomfort, cool cloths, nonscented lotions, and soft, loose clothing are helpful (Anderson and Thibault, 1981). During the acute phase, mouth care, including lubricating ointment to the lips, is important for the mucosal inflammation. Clear liquids and soft foods can be offered. Elevated temperatures need to be carefully monitored. Acetaminophen can be given for fever. Cool cloths and light clothing may also help (see Controlling Elevated Temperatures, Chapter 27). If arthritis develops, passive range of motion may be indicated and can be done most easily during the child's bath.

The administration of gamma globulin should follow the same guidelines as for any blood product, with frequent monitoring of vital signs. Patients must be watched for allergic reactions (see Table 35-2). Cardiac status needs monitoring because of the large volume being administered to patients with myocarditis and diminished left ventricular function. Intravenous patency is checked because extravasation can result in tissue damage. Hypercoagulability and venous fragility often make it difficult to maintain intravenous access in children with KD (McEnhill and Vitale, 1989).

Patient irritability is perhaps the most challenging problem. These children need to be placed in a quiet environment that promotes adequate rest. Their parents need to be supported in their efforts to comfort an often inconsolable child. They may need time away from their child, and nurses can often provide respite care for the family. Parents need to understand that irritability is a hallmark of KD and that they need not feel guilty or embarrassed about their child's behavior.

Discharge teaching. Parents need accurate information about the progression of KD, including the importance of follow-up monitoring and when they should contact their practitioner. Irritability is likely to persist for up to 2 months after the onset of symptoms. Peeling of the hands and feet is painless and occurs primarily in the second and third weeks. Arthritis, especially of the larger weight-bearing joints, may persist for several weeks. Children are typically most stiff in the mornings, during cold weather, and after naps. Passive range of motion in the bathtub is often helpful in increasing flexibility. Any live immunizations (e.g., measles-mumps-rubella) should be deferred for 3 months after the administration of gamma globulin, since the body might not produce the appropriate amount of antibodies.

A few children develop recurrent fever symptoms, and a small number may have a recurrence of KD. Temperature should be recorded after discharge until the child has been afebrile for several days. Parents should be educated about the signs and symptoms of KD; if any occur together with a temperature of 38.4° C (101° F) or above, they are instructed to notify their practitioner.

Parents also need to be instructed about the administration of salicylates and made aware of the signs of aspirin toxicity—ringing in the ears (tinnitus), headache, dizziness, and confusion. In addition, the aspirin should be stopped and the practitioner notified if the child is exposed to chickenpox or influenza, since the drug is associated with Reye syndrome.

All parents should understand the unlikely but real possibility of myocardial infarction as well as the signs and symptoms of cardiac ischemia in a child. At discharge the ultimate cardiac sequela is generally not known, since changes occur up to a month after the onset of KD. In addition, the parents of children with known severe coronary artery sequelae may be taught cardiopulmonary resuscitation.*

SYSTEMIC HYPERTENSION

Hypertension is the consistent elevation of the blood pressure beyond values considered the upper limits of normal. The two major categories of hypertension are *essential,* or *primary* (no identifiable cause), and *secondary* (subsequent to an identifiable cause) hypertension. Traditionally, primary hypertension has been considered a disease of middle-aged or older persons and is a major health problem. Hypertension is the most common cause of cerebrovascular accident and is a major risk factor in myocardial infarction. However, in recent years there has been increasing interest in this disorder as it occurs in adolescents and children, particularly in terms of prevention of fatal consequences in adulthood.

Routine blood pressure measurements of children have detected hypertension similar to primary hypertension in adults with surprising frequency in asymptomatic children, especially teenagers. A conservative estimate suggests at least 1% to 2% incidence of sustained hypertension in the age-groups under 20 years (Cranwell, 1984), although many authorities believe that the incidence is considerable higher (Rocchini, 1984). There is accumulating evidence that the primary hypertension of adulthood may have its origin in childhood; thus its early detection has significance for prevention and treatment.

Etiology

Most instances of hypertension observed in young children occur secondary to a structural abnormality or an underlying pathologic process, although this is being challenged by screening programs of relatively healthy children. The most common cause of secondary hypertension is renal disease (80%), followed by cardiovascular, endocrine, and some neurologic disorders. Miscellaneous conditions such as lead poisoning and ingestion of excessive amounts of licorice are causes unique to children. As a rule, the younger the child and the more severe the hypertension, the more likely it is to be secondary. The conditions associated with secondary hypertension in children and adolescents are listed in Box 34-8.

The causes of primary hypertension are undetermined. There is evidence that both genetic and environmental factors play a role. In younger children hypertension is most commonly due to secondary causes; however, in adolescents primary hypertension is seen more often than the secondary forms (Loggie and others, 1984). The incidence of hypertension is greater in children with a family history of hypertension. American blacks have a higher incidence of hypertension than whites. In the black population hypertension develops earlier and is frequently more severe, resulting in mortality at an earlier age. Environmental factors that contribute to the risk of developing hypertension include obesity, salt ingestion, smoking, and stress.

Clinical Manifestations

Although clinical manifestations associated with hypertension depend largely on the underlying cause, some observations can provide clues to the practitioner that an elevated blood pressure may be a factor. Adolescents and older children with hypertension complain of frequent headaches, dizziness, and/or changes in vision. In infants or young children who cannot communicate symptoms, observation of behavior provides clues, although gross behavioral changes may not be apparent until complications are present. Parents of infants and small children who have been treated for hypertension report that their child had previously been irritable, often indulged in an abnormal degree of head banging or rubbing, and may have wakened screaming in the night (when blood pressure tends to be highest).

*Home care instructions are available in Wong, D.L., and Whaley, L.F.: Clinical manual of pediatric nursing, ed. 3, St. Louis, 1990, Mosby–Year Book, Inc.

Box 34-8 CONDITIONS ASSOCIATED WITH SECONDARY HYPERTENSION IN CHILDREN

Renal Disorders
Congenital defects
- Polycystic kidney, ectopic kidney, horseshoe kidney, etc.
- Obstructive anomalies
- Hydronephrosis

Renal tumor
- Wilms tumor
- Renovascular

Abnormalities of renal arteries
Renal vein thrombosis
Acquired disorders
- Glomerulonephritis—acute or chronic
- Pyelonephritis
- Nephritis associated with collagen disease

Cardiovascular Disease
Coarctation of aorta
Arteriovenous fistulas
Patent ductus arteriosus
Aortic or mitral insufficiency

Metabolic and Endocrine Diseases
Adrenal tumors
- Adenoma
- Pheochromocytoma
- Neuroblastoma
- Cushing syndrome
- Adrenogenital syndrome
- Hyperthyroidism
- Aldosteronism
- Hypercalcemia
- Diabetes mellitus

Neurologic Disorders
Space-occupying lesions of cranium (increased intracranial pressure)
- Tumors, cysts, hematoma
- Cerebral edema
- Encephalitis (including Guillain-Barré and Reye syndromes)

Miscellaneous Causes
Drugs (corticosteroids, oral contraceptives, pressor agents, amphetamines)
Burns
Genitourinary surgery
Trauma (e.g., stretching of femoral nerve with leg traction)
Insect bites (e.g., scorpion)
Intravascular overload (blood, fluid)
Hypernatremia
Toxemia of pregnancy
Heavy metal poisoning

Table 34-7 Classification of hypertension by age-group

AGE-GROUP	SIGNIFICANT HYPERTENSION (mm Hg)	SEVERE HYPERTENSION (mm Hg)
Newborn		
(7 days)	Systolic BP ≥ 96	Systolic BP ≥ 106
(8-30 days)	Systolic BP ≥ 104	Systolic BP ≥ 110
Infant (<2 years)	Systolic BP ≥ 112 Diastolic BP ≥ 74	Systolic BP ≥ 118 Diastolic BP ≥ 82
Children (3-5 years)	Systolic BP ≥ 116 Diastolic BP ≥ 76	Systolic BP ≥ 124 Diastolic BP ≥ 84
Children (6-9 years)	Systolic BP ≥ 122 Diastolic BP ≥ 78	Systolic BP ≥ 130 Diastolic BP ≥ 86
Children (10-12 years)	Systolic BP ≥ 126 Diastolic BP ≥ 82	Systolic BP ≥ 134 Diastolic BP ≥ 90
Adolescents (13-15 years)	Systolic BP ≥ 136 Diastolic BP ≥ 86	Systolic BP ≥ 144 Diastolic BP ≥ 92
Adolescents (16-18 years)	Systolic BP ≥ 142 Diastolic BP ≥ 92	Systolic BP ≥ 150 Diastolic BP ≥ 98

From American Academy of Pediatrics: Report of the Second Task Force on Blood Pressure Control in Children—1987, Pediatrics 79(1):1-25, 1987.

Diagnostic Evaluation

It is clear from the increasing numbers of hypertensive or potentially hypertensive children and adolescents being identified that a blood pressure determination should be a routine part of annual assessment in children 3 years of age and older. In addition, any child who is ill should have blood pressures measured, since the signs and symptoms of hypertension in children are often vague. The blood pressure of children at any age should be measured if they are diagnosed as having or suspected of having coarctation of the aorta, unexplained heart failure, unexplained heart murmurs, unexplained seizures or other neurologic signs, an abdominal mass or masses, edema, ascites, and/or evidence of renal failure, hypernatremia, failure to thrive, respiratory distress, and hyperlipidemia.

No definitive cutoff values are used in the diagnosis of hypertension in the pediatric patient. The American Academy of Pediatrics (1987) has suggested the classification in Table 34-7. *Significant hypertension* is considered a blood pressure persistently between the 95th and 99th percentiles for age and sex. *Severe hypertension* is a blood pressure persistently at or above the 99th percentile for age and sex. It is important to note that a child who is large for age may normally have a higher blood pressure than a child who is of average size.

Before a diagnosis is made, blood pressure should be measured on at least three separate occasions. To obtain an accurate reading, care is taken to quiet the child or relax the adolescent while the measurement is recorded to avoid false readings caused by excitement. The chief cause of falsely elevated blood pressure readings is the use of improperly fitting, narrow cuffs. Therefore attention to correct measurement technique is essential (see Blood Pressure, Chapter 7). Twenty-four-hour blood pressure monitoring devices are currently available to detect changes in blood pressure throughout the day, thus giving a more realistic picture. These devices are best used with older children who are able to tolerate being attached to an ambulatory monitor.

In children with suspected primary hypertension, initial

laboratory data are also obtained. This generally includes a urinalysis, renal function studies such as a creatinine and blood urea nitrogen, a lipid profile, complete blood count, and electrolytes. More intensive tests may be indicated for those with probable secondary hypertension.

Therapeutic Management

Therapy for secondary hypertension involves diagnosis and treatment of the underlying cause. In those cases amenable to surgical repair, the nature of the condition, the type of surgery, and the age of the child are all important considerations. Children or adolescents with consistently elevated blood pressure readings from no known cause or those with secondary hypertension not amenable to surgical correction may be treated with a combination of nonpharmacologic and pharmacologic interventions. Dietary practices and life-style changes are important in the control of hypertension both for children and for adults. Nonpharmacologic measures, such as limitation of dietary salt, weight control, increased exercise, and avoidance of stress and smoking, carry no risk and should be instituted first, except in severe cases. Since the long-term effects of antihypertensive agents on children are not known, drug treatment of asymptomatic children with mild or borderline hypertension is not recommended.

Since overweight and hypertension are closely related, a weight reduction program is recommended for overweight youngsters. In salt-sensitive children, high salt intake increases the risk of hypertension for those genetically predisposed and aggravates existing hypertension unless salt intake is limited. Modifying salt in children is difficult and takes time and support. Regular exercise augments weight reduction and alone has been shown to normalize blood pressure. The exercise regimen should be tailored to the child's interest. Aerobic exercise such as swimming, running, or cycling is highly recommended. Stress reduction strategies may be beneficial and include biofeedback and relaxation. Smoking is discouraged. If the adolescent is taking oral contraceptives, these need to be discontinued and other contraceptive options provided.

Drug therapy in children is instituted with caution. Indications for hypotensive drug therapy are consistent, significant elevations of blood pressure resistant to nonpharmacologic intervention. The American Academy of Pediatrics Second Task Force on Blood Pressure Control in Children (1987) recommends beginning with one drug and adding other drugs only if control is not obtained. Compliance with antihypertensive drug regimens is extremely difficult.

The oral antihypertensive drugs used most often in children include the beta blockers (propranolol), ACE inhibitors, diuretics, and occasionally a vasodilator (hydralazine). Calcium channel blockers remain controversial for the pediatric population. The drug is tailored to meet the needs of individual children and is determined by the hypotensive effect produced and appearance of any side effects. The goal is to achieve a normotensive state throughout the day without accompanying side effects. With many antihypertensive drugs, minimum data are available regarding their side effects in children. Therefore any behavioral or physical changes that occur after institution of therapy should be considered a possible effect, and therapy may need to be revised.

Nursing Considerations

The nurse is a valuable link in the health care delivery system in relation to hypertension in the pediatric age-group. Active in detection, diagnosis, and therapy in any setting—hospital, school, clinic, private office, public health services, and private practice—nurses are frequently the persons who operate well-child care and follow-up units and are usually the primary contact between health services and the child and family.

A blood pressure measurement should always be a part of the routine assessment of infants and children. In carrying out the procedure, it is important to use the correct cuff size. Any questionable reading should be repeated. When an elevated pressure is detected, the procedure should be carried out in the supine, sitting, and standing positions as feasible. In addition, comparisons should be made between the upper and lower extremities.

Nursing counseling and guidance of affected children is a challenge. Education aimed at the understanding of hypertension and its implication over the life span is essential in promoting patient and family compliance with both nonpharmacologic and pharmacologic therapies (see Compliance, Chapter 27).

Home blood pressure measurements can facilitate surveillance in youngsters with chronic hypertension and can document effectiveness of therapy. A family member can be instructed in how to take and record accurate blood pressure measurements, thus decreasing the number of trips to a health care facility. This individual needs to understand when to contact the practitioner regarding elevated values. When this option is not feasible, the school nurse can often be a valuable resource in monitoring blood pressures.

The nurse plays an important role in assessing individual families and providing targeted information regarding nonpharmacologic modes of intervention, such as diet, weight loss, smoking, and exercise programs. If extensive dietary counseling is required, the child should be referred to a registered nutritionist with expertise in working with children and adolescents. Exercise regimens should be individualized. School children and young adolescents generally prefer team sports rather than individual training, which they may view as a burden rather than an enjoyable activity. If peers and family members can be encouraged to participate in any of the management strategies, the child's compliance is likely to be greater.

Young hypertensive women should avoid oral contraceptives because of their pressor effects. Other options need to be presented before this form of birth control is discontinued (see Contraception, Chapter 20).

If drug therapy is prescribed, the nurse needs to provide information to the family regarding the reasons for drug therapy, how the drug works, and possible side effects (Box 34-9). It is important to explain that the drug needs to be

Box 34-9 ANTIHYPERTENSIVE DRUGS COMMONLY USED IN THE TREATMENT OF PEDIATRIC HYPERTENSION, WITH NURSING INTERVENTIONS*

Beta Blockers

Actions: Blocks response to beta stimulation
Depresses renin output

Propranolol (Inderal)
- Monitor pulse and blood pressures (can cause bradycardia and hypotension).
- Instruct to take with meals.
- Advise that drug may cause fatigue, a decrease in exercise tolerance, weakness, and cold extremities.
- Warn males of possible impotence.

Atenolol (Tenormin)
- Monitor pulse and blood pressures (can cause bradycardia and hypotension).
- Advise that drug can be given once a day.
- Instruct patients not to discontinue abruptly (needs to be withdrawn over a 2-week period).

ACE Inhibitors

Action: Acts primarily by interfering with the production of angiotensin II, a potent vasoconstrictor

Captopril (Capoten)
- Monitor blood pressure and pulse.
- Instruct to take 1 hour before meals to increase absorption.
- Instruct patient to report any evidence of infection.
- Advise to avoid position changes (can initially cause dizziness).

Enalapril (Vasotec)
- Monitor blood pressure and pulse (may cause hypotension).
- Instruct to report any swelling of face or lips and difficulty breathing (may rarely cause laryngeal edema).
- Instruct to report any evidence of infection.
- Advise not to use potassium supplements (can increase serum levels).

Vasodilator

Actions: Acts on vascular smooth muscle
Thought to produce its effect by direct action on blood vessels to cause arterial vasodilation

Hydralazine (Apresoline)
- Instruct to take with meals.
- Advise that drug may cause drowsiness and to use caution operating machinery or doing other hazardous activity.
- Instruct to report if sore throat, fever, muscle and joint aches, or skin rash develops.

Diuretics (see Table 34-5)

*For the use of all drugs, instruct child or adolescent (and family) to:
- Rise slowly from a horizontal position and avoid sudden position changes.
- Take drug as prescribed.
- Notify practitioner if unpleasant side effects occur, but do not discontinue drug.
- Avoid alcohol and stay on prescribed diet.

taken consistently to achieve any prolonged control of blood pressure. The need for follow-up is stressed, especially since antihypertensive therapy can sometimes be safely discontinued if blood pressure remains under control over time.

Learning needs vary greatly depending on developmental levels and individual differences. Some children and families require a great deal of support, education, and guidance, whereas others need only education and periodic follow-up. A positive approach is essential; negative feedback will serve only to alienate the family. Exploring the reasons for difficulty in compliance can often provide realistic alternatives. Continued education, support, and reinforcement for positive behavior is a major nursing responsibility.

HYPERLIPIDEMIA (HYPERCHOLESTEROLEMIA)

Hyperlipidemia is a general term for excessive lipids (fat and fatlike substances); *hypercholesterolemia* refers to excessive cholesterol in the blood. High lipid or cholesterol levels are believed to play an important role in producing atherosclerosis (fatty plaques on the arteries), which eventually can lead to coronary heart disease, a primary cause of morbidity and mortality in the adult population. The risk of premature coronary heart disease has been shown to increase directly with plasma concentrations of total cholesterol and certain types of lipids. Interventions that decrease low-density lipoproteins (LDLs) and high-density lipoproteins (HDLs) have been shown to lower the risk for coronary heart disease (LaRosa and others, 1990). Current research indicates that a presymptomatic phase of atherosclerosis begins in childhood. Fatty streaks in the coronary arteries may be detected in children as young as 10 to 14 years of age and appear in almost all individuals over the age of 20 years (Stary, 1987). As a result, a new initiative in preventive cardiology focuses on the screening and management of lipid levels in childhood. The goal is to identify those children at high risk and intervene early.

The rationale for lipid management in children is evolving, as lipid levels have been followed from childhood into adulthood. Children who demonstrate cholesterol levels in the upper percentiles seem to have an increased risk of remaining in the upper percentiles into adulthood. On the other hand, children in the lower percentiles are unlikely to have high cholesterol levels as adults. Cholesterol in childhood appears to be a major population predictor for adult cholesterol levels (Newburger, 1990). From known data on lipid levels and their relationship to cardiovascular disease in adults, some experts believe that children with hypercholesterolemia may suffer an increased risk of cardiovascular disease in adulthood.

To date, no definitive studies can predict the long-term risk of heart disease for children with hyperlipidemia. Research in this area is logistically difficult to complete because of the long period of clinical follow-up extending over 40 to 60 years. As a result, many pediatric guidelines are inferred from adult data. Life-style habits, including diet, exercise patterns, and smoking, all known to be potential risk factors for cardiovascular disease, are normally established at a young age.

Cholesterol, a fatlike steroid alcohol, is part of the lipoprotein complex in plasma that is essential for cellular metabolism. Triglycerides, natural fats synthesized from carbohydrates, are used for energy. Both are major lipids transported on lipoproteins, a combination of lipids and proteins. There are four classes of lipoproteins:

Chylomicrons—produced in the intestine in response to the intake of dietary fat. These are the principal transporters of dietary fat (triglycerides) from the intestine to the blood and ultimately to the fatty tissue. Chylomicrons are usually not present in the blood after a 12- to 14-hour fast.

Very-low-density lipoproteins (VLDLs)—contain high concentrations of triglycerides, moderate concentrations of cholesterol, and little protein.

Low-density lipoproteins (LDLs)—contain low concentrations of triglycerides, high levels of cholesterol, and moderate levels of protein. The end-product of VLDL synthesis, LDL, is the major carrier of cholesterol to the cells. Cells use cholesterol for synthesis of membranes and steroid production. Elevated circulating LDL is a strong risk factor in cardiovascular disease.

High-density lipoproteins (HDLs)—contain very low concentrations of triglycerides, relatively little cholesterol, and high levels of protein. Transport free cholesterol to the liver for secretion in the bile. High levels of HDL are thought to protect against cardiovascular disease.

The formula used for a standard fasting lipid profile that reflects total cholesterol (TC) is:

$$TC = LDL + HDL + \frac{\text{Triglycerides}}{5}$$

LDL concentration can be calculated from this formula. It is considered accurate as long as the fasting triglyceride level is <400 mg/dl.

$$LDL = TC - \left(HDL + \frac{\text{Triglycerides}}{5}\right)$$

Diagnostic Evaluation

Diagnosis of hyperlipidemia is based on analysis of blood for a full lipid profile. However, normal serum cholesterol values for children are not universally defined. The mean cholesterol levels for children ages 1 to 19 years are reported as 160.9 to 166.4 mg/dl (Resnicow, Morley-Kotchen, and Wynder, 1989). Cutoff values for determining risk for future coronary heart disease in children are inconsistent. The American Academy of Pediatrics, Committee on Nutrition (1989) recommends a cutoff value of 176 mg/dl (75th percentile) for children up to 19 years of age. The National Institutes of Health recommends using 170 mg/dl as the cutoff for moderate risk and 185 mg/dl for high risk (Consensus, 1985). LDL levels may be even more important than TC levels, but cutoff levels have not been defined (Dennison and others, 1990). Lipid concentrations during childhood are listed in Table 34-8.

Before a diagnosis of hyperlipidemia can be made, two or three consecutive samples drawn in the fasting state (12 to 14 hours) should be analyzed. Blood samples should be collected after having the patient sit for 5 minutes, and the tourniquet should be applied immediately before the needle stick, since posture and vascular stasis may affect results. Screening of children for hypercholesterolemia is currently a controversial and unresolved issue (see Questions and Controversies, p. 1592).

Therapeutic Management

In treating hyperlipidemia, it is important to rule out secondary systemic causes, including endocrine, metabolic, hepatic, and renal disorders. In addition, oral contraceptives, alcohol, other medications, acute illness, ongoing weight loss, and biologic variation may affect lipid values. When no organic cause is found, treatment involves dietary changes with or without drug therapy.

Dietary management is the cornerstone of therapy for pediatric hyperlipidemia. The National Institutes of Health, the American Heart Association, and the American Academy of Pediatrics currently recommend a prudent low-fat, low-cholesterol diet for children over 2 years of age. It is beneficial to begin preventive practices in childhood before poor di-

Table 34-8 Normal plasma lipid concentrations in the first 2 decades of life (mg/dl)

AGE (YEARS)	CHOLESTEROL			TRIGLYCERIDES			HDL CHOLESTEROL			LDL CHOLESTEROL		
	5th	MEAN	95th	5th	MEAN	95th	5th	MEAN	95th	5th	MEAN	95th
0-4												
Males	114	155	203	29	56	99	—	—	—	—	—	—
Females	112	156	200	34	64	112	—	—	—	—	—	—
5-9												
Males	121	160	203	30	56	101	38	56	75	63	93	129
Females	126	164	205	32	60	105	36	53	73	68	100	140
10-14												
Males	119	158	202	32	66	125	37	55	74	64	97	133
Females	124	160	201	37	75	131	37	52	70	68	97	136
15-19												
Males	113	150	197	37	78	148	30	46	63	62	94	130
Females	120	158	203	39	75	132	35	52	74	59	96	137

Modified from The Lipid Research Clinics population studies data book. Vol. I. The prevalence study, NIH Pub. No. 80-1527, Lipid Metabolism Branch, Division of Heart and Vascular Diseases, National Heart, Lung, and Blood Institute, U.S. Department of Health and Human Services, Public Health Service, National Institutes of Health, Washington, DC, 1980, U.S. Government Printing Office.

QUESTIONS AND CONTROVERSIES

Should all children be screened for high cholesterol levels?

Practitioners' opinions differ regarding lipid screening in childhood. The American Heart Association (A Joint Statement, 1986), the American Academy of Pediatrics (1989), and the National Institutes of Health (Consensus, 1985) all recommend selected screening for children with a family history of hyperlipidemia, xanthomas, sudden death, early angina, or myocardial infarction (less than 50 years of age for males, less than 60 years for females) in siblings, parents, uncles, aunts, or grandparents. In addition, children with nonfamilial risk factors should also be screened. This would include children with a history of KD, obesity, and diabetes.

Advocates of selective screening oppose universal screening for various reasons. Screening is costly, and the laboratory data may vary significantly from center to center, resulting in inappropriate diagnosis. Since a prudent diet is now recommended for children over 2 years of age, universal screening will not alter management for most, and no valid evidence indicates that cholesterol-lowering diets prevent death from heart disease in adults (Feldman, 1990; Finberg, 1990).

Those favoring universal screening believe that selective screening is too limited and overlooks many children with hyperlipidemia. With varying family constellations a common situation today, family history may be incomplete. In addition, a negative history from a parent may be inaccurate, since approximately half of well-educated adults do not know their own cholesterol levels (Strong and Dennison, 1988). In a study of children from eight pediatric practices in the Chicago area, family history did not identify half the children with elevated LDL, and it did not selectively identify the most severely affected children (Griffin and others, 1989). Other researchers have found similar results (Garcia and Moodle, 1989; Resnicow, Morley-Kotchen, and Wynder, 1989).

Universal screening would identify most children with hyperlipidemia. However, whether long-term survival would increase with early treatment to lower blood lipid levels is unknown. For the present, nurses play an important role in identifying children who meet the criteria for selective screening.

etary habits are formed. These authorities further state that children with TC values above the 75th percentile should have dietary counseling. For children with hyperlipidemia, the American Heart Association recommends a two-step dietary approach that restricts the intake of cholesterol and fat. A "step one" diet restricts cholesterol intake to no more than 300 mg/day and fat intake to 30% of the daily calories, equally divided between saturated, polyunsaturated, and monounsaturated fats. A "step two" diet further restricts saturated fats to less than 7% and dietary cholesterol to less than 200 mg/day.

For the most benefit to the child and family, formal dietary counseling with a nutritionist experienced in pediatric lipids is recommended. In this way dietary information can be targeted specifically for the individual family. Interactive group sessions geared to children and their families, along with individual follow-up, is most beneficial. Most patients should be given a trial of at least 6 months of dietary management before initiation of pharmacologic therapy. The available data on dietary therapy for hyperlipidemia in children suggest that a 10% to 15% reduction in total and LDL cholesterol can be achieved. Increases in HDL cholesterol are affected most by regular aerobic exercise, weight loss, cessation of smoking, and the addition of monounsaturated fats to the diet (e.g., olive and canola oil). Children in the highest percentiles may not respond adequately to diet alone and may need adjunct medication.

For children with severe hyperlipidemia who fail to respond to diet modification and aerobic activity, drug therapy may be necessary. The two drugs most often used in pediatric patients are bile acid–binding resins and niacin.

The *bile acid–binding resins,* cholestyramine (Questran) and colestipol, are two resins frequently prescribed for children to reduce their LDL cholesterol level. These drugs are taken orally but are not absorbed systemically. They have been shown to be safe and effective for pediatric use. Cholestyramine is available as both a powder, to be mixed with juice, and a solid bar (Cholybar). A pill is currently being developed. Some patients cannot tolerate this medication because of the taste and the side effects, the most significant being constipation, abdominal pain, gastrointestinal bloating, flatulence, and nausea. Patients often complain of the "gritty" consistency of the medication. The average dose for a child is 4 g three times daily or 6 g twice daily.

Patients should be instructed to take one multivitamin with iron daily, since cholestyramine may interfere with the absorption of fat-soluble vitamins. It may also interfere with the absorption of other medications, which should be given earlier than 1 hour before or 6 hours after the resin-binding agent is ingested. The results of liver function tests, a complete blood count, chloride and folate levels, and serum concentrations of vitamins A, D, and E should be evaluated yearly.

Niacin (nicotinic acid) decreases TC and triglycerides and increases HDL cholesterol. It is generally administered to older children who do not tolerate resin-binding agents well or whose lipid profiles show a high triglyceride and low HDL cholesterol levels. Some patients require adjunct therapy with bile acid–binding resins. Patients taking niacin often complain of itching, gastrointestinal distress, and flushing episodes, especially when initially taking the drug. Flushing can be avoided if the patient is premedicated with one aspirin (300 mg) approximately ½ hour before the dose. The initial dose of niacin for children, using a time-release or long-acting preparation, is 125 to 250 mg twice daily. This can be increased to 25 to 75 mg/kg/day. Side effects are uncommon in patients taking less than 1500 g/day. Patients taking nicotinic acid need to have liver function tests, glucose levels, uric acid concentrations, and blood counts monitored every 6 months. Niacin should not be given in the presence of liver disease or ulcers.

Nursing Considerations

Nurses play an important role in the screening, education, and support of children with hyperlipidemia and their families. When a child is referred to a lipid clinic, it is essential that the family be adequately prepared for the first visit. Generally the parents will be asked to keep a dietary history of the child before this visit. Sometimes they will need to complete a questionnaire regarding the child's normal dietary habits over the preceding year. Families should be instructed to keep their child fasting for at least 14 hours before screening. Therefore it is important to schedule the blood test early in the morning and to arrange for nourishment immediately thereafter. At the visit a full family history should be taken, including the health of both parents and all first-degree relatives. Specific questions should be asked regarding early heart disease, hypertension, strokes (CVAs), sudden death, hyperlipidemia, diabetes, and endocrine abnormalities. Nurses may also uncover risk factors when obtaining a health history for other purposes. It is therefore important that nurses be familiar with current screening practices and the availability of resources for children with positive family histories.

Parents and extended families should be informed about cholesterol and hyperlipidemia. This education should include a brief introduction to the different lipoprotein categories, including cholesterol, HDL, LDL, VLDL, and triglycerides. Also, behavioral risk factors for heart disease, such as smoking and exercise, should be reviewed. For management to be effective, parents need to understand the rationale for dietary and/or pharmacologic intervention. The key is prevention of future cardiovascular disease.

Stringent dietary guidelines may become an issue of control and a source of great stress for many families. Children should not be viewed as having a disease. Rather, the positive aspects of healthy eating, regular exercise, and avoiding smoking should be emphasized. Basic dietary changes should be encouraged for the whole family so that the affected sibling is not singled out. The focus should be positive, with emphasis on what can be eaten, such as substituting chicken and fish for hot dogs and hamburgers and frozen yogurt for ice cream (Table 34-9). Cultural differences must be considered and recommendations individualized. For example, it is more realistic to suggest frying food in a monounsaturated oil such as canola than to forbid fried food altogether in families where this is common practice. Substitution rather than elimination needs to be emphasized. Visual aids are often helpful, especially for the children (e.g., test tubes depicting the amount of fat in a hot dog). Diets should be flexible and individually tailored by a nutritionist experienced in combining recommendations that meet both the nutritional demands of the growing child and lipid modifications. Parents should be encouraged to participate in dietary and educational sessions, ask questions, and share ideas and experiences.

Parents often feel guilty about the hereditary component of hyperlipidemia. Many of these same parents believe they have failed if the diet alone is not making a significant difference in their child's lipid profile. They need to be reassured that a dietary approach alone is often not sufficient, especially for children with values greater than the 95th percentile.

Table 34-9 Low-cholesterol substitutes for common foods

COMMON FOODS HIGH IN CHOLESTEROL AND SATURATED FAT	SUBSTITUTES LOW IN CHOLESTEROL AND SATURATED FAT
Ice cream	Nonfat frozen yogurt Frozen fruit juice bars Sherbet
Processed luncheon meats	Turkey breast
Hot dogs	Chicken
Bologna	Lean ham
Salami	Turkey ham, turkey pastrami
Whole milk	Nonfat milk
Cheddar cheese	Mozarella cheese
American cheese	String cheese Lowfat cottage cheese
Snack crackers	Popcorn (unbuttered), pretzels
Chips	Fresh fruit, vegetable sticks
Butter	Margarine
Pepperoni or sausage pizza	Cheese pizza with vegetables and lean ham
Sirloin or ribeye steak	Flank or round steak
Spareribs	London broil
Hamburger	Ground turkey burger
Fried chicken	Skinless chicken or turkey

From Davidson, D.M., Smith, R.M., and Qaqundah, P.Y.: Cholesterol screening in children during office visits, J. Pediatr. Health Care 4(1):11-17, 1990.

Parents of children who require pharmacologic therapy need to understand the purpose, dosage, and possible side effects of the various drugs. Medication schedules should remain flexible and should not interfere with the child's daily activities. As an example, children of elementary school age may have better compliance if they take a resin-binding agent (e.g., cholestyramine, colestipol) twice a day (i.e., before school and at night) rather than the standard three times a day. Follow-up phone calls by the nurse between visits allow parents to discuss their concerns and ask any questions that have arisen.

CARDIOMYOPATHY

Cardiomyopathy refers to abnormalities of the myocardium in which the cardiac muscles' ability to contract is impaired. Although the incidence of cardiomyopathy in infants and children is small, it accounts for 4.8% of all cardiac deaths in childhood, and about one half the survivors have chronic cardiac disability (Tripp, 1984). Possible etiologic factors include familiar genetic causes, infection, deficiency states, metabolic abnormalities, and collagen vascular diseases (Hohn and Stanton, 1987). Most cardiomyopathies in children are considered primary or idiopathic, in which the cause is unknown and the cardiac dysfunction is not associated with systemic disease. Some of the known causes of secondary cardiomyopathy are anthracycline toxicity (the antineoplastic agents doxorubicin [Adriamycin] and daunomycin), hemochromatosis (from excessive iron storage), Duchenne muscular dystrophy, Kawasaki disease, collagen diseases, and thyroid dysfunction (French, 1981; Tripp, 1984).

Cardiomyopathies can be divided into three broad clinical categories according to the type of abnormal structure and dysfunction present: dilated cardiomyopathy, hypertrophic cardiomyopathy, and restrictive cardiomyopathy (Brandenburg and others, 1981). *Dilated cardiomyopathy* is characterized by ventricular dilatation and greatly decreased contractility resulting in symptoms of CHF. This is the most common type of cardiomyopathy in children. Its cause is often unknown, although carnitine and selenium deficiency, metabolic diseases, drug toxicities, dysrhythmias, and infection causing myocarditis should be considered. The clinical findings are of CHF with tachycardia, dyspnea, hepatosplenomegaly, fatigue, and poor growth. Dysrhythmias may be present and may be more difficult to control with worsening heart failure. Chest radiography demonstrates cardiomegaly and congested lung fields. The echocardiogram demonstrates poor ventricular contractility, dilated left ventricle, and reduced shortening and ejection fraction. Cardiac catheterization with endomyocardial biopsy is usually done to assist with diagnosis and identify a possible infectious cause.

Hypertrophic cardiomyopathy is characterized by an increase in heart muscle mass without an increase in cavity size, usually occurring in the left ventricle and associated with abnormal diastolic filling. A large subgroup of this category is idiopathic hypertrophic subaortic stenosis, or obstructive cardiomyopathy, which has a familial association. Infants of diabetic mothers may have a hypertrophic cardiomyopathy that resolves with time (Lees and King, 1989). Clinical findings may include signs of CHF, especially in infants, and anginal chest pain. Dysrhythmias and syncope are also seen, and sudden death is a possibility. Chest radiography shows a mildly enlarged heart; the ECG demonstrates left ventricular hypertrophy, often with ST-T changes. The echocardiogram is most helpful and demonstrates asymmetric septal hypertrophy and an increase in left ventricular wall thickness, with a small left ventricular cavity.

Restrictive cardiomyopathy, rare in children, describes a restriction to ventricular filling caused by endocardial or myocardial disease or both. It is characterized by diastolic dysfunction and absence of ventricular dilatation or hypertrophy (Hohn and Stanton, 1987). Symptoms are of CHF.

Therapeutic Management

Treatment is directed toward correcting the underlying cause whenever feasible. However, in most affected children this is not possible, and treatment is aimed at managing CHF (see p. 1543) and dysrhythmias (see at right). Digoxin, diuretics, and aggressive use of afterload reduction agents have been found helpful in managing symptoms in those with dilated cardiomyopathy. Digoxin and inotropic agents are usually not helpful in the other forms of cardiomyopathy, since increasing the force of contraction may exacerbate the muscular obstruction and actually impair ventricular ejection. Beta blockers such as propranolol (Inderal) or calcium channel blockers such as verapamil (Calan) have been used to reduce left ventricular outflow obstruction and improve diastolic filling in those with hypertrophic cardiomyopathy.

Careful monitoring and treatment of dysrhythmias are essential. Anticoagulants may be given to reduce the risk of thromboemboli, a complication of the sluggish circulation through the heart. For worsening heart failure and signs of poor perfusion, intravenous inotropic support with dobutamine for several days appears useful in adults, with symptomatic improvement lasting beyond the infusion (Liang and others, 1984), and has been successfully used in children. Severely ill children may benefit from mechanical ventilation, oxygen administration, and intravenous afterload reduction agents such as nitroprusside or amrinone. Heart transplantation may be a treatment option for patients who have worsening symptoms despite maximum medical therapy (see p. 1570).

Nursing Considerations

Because of the poor prognosis in most children with cardiomyopathy, nursing care is consistent with that for any child with a life-threatening disorder (see Chapter 23). One of the most difficult adjustments for the child may be the realization of failing health and the need for restricted activity, especially the normally active youngster with idiopathic hypertrophic subaortic stenosis. The child should be included in decisions regarding activity and allowed to discuss feelings, particularly if the disease follows a progressively fatal course. Once symptoms of CHF or dysrhythmias develop, the same nursing interventions are implemented as discussed on pp. 1548 and 1596. If cardiac transplantation is considered, the needs of the child and family are great in terms of psychological preparation and postoperative care. The nurse plays an important role in assessing the family's understanding of the procedure and long-term consequences. Children of school age and older should be fully informed to give their assent to the procedure (see Informed Consent, Chapter 27).

CARDIAC DYSRHYTHMIAS

Cardiac dysrhythmias, or abnormal heart rhythms, occur less frequently in children than adults; however, they are not rare and the incidence is rising. This increase may be attributed to two major factors. First, the survival rate of children undergoing complex cardiac surgical procedures is higher, and conduction system damage may be a complication. Second, pediatricians are more aware that certain cardiac dysrhythmias in otherwise normal children are important.

Classification

Dysrhythmias can be classified according to various criteria, such as effect on heart rate and rhythm:

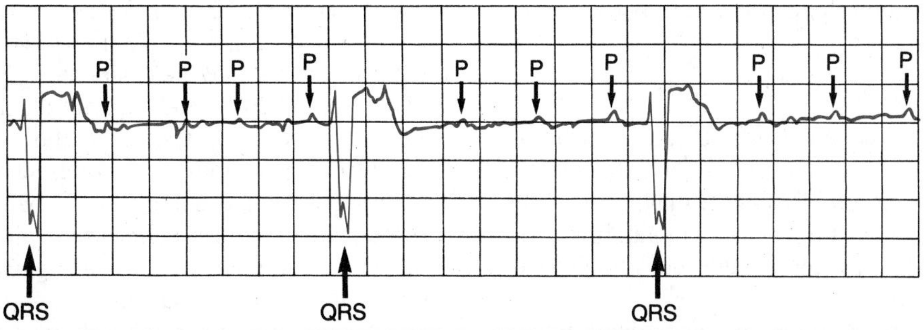

Fig. 34-29. Complete heart block. Note slow rhythm and several P waves not followed by a QRS complex.

Bradydysrhythmias—abnormally slow rate
Tachydysrhythmias—abnormally rapid rate
Conduction disturbances—irregular heart rate

Before classifying an infant or child with an abnormal rate, nurses must be familiar with the standards of normal heart rate for the particular age-group (see inside front cover). Heart rate variations considered normal for a particular child can vary tremendously.

Bradydysrhythmias. The most common bradydysrhythmia in children is *complete atrioventricular block (A-V block),* also referred to as complete heart block (Fig. 34-29). This can be either congenital or acquired, as seen in postoperative patients following surgery in the area of the A-V valves and ventricular septum.

Sinus bradycardia in children can be due to the influence of the autonomic nervous system, as with hypervagal tone, or in response to hypoxia and hypotension. Once the infant receives adequate oxygenation and any acidosis is eliminated, the heart rate will often return to baseline. Sinus bradycardias are also known to develop after atrial inversion (baffle) procedures (Mustard or Senning).

Not all bradycardias originate in the sinus node. *Junctional* or *nodal rhythms* are common in the postoperative patient. The impulse for these rhythms originates further down the conduction system, in the A-V node. Identification is marked by absence of P waves on the ECG, and often little change occurs in the heart rate or cardiac output. If there is no significant compromise to the patient's cardiac status, no treatment is necessary.

Tachydysrhythmias. Sinus tachycardia secondary to fever, anxiety, pain, anemia, dehydration, or any other etiologic factor requiring increased cardiac output should be ruled out first before diagnosing an increased heart rate as pathologic. *Supraventricular tachycardia* (SVT) is one of the most common dysrhythmias found in children and refers to a rapid regular heart rate of 200 to 300 beats/minute (Fig. 34-30). The onset of SVT is often sudden, and the duration is variable. Infants and young children with SVT may be unable to communicate the rapid heart rate, and the clinical course can progress to CHF. Important signs in the infant and young child are poor feeding, extreme irritability, and pallor.

Junctional ectopic tachycardia is a tachydysrhythmia that

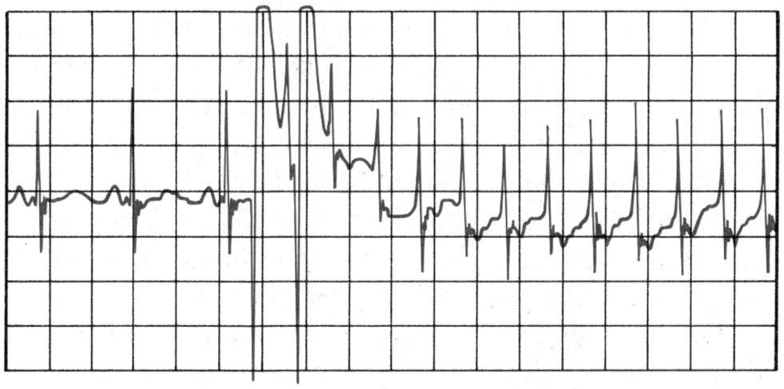

Fig. 34-30. Supraventricular tachycardia (SVT). Note normal sinus rhythm (three PQRST complexes) on the left and the abrupt onset of a very fast rhythm (SVT) on the right.

can result in significant compromise in the pediatric patient. Often the ventricular rate will exceed 250 beats/minute. The onset is characterized by a progressive increase in heart rate, and the duration can range from hours to several days.

Wolff-Parkinson-White syndrome is the result of an accessory pathway that manifests as a tachydysrhythmia. The refractory period in the accessory pathway is shorter than that in the normal conduction pathway. The electrical impulse is diverted to the accessory pathway, resulting in a rapid reentry SVT.

Wide-complex tachycardias are seldom found in the pediatric population but can be potentially serious. The site of origin either can be supraventricular, with ventricular aberration below the bundle of His, or can be a true ventricular tachycardia. Treatment and outcome depend on which type of complex is diagnosed. The presence of either, however, requires immediate attention.

Conduction disturbances. Most rhythm disturbances are seen postoperatively in the child undergoing cardiac surgery and are of little significance. A-V blocks are most often related to edema around the conduction system and resolve without treatment. Temporary epicardial wires are placed in most patients at surgery; if a rhythm disturbance occurs, temporary pacing can be employed. Just before discharge, the surgeon removes the wires by pulling slowly and deliberately down on them from the site of insertion.

Premature contractions can occur from an atrial, ventricular, or junctional focus. Their significance depends on the degree of compromise and the presence or absence of underlying CHD.

Diagnostic Evaluation

Several advances in the diagnosis of cardiac dysrhythmias have greatly improved the understanding and treatment of these conditions in children. The basic diagnostic procedure is the ECG, including 24-hour Holter monitoring. However, more definitive procedures include both noninvasive and invasive techniques.

An invasive procedure performed in the cardiac catheterization room allows for precise identification of the conduction disturbance and immediate investigation of drugs that are effective in halting the dysrhythmia. Electrode catheters are introduced transvenously and directed toward the right side of the heart. The heart is then selectively stimulated to induce dysrhythmias. Once a dysrhythmia occurs, different antidysrhythmic drugs are administered intravenously to monitor which pharmacologic agent is most successful in terminating the dysrhythmia. Patients and families undergoing this procedure are prepared in the same manner as any patient undergoing cardiac catheterization (see p. 1538).

Another procedure that may be employed is *transesophageal recording.* An electrode catheter is passed to the lower esophagus and, when in position at a point proximal to the heart, is used to stimulate and record dysrhythmias.

Therapeutic Management

Treatment of dysrhythmias depends on the cause and severity. Whenever possible, the underlying cause is treated. However, in some cases it is necessary to use antidysrhythmic drugs, with the goal being control, not cure. A permanent pacemaker may be needed in some children, such as those with postsurgical A-V block or, less frequently, congenital A-V block. The pacemaker takes over or assists in the conduction function of the heart. The surgical implantation of a pacemaker is usually a low-risk procedure. Once the wire has been introduced, a small incision is made and a pocket formed under the muscle to house and protect the generator. Continuous ECG monitoring is necessary during the recovery phase to assess pacemaker function. The nurse should be aware of the programmed rate and expected individual generator variations. A baseline ECG strip should be documented for future comparison.

Pacemaker functions have become dramatically more sophisticated; the capabilities are no longer limited to fixed rates. Today generators can control heart rate according to activity, cardiac output, and respirations. In addition, some models can be programmed for overdrive pacing or cardioversion when the generator detects accelerated rates beyond established normal values.

The treatment of SVT depends on the degree of compromise imposed by the dysrhythmia. In some instances, vagal maneuvers, such as applying ice to the face, massaging the carotid artery (on *one* side of the neck only), or having an older child perform a Valsalva maneuver (e.g., exhaling against a closed glottis, blowing on the thumb as if it were a trumpet for 30 to 60 seconds), have reversed the SVT. If the infant or child is minimally symptomatic, pharmacologic measures may be adequate. Digitalization of the patient should be undertaken, with careful monitoring of vital signs and patient response to the intervention. If cardiac output is significantly compromised or signs of CHF exist, pharmacologic measures will not be adequate. Esophageal overdrive pacing or synchronized cardioversion can be employed in the intensive care setting. *Overdrive pacing* is accomplished through placement of a protected lead into the esophagus, behind the left atrium of the heart. The lead is then attached to a stimulator capable of pacing at very rapid rates to interrupt the tachydysrhythmia. *Cardioversion* is the timed delivery of a preset amount of energy in an attempt to reestablish an organized rhythm. Cardioversion is contraindicated when recent digitalization has occurred, since it may result in ventricular fibrillation.

Junctional ectopic tachycardia is rarely responsive to conservative therapy. Initial management should be directed toward establishing A-V synchrony through atrial pacing. If cardiac output of the postoperative patient is compromised, core cooling to 35° C (95° F) using a cooling blanket and the initiation of a procainamide drip is the recommended therapy (Sholler and others, 1988).

Wolff-Parkinson-White syndrome requires careful supervision by a pediatric cardiologist. The majority of these patients can be managed with digoxin; however, there have been reports of shortened refractory times and sudden death from ventricular fibrillation (Gillette, 1981). For patients who are unresponsive to pharmacologic management and have frequent symptomatic episodes, isolation and surgical ablation of the accessory pathway may be indicated.

Nursing Considerations

An initial nursing responsibility is recognition of an abnormal heartbeat, either in rate or rhythm. When a dysrhythmia is suspected, the apical rate is counted for 1 full minute and compared with the radial rate. Consistently high or low heart rates should be regarded as suspicious. Accurate nursing assessment, especially in regard to cardiac output, is essential.

The onset and diagnosis of a cardiac dysrhythmia are frightening experiences for parents and the older child. Sometimes the dysrhythmia rapidly leads to heart failure and an emergency medical crisis. In this situation parents need much support to express their feelings, understand the diagnosis, and comply with home therapy, such as daily drug administration. In working with the family, the nurse must not forget the impact of the diagnosis of a heart problem. As one mother stated, "The heart is the body"; there is acute awareness of the necessity of the heart as a vital organ. Often an unspoken fear of potential death exists even if the dysrhythmia is benign, and repeated explanations are needed to allay the anxiety. In dealing with parents of an infant diagnosed with a dysrhythmia, the nurse must be sensitive to the care needed by parents facing the birth of a child with a congenital anomaly (see Chapter 11).

A primary focus of nursing care is education of the family regarding the specific treatment of the dysrhythmia. Following the first episode of SVT, parents should be taught to take a pulse for 1 full minute. If medication is prescribed, instructions regarding accurate dosage and the importance of administering the correct dose at specified intervals are stressed.

When a pacemaker is implanted, the education of the parents and child includes an explanation of the device, a description of the component parts, the surgical procedure, and discharge teaching. The pacemaker is comprised of two basic parts, the pulse generator and the lead. The pulse generator is composed of the battery and the electronic circuitry. The function is to produce the electrical impulse sent to the heart and to receive and respond to signals produced by the heart. The lead is an insulated, flexible wire that conducts the electrical impulse from the pulse generator to the heart. Two types of leads are available, transvenous and epicardial. The child's size and the heart's structure determine which lead is more appropriate. *Transvenous leads* are inserted into a large vein, often the subclavian, and advanced into the right side of the heart. Placement is secured by engaging a small corkscrew or fish-hook attachment at the end of the lead into the endocardium. *Epicardial leads* are directly attached to the epicardial layer of the heart. Parents should be aware of which type of lead their child has in place.

Discharge teaching includes information about the signs and symptoms of infection, general wound care, and any specific limitations to activity. Instructions for telephone transmission of ECG readings are also given. Telephone transmission can be used to transmit ECG strips and also to monitor battery life and pacemaker function. Children with pacemakers should wear a medical alert device, and their parents should have a pacer identification card with specific pacer data in case of an emergency.

In life-threatening dysrhythmias, the family needs support and concise information regarding the medical interventions. Most important, families need to be assured that effective pain management will be employed during cardioversion. Following the child's conversion to normal rhythm, the family may need to learn cardiopulmonary resuscitation.*

*Home care instructions are available in Wong, D.L., and Whaley, L.F.: Clinical manual of pediatric nursing, ed. 3, St. Louis, 1990, Mosby–Year Book, Inc.

KEY POINTS

- Congenital heart disease is the most common form of cardiac disease in children.
- Major categories to investigate in the cardiac history are poor weight gain, poor feeding habits, and fatigue during feeding; frequent respiratory infections and difficulties; and evidence of exercise intolerance.
- The most common tests used in assessing cardiac function are radiography, electrocardiography, echocardiography, and cardiac catheterization.
- Cardiac catheterization procedures can be divided into two groups: (1) diagnostic procedures, including angiography, that measure pressures and saturations to establish cardiac diagnosis and (2) interventional procedures, in which catheters or balloon devices are used to correct cardiac defects.
- Cardiac catheterization provides important information about oxygen saturation of blood within the chambers and great vessels, pressure changes, changes in cardiac output or stroke volume, and anatomic abnormalities.
- Several prenatal factors may predispose children to congenital heart disease: maternal rubella during pregnancy, maternal alcoholism, maternal age above 40 years, and maternal insulin-dependent diabetes.
- Congenital heart defects can be divided into four main groups, as determined by hemodynamic patterns: (1) defects that result in increased pulmonary blood flow, (2) obstructive defects, (3) defects that result in decreased pulmonary blood flow, and (4) mixed defects.
- Cardiac output is determined by the interaction of several factors: preload, afterload, contractility, and heart rate.
- Clinical consequences of congenital heart defects include congestive heart failure (CHF) and hypoxemia. A child can have both hypoxemia and CHF although usually they occur independently.
- Nursing measures in the care of a child with CHF are to assist in improving cardiac function, decrease cardiac demands, reduce respiratory distress, maintain nutritional status, promote fluid loss, and provide family support.
- Clinical manifestations of hypoxemia are cyanosis, polycythemia, clubbing, and delayed growth and development. The child is at increased risk for hypercyanotic spells, cerebrovascular accidents, brain abscess, and bacterial endocarditis.
- Heart transplantation has been extended to infants and children with cardiomyopathy and complex congenital heart defects involving ventricular dysfunction, such as hypoplastic left heart syndrome.
- Caring for the child with congenital heart disease (CHD) and the family requires helping them adjust to the disorder and cope with the effects of the defect and fostering growth-promoting family relationships.
- Preoperative care of the child with a congenital defect involves introducing the child and family to the hospital and preparing them for preoperative and postoperative procedures.
- Providing postoperative care includes observing vital signs and arterial/venous pressures, maintaining respiratory status, allowing maximum rest, providing comfort, monitoring fluids, planning for progressive activities, giving emotional support, observing for complications of surgery, and planning for discharge and home care.
- Acquired cardiovascular disorders include bacterial endocarditis, rheumatic fever, systemic hypertension, cardiac dysrhythmias, Kawasaki disease, cardiomyopathy, and hyperlipidemia.

- Clinical manifestations of CHF are impaired myocardial function (tachyardia, cardiomegaly), pulmonary congestion (dyspnea, tachypnea, orthopnea, cyanosis), and systemic congestion (hepatosplenomegaly, edema, distended veins).
- Prevention of bacterial endocarditis in certain children with CHD involves administration of prophylactic antibiotics when specific procedures are performed.
- Acute rheumatic fever is a systemic inflammatory disease that can damage the cardiac valves and is associated with previous group A streptococcal infection. Its incidence has increased in some areas of the United States.
- Kawasaki disease is an extensive inflammation of small vessels and capillaries that may progress to involve the coronary arteries, causing aneurysm formation. The administration of gamma globulin is an important aspect of treatment.
- Education of the child and family with hypertension focuses on drug therapy, diet control, and appropriate exercise.
- Cholesterol screening in children is controversial; currently, children with known risk factors for hyperlipidemia are screened and treated as needed. The influence of childhood cholesterol levels on later development of coronary artery disease is under investigation.
- Cardiomyopathy, or abnormality of the myocardium, is a serious, often fatal, disorder. Heart transplantation may offer more favorable options for some children than drug or other regimens.
- Common dysrhythmias in children include slow rhythms (bradycardias, heart block) and fast rhythms (sinus tachycardia, supraventricular tachycardia).

REFERENCES

Adams, F.H., Emmanouilides, G.C., and Riemenschneider, T.A., editors: Moss' heart disease in infants, children, and adolescents, ed. 4, Baltimore, 1989, Williams & Wilkins.

Agamalian, B.: Pediatric cardiac catheterization, J. Pediatr. Nurs. 1(2):73-79, 1986.

Aisenberg, R.B., and others: Developmental delay in infants with congenital heart disease, Pediatr. Cardiol. 3(2):133-137, 1982.

American Academy of Pediatrics: Report of the Second Task Force on Blood Pressure Control in Children—1987, Pediatrics 79(1):1-25, 1987.

American Academy of Pediatrics, Committee on Nutrition: Indications for cholesterol testing in children, Pediatrics 83(1):141-142, 1989.

Anderson, D.J., and Thibault, J.: Nursing management of the pediatric patient with Kawasaki's disease, Issues Compr. Pediatr. Nurs. 5(1):1-10, 1981.

Anthony, C., and Thibodeau, G.: Textbook of anatomy and physiology, ed. 11, St. Louis, 1983, Mosby–Year Book, Inc.

Bailey, L.L., and Gundry, S.R.: Hypoplastic left heart syndrome, Pediatr. Clin. North Am. 37(1):137-149, 1990.

Bailey, L., and others: Method of heart transplantation for treatment of hypoplastic left heart syndrome, J. Thorac. Cardiovasc. Surg. 92:1-5, 1986.

Berne, R.M., and Levy, M.N.: Cardiovascular physiology, ed. 5, St. Louis, 1986, Mosby–Year Book, Inc.

Bland, E.F.: The way it was, Circulation 76:1190-1195, 1987.

Brandenburg, R.O., and others: Report of the WHO/ISLF Task Force on Definition and Classification of Cardiomyopathies, Circulation 64(2):437-438, 1981.

Castaneda, A.R.: Correction of transposition: arterial switch procedure. In Grillo, H., editor: Current therapy in cardiothoracic surgery, Toronto, 1989, B.C. Decker, Inc.

Consensus conference: Lowering blood cholesterol to prevent heart disease, JAMA 253:2080-2086, 1985.

Cranwell, P.D.: Blood pressure teaching and screening programs for school children in grades 5-8, Home Healthcare Nurse 2(3):42-46, 1984.

Dajani, A.S., and others: Prevention of bacterial endocarditis: recommendations by the American Heart Association, JAMA 264(22): 2919-2922, 1990.

de Leval, M.R., and others: Total cavopulmonary connection: a logical alternative to atriopulmonary connection for complex Fontan operations, J. Thorac. Cardiovasc. Surg. 96:682-695, 1988.

Dennison, B.A., and others: Serum total cholesterol screening for the detection of elevated low-density lipoprotein in children and adolescents: the Bogalusa heart study, Pediatrics 85(4):472-479, 1990.

Driscoll, D.J.: Evaluation of the cyanotic newborn, Pediatr. Clin. North Am. 37(1):1-23, 1990.

Feldman, W.: Routine cholesterol surveillance in childhood (letter), Pediatrics 86(1):150-151, 1990.

Few, B.J.: Digoxin immune Fab, MCN 12(6):431, 1987.

Finberg, L.: Pediatrics, JAMA 263(19):2672-2673, 1990.

Freed, M.D.: Recreational and sports recommendations for the child with heart disease, Pediatr. Clin. North Am. 31(6):1307-1320, 1984.

French, J.W.: Diseases of the myocardium. In Kelley, V.C., editor: Practice of pediatrics, Philadelphia, 1981, Harper & Row, Publishers, Inc.

Fyler, D.F.: Rheumatic fever. In Fyler, D.F., editor: Nadas' pediatric cardiology, Philadelphia, 1990, Hanley & Belfus, Inc.

Garcia, R.E., and Moodle, D.S.: Routine cholesterol surveillance in childhood, Pediatrics 84(5):751-755, 1989.

Gersony, W.M.: Patent ductus arteriosus in the neonate, Pediatr. Clin. North Am. 33(3):545-560, 1986.

Gillette, P.C.: Cardiac dysrhythmias in infants and children, Cardiovasc. Clin. 11(2):79-95, 1981.

Griffin, T., and others: Family history evaluation as a predictive screen for childhood hypercholesterolemia, Pediatrics 84(2):365-373, 1989.

Hastreiter, A.R., and others: Maintenance digoxin dosage and steady-state plasma concentration in infants and children, J. Pediatr. 107(1):140-146, 1985.

Hazinski, M.F.: Nursing care of the critically ill child, St. Louis, 1984, Mosby–Year Book, Inc.

Hoffman, J.I.: Congenital heart disease: incidence and inheritance, Pediatr. Clin. North Am. 37(1):31, 1990.

Hohn, A.R., and Stanton, R.E.: Myocarditis in children, Pediatr. Rev. 9(3):83-88, 1987.

A Joint Statement for Physicians by the Committee on Atherosclerosis and Hypertension in Childhood, Council on Cardiovascular Disease in the Young and the Nutrition Committee, American Heart Association: Diagnosis and treatment of primary hyperlipidemia in childhood, Circulation 74(5):1181A-1188A, 1986.

Jonas, R.A., and Lang, P.: Open repair of cardiac defects in neonates and young infants, Clin. Perinatol. 15(3):659-680, 1988.

Jonas, R., and others: Normothermic caval inflow occlusion, J. Thorac. Cardiovasc. Surg. 89(5):780-786, 1985.

Kaden, G.G., and others: Physician-patient communication: understanding congenital heart disease, Am. J. Dis. Child. 139(10):995-999, 1985.

Kaplan, E.L.: The startling comeback of rheumatic fever, Contemp. Pediatr. 4(11):20-34, 1987.

Kaplan, E.L.: Myocarditis, pericarditis, and infective endocarditis. In Moeller, J.H., and Neal, W.A., editors: Fetal, neonatal, and infant cardiac disease, Norwalk, CT, 1990, Appleton & Lange.

Kaplan, E.L., and Shulman, S.T.: Infective endocarditis. In Adams, F.H., Emmanouilides, G.C., and Riemenschneider, T.A., editors: Moss' heart disease in infants, children, and adolescents, ed. 4, Baltimore, 1989, Williams & Wilkins.

Kashani, I.A.: Acute rheumatic fever: a review of pathogenesis, diagnosis, and a modified approach to Jones criteria and management, Paediatrician 10:158-176, 1981.

Kato, H., Ichinose, E., and Kawasaki, T.: Myocardial infarction in Kawasaki disease: clinical analyses in 195 cases, J. Pediatr. 108(6):923-927, 1986.

Koren, G., and others: Kawasaki disease: review of risk factors for coronary aneurysms, J. Pediatr. 108(3):388-392, 1986.

Kriett, J.M., and Kaye, M.P.: The registry of the International Society for Heart Transplantation: seventh official report—1990, J. Heart Transplant. 9(4):323-330, 1990.

LaRosa, J.C., and others: The cholesterol facts: a joint statement by the American Heart Association and the National Heart, Lung, and Blood Institute, Circulation 81(5):1721-1733, 1990.

Lees, M.H., and King, D.H.: Heart disease in the newborn. In Adams, F.H., Emmanouilides, G.C., and Riemenschneider, T.A., editors: Moss' heart disease in infants, children, and adolescents, ed. 4, Baltimore, 1989, Williams & Wilkins.

Liang, C.S., and others: Sustained improvement of cardiac function in patients with congestive heart failure after short term infusion of dobutamine, Circulation 69(1):113-119, 1984.

Lock, J.E., Keane, J.F., and Fellows, K.E.: Diagnostic and interventional catheterization in congenital heart disease, Boston, 1987, Martinus Nijhoff Publishing.

Loggie, J.M.H., and others: Juvenile hypertension: highlights of a workshop, J. Pediatr. 104(5):657-663, 1984.

Lowrey, G.: Growth and development of children, ed. 8, St. Louis, 1986, Mosby–Year Book, Inc.

Maguire, D.P., and Maloney, P.: A comparison of fentanyl and morphine use in neonates, Neonatal Network 7(1):27-35, 1988.

Martin, G.R., Perry, L.W., and Ferencz, C.: Increased prevalence of ventricular septal defect: epidemic or improved diagnosis, Pediatrics 83(2):200-203, 1989.

McEnhill, M., and Vitale, K.: Kawasaki disease: new challenges in care, MCN 14:406-410, 1989.

Mills, L.J., and others: Cardiothoracic surgery: perioperative principles. In Levin, D.L., Morriss, F.C., and Moore, G.C., editors: A practical guide to pediatric intensive care, ed. 2, St. Louis, 1984, Mosby–Year Book, Inc.

Moller, J.H., and Neal, W.A., editors: Fetal, neonatal, and infant cardiac disease, Norwalk, CT, 1990, Appleton & Lange.

Naylor, D., Coates, T.J., and Kan, J.: Reducing distress in pediatric cardiac catheterization, Am. J. Dis. Child. 138(8):726-729, 1984.

Newburger, J.: Management of dyslipidemia in childhood and adolescence. In Fyler, D.F., editor: Nadas' pediatric cardiology, Philadelphia, 1990, Hanley & Belfus, Inc.

Newburger, J.W., and Burns, J.C.: Kawasaki syndrome, Cardiol. Clin. 7(2):453-465, 1989.

Newburger, J.W., and others: Cognitive function and age at repair of transposition of great arteries in children, N. Engl. J. Med. 310:1495-1499, 1984.

Newburger, J.W., and others: The treatment of Kawasaki syndrome with intravenous gamma globulin, N. Engl. J. Med. 315:341-347, 1986.

Newburger, J.W., and others: Preliminary results of multicenter trial on IVGG treatment of Kawasaki disease with single-infusion vs. 4-infusion regimen, Pediatr. Res. 27(4, pt. 2):A119, 1990.

Noonan, J.A.: Association of congenital heart disease with syndromes or other defects, Pediatr. Clin. North Am. 25(4):797-816, 1978.

Norton, S.J.: Aftereffects of morphine and fentanyl analgesia: a retrospective study, Neonatal Network 7(3):25-28, 1988.

Norwood, W.I.: Hypoplastic left heart syndrome, Cardiol. Clin. 7(2):377-385, 1989.

O'Dougherty, M., and others: Later competence and adaptation in infants who survive severe heart defects, Child Dev. 54:1129-1142, 1983.

Opie, L.H., editor: Drugs for the heart, Philadelphia, 1987, W.B. Saunders Co.

Pacifico, A.D.: Surgical treatment of complex atrioventricular septal defects, Cardiol. Clin. 7(2):399-410, 1989.

Parness, I.A., and Nadas, A.S.: Cardiac transplantation in children, Pediatr. Rev. 10(4):111-117, 1988.

Perry, S.B., and others: Interventional catheterization of left heart lesions, including aortic and mitral valve stenosis and coarctation of the aorta, Cardiol. Clin. 7(2):341-349, 1989.

Radtke, W., and Lock, J.E.: Balloon dilation, Pediatr. Clin. North Am. 37(1):193-214, 1990.

Rauch, A.M.: Kawaski syndrome: critical review of U.S. epidemiology, Prog. Clin. Biol. Res. 250:33-44, 1987.

Reif, K.: A heart makes you live, Am. J. Nurs. 72(6):1085, 1972.

Resnicow, K., Morley-Kotchen, J., and Wynder, E.: Plasma cholesterol levels of 6585 children in the United States: results of the Know Your Body screening in five states, Pediatrics 84(6):969-976, 1989.

Roberts, P.J.: Caring for patients undergoing therapeutic cardiac catheterization, Crit. Care Nurs. Clin. North Am. 1(2):275-288, 1989.

Rocchini, A.P.: Childhood hypertension: etiology, diagnosis, and treatment, Pediatr. Clin. North Am. 31(6):1259-1273, 1984.

Rocchini, A.P., and others: Balloon angioplasty in the treatment of pulmonary valve stenosis and coarctation, Tex. Heart Inst. J. 13(3):377-385, 1986.

Rose, V., and others: A possible increase in the incidence of congenital heart defects among the offspring of affected parents, J. Am. Coll. Cardiol. 6:376-382, 1985.

Rosen, K.R., and Rosen, D.A.: Caudal epidural morphine for control of pain following open heart surgery in children, Anesthesiology 70(3):418-421, 1989.

Rosenthal, A.: Care of the postoperative child and adolescent with congenital heart disease. In Barness, L.A., editor: Advances in pediatrics, vol. 30, St. Louis, 1983, Mosby–Year Book, Inc.

Rosenthal, A.: How to distinguish between innocent and pathologic murmurs in childhood, Pediatr. Clin. North Am. 31(6):1229-1240, 1984.

Rosenthal, A., and Dick, M.: Tricuspid atresia. In Adams, F.H., Emmanouilides, G.C., and Riemenschneider, T.A., editors: Moss' heart disease in infants, children, and adolescents, ed. 4, Baltimore, 1989, Williams & Wilkins.

Rotondi, P., editor: Neonatal and pediatric cardiovascular nursing, Crit. Care Nurs. Clin. North Am. 1(2):195-305, 1989.

Rushton, C.H.: Preparing children and families for cardiac surgery: nursing interventions, Issues Compr. Pediatr. Nurs. 6:235-248, 1983.

Sade, R.M., and Fyfe, D.A.: Tricuspid atresia: current concepts in diagnosis and treatment, Pediatr. Clin. North Am. 37(1):151, 1990.

Sholler, G.F., and others: Evaluation of a staged treatment protocol for postoperative rapid junctional ectopic tachycardia (abstract), Circulation 78(4):597, 1988.

Snider, A.R.: Use and abuse of echocardiogram, Pediatr. Clin. North Am. 31(6):1345-1366, 1984.

Starnes, V.A., and others: Cardiac transplantation in children and adolescents, Circulation 76(suppl. 5):43-47, 1987.

Stary, H.C.: Evolution and progression of atherosclerosis in the coronary arteries of children and adults. In Bates, S.R., and Gangloff, E.C., editors: Atherogenesis and aging, New York, 1987, Springer-Verlag, New York, Inc.

Strong, W.B., and Dennison, B.A.: Pediatric preventive cardiology: atherosclerosis and coronary heart disease, Pediatr. Rev. 9(10):303-314, 1988.

Takahashi, M., and others: Regression of coronary aneurysms in patients with Kawasaki syndrome, Circulation 75:387-394, 1987.

Trento, A., and others: Lessons learned in pediatric heart transplantation, Ann. Thorac. Surg. 48(4):617-623, 1989.

Tripp, M.E.: Congestive cardiomyopathy of childhood, Adv. Pediatr. 31:179-206, 1984.
van Breda, A.: Postoperative care of infants and children who require cardiac surgery, Heart Lung 14(3):205-208, 1985.
Whittemore, R., Hobbins, J.C., and Engle, M.A.: Pregnancy and its outcome in women with and without surgical treatment of congenital heart disease, Am. J. Cardiol. 50(3):641-651, 1982.
Yeager, S.B., and others: Primary surgical closure of VSDs in the first year of life, J. Am. Coll. Cardiol. 3(5):1269-1276, 1984.
Zabriskie, J.B.: Rheumatic fever: a streptococcal induced autoimmune disease? Pediatr. Ann. 11:383-396, 1985.
Ziemer, G., and others: Surgery for coarctation of the aorta in the neonate, Circulation 74(3, suppl. 1):25-31, 1986.
Zuberbuhler, J.R., Fricker, F.J., and Griffith, B.P.: Cardiac transplantation in children, Cardiol. Clin. 7(2):411-418, 1989.

BIBLIOGRAPHY

Diagnostic Procedures

Benson, L.N., and Freedom, R.M.: Interventional cardiac catheterization, Curr. Opin. Pediatr. 1(1):106-109, 1989.
Caire, J.B., and Erickson, S.: Reducing distress in pediatric patients undergoing cardiac catheterization, Child. Health Care 14(3):146-152, 1986.
Elixson, E.M.: Hemodynamic monitoring modalities in pediatric cardiac surgical patients, Crit. Care Nurs. Clin. North Am. 1(2):263-274, 1989.
Fahey, V.A., and Finkelmeier, B.A.: Iatrogenic arterial injuries, Am. J. Nurs. 84(4):448-451, 1984.
Glasier, C.M., and others: Extracardiac chest ultrasonography in infants and children: radiographic and clinical implications, J. Pediatr. 114(4, pt. 1):540-544, 1989.
Haughey, C.W.: Preparing your patient for echocardioagraphy, Nursing '84 14(5):68-71, 1984.
Laird, W.P.: Echocardiography. In Levin, D.L., Moriss, F.C., and Moore, G.C., editors: A practical guide to pediatric intensive care, ed. 2, St. Louis, 1984, Mosby–Year Book, Inc.
Malinowski, L.M., and Doyle, J.E.: Cardiac catheterization of the neonate, Am. J. Nurs. 85(1):60-62, 1985.
McConnell, J.R., and others: Magnetic resonance imaging of the brain in infants and children before and after cardiac surgery, Am. J. Dis. Child. 144(3):374-378, 1990.
Reidy, S.J., O'Hara, P.A., and O'Brien, P.: Streptokinase use in children undergoing cardiac catheterization, J. Cardiovasc. Nurs. 4(1):46-56, 1989.
Sherman, F.S., and Sahn, D.J.: Pediatric doppler echocardiography 1987: major advances in technology, J. Pediatr. 110(3):333-342, 1987.
Smith, P.A.: Current diagnostic and therapeutic catheterization techniques, Crit. Care Q. 9(2):24-39, 1986.
Sondheimer, H.M.: Cardiac catheterization—a new role in the 90s, Contemp. Pediatr. 7(3):91-106, 1990.
Sumner, S.M., and Grau, P.A.: Guidelines for running a 12-lead E.K.G., Nursing '85 15(12):30-33, 1985.
Tonkin, I.L., Stapleton, F.B., and Shane, R.: Digital subtraction angiography in the evaluation of renal vascular hypertension in children, Pediatrics 81(1):150-158, 1988.
Williams, R.G.: Echocardiography in the neonate and young infant, J. Am. Coll. Cardiol. 5:30S-36S, 1985.
Zellers, T., and Gutgesell, H.P.: Noninvasive estimation of pulmonary artery pressure, J. Pediatr. 114(5):735-741, 1989.

Congestive Heart Failure

Dahlmann, A.R.: Captopril, Neonatal Network 7(5):41-43, 1989.
Faxon, D.P.: ACE inhibition for the failing heart: experience, Am. Heart J. 115(5):1085-1093, 1988.
Friedman, W.F., and George, B.L.: New concepts and drugs in the treatment of congestive heart failure, Pediatr. Clin. North Am. 31(6):1197-1227, 1984.
Friedman, W.F., and George, B.L.: Treatment of congestive heart failure by altering loading conditions of the heart, J. Pediatr. 106(5):697-706, 1985.
Koren, G.: Interaction between digoxin and commonly coadministered drugs in children, Pediatrics 75(6):1032-1037, 1985.
Linday, L., and others: Digoxin inactivation by the gut flora in infancy and childhood, Pediatrics 79(4):544-548, 1987.
Norsen, L.H., and Fox, G.B.: Understanding cardiac output—and the drugs that affect it, Nursing '85 15(4):34-41, 1985.
Shaddy, R.E., Teitel, D.F., and Brett, C.: Short-term hemodynamic effects of captopril in infants with congestive heart failure, Am. J. Dis. Child. 142:100-105, 1988.
Zalzstein, E., and others: Once-daily versus twice-daily dosing of digoxin in the pediatric age group, J. Pediatr. 116(1):137-139, 1990.

Congenital Heart Disease

Arfken, C.L., and others: Mitral valve prolapse: associations with symptoms and anxiety, Pediatrics 85(3):311-315, 1990.
Beekman, R.H., Rocchini, A.P., and Rosenthal, A.: Therapeutic cardiac catheterization for pulmonary valve and pulmonary artery stenosis, Cardiol. Clin. 7(2):331-340, 1989.
Benson, D.W.: Changing profile of congenital heart disease, Pediatrics 83(5):790-791, 1989.
Carey, B.E.: Prostaglandin E1 treatment for neonatal heart defects, Dimens. Crit. Care Nurs. 1(5):275-283, 1982.
Castaneda, A.R., and others: Transposition of the great arteries: the arterial switch operation, Cardiol. Clin. 7(2):369-376, 1989.
Clark, E.B.: Cardiac embryology: its relevance to congenital heart disease, Am. J. Dis. Child. 140(1):41-44, 1986.
Cleary, J.D.: Two inotropic agents: dopamine and dobutamine, Pediatr. Nurs 14(5):414, 1988.
Cloutier, J., and Measel, C.P.: Home care for the infant with congenital heart disease, Am. J. Nurs. 82(1):100-103, 1982.
Cohen, M.A.: The use of prostaglandins and prostaglandin inhibitors in critically ill neonates, MCN 8:194-199, 1983.
Deanfield, J.E.: Transposition of the great arteries: to switch or not to switch? Curr. Opin. Pediatr. 1(1):85-89, 1989.
Deleon, S.Y., and others: Fontan type operation for complex lesions, J. Thorac. Cardiovasc. Surg. 92:1029, 1986.
Elixson, E.M., editor: Cardiovascular surgery update: pediatrics, Crit. Care Q. 9(2):entire issue, 1986.
Ferencz, C., and others: Congenital cardiovascular malformations associated with chromosome abnormalities: an epidemiologic study, J. Pediatr. 114(1):79-85, 1989.
Ferry, P.C.: Neurologic sequelae of open-heart surgery in children, Am. J. Dis. Child. 144(3):369-373, 1990.
Freed, M.D., and others: Prostaglandin E1 in infants with ductus arteriosus–dependent congenital heart disease, Circulation 64(5):899-904, 1981.
Freedom, R.M.: The hypoplastic left heart syndrome: evolving trends in therapy and present concerns, Curr. Opin. Pediatr. 1(1):90-93, 1989.
Gersony, W.M., and others: Effects of indomethacin in premature infants with patent ductus arteriosus: results of a national collaborative study, J. Pediatr. 102(6):895-905, 1983.
Givens, L., and Ricks, J.: Assessment of clinical manifestations of cyanotic and acyanotic heart disease in infants and children, Heart Lung 14(3):200-204, 1985.
Harlan, J.L., and others: Coarctation of the aorta in infants, J. Thorac. Cardiovasc. Surg. 88:1012-1019, 1984.
Hedenkamp, E.A.: Hypoplastic left heart syndrome—options for the infant and family, Prog. Cardiovasc. Nurs. 2(3):80-85, 1987.
Hellenbrand, W.E., and Mullins, C.E.: Catheter closure of congenital cardiac defects, Cardiol. Clin. 7(2):351-368, 1989.

Hudgins, R.J., and others: Natural history of fetal ventriculomegaly, Pediatrics 82(5):692-697, 1988.

Kaden, G.G., and others: Physician-patient communication: understanding congenital heart disease, Am. J. Dis. Child. 139(10):995-999, 1985.

Kern, L.S., and O'Brien, P.: The Fontan procedure, Heart Lung 14(5):457-469, 1985.

Kirklin, J., and Barret-Boyes, B.: Cardiac surgery, New York, 1986, John Wiley & Sons, Inc.

Latson, L.A., and others: Transcatheter closure of patent ductus arteriosus in pediatric patients, J. Pediatr. 115(4):549-553, 1989.

Lewis, A.B., and others: Side effects of therapy with prostaglandin E1 in infants with critical congenital heart disease, Circulation 64(5):893-898, 1981.

Lin, A., and Garver, K.: Genetic counseling for congenital heart defects, J. Pediatr. 113(6):1105-1108, 1988.

Mair, D.D.: The Fontan procedure: the first 20 years, Curr. Opin. Pediatr. 1(1):94-99, 1989.

Mayer, J.E., Jr., and others: Extending the limits for modified Fontan procedures, J. Thorac. Cardiovasc. Surg. 92:1021-1028, 1986.

Natowics, M., and others: Genetic disorders and major extracardiac anomalies associated with the hypoplastic left heart syndrome, Pediatrics 82(5):698-706, 1988.

Nora, J.J.: Chance and ventricular septal defect (letter), Pediatrics 77(6):930-931, 1986.

Page, G.G.: Patent ductus arteriosus in the premature neonate, Heart Lung 14(2):156-163, 1985.

Page, G.G.: Tetralogy of Fallot, Heart Lung 15:390-399, 1986.

Perloff, J.K.: The clinical recognition of congenital heart disease, ed. 3, Philadelphia, 1987, W.B. Saunders Co.

Rao, P.S.: Balloon angioplasty for coarctation of the aorta in infancy, J. Pediatr. 110(5):713-718, 1987.

Rao, P.S.: Balloon valvuloplasty and angioplasty in infants and children, J. Pediatr. 114(6):907-914, 1989.

Rigby, M.L.: The trend to primary repair of congenital heart defects in the first 3 months of life, Curr. Opin. Pediatr. 1(1):82-84, 1989.

Rubin, J.D., and Ferencz, C.: Subsequent pregnancy in mothers of infants with congenital heart disease, Pediatrics 76(3):371-374, 1985.

Salzer, H.R., and others: Growth and nutritional intake of infants with congenital heart disease, Pediatr. Cardiol. 10(1):17-23, 1989.

Siebert, J.R., and others: Ebstein's anomaly and extracardiac defects, Am. J. Dis. Child. 143:570-572, 1989.

Smith, J.B., and Vernon-Levett, P.: Hypoplastic left heart syndrome: treatment options, MCN 14:180-183, 1989.

Smith, M.S., and others: Symptomatic mitral valve prolapse in children and adolescents: catecholamines, anxiety, and biofeedback, Pediatrics 84(2):290-295, 1989.

Spevak, P., and others: Valve replacement in children less than five years of age, J. Am. Acad. Cardiol. 8(4):901-908, 1986.

Swetnam, S.M., Yabek, S.M., and Alverson, D.C.: Hemodynamic consequences of neonatal polycythemia, J. Pediatr. 110(3):443-447, 1987.

Vet, T.W., and Ottenkamp, J.: Correction of atrioventricular septal defect, Am. J. Dis. Child. 143:1361-1365, 1989.

Vincent, R.N., and Collins, G.F.: Cardiac embryology and fetal cardiovascular physiology, Crit. Care Q. 9(2):1-5, 1986.

Heart Transplantation

Addonizio, L.J., and Rose, E.A.: Cardiac transplantation in children and adolescents, J. Pediatr. 3:1034-1038, 1987.

Bailey, L.L., and others: Cardiac allotransplantation in newborns as therapy for hypoplastic left heart syndrome, N. Engl. J. Med. 315:949-963, 1986.

Boucek, M.M., and others: Cardiac transplantation in infancy: donors and recipients, J. Pediatr. 116(2):171-176, 1990.

Cardin, S., and Clark, S.: A nursing diagnosis approach to the patient awaiting cardiac transplantation, Heart Lung 14(5):499-504, 1985.

Fricker, F.J., and others: Experience with heart transplantation in children, Pediatrics 79(1):138-146, 1987.

Funk, M.: Heart transplantation: postoperative care during the acute period, Crit. Care Nurse 6:27-45, 1986.

Gold, L., and others: Psychosocial issues in pediatric organ transplantation: the parents' perspective, Pediatrics 77:738-743, 1986.

Gunderson, L.: Teaching the transplant recipient, J. Heart Transplant. 4:226-227, 1985.

Harwood, C.H., and Cook, C.V.: Cyclosporine in transplantation, Heart Lung 14:529-540, 1985.

Hutchings, S.M., and Monett, Z.J.: Caring for the cardiac transplant patient, Crit. Care Nurs. Clin. North Am. 1(2):245-262, 1989.

Kaman, B.D.: Immunosuppressive therapy with cyclosporine for cardiac transplantation, Circulation 75:40-56, 1987.

Kauffman, R.E.: Cardiac transplantation in infants and children, J. Pediatr. 116(2):266-268, 1990.

Marsden, C.: Ethical issues in a heart transplant program, Heart Lung 14:495-498, 1985.

McAleer, M.J., and others: Psychological aspects of heart transplantation, J. Heart Transplant. 4(2):232-233, 1985.

Muirhead, J.: Heart and heart-lung transplantation, Nurs. Clin. North Am. 24(4):865-880, 1989.

Murdock, D.K., and others: Rejection of the transplanted heart, Heart Lung 16:237-245, 1987.

O'Brien, V.C.: Psychological and social aspects of heart transplantation, J. Heart Transplant. 4(2):229-231, 1985.

Pahl, E., and others: Coronary arteriosclerosis in pediatric heart transplant survivors: limitation of long-term survival, J. Pediatr. 116(2):177-183, 1990.

Painvin, G.A., and others: Cardiac transplantation: indications, procurement, operation, and management, Heart Lung 14(5):484-489, 1985.

Radley-Smith, R.C.: Cardiac transplantation in the management of congenital and acquired heart disease, Curr. Opin. Pediatr. 1(1):100-102, 1989.

Rimar, J.: Cyclosporine for organ transplantation, MCN 10:237, 1985.

Schnepf, C.A.: The pediatric heart transplant patient: immunosuppressive drugs and organ rejection, J. Pediatr. Health Care 1(2):91-97, 1987.

Wiles, H.B., and others: Repeated endomyocardial biopsy without complication in an infant after heart transplantation, J. Thorac. Cardiovasc. Surg. 91(4):637-638, 1986.

Nursing Care

Fisk, R.: Management of the pediatric cardiovascular patient after surgery, Crit. Care Q. 9(2):75-82, 1986.

Foldy, S.M., and Gorman, J.B.: Perioperative nursing care for congenital cardiac defects, Crit. Care Nurs. Clin. North Am. 1(2):289-296, 1989.

Kashani, I.A., and Higgins, S.S.: Counseling strategies for families of children with congenital heart disease, Pediatr. Nurs. 12(1):38-40, 1986.

Malinowski, P., and Yablonski, C.: Congenital heart disease in infants: nursing assessment, Crit. Care Q. 9(2):6-23, 1986.

Myrer, M.L.: Respiratory care of the postoperative cardiac surgery patient, Crit. Care Q. 9(2):64-74, 1986.

O'Brien, P., and Boisvert, J.T.: Discharge planning for children with heart disease, Crit. Care Nurs. Clin. North Am. 1(2):297-305, 1989.

Rotondi, P.: Intensive care unit management of the postoperative cardiac surgery patient, Crit. Care Q. 9(2):49-63, 1986.

Uzark, K., Messiter, E., and Rosenthal, A.: Promoting dental health care in children with congenital heart disease, Pediatr. Nurs. 12(2):96-99, 1986.

Vincent, R.N., and Elixson, E.M.: Hemodynamic monitoring, Crit. Care Q. 9(2):40-48, 1986.

Bacterial Endocarditis

Dajani, A.S.: Prevention of bacterial endocarditis, Pediatr. Infect. Dis. 4(4):349-352, 1985.

Guntheroth, W.G.: How important are dental procedures as a cause of infective endocarditis? Am. J. Cardiol. 54:797-801, 1984.

Jenkins, J.: Infective endocarditis: a clinical overview, Crit. Care Update 10(5):42-47, 1983.

Scrima, D.A.: Infective endocarditis: nursing considerations, Crit. Care Nurse 7:47-56, 1987.

Special statement: prevention of bacterial endocarditis, Pediatrics 75(3):603-607, 1985.

Wensley, K.T., and others: Infective endocarditis in children with congenital heart disease: comparison of selected features in patients with surgical correction of palliation and those without, Br. Heart J. 58:57-65, 1987.

Rheumatic Fever

Ayoub, E.M.: Prophylaxis in patients with rheumatic fever: every three or every four weeks? (letter), J. Pediatr. 115(1):89-91, 1989.

Bisno, A.L.: The rise and fall of rheumatic fever, JAMA 254(4):538-541, 1985.

Bisno, A.L.: Acute rheumatic fever: forgotten but not gone, N. Engl. J. Med. 316(8):476-478, 1987.

Chun, L.T., Reddy, D.V., and Yamamoto, L.G.: Rheumatic fever in children and adolescents in Hawaii, Pediatrics 79(4):549-552, 1987.

Congeni, B., and others: Outbreak of acute rheumatic fever in northeast Ohio, J. Pediatr. 111:176-179, 1987.

Hosier, D.M., and others: Resurgence of acute rheumatic fever, Am. J. Dis. Child. 141:730-733, 1987.

Kaplan, E.L.: Return of rheumatic fever: consequences, implications, and needs (letter), J. Pediatr. 111(2):244-246, 1987.

Kaplan, E.L.: Pharmacokinetics on benzathine penicillin G: serum levels during the 28 days after intramuscular injection of 1,200,000 units, J. Pediatr. 115(1):146-150, 1989.

Lue, H., and others: Rheumatic fever recurrences: controlled study of 3-week versus 4-week benzathine penicillin prevention programs, J. Pediatr. 108(2):229-304, 1986.

Nordin, J.D.: Recurrence of rheumatic fever during prophylaxis with monthly benzathine penicillin G, Pediatrics 73(4):530-531, 1984.

Tolaymat, A., and others: Acute rheumatic fever in north Florida, South. Med. J. 77:819-823, 1984.

Veasy, L.G., and others: Resurgence of acute rheumatic fever in the intermountain area of the United States, N. Engl. J. Med. 316:421-427, 1987.

Kawasaki Disease

American Academy of Pediatrics, Committee on Infectious Diseases: Intravenous γ-globulin use in children with Kawasaki disease, Pediatrics 82(1):122, 1988.

Anderson, T.M., Meyer, R., and Kaplan, S.: Long-term echocardiographic evaluation of cardiac size and function in patients with Kawasaki disease, Am. Heart J. 110(1, pt. 1):107-115, 1985.

Bierman, F.Z., and Gersony, W.M.: Kawasaki disease: clinical perspective, J. Pediatr. 3(5):789-793, 1987.

Burns, J.C.: Kawasaki disease, Curr. Opin. Pediatr. 1:13-15, 1989.

Fatica, N.S., and others: Rug shampoo and Kawasaki disease, Pediatrics 84(2):231-234, 1989.

Fujita, Y., and others: Kawasaki disease in families, Pediatrics 84(4):666-669, 1989.

Glode, M.P., and others: Effect of intravenous immune globulin on the coagulopathy of Kawasaki syndrome, J. Pediatr. 115(3):469-473, 1989.

Ichida, F., and others: Coronary artery involvement in Kawasaki syndrome in Manhattan, New York: risk factors and role of aspirin, Pediatrics 80(6):828-835, 1987.

Ichida, F., and others: Epidemiologic aspects of Kawasaki disease in a Manhattan hospital, Pediatrics 84(2):235-241, 1989.

Koike, K., and Freedom, R.M.: Kawasaki disease, with a focus on cardiovascular manifestations, Curr. Opin. Pediatr. 1(1):135-141, 1989.

Morens, D.M., Anderson, L.J., and Hurwitz, E.S.: National surveillance of Kawasaki disease, Pediatrics 65(1):21-25, 1980.

Nakano, H., and others.: Clinical characteristics of myocardial infarction following Kawasaki disease: report of 11 cases, J. Pediatr. 108(2):198-203, 1986.

Nash, D.J.: Kawasaki disease: application of the Roy adaptation model to determine interventions, J. Pediatr. Nurs. 2(5):308-315, 1987.

Rowley, A.H., Duffy, C.E., and Shulman, S.T.: Prevention of giant coronary artery aneurysms in Kawasaki disease by intravenous gamma globulin therapy, J. Pediatr. 113(2):290-294, 1988.

Suzuki, A., and others: Aortocoronary bypass surgery for coronary arterial lesions resulting from Kawasaki disease, J. Pediatr. 116(4):567-573, 1990.

Turner-Gomes, S., and others: High persistence rate of established coronary artery lesions secondary to Kawasaki disease among a panethnic Canadian population, J. Pediatr. 108(6):928-932, 1986.

Yanagawa, H., Kawasaki, T., and Shigematsu, I.: Nationwide survey on Kawasaki disease in Japan, Pediatrics 80(1):58-62, 1987.

Yanagawa, H., and others: A nationwide incidence survey of Kawasaki disease in 1985-1986 in Japan, J. Infect. Dis. 158(6):1296-1301, 1988.

Systemic Hypertension

De Swiet, M., and Dillon, M.J.: Hypertension in children, Br. Med. J. 299(6697):469-470, 1989.

Falkner, B.: Essential hypertension in children, Curr. Opin. Pediatr. 1(1):131-134, 1989.

Grimm, R.H., Jr., and Hunninghake, D.B.: Lipids and hypertension: implications of new guidelines for cholesterol management in the treatment of hypertension, Am. J. Med. 80(suppl. 2A):56-63, 1986.

Gruskin, A.B.: The adolescent with essential hypertension, Am. J. Kidney Dis. 6(2):86-90, 1985.

Inglefinger, J.: Systemic hypertension. In Adams, F.H., Emmanouilides, G.C., and Riemenschneider, T.A., editors: Moss' heart disease in infants, children, and adolescents, ed. 4, Baltimore, 1989, Williams & Wilkins.

Jorde, L.B., and Williams, R.R.: Innovative blood pressure measurements yield information not reflected by sitting measurements, Hypertension 14(4):252-257, 1986.

Olson, R.E.: Mass intervention vs screening and selective intervention for the prevention of coronary heart disease, JAMA 255(16):2204-2207, 1986.

Rocchini, A.P., and others: Blood pressure in obese adolescents: effect of weight loss, Pediatrics 82(1):16-23, 1988.

Roy, C.C., and Galeano, N.: Childhood antecedents of adult degenerative disease, Pediatr. Clin. North Am. 32(2):517-533, 1985.

Shear, C.L., and others: Value of childhood blood pressure measurements and family history in predicting future blood pressure status: results from 8 years of follow-up in the Bogalusa heart study, Pediatrics 77(6):862-869, 1986.

Sinaiko, A.R., Gomez-Marin, O., and Prineas, R.J.: Prevalence of "significant" hypertension in junior high school-aged children: the children and adolescent blood pressure program, J. Pediatr. 114(4, pt. 1):664-669, 1989.

Whincup, P.H., Cook, D.G., and Shaper, A.G.: Early influences on blood pressure: a study of children aged 5-7 years, Br. Med. J. 299:587-591, 1989.

Hyperlipidemia (Hypercholesterolemia)

Cardiovascular risk factors from birth to 7 years of age: the Bogalusa heart study, Pediatrics 80(5):entire issue, 1987.

Cortner, J.A., Coates, P.M., and Gallagher, P.R.: Prevalence and expression of familial combined hyperlipidemia in childhood, J. Pediatr. 16(4):514-519, 1990.

Cresanta, J.L., and others: Prevention of atherosclerosis in childhood, Pediatr. Clin. North Am. 33(4):835-858, 1986.

Davidson, D.M., Smith, R.M., and Qaqundah, P.Y.: Cholesterol screening in children during office visits, J. Pediatr. Health Care 4(1):11-17, 1990.

Davidson, D.M., and others: School-based blood cholesterol screening, J. Pediatr. Health Care 3(1):3-8, 1989.

Dennison, B.A., and others: Parental history of cardiovascular disease as an indication for screening for lipoprotein abnormalities in children, J. Pediatr. 115(2):186-194, 1989.

Glueck, C.J., and others: Safety and efficacy of long-term diet and diet plus bile acid–binding resin cholesterol-lowering therapy in 73 children heterozygous for familial hypercholesterolemia, Pediatrics 78(2):338-348, 1986.

Granot, E., and Deckelbaum, R.J.: Hypocholesterolemia in childhood, J. Pediatr. 115(2):171-185, 1989.

Hayman, L.L., and others: Reducing risk for heart disease in children, MCN 13:442-448, 1988.

Hayman, L.L., and others: Which child is at risk for heart disease? MCN 13:328-333, 1988.

Jacobson, M.S., and Lillienfeld, D.E.: The pediatrician's role in atherosclerosis prevention, J. Pediatr. 112(5):836-841, 1988.

Kwiterovich, P.O.: Biochemical, clinical, epidemiologic, genetic, and pathologic data in the pediatric age group relevant to the cholesterol hypothesis (letter), Pediatrics 78(2):349-361, 1986.

LaRosa, J., and Finberg, L.: Preliminary report from a conference entitled "prevention of adult atherosclerosis during childhood" (letter), J. Pediatr. 112:1317-1318, 1988.

Lauer, R.M., and Clarke, W.R.: Childhood risk factors for high adult blood pressure: the Muscatine study, Pediatrics 84(4):633-641, 1984.

Lauer, R.M., Lee, J., and Clarke, W.R.: Factors affecting the relationship between childhood and adult cholesterol levels: the Muscatine study, Pediatrics 82(3):309-318, 1988.

Lee, J., Lauer, R.M., and Clarke, W.R.: Lipoproteins in the progeny of young men with coronary artery disease: children with increased risk, Pediatrics 78(2):330-337, 1986.

Lifshitz, F., and Moses, N.: A complication of dietary treatment of hypercholesterolemia, Am. J. Dis. Child. 143:537-542, 1989.

Mistretta, E.F., and Stroud, S.: Hypercholesterolemia in children: risk and management, Pediatr. Nurs. 16(2):152-154, 1990.

Nader, P.R., and others: Adult heart disease prevention in childhood: a national survey of pediatricians' practices and attitudes, Pediatrics 79(6):843-850, 1987.

Schifman, V., and Hannaman, K.N.: Cholesterol: a practical teaching plan for children and adolescents, Issues Compr. Pediatr. Nurs. 12(5):359-369, 1989.

Stoy, D.B.: Controlling cholesterol with diet, Am. J. Nurs. 89(12):1625-1627, 1989.

Cardiomyopathy

Gillum, R.F.: Idiopathic cardiomyopathy in the United States, 1970-1982, Am. Heart J. 111(4):752-755, 1986.

Hanukoglu, A., Fried, D., and Somekh, E.: Inheritance of familial primary endocardial fibroelastosis, Clin. Pediatr. 25(5):272-275, 1986.

Hazinski, M.F.: Sudden cardiac death in children, Crit. Care Q. 7(2):59-70, 1984.

Maron, B.J.: Cardiomyopathies. In Adams, F.H., Emmanouilides, G.C., and Riemenschneider, T.A., editors: Moss' heart disease in infants, children, and adolescents, ed. 4, Baltimore, 1989, Williams & Wilkins.

Purcell, J.A.: Cardiomyopathy, Am. J. Nurs. 89(1):57-75, 1989.

Rao, P.S.: Chronic afterload reduction in infants and children with primary myocardial disease, J. Pediatr. 108(4):530-534, 1986.

Ino, T., and others: Dilated cardiomyopathy with neutropenia, short statures, and abnormal carnitine metabolism, J. Pediatr. 113(3):511-514, 1988.

Vetter, V.L.: Sudden death in infants, children, and adolescents, Cardiovasc. Clin. 15(3):310-313, 1985.

Cardiac Dysrhythmias

Alpern, D., Uzark, K., and Dick, M.: Psychosocial responses of children to cardiac pacemakers, J. Pediatr. 114(3):494-501, 1989.

Campbell, R.M.: and others: Atrial overdrive pacing for conversion of atrial flutter in children, Pediatrics 75(4):730-736, 1985.

Campbell, R.M., and others: Surgical treatment of pediatric cardiac arrhythmia, J. Pediatr. 110(4):501-508, 1987.

Case, C.L., Trippel, D.L., and Gillette, P.C.: New antiarrhythmic agents in pediatrics, Pediatr. Clin. North Am. 36(5):1293-1320, 1989.

Curley, M.A.: Pediatric cardiac dysrhythmias, Bowie, MD, 1985, Brady Communications Co., Inc.

Danaher, R.R.: Complete congenital heart block: a case study, Neonatal Network 5(4):19-23, 1987.

Dick, M., II, and Campbell, R.M.: Advances in the management of cardiac arrhythmias in children, Pediatr. Clin. North Am. 31(6):1175-1195, 1984.

Dunnigan, A., Benson, D.W., Jr., and Benditt, D.G.: Atrial flutter in infancy: diagnosis, clinical features, and treatment, Pediatrics 75(4):725-729, 1985.

Garson, A.: Medicolegal problems in the management of cardiac arrhythmias in children, Pediatrics 79(1):84-88, 1987.

Gillette, P.C., and others: Dysrhythmias. In Adams, F.H., Emmanouilides, G.C., and Riemenschneider, T.A., editors: Moss' heart disease in infants, children, and adolescents, ed. 4, Baltimore, 1989, Williams & Wilkins.

Higgins, S.S., Hardy, C.E., and Higashino, S.M.: Should parents of children with congenital heart disease and life-threatening dysrhythmias be taught cardiopulmonary resuscitation? (letter), Pediatrics 84(6):1102-1104, 1989.

Johnson, D.L.: Pediatric arrhythmias: a nursing approach, Dimens. Crit. Care Nurs. 2(3):147-157, 1983.

Luckstead, E.F.: Sudden death in sports, Pediatr. Clin. North Am. 29(6):1355-1362, 1982.

Mahoney, L.T., and others: Pacemaker management for acute onset of heart block in childhood, J. Pediatr. 107(2):207-211, 1985.

Mofenson, H.C., Caraccio, T.R., and Schauben, J.: Poisoning by antidysrhythmic drugs, Pediatr. Clin. North Am. 33(3):723-738, 1986.

Moser, S., and Flaker, G.: Get ready: the new antiarrhythmics are coming, Nursing '85 15(9):56-58, 1985.

CHAPTER 35

The Child with Hematologic or Immunologic Dysfunction

RELATED TOPICS

Administration of medication, Ch. 27
Bone marrow aspiration/biopsy, Ch. 27
Bone marrow transplantation, Ch. 36
Collection of specimens, Ch. 27
Compliance, Ch. 27
Hemolytic disease of the newborn, Ch. 9
Human immunodeficiency virus encephalopathy, Ch. 37
Human immunodeficiency virus infection and acquired immune deficiency syndrome, Ch. 20
Immunizations, Ch. 12
Infection control, Ch. 27
Leukemias, Ch. 36
Lymphomas, Ch. 36
Pain assessment; pain management, Ch. 26
Physical examination: skin, Ch. 7
Preparation for procedures, Ch. 27

GLOSSARY

AIDS Acquired immune deficiency syndrome
ALG Antilymphocyte globulin
ANC Absolute neutrophil count
anemia Reduction of red blood cells or hemoglobin concentration below normal
Antigen Substance the body recognizes as foreign that triggers the manufacture of specific antibodies
ATG Antithymocyte globulin
AZT Azidothymidine, Zidovudine (Retrovir)—drug used in the treatment of AIDS
B-lymphocyte Type of lymphocyte that produces antibodies
bands Slightly immature forms of granulocytes
basophil Granular leukocyte
BMT Bone marrow transplantation
CBC Complete blood count
coagulation Process of clotting
complement Series of proteins that function in an interrelated manner that enhances chemotaxis and the inflammatory response
DDAVP 1-Desamino-8-D-arginine vasopressin (desmopressin)
DIC Disseminated intravascular coagulation
eosinophil Granular leukocyte
erythrocyte Red blood cell
erythropoiesis Process of RBC manufacture
FVIII-c Factor VIII coagulant activity
FVIII R:Ag Factor VIII–related antigen
granulocyte (polymorphonuclear leukocyte) One of the major groups of WBCs
hematocrit (Hct) Percent of RBCs in total blood volume
hemoglobin (Hgb) Oxygen-carrying, iron-containing pigment in red blood cells

hemolysis The destruction of RBCs
hemostasis Process whereby bleeding from an injured vessel is stopped
HIV Human immunodeficiency virus
HSP Henoch-Schönlein purpura
ITP Idiopathic thrombocytopenic purpura
leukocyte General term for the group of cells in the body active in the immune process
lymphocyte One of the major groups of WBCs
mean corpuscular hemoglobin (MCH) Average quantity of Hgb in a RBC
mean corpuscular hemoglobin concentration (MCHC) Average concentration of Hgb in an RBC
mean corpuscular volume (MCV) Average size of RBCs
monocyte Cells active in the immune process that develop into macrophages that are highly effective phagocytes
neutrophil Granulocyte that phagocytizes bacteria
phagocytosis Process of ingesting and digesting foreign proteins
plasma Liquid portion of blood
platelet Cellular fragment involved in coagulation
PT Prothrombin time
PTT Partial thromboplastin time
PWA People with AIDS
RBC Red blood cell
reticulocyte Immature RBC
SCIDS Severe combined immunodeficiency syndrome
serum Remaining plasma after coagulation has taken place
T-lymphocyte Type of lymphocyte active in cellular immunity
thrombocyte Platelet
WBC White blood cell

Disorders related to the blood and/or blood-forming organs in childhood encompass a wide range of diseases and pathologic states. Since the blood is a multipurpose fluid involved in the functions of so many tissues and organs, either primary or secondary changes in the blood are reflected in the essential functions of these structures. Hematologic disorders in childhood include the anemias, defects in hemostasis, and the immunologic disorders. Nonneoplastic white blood cell disorders do occur, but rarely in pediatrics. Therefore they are not discussed. Related neoplastic disorders—the leukemias and lymphomas—are discussed in Chapter 36.

THE HEMATOLOGIC SYSTEM AND ITS FUNCTION

The hematologic system, composed of the blood and blood-forming tissues, is responsible for a complex system of homeostatic mechanisms that produces cells with specific functions and provides for oxygenation and distribution of nutrients and other chemicals to the cells, collection of wastes from the cells, immune protection (defense, homeostasis, and surveillance), clotting, and regulation of heat. Any disturbance within this system can result in widespread alteration of function almost anywhere in the body, including rapid death from acute loss of blood. The following is an overview of the formation of the various elements of the blood and a brief discussion of assessment of hematologic function. More detailed information is provided when specific disorders are presented.

ORIGIN OF FORMED ELEMENTS

Blood has two major components: a fluid portion called plasma and a cellular portion known as the formed elements of the blood. The two components are approximately equal in volume. Plasma is about 90% water and 10% solutes. The principal solutes are albumin, electrolytes, and proteins. Among the proteins are clotting factors, globulins, circulating antibodies, and fibrinogen. The cellular elements are red blood cells (RBCs, *erythrocytes*), white blood cells (WBCs, *leukocytes*), and platelets *(thrombocytes)*.

The major blood-forming (hemopoietic) organs of the body are the red bone marrow (myeloid tissue) and lymphatic system, which consists of lymph (fluid), lymphatic vessels, and lymphoid structures—the lymph nodes, spleen, thymus, and tonsils. Although the lymphatic system plays an important role in regulating blood cells, the lymph vessels and fluids do not produce cells. The lymph nodes regulate the manufacture of WBCs. The spleen and liver are prime organs for hematopoiesis in the young fetus and cell removal in postnatal life. Macrophages (formerly called reticular cells) are cells of mesodermal origin that are widely dispersed in the lining of the vascular and lymph channels. Macrophages form a network and are capable of phagocytosis (ingestion and digestion of foreign substances), formation of immune bodies, and differentiation into other cells, such as hemocytoblasts, myeloblasts, or lymphoblasts.

All of the formed elements of the blood, except to some extent the agranulocytes, are believed to be formed in myeloid tissue during postnatal life. During embryonic development the mesenchyme, spleen, liver, thymus, and yolk sac serve as additional sites of blood cell formation. In certain blood disorders these sites, particularly the spleen, can be stimulated to produce blood cells, and constitute *extramedullary hemopoiesis.* In infants and young children all of the bone contains red marrow (so called because of its color from formation of erythrocytes), but as bone growth ceases near the end of adolescence, only the ribs, sternum, vertebrae, and pelvis continue to produce blood cells. The remainder of the bone marrow becomes yellow from deposition of fat. However, in conditions of increased demand

Christina Algiere Kasprisin, R.N., M.S., assisted in the revision of this chapter.

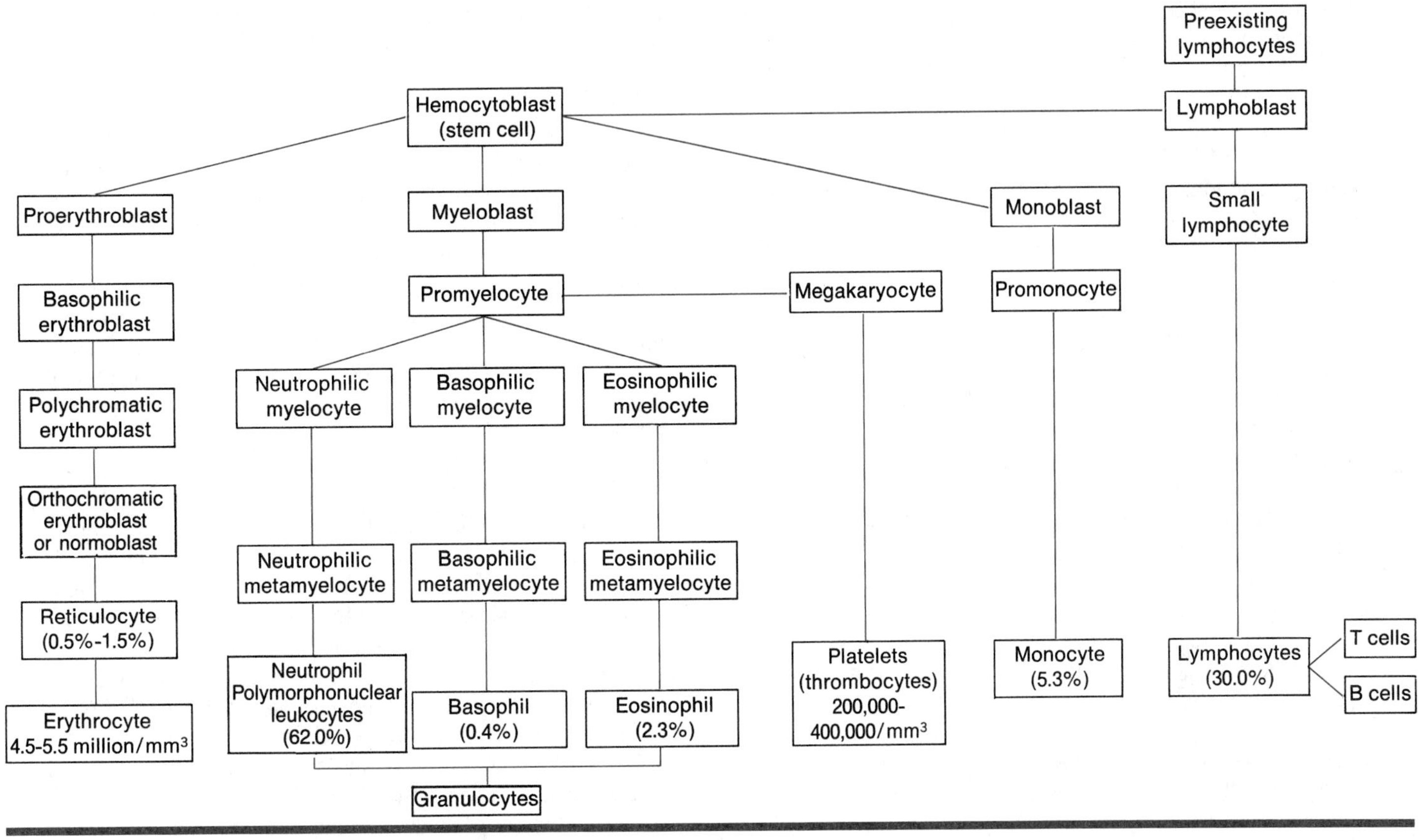

Fig. 35-1. Formation of blood cells. Erythrocyte values are averages for older children. (For blood values at each age, see Appendix D.)

for blood cells, the yellow marrow can revert to red marrow as another hemopoietic source.

Although the progressive development of each blood cell is fairly well delineated, there is considerable controversy regarding the origin of the blood cell. One of the most widely held theories (monophyletic) is that each blood cell originates from a primordial (primitive) cell called a *blast,* or *stem,* cell. This *hemocytoblast* in turn gives rise to the erythroblast, myeloblast, monoblast, lymphoblast, and megakaryoblast (Fig. 35-1).

Erythrocytes

The erythrocyte is formed from the hemocytoblast in the red bone marrow. As illustrated in Fig. 35-1, the *hemocytoblast* forms the proerythroblast. The initial cells of this series has a deep blue (basophilic) staining cytoplasm and therefore is called a *basophilic erythroblast.* The chief change in the erythroblast is accumulation of hemoglobin in the cytoplasm. As the basophilic material decreases and the amount of hemoglobin increases, the cell is called a *polychromatic erythroblast,* which describes its mixture of staining properties. At the same time as the nucleus is decreasing in size, the basophilic material disappears, so that the cell is uniformly stained by eosin dye, hence the name *orthochromatic erythroblast,* or *normoblast.* Finally the normoblast completely loses its nucleus by a process of extrusion as it squeezes through the pores of the membrane into the capillary. As a result of losing its nucleus, the cell caves in on both sides, giving the mature *erythrocyte* its characteristic appearance as a biconcave disk. During each of these stages the different cells continue to undergo mitosis so that increasingly greater numbers of cells are produced. Since the mature RBC does not have a nucleus, it is unable to multiply.

The *reticulocyte* is the last stage of development before the mature erythrocyte. Reticulocytes are slightly larger than erythrocytes and are used as an indicator of active erythropoiesis. Ordinarily the total proportion of circulating reticulocytes (known as the reticulocyte count) is between 0.5% and 1.5%. A change in the number of reticulocytes is an indicator of increased *RBC* production or hyperfunctioning of the bone marrow. The *reticulocyte* (or "retic") *count* is a simple laboratory test frequently used to indirectly analyze hemopoiesis.

Regulation of erythrocyte production. The usual life span of the mature erythrocyte is 120 days. Apparently as RBCs grow old, their membranes become fragile and eventually rupture. The contents of the cell fragment as they circulate through the blood vessels and are phagocytized by the macrophages in the spleen, liver, and bone marrow. The hemoglobin is broken down into the iron-containing pigment hemosiderin and the bile pigments biliverdin and bilirubin. Most of the iron is reused by the bone marrow for production of new RBCs or stored in the liver and other tissues for future use. The bile pigments are excreted by the liver in bile.

Normally there is a homeostatic balance between the regulation of RBC production and destruction. This balance ensures adequate tissue oxygenation and a blood viscosity that allows the blood to flow freely through the vessels. The basic regulator of erythrocyte production is believed to be tissue oxygenation and renal production of erythropoietin. In states of tissue hypoxia, *erythropoietin* (also called *erythropoietic stimulating factor*) is released by the kidneys into the bloodstream. As a result, the bone marrow is stimulated to produce new RBCs. The major activity seems to be an increase in both the maturation rate and mitosis of all stages of erythrocyte production, but primarily at the stem cell level.

During this rapid increase of RBC production, the circulating erythrocytes may not be totally mature. Consequently, the number of reticulocytes may increase dramatically (as high as 30% or more of the total red blood cell count). Even normoblasts may appear in the blood. If this rise in erythrocyte and reticulocyte count does not occur, it may indicate bone marrow failure.

Once tissue oxygenation is adequate, the production of erythropoietin ceases. Thus tissue oxygen requirements control both the stimulation and termination of erythrocyte production. It is important to note that it is the ability of RBCs to transport oxygen to the tissues in response to their needs, not the circulating numbers of erythrocytes, that is the basic regulatory mechanism. Oxygen transport depends on both the number of circulating RBCs and the amount of normal hemoglobin in the cell. This explains why *polycythemia* (increase in the number of erythrocytes) occurs in conditions of prolonged tissue hypoxia, such as cyanotic heart defects (see Chapter 34). If the circulating numbers of erythrocytes controlled erythropoietin release, this feedback mechanism would control erythrocyte production at a constant level (4.5 to 5.5 million/mm^3 of blood) regardless of existing tissue hypoxia.

Synthetic erythropoietin is currently being used for several clinical indications. The most dramatic results have been achieved with children who are anemic secondary to chronic renal failure. The synthetic erythropoietin is able to induce an increase in hematocrit sufficient to eliminate the need for red cell transfusions. Current research is investigating the use of synthetic erythropoietin in the anemia of prematurity, hemoglobinopathies, and, with synthetic colony-stimulating factor (WBC), to minimize the bone marrow depression of chemotherapy (Shannon, 1990).

Functions of erythrocytes. The major function of RBCs is to transport hemoglobin, which in turn carries oxygen to all cells of the body. However, erythrocytes have other significant functions: (1) they contain quantities of carbonic anhydrase, an enzyme that catalyzes the reaction between carbon dioxide and water, allowing large quantities of carbon dioxide to react with blood for transportation to the lungs, and (2) the hemoglobin, a protein, serves as an acid-base buffer, which, in combination with CO_2, maintains the blood pH at a constant level.

Hemoglobin

Hemoglobin (Hgb) is a complex molecule composed of four globin chains. The type of Hgb in the cells depends on both the stage of life and any abnormalities in the genes that regulate the production of hemoglobin. Fetal Hgb, composed of two alpha and two gamma chains, has a greater affinity for oxygen and is best suited to the fetal environment. During the latter part of pregnancy, the fetus begins developing adult Hgb (two alpha and two beta chains). When a defect in Hgb synthesis is present (e.g., sickle cell disease or thalassemia), fetal Hgb may be produced into adulthood.

Leukocytes

The leukocytes (white blood cells [WBCs]) refer to a number of cells with similar yet distinct functions. They are divided into two major classifications—granulocytes and agranulocytes—based on the presence or absence, respectively, of granules within the cytoplasm of the cells.

Granulocytes. There are three types of granulocytes: *neutrophils, basophils,* and *eosinophils.* The name of each of these refers to the characteristic staining property of the granule during laboratory analysis. Neutrophils stain neutral to the dyes, whereas basophils stain a purple color to the basic methylene blue dye, and eosinophils take on a red color to the acidic eosin dye. Because the nuclei of neutrophils have two or more lobules that are connected by fine chromatin strands, the term *polymorphonuclear* (meaning "many-formed nuclei") *leukocytes,* or simply "polys," "segs" (segmented or mature neutrophils), and "bands" (immature neutrophils with the nuclei connected), may be used collectively to refer to the neutrophils.

The granulocytes, like erythrocytes, are produced in the bone marrow. For this reason these cells are sometimes referred to as *myelogenous leukocytes.* It is believed that these cells originate from primitive stem cells, which develop into myeloblasts. As Fig. 35-1 illustrates, the genesis of neutrophils, basophils, and eosinophils is similar to the stages observed during erythrocyte production. The differentiation of myeloblasts into various mature WBCs is primarily the result of specialization within the cytoplasm and degeneration of the nucleus. Unlike the erythrocyte, however, all of the WBCs are nucleated.

Increased numbers of bands in the peripheral circulation (referred to as a "shift to the left" on the complete blood count) indicate an accelerated production of granulocytes to meet the body's needs, such as in bacterial infection. The absolute neutrophil count (ANC) reflects the body's ability to handle bacterial infections. If the ANC is less than 1000, there is a serious risk of infection; if it is less than 500, a severe risk of infection is present.

Agranulocytes. The agranulocytes comprise two cell types, the *monocytes* and *lymphocytes.* Characteristically these cells do not develop granules, and the nuclei are not lobulated. They are believed to have their origin in various lymphogenous organs and for this reason are sometimes referred to as *lymphogenous leukocytes.* However, since stem cells and reticular cells are capable of differentiating into monocytes or lymphocytes, the origin of these cells is frequently designated as the *lymphomyeloid complex,* which includes the bone marrow, lymph nodes, spleen, liver, thymus, subepithelial lymphoid tissue (tonsils, vermiform appendix, and intestinal lymphoid tissues), and connective tissues (mesenchymal cells of the reticuloendothelial system).

The monocytes follow the same sequence of development from the stem cell as the granulocytes (see Fig. 35-1). The monocytes, in turn, have the ability to exit the vessels and develop into *macrophages,* large cells that are highly effective phagocytes. *Kupfer cells* are macrophages located in the liver. *Histiocytes* are macrophages in the connective tissue. These names are remnants of the old reticular endothelial system.

Lymphocyte formation *(lymphocytopoiesis)* is believed to take place anywhere in the lymphomyeloid complex. Lymphocytes develop from blast (stem) cells (see Fig. 35-1). The lymphocyte has the potential to develop into other cells. For example, lymphocytes may become T-cells or B-cells (see p. 1643).

Regulation of leukocyte production. The exact life span of the leukocytes is not as clearly defined as that of the erythrocytes, because their existence in the circulation is primarily for transportation to extravascular areas, where they reside in reservoirs or where they are needed to resist infection. Therefore their survival rate has been divided into three phases: (1) the *hemopoietic phase,* extending from the development of the blast cell to the delivery of the mature leukocyte into the circulation, (2) the *intravascular phase,* or the period within the circulation, and (3) the *extravascular phase,* or the time spent in the viscera or tissues.

Granulocytes have a half-life of 6 to 8 hours in the blood and, after entering the tissues, die over 4 to 5 days. Agranulocytes live for an extended period because they remain in inflamed tissue areas longer than the granulocytes. Because monocytes wander back and forth between the blood and tissues and are capable of becoming macrophages, their half-life in the blood is 8 to 10 hours, but the half-life in the tissue is 60 to 90 days.

The regulation of leukocytes is based on the body's need for them. Tissue damage from bacterial or viral agents promotes leukocyte circulation and production. However, *leukocytosis* (increase in leukocytes) results from tissue destruction from almost any factor, such as hemorrhage, neoplastic disease, toxicity, operative procedures, chemical and thermal injury, or tissue ischemia.

The leukocytes probably die as a result of their activity at the site of injury and are phagocytized by other newly formed WBCs. Effective control of the inflammatory process with subsequent tissue recovery most likely results in a feedback mechanism to the bone marrow and causes lymphogenous organs to cease increased production of WBCs.

Functions of leukocytes. Although all of the leukocytes play some role in the immune process, each of the WBCs plays a specific role. Neutrophils and monocytes are effective phagocytes and as a result are primarily involved in inflammatory reactions. *Neutrophilia* (increased numbers of neutrophils) is most evident in an acute inflammation, whereas *monocytosis* (increased number of monocytes) is more evident in chronic conditions. The reason for this is that as the affected area becomes acidic from tissue necrosis, neutrophils, which prefer a neutral environment, become less efficient, and the monocytes, which become macrophages, become more powerful. These cells also increase during chronic inflammation. The other functions of lymphocytes in terms of the immune process are discussed on p. 1643.

The function of eosinophils is still not completely known. They seem to have parasiticidal properties because they can selectively destroy parasites. They may also function in the immediate type of allergic or anaphylactic hypersensitivity reactions, since *eosinophilia* (increased numbers of eosinophils) is well documented in such conditions. Eosinophils also are thought to release a substance called *profibrinolysin,* which, when activated to form fibrinolysin, digests *fibrin,* thereby helping dissolve a clot.

The function of basophils is also not completely understood, although *basophilia* (increased numbers of basophils) occurs during the healing phase of inflammation and during prolonged inflammation. Basophils in the blood exit the vessels and become mast cells in the tissue. They are responsible for histamine release, resulting in increased permeability of the vessels to allow WBCs to exit the vessels at the site of injury.

Platelets

Platelets are actually small fragments of cells. They are smaller than blood cells, do not possess a cellular structure, and consist of a clear substance containing granules. The origin of platelets is the megakaryocyte, which is part of the myelogenous group of WBCs (see Fig. 35-1). Platelets are formed when the megakaryocytic membrane invaginates, fuses within the cell to separate the cytoplasm, and then fragments.

Regulation of platelet production. The life span of platelets has been estimated as 8 to 10 days. Apparently the body regulates platelets to maintain a fairly constant level (between 200,000 and 400,000/mm^3). Platelet production is probably regulated by a hormone, thrombopoietin, but the source and mode of action of this substance are unknown. Old platelets are most likely removed by the liver and spleen.

Function of platelets. The term *thrombocyte* means "clot" (thrombo) and "cell" (cyte) and accurately describes the main function of platelets. When there is a break in the continuity of a blood vessel, the platelets, which are normally round or oval disks, come in contact with the wet vessel surface and dramatically change their shape to become swollen spheres with long irregular projections called *pseudopodia* (false feet). As a result, the platelets begin to adhere to the wet endothelium and to each other. The initial platelets at the site of injury release substances that attract other thrombocytes to the area. This causes a layering of platelets, which eventually forms a plug. This plug is large enough to partially or totally occlude the opening in the vessel wall but small enough to allow blood flow to continue unimpaired through the vessel.

In small vessel tears, the platelet plug is sufficient to produce hemostasis, and additional blood coagulation is not necessary. However, when platelet counts are low, these numerous small ruptures, which occur continually in the body as a result of general functioning, are not repaired. Consequently, small hemorrhagic areas called *petechiae* form under the skin. Their appearance is similar to reddish freckles or spiderwebs.

Platelets also influence hemostasis by releasing a substance called *serotonin* at the site of injury. This substance is a vasoconstrictor that produces vascular spasm to decrease the amount of blood flow to the injured area.

ASSESSMENT OF HEMATOLOGIC FUNCTION

Several tests can be performed to assess hematologic function, including additional procedures to identify the cause of the dysfunction. The following discussion is limited to a description of the most common and one of the most valuable tests, the complete blood count (CBC). Other procedures, such as those related to iron, coagulation, and immune status, are discussed throughout the chapter as appropriate.

The CBC consists of the following determinations: RBC count, WBC count, hematocrit (Hct), hemoglobin (Hb or Hgb), differential WBC, RBC indices (mean corpuscular volume [MCV], mean corpuscular hemoglobin [MCH], mean corpuscular hemoglobin concentration [MCHC]), and peripheral smear. Additional tests may be included, such as the reticulocyte count, RBC volume distribution width (RDW), and platelet count. Each of these is summarized in Table 35-1. Most of the determinations can be performed on a small quantity of blood (micromethod) and are automatically computed. The nurse should be familiar with the significance of the findings from the CBC and aware of normal values for age, which are listed in Appendix D.

As with any other disorder, the history and physical examination are essential to identification of hematologic dysfunction, and the nurse is often the first person to suspect a problem based on information from these sources. Comments by the parent regarding the child's lack of energy, food diary of poor sources of iron, frequent infections, and bleeding that is difficult to control offer clues to the more common disorders affecting the blood. A careful physical appraisal, especially of the skin, can reveal findings such as pallor, petechiae, or bruising that may indicate minor or serious hematologic conditions. Nurses need to be aware of the clinical manifestations of blood diseases in order to assist in recognizing symptoms and establishing a diagnosis.

■ RED BLOOD CELL DISORDERS

The most common disorders affecting the blood are those that in some way alter the functino or production of RBCs. In broad terms all of the disorders produce anemia, but the causes of reduction in erythrocyte volume or hemoglobin production vary tremendously. The following presents an overview of anemia in general and specific disorders in children that produce an anemic state.

ANEMIA

Anemia is defined as reduction of red cell volume or hemoglobin concentration to levels below normal. It is not a disease itself but a manifestation of an underlying pathologic process. The anemias are the most common hematologic disorders of infancy and childhood. The following discussion is primarily concerned with an overview of the classification of anemia. Specific anemic conditions such as iron deficiency anemia, the hemoglobinopathies, and aplastic anemia are then presented in greater detail.

Classification

Anemias can be classified using two basic approaches: (1) etiology or physiology, the causes of erythrocyte and hemoglobin depletion, or (2) morphology, the characteristic changes in red cell size, shape, and color. While the morphologic classification is more useful in terms of laboratory evaluation of the anemia, the etiologic approach is more relevant to nurses because it helps direct the planning of nursing care. In anemia caused by decreased red cell production, the etiology may be dietary deficiency of iron, and the principal intervention is replenishing iron stores.

Etiology. The basic causes of anemia are (1) excessive blood loss, (2) increased destruction of RBCs, or (3) impaired or decreased rate of production. Each of these causes affects the amount of hemoglobin that is available to carry oxygen to the cells. An etiologic classification is based on the various conditions that can result from any of these physiologic changes.

Blood loss. Acute or chronic hemorrhage results in loss of plasma and all formed elements of the blood. After acute hemorrhage the body replaces plasma within 1 to 3 days, maintaining blood volume. However, this results in a low concentration of RBCs, which are gradually replaced within 3 to 4 weeks. During this period there is usually a normocytic (normal size), normochromic (normal color) anemia, provided there are sufficient iron stores for hemoglobin synthesis.

In chronic blood loss the actual number of RBCs may be normal because of continual replacement. However, insufficient iron is available to form hemoglobin as quickly as it is lost. As a result, erythrocytes are usually small in size (microcytic) and pale in color (hypochromic).

Excessive destruction. Excessive destruction or hemolysis of erythrocytes can occur from a variety of causes. One of the most common is a result of a defect within the RBC (intracorpuscular) that shortens the life span of the cell so

Table 35-1 Tests performed as part of the complete blood count

TEST (AVERAGE VALUE)*	DESCRIPTION	COMMENTS
Red blood cell (RBC) count (4.5-5.5 million/mm^3)	Number of RBCs/mm^3 of blood	Indirectly estimates Hgb content of blood Reflects function of bone marrow
Hemoglobin (Hgb) determination (11.5-15.5 g/dl)	Amount of Hgb/dl of whole blood	Total blood Hgb primarily depends on number of circulating RBCs, but also on amount of Hgb in each cell
Hematocrit (Hct) (35%-45%)	Percentage or volume of packed RBCs to whole blood	Indirectly measures Hgb content Is approximately three times Hgb content
RBC indices		
Mean corpuscular volume (MCV) (77-95 μm^3)	Average of mean volume (size) of a single RBC $MCV = \frac{Hct\ (\%) \times 10}{RBC\ count\ (millions/mm^3)}$	MCV and MCH depend on accurate counts of RBCs, whereas MCHC does not; therefore, MCHC is often more reliable All indices depend on *average* cell measurements and do not show individual RBC (anisocytosis) variations MCV values expressed as cubic microns (μm^3) or femtoliters (fl)
Mean corpuscular hemoglobin (MCH) (25-33 pg/cell)	Average or mean quantity (weight) of Hgb of a single RBC $MCH = \frac{Hgb\ (g)/dl \times 10}{RBC\ count\ (millions/mm^3)}$	MCH values expressed as picograms (pg) or micromicrograms ($\mu\mu g$)
Mean corpuscular hemoglobin concentration (MCHC) (31%-37% Hgb (g)/dl RBC)	Average concentration of Hgb in a single RBC $MCHC = \frac{Hgb\ (g)/dl \times 100}{Hct\ (\%)}$	MCHC values expressed as % Hgb (g)/cell or Hgb (g)/dl RBC
RBC volume distribution width 13.4% ± 1.2%		Average size of RBCs
Reticulocyte count (0.5%-1.5% erythrocytes)	% Reticulocytes to RBCs	Index of production of mature RBCs by red bone marrow Decreased count indicates depressed bone marrow function Increased count indicates erythrogenesis in response to some stimulus When reticulocyte count is extremely high, other forms of immature RBCs (normoblasts, even erythroblasts) may be present Indirectly estimates hypochromic anemia
White blood cell (WBC) count (4.5-13.5 × 10^3 cells/mm^3)	Number of WBCs/mm^3 of blood	Total number of WBCs less important than differential count
Differential WBC count	Inspection and quantification of WBC types present in peripheral blood	Values are expressed as percentages; to obtain absolute number of any type of WBCs, multiply its respective percentage by total number of WBCs
Neutrophils (polys) (54%-62%) (3.0-5.8 × 10^3 cells/mm^3)		Primary defense in bacterial infection; capable of phagocytizing and killing bacteria
Bands (3%-5%) (0.15-0.4 × 10^3 cells/mm^3)		Immature neutrophil Increased numbers in bacterial infection Also capable of phagocytosis and killing
Eosinophils (1%-3%) (0.05-0.25 × 10^3 cells/mm^3)		Named for their staining characteristics with eosin dye Increased in allergic disorders, parasitic diseases, certain neoplasms, and other diseases
Basophils (0.075%) (0.015-0.030 cells/mm^3)		Named for their characteristic basophilic stippling Contain histamine, but their function is unknown

*See Appendix D for normal values according to ages.

Continued.

Table 35-1 Tests performed as part of the complete blood count—cont'd

TEST (AVERAGE VALUE)	DESCRIPTION	COMMENTS
Differential WBC count—cont'd		
Lymphocytes (25%-33%; 1.5-3.0 × 10^3 cells/mm^3)		Involved in development of antibody and delayed hypersensitivity
Monocytes (3%-7%)		Large phagocytic cells that are involved in early stage of inflammatory reaction
Absolute neutrophil count (ANC) (>1000)	% neutrophils × WBC	Indicates body's capability to handle bacterial infections
Platelet count (150-400 × 10^3/mm^3)		Cellular fragments that are necessary for clotting to occur
Stained peripheral blood smear	Visual estimation of amount of Hgb in RBCs and overall size, shape, and structure of RBCs	Various staining properties of RBC structures may be evidence of immature forms of erythrocyte Shows variation in size and shape of RBCs—microcytic, macrocytic, poikilocytic (variable sizes)

that production cannot keep pace with destruction. The two examples discussed in this chapter, sickle cell anemia and thalassemia, have decreased erythrocyte life spans because of a hemoglobin defect.

Extracorpuscular factors are those conditions that cause hemolysis in otherwise normal RBCs. A classic example is blood group incompatibility, such as hemolytic disease of the newborn or consequent to mismatched blood transfusion. Other causes can be toxic drugs, burns, poisonings (such as from lead), infections such as malaria, and splenic sequestration (hypersplenism).

Impaired or decreased production. Production of RBCs can occur as a result of either bone marrow failure or deficiency of essential nutrients. Bone marrow failure may be caused by (1) replacement of bone marrow by fibrosis or by neoplastic cells, such as in leukemia, (2) depression of marrow activity from irradiation, chemicals, or drugs, or (3) interference with bone marrow activity from other systemic diseases, such as severe infection, chronic renal disease, widespread malignancy (without marrow infiltration), collagen diseases, or hypothyroidism. When depression of the hematologic system is extensive, aplastic anemia develops.

The reason for various systemic disorders affecting erythrocyte production varies according to the condition. For example, in severe chronic infection there is evidence that depression of erythropoiesis is caused by a defect in the conversion of protoporphyrin into hemoglobin. In addition, there is some degree of hemolysis, although the exact mechanism is not known.

The most common childhood anemia is a result of deficient iron supply. Besides iron as an essential component of hemoglobin synthesis, RBC production depends on amino acids, vitamins B_6, B_{12}, and C, folic acid, copper, and possibly cobalt. Chronic malnutrition causes anemia as a result of generalized protein, mineral, and vitamin deficiencies.

Pernicious anemia develops when the gastric mucosa fails to secrete sufficient amounts of intrinsic factor, which is essential for absorption of vitamin B_{12}. This type of anemia is common in the elderly as a result of physiologically decreased gastric secretions. Deprived of vitamin B_{12}, the bone marrow produces fewer but larger (macrocytic) RBCs. The erythrocytes are usually immature and, because of their extremely fragile cell membranes, are more rapidly destroyed during circulation.

Morphology. The morphologic classification provides an orderly method for ruling out certain diagnoses when establishing a cause for a particular anemia. The major characteristics of the RBC that are affected are (1) its size—which may be *normocytic* (normal), *microcytic* (small), or *macrocytic* (large)—and (2) its color—*normochromic* (normal) or *microchromic* (pale), which reflects reduced hemoglobin in the cell. These changes are also reflected in tests that measure the average or mean volume of a single RBC (mean corpuscular volume [MCV]), the mean quantity of hemoglobin in a single RBC (mean corpuscular hemoglobin [MCH]), and the mean concentration of hemoglobin in a single RBC (mean corpuscular hemoglobin concentration [MCHC]) (see Table 35-1). For example, a hypochromic microcytic anemia is characterized by a reduced MCV and MCH.

Pathophysiology and Clinical Manifestations

The basic physiologic defect caused by anemia is a decrease in the oxygen-carrying capacity of blood and consequently a reduction in the amount of oxygen available to the tissues. When the anemia has developed slowly, the child usually adapts to the declining hemoglobin level, and most children seem to have a remarkable ability to function quite well despite low levels of hemoglobin. Also, compensatory mechanisms such as a shift in the oxyhemoglobin dissociation curve may delay the development of any obvious signs.

When the hemoglobin falls sufficiently to produce clinical manifestations, the signs and symptoms are directly attributable to tissue hypoxia. Muscle weakness and easy fatigability are common. The skin is usually pale and may take on a waxy pallor in severe anemia. Cyanosis is typically not evident, because it is the result of the quantity of deoxygenated hemoglobin in arterial blood. Hemoglobin levels generally must *exceed* 5 g/dl before cyanosis is evident. Anemia is caused by decreased hemoglobin and/or RBCs, not inadequate oxygen saturation of existing hemoglobin.

Central nervous system manifestations include headache, dizziness, light-headedness, irritability, slowed thought processes, decreased attention span, apathy, and depression. Growth retardation resulting from decreased cellular metabolism and coexisting anorexia is a common finding in chronic severe anemia. It is frequently accompanied by delayed sexual maturation in the older child.

The effects of anemia on the circulatory system can be profound. A reduction in hemoglobin concentration that results in decreased oxygen-carrying capacity of the blood is associated with a compensatory increase in heart rate and cardiac output. Initially this greater cardiac output compensates for the lower oxygen-carrying capacity of the blood, since blood replenished with oxygen returns to the tissues at a faster than normal rate. However, if the body's demand on the pumping action of the heart increases, such as during exercise, infection, or emotional stress, cardiac failure may ensue.

Diagnostic Evaluation

The diagnosis depends largely on the cause of the anemia. In general, anemia may be suspected from findings on the history and physical examination, such as lack of energy, easy fatigability, and pallor, but unless the anemia is severe, the first clue to the disorder may be alterations in the CBC, such as decreased RBCs, hemoglobin, and hematocrit levels. Although some authorities define anemia by a hemoglobin below 10 or 11 g/dl, this arbitrary cutoff is inappropriate for all children, because hemoglobin levels normally vary with age (see Appendix D).

Various findings on the CBC are also significant, such as increased reticulocytes, which indicate the body's increased demand for RBCs, such as in severe anemia hemolysis. A peripheral smear may demonstrate significant changes in the shape of RBCs, such as sickled cells. As mentioned previously, tests to measure the amount of hemoglobin in a single cell are helpful in determining the cause of the anemia (Table 35-1). Rarely, a bone marrow aspiration may be necessary to evaluate the body's ability to produce normal cells, such as in leukemia and aplastic anemia. In leukemia the bone marrow is hyperplastic (producing increased numbers of cells), whereas in aplastic anemia the bone marrow is hypoplastic (producing decreased numbers of cells) or aplastic (producing no cells).

Tests for hematologic function do not always reflect the *immediate* changes occurring in the blood. For example, in acute massive hemorrhage the hemoglobin and hematocrit may not be reliable, since the plasma volume may not reequilibrate for several hours. Without the hemodilution caused by the reexpansion of the vascular space, the RBC loss may not be apparent in these laboratory tests. Consequently, assessing the quantity of blood loss in a seriously ill child may be difficult. The estimated volume of blood loss must be analyzed in conjunction with the total blood volume of the child to determine the percent of blood loss. Blood specimens obtained from central lines may more accurately reflect the patient's status than specimens obtained from an extremity, because of the vasoconstriction of the peripheral vasculature. Blood pressure changes may be a late symptom because of the compensatory mechanisms.

Therapeutic Management

The objective of medical management is to reverse the anemia by treating the underlying cause. For example, in nutritional anemias the specific deficiency is replaced. In blood loss from acute hemorrhage, RBC transfusion may be given. In instances of severe anemia, supportive medical care may include oxygen therapy, restoration of adequate blood volume, intravenous fluids, and bed rest. In addition to these general measures, more specific interventions may be implemented depending upon the cause, and these are discussed in the next sections.

Nursing Considerations

Since anemia is not a disorder but a symptom of some underlying problem, nursing care is related to determining the cause, fostering appropriate supportive and therapeutic treatments, and decreasing tissue oxygen requirements.

Assessment

The assessment of anemia includes basic techniques that are applicable to any condition. Although the physical examination yields valuable evidence regarding the severity of the anemia and some indication of its possible etiology, diagnosis primarily rests on hematologic blood studies and a careful history. In interviewing parents the nurse stresses the following areas that include tentative information regarding common causes of childhood anemia: (1) nutrition, especially dietary intake of iron, (2) past history of chronic, recurrent infection, (3) eating habits, particularly pica and ingestion of lead-based paint or other toxic agents, (4) bowel habits and presence of frank blood in stools or black, tarry stools, and (5) familial history of hereditary diseases, such as sickle cell disease or thalassemia.

The nurse should also be aware of the significance of blood tests. For example, if the blood studies show a microcytic, hypochromic anemia suggestive of iron deficiency but the parent reports an iron-rich diet, the nurse needs to pursue the nutritional history for possible discrepancies.

Nursing Diagnoses

A variety of nursing diagnoses may be evident following assessment of anemia. Some of the general aspects of nursing management are included in the Nursing Care Plan on p. 1615. Others become apparent in specific situations.

Planning

The goals of nursing care for the infant or child with anemia depend on the severity of the condition and the cause. Most children tolerate anemia well, and a priority goal is preparing them for diagnostic tests and possible transfusion. In this situation goals of care are:

1. Provide support and education to child and family.
2. Decrease tissue oxygen needs.
3. Implement safety precautions.
4. Observe for complications.

Implementation

The nursing care of an infant or child with anemia may involve a number of modalities. One of the most important is patient education about the diagnostic process and nutritional therapy if indicated. Other nursing responsibilities include administration of medications, as well as blood or blood products (usually packed RBCs).

Prepare child for laboratory tests. Usually a battery of blood tests are ordered, but, since they are generally done sequentially rather than at one time, the child is subjected to multiple finger sticks and/or venipunctures. Laboratory technicians frequently are not aware of the trauma that repeated punctures represent to a child. Therefore it is the nurse who has the responsibility of preparing the child for the tests by (1) explaining the significance of each test, particularly why the tests are not done at one time, (2) physically being with the child during the procedure whenever possible, and (3) allowing the child to play with the equipment on a doll and/or participate in the actual procedure, for example, by cleansing the finger with an alcohol swab. Older children may appreciate the opportunity to observe the blood cells under a microscope or in photographs. This is an especially important consideration if a serious blood disorder, such as leukemia, is suspected, since it serves as a foundation for explaining the pathophysiology of the disorder.

Bone marrow aspiration is not a routine hematologic test but is essential for definitive diagnosis of the leukemias, lymphomas, and certain anemias. Suggested explanations for teaching children about blood components are described in the Nursing Tip.

NURSING TIP: EXPLAINING BLOOD COMPONENTS TO CHILDREN

Red blood cells—carry the oxygen you breathe from your lungs to all parts of your body.
White blood cells—help keep germs from causing infection.
Platelets—small parts of cells that help to make bleeding stop; platelets help your body stop bleeding by forming a clot (scab) over the hurt area.
Plasma—the liquid portion of blood; has clotting factors that help make the bleeding stop.

Decrease tissue oxygen needs. Since the basic pathology in anemia is a decrease oxygen-carrying capacity in the RBCs, a nursing responsibility is to minimize tissue oxygen needs when anemia is severe enough to affect the child's energy level. In most instances of anemia this is not necessary, but when it is, several important interventions should be implemented. The child's level of tolerance for activities of daily living and play is assessed, and adjustments are made to allow as much self-care as possible without undue exertion. During periods of rest the nurse takes vital signs and observes behavior to establish a baseline of nonexertion energy expenditure. During periods of activity the nurse repeats these measurements and observations to compare them with resting values. Signs of exertion include tachycardia, palpitations, tachypnea, dyspnea, shortness of breath, hyperpnea, breathlessness, dizziness, light-headedness, diaphoresis, and change in skin color. The child looks fatigued (sagging, limp posture; slow, strained movements; inability to tolerate additional activity).

Once a baseline of physical tolerance has been established, the nurse anticipates those activities that are physically taxing, such as dressing, feeding, or getting out of bed, and allows for conservation of energy by assisting the child as needed. However, since dependency can be threatening, the child is allowed as much control in the environment as possible. For example, a child with severe anemia may be unable to walk to the bathroom but may be able to use a bedside commode or be transported in a wheelchair to the lavatory rather than having to use a bedpan. Scheduling activities throughout the day with planned rest periods in between maximizes the child's energy potential without causing undue exertion.

Diversional activities are planned that promote rest but prevent boredom and withdrawal. Since short attention span, irritability, and restlessness are common in anemia and increase stress demands on the body, appropriate activities are planned, such as listening to music; using a tape recorder; watching television; reading or listening to stories or comics; continuing a favorite hobby, such as stamp collecting, coloring, or drawing; playing board and card games; or being wheeled in a carriage or chair. Choosing the appropriate roommate, such as a child of similar age with a diagnosis that also requires restricted activity, is a major asset in preventing the boredom of imposed bed rest.

If infants or young children are hospitalized, the importance of preventing separation from parents must be considered. Crying and fretfulness place increased stress demands on the body, which increases oxygen needs. Parents need help in understanding the importance of their presence, even though the child may be less responsive than usual. The nurse also explains the reason for mood changes and the necessity of allowing the child's dependency.

Children with anemia are prone to infection because tis-

NURSING CARE PLAN
The Child with Anemia

NURSING DIAGNOSIS: Anxiety/fear related to diagnostic procedures/transfusion

GOAL 1

Support and educate child and family

INTERVENTIONS

Prepare child for tests
Remain with child during tests and initiation of transfusion
Explain purpose of blood components

EXPECTED OUTCOMES

Child and family display minimal anxiety
Child and family demonstrate an understanding of the disorder, diagnostic tests, and treatment

NURSING DIAGNOSIS: Activity intolerance related to generalized weakness, diminished oxygen delivery to tissues

GOAL 1

Minimize physical exertion

INTERVENTIONS

Anticipate and assist in those activities of daily living that may be beyond child's tolerance
Provide diversional play activities that promote rest and quiet but prevent boredom and withdrawal
Choose appropriate roommate of similar age and interests who requires restricted activity
Plan nursing activities to provide sufficient rest
Assist with activities requiring exertion

EXPECTED OUTCOME

Child plays and rests quietly and engages in activities appropriate to capabilities

GOAL 2

Increase oxygen to tissues

INTERVENTIONS

Position for optimum air exchange
Administer supplemental oxygen if needed

EXPECTED OUTCOME

Patient breathes easily; respiratory rate and depth normal (see inside front cover)

GOAL 3

Minimize emotional stress

INTERVENTIONS

Anticipate child's irritability, short attention span, and fretfulness by offering to assist child in activities rather than waiting for request for help
Encourage parents to remain with child

*Dependent nursing action.

EXPECTED OUTCOME

Child remains calm and quiet

GOAL 4

Help replace blood elements

INTERVENTIONS

*Administer blood, packed cells, platelets as prescribed (Table 35-2)

EXPECTED OUTCOME

Child receives the appropriate blood elements without incident

NURSING DIAGNOSIS: Altered nutrition: less than body requirements related to reported inadequate iron intake (less than RDA); knowledge deficit regarding iron-rich foods

GOAL 1

Promote adequate intake of iron-rich foods

INTERVENTIONS

Provide diet counseling to caregiver, especially in regard to
- Food sources of iron, e.g., meat, liver, fish, egg yolks, green leafy vegetables, legumes, nuts, whole grains, including iron-fortified infant cereal and dry cereal (see also Chapter 12)
- Feed milk as supplemental food in infant's diet after solids are begun

EXPECTED OUTCOME

Child receives at least minimum daily requirement of iron

GOAL 2

Increase body iron stores

INTERVENTIONS

*Administer iron preparations as prescribed
Instruct family regarding correct administration of oral iron preparation
- Give in divided doses (specify)
- Give between meals
- Administer with fruit juice or multivitamin preparation
- Do not give with milk or antacids

*Administer the liquid preparation with dropper, syringe, or straw to avoid contact with teeth

EXPECTED OUTCOMES

Family relates a diet history that verifies that the child complies with these suggestions
Child is given iron supplement as evidenced by green, tarry stools
Child takes medication appropriately

See also Nursing Care Plan: The Family of the Ill or Hospitalized Child, Chapter 26 sue hypoxia causes cellular dysfunction and the disturbed metabolic processes weaken the host's defenses against foreign agents. Infection also worsens the anemia by increasing metabolic needs and in instances of chronic infection also interferes with erythropoiesis and shortens the survival time of RBCs. All the usual precautions are taken to prevent infection, such as practicing thorough handwashing, appropriate room selection in a noninfectious area, restricting visitors or hospital personnel with active infection, and maintaining adequate nutrition. The nurse also observes for signs of infection, particularly temperature elevation and leukocytosis. However, an elevated WBC count sometimes occurs in anemia without the presence of systemic or local infection.

Implement safety precautions. Children with chronic anemia usually adjust to the low levels of hemoglobin remarkably well. Often it is difficult for others unfamiliar with the child's condition to recognize the actual degree of physical tolerance. The nurse needs to inform all health personnel caring for the child to be alert to signs of overexertion and to anticipate the need for assistance, particularly when getting out of bed or going for a walk. Since young children cannot verbalize their fatigue or weakness, others must rely on observation to prevent accidental injuries. The importance of safety measures such as raised side rails or the use of restraints when the young child is in a high chair or stroller should be emphasized.

Observe for complications. Multiple blood samples may present a problem with cumulative blood loss, necessitating blood replacement. This situation occurs most often in infants or young children with severe anemia. To prevent this, blood may be withdrawn through a continuous intravenous line and replaced after the exact amount needed has been tested and discarded. As a precaution, a record should be kept of the volume of blood being withdrawn. Another measure is to use micromethods of testing whenever possible to minimize the amount of blood required for the test. The nurse needs to observe for cumulative effects of blood loss, particularly signs of shock and increased hypoxia, and to explain to parents the necessity of multiple blood samples and the reason for blood replacement.

The main complication of anemia is cardiac decompensation, which can result from excessive demands on the heart as a result of increased metabolic needs or of cardiac overload during rapid blood transfusion. Signs and symptoms of heart failure are tachycardia, dyspnea, rales, moist respirations, cough, shortness of breath, and sweating. Obviously, preventing heart failure through minimizing hypoxia and transfusing blood slowly is of first priority. Packed RBCs are usually administered to prevent circulatory hypervolemia. When blood transfusions are required in severe anemia to increase the hemoglobin level, all the usual precautions for administering blood and observing for signs of transfusion reactions are instituted (Table 35-2). Technologic advances in blood banking and transfusion medicine enable the administration of only the blood component needed by the child (Table 35-3).

Oxygen may be administered to provide optimum envi-

Table 35-2 Nursing care of the child receiving blood transfusions

COMPLICATION	SIGNS/SYMPTOMS	PRECAUTIONS/NURSING RESPONSIBILITIES
▪ Immediate reactions		
Hemolytic reactions		
Most severe type, but rare Incompatible blood Intradonor incompatibility in multiple transfusions	Chills Shaking Fever Pain at needle site and along venous tract Nausea/vomiting Sensation of tightness in chest Red or black urine Headache Flank pain Progressive signs of shock and/or renal failure	Identify donor and recipient blood types and groups before transfusion is begun; verify with one other nurse or physician Transfuse blood slowly for first 15 to 20 minutes and/or initial ⅕ volume of blood; remain with patient Stop transfusion immediately in event of signs or symptoms, maintain patent intravenous line, and notify physician Save donor blood to re-crossmatch with patient's blood Monitor for evidence of shock Insert urinary catheter and monitor hourly outputs Send sample of patient's blood and urine to laboratory for presence of hemoglobin (indicates intravascular hemolysis) Observe for signs of hemorrhage resulting from disseminated intravascular coagulation (DIC) Support medical therapies to reverse shock
Febrile reactions		
Leukocyte or platelet antibodies Plasma protein antibodies	Fever Chills	May give acetaminophen for prophylaxis Leukocyte-poor RBCs are less likely to cause reaction Stop transfusion immediately; report to physician for evaluation

Table 35-2 Nursing care of the child receiving blood transfusions—cont'd

COMPLICATION	SIGNS/SYMPTOMS	PRECAUTIONS/NURSING RESPONSIBILITIES
Allergic reactions		
Recipient reacts to allergens in donor's blood	Urticaria Flushing Asthmatic wheezing Laryngeal edema	Give antihistamines for prophylaxis to children with tendency toward allergic reactions Stop transfusions immediately Administer epinephrine for wheezing or anaphylactic reaction
Circulatory overload		
Too rapid transfusion (even a small quantity) Excessive quantity of blood transfused (even slowly)	Precordial pain Dyspnea Rales Cyanosis Dry cough Distended neck veins	Transfuse blood slowly Prevent overload by using packed RBCs or administering divided amounts of blood Use infusion pump to regulate and maintain flow rate Stop transfusion immediately if signs of overload Place child upright with feet in dependent position to increase venous resistance
Air emboli		
May occur when blood is transfused under pressure	Sudden difficulty in breathing Sharp pain in chest Apprehension	Normalize pressure before container is empty when infusing blood under pressure Clear tubing of air by aspirating air with syringe at the nearest Y connector if air is observed in tubing; disconnect tubing and allow blood to flow until air has escaped only if a Y connector is not available
Hypothermia	Chills Low temperature Irregular heart rate Possible cardiac arrest	Allow blood to warm at room temperature (less than 1 hour) Use an electric warming coil to rapidly warm blood Take temperature if patient complains of chills; if subnormal, stop transfusion
Electrolyte disturbances		
Hyperkalemia (in massive transfusions or in patients with renal problems)	Nausea, diarrhea Muscular weakness Flaccid paralysis Paresthesia of extremities Bradycardia Apprehension Cardiac arrest	Use washed RBCs or fresh blood if patient at risk
▪ **Delayed reactions**		
Transmission of infection		
Hepatitis AIDS Malaria Syphilis Bacteria or viruses Other	Signs of infection, e.g., jaundice Toxic reaction: high fever, severe headache or substernal pain, hypotension, intense flushing, vomiting/diarrhea	Blood is tested for antibodies to HIV, HTLVI, hepatitis C virus, hepatitis B core antigen. In addition, blood is tested for hepatitis B surface antigen (HBsAg), alanine aminotransferase (ALT), and a serology test is performed for syphilis. Positive units are destroyed. Individuals at risk for carrying certain viruses are deferred from donation Report any sign of infection, and, if occurring during transfusion, stop transfusion immediately, send sample for culture and sensitivity tests, and notify physician
Alloimmunization		
(Antibody formation) Occurs in patients receiving multiple transfusions	Increased risk of hemolytic, febrile, and allergic reactions	Use limited number of donors Observe carefully for signs of reactions
Delayed hemolytic reaction	Destruction of RBCs and fever 5 to 10 days after transfusion	Observe for posttransfusion anemia and decreasing benefit from successive transfusions

Table 35-3 Description of blood components

COMPONENT	APPROXIMATE VOLUME (ML/U)	INDICATIONS	DOSE
Whole blood	500	Symptomatic anemia with large volume deficit	Volume of whole blood = weight (kg) × change in Hct desired × 2
RBCs	300	Symptomatic anemia	Volume PRBC = weight (kg) × change in Hct desired
RBCs, leukocytes removed	275-300	Symptomatic anemia, febrile reactions from leukocyte antibodies	Same as for RBCs
Fresh frozen plasma	150	Deficit of labile and stable plasma coagulation factors and thrombotic thrombocytopenic purpura (TTP)	Varies
Cryoprecipitate with antihemophilic factor (AHF)	15—containing 80 or more units of factor VIII (FVIII-c) and at least 150 mg of fibrinogen	Hemophilia A von Willebrand disease Hypofibrinogenemia Factor XIII deficiency	Varies
Platelets—single donor	40-70	Bleeding from thrombocytopenia or platelet function abnormality	0.1 U/kg will raise the count by 40,000/mm^3 at 1 hour
Platelets can also be produced by pheresis	200-500		
Granulocytes (pheresis)	200-300	Neutropenia with infection	
Factor VIII concentrate	Varies	Hemophilia A	1 U/kg body weight for each 0.02 U/ml (2%) increase
Prothrombin complex (factors II, VII, IX, and X)	Varies	Hereditary II, VII, IX, X deficiency Hemophilia B (IX deficiency)	

ronmental conditions for hemoglobin saturation. However, oxygen is of limited value because each gram of hemoglobin is able to carry a limited amount of the gas. In addition, prolonged supplemental oxygen can decrease erythropoiesis. Therefore the child is monitored closely for evidence of decreasing benefit from oxygen. One of the first signs of hypoxia is restlessness.

Observe for complications of blood transfusions. Any blood transfusion carries attendant risks. Since the child may require multiple transfusions for several years, the possibility of complications is increased. It is critical for the nurse assisting in this procedure always to be suspicious for signs indicative of a reaction. Table 35-2 summarizes the major hazards of transfusions, the signs and symptoms commonly associated with each, and nursing responsibilities.

Although hemolytic reactions are rare, ABO incompatibility remains the most common cause of death from blood transfusion, and human error is usually responsible (administration of wrong type to patient or mislabeling of blood product) (Kasprisin, 1986). Blood is usually matched between the donor and recipient for blood groups (A, B, AB, or O) and Rh factors (positive or negative). (See Chapter 9 for a discussion of blood groups and ABO and Rh incompatibility.) When blood is mismatched, the A or B antiagglutinin is mixed with RBCs containing A or B agglutinogens, respectively, and agglutination of the RBCs occurs. The agglutinins, which are bivalent, attach themselves to two different erythrocytes at the same time, causing the cells to clump together and clog small blood vessels. Over a few hours to days, the entrapped cells degenerate and hemolyze, liberating excessive quantities of hemoglobin into the circulation. The eventual hemolysis of large numbers of RBCs decreases the blood volume, causing circulatory failure and *shock*. Treatment is aimed at replacing lost blood and using plasma volume expanders.

Acute kidney shutdown and eventual *renal failure* are the result of renal vasoconstriction from antigen-antibody complexes derived from the red cell surface. The greatly reduced blood flow causes complete renal failure and death within 7 to 12 days. Treatment involves promoting diuresis with rapid dilute intravenous fluids and diuretics, such as furosemide and mannitol, and alkalinizing body fluids, which render hemoglobin more soluble.

Another consequence of hemolysis is the release of large quantities of phospholipids, which are capable of stimulating disseminated intravascular coagulation (DIC) (p. 1641). As a result, the plasma is depleted of the necessary coagulation factors needed to prevent hemorrhage. Without treatment with heparin to prevent the coagulation and blood components to initiate clotting, death from generalized hemorrhage can occur.

Besides the nursing precautions and responsibilities outlined in Table 35-2, some general guidelines that apply to all transfusions include:

1. Take vital signs and blood pressure *before* administering blood to establish baseline data for posttransfusion comparison, then every 15 minutes for 1 hour while blood is infusing.
2. Check the identification of the recipient with the donor's blood group and type, regardless of the blood product used.
3. Administer the first 50 ml of blood or ⅕ volume (whichever is smaller) *slowly* and stay with the child.
4. Administer with normal saline on a piggyback setup.
5. Administer blood through an appropriate filter to eliminate particles in the blood and prevent the precipitation of formed elements.
6. Use blood within 30 minutes of its arrival from the blood bank; if it is not used, return to blood bank—do not store in regular unit refrigerator.
7. If a reaction of any type is suspected, stop the transfusion, maintain a patent intravenous line with normal saline and new tubing, notify the physician, and do not restart the blood until the child's condition has been medically evaluated.

When the blood is started, the filter chamber is filled to allow the total filter to be used. The drip chamber is partially filled with blood to permit counting of the drops. In adjusting the flow rate, it is important to remember that blood administration sets do not use microdrops (60 drops/ml) but regular drops (usually 10 or 15 drops/ml). Therefore, when administering the first 50 ml of blood, the nurse adjusts the flow rate to 16 drops per minute to infuse this amount in 30 minutes. If no reaction occurs, the flow rate is increased accordingly to infuse the remainder of blood within 2 hours. For example, if a unit of 275 ml of blood is to be given, a flow rate of 19 drops per minute permits the remaining 225 ml to be infused in 2 hours. (These calculations are based on 10 drops/ml.) A unit of blood should be infused within 4 hours. If the infusion will exceed this time, the blood should be divided by the blood bank and the unused portion refrigerated under controlled conditions.

Evaluation

The effectiveness of nursing interventions is determined by continual reassessment and evaluation of care based on the following observational guidelines and expected outcomes:

1. Provide support and education to child and family.
2. Monitor effectiveness of therapeutic interventions, especially child's activity tolerance.
3. Observe environment for appropriate safety measures.
4. Monitor child for reactions to blood transfusions or signs of worsening conditions.

Expected outcomes:
See Nursing Care Plan, p. 1615.

IRON DEFICIENCY ANEMIA

Anemia caused by an inadequate supply of dietary iron is the most prevalent nutritional disorder in the United States and the most common mineral disturbance. It most frequently occurs in children between 6 and 36 months of age with a peak between 10 to 15 months (Lanzkowsky, 1985). Adolescents are also at risk because of their rapid growth rate combined with poor feeding or eating habits. Premature infants are especially at risk because of their reduced fetal iron supply.

Reports on the prevalence of iron deficiency vary widely and are complicated by the lack of acceptable definitions of anemia. However, using a diagnosis of anemia as hemoglobin level below 10 g/dl, the reported incidence of iron deficiency in children between 6 and 36 months varies from 17% to 44% (Lanzkowsky, 1985). In general, iron deficiency anemia is more common in black children and in children from inner city areas attending clinics than in children from private practice settings (Lukens, 1984). Although no socioeconomic group is spared, this difference probably reflects the influence of socioeconomic status on adequate nutritional intake. However, this is changing; the prevalence of iron deficiency anemia has declined from 7.8% in 1975 to 2.9% in 1985 (Yip and others, 1987a). This decline is attributed primarily to supplemental programs, such as Women, Infants, and Children (WIC), which improve the iron intake in infants by altering feeding patterns (increased breastfeeding and use of commercial formula rather than whole cow's milk) (Miller, Swaney, and Deinard, 1985; Ryan and Martinez, 1985).

Etiology

Iron deficiency anemia can be caused by any number of factors that decrease the supply of iron, impair its absorption, increase the body's need for iron, or affect the synthesis of hemoglobin (Box 35-1). Although the clinical manifestations and diagnostic evaluation are quite similar regardless of the cause, the therapeutic and nursing considerations depend on the specific reason for the iron deficiency. The following discussion is limited to iron deficiency anemia resulting from inadequate iron in the diet.

At birth the full-term infant's supply of iron is approximately 300 mg, or 75 mg/kg of body weight. The majority of iron has been transferred from the mother at the rate of 4 mg per day during the last trimester. The bulk of the iron is stored in the circulating hemoglobin of the erythrocytes; the rest is deposited in the liver, spleen, and bone marrow. Maternal iron stores are adequate for the first 5 to 6 months of age in the full-term infant but only for about 2 to 3 months in premature infants or infants of multiple births. When exogenous sources of iron are not supplied to meet the infant's growth demands following depletion of fetal iron stores, iron deficiency anemia results. Physiologic anemia should not be confused with iron deficiency anemia resulting from nutritional causes (see Chapter 12).

Box 35-1 CAUSES OF IRON DEFICIENCY ANEMIA

1. Inadequate supply of iron
   a. Deficient dietary intake
      (1) Rapid growth rate
      (2) Excessive milk intake, delayed addition of solid foods
      (3) Poor general eating habits
   b. Inadequate iron stores at birth
      (1) Low birth weight, premature, multiple births
      (2) Severe iron deficiency in mother (hemoglobin level below 9 g/dl)
      (3) Fetal blood loss at or before delivery
2. Impaired absorption
   a. Presence of iron inhibitors
      (1) Phytates, phosphates, or oxalates
      (2) Gastric alkalinity
   b. Malabsorptive disorders
   c. Chronic diarrhea
3. Blood loss
   a. Acute or chronic hemorrhage
   b. Parasitic infestation
4. Excessive demands for iron required for growth
   a. Prematurity
   b. Adolescence
   c. Pregnancy
5. Inability to form hemoglobin
   a. Lack of vitamin B_{12} (pernicious anemia)
   b. Folic acid deficiency

Pathophysiology

Iron is required for the production of hemoglobin. One hemoglobin molecule consists of protein (globin) combined with four molecules of a pigmented compound (heme). Each molecule of heme contains one atom of iron. When iron stores are deficient, the production of hemoglobin is reduced. Consequently, the main effect of iron deficiency is decreased hemoglobin and reduced oxygen-carrying capacity of the blood.

Clinical Manifestations

The clinical manifestations are directly attributed to the reduction in the amount of oxygen available to tissues and resemble those seen in any type of anemia. Usually the signs are insidious and obscure, and the severity is directly related to the duration of the dietary deficiency.

Although the majority of infants with iron deficiency anemia are underweight, many are overweight because of excessive milk ingestion (known as *milk baby*). These children become anemic for two reasons. Milk, a poor source of iron, is given almost to the exclusion of solid foods, and some infants fed cow's milk have an increased fecal loss of blood. This asymptomatic loss can be large enough to cause iron deficiency (Ziegler and others, 1990). Although chubby, these infants are pale, usually demonstrate poor muscle development, and are prone to infection. The skin color may be described as porcelain-like.

Although the mechanism is unknown, iron deficiency anemia enhances the leakage of plasma proteins in infants, causing edema, retarded growth, and decreased serum concentration of the proteins albumin, gamma globulin, and transferrin, a protein that binds iron and transports it through the plasma. Other less common manifestations of iron deficiency include glossitis, angular stomatitis, and koilonychia (concave or "spoon" fingernails). The precise relationship of iron deficiency anemia to behavioral and intellectual functioning is not clear, but increasing evidence suggests that iron deficiency, alone or with anemia, results in impaired cognitive skills that may or may not reverse after correction of the iron-deficient state (Deinard and others, 1986; Lozoff and others, 1987; Walter and others, 1989).

Diagnostic Evaluation

Since iron deficiency primarily affects hemoglobin synthesis, laboratory tests that measure or describe hemoglobin, the morphologic changes in the RBC, and iron concentration are usually performed. The RBC count may be normal, borderline, or moderately reduced. Typically the almost normal number of erythrocytes is strikingly out of proportion to the hemoglobin concentration, which is below normal for the child's age. Although the RBC count may be normal, RBCs are typically small in size. Consequently, this alteration is expressed in a lowered hematocrit level (usually below 33%), since the microcytic RBCs pack together into a smaller volume, regardless of their actual number. The mean corpuscular volume is decreased, since the size of the RBC is affected. For infants near 1 year of age, a mean corpuscular volume below 70 μm^3 is considered diagnostic, whereas in the preschool and older child an MCV of 75 μm^3 is usually the lower limit of normal.

The reticulocyte count is usually normal or slightly reduced because of decreased stores of iron. However, in severe anemia when tissue hypoxia exerts an erythropoietic response, the reticulocyte count may be elevated to 3% or 4%. The level of erythrocyte protoporphyrin (EP), the immediate precursor of heme, becomes elevated in red blood cells whenever heme synthesis is disturbed. An EP level of 35 μg/dl or above can be used as a screening test for anemia (Yip, Schwartz, and Deinard, 1983).

In terms of differential diagnosis, a stool analysis for occult blood (guaiac test) is commonly performed to confirm or rule out the possibility of chronic fecal blood loss, especially from milk intolerance or structural anomalies such as diverticulitis.

Iron studies. In addition to those tests that indirectly indicate the level of iron by the effects of iron deficiency on the RBC, several other tests are usually performed that more directly measure the amount of circulating iron. The serum-iron concentration (SIC) measures the amount of circulating iron and normally is about 70 μg/dl in infants and slightly higher in older children. Lower limits of serum iron vary not only with age but also with time of day; they are highest in the morning, when the test should be performed (Lanzkowsky, 1985).

The total iron-binding capacity (TIBC) measures the amount of transferrin or iron-binding globulin, which is necessary for the transport of iron in the bloodstream. When combined with transferrin, the iron is loosely bound to the globulin molecule so that it can be released easily to tissue cells anywhere in the body. In iron deficiency anemia the TIBC is elevated above the normal range of 350 μg/dl (6 months to 2 years) or 450 μg/dl (children older than 2 years and adults). The elevated TIBC represents the body's compensatory mechanisms to absorb more exogenous sources of iron during states of deficiency than normally. The combination of a reduced SIC and an elevated TIBC is of significant diagnostic value because it is not found in any other condition, except hypochromic, microcytic anemia caused by inadequate intake or absorption of iron. The transferrin saturation is calculated by dividing the SIC by the TIBC and multiplying the result by 100 to express the value as a percentage. A transferrin saturation of 10% suggests anemia.

Therapeutic Management

Prevention is the primary goal and is achieved through optimum nutrition and appropriate iron supplementation. In infants the American Academy of Pediatrics has set forth guidelines to prevent iron deficiency (Box 35-2). The recommendations for feeding include iron supplementation primarily through food sources, except for preterm breast-fed infants, whose iron needs may exceed those supplied through human milk. In formula-fed infants the most convenient and best sources of supplemental iron are iron-fortified commercial formula and iron-fortified infant cereal. Iron-fortified formula provides a relatively constant and predictable amount of iron and is not associated with an increased incidence of gastrointestinal symptoms, such as colic, diarrhea, or constipation. Children receiving cow's milk formula should be given heat-treated milk products such as evaporated milk rather than fresh cow's milk to decrease the possibility of iron deficiency from gastrointestinal blood loss occurring from allergy to the milk protein.

Past infancy, prevention is accomplished through sound nutritional practices. Unfortunately, this becomes increasingly difficult to ensure during adolescence, when the growth rate is increased and the food practices of these youngsters are less than ideal. Consequently, daily iron supplementation may be needed, especially in menstruating girls, to prevent the development of iron deficiency.

Iron deficiency anemia is usually treated with oral iron supplements. Dietary addition of iron-rich foods is usually inadequate to provide sufficient supplemental quantities of iron. Ferrous iron is more readily absorbed than ferric iron, resulting in higher hemoglobin levels. Ingested iron is absorbed largely from the duodenum, and absorption is facilitated by an acid environment. Children absorb an average of 10% to 20% of oral iron supplements, but during periods of iron deficiency they absorb an additional 5% to 10%. Oral iron supplements are prescribed in daily doses of 10 to 15 mg for approximately 4 months to replace body stores. Ideally the daily dose of iron should be given in two or three divided doses between meals. Side effects of oral iron therapy include nausea, gastric irritation, diarrhea or constipation, and anorexia, but they occur infrequently, especially in infants (Reeves and Yip, 1985). If the iron produces vomiting and diarrhea, it should be administered with meals and in gradually increasing doses.

Response to oral iron therapy is reflected in a peak increase in reticulocyte count by the fifth to the tenth day of administration. Following the reticulocyte rise, the hemoglobin and hematocrit levels and RBC count increase. The hemoglobin level rises an average of 0.17 to 0.25 g/dl/day; therefore a substantial increase should occur by the end of 1 month.

Parenteral iron therapy may be used if hemoglobin levels fail to raise after 1 month of oral therapy. The most common cause of failure of oral iron therapy is noncompliance. Since parenteral iron can cause a fatal anaphylactic reaction, every attempt should be made to encourage adequate therapy with oral supplements. If iron dextran (Imferon) is ordered, it must be injected deeply into a large muscle mass using the Z-tract method to minimize skin staining and irritation or administered intravenously.

Transfusions are indicated for the severest degree of anemia, in cases of serious infection, cardiac dysfunction, or surgical emergency when anesthesia is required. Packed red cells, not whole blood, should be used to minimize the chance of circulatory overload. Supplemental oxygen is administered when tissue hypoxia is severe.

Box 35-2 RECOMMENDATIONS FOR INFANT FEEDING TO PREVENT IRON DEFICIENCY ANEMIA

Begin iron supplementation (preferably iron-fortified commercial formula or in breast-fed infants, iron-fortified infant cereal) to provide 1 mg/kg/day of iron by 4 to 6 months of age in full-term infants and by 2 months in preterm infants.

Administer iron (ferrous sulfate) drops at a dose of 2 to 3 mg/kg/day to a maximum of 15 mg/day to breast-fed preterm infants after 2 months of age and iron-fortified infant cereal when solid foods are introduced.

Use commercial infant formula or other sterilized milk products, rather than fresh whole cow's milk, as substitutes for breast milk during first 9 to 12 months.

Limit amount of milk or formula feeding to no more than 1 L/day to encourage intake of iron-rich solid foods.

Modified from Committee on Nutrition: Pediatric nutrition handbook, ed. 2, Elk Grove Village, IL, 1985, American Academy of Pediatrics.

Nursing Considerations

The main nursing objective is prevention of nutritional anemia through parent education. Nurses need to be aware of recommendations regarding iron supplementation during infancy and appropriate sources of dietary iron. One of the difficulties in terms of infant feeding is encouraging parents to limit the quantity of milk, use iron-fortified infant formulas, and introduce solid foods when they believe milk is best for the infant and equate the resultant weight gain with a "healthy child." Although milk is an excellent food, it is deficient in iron, vitamin C, zinc, and fluoride. Sources of each of these nutrients and the role they play in preventing deficiencies need to be discussed with the family, especially the person who is responsible for feeding the infant. For example, the mother may have less decision-making power regarding feeding than the grandmother who cares for the child.

It is also stressed that overweight is not synonymous with good health. If the infant has obvious signs of anemia such as pallor, listlessness, frequent infections, and muscular weakness, they are pointed out as evidence of suboptimum health. In some instances it is helpful to chart the hemoglobin or hematocrit values to visually impress on parents the change in iron levels. Often increased blood values correspond to improved physical status and reinforce the benefit of dietary or oral iron supplementation.

Instructing parents regarding proper administration of oral iron supplements is an essential nursing responsibility. Several factors affect the absorption of iron, such as stomach acidity (see Table 13-2). Ideally iron supplements are administered in two divided doses between meals when the presence of free hydrochloric acid is greatest and are accompanied with a citrus fruit or juice, which helps reduce iron to its most soluble state. An inadequate dietary intake of calcium helps bind and remove agents such as phosphates and phytates that react with iron to render it insoluble. In cultures in which tea is drunk as a common beverage, iron should be administered with some other liquid, because the tannins in tea form an insoluble complex with iron from foods other than meat (Merhav and others, 1985). When adequate dosage is reached, the stools usually turn a tarry green color. The nurse advises parents of this normally expected change and inquires about its occurrence on follow-up visits. Absence of the greenish-black stool may be a clue to poor compliance. If compliance is an issue, every effort should be made to institute strategies to improve adherence to the medication regimen, such as administering the drug once a day at the most convenient time (see Compliance, Chapter 27).

Oral iron supplements are available in liquid or tablet form. Since liquid preparations may temporarily stain the teeth, the medication should be taken through a straw or given through a syringe or medicine dropper placed toward the back of the mouth. Brushing the teeth after administration of the drug lessens the discoloration. Because iron ingested in excessive quantities is toxic, even fatal, parents should keep no more than a 1-month supply in the home and store it safely away from the reach of children.

Counseling families whose children are anemic is often a difficult and challenging task. Meal planning must be based on their budget, cultural pattern, and food preferences. Often this requires more than a brief discussion with the mother or usual caregiver about foods high in iron (see Table 13-2). For teaching to be effective, the nurse may need to offer recipes, assist in planning a shopping list, and investigate food prices for economy. Since the physical effects of anemia are insidious, parents may not consider their child ill and consequently may view the medication and diet changes as unnecessary. Stressing what the physical and behavioral improvements will be and what effect the improved diet will have on all family members may encourage parents to adhere to the treatment plan.

SICKLE CELL DISEASE

Sickle cell disease is part of a group of diseases called *hemoglobinopathies.* In these diseases the normal adult hemoglobin (hemoglobin A or HbA) is partly or completely replaced by a hemoglobin variant, including fetal hemoglobin (HbF). Sickle cell disease includes all those hereditary disorders, the clinical, hematologic, and pathologic features of which are related to the presence of sickle hemoglobin (HbS).

In the United States the most common forms of sickle cell disease are:

1. Sickle cell trait, the heterozygous form of the disease (HbA and HbS or HbSA)
2. Sickle cell anemia, the homozygous form of the disease (HbSS)
3. Sickle cell–hemoglobin C disease, a variant of sickle cell anemia including both HbS and HbC
4. Sickle cell–hemoglobin E disease, a variant of sickle cell anemia in which glutamic acid has been substituted for lysine in the number 26 position of the beta chain
5. Sickle cell–thalassemia disease, a combination of sickle cell trait and β-thalassemia trait

Sickle cell disease is found primarily in the black race, although infrequently it affects whites, especially those of Mediterranean descent. The incidence of the disease varies in different geographic locations. Among American blacks, the incidence of sickle cell trait is about 8%. In West Africa the incidence is reported to be as high as 40% among native blacks. The high incidence of sickle cell trait in these individuals is believed by some to be the result of selective protection of trait carriers against malaria caused by *Plasmodium falciparum* (Pearson, 1984).

Of the sickle cell diseases, sickle cell anemia is the most common form in black Americans in the United States, followed by sickle cell–hemoglobin C disease. Another beta chain variant, hemoglobin E, is found primarily in people of Southeast Asian origin. People who carry the trait for hemoglobin E are completely asymptomatic, but those who are homozygous exhibit a disease clinically similar to hemoglobin C disease.

Mode of Transmission

Sickle cell disease is an autosomal disorder. The expected pattern of transmission from two parents who carry the heterozygous gene HbSA is illustrated in Fig. 5-4. In the United States it is estimated that one in 12 black persons carries the trait; therefore the risk of two black parents having a child with the disease is 0.7%. The occurrence of other forms of sickle cell disease is the result of union between two individuals who carry the heterozygous form of variants of sickle cell trait.

Basic Defect

The basic defect responsible for the sickling effect of erythrocytes is in the globin fraction of hemoglobin, which is composed of 574 amino acids. Hemoglobin S differs from hemoglobin A in the substitution of only one amino acid (valine) for another (glutamine) at the sixth position of the β-polypeptide chain. Under conditions of decreased oxygen tension and lowered pH, the relatively insoluble hemoglobin S changes its molecular structure to form long, slender crystals. The rapid growth of these filamentous crystals causes tenting of the cell membrane and the formation of crescent- or sickle-shaped red blood cells. The filamentous forms are associated with much greater viscosity than the normal holly-leaf structure of hemoglobin A.

The tendency to sickle is also related to the concentration of hemoglobin within the cell. Since hypertonicity of the blood plasma increases the intracellular concentration of hemoglobin, dehydration promotes sickling. In most instances the sickling response is reversible under conditions of adequate oxygenation and hydration. During this time the red blood cells are indistinguishable from normal erythrocytes on peripheral examination.

Although the defect is inherited at the time of conception, the sickling phenomenon is usually not apparent until later in infancy because of the presence of fetal hemoglobin (HbF). HbF is composed of two alpha and two gamma polypeptide chains. At 32 weeks' gestation, the production of beta and delta chains begins. These combine with alpha chains to form the major adult hemoglobins, HbA (two alpha and two beta chains) and HbA_2 (two alpha and two delta chains). As long as HbF persists, sickling does not occur, because there are no beta chains carrying the defect. The newborn has from 60% to 80% fetal hemoglobin, but this rapidly decreases during the first year, so that sickling becomes apparent after 4 months of age.

Sickle cell trait. Persons with sickle cell trait have the same basic defect, but only about 34% to 45% of the total hemoglobin is hemoglobin S (Pearson, 1984). The remainder is HbA. Normally these individuals are asymptomatic. However, under conditions of extreme or prolonged deoxygenation, such as strenuous physical exercise, anesthesia, infection, pulmonary disease, anemia, high-altitude environments, underwater swimming, or pregnancy, sickling crises may occur. The higher the percentage of hemoglobin S, the more likely the occurrence of symptomatic responses.

Pathophysiology and Clinical Manifestations

The pathologic changes in sickle cell anemia are primarily the result of (1) increased blood viscosity and (2) increased red blood cell destruction (Fig. 35-2). The entanglement and enmeshing of rigid sickle-shaped cells with one another increases the internal friction of the suspension, thus increasing blood viscosity. The thickened blood slows the circulation, causing capillary stasis, obstruction by elongated and pointed erythrocytes, and thrombosis. Eventually tissue ischemia and necrosis result with pathologic changes in the following sites.

Spleen. Initially the spleen becomes enlarged from congestion and engorgement with sickled cells. Eventually the sinuses are compressed and infarctions result. The functioning cells are gradually replaced with fibrotic tissue, until eventually in severe stages of the disease the spleen is decreased in size and totally replaced by a fibrous mass, resulting in functional asplenia. Without the spleen to filter bacteria and to promote the release of large numbers of phagocytic cells, these individuals are highly susceptible to infection.

Liver. The liver is also altered in form and function. Liver failure and necrosis are the result of severe impairment of hepatic blood flow from anemia and capillary obstruction. The liver is usually enlarged as a result of blood stasis and is occasionally tender. With progressive focal necrosis and subsequent scarring, cirrhosis eventually occurs.

Kidney. Kidney abnormalities are probably the result of the same cycle of congestion of glomerular capillaries and tubular arterioles with sickle cells and hemosiderin, tissue necrosis, and eventual scarring. The principal results of kidney ischemia are hematuria, inability to concentrate urine, enuresis, and occasionally nephrotic syndrome.

Bones. The hyperplasia and congestion of the bone marrow result in osteoporosis, widening of the medullary spaces, and thinning of the cortices. As a result of the weakening of bone, especially in the lumbar and thoracic regions, skeletal deformities, particularly lordosis and kyphosis, may occur. From chronic hypoxia, the bone becomes susceptible to osteomyelitis, frequently from *Salmonella.* Aseptic necrosis of the femoral head from chronic ischemia is an occasional problem.

Vaso-occlusive crises can result in a variety of skeletal problems. One of the more frequent is the *hand-foot syndrome,* which occurs primarily in young children ages 6 months to 2 years. It is caused by infarction of short tubular bones and is characterized by pain and swelling of the soft tissue over the hands and feet. It usually resolves spontaneously within a couple of weeks. Localized swelling over joints with arthralgia can occur from erythrostasis with sickle cells.

Central nervous system. Changes in the central nervous system are primarily vascular from the same cyclic reaction of stasis, thrombosis, and ischemia. Stroke or cerebrovascular accident is a major complication and can result in permanent paralysis or death. Any number of neurologic symptoms can herald a minor cerebral insult, such as headache, aphasia, weakness, convulsions, or visual disturbances. Loss of vision is usually the result of progressive retinopathy and retinal detachment. One study suggests cognitive impairment from sickle cell anemia. Affected children scored 1 standard deviation (SD) below siblings on most cognitive measures (Swift and others, 1989).

Heart. Cardiac problems are mainly attributable to the stress of chronic anemia, which can eventually result in decompensation and failure. Myocardial infarctions may also occur from stasis and thrombosis.

Blood. With the formation of sickled erythrocytes, mechanical fragility is increased, thereby decreasing the red blood cell's life span. Hemolysis occurs both during intravascular circulation and as a result of stagnation of sickled cells in the congested spleen. Although the body attempts to compensate through stimulated erythropoietic activity, as evidenced by a hyperplastic bone marrow, the rate of destruction exceeds the rate of production. A normocytic, nor-

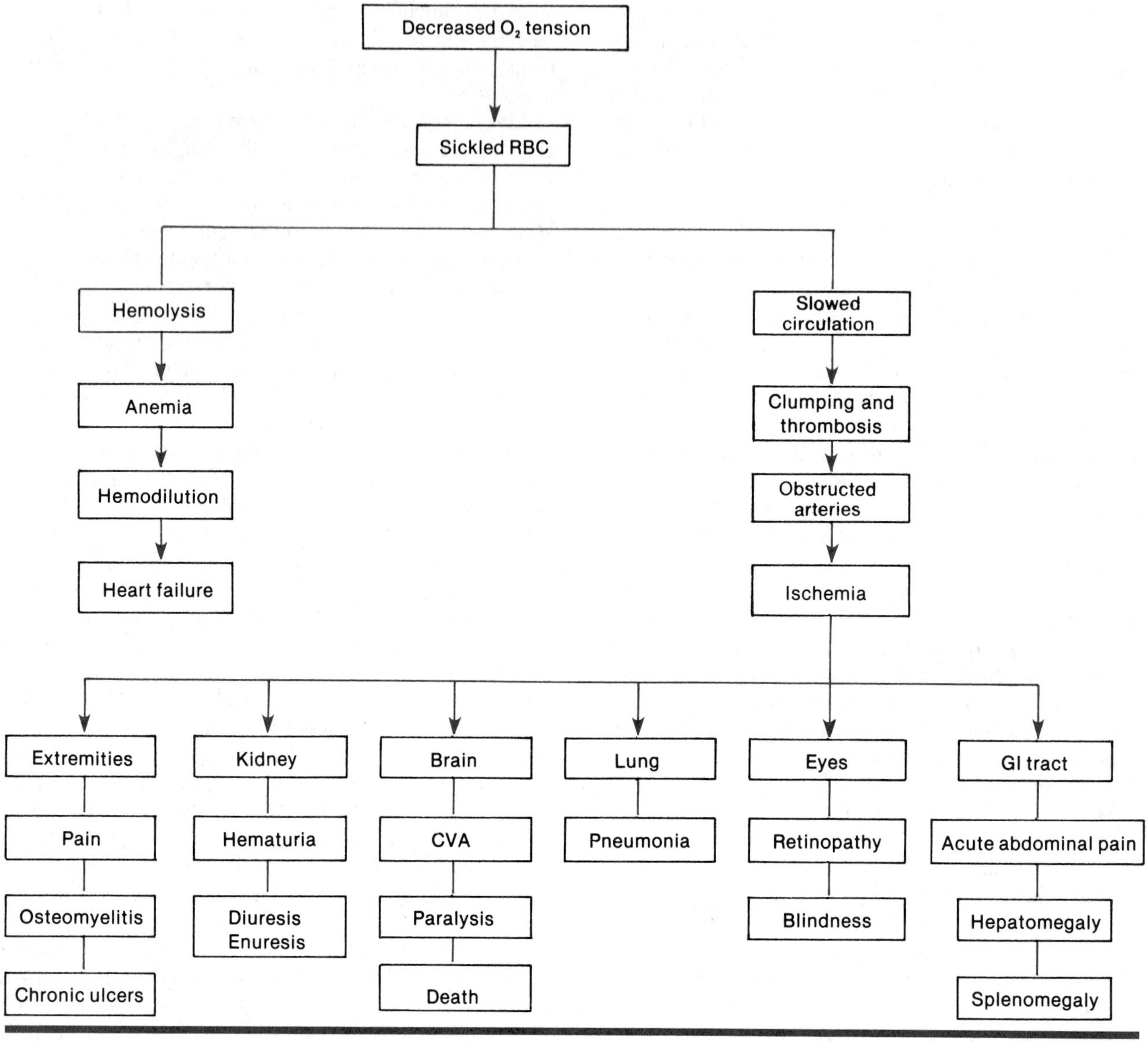

Fig. 35-2. Tissue effects of sickle cell anemia.

mochromic anemia results. With increased hemolysis, hemosiderosis (increased storage of iron) is present in the liver, spleen, bone marrow, kidneys, and lymph nodes (see p. 1631).

Other signs and symptoms. In addition to the effects of sickling on various organ structures, the child with sickle cell anemia may have a variety of complaints, such as weakness; anorexia; joint, back, and abdominal pain; fever; and vomiting. Chronic leg ulcers are common in adolescents and adults and are thought to be the result of thrombosis and decreased peripheral circulation. Other generalized effects include growth retardation in both height and weight, delayed sexual maturation, decreased fertility, and priapism (constant penile erection). If the child reaches adulthood, sexual development and adult height are usually achieved.

Sickle cell crisis. The clinical manifestations of sickle cell anemia vary markedly in severity and frequency. The most acute symptoms of the disease occur during periods of exacerbation called *crises,* which are usually precipitated by infection. There are four types of episodic crises—vaso-occlusive, splenic sequestration, aplastic, and hyperhemolytic.

Vaso-occlusive crises are the most common and the only painful ones. They are the result of sickled cells obstructing the blood vessels, causing occlusion, ischemia, and potentially necrosis. The major symptoms of this crisis are fever, acute abdominal pain from visceral hypoxia, hand-foot syndrome, and arthralgia, without an exacerbation of anemia.

Splenic sequestration crises are caused by the spleen sequestering (pooling) large quantities of blood, causing a precipitous drop in blood volume and ultimately shock. The crisis may be acute or chronic. The chronic manifestation is termed *functional asplenia.* The acute form occurs most commonly in children between 8 months and 5 years of age and may result in death from profound anemia and cardiovascular collapse.

Aplastic crisis is diminished red blood cell production, usually triggered by a viral (especially the human parvovirus) or other infection (Gowda and others, 1987). When it is superimposed on the existing rapid destruction of red blood cells, a profound anemia results.

Another type of bone marrow crisis is *megaloblastic anemia,* which is attributed to an excessive nutritional need for folic acid and/or vitamin B_{12} during periods of pronounced erythropoiesis. Since infection is not always antecedent to aplastic or hypoplastic crises, it is possible that folic acid deficiency is a causative agent.

Hyperhemolytic crisis occurs when there is an even greater rate of red blood cell destruction characterized by anemia, jaundice, and reticulocytosis. It is a rare complication and frequently suggests other coexisting abnormalities, such as glucose-6-phosphate dehydrogenase (G6PD) deficiency, which is also common in black persons.

Diagnostic Evaluation

Although sickle cell anemia has been reported during the neonatal period and early part of infancy, it may not be recognized until the toddler and preschool period, during a crisis precipitated by an acute upper respiratory or gastrointestinal infection. However, early diagnosis (before 3 months of age) facilitates initiation of appropriate interventions to minimize complications. Several tests are available for detecting sickle cell disease. Although most of the routine hematologic tests described in Table 35-1 are done primarily to evaluate the anemia, this discussion focuses on the tests specifically used to detect the homozygous or heterozygous form of the disease.

For screening purposes the Sickledex is commonly used. If the test is positive, hemoglobin electrophoresis is necessary to distinguish between those children with the trait and those with the disease. Screening for sickle cell trait has become a controversial subject, especially among the black community, since there is no method of preventing the disease other than selective birth procedures. This subject is discussed in more detail under Nursing Considerations.

Stained blood smear. Examination of the stained smear of blood may reveal a few sickled red blood cells. However, since the erythrocyte assumes its normal discoid shape under adequate oxygenation, no sickled cells may be present even in the homozygous form of the disease. Whenever sickle cells are found, the diagnosis is usually positive for sickle cell anemia, not sickle cell trait.

Sickle-turbidity test (Sickledex). In this test anticoagulated blood is mixed with a special solution. Since hemoglobin S is normally much less soluble than hemoglobin A or F (as well as other variants), when mixed with this solution it is insoluble and forms a cloudy or turbid mixture. All other forms of hemoglobin result in a clear suspension. This test is a reliable screening method because it can be done on blood from a fingerstick and yields accurate results in 3 minutes. However, it is not specific for the trait or disease and yields false negatives in children whose hemoglobin is less than 10 g/dl or in infants less than 4 to 6 months of age who have not completely converted to adult hemoglobin.

Hemoglobin electrophoresis ("fingerprinting"). In this test the blood is specially prepared and separated into various hemoglobins by high-voltage electrophoresis. The resulting pattern of the separated peptides as it appears on paper is referred to as "fingerprinting" of the protein. This test is accurate, rapid, and specific for detecting the homozygous and heterozygous forms of the disease, as well as the percentages of the various hemoglobins.

Newborn screening. Screening for sickle cell anemia in the newborn period can identify children with hemoglobinopathies. Early diagnosis can facilitate parent education and medical intervention. There has been a decrease in the death rate from splenic sequestration. Parents are taught to palpate the child's abdomen and seek medical attention if splenic enlargement is present (Leiken and others, 1989; Pappo and Buchanan, 1989).

Therapeutic Management

There is no cure for sickle cell anemia. The aims of therapy are (1) to prevent the sickling phenomenon, which is responsible for the pathologic sequelae, and (2) to treat the medical emergency of sickle cell crisis.

Prevention of sickling. Prevention of sickling involves promoting adequate oxygenation and maintaining hemodilution. The successful implementation of these two goals often depends more on nursing intervention than on medical therapies. Research is investigating antisickling agents such as ethacrynic acid analogs and the induction of hyponatremia to induce hydration (Charache, 1986).

Treatment of crisis. More often medical management is directed at supportive and symptomatic treatment of crises. Although specific treatments are warranted in different types of crises, the main general objectives include (1) bed rest to minimize energy expenditure and oxygen utilization at the child's discretion, (2) hydration for hemodilution through oral and intravenous therapy, (3) electrolyte replacement, since hypoxia results in metabolic acidosis, which also promotes sickling, (4) analgesics for the severe abdominal and joint pain (see Nursing Considerations), (5) blood replacement to treat anemia and to reduce the viscosity of the sickled blood, and (6) antibiotics to treat any existing infection. The administration of pneumococcal, *Haemophilus influenzae* type b, and meningococcal vaccines is recommended for these children because of their susceptibility to infection from asplenia (see Immunizations, Chapter 12). In addition, it is recommended that they receive prophylaxis with oral penicillin by 4 months of age (Gaston and others, 1986).

Short-term oxygen therapy may be helpful in severe crises, especially in children with cardiac failure. Although oxygen may prevent more sickling, it usually is not effective in reversing sickling, because with the vessels clogged with cells, the oxygen is not able to reach the enmeshed sickled erythrocytes. In addition, prolonged administration of oxygen can depress bone marrow activity, further aggravating the anemia.

The use of blood transfusions is another important component of care. Exchange transfusions have been successful in reducing the number of circulating sickle cells and therefore slowing down the vicious cycle of hypoxia, thrombosis, tissue ischemia, and injury. They are used in aplastic, hyperhemolytic, and sequestration crises, as well as after a stroke to prevent recurrence and further cerebral damage. Routine transfusions to maintain the hemoglobin above 10 g/dl in children with central nervous system disease can minimize the chances of further neurologic problems. In the event of surgery, preoperative exchange or partial exchange transfusions are given to prevent anoxia and suppress the formation of new sickle cells and postoperatively to replace lost blood. However, multiple transfusions carry the risk of hepatitis, hemosiderosis, and transfusion reactions (Charache, Lubin, and Reid, 1989).

In children with recurrent splenic sequestration, splenectomy may be a lifesaving measure. However, because the spleen usually atrophies on its own through progressive fibrotic changes, routine splenectomy is not recommended, especially since any surgical procedure has increased risk for these children. Warranted surgical or autosplenectomy has several advantages, since the spleen is the major site of sickling, sequestration, and destruction of red blood cells.

Priapism, a painful condition, may be treated with aspiration of the corpora cavernosum. This complication is particularly frequent in vaso-occlusive crises.

Nursing Considerations

Nursing management of the child with sickle cell anemia is largely related to teaching and supporting the family and providing comfort and pain relief to the child during a sickle cell crisis. The disease is usually first recognized when the child is a toddler, and the lifelong care begins with the diagnosis. This requires awareness of factors that precipitate reactions and active measures to prevent crises.

Assessment

Many nurses are involved in screening programs for sickle cell anemia to identify persons with the abnormal hemoglobin in order to implement therapy for homozygotes and provide genetic counseling for heterozygotes. Young children from families of at-risk racial or geographic origins who exhibit any of the signs previously described are advised to seek medical attention immediately.

Assessment of the child in sickle cell crisis involves all areas and systems that can be affected by circulatory obstruction, including vital signs, neurologic signs, vision, and hearing, as well as the respiratory, gastrointestinal, renal, and musculoskeletal systems. It is also important to assess the location and intensity of pain.

Nursing Diagnoses

Nursing diagnoses are derived from observation and assessment of children at risk or who demonstrate evidence of sickle cell disease. Some of the general aspects of nursing management are included in the Nursing Care Plan on pp. 1627-1628. Others will be apparent, depending on the state of the child's health, the organs involved, and the individual needs of the child and family.

Planning

The primary nursing goals are as follows:

1. Minimize the effects of sickling.
2. Encourage genetic counseling.
3. Educate family and child (when appropriate) regarding the sickling phenomenon and possible consequences.
4. Help the child and parents adjust to a lifelong, potentially fatal hereditary disease.

Implementation

Many of the measures that prevent sickling are also appropriate when a crisis occurs. In addition, special cautions are mandatory when the child undergoes surgery of any kind. Nurses may also be faced with the dilemmas of sickle cell screening and their role in genetic counseling. Taking time to establish a sound basis of understanding why certain measures are beneficial to the child encourages parents to practice them.

Prevent tissue deoxygenation. Anything that increases cellular metabolism also results in tissue hypoxia. For the child this includes avoiding (1) strenuous physical activity (especially contact sports if the spleen is enlarged, since rupture will cause massive internal hemorrhage), (2) emotional stress, (3) environments of low oxygen concentration, such as high altitudes or nonpressurized airplane flights, and (4) known sources of infection. If the child has even a mild infection, the parents must seek medical attention at once.

Promote hydration. The importance of hemodilution in preventing sickling and later in delaying the stasis-thrombosis-ischemia cycle has already been discussed. The nurse calculates the child's fluid requirements (approximately 150 ml/kg/day), which is the minimum daily fluid intake (Charache, Lubin, and Reid, 1989). The nurse also assesses the child's usual fluid consumption to evaluate its adequacy and makes adjustments based on this knowledge. It is not sufficient to advise parents to "force fluids" or "encourage drinking." They need specific instructions on how many glasses or bottles of fluid are required. Many foods are also a source of fluid, particularly soups, gelatin, and puddings, and these can be included as liquid sources.

Children can be encouraged to drink by giving them a "special" cup or glass, using a straw, taking advantage of thirsty times, such as on awakening or after playing, serving frequent, small portions, and leaving the cup in easy reach for self-service. Frozen popsicles, crushed ice "slurpies," and flavored ice cubes are sources of fluid commonly accepted by children.

Since the kidneys' ability to concentrate urine is impaired, the child is especially prone to dehydration. Dilute urine or low specific gravity is no longer a valid sign of ad-

NURSING CARE PLAN
The Child with Sickle Cell Disease

NURSING DIAGNOSIS: Potential for injury related to abnormal hemoglobin, decreased ambient oxygen, dehydration

GOAL 1

Increase tissue oxygenation and prevent sickling

INTERVENTIONS

Explain preventive measures
- Avoid strenuous physical exertion
- Avoid emotional stress
- Prevent infection
- Avoid low oxygen environment

EXPECTED OUTCOME

Child avoids situations that reduce tissue oxygenation

GOAL 2

Promote hydration

INTERVENTIONS

Calculate recommended daily fluid intake and base child's fluid requirements on this *minimum* amount (specify)
Give parents written instructions regarding specific quantity of fluid required
Encourage child to drink
Teach family signs of dehydration (see Chapter 28)
Stress importance of avoiding overheating as source of fluid loss

EXPECTED OUTCOME

Child drinks an adequate amount of fluid and shows no signs of dehydration

GOAL 3

Prevent infection

INTERVENTIONS

Stress importance of adequate nutrition, protection from known sources of infection, and frequent medical supervision
Report any sign of infection to physician immediately
Promote compliance with antibiotic therapy

EXPECTED OUTCOME

Child remains free of infection

GOAL 4

Decrease risks associated with a surgical procedure

INTERVENTIONS

Explain reason for preoperative blood transfusion
Keep child well hydrated
Decrease fear through appropriate preparation
Avoid unnecessary exertion
Promote pulmonary hygiene postoperatively
Use passive range of motion exercises to promote circulation
*Administer oxygen, if prescribed
Monitor for evidence of infection

EXPECTED OUTCOME

Child undergoes a surgical procedure without crisis

NURSING DIAGNOSIS: Altered family processes related to a child with potentially life-threatening disease

GOAL 1

Increase understanding of disease

INTERVENTIONS

Teach family and older children characteristics of basic defect and measures to prevent sickling
Stress importance of informing significant health personnel of child's disease
Explain signs of developing crisis, especially fever, pallor, and pain
Reinforce basics of trait transmission
Refer to genetic counseling services

EXPECTED OUTCOME

Child and family demonstrate an understanding of the disease, its etiology, and its therapies

GOAL 2

Support family

INTERVENTIONS

Refer to special organizations and agencies
Refer child to comprehensive sickle cell clinic for ongoing medical care
Be especially alert to family's needs when two or more members are affected
See Nursing Care Plan: The Child with a Chronic Illness or Disability, Chapter 22

EXPECTED OUTCOMES

Family takes advantage of community services (specify)
Child receives ongoing care from appropriate facility

*Dependent nursing action.

Continued.

NURSING CARE PLAN
The Child with Sickle Cell Disease—cont'd

Sickle cell crisis

NURSING DIAGNOSIS: Altered tissue perfusion related to generalized sickling

GOAL 1
Increase tissue oxygenation

INTERVENTIONS

*Administer oxygen as prescribed
Promote circulation through passive range of motion exercises

EXPECTED OUTCOME

Child exhibits no evidence of sickling

NURSING DIAGNOSIS: Pain related to tissue anoxia

GOAL 1
Relieve pain

INTERVENTIONS AND EXPECTED OUTCOMES

See Nursing Care Plan: The Child in Pain, Chapter 26

See also:
Nursing Care Plan: The Child in the Hospital, Chapter 26
Nursing Care Plan: The Family of the Ill or Hospitalized Child, Chapter 26

equate hydration. Parents are taught to observe for other indications of fluid loss, such as dry mucous membranes, weight loss, and sunken fontanel in infants. In addition, without the ability to conserve water by concentrating urine, the child is prone to dehydration from environmental factors, particularly overheating. The nurse alerts parents to the need for wearing proper indoor and outdoor clothing and avoiding excess exposure to the sun.

Forced fluids combined with renal diuresis result in the problem of enuresis. Parents who are unaware of this fact frequently employ the usual measures to discourage bedwetting, such as limiting fluids at night, and many revert to punishment and shame to force bladder control. The nurse discusses this problem with parents, stressing the child's inability to master prolonged control. Reminding the child to urinate frequently is helpful during the day, and waking him once during the night may prove beneficial if the child's sleep patterns are not disturbed. Parents who are toilet training their toddlers should be aware of the more frequent pattern of urination and increased difficulty in learning control. It is advisable to treat the enuresis as a complication of the disease, such as joint pain or some other symptom, in order to alleviate parental pressure on the child and to prevent any fluid restriction.

Prevent crises. Since infection is the major predisposing factor toward development of a crisis and the body's natural ability to resist infection is compromised, the nurse stresses to parents the importance of adequate nutrition, frequent medical supervision, proper handwashing, and isolation from known sources of infection. The last measure must be tempered with an awareness of the child's need for living a normal life. Overprotection can be equally as devastating emotionally as an infection is physically. Parents need to be aware of the necessity of seeking prompt medical care at the first sign of any infection.

The family should be taught the signs and symptoms of crises and advised to seek medical attention immediately. There is some evidence that teaching parents spleen palpation for earlier detection of splenic sequestration can reduce mortality from this serious complication (Emond and others, 1985).

Promote supportive therapies during crises. The success of many of the medical therapies relies heavily on nursing implementation. Management of pain is an especially difficult problem and often involves experimenting with various analgesics, including narcotics, and schedules before relief is achieved. Unfortunately, these children tend to be undermedicated, resulting in "clock watching" and demands for additional doses sooner than might be expected. Often this incorrectly raises suspicions of drug addiction, when in fact the problem is one of improper dosage. In choosing and scheduling analgesics, the goal should be *prevention* of pain.

The most frequent problem for patients with sickle cell disease is pain from vaso-occlusive crises. The chronic nature of this pain can greatly affect the child's development. A multidisciplinary approach is best for its management. When mild to moderate pain is reported, acetaminophen is initially used. If acetaminophen is not effective alone, codeine can be added. The dosages of both drugs are titrated to a therapeutic level. Opioids such as immediate- and sustained-release morphine, oxycodone, hydromorphone, and methadone can be administered parenterally or orally for severe pain and are administered around the clock (Shapiro, 1989). Meperidine (pethidine [Demerol]) is not recommended. Normeperidine, a metabolite of meperidine, is a central nervous system stimulant that produces anxiety, tremors, myoclonus, and generalized seizures when it accumulates with repetitive dosing. Patients with sickle cell disease are particularly at risk for normeperidine-induced seizures (American Pain Society, 1989). Medication given by mouth can be as effective as by the intravenous route when equianalgesic dosages are prescribed (see Chapter 26). Protocols for the comprehensive pharmacologic management of pain are available (Morrison and Vedro, 1989).

Any pain program should be combined with psychologic support to help the child deal with the depression, anxiety, and fear that accompany the disease. This includes regular visits with the child to discuss his concerns during the hospitalization and positive reinforcement of adaptive coping skills, such as successful methods of dealing with the pain and compliance with treatment prescriptions.

Frequently heat to the affected area is soothing. Cold compresses are not applied to the area, because this enhances sickling and vasoconstriction. Bed rest is usually well tolerated during a crisis, although actual rest depends a great deal on pain alleviation and organized schedules of nursing care. Although the objective of bed rest is to minimize oxygen consumption, some activity, particularly passive range of motion exercises, is beneficial to promote circulation. Usually the best course of action is to let the child dictate his activity tolerance.

If blood transfusions or exchange transfusions are given, the nurse has the responsibility of observing for signs of transfusion reaction (see Table 35-2). Since hypervolemia from too rapid transfusion can increase the workload of the heart, the nurse also is alert to signs of cardiac failure.

In splenic sequestration the size of the spleen is gently measured, since increasing splenomegaly is an ominous sign. A decreasing spleen denotes response to therapy. Vital signs and blood pressure are also closely monitored for impending shock. Anemia is typically not a presenting complication in vaso-occlusive crises but is a critical problem in other types of crises. The nurse monitors for evidence of increasing anemia and institutes appropriate nursing intervention.

Oxygen is not beneficial in vaso-occlusive episodes, unless hypoxemia is present (Charache, Lubin, and Reid, 1989). However, since prolonged oxygen can aggravate the anemia, signs of lack of therapeutic benefit, such as restlessness, increased pallor, and continued pain, are reported.

Intake, especially of intravenous fluids, and output are recorded. The child's weight should be taken on admission, since it serves as a baseline for evaluating hydration. Since diuresis can result in electrolyte loss, the nurse also observes for signs of hypokalemia and should be familiar with normal serum electrolyte values to report changes.

Decrease surgical risks. The main surgical risk is hypoxia from anesthesia. However, emotional stress, the demands of wound healing, and the possibility of infection potentially increase the sickling phenomenon, both in children with the disease and in those with the trait. The primary nursing objectives are aimed at minimizing each of these threats preoperatively and postoperatively by keeping the child well hydrated, preparing the child psychologically, and preventing infection.

Provide screening and genetic counseling. Screening is recommended during the neonatal period, since early diagnosis allows earlier, more prevention-oriented treatment, such as prophylactic antibiotic therapy and parent education about potential complications. The advantages of trait identification lie in selective reproduction of offspring not afflicted with hemoglobin SS. Alternate methods of childbearing include artificial insemination, adoption, or abortion of afflicted fetuses. However, these alternatives may be viewed as unacceptable.

To be effective, screening must be combined with genetic counseling and long-term follow-up. The nurse can be instrumental in such programs by conducting parent education sessions, following the family in the home, disseminating correct information about the disease and trait to the community, and rendering support to parents of newly diagnosed children. A primary consideration in genetic counseling is informing parents who both carry the trait of the chances of having a child with the disease (see Chapter 5).

Prenatal diagnosis is possible through amniocentesis or fetoscopy and fetal blood sampling. Analysis of amniotic cells for a DNA fragment associated with the gene responsible for sickled β-globulin chain synthesis can be done at the sixteenth week of gestation. In the event of an affected fetus, the decision regarding termination of the pregnancy should be left to the couple rather than viewed as an automatic selection of abortion.

Explain the disease. Since sickle cell anemia is first recognized when the child is a toddler, most of the nurse's counseling is with parents. The nurse explains to parents the basic effect of tissue hypoxia on red blood cells and the effect of sickling on circulation (Fig. 35-3). One simple yet graphic way of illustrating the difference between normal discoid red blood cells and sickle cells is to roll round or oval objects, such as marbles, through a tube to demonstrate normal blood cell circulation and then roll pointed objects such as screws or jacks through the tube. The effect of sickling and clumping of the pointed objects is especially noticeable at a bend or slight narrowing of the tube. This same idea can be expanded to discuss the importance of increased fluid in keeping the pointed objects suspended away from each other to prevent concentration. Taking time to establish a sound basis of understanding why certain measures are beneficial to the child encourages parents to practice them.*

Parents are advised to inform all treating practitioners of the child's condition. The use of a Medic Alert bracelet is another way of ensuring awareness of the disease. Some people view such identification as "negative labeling." The nurse can stress the benefits of displaying this information, especially in emergencies when the use of anesthesia may be required.

Support the family. Parents need the opportunity to discuss their feelings regarding transmitting a potentially fa-

*A Sickle Cell Home Study Kit for Families is available from the **National Association for Sickle Cell Disease, Inc.,** 3345 Wilshire Blvd., Ste. 1106, Los Angeles, CA 90010-1880; (213) 736-5455 or (800) 421-8453. Additional resources are **Howard University,** Center for Sickle Cell Disease, 2121 Georgia Ave., N.W., Washington, DC 20059, (202) 806-7930; **National Heart, Lung, and Blood Institute,** 9000 Rockville Pike, Building 31, Room 4A-21, Bethesda, MD 20892, (301) 496-4236.

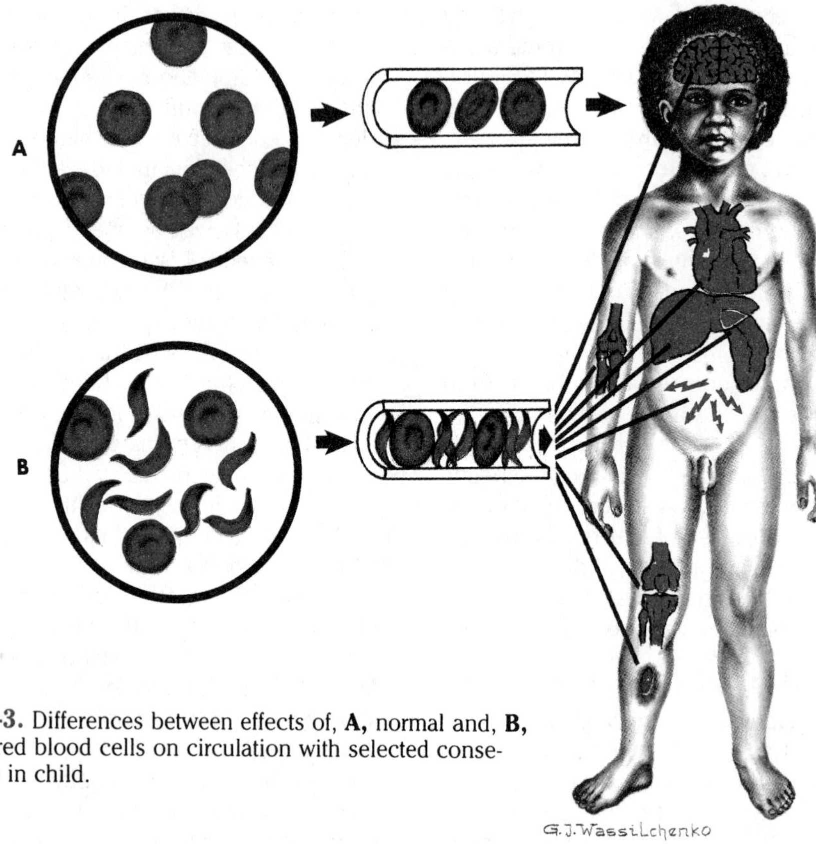

Fig. 35-3. Differences between effects of, **A,** normal and, **B,** sickled red blood cells on circulation with selected consequences in child.

tal, chronic illness to their child. Some parents are able to cope with this fact; some feel great guilt and remorse for giving their child the disease, whereas others regret not knowing that they carried the trait. For many parents the decision regarding subsequent pregnancies is viewed with doubt and ambivalence.

Because of the sometimes poor prognosis for children with sickle cell anemia, many parents express their fear of death. Prognosis varies; with early diagnosis and treatment these children are living longer. However, since there is no way to predict which child will follow a favorable course, the nurse should care for the family as she would for any family with a child who has a chronic and life-threatening illness, with particular emphasis on the siblings' reactions, the stress on the marital relationship, and the childrearing attitudes displayed toward the child (see Chapters 22 and 23).

Evaluation

The effectiveness of nursing interventions is determined by continual reassessment and evaluation of care based on the following observational guidelines and expected outcomes:

1. Observe the child for any evidence of sickling; monitor preventive strategies and therapies.
2. Interview family regarding genetic counseling.
3. Interview the family regarding their understanding of the disease, the sickling phenomenon, and its consequences.
4. Interview and observe the child and family regarding the way in which the disease has affected their lives.

Expected outcomes:
See Nursing Care Plan, pp. 1627-1628.

β-THALASSEMIA

The term *thalassemia* comes from the Greek word *thalassa,* meaning "sea," and is applied to a variety of inherited blood disorders characterized by deficiencies in the rate of production of specific globin chains in hemoglobin. The name appropriately refers to those people living near the Mediterranean Sea who have the highest incidence of the disease, namely, Italians, Greeks, and Syrians. There is evidence to suggest that the high incidence of the disorder among these groups is a result of selective advantage of the trait to malaria, as is postulated in sickle cell disease. However, the disorder has a wide geographic distribution, probably as a result of genetic migration through intermarriages or possibly as a result of spontaneous mutation.

The thalassemias are classified according to the hemoglobin chain affected and by the amount of the globin chain that is synthesized; for example, if alpha chains are affected, α-thalassemia. Each of the abnormal genes that cause thalassemia is seen in particular populations; for example, β-thalassemia, Greeks, Italians, and Syrians; α-thalassemia, Chinese, Thai, African, and Mediterranean peoples.

β-Thalassemia is the most common form, and it is the entity that will be discussed further. *Silent carriers* are individuals who carry the gene but demonstrate no clinical symptoms. Persons with *thalassemia trait,* the heterozygous form, usually have mild anemia, hypochromic and microcytic cells, and elevated HbA_2 and/or HbF. *Thalassemia intermedia* presents with splenomegaly and severe anemia. Skeletal deformities, frequent fractures, and arthritis complicate the clinical course. The homozygous form, *thalassemia major* (formerly referred to as *Cooley anemia*), results in a severe anemia that is not compatible with life unless transfusion support is given. Ordinarily homozygous α-thalassemia results in hydrops fetalis, which usually ends in death in utero. However, supportive therapy has resulted in live births and survival through the neonatal period (Beaudry and others, 1986; Bianchi and others, 1986).

Mode of Transmission

Thalassemia is an autosomal-recessive disorder with varying expressivity. Sometimes the trait is found in only one parent of a child with severe thalassemia. In this situation the likelihood is that the other parent carries a gene for some variant of sickle cell anemia or other hemoglobinopathy. The exact mode of transmission between parents who are heterozygous for thalassemia is illustrated in Fig. 5-4.

Pathophysiology

Normal postnatal hemoglobin (HbA) is composed of two α- and two β-polypeptide chains. In β-thalassemia there is a partial or complete deficiency in the synthesis of the β-chain of the hemoglobin molecule. Consequently, there is a compensatory increase in the synthesis of α-chains, and γ(gamma)-chain production remains activated, resulting in defective hemoglobin formation. This unbalanced polypeptide unit is very unstable, disintegrates, and damages the red blood cells, causing severe anemia. To compensate for the hemolytic process, an overabundance of red blood cells is formed. The body also attempts to balance the low level of circulating hemoglobin A by producing large concentrations of fetal hemoglobin, which does not contain β-chains.

Clinical Manifestations

The clinical effects of thalassemia major are primarily attributable to (1) defective synthesis of hemoglobin A, (2) structurally impaired red blood cells, and (3) shortened life span of the erythrocyte. The major consequences of thalassemia are caused by the pathologic condition, resultant chronic hypoxia, and the supportive treatment of multiple blood supplements (Fig. 35-4). The onset is usually insidious and not recognized until the latter half of infancy. Signs of anemia, unexplained fever, poor feeding, and a markedly enlarged spleen, particularly in a child of Mediterranean extraction, are descriptive.

Anemia. Anemia results from the body's inability to maintain a level of erythropoiesis commensurate with hemolysis. The bone marrow compensates by increasing production of large numbers of immature cells, such as normoblasts and erythroblasts, large cells that are extremely thin and form bizarre shapes, and nonspecific macrocytes called *target cells,* which have abnormal staining properties. As a result of the excessive production of abnormal red blood cells, their life span is severely shortened.

Anemia also is exaggerated by aplastic crises after infection, folic acid deficiencies from demands of bone marrow hyperplasia, splenic sequestration, and progressive hemolysis from repeated blood transfusions. The spleen becomes greatly enlarged as a result of extramedullary hemopoiesis, rapid destruction of the defective erythrocytes, and, rarely, progressive fibrosis from hemochromatosis. Splenomegaly may progress until the organ's very size interferes with the function of other abdominal organs and respiratory expansion.

With progressive anemia, signs of chronic hypoxia, namely, headache, precordial and bone pain, decreased exercise tolerance, listlessness, and anorexia, may develop. Another common symptom in these children is frequent epistaxis, although the exact reason is unknown. Hyperuricemia and gout from rapid cellular catabolism are also seen.

Hemosiderosis and hemochromatosis. *Hemosiderosis* is excess iron storage in various tissues of the body, especially the spleen, liver, lymph glands, heart, and pancreas, but without associated tissue injury. *Hemochromatosis* refers to excess iron storage with resultant cellular damage. Although the exact mechanism for the conversion of iron storage to tissue destruction is not known, chronic hypoxia is believed to be an important contributing factor.

In thalassemia, excess hemosiderin, the iron-containing pigment from the breakdown of hemoglobin, results from decreased hemoglobin synthesis and increased hemolysis of transfused erythrocytes. Decreased production of hemoglobin results in an excess supply of available iron. In addition, the body probably responds to the anemia by increasing the rate of gastrointestinal absorption of dietary iron, since ineffective erythropoiesis is a potent controlling factor regarding exogenous iron use. However, the primary source of additional iron is from the hemolysis of supplemental erythrocytes and rapid destruction of defective red blood cells. With the prophylactic use of deferoxamine to minimize excess iron storage, the characteristic changes in body structures from hemochromatosis have been greatly reduced.

Growth and sexual maturation. Retarded growth and especially delayed sexual maturation are common findings. There is evidence that both may also be caused by pituitary failure, although the exact reasons for this are unclear, but the impaired growth is probably related to hemochromatosis. It is possible that the endocrine glands are extremely sensitive to iron toxicity and that even small amounts of deposited iron can produce organ dysfunction. Children with severe disease usually achieve normal growth rates until puberty, when height becomes markedly retarded. Secondary sexual characteristics are delayed or absent in as many as 40% of adolescents (Borgna-Pignatti and others, 1985).

Diagnostic Evaluation

The classic picture of β-thalassemia in a child of Mediterranean background provides ample evidence of the disease. Hematologic studies reveal the characteristic changes in the red blood cell, that is, microcytosis, hypochromia, anisocytosis, poikilocytosis, target cells, and basophilic stip-

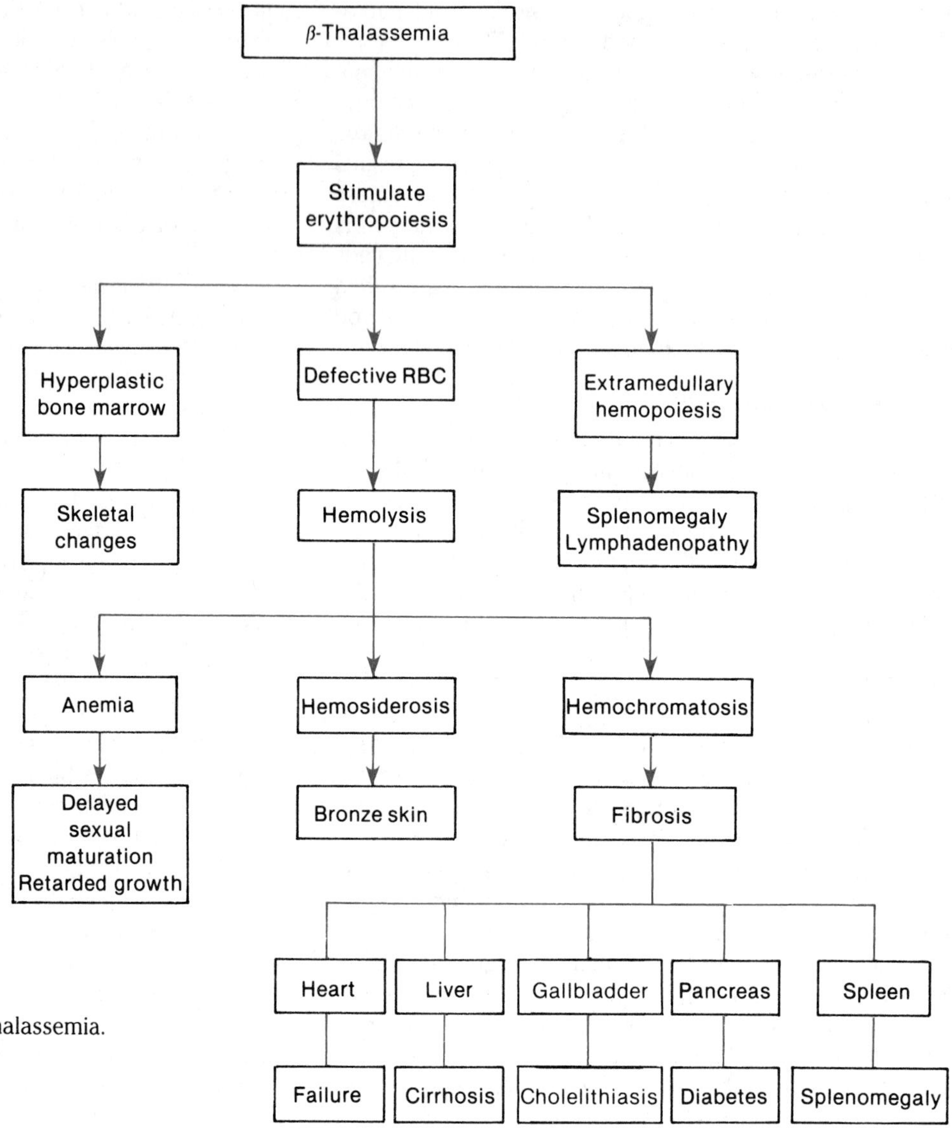

Fig. 35-4. Effects of thalassemia.

pling of immature erythrocytes of various stages. Low hemoglobin and hematocrit levels are seen in severe anemia, although they are typically lower than the reduction in red blood cell count because of the proliferation of immature erythrocytes.

Hemoglobin electrophoresis is very helpful in diagnosing the type and severity of the various thalassemias because it analyzes the quantity and specific hemoglobin variants found in blood. In β-thalassemia, hemoglobins F and A_2 (a type of normal adult hemoglobin) are elevated because neither depends on β-chain polypeptides for synthesis.

Therapeutic Management

There is no known cure for children with thalassemia major. The objective of supportive therapy is to maintain sufficient hemoglobin levels to prevent tissue hypoxia. Transfusions are the foundation of medical management. Recent studies have evaluated the benefits of maintaining the child's hemoglobin level above 10 g/dl, a goal that may require transfusions as often as every 3 weeks. The advantages of this therapy include (1) improved physical and psychologic well-being because of the ability to participate in normal activities, (2) decreased cardiomegaly and hepatosplenomegaly, (3) fewer bone changes, (4) normal or near normal growth and development until puberty, and (5) fewer infections (Festa, 1985).

One of the potential complications of frequent blood transfusions is iron overload. Since the body has no effective means of eliminating the excess iron, the mineral is deposited in body tissues. To minimize the development of hemosiderosis, deferoxamine (Desferal), an iron-chelating agent, is given. To be effective, it must be administered parenterally. The preferred routes are intravenous or subcutaneous, and the regimen may include subcutaneous administration via portable infusion pump over 8 to 10 hours (usually during sleep) for 6 days a week and intravenous administration over 8 hours at the time of blood transfusion (Festa, 1985). Significant liver fibrosis and growth impairment may be prevented if chelation therapy is initiated before age 3 years (Maurer and others, 1988).

In some children with severe splenomegaly who require repeated transfusions, a splenectomy may be necessary to decrease the disabling effects of abdominal pressure and to increase the life span of supplemental red blood cells. With repeated blood transfusions, a hemolytic factor develops in the spleen that increases the rate of erythrocyte destruction. After a splenectomy children generally require fewer transfusions, although the basic defect in hemoglobin synthesis remains unaffected. A major postsplenectomy complication is severe and overwhelming infection. Therefore these children are kept on prophylactic antibiotics with close medical supervision for many years and should receive the pneumococcal, meningococcal, and *Haemophilus influenzae* vaccines (see Immunizations, Chapter 12).

A promising treatment for some children is bone marrow transplantation (BMT). In one study children under 16 years who underwent allogeneic BMT had a high rate of complication-free survival (Lucarelli and others, 1990).

Nursing Considerations

The objectives of nursing care are to (1) assist the child in coping with the effects of the illness, (2) foster the parents' and child's adjustment to a chronic life-threatening illness, and (3) observe for complications of multiple blood transfusions (see Table 35-2).

Basic to each of these goals is explaining to parents and older children the defect responsible for the disorder and its effect on red blood cells. Since the incidence of this condition is high among families of Mediterranean descent, the nurse also inquires regarding the family's previous knowledge about thalassemia. All families with a child with thalassemia should be tested for the trait and referred for genetic counseling. (See also Nursing Care Plan: The Child with Beta-Thalassemia [Cooley Anemia].*)

Assist in coping with effects of disorder. Body image alterations, decreased growth, and sexual immaturity are frequently difficult adjustment problems for older children. These children feel different from their peers, and the delayed sexual development with ramifications on sexual function is a major issue for the maturing adolescent with an improved life expectancy. Adolescents need an opportunity to express their thoughts and feelings about these complex issues. They can learn grooming aids that make them appear more sexually mature, such as up-to-date clothing, new hairstyles, and well-applied makeup. Children with the characteristic bone changes may benefit from surgery or orthodontic appliances to improve facial structure.

With frequent transfusion therapy there is less restriction imposed on physical activity because of severe anemia, and these children should be encouraged to pursue activities commensurate with their exercise tolerance. However, the frequency of treatment can interfere with a normal life-style. To minimize disruptions, the nurse can be instrumental in arranging for blood transfusions and medical supervision at times that interfere least with the child's regular activities, especially school. In addition, children are more likely to cooperate with medical treatments that do not interfere significantly with their routine.

*In Wong, D.L., and Whaley, L.F.: Clinical manual of pediatric nursing, ed 3, St. Louis, 1990, Mosby–Year Book, Inc.

Support the family. As with any chronic, life-threatening illness, the needs of the family must be met for optimum adjustment to the stresses imposed by the disorder. These needs are discussed in Chapter 22. A source of information for the family is the **Cooley's Anemia Foundation.*** Genetic counseling for the parents and fertile offspring is mandatory, and both prenatal diagnosis using amniocentesis at 10 weeks or fetal blood sampling at 20 weeks' gestation (Alter, 1985) and screening for thalassemia trait are available. There has been a marked decrease in the number of new cases of thalassemia in the United States and Canada. This is thought to be a result of education and testing of parents (Pearson and others, 1987).

Even though the prognosis for children with thalassemia major is improving and will probably continue to improve, a proportion of these children die before adulthood, and for the survivors the life expectancy is significantly reduced. The chief cause of death is heart failure, followed by infection, liver disease, and malignancy (Zurlo and others, 1989). Unfortunately, it is not possible to predict which severely afflicted child will follow a more favorable course. The nurse must care for families of these children in light of this knowledge, be willing to discuss the future prospects with the parents and child as appropriate, and plan realistic goals for the thalassemic child. (See also Chapter 23.)

APLASTIC ANEMIA

Aplastic anemia refers to a condition in which all formed elements of the blood are simultaneously depressed. The peripheral blood smear demonstrates pancytopenia or the triad of profound anemia, leukopenia, and thrombocytopenia. *Hypoplastic anemia* is characterized by a profound depression of erythrocytes but normal or slightly decreased white blood cells and platelets.

A type of hypoplastic anemia is pure red cell aplasia, a congenital condition marked by complete or almost complete absence of all cells of the erythroid series with normal production of the other myeloid cells. Its treatment, which consists of transfusions, splenectomy, and administration of corticosteroids, is similar to that of other diseases, such as the thalassemias, that result in profound anemia. Prognosis varies, although long-term survival is possible. The principal causes of death are cardiac failure, hepatitis from transfusion therapy, and sepsis. Hemosiderosis and hemochromatosis (p. 1631) also affect vital tissues necessary for survival.

Acquired hypoplastic anemia can result from several factors, including suppressed erythropoiesis from multiple tranfusion therapy, hemolytic syndromes, such as sickle cell anemia, infections, toxic substances, drugs, and autoimmune or allergic states. The following discussion, however, focuses on aplastic anemia, which carries a much poorer prognosis and follows a more rapidly fatal course.

*105 E. 22nd St., New York, NY 10010; (212) 598-0911.

Etiologic Factors

Aplastic anemia can be primary (congenital) or secondary (acquired). Of the congenital variety, one of the best known disorders of which aplastic anemia is an outstanding feature is *Fanconi syndrome.* Besides pancytopenia, the condition is associated with a large number of congenital anomalies, including microcephaly; dwarfism; mental retardation; anomalies of ears, skeleton, kidneys, and heart; strabismus; ptosis; nystagmus; deafness; and excess deposits of melanin in areas of the skin. The syndrome appears to be inherited as an autosomal-recessive trait with varying penetrance; therefore affected siblings may demonstrate several different combinations of defects. The treatment is the same as for other causes of aplastic anemia. Prognosis is variable but is better than for acquired types.

The most common causes of acquired aplastic anemia are:

1. Infection with the human parvovirus (HPV), hepatitis, or overwhelming infection
2. Irradiation
3. Drugs, such as the chemotherapeutic agents and several antibiotics, one of the most notable being chloramphenicol
4. Industrial and household chemicals, including benzene and its derivatives, which are found in petroleum products, dyes, paint remover, shellac, and lacquers
5. Infiltration and replacement of myeloid elements, such as in leukemia or the lymphomas
6. Idiopathic, in which no identifiable precipitating cause can be found

The anemia will not be clinically evident until 6 to 8 weeks after the bone marrow insult. Therefore it may be difficult to identify the cause.

Clinical Manifestations and Diagnosis

The clinical manifestations, which include anemia, leukopenia, and decreased platelet count, are usually insidious. The onset is not unlike that seen in leukemia. Definitive confirmation is based on bone marrow aspiration or biopsy, which demonstrates the conversion of red bone marrow to yellow, fatty bone marrow.

Therapeutic Management

The objectives of treatment are based on the recognition that the underlying disease process is failure of the bone marrow to carry out its hematopoietic functions. Therefore therapy is directed at restoring function to the marrow and involves two main approaches: (1) immunosuppressive therapy to remove the presumed immunologic functions that prolong aplasia and/or (2) replacement of the bone marrow through transplantation (Gordon-Smith, 1985). Bone marrow transplantation is the treatment of choice in severe aplastic anemia when a compatible donor exists.

Currently, antilymphocyte globulin (ALG) or antithymocyte globulin (ATG) is the principal drug treatment for aplastic anemia. The specific globulin is prepared by immunizing suitable animals, usually horses or rabbits, with lymphocytes (ALG) obtained from patients undergoing surgery or with lymphocytes obtained by thymectomy (ATG). The cells are then harvested and commercially prepared. ALG and ATG are similar products; therefore the terms are used interchangeably. The rationale for using ATG is based on the theory that aplastic anemia may be the result of autoimmunity. ATG suppresses T-cell-dependent autoimmune responses but does not cause bone marrow suppression. The optimum schedule for ATG administration is still under investigation. It is usually given intravenously over 12 to 16 hours, after a test dose to check for hypersensitivity. Subsequent doses are given depending on the reduction in circulating lymphocytes.

Androgens may be used with ATG to stimulate erythropoiesis, although the exact mechanism of erythropoietic action is unclear. Cyclosporine may also be administered in children who fail to respond to ATG, and success has also been achieved using high-dose methylprednisolone.

Response to immunosuppressive therapy is gradual. Elevations in hemoglobin and red blood cells may take as long as 3 to 6 months. During this period the child must be protected from infection and hemorrhage and treated for the pancytopenia with transfusions. Published studies report a favorable prognosis in 50% or more of children treated with ATG, with slightly better reponses from the addition of cyclosporine (Werner and others, 1989).

Because of the relatively poor prognosis in aplastic anemia treated with drug therapy, bone marrow transplantation should be considered *early* in the course of the disease if a compatible donor can be found. Transplantation is more successful when performed before multiple transfusions have sensitized the child to leukocyte and HLA antigens. Children who are eligible for transplantation should be transferred to one of the medical centers that specialize in this procedure. For nontransfused patients, pretransplantation immunosuppressive therapy consists of administration of near lethal doses of cyclophosphamide. Those patients who have received transfusions undergo total body irradiation with immunosuppressives (e.g., cyclophosphamide, ATG, or cyclosporine). Bone marrow transplantation is associated with a 60% to 80% survival rate (Kamani, 1985; Werner and others, 1989).

Nursing Considerations

The care of the child with aplastic anemia is similar to that of the child with leukemia, that is, preparing the family for the diagnostic and therapeutic procedures, preventing complications from the severe pancytopenia, and emotionally supporting them in terms of a potentially fatal outcome (Chapters 23 and 36). Since each of these has already been discussed, only the exceptions are presented here. Bone marrow transplantation is discussed in Chapter 36.

During administration of ATG, vigilant attention must be directed to the intravenous infusion to prevent extravasation. To prevent sclerosing from extravasation, a central vein should be used. Because of the child's susceptibility to infection, meticulous care of the venous access catheter is essential. Although anaphylactic reactions to ATG are rare, emergency preparations should be planned in advance, with epinephrine readily available. The nurse should observe for other reactions. Immediate reactions to ATG are common and include fever and skin rash. Delayed reactions (serum sickness) may also occur within 7 to 14 days of a course of ATG, and the manifestations are similar to immediate reactions. The symptoms are reversed and in the case of serum sickness may be prevented with corticosteroids.

Since chemotherapeutic agents may be used, many of the reactions, such as nausea and vomiting, alopecia, and mucosal ulceration, can be encountered. In addition, extensive ecchymotic areas of the oral mucosa from thrombocytopenia require meticulous mouth care to prevent breakdown, bleeding, and infection. Fortunately, these lesions, which look painful, cause little or no discomfort. Local anesthetics are not necessary, but anorexia is still a consequence because of the edematous nature of the lesions. Liquid, bland, and soft diets are usually tolerated best.

DEFECTS IN HEMOSTASIS

Hemostasis is the process that stops bleeding when a blood vessel is injured. Vascular and plasma clotting factors, as well as platelets, are required. A complex system of clotting, anticlotting, and clot breakdown (fibrinolysis) mechanisms exists in equilibrium to ensure clot formation only in the presence of blood vessel injury and to limit the clotting process to the site of vessel wall injury. Dysfunction in these systems will lead to bleeding or thrombosis. The following discussion focuses on the major conditions that require nursing intervention. The reader is urged to apply these principles to other medical conditions that involve similar nursing considerations.

MECHANISMS INVOLVED IN NORMAL HEMOSTASIS

To understand the role that factor deficiencies play in promoting bleeding tendencies, it is necessary to review the normal coagulation process of the blood. Although the process is complex, clotting depends on three factors:

1. Vascular influence
2. Platelet role
3. Clotting factors

Vascular Influence

At the time of injury, several events occur at the site of injury to initiate hemostasis. There is local vasoconstriction, compression of the blood vessels by extravasated blood, release of von Willebrand factor (vWF) by endothelial walls, and the presence of collagen in exposed subendothelial cells that acts as a site for platelet adhesion.

Platelet Role

Normally the platelets do not adhere to each other or to normal endothelium. However, at the time a blood vessel is injured, the following occur. Platelet adhesion occurs at the site of the injury, providing a plug. The platelets change shape, develop pseudopods, and release a variety of chemicals to stimulate vasoconstriction, vessel repair, and activate and recruit more platelets to the injury site. Receptor sites are located on the platelets for fibrinogen and other adhesive proteins, causing the platelets to stick together (aggregation). As the membrane of the platelet changes, the phospholipids necessary for blood coagulation are exposed, resulting in fibrin production, which secures the platelet plugs to the site. Finally, the clot compresses and is secured to the injury.

Table 35-4 Blood-clotting factors

FACTOR NUMBER	SYNONYMS
I	Fibrinogen
II	Prothrombin
III	Platelet factor 3, thromboplastin
IV	Calcium
V	Labile factor, proaccelerin, Ac globulin
VII	Serum prothrombin conversion accelerator (SPCA), proconvertin, stable factor
VIII	Antihemophilic factor (AHF), antihemophilic globulin (AHG)
IX	Plasma thromboplastin component (PTC), Christmas factor
X	Stuart-Prower factor
XI	Plasma thromboplastin antecedent (PTA)
XII	Hageman factor
XIII	Fibrin-stabilizing factor (FSF)

Clotting Factors

The clotting factors (Table 35-4) are activated in sequence to develop a fibrin clot. Two mechanisms exist that can generate prothrombin activator complex to produce thrombin from prothrombin:

1. **Intrinsic pathway.** Factor XII, high-molecular-weight kininogen (HMK, Fitzgerald factor), and prekallikrein (KAL, Fletcher factor) react on a negative-charged surface (contact activation reaction) to activate factor XI (PTA, plasma thromboplastin antecedent). The partial thromboplastin time (PTT) measures abnormalities in the intrinsic pathway (abnormalities in factors XII; HMK; KAL; IX, VIII, X; V; II; I).
2. **Extrinsic pathway.** A lipoprotein tissue factor stimulates activation of factor VII. The prothrombin time (PT) measures abnormalities of the extrinsic pathway (abnormalities in factors V, VII, X, II, I).

Laboratory tests to assess hemostasis are presented in Table 35-5.

HEMOPHILIA

Hemophilia refers to a group of bleeding disorders in which there is a deficiency of one of the factors necessary for coagulation of the blood. Although the symptomatology is similar despite the missing factor, the identification of spe-

Table 35-5 Laboratory tests for hemostasis*

TEST	DESCRIPTION	COMMENTS
▪ Platelet function		
Bleeding time	Measures time interval for bleeding from small superficial wound to cease	Function depends on platelet aggregation and vasoconstriction; two common methods used: Ivy (incision made on forearm) and Duke (incision made on earlobe)
Tourniquet test	Measures platelet function and capillary fragility; apply pressure to forearm with tourniquet for 5 to 10 minutes	Normal response is absence of petechiae or fewer than 10 Abnormal in platelet and connective tissue disorders
Clot retraction test	Measures degree to which clot shrinks and expresses serum	Depends on platelet function
▪ Blood clotting mechanisms		
Whole blood clotting time	Measures time it takes for clot to form *within* blood	Prolonged clotting time indicates problem in thrombin-to-fibrin phase or in any factor in intrinsic clotting mechanism; difficult test to standardize; therefore often unreliable results
Prothrombin time (PT)	Measures activity of prothrombin, as well as factors necessary for its conversion to thrombin and fibrinogen	Actually does not measure prothrombin levels, but activity; since it bypasses intrinsic-extrinsic mechanism, detects deficiencies of factors V, VII, X, and fibrinogen, as well as prothrombin
Partial thromboplastin time (PTT) test	Similar to PT but measures activity of thromboplastin, which depends on intrinsic clotting factors	Specific for factor deficiencies, except factor VII, which results in a normal PTT but prolonged PT
Thromboplastin generation test (TGT)	Measures blood's ability to generate thromboplastin	Allows for determination of specific factor deficiencies, especially distinguishing between factors VIII and IX
Prothrombin consumption test	Indirectly measures thromboplastin generation and prothrombin response	Normally, as blood clots, prothrombin is converted to thrombin so that serum is depleted of prothrombin; if thromboplastin is decreased (as a result of extrinsic factor deficiencies), not all prothrombin will be converted and removed from serum
Fibrinogen level	Directly measures fibrinogen levels in blood	Not dependent on phase I or II deficiencies

*Normal values are listed in Appendix D.

cific factor deficiencies has allowed definitive treatment with replacement agents. The two most common forms of the disorder are *classic hemophilia* (hemophilia A or factor VIII deficiency) and *Christmas disease* (hemophilia B or factor IX deficiency). The following discussion is primarily concerned with the classic form, which accounts for about 75% of all cases.

A major feature of hemophilia is that its expression varies markedly in the degree of bleeding severity. Hemophilia is generally classified into three groups according to the severity of factor deficiency as described below; approximately 60% to 70% of children with hemophilia demonstrate the severe form of the disorder:

Clinical severity	Factor VIII activity	Bleeding tendency
Severe	1%	Spontaneous bleeding without trauma
Moderate	1%- 5%	Bleeding with trauma
Mild	5%-50%	Bleeding with severe trauma or surgery

Modes of Transmission

Hemophilia is transmitted as an X-linked recessive disorder; however, only about 60% of affected children have a positive family history for the disease. As many as one third of the cases of hemophilia may be caused by gene mutation (Karayalcin, 1985). The most frequent pattern of transmission is between an unaffected male and a trait-carrier female (see Fig. 5-6). With improved treatment for persons with hemophilia, it is important to consider the results of mating between an affected male and a normal female or a carrier female. For example, the mating of an affected male with a carrier female results in a 1:4 chance of producing either an affected son or daughter, a carrier daughter, or a normal son. This is one of the few ways in which a female inherits the disorder. Other mechanisms responsible for female expression of the disease include a symptomatic carrier of classic hemophilia with a moderate defect of factor VIII and a female with an autosomal dominant transmitted form of factor VIII deficiency, such as von Willebrand disease.

Pathophysiology

In hemophilia A the factor VIII molecule is present but is defective in its clotting function. Factor VIII–related antigen (FVIII R:Ag) is normal. In hemophilia B there may be a defect or a deficiency of factor IX.

Clinical Manifestations

The effect of hemophilia is prolonged bleeding anywhere from or in the body. With severe factor deficiencies, hemorrhage can occur as a result of minor trauma, such as after circumcision, during loss of deciduous teeth, or as a result of a slight fall or bruise. In children with less severe deficiencies the bleeding tendency may not be noted until onset of walking.

Subcutaneous and intramuscular hemorrhages are common. *Hemarthrosis,* which refers to bleeding into the joint cavities, especially the knees, elbows, and ankles, is the most frequent form of internal bleeding and often results in bone changes and consequently crippling, disabling deformities. Early signs of hemarthrosis are a feeling of stiffness, tingling, or ache in the joint, followed by a decrease in the ability to move the affected joint. Obvious signs and symptoms are warmth, redness, swelling, and severe pain with considerable loss of movement. Spontaneous hematuria is not uncommon. Epistaxis may occur but is not as frequent as other kinds of hemorrhage. Petechiae are uncommon in persons with hemophilia because repair of small hemorrhages depends on platelet function, not on blood-clotting mechanisms.

Bleeding into the tissue can occur anywhere but is serious if it occurs in the neck, mouth, or thorax, since the airway can become obstructed. Intracranial hemorrhage can have fatal consequences and is one of the major causes of death. Hemorrhage anywhere along the gastrointestinal tract can lead to obstruction, and bleeding into the retroperitoneal cavity is especially hazardous because of the large space for blood to accumulate. Hematomas in the spinal cord can cause paralysis.

Diagnostic Evaluation

The diagnosis is usually made on a history of bleeding episodes, evidence of X-linked inheritance, and laboratory findings. To understand the significance of various tests of hemostasis, it is helpful to recall the usual mechanisms to control bleeding, that is, the function of platelets and of clotting factors. Tests that measure platelet function, such as the bleeding time, tourniquet test, and clot retraction test, are all normal in persons with hemophilia, whereas tests that assess clotting factor function may be abnormal (Table 35-5). The tests specific for hemophilia are those that depend on specific factors for a reaction to occur, such as the partial thromboplastin time test, thromboplastin generation test, and prothrombin consumption test. Specific determination of factor deficiencies requires assay procedures normally done by specialized laboratories.

Carrier detection is possible in classic hemophilia and is an important consideration in families in which female offspring may have inherited the trait. The test involves an assay and comparison of factor VIII coagulant activity (FVIII-c) and factor VIII-related antigen (FVIII R:Ag), a protein found in the plasma that is antigenically similar to FVIII-c but has no measurable coagulant activity. To increase the accuracy of the test, DDAVP (1-desamino-8-D-arginine vasopressin), a synthetic derivative of vasopressin, may be given intravenously. In unaffected individuals, DDAVP produces an increase in FVIII-c and FVIII R:Ag, but in carriers the increase in FVIII-c, not FVII R:Ag, is less pronounced, thus increasing the difference in the ratio between the two factors (Kobrinsky and others, 1984). Prenatal diagnosis includes sex determination through amniocentesis or fetal blood sampling to detect FVIII R:Ag.

Therapeutic Management

The primary therapy for hemophilia is preventing spontaneous bleeding by replacement of the missing factor. Vigorous therapy is instituted to prevent chronic crippling effects from joint bleeding. Table 35-6 summarizes the adjunctive therapy for hemophilia.

One of the major concerns with the use of factor replacement is the risk of hepatitis and, especially, acquired immune deficiency syndrome (AIDS). Improved processing has significantly decreased the risk of disease transmission. Factor VIII manufactured by recombinant DNA is currently in clinical trials and will be commercially available in 1991 (Lusher, 1989) (see p. 1645). Since the risk of infections is lower with the use of cryoprecipitate or fresh frozen plasma than with factor concentrates, these products should be used whenever possible, especially in children under age 4. Individuals with hemophilia diagnosed and treated with fac-

Table 35-6 Adjunctive therapy for hemophilia A

Acute hemarthrosis Early Late	Ice packs, non-weight-bearing sling or lightweight splint may be helpful; rarely, joint aspiration
Intramuscular hemorrhage	Non-weight-bearing support; complete bed rest for hemorrhage in muscles of the lower spine attaching to the trochanter of the femur
Tongue and mouth lacerations	An antifibrinolytic agent (tranexamic acid or EACA), sedation, NPO in small child; local application of oradhesive gauze may be beneficial for gum bleeding
Extractions of permanent teeth	Antifibrinolytic agent beginning 1 day before surgery; continue 7-10 days
Painless spontaneous gross hematuria	Increased PO fluids; corticosteroids and/or factor VIII are used by some

*Modified from Lusher, J.M.: Management of hemophilia. In Westphal, R.G., and Smith, D.M., editors: Treatment of hemophilia and von Willebrand's disease: new developments, Arlington, VA, 1989, American Association of Blood Banks.

tor concentrates since 1989 are probably at low risk for developing human immunodeficiency (HIV) infection (Pierce and others, 1989). However, it is estimated that 70% to 90% of adolescents with hemophilia are HIV antibody positive (Overby, Lo, and Lett, 1989). As these individuals become sexually active, the issue of sexual transmission of HIV becomes increasingly important. The adolescent must be knowledgeable regarding high-risk sexual behavior.

A number of other drugs may be included in the therapy plan, depending on the source of the hemorrhage. Corticosteroids are administered to reduce inflammation in the joints; nonsteroidal antiinflammatory drugs (NSAIDs), such as aspirin, indomethacin (Indocin), and phenylbutazone (Butazolidin) should not be used because they inhibit platelet function. Ibuprofen (Motrin, Advil, or Nuprin) has been demonstrated to be safe despite its anti–platelet aggregation effect (Karayalcin, 1985). DDAVP is helpful in children with mild to moderate hemophilia because of the transient rise in FVIII-c. Local application of epsilon aminocaproic acid (EACA, Amicar) prevents clot destruction; however, its use is limited to mouth or trauma surgery.

A regular program of exercise and physical therapy is an important aspect of management. Physical activity, within reasonable limits, strengthens muscles around joints, which helps control bleeding in the area. Pain management with appropriate nonnarcotic and narcotic drugs, such as acetaminophen with or without codeine, is essential to ensure compliance with the physical therapy plan.

Treatment without delay results in more rapid recovery and a decreased likelihood of complications; therefore most children are treated at home. The family is taught the technique of venipuncture and the administration of the replacement factor to children over 3 years of age. The child learns the procedure for self-administration between ages 9 and 12. Home treatment is highly successful, and the rewards, in addition to the immediacy of treatment, are less disruption of family life, fewer school or work days missed, and enhancement of the child's independence and self-esteem.

Nursing Considerations

The objectives for nursing care can be divided into immediate needs and long-term goals. Obviously, the most immediate consideration is control of bleeding episodes. However, the ultimate adjustment and prognosis for the child rely heavily on the family's ability to cope with the disorder, to learn effective methods of control and prevention, and to temper childrearing practices with judicious protection from injury while fostering independence and development.

Prevent bleeding by decreasing risk of injury. Prevention of bleeding through control of behavior is no easy task. During infancy and toddlerhood the normal acquisition of motor skills creates innumerable opportunities for falls, bruises, and minor wounds. Restraining the child from mastering motor development can herald more serious long-term problems than allowing the behavior. However, the environment can be made as safe as possible to minimize the incidental injuries, with close supervision maintained during playtime.

For older children the family usually needs assistance in preparing for school. A nurse who knows the family can be instrumental in discussing the situation with the school nurse and in jointly planning an appropriate schedule of activity. Since almost all persons with hemophilia are boys, the physical limitations in regard to active sports are a difficult adjustment, and activity restrictions must be tempered with sensitivity to the child's emotional as well as physical needs. Noncontact sports, especially swimming, are suitable activities and should be encouraged.

To prevent oral bleeding, some readjustment in terms of dental hygiene may be needed to minimize trauma to the gums. For example, the nurse can recommend the use of a water irrigating device, softening the toothbrush in warm water before brushing, or using a sponge-tipped disposable toothbrush available in many drugstores. A regular toothbrush should be soft bristled and small in size. Adolescents also need to be advised of the dangers of shaving with razor blades and encouraged to use an electric shaver.

Since any trauma can lead to a bleeding episode, all persons caring for these children must be aware of their disorder. These children should wear Medic Alert identification, and older children should be encouraged to recognize situations in which disclosing their condition is important, such as dental extraction or injections. Health personnel need to take special precautions to prevent the use of procedures such as intramuscular injections or venipunctures. A peripheral fingerstick is better for blood samples, and the subcutaneous route is substituted for intramuscular injections. Neither aspirin nor any aspirin-containing compound should be used. Acetaminophen (Tylenol) is a suitable aspirin substitute, especially for use during control of pain at home. Another common drug that should not be used is glyceryl guaiacolate (guaifenesin), an expectorant found in several over-the-counter cough preparations.

Recognize and manage bleeding. The earlier a bleeding episode is recognized, the more effectively it can be treated. Children are often aware of internal bleeding before clinical manifestations are evident, and they must be taken seriously when they report their concerns. In addition to the signs of hemarthrosis that have been discussed, the family also needs to be aware of signs and symptoms indicating internal tissue bleeding, such as headache, slurred speech, and loss of consciousness from bleeding within the brain and black tarry stools, hematemesis, and loss of consciousness from gastrointestinal bleeding, which require immediate medical attention.

Factor replacement therapy should be instituted according to established medical protocol and supportive measures implemented, such as (1) applying pressure to the area for at least 10 to 15 minutes to allow clot formation, (2) immobilizing and elevating the area above the level of the heart to decrease blood flow, and (3) applying cold to promote vasoconstriction. When parents and older children are taught such measures beforehand, they can be prepared to initiate immediate treatment before blood loss is excessive. Plastic bags of ice or commercial cold packs* should

*Manufactured by 3M Co., Medical-Surgical Division, P.O. Box 33600, St. Paul, MN 55133-3600; (800) 288-3957.

be kept in the freezer for such emergencies. However, such measures should not take the place of factor replacement.

Prevent crippling effects of joint degeneration. From repeated hemarthrosis, incompletely absorbed blood in the joints, and limitation of motion, bone and muscle changes occur that result in flexion contractures and joint fixation. Obviously, prevention of bleeding is the ideal goal. However, since spontaneous bleeding is not uncommon in persons with severe hemophilia, definitive measures, including replacement therapy and physical therapy, are necessary to limit joint damage.

During bleeding episodes the joint is elevated and immobilized. Passive range of motion exercises are usually instituted after the acute phase. Physical therapy is beneficial to promote maximum function of the joint and unaffected body parts. Success of a physical therapy plan involves control of pain by administering analgesics before therapy and adjusting the dose to provide maximum benefit.

If an exercise program is instituted in the home, a physical therapist or public health nurse may need to supervise compliance with the regimen. Occasionally orthopedic intervention such as casting, application of traction, or aspiration of blood may be necessary to preserve joint function. Diet is also an important consideration, since excessive body weight can increase the strain on affected joints, especially the knees, and predispose to hemarthrosis. Consequently, calories need to be supplied in accordance with energy requirements.

Since many individuals are unaware of the serious effects of joint involvement, the nurse has the responsibility of educating the child and family concerning the long-range consequences of this complication. Surgical joint replacement in instances of total disability offers new hope to some persons with hemophilia.

Prepare for home care. The discovery of factor concentrates has greatly changed the outlook for these children. With scheduled infusions of the missing factor, bleeding can be prevented, and the child can live a more normal, unrestricted life. To foster maximum independence, home-care programs that teach the parent and/or child to administer the drug have been instituted. The same principles discussed in Chapter 26 regarding preparing families for home management apply here. The nurse skilled in venipuncture techniques is often the person who teaches the families to administer antihemophilic factor concentrates.

In addition, the nurse must be familiar with the properties of the concentrates and their preparation. For example, to hasten the mixing process of reconstituting dried antihemophilic factor with diluent, the solution may be warmed, or the vial gently rotated. Excessive heating or shaking of the container will result in loss of active antihemophilic factor. A filtered intravenous setup is usually supplied with the drug to filter any particles in the solution. If the solution is not thoroughly mixed before administration, the filter will also remove the active factor.

Transfusion reactions and infection with viral hepatitis and AIDS are potential complications from replacement products. The nurse teaches the parents and/or child the signs of transfusion reactions or hepatitis and stresses the necessity of notifying a physician of their occurrence. If the child tests positive for AIDS, the family may need additional support in dealing with this diagnosis and the often unsympathetic responses of the community (see also p. 1648).

Not all children with hemophilia are eligible for or have the opportunity of a home-care program. For these children, repeated hospitalizations may be needed to control the bleeding episodes. Ideally a core of nurses should work with these children to maintain consistency of care during each hospitalization. Besides the physical goals of controlling bleeding and preventing disability, the nursing objectives should include fostering independence and self-care, providing an opportunity for the children to discuss their feelings regarding the disease, and a continuous reevaluation of those factors that may influence a bleeding episode. Every effort is made to discharge the child as soon as possible and continue treatment on an outpatient basis.

Support the family. Not only is hemophilia a chronic, potentially fatal, hereditary condition, it is also one of unpredictable emergencies that impose additional emotional stress on family members. Children with the moderate or mild form may be undiagnosed until an accident occurs or elective medical procedure is performed. Then, coping with the diagnosis may be hindered by the circumstances surrounding its discovery. At other times parents are aware of the severity of the defect from birth and are immediately faced with the birth of a defective child. Whatever the situation, constructive teaching about the disease and measures to control or prevent bleeding must follow a period of parental adjustment to the diagnosis. For the nurse this involves (1) carefully listening to the parents' statements regarding their understanding of the condition, (2) awareness of the parents' feelings, particularly those of the mother concerning transmitting the disorder, and (3) an assessment of those factors that promote or retard coping with a crisis, such as marital stability, previous patterns of coping, and the ability to seek out and use help (see Chapter 22).

Genetic counseling as soon as possible after diagnosis is essential and must include evaluation of parental understanding and counseling about feelings as well as transmission of information. Unlike many other disorders in which both parents carry the trait, the feeling of responsibility for this condition rests on the mother.

The needs of the family are best met through a comprehensive team approach of physicians (pediatrician, hematologist, orthopedist), nurse, social worker, and physical therapist. Parent-group discussions are beneficial in addressing those needs often best met by similarly affected families. For example, with the improved prognosis for these children, adolescents with hemophilia are faced with vocational, employment, and financial problems (see Questions and Controversies, p. 1025). Further, factor replacement therapy and other treatments for the child with severe hemophilia can cost in excess of $10,000 a year. The **National Hemophilia Foundation*** and the **Canadian He-**

*110 Greene St., Room 406, New York, NY 10012; (212) 219-8180.

mophilia Society* provide numerous services and publications for both health providers and families. (See also Nursing Care Plan: The Child with Hemophilia.†)

VON WILLEBRAND DISEASE

von Willebrand disease is a hereditary bleeding disorder characterized by a moderate to severe factor VIII deficiency and low levels of factor VIII–related antigen (FVIII R:Ag). In addition, the functional component of the factor VIII molecule that is required for platelet adhesion to vascular subendothelium (known as von Willebrand factor or ristocetin cofactor) is reduced. This results in prolonged bleeding time because the platelets fail to adhere to the walls of the ruptured vessel to form a platelet plug.

The most characteristic clinical feature of von Willebrand disease is an increased tendency toward bleeding from mucous membranes. The most common symptom is frequent nosebleeds, followed by gingival bleeding, easy bruising, and menorrhagia in females. Unlike hemophilia, it affects both males and females because its inheritance is autosomal dominant. However, the treatment and final outcome are similar in both disorders. Treatment of bleeding is with cryoprecipitate or fresh frozen plasma.

Nursing Considerations

The nursing goals are similar to those for hemophilia with special considerations related to epistaxis (p. 1642) and menorrhagia. Replacement therapy may be beneficial before the menstrual cycle to lessen the flow. Teaching the adolescent methods to prevent embarrassing accidents during menstruation, such as wearing plastic-lined underpants and using double sanitary pads, helps her adjust to the inconvenience. Interestingly, these females frequently do not experience excessive bleeding at the time of delivery. This is thought to be because of increased levels of factor VIII during pregnancy. Decisions regarding childbearing are difficult because of the dominant pattern of inheritance.

IDIOPATHIC THROMBOCYTOPENIC PURPURA

Idiopathic thrombocytopenic purpura (ITP) is an acquired hemorrhagic disorder that results from excessive destruction of platelets. Although the exact cause is unknown, it is believed to be an autoimmune response to disease-related antigens and is the most commonly occurring thrombocytopenia of childhood.

Clinical Manifestations

ITP occurs in one of two forms: an acute, self-limiting course or a chronic condition interspersed with remissions. The acute form is most commonly seen after upper respiratory infections or the childhood diseases measles, rubella, mumps, and chickenpox. The most common clinical manifestations of either type include (1) easy bruising with petechiae and/or ecchymoses, particularly over bony prominences, (2) bleeding from mucous membranes, such as epistaxis, bleeding gums, and internal hemorrhage with evidence of hematuria, hematemesis, melena, hemarthrosis, and menorrhagia, and (3) hematomas over the lower extremities that may result in chronic leg ulcers.

Diagnostic Evaluation

In ITP the platelet count is reduced to below 20,000 mm^3/dl; therefore tests that depend on platelet function are abnormal, such as the tourniquet test, bleeding time, and clot retraction. Although there is no definitive test on which to establish a diagnosis of ITP, several tests are usually performed to rule out other disorders in which thrombocytopenia is a manifestation, such as systemic lupus erythematosus, lymphoma, or leukemia.

Therapeutic Management

Management is primarily supportive, because the course of the disease is self-limited in the majority of cases. Activity is restricted at the onset while the platelet count is low and active bleeding or progression of lesions is occurring. This restriction is most easily accomplished in the hospital. Corticosteroids are used for children with the highest risk for serious bleeding (platelet count less than 30,000); it is hypothesized that steroids inhibit removal of sensitized platelets by the reticuloendothelial system. The use of intravenous gamma globulin has also been advocated and has demonstrated some effectiveness in increasing platelet production until spontaneous recovery takes place, although the mechanism of action is unknown. Splenectomy is reserved for symptomatic children who do not respond to drug therapy and who have life-threatening hemorrhage. Any child undergoing splenectomy is at risk for overwhelming sepsis and should receive the pneumococcal and meningococcal vaccines and antibiotic therapy.

Nursing Considerations

Nursing care is largely supportive and directed toward restricting the activity of an otherwise normal child. Children and parents need careful explanations of the rationale behind the therapies used and support in their efforts to comply. As in any condition with an uncertain outcome, the family needs emotional support, especially during periods of hospitalization.

The nursing considerations of controlling bleeding, preventing bruising, and preventing crippling effects of hemarthrosis are similar to those discussed for hemophilia. The deleterious effects of using aspirin to control joint pain are critical for these children; therefore salicylate substitutes should always be used. The family also needs to be aware of signs and symptoms indicating internal bleeding, which, although rare, requires immediate medical attention.

HENOCH-SCHÖNLEIN PURPURA

Henoch-Schönlein purpura (HSP) (Schönlein-Henoch vasculitis, allergic purpura, anaphylactoid purpura) is a relatively common acquired disorder in children characterized

---

*1450 City Councillors, Ste. 840, Montreal, Quebec H3A 2E6; (514) 848-0503.

†In Wong, D.L., and Whaley, L.F.: Clinical manual of pediatric nursing, St. Louis, 1990, Mosby–Year Book, Inc.

by a nonthrombocytopenic purpura, arthritis, nephritis, and abdominal pain.

No primary hemostatic defect is involved, but because the chief sign is purpura, the disorder is discussed in this section. The etiology is unknown, but the disease often follows an upper respiratory infection, and allergy or drug sensitivity plays a role in some instances. The disease occurs in children aged 6 months to 16 years but more frequently between ages 2 to 8 years. It is observed more often in white children than in other races and in boys three times more often than in girls.

Pathophysiology

The disease is characterized by inflammation of small blood vessels, and the manifestations observed are influenced by the size and distribution of the affected vessels. A generalized vasculitis of dermal capillaries (and to a lesser extent small arterioles and veins) causing extravasation of red blood cells produces the petechial skin lesions. Inflammation and hemorrhage may also occur in the gastrointestinal tract, synovium, glomeruli, and central nervous system.

Clinical Manifestations

The onset of the disease may be abrupt with simultaneous appearance of several manifestations or gradual with sequential appearance of different manifestations. The primary feature, however, is a symmetric purpura that involves the buttocks and lower extremities but may extend to include the extensor surfaces of the upper extremities and, less commonly, the upper trunk and face (see Color Plate 6). The rash may be associated with maculopapular lesions, urticaria, and erythema. There is often marked edema of scalp, eyelids, lips, ears, and dorsal surfaces of hands and feet—especially in infants and younger children.

Arthritic effects are evident in two thirds of affected children and range from asymptomatic swelling around a single joint to painful tender swelling of several joints, most often the knees and ankles. The involvement is periarticular and resolves in a few days without permanent damage or deformity.

Two thirds of the children have gastrointestinal involvement manifested by recurrent colicky midabdominal pain often associated with nausea and vomiting. The stools contain gross or occult blood and mucus.

Renal involvement occurs in up to 50% of affected children and is potentially the most serious long-term complication. Initially the nephritis is manifested as hematuria, casts, and proteinuria. Although the majority of children with renal involvement recover completely, some develop chronic renal disease with eventual renal failure.

Diagnostic Evaluation

Diagnosis is usually established on the basis of clinical manifestations. Laboratory tests are used to assess gastrointestinal and renal involvement and to determine adequacy of hemostatic function. Although no test is diagnostic, increased levels of immunoglobin A are a frequent finding (Saulsbury, 1986).

Therapeutic Management

Management is primarily supportive with close observation for signs of renal or gastrointestinal manifestations. Edema, rash, malaise, and arthralgia are usually managed with appropriate analgesics, such as acetaminophen, and mild sedation if necessary. Corticosteroids may be prescribed for relief of more severe edema, arthralgia, and colicky abdominal pain but are not warranted in all cases.

The majority of children recover without the need for hospitalization, and in most instances a single acute episode clears spontaneously within a month. Others may have periodic recurrences for as long as 2 to 3 years before permanent remission from symptoms. Rarely death occurs from severe gastrointestinal complications, acute renal failure, or central nervous system involvement.

Nursing Considerations

Nursing care of the child hospitalized with HSP is primarily supportive with vigilant observation for signs of complications. Vital signs are taken and recorded at regular intervals, specimens are obtained for laboratory examination, and medication is administered as prescribed. Urine and stools are carefully observed for fresh and occult blood.

If the child suffers from joint pain, positioning, careful movement, and administration of analgesics help reduce discomfort. Nonnarcotic analgesics also relieve the discomfort of fever and malaise. More severe involvement such as gastrointestinal symptoms and nephritis is managed as for any such disorder (see appropriate nursing care).

Concern about the unsightly appearance of the rash is common. The child and parents can be reassured that it is only a temporary phenomenon, and he can be encouraged to wear clothing that helps hide the rash, such as long sleeves, pants, and robe. Emphasizing good grooming and attractive apparel helps promote a more positive self-image.

DISSEMINATED INTRAVASCULAR COAGULATION

Disseminated intravascular coagulation (DIC), also known as *consumption coagulopathy,* is not a primary disease but a secondary disorder of coagulation that complicates a number of pathologic processes (such as hypoxia, acidosis, shock, and endothelial damage [burns]) and many severe systemic disease states (such as congenital heart disease, necrotizing enterocolitis, gram-negative bacterial sepsis, rickettsial infections, and some severe viral infections). The disease is characterized by inappropriate systemic activation and acceleration of the normal clotting mechanism.

Pathophysiology

DIC occurs when the first stage of the coagulation process is abnormally stimulated. Although there is no well-defined sequence of events, two distinct phases can be identified. First, when the clotting mechanism is triggered in the circulation, thrombin is generated in greater amounts than can be neutralized by the body. Consequently, there is rapid conversion of fibrinogen to fibrin with aggregation and destruction of platelets. If local and widespread fibrin deposi-

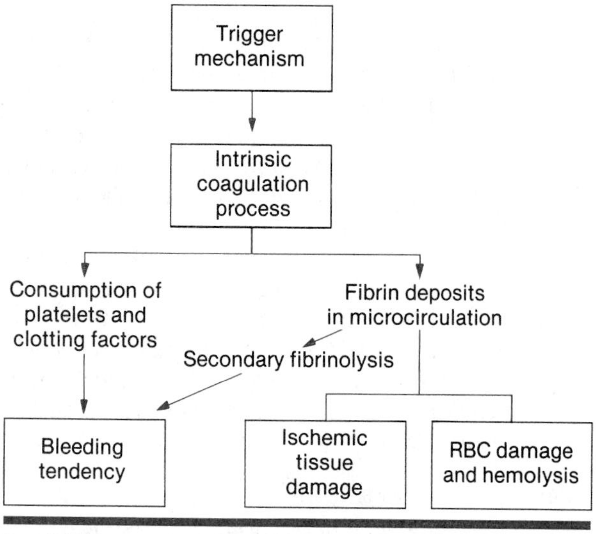

Fig. 35-5. Effects of disseminated intravascular coagulation.

tion in blood vessels takes place, obstruction and eventual necrosis of tissues occur. Second, the fibrinolytic mechanism is activated, causing extensive destruction of clotting factors. With a deficiency of clotting factors the child is vulnerable to uncontrollable hemorrhage into vital organs. An additional complication is damage and hemolysis of red blood cells (Fig. 35-5).

Clinical Manifestations

Signs of DIC are those of many other diseases, which often confuses the diagnosis. There is evidence of bleeding—petechiae, purpura, bleeding from openings in the skin (e.g., a venipuncture site or surgical incision), hypotension, and dysfunction of organs from infarction and ischemia.

Diagnostic Evaluation

DIC is suspected when there is an increased tendency to bleed, as from venipuncture or blood taken from the heel, and bleeding from the umbilicus, trachea, or gastrointestinal tract. Hematologic findings include prolonged prothrombin (PT), partial thromboplastin (PTT), and thrombin times. There is a profoundly depressed platelet count, fragmented red blood cells, and depleted fibrinogen.

Therapeutic Management

Treatment is directed toward control of the underlying or initiating cause, which in most instances stops the coagulation problem spontaneously. Platelets and fresh frozen plasma may be needed to replace lost plasma components, especially in the child whose underlying disease remains uncontrolled. The very ill newborn infant may require exchange transfusion with fresh blood. The administration of heparin to inhibit thrombin formation is most often restricted to severe cases.

Nursing Considerations

The goals of nursing care are to be aware of the possibility of DIC in the severely ill child and to recognize signs that might indicate its presence. The skills needed to monitor intravenous infusion and blood transfusions and to administer heparin are the same as for any child receiving these therapies. Since the child is usually cared for in an intensive care unit, the special needs of the family must be considered (see Chapter 26).

EPISTAXIS (NOSEBLEEDING)

Isolated and transient episodes of epistaxis, or nosebleeding, are common in childhood. The nose is a highly vascular structure, and bleeding usually results from direct trauma, including blows to the nose, foreign bodies, and nose picking, or from mucosal inflammation associated with allergic rhinitis and upper respiratory tract infections or drying of the mucous membranes in environments with low humidity (Katsanis and others, 1988). Ordinarily the bleeding stops spontaneously or with minimal pressure and requires no medical evaluation or therapy.

Recurrent epistaxis and severe bleeding may indicate an underlying disease, particularly vascular abnormalties, leukemia, thrombocytopenia, and clotting factor deficiency diseases such as hemophilia and von Willebrand disease. Sometimes nosebleeds are associated with administration of aspirin, even in normal amounts. Persistent nosebleeding requires medical evaluation.

Nursing Considerations

Nosebleeds are often a frightening experience for the child and parents. A calm, reassuring manner can alleviate anxiety and promote the child's cooperation. Since most of the nosebleeding originates in the anterior part of the nasal septum, bleeding can be controlled by applying pressure to the nose with the thumb and forefinger (see Emergency Treatment). During this time the child breathes through the mouth.

In the event that hemorrhage continues, the child should be evaluated by a practitioner, who may pack the nose with epinephrine-soaked gauze. After a nosebleed, petroleum or water-soluble jelly can be inserted into each nostril to prevent crusting of old blood and to lessen the likelihood of the child's picking at his nose and restarting the hemorrhage. Whenever possible, factors believed to increase the likelihood of epistaxis are eliminated, such as discouraging nose picking or altering the household humidity by placing a cool-mist vaporizer in the child's room.

■ IMMUNOLOGIC DEFICIENCY DISORDERS

A number of disorders can cause profound, often life-threatening alterations within the body's immune system. The most serious are those conditions that completely depress immunity, such as severe combined immunodeficiency disease. However, the one disorder that generates the most anxiety, within both the family and the community at large, is acquired immune deficiency syndrome (AIDS).

Several classifications of immune dysfunction exist.

AIDS, severe combined immunodeficiency syndrome (SCIDS), and Wiskott-Aldrich syndrome are the inability of the body to react. An allergy is the overreaction of the immune system to a relatively harmless antigen. The immune response can also be misdirected. In autoimmune disorders, antibodies, macrophages, and lymphocytes attack healthy cells. Some disorders and their target organs include myasthenia gravis, muscle cells; Graves disease, thyroid cells; and type I diabetes, B-cells in the pancreas. With the exception of AIDS, SCIDS, and Wiskott-Aldrich syndrome, the other disorders are discussed elsewhere in the book.

To enhance understanding of immunologic deficiency disorders, the following overview is presented of the body's immune system.

EMERGENCY TREATMENT
Epistaxis

1. Have child sit up and lean forward (not lying down).
2. Apply continuous pressure to nose with thumb and forefinger for at least 10 minutes.
3. Insert cotton or wadded tissue into each nostril and apply ice or cold cloth to bridge of nose if bleeding persists.
4. Keep child calm and quiet.

MECHANISMS INVOLVED IN IMMUNITY

In simple terms, the function of the immune system is to recognize "self" from "non-self" and to initiate responses to eliminate the non-self or the foreign substance known as *antigen.* However, the specific processes involved in this function are complex and interrelated, and advances in the understanding of immunologic mechanisms are helping to further elucidate the intricacies of this system.

The protective mechanisms of the body consist of complex, overlapping defense systems. Intact skin serves as the first line of protection for the body. Body secretions such as saliva, sweat, and tears contain chemicals that can kill many organisms. The stomach contains acids that can destroy swallowed pathogens as they adhere to the mucus of the nose and mouth. Organisms trapped in these areas are expelled by sneezing or coughing. If the foreign substance has penetrated these barriers, cellular elements are mobilized.

The immune system includes the *primary lymphoid organs* (thymus, bone marrow, and probably liver) and the *secondary lymphoid organs* (lymph nodes, spleen, and gut-associated lymphoid tissue [GALT]). The functions of the immune system are basically of two types: nonspecific and specific (Fig. 36-6). *Nonspecific immune defenses* are activated on exposure to any foreign substance but react similarly regardless of the type of antigen; they are unable to identify the antigen, except to know that it is "non-self." The principal activity of this system is *phagocytosis,* the process of ingesting and digesting foreign substances. Phagocytic cells include neutrophils and monocytes (see 1608). Specific defenses are discussed in the following paragraphs.

Specific Immune Mechanisms

Specific (adaptive) defenses are those that have the ability to recognize the antigen and respond selectively. The components of adaptive immunity are *humoral immunity* and *cell-mediated immunity.* The cells responsible for these two forms of immunity are the lymphocytes, specifically B-lymphocytes and T-lymphocytes.

Humoral Immunity

Humoral immunity is involved with antibody production and complement and is concerned with immune processes occurring *outside* the cells, such as on cell surfaces or in body fluids. The principal cell involved in antibody production is the B-lymphocyte. In humans the exact site of production of the B-lymphocyte is speculative, although it is probably the bone marrow. In chickens the site is clearly identified as a hind-gut organ known as the bursa of Fabricius, hence the term "B-lymphocyte," or "B-cell." When challenged with an antigen, B-cells divided and differentiate into *plasma cells.* The plasma cells produce and secrete large quantities of antibodies specific to the antigen. Five classes of antibodies of immunoglobulins (Ig) have been identified: G, M, A, D, and E, each serving a specific function.

On initial exposure to an antigen, the B-lymphocyte system begins to produce antibody, predominantly IgM, which appears in 2 to 3 days. This process is referred to as the *primary antibody response.* With subsequent exposure to the antigen, a *secondary antibody response* occurs. Specific IgG antibodies are formed within 4 to 10 days. An example of the secondary response is consecutive administration of immunizations, often called boosters. Memory B-cells allow the immune system to recognize the same antigen for months or years.

When antibody reacts with antigen, they bind to form an antigen-antibody complex. This binding serves several functions. Antibody aids in the phagocytosis of antigen by sensitizing it in such a manner that it is more readily destroyed by phagocytes, a process known as *opsonization.*

Antibody also activates or fixes complement, the second component of humoral immunity. The complement system is a series of proteins (C_1 to C_9) present in serum that results in a cascade of enzymatic actions and death of a viable antigen. After being activated by antibody, complement produces a chemotactic factor that summons T-lymphocytes and macrophages to the antigen site.

Cell-Mediated Immunity

Cell-mediated immunity is involved in a variety of specific functions mediated by the T-lymphocyte and occurs *within* the cell. The T-lymphocyte is so named because it passes through the thymus during the differentiation process, which leads to the mature T-cell. T-lymphocytes do not carry typical immunoglobulins on their surfaces as do the B-cells. However, they are functionally heterogeneous in that several subsets have been identified, including cytotoxic T-cells, helper T-lymphocytes, and suppressor T-lymphocytes. T-cells may also be classified structurally by their

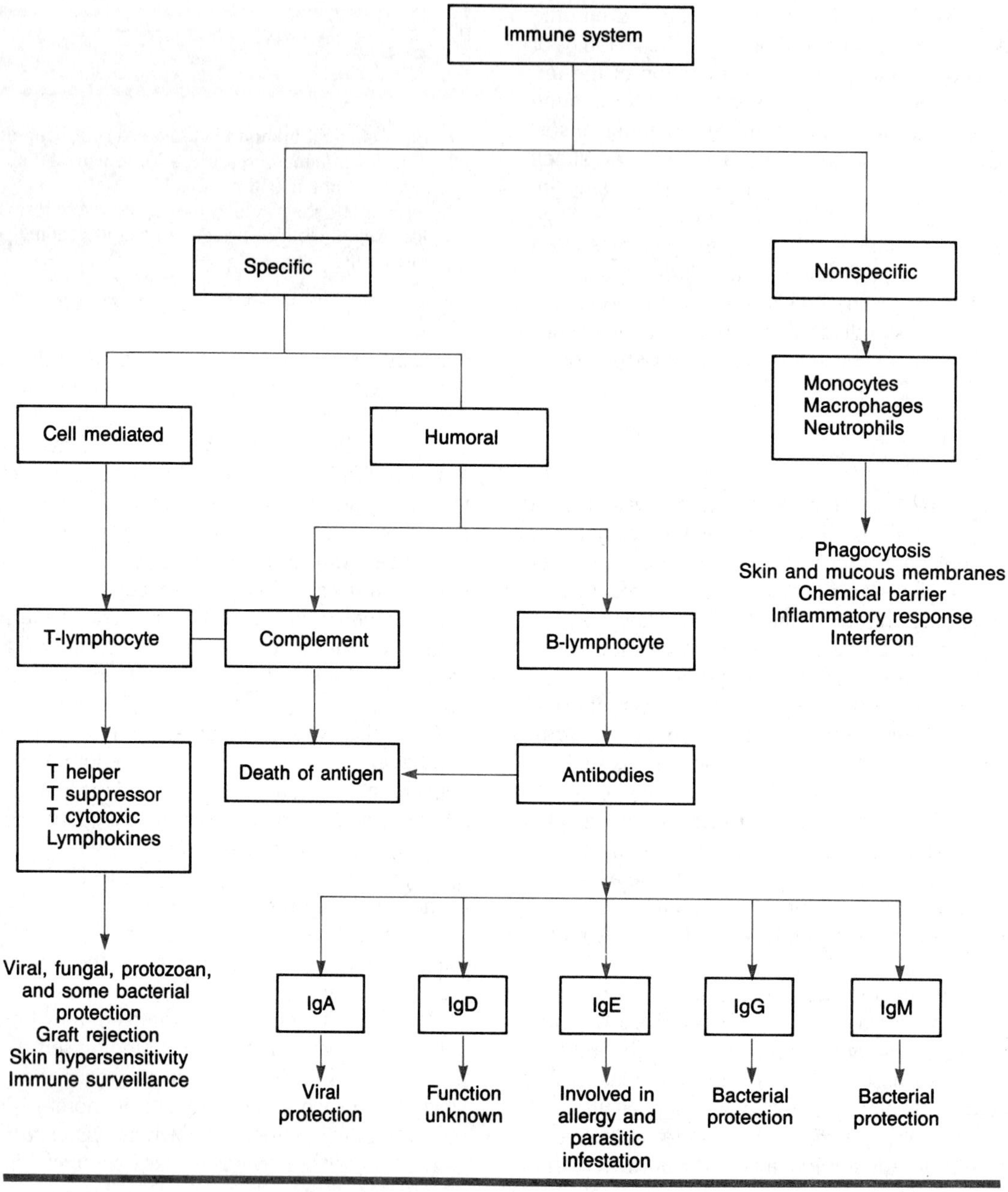

Fig. 35-6. Components of immune system.

surface antigens. Once mature, T-cells display either the T_4 or the T_8 antigen. The T_4, which comprises 60% to 70% of circulating T-cells, consists mainly of helper/inducer cells, whereas the T_8 subset contains cytotoxic/suppressor cells.

Specific functions of T-lymphocytes include: (1) protection against most viral, fungal, and protozoan infections and slow-growing bacterial infections, such as tuberculosis, (2) rejection of histoincompatible grafts, (3) mediation of cutaneous delayed hypersensitivity reactions, such as in tuberculin testing, and (4) probably immune surveillance for malignant cells. In addition, they also have regulatory functions within the immune system. For example, helper T-lymphocytes assist B-lymphocytes and other types of T-cells to mount an optimum immune response.

The cellular immune response is initiated when a T-lymphocyte is sensitized by antigen. In response to this contact the T-cell releases numerous humoral factors called *lymphokines,* which eventually bring about death of the antigen. For example, *chemotactic factor* promotes the migration of phagocytes and other T-lymphocytes to the antigenic area, *migratory inhibitor factor* prevents their leaving the site, *transfer factor* transforms nonsensitized T-cells into sensitized T-lymphocytes, *blastogenic factor* initiates the rapid mitosis of sensitized T-cells, and *macrophage activation factor* transforms local macrophages to highly phagocytic cells. Another lymphokine is *interferon,* which nonspecifically inhibits viral replication, promotes phagocytosis, and stimulates the killer activity of sensitized lymphocytes.

ACQUIRED IMMUNE DEFICIENCY SYNDROME

Acquired immune deficiency syndrome (AIDS) is a recently recognized disorder that has generated intense medical investigation and even greater public concern and fear. The first published reports of unusual opportunistic infections in previously healthy individuals appeared in 1981; retrospective analysis of data demonstrated the existence of cases since 1978, with the first case diagnosed in a child. In 1983 and 1984, a retrovirus (RNA virus) found in AIDS patients was characterized and named. The French researchers named the virus *Lymphadenopathy Associated Virus (LAV)*, and the United States team labeled it *Human T-cell Lymphotrophic Virus Type III (HTLV-III)*. These viruses are one and the same; the term *human immunodeficiency virus (HIV) type I* is now the official name for the virus.

Etiology and High-Risk Groups

HIV is the causative agent for AIDS. The virus has been found in blood and almost all body fluids (semen, saliva, vaginal secretions, urine, breast milk, and tears), but to date there is evidence that the virus is transmitted only through direct contact with blood or blood products, including sharing of intravenous needles for drug use and intimate sexual contact. There is no evidence that *casual* contact between affected and unaffected individuals can spread the virus (Centers for Disease Control, 1986; Kaplan and others, 1985).

Initially AIDS was identified in sexually active homosexual males; since then additional high-risk groups have been identified, which include bisexual males, intravenous drug users, recipients of multiple transfusions (e.g, people with hemophilia), sexual partners of risk-group members, and newborns of infected mothers (e.g., resulting from intravenous drug use in mother or father, maternal promiscuity). People with AIDS (PWA) are a diverse group. In the pediatric age-group, three populations are primarily affected—children who are exposed in utero to an infected mother, children who have received blood products, especially children with hemophilia, and, recently, adolescents who are infected after engaging in high-risk behaviors. Each group has unique needs relative to the origin of the infection. The majority of children with AIDS are less than 2 years of age and constitute a small percentage of the AIDS population. Approximately 77% of these cases resulted from perinatal transmission, and 14% from blood transfusions. Before donor blood was routinely tested for HIV (March, 1985), children with hemophilia were especially at risk because factor concentrates are prepared from pooled plasma that is obtained from as many as 20,000 donors, thus exposing these children to tens of thousands of blood donors (Speck, 1983). Recent advances in the preparation of concentrates and screening for the antibody to HIV in blood products are reducing the risk to these children and other children who require frequent blood transfusions.

The third pediatric population, adolescents who place themselves at risk because of their life-style, is rapidly increasing (Hein, 1989). The rising incidence of the disorder is of major concern. In the United States the current doubling time for cases is 11 to 12 months. More than 50% of risk-group members in certain areas of the country have been infected with the virus; it is estimated that between 1 and 2 million people (mostly adults) have already been exposed to the virus, with perhaps 1000 new cases a day (Selwyn, 1986). Nearly 1000 infected children under age 13 have been identified in the United States. The largest numbers of cases occur in New York City; Newark, New Jersey; and Miami, Florida (Nicholas and others, 1989). It is estimated that by 1991 there will be over 3000 cases of pediatric HIV infection (Falloon and others, 1989). Although individuals exposed to the virus may demonstrate a positive antibody test to HIV, it is uncertain who are carriers of the virus and who will eventually develop the clinical syndrome of AIDS.

Pathophysiology

AIDS is characterized by a generalized dysfunction of the immune system. In adult-onset AIDS, the primary immunologic abnormality includes helper T-cells. HIV attacks helper T-cells, where it can either lie dormant or proliferate more virus and eventually inactivate the immune role of the cell in which it resides. HIV can also attack macrophages. It does not kill this cell, however, but uses it as a vehicle to cross the blood-brain barrier to spread the virus to the brain. In normal individuals there are more helper than suppressor T-cells (T_8 subset), but in AIDS victims there is a reverse helper-to-suppressor ratio. There is also cutaneous anergy to delayed hypersensitivity antigens. Similar pathologic findings are found in children with AIDS, but they occur later in the disease course.

Abnormal B-cell function is apparent early in pediatric AIDS. Because the helper T-cell controls B-cell functioning, young children with AIDS are deficient in both cellular and humoral systems. Often there are increased numbers of B-cells and increased levels of IgG, IgM, and IgA, but deficiencies of IgG subclasses have been identified. Despite the hypergammaglobulinemia, the immunoglobulins are nonfunctional, leaving the body defenseless to many opportunistic infections (Iazzetti, 1986).

Clinical Manifestations

The majority of children with perinatally acquired AIDS appear normal at birth but develop symptoms within the first 24 months of life. The clinical manifestations include lymphadenopathy, hepatosplenomegaly, parotitis, opportunistic infections, such as recurrent upper respiratory infections and persistent oral candidiasis, and chronic or recurrent diarrhea. Neurologic involvement occurs in 50% of the children with HIV infection. It is usually manifested as a progressive encephalopathy (see Chapter 37). The neurologic manifestations are characterized by a developmental delay, or, after achieving normal developments, loss of motor milestones. There is decreased brain growth as evidenced by microcephaly and abnormal neurologic examination findings. Many of these children are excessively irritable and difficult to console (Cooper, Pelton, and LeMay, 1988).

A small number of HIV-infected infants have craniofacial dysmorphic features. At this time it is not known if this is related to the infection or to other factors. Kaposi sarcoma, one of the hallmarks of the adult disease, is found in less than 10% of the affected children. Clinical and laboratory signs of AIDS in children with maternal transmission usually occur between 3 months and 3 years.

Diagnostic Evaluation

The Centers for Disease Control (CDC) have defined specific criteria for the diagnosis of AIDS in children less than 13 years old. Children less than 13 months old have one of the following:

1. Confirmed HIV in blood or tissues
2. Symptoms meeting CDC case definition
3. HIV antibody and evidence of both cellular and humoral deficiency and symptoms

Older children have one of the following:

1. Confirmed HIV in blood or tissues
2. HIV antibody
3. Symptoms meeting CDC case definition (Recommendation, 1988)

Because of the number of disorders that may mimic AIDS, such as severe combined immunodeficiency disease and Wiskott-Aldrich syndrome, the diagnosis is often one of ruling out other probable causes, demonstrating the principal immunologic abnormalities in AIDS, and establishing a positive antibody to HIV. A positive HIV antibody test is not sufficient to establish a diagnosis of AIDS, because HIV virus infections result in a spectrum of responses, from asymptomatic seroconversion to complete immunologic incompetence (Church, Allen, and Stiehm, 1986).

Therapeutic Management

Currently there is no cure for AIDS, and the disease is uniformly fatal. AIDS is the ninth leading cause of death among children 1 to 4 years of age and the seventh in young people between 15 and 24 years of age (Novello and others, 1989). Sixty-five percent of children with perinatally transmitted AIDS die within the first 24 months of age (Task Force on Pediatric AIDS, 1988). Zidovudine (AZT (Retrovir)) has been approved for use in pediatrics. Although not a cure, this drug appears to control disease progression. Clinical improvements include weight gain in children with previous growth retardation, a reduction in the size of enlarged livers and spleens, improvements in IQ scores and other measures of brain function, and improvement in immune system function (Progress, 1990). Treatment is also directed at the prevention and management of the opportunistic infections. The most common infections are chronic candidiasis and interstitial pneumonia, especially *Pneumocystis carinii,* which occurs in greater than 70% of affected children. Combination therapy for *P. carinii* includes trimethoprim/sulfamethoxazole (Bactrim, Septra) and pentamidine. If a skin reaction, fever, or cytopenia occurs secondary to the trimethoprim/sulfamethoxazole, the drug is discontinued.

Gamma globulin administration may be helpful to compensate for the deficiency of B-lymphocytes. Ongoing studies are investigating the benefits of periodic administration of intravenous gamma globulin. Preliminary results suggest that the treated group may have fewer episodes of bacterial infection (Rubinstein and others, 1986).

Disease prevention is of great importance for these children, and immunization against common childhood illnesses is recommended for all children with HIV infection. The only change in the schedule is the use of inactivated poliovirus (IPV) rather than oral poliovirus (OPV) for these children and their close contacts. For children with AIDS, the pneumococcal and influenza vaccines are recommended (Recommendations, 1988).

Nursing Considerations

Nursing considerations are primarily directed at preventing the transmission of the virus, caring for the child with AIDS, and educating the public regarding the *realistic* concerns in terms of communicability of the virus. Recommendations for preventing spread of the virus consist of Universal Precautions, which are the same guidelines for preventing the transmission of other blood-borne diseases, such as hepatitis B virus (see Infection Control, Chapter 27). These precautions should be routinely enforced, regardless of whether the child is a known carrier.

The nursing care of the child with AIDS is primarily supportive, both physiologically and psychologically. The physiologic care of the AIDS patient is directed at minimum exposure to infections, nutritional support, comfort measures, and assessment and recognition of changes in status that may indicate impending sepsis or other complications. Fever is a cardinal sign of infection, especially since other responses to infection are usually absent. The psychologic interventions will vary with the etiology of the infection.

The family of the child infected in utero usually is faced with multiple problems. The mother is infected. Her most likely exposure occurred through either intravenous drug use, prostitution, or sex with a bisexual partner. Since the mother is carrying the virus, she may be ill or dying and therefore unable to care for a child. Often grandparents or other relatives may have to assume responsibility for the care of the child. If no extended family is available, the child may become a ward of the state, often a long-term boarder in an acute care hospital.

Since these children are frequently ill, they may spend most of their lives in a hospital. Foster care is difficult to arrange because of the nature of the illness and the fear of disease transmission. These children have many symptoms, including diarrhea, lung infections, failure to thrive, and encephalopathy. They are often irritable, with a shrill cry, and difficult to console. If there is family involvement, nursing considerations are directed at supporting the family. Whenever possible, social services and home health and nutritional services such as Women, Infants, and Children (WIC) should be made available. Since the disease is congenitally acquired, the parents must deal with feelings of guilt. They will need support during the disease progression and terminal phase (Box 35-3).

Children with hemophilia represent the second major population with AIDS in the pediatric age-group. They are infected with the virus secondary to treatment of their pri-

NURSING CARE PLAN
The Child with AIDS

NURSING DIAGNOSIS: Potential for infection related to impaired body defenses, presence of infective organisms

GOAL 1
Prevent infection

INTERVENTIONS

Promote good health practices
- Maintain adequate nutrition
- Maintain good hygienic habits

Protect child from contact with infected persons
Observe thorough handwashing
Place child in room with noninfectious children; restrict visitors with active illnesses
Advise visitors (and hospital personnel) to practice good handwashing
Restrict contact with persons who have infections, including family, other children, friends, and members of staff
Observe medical asepsis
Keep child dry and warm
*Administer medications as prescribed
*Administer appropriate immunizations as prescribed

EXPECTED OUTCOMES

Child and family apply good health practices
Child exhibits no evidence of infection

GOAL 2
Prevent spread of infection to others

INTERVENTIONS

Employ infection control (see Chapter 27)
Instruct others (parents, members of staff) in appropriate precautions
Teach affected children protective methods to prevent spread of infection, for example, handwashing, handling genital area, care after using bedpan or toilet
Endeavor to keep infants and small children from placing hands and objects in contaminated areas
Assess home situation and implement protective measures as feasible in individual circumstances
*Administer antimicrobial medications if prescribed
Support body's natural defenses, e.g., good nutrition

EXPECTED OUTCOME

Others remain free from infection

NURSING DIAGNOSIS: Potential for infection related to risk factors for AIDS

GOAL 1
Prevent AIDS

*Dependent nursing action.
*Dependent nursing action.

INTERVENTIONS

Educate children and youth regarding the prevention of transmission of AIDS
Attempt to discourage youth from engaging in intimate sexual contacts (especially casual contacts), including homosexual pairings
Educate sexually active youth regarding use of condoms to minimize exposure to genital mucous membranes and secretions
Educate IV drug users regarding dangers of sharing needles and IV equipment (if unable to prevent IV drug use)
Check all blood products for evidence of AIDS testing before administration

EXPECTED OUTCOME

Children and youth do not contract AIDS infection

GOAL 2
Prevent transmission of disease to others

INTERVENTIONS

See above
Implement and carry out Universal Precautions, especially body substance isolation (see Infection Control Chapter 27)
Place restrictions on behaviors and contacts for affected children who bite or who do not have control of their bodily secretions

EXPECTED OUTCOME

Others do not acquire the disease

NURSING DIAGNOSIS: Altered family processes related to having a child with a dreaded and life-threatening disease

GOAL 1
Support family

INTERVENTIONS AND EXPECTED OUTCOMES

See Nursing Care Plan: The Family of the Ill or Hospitalized Child, Chapter 26

NURSING DIAGNOSIS: Anticipatory grief related to having a child with a potentially fatal illness

See Nursing Care Plan: The Child Who Is Terminally Ill or Dying, Chapter 23

NURSING CARE PLAN
The Child with AIDS—cont'd

NURSING DIAGNOSIS: Impaired social interaction

GOAL 1

Maintenance of peer group

INTERVENTIONS

Assist child in identifying personal strengths
Educate school personnel and classmates about AIDS
Encourage child to participate in activities with other children

EXPECTED OUTCOME

Child participates in activities with peer group and family

NURSING DIAGNOSIS: Altered sexuality pattern

GOAL 1

Adolescent identifies safe, healthy expression of sexuality

INTERVENTIONS

Educate adolescent about:
- Sexual transmission
- Risks of perinatal infection
- Dangers of promiscuity
- Abstinence, use of condoms
- Avoidance of high-risk behaviors

EXPECTED OUTCOMES

Adolescent exhibits a positive sexual identity
Adolescent does not infect other individuals

Box 35-3 VARIABLES UNIQUE TO PEDIATRIC AIDS AND GRIEF

Secrecy regarding the diagnosis
Isolation
Lack of support
Fear/worry about disclosure of the diagnosis
Prior feelings of guilt, anger, and/or denial may return
Siblings and family members may be unaware of the diagnosis
Parent may be ill or dying from HIV/AIDS

From Boland, M., Mahan-Rudolph, P., and Evans, P.: Special issues in the care of the child with HIV infection/AIDS. In Martin, B, editor: Pediatric hospice care: what helps, Los Angeles, CA, 1989, LA Children's Hospital, p. 132.

mary illness. Since hemophilia is a genetically transmitted disease, the parents experience guilt, as well as the probable loss of their child. These children are usually older and must deal with peer groups, schools, and the usual developmental tasks of childhood. Other children and families often fear possible disease transmission. The nurse must provide the education to dispel the myth that HIV is spread through casual contact. As these individuals become adolescents and possibly sexually active, they must be taught responsible sexual behavior. Many states have required AIDS education programs in schools.

A third group of individuals increasingly infected with HIV is adolescents. As the young people engage in the high-risk behaviors associated with AIDS, the possibility of infection increases. Adolescents must be taught about the risk factors, including intravenous drug use and high-risk sexual practices, including promiscuity and anal intercourse (see Human Immunodeficiency Virus Infection and Acquired Immune Deficiency Syndrome, Chapter 20). Numerous AIDS educational materials are available (Hobbie, 1988).

One of the most pressing concerns in caring for PWA is protection for the caregiver. Because of the uniformly fatal nature of this disease, limiting exposure of the HIV to uninfected persons is of crucial importance. Universal Precautions (see Chapter 27) must be used in caring for all patients. Unfortunately, the public is also very fearful of contracting the disease from AIDS victims, and criticism and ostracism of the child and family are common. In an effort to protect the child and deal with the community's fear, the family may keep the child at home in an atmosphere of overprotection. While certain precautions are justified in limiting exposure to sources of infection, they must be tempered with concern for the child's normal developmental needs. Both the family and the community need education about AIDS virus to dispel many of the myths that have been perpetuated by the uninformed.*

Of major concern for both family and community has been school attendance for children with AIDS. Both the Centers for Disease Control (1985) and the American Academy of Pediatrics (1986) have published guidelines regarding school attendance, which include the following:

1. Unrestricted school attendance for most school-aged children and adolescents, with the approval of their personal physician, is recommended, including children with AIDS or AIDS-related complex, or who have antibody to the virus.

*Information is available from the AIDS hotline: (800) 342-2437 (AIDS).

2. Students who do not have control of their bodily secretions, who display behaviors such as biting, or who have open sores that cannot be covered may present a greater risk and should be given a more restricted school environment until more is known about the disease.

Nurses need to be knowledgeable of these guidelines and of changes that may occur as additional information about the virus is known. School nurses, in particular, play a vital role in educating the public and in monitoring the needs of the affected child. Confidentiality is a major factor—the number of personnel aware of the child's condition should be kept to a minimum. In addition, school personnel must be aware of sanitary practices to prevent spread of the virus, including proper disposal of items contaminated with blood, for example, sanitary napkins, tissues from caring for a bloody nose, or bandages used in cleaning a wound. Nursing care of the child with AIDS is summarized in the Nursing Care Plan on pp. 1647-1648.

SEVERE COMBINED IMMUNODEFICIENCY DISEASE

Severe combined immunodeficiency disease (SCID) is a defect characterized by absence of both humoral and cell-mediated immunity. The terms *Swiss-type lymphopenic agammaglobulinemia,* an autosomal-recessive form of the disease, and *X-linked lymphopenic agammaglobulinemia* have been used to describe this disorder, which, as the names imply, can follow either mode of inheritance.

Pathophysiology

The exact cause of SCID is unknown. The theories include (1) a defective stem cell that is incapable of differentiating into B- or T-cells, (2) defective organs responsible for the differentiating process, primarily the thymus and lymphoid complex, or (3) an enzymatic defect that suppresses lymphocytic cell function.

The consequence of the immunodeficiency is an overwhelming susceptibility to infection and to the *graft-vs-host* reaction, which can occur when any histoincompatible (unmatched) tissue from an immunocompetent donor is infused into the immunodeficient recipient. Because of its immunodeficiency, the body is unable to reject the foreign incompatible tissue. Therefore the antigenic donor cells attack the host's tissues. The graft-vs-host reaction is a serious complication in the only known treatment for SCID, bone marrow transplantation.

Clinical Manifestations

The most common manifestation is susceptibility to infection early in life, most often by 3 months of age when prenatal acquired immunity is exhausted. Specifically, the disorder in children is characterized by chronic infection, failure to completely recover from an infection, frequent reinfection, and infection with unusual agents. In addition, the history reveals no logical source of infection. Failure to thrive is a consequence of the persistent illnesses.

If the child should receive a foreign tissue, such as blood supplements, signs of graft-vs-host reaction, such as fever, skin rash, alopecia, hepatosplenomegaly, and diarrhea, are expected. Since the reaction requires 7 to 20 days for tissue damage to become evident, the symptoms may be mistaken for an infection. However, the presence of a graft-vs-host reaction increases the child's susceptibility to overwhelming infection and therefore is a grave complication.

Diagnostic Evaluation

Diagnosis is usually based on a history of recurrent, severe infections from early infancy, a familial history of the disorder, and specific laboratory findings, which include lymphopenia, lack of lymphocyte response to antigens, and absence of plasma cells in the bone marrow. Documentation of immunoglobulin deficiency is difficult during infancy because of the normally delayed response of the infant to produce his own immunoglobulins and maternal transfer of immunoglobulin G.

Therapeutic Management

The only definitive treatment is a histocompatible bone marrow transplant. The most suitable donor is a sibling with a matched HLA bone marrow. Because SCID is inherited, an identical twin, who usually is a perfect donor, is not a candidate, since that offspring would also display the disorder. Since the host's immunologic system is incompetent, graft rejection is not a problem. However, a graft-vs-host reaction is always a possibility, and once it occurs, little can be done to reverse the process.

Other approaches to SCID are providing passive immunity with intravenous immunoglobulin and maintaining the child in a sterile environment. The latter is effective only if instituted before the existence of any infectious process in the infant, and it represents an extreme effort to prevent life-threatening infections. Other investigational transplant procedures include nonidentical HLA bone marrow grafts and fetal liver or thymus transplants. However, the results are still uncertain, although they provide potential hope for future children born with the disorder.

Nursing Considerations

Nursing care depends on the type of therapy used. If bone marrow transplantation is attempted, the care is consistent with that needed for bone marrow transplantation for any condition (see Chapter 36). To prevent infection, all interventions aimed at protecting the immunocompromised child are implemented (see Nursing Care Plan: The Child with AIDS, p. 1647). However, even with exacting environmental control, these children are prone to opportunistic infection. Chronic fungal infections of the mouth and nails with *Candida albicans* are frequent problems despite vigorous efforts at prevention or treatment. A hoarse voice may result from repeated esophageal and vocal cord erosions from the fungus. It is important to stress to parents that such conditions are not a result of laxity on their part in preventing them but are the result of the severe immunologic disorder. Parents should be encouraged to immediately notify a physician regarding any evidence of a worsening infection.

Since the prognosis for SCID is very poor if a compatible

bone marrow donor is not available, nursing care is directed at supporting the family in caring for a child with a life-threatening illness (see Chapter 23). Genetic counseling is essential because of the modes of transmission in either form of the disorder.

WISKOTT-ALDRICH SYNDROME

The Wiskott-Aldrich syndrome is an X-linked recessive disorder characterized by a triad of abnormalities: (1) thrombocytopenia, (2) eczema, and (3) immunodeficiency of selective functions of B- and T-lymphocytes.

Pathophysiology

The exact defect is unknown. A variety of pathologic findings are evident. The platelets are abnormally small in size and have a shortened life span, possibly because of a met abolic defect in their synthesis. The primary immunologic defect consists of the inability of phagocytes (macrophages) to process foreign antigens, particularly polysaccharides such as pneumococcus. As a result, immunologically competent cells fail to produce normal immunoglobulin patterns. Early in life the immunoglobulin levels may be normal, but later low levels of IgM are observed. Typically isohemagglutinins (anti-A and anti-B agglutinins in the blood) are decreased or absent.

The thymus and lymph nodes are normal at birth but become progressively dysfunctional with age until a profound cellular immunodeficiency results. Consequently, these children are highly susceptible to infection and malignancy, especially lymphoma and leukemia.

Clinical Manifestations

At birth the major effect of the disorder is bleeding because of the thrombocytopenia. As the child grows older, recurrent infection and eczema become more severe, and the bleeding becomes less frequent.

Eczema is typical of the allergic type and readily becomes superinfected. Chronic infection with herpes simplex is a frequent problem and may lead to chronic keratitis with loss of vision. From infection, chronic pulmonary disease, sinusitis, and otitis media result. In those children who survive the bleeding episodes and overwhelming infections, malignancy presents an additional threat to survival.

Diagnostic Evaluation

Diagnosis can usually be made during the neonatal period because of the thrombocytopenia. Specific tests for immunologic function confirm the diagnosis. Carrier detection is also possible.

Therapeutic Management

Medical treatment mainly involves (1) counteracting the bleeding tendencies with platelet transfusions, (2) using intravenous immunoglobulin to provide passive immunity, and (3) administering prophylactic antibiotics to prevent and control infection. Splenectomy may be performed to reverse the thrombocytopenia, but asplenia imposes the additional risk of fulminant infection. These children require the same prophylactic measures as any child with asplenia—appropriate immunizations and continuous antibiotics—and, despite their immune deficiency, they are able to mount an adequate immunologic response to the inactivated vaccines. When an HLA-matched donor exists, bone marrow transplantation is the treatment of choice.

Nursing Considerations

Because of the grave prognosis for these children, the main nursing consideration is supporting the family in the care of a child with a life-threatening illness (see Chapter 23). Physical care is directed at controlling the problems imposed by the disorder. The measures used to control bleeding are similar to those discussed under hemophilia and epistaxis. Another major goal is related to preventing or controlling infection. Since eczema is a troublesome problem, nursing measures specific to this condition are especially important.

The genetic implications of this X-linked recessive disorder differ little from those of hemophilia. However, because of the multiplicity of defects, the emotional adjustment and physical care required for these children are greater than those of many other conditions. The nurse can be especially supportive by providing short-term goals during periods of hospitalization and by focusing on long-range needs through coordinated efforts with a public health nurse.

KEY POINTS

- Major functions of the hematologic system include production of cells, oxygenation, nutrient distribution to the cells, immune protection, collection of wastes from the cells, and heat regulation.
- The major blood-forming organs of the body are red bone marrow, lymphatic system, and reticuloendothelial system.
- Anemia is defined as reduction of red cell volume or hemoglobin concentration to levels below normal; disorders are classified either by etiology/physiology or by morphology.
- The nurse's role in treatment of anemia is to assist in establishing a diagnosis, prepare the child for laboratory tests, decrease tissue oxygen needs, implement safety precautions, and observe for complications.
- The main nursing goal in prevention of nutritional anemia is parent education regarding correct feeding practices.
- Four types of sickle cell crisis are: vaso-occlusive, splenic sequestration, aplastic, and hyperhemolytic.
- Nursing care of the child with sickle cell disease is aimed at teaching the family how to recognize and prevent sickling, managing pain during splenic crises, and helping the child and parents adjust to lifelong, potentially fatal disease.
- Nursing care of the child with thalassemia entails observing for complications of multiple blood transfusions, assisting the child to cope with the effects of illness, and fostering parent-child adjustment to long-term illness.

- Common causes of aplastic anemia include irradiation, drugs, industrial and household chemicals, infections, infiltration and replacement of myeloid elements, and idiopathic conditions.
- Nursing care of the child with hemophilia involves preventing bleeding by decreasing the risk of injury, recognizing and managing bleeding, preventing the crippling effects of joint degeneration, and preparing and supporting the child and family for home care.
- Pediatric clinical manifestations of AIDS include failure to thrive, interstitial pneumonitis, and hepatosplenomegaly.

REFERENCES

Alter, B.P.: Antenatal diagnosis of thalassemia: a review. In Bank, A., Anderson, W.F., and Zaino, E.C., editors: Fifth Cooley's anemia symposium, vol. 445, New York, 1985, Ann. N.Y. Acad. Sci.

American Academy of Pediatrics, Committee on School Health, and Committee on Infectious Diseases: School attendance of children and adolescents with human T lymphotropic virus III/lymphadenopathy-associated virus infection, Pediatrics 77(3):430-432, 1986.

American Pain Society: Principles of analgesic use in the treatment of acute pain and chronic cancer pain, ed. 2, Skokie, IL, 1989, The Society.

Beaudry, M.A., and others: Survival of a hydropic infant with homozygous α-thalassemia-1, J. Pediatr. 108(5):713-716, 1986.

Bianchi, D.W., and others: Normal long-term survival with α-thalassemia, J. Pediatr. 108(5):716-718, 1986.

Borgna-Pignatti, C., and others: Growth and sexual maturation in thalassemia major, J. Pediatr. 106(1):150-155, 1985.

Centers for Disease Control: Apparent transmission of HTLV-III/LAV from a child to a mother providing health care, MMWR 35(5):76-79, 1986.

Centers for Disease Control: Education and foster care of children infected with human T-lymphotropic virus type III/lymphadenopathy-associated virus, MMWR 34(34):517-521, 1985.

Charache, S.: Advances in the understanding of sickle cell anemia, Hosp. Pract. 21(2):173-190, 1986.

Charache, S., Lubin, B., and Reid, C.D.: Management and therapy of sickle cell disease, U.S. Department of Health and Human Services, Public Health Service, National Institutes of Health, Pub. No. 89-2117, Washington, DC, 1989.

Church, J.A., Allen, J.R., and Stiehm, E.R.: New scarlet letter(s), pediatric AIDS, Pediatrics 77(3):423-427, 1986.

Cohen, F.: Clinical genetics in nursing practice, Philadelphia, 1984, J.B. Lippincott Co.

Cole, T.B., and others: Intravenous narcotic therapy for children with severe sickle pain crisis, Am. J. Dis. Child. 40:1255-1259, 1986.

Cooper, E.R., Pelton, S.I., and LeMay, M.: Acquired immunodeficiency syndrome: a new population of children at risk, Pediatr. Clin. North Am. 35(6):1365, 1988.

Deinard, A.S., and others: Cognitive deficits in iron-deficient and iron-deficient anemic children, J. Pediatr. 108(1):681-689, 1986.

Emond, A.M., and others: Acute splenic sequestration in homozygous sickle cell disease: natural history and management, J. Pediatr. 107(2):201-206, 1985.

Falloon, J., and others: Human immunodeficiency virus infection in children, J. Pediatr. 114(1):1, 1989.

Festa, R.S.: Modern management of thalassemia, Pediatr. Ann. 14(9):597-606, 1985.

Frank, A.L., and others: *Haemophilus influenzae* type b immunization of children with sickle cell diseases, Pediatrics 82(4):571-575, 1988.

Gordon-Smith, E.C.: Treatment of aplastic anemias, Hosp. Pract. 20(5):69-84, 1985.

Gowda, N., and others: Human parvovirus infection in patients with sickle cell disease with and without hypoplastic crisis, J. Pediatr. 110(1):81-84, 1987.

Hein, K.: Commentary on adolescent acquired immunodeficiency sydrome: the next wave of the human immunodeficiency virus epidemic? J. Pediatr. 114(1):144-149, 1989.

Hein, K.: Adolescent acquired immunodeficiency syndrome: a paradigm for training in early intervention and care, Am. J. Dis. Child. 144(1):46-48, 1990.

Hobbie, C.: AIDS educational materials, J. Pediatr. Health Care 2(2):109-110, 1988.

Iazzetti, L.: Nursing management of the pediatric AIDS patient, Issues Compr. Pediatr. Nurs. 9(2):119-129, 1986.

Kamani, N.: Marrow transplantation in pediatric hematologic disorders, Pediatr. Ann. 14(9):661-670, 1985.

Kaplan, J.E., and others: Evidence against transmission of human T-lymphotropic virus/lymphadenopathy-associated virus (HTLV-III/LAV) in families of children with the acquired immunodeficiency syndrome, Pediatr. Infect. Dis. 4(5):468-471, 1985.

Karayalcin, G.: Current concepts in the management of hemophilia, Pediatr. Ann. 14(9):640-659, 1985.

Kasprisin, C.A.: Recipient considerations. In Reynolds, A.W., and Steckler, D., editors: Practical aspects of blood administration, Arlington, VA, 1986, American Association of Blood Banks.

Katsanis, E., and others: Prevalence and significance of mild bleeding disorders in children with recurrent epistaxis, J. Pediatr. 113(1, pt. I):73-76, 1988.

Kobrinsky, N.L., and others: Improved hemophilia A carrier detection by DDAVP stimulation of factor VIII, J. Pediatr. 104(5):718-724, 1984.

Lanzkowsky, P.: Problems in diagnosis of iron deficiency anemia, Pediatr. Ann. 14(9):618-636, 1985.

Leikin, S.L., and others: Mortality in children and adolescents with sickle cell disease, Pediatrics 84(3):500-507, 1989.

Lozoff, B., and others: Iron deficiency anemia and iron therapy effects on infant developmental test performance, Pediatrics 79(6):981-995, 1987.

Lucarelli, G., and others: Bone marrow transplantation in patients with thalassemia, N. Engl. J. Med. 322(7):417-421, 1990.

Lukens, J.N.: Iron metabolism and iron deficiency anemia. In Miller, D.R., and others, editors: Blood diseases of infancy and childhood, ed. 5, St. Louis, 1984, Mosby–Year Book, Inc.

Lusher, J.M.: Management of hemophilia. In Westphal, R.G., and Smith, D.M., editors: Treatment of hemophilia and von Willebrand's disease: new developments, Arlington, VA, 1989, American Association of Blood Banks.

Maurer, H.S., and others: A prospective evaluation of iron chelation therapy in children with severe beta-thalassemia: a six-year study, Am. J. Dis. Child. 142(3):287-292, 1988.

McLaughlin, M., and others: Live virus vaccines in human immunodeficiency virus–infected children: a retrospective survey, Pediatrics 82(2):229-233, 1988.

Merhav, H., and others: Tea drinking in infants may cause anemia, Am. J. Clin. Nutr. 41(6):1210-1213, 1985.

Miller, V., Swaney, S., and Deinard, A.: Impact of the WIC program on the iron status of infants, Pediatrics 75:100-150, 1985.

Morrison, R.A., and Vedro, D.A.: Pain management in the child with sickle cell disease, Pediatr. Nurs. 15(6):595-599, 613, 1989.

Nicholas, S.W., and others: Human immunodeficiency virus infection in childhood, adolescence, and pregnancy: a status report and national research agenda, Pediatrics 83(2):293-308, 1989.

Novello, A.C., and others: Final report of the United States Department of Health and Human Services Secretary's work group on pediatric human immunodeficiency virus infection and disease: content and implications, Pediatrics 84(3):547-555, 1989.

Overby, K.J., Lo, B., and Litt, I.F.: Knowledge and concerns about acquired immunodeficiency syndrome and their relationship to behavior among adolescents with hemophilia, Pediatrics 83(2):204-209, 1989.

Pappo, A., and Buchanan, G.: Acute splenic sequestration in a 2-month-old infant with sickle cell anemia, Pediatrics 84(3):578, 1989.

Pearson, H.A.: Sickle cell syndromes and other hemoglobinopathies. In Miller, D.R., and others, editors: Blood diseases of infancy and childhood, ed. 5, St. Louis, 1984, Mosby–Year Book, Inc.

Pearson, H.A., and others: Patient age distribution in thalassemia major: changes from 1973 to 1985, Pediatrics 80(1):53-57, 1987.

Pierce, G.F., and others: The use of purified clotting factor concentrates in hemophilia: influence of viral safety, cost, and supply on therapy, JAMA 261(23):3434-3438, 1989.

Progress in the use of Zidovudine, FDA Drug Bull., p. 6, April 1990.

Recommendations of the immunization practices advisory committee (ACIP): Immunization of children infected with human immunodeficiency virus—supplementary ACIP statement, MMWR 37(12):181-183, 1988.

Reeves, J.D., and Yip, R.: Lack of adverse side effects of oral ferrous sulfate therapy in 1-year-old infants, Pediatrics 75(2):352-355, 1985.

Rubinstein, A., and others: Periodic intravenous gammaglobulin in children with AIDS or AIDS related complex (ARC), Pediatr. Res. 20(4):299A, 1986.

Ryan, A.S., and Martinez, G.A.: Iron intake in the United States during the first year of life according to demographic characteristics, Ecology Food Nutr. 16:21-32, 1985.

Saulsbury, F.: IgA rheumatoid factor in Henoch-Schonlein purpura, J. Pediatr. 108(1):71-76, 1986.

Selwyn, P.A.: AIDS: what is now known. II. Epidemiology, Hosp. Pract. 21(6):127-164, 1986.

Shannon, K.M.: Recombinant erythropoietin in pediatrics: a clinical perspective. Pediatr. Ann. 19(3):197-206, 1990.

Shapiro, B.S.: The management of pain in sickle cell disease, Pediatr. Clin. North Am. 36(4):1029-1043, 1989.

Speck, W.: Acquired immune deficiency syndrome, J. Pediatr. 103(1):161-163, 1983.

Swift, A.V., and others: Neuropsychologic impairment in children with sickle cell anemia, Pediatrics 84(6):1077-1085, 1989.

Task Force on Pediatric AIDS: Perinatal human immunodeficiency virus infection, Pediatrics 62(6):941-944, 1988.

Walter, T., and others: Iron deficiency anemia: adverse effects on infant psychomotor development, Pediatrics 84(1):7-17, 1989.

Werner, E.J., and others: Immunosuppressive therapy versus bone marrow transplantation for children with aplastic anemia, Pediatrics 83(1):61-65, 1989.

Yip, R., Schwartz, S., and Deinard, A.S.: Screening for iron deficiency with the erythrocyte protoporphyrin test, Pediatrics 72(2):214-219, 1983.

Yip, R., and others: Declining prevalence of anemia among low-income children in the United States, JAMA 258(12):1619-1623, 1987a.

Yip, R., and others: Declining prevalence of anemia in childhood in a middle-class setting: a pediatric success story? Pediatrics 80(3):330-334, 1987b.

Ziegler, E.E., and others: Cow milk feeding and GI blood loss, J. Pediatr. 116:11-18, 1990.

Zurlo, M.G., and others: Survival and causes of death in thalassemia major, Lancet 1(8653):27-29, 1989.

BIBLIOGRAPHY

Anemia/Iron Deficiency Anemia

Barbara, J.A.J.: Infectious complications of blood transfusion: viruses, Br. Med. J. 300:450-453, 1990.

Contreras, M., and Mollison, P.L.: Immunological complications of transfusion, Br. Med. J. 300:173-176, 1990.

Dallman, P.R., and Yip, R.: Changing characteristics of childhood anemia, J. Pediatr. 114(1):161-164, 1989.

Groopman, J.E., Molina, J.M., and Scadden, D.T.: Hematopoietic growth factors: biology and clinical applications, N. Engl. J. Med. 321(21):1449-1459, 1989.

Kasprisin, D.O., and Luban, N.L.C.: Pediatric transfusion medicine, vol. 2, Boca Raton, FL, 1987, CRC Press, Inc.

Looker, A.C., and others: Iron status: prevalence of impairment in three Hispanic groups in the United States, Am. J. Clin. Nutr. 49:553-558, 1989.

Miller, D.R.: Anemias: general considerations. In Miller, D.R., and others, editors: Blood diseases of infancy and childhood, ed. 5, St. Louis, 1984, Mosby–Year Book, Inc.

Milne, R.I.G.: Assessment of care of children with sickle cell disease: implications for neonatal screening programmes, Br. Med. J. 300:371-374, 1990.

Monzon, C.M., Beaver, B.D., and Dillon, T.D.: Evaluation of erythrocyte disorders with mean corpuscular volume (MCV) and red cell distribution width (RDW), Clin. Pediatr. 26:632-638, 1987.

Oski, F.A.: Iron deficiency—facts and fallacies, Pediatr. Clin. North Am. 32(2):493-497, 1985.

Patterson, K.L.: The childhood anemias, Pediatr. Nurs. Update 1(4):2-7, 1985.

Pekrun, A., and Gratzer, W.: Disorders of the red-cell membrane, Curr. Opin. Pediatr. 2(1):116-120, 1990.

Reeves, J.D., and others: Iron deficiency in infants: influence of mild antecedent infection, J. Pediatr. 105(6):874-879, 1984.

Rutman, R.C., and others: Blood transfusions, Am. J. Nurs. 84(4):486-489, 1989.

Waskerwitz, M.J.: Iron deficiency anemia in children, Issues Compr. Pediatr. Nurs. 6(5-6):283-294, 1983.

Sickle Cell Disease

Anglin, D.L., and others: Effect of penicillin prophylaxis on nasopharyngeal colonization with *Streptococcus pneumoniae* in children with sickle cell anemia, J. Pediatr. 104(1):18-22, 1984.

Burghardt-Fitzgerald, D.C.: Pain-behavior contracts: effective management of the adolescent in sickle-cell crisis, J. Pediatr. Nurs. 4(5):320-324, 1989.

Evans, J.P.M., and Rogers, D.W.: Sickle cell disease and thalassemia, Curr. Opin. Pediatr. 2(1):121-123, 1990.

Gigliotti, F., and others: Immunization of young infants with sickle cell disease with a *Haemophilus influenzae* type b saccharide-diphtheria CRM_{197} protein conjugate vaccine, J. Pediatr. 114(6):1006-1010, 1989.

Gradolf, B.: Sickle cell anemia in children, Issues Compr. Pediatr. Nurs. 6(5-6):295-306, 1983.

Hathaway, G.: The child with sickle cell anemia: implications and management, Nurse Pract. 9(10):16-22, 1984.

Johnson, F.L., and others: Bone marrow transplantation in patients with sickle cell anemia, N. Engl. J. Med. 311:780-783, 1984.

Lamb, C., editor: Managing sickle cell emergencies, Patient Care 19(1):92-141, 1985.

Miller, S.T., and others: Cerebrovascular accidents in children with sickle-cell disease and alpha-thalassemia, J. Pediatr. 113(5):847-850, 1988.

National Institutes of Health Consensus Development Conference Statement: Newborn screening for sickle cell disease and other hemoglobinopathies, vol. 6, no. 9, pp. 1-8, April 6-8, 1987.

Pearson, H.A., and others: Developmental pattern of splenic dysfunction in sickle cell disorders, Pediatrics 76(3):392-397, 1985.

Phebus, C.K., Glonger, M.F., and Maciak, B.J.: Growth patterns by age and sex in children with sickle cell disease, J. Pediatr. 105(1):28-33, 1984.

Richardson, E.A.W., and Milne, L.S.: Sickle-cell disease and the childbearing family: an update, MCN 8:417-422, 1983.

Rubin, L.G., Voulalas, D., and Carmody, L.: Immunization of children with sickle cell disease with *Haemophilus influenzae* type b polysaccharide vaccine, Pediatrics 84(3):509-512, 1989.

Whitten, C.F., and Bertles, J.F.: Sickle cell disease, vol. 565, New York, 1989, New York Academy of Sciences.

Williams, S., Maude, G.H., and Serjeant, G.R.: Clinical presentation of sickle cell-hemoglobin C disease, J. Pediatr. 109:586-589, 1986.

Thalassemia

Cohen, A.R., Mizanin, J., and Schuartz, E.: Rapid removal of excessive iron with daily high dose intravenous chelation therapy, J. Pediatr. 115(1):151-155, 1989.

Giordano, V.: Psychosocial impacts on a thalassemic patient's life. In Bank, A., Anderson, W.F., and Zaino, E.C., editors: Fifth Cooley's anemia symposium, vol. 445, New York, 1985, Ann. N.Y. Acad. Sci.

Maurer, H.S., and others: A prospective evaluation of iron chelation therapy in children with severe β-thalassemia: a six-year study, Am. J. Dis. Child. 142:287-292, 1988.

Modell, B., and others: Effect of fetal diagnostic testing on birth rate of thalassemia major in Britain, Lancet 2:1383-1386, 1984.

Pearson, H.W., and others: Low risk of hepatitis B from blood transfusions in thalassemic patients in Connecticut, J. Pediatr. 108(2):252-253, 1986.

Piomelli, S., and others: Current strategies in the management of Cooley's anemia. In Bank, A., Anderson, W.F., and Zaino, E.C., editors: Fifth Cooley's anemia symposium, vol. 445, New York, 1985, Ann. N.Y. Acad. Sci.

Sherman, M., and others: Thalassemic children's understanding of illness: a study of cognitive and emotional factors. In Bank, A., Anderson, W.F., and Zaino, E.C., editors: Fifth Cooley's anemia symposium, vol. 445, New York, 1985, Ann. N.Y. Acad. Sci.

Wolfe, L., Sallan, D., and Nathan, D.G.: Current therapy and new approaches to the treatment of thalassemia major. In Bank, A., Anderson, W.F., and Zaino, E.C., editors: Fifth Cooley's anemia symposium, vol. 445, New York, 1985, Ann. N.Y. Acad. Sci.

Aplastic Anemia

Glader, B.E.: Red blood aplasias in children, Pediatr. Ann. (19)3:168-176, 1990.

Griner, P.F.: A survey of the effectiveness of cyclophosphamide in patients with severe aplastic anemia, Am. J. Hematol. 8:55-60, 1980.

Heimpel, H., and Heit, W.: Drug-induced aplastic anaemia: clinical aspects, Clin. Haematol. 9(3):641-662, 1980.

Hunter, R.F., Roth, P.A., and Huang, A.T.: Predictive factors for response to anti-thymocyte globulin in acquired aplastic anemia, Am. J. Med. 79(1):73-78, 1985.

Sanders, J.E., and others: Bone marrow transplantation experience for children with aplastic anemia, Pediatrics 77(2):179-186, 1986.

Weinblatt, M.E., Higgins, G., and Ortega, J.A.: Aplastic anemia in Down's syndrome, Pediatrics 67(6):896-897, 1981.

Defects in Hemostasis

Aledort, L.M.: New approaches to management of bleeding disorders, Hosp. Pract. 24(2):207-226, 1989.

Buchanan, G.R., and others: Hepatitis in household contacts of patients with hemophilia who have received multiple transfusions, J. Pediatr. 108(6):937-939, 1986.

Bussel, J.B.: Thrombocytopenia in newborns, infants, and children, Pediatr. Ann. 19(3):181-193, 1990.

Bussel, J.B., and others: Treatment of acute idiopathic thrombocytopenia of childhood with intravenous infusions of gammaglobulin, J. Pediatr. 106(6):886-890, 1985.

Diethorn, M.L., and Weld, L.M.: Physiologic mechanisms of hemostasis and fibrinolysis, J. Cardiovasc. Nurs. 4(1):1-10, 1989.

Dubansky, A.S., and Oski, F.A.: Controversies in the management of acute idiopathic thrombocytopenic purpura: a survey of specialists, Pediatrics 77(1):49-52, 1986.

Gaddy-Cohen, D.: Idiopathic thrombocytopenic purpura in children, Issues Compr. Pediatr. Nurs. 6(5-6):307-316, 1983.

Gill, J.C., and others: HTLV-III serology in hemophilia: relationship with immunologic abnormalities, J. Pediatr. 108(4):511-516, 1986.

Karpatkin, M.: Screening tests in hemostasis, Pediatr. Clin. North Am. 27(4):831-841, 1980.

Persky, M.S.: Stanching a nasal bleed, Emerg. Med. 14(1):108-115, 1982.

Rosenblum, N., and Winter, H.: Steroid effects on the course of abdominal pain in children with Henoch-Schonlein purpura, Pediatrics 79(6):1018-1021, 1987.

Sergis-Deavenport, E., and Varni, J.W.: Behavioral techniques in teaching hemophilia factor replacement procedures to families, Pediatr. Nurs. 8(6):416-419, 1982.

Shende, A.: Idiopathic thrombocytopenic purpura in children, Pediatr. Ann. 14(9):609-616, 1985.

Stuart, M.J., and others: Bleeding time in hemophilia A: potential mechanisms for prolongation, J. Pediatr. 108(2):215-218, 1986.

Walker, R.W., and Walker, W.: Idiopathic thrombocytopenia: initial illness and long-term follow-up, Arch. Dis. Child. 59:316-322, 1984.

Immunologic Deficiency Disorders

American Academy of Pediatrics: Acquired immunodeficiency syndrome education in schools, Pediatrics 82(2):278-280, 1988.

American Red Cross: AIDS and children: information for teachers and school officials, October 1986, U.S. Public Health Service.

Barrett, D.J.: The clinician's guide to pediatric AIDS, Contemp. Pediatr. 5:24-47, 1988.

Chanock, S.J., and McIntosh, K.: Selected issues in pediatric infection with human immunodeficiency virus, Curr. Opin. Pediatr. 1:16-21, 1989.

Committee on Infectious Diseases: Health guidelines for the attendance in daycare and foster care settings of children infected with human immunodeficiency virus, Pediatrics 79(3):466-471, 1987.

Durandy, A., and others: Prenatal diagnosis of severe combined immunodeficiency, J. Pediatr. 101(6):995-997, 1982.

Epstein, L.G.: Human immunodeficiency virus infection in children: neurologic manifestations and pathogenetic mechanisms, Curr. Opin. Pediatr. 1:290-295, 1989.

Fischer, G.W.: Therapeutic uses of intravenous gammaglobulin for pediatric infections, Pediatr. Clin. North Am. 35(3):517-533, 1988.

Flaskerud, J.H.: AIDS/HIV infection: a reference guide for nursing professionals, Philadelphia, 1989, W.B. Saunders Co.

Goodman, E., and Cohall, A.T.: Acquired immunodeficiency syndrome and adolescents: knowledge, attitudes, beliefs, and behaviors in a New York City adolescent minority population, Pediatrics 84(1):36-42, 1989.

Guidelines for effective school health education to prevent the spread of AIDS, MMWR 37(S-2):1-13, 1988.

Guidelines for prevention of transmission of human immunodeficiency virus and hepatitis B virus to health-care and public-safety workers, MMWR 38(S-6), June 23, 1989.

Gurka, A.M.: The immune system: implications for critical care nursing, Crit. Care Nurse 9(7):24-36, 1989.

Henley, W.L.: Mechanisms of autoimmunity, Pediatr. Ann. 11(3):293-300, 1982.

Jason, J.M., and others: Human immunodeficiency virus infection in hemophilic children, Pediatrics 82(4):565-569, 1988.

Jemison-Smith, P., and Hamm, P.: Immune responses, Crit. Care Update 10(8):45-46, 1983.

Meuwissen, H.J., and others: Long-term survival after bone marrow transplantation: a 15-year follow-up report of a patient with Wiskott-Aldrich syndrome, J. Pediatr. 105(3):365-369, 1984.

Selekman, J.: The multiple faces of immune deficiency in children, Pediatr. Nurs. 16(4):351-355, 361, 1990.

Steiner, J.D., and others: Are adolescents getting smarter about acquired immunodeficiency syndrome? Am. J. Dis. Child. 144(3):302-306, 1990.

Stiehm, E.R.: Clinical and laboratory evaluation of the child with suspected immunodeficiency, Pediatr. Rev. 7(2):53-61, 1985.

Task Force on Pediatric AIDS: Pediatric guidelines for infection control of human immunodeficiency virus (acquired immunodeficiency virus) in hospitals, medical offices, schools, and other settings, Pediatrics 82(5):801-807, 1988.

Taylor, D.L.: Immune response: physiology, signs, and symptoms, Nursing '84 14(5):52-54, 1984.

Todd, J.: A most intimate foe: how the immune system can betray the body it defends, Science 30(2):20-27, 1990.

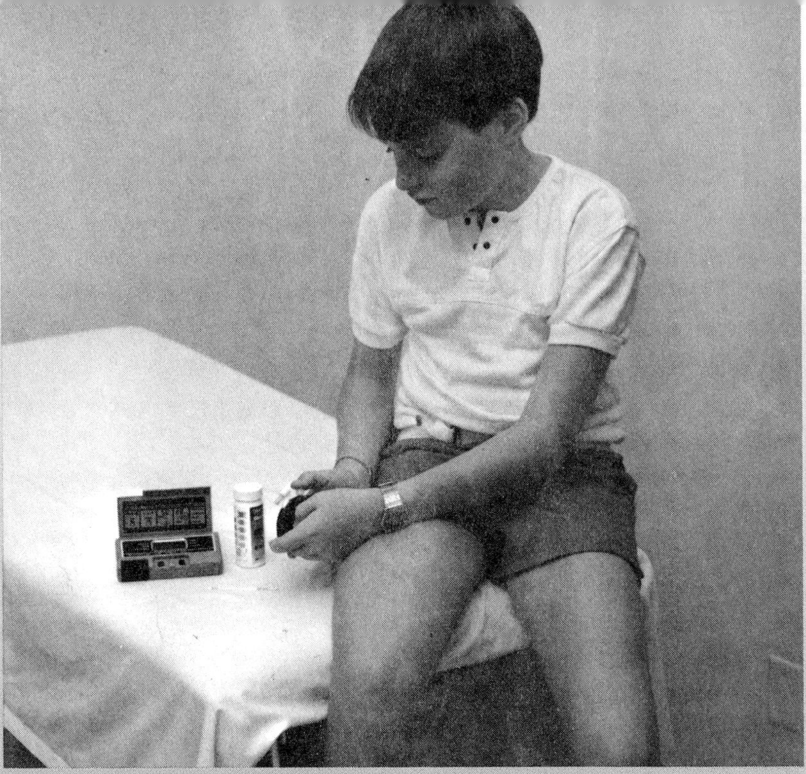

The Child with a Disturbance of Regulatory Mechanisms

UNIT

XIII

In an organism such as a human being, the maintenance of dynamic equilibrium involves a complex interaction of many systems and subsystems. All the activities within the individual cells, tissues, and organs that comprise these systems depend on the function of other systems, and, like all systems, each component has one or more factors that act on it or affect it. A change in one component can affect all other components.

Regulation enables the organism to maintain the function of cells, tissues, organs, and systems within the parameters described as normal for that system despite changes in the internal or external environment. Communication between the various systems and subsystems is carried by chemical or neural mechanisms. Disturbances in the regulatory processes can create disturbances in one or more of the interrelated components of the system with consequences that affect other systems and the organism as a whole.

The major regulatory mechanisms of the body are the endocrine and neural systems. Dysfunction in the central nervous system is discussed in Chapter 37, *The Child with Cerebral Dysfunction.* Defects in the integrity of the peripheral nervous system are elaborated in Unit XIV. It is sometimes difficult to determine if dysfunctions in this interrelated system are caused by impaired function in the target glands that secrete the hormones, the pituitary tropic substances that stimulate the target glands to secrete hormones, or the portions of the midbrain that produce releasing factors that stimulate the pituitary gland. Defects within the complex neuroendocrine regulatory system and the pancreatic hormones are discussed in Chapter 38, *The Child with Endocrine Dysfunction.*

Chapter 36, *The Child with Cancer,* is concerned with disordered cell proliferation. Although the mechanism is unknown, it is believed that altered cell regulation may be caused by a genetic abnormality, which is in some way provoked by environmental or other influences into initiating uncontrolled abnormal cell proliferation—the malignant process. It is speculated that some regulatory mechanism is affected, probably the immune response.

CHAPTER 36

The Child with Cancer

RELATED TOPICS

GLOSSARY

ALL Acute lymphocytic leukemia
ANLL Acute nonlymphocytic leukemia
B-cell B-lymphocyte
biopsy Removal of tissue for examination
biotherapy Treatment that uses BRM to combat malignancy
BMT Bone marrow transplantation
BRM Biologic response modifier
CALLA Common acute lymphoblastic leukemic antigen

carcinogen Substance that causes cancer
chemotherapy Treatment with chemical substances having a specific effect on a disease
classification Identification of specific characteristics of a disease
CT Computer tomography
FAB French-American-British system
GVHD Graft-versus-host disease
immunosuppression Inhibition of antibodies to antigens that may be present
limb salvage Preservation of the limb with removal of a tumor
LP Lumbar puncture
malignancy A cancerous condition
metastasis A second lesion developing away from the primary lesion
MRI Magnetic resonance imaging
myelosuppression Reduction in the blood-forming cells made in the bone marrow
neoplasm A mass of newly formed tissue
NHL Non-Hodgkin lymphoma
oncology The study of cancer
protocol Written statement of a specific treatment plan
radiotherapy Treatment by means of irradiation
staging Defining the phase of a disease
SVCS Superior vena cava syndrome
T-cell T-lymphocyte
tumor lysis Rapid breakdown of malignant cells

There are few situations in nursing that exceed the challenges of caring for a child with cancer. Despite the dramatic improvements in survival rates for these children, the needs of the family are tremendous as they cope with a serious physical illness as well as the fear that the child will not be cured. This chapter is concerned primarily with the physical problems associated with several types of childhood cancer. The general psychologic needs of these children and their families are discussed in Chapter 22 in terms of chronic illness and in Chapter 23 for situations when the outcome becomes life-threatening and death is a possibility. Except for specific emotional concerns of the family that are unique to the type of cancer, the interventions thoroughly explored in these earlier chapters are not repeated here. Nurses are encouraged to apply the psychologic principles of care whenever they are involved with these children and their families. The child's future, not just the cancer, must be viewed as the priority. If a cured child is a possible outcome, then a *truly cured child* is an essential outcome—that is, a child who is not just free of disease but who is developmentally commensurate with age and well adjusted to the experience of having cancer (van Eys, 1977).

The purpose of discussing types of childhood cancer in one chapter is to present a comprehensive model of the nursing care that applies to these diseases. In addition, since many of the diagnostic procedures and medical therapies differ little from one type of malignancy to another, discussing them together allows for a detailed exploration without undue repetition.

CANCER IN CHILDREN

Cancer is the leading cause of death from disease in children ages 3 to 15 years and the second cause of death from all causes, exceeded only by injuries. The incidence of cancer in this age-group is approximately 12.9 per 100,000 white children and 10.1 per 100,000 black children (Miller, 1989). If the present rates continue, the projected number of new cases will be about 7600 per year in the United States, with an estimated 1600 deaths in 1990 (Cancer facts, 1990).

For children in all age-groups, leukemia is the most frequent cancer, followed by brain tumors and lymphomas (Table 36-1). However, there are some important differences between groups. Tumors of the kidney and soft tissue are more common in blacks, whereas tumors of the bone are more common in whites. Males are affected more often by cancer than females (ratio of 1.2:1), although this varies with the type of cancer. The most frequent forms of cancer occur in more males, but tumors of the skin and gonads are found in more females (Cancer facts, 1990).

Probably the most significant aspect of childhood cancer is the improved prognosis during the last 3 decades. Mortality among children with cancer has declined from 8.3 per 100,000 in 1950 to 3.5 per 100,000 in 1986 (Cancer facts, 1990). Currently, more than 50% of all children with malignant neoplasms treated at major cancer centers will become long-term survivors. The cancers demonstrating the greatest improvement in survival rates are acute leukemia,

Table 36-1 Cancer incidence by site for children under 15, SEER program 1982-1986

SITE	PERCENT OF TOTAL	RATE PER 1,000,000 CHILDREN
Leukemia	30.5	39.7
Brain and nervous system	20.1	27.0
Lymphoma	10.5	15.1
Kidney	7.0	8.8
Soft tissue	6.3	8.2
Bone	4.8	7.1
Eye	3.7	4.8
Liver	1.7	2.0
All other	15.4	20.0
All sites	100.0	132.7

Data from Cancer Statistics Branch, National Cancer Institute.

Marilyn Hockenberry-Eaton, R.N., M.S.N., P.N.P., assisted in the revision of this chapter.

lymphomas, Wilms tumor, rhabdomyosarcoma, osteosarcoma, and Ewing sarcoma (Miller, 1989). However, black children with cancer do more poorly than white children (Cancer facts, 1990).

Although survival is discussed in terms of "cure," the term *biologic cure* is not absolute, since it is not possible to demonstrate definitively complete eradication of all cancer cells, and late recurrences do occur. The definition of cure includes the criteria of (1) cessation of therapy, (2) continuous freedom from clinical and laboratory evidence of cancer, and (3) minimum or no risk of relapse, as determined by previous experience with the disease. The time that must elapse before a child clinically free of cancer is considered cured varies with each type of cancer but typically ranges from 2 to 5 years.

ETIOLOGIC FACTORS

The cause of cancer is not known. While there are numerous hypotheses concerning its origin, the most enduring theory is that some genetic alteration results in the unregulated proliferation of cells. Recent studies have demonstrated the existence of genes activated in human tumors that are capable of causing uncontrolled proliferation of cells when transmitted to normal cells. Genes having the potential to transform normal cells into malignant ones are called *oncogenes.* What causes the induction of cell transformation is speculative, but RNA tumor viruses (also called retroviruses, because they have the ability to translate RNA back to DNA) may play a role in the transfer of DNA from a malignant cell to a normal cell (Stine, 1989). The identification of the human T-cell leukemia-lymphoma virus (HTLV) in some forms of adult leukemia and lymphoma and the Epstein-Barr (EB) virus, a type of herpes virus, in Burkitt lymphoma has lent support to this theory (Li and others, 1988). While these viruses have been isolated, there is no firm evidence that childhood cancer is communicable.

Despite the lack of knowledge about the origin of cancer, there is considerable information on risk factors that increase the likelihood of children developing specific types of cancer. The following is a brief overview of some of the etiologic factors implicated in childhood cancer.

Several environmental agents that are carcinogenic (capable of producing cancer) in adults have been described, but only one of these—ionizing radiation—has been implicated in children. Low doses of radiation have been known to cause thyroid cancer and leukemia. There is some evidence that exposing pregnant women to diagnostic radiographic procedures increases the occurrence of leukemia and other forms of cancer among their children (Li and others, 1988).

Although drugs, particularly those containing radioisotopes and immunosuppressive agents, can increase the risk of developing childhood cancer, the one drug most notably recognized for its carcinogenic effect is diethylstilbestrol. Large doses of this hormone given to pregnant women to prevent abortion cause adenocarcinoma of the vagina in a significant proportion of the female offspring when they reach adolescence and early adulthood.

Some childhood cancers, in particular retinoblastoma, Wilms tumor, and neuroblastoma, may demonstrate patterns of inheritance that suggest a genetic basis for the disorder.

The Philadelphia chromosome was the first chromosomal abnormality to be found in a malignancy. It occurs as a result of a translocation between chromosomes 9 and 22 and is observed in almost all individuals with chronic myelogenous leukemia (Rubin, 1988). Chromosomal abnormalities have been found in children with acute leukemia as well as Ewing sarcoma, neuroblastoma, and rhabdomyosarcoma (Hayashi and others, 1988; 1989; Moss, 1989; Rubin, 1988). Bilateral Wilms tumor is associated with increased incidence of congenital anomalies, which include aniridia, hemihypertrophy, and urogenital anomalies (Coppes and others, 1989). In addition, children with certain types of chromosomal abnormalities, especially those syndromes caused by abnormal numbers of chromosomes, have an increased incidence of cancer. For example, in children with Down syndrome the probability of developing leukemia is about 15 times greater than the normal rate for whites (Poplack, 1989). Other chromosome syndromes associated with a predisposition to cancer are Fanconi syndrome (a deficiency of all cellular elements of the blood), Bloom syndrome (dwarfism and skin changes), ataxia-telangiectasia (progressive cerebellar ataxia and oculocutaneous vascular lesions), and Klinefelter syndrome.

Children with immune deficiencies, such as Wiskott-Aldrich syndrome or acquired immune deficiency syndrome, or children whose immune system has been suppressed, such as following transplant procedures, are at a greater risk for developing various cancers. Of major concern is the increased risk of secondary cancers in some children successfully treated for their primary malignancy.

A familial tendency of clustering of cancer also occurs. For example, there are some families who have a higher than expected incidence of cancer, although no environmental or host factor can explain the event. When cancer has occurred in one child, the risk of cancer in the remaining siblings is two times the expected risk for the general population, but the actual risk is considered low because of the rarity of childhood cancer (Li and others, 1988). However, in leukemias the risk among monozygous twins is extremely high—almost 100% if the disease is diagnosed in the twin before 1 year of age. This decreases beyond the first year to approach the same risk of other family members by 6 years of age (Mulvihill, 1989).

Clustering of cases of cancer within a geographic location that exceeds the incidence expected by chance also occurs, but it is thought that these are unusual, random events. Unfortunately, such situations can cause considerable concern and even panic in the community.

Prevention

Knowledge of the risk factors that increase the likelihood of cancer holds the promise of prevention. Unfortunately, in children the known carcinogens are limited to radiation and a few drugs given to the mother during pregnancy. Therefore at present there is really no known prevention.

Table 36-2 Cardinal symptoms of cancer in children

SYMPTOM	PROBABLE MALIGNANCY
Fever	Leukemia, lymphoma, neuroblastoma, Wilms tumor
Pain	Leukemia, bone tumors, brain tumors (headache)
Mass	Wilms tumor, neuroblastoma, lymphoma
Purpura	Leukemia, neuroblastoma
Changes in balance, gait, or personality	Brain tumors
Changes in eye	Retinoblastoma

Modified from Fernbach, D.: The role of the family physician in the care of the child with cancer, CA 35(5):258-270, 1985.

Health professionals do have two roles, however. One is aimed at preventing adult-type cancers by educating parents and children about the hazards of known carcinogens, particularly the effects of cigarette smoking and excessive exposure to sunlight. Lung cancer is the leading cause of death from cancer in adults, and malignant melanoma is the leading cause of death from diseases of the skin. Children at higher risk for skin cancer are those with light-colored eyes, complexion, and hair, those who sunburn easily, and those who live near the equator (Weinstock and others, 1989; Williams and Sagebiel, 1989). Not only these children but all children should be protected from overexposure to the sun (see Chapter 18). In addition, to prevent other types of cancer, males should be taught testicular self-examination; female adolescents should be taught breast self-examination and encouraged to seek periodic health examinations, including a Papanicolaou (Pap) smear.*

Second, health professionals need to be aware of the cardinal symptoms of childhood cancer (Table 36-2). Unfortunately, fever and pain are manifestations of common childhood disorders, and without a high index of suspicion, they may be attributed to minor ailments. The other signs are subtle and easily missed. If parents suspect an abnormality, their concerns must be taken seriously. The greatest weapons against all forms of cancer are early detection and treatment.

PROPERTIES OF MALIGNANT CELLS

Malignant or cancer cells are cells that have the specific properties of anaplasia, invasion, and metastasis. An appreciation of the unique properties of these abnormal cells facilitates an understanding of the pathologic changes that occur in cancer (Box 36-1).

Neoplasms are any new and abnormal growth and may be benign or malignant. Benign neoplasms do not demonstrate the degree of anaplasia or metastasis that malignant neoplasms do, but they may still be serious, especially when they occur in confined spaces, such as the brain. Malignant neoplasms can arise from any tissue of the body and are classified according to tissue and cell type (Box 36-2).

Childhood cancers occur most frequently in rapidly growing tissue, especially the bone marrow. Carcinoma and adenocarcinoma are primarily adult types of cancer and may result from prolonged contact with various carcinogens, such as excessive sunlight on the skin or tobacco products in the lungs.

Box 36-1 PROPERTIES OF TUMOR CELLS

Growth rate—usually very rapid, in contrast to other cells of the body, which divide slowly

Anaplasia—loss of orderly differentiation and organization of cells to perform a specific function

Competition—rapidly proliferating, nonfunctional cells compete with normal cells for essential nutrients, until eventually the normal cells die and are replaced by cancer cells

Expansion—abnormal, unrestricted growth of cancer cells produces organ damage by compressing adjacent tissues, until the tissues' normal functions are altered

Invasion—malignant cells invade adjacent tissues, and eventually the normal cells may be replaced by cancer cells that are incapable of performing the original cells' functions

Metastasis—the ability to spread to distant sites within the body and establish secondary colonies of malignant growth; may occur by natural seeding via the bloodstream or lymph system or iatrogenically, such as during surgery or needle biopsy, when cancer cells are dislodged and implant elsewhere in the body

Box 36-2 MAJOR CLASSIFICATIONS OF MALIGNANT NEOPLASMS

Embryonal tumor—arising from embryonic tissue, such as the blastomas

Lymphomas—arising from the lymphatic system

Leukemias—arising from the blood-forming organs

Sarcoma—derived from connective and supporting tissue, such as bone, cartilage, nerve, and fat

Carcinoma—derived from epithelial tissue such as skin and lining of the body cavities

Adenocarcinoma—a carcinoma of glandular tissue, such as the breast or prostate

ASSESSMENT OF MALIGNANCY AND METASTASIS

When a child is suspected of having cancer, extensive diagnostic procedures are carried out to locate the primary (original) site and any evidence of metastasis. In addition to the initial workup, diagnostic tests are repeated regularly to assess the effectiveness of treatment. Consequently, the

*Information on self-instructional materials on testicular and breast self-examination is available from the local chapters of the American Cancer Society, Inc., or the national office, 1599 Clifton Rd., Atlanta, GA 30329; (404) 329-7617.

child is subjected to numerous noninvasive and invasive procedures, many of which cause considerable pain and anxiety. The following is an overview of the more typical diagnostic procedures employed to assess a malignancy and metastasis and the nursing interventions needed to support the child and family. Specific tests and nursing considerations that are unique to a particular type of cancer are discussed later in the chapter.

History and Physical Examination

The history and physical examination often yield the first clues to the presence of cancer. Vague complaints, such as fatigue, pain in a limb, night sweating, lack of appetite, headache, and general malaise, may be the earliest clues and need to be taken seriously. Most children have a great deal of energy and if sick with a cold or other childhood affliction recover quickly and completely. Any evidence of a lingering disorder is often the first sign of leukemia. Parents are often the first persons to detect physical signs, such as enlarged lymph nodes (lymphoma), a strange glint in the eye (retinoblastoma), or an abdominal mass (Wilms tumor). Any such complaints must be thoroughly followed with a complete examination (see also p. 1671).

Laboratory Tests

Any number of laboratory tests may be performed, but most often a complete blood count and chemistry and urinalysis will be done. Malignancies of the blood-forming organs manifest signs early, and these frequently cause decreased elements of the blood, increased production of immature cells, and/or overproduction of some cells, such as leukocytosis. Since many of the chemotherapeutic agents depress bone marrow function, repeated blood counts are a constant feature of follow-up care.

Blood chemistry yields important information concerning renal and liver function and electrolyte balance. Evaluation of renal and liver function is important not only for detection of cancer or metastasis to these organs, but also for monitoring during treatment because of the extra burden placed on these systems to metabolize and excrete the chemotherapeutic drugs. Consequently, regular blood chemistries and urinalysis are standard procedures through the course of the disease.

A lumbar puncture (LP) is a routine test employed in leukemia, brain tumors, and other cancers that may metastasize to the spinal cord and brain. An LP is also performed to administer intrathecal drugs, such as methotrexate and cytosine arabinoside, when this mode of administration is part of the treatment protocol.

Imaging Techniques

Advances in imaging procedures have greatly aided in the diagnosis of solid tumors and have minimized the need for invasive techniques. Depending on the suspected site of the malignancy, initial preliminary radiologic studies include conventional films of the chest, abdomen, bone, and skull and more specialized tests such as the intravenous pyelogram for kidney involvement. However, these radiographs are generally followed by much more sophisticated imaging procedures, including computed tomography (CT), ultrasound, nuclear scan, and magnetic resonance imaging (MRI) (see Table 37-4).

Biopsy

As part of the diagnostic evaluation, biopsies are essential to determine the classification and stage of the disease. *Classification* refers to the biologic characteristics of the tumor in relation to the tumor (T) itself, the involvement of regional lymph nodes (N), and the presence of metastasis (M). *Staging* refers to the extent of the disease at the time of diagnosis in regard to TNM (DeVitta, 1989). While the classification of the tumor may not change, the stage frequently does and is usually directly related to prognosis (the higher the stage, the poorer the prognosis).

Biopsies may be performed during surgical removal of the tumor, or in the case of lymphomas, surgery may be performed specifically to obtain tissue samples of the spleen and involved lymph nodes. Easily accessed nodes, such as those in the cervical or axillary region, may be removed for biopsy. Whenever there is concern for metastasis to the hematologic system or when the primary site is the blood-forming organs, bone marrow studies are performed.

Access to the bone marrow may be accomplished by (1) *aspiration,* obtaining marrow through a large- or fine-bore needle, or (2) *biopsy,* obtaining a piece of bone through a special type of needle. Aspiration is the procedure of choice, unless the cells are so tightly packed that suction is inadequate to remove a sample. In that case a biopsy is performed. Examination of bone marrow is used to determine the extent of involvement by malignant cells. In leukemia, this is classified by the percentage of leukemia cells present in bone marrow, where M_1 is less than 5%, M_2 is greater than 5% but less than 25%, and M_3 is greater than 25% (Poplack, 1989).

MODES OF THERAPY

Several advances in the understanding of cancer and improvements in technical procedures have greatly influenced present modes of therapy, including (1) surgery, (2) chemotherapy, (3) radiotherapy, (4) immunotherapy, and (5) bone marrow transplantation. While there have been significant developments in new modes of treatment, one of the major reasons for more effective treatment regimens has been the use of clinical trials and protocols. Because of the relatively small number of children with cancer, the National Cancer Institute (NCI) set up cooperative groups of pediatric oncologists (physicians specializing in the care of children with cancer) from different regions of the United States to systematically pool their information regarding treatment and other aspects of cancer care (Guidelines, 1986). Based on the evaluation of success from different types of treatment, these experts plan and initiate *comparative clinical trials.* Although clinical trials may involve any aspect of cancer care (prevention, treatment, or long-term effects), they are frequently concerned with evaluating investigational drugs. For example, one group of patients (control group) typically receives the best possible treatment presently known. The experimental group(s) receives the same treatment plus another form of treatment that is believed to be even better. The formalized outline of the clinical study, which among other details includes the treatment plan (administration and evaluation), is called a *protocol.*

Over the past 30 years the use of clinical trials and protocols has been responsible for major changes in the approaches to cancer treatment. Some of the recent strategies include reduction of toxicity with prolonged and continuous rather than intermittent intravenous infusion; shortening of duration of maintenance therapy; the use of intensive combination therapy; and the administration of as many effective agents as possible in the highest doses possible during the initiation of therapy. The following is an overview of the major modes of therapy. In addition, specific aspects of therapy are discussed later in the chapter when applicable to the individual type of cancer.

Surgery

The main goal of surgery, besides obtaining biopsies, is to remove all traces of tumor and restore normal body functioning. Surgery is most successful when the tumor is encapsulated and localized (confined to the site of origin). It may only be palliative when the cancer is regional (metastasized to an area adjacent to the original site) or advanced (widespread throughout the body). Obviously, the best prognosis is directly related to early detection of the tumor.

The recent trend is toward more conservative surgical excision. For example, in some types of bone cancer, such as osteosarcoma, patients are successfully treated with resection of the diseased portion of the bone rather than amputation. There is an increasing emphasis on the use of combination drug therapy and radiotherapy after limited surgical intervention.

Chemotherapy

Chemotherapy, the use of drugs with antineoplastic capabilities, may be the primary form of treatment, or it may be used as an adjunct to surgery and/or radiotherapy. Although several agents have been found effective in treating different forms of cancer, the remarkable survival rates have been the result of improved combination-drug regimens. Combining drugs allows for optimum cell-cycle destruction with minimum toxic effects and decreased resistance by the cancer cells to the agent. For example, the combination MOPP (mechlorethamine [Mustargen], vincristine [Oncovin], procarbazine, and prednisone) combines complementary cytotoxic effects with nonsimilar side effects. Mechlorethamine and procarbazine are myelosuppressive, vincristine is neurotoxic, and prednisone produces mild bone marrow depression with beneficial effects of improved appetite and a feeling of well-being.

In addition to more effective combinations of drugs, several advances in the administration of chemotherapy have permitted continuous or intermittent intravenous administration without multiple venipunctures. The use of venous access devices, especially indwelling atrial catheters (Hickman/Broviac catheters) and implantable infusion ports, has greatly facilitated safe and effective drug administration with minimum discomfort for the child (see Chapter 28). Continuous infusions over an extended period using syringe pumps have made possible the administration of certain drugs, such as cytosine arabinoside, in higher doses with less toxicity than when the drug is administered intermittently (Mioduszewski and Zarbo, 1987).

Another advance in intrathecal administration is the *Ommaya reservoir,* which eliminates the need for repeated lumbar punctures. In this procedure a silicone rubber tube is surgically inserted into one of the ventricles and connected to a reservoir placed beneath the scalp. To instill medication, the area of scalp covering the reservoir is cleansed with an antiseptic and a small needle is inserted through the skin into the reservoir. The drug is then injected into the reservoir and, by gentle compression of the skin over this site, is pumped into the ventricles. If no complications develop, such as a misplaced reservoir or infection that does not respond to treatment, the device can function for months and in some instances for years (Rahr, 1986). In addition to facilitating the administration of chemotherapy, venous access devices and the Ommaya reservoir can be used to obtain blood or cerebrospinal fluid, respectively, and to administer other drugs, such as antibiotics and analgesics.

Chemotherapeutic agents are classified according to their cytotoxic action. The agents are discussed in the following paragraphs, and the principal drugs used in treatment of childhood cancer are summarized in Table 36-3. An understanding of drugs' actions and side effects is essential to nursing care of children with cancer. Unfortunately, the drugs are not selectively cytotoxic for malignant cells, and other cells with a high rate of proliferation, such as the bone marrow elements, hair, skin, and epithelial cells of the gastrointestinal tract, are also affected. Frequently the problems related to the destruction of these normal cells require more nursing care than the disease itself.

Alkylating agents. Alkylation is the replacement of a hydrogen atom of a molecule by an alkyl group. The irreversible combination of alkyl groups with nucleotide chains, particularly DNA, causes unbalanced growth of unaffected cell constituents so that the cell eventually dies. They are radiomimetic, in that their action is similar to irradiation.

Antimetabolites. These agents resemble essential metabolic elements needed for cell growth but are sufficiently altered in molecular structure to inhibit further synthesis of DNA and/or RNA.

Plant alkaloids. These agents arrest cells in metaphase (a phase of mitosis) by binding to microtubular protein needed for spindle formation.

Antitumor antibiotics. These agents are natural products that interfere with cell division by reacting with DNA in such a way as to prevent further replication of DNA and transcription of RNA.

Hormones. Both adrenal and gonadal hormones have antineoplastic properties. The precise mechanism of action is still unclear. Adrenocorticosteroids are thought to bind with DNA and alter the transcription process. Although there are a number of cortisone preparations, prednisone is

Table 36-3 Summary of chemotherapeutic agents used in the treatment of childhood cancers*

AGENT/ADMINISTRATION	SIDE EFFECTS AND TOXICITY	COMMENTS AND SPECIFIC NURSING CONSIDERATIONS
▪ Alkylating agents		
Mechlorethamine (nitrogen mustard, Mustargen) IV, IT†	N/V‡ (½-8 hours later) (severe) BMD§ (2-3 weeks later) Alopecia Local phlebitis	Vesicant‖
Cyclophosphamide (Cytoxan, CTX,¶ Neosar) PO, IV, IM†	N/V (3-4 hours later) (severe at high doses) BMD (10-14 days later) Alopecia Hemorrhagic cystitis Severe immunosuppression Stomatitis (rare) Hyperpigmentation Transverse ridging of nails Infertility	BMD has platelet-sparing effect Give dose early in day to allow adequate fluids afterward Force fluids before administering drug and for 2 days after to prevent chemical cystitis; encourage frequent voiding even during night Warn parents to report signs of burning on urination or hematuria to practitioner
Chlorambucil (Leukeran) PO	N/V (mild) BMD (7-14 days later) Diarrhea Dermatitis Less commonly may be hepatotoxicity	Usually slow onset of side effects; side effects related to high doses
▪ Antimetabolites		
Cytosine arabinoside (Ara-C, Cytosar, Cytarabine, arabinosyl cytosine) IV, IM, SC,† IT	N/V (mild) BMD (7-14 days later) Mucosal ulceration Immunosuppression Hepatitis (usually subclinical)	Crosses blood-brain barrier Use with caution in patients with hepatic dysfunction
5-Azacytidine (5-AzaC) IV	N/V (moderate) BMD (7-14 days later) Diarrhea	Infuse slowly via IV drip to decrease severity of N/V
Mercaptopurine (6-MP, Purinethol) PO	N/V (mild) Diarrhea Anorexia Stomatitis BMD (4-6 weeks later) Immunosuppression Dermatitis Less commonly may be hepatic dysfunction	6-MP is an analog of xanthine; therefore allopurinol (Zyloprim) delays its metabolism and increases its potency, necessitating a lower dose (⅓ to ¼) of 6-MP
Methotrexate (MTX, Amethopterin) PO, IV, IM, IT May be given in conventional doses (mg/m^2) or high doses (g/m^2)	N/V (severe at high doses) Diarrhea Mucosal ulceration (2-5 days later) BMD (10 days later) Immunosuppression Dermatitis	Side effects and toxicity are dose related Potency and toxicity increased by reduced renal function, salicylates, sulfonamides, and aminobenzoic acid; avoid use of these substances, such as aspirin

*Table includes principal drugs used in the treatment of childhood cancers. Several other conventional and investigational chemotherapeutic agents may be employed in the treatment regimen.
†IV, Intravenous; IT, intrathecal; PO, by mouth; IM, intramuscular; SC, subcutaneous.
‡N/V, Nausea and vomiting. Mild = <20% incidence; moderate = 20% to 70% incidence; severe = >75% incidence.
§BMD, Bone marrow depression.
‖Vesicants (sclerosing agents) can cause severe cellular damage if even minute amounts of the drug infiltrate surrounding tissue. Only nurses experienced with chemotherapeutic agents should administer vesicants. These drugs must be given through a free-flowing intravenous line. The infusion is stopped *immediately* if any sign of infiltration (pain, stinging, swelling, or redness at needle site) occurs. Interventions for extravasation vary, but each nurse should be aware of the institution policies and implement them at once.
¶Abbreviations stand for chemical compound.

Table 36-3 Summary of chemotherapeutic agents used in the treatment of childhood cancers—cont'd

AGENT/ADMINISTRATION	SIDE EFFECTS AND TOXICITY	COMMENTS AND SPECIFIC NURSING CONSIDERATIONS
▪ Antimetabolites—cont'd		
Methotrexate—cont'd	Photosensitivity Alopecia (uncommon) Toxic effects include: Hepatitis (fibrosis) Osteoporosis Nephropathy Pneumonitis (fibrosis) Neurologic toxicity with IT use—pain at injection site, meningismus (signs of meningitis without actual inflammation), especially fever and headache; potential sequelae—transient or permanent hemiparesis, convulsions, dementia, death	High-dose therapy: Citrovorum factor (folinic acid or leucovorin) decreases cytotoxic action of MTX; used as an antidote for overdose and to enhance normal cell recovery following high-dose therapy; avoid use of vitamins containing folic acid during MTX therapy unless prescribed by physician IT therapy: Drug *must* be mixed with preservative-free diluent Report signs of neurotoxicity immediately
6-Thioguanine (6-TG, Thioguan) PO	N/V (mild) BMD (7-14 days later) Stomatitis Rarely: Dermatitis Photosensitivity Liver dysfunction	Side effects are unusual
▪ Plant alkaloids		
Vincristine (Oncovin) IV	Neurotoxicity—paresthesia (numbness); ataxia; weakness; footdrop; hyporeflexia; constipation (adynamic ileus); hoarseness (vocal cord paralysis); abdominal, chest, and jaw pain; mental depression Fever N/V (mild) BMD (minimal; 7-14 days later) Alopecia	Vesicant Report signs of neurotoxicity because may necessitate cessation of drug Individuals with underlying neurologic problems may be more prone to neurotoxicity Monitor stool patterns closely; administer stool softener Excreted primarily by liver into biliary system; administer cautiously to anyone with biliary disease
Vinblastine (Velban) IV	Neurotoxicity (same as for vincristine but less severe) N/V (mild) BMD (especially neutropenia; 7-14 days later) Alopecia	Same as for vincristine
VP-16-213 (Etoposide, VePesid)	N/V (mild to moderate) BMD (7-14 days later) Alopecia Hypotension with rapid infusion Bradycardia Diarrhea (infrequent) Stomatitis (rare) May reactivate erythema of irradiated skin (rare) Allergic reaction with anaphylaxis possible	Give slowly via IV drip with child recumbent Have emergency drugs available at bedside*

*Emergency drugs include oxygen and parenteral preparations of epinephrine 1:1000, diphenhydramine or similar antihistamine, aminophylline, corticosteroids, and vasopressors.

Continued.

Table 36-3 Summary of chemotherapeutic agents used in the treatment of childhood cancers—cont'd

AGENT/ADMINISTRATION	SIDE EFFECTS AND TOXICITY	COMMENTS AND SPECIFIC NURSING CONSIDERATIONS
Antibiotics		
Actinomycin-D (Dactinomycin, Cosmegen, ACT-D) IV	N/V (2-5 hours later) (moderate) BMD (especially platelets; 7-14 days later) Immunosuppression Mucosal ulceration Abdominal cramps Diarrhea Anorexia (may last few weeks) Alopecia Acne Erythema or hyperpigmentation of previously irradiated skin Fever Malaise	Vesicant Enhances cytotoxic effects of radiation therapy but increases toxic effect May cause serious desquamation of irradiated tissue
Doxorubicin (Adriamycin, Doxyrubicin) IV	N/V (moderate) Stomatitis BMD (7-14 days later) Fever, chills Local phlebitis Alopecia Cumulative-dose toxicity includes: Cardiac abnormalities ECG changes Heart failure	Vesicant (extravasation may *not* cause pain) Use only sterile distilled water as a diluent Observe for any changes in heart rate or rhythm and signs of failure Cumulative dose must not exceed 550 mg/m^2 Warn parents that drug causes urine to turn red (for up to 12 days after administration); this is normal, not hematuria
Daunorubicin (Daunomycin, Rubidomycin) IV	Similar to doxorubicin	Similar to doxorubicin
Bleomycin (Blenoxane) IV, IM, SC	Allergic reaction—fever, chills, hypotension, anaphylaxis Fever (nonallergic) N/V (mild) Stomatitis Cumulative dose effects include: Skin—rash, hyperpigmentation, thickening, ulceration, peeling, nail changes, alopecia Lungs—pneumonitis with infiltrate that can progress to fatal fibrosis	Should give test dose (SC) before therapeutic dose administered Have emergency drugs* at bedside Hypersensitivity occurs with first one to two doses May give acetaminophen before drug to reduce likelihood of fever Concentration of drug in skin and lungs accounts for toxic effects
Hormones		
Corticosteroids (prednisone most frequently used; many proprietary names such as Meticorten, Deltasone, Paracort) PO; also IM or IV but rarely used	For short-term use, no acute toxicity Usual side effects are mild; moon face, fluid retention, weight gain, mood changes, increased appetite, gastric irritation, insomnia, susceptibility to infection	Explain expected effects, especially in terms of body image, increased appetite, and personality changes Monitor weight gain Recommend moderate salt restriction Administer with antacid and early in morning (sometimes given every other day to minimize side effects) May need to disguise bitter taste (crush tablet and mix with syrup, jam, ice cream, or other highly flavored substance; use ice to numb tongue before administration; place tablet in gelatin capsule if child can swallow it) Observe for potential infection sites; usual inflammatory response and fever are absent

*Emergency drugs include oxygen and parenteral preparations of epinephrine 1:1000, diphenhydramine or similar antihistamine, aminophylline, corticosteroids, and vasopressors.

Table 36-3 Summary of chemotherapeutic agents used in the treatment of childhood cancers—cont'd

AGENT/ADMINISTRATION	SIDE EFFECTS AND TOXICITY	COMMENTS AND SPECIFIC NURSING CONSIDERATIONS
▪ Hormones—cont'd		
Corticosteroids—cont'd	Long-term effects of chronic steroid administration are mood changes, hirsutism, trunk obesity (buffalo hump), thin extremities, muscle wasting and weakness, osteoporosis, poor wound healing, bruising, potassium loss, gastric bleeding, hypertension, diabetes mellitus, growth retardation	Same as for short-term use; in addition, encourage foods high in potassium (bananas, raisins, prunes, coffee, chocolate) Test stools for occult blood Monitor blood pressure Test blood for sugar and urine for acetone Observe for signs of abrupt steroid withdrawal; flulike symptoms, hypotension, hypoglycemia, shock
▪ Enzymes		
L-Asparaginase (Elspar) IV, IM	Allergic reactions (including anaphylactic shock) Fever N/V (mild) Anorexia Weight loss Arthralgia Toxicity: Liver dysfunction Hyperglycemia Renal failure Pancreatitis	Have emergency drugs at bedside* Record signs of allergic reaction, such as urticaria, facial edema, hypotension, or abdominal cramps Check weight daily Normally, blood urea nitrogen (BUN) and ammonia levels rise as a result of drug; not evidence of liver damage Check urine for sugar and blood amylase
▪ Nitrosoureas		
Carmustine (BCNU) IV Lomustine (CCNU) PO	N/V (2-6 hours later) (severe) BMD (3-4 weeks later) Burning pain along IV infusion (usually due to alcohol diluent) BCNU—flushing and facial burning on infusion	Prevent extravasation; contact with skin causes brown spots Oral form—give 4 hours after meals when stomach is empty Reduce IV burning by diluting drug and infusing slowing via IV drip Crosses blood-brain barrier
▪ Other agents		
Hydroxyurea (Hydrea) PO	N/V (mild) Anorexia Less commonly: Diarrhea BMD Mucosal ulceration Alopecia Dermatitis	Must be given cautiously in patients with renal dysfunction
Procarbazine (Matulane) PO	N/V (moderate) BMD (3-4 weeks later) Lethargy Dermatitis Myalgia Arthralgia Less commonly: Stomatitis Neuropathy Alopecia Diarrhea	Central nervous system depressants (phenothiazines, barbiturates) enhance central nervous system symptoms Monoamine oxidase (MAO) inhibition sometimes occurs; therefore all other drugs are avoided unless medically approved; red wine, fava beans, and broad bean pods are avoided

Continued.

Table 36-3 Summary of chemotherapeutic agents used in the treatment of childhood cancers—cont'd

AGENT/ADMINISTRATION	SIDE EFFECTS AND TOXICITY	COMMENTS AND SPECIFIC NURSING CONSIDERATIONS
Dacarbazine (DTIC-Dome) IV	N/V (especially after first dose) (severe) BMD (7-14 days later) Alopecia Flulike syndrome Burning sensation in vein during infusion (not extravasation)	Vesicant (less sclerosive) Must be given cautiously in patients with renal dysfunction Decrease IV rate or use warm moist towels on IV site to decrease burning
Cisplatin (Platinol) IV	Renal toxicity (severe) N/V (1-4 hours later) (severe) BMD (mild, 2-3 weeks later) Ototoxicity Neurotoxicity (similar to that for vincristine) Electrolyte disturbances, especially hypomagnesium, hypocalcemia, hypokalemia, and hypophosphatemia Anaphylactic reactions may occur	Renal function (creatinine clearance) must be assessed before giving drug Must maintain hydration before and during therapy (specific gravity of urine is used to assess hydration) Mannitol may be given IV to promote osmotic diuresis and drug clearance Monitor intake and output Monitor for signs of ototoxicity (e.g., ringing in ears) and neurotoxicity; report signs immediately; ensure that routine audiogram is done before treatment for baseline and routinely during treatment Do not use aluminum needle; reaction with aluminum decreases potency of drug Monitor for signs of electrolyte loss, i.e. hypomagnesium—tremors, spasm, muscle weakness, lower extremity cramps, irregular heartbeat, convulsions, delirium Have emergency drugs at bedside*

*Emergency drugs include oxygen and parenteral preparations of epinephrine 1:1000, diphenhydramine or similar antihistamine, aminophylline, corticosteroids, and vasopressors.

most frequently used. Androgens and estrogens are effective against certain cancers usually found in adults, such as prostate and breast cancers. Consequently, they have little applicability in childhood cancer.

Miscellaneous agents. A number of agents are not categorized according to the preceding classifications. The most commonly used ones are described in the following:

L-*Asparaginase* is an enzyme isolated from extracts of bacterial cultures of *Escherichia coli* or *Erwinia carotovora*. It hydrolyzes L-asparagine, an amino acid, to L-aspartic acid, which prevents the cell from synthesizing protein needed for DNA and RNA synthesis.

L-Asparaginase is unique because it is selectively cytotoxic only for certain cancer cells. L-Asparagine is synthesized by normal cells but must be exogenously supplied to certain leukemic and lymphoma cells. Administration of the enzyme L-asparaginase destroys the essential exogenous supply while sparing normal cells of untoward effects.

Hydroxyurea, a cell-cycle dependent agent, inhibits ribonucleotide reduction to deoxyribonucleotide. DNA synthesis is impaired, but protein and RNA synthesis is less affected; therefore the unbalanced growth results in eventual cellular death.

Nitrosoureas, of which a number of compounds are available, act similarly to alkylating agents and are sometimes classified as such because they replace an essential DNA molecule, thus inhibiting DNA, RNA, and protein synthesis. One of their unique properties is the ability to cross the blood-brain barrier.

Procarbazine is a weak monoamine oxidase (MAO) inhibitor. (MAO is an enzyme that destroys the neurohormones epinephrine, norepinephrine, and serotonin. MAO inhibitors act as psychic energizers.) Its exact cytotoxic action is not known, although it inhibits DNA, RNA, and protein synthesis.

Dacarbazine is an analog of aminoimidazole carboxamide. It interferes with purine synthesis and also exhibits alkylating properties in DNA synthesis. It has shown significant antitumor activity when combined with other drugs, especially doxorubicin.

Cisplatin is a heavy-metal derivative containing central platinum atom bounded by ammonia and chloride groups. It inhibits DNA synthesis by the formation of intrastrand and interstrand cross-links, similar to alkylating agents.

Precautions in administering and handling chemotherapeutic agents. Many chemotherapeutic agents are vesicants (sclerosing agents) that can cause severe cellular damage if even minute amounts of the drug infiltrate surrounding tissue. Only nurses experienced with chemotherapeutic agents should administer vesicants. Guidelines are available* and must be followed meticulously to prevent tissue damage to patients. Interventions for extravasation vary, but each nurse should be aware of the institution's policies and implement them at once.

✦ **NURSING ALERT** Chemotherapeutic drugs must be given through a free-flowing intravenous line. The infusion is stopped *immediately* if any sign of infiltration (pain, stinging, swelling, or redness at needle site) occurs.

In addition to extravasation, a potentially fatal complication is anaphylaxis, especially from L-asparaginase, bleomycin, cisplatin, and etoposide (see Chapter 29). Nursing responsibilities include prevention of, recognition of, and preparation for serious reactions. Prevention begins with a careful history for known allergy (see Chapter 6) (Hammond, 1988).

✦ **NURSING ALERT** When chemotherapeutic and immunologic agents are given, the child must be observed for 20 minutes after the infusion for signs of anaphylaxis (cyanosis, hypotension, wheezing, severe urticaria). Emergency equipment (especially blood pressure monitor and bag-valve-mask) and emergency drugs (especially oxygen, epinephrine, antihistamine, aminophylline, corticosteroids, and vasopressors) must be available.

If a reaction is suspected, the drug is discontinued, the intravenous line is flushed with saline, and the child's vital signs and subsequent responses are monitored.

In addition to the many responsibilities nurses must have in regard to the child and family, they must also use safeguards to protect themselves. Handling chemotherapeutic agents may present risks to handlers and to their offspring, although the exact degree of risk is not known.

The Oncology Nursing Society has published comprehensive guidelines for safe practice issues related to administration of chemotherapy.† Safe management procedures for chemotherapy administered in the home have also been established (Blecke, 1989; Sansievero and Murray, 1989). Basic nursing guidelines are listed in Box 36-3.

Box 36-3 GUIDELINES FOR HANDLING CHEMOTHERAPEUTIC AGENTS

Use utmost care and strict aseptic technique in handling chemotherapeutic agents to prevent any physical contact with the substance.

Prepare drugs in a properly ventilated room or biologic safety cabinet (incorporates protective front panel and vertical laminar air flow to reduce potential for inhalation during preparation).

Wear disposable gloves and protective clothing and discard in special container after each use.

Use a sterile gauze pad when priming IV tubing, connecting and disconnecting tubing, inserting syringes into vials, breaking glass ampules, or any other procedure in which antineoplastic drugs may be inadvertently discharged.

Dispose of all contaminated needles, syringes, IV tubing, and other contaminated equipment in a leakproof and puncture-resistant container; do not recap or break needles.

Radiotherapy

Radiotherapy is frequently used in the treatment of childhood cancer, usually in conjunction with chemotherapy and/or surgery. It can be used for curative purposes and is often employed for palliation to relieve symptoms by shrinking the size of the tumor. Recent advances in radiation therapy have optimized its beneficial effects and minimized many of the undesirable side effects, although high-dose radiation is associated with many serious late effects.

Ionizing radiation is cytotoxic in at least three different ways: (1) damaging the pyrimidine bases cytosine, thymine, and uracil needed for the synthesis of nucleic acids, (2) causing single-strand breaks in the DNA or RNA molecule, or (3) causing double helical–strand breaks in these molecules. The effect of disturbing cellular metabolic and reproductive functions is either sublethal or lethal damage.

Lethal damage refers to the death of the cell. *Sublethal* damage refers to injured cells that may subsequently be repaired. Many of the acute side effects are the result of lethal damage to radiosensitive tissue, particularly proliferating cells such as those of the bone marrow, gastrointestinal tract, and hair follicles. Late effects are usually the result of cell death.

The acute untoward reactions from radiotherapy depend primarily on the area to be irradiated. Total-body irradiation (TBI) is associated with the most severe reactions and is employed to prepare the immune system for bone marrow transplantation. Table 36-4 summarizes the acute effects of radiation therapy and nursing interventions that may be helpful in lessening or preventing them.

Biotherapy

In recent years much research has focused on biotherapy—the use of biologic response modifiers (BRMs) to treat cancer. BRMs are agents or interventions that modify the relationship between tumor and host by therapeutically changing the host's biologic response to tumor cells. BRMs may affect the host's immunologic mechanisms (immunotherapy), have direct antitumor activity, or have other biologic effects (Abernathy, 1987).

To date there have been many disappointments in the development of specific BRMs, such as interferon, in acting selectively against tumor cells. Much of the current work in biotherapy is directed toward the use of *monoclonal antibodies* in diagnosis and treatment of cancers. Through a complex process, special cells are fused to form a hybrid clone or hybridoma that produces antibodies that recognize a single specific antigen, hence the term *monoclonal antibody* ("mono" meaning one and "clone" meaning exact

**Giving Cancer Drugs Intravenously: Some Guidelines* is available from the American Cancer Society, 1599 Clifton Rd., Atlanta, GA 30329; (404) 329-7617.

†*Cancer Chemotherapy Guidelines* can be obtained from Oncology Nursing Society, 501 Holiday Dr., Pittsburgh, PA 15220-2749; (412) 921-7373.

Table 36-4 Early side effects of radiotherapy

SITE/EFFECTS	NURSING INTERVENTIONS
▪ Gastrointestinal tract	
Nausea/vomiting	Give antiemetic around the clock Measure amount of emesis to prevent dehydration
Anorexia	Encourage fluids and foods best tolerated, usually light, soft diet and small, frequent meals Monitor weight loss
Mucosal ulceration	Use frequent mouthwashes and oral hygiene to prevent mucositis
Diarrhea	Can be controlled with antispasmodics and kaolin pectin preparations Observe for signs of dehydration
▪ Skin	
Alopecia (within 2 weeks; begins to regrow by 3-6 months)	Introduce idea of wig Stress necessity of scalp hygiene and need for head covering in cold weather
Dry or moist desquamation	Do not refer to skin change as a "burn" (implies use of too much radiation) Keep skin clean Wash daily, using soap (e.g., Tone, Dove) sparingly Do not remove skin marking for radiation fields Avoid exposure to sun For dryness, apply lubricant For desquamation, consult practitioner for skin hygiene and care
▪ Head	
Nausea/vomiting (from stimulation of vomiting center in brain)	Same as for gastrointestinal tract
Alopecia	Same as for skin Encourage regular dental care, fluoride treatments
Potential effects	
Parotitis	May need analgesics to relieve discomfort
Loss of taste	
Xerostomia (dry mouth)	Combat severe dryness of mouth with oral hygiene and liquid diet
▪ Urinary bladder	
Rarely cystitis	More likely to occur with concomitant use of cyclophosphamide Encourage liberal fluid intake and frequent voiding Evaluate for hematuria
▪ Bone marrow	
Myelosuppression	Observe for fever (temperature above 101° F) Initiate workup for sepsis as ordered Administer antibiotics as prescribed Avoid use of suppositories, rectal temperatures Institute bleeding precautions Observe for signs of anemia

duplicate). These clones are then frozen, maintained in culture, or grown as tumors in mice to produce large quantities of the antibody in ascites fluid (Weinberg and Parkman, 1989). While there are many prospective uses for monoclonal antibodies, their current role has been in diagnosing subclasses of leukemia cells to enhance understanding of which types of leukemia respond to different treatments and to determine if the subclass is related to prognosis. Monoclonal antibodies have also been used to deplete allogeneic bone marrows of T-cells to reduce graft-versus-host disease and to selectively eliminate malignant cells from autologous marrow for transplanting back into the patient (Poplack, 1989). Results from these studies have been encouraging, but further work is needed to define the role monoclonal antibodies and other BRMs will have in cancer care.

Bone Marrow Transplantation

Another approach to the treatment of childhood cancer is bone marrow transplantation (BMT). Candidates for transplantation are children who have malignancies that are unlikely to be cured by other means. BMT allows for lethal doses of chemotherapy, often combined with radiation therapy, to be given in order to rid the body of all cancer cells (Yeager, 1988). Once the body is free of malignant cells and the immune system is suppressed to prevent rejection of the transplanted marrow, the donor marrow cells or the cells previously stored from the patient's own marrow are given to the patient by intravenous transfusion. The newly transfused marrow will begin to produce functioning nonmalignant blood cells. In essence, a new blood-forming organ will be accepted by the recipient.

Presently three types of bone marrow transplants may be done:

Allogeneic, which involves the matching of a histocompatible donor, usually a sibling, with the recipient; may also involve an unmatched donor

Autologous, which uses the patient's own marrow that was collected from disease-free tissue and frozen

Syngeneic, which uses marrow from an identical twin

The most common type of bone marrow transplantation is allogeneic. The selection process of a suitable donor and the potential complications in transplantation are related to the human leukocyte antigen (HLA) system complex (see p. 167). Some of the major HLA antigens are A, B, C, D, and DR. There is a wide diversity for each of these HLA loci. There are more than 20 different HLA-A antigens that can be inherited and more than 40 different HLA-B antigens.

The genes are inherited as a single unit or haplotype. A child inherits one unit from each parent; thus a child and each parent have one identical and one nonidentical haplotype. Since the possible haplotype combinations among siblings follow the laws of Mendelian genetics, there is a one in four chance that two siblings have two identical haplotypes and are perfectly matched at the HLA loci. Since many patients have more than one sibling and certain HLA genotypes are more common among families prone to leukemia, approximately 35% of leukemia patients have a matched sibling (World of Children's Hospital, 1988).

The importance of HLA matching is to prevent the serious complication known as *graft-versus-host disease (GVHD)*. Since the child's immune system is essentially rendered nonfunctional prior to surgery, there is little difficulty with bone marrow rejection by the recipient. However, the donor's marrow may contain antigens not matched to the recipient's antigens, which begin attacking body cells. The more closely the HLA systems match, the less likely GVHD is to develop. However, it can occur even with a perfect HLA match, because there are as yet unidentified and thus unmatched histocompatibility antigens (Vega and others, 1987). GVHD is not a complication in autologous BMT, used in many children with solid tumors who have a poor prognosis (Wiley and House, 1988).

Although the actual transplant procedure is simple and involves harvesting several bone marrow specimens from the donor (which is done under general anesthesia) and diluting the marrow and administering it intravenously similar to any blood product to the recipient, the preoperative and postoperative care is complex. The first stage is identifying a compatible donor in the case of an allogeneic transplant. The second phase is cytoreduction to produce a totally aleukemic immunosuppressed state, which involves intense chemotherapy and total-body irradiation (Vega and others, 1987).

The third phase is preventing complications. During the preoperative aplastic phase and for the 10- to 20-day period after transplantation before the new marrow begins adequately replacing granulocytes, the child is extremely susceptible to infection. Interstitial or nonbacterial pneumonia is another serious complication with a high mortality rate. However, the most common complication in allogeneic transplants is GVHD, which can affect the skin, gastrointestinal tract, liver, heart, lungs, lymphoid tissue, and marrow. GVHD is characterized by a hardening of the tissues and drying of the mucous membranes. The severity of the manifestations varies, but once vital organs are affected, death can ensue. Treatment involves the use of steroids and/or azathioprine (Imuran) or cyclosporine. However, these immunosuppressive drugs further increase the risk of infection. All blood products should be irradiated to minimize the introduction of additional antigens (Kelleher, 1986). Another unfortunate posttransplant possibility is recurrence of the malignancy after engraftment.

Supportive Therapies

Cancer care encompasses more than treatments aimed at eliminating the malignant cells. Because of the delicate balance between killing malignant cells and preserving functional cells, supportive therapy is frequently needed during those times that serious damage occurs to normal body tissues. For example, infection is a constant threat from the immunosuppressant effects of antineoplastic agents. Prophylactic antibiotics, such as trimethoprim/sulfamethoxazole (Bactrim, Septra) and clotrimazole or amphotericin B, may be given to reduce the incidence of serious infection (Mitchell, 1988).

Other supportive therapies include replacement of blood elements as needed in anemia, agranulocytopenia, and thrombocytopenia. However, the use of granulocyte transfusions and preventive infusions of platelets is controversial because of the lack of documented effectiveness and the risk of developing antibodies to the foreign antigens, respectively (Darbyshire, 1988; Mitchell, 1988).

Allopurinol, a xanthine-oxidase inhibitor, may be administered to prevent renal damage in the newly diagnosed or relapsed patient. Massive cellular damage from cytotoxic therapy releases large amounts of uric acid, which can accumulate and precipitate in the renal tubules, eventually causing tubular obstruction. Allopurinol prevents the metabolic breakdown of xanthine to uric acid. Other supportive measures include alkalinization of the urine and adequate hydration.

Nutritional support has been increasingly recognized as a significant component of cancer treatment. Optimum nutrition promotes the body's tolerance to antineoplastic agents and preserves immunologic responsiveness. Excellent nutrition before intensive therapy provides nutrient stores during periods of anorexia, nausea, and vomiting. The most common nutritional problem is children's unwillingness to consume sufficient food to maintain a nutritional balance. Oral supplementation with fortified foods, such as commercial preparations (Ensure), may be helpful, but nonoral routes may be necessary (e.g., nasogastric tube feedings, gastrostomy, parenteral alimentation) (Drakeford, 1988).

A final supportive therapy is the effective use of analgesics, especially the use of opioids when pain is severe. Dosages of analgesics are *titrated to the child's needs* and administered *around the clock* for optimum pain control. Nonpharmacologic strategies should be implemented as needed but should not be regarded as substitutes for pharmacologic management. The reader is encouraged to review the principles of pain assessment and management presented in Chapter 26 in caring for the child with cancer.

COMPLICATIONS OF THERAPY

Although tremendous advances have been achieved through current modes of cancer therapy, the successes are not without consequences. Numerous side effects are expected with chemotherapy and radiotherapy, and these are discussed under Nursing Care of the Child with Cancer. However, other complications that are less frequently seen but generally more serious and possibly permanent are described here.

Pediatric Oncologic Emergencies

Life-threatening conditions may develop in children with cancer as a result of aggressive treatment modalities or from the malignancy itself. Acute tumor lysis syndrome is caused by the rapid release of intracellular metabolites during the initial treatment of malignancies such as Burkitt and T-cell lymphomas and acute leukemia. Rapid tumor lysis leads to hyperuricemia, hypocalcemia, hyperphosphatemia, and hyperkalemia (Patterson and Klopovich, 1987).

Obstruction may create an oncologic emergency for a child with cancer. Space-occupying lesions, especially from Hodgkin disease and non-Hodgkin lymphoma (NHL), located in the chest may cause superior vena cava syndrome (SVCS) (compression of mediastinal structures), leading to airway compromise and potentially to respiratory failure. SVCS has also been reported with central venous catheters from formation of a thrombus or a fibrotic reaction (Faro, 1987). Children may have a mass obstructing the spinal cord, as manifested by symptoms ranging from tingling to paresthesias and loss of bowel and bladder control. Children with brain tumors may develop symptoms ranging from increased intracranial pressure to respiratory compromise and herniation, depending on the location and size of the tumor (Heideman and others, 1989).

Infections in the immunocompromised child constitute an emergency situation. Gram-negative sepsis can result in numerous complications, including disseminated intravascular coagulation (DIC), created by bacteria or fungus causing damage to the endothelial system. Life-threatening hemorrhage can occur from DIC, thrombocytopenia (platelet count $< 20,000/mm^3$), and leukocytosis (leukocyte count $> 100,000/mm^3$). Leukocytosis may cause intracranial bleeding from increased viscosity of the blood. The resulting leukocytosis leads to vascular damage and subsequent hemorrhage (Happ, 1987).

Long-Term Sequelae of Treatment

Vigorous treatment of childhood cancers has resulted in dramatically improved survival rates. However, treatment programs combining surgery, irradiation, and chemotherapy are not without their complications. Some may occur immediately, such as loss of a limb from surgical amputation or asplenia from splenectomy in Hodgkin disease. However, current concern is with late effects—adverse changes related to treatment modalities, interactions between modes of treatment, individual characteristics of the child, and the disease process that may appear months to years after lifesaving treatment (Raymond, 1988). Because of the greater number of children who are cured and surviving into adulthood, increasing documentation of late effects is emerging (see Table 36-5). Almost no organ is exempt, and almost every antineoplastic agent and especially irradiation are responsible for some adverse effect. Although many factors influence the development of late effects from radiation, some of the more important ones include the total cumulative dose given, the age of the child (the younger the child, the more radiosensitive the body organs are), and the location of the tumor.

In addition to physical effects, there is also concern for the psychologic sequelae of surviving cancer (see Questions and Controversies). Regardless of the level of functioning at the time of cure, having cancer is a stressful experience, and nurses can play an important part in ameliorating many of the frightening and painful aspects of care.

QUESTIONS AND CONTROVERSIES

Are there long-term psychologic consequences of surviving childhood cancer?

With increasing numbers of children surviving childhood cancer, there is concern for their emotional as well as their physical health. Studies involving young adults who are childhood cancer survivors suggest the majority of persons are functioning well, with only 10% to 20% showing signs of psychologic distress (Fobair and others, 1986; Lansky, List, and Ritter-Stern, 1986; Wasserman and others, 1987).

Long-term survivors have reported that their illness disrupted school attendance, resulted in academic difficulties, and altered future plans and peer relationships. While most youngsters adapted well, some developed emotional problems, specifically, symptoms related to depression and/or alcoholism (Lansky and others, 1985).

Factors related to fewer adjustment problems included (1) young age at time of diagnosis, (2) short treatment course with minimum side effects, (3) absence of relapse or recurrence of the disease, and (4) absence of unresolved concerns about the outcome of the disease (Koocher and O'Malley, 1981).

An older age at evaluation, treatment with cranial radiation, and residence in a single-parent household were associated with increased risk of psychologic problems (Deasy-Spinetta, Spinetta, and Oxman, 1988; Mulhern and others, 1989). Of primary importance is the role played by the family in adaptation to childhood cancer survival (Greenberg, Kazak, and Meadows, 1989).

NURSING CARE OF THE CHILD WITH CANCER

The child with cancer presents a challenge to the nurse providing care for the hospitalized child as well as the child returning to the outpatient setting. This section presents an overview of general nursing concepts that apply to most cancers. Specific nursing care for the child with a particular type of cancer is discussed under each disease section later in this chapter. The focus of this discussion is on the physical aspects of care. Emotional aspects are presented in Chapter 22 (chronic illness) and in Chapter 23 (terminal illness).

Assessment

Three major areas of assessment for nurses caring for children with cancer are (1) signs and symptoms associated with the onset of childhood cancer, (2) the child at risk for complications of treatment for cancer, and (3) the child who is a survivor of cancer. Essential physical assessment skills are discussed in Chapter 7.

Signs and Symptoms of Cancer in Children

Early detection is critical to early treatment and eventual cure. Cancers in children are often difficult to recognize. Therefore, being alert to the persistence of unusual symptoms is essential (Box 36-4). Some of the more significant clues to pediatric cancer are discussed here.

Pain may be an early or late initial sign of cancer and requires a careful history of its onset, characteristics, location, intensity, and alleviating factors. Pain may be generalized or present at a specific location. For example, bone pain occurs in approximately 20% of children with leukemia. Pain, swelling, and tenderness at the tumor site may be the initial sign in bone tumors.

Fever is a frequent occurrence during childhood and is caused by numerous illnesses, including cancer. Fever is most often caused by infection secondary to the malignant process.

A careful skin assessment will reveal signs and symptoms of a low platelet count. Ecchymosis and petechiae are most commonly found on the child's extremities, and nose bleeding may occur when the platelet count falls below $40,000/mm^3$.

The child with malignant invasion of the bone marrow often appears pale with symptoms of lethargy, weight loss, and generalized malaise. These symptoms may be attributed to the development of anemia caused by the replacement of normal cells with malignant cells in the bone marrow. The nurse should assess for signs and symptoms of anemia, as discussed in Chapter 35.

An abdominal mass is a typical finding in children with Wilms tumor and neuroblastoma. The presence of an abdominal mass in a child must be evaluated for a malignancy.

Swollen lymph glands are another common finding in children. However, enlarged, firm, lymph nodes in a child with fever for more than 1 week, a recent history of weight loss, and/or an abnormal chest x-ray film may indicate a serious disease and should be evaluated further.

The presence of a white reflection as opposed to the normal red pupillary reflex in the pupil of a child's eye is the classic sign of retinoblastoma. The presence of squinting, strabismus, or swelling can indicate other solid tumors of the eye.

The child with a brain tumor will develop signs and symptoms according to the exact area of the brain involved. The nurse must perform a thorough assessment to identify the specific area of tumor involvement (see Table 36-7).

Box 36-4 CARDINAL SYMPTOMS OF CANCER IN CHILDREN

Unusual mass or swelling
Unexplained paleness and loss of energy
Sudden tendency to bruise
Persistent, localized pain or limping
Prolonged, unexplained fever or illness
Frequent headaches, often with vomiting
Sudden eye or vision changes
Excessive, rapid weight loss

From Cancer facts and figures, 1990, Atlanta, 1990, American Cancer Society.

The Child Undergoing Treatment for Cancer

A major concern for the child receiving treatment for cancer is the risk for the development of complications secondary to cancer treatment. Major complications include fever, bleeding, and anemia.

The nurse caring for the child with fever must be aware of the signs and symptoms for septic shock, as discussed in Chapter 29. The child with fever who has an absolute granulocyte count less than $500/mm^3$ is at risk for the following:

- Overwhelming infection
- General malaise
- Dehydration
- Seizures (young infants and children)
- Invasion of organisms producing secondary infections

The child with fever is evaluated for potential sites of infection, such as from a needle puncture, mucosal ulceration, minor abrasion, or skin tears (e.g., a hangnail). Although the body may not be able to produce an adequate inflammatory response to the infection and the usual clinical signs of infection may be partially expressed or absent, fever will occur. Therefore, temperature is monitored closely. To identify the source of infection, blood, stool, urine, and nasopharyngeal cultures and chest x-ray films are taken.

The child with a platelet count less than $40,000/mm^3$ is assessed closely for signs of active bleeding, especially those common sites where bleeding occurs in the child with thrombocytopenia—the nose, mouth, conjunctiva, and ears. Petechiae and areas of ecchymoses are documented to determine areas of new bleeding under the skin. The child's urine and stool are observed and tested for the presence of blood.

The child undergoing cancer treatment may develop anemia caused by aggressive therapy regimens preventing the bone marrow from producing red blood cells. The nurse should assess closely for changes in vital signs and physical symptoms that may reflect the presence of anemia, as described in Chapter 35.

The Childhood Cancer Survivor

It is estimated that by the year 2000, one individual in 1000 will have survived cancer. Such children are at risk for the development of numerous late effects caused by the cancer or its treatment. These complications are defined as post-therapeutic disabilities, ranging from impaired cognitive development to the onset of second malignancies.

Psychosocial, cognitive, emotional, and physical devel-

Table 36-5 Late effects of cancer treatment

SYSTEMIC EFFECTS/CLINICAL MANIFESTATIONS	ASSOCIATED MODE OF TREATMENT
▪ Central nervous system (CNS)	
Leukoencephalopathy (syndrome ranging from lethargy, dementia, and seizures to quadriplegia and death)	Methotrexate and/or CNS irradiation
Mineralizing microangiopathy (headaches, focal seizures, incoordination, gate abnormalities)	Methotrexate and/or CNS irradiation
Peripheral neuropathy (footdrop, incoordination)	Vincristine
Cognitive deficits (intelligence, nonlanguage skills)	Intrathecal chemotherapy and/or cranial irradiation (especially before age 3 years)
▪ Cardiovascular	
Cardiomyopathy (tachycardia, tachypnea, dyspnea, shortness of breath, edema, palpitations)	Anthracyclines (doxorubicin and daunorubicin) and/or irradiation to heart High-dose cyclophosphamide
Pericardial damage (pleural effusion, cardiomegaly)	Mediastinal irradiation
▪ Respiratory	
Pneumonitis (dyspnea, nonproductive cough, fever) Pulmonary fibrosis (dyspnea, restrictive ventilation, decreased exercise tolerance)	Lung irradiation, alkylating agents, possibly bleomycin, vinblastine, cisplatin
▪ Gastrointestinal	
Chronic enteritis (colic, abdominal pain, vomiting, diarrhea, obstipation, bleeding)	Abdominal irradiation, methotrexate, cytosine arabinoside
Hepatic fibrosis (jaundice, hepatomegaly)	Methotrexate, 6-mercaptopurine
▪ Urinary	
Hemorrhagic cystitis (chronic microscopic hematuria to gross hemorrhage) Bladder fibrosis (decreased bladder capacity, ureteral reflux) Tubular necrosis (decreased creatinine clearance)	Cyclophosphamide; cisplatin; irradiation, especially with radiomimetic chemotherapeutic agents (i.e., doxorubicin and daunorubicin)
▪ Endocrine	
Growth retardation (abnormal growth velocity) Thyroid dysfunction (see Chapter 38) Gonadal dysfunction (see Reproductive)	Irradiation to the thyroid, pituitary gland
▪ Reproductive	
Possible gonadal damage—both sexes (amenorrhea, decreased sperm counts, increased follicle-stimulating and luteinizing hormones [FSH, LH], decreased testosterone/estrogen)	Alkylating agents Irradiation to the pituitary gland, testes, ovaries
▪ Skeletal	
Linear growth retardation (short stature)	Irradiation, long-term steroids
Spinal deformities, scoliosis, kyphosis, asymmetric growth, pathologic fractures	Irradiation
▪ Immune	
Asplenia (overwhelming infection, fever)	Splenectomy (Hodgkin disease)
▪ Sensory organs	
Cataracts (opacity over pupil)	Cranial irradiation, high-dose steroids
Hearing (decreased hearing associated with high-frequency loss)	Cisplatin
▪ Additional effects	
Dental problems	
Increased caries, periodontal disease, hypoplastic teeth, hypodontia (delayed or absent tooth development)	Irradiation to maxilla and mandible
Second malignancies	
Bone and soft tissue tumors Leukemia Nonlymphocytic leukemia	Irradiation, alkylating agents

opment may be affected by treatment as well as the disease. Table 36-5 describes the systemic late effects caused by cancer treatment that require careful nursing assessment.

All tissues and organs are susceptible to the toxicity of cancer treatment. Many of the problems observed from the treatment for childhood cancer relate to the effects on developing tissues. As a general principle, cytotoxic therapy is more harmful to rapidly growing tissue than to slowly growing tissue.

Four systems that have the potential to develop complications unique to children require careful assessment following therapy for cancer. These are the central nervous, endocrine, reproductive, and skeletal systems.

Nurses caring for young children with cancer must be aware of the impairment caused by treatment with cranial irradiation and intrathecal chemotherapy. Intellectual and motor function may be impaired because of interference with neural development before maturation of the brain is complete. Children under the age of 3 years are at the highest risk for this complication. Assessment of children who have received cranial radiation and intrathecal chemotherapy must incorporate an extensive neurologic evaluation that includes cognitive function.

Radiation therapy to growing bones or reproductive glands responsible for growth-related hormones can delay or stunt growth. Nurses must document growth by assessing height and weight at each visit. Any decrease in growth velocity should be further evaluated. Further assessment includes documenting parental heights, obtaining a wrist x-ray film to predict further growth potential, and assessing gonadal development and pituitary function.

Radiation therapy and the alkylating agents can cause hormonal dysfunction, decreased fertility, and sterility. The potential for gonadal dysfunction depends on the child's age, sex, type of treatment, and the duration and total doses of treatment. Nursing assessment must begin with careful documentation of the child's sexual development using the Tanner staging scale (see Sexual Maturation, Chapter 19). Assessment of delayed or absent sexual development is discussed in Chapter 20.

Radiation therapy to developing bone and cartilage may cause numerous abnormalities. Assessment includes close observations of the irradiated bone for defects, such as spinal kyphoscoliosis, leg length discrepancy, and skull and facial disfigurement.

Irradiated bones are more fragile and may fracture easily, have functional limitations, and heal slowly in the presence of infection. Osteoporosis may develop. Children who have received radiation therapy to the mandibular area are at risk for dental caries, arrested tooth development, and incomplete dental calcification. A careful assessment of the oral cavity in children who have received radiation therapy to the mandible is performed at each clinic visit.

Nursing Diagnoses

A number of nursing diagnoses become apparent following an assessment of the child with cancer and the family. Some are considered in the Nursing Care Plan on pp. 1674-1678. Others are identified here in specific situations.

Planning

The goals of nursing care of the child with cancer and the family include:

1. Promote general health.
2. Prepare the child and family for diagnostic and therapeutic procedures.
3. Prevent complications of myelosuppression.
4. Manage problems of irradiation and drug toxicity.
5. Provide child and family education.

Implementation

Nursing care of the child with cancer is directly related to the regimen of therapy. Nurses working with families of children with cancer have a significant supportive role in helping them understand the various therapies, preventing or managing expected side effects or toxicities, observing for late effects of treatment, and helping the child and family live as normal and healthy a life as possible and cope with the emotional aspects of the disease. Education is a constant feature of the nursing role, especially in terms of new treatments, clinical trials, and home care.

Health Promotion

Children with cancer require the same basic health supervision as any child. Sometimes the overwhelming needs and demands placed on the family coupled with the singular concern focused on the cancer by both family and practitioners result in a lack of attention to normal health care needs. Nurses should monitor the type of primary care the child receives, using as a guideline recommendations for health supervision (see Chapter 7). As discussed under the Assessment section, areas of particular concern are growth, physical and cognitive development, and neurologic status. Two other areas are also important: (1) dental care, because of potential side effects from treatment; and (2) immunizations, because of concern with live virus vaccines and immunosuppression.

Dental care. Irradiation to the head and neck can cause a number of late complications (Niehaus and others, 1987). Some are irreversible, such as facial asymmetry, but those affecting the teeth and gums (caries, periodontal disease) benefit from excellent oral hygiene, including regular use of systemic and topical fluoride (see Dental Health, Chapter 14). There is also evidence of delayed or absent development of the permanent teeth (Halperin, 1986). Depending on the child's age, this can be a source of acute psychologic distress, especially during early school-age years when "losing a tooth" is a status symbol. Therefore children need to be aware of this possibility and helped to explain the delay to peers.

Daily toothbrushing and flossing is encouraged in children with granulocyte counts in excess of 500/mm^3 and platelet counts above 40,000/mm^3 (Berkowitz, Feretti, and

NURSING CARE PLAN
The Child with Cancer

NURSING DIAGNOSIS: Potential for injury related to malignant process

GOAL 1

Help eradicate malignancy

INTERVENTIONS

*Administer chemotherapeutic agents as prescribed
Assist with radiotherapy as ordered
Assist with procedures for administration of chemotherapeutic agents (e.g., lumbar puncture for intrathecal administration)
Prepare child and family for surgical procedure.

EXPECTED OUTCOME

Child achieves a remission from disease

NURSING DIAGNOSIS: Potential for infection related to depressed body defenses

GOAL 1

Minimize risk of infection

INTERVENTIONS

Place child in private room
Advise all visitors and staff to practice handwashing
Screen all visitors and staff for signs of infection
Use scrupulous aseptic technique for all invasive procedures
Evaluate child for any potential sites of infection (needle punctures, mucosal ulceration, minor abrasions, dental problems)
Provide nutritionally complete diet for age
*Administer antibiotics as prescribed

EXPECTED OUTCOMES

Child does not come in contact with infected persons or contaminated articles
Child consumes diet appropriate for age (specify)

NURSING DIAGNOSIS: Potential for injury (hemorrhage, hemorrhagic cystitis) related to interference with cell proliferation

GOAL 1

Prevent hemorrhage

INTERVENTIONS

Use all measures to prevent infection, especially in ecchymotic areas
Use local measures to stop bleeding
Restrict strenuous activity that could result in accidental injury
Involve child in responsibility for limiting activity when platelet count drops
*Administer platelets as prescribed

EXPECTED OUTCOME

Child exhibits no evidence of bleeding

GOAL 2

Prevent hemorrhagic cystitis

INTERVENTIONS

Observe for signs (burning and pain or urination)
Give liberal (3000 ml/m^2/day) fluid intake
Encourage frequent voiding, including during nighttime

EXPECTED OUTCOMES

Child voids without discomfort
No hematuria is present

GOAL 3

Prevent or reduce the effects of anemia

INTERVENTIONS AND EXPECTED OUTCOMES

See Nursing Care Plan: The Child with Anemia, Chapter 35

NURSING DIAGNOSIS: Potential fluid volume deficit related to nausea and vomiting

GOAL 1

Prevent vomiting

INTERVENTIONS

*Administer initial dose of antiemetic before onset of nausea and vomiting
*Administer antiemetic around the clock for as long as nausea and vomiting typically last
Avoid foods with strong odors

EXPECTED OUTCOME

Child retains food and fluid

*Dependent nursing action.

NURSING CARE PLAN
The Child with Cancer—cont'd

NURSING DIAGNOSIS: Altered mucous membranes related to administration of chemotherapeutic agents

GOAL 1
Prevent or reduce effects of oral ulceration

INTERVENTIONS
Inspect mouth daily for oral ulcers; avoid oral temperatures
Institute meticulous oral hygiene as soon as a drug is used that caused oral ulcers
- Use soft-sponge toothbrush, cotton-tipped applicator, or gauze-wrapped finger
- Administer frequent (at least every 4 hours and after meals) mouthwashes (normal saline)

Apply local anesthetics to ulcerated areas before meals and as needed
Serve bland, moist, soft diet
Encourage fluids; use a straw to help bypass painful areas
Report evidence of ulcers to practitioner
Avoid juices containing ascorbic acid, lemon swabs, and hot or cold food
*Administer antiinfective medication as ordered

EXPECTED OUTCOMES
Mucous membranes remain intact
Ulcers show evidence of healing

GOAL 2
Prevent or reduce effects of rectal ulceration

INTERVENTIONS
Wash perianal area after each bowel movement
Use warm sitz baths or tub baths as frequently as necessary for comfort
Apply protective skin barriers (transparent film dressings, occlusive ointment) to perineal area
Expose ulcerated area to warm heat to hasten healing
Observe for constipation resulting from child's voluntary refusal to defecate or from chemotherapy
Avoid rectal temperatures and suppositories
Record bowel movements; use stool softener to prevent constipation; may need stimulants for evacuation

EXPECTED OUTCOMES
Rectal mucosa remains clean and intact
Ulcerated areas heal without complications
Child has regular bowel movements

*Dependent nursing action.

NURSING DIAGNOSIS: Altered nutrition: less than body requirements related to loss of appetite

GOAL 1
Stimulate appetite

INTERVENTIONS
Encourage parents to relax pressures placed on eating; stress legitimate nature of loss of appetite
Allow child *any* food tolerated; plan to improve quality of food selections when appetite increases
Stress expected increase in appetite from steroids
Take advantage of any hungry period; serve small "snacks"
Fortify foods with nutritious supplements, such as powdered milk or commercial supplements
Allow child to be involved in food preparation and selection
Make food appealing
Remember usual food practices of children in each age-group, such as food jags in toddlers or normal occurrence of physiologic anorexia
Assess family for additional problems (e.g., use of food by child as a control mechanism if appetite does not improve despite improved physical status)

EXPECTED OUTCOME
Nutritional intake is adequate

NURSING DIAGNOSIS: Impaired skin integrity related to administration of chemotherapeutic agents, radiotherapy, immobility

GOAL 1
Maintain skin integrity

INTERVENTIONS AND EXPECTED OUTCOMES
See Nursing Diagnosis: Potential impaired skin integrity in Nursing Care Plan: The Child with a Skin Disorder, Chapter 18

GOAL 2
Reduce undesirable effects of therapy

INTERVENTIONS
Suggest and/or implement measures to reduce discomfort from radiotherapy
- Select loose-fitting clothing over irradiated area to minimize additional irritation
- Protect area from sunlight and sudden changes in temperature (avoid ice packs, heating pads)

EXPECTED OUTCOME
Child and family comply with suggestions (specify)

Continued.

NURSING DIAGNOSIS: Impaired physical mobility related to neuromuscular impairment (neuropathy)

GOAL 1

Reduce effects of peripheral neuropathy

INTERVENTIONS

Encourage ambulation when child is able
Alter activity to prevent accidents if weakness occurs, including school attendance
Use footboard to prevent footdrop
Provide fluids and soft foods to lessen chewing movements with jaw pain

EXPECTED OUTCOMES

Child ambulates without incident or difficulty
Nutritional intake is adequate

NURSING DIAGNOSIS: Body image disturbance related to loss of hair, moon face, debilitation

GOAL 1

Help child and family cope with hair loss

INTERVENTIONS

Introduce idea of wig before hair loss
Administer good scalp hygiene
Provide adequate covering during exposure to sunlight, wind, or cold
Suggest keeping thin hair clean, short, and fluffy to camouflage partial baldness
Stress that hair begins to regrow in 3 to 6 months and may be a slightly different color or texture
Stress that alopecia during a second treatment with same drug may be much less severe
Encourage good hygiene, grooming, and sex-appropriate items to enhance appearance, such as wig, scarves, hats, makeup, attractive sex-appropriate clothing

EXPECTED OUTCOMES

Child verbalizes concern regarding hair loss
Child helps determine methods to reduce effects of hair loss and applies these methods
Child appears clean, well-groomed, and attractively dressed

GOAL 2

Promote adjustment to altered facial appearance

INTERVENTIONS

Encourage rapid reintegration with peers to lessen contrast of changed facial appearance
Stress that this reaction is temporary
Evaluate weight gain carefully (in weight gain resulting from administration of steroids, extremities remain thin)
Encourage visits from friends before discharge to prepare child for reactions and questions
Encourage early and consistent interaction with peers

EXPECTED OUTCOMES

Family demonstrates understanding of consequences of therapies
Child resumes former activities and relationships within capabilities

GOAL 3

Encourage expression of feelings

INTERVENTIONS

Provide opportunities for child to discuss feelings and concerns
Provide materials for nonverbal expression (e.g., play, art)

EXPECTED OUTCOME

Child expresses feelings regarding altered body in words, play, art (specify)

NURSING DIAGNOSIS: Pain related to diagnosis, treatment, and physiologic effects of neoplasia

GOAL 1

Relieve pain

INTERVENTIONS

Assess need for pain management (see Chapter 26)
During terminal stage, appreciate that pain control is necessary component of physical and emotional care
Avoid excessive noise or light
Place all commodities within easy reach
Use gentle, minimal physical manipulation
Avoid pressure (bedclothes, sheets) on painful areas
Experiment with using heat or cold on painful areas (use cautiously because of easy skin breakdown)
Whenever possible, make use of procedures that minimize discomfort, such as a venous access device (Broviac catheter, implanted port) or Ommaya reservoir
Change position frequently; if difficult for child, coordinate with pain relief from analgesics
Avoid pressure on bony prominences or painful sites (water bed, bean bag chair, flotation mattress); ensure good body alignment
Evaluate effectiveness of pain relief with degree of alertness vs sedation
Implement appropriate nonpharmacologic pain reduction techniques
*Administer analgesics as prescribed
  Avoid aspirin or any of its compounds
*Administer drugs on preventive schedule
Monitor effectiveness of therapy on pain assessment record (Chapter 26)
See also Nursing Care Plan: the Child in Pain, Chapter 26

EXPECTED OUTCOME

Child rests quietly, exhibits no evidence of discomfort, verbalizes no complaints of discomfort

*Dependent nursing action.

NURSING DIAGNOSIS: Fear related to diagnostic tests, procedures, and treatments

GOAL 1

Reduce fear related to diagnostic procedures and tests

INTERVENTIONS

Explain procedure carefully at the child's level of understanding
Explain what will take place and what the child will feel, see, and hear
Use recall of each step as method of distraction
Explain responsibility of child (e.g., need to remain motionless during test and/or radiotherapy)
Provide the child with some means for involvement with the procedure (e.g., holding a piece of equipment, such as bandage or tape, counting with the operator, answering questions)
Implement distracting techniques and pain reduction techniques as indicated (see Nursing Care Plan: The Child in Pain, Chapter 26)
See also Preparation for Procedures, Chapter 27

EXPECTED OUTCOMES

Child readily responds to verbal directives
Child repeats information accurately

NURSING DIAGNOSIS: Fear related to diagnosis and prognosis

See Nursing Care Plan: The Child Who Is Terminally Ill or Dying, Chapter 23

NURSING DIAGNOSIS: Diversional activity deficit related to restricted environment (private room)

GOAL 1

Provide diversion

INTERVENTIONS

Provide age-appropriate toys that can be properly cleaned
Involve child life specialist or other supportive services in planning diversional activities

EXPECTED OUTCOMES

Child engages in activities appropriate for age and interests
Suitable toys are provided

NURSING DIAGNOSIS: Altered family processes related to having a child with a life-threatening disease

GOAL 1

Prepare family for diagnostic/therapeutic procedures

INTERVENTIONS

Explain reason for each test and procedure
Whenever possible, make use of procedures that minimize discomfort, such as a venous access device (Broviac catheter, implanted port) or Ommaya reservoir
Explain reason for radiotherapy
Explain operative procedure honestly (if appropriate)
Avoid overemphasis on benefits, which may not be evident for several days postoperatively
See also Preparation for Procedures, Chapter 27

EXPECTED OUTCOME

Child and family demonstrate understanding of procedures (specify learning and manner of demonstration)

GOAL 2

Support family

INTERVENTIONS

Teach parents about disease process
Explain all procedures that will be done to child
Schedule time for family to be together, without interruptions from staff
Help family plan for future, especially toward helping child live a normal life
Encourage family to discuss feelings regarding child's course prior to diagnosis and child's prospects for survival
Discuss with family how they will tell child about outcome of surgery and need for additional treatment (if appropriate)
Refer to local chapter of American Cancer Society or other organizations

EXPECTED OUTCOMES

Family demonstrates knowledge of child's disease and treatments (specify methods of learning and evaluation)
Family expresses feelings and concerns and spends time with child
See also:
Nursing Care Plan: The Child in the Hospital, Chapter 26
Nursing Care Plan: The Family of the Ill or Hospitalized Child, Chapter 26

Continued.

NURSING CARE PLAN
The Child with Cancer—cont'd

NURSING DIAGNOSIS: Altered family processes related to a child undergoing therapy

GOAL 1

Prepare family for side effects and/or complications of chemotherapy or radiotherapy

INTERVENTIONS

Advise family of expected therapy side effects vs toxicities; clarify which demand medical evaluation (mucosal ulceration, hemorrhagic cystitis, peripheral neuropathy, evidence of infection or dehydration)
Reassure family that such reactions are not caused by return of cancer cells
Interpret prognostic statistics carefully, realizing family's temporary need to interpret them as they see necessary
Prepare family for expected mood changes from steroids
Interpret mood changes based on drugs or reactions to disease/treatment

EXPECTED OUTCOMES

Family demonstrates knowledge of instructions (specify methods of learning and evaluation)
Family demonstrates an understanding of behavior changes

GOAL 2

Support child during treatment for myelosuppression

INTERVENTIONS

Explain reason for antibiotics and/or transfusions, particularly why platelets are reserved for acute, uncontrolled bleeding episodes
Observe for signs of transfusion reaction (see Table 35-2)
Record approximate time for hemostasis to occur after administration of platelets

EXPECTED OUTCOME

Child demonstrates understanding of procedures and tests (specify method and learnings)

GOAL 3

Prepare family for home care

INTERVENTIONS

Teach preventive measures as discharge (handwashing and isolation from crowds)
Stress importance of isolating child from any known cases of chickenpox or other childhood diseases; work with school nurse and physician to determine optimum time for school reattendance

EXPECTED OUTCOME

Family demonstrates the ability to provide home care for the child

NURSING DIAGNOSIS: Anticipatory grief related to perceived potential loss of a child

GOAL 1

Help family face possibility of child's death

INTERVENTIONS

Provide consistent contact with family
Clarify, refocus, and supply information as needed
Help family plan care of child, especially at terminal stage (e.g., extent of extraordinary lifesaving measures)
Provide or help arrange for hospice care if family desires
Arrange for spiritual support in accordance with family's beliefs and/or affiliations

EXPECTED OUTCOMES

Family remains open to counseling and nursing contacts
Family and child discuss their fears, concerns, needs, and desires at terminal stage
Family investigates hospice care
Appropriate religious representative is contacted (specify)

GOAL 2

Support family

INTERVENTIONS AND EXPECTED OUTCOMES

See Nursing Care Plan: The Child Who Is Terminally Ill or Dying, Chapter 23

Berg, 1987). Fluoride rinses are used as discussed in Chapter 14. Oral hygiene for children whose counts are below these parameters is limited to wiping the teeth with moistened gauze sponges or Toothettes.

Immunizations. Viral replication following the administration of live vaccine for polio, measles, rubella, and mumps can cause serious disease in immunocompromised children who receive these vaccines. The inactivated poliovirus vaccine (IPV) should be given to immunosuppressed children and their household contacts in place of the routine immunization with the oral poliovirus. Children who have not received chemotherapy for at least 3 months can be given live vaccines (U.S. Department of Health and Human Services, 1989). Children who are immunosuppressed can receive the varicella (chickenpox) vaccine, which has been shown to be effective in preventing varicella in high-risk children (Brunell and others, 1987; Feldman and Lott, 1987; Gershon, 1987).

✦ **NURSING ALERT** Children receiving chemotherapy should not be given live vaccines.

A very important indication for isolation is an outbreak of childhood disease, especially chickenpox. The child is confined from all known sources of the infection, such as schoolmates, until the epidemic is over. Ideally the school nurse should work with the treating practitioner to decide the optimum time for school reattendance. If the child has been exposed to the varicella virus, varicella-zoster immune globulin (VZIG) given within 96 hours may favorably alter the course of the disease, or antiviral agents, such as acyclovir, may be given if the child develops varicella (Caul and Roome, 1988). These antiviral agents are very effective in preventing serious disease if given during the first 3 days of the appearance of symptoms (U.S. Department of Health and Human Services, 1989). Without treatment, death from disseminated varicella (about 7%) is usually caused by pneumonia; other serious although nonfatal complications include hepatitis, pancreatitis, meningitis, and bacterial skin infections (see also Immunizations, Chapter 12).

Preparation for Procedures

Children in particular need psychologic preparation for the various treatment modalities, which often involve surgery, intravenous injections, bone marrow aspiration, and lumbar punctures. The diagnostic procedures initially employed to confirm the diagnosis and those that are repeated to monitor treatment are often a source of discomfort and stress to the child and family. Even noninvasive procedures such as radiologic tests are frightening to a young child. Many of these tests require the child to lie absolutely motionless for a prolonged time in a confined space with little or no communication with a supportive adult. Consequently, infants and young children are usually sedated, and older children need an explanation of what to expect and reminders during the test of how much longer they must remain still. The same principles for preparing children for procedures that are discussed in Chapter 27 apply here, including the option of having parents stay with the child whenever possible (see Questions and Controversies, p. 1191). It is a mistake to assume that children who undergo repeated tests do not need additional preparation or emotional support. Children are more likely to become conditioned to the discomfort and to experience *increasing*, not decreasing, levels of stress (Dolgin and others, 1989; Zeltzer, Jay, and Fisher, 1989).

Two procedures, bone marrow studies and lumbar punctures, are so commonly employed in many types of childhood cancer that they deserve special consideration in preparing children. Both tests can be frightening to children because they are done behind the child's field of vision. In some institutions sedation is administered before the test, but sedatives provide no analgesia. The child may arrive to the treatment room asleep, but once the procedure begins, the pain wakens the child. Typically (but not always) the puncture site is anesthetized with a local anesthetic, which may be given by subcutaneous injection or with a pressurized air gun. (As of this printing a topical preparation, EMLA [eutectic mixture of local anesthetics], is pending approval for use in the United States. Studies support its effectiveness in reducing local pain from invasive procedures [Juhlin and Evers, 1990].) In a lumbar puncture, when a local anesthetic is given, this is the only discomfort the child feels. However, in a bone marrow test, the insertion of the needle into the bone as it passes through the periosteum and the withdrawal of the marrow also cause pain. In addition, pressure must be exerted to facilitate entry through the bone, which is upsetting to some children. (See discussion on pharmacologic pain management in Chapter 26.)

Although it is an infrequent practice, some institutions are recognizing the extreme stress associated with these invasive procedures and are offering children the option of having general anesthesia on an outpatient basis. Parents are allowed to stay with the child from induction of anesthesia through recovery. Preliminary results indicate that children choose to have the procedure performed under general anesthesia and that the technique is safe (Forlini, Morin, and Treacy, 1987; Perin and Frase, 1985; Zeltzer, Jay, and Fisher, 1989).

For both procedures, children of preschool age and beyond should be prepared beforehand. If this is not possible, the nurse should explain each step of the procedure as it occurs, stressing what will be done and what it will feel like. If each step is explained beforehand, having the child recall the next step during the procedure can be a distraction mechanism.

Physical care after the procedures is minimal. A small pressure bandage is applied to the bone marrow puncture site, and an adhesive bandage is applied to the lumbar puncture site. No activity restriction is necessary after the bone marrow test, although the site is usually sore and the child may prefer to remain quiet. Recommendations after the lumbar puncture vary. If medication was instilled, the child may be placed in a slight Trendelenburg position to facilitate circulation of the medicated spinal fluid.

Prevention of Complications of Myelosuppression

Some types of malignancies (leukemia, lymphoma) and most of the chemotherapeutic agents cause myelosuppression. The reduced numbers of blood cells result in secondary problems of infection, bleeding tendencies, and anemia. Supportive care involves both medical and nursing management. Because they are so closely linked, they are discussed together rather than separately.

Infection. A frequent cause of death from childhoo
cancer is overwhelming infection secondary to neutrope
(defined as an absolute neutrophil count below 1000/m
(Darbyshire, 1988).

The child is most susceptible to overwhelming inf
during three phases of the disease: (1) at the time c
nosis and relapse when the cancer process has r
normal leukocytes, (2) during immunosuppressive
and (3) after prolonged antibiotic therapy, whi
poses the child to the growth of resistant organi

The first defense against infection is preve
the child is hospitalized, all measures to con
infection are instituted, such as the use of
restriction of all visitors and health personn
fection, and strict handwashing technique
tic solution. The use of protective (revers
troversial; however, research provides e

tive isolation does *not* decrease the risk of infection nor improve survival (Zaia and Forman, 1987). Therefore any decision to implement protective isolation must be seriously evaluated in terms of its doubtful benefit and the psychologic stress it imposes on the child.

The organisms most lethal to these children are (1) viruses, particularly varicella (chickenpox), herpes zoster, herpes simplex, measles, rubella, mumps, and poliomyelitis; (2) *Pneumocystis carinii* (a protozoan); (3) fungi, especially *Candida albicans;* (4) gram-negative bacteria, such as *Pseudomonas aeruginosa, Escherichia coli, Proteus,* and *Klebsiella;* and (5) gram-positive bacteria, especially *Staphylococcus aureus, S. epidermidis,* and group A β-hemolytic streptococcus (Viscoli, 1988; Wagner, 1988). As prophylaxis against these various organisms, broad-spectrum antibiotics are usually prescribed. Ensuring compliance with this long-term regimen is an important nursing responsibility.

Once infection is suspected, broad-spectrum intravenous antibiotic therapy is begun before the organism is identified and continued for the usual 7- to 10-day period, regardless of whether a specific agent is isolated. If the child does not have a venous access device, a heparin lock should be inserted to prevent the inconvenience of multiple venipunctures in maintaining a patent intravenous line and to prevent limited activity imposed by an immobilized body part.

Prevention of infection continues as a priority after discharge from the hospital. However, rigid social restriction must be tempered with the child's need for resuming normal activity. Ordinarily the child can return to school when the absolute neutrophil count is above $500/mm^3$. If the level falls below this value, cautious isolation from crowded areas, such as shopping centers or subways, is advisable. At all times family members are encouraged to practice good handwashing to prevent introducing pathogens into the home.

Nutrition is another important component of infection prevention. An adequate protein-calorie intake provides the child with better host defenses against infection and increased tolerance to chemotherapy and irradiation. However, providing optimum nutrition during periods of anorexia and vomiting from chemotherapy is a tremendous challenge. Every effort is made to encourage the child to eat (see Feeding the Sick Child, Chapter 27), and if nonoral feedings are instituted, meticulous care in terms of the feeding procedure is implemented to prevent infection.

Hemorrhage. Before the use of transfused platelets, hemorrhage was a leading cause of death in children with some types of cancer. Now most bleeding episodes can be prevented or controlled with judicious administration of platelet concentrates or platelet-rich plasma. Severe spontaneous internal hemorrhage usually does not occur until the platelet count is $20,000/mm^3$ (Greenbaum and Herman, 1988).

Since infection increases the tendency toward hemorrhage, and bleeding sites become more easily infected, special care is taken to avoid performing skin punctures whenever possible. When fingersticks, venipunctures, intramuscular injections, and bone marrow aspirations are performed, aseptic technique must be employed with continued observation for bleeding. Meticulous mouth care is essential, since gingival bleeding with resultant mucositis is a frequent problem. Since the rectal area is prone to ulceration from various drugs, hygiene is essential. To prevent additional trauma, rectal temperatures and suppositories are avoided. Frequent turning, the use of a flotation or alternating-pressure mattress, and sheepskin under bony prominences prevent development of pressure areas and decubital ulcers.

Platelet transfusions are generally reserved for active bleeding episodes that do not respond to local treatment and that may occur during induction or relapse therapy. Epistaxis and gingival bleeding are the most common. The nurse teaches parents and older children measures to control nose bleeding (see Epistaxis (nosebleeding), Chapter 35). Pressure at the site without disturbing clot formation is the general rule.

Two of the problems with multiple platelet transfusions are the risk of febrile reactions and decreased life span of the platelets. Platelet concentrates normally do not have to be crossmatched for blood group or type. However, because platelets contain specific antigen components similar to blood group factors, children who receive multiple transfusions may become sensitized to a platelet group other than their own. Therefore it is advisable to crossmatch platelets with the donor's blood components whenever this is possible.

Transfused platelets generally survive in the body for 1 to 3 days. The peak effect is reached in about 2 hours and decreased by half in 24 hours. Therefore after a transfusion the nurse observes and records the approximate time when hemostasis of bleeding sites occurs. Delayed hemostasis is evidence of platelet destruction. For long-term patients, multiple transfusion therapy becomes progressively less effective.

During bleeding episodes the parents and child need much emotional support. The sight of oozing blood is very upsetting. Often parents will request a platelet transfusion, unaware of the necessity of trying local measures first. The nurse can be instrumental in allaying anxiety by explaining the reason for delaying a platelet transfusion until absolutely necessary. Since compatible donors decrease the risk of antigen formation in the recipient, the nurse should encourage parents to locate suitable donors for eventual blood use.

Children at home who have low platelet counts (usually below $100,000/mm^3$) are advised to avoid those activities that might cause injury or bleeding, such as riding bicycles or skateboards, roller skating, and contact sports such as football or soccer. These restrictions can be terminated once the platelet count rises, such as after platelet transfusion. In addition, parents are cautioned to avoid aspirin and aspirin-containing products; for mild pain or significantly elevated temperature, acetaminophen is substituted.

Anemia. Initially anemia may be profound from complete replacement of the bone marrow by cancer cells. During induction therapy, blood transfusions with packed red cells may be necessary to raise hemoglobin to levels approaching 10 g. The usual precautions in caring for the child are instituted (see Chapter 35).

Anemia is also a consequence of drug-induced myelosuppression. Although not as severely affected as the white blood cells, erythrocyte production may be delayed. Since children have an amazing capacity to withstand low hemoglobin levels, the best approach is to allow the child to regulate activity with reasonable adult supervision. It may be necessary for the parents to alert the schoolteacher to the child's physical limitations, particularly in terms of strenuous activity.

Management of Problems Related to Irradiation and Drug Toxicity

Irradiation and chemotherapy present several challenges to providing effective care. The complexity of the treatment protocols alone is often overwhelming to families, who can benefit from receiving a monthly calendar of anticipated treatment dates. In addition, each therapy is associated with a number of predictable side effects (see Tables 36-3 and 36-4). The following is a discussion of these reactions and appropriate interventions.

Nausea and vomiting. The nausea and vomiting that occur shortly after administration of several of the drugs and as a result of cranial radiation can be profound. Although a number of antiemetic agents are available, no product is uniformly successful in controlling the vomiting. For mild to moderate vomiting, antiemetics such as promethazine (Phenergan), chlorpromazine (Thorazine), prochlorperazine (Compazine), or trimethobenzamide (Tigan) may be effective. Metoclopramide (Reglan) is a more effective antiemetic for severe vomiting (Craig and Powell, 1987). Unfortunately, the drug causes a number of side effects in children, particularly extrapyramidal reactions, such as muscle tremors or twitching, agitation, grimacing, dysarthria, and oculogyric crisis (fixation of eyes in one position for minutes or hours) (Sridhar and Donnelly, 1988). The incidence of extrapyramidal reactions is dose and age related—increased in older children and at higher doses (Craig and Powell, 1987). Metoclopramide used in conjunction with benztropine, dexamethasone, diphenhydramine, and/or lorazepam has been shown to significantly decrease nausea and vomiting as well as the untoward side effects of metoclopramide (Kris and others, 1987; Marshall and others, 1989; Sridhar and Donnelly, 1988).

Another drug that has yielded promising results is THC (delta-9-tetrahydrocannabinol), the active component of marijuana. Synthetic cannabinoids are now being used in children undergoing chemotherapy. Nabilone was developed to overcome the problems associated with the naturally occurring cannabinoids. Nabilone has shown to be superior to placebo, prochlorperazine, and low-dose metoclopramide both as an antiemetic and in terms of patient preference (Few, 1988).

The most beneficial regimen for antiemetic control has been the administration of the antiemetic *before* the chemotherapy begins (30 minutes to 1 hour before) and regular (not PRN) administration every 2, 4, or 6 hours for at least 24 hours after chemotherapy (Yasko, 1985). There is some evidence that beginning antiemetic therapy up to 24 hours before the chemotherapy adds additional effectiveness (Williams and others, 1989). The goal is to prevent the child from ever experiencing nausea or vomiting, since this can prevent the development of anticipatory symptoms (the conditioned response of developing nausea and vomiting before receiving the drug) (Dolgin and others, 1985). Other nonpharmacologic interventions (similar to those discussed for pain management in Chapter 26) can be useful in controlling posttherapy and anticipatory nausea and vomiting (Hockenberry, 1988; Yasko, 1985). Giving the antineoplastic drug with a mild sedative at bedtime is also helpful for some children, and there is evidence that nighttime administration of drugs such as methotrexate and 6-mercaptopurine may be more effective cytotoxically than morning administration (Evans and others, 1989).

Anorexia. Loss of appetite is a direct consequence of the chemotherapy and/or irradiation. It is a major problem for parents because it is the one area they feel responsible for, particularly when so many other facets of care are outside their control. There are no universally successful techniques for encouraging a sick child to eat. However, the guidelines in Box 27-9 may help during the anorexic period and also during the remission.

Some children still do not eat despite these approaches. The following theories have been postulated to explain persistent anorexia: (1) a physical cause related to the cancer that is nonspecific; (2) a conditioned aversion to food from nausea and vomiting during treatment; (3) stress in the environment, related to eating and/or to the child's condition; (4) depression; (5) a control mechanism when so much else has been imposed on the child; and (6) an opportunity to express anger at parents and punish them for "allowing" the child to become sick. When loss of appetite and weight persists, the nurse should investigate the family situation to determine if any of these variables are contributing to the problem. To prevent conditioned aversion to food, it is best to offer few foods and no favorite foods before chemotherapy. Meats and proteins are more apt to trigger learned food aversions. A light, low-protein meal, followed by candy of a distinctive flavor before a chemotherapy treatment, proved to be effective in decreasing food aversions in one study (Broberg and Bernstein, 1987).

Mucosal ulceration. One of the most distressing side effects of several drugs is gastrointestinal mucosal cell damage, which results in ulcers anywhere along the alimentary tract. Oral ulcers (stomatitis) are red, eroded, painful areas in the mouth and/or pharynx (see also Stomatitis, Chapter 16). Similar lesions may extend along the esophagus and frequently occur in the rectal area. They greatly compound anorexia, because eating is extremely uncomfortable. When oral ulcers develop, the following interventions are helpful: (1) a bland, moist, soft diet; (2) use of soft sponge toothbrush (Toothette)* or cotton-tipped applicator; (3) frequent mouthwashes with normal saline (using a solution of 1 teaspoon of table salt and 1 pint of water) or sodium bicarbonate and salt mouthrinses (using a solution of 1 teaspoon of baking soda and ½ teaspoon of table salt in 1

*Manufactured by Halbrand, Inc., Willoughby, OH.

quart of water); and (4) local anesthetics such as Chloraseptic lozenges or nonprescription preparations without alcohol such as Orabase (Berkowitz, Feretti, and Berg, 1987). Although local anesthetics are effective in temporarily relieving the pain, many children dislike the taste and numb feeling they produce.

✦ **NURSING ALERT** Viscous lidocaine is not recommended for young children; if applied to the pharynx, it may depress the gag reflex, increasing the risk of aspiration. Seizures have also been associated with the use of oral viscous lidocaine (Hess and Walson, 1988).

Protocols for oral care during myelosuppression vary according to the institution. For example, Ulcerase is free of sugar, alcohol, and dyes and has been used to soothe mucositis and gum irritations. Moi-Stir swabs have been shown to be effective in decreasing dryness and improving xerostomia (Poland, 1987). Chlorhexidine gluconate (Peridex) is used at many institutions because of its dual effectiveness against candidal as well as bacterial infections (Samaranayake and others, 1988). *Candida* prophylaxis using antifungal troches (lozenges) or mouthwash is typically used in patients with myelosuppression, especially for children who have undergone BMT (Berkowitz, Feretti, and Berg, 1987).

Sucralfate (Carafate) has not been found to be effective in preventing or treating mucositis, although it helps relieve oral pain and has an antimicrobial effect on the bowel (Shenep and others, 1988). Agents such as lemon glycerin swabs, hydrogen peroxide, and milk of magnesia are avoided because of the drying effects on the mucosa. In addition, lemon may be irritating to eroded tissue and can decay the teeth (Poland, 1987).

A strategy that may be helpful in reducing oral pain is massaging the area on the backs of both hands between the thumb and index finger with an ice cube for 5 to 7 minutes until the area becomes numb (Melzack, Guite, and Gonshor, 1980).

Administering mouth care is particularly difficult in infants and toddlers. A satisfactory method of cleaning the gums is to wrap a piece of gauze around a finger, soak it in saline or plain water, and swab the gums, palate, and inner cheek surfaces with the finger. Mouthwashes are best accomplished with plain water or saline, because the child cannot gargle or spit out excess fluid. Mouth care should be done routinely before and after any feeding and as often as every 2 to 4 hours to rid mucosal surfaces of debris, which becomes an excellent medium for bacterial and fungal growth.

Dental hygiene can become a serious problem if the child wears an orthodontic appliance. The accumulated debris on braces is difficult to remove without vigorous brushing, and the appliance itself traumatizes the gums. Sometimes braces are removed to allow chemotherapy to continue.

Difficulty in eating is a major problem with stomatitis and may warrant hospitalization if the child refuses fluids. The child will usually choose the foods that are best tolerated. Surprisingly, some children prefer salty foods to more bland ones. Drinking can usually be encouraged if a straw is used to bypass the ulcerated oral mucosa. The nurse should encourage parents to relax any eating pressures, because the anorexia accompanying stomatitis is well justified. In addition, since it is a temporary condition, once the ulcers heal the child can resume good food habits. Ordinarily, severe mucosal ulceration indicates a need for decreased chemotherapy until complete healing takes place, usually within a week. Analgesics, including opioids, may be needed when treatment cannot be altered, such as during BMT.

If rectal ulcers develop, meticulous toilet hygiene, warm sitz baths after each bowel movement, and periodic exposure of the ulcerated area to warm heat promote healing, and the use of stool softeners is necessary to prevent further discomfort. Sometimes a rectal ulcer can be so uncomfortable that the child prefers to spend as much time as possible in the bathtub. Parents should be advised to record bowel movements, since the child may voluntarily avoid defecation to prevent discomfort. Rectal temperatures and suppositories are avoided because they may further traumatize the area.

Neurologic problems. Vincristine and to a lesser extent vinblastine can cause various neurotoxic effects, one of the more common of which is severe constipation from decreased bowel innervation. Constipation is further aggravated by opioids. The nurse advises parents to record bowel movements and to notify the practitioner of a change in stool habits. Physical activity and stool softeners are helpful in preventing the problem, but laxatives, such as Peri-Colace, or enemas are often necessary to stimulate evacuation. Dietary changes such as increased fiber are not advised, because the increased bulk tends to increase fecal distention and discomfort without producing the necessary mechanical stimulation (Cimprich, 1985).

Footdrop, weakness, and numbing of the extremities may cause difficulty in walking or fine hand movement. The nurse should look for these problems and warn parents of these side effects, which are reversible once the drug is stopped. If the child is on bed rest, a footboard should be used to preserve proper alignment. If weakness occurs while the child is attending school, a temporary alteration of activity may be necessary. The teacher should be apprised of the situation so that unrealistic expectations of the child's abilities are not made.

Another side effect that can be severe is jaw pain. Analgesics may be necessary to relieve the discomfort. Avoiding movement by not talking or chewing is usually self-imposed, although continuous chewing, such as with gum, may actually reduce the pain. Since the pain is temporary, usually lasting for a day or two, the child can be given fluids through a straw.

A neurologic syndrome (postirradiation somnolence) may develop 5 to 8 weeks after central nervous system irradiation and may last for 4 to 15 days. It is characterized by somnolence with or without fever, anorexia, and nausea and vomiting. Parents should be warned of the possibility of such symptoms and encouraged to seek medical evaluation, since somnolence may be an early indicator of long-term neurologic sequelae after cranial irradiation (Halperin, 1986).

Hemorrhagic cystitis. Sterile hemorrhagic cystitis is a side effect of chemical irritation to the bladder from chemotherapy and/or radiation therapy. It can be prevented by (1) a liberal oral and/or parenteral fluid intake (at least one and one-half times the recommended daily fluid requirement [2 liters/m^2 per day]), (2) frequent voiding immediately after feeling the urge, including immediately before bed and after arising (may include one nighttime void), and (3) administering the drug early in the day to allow for sufficient fluids and frequent voiding.

✦ **NURSING ALERT** If signs of cystitis such as burning on urination occur, prompt medical evaluation is needed. Hemorrhagic cystitis warrants cessation of the drug.

In some cases intravenous fluids are given before, during, and after the drug to ensure adequate hydration, thereby eliminating the need for the child's drinking large amounts of fluid. If oral home administration is prescribed, the family needs *specific* instructions on exactly how much fluid the child must have.

Alopecia. Hair loss is a side effect of several chemotherapeutic drugs and cranial irradiation. Not all children lose their hair during drug therapy; however, retaining hair is the exception rather than the rule. It is better to warn children and parents of this side effect than to allow them to think that it is only a remote possibility.

The family should know that the hair falls out in clumps, causing patchy baldness. To lessen the trauma of seeing large amounts of hair on bed linen or clothing, the child can wear a disposable surgical cap to collect the shed hair during the period of greatest hair loss or cut the hair short. Families should also be aware that wigs are tax deductible and that hair regrows in 3 to 6 months. The hair frequently is darker, thicker, and curlier than before.

If the child chooses not to wear a wig, attention to some type of head covering is important, especially in cold or sunny climates. Scalp hygiene is also important. The scalp should be washed regularly as with any other body part.

Many children demonstrate increased tolerance to hair loss on reinduction therapy. Rather than complete baldness, the child may experience thinning of the hair. If the hair is cut short, kept clean, and blow-dried with an electric hair drier, it usually can look full enough to make a wig unnecessary. This can be a tremendous psychologic boost to the child who is already depressed about learning of a relapse and the need for additional chemotherapy.

NURSING TIP: CHOOSING A WIG

Encouraging children to choose a wig similar to their own hairstyle and color *before* the hair falls out is helpful in fostering later adjustment to hair loss.

Moon face. Short-term steroid therapy produces no acute toxicities and often results in two beneficial reactions—increased appetite and a sense of well-being. However, it does produce alterations in body image, which, although not clinically significant, can be extremely distressing to older children. One of these is moon face. The child's face becomes rounded and puffy (see Fig. 38-3). Unlike hair loss, little can be done to camouflage this obvious change, although careful avoidance of salt and salt-containing foods can help reduce fluid accumulation. It is not unusual for other children to make fun of the child with such remarks as "Porky-Pig" or "fat face." For the child who experiences such name-calling, it is helpful to reassure him or her that after cessation of the drug the facial contours will return to normal. If the child resumes activity early in the course of treatment, the change may be less noticeable to peers than after a long absence. Also, the use of loose-fitting clothes, such as warm-up outfits, can help camouflage the change in weight.

In contrast, parents may appreciate the full-rounded appearance because it simulates the look of a well-nourished, healthy child. Because of their own needs, they may be less able to understand the child's misery over altered body image. The nurse can foster a better understanding between the parents and child if both parties are encouraged to openly discuss their feelings.

Children on steroid therapy do look healthy. The moon face, red cheeks, supraclavicular fat pads, protuberant abdomen, and fluid retention indicate weight gain. However, the actual weight gain resulting from increased muscle mass and subcutaneous tissue may be small. Therefore the nurse should evaluate weight gain carefully during steroid therapy to make certain that some of it is a result of increased dietary intake. This is done by observing the extremities and measuring skinfold thickness and arm circumference.

Mood changes. Shortly after beginning steroid therapy, children may experience a number of mood changes, which range from feelings of well-being and euphoria to depression and irritability. If parents are unaware of these drug-induced changes, they may become unduly concerned. Therefore the nurse should warn them of the reactions and encourage them to discuss the behavioral changes with each other and the child.

Bone Marrow Transplantation

The needs of the family are great when bone marrow transplantation is expected. These children may be hospitalized from 30 to 60 days and are usually in a medical center that specializes in this procedure. Because of the risk of infection, the unit may employ strict protective isolation, including laminar air flow to sterilize the air. Consequently, the child is faced with the additional trauma of isolation (see also Chapter 26). The cost/benefit ratio of conventional isolation compared with laminar flow rooms remains controversial. Survival rates of patients undergoing BMT in both types of isolation are comparable (Zaia and Forman, 1987).

Numerous procedures are performed, such as use of a venous access device (if not already performed), intensive chemotherapy and irradiation, and meticulous personal hygiene. In addition, side effects and complications may occur after the preoperative cytotoxic regimen and include development of infection, severe mucositis, parotitis, nausea, vomiting, diarrhea, syndrome of inappropriate antidiuretic hormone (SIADH), nephropathy, and heart failure (Wiley and House, 1988). Skin breakdown and delayed wound healing occur frequently in the patient undergoing BMT. Preventive interventions to minimize pressure on dependent areas of the skin include the use of Egg-crate mattresses, air mattresses, and/or sheepskin. Measures to promote healing when breakdown occurs include frequent sitz baths for the perianal area; transparent dressings, such as Tegaderm, over bony prominences; and protective skin barriers, such as ointments (Abramovitz and Baache, 1988). Throughout this long ordeal involved in BMT, there is the family's concern for successful engraftment and fear of fatal complications. Consequently, nurses involved with the child and family need to provide sensitive care and maintain a supportive attitude during the many crises that may arise. If the procedure is not successful, the care needed by these families is consistent with that required by the family of any child with a life-threatening disorder (see Chapter 23).

Cessation of Therapy

Care does not end when the child completes therapy. With the increasing awareness of late effects, nurses play an important role in the assessment of the child for problems such as delayed growth, secondary malignancies, and disturbances in any body system. These children require regular follow-up, and the family needs to be aware of the importance of continued medical supervision. Other health care professionals caring for the child, such as school nurses, family physicians, and dentists, should be informed of the child's previous diagnosis of cancer. As children reach adulthood, they may benefit from genetic counseling regarding cancers that are likely to be inherited. If the possibility of sterility exists, pretreatment sperm banking may be offered to adolescent boys, which allows additional options regarding family planning in adulthood (Moshang and Lee, 1988).

Family Education

Nurses working with children who have cancer have a significant supportive role in helping the family understand the various therapies, preventing or managing expected side effects or toxicities, and observing for late effects of treatment. Education is a constant feature of the nursing role, especially in terms of new treatments, clinical trials,* and home care. Because of the anxiety generated by the diagnosis of cancer, some families may resort to unproven methods of treatment that are frequently referred to as "cancer quackery." These unorthodox approaches may produce unnecessary harm by themselves or, if benign, render injury because other proven modes of therapy are avoided. In many instances this causes financial burden and emotional strife among family members.

Nurses can be instrumental in working against cancer quackery by being aware of factors that increase a family's likelihood of seeking unproven remedies, such as social pressure to "leave no stone unturned" and feelings of depression, helplessness, and hopelessness (Lichter, 1987). Communicating effectively with families about the diagnosis and forms of therapy and providing all possible support and reassurance during treatment are also important interventions to counteract the factors that lead to dissatisfaction with conventional care. Nurses must be fortified with knowledge to substantiate present treatment protocols and to discredit unauthorized methods. The American Cancer Society and local and state medical societies are reliable sources of information concerning research on investigational vs quack methods of cancer therapy.

Instruction regarding home care frequently involves teaching about medication schedules, observation for side effects or toxicities that require further evaluation, measures to prevent or manage these problems, and care of special devices such as central venous catheters.* Compliance is a very important issue, since poor adherence to drug regimens can result in a relapse. Every effort must be made to ensure that the family understands the importance of adhering to the prescribed treatment schedule and measures to improve compliance (see Chapter 27).

Evaluation

The effectiveness of nursing interventions is determined by continual reassessment and evaluation of care based on the following observational guidelines and expected outcomes:

1. Compare number of visits for primary health with recommended schedule of health supervision.
2. Monitor growth, development, and other aspects of regular health assessment; check mouth for adequacy of dental hygiene; review immunization record for age-appropriate vaccines and use of non–live virus preparations.
3. Interview child and family regarding their understanding of treatments and diagnostic tests.
4. Employ pain assessment techniques for procedural pain.
5. Make careful observations of physical status:
   - Take vital signs regularly.
   - Observe for evidence of bleeding, infection, neuropathy, cystitis, and mucosal ulceration.
   - Observe and record intake and output.
6. Interview child and family and observe behaviors as a result of complications of therapies.
7. Interview child and family and observe behaviors that provide clues to their response to the disease, its therapy, and nursing interventions.

*A helpful resource is *What Are Clinical Trials All About?*, which is available at no cost from the Office of Cancer Communications, National Cancer Institute, Bldg. 31, Room 10A24, Bethesda, MD 20892; (800) 4-CANCER.

*Home care instructions on giving medications to children and caring for a central venous catheter are available in Wong, D., and Whaley, L.: Clinical manual of pediatric nursing, ed. 3, St. Louis, 1990, Mosby–Year Book, Inc.

Expected outcomes:
See Nursing Care Plan, pp. 1674-1678.

CANCERS OF THE BLOOD AND LYMPH SYSTEMS

Three of the most common cancers in children, leukemia, Hodgkin disease, and non-Hodgkin lymphoma, arise in the blood and lymph systems. Children with all of these cancers have benefited from improved methods of treatment in recent years, and a significant portion of affected children will be long-term survivors.

LEUKEMIAS

Leukemia, cancer of the blood-forming tissues, is the most common form of childhood cancer. The annual incidence in white children under 15 years of age is 4.2 per 100,000 and in black children is 2.4 per 100,000 (Poplack, 1989). It occurs more frequently in males than females after age 1 year, and the peak onset is between 2 and 6 years. It is one of the forms of cancer that have demonstrated dramatic improvements in survival rates. Before the use of antileukemic agents in 1948, a child with acute lymphocytic leukemia (ALL) lived 2 to 3 months. Current 5-year survival rates for children with ALL exceed 60% in major research centers, and the majority of these children may be cured (Steinherz, 1987).

Classification

Leukemia is a broad term given to a group of malignant diseases of the bone marrow and lymphatic system. Current research has revealed that it is a complex disease of varying heterogeneity. Consequently, classification has become increasingly complex, sophisticated, and essential, since identification of the subtype of leukemia has therapeutic and prognostic implications. The following is an overview of the major classification systems currently being used.

Morphology. Leukemia is classified according to its predominant cell type and level of maturity, as described by the following:

Lympho—for leukemias involving the lymphoid or lymphatic system
Myelo—for those of myeloid (bone marrow) origin
Blastic and acute—for those involving immature cells
Cytic and chronic—for those involving mature cells

Prior to modern treatment, the classifications of acute or chronic were applied to the cells' level of maturity, because they correlated with the course of the disease—the immature form of the disease demonstrated a rapid or acute course of deterioration. Now this distinction is less likely to be seen, and the acute disease refers primarily to the presence of immature blast cells that accumulate and inhibit production of normal functioning cells (Neglia and Robison, 1988). (For a review of the origin and development of blood cells, see Chapter 35.)

In children two forms are generally recognized: *acute lymphoid leukemia (ALL)* and *acute nonlymphoid (myelogenous) leukemia (ANLL* or *AML)*. Synonyms for ALL include lymphatic, lymphocytic, lymphoblastic, and lymphoblastoid leukemia. Usually the terms *stem cell* or *blast cell leukemia* also refer to the lymphoid type of leukemia. Synonyms for the ANLL type include granulocytic, myelocytic, monocytic, myelogenous, monoblastic, and monomyeloblastic. There are also much rarer forms of leukemia that are named for the specific cell involved, such as basophilic or eosinophilic leukemia.

Because of the confusion and inconsistency in classifying the leukemias, acute lymphoblastic and acute nonlymphoblastic leukemias are further subdivided according to another system known as the *French-American-British (FAB) system.* In the FAB system the subtypes are determined after a thorough study of the morphology (structure) and cytochemical reactivity of the leukemic cells. Accordingly, ALL is divided into three subtypes: L_1, L_2, and L_3. L_1 morphology is the most common subtype, accounts for 84% of children with ALL, and has the best prognosis (Poplack, 1989). ANLL is classified into six subtypes that comprise 10% to 20% of leukemias in children. The subtypes of ANLL are not clearly related to prognosis as is the case with ALL.

Cytochemical markers. Leukemic cells demonstrate different reactions when they are exposed to certain chemicals. For example, terminal deoxynucleotidyl transferase is able to provide excellent differentiation between ALL and ANLL. Several other chemicals are available to further differentiate various cell types.

Chromosomal studies. Chromosomal analysis has become an important tool in the diagnosis of acute lymphoblastic leukemia. For example, children with trisomy 21 have 15 times the risk of developing ALL as other children (Poplack, 1989). Translocation or inversion of chromosomes 7 and 14 have been observed in many children with ALL at diagnosis. Children whose bone marrow contains only genetically abnormal cells have much poorer prognoses and higher treatment complications than those whose marrow contains mixed or genetically normal cells (Lovejoy and Halliburton, 1989).

Cell-surface immunologic markers. A number of cell-surface antigens have permitted differentiation of ALL into three broad classes: T-lymphocytes (T-cells), B-lymphocytes (B-cells), and "null" cells, those cells that lack T- or B-cell characteristics. Within the null cell category are those that react with an antigen called the common acute lymphoblastic leukemia antigen (CALLA). This further classification of lymphocytic leukemia appears to have prognostic importance in that persons with leukemias of the "null" category (about 85% of ALL), especially those who are CALLA-positive, demonstrate better survival rates (Steinherz, 1987). At present, cell-surface markers for ANLL are still rudimentary, although there is current research with monoclonal antibodies that may provide significant information about the nonlymphoid cells.

Pathologic and Related Clinical Manifestations

Leukemia is an unrestricted proliferation of immature white blood cells in the blood-forming tissues of the body. Al-

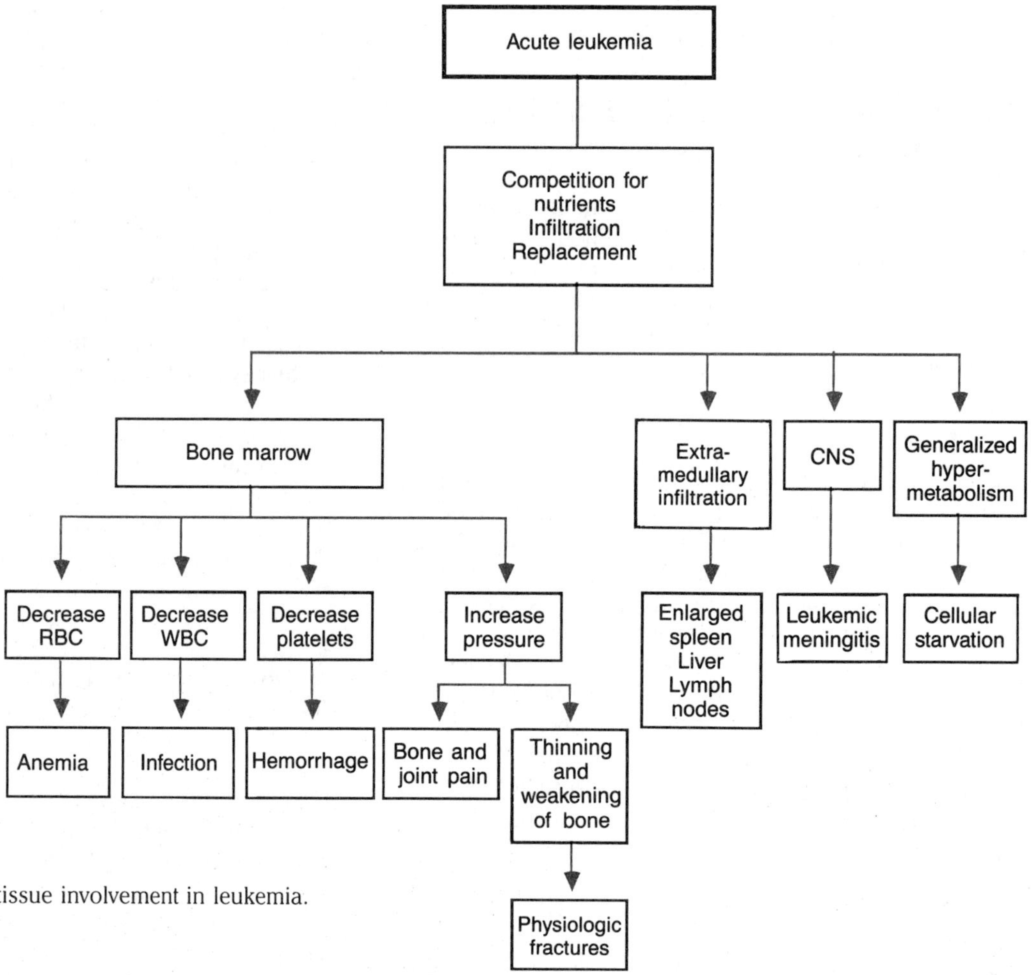

Fig. 36-1. Principal sites of tissue involvement in leukemia.

though not a "tumor" as such, the leukemic cells demonstrate the neoplastic properties of solid cancers. Therefore the resultant pathology and clinical manifestations of the disease are caused by infiltration and replacement of any tissue of the body with nonfunctional leukemic cells. Highly vascular organs, such as the spleen and liver, are most severely affected.

In order to understand the pathophysiology of the leukemic process, it is important to clarify two common misconceptions. First, although leukemia is an overproduction of white blood cells, most often in the acute form the leukocyte count is low. Instead, the peripheral blood smear and, more definitively, the bone marrow examination reveal greatly elevated counts of immature cells or "blasts." Second, these immature cells do not deliberately attack and destroy the normal blood cells or vascular tissues. Cellular destruction is by the process of infiltration and subsequent competition for metabolic elements. The following discussion elaborates on the pathologic process and related clinical manifestations in the most susceptible organs of the body (Fig. 36-1).

Bone marrow dysfunction. In all types of leukemia the proliferating cells depress bone marrow production of the formed elements of the blood by competing for and depriving the normal cells of the essential nutrients for metabolism. The three main consequences are (1) *anemia* from decreased erythrocytes, (2) *infection* from neutropenia, and (3) *bleeding tendencies* from decreased platelet production.

The invasion of the bone marrow with leukemic cells gradually causes a weakening of the bone and a tendency toward fractures. As leukemic cells invade the periosteum, increasing pressure causes severe pain.

The most frequent presenting signs and symptoms of leukemia are a result of infiltration of the bone marrow. These include fever, pallor, fatigue, anorexia, hemorrhage (usually petechiae), and bone and joint pain. In the presence of neutropenia the body's normal bacterial flora can become aggressive pathogens. Any break in the skin is a potential site of infection. Frequently, vague abdominal pain is caused by areas of inflammation from normal flora within the intestinal tract.

Disturbance of involved organs. The spleen, liver, and lymph glands demonstrate marked infiltration, enlargement, and eventually fibrosis. Hepatosplenomegaly is typically more common than lymphadenopathy.

The next most important site of involvement is the central nervous system. Initially, leukemic cells do not tend to invade this area, probably as a result of the protective blood-brain barrier. However, this normal protective mechanism also prevents the antileukemic drugs, with the exception of a few agents, from entering the brain in sufficient therapeutic doses to be effective. Before prophylactic use of cranial irradiation and intrathecal methotrexate, central nervous system involvement was frequent in children who survived 6 months or more. However, newer modes of therapy have significantly changed the course of the disease, although central nervous system complications still occur, even during bone marrow remission.

The usual effect of leukemic infiltration of the meninges is increased intracranial pressure. The pathogenesis is presumably attributable to invasion of the arachnoid by proliferating cells, which then interfere with the flow of cerebrospinal fluid in the subarachnoid space and at the base of the brain. The increased fluid pressure causes dilation of all four ventricles and consequently the signs and symptoms normally associated with this condition, such as severe headache, vomiting, papilledema, irritability, lethargy, and eventually coma. Irritation of the meninges also causes pain and stiffness in the neck and back.

Additional sites of involvement may be the cranial nerves, most often cranial nerve VII, or the facial nerve, and spinal nerves, particularly of the lumbosacral plexus, hypothalamus, and cerebellum. Clinical manifestations for these sites are directly related to the area involved. For example, with lumbosacral invasion, there is weakness in the lower extremities, pain radiating down the legs to the feet, and difficulty in voiding. Although such signs may suggest a brain tumor, the absence of localized signs often leads to the discovery of central nervous system involvement in leukemia.

Other sites that may become invaded with leukemic cells include the kidneys, testes, prostate, ovaries, gastrointestinal tract, and lungs. With long-term survivors becoming increasingly common, such extramedullary sites of leukemic invasion, especially the testes, are becoming more important clinically.

Hypermetabolism. The immense metabolic needs of proliferating leukemic cells eventually deprive all body cells of nutrients necessary for survival. Muscle wasting, weight loss, anorexia, and fatigue are natural consequences. Obviously, in addition to the risk of death from infection and hemorrhage, uncontrolled growth of leukemic cells can terminate in metabolic starvation.

Onset

The precise onset of leukemia is unknown. Its clinical appearance varies markedly from acute to insidious. In most instances the child displays remarkably few symptoms. For example, it is quite typical for leukemia to be diagnosed when a minor infection, such as a cold, fails to completely disappear. The child continues to be pale, listless, irritable, febrile, and anorexic. Parents often suspect some underlying problem when they observe the weight loss, petechiae, bruising without cause, and continued complaints of bone and joint pain.

At other times leukemia is diagnosed after an extended history of signs and symptoms mimicking such conditions as rheumatoid arthritis or mononucleosis. There are also occasions when the diagnosis of leukemia accompanies some totally unrelated event, such as a routine physical examination or accidental injury.

The history not only yields valuable medical information regarding the subsequent course of the illness but also bears heavily on the parents' emotional reaction to the discovery of the diagnosis. In most instances the diagnosis is an unexpected revelation of catastrophic proportion.

Staging and Prognostic Factors

There is general agreement among researchers that the most important prognostic factors in determining long-term survival for children with ALL are the initial white blood count (WBC) and the patient's age at diagnosis, followed by the histologic type of the disease and sex, which favors females. These factors are identified by specific criteria found in Table 36-6.

No such staging exists with ANLL, and prognostic indicators are less clearly defined. Initial evidence suggests that high myeloblast count and age below 2 years are associated with a poorer prognosis (Preisler, 1987).

From the time of establishment of the diagnosis, the nurse has some idea of the expected course the child will follow. However, in some instances, because of the variety of cell types observed and the marked undifferentiation of immature cells, a definitive classification cannot be made or the diagnosis may be changed. The nurse should be aware of the importance of such events in counseling and supporting family members.

Diagnostic Evaluation

Leukemia is usually suspected from the history, physical manifestations, and a peripheral blood smear that contains immature forms of leukocytes, frequently combined with low blood counts. Definitive diagnosis is based on bone marrow aspiration or biopsy. Typically the bone marrow is hypercellular with primarily blast cells. Once the diagnosis is confirmed, a lumbar puncture is performed to determine if there is any central nervous system involvement, although

Table 36-6 Favorable prognostic factors for acute lymphoblastic leukemia

FACTOR	CRITERIA
Leukocyte count	$<50,000/mm^3$
Age	>2 and <10 years
Immunologic subtype	CALLA-positive
FAB morphology	L_1
Cytogenetics	Absence of ploidy (additional chromosome, e.g., trisomy 21) or translocation
Sex	Female
Serum immunoglobulin	Normal
Race	White
Leukemia cell burden	Minimal

Data from Poplack, D.G.: Acute lymphoblastic leukemia. In Prizzo, P.A., and Poplack, D.G.: Principles and practice of pediatric oncology, Philadelphia, 1989, J.B. Lippincott Co.

a very small number of children have central nervous system involvement and most are asymptomatic.

Therapeutic Management

Treatment of leukemia involves the use of chemotherapeutic agents with or without cranial irradiation in three phases: (1) *induction*, which achieves a complete remission or disappearance of leukemic cells; (2) *sanctuary therapy*, which prevents leukemic cells from invading or destroys leukemic cells in those areas of the body normally protected from cytotoxic drug levels; and (3) *maintenance*, which serves to maintain the remission phase. Although the combination of drugs and radiation may vary according to the institution, the prognostic or risk characteristics of the patient, and the type of leukemia being treated, the following general principles for each phase are consistently employed.

Remission induction. Almost immediately after confirmation of the diagnosis, induction therapy is begun and lasts for 4 to 6 weeks (van Eys and others, 1989). The principal drugs used for induction in ALL are the corticosteroids (especially prednisone), vincristine, and L-asparaginase, with or without doxorubicin (see Table 36-3). Oral steroids are administered daily in divided doses to maintain consistently high blood levels. Vincristine is given by intravenous infusion once a week for a total of four to six doses, and L-asparaginase or doxorubicin is given at various schedules. Some treatment regimens include a period of *consolidation* or *intensification therapy* with one or more of the usual remission drugs. A complete remission is determined by the absence of clinical signs or symptoms of the disease and the presence of less than 5% blast cells in the bone marrow (may be described as an M_1-type bone marrow).

With AML the drug therapies differ from those used for lymphoid leukemia. The principal drugs used for induction therapy in AML are doxorubicin or daunomycin and cytosine arabinoside; various other drugs may be added.

Since many of the drugs also cause myelosuppression of normal blood elements, the period immediately following a remission can be critical; the body is defenseless against invading organisms (especially normal bacterial flora) and highly susceptible to spontaneous hemorrhage. Consequently, supportive therapy during this time is essential.

Sanctuary therapy. Sanctuary therapy refers to treatment directed at those anatomic areas that are protected to some degree from systemic chemotherapy—the central nervous system (protected by the blood-brain barrier) and the testes (lie outside the body). The second phase involves prophylactic treatment of the central nervous system with cranial irradiation and/or intrathecal administration of methotrexate. Because of the concern regarding late effects of cranial irradiation, this mode of therapy is generally reserved for high-risk patients and/or those with central nervous system disease. Therapy is usually begun during the first 6 to 8 weeks after diagnosis and may consist of daily high-dose radiation treatments for about 2 weeks and weekly or twice weekly doses of methotrexate for a total of five to six injections. Another approach is intrathecal chemotherapy, such as a combination of methotrexate, cytosine arabinoside, and steroids, without irradiation.

A second site that is resistant to chemotherapy and is responsible for leukemic relapse is the testes. A minority of males experience relapse during maintenance therapy or have occult disease after cessation of therapy. Most authorities believe in routine bilateral testicular biopsies at the time of terminating treatment to identify occult disease, followed by aggressive treatment for affected males, including bilateral testicular irradiation, intensive systemic chemotherapy, and central nervous system reinforcement therapy (Steinherz, 1987).

Maintenance. Maintenance, or continuation, therapy is begun after completion of successful induction and sanctuary therapy to preserve the remission and further reduce the number of leukemic cells. It begins when blood values start to approach normal levels. As with induction therapy, combined-drug regimens have been more successful in maintaining remissions and preventing drug resistance. Although a variety of combinations are used, a frequent schedule includes daily doses of oral 6-mercaptopurine and weekly doses of oral methotrexate. Intermittent short-term intensified therapy with prednisone and vincristine may be included. Depending on the type of leukemia and the risk factors of the child, several other drugs may be added to the intensification protocol, including intravenous methotrexate and cytosine arabinoside.

During maintenance therapy, weekly or monthly complete blood counts are taken to evaluate the marrow's response to the drugs. If myelosuppression becomes severe (usually indicated by an absolute neutrophil count below $1000/mm^3$) or toxic side effects occur, therapy is temporarily stopped or the dose decreased.

Duration of therapy has been based on clinical experience comparing survival rates for various time intervals and is concerned with preventing deleterious effects of excessive treatment. While the optimum time for discontinuing therapy is not known, current research indicates that girls do not need therapy for longer than 1.5 years. Because of the risk of testicular relapse in boys, some centers favor longer maintenance programs, but in general the additional maintenance therapy appears to delay, not prevent, relapses (Gale, 1989). All children after cessation of therapy require regular medical evaluation for surveillance of relapse and long-term sequelae of treatment. Most relapses (16%) occur during the first year off therapy, about 2% to 3% of the relapses occur during each of the next 3 years, and very few relapses occur after 6 years (Poplack, 1989).

Reinduction. For many children additional therapy becomes necessary when a relapse occurs, as evidenced by the presence of leukemic cells within the bone marrow. Usually reinduction for ALL includes the use of prednisone and vincristine with a combination of other drugs not previously used. Sanctuary and maintenance therapy follow as already outlined if a remission is induced. Although remissions may be achieved after more than one relapse, each relapse heralds an increasingly poor prognosis. However, more long-term second and subsequent remissions are occurring, and these may have better outlooks than previously thought (Musgrave, Dickerman, and Land, 1986).

Bone marrow transplantation. Bone marrow transplants have been used successfully in treating some children with ALL and ANLL. In general, bone marrow transplantation is not recommended for children with acute lymphocytic leukemia (ALL) during the first remission because of the excellent results possible with chemotherapy. The group with the best results have been those with ALL who receive the graft during the second remission (Poplack, 1989). Because of the poorer prognosis in children with acute nonlymphocytic leukemia (ANLL), transplantation may be considered during the first remission when a suitable donor is available (Vega and others, 1987).

Prognosis after transplantation varies with the timing of the procedure and the type of leukemia; reported ranges for long-term survival are between 25% and 50% (Vega and others, 1987). However, many of the transplanted children faced almost certain death without transplantation, so that even these low figures represent a major advance in eliciting a cure.

Nursing Considerations

Nursing care of the child with leukemia is directly related to the regimen of therapy. Secondary complications that necessitate supportive physical care are caused by myelosuppression, drug toxicity, and leukemic infiltration. This discussion focuses on supportive interventions for the child with leukemia and the family. General aspects of care appropriate for the child with leukemia have been discussed under Nursing Care of the Child with Cancer. (See also Nursing Care Plan: The Child with Leukemia.*) Psychologic interventions appropriate for children with leukemia during significant phases of therapy are discussed in Chapter 23.

Prepare the family for diagnostic/therapeutic procedures. From the time before diagnosis to cessation of therapy, children must undergo several tests, the most traumatic of which are bone marrow aspiration or biopsy and lumbar punctures. Multiple finger sticks and venipunctures for blood analysis and drug infusion are common occurrences for several years after the diagnosis. Therefore the child needs an explanation of why each procedure is done and what can be expected (see also Preparation for Procedures, Chapter 27).

Depending on the age of the child, one way of beginning such preparation is to explain the basic elements of the blood.† Using a drawing or letting the child look at a drop of blood under a microscope not only teaches but also encourages trust between the nurse and child. It also allows the nurse to assess the child's level of understanding. An error many health professionals make is to overestimate children's knowledge about their bodies. For example, a bone marrow aspiration makes sense only when it is clarified that the center of a bone is hollow and contains the cells that later become "working" blood cells or leukemic cells.

Provide continued emotional support. Nursing care of the child with leukemia is based on typical problems with which the family is confronted during the treatment phases. It is not unusual for a child who discontinues therapy after 2 or 3 years and maintains a permanent remission to experience many of these side effects. Therefore the nurse's role is continually one of support, guidance, clarification, and judgment. Parents need to know how to recognize symptoms that demand medical attention. Although some of the reactions discussed are expected, parents still should report them to their practitioner. Warning parents of their possible occurrence beforehand also allows parents the opportunity to prepare for them. At the same time it reassures them that these reactions are not caused by a return of leukemic cells.

The nurse must also use judgment in recognizing which side effects are normal reactions and which indicate toxicity. Frequently it is the office or clinic nurse who screens such telephone calls and gives advice when appropriate. Usually nausea and vomiting are not indications for drug cessation. However, severe vomiting may require immediate intervention to prevent dehydration. Signs of infection, mucosal ulceration, hemorrhagic cystitis, peripheral neuropathy, and obstipation require medical evaluation.

Another aspect of continued emotional support involves prognosis. Certainly, leukemia can no longer be defined as invariably fatal. However, present statistics must also be correctly interpreted; while more than 95% of children with ALL will achieve an initial remission and as many as 60% of them will live 5 years or longer, it must be remembered that these are *average* estimates and apply to those children treated with the latest protocols since diagnosis (Poplack, 1989). For the low-risk child the chances may be better, but for the high-risk child they may be significantly poorer. Of those who do survive after discontinuing therapy, a portion will relapse. At present only the passage of time is positive confirmation of the child who is "cured" of the disease.

The nurse must be familiar with these statistics in order to interpret them correctly to parents. At the same time the nurse must realize that a realistic understanding of the chances for survival requires an adjustment period. For example, it is not unusual for parents to interpret the "95% remission" as the probability for a cure. When a relapse occurs, parents may for the first time be able to "hear" the correct facts.

Statistics are numbers. Sometimes they bring hope and at other times despair. Although very important in terms of research, better treatment, and identification of high- or low-risk populations, they present a general picture of what to expect. The nurse who is working with family members must individualize the "numbers" to relate to the people. An understanding of each member's emotional needs, as well as competent care of physical ones, is essential to the positive, growth-promoting support of the family. Comprehensive emotional support for the family through all phases of the illness is discussed in Chapter 23.

---

*In Wong, D.L., and Whaley, L.F.: Clinical manual of pediatric nursing, ed. 3, St. Louis, 1990, Mosby–Year Book, Inc.

†Especially recommended is the book by Baker, L.: You and leukemia: a day at a time, Philadelphia, 1988, W.B. Saunders Co.

LYMPHOMAS

The lymphomas are a group of neoplastic diseases that arise from the lymphoid and hemopoietic systems. They are usually divided into Hodgkin disease and non-Hodgkin lymphoma (NHL) and subdivided according to tissue type and extent of disease (staging). In children non-Hodgkin lymphoma, which has been called lymphosarcoma, reticulum cell sarcoma, and giant follicular lymphoma, is more common than Hodgkin disease. Although Hodgkin disease is extremely rare before 5 years of age, there is a striking increase in children 15 to 19 years, when it occurs with almost the same frequency as leukemia.

HODGKIN DISEASE

Hodgkin disease affects about 5 per million children, mostly adolescents. The malignancy originates in the lymphoid system and primarily involves the lymph nodes. It predictably metastasizes to nonnodal or extralymphatic sites, especially the spleen, liver, bone marrow, lungs, and mediastinum (mass of tissues and organs separating the lungs; includes heart and its vessels, trachea, esophagus, thymus, and lymph nodes), although no tissue is exempt from involvement (Fig. 36-2). It is classified according to four histologic types: (1) lymphocytic predominance, (2) nodular sclerosis, (3) mixed cellularity, and (4) lymphocytic depletion. With present treatment protocols, the histologic stage of the disease has less prognostic significance than previously, although children with the lymphocyte-depleted histology are likely to do poorly (Sullivan, 1987).

Clinical Staging and Prognosis

Accurate staging of the extent of disease is the basis for treatment protocols and expected prognoses (Box 36-5).

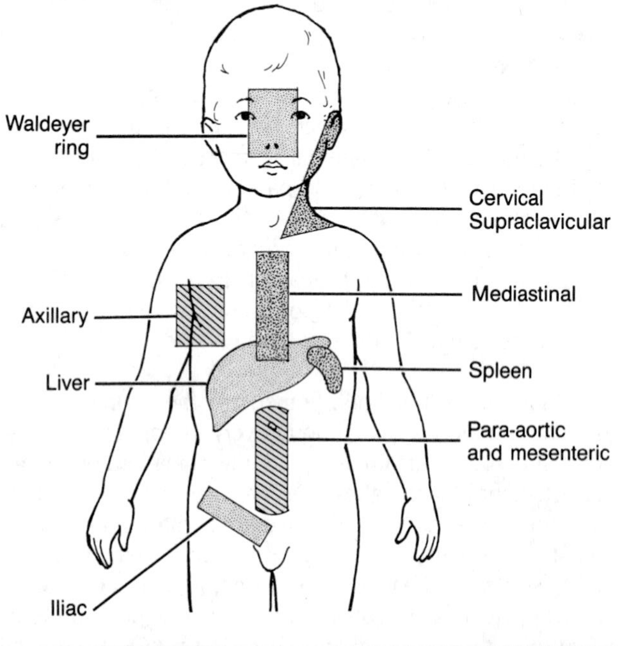

Fig. 36-2. Main areas of lymphadenopathy and organ involvement in Hodgkin disease.

Box 36-5 STAGES OF HODGKIN DISEASE

Stage I: Lesions are limited to one lymph node area or only one additional extralymphatic site (IE), such as the liver, lungs, kidney, or intestines.
Stage II: Two or more lymph node regions on the same side of the diaphragm or one additional extralymphatic site or organ (IIE) on the same side of the diaphragm is involved.
Stage III: Lymph node regions on both sides of the diaphragm are involved, or one extralymphatic site (IIIE), spleen (IIIS), or both (IIISE).
Stage IV: Cancer has metastasized diffusely throughout the body to one or more extralymphatic sites with or without involvement of associated lymph nodes.

Each stage is further subdivided into A or B. *A* denotes absence of associated general symptoms. *B* indicates presence of symptoms such as night sweats, fever, or weight loss of 10% or more during the preceding 6 months. In stages II and III, subtype B has a significantly poorer prognosis than subtype A.

Prognosis for patients with Hodgkin disease has improved dramatically in the past few years, largely as a result of the systematic staging procedure and improved treatment protocols. The prognosis is excellent in children with localized disease. Even in those with disseminated disease, long-term remissions are possible in more than half of the patients. For example, in one study 81% of children in stage I, 76% in stage II, 74% in stage III, and 69% in stage IV were without evidence of disease 5 years after diagnosis (Sullivan, 1987). Unfortunately, a number of children may have late recurrences of the original disease or develop a second malignancy, especially osteosarcoma, soft tissue sarcoma, thyroid carcinoma, or leukemia.

Clinical Manifestations

Hodgkin disease is characterized by painless enlargement of lymph nodes. The most common finding is enlarged, firm, nontender, movable nodes in the supraclavicular area. In children the "sentinel" node located near the left clavicle may be the first enlarged node. Enlargement of axillary and inguinal lymph nodes is less frequent (see Fig. 36-2).

Other signs and symptoms depend on the extent and location of involvement. Mediastinal lymphadenopathy may cause a persistent nonproductive cough. Enlarged retroperitoneal nodes may produce unexplained abdominal pain. Systemic symptoms include low-grade and/or intermittent fever (Pel-Ebstein disease), anorexia, nausea, weight loss, night sweats, or pruritus. Generally such symptoms indicate advanced lymph node and extralymphatic involvement.

Diagnostic Evaluation

The history and physical examination often yield important clues to the disease, such as fevers, night sweats, or weight loss, and enlarged lymph nodes, spleen, or liver. Because of the multiple organs that can become involved, diagnosis consists of several tests to confirm the presence of Hodgkin disease and to assess the extent of involvement for accurate staging. Tests include complete blood count, uric acid levels, liver function tests, urinalysis, and erythrocyte sedimentation rate. Computed tomography (CT) of the chest, liver, spleen, and bone is done to detect metastasis.

With the advent of CT, a special procedure, lymphangiography, may not be needed, although elimination is controversial. A lymphangiogram involves the intradermal injection of a contrast material (usually alphazurine) in the first interdigital space of each foot for visualization of the lymphatic vessels to determine the presence of disease in various lymph node regions. One or more vessels are then chosen for catheterization, and a radiopaque medium, usually ethiodized oil (Ethiodol), is injected under pressure to visualize the entire lymphatic chain in the lower extremities, groin, iliopelvic and abdominal-aortic regions, and the thoracic duct. If the axillary, periclavicular, and supraclavicular lymph nodes must be examined, the same procedure is performed in the hands.

Biopsy is essential to diagnosis and staging. The enlarged lymph node is excised and analyzed for histologic type and evidence of the *Sternberg-Reed cell,* a giant cell with a dark-staining nucleolus. Although the cell is considered diagnostic of Hodgkin disease because it is absent in the other lymphomas, it may occur in infectious mononucleosis. A bone marrow aspiration or biopsy is also usually performed. A laparotomy is recommended for definitive pathologic staging and the spleen is removed, although it remains a controversial practice because of the risk of overwhelming infections from asplenia. During this procedure the entire abdomen is examined for evidence of disease; samples of the liver are taken for microscopic study. Biopsies of any involved lymph nodes and the spleen are performed. During surgery, metal clips are placed to outline margins of involved sites for irradiation and to monitor any disease progression. The ovaries may be moved out of the radiation field (oophoropexy) to protect them from irradiation damage.

Therapeutic Management

The primary modalities of therapy are radiation and chemotherapy. Each may be used alone or in combination. The decision is based on the clinical staging. The goal of treatment is obviously a cure; however, aggressive therapy increases the chances of complications in the disease-free state and can seriously compromise the quality of life. Consequently, numerous research studies are presently investigating treatment options to minimize long-term sequelae. Based on the diversity of approaches to treatment, the following is an overview of general principles that may or may not apply to all children. One of the major concerns with combined radiation and antineoplastic drug therapy is the serious late effects in children with an excellent prognosis.

Children with favorable stage I disease may receive only involved field (IF) radiation. Those with stage II or III disease are candidates for extended field (EF) radiation (involved areas plus adjacent nodes) or total nodal irradiation (TNI) (the entire axial lymph node system). Chemotherapy is usually combined with radiation. In stage IV, chemotherapy is the primary form of treatment, although limited radiation may be given to areas of bulky disease. The most widely used drug regimen is MOPP (mechlorethamine [Mustargen], vincristine [Oncovin], prednisone, and procarbazine). Several other drug combinations may be used, such as adriamycin, bleomycin, vinblastine, and decarbazine (ABVD).

Follow-up care of children taken off therapy is essential to identify relapse, as well as second malignancies (Tucker and others, 1988). In children with asplenia, prophylactic antibiotics are administered for an indefinite period, and immunizations against pneumococci and meningococci are recommended (see Chapter 12).

Nursing Considerations

Nursing care involves the same objectives as for patients with other types of cancer, namely, (1) preparation for diagnostic and operative procedures, (2) explanation of treatment side effects, and (3) family support (see Chapters 22 and 23). The specific care plan is based on the clinical stage of the disease. Since this is most often a disease of adolescents and young adults, the nurse must have an appreciation of their psychologic needs and reactions during the diagnostic and treatment phases.

Prepare the family for diagnostic/operative procedures. Once the child is hospitalized for suspected Hodgkin disease, a battery of diagnostic tests is ordered. The family needs an explanation of why each test is performed, since many of them, such as bone marrow aspiration (see Chapter 27), are not routine. If lymphangiography is performed, the child needs to be prepared for the test, and particularly told that the length of the procedure is anywhere from 2 to 10 hours and frequently averages 4 to 5 hours. Although the feet are anesthetized, the initial injections are painful. Immobilization of the feet during lymphatic vessel catheterization may be uncomfortable and tiresome, especially since the child must remain still for long periods. Whenever possible the child is encouraged to sleep or diversions should be provided, such as listening to music, reading, or talking. Ideally a family member should be allowed to accompany the child. Fluids and food are not necessarily restricted. If allowed, provisions are made for the child to have a favorite drink or snack.

The procedure is not without complications, the most serious of which is pulmonary embolism from the oil-based dye ethiodized oil (Ethiodol). Fine pulmonary emboli produce symptoms of slight fever, chills, pleuritic pain, mild dyspnea, and a dry cough. Acetaminophen is helpful to reduce the fever and relieve the pain. The symptoms usually subside within 24 to 48 hours.

Severe oil embolism may occur if the contrast medium has been infused too rapidly. Signs of this complication include cyanosis, distended neck veins, hypotension, liver tenderness, and edema in the lower extremities from increased venous resistance. Emergency medical treatment usually involves supplemental oxygen and antihypotensive drugs. The child may become very apprehensive and need considerable reassurance. Usually sedation is avoided, because it may depress the respiratory center.

Expected reactions to the contrast medium include abnormal taste sensations, retrosternal burning, headache, sleeplessness, diarrhea, and elevated temperature. The alphazurine turns the urine and skin of the feet and/or hands bluish green. Although the urine clears rapidly, the discoloration of skin may last for months. Adolescents may be very self-conscious about the staining, especially in the hands.

Since a cutdown procedure is done for vessel catheterization, a pressure bandage may be in place. The area(s) is observed for signs of bleeding and subsequent infection. Sutures are usually removed in 7 to 10 days. Ordinarily the child has no restrictions on activity after the test. However, the child is cautioned to keep the wound clean and to avoid excessive irritation from shoes.

Preparation for a laparotomy is similar to that for any other surgery. One special area of concern for families is the effects of the splenectomy on bodily functions. Although not a vital organ, the spleen does have an important role in resisting infection, particularly in young children. The family needs to be aware of the benefits of the procedure in terms of staging and potential risks. Compliance is a major issue with indefinite administration of antibiotics, and every effort should be made to employ strategies that enhance compliance (see Chapter 27).

Explain treatments and side effects. Explanations of chemotherapeutic reactions vary with the specific drug regimen. Drugs commonly used are outlined in Table 36-3, and the most common side effects, such as nausea and vomiting, body image changes, neuropathy, and mucosal ulceration, are discussed under Nursing Care of the Child with Cancer.

Involved field radiation results in few side effects, sometimes consisting only of a mild skin reaction. With extended field radiation to the chest and abdomen, nausea and vomiting, weight loss, and mucosal ulceration (esophagitis, gastric ulcers) are common. The usual measures for providing relief have been discussed on p. 1681 and are outlined in Table 36-4.

The most common side effect of extensive radiation is malaise, which may result from damage to the thyroid gland, causing hypothyroidism. Lack of energy is particularly difficult for adolescents, because it prevents them from keeping up with their peers. Sometimes adolescents will push themselves to the point of physical exhaustion rather than admit fatigue and succumb to the decreased activity tolerance. Parents are advised to observe for such behavior, such as extreme fatigue at the end of the day, falling asleep at the dinner table, inability to concentrate on homework, or an increased susceptibility to infection. Regular bedtimes and periodic rest times are important for these children, especially during chemotherapy when myelosuppression increases the risk of infection and debilitation. Before discharge the nurse should discuss a feasible school schedule with the parents and child. If alterations are necessary, such as elimination of strenuous physical education, they are discussed with the teacher, nurse, and principal. Follow-up care is essential to diagnose hypothyroidism early and institute thyroid replacement.

An area of concern for adolescents is the high risk of sterility from irradiation and chemotherapy. Both irradiation to the gonads and drugs, particularly procarbazine and alkylating agents, may lead to infertility. Younger patients with a greater complement of oocytes are more likely to retain ovarian function (Waskerwitz and Fergusson, 1986).

Although sexual function is not altered, the appearance of secondary sexual characteristics and menstruation may be delayed in the pubescent child. Adolescents should be informed of these side effects early in the course of the diagnosis and treatment. Delayed sexual maturation may be an extremely sensitive and painful area for children (see Chapter 20). It is important for the nurse to respect their concern and refrain from casually placating them with expressions such as, "You'll catch up someday."

NON-HODGKIN LYMPHOMA

Non-Hodgkin lymphoma (NHL) occurs in between 7 and 8 children per million under age 15 and has about one and one-half times the incidence of Hodgkin disease. Histologic classification of childhood NHL is strikingly different from that of Hodgkin disease and adult NHL in several respects (Magrath, 1987):

- The disease is usually diffuse rather than nodular.
- The cell type is either undifferentiated or poorly differentiated.
- Dissemination occurs earlier, more often, and more rapidly.
- Mediastinal involvement and invasion of meninges typically occur.

Staging and Prognosis

NHL is heterogeneous, exhibiting a variety of morphologic, cytochemical, and immunologic features, not unlike the diversity seen in leukemia. Classification is based on the pattern of histologic presentation, namely, nodular (circumscribed) or diffuse (spread out). Immunologically these cells are also classified as T-cells, B-cells (an example of which is Burkitt lymphoma), or null cells, which lack specific immunologic properties.

The clinical staging system used in Hodgkin disease is of little value in NHL, although that system has been modified for NHL and other systems have been developed. Favorable prognosis is defined by (1) lymph node involvement only and limited to one or two adjacent lymphatic regions (excluding the mediastinum); (2) an extranodal site in the nasopharynx, oropharynx, or other isolated extranodal site, with or without regional lymphadenopathy; or (3) gastrointestinal involvement, with or without regional lymphadenopathy, limited to the mesentery (Magrath, 1989). The most commonly used staging system is presented in Box 36-6. The use of aggressive combination chemotherapy has had a major impact on the survival rates of children with NHL. The most effective treatment regimens result in cure in almost all children with limited disease involvement;

Box 36-6 STAGING SYSTEM FOR NON-HODGKIN LYMPHOMA

Stage I: Single tumor at a single site
Stage II: Single tumor with regional involvement on same side of abdomen
Stage III: Tumor on both sides of abdomen; also, all primary thoracic, intraabdominal, and paraspinal or epidural tumors
Stage IV: Any of the involvement in stages I and II, with central nervous system and/or bone marrow involvement

50% to 75% of children with extensive disease are cured (Magrath, 1987).

Clinical Manifestations

Clinical manifestations depend on the anatomic site and extent of involvement. Many of those seen in Hodgkin disease may be present in NHL, although rarely does a single symptom give rise to the diagnosis. Rather, metastasis to the bone marrow or central nervous system may produce signs and symptoms typical of leukemia. Lymphoid tumors compressing various organs may cause intestinal or airway obstruction, cranial nerve palsies, or spinal paralysis.

The exception to the usual presentation of NHL is Burkitt lymphoma, a type of cancer that is rare in the United States but endemic in parts of Africa. It is a rapidly growing neoplasm that is most commonly seen as a mass in the jaw, abdomen, or orbit. However, no anatomic site appears exempt from involvement. Peripheral lymphadenopathy, hepatosplenomegaly, or signs of conversion to leukemia are rarely seen.

Diagnostic Evaluation

Since widespread disease exists in most children with NHL at presentation, thorough pathologic staging is unnecessary. Current recommendations for staging include a surgical biopsy for histopathologic confirmation of disease with cytochemical and immunologic evaluation; bone marrow aspiration; radiologic studies, especially CT scans of the lungs and gastrointestinal organs; and lumbar puncture.

Therapeutic Management

The present treatment protocols for NHL include an aggressive approach using irradiation and chemotherapy. Similar to leukemic therapy, the protocols include induction, consolidation, and maintenance phases, some with intrathecal methotrexate and/or cranial irradiation. At present the differentiation between lymphoblastic lymphoma and all other lymphomas is widely used as a way to categorize patients for specific treatment regimens (Magrath, 1989). Children with lymphoblastic lymphoma are treated wth several drug protocols, most containing several chemotherapeutic agents. One of the most commonly used regimens, known as the LSA_2-L_2 protocol, includes cyclophosphamide, vincristine, intrathecal methotrexate, prednisone, daunomycin, 6-thioguanine, cytosine arabinoside, BCNU, and L-asparaginase with or without radiotherapy.

Children with nonlymphoblastic lymphoma are treated with cyclic drug combinations, including cyclophosphamide and intermediate-dose or high-dose methotrexate (Magrath, 1989). Most protocols also include an anthracycline. These children receive central nervous system prophylaxis with cranial radiation and combination intrathecal chemotherapy (Meadows and others, 1989). These multiagent regimens are administered for 6 to 24 months.

Nursing Considerations

Nursing care of the child with NHL is very similar to the care discussed in the section, Nursing Care of the Child with Cancer. Because of the intensive chemotherapy protocol, nursing care is primarily directed toward managing the side effects of these agents.

NERVOUS SYSTEM TUMORS

Two major forms of childhood cancer are derived from neural tissue. Brain tumors are the most common solid tumors that occur in children and are second only to leukemia as a form of cancer. Neuroblastomas are the most common malignant tumors of infancy and are second only to brain tumors as the type of solid malignancy seen during the first 10 years (Cohn, 1988). Both of these tumors have presented difficulties in identifying successful modes of treatment and have not demonstrated the dramatic improvements in survival seen in many other forms of cancer.

BRAIN TUMORS

Tumors of the central nervous system account for about 20% of all childhood cancers and have an annual incidence of 2.4 per 100,000 children under 15 years. The majority of tumors (about 60%) are *infratentorial* (below the tentorium cerebelli), which means that they occur in the posterior third of the brain, primarily in the cerebellum or brainstem. This anatomic distribution accounts for the frequency of symptoms resulting from increased intracranial pressure. A smaller number are *supratentorial,* or within the anterior two thirds of the brain, mainly the cerebrum. Box 36-7 lists major brain tumors of childhood.

Because the neoplasms can arise from any cell within the cranium, it is possible to have tumors originating from the nerve cells, neuroepithelium, glia, cranial nerves, blood vessels, pineal gland, and hypophysis. Within each of these structures, specific cells may be involved to provide a histologic classification of the major tumors found in children.

Clinical Manifestations

The signs and symptoms of brain tumors are directly related to their anatomic location and size and to some extent the age of the child. In infants, whose sutures are still open, virtually no early detectable symptoms develop. It is not until spinal fluid obstruction causes markedly increased head

Box 36-7 MAJOR BRAIN TUMORS OF CHILDHOOD

Medulloblastoma
Most common tumor (20% of brain tumors)
Fast growing, highly malignant
Characteristic presenting signs include headache, vomiting, ataxia
Improved survival rates with irradiation and excision of most or all of tumor
Overall survival rate is approximately 77%

Cerebellar Astrocytoma
Accounts for about 17% of brain tumors
Benign, cystic, and slow growing
Characteristic presenting signs include clumsiness (usually one hand), awkward gait (stumbling to one side), headache, vomiting
Surgical excision associated with high rate of cure (94%) in well-differentiated-type tumors but low rate (38%) in diffuse type

Brainstem Glioma
Accounts for about 10% to 15% of brain tumors
Often grows to a very large size before causing symptoms
Characteristic presenting signs include diplopia, facial weakness, and difficulty walking (headache and vomiting are uncommon)
Surgical excision is very difficult because of tumor location in vital brain centers; removal is attempted whenever possible
Palliative therapy with irradiation shrinks tumor to prolong survival
Overall 5-year survival rate is 20% to 30%

Ependymoma
Accounts for about 9% of brain tumors
Demonstrates varying rates of growth
Most invade ventricles, obstructing flow of cerebrospinal fluid
Characteristic presenting signs include headache, vomiting, and ataxia
Goal of surgery is gross total resection
Role of radiotherapy and chemotherapy is controversial
Overall 5-year survival rate is 25%

Data from Walker, R., and Allen, J.: Pediatric brain tumors, Pediatr. Ann. 12(5):383-391, 1983.

size that a lesion may be suspected. Head circumference allows for detection of increased intracranial pressure. Because the tumor typically grows to a large size before being diagnosed, prognosis in infants is generally poorer than in older children.

Even in older children, clinical manifestations are nonspecific. However, the most common symptoms are headache, especially on awakening, and vomiting that is not related to feeding and is attributable to increased intracranial pressure. The common presenting symptoms of brain tumors are presented in Table 36-7.

Diagnostic Evaluation

Diagnosis of a brain tumor is based subjectively on presenting clinical signs and objectively on neurologic tests. Because the signs and symptoms are vague and easily overlooked, early diagnosis necessitates a high index of suspicion during history taking. A number of tests may be employed in the neurologic evaluation (see Table 37-4), but the most common diagnostic procedure is computed tomography (CT). It permits direct visualization of the brain parenchyma, ventricles, and surrounding subarachnoid space. By the intravenous injection of radiographic contrast agents, intracranial blood vasculature can be demonstrated (Finlay and others, 1987).

When a positive CT scan is obtained, angiography may be done to provide information about the tumor's blood supply and degree of vascularity, which may assist the surgeon in planning the operative approach. Other tests (e.g., electroencephalography or lumbar puncture) may be performed, although the latter is dangerous in the presence of increased intracranial pressure.

Magnetic resonance imaging (MRI) permits early diagnosis of brain tumors, as well as assessment of tumor growth during or following treatment. The advantages of MRI include superior resolution in parts of the central nervous system surrounded by bone, easy manipulation of the image plane, and avoidance of radiation exposure (Kadota and others, 1989).

Definitive diagnosis is based on tissue specimens obtained during surgery. Occasionally special techniques are required for determining the cell type. This period of waiting is one of anxiety for the family, who are aware of its relevance to prognosis.

Therapeutic Management

Treatment may involve the use of surgery, radiotherapy, and chemotherapy. All three may or may not be used, depending on the type of tumor. The treatment of choice is total removal of the tumor without residual neurologic damage. Patients with the most complete tumor removal have the greatest chance of survival. Several surgical advances have allowed the biopsy and removal of tumors in areas previously considered too dangerous for traditional operative techniques. *Stereotactic surgery* involves the use of CT and MRI in conjunction with other special computer techniques to reconstruct the tumor in three dimensions. With computer-assisted instruments, removal is sometimes possible. Other procedures include the use of *lasers* to vaporize tumor tissue and *brain mapping* to determine the precise location of critical brain areas that are avoided during surgery.

Radiotherapy is used to treat most tumors and to shrink the size of the tumor before attempting surgical removal. The use of chemotherapy is controversial and has not demonstrated significant improvement in survival. The drugs most commonly used are nitrosoureas (CCNU), vincristine, methotrexate, and cisplatin (Heideman and others, 1989). In addition, other drugs, such as corticosteroids, may be needed to manage complications, such as brain edema.

The problems of treatment and relatively poor prognosis are compounded by the serious late effects of all three modes of therapy. Surgery may cause injury to important areas of brain, especially when attempting to remove invasive tumors. Radiation has serious long-term consequences, including radiation somnolence syndrome (see p. 1682), brain

Table 36-7 Clinical manifestations and assessment of brain tumors

SIGNS AND SYMPTOMS	ASSESSMENT
▪ Headache	
Recurrent and progressive In frontal or occipital areas Worse on arising, less during day Intensified by lowering head and straining, such as during bowel movement, coughing, sneezing	Record location, severity, and duration Use pain rating scale to assess severity of pain (see Chapter 26) Note changes in relation to time of day and activity Observe changes in behavior in infants (persistent irritability, crying, head rolling)
▪ Vomiting	
With or without nausea or feeding Progressively more projectile More severe in morning Relieved by moving about and changing position	Record time, amount, and relationship to feeding, nausea, and activity
▪ Neuromuscular changes	
Incoordination or clumsiness Loss of balance (use of wide-based stance, falling, tripping, banging into objects) Poor fine motor control Weakness Hyporeflexia or hyperreflexia Positive Babinski sign Spasticity Paralysis	Test muscle strength, gait, coordination, and reflexes (see Chapter 7)
▪ Behavioral changes	
Irritability Decreased appetite Failure to thrive Fatigue (frequent naps) Lethargy Coma	Observe behavior regularly Compare observations with parental reports of normal behavioral patterns Monitor growth and food intake Monitor activity and sleep
▪ Cranial nerve neuropathy	
Cranial nerve involvement varies according to tumor location Most common signs Head tilt Visual defects (nystagmus, diplopia, strabismus, episodic "graying out" of vision, visual field defects)	Assess cranial nerves, especially VII (facial), IX (glossopharyngeal), X (vagus), V (trigeminal, sensory roots), and VI (abducens) (see Chapter 7) Assess visual acuity, binocularity, and peripheral vision (see Chapter 7)
▪ Vital sign disturbances	
Decreased pulse and respiration Increased blood pressure Decreased pulse pressure Hypothermia or hyperthermia	Measure vital signs frequently Monitor pulse and respirations for 1 full minute Record pulse pressure (difference between systolic and diastolic blood pressure)
▪ Other signs	
Seizures Cranial enlargement* Tense, bulging fontanel at rest* Nuchal ridigity Papilledema (edema of optic nerve)	Record seizure activity (see Chapter 37) Measure head circumference daily (infant and young child) Perform funduscopic examination if skilled in procedure

*Present only in infants and young children.

necrosis, endocrine dysfunction, and behavioral/intellectual deficits. Chemotherapy is also not without harmful effects (see Table 36-5).

Nursing Considerations

Nursing care of the child with a brain tumor involves (1) assessing for signs and symptoms related to the tumor, (2) preparing the child and parents for the diagnostic tests and operative procedure, (3) preventing postoperative complications, (4) planning for discharge, and (5) promoting a return to optimum functioning. The principles of care are similar regardless of the type of intracranial lesion. Since a brain tumor is a potentially fatal diagnosis, the reader is urged to incorporate the psychologic interventions discussed in Chapter 23 with those elaborated in this section.

Assess for signs and symptoms. A child admitted to the hospital with neurologic dysfunction is often suspected of having a brain tumor, although the actual diagnosis is as yet unconfirmed. Establishing a baseline of data on which to compare preoperative and postoperative changes is an essential step toward planning physical care and preventing complications. It also allows the nurse to assess the degree of physical incapacity and the family's emotional reaction to the diagnosis. For example, children with cerebellar astrocytoma may have displayed vague cerebellar symptoms for several years before a tumor is suspected. For these parents the revelation of a neoplasm may be more of a shock than for those who have witnessed a rapid deterioration in their child's abilities. Common presenting signs and assessment procedures to document significant changes in the child's condition are summarized in Table 36-7.

Prepare the family for diagnostic/operative procedures. The suspected diagnosis of a brain tumor is always a crisis event. Despite the fact that some tumors are removed with excellent results, the physician can rarely give definitive answers regarding prognosis until after surgery. Therefore parents and older children require much emotional support to face the diagnostic procedures and a craniotomy.

How the child is prepared for the dignostic tests depends on age and previous experience. Since most of the tests involve x-ray equipment, the child may be familiar with the procedure. Preparing children for a CT scan is discussed in Chapter 37. Once surgery is scheduled, the child needs an explanation of what to expect. By the time most children are late preschoolers, they know that the head and brain are important parts of their body. It may be helpful to have children draw their concept of the brain in order to clarify misconceptions and base the explanation on their level of understanding.

Although the temptation is to justify the need for surgery by stating that removing the tumor will take away various symptoms, the nurse should refrain from emphasizing this point too strenuously. Postsurgical headaches and cerebellar symptoms, such as ataxia, may be aggravated rather than improved. Surgery may not improve vision. With optic gliomas the child will be blind in one eye. Finally, surgical removal of the mass may be impossible, and after surgery there may be temporary deterioration of functioning. Being honest before surgery most often makes honesty after the procedure easier because no false hopes were created.

Honesty does not negate instilling hope. A truthful explanation regarding the surgery is: "The surgeon will see exactly where the tumor is. If it is small and in one place, it will be removed. If it is large, as much of it as possible will be removed so that some of your symptoms will go away." It is best to deliver information in small amounts to let the child pursue additional answers. For example, some children will ask about what happens when part of the tumor is left in. An honest reply is that, after surgery, the practitioner will try to shrink the tumor with a special radiation machine and/or drugs. A further explanation of radiation or chemotherapy should be delayed until a decision regarding these treatments is made.

The hair is shaved in the operating room just before surgery, or in the child's room, usually the night before surgery. When shaving is done with the child awake, the procedure is approached in a sensitive, positive way. If the child's hair is long, it should be braided so that the long swatch can be saved. Showing children how they look at different stages of the process helps them prepare for the final appearance.

Once the hair is clipped very short or shaved, the child can be given a cap or scarf to wear in order to camouflage the baldness. Every precaution is taken to provide privacy during the procedure and to protect the child from teasing or ridicule by other children before surgery. It is also emphasized that the hair will regrow shortly after surgery. Depending on the child's immediate adjustment to the hair loss, the nurse may introduce the idea of wearing a wig until the hair is grown in, particularly if additional irradiation or chemotherapy is anticipated.

Children are also told about the size of the dressing. Usually the entire scalp is covered to maintain a tight wound closure, even if a small incision is made. Infratentorial head dressings may be attached to the upper back and extend forward to the neck in order to maintain slight extension and alignment as a precaution against wound rupture. Applying a similar dressing or "special hat" to a doll is often a less traumatic way of demonstrating the physical appearance.

Children also need a brief explanation of how they will feel after surgery and where they will be. Ordinarily they will return to a special intensive care unit, which they may visit beforehand depending on hospital policy. They should be aware that they may be sleepy for some time after surgery and that a headache is likely, although it should last only a few days.

Parents need similar explanations before surgery, especially in terms of special equipment used in the intensive care unit, dressings, and their child's behavior. For example, they should know that it is not unusual for the child to be comatose or lethargic for a few days after surgery. The nurse may wish to encourage less frequent visiting during this period so that parents can rest and be able to support their child when awake.

It is also advisable for the nurse to participate in preoperative conferences with the physician and parents. The nurse needs to know what information the parents have been given in order to be able to give further explanations or emotional support when necessary.

Prevent postoperative complications. Usually the surgeon will prescribe specific orders for vital signs, positioning, fluid regulation, and medication. These vary somewhat, depending on the location of the craniotomy. The following are general principles of care for infratentorial or supratentorial surgery. Additional aspects of care are discussed in Chapter 37, such as care of the child with seizures and care of the unconscious child in terms of respiratory status and neurologic assessment.

Assessment. Vital signs are taken as frequently as every 15 to 30 minutes until stable. Temperature measurement is particularly important because of hyperthermia resulting from surgical intervention in the hypothalamus or brainstem and from some types of general anesthesia. To prepare for this reaction, a cooling blanket should be placed on the bed *before* the child returns to the unit so that it is ready for use when needed. Since the temperature control centers are affected, the nurse monitors body temperature often when any cooling measures are employed, because hypothermia can occur suddenly.

When temperature is elevated, an infectious process must always be suspected, particularly if the febrile state occurs 1 to 2 days after surgery. The most likely types of infection are meningitis and respiratory tract infection. The probable cause of meningitis is wound contamination. Signs of meningitis, such as opisthotonos, Kernig and Brudzinski signs (see Chapter 7), and nuchal rigidity (see Chapter 37), are very similar to those of increased intracranial pressure and must be carefully evaluated to determine whether they indicate an infection.

The risk of respiratory infections is high because of the imposed immobility, danger of aspiration, and possible depression from the brainstem, and the usual precautions in terms of deep breathing and turning as allowed are instituted. Regular pulmonary assessments should be performed to identify adventitious sounds or any areas of diminished or absent breath sounds. Blood pressure is also taken at frequent intervals. The deflated cuff is left on the arm between readings to allow for the least movement and disturbance of the child. Ocular signs are recorded at least every hour. Sluggish, dilated, or unequal pupils are reported to the practitioner, since they may indicate increased pressure.

Observations for function are not instituted until the child regains consciousness. However, as soon as possible the nurse should begin testing reflexes, handgrip, and functioning of the cranial nerves. Muscle strength is usually less after surgery from general weakness but should improve daily. Ataxia may be significantly worse with cerebellar intervention, but it will slowly improve. Edema near the cranial nerves may depress important functions such as the gag, blink, or swallowing reflex.

The nurse records behavior at regular intervals, noting sleep patterns, response to stimuli, and level of consciousness. Although children may be comatose for a few days, once they regain consciousness there should be a steady increase in alertness. Regression to a lethargic, irritable state indicates increasing pressure, possibly caused by meningitis.

Dressings are observed for evidence of drainage. If soiled, the dressing is not removed but reinforced with dry sterile gauze. The approximate amount of drainage is estimated and recorded.

✦ **NURSING ALERT** To keep an accurate account of drainage, the soiled area is circled with a pen every hour or so. In this way continuous bleeding is easily recognized. The presence of colorless drainage is reported immediately, since it most likely is cerebrospinal fluid from the incisional area. A foul odor from the dressing may indicate an infection. Such a finding is reported, and a culture is taken.

Once the younger child is alert, the arms may need to be restrained to preserve the dressing. Even a child who has been cooperative before surgery must be closely supervised during the initial stages of regaining consciousness, when disorientation and restlessness are common. Elbow restraints are satisfactory to prevent the hands from reaching the head, although additional restraint may be necessary to preserve an infusion line and maintain a specific position.

Positioning. Correct positioning after surgery is critical to prevent pressure against the operative site, reduce intracranial pressure, and avoid the danger of aspiration. If a large tumor was removed, the child is not placed on the operative site, since the brain may suddenly shift to that cavity, causing trauma to the blood vessels, linings, and the brain itself. The nurse confers with the surgeon to be certain of the correct position, including degree of neck flexion. The first 24 to 48 hours after brain surgery are critical. If position is restricted, notice of this is posted above the head of the bed. When the child is turned, every precaution is used to prevent jarring or malalignment in order to prevent undue strain on the sutures. Two nurses, one supporting the head and the other the body, are needed. The use of a turning sheet may facilitate turning a heavy child.

The child with an infratentorial procedure is usually positioned flat and on either side. Pillows should be placed against the child's back, not head, to maintain the desired position. Ordinarily the head and neck are kept in midline with the body and slightly extended. In a supratentorial craniotomy the head is usually elevated above the heart to facilitate cerebrospinal fluid drainage and decrease excessive blood flow to the brain to prevent hemorrhage.

✦ **NURSING ALERT** Trendelenburg position is contraindicated in both infratentorial and supratentorial surgeries because it increases intracranial pressure and the risk of hemorrhage. If shock is impending, the practitioner is notified immediately, before the head is lowered.

Fluid regulation. With an infratentorial craniotomy the child is allowed nothing by mouth for at least 24 hours and longer if the gag and swallowing reflexes are depressed or the child is comatose. With a supratentorial procedure, feeding may be resumed soon after the child is alert, sometimes within 24 hours. Clear water is always started first because of the danger of aspiration. If the child vomits, oral liquids are stopped. Vomiting not only predisposes to aspiration but also increases intracranial pressure and incisional rupture.

Intravenous fluids are continued until fluids are well tolerated. Because of the cerebral edema postoperatively and danger of increased intracranial pressure, fluids are carefully monitored. If drugs, such as prophylactic antibiotics, are given intravenously, the medication amount is calculated as part of the intravenous fluid. For example, if the child is to receive 20 ml per hour and the diluted drug is 5 ml, the intravenous solution is reduced to 15 ml for that hour.

A hypertonic solution such as mannitol or dextrose may be necessary to remove excess fluid. These drugs cause rapid diuresis. After surgery the child may have a Foley catheter. Urine output is monitored after administration of these drugs to evaluate their effectiveness.

When able to take fluids, the child should be fed to conserve strength and minimize movement. If there is any sign of facial paralysis, the child is fed slowly to prevent choking or aspiration. Scrupulous mouth care is essential to prevent oral infection. Sometimes gavage feeding is necessary when bodily functions are too depressed to permit safe oral feedings or the child refuses to eat or drink. In the latter instance the nurse should employ every measure to encourage acceptance of fluids or solids. (See Chapter 27 for nursing interventions.)

Comfort measures. Although used after most other types of surgery, postoperative analgesics may not be routinely prescribed, because they may mask signs of altered consciousness or body functioning. However, this varies, and if analgesics are ordered they should be used effectively, preferably on a preventive basis and in sufficient doses (see Pain Management, Chapter 26).

Headache may be severe and is largely the result of cerebral edema. Measures to relieve some of the discomfort include providing a quiet, dimly lit environment, restricting visitors to a minimum, preventing any sudden jarring movement, such as banging into the bed, and preventing an increase in intracranial pressure. The last is most effectively achieved by proper positioning and prevention of straining, such as during coughing, vomiting, or defecating. Bowel movements are monitored to prevent constipation. Stool softeners may be given as soon as liquids are tolerated to facilitate easy passage of stool. Placing an ice bag on the forehead may also provide some headache relief, especially if facial edema is severe.

Brain edema may also severely depress the gag reflex, necessitating suctioning of oral secretions. Facial edema may also be present, necessitating eye care if the lids remain partially open. Ice compresses applied to the eyes for short periods help in relieving the edema. A depressed blink reflex also predisposes to corneal ulceration. Irrigating the eyes with saline drops and covering them with eye dressings are important steps in preventing this complication.

Support the family. The emotional needs of the family are great when the diagnosis is a brain tumor, and feelings are influenced by the extent of surgery, any neurologic deficits, expected prognosis, and additional therapy. Since few definitive answers can be given before surgery, the surgeon's report is a significant finding that can vary from a completely benign, resected neoplasm to a highly malignant, invasive, and only partially removed tumor. Although parents try to prepare themselves for a potentially fatal diagnosis, it is a shock for them.

Ideally a nurse should be with the family when the physician discusses with parents the expected prognosis and plan of therapy. Although parents may hear only a fraction of what they are told, they can begin to put the future into perspective. While some children will be cured, those with residual tumor may die within a relatively short time or live for several years. Regardless of the future prospects, the parents' thinking must be directed toward helping the child recover and resume a normal life to his or her fullest potential.

It is also a time to encourage parents to verbalize their feelings about the diagnosis. Often they express tremendous guilt for attributing the insidious onset of symptoms, such as ataxia, visual difficulty, or headache, to minor "complaints" by the child. Parents may have punished their child for clumsiness, mistaking it for carelessness. The nurse listens to such statements, emphasizing the normalcy of the parents' reactions. Sometimes it may be helpful to precipitate such a discussion with a statement such as, "It is difficult to know when a child's complaints are significant, because so often they are caused by minor ailments." Any comments that insinuate that the parents should have sought medical advice sooner are avoided, since such remarks only add to the parents' guilt feelings.

During this period the nurse should also discuss with parents what they plan to tell the child. If the child was prepared honestly as described previously, the diagnosis can be expressed in a similar manner, such as, "The surgeon removed most of the tumor, and the rest will be treated with special drugs and x-ray treatments." During the recovery, the child will need additional explanation about the treatment as well as the reason for residual neurologic effects, such as ataxia or blindness. Since the hair was shaved before surgery, hair loss is less of a concern from treatment, although its regrowth will be delayed by 3 to 6 months, depending on length of therapy. At this point it is advisable to reinforce the idea of a wig.

Promote return to optimum functioning. The ultimate goal is a cured child who has maximum functioning. As soon as possible the child should resume usual activities within tolerable limits, especially returning to school.* Until the skull is completely healed, the child may need to wear a helmet when engaging in any active sport. The

*Excellent publications, including the pamphlet *When Your Child Is Ready to Return to School,* are available from the Association for Brain Tumor Research, 3725 N. Talman Ave., Chicago, IL 60618; (312) 286-5571.

school nurse and teacher should confer with the parents to discuss activity restrictions, such as physical education, and the reactions of schoolmates to the child's appearance. Since children often equate brain surgery with "going crazy," it is important to prepare the child for possible remarks to this effect. As one child told a classmate, "It's *your* head they should have fixed, because you're crazy. Can't you see that I'm all better?"

After discharge the family needs continuing medical and emotional support from health personnel. Even with children who are long-term survivors after treatment for a brain tumor, residual disabilities, such as growth retardation, cranial nerve palsies, sensory defects, motor abnormalities (especially ataxia), intellectual deficits, dysphagia, dysgraphia, and behaviorial problems, may occur (Heideman and others, 1989). It is difficult to assess the exact cause of the nonphysical disabilities, since numerous variables influence the total rehabilitation of the child. However, the high frequency of late effects attests to the tremendous need for follow-up care despite successful treatment of the tumor.

The realm of possible consequences following the diagnosis of a brain tumor is vast. They are not discussed here. Rather, the reader is urged to refer to other sections of the text that deal with possible outcomes, such as the paralyzed, visually impaired, or unconscious child or the care of a child with a ventricular shunt, seizure disorder, or meningitis. Numerous physical problems can occur with progression of the tumor that may necessitate additional procedures. For example, frequent vomiting, anorexia, and nausea may require nonoral routes of feeding, such as gastrostomy or parenteral alimentation. Trials with chemotherapy may necessitate the use of central venous access devices. Whenever these procedures are instituted, the nurse may be responsible for teaching the family appropriate home care to allow the child the highest quality of life for the longest period of time. (See discussion of discharge planning and home care in Chapter 26 and Nursing Care Plan: The Child with a Brain Tumor*).

NEUROBLASTOMA

Neuroblastoma occurs in about 1 in 10,000 live births, with a slightly higher incidence in males. About half the cases occur in children under 2 years of age, and another fourth occur in children under age 4. These tumors originate from embryonic neural crest cells that normally give rise to the adrenal medulla and the sympathetic ganglia. Consequently, the majority of the tumors arise from the adrenal gland or from the retroperitoneal sympathetic chain. Therefore the primary site is within the abdomen. Other sites may be within the head, neck, chest, or pelvis.

Clinical Manifestations

The signs and symptoms of neuroblastoma depend on the location and stage of the disease. Most presenting signs are caused by compression of adjacent structures. With abdominal tumors the most common presenting sign is a firm, nontender, irregular mass in the abdomen that crosses the midline (in contrast to Wilms tumor, which is usually confined to one side). Compression of the kidney, ureter, or bladder may cause urinary frequency or retention.

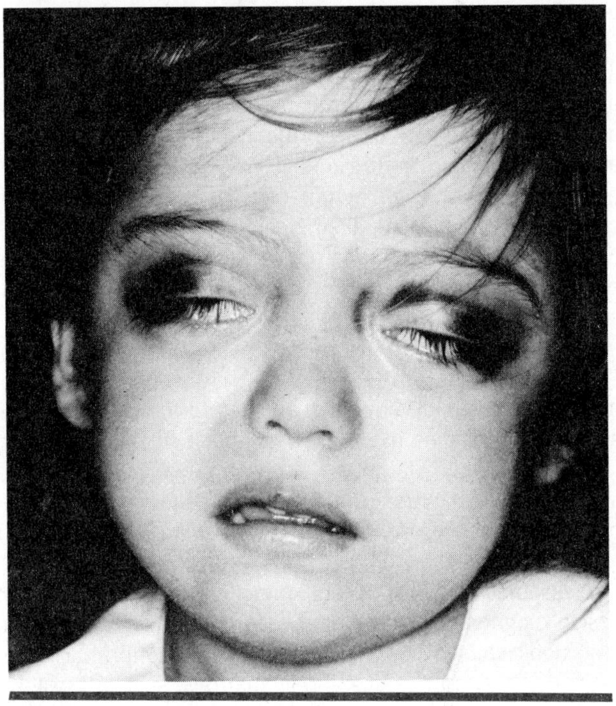

Fig. 36-3. Supraorbital ecchymoses associated with periorbital metastases.

Courtesy Howard A. Britton. From Sutow, W.W., Vietti, T.J., and Fernbach, D.J., editors: Clinical pediatric oncology, ed. 2, St. Louis, 1977, Mosby–Year Book, Inc.

Distant metastasis frequently causes supraorbital ecchymosis, periorbital edema, and proptosis (exophthalmos) from invasion of retrobulbar soft tissue (Fig. 36-3). Lymphadenopathy, especially in the cervical and supraclavicular areas, may also be an early presenting sign. Bone pain may or may not be present with skeletal involvement. Vague symptoms of widespread metastasis include pallor, weakness, irritability, anorexia, and weight loss.

Other primary tumors may cause significant clinical effcts, such as neurologic impairment from an intracranial lesion, respiratory obstruction from a thoracic mass, or varying degrees of paralysis from compression of the spinal cord. Infrequently a child may have symptoms of increased catecholamine excretion, such as flushing, hypertension, tachycardia, and diaphoresis (Blatt and Lee, 1988).

Diagnostic Evaluation

Diagnostic evaluation is aimed at locating the primary site and areas of metastasis. A skeletal survey; skull, neck, chest, abdominal, and bone CT scans; and a bone marrow test are used to locate a tumor mass and/or metastasis. With an adrenal neuroblastoma an intravenous pyelogram often demonstrates a downward displacement of the af-

*In Wong, D.L., and Whaley, L.F.: Clinical manual of pediatric nursing, ed. 3, St. Louis, 1990, Mosby–Year Book, Inc.

fected kidney but normal renal function. Neuroblastomas, particularly those arising on the adrenal glands or from a sympathetic chain, excrete the catecholamines epinephrine and norepinephrine. Analyzing the breakdown products that are normally excreted in the urine, namely, vanillylmandelic acid (VMA), homovanillic acid (HVA), dopamine, and norepinephrine, permits detection of a suspected tumor both before and after medical/surgical intervention. Amplification of the N-myc gene and abnormalities in chromosomes have been associated with a poorer prognosis (Finklestein, 1987; Hayashi and others, 1989).

Staging and Prognosis

In recent years there has been an attempt to classify tumors according to stages in order to establish improved criteria for treatment and prognosis at the time of diagnosis and surgery. A new international system of staging for neuroblastoma has been developed (Brodeur and others, 1988) (Box 36-8).

Neuroblastoma is a "silent" tumor. In more than 70% of cases, diagnosis is made after metastasis occurs, with the first signs caused by involvement in the nonprimary site, usually the lymph nodes, bone marrow, skeletal system, skin, or liver. Because of the frequency of invasiveness, prognosis for neuroblastoma is poor.

The age of the child and the stage of the disease at diagnosis are important prognostic factors. Survival is inversely correlated with age. If all stages are grouped together, the survival rates are 72% for birth to age 11 months, 28% for ages 12 to 23 months, and 12% for ages 2 years or more. This marked difference in survival rates by age is partly accounted for by the larger proportion of very young children with stage I, II, or IV-S disease (Brodeur and others, 1988). However, survival expectancy improves for children over 6 years of age. Infants who remain free of disease for 1 year after treatment are usually cured, but older children have experienced relapses several years after cessation of treatment (Hayes and Smith, 1989). Neuroblastoma is one of the few tumors that demonstrate spontaneous regression (especially stage IV-S), possibly as a result of maturity of the embryonic cell or development of an active immune system.

Box 36-8 STAGING SYSTEM FOR NEUROBLASTOMA

Stage I: Localized tumor confined to the area of origin; local excision with or without microscopic disease; negative lymph nodes

Stage II: Unilateral tumor with incomplete gross excision; lymph nodes negative

Stage III: Tumor infiltrating across the midline with or without regional lymph node involvement; unilateral tumor with regional involvement; midline tumor with bilateral regional lymph node involvement

Stage IV: Dissemination of tumor to distant lymph nodes, bone, bone marrow, liver, and/or other organs

Stage IV-S: Localized primary tumor as defined for stage I or II with dissemination limited to liver, skin, and/or bone marrow

In recent years considerable controversy has developed regarding the use of mass screening for neuroblastoma in infants (Mauer, 1988; Tuchman and others, 1989; Woods and Tuchman, 1987). Whether the cost/benefit ratio of screening for this rare tumor in infants is actually worthwhile remains to be seen.

Therapeutic Management

Accurate clinical staging is important for establishing initial treatment. Therefore surgery is employed both to remove as much of the tumor as possible and to obtain biopsies. In stages I and II, complete surgical removal of the tumor is the treatment of choice. If the tumors are large, partial resection is attempted, with a course of irradiation postoperatively to shrink the tumor in the hope of complete removal at a later date. Surgery is usually limited to biopsy in stages III and IV because of the extensive metastasis, although the use of additional surgery to assess tumor regression or remove a regressed tumor is not unlikely.

The precise role of radiotherapy is unclear. It does not appear to be of any benefit in children with stage I and II disease; it is commonly used with stage III disease although it may not improve survival expectancy; and it may make a large tumor operable. It offers palliation for metastatic lesions in bones, lungs, liver, or brain.

Chemotherapy is the mainstay of therapy for extensive local or disseminated disease. The drugs of choice are vincristine, doxorubicin, cyclophosphamide, adriamycin, cisplatin, and VM-26 (a podophyllin derivative that works similarly to vincristine). They are administered in a variety of combinations, but none has proved superior.

Nursing Considerations

Nursing considerations are similar to those discussed previously in the section, Nursing Care of the Child with Cancer, including psychologic and physical preparation for diagnostic and operative procedures, prevention of postoperative complications for abdominal, thoracic, or cranial surgery, and explanation of chemotherapy and radiotherapy and their side effects (see Tables 36-3 and 36-4).

Since this tumor carries a poor prognosis for many children, every consideration must be given the family in terms of coping with a life-threatening illness (see Chapter 23). Because of the high degree of metastasis at the time of diagnosis, many parents suffer much guilt for not having recognized signs earlier. Often the guilt is expressed as anger toward professionals for not diagnosing it sooner. Parents need much support in dealing with these feelings and expressing them to the appropriate people.

BONE TUMORS

Malignant bone tumors represent less than 1% of all malignant neoplasms but are more common in children than adults. The peak ages during childhood are 15 to 19 years. The sexes are affected equally until puberty, at which time the ratio approaches 2:1 in favor of males. This propensity for males with a peak incidence during adolescence is thought to result from the accelerated growth rate of osseous tissue.

GENERAL CONSIDERATIONS

Neoplastic disease can arise from any tissues involved in bone growth, such as osteoid matrix, bone marrow elements, fat, blood and lymph vessels, nerve sheath, and cartilage. In children the two types that account for 85% of all primary malignant bone tumors are osteogenic sarcoma and Ewing sarcoma. They have several characteristics in common, which are discussed in the following sections. Specific information about each tumor is then elaborated on further.

Clinical Manifestations

Most malignant bone tumors produce localized pain in the affected site, which may be severe or dull and may be attributed to trauma or the vague complaint of "growing pains." The pain is often relieved by a flexed position, which relaxes the muscles overlying the stretched periosteum. Frequently it draws attention when the child limps, curtails physical activity, or is unable to hold heavy objects.

Diagnostic Evaluation

Diagnosis begins with a thorough history and physical examination. A primary objective is to rule out causes such as trauma or infection. Careful questioning regarding pain is essential in attempting to determine the duration and rate of tumor growth. Physical assessment focuses on functional status of the affected area, signs of inflammation, size of the mass, involvement of regional lymph nodes, and any systemic indication of generalized malignancy, such as anemia, weight loss, and frequent infection.

Definitive diagnosis is based on radiologic studies, particularly CT, to determine the extent of the lesion; radioisotope bone scans to evaluate metastasis; and either needle or surgical bone biopsy to determine the histologic pattern. Radiologic findings are characteristic for each type of tumor. In osteogenic sarcoma, needlelike new bone formation growing at right angles to the diaphysis (shaft) produces a "sunburst" appearance. In Ewing sarcoma, the deposits of new bone in layers under the periosteum produce an "onionskin" appearance. In both types of bone tumors, soft tissue infiltration may be apparent.

At present there is no reliable biochemical test for bone cancers. Elevated alkaline phosphatase levels may occur in osteoid tumors. Several tests may be done for differential diagnosis in terms of secondary bone metastasis from Wilms tumor, neuroblastoma, retinoblastoma, rhabdomyosarcoma, lymphoma, or leukemia. Lung tomography is usually a standard procedure, since pulmonary metastasis is the most common complication of primary bone tumors. Bone marrow aspiration is helpful in diagnosing Ewing sarcoma in the rare event that the child has bone marrow metastasis.

Prognosis

A better understanding of the biology of neoplastic growth has resulted in more aggressive treatment and improved prognosis. The natural history of osteogenic sarcoma and Ewing sarcoma suggests that multiple submicroscopic foci of metastatic disease are present at the time of diagnosis despite clinical evidence of localized involvement. Before the use of aggressive multimodal therapy, pulmonary metastasis invariably appeared in 6 to 24 months in patients with osteogenic sarcoma who were treated with surgical excision of the tumor. Now, with surgery for osteosarcoma or intensive radiotherapy for Ewing sarcoma combined with chemotherapy, survival statistics are improving for both types of bone cancer. Survival rates differ according to the specific treatment protocols and are influenced by a number of factors, such as site of primary tumor, especially in Ewing sarcoma, and the presence or absence of metastatic disease at diagnosis. However, approximately 50% of children with either type of bone cancer can be expected to be long-term survivors, and various cancer centers are reporting higher figures (Meyers, 1987).

OSTEOGENIC SARCOMA

Osteogenic sarcoma (osteosarcoma) is the most common bone cancer in children. Its peak incidence is between 10 and 25 years of age. It presumably arises from bone-forming mesenchyme, which gives rise to malignant osteoid tissue. Most primary tumor sites are in the metaphysis (wider part of the shaft, adjacent to the epiphyseal growth plate) of long bones, especially in the lower extremities. More than half occur in the femur, particularly the distal portion, with the rest involving the humerus, tibia, pelvis, jaw, and phalanges.

Therapeutic Management

Optimum treatment of osteosarcoma is controversial. The traditional approach has consisted of radical surgical resection or amputation of the affected area followed by intensive chemotherapy. Depending on the tumor site, surgery includes amputation of the affected extremity at least 7.5 cm (3 inches) above the proximal tumor margin or above the joint proximal to the involved bone. With tumors of the distal femur, preservation of the hip joint may be possible. Other procedures include an above-the-knee amputation for tumors of the tibia or fibula, a hemipelvectomy for tumors of the innominate (hip) bone, and a forequarter amputation (removal of arm, scapula, and portion of the clavicle on the affected side) for tumors of the upper humerus. Another surgical approach for selected patients is the limb salvage procedures, which involve en bloc resection of the primary tumor with prosthetic replacement of the involved bone. For example, with osteosarcoma of the distal femur, a total femur and joint replacement is performed. Frequently children undergoing a limb salvage procedure will receive preoperative chemotherapy in an attempt to decrease tumor size and make surgery more manageable (Simon, 1988; Stine and others, 1989).

Chemotherapy now plays a vital role in treatment. Antineoplastic drugs, such as high-dose methotrexate with citrovorum factor rescue, adriamycin, bleomycin, actinomycin, cyclosphosphamide, and cisplatin, may be administered singly or in combination and may be employed both before and after surgery. When pulmonary metastasis is found, thoracotomy and chemotherapy have resulted in prolonged survival and potential cure. These combined-modal-

THERAPEUTIC DIALOGUE

Amputation

Nurse returns to the room of a 17-year-old adolescent with osteogenic sarcoma who has earlier learned that his leg will be amputated tomorrow.

NURSE: I thought that we might talk a bit about the doctor's visit earlier today and your surgery tomorrow.
ADOLESCENT: (with anger in his voice): What is there to talk about? I am going to have my leg cut off and be a cripple.
NURSE: You feel angry because your leg will be amputated (nurse uses facilitative responding).
ADOLESCENT: Yes. How would you feel if you knew your leg had to come off?
NURSE: Probably angry, sad, and confused.
ADOLESCENT: Right.
NURSE: That's why I am here. Sometimes talking helps.

SUMMARY

At this time the adolescent was not ready to talk, but after the surgery he asked the nurse several questions about wearing a prosthesis.

ity approaches have significantly improved the prognosis in osteosarcoma.

Nursing Considerations

Nursing care depends on the type of surgical approach. Obviously, the family may have more difficulty adjusting to an amputation than a limb salvage procedure. In either instance, preparation of the child and family is critical. Straightforward honesty is essential in gaining the cooperation and trust of the child. The diagnosis of cancer should not be disguised with falsehoods such as "infection." To accept the need for radical surgery, the child must be aware of the lack of alternatives for treatment. While the responsibility of telling the child is generally left to the physician, the nurse should be present at the discussion or be aware of exactly what is said to the child. The child should be told a few days before surgery to allow time to think about the diagnosis and consequent treatment and to ask questions. (see Nursing Care Plan: The Child with a Bone Tumor.*)

Sometimes children have many questions about the prosthesis, limitations on physical ability, and prognosis in terms of cure. At other times they react with silence or with a calm manner that belies their concern and fear. Either response must be accepted, because it is part of the grieving process of a loss. For those who wish information, it may be helpful to introduce them to another amputee before surgery or to show them pictures of the prosthesis.† However, the nurse must be careful not to overwhelm children with information. A sound approach is to answer their questions without offering additional information. For those who do not pursue additional information, the nurse expresses a willingness to talk (see Therapeutic Dialogue).

The child is also informed of the need for chemotherapy. Although it is best to introduce this subject before surgery, since treatment begins as soon as possible postoperatively, caution must be exercised in offering too much information at one time. It is wise to discuss hair loss with emphasis on positive aspects, such as wearing a wig. Since bone tumors affect adolescents and young adults, it is not unusual for them to become angry over all the radical body alterations.

If an amputation is performed, the child is usually fitted with a temporary prosthesis immediately after surgery, which permits early functioning and fosters psychologic adjustment. If this is not done, the child requires stump care, which is the same as for any amputee. A permanent prosthesis is usually fitted within 6 to 8 weeks. During hospitalization the child begins physical therapy to become proficient in the use and care of the device.

Phantom limb pain may develop following amputation. This symptom is characterized by sensations such as tingling, itching, and more frequently pain felt in the amputated leg. Amitriptyline (Elavil) has been used successfully in children to decrease the pain (Rogers, 1989).

Discharge planning must begin early during the postoperative period. Once the child has begun physical therapy, the nurse should consult with the therapist and practitioner to evaluate the child's physical and emotional readiness to reenter school. It is an opportune time to involve a community nurse in the home care of the child. Every effort is made to promote normalcy and gradual resumption of realistic preamputation activities.* Role playing in anticipation of such experiences is very beneficial in preparing the child for the inevitable confrontation by others. Environmental barriers, such as stairs, are assessed in terms of the accessibility of the school and/or home, especially since the child may need to use crutches or a wheelchair before com-

---

*In Wong, D.L., and Whaley, L.F.: Clinical manual of pediatric nursing, ed. 3, St. Louis, 1990, Mosby–Year Book, Inc.

†A source of information is the National Amputation Foundation, Inc., 12-45 150th St., Whitestone, NY 11357; (718) 767-0596.

*Information about special programs for children with amputations, such as "Sunshine Skiers," is available from the Candlelighters Childhood Cancer Foundation, 1901 Pennsylvania Ave., N.W., Washington, DC 20006; (202) 659-5136.

plete healing and prosthetic competency are achieved.

The nurse encourages the child to select clothing that best camouflages the prosthesis, such as pants or long-sleeved shirts. Well-fitted prostheses are so natural looking that girls can usually wear sheer stockings without revealing the device. Emphasizing feminine or masculine apparel helps the child regain a feeling of self-identity. Even during the postoperative period, encouraging the child to wear blue jeans and a shirt may distract attention from the deformity and focus it on familiar aspects of appearance.

The family and child need much support in adjusting not only to a life-threatening diagnosis but also to alteration in body form and function. Since loss of a limb constitutes a grieving process, those caring for the child need to recognize that the reactions of anger and depression are normal and necessary. Often parents view the anger as a direct affront to them for allowing the amputation to occur, or they see the depression as rejection. On the contrary, these are not interpersonal attacks but self-attempts to cope with a loss.

EWING SARCOMA

Ewing sarcoma arises in the marrow spaces of the bone rather than from osseous tissue. The tumor originates in the shaft of long and trunk bones, most often affecting the femur, tibia, fibula, humerus, ulna, vertebra, scapula, ribs, pelvic bones, and skull. It occurs almost exclusively in individuals under age 30, with the majority between 4 and 25 years of age.

Therapeutic Management

Surgical amputation is not routinely recommended but may be considered when the results of radiotherapy render the extremity useless or deformed (e.g., from retarded growth in young children) or the tumor appears resectable. The treatment of choice is intensive irradiation of the involved bone combined with chemotherapy. A widely used drug regimen includes vincristine, actinomycin D, cyclophosphamide, and adriamycin (often referred to as VACA).

Nursing Considerations

The psychologic adjustment to Ewing sarcoma is typically less traumatic than to osteogenic sarcoma because of the preservation of the affected limb. Many families accept the diagnosis with a sense of relief in knowing that this type of bone cancer does not necessitate amputation, and initially they may not be aware of the damaging effects on the irradiated site. Consequently, they need preparation for the various diagnostic tests, including bone marrow aspiration and surgical biopsy, and adequate explanation of the treatment regimen. High-dose radiotherapy often causes a skin reaction of dry or moist desquamation followed by hyperpigmentation. The child should wear loose-fitting clothes over the irradiated area to minimize additional skin irritation. Because of increased sensitivity, the area is protected from sunlight and sudden changes in temperature, such as from heating pads or ice packs. The child is encouraged to use the extremity as tolerated. Occasionally an active exercise program may be planned by the physical therapist to preserve maximum function.

The child needs the same considerations for adjusting to the effects of chemotherapy as any other patient with cancer. The drug regimen usually results in hair loss, severe nausea and vomiting, peripheral neuropathy, and possibly cardiotoxicity. Every effort should be made to outline a treatment plan that allows the child maximum resumption of a normal life-style and activities.

■ OTHER SOLID TUMORS

In addition to the cancers already discussed, several other types of solid tumors may occur in children. Wilms tumor, rhabdomyosarcoma, and retinoblastoma are unique in that they tend to be diagnosed early, typically before 5 years of age. Wilms tumor and retinoblastoma are also unusual in that they are among the few types of cancer that may occur in both hereditary and nonhereditary forms.

WILMS TUMOR

Wilms tumor, or nephroblastoma, is the most frequent intraabdominal tumor of childhood and the most common type of renal cancer. Its frequency is estimated to be 1 per 200,000 to 250,000 children. The peak incidence is at 3 years of age. Wilms tumor is one of the childhood cancers that show an increased incidence among siblings and identical twins, reflecting evidence of genetic inheritance. The mode of inheritance in familial cases, which accounts for less than 2% of all Wilms tumors, is autosomal dominant with variable penetrance (estimated at 63%) and expressivity. Thus gene carriers may develop no tumors (37%), unilateral tumors (48%), or bilateral tumors (15%). Wilms tumor is heritable in about 30% of all cases, including some unilateral sporadic cases (Li and others, 1988). Unfortunately, there is no method of identification of gene carriers.

Wilms tumor is also associated with several congenital anomalies; the most common are aniridia, hemihypertrophy, and genitourinary anomalies, such as hypospadias, cryptorchidism, and ambiguous genitalia (Ganick, 1987). Other less common anomalies are microcephaly, pigmented and vascular nevi, pinna deformities, and mental and growth retardation.

Clinical Manifestations

The most common presenting sign is a swelling or mass within the abdomen. The mass is characteristically firm, nontender, confined to one side, and deep within the flank. If it is on the right side, it may be difficult to distinguish from the liver, although, unlike that organ, it does not move with respiration. Parents usually discover the mass during routine bathing or dressing of the child.

Other clinical manifestations are the result of compression from the tumor mass, metabolic alterations secondary to the tumor, or metastasis. Hematuria occurs in less than one fourth of children with Wilms tumor. Anemia, usually secondary to hemorrhage within the tumor, results in pallor, anorexia, and lethargy. Hypertension, probably caused by secretion of excess amounts of renin by the tumor, occurs occasionally. Other effects of malignancy include weight loss and fever. If metastasis has occurred, symptoms of lung involvement, such as dyspnea, cough, shortness of breath, and pain in the chest, may be evident.

Diagnostic Evaluation

In a child suspected of having Wilms tumor, special emphasis is placed on the history and physical examination for presence of congenital anomalies, family history of cancer, and signs of malignancy, such as weight loss, size of liver and spleen, indications of anemia, and lymphadenopathy. Specific tests include radiographic studies, including intravenous pyelogram, CT, hematologic studies (polycythemia is sometimes present if the tumor secretes excess erythropoietin), biochemical studies, and urinalysis. Studies to demonstrate the relationship of the tumor to the ipsilateral kidney and the presence of a normal functioning kidney on the contralateral side are essential. If a large tumor is present, an inferior venacavagram is necessary to demonstrate possible tumor involvement adjacent to the vena cava. A bone marrow aspiration is electively performed to rule out metastasis.

Staging and Prognosis

Wilms tumor probably arises from a malignant, undifferentiated metanephrogenic blastoma (a cluster of primordial cells capable of initiating the regeneration of an abnormal structure). Its occurrence slightly favors the left kidney, which is advantageous because surgically this kidney is easier to manipulate and remove. Although the tumor may become quite large, it remains encapsulated for an extended period. During surgery the tumor is staged to maximize the effectiveness of treatment protocols (Box 36-9).

The histology of the tumor cells is also identified and classified according to two groups: favorable histology (FH) and unfavorable histology (UH). Only about 12% of Wilms tumors demonstrate UH, which is associated with a poorer prognosis and demands a more aggressive treatment protocol, regardless of the clinical stage.

Survival rates for Wilms tumor are the highest among all childhood cancers. Children with localized tumor (stages I and II) have a 90% chance of cure with multimodal therapy. FH of the tumor, first complete remission being greater than 12 months from relapse, and nonabdominal relapse sites are each associated with a significantly better survival expectancy (D'Angio and others, 1989; Grundy and others, 1989).

Box 36-9 STAGING OF WILMS TUMOR

Stage I: Tumor is limited to kidney and completely resected.
Stage II: Tumor extends beyond kidney but is completely resected.
Stage III: Residual nonhematogenous tumor is confined to abdomen.
Stage IV: Hematogenous metastases; deposits are beyond stage III, namely, to lung, liver, bone, and brain.
Stage V: Bilateral renal involvement is present at diagnosis.

Therapeutic Management

The remarkable survival rates for children with Wilms tumor have been the result of a cooperative group of specialists who formed the National Wilms Tumor Study (NWTS) to systematically investigate optimum treatment protocols, including surgery, radiation, and chemotherapy. Combined treatment of surgery and chemotherapy with or without radiation is based on the clinical stage and histologic pattern.

In unilateral disease a large transabdominal incision is performed for optimum visualization of the abdominal cavity; the tumor, affected kidney, and adjacent adrenal gland are removed. Great care is taken to keep the encapsulated tumor intact, since rupture can seed cancer cells throughout the abdomen, lymph channel, and bloodstream. The contralateral kidney is carefully inspected for evidence of disease or dysfunction. Regional lymph nodes are inspected and a biopsy is performed when indicated. Any involved structures, such as part of the colon, diaphragm, or vena cava, are removed. Metal clips are placed around the tumor site for exact marking during radiotherapy.

If both kidneys are involved, the child may be treated with radiotherapy and/or chemotherapy preoperatively to shrink the tumor, allowing more conservative therapy. In some cases a partial nephrectomy is performed on the less affected kidney, with a total nephrectomy on the opposite side. When a transplant is feasible, such as from a twin, sibling, or parent, bilateral nephrectomy is considered as a last resort.

Postoperative radiotherapy is indicated for all children with Wilms tumor except those with stage I disease and FH. Chemotherapy is indicated for all stages. The most effective agents for treating Wilms tumor are actinomycin D and vincristine, sometimes combined with adriamycin. Duration of therapy varies, ranging from 6 to 15 months.

Nursing Considerations

The nursing care of the child with Wilms tumor is similar to that of other cancers treated with surgery, irradiation, and chemotherapy. However, some significant differences are discussed for each phase of nursing intervention. (See also Nursing Care Plan: Care of the Child with Wilms Tumor.*)

Preoperative care. As with many of the other cancers, the diagnosis of Wilms tumor is a shock. Frequently the child has no physical indication of the seriousness of the disorder other than a palpable abdominal mass. Since it is the parents who usually discover the mass, the nurse needs to take into account their feelings regarding the diagnosis. Whereas some parents are grateful for their detection of the tumor, others feel guilty for not finding it sooner or anger toward the practitioner for missing it on earlier examinations.

The preoperative period is one of swift diagnosis. Typi-

*In Wong, D.L., and Whaley, L.F.: Clinical manual of pediatric nursing, ed. 3, St. Louis, 1990, Mosby–Year Book, Inc.

cally surgery is scheduled within 24 to 48 hours of admission. The nurse is faced with the challenge of preparing the child and parents for all laboratory and operative procedures. Because of the little time available, explanations should be kept simple and repeated often with attention to what the child will experience. Besides usual preoperative observations, blood pressure is monitored, since hypertension from excess renin production is a possibility.

There are several special preoperative concerns, the most important of which is that the tumor is not palpated unless absolutely necessary, since manipulation of the mass may cause dissemination of cancer cells to adjacent and distant sites.

✦ **NURSING ALERT** To reinforce the need for caution, it may be necessary to post a sign on the bed that reads "DO NOT PALPATE ABDOMEN." Careful bathing and handling are also important in preventing trauma to the tumor site.

Since radiotherapy and chemotherapy are usually begun immediately after surgery, parents need an explanation of what to expect, such as major benefits and side effects, although the timing of the information should be considered to avoid overwhelming the family. Ideally the nurse should be present during physician-parent conferences to answer questions as they arise. It is usually better to reserve telling the child about these side effects until after surgery. Alopecia, usually of most concern to older children, does not occur until 2 weeks after the initial treatment regimen. Therefore the child can be prepared for the hair loss postoperatively.

Postoperative care. Despite the extensive surgical intervention necessary in many children with Wilms tumor, the recovery period is usually rapid. The major nursing responsibilities are those following any abdominal surgery (see Nursing Care Plan: The Child Undergoing Surgery, Chapter 27). Since these children are at risk for intestinal obstruction from vincristine-induced adynamic ileus, radiation-induced edema, and postsurgical adhesion formation, gastrointestinal activity, such as bowel movements, bowel sounds, distention, and vomiting, is monitored. Other considerations are frequent evaluation of blood pressure and observation for signs of infection, especially during chemotherapy. Because of the myelosuppression from the drugs, pulmonary hygiene measures are instituted in the immediate postoperative period to prevent complications.

Support the family. The postoperative period is frequently difficult for parents. The shock of seeing their child immediately after surgery may be the first realization of the seriousness of the diagnosis. It also marks the confirmation of the stage of the tumor. During this period the nurse should again be with parents to assure them of the child's recovery after surgery and to assess their understanding of the pathology report.

Older children need an opportunity to deal with their feelings concerning the many procedures to which they have been subjected in rapid succession. Play therapy with dolls, puppets, or drawing can be extremely beneficial in helping them adjust to the surgery and hair loss. It is not unusual for children to feel betrayed because they were not adequately prepared for the extent of surgery, the need for additional therapy, or the seriousness of the disorder.

Because the child is left with only one kidney, certain precautions are recommended to prevent injury to the organ, such as avoiding contact sports or any other activity that has a high risk potential. Urinary tract infections should be prevented with good hygiene, especially in girls, and adequate fluid intake. Prompt detection and treatment of any genitourinary signs or symptoms is mandatory.

RHABDOMYOSARCOMA

Soft tissue sarcomas are the fourth most common type of solid tumors in children. These malignant neoplasms originate from undifferentiated mesenchymal cells in muscles, tendons, bursae, and fascia, or fibrous, connective, lymphatic, or vascular tissue. They derive their name from the specific tissue(s) of origin, such as myosarcoma (*myo*—muscle). Rhabdomyosarcoma (*rhabdo*—striated) is the most common soft tissue sarcoma in children. Because striated (skeletal) muscle is found almost anywhere in the body, these tumors occur in many sites, the most common of which are the head and neck, especially the orbit. The disease occurs in children in all age-groups but most commonly in children younger than 5 years of age. Its incidence is approximately 4.4 per million for white children under age 15, but only 1.3 per million for black children in this age-group.

Rhabdomyosarcoma arises from embryonic mesenchyme. Four subtypes are recognized and described in Box 36-10.

Clinical Manifestations

The initial signs and symptoms are related to the site of the tumor and compression of adjacent organs (Table 36-8). Some tumor locations, particularly the orbit, produce symptoms early in the course of the illness and contribute to rapid diagnosis and improved prognosis. Other tumors, such as those of the retroperitoneal area, produce no symptoms until they are large, invasive, and widely metastasized. In some instances a primary tumor site is never identified.

Box 36-10 SUBTYPES OF RHABDOMYOSARCOMA

Embryonal—most common type; most frequently found in the head, neck, abdomen, and genitourinary tract
Alveolar—second most common type; most often seen in deep tissues of the extremities and trunk
Botryoid—third most common type; appears as multiple grapelike clusters or polyps, usually found in cavities such as the vagina, urinary bladder, ear, and nasopharynx
Pleomorphic—rare in children (adult form); most often occurs in soft parts of extremities and trunk

Table 36-8 Clinical manifestations of rhabdomyosarcoma according to tumor site

LOCATION	SIGNS AND SYMPTOMS
Orbit	Rapidly developing unilateral proptosis Ecchymosis of conjunctiva Loss of extraocular movements (strabismus)
Nasopharynx	Stuffy nose (earliest sign) Nasal obstruction—dysphagia, nasal voice (obstruction of posterior nasal conchae), serous otitis media (obstruction of eustachian tube) Pain (sore throat and ear) Epistaxis Palpable neck nodes Visible mass in oropharynx (late sign)
Paranasal sinuses	Nasal obstruction Local pain Discharge Sinusitis Swelling
Middle ear	Signs of chronic serous otitis media Pain Sanguinopurulent drainage Facial nerve palsy
Retroperitoneal area (usually a "silent" tumor)	Abdominal mass Pain Signs of intestinal or genitourinary obstruction
Perineum	Visible superficial mass Bowel or bladder dysfunction (from tumor compression)

Diagnostic Evaluation

Unfortunately, many of the signs and symptoms attributable to rhabdomyosarcoma are vague and frequently suggest a common childhood illness, such as "earache" or "runny nose." However, diagnosis begins with a careful examination of the head and neck area, particularly palpation of a nontender, firm, hard mass. The nasopharynx and oropharynx are inspected for any evidence of a visible mass.

Radiographic studies to isolate a tumor site are performed, accompanied by chest x-ray examinations, lung tomograms, bone surveys, and bone marrow aspiration to rule out metastasis. A lumbar puncture is indicated for head and neck tumors. An excisional biopsy is done to confirm histologic type.

Staging and Prognosis

Careful staging is extremely important for planning treatment and determining prognosis. The Intergroup Rhabdomyosarcoma Study has established clinical staging (Ruymann, 1987) (Box 36-11).

Box 36-11 STAGING OF RHABDOMYOSARCOMA

Group I: Localized disease; tumor completely resected and regional nodes not involved
Group II: Localized disease with microscopic residual, or regional disease with no residual or with microscopic residual
Group III: Incomplete resection or biopsy with gross residual disease
Group IV: Metastatic disease present at diagnosis

With the change in treatment from radical surgery or radiotherapy to a multimodal approach, survival rates for all stages have increased considerably. Overall cure rate is 65% for children with rhabdomyosarcoma (Ruymann, 1987). Two-year survival rates from the most recent national study vary for each clinical group: 92% to 100% for group I, 79% to 94% for group II, 71% to 79% for group III, and 37% to 40% for group IV (Raney and others, 1989; Ruymann, 1987).

Data suggest that children who remain disease free for 2 years are probably cured; however, if relapse occurs, the prognosis for long-term survival is extremely poor (Ruymann, 1987).

Therapeutic Management

Since this tumor is highly malignant, with metastasis frequently occurring at time of diagnosis, aggressive multimodal therapy is recommended. In the past, radical surgical removal of the tumor was the treatment of choice, but with improved survival from combined chemotherapy and radiation, surgery plays a lesser role. Complete removal of the primary tumor is advocated whenever possible. However, biopsy only is required in certain tumor locations, such as those of the orbit when followed by radiation and chemotherapy. This is a fortunate change, because it avoids the devastating effects of enucleation, amputation, or pelvic exenteration.

High-dose irradiation to the primary tumor is recommended, except in group I tumors. Chemotherapy plays a major role in treatment of all groups. Drugs that are cytotoxic for rhabdomyosarcoma are vincristine, actinomycin D, and cyclophosphamide (collectively known as VAC), with or without adriamycin, for 1 to 2 years depending on the stage of the disease (Ruymann, 1987).

Nursing Considerations

The nursing responsibilities are similar to those for other types of cancer, especially the solid tumors when surgery is employed. Specific objectives include (1) careful assessment for signs of the tumor, especially during well-child examinations; (2) preparation of the child and family for the multiple diagnostic tests (see p. 1679); and (3) supportive care during each stage of multimodal therapy. The reader is urged to review the Nursing Considerations section for cancer and Chapter 23 for emotional support of the family in the event of a poor prognosis.

RETINOBLASTOMA

Retinoblastoma is a congenital malignant tumor arising from the retina. It is a relatively rare tumor in the United States and occurs less frequently than any of the cancers previously discussed, with an incidence of 3.4 per million in children under 15 years. As with Wilms tumor, it can be inherited, and it may be present at birth or may arise in the retina during the first 2 years of life. The average age of the child at the time of diagnosis is 17 months; it is usually diagnosed earlier in hereditary cases and later in nonhereditary types.

Retinoblastoma may be caused by (1) a somatic mutation, (2) a germinal mutation, or (3) a chromosomal aberration. *Somatic mutations* (those occurring in the general body cells, as opposed to the germ cells or gametes) are a sporadic event and consequently are nonhereditary. They are always unilateral. *Germinal mutations* are passed to future generations. All bilateral retinoblastomas are considered hereditary, and 10% to 15% of individuals with unilateral disease have the hereditary form (Donaldson and Smith, 1989). Hereditary retinoblastomas are transmitted as an autosomal dominant trait, with an 80% penetrance. Consequently, 20% of gene carriers remain unaffected.

Retinoblastoma has also been associated with partial deletion of the long arm of a group D chromosome (number 13) and chromosomal polyploidy (excessive numbers of chromosomes), such as trisomy 21. In children who have chromosomal aberrations and retinoblastoma, there is often an increased incidence of mental retardation and congenital malformations, although the vast majority of children with retinoblastomas apparently have normal chromosomes and intelligence.

Clinical Manifestations

Retinoblastoma has few grossly obvious signs. Typically it is the parent who first observes a whitish "glow" in the pupil, known as the *cat's eye reflex* or *leukokoria.* The reflex represents visualization of the tumor as the light momentarily falls on the mass (Fig. 36-4). When a tumor arises in the macular region (area directly at the back of the retina when the eye is focused straight ahead), a white reflex may be seen when the tumor is quite small. It is best observed when a bright light is shining toward the child as the child looks forward. It is sometimes accidentally discovered by parents when taking a photograph of their child using a flash attachment.

When the tumor arises in the periphery of the retina, it must grow to a considerably large size before light can strike it sufficiently to produce the cat's eye reflex. In this situation it is seen only when the child looks in certain directions (sideways) or if the observer stands at an oblique angle to the child's face as the child looks straight ahead. The fleeting nature of the reflex often results in a delayed diagnosis, because health professionals fail to appreciate the ominous significance of the parents' findings.

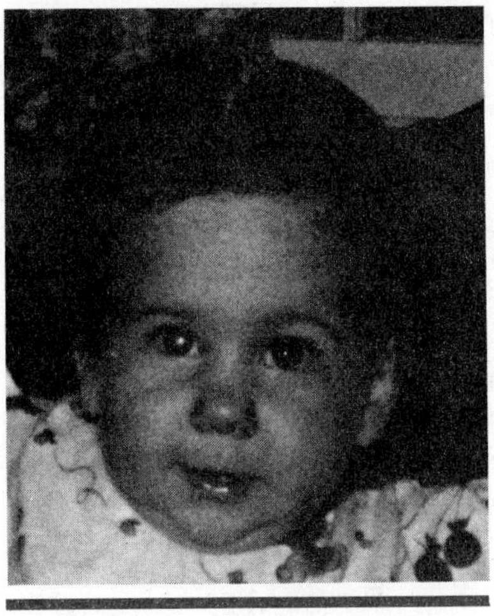

Fig. 36-4. Cat's eye reflex. Whitish appearance of lens is produced as light falls on tumor mass in right eye.

The next most common sign is strabismus resulting from poor fixation of the visually impaired eye, particularly if the tumor develops in the macula, the area of sharpest visual acuity. Blindness is usually a late sign, but it frequently is not obvious unless the parent consciously observes for behaviors indicating loss of sight, such as bumping into objects, slowed motor development, or turning of the head to see objects lateral to the affected eye.

Another common presenting sign is a red, painful eye, often accompanied by glaucoma. Other common clinical manifestations include orbital cellulitis, unilateral mydriasis, a change in the color of the iris, hyphema, white spots on the iris, nystagmus, and complaints indicating systemic metastasis, such as weight loss, poor appetite, or fatigue.

Diagnostic Evaluation

The first step in diagnosis is carefully listening to and recognizing the significance of reports from family members regarding suspected abnormalities within the eye. Parental remarks that in any way suggest the presence of such findings must be taken seriously and further investigated. For example, if the parent indicates that the child has a strange expression or an unusual glow in the eye, every attempt is made to duplicate the circumstances necessary to observe these changes. Children suspected of having this disorder are referred to an ophthalmologist. Definitive diagnosis is usually based on indirect ophthalmoscopy employing scleral indentation, which is done under general anesthesia with maximum dilation of the pupils.

A potentially useful test is catecholamine excretion by measuring vanillylmandelic or homovanillic acid in the urine. These substances are excreted by some retinoblastomas as well as by neuroblastomas. If distant metastasis is suspected, a bone marrow aspiration, bone survey, and lumbar puncture may be performed.

Box 36-12 STAGING OF RETINOBLASTOMA

Group I: Very favorable
Solitary tumor, less than 4 DD, at or behind the equator
Multiple tumors, none greater than 4 DD, all at or behind the equator
Group II: Favorable
Solitary tumors, 4 to 10 DD, at or behind the equator
Multiple tumors, 4 to 10 DD, behind the equator
Group III: Doubtful
Any lesion anterior to the equator
Solitary tumors larger than 10 DD behind the equator
Group IV: Unfavorable
Multiple tumors, some larger than 10 DD
Any lesion extending anteriorly to the ora serrata
Group V: Very unfavorable
Massive tumors involving more than half the retina
Vitreous seeding

Staging and Prognosis

Staging of retinoblastomas is done under indirect ophthalmoscopy before surgery to determine accurately tumor size (measured in disc diameters—DD) and location (according to an imaginary line called the equator drawn on the midplane of the eye) (Grabowski, and Abramson, 1987). The classification by Reese-Ellsworth is commonly used (Box 36-12).

The classification system has been used to define cure in terms of numbers of years free of disease and in terms of preservation of useful vision in the affected eye (favorable, doubtful, or unfavorable). Cure rates for survival are much better than for retention of useful vision. The overall 5-year survival rate is 85% to 90% for unilateral and bilateral tumors; most of the deaths occur in children with group V disease (Donaldson and Smith, 1989). Retinoblastoma is one of the tumors that may spontaneously regress.

Of major concern in long-term survivors is the development of secondary tumors, especially osteogenic sarcoma. Children with bilateral disease (hereditary form) are more likely to develop secondary cancers than children with unilateral disease. It is thought that these individuals are predisposed to developing cancer, and radiation increases their risk.

Therapeutic Management

Treatment of retinoblastoma depends chiefly on the stage of the tumor at diagnosis. In general, unilateral retinoblastomas in stages I, II, and III are treated with irradiation. The aim of radiotherapy is to preserve useful vision in the affected eye and eradicate the tumor.

Other approaches toward treating small, localized tumors involve (1) *cobalt plaque applicators* (surgical implantation of a cobalt 60 applicator on the sclera until the maximum radiation dose has been delivered to the tumor), (2) *light coagulation* (use of a laser beam to destroy retinal blood vessels that supply nutrition to the tumor), and (3) *cryotherapy* (freezing of the tumor, which destroys the microcirculation to the tumor and the cells themselves through microcrystal formation). One of the reasons for investigating treatments other than radiotherapy is to minimize the risk of radiation-induced malignancies later in life.

With advanced tumor growth, especially optic nerve involvement, enucleation of the affected eye is the treatment of choice. The use of chemotherapy in advanced disease, even in group V, is controversial and has not shown improved survival. Drugs that may be used in the treatment of metastatic disease include vincristine, cyclophosphamide, actinomycin, and adriamycin. In the case of central nervous system disease, intrathecal methotrexate or a combination of methotrexate, cytosine arabinoside, and hydrocortisone may be administered (Donaldson and Smith, 1989).

With bilateral disease, every attempt is made to preserve useful vision in the less affected eye with enucleation of the severely diseased eye. When bilateral tumors are found very early, enucleation may be prevented with only the use of radiotherapy to both eyes.

Nursing Considerations

The care of the child with retinoblastoma involves much attention to individual aspects of diagnosis, treatment protocols, and possible hereditary factors. Nursing objectives include (1) identifying signs of retinoblastoma, (2) preparing the family for diagnostic/therapeutic procedures and home care, and (3) providing emotional support. The importance of recognizing possible early signs and appreciating their significance has already been discussed.

Prepare the family for diagnostic/therapeutic procedures and home care. Since the tumor is usually diagnosed in infants or very young children, most of the preparation for diagnostic tests and treatment involves parents. After indirect ophthalmoscopy the child may not see very clearly, or the eyes may be sensitive to light because of pupillary dilation. Parents are made aware of these normal reactions before the procedure.

Once the disease is staged, the physician confers with the parents regarding treatment. Unless the diagnosis is made very early, an enucleation is performed. Parents are told about the procedure as well as about the benefits of a prosthesis. Parents often believe the procedure is bloody and mutilating, envisioning that the eye is "ripped out of its socket." Actually, the surgery is very similar to scooping a nut out of its shell. All the adnexal structures of the eye, such as the lids, lashes, and tear glands, are left undisturbed.

Showing parents pictures of another child with an artificial eye may be very helpful in their adjustment to the thought of disfigurement (Fig. 36-5). Although the idea of loss of vision is a very distressing one, most parents seem to realize that there is no alternative. The facts that the unaffected eye retains normal vision and that the affected eye is probably already blind are particularly helpful in promoting acceptance of the imposed impairment and should be emphasized.

After surgery, the parents need to be prepared for the child's facial appearance. An eye patch is in place, and the child's face may be edematous or ecchymotic. Parents often fear seeing the surgical site because they imagine a cavity

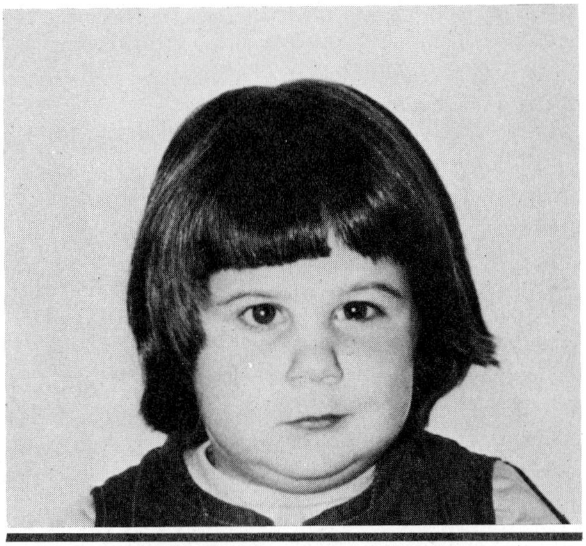

Fig. 36-5. Preschooler with right prosthetic eye.

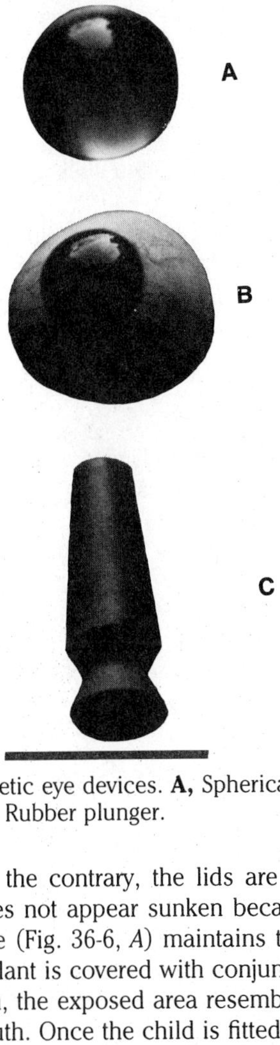

Fig. 36-6. Prosthetic eye devices. **A,** Spherical implant. **B,** Prosthetic eye. **C,** Rubber plunger.

in the skull. On the contrary, the lids are usually closed, and the area does not appear sunken because a surgically implanted sphere (Fig. 36-6, *A*) maintains the shape of the eyeball. The implant is covered with conjunctiva, and when the lids are open, the exposed area resembles the mucosal lining of the mouth. Once the child is fitted for a prosthesis (Fig. 36-6, *B*), usually within 3 weeks, the facial appearance returns to normal.

After an uneventful recovery from enucleation, plans can be made for discharge from the hospital, usually within 3 to 4 days postoperatively. Parents need instruction regarding care of the surgical site and preparation for any additional therapy. They should be given the opportunity to see the socket as soon after surgery as possible. A good time to do this without unduly pressuring them is during dressing changes. They should then be encouraged to participate in the dressing changes.

Care of the socket is minimal and easily accomplished. The wound itself is clean and has little or no drainage. If an antibiotic ointment is prescribed, it is applied in a thin line on the surface of the tissues of the socket. To cleanse the site, an irrigating solution may be ordered and is instilled daily or more frequently if necessary, *before* application of the antibiotic ointment. The dressing consists of an eye pad taped over the surgical site with nonirritating tape; it is changed daily. Self-adhesive eye pads can also be used as dressings. Once the socket has healed completely, a dressing is no longer necessary, although there are several reasons for continuing to have the child wear the eye patch. Infants and toddlers explore their environment with their hands, and the socket is available to exploring fingers without an eye patch in place. Although there is little danger of the child injuring the socket, parents may feel more secure with the socket covered. This also helps prevent infection.

Initial instructions for care of the prosthesis are given by the ocularist, who fits and manufactures the device. Once in place, the prosthesis need not be removed unless cleaning is necessary, in which case it is taken out by gently pulling down on the lower lid, which frees the lower edge of the prosthesis, and applying pressure to the upper lid. If the child resists by forcing the lids shut, a small rubber instrument resembling a plunger (Fig, 36-6, *C*) can be used to facilitate removal and reinsertion. The end of the plunger is moistened and placed on top of the prosthetic iris. The lower eyelid is retracted, and the prosthesis is pulled out with a downward motion.

The prosthesis is cleaned by placing it in hot water and soaking it for several minutes. Reinsertion is easier if the prosthesis remains wet. To reinsert the prosthesis, the lids are separated, and with the prosthesis held in the correct position (it should be marked to indicate the nasal side), it is pushed up under the upper lid, allowing the lower lid to cover its lower edge.

Because the prosthesis is easily removed, the child may accidentally cause it to dislodge. Reactions of children vary from fear that they have "lost" their eye to matter-of-fact acceptance. The first time can be disturbing to both parents and child, but it is just one part of the child's adjusted lifestyle. If children are old enough to understand, parents can explain that they have a "special" eye that can accidentally fall out but that can also be quickly put back in place.

Safety is a major concern to prevent damage to the unaffected eye. Safety measures such as those presented in Box 25-5 should be practiced at all times, and rough contact sports should be avoided or protective eye wear worn during such activity.

Support the family. The diagnosis of retinoblastoma presents some special concerns in addition to those created by any type of cancer. Families with a history of the

Table 36-9 Recurrence risks of retinoblastoma in families with an affected child

TYPE OF TUMOR	RISK TO SUBSEQUENT SIBLINGS	RISK TO AFFECTED CHILD'S OFFSPRING
Unilateral*	1%	5%-6%
Bilateral†	6%	50%

Data from Donaldson, S.S., and Egbert, P.R.: Retinoblastoma. In Pizzo, P.A., and Poplack, D.G.: Principles and practice of pediatric oncology, Philadelphia, 1989, J.B. Lippincott Co.
*Refers only to families with negative family history.
†Regardless of family history.

disorder may feel great guilt for transmitting the defect to their offspring, especially if they knowingly "played the odds" and parented an affected child. Conversely, when parents are aware of the probability and have an affected child, early treatment results in such favorable outcomes that parental adjustment may be rapid. In families with no history of retinoblastoma, the discovery of the diagnosis is a shock, frequently complicated by guilt for not having found it sooner. Since parents frequently are the first to observe the cat's eye reflex, they may feel angry at themselves or others, especially professionals, for delaying a more thorough examination. Each of these variables needs to be considered in offering supportive care to the family.

Other concerns are also related to the hereditary aspects of the disease. Of great importance to parents is the recurrence risk of retinoblastoma in their subsequent offspring and in the offspring of the surviving affected child (Table 36-9). With improving prognosis for these children, the necessity of genetic counseling to prevent transmission of the disease is assuming greater importance. (See Chapter 5 for a discussion of the nurse's role in genetic counseling.) Determining the risk of transmission is possible through DNA/RNA studies of the tumor cells. If a germinal mutation is found, blood samples from family members can be analyzed to see if they carry the mutation (Dryja, 1989).

These families are also encouraged to seek regular follow-up care for the affected child to detect secondary tumors, and all subsequent offspring of unaffected parents and survivors should undergo regular indirect ophthalmoscopy under anesthesia to detect retinoblastoma at its earliest stage.

KEY POINTS

- Criteria used to determine cure of cancer include cessation of therapy, continuous freedom from clinical and laboratory evidence of cancer, and minimum or no risk of relapse, as determined by previous experience with disease.
- Although the cure rate for most types of childhood cancer has improved, the late effects of treatment are of increasing concern.
- Determination of malignancy and metastasis is made by history and physical examination, laboratory tests, imaging techniques, and biopsy.
- The major modes of cancer therapy are surgery, chemotherapy, radiotherapy, immunotherapy, and bone marrow transplantation.
- Chemotherapeutic agents are classified according to their cytotoxic action: alkylating agents, antimetabolites, plant alkaloids, antitumor antibiotics, and hormones.
- Types of bone marrow transplants are allogeneic, autologous, and syngeneic.
- Treatment of leukemia follows four phases: remission induction, sanctuary therapy, maintenance therapy, and reinduction.
- Nursing goals in the care of the child with cancer are to prepare the family for diagnostic and therapeutic procedures, prevent complications of myelosuppression (infection, hemorrhage, anemia), manage problems of irradiation and drug toxicity (nausea and vomiting, anorexia, mucosal ulceration, neuropathy, hemorrhagic cystitis, alopecia, moon face, mood changes), and provide continued emotional support.
- Leukemia is the most common form of childhood cancer. Current 5-year survival rates exceed 60% in major research centers, and the majority of these children will be cured.
- The lymphomas include Hodgkin disease and non-Hodgkin lymphoma; Hodgkin disease affects primarily adolescents.
- Nursing care of the child with a brain tumor includes observing for signs and symptoms related to the tumor, preparing the child and family for diagnostic tests and operative procedures, preventing postoperative complications, planning for discharge, and promoting a return to optimum health.
- The traditional approach to treatment of osteosarcoma has been radical surgical resection or amputation followed by chemotherapy. Limb preservation to prevent amputation is now playing an increasing role.
- Wilms tumor shows an increased incidence among siblings and identical twins, demonstrating a hereditary predisposition.
- Rhabdomyosarcoma may occur almost anywhere in the body, but the most common sites are the head and neck.
- Common presenting signs in retinoblastoma are cat's eye reflex, strabismus, and red, painful eye.

REFERENCES

Abernathy, E.: Biotherapy: an introductory overview, Oncol. Nurs. Forum 14(suppl. 6):13-15, 1987.
Abramovitz, L.Z., and Baache, B.: Management of skin care complications in pediatric bone marrow transplant patients: a nursing challenge, J. Assoc. Pediatr. Oncol. Nurs. 5(1):37, 1988.
Berkowitz, R.J., Feretti, G.A., and Berg, J.H.: Dental management of children with cancer, Pediatr. Ann. 17(11):715-725, 1987.
Blatt, J., and Lee, P.A.: Neuroblastoma associated with adrenocortical defects, Pediatrics 82(5):790-792, 1988.

Blecke, C.: Home chemotherapy safety procedures, Oncol. Nurs. Forum 16(5):719-721, 1989.

Broberg, D.J., and Bernstein, B.D.: Candy as a scapegoat in the prevention of food aversions in children receiving chemotherapy, Cancer 60(9):2344-2347, 1987.

Brodeur, G.M., and others: International criteria for diagnosis, staging, and response to treatment in patients with neuroblastoma, J. Clin. Oncol. 6(12):1874-1881, 1988.

Brunell, P.A., and others: Varicella-like illness caused by live varicella vaccine in children with acute lymphocytic leukemia, Pediatrics 79(6):922-927, 1987.

Cancer facts and figures, 1990, New York, 1990, American Cancer Society.

Caul, O., and Roome, A.: Viral infection. In Oakhill, A.: The supportive care of the child with cancer, Boston, 1988, Butterworth & Co.

Cimprich, B.: Symptom management: constipation, Cancer Nurs. 8(suppl.1):39-43, 1985.

Cohn, S.L.: Neuroblastoma update: prognostic factors, J. Assoc. Pediatr. Oncol. Nurs. 5:28-29, 1988.

Coppes, M.J., and others: Bilateral Wilms' tumor: long-term survival and some epidemiological features, J. Clin. Oncol. 7(3):310-315, 1989.

Craig, J.B., and Powell, B.L.: Review: the management of nausea and vomiting in clinical oncology, Am. J. Med. Sci. 29(1):34-44, 1987.

D'Angio, G.J., and others: Wilms' tumor. In Pizzo, P.A., and Poplack, D.G.: Principles and practice of pediatric oncology, Philadelphia, 1989, J.B. Lippincott Co.

Darbyshire, P.J.: Bacterial infections. In Oakhill, A.: The supportive care of the child with cancer, Boston, 1988, Butterworth & Co.

Deasy-Spinetta, P., Spinetta, J.J., and Oxman, J.B.: The relationship between learning deficits and social adaptation in children with leukemia, J. Psychosoc. Oncol. 6(3/4):109-121, 1988.

DeVitta, V.: Cancer: principles of oncology, Philadelphia, 1989, J.B. Lippincott Co.

Dolgin, M.J., and others: Anticipatory nausea and vomiting in pediatric cancer patients, Pediatrics 75(3):547-552, 1985.

Dolgin, M.J., and others: Behavioral distress in pediatric patients with cancer receiving chemotherapy, Pediatrics 84(1):103-110, 1989.

Donaldson, S.S., and Egbert, P.R.: Retinoblastoma. In Pizzo, P.A., and Poplack, D.G.: Principles and practice of pediatric oncology, Philadelphia, 1989, J.B. Lippincott Co.

Donaldson, S.S., and Smith, L.M.: Retinoblastoma: biology, presentation, and current management, Oncology 3(4):45-51, 1989.

Drakeford, J.D.: Nutrition. In Oakhill, A.: The supportive care of the child with cancer, Boston, 1988, Butterworth & Co.

Dryja, T.: Genetics of retinoblastoma, Curr. Opin. Pediatr. 1:413-420, 1989.

Evans, W.E., and others: Clinical pharmacology of cancer chemotherapy in children, Pediatr. Clin. North Am. 36(5):1199, 1989.

Faro, V.: Superior vena cava syndrome in pediatric oncology, J. Assoc. Pediatr. Oncol. Nurs. 4(3/4):32-35, 1987.

Feldman, S., and Lott, L.: Varicella in children with cancer: impact of antiviral therapy and prophylaxis, Pediatrics 80(4):465-472, 1987.

Few, B.J.: MCN pharmacopoeia: nabilone as an antiemetic for children undergoing chemotherapy, MCN 13:209, 1988.

Finklestein, J.Z.: Neuroblastoma: the challange and frustration, Hematol. Oncol. Clin. North Am. 1(4):675-694, 1987.

Finlay, J.L., and others: Progress in the management of childhood brain tumors, Hematol. Oncol. Clin. North Am. 1(4):753-776, 1987.

Fobair, P., and others: Psychosocial problems among survivors of Hodgkin's disease, J. Clin. Oncol. 4:805-814, 1986.

Forlini, J., Morin, D.M., and Treacy, S.: Painless peds procedures, Am. J. Nurs. 87(3):321-323, 1987.

Gale, R.P.: The management of acute leukemias, Clin. Adv. Oncol. Nurs. 1(3):1-9, 1989.

Ganick, D.J.: Wilms' tumor, Hematol. Oncol. Clin. North Am. 1(4):695-719, 1987.

Gershon, A.: Live attenuated varicella vaccine, J. Pediatr. 110(1):154-156, 1987.

Grabowski, E.F., and Abramson, D.H.: Intraocular and extraocular retinoblastoma, Hematol. Oncol. Clin. North Am. 1(4):721-735, 1987.

Greenbaum, B.F., and Herman, J.H.: Transfusion therapy in pediatric oncology, Pediatr. Ann. 17(11):687-693, 1988.

Greenberg, H.S., Kazak, A.E., and Meadows, A.T.: Psychologic functioning in 8- to 16-year-old cancer survivors and their parents, J. Pediatr. 114(3):488-493, 1989.

Grundy, P., and others: Prognostic factors for children with recurrent Wilms' tumor: results from the second and third national Wilms' tumor study, J. Clin. Oncol. 7(5):638-647, 1989.

Guidelines for the pediatric cancer center and role of such centers in diagnosis and treatment, Pediatrics 77(6):916-917, 1986.

Halperin, E.C.: Radiation therapy. In Hockenberry, M.J., and Coody, D.K.: Pediatric oncology and hematology: perspectives on care, St. Louis, 1986, Mosby–Year Book, Inc.

Hammond, E.: Anaphylactic reactions to chemotherapeutic agents, J. Assoc. Pediatr. Oncol. Nurs. 5(3):16-19, 1988.

Happ, M.: Life threatening hemorrhage in children with cancer, J. Assoc. Pediatr. Oncol. Nurs. 4(3/4):36-40, 1987.

Hayashi, Y., and others: Chromosome findings and prognosis in 15 patients with neuroblastoma found by VMA mass screening, J. Pediatr. 112(4):567-571, 1988.

Hayashi, Y., and others: Similar chromosomal patterns and lack of N-myc gene amplication in localized and IV-S stage neuroblastomas in infants, Med. Pediatr. Oncol. 17:111-115, 1989.

Hayes, F.A., and Smith, E.I.: Neuroblastoma. In Pizzo, P.A., and Poplack, D.G.: Principles and practice of pediatric oncology, Philadelphia, 1989, J.B. Lippincott Co.

Heideman, R.L., and others: Tumors of the central nervous system. In Pizzo, P.A., and Poplack, D.G.: Principles and practice of pediatric oncology, Philadelphia, 1989, J.B. Lippincott Co.

Hess, G., and Walson, P.: Seizures secondary to oral viscous lidocaine, Ann. Emerg. Med. 17:725-727, 1988.

Hockenberry, M.J.: Relaxation techniques in children with cancer: the nurse's role, J. Pediatr. Oncol. Nurs. 5(1/2):7-11, 1988.

Hockenberry, M.J., and Lane, B.: Limb salvage procedures in children with osteosarcoma, Cancer Nurs. 11(1):2-8, 1988.

Juhlin, L., and Evers, H.: EMLA: a new topical anesthetic, Adv. Dermatol. 5:75-92, 1990.

Kadota, R.P., and others: Brain tumors in children, J. Pediatr. 114(4, pt. 1):511-519, 1989.

Kelleher, J.: Bone marrow transplantation. In Hockenberry, M.J., and Coody, D.K.: Pediatric oncology and hematology: perspectives on care, St. Louis, 1986, Mosby–Year Book, Inc.

Koocher, G.P., and O'Malley, J.E.: The Damocles syndrome: psychosocial consequences of surviving cancer, New York, 1981, McGraw-Hill Book Co.

Kris, M.G., and others: Antiemetic control and prevention of side effects of anticancer therapy with lorazepam or diphenhydramine when used in combination with metoclopramide plus dexamethesone, a double blind randomized trial, Cancer 60(11):2816-2822, 1987.

Lansky, S., List, M, and Ritter-Stern, C.: Psychosocial consequences of cure, Cancer 58:529-533, 1986.

Lansky, S.B., and others: Late effects: psychosocial, Clin. Oncol. 4(2):239-246, 1985.

Li, F.P., and others: Heritable fraction of unilateral Wilms' tumor, Pediatrics 81(1):147-149, 1988.

Lichter, I.: Communication in cancer care, New York, 1987, Churchill Livingstone, Inc.

Lovejoy, N.C., and Halliburton, P.: Pediatric tumor markers, J. Pediatr. Nurs. 4(5):357-369, 1989.

Magrath, I.T.: Malignant non-Hodgkin's lymphomas in children, Hematol. Oncol. Clin. North Am. 1(4):577-602, 1987.

Magrath, I.T.: Malignant non-Hodgkin lymphomas. In Pizzo, P.A., and Poplack, D.G.: Principles and practice of pediatric oncology, Philadelphia, 1989, J.B. Lippincott Co.

Marshall, G., and others: Antiemetic therapy for chemotherapy-induced vomiting: metoclopramide, benztropine, dexamethasone, and lorazepam regimen compared with chlorpromazine alone, J. Pediatr. 115:156-160, 1989.

Mauer, A.M.: Screening for neuroblastoma, J. Pediatr. 112(4):576-577, 1988.

Meadows, A.T., and others: Similar efficacy of 6 and 18 months of therapy with four drugs (COMP) for localized non-Hodgkin's lymphoma of children: a report from the Children's Cancer Study Group, J. Clin. Oncol. 17(1):92-99, 1989.

Melzack, R., Guite, S., and Gonshor, A.: Relief of dental pain by ice massage of the hand, Can. Med. Assoc. J. 122:189-191, 1980.

Meyers, P.: Malignant bone tumors in children: osteosarcoma, Hematol. Oncol. Clin. North Am 1(4):655-665, 1987.

Miller, D.S.: Frequency and environmental epidemiology of childhood cancer. In Pizzo, P.A., and Poplack, D.G.: Principles and practice of pediatric oncology, Philadelphia, 1989, J.B. Lippincott Co.

Mioduszewski, J., and Zarbo, A.G.: Ambulatory infusion pumps: a practical view at an alternative approach, Semin. Oncol. Nurs. 3(2):106-111, 1987.

Mitchell, C.D.: Management of infections in the neutropenic child with cancer, Pediatr. Ann. 17(11):677-686, 1988.

Moshang, Jr., T., and Lee, M.M.: Late effects: disorders of growth and sexual maturation associated with the treatment of childhood cancer, J. Assoc. Pediatr. Oncol. Nurs. 5(4):14-19, 1988.

Moss, J.: Alfred Knudson, M.D. works to unravel the cancer puzzle, Cope 3(5):25-26, 1989.

Mulhern, R.K., and others: Social competence and behavioral adjustment of children who are long-term survivors of cancer, Pediatrics 83(1):18-25, 1989.

Mulvihill, J.: Clinical genetics of pediatric nursing. In Pizzo, P.A., and Poplack, D.G.: Principles and practice of pediatric oncology, Philadelphia, 1989, J.B. Lippincott Co.

Musgrave, S., Dickerman, J.D., and Land, V.J.: Second or subsequent remission with a disease-free survival of 5 years or longer in acute lymphocytic leukemia of childhood: results of a national survey, Pediatrics 77(5):765-769, 1986.

Neglia, J.P., and Robison, L.L.: Epidemiology of the childhood acute leukemias, Pediatr. Clin. North Am. 35(4):675-692, 1988.

Niehaus, C.S., and others: Oral complications in children during cancer therapy, Cancer Nurs. 10(1):15-20, 1987.

Oncology Nursing Society: Cancer chemotherapy guidelines, Pittsburgh, 1988, The Society.

Patterson, K.L., and Klopovich, P.: Metabolic emergencies in pediatric oncology: the acute tumor lysis syndrome, J. Assoc. Pediatr. Oncol. Nurs. 4(3/4):19-24, 1987.

Perin, G., and Frase, D.: Development of a program using general anesthesia for invasive procedures in a pediatric outpatient setting, J. Assoc. Pediatr. Oncol. Nurs. 3(4):8-10, 1985.

Poland, J.: Comparing Moi-Stir to lemon-glycerin swabs, Am. J. Nurs. 87(4):422-424, 1987.

Poplack, D.G.: Acute lymphoblastic leukemia. In Pizzo, P.A., and Poplack, D.G.: Principles and practice of pediatric oncology, Philadelphia, 1989, J.B. Lippincott Co.

Preisler, H.: Acute nonlymphocytic leukemias, Issues Oncol. 4(3):1, 6-7, 1987.

Rahr, V.: Giving intrathecal drugs, Am. J. Nurs. 86(7):829-831, 1986.

Raney, R.B., and others: Rhabdomyosarcoma and the undifferentiated sarcomas. In Pizzo, P.A., and Poplack, D.G.: Principles and practice of pediatric oncology, Philadelphia, 1989, J.B. Lippincott Co.

Raymond, C.A.: Childhood cancers' improved survival rates can exact a price in late effects of therapy, JAMA 260(23):3400-3401, 1988.

Rogers, A.G.: Use of amitriptyline (Elavil) for phantom limb pain in younger children, J. Pain Symptom Manag. 4(2):96, 1989.

Rubin, C.M.: Chromosomal abnormalities in pediatric malignancies, J. Assoc. Pediatr. Oncol. Nurs. 5(1/2):33, 1988.

Ruymann, F.B.: Rhabdomyosarcoma in children and adolescents: a review, Hematol. Oncol. Clin. North Am. 1(4):621-654, 1987.

Samaranayake, L.P., and others: The effect of chlorhexidine and benzydamine mouthwashes on mucositis induced therapeutic irradiation, Clin. Radiol. 39:291-294, 1988.

Sansievero, G.E., and Murray, S.A.: Safe management of chemotherapy at home, Oncol. Nurs. Forum 16(5):711-713, 1989.

Shenep, J.L., and others: Efficacy of oral sucralfate suspension in prevention and treatment of chemotherapy-induced mucositis, J. Pediatr. 113:758-763, 1988.

Simon, M.A.: Limb salvage for osteosarcoma, J. Bone Joint Surg. 70A:307-310, 1988.

Sridhar, K.S., and Donnelly, E.: Combination antiemetics for cisplatin chemotherapy, Cancer 61:1508-1517, 1988.

Steinherz, P.G.: Acute lymphoblastic leukemia of childhood, Hematol. Oncol. Clin. North Am. 1(4):549-575, 1987.

Stine, G.J.: The new human genetics, Dubuque, IA, 1989, Wm. C. Brown Group.

Stine, K.C., and others: Systemic doxorubicin and intraarterial cisplatin preoperative chemotherapy plus postoperative adjuvant chemotherapy in patients with osteosarcoma, Cancer 63:848-853, 1989.

Sullivan, M.P.: Hodgkin's disease in children, Hematol. Oncol. Clin. North Am. 1(4):603-620, 1987.

Tuchman, M., and others: Feasibility study for neonatal neuroblastoma screening in the United States, Med. Pediatr. Oncol. 17:258-264, 1989.

Tucker, M.A., and others: Risk of second cancers after treatment for Hodgkin's disease, N. Engl. J. Med. 318(2):76-81, 1988.

U.S. Department of Health and Human Services: Recommendations of the immunization practices advisory committee: general recommendations on immunization, Centers for Disease Control, MMWR 38(13):205-227, 1989.

van Eys, J., editor: The truly cured child: the new challenge in pediatric cancer care, Baltimore, 1977, University Park Press.

van Eys, J., and others: Treatment intensity and outcome for children with acute lymphocytic leukemia of standard risk, Cancer 63(8):1466-1471, 1989.

Vega, R.A., and others: Bone marrow transplantation in the treatment of children with cancer: current status, Hematol. Oncol. Clin. North Am. 1(4):777-800, 1987.

Viscoli, C.: Aspects of infections in children with cancer, Recent Results Cancer Res. 108:71-81, 1988.

Wagner, H.P.: Supportive care in pediatric oncology, Recent Results Cancer Res. 108:301-305, 1988.

Walker, R., and Allen, J.: Pediatric brain tumors, Pediatr. Ann. 12(5):383-391, 1983.

Waskerwitz, M.J., and Fergusson, J.H.: Late effects of cancer treatment in children. In Hockenberry, M.J., and Coody, D.K.: Pediatric oncology and hematology: perspectives on care, St. Louis, 1986, Mosby–Year Book, Inc.

Wasserman, A., and others: The psychological status of survivors of childhood/adolescent Hodgkin's disease, Am. J. Dis. Child. 141:626-631, 1987.

Weinberg, K.I., and Parkman, R.: Interface between immunodeficiency and pediatric cancer. In Pizzo, P.A., and Poplack, D.G.: Principles and practice of pediatric oncology, Philadelphia, 1989, J.B. Lippincott Co.

Weinstock, M.A., and others: Nonfamilial cutaneous melanoma incidence in women associated with sun exposure before 20 years of age, Pediatrics 84(2):199-204, 1989.

Wiley, F.M., and House, K.U.: Bone marrow transplant in children, Semin. Oncol. Nurs. 4(1):31-40, 1988.

Williams, C.J., and others: Comparison of starting antiemetic treatment 24 hours before or concurrently with cytotoxic chemotherapy, Br. Med. J. 298:430-431, 1989.

Williams, M.L., and Sagebiel, R.W.: Sunburns, melanoma, and the pediatrician, Pediatrics 84(2):381-382, 1989.

Woods, W.G., and Tuchman, M.: Neuroblastoma: the case for screening infants in North America, Pediatrics 79(6):869-873, 1987.

World of Children's Hospital: Autologous transplant program boosts survival rates for children with leukemia and other cancers, World of Children's Hospital, Los Angeles, June 1-11, 1988.

Yasko, J.M.: Holistic management of nausea and vomiting caused by chemotherapy, Top. Clin. Nurs. 7(1):26-38, 1985.

Yeager, A.M.: Bone marrow transplantation in children, Pediatr. Ann. 17(11):694-714, 1988.

Zaia, J.A., and Forman, S.J.: Management of the bone marrow transplant recipient. In Parillo, J.e., and Masur, H., editors: The critically ill immunosuppressed patient: diagnosis and management, Rockville, MD, 1987, Aspen Systems Corp.

Zeltzer, L.K., Jay, S.M., and Fisher, D.M.: The management of pain associated with pediatric procedures, Pediatr. Clin. North Am. 36(4):941-964, 1989.

BIBLIOGRAPHY

Cancer in Children

Aaronson, N.K., and Beckmann, J.H.: The quality of life of cancer patients, New York, 1987, Raven Press.

Association of Pediatric Oncology Nurses: Scope of practice, J. Assoc. Pediatr. Oncol. Nurs. 7(1):22-23, 1990.

Baker, H.W.: Classic in oncology: needle aspiration biopsy; an introduction, CA 36(2):69-70, 1986.

Ceccarelli, C., and others: Thyroid cancer in children and adolescents, Surgery 104:1143-1148, 1988.

Chandra, R.K.: Nutrition and immunity—basic considerations, part 1, Contemp. Nutr. 11(11), 1986.

Chandra, R.K.: Nutrition and immunity—basic considerations, part 2, Contemp. Nutr. 11(12), 1986.

Civin, C.I., Vogel, V.G., and Strauss, L.C.: Tumor markers and their significance in adolescent oncology. In Tebbi, C.K., editor: Major topics in adolescent oncology, New York, 1987, Futura Publishing Co., Inc.

Crom, D.B., and others: Malignancy in the neonate, Med. Pediatr. Oncol. 17:101-104, 1989.

DiMario, F.J., and Packer, R.J.: Acute mental status changes in children with systemic cancer, Pediatrics 85(3):353-360, 1990.

Dowell, R.E., Copeland, D.R., and van Eys, J., editors: The child with cancer in the community, Springfield, Ill., 1988, Charles C Thomas, Publisher.

Faulkenberry, J.E., and others: Cancer prevention and early detection, Fam. Community Health 10(3):9-17, 1987.

Fones, M.: Patient history plays an important role in care, Cope 3(4):44, 1989.

Frank-Stromberg, M., and others: Carcinogens: are some risks acceptable? Am. J. Nurs. 86(7):814-817, 1986.

Hockenberry, M.J., and Coody, D.K.: Pediatric oncology and hematology: perspectives on care, St. Louis, 1986, Mosby–Year Book, Inc.

Johnson, C.C.: The epidemiology of cancer, Fam. Community Health 10(3):1-7, 1987.

Marino, L.B., and Levy, S.M.: Primary and secondary prevention of cancer in children and adolescents: current status and issues, Pediatr. Clin. North Am. 33(4):975-993, 1986.

Markman, M.: The ethical dilemma of phase 1 clinical trials, CA 36(6):367-369, 1986.

Martin, H.E., and Ellis, E.B.: Classics in oncology: biopsy by needle puncture and aspiration, CA 36(2):71-82, 1986.

Miller, D.S.: Intravenous immune globulin for treating primary immunodeficiency disease, MCN 12(4):244-248, 1987.

Outcome standards of pediatric oncology nursing practice, J. Assoc. Pediatr. Oncol. Nurs. 7(1):24-30, 1990.

Pizzo, P.A.: Childhood cancer: advances in the past decade, J. Assoc. Pediatr. Oncol. Nurs. 4(1/2):34-35, 1987.

Pizzo, P.A., and Poplack, D.G.: Principles and practice of pediatric oncology, Philadelphia, 1989, J.B. Lippincott Co.

Plaschkes, J.: Surgical supportive care in pediatric oncology, Recent Results Cancer Res. 108:148-153, 1988.

Souba, W.W., and Copeland, E.M., III: Hyperalimentation in cancer, CA 39(2):105-114, 1989.

Tebbi, C.K., editor: Major topics in adolescent oncology, New York, 1987, Futura Publishing Co., Inc.

Vaz, R.M., and others: Clinical and laboratory observations, evaluations of a testicular cancer curriculum for adolescents, J. Pediatr. 114(1):150-153, 1989.

Chemotherapy

Balis, F.: The pharmacology of antineoplastic agents in children. In Poplack, D.G., and others, editors: The role of pharmacology in pediatric oncology, Boston, 1987, Martinus Nijhoff, Publishing.

Balis, F.M.: Pharmacologic considerations in the treatment of acute lymphoblastic leukemia, Pediatr. Clin. North Am. 35(4):835-852, 1988.

Betcher, D.L., and Burnham, N.: Leucovorin, J. Assoc. Pediatr. Oncol. Nurs. 6(3):102-104, 1989.

Chabner, B.A., Browne, M.J., and Boyd, M.R.: The future for chemotherapy, Cancer Nurs. 10(suppl. 1):40-46, 1987.

Dolgin, M.J., and Katz, E.R.: Conditioned aversion in pediatric cancer patients receiving chemotherapy, J. Dev. Behav. Pediatr. 9(2):82-85, 1988.

Fischer R.G.: Handling antineoplastic drugs, Pediatr. Nurs. 12(1):59, 1986.

Fischetti, L.F.: Interaction between nonsteroidal anti-inflammatory drugs and high-dose methotrexate: a literature review, J. Assoc. Pediatr. Oncol. Nurs. 7(1):14-16, 1990.

Garvey, E.C.: Current and future nursing issues in the home administration of chemotherapy, Semin. Oncol. Nurs. 3(2):142-147, 1987.

Hagle, M.E.: Implantable devices for chemotherapy: access and delivery, Semin. Oncol. Nurs. 3(2):96-105, 1987.

Hayes, J.D.: Economics of chemotherapy, Semin. Oncol. Nurs. 3(2):148-153, 1987.

Hughes, C.B.: Giving cancer drugs. IV. Some guidelines, Am. J. Nurs. 86(1):34-38, 1986.

Krakoff, I.: Cancer chemotherapeutic agents, CA 37(2):93-105, 1987.

Krementz, E.T.: Regional perfusion, current sophistication, what next? Cancer 57:416-432, 1986.

LeBaron, S., and others: Chemotherapy side effects in pediatric oncology patients: drugs, age, and sex as risk factors, Med. Pediatr. Oncol. 16(4):263-268, 1988.

Lind, J., and Bush, N.J.: Nursing's role in chemotherapy administration, Semin. Oncol. Nurs. 3(2):83-86, 1987.

McNamara, J., and Komp, D.M.: Interleukin-2: a major lymphokine, J. Pediatr. 114(3):420-421, 1989.

Nishikawa, A., and others: Acute monocytic leukemia in children: response to VP-16-213 as a single agent, Cancer 60(9):2146-2149, 1987.

Ozols, R.F.: Intraperitoneal chemotherapy, Mediguide Oncol. 5(4):1-5, 1986.

Pasut, B.: Home administration of medications in pediatric oncology patients: use of the Travenol infusor, J. Assoc. Pediatr. Oncol. Nurs. 6(4):139-142, 1989.

Rogers, B., and Emmett, E.A.: Handling antineoplastic agents: urine mutageneity in nurses, Image J. Nurs. Scho. 19(3):108-113, 1987.

Taylor, B., and others: Recombinant interleukin-2 in the treatment of refractory solid tumors in pediatric oncology patients: nursing implications, J. Assoc. Pediatr. Oncol. Nurs. 6(3):98-101, 1989.

Bone Marrow Transplantation

Anasetti, C.: Effect of HLA compatibility on engraftment of bone marrow transplants in patients with leukemia or lymphoma, N. Engl. J. Med. 320(4):197-204, 1989.

Atkins, D.M., and Patenaude, A.F.: Psychosocial preparation and follow-up for pediatric BMT patients, Am. J. Orthopsychiatry 57(2):246-252, 1987.

Bracken, J.D., and DeCuir-Whalley, S.: Continuous bladder irrigation for children receiving high-dose cyclophosphamide before bone marrow transplantation, J. Assoc. Pediatr. Oncol. Nurs. 6(3):105-107, 1989.

Brochstein, J.A.: Critical care issues in BMT, Crit. Care Clin. 4(1):147-166, 1988.

Corcoran-Buchsel, P.: Long term complications of allogeneic bone marrow transplantation: nursing implications, Oncol. Nurs. Forum 13(6):61-70, 1986.

Corcoran-Buchsel, P., and Parchem, C.: Ambulation care of the bone marrow transplant patient, Semin. Oncol. Nurs. 4(1):41-46, 1988.

Durbin, M.: Bone marrow transplantation: economic, ethical, and social issues, Pediatrics 82(5):774-783, 1988.

Engelhard, D., Marks, M.I., and Good, R.A.: Infections in bone marrow transplant recipients, J. Pediatr. 108(3):335-346, 1986.

Freedman, S.E.: An overview of bone marrow transplant, Semin. Oncol. Nurs. 4(1):55-59, 1988.

Freund, B.L., and Siegal, K.: Problems in transition following bone marrow transplantation: psychosocial aspects, Am. J. Orthopsychiatry 56(2):244-252, 1986.

Gottlieb, S.E., and Portnoy, S.: The role of play in a pediatric bone marrow transplantation unit, Child. Health Care 16(3):177-181, 1988.

Hann, I.M.: Bone marrow transplantation, Curr. Opin. Pediatr. 2:143-150, 1990.

Hare, J., Skinner, D., and Kliewer, D.: Family systems approach to pediatric bone marrow transplantation, Child. Health Care 18(1):30-36, 1989.

Kaleita, T.A., and others: Normal neurodevelopment in four young children treated with bone marrow transplantation for acute leukemia or aplastic anemia, Pediatrics 93(5):753-757, 1989.

Kinrade, L.: Preparation of a sibling donor for bone marrow harvest procedure, Cancer Nurs. 10(2):77-81, 1987.

McConn, R.: Skin changes following bone marrow transplantation, Cancer Nurs. 10(2):82-84, 1987.

McCord, D.J., and Hathaway, G.: Autologous bone marrow transplantation in childhood cancer, Pediatr. Nurs. 14(6):454-456, 1988.

Nims, J.W., and Strom, S.: Late complications of bone marrow transplant recipients: nursing care issues, Semin. Oncol. Nurs. 4(1):47-54, 1988.

O'Quin, J., and Moravel, C.: The critically ill BMT patient, Semin. Oncol. Nurs. 4(1):25-30, 1988.

Rubin, C.M., and others: Bone marrow transplantation for children with acute leukemia and Down's syndrome, Pediatrics 78(4):688-691, 1986.

Schryber, S., and others: Autologous bone marrow transplantation, Oncol. Nurs. Forum 14(4):74-78, 1987.

Stutzer, C.A.: Work-related stresses of pediatric bone marrow transplant nurses, J. Assoc. Pediatr. Oncol. Nurs. 6(3):70-78, 1989.

Thomas, E.D.: Bone marrow transplantation, CA 37(5):291-301, 1987.

Thomas, E.D.: The future of marrow transplantation, Semin. Oncol. Nurs. 4(1):74-78, 1988.

Trigg, M.E.: Bone marrow transplantation for treatment of leukemia in children, Pediatr. Clin. North Am. 35(4):933-948, 1988.

Truog, A.W., and Wozniak, S.P.: Cyclosporine-A as prevention for graft-versus-host disease in pediatric patients undergoing bone marrow transplants, Oncol. Nurs. Forum 17(1):39-44, 1990.

Long-Term Sequelae of Treatment

D'Angio, G.: Cure is not enough: late consequences associated with radiation treatment, J. Assoc. Pediatr. Oncol. Nurs. 5(4):20-23, 1988.

Fergusson, J., Ruccione, K., and Hobbie, W.L.: The effects of the treatment for cancer in childhood growth and development, J. Assoc. Pediatr. Oncol. Nurs. 3(4):13-21, 1986.

Gallagher, J.A.: Acute lymphocytic leukemia treatment: effects on learning, J. Pediatr. Health Care 3(5):257-258, 1989.

Green, D.M.: Long term complications of therapy for cancer in childhood and adolescence, Baltimore, 1989, Johns Hopkins University Press.

Hobbie, W.L.: The role of the pediatric nurse specialist in a follow-up clinic for long term survivors of childhood cancer, J. Assoc. Pediatr. Oncol. Nurs. 3(4):9-12, 1986.

Hoffman, B.: Cancer survivors at work: job problems and illegal discrimination, Oncol. Nurs. Forum 16(1):39-42, 1989.

Hutter, J.: Late effects of children with cancer, Am. J. Dis. Child. 140(1):17-19, 1986.

McCalla, J.L.: A multidisciplinary approach to identification and remedial intervention for adverse late effects of cancer therapy, Nurs. Clin. North Am. 20(1):117-130, 1985.

Meadows, A.T.: Second malignant neoplasms in childhood cancer survivors, J. Assoc. Pediatr. Oncol. Nurs. 6(1):7-11, 1989.

Moore, I.M., Kramer, J., and Ablin, A.: Late effects of central nervous system prophylactic leukemia therapy on cognitive functioning, Oncol. Nurs. Forum 13(4):45-51, 1986.

Oberfield, S.E., and others: Long-term endocrine sequelae after treatment of medulloblastoma: a prospective study of growth and thyroid function, J. Pediatr. 108(2):219-223, 1986.

Ochs, J., and Mulhern, R.K.: Late effects of antileukemic treatment, Pediatr. Clin. North Am. 35(4):815-834, 1988.

Peckham, V.C.: Learning disorders associated with the treatment of cancer in childhood, J. Assoc. Pediatr. Oncol. Nurs. 5(4):10-13, 1988.

Peckham, V.C., and others: Educational late effects in long-term survivors of childhood acute lymphocytic leukemia, Pediatrics 81(1):127-133, 1988.

Robison, L.L.: Late effects in successfully treated children with cancer, Curr. Concepts Oncol. 8(4):18-23, 1986.

Takaue, Y., and others: Second malignant neoplasms in treated Hodgkin's disease, Am. J. Dis. Child. 140(1):49-51, 1986.

Vanderwal, R., Nims, J., and Davies, B.: Bone marrow transplantation in children: nursing management of late effects, Cancer Nurs. 11(3):132-143, 1988.

Symptom Management*

Adams, J.: Pediatric pain assessment: trends and research directions, J. Assoc. Pediatr. Oncol. Nurs. 6(3):79-85, 1989.

Albano, E.A., and Pizzo, P.A.: Infectious complications in childhood acute leukemias, Pediatr. Clin. North Am. 35(4):873-902, 1988.

Babani, L., and others: Comprehensive assessment of long-term therapeutic adherence and recurrent pain in children and adolescents, Educ. Treat. Child. 10(1):7-18, 1987.

Barbour, L.A., McGuire, D.B., and Kirchhoff, K.T.: Nonanalgesic methods of pain control used by cancer outpatients, Oncol. Nurs. Forum 13(6):56-60, 1986.

Bendorf, K., and Meehan, J.: Home parenteral nutrition for the child with cancer, Issues Compr. Pediatr. Nurs. 12(2/3):171-186, 1989.

Beyer, J.E. and Levin, C.R.: Issues and advances in pain control in children, Nurs. Clin. North Am. 22(3):661-676, 1987.

Brescia, F.J.: An overview of pain and symptom management in advanced cancer, J. Pain Symptom Manag. 2(suppl. 2):S7-S11, 1988.

Broome, M.E.: Implementation of a clinical study of a pain management program for pediatric oncology patients, J. Pediatr. Nurs. 4(1):54-56, 1989.

Carl, W.: Oral and dental care of the adolescent oncology patient. In Tebbi, C.K., editor: Major topics in adolescent oncology, New York, 1987, Futura Publishing Co., Inc.

*See Chapter 26 for additional references on pain.

Cleeland, C.S.: Nonpharmacological management of cancer pain, J. Pain Symptom Manag. 2(suppl. 2):S23-S28, 1987.
Cotanch, P.H., Harrison, M., and Roberts, J.: Hypnosis as an intervention for pain control, Nurs. Clin. North Am. 22(3):699-704, 1987.
Cotanch, P.H., and Strum, S.: Progressive muscle relaxation as antiemetic therapy for cancer patients, Oncol. Nurs. Forum 14(1):33-37, 1987.
Cuzzell, J.Z., and Willey, T.: Wound care forum: pressure relief perennials, Am. J. Nurs. 87(9):1157-1159, 1987.
D'Agostino, N.S.: Managing nutrition problems in advanced cancer, Am. J. Nurs. 89(1):50-56, 1989.
Dorrepaal, K.L., Aaronson, N.K., and van Dam, F.: Pain experience and pain management among hospitalized cancer patients, Cancer 63:593-598, 1989.
Dothage, J.A., Arndt, C., and Miser, A.W.: Use of a continuous intravenous morphine infusion for pain control in an infant with terminal malignancy, J. Assoc. Pediatr. Oncol. Nurs. 3(4):22-24, 1986.
Eland, J.M.: Pharmacologic management of acute and chronic pediatric pain, Issues Compr. Pediatr. Nurs. 11:93-111, 1988.
Foley, K.M.: Cancer pain syndromes, J. Pain Symptom Manag. 2(suppl. 2):S13-S17, 1988.
Frick, S.B., and others: Chemotherapy-associated nausea and vomiting in pediatric oncology patients, Cancer Nurs. 11(2):118-124, 1988.
Hamner, S.B., and Miles, M.S.: Coping strategies in children with cancer undergoing bone marrow aspirations, J. Assoc. Pediatr. Oncol. Nurs. 5(3):11-15, 1988.
Harrison, M., and Cotanch, P.H.: Pain: advances and issues in critical care, Nurs. Clin. North Am. 22(3):691-697, 1987.
Higby, D.J.: Supportive care of the adolescent oncology patient: transfusions, pain, and emesis. In Tebbi, C.K., editor: Major topics in adolescent oncology, New York, 1987, Futura Publishing Co., Inc.
Iazzetti, L.: The air-fluidized bed: use in pediatrics, Issues Compr. Pediatr. Nurs. 10:195-198, 1987.
Kanner, R.M.: Pharmacological management of pain and symptom control in cancer, J. Pain Symptom Manag. 2(suppl. 2):S19-S22, 1987.
Kinrade, L.C.: Typhlitis: a complication of neutropenia, Pediatr. Nurs. 14(4):291-295, 1988.
Lawson, K.: Oral-dental concerns of the pediatric oncology patient, Issues Compr. Pediatr. Nurs. 12(2/3):199-206, 1989.
Lever, S.A., Dupuis, L.L., and Chan, H.S.L.: Comparative evaluation of benzydamine oral rinse in children with antineoplastic-induced stomatitis, Drug Intell. Clin. Pharm. 21:359-361, 1987.
Levick, S., and others: Naproxen sodium in treatment of bone pain due to metastatic cancer, Pain 35:253-258, 1988.
Mason, C.A.: Septic shock, J. Assoc. Pediatr. Oncol. Nurs. 4(3/4):25-31, 1987.
Morrow, G.R.: Chemotherapy-related nausea and vomiting: etiology and management, CA 39(2):89-104, 1989.
Novotny, M.P.: Body image changes in amputee children: how nursing theory can make a difference, J. Assoc. Pediatr. Oncol. Nurs. 3(2):8-13, 1986.
Ohanian, N.A.: Informational needs of children and adolescents with cancer, J. Assoc. Pediatr. Oncol. Nurs. 6(3):94-97, 1989.
Pack, B., and Maria, B.L.: Neurological emergencies in pediatric oncology, J. Assoc. Pediatr. Oncol. 4(3/4):8-18, 1987.
Redd, W.H., and others: Cognitive/attentional distraction in the control of conditioned nausea in pediatric cancer patients receiving chemotherapy, J. Consult. Clin. Psychol. 55(3):391-395, 1987.
Rhodes, V.A., and others: Patterns of nausea, vomiting, and distress in patients receiving antineoplastic drug protocols, Oncol. Nurs. Forum 14(4):35-44, 1987.
Robertson, Jr., W.W.: Orthopedic interventions for problems associated with the treatment of cancer in childhood, J. Assoc. Pediatr. Oncol. Nurs. 6(1):12-14, 1989.
Schechter, N.L., Altman, A., and Weisman, S., editors: Report of the Consensus Conference on the Management of Pain in Childhood Cancer, Pediatrics 86(5, suppl.): 813-834, 1990.
A short course on the management of cancer pain, J. Pain Symptom Manag. 2(suppl. 2), 1987.
Triozzi, P.L., and Laszlo, J.: Optimum management of nausea and vomiting in cancer chemotherapy, Drugs 34(1):136-149, 1987.
van Hoff, J., and Olszewski, D.: Lorazepam for the control of chemotherapy-related nausea and vomiting in children, J. Pediatr. 113(1, pt. 1):146-149, 1988.
Wickham, R.: Managing chemotherapy-related nausea and vomiting: the state of the art, Oncol. Nurs. Forum 16(4):563-574, 1989.
Wolfe, V.V., and others: Nurses' perception of stress reduction techniques in pediatric oncology, J. Assoc. Pediatr. Oncol. Nurs. 4(1/2):9-13, 1987.
Yasko, J.M.: Control of anticipatory nausea and vomiting, Issues Oncol. Nurs. 4(3):4-5, 7, 1987.
Yasko, J.M., and Greene, P.: Coping with problems related to cancer and cancer treatment, CA 37(2):106-125, 1987.
Young, J.A., Eslinger, P., and Galloway, M.: Radiation treatment for the child with cancer, Issues Compr. Pediatr. Nurs. 12(2/3):159-170, 1989.

Leukemias/Lymphomas

Altman, A.J.: Chronic leukemias of children, Pediatr. Clin. North Am. 35(4):765-788, 1988.
Champlin, R.: Acute myelogenous leukemia: biology and treatment, Mediguide Oncol. 8(4):1-4, 6, 9, 1988.
Chessells, J.M.: The management of childhood leukemia, Practitioner 229(1407):803-807, 1985.
Cramer, P., and Andrieu, J.M.: Hodgkin's disease in childhood and adolescents: results of chemotherapy-radiotherapy in clinical stages IA-IIB, J. Clin. Oncol. 3:1495-1502, 1985.
Gaynon, P.S., and others: Intensive therapy for children with acute lymphoblastic leukaemia and unfavourable presenting features, Lancet 2(8617):921-923, 1988.
Hammond, E.: Herpes-zoster infection in children with Hodgkin's disease, J. Assoc. Pediatr. Oncol. Nurs. 4(1/2):23-29, 1987.
Kinlen, L.: Evidence for an infective cause of leukemia: comparison of a Scottish new town with nuclear reprocessing sites in Britain, Lancet 2(8624):1323-1326, 1988.
Kirsh, I.L.: Molecular biology of the leukemias, Pediatr. Clin. North Am. 35(4):693-722, 1988.
Lampkins, B.C., and others: Biologic characteristics and treatment of acute nonlymphocytic leukemia in children, Pediatr. Clin. North Am. 35(4):743-764, 1988.
Look, T.: The cytogenics of childhood leukemia: clinical and biologic implications, Pediatr. Clin. North Am. 35(4):723-742, 1988.
Paolucci, G., and others: Treating childhood acute lymphoblastic leukemia (ALL): summary of ten years experience in Italy, Med. Pediatr. Oncol. 17:83-91, 1989.
Pate, L.H.: Therapy-related acute leukemia, an overview, Cancer Nurs. 11(5):295-302, 1988.
Poland, J.M.: Oropharyngeal HSV infections and leukemia, Nurs. Acumen 1(2):3, 5, 1989.
Reaman, G., and others: Acute lymphoblastic leukemia in infants less than one year of age: a cumulative experience of the Children's Cancer Study Group, J. Clin. Oncol. 3:1513-1521, 1985.
Ridgway, D., and Borzy, M.S.: Elevated production of interleukin-2 by lymphocytes from children with acute leukemia, J. Pediatr. 114(3):384-391, 1989.
Ridgway, D., and others: Unsuspected non-Hodgkin's lymphoma of the tonsils and adenoids in children, Pediatrics 79(3):399-401, 1987.
Ritter, J., and others: Prognostic significance of Auer rods in childhood acute myelogenous leukemia: results of the studies AML-BFM-78 and -83, Med. Pediatr. Oncol. 17:202-204, 1989.
Rosenberg, S.A.: Cure of Hodgkin's disease and other lymphomas, Issues Oncol. 4(3):2-3, 8, 1987.
Saral, R.: Herpes simplex virus reactivation in the leukemic patient, Nurs. Acumen 1(2):4, 1989.
Stagner, S.: Congenital leukemia: an overview, J. Assoc. Pediatr. Oncol. Nurs. 3(1):19-21, 1986.
Strohl, R.A.: Lymphoma: an overview, Nurs. Acumen 1(3):1, 4, 1989.

van Eys, J., and others: A comparison of two regimens for high-risk acute lymphocytic leukemia in childhood, Cancer 63:23-29, 1989.

Volker, D.L.: Varicella-zoster virus infection in lymphoma patients, Nurs. Acumen 1(3):1, 6, 1989.

Whedon, M.B.: Care of the patient with leukemia: nursing challenges, Nurs. Acumen 1(2):1, 6, 1989.

Nervous System Tumors

Bleyer, W.A.: Central nervous system leukemia, Pediatr. Clin. North Am. 35(4):789-814, 1988.

Davidson, G.S., and Hope, J.K.: Meningeal tumors of childhood, Cancer 63:1205-1210, 1989.

Flores, L., and others: Delay in the diagnosis of pediatric brain tumors, Am. J. Dis. Child. 140(7):684-686, 1986.

Halperin, E.C., and others: Selection of a management strategy for pediatric brainstem tumors, Med. Pediatr. Oncol. 17:116-125, 1989.

Kelly, J.U.: The use of an investigational radiopharmaceutical in neuroblastoma: a nursing perspective, J. Assoc. Pediatr. Oncol. Nurs. 6(4):133-138, 1989.

Packer, R.J.: Primary childhood central nervous system tumors and neurologic complications of systemic childhood cancer and its treatment, Curr. Opin. Pediatr. 1(2):257-268, 1989.

Phillips, P.C., and Allen, J.C.: Brain tumors in adolescence: treatment of initial and recurrent disease. In Tebbi, C.K., editor: Major topics in adolescent oncology, New York, 1987, Futura Publishing Co., Inc.

Squires, R.H., Jr.: Intracranial tumors: vomiting as a presenting sign: a gastroenterologist's perspective, Clin. Pediatr. 28(8):351-354, 1989.

Tuchman, M., and others: Three years of experience with random urinary homovanillic and vanillylmandelic acid levels in the diagnosis of neuroblastoma, Pediatrics 79(2):203-205, 1987.

van Eys, J.: Medical and oncological management of pediatric brain tumors, Prog. Exp. Tumor Res. 29:235-248, 1985.

Bone Tumors

Bohm, P., Wirth, C.J., and Jansson, V.: Limb-preserving operations in the treatment of malignant bone tumors, Arch. Orthop. Trauma Surg. 108:218-224, 1989.

Carrasco, C.H., and others: Arteriographic prediction of tumor necrosis after primary treatment of osteosarcoma in adults (abstract), Proc. Am. Soc. Clin. Oncol. 6:129, 1987.

Haddy, T.B., and others: Bone involvement in young patients with non-Hodgkin's lymphoma: efficacy of chemotherapy without local radiotherapy, Blood 72(4):1141-1147, 1988.

Jaffe, N.: Advances in the management of malignant bone tumors in children and adolescents, Pediatr. Clin. North Am. 32(3):801-810, 1985.

Jaffe, N., and others: Pathologic fractures in osteosarcoma; impact of chemotherapy on primary tumor and survival, Cancer 59:701-709, 1987.

Kumpan, W., and others: The angiographic response of osteosarcoma following pre-operative chemotherapy, Skeletal Radiol. 15:96-102, 1986.

Link, M.P., and others: The effect of adjuvant chemotherapy on relapse-free survival in patients with osteosarcoma of the extremity, N. Engl. J. Med. 314:1600-1606, 1986.

Winkler, K., and others: Prediction of tumor response during neoadjuvant chemotherapy (NCT) of osteosarcoma (OS) by 99m TC-MDP sequential bone scan digital analysis (BSA) (abstr.), Proc. Am. Soc. Clin. Oncol. 6:220, 1987.

Solid Tumors

Albert, D.M.: Historic review of retinoblastoma, Ophthalmology 94(6):654-662, 1987.

Bonilla, J.A., and Healy, G.B.: Management of malignant head and neck tumors in children, Pediatr. Clin. North Am. 36(6):1443-1450, 1989.

Burgert, Jr., E.O.: Ewing's sarcoma, Curr. Concepts Oncol. 8(4):11, 15-17, 1986.

Friedman, A.L.: Wilms' tumor detection in patients with sporadic aniridia, Am. J. Dis. Child. 140(2):173-174, 1986.

Glassberg, K.: Annual meeting of the section on pediatric urology, Pediatrics 80(1):111-117, 1987.

Hays, D.M.: Rhabdomyosarcoma: management in children and young adults, Curr. Concepts Oncol. 8(4):3-10, 1986.

Kyritsis, A.P., Tsokos, M., and Chader, G.J.: Control of retinoblastoma cell growth by differentiating agents: current work and future directions, Anticancer Res. 6(3, pt. B):465-473, 1986.

Loughlin, K.R., and others: Genitourinary rhabdomyosarcoma in children, Cancer 63:1600-1606, 1989.

Manival, J.C., and others: Pleuropulmonary blastoma, the so-called pulmonary blastoma of childhood, Cancer 62:1516-1526, 1988.

Potluri, V.R., and others: Chromosomal abnormalities in human retinoblastoma: a review, Cancer 58(3):663-671, 1986.

Rofary, C., Flament, F., and Donaldson, S.S.: An attempt to use a common staging system in rhabdomyosarcoma: a report of an international workshop initiated by the International Society of Pediatric Oncology, Med. Pediatr. Oncol. 17:210-215, 1989.

Rootman, J., Carruthers, J.D., and Miller, R.R.: Retinoblastoma, Perspect. Pediatr. Pathol. 10:208-258, 1987.

Shamberger, R.C., and others: Chest wall tumors in infancy and childhood, Cancer 63:774-785, 1989.

Shields, J.A., Augsburger, J.J., and Donoso, L.A.: Recent developments related to retinoblastoma, J. Pediatr. Ophthalmol. Strabismus 23(3):148-152, 1986.

CHAPTER 37

The Child with Cerebral Dysfunction

RELATED TOPICS

Administration of medication, Ch. 27
Anencephaly, Ch. 11
Brain tumors, Ch. 36
Cranial deformities, Ch. 11
High risk related to neurologic disturbance, Ch. 10
Hydrocephalus, Ch. 11
Infection control, Ch. 27
Injuries—the leading killer, Ch. 1
Neurologic assessment, Chs. 7 and 8
Pain assessment; pain management, Ch. 26
Preparation for procedures, Ch. 27

GLOSSARY

ACTH Adrenocorticotropic hormone
aura A sensation, as of warmth or light, that may precede an attack of migraine or an epileptic seizure
BBB Blood-brain barrier
CBF Cerebral blood flow
CN Cranial nerve
CNS Central nervous system
convulsion Involuntary muscular contraction and relaxation
CPP Cerebral perfusion pressure
CSF Cerebrospinal fluid
CT Computed tomography
DI Diabetes insipidus
EEG Electroencephalogram
GCS Glasgow Coma Scale
ICP Intracranial pressure
LOC Level of consciousness
MAP Mean arterial pressure
MRI Magnetic resonance imaging

Pa_{CO_2} Arterial carbon dioxide pressure
Pa_{O_2} Arterial oxygen pressure
postictal Period following a seizure
RS Reye syndrome
seizure A sudden attack
SIADH Syndrome of inappropriate antidiuretic hormone
TB Tuberculosis

Neural control between children and their environment is made possible by the nervous system. Any disturbance in this central communication system can produce alterations in the way in which the system receives, integrates, and responds to stimuli entering the system. These disturbances are reflected in a variety of clinical manifestations, depending on the focus of the disturbance and the integrity of the conducting mechanism. Moreover, children are constantly changing as their systems develop and mature, and neurodevelopmental milestones represent the transition of immature primitive reflexes to mature activity. This chapter is concerned primarily with alterations in consciousness caused by trauma, hypoxia, infectious processes, and seizure activity.

CEREBRAL STRUCTURE AND FUNCTION

The nervous system is composed of three intimately connected and functioning parts: (1) the central nervous system (CNS), composed of two cerebral hemispheres, the brainstem, the cerebellum, and the spinal cord; (2) the peripheral nervous system, which consists of the cranial nerves that arise from or travel to the brainstem and the spinal nerves that travel to or from the spinal cord, which may be motor (efferent) or sensory (afferent); and (3) the autonomic nervous system (ANS), composed of the sympathetic and parasympathetic systems, which provide automatic control of vital functions.

Since this chapter is concerned primarily with disturbances of the brain, the major emphasis is placed on this system. The structure and function of the spinal cord and ANS are elaborated in Chapter 40.

DEVELOPMENT OF THE NEUROLOGIC SYSTEM

In contrast to other body tissues, which grow rapidly after birth, the nervous system grows proportionately more rapidly before birth. Two periods of rapid brain cell growth occur during fetal life. There is a dramatic increase in the number of neurons between 15 and 20 weeks of gestation, and another increase in rate begins at 30 weeks of gestation and extends to 1 year of age. This rapid growth during infancy continues during early childhood, then slows to a more gradual rate during later childhood and adolescence. Brain volume is readily reflected in head circumference, which increases six times as much during the first year as in the second year of life. One half of the postnatal brain growth is achieved by age 1 year, 75% by age 3, and 90% by age 6.

The brain growth and final form depend on the development and multiplication of neurons. Creation of new cells is believed to occur only during the first 100 days of gestation. During the remainder of gestation, cells divide and multiply at the astonishing rate of 250,000 per minute (Restak, 1984). It is believed that no new nerve cells appear after the sixth month of fetal life. Postnatal growth consists of increasing the amount of cytoplasm around the nuclei of the 10 billion existing cells, increasing the number and intricacy of communications with other cells, and advancing their peripheral axons to keep pace with expanding body dimensions.

The brain comprises 12% of the body weight at birth. It doubles this weight in the first year, and by age 5 or 6 years its weight at birth has tripled. Thereafter growth slows until in adulthood the brain is only about 2% of the total body weight. The surface configuration also changes with development. The early embryonic brain surface is smooth, but with advancing development the sulci deepen. This process continues throughout childhood. At birth the cortex is only about one half of its adult thickness, although all the major surface features are present. There is very little cortical control over body movements at birth, with the movements guided principally by primitive reflexes (see Chapter 8). With advancing development and maturation, the brain, through association pathways, exercises increasing control over much of the reflex activity. This allows the growing child to perform progressively complex tasks requiring coordinated movements. Persistence of primitive reflexes may suggest defective cortical development.

Cortical control is closely associated with the acquisition of a myelin coating on the nerves. Although nerve fibers are able to conduct impulses without this myelin sheath, the impulses travel at a slower rate and with more likelihood of diffusion. Myelinization of the various nerve tracts in the CNS, which allows progressive neuromotor function, follows the cephalocaudal and proximodistal sequence. It appears first with the fibers of the spinal cord and cranial nerves, then in the brainstem and corticospinal tracts.

Development of the nervous system proceeds on a continuum. The brain and spinal cord are among the first of the major organ systems to be recognized in the embryo and one of the last to finish significant development after birth.

Jeanne O'Connor Egan, R.N., M.S.N., assisted in the revision of this chapter.

The rate of myelogenesis accelerates rapidly after birth. In general, the pathways concerned with sensation are myelinated early, before the motor pathways. The acquisition of motor skills depends on the maturation and myelination of the nervous system, and no amount of special training or practice will hasten the process. Most of the advancing performance in an infant is a direct result of brain development and only depends indirectly on environmental stimuli.

CENTRAL NERVOUS SYSTEM

The bony skull forms the strongest covering and provides the primary protection to the brain. It is an expansible structure in the infant and young child but becomes rigid in the older child and adolescent. Blood is supplied to the dura mater by the middle meningeal artery, a branch of the external carotid artery. It enters the skull at a point inferior to the temporal bone, then branches over the surface of the dura, usually encased in a groove in the temporal and parietal bones. Damage to this artery or its branches is a frequent cause of an epidural hematoma.

Brain Coverings

Within the skull the brain is covered and protected further by three membranes, the *meninges*—the dura mater, arachnoid membrane, and pia mater (Fig. 37-1). The tough outer membrane, the *dura mater,* is a double layer that serves as the outer meningeal layer and the inner periosteum of the cranial bones separated by the *epidural space.* The dura is closely attached to the skull in infancy, causing slower spread of blood in epidural hemorrhage. This adherence explains why epidural hemorrhages are uncommon in the first 2 years of life.

Between these layers of dura inside the skull lie large venous sinuses. Sheets of the dura mater also extend downward and inward to form partitions within the cranium. Projecting downward into the longitudinal fissure is the sheet of dura called the *falx cerebri,* separating the cerebral hemispheres, and the *falx cerebelli,* separating the cerebellar hemispheres. Another segment is a tentlike structure, the *tentorium,* which separates the cerebellum from the occipital lobe of the cerebrum. The large gap through which the brainstem passes is the tentorial hiatus, the site of herniation in untreated intracranial pressure.

The middle meningeal layer, the *arachnoid membrane,* is a delicate, avascular, weblike structure that loosely surrounds the brain. Between the arachnoid and the dura mater lies the *subdural area,* a potential space that normally contains only enough fluid to prevent adhesion between the two membranes. During cerebral trauma, however, the fine blood vessels that bridge the subdural space are stretched and ruptured, causing venous blood to escape and spread freely. The subdural space is small in children; therefore small amounts of blood can increase intracranial hemorrhage significantly.

The innermost covering layer, the *pia mater,* is a delicate transparent membrane that, unlike the other coverings, adheres closely to the outer surface of the brain, conforming

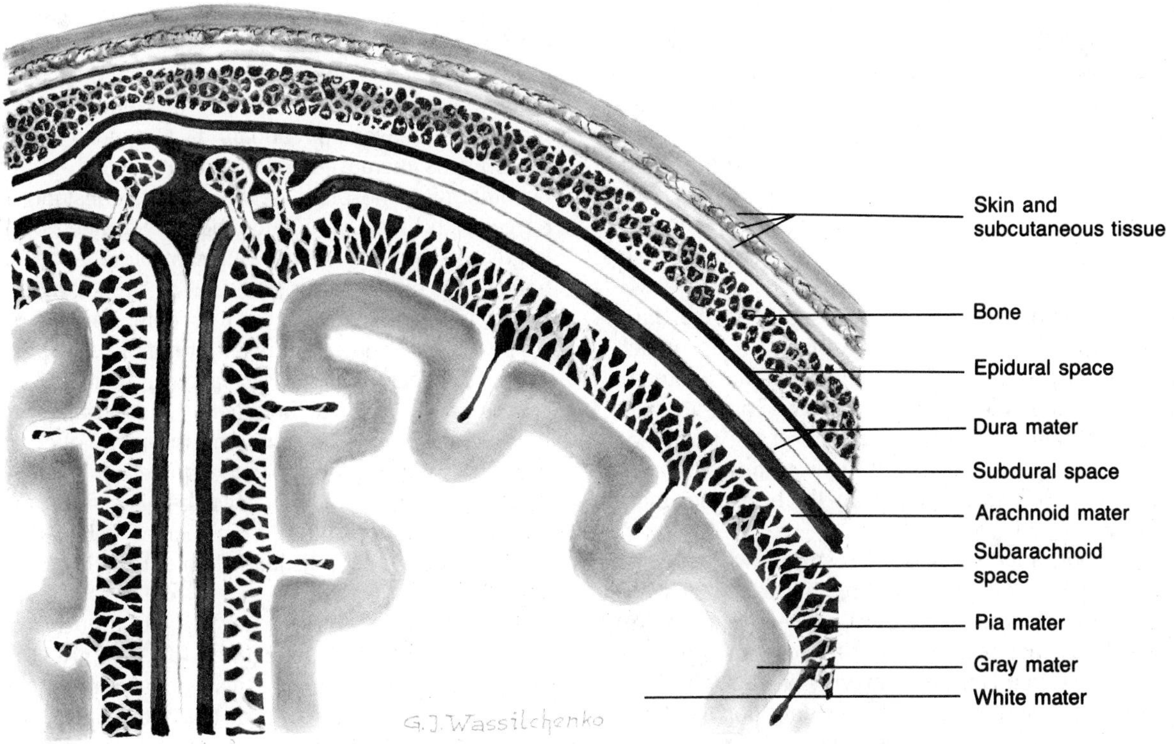

Fig. 37-1. Protective coverings of the brain.

to the folds (gyri) and furrows (sulci). Within the pial layer lie the arteries and veins of the brain. Between the pia mater and the arachnoid membrane is the *subarachnoid space.* Cerebrospinal fluid (CSF) fills the entire subarachnoid space surrounding the brain and spinal cord, which acts as a protective cushion for the brain tissue. Further protection is provided by fibrous filaments known as *arachnoid trabeculae,* which help anchor the brain. When the head receives a blow, these attachments allow the arachnoid to slide on the dura, preventing excessive movement.

The Brain

Each section of the brain plays a vital role in regulation and control of body function. Each hemisphere is artificially divided into lobes. Pressure on or damage to these lobes produces observable signs or symptoms directly related to the area of pathology, which provides clues to the location of the damage. The major structures of the brain and their functions are briefly outlined in Table 37-1.

The two large cerebral hemispheres that occupy the anterior and medial fossae of the skull are separated in the upper part by the *longitudinal fissure.* This separation is complete anteriorly and posteriorly, but centrally the hemispheres are joined by the block of fibers known as the *corpus callosum,* the largest fiber bundle in the brain. These fibers interconnect cortical areas of the right and left hemispheres. Destruction of the corpus callosum causes hemispheric independence, or "split brain."

Situated deeply within each hemisphere and on each side of the midline are the *basal ganglia* (or cerebral nuclei), which serve as vital sorting areas for messages passing to and from the hemispheres. Connected to the hemispheres by thick bunches of nerve fibers is the *brainstem,* through which all the nerve fibers traverse as they pass from the hemispheres to the cerebellum and spinal cord. The brainstem extends from the base of the hemispheres through the foramen magnum, where it is continuous with the spinal cord. Within the cranium and behind the brainstem is the cerebellum. Any pressure exerted on the intracranial structures can cause compression of the brainstem and prolapse of the cerebellum through the foramen magnum.

Cerebral blood flow. The blood supply to the brain tissue is carried by the internal carotid arteries, which branch to supply the various brain segments. The volume of blood to the brain, which constitutes only 17% of the cardiac output, supplies the brain with 20% of the body oxygen. The brain, an "inactive" organ, uses 10 times the oxygen used by the body as a whole. Only the heart uses more oxygen per gram of tissue.

Cerebral blood flow (CBF) is the result of two opposing forces—cerebral blood pressure (the difference between systemic arterial pressure and cerebral venous pressure) and cerebral vascular resistance. At a blood pressure between 50 and 150 mm Hg, CBF remains constant. Since cerebral venous pressure is usually very low and relatively constant, the cerebral blood pressure is determined mainly by systemic arterial pressure.

Autoregulation. One of the most important factors in the control of CBF is *autoregulation,* the unique ability of cerebral arterial vessels to change their diameter in response to fluctuating cerebral perfusion pressure (CPP). The CPP is the mean arterial pressure (MAP) minus the intracranial pressure (ICP):

$$\text{CPP} = \text{MAP} - \text{ICP}$$

As a result, cerebral vessels maintain a constant blood flow during alterations in blood pressure and perfusion caused by body posture, increased ICP, decreased cardiac output, or narrowing or occlusion in the major blood vessels of the neck. Autoregulation fails when the limits of cerebrovascular dilatation are reached; then CBF decreases, causing clinical symptoms of ischemia (nausea, fainting, dizziness, dim vision). Conversely, increased MAP leads to "breakthrough of autoregulation," with increased CBF leading to microhemorrhages and cerebral edema. Autoregulation may be impaired locally or globally as a result of trauma or ischemia.

Changes in arterial oxygen pressure (Pa_{O_2}) or arterial carbon dioxide pressure (Pa_{CO_2}) have a profound effect on autoregulation. Hypercapnia (Pa_{CO_2} over 40 mm Hg) or increased levels of lactic acid have a pronounced dilating effect on cerebral arterioles that increases CBF and thus cerebral volume. Hypocapnia (Pa_{CO_2} 25 to 30 mm Hg) constricts cerebral arterioles and decreases CBF. Changes in Pa_{O_2} between 70 and 100 mm Hg have little effect on the cerebrovascular system. However, profound hypoxia (Pa_{O_2} below 50 mm Hg) dramatically increases CBF. Consequently, maintenance of the airway and effective ventilation are of primary importance in the initial management of the neurologically impaired patient.

Oxygen. Metabolic requirements for oxygen by the brain are not affected by rest or sleep, although they are reduced by narcosis and coma and altered by changes in temperature. CBF is not altered when body temperature is maintained between 35° and 40° C. Oxygen consumption of the brain is increased by hyperthermia and decreased by hypothermia. The brain depends on a constant supply of oxygen-rich blood, and since the oxygen need of the brain is great in relation to the volume of blood supplied, it extracts more oxygen from each unit of circulating blood.

Oxygen supply to the brain is compromised when the supply is inadequate as a result of impaired respiration, hypotension, increased ICP or vascular damage, spasm, or compression. Neurons are highly susceptible to elevated Pa_{CO_2} (a potent vasodilator), and the metabolic damage to brain tissue caused by an inadequate supply of well-oxygenated blood can often exceed the effects of trauma. Respiratory acidosis resulting from increased Pa_{CO_2} levels can produce symptoms indistinguishable from those of head injury.

Blood-brain barrier. The blood-brain barrier (BBB) is an anatomic-physiologic feature of the brain that separates the brain parenchyma from the blood. Cerebral capillaries, unlike those in other parts of the body, have no fenestrations or pores. The tight junctions of the vascular endothelium are thought to be responsible for the selective nature

Table 37-1 Structure and function of the brain

STRUCTURE	DESCRIPTION	FUNCTION	DYSFUNCTION
Cerebrum	Two hemispheres divided artificially into lobes Upper parts divided anteriorly and posteriorly by longitudinal fissure Lower parts joined centrally by block of fibers, the corpus callosum	Center for consciousness, thought, memory, sensory input, motor activity	Pressure or damage produces signs and symptoms specific to involved areas
Frontal lobes	Most anteriorly located of all lobes that end posteriorly at fissure of Rolando	Posterior portion contains cells that control motor activity throughout body Basis for social interaction Recognition of cause-and-effect relationships, abstract thinking, expressive language	Injury or damage to anterior portion may cause personality changes, altered intellectual functioning Impaired movement of body part directly related to motor center for that part Memory deficits Language deficits
Parietal lobes	Situated posterior to fissure of Rolando	Important for appreciation of sensation, somatic interpretation and integration	Language dysfunction Aphasia, apraxia, motor and sensory loss to lower extremities, atopognosia
Occipital lobe	At posterior base of skull Most posteriorly placed lobe	Receives stimuli for vision Spatial orientation Visual recognition	Injury produces impaired vision, functional blindness
Temporal lobes	Situated anterior to occipital lobe and inferior to parietal lobes	Receives and interprets stimuli for taste, vision, sound, smell Converts crude visual impressions into recognizable images	Injury or destruction causes inability to interpret meanings of sensory experiences
	Point where temporal, parietal, and occipital lobes converge	Primary interpretive area	Impairment causes inability to interpret sensory stimuli; difficulty in understanding higher levels of meaning of body sensory experiences
	Point where temporal, parietal, and frontal lobes converge	Center for speech, hearing, receptive language	Impairment produces aphasia Hearing dysfunction
Cerebellum	Located just below posterior part of cerebrum and separated from it by tentorium Contains two lateral lobes joined by midline portion, the vermis	Necessary for refinement and coordination of all muscle movements, including walking, talking, control of muscle tone and balance	Dysmetria, ataxia, dysarthria, hypotonia, nystagmus, dystonia Rest tremor
Basal ganglia	Situated deeply within cerebral hemispheres on either side of midline	Unconscious or automatic control of lower motor centers Excitation causes inhibition of muscle tone throughout body	Chorea, athetosis Dystonia Rest tremor
Diencephalon	Situated between cerebrum and mesencephalon	Contains diffuse fibers that compose reticular activating system	Stupor
Thalamus	Rounded mass forms most of lateral wall of third ventricle and part of floor of lateral ventricles	Major relay station for sensory impulses to cerebral cortex Activates cerebral cortex	Impaired consciousness

Continued.

Table 37-1 Structure and function of the brain—cont'd

STRUCTURE	DESCRIPTION	FUNCTION	DYSFUNCTION
Diencephalon—cont'd			
Hypothalamus	Lies beneath thalamus Forms floor of third ventricle	Vital control center for involuntary functions (e.g., blood pressure, satiety, hunger, rage, feeding, water conservation, temperature, sleep regulation, libido) Controls secretion of tropic hormones	Impairment causes alterations in vegetative functions Somnolence, coma Anorexia, loss of weight, fever, diabetes insipidus, loss of libido Endocrine disorders
Brainstem	Extends from cerebral hemisphere to spinal cord	All cranial nerves (except I) arise from brainstem	Stupor, coma
Mesencephalon (midbrain)	Lies below inferior surface of cerebellum and above pons	Main connection between forebrain and hindbrain Contains nuclei for cranial nerves III, IV, part of V	Impaired consciousness No independent movement or verbal response Decerebrate posturing Neurologic hyperventilation
	Ventral portion composed of cerebral peduncles	Control of eye movement	Impaired function of muscles supplied by these nerves
Pons	Located just above medulla oblongata	Contains pneumotaxic center—control of respiration	Deep, rapid, or periodic breathing
		Cranial nerves V through VIII	Impaired function of muscles supplied by these nerves
Medulla	Forms attachment of brain to spinal cord Separated from pons by horizontal groove	Contains vital centers, including respiratory and vasomotor cranial nerves IX, X, XI, XII	Impaired vital functions No response to any stimuli Ataxic (Biot) breathing Flaccid muscle tone Deep tendon, gag, corneal reflexes absent

of the BBB. The mature BBB allows facilitated diffusion of glucose and passive diffusion of water and carbon dioxide but is impermeable to protein and does not permit passage of many active substances. However, the BBB of the fetus and newborn is normally indiscriminately permeable, allowing protein and other large and small molecules to pass freely between the cerebral vessels and the brain. Conditions that cause cerebrovascular dilatation (hypertension, hypercapnia, hypoxia, acidosis) disrupt the BBB, as do hyperosmotic fluids, which cause shrinkage of vascular endothelium and widen the vascular junctions.

INCREASED INTRACRANIAL PRESSURE

The brain, tightly enclosed in the solid bony cranium, is well protected but highly vulnerable to pressure that may accumulate within the enclosure. Its total volume—brain (80%), CSF (10%), and blood (10%)—must remain approximately the same at all times. A change in the proportional volume of one of these components (e.g., increase or decrease in intracranial blood) must be accompanied by a compensatory change in another (e.g., decrease or increase in CSF)—the Monro-Kellie hypothesis. In this way the volume and pressure normally remain constant. Examples of compensatory changes are reduction in blood volume, decrease in production of CSF, increase in CSF absorption, or shrinkage of brain mass by displacement of intracellular and extracellular fluid.

In children with open fontanels, compensation may take place by skull expansion and widened sutures. However, at any age the capacity for spatial compensation is limited. An increase in ICP may be caused by tumors or other space-occupying lesions, accumulation of fluid within the ventricular system, bleeding, or edema of cerebral tissues. Once compensation is exhausted, any further increase in volume will result in a rapid rise in ICP.

Early signs and symptoms of increased ICP are often subtle and assume many patterns, such as personality changes, irritability, and fatigue (Box 37-1). In older children subjective symptoms are headache, especially when lying flat (e.g., on awakening in the morning) or when coughing, sneezing, or bending over, and nausea and vomiting. The child may complain of double vision or blurred vision with movement of the head. Seizures are not uncommon. In chil-

Box 37-1 SIGNS OF INCREASED INTRACRANIAL PRESSURE (ICP) IN INFANTS AND CHILDREN

Infants
Tense, bulging fontanel; lack of normal pulsations
Separated cranial sutures
Macewen (cracked-pot) sign
Irritability
High-pitched cry
Increased occipitofrontal circumference (OFC)
Distended scalp veins
Changes in feeding
Cries when held or rocked
"Setting sun" sign

Children
Headache
Nausea
Vomiting—often without nausea
Diplopia, blurred vision
Seizures

Personality and Behavior Signs
Irritability (toddlers), restlessness
Indifference, drowsiness, or lack of interest
Decline in school performance
Diminished physical activity and motor performance
Increased complaints of fatigue, tiredness; increased time devoted to sleep
Significant weight loss possible from anorexia and vomiting
Memory loss if pressure is greatly increased
Inability to follow simple commands
Progression to lethargy and drowsiness

Late Signs
Lowered level of consciousness
Decreased motor response to command
Decreased sensory response to painful stimuli
Alterations in pupil size and reactivity
Sometimes decerebrate or decorticate posturing
Cheyne-Stokes respirations
Papilledema

dren whose cranial sutures have not closed, there is an increase in the head circumference and bulging fontanels. Cranial sutures may become diastatic, or split, and head circumference can enlarge until the child is 5 years of age if the pathology progresses slowly. As pressure increases, pupils become progressively sluggish in reaction, eventually to become fixed and dilated, sometimes referred to as "blown." The level of consciousness progressively deteriorates from drowsiness to eventual coma. Problems related to increased ICP are discussed later in this chapter in relation to head injury. (See also Brain Tumors, Chapter 36, and Hydrocephalus, Chapter 11).

Physiologic and biochemical changes within the cerebral vasculature serve to complicate the primary causes of increased ICP. Initially, especially in cases of trauma, there is often increased blood flow as a result of venous congestion or vasomotor paralysis. If cerebral hypoxia is associated with the cerebral dysfunction, the compensatory vasodilatation caused by oxygen deficiency will tend to increase the cerebral flow. However, as ICP progressively increases, blood flow is reduced with diminished blood supply to the brain tissues. The classic responses observed in adults (widening pulse pressure, increased blood pressure) are rarely seen in children and, if so, are very late signs. Breathing characterized by periods of hyperpnea that alternate with apnea (Cheyne-Stokes respirations) is seen in brainstem damage.

■ EVALUATION OF NEUROLOGIC STATUS

Dysfunction of the central nervous system (CNS) can be manifest in almost any body system and may result from various causes. Earlier chapters discuss methods used to evaluate neurologic function in relation to numerous aspects of child care. The neurologic examination is an integral part of the health assessment (see Chapter 7) and newborn assessment (see Chapter 8). Some of the tests used to differentiate neuromuscular disorders are discussed in Chapter 40. The assessment tools and examinations in this chapter are primarily those used to assess intracranial integrity. An overall discussion of some factors that influence assessment is followed by some general observations. More specific techniques are discussed in relation to assessment of level of consciousness.

ASSESSMENT: GENERAL ASPECTS

Children younger than 2 years require special evaluation, since they are unable to respond to directions designed to elicit specific responses in infants neurologically. Early neurologic responses in infants are primarily reflexive; these responses are gradually replaced by meaningful movement in the characteristic cephalocaudal direction of development. This evidence of progressive maturation reflects more extensive myelinization and changes in neurochemical and electrophysiologic properties.

Most information about infants and small children is gained through observation of their spontaneous and elicited reflex responses, by their development of increasingly complex locomotor and fine motor skills, and by eliciting progressively sophisticated communicative and adaptive behaviors. Delay or deviation from expected milestones helps identify high-risk children. Persistence or reappearance of reflexes that normally disappear indicates pathology. In evaluating the infant or young child, it is also important to obtain the pregnancy and delivery history to determine the possible effect of intrauterine environmental influences known to affect the orderly maturation of the CNS. These influences include maternal infections, chemicals, trauma, and metabolic insults.

History

A family history can sometimes offer clues regarding possible genetic disorders with neurologic manifestations. A review of family members often identifies conditions that might otherwise be overlooked, especially siblings who have died or relatives whose conditions have been hidden from memory. Questions regarding specific neurologic problems are mentioned, such as mental retardation, deafness, epilepsy, blindness, unusual movements, weakness, ataxia, and progressive mental deterioration.

A history is very important because it provides valuable clues regarding the cause of unconsciousness. There may have been an injury or short febrile illness, or the child may be known to have diabetes. A history of any event that led to the health care assessment is probed, especially when it involves injury, encounter with an animal or insect, ingestion of neurotoxic substances, inhalation of chemicals, or past illness. Sudden or progressive alterations in movement or mental abilities may provide clues for investigation.

Physical Examination

Physical evaluation includes observation of the size and shape of the *head,* spontaneous *activity* and postural *reflex activity,* and *sensory responses.* The attitude is observed. It is noted whether the infant assumes a normal flexed posture or one of extreme extension, opisthotonos, or hypotonia. Extremities are observed for symmetry of *movement.* Excessive tremulousness or frequent twitching movements may be significant signs indicating the onset of a seizure disorder. Seizure activity is suspected if holding the extremity snugly does not stop the activity.

Skin and hair texture may be important factors in detecting certain neurologic diseases. Facial features may suggest a specific syndrome, and a high-pitched, piercing cry is associated with CNS disorders. Abnormal eye movements, inability to suck or swallow, lip smacking, asymmetric contraction of facial muscles, and yawning may indicate *cranial nerve (CN)* involvement. An abnormal respiratory cycle such as prolonged apnea, ataxic breathing, paradoxic chest movement, and hyperventilation (central neurogenic) may be the result of a neurologic problem.

Older children can be evaluated by the usual methods employed in a neurologic examination. In addition, an estimation of the *level of development* provides essential information about neurologic function. These accomplishments are discussed throughout the book in relation to evaluation for specific disorders such as mental retardation, failure to thrive, attention deficit disorder, cerebral palsy, cerebral tumors, and other physical or behavioral problems. Developmental screening tests (see Appendix B) can be used to assess developmental progress in the young child.

Muscular activity. Muscular activity and coordination, including ocular movements and gait, are valuable sources of information. Ocular movements, pupillary response, facial movements, and mouth functions provide clues regarding CN involvement or impingement. (See Chapter 7 for CN and reflex testing.) Testing reflexes, strength, and coordination, and for the presence and location of tremors, twitching, tics, or other unusual movements (Table 37-2) are also aspects of the neurologic assessment. Abnormalities of gait that indicate cerebral dysfunction are described in Box 37-2.

Table 37-2 Description of abnormal involuntary muscular movements

TERM	DESCRIPTION
Ataxia	Gross incoordination that may become worse with the eyes closed
Spasm	Involuntary contraction of a muscle mass; cramp (if painful), convulsion (if violent)
Spasticity	Prolonged and steady contraction of a muscle characterized by clonus (alternating relaxation and contraction of the muscle) and exaggerated reflexes
Rigidity	Inability to flex a joint
Tremors	Constant small involuntary movements
Twitching	Spasmodic movements of short duration
Tic	Involuntary, compulsive, stereotyped movement of an associated group of muscles
Choreiform movements	Quick, jerky, grossly incoordinated, irregular movements that may disappear on relaxation
Athetosis	Slow, writhing, wormlike, constant, grossly incoordinated movements that increase on voluntary activity and decrease on relaxation
Dystonia	Slow twisting movements of limbs or trunk
Associated movements	Voluntary movement of one muscle accompanied by involuntary movement of another muscle
Mirroring movements	Same as associated movements except with symmetric muscle groups

Box 37-2 ABNORMALITIES OF GAIT THAT INDICATE CEREBRAL DYSFUNCTION

Ataxia—impaired ability to coordinate movements; staggering gait and postural imbalance.

Spastic paraplegic gait—narrow-based gait with a tendency to walk on the toes, along with flexion at the knees and hips, and shuffling. Thighs adducted, and knees may strike each other with each step; in younger children a "scissoring" position results when lower limbs cross because of increased adductor tone. Patients walk stiffly and take slow, deliberate steps. Increased difficulty when attempting to walk on heels or run.

Spastic hemiplegic gait—involved leg extended, circumducted, plantar flexed, and does not swing naturally at the knee or hip.

Cerebellar gait—staggering, irregularity, unsteadiness, wide-based lurching movement in any direction, and tendency to veer in one lateral direction (hemispheric lesion).

Extrapyramidal gait—rigidity, few automatic movements, and bradykinesia (slowness of all movements) with associated bending of trunk and head, arms adducted at shoulders and flexed at elbows and wrists, fingers extended; festination (upper body moves forward in advance of lower part), causing more rapid steps and risk of falling.

ALTERED STATES OF CONSCIOUSNESS

Consciousness implies awareness—the ability to respond to sensory stimuli and have subjective experiences. There are two aspects of consciousness: *alertness,* an arousal-waking state including the ability to respond to stimuli, and *cognitive power,* including the ability to process stimuli and produce verbal and motor responses (Plum and Posner, 1980).

An altered state of consciousness usually refers to varying states of unconsciousness that may be momentary or may last for hours, days, or indefinitely. *Unconsciousness* is depressed cerebral function—the inability to respond to sensory stimuli and have subjective experiences. *Coma* is defined as a state of unconsciousness from which the patient cannot be aroused even with powerful stimuli.

The seat of consciousness, or *alerting area,* of the brain is in the reticular formation—the central core of the brainstem. The reticular formation extends from the midbrain to the medulla. The *reticular activating system (RAS)* receives collaterals from and is stimulated by *every* major somatic and special sensory pathway in the brain. Disturbances of consciousness may occur when any part of the reticular, thalamic, hypothalamic, and cortical circuits is sufficiently impaired. However, the effects may vary according to the areas involved. For example, small lesions of the reticular or hypothalamic regions will produce a profound effect, whereas extensive impairment of the cortex is required to produce quantitatively similar results.

Etiology

An altered state of consciousness may be the outcome of several processes that affect the CNS. Impaired neurologic function can result from a direct or indirect cause. Some altered states, such as the diffuse changes observed in encephalitis, are directly related to cerebral insult; others are the result of dysfunction to other organs or processes manifest by CNS signs. For example, biochemical changes can impair neurologic function without morphologic findings, as in hypoglycemia.

Level of Consciousness

Assessment of level of consciousness (LOC) remains the earliest indicator of improvement or deterioration in neurologic status. LOC is determined by observations of the child's responses to the environment. Other diagnostic tests, such as motor activity, reflexes, and vital signs, are more variable and do not necessarily directly parallel the depth of the comatose state. The most consistently used terms are described in Table 37-3.

Coma Assessment

Diminished alertness as a result of pathologic conditions occurs as a continuum and is designated as the *comatose state,* which extends from somnolence at one end to deep coma at the other. To produce coma, one of the following must occur: (1) extensive, diffuse, *bilateral* cerebral hemispheric destruction (the brainstem may be intact); (2) a lesion in the diencephalon; or (3) destruction of the brainstem down to the level of the lower pons.

Table 37-3 Levels of consciousness

STATE	DESCRIPTION AND CHARACTERISTICS
Sleep (normal unconsciousness)	Cyclic (regularly recurring) physiologic state Reversible by auditory, visual, or tactile stimuli Immobile posture Absence of alertness, cognition, voluntary movement Body processes partially suspended Intermittent dreaming; may be able to recall dream
Confusion	Fails to comprehend surroundings Appears to lose proper bearings Unable to estimate direction or location Likely to be disoriented in time May misidentify people Short attention span, difficulty in following even simple directions Tends to misinterpret events May be hyperactive or apathetic and immobile Usually able to give relevant answers to simple questions about age or location of pain Gives irrelevant and inaccurate answers to more complex questions Alert; arousal responses intact
Delirium	Confusion, disorientation, fear, irritability, agitation, hyperactivity Illusions—false interpretation of sensory perceptions Hallucinations—false sensory perceptions Delusions—false ideas Typically loud, talkative, suspicious, agitated Often associated with high fever, toxic substances, shock states Tremulousness, sweating Frequently responds with a "startle" reaction to unexpected stimuli
Pseudowakeful states (akinetic mutism, apallic syndrome)	Sits or lies with eyes open but fails to follow objects or lights Does not turn eyes toward a noise Does not speak May follow objects or persons with eyes, may turn slowly toward a sound and appear about to speak, but remains silent (reptilian stare) Response to external stimuli similar to that of stupor or light coma May be restless and hyperkinetic May remain motionless and speechless
Comatose states	Diminished alertness Occurs as a continuum Extends from somnolence to deep coma

NEUROLOGIC ASSESSMENT

GLASGOW COMA SCALE

Pupils	Right	Size		
		Reaction		
	Left	Size		
		Reaction		
Eyes open	Spontaneously	4		
	To speech	3		
	To pain	2		
	None	1		
Best motor response	Obeys commands	6		
	Localizes pain	5		
	Flexion withdrawal	4		
	Flexion abnormal	3		
	Extension	2		
	None	1		
Best response to auditory and/or visual stimulus	>2 years			<2 years
	Orientation	5		5 Smiles, listens, follows
	Confused	4		4 Cries, consolable
	Inappropriate words	3		3 Inappropriate persistent cry
	Incomprehensible words	2		2 Agitated, restless
	None	1		1 No response
	Endotracheal tube or trach	T		
COMA SCALE TOTAL				

++ = Brisk
+ = Sluggish
– = No reaction
C = Eye closed by swelling

Usually record best arm or age-appropriate response

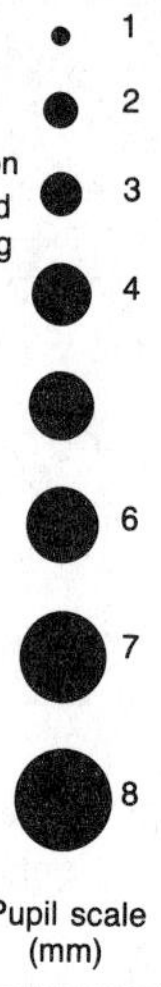

HAND GRIP:
Equal
Unequal
R_____L
Weakness

MUSCLE TONE:
Normal
Arching
Spastic
Flaccid
Weak
Decorticate
Decerebrate
Other ________

FONTANEL/ WINDOW:
Soft
Flat
Sunken
Tense
Bulging
Closed
Other ________

LOC:
Alert/oriented ×4
Sleepy
Irritable
Comatose
Disoriented
Combative
Lethargic
Awake
Sleeping
Drowsy
Agitated

EYE MOVEMENT:
Normal
Nystagmus
Strabismus
Other ________

MOOD/AFFECT:
Happy
Content
Quiet
Withdrawn
Sad
Flat
Hostile

Fig. 37-2. Pediatric coma scale.

Several scales have been devised in an attempt to standardize the description and interpretation of the degree of depressed consciousness. The most popular of these is the Glasgow Coma Scale (GCS), which consists of a three-part assessment: eye opening, verbal response, and motor response. The GCS requires observational skills and is readily reproducible between observers. A pediatric version recognizes that expected verbal and motor responses must be related to the child's age, and although not widely used, the assessments are reasonably consistent. The scale with variations adapted to the young patient is provided in Fig. 37-2. When assessing LOC in young children, it is often useful to have a parent present to help elicit a desired response. An infant or child may not respond in an unfamiliar environment or to unfamiliar voices. Children over 3 years of age should be able to give their name, although they may not be cognizant of place or time.

Numerical values, 1 to 5, are assigned to the levels of response in each category. The sum of these numerical values provides an objective measure of the patient's LOC. The lower the score, the deeper is the coma. A normal person would score the highest, 15; a score of 8 or below is generally accepted as a definition of coma; the lowest score, 3, indicates deep coma or death.

The GCS in itself is not sufficient to determine the responses of all children. For example, a quadriplegic child can score very low but be cerebrally intact because the child cannot respond to commands physically. However, the GCS provides a more objective method for evaluating the state of consciousness in most cases. Any child less than 3 years of age who cries is assigned a full verbal score. Severely injured children (GCS of 8 or less) may have a consistent grading of motor response, verbal response, and eye opening.

Irreversible coma. There is no precise diagnosis for clinical death. Different tissues undergo permanent damage after varying periods of exposure to an ongoing insult; therefore the brain (especially the cerebrum) has become the tissue of most importance in determining the time of death. The current concept of dying is a process that takes place over a finite interval of time, rather than an event that occurs spontaneously. The patient who meets the criteria for brain death will eventually suffer cardiovascular collapse (usually within hours).

Organ transplantation has created a need to subdivide the process of death in order to obtain viable tissues at a time when the brain is already dead. The clinical criteria for brain death must be so constituted that there is *no error.* Although the legal status of the concept of death varies among individual states and communities in the United States, The Task Force for the Determination of Brain Death in Children has established physical examination criteria (Box 37-3). (See also Tissue Donation/Autopsy, Chapter 23.)

NEUROLOGIC EXAMINATION

The purpose of the neurologic examination is to establish an accurate, objective baseline of neurologic function. Therefore it is essential that the neurologic examination be documented in a fashion that is *reproducible.* In this way a comparison of baseline, previous, and current findings allows the observer to detect subtle changes in the neurologic status that might not be evident otherwise. Descriptions of behaviors should be simple, objective, and easily interpreted: "Drowsy but awake and conversationally rational/oriented," "Sleepy but arousable with vigorous physical stimuli. Pressure to nail base of right hand results in upper extremity flexion/lower extremity extension."

Vital signs, observation of posture and movement (both spontaneous and elicited), eye examination, CN testing, and reflex testing all provide valuable clues regarding the

Box 37-3 GUIDELINES FOR ESTABLISHING BRAIN DEATH IN CHILDREN

1. Coma and apnea must coexist. Child must exhibit complete loss of consciousness, vocalization, and vocational activity.
2. Brainstem function must be absent, as defined by:
   a. Midposition or fully dilated pupils that do not respond to light. Drugs may influence and invalidate pupillary assessment.
   b. Absence of spontaneous eye movements and those induced by oculocephalic and caloric (oculovestibular) testing.
   c. Absence of movement of bulbar musculature, including facial and oropharyngeal muscles. The corneal, gag, cough, sucking, and rooting reflexes are absent.
   d. Respiratory movements are absent when child is removed from respirator. Apnea testing using standardized methods can be performed but is done after other criteria are met.
3. Child must not be significantly hypothermic or hypotensive for age.
4. Flaccid tone and absence of spontaneous or induced movements, including spinal cord events such as reflex withdrawal or spinal myoclonus, should exist.
5. Examination should remain consistent with brain death throughout the observation and testing period.
6. Observation periods according to age:

7 days to 2 months	Two examinations and EEGs, separated by at least 48 hours
2 months to 1 year	Two examinations and EEGs, separated by at least 24 hours
Over 1 year	Observation period of at least 12 hours
	If irreversible cause exists, no laboratory testing needed
	If difficult to assess extent of reversibility of brain damage, observation indicated for at least 24 hours

Modified from Task Force for the Determination of Brain Death in Children: Ann. Neurol. 21:616, 1987.

LOC, the site of involvement, and the probable cause, although they do not necessarily parallel the depth of a comatose state.

Vital Signs

Pulse, respiration, and *blood pressure* provide information regarding the adequacy of circulation and the possible underlying cause of altered consciousness. *Autonomic activity* is most intensively disturbed in deep coma and in brainstem lesions. *Body temperature* is often elevated, and sometimes the elevation may be extreme. Coma of a toxic origin may produce hypothermia. High temperature is most frequently a sign of an acute infectious process or heat stroke but may be caused by ingestion of some drugs, especially salicylates, alcohol, and barbiturates, or intracranial bleeding. A fever sometimes follows a cerebral seizure.

The pulse is variable and may be rapid, slow and bounding, or feeble. Blood pressure may be normal, elevated, or at shock levels. The Cushing reflex or pressor response that causes a slowing of the pulse and an increase in blood pressure is uncommon in children; when it occurs, it is a very late sign. Vital signs are also affected by medications. For assessment purposes *changes* in pulse and blood pressure are more important than the direction.

Respirations are more often slow, deep, and irregular. Slow and deep breathing is often seen in the heavy sleep caused by sedatives, after seizures, or in cerebral infections. Slow, shallow breathing may result from sedatives or narcotics. Hyperventilation (deep and rapid respirations) is usually the result of metabolic acidosis or abnormal stimulation of the respiratory center in the medulla caused by salicylate poisoning, hepatic coma, or Reye syndrome.

Breathing patterns have been described with a number of terms (e.g., apneustic, cluster, ataxic, Cheyne-Stokes). However, it is better to describe what is being observed rather than placing a label on it. The terms are often used and interpreted incorrectly. Periodic and irregular breathing are signs of brainstem (especially medullary) dysfunction. This is an ominous sign that often precedes complete apnea. The odor of the breath may provide additional clues, for example, the fruity, acetone odor of ketosis, the foul odor of uremia, the fetid odor of hepatic failure, or the odor of alcohol.

Skin

The skin may offer clues to the cause of unconsciousness. The body surface should be examined for the presence of injury, needle marks, petechiae, bites, and ticks. Evidence of toxic substances may be found on the hands, face, mouth, and clothing—especially in small children.

Eyes

Pupil size and reactivity are assessed (Fig. 37-3). Pupils either react or do not react to light. Pinpoint pupils are commonly observed in poisoning, such as opiate or barbiturate poisoning, or in brainstem dysfunction. Widely dilated and reactive pupils are often seen after seizures and may involve only one side. Dilated pupils may also be caused by eye trauma. Widely dilated and fixed pupils suggest paralysis of CN III secondary to pressure from herniation of the brain through the tentorium. A unilateral fixed pupil usually suggests a lesion on the same side. Bilateral fixed pupils usually imply brainstem damage if present for more than 5 minutes. Dilated and nonreactive pupils are also seen in hypothermia, anoxia, ischemia, poisoning with atropine-like substances, or prior instillation of mydriatic drugs.

NURSING ALERT The sudden appearance of a fixed and dilated pupil is a neurosurgical emergency.

Some of the therapies used (e.g., barbiturates) can alter pupil size and reaction. The description of eye movements should indicate whether one or both eyes are involved and how the reaction was elicited. The parents should be asked if the child has a strabismus. A preexisting strabismus will cause the eyes to appear normal under compromise.

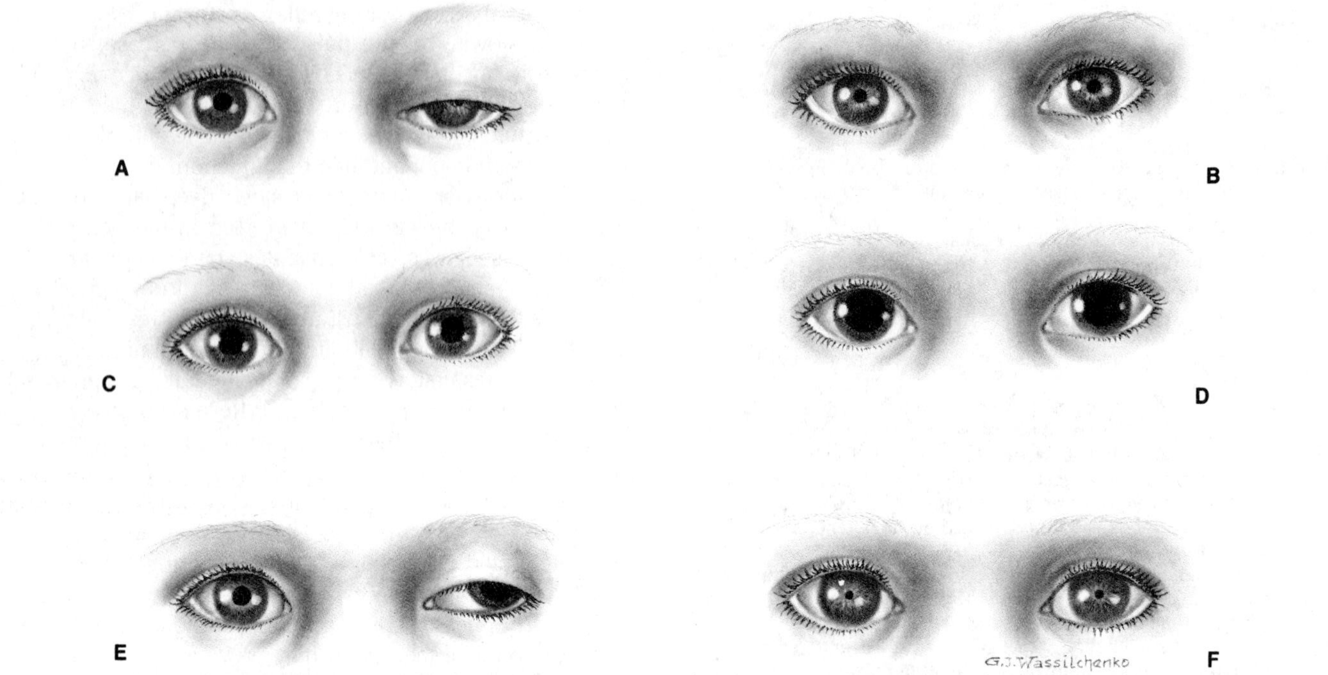

Fig. 37-3. Variations in pupil size with altered states of consciousness. **A,** Ipsilateral pupillary constriction with slight ptosis. **B,** Bilateral small pupils. **C,** Midposition, light fixed to all stimuli. **D,** Bilateral dilated and fixed pupils. **E,** Dilated pupil, left eye abducted with ptosis. **F,** Pinpoint pupils.

Blinking observed at rest or in response to a sudden loud noise or bright light implies that the pontine reticular formation is intact. The *corneal reflex,* blinking of the eyelids when the cornea is touched with a wisp of cotton or a camel hair pencil, is used to test the integrity of the ophthalmic division of CN V. A posttraumatic strabismus indicates CN VI damage.

Eye movements are assessed by the *doll's head maneuver,* in which the child's head is rotated quickly to one side and then to the other. When brainstem centers for eye movement are intact, there is conjugate (paired or working together) movement of the eyes in the direction opposite to the head rotation. Absence of this response suggests dysfunction of the brainstem or oculomotor nerve (CN III). Downward or lateral deviation is frequently observed in association with pupillary dilation in dysfunction of CN III because of tentorial herniation. This assessment is not attempted until after cervical spine injury has been ruled out for the child who is suspected of or has sustained a traumatic injury.

The caloric test, or *oculovestibular response,* is elicited by irrigating the external auditory canal with ice water (head of the bed elevated at a 30-degree angle). This normally causes conjugate movement of the eyes toward the side of stimulation. This is lost when the pontine centers are impaired, thus providing important information in assessment of the comatose patient.

✦ **NURSING ALERT** This painful test is never performed on the awake child.

Funduscopic examination reveals additional clues. *Papilledema,* if it develops at all, will not be evident early in the course of unconsciousness because papilledema takes 24 to 48 hours to develop. The presence of preretinal (subhyaloid) hemorrhages in children is almost invariably the result of acute trauma with intracranial bleeding, usually subarachnoid or subdural hemorrhage.

Motor Function

Observation of spontaneous activity, posture, and response to painful stimuli provides clues to the location and extent of cerebral dysfunction. Even subtle movements (e.g., the out-turning of a hip) should be noted and the child observed for other signs. Asymmetric movements of the limbs or absence of movement suggests paralysis. In hemiplegia the affected limb lies in external rotation and will fall uncontrollably when lifted and allowed to drop. These observations should be described rather than labeled. In the deeper comatose states there is little or no spontaneous movement and the musculature tends to be flaccid. There is considerable variability in the motor behavior in lesser degrees of coma. For example, the child may be relatively immobile or restless and hyperkinetic; muscle tone may be increased or decreased. Tremors, twitching, and spasms of muscles are common observations. The patient may display purposeless plucking or tossing movements. Combative or negativistic behavior is not uncommon. Hyperactivity is more common in acute febrile and toxic states than in cases of increased ICP. Convulsions are common in children and may be present in coma as a result of any cause.

Any repetitive or convulsive movements should be described.

Posturing

As cortical control over motor function is lost in brain dysfunction, primitive postural reflexes emerge. These are evident in posturing and motor movements directly related to the area of the brain involved. Posturing reflects a balance between the lower exciting and the higher inhibiting influences, and strong muscles overcome weaker ones. *Decorticate posturing* (Fig. 37-4, *A*) is seen when there is severe dysfunction of the cerebral cortex. Typical decorticate posturing includes adduction of arms at the shoulders, the arms being flexed on the chest with the wrists flexed and the hands fisted, and the lower extremities being extended and adducted. *Decerebrate posturing* (Fig. 37-4, *B*), a sign of dysfunction at the level of the midbrain, is characterized by rigid extension and pronation of the arms and legs. Unilateral decerebrate posturing is often caused by tentorial herniation.

The posturing may not be evident when the child is quiet but can usually be elicited by applying painful stimuli, such as a blunt object pressed on the base of the nail. Nurses should avoid applying thumb pressure to the supraorbital region of the frontal bone (risk of orbital damage) or knuckle pressure to the sternum (risk of bruising). Noxious stimuli, such as suctioning, will elicit a response, as may turning or touching. When describing posturing, the stimulus needed to provoke the response is as important as the reaction.

Reflexes

Testing of some reflexes may be of limited value, such as those present in an intact spinal cord (see Chapter 40). In general, the corneal, pupillary, muscle-stretch, superficial, and plantar reflexes tend to be absent in deep coma. The state of reflexes is variable in lighter grades of unconsciousness and depends on the underlying pathologic process and the location of the lesion. The doll's eye reflex maneuver, described previously, reflects paralysis of CN III. Absence of corneal reflexes and presence of a tonic neck reflex are associated with severe brain damage. Babinski reflex, in which the lateral portion of the foot is stroked, may be of value if it is found to be present consistently in children older than 1 year. A positive Babinski reflex is significant in assessment of pyramidal tract lesions when it is unilateral and associated with other pyramidal signs. A fluctuating Babinski reflex is often observed after seizures (see Fig. 8-10, *B*).

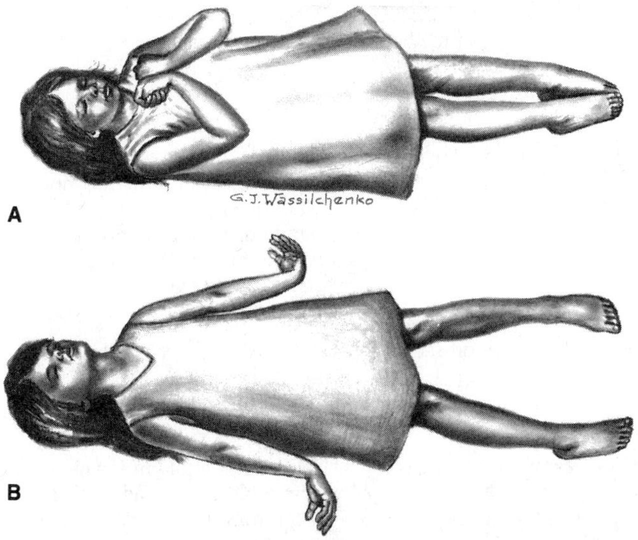

Fig. 37-4. A, Decorticate posturing. **B,** Decerebrate posturing.

✦ **NURSING ALERT** Three key reflexes that demonstrate neurologic health in young infants are the Moro, tonic neck, and withdrawal reflexes.

SPECIAL DIAGNOSTIC PROCEDURES

Numerous diagnostic procedures are used for assessment of cerebral function. Laboratory tests that may help to delineate the cause of unconsciousness include blood glucose, urea nitrogen, and electrolyte (pH, sodium, potassium, chloride, calcium, and bicarbonate) tests; clotting studies, hematocrit, and a complete blood count; liver function tests; blood cultures if there is fever; and sometimes studies to detect lead or other toxic substances, such as drugs.

An electroencephalogram (EEG) may provide important information. For example, generalized random slow activity suggests suppressed cortical function; localized slow activity suggests a focal lesion, such as a mass; and generalized projected patterns suggest brainstem involvement. A flat tracing is one of the criteria used as evidence of brain death. Examination of spinal fluid is carried out when toxic encephalopathy or infection is suspected. Lumbar puncture is ordinarily delayed if intracranial hemorrhage is suspected and is contraindicated in the presence of ICP because of the potential for tentorial herniation (see p. 1743).

Auditory and visual evoked potentials are sometimes used in neurologic diagnosis of very young children. Auditory evoked potential (AEP) and visual evoked potential (VEP) testing demonstrate brainstem integrity and transmission of stimuli to cortical centers (Taylor and Farrell, 1989). Brainstem auditory evoked potentials are useful for evaluating the continuity of brainstem auditory tracts and are particularly useful for detecting demyelinating disease and neoplasms of the brainstem and distinguishing between brainstem and cortical lesions. For example, a normal evoked potential in a comatose patient suggests involvement of the cerebral hemispheres.

Highly sophisticated tests are carried out with specialized equipment by skilled personnel. Two imaging techniques, computed tomography (CT) (Fig. 37-5) and magnetic resonance imaging (MRI), assist in diagnosis by scanning soft tissues as well as solid matter. Most of these tests are outlined in Table 37-4. Because such tests can be threatening to children, a child will need preparation for, and support and reassurance during, the tests. (See Preparation for Procedures, Chapter 27.)

Children who are old enough to understand require care-

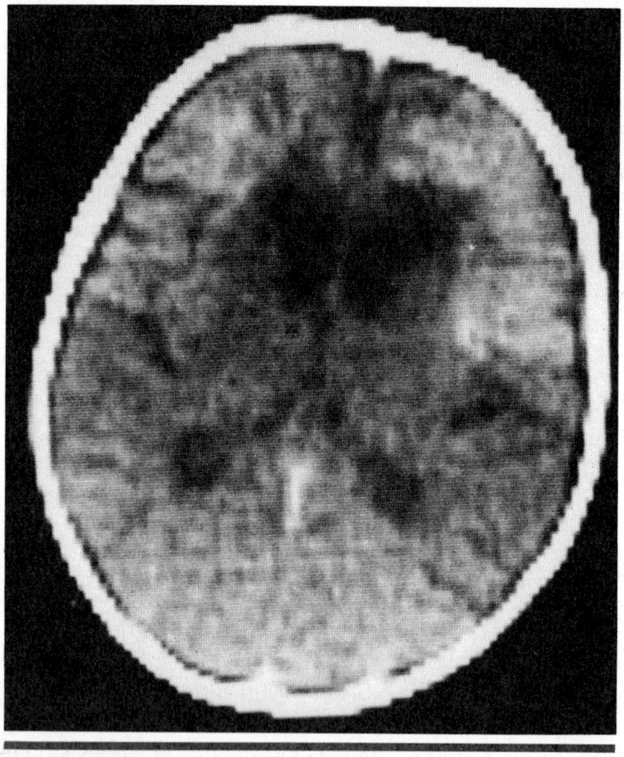

Fig. 37-5. CT scan of 5-month-old with *H. influenzae* meningitis, seizures, and coma. Note bilateral cortical enhancement.
From Swaiman, K.F.: Pediatric neurology, St. Louis, 1989, Mosby–Year Book, Inc.

ful explanation of the procedure, why it is being done, what they will experience, and how they can help. School-age children usually appreciate a more detailed description of why contrast material is injected. The importance of lying still for tests, particularly CT, needs to be stressed. Children unfamiliar with the machines can be shown a picture beforehand. Although radiographic examinations are not painful, the machinery is often so frightening in appearance that the child protests because of anxiety.

This is especially true of CT and MRI, which require that the child's head be placed within a special immobilizing device. Chin and cheek pads are sometimes used to prevent the slightest head movement, and straps are applied to the body to prevent a slight change in body position. The nurse can explain these events to a frightened child by comparing them to an astronaut's preparation for a space flight. It is very important to emphasize to the child that at no time is the procedure painful. Young children who are unable to cooperate require sedation.

It is helpful for nurses to become acquainted with the equipment and the general environment in which the test will take place so that they can better explain the procedure to children at their level of understanding. Written material describing the procedure should be available for parents and may be appropriate to share with children. Equipment is often strange and ominous to children and may be perceived as a frightening monster. It is especially frightening to young children to experience a large mechanical device

Table 37-4 Neurologic diagnostic procedures

TEST	DESCRIPTION	PURPOSE	COMMENTS
Lumbar puncture (LP)	Long needle is inserted between L3 and L4 vertebrae into subarachnoid space; cerebrospinal fluid (CSF) pressure is measured, and sample is collected for examination	Diagnostic—measures spinal fluid pressure, obtains CSF for visualization and laboratory analysis Therapeutic—injection of medication, spinal anesthesia	Contraindicated in patients with increased intracranial pressure (ICP) or infected skin over puncture site
Subdural tap	Needle is inserted into anterior fontanel or coronal suture (midline to pupil)	Helps rule out subdural effusions Relieves ICP	Requires shaving scalp Infant placed in semierect position after subdural tap to minimize leakage from site; avoid crying if possible Check site frequently for evidence of leakage
Ventricular puncture	Needle is inserted into lateral ventricle via coronal suture (midline to pupil)	Removes CSF to relieve pressure	Used if LP unsuccessful or contraindicated Risk of intracerebral or ventricular hemorrhage
Transillumination	Flashlight with rubber adapter is held snugly against infant's head in totally darkened room	Varying degrees of localized glowing may be seen in abnormal fluid accumulation in various areas of head	Normally in full-term infant, a halo of light extends 1 to 2 cm from rim of light source

Table 37-4 Neurologic diagnostic procedures—cont'd

TEST	DESCRIPTION	PURPOSE	COMMENTS
Electroencephalography	Records changes in electric potential of brain Electrodes are placed at various points on scalp and amplified Impulses are recorded by electromagnetic pen	Measures electric activity of cerebral cortex Detects electric abnormalities—diagnosis of seizures Used to determine brain death	Patient should rest quietly during procedure May require sedation Reduce external stimuli to a minimum during procedure
Nuclear brain scan	Intravenous (IV) injection of radioactive material that is counted and recorded after fixed time interval	Test material accumulates in areas where blood-brain barrier is defective Identifies focal brain lesions (e.g., tumors, abscesses) Positive uptake of material with encephalitis and subdural hematoma Visualizes CSF pathways	Requires sedation in young or uncooperative children and IV infusion In normal children or noncommunicating hydrocephalus there is no retrograde filling of ventricles Areas of concentrated uptake of material are termed "hot spots"
Echoencephalography	Pulses of ultrasonic waves are beamed through head; echoes from reflecting surfaces are recorded graphically	Identifies shifts in midline structures from their normal positions as a result of intracranial lesions May show ventricular dilatation	Simple, safe, rapid procedure Fontanel must be patent
Real-time ultrasonography (RTUS)	Similar to CT but uses ultrasound instead of ionizing radiation	Allows high-resolution anatomic visualization in variety of imaging planes	Produces images similar to CT scan Especially useful in neonatal CNS problems Anterior fontanel must be patent
Radiography	Skull films are taken from several projections—lateral, posterolateral, axial (submentoventricular), half-axial	Shows fractures, dislocations, spreading suture lines, craniostenosis Shows degenerative changes, bone erosion, calcifications	Simple, noninvasive procedure
Computed tomography (CT scan)	Pinpoint x-ray beam is directed on horizontal or vertical plane to provide series of "cuts" or "slices" that are fed into computer and assembled in image displayed on video screen and transferred to permanent record	Visualized horizontal and vertical cross section of brain at any axis Distinguishes density of various intracranial tissues and structures—congenital abnormalities, hemorrhage, tumors, demyelinating and inflammatory processes	Noninvasive procedure Requires sedation Can be done on outpatient basis Rapid, relatively safe and accurate
Magnetic resonance imaging (MRI) or nuclear magnetic resonance (NMR)	Produces radiofrequency emissions from elements (e.g., hydrogen, phosphorus), which are converted to visual images by computer	Permits visualization of morphologic features of target structures Permits tissue discrimination unavailable with many techniques	Noninvasive No exposure to radiation Requires heavy sedation for lengthy immobilization Parent or attendant can remain in room with child Does not visualize bone detail or calcifications No metal can be present in the scanner
Positron emission transaxial tomography (PETT) or positron emission tomography (PET)	IV injection of positron-emitting radionucleotide; local concentrations are detected and transformed into a visual display by computer	Detects and measures blood volume and flow in brain, metabolic activity, biochemical changes within tissues, etc.	Requires lengthy period of immobility Minimum exposure to radiation
Digital subtraction angiography (DSA)	Contrast dye injected IV; computer "subtracts" all tissues without contrast medium, leaving clear image of contrast medium in vessels studied	Visualizes vasculature of target tissue Visualizes finite vascular abnormalities	Safe alternative to angiography Patient must remain still during procedure

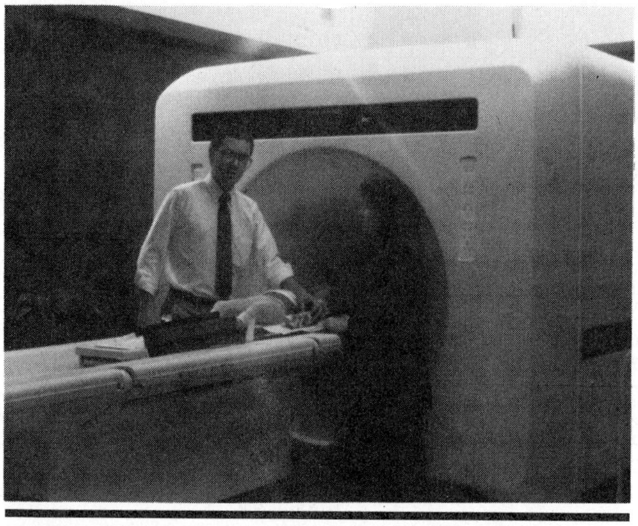

Fig. 37-6. This child requires sedation for his MRI scan. Parents may remain at his side until he is asleep and be present when he awakens.

coming toward them as if to crush or devour them. They need constant reassurance from a trusted companion (Fig. 37-6). Since children are particularly frightened of needles, they need to be informed of any medication or contrast media to be administered by this route.

Physical preparation may involve administration of a sedative. If so, children should be helped through the preparation and administration and assured that someone will remain with them (if this is possible). Children need continual support and reinforcement during the procedures in which they remain conscious. Vital signs and physiologic response to the procedure are monitored throughout. Many diagnostic procedures performed on an outpatient basis require sedation, and children need recovery time and observation.

Children who have undergone a procedure with general anesthesia require postanesthesia care, including positioning to prevent aspiration of secretions and frequent assessment of vital signs and LOC. In addition, other neurologic functions, such as pupillary responses, motor strength, and movement, are tested at regular intervals. Any surgical wound resulting from the test is checked for bleeding, CSF leakage, and other complications. Children who undergo repeated subdural taps should have their hematocrit measured daily to detect any blood loss from the procedure.

Children's emotional reaction to the procedure is also considered. They should be allowed to express their feelings about the experience through verbal expression and the use of therapeutic play. Parents also seek and are entitled to an explanation of results of tests and procedures performed on their children. Nurses are in a unique position to provide support and education to parents regarding procedures.

THE CHILD WITH CEREBRAL COMPROMISE

The child who has sustained some manner of cerebral compromise as a result of physical injury, infection, near-drowning, or toxic injury is usually in varying states of consciousness. No matter what the etiologic factor, the nursing efforts are directed primarily toward detection of possible alterations in condition and preventing further damage to the various systems and tissues. The outcome and recovery of the unconscious child may depend on the level of nursing care and observational skills.

NURSING CARE OF THE UNCONSCIOUS CHILD

The unconscious child requires continuous nursing attendance with observation, recording, and evaluation of changes in objective signs. These observations provide valuable information regarding the patient's progress. Often they serve as a guide to diagnosis and treatment. Therefore careful and detailed observations are essential for the patient's welfare. In addition, vital functions must be maintained and complications prevented through conscientious and meticulous nursing care. The outcome of unconsciousness may be early and complete recovery, death within a few hours or days, persistent and permanent unconsciousness, or recovery with varying degrees of residual mental and/or physical disability.

Emergency measures are directed toward assuming a patent airway, treatment of shock, and reduction of ICP (if present). Delayed treatment often leads to increased damage. As soon as emergency measures have been implemented—in many cases concurrently—therapies for specific causes are begun. Because nursing care is closely related to the medical management, both are considered here.

Assessment

Continual observation of level of LOC, pupillary reaction, and vital signs is essential to management of CNS disorders. Regular assessment of neurologic signs is a vital part of nursing comatose children. Vital signs are taken and recorded regularly. The frequency depends on the cause of coma, the status, and the progression of cerebral involvement. Intervals may be as frequent as every 15 minutes or as long as every 2 hours. Significant alterations are reported immediately. Temperature is taken every 2 to 4 hours, depending on the patient's condition.

An elevated temperature may occur in children with CNS dysfunction; therefore a light covering is sufficient. Vigorous efforts, such as tepid sponge baths or application of a hypothermia blanket, are needed to prevent brain damage if temperature exceeds 40° C (104° F) rectally.

The LOC is assessed periodically, including size, equality, and reaction of pupils to light and signs of meningeal irritation, such as nuchal rigidity. This also includes response to vocal commands, spontaneous behavior, resistance to care, and response to painful stimuli. Motions of any type, changes in muscle tone or strength, and body position are noted. Seizure activity is described according to type and length of seizure and body areas involved (see Box 37-9).

Pain management for the comatose child requires astute nursing observation and management. Signs of pain include changes in behavior (e.g., increased agitation and rigidity, and alterations in physiologic parameters); usually increased heart rate, respiratory rate, and blood pressure; and decreased oxygen saturation. Since these findings are not specific for pain, the nurse should observe for their appearance during times of induced or suspected pain and their disappearance following the inciting procedure or the administration of analgesia. A pain assessment record should be used to document indications of pain and the effectiveness of interventions (see Pain Assessment, Chapter 26).

Sedatives are usually avoided but may be indicated when extreme agitation or restlessness may result in further damage. If so, chloral hydrate or diphenhydramine (Benadryl) are preferred. These drugs are less likely to produce respiratory depression but produce no analgesia. However, favorable results are achieved with the administration of codeine and acetaminophen, which are analgesics.

NURSING ALERT When codeine is used, bowel elimination must be closely monitored because of the constipating effect of codeine. A stool softener should be given regularly.

Anticonvulsants, primarily phenytoin (Dilantin) or phenobarbital, are ordered for control of seizure activity.

Nursing Diagnoses

Based on a thorough assessment, several nursing diagnoses are identified. The more common diagnoses for the unconscious child are included in the Nursing Care Plan on pp. 1734-1736. Others may apply in specific situations.

Planning

Nursing objectives for the unconscious child include the following:

1. Maintain respiratory integrity.
2. Prevent increasing ICP.
3. Provide for basic needs—hygiene, nutrition, hydration, elimination.
4. Prevent complications of immobility.
5. Support and educate the family.

Implementation

Respiratory Management

Respiratory effectiveness is the primary concern in care of the unconscious child, and establishment of an adequate airway is *always* the first priority. Carbon dioxide has a potent vasodilating effect and will increase CBF and ICP. Cerebral hypoxia that extends longer than 4 minutes nearly always causes irreversible brain damage.

Children in lighter stages of coma may be able to cough and swallow, but those in deeper states of coma are unable to handle secretions, which tend to pool in the throat and pharynx. Dysfunction of CN IX and X place the child at risk of aspiration and cardiac arrest; therefore the child is positioned to prevent aspiration of secretions, and the stomach is emptied to reduce the likelihood of vomiting. In infants, blockage of air passages from secretions can happen in seconds. In addition, upper airway obstruction from laryngospasm is a frequent complication in comatose children.

A temporary airway can be used for the child who is suffering a temporary loss of consciousness, such as after a seizure or anesthesia. For children who remain unconscious for a time, a nasotracheal or orotracheal tube is inserted to maintain the open airway and facilitate removal of secretions. A tracheostomy is performed in cases in which laryngoscopy for introduction of an endotracheal tube would be difficult or dangerous. Suctioning is used as often as needed to clear the airway, exerting care to prevent increasing ICP. Respiratory status is observed and evaluated regularly. Signs of respiratory embarrassment may be an indication for ventilatory assistance.

When the respiratory center is involved, mechanical ventilation is usually indicated (see Chapter 31). Blood gas analysis is performed regularly, and oxygen is administered when indicated. Moderately severe hypoxia and respiratory acidosis are often present but not always evident from clinical manifestations. Hyperventilation frequently accompanies unconsciousness and may lead to respiratory alkalosis, or it may represent the body's attempt to compensate for metabolic acidosis. Therefore blood gas and pH determinations are essential guides for electrolyte therapy. Chest physiotherapy is carried out on a regular basis, and the child's position is changed at least every 2 hours to prevent pulmonary complications.

Increased Intracranial Pressure Monitoring

Prompt intervention is lifesaving in the comatose patient who has evidence of marked increase in ICP. When increased ICP is the result of accumulation of CSF from obstruction of CSF flow, a ventricular tap will provide relief quickly and effectively. Evacuation of a hematoma reduces pressure from this source. Indications for inserting an ICP monitor are (1) Glasgow Coma Scale (GCS) evaluation of less than 7, (2) Glasgow Coma Scale (GCS) evaluation of less than 8 with respiratory assistance, (3) deterioration of condition, and (4) subjective judgment regarding clinical appearance and response.

Four major types of ICP monitors are (1) intraventricular catheter with fibroscopic sensors attached to a monitoring system, (2) subarachnoid bolt (Richmond screw), (3) epidural sensor, and (4) anterior fontanel pressure monitor. Transducers for both ventricular and subarachnoid

NURSING CARE PLAN
The Unconscious Child

NURSING DIAGNOSIS: Potential for suffocation (aspiration): ineffective airway clearance related to depressed sensorium, impaired motor function

GOAL 1

Maintain patent airway

INTERVENTIONS

Position for optimum ventilation
Remove accumulated secretions promptly
Administer care of endotracheal tube or tracheostomy if appropriate; have equipment available for emergency insertion if indicated for respiratory distress
Monitor artificial ventilation

EXPECTED OUTCOME

Aiway remains patent

NURSING DIAGNOSIS: Potential for injury related to physical immobility, depressed sensorium, intracranial pathology

GOAL 1

Minimize intracranial pressure (ICP)

INTERVENTIONS

Elevate head of the bed 15 to 30 degrees
Avoid positions or activities that increase ICP
- Pressure on neck veins
- Flexion or extension of neck
- Head rotation
- Valsalva maneuver
- Painful stimuli
- Respiratory procedures (especially suctioning)

Prevent constipation
Provide:
- Quiet, subdued environment
- Pleasant auditory experiences
- Therapeutic touch
- Avoid emotionally stressful conversation (e.g., about pain, condition, prognosis)

*Administer paralyzing agents if prescribed

EXPECTED OUTCOMES

ICP remains within safe limits
Child shows no evidence of increased ICP

GOAL 2

Prevent cerebral hypoxia

INTERVENTIONS

Position for maximum ventilation
Maintain patent airway
- Position to prevent aspiration: semiprone position, side-lying position
- Aspirate airway as needed
- Insert oral airway if indicated
- Avoid neck hyperextension

Provide oxygen as indicated by objective signs or as ordered
Hyperventilate at prescribed intervals, if ordered
If on mechanical ventilation:
- Monitor for correct settings, proper functioning
- Prepare to provide artificial ventilation in case of ventilatory failure, have manual resuscitation (Ambu) bag at hand

*Administer medications as ordered to prevent cerebral edema and improve cerebral circulation

EXPECTED OUTCOME

Child breathes easily; respirations are within normal limits (see inside front cover)

GOAL 3

Prevent cerebral edema

INTERVENTIONS

Elevate head of bed to 15 to 30 degrees
Maintain intravenous fluids as prescribed
*Administer hyperosmolar fluids as prescribed
*Administer corticosteroids as ordered

EXPECTED OUTCOME

Child exhibits no signs of increased ICP

GOAL 4

Prevent seizures

INTERVENTIONS

Avoid stimulation that precipitates undesirable responses
*Administer sedatives or anticonvulsants as prescribed
Schedule nursing activities for minimum disturbance

EXPECTED OUTCOME

Child exhibits no seizure activity or undue restlessness and agitation

GOAL 5

Prevent or control hyperthermia

INTERVENTIONS

Remove excess coverings
*Administer antipyretics, if prescribed
Apply and monitor hypothermia blanket if indicated or ordered; administer antishivering agents if ordered

EXPECTED OUTCOME

Body temperature remains within safe limits (see inside front cover)

*Dependent nursing action.

GOAL 6

Prevent respiratory infection

INTERVENTIONS

Turn frequently—at least every 2 hours
Avoid contact with persons with upper respiratory infection
Provide good oral hygiene
Perform chest physiotherapy as prescribed and as tolerated

EXPECTED OUTCOME

Child exhibits no evidence of pulmonary dysfunction

GOAL 7

Prevent corneal irritation

INTERVENTIONS

Patch eyes if indicated
Keep lids completely closed
Instill "artificial tears"

EXPECTED OUTCOME

Corneas remain clear and moist

GOAL 8

Prevent drying and caking of mucous membranes

INTERVENTION

Provide meticulous mouth care

EXPECTED OUTCOME

Mucous membranes remain clean, moist, and free of irritation

GOAL 9

Protect from physical injury

INTERVENTIONS

Keep siderails up
Pad hard surfaces that may injure extremities during spontaneous or involuntary movement

EXPECTED OUTCOME

Child remains free of physical injury

GOAL 10

Maintain limb flexibility and functions

INTERVENTIONS

Perform passive range of motion exercises
Position to reduce contractures—splint contracting joints if needed

EXPECTED OUTCOME

Joints remain flexible and retain full range of motion

NURSING DIAGNOSIS: Potential impaired skin integrity related to immobility, body secretions, invasive procedures

GOAL 1

Maintain skin integrity

INTERVENTIONS

Place child on sheepskin, Egg-crate pad, or other resilient surface
Change position frequently unless contraindicated by increased ICP
Protect pressure points (e.g., trochanter, sacrum, ankle, shoulder, occiput)
Inspect skin surfaces regularly for signs of irritation, redness, evidence of pressure
Cleanse skin regularly, at least once daily
Protect skinfolds and surfaces that rub together
Keep clothing and linen clean and dry
Carry out good perineal care under urine collection device
Stimulate circulation by gentle rubbing with lotion or other lubricating substance
Protect lips with cream or ointment

EXPECTED OUTCOME

Skin remains clean, intact, and free of irritation

NURSING DIAGNOSIS: Feeding, bathing/hygiene, toileting self-care deficits (level 4) related to physical immobility, perceptual and cognitive impairment

GOAL 1

Ensure adequate nutritional intake

INTERVENTIONS

Provide nourishment in manner suitable to child's condition
Monitor intravenous feedings when ordered
*Feed prescribed formula by means of nasogastric or gastrostomy tube

EXPECTED OUTCOME

Child obtains sufficient nourishment

GOAL 2

Provide hygienic care

INTERVENTIONS

Bathe daily or more often, if indicated
Dress appropriately
Keep hair combed and styled

EXPECTED OUTCOME

Child appears clean and as well groomed as possible within limitations of condition

*Dependent nursing action.

Continued.

NURSING CARE PLAN
The Unconscious Child—cont'd

GOAL 3

Provide toileting and ensure adequate elimination

INTERVENTIONS

Provide sufficient liquid intake, unless contraindicated by cerebral edema or if overhydration is a threat
Apply urine collecting device or insert indwelling catheter (if ordered)
Provide proper care of catheter
Use collection appliances, if feasible
Clean skin well after each elimination
Diaper as needed
Check abdomen for evidence of distention
Measure abdominal girth
*Administer stool softener
*Administer suppositories or enema as indicated

EXPECTED OUTCOMES

Child eliminates sufficient urine (specify)
Bowel is evacuated daily
Child's diaper area remains clean and free of irritation

NURSING DIAGNOSIS: Sensory/perceptual alterations (visual, auditory, kinesthetic, gustatory, tactile, olfactory) related to central nervous system impairment, bed rest

GOAL 1

Provide sensory stimulation

INTERVENTIONS

Provide tactile stimulation (if it does not evoke undesirable muscle response, e.g., seizures)
Provide auditory stimulation by voice, radio, muscle box, etc.
Provide visual stimuli appropriate for age
Provide proprioceptive stimulation by rocking, cuddling, etc.

EXPECTED OUTCOMES

Child receives sensory stimulation appropriate to age and condition
Child appears relaxed and rests quietly

GOAL 2

Relieve discomfort

INTERVENTIONS

Assess for evidence of pain
*Administer pain medication as needed

EXPECTED OUTCOME

Child exhibits no evidence of pain
See Nursing Care Plan: The Child in Pain, Chapter 26

NURSING DIAGNOSIS: Altered family processes related to a child hospitalized with a potentially fatal condition or permanent disability

GOAL 1

Support family

INTERVENTIONS AND EXPECTED OUTCOMES

See Nursing Care Plan: The Family of the Ill or Hospitalized Child, Chapter 26

GOAL 2

Assist in child placement, if indicated

INTERVENTIONS

Provide needed information
Answer family's questions; encourage expression of feelings
Refer to persons or agencies for further information and clarification
Support parent's decisions

EXPECTED OUTCOME

Family verbalizes feelings and concerns

*Dependent nursing action.

monitoring should be set up without the use of a flush device.

The catheter method involves introduction of a catheter into the lateral ventricle on the nondominant side, if known, or placement in the subdural space. The catheter has the advantage of providing a means of extraventricular (or continuous) drainage to reduce pressure. A drainage bag attached to the system is kept at the level of the ventricles and can be lowered to decrease ICP.

In the bolt method the end of the bolt is placed into the subarachnoid space. The bolt cannot be adequately secured in a small child's pliant skull, although special modifications have been developed for children under 6 years of age.

✦ **NURSING ALERT** The bolt is stabilized with dressings, but these are not changed or disturbed, even to check the site.

The placement of the bolt is not adjusted by anyone except the neurosurgeon who placed the device. The neurosurgeon is notified if a satisfactory wave form is not observed.

An epidural sensor can be placed between the dura and the skull through a burr hole, and connected to a stopcock assembly and a transducer, which provides a readout of the pressure. Although less invasive, correlation of pressure readings may be inconsistent. In infants a fontanel transducer can be used to detect impulses from a pressure sensor and convert them to electrical energy. The electrical energy is then converted to visible waves or numerical readings on an oscilloscope. ICP measurement from the anterior fontanel, although noninvasive, may prove to be inaccurate if the equipment is poorly placed or inconsistently recalibrated.

ICP can be increased by instillation of solutions; therefore antibiotics are administered sytemically if a positive CSF culture is obtained. However, intravenous ICP monitoring rarely causes infection. Since CSF is a body fluid, isolation precautions may be implemented according to hospital policy (see Infection Control, Chapter 27).

Nurses caring for patients with intracranial monitoring devices must be acquainted with the system, assist with insertion, interpret the monitor readings, and be able to distinguish between danger signals and mechanical dysfunction.

For increased ICP resulting from cerebral edema, several medical measures are available. Osmotic diuretics may provide rapid relief in emergency situations. Although their effect is transient, lasting only about 6 hours, they can be lifesaving in emergencies. These substances are rapidly excreted by the kidneys and carry with them large quantities of sodium and water. Mannitol (or sometimes urea) administered intravenously is the drug most frequently employed for rapid reduction. The infusion is generally given slowly but may be pushed rapidly if there is herniation or impending herniation. Because of the profound diuretic effect of the drug, an indwelling catheter is inserted to ensure bladder emptying. Adrenocorticosteroids are not recommended for cerebral edema secondary to head trauma. $Paco_2$ should be maintained at 25 to 30 mm Hg to produce vasoconstriction, which reduces CBF, thereby decreasing ICP.

Nursing activities. In cases of high levels of increased ICP, nursing procedures tend to trigger reactive pressure waves in many patients. For example, increased intrathoracic or abdominal pressure will be transmitted to the cranium. Particular care should be taken in positioning these patients to avoid neck vein compression, which may further increase ICP by interfering with venous return.

✦ **NURSING ALERT** The head of the bed is elevated 15 to 30 degrees and the child positioned so that the head is maintained in a midline to facilitate venous drainage and avoid jugular compression. Turning side to side is contraindicated because of the risk of jugular compression.

The child can be propped to one side or the other, and the use of an alternating-pressure or Egg-crate mattress reduces the chance of prolonged pressure to vulnerable areas. Frequent clinical assessment of the child cannot be replaced by an ICP monitoring device.

It is important to avoid activities that may increase ICP by causing pain, emotional stress, or crying or those that might trigger a convulsive seizure. Gentle range of motion exercises can be carried out but should not be performed vigorously. Nontherapeutic touch can cause an increase in ICP. Any disturbing procedures to be performed should be scheduled to take advantage of therapies that reduce ICP, such as osmotherapy and sedation. Efforts are taken to minimize or eliminate environmental noise (see Nursing Tip). Assessment and intervention to relieve pain are important nursing functions to decrease ICP.

Suctioning. Suctioning and percussion are poorly tolerated and are therefore contraindicated unless there are concurrent respiratory problems. Hypoxia and the Valsalva maneuver associated with cough both acutely elevate ICP. Vibration, which does not increase ICP, accomplishes excellent results and should be tried first if treatment is needed. If suctioning is necessary, it should be used judiciously and preceded by hyperventilation with 100% oxygen, which can be monitored during suctioning with a pulse oxygen sensor reading to determine oxygen saturation.

Nutrition and Hydration

Fluids and calories are supplied initially by the intravenous route (see Chapter 28). An intravenous infusion is started early, and the type of fluid administered is determined by the general condition of the patient. Fluid therapy requires careful monitoring and adjustment based on neurologic signs and electrolyte determinations. Often comatose children are unable to cope with the same amounts of fluid they could tolerate at other times, and overhydration must be avoided to prevent fatal cerebral edema.

Later, nutrition is provided in a balanced formula given by nasogastric or gastrostomy tube. The nasogastric tube is usually taped in place with care to prevent pressure on the nares. Most children have continuous feedings, but if bolus feedings are used, the tube is rinsed with water after each feeding. Tubes are replaced according to unit policy. Nostrils are alternated with each replacement to prevent nasal irritation and pressure. Overfeeding should be avoided to prevent vomiting with its attendant danger of aspiration. Stomach contents are aspirated and measured before feeding to ascertain the amount remaining in the stomach. If the residual volume is excessive (depending on the size of the child), the dietitian and physician should be consulted regarding alteration of the formula composition to provide the

NURSING TIP: ENVIRONMENTAL NOISE

Placing earphones over a child's ears has been shown to lower ICP, heart rate, and blood pressure significantly. A greater net decline was achieved when soothing music was played through the earphones (Wincek, as reported by Wong, 1988).

Table 37-5 Effects of altered pituitary secretion

MEASUREMENT	DI	SIADH
Urine output	Increased	Decreased
Specific gravity	Decreased	Increased
Serum sodium	Increased (hypernatremia)	Decreased (hyponatremia)

needed calories and nutrients in a smaller volume. The aspirated contents should always be refed.

Hydration is maintained in the same manner. When cerebral edema is a threat, fluids may be restricted to reduce the chance of fluid overload. Skin and mucous membranes are examined for signs of dehydration. Observation for signs of altered fluid balance related to abnormal pituitary secretions is a part of nursing care.

Altered pituitary secretion. An altered ability to handle fluid loads is attributed in part to the syndrome of inappropriate antidiuretic hormone (SIADH) and diabetes insipidus (DI) resulting from hypothalamic dysfunction (see Chapter 38). SIADH frequently accompanies CNS diseases such as head injury, meningitis, encephalitis, brain abscess, brain tumor, and subarachnoid hemorrhage. In the patient with SIADH, scant quantities of urine are excreted, electrolyte analysis reveals hyponatremia and hyposmolality, and manifestations of overhydration are evident. It is important to evaluate all parameters, since the reduced urine output might be erroneously interpreted as a sign of dehydration.

The treatment of SIADH consists of restriction of fluids until serum electrolytes and osmolality return to normal levels. Since SIADH frequently occurs with meningitis in children, fluid restriction is often prescribed. Likewise, DI may occur following intracranial trauma. There is increased urine volume and the accompanying danger of dehydration (see Table 37-5 for comparison of fluid changes in SIADH and DI). Adequate replacement of fluids is essential, and observation of electrolyte balance is necessary to detect signs of hypernatremia and hyperosmolality. Exogenous vasopressin may be administered.

Medications

The cause of unconsciousness determines specific drug therapies. Children with infectious processes are given antibiotics appropriate to the disease and the infecting organism, and corticosteroids are prescribed for inflammatory conditions and edema. Cerebral edema is an indication for osmotherapy with osmotic diuretics (e.g., mannitol), diuretics (e.g., furosemide), and/or hypertonic glucose solution. Sedatives are often indicated for extreme restlessness, agitation, and hyperresponsiveness to stimuli. Sedatives or anticonvulsants are prescribed for seizure activity. Analgesics are prescribed to control pain.

✦ **NURSING ALERT** When used for seizures, phenytoin should be administered slowly but infused completely in 1 hour (the drug tends to precipitate). Too rapid administration may cause cardiac dysrhythmias.

Deep coma, induced by administration of barbiturates, is controversial in the management of ICP. Barbiturate coma requires extensive monitoring, cardiovascular and respiratory support, and ICP monitoring to assess response to therapy. Paralyzing agents, such as pancuronium (Pavulon) also may be needed to aid in performing diagnostic tests, improving effectiveness of therapy, and reducing risks of secondary complications. Elevation of ICP and/or heart rate of patients who are being given paralyzing agents or are under sedation may indicate the need for another dose of either or both medications.

Thermoregulation

Hyperthermia often accompanies cerebral dysfunction, and if present, measures are implemented to reduce the temperature to prevent brain damage from hyperthermia and to reduce metabolic demands generated by the increased body temperature. Antipyretics are the method of choice for fever reduction; cooling devices are used for hyperthermia. Laboratory tests and other methods are used in an attempt to determine the cause, if any, of the hyperthermia. Shivering responses triggered by a cooling blanket can often be alleviated by lukewarm to warm sponging. Treatment with hypothermia and barbiturates increases the risk of iatrogenic complications.

Elimination

A retention catheter is usually inserted in the older child, and a plastic collection bag is placed on the infant or small child. Long-term use of collection bags creates excoriation problems, however. The child who formerly had bowel and bladder control is generally incontinent. The collecting devices help keep the skin clean and provide a means for obtaining an accurate intake and output measurement. If the child remains comatose for a long period, the indwelling catheter may be removed and periodic bladder emptying accomplished by intermittent catheterization. Stool softeners are usually sufficient to maintain bowel function, but suppositories or enemas may be needed occasionally for adequate elimination.

Hygienic Care

Routine measures for cleansing and maintaining skin integrity are an integral part of nursing care of the unconscious child. Skinfolds require special attention to prevent excoriation. The child who is unable to move is prone to develop tissue breakdown and pressure necrosis; therefore the child is placed on a sheepskin, Egg-crate pad, or other resilient appliance (alternating-pressure and water-filled mattresses are also used) to prevent pressure on prominent areas of the body. The goal is prevention by regular change of position and inspection of vulnerable areas, such as the ankle, trochanter, and shoulder. Since unconscious children undergo numerous invasive procedures, these skin sites require special assessment and intervention to promote healing and to prevent infection. Bed linen and any clothing are kept dry and free of wrinkles. Rubbing the back and extremities with lotion or other lubricating preparation stimulates circulation and helps prevent drying of the skin. If the child requires surgery or radiography, the nurse checks all dressings, bony sites, catheters, and intravenous access lines.

Mouth care is performed at least twice daily, since the mouth tends to become dry or coated with mucus. The teeth are carefully brushed with a soft toothbrush or cleaned with gauze saturated with saline. Commercially prepared cleansing devices, such as Toothettes, are convenient for cleansing the mouth and teeth. Lips are coated with ointment, or other preparations to protect them from drying, cracking, or blistering.

The deeply comatose child is also prone to eye irritation. The corneal reflexes are absent; therefore the eyes are easily irritated or damaged by linen, dust, or other substances that may come in contact with them. There is excessive dryness as a result of decreased secretions, especially if the child is undergoing osmotherapy to reduce or prevent brain edema, and incomplete closure of the eyes.

✦ **NURSING ALERT** The eyes should be examined regularly and carefully for early signs of irritation or inflammation. Artificial tears (methylcellulose) are placed in the eyes every 1 to 2 hours. Sometimes eye dressings may be needed to protect the eyes from possible damage.

The hair is combed and styled neatly. Long hair is usually braided and secured with rubber bands. The scalp should be kept clean with dry or wet shampoos as needed. The child's head may be shaved for tests or surgical procedures. If so, the hair is saved if possible and given to the family.

Positioning and Exercise

The unconscious child is positioned to prevent aspiration of saliva, nasogastric secretions, and vomitus and to minimize ICP. The head of the bed is elevated, and the child is placed in a side-lying or semiprone position. A small, firm pillow is placed under the head, and the uppermost limbs are flexed and supported with pillows. The weight of the body should not rest on the dependent arm. In the semiprone position the child lies with the dependent arm at the side behind the body, the opposite side supported on pillows, and the uppermost arm and leg flexed and resting on the pillows. This position prevents undue pressure on the dependent extremities. The dependent position of the face encourages drainage of secretions and prevents the flaccid tongue from obstructing the airway.

Normal range of motion exercises help to maintain function and prevent contractures of joints. Exercises should be done gently and with full range of motion. A small rolled pad can be placed in the palms to help maintain proper position of fingers; footboards or boots can be used to help prevent footdrop; splinting may be needed to prevent severe contractures of wrist, knee, or ankle in decerebrate children.

Stimulation

Sensory stimulation is important in the care of the unconscious child, just as it is in the care of the alert child. For the temporarily unconscious or semiconscious child, sensory stimulation helps to arouse the child to the conscious state and orient the child in terms of time and place. Auditory and tactile stimulation are especially valuable. Tactile stimulation is not appropriate for the child in whom it may elicit an undesirable response. However, for other children tactile contact often has a relaxing and calming effect. When the child's condition permits, holding or rocking the child has a soothing effect and provides the body contact needed by young children.

The auditory sense is often present in a state of coma. Hearing is the last sense to be lost and the first one to be regained; therefore the child should be spoken to as any other child. Conversation around the child should not include thoughtless or derogatory remarks. A radio playing soft music, a music box, or a record player is frequently used to provide auditory stimulation. Singing the child's favorite songs or reading a favorite story is a tactic used to maintain the child's contact with a familiar world. Having parents tape songs or stories provides a continuous source of familiar stimulation. Above all, it is important to remember that this is a child who has all the needs of any ill child.

Family Support

Dealing with the parents of an unconscious child is especially difficult. They may demonstrate all the guilt, fear, hostility, and anxiety of any parent of a seriously ill child (see Chapter 23). In addition, these parents are faced with the uncertain outcome of the cerebral dysfunction. The fear of death, mental retardation, or other permanent disability is present. Nursing intervention with parents depends on the nature of the pathologic condition, the personality of the parents, and the parent-child relationship before injury or illness.

The child may regain consciousness within a short time. If there is little or no residual effect, the child will be dismissed to home care fairly soon. The parents need the most intensive nursing intervention during the period of crisis and uncertainty. During the recovery phase they are given information, information is clarified, and they are encouraged to become involved in the child's care. Often the child's hospitalization is brief; however, some children require extended hospitalization for intensive therapy and rehabilitation.

The parents of children who die within hours or days require the support and guidance that the parents of any dying child would need in coping with the reality of the death and resolving their grief (see Chapter 23).

Probably the most difficult situations are those that involve children who are unconscious permanently or for an indefinite period. Unlike parents who lose a child through death, the finality is lacking for these parents, often leaving them in a state of suspended grief. The presence of the child renders the parents unable to resolve the loss. Like parents of dying children, parents of the comatose child search for any signs of hope. Well-meaning friends and relatives relate instances of miraculous recoveries. The parents seek confirmation and support for such possibilities and assign erroneous meanings to any sign in the child, such as reflexive muscle contractions, that might be interpreted as evidence of recovery.

Like parents who lose a child through death, the parents of the child lost to their world attempt to reconstitute a representation of the child. They bring items that belong to the child, such as favorite toys, music, and other objects cherished by the child. This is interpreted as an attempt to provide stimulation for the child in the hope of eliciting a response, to let the hospital staff know the child as the unique individual he or she was so that the parents' distress can be better appreciated, and to reconstitute an image of the child "lost" to them and for whom they mourn. An awareness of these behaviors and coping mechanisms provides nurses with the understanding that helps them support the parents in their grief process.

Superimposed on the process of grieving for the "lost" child, parents may be faced with difficult decisions. First, there is the child whose brain is so severely damaged that vital functions must be maintained by artificial means. The parents must make the final decision to remove life-support systems. Since the decision is so difficult for parents, the practitioner is frequently placed in a position of making the decision indirectly. After providing the parents with all the information, the physician will suggest that the child be removed from the life support to "see if the child can make it without help." The approach relieves the parents of the decision and can be effective, but it is based on an evaluation of the parents' intellectual level and emotional state. Sometimes parents may even choose to refuse treatment if they believe it to be best for the child and the family (informed dissent). At other times parents request that "everything possible" be done for the child.

The nurses can be instrumental in providing guidance and clarifying information—a valued but demanding undertaking. It is not unusual for the family to ask the same questions and to compare responses elicited from different staff members. A child's death is an intensely personal issue that deserves direct involvement by the nurse and auxiliary support systems.

There is also the child who has survived the illness or injury that produced the brain damage but is left unconscious permanently. In such a situation the parents must decide whether to place the child in a chronic care facility or make arrangements to care for the child at home. During these decisions the nurse can listen to the parents' discussions regarding alternatives, provide information where appropriate, and support the family in their decision. The nurse can help the family prepare for the transfer of the child and make referrals to persons or agencies that can provide additional assistance.

There is also the child who survived the cerebral insult, who is not comatose, but whose physical and/or mental capacity is limited, either minimally or severely. Families of such children must cope with the long and tedious rehabilitation process and uncertain outcome. The drain on financial, emotional, and social resources can be enormous.

For parents who choose to care for their child at home, planning for home care begins early in the process of recovery. The family should become involved with the care of the child as soon as they indicate an interest and ability to do so. They will need education and support in learning to care for the child, regular follow-up observation and assessment of the home management, and planning for some respite care of the child. Parents need to understand that it is important to plan for periodic relief from the continual care of the child (see Discharge Planning and Home Care, Chapter 26).

Evaluation

The effectiveness of nursing interventions for the unconscious child is determined by continual reassessment and evaluation of care based on the following observational guidelines and expected outcomes:

1. Monitor the child's neurologic signs, vital signs, and behavior.
2. Observe the child's response to nursing activities, therapies, and diagnostic procedures; monitor ICP.
3. Observe the child's color, position, and motor activity; measure fluid and nutritional intake and output.
4. Monitor status of the child's respiratory, renal, and gastrointestinal systems and skin.
5. Observe family behaviors and interview members regarding their understandings and their feelings and concerns.

Expected outcomes:
See Nursing Care Plan, pp. 1734-1736.

HEAD INJURY

Head injury can be defined as any pathologic process involving the scalp, skull, meninges, or brain as a result of mechanical force. Accidental injury is the leading cause of death in children under 15 years of age. According to the Head Injury Foundation (1989), 40% of head injuries occur in children and result in 200,000 hospital admissions, including 20,000 severely brain-injured children. Most of these injuries are the result of CNS trauma. Rarely does a child attain adulthood without having sustained a significant bump or blow to the head. Ten of every 100,000 children in the United States between infancy and 14 years of age die each year from head trauma.

Etiology

Falls are the leading cause of head injury, and almost 67% of children less than 5 years of age who died from a fall did so at home (Deaths, 1988). Motor vehicle–related accidents constitute the major cause of severe and fatal head injury at all ages. Child abuse is a cause of severe head injury in children less than 1 year of age. Vigorous shaking of an infant can cause CNS damage, especially a whiplash type of injury and subdural hematoma. Unrestrained children from age 2 to 10 years sustain head injuries in motor vehicles. Unhelmeted children on bicycles and impact injuries in sports are the causes of a significant number of injuries in children over 12 years of age. Adolescents are most often injured in motor vehicle accidents.

The exposed nature of the head renders it particularly vulnerable to external violence, and many of the physical characteristics of children predispose them to craniocerebral trauma. For example, infants are frequently left unattended on beds, in high chairs, and in other places from which they can fall. Because the head of an infant or toddler is proportionately large and heavy in relation to other body parts, it is the most likely to be injured. Incomplete motor development contributes to falls at young ages, and the natural curiosity and exuberance of children frequently place them in situations in which they are likely to incur an injury.

Pathophysiology

The pathology of brain injury is directly related to the force of impact. Intracranial contents (brain, blood, CSF) are damaged because the force is too great to be absorbed by the skull and musculoligamentous support of the head. The elastic, pliable skulls of infants and young children absorb much of the direct energy of physical impact to the head and afford some protection to intracranial structures. Although nervous tissue is delicate, it usually requires a severe blow to cause significant damage.

A child's response to head injury is different from that of adults. The larger head size and insufficient musculoskeletal support render the very young child particularly vulnerable to acceleration-deceleration injuries. The surface area of the child's scalp is large with remarkable vascularity; therefore a child can bleed to death from a severe scalp laceration.

Primary head injuries are those that occur at a time of trauma and include skull fracture, contusions, intracranial hematoma, and diffuse injury. Subsequent complications include hypoxic brain damage, ICP, infection, and cerebral edema. The predominant feature of a child's brain injury is the diffuse amount of swelling that occurs. Hypoxia and hypercapnia threaten the energy requirements of the brain and increase CBF. The added volume across the blood-brain barrier plus the loss of autoregulation exacerbates cerebral edema. Pressure inside the skull greater than arterial pressure results in inadequate perfusion.

Cerebral hyperemia occurs more often in children, and this volume expansion may account for children's tendency to develop intracranial hypertension (Johnson, 1989). However, because the cranium of very young children has the ability to expand and the thin skull is more compliant, they may tolerate increases in ICP better than older children and adults. Children have a significantly higher percentage of good outcomes and a lower mortality rate, as well as a lower incidence of surgical mass lesions after severe head trauma. Their thinner, softer brain, however, may sustain greater long-term damage than previously suggested.

Physical forces act on the head through *acceleration, deceleration,* or *deformation.* Acceleration or deceleration is more descriptive of the circumstances responsible for most head injuries. When the stationary head receives a blow, the sudden acceleration causes deformation of the skull and mass movement of the brain. Continued movement of

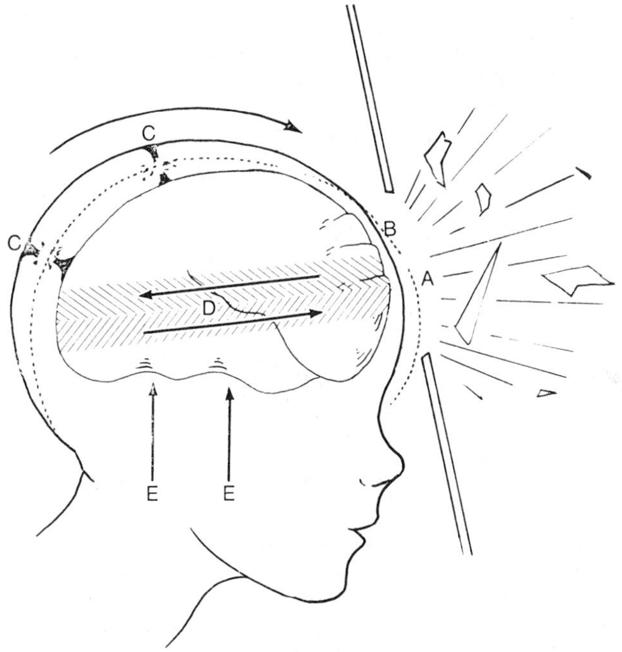

Fig. 37-7. Mechanical distortion of cranium during closed head injury. **A,** Preinjury contour of skull. **B,** Immediate postinjury contour of skull. **C,** Torn subdural vessels. **D,** Shearing forces. **E,** Trauma from contact with floor of cranium.

Redrawn from Grubb, R.L., and Coxe, W.S.: Central nervous system trauma: cranial. In Eliasson, S.G., Presky, A.L., and Hardin, W.B., Jr., editors: Neurological pathophysiology, New York, 1974, Oxford University Press, Inc.

the intracranial contents allows the brain to strike parts of the skull (e.g., the sharp edges of the sphenoid or the irregular surface of the anterior fossa) or the edges of the tentorium.

Although the brain volume remains unchanged, significant distortion and cavitation take place as the brain changes shape in response to the force transmitted from the impact to the skull. This deformation can cause bruising at the point of impact *(coup)* and/or at a distance as the brain collides with the unyielding surfaces far removed from the point of impact *(contrecoup)* (Fig. 37-7). Some of the changes related to this phenomenon may be a result of a momentary increased pressure that produces a temporary negative pressure with cavitation and vaporization contralaterally. Thus a blow to the occipital region can cause severe injury to the frontal and temporal areas of the brain. Sudden deceleration, as takes place during a fall, causes the greatest cerebral injury at the point of impact.

Another effect of brain movement is shearing stresses, which are caused by unequal movement or different rates of acceleration at various levels of the brain. A shearing force may tear small arteries that travel from the cerebral surfaces through the meninges to the dural sinuses to cause subdural hemorrhages. Shearing or stretching effects can also be transmitted to nerve fibers. Maximum stress from the shearing force occurs at the interface between structures of different density so that the gray matter (cell body) rapidly accelerates while the white matter (axons) tends to lag behind. Although shearing forces are maximum at the cerebral surface and extend toward the center of rotation within the brain, the most serious effects are frequently in the area of the brainstem.

Another source of damage occurs when severe compression of the skull causes the brain to be forced through the tentorial opening. This can produce irreparable damage to the brainstem (see Fig. 37-8). Since the uncus of the temporal lobe is the presenting part, this complication is usually referred to as uncal herniation.

As a whole, head injuries can be regarded as localized or generalized. In localized injuries the force is spent on a local area of both skull and underlying tissues; in generalized injuries the force is transmitted to the entire skull, causing widespread movement, distortion, and damage. Local injuries frequently cause hemorrhage and infection, but generalized trauma is associated with a higher mortality. Many head injuries involve both localized and generalized disorders. Patients with mild head injuries have a GCS evaluation of 13 to 15; those with moderate head injuries have a GCS of 9 to 12; and a GCS of 8 or less indicates severe injury.

Concussion. The most common head injury is concussion, a transient and reversible neuronal dysfunction with instantaneous loss of awareness and responsiveness from trauma to the head that persists for a relatively short time, usually minutes or hours. It is generally followed by amnesia for the moment of the injury and a variable period before the injury. This posttraumatic amnesia is characteristic and reflects the extent and severity of injury to the brain after blunt trauma. Posttraumatic amnesia consists of two parts: (1) retrograde amnesia, the period of time before impact for which the patient has no memory, and (2) anterograde amnesia, the period of memory loss after injury. Amnesia in both these periods tends to lessen with time, although there is some permanent amnesia.

The pathogenesis of concussion is still unclear but may be a result of shearing forces that cause stretching, compression, and tearing of nerve fibers, particularly in the area of the central brainstem, the seat of the reticular activating system. It has also been suggested that the anatomic alterations of nerve fibers cause the release of large quantities of acetylcholine into the CSF and a reduction in oxygen consumption with increased lactate production.

Contusion and laceration. The terms *contusion* and *laceration* are used to describe visible bruising and tearing of cerebral tissue. Contusions represent petechial hemorrhages along the superficial aspects of the brain at the site of impact (coup injury) and/or a lesion remote from the site of direct trauma (contrecoup injury). In serious accidents there may be multiple sites of injury.

The major areas of the brain susceptible to contusion or laceration are the occipital, frontal, and temporal lobes. Also, the irregular surfaces of the anterior and middle fossae at the base of the skull are capable of producing bruises or lacerations on forceful impact. Contusions may cause focal disturbances in strength, sensation, or visual awareness. The degree of brain damage in the contused areas varies according to the extent of vascular injury. Signs will vary from mild, transient weakness of a limb to prolonged unconsciousness and paralysis. However, the signs and symptoms may be clinically indistinguishable from concussion.

As a rule, contusions are less common in infants and young children than in adults with comparable trauma, and contrecoup injuries are relatively rare in infants. However, infants who are roughly shaken (whiplash-shake syndrome) can sustain profound neurologic impairment, seizures, retinal hemorrhages, and intracranial subarachnoid or subdural hemorrhages. In addition to these classic injuries, high cervical spinal cord hemorrhages and contusions can occur (Hadley and others, 1989).

Cerebral lacerations are generally associated with penetrating or depressed skull fractures. However, they may occur without fracture in small children. When brain tissue is actually torn, with bleeding into and around the tear, usually more severe and prolonged unconsciousness and paralysis occur, leaving permanent scarring and some degree of disability.

Fractures. Skull fractures are found in over 25% of children who are seen with head injuries (Mealey, 1988). However, the immature skull, because of its flexibility, is able to sustain a greater degree of deformation than the adult skull before it incurs a fracture. It requires a great deal of force to produce a fracture in the skull of an infant. A fracture may occur with little or no brain damage, or severe and fatal brain injury can take place without fracture. The undersurface of the skull contains grooves in which the meningeal arteries lie. A fracture that runs through one of these grooves may tear the artery and produce severe and damaging hemorrhage. The types of fractures that occur are linear, depressed, compound, basilar, and diastatic. As a rule, the faster the blow, the greater the likelihood of a depressed fracture; a low-velocity impact tends to produce a linear fracture.

Linear fractures comprise about 75% of childhood skull fractures (Mealey, 1988). The lines of the fracture are predetermined by the site and velocity of the impact as well as the strength of the bone. Linear fractures are often asymptomatic in older children and heal in 3 to 4 months without special treatment, unless they involve a blood vessel, enter the paranasal sinuses, or impinge on the brainstem or cranial nerves. The location of the fracture often provides clues to the possibility of such complications. For example, a fracture that extends through the squamous portion of the temporal bone is more apt to be associated with laceration of the middle meningeal artery, and fractures extending through the base of the skull may cause leakage of CSF and/or blood into either the auditory or the nasal passages. In infants the uneven ossification and the absence of buttresses cause fracture lines to be irregular, following no predictable pattern.

Depressed fractures are those in which the bone is locally broken, usually into several irregular fragments that are pushed inward, causing pressure on the brain. This pressure constitutes a neurosurgical emergency requiring surgical intervention to elevate the fracture. The inner portion of the bone is more extensively fragmented than the outer portion, which almost invariably produces tears in the dura. Depressed skull fractures may be associated with direct underlying parenchymal damage. Both linear and comminuted (fracture consisting of several breaks in the bone) depressed fractures are uncommon before 2 to 3 years of age. In infants and very young children, the soft, malleable bone may become dented in a peculiar rounded or "ping-pong ball" depression without laceration of either skin or dura. This effect is encountered occasionally in difficult deliveries, resulting from either pressure of the head against the pelvis or incorrect application of forceps.

Compound fractures consist of laceration of skin that extends to the site of the bony fracture, which can be linear, depressed, or comminuted. Prompt surgical debridement is needed (unless contraindicated by the child's clinical condition), as is reduction of the fracture, either elevating or removing fragmented bone. Antibiotic and antitetanus therapy is implemented.

Basilar fractures involve the basilar portion of the frontal, ethmoid, sphenoid, temporal, or occipital bones. The diagnosis of basilar fractures is difficult to make from radiographs because of the complex structure of the base of the skull. Because of the proximity of the fracture line to structures surrounding the brainstem, basal skull fracture is a serious head injury. Clinical features include hemorrhage into the nose, nasopharynx, or middle ear (hemotympanum if it occurs behind the eardrum). Effusion of blood is seen on the posterior neck and under and posterior to the ear (Battle sign). Anterior basal fracture produces the characteristic hemorrhage about the eyes ("raccoon eyes"). CN palsies may occur involving primarily CN I, VIII, and VII in order of decreasing frequency.

✦ **NURSING ALERT** Posttraumatic meningitis should be suspected in children with increasing drowsiness and fever who also have basilar skull fractures.

Diastatic fractures are traumatic separation of cranial sutures. These most frequently affect the lambdoid suture and are rarely seen beyond the first 4 years of life. They require no specific treatment but should be observed for "growing fractures," development of a fluid-filled cyst, or cephalhydrocele. This occurs as a result of a tear in the dura and arachnoid membrane or because a piece of arachnoid is entrapped between bone fragments, causing CSF to accumulate beneath the scalp.

Complications

The major complications of trauma to the head are hemorrhage, infection, edema, and herniation through the tentorium. Infection is always a hazard in open injuries, and edema is related to tissue trauma. Vascular rupture may occur even in minor head injuries, causing hemorrhage between the skull and cerebral surfaces. Compression of the underlying brain produces effects that can be rapidly fatal or insidiously progressive.

Epidural hemorrhage. Epidural (extradural) hemorrhage is usually secondary to rupture of the middle meningeal artery, most often as a result of skull fracture that penetrates the groove in the skull occupied by the artery. However, a child's skull can be indented with sufficient force to tear the middle meningeal artery and then rebound intact without causing a fracture. Hemorrhage can also derive from dural veins or the dural sinuses, especially in infants and small children, in whom fracture is less likely to occur. In 20% to 40% of children a skull fracture is not detectable.

The blood accumulates between the dura and the skull to form a hematoma, which, because of the difficulty with which dura is stripped from bone, forces the underlying brain contents downward and inward as it expands (Fig. 37-8, *A*). Since bleeding is generally arterial, brain compression occurs rapidly. Most often the expanding hematoma is located in the parietotemporal region, forcing the medial portion of the temporal lobe under the edge of the tentorium, where it causes pressure on nerves and blood vessels. Pressure on the arterial supply and venous return to the reticular formation causes loss of consciousness; pressure on CN III (oculomotor nerve) produces dilation and (later) fixation of the ipsilateral pupil. Pressure on the fibers of the pyramidal tract is evidenced by contralateral weakness or paralysis and increased deep tendon reflexes. Extreme pressure may extend to the brainstem to cause decerebrate signs and disturbances in the respiratory and other vegetative centers.

The classic clinical picture of epidural hemorrhage (mo-

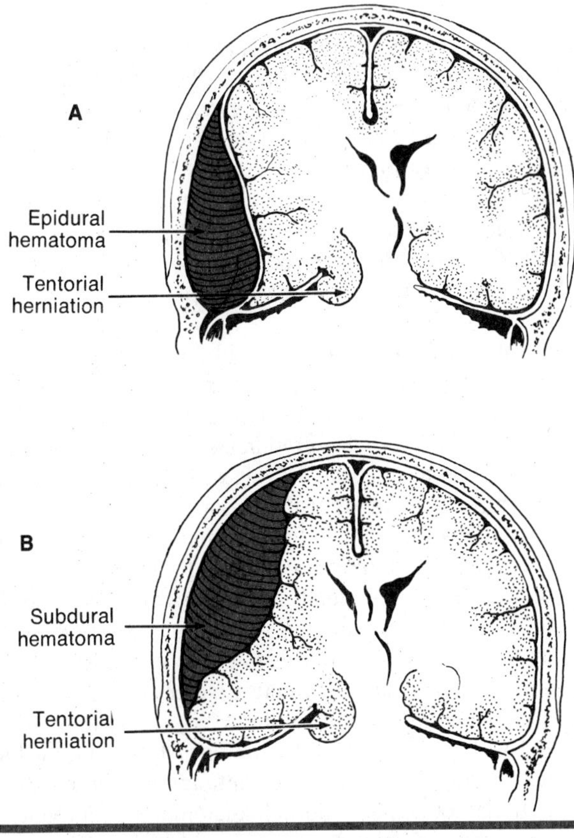

Fig. 37-8. A, Epidural (extradural) hematoma and compression of temporal lobe through tentorial hiatus. **B,** Subdural hematoma.

Table 37-6 Clinical features of acute epidural and acute subdural hematomas

	EPIDURAL	SUBDURAL
▪ Supratentorial		
Frequency	Less	5 to 10 times greater
Skull fracture	70%	30%
Source of hemorrhage	Usually arterial	Almost always venous
Age	Usually older than 2 years	Usually younger than 1 year
Laterality	Usually unilateral	Usually bilateral
Seizures	Less than 25%	75%
Preretinal or retinal hemorrhages	Uncommon	Very frequent
Increased intracranial pressure	Present	Present
CT configuration	Usually lenticular	Usually crescentic
Mortality	As high as 25%	Low
Morbidity	Low	High
▪ Infratentorial		
Frequency	2 to 3 times greater	Less
Skull fracture	Almost always	Usually
Source of hemorrhage	Venous	Venous
Impaired consciousness	Frequent	Frequent
Altered respiration	Often	Often

From Swaiman, K.F.: Pediatric neurology, St. Louis, 1989, Mosby–Year Book, Inc.

mentary unconsciousness followed by a normal period, then lethargy or coma) is seldom evident in children. The period of impaired consciousness is frequently lacking, and the symptom-free period is atypical because of nonspecific complaints such as irritability, headache, and vomiting. The symptom-free period frequently lasts longer than 48 hours. Clinically significant epidural hematomas are uncommon in children younger than 4 years of age. These differences may be caused by the decreased tendency of the resilient skull to fracture; the ability of blood to escape through widened sutures, an open fontanel, or a fracture; bleeding from smaller vessels with less rapid and massive bleeding; lower systolic blood pressure in children; and possibly the brain being less susceptible to pressure changes in children. See Table 37-6 for a comparison between epidural and subdural hematomas.

Subdural hemorrhage. A subdural hemorrhage is bleeding between the dura and the cerebrum, usually as a result of rupture of cortical veins that bridge the subdural space (Fig. 37-8, *B*). Unlike epidural hemorrhage, which develops inwardly against the less resistant brain tissue, subdural hemorrhage tends to develop more slowly and spreads thinly and widely until it is limited by the dural barriers—the falx and tentorium. Subdural hematoma is fairly common in infants, frequently as the result of birth trauma. The small subdural space and dura firmly attached to the skull in this area are highly vulnerable to increased ICP.

Subdural hemorrhage can cause either acute or chronic subdural hematoma. Acute subdural hematoma may be associated with contusions or lacerations. It develops within minutes or hours of injury and, although the mortality is less than that for acute epidural hematoma, the morbidity is greater because of injury to the underlying brain (Swaiman, 1989). Chronic subdural hematoma is more common. The clinical course and manifestations are variable and depend on the damage sustained by the brain substance and the age of the child. Delayed symptoms are common in children with open fontanels and sutures. The most common presenting manifestations in children are seizures, vomiting, and irritability, drowsiness, increased head circumference, or other personality changes. Older children may complain of headache. Less common signs are developmental retardation and failure to thrive.

Presenting signs of acute hematoma include evidence of increased ICP, such as increased head size and bulging fontanels (in the infant), retinal hemorrhages, extraocular palsies (especially CN VI), hemiparesis, quadriplegia, and sometimes elevated temperature. Older children may display an unsteady gait, and papilledema is usually present. Since papilledema is a late sign of increased ICP, it constitutes an emergency. In infants the bleeding may be extensive enough to lower the hematocrit significantly and may be observed before any change in LOC in fast-expanding lesions.

Repeated subdural taps often provide relief in the infant. Surgical evacuation of the hematoma is the treatment of choice in the older child and is frequently required in infants.

Other hemorrhagic lesions. Subarachnoid and intracerebral hemorrhages may occur as the result of head injury. Seizures, nuchal rigidity, and altered consciousness are features of subarachnoid hemorrhage. Manifestations of intracranial bleeding depend on the size and location of the resulting hematoma.

Cerebral edema. Some degree of brain edema is expected after craniocerebral trauma and often accompanies any of the previously mentioned disorders. Cerebral edema peaks at 24 to 72 hours following injury and may account for changes in a child's neurologic status. Cerebral edema caused by direct cellular injury or vascular injury induces vascular stasis, anoxia, and further vasodilatation. Increased tissue pressure within the skull causes venules to collapse, which leads to venous stasis and tissue anoxia. This results in loss of selective permeability of tissue membranes with increased loss of fluid from the vascular compartment to the cerebral tissues, thereby increasing cerebral edema. Thus a self-perpetuating sequence of events is repeated. If this progression continues unchecked, ICP exceeds arterial pressure and fatal anoxia ensues and/or the pressure causes herniation of a portion of the brain over the edge of the tentorium, compressing the brainstem and occluding the posterior cerebral arteries.

Posttraumatic syndromes. *Postconcussion syndrome* is a common sequela to brain injury, and the manifestations vary with the age of the child. Most often there are behavioral disturbances (e.g., aggressiveness, withdrawal, regression), sleep disturbances, phobias, emotional lability, irritability, and alterations in school performance. The younger the child with severe head trauma, the higher is the risk of late behavioral and emotional sequelae.

Postconcussion syndrome occurs very frequently in children under 1 year of age. Within minutes to an hour after a minimum head injury a child sweats; becomes pale, irritable, and sleepy; and may vomit. The syndrome requires no treatment. In children beyond 1 year of age a severe degree of concussion causes acute brain swelling, which may progress to coma with pupillary changes, apnea, and even death. Death from concussion is preventable unless overwhelming secondary brain injury has occurred (Bruce and Schut, 1989).

✦ **NURSING ALERT** If a child loses consciousness or vomits more than three times, medical attention should be sought.

The adolescent syndrome, similar to that of adults, includes headache, dizziness, irritability, and impaired concentration. The symptoms are self-limited and relatively mild. Postconcussion syndrome in children is unique. It consists of behavior changes that may include aggression, disobedience, regressive behavior, and anxiety. Manifestations that continue for more than 1 month require follow-up evaluation (Box 37-4).

Posttraumatic seizures occur in a number of children who survive a head injury. They are more common in young children and in those who sustain cerebral lacerations. The onset may be in the first 24 hours, usually within the first year, and in most cases within 2 years after the injury. Prophylactic anticonvulsants are recommended for children at high risk for seizures. Situations that increase the likelihood of posttraumatic seizures include diffuse cerebral edema, acute subdural hematoma, open depressed skull fracture with parenchymal damage, or severe head injury (GCS of 8 or less) (Hahn and others, 1988). Seizure activity may mimic brainstem herniation signs in children following head injuries.

Box 37-4 CLINICAL MANIFESTATIONS OF POSTTRAUMATIC SYNDROME

Infants
Pallor
Sweating
Irritability
Sleepiness
Possible vomiting

Children
Behavioral disturbances
- Aggressiveness
- Disobedience
- Withdrawal
- Regression
- Anxiety

Sleep disturbances
Phobias
Emotional lability
Irritability
Altered school performance
Seizures

Adolescents
Headache
Dizziness
Impaired concentration

Structural Complications
Hydrocephalus
Focal deficits
- Optic atrophy
- Cranial nerve palsies
- Motor deficits
- Diabetes insipidus
- Aphasia

Structural complications may occur as the result of head injuries. Hydrocephalus is seen when there has been subarachnoid hemorrhage or infection. Focal deficits, including optic atrophy, CN palsies, motor deficits, diabetes insipidus, or aphasia, may be seen. The type of residual effect depends on the location and nature of the trauma. True mental retardation occurs only after severe injuries.

Diagnostic Evaluation

A detailed history, both past and present, is essential in evaluating the child with craniocerebral trauma. It is important to know whether the child suffers from disorders such as drug allergies, hemophilia, diabetes mellitus, or epilepsy; such information may assist in diagnosis. In addition, events surrounding the injury often supply significant data. For example, if a child stumbles and falls while running and strikes the head on the sidewalk, it is usually safe to assume that the neurologic manifestations are a direct result of the injury. However, if a child sinks to the sidewalk and in doing so strikes the head, there may be other causes that contributed to the injury. Sometimes a traumatic injury, even a minor one, will aggravate a preexisting disease process, thereby producing neurologic signs out of proportion to the injury.

Whether or not the infant or child exhibited alterations in consciousness must be determined. Usually this information is easily elicited from older children, but in young children it may be difficult to differentiate between a breath-holding spell and a seizure. The parents are asked if the infant cried immediately after the injury. After a minor injury, initial unconsciousness (if present) is brief and the child will ordinarily exhibit a transient period of confusion, somnolence, and listlessness, most often accompanied by irrita-

Box 37-5 CLINICAL MANIFESTATIONS OF ACUTE HEAD INJURY

Minor Injury
May or may not lose consciousness
Transient period of confusion
Somnolence
Listlessness
Irritability
Pallor
Vomiting (one or more episodes)

Signs of Progression
Altered mental status (e.g., difficulty rousing child)
Mounting agitation
Development of focal lateral neurologic signs
Marked changes in vital signs

Severe Injury
Signs of increased ICP (see Box 37-1)
- Increased head size (infant)
- Bulging fontanel (infant)

Retinal hemorrhage
Extraocular palsies (especially CN VI)
Hemiparesis
Quadriplegia
Elevated temperature (sometimes)
Unsteady gait (older child)
Papilledema (older child)

Associated Signs
Skin injury (to area of head sustaining injury)
Other injuries (e.g., to extremities)

bility, pallor, and one or more episodes of vomiting.

A severe head injury, such as one sustained in a fall from a significant height or a motor vehicle accident, requires prompt evaluation and treatment. Since head injuries are frequently accompanied by injuries in other areas (spine, viscera, extremities), the examination is performed with care to avoid further damage. Box 37-6 lists manifestations of head injury.

Initial assessment. Priorities in the initial phase in the care of a child with a head injury include assessment of the ABCs (airway, breathing, circulation); evaluation for shock; a neurologic examination, especially LOC; pupillary symmetry and response to light; and seizures. The assessment is carried out quickly in relation to vital signs (see Emergency Treatment). Excited and irritable children may have a rapid pulse, hyperventilate, appear pale, and feel clammy shortly after an injury.

✦ **NURSING ALERT** Deep, rapid, periodic, or intermittent and gasping respirations, wide fluctuations or noticeable slowing of the pulse, and widening pulse pressure or extreme fluctuations in blood pressure are signs of brainstem involvement. It is important to note that marked hypotension may represent internal injuries.

Ocular signs such as fixed and dilated pupils, fixed and constricted pupils, and pupils that are poorly reactive or unreactive to light and accommodation indicate increased ICP or brainstem involvement. It is important to remain with the patient who demonstrates fixed and dilated pupils, since these are ominous signs with the probability of respiratory arrest. Dilated, nonpulsating blood vessels indicate increased ICP before the appearance of papilledema. Retinal hemorrhages are seen in acute head injuries.

✦ **NURSING ALERT** Observation of asymmetric pupils or one dilated, unreactive pupil in a comatose child is a neurosurgical emergency that may require evacuation of an epidural hematoma.

Ophthalmosopy should be performed routinely to detect retinal hemorrhages in a child with CNS dysfunction. Cortical blindness, defined as a complete bilateral visual loss associated with normal pupillary responses to light, can be a brief or transient consequence of head trauma. Theories of possible etiologies are vasospasm or localized cerebral edema. Transient blindness following mild head trauma may not be obvious in children unless this diagnosis is considered and evaluated.

Less urgent but important additional assessments include examination of the scalp for lacerations and palpation for depressed skull fractures, widely separated sutures, and the size and tension of fontanels, which indicate intracranial hemorrhage or rapidly developing cerebral edema. However, a significant amount of blood loss can occur from scalp lacerations.

✦ **NURSING ALERT** Bleeding from the nose or ears (although uncommon in children) needs further evaluation, and a watery discharge from the nose (rhinorrhea) that is positive for glucose (as tested with Dextrostix) suggests leaking of CSF from a skull fracture.

Injury to the skin, extremities, and abdomen may occur after severe blunt head trauma and must be ruled out by sensory examination in children with altered motor function. Testing reflexes provides information about cerebral and pyramidal involvement, although transient abnormalities of the abdominal reflexes and Babinski sign may be present in children with mild head trauma. Conscious, cooperative children are examined for cerebellar signs such as ataxia. Children may display unsteadiness, clumsiness, or tremor with intentional movement after head injury.

Temperature may be moderately elevated for 1 or 2 days following an initial mild hypothermia after injury. A persistent fever may indicate subarachnoid hemorrhage or infection.

An accurate assessment of these various clinical signs provides baseline information. Serial evaluations, preferably by a single observer, help to detect changes in the neurologic status. Alterations in mental status, evidenced by increased difficulty in rousing the child, mounting agitation, development of focal lateral neurologic signs, or marked changes in vital signs, usually indicate extension or progression of the basic pathologic process.

Special tests. After a thorough clinical examination, a

variety of diagnostic tests are helpful in providing a more definitive diagnosis of the type and extent of the trauma. Where available, CT is especially valuable in diagnosis of neurologic trauma and usually makes other diagnostic procedures unnecessary. CT is indicated for a deteriorating state while the patient is under observation, for persistent somnolence, or for vomiting that does not abate within 12 hours.

MRI and neurobehavioral assessment following early head injury may be useful in documenting cognitive impairment in relation to structural alterations in the young brain. MRI has been shown to be superior to other techniques for detection of intracranial injury caused by shaking and may help document milder cases of this form of child abuse (Alexander and others, 1986). Where available, MRI has replaced cerebral angiography.

Skull films and other radiographic tests may be indicated. Echoencephalography may contribute to diagnosis and management. Electroencephalography is not particularly helpful for early diagnosis but is useful for defining seizure activity or focal destructive lesions after the acute phase of illness. Lumbar puncture is rarely employed in craniocerebral trauma and is contraindicated in the presence of increased ICP.

In the infant or small child a subdural tap through a fontanel or coronal suture may establish the diagnosis of subdural or epidural hemorrhage. In some centers monitoring ICP is part of the assessment.

Therapeutic Management

The majority of children with mild to moderate concussion who have not lost consciousness can be cared for and observed at home after careful examination reveals no serious intracranial injury. The parents are instructed to check the child every 2 hours to determine any changes in responsiveness. The sleeping child should be wakened to see if the child can be roused normally. Parents are advised to maintain contact with the attending physician, who usually wishes to examine the child again in 1 or 2 days. The manifestations of epidural hematoma in children do not generally appear until 24 hours or more after injury.

Maintaining contact with the parents for continued observation and reevaluation of the child, when indicated, facilitates early diagnosis and treatment of possible complications such as hematoma, hydrocephalus, cysts, and posttraumatic seizures. Children with minor injuries who live far from medical facilities or whose parents or caregivers are not deemed reliable in observing their condition are generally hospitalized for 24 to 48 hours for observation.

Children with severe injuries, those who have lost consciousness for more than a few minutes, and those with prolonged and continued seizures or other focal or diffuse neurologic signs must be hospitalized until their condition is stable and their neurologic signs have diminished. The child is maintained on nothing by mouth or restricted to clear liquids, if able to take fluids by mouth, until it is determined that vomiting will not occur. Intravenous fluids are indicated for the child who is comatose or displays dulled sensorium and for the child with persistent vomiting.

EMERGENCY TREATMENT
Head Injury

1. Assess child:
   A—airway
   B—bleeding
   C—circulation
2. Clean any abrasions with soap and water.
   Apply clean dressing.
   If bleeding, apply ice for 1 hour to relieve pain and swelling.
3. Give only clear liquids until no vomiting for at least 6 hours.
4. Give no analgesics.
5. Check pupil reaction every 4 hours (including twice during night) for 48 hours.
6. Awaken two times during night to check level of consciousness.
7. Seek medical attention if there is any of the following:
   Injury sustained
   —at high speed (e.g., auto)
   —fall from a significant distance (e.g., roof, tree)
   —from great force (e.g., baseball bat)
   —under suspicious circumstances
   Child less than 6 months of age
   Unconscious more than 5 seconds
   Discomfort (crying) more than 10 minutes after injury
   Headache that is severe, worsening, interferes with sleep
   Vomiting three or more times
   Swelling in front of or above earlobe or swelling that increases in size
   Confused or not behaving normally
   Difficult to rouse from sleep
   Difficulty with speaking
   Blurring of vision or seeing double
   Unsteady gait
   Difficulty using upper extremities
   Neck pain
   Pupils dilated or fixed
   Infant with bulging fontanel

The volume of intravenous fluid is carefully monitored to avoid aggravating any cerebral edema and to minimize the possibility of overhydration in case of SIADH. However, damage to the hypothalamus or pituitary gland may produce diabetes insipidus with its accompanying hypertonicity and dehydration. Fluid balance is closely monitored by daily weight, accurate intake and output measurement, and serum osmolality to detect early signs of water retention, excessive dehydration, and states of hypertonicity or hypotonicity.

Restlessness can be satisfactorily managed, if necessary, with diphenhydramine (Benadryl) or chloral hydrate, and headache is usually controlled with acetaminophen (Tylenol). Anticonvulsants are used for seizure control and frequently in cases of suspected contusion or laceration. Antibiotics are administered if there are lacerations, CSF leakage, or excessive cerebral tissue damage. Prophylactic tetanus toxoid is given as appropriate (see Chapter 12). Cerebral edema is managed as described for the unconscious child. Hyperthermia is controlled with tepid sponges or a hypothermia blanket.

Surgical therapy. Scalp lacerations are sutured after careful examination of underlying bone. Torn dura is sutured as well. Depressed fractures require surgical reduction and removal of bone fragments. A skull fracture depressed more than the thickness of the skull or an intracranial hematoma causing more than 5 mm midline shift are indications for surgery. "Ping-pong ball" skull fractures in very young infants can correct themselves within a few weeks or may require surgical elevation.

Prognosis. The outcome of craniocerebral trauma depends on the extent of injury and complications. However, the outlook is generally more favorable for children than for adults. Over 90% of children with concussions or simple linear fractures recover without symptoms after the initial period. The incidence of fatalities and neurologic sequelae is lower in children, even in those with severe head injuries. The prognosis for recovery is primarily related to the duration of coma and the degree of injury (Eiben and others, 1984).

The concern regarding outcome is increasingly focused on cognitive, emotional, and/or mental problems. Recent studies indicate that children experience a higher frequency of psychologic disturbances following head injury, whereas adults are more prone to complaints of a physical nature. Children who suffer even minor head injuries exhibit unacceptable behavior, poor attention span, impaired self-control, difficulty managing stress or frustration, oversensitivity, irritability, mental inconsistency, personality changes, headaches, and memory impairment (Boll, 1985; Eisenberg and Briner, 1989; Jacobson and others, 1986).

Nursing Considerations

The hospitalized child requires careful neurologic assessment and evaluation (see p. 1723). Frequent nursing assessments can provide information needed to establish a correct diagnosis, identify signs and symptoms of increased ICP, determine clinical management, and prevent many complications.

The child is placed on bed rest, usually with the head of the bed elevated slightly. Appropriate safety measures, such as siderails kept up for older children and seizure precautions for children of all ages, are implemented. The extremely restless child may require that hard surfaces be padded and restraint used to prevent the possibility of further injury. Care is individualized according to the specific needs of the child. The unconscious child is managed as described in the previous section, but most childhood head injuries are those causing momentary stunning or temporary unconsciousness. Children may be restless and irritable, but more often their reaction is to fall asleep when left undisturbed. A quiet environment helps reduce the restlessness and irritability. Bright lights shining directly into the child's face are irritating. This often makes checking the ocular responses more difficult to perform and more aggravating to the child.

Frequent examinations of vital signs, neurologic signs, and LOC are extremely important nursing observations. When possible, they should be performed by a single observer in order to better detect subtle changes that may indicate worsening of neurologic status. Pupils are checked for size, equality, reaction to light, and accommodation. After the initial elevations usually seen after injury, the vital signs generally return to normal unless there is brainstem involvement. An axillary temperature is the safest method of measuring temperature, since seizures are not uncommon and vomiting is a frequent response in children, especially when the child is disturbed.

The most important nursing observation is assessment of the child's LOC. Alterations in consciousness appear earlier in the progression of an injury than alterations of vital signs or focal neurologic signs (see p. 1725 for evaluation of responsiveness). Some expected responses may be misinterpreted as deviations from the normal. Frequent examinations of alertness are fatiguing to the child; therefore the child often desires to fall asleep, which may be confused with depressed consciousness. When left alone, the child promptly dozes. It is not uncommon to observe ocular divergence through the partially closed eyelids.

Observations of position and movement provide additional information. Any abnormal posturing is noted, as well as whether or not it occurs continuously or intermittently. Questions nurses might ask themselves include:

Are the child's hand grips strong and equal in strength?
Are there any signs of decerebrate or decorticate posturing?
What is the child's response to stimulation?
Is movement purposeful, random, or absent?
Are movement and sensation equal on both sides or restricted to one side only?

The child may complain of headache or other discomfort. The child who is too young to describe a headache will be fussy and resist being handled. The child who suffers from vertigo will often assume a position and vigorously resist being moved. Forcible movement causes the child to vomit and display spontaneous nystagmus. Seizures, relatively common in children at the time of injury, may be of any type but are more often generalized regardless of the type of injury. Any seizure activity should be carefully observed and described in detail (see Box 37-9). Children in postictal states are more lethargic with sluggish pupils.

Drainage from any orifice is noted. Bleeding from the ear suggests the possibility of a basal skull fracture. The amount and characteristics of the drainage are observed, and since the auditory canal may be a source of infection, dry, sterile cotton can be placed loosely at the orifice and changed when soiled.

✦ NURSING ALERT Suctioning through the nares is contraindicated, since there is a high risk of secondary infection and the probability of the catheter entering the brain substance through a fracture.

Head trauma is frequently accompanied by other undetected injuries; therefore any bruises, lacerations, or evidence of internal injuries or fractures of the extremities are noted and reported. Associated injuries are evaluated and treated appropriately.

The child with normal LOC is usually allowed clear liquids unless fluid is restricted. If the child has an intravenous infusion, it is maintained as prescribed. The diet is advanced to that appropriate for the child's age as soon as the condition permits. Intake and output are measured and recorded, and any incontinence of bowel or bladder is noted in the child who has been toilet trained.

The child should be observed for any unusual behavior, but interpretation of behavior should be made in relation to the child's normal behavior. For example, urinary incontinence during sleep would be of no consequence in a child who routinely wets the bed but would be highly significant for one who is always dry. In addition, a child who is subject to nightmares might cry out and demonstrate agitated behavior at night. Parents are valuable resources in evaluating objective behaviors of their children. Information obtained from parents at or shortly after admission is helpful in evaluating the child's behavior, for example, the ease with which the child is roused normally, the usual sleeping position, how much the child sleeps during the day, motor activity the child is capable of (rolling over, sitting up, climbing), hearing and visual acuity, appetite, and manner of eating (spoon, bottle, cup). There would be less concern about a child who falls asleep several times during the day if this particular type of behavior is consistent with the child's usual behavior.

When the child is discharged, the parents are advised of probable posttraumatic symptoms that may be expected, such as behavioral changes, sleep disturbances, phobias, and seizures. They should understand observations that should be made and how to contact the physician, nurse, or health facility in case the child develops any unusual signs or symptoms. The importance of follow-up evaluation should be emphasized. It is often advisable to refer the family to a public health agency for home follow-through care to ensure that the child receives posthospital evaluation.

The rehabilitation and management of the child with permanent brain injury are beyond the scope of this discussion, but it is an important aspect of care. Rehabilitation of brain-injured children is begun as soon as feasible and usually involves the family and a rehabilitation team. Careful assessment of the child's capabilities, limitations, and probable potential is made as early as possible and appropriate interventions are implemented to maximize the residual capacities. The **National Head Injury Foundation*** "arose from the mutual frustration and sense of hopelessness experienced by families in their search for appropriate facilities and support to return head-injured loved ones to their maximum functioning potential." It provides information and listings of rehabilitation services and support groups throughout the country.†

Prevention. Preventive strategies are underused in almost all cases of accidental childhood injury. Head injuries are involved in most serious accidental injuries—especially motor vehicle accidents, sports, and falls. For extensive discussions of childhood injuries, see the discussions on injury prevention in Chapters 12, 14, 15, 17, and 19. See also Injuries—The Leading Killer, Chapter 1.

NEAR-DROWNING

Drowning ranks second as a cause of accidental death in children. Most cases usually involve children who are helpless in water, such as inadequately attended children in or near swimming pools or infants in bathtubs; small children who fall into ponds, streams, and flooded excavations, usually near home (Fig. 37-9); occupants of pleasure boats who fail to wear life preservers; children who have diving accidents; and children who are able to swim but overestimate their endurance.

Accidental drowning occurs more than four times more frequently in males than in females; in 89% of all cases, supervision is absent (Quan and others, 1989). Most of the drownings are related to the characteristics of specific age-groups. For example, infants drown in bathtubs, preschool children in swimming pools, and teenagers in lakes and rivers. The largest proportion of drownings for all children occur in private swimming pools, with the highest rate among children 2 to 3 years of age. Drowning as a form of fatal child abuse has also been recognized as a problem. Homicidal drownings are unwitnessed, usually occur in the home, and the victims are either infants or toddlers (Griest and Zumwalt, 1989).

Drowning can take place in any body of water, including such unlikely places as a pail of water. Top-heavy toddlers fall headfirst into a pail of water, their arms become trapped, and they are unable to free themselves. Hot tubs and whirlpool spas have been implicated in childhood drowning injury. The suction created at the outlet is strong

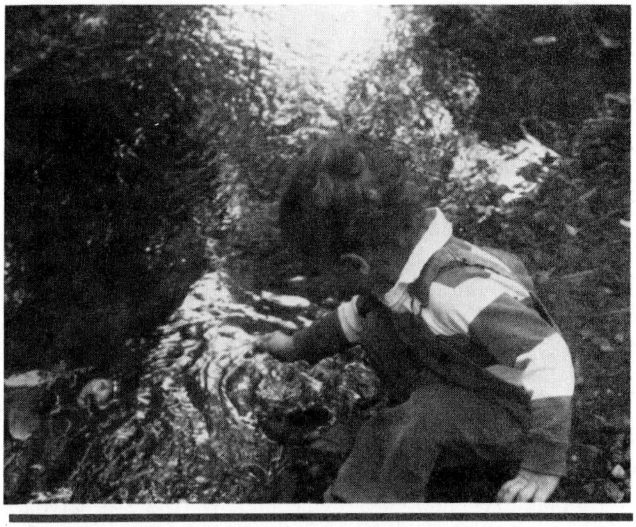

Fig. 37-9. Water is fascinating for children; however, drowning is the second leading cause of accidental death in unsupervised situations.

*333 Turnpike Rd., Southborough, MA 01772; (508) 485-9950. In Canada: **Association for the Rehabilitation for the Brain Injured,** 97 Warwick Dr., Calgary, Alberta T3C 2R5.

†See Nursing Care Plan: The Child with a Head Injury in Wong, D.L., and Whaley, L.F.: Clinical manual of pediatric nursing, ed. 3, St. Louis, 1990, Mosby–Year Book, Inc.

Box 37-6 TERMS DESCRIBING DROWNING INJURY

Drowning—death from asphyxia while submerged, regardless of whether fluid has entered the lungs.
Near-drowning—survival at least 24 hours after submersion in a fluid medium.

These can be further described as:

Drowning without aspiration—death from respiratory obstruction and asphyxia while submerged, usually as a result of prolonged laryngospasm. This is also called *dry drowning* (approximately 10% of drownings).
Drowning with aspiration—death from the combined effects of asphyxia and changes secondary to fluid aspiration while submerged.
Near-drowning without aspiration—survival, at least temporarily, following asphyxia after submersion in a fluid medium.
Near-drowning with aspiration—survival, at least temporarily, following aspiration of fluid while submerged.
Delayed death caused by drowning—death as the result of complications subsequent to successful resuscitation following submersion.

enough to trap even larger children underwater, and rapidly proliferating *Pseudomonas aeruginosa* have been reported as complicating hot tub submersion injury (Tron, Baldwin, and Price, 1985).

With expeditious treatment many children can and are being saved. See Box 37-6 for terms describing drowning and near-drowning.

Pathophysiology

The major pulmonary changes that occur in drowning are directly related to the length of submersion (regardless of the type and amount of fluid aspirated), the physiologic response of the victim, and the development and degree of immersion hypothermia. In addition, cerebral recovery depends on the effectiveness of initial resuscitation and subsequent critical care measures to support cerebral salvage.

Physiologic factors that influence the extent of damage from immersion include resistance to asphyxia and anoxia, which shows some individual variation. There is greater resistance with diminishing age; young children can withstand longer periods of submersion. More important is the drowning, or diving, reflex. This neurologic response is triggered by immersion of the face in cold water. Blood is shunted away from the periphery, and the flow is concentrated to the brain and heart predominantly. There is a profound bradycardia, but the diminishing supply of oxygen is delivered to these essential organs. Consequently, although the brain may appear to be severely damaged, some victims have the potential for recovery even after lengthy submersion.

Submerged children struggle initially. There is laryngospasm, and they swallow water and frequently vomit. This is followed by terminal gasping and aspiration. Cardiopulmonary arrest is secondary to asphyxia after about 4 to 6 minutes of complete submersion. The problems created by near-drowning are (1) hypoxia and asphyxiation, (2) aspiration, and (3) hypothermia (except near-drowning in hot tubs).

Hypoxia is the primary problem because it results in global cell damage, and different cells tolerate variable lengths of anoxia. Neurons, especially cerebral cells, sustain irreversible damage after 4 to 6 minutes of submersion. The heart and lungs can survive up to 30 minutes. Regardless of the amount of water aspirated, there is arterial hypoxemia (resulting from atelectasis with shunting of blood through the nonventilated alveoli) and a combined respiratory acidosis (resulting from retained carbon dioxide) and metabolic acidosis (caused by buildup of acid metabolites due to anaerobic metabolism). Although electrolyte imbalances are contributing factors, they are not the major causes of morbidity and mortality, as had been previously thought. The pathologic events are directly related to the duration of submersion. The major difficulty is acute ventilatory insufficiency. Approximately 10% of drowning victims die without aspirating fluid but succumb from acute asphyxia as a result of prolonged reflex laryngospasm.

Aspiration of fluid occurs in the majority of drownings. The aspirated fluid results in pulmonary edema, atelectasis, airway spasm, and pneumonitis, which aggravates the hypoxia. It was previously thought that submersion in salt water and fresh water altered the physiologic response to near-drowning. However, there is no clinically significant difference in human survivors, and type of water does not alter the therapy or outcome.

Immersion in cold water (at or less than 20° C, or 68° F) produces a significant and slow fall in body temperature; but in very cold water (at or less than 5° C, or 41° F), however, body temperature falls at an incredibly rapid rate as a result of cutaneous capillary paralysis and accelerated heat loss (Orlowski, 1987). Hypothermia occurs rapidly in infants and children, partly because of their large surface area relative to size and partly as a result of the cold water itself. Water is an excellent heat conductor, and the contact with the skin is increased by struggling. Body heat loss in water is approximately 30 times greater than in air (Robinson and Seward, 1987). Hypothermia may make resumption or maintenance of cardiac function possible if body temperature is less than 30° C (86° F). Profound hypothermia is usually evidence of lengthy submersion.

Clinical Manifestations

Clinical manifestations are directly related to the degree of consciousness following rescue and resuscitation. The manifestations and management are categorized in Table 37-7.

Therapeutic Management

Resuscitative measures should begin at the scene of a drowning and the victim should be transported to the hospital with maximum ventilatory and circulatory support. Many victims need care for some time after aspiration of fluid. In the hospital, intensive pulmonary care is implemented and continued according to the needs of the patient.

Table 37-7 Clinical manifestations and management of near-drowning related to degree of consciousness

CATEGORY	CHARACTERISTICS	MANAGEMENT
A	Awake, minimum injury Fully conscious; may have mild hypothermia, mild chest radiograph changes, mild arterial blood gas abnormalities	Symptomatic treatment with oxygen administration and warming Laboratory assessment of electrolytes Usually well enough to be discharged in 12 to 24 hours
B	Blunted sensorium, moderate injury Obtund, stuporous, purposeful response to painful stimuli, mild to moderate hypothermia, frequently respiratory distress, chest radiographs abnormal, arterial blood gas abnormalities	Symptomatic, as for category A Regular monitoring of neurologic and respiratory status Correction of acidosis Furosemide to stimulate diuresis
C	Comatose, severe anoxia Patient unarousable, abnormal response to pain, abnormal respiratory pattern, seizures, shock, marked arterial blood gas abnormalities, abnormal chest radiographs, dysrhythmias, metabolic acidosis, hyperkalemia, hyperglycemia, disseminated intravascular coagulation	Invasive life-support measures Mechanical ventilation for at least 12 to 24 hours (to reduce energy expenditure) More severely affected children managed as any unconscious child Increased ICP usually not a problem in children who do well, but when present (even with treatment), associated with death or significant neurologic damage
C1	Decorticate, Cheyne-Stokes respirations	Symptomatic management
C2	Decerebrate, central hyperventilation	
C3	Flaccid, apneustic or cluster breathing	
C4	Flaccid, apneic, no detectable circulation	

In general, the management of the near-drowning victim is based on the degree of cerebral insult. The first priority is to restore oxygen delivery to the cells and prevent further hypoxic damage. A spontaneously breathing child will do well in an oxygen-enriched atmosphere; the more severely affected child will require endotracheal intubation and mechanical ventilation. Blood gases and pH are monitored frequently as a guide to oxygen, fluid, and electrolyte therapies.

Because of the frequency of complications after near-drowning, any patient should be hospitalized for 12 to 48 hours for observation. Aspiration pneumonia is a frequent complication that occurs about 48 to 72 hours after the episode. Bronchospasm, alveolar-capillary membrane damage, atelectasis, abscess formation, and hyaline membrane disease are other complications that occur after aspiration of fluid.

Prognosis. If the victim is one of the 10% who do not aspirate water, is rescued and resuscitated before circulatory arrest, and does not suffer CNS damage, recovery should be complete. The outcome for near-drowning is excellent for most category C1 and C2 patients if they are resuscitated and receive intensive care (see Table 37-7). The poorest outlook is for children in category C4, especially when associated with complications such as disseminated intravascular coagulation, intestinal sloughing, shock, and dysrhythmias.

Nursing Considerations

Nursing care depends on the condition of the child. A child who survives may need intensive respiratory nursing care with attention to vital signs, mechanical ventilation and/or tracheostomy, blood gas determination, chest therapy, and intravenous infusion. Frequently the child is comatose for an indefinite period and requires the same care as an unconscious child.

Probably the most difficult aspect in the care of the child victim of near-drowning is dealing with the parents, whose guilt reactions are severe. The magnitude of the event is so great that efforts to provide comfort and support are of only limited success. Parents need to hear that everything possible is being done to treat the child, and this message needs to be repeated often.

Most drownings, particularly of infants or small children, could have been prevented with adequate supervision. If the child dies, the sudden, unexpected nature of the death and the particular circumstances of the accident, especially in terms of guilt for not preventing it, compound the grief for these individuals (see Chapter 23). The parents of the child who is saved from death are faced with the anxiety of not knowing what the outcome will be and sometimes wish for the death of the child. Because their situation generates such intense feelings of loneliness, it is important for families to know that they are not alone. They need to be reminded frequently that there are caring people to assist them both during the crisis and later. Additional sources of support that can be recommended are psychiatric and social work consultants, community services, and religious support. Self-help groups are excellent if these are available in the community.

Nurses often have difficulty relating to the parents if obvious neglect has precipitated the accident and subsequent problems; therefore it is important for those who care for these children and their families to assess their own feelings about the situation, as well as the coping abilities and resources of the family. Caring for near-drowning victims and their families requires the nurse to be sensitive to the needs of the child and the family and to recognize his or her own reactions and emotions.

Prevention. All children should be taught to handle themselves in the water. Even very young children can learn to do so sufficiently to avoid panic and propel themselves to safety until they can be removed from the water. The American Academy of Pediatrics supports the recommendations of the YMCA regarding guidelines for swimming instruction for children less than 3 years of age. The programs recommended for older infants and toddlers are not those that promise to "waterproof" or "drownproof" the child, which can lead to complacency on the part of parents who believe the child can "swim." Those that offer water enrichment and emphasize water familiarization and water fun, and stress water safety and parent participation are best for very young children. These programs train both parent and child in swimming instruction, safety precautions, and risk awareness.

Water safety and survival training should be required for all school-age children, and nurses can be active advocates in their communities. Nurses are also in a position to emphasize the importance of adequate adult supervision when children are in the water. Young children should never be left unattended when in the water. Regulations requiring fencing of water areas such as swimming pools must be enforced to prevent drowning.

INTRACRANIAL INFECTIONS

The nervous system and its coverings are subject to infection by the same organisms that affect other organs of the body. However, the nervous system is limited in the ways in which it responds to injury. Infectious processes share virtually the same clinical and pathologic features. They differ primarily in the growth and virulence of the specific organism. It is generally difficult to distinguish between the various etiologic agents from clinical manifestations. Laboratory studies are needed to identify the causative agent. The inflammatory process can affect the meninges *(meningitis)*, brain *(encephalitis)*, or spinal cord *(myelitis)*.

The most common infection of the CNS is meningitis. It can be caused by a variety of organisms, but the three main types are:

1. **Bacterial,** or pyogenic, caused by pus-forming bacteria, especially the meningococcus, pneumococcus, and influenza bacillus
2. **Tuberculous,** caused by the tubercle bacillus
3. **Viral,** or aseptic, caused by a wide variety of viral agents

BACTERIAL MENINGITIS

Bacterial meningitis is a potentially fatal disease, and although the advent of antimicrobial therapy has had a marked effect on the course and prognosis, it remains a significant cause of illness in the pediatric age-groups. Its importance lies primarily in the frequency with which it occurs in infancy and childhood and the unnecessarily high death rates and residual damage caused by undiagnosed and untreated or inadequately treated cases. Ninety percent of cases occur in children between the ages of 1 month and 5 years; infants 6 to 12 months of age are at greatest risk (Krugman and others, 1985).

Etiology

Bacterial meningitis can be caused by any of a variety of bacterial agents. *Haemophilus influenzae* (type B), *Streptococcus pneumoniae,* and *Neisseria meningitidis* (meningococcus) organisms are responsible for bacterial meningitis in 95% of children older than 2 months. *H. influenzae* is the predominant organism in children 3 months to 3 years of age but is rare in infants younger than 3 months, who are apparently protected by passively acquired bactericidal substances, and in children older than 5 years, who are beginning to acquire this protection (Krugman and others, 1985).

Other organisms are the β-hemolytic streptococcus, *Staphylococcus aureus,* and *Escherichia coli.* The leading causes of neonatal meningitis are the group B streptococci and *E. coli* organisms. *E. coli* infection is seldom seen beyond infancy. Meningococcic (epidemic cerebrospinal) meningitis occurs in epidemic form and is the only type readily transmitted by droplet infection from nasopharyngeal secretions. Although this condition may develop at any age, the risk of meningococcal infection increases with the number of contacts; therefore it occurs predominantly in school-age children and adolescents.

There appear to be some seasonal variations. Meningitis caused by *H. influenzae* is a disease that primarily occurs in autumn or early winter. Pneumococcal and meningococcal infections can occur at any time but are more common in later winter or early spring. The increased incidence of *H. influenzae* in certain ethnic groups and in families suggests that there may be a genetic susceptibility to the disease (Hill, 1983).

Several factors may predispose the child to the development of bacterial meningitis. Males are affected more often than females, and this is somewhat more pronounced in the neonatal period. The greatest morbidity after meningitis appears to involve children who were afflicted between birth and 4 years of age. Maternal factors, such as premature rupture of fetal membranes and maternal infection during the last week of pregnancy, are major causes of neonatal meningitis.

Deficiencies in the immune mechanisms and decreased leukocyte activity may influence the incidence in newborns, children with immunoglobulin deficiencies, and children receiving immunosuppressant drugs. Meningitis appears to occur as an extension of a variety of bacterial infections, probably as a result of the lack of acquired resistance to the various etiologic organisms. Preexisting CNS anomalies, neurosurgical procedures or injuries, sickle cell disease, or primary infections elsewhere in the body are factors related to an increased susceptibility.

Pathophysiology

The most common route of infection is vascular dissemination from a focus of infection elsewhere. For example, organisms from the nasopharynx invade the underlying blood vessels and enter the cerebral blood supply or form local thromboemboli that release septic emboli into the bloodstream. Invasion by direct extension from infections in the paranasal and mastoid sinuses is less common. Organisms also gain entry by direct implantation after penetrating wounds, skull fractures that provide an opening into the skin or sinuses, lumbar puncture or surgical procedures, and anatomic abnormalities such as spina bifida or foreign bodies such as a ventricular shunt. Once implanted, the organisms spread into the CSF, by which the infection spreads throughout the subarachnoid space. (See Nursing Alert, p. 1743)

The infective process is that seen in any bacterial infection—inflammation, exudation, white blood cell accumulation, and varying degrees of tissue damage. The brain becomes hyperemic and edematous, and the entire surface of the brain is covered with a layer of purulent exudate, which varies with the type of organism. For example, meningococcal exudate is most marked over the parietal, occipital, and cerebellar regions; the thick, fibrinous exudate of pneumococcal infection is confined chiefly to the surface of the brain, particularly the anterior lobes; and the exudate of streptococcal infections is similar to that of pneumococcal infections, but thinner.

Clinical Manifestations

The clinical manifestations of acute bacterial meningitis depend to a large extent on the age of the child. The picture is also influenced to some degree by the type of organism, the effectiveness of therapy for antecedent illness, and whether it occurs as an isolated entity or as a complication of another illness or injury.

Children and adolescents. The illness is likely to be abrupt, with fever, chills, headache, and vomiting that are associated with or quickly followed by alterations in sensorium. Often the initial sign is a seizure, which may recur as the disease progresses. The child is extremely irritable and agitated and may develop photophobia, delirium, hallucinations, aggressive or maniacal behavior, or drowsiness, stupor, and coma. Sometimes the onset is slower, frequently preceded by several days of respiratory or gastrointestinal symptoms. Occasionally a prior infection treated with antibiotics masks or delays the signs of meningitis.

The child resists flexion of the neck, and as the disease progresses, the neck stiffness becomes marked until the head is drawn into extreme overextension (opisthotonos). Kernig and Brudzinski signs are positive. Reflex responses are variable, although they show hyperactivity. The skin may be cold and cyanotic with poor peripheral perfusion.

Other signs and symptoms may appear that are peculiar to individual organisms. Petechial or purpuric rashes usually indicate a meningococcal infection, especially when the eruption is associated with a shocklike state. Joint involvement is seen in meningococcic and *H. influenzae* infection. A chronically draining ear commonly accompanies pneumococcal meningitis. *E. coli* infection may be associated with a congenital dermal sinus that communicates with the subarachnoid space.

Infants and young children. The classic picture of meningitis is rarely seen in children between 3 months and 2 years of age. The illness is characterized by fever, poor feeding, vomiting, marked irritability, and frequent seizures, which are often accompanied by a high-pitched cry. A bulging fontanel is the most significant finding, and nuchal rigidity may or may not be present. Brudzinski and Kernig signs are not usually helpful in diagnosis, since they are difficult to elicit and evaluate in children in this age-group.

Neonates. Meningitis in newborn and premature infants is extremely difficult to diagnose. The vague and nonspecific manifestations, characteristic of all neonatal sepsis, bear little resemblance to the findings in older children. These infants are usually well at birth but within a few days begin to look and behave poorly. They refuse feedings, have poor sucking ability, and may vomit or have diarrhea. They display poor tone, lack of movement, and a poor cry. Other nonspecific signs that may be present include hypothermia or fever (depending on the maturity of the infant), jaundice, irritability, drowsiness, seizures, respiratory irregularities or apnea, cyanosis, and weight loss. The full, tense, and bulging fontanel may or may not be present until late in the course of the illness, and the neck is usually supple. Untreated, the child's condition will decline to cardiovascular collapse, seizures, and apnea.

Complications. The incidence of complications from acute bacterial meningitis has been significantly reduced with early diagnosis and vigorous antimicrobial therapy. If infection extends to the ventricles, thick pus, fibrin, or adhesions may occlude the narrow passages, thereby obstructing the flow of CSF to cause obstructive hydrocephalus. Subdural effusions occur frequently, and thrombosis may occur in meningeal veins or venous sinuses. Destructive changes may take place in the cerebral cortex, and brain abscesses may form by direct extension of the infection or by vascular dissemination. Extension of the infection to the areas of the cranial nerves or compression necrosis from increased pressure may cause deafness, blindness, or weakness or paralysis of facial or other muscles of the head and neck.

One of the most dramatic and serious complications usually associated with meningococcal infections is peripheral circulatory collapse, known as the Waterhouse-Friderichsen syndrome, which if untreated is rapidly fatal. Extensive and diffuse intravascular coagulation with marked thrombocytopenia occurs with any form but is most common in meningococcic (epidemic cerebrospinal) meningitis.

Other acute complications of meningitis include the syndrome of inappropriate antidiuretic hormone (SIADH) (see Chapter 38), subdural effusions, seizures, cerebral edema and herniation, and hydrocephalus. Obstruction to the flow of CSF occurs in the acute phase of illness by clumping of purulent material in the drainage channels and in the chronic phase by adhesive arachnoiditis or fibrotic obstruction through any of the ventricular foramina. Postmeningitic complications in neonates include ventriculitis, resulting in cystic, walled-off areas of the brain with fluid accumulation and pressure.

Extension of the inflammation to cranial nerves or compression and destruction of the nerves from ICP can produce permanent impairment of vision or hearing and other nerve palsies. Auditory nerve damage is usually followed by permanent deafness. Other long-term complications include cerebral palsy, mental retardation, seizures, learning disorder, and attention deficit disorder.

Hemiparesis and quadriparesis may result from damage caused by arteritis and/or thrombosis or other mechanisms. Behavioral changes are noted in some children. Also, evidence indicates that psychometric and behavioral defects may be a significant concomitant sign of meningitis in childhood, although it is difficult to determine the degree to which meningitis affects the intelligence quotient of children.

Diagnostic Evaluation

A diagnosis of acute bacterial meningitis cannot be made on the basis of clinical manifestations. A definitive diagnosis is made only by examination of the CSF by means of a lumbar puncture. The fluid pressure is measured and samples are obtained for culture, Gram stain, blood cell count, and determination of glucose and protein content. The findings are usually diagnostic. Culture and stain are needed to identify the causative organism. Spinal fluid pressure is usually elevated, but interpretation is often difficult when the child is crying.

There is generally an elevated white blood cell count, predominantly polymorphonuclear leukocytes, but it may be extremely variable. The glucose level is reduced, generally in proportion to the duration and severity of the infection. The relationship between the CSF glucose and serum glucose levels is important in evaluating the glucose content of CSF; therefore a serum glucose sample is drawn approximately ½ hour before the lumbar puncture. Protein concentration is usually increased.

A blood culture is advisable for all children suspected of meningitis and occasionally proves positive when CSF culture is negative. Nose and throat cultures may provide helpful information in some cases. Several newer techniques for diagnosing or differentiating meningitis are also available.

Therapeutic Management

Acute bacterial meningitis is a medical emergency that requires early recognition and immediate institution of therapy to prevent death and avoid residual disabilities. The initial therapeutic management includes:

- Isolation precautions
- Initiation of antimicrobial therapy
- Maintenance of optimum hydration
- Maintenance of ventilation
- Reduction of increased ICP
- Management of bacterial shock
- Control of seizures
- Control of extremes of temperature
- Correction of anemia
- Treatment of complications

The child is isolated from other children, usually in an intensive care unit for close observation. An intravenous infusion is started as soon as the lumbar puncture has been completed in order to facilitate the administration of antimicrobial agents, fluids, anticonvulsive drugs, and blood if needed. The child is placed on a cardiac monitor.

Drugs. Until the causative organism is identified, the choice of antibiotic is based on the known sensitivity of the organism most likely to be the infective agent in any given situation and the probable interactions with the specific patient. Except under special circumstances, the drugs are administered intravenously throughout the course of treatment. The drugs are given in large doses, and the period of therapy is determined by CSF findings and the child's clinical condition. Appropriate antibiotics are administered following identification of the causative organism.

Nonspecific measures. Maintaining hydration is a prime concern, and intravenous fluids and the type and amount of fluid are determined by the patient's condition. The optimum hydration involves correction of any fluid deficits followed by low maintenance levels to prevent cerebral edema. If indicated, measures are employed to reduce ICP, as described previously (see p. 1737). Increased ICP seen with CNS infections commands attention because of the severe reduction of cerebral perfusion pressure (CPP) in children suffering from bacterial meningitis in the early period, herpes encephalitis, and postinfectious encephalitis with severe status epilepticus.

Complications are treated appropriately, such as aspiration of subdural effusion in infants and heparin therapy for children who develop disseminated intravascular coagulation syndrome. Shock, if it occurs in the child, is managed by restoration of blood volume and maintenance of electrolyte balance. Seizures occur in about 30% of affected children during the first few days of treatment (Feigin and Neglia, 1986). These are controlled with appropriate anticonvulsants.

Lumbar puncture is carried out as needed to determine the effectiveness of therapy. The patient is evaluated neurologically during the convalescent period and at regular intervals during the succeeding year.

Prognosis. The age of the child, the rapidity of diagnosis after onset, and the adequacy of therapy are important in the prognosis of bacterial meningitis. The mortality of neonatal meningitis is approximately 50%, although late-onset β-hemolytic streptococcal meningitis carries a 15% to 20% case fatality. With *H. influenzae* disease and meningococcal meningitis, the mortality rate is 5% to 10%, and with pneumococcal meningitis in infancy and childhood, about 20%.

Sequelae of bacterial meningitis are seen most frequently when the disease occurs in the first 2 months of life and least often in children with meningococcal meningitis. The residual deficits in infants are primarily a result of communicating hydrocephalus and the greater effects of cerebritis on the immature brain. In older children the residual effects are related to the inflammatory process itself or result from vasculitis associated with the disease. Evaluation of CN VIII is needed for at least a 6-month follow-up period to assess for possible hearing loss.

Prevention. Vaccines are now available for types A, C, Y, and W-135 meningococci and *H. influenzae* type B. At present, type A is effective in children ages 3 months and older. For children less than 18 months of age, two doses 3 months apart have been given to control an epidemic. Quadrivalent vaccine given to infants may cause poor response to other types. Group C vaccine is effective in children ages 2 years and older. Duration of protection is not established but is likely to be less than 3 years for group A in children immunized at less than 4 years of age. Routine meningococcal vaccination of children is not recommended (see Table 12). As of this writing, routine vaccinations for *H. Influenzae* type B is recommended for all children beginning at 2 months of age (see Appendix G).

Nursing Considerations

Nurses should take necessary precautions to protect themselves and others from possible infection. Parents are taught the proper procedures and supervised in their application.

✦ **NURSING ALERT** The first priority of nursing care of a child suspected of having meningitis is to administer the antibiotic as soon as it is ordered. The child is also placed on respiratory isolation for at least 24 hours after implementation of antimicrobial therapy.

The room should be kept as quiet as possible and environmental stimuli kept at a minimum, since most affected children are sensitive to noise, bright lights, and other external stimuli. Most children are more comfortable without a pillow and with the head of the bed slightly elevated. A side-lying position is more often assumed because of nuchal rigidity. The nurse should avoid actions, such as lifting the child's head, that cause pain or increase discomfort. Measures are employed to ensure safety, since the child is often restless and subject to seizures.

The nursing care of the child with meningitis is determined by the child's symptoms and treatment. Observation of vital signs, neurologic signs, level of consciousness, urine output, and other pertinent data is carried out at frequent intervals. The child who is unconscious is managed as described previously (see p. 1732), and all children are observed carefully for signs of complications just described, especially signs of increased ICP, shock, or respiratory distress.

Fluids and nourishment are determined by the child's status. The child with dulled sensorium is usually given nothing by mouth. Other children are allowed clear liquids initially and progressed to a diet suitable for their age. Careful monitoring and recording of intake and output are needed to determine deviations that might indicate impending shock or increasing fluid accumulation, such as cerebral edema or subdural effusion.

One of the most difficult problems in nursing care of children with meningitis is maintaining the intravenous infusion for the length of time needed to provide adequate antimicrobial therapy (usually 10 days). Since continuous intravenous fluids are usually not necessary, a heparin lock device is used. In some cases, children who are recovering uneventfully are sent home with the device, and parents are taught intravenous drug administration.*

Family support. The sudden nature of the illness makes emotional support of the child and parents extremely important. Parents are very upset and concerned about their child's condition and frequently feel guilty for not having suspected the seriousness of the illness sooner. They need much reassurance that the natural onset of meningitis is sudden and that they acted responsibly in seeking medical assistance when they did. The nurse encourages them to openly discuss their feelings to minimize blame and guilt. They also are kept informed of the child's progress and of all procedures and treatments. In the event that the child's condition worsens, they need the same psychologic care as parents facing the possible death of their child (see Chapter 23).

TUBERCULOUS MENINGITIS

Tuberculous (TB) meningitis must be considered, especially in persons traveling or living in developing countries and in immigrants from Third World areas. Ischemic infarction can occur with TB meningitis. The most frequent clinical findings are meningeal signs, fever, alteration of consciousness, CN involvement, seizures, and focal neurologic deficit. Hydrocephalus is a frequent complication of TB meningitis.

NONBACTERIAL (ASEPTIC) MENINGITIS

Aseptic meningitis is caused by a number of agents, principally viruses, and is frequently associated with other diseases, such as measles, mumps, herpes, and leukemia. Enteroviruses and mumps viruses account for a large number of cases.

The onset may be abrupt or gradual. The initial manifestations are headache, fever, malaise, gastrointestinal symptoms, and signs of meningeal irritation that develop 1 or 2 days after the onset of illness. Abdominal pain and nausea and vomiting are common; back and leg pain, sore throat,

*See Nursing Care Plan: The Child with Acute Bacterial Meningitis and home care instructions for caring for a heparin lock in Wong, D.L., and Whaley, L.F.: Clinical manual of pediatric nursing, ed. 3, St. Louis, 1990, Mosby–Year Book, Inc.

photophobia, chest pain, and generalized muscular aches or pains are found occasionally. Onset is more insidious in infants and toddlers. Parents may report a change in the child's level of activity and responsiveness. They suspect a minor illness until meningeal signs appear. There may be a maculopapular rash. These symptoms usually subside spontaneously and rapidly, and the child is well in 3 to 10 days with no residual effects.

Diagnosis is based on clinical features and CSF findings, which include increased lymphocytes, predominantly mononuclear cells. It is important to differentiate this self-limited disorder from the more serious form of meningitis and to diagnose and treat any disease of which it is a manifestation.

Treatment is primarily symptomatic, such as acetaminophen for headache, moist heat for muscle aches and pains, and positioning for comfort. Antimicrobial agents may be administered and isolation enforced until a definitive diagnosis is made as a precaution against the possibility that the disease might be of bacterial origin.

BRAIN ABSCESS

Brain abscesses are the most common form of intracranial suppurative process in children. They may be multiple or single, are identified less often in infancy than in later childhood, and are two to three times more common in boys than in girls (Strauss, 1986). Intracerebral abscesses form when pyogenic organisms gain access to neural tissue by way of the bloodstream from foci of infection or from direct inoculation of organisms from meningitis, penetrating trauma, or surgical procedures. The majority of cases spread from secondary ear, nose, and throat sources; meningitis; sepsis; or cyanotic congenital heart disease. However, a large number of children with brain abscesses have no discernible source of infection.

The most common sites of intracerebral abscesses are the temporal and frontal lobes between the gray and white matter, and the most frequently demonstrated organisms are the streptococci, pneumococci, and staphylococci. Early signs of the disease are vague, and the insidious onset often includes vomiting, lethargy, fever, seizures, and progression to coma. Specific neurologic signs are related to the area invaded by the infectious process and, as this area enlarges, resemble those produced by an intracranial tumor. Cerebellar abscesses produce signs associated with any posterior fossa mass (see Brain Tumors, Chapter 36).

Antibiotic therapy is effective during abscess formation. Successful management consists of surgical drainage of a loculated infection and antibiotic therapy. The child is treated symptomatically with frequent CT scans to monitor the progress of the abscess. Where possible, the source of the infection is eradicated. Children may experience seizure disorders as a long-term complication.

ENCEPHALITIS

Encephalitis is an inflammatory process of the CNS producing altered function of various portions of the brain and spinal cord. Encephalitis can be caused by a variety of organisms, including bacteria, spirochetes, fungi, protozoa, helminths, and viruses. Most infections are associated with viruses, and this discussion is limited to these agents.

Etiology

Encephalitis can occur as the result of (1) direct invasion of the CNS by a virus or (2) postinfectious involvement of the CNS after a viral disease. Often the specific type of encephalitis in a particular patient may not be identified for some time or not at all. The cause of over half the cases reported in the United States is unknown. The majority of cases of known etiology are associated with the childhood diseases of measles, mumps, varicella, and rubella and, less often, with the enteroviruses and herpes viruses. Vaccination programs have greatly reduced the incidence of encephalitis in children.

Herpes simplex encephalitis is an uncommon disease, but 30% of cases involve children (Kohl, 1988). The initial clinical findings are nonspecific (fever, altered mental status), but most cases evolve to demonstrate focal neurologic signs and symptoms. Children may experience focal seizures. The CSF is abnormal in most cases. Because of a rise in the number of children with herpes simplex virus encephalitis, suspected cases require prompt attention, especially since the diagnosis can be difficult. The clinical diagnosis can be confirmed by the rapid appearance of IgM antibody to herpes simplex virus type 1 in CSF and serum. The early use of intravenous acyclovir reduces mortality and morbidity.

The multiplicity of causes of viral encephalitis makes diagnosis difficult. Most are those involved with arthropod vectors (togaviruses and bunyaviruses) and those associated with hemorrhagic fevers (arenaviruses, filoviruses, Hantaan viruses). The vector reservoir for most agents pathogenic for humans and detected in the United States is the mosquito; therefore most cases of encephalitis appear during the hot summer months and subside during the autumn. One type found along the United States–Canadian border is carried by ticks.

Clinical Manifestations

The clinical features of encephalitis are similar regardless of the agent involved. Manifestations can range from a mild benign form that resembles aseptic meningitis, lasting a few days and being followed by rapid and complete recovery, to a fulminating encephalitis with severe CNS involvement. The onset may be sudden or gradual with malaise, fever, headache, dizziness, apathy, stiffness of the neck, nausea and vomiting, ataxia, tremors, hyperactivity, and speech difficulties. In severe cases there is high fever, stupor, seizures, disorientation, spasticity, and coma that may proceed to death. Ocular palsies and paralysis also may occur.

Diagnostic Evaluation

The diagnosis is made on the basis of clinical findings, circumstances associated with the disease, and, where possible, identification of the specific virus. A diagnostic evaluation of encephalitis may include a brain biopsy, usually from the temporal lobe area. Togaviruses (some of which were formerly labeled arboviruses) are rarely detected in the blood or spinal fluid, but viruses of herpes, mumps, measles, and enteroviruses may be found in CSF. Serologic diagnosis may be reached by means of a variety of antibody tests. The first should be drawn as soon after onset as possible and the second 2 or 3 weeks later.

Therapeutic Management

Patients suspected of having encephalitis are hospitalized promptly for skilled nursing care and observation. Treatment is primarily supportive, including conscientious nursing care, control of cerebral manifestations, and adequate nutrition and hydration, with observations and management as for other disorders involving cerebral injury. Follow-up care with periodic reevaluation and rehabilitation are important for survivors with residual effects of the disease.

Nursing Considerations

Nursing care of the child with encephalitis is the same as for any unconscious child and for the child with meningitis. Neurologic monitoring, administration of medications, and support of the child and parents are the major aspects of care.

RABIES

Rabies is an acute infection of the nervous system caused by a virus that is almost invariably fatal if left untreated. It is transmitted to humans by the saliva of an infected mammal introduced through a bite or skin abrasion. After entry into a new host the virus multiplies in muscle cells and is spread through neural pathways without stimulating a protective host immune response.

Approximately 88% of rabies cases come from wild animals and 12% from domestic animals. The most commonly reported wildlife species include skunks, raccoons, bats, and foxes. Domestic animals that may cause rabies are cats, cattle, and dogs. Although domestic animals account for only a small percentage of all rabid animals, they account for 64% of all exposures requiring rabies treatment (Rabies surveillance, 1989).

The domestic dog, formerly considered a prime source, is relatively well controlled by rabies vaccination programs. Cats are now the most common rabid domestic animals and should be the target of rabies vaccination programs. The circumstances of a biting incident are important. An unprovoked attack is more likely to indicate a rabid animal than a provoked attack. Bites inflicted on a child attempting to feed or handle an apparently healthy animal can generally be regarded as provoked. Any child bitten by a wild animal is assumed to be exposed to rabies.

✦ **NURSING ALERT** Unusual behavior in an animal is cause for suspicion; children should be warned to beware of wild animals that appear to be friendly.

The disease is uncommon in humans, but the highest incidence occurs in children under 15 years. The incubation period usually ranges from 1 to 3 months but may be as short as 10 days or as long as 8 months. Only 10% to 15% of persons bitten develop the disease, but once symptoms are present, rabies progresses inexorably to a fatal outcome. The disease is characterized by a period of general malaise, fever, and sore throat followed by a phase of excitement featuring hypersensitivity and increased reaction to external stimuli, convulsions, maniacal behavior, and choking. Attempts at swallowing may cause such severe spasm of respiratory muscles that apnea, cyanosis, and anoxia are produced—the characteristics from which the term *hydrophobia* was derived. Diagnosis is made on the basis of history and clinical features. Once symptoms appear, treatment is of little avail, but the long incubation period allows time for induction of active and passive immunity before the onset of illness.

Therapeutic Management

Two types of immunizing products are available for use in humans: (1) the inactivated rabies vaccines, which induce an active immune response, and (2) the globulins, which contain preformed antibodies. The two types of products should be used concurrently for rabies postexposure treatment when prophylaxis is indicated.

The current therapy for a rabid animal bite consists of thorough cleansing of the wound and passive immunization with human rabies immune globulin (HRIG) as soon as possible after exposure to provide rapid, short-term passive immunity (Wilson, 1990).

Postexposure active immunity is conferred by administration of the human diploid cell rabies vaccine (HDCV). The first dose of the vaccine is given at the same time as the immune globulin and followed by intramuscular injections at 3, 7, 14, and 28 days after the first dose. An additional dose in 90 days is recommended by the World Health Organization. Before initiating antirabies prophylaxis, the local or state health department should be consulted.

Nursing Considerations

Parents, as well as children, are frightened by the urgency and seriousness of the situation. They need anticipatory guidance for the therapy and support and reassurance regarding the efficacy of the preventive measures for this dreaded disease. The vaccine is well tolerated by children, but mass immunization is unnecessary and unlikely to be implemented. In areas in which rabies is rare, the schedule given is sufficient. However, certain circumstances may warrant preexposure vaccination, such as when a child is being taken to an area of the world where rabies in stray dogs is still a problem.

REYE SYNDROME

Reye syndrome (RS) is a disorder defined as toxic encephalopathy associated with other characteristic organ involvement. It is characterized by fever, profoundly impaired consciousness, and disordered hepatic function.

The etiology of the disorder is obscure, but most cases of RS follow a common viral illness, most frequently influenza or varicella. The American Academy of Pediatrics, Committee on Infectious Diseases (1982) has recommended that aspirin should not be prescribed under usual circumstances for children with varicella or those suspected of having influenza. Recent studies confirm an association between aspirin administration and RS. Changing epidemiology of the disease in the United States lends support to the success of public education (Hurwitz, 1988). A decline of 91% in the number of cases in children less than 5 years of age and a decline of 75% in children over age 5 years is impressive (Reye's syndrome, 1989).

RS has been defined by the Centers for Disease Control as an acute noninflammatory encephalopathy and hepatopathy, with no reasonable explanation for the cerebral and hepatic abnormalities. The pathology of RS is a mitochondrial insult induced by different viruses, drugs, exogenous toxins, and genetic factors. Elevated ammonia levels tend to correlate with the clinical manifestations and prognosis. Definitive diagnosis is established by liver biopsy. (See Box 37-7 for staging of Reye Syndrome).

The most important aspect of successful management of the child with RS is early diagnosis and aggressive therapy. Rapid progression through coma stages and high peak ammonia concentrations are associated with a more serious prognosis. Cerebral edema with increased ICP represents the most immediate threat to life. Recovery from RS is rapid and usually without sequelae if there has been early diagnosis and implementation of therapy.

Nursing Considerations

The child who is acutely ill with RS requires continuous and intensive nursing care. In addition to an appraisal of vital functions and neurologic status, the nurse assists with a lumbar puncture, obtains blood for laboratory examination, and inserts various intravenous lines such as peripheral, arterial, and central venous pressure. A retention catheter and a nasogastric tube are inserted, and when respirations are compromised, an endotracheal tube is inserted and attached to a respirator for controlled respirations.

Care and observations are implemented as for any child with an altered state of consciousness (see p. 1732) and increasing ICP. Accurate and frequent monitoring of intake and output is essential for adjusting fluid volumes to prevent both dehydration and cerebral edema. The child who is paralyzed and in a drug-induced coma is totally dependent on the caregivers, and meticulous vigilance and attention to all biologic needs are mandatory. Since hypovolemic shock is a constant danger in children with controlled fluid intake and osmotic diuresis, vital signs, including central venous pressure and/or cardiac output (Swan-Ganz catheter), are monitored frequently. Because of related liver dysfunction, the nurse must observe for signs of impaired coagulation such as prolonged bleeding time.

Children often awaken from the coma puzzled by the surroundings and the appearance of other children. Nurses can help them deal with their stress by orienting them to where they are and the circumstances of their being there, describing what is expected of them, and giving them a sense of control whenever possible. Play therapy is a valuable tool for assessment and intervention in postcomatose children. Encouraging parents to visit and providing items associated with home, such as a favorite toy, a photograph, or other item, help them maintain a link with their lives outside the confines of the critical care environment. Understanding and individualized care help children to cope with the stresses and tension of this period of crisis.

Parents of children with RS need a great deal of emotional support. They are usually frightened by the child's appearance, the treatment, and the life-threatening severity and suddenness of the illness. Their distress is increased if they believe that their actions may have contributed to a delay in diagnosis. They need to be kept informed regarding the child's progress, to have diagnostic procedures and therapeutic management explained, and to be given concerned and sympathetic support.

It is important for nurses to continue to discourage the use of aspirin as an analgesic and antipyretic. Research data support the suggestion that continuing decline in aspirin use may be related to the continuing decline in reported number of cases of RS (Arrowsmith and others, 1987). Families need to be aware that salicylate, the offending ingredient in aspirin, is contained in other products (e.g., over-the-counter products such as Pepto-Bismol, a popular antacid) (Szap, Schwartz, and Schwartz, 1989). They should refrain from administering any product for influenza-like symptoms without first checking the label for "hidden" salicylates.

The **National Reye's Syndrome Foundation*** has been established by the parents of a child who died from this disease in hope of encouraging research on the disease and of educating parents and health professionals.

*P.O. Box 829, Bryan, OH 43506; (419) 636-2679.

Box 37-7 STAGING CRITERIA FOR REYE SYNDROME

Stage I	Vomiting, lethargy, and drowsiness; liver dysfunction; type I EEG, follows commands, pupillary reaction brisk
Stage II	Disorientation, combativeness, delirium, hyperventilation, hyperactive reflexes, appropriate responses to painful stimuli; evidence of liver dysfunction; type I EEG, pupillary reaction sluggish
Stage III	Obtunded, coma, hyperventilation, decorticate rigidity, preservation of pupillary light reaction and oculovestibular reflexes (although sluggish); type II EEG
Stage IV	Deepening coma, decerebrate rigidity, loss of oculocephalic reflexes, large and fixed pupils, loss of doll's eye reflex, loss of corneal reflexes; minimum liver dysfunction; type III or IV EEG, evidence of brain stem dysfunction
Stage V	Seizures, loss of deep tendon reflexes, respiratory arrest, flaccidity; type IV EEG; usually no evidence of liver dysfunction

HUMAN IMMUNODEFICIENCY VIRUS ENCEPHALOPATHY

Children with human immunodeficiency virus (HIV) encephalopathy, a complication of acquired immune deficiency syndrome (AIDS), present a nursing challenge. Progressive encephalopathy occurs in 30% to 50% of infants and children infected with HIV; 82% are less than 5 years of age, and 78% of infections are maternally acquired (AIDS, 1989). Epidemiologic data predict increasing numbers of HIV-infected women and children.

Neurologic manifestations in children suggest that the progressive encephalopathy is the result of primary and persistent infection of the brain with the virus. Unexplained neurodevelopmental regression and focal seizures are the dominant clinical features of the disorder. Others include progressive motor dysfunction and atypical CNS infections. These manifestations indicate a poor prognosis and, almost invariably, a fatal outcome. However, earlier implementation of therapies for AIDS may allow for slower progression of these neurologic complications.

Appropriate precautions should be respected by nurses when caring for these unfortunate children. Careful handling of the child is a hallmark of excellent nursing, since these children may experience pain, isolation, social stigma, susceptibility to infection, and abandonment resulting in less than minimum sensorimotor stimulation. Nursing assessment and intervention warrant planning time to meet developmental needs, especially if it means holding, rocking, and comforting the child. (See Chapter 35 for a more extensive discussion of AIDS.)

■ SEIZURE DISORDERS

Convulsive phenomena are among the most frequently observed neurologic dysfunctions in children and can occur with a wide variety of conditions involving the CNS. Generally a *convulsion* is defined as involuntary muscular contractions and relaxation; a *seizure* is a sudden attack. Persons who have a tendency to experience seizures are said to have *epilepsy*. The words are all used synonymously. More specifically, seizure phenomena are characterized by a single attack or recurrent transient attacks of involuntary loss of consciousness, altered motor activity and/or autonomic function, disturbed feelings, or behavior associated with excessive neuronal discharges. These discharges may be focal or diffuse, and the sites of the discharges determine the clinical manifestations observed during the attack.

EPILEPSY: GENERAL CONCEPTS

Seizures are a symptom complex resulting from paroxysmal discharges in cortical neurons. The course and prognosis for children with seizures depend on the etiology, the type of seizure, age of onset, and family and medical histories.

Etiology

Seizures in children have many different causes and histories. Most seizures are *idiopathic*. Although the cause of idiopathic epilepsy is unknown, it may indicate genetic factors that in some way alter the seizure threshold to influence neuronal discharge. Congenital defects and some genetic disorders (e.g., tuberous sclerosis) have seizures as a manifestation. Febrile and breath-holding seizures are related to a lowered seizure threshold that tends to have a higher incidence in certain families. Hereditary EEG abnormalities have been detected in some families, and there is a higher incidence of seizures among relatives of children with idiopathic convulsive disorders.

A seizure disorder also can be *acquired* as a result of brain injury during prenatal, perinatal, or postnatal periods. This injury may be caused by trauma, hypoxia, infections, exogenous or endogenous toxins, and a variety of other factors. Biochemical events (e.g., hypoglycemia, hypocalcemia, certain nutritional deficiencies) produce seizure activity. A partial list of causative factors is presented in Box 37-8.

The incidence of causative factors associated with childhood seizures is frequently related to the age of the child. Seizures are more common during the first 2 years of life than during any other period of childhood. In very young infants the most frequent causes are birth injuries, that is, intracranial trauma, hemorrhage, or anoxia and congenital

Box 37-8 ETIOLOGY OF SEIZURES IN CHILDREN

Nonrecurrent (Acute)	**Recurrent (Chronic)**
Febrile episodes	Idiopathic epilepsy
Intracranial infection	Epilepsy secondary to:
Intracranial hemorrhage	Trauma
Space-occupyng lesions (cyst, tumor)	Hemorrhage
Acute cerebral edema	Anoxia
Anoxia	Infections
Toxins	Toxins
Drugs	Degenerative phenomena
Tetanus	Congenital defects
Lead encephalopathy	Parasitic brain disease
Shigella, Salmonella	Hypoglycemia injury
Metabolic alterations	Epilepsy—sensory stimulus
Hypocalcemia	Epilepsy-stimulating states
Hypoglycemia	Narcolepsy and catalepsy
Hyponatremia or hypernatremia	Psychogenic
Hypomagnesemia	Tetany from hypocalcemia, alkalosis
Alkalosis	Hypoglycemic states
Disorders of amino acid metabolism	Hyperinsulinism
Deficiency states	Hypopituitarism
Hyperbilirubinemia	Adrenocortical insufficiency
	Hepatic disorders
	Uremia
	Allergy
	Cardiovascular dysfunction or syncopal episodes
	Migraine

defects of the brain. Acute infections are a frequent cause of seizures in late infancy and early childhood but become an infrequent cause in middle childhood. In children older than 3 years the most common cause is idiopathic epilepsy.

Other contributing factors are fatigue, undue excitement, and stressful situations at home or school. Excessive fluid intake or fluid retention, such as occurs during premenstrual tension, produces alterations in the serum (and brain) concentrations of sodium, potassium, and water, which may precipitate seizures. There appear to be periods of functional instability of the brain, normally when falling asleep or awakening from sleep. At these times seizures are more likely to occur. The hormonal and metabolic changes associated with adolescence can alter the convulsive threshold. Photogenic stimulation by such commonplace things as television, video games, rays of the sun, or certain kinds of music in susceptible children have been implicated in precipitating seizures in some instances.

Pathophysiology

Regardless of the etiologic factor or the type of seizure, the basic mechanism is the same. There are electric discharges that (1) may arise from central areas in the brain that affect consciousness immediately; (2) may be restricted to one area of the cerebral cortex, producing manifestations characteristic of that particular anatomic focus; or (3) may begin in a localized area of the cortex and spread to other portions of the brain, which, if sufficiently extensive, produce generalized neurologic manifestations.

Seizure activity is believed to be caused by spontaneous electric discharge initiated by a group of hyperexcitable cells referred to as the *epileptogenic focus.* These cells display increased electric excitability but may remain quiescent over a time while discharging intermittently, as evidenced on EEG tracings. Normally these discharges are restrained from spreading beyond the focal area by normal inhibitory mechanisms.

In response to any of a variety of physiologic stimuli, such as cellular dehydration, abnormal blood sugar levels, electrolyte imbalance, fatigue, emotional stress, and endocrine changes, these hyperexcitable cells activate normal cells in surrounding areas and in distant, synaptically related cells. When the neuronal excitation from the epileptogenic focus spreads to the brainstem, particularly the midbrain and reticular formation, a generalized seizure develops. These centers within the brainstem, known as the centrencephalic system, are responsible for the spread of the epileptic potentials. The discharges can originate spontaneously in the centrencephalic system or be triggered by a focal area in the cortex. Seizures are designated as focal, focal with rapid generalization, and generalized, on the basis of these characteristic neuronal discharges, as recorded by the EEG. In a large proportion of children focal seizures spread to other areas, ultimately becoming generalized with loss of consciousness.

Clinical Manifestations

A number of observations provide information to identify the type of seizure and the area of the brain where the neuronal discharges originate. Some clues that distinguish epileptic seizures from other seizure episodes are abrupt onset, genuine loss of awareness, brief duration, rapid recovery, and stereotypic episodes. Some clinical entities that mimic seizures are migraine, toxic effects of drugs, syncope, hyperventilation, transient ischemic attacks, breath-holding spells in infants, and brainstem herniation.

Cocaine intoxication should be considered in the differential diagnosis of new-onset seizure activity in children. Those exposed to smoke of freebase cocaine (crack) used by adult caretakers may have neurologic symptoms of drowsiness, unsteady gait, and seizures (Ernst and Sanders, 1989). Passive cocaine inhalation is evident from isolation of its principal metabolite, benzoyl ecgonine, in the urine (Bateman and Heagarty, 1989). In this situation child protection agencies must be consulted because of the possibility of abuse or neglect.

A seizure is a finite event and consists of a limited number of clinical manifestations. In most cases these can be reduced to commonalities. Generalized seizures without a focal onset may occur at any age and at any time, day or night. The interval between attacks may be minutes, weeks, or even years. Children, in contrast to adults, seldom report an aura or warning.

There are several features that may be observed during various seizures. A clear description of these phenomena is a valuable aid in localizing the area involved and frequently suggests the underlying pathology. The initial event may provide the best clue for assessing the type of seizure and its localization. These include sensory-hallucinatory phenomena, motor effects, sensorimotor effects, and loss of consciousness. The duration of a seizure is determined by separating the active portion of the seizure from the manifestations following the episode.

Sensory-hallucinatory phenomena. An *aura* is the peculiar sensation experienced by some persons just before the onset of a seizure. The aura serves two useful purposes. It warns persons of the impending attack so that they are able to seek privacy and a safe place to lie down before the seizure begins. The nature of the sensation can also provide the most reliable clue to help localize the origin of the discharge. The most common epileptic aura is a sensation of dizziness or an unusual feeling of ascending abdominal discomfort. Other sensations are those described as sensorimotor.

Motor effects. Sometimes there will be only minimal effects with little interference with activity; single groups of muscles may be activated; there can be complex reactive movement patterns or repetitive, stereotypic movements described as automatisms (e.g., lip-smacking, swallowing, chewing). *Eye movement* provides clues to the focus of the seizure. Discharges in the cortex of one hemisphere tend to cause the eyes to deviate to the opposite side. Bilateral discharges tend to cause the eyes to move upward or straight ahead. However, after the seizure, the eyes will often deviate in the opposite direction. When the child's eyes are closed during the attack, a gentle attempt to open them may provide valuable information.

Muscle contraction during the seizure can be one of

three types: *clonic, tonic,* or *jacksonian.* Clonic contractions are those in which opposing muscles contract and relax alternately, producing rhythmic movements. Tonic contractions are those in which all the muscles are maintained in a contraction for a time, causing the person to become rigid. Jacksonian contractions are those in which muscular twitchings begin in one area and spread to another.

Laterality of seizure activity is an important observation. Motor activity may involve the entire body, one side, or one or more body parts. The body part or side involved implies an electric discharge in the corresponding area of the opposite cerebral cortex. *Complex motor activity* is observed in some types of seizures. Seizures may begin with or consist of complex, stereotypic, or repetitive activities. These are often associated with lesions in the temporal lobe.

Sensorimotor effects. Various sensorimotor sensations may accompany a seizure; these may include a tingling or prickling sensation, hallucinations or light flashes, tastes, smells, or sounds. The focal areas implicated are visual hallucinations (occipital or temporal lobe), verbal phenomena (the dominant hemisphere), and unusual tastes, odors, visceral sensations, or dreamy feelings (temporal lobe). Autonomic activity may include pallor, sweating, flushing, piloerection, and pupillary dilation.

Alteration of consciousness. Consciousness may be unaffected, lost completely, or altered but not lost. Persons who do not lose consciousness usually have some degree of reactivity and may even talk, but activity is incomplete, inappropriate, bizarre, or automatic with impaired memory for the event.

Loss of consciousness causes amnesia for the attack and indifference to the environment with no response to stimuli. Loss of consciousness commonly accompanies a seizure and indicates generalized cortical or centrencephalic involvement. The loss of consciousness is frequently shown by various manifestations such as incontinence or injury.

Other observations. In addition to the initial event, which helps localize the cerebral site of origin and is usually stereotypic for a given patient, the circumstances that precipitated the attack or in which the attack occurred are important. The *postictal state,* the period following a seizure, may be varied. The child may be drowsy, be uncoordinated, have transient aphasia or confusion, and display some sensory or motor impairment. Neurologic changes are important to document. Weakness, hypotonia, or inactivity of a body part may be an indication of an epileptogenic focus in the corresponding contralateral cortical region.

EPILEPSY: CLASSIFICATION

There are many different types of epileptic seizures, and each has unique characteristics. They are classified on the basis of careful clinical description of the attacks in conjunction with results of physical examination and EEG analysis. The onset of a seizure is abrupt, paroxysmal, and transitory, and signs are highly variable, as evidenced by the previous discussion. The International Classification of Epileptic Seizures divides seizures into two major categories: partial seizures and generalized seizures (Box 37-9).

Box 37-9 INTERNATIONAL CLASSIFICATION OF EPILEPTIC SEIZURES

I. Partial seizures (seizures beginning locally)
  A. Simple partial seizures (with elementary symptomatology; consciousness unimpaired)
    1. With motor symptoms
    2. With somatosensory or special sensory symptoms
    3. With autonomic symptoms
    4. Compound forms (with psychic symptoms)
  B. Complex partial symptomatology (temporal lobe or psychomotor seizures; generally with impaired consciousness)
    1. With impairment of consciousness only
    2. With cognitive symptomatology
    3. With affective symptomatology
    4. With psychosensory symptomatology
    5. With psychomotor symptomatology
    6. Compound forms
  C. Partial seizures, secondarily generalized
II. Generalized seizures (bilaterally symmetric; without local onset; with impairment of consciousness)
  A. Tonic-clonic (grand mal) seizures
  B. Tonic seizures
  C. Clonic seizures
  D. Absence (petit mal) seizures
  E. Atonic seizures
  F. Myoclonic seizures
  G. Infantile spasms
  H. Akinetic seizures
III. Unilateral seizures (those involving one hemisphere)
IV. Unclassified epileptic seizures (due to incomplete data)

Modified from Commission on Classification and Terminology of the International League Against Epilepsy: Proposal for revised clinical and electroencephalographic classification of epileptic seizures, Epilepsia 22:489-501, 1981.

Partial Seizures

Partial seizures are caused by abnormal electric discharges from epileptogenic foci limited to a more or less circumscribed region of the cerebral cortex. There is usually evidence that the irritating focus of the seizure is secondary to an underlying condition that causes damage to brain tissue. Focal lesions include scars from previous craniocerebral trauma, atrophy, malformations, or tumors. Focal seizures may arise from any area of the cerebral cortex, but the frontal, temporal, and parietal lobes are the ones most often affected. The area of cerebral involvement is reflected by clinical manifestations.

Partial seizures are categorized as (1) those with elementary or simple symptoms, (2) those with associated impairment of consciousness, and (3) those with impaired consciousness and that spread to become generalized. The hallmark of partial seizures is the onset in a portion of one cerebral hemisphere, as evidenced by focal spikes or sharp waves on the EEG.

Simple partial seizures. Focal seizures are characterized by localized motor symptoms; somatosensory, psychic, autonomic symptoms; or a combination of these. The abnormal discharges remain unilateral. The most common motor seizure in children is the aversive seizure, in which the eye or eyes and head turn away from the side of the focus. In some children the upper extremity toward which the head turns is abducted and extended and the fingers are clenched, giving the impression that the child is looking at the closed fist. The child may be aware of the movement or lose consciousness simultaneously with assuming the position.

A common form is the sylvian seizure, in which there are tonic-clonic movements involving the face, salivation, and arrested speech. These are most common during sleep. On rare occasions children display the *jacksonian* march, an orderly, sequential progression of clonic movements that begin in a foot, hand, or face and, as electric impulses spread from the irritable focus to contiguous regions of the cortex, move or "march" body parts activated by these cerebral regions. Motor seizures are particularly common in hemiplegic children. The movements, which are usually clonic, begin in the hemiplegic hand, spread to the entire affected side and, in many cases, become generalized seizures. Postictal weakness is common after this type of seizure.

Special sensory seizures are characterized by various sensations, including numbness, tingling, prickling, paresthesia, or pain that originates in one area (e.g., face or extremities) and spreads to other parts of the body. Visual sensations or formed images may be manifestations. Motor phenomena such as posturing or hypertonia may accompany sensory seizures. Special sensory seizures are uncommon in children under 8 years of age.

Complex partial seizures. Partial seizures with complex symptoms are the most difficult to recognize and are among those most difficult to control. Because they involve more organized and higher-level cerebral function as well as sensory and motor function, they have been termed *psychomotor seizures.* The attack is characterized by a period of altered behavior for which the individual is amnesic and during which he or she is unable to respond to the environment. Although children do not lose consciousness during an attack, they have no recollection of their behavior during the seizure. Drowsiness or sleep usually follows the seizure. Confusion and amnesia may be prolonged.

Psychomotor seizures are observed more often in children from 3 years of age through adolescence and are more common in adults than in children. The seizures are most characteristically associated with focal lesions of the temporal lobe and are sometimes referred to as temporal lobe seizures.

Complex sensory phenomena associated with the beginning of a seizure reflect the complicated connections and integrative functions of that area of the brain. The most frequent sensation is a strange feeling in the pit of the stomach that rises toward the throat. This feeling is often accompanied by odd or unpleasant odors or tastes, complex auditory or visual hallucinations, or ill-defined feelings of elation or strangeness (e.g., *déjà vu,* a feeling of familiarity in a strange environment). Small children may emit a cry or attempt to run for help as a manifestation of an aura. Strong feelings of fear and anxiety and a distorted sense of time and self may be mental symptoms associated with an episode.

A variety of patterns of motor behavior may be observed during a psychomotor attack. The attacks are usually stereotypic and recur in a similar manner with each subsequent seizure. It is sometimes difficult to determine whether the manifestations are related to a seizure disorder or to a nonconvulsive behavioral disturbance. The child may suddenly cease activity, appear dazed, stare into space, become confused and apathetic, and become limp, stiff, or display some form of posturing. The primary feature may be confusion, and the child may perform purposeless, complicated activities in a repetitive manner (automatisms), such as walking, running, kicking, laughing, or speaking incoherently, most often followed by postictal confusion or sleep. The predominant observations may be oropharyngeal activities (e.g., smacking, chewing, drooling, swallowing) and nausea or abdominal pain followed by stiffness, a fall, and postictal sleep. Rarely children manifest auras such as rage or temper tantrums, and aggressive acts are uncommon during a seizure. See Table 37-8 for a comparison of simple partial, complex partial, and absence seizures.

Generalized Seizures

Generalized seizures without a focal onset appear to arise in the reticular formation, and the clinical observations indicate that the initial involvement is from both hemispheres. Loss of consciousness occurs and is the initial clinical manifestation. Unlike partial seizures that become generalized, there is no aura. Attacks occur at any time, day or night, and the interval between attacks may be minutes, hours, weeks, or even years. Most affected persons first experience seizures in childhood, and children whose seizures begin before age 4 years have mental retardation and behavioral and learning problems more frequently than those whose seizures begin after age 4.

Tonic-clonic seizures. The generalized tonic-clonic seizure, traditionally known as *grand mal,* is the most common and most dramatic of all seizure manifestations of childhood. The seizure usually occurs without warning. There is a rolling of the eyes upward and immediate loss of consciousness. If the child is standing, he or she falls to the floor or ground. The child stiffens in a generalized and symmetric tonic contraction of the entire body musculature. The arms usually flex, whereas the legs, head, and neck extend. The child may utter a peculiar piercing cry produced as the jaws clap shut and the thoracic and abdominal muscles contract, forcing air through tightly closed vocal cords. This tonic phase lasts approximately 10 to 20 seconds, during which the child is apneic and may become cyanotic. Autonomic stimulation causes increased salivation.

The tonic rigidity is replaced by violent jerking movements as the trunk and extremities undergo rhythmic contraction and relaxation of the clonic phase. During this time the child may foam at the mouth and be incontinent of urine and feces. As the attack ends, the movements become less intense and occur at longer intervals until they cease entirely. The clonic phase generally lasts about 30 seconds

Table 37-8 Comparison of simple partial, complex partial, and absence seizures

CLINICAL MANIFESTATIONS	SIMPLE PARTIAL	COMPLEX PARTIAL	ABSENCE
Age of onset	Any age	Uncommon before age 3 years	Uncommon before age 3 years
Frequency (per day)	Variable	Rarely over 1-2 times	Multiple
Duration	Usually less than 30 seconds	Usually over 60 seconds, rarely less than 10 seconds	Usually less than 15 seconds, rarely more than 30 seconds
Aura	May be sole manifestation of seizure	Frequently	Never
Impaired consciousness	Never	Always	Always, but may be brief
Automatisms	No	Frequently	Frequently
Clonic movements	Frequently	Occasionally	Occasionally
Postictal impairment	Occasionally	Frequently	Never
Mental disorientation	Frequently	Common	Unusual

but can vary from only a few seconds to a half hour or longer. A series of seizures at intervals too brief to allow the child to regain consciousness between the time one attack ends and the next begins is known as *status epilepticus.* This requires emergency intervention. A succession of interrupted seizures can lead to exhaustion, respiratory failure, and death.

In the postictal state children appear to relax but may remain semiconscious and difficult to rouse. They may awaken in a few minutes but remain confused for several hours. They are poorly coordinated, with mild impairment of fine motor movements. Children may have visual and speech difficulties and may vomit or complain of severe headache. When left alone, they usually sleep for several hours. On awakening they are fully conscious but usually feel tired and complain of sore muscles and headache but have no recollection of the entire event.

Absence seizures. Absence seizures, traditionally called *petit mal* or *lapses,* are characterized by a brief loss of consciousness with minimal or no alteration in muscle tone and may go unrecognized because the child's behavior is changed very little. Attacks almost always first appear during childhood. In most instances the onset occurs between 4 and 12 years of age. Attacks are rarely detected before age 5, usually cease at puberty, but may be seen in adults. They are more common in girls than in boys.

The onset of absence seizures is abrupt, and the child suddenly develops 20 or more attacks daily. Characteristically the brief loss of consciousness appears without warning or aura and usually lasts about 5 to 10 seconds. Slight loss of muscle tone may cause the child to drop objects, but the child is able to maintain postural control and seldom falls. There are frequently minor movements such as lip smacking, twitching of eyelids or face, or slight hand movements. The sudden arrest of activity and consciousness is not accompanied by incontinence, and the child is amnesic for the episode but may need to reorient to the previous activity. An attack is often mistaken for inattentiveness or daydreaming. Frequent attacks can result in slowed intellectual processes and deterioration in schoolwork and behavior, which is sometimes the first indication of the problem. Attacks can be precipitated by hyperventilation, hypoglycemia, stresses (emotional and physiologic), fatigue, or sleeplessness (see Table 37-8).

Atonic and akinetic seizures. Akinetic and atonic seizures are manifest as a sudden, momentary loss of muscle tone and postural control. *Atonic* refers to loss of muscle tone; *akinetic* is loss of movement. The onset is usually between 2 and 5 years of age. The sudden loss of postural tone and reflexes causes the child to fall to the floor violently. The child is unable to break the fall by putting out the hand and may incur a serious injury to the face, head, or shoulder. Loss of consciousness is only momentary. Akinetic attacks recur frequently during the day, particularly in the morning hours and shortly after the child awakens. Atonic seizures are also known as *drop attacks.*

Myoclonic seizures. Myoclonic seizures include a variety of convulsive episodes characterized by sudden, brief contractures of a muscle or group of muscles, occurring singly or repetitively without loss of consciousness or postictal state. The seizure may or may not be symmetric and may be isolated as benign essential myoclonus or may occur in association with other seizure forms. Myoclonus frequently appears normally in the course of falling asleep or is observed as a nonspecific symptom in many diseases of the nervous system, such as viral encephalitis, uremic encephalopathy, and degenerative diseases of the cerebrum.

Infantile spasms. Infantile spasms refer to a rare disorder with onset within the first 6 to 8 months of life. A large percentage of children with this disorder (85% to

90%) show various degrees of retardation (Hrachovy and Frost, 1989). The pathophysiology is unknown, but recent evidence suggests that certain regions in the brainstem associated with sleep cycling are involved. The underlying cause may be a disturbance of the central neurotransmitter regulation at a specific phase of brain development.

Other terms for this disorder are infantile myoclonus, massive spasms, hypsarrhythmia, salaam attacks, or infantile myoclonic spasms. They are twice as common in males as in females. In infants who are able to sit but not stand, the seizure is observed as a sudden dropping forward of the head and neck with trunk flexed forward and knees drawn up—the "salaam" or "jackknife" seizure. The attack may consist of a series of sudden, brief, symmetric, muscular contractions by which the head is flexed, the arms are extended, and the legs are drawn up. The eyes may roll upward or inward, and the seizure may be preceded or followed by a cry or giggling. There may or may not be loss of consciousness, and the infant will sometimes flush, turn pale, or become cyanotic. The child may have numerous seizures during the day without postictal drowsiness or sleep.

Less often, alternate clinical forms are observed and include extensor spasms rather than flexion of arms, legs, and trunk and head nodding. Lightning attacks, which involve a single, momentary, shocklike contraction of the entire body, are another variant.

Infantile spasms are frequently associated with cerebral abnormalities, such as structural malformations, severe anoxic brain damage, phenylketonuria, and degenerative changes. Microcephaly, choreoathetoid or tonic posture, and abnormal movements are frequently present. There may be a history of maternal infection, prematurity, or birth injury, and development is retarded before the onset of seizures. At present the only effective treatment is administration of adrenocorticotropic hormone (ACTH) or corticosteroids. The long-term prognosis is poor, both mentally and developmentally.

EPILEPSY: MANAGEMENT

The management of epilepsy requires a well-organized approach. It involves diagnosis, therapy, and monitoring of progress to ensure the efficacy of therapy. Parental involvement is essential, and education and support are vital to the success of any therapeutic plan.

Diagnostic Evaluation

Establishing a diagnosis is critical. The process of diagnosis in a child with a convulsive disorder has two major foci: (1) to ascertain the type of seizure the child has experienced and (2) to attempt to understand the cause of the attacks. The assessment and diagnosis rely heavily on a thorough history, skilled observation, and employment of several diagnostic tests.

It is especially important to differentiate epilepsy from other brief alterations in consciousness and/or behavior. Epilepsy results from a wide range of etiologic factors. It is unusual to observe the child during a seizure in the assessment process. A complete, accurate, and detailed history should be obtained from a reliable and knowledgeable informant. This history involves prenatal, perinatal, and neonatal periods, including any instances of infection, apnea, colic, or poor feeding, and information regarding any previous accidents or serious illnesses. If the diagnosis is clear, the seizure can be identified as an isolated event and unlikely to recur (e.g., a febrile seizure) or as a symptom of an underlying and potentially lethal disease (e.g., a brain tumor).

History of the seizure(s) should be equally detailed, including the type of seizure or description of the child's behavior during the attack(s), the age at onset, and the time at which the seizure occurs (i.e., early morning, before meals, while awake, or during sleep). Any factors that may have precipitated the seizure are important, including fever, infection, falls that may have caused trauma to the head, anxiety, fatigue, and activity (e.g., hyperventilation or exposure to strong stimuli such as bright flashing lights or loud noises). If the child can describe any sensory phenomena, these are recorded. The duration and progression of the seizure (if any) and the postictal feelings and behavior, such as confusion, inability to speak, amnesia, headache, and sleep, are recorded. The ability to identify seizure types accurately has resulted from the technologic advances in video recording and long-term EEG monitoring.

A complete physical and neurologic examination, including developmental assessment of language, learning, behavior, and motor abilities, often provides clues to neurologic disturbances. A family history can offer clues to paroxysmal disorders such as migraine, breath-holding spells, febrile convulsions, or neurologic diseases that may be related to the convulsive disorder.

Laboratory studies that may prove to be of value include a complete blood cell count (for evidence of lead poisoning) and white blood cell count for signs of infection. Blood and CSF glucose may give evidence of hypoglycemic episodes, and serum electrolytes, blood urea nitrogen, calcium, and other blood studies might indicate metabolic disturbances. Lumbar puncture can confirm a suspected diagnosis of cerebrospinal infection or trauma.

Skull radiographs, CT, echoencephalograms, brain scans, and other studies help to identify skull abnormalities, separation of sutures, and intracranial calcifications. Invasive techniques are rarely indicated. Focal seizures in children less than 1 year of age are indications for a diagnostic CT scan to rule out a supratentorial tumor (see Brain Tumors, Chapter 36).

The EEG is obtained for all children with convulsive manifestations and is the most useful tool for evaluating seizure disorders. The EEG is carried out under varying conditions—with the child asleep, awake, awake with provocative stimulation (flashing lights, noise), and hyperventilating. Stimulation elicits abnormal electrical activity, which is recorded on the EEG. Various seizure types produce characteristic EEG patterns—high-voltage spike discharges are seen in grand mal seizures, with abnormal patterns in the intervals between seizures; a three-per-second spike and wave pattern is observed in a petit mal seizure; and absence of electrical activity in an area suggests a large lesion, such as an abscess or subdural collection of fluid.

Variations of the EEG are video recordings of the patient during waking and/or sleeping. The full body image is displayed on half of the video screen, the facial image is shown on one fourth, and selected EEG channels are displayed on the remaining one fourth. Split-screen capabilities allow modification and arrangement of a larger number of channels and images. Polygraph equipment is also used to monitor physiologic data such as respiratory effort, eye movements, heart rate, and systemic blood pressure. These techniques can be used concurrently and are especially valuable in differentiating epileptic activity from paroxysmal behavior or nonepileptic motor events.

Therapeutic Management

The objective of treatment of convulsive disorders is to control the seizures or to reduce their frequency, discover and correct the cause when possible, and help the child who has recurrent seizures to live as normal a life as possible. Seizures of a recurrent nature are treated as soon as the diagnosis is established. If the seizure activity is a manifestation of an infectious, traumatic, or metabolic process, the seizure therapy is instituted as a part of the general therapeutic regimen. Seizure control is considered to prevent secondary brain cell injury from the neuronal discharge and hypoxia.

Drug therapy. It is known that persons predisposed to epilepsy have seizures when their basal level of neuronal excitability exceeds a critical point or threshold; no attack occurs if the excitability is maintained below this threshold. The administration of anticonvulsant drugs serves to raise this threshold and prevent seizures. Consequently the primary therapy for convulsive disorders is the administration of the appropriate anticonvulsant drug or combination of drugs in a dosage that provides the desired effect without causing undesirable side effects or toxic reactions. Anticonvulsant (antiepileptic) drugs are believed to exert their effect primarily by reducing the responsiveness of normal neurons to the sudden, high-frequency nerve impulses that arise in the epileptogenic focus. Thus the convulsive seizure is effectively suppressed; the abnormal brain waves may or may not be altered. Complete control can be achieved in only 50% to 75% of children with epilepsy, however, even with careful attention to details of therapy. The anticonvulsant drugs used for control of seizures are outlined in Table 37-9. Some success has been achieved in treating infantile spasms with ACTH. Hyperkalemia can be a late side effect of this therapy.

Therapy is begun with a single drug known to be effective for the child's particular type of seizure, and the dosage is gradually increased until the seizures are controlled or the child develops signs of toxicity. If the drug is effective but does not sufficiently control the seizures, a second drug is added in gradually increasing doses. Once seizures are controlled, the drug or drugs are continued for a prolonged time.

Periodic reevaluation of the drug is important to assess the continued effectiveness and to alter the dosage if indicated. The dosage will need to be increased as the child grows. Blood levels often prove valuable in determination of optimum dosage levels. Blood cell counts, urinalysis, and liver function tests are obtained at frequent intervals in children receiving particular anticonvulsant medications. Repeat EEGs are generally obtained every 1½ to 2 years.

Withdrawal of antiepileptic therapy follows a predesigned protocol, usually begun when the child has been seizure-free for at least 2 years with a normal EEG. Relapse in children may be related to factors such as neurologic deficit or a positive family history for epilepsy. Recurrence is most likely within the first year after discontinuance of the medication.

When a medication is discontinued, the dosage should be reduced gradually over 1 to 2 weeks. Sudden withdrawal of a drug can cause an increase in the number and severity of seizures, often precipitating status epilepticus. If the time for reducing the medication coincides with puberty or, in younger children, occurs during periods when the child is subject to frequent infections, the drug is continued for a longer period.

Complications of drug therapy. Side effects of continued use of anticonvulsant medications are sometimes distressing to the child and the family. Most side effects are transient and dose related but warrant immediate attention of health care personnel. Drug reactions require clinical evaluation and serum drug levels. Combination therapy, such as with barbiturates and carbamazepine, can potentiate drug levels. Careful monitoring is necessary to avoid toxicity. It is also important to be aware that phenytoin (Dilantin) causes gingival hyperplasia, which can be cosmetically undesirable. Frequent gum massage and careful attention to good oral hygiene are recommended. Ataxia and rashes often disappear when drug dosages are reduced. Depression, which has been reported in children with epilepsy who are taking barbiturate anticonvulsants, can be relieved by changing drugs.

More troublesome, however, is the accumulating evidence indicating that anticonvulsant therapy may have detrimental effects on behavior and mental function (Engel, 1989). The American Academy of Pediatrics, Committee on Drugs (1985), stresses that physicians prescribe the appropriate drug and be alert to reports of side effects. The committee also encourages development of screening tests to detect subtle intellectual and behavioral side effects and studies to evaluate and compare the effects of anticonvulsant therapy.

Surgical therapy. When seizure activity is determined to be caused by a hematoma, tumor, or other progressive cerebral lesion, surgical removal is the treatment. When medication is unsuccessful and accumulated evidence indicates a single, distinct epileptogenic focus in a surgically removable and functionally silent area of the brain, excision of the involved tissue is sometimes considered. With children, surgery is reserved for those who suffer from repetitive, incapacitating seizures that are caused by a focal brain abnormality. Surgical treatment for intractable seizures should be instituted before the age of 12 years if focality and intractability can be determined. Assessment of speech

Table 37-9 Major drugs used for control of seizures

DRUG	COMMENTS	SIDE EFFECTS
▪ Partial seizures and/or generalized tonic-clonic seizures		
Primary agents		
Carbamazepine (Tegretol)	Relatively free from unwanted side effects; fewer sedative properties	Side effects: blurred vision, diplopia, drowsiness, vertigo, headache Toxic effects: Leukopenic aplastic anemia
Phenytoin (Dilantin)	Generally effective and safe May cause behavioral disturbances in children May aggravate absence and myoclonic seizures May induce folate deficiency	Side effects: gum hyperplasia, hirsutism, ataxia, nystagmus, diplopia, anorexia, nausea, nervousness Toxic effects: Stevens-Johnson syndrome (erythema multiforme), thrombocytopenia
Mephenytoin	Effective anticonvulsant Regular monitoring of blood count	Side effects: rash, drowsiness, ataxia Toxic effect: aplastic anemia, granulocytosis
Secondary agents		
Clorazepate (Tranxene)	Few side effects	Some drowsiness
Primidone* (Mysoline)	Effective with phenobarbital in mixed-type seizure patterns	Side effects: drowsiness, ataxia, diplopia
Phenobarbital (Luminal)	Safest overall drug Most useful in combination with other drugs May interfere with concentration and motor speed May cause vitamin D and folic acid deficiencies	Side effects: drowsiness, irritability, hyperactivity, skin rash, mild ataxia, hyperpyrexia, diminished cognitive performance
Valproic acid (Depakene)	Relatively free from unwanted effects Frequently given in association with other anticonvulsants Potentiates action of phenobarbital and phenytoin Excessively sweet taste may aggravate nausea; give with food	Side effects: anorexia, nausea, drowsiness
Ethosuximide (Zarontin)	Occasionally aggravates generalized seizures Administer with food	Side effects: nausea, gastric discomfort, anorexia, headache, drowsiness
Methsuximide (Celontin)	May induce folate deficiency	Side effects: drowsiness, nausea, headache, vertigo
Phensuximide	Less effective than others; used when others fail Slight nephrotoxicity; monthly urinalysis	Side effects: drowsiness, headache, vertigo, nausea
Ancillary agents		
Dextroamphetamine (Dexadrine)	Given to counteract drowsiness and lethargy	
Acetazolamide (Diamox)	Given to reduce fluid accumulation	
▪ Absence seizures		
Primary agents		
Ethosuximide	Drug of choice for absences	
Valproic acid	See above	
Methsuximide	See above	
Phenobarbital	See above	
Clonazepam (Clonopin)	Usually given as adjunct to other anticonvulsants	Side effects: lethargy, ataxia, hyperactivity, agitation, nystagmus, slurred speech, rhinorrhea

*May be used as a primary agent.

Table 37-9 Major drugs used for control of seizures—cont'd

DRUG	COMMENTS	SIDE EFFECTS
Primary agents—cont'd		
Trimethadione (Tridione)	May aggravate generalized seizures Monthly blood counts and urinalysis	Side effects: rash, photophobia, nausea, irritability, drowsiness Toxic effects: leukopenia, agranulocytosis, nephrosis
Ancillary agents	See above	
▪ Atonic, akinetic, and myoclonic seizures		
Combinations of agents		
▪ Status epilepticus (convulsive)		
Diazepam (Valium)	Administer intravenously Rapid onset of action but short duration; unless followed by longer-acting anticonvulsants, seizures usually recur in 20 to 30 minutes	
Lorazepam (Ativan)	Longer acting than diazepam	
Phenytoin (Dilantin)	Longer-acting drug; little additional hypnotic effect Effective in controlling tonic-clonic status	
Phenobarbital (Luminal)	Slowly absorbed by brain parenchyma; requires 10 to 20 minutes for antiepileptic effect	
Paraldehyde	Use in controversial Used if other drugs are ineffective	
General anesthesia	Used if anticonvulsants are ineffective	

dominance and memory function is a preoperative requirement (Vries and others, 1989). Surgical excision of the epileptogenic focus does not eliminate the need for continuation of drug therapy. Drug administration is restarted as soon as the patient regains consciousness and is continued until the patient is free of seizures.

Status epilepticus. Status epilepticus is defined as a continuous seizure that lasts more than 30 minutes or as serial seizures from which the child does not regain a premorbid level of consciousness. The initial treatment is directed toward support and maintenance of vital functions, including maintaining an adequate airway, administration of oxygen, and hydration, and followed by intravenous administration of either diazepam or phenobarbital. Lorazepam may be replacing diazepam as a drug of choice. It has a longer duration of action and causes less respiratory distress in children over 2 years of age. Concurrent intravenous loading with phenytoin is usually necessary for sustained control of seizures.

The child must be closely monitored during administration to detect early alterations in vital signs that may indicate impending cardiac arrest or respiratory depression. When diazepam is ineffective, phenobarbital, often in extremely high levels that may require respiratory support, is given intravenously as the initial medication. Patients who do not respond to drug therapy may require the use of intravenous lidocaine, general anesthesia, or a potent skeletal muscle relaxant such as curare. This should be administered by an anesthesiologist.

Status epilepticus is a medical emergency requiring immediate intervention to prevent permanent injury to the brain. Equally imperative to halting the tonic-clonic movement is correct diagnosis of the underlying problem. The outcome is related to the etiology and duration of the status epilepticus.

Nursing Considerations

Nursing care of the child with a convulsive disorder involves both acute care during a seizure and long-term management. A child with epilepsy and the family require continuous and consistent support in dealing with the stigma associated with a seizure disorder. Education can decrease

Box 37-10 OBSERVATIONS: THE CHILD DURING A GENERALIZED CONVULSIVE SEIZURE

Observe seizure

Describe
Only what is actually observed
Order of events
Duration of seizure

Onset
Significant preseizure events—bright lights, noise, excitement, emotional outbursts
Behavior
- Change in facial expression, such as for fear
- Cry or other sound
- Stereotypic or automatous movements
- Random activity

Position of head, body, extremities
- Unilateral or bilateral posturing of one or more extremities
- Body deviation to side

Time of onset

Movement
Change of position, if any
Site of commencement—hand, thumb, mouth, generalized
Tonic phase, if present—length, parts of body involved
Clonic phase—twitching or jerking movements, parts of body involved, sequence of parts involved, generalized, change in character of movements
Lack of movement of any extremity

Face
Color change—pallor, cyanosis, flushing
Perspiration
Mouth—position, deviating to one side, teeth clenched, tongue bitten, frothing at mouth, flecks of blood or bleeding

Eyes
Position—straight ahead, deviation upward, deviation outward, conjugate or divergent
Pupils (if able to assess)—change in size, equality, reaction to light and accommodation

Respiratory effort
Presence and length of apnea
Presence of stertor

Other
Involuntary urination
Involuntary defecation

Observe postictally
Method of termination
State of consciousness—unresponsiveness, drowsiness, confusion
Orientation to time, persons, etc.
Sleeping but able to be aroused
Motor ability
- Any change in motor power
- Ability to move all extremities
- Any paresis or weakness
- Ability to whistle (if appropriate to age)

Speech—changes, peculiarities, type and extent of any difficulties
Sensations
- Complaint of discomfort or pain
- Any sensory impairment of hearing, vision
- Recollection of preseizure sensations, warning of attack
- Awareness that attack was beginning

Promote rest
- Make child comfortable
- Allow child to rest after seizure
- Reduce sensory stimuli
- Record length of postictal sleep
- Notify physician if seizure is followed by other seizures in rapid succession or if duration of seizure is excessive

Reduce anxiety
- Provide calm, relaxed atmosphere

the psychologic conflicts that persist with the burden of epilepsy. Educating the child, family, and community are key nursing functions.

Assessment

An important nursing function during a seizure is observing the seizure and describing its pertinent features. Any alterations in behavior and characteristics of the attack, such as sensory-hallucinatory phenomena (e.g., an aura), motor effects (e.g., eye movements, muscular contractions, laterality, complex activities), alterations in consciousness, and postictal state, are noted and recorded (Box 37-10).

Generalized seizures and others with dramatic manifestations are easily detected, but absence seizures present more difficulties. They are easily misinterpreted as inattention. Any unusual behavior, even seemingly inconsequential behavior such as a momentary interruption of activity, staring, or mental blankness, should be described. The more detailed these descriptions, the more valuable they are for assessment. The nurse notes the time that the seizure began and times the length of the seizure. This is especially important if the child becomes cyanotic.

History taking is a vital tool for helping to identify factors that aid in establishing a cause of the seizures. Interviewing the child and the family helps to elicit problems related to the psychologic impact of the disorder on their lives.

Nursing Diagnoses

Based on a thorough assessment, several nursing diagnoses are identified. The more common diagnoses for the child with a convulsive disorder are included in the Nursing Care Plan on p. 1769. Others may apply in specific situations.

Planning

Nursing objectives for the child with a convulsive disorder include the following:

NURSING CARE PLAN
The Child with Epilepsy

NURSING DIAGNOSIS: Potential for injury related to sudden and unexpected loss of consciousness

GOAL 1

Prevent physical injury during seizure

INTERVENTIONS

Protect child during a seizure
- Do not attempt to restrain child or use force
- If child is standing or sitting in wheelchair at beginning of attack, ease child down so that he or she will not fall; when possible, place cushion or blanket under child
- Do not put anything in child's mouth
- Loosen restrictive clothing
- Prevent child from hitting hard or sharp objects that might cause injury during uncontrolled movements
  - Remove object(s)
  - Pad object(s)
  - Move furniture out of way
  - Allow seizure to end without interference

Educate parents and child regarding appropriate activities for the child
- Age appropriate
- Avoid contact sports
- Avoid situations that pose a danger during a seizure (e.g., climbing trees, play apparatus)
- Provide companionship during permissible activities such as swimming, bicycling

Educate teachers and other persons who are associated with the child regarding correct behavior during a seizure

EXPECTED OUTCOME

Child exhibits no evidence of physical injury

GOAL 2

Prevent or control seizure activity

INTERVENTIONS

*Administer anticonvulsants
Teach family the administration of medications†
Stress importance of complying with therapeutic regimen
Avoid situations that are known to precipitate a seizure (e.g., blinking lights, emotional stress)

EXPECTED OUTCOME

Child remains free of seizure activity

GOAL 3

Prevent complications from medication

INTERVENTIONS

Be aware of and teach family to recognize unfavorable reactions to medications
Encourage periodic physical and laboratory assessment to determine possible deviations from normal findings

EXPECTED OUTCOME

Child and family demonstrate an understanding of possible unfavorable responses to medications and the appropriate intervention (specify)

NURSING DIAGNOSIS: Altered family processes related to a child with a chronic illness

GOAL 1

Support family

INTERVENTIONS

See Nursing diagnosis: Altered family processes in Nursing Care Plan: The Child with a Chronic Illness or Disability, Chapter 22
*Refer to special support groups and agencies

EXPECTED OUTCOME

Family becomes involved with special group

See also:
Nursing Care Plan: The Child with a Chronic Illness or Disability, Chapter 22
Nursing Care Plan: The Unconscious Child, p. 1734

*Dependent nursing action.
†Home care instructions are available in Wong, D.L., and Whaley, L.F.: Clinical manual of pediatric nursing, ed. 3, 1990, Mosby-Year Book, Inc.

1. Protect the child during a seizure.
2. Prevent seizures if possible.
3. Help the child and family cope with the stigma often associated with the disorder.
4. Promote a positive self-image in the child.

IMPLEMENTATION

Nurses, when they first witness a child in a generalized cerebral seizure, are often frightened, puzzled, and immobilized. These reactions are normal but can reduce the effectiveness of care for the child and interfere with observations of the event. The child must be protected from injury during the seizure, and nursing observations made during the attack provide valuable information for diagnosis and management of the disorder (see Emergency Treatment).

It is impossible to halt a seizure once it has begun, and no attempt should be made to do so. The nurse must remain calm, stay with the child, and prevent the child from sustaining any harm during the attack. If possible, the child should be isolated from the view of others by closing a door or pulling screens. A seizure can be very upsetting to the child, other visitors, and their families. If other persons are present, they should be assured that the affected child is in no danger, and after the attack they can be provided with a simple explanation to meet their needs.

The convulsing child should not be moved or forcefully restrained, and force should not be exerted in an attempt to place a solid object between the teeth. A standing child whom the nurse is able to reach in time, or a child who is seated in a chair (including a wheelchair), should be eased to the floor immediately. After the attack the child should be placed on the side in bed or a similar place to allow the child to sleep. A side-lying position can prevent a hypotonic tongue from occluding the airway. If the child is at school or away from home, the parents should be contacted so that the child can be taken home to rest.

Children who are known to have convulsive attacks or who are under observation for seizures will require special precautions. The extent of these measures will depend on the type and frequency of the seizure. Children who are subject to daily seizures should not be permitted to engage in activities in which they might be injured, such as climbing. If necessary, additional protection can be provided by lightweight bicycle helmets. These children should have siderails on beds with the hard surfaces padded if there is danger that they could hurt themselves.

Children who have infrequent seizures or who are relatively free of seizures will have few restrictions on their activities.

✦ **NURSING ALERT** When a child is hospitalized, appropriate precautions should be implemented, such as siderails kept up when the child is sleeping or resting, especially if the seizures are of the grand mal variety, since many of these children are subject to nocturnal attacks.

However, some precautions are implemented, for example, the bed should be protected with a waterproof mattress or sheeting.

Long-term care. Care of the child with a recurrent convulsive disorder involves the physical care and instruction regarding the importance of the drug therapy and, probably more significant, the problems related to the emotional aspects of the disorder. There are few diseases that generate as much anxiety among relatives as epilepsy. Fears and misconceptions about the disease and its treatment abound in the layperson's mind. For many it represents the archetype of severe hereditary affliction. Therefore the foci of nursing care are directed toward helping the child and the family to deal with the psychologic and sociologic problems related to the disorder and to educate the child, the family, peers, and the public toward a more realistic and liberal view of the disease.

Physical aspects. Children subject to seizures are prescribed some type of drug therapy. The nurse can help the parents plan the administration of the medication at convenient times in order to disrupt the family routine as little as possible. Once a sufficient blood level of the drug has been achieved, the daily dosage can be given at less frequent intervals to reduce the interruptions in the parents' and the child's daily activities. This also increases the likelihood of compliance. The most convenient times for administration seem to be with meals or at bedtime. Although the anticonvulsant drugs are available in liquid extracts or emulsions, the tablet form is preferred by neurologists. The unequal distribution of the drug in the solute and the increased likelihood of inaccurate measurements make liquid medication less desirable. For small children the tablet of the proper dosage can be crushed and administered in syrup, jelly, or other palatable substances. Children taking phenobarbital and/or phenytoin should receive adequate vitamin D and folic acid, since deficiencies have been associated with these drugs. Phenytoin should not be taken with milk.

It is important to impress on the family the necessity of continuing the medication regularly without interruption for as long as required. This is usually 2 to 3 years after the last seizure, at which point the drug is discontinued slowly over a period of weeks to avoid the possibility of precipitating a seizure. Planning ahead to replace a nearly empty bottle will prevent the risk of running out of the medication. It is sometimes easy to skip doses or omit them for any of a variety of reasons, especially when the child is free of seizures most of the time. This is particularly so when the child is older and assumes the responsibility for the medication. Parents should notify the health professional if the child has an illness, including vomiting or fever. Vomiting can interfere with drug absorption; fever may increase metabolic requirements. Both can precipitate seizure activity.

Rectal preparations of some anticonvulsant medications are highly useful and effective when a child is unable to take oral medications because of repeated vomiting, gastrointestinal surgery, or status epilepticus. Administration of rectal anticonvulsants can be learned by parents for home treatment during a seizure.* Rectal diazepam is useful adjunctive home treatment for children at risk for prolonged seizures. Hospitalization is minimized and parental confidence enhanced (Camfield and others, 1989).

Nurses need to educate the child and parents of the possible adverse reactions to the medications used to treat seizure disorders in children. They should understand the common side effects so that they can report any unusual observations that might indicate unfavorable reactions. These should be known in detail. Parents should understand that the child needs periodic physical assessment and laboratory studies if the child is taking phenytoin, prim-

*Home care instructions for administration of medications are available in Wong, D.L., and Whaley, L.F.: Clinical manual of pediatric nursing, ed. 3, St. Louis, 1990, Mosby–Year Book, Inc.

idone, ethosuximide, or methsuximide. Possible adverse effects on the hematopoietic system, liver, and kidneys may be reflected in symptoms such as fever, sore throat, enlarged lymph nodes, jaundice, and bleeding manifestations (e.g., easy bruising, petechiae, ecchymoses, epistaxis). A common factor in status epilepticus is indequate blood levels of anticonvulsants.

Parents need to be warned of possible behavioral changes as the convulsions are controlled in children taking primidone, phenobarbital, or phenytoin. Changes in personality, indifference to school activities and family, hyperactivity, or even psychotic behavior may sometimes be observed. The potential effects of anticonvulsants on learning and behavior should be considered. Progressive intellectual deterioration in a child with epilepsy requires investigation of present medication plus the role of the underlying cerebral pathology.

The degree to which activities are restricted is individualized for each child and depends on the type, frequency, and severity of the seizures; the child's response to therapy; and the length of time the seizures have been controlled. Normal healthy activities are encouraged for children, and participation in competitive sports is determined on an individual basis. With encouragement most older children can accept the restrictions placed on activities. Climbing trees or structures from which the child might fall and be seriously injured is not usually permitted. The well-controlled child can ride a bicycle or swim if accompanied by a companion. Few other restrictions should be placed on children regarding sports and peer activity to reduce the likelihood of needlessly accentuating differences.

Because the child is encouraged to attend school, camp, and other normal activities, the school nurse and the teacher should be made aware of the child's condition and the therapy. They can help to ensure regularity of medication and any special care the child might need. The child's teacher should be instructed regarding care of the child during a seizure so that he or she can act in a calm manner to ensure the child's welfare and to influence the attitude of the child's classmates.

Parents of the child with epilepsy. Parental attitudes and management of a child with a convulsive disorder are as varied as those of other parents of children with a chronic disorder, and they are subject to the same long-term problems (see Chapter 22). Whether the seizures result from illness, injury, or unknown etiology, the parents may feel guilt, anxiety, and often humiliation. In the past, epilepsy has had a derogatory connotation. The parents want to know if it will affect the child's mental capacities. Many persons erroneously associate epilepsy with mental deficiency. Seizures do frequently accompany other manifestations of severe brain damage from disease or injury, but most children with seizures, as in any population of healthy children, display a wide range of intelligence.

Parents also wonder how the illness will affect the child's future and need reassurance that the illness will not shorten the life of the child and that the child can attend school, marry, and elect to have children. The child will need vocational guidance, and the parents will need to become familiar with the laws in their state regarding any limitations that might be imposed on the child because of the disorder. It should be emphasized that the seizures can be controlled or greatly reduced in the large majority of affected children and that new studies hold the promise of progress in future treatment. Parents need reassurance that in this enlightened day and age there is less stigma attached to the disease than in the past.

It is important to encourage a healthy attitude toward the child and the disease and to help the parents feel competent in their ability to meet their responsibilities to the child. The child should be reared as any normal child, with natural concern tempered by the understanding of the need not to be overprotected. Many parents refrain from correcting or punishing the child, especially if they have had the experience of such an emotional stress precipitating an attack. The child must not be made to feel different in any way. Parents should be encouraged to be honest and open about the disorder with the child and to others. Some parents are tempted to try to conceal the nature of the child's illness because of their belief that the disorder is shameful or a disgrace to the family.

Restrictions on the child's activities will be necessary for safety, but this area can be approached in a positive way in terms of what the child *can* do rather than what cannot be done. Sometimes parents curtail the child's activities more than necessary. Educational materials and support groups may prove beneficial for families. The child needs to experience the maturing influences of play and work. The **Epilepsy Foundation of America*** is a national organization that works toward and for the welfare of persons with epi-

EMERGENCY TREATMENT
Seizure

Do not attempt to restrain child or use force.
Protect child during seizure.
If child is standing or sitting in wheelchair at beginning of attack, ease child down so that he or she will not fall; when possible, place cushion or blanket under child.
Do not put anything in child's mouth.
Loosen restrictive clothing.
Prevent child from hitting hard or sharp objects that might cause injury during uncontrolled movements.
Remove object(s).
Pad object(s).
Move furniture out of way.
Allow seizure to end without interference.
When seizure has stopped, check for breathing.
If not present, open airway and use mouth-to-mouth resuscitation.
Check around mouth for evidence of burns or suspicious substances that might indicate poisoning.
Remain with child.
When child is able to move, seek help.

EMERGENCY TREATMENT

*4351 Garden City Dr., Landover, MD 20785; (301) 459-3700. In Canada: **Epilepsy Canada,** 2099 Alexandre De Seve, Bureau 27, Montreal, Quebec H2L 4R8.

lepsy and their families, helps with employment and legal problems, and provides education to patients, families, and communities.

The child with epilepsy. The child who is provided the security of a loving family, rewards and punishments no different from those of other children, and support in acquiring self-esteem is more apt to have a positive attitude toward the disease. Development of normal emotional maturity is inhibited by parental overprotection, indulgence, and restrictions. Maladaptation and a negative self-image are stimulated by peer and family rejection, embarrassment and humiliation, teasing by playmates, and social segregation.

Children derive their self-concept and self-esteem from the observations of others' reactions to them and their own perception of their capabilities. When others consider children to be different, inferior, or an object of ridicule, they come to view themselves as different, inferior, and incapable. They may become frustrated because their activities are limited or because they are excluded from activities in which they feel capable of participating but are segregated from by others, including their family. Such children are encouraged in dependency.

Behavioral problems are common in children with epilepsy and can become a more serious problem than the seizures. Much of the behavioral difficulty, especially aggressive or delinquent behavior, has been attributed to a child's reaction to parental rejection. Feelings of guilt, frustration, depression, and self-negation can contribute to antisocial behavior.

The suddenness and unpredictability of the attacks and the reactions of others further influence children's feelings. They need to learn about the disease and the role that medication plays in contributing to their prolonged well-being. As soon as they are old enough, children should assume responsibility for taking their own medication. They should be advised to carry a card or a Medic-Alert bracelet with pertinent information about the condition. Planning activities with children and emphasizing those in which they can engage rather than those in which they cannot participate help children to succeed and to gain satisfaction in their achievements. Children should be offered opportunities and encouraged to exercise judgment in their daily lives.

The adolescent period may prove to be a difficult time for children with epilepsy. The normal changes and emotional responses may be confused with symptoms of the disease. Normal rebellious attitudes and behavior may cause more insecure adolescents, angry at being different, to stop taking medication. Sudden withdrawal of the drug together with the accelerated metabolic needs and the increased stress of this period of life will often cause a resumption of, or an increase in, seizures. Normally adolescents with a convulsive disorder will need their dosage increased to meet the new growth needs. Limits imposed on activities at a time when young persons desire freedom and independence may bring the disability into sharp focus. For example, some states do not allow persons with epilepsy to obtain a driver's license, even when the disease is controlled; in others there are restrictions on employment, insurance, and, in a few isolated instances, a marriage license.

Epilepsy should not be a severe disability to most youngsters. The nurse, by assuming the role of patient advocate, helping to educate the public regarding the disease, working toward making opportunities available to persons with the disorder, and lobbying for legislation that recognizes the needs of the individual with a seizure disorder, can help to erase the stigma that still remains regarding the disease.

Evaluation

The effectiveness of nursing interventions for the child with epilepsy is determined by continual reassessment and evaluation of care based on the following observational guidelines and expected outcomes:

1. Observe the child's behavior for evidence of seizure activity and assess the environment for situations that could cause injury to the child in the event of a seizure; interview the family regarding managment of the child during a seizure.
2. Interview the child and family regarding compliance with the medication regimen.
3. Observe and interview the famly regarding their feelings and concerns and their understanding of the child's disease.
4. Observe the child's interactions with others and interview the child about any feelings or concerns about the disease.

Expected outcomes:
See Nursing Care Plan, p. 1769.

FEBRILE SEIZURES

Febrile convulsions are transient disorders of children that occur in association with a fever. They are one of the most common neurologic disorders of childhood, affecting 3% to 5% of children. Most febrile convulsions occur after 6 months of age and usually before age 3 years, with increased frequency in children younger than 18 months. They are unusual after 5 years of age. Boys are affected about twice as often as girls, and there appears to be an increased susceptibility in families, indicating a possible genetic predisposition.

The cause of febrile seizures is still uncertain. They are associated with disease outside the CNS and are usually generalized, brief, and self-limited. A history and physical assessment usually rule out CNS disease. In most children the height and rapidity of the temperature elevation seem to be factors. The fever usually exceeds 38.8° C (101.8° F) and occurs during the temperature rise rather than after a prolonged elevation. Sometimes it constitutes the dramatic beginning of an illness. Febrile seizures usually accompany an upper respiratory or gastrointestinal infection, and 25% of children with simple febrile seizures have a recurrence of the seizure with subsequent infections. Since fevers are almost impossible to prevent in children, efforts are directed toward preventing an increase in the temperature.

Treatment consists of controlling the seizure with phenobarbital or diazepam (Valium) in appropriate dosage and reducing the temperature by administration of acetaminophen (Tylenol). Whether or not to implement continuous prophylactic anticonvulsant therapy in children who have experienced their initial febrile convulsion is still controversial. At present, anticonvulsant therapy is recommended for those children with febrile seizures who are at increased risk for developing sequelae. Little risk of neurologic deficit, mental retardation, or altered behavior has been observed as sequelae of febrile seizures.

Febrile seizures are divided into two categories: simple and complex. Simple febrile seizures are brief, last from 10 to 15 minutes, and are generalized. Complex febrile seizures are prolonged and may have focal features. The chance of developing chronic seizure disorder is increased in children who have a prolonged convulsion, those with focal seizures, those who have a near relative who experiences convulsions, and those with an abnormal EEG. Recurrences are more likely when the first seizure occurs in the first year of life. Seventy-five percent of recurrences take place within 1 year of the first febrile seizure and almost 90% within 2 years of onset.

BREATH-HOLDING SPELLS

Breath-holding spells (reflex hypoxic crisis) are readily recognized and follow a distinct clinical pattern. Not a true convulsive disorder, the typical attack has its onset in infants between the ages of 6 and 18 months and may occur up to 4 years of age. The episode is characterized by violent crying and cessation of breathing that is precipitated by fright, frustration, or anger. The breath is usually held on expiration, and the child becomes cyanotic, loses consciousness, and may display a few clonic convulsions of the extremities. The episode ends with a gasp and the color returns promptly. The frequency of attacks varies considerably, but they almost always disappear by 5 to 6 years of age.

Breath-holding spells are a benign entity, and drug therapy is generally not indicated. Family therapy may be beneficial, since many children appear to use an attack or the threat of an attack to assert themselves and to express anger. Parents need reassurance that the attacks do not represent a danger to the child, and this knowledge may even help to decrease or eliminate the incidence of attacks.

HEADACHE

Headaches are one of the most frequent neurologic complaints of children. Headaches can be caused by extracranial disease, intracranial disease, vascular disease, or psychologic problems (Table 37-10).

Assessment

It is important to determine the pattern of the headache—single acute episode, paroxysmal, recurrent and acute, chronic and progressive, or chronic and nonprogressive. Other assessment information includes whether or not the headache is associated with seizures, ataxia, lethargy, weakness, unexplained nausea or vomiting, or any personality changes. Factors that might be pertinent to the headache are related to early development and past illnesses.

Table 37-10 Headache syndromes in children

TYPE OF HEADACHE	CHARACTERISTICS
▪ Acute extracranial	
Sinusitis	Frontal sinus most frequently involved
Ocular abnormalities	Usually frontal and precipitated by television viewing or schoolwork
Dental disorders	Frontal or temporal headaches caused by malocclusion, caries, abscess, temporomandibular joint dysfunction
Respiratory infections (pharyngitis, otitis media)	Pain localized to affected structures
Trauma	Localized to area of trauma; related to nerve and tissue injury Postconcussion syndrome (see Posttraumatic Syndromes, p. 1745)
▪ Acute recurrent	
Vascular: migraine syndrome	Intermittent attacks of vasoconstriction Paroxysmal Positive family history Triggered by stress, fatigue, trauma, exercise, illness, diet, menses, medication
▪ Chronic progressive	
Intracranial abnormalities	Symptoms of increased ICP
Tumors	Frontal: supratentorial tumors Occipital: infratentorial tumors
Hydrocephalus	Rapid head enlargement, suture splitting (infants, young children)
Subdural hematoma	Usually results from trauma Seizures and focal neurologic deficits more common than headaches
Brain abscess	More often associated with ear infections and cyanotic heart disease
Pseudotumor cerebri	Increased ICP without obstruction of CSF
▪ Chronic nonprogressive (psychogenic)	Common in children Adjustment reaction, anxiety Sign of depression Conversion hysteria (anxiety converted to somatic symptoms)

Family history may provide clues to the etiologic factor, including those related to the home or social situation (e.g., alcoholism, divorce, separation). Specific questions to ask in order to elicit needed information are listed in Box 37-11.

Box 37-11 QUESTIONS FOR EVALUATING HEADACHE

How did the headache begin?
How long has it been present?
Are the symptoms progressive or static?
How frequently does it occur?
How long does it last?
Does it occur at any special time or under any special circumstances?
Are there warning symptoms?
Where does it hurt?
What is the quality of the pain?
Are there associated symptoms (nausea, vomiting, photophobia)?
Does it require cessation of activity?
Does anything make it go away?
Does anyone else in the family have headaches?

Modified from Rothner, A.D.: Headache. In Swaiman, K.F.: Pediatric neurology: principles and practice, St. Louis, 1989, Mosby–Year Book, Inc.

Thorough physical and neurologic examinations are carried out, and special diagnostic tests (e.g., radiographs, EEG, CT, MRI) may be indicated.

Migraine Headache

Migraine is the most common paroxysmal disorder that affects the brain and is particularly prevalent among teenagers. It is characterized by chronic recurrent headache, often preceded by visual disturbances and accompanied by nausea and vomiting. The cause is unknown, although attacks may be precipitated by stress, fatigue, stroboscopic stimulation, anxiety, conflict, or certain foods. Emotional factors may play a part.

There are two phases in the pathologic development of migraine, both caused by a functional disturbance of intracerebral circulation. Initially there is a prodromal phase caused by vasoconstriction of intracranial vessels followed by dilatation of the extracranial vessels, which produces a throbbing, pulsating, and pounding headache. Characteristics of several patterns of migraine headache are described in Box 37-12.

A family history of migraine is elicited in over 50% of patients, and some observers have noted that children often display a characteristic personality. They tend to be meticulous, compulsive, unusually mature for their age, and high achievers in school and strive to please the family at home. They have difficulty in expressing anger or rage. Boys are affected twice as often as girls.

The diagnosis is seldom made until the child is old enough to relate the symptoms, although one in five children has a first attack before age 5 years. Early in life the symptoms are nonspecific, such as recurrent abdominal pain, car sickness, and restlessness, and the child may display head banging or sudden alterations in personality. The typical attack of migraine begins early in the day, often awakening the child. The prodromal symptoms, induced by vasoconstriction, consist of transient visual disturbances or other neurologic disabilities. In a few minutes or sometimes a few hours, the aura is followed by throbbing unilateral head pain accompanied by nausea and vomiting. Sleep ordinarily terminates an attack.

Box 37-12 MIGRAINE PATTERNS

Classic Migraine
Vasoconstriction (prodromal) phase:
- Visual symptoms—blindness, blurring, visual field cuts, scotoma, micropsia or macropsia
- May include (less frequently) weakness, inability to speak, sensory abnormalities

Dilatation phase:
- Throbbing, unilateral or frontal pain
- Onset of pain followed by vomiting and abdominal pain, photophobia, phonophobia, desire to sleep
- On awakening, child usually well

Common Migraine
More variable symptoms than classic migraine; aura less pronounced
Prodromal: malaise, personality change, or depression
Headache, nausea, vomiting
Course similar to classic migraine

Cluster Headaches
Unilateral, orbital pain; tearing; rhinorrhea; nasal stuffiness
Pain severe and recurrent for weeks at a time
Rare in childhood

Ophthalmoplegic Migraine
Eye pain
Complete or incomplete CN III palsies
Unilateral pupillary dilatation, ptosis, outward deviation of eyes

Hemiplegic Migraine
Associated with recurrent paralysis
Hemiplegia may precede or follow headache
May be familial

Basilar Migraine
Recurrent attacks
Symptoms and signs referable to brainstem and cerebellum
- Paroxysmal acute ataxia, alternating weakness, vertigo, (occasionally) loss of consciousness

More common in girls

Paroxysmal Vertigo
Episodes of vertigo in very young child (ages 2 to 4 years)
Retained consciousness, inability to maintain posture, nystagmus
Headaches may or may not be present
May be related to basilar migraine

Confusional State
Disturbed sensorium, retained consciousness, agitation
Paroxysmal occurrence
Headaches may or may not be present

Cyclic Vomiting
Unexplained recurrent episodes of vomiting
Abdominal pain usually present
Headache absent

Epilepsy Equivalent Syndrome
Episodes of paroxysmal headache, nausea, vomiting
May be interpreted as seizures in some children

Although serious intracranial disease needs to be ruled out, in most cases *chronic recurrent headache of childhood* represents migraine. The difference between migraine and seizures in children must be determined. The diagnosis can be confusing and frustrating for families. Migraine headaches may be confused with other types of headache (e.g., those caused by tension or organic disorders), but several features often set them apart, including a family history for migraine and nausea and vomiting.

Treatment is symptomatic. For most patients the vasoconstrictor ergotamine tartrate taken at the onset of symptoms provides relief. Simple analgesics such as acetaminophen may be effective and are usually the preferred medication. Other modalities, such as biofeedback, diet, and stress management techniques, may help. Stress management includes a headache diary, progressive relaxation, cognitive restructuring, distraction or attention focusing, mental activities, thought stopping, imaging, behavior rehearsal, assertiveness, and problem solving (Lascelles and others, 1989). (For a description of many of these techniques, see Nonpharmacologic Pain Management, Box 26-6.)

The outlook for the child with migraine is good, but the child and parents should be informed that predisposition to the headaches is lifelong, although benign, and should not interfere with normal activities. Historically, children improve over time regardless of treatment (Hanson, 1988.)

KEY POINTS

- The central nervous system (CNS) is composed of the brain and spinal cord. Brain, blood, and cerebrospinal fluid (CSF) maintain an equilibrium inside the skull; and disturbance of these components creates disequilibrium.
- Gait abnormalities that may indicate cerebral dysfunction include a change in ambulatory function such as ataxia, spastic paraplegic gait, hemiplegic gait, cerebellar gait, and extrapyramidal gait.
- Level of consciousness (LOC) is the most important indicator of neurologic health; altered levels include sleep, confusion, delirium, pseudowakeful states, and comatose states.
- Complete neurologic examination includes LOC; posture; motor, sensory, cranial nerve (CN), and reflex testing; and vital signs.
- Nursing care of the unconscious child focuses on respiratory management, neurologic assessment, increased intracranial pressure (ICP) monitoring, supplying adequate nutrition and hydration, drug therapy, promoting elimination, hygienic care, positioning and exercise, stimulation, and family support.
- Primary head injury involves features that occur at the time of trauma, including fractured skull, contusions, intracranial hematoma, and diffuse injury. Secondary complications include hypoxic brain damage, increased ICP, infection, cerebral edema, and posttraumatic syndromes.
- The young child's response to head injury is different because of the following features: larger head size, expandable skull, larger amount of blood volume to the brain, small subdural spaces, and thinner, softer brain tissue.
- Fractures resulting from head injuries may be classified as linear, depressed, compound, basilar, and diastatic.
- Problems resulting from near-drowning include hypoxia and asphyxiation, aspiration, and hypothermia.
- Nursing care of the child with meningitis includes administration of antibiotics, prevention of self-infection, removal of environmental stimuli, correct positioning, vital signs monitoring, intravenous therapy, and promoting fluid, nutritional status, and supportive care of the family.
- Encephalitis may result from direct invasion of the CNS by a virus or from postinfectious involvement of the CNS after viral disease.
- A seizure is a symptom of underlying pathology and is manifest by sensory-hallucinatory phenomena, motor effects, sensorimotor effects, and loss of consciousness.
- Partial seizures are categorized as simple, with associated impairment of consciousness and as those with impaired consciousness that spread to become generalized.
- Generalized seizures are categorized as tonic-clonic, absence, atonic and akinetic, myoclonic, and infantile spasms.
- Long-term care of the child with recurrent convulsive disorders includes physical care and education regarding the importance of drug therapy and problems related to emotional aspects of the disorder.

REFERENCES

AIDS and human immunodeficiency virus infection in the United States, 1988 update, MMWR 38:S-4, 1989.

Alexander, R.C., and others: Magnetic resonance imaging of intracranial injuries in child abuse, J. Pediatr. 109:975-979, 1986.

American Academy of Pediatrics, Committee on Drugs: Behavioral and cognitive effects of anticonvulsant therapy, Pediatrics 76:644-647, 1985.

American Academy of Pediatrics, Committee on Infectious Diseases: Aspirin and Reye syndrome, Pediatrics 69:810-812, 1982.

American Academy of Pediatrics: Report of the committee on infectious diseases, Elk Grove, IL, 1988, The Academy.

Arrowsmith, J.B., and others: National patterns of aspirin use and Reye syndrome reporting, United States, 1980 to 1985, Pediatrics 79:858-863, 1987.

Bateman, P.A., and Heagarty, M.C.: Passive freebase cocaine inhalation by infants and toddlers, Am. J. Dis. Child. 143:25-27, 1989.

Boll, T.: Minor head injury in children, out of sight but not out of mind, J. Clin. Child Psychol. 12:74-80, 1985.

Bruce, D., and Schut, L.: Concussion and contusion following pediatric head trauma. In McLaurin, R., editor: Pediatric neurosurgery, Philadelphia, 1989, W.B. Saunders Co.

Camfield, C.S., and others: Home use of rectal diazepam to prevent status epilepticus in children with convulsive disorders, J. Child Neurol. 4:125-126, 1989.

Deaths from falls, 1978-1984, MMWR 137 (suppl. 1): 21-26, 1988.

Eiben, C.F., and others: Functional outcome of closed head injury in children and young adults, Arch. Phys. Med. Rehabil. 65:168-170, 1984.

Eisenberg, H., and Briner, A.: Late complication of head injury. In McLaurin, R., editor: Pediatric neurosurgery, Philadelphia, 1989, W.B. Saunders Co.
Engel, J.: Seizures and epilepsy, Philadelphia, 1989, F.A. Davis Co.
Ernst, A.A., and Sanders, W.M.: Unexpected cocaine intoxication presenting as seizures in children, Ann. Emerg. Med. 18:747-749, 1989.
Feigin, R.D., and Neglia, J.P.: Bacterial meningitis and septicemia beyond the neonatal period. In Gellis, S.S., and Kagan, B.M.: Current pediatric therapy 12, Philadelphia, 1986, W.B. Saunders Co.
Griest, K.J., and Zumwalt, R.E.: Child abuse by drowning, Pediatrics 83:41-46, 1989.
Hadley, M.N., and others: The infant whiplash-shake injury syndrome, Neurosurgery 24:536-540, 1989.
Hahn, Y., and others: Factors influencing post-traumatic seizures in children, Neurosurgery 22:864-867, 1988.
Hanson, R.R.: Headache in children, Semin. Neurol. 8:51-60, 1988.
Head Injury Foundation, Personal communication, 1989.
Hill, J.C.: Summary of a workshop on *Haemophilus influenzae* type B vaccines, J. Infect. Dis. 148:167-175, 1983.
Hrachovy, R.A., and Frost, J.D., Jr.: Infantile spasms, Pediatr. Clin. North Am. 36:311-329, 1989.
Hurwitz, E.S.: The changing epidemiology of Reye's syndrome, JAMA 260:3178-3180, 1988.
Jacobson, M.S., and others: Follow-up of adolescent trauma victims: a new model of care, Pediatrics 77:236-241, 1986.
Johnson, D.: Head injury. In Eichelberger, M., and Paatsch, G., editors: Pediatric trauma care, Rockville, MD, 1988, Aspen Publishers, Inc.
Kohl, S.: Herpes simplex virus encephalitis in children, Pediatr. Clin. North Am. 35:465-483, 1988.
Krugman, S., and others: Infectious diseases of children, ed. 8, St. Louis, 1985, Mosby–Year Book, Inc.
Lascelles, M.A., and others: Teaching coping strategies to adolescents with migraine, J. Pain Symptom Manag. 4:135-144, 1989.
Mealey, J.: Skull fractures. In Eichelberger, M., and Paatsch, G., editors: Pediatric trauma care, Rockville, MD, 1988, Aspen Publishers, Inc.
Orlowski, J.P.: Drowning, near-drowning, and ice-water submersions, Pediatr. Clin. North Am. 34:75-92, 1987.
Plum, F., and Posner, J.: Diagnosis of stupor and coma, Philadelphia, 1980, F.A. Davis Co.
Quan, L., and others: Ten year study of pediatric drownings and near drownings, Pediatrics 83:1035-1040, 1989.
Rabies surveillance, U.S., 1988, MMWR 38:1-19, 1989.
Restak, R.M.: The brain, New York, 1984, Bantam Books.
Reye's syndrome, MMWR 38:325-327, 1989.
Robinson, M.D., and Seward, P.N.: Submersion injury in children, Pediatr. Emerg. Care 3:44-49, 1987.
Strauss, R.H.: Brain abscess. In Gellis, S.S., and Kagan, B.M.: Current pediatric therapy 12, Philadelphia, 1986, W.B. Saunders Co.
Swaiman, K.F.: Pediatric neurology, St. Louis, 1989, Mosby–Year Book, Inc.
Szap, M.D., Schwartz, A, and Schwartz, M.: Hidden salicylates (letter), Am. J. Dis. Child. 143:142, 1989.
Taylor, M.J., and Farrell, E.J.: Comparison of the prognostic utility of VEP's and SEP's in comatose children, Pediatr. Neurol. 5:145-150, 1989.
Tron, V.A., Baldwin, V.J., and Price, G.E.: Hot tub drownings, Pediatrics 75:789-790, 1985.
Vries, J., and others: Epilepsy surgery in childhood. In McLaurin, R., editor: Pediatric neurosurgery, Philadelphia, 1989, W.B. Saunders Co.
Wilson, M.H.: Immunization. In Aski, F.A., and others, editors: Principles and practice of pediatrics, J.B. Lippencott Co.
Wong, D.: Changing what children hear in the ICU can lower intracranial pressure, Am. J. Nurs. 88:279-280, 1988.

BIBLIOGRAPHY

General

Davies, C.: Neurologic outcome following pediatric resuscitation, J. Neurosci. Nurs. 19:205-210, 1987.
Hazinski, M.F.: Nursing care of the critically ill child, St. Louis, 1984, Mosby–Year Book, Inc.
James, H.E.: Neurologic evaluation and support in the child with an acute brain insult, Pediatr. Ann. 15:16-22, 1986.
Joy, C.: Pediatric trauma nursing, Rockville, MD, 1989, Aspen Publishers, Inc.
Kelly, S.: Pediatric emergency nursing, Norwalk, CN, 1988, Appleton & Lange.
McKellar, A.: Head injuries in children and implication for their prevention, J. Pediatr. Surg. 24:577-579, 1989.
Molmar, G.E., and others: Pediatric rehabilitation: brain damage causing disability, Arch. Phys. Med. Rehabil. 70:166-169, 1989.
Rimar, J.M.: Pancuronium bromide, MCN 10:65, 1985.
Volpe, J.J.: Neurology (editorial overview), Curr. Opin. Pediatr. 1:253-256, 1989.

Neurologic Assessment

Engler, M.B., and Engler, M.M.: The hazards of magnetic resonance imaging, Am. J. Nurs. 86:650, 1986.
Esposito, N., and Westgate, P.: Continuous EEG monitoring in the PICU, J. Pediatr. Nurs. 2:272-277, 1987.
Fisher, J.: What you need to know about neurological testing, RN 50(1):47-53, 1987.
Hanigan, W.C., Wright, S.M., and Wright, R.M.: Clinical utility of magnetic resonance imaging in pediatric neurosurgical patients, J. Pediatr. 108:522-529, 1986.
Hellier, A., Ptak, H., and Cerrito, M.: CATS inside my brain: children's understanding of the cerebral computed tomography scan procedure, Child. Health Care 14:211-217, 1986.
Hershey, B.L., and Zimmerman, R.A.: Pediatric brain computed tomography, Pediatr. Clin. North Am. 32:1477-1508, 1985.
Kryba, F.N., Ogburn-Russell, L., and Rutledge, J.N.: Magnetic resonance imaging: the latest in diagnostic technology, Nursing '87 17(1):45-47, 1987.
Levin, H.S., and others: Magnetic resonance imaging after closed head injury in children, Neurosurgery 24:223-227, 1989.
Mills, G.C.: Preparing children and parents for cerebral computed tomography, MCN 5:403-407, 1980.
Mizrahi, E.M., and Kellaway, P.: Cerebral concussion in children: assessment of injury by electroencephalography, Pediatrics 73:419-425, 1984.
Moore, P.C.: When you have to think small for a neurological exam, RN 51(6):38-44, 1988.
Oliphant, M., and Berne, A.S.: An integrated look at pediatric imaging, Contemp. Pediatr. 7(1):61-78, 1990.
Reilly, P.L., and others: Assessing the conscious level in infants and young children, Childs Nerv. Syst. 4:31-33, 1988.
Scherer, P.: Assessment: the logic of coma, Am. J. Nurs. 86:541-550, 1986.
Stolarik, A.: What the comatose patient can tell you, RN 48(4):26-33, 1985.
Zegeer, L.: Oculocephalic and vestibulo-ocular responses: significance for nursing care, J. Neurosci. Nurs. 21:46-55, 1989.

Increased Intracranial Pressure

American Academy of Pediatrics, Committee on Drugs, Section on Anesthesiology: Guidelines for the elective use of conscious sedation, deep sedation, and general anesthesia in pediatric patients, Pediatrics 77:754, 1986.
Boortz-Marx, R.: Factors affecting intracranial pressure: a descriptive study, J. Neurosurg. Nurs. 17:89-94, 1985.

Hinkle, J.L.: Treating traumatic coma, Am. J. Nurs. 86:551-556, 1986.

Jess, L.W.: Assessing your patient for increased ICP, Nursing '87 17(6):34-41, 1987.

Rebaud, P., and others: Intracranial pressure in childhood CNS infections, Intensive Care Med. 14:522-555, 1988.

Robinet, K.: Increased intracranial pressure: management with an intraventricular catheter, J. Neurosurg. Nurs. 17:95-104, 1985.

Brain Death

Elliott, J., and Smith, D.R.: Meeting family needs following severe head injury: a multidisciplinary approach, J. Neurosurg. Nurs. 17:111-113, 1985.

Fackler, J.C., Troncoso, J.C., and Gioia, F.R.: Age-specific characteristics of brain death in children, Am. J. Dis. Child. 142:999-1003, 1988.

Freeman, J.M., and Ferry, P.C.: New brain death guidelines in children: further confusion (editorial), Pediatrics 81:301-303, 1988.

Murphy, P.: When a non-death death occurs, Nursing '86 16(7):34-39, 1986.

Myer, E.C.: Determination of brain death in infants and children, Curr. Opin. Pediatr. 1:315-317, 1989.

Report of Special Task Force: Guidelines for the determination of brain death in children, Pediatrics 80:298-300, 1987.

Rowland, T.W., Donnelly, J.H., and Jackson, A.H.: Apnea documentation for determination of brain death in children, Pediatrics 74:505-508, 1984.

Head Injury

Alberico, A.M., and others: Outcome after severe head injury, J. Neurosurg. 67:648-656, 1987.

Bagnato, S.J., and Feldman, H.: Closed head injury in infants and preschool children: research and practice issues, Inf. Young Child. 2(1):1-13, 1989.

Billmire, M.E., and Myers, P.A.: Serious head injury in infants: accident or abuse? Pediatrics 75:340-342, 1985.

Casey, R., Ludwig, S., and McCormick, M.C.: Minor head trauma in children: an intervention to decrease functional morbidity, Pediatrics 80:159-164, 1987.

Derechin, M.E.: Pediatric head injury, Crit. Care Nurs. Q. 10(3):12-24, 1987.

Gordon, V.L.: Recovery from a head injury: a family process, Pediatr. Nurs. 15:131-133, 1989.

Hennes, H., and others: Clinical predictors of severe head trauma in children, Am. J. Dis. Child. 142:1045-1047, 1988.

Hobdell, E.F., and others: The effect of nursing activities on the intracranial pressure of children, Crit. Care Nurse 9(6):75-79, 1989.

Hochstetler, K., and Beals, R.D.: Transient cortical blindness in a child, Ann. Emerg. Med. 16:218-219, 1987.

Kraus, J.F., Fife, D., and Conroy, C.: Pediatric brain injuries: the nature, clinical course, and early outcomes in a defined United States' population, Pediatrics 79:501-507, 1987.

Martin, K.M.: Predicting short-term outcome in comatose head-injured children, J. Neurosci. Nurs. 19:9-13, 1987.

Nikas, D.L: Critical aspects of head trauma, Crit. Care Nurs. Q. 10(1):19-43, 1987.

Reilly, A.N.: Head trauma in children: the stages to cognitive recovery, MCN 12:405-412, 1987.

Rosenthal, B.W., and Bergman, I.: Intracranial injury after moderate head trauma in children, J. Pediatr. 115:346-350, 1989.

Rosman, N.P.: Pediatric emergencies: managing acute head trauma, Contemp. Pediatr. 3(11):24-46, 1986.

Sherman, D.W.: Managing acute head injury, Nursing '90 20(4):47-51, 1990.

Worthington, J.: The impact of adolescent development on recovery from traumatic brain injury, Rehabil. Nurs. 14:118-122, 1989.

Near-Drowning

Brill, J.E.: Dispelling the myth of the "drownproof" child, Contemp. Pediatr. 4(6):30-43, 1987.

Brooks, J.G.: Near drowning, Pediatr. Rev. 10:5-10, 1988.

Butler, S.: Out of the water, but not out of the woods, RN 51(6):26-29, 1988.

Frank, B.S.: Hypokalemia following fresh-water submersion injuries, Pediatr. Emerg. Care 3:158-159, 1987.

Hartsell, M.B.: New technology for safety and research, J. Pediatr. Nurs. 2:212-213, 1987.

Orlowski, J.P.: Drowning, near-drowning, and ice-water drowning, JAMA 260:390-391, 1988.

Robinson, M.D., and Seward, P.N.: Submersion injury in children, Pediatr. Emerg. Care 3:44-49, 1987.

Rogers, M.C.: Near-drowning: cold water or a hot topic? J. Pediatr. 106:603-604, 1985.

Shinaberger, C.S., and others: Young children who drown in hot tubs, spas, and whirlpools in California: a 26 year survey, Am. J. Public Health 80:613-614, 1990.

Shovein, J., and others: Near drowning, Am. J. Nurs. 89:680-686, 1989.

Wintemute, G.J., and Wright, M.A.: Swimming pool owners' opinions of strategies for prevention of drowning, Pediatrics 85:63-69, 1990.

Wintemute, G.J., and others: Drowning in childhood and adolescence: a population based study, Am. J. Public Health 77:830-832, 1987.

Intracranial Infections

American Academy of Pediatrics, Committee on Infectious Diseases: Treatment of bacterial meningitis, Pediatrics 81:904-907, 1988.

Baer, G.M., and Fishbein, D.B.: Rabies post-exposure prophylaxis, New Engl. J. Med. 316:1270-1271, 1987.

Bonadio, W.A., Mannenbach, M., and Krippendorf, R.: Bacterial meningitis in older children, Am. J. Dis. Child. 144:463-465, 1990.

Coderre, C.: Meningitis: danger when the diagnosis is viral, RN 52(8):50-54, 1989.

Dagbjartsson, A., and Ludvigsso, P.: Bacterial meningitis: diagnosis and initial antibiotic therapy, Pediatr. Clin. North Am. 34:219-230, 1987.

Edwards, M.S., and others: Long-term sequelae of group B streptococcal meningitis in infants, J. Pediatr. 106:717-722, 1985.

Epstein, L., and others: Neurological and neuropathological features of human immunodeficiency virus infection in children, Ann. Neurol. 23(suppl.):S19-23, 1988.

Feldman, H.M., and Michaels, R.H.: Academic achievement in children ten to 12 years after *Haemophilus influenzae* meningitis, Pediatrics 81:339-344, 1988.

Greene, C.L., Blitzer, M.G., and Shapira, E.: Inborn errors of metabolism and Reye syndrome: differential diagnosis, J. Pediatr. 113:156-159, 1988.

Harteman, E.: Reye's syndrome: a current entity which remains enigmatic, Pediatrics 43:499-507, 1988.

Johnson, D.L., and others: Treatment of intracranial abscesses associated with sinusitis in children and adolescents, J. Pediatr. 113:15-23, 1988.

Lebel, M.H., and McCracken, G.H.: Delayed cerebrospinal fluid sterilization and adverse outcome of bacterial meningitis in infants and children, Pediatrics 83:161-167, 1989.

Lebel, M.H., and others: Dexamethasone therapy for bacterial meningitis: results of two double-blind, placebo-controlled trials, N. Engl. J. Med. 319:964-971, 1988.

Lebel, M.H., and others: Magnetic resonance imaging and dexamethasone therapy for bacterial meningitis, Am. J. Dis. Child. 143:301-306, 1989.

Orlowski, J.P., Gillis, J., and Kilham, H.A.: A catch in the Reye, Pediatrics 80:638-642, 1987.

Patrick, C., and Kaplan, S.: Current concepts in the pathogenesis and management of brain abscesses in children, Pediatr. Clin. North Am. 35:625-636, 1989.

Pinsky, P., and others: Reye's syndrome and aspirin: evidence for a dose-response effect, JAMA 260:657-661, 1988.
Spaniolo, A.M., and Van Antwerp, C.: Case study of a child with meningococcemia, J. Pediatr. Nurs. 1:396-403, 1986.
Visudhiphan, P., and Chiemchanya, S.: Tuberculous meningitis in children: treatment with isoniazid and rifampin for twelve months, J. Pediatr. 114:875-879, 1989.
Wald, E.R., and others: Long-term outcome of group B streptococcal meningitis, Pediatrics 77:217-221, 1986.
Yogev, R.: Cerebrospinal fluid shunt infections: a personal view, Pediatr. Infect. Dis. 4:113-118, 1985.

Epilepsy

Ashkenasi, A., and Snead, O.C., III: Epileptic syndromes in children and their therapy, Curr. Opin. Pediatr. 1:269-277, 1989.
Austin, J.K.: Predicting parental anticonvulsant medication compliance, J. Pediatr. Nurs. 4:88-95, 1989.
Austin, J.K., and McDermott, N.: Parental attitude and coping behavior in families of children with epilepsy, J. Neurosci. Nurs. 20:174-179, 1988.
Brent, D.A., and others: Phenobarbital treatment and major depressive disorder in children with epilepsy, Pediatrics 80:909-917, 1987.
Callaghan, N., Garrett, A., and Goggin, T.: Withdrawal of anticonvulsant drugs in patients free of seizures for two years, N. Engl. J. Med. 318:942-946, 1988.
Dodson, W.E.: Medical treatment and pharmacology of antiepileptic drugs, Pediatr. Clin. North Am. 36:421-433, 1989.
Dreyfuss, F.E.: Classification of epileptic seizures, Pediatr. Clin. North Am. 36:265-279, 1989.
Duchowny, M.S.: Surgery for intractable epilepsy: issues and outcome, Pediatrics 84:886-894, 1989.
Dunn, D.W.: Anticonvulsants: when to start, what to use, and when to stop, Contemp. Pediatr. 3(9):50-68, 1986.
Egger, J., and others: Oligoantigenic diet treatment of children with epilepsy and migraine, J. Pediatr. 114:51-58, 1989.
Esposito, N., and Westgate, P.: Continuous EEG monitoring in the PICU, J. Pediatr. Nurs. 2:272-277, 1987.
Frank, J., and Fischer, R.G.: Drug interactions with carbamazepine, Pediatr. Nurs. 13:54-55, 1987.
Freeman, J.M.: A clinical approach to the child with seizures and epilepsy, Epilepsia 28(suppl. 1):103-109, 1987.
Freeman, J.M., and others: Benign epilepsy of childhood: a speculation and its ramifications, Pediatrics 79:864-868, 1987.
Friedman, D.: Taking the scare out of caring for seizure patients, Nursing '88 18(2):52-59, 1988.
Hidrtz, D.G.: Generalized tonic-clonic and febrile seizures, Pediatr. Clin. North Am. 36:365-382, 1989.
Lacey, D.J.: Status epilepticus, J. Clin. Psychiatry 49:33-36, 1988.
Lockman, L.A.: Absence myoclonic and atonic seizures, Pediatr. Clin. North Am. 36:331-342, 1989.
Maytal, J., and others: Low morbidity and mortality of status epilepticus in children, Pediatrics 83:323-331, 1989.
Pellock, J.M.: Efficacy and adverse effects of antiepileptic drugs, Pediatr. Clin. North Am. 36:435-448, 1989.
Schwartz, R., and others: Ketogenic diets in the treatment of epilepsy: short-term clinical effects, Dev. Med. Child Neurol. 31:145-149, 1989.
Shields, W.D.: Status epilepticus, Pediatr. Clin. North Am. 36:383-393, 1989.
Tse, A.M.: Seizures and societal attitudes: a teaching tool for children, siblings, classmates, parents, and classroom teachers, Issues Compr. Pediatr. Nurs. 9:299-303, 1986.
Vining, E.P.: Educational, social, and life-long effects of epilepsy, Pediatr. Clin. North Am. 36:449-461, 1989.
Vining, E.P.G., and others: Psychologic and behavioral effects of antiepileptic drugs in children: a double-blind comparison between phenobarbital and valproic acid, Pediatrics 80:165-174, 1987.
Woody, R.C., and Laney, S.M.: Rectal anticonvulsants in pediatric practice, Pediatr. Emerg. Care 4:112-116, 1988.
Wyllie, E.: Corpus callosotomy for intractable generalized epilepsy, J. Pediatr. 113:255-261, 1988.
Wyllie, E., Rothner, A.D., and Lüders: Partial seizures in children, Pediatr. Clin. North Am. 36:343-364, 1989.
Wyllie, E., and others: Psychogenic seizures in children and adolescents: outcome after diagnosis by ictal video and electroencephalographic recording, Pediatrics 85:480-484, 1990.

Other Seizures

Anderson, A.B., and others: Duration of fever prior to onset of a simple febrile seizure, Pediatr. Emerg. Care 5:12-15, 1989.
Annegers, J.F., and others: Factors prognostic of unprovoked seizures after febrile convulsions, N. Engl. J. Med. 316:493-498, 1987.
Berg, A.T., and others: Predictors of recurrent febrile seizures: a metaanalytic review, J. Pediatr. 116:329-337, 1990.
Bonadia, W.A.: Febrile convulsion is a common pediatric disorder, Pediatr. Emerg. Care 4:229, 1988.
Glaze, D.G., and others: Prospective study of outcome of infants with infantile spasms treated during controlled studies of ACTH and prednisone, J. Pediatr. 112:389-396, 1988.
Hirtz, D.G.: Generalized tonic-clonic and febrile seizures, Pediatr. Clin. North Am. 36:365-382, 1989.
Hobdell, E.F.: Infantile spasms, Pediatr. Nurs. 145:207-209, 1988.
Rosman, N.P.: Evaluation and management of febrile seizures, Curr. Opin. Pediatr. 1:318-323, 1989.
Vining, E.P.G., and Freeman, J.M.: Paroxysmal events which are not seizures, Pediatr. Ann. 14:726-727, 1985.

Migraine

Cooper, P.J., and others: Anxiety and life events in childhood migraine, Pediatrics 79:999-1004, 1987.
Golden, G.: Management of headaches in children, Nurs. Pract. 12(6):38-41, 1987.
Kandt, R.S., and Levine, R.M.: Headache and acute illness in children, J. Child Neurol. 2:22-27, 1987.
Lascelles, M.A., and others: Helping adolescents manage migraine headaches, Am. J. Nurs. 89:1215-1216, 1989.
Linet, M.S., and others: An epidemiologic study of headache among adolescents and young adults, JAMA 261:2211-2216, 1989.
Olness, K., and MacDonald, J.T.: Recurrent headaches in children: diagnosis and treatment, Pediatr. Rev. 8:307-311, 1987.
Olness, K., MacDonald, J.T., and Uden, D.L.: Comparison of self-hypnosis and propranolol in the treatment of juvenile classic migraine, Pediatrics 79:593-597, 1987.
Rapoff, M., Walsh, D., and Engel, J.M: Assessment and management of chronic pediatric headaches, Issues Compr. Pediatr. Nurs. 11:159-178, 1988.
Womack, W.M., and others: Behavioral management of childhood headaches: a pilot study and case history report, Pain 32:279-283, 1988.

CHAPTER 38

The Child with Endocrine Dysfunction

RELATED TOPICS

Aberrant sexual development, Ch. 11
Alterations in growth and maturation, Ch. 20
Biologic development (adolescence), Ch. 19
Congenital hypothyroidism, Ch. 9
Genetic counseling, Ch. 5
Hypocalcemia, Ch. 9
Hypoglycemia, Ch. 9
Monogenic (single-gene) disorders, Ch. 5

GLOSSARY

ACTH Adrenocorticotropic hormone
ADH Antidiuretic hormone
allele The different forms of a gene; alleles that occur at the same position on a chromosome pair may produce different effects during development
Chvostek sign Facial muscle spasm elicited by tapping the facial nerve in the region of the parotid gland
CNS Central nervous system
CRF Corticotropin-releasing factor
DI Diabetes insipidus
DKA Diabetic ketoacidosis
DM Diabetes mellitus
GH Growth hormone
gluconeogenesis Formation of glucose from molecules that are not themselves carbohydrates (e.g., amino acids, lactate, and glycerol portion of fats)
glycogenolysis Breakdown of glycogen to glucose
HGBM Home glucose blood monitoring
hGH Human growth hormone
HLA Human lymphocyte antigen
ICA Islet cell antibodies
IDDM Insulin-dependent diabetes mellitus
MODY Maturity-onset diabetes of youth
NIDDM Non-insulin-dependent diabetes mellitus
PTH Parathormone
SIADH Syndrome of inappropriate ADH
T_3 Triiodothyronine
T_4 Thyroxine
TH Thyroid hormone
TRF Thyroid-releasing factor
Trousseau sign Carpal spasm elicited by pressure applied to nerves of the upper arm
TSH Thyroid-stimulating hormone

The major chemical regulators of the body are internal secretions and their secreting cells, which are collectively known as the endocrine system. The function of the endocrine system is to secrete intracellularly synthesized hormones into the circulation, where they are transported to nearby or distant sites to stimulate, catalyze, or serve as pacemaker substances for metabolic processes. Together with the closely related but more rapidly reacting nervous system, the endocrine system serves to integrate the various physiologic functions of the organism in adjusting to external and internal environmental demands. Endocrine substances, even in extremely small concentrations, are effective in modifying metabolism, behavior, and development.

This chapter is primarily concerned with problems associated with oversecretion or undersecretion of the major hormones or defective responses in those organs and tissues sensitive to these hormones. The initial discussion is devoted to disorders of the large, interrelated neuroendocrine system. The most common endocrine disturbance in childhood, diabetes mellitus—caused by defective pancreatic hormone (insulin) secretion—is discussed at length.

THE ENDOCRINE SYSTEM

The endocrine system consists of three components: (1) the *cell,* which sends a chemical message by means of a hormone; (2) the *target cells,* or *end organs,* which receive the chemical message; and (3) the *environment* through which the chemical is transported (blood, lymph, extracellular fluids) from the site of synthesis to the sites of cellular action. The endocrine system controls or regulates metabolic processes governing energy production, growth, fluid and electrolyte balance, response to stress, and sexual reproduction.

The endocrine glands, which are distributed throughout the body, are listed in Box 38-1, including several additional structures sometimes considered as endocrine glands, although they are not usually included.

Box 38-1 ENDOCRINE GLANDS

Pituitary gland (hypophysis cerebri)—a pea-sized gland that lies within a deep bony depression at the base of the cranium, the sella turcica, and is attached to the hypothalamus on the undersurface of the brain by a slender infundibulum or pituitary stalk
Thyroid gland—two large lateral lobes and a connecting portion, the isthmus, situated on the anterior aspect of the neck just below the larynx
Parathyroid glands—four or five (there may be more or less) small round bodies attached to the posterior surfaces of the lateral lobes of the thyroid gland
Adrenal glands—pyramid-shaped glands situated atop the kidneys, fitting like caps over these organs
Ovaries—glands located in the female pelvis on each side of the uterus at the fimbriated end of the fallopian tubes
Testes—oval-shaped glands situated within the male scrotum
Islands of Langerhans—small clusters of endocrine cells within the pancreas situated between the acinar or exocrine-secreting portions of the gland

Structures Sometimes Considered Endocrine Glands
Pineal body (epiphysis cerebri)—a gland located in the cranial cavity behind the midbrain and third ventricle, the functions of which are largely speculative
Thymus—a gland situated behind the sternum and below the thyroid gland; plays an important role in immunity but only during fetal life and early childhood
Gastrointestinal glands—mucosal lining of the gastrointestinal tract containing cells that produce hormones that play important roles in controlling and coordinating secretory and motor activities of digestion
Placenta—a body that secretes ovarian hormones and chorionic gonadotropin during gestation; only a temporary endocrine gland

HORMONES

A hormone is a complex chemical substance produced and secreted into body fluids by a cell or group of cells that exerts a physiologic controlling effect on other cells. Some are *local hormones* creating their effect near the point of secretion. For example, acetylcholine, released at the parasympathetic and skeletal nerve endings, mediates the synaptic activity of the nervous system; secretin, a digestive hormone secreted by certain cells lining the duodenum, stimulates the pancreas to release a watery secretion; and the prostaglandins, or tissue hormones, secreted by a wide variety of organs (including the seminal vesicles, kidneys, lungs, iris, brain, and thymus), usually diffuse only a short distance to integrate activities of neighboring cells.

General hormones are produced in one organ or part of the body and are carried through the bloodstream to a distant part, or parts, of the body where they initiate or regulate physiologic activity of an organ or group of cells. Some of these hormones (such as thyroid hormone and growth hormone) affect most cells of the body, whereas others (such as the tropic hormones) produce their effects on specific tissues. The tissues affected by this specific action are called *target tissues.* For example, the pituitary hormones stimulate the adrenal glands and the thyroid gland to secrete adrenocorticotropin and thyrotropic hormone, respectively.

Control of Hormone Secretion

Hormones are released by endocrine glands into the bloodstream, where they are carried to responsive tissues. These responsive, or target, tissues may be another endocrine gland, an organ, or tissue. Regulation of hormonal secretion is based on negative feedback. As a general rule, endocrine glands have a tendency to oversecrete their particular hormones. However, once the physiologic effect of the hormone has been achieved, this information is transmitted to the producing gland, either directly or indirectly, to inhibit further secretion. If the gland undersecretes, the inhibition is relieved, and the gland increases production of the hor-

Marilyn Cox Borgersen, R.N., M.S.N., C.D.E., assisted in the revision of this chapter.

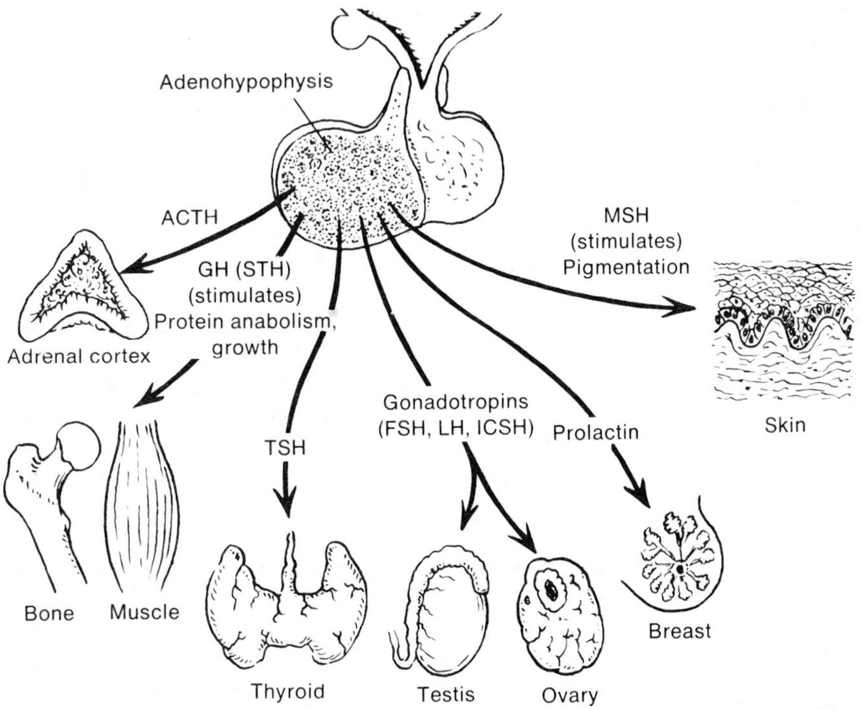

Fig. 38-1. Anterior pituitary hormones and their target organs and tissues. See text for discussion.
From Anthony, C.P., and Thibodeau, G.A.: Textbook of anatomy and physiology, ed. 10, St. Louis, 1979, Mosby–Year Book, Inc.

mone. As a result, the hormone is secreted according to the amount needed. This is the primary function of the tropic hormones.

The endocrine gland primarily responsible for stimulation and inhibition of target glandular secretions is the *anterior pituitary,* or "master gland." *Tropic* (which literally means "turning") hormones secreted by the anterior pituitary regulate the secretion of hormones from various target organs (Fig. 38-1). As blood concentrations of the target hormones reach normal levels, a negative message is sent to the anterior pituitary to inhibit release of the tropic hormone. For example, thyroid-stimulating hormone (TSH) responds to low levels of circulating thyroid hormone (TH). As blood levels of thyroid hormone reach normal concentrations, a negative feedback message is sent to the anterior pituitary, resulting in diminished release of thyroid-stimulating hormone.

The pituitary gland is, in turn, controlled by either hormonal or neuronal signals from the hypothalamus. Two types of substances are secreted from the hypothalamus: (1) *releasing hormones* and (2) *inhibitory hormones,* which are secreted within the hypothalamus and transported by way of the pituitary portal system to the anterior pituitary, where they stimulate the secretion of tropic hormones. An example of this is the secretion of corticotropin-releasing factor (CRF) by the hypothalamus, which stimulates the pituitary to secrete adrenocorticotropic hormone (ACTH). In this instance the anterior pituitary is the target of the hypothalamus and secondarily effects a response from another target gland, the adrenals. The adrenals in turn secrete glucocorticoids, which have multiple target sites throughout the body. Pituitary hormones that lack feedback control from the product of a target tissue (growth hormone, prolactin, and melanocyte-stimulating hormone) require hypothalamic inhibitors and stimulators for their control.

Not all hormones depend on other hormones for their release. For example, insulin is secreted in response to blood glucose concentrations. Other glandular hormones that are not under the control of the pituitary gland are glucagon, parathyroid hormone (PTH), antidiuretic hormone (ADH), and aldosterone.

NEUROENDOCRINE INTERRELATIONSHIPS

Homeostasis is maintained by two regulatory systems: the endocrine and the autonomic nervous systems (collectively known as the *neuroendocrine system).* The *autonomic nervous system* consists of the sympathetic and parasympathetic systems that control nonvoluntary functions, specifically of smooth muscle, myocardium, and glands. The *parasympathetic system,* in particular, is primarily involved in regulating digestive processes, whereas the *sympathetic system* functions to maintain homeostasis during stress.

The higher autonomic centers, located in the hypothalamus and limbic system, help control the functioning of both autonomic systems. Both the sympathetic and parasympathetic nerve fibers secrete neurotransmitting substances—acetylcholine, released by cholinergic fibers, and norepinephrine, released by adrenergic fibers. Neural release of norepinephrine into the plasma produces the same effects as secretion of this substance by the adrenal medulla. This similarity in chemical activity demonstrates the interrelatedness between the two systems.

The neuroendocrine system acts by synthesizing and releasing various chemical substances that regulate body functions. Information is carried by means of neural impulses in the autonomic system and by the blood in the endocrine system. In general, neural responses are more rapid and localized; endocrine responses are more lasting and widespread. The two systems function synergistically because neural impulses transmitted to the central nervous system stimulate the hypothalamus to manufacture and release several *releasing* or *inhibiting* factors.

Because of the interdependent relationship of these glands, a malfunction in one gland produces effects elsewhere in the body. Endocrine dysfunction may result because of an intrinsic defect in the target gland (primary) or because of a diminished or elevated level of tropic hormones (secondary). Endocrine problems occur from hypofunction or hyperfunction of the glands. Primary hypofunction is usually associated with a more profound deficiency of the target gland hormone because little or no hormone is secreted. In secondary dysfunction the target glands secrete some of their hormones but in smaller amounts and less rapidly.

Hyperfunction or hypofunction may also be the result of an increase or a decrease in secretion of the tropic hormones (primary) with a consequent increase in the target gland hormones (secondary) or a hypersecretion or hyposecretion of the target glands. A summary of the endocrine glands, their functions, and the primary effects of oversecretion or undersecretion is given in Table 38-1.

Table 38-1 Summary of the endocrine system

GLAND/HORMONE	EFFECT	HYPOFUNCTION	HYPERFUNCTION
Adenohypophysis (anterior pituitary)*			
Somatotropic hormone (STH) or growth hormone (GH) (somatotropin) Target tissue: bones	Promotes growth of bone and soft tissues Has main effect on linear growth Maintains a normal rate of protein synthesis Conserves carbohydrate utilization and promotes fat mobilization Is essential for proliferation of cartilage cells at epiphyseal plate Is ineffective after epiphyseal closure Has hyperglycemic effect (antiinsulin action)	Epiphyseal fusion with cessation of growth Prepubertal dwarfism Pituitary cachexia (Simonds disease) Generalized growth retardation Hypoglycemia	Prepubertal gigantism Acromegaly (after full growth is attained) Diabetes mellitus Postpubertal hypoproteinemia
Thyrotropin (thyroid-stimulating hormone [TSH]) Target tissue: thyroid gland	Promotes and maintains growth and development of thyroid gland Stimulates thyroid hormone secretion	Hypothyroidism Marked delay of puberty Juvenile myxedema	Hyperthyroidism Thyrotoxicosis Graves disease
Adrenocorticotropic hormone (ACTH) Target tissue: adrenal cortex	Promotes and maintains growth and development of adrenal cortex Stimulates adrenal cortex to secrete glucocorticoids and androgens	Acute adrenocortical insufficiency (Addison disease) Hypoglycemia Increased skin pigmentation	Cushing syndrome
Gonadotropins Target tissue: gonads	Stimulate gonads to mature and produce sex hormones and germ cells	Absent or incomplete spontaneous puberty	Precocious puberty Early epiphyseal closure
Follicle-stimulating hormone (FSH) Target tissue: ovaries, testes	Male: Stimulates development of seminiferous tubules Initiates spermatogenesis Female: Stimulates graafian follicles to mature and secrete estrogen	Hypogonadism Sterility Loss of secondary sex characteristics Amenorrhea	Precocious puberty Primary gonadal failure Hirsutism Polycystic ovary Early epiphyseal closure

*For each anterior pituitary hormone there is a corresponding hypothalamic-releasing factor. A deficiency in these factors caused by inhibiting anterior pituitary hormone synthesis produces the same effects (see text for more detailed information).

Table 38-1 Summary of the endocrine system—cont'd

GLAND/HORMONE	EFFECT	HYPOFUNCTION	HYPERFUNCTION
Adenohypophysis (anterior pituitary)—cont'd			
Luteinizing hormone (LH)* Target tissue: ovaries, testes	Male: Stimulates differentiation of Leydig cells, which secrete androgens, principally testosterone Female: Produces rupture of follicle with discharge of mature ova Stimulates secretion of progesterone by corpus luteum	Hypogonadism Sterility Impotence Loss of secondary sex characteristics Ovarian failure Eunuchism	Precocious puberty Primary gonadal failure Hirsutism Polycystic ovary Early epiphyseal closure
Prolactin (luteotropic hormone) Target tissue: ovaries, breasts	Stimulates milk secretion Maintains corpus luteum and progesterone secretion during pregnancy	Inability to lactate Amenorrhea	Galactorrhea Functional hypogonadism
Melanocyte-stimulating hormone (MSH) Target tissue: skin	Promotes pigmentation of skin	Diminished or absent skin pigmentation	Increased skin pigmentation
Neurohypophysis (posterior pituitary)			
Antidiuretic hormone (ADH) (vasopressin) Target tissue: renal tubules	Acts on distal and collecting tubules, making them more permeable to water, thus increasing reabsorption and decreasing excretion of urine	Diabetes insipidus	Syndrome of inappropriate secretion of ADH Fluid retention Hyponatremia
Oxytocin Target tissue: uterus, breasts	Stimulates powerful contractions of uterus Causes ejection of milk from alveoli into breast ducts (letdown reflex)		
Thyroid			
Thyroxine (T_4) and triiodothyronine (T_3)	Regulates metabolic rate; controls rate of growth of body cells Especially important for growth of bones, teeth, and brain Promotes mobilization of fats and gluconeogenesis	Hypothyroidism Myxedema Hashimoto thyroiditis General growth is greatly reduced; extent depends on age at which deficiency occurs	Exophthalmic goiter (Graves disease) Accelerated linear growth Early epiphyseal closure
Thyrocalcitonin	Regulates calcium and phosphorus metabolism Influences ossification and development of bone		
Parathyroid glands			
Parathyroid hormone (PTH)	Promotes calcium reabsorption from blood, bone, and intestines Promotes excretion of phosphorus in kidney tubules	Hypocalcemia (tetany)	Hypercalcemia (bone demineralization) Hypophosphatemia

*In the male, LH is sometimes known as interstitial cell–stimulating hormone (ICSH).

Continued.

Table 38-1 Summary of the endocrine system—cont'd

GLAND/HORMONE	EFFECT	HYPOFUNCTION	HYPERFUNCTION
■ Adrenal cortex			
Mineralocorticoids Aldosterone	Stimulate renal tubules to reabsorb sodium, thus promoting water retention but potassium loss	Adrenocortical insufficiency	Electrolyte imbalance Hyperaldosteronism
Sex hormones (androgens, estrogens, progesterone)	Influence development of bone, reproductive organs, and secondary sexual characteristics	Male feminization	Adrenogenital syndrome
Glucocorticoids Cortisol (hydrocortisone and compound F) Corticosterone (compound B)	Promote normal fat, protein, and carbohydrate metabolism In excess, tend to accelerate gluconeogenesis and protein and fat catabolism Mobilize body defenses during period of stress Suppress inflammatory reaction	Addison disease Acute adrenocortical insufficiency Impaired growth and sexual function	Cushing syndrome Severe impairment of growth with slowing of skeletal maturation
■ Adrenal medulla			
Epinephrine (adrenaline), norepinephrine (noradrenaline)	Produces vasoconstriction of heart and smooth muscles (raises blood pressure) Increases blood sugar via glycolysis Inhibits gastrointestinal activity Activates sweat glands		Hyperfunction caused by: Pheochromocytoma Neuroblastoma Ganglioneuroma
■ Islands of Langerhans of pancreas			
Insulin (β-cells)	Promotes glucose transport into the cells Increases glucose utilization, glycogenesis, and glycolysis Promotes fatty acid transport into cells and lipogenesis Promotes amino acid transport into cells and protein synthesis	Diabetes mellitus	Hyperinsulinism
Glucagon (α-cells)	Acts as antagonist to insulin, thereby increasing blood glucose concentration by accelerating glycogenolysis Able to inhibit secretion of both insulin and glycogen		Hyperglycemia May be instrumental in genesis of DKA in diabetes mellitus
Somatostatin (δ-cells)	Able to inhibit secretion of both insulin and glycogen		
■ Ovaries			
Estrogen	Accelerates growth of epithelial cells, especially in uterus following menses Promotes protein anabolism Promotes epiphyseal closure of bones Promotes breast development during puberty and pregnancy Plays role in sexual function Stimulates water and sodium reabsorption in renal tubules Stimulates ripening of ova	Lack of or repression of sexual development	Precocious puberty, early epiphyseal closure

Table 38-1 Summary of the endocrine system—cont'd

GLAND/HORMONE	EFFECT	HYPOFUNCTION	HYPERFUNCTION
Ovaries—cont'd			
Progesterone	Prepares uterus for nidation of fertilized ovum and aids in maintenance of pregnancy Aids in development of alveolar system of breasts during pregnancy Inhibits myometrial contractions Has effect on protein catabolism Promotes salt and water retention, especially in endometrium		
Testes			
Testosterone	Accelerates protein anabolism for growth Promotes epiphyseal closure Promotes development of secondary sex characteristics Plays role in sexual function Stimulates testes to produce spermatozoa	Delayed sexual development or eunuchoidism	Precocious puberty, early epiphyseal closure

DISORDERS OF PITUITARY FUNCTION

Deficiencies of the anterior pituitary hormones may be the result of organic defects or of idiopathic etiology and may occur as a single hormonal problem or in combination with other hormonal deficiencies. The clinical manifestations depend on the hormones involved and the age of onset. If the tropic hormones are involved, the resulting disorder reflects the altered stimulus to the target gland. For example, if thyroid-stimulating hormone is deficient, thyroid hormone is also deficient, and the child displays the manifestations of hypothyroidism.

An overproduction of the anterior pituitary hormones can result in gigantism (caused by excess growth hormone production during childhood), hyperthyroidism, hypercortisolism (Cushing syndrome), and precocious puberty from excessive gonadotropins. Overproduction is thought to be caused by hyperplasia of the pituitary cells—which may eventually progress to a tumor (adenoma)—or a primary hypothalamic defect that results in excess of the hormone's respective releasing factor. Although the initial clinical manifestations are a result of pituitary hypersecretion, eventually pituitary insufficiency occurs, and the signs of panhypopituitarism become evident.

HYPOPITUITARISM

Hypopituitarism is diminished or deficient secretion of pituitary hormones. The consequences of the condition depend on the degree of dysfunction and lead to gonadotropin deficiency with absence or regression of secondary sex characteristics; somatotropin deficiency, in which children display retarded somatic growth; thyrotropin deficiency that produces hypothyroidism (p. 1792); and corticotropin deficiency, which results in manifestations of adrenal hypofunction (p. 1800). Hypopituitarism can result from any of the conditions listed in Box 38-2.

The most common organic cause of pituitary hyposecretion is tumors in the pituitary or hypothalamic region, especially the craniopharyngiomas. These tumors usually invade the anterior and posterior pituitary lobes and the hypothala-

Box 38-2 ETIOLOGY OF HYPOPITUITARISM

- Aplasia or hypoplasia
  - Developmental defects
  - Idiopathic—sporadic; genetic
- Destructive lesions
  - Trauma—perinatal; child abuse; basal skull fracture
  - Infiltrative lesions—tumors; tuberculosis; toxoplasmosis; hemochromatosis; sarcoidosis
- Irradiation—CNS; eye; middle ear
- Autoimmune hypophysitis
- Surgery—removal of pharyngeal pituitary; ablation of craniopharyngioma or other tumor
  - Vascular—aneurysm; infarct
- Functional deficiency
  - Psychosocial dwarfism
  - Anorexia nervosa

Box 38-3 EFFECTS OF PANHYPOPITUITARISM

Growth Hormone (GH)
Short stature but proportional height and weight
Delayed epiphyseal closure
Retarded bone age proportional to height
Premature aging
Increased insulin sensitivity

Thyroid-Stimulating Hormone (TSH)
Short stature with infantile proportions
Dry, coarse skin, yellow discoloration, pallor
Cold intolerance
Constipation
Somnolence
Bradycardia
Dyspnea on exertion
Delayed dentition, loss of teeth

Gonadotropins
Absence of sexual maturation or loss of secondary sex characteristics
Atrophy of genitalia, prostate gland, breasts
Amenorrhea without menopausal symptoms
Decreased spermatogenesis

Adrenocorticotropic Hormone (ACTH)
Severe anorexia, weight loss
Hypoglycemia
Hypotension
Hyponatremia, hyperkalemia
Adrenal apoplexy, especially in response to stress
Circulatory collapse

Antidiuretic Hormone (ADH)
Polyuria
Polydipsia
Dehydration

Melanocyte-Stimulating Hormone (MSH)
Decreased pigmentation

mus, causing panhypopituitarism, a generalized disorder involving multiple systems (Box 38-3). The child may evidence growth retardation for quite some time before developing any symptoms or signs of increased intracranial pressure, local compression, or the destructive effects of the tumor. Other causes of panhypopituitarism sometimes include encephalitis, head trauma (rarely), and congenital hypoplasia of the hypothalamic area.

Idiopathic hypopituitarism is usually related to growth hormone (GH) deficiency, which inhibits somatic growth in all cells of the body. Although children with hypopituitarism are normal at birth, they show growth patterns that progressively deviate from the normal growth rate, often beginning in infancy. The chief complaint in most instances is short stature. Of those who seek help, boys outnumber girls three to one. The extent of idiopathic GH deficiency may be complete or partial, but the cause is unknown. It is frequently associated with other pituitary hormone deficiencies, such as deficiencies of TSH and ACTH; thus it is theorized that the disorder is probably secondary to hypothalamic deficiency. It has also been observed that there is a higher than average frequency in some families, which indicates a possible genetic etiology in a number of instances.

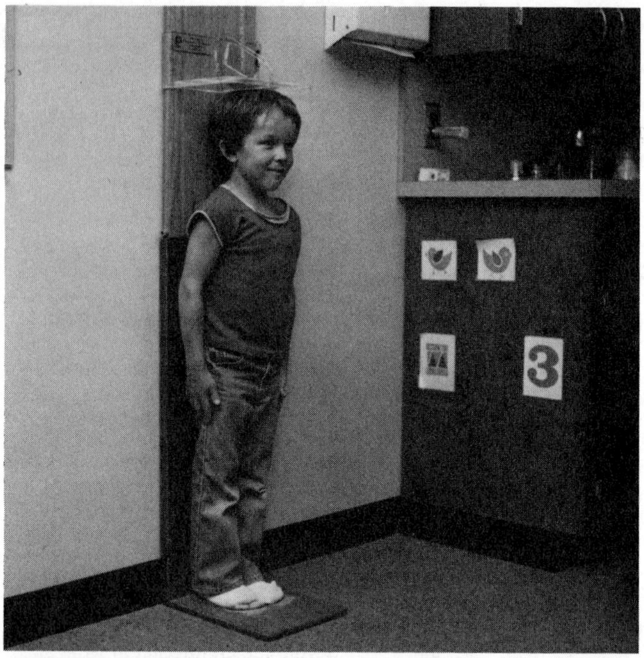

Fig. 38-2. Ten-year-old child with growth hormone deficiency. Height is 42.5 inches.

Clinical Manifestations

The usual presenting complaint with dwarfism is short stature. These children generally grow normally during the first year and then follow a slowed growth curve that is below the third percentile. In children with a partial GH deficiency, the growth retardation is less marked than in children with complete GH deficiency. Height may be retarded more than weight because, with good nutrition, these children can become overweight or even obese. Their well-nourished appearance is an important diagnostic clue to differentiation from other disorders such as failure to thrive.

Skeletal proportions are normal for the age, but these children appear younger than their chronologic age (Fig. 38-2). However, later in life premature aging is common. The appearance of fine wrinkles about the eyes and mouth gives these children a peculiar impression of immaturity combined with presenility. They are no less active than other children if directed to size-appropriate sports such as swimming, wrestling, gymnastics, soccer, or ballet. Bone age is nearly always retarded but is closely related to height age—the degree of retardation depends on the duration and extent of the hormonal deficiency. Children with diminished function of recent onset may show little retardation in skeletal age, whereas children with a long-standing deficiency may evidence a skeletal age only 40% to 50% of their chronologic age. It is difficult to predict their eventual height. Because the period of growth is prolonged past adolescence into the third or fourth decade, many of them reach a permanent height of 4 to 5 feet.

Usually primary teeth appear at the expected age, but the eruption of the permanent teeth is delayed. Because of the underdeveloped jaw, the teeth are overcrowded and malpositioned. Sexual development is usually delayed but is otherwise normal. Even without growth hormone replacement, dwarf adults are able to reproduce normal offspring. However, if the gonadotropins are deficient, sexual maturation is absent.

Most of these children have normal intelligence. In fact, during early childhood they often appear precocious in their learning because their ability seems to exceed their small size. However, emotional problems are not uncommon, especially as they near puberty, when their smallness becomes increasingly apparent compared with their peers. Also, academic problems are not uncommon. A history will often reveal repeated classes or enrollment in classes for children with learning disabilities. These children are usually not pushed to perform at their chronologic age but at their height age.

Diagnostic Evaluation

Only a small number of children with delayed growth or short stature have hypopituitary dwarfism. In the majority of instances the cause is constitutional delay (see Chapter 20). Diagnostic evaluation is aimed at isolating organic causes, which, in addition to GH deficiency, may include hypothyroidism, hypersecretion of cortisol, gonadal aplasia, chronic illness, or nutritional inadequacy.

A complete diagnostic evaluation should include a family history, a history of the child's growth patterns and previous health status, physical examination, radiographic surveys, and endocrine studies.

Family history. A family history is of utmost importance in relating short stature to genetic background. Children with constitutional delays frequently are the products of parents who experienced similar slow growth patterns and delayed sexual maturation. A small percentage of those with hypopituitarism demonstrate an autosomal-recessive inheritance pattern. Height and weight of siblings should be compared with the child's growth patterns at comparable age periods.

Child's history. The child's history should include a thorough prenatal history to rule out maternal disorders that may have influenced growth, such as malnutrition. Birth height and weight should be compared with gestational age. Children with hypopituitarism are usually of normal size and gestational age at birth.

The child's past health history is investigated for evidence of chronic illness that may have influenced growth patterns, although a chronic illness, such as congenital heart disease, malabsorptive disorders, severe anemia, or neurologic impairments, usually has been identified long before the growth problem becomes a concern. Signs and symptoms suggesting a tumor, such as visual disturbances, headache, and signs of increasing intracranial pressure, are important. Such symptoms often precede retarded growth but may not have been regarded as significant. With lesions involving the hypothalamus, the history may also reveal characteristic manifestations of dysfunction such as somnolence, thermodysregulation, epilepsy, and hyperphagia, resulting in obesity. Since a craniopharyngioma can affect the secretion of any of the pituitary hormones, assessment for hypothyroidism, hypoadrenalism, and hypoaldosteronism should also be included.

Whenever possible, the child's growth patterns since birth should be evaluated, especially growth velocity, as compared with standard measurements. Age of onset of short stature provides a significant diagnostic clue. Progressive retardation in height and weight since early childhood suggests idiopathic hypopituitary dwarfism, whereas a recent change from normal growth is more characteristic of a tumor. In addition, these children are usually well nourished, ruling out other causes of growth failure.

Physical examination. Accurate measurement of height and weight and comparison with standard growth charts are essential. Other measurements may include crown-to-pubis and pubis-to-heel length to compare body proportions, and sexual development should be assessed and compared with age-appropriate development. Observation of general appearance yields valuable clues, especially signs of premature aging and infantile facial features. A funduscopic examination and testing for visual acuity should be performed to detect evidence of ocular damage from a tumor.

Radiographic surveys. A skeletal survey in children less than 3 years of age and radiographic examination of the wrist for centers of ossification in older children are important in evaluating growth. Epiphyseal maturation is retarded in hypopituitarism but consistent with retardation in height. This is in contrast to hypothyroidism, in which bone maturation is greatly retarded, or gonadal dysplasia, such as Turner syndrome, in which bone age is near normal. Radiographic studies should also include a skull series, which helps in identifying abnormalities such as an abnormally small sella turcica or evidence of a space-occupying lesion such as craniopharyngioma. Computed tomography, radionuclear scans, or carotid angiograms may be needed to establish diagnosis and localization of lesions.

Endocrine studies. Definitive diagnosis is based on absent or subnormal reserves of pituitary GH. Since GH levels are normally so low in children that differentiation from abnormal concentrations is unreliable, GH secretion should be stimulated followed by measurement of blood levels. Exercise is a natural and benign stimulus for GH release, and elevated levels can be detected after 20 minutes of strenuous exercise in normal children. Also, GH levels are elevated 45 to 90 minutes following the onset of sleep.

If physiologic methods are inconclusive, GH release can be stimulated pharmacologically, which is a method used to identify children who do not respond to treatment with GH. Agents used to provoke GH are L-dopa, insulin-arginine, and glucagon. Tests with two or more agents may be required. GH levels below 10 ng/ml after two provocative tests establish the diagnosis. Somatomedin-C levels, compared with age- and sex-matched controls, are also used to detect GH deficiency. Levels are very low in children with GH deficiency but, in most cases, rise significantly within 16 to 28 hours of GH administration (DiGeorge, 1987).

Since retarded growth may be caused by other endocrine disorders (such as hypothyroidism or gonadotropic deficiency), Turner syndrome, or emotional deprivation or may be associated with other forms of delayed growth (such as tissue unresponsiveness to GH or primordial dwarfism), tests for these conditions are often performed.

Therapeutic Management

Treatment of GH deficiency caused by organic lesions is directed toward correction of the underlying disease process (e.g., surgical removal or irradiation of a tumor). The definitive treatment of GH deficiency is replacement of GH and is successful in 80% of affected children. Human-derived GH (hGH), obtained from human cadavers, is no longer available because of some reported adverse effects (Brown, 1988; Rappaport, 1987; Rappaport and others, 1986). Creutzfeldt-Jakob disease, a rare neurodegenerative condition, was reported in some patients after administration of the natural form of GH (Brown, Gajdusek, and Gibbs, 1985). Biosynthetic GH prepared by recombinant DNA technology is now available and is the therapy of choice, without the risk of Creutzfeldt-Jakob disease.

Children who respond to the therapy typically increase their growth rate from 3.5 to 4 cm/year before treatment to 8 to 10 cm/year during the first year of therapy. Young children usually respond better than adolescents, obese children better than thin children, and severely GH-deficient children better than those with partial deficiencies (Underwood, 1986). Although treated children display initial rapid catch-up growth, treatment does not appear to make up a deficit in *prognosis* of eventual height that is already present at diagnosis; however, it does prevent further loss of stature (Bundak and others, 1988). Therefore early diagnosis is important to successful therapy.

The decision to stop GH therapy is made jointly by the child, family, and health care team. Radiologic evidence of epiphyseal closure is a criterion for ending therapy. Dosage is increased as the time of epiphyseal closure nears in order to gain the best advantage of the GH. Children with other hormone deficiencies require replacement therapy to correct the specific disorders. This may involve administration of thyroid extract, cortisone, testosterone, or estrogens and progesterone. The sex hormones are usually begun during adolescence to promote normal sexual maturation.

Nursing Considerations

The principal nursing consideration is identifying children with growth problems. Despite the fact that the majority of growth problems are not a result of organic causes, any delay in normal growth and sexual development poses special emotional adjustments for these children (see also Chapter 20).

The nurse may be a key person in helping to establish a diagnosis. For example, if serial height and weight records are not available, the nurse can question parents about the child's growth in comparison with that of siblings, peers, or relatives. Investigating clothing sizes is often helpful in determining growth at different ages. Parents of these children frequently comment that the child wore out clothes before growing out of them or that, if the clothing fit the body, it often was too long in the sleeves or legs.

Because the behavioral or physical changes that suggest a tumor are insidious, they are frequently overlooked. It is important to correlate the onset of any positive findings with the initial evidence of growth retardation. For example, visual problems and headache are not uncommon in school-age children and can coincidentally occur after a growth problem is recognized. In fact, headache may represent the emotional trauma caused by short stature rather than be a symptom of a tumor. This line of questioning should be pursued cautiously to avoid alarming parents unduly about the possibility of a brain tumor.

Part of a nurse's role in helping establish a diagnosis is assisting with diagnostic tests. Preparation of child and family is especially important if a number of tests are being performed, and the child will require particular attention during provocative testing. Blood samples are usually taken every 30 minutes for a 3-hour period. Children also have difficulty overcoming hypoglycemia generated by tests with insulin, so they must be observed carefully for signs of hypoglycemia. Thin children under 5 years of age are at particular risk, especially those with low fasting-glucose levels (DiGeorge, 1987).

Child and family support. Once a diagnosis is made confirming an organic cause of the problem, the parents and child need an opportunity to express their thoughts and feelings. Not infrequently a growth problem that was present since birth is missed until adolescence, at which time the child's difference in body development becomes dramatically evident when compared with peers. Family members may feel anger and resentment toward members of the health staff for not detecting the problem sooner. Parents may experience guilt for not seeking medical attention earlier, especially if the child had been miserable from experiencing ridicule and criticism from associates. Each family member needs a sympathetic listener who is aware of his or her needs and realizes the importance of remaining objective and not defensive or overly apologetic. Appropriate emotional support from the nurse can include an affirmation of each person's justified feelings, such as anger or guilt, and emphasis on the treatment plan and prospects for improvement in the future.

Children undergoing hormone replacement require additional support. Therapy for GH deficiency requires daily subcutaneous injections. Nursing functions include family education concerning medication preparation and storage, injection sites, injection technique, and syringe disposal (see Chapter 27). Administration of GH is facilitated by family routines that include a specific time of day for the injection. Younger children may enjoy using a calendar and colorful stickers to designate received injections.

Even when hormone replacement is successful, these children attain their eventual adult height at a slower rate than their peers; therefore they need assistance in setting realistic expectations regarding improvement. For example, increases in height of 3 to 5 inches are common during the first year of therapy, but increases are less dramatic during subsequent years. Both sexes, but especially males, need guidance toward appropriate vocational goals. For example, children with aspirations for athletic sports such as basketball would be better advised to explore other activities not so dependent on excessive height.

Since these children appear younger than their chronologic age, others frequently relate to them in infantile or childish ways. Children having school problems will need special counseling. Parents and teachers benefit from guidance directed toward setting realistic expectations for the child based on age and abilities. For example, in the home such children should have the same age-appropriate responsibilities as their siblings. As they approach adolescence, they should be encouraged to participate in group activities with their peers. They should wear styles that accentuate their actual age, not their size. If abilities and strengths are emphasized rather than physical size, such children are more likely to develop a positive self-image.

Professionals and families may find education and support from the **Human Growth Foundation.*** The treatment is expensive—up to $15,000 to $25,000 per year, depending on dosage. Usually the cost is partially covered by insurance if the child has a *documented* deficiency. Children with panhypopituitarism should be advised to wear a Medic-Alert tag at all times.

PITUITARY HYPERFUNCTION

Excess growth hormone before closure of the epiphyseal shafts results in proportional overgrowth of long bones, until the individual reaches a height of 8 feet or more. Vertical growth is accompanied by rapid and increased development of muscles and viscera. Weight is increased but is usually in proportion to height. Proportional enlargement of head circumference also occurs and may result in delayed closure of the fontanels in young children. Children with a pituitary secreting tumor may also demonstrate signs of increasing intracranial pressure, especially headache.

If hypersecretion of GH occurs after epiphyseal closure, growth is in the transverse direction, producing a condition known as *acromegaly.* Typical facial features include overgrowth of head, lips, nose, tongue, jaw, and paranasal and mastoid sinuses; separation and malocclusion of the teeth in the enlarged jaw; disproportion of the face to the cerebral division of the skull; increased facial hair; thickened, deeply creased skin; and increased tendency toward hyperglycemia and diabetes mellitus.

Diagnostic Evaluation

Diagnosis is based on a history of excessive growth during childhood and evidence of increased levels of GH. Radiographic studies may reveal a tumor in an enlarged sella turcica, normal bone age, enlargement of bones (such as the paranasal sinuses), and evidence of joint changes. Endocrine studies to confirm excess of other hormones, specifically thyroid, cortisol, and sex hormones, should also be included in the differential diagnosis.

*4720 Montgomery Lane, Bethesda, MD 20814; (800) 451-6434.

Therapeutic Management

If a lesion is present, surgical treatment by cryosurgery or hypophysectomy is performed to remove the tumor whenever feasible. Other therapies aimed at destroying pituitary tissue include external irradiation and radioactive implants. Depending on the extent of surgical extirpation and the degree of pituitary insufficiency, hormone replacement with thyroid extract, cortisone, and sex hormones may be necessary.

Nursing Considerations

The primary nursing consideration is early identification of children with excessive growth rates. Although medical management is unable to reduce growth already attained, further growth can be retarded, and the earlier the treatment, the more control there is in predetermining a normal adult height. Nurses in ambulatory settings who are frequently involved in growth screening should refer children who demonstrate excessive linear growth for a medical evaluation. They should also observe for signs of a tumor, especially headache, and evidence of concurrent hormonal excesses, particularly the gonadotropins, which cause sexual precocity.

Children with excessive growth rates require as much emotional support as those with short stature. However, girls may suffer from the effects of excessive height much more than boys (see Tall Stature, Chapter 20). In fact, males may find the tallness an asset when pursuing sports such as basketball. Children and their parents need an opportunity to express their thoughts. A compassionate nurse can be very supportive to these children, especially before adolescence when they are larger than their peers. The nurse can emphasize to a tall girl that as boys grow older they become taller and that she will not always be looking down at them. Since early adolescence is a time of idol worship, the nurse can point out marriages of celebrities in which the woman is taller than the man to help the girl gain a perspective that not all heterosexual relationships must follow stereotypic models.

PRECOCIOUS PUBERTY

Manifestations of sexual development before age 10 in boys or age 8½ in girls are considered precocious and should be investigated. Early sexual development can have a number of causes and may result from a disorder of the gonad, the adrenal gland, or the hypothalamic-pituitary gonadal axis. The disorder is nine times more common in girls than in boys (Silver, Gotlin, and Klingensmith, 1984). A familial incidence of male sexual precocity has been observed in some families, but sexual precocity occurs as an isolated event in girls.

Normally the hypothalamic-releasing factors stimulate secretion of the gonadotropic hormones from the anterior pituitary at the time of puberty. In the male, interstitial cell–stimulating hormone stimulates Leydig cells of the testes to secrete testosterone; in the female follicle-stimulating hormone and luteinizing hormone stimulate the ovarian follicles to secrete estrogens. This sequence of events is known as the *hypothalamic-pituitary-gonadal axis.* If for some reason there is premature activation of this cycle, the child will display evidence of advanced or precocious puberty.

True Precocious Puberty

True, or complete, precocious puberty is always isosexual and results from premature activation of the hypothalamic-pituitary-gonadal axis, which produces early maturation and development of the gonads with secretion of sex hormones, development of secondary sex characteristics, and sometimes production of mature sperm or ova. True precocious puberty may be caused by a variety of organic brain lesions, such as tumors, congenital lesions, or postinflammatory disorders, but in most instances no cause can be identified. These cases are termed *functional idiopathic* or *constitutional precocious puberty.* They may occur at any time during childhood and are explained only as an unusually early activation of the maturation process regarded as a normal course of events at a later age. There is early acceleration of linear growth with early epiphyseal fusion and ultimate height less than would have been anticipated with later pubertal onset.

Precocious Pseudopuberty

Precocious pseudopuberty, or incomplete puberty (also called pseudosexual precocious puberty), differs from true sexual precocity in that there is no early secretion of gonadotropin. Most cases result from early overproduction of sex hormone, usually caused by a tumor of the ovary or testis, a tumor or hyperplasia of the adrenal gland, or exogenous sources of androgens or estrogens. There is no maturation of the gonads, but there is appearance of secondary sex characteristics. Unlike true sexual precocity, precocious pseudopuberty may be heterosexual. A tumor of the adrenal gland in a girl can cause early and inappropriate female development (e.g., clitoral enlargement and masculinization).

Isolated manifestations that are usually associated with puberty may be seen as variations in normal sexual development. They appear without other signs of pubescence and are probably caused by unusual end organ sensitivity to prepubertal levels of estrogen or androgen. Included are:

Premature thelarche—development of breasts in prepubertal females

Premature pubarche (premature adrenarche)—early development of sexual hair

Therapeutic Management

Treatment of precocious pseudopuberty is directed toward the specific cause when known. Precocious puberty of central (hypothalamic-pituitary) origin is managed with daily subcutaneous or monthly injections of a synthetic analog of luteinizing hormone–releasing hormone (LHRH), which regulates pituitary secretions. This therapy slows the prepubertal growth to normal rates in affected children. The children receiving LHRH therapy will need preparation for the regular injections, especially those with daily therapy. Treatment is discontinued at a chronologically appropriate time, allowing pubertal changes to resume.

Treatment is seldom helpful for idiopathic true precocious puberty. In females, administration of medroxyprogesterone acetate may arrest and reverse the condition, either by inhibiting gonadotropin production or by a direct effect on the ovary. Some cases of precocious puberty have responded to the administration of luteinizing hormone–releasing hormone (Pescovitz and others, 1986). Psychologic management of the patient and family is an important aspect of care.

Nursing Considerations

Psychologic support and guidance of the child and family are the most important aspects of management. Although the majority of children do not display behavior problems, girls with true precocious puberty have a high incidence of problem behavior, primarily social difficulties related to age/appearance dyssynchrony and moodiness (Sonis and others, 1985).

Parents need a detailed explanation and reassurance of the benign nature of the condition. Dress and activities for the physically precocious child should be appropriate to the chronologic age. Heterosexual interest is not usually advanced beyond the child's chronologic age, and parents need to understand that the child's mental age is congruent with the chronologic age and that the child's normal, overt manifestations of affection are age appropriate and do not represent sexual advances.

Despite the early sexual development, maturation of the gonads and the appearance of secondary sexual characteristics proceed normally. The most difficult time for the child is usually the school years before adolescence. After puberty, physical differences from peers are no longer present.

Although the child's heterosexual behavior is appropriate for the chronologic age, the nurse should emphasize to parents that the child is fertile. Usually no form of contraception is necessary, unless the child is sexually active. In this situation proper counseling is important because forms of birth control such as estrogen pills will prematurely initiate epiphyseal closure, resulting in stunted linear growth.

DIABETES INSIPIDUS

The principal disorder of posterior pituitary hypofunction is diabetes insipidus (DI) (sometimes called neurogenic DI) resulting from hyposecretion of antidiuretic hormone (ADH), or vasopressin, and producing a state of uncontrolled diuresis. This disorder is not to be confused with nephrogenic DI, a rare hereditary disorder affecting primarily males, caused by unresponsiveness of the renal tubules to the hormone (see Chapter 30).

Neurogenic DI may result from a number of different causes. Primary causes are familial or idiopathic; of the total groups, approximately 45% to 50% are idiopathic. Secondary causes include trauma (accidental or surgical), tumors, granulomatous disease, infections (meningitis or encephalitis), or vascular anomalies (aneurysm). Certain drugs, such as alcohol or phenytoin diphenylhydantoin, can cause a transient polyuria.

Clinical Manifestations

The cardinal signs of DI are polyuria and polydipsia. In the older child excessive urination accompanied by a compensatory insatiable thirst may be so intense that the child does little more than go to the toilet and drink fluids. Not infrequently the first sign is enuresis. In the infant the initial symptom is irritability that is relieved with feedings of water but not milk. The infant is also prone to dehydration, electrolyte imbalance, hyperthermia, azotemia, and potential circulatory collapse.

Dehydration is usually not a serious problem in older children who are able to drink larger quantities of water. However any period of unconsciousness, such as after trauma or anesthesia, may be life threatening because the voluntary demand for fluid is absent. During such instances careful monitoring of urine volumes, blood concentration, and intravenous fluid replacement is essential to prevent dehydration.

Diagnostic Evaluation

The simplest test used to diagnose this condition is restriction of oral fluids and observation of consequent changes in urine volume and concentration. Normally reducing fluids results in concentrated urine and diminished volume. In DI fluid restriction has little or no effect on urine formation but causes weight loss from dehydration. Accurate results from this procedure require strict monitoring of fluid intake, urine output, measurement of urine concentration (specific gravity or osmolality), and frequent weight checks. A weight loss between 3% and 5% indicates significant dehydration and requires termination of the fluid restriction.

✦ **NURSING ALERT** Small children require close observation during fluid deprivation to prevent them from drinking, even from toilet bowls, plants, or other unlikely sources of fluid.

If this test is positive, the child should be given a test dose of injected aqueous vasopressin (Pitressin), which should alleviate the polyuria and polydipsia. Unresponsiveness to exogenous vasopressin usually indicates nephrogenic DI.

An important diagnostic consideration is to differentiate DI from other causes of polyuria and polydipsia, especially diabetes mellitus. Other tests used in the diagnostic evaluation include a skull x-ray film to detect a tumor, kidney function tests and blood electrolyte levels to assess renal failure, and specific endocrine studies to isolate associated problems. In rare instances a psychologic consultation may be warranted to confirm the possibility of compulsive water drinking related to psychogenic causes.

Therapeutic Management

The usual treatment is hormone replacement, either with an intramuscular or subcutaneous injection of vasopressin tannate in peanut oil or with nasal sprays of aqueous lysine vasopressin. The injectable form has the advantage of lasting for 48 to 72 hours, which affords the child a full night's sleep. However it has the disadvantages of requiring frequent injections as well as proper preparation of the drug.

✦ **NURSING ALERT** To be effective, the active material must be thoroughly resuspended in the oil by being held under warm running water for 10 to 15 minutes and shaken vigorously before being drawn into the syringe. If not, the oil may be injected minus the antidiuretic hormone. Small brown particles, which indicate drug dispersion, must be seen in the suspension.

The nasal spray has the benefit of being a simple, painless route of administration. However, applications must be repeated every 8 to 12 hours to prevent recurrence of symptoms. To provide longer relief during the night, a cotton pledget moistened with the spray can be inserted into the nostril. However, mucous membrane irritation caused by a cold or allergy renders this route unreliable. Although the vaginal and buccal mucosae are substitute routes for the spray, they can be inconvenient. Desmopressin acetate (DDAVP), a new long-acting analog of arginine vasopressin, is available and administered intranasally by way of a flexible tube to achieve adequate control. It is usually administered twice daily—at bedtime to allow the child to sleep through the night and in the morning to allow fewer interruptions in the school day. Some "breakthrough" urination is allowed during the evening hours as a precaution against overmedication. The drug is also available for parenteral administration.

Nursing Considerations

The initial objective is identification of the disorder. Since an early sign may be sudden enuresis in a child who is toilet trained, excessive thirst with bed-wetting is an indication for further investigation. Another clue is persistent irritability and crying in an infant that is relieved only by bottle-feedings of water. Following head trauma or certain neurosurgical procedures, the development of DI can be anticipated; therefore these patients must be closely monitored for signs of the disorder.

Observations include body weight, serum electrolytes, blood urea nitrogen, hematocrit, and urine specific gravity taken before surgery and every other day following the procedure. Fluid intake and output should be carefully measured and recorded. Alert patients are able to adjust intake to urine losses, but unconscious or very young patients will require closer fluid observation. In children who are not toilet trained, collection of urine specimens may require application of a urine-collecting device.

After confirmation of the diagnosis, parents need a thorough explanation regarding the condition with specific clarification that DI is a different condition from diabetes mellitus. They must realize that treatment is lifelong. If children are to receive the injectable vasopressin (Pitressin), ideally both parents should be taught the correct procedure for preparation and administration of the drug. Once children are old enough, they should be encouraged to assume full responsibility for their care. (See the discussion of diabetes mellitus on p. 1807 for ways to help children learn to give their own injections.)

For emergency purposes these children should wear Medic-Alert tags. Older children should carry the nasal spray with them for temporary relief of symptoms. School personnel need to be aware of the problem in order that they can grant children unrestricted use of the lavatory. Failure to permit this may result in embarrassing accidents that often result in a child's unwillingness to attend school.

Children receiving DDAVP need to be observed for possible overdose of the drug. The signs of overdosage are those of water intoxication and similar to manifestations of inappropriate secretion of antidiuretic hormone (see next section).

SYNDROME OF INAPPROPRIATE ANTIDIURETIC HORMONE

The disorder that results from hypersecretion of the posterior pituitary hormone, or antidiuretic hormone (ADH, vasopressin), is known as the *syndrome of inappropriate ADH (SIADH).* SIADH is observed with increased frequency in a variety of conditions, especially those involving infections, tumors, or other central nervous system disease and trauma to the central nervous system.

The manifestations are directly related to fluid retention and hypotonicity. Serum osmolality is low, and urine osmolality is inappropriately elevated. When serum sodium levels are diminished to 110 mEq/L, affected children display anorexia, nausea (and sometimes vomiting), stomach cramps, irritability, and personality changes. With progressive reduction in sodium, other neurologic signs, stupor, and convulsions may be evident. The symptoms usually disappear when the underlying disorder is corrected.

The immediate management consists of restricting fluids. Subsequent management depends on the cause and severity. Fluids continue to be restricted to one-fourth to one-half maintenance. When there are no fluid abnormalities but SIADH can be anticipated, fluids are often restricted expectantly at two-thirds to three-fourths maintenance.

Nursing Considerations

The first goal of nursing management is recognizing the presence of SIADH from symptoms described in patients at risk, especially those in the pediatric intensive care unit (PICU). Accurately measuring intake and output, noting daily weight, and observing for signs of fluid overload are primary nursing functions, especially in the child receiving intravenous fluids. Seizure precautions are implemented, and the child and family need education regarding the rationale for fluid restrictions. The rare child with chronic SIADH will be placed on long-term ADH-antagonizing medication and require instructions for its administration.

DISORDERS OF THYROID FUNCTION

The thyroid gland secretes two types of hormones: (1) *thyroid hormone,* which consists of the hormones *thyroxine* (*T_4*) and *triiodothyronine* (*T_3*), and (2) *thyrocalcitonin.* The secretion of thyroid hormones is controlled by thyroid-stimulating hormone (TSH) from the anterior pituitary, which in turn is regulated by thyrotropin-releasing factor (TRF) from the hypothalamus as a negative feedback response. Consequently, hypothyroidism or hyperthyroidism may result from a defect in the target gland or from a disturbance in the secretion of TSH or TRF. Since the functions of T_3 and T_4 are qualitatively the same, the term *thyroid hormone (TH)* will be used throughout the discussion.

The synthesis of TH depends on available sources of dietary iodine and tyrosine. The thyroid is the only endocrine gland capable of storing excess amounts of hormones for release as needed. During circulation in the bloodstream, T_4 and T_3 are bound to carrier proteins (thyroxine-binding globulin [TBG]). They must be unbound before they are able to exert their metabolic effect.

The main physiologic action of thyroid hormone is to regulate the basal metabolic rate and thereby control the processes of growth and tissue differentiation, as outlined in Box 38-4. Unlike GH, TH is involved in many more diverse activities that influence the growth and development of body tissues. Therefore a deficiency of TH exerts a more profound effect on growth than that seen in hypopituitarism.

Thyrocalcitonin helps maintain blood calcium levels by decreasing the calcium concentration. Its effect is the opposite of parathormone in that it inhibits skeletal demineralization and promotes calcium deposition in the bone.

JUVENILE HYPOTHYROIDISM

Hypothyroidism is one of the most common endocrine problems of childhood. It may be either congenital (see Chapter 9) or acquired and represents a deficiency in secretion of thyroid hormones. Hypothyroidism from dietary insufficiency of iodine is now rare in the United States because the use of iodized salt has permitted a readily available source of the nutrient.

Beyond infancy primary hypothyroidism may be caused by a number of defects. For example, a congenital hypoplastic thyroid gland may provide sufficient amounts of TH during the first year or two but be inadequate when rapid body growth increases demands on the gland. Partial or complete thyroidectomy for cancer or thyrotoxicosis can leave insufficient thyroid tissue to furnish hormones for body requirements. Irradiation for Hodgkin disease or other malignancies causes thyroid dysfunction in approximately one third of children and adolescents (DiGeorge, 1987). Infectious processes may be a cause of hypothyroidism. It can also occur when dietary iodine is deficient.

Clinical manifestations depend on the extent of dysfunction and the age of the child at the onset. The presenting

Box 38-4 PHYSIOLOGIC EFFECTS OF THYROID HORMONE

Regulates metabolic rate of all cells; protein, fat, and carbohydrate catabolism; and nitrogen excretion
Regulates body heat production and heat-dissipating mechanisms
Regulates protein synthesis and catabolism, amino acid incorporation into protein, and transcription of messenger RNA
Increases gluconeogenesis and peripheral utilization of glucose
Maintains appetite and secretion of gastrointestinal substances
Maintains calcium mobilization
Stimulates cholesterol synthesis and hepatic mechanisms that remove cholesterol from the circulation; stimulates lipid turnover and free fatty acid release
Regulates hepatic conversion of carotene to vitamin A
Maintains growth hormone secretion, skeletal maturation, and tissue differentiation
Is necessary for muscle tone and vigor and normal skin constituents
Maintains cardiac rate, force, and output
Affects respiratory rate, depth of oxygen utilization, and carbon dioxide formation
Affects central nervous system development and cerebration during first 2 to 3 years
Affects milk production during lactation and menstrual cycle fertility
Maintains sensitivity to insulin and insulin degradation
Affects red cell production
Affects cortisol secretion, probably caused by direct effect on adrenal glands and by increasing ACTH secretion

symptoms are decelerated growth from chronic deprivation of thyroid hormone or thyromegaly. Impaired growth and development are less when hypothyroidism is acquired at a later age and, since brain growth is nearly complete by 2 to 3 years of age, mental retardation or neurologic sequelae are not associated with juvenile hypothyroidism. Other manifestations are myxedematous skin changes (dry skin, puffiness around the eyes, sparse hair), constipation, sleepiness, and mental decline.

Therapy is thyroid hormone replacement, the same as hypothyroidism in the infant, although the prompt treatment needed in the infant is not required in the child. In children with severe symptoms, the restoration of euthyroidism is achieved more gradually with administration of increasing amounts of L-thyroxine over 4 to 8 weeks to avoid symptoms of hyperthyroidism that can occur with treatment of chronic hypothyroidism.

Nursing Considerations

The importance of early recognition in the infant has already been discussed in Chapter 9. Cessation or retardation in growth in a child whose growth has previously been normal should alert the observer to the possibility of hypothyroidism. Following diagnosis and implementation of thyroxine therapy, the importance of compliance and periodic monitoring of response to therapy should be stressed to parents. Children should learn to take responsibility for their own health as soon as they are old enough, about 9 to 10 years of age.

GOITER

A goiter is an enlargement or hypertrophy of the thyroid gland. It may occur in deficient (hypothyroid), excessive (hyperthyroid), or normal (euthyroid) thyroid hormone secretion. It can be congenital or acquired and can be palpated in about 5% of school-age children (Mahoney, 1987). Congenital disease usually occurs as a result of maternal administration of antithyroid drugs and/or iodides during pregnancy. Acquired disease can result from increased secretion of pituitary TSH in response to decreased circulating levels of TH or from infiltrative neoplastic or inflammatory processes. In areas where dietary iodine (essential for TH production) is deficient, goiter can be endemic.

Enlargement of the thyroid gland can be mild and noticeable only when there is an increased demand for TH (e.g., during periods of rapid growth). Where iodine deficiency is severe, a large percentage of the population display goiters. Enlargement of the thyroid at birth can be sufficient to cause severe respiratory distress. Sporadic goiter is usually caused by lymphocytic thyroiditis, and intrinsic biochemical defects in synthesis of the hormones are associated with goiters. Thyroid hormone replacement is necessary to treat the hypothyroidism and reverse the thyroid-stimulating hormone effect on the gland.

Nursing Considerations

Identification of large goiters is facilitated by their obvious appearance. Smaller nodules may be evident only on palpation. Nurses in ambulatory settings need to be aware of the possibility of goiters and report such findings to a physician. Benign enlargement of the thyroid gland may occur during adolescence and should not be confused with pathologic states. Nodules rarely are caused by a cancerous tumor but always require evaluation. Since they are frequently associated with a history of exposure to irradiation of the neck or upper thorax, inquiry about this possibility is part of the assessment.

✦ **NURSING ALERT** If an infant is born with a goiter, immediate precautions are instituted for emergency ventilation, such as supplemental oxygen and a tracheostomy set. Positioning the child with the neck hyperextended often facilitates breathing.

Immediate surgery to remove part of the gland may be lifesaving in infants born with a goiter. When thyroid replacement is necessary, parents have the same needs regarding its administration as discussed for the parents of children who have hypothyroidism (see Chapter 9).

LYMPHOCYTIC THYROIDITIS

Lymphocytic thyroiditis (Hashimoto disease, juvenile autoimmune thyroiditis) is the most common cause of thyroid disease in children and adolescents and accounts for the largest percentage of juvenile hypothyroidism. It accounts for many of the enlarged thyroid glands formerly designated as thyroid hyperplasia of adolescence or "adolescent goiter." The disease is four to seven times more common in girls than in boys and four times more common in white than in black persons (Fink and Beall, 1982). Although it can occur during the first 3 years of life, it more frequently appears after age 6. It reaches a peak incidence at adolescence (DiGeorge, 1987), and there is evidence that the disease is self-limited.

Pathophysiology

There is a strong genetic predisposition to the development of autoimmune thyroiditis, although no mode of inheritance has been delineated and the basic stimulus or autoimmune defect is unknown. There is a close relationship between this disease and other thyroid disorders (Graves disease, idiopathic hypothyroidism, idiopathic myxedema) and autoimmune disorders (pernicious anemia, Addison disease, type I diabetes mellitus, and hypoparathyroidism) in families. An increased incidence of the histocompatibility antigens HLA-DR3 and HLA-DR5 has been observed in patients with autoimmune thyroiditis (Sack and others, 1983).

The disease is characterized by lymphocytic infiltration of the gland, germinal-center inflammation, and, in many patients, replacement with fibrous tissue. In the early stages there may be only hyperplasia. A defect in autoregulation allows the persistence of a T-cell clone, which induces a cell-mediated immune response. Several antithyroid antibodies have been recognized in patients with thyroiditis.

Clinical Manifestations

The presence of the enlarged thyroid gland is usually detected by the physician or pediatric nurse practitioner during a routine examination, although it may be noted by parents when the youngster swallows. In most children the entire gland is enlarged symmetrically (but may be asymmetric), firm, freely movable, and nontender. There may be manifestations of moderate tracheal compression (sense of fullness, hoarseness, and dysphagia), but it is extremely rare for nontoxic diffuse goiter to enlarge to the extent that its size causes mechanical obstruction. Most children are euthyroid, but some display symptoms of hypothyroidism. Others have signs suggestive of hyperthyroidism, such as nervousness, irritability, increased sweating, or hyperactivity.

Diagnostic Evaluation

Thyroid function tests are usually normal, although TSH levels may be slightly or moderately elevated. With progressive disease the T_4 decreases followed by a decrease in T_3 levels and an increase in TSH. A variety of abnormalities in radioactive iodine uptake may be noted. The majority of children have serum antibody titers to thyroid antigens, but fewer children have a positive red blood cell hemagglutination test. When both tests are used, almost all children with thyroid autoimmunity are detected. However, levels in children are lower than in adults; therefore repeated measurements may be needed in doubtful cases because titers may increase later in the disease (DiGeorge, 1987).

Therapeutic Management

In many cases the goiter is transient and asymptomatic and regresses spontaneously within a year or two. Therapy of nontoxic diffuse goiter is usually simple, uncomplicated, and effective. Oral administration of TH will decrease the size of the gland significantly. It provides the feedback needed to suppress TSH stimulation, and the hyperplastic thyroid gland gradually regresses in size. Surgery is contraindicated in this disorder. Untreated patients should be evaluated periodically.

Nursing Considerations

Nursing care consists of identifying the youngster with thyroid enlargement, reassuring the child that the condition is probably only temporary, and reinforcing instructions for thyroid therapy.

HYPERTHYROIDISM

The largest percentage of hyperthyroidism in childhood is caused by Graves disease, usually associated with an enlarged thyroid gland and exophthalmos. Most cases of Graves disease occur in children ages 6 to 15, with a peak at 12 and 14 years of age, but may be present at birth in children of thyrotoxic mothers. The incidence is five times higher in girls than in boys.

The hyperthyroidism of Graves disease is apparently caused by an autoimmune response to TSH receptors, but no specific etiology has been identified. There is definitive evidence for familial association with a high concordance incidence in twins. A large number of persons (approximately 80%) with the disease possess the histocompatibility antigen HLA-B8.

Clinical Manifestations

The development of manifestations is highly variable. Signs and symptoms develop gradually, with an interval between onset and diagnosis of approximately 6 to 12 months. The principal clinical features are excessive motion—irritability, hyperactivity, short attention span, tremors, insomnia, and emotional lability. Gradual weight loss despite a voracious appetite is observed in half of the cases. Linear growth and bone age are usually accelerated. Muscle weakness often occurs. Hyperactivity of the gastrointestinal tract may cause vomiting and frequent stooling. Cardiac manifestations include a rapid, pounding pulse even during sleep, widened pulse pressure, systolic murmurs, and cardiomegaly. Dyspnea occurs during slight exertion, such as climbing stairs. The skin is warm, flushed, and moist. Heat intolerance may be severe and is accompanied by diaphoresis. The hair is unusually fine and unable to hold a wave.

Exophthalmos (protruding eyeballs), observed in many children, is accompanied by a wide-eyed staring expression, increased blinking, lid lag, lack of convergence, and absence of wrinkling of the forehead when looking upward. As protrusion of the eyeball increases, the child may not be able to completely cover the cornea with the lid. Visual disturbances may include blurred vision and loss of visual acuity.

Diagnostic Evaluation

Presence of a thyroid mass in a child requires a thorough history, including inquiry into prior irradiation to the head and neck and exposure to a goiterogen. Diagnosis is established on the basis of increased levels of T_4 and T_3. Thyrotropin (TSH) is suppressed to unmeasurable levels. Other tests are rarely indicated.

Therapeutic Management

Therapy for hyperthyroidism is controversial, but all methods are directed toward retarding the rate of hormone secretion. The three acceptable modes available are (1) the antithyroid drugs, which interfere with the biosynthesis of thyroid hormone, including propylthiouracil (PTU) and methimazole (MTZ, Tapazole), (2) subtotal thyroidectomy, and (3) ablation with radioiodine (^{131}I-iodide). Each is effective, but each has advantages and disadvantages (Foley, 1986).

While affected children exhibit signs and symptoms of hyperthyroidism (i.e., increased weight loss, pulse, pulse pressure, and blood pressure), their activity should be limited to classwork only. Vigorous exercise is restricted until thyroid levels are decreased to normal or near normal values.

Drug therapy. Most centers favor drugs as an initial therapy. An effective response to these drugs occurs after a latent period, since they inhibit production of additional thyroid hormone but do not retard secretion of stored supplies. Generally, some improvement is noted within the first 2 weeks, with evidence of decreased nervousness, less fatigue, increased strength, a lowered pulse, and weight gain. In many children an initial treatment course of 1 to 2 years will be followed by a complete remission of the disorder. Those who relapse may benefit from a second course of therapy but may also be candidates for surgical intervention.

Disadvantages include toxic drug reactions requiring alternate therapy, chronic dependency on the drug, and failure to produce remission in a large number of patients. The most serious side effect of these antithyroid drugs is agranulocytosis (pronounced leukopenia), which generally occurs within the initial weeks or months of therapy. It is usually accompanied by a sore throat and fever. Treatment involves immediate discontinuation of the drug, isolation of the child, and administration of antibiotics and glucocorticoids.

Thyroidectomy. Surgical treatment involves surgical ablation of the thyroid (thyroidectomy). Although this approach has the advantage of being a long-lasting form of therapy without the need for multiple-dose drug therapy, it has a number of serious disadvantages, including the increased incidence of hypothyroidism and the need for thyroxine therapy, infrequent recurrent laryngeal nerve palsy and permanent hypoparathyroidism, keloid formation of the anterior cervical scar in susceptible individuals, and (rarely) surgical mortality. Therefore surgery in most centers is reserved for children who do not respond to or comply with the use of antithyroid drugs or who are prone to recurrences.

Radioiodine therapy. Radioiodine therapy is not recommended for children because of the increased risk of subsequent carcinoma of the thyroid and the possibility of genetic damage.

Thyrotoxicosis. Thyrotoxicosis (thyroid "crisis" or thyroid "storm") may occur from sudden release of the hormone. Although unusual in children, a crisis can be life-threatening. These "storms" are evidenced by acute onset of severe irritability and restlessness, vomiting, diarrhea, hyperthermia, hypertension, severe tachycardia, and prostration. There may be rapid progression to delirium, coma, and even death. A crisis may be precipitated by acute infection, surgical emergencies, or discontinuation of antithyroid therapy. Treatment in addition to antithyroid drugs is administration of β-adrenergic blocking agents (propranolol), which provide relief from the adrenergic hyperresponsiveness that produces the disturbing side effects of the reaction. Therapy is usually required for 2 to 3 weeks.

Nursing Considerations

The initial nursing objective is identification of children with hyperthyroidism. Since the clinical manifestations often appear gradually, the goiter and ophthalmic changes may not be noticed, and the excessive activity may be attributed to behavioral problems. Nurses in ambulatory settings, particularly those caring for children in school, need to be alert to signs that suggest this disorder, especially weight loss despite an excellent appetite, academic difficulties resulting from short attention span and inability to sit still, unexplained fatigue and sleeplessness, and difficulty with fine motor skills, such as writing.

Much of children's care is related to treating physical symptoms before a response to drug therapy is achieved. These children need a quiet, unstimulating environment that is conducive to rest. Sometimes hospitalization is necessary during the immediate treatment phase to remove a child from a troubled home. A regular routine is beneficial in providing frequent rest periods, minimizing the stress of coping with unexpected demands, and meeting the children's needs promptly. Physical activity is restricted. For example, school physical performance classes are discontinued.

Since the nervous manifestations often interfere with schoolwork, a consultation with the child's teachers is important in advising them of the medical reason for the problem and suggesting ways of helping the child adjust. For example, the child may benefit from a shortened school day or at least study periods in a quiet area. Limiting demands on the child such as reciting in class or participating in extracurricular activities may help conserve strength for academic studies. Despite the excessive activity of these children, they tire easily, experience muscle weakness, and are unable to relax to recoup their strength.

Emotional lability is often manifest by sudden episodes of crying or elation. Such behavior, coupled with irritability, disrupts interpersonal relationships, creating difficulties within and outside the home. Parents need help in understanding the uncontrollable nature of these outbursts and ways of minimizing them through decreased environmental stimulation, stress, and frustration. The child should be encouraged to express feelings about behavior and the effect that it has on others. The nurse can encourage the child to concentrate on friendships with one special peer rather than a group until such time as the condition is stabilized.

Heat intolerance may produce considerable family conflict. Preferring a cooler environment than others, the child is likely to open windows, complain about the heat, wear minimal clothing, and kick off blankets while sleeping. Although the child should dress in accordance with climatic conditions, the use of light cotton clothing in the home, good ventilation, frequent baths, and adequate hydration is helpful in providing comfort. Hygiene should be stressed because of excessive sweating.

Dietary requirements should be adjusted to meet the child's increased metabolic rate. Although the need for calories is increased, these should be provided in wholesome foods rather than "junk" foods. The child may require vitamin supplements to meet the daily requirement. Rather than three large meals, the child's appetite may be better satisfied by five or six moderate meals throughout the day. Family members should refrain from making remarks about the child's appetite, since the child may voluntarily restrict his or her eating to avoid such attention.

Once therapy is instituted, the drug regimen is explained, emphasizing the importance of observing for side effects of antithyroid drugs. Untoward effects of propylthiouracil and related compounds include urticarial rash, fever, arthritis, or arthralgia. There may be enlargement of the salivary and cervical lymph glands, diminished sense of taste, hepatitis, and edema of the lower extremities. Since sore throat and fever accompany the grave complication of leukopenia, these children should be seen by a practitioner if these symptoms occur. Parents should also be aware of the signs of hypothyroidism, which can occur from overdose of the drugs. The most common indications are lethargy and somnolence.

Surgical care. If surgery is anticipated, iodine is usually administered for a few weeks before the procedure. Since oral iodine preparations are unpalatable, they should be mixed with a strong-tasting fruit juice, such as grape or punch flavors, and be given through a straw. Compliance with iodine therapy is essential to avoid the danger of thyroid crisis after sudden discontinuation.

Psychologic preparation of children for thyroidectomy is similar to that for any other surgical procedure (see Chapter 27). However, of special consideration is the site of the incision. The fear of having the throat cut is very real and in older children is associated with death. The nurse should explain that the throat is not cut, only the skin, to allow for removal of the gland. Showing children a picture of the anatomic location of the thyroid around the trachea is often helpful. Children should be prepared for the dressing around the neck and the possibility of an endotracheal or "breathing" tube after surgery.

Postoperative care involves positioning with the neck slightly flexed to avoid strain on the sutures and observation for bleeding and complications. The children are taught to support the neck in this position when they sit up. Damage to the recurrent laryngeal nerve is evidenced by severe stridor and/or hoarseness, although some hoarseness is expected.

✦ **NURSING ALERT** The earliest indication of hypoparathyroidism may be anxiety and mental depression, followed by paresthesia and evidence of heightened neuromuscular excitability, such as *Chvostek* and *Trousseau* signs and *carpopedal spasm* (tetany).

DISORDERS OF PARATHYROID FUNCTION

The parathyroid glands secrete parathormone (PTH), the main function of which, along with vitamin D and calcitonin, is homeostasis of serum calcium concentration. The effect of PTH on calcium is opposite that of thyrocalcitonin. The principal effects of PTH on its target sites are listed in Box 38-5.

The net result of the integrated action of PTH and vitamin D is maintenance of serum calcium levels within a narrow normal range and the mineralization of bone. Secretion of PTH is controlled by a negative feedback system involving the serum calcium ion concentration. Low ionized calcium levels stimulate PTH secretion, causing absorption of calcium by the target tissues; high ionized calcium concentrations suppress PTH.

HYPOPARATHYROIDISM

Two classic forms of hypoparathyroidism are observed during childhood: *autoimmune hypoparathyroidism,* in which there is deficient production of PTH, and *pseudohypoparathyroidism,* in which production of PTH is increased but end-organ responsiveness to the hormone is deficient. The presenting signs or symptoms are similar.

Autoimmune hypoparathyroidism may occur as a component of multiglandular failure, usually related to autoimmune phenomena. Familial hypoparathyroidism is inherited as an autosomal recessive trait, with early onset, usually in the first month of life.

Box 38-5 PHYSIOLOGIC EFFECTS OF PARATHYROID HORMONE

Bones—increases osteoclastic activity, causing phosphate-producing bone demineralization
Kidneys—increases absorption of calcium and excretion of phosphate
Gastrointestinal tract—promotes calcium absorption

Hypoparathyroidism can also occur secondary to other causes. Postoperative hypoparathyroidism may follow thyroidectomy with acute or gradual onset and be transient or permanent. Two forms of transient hypoparathyroidism may be present in the newborn, both of which are the result of a relative PTH deficiency. One type is caused by maternal hyperparathyroidism or maternal diabetes mellitus. A more common, later, form appears almost exclusively in infants fed a milk formula with a high phosphate to calcium ratio (see Chapter 9).

Clinical Manifestations

Children with pseudohypoparathyroidism are short with round faces, short thick necks, and short and stubby fingers and toes with dimpling of the skin over the knuckles. None of these are observed in hypoparathyroidism. In both types the skin can be dry, scaly, and coarse with skin eruptions, the hair is often brittle, and the nails are thin and brittle with characteristic transverse grooves. Subcutaneous soft tissue calcifications appear in pseudohypoparathyroidism but not in idiopathic hypoparathyroidism. Dental and enamel hypoplasia occurs in both types.

Tetany, convulsions, carpopedal spasm, muscle cramps and twitching, paresthesias, and laryngeal stridor are often the initial symptoms in both types. Mental retardation is a prominent feature of pseudohypoparathyroidism and may also occur in idiopathic hypoparathyroidism but is less frequent in later onset disease and early diagnosis and treatment. Swings of emotion, loss of memory, depression, and confusion can occur. Papilledema may be seen in the idiopathic disease but is rare in pseudohypoparathyroidism. Since hypoparathyroidism results in decreased bone resorption and inactive osteoclastic activity, skeletal growth is retarded.

Diagnostic Evaluation

The diagnosis of hypoparathyroidism is made on the basis of clinical manifestations associated with decreased serum calcium and increased serum phosphorus. Levels of plasma PTH are low in idiopathic hypoparathyroidism but high in pseudohypoparathyroidism. End-organ responsiveness is tested by the administration of PTH with measurement of urinary cyclic AMP. Kidney function tests are included in the differential diagnosis to rule out renal insufficiency. Although bone radiographs are usually normal, they may demonstrate increased bone density and suppressed growth.

Therapeutic Management

The objective of treatment is to maintain normal serum calcium and phosphate levels with minimum complications. Acute or severe tetany is corrected immediately by intravenous and oral administration of calcium gluconate and follow-up daily doses to achieve normal levels. Twice-daily serum calcium measurements are taken to monitor the efficacy of therapy and prevent hypercalcemia. When diagnosis is confirmed, vitamin D therapy is begun. Vitamin D therapy is somewhat difficult to regulate because the drug has a prolonged onset and a long half-life. Some advocate beginning with a lower dose with stepwise increases and careful monitoring of serum calcium until stable levels are achieved. Others prefer rapid induction with higher doses and rapid reduction to lower maintenance levels.

Long-term management consists of administration of massive doses of vitamin D, and oral calcium supplementation may be useful in maintaining adequate serum calcium levels, although it is not essential. Blood calcium and phosphorus are monitored frequently until the levels have stabilized; they are then monitored monthly and less often until the child is seen at 6-month intervals. Renal function, blood pressure, and serum vitamin D levels are measured every 6 months. Serum magnesium levels are measured every 3 to 6 months to permit detection of hypomagnesemia, which may raise the requirement for vitamin D.

Nursing Considerations

The initial objective is recognition of hypocalcemia. Unexplained convulsions, irritability (especially to external stimuli), gastrointestinal symptoms (diarrhea, vomiting, cramping), and positive signs of tetany should lead the nurse to suspect this disorder. Much of the initial nursing care is related to the physical manifestations and includes institution of seizure and safety precautions, reduction of environmental stimuli (e.g., avoiding sudden or loud noise, bright lights, stimulating activities), and observation for signs of laryngospasm, such as stridor, hoarseness, and a feeling of tightness in the throat. A tracheostomy set and injectable calcium gluconate should be placed near the bedside for emergency use. The administration of calcium gluconate requires precautions against extravasation of the drug.

After initiation of treatment, the nurse discusses with the parents the need for continuous daily administration of calcium salts and vitamin D. Because vitamin D toxicity can be a serious consequence of therapy, parents are advised to watch for signs that include weakness, fatigue, lassitude, headache, nausea, vomiting, and diarrhea. Early renal impairment is manifest by polyuria, polydipsia, and nocturia.

HYPERPARATHYROIDISM

Hyperparathyroidism is rare in childhood but can be be primary or secondary. The most common cause of primary hyperparathyroidism is adenoma of the gland. The most common causes of secondary hyperparathyroidism are chronic renal disease, renal rickets, and congenital anomalies of the urinary tract. The common factor is hypercalcemia.

Clinical Manifestations

The manifestations of primary hyperparathyroidism are conveniently grouped according to the system involved (Box 38-6).

Diagnostic Evaluation

Blood studies to identify any alterations in calcium/phosphorus ratio are routinely performed. Measurement of PTH, as well as several tests to isolate the cause of the hypercalcemia, such as renal function studies, should be included. Other procedures used to substantiate the physiologic con-

Box 38-6 MANIFESTATIONS OF PRIMARY HYPERPARATHYROIDISM

Gastrointestinal—nausea, vomiting, abdominal discomfort, and constipation
Central nervous system—delusions, confusion, hallucinations, impaired memory, lack of interest and initiative, depression, and varying levels of consciousness
Neuromuscular—weakness, easy fatigability, muscle atrophy (especially proximal muscles of the lower limbs), twitching of the tongue, paresthesias in extremities
Skeletal—vague bone pain, subperiosteal resorption of phalanges, spontaneous fractures, and absence of lamina dura around the teeth
Renal—polyuria and polydipsia, renal colic, and hypertension

sequences of the disorder include electrocardiography and radiographic bone surveys.

Therapeutic Management

Treatment depends on the cause of hyperparathyroidism. The treatment of primary hyperparathyroidism is surgical removal of the tumor or hyperplastic tissue. Treatment of secondary hyperparathyroidism is directed at the underlying contributing cause, which subsequently restores the serum calcium balance. However, in some instances the underlying disorder is irreversible, such as in chronic renal failure. In this instance treatment is aimed at raising serum calcium levels in order to inhibit the stimulatory effect of low levels on the parathyroids. This includes oral administration of calcium salts, high doses of vitamin D to enhance calcium absorption, a low-phosphorus diet, and administration of a phosphorus-mobilizing aluminum hydroxide to reduce phosphate absorption.

Nursing Considerations

The initial nursing objective is recognition of the disorder. Since secondary hyperparathyroidism is a consequence of chronic renal failure, the nurse is always alert to signs that suggest this complication, especially bone pain and fractures. Since urinary symptoms are the earliest indication, assessment of other body systems for evidence of high calcium levels is indicated when polyuria and polydipsia coexist. Change in behavior, especially inactivity, unexplained gastrointestinal symptoms, and cardiac irregularities provide clues to the possibility of hyperparathyroidism.

Much of the initial nursing care is related to the physical symptoms and prevention of complications. To minimize renal calculi formation, hydration is essential. Fruit juices that maintain a low urinary pH, such as cranberry or apple juice, are encouraged, since acidity of body fluids promotes calcium absorption. All urine should be strained for evidence of renal casts.

Safety precautions, such as side rails in place at all times and assistance with ambulation, are instituted because of the tendency toward fractures and muscular weakness. Children with renal rickets (osteodystrophy) may wear braces to minimize skeletal deformities. These should be worn as prescribed. If the child is confined to bed, the nurse should consult with the physical therapist regarding proper use of orthopedic appliances.

Vital signs should be taken frequently, and the pulse counted for 1 full minute to detect irregularities. A decrease in pulse rate should be reported, since it may signal severe bradycardia and cardiac arrest. The diet needs supervision to ensure compliance with low-phosphate foods, particularly dairy products. The nurse should instruct parents regarding foods that need to be avoided and the necessity of administering calcium and vitamin D.

If surgery is anticipated, care is similar to that discussed for the child with hyperthyroidism (p. 1795). Since hypocalcemia is a potential complication, observation for signs of tetany, institution of seizure precautions, and having calcium gluconate available for emergency use are part of the nursing plan.

DISORDERS OF ADRENAL FUNCTION

The adrenal glands consist of two distinct portions: the cortex, or outer section, and the medulla, or inner core, each of which produces different hormones.

ADRENAL HORMONES

The adrenal cortex secretes the hormones, collectively known as steroids, that are essential to life. The medulla produces the catecholamines epinephrine and norepinephrine. Since these chemicals are also produced by the sympathetic nervous system, absence of the adrenal supply is not incompatible with life.

Adrenal Cortex

The cortex secretes three groups of hormones that are classified according to their biologic activity: (1) glucocorticoids (cortisol, corticosterone), (2) mineralocorticoids (aldosterone), and (3) sex steroids (androgens, estrogens, and progestins). The glucocorticoids and mineralocorticoids influence metabolic regulation and stress adaptation. The sex steroids influence sexual development but are not essential because the gonads secrete the major supply of these hormones.

Glucocorticoids. The most important glucocorticoids in humans are cortisol and corticosterone, the principal effects of which are outlined in Box 38-7. The secretion of the glucocorticoids is controlled by adrenocorticotropic hormone (ACTH) from the anterior pituitary. That means that a decrease in circulating levels of cortisol results in an increased secretion of adrenocorticotropic hormone, which stimulates the adrenal cortex to secrete additional glucocorticoids.

In times of stress the anterior pituitary is stimulated by corticotropin-releasing factor from the hypothalamus, which causes the release of increased amounts of ACTH. Stressful stimuli capable of provoking this response include trauma, anesthesia, surgical intervention, sepsis, acute anoxia, hy-

Box 38-7 PHYSIOLOGIC EFFECTS OF GLUCOCORTICOIDS

Stimulation of gluconeogenesis by the liver (a hyperglycemic effect)
Increased protein catabolism with resulting reduction in protein stores (except in the liver)
Increased mobilization and utilization of fatty acids for energy
Increased storage of adipose tissue in certain sites
Decreased inflammatory and allergic actions
Regulation of fluid and electrolytes by promoting sodium retention and potassium excretion by the kidneys and by water diuresis through direct antagonistic action against antidiuretic hormone
Increased gastric acid and pepsin production
Suppression of lymphocytes, eosinophils, and basophils, but elevation of neutrophils, erythrocytes, and thrombocytes

pothermia, hypoglycemia, and emotional states, especially panic, anxiety, or anger.

Secretion of the glucocorticoids is also regulated by body rhythms. Blood levels of cortisol demonstrate a typical diurnal or circadian pattern. In individuals who follow a regular routine of nighttime sleeping, cortisol levels are highest in the early morning hours after arising and lowest in the evening hours before bedtime.

Mineralocorticoids. The most important mineralocorticoid is aldosterone. Like cortisol, it promotes sodium retention, as do the anions chloride and bicarbonate, and potassium excretion in the renal tubules. However, its effect is many times more potent than that of the glucocorticoids in maintaining extracellular fluid volume, acid-base balance, and normal potassium levels.

Aldosterone secretion is primarily under control of the renin-angiotensin system. The juxtaglomerular cells of the kidney respond to decreased arterial pressure and/or blood volume and to decreased sodium concentrations by secreting the enzyme renin into the blood. Renin in turn converts angiotensinogen to angiotensin I and then to angiotensin II. Increased levels of angiotensin stimulate the adrenal cortex to secrete aldosterone, which preserves sodium, thereby retaining water. The renin-angiotensin mechanism also results in increased blood pressure.

Sex steroids. Except for the first few days of life, the sex hormones are normally secreted in only minimum amounts until adolescence, at which time they play a role in pubertal changes. Their actions are the same as those of the gonadal hormones on internal and external sexual structures and skeletal growth.

Adrenal Medulla

The adrenal medulla secretes the catecholamines epinephrine and norepinephrine. Both hormones have essentially the same effects on different organs as those caused by direct sympathetic stimulation, except that the hormonal effects last several times longer. Their major actions are outlined in Box 38-8.

Box 38-8 PHYSIOLOGIC EFFECTS OF CATECHOLAMINE SECRETION

Increased cardiac activity
Vasoconstriction of blood vessels (elevation of blood pressure)
Increased rate and depth of respirations
Bronchial dilation
Inhibition of gastrointestinal activity
Increased muscular contraction
Pupillary dilation
Increased metabolic rate
Heightened sensory awareness
Diaphoresis

Although the catecholamines evoke similar responses from target sites, there are some important differences. Epinephrine has a greater effect on cardiac activity than norepinephrine, but it causes only weak constriction of the blood vessels of muscles in comparison to the effect of norepinephrine. As a result, norepinephrine elevates blood pressure, whereas epinephrine increases cardiac output. Another important difference is their effect on metabolism. Epinephrine increases the metabolic rate to a much greater extent than norepinephrine. These differences in action have been attributed to the catecholamines' effects on α- or β-adrenergic receptors. Supposedly norepinephrine can only affect those effector cells that contain α-receptors, which are mostly excitatory in nature (constriction and contraction). Epinephrine, however, can affect both α- and β-receptors, and β-receptors are mostly inhibitory (dilation and relaxation).

Control of secretion of catecholamines, primarily in response to physiologic or emotional stress, is through the hypothalamus. Also, stimulation of the sympathetic nervous system results in the release of epinephrine and norepinephrine from the sympathetic nerves and adrenal medulla. Both systems support each other, and one can be substituted for the other. For this reason there is no condition attributable to hypofunction of the adrenal medulla. Even in bilateral adrenalectomy, catecholamine replacement is not necessary because the sympathetic release of these chemicals is sufficient to meet all the physiologic functions required to cope with stressful events.

Catecholamine-secreting tumors are the primary cause of adrenal medullary hyperfunction. In children the most common neoplasms of this type are pheochromocytoma, neuroblastoma, and ganglioneuroma. Ganglioneuromas are thought to be neuroblastomas that have undergone maturation into a benign tumor composed of ganglion cells. These tumors are associated with less abnormal catecholamine secretion than the other two types, but persons with ganglioneuromas may have a clinical picture of chronic diarrhea, failure to thrive, skin rash, hypokalemia, persistent cough, and abdominal distention. The exact reason for these symptoms is unknown, although they are attributable to the tumor because they disappear after surgical extirpation of the mass.

ACUTE ADRENOCORTICAL INSUFFICIENCY

The acute form of adrenocortical insufficiency (adrenal crisis) may result from a number of causes during childhood. Although a rare disorder, some of the more common etiologic factors include hemorrhage into the gland from trauma, which may be caused by a prolonged, difficult labor; fulminating infections, such as meningococcemia, which result in hemorrhage and necrosis (Waterhouse-Friderichsen syndrome); abrupt withdrawal of exogenous sources of cortisone or failure to increase exogenous supplies during stress; or as a result of congenital adrenogenital hyperplasia of the salt-losing type.

Clinical Manifestations

Early symptoms of adrenocortical insufficiency include increased irritability, headache, diffuse abdominal pain, weakness, nausea and vomiting, and diarrhea. Generalized hemorrhagic manifestations are present in the Waterhouse-Friderichsen syndrome. Fever increases as the condition worsens and is accompanied by signs of central nervous system involvement, such as nuchal rigidity, convulsions, stupor, and coma. The child is in a shocklike state with a weak, rapid pulse, decreased blood pressure, shallow respirations, cold clammy skin, and cyanosis. Circulatory collapse is the terminal event.

In the newborn, adrenal crisis is accompanied by extreme hyperpyrexia, tachypnea, cyanosis, and convulsions. Usually there is no evidence of infection or purpura. However, hemorrhage into the adrenal gland may be evident as a palpable retroperitoneal mass.

Diagnostic Evaluation

There is no rapid, definitive test for confirmation of acute adrenocortical insufficiency. Routine procedures such as measurement of plasma cortisol levels are too time-consuming to be practical. Therefore diagnosis is usually made based on clinical presentation, especially when a fulminating sepsis is accompanied by hemorrhagic manifestations and signs of circulatory collapse despite adequate antibiotic therapy. Since there is no real danger in administering a cortisol preparation for a short period, treatment should be instituted immediately. Improvement with this therapy confirms the diagnosis.

Therapeutic Management

Treatment involves replacement of cortisol, replacement of body fluids to combat dehydration and hypovolemia, administration of glucose solutions to correct hypoglycemia, and specific antibiotic therapy in the presence of infection. Initially, intravenous hydrocortisone (Solu-Cortef) is administered. Normal saline containing 5% glucose is given parenterally to replace lost fluid, electrolytes, and glucose. If hemorrhage has been severe, whole blood may be replaced. In the event that these measures do not reverse the circulatory collapse, vasopressors are used for immediate vasoconstriction and elevation of blood pressure.

Once the child's condition is stabilized, oral doses of cortisone, fluids, and salt are given, similar to the regimen used for chronic adrenal insufficiency. To maintain sodium retention, aldosterone is replaced by synthetic salt-retaining steroids.

Nursing Considerations

Because of the abrupt onset and potentially fatal outcome of this condition, prompt recognition is essential. Vital signs and blood pressure are taken every 15 minutes to monitor the hyperpyrexia and shocklike state. Seizure precautions are instituted, since convulsions from the elevated temperature are not uncommon. As soon as therapy is instituted, the nurse should monitor the child's response to fluid and cortisol replacement. Too rapid administration of fluids can precipitate cardiac failure, whereas overdosage with cortisol produces hypotension and a sudden fall in temperature. The nurse should regulate intravenous infusions carefully to guard against too rapid administration of drugs. Intake and urinary output should be recorded.

Once the acute phase is over and the hypovolemia is corrected, the child is started on oral fluids, such as small quantities of ginger ale, fruit juice, or salted broth. Too rapid ingestion of oral fluids may induce vomiting, which increases dehydration. Therefore the nurse should plan a gradual schedule for reintroducing liquids. For children who refuse to drink, the prospect of having the intravenous infusion removed once oral fluids are increased is often a motivating factor.

An ascending flaccid paralysis may occur on the second to third day of treatment because of an abnormally low serum potassium level secondary to overtreatment with cortisol and sodium chloride. The nurse should observe for signs of hypokalemia, such as cardiac irregularities and poor muscle control, and should evaluate serum electrolyte levels. The condition is rapidly corrected with intravenous and oral potassium replacement.

The sudden, severe nature of this disorder necessitates a great deal of emotional support for the child and family. The child may be placed in an intensive care unit where the surroundings are strange and frightening. Despite the need for emergency intervention, the nurse must be sensitive to the family's psychologic needs and prepare them for each procedure, even if this is as brief as a statement, such as, "The intravenous infusion is necessary to replace fluid that the child is losing." Since recovery within 24 hours is often dramatic, the nurse should keep the parents apprised of the child's condition, emphasizing signs of improvement such as a lowered temperature and elevated blood pressure. If paralysis occurs, the nurse should assure them that this condition is temporary and quickly reversed.

If treatment needs to be continued past the acute stage,

NURSING TIP: ADMINISTRATION OF ORAL POTASSIUM

When the oral preparation is given, it should be mixed with a small amount of strongly flavored fruit juice to disguise its bitter taste.

parents require the same preparation as those of children with chronic adrenal insufficiency. Preparation for discharge should begin as soon as possible after the child's condition has stabilized.

CHRONIC ADRENOCORTICAL INSUFFICIENCY

Chronic adrenocortical insufficiency (Addison disease) is rare in children. When it does occur, it is usually caused by a destructive lesion of the adrenal glands, neoplasms, or an idiopathic cause. At one time generalized tuberculosis was the leading cause of adrenal gland destruction.

Evidence of this disorder is usually gradual in onset, since 90% of adrenal tissue must be nonfunctional before signs of insufficiency are manifest. However, during periods of stress when demands for additional cortisol are increased, symptoms of acute insufficiency may appear in a previously well child. The cardinal signs and symptoms are listed in Box 38-9.

Definitive diagnosis is based on measurements of functional cortisol reserve. The cortisol and urinary 17-hydroxycorticosteroid levels are low and fail to rise while plasma ACTH levels are elevated with corticotropin (ACTH) stimulation, the definitive test for the disease.

Therapeutic Management

Treatment involves replacement of glucocorticoids (cortisol) and mineralocorticoids (aldosterone). Some children are able to be maintained solely on oral supplements of cortisol (cortisone or hydrocortisone preparations) with a liberal intake of salt. During stressful situations, such as infection, emotional upset, or surgery, the dosage must be tripled to accommodate the body's increased need for glucocorticoids. Failure to meet this requirement will precipitate an acute crisis. Overdosage produces appearance of cushingoid signs.

Children with more severe states of chronic adrenal insufficiency require mineralocorticoid replacement to maintain fluid and electrolyte balance. Other forms of therapy include monthly injections of desoxycorticosterone acetate or implantation of desoxycorticosterone acetate pellets subcutaneously every 9 to 12 months.

Box 38-9 CARDINAL SIGNS OF CHRONIC ADRENOCORTICAL INSUFFICIENCY

- Muscular weakness and mental fatigue, which are aggravated by slight additional exertion or minor illness
- Pigmentary changes of previous scars, palmar creases, mucous membranes, and hair; hyperpigmentation over pressure points (elbows, knees, or waist); or, less frequently, loss of pigmentation (vitiligo)
- Weight loss resulting from dehydration and anorexia from impaired gastrointestinal functioning (decreased hydrochloric acid)
- Hypotension and small heart size, which predispose to dizziness and syncopal (fainting) attacks
- Irritability, apathy, and negativism
- Signs of hypoglycemia, such as headache, hunger, weakness, trembling, and sweating; other signs seen in some children are recurrent unexplained convulsions, an intense craving for salt, and acute abdominal pain

Nursing Considerations

Once the disorder is diagnosed, parents need guidance concerning drug therapy. They must be aware of the continuous need for cortisol replacement. Sudden termination of the drug because of inadequate supplies or inability to ingest the oral form because of vomiting places the child in danger of an acute adrenal crisis. Therefore parents should always have a spare supply of the medication in the home. Ideally they should have a prefilled syringe of hydrocortisone in the home and be instructed in proper technique for intramuscular administration of the drug in case of a crisis. As was mentioned earlier, unnecessary administration of cortisone will not harm the child but, if needed, may be lifesaving. Any evidence of acute insufficiency should be reported to the practitioner immediately.

Parents also need to be aware of side effects of the drugs. Undesirable side effects of cortisone include gastric irritation, which is minimized by ingestion with food or the use of an antacid, increased excitability and sleeplessness, weight gain that may require dietary management to prevent obesity, and, rarely, behavioral changes, including depression or euphoria. Parents should be aware of signs of overdose (see Table 38-2) and report these to the practitioner. In addition, the drug has a very bitter taste, which creates a challenge for nurses and parents in its administration.

The side effects of mineralocorticoids are primarily caused by overdosage and include generalized edema, which is first noticed around the eyes; hypertension, which may cause headaches; cardiac arrhythmias; and signs of hypokalemia. Ideally the child should be evaluated periodically for evidence of excessive medication. Emphasizing the importance of routine follow-up care is a significant nursing responsibility.

Since the body cannot supply endogenous sources of cortical hormones during times of stress, the home environment should be stable and relatively unstressful. Parents need to be aware that during periods of emotional or physical crisis the child requires additional hormone replacement. The child should wear a Medic-Alert tag to permit medical personnel to adjust requirements during emergency care.

CUSHING SYNDROME

Cushing syndrome is a characteristic group of manifestations caused by excessive circulating free cortisol. It can result from a variety of etiologies, which generally fall into one of four categories (Box 38-10).

Cushing syndrome is uncommon in children. When seen, it is often caused by excessive or prolonged steroid therapy that produces a cushingoid appearance. This condition is reversible once the steroids are gradually discontin-

Box 38-10 ETIOLOGY OF CUSHING SYNDROME

Pituitary—Cushing syndrome with adrenal hyperplasia, usually attributed to an excess of ACTH
Adrenal—Cushing syndrome with hypersecretion of glucocorticoids, generally the result of adrenocortical neoplasms
Ectopic—Cushing syndrome with autonomous secretion of ACTH, most often caused by extrapituitary neoplasms
Iatrogenic—Cushing syndrome, frequently the result of administration of large amounts of exogenous corticosteroids

ued. Abrupt withdrawal will precipitate acute adrenal insufficiency. Gradual withdrawal of exogenous supplies is necessary to allow the anterior pituitary an opportunity to secrete increasing amounts of adrenocorticotropic hormone to stimulate the adrenals to produce cortisol.

Clinical Manifestations

Because the actions of cortisol are widespread, clinical manifestations are equally profound and diverse (Table 38-2 and Fig. 38-3). Those symptoms that produce changes in physical appearance occur early in the disorder and are of considerable concern to older children. The physiologic disturbances, such as hyperglycemia, susceptibility to infection, hypertension, and hypokalemia, may have life-threatening consequences unless recognized early and treated successfully.

Diagnostic Evaluation

Several tests are helpful in confirming excess cortisol levels. They include fasting blood glucose levels for hyperglycemia, serum electrolyte levels for hypokalemia and alkalosis, 24-hour urinary levels of elevated 17-hydroxycorticoids and 17-ketosteroids, and radiographic studies of bone for evidence of osteoporosis and of the skull for enlargement of the sella turcica. Another procedure used to establish a more definitive diagnosis is the dexamethasone (cortisone) suppression test. Administration of an exogenous supply of cortisone normally suppresses adrenocorticotropic hormone production. However, in individuals with Cushing syndrome, cortisol levels remain elevated. This test is helpful in differentiating between children who are obese and those who appear to have cushingoid features.

Therapeutic Management

Treatment depends on the cause. In most cases surgical intervention involves bilateral adrenalectomy and postoperative replacement of the cortical hormones (the therapy for this is the same as that outlined for chronic adrenal insufficiency). If a pituitary tumor is found, surgical extirpation or irradiation may be chosen. In either of these instances, treatment of panhypopituitarism with replacement of growth hormone, thyroid extract, antidiuretic hormone, gonadotropins, and steroids may be necessary for an indefinite period.

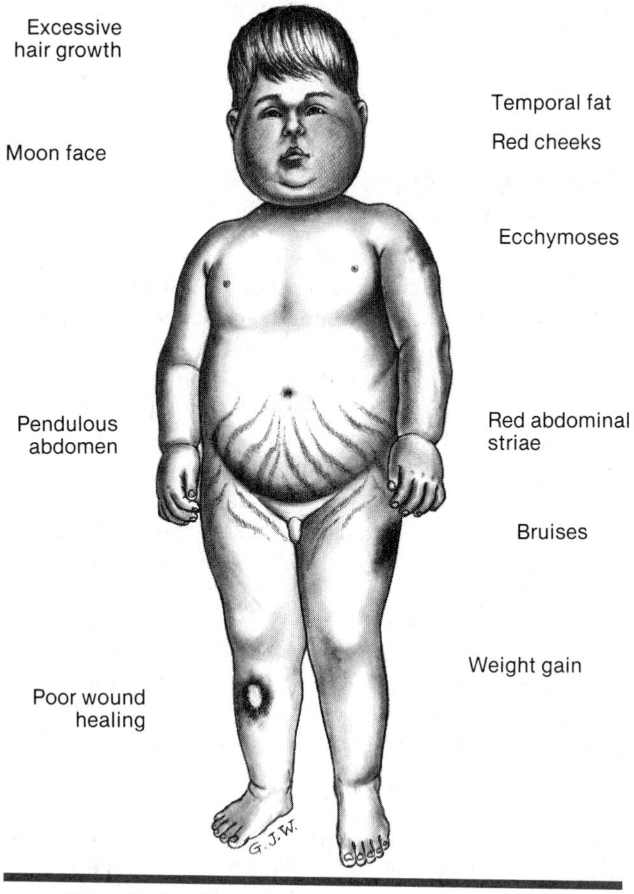

Fig. 38-3. Characteristics of Cushing syndrome.

Nursing Considerations

Nursing care also depends on the cause. When cushingoid features are caused by steroid therapy, the effects may be lessened with administration of the drug early in the morning and on an alternate-day basis. Giving the drug early in the day maintains the normal diurnal pattern of cortisol secretion. If given during the evening, it is more likely to produce symptoms because endogenous cortisol levels are already low and the additional supply exerts more pronounced effects. An alternate-day schedule allows the anterior pituitary an opportunity to maintain more normal hypothalamic-pituitary-adrenal control mechanisms.

If an organic cause is found, nursing care is related to the treatment regimen. Although a bilateral adrenalectomy permanently solves one condition, it reciprocally produces another syndrome. Before surgery parents need to be adequately informed of the operative benefits and disadvantages. Postoperative teaching regarding drug replacement is the same as discussed in the previous section.

Postoperative complications of adrenalectomy are related to the sudden withdrawal of cortisol. The nurse should observe for signs of a shocklike state, especially hypotension and hyperpyrexia. Anorexia and nausea and vomiting are very common and may be improved with the use of nasogastric decompression. Muscle and joint pain may be

Table 38-2 Clinical manifestations of Cushing syndrome

SIGNS/SYMPTOMS	PHYSIOLOGIC CAUSE	SIGNS/SYMPTOMS	PHYSIOLOGIC CAUSE
Centripetal fat distribution Truncal obesity Supraclavicular fat pads Fat pads on neck and back ("buffalo hump") Rounded or "moon" face	Increased appetite and deposition of fat	Osteoporosis Compression fractures of vertebrae Kyphosis Backache Retarded linear growth (short stature)	Increased glomerular filtration rate and excretion of calcium and decreased absorption of calcium from intestinal tract
Muscular wasting Thin extremities Pendulous abdomen Muscle weakness Thin skin and subcutaneous tissue Poor wound healing	Increased protein catabolism resulting in negative nitrogen balance	Hypercalciuria—renal calculi	
Increased susceptibility to infection Decreased inflammatory response	Decreased production and circulating levels of antibodies by lysis of fixed plasma cells and lymphocytes	Psychoses Irritability Insomnia Euphoria Depression Frank psychoses	Cause unknown
Excessive bruising Petechial hemorrhages	Capillary weakness resulting from loss of protein	Peptic ulcer	Increased production of hydrochloric acid and pepsin and decreased gastric mucus production
Facial plethora ("red cheeks") Reddish purple abdominal striae	Thin skin that allows capillary blood to be visible, increased color from polycythemia	Hyperglycemia Glycosuria	Increased gluconeogenesis by liver and decreased rate of glucose utilization by cells
Hypertension—arteriosclerosis	Increased salt and water retention (hypervolemia)	Latent or overt diabetes	Overstimulation of islets of Langerhans
Hypokalemia Alkalosis	Increased excretion of potassium and hydrogen ions	Virilization Hirsutism Acne Deepening of voice Clitoral enlargement Tendency toward male physique in female Amenorrhea Impotence	Excess production of androgens

severe, requiring use of analgesics. The psychologic depression can be profound and may not improve for months. Parents should be aware of the physiologic reasons behind these symptoms in order to be supportive of the child. Facial changes that occur rapidly often help to improve family members' disposition but may not affect the child's behavior until the child's physiologic state is stabilized.

CONGENITAL ADRENOGENITAL HYPERPLASIA

Disorders caused by excessive secretion of androgens by the adrenal cortex are known variously as *congenital adrenogenital hyperplasia (CAH), adrenocortical hyperplasia (ACH), adrenogenital syndrome (AGS),* and *congenital adrenocortical hyperplasia (CAH).* Although hyperfunction of the adrenal gland can occur from a number of causes, such as a virilizing adrenal tumor, in children the most common cause is congenital adrenogenital hyperplasia, an inborn deficiency of various enzymes necessary for the biosynthesis of cortisol. Congenital adrenogenital hyperplasia is inherited as an autosomal-recessive disorder or may result from a tumor or maternal ingestion of steroids.

Pathophysiology

Interference in the biosynthesis of cortisol during fetal life results in an increased production of adrenocorticotropic hormone, which stimulates hyperplasia of the adrenal gland. Depending on the enzymatic defect, increased quantities of cortisol precursors and androgens are secreted. There are six major types of biochemical defects. The most common is partial or complete *21-hydroxylase deficiency.* With partial deficiency, enough aldosterone is produced to preserve sodium, and adequate cortisol is produced to prevent signs of adrenocortical insufficiency.

In the complete or salt-losing form, insufficient amounts of aldosterone and cortisol are produced, so that circulatory collapse occurs without immediate replacement of the mineralocorticoids and glucocorticoids. In *11-hydroxylase deficiency* there is an increase in the mineralocorticoid 11-desoxycorticosterone, which leads to hypertension. In each of these types there is excess production of androgens, which causes ambiguous female genitalia in females and precocious genital development in males. Other forms of congenital adrenogenital hyperplasia do not result in excess production of androgens but cause various degrees of hypoaldosteronism or hyperaldosteronism.

Clinical Manifestations

Excessive androgens cause masculinization of the urogenital system during the twelfth and twentieth weeks of fetal development. The most pronounced abnormalities occur in the female, who is born with varying degrees of ambiguous genitalia (pseudohermaphroditism). Masculinization of external genitalia causes the clitoris to enlarge so that it appears as a small phallus. Fusion of the labia produces a saclike structure resembling the scrotum without testes. However, no abnormal changes occur in the internal sexual organs, although the vaginal orifice is usually closed by the fused labia (see also Aberrant Sexual Development, Chapter 11).

In the male, enlargement of the genitals (macrogenitosomia precox) and frequent erections are the principal signs. When androgen production is not excessive, virilizing effects in the female may be minimal or absent, and the male may have evidence of pseudohermaphroditism, such as microphallus, hypospadias, and incompletely fused scrotum.

Untreated congenital adrenogenital hyperplasia results in early sexual maturation, with enlargement of the external sexual organs; development of axillary, pubic, and facial hair; deepening of the voice; acne; and marked increase in musculature with changes toward an adult male physique. However, in contrast to precocious puberty, breasts do not develop in the female, and she remains amenorrheic and infertile. In the male the testes remain small, and spermatogenesis does not occur. In both sexes linear growth is accelerated, and epiphyseal closure is premature, resulting in short stature by the end of puberty.

Diagnostic Evaluation

Clinical diagnosis is initially based on congenital abnormalities that lead to difficulty in assigning sex to the newborn and on signs and symptoms of adrenal insufficiency or hypertension. Definitive diagnosis is confirmed by evidence of increased 17-ketosteroid levels in most types of congenital adrenogenital hyperplasia. Usually the level of 17-hydroxycorticoids is low or near normal. In complete 21-hydroxylase deficiency, blood electrolytes demonstrate loss of sodium and chloride and elevation of potassium. In older children bone age is advanced, and linear growth is increased. Chromosome typing for positive sex determination and to rule out any other genetic abnormality (e.g., Turner syndrome) is always done in any case of ambiguous genitalia.

Another test that can be used to visualize the presence of pelvic structures is ultrasonography, a noninvasive, painless imaging technique that does not require anesthesia or sedation. It is especially useful in congenital adrenogenital hyperplasia because it readily identifies the absence or presence of female reproductive organs in a newborn or child with ambiguous genitalia. Because it yields immediate results, it has the advantage of determining the child's gender long before the more complex laboratory results for chromosomal analysis or steroid levels are available.

Therapeutic Management

The initial medical objective is to confirm the diagnosis and assign a sex to the child, usually according to the genotype. In both sexes cortisone is administered to suppress the abnormally high secretions of adrenocorticotropic hormone. If this is begun early enough, it is very effective. Cortisone depresses the secretion of adrenocorticotropic hormone by the adenohypophysis, which in turn inhibits the secretion of adrenocorticosteroids, which stems the progressive virilization. The signs and symptoms of masculinization in the female gradually disappear, and excessive early linear growth is slowed. Puberty occurs normally at the appropriate age.

The recommended oral dosage is divided to simulate the normal diurnal pattern of adrenocorticotropic hormone secretion. Since these children are unable to produce cortisol in response to stress, it is necessary to increase the dosage during episodes of infection, fever, or other stresses. Acute emergencies require immediate intravenous or intramuscular administration. Emergency situations include bacterial and viral infections, vomiting, surgery, fractures, major injuries, and sometimes insect stings. Children with the salt-losing type of congenital adrenogenital hyperplasia require aldosterone replacement, as outlined under chronic adrenal insufficiency, and supplementary dietary salt. Frequent laboratory tests are conducted to assess the effects on electrolytes, hormonal profiles, and renin levels. These are tapered from weekly, to every 2 weeks, to monthly, then every 3 months.

Depending on the degree of masculinization in the female, reconstructive surgery may be required to reduce the size of the clitoris, separate the labia, and create a vaginal orifice. This should be done after the infant is physically able to withstand the procedure and before she is old enough to be aware of the abnormal genitalia. Plastic surgery is generally done in stages and yields excellent cosmetic results. Reports concerning sexual satisfaction after partial clitoridectomy indicate that the capacity for orgasm and sexual gratification is not necessarily impaired.

Unfortunately not all children with congenital adrenogenital hyperplasia are diagnosed at birth and raised in accordance with their genetic sex. Particularly in the case of affected females, masculinization of the external genitalia may have led to sex assignment as a male. In males diagnosis is usually delayed until early childhood, when signs of virilism appear. In these situations it is advisable to continue rearing the child as a male in accordance with assigned sex and phenotype. Hormonal replacement may be required to permit linear growth and to initiate male pubertal changes. Surgery is usually indicated to remove the female organs and reconstruct the phallus for satisfactory sexual relations. These individuals are not fertile.

Nursing Considerations

Of major importance is recognition of ambiguous genitalia in newborns. If there is any question regarding assignment of sex, the parents need to be told immediately to prevent the embarrassing situation of informing family members of the child's sex and then having to change the announcement. As with any congenital defect, the parents require an adequate explanation of the condition and a period of time to grieve for the loss of perfection. In this instance they may also need to grieve for the loss of the desired-sex child. For example, the birth of a phenotypically male infant may fulfill their wish for a son. Knowledge of the child's actual sex may leave them disappointed. Such situations may also lead them to discuss the possibility of raising the child as a male despite the actual sex. This is a difficult question that requires thoughtful discussion among the parents and members of the health team.

In general, rearing the genetically female child as a female is preferred because of the success of surgical intervention and the satisfactory results with hormones in reversing virilism and providing a prospect of normal puberty and the ability to conceive. This is in contrast to the choice of rearing the child as a male, in which case the child is sterile and may never be able to function satisfactorily in heterosexual relationships. If the parents persist in their decision to assign a male sex to a genetically female child, a psychologic consultation should be requested to explore their motivations and ensure their understanding of the child's future consequences.

Parents need an explanation regarding this disorder that facilitates their explaining it to others. Before confirmation of the diagnosis and sex of the child, the nurse should refer to the infant as "child" or "baby" rather than "he" or "she" and definitely not "it." When referring to the external genitalia, it is preferable to refer to them as sex organs and to emphasize the similarity between the penis/clitoris and scrotum/labia during fetal development. In this way it can be explained that the sex organs were overdeveloped because of too much male hormone secretion. Using a correct vocabulary allows parents to explain the abnormalities to others in a straightforward manner, just as if the defect involved the heart or an extremity.

It is also important to stress that sex assignment and rearing depend on psychosocial influences, not on genetic sex hormonal influences during fetal life. Parents often fear that the infant will retain "male behavioral characteristics" because of prenatal masculinization and will not be able to develop female characteristics. Using the word "hermaphrodite" often confuses parents because they interpret this term to mean that the child is "half male–half female." Since the prognosis for normal sexual development is excellent after early treatment, the nurse should foster identification with the child as one sex only. It is also beneficial to mention that ambiguous genitalia have no relationship with homosexual or bisexual activity later in life.

As soon as the sex is determined, parents should be informed of the findings and encouraged to choose an appropriate name, and the child should be identified as a male or female, with no reference to ambiguous sex. If the appearance of the enlarged genitalia in a female child concerns the parents, they should be encouraged to discuss their feelings. Suggesting ways to avoid questioning remarks from visitors, such as diapering the child in a separate room, is also helpful. If surgery is anticipated, showing parents before and after photographs of reconstruction helps to reinforce the expected cosmetic benefits.

Nursing considerations regarding cortisol and aldosterone replacement are the same as those that are discussed for chronic adrenocortical insufficiency. However, since parents may be overwhelmed with the diagnosis and obvious abnormalities at the time of birth, they may not hear all the discharge instructions regarding the medication schedule. A follow-up visit by a public health nurse may be desirable to ensure that parents understand and comply with the treatment regimen. Likewise, nurses in well-child facilities should assume responsibility for guidance and supervision regarding this aspect of care during each visit.

Since infants are especially prone to dehydration and salt-losing crises, parents need to be aware of signs of dehydration and the urgency of immediate medical intervention to stabilize the child's condition. Parents, and later the child, need to understand that the medical regimen must be a lifelong commitment; therefore, they should be provided with the education and counseling that is most likely to ensure informed and willing compliance. They also need to know that growth retardation that may have occurred before therapy cannot be overcome and that normal stature is not a realistic expectation, even though growth velocity may improve with medication. The parents are also taught to give necessary injections (see Chapter 27).*

In the unfortunate situation in which the sex is erroneously assigned and the correct sex determined later, parents need a great deal of help in understanding the reason for the incorrect sex identification and the options for sex reassignment and/or medical/surgical intervention. Since children become aware of their sexual identity by 18 months to 2 years of age, it is believed that any reassignment after this period can cause tremendous psychologic conflicts in the child. Therefore sex rearing should be continued as previously established with medical/surgical intervention as required.

A dilemma often arises, however, regarding what these children should know about their condition, especially gender identification. Because the knowledge that one has been reared opposite to the genetic gender can initiate profound psychologic problems, it is recommended that children not be told this fact but rather be given an explanation regarding their physical disabilities, such as infertility, and the need for hormone replacement and plastic surgery. Parents, in turn, must believe that these children have been raised according to their "true sex," which is absolutely honest, since sex is not solely a biologic entity but an expression of multiple environmental influences.

Since the hereditary form of adrenogenital hyperplasia is an autosomal-recessive disorder, parents should be referred for genetic counseling before conceiving another child. The nurse's role is to ensure that parents understand the proba-

*Home care instructions are available in Wong, D.L., and Whaley, L.F.: Clinical manual of pediatric nursing, ed. 3, St. Louis, 1990, Mosby–Year Book Inc.

bility of transmitting the trait or disorder with each pregnancy. Affected offspring also require genetic counseling, since both sexes are generally able to reproduce. (See Chapter 5 for recurrence risks and genetic counseling.)

HYPERALDOSTERONISM

Excessive secretion of aldosterone may be caused by an adrenal tumor or, in some types of adrenogenital syndromes, may be the result of enzymatic deficiency. The signs and symptoms are caused by increased sodium levels, water retention, and potassium loss. Hypervolemia causes hypertension and resultant headaches. Paradoxically, funduscopic changes resulting from increased blood pressure and edema from water retention are minimal. Hypokalemia results in muscular weakness, paresthesia, episodes of paralysis, and tetany and may be responsible for polyuria and consequent polydipsia.

The clinical diagnosis is suspected when there are findings of hypertension, hypokalemia, and polyuria that fail to respond to antidiuretic hormone administration. Renin and angiotensin titers are abnormally low. Urinary levels of 17-hydroxycorticosteroids and 17-ketosteroids are normal in primary hyperaldosteronism caused by an aldosterone-secreting tumor but are usually abnormal in adrenogenital syndrome.

Therapeutic Management

Temporary treatment of the disorder involves replacement of potassium and administration of spironolactone (Aldactone), a diuretic that blocks the effects of aldosterone, thereby promoting excretion of sodium and water while preserving potassium. Definitive treatment is similar to that for chronic adrenocortical insufficiency.

Nursing Considerations

An important nursing consideration is recognition of the syndrome, particularly in children who demonstrate high blood pressure. Other clues include bed-wetting, excessive thirst, and unexplained weakness. After the diagnosis, nursing care should be related to the treatment regimen. If diuretics are used, they should be administered in the morning to avoid accidents during the night. Children need unrestricted lavatory privileges at school. Potassium supplements should be mixed with fruit juice to increase their acceptability, and potassium-rich foods should be encouraged. Parents need to be aware of the signs of hypokalemia and hyperkalemia.

After an adrenalectomy, nursing care is similar to that for chronic adrenocortical insufficiency.

PHEOCHROMOCYTOMA

Pheochromocytoma is an adrenal tumor characterized by secretion of catecholamines. The tumor most commonly ...es from the chromaffin cells of the adrenal medulla but ...ccur wherever these cells are found, such as along ...anglia of the aorta or thoracolumbar sympathetic ...oximately 10% of these tumors are located in extraadrenal sites. In children they are frequently bilateral or multiple and are generally benign. Often there is a familial transmission of the condition as an autosomal-dominant trait that tends to favor males.

Clinical Manifestations

The clinical manifestations of pheochromocytoma are caused by an increased production of catecholamines, producing hypertension, tachycardia, headache, decreased gastrointestinal activity with resultant constipation, increased metabolism with anorexia, weight loss, hyperglycemia, polyuria, polydipsia, hyperventilation, nervousness, and diaphoresis. In severe cases signs of congestive heart failure are evident.

Diagnostic Evaluation

The clinical manifestations mimic those of other disorders, such as hyperthyroidism, diabetes mellitus, or functional hyperventilation. Therefore several tests specific to these conditions may be performed as part of the differential diagnosis. In only a small number of instances is a palpable tumor suggestive of the diagnosis. Definitive tests include measurement of urinary levels of the catecholamine metabolites, histamine stimulation, which will provoke a hypertensive attack from sudden release of large amounts of catecholamines, and alpha-blocking agents, which will produce a hypotensive episode by inhibiting the action of circulating catecholamines.

Therapeutic Management

Definitive treatment consists of surgical removal of the tumor. In children the tumors may be bilateral, requiring a bilateral adrenalectomy and lifelong glucocorticoid and mineralocorticoid therapy. The major complications that can occur during surgery are severe hypertension, tachyarrhythmias, and hypotension. The first two are caused by excessive release of catecholamines during manipulation of the tumor, and the latter from catecholamine withdrawal and hypovolemic shock (New, Levine, and Temeck, 1986).

Preoperative preparation is implemented beginning 1 to 3 weeks before surgery to prevent these complications. This consists of medication to inhibit the effects of catecholamines. The major group of drugs used is the α-adrenergic blocking agents with or without β-adrenergic blocking agents. The most commonly used α-adrenergic blocker is phenoxybenzamine (Dibenzyline), a longer-acting medication given orally every 12 hours. The shorter-acting phentolamine (Regitine) is equally effective but less satisfactory for long-term use, although it is useful for acute hypertension. To control catecholamine release when α-adrenergic blocking agents are inadequate, the child is given β-adrenergic blocking agents.

Success of therapy is judged by lowering of blood pressure to normal, absence of hypertensive attacks (flushing or blanching, fainting, headache, palpitations, tachycardia, nausea and vomiting, profuse sweating), decrease in perspiration, and disappearance of hyperglycemia. A disadvantage of these drugs is their inability to block the effects of catecholamines on beta-receptors.

Nursing Considerations

An initial nursing objective is identification of children with this disorder. Outstanding clues are hypertension and hypertensive attacks. Because of behavioral changes (nervousness, excitability, overactivity, even psychosis), increased cardiac and respiratory activity may appear to be related to an acute anxiety attack. Therefore a careful history of the onset of symptoms and association with stressful events is helpful in distinguishing between an organic and a psychologic cause for the symptoms.

Preoperative nursing care involves frequent monitoring of vital signs and observing for evidence of hypertensive attacks and congestive heart failure. Therapeutic effects are evidenced by normal vital signs and absence of glycosuria. Daily blood glucose levels, urine acetone, and any signs of hyperglycemia are noted and reported immediately.

The environment is made conducive to rest and free of emotional stress. This requires adequate preparation during hospital admission and before surgery. Parents are encouraged to room-in with their child and to participate in daily care. Play activities need to be tailored to the child's energy level but not be overly strenuous or challenging, since these can increase metabolic rate and promote frustration and anxiety.

After surgery the child is usually admitted to the PICU for 2 to 3 days postoperatively to observe and monitor for signs of shock from removal of excess catecholamines. If a bilateral adrenalectomy was performed, the nursing interventions are those discussed for chronic adrenocortical insufficiency.

DISORDERS OF PANCREATIC HORMONE SECRETION

The islets of Langerhans of the pancreas have three major functioning cells: the alpha cells, which produce glucagon, the beta cells, which produce insulin, and the delta cells, which produce somatostatin. Glucagon causes an increase in the blood glucose by stimulating the liver and other cells to release stored glucose (glycogenolysis). Glucagon acts as an emergency supplier of glucose whenever the blood glucose falls too low and is believed to function more independently when insulin is lacking. Somatostatin, although secreted by the islet cells, is found in greater supply in the hypothalamus, where it prevents the release of growth hormone. In the islets of Langerhans somatostatin is believed to regulate the release of insulin and glucagon. This discussion of disorders of pancreatic hormone secretion is limited to diabetes mellitus.

DIABETES MELLITUS

Diabetes mellitus (DM) is a chronic disorder of metabolism characterized by a deficiency (relative or absolute) of the hormone insulin. It is the most common metabolic disease, resulting in metabolic adjustment or physiologic change in almost all areas of the body. DM affects approximately 10 to 12 million persons in the United States, and although estimates of prevalence in the United States vary, most sources report a rate of 1.2 to 1.9 cases per 1000 children and adolescents (Plotnick, 1990).

The disease is rarely diagnosed in infancy, and children younger than school age have a lower incidence of the disease than school-age children. The peak incidence is reached during early adolescence and then declines through the remainder of adolescence. It can be manifest at any age, but over 80% of diagnosed cases are in the adult population; therefore, the older the individual, the greater the chance of developing some type of diabetes.

DM is more prominent in whites and rare in African blacks, Asians, Native Americans, and Eskimos. The incidence in black Americans corresponds with the percentage of white genes in the black population (MacDonald, 1983).

Classification

DM can be classified as *idiopathic* or *secondary*. Secondary DM can be precipitated by exogenous factors and is usually (but not always) reversible when the primary disorder is treated. These include pancreatic trauma, disease (cystic fibrosis, carcinoma), or resection; hormones (Cushing syndrome, primary aldosteronism, pheochromocytoma), drugs or chemicals (some diuretics, hormones, psychoactive agents, catecholamines, antineoplastic agents); insulin receptor abnormalities; and a variety of genetic syndromes that are associated with glucose intolerance or frank diabetes. Gestational diabetes is the appearance of DM or abnormalities of glucose tolerance for the first time during pregnancy.

Idiopathic DM can be classified into two major groups and one newly described type (Box 38-11), and characteristics of insulin-dependent DM (IDDM) and non-insulin-dependent DM (NIDDM) are outlined in Table 38-3. Because DM of childhood is, with few exceptions, the IDDM, or type I form, the remainder of the discussion is devoted to this important cause of long-term health problems. However, NIDDM is included as appropriate for comparison throughout.

Box 38-11 CLASSIFICATION OF DIABETES MELLITUS

Insulin-dependent (IDDM), or type I—characterized by catabolism and the development of ketosis in the absence of insulin replacement therapy; onset is typically in childhood and adolescence but can be at any age

Non-insulin-dependent (NIDDM), or type II—appears to involve resistance to insulin action and defective glucose-mediated insulin secretion; onset is usually after age 40, and there appears to be considerable heterogeneity; affected persons may or may not require daily insulin injections

Maturity-onset diabetes of youth (MODY)—transmitted as an autosomal dominant disorder in which there is formation of structurally abnormal insulin that has decreased biologic activity

Table 38-3 Comparison of characteristics of types I and II diabetes mellitus

CHARACTERISTIC	TYPE I (IDDM)	TYPE II (NIDDM)
Age on onset	Less than 20 years	Over 40 years
Type of onset	Abrupt	Gradual
Sex ratio	No sex difference	Females outnumber males
Percentage of population	5%-8%	85%-90%
Heredity:		
Family history	Sometimes	Frequency
HLA	Associations	No associations
Twin concordance	25%-50%	90%-100%
Ethnic distribution	Primarily whites	Common to all, especially American Indians
Presenting symptoms	Three Ps* common	May be none
Nutritional status	Underweight	Overweight
Insulin (natural):		
Pancreatic content	Usually 0	Over 50% normal
Serum insulin	Low to absent	High or low
Primary resistance	Minimum	Marked
Islet cell antibodies	80%-85%	Less than 5%
Metabolic control	Difficult	Usually easy
Stability	Unstable	Stable
Therapy:		
Insulin	Always	20%-30% of patients
Oral agents	Ineffective	Often effective
Diet only	Ineffective	Often effective
Chronic complications	Greater than 80%	Variable
Ketoacidosis	Common	Infrequent

*Polyuria, polydipsia, and polyphagia.

Etiology

The clinical syndrome of DM results from a large variety of etiologic and pathogenic mechanisms. IDDM is now believed to be an autoimmune disease that arises when a person with a genetic predisposition is exposed to a precipitating event, usually a viral infection. NIDDM is more likely to be influenced by stronger, but as yet unknown, genetic factors.

Genetic factors. IDDM is not inherited, but heredity is unquestioned as a prominent factor in the etiology. There are more than 40 rare genetic syndromes of which diabetes is a major feature (Nora and Fraser, 1989). No simple Mendelian pattern is found for DM. A variety of genetic mechanisms have been proposed, but it appears that susceptibility to DM depends on a locus within the human lymphocyte antigen (HLA) complex. The HLA alleles are situated on the number 6 chromosome at the loci designated A, B, C, and D. From 8 to 30 possible antigens are coded for each locus, and some have alternate types (e.g., D and DR) or subtypes (e.g., A1, A2). HLA-DR3 appears to be transmitted in an autosomal recessive–like pattern, whereas DR4 is dominant or intermediate (Thompson and others, 1988). It is also suggested that one allele predisposes to the autoimmune form of IDDM and is DR3 associated; a second predisposes to a form with antiinsulin antibodies and is associated with DR4 (Nora and Fraser, 1989). Many persons with DR3 and DR4 antigens never develop DM. D2 and DR2 antigens seem to afford a protection against DM and are rarely found in patients with IDDM.

The genetic influence in NIDDM and IDDM appears to differ in several ways. Nearly 100% of offspring of parents who both have NIDDM develop that type of diabetes, but only 45% to 60% of the offspring of both parents who have IDDM will develop the disease. The incidence doubles with every 20% of excess weight, and this figure applies to the young as well as to the older diabetic person.

Autoimmune mechanisms. It is now accepted that antibodies to some aspect of islet tissue are regularly present at the time of diagnosis of IDDM. Pancreatic islet cell antibodies (ICAs) are found in about 70% to 85% of patients newly diagnosed with IDDM (Drash, 1989). The antibodies disappear by 1 year after diagnosis in most persons, but in some they may persist for years. The current theory is that the presence of the HLA genes causes a defect in the immune system that renders the possessor susceptible to a trigger event, which can be a virus (usually), bacteria, or a chemical irritant (Eisenbarth, 1987). In DR3-positive persons the virus invades the beta cells and initiates an autoimmune process that gradually destroys them. Without beta cells no insulin can be produced. It is unclear whether the ICAs are the result of the inflammatory process or a significant aspect of the beta cell destruction. Controversy exists regarding whether the autoimmune response is primarily mediated by the lymphocyte response or the humoral (antibody) response or is a result of the two.

There is a strong association between IDDM and other autoimmune endocrine disorders. An increased incidence of other autoimmune endocrine disorders, such as thyroiditis and Addison disease, has been found in families of children with DR3-associated IDDM.

It has also been found that anti–islet cell antibodies are detected in a number of unaffected first-degree relatives of children with IDDM (Drash, 1989). These findings offer hope of identifying persons at risk for diabetes with the eventual possibility of screening and implementation of immunotherapy. Immunosuppression therapy is controversial and has been attempted only in controlled situations with selected persons. The effects of lifelong immunosuppression must be carefully weighed against the lifelong effects of diabetes.

Viruses. A variety of viruses have been implicated as the prime environmental factor in the etiology of DM. Islet cells appear to be particularly susceptible to either direct viral damage or chemical insult. The body reacts to this damaged or changed tissue in an autoimmune phenomenon. Therefore the virus serves as a precipitating factor or "trigger." A viral etiology also helps explain the seasonal variation in the onset of DM. Although this seasonal variation is not evident in children under 5 years of age, the marked increase in older children during the winter months strongly suggests an infectious disease relationship in either the etiology or expression of diabetes in children.

Type II diabetes. Although IDDM is the predominant form of diabetes in the pediatric age-group, NIDDM, or type II diabetes, can also occur in children. NIDDM can be further classified as obese and nonobese, which are also subgrouped into those who require insulin and those who do not. The disturbed carbohydrate metabolism of NIDDM may be a result of a sluggish or insensitive secretory response in the pancreas or a defect in body tissues that requires unusual amounts of insulin, or it may be the case that the insulin secreted is rapidly destroyed, inhibited, or inactivated in affected persons.

Pathophysiology

Insulin is needed to support the metabolism of carbohydrates, fats, and proteins, primarily by facilitating the entry of these substances into the cell. Insulin is needed for the entry of glucose into the muscle and fat cells, prevention of mobilization of fats from fat cells, and storage of glucose as glycogen in the cells of liver and muscle. Insulin is not needed for the entry of glucose into nerve cells or vascular tissue. The chemical composition and molecular structure of insulin are such that it fits into receptor sites on the cell membrane. Here it initiates a sequence of poorly defined chemical reactions that alter the cell membrane to facilitate the entry of glucose into the cell and stimulate enzymatic systems outside the cell that metabolize the glucose for energy production.

With a deficiency of insulin, glucose is unable to enter the cell, and its concentration in the bloodstream increases. The increased concentration of glucose *(hyperglycemia)* produces an osmotic gradient that causes the movement of body fluid from the intracellular space to the interstitial space then to the extracellular space and into the glomerular filtrate in order to "dilute" the hyperosmolar filtrate. Normally the renal tubular capacity to transport glucose is adequate to reabsorb all the glucose in the glomerular filtrate. When the glucose concentration in the glomerular filtrate exceeds the threshold (160 to 180 mg/dl), glucose "spills" into the urine along with an osmotic diversion of water *(polyuria),* a cardinal sign of diabetes. The urinary fluid losses cause the excessive thirst *(polydipsia)* observed in diabetes. As might be expected, this water washout results in a depletion of other essential chemicals, especially potassium.

Protein is also wasted during insulin deficiency. Since glucose is unable to enter the cells, protein is broken down and converted to glucose by the liver (glucogenesis); this glucose then contributes to the hyperglycemia. These mechanisms are similar to those seen in starvation when substrate (glucose) is absent. The body is actually in a state of starvation during insulin deficiency. Without the use of carbohydrates for energy, fat and protein stores are depleted as the body attempts to meet its energy needs. The hunger mechanism is triggered, but the increased food intake *(polyphagia)* enhances the problem by further elevating the blood glucose (Fig. 38-4).

Ketoacidosis. When insulin is absent, glucose is unavailable for cellular metabolism, and the body chooses alternate sources of energy, principally fat. Consequently, fats break down into fatty acids, and glycerol in the fat cells is converted by the liver to ketone bodies (β-hydroxybutyric acid, acetoacetic acid, acetone). The ketone bodies can be used as an alternative source of fuel for glucose, but they are used in the cells at a limited rate. Any excess is eliminated in the urine (ketonuria) or the lungs (acetone breath). The ketone bodies are strong acids that lower serum pH, producing *ketoacidosis.*

Ketones are organic acids that readily produce excessive quantities of free hydrogen ions, causing a fall in plasma pH. Then chemical buffers in the plasma, principally bicarbonate, combine with the hydrogen ions to form carbonic acid, which readily dissociates into water and carbon dioxide. The respiratory system attempts to eliminate the excess carbon dioxide by increased depth and rate—Kussmaul respirations, or the hyperventilation characteristic of metabolic acidosis. The ketones are buffered by sodium and potassium in the plasma. The kidney attempts to compensate for the increased pH by increasing tubular secretion of hydrogen and ammonium ions in exchange for fixed base, thus depleting the base buffer concentration.

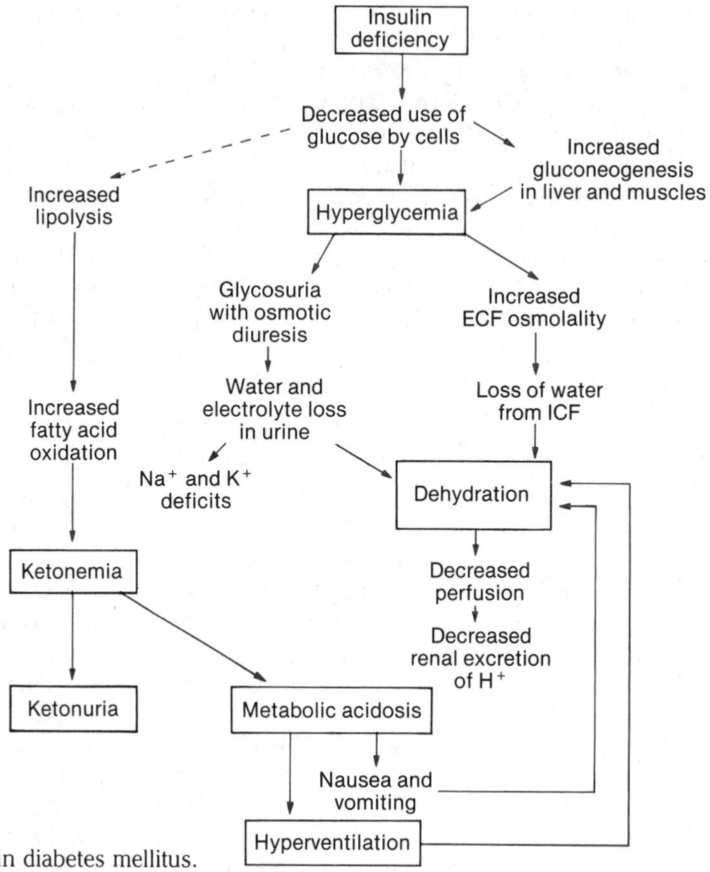

Fig. 38-4. Pathophysiology of acidosis in diabetes mellitus.

Potassium levels are also a problem and were once the cause of unexplained deaths shortly after insulin therapy was instituted. With cellular death, potassium is released from the cell into the bloodstream and excreted by the kidney where the loss is accelerated by the osmotic diuresis. The total body potassium is then decreased, even though the serum potassium level may be elevated as a result of the decreased fluid volume in which it circulates. Alteration in serum and tissue potassium can make cardiac arrest a potential problem.

If these conditions are not reversed by insulin therapy in combination with correction of the fluid deficiency and electrolyte imbalance, progressive deterioration occurs with dehydration, electrolyte imbalance, acidosis, coma, and death. Diabetic ketoacidosis should be diagnosed promptly in a seriously ill patient, and therapy instituted.

Long-term complications. Long-term complications of diabetes involve both the microvasculature and macrovasculature. The principal microvascular complications are nephropathy, retinopathy, and neuropathy. Retinopathy appears more frequently in teenage females with IDDM who have both HLA DR3 and DR4 (Malone and others, 1984). Microvascular disease develops in the first 30 years of diabetes, beginning in the first 10 to 15 years with renal involvement evidenced by proteinuria and clinically apparent retinopathy.

With poor diabetic control, vascular changes appear as early as 2½ to 3 years after diagnosis; however, with good to excellent control, changes have been postponed for 20 or more years. Changes before puberty are uncommon, but after puberty the poorer the control, the more rapid the vascular changes. The process appears to be one of *glycosylation,* wherein proteins from the blood become deposited in the walls of small vessels (e.g., glomeruli) where they become trapped by "sticky" glucose compounds (glycosyl radicals). The buildup of these substances over time causes narrowing of the vessels, with subsequent interference with microcirculation to the affected areas (Starkman and others, 1986). Macrovascular disease develops after 25 years of diabetes and creates the predominant problems in patients with NIDDM.

Other complications have been observed in children with IDDM. Hyperglycemia appears to influence thyroid function, and altered function is frequently observed at the time of diagnosis, as well as in poorly controlled diabetes. Limited mobility of small joints of the hand occurs in 30% of 7- to 18-year-old children with IDDM and appears to be related to changes in the skin and soft tissues surrounding the joint as a result of glycosylation.

Clinical Manifestations

The symptomatology of diabetes is more readily recognizable in children than in adults, so it is surprising that the diagnosis may sometimes be missed or delayed. Diabetes is a great imitator; influenza, gastroenteritis, and appendicitis are the conditions most often diagnosed, only to find that the disease was really diabetes. Diabetes should be suspected in those families with a strong family history of diabetes, especially if there is one child in the family with diabetes.

The sequence of chemical events described previously results in hyperglycemia and acidosis, which in turn produce weight loss and the three "polys" of diabetes—polyphagia, polydipsia, and polyuria—the cardinal symptoms of the disease. In NIDDM diabetes (which has also been found in older children), the insulin values are found to be elevated, 80% to 90% of this population have been found to be overweight, and fatigue and frequent infections (such as monilial infections in females) are often present.

NURSING ALERT Recurrent *Candida* is often an early sign of diabetes, especially in adolescents. *Candida* likes sugar.

The variability of clinical manifestations in IDDM at diagnosis is best understood if the autoimmune destruction of islet cells is considered an ongoing process. Symptoms of hyperglycemia may be apparent only during stress (such as an illness) in early stages of disease because of near normal levels of insulin production. Progressive islet cell destruction of later stages produces more obvious signs and symptoms. Eighty percent to 90% of islet cell function has been destroyed at the time of overt diabetic symptoms (Eisenbarth and others, 1987). Frequently identified symptoms of overt diabetes include enuresis, irritability, and unusual fatigue.

Abdominal discomfort is common. Weight loss, though quite observable on the charts, may be a less frequent presenting complaint because of the fact that the family might not have noticed the change. Another outstanding feature of diabetes is thirst. One couple reported that their child, during a trip from California to Kansas, drank the contents of a gallon jug of water between each gas station stop. As abdominal discomfort and nausea increase, the child may actually refuse fluid and food, adding to the increasing state of dehydration and malnutrition. Other symptoms include dry skin, blurred vision, and sores that are slow to heal. More commonly in children, fatigue and bed-wetting are the chief complaints that prompt parents to take their child for evaluation.

At diagnosis, the child may be *hyperglycemic,* with elevated blood glucose levels and glucose in the urine; *ketotic,* with ketones measurable in the blood and urine, with or without dehydration; or suffering from *diabetic ketoacidosis,* with dehydration, electrolyte imbalance, and acidosis.

Diagnostic Evaluation

Three groups of children who should be considered as possibly diabetic are (1) children who have glycosuria, polyuria, and a history of weight loss or failure to gain despite a voracious appetite; (2) those with transient or persistent glycosuria; and (3) those who display manifestations of metabolic acidosis, with or without stupor or coma. In every case diabetes must be considered if there is glycosuria, with or without ketonuria, in association with otherwise unexplained hyperglycemia.

Glycosuria by itself is not diagnostic of diabetes. Other sugars, such as galactose, can produce a positive Clinitest, and other conditions may cause a mild degree of glycosuria. These are infection, trauma, emotional or physical stress, hyperalimentation, and some renal or endocrine diseases.

A fasting blood sugar greater than 120 mg/dl or a random blood glucose of ≥ 200 accompanied by classic signs of diabetes is almost certain to be caused by diabetes. Postprandial blood glucose determinations and the traditional oral glucose tolerance tests have yielded low detection rates in children and are not usually necessary for establishing a diagnosis. Serum insulin levels may be normal or moderately elevated at the onset of diabetes; delayed insulin response to glucose indicates the presence of prediabetes.

Ketoacidosis must be differentiated from other causes of acidosis or coma, including hypoglycemia, uremia, gastroenteritis with metabolic acidosis, salicylate intoxication, encephalitis, and other intracranial lesions. Diabetic ketoacidosis is determined by the presence of hyperglycemia (blood glucose measurement equal to or greater than 300 mg/dl), ketonemia (strongly positive), and acidosis (pH less than 7.3 and bicarbonate less than 15 mEq/L).

Therapeutic Management

The management of the child with IDDM consists of a multidisciplinary approach involving the family, the child (when appropriate), and professionals, including a pediatrician, diabetes nurse educator, and nutritionist. Sometimes psychologic support from a mental health professional is also needed. Communication among the team members is essential and extends to other individuals in the child's life, such as teachers, the school nurse, school guidance counselor, and coach.

The definitive treatment is replacement of insulin that the child is unable to produce. However insulin needs are also affected by emotions, nutritional intake, activity, and other life events, such as illnesses and puberty. The complexity of the disease and its management requires that the child and family incorporate diabetes needs into their life-style. Medical and nutritional guidance are primary, but management also includes continuing diabetes education, family guidance, and emotional support.

Maturity-onset diabetes of youth (MODY), a form of type II diabetes with childhood onset, is usually seen in the obese teenager and can often be controlled with diet restriction.

Insulin therapy. Insulin replacement is the cornerstone of management of IDDM. Insulin dosage is tailored to each child based on home blood glucose monitoring. The goal of insulin therapy is maintaining near normal blood glucose values while avoiding too frequent episodes of hypoglycemia. Insulin is administered as two or more injections per day or as continuous subcutaneous infusion using a portable insulin pump.

Healthy pancreatic cells secrete insulin at a low but

steady basal rate with superimposed bursts of increased secretion that coincide with intake of nutriments. Consequently, insulin levels in the blood increase and decrease coincident with rises and falls in blood glucose levels. In addition, insulin is secreted directly into the portal circulation; therefore the liver, which is the major site of glucose disposal, receives the largest concentration of insulin. No matter which method of insulin replacement is used, this normal pattern cannot be duplicated. Subcutaneous injection results in absorption of the drug into the general circulation, thus reducing the concentrations of insulin to which the liver is exposed.

Insulin preparations. Insulin is available in highly purified beef, pork, and beef-pork preparations, and in human insulin manufactured by gene-splicing techniques. Human and pork varieties are less allergenic than beef preparations, and the animal insulins are less expensive than the synthetic human insulins. Insulin is available in rapid-, intermediate-, and long-acting preparations, and all are packaged in the strength of 100 U/ml. Other dosages are available when extraordinarily large or small dosages are required.

Dosage. Most children can be controlled satisfactorily with a twice-daily insulin regimen consisting of a combination of rapid-acting (regular) and intermediate-acting (NPH or Lente) insulin drawn up into the same syringe and injected before breakfast and before the evening meal. The amount of morning regular insulin is determined by the previous day's late morning and lunchtime blood glucose values. The morning intermediate-acting dosage is determined by the previous day's late afternoon and supper blood glucose values. Hence, the morning blood glucose is controlled by the previous evening dose of intermediate insulin, and the bedtime blood glucose value determines the supper dosage of regular insulin. For some children, better morning glucose control is achieved by a later (bedtime) injection of intermediate-acting insulin.

Regular insulin is best administered at least 30 minutes before meals. This allows sufficient time for absorption and results in a significantly more reduced postprandial rise in blood glucose than if the meal were eaten immediately following the insulin injection. Some authorities advocate multiple injections throughout the day rather than the twice-daily regimen, that is, a once-daily dose of long-acting (Ultralente) insulin to simulate the basal insulin secretion and injections of rapid-acting insulin before each meal. A multiple daily injection (MDI) program is particularly suitable for the child whose DM is difficult to manage.

The precise dose of insulin needed cannot be predicted. Therefore the total dosage and percentage of regular- to intermediate-acting insulin should be determined empirically for each child. Usually 60% to 75% of the total daily dose is given before breakfast, and the remainder before the evening meal. Furthermore, insulin requirements do not remain constant but change continuously during growth and development, and the need varies according to the child's activity level. For example, less insulin is required during the active spring and summer months. Illness also alters insulin requirements. Some children require more frequent insulin administration. This includes children with difficult-to-control diabetes and during the adolescent growth spurt.

Methods of administration. Daily insulin is administered subcutaneously by twice-daily injections, by multiple dose injections, or by means of a portable pump. The pump is an electromechanical device designed to deliver fixed amounts of a dilute solution of regular insulin continuously, thereby more closely imitating the release of the hormone by the islet cells. Humulin BR insulin is manufactured specifically for use with a pump.

The system consists of a syringe to hold the insulin, a plunger, and a mechanism to drive the plunger. The insulin flows from the syringe through a catheter to a needle inserted into subcutaneous tissue (the abdomen or thigh), and the lightweight device is worn on a belt or a shoulder holster. The needle and catheter are changed every 48 hours by the child or parent, using aseptic technique, and taped in place.

Although the pump provides more even insulin release, it has certain disadvantages. It cannot be removed for more than 1 hour, which limits some activities, such as bathing and swimming (it is damaged by water), and like any other mechanical device, it is subject to malfunction. Problems with abscess formation at the needle site and the need for more sophisticated control from the user have made this a rarely used option.

Researchers are experimenting with a new approach to insulin administration—intranasal. When insulin is combined with bile salts, the mixture can be administered by way of an aerosol pump. The insulin is able to cross the nasal mucosa to increase serum levels. The duration of action is not long enough to be a total replacement for injections but may be of value as insulin supplementation at mealtime. Patients are cautioned not to attempt to inhale standard insulin because it is not absorbed through the mucosa without an appropriate transport medium.

Monitoring. Monitoring the effectiveness of insulin therapy is a vital part of management. It is the only way in which to determine the amount of insulin needed by a child at any given time. Several measurements are used to evaluate the glucose levels as a basis for insulin administration and regulation.

Urine. Urine testing has been a mainstay of diabetic management in the past, but urine tests for glucose have many limitations. There is poor correlation between simultaneous glycosuria and blood glucose concentration. Even the double-voided specimens may not accurately reflect the concurrent level of blood glucose. Glucose does not appear in the urine until the blood glucose concentration is well above the optimum range. However, urine testing for ketones remains a cornerstone of home management. It is recommended that urine be tested for ketones during an illness and whenever blood glucose is 250 mg/dl or higher when measured twice in a row 4 to 6 hours apart.

Blood glucose. Home blood glucose monitoring (HBGM) has improved diabetes management and is used successfully by children from the onset of their diabetes. By testing their own blood, children are able to change their insulin regimen to maintain their glucose level in the euglycemic range of 80 to 120 mg/dl. Diabetes management depends to a great extent on home glucose monitoring. In general, children tolerate the testing well.

Glycosylated hemoglobin. The measurement of glycosylated hemoglobin (hemoglobin A_{1c}) levels is a satisfactory method for assessing the control of the difficult-to-control diabetic patient. As red blood cells circulate in the bloodstream, glucose molecules gradually attach to the hemoglobin A molecules and remain there for the lifetime of the red blood cell, approximately 120 days. The attachment is not reversible; therefore this glycosylated hemoglobin serves as a reflection of the average blood glucose levels that have taken place during the previous 2 to 3 months. The test is a satisfactory method for assessing control, detecting incorrect testing, monitoring effectiveness of changes in treatment, defining patients' goals, and detecting nonadherence.

Nutrition. Essentially the nutritional needs of children with diabetes are no different from those of healthy children, except for deletion of concentrated sugar. Children with diabetes need no special foods or supplements. They need sufficient calories to balance daily expenditure for energy and to satisfy the requirement for growth and development. Unlike the healthy child whose insulin is secreted in response to food intake, insulin injected subcutaneously has a relatively predictable time of onset, peak effect, duration of action, and absorption rate depending on the type of insulin used. Consequently, the timing of food consumption must be regulated to correspond to the time and action of the insulin prescribed.

Meals and snacks must be eaten at the same times each day, and the total number of calories and proportions of basic nutrients must be consistent from day to day. The constant release of insulin into the circulation makes the child prone to hypoglycemia between the three daily meals unless a snack is provided between meals and at bedtime. The distribution of calories should be calculated to fit the activity pattern of each child. For example, a child who is more active in the afternoon will need the larger snack at that time. This larger snack might also be split to allow some food at school and some food after school. Alterations in food intake should be made so that food, insulin, and exercise are balanced. Extra food is needed for increased activity.

The food intake may be planned in a variety of ways but is based on a balanced diet that incorporates six basic food groups: milk, meat, vegetables, fat, fruit, and starch. The family may follow the exchange system approved by the American Diabetes Association (ADA) or the point system, based on 75 kcal equaling 1 point. The exchange system indicates the amount (portion size) of each food by volume or weight and is prescribed in terms of the number of exchanges from each food group that constitutes each meal and snack. This ensures day-to-day consistency in total calories, protein, fat, and carbohydrate while allowing a choice from a wide variety of foods.

Concentrated sweets are eliminated and, because of the increased risk for atherosclerosis in persons with DM, fat is reduced to 30% or less of the total caloric requirement. Dietary fiber has become increasingly important in dietary planning because of its influence on digestion, absorption, and metabolism of many nutrients. It has been found to diminish the rise in blood sugar after meals.

Correctly used, the diet allows for flexibility and the incorporation of preferred foods in most instances. For the growing child, food restriction should never be used for diabetic control, although calorie restrictions may be imposed for weight control if the child is overweight. In general, the child's appetite should be the guide for the amount of calories needed, with the total calorie intake adjusted to appetite and activity. Basic principles of diet management are outlined in Box 38-12.

Box 38-12 NUTRITIONAL PRINCIPLES IN TYPE I DIABETES

1. Develop a basic daily meal plan that is relatively consistent in terms of:
   - Total energy (calorie) intake
   - Balance of energy-yielding nutrients (carbohydrates, fats, and proteins)
2. Provide for compensatory changes for nonbasal circumstances:
   - Extra food for extra activity
   - Extra insulin or activity for extra food
3. Avoid hyperglycemia by:
   - Omitting rapidly absorbed simple sugars from regular meal planning
4. Avoid hypoglycemia by:
   - Reasonably consistent meal timing
   - Provision of snacks

From Skyler, J.S.: Dietary planning in insulin-dependent diabetes mellitus, Pediatr. Ann. 12:652-657, 1983.

Exercise. Exercise is encouraged and never restricted unless indicated by other health conditions. Exercise lowers blood sugar levels, depending on the intensity and duration of the activity. Consequently, exercise should be included as part of diabetic management, and the type and amount of exercise should be planned around the child's interests and capabilities. However, in most instances children's activities are unplanned, and the resulting decrease in blood sugar can be compensated for by providing extra snacks before (and, if prolonged, during) the activity. Insulin should not be reduced unless the needed increase in food cannot be tolerated. In addition to a feeling of well-being, regular exercise aids in utilization of food and often results in a reduction of insulin requirements.

Physical training tends to increase tissue sensitivity to insulin, even in the resting state. Consequently, it is especially important to understand the relationship between the activity and the diabetic regimen. Vigorous muscular contraction increases regional blood flow and accelerates the absorption and circulation of insulin that is injected into the area, which can contribute to development of hypoglycemia. If exercise involving leg muscles is planned, it is recommended that nonexercised sites (arm or abdomen) should be used for insulin injection. This practice may replace the need for further increased carbohydrate intake or reduced insulin dose (or both) to avoid exercise-induced hypoglycemia.

Children with poorly controlled diabetes are particularly at risk for hypoglycemia with exercise or may actually stimulate ketoacid production. Therefore the child who has marked hyperglycemia and ketonuria should be discouraged from strenuous physical activity until satisfactory control of the diabetes is achieved by appropriate adjustments of insulin and diet (Wolfsdorf, 1986).

Athletes and those youngsters who regularly participate in organized sports are advised to adjust their insulin dosage in anticipation of sustained physical activity during the part of the day devoted to strenuous exercise. For example, the morning dose of intermediate-acting insulin may need to be reduced to compensate for after-school sports activity. Optimum adjustments for each child are determined primarily by trial and error. Nutritional needs of the athlete are subject to those dietary needs discussed for sports participation in Chapter 39, as well as the diabetic dietary management.

Hypoglycemia. Occasional episodes of hypoglycemia are an integral part of insulin therapy, and an objective of diabetic management is to achieve the best possible glycemic control while minimizing the frequency and severity of hypoglycemia. Even with good control, a child may frequently experience mild symptoms of hypoglycemia. If the signs and symptoms are recognized early and promptly relieved by appropriate therapy, the child's activity should be interrupted for no more than a few minutes.

The most common causes of hypoglycemia are bursts of physical activity without additional food, or delayed, omitted, or incompletely consumed meals. Sometimes the reaction from sustained exercise may occur several hours after the exercise. Occasionally hypogylcemic reactions occur unexpectedly and without apparent cause. They may be the result of an inadvertent or deliberate error in insulin administration.

Gastroenteritis, in which there is a gastric stasis, may impede the absorption of food, even though the child is eating reasonably well. It can also occur when the blood glucose level is so low it causes stasis. Then the child may eat a meal or snack and still have an insulin reaction. Continued feeding does not seem to alter the blood glucose level, because the simple glucose or sugar remains in the stomach.

The signs and symptoms of hypoglycemia are caused by both increased adrenergic activity and impaired brain function. The increased adrenergic nervous system activity plus increased secretion of catecholamines produce nervousness, pallor, tremulousness, palpitations, sweating, and hunger. Weakness, dizziness, headache, drowsiness, irritability, loss of coordination, convulsions, and coma are more severe responses and reflect central nervous system glucose deprivation and the body's attempts to elevate the serum glucose levels (Fig. 38-5).

It is often difficult to distinguish between hyperglycemia and a hypoglycemic reaction (Table 38-4). Since the symptoms are similar and usually begin with changes in behavior, the simplest way to differentiate between the two is to test the blood glucose level. Blood glucose is low in hypoglycemia, whereas in hyperglycemia the glucose content will be significantly elevated. Urinary ketones may be present following hypoglycemia due to starvation ketone production. In doubtful situations it is safer to give the child some simple carbohydrate. This will help alleviate the symptoms in the case of hypoglycemia but will do little harm if the child is hyperglycemic.

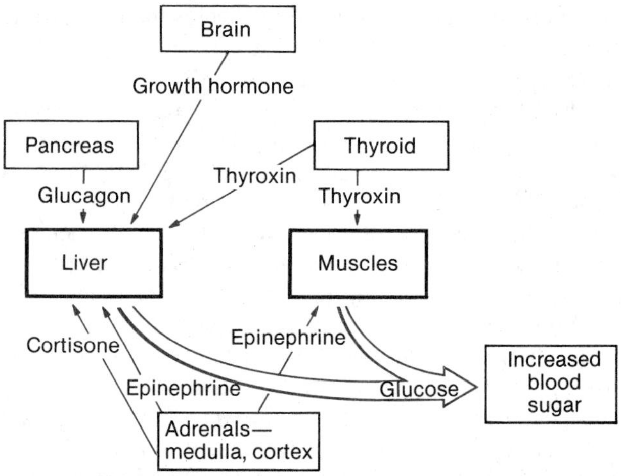

Fig. 38-5. Body systems respond to hypoglycemia in various ways to increase blood sugar level.

Children are usually able to detect the onset of hypoglycemia, but some are too young to implement treatment. Parents should become adept at recognizing the onset of symptoms—for example, a change in a child's behavior such as tearfulness or euphoria. In the majority of cases, 10 to 15 g of simple carbohydrate, such as honey, will elevate the blood glucose level and alleviate the symptoms. The simpler the carbohydrate, the more rapidly it will be absorbed (8 oz milk = 15 g carbohydrate). The rapid-releasing sugar is followed by a complex carbohydrate such as a slice of bread or a cracker.

For a mild reaction, milk or fruit juice is a good food to use in children. Milk supplies them with lactose or milk sugar, as well as a more prolonged action from the protein and fat (aids in decreased absorption). Other glucose sources include Insta-glucose (cherry-flavored glucose), carbonated drink (not sugarless), sherbet, gelatin, cottage cheese, or cake icing. All children with diabetes should carry with them glucose tabs, Insta-glucose, or sugar-containing candy, such as Life Savers or Charms, or some sugar cubes. A difficulty with candies or icing is that the child may learn to fake a reaction to get the sweets; therefore, Insta-glucose is the preferred treatment.

It is better to overtreat than to undertreat, but overtreatment should be kept to a minimum whenever possible. The treatment may be repeated in 10 to 15 minutes if the initial response is not satisfactory. With positive response to the simple carbohydrate, the pulse rate should show a noticeable change in 2 to 3 minutes. Rest and the addition of food should be part of the plan.

An insulin reaction is often the most feared aspect of diabetes, since severe brain symptoms may develop. In a se-

Table 38-4 Comparison of manifestations of hypoglycemia and hyperglycemia

VARIABLE	HYPOGLYCEMIA	HYPERGLYCEMIA
Onset	Rapid (minutes)	Gradual (days)
Mood	Labile, irritable, nervous, weepy	Lethargic
Mental status	Difficulty concentrating, speaking, focusing, coordinating	Dulled sensorium Confused
Inward feeling	Shaky feeling, hunger Headache Dizziness	Thirst Weakness Nausea/vomiting Abdominal pain
Skin	Pallor Sweating	Flushed Signs of dehydration
Mucous membranes	Normal	Dry, crusty
Respirations	Shallow	Deep, rapid (Kussmaul)
Pulse	Tachycardia	Less rapid, weak
Breath odor	Normal	Fruity, acetone
Neurologic	Tremors Late: hyperreflexia, dilated pupils, convulsion	Diminished reflexes Paresthesia
Ominous signs	Shock, coma	Acidosis, coma
Blood:		
Glucose	Low: below 60 mg/dl	High: 250 mg/dl or more
Ketones	Negative/trace	High/large
Osmolarity	Normal	High
pH	Normal	Low (7.25 or less)
Hematocrit	Normal	High
HCO_3	Normal	Less than 20 mEq/L
Urine:		
Output	Normal	Polyuria (early) to oliguria (late)
Sugar	Negative	High
Acetone	Negative/trace	High

vere reaction the various areas of the brain respond in sequence: the forebrain with increased drowsiness and perspiration, the hypothalamus and thalamus with tachycardia and loss of consciousness, the midbrain with seizure activity that may be started from stimulation initially from the hypothalamus, and finally the hindbrain with responses of deeper coma and decreasing reflexes. The treatment of choice for severe hypoglycemia is 50% glucose administered intravenously.

Glucagon is sometimes prescribed for home treatment of hypoglycemia. It is packaged as an emergency kit containing a prefilled syringe of diluent and a vial of powder. When reconstituted, the diluent syringe is used to inject the glucagon. It is administered intramuscularly or subcutaneously. It functions by releasing stored glycogen from the liver and requires about 15 to 20 minutes to elevate the blood glucose level. Once the child is responsive, the lost glycogen stores are replaced by small amounts of sugar-containing fluid administered frequently until the child feels comfortable about trying solid foods.

Somogyi effect. Somogyi effect should be recognized as a separate response and can be a cause of poor glycemic control. This phenomenon is a physiologic reflex response to a decreased blood glucose level, which results in release of counterregulatory hormones (epinephrine, growth hormone, and corticosteroids) and a rebound hyperglycemia. The condition should be suspected in children whose blood or urine glucose levels are high and who are receiving a relatively large dose of insulin. More frequent blood monitoring (especially at times of anticipated peak insulin action) will usually identify this condition. Trace amounts of urinary ketones aid in identifying undetected hypoglycemia. Treatment consists of increasing the amount of food eaten and/or decreasing the insulin. Hyperglycemia and glycosuria will subside as hypoglycemia and the counterregulatory hormonal response subside.

Illness management. Illness alters diabetes management, and maintaining control is usually related to the seriousness of the illness. In the well-controlled child an illness will run its course as it does in the unaffected child. The goal during an illness is to maintain some euglycemia while recognizing and treating urinary ketones. Frequent monitoring of blood glucose and urine for ketones is important. Some hyperglycemia and ketonuria are expected in most illnesses, even with diminished food intake, and are an indication for increased insulin. Insulin should never be omitted during an illness, although dosage requirements may increase, decrease, or remain unchanged, depending on the severity of the illness and the child's appetite. In the presence of nausea or decreased appetite, simple carbohydrates may be substituted for carbohydrate-containing exchanges in the meal plan. Fluids are encouraged to prevent dehydration and to flush out ketones.

New data support the concept that life expectancy in the child with diabetes is lengthened if the body is maintained in as normal a physiologic state as possible. Promotion of good health, a balance of adequate rest and exercise, and good nutrition along with close management of the disease will allow the person with diabetes to live as long as, if not longer than, the person without the disease who may not develop health and nutrition habits as good as those of the properly managed person with DM.

Surgery. The physiologic and emotional stresses related to surgery require careful adjustment of insulin. Since the child receives intravenous glucose during surgery and the stress of the surgery itself will also raise the blood glucose level, the risk of an insulin reaction is very slight. Regular insulin should be continued until the child is able to tolerate oral feedings and a return to the routine pattern of insulin administration.

Islet cell transplantation. There has been some experimentation with islet cell transplants. Viable insulin-producing cells are injected into the portal vein where they take root in the liver and eventually produce up to two thirds of the needed insulin. Some persons have received whole pancreas transplants and need no insulin supplementation. However, because it is an allograft, persons receiving islet cell transplants require immunosuppression, which in itself is a risk factor. The major use of transplants has been in persons who have serious complications, particularly those whose deteriorating kidneys have required renal transplants and who are necessarily on immunosuppression. Islet transplants may eventually be made more effective and possible without the need for powerful immunosuppressants.

Prevention. Major advances have been made in the ability to detect susceptibility of IDDM, and animal studies indicate that the disease can be prevented by various immunologic interventions (Bach, 1987). Recent sources also indicate that early immunosuppression may preserve long-term endogenous insulin secretion in individuals with IDDM. Cyclosporine, used extensively in transplant patients, continues to undergo trials in newly diagnosed patients with diabetes. Its administration has achieved short-term control in some patients (Stiller and others, 1987). However, long-term effects are unknown, and it is questionable whether long-term dependence on the drug is of greater benefit than long-term dependence on insulin.

Therapeutic Management: Diabetic Ketoacidosis

Diabetic ketoacidosis (DKA), the most complete state of insulin deficiency, is a life-threatening situation. Management consists of rapid assessment, adequate insulin to reduce the elevated blood glucose level, fluids to overcome dehydration, and electrolyte replacement (especially potassium and bicarbonate).

Diabetic ketoacidosis constitutes an emergency situation; therefore the child should be admitted to an intensive care facility for management. The priority is to obtain a venous access for administration of fluids, electrolytes, and insulin. The child should be weighed, measured, and placed on a cardiac monitor. Blood glucose and ketone levels are determined at the bedside, and samples obtained for laboratory measurements of glucose, electrolytes, blood urea nitrogen, arterial pH, Po_2, Pco_2, hemoglobin, hematocrit, white blood count and differential, and calcium and phosphorus.

Oxygen may be administered to patients who are cyanotic and in whom arterial oxygen is less than 80%. Gastric suction is applied to unconscious children to avoid the possibility of pulmonary aspiration. Antibiotics may be administered to febrile children after appropriate specimens are obtained for culture. A Foley catheter may or may not be inserted for urine samples and measurement. Unless the child is unconscious, a collection bag is usually sufficient for accurate assessments.

Fluid and electrolyte therapy. All patients with diabetic ketoacidosis suffer from dehydration (10% of total body weight in severe ketoacidosis) due to the osmotic diuresis, accompanied by depletion of electrolytes, sodium, potassium, chloride, phosphate, and magnesium. Serum pH and bicarbonate reflect the degree of acidosis. Prompt and adequate fluid therapy restores tissue perfusion and suppresses the elevated levels of stress hormones.

The initial hydrating solution is isotonic saline solution. Even normal saline is hypotonic relative to the patient's serum hyperosmolality; therefore a gradual decline in osmolality is desirable because too rapid reduction in osmolality predisposes the child to cerebral edema, the most serious complication of therapy (Sperling, 1984). The intravenous saline is followed by 5% dextrose when blood glucose levels are sufficiently reduced. Present evidence indicates that sodium bicarbonate neither hastens resolution of acidosis nor improves survival (Lever and Jaspan, 1983). However, it may be given to improve cardiac contractility and enhance peripheral vascular responsiveness to catecholamines (Wolfsdorf, 1986).

Serum potassium levels may be normal on admission, but, following fluid and insulin administration, the rapid return of potassium to the cells can seriously deplete serum levels, with the attendant risk of cardiac arrhythmias. As soon as the child has established renal function (is voiding at least 25 ml/hour) and insulin has been given, vigorous potassium replacement is implemented. The cardiac monitor is used as a guide to therapy, and configuration of T waves should be followed every 30 to 60 minutes to determine changes that might indicate alterations in potassium concentration (widening of the QT interval and the appearance of a U wave following a flattened T wave indicate hypokalemia; an elevated and spreading T wave and shortening of the QT interval indicate hyperkalemia).

Insulin. The preferred method for administering insulin to the child with ketoacidosis is a continuous infusion of low-dose insulin consisting of a 0.1 U/kg priming dose followed by 0.1 U/kg/hour. This appears to be an efficient, simple, and physiologically sound form of therapy (Sperling, 1984). The insulin is added to 0.5% normal saline, and some of the mixture is run through the intravenous tubing to saturate the insulin-binding sites that exist on the plastic tubing. It has been found that plastic tubing and in-line filters can chemically bind to significant amounts of insulin, thereby reducing the amount of the medication reaching the bloodstream. The infusion is titrated to lower the blood glucose about 100 mg/dl/hour to obtain a blood glucose level of approximately 200 mg/dl. As 5% dextrose is added to the fluid replacement, the insulin infusion is then continued until the pH and serum bicarbonate are normal. Subcutaneous insulin is then instituted.

Nursing Considerations: Acute Care

Children with DM may be admitted to the hospital at the time of their initial diagnosis, during illness or surgery, or for episodes of ketoacidosis, which may be precipitated by any of a variety of factors. Most children are able to keep the disease under control with periodic assessment and adjustment of insulin, diet, and activity as needed under the supervision of a physician. Under most circumstances these children can be managed very well at home and require hospitalization only for a serious illness or upset.

However, a small number of children with diabetes exhibit a degree of metabolic lability and have repeated episodes of diabetic ketoacidosis that require hospitalization, which interferes with education and social development. These children appear to display a characteristic personality structure. They tend to be unusually passive and nonassertive and to come from families that are inclined to smooth over conflicts without resolution. Children in this type of setting experience emotional arousal with little, if any, opportunity or ability to bring about its termination. Other children from psychosocially dysfunctional families display behavioral and personality problems. This emotional stress causes an increased production of endogenous catecholamines, which stimulates fat breakdown leading to ketonemia and ketonuria.

Loving discipline is a supportive measure for any child; however, children with poorer diabetic control come from predominantly disruptive family units with little or no discipline as part of the family life-style. Lack of control is psychologically harmful. Since many of the psychosocial problems are not immediately apparent, psychosocial assessment and involvement by professionals are required, together with ongoing emotional support and counseling to reverse the patterns of ketoacidosis (White and others, 1984).

Hospital management. The child with diabetic ketoacidosis requires intensive nursing care. Vital signs should be observed and recorded frequently. Hypotension caused by the contracted blood volume of the dehydrated state may cause decreased peripheral blood flow, which can be particularly hazardous to the heart, lungs, and kidneys. An elevated temperature may indicate the presence of infection and should be reported so that treatment can be implemented immediately.

Careful and accurate records should be maintained, including vital signs (pulse, respiration, temperature, blood pressure), intravenous fluids, electrolytes, insulin, blood glucose level, and intake and output. A urine collection device or retention catheter is used to obtain the urine measurements, which include volume, specific gravity, and glucose and ketone values. The volume relative to the glucose content is important, since 5% glucose in a 300 ml sample is a significantly greater amount than a similar reading from a 75 ml sample. A diabetic flow sheet maintained at the bedside provides an ongoing record of the vital signs, urine and blood tests, amount of insulin given, and intake and output of the patient. The level of consciousness is assessed and recorded at frequent intervals. The comatose child generally regains consciousness fairly soon after initiation of therapy but is managed as any unconscious child during that time.

When the critical period is over, the task of regulating insulin dosage to diet and activity is begun. The same meticulous records of intake and output, urine glucose and acetone levels, and insulin administration are maintained. Capable children should be actively involved in their own care and are given responsibility for keeping the intake and output record, testing the blood and urine, and, when appropriate, administering their own insulin—all under the supervision and guidance of the nurse.

Nursing Considerations: General Care

Nurses play a prominent role in diagnosis and management of children with IDDM. Assessing and educating the child and family are almost exclusively a nursing function.

Assessment

Diabetic management involves a constant state of assessment. Daily monitoring of blood glucose levels, periodic urinalysis for ketones, and observation for signs of hypoglycemia, hyperglycemia, or other complications is part of the daily life of children with diabetes and their families. Diabetes can be suspected in any child who exhibits the manifestations of hypoglycemia or hyperglycemia (see Table 38-4), and the child should be referred for further assessment and appropriate testing.

The nurse should be alert to evidence of complications, although these are usually not manifest until adulthood. Assessment of skin for evidence of breakdown is important in order that appropriate care can be implemented to facilitate healing and prevent infection. Because illnesses, such as respiratory infections or gastrointestinal upsets, complicate the diabetes management, they should be detected early.

Nursing Diagnoses

Based on a thorough assessment, several nursing diagnoses are identified. The more common diagnoses for the child with DM are included in the Nursing Care Plan on pp. 1818-1820. Others may apply in specific situations.

Planning

Nursing objectives for the child with DM include the following:

1. Educate the child and family about the disease, assessment techniques, and therapy.
2. Prevent ill effects from complications of diabetes.
3. Promote a positive self-image in the child.
4. Provide support to child and family.

Implementation

Education is the cornerstone of diabetes management and the major responsibility in diabetes nursing care. This includes education and reinforcement of information for the family and for children who are old enough to participate in self-management of the disease. With younger children, parents must supervise and manage their therapeutic program, but children should assume responsibility for self-management as soon as they are capable. Children can assist with blood glucose testing at a relatively young age, and most should be able to administer their own insulin at about 9 years of age. In situations in which the parents are inconsistent and/or unreliable, the child should be taught self-care at an earlier age. It must be understood, however,

NURSING CARE PLAN
The Child with Diabetes Mellitus

Hospital care

NURSING DIAGNOSIS: Potential for injury related to insulin deficiency

GOAL 1
Replace insulin deficit

INTERVENTIONS

Obtain serum glucose level
*Administer insulin as prescribed
Understand the action of insulin
  Understand the differences in composition, time of onset, and duration of action for the various insulin preparations
Employ insulin techniques when preparing and administering insulin
  Subcutaneous injection
  Rotation of sites

EXPECTED OUTCOME

Child demonstrates reduced blood glucose levels

NURSING DIAGNOSIS: Potential for injury related to hypoglycemia

GOAL 1
Elevate blood glucose level

INTERVENTIONS

Recognize signs of hypoglycemia early
  Be particularly alert at times when blood glucose levels are lowest
  Test blood glucose
Offer 10 to 15 g of readily absorbed carbohydrates, such as orange juice, hard candy, or milk
Follow with complex carbohydrate, such as bread or cracker
*Administer glucagon, if prescribed

EXPECTED OUTCOMES

Child ingests an appropriate carbohydrate
Child displays no evidence of hypoglycemia

Preparation for home care

NURSING DIAGNOSIS: Knowledge deficit (diabetes management) related to care of a child with newly diagnosed diabetes mellitus

GOAL 1
Educate parents and child regarding diabetic management

INTERVENTIONS

Select methods, vocabulary, and content appropriate to the level of the learner
Allow 3 or 4 days for family and child to begin to adjust to the initial impact of the diagnosis
Select an environment conducive to learning
Allow ample time for the education process
Restrict length of teaching sessions
  Child—15-20 minutes
  Parents—45-60 minutes
Involve all senses and employ a variety of teaching strategies
Provide pamphlets or other supplementary materials

EXPECTED OUTCOME

Child and/or family display attitudes conducive to learning

GOAL 2
Teach child and family nature of the disease

INTERVENTIONS

Provide information regarding the pathophysiology of diabetes and the function and actions of insulin and glucagon in relation to caloric intake and exercise
Answer questions and clarify misconceptions
Explain function and expected effects of procedures and tests

EXPECTED OUTCOME

Child and/or family demonstrate an understanding of the disease and its therapy (specify indicators)

GOAL 3
Teach child and family meal planning

INTERVENTIONS

Enlist the services of a dietitian
Emphasize the relationship between normal nutritional needs and the disease
Become familiar with the family's food preferences
Teach or reinforce the learners' understanding of the basic food groups and the diet plan prescribed (e.g., exchange diet)
Help the child and family estimate food weights by volume
Suggest low-carbohydrate snack items
Guide family in assessing the labels of food products for carbohydrate content
Teach or reinforce an understanding of the concept of exchanges
Relate constant carbohydrate equivalents to familiar foods
Retain cultural patterns and family preferences as much as possible

EXPECTED OUTCOME

Child and/or family demonstrate an understanding of diet planning and food selection (specify indicators)

*Dependent nursing action.

NURSING CARE PLAN
The Child with Diabetes Mellitus—cont'd

GOAL 4
Teach characteristics of and administration of insulin

INTERVENTIONS

Teach child and family the characteristics of the insulins prescribed for the child
Teach the proper mixing of insulins and acceptable substitutions (when the family brand is unavailable)
Teach injection procedure
- Impress upon the learners that the procedure will be a routine part of the child's life
- Involve caregivers and the child, if old enough
- Teach basic techniques using an orange or similar item
- Use demonstration and return demonstration techniques on another before injecting the child
- Help families and child work out a set rotational pattern
- Teach proper care of insulin and equipment

Teach management of continuous infusion pump (if used)

EXPECTED OUTCOMES

Child and/or family demonstrate an understanding of insulin, its various forms, and action (specify indicators)
Child and/or family demonstrate injection technique correctly
Child and/or family develop a rotation plan
Child and/or family demonstrate correct use of pump and care of injection site

GOAL 5
Teach blood glucose testing

INTERVENTIONS

Teach:
- Blood glucose monitoring and/or use of equipment selected for use
- Interpretation of results
- Care and maintenance of equipment

EXPECTED OUTCOME

Child and/or family demonstrate the correct use of the glucose monitoring equipment

GOAL 6
Teach urine testing

INTERVENTIONS

Teach:
- Urine ketone testing and interpretation of results
- Proper care of test strips

EXPECTED OUTCOME

Child and/or family demonstrate urine testing and interpretation

GOAL 7
Teach importance of hygiene

INTERVENTIONS

Emphasize the importance of personal hygiene
Encourage regular dental care and yearly ophthalmologic examinations
Teach proper care of cuts and scratches
Teach proper foot care

EXPECTED OUTCOME

Child and family demonstrate an understanding of the importance of proper hygiene

GOAL 8
Teach importance of exercise

INTERVENTIONS

Arrange for occupational therapy program that includes physical activity
Work with child, family, and others (e.g., coaches) to help plan a home exercise program
Reiterate practitioner's instructions regarding adjustment of food and/or insulin to meet the child's activity pattern; reinforce with examples

EXPECTED OUTCOME

Child and family helps child outline and carry out a regular exercise program

GOAL 9
Teach child and family recognition and management of hyperglycemia and hypoglycemia

INTERVENTIONS

Instruct learners in how to recognize signs of hyperglycemia and hypoglycemia (especially hypoglycemia)
Explain the relationship of insulin needs to illness, activity, and intense emotion (either positive or negative)
Teach how to adjust food, activity, and insulin at times of illness and during other situations that alter blood sugar levels
Suggest carrying source of carbohydrate, such as sugar cubes or hard candy, in pocket or handbag
Instruct parents and child in how to treat hypoglycemia with food, simple sugars, or glucagon

EXPECTED OUTCOME

Child and family demonstrate an understanding of the signs and management of a hypoglycemic reaction (specify)

GOAL 10
Teach importance of identification

INTERVENTIONS

Encourage the acquisition of a means of identification, such as an identification bracelet, that explains the child's condition in case of emergency

EXPECTED OUTCOME

Family acquires and child wears identification bracelet

Continued.

NURSING CARE PLAN
The Child with Diabetes Mellitus—cont'd

GOAL 11

Teach record keeping

INTERVENTIONS

Help child and family to design a form for keeping records of:
- Insulin administered
- Blood and urine tests
- Food intake
- Marked variation in exercise
- Illness

EXPECTED OUTCOME

Family and child keep an accurate record of insulin administration, glucose testing, etc.

GOAL 12

Facilitate self-management

INTERVENTIONS

Encourage honesty in recording, such as eating a forbidden candy bar

Encourage independence in applying the concepts learned in teaching sessions

Instruct when to seek assistance from medical personnel

EXPECTED OUTCOME

Child takes responsibility for management of disease commensurate with age and capabilities

NURSING DIAGNOSIS: Altered family processes related to situational crisis (child with a chronic disorder)

See Nursing Care Plan: The Child with a Chronic Illness or Disability, Chapter 22

that education programs cannot be conducted as one-time activities with the expectation that they will achieve permanent behavior changes. Education is a long-term nursing activity as family and patient needs change and new findings are applied.

Concepts of child and family education. Children and their families vary in educational background and the capacity to learn and understand the various aspects of the therapeutic program. Some families respond best to very simple explanations and directions, whereas others expect thorough, in-depth information about the physiologic processes and responses associated with the disease and its therapy. All the principles of teaching and learning are applied in the educational process; therefore, before beginning, the nurse must determine the optimum time, place, method, and content to be taught. Self-management, the ultimate goal for children with diabetes, is more likely to occur when they understand the disease and the care it requires. Properly educated, any family should be able to follow a program of regulated control satisfactorily.

When to teach a family is best judged by the psychologic state of the family and/or the child and the time of initial diagnosis. If a child is newly diagnosed, the psychologic adjustment to the disease can block the learning process completely—for example, members of the family may in a follow-up visit state that it is the first time that they have heard a certain bit of information when, in reality, the specific material had been covered several times in the course of teaching.

Certainly, the first 3 or 4 days after diagnosis is not an optimum time for learning. In fact, the later the more complex material is presented, the better. For example, one successful program teaches only essential, or survival, information first and intense information a month later. Another program advocates as a choice of time for teaching 1 week after diagnosis followed by a review of survival techniques 2 weeks after discharge. Probably the most inopportune and ineffective time for teaching is the day or so after diagnosis when the education must be compressed into a few hours or days so that the child can be discharged early. Whether teaching is conducted on an outpatient basis or in a preparatory, in-depth manner on an inpatient basis, the ability of the individuals involved to learn must be accurately assessed. This includes assessment of the educational background and emotional stability of the individual(s) involved and the use of appropriate measurement tools, such as a pretest or an objective assessment of the learner's educational level.

The setting for the educational process can facilitate the learning process. An environment that is too hot or too cold or one in which there is too much noise will distract the learner. Bedside education may be necessary in some cases, but the coming and going of a number of people are distracting. There are times in the educational process when individual instruction is needed, but contact with other children and/or parents can assist in adjustment to the reality of the disease and the implications of having a chronic condition. Supplementary material such as audiovisual aids enhances the learning process and promotes retention of information.

A child learns best when sessions are kept short, no more than 15 to 20 minutes. The parents do best in periods of 45 to 60 minutes, or longer if they are inquisitive. Education should involve all the senses, and although visual aids are valuable tools, participation is the most effective method for learning. For example, to teach urine testing, the technique is explained, the procedure is demonstrated, and the learner is allowed to perform the procedure followed by a review of the material by visual aids, with learning validated by some testing method that includes a feedback. A variety of teaching methods and teaching aids can be used. Some visual aids may be beautifully illustrated but miss a major point; therefore materials should be previewed for accuracy and appropriateness. Varying the presentation with a variety of audiovisual materials, including films, slide-tape programs, and books, stimulates the senses and helps the individual to learn.

Several organizations are prepared to assist with education and dissemination of knowledge about diabetes. The **American Diabetes Association, Inc.,* Canadian Diabetes Association,† Juvenile Diabetes Foundation International,‡** the **Juvenile Diabetes Foundation International—Canada,§** and the **American Association of Diabetes Educators‖** are valuable resources for a wide variety of educational materials. The **National Diabetes Information Clearinghouse¶** publishes a number of comprehensive annotated bibliographies, including *Educational Materials for and about Young People with Diabetes,* a compilation of resource materials for children, siblings, parents, teachers, and health professionals, and *Sports and Exercise for People with Diabetes.*

The content of the educational course must include all aspects of the disease as they specifically relate to the individual child. There are many aspects of the disease that may not be covered in an initial educational course but can be postponed until subsequent office or clinic visits or can be done through referral sources such as the American Diabetes Association. The minimal information needed is that which will help the family manage from one day to the next; expanded information helps the individual with the biopsychosocial adjustment basic to in-depth knowledge about the disease. The more the family understands about the disease in relation to body needs, the better they are able to maintain a high degree of control. Important content needed for minimum management is discussed briefly in the following segments.

Identification. One of the first things that should be called to the attention of the parents is the need for the child to wear some means of medical identification. Usually recommended is the Medic-Alert identification, a stainless steel, silver, or gold-plated identification bracelet or necklace that is visible and immediately recognizable. It contains a collect telephone number that medical personnel can call around the clock for medical records and personal information.

Nature of diabetes. The better the parents understand the pathophysiology of diabetes and the function and action of insulin and glucagon in relation to calorie intake and exercise, the better will be their understanding of the disease and its effect on the child. Parents need answers to a number of questions (voiced or unvoiced) because those answers can provide them an increased feeling of security in coping with the disease. For example, they may want to know about the various procedures performed on their child and treatment rationale, such as what is being put in the intravenous bottle and the expected effect.

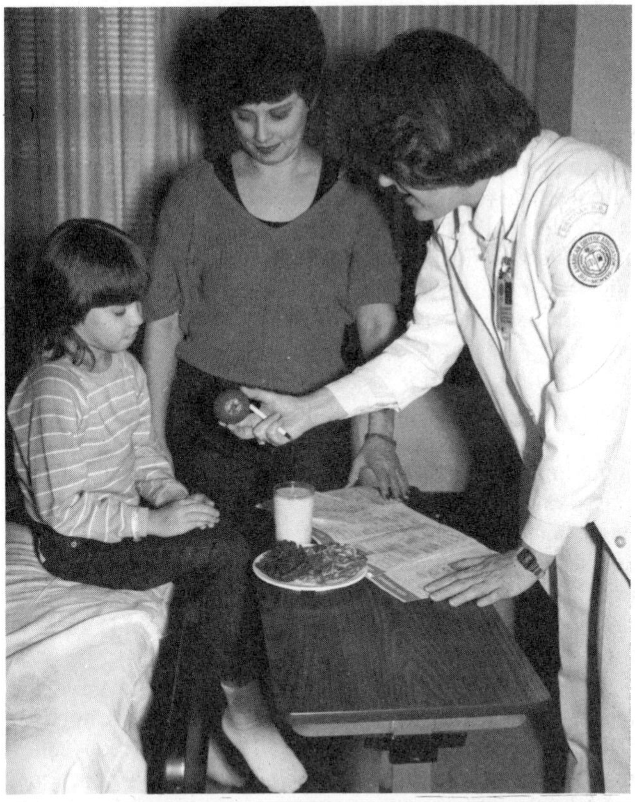

Fig. 38-6. Nutritionist instructs child and family using food models to explain food exchanges.

Meal planning. Normal nutrition is a major aspect of the family education program. Diet instruction is usually conducted by the nutritionist, with reinforcement and guidance from the nurse (Fig. 38-6). The emphasis is on adequate intake for age, constant menus, complex carbohydrates, and consistent eating times. The family is taught how the meal plan relates to the requirements of growth and development, the disease process, and the insulin regimen. Meals and snacks are modified around the child and the present food menu, preserving cultural patterns and preferences as much as possible. Extensive exchange lists are available that include foods that are compatible with most life-styles.

Learning about foods within specific food groups helps in making choices. Weights and measures of foods are used as eye-training devices for defining food volumes and should be practiced for about 3 months, with gradual progression to estimation of food portions. Even when the

*1660 Duke St., Alexandria, VA 22314; (800) 232-3472. In Virginia or Washington, DC: (703) 549-1500.

†123 Edward St., Suite 601, Toronto, Ontario, Canada M5G 1E2.

‡432 Park Ave. South, New York, NY; (212) 889-7575, Hotline: (800) 223-1138.

§4632 Yonge St., Suite 201, Willowdale, Ontario, Canada M2N 5M1.

‖Suite 1400, 500 North Michigan Ave., Chicago, IL 60611; (708) 661-1700.

¶Box NDIC, 9000 Rockville Pike, Bethesda, MD 20892; (301) 468-2162.

child and/or family become competent in estimating food volumes, reassessment should take place weekly or monthly and when there is any change of brands. Members of the family should also be guided in reading labels for the nutritional value of foods and food contents.

Family members should also become familiar with the carbohydrate content of food groups. Substitutions with foods of equal carbohydrate content is occasionally acceptable without affecting blood glucose control. Substitution might be necessary if a food is not available in sufficient quantity or for the teen who wishes to eat fast food with peers.

Educating children or teenagers to make healthy food choices is an ongoing task. Younger children might be taught to choose from a special treat box stocked with sugar-free items when high-sugar treats are brought to the classroom by others. Discussions with school-age children might include situations encountered at school or parties, such as choosing food in the cafeteria or bringing substitute treats to parties. Role-playing and discussion help teenagers deal with food choices when on dates, with friends, or on a food break after school.

Lists of popular fast-food items and items served at the major fast-food chains can be obtained from the **American Dietetic Association (ADA)*** to help guide food selections. It is important that the child know the nutritional value of these items (the major chains are remarkably uniform), but the child should be cautioned to avoid high-fat and high-sugar items, for example, choosing a plain hamburger instead of a double cheeseburger. (See Table 38-5 for a small sample of some popular fast-food items.)

Children should be advised to use sugar substitutes with moderation in items such as soft drinks. Artificial sweeteners have been shown to be safe, but if there is any question about amounts, the physician, dietitian, or nurse specialist can provide guidelines based on body weight. "Sugar-free" chewing gum and candies made with sorbitol are not usually recommended for children with DM. Although sorbitol is less cariogenic than other varieties of sugar substitutes, it is an alcohol sugar that is metabolized to fructose and then to glucose. Furthermore, large amounts can cause osmotic diarrhea. Most dietetic foods contain sorbitol. They are more expensive than regular foods, and careful reading of labels reveals that the caloric content is the same.

Traveling requires advance planning, especially when a trip involves crossing time zones. A number of tips are included in pamphlets available free of charge from the local chapter of the ADA or the publishers.* Suggestions for traveling include what will be needed from the doctor before leaving, what and how much to take along, planning for needs in transit, what to consider at the destination, and planning for when the child returns home. Planning is needed no matter what type of travel is considered—automobile, plane, bus, or train. The ADA also has a computer service that can provide a vacation schedule of insulin and meals based on the accustomed regimen and the anticipated changes.

Insulin. Families need to understand the treatment method and the insulin prescribed, including the effective duration, onset, and peak action. They also need to know the characteristics of the various types of insulins, the proper mixing and dilution of insulins, and how to substitute another type when their usual brand is not available (insulin is a nonprescription drug). Insulin need not be refrigerated but should be maintained at a temperature between 15° C (59° F) and 29.4° C (85° F). Freezing renders insulin inactive. An extra supply can be kept in the refrigerator.

Injection procedure. Learning to give the insulin injections is a source of anxiety for both the parents and children. It is helpful for the learner to know that this important aspect of care will become as routine as brushing the teeth.

*208 South La Salle St., Suite 1100, Chicago, IL 60604-1003; (312) 899-0040.

**Vacations, Travel, and Diabetes,* available from Becton, Dickson & Co., Rochelle Park, NJ 07662. *Vacationing with Diabetes,* available from E.R. Squibb, P.O. Box 4000, Princeton, NJ 08540.

Table 38-5 Exchange equivalents for selected fast-food items

	EXCHANGE EQUIVALENTS			
FOOD	LEAN-MED. MEAT	STARCH/ BREAD	FAT	VEGETABLE
Arby's roast beef sandwich (regular)	2½	2	½	—
Burger King "Whopper"	3	3	3½	1
Kentucky Fried				
Original dinner (2 pieces chicken, potatoes, gravy, cole slaw, roll)	3½	3	3	2
McDonald's "Big Mac"	3	2	3	2
Pizza Hut cheese pizza (½ of 10-inch)	2	3	1	2
Taco Bell				
Taco	2	1	1	—
Beef burrito	3	2	1	2
Wendy's cheeseburger (single)	4	2	2	—

First, the basic injection technique is taught, using an orange or similar item and sterile normal saline for practice.* To gain children's confidence, the nurse can demonstrate the technique by giving a skillful injection to the parent and then having the parent return the demonstration by giving the nurse an injection. With practice and confidence the parents soon are able to give the insulin injection to their children, and their children will trust them. Another effective strategy is to instruct the children and then have them teach the technique to the parents while the nurse observes. Both parents should participate, and as little time as possible should elapse between instruction and the actual injection, especially with parents and teenage learners.

Insulin can be injected into any area in which there is tissue over muscle. The drug is injected at a 45-degree angle, and the depth of injection is altered according to the thickness of the layer of adipose tissue. Newly diagnosed children may have lost adipose tissue, and care should be exerted not to inject intramuscularly. The pinch technique is the most effective method for obtaining skin tightness to allow easy entrance of the needle to subcutaneous tissues in children. The site selected will sometimes depend on whether children or parents administer the insulin. The arms, thighs, hips, and abdomen are usual injection sites for insulin. The children can reach the thighs, abdomen, and part of the hip and arm easily but may require help to inject other sites. For example, a parent can pinch a loose fold of skin of the arm while the child injects the insulin.

The parents and child are helped to work out a rotation pattern to various areas of the body to enhance absorption, since insulin absorption is slowed by the fat pads that develop in overused injection areas (Young and others, 1984). The most efficient rotation plan involves giving about 4 to 6 injections in one area (each injection about 1 inch [2.5 cm] apart or the diameter of the insulin vial from the previous injection) and then moving to another area.

It is important to remember that the absorption rate varies in different parts of the body. Absorption has been demonstrated to be more rapid in the arm, less rapid in the abdomen, and slowest when injected into the thigh (Binder and others, 1984). The methodical use of one anatomic area and then moving to another (as described in the previous paragraph) minimizes variation in absorption rates. However, absorption is also altered by vigorous exercise, which enhances absorption from exercised muscles. Therefore it is recommended that excess exercise be avoided during the time the insulin is expected to peak (Thatcher, 1985).

Injection sites for an entire month can be determined in advance on a simple chart. For example, the "paper doll" (body outline) described in Box 7-2 can be constructed and insulin sites marked by the child. After injection, the child places the date on the appropriate site. In order to keep in practice, it is a good idea for the parent to give two or three injections a week in the areas that are difficult for the child to reach.

The same basic methodology is used when teaching children to give their own insulin injections (Fig. 38-7). They should practice first on an orange or a doll, building courage gradually. The first attempt will undoubtedly be awkward, since children tend to slowly push the needle through the skin rather than using a quick approach. It is best not to pressure them into assuming this responsibility until they are ready. When children participate in a group-learning situation or have an opportunity to observe their peers giving their own injections, they may become more strongly motivated. Parents should be warned that at some time children will give themselves an uncomfortable injec-

*Home care instructions on subcutaneous injection are available in Wong, D.L., and Whaley, L.F.: Clinical manual of pediatric nursing, ed. 3, St. Louis, 1990, Mosby–Year Book, Inc.

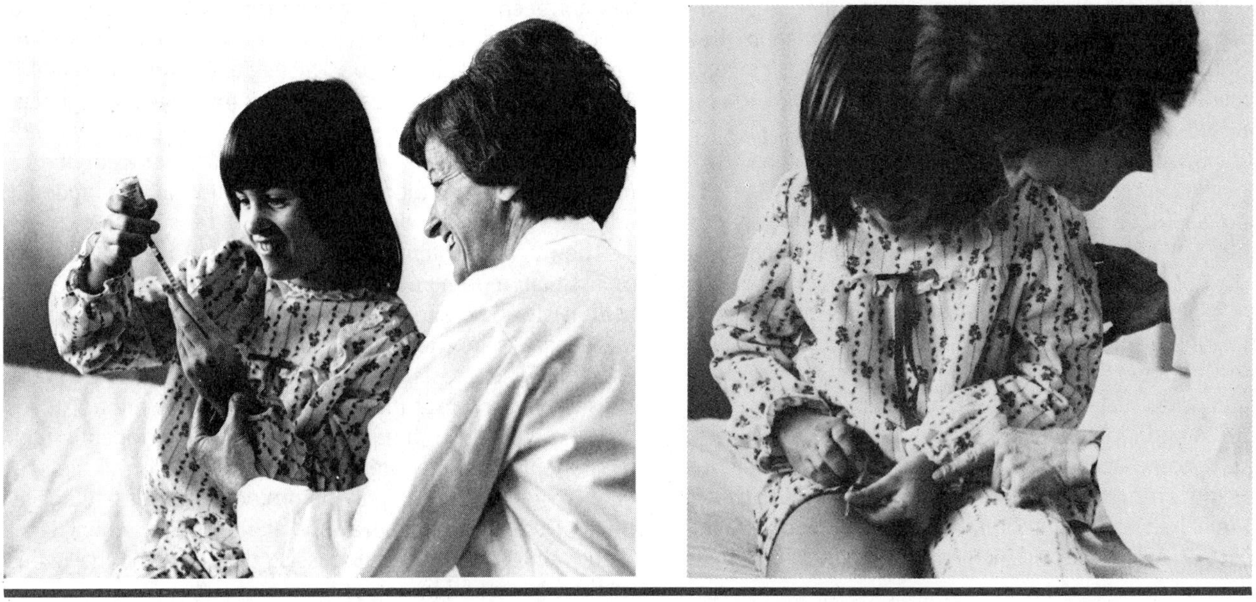

Fig. 38-7. School-age children are able to administer their own insulin.

tion at home and that they will need parental support and encouragement. Otherwise children may not wish to give themselves injections for some time. Occasionally children are taught to use a syringe-loaded injector (Injectease), especially those who are fearful of puncturing their skin. With the device, puncture is always automatic. Adolescents respond well to a self-contained and compact device resembling a fountain pen (NovoPen*), which eliminates conventional vials and syringes.

Teaching includes the proper way to equalize pressure in the bottle by injecting an amount of air equal to the amount of solution withdrawn and how to remove air bubbles from the syringe. When insulin dosages are small, an air bubble in the syringe can displace a significant amount of medication. Since the introduction of the 5/10 ml and 3/10 ml syringes, the risk of incorrect dosage has diminished. Patients who have small doses of mixed insulins should be advised and instructed to use one of these syringes. Insulin syringes should be compared for accuracy, comfort, and strength. The family and/or child should be able to choose both "their" insulin and "their" syringe from a variety of samples. Use of the same type of syringe (even during hospitalization) is recommended to prevent errors in dosage caused by varying amounts of dead space among syringes (Wong, 1982). The needle length and gauge are also factors to consider from the point of view of comfort (e.g., use the smallest gauge needle available). Some brands of syringes may be more comfortable than others.

When the child's dosage requires the injection of both short- and intermediate-acting insulin at the same time, most families prefer to mix the two and use a single injection. However, some problems are associated with this accepted practice, and the family should understand what happens when insulins are mixed. Longer-acting insulins contain ingredients that bind to insulin, allowing for gradual release after injection. Some brands contain extra binding compounds that can bind with regular insulin, converting it to the longer-acting type, thus altering the effect on blood glucose. The degree of alteration depends on the type of longer-acting insulin, the ratio of short–to–longer-acting insulin, and how long the mixture is allowed to remain unused.

To obtain maximum benefit from mixing insulins, the recommended practice is to (1) inject the measured amount of air (equivalent to the dosage) into the longer-acting insulin, (2) inject the measured amount of air into the regular insulin and, without removing the needle, (3) withdraw the regular insulin, and (4) insert the needle (already containing the regular insulin) into the longer-acting insulin and then withdraw the desired amount. The mixture should be injected immediately—in less than 5 minutes after mixing (Jenkins and Molitch, 1986).

It has become acceptable practice to reuse disposable needles and syringes for 3 to 7 days. Research indicates that no infection has resulted and that there is a considerable cost saving (Poteet, Reinert, and Ptak, 1987). If this method is approved, it is essential to stress the importance of vigorous handwashing before handling any equipment, as well as capping the syringe immediately after use and storing it in the refrigerator to reduce the possibility of infection. Nurses should also teach proper disposal of equipment after use in the home. Although not standard practice in the hospital, use of a needle clipper is recommended to safely remove and house the used needle. In addition, the syringe plunger can be broken before disposal. An excellent means for syringe disposal is in an opaque, puncture-resistant container such as an empty coffee can, bleach bottle, or milk carton, any of which can be discarded with household trash.

Continuous subcutaneous insulin infusion. Some children are considered candidates for use of a portable insulin pump, and even some young children with unsatisfactory metabolic control can benefit from its use. The child and the parents are taught to operate the device, including the mechanics of the pump, battery changes, and alarm systems. A number of devices are available on the market that vary in the basal rates they are able to deliver and in the cost of the equipment. Most children can be adequately controlled with one of the simpler models (Rosenstock, Strowig, and Raskin, 1985). Families can investigate the various devices at the local chapter of the ADA and select the model that best suits their needs.

Parents and child learn (1) the technical aspects of the pump and self-monitoring of blood glucose; (2) how to prevent and treat hyperglycemia, sick-day management, and diet planning; (3) effects of exercise, stress, and diet on blood glucose levels; and (4) decision-making strategies to evaluate blood glucose patterns and how to make adjustments in all aspects of the regimen. The child may be hospitalized for regulation and instruction.

Since numerous blood glucose measurements (at least four times per day) are an essential part of infusion pump use, families must acquire a monitor and learn its use if this has not been a part of their regular management. Intensive education and supervision are critical to obtaining maximum efficiency and control. This is particularly important if the family has been accustomed to a fixed insulin regimen. They must realize that simply wearing the pump will not normalize blood glucose. It is merely a tool for using the information from self blood-glucose monitoring as a guide for adjusting the insulin delivery.

The major problem with the use of the insulin pump is inflammation from an allergic reaction or infection at the insertion site. The site should be cleaned thoroughly before the needle is inserted and then covered with a transparent dressing. The site is changed and rotated every 48 hours (this may vary) or at the first sign of inflammation. Nurses working where the pumps are part of the therapeutic regimen should become familiar with the operation of the specific device being used and the protocol of disease management. Others should be aware of this management technique and be prepared to assist patients who have this method in operation.

Monitoring. Nurses should also be prepared to teach and supervise blood glucose monitoring. Home blood glu-

*Squibb-Novo, Inc., Princeton, NJ.

cose monitoring (HBGM) is associated with very few complications, and although it does not necessarily lead to improved metabolic control, it provides a more accurate assessment of blood glucose levels than the traditional urine testing. Blood glucose monitoring has the added advantage that it can be performed anywhere.

Blood for testing can be obtained by two different methods: manually or with a mechanical bloodletting device. A mechanical device is recommended for children, although the child and family should learn to use both methods in the event of mechanical failure. Several lancet devices are available from which to choose, and each provides a means for obtaining a large drop of blood for testing (Fig. 38-8). Children are cautioned not to allow anyone else to use their lancet because of the danger of contracting hepatitis or other blood-borne diseases. Any signs of redness and soreness at the site of finger puncture should be examined by the health professional. It may be evidence of poor technique or poor skin healing relative to poor control.

Many types of blood testing meters are available for home use. Meter size and ease of use has been greatly improved with newer technology. The family should be shown features of several meters, including advantages and disadvantages, and allowed to choose equipment that best meets their needs.

The least expensive testing method uses a reagent strip to which blood is applied. After blotting, the color change is compared against a color scale for an estimation of blood glucose level. The strips can be cut in half (although this is not recommended by all professionals) to obtain two readings per strip. This method might be ideal for use at school where expensive equipment can be lost or broken.

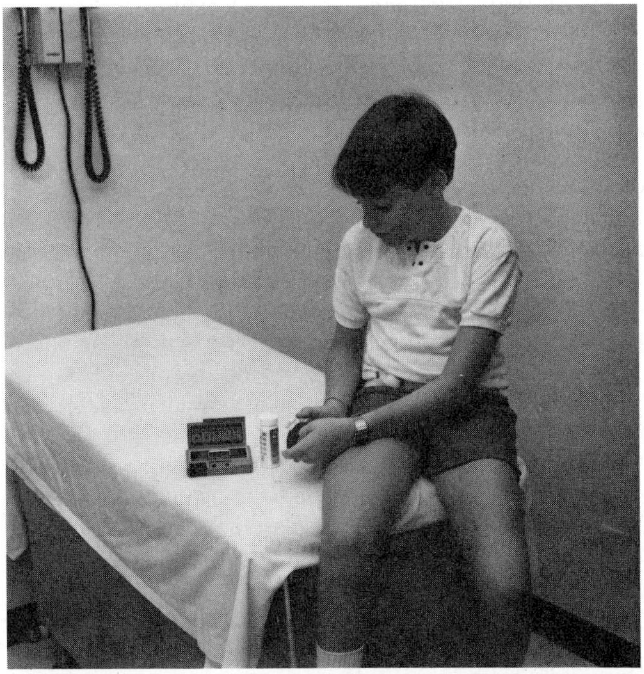

Fig. 38-8. Child using device to obtain blood sample.

NURSING TIPS: FINGER STICK

- To enhance blood flow to the finger, hold it under warm water for a few seconds before the stick.
- When obtaining blood samples, use the ring finger or thumb (blood flows more easily to these areas), and stick the finger just to the side of the finger pad (more blood vessels and fewer nerve endings).
- To prevent a deep puncture, press lancet device lightly against the skin and avoid steadying finger against a hard surface.

Urine testing. Testing for urinary ketones is recommended during times of illness or when blood glucose values are elevated. Information on a specific ketone testing product should include correct procedure, storage, and product expiration. Families need a clear understanding of home management of ketones: fluids and additional insulin as directed by the health care team.

Shopping. Diabetic maintenance is not an inexpensive necessity. Families are advised to investigate all sources of obtaining supplies for managing the disease. Prices are often lower when supplies are purchased in volume; however, it is not advisable to buy bulk items that are unfamiliar or untried, since the new items may not be satisfactory for the individual child. Costs vary considerably among pharmacies and other suppliers, including the numerous discount mail-order establishments. When buying by mail, it is important to find one that responds to the family's satisfaction and that allows the family ample time for delivery to avoid running out of supplies. Parents are also cautioned not to substitute insulins or the type of insulin syringe (e.g., a 1 ml syringe for the low-dose type) simply to save money. Parent groups and the local ADA can offer some suggestions for investigation.

Hyperglycemia. Severe hyperglycemia is most often caused by illness, growth, or emotional upset. With careful glucose monitoring, any elevation can be managed by adjustment of insulin or food intake. Parents should understand how to adjust food, activity, and insulin at the time of illness or when the child is treated for an illness with a medication known to raise the blood glucose level. The hyperglycemia is managed by increasing insulin soon after the increased glucose is noted.

Hypoglycemia. Hypoglycemia is caused by imbalances of food intake, insulin, and activity. Ideally hypoglycemia should be prevented, and parents need to be prepared to prevent, recognize, and treat the problem. They should be familiar with the signs of hypoglycemia and instructed in treatment, including care of the child with seizures (see Chapter 37). Early signs are *adrenergic,* including sweating and trembling, which help raise the blood sugar, much like the reaction when an individual is startled or anxious. The second set of symptoms that follow an untreated adrenergic reaction are *neuroglycopenic* (also called brain hypoglycemia). They typically include difficulty with

NURSING TIP: ADMINISTER CARBOHYDRATE

Commercial glucose gel, cake frosting, or honey can be rubbed on the gums and buccal mucosa of the unconscious, hypoglycemic child if glucagon is not available. Caution: keep the gel in the cheek to avoid occluding the airway.

balance, memory, attention, and/or concentration; dizziness, lightheadedness; and slurred speech. Severe and prolonged blood sugar leads to convulsions, coma, and possible death (Cox, Carter, and Gonder-Frederick, 1986). Hypoglycemia can be managed effectively as outlined in Emergency Treatment: Hypoglycemia.

It is advisable for parents to plan for anticipated excitement or exercise. In addition, gastroenteritis may decrease insulin needs slightly as a result of poor appetite, vomiting, and/or diarrhea. If the blood glucose level is low but urinary ketones are present, the family should be aware of the increased need for simple carbohydrates and liquids.

Hygiene. All aspects of personal hygiene should be emphasized for the child with diabetes. The child has not had time to develop the blood vessel disease that causes a decrease in peripheral circulation; therefore, foot care is not as important in the child as it is in the adult with diabetes. However, the child should be cautioned against wearing shoes without socks, wearing sandals, or walking barefoot. Correct nail and extremity care instituted for each particular child (with the guidance of a podiatrist) can begin health practices that last a lifetime. Eyes should be checked once a year unless the child wears glasses and then as directed by the ophthalmologist. Regular dental care is emphasized, and cuts and scratches should be treated with plain soap and water unless otherwise indicated.

Exercise. Exercise should be planned, as may be necessary for the sedentary teenager, or observed, as is found in most active children. If the child is more active at one time of the day than another, food and/or insulin can be altered to meet the activity pattern of the individual child. Food should be increased in the summer when children tend to be more active. Decreased activity on return to school may require a decrease in food intake and/or increase in insulin dosage. The child who is active in team sports will need additional food intake in the form of a snack about ½ hour before the anticipated activity. Races or other competition may call for a slightly higher food intake than practice times.

Food will usually need to be repeated for prolonged activity periods, often as frequently as every 45 minutes to 1 hour. Families should be informed that if increased food is not tolerated, decreased insulin is the next course of action. If the timing of the exercise is changed so that the supper meal is delayed, the insulin in the second or third dose of the day may be moved back to precede the mealtime. Sugar may sometimes be needed during exercise periods for quick response. Elevated blood glucose levels following extreme activity may represent the Somogyi reflex (see p. 1815).

Record keeping. Home records are an invaluable aid to diabetes self-management. The nurse and family devise a method to chart insulins administered, blood glucose values, urine ketone results, and other factors and events that affect diabetes control. Variations in diet and exercise are recorded, including ketone results, temperature, and intake. The child and family are encouraged to observe for patterns of blood glucose responses to events such as exercise. If lapses in management occur (such as eating a candy bar), the child should be encouraged to note this and not be condemned for the transgression.

Complications. It is debatable whether or not knowledge of potential hazards of poor control should be shared with the family and child. If so, the implications of the disease should be presented in a tactful, clear, and nonfearful manner. Knowledge of the complications of diabetes and their relationship to control provides a basis for knowledgeable decision-making. Eye and kidney disease are the greatest threats, with neurologic complications close behind. Clear explanations of these problems clarify false information often given by well-meaning friends. By this time the nurse has developed a rapport with the patient and family and knows at what level and how openly the problem can be discussed. The information should include discussion of research so that the family is left with the positive impression that others are concerned about finding answers and preventing complications. It also gives them hope that somehow, some way, a prevention and/or cure is possible.

Self-management. Self-management is the key to close control. Being able to make changes at the time they are needed rather than waiting until the next contact with health professionals is important for self-management and gives the individual and family the feeling that they have control over the disease. Psychologically this helps the family members feel that they are useful and participating members of the team. Learning to look at records objectively gives the child support. As children grow and assume more and more responsibility for self-management, they develop confidence in their ability to manage their disease and in themselves as persons. They grow to respond to the disease and to make more accurate interpretations and changes in self-management when they become adults.

Self-management techniques to be mastered are the testing and adjustment of insulin and diet with alterations in day-to-day activities and unusual occurrences. However, limitations should be set regarding how many alterations can be made without consulting with the health professionals. The degree of control before the illness is a determining factor in seeking medical help during illness. In an individual with poor control, it takes only a few hours before the trouble is severe, whereas, if control is good before the illness, several days may elapse before help is needed. Patients and families are cautioned to seek assistance if glucose levels are elevated and urine has not cleared of ketones after 24 hours of self-management.

NURSING TIP: ADHERENCE

Ongoing motivation to adhere to a regimen is difficult. An older child and parent may enjoy negotiating a day off when the responsibility for testing and recording blood glucose is delegated from the child to the parent (or vice-versa).

Child and family support. The parents and other family members of the child with newly diagnosed DM experience various emotional responses to the crises just as the physiologic responses affect the child. Care in the acute setting is short but may create fears and frustrations. The prospect of a chronic illness in their child engenders all the feeling and concerns that are faced by parents of children with other chronic illnesses (see Chapter 22). The threat of complications and death is always present, as well as the continuing drain on emotional and financial resources.

Certain fears may develop as a result of past experiences with the disease. A severe insulin reaction with seizures is certainly one experience that contributes to fear of repetition. Once parents experience a seizure or the adolescent has one in a public place, the desire to maintain better control is reinforced. They must understand how to prevent problems and how to handle problems calmly and coolly if they occur and understand the complexities of the body, the disease, and its complications. Young children usually adjust well to problems related to the disease. With toddlers and preschoolers, insulin injections and glucose testing may be difficult at first. However, they usually accept the procedures when the parents use a matter-of-fact approach without calling attention to a "hurt" and treat the procedure like any other routine part of a child's life. Following the injection, time with some special and positive attention such as reading, talking, or other pleasant activity is one way to convert children who initially refuse injections to those who accept them.

Children in the years before adolescence probably accept their condition most easily. They are able to understand the basic concepts related to their disease and its treatment. They are able to test blood glucose and urine, recognize food groups, give injections, keep records, and distinguish between feelings of fear, excitement, and hypoglycemia. They understand how to recognize, prevent, and treat hypoglycemia. However, they still need considerable parental involvement.

Adolescents appear to have most difficulty in adjusting. Adolescence is a time when there is much stress toward being perfect and being like their peers and, no matter what others say, having diabetes is being different. Some youngsters are more upset about not being able to have a candy bar than about injections, diet, and other aspects of management. If children can accept the difference as a part of life, in other words, that each person is different in some way, then with adequate parental support they should be able to adjust well.

EMERGENCY TREATMENT
Hypoglycemia

Mild reaction: adrenergic symptoms

Give child 10 to 15 g simple, high carbohydrate (preferably liquid, e.g., 3 to 6 oz orange juice).
Follow with starch-protein snack.

Moderate reaction: neuroglycopenic symptoms

Give child 10 to 15 g simple carbohydrate as above.
Repeat in 10 to 15 minutes if symptoms persist.
Follow with larger snack.
Watch child closely.

Severe reaction: unresponsive, unconscious, and/or seizures

Administer glucagon as prescribed.
Follow with planned meal or snack when child is able to eat, or add a snack of 10% of daily calories.

Nocturnal reaction

Give child 10 to 15 g simple carbohydrate.
Follow with snack of 10% of daily calories.

Problems of adjustment to diabetes are especially difficult for the youngster whose disease is diagnosed in adolescence. Denial is sometimes expressed by omitting insulin, not performing tests, and eating incorrectly, although denial of the disease usually diminishes during this period as the youngster with DM begins to feel competent and worthy. This is the age when greatest falsification of records occurs. Diabetes makes the youngster different when conformity and sameness are desired; having the disease emphasizes vulnerability and imperfection when the search for identity is the foremost developmental task. It is often difficult for the adolescent to know what to tell friends who doubt that they have the disease.

Camping and other special groups are very useful. At diabetes camp children learn that they are not alone. As a result, they become more independent and resourceful in the nondiabetes camp setting, especially if they have had experience in a diabetes camp. Useful information about such camps and organizations can be obtained from the American Diabetes Association (ADA). A free list of accredited camps specifically for children and teens with diabetes is also available.*

Puberty is associated with decreased sensitivity to insulin that normally would be compensated by an increased insulin secretion. In youngsters with IDDM an approximately 30% increase in insulin dosage should be anticipated with the onset of puberty (Bloch, Clemons, and Sperling, 1987).

Eating disorders, such as bulimia or anorexia nervosa, in the teenager with IDDM (see Chapter 21) pose a serious health hazard. The nurse should be alert to a history of preoccupation with weight, food faddism, excessive calorie restriction, and/or unexplained hypoglycemia. Moreover, in-

*Camp Directory, 1660 Duke St., Alexandria, VA 22314; (800) 232-3472.

sulin manipulation or omission has been identified as a weight loss tool used by some female adolescents (Rodin, Craven, and Daneman, 1989).

Inaccurate doses of insulin may occur inadvertently or, if they occur frequently, as an attention-seeking device, or in a number of cases as a subconscious but socially accepted method of suicide. Excessive intake of food leads to obesity, which may also represent a subconscious death wish. Psychiatric counseling may be needed if suicidal tendencies are amplified by the diabetes.

Rehospitalizations are most often related to poor control of the disease, although it is also possible that they are indirectly related to noncoping and are a method of avoiding the pressures caused by family and peers. The hospital may represent an environment that is peaceful and free of stress. The goal for this problem is to determine the cause of the hospitalization. It may be related to poor control, poor self-management, or the need for better supportive management at home. Evaluation should be based on the physiologic and psychologic adjustment of the child and the family.

Parents. Parents develop guilt feelings when they have a child with any chronic disease, especially one with a hereditary component. They cope with these feelings in a number of ways. For example, they may be overprotective or neglectful. Guilt-ridden parents may blame themselves for the disease, consciously or subconsciously. Nevertheless, they must come to realize through education and counseling that there was nothing they could have done to prevent the disease and that it was not their fault, since environmental as well as hereditary factors may be involved in the development of the disease.

Parents who are overprotective suffer from feelings of guilt, as well as fear of the unknown. Overprotection is a mechanism that alters the guilt responses to justify their own needs—for example, "If the child is in my sight, nothing worse will happen than has already happened by the child getting diabetes. Therefore, I am going to watch this child every single minute so that nothing further can happen to him." The overprotective parent becomes the smothering parent, one that hampers the growth, development, and maturation of the affected child.

The neglectful parent, on the other hand, has a different problem. This response is a mechanism developed to block feelings that give pain and provide relief from feelings of guilt—"This is your disease and I have no responsibilities related to your disease; therefore if anything bad happens to you as a result of your having this disease, it is not my fault." The neglectful parent assigns responsibilities to the child before the child is mature enough to accept a more adult role.

Threatened parents look at the disease as a way to keep the child tied to them. If the child learns to be independent, as is expected of the child in a camping experience, the parent may feel threatened and place obstacles in the child's path to independent development. Problems in the parental response provide a challenge for the nurse to assist by counseling or, if severe enough, to appropriately refer the parents to resources designed to help them alter their behavior.

Children who are sufficiently mature may be seen alone by the health professional, although the parents should not be made to feel that they are being left out. Times should be set aside during the child's health visit or afterward to meet the needs of the parents. They should also be included in special sessions to keep them abreast of the child's management, to help them continue to participate in the child's care, and to provide them with an opportunity to express their own feelings concerning their own or their child's adjustment to the disease. The amount of information that they offer at this time can give clues to their level of support of the child and help assist in decisions concerning the therapeutic management of the child. This helps guide the child through the most disruptive time of life—the teenage years.

Health professionals must be aware of parents who voice support and appear to be supporting the child to the optimum level but who, upon deeper interview techniques, are found to be supporting the child in word but not by action. These parents seldom see the need for following through from verbalizing to fulfilling the real needs of the child, and they unknowingly place obstacles in the child's path. They may be helping the child grow up too fast and therefore insecurely. Counseling is urgently needed for these parents who need to realize how their behavior affects the child. The classroom experience, group therapy, or parenting programs can help guide the parents' relationships with their children. All parents should be made to recognize that as children grow and develop they are children first and children with diabetes second. The ultimate goal for these parents is to be supportive of their children, to communicate more effectively, and to help their children develop in a more acceptable manner.

Evaluation

The effectiveness of nursing interventions is determined by continual reassessment and evaluation of care based on the following observational guidelines and expected outcomes:

1. Interview the family to determine their understanding of the disease; have the child and family demonstrate and discuss the needed assessment and therapeutic techniques.
2. Interview the family regarding their understanding of tight control; analyze and evaluate management records.
3. Discuss the disease with the child.
4. Interview the family and child regarding their feelings and concerns about the disease.

Expected outcomes:
See Nursing Care Plan, pp. 1818-1820.

KEY POINTS

- The endocrine system has three components: the cell, which sends a chemical message via a hormone; target cells, which receive the message; and the environment through which the chemical is transported from the site of synthesis to the sites of cellular action.

- Pituitary dysfunction is manifest primarily by growth disturbance.
- The main physiologic action of thyroid hormone is to regulate the basal metabolic rate and control the processes of growth and tissue differentiation.
- Disorders of thyroid function include hypothyroidism, autoimmune thyroiditis, goiter, and hyperthyroidism.
- Therapy for hyperthyroidism is directed at retarding the rate of hormone secretion and may include drug therapy, thyroidectomy, or radioiodine therapy.
- Classic forms of hypoparathyroidism in childhood are idiopathic—deficient production of PTH—and pseudohypoparathyroidism—increased PTH production with end organ unresponsiveness to PTH.
- The adrenal cortex secretes three important groups of hormones: glucocorticoids, mineralocorticoids, and sex steroids.
- Disorders of adrenal function include acute adrenocortical insufficiency, chronic adrenocortical insufficiency, Cushing syndrome, congenital adrenogenital hyperplasia, and hyperaldosteronism.
- Four categories of Cushing syndrome are pituitary, adrenal, ectopic, and iatrogenic.
- Management of congenital adrenogenital hyperplasia includes assignation of a sex according to genotype, administration of cortisone, and, possibly, reconstructive surgery.
- Childhood diabetes mellitus is categorized as insulin-dependent, non-insulin-dependent, and maturity-onset diabetes of youth.
- The focus of diabetes management is insulin replacement, diet, and exercise.
- Education of families includes explanation of diabetes, meal planning, administering insulin injection, monitoring, general hygienic practices, promoting exercise, record keeping, and observing for complications.

REFERENCES

Bach, J.: Cyclosporine in insulin-dependent diabetes mellitus, J. Pediatr. 111:1073-1074, 1987.

Binder, C., and others: Insulin pharmacokinetics, Diabetes Care 7:188-199, 1984.

Bloch, C.A., Clemons, P., and Sperling, M.A.: Puberty decreases insulin sensitivity, J. Pediatr. 110:481-487, 1987.

Brown, P.: Human growth hormone therapy and Creutzfeldt-Jakob disease: a drama in three acts, Pediatrics 81:85-89, 1988.

Brown, P., Gajdusek, D.C., and Gibbs, C.J.: Potential epidemic of Creutzfeldt-Jakob disease from human growth hormone therapy, N. Engl. J. Med. 313:728-731, 1985.

Bundak, R., and others: Long-term auxologic effects of human growth hormone, J. Pediatr. 112:875-879, 1988.

Cox, D.J., Carter, W.R., and Gonder-Frederick, L.: Without warning, Diabetes Forecast 39:41-43, 1986.

DiGeorge, A.M.: The endocrine system. In Behrman, R.E., and Vaughan, V.C., III: Textbook of pediatrics, ed. 13, Philadelphia, 1987, W.B. Saunders Co.

Drash, A.L.: Insulin-dependent diabetes mellitus in children and adolescents: genetics and etiology, Curr. Opin. Pediatr. 1:61-73, 1989.

Eisenbarth, G.: Immunology: new knowledge and new horizons, JDF Countdown 8(1):8-14, 1987.

Eisenbarth, G.S., and others: The natural history of type I diabetes, Diabetes Metab. Rev. 3:873-891, 1987.

Fink, J.N., and Beall, G.N.: Immunologic aspects of endocrine diseases, JAMA 248:2696-2700, 1982.

Foley, T.P.: Thyroid disease. In Gellis, S.S., and Kagan, B.M.: Current pediatric therapy 12, Philadelphia, 1986, W.B. Saunders Co.

Jenkins, C.A., and Molitch, M.E.: Get the most out of mixing insulin, Diabetes Forecast 39(1):13-14, 1986.

Lever, E., and Jaspan, J.: Sodium bicarbonate therapy in severe diabetic ketoacidosis, Am. J. Med. 75:263-268, 1983.

MacDonald, M.J.: Etiology and classification of diabetes in children, Prim. Care 10:531-551, 1983.

Mahoney, C.P.: Differential diagnosis of goiter, Pediatr. Clin. North Am. 34:891-905, 1987.

Malone, J.I., and others: Risk factors for diabetic retinopathy in youth, Pediatrics 73:756-761, 1984.

New, M.I., Levine, L.S., and Temeck, J.W.: Disorders of the adrenal gland. In Gellis, S.S., and Kagan, B.M.: Current pediatric therapy 12, Philadelphia, 1986, W.B. Saunders Co.

Nora, J.J., and Fraser, F.C.: Medical genetics, Philadelphia, 1989, Lea & Febiger.

Pescovitz, O.H., and others: The NIH experience with precocious puberty diagnostic subgroups and response to short-term luteinizing hormone–releasing hormone analogue therapy, J. Pediatr. 108:47-54, 1986.

Plotnick, L.P.: Insulin-dependent diabetes mellitus. In Oski, F.A., and others, editors: Principles and practice of pediatrics, Philadelphia, 1990, J.B. Lippincott Co.

Poteet, G., Reinert, B., and Ptak, H.: Outcome of multiple usage of disposable syringes in the insulin-requiring diabetic, Nurs. Res. 36:350-352, 1987.

Rappaport, E.: Iatrogenic Creutzfeldt-Jakob disease, Neurology 37:1520-1526, 1987.

Rappaport, R., and others: Suppression of immune function in growth hormone–deficient children during treatment with human growth hormone, J. Pediatr. 109:434-439, 1986.

Reiter, E.O., and others: Childhood thyromegaly: recent developments, J. Pediatr. 99:507-518, 1981.

Rodin, G., Craven, J., and Daneman, D.: Eating disorders and insulin manipulation in adolescent females with insulin-dependent diabetes mellitus, Psychosom. Med. 51:244-266, 1989.

Rosenstock, J., Strowig, S., and Raskin, P.: Insulin pump therapy: a realistic appraisal, Clin. Diabetes 3:1, 27-30, 1985.

Sack, J., and others: Association of automimmune thyroiditis and HLA-DR5 in multiple family members, J. Pediatr. 103:758-760, 1983.

Silver, H.K., Gotlin, R.W., and Klingensmith, G.J., editors: Endocrine disorders. In Kempe, C.H., Silver, H.K., and O'Brien, D.: Current pediatric diagnosis and treatment, ed. 8, Los Altos, CA, 1984, Lange Medical Publications.

Sonis, W.A., and others: Behavior problems and social competence in girls with true precocious puberty, J. Pediatr. 106:156-160, 1985.

Sperling, M.A.: Diabetic ketoacidosis, Pediatr. Clin. North Am. 31:591-610, 1984.

Sperling, M.A.: Diabetes mellitus. In Behrman, R.E., and Vaughan, V.C., III: Textbook of pediatrics, ed. 13, Philadelphia, 1987, W.B. Saunders Co.

Starkman, H., and others: Limited joint mobility (LJM) of the hand in patients with diabetes mellitus: relation to chronic complications, Ann. Rheum. Dis. 4:130-151, 1986.

Stiller, C.R., and others: Effects of cyclosporine in recent-onset juvenile type 1 diabetes: impact of age and duration of disease, J. Pediatr. 111:1069-1072, 1987.

Thatcher, G.: Insulin injections: the case against random rotation, Am. J. Nurs. 85:690-692, 1985.

Thompson, G., and others: Genetic heterogeneity, modes of inheritance, and risk estimates for a joint study of Caucasians with insulin-dependent diabetes mellitus, Am. J. Hum. Genet. 43:799-816, 1988.

Underwood, L.E.: Endocrine system. In Gellis, S.S., and Kagan, B.M.: Current pediatric therapy 12, Philadelphia, 1986, W.B. Saunders Co.
White, K., and others: Unstable diabetes and unstable families: a psychosocial evaluation of diabetic children with recurrent ketoacidosis, Pediatrics 73:749-755, 1984.
Wolfsdorf, J.I.: Diabetes mellitus. In Gellis, S.S., and Kagan, B.M.: Current pediatric therapy 12, Philadelphia, 1986, W.B. Saunders Co.
Wong, D.L.: The significance of dead space in syringes, Am. J. Nurs. 82:1237, 1982.
Young, R.J., and others: Diabetic lipohypertrophy delays insulin absorption, Diabetes Care 7:479-480, 1984.

BIBLIOGRAPHY

Pituitary Dysfunction

Bercu, B.B.: Growth hormone treatment and the short child: to treat or not to treat? J. Pediatr. 110:991-994, 1987.
Bundak, R., and others: Long-term auxologic effects of human growth hormone, J. Pediatr. 112:875-879, 1987.
Costin, G., and Kaufman, F.R.: Growth hormone secretory patterns in children with short stature, J. Pediatr. 110:362-368, 1987.
Genentech Collaborative Study: Idiopathic short stature: results of a one-year controlled study of human growth hormone treatment, J. Pediatr. 15:713-719, 1989.
Jackson, P.L., and Ott, M.J.: Precocious puberty: the role of the school nurse, School Nurse 6(1):16-18, 1990.
Kappy, M.S., Stuart, T., and Perelman, A.: Efficacy of leuprolide therapy in children with central precocious puberty, Am. J. Dis. Child. 142:1061-1064, 1988.
Lee, P.A., Page, J.G., and Leuprolide Study Group: Effects of leuprolide in the treatment of central precocious puberty, J. Pediatr. 114:321-324, 1989.
Lippe, B.M.: Short stature in children: evaluation and management, J. Pediatr. Health Care 1:313-322, 1987.
Manasco, P.K., and others: Resumption of puberty after long-term luteinizing hormone–releasing hormone agonist treatment of central precocious puberty, J. Clin. Endocrinol. Metab. 67:368-372, 1988.
McElroy, D.B., and Davis, G.T.: SIADH and the acutely ill child, MCN 11:193-196, 1986.
Parks, B.R., and Fischer, R.G.: Growth hormone, Pediatr. Nurs. 12:302, 1986.
Root, A.W., Diamond, F.B., and Bercu, B.B.: Short stature: when is growth hormone indicated? Contemp. Pediatr. 4(2):26-56, 1987.
Ross, J.L., and others: Growth hormone secretory dynamics in children with precocious puberty, J. Pediatr. 110:369-372, 1987.
Saggese, G., and Cesaretti, G.: Criteria for recognition of the growth-inefficient child who may respond to treatment with growth hormone, Am. J. Dis. Child. 143:1287-1293, 1989.
Schwartz, I.D., and Root, A.W.: Puberty in girls: early, incomplete, or precocious? Contemp. Pediatr. 7(1):147-156, 1990.
Stern, M., and Zaiken, H.: Assessing the child with short stature, Pediatr. Nurs. 11:106-110, 1985.
Stewarts, M.L.K.: When patient has the "other" diabetes, RN 48(5):54-58, 1985.
Usala, A, and Blumer, J.L.: Pharmacology of new hormonal therapies in the treatment of pediatric endocrine disorders, Pediatr. Clin. North Am. 36:1157-1182, 1989.
Zucker, A.R., and Chernow, B.: Diabetes insipidus and the syndrome of inappropriate antidiuretic hormone release, Crit. Care Q. 6(3):63-74, 1983.

Disorders of Thyroid Function/Disorders of the Parathyroid Gland

Arcangelo, V.P.: Simple goiter, Nursing '83 13(3):47, 1983.
Bachrach, L.K., and others: Use of ultrasound in childhood thyroid disorders, J. Pediatr. 103:547-552, 1983.
Fisher, D.A., Pandian, M.R., and Carlton, E.: Autoimmune thyroid disease: an expanding spectrum, Pediatr. Clin. North Am. 34:907-918, 1987.
Gorton, C., Sadeghi-Nejd, A, and Senior, B.: Remission in children with hyperthyroidism treated with propylthiouracil, Am. J. Dis. Child. 141:1084-1086, 1987.
Mäenpää, J., and others: Natural course of juvenile autoimmune thyroiditis, J. Pediatr. 107:898-904, 1985.

Adrenal Dysfunction

Camunas, C.: Surviving pheochromocytoma, Am. J. Nurs. 83:887-891, 1983.
Darland, N.W.: Congenital adrenocortical hyperplasia: supportive nursing interventions, J. Pediatr. Nurs. 1(2):117-123, 1986.
Larson, C.A.: The critical path of adrenocortical insufficiency, Nursing '84 14(10):66-69, 1984.
Lee, P.D.K., Winter, R.J., and Green, O.C.: Virilizing adrenocortical tumors in childhood: eight cases and a review of the literature, Pediatrics 76:437-444, 1985.
New, M.I., and Levine, L.S.: New developments in congenital adrenal hyperplasia, Pediatr. Ann. 10:346-355, 1981.
Sanford, S.J.: Dysfunction of the adrenal gland: physiologic considerations and nursing problems, Nurs. Clin. North Am. 15:481-498, 1980.

Diabetes Mellitus: General

Aziz, S.: Recurrent use of disposable syringe-needle units in diabetic children, Diabetes Care 7:118-120, 1984.
Brouhard, B.H.: Control and monitoring for the child with insulin-dependent diabetes mellitus, Am. J. Dis. Child. 137:787-794, 1983.
Brouhard, B.H.: Management of the very young diabetic, Am. J. Dis. Child. 139:446-447, 1985.
Caprio, S., and others: Increased insulin secretion in puberty: a compensatory response to reductions in insulin sensitivity, J. Pediatr. 114:963-967, 1989.
Chase, H.P., and others: Diagnosis of pre-type I diabetes, J. Pediatr. 111:807-812, 1987.
Christensen, K.S.: Self-management in diabetic children, Diabetes Care 6:552-555, 1983.
Cunningham, L.: Sports nutrition for the serious athlete, Diabetes Forecast 39(1):63-64, 1986.
DiFlorio, I.A., and Duncan, P.: Design for successful patient teaching, MCN 11:246-249, 1986.
Donohue-Porter, P.: Insulin-dependent diabetes mellitus, Nurs. Clin. North Am. 20:191-198, 1985.
Haire-Joshu, D., Flavin, K., and Clutter, W.: Contrasting type I and type II diabetes, Am. J. Nurs. 86:1240-1243, 1986.
Ingersoll, G.M., and others: Cognitive maturity and self-management among adolescents with insulin-dependent diabetes mellitus, J. Pediatr. 108:620-623, 1986.
Jackson, R.L.: Growth and maturation of children with insulin-dependent diabetes mellitus, Pediatr. Clin. North Am. 31:545-567, 1984.
Leslie, N.D., and Sperling, M.A.: Relation of metabolic control to complications in diabetes mellitus, J. Pediatr. 108:491-497, 1986.
Lipman, T.H.: What causes diabetes? MCN 13:40-43, 1988.
Rossini, A.A., Mordes, J.P., and Handler, E.A.S.: A tumbler hypothesis: the autoimmunity of insulin-dependent diabetes mellitus, Diabetes Spectrum 2:195-200, 1989.
Rotter, J., and others: HLA genotype study of insulin-dependent diabetes, Diabetes 32:169-174, 1983.
Skyler, J.S., and Rabinovitch, A.: Etiology and pathogenesis of insulin dependent diabetes mellitus, Pediatr. Ann. 16:682-692, 1987.
Tamborlane, W.V.: Teenage trouble with glucose control: it's not all in their heads, JDF Countdown 8(2):14-17, 1987.
Travis, L.B., Brouhard, B.H., and Schriener, B.: Diabetes mellitus in children, Philadelphia, 1987, W.B. Saunders Co.

Diabetes Mellitus: Testing and Monitoring

Belsey, R., and others: Managing bedside glucose testing in the hospital, JAMA 258:1634-1638, 1987.

Clarson, C., and others: Self-monitoring of blood glucose: how accurate are children with diabetes at reading Chemstrip bG? Diabetes Care 8:354-358, 1985.

Connors, M.H.: Blood glucose monitoring in childhood diabetes, Nurse Pract. 9:30-32, 62, 1984.

Daneman, D., and others: The role of self-monitoring of blood glucose in the routine management of children with insulin-dependent diabetes mellitus, Diabetes Care 8:1-4, 1985.

Davis, S.G., and others: In-hospital bedside blood glucose monitoring: the importance of a quality control program, J. Pediatr. Nurs. 4:353-356, 1989.

Fow, S.M.: Home blood glucose monitoring in children with insulin-dependent diabetes mellitus, Pediatr. Nurs. 9:439-442, 1983.

Furberg, H., Jensen, A.K., and Salbu, B.: Effect of pretreatment with 0.9% sodium chloride on insulin solutions on the delivery of insulin from an infusion system, Am. J. Hosp. Pharm. 43:2209-2212, 1986.

Hahn, K.: Testing blood glucose levels, Nursing '89 19(12):66, 1989.

Loman, D., and Galgani, C.: Monitoring diabetic children's blood-glucose levels at home, MCN 9:192-196, 1984.

Lombrail, P., and others: Abnormal color vision and reliable self-monitoring of blood glucose, Diabetes Care 7:318-321, 1984.

Miller, V.G.: Diabetes: let's stop testing urine, Am. J. Nurs. 86:54, 1986.

Montana, J.A.: Glucose meters, J. Pediatr. Nurs. 4:132-136, 1989.

Riley, W.J., Winter, W.E., and Maclaren, N.K.: Identification of insulin-dependent diabetes mellitus before the onset of clinical symptoms, J. Pediatr. 112:314-316, 1988.

Robertson, C.: How to teach patients to monitor blood glucose, RN 48(12):24-25,1985.

Robertson, C.: Interpreting blood glucose studies, Nursing '86 16(8):64, 1986.

Strumph, P.S., Odoroff, C.L., and Amatruda, J.M.: The accuracy of blood glucose testing by children, Clin. Pediatr. 27:188-194, 1988.

Diabetes Mellitus: Therapeutic Management

Alli, C.R., and Crapo, P.A.: Sweetener safety: the bitter debate, Diabetes Forecast 38(3):34-37, 1985.

Arky, R.A.: Nutrition therapy for the child and adolescent with type I diabetes mellitus, Pediatr. Clin. North Am. 31:711-719, 1984.

Bates, S., and Ahern, J.A.: Tight control: what does it mean? Am. J. Nurs. 86:1256-1258, 1986.

Borders, L., Bingham, P., and Riddle, M.: Traditional insulin-use practices and the incidence of bacterial contamination and infection, Diabetes Care 7:121, 1984.

Byrnes, C.A.: What's new in the diabetic diet, Nursing '87 17(8):58-59, 1987.

Chait, A.: Dietary management of diabetes mellitus, Contemp. Nutr. 9(2):1-2, 1984.

Chase, H.P, and others: Cyclosporine A for the treatment of new-onset insulin-dependent diabetes mellitus, Pediatrics 85:241-245, 1990.

Clark, L.M., and Plotnick, L.P.: Insulin pumps in children with diabetes, J. Pediatr. Health Care 4:3-10, 1990.

Dicenso, A.M.: Eating out, Diabetes Forecast 41:82, 1988.

Doner, K.: Exercise and diabetes, JDF Internat. Countdown 10(4):16-20, 1989.

Fishman, P.B.: Teaching children to buy food, Diabetes Forecast 39:12-15, 1986.

Flavin, K., and Haire-Joshu, D.: The pharmacologic repertoire, Am. J. Nurs. 86:1244-1249, 1986.

Franz, M.J.: An exchange list for the 80s, Diabetes Forecast, p. 61, Oct. 1986.

Franz, M.J.: Fast food: where's the nutrition? Diabetes Forecast 38(6):31-34, 1985.

Gavin, J.R., III: Diabetes and exercise, Am. J. Nurs. 88:178-180, 1988.

Hahn, K.: Teaching patients to administer insulin, Nursing '90 20(4):70, 1990.

Haire-Joshu, D., Flavin, K., and Santiago, J.V.: Intensive conventional insulin therapy, Am. J. Nurs. 88:1251-1253, 1986.

Heins, J.M., Wylie-Rosett, and Davis, S.G.: The new look in diabetic diets, Am. J. Nurs. 87:196-198, 1987.

Hurxthal, K.: Quick! Teach this patient about insulin, Am. J. Nurs. 88:1097-1100, 1988.

Institute of Food Technologists' Expert Panel on Food Safety and Nutrition: Sweeteners: nutritive and nonnutritive, Contemp. Nutr. 12(9), 1987.

Kruger, D.F., Treacy, M., and Whitehouse, F.W.: Jet injection comes of age, Diabetes Forecast 41:17-18, 1988.

LaPorte, R.E., and others: Pittsburgh insulin-dependent diabetes mellitus morbidity and mortality study: physical activity and diabetic complications, Pediatrics 78:1027-1033, 1986.

Lockwood, D.N., Trand, M.J., and Mather, H.M.: Is injecting air into insulin bottles necessary? Br. Med. J. 297:1315-1316, 1988.

Lorenz, R.A., Christensen, N.K., and Pichert, J.W.: Diet-related knowledge, skill, and adherence among children with insulin-dependent diabetes mellitus, Pediatrics 75:872-876, 1985.

Marrero, D.G., Fremion, A.S., and Golden, M.P.: Inproving compliance with exercise in adolescents with insulin-dependent diabetes mellitus: results of a self-motivated home exercise program, Pediatrics 81:519-525, 1988.

Maryniuk, M.D.: Eating out, Diabetes Forecast 41:57-58, 1988.

Price, J., and others: Evaluation of the insulin jet injector as a potential source of infection, Am. J. Infect. Control 17:257-263, 1989.

Rowland, T.W., and others: Glycemic control with physical training in insulin-dependent diabetes mellitus, Am. J. Dis. Child. 139:307-309, 1985.

Schiffrin, A.: Management of childhood diabetes, Pediatr. Ann. 16:694-710, 1987.

Schiffrin, A., and others: Feasibility of strict diabetes control in insulin-dependent diabetic adolescents, J. Pediatr. 103:522-527, 1983.

Sperling, M.A.: Outpatient management of diabetes mellitus, Pediatr. Clin. North Am. 34:919-934, 1987.

Stein, R., and others: Exercise and the patient with type I diabetes mellitus, Pediatr. Clin. North Am. 31:665-673, 1984.

Sutherland, D.E.R., and others: Pancreas transplantation, Pediatr. Clin. North Am. 31:735-750, 1984.

Diabetes Mellitus: Complications

Bailie, M.D.: Heading off the complications of diabetes, Contemp. Pediatr. 6(1):87-102, 1989.

Chase, H.P., and others: Glucose control and the renal and retinal complications of insulin-dependent diabetes, JAMA 261:1155-1160, 1989.

Chipman, J.J., and Marks, J.F.: Diabetic ketoacidosis. In Levin, D.L., Morriss, F.C., and Moore, G.C., editors: A practical guide to pediatric intensive care, ed. 3, St. Louis, 1988, Mosby–Year Book, Inc.

Daneman, D., and others: Severe hypoglycemia in children with insulin-dependent diabetes mellitus: frequency and predisposing factors, J. Pediatr. 681-685, 1989.

Gill, G.V., and Alberti, K.G.G.M.: The ups and downs of brittle diabetes, Diabetes Forecast 39(1):45-46, 50, 1986.

Golden, M.P., Herrold, A.J., and Orr, D.P.: An approach to prevention of recurrent diabetic ketoacidosis in the pediatric population, J. Pediatr. 107:195-200, 1985.

Hernandez, C.M.G.: Surgery and diabetes: minimizing the risks, Am. J. Nurs. 7:788-792, 1987.

Krane, E.J.: Diabetic ketoacidosis, Pediatr. Clin. North Am. 34:935-960, 1987.

LaFranchi, S.: Hypoglycemia of infancy and childhood, Pediatr. Clin. North Am. 34:961-982, 1987.

Lipman, T.H.: Assessment of the child with diabetic ketoacidosis, Dimens. Crit. Care Nurs. 6:82-93, 1987.

Malone, J.I., and others: Hypercalciuria, hyperphosphaturia, and growth retardation in children with diabetes mellitus, Pediatrics 78:298-304, 1986.

Narins, B.: Products to help with insulin reactions, Diabetes Forecast 39(5):26, 1986.

Ransey, P.W.: Hyperglycemia at dawn, Am. J. Nurs. 87:1424-1426, 1987.

Ryan, J.R.: Nonprescription drugs: caution prescribed, Diabetes Forecast 39:33-34, 1986.

Sabo, C.E., and Michael, S.R.: Managing D.K.A. and preventing a recurrence, Nursing '89 19(2):50-56, 1989.

Stock, P.L.: Action stat! insulin shock, Nursing '85 15(4):53, 1985.

Diabetes Mellitus: Child and Family

Ahlfield, J.E., Soler, N.G., and Marcus, S.D.: Adolescent diabetes mellitus: parent/child perspectives of the effect of the disease on family and social interactions, Diabetes Care 6:393-398, 1983.

Armstrong, N.: Coping with diabetes mellitus, Nurs. Clin. North Am. 22:559-568, 1987.

Balik, B., Haig, B., and Moynihan, P.M.: Diabetes and the school-aged child, MCN 11:324-330, 1986.

Banion, C.R., Miles, M.S., and Carter, M.C.: Problems of mothers in management of children with diabetes, Diabetes Care 6:548-551, 1983.

Beck, S.J.: Adjustment and compliance of the child with diabetes, Feelings Med. Signif. 28:25-28, 1986.

Betschart, J.: Back to school, Diabetes Forecast 40:48-52, 1987.

Brown, A.J.: School-age children with diabetes: knowledge and management of the disease, and adequacy of self-concept, Matern. Child Nurs. J. 14(1):47-61, 1985.

Cerreto, M.C., and Travis, L.B.: Implications of psychological and family factors in the treatment of diabetes, Pediatr. Clin. North Am. 31:689-710, 1984.

Dunning, D.: Safe travel tips for the diabetic patient, RN 52(4):51-54, 1989.

Edwards, D.R.: Initial psychosocial impact of insulin-dependent diabetes mellitus on the pediatric client and family, Issues Compr. Pediatr. Nurs. 10:199-207, 1987.

Ferrari, M.: The diabetic child and well sibling: risks to the well child's self-concept, Child. Health Care 15:141-148, 1987.

Frey, M.A., and Denyes, M.J.: Health and illness self-care in adolescents with IDDM: a test of Orem's theory, Adv. Nurs. Sci. 12(1):67-75, 1989.

Gallo, A.M.: Family management style in juvenile diabetes: a case illustration, J. Pediatr. Nurs. 5:23-32, 1990.

Ginsberg-Fellner, F.: Balancing the scales: weight control for teens is a delicate problem, JDF Countdown 8(3):22-23, 1987.

Harrigan, J.F., and others: The application of locus of control to diabetes education in school-aged children, J. Pediatr. Nurs. 2:236-243, 1987.

Hodges, L.C., and Parker, J.: Concerns of parents with diabetic children, Pediatr. Nurs. 13:22-24, 68, 1987.

Jacobson, A.M., and others: Psychologic predictors of compliance in children with recent onset of diabetes mellitus, J. Pediatr. 110:805-811, 1987.

Kovacs, M., and others: Initial coping response and psychosocial characteristics of children with insulin-dependent diabetes mellitus, J. Pediatr. 106:827-834, 1985.

La Greca, A., and Satin, W.: Peer pressure, Diabetes Forecast 41:67-72, 1988.

Lipman, T.H., and others: A developmental approach to diabetes in children: birth through preschool, MCN 14:255-259, 1989.

Lipman, T.H., and others: A developmental approach to diabetes in children: school age—adolescence, MCN 14:330-332, 1989.

Lowe, E., and Arsham, G.: "I know how you feel," Diabetes Forecast 38(11):56-62, 1985.

Maiuri, S.: Overcoming the road blocks, Diabetes Forecast 40:48-49, 1987.

Margalit, M.: Mothers' perceptions of anxiety of their diabetic children, Dev. Behav. Pediatr. 7:27-30, 1986.

Moffatt, M.E.K., and Pless, I.B.: Locus of control in juvenile diabetic campers: changes during camp, and relationship to camp staff assessments, J. Pediatr. 103:146-150, 1983.

Moran, M.M.: Diabetes camps: management guidelines, Pediatr. Nurs. 11:183-186, 1985.

Pless, I.B., and others: Expected diabetic control in childhood and psychosocial functioning in early adult life, Diabetes Care 11:387-392, 1988.

Rovet, J.F., and Ehrlich, R.M.: Effect of temperament on metabolic control in children with diabetes mellitus, Diabetes Care 11:77-82, 1988.

Ryan, C., Vega, A., and Drash, A.: Cognitive deficits in adolescents who developed diabetes early in life, Pediatrics 75:921-927, 1985.

Saucier, C.P.: Self-concept and self-care management in school-age children with diabetes, Pediatr. Nurs. 10:135-138, 1984.

Schreiner, B.J., and Travis, L.B.: When your child has diabetes: the preteen years, Diabetes Forecast 40:37-41, 1987.

Smith, K.E., and others: Issues of managing diabetes in children and adolescents: a multifamily group approach, Child. Health Care 18:49-52, 1989.

Snyder, A.: The role of school personnel in caring for the child with diabetes, School Nurse 40:9-17, 1987.

Stenger, P.: Babysitter blues, Diabetes Forecast 41:53-54, 1988.

Tattersall, R.: Psychosocial aspects of diabetes in childhood and adolescence, Pediatr. Ann. 16:728-740, 1987.

Thorner, N.: Family vacations, Diabetes Forecast 40:45-46, 1987.

Zimmerman, E., and others: Diabetic camping: effect on knowledge, attitude, and self-concept, Issues Compr. Pediatr. Nurs. 10:99-111, 1987.

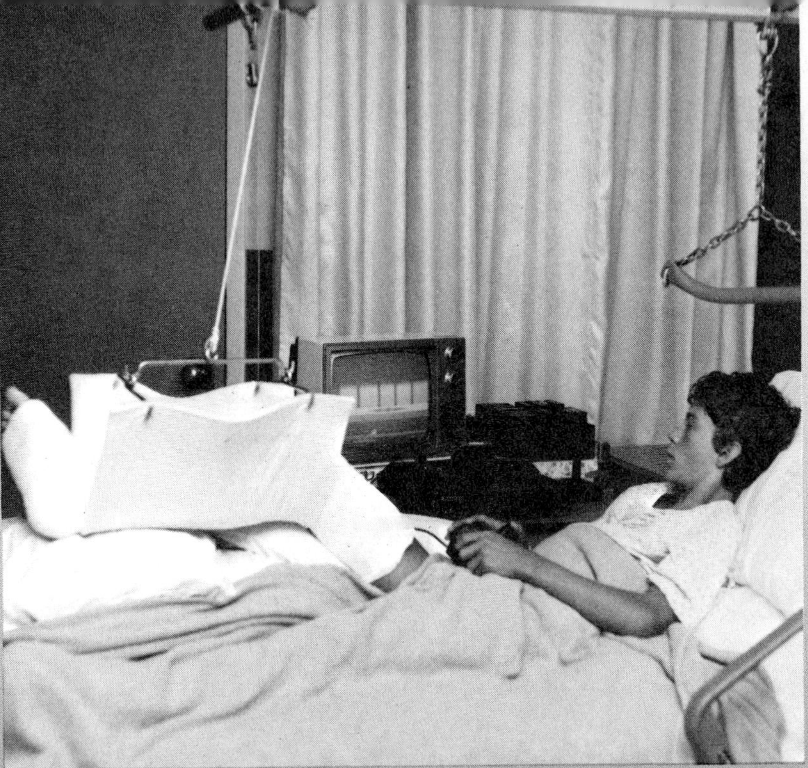

The Child with a Problem That Interferes with Physical Mobility

UNIT XIV

Childhood is the age of onset for a variety of physically disabling conditions of hereditary, infectious, or traumatic etiologies. Impaired mobility can be associated with diseases or deficits in the supporting structures (the skeleton), the movement-producing structures (muscles or their innervation), or the articulating structures (joints) of the body. Many disorders that interfere with movement are present at birth; a few of these have been discussed previously, including congenital defects such as myelomeningocele, dislocation of the hip, and foot deformities (see Chapter 11). Others appear later in childhood. Some of these can occur at any age, such as fractures; others make their appearance at ages characteristic for the specific condition, such as muscular dystrophy during early childhood and slipped femoral capital epiphysis at puberty.

Some locomotor disabilities are acquired in an instant, such as amputation or spinal cord injury, whereas others develop over an extended period, such as tuberculosis or progressive muscular atrophy. Some, including fractures, need only short-term therapy; others, such as spinal cord injuries and cerebral palsy, require long-term therapy and a longer period of adjustment and involve the whole problem of daily living activities.

The physical limitations may involve only temporary inconvenience, or they may be permanent and require an alternative form of locomotion. Some are helped by specific treatments; for others therapy is merely supportive. A large number of these disabilities require a health team approach with contributions from a variety of specialists. Concomitant problems associated with permanent disabilities, particularly those acquired in later childhood, are emotional adjustment and alterations in self-image.

Chapter 39, *The Child with Musculoskeletal or Articular Dysfunction,* is concerned with problems related to the supporting and articular structures of the body, primarily bones, ligaments, and articular surfaces. Chapter 40, *The Child with Neuromuscular Dysfunction,* deals with congenital or acquired disorders involving neurologic and muscular function. The coverage is by no means comprehensive, but representative examples are used to illustrate specific problems.

CHAPTER 39

The Child with Musculoskeletal or Articular Dysfunction

RELATED TOPICS

Birth injuries, Ch. 9
Congenital clubfoot, Ch. 11
Congenital hip dysplasia, Ch. 11
Injuries—the leading killer, Ch. 1
Injury prevention: infant, Ch. 12; toddler, Ch. 14; preschooler, Ch. 15; school-age child, Ch. 17; and adolescent, Ch. 19.
Physical activity, Ch. 17

GLOSSARY

JA Juvenile arthritis
JRA Juvenile rheumatoid arthritis
LCPD Legg-Calvé-Perthes disease
LE Lupus erythematosus
NSAID Nonsteroidal antiiflammatory drugs
OI Osteogenesis imperfecta
SAARD Slower-acting antirheumatic drugs
SFCE Slipped femoral capital epiphysis
SLE Systemic lupus erythematosus

The musculoskeletal system is composed of a variety of structures. Each component of the system is essential for the mobility needed to perform activities of daily living, such as walking, feeding, dressing, and playing. The skeleton, or bony framework, provides the support; the muscles, tendons, ligaments, and joints allow for active movement. Muscles are attached to bones by tendons, and strong, fibrous bands (ligaments) attach the bone ends to an articulated joint. Muscles are innervated by sensory and motor fibers from the central nervous system. The bulk of musculoskeletal problems are related to traumatic injuries, which are common in childhood. Degenerative conditions of bone usually involve lengthy treatment. The first part of this chapter is devoted to the problem of immobility and trauma, particularly musculoskeletal trauma. The remainder of the chapter deals with less common skeletal and articular disorders.

■ THE CHILD AND TRAUMA

Trauma is the leading cause of death in children over age 1 year (see Chapter 1) and an important cause of disability during childhood and adolescence. Most injuries are relatively minor and cause little disruption in the daily life of the child and produce only minor discomfort. However, accidental injury is the leading cause of death in the pediatric age-group. Every year thousands of children die and many thousands more are permanently disabled as a result of trauma. Any or all musculoskeletal structures can be involved in a traumatic injury and may alter the course of healing in certain situations. Some skeletal injuries heal in a short time; others, such as fractured femurs, take much longer.

TRAUMA MANAGEMENT

In order to provide optimum care for trauma victims, community resources for children must be available and appropriately organized for rapid transit, skilled care, and specialized facilities. With such a system of care for pediatric patients, the mortality and morbidity can be minimized (Ramenofsky and Morse, 1983).

Epidemiology of Trauma

In many ways childhood trauma differs little from trauma in adults. However, many aspects of injury are affected by the developmental stage of the child in both the type of injury that is incurred and the physiologic response to injury.

Accidental injury. Among the leading causes of morbidity in children are medical problems resulting from traumatic injury at home, at school, in an automobile, or associated with recreational activities. Children's everyday activities include vigorous play, such as climbing, falling, running into immovable objects, and receiving blows to any part of their bodies. All of these activities make them prone to injury. School-age children and adolescents are vulnerable to multiple and severe trauma because they are mobile on bikes and motorcycles and in automobiles; they are also active in sports. Speed and congested surroundings often intensify the chance of injury.

Young children and teenagers usually do not calculate risks as they learn to manipulate their environment and achieve developmental goals. Therefore accidents are a part of most childhood experiences. Fortunately, when children fall or are hit, their body resilience protects them from incurring serious damage to soft tissue, the musculoskeletal system, or other body organs. Their bones are more flexible and therefore do not offer the rigid resistance to external forces that are likely to cause fractures (as occurs in more mature bones).

Child abuse injury. Unfortunately, careless handling of an infant or child (in some instances intentional physical abuse) is not uncommon in our society. A multitude of different types of bone and soft tissue injuries are inflicted on children by adults, and smaller children who are unable to protect themselves are most vulnerable. It is estimated that perhaps 25% of fractures in children under 3 years of age are the result of child abuse. Emergency room and pediatric office personnel should be alert to situations in which the child's injuries are not congruent with the parent's description of the incident; in which the child's behavior, such as lack of crying or fearful mannerisms, are not the expected ones; or in which x-ray films show multiple healed fractures. For example, toddlers do not readily fall and break bones or catch a leg in the crib and break it. Reporting these incidents will aid in securing help for the child and family. A traumatic incident that produces physical injury to an infant or child may be the outcome of an accident that was no one's fault or may be associated with child abuse. A well-documented history is essential to determine the cause of the injury. (See Physical Abuse, Chapter 16.)

Birth injuries. During the birth process, fractures, dislocations, and/or nerve damage may be sustained. These injuries most often occur when the baby is large, the presentation is breech, or forceful extraction is used because of fetal distress. The two most common types of musculoskeletal injuries incurred during birth are fractured clavicle and brachial plexus injury. The presence of a qualified person at delivery will aid in reducing the complications of a difficult delivery. Complete postdelivery assessment of the newborn is essential for early detection of neurologic and/or musculoskeletal problems. (See also Birth Injuries, Chapter 9.)

Childhood characteristics. Certain developmental characteristics of children at various ages render them more susceptible to injury. For example, the large head of infants and toddlers predisposes them to head injury, especially in falls. Also, the relatively large spleen and liver and the broad costal arch make these organs prone to direct trauma. Because of their light weight and small size, infants and small children are easily thrown around in a moving vehicle. Their natural curiosity and propensity for using large muscles lure them to attempt potentially hazardous activities.

Later, in school-age children and adolescents, whose bone growth outstrips muscle growth, difficulty controlling movement can contribute to physical injury. It is also a time when many of these youngsters are attempting to engage in activities beyond their capabilities to keep up with more agile companions. They are also vulnerable to a "dare." Risk taking compounded by a feeling of invulnerability is also characteristic of adolescence.

Prevention of Injury

Hazardous environmental factors play a major role in the number of serious accidents incurred by children. Stairways without handrails or a gate at the top, cluttered walkways, waxed floors, or throw rugs can contribute to a severe fall. Playground equipment should be checked periodically for hazards, and play areas should be supervised. Adults in charge of sports activities are encouraged to promote the use of safety-tested equipment and to follow game rules to prevent trauma and overplaying of a young athlete whose immature musculoskeletal system and lack of coordination cannot tolerate excessive abuse.

Musculoskeletal trauma is most likely to occur in contact sports, with sprains being common. Certain contact sports, such as football, tend to produce joint damage, especially knee injuries. Severe hyperflexion of the neck from diving, trampoline activities, or football produces spinal cord injury and quadriplegia. Protective head and shoulder gear is helpful, but youngsters usually do not consistently wear appropriate protection unless they are well supervised (see Injuries and Health Problems Related to Sports Participation, p. 1871).

For children riding in a car, an effective infant or child car seat is a must to avoid their being thrown during a sudden stop or collision (see Chapters 12 and 14). If this practice is begun when the child is an infant, the young child will be more likely to develop the habit of securing safety belts before the engine is started. In their everyday life observant nurses are a valuable community resource in giving suggestions to parents and schools that might prevent at least some very serious injuries. (See also injury prevention segments in sections on health promotion during various age-groups.) *Safe and Sound,* a book written by Bosque and Watson of Babysavers CPR, Inc.,* is designed to teach parents, baby-sitters, and other caretakers how to deal with common childhood emergencies, including trauma.

ASSESSMENT OF TRAUMA

The site of the injury usually influences the order of priority of interventions when instituting emergency care. The safety of both the victim and the "Good Samaritan" rescuers must be considered in order to prevent further injury. For example, removing a child from a burning building or the bottom of a swimming pool is the obvious action to the logically thinking person, but anxious rescuers may not consider their safety to be of prime importance. The major reason for thinking through steps to be taken in an emergency before the actual incident occurs is to have a mental repertory of preplanned actions available at a stimulus-response level.

Emergency Management

Guidelines for care of the child at the scene of the injury are outlined under Emergency Treatment. The first concerns are always for *airway, breathing,* and *circulation,* after which other injuries are managed as indicated by the assessment. Severe bleeding is treated by removing gross debris from the wound, such as glass, but not if a large object is impaled in the victim. In this situation the wound is covered with a sterile or clean dressing, and direct pressure is applied over the wound or at appropriate pressure points. (See management of specific injuries in the remainder of this chapter.)

Assessment of the child involves observation from head to toes because infants and young children are unable to communicate except by crying and other behaviors. Therefore pinpointing areas of pain is very difficult. To check for any motor or sensory dysfunction in extremities, the nurse should note any spontaneous movement, which provides the best clue in infants and young children. Older children are able to follow directions for wiggling toes or fingers. The child is not encouraged to move all extremities until after it is determined that no spinal injury is present.

A spinal cord injury is suspected if there is loss of sensation or motor function. In this case a child is moved only if remaining in the present position is a threat to safety; if so, the child is carried in log fashion with the head and neck held firmly in a neutral position. No attempt should be made to transport the child until adequate help can be obtained to keep the body in straight alignment throughout and after the repositioning.

✦ **NURSING ALERT** Pain at the level of the injury, local muscle spasms, and sensorimotor loss are the outstanding features of spinal cord injury.

The child should be identified as soon as feasible by anyone who knows the child. It is important to determine if the child has any existing health problems that might have implications for the circumstances of the injury and for therapeutic management. Any witnesses are asked for details about the incident to aid in assessment of the child's emotional responses.

In situations of severe injury the emergency medical team will be needed to treat for shock and to transport the child adequately to the nearest emergency facility. Hospital emergency departments have protocols for managing injuries, including establishing an intravenous line, ventilatory assistance, and monitoring vital signs, as well as radiography, laboratory, and other diagnostic services.

Systematic Assessment

There are several factors that can affect a child's response to trauma. An undetected congenital anomaly can contribute to a complicated injury. Acute gastric distention is a frequent occurrence in children because of the crying and

*Published by St. Martin's Press, 175 Fifth Ave., New York, NY 10010; (212) 674-5151.

BOX 39-1 GUIDELINES FOR ASSESSING TRAUMA

Head

Observe for level of consciousness.
Feel the head—palpate for depression or swelling over the cranium; feel the facial bones for depression or pain.
Observe for bruises, petechiae of skin and conjunctiva, singed hair, extraocular movement, pupil size and reactivity.
Observe the palate and mobility of the maxilla if child is cooperative.
Observe for drainage from ears and nose.

Neck

Observe status of neck veins (distended with chest injury), swelling, bruising, deformity of thyroid cartilage, penetrating wounds.
Palpate cervical spine (maintaining traction and neutral position), thyroid for tenderness, position of trachea, evidence of subcutaneous emphysema, carotid pulses.
Auscultate for bruits.

Chest

Observe symmetry of respiratory movement, flail segment, bruising, penetrating wounds.
Palpate clavicles, sternum, thoracic spine, subcutaneous emphysema; compress rib cage for local tenderness.
Auscultate for diminished breath sounds (hemothorax or pneumothorax), shifted or muffled heart sounds, pericardial rub.

Abdomen

Observe for distention, bruising, penetrating wounds, blood at the meatus or perineum.
While patient is quiet, palpate the bladder gently; compress the pelvic brim.
Auscultate for diminished bowel sounds, bruits.

Extremities

Observe for perfusion, gross deformity, spontaneous movement.
Palpate pulses at ankles, wrists, groin; palpate for local bone tenderness and sensation.

screaming that accompany an injury. The temperature of young children is unstable because of their large surface area related to body mass, and temperature maintenance is critical in trauma management. Children also experience rapid metabolic changes. When they are ill, children are really ill; but, as they recover, they change very rapidly. In addition, children have a small amount of blood volume in the absolute sense. Whereas blood volume is 60% of total body weight in the adult, it is 70% to 85% in the child.

The first priority on admission to an emergency facility is rapid assessment of the ABC status (airway, breathing, and circulation). Since the overwhelming majority of childhood injuries are the result of blunt-impact trauma, multiple organ involvement is a common finding; therefore it is essential to perform a systematic assessment of the trauma victim. The most efficient method consists of a head-to-toe assessment (Box 39-1).

EMERGENCY TREATMENT
Trauma

Make certain that the child and rescuer are not in immediate danger of additional trauma.
- Do not move child unless absolutely necessary.
- Keep child flat unless injury or symptoms specifically indicate otherwise:
  - Head injury—elevate head slightly.
  - Vomiting—carefully turn head to side.

Apply ABCs of emergency management;
- Airway—ensure open airway.
- Breathing—promote breathing; if not breathing, begin pulmonary resuscitation (see Chapter 31).
- Circulation—check pulse; if no pulse, begin chest compression (see Chapter 31).

Assess for extent of injury.
Stop bleeding with direct pressure to the wound or at appropriate bleeding point(s):
- Elevate injured part.
- Apply sterile or clean dressing.
- Use tourniquets only when bleeding cannot be stopped by any other means:
  - Release tourniquet pressure every 15 to 20 minutes.
  - Notify person(s) taking over care of the child of the presence of tourniquet(s).
  - Do not remove tourniquet until a physician is present.

Assess for further injury.
Determine state of consciousness:
- Talk to child.
- Observe child's behavior.

If present, do not remove objects protruding from child's body.
Check for evidence of decreased motor or sensory function in extremities:
- Infant and young child—observe spontaneous movement in extremities.
- Older child—ask if able to wiggle extremities.

Evaluate pain—present, absent; severe, mild.
- Attempt to alleviate with nonpharmacologic techniques.

Assess pulses in extremity distal to the injury.
- Check color and temperature of extremities.

Manage any injuries appropriately (e.g., splint fractures) (see Emergency Treatment: Fracture, p. 1859).
Identify child.
Obtain information regarding the injury from witnesses, if any.
Call Emergency Transport Team (Service) or transport to nearest facility.

NOTE: If spinal cord injury is suspected, do not move child unless absolutely necessary for the child's safety.

EMERGENCY TREATMENT

THE IMMOBILIZED CHILD

Immobilization is a major therapy for injuries to soft tissues, long bones, ligaments, vertebrae, and joints. Restriction of motion for a period of time at the site at which muscle or bone integrity has been disrupted allows tissue and bone to heal. However, prolonged immobilization, whether for therapy or because of disability, can produce severe complications, many of which are preventable. The nurse's awareness and implementation of appropriate actions during this restrictive state can significantly reduce the adverse effects of immobilization. Thus nursing care plans must focus not only on tissue and bone healing but also on regaining functional use of the injured part to the greatest extent possible and preventing complications.

IMMOBILIZATION

One of the most difficult aspects of illness is the immobility it often imposes on a child. Children's natural tendency to be mobile influences all elements of growth and development—physical, social, psychologic, and emotional. It is also important for expression and for dealing with anxiety and frustration. For these reasons children are immobilized only when necessary and for the shortest time possible.

Etiology of Immobilization

The usual reason for immobilizing or restricting the activity of a child is illness or injury. Bed rest or mechanical restraining devices are frequently prescribed to aid in the healing and restorative processes. When children are ill, they are content to remain quiet, and most of them instinctively reduce their activity. It is children who are forced to remain inactive because of physical limitations or therapy who display the multiple effects of restricted movement. The most frequent reasons for immobility are congenital defects (e.g., spina bifida), degenerative disorders (e.g., muscular dystrophy), and infections or accidents that impair the integumentary system (severe burns), the musculoskeletal system (fractures or osteomyelitis), or the neurologic system (spinal cord injury, polyneuritis, or head injury). Sometimes therapies, such as traction and spinal fusion, are responsible for prolonged immobilization.

Physiologic Effects of Immobilization

Although the bulk of information about the effects of immobility has been obtained from studies on adults, it is assumed that similar results occur in children. Many clinical studies, including space program research, have documented predictable consequences that occur following immobilization and the absence of gravitational force. Functional and metabolic responses to restricted movement can be noted in most of the body systems, all of which have a direct influence on the child's growth and development, because homeostatic mechanisms thrive on normal use and need feedback to maintain dynamic equilibrium. Inactivity leads to a decrease in the functional capabilities of the whole body as dramatically as the lack of physical exercise leads to muscle weakness.

Most of the pathologic changes that take place during immobilization arise from decreased muscle strength and mass, decreased metabolism, and bone demineralization, which are closely interrelated with one change leading to or affecting another. Some results of immobilization are primary and produce a direct effect; other pathophysiologic consequences occur frequently but seem to be more indirect and are therefore secondary effects. Many pathophysiologic changes affect more than one body system, with the primary or secondary effect being demonstrated in both systems.

Children who are confined to bed during a disease process or who are immobilized with an injury are usually restricted in movement for a relatively short time or are sufficiently active to avoid the physical consequences of immobility. Most physical and biologic effects of immobilization are the result of complete immobility, usually as a result of paralysis caused by nervous system infection (e.g., poliomyelitis, encephalitis, or polyneuritis) or trauma to the brain or spinal cord. Partial paralysis or weakness may be caused by birth defects (usually myelomeningocele), trauma, infection, or degenerative disease, such as muscular dystrophy or muscular atrophy.

The major effects of immobilization (Fig. 39-1) are related directly or indirectly to decreased muscle activity, which produces numerous primary changes in both muscular and bone structures with secondary alterations in the cardiovascular, respiratory, metabolic, and renal systems. The major consequences are:

1. Significant loss of muscle strength, endurance, and muscle mass (atrophy)
2. Bone demineralization leading to osteoporosis
3. Loss of joint mobility and contractures

The larger the portion of the body immobilized and the longer the immobilization, the greater the hazards of immobility.

Muscular system. Inactive muscle loses strength at the rate of 3% per day and, in instances without primary neuromuscular deficit, sometimes requires several weeks or months to regain function. A stretching can occur as muscle loses its tone or as excessive strain is put on weakened muscle, for example, stretching by tight bed covers or poor body position that produces wristdrop or footdrop experienced by debilitated children. The disuse leads to tissue breakdown and loss of the muscle mass (atrophy). The chief intracellular muscle enzyme, creatine, is released into the serum as the muscle atrophies; therefore serum levels provide an indication of the amount of muscle mass undergoing degeneration. Inactive muscle also affects the cardiovascular system by decreasing venous return and cardiac output.

Skeletal system. The daily stresses on bone created by motion and weight bearing maintain the balance between bone formation (osteoblastic activity) and bone resorption (osteoclastic activity). When these stresses are diminished, bone formation ceases, whereas the bone destruction continues, thus disrupting the state of equilibrium. Bone calcium becomes severely depleted, and there is increased secretion of phosphorus and nitrogen. This demineralization of the bone (osteoporosis) makes the skeletal structures prone to pathologic fractures and increases calcium ion concentration in the blood (hypercalcemia).

In children who are unable to move, such as the child who is unconscious or paralyzed or the child with rheumatoid arthritis, joint mobility becomes restricted. In the ab-

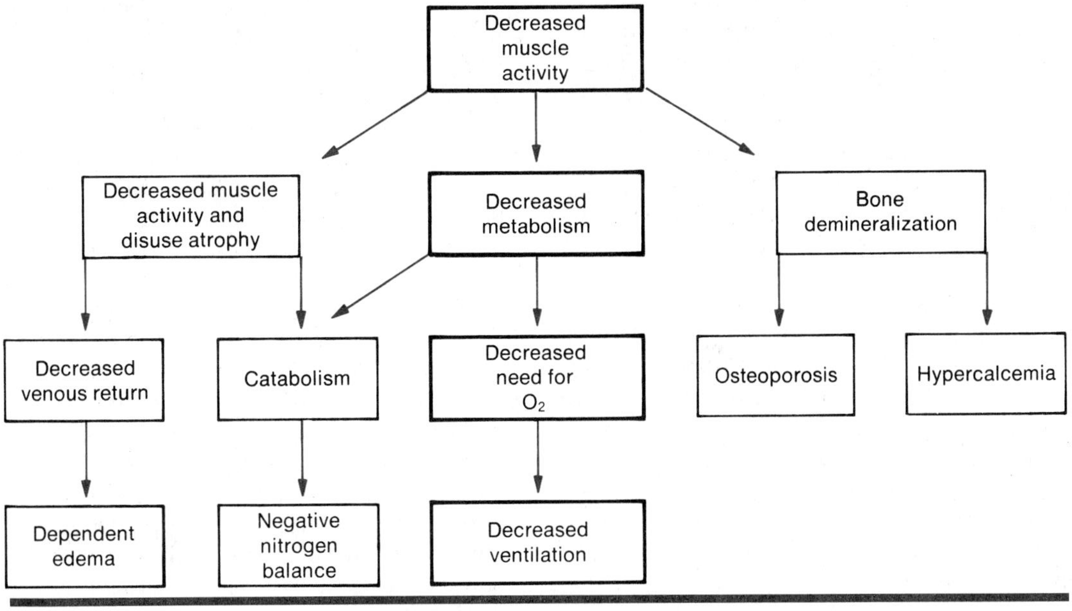

Fig. 39-1. Effects of immobilization.

sence of normal structural stretching, collagen fibers generated within the joint become fibrotic and further limit movement. This tissue fibrosis creates a shortening of the muscles and a contracture of the joint. Any decrease in circulation to the joint by edema, inflammation, or restrictive positioning will contribute to further fibrotic changes. The problem rapidly becomes cyclic as the contracture leads to muscle fatigue and pain, which causes the child to splint the site, thus leading to more fibrosis. This process is further exaggerated because body flexor muscles are stronger than the extensor muscles, and unless range of motion is instituted within 3 to 7 days, contractures will develop. Frequent disabling contractures are hip flexion, knee flexion, shoulder stiffness, and plantar flexion of the feet.

Cardiovascular system. There are three major cardiovascular consequences of immobility: orthostatic hypotension, increased workload of the heart, and thrombus formation. During movement, muscle contraction causes pressure on peripheral veins, which in turn causes the venous valves to close, thus assisting return of the blood to the heart when the individual is in an upright position. In the absence of this assistance, blood tends to pool in the dependent areas, reducing the blood supply to trunk and brain. In addition, direct reflex stimulation to the splanchnic and peripheral vessels causes them to constrict when a person is upright. Impairment of this neurovascular orthostatic reflex activity from lack of motion causes further interference with venous return. The individual displays signs of excessive autonomic activity, that is, pallor, sweating, and restlessness, which are frequently followed by fainting. The child with a spinal cord injury has unique problems with orthostatic hypotension, which is discussed in Chapter 40.

Changes in vascular resistance caused by the horizontal position and immobility alter the distribution of blood within the body. The reduction in gravity pressure to the extremities causes much of the total blood volume to be redistributed from the lower extremities to other parts of the body. Consequently there is an increase in the venous return and the volume of blood to be handled by the heart, which is reflected in an elevated blood pressure. Therefore the cardiac output and stroke volume are increased, and a progressive increase in heart rate occurs. When immobilization extends over a period of time, there is a compensatory decrease in blood volume and a decrease in heart rate and blood pressure.

Without muscle contraction the venous stasis and increased intravascular pressure in the extremities lead to dependent edema. If undue pressure is exerted on the major veins by positioning or mechanical devices, the likelihood of interstitial edema is increased. Most frequently this situation is seen when a child is placed on the side with one leg resting on the other or when the youngster is permitted to sit for a long time with pressure on the large veins behind the knee and in the groin. Edematous tissue is prone to infection and trauma, especially tissue located over an area that receives much of the body's weight.

Circulatory stasis combined with hypercoagulability of the blood, resulting from factors such as increased serum calcium or damage to the inner walls of blood vessels by trauma or infection, can lead to thrombus and embolus formation. Bed rest alone will not produce the blood-clotting problems, but debilitated persons often have one or more of these other contributing factors.

✦ **NURSING ALERT** Sudden chest pain and dyspnea, the symptoms of pulmonary edema, or pain and swelling in the lower extremities, which indicate deep vein thrombosis, are constant concerns of the nurse.

The deconditioned state of cardiac function, caused by skeletal muscle inactivity, can produce a variety of secondary problems in other systems. However, the major clinical manifestation is increased pulse and heart rate in response to an active exercise program. After prolonged immobility the child should build up activity tolerance slowly to allow the heart to regain its optimum capabilities.

Respiratory system. Initially the effects of immobilization are compensatory or adaptive. The basal metabolic rate is decreased because with reduced expenditure of energy the cells require less oxygen and produce less carbon dioxide. Lessened demand for oxygen–carbon dioxide exchange causes the respirations to become slower and more shallow. Chest expansion may be limited by the supine posture; by abdominal distention caused by accumulation of feces, gas, or fluid; and by mechanical restriction such as a body cast, brace, or tight binders. Reduced muscle power and coordination secondary to altered innervation can also hinder respiratory movement. More effort is required to expand the lungs in the supine position (see Fig. 31-3).

Prolonged immobility also reduces the normal movement of secretions from the tracheobronchial tree, particularly in the presence of impaired muscle function and positional changes that normally facilitate removal of secretions. A weak and ineffectual cough reflex contributes to stasis of secretions and the possibility of airway obstruction. Shallow respirations and obstruction of the airway with thick mucus contribute to the development of secondary complications such as atelectasis, hypostatic pneumonia, and respiratory acidosis.

Gastrointestinal system. Prolonged immobility produces a state of negative nitrogen balance resulting from the increased catabolic activity related to muscle atrophy. This and the reduced energy requirements contribute to a diminished appetite and a resulting decrease in ingestion of nutrients. The mechanisms of eating and feeding become more difficult with immobility, and the risk of aspiration is increased. Intake is further influenced by associated psychologic factors.

The process of elimination depends on the integration of smooth and skeletal muscle activity and on visceral reflex patterns. Immobility may interfere with these mechanisms as well as with the gravitational effect on stool passing through the intestines. Slowing of stool in the colon causes the feces to become hard, and the bowel wall is not stimulated to further its peristaltic movement down the tract to the rectum. Weakened muscles used in defecation (diaphragmatic and abdominal muscles) are unable to produce the intraabdominal pressure needed for elimination. Sometimes embarrassment in using the bedpan may be the cause of not responding to the urge to defecate.

Urinary system. The structure of the urinary system is designed to function in an upright posture. When the gravitational force is altered by the reclining position, the peristaltic contractions of the ureters are insufficient to overcome gravitational resistance. Consequently there may be stasis of urine in the kidney pelves, and any particulate matter that settles in the calyces may serve as nuclei for calculi formation or as foci for infection.

In the horizontal position the individual has difficulty in relaxing the perineal musculature and external sphincter sufficiently to initiate the integrated reflex micturition mechanism that involves the external sphincter, the internal sphincter, and the detrusor muscle of the bladder wall. If adequate intraabdominal pressure is exerted, voiding can occur, but if the individual does not respond to the sensation to void, bladder distention leads to stasis and its complications add to overflow incontinence, a source of embarrassment. In time, reflex and back pressure may impair renal function, and urinary tract infection is always a hazard with urine retention.

Normally the kidney is able to handle the increased metabolites from protein breakdown and bone demineralization. However, the increased level of calcium excreted may predispose to the formation of calculi. Calculi formation is further favored by urinary stasis, infection, and an alkaline urine caused by the decreased production of the acid byproducts of metabolism. Painless hematuria may be the only clue to diagnosis.

Metabolism. Immobility or severe restriction of activity is often accompanied by decreased or inappropriate nutritional intake, which frequently leads to decreased basal metabolic rate, a negative nitrogen balance associated with catabolism, and a high calcium serum level.

All body systems are influenced by a decrease in metabolism. The altered energy level leads to further fatigue and lack of motivation for moving. Although less of a problem in children, immobilized persons often feel sluggish and have a poor appetite, particularly for protein foods. The protein breakdown in the body related to a loss of muscle and other tissues is more apt to be severe after injury or surgery. Protein breakdown produces nitrogenous wastes, and on the fifth or sixth day of catabolic protein metabolism, an increase in urinary nitrogen develops that contributes to anemia and delayed healing.

Another metabolic problem is hypercalcemia associated with bone catabolism. Completely immobilized youngsters are especially prone to hypercalcemia. Symptoms that include nausea and vomiting, polydipsia, polyuria, and lethargy usually appear 4 to 8 weeks after immobilization. In quadriplegia symptoms may occur within 10 days and last for as long as 6 months. The accelerated rates of bone metabolism in youngsters make the bone demineralization a greater hazard. Larger amounts of calcium are released into the blood than the kidney can excrete, and calcium continues to accumulate in the serum. High levels of serum calcium decrease neuronal permeability, which can lead to a depression of the central and peripheral nervous systems. Symptoms, including smooth and skeletal muscle fatigue, diminished reflexes, and atony of the gastrointestinal tract, are the result of the depressed nervous system.

Medical treatment for hypercalcemia consists of restricting dietary calcium, increasing weight bearing when this is possible, and most importantly vigorous hydration (e.g., 3000 to 4000 ml/day of fluid for a teenager). Electrolyte imbalances are corrected, and diuretics are administered to promote removal of calcium. Sometimes pharmacologic agents, such as corticosteroids, oral phosphates, and thyrocalcitonin, may be used to lower serum calcium levels. Any urinary tract infection is treated.

A child with bone demineralization may not develop hypercalcemia, but the excess amount of calcium that the kidneys are required to excrete may produce a negative calcium balance with more calcium than citric acid lost in the urine. This imbalance causes the urine to become alkaline with the potential danger of renal calculi, especially if there is an accompanying retention of urine.

Integumentary system. Circulation to the skin is reduced during inactivity and may be further impeded by dependent edema. Circulation is especially compromised in places where the bone surface is near the skin, such as areas over the sacrum, occiput, trochanter, and ankle, and continued impairment causes rapid necrosis with ulcer formation. Mechanical irritation from appliances, such as straps, rods, and ropes, and the friction of bedclothes during turning or other movement can produce skin breakdown. Healing capacity is also impaired by poor circulation, negative nitrogen balance, and anemia. Immobilization often makes it difficult to carry out adequate cleansing and hygienic measures, which may also contribute to tissue breakdown in areas that are difficult to reach. Children with neurologic deficit should be guarded against extremes of heat and cold in direct contact with the skin.

Cellular breakdown caused by prolonged pressure can be identified by several characteristics. Normally when pressure is applied to the skin, the skin appears pale but becomes very red, or hyperemic, after pressure is removed. This reactive hyperemia should disappear within 5 to 15 minutes. Prolonged redness (over 30 minutes) indicates that a pressure area is developing and treatment should be instituted. Other manifestations of tissue ischemia include an increase in temperature in the area, blistering, swelling, or dark purple or black areas. The pressure area may be limited to the skin and subcutaneous layers or may be deeper and more extensive. The skin changes observed may represent the top of a cone-shaped area with widespread tissue destruction, beneath which tissue rapidly ulcerates and creates a large hole that sometimes extends to the bone. The skin may be broken, and there may even be a purulent drainage. Fig. 39-2 illustrates the sequence of events in tissue breakdown.

Neurosensory system. Studies indicate that immobilization does not produce neurosensory consequences directly; however, two occurrences—loss of innervation and sensory and perceptual deprivation—are common.

Peripheral nerves, in contrast to skeletal muscles, do not degenerate with disuse, but loss of innervation takes place if nerves are damaged by pressure or if their blood supply is disrupted. Improper body positioning or poorly applied casts or restraints can place unwarranted pressure on nerves and blood vessels that can lead to ischemia and nerve degeneration. Frequent sites of this compression phenomenon are pressure on the peroneal nerve, resulting in footdrop, or on the radial nerve, leading to wristdrop. These complications significantly interfere with attempts to regain functional use of extremities, but they can be prevented by conscientious nursing assessment and intervention. Preventing pressure on vulnerable areas and avoiding unnatural positions of flexion and extension that apply inappropriate pressure on nerves and blood vessels reduce the likelihood of compression injury. Periodic plantar flexion and dorsiflexion of the feet and hands will stimulate circulation

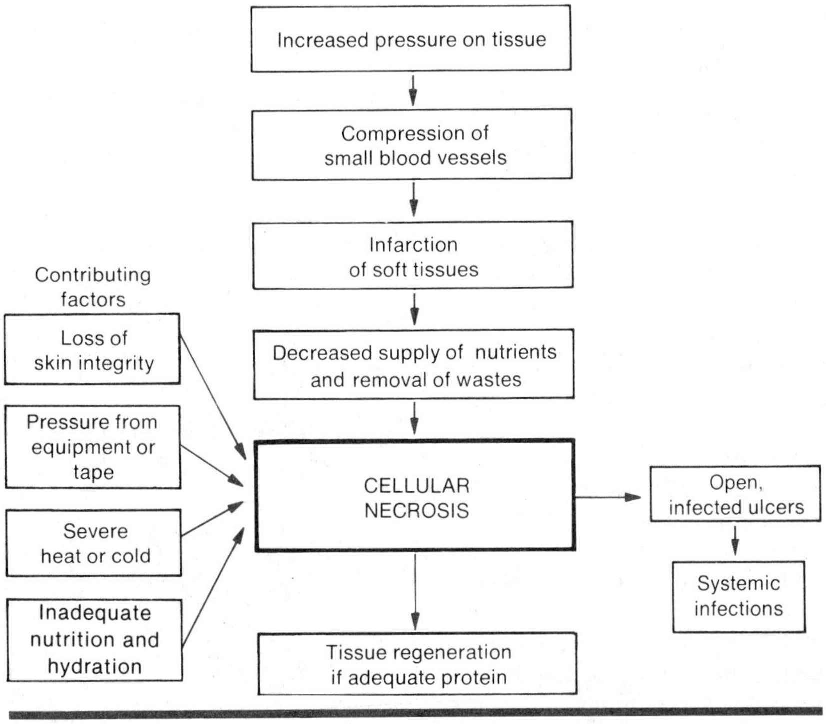

Fig. 39-2. Sequence of events in tissue breakdown.

and keep nerves from becoming pinched.

NURSING ALERT Numbness and tingling are symptoms of neurologic impairment and should be evaluated immediately.

Psychologic Effects of Immobilization

For children one of the most difficult aspects of illness is immobilization. Throughout childhood physical activity is an integral part of daily life and is essential for physical growth and development. It also serves children as an instrument for communication and expression and as a means for learning about and understanding their world. It helps them deal with a variety of feelings and impulses and provides a mechanism by which they can exert control over inner tensions. Children respond to anxiety with increased activity. Removal of this power deprives them of necessary input and a natural outlet for their feelings and fantasies. Through movement children also gain sensory input, which provides an essential element for developing and maintaining a body image.

In daily life children's activity is restricted in many ways: limits are set on behavior and expression, activity is restricted by physical and verbal barriers, and neuromuscular function is affected directly by disease or injury. Children perceive restraint by persons or inanimate objects as either comforting or stressful. Adult controls on behavior often provide children with a sense of security in frightening situations or when they fear loss of control. On the other hand, forced inactivity deprives them of one of their most valuable means for dealing with stress. Children who are confined to bed may become victims of their fears and fantasies without the physical means for stress reduction. Sometimes children will impose restrictions on themselves, particularly in interaction with others, by confining themselves to bed with blankets pulled about them or by retreating into sleep in the presence of stimulation.

Active children have many opportunities for input from a wide variety of settings. When they are immobilized by disease or as a part of a treatment regimen, they experience diminished environmental stimuli with a loss of tactile input and an altered perception of themselves and their environment. Sudden or gradual immobilization narrows the amount and variety of environmental stimuli they receive by means of all their senses: touch, sight, hearing, taste, smell, and proprioception—a feeling of where they are in their environment. This sensory deprivation frequently leads to a feeling of isolation, boredom, and being forgotten, especially by peers.

Sensorimotor activity is a predominant mode of activity in infants; even newborns respond with rage when they are physically restrained. Physical interference with the activity of infants and young children gives them a feeling of helplessness. It has also been found that speech and language skills require sensorimotor activity and experience. There appears to be a significant relationship between physical restraint and the incidence of language problems. Children who are restrained by casts, splints, or straps during the first 3 years of life have more difficulty with language than children whose activities were unrestricted. Language delay is even more marked in children with neurologic impairment (Sibinga and Freedman, 1971).

Observations of children's behavior during restraint indicate some differences between infants and older children. Initially infants temporarily freed from physical restraint remain immobile and then submit without protest to restoration of restraint. However, with subsequent release, their activity level progressively increases, as does their protesting behavior after reapplication of restraints. In contrast, toddlers and preschool children show a decrease in protest with each subsequent removal and restoration of restraint. It is uncertain whether this diminished protest in these children reflects inhibitions developed as a result of frustration or a development of trust that the nurse will return to release the restraints.

The struggle for independence is thwarted by imposed immobility. For toddlers, exploration and imitative behaviors are essential to developing a sense of autonomy; preschoolers' expression of initiative is evidenced by their penchant for vigorous physical activity; school-age children's development is strongly influenced by physical achievement and competition; and adolescents rely on mobility to achieve independence. The quest for mastery at every stage of development is related to mobility. To children the inability to move is threatening to self-preservation and reactivates the struggle between activity and passivity and between dependence and independence.

Behavioral changes are noted when children experience prolonged sensory deprivation. Some of these behaviors are demonstrated by a higher than normal level of anxiety (Box 39-2). Children are likely to become depressed over their loss of ability to function or the marked changes in body image. Significant others are apt to notice regressive behavior and a greater reliance on them for tasks the children are able to perform. Children seek their attention by reverting to earlier developmental behaviors, such as wanting to be fed,

BOX 39-2 BEHAVIORAL CHANGES IN IMMOBILIZED CHILDREN

Higher than normal level of anxiety leads to:
- Restlessness
- Difficulty with problem solving
- Inability to concentrate on activities
- Depression
- Regression
- Egocentrism

Monotony leads to:
- Sluggish intellectual responses
- Sluggish psychomotor responses
- Decreased communication skills
- Increased fantasizing
- Hallucinations
- Disorientation

bed-wetting, and baby talk. In many ways immobilized children are realistically dependent on others; therefore intelligent and sensitive care is required to prevent major developmental regressions during the period of immobility.

Limbs in casts or traction transmit less than normal sensory data. The presence of sensory impairment may be a concomitant problem of the involved part. Numbness or loss of feeling markedly alters proprioception. Children who have limited ability to feel others touching them not only experience less tactile stimuli in a physical sense but are also deprived of warm, loving feelings that arise from being touched. The loss of feeling derived from touch can further add to their sense of being isolated and unwanted.

The type and extent of immobilization influence the emotional response. When children are able to see the reason for their restraint (e.g., a cast), they are less likely to be resistant. The child whose activity is restricted because of a nonvisible disorder (e.g., rheumatic fever) finds it difficult to understand the reason for adult restrictions on activity, imagines the worst, and may react with noncompliance and overactivity when unobserved. Children may react to immobility by active protest, anger, and aggressive behavior, or they may become quiet, passive, and submissive. Often children believe that the immobilization is a justified punishment for misbehavior. Children should be allowed to discharge their anger, but it should be within the limits of safety to their self-esteem and not damaging to the integrity of others. For example, providing an object to attack rather than a person or a valued possession is safe and therapeutic.

Unfortunately most adults resent and find it difficult to deal with the acting-out behavior of children. Too often this behavior is considered "bad" even when it is obviously a release of tension. In some cases, such as the paralyzed child, nurses may feel inadequate to cope with the child's profound distress and feelings of hopelessness, and the professional help of a psychologist or psychiatrist is needed.

The most difficult situations are those involving major injuries and diseases that produce a disfigurement or a severe loss of function that directly affects children's self-image, such as burns, amputation, or the sudden catastrophic effects of an accident that leaves healthy, athletic children paralyzed for life. Feelings of anger and hostility are difficult for children to express when they are at the mercy of the environment. They dare not speak out against or defy the authorities on whom they depend so completely. Consequently their aggression may be masked by cheerfulness or rigidity. When they are unable to express their anger, the aggression is often displayed inappropriately through regressive behavior and outbursts of crying or temper tantrums over insignificant irritations, such as warm milk, a wrinkled collar, or a delay in routine.

Effect on Families

Brief periods of immobilization have few effects on the family; however, catastrophic illness or disability severely taxes the resources of the family. In general, emotionally mature families with financial resources and satisfactory problem-solving skills handle the crises well. Their needs are often very specific, primarily in the areas of instruction concerning medical and nursing care, community resources to contact, and emotional support as they go through the grief process. However, many families are unstable, are already plagued by unmet needs, operate from crisis to crisis, and are often unable to use outside help appropriately. For these families the new situation can disrupt the entire family; therefore the rehabilitation team must help the family members identify unmet needs and actively help in the family's problem-solving process. The following are commonly occurring problems:

1. Financial strains may decrease or totally eliminate the family's resources.
2. The focus of attention is placed, at least temporarily, on the affected member; therefore other members of the family may feel neglected or their needs may not be met.
3. The family may have difficulty in accepting the child's altered body image.
4. Individual family members may be unable to express their feelings and become immobilized in the face of the crisis.

The family's needs can often be met by the physician and nurse but may also require the services of other professionals, such as a social worker, psychiatrist, or marriage counselor. In preparation for discharge, home visits are advisable and home management is frequently planned weeks in advance of the actual discharge, including special considerations for cultural, economic, physical, and psychologic needs. A child with a severe disability is very dependent, and caregivers need rest periods to revitalize themselves. Individual and group counseling is beneficial for preproblem-solving situations and provides an emotional support system. Parent groups are also helpful and often allow nonthreatening social contact. The families of children with permanent disabilities need long-term resources, since some of the most difficult problems arise as they try to sustain high-quality care for many years (see Chapter 22).

Nursing Considerations

The effects of immobilization can be minimized and in many instances prevented by conscientious nursing care. The major goals in care of the immobilized child are to prevent the pathophysiologies associated with immobility and to use measures for regaining function and remobilization within the limitations of the therapeutic regimen or the physical disabilities of the child.

Assessment

Assessment of the child who is immobilized as a result of an injury or a degenerative disease not only includes the injured part (e.g., fracture or damaged joint), but also the functioning of other systems that may be affected secondarily—the circulatory, renal, respiratory, muscular, and gastrointestinal systems. In long-term immobilization there may also be neurologic impairment and metabolic changes in electrolytes (especially calcium), nitrogen balance, and general metabolic rate.

Nursing Diagnoses

Based on a thorough assessment, several nursing diagnoses are identified. The more common diagnoses for the immobilized child are included in the Nursing Care Plan on p. 1845. Others may apply in specific situations.

Planning

Nursing objectives for the immobilized child include the following:

1. Prevent physical complications.
2. Prevent psychologic complications.
3. Provide appropriate diversional activities.
4. Support child and family.

Implementation

Frequent position changes help to prevent dependent edema and fluid movement to third spaces and to stimulate circulation, respiratory function, gastrointestinal motility, and neurologic sensations. When the condition allows, the child can periodically assume the upright position on a tilt table or similar device to stimulate gastrointestinal and renal function and increase the stress on bones.

Each metabolic disturbance is treated specifically. Metabolism is increased by activity within the limitations of the disability and capabilities of the child. High-protein, high-calorie foods are encouraged for correction of negative nitrogen balance. This may be difficult to correct by diet, especially if anorexia is present. It is desirable to determine the child's favorite foods and to allow the family to bring special foods from home. This is especially helpful for children from varied cultural backgrounds. Stimulating the appetite with small servings of attractively arranged preferred foods may be sufficient. Sometimes supplementary nasogastric feedings or hyperalimentation may be needed.

Diet modification for the child with increased serum calcium presents problems, because the dairy foods that children often desire are high in this mineral. Acid ash foods such as cereals, meats, poultry, fish, and cranberry or apple juice are encouraged. Lying in a prone position may precipitate problems with swallowing or self-feeding. Therefore offering small bites, controlling swallowing with semisolid food, and using a straw for fluids are nursing behaviors that will prevent choking. A suction machine should be in the vicinity for emergencies. The primary nursing measure for hypercalcemia is conscientious hydration and active remobilization as soon as possible.

Adequate hydration promotes bowel and kidney function and helps prevent complications in these systems. A knowledge of previous bowel habits and of a method to get the child to a commode helps promote elimination and will be valuable data if needed for a bowel program. It is important to determine the words the child uses for elimination. Embarrassment can be avoided by a mutually satisfactory communication system. Whenever possible, the child should be helped into a sitting position to use a fracture urinal or a bedpan. Providing privacy for toileting and encouraging the child to participate in solving toileting problems will increase the chances of a successful program.

Children should be encouraged to be as active as their condition and restrictive devices allow. This poses few problems for children, whose innate ingenuity and natural inclination toward mobility provide them with the impetus for physical activity. They need the opportunity, the materials or objects to stimulate activity, and the encouragement and participation of others. Those who are unable to move will need passive exercise and movement.

Whenever possible, transporting the child by stretcher, stroller, or wagon outside the confines of the room will increase environmental stimuli and provide social contact with others. While hospitalized, the child will benefit from frequent visitors, clocks and calendars, and a program of diversional therapy, which will help the child to function in a more normal way. As soon as possible, the child should wear "street clothes" and resume school and preinjury hobbies. Play is the most useful tool of nursing (see Chapter 26), and activities, which are selected on the basis of interest, ability, and limitations, should include some form of physical activity that encourages the use of uninvolved muscles and joints. Any activity that is tolerated (e.g., turning in bed or changing position of a bed in the room) helps to alter the monotony of immobilization and dissipates tension and frustration (Fig. 39-3).

Using dolls to illustrate and explain the restraining method is a valuable tool for small children. Placing a cast, tubing, or other restraining equipment on the doll offers the

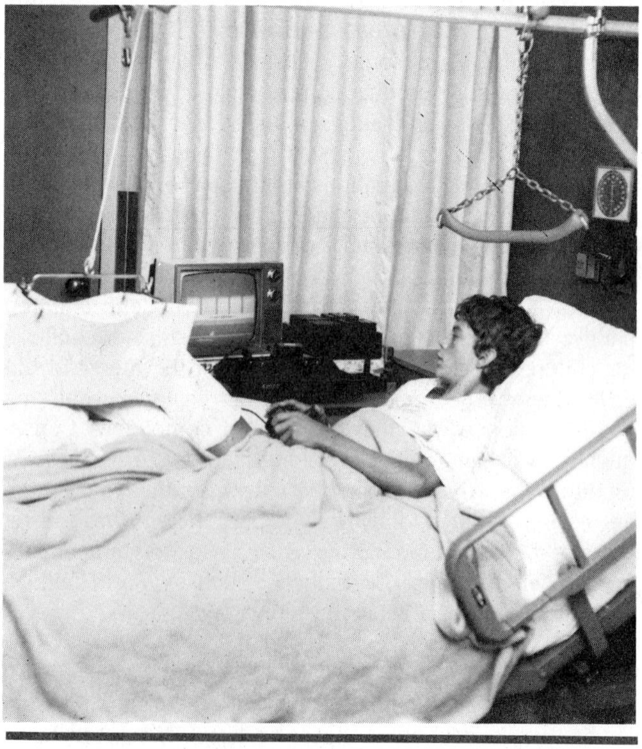

Fig. 39-3. Immobilized child playing a video game.

NURSING CARE PLAN
The Child Who Is Immobilized

NURSING DIAGNOSIS: Impaired physical mobility related to mechanical restrictions, physical disability (specify level)

GOAL 1
Provide mobilization (if appropriate)

INTERVENTIONS

Transport child by gurney, stroller, wagon, bed, or other conveyance from confines of room

EXPECTED OUTCOME

Child moves from confines of room

GOAL 2
Promote autonomy

INTERVENTIONS

Provide mobilizing devices (braces, crutches, wheelchair)
Assist with acquisition of specialized equipment
Instruct in use of equipment
Encourage activities that require mobilization
Allow as much freedom of movement as possible and encourage normal activites

EXPECTED OUTCOMES

Child moves about without assistance
Child engages in activites appropriate to limitations and developmental level

NURSING DIAGNOSIS: Potential impaired skin integrity related to immobility, therapeutic appliances

GOAL 1
Prevent skin irritation or breakdown

INTERVENTIONS

Place child on sheepskin, Egg-crate pad, or other resilient surface
Change position frequently
Protect pressure points, for example, trochanter, sacrum, ankle, shoulder, occiput
Inspect skin surfaces regularly for signs of irritation, redness, evidence of pressure
Eliminate mechanical factors causing pressure, friction, or irritation
Maintain meticulous skin cleanliness
Stimulate circulation by gentle rubbing with lotion or other lubricating substance

EXPECTED OUTCOME

Skin remains clean and intact with no evidence of irritation

NURSING DIAGNOSIS: Potential for trauma related to impaired mobility

GOAL 1
Prevent falls

INTERVENTIONS

Teach correct use of mobilizing devices and/or apparatus
Assist with moving and/or ambulating as needed
Remove hazards from environment (specify)
Modify environment as needed (specify)
Keep call button within reach
Keep siderails up at all times
Assist child to use bathroom or commode if possible

EXPECTED OUTCOME

Child remains free of injury

GOAL 2
Prevent other injuries (specify)

INTERVENTIONS

Implement safety measures appropriate to child's developmental age (specify)

EXPECTED OUTCOME

Child exhibits no signs of injury

NURSING DIAGNOSIS: Diversional activity deficit related to impaired mobility, musculoskeletal impairment, confinement to hospital or home

INTERVENTIONS AND EXPECTED OUTCOMES

See Nursing Care Plan: The Child in the Hospital, Chapter 26

NURSING DIAGNOSIS: Altered family processes related to a child with disability

GOAL 1
Support family

INTERVENTIONS AND EXPECTED OUTCOMES

See Nursing Care Plan: The Family of the Ill or Hospitalized Child Chapter 26 child a nonthreatening opportunity to express, through the doll, feelings concerning the restrictions and feelings toward the nurse and other health providers. It also provides a means for anticipatory teaching and explanation of needed restraining devices.

One of the most useful interventions to help children cope with immobility is participation in their own care. Self-care to the maximum extent is usually well received by children. They can help plan their daily routine, select their diet (when possible), and choose the clothes they are to wear, including innovative adornment, such as a baseball cap, brightly colored stockings, or other items of apparel that express each child's autonomy and individuality. They should be encouraged to do as much for themselves as they are able in order to keep muscles active and their interest alive. If feasible, they should be placed where they can benefit from the company of other children who are immobilized, which assures them that they are not singled out for this treatment.

It is important for children to understand behavioral limitations or rules, and their questions should be answered. For example, they need to know the reasons for medical, nursing, occupational, and physical therapy and to know that schedules are necessary. In some areas they have a choice; in others they do not. They may or may not be permitted to sleep late, but they can choose their own clothing. Most of children's activity of daily living is play; therefore therapies that incorporate this concept are more apt to gain their cooperation.

Visits from significant persons, such as family members and friends, offer occasions for emotional support and also provide opportunities for learning how to care for the child. The needs of a child with severe disability can be very complex, and family members require time to assimilate the teachings and demonstrations needed to understand their child's situation and care.

Some privacy is needed, particularly by the teenager, and most long-term health care facilities recognize that rooms shared by two to four youngsters are better environments for habilitation or rehabilitation. When roommates are selected according to age and companionship, a chance is available to test out thoughts and feelings safely with others. If a traumatic incident caused the child's disability, guilt feelings may be displayed overtly or masked behind regressive or aggressive behavior. The feeling that "I must have been bad to receive this fate" is common, and honest feedback stating, "It just happened—it was an accident," needs repeating many times. Additional aspects of grieving are involved if there was a loss of another in the accident. All these feelings need to be brought out and dealt with. In addition, professional persons working with these children must not baby or overprotect them but must help them to cope with their altered body image and reestablish their self-esteem.

For a child with greatly restricted movement, for example, a child with quadriplegia or a child with a large bilateral hip spica cast, nursing care is a challenge. These situations require long-term care either in the hospital or at home, but, wherever the care occurs, consistent planning and coordination of activities with professionals and significant others are vital. Nursing assessment includes psychosocial data as well as physical manifestations, since long-term immobilization has a profound effect on the child and the family. Nursing approaches are evaluated frequently and continued, discontinued, or modified to meet the changing problems and goals. Physical effects of immobilization and appropriate nursing considerations are summarized in Table 39-1.

Evaluation

The effectiveness of nursing interventions is determined by continual reassessment and evaluation of care based on the following observational guidelines and expected outcomes:

1. Observe vital signs, neurologic signs, and respiratory, gastrointestinal, and renal functioning; inspect skin; observe effects of correct functioning of equipment and appliances (restraints, traction, cast, braces).
2. Observe child's behavior; engage in dialogue to elicit feelings, concerns, and interests.
3. Observe the child's activities and interests.
4. Interview child and family regarding their feelings and concerns; observe family interaction at home, if possible.

Expected outcomes:
See Nursing Care Plan, p. 1845.

MOBILIZATION DEVICES

Children usually respond well to mobilization and require little encouragement, but they need instruction in correct use of appliances, their operation, and precautions for their safe usage.

Braces

Paralyzed or markedly weakened extremities can sometimes be stabilized by metal braces that facilitate walking. Some are designed to stabilize the extremities and offer support during ambulation. Special joint hinges permit the hip, knee, and ankle to flex during sitting, whereas the leg is held rigid during ambulation. Meticulous skin care and the wearing of protective clothing under the brace are necessary. Well-fitted braces promote ambulation, whereas ill-fitting braces are dangerous to the balance of the child and frequently cause muscle stress and tissue breakdown. Braces for the growing child will need frequent adjusting and replacement by the orthotist if long-term use is necessary.

The Jewett-Taylor brace is frequently used to support the spine and trunk during ambulation in conditions such as scoliosis and spinal cord injury. The brace must fit each body curvature to avoid undue pressure on tissues and imbalance between muscle groups. Bony prominences where the brace has contact, such as along the spine, chin, and iliac crests, are observed closely for pressure or irritation and are padded as necessary. A corset with metal stays may provide the needed torso support, especially for a paraple-

Table 39-1 Summary of physical effects of immobilization with nursing interventions*

PRIMARY EFFECTS	SECONDARY EFFECTS	NURSING CONSIDERATIONS
▪ Muscular system		
Decreased muscle strength, tone, and endurance	Decreased venous return and decreased cardiac output Decreased metabolism and need for oxygen Decreased exercise tolerance Bone demineralization	Use elastic stockings or wrap legs with Ace bandages to promote venous return Plan play activities to use uninvolved extremities Place in upright posture when possible
Disuse atrophy and loss of muscle mass	Catabolism Loss of strength	Perform range of motion, active, passive, and stretching exercises
Loss of joint mobility	Contractures, ankylosis of joints	Maintain correct body alignment Use joint splints as indicated to prevent further deformity
Weak back muscles	Secondary spinal deformities	Maintain body alignment
Weak abdominal muscles	Impaired respiration	See nursing considerations for respiratory system
▪ Skeletal system		
Bone demineralization—osteoporosis, hypercalcemia	Negative calcium balance Pathologic fractures Calcium deposits Extraosseous bone formation, especially at hip, knee, elbow, and shoulder Renal calculi	In paralysis, use upright posture on tilt table Handle extremities carefully when turning and positioning Administer calcium-mobilizing drugs (diphosphonates) if ordered Ensure adequate intake of fluid; monitor output Acidify urine Promptly treat urinary tract infections
Negative calcium balance	Life-threatening electrolyte imbalance	Monitor blood levels of calcium electrolytes Provide electrolyte replacement as indicated
▪ Metabolism		
Decreased metabolic rate	Slowing of all systems Decreased food intake	Mobilize as soon as possible Perform active and passive resistance and deep breathing exercises Ensure adequate food intake Provide a high-protein diet
Negative nitrogen balance	Decline in nutritional state Impaired healing	Encourage small, frequent feedings with protein and preferred foods Prevent pressure areas
Hypercalcemia	Electrolyte imbalance	See nursing considerations for skeletal system
Decreased production of stress hormones	Decreased physical and emotional coping capacity	Identify etiologies of stress Implement appropriate interventions to lower physical and psychosocial stresses
▪ Cardiovascular system		
Decreased efficiency of orthostatic neurovascular reflexes	Inability to adapt readily to upright position Pooling of blood in extremities in upright posture	Monitor peripheral pulses and skin temperature changes Wrap legs in elastic bandage or stockings to decrease pooling when upright
Diminished vasopressor mechanism	Orthostatic hypotension with syncope—hypotension, decreased cerebral blood flow, tachycardia	Provide abdominal support In severe cases, use antigravitational suit Administer peripheral sympathetic stimulating agents such as ephedrine if ordered Position horizontally
Altered distribution of blood volume	Decreased cardiac work load Decreased exercise tolerance	Monitor hydration and urine output

*Use measures that apply. Not all problems will be applicable in every situation.

Continued.

Table 39-1 Summary of physical effects of immobilization with nursing interventions—cont'd

PRIMARY EFFECTS	SECONDARY EFFECTS	NURSING CONSIDERATIONS
Venous stasis	Pulmonary emboli and/or thrombi	Have frequent position changes Elevate extremities without knee flexion Ensure adequate fluid intake Perform active or passive exercises or movement, if ordered Prescribe routine wearing of antiembolic stockings or wrap lower extremities from metatarsus to gluteal folds Measure circumference of extremities periodically Give anticoagulant drugs if ordered until mobilization possible Promptly intervene to maintain adequate oxygen if signs and symptoms of pulmonary emboli
Dependent edema	Tissue breakdown and susceptibility to infection	Administer good skin care Turn every 2 hours Monitor skin color, temperature, and integrity
▪ Respiratory system		
Decreased need for oxygen	Altered oxygen–carbon dioxide exchange and metabolism	Exercise as tolerated Use position for optimum chest expansion
Decreased chest expansion and diminished vital capacity	Diminished oxygen intake Dyspnea and inadequate arterial oxygen saturation; acidosis	Use prone positioning without pressure on abdomen to allow gravity to aid in diaphragm excursion When sitting, maintain proper alignment to prevent pressure on respiratory mechanism
Poor abdominal tone and distension	Interference with diaphragmatic excursion	Avoid restriction of chest and abdominal musculature Supply torso support to promote chest expansion
Mechanical or biochemical secretion retention	Hypostatic pneumonia Bacterial and viral pneumonia Atelectasis	Change position frequently Carry out percussion, vibration, and drainage (or suctioning) as necessary Monitor breath sounds
Loss of respiratory muscle strength	Poor cough	Encourage coughing and deep breathing Support chest wall when coughing Use special devices such as a rocking bed, breathing bag, incentive spirometers, intermittent positive-pressure breathing Observe for signs of acute respiratory distress with blood gas levels measured as necessary
	Upper respiratory infection	Avoid contact with infected persons Provide adequate hydration
▪ Gastrointestinal system		
Distention caused by poor abdominal muscle tone	Interference with respiratory movements	Use abdominal binder if indicated Monitor bowel sounds Encourage small, frequent feedings
	Difficulty in feeding in prone position	Sit in upright position if possible
No specific primary effect	Gravitation effect on feces through ascending colon or weakened smooth muscle tone may cause constipation	Carry out bowel training program with hydration, stool softeners, and mild laxatives if necessary
	Anorexia	Stimulate appetite with favored foods

Table 39-1 Summary of physical effects of immobilization with nursing interventions—cont'd

PRIMARY EFFECTS	SECONDARY EFFECTS	NURSING CONSIDERATIONS
▪ Urinary system		
Alteration of gravitational force	Difficulty in voiding in prone position	Position as upright as possible to void
Impaired ureteral peristalsis	Urinary retention in calyces and bladder Infection Renal calculi	Hydrate to ensure adequate urinary output for age Collect specimens as needed Stimulate bladder emptying with warm water, running water, striking suprapubic area Catheterize only for severe retention Administer urinary tract antiseptics as indicated
▪ Integumentary system		
No specific primary effect	Decreased circulation and pressure leading to tissue injury Difficulty with personal hygiene	Turn and position at least every 2 hours Frequently inspect total skin surface Eliminate mechanical factors causing pressure, friction, or irritation Assess ability to perform hygienic care and assist with bathing, grooming, and toileting as needed

Use measures that apply. Not all problems will be applicable in every situation.

gic child. Generally the corset is more comfortable than the metal and leather brace and presents fewer problems with dressing. Specialized devices can be used to provide upright mobility in small children with lower limb paralysis who shift body weight to achieve locomotion.

Parallel bars. Parallel bars provide secure handrails on both sides of children as they learn to walk again with or without braces. As they become more proficient, a walker with or without wheels is substituted for the bars and children are no longer confined to a limited territory. Children then progress to crutches if their age and condition permit.

Crutches and Canes

Crutches are used when children are not allowed to bear weight or can only place part of their body weight on an extremity, such as most lower leg injuries. A variety of crutches can be employed, and the selection is determined by the individual needs of the child. *Axillary* crutches are used most frequently as temporary assistance. *Forearm* crutches are the usual selection for children who anticipate permanent use, such as paraplegic children who are able to use braces. For children with limited hand and arm strength or function, *trough* crutches allow the weight to be assumed by the elbow. For habilitating small children who have not yet learned to walk or who are unsteady, special crutches stabilized with three or four legs provide needed stability for a child to maintain an upright position and learn to walk.

Children must be properly fitted for the crutch or cane to prevent poor posture and crutch pressure on the axilla dur-

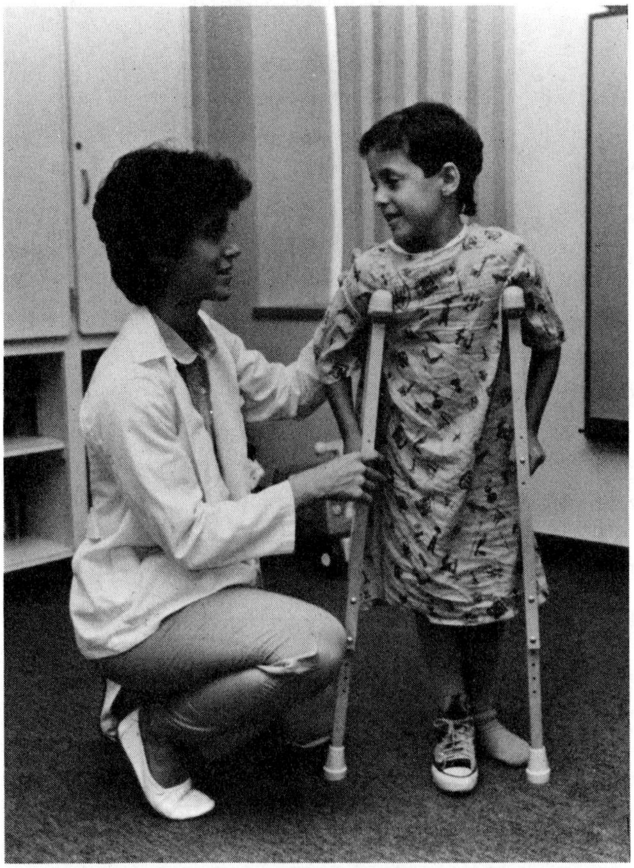

Fig. 39-4. Child learning to walk with crutches.

ing ambulation. Measuring for crutches and teaching crutch and cane use are usually assumed by the physical therapist in most institutions; however, nurses are the persons who supervise the use of crutches in pediatric units and in the home (Fig. 39-4). The type of crutch gait taught to children depends on their degree of stability, whether or not the knees can be flexed, and the specific goal established for each child.

Bed exercises for strengthening arms and shoulders are important if immobilization has been prolonged. The youngster gains confidence in ambulating by wearing a safety belt held by the therapist. The types of gaits used and instructions to children are similar to those given adults. They are conveyed with language children understand and with demonstration. Most children grasp the techniques readily.

Special Beds

Older quadriplegic children often require a special bed to immobilize the head and spine during the early phases of spinal cord injury care. Some rehabilitation units use a regular bed for the patient in cervical traction, whereas others use a Stryker frame or one of the Roto-Rest beds. Whatever special bed is used, the success of its use is greatly influenced by the preparation of the child. Explanations of how the bed works (and, when possible, showing the child someone being turned in the bed) are needed. Nursing personnel need in-service practice in the operation of these beds to ensure the safe handling of the equipment.

A Stryker frame employs two frames, one anterior and one posterior, to turn the child horizontally. The Stryker wedge frame was designed to allow prone-supine turning by one person, but for safety, two people are used for turning a child in a Stryker frame. Cervical traction can easily be attached to the stationary frame and presents no discomfort when turning as long as the weights are prevented from swinging. Before turning, the child's arms and legs are aligned within the frame and straps are wrapped around the entire "sandwich" of frames. All of the skin areas should be checked with each turning.

The Roto-Rest bed operates electrically; with the entire body securely immobilized by firm bolsters, the person is slowly and constantly rotated from side to side. Traction can be attached to this bed, and various parts can be removed to permit care and physical therapy. The continuous changes of position decrease the problems of pressure areas and promote venous circulation. The bed has a major advantage over a Stryker frame for teenagers with trache-

A

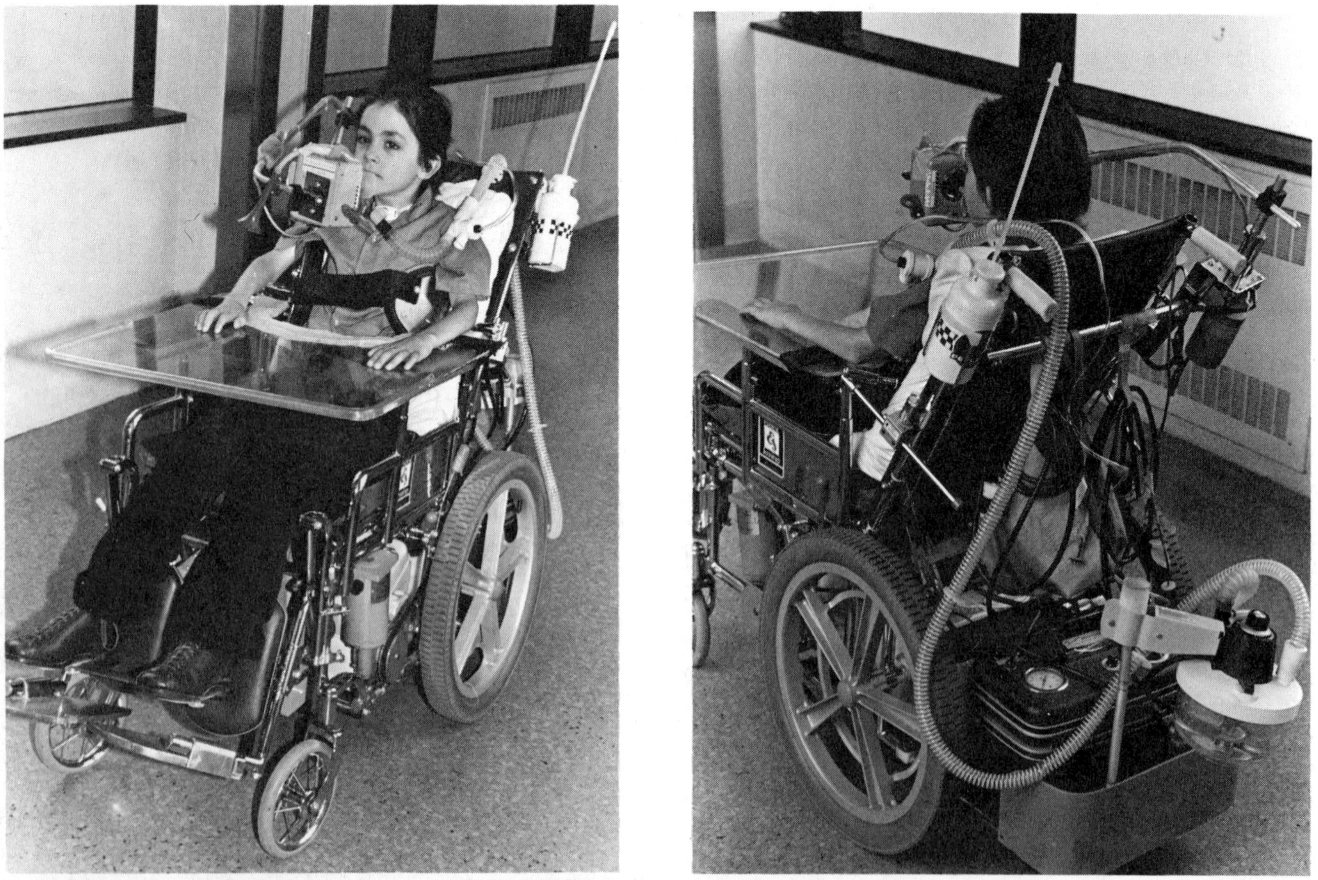

B

Fig. 39-5. Motorized wheelchair for quadriplegic child. **A,** Front view. **B,** Back view. Note portable respirator.

ostomies or other conditions that do not allow placing them in the prone position. The bed is made in an adult size and is suited only for large children.

Wheelchairs

Wheelchairs are used temporarily or permanently as a means of transportation. For temporary use, a wheelchair should fit the child and contain any adaptations needed, such as an elevating leg rest or reclining back. The child is taught how to transfer in and out of the chair and how to propel it safely. Prescribing a wheelchair for permanent use is the joint responsibility of physician and therapist after an assessment of home and surroundings. A wheelchair should be neither too small nor too large, preferably one that can be adapted to the child's growth needs. Detachable or rotating armrests, which permit easy transfer in and out, are needed for children with spinal cord injuries.

Other desirable features are detachable and swing-away footrests and detachable desk arms. Elevating leg rests are required for children who are prone to contractures, and a reclining back rest is needed for those who may have poor trunk balance. A proper cushion with adequate padding should be provided for the child who has decreased sensation. Hand rim and brake lever projections are helpful for the child with upper extremity weakness. Children with paraplegia will require upper arm strengthening exercises and instruction on transfer techniques before wheelchair mobilization. Often a tilt table must be used to overcome the problems of orthostatic hypotension before wheelchair sitting can be tolerated.

Various motorized chairs are available for marked upper extremity weakness, and mouth- or cheek-operated models are available for children who do not have the use of upper extremities so that children can operate them independently (Fig. 39-5). Very small children who have permanent paralysis of lower extremities are provided with specially designed units that allow independent mobility (Fig. 39-6). A detachable handle on these units permits their conversion to strollers.

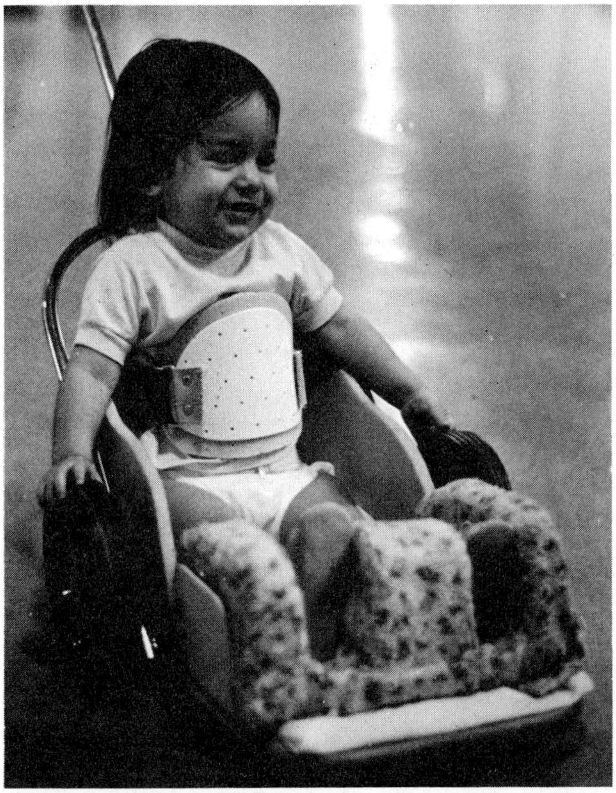

Fig. 39-6. Mobilization device for toddler.

THE CHILD WITH A FRACTURE

The musculoskeletal system, like all the body systems of the newborn, is immature, and the specific functions of the system develop slowly so that the muscles, bones, tendons, and ligaments can function in an integrated fashion to perform complex tasks. The process of ossification, the gradual conversion of precursor substances (namely cartilage) to bony structures, begins in the embryo and continues until the child is 18 to 21 years of age. In long bones this process progresses outwardly from the diaphysis, the hard shaftlike portion that constitutes the major portion of the bone. Within this hard, compact shaft is the hollow medullary canal composed of the bone marrow.

The epiphysis, located at the ends of long bones, consists of layers of cartilage, subchondral bone, and spongelike cancellous bone. Situated between the diaphysis and epiphysis is the epiphyseal plate, which plays a major role in the longitudinal growth of the developing child. The periosteum, the thin, tough membrane covering all bones, contains blood vessels that nourish the living bone (Fig. 39-7). Damage to this thin membrane can be a major problem in bone growth and healing.

FRACTURES

Bones fracture when the resistance of the bone against the stress being exerted yields to the stress force. Fractures are a common injury at any age but are more likely to occur in children and aged persons. The natural tendency toward active mobility and their limited gross motor coordination make children more susceptible to physical injury.

Etiology

The causes of fracture injuries in children are those described for general traumatic injuries in childhood. Fractures in infancy are more often the result of birth trauma, injury, or child abuse. Aside from motor vehicle accidents, true accidents rarely occur in infancy; therefore injury in children in that age-group warrants further investigation. In any small child radiographic evidence of fractures at various stages of healing is, with few exceptions, an indication of physical abuse. Most often early bone trauma in infants

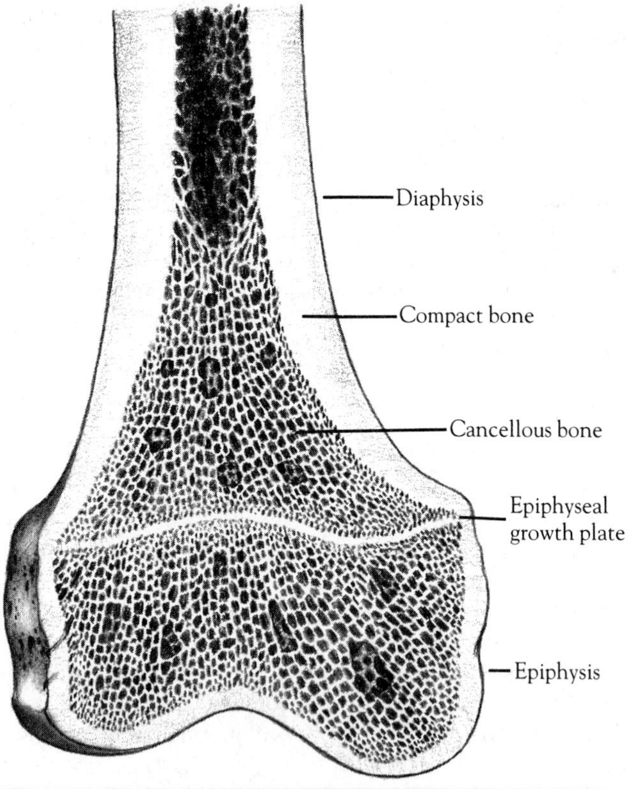

Fig. 39-7. Bone showing relationships of compact and cancellous bone, epiphysis, epiphyseal plate, and diaphysis.
From Thompson, J.M., and others: Mosby's manual of clinical nursing, ed. 2, St. Louis, 1989, Mosby–Year Book, Inc.

consists of periosteal bleeding in the long bones of arms and legs, usually caused by rough handling, twisting, and pulling, which is not evident on radiographic examination until 3 to 6 weeks after the injury.

Fractures of the forearm are common bone injuries in childhood and are usually caused when the child extends the palm of the hand to break a fall. The force resulting from a fall on the outstretched hand progresses up the length of the extremity with the possibility of injury to finger, wrist, elbow, shoulder, and/or clavicle (Fig. 39-8). The clavicle is probably the bone most frequently broken in children; approximately half of clavicle fractures occur in children under 10 years of age. Many occur at birth. Hip fractures are rare in children and require a great deal of violence to produce. A femoral neck fracture may be sustained in children 6 or 7 years of age as a result of pedestrian-automobile accidents because their hip height is on the same level as an automobile bumper. In older children the femur is the most likely target; in adolescents knee injuries are common.

Children fall from heights (e.g., trees, roofs) as their insatiable curiosity and immature judgment lure them to places of danger. Fractures in school-age children are often the result of bicycle-automobile accidents or skateboard injury. At all ages motor vehicle accidents are a frequent cause of bone injury. Most children who are hit by an automobile are between 4 and 7 years of age and sustain a triad of injuries, which must be kept in mind when making an assessment of injuries: (1) the child's femur, which is at the level of the bumper, is fractured; (2) the hood of the automobile produces injuries to the child's trunk; and (3) a contralateral head injury is usually sustained when the child is thrown to the ground by the impact (Fig. 39-9). Therefore a child with any of these injuries who was struck by an automobile should be examined for evidence of the other two.

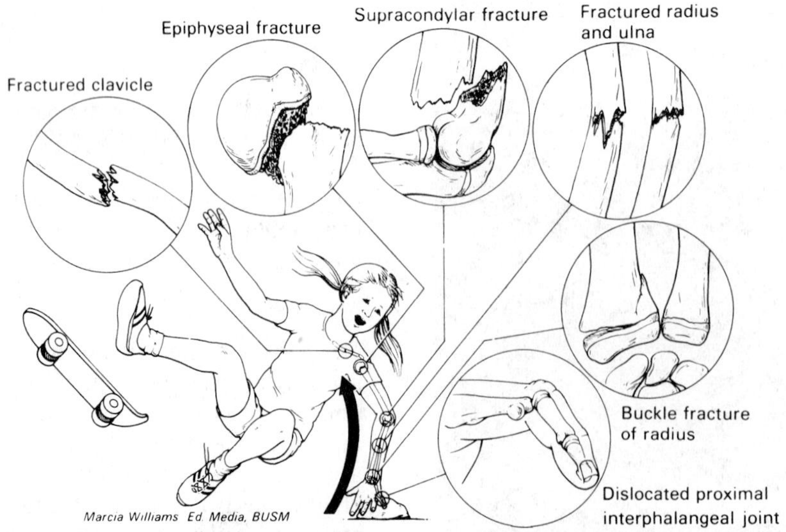

Fig. 39-8. Trauma resulting from progression of force in fall on outstretched hand.
From Segal, D.: Pediatr. Clin. North Am. 26:793-802, 1979.

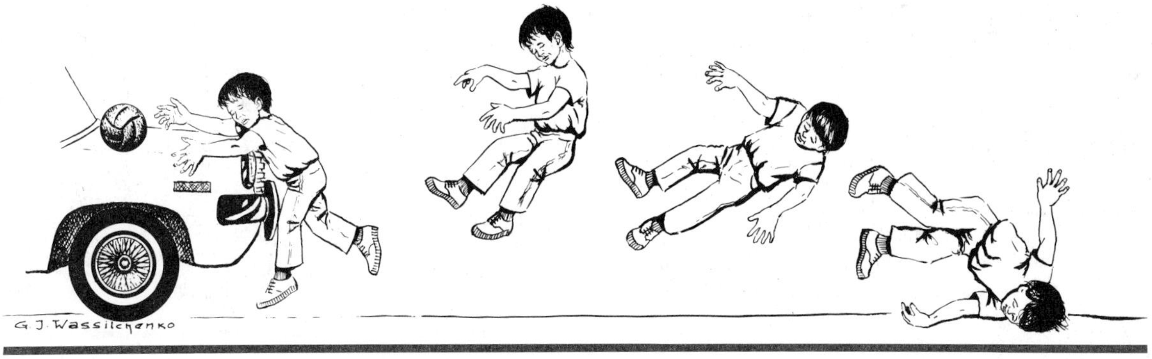

Fig. 39-9. Triad of injuries sustained when a child is struck by automobile.

Pathophysiology

The anatomic, biomechanical, and physiologic nature of children's skeletons causes differences in the pattern of fractures, the problems of diagnosis, and the methods of treatment. The bones of the adult are strong and require a violent traumatic force to fracture, which is accompanied by massive injury to surrounding soft tissues. In children the bones are more easily injured, and fractures may result from minor falls or twists and thus are less likely to be accompanied by damage. Features of children's fractures not observed in the adult are outlined in Box 39-3.

BOX 39-3 FEATURES OF FRACTURES IN CHILDREN

1. The growth plate, a thick, elastic portion of bone where growth takes place, serves to absorb shock and protect joint surfaces from injury and is the means by which the limb is able to grow and to straighten itself. Growth is stimulated by a fracture in the diaphysis, whereas damage to the growth plate can cause shortening and often a progressive angular deformity.
2. The periosteum of a child's bone is thicker, stronger, and has more active osteogenic potential compared with the adult.
3. The pliable bones of growing children are more porous than those of the adult, which allows them to bend, buckle, and break in a "greenstick" manner. The greater porosity increases the flexibility of the bone and dissipates and absorbs a significant amount of the force on impact.
4. Healing is more rapid in children, and the rapidity is inversely related to the age of the child. The younger the child, the more rapid is the healing process. Nonunion of bone fragments is almost unknown in children.
5. Stiffness is unusual and, unlike in adults, an uninjured joint in a child can be immobilized for a long period without producing stiffness that lasts longer than a few minutes. Injured joints do become stiff, however, and the current trend is toward early mobilization and active range of motion exercises as preventive measures.
6. Children only complain when something is wrong. Unreasonable crying, restlessness, and calling for the parents are usually indications that something is amiss and requires investigation.

Types of fractures. A fractured bone consists of fragments—the fragment closer to the midline, or the proximal fragment, and the fragment farthest from the midline, or the distal fragment. When fracture fragments are separated, the fracture is *complete;* when fragments remain attached, it is said to be *incomplete.* The fracture line can be:

Transverse—crosswise, at right angles to the long axis of the bone
Oblique—slanting but straight, between a horizontal and a perpendicular direction
Spiral—slanting and circular, twisting around the bone shaft

All fractures affect the entire cross-section of the bone. The twisting of an extremity while the bone is breaking results in the spiral break. If the fracture does not produce a break in the skin, it is a *simple,* or *closed,* fracture. *Open,* or *compound,* fractures are those with an open wound through which the bone is or has protruded. If the bone fragments cause damage to other organs or tissues (e.g., the lung or bladder), the injury is said to be *complicated.* When small

BOX 39-4 TYPES OF FRACTURES IN CHILDREN

Bends—a child's flexible bone can be bent 45 degrees or more before breaking. However, if bent, the bone will straighten slowly, but not completely, to produce some deformity but without the angulation that exists when the bone breaks. Bends occur more commonly in the ulna and fibula, often associated with fractures of the radius and tibia.
Buckle fracture—compression of the porous bone produces a *buckle,* or *torus,* fracture. This appears as a raised or bulging projection at the fracture site. Torus fractures occur in the most porous portion of the bone near the metaphysis (the portion of the bone shaft adjacent to the epiphysis) and are more common in young children.
Greenstick fracture—occurs when a bone is angulated beyond the limits of bending. The compressed side bends and the tension side fails, causing an incomplete fracture similar to the break observed when a green stick is broken.
Complete fracture—divides the bone fragments. They often remain attached by a periosteal hinge, which can aid or hinder reduction.

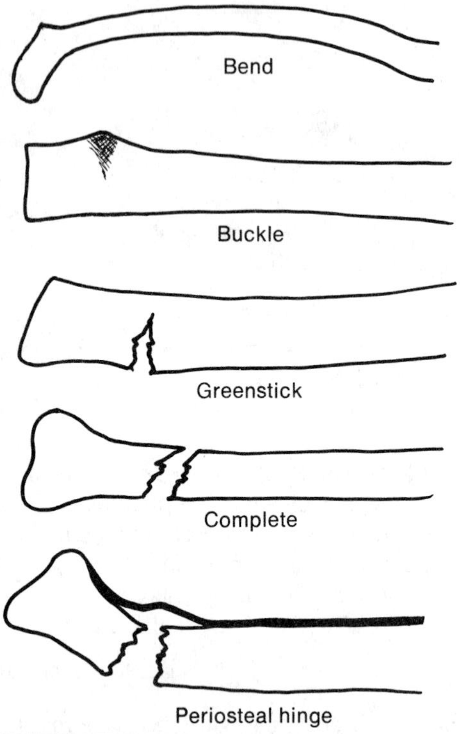

Fig. 39-10. Types of fractures in children.

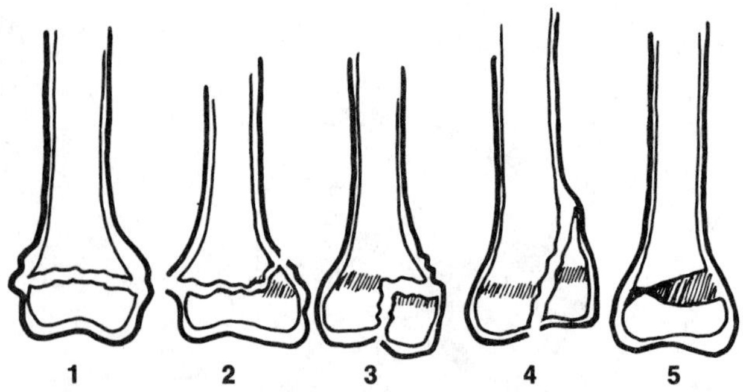

Fig. 39-11. Types of epiphyseal injuries in order of increasing risk.

fragments of bone are broken from the fractured shaft and lie in the surrounding tissue, the fracture is called *comminuted.* This type of fracture is rare in children. The types of fractures that occur most often in children are shown in Fig. 39-10 and described in Box 39-4.

Epiphyseal injuries. The weakest point of long bones is the cartilage growth plate or epiphyseal plate. Consequently this is a frequent site of damage during trauma. Under most conditions, fractures in this area proceed along the zone of degenerating cartilage cells, before the cartilage begins to ossify, without damage to the growth plate, thus causing little damage. Healing is usually prompt. When fracture lines deviate from a transverse direction through the degenerating cells, more serious damage to the epiphysis and the plate may occur. Fig. 39-11 illustrates the types of epiphyseal injuries in order of increasing risk of permanent epiphyseal damage and possible growth disturbance.

Detection of epiphyseal injuries is sometimes difficult, and they may be mistaken for dislocations or ligamentous injuries. Fractures involving the epiphysis or epiphyseal plate present special problems in determining whether or not bone growth will be affected. Early and correct assessment is essential to minimize the incidence of longitudinal growth problems and angular deformities. The medical management of these injuries is different than that for other fractures because open reduction and internal fixation are often employed to prevent complications. If the affected limb is shorter, epiphyseal surgery is done either to stimulate the involved epiphysis or to retard growth in the unaffected leg.

Associated problems. Immediately after a fracture occurs, the muscles contract and physiologically splint the injured area. This phenomenon accounts for the muscle tightness observed over a fracture site and the deformity that is produced as the muscles pull the bone ends out of alignment. This muscle response must be overcome by traction or complete muscle relaxation, that is, anesthesia, in order to realign the distal bone fragment to the proximal bone fragment.

Contusions of the soft tissues frequently accompany fractures, especially of femurs, and severe hemorrhage into the tissues is not uncommon. Both the bleeding and the pain are major contributors to shock associated with this injury; therefore suspected musculoskeletal injury should be treated as a fracture until radiographic confirmation can be made. The surrounding tissue will be swollen, and a hematoma is usually present. The soft tissue injury must be treated as any contusion. Since the injury may cause damage to essential structures, the circulatory and neurologic status of tissues distal to the fracture is carefully assessed, especially for fractures of the femur and supracondylar fractures of the elbow.

Clinical Manifestations

Children demonstrate the usual signs of injury—generalized swelling, pain or tenderness, and diminished functional use of the affected part. There may be bruising, severe muscular rigidity, and sometimes crepitus (a grating sensation at the fracture site), which are also frequent signs in adults. More often the fracture is remarkably stable because of the usually intact periosteum. The child may even be able to use an affected arm or walk on a fractured leg.

✦ **NURSING ALERT** A fracture should be strongly suspected in a small child who refuses to walk.

Although neurologic and vascular damage is much less frequent in children than in adult patients, the integrity of these structures must be accurately assessed. This is often difficult in infants and young children who are unable to cooperate. Vascular injury is most likely to occur with supracondylar fractures of the humerus and femur. Femoral and popliteal vessels and the sciatic nerve are prone to trauma in femoral fractures; humeral fractures may cause damage to the medial, ulnar, or radial nerves and to the brachial artery.

✦ **NURSING ALERT** The five "Ps" of ischemia from a vascular injury—*pain, pallor, pulselessness, paresthesia,* and *paralysis*—should be kept in mind when making an assessment.

Diagnostic Evaluation

A medical history is often lacking for childhood injuries. Infants are unable to communicate, and older children are unreliable informants and seldom volunteer information (even under direct questioning) when the injury occurred during forbidden activities. Unless they are witnesses to the injury, parents may misinterpret what the child is trying to say. In cases of child abuse parents may give false information deliberately in order to protect themselves.

Radiography. Radiographic examination is the most useful diagnostic tool for assessing skeletal trauma. The calcium deposits in bone make the entire structure radiopaque. However, in normal growth and development bony structures ossify from precursor substances, usually cartilage, to form true bone from the shaft or diaphysis toward the epiphysis. This ossification process begins in the embryo and continues until bone formation is completed by 18 to 21 years of age. Ossification centers alter the appearance of the bone, and much of the skeleton of infants and young children is composed of radiolucent growth cartilage that does not appear on radiograms. In addition, the epiphyseal cartilage and undisplaced separations of the epiphysis, which often occur, are not easily detected on x-ray films. It has been observed that radiographs are less reliable in predicting extremity fractures than are gross deformity and point tenderness (Rivara, Parish, and Mueller, 1986).

Many practitioners obtain a film of the uninjured limb for a direct comparison to help identify minor alterations in alignment and configuration of the epiphysis and associated injuries that might be missed. Radiographic films are taken after fracture reduction and in some situations may be taken during the healing process to determine satisfactory progress.

Blood studies. Severe soft tissue, muscle, and bone injury often results in a destruction of red blood cells with a rise in bilirubin and a fall in the hemoglobin or hematocrit reading. The child's homeostatic mechanisms are activated to correct the problem, and generally only supportive therapy with a high-protein diet and iron replacement is needed. When muscle integrity is disrupted, enzymes normally contained within muscles are released into the bloodstream. Serum levels of creatine, alkaline phosphatase, serum glutamic-oxaloacetic transaminase (SGOT), and lactic dehydrogenase (LDH) may increase in proportion to the amount of muscle damage.

A normal physiologic response to tissue injury is the inflammatory process with a slight elevation of white blood cells, especially neutrophils. When infection occurs, the rise in leukocytes is anticipated and the accompanying symptoms of fever and lethargy develop.

Therapeutic Management

The majority of children's fractures heal well, and nonunion is rare. Most are readily reduced by simple traction and immobilization until healing takes place. The goals of fracture management are:

1. To regain alignment and length of the bony fragments (reduction)
2. To retain alignment and length (immobilization)
3. To restore function to the injured parts

In children the bone fragments are usually realigned and immobilized by traction or by closed manipulation and casting until adequate callus is formed. Weight bearing and active movement for the purpose of regaining function can begin after the fracture site is stable. The child's natural tendency to be active is usually sufficient to restore normal mobility, and physical therapy is rarely needed. Open reduction is seldom required and is limited to fractures that cannot be maintained by conservative methods and when there is interposed tissue or injury to arteries or nerves. However, surgical reductions are more apt to delay normal healing and often predispose to nonunion. In the majority of cases children's fractures can be managed by closed reduction and plaster immobilization, which is often provided on an outpatient basis with reevaluation in 7 to 10 days.

Children are most frequently hospitalized for fractures of the femur and the supracondylar area of the distal humerus. If simple reductions cannot be achieved or a neurovascular problem is detected after injury, observation in a hospital unit is indicated. Severe contusions with profound swelling cannot be treated with a cast, which would act as a tourniquet on the extremity, and badly malaligned fractures require traction for a time before a cast is applied. The method of fracture reduction is determined by several criteria (Box 39-5).

Some problems that are associated with fracture injury involve both the physician and the nurse in their management (Box 39-6). Specific interventions and nursing responsibilities in the general management directed toward restoring bone integrity and functional use are discussed in relation to the major modalities of fracture immobilization—casting and traction.

Surgical intervention. When surgical intervention is necessary to realign a fracture, the child needs physical and psychologic preparation. The preoperative teaching is the same as for any other surgical procedure, except that ortho-

BOX 39-5 CRITERIA FOR DETERMINING USE OF REDUCTION METHOD FOR FRACTURES

Age of child
Degree of displacement
Amount of overriding
Degree of edema
Condition of skin and soft tissue
Sensation and circulation distal to fracture

BOX 39-6 PROBLEMS ASSOCIATED WITH FRACTURE INJURY

Control of pain, hemorrhage, and edema
Relief of muscle spasms
Realignment of fracture fragments
Promotion of bone healing
Immobilization of fracture until adequate healing has begun
Prevention of secondary complications
Limitation of disuse syndrome
Restoration of function

pedic surgery uses a variety of rods, screws, staples, and plates and the child needs to know about these unfamiliar objects and how they will appear when he returns from the procedure. The fixating devices are made of substances that do not act as foreign proteins to the body and therefore are not rejected. Usually the rods are driven down the shaft of the long bones, whereas screws and plates are attached to the side of the bone shaft. Postoperatively the bone healing takes place with callus formation as it does in a new fracture. Generally the child with an internal fixation device sits in a chair and walks with a walker or crutches within a few hours or days. The most common postoperative complication is infection. The nurse's responsibility includes close monitoring of neurovascular changes in the involved extremity and the prevention of postanesthesia problems.

Bone Healing and Remodeling

Bone healing follows a patterned sequence. Fig. 39-12 shows three broad overlapping phases: inflammatory, restorative, and remodeling. Bone healing is described more definitively in five stages (Table 39-2). When the bone breaks, the envelope of subcutaneous tissue, muscle, and periosteal tissue surrounding the site is torn, blood vessels rupture, and a hematoma forms. The ends of the fractured bone segments, deprived of circulation, die as far back as the nearest collateral circulation. Necrotic tissue accumulates, and an inflammatory response takes place at the site with its characteristic vasodilation, plasma exudation, and edema. The organization and resorption of the hematoma proceeds, and the restorative phase begins with the reestablishment of local circulation. Repair requires an adequate blood supply and immobilization of the fracture fragments.

When there is a break in the continuity of bone, the periosteal and intraosseous osteoblasts are in some way stimulated to maximum activity. New osteoblasts are formed in immense numbers almost immediately after the injury and begin building a bridge, as evidenced by a bulging growth of osteoblastic tissue and new bone matrix between the fractured bone fragments. This is followed by deposition of calcium salts to form *callus,* which provides stability (Fig. 39-13, *B*).

Bone healing is characteristically rapid in children because of the thickened periosteum and generous blood supply. In the young child, for example, there is frequently a

Table 39-2 Stages of bone healing

TIME*	PHYSIOLOGIC EVENTS
▪ Stage 1: hematoma formation	
Impact	Fracture Injury to soft tissue envelops site Periosteal tissue torn Vessels rupture
3-5 minutes	Bleeding from bone and tissues into area between and around bone fragments
First 24 hours	*Hematoma* forms and clots; fibrin assists in clotting periosteal membrane to aid in repair Clot provides fibrin network for cellular invasion Granulation tissue forms by fibroblasts and new capillaries Osteoblastic activity stimulated
▪ Stage 2: cellular proliferation	
After 24 hours	Blood supply increases, bringing available calcium, phosphate, and fibroblasts Cells proliferate at ends of bone fragments and differentiate into cartilage and connective tissue
Next few days	Hematoma becomes *granulation tissue,* which forms into a framework for bone-forming substances Fibroblasts convert to osteoblasts (bone-forming cells)
2-3 days	*Halisteresis* (softening of bone ends) ⅛- ¼-inch; absorption of bone cells
▪ Stage 3: callus formation	
6-10 days	Fibroblasts form in granulation tissue; form bone in areas adjacent to surface of bone shaft; form cartilage at surfaces more distal to blood supply *Provisional callus* develops, bridging fracture ends; holds bone together but will not support body weight
14-21 days	*True callus* develops, seen on radiographs; forms more than needed, but with remodeling, excess callus absorbs Cartilage differentiates to bone tissue
▪ Stage 4: ossification	
3-10 weeks	Callus forms into bone, which grows beneath periosteum of fragments; fuses fracture defect (knits together) Also called the *union stage*
▪ Stage 5: consolidation and remodeling	
After 9 months	Bone marrow cavity restored Compact bone formed according to stress patterns Remodeling according to Wolff's law Fracture line always visible on radiographs

*Healing time more rapid in infants and in cancellous (spongy) bone and delayed with complications.

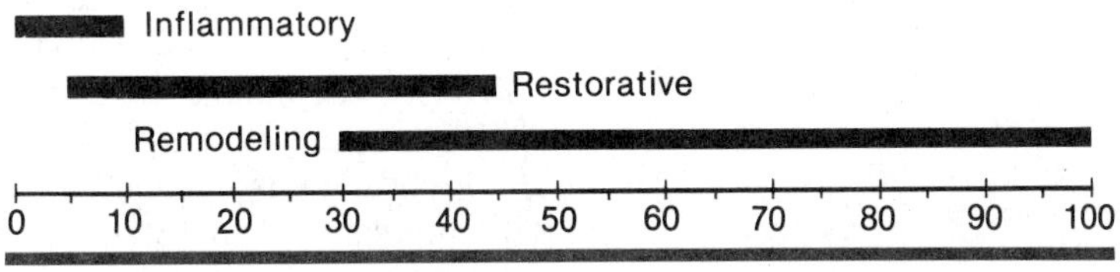

Fig. 39-12. Approximate time devoted to inflammatory, restorative, and remodeling phases of bone healing. Scale indicates percentage of healing time.

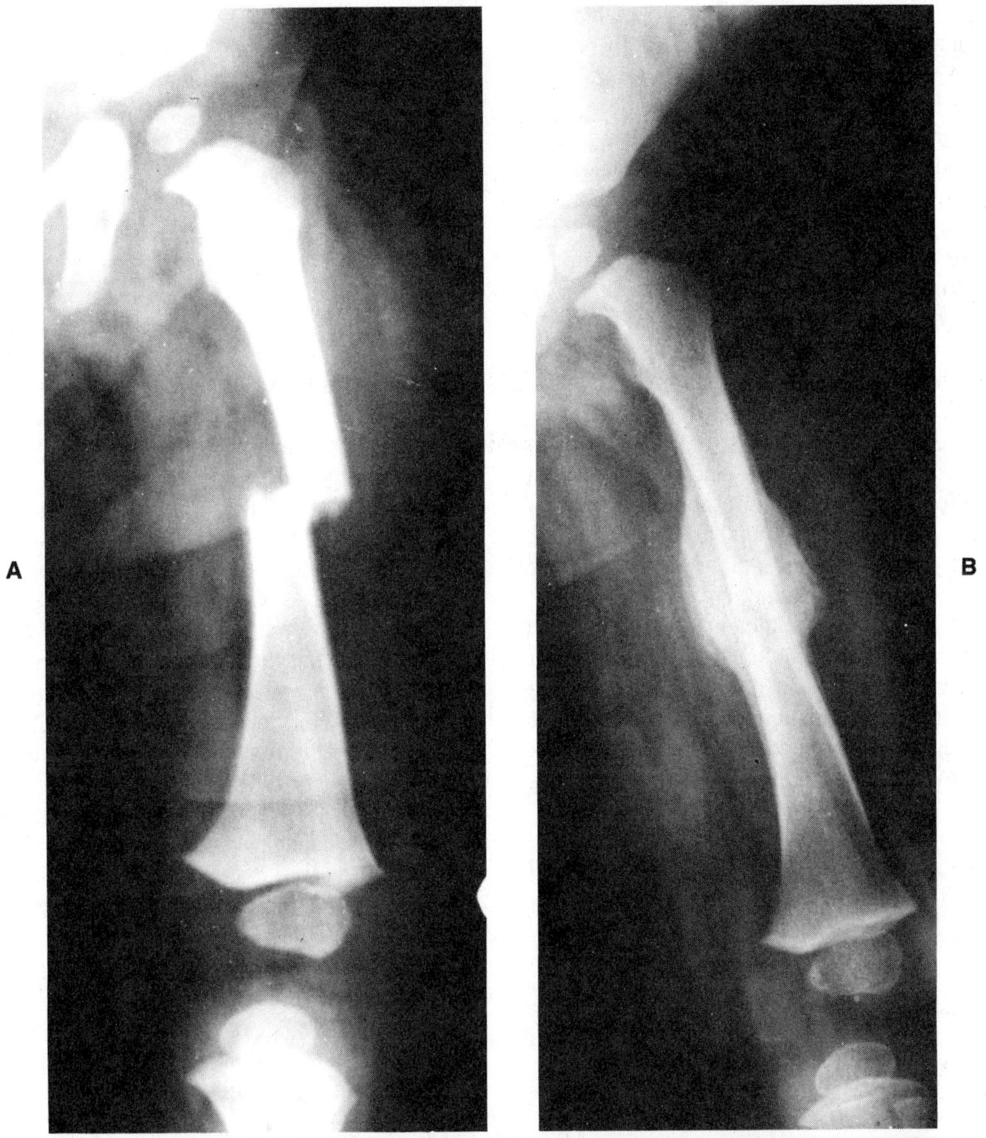

Fig. 39-13. Fractured femur. Most fractured femurs in childhood are of spiral type shown here. Note comparison of, **A,** original x-ray film with, **B,** 6-month postfracture film showing callus formation.

Courtesy Henrietta Egleston Hospital for Children, Atlanta, GA. From Hilt, N.E., and Schmitt, E.W.: Pediatric orthopedic nursing, St. Louis, 1975, Mosby–Year Book, Inc.

solid union of the femoral shaft in 3 to 4 weeks, whereas in the adult, callus sufficient to avoid deformities from constant muscle contraction associated with movement may not take place in less than 10 to 16 weeks. The approximate healing times for a femoral shaft are:

Neonatal period—2 to 3 weeks
Early childhood—4 weeks
Later childhood—6 to 8 weeks
Adolescence—8 to 12 weeks

Remodeling is a unique process that occurs in the healing of fractures of long bone before epiphyseal closure. When a bone remodels, the irregularities produced by the fracture become indistinct, as hollows are filled in and angles are rounded off in the healing process, which gives the bone a straighter appearance. It does not alter the alignment of the bone. The buildup of new bone or callus will restore a portion of the normal bone structure in most cases despite observable malalignment. The younger the child and the closer the proximity of the fracture to the growth plate, the more likely it is that spontaneous correction will take place. In some instances a 90-degree angle will straighten in a year, but rotational deformities do not correct themselves. Various factors such as the type and location of the fracture, the age of the child, and the amount of fragment angulation or rotation will influence the degree of correction in alignment that can be obtained by remodeling.

The position of the bone fragments in relation to one another influences the rapidity of healing and the residual deformity. A gap between fragments delays (or prevents) healing (Fig. 39-14, *A*). Healing is prompt and complete with end-to-end apposition (Fig. 39-14, *B*), but the fracture stimulates accelerated growth of the neighboring epiphysis, which causes bony overgrowth and increased length of the extremity. When the fragments overlap in a bayonet-type reduction (Fig. 39-14, *C*), there is sufficient bone contact to allow for rapid healing, and the lost length compensates for overgrowth as a result of epiphyseal stimulation. The length that can be compensated for depends on the age of the child. Approximately 1 cm of overlap can be allowed in a young child, but in a child who is near the end of the growth period, correction will be less and therefore overlap must be less. Angulation deformity caused by an incomplete fracture (Fig. 39-14, *D*) may remodel in the young child, but the degree of residual deformity depends on the relationship of the angulation of the bone fragments to the angle of the joint. This requires careful evaluation and reduction to prevent permanent deformity.

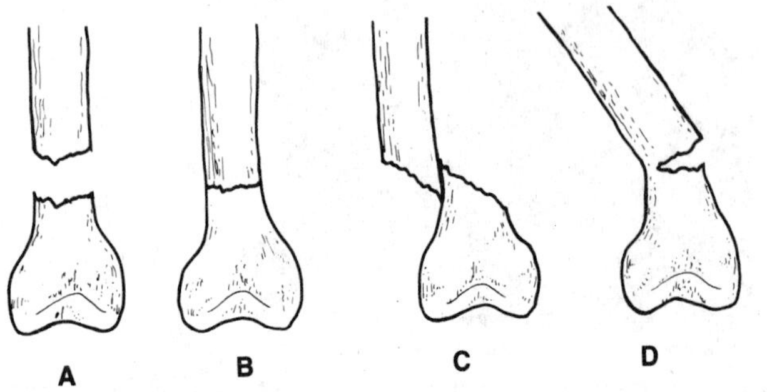

Fig. 39-14. Relationships of fracture fragments. **A,** Gap between fragments. **B,** End-to-end apposition. **C,** Bayonet apposition or overlap. **D,** Angulation of incomplete fracture.

Wolff's law is applied to treating children with orthopedic problems. Paraphrased, it states that bone will grow in the direction in which stress is placed on it. Examples of the use of this law are the hip spica cast with an abduction bar for treating congenital hip disorders or application of casts or traction at a selected angle to influence the direction of bone healing.

Bone healing in persons of any age-group is greatly influenced by the general health of the traumatized person. The child with a fracture requires adequate nutrition, including supplementary vitamins. No special dietary changes need to be made except to correct nutritional deficiencies. Monitoring of fluid and electrolyte balance, renal function, and possible anemia is equally important to promote wellness of the child.

THE CHILD IN A CAST

Nurses are frequently in a position where they must make the initial assessment of a child with a suspected fracture (see Emergency Treatment). The child and the parents are frightened and upset, the child is in pain, and since most fractures are obvious, the parents and frequently the child are already convinced of the diagnosis. Therefore if the child is alert and there is no evidence of hemorrhage, the initial nursing interventions are directed toward calming and reassuring the child and parents so that an extensive assessment can be more easily accomplished.

Maintaining a calm manner and speaking in a quiet voice, the nurse can ask the parents to describe what happened and what they think about it. Since children usually arrive with the limb supported in some manner, this minute or two does not delay or endanger the treatment. It is best not to touch children initially but to ask them to point to the painful area and wiggle their fingers or toes. By this time they usually feel relatively safe and will allow someone to touch them gently to feel the pulse and test for sensation. A child's anxiety is greatly influenced by previous experiences with injury and health personnel. However, children need to be told what will happen and what they can do to help. The affected limb need not be palpated and should not be moved unless properly splinted. If the child is at home or if the practitioner is not present to examine the child, some type of splint should be applied carefully for transport to the hospital and to the radiography department and cast room.

The Cast

The completeness of the fracture, the type of bone involved, and the amount of weight that can be placed on the limb influence how much of the extremity must be included in the cast to immobilize the fracture site completely. In most situations the joints above and below the fracture are immobilized to eliminate the possibility of movement that might cause displacement at the fracture site. Four major categories of casts are used for immobilization of fractures: *upper extremity* to immobilize wrist and/or elbow, *lower extremity* to immobilize ankle and/or knee, *spinal* and *cervical* for immobilization of the spine, and *spica casts* to immobilize the hip and knee.

Casting materials. Casts are constructed from gauze strips and bandages impregnated with plaster of Paris or synthetic lighter-weight and water-resistant materials (e.g., fiberglass and polyurethane resin). The lightweight casts are satisfactory for arms and hip spicas on infants and very young children and are even available in colors. Plaster is better for large hip spicas and legs. Table 39-3 compares the relative merits of plaster and synthetic casts.

Cast application. When a cast is to be applied by the operator, it is often the nurse's role to set up the cast materials and hold the extremity in alignment (Fig. 39-15). Special cast tables that hold the child's body are used for applying large hip spica casts. If possible, children should be allowed to play with a small doll that has a cast so that they understand what will be done. Before the cast is applied, the extremities are checked for any abrasions, cuts, or other alterations in the skin surface and for the presence of rings

EMERGENCY TREATMENT
Fracture

Assess extent of injury—5"Ps":
- Pain and point of tenderness
- Pulse—distal to the fracture site
- Pallor
- Paresthesia—sensation distal to the fracture site
- Paralysis—movement distal to the fracture site

Determine the mechanism of injury.

Move injured part as little as possible.
- Cover open wounds with sterile or clean dressing.

Immobilize the limb, including joints above and below fracture site; do not attempt to reduce fracture or push protruding bone under the skin.
- Soft splint (pillow or folded towel)
- Rigid splint (rolled newspaper or magazine)
- Uninjured leg can serve as splint for leg fracture if no splint available

Reassess neurovascular status.

Apply traction if circulatory compromise is present.

Elevate the injured limb if possible.

Apply cold to the injured area.

Call Emergency Transport Team (Service) or transport to medical facility.

A

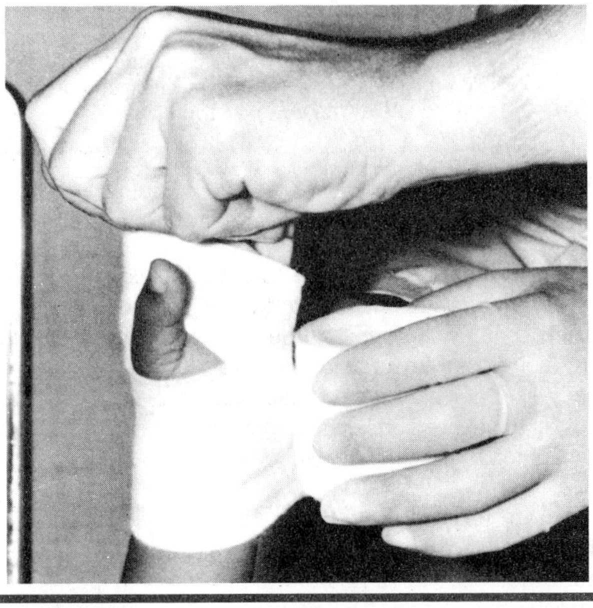

B

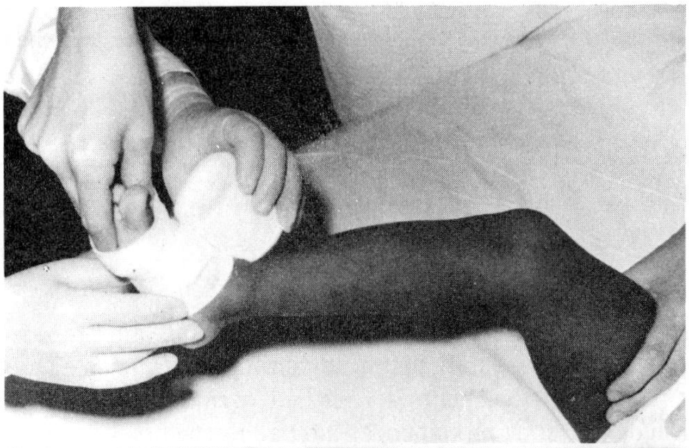

C

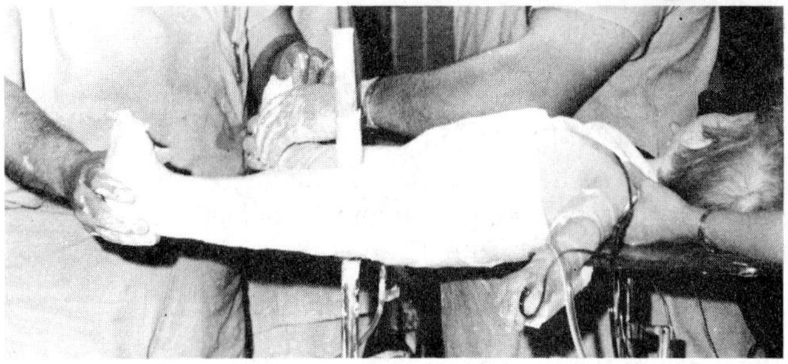

Fig. 39-15. Proper methods of holding child for cast application. **A,** Arm cast: arm should be held by fingers (and upper arm, if necessary) and off side of table or bed to permit exposure of entire arm. **B,** Leg cast: foot and toes are grasped with one hand as shown, and upper thigh with other hand; maintaining knee in flexion will discourage kicking. **C,** Hip spica cast: one individual maintains desired leg position; another individual pushes child at shoulder level toward perineal post; child's shoulders and pelvis should remain level.

From Hilt, N.E., and Schmitt, E.W.: Pediatric orthopedic nursing, St. Louis, 1975, Mosby–Year Book, Inc.

Table 39-3 Comparison of plaster of Paris and synthetic cast

	PLASTER OF PARIS	SYNTHETIC
Composition and preparation	Cotton tape permeated with calcium sulfate crystals that interlock as tape dries (tepid water–activated)	1. Polyester/cotton tape permeated with polyurethane resin (cool water–activated) 2. Knitted fiberglass tape with polyurethane resin (tepid water–activated or photoactivated) 3. Knitted thermoplastic polyester fabric (hot water–activated)
Setting time	3 to 8 minutes	3 to 15 minutes
Drying time	10 to 72 hours (varies with cast size)	5 to 30 minutes (varies with type of cast)
Indentations	Slow drying time increases possibility	Rapid drying time reduces likelihood of indentations; allows rapid use
Weight	Relatively heavy; bulky; difficulty wearing regular clothing	Lightweight; less bulky; can wear with regular clothing; allows for greater range of activity
Conformity	Molds readily to body part	Does not mold easily to body parts; unsuitable for small children or severely displaced fractures
Surface	Smooth exterior; does not scratch clothing or furniture	Rough exterior; can snag clothing or furniture; abrasive to skin
Cost	Relatively inexpensive; an advantage if cast changes anticipated	Expensive; cost three to seven times that of plaster casts
Stability	Relatively stable; must keep cast dry; clean with damp cloth and a dry, low-abrasive cleanser	May get cast wet or immerse in water with permission from practitioner (with use of nonabsorbent synthetic lining); clean with small amount of mild soap and water; dry with towel followed by blow dryer on cool or warm setting
Miscellaneous	Child may feel uncomfortable warming or burning sensation under cast while drying (chemical reaction) Skin under cast may become irritated Cast must be protected when around water (bathing)	Special aids may be required for application or removal of some types Increased activity may displace fracture Skin under cast may become macerated from inadequate drying after water immersion

Data from Lane, P.L., and Leem, M.M.: Special care for special casts, Nursing '83 13(7):50, 1983; Wise, L.B.: A comparison of orthopedic casts: breaking the mold, MCN 11:174-176, 1986.

or other items that might cause constriction from swelling; such objects are removed. Identification bands are placed on a noninjured extremity if hospitalization is anticipated.

A tube of stockinette is stretched over the area to be casted, and bony prominences are padded with soft cotton sheeting. Dry rolls of gauze impregnated with plaster of Paris are immersed in a pail of cold water with the open end of the roll downward to allow soaking of the bandage. The wet plaster rolls are put on in a bandage fashion and molded to the extremity. A heat-producing chemical reaction occurs between the plaster and water as the plaster becomes a crystalline gypsum. During application of the cast the underlying stockinette is pulled over the raw edges of the cast and secured with a layer of wet plaster ½ to 1 inch below the rim to form a smooth, padded edge to protect the skin.

If the operator does not form such a protective edge with stockinette, the raw edges of the cast can be protected by a "petaled" edge. Small pieces approximately 2 to 3 inches long are cut from 1- or 1½-inch wide adhesive tape. The edges are rounded with scissors, and each of these "petals" is placed over the edge of the cast, each petal slightly overlapping the previous petal to form a smooth, neat edge. It is easier to apply the petal to the underside of the cast first and then bring the unadhered edge to the front, pressing firmly so that the edges remain securely attached. Band-Aids can be used instead of the tape petals for quicker preparation and a slightly padded cast edge.

Nursing Considerations

The complete evaporation of the water from the hip spica cast can take 24 to 72 hours when traditional types of plaster materials are used. Drying occurs within 30 minutes with new quick-drying substances. Turning the child at least every 2 hours will help to dry the cast evenly. The cast must remain uncovered to allow it to dry from the inside out. A regular fan to circulate air may be helpful during high-humidity weather. Heated fans or dryers are discouraged because they cause the cast to dry on the outside while remaining wet beneath and can cause burns from heat conduction by way of the cast to the underlying tissue. If dryers are used, they should be set at cool or the lowest heat.

A wet cast should be supported by a pillow covered with plastic and handled by the palms of the hands to prevent indenting the cast and creating pressure areas. A dry plaster of Paris cast produces a hollow sound when tapped with the finger. If "hot spots" are felt on the cast surface (usually indicating infection beneath the area), this should be reported so a window can be made in the cast to observe the site.

During the first few hours after a cast is applied, the chief concern is that the extremity may continue to swell to the extent that the cast becomes a tourniquet, shutting off circulation and producing neurovascular complications. A measure for reducing the likelihood of this potential problem is to elevate the body part, thereby increasing venous return. If edema is excessive, casts are bivalved, that is, cut to make anterior and posterior halves that are held together with an elastic bandage. The cast and the involved extremity are observed frequently for neurovascular integrity and any signs of compromise. Permanent muscle and tissue damage can occur within 6 to 8 hours (McCullough and Evans, 1985), for which nurses can be held liable (Northrup and Kelly, 1987).

PARENT GUIDELINES
Cast Care

- Keep the casted extremity elevated on pillows or similar support for the first day, or as directed by the health professional.
- Avoid indenting the cast until it is thoroughly dry.
- Observe the extremities (fingers or toes) for any evidence of swelling or discoloration (darker or lighter than a comparable extremity) and contact the health professional if noted.
- Check movement and sensation of the visible extremities frequently.
- Follow health professional's orders regarding any restriction of activities.
- Restrict strenuous activities for the first few days.
  - Engage in quiet activities but encourage use of muscles.
  - Move the joints above and below the cast on the affected extremity.
- Encourage frequent rest for a few days, keeping the injured extremity elevated while resting.
- Avoid allowing the affected limb to hang down for any length of time.
  - Keep an injured upper extremity elevated (e.g., in a sling) while upright.
  - Elevate a lower limb when sitting and avoid standing for too long.
- Do not allow the child to put anything inside the cast.
  - Keep small items that might be placed inside the cast away from small children
- Keep a clear path for ambulation.
  - Remove toys, hazardous floor rugs, pets, or other items over which the child might stumble.
- Use crutches appropriately if lower limb fracture.
  - The crutches should fit properly, have a soft rubber tip to prevent slipping, and be well padded at the axilla.

NURSING ALERT Observations such as pain, swelling, discoloration (pallor or cyanosis) of the exposed portions, lack of pulsation and warmth, or the inability to move the exposed part(s) are reported immediately.

When casting an extremity that has sustained an open fracture, a window is often left over the wound area to allow for observation and for dressing of the wound. A surgical reduction is usually casted as for a closed fracture. For the first few hours after surgery there may be substantial bleeding that will soak through the cast. Periodically the circumscribed blood-stained area should be outlined with a ballpoint pen or pencil and the time indicated to provide a guide for assessing the amount of bleeding.

Usually the child is discharged to home care after a cast is applied in the emergency room or clinic. Parents need instructions on drying and caring for the cast and checking for signs and symptoms that indicate the cast is too tight (see Parent Guidelines). They should also be told to take the child to the health professional for attention if the cast becomes too loose, since a loose cast no longer serves its purpose. A cast is a badge of honor for the child and serves as visible evidence of an otherwise invisible injury (Fig. 39-16).

Cast removal. Cutting the cast to remove it or to relieve tightness is frequently a frightening experience for children. They fear the sound of the cast cutter and are terrified that their flesh, as well as the cast, will be cut. Since it works by vibration, a cast cutter cuts only the hard surface of the cast. This can be demonstrated on the nurse or person removing the cast. The oscillating blade vibrates very rapidly back and forth and will not cut when placed lightly on the skin. Children have described it as producing a "tickly" sensation. The vibration also generates heat that

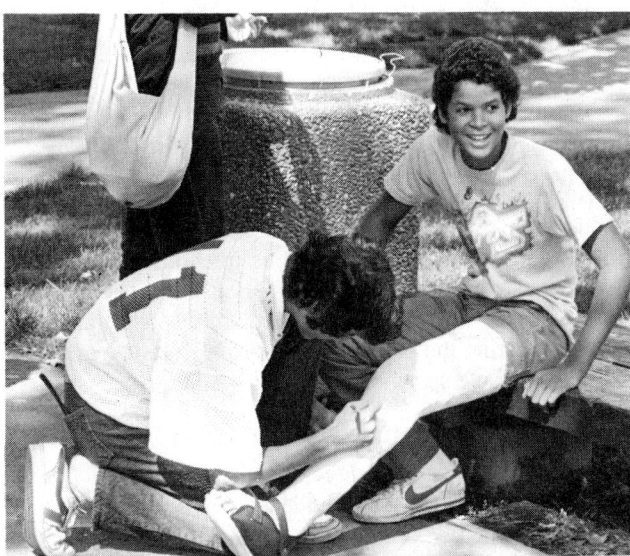

Fig. 39-16. A cast serves as an excellent medium for collecting autographs and assorted graffiti.

may be felt by the child. Both these feelings should be explained.

Preparation for the procedure will help reduce anxiety, especially if a trusting relationship has been established between the child and the nurse. Many young children come to regard the cast as part of themselves, which intensifies their fear of removal. Using the analogy of having fingernails or hair cut sometimes helps reduce their anxiety. They need continual reassurance that all is going well and that their behavior is accepted.

Home care for children in casts creates problems of various magnitude, especially with large casts (e.g., a hip spica). Commonplace situations become problematic, for example, returning the child home safely and comfortably. Standard seat belts and car seats are not readily adapted for use by children in casts (see Congenital Hip Dysplasia, Chapter 11, and Educate About the Disorder and General Health Care, Chapter 22). Sitting can be impossible in a spica cast, and leg casts require extra space in a small room, under a table, or in a bathroom. Children in spica casts usually find the prone position easier for self-feeding from a small table placed next to the dining table or on the floor. The conventional toilet is almost impossible for a child in a spica cast. Small bedpans or other containers offer alternatives for elimination.

Nurses can help families adapt the child's environment to meet the temporary encumbrance of a cast, for example, devising plastic wraps for waterproofing casts for a shower. Baths are possible only if the plaster cast is kept out of the water and covered to prevent it from becoming wet from splashes. Some synthetic casts are waterproof, but skin can become irritated from water that collects beneath the cast.

After the cast is removed, the skin surface will be caked with desquamated skin and sebaceous secretions. Simple soaking in a bathtub is usually sufficient for their removal but may require several days to eliminate the accumulation completely. Application of olive oil or lotion may provide comfort. Parents and child should be instructed not to pull or forcibly remove this material with vigorous scrubbing because it may cause excoriation and bleeding.*

THE CHILD IN TRACTION

Bone fragments that cannot be aligned initially by simple traction and stabilization with a cast require the extended pulling force offered by continuous traction. Traction also may be used for other purposes (Box 39-7). In some of these cases the skin traction is applied at night and intermittently during the day. Muscle relaxants may be administered for muscle spasms.

Purposes of Traction

When forces having both direction and magnitude act on an object at the same point simultaneously from opposite directions, the object either changes its state of rest or motion or remains in equilibrium. The use of traction in the management of fractures is the direct application of these forces to produce equilibrium at the fracture site. A forward force (traction) is produced by attaching weight to the distal bone fragment, which is balanced by the backward force of the muscle pull (countertraction) and the frictional force between the patient and the bed. Thus the three essential components of traction management are traction, countertraction, and friction (Fig. 39-17).

BOX 39-7 PURPOSES OF TRACTION

To realign bone fragments
To provide rest for an extremity
To help prevent or improve contracture deformity
To correct a deformity
To treat a dislocation
To allow preoperative or postoperative positioning and alignment
To provide immobilization of specific areas of the body
To reduce muscle spasms (rare in children)

To reduce or realign a fracture site, traction is provided by weights applied to the distal bone fragment; body weight provides countertraction. By adjusting the line of pull upward or downward or by adducting or abducting the extremity, the operator uses these forces to align the distal and proximal bone fragments. To attain equilibrium, the amount of forward force is adjusted by adding weight to or subtracting weight from the traction, and/or countertraction can be increased by elevating the foot of the bed to create a greater gravitational pull to the backward force. A bed board placed under the mattress of heavy children prevents sagging, which might otherwise change the direction of the forces applied to the fracture.

The three primary purposes of traction for reduction of fractures are:

1. To fatigue the involved muscle and reduce muscle spasm so that bones can be realigned
2. To position the distal and proximal bone ends in desired realignment to promote satisfactory bone healing
3. To immobilize the fracture site until realignment has been achieved and sufficient healing has taken place to permit casting or splinting

Fatiguing of a muscle is accomplished by applying constant stress to the muscle so that the buildup of lactic acid will produce muscle relaxation. The all-or-none law, characteristic of muscle contractility, influences the complete relaxation. When muscle is stretched, muscle spasm ceases and permits the realignment of the bone ends. The continuous maintenance of traction is important during this phase because releasing the traction allows the muscle's normal contracting ability to again cause a malpositioning of the bone ends.

The realignment of the fragments is a gradual process

*See Nursing Care Plans: The Child with a Fracture and the Child in a Cast; and home care instructions for the child in a cast in Wong, D.L. and Whaley, L.F.: Clinical manual of pediatric nursing, ed. 3, St. Louis, 1990, Mosby–Year Book, Inc.

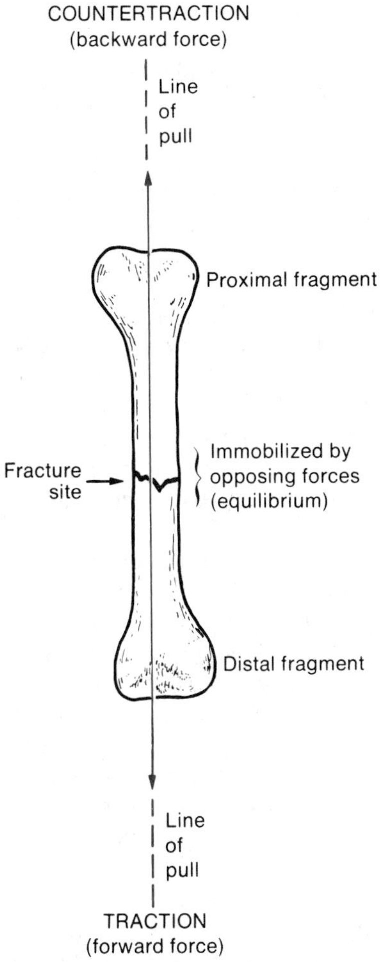

Fig. 39-17. Application of traction for maintaining equilibrium.

that is achieved more rapidly in infants, who have limited muscle tone, than in muscular teenagers. The desired line of pull and callus formation are checked periodically by radiographic examination. The traction pull to some degree immobilizes the fracture site; however, adjunctive immobilizing devices such as splints or casts are sometimes used with skeletal traction. In injuries in which there is severe soft tissue swelling or vascular and nerve damage, it is customary to use traction until these complications have been resolved and it is safe to apply a cast. Immobilization with traction will be maintained until the bone ends are in satisfactory realignment, after which a less-confining type of immobilization, usually a cast, will be applied.

Types of Traction (General)

The pull needed for traction can be applied to the distal bone fragment in several ways (Box 39-8). *Manual traction* is used by the operator in uncomplicated arm or leg fractures in which there is little overriding of the bones and minimum muscle pull to overcome. Manual traction is used to realign bone fragments for immediate cast application.

BOX 39-8 TYPES OF TRACTION

Manual traction—traction applied to the body part by the hand placed distally to the fracture site. Nurses frequently provide manual traction during cast application.
Skin traction—pull applied directly to the skin surface and indirectly to the skeletal structures. The pulling mechanism is attached to the skin with adhesive material or an elastic bandage. Both types are applied over soft foam-backed traction straps to distribute the traction pull.
Skeletal traction—pull applied directly to the skeletal structure by a pin, wire, or tongs inserted into or through the diameter of the bone distal to the fracture.

Skin traction is applied when there is minimum displacement and little muscle spasticity but is contraindicated when there is associated skin damage. Skin traction has specific limits of weight that it can pull without causing tissue breakdown. *Skeletal traction* is employed when significant traction pull must be applied in order to achieve realignment and immobilization. By inserting a pin or wire into the bone, the stress is placed on the bone and not on the surrounding tissue.

The type of traction applied is determined primarily by the age of the child, the condition of the soft tissues, and the type and degree of displacement of the fracture. Fractures most commonly treated by application of traction are those involving the humerus, femur, and vertebrae. The major types of traction for specific fractures are discussed in the following sections.

Upper Extremity Traction

Treatment of fractures of the humerus by traction is accomplished either (1) by overhead suspension, in which the arm, bent at the elbow, is suspended vertically by skin or skeletal attachment and traction is applied to the distal end of the humerus, or (2) by Dunlop traction. With Dunlop traction the arm is suspended horizontally, using either skin or skeletal attachment.

When skin traction is used, straps are placed on the lower and upper arm with the arm flexed to accomplish pull in two directions: one along the longitudinal direction of the upper arm and one to maintain alignment of the lower arm. In instances such as supracondylar fractures, the amount of traction pull needed to align the site more critically requires a skeletal wire placed in the upper arm to allow the additional weight.

Fractures of the humerus, which are usually the result of a fall with the arm in extension, frequently involve the supracondylar portion. There are three major complications associated with this injury: Volkmann contractures (p. 1869); traumatic injury to the median, ulnar, or radial nerves; and angulation deformities. The fracture must be carefully reduced, sometimes with the child under anesthesia, and because of the danger of complications, children with closed reduction of supracondylar fractures are often hospitalized for observation. In severely malaligned fractures, closed reduction with the child under anesthesia is followed by application of skeletal traction for 2 to 3 weeks, after which a long arm cast is applied for an additional 2 to 3 weeks.

Lower Extremity Traction

The frequent site for a femoral fracture is in the middle one third of the shaft, as pictured by the radiograph in Fig. 39-13, *A*. With this fracture there is significant overriding but minimum displacement. In a fracture in the lower one third of the shaft, the pull of the gastrocnemius muscle causes the distal fragment to become downwardly displaced. The severity of the fracturing force and the ability of the muscles to hold the fracture out of alignment will determine the fracture type and the amount of overriding of the fragments. The periosteum may remain intact, which helps maintain alignment.

Fractures of the femur can often be reduced with early application of a hip spica cast in young children. When traction is required, several types may be employed, based on the initial assessment.

Bryant traction. When a traction pulls only in one direction, it is called *running traction.* Bryant traction is this type of traction (Fig. 39-18). Adhesive traction strips are applied to the child's legs and secured with elastic bandages wrapped from the foot to the groin. Both of the child's hips are flexed at a 90-degree angle with the knees in extension and the legs suspended by pulleys and weights. The child's weight supplies the countertraction; therefore the buttocks are slightly elevated off the bed. By applying the same amount of traction to both legs and restraining the torso, the pelvis and hips are prevented from rotating and equal stress is placed on the growing extremities. The ankle bones are protected with stockinette or cotton wadding. This type of traction is used for children younger than 2 years of age whose weight is not sufficient to provide adequate countertraction without the additional gravitational force. Both legs are suspended, even though only one may be involved.

Bryant traction is unsuitable for older children and is usually limited to children who weigh less than 12 to 14 kg (26 to 30 pounds) because of the risk of postural hypertension and to children without spasticity or contractures of the hamstring muscles. The child's position needs to be monitored, and the alignment of the fracture is checked by periodic x-ray films with needed traction adjustments made by the operator. Remodeling and callus formation occur rapidly within 2 to 3 weeks, after which the child is placed in a hip spica cast for an additional 3 to 9 weeks.

A specific complication of overhead traction is impairment of circulation. This is especially a problem in Bryant traction because of the gravitational vascular draining of the elevated extremities, the possible tourniquet effect of the bandages, and the effect of the traction, which can trigger vasospasms.

A child younger than 2 years of age normally has the hips in flexion most of the time; therefore the mild contracture that might develop from this position is easily corrected. The youngster is permitted sufficient room between the foot and the traction foot plate to move the foot and prevent ankle problems. The legs must be maintained perpendicular to the trunk, and the buttocks should not be allowed to rest on the mattress. Sometimes the child, especially the very active child, is placed in a jacket restraint to prevent turning and twisting out of alignment.

Buck extension. Buck extension (Fig. 39-19) is a type of skin traction with the legs in an extended position, but it differs from Bryant traction in that the hips are not flexed. The postural hypertension that could develop as a result of Bryant traction is avoided, and this traction allows for greater mobility. Turning from side to side is permitted (except for fractures) with care to maintain the involved leg in alignment. Buck extension is used primarily for short-term immobilization or frequently for correcting contracture or bone deformities such as Legg-Calvé-Perthes disease.

Russell traction. Russell traction (Fig. 39-20) uses skin traction on the lower leg and a padded sling under the knee. Two lines of pull, one along the longitudinal line of the lower leg and one perpendicular to the leg, are produced. This combination of pulls allows realignment of the lower extremity and immobilizes the hip and knee in a flexed position. The hip flexion must be kept at the prescribed angle to prevent fracture malalignment, since there is no direct support under the fracture and the skin traction may slip. Because the traction is set up to have two ropes

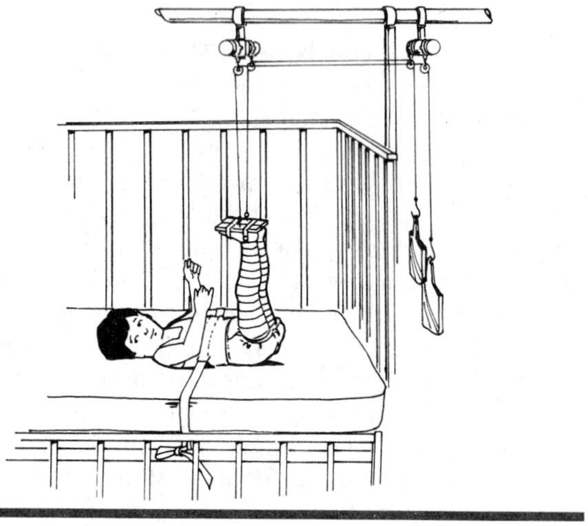

Fig. 39-18. Bryant traction.

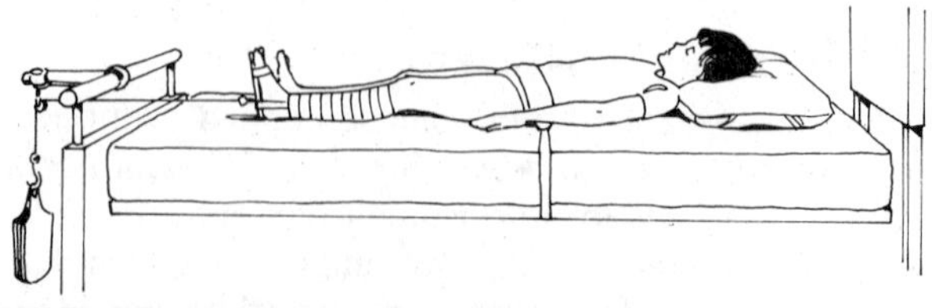

Fig. 39-19. Buck extension traction.

pulling in the same direction at the foot plate, the traction pull will be twice the amount of weight at the end of the bed. For example, 5 pounds of weight produces 10 pounds of pull. Special nursing measures include carefully checking the position of the traction so that the amount of desired hip flexion is maintained and damage to the common peroneal nerve under the knee does not produce footdrop.

"90-90" traction. The most common skeletal traction is 90-degree–90-degree traction (90-90 traction) (Fig. 39-21). The lower leg is put in a boot cast or supported in a sling, and a skeletal Steinmann pin or Kirschner wire is placed in the distal fragment of the femur. From a nursing standpoint this traction easily facilitates position changes, toileting, and prevention of traction complications. This traction also:

Achieves the desired line of pull for reducing the fracture by means of the skeletal traction
Allows a 90-degree flexion of both the hip and the knee
Supports the lower extremity in a desired position with good venous return
Provides adequate immobilization of the fracture site

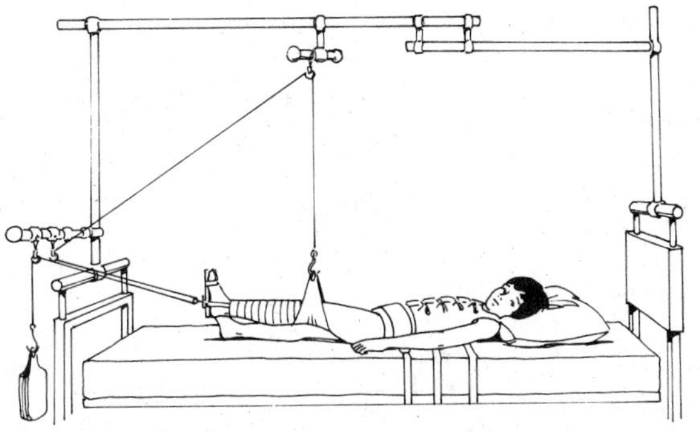

Fig. 39-20. Russell traction.

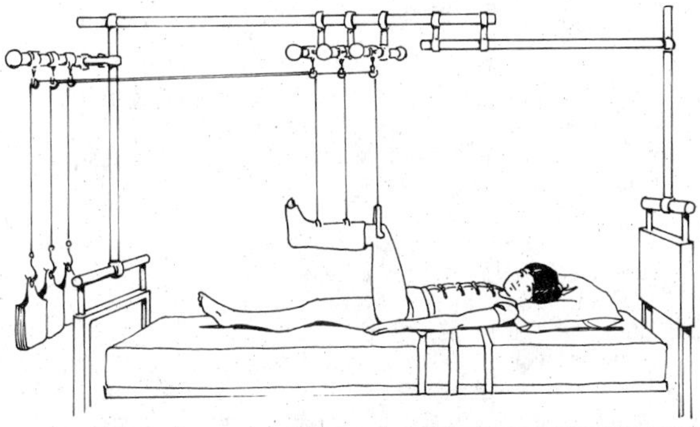

Fig. 39-21. "90-90" traction.

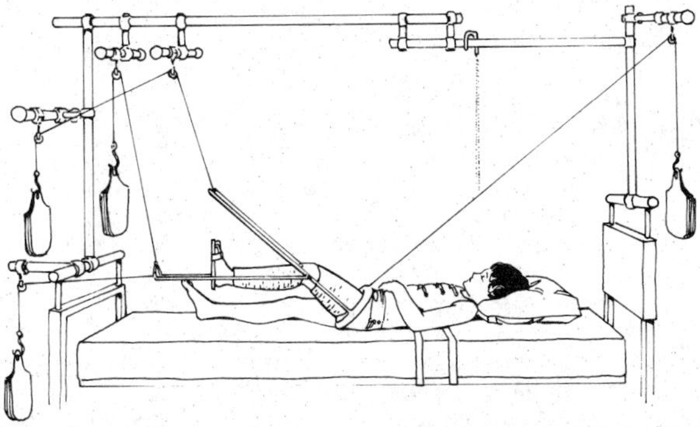

Fig. 39-22. Balance suspension with Thomas ring splint and Pearson attachment.

Balance suspension traction. Balance suspension traction (Fig. 39-22) may be used with or without skin or skeletal traction. Unless used with another traction, the balanced suspension merely suspends the leg in a desired flexed position to relax the hip and hamstring muscles and does not exert any traction directly on a body part. A Thomas splint extends from the groin to midair above the foot, and a Pearson attachment supports the lower leg. Towels or pieces of felt covered with stockinette are clipped or pinned to the splints for leg support. Note that the ropes are attached to create a balanced traction. When the child is lifted from the bed, the traction lifts as well with no loss of alignment.

The Pearson attachment will stay wherever positioned. Many times the practitioner will put a rope between the end of the Pearson attachment and the end of Thomas splint to prevent any knee flexion alteration while the child is moved. This traction requires very careful checking of splints and ropes to make certain that no slippage or fraying has occurred. The traction is of great value in an older and heavier child when lifting the patient for care is essential.

Cervical Traction

The cervical area is a vulnerable site for flexion or extension injuries to muscle, vertebrae, and/or the spinal cord. Cervical muscle trauma without other complications is treated with a cervical soft or hard collar to relieve the weight of the head from the fracture site. Intermittent cervical skin traction might be employed with a head halter and weight to decrease muscle spasms (Fig. 39-23). Injuries limited to cervical muscles can be very uncomfortable but, with prompt medical care, usually resolve with conservative treatment.

When a child displaces or fractures a cervical vertebra, it is necessary to reduce and immobilize the site with cervical skeletal traction. The spinal cord runs through the intravertebral canal, and dislocation or fracture of the vertebrae can also cause spinal cord trauma.

Physical examination, especially a neurologic assessment, and radiographic studies are essential diagnostic aids to determine:

Presence of vertebral fracture
Degree of vertebral dislocation
Displacement of intravertebral disk
Compression of spinal cord and other neurologic structures
Sensory, motor, and autonomic nerve deficits

Cervical traction is usually accomplished by insertion of Crutchfield or Barton tongs through burr holes in the skull.

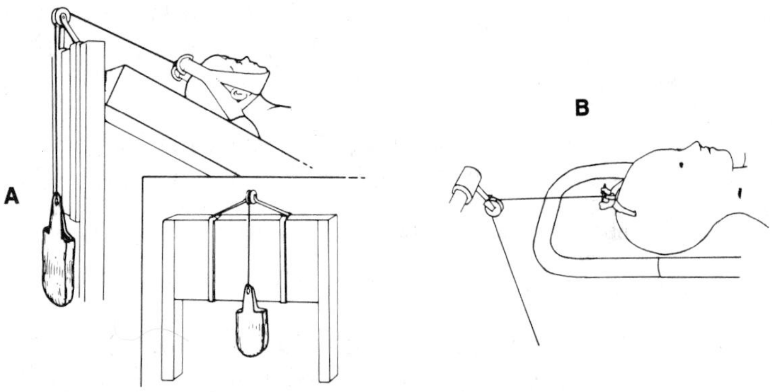

Figs. 39-18 to 39-23 from Hilt, N.E., and Schmitt, E.W.: Pediatric orthopedic nursing, St. Louis, 1975, Mosby–Year Book, Inc.

Fig. 39-23. **A,** Cervical traction. **B,** Crutchfield tong traction.

The head is placed in a hyperextended position, and, as the neck muscles fatigue with constant traction pull, the vertebral bodies gradually are pulled apart and the cord is no longer pinched between the vertebrae. Immobilization until fracture healing can occur is an essential goal of cervical traction. If the injury has been limited to a vertebral fracture without neurologic deficit, a halo cast can be applied to permit earlier ambulation.

Nursing Considerations

Traction is a valuable therapy if the purposes for the traction are achieved without complications. Generally the child in traction is hospitalized under the direct care of nurses, who develop individualized nursing care plans based on an understanding of correct traction management.

Assessment

To assess the child in traction, it is essential to know the purpose for which the traction is applied. Regular assessment of both the child and the traction apparatus is required, as outlined in Box 39-9. The child is also assessed for evidence of adverse effects of immobilization (see p. 1838).

Nursing Diagnoses

Based on a thorough assessment, several nursing diagnoses are identified. The more common diagnoses for the child in traction are included in the Nursing Care Plan on pp. 1867-1868. Others may apply in specific situations.

Planning

Nursing objectives for the child in traction include the following:

1. Maintain bone alignment.
2. Prevent complications.
3. Provide diversion.
4. Support child and family.

BOX 39-9 GUIDELINES FOR ASSESSMENT OF TRACTION

Check desired line of pull and relationship of distal fragment to proximal fragment.
- Check whether fragment is being directed upward, adducted, or abducted.

Check function of each component:
- Position of bandages, frames, splints
- Ropes—in center tract of pulley, taut, no fraying, knots tied securely
- Pulleys
  - In original position on attachment bar; have not slid from original site
  - Wheels freely movable
- Weights
- Correct amount of weight
  - Hanging freely
  - In safe location

Check bed position—head or foot elevated as directed for desired amount of pull and countertraction.

Assess child's behavior to determine if traction causes pain or discomfort.

Skin traction:
- Replace nonadhesive straps and/or Ace bandage on skin traction *when permitted* and/or absolutely necessary, but make certain that traction on limb is maintained by someone during procedure.
- Assess bandages to ascertain if they are correctly applied (diagonal or spiral), not too loose or too tight, which could cause slippage and malalignment of traction.

Skeletal traction:
- Check pin sites frequently for signs of bleeding, inflammation, or infection.
- Check pin screws to be certain that screws are tight in metal clamp that attaches traction apparatus to pin.
- Note pull of traction on pin; pull should be even.

Observe for correct body alignment with emphasis on alignment of shoulders, hip, and leg(s).

Check after child has moved.

Assess any circular dressing for excessive tightness.

Assess restraining devices, if prescribed.
- Make certain that they are not too loose or too tight.
- Remove periodically and check for pressure areas.

Note if any tightness, weakness, or contractures are developing in uninvolved joints and muscles.

Note any neurovascular changes, such as:
- Color in skin and nail beds
- Alterations in sensation
- Alterations in motor ability

Check beneath the child for small objects (e.g., foods, toys).

NURSING CARE PLAN
The Child in Traction

NURSING DIAGNOSIS: Potential for injury related to immobility and traction apparatus

GOAL 1

Prevent complications

INTERVENTIONS

Encourage deep breathing frequently with maximum inspiratory chest expansion
Apply restraints when indicated
Maintain correct angles at joints
Carry out passive, active, or active-with-resistance exercises of uninvolved joints
Take measures to correct or prevent further development of deformity, such as applying foot plate to prevent footdrop
*Cleanse and dress pin sites on skeletal traction as ordered
*Apply topical antiseptic or antibiotic daily as ordered
Cover ends of pins with protective cord or padding to prevent child from being scratched by pin
Do not remove skeletal traction or adhesive traction straps on skin traction
Understand purpose of traction
Understand function of traction in each specific situation
*Administer stool softeners as indicated
*Administer rectal suppository or mild laxative if indicated
Make certain that child ingests sufficient amount of calcuim-rich foods

EXPECTED OUTCOMES

Circulation in extremities remains satisfactory; movement, good (pink) color, sensation present
Child exhibits no signs of complications

NURSING DIAGNOSIS: Pain related to physical injury

GOAL 1

Relieve pain
See Nursing Care Plan: The Child in Pain, Chapter 26

NURSING DIAGNOSIS: Potential impaired skin integrity related to immobility, traction apparatus

GOAL 1

Prevent skin breakdown

INTERVENTIONS

Provide sheepskin, Egg-crate, or alternating pressure mattress underneath hips and back
Make total body skin checks for redness or breakdown, especially over areas that receive greatest pressure
Wash and dry skin at least twice daily
Stimulate circulation with gentle massage over pressure areas
Change position at least every 2 hours to relieve pressure, if possible
Check for small objects (e.g., toys, food) under child

EXPECTED OUTCOME

Skin remains clean and intact with no evidence of irritation

NURSING DIAGNOSIS: Impaired physical mobility (specify level) related to musculoskeletal impairment

GOAL 1

Maintain limb function

INTERVENTIONS

Provide apparatus (e.g., overhead trapeze) and encourage child in activities that provide exercise for uninvolved muscles and joints

EXPECTED OUTCOME

Joints remain flexible; muscles retain tone

NURSING DIAGNOSIS: Fear related to discomfort, unfamiliar apparatus, strange environment

GOAL 1

Decrease anxiety and gain cooperation

INTERVENTIONS

Explain traction apparatus to child
Explain to child what nursing care will be
Determine with child ways to participate in own care
Make certain that child knows how to call for help
Provide assurance that the child will not be left totally helpless
Have family bring child's favorite toy and/or security object

EXPECTED OUTCOME

Child cooperates throughout procedures

GOAL 2

Relieve discomfort

INTERVENTIONS

Use pads, pillows, and rolls to position for comfort
See also Nursing Care Plan: The Child in Pain, Chapter 26

EXPECTED OUTCOMES

Child plays and interacts readily
Child exhibits no signs of discomfort

*Dependent nursing action.

Continued.

NURSING CARE PLAN
The Child in Traction—cont'd

NURSING DIAGNOSIS: Bathing/hygiene, feeding, dressing/grooming, toileting self-care deficits related to impaired mobility

GOAL 1
Promote maximum self-help

INTERVENTIONS

Devise means to facilitate self-help in daily activities
Assist with self-care activities where needed, for example, bathe inaccessible parts, make food easy to eat without assistance, provide grooming

EXPECTED OUTCOME

Child assists with self-care activities: feeds self, washes reachable areas, attends to grooming within child's capabilities (specify)

GOAL 2
Facilitate elimination

INTERVENTIONS

Determine child's words for elimination needs
Provide privacy
Use fracture pan for bowel movements and voiding for females
Check frequency and consistency of bowel movements
Adjust fluid and food intake according to stools, for example, increase fluids, fruits, grains for constipation

EXPECTED OUTCOMES

Elimination is managed with minimum difficulty
Child has regular bowel movements

See also:
Nursing Care Plan: The Child in the Hospital, Chapter 26
Nursing Care Plan: the Family of the Ill or Hospitalized, Child Chapter 26

Implementation

Evaluating the therapeutic effects and possible negative consequences is essential to good patient care. Many of the nursing problems associated with a child in traction are related to immobility. However, there are a number of physical needs that require attention and vigilance.

NURSING ALERT Skeletal traction is never released by the nurse. This includes not lifting weights (e.g., for moving the child in bed, for repositioning) that are applying traction.

However, the nurse may remove nonadhesive skin traction. In these cases intermittent traction is periodically released and reapplied as ordered. When skin traction must be constantly maintained, such as in fractures, nurses may occasionally remove and reapply the Ace bandage if this is approved by the attending physician, provided that *someone manually maintains the traction during the rewrapping process.* A child may have several types of traction at one time, and each traction must be assessed separately to avoid problems.

In addition to routine skin observation and care (see The Immobilized Child, p. 1837), children in skeletal traction will need special skin care at the pin site according to hospital policy or practitioner preference. A sheepskin or alternating pressure mattress placed beneath hips and back reduces the chance of skin breakdown in these vulnerable areas. (See Nursing Care Plan, p. 1867 and above, for additional nursing measures.)

When children are first placed in traction, they may have increased discomfort as a result of the traction pull fatiguing the muscle. Analgesics and muscle relaxants should be given during this phase of care, but helping children cope with the confinement and new experience requires more than medications. An explanation should be given according to each child's level of development about what is happening and why the child must remain in the device. They should be reassured that someone will always be available to aid them in adjusting to the traction and to cope with the problems of immobilization.

Some devices assist children in performing activities independently. An overhead trapeze, which they can use to help lift themselves, facilitates hygiene and repositioning and provides exercise for uninvolved muscles. Specific nursing responsibilities for care of the patient in cervical traction are included in the Nursing Care Plan on p. 1867 and above. For helping the child and family cope with immobility, see Nursing Care Plan, p. 1845.

Evaluation

The effectiveness of nursing interventions is determined by continual reassessment and evaluation of care based on the following observational guidelines and expected outcomes:

1. Perform routine assessment of the child and traction, as described in Box 39-9.
2. Perform assessment for circulation, skin integrity, neurologic function, and evidence of infection.
3. Observe types of activity in which child engages; observe for visitors and interaction with other patients and staff.
4. Interview child and family regarding feelings and concerns.

Expected outcomes:
See Nursing Care Plan, pp. 1867-1868.

FRACTURE COMPLICATIONS

Complications associated with fractures and immobilization are varied and have some problems in common. In addition to problems related to immobilization, the major complications of fractures include the following areas.

Circulatory Impairment

If the trauma or immobilizing device restricts veins or arteries in the affected extremity, bone healing will be seriously impaired. Careful assessment of the pulses, skin color, and temperature is an important nursing responsibility. After injury, swelling of tissues occurs more rapidly in the child than in the adult. In the upper extremity, brachial, radial, ulnar, and digital pulses are felt. In the leg, femoral, popliteal, posterior tibial, and dorsalis pedis pulses are checked.

✦ **NURSING ALERT** When circulatory impairment is evident (absence of pulse, discoloration, swelling, pain), the nurse takes quick action to relieve the problem by reporting the situation immediately. If the practitioner is unable to come and release the pressure, the nurse must be able to cut the cast in half to form a bivalve cast or make a large window in it to decrease the pressure.

Closely associated with an inadequate blood supply is a low hematocrit value, which can result from the initial blood loss or surgically induced anemia. Although the blood flow may be adequate, a lowered amount of hemoglobin will not provide a sufficient supply of oxygen for tissue repair.

Nerve Compression Syndromes

Nerve damage can take place at the time of injury, develop in the process of realignment, or be a complication of an immobilizing apparatus. The syndromes are classified according to the anatomic area affected and can involve the median (carpal tunnel syndrome), ulnar (at wrist or elbow), radial, posterior tibial (tarsal tunnel syndrome), common peroneal, or sciatic nerves. Peroneal nerve damage can result in footdrop, and radial nerve impairment produces wristdrop. Both of these disabilities can significantly interfere with activities of daily living.

Sensory testing with touch and pinprick and evaluating motor strength by asking the child to move the unaffected joint distal to the injury are common means of determining neurologic involvement. Subjective symptoms are pain or discomfort, muscular weakness, a burning sensation, limitation of motion, and altered sensation. Because the fear of pain limits the child's cooperation, play can be the nurse's most valuable tool.

Treatment is alleviation of pressure on the nerve. The practitioner determines whether correcting the alignment will alleviate pressure on the nerve or if surgical intervention is necessary. At times sensory or motor changes indicate ischemia, and the treatment is correction of the vascular disturbance.

Compartment Syndromes

A *compartment* is a group of muscles surrounded by tough, inelastic fascial tissue. The compartment syndrome occurs when increased pressure within this closed space rises and compromises circulation to the muscles and nerves within the space. Muscles and nerves of both upper and lower extremities are enclosed within such compartments. The most frequent causes of compartment syndrome are tight dressings or casts, hemorrhage, trauma, burns, and surgery.

Signs and symptoms of compartment syndrome reflect a deficit or deterioration of neuromuscular status in the anatomic area surrounding the involved structures. These include motor weakness and pain or discomfort out of proportion to the injury and unrelieved by pain medication. Tenseness may be noted on palpation of the area. Because early detection is important in preventing permanent damage to tissues, specialists recommend continuous monitoring of compartment pressures by way of a small, slit-tip catheter inserted into the compartment. Treatment of compartment syndrome is immediate relief of pressure, which sometimes requires fasciotomy.

Volkmann contracture. Volkmann contracture (ischemic muscular atrophy) is a serious, persistent flexion contraction of the forearm and hand caused by massive infarction of muscle. Pressure from a cast, a tight bandage, or from swelling from the injury in the area of the elbow begins with arterial occlusion and then progresses to muscle anoxia and reflex vasospasms. Finally the lack of blood supply leads to muscle necrosis and replacement with fibrous tissue, which produces paralysis and a clawlike hand contracture. Any fracture that requires excessive traction can be complicated by Volkmann contracture; however, it occurs most often in the elbow.

The neuromuscular symptoms are severe pain (although pain is not always a manifestation), pallor or cyanosis, edema, absence of pulses in the extremity, and loss of sensitivity. Unrelieved, the occlusive hypoxic process can cause some contracture if ischemia lasts as little as 6 hours. A great deal of muscle damage occurs after 12 to 24 hours; 48 hours of ischemia produces severe deformity, with muscle fibrosis and contractures in 5 to 10 days. If not treated, the contracture leads to severe deformity and paralysis.

The immediate treatment is to remove any mechanically obstructive materials, such as tight bandages, and extend the joint to free blood vessels. If the symptoms do not improve within a few hours, arteriography is done in anticipation that surgery may be needed to decrease arterial spasms and to improve the blood supply by separation of the fascial sheaths of the involved muscles.

Epiphyseal Damage

Growth of bone originates from the epiphyseal plate, and damage to this structure could result in an unequal extremity length. Surgical intervention to the epiphysis on the affected extremity or to the epiphyseal line on the opposite extremity is the usual treatment.

Nonunion

Bone healing and callus formation can span and repair only a limited space between fragments. When inadequate reduction, poor immobilization, or a damaged or softened cast cannot maintain the bone fragments in correct alignment for repair, bone healing is impaired. Based on the physiologic needs for bone healing, the factors most likely to interfere with bone healing and cause delayed union or nonunion are listed in Box 39-10.

The hematoma, which becomes the matrix for bone deposition in the break, must be free of infection or bits of adipose or connective tissue. The constant supply of nutrients and bone-forming cells brought to the area by way of the bloodstream provides the vital ingredients for repair.

Sometimes artificial means are employed to facilitate bone healing. Bone grafting becomes necessary when bone nonunion occurs. The donor sites are usually the tibia or the iliac crest. Bleeding of bone ends may need to be artificially stimulated, and at times holes are drilled near the bone ends in an attempt to increase circulation. Postsurgical immobilization of the recipient area is crucial to a successful graft.

Malunion

Malunion is fracture union with increased angulation or deformity at the fracture site. It can be detected at any stage in the healing process or after complete healing. Unsatisfactory reduction is the usual reason for malunion. A cast or splint that allows fracture movement will also likely result in malunion. Periodic radiographic examinations will help detect this complication and avoid its becoming a major problem over a long period.

Excessive deformity can be corrected during the healing process through realignment and reimmobilization. However, attempts at correction may cause delayed union or nonunion; therefore the degree of deformity is carefully evaluated in light of these complications. The probability of sufficient spontaneous alignment that occurs with growth and continuation of the healing process also is considered. Correction of the malunion when healing is near completion requires surgical intervention.

BOX 39-10 FACTORS THAT INTERFERE WITH BONE HEALING

- Separation of bone fragments at fracture site
- Loss of hematoma
- Interposition of tissue between bone fragments
- Loss of bone tissue, especially from necrosis
- Infection
- Poor nutrition
- Interruption of blood supply
- Diseases that influence calcium metabolism (e.g., thyroid disorder)
- Cancer of bone
- Administration of steroids

Infection

Osteomyelitis, infection of the bone, is often secondary to a bloodstream infection but is a potential problem in open fractures or when bone surgery has been performed. Any bacterial organism can cause this infectious process; however, *Staphylococcus aureus* is the most frequent pathogen. (See p. 1895 for a discussion of osteomyelitis.)

Kidney Stones

Although uncommon in children, renal calculi are a potential risk whenever the child has a limb that is non–weight bearing for a long time, especially if the circumstances also produce urinary stasis. Preventive measures for renal calculi are to maintain good hydration, to mobilize the child as much as possible, and to check closely the amount and characteristics of urinary output. Any urinary tract infection should be treated promptly with appropriate antimicrobials and urine acidification because the nucleus of the calculi is often composed of bacterial debris or calcium and the buildup of stone is precipitated by alkaline urine. An associated problem, hypercalcemia, is reviewed under problems of the immobilized child.

Pulmonary Emboli

Blood, air, or fat emboli can be a hazard to the child with a fracture. As postinjury bleeding and clotting occur, a small piece of the clot can travel to vital organs, such as the lung, heart, or brain, and produce a life-threatening vascular obstruction and ischemia. Generally the pulmonary system is the most frequent site for emboli deposition, but it may not occur until 6 to 8 weeks after the injury.

Fat emboli are the greatest threat to an individual with multiple fractures, particularly in fractures of the long bones such as the femur. Fat droplets from the marrow are transferred to the general circulation by means of the venous-arterial route, where they can be transported to the lung or brain. This type of emboli phenomenon occurs within the first 24 hours, generally in the second 12 hours after the injury occurs. Adolescents are the usual victims in the pediatric age-groups.

Emboli in the vital organs produce the classic symptoms of shock. Petechial hemorrhages of the chest and shoulders are the outstanding signs that differentiate this condition from other kinds of shock. Deep breathing, coughing, and mechanical respiratory assistance are important to maintain adequate alveolar gas exchange. An intravenous infusion is established to treat the shock and administer medications such as heparin and corticosteroids.

NURSING ALERT In the immobilized child who suddenly develops chest pain and dyspnea when turned, pulmonary embolism should be suspected.

The severe dyspnea must be treated immediately by elevating the head when possible and administering oxygen by means of mask, cannula, or hood.

AMPUTATION

A child may be born with the congenital absence of a body part, have a traumatic loss of an extremity, or need a surgical amputation for a pathologic condition such as osteogenic sarcoma. With today's surgical technology and the quick thinking of bystanders who save a traumatically amputated body part, some children have had fingers and arms sewn back on with variable degrees of functional use regained. A severed part should be wrapped lightly in a clean cloth or gauze saturated with normal saline and sealed in a watertight plastic bag. One should avoid using ice, which might come in contact with the tissue and make implantation impossible. The bag should be labeled with the child's name, the date, and the time and taken to the hospital with the child.

Surgical amputation or the surgical repair of a permanently severed limb focuses on constructing an adequately nourished stump. A smooth, healthy, padded stump, free of nerve endings, is important in prosthesis fitting and subsequent ambulation. In some situations in which there is no vascular or neurologic deficit, a cast is applied to the stump immediately after the procedure, and a pylon, metal extension, and artificial foot are attached so that the patient can walk on the temporary prosthesis within a few hours.

Nursing Considerations

Stump shaping is done postoperatively with special elastic bandaging using a figure-8 bandage, which applies pressure in a cone-shaped fashion. This technique decreases stump edema, controls hemorrhage, and aids in developing desired contours so that the child will bear weight on the posterior aspect of the skin flap rather than on the end of the stump. Stump elevation may be used during the first 24 hours, but after this time the extremity should not be left in this position because contractures in the proximal joint will develop and seriously hamper ambulation. Monitoring proper body alignment will further decrease the risk of flexion contractures.

For older children and adolescents, arm exercises and bed pushups, as well as parallel bars, which are used in prosthesis-training programs, help to build up the arm muscles necessary for walking with crutches. Full range of motion exercises of joints above the amputation must be performed several times daily, using active and isotonic exercises. Young children are spontaneously active and require little encouragement.

Depending on the age, children or their parents will need to learn stump hygiene, including careful soap and water washing every day and checking for skin irritation, breakdown, or infection. A tube of stockinette or talcum powder is used to slide the prosthesis on more easily. A careful skin check must be done every time the prosthesis is removed, and prosthesis tolerance time must be adjusted to prevent skin breakdown.

For children who have had an amputation, phantom limb sensation is an expected experience because the nerve-brain connections are still present. Gradually these sensations fade. Preoperative discussion of this phenomenon will aid a child to understand these "unusual feelings" and not to hide the experiences from others. Limb pain, especially pain that increases with ambulation, should be evaluated for the possibility of a neuroma at the free nerve endings in the stump. Psychogenic phantom limb pain is a complex problem that involves the child's response to the altered body image and the coping mechanisms used to handle the new experience. The problems of amputation, particularly the psychologic aspects, are discussed in Chapter 36.

■ INJURIES AND HEALTH PROBLEMS RELATED TO SPORTS PARTICIPATION*

Adolescents probably spend more time and energy practicing and participating in sports activities than members of any other age-group. The practice of sports and games contributes significantly to growth and development, to the education process, and to better health. It provides exercise for growing muscles, interactions with peers, and a socially acceptable means to enjoy stimulation and conflict. In addition, competitive activities help the teenager in the process of self-appraisal, development of self-respect, and concern for others.

Every sport has some potential for injury to the participant—whether the youngster engages in serious competition or participates for pure enjoyment. Serious injury is not limited to the athlete who competes in rough contact sports; a large number of severe or fatal injuries occur to persons who are not physically prepared for the activity. For example, a body build may not be suited to the sport, muscles and support systems (respiratory and cardiovascular) may not have not been sufficiently conditioned to withstand the rigors of the physical stress, or youngsters may not possess insight and judgment to recognize when an activity is beyond their capabilities. Rapidly growing bones, muscles, joints, and tendons are especially vulnerable to unusual strain.

The awkward and inexperienced youngster suffers more injury than the more skilled and experienced one; strong muscles are less easily damaged than weak ones and will provide better protection to the joints they cross, and fatigue significantly impairs muscle function and judgment. More injuries occur during recreational sports participation than in organized athletic competition. The increase in strength and vigor in adolescence may tempt youngsters to

*Jeanette M. Broering, R.N., M.S., C.P.N.P., assisted in the revision of this section.

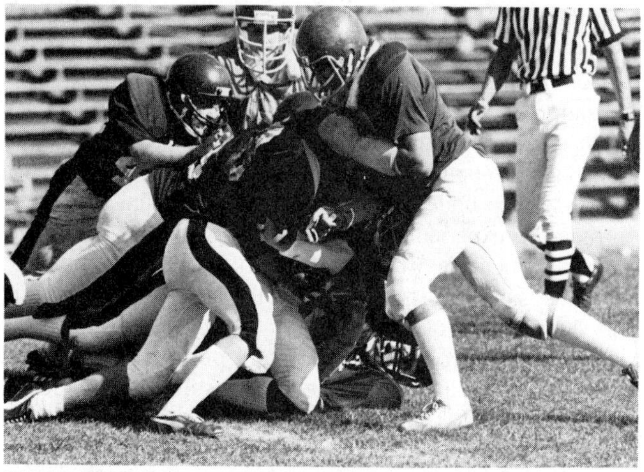

Fig. 39-24. Football is an example of a strenuous collision sport.

overextend themselves, especially boys who are egged on by teammates or are stimulated by the admiration of female observers.

Not only does the activity itself pose a hazard of greater or lesser degree (Fig. 39-24), but the environment and the sports or recreational equipment present additional risks. Adolescents participate in physical activity in a variety of environments, both indoors and outdoors, on floors, on the ground, on snow, on or beneath water surfaces, and sometimes in free air space. These activities frequently involve equipment that intensifies the risk factor.

BOX 39-11 CLASSIFICATION OF SPORTS

Contact Sports

Contact/collision
- Boxing
- Field hockey
- Football
- Ice hockey
- Lacrosse
- Martial arts
- Rodeo
- Soccer
- Wrestling

Limited contact/collision
- Baseball
- Basketball
- Bicycling
- Diving
- Field
  - High jump
  - Pole vault
- Gymnastics
- Handball
- Horseback riding
- Skating (ice and roller)
- Skiing
  - Cross-country
  - Downhill
  - Water
- Softball
- Squash
- Volleyball

Noncontact Sports

Strenuous
- Aerobic dancing
- Crew
- Fencing
- Field
  - Discus
  - Javelin
  - Shot put
- Running
- Swimming
- Tennis
- Track
- Weight lifting

Moderately strenuous
- Badminton
- Curling
- Table tennis

Nonstrenuous
- Archery
- Golf
- Riflery

Modified from American Academy of Pediatrics, Committee on Sports Medicine: Recommendations for participation in competitive sports, Pediatrics 81:737-739, 1988.

PREPARATION FOR SPORTS

The degree of physical maturation varies greatly among adolescents of the same age, and many of the physical characteristics important in sports are related to hormone production. Consequently, physical strength, coordination, endurance, and size vary considerably among youngsters who wish to compete against each other. Sports competition between young people who differ markedly in strength and agility is unfair and hazardous. Matching of candidates for sports should be made relative to physical maturity, height, weight, and physical fitness and skills, particularly in a sport involving rigorous body contact. Age is a less important consideration.

The American Academy of Pediatrics, Committee on Sports Medicine (1988) has devised a classification that divides sports according to strenuousness and probability of collision (Box 39-11 and Fig. 39-25). The Academy also has prepared a table that provides criteria for determining inclusion or exclusion of the young athlete relative to common medical and surgical conditions and relative risks in various sports categories. This serves as a useful guideline for the health professional in counseling youth for activities. Other factors to consider in determining sports participation are (Cook and Gustafson, 1986):

1. The level on which the youth will participate (e.g., Little League, intramural, sandlot, varsity sports program)
2. The facilities available to the athlete
3. The expertise of the coaches
4. The desire of the athlete to participate

The role of health professionals in relation to sports injuries is directed toward prevention, treatment, and rehabilitation. Of these, the area of prevention is perhaps the most important. To this end, those youth who are actively involved in athletic programs need medical evaluation as a prerequisite to participation; education in sports skills with correct training and conditioning methods; omission of those tactics that are dangerous beyond the ordinary risk associated with the specific sport; use of appropriate protective equipment, properly maintained and suited to the individual; and an environment with maximum provision for safety and availability of first-aid and medical services.

The same protective principles apply to noncompetitive sports enthusiasts. They need the same education in basic safety precautions, encouragement to acquire proper instruction in the skills required for performance of the activ-

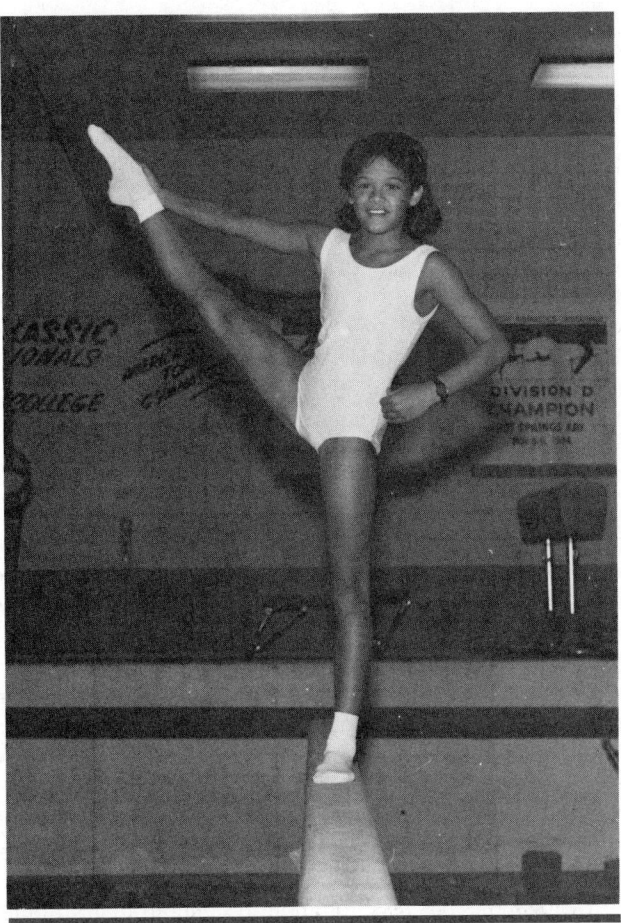

Fig. 39-25. Gymnastics is an example of a strenuous non-contact sport.

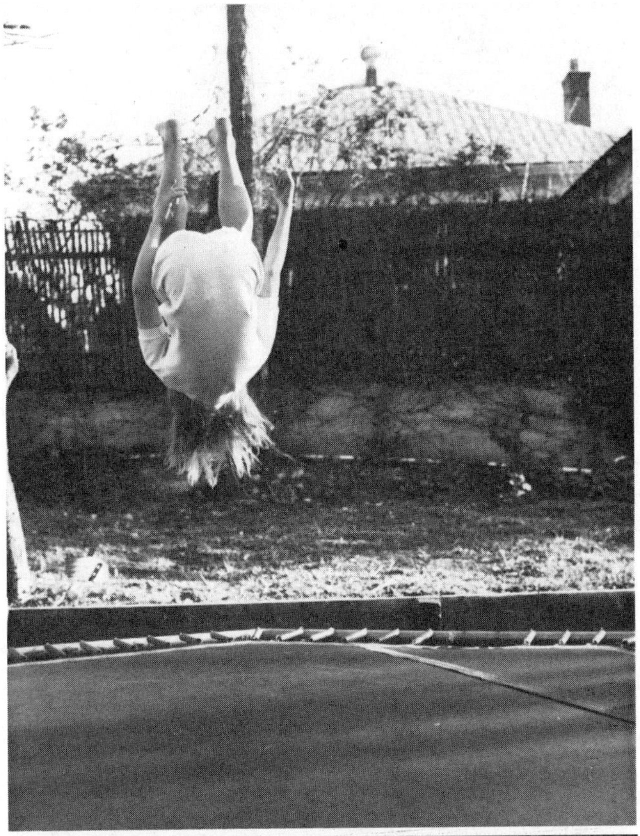

Fig. 39-26. Trampolines are not recommended for home or recreational use.

ity (instruction in water safety, skiing techniques, and so on), and proper maintenance of equipment.

TYPES OF INJURY

The injuries sustained in sports or recreational activities can involve any part of the body and extend from relatively minor cuts, bruises, and abrasions to totally incapacitating central nervous system injuries or death. Some of these injuries are discussed in chapters devoted to the major topic, for example, spinal cord injuries (Chapter 40) and head injuries (Chapter 37). Fractures are discussed earlier in this chapter.

There are some sports that are particularly dangerous for children. Some time ago the American Academy of Pediatrics, Committee on Accident and Poison Prevention issued a statement calling for a ban on the use of trampolines in schools because of the high incidence of quadriplegic injuries caused by the apparatus but has since modified the statement to allow some controlled use (American Academy of Pediatrics, Committee on Pediatric Aspects of Physical Fitness, Recreation, and Sports, 1981). However, the Academy states that trampolines should not be part of a physical education program or competitive sports and should *never* be used in home or recreational settings (Fig. 39-26). The Academy also opposes boxing in any sports program for *any* child or young adult (American Academy of Pediatrics, Committee on Sports Medicine, 1984) because of the potential for progressive brain injury. The "accumulated destructive effects of repeated blows even when consciousness and posture are not lost are well known and accepted" (Van Allen, 1983).

A variety of injuries can result when an external force is exerted with severe stress on tissue, muscle, and skeletal structures. The body structures attempt to accommodate the force, but when they are unable to do so, injuries occur. Two general types of injury are recognized: (1) *acute overload,* which includes injuries such as dislocations, sprains, and muscle pulls, and (2) *chronic overload (overuse syndrome),* which includes stress fractures, tendinitis, bursitis, and fasciculitis. More than 95% of sports injuries involve the soft tissues, not the bony skeleton. About two thirds of these consist of strains and sprains, and most injuries involve the extremities (American Academy of Pediatrics, Committee on Sports Medicine, 1983).

Acute overload injuries are those that occur suddenly during an activity and produce immediate symptoms. They can be caused by a blow or overstretching, twisting, or otherwise causing a sudden stress to tissues (Fig. 39-27).

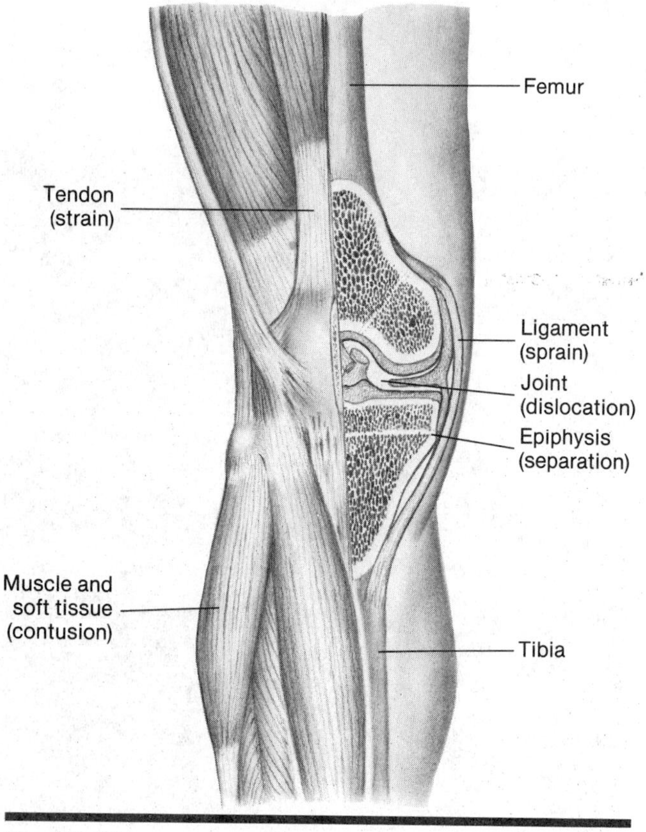

Fig. 39-27. Sites of injuries to bones, joints, and soft tissues.

CONTUSIONS

Contusions are probably the most common of sports injuries and often considered to be "part of the game." A contusion is damage to the soft tissue, subcutaneous structures, and muscle. The tearing of these tissues and small blood vessels and the inflammatory response lead to hemorrhage, edema, and associated pain when the youngster attempts to move the injured part. The escape of blood into the tissues will be observed as *ecchymosis,* a black-and-blue discoloration.

The most serious contusions are those involving the quadriceps and are common in strenuous, collision-type sports, usually as a result of getting kicked or "kneed" in the thigh. Large contusions cause gross swelling, pain, and disability and usually receive immediate attention from health personnel. The less spectacular smaller injuries may go unnoticed, allowing continued participation. However, they can become disabling after rest because of pain and muscle spasm. The young athlete is frequently instructed to work it out or disregard the pain. Unfortunately, this can result in myositis ossificans, which requires a lengthy recovery.

Immediate treatment consists of cold application, as in the treatment of sprains described on p. 1875. Return to participation is allowed when the strength and range of motion of the affected extremity are equal to those of the opposite extremity.

Although not always directly related to sports, crush injuries occur in children when they slam their fingers (in doors, folding chairs, or equipment) or hit their fingers (as when hammering a nail). A severe crush injury involves the bone, with swelling and bleeding beneath the nail (subungual) and sometimes laceration of the pulp of the distal phalanx. The subungual hematoma can be released by drilling holes at the proximal end of the nail. The time-honored method of applying a heated paper clip or needle to melt the nail is highly effective and causes few problems. However, any procedure should be performed with aseptic technique. If the bone is fractured, any communication with the skin essentially renders it an open fracture.

DISLOCATIONS

Long bones are held in approximation to one another at the joint by ligaments. Joints can be tight or loose, and loose joints are more likely to be dislocated. For certain sports the joints need to be limber (e.g., gymnastics and acrobatic dancing); a tight joint is needed for sports like football. One of the most vulnerable joints is the shoulder, which is structurally insecure, having only a rotator cuff to maintain the shoulder in place. The joint is shallow with relatively little muscle protection; therefore, the capsule becomes stretched and the joint dislocates easily. There is a high incidence of shoulder injuries in male gymnasts.

Dislocations are less common in children than in older persons, but some types are peculiar to the younger age-groups. Before final closure of the epiphyses, injuries to the joints are more likely to cause epiphyseal separation than dislocation. For example, shoulder dislocation occurs most often in older adolescents, and dislocation unaccompanied by fracture is rare. Dislocation of the phalanges is the most common type seen in children, followed by elbow dislocations. Injury to the hip causes dislocation more frequently than femoral neck fracture (often experienced by persons in the older age-groups).

In children younger than 5 years of age the hip is usually dislocated by a fall, but trauma is minimal because of the largely cartilaginous acetabulum and general joint laxity. Children with naturally lax joints, such as children with Down syndrome, are more prone to recurrent dislocation of the hip.

A dislocation occurs when the force of stress on the ligament is so great as to displace the normal position of the opposing bone ends or the bone end to its socket. The predominant symptom is pain that increases with attempted passive or active movement of the extremity. In dislocations there may be an obvious deformity and inability to move the joint. Temporary restriction of the joint, with a sling or bandage that secures the arm to the chest in a shoulder dislocation, provides sufficient comfort and immobilization until the youngster can receive medical help.

Simple dislocations should be reduced as soon as possible with the child under sedation and often local anesthesia. An unreduced dislocation will be complicated by increased swelling, making reduction difficult and increasing the risk of neurovascular problems. Reduction is accomplished by simple traction and slight flexion followed by immobilization in a splint for 10 to 16 days or up to 3 weeks or more for healing of torn ligaments.

Patella

Dislocation of the patella is a recurrent episode in some children; in others it is the result of injury. It is common among adolescent girls. The patella is always dislocated laterally. Most dislocations are reduced either spontaneously or by a companion before the child is seen by a physician. Therapy is immobilization for 3 to 4 weeks. Surgery may be needed for recurrent dislocations.

Radial Head

The most common dislocation injury, often handled by a nonspecialist, is subluxation or partial dislocation of the head of the radius in the elbow, also called "pulled elbow" or "nursemaid's elbow." In about 90% of cases the injury occurs in a child between ages 1 and 5 years who receives a sudden longitudinal pull or traction at the wrist while the arm is fully extended and the forearm pronated (Nichols, 1988). It usually occurs when an adult who is holding the child by the hand or wrist gives a sudden jerk to prevent a fall. The child has an anxious expression, whines, complains of pain in the elbow and wrist, refuses to move the arm, and holds it with the opposite hand and in a slightly flexed and pronated position.

The practitioner manipulates the arm by applying firm finger pressure to the head of the radius and then supinates and flexes the forearm to return the bone structures to normal alignment. A click is heard, and functional use of the arm returns within 30 minutes. However, the longer the subluxation is present, the longer it takes for the child to recover mobility after treatment.

SPRAINS AND STRAINS

Strains and sprains are some of the most common athletic injuries and result in variable degrees of tissue involvement and damage. Both are graded according to degree of severity.

Sprains

A sprain occurs when trauma to a joint is so severe that a ligament is partially or completely torn or stretched by the force created as a joint is twisted or wrenched, often accompanied by damage to associated blood vessels, muscles, tendons, and nerves. As a guideline for management and prognosis, sprains are classified according to degree of injury (Box 39-12).

The presence of joint laxity is the most valid indicator of the severity of a sprain. In a severe injury the athlete complains of the joint "feeling loose" or as if "something is coming apart" and may describe hearing a "snap," "pop," or "tearing." Pain is seldom the principal subjective symptom. There is a rapid onset with swelling, often diffuse, accompanied by immediate disability and appreciable reluctance to use the injured joint.

BOX 39-12 CLASSIFICATION OF SPRAINS

Grade I: Mild injury; involves overstretching or microscopic tearing but without hemorrhage or increased instability of the involved joint. Swelling may develop later.

Grade II: Moderate injury; involves partial, overt tearing of the ligament with at least some ligamentous continuity remaining; usually immediate pain and swelling with decreased function.

Grade III: Severe injury; total loss of ligamentous continuity, that is, disruption of one or more ligaments or the musculotendinous unit. Pain is immediate but subsides because none of the pain fibers is being stretched. Swelling may be minimal because hemorrhage extravasates outside of the area into soft tissues.

Strains

A strain is a microscopic tear to the musculotendinous unit and has features in common with sprains. The area is painful to touch and swollen. The severity is evaluated in grades I, II, and III except that the degree of laxity does not apply. Even with severe grade III injuries complaints of laxity are rare. Most strains are incurred over time rather than suddenly, and the rapidity of the appearance provides clues regarding severity. In general, the more rapidly the strain occurs, the more severe the injury. When the strain involves the muscular portion there is more bleeding, often palpable soon after injury and before edema obscures the hematoma.

Therapeutic Management

The first 6 to 12 hours is the most critical period for virtually all soft tissue injuries. Basic principles of managing sprains and other soft tissue injuries are summarized in the acronyms RICE or ICES:

R—rest	I—ice
I—ice	C—compression
C—compression	E—elevation
E—elevation	S—support

Soft tissue injuries should be iced immediately (see Nursing Tip, p. 1876). This is best accomplished with crushed ice wrapped in a towel or encased in a screw-top ice bag or plastic bag (e.g., a resealable storage bag). A wet elastic wrap is applied to provide compression and to keep the ice pack in place. A single layer of the wrap is placed over the injured area to protect the skin under the ice pack, and the remainder of the bandage secures the pack in place. The wet wrap transfers the cold better than a dry wrap. Some athletic trainers keep wet elastic wraps refrigerated for ready use. There is still controversy regarding the use of heat or ice during the rehabilitative phase of manage-

> **NURSING TIP: ICE APPLICATION**
>
> A plastic bag of frozen vegetables, such as peas, serves as a convenient ice pack for soft tissue injuries. It is clean, watertight, and easily molded to the injured part.

ment. Regardless of the method used, it is accompanied by appropriate exercise, depending on the severity of the injury, and carried out under the direction of a competent professional experienced in care of sports injuries.

Ice has a rapid cooling effect on tissues that reduces the pain threshold and the magnitude of the stretch reflex by decreasing muscle spindle response, afferent nerve discharge, and the afferent loop response (monosynaptic reflex). Secondary effects are achieved by vasoconstriction, slowing muscle nerve velocity, and increasing muscle viscosity. Also, the decreased temperature slows metabolism, thus reducing tissue oxygen requirements. Edema formation is reduced when fewer histamine-like substances are released. Nine to 15 minutes of ice exposure produces a deep-tissue vasodilation without increased metabolism. Ice therapy should never be applied for more than 30 minutes (Dyment, 1988). However, the effects last up to 7 hours.

Elevating the extremity uses gravity to facilitate venous return and reduce edema formation in the damaged area. The point of injury should be kept several inches above the level of the heart for therapy to be effective (Fig. 39-28). Several pillows can be used effectively for elevation. Allowing the extremity to be dependent causes excessive fluid accumulation in the area of injury, delaying healing and causing painful swelling.

Major sprains or tears to the ligamentous tissue rarely occur in growing children. Ligaments are stronger than bone, and the epiphysis and growth plate are the weakest areas of the bone; therefore the more usual sites of injury are at the growth plate (see Fractures, p. 1851). Torn ligaments, especially those in the knee, are usually treated by immobilization with a cast for 3 to 4 weeks or strapping of the joint with adhesive or Elastoplast bandage. Passive leg exercises, gradually increased to active ones, are begun as soon as sufficient healing has taken place. Parents and adolescents should be cautioned against using any form of liniment or other heat-producing preparation before examination. If the injury requires casting or splinting, the heat generated in the enclosed space can cause extreme discomfort and may even cause tissue damage.

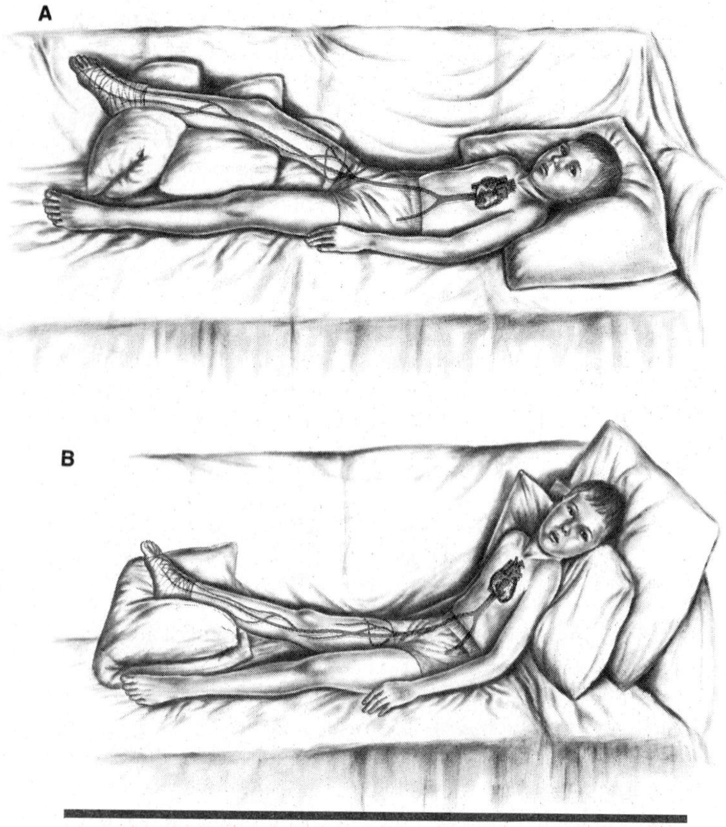

Fig. 39-28. Correct method for elevating a lower extremity. **A,** Lower leg elevated on pillows; ankle above heart level. **B,** Incorrect positioning; ankle below level of heart.

OVERUSE SYNDROME

To excel in sports, the young athlete is forced to train longer, harder, and earlier in life than previously. The rewards are increased level of fitness, better performances, faster times, and the satisfaction of attaining a personal goal. However, the risk of overuse injury is always present and can be related to several factors: training errors, muscle-tendon imbalance, anatomic malalignment (i.e., femoral anteversion, excessive lumbar lordosis, or tibial torsion), incorrect footwear or playing surface, an associated disease state, and growth (growth cartilage is less resistant to microtrauma).

The common feature in overuse injuries is the repetitive microtrauma that occurs to a particular anatomic structure. Performing the same movements time and again sometimes causes several types of injury: (1) frictional—rubbing of one structure against another, (2) tractional—repeated pull on a ligament or tendon, or (3) cyclic loading of impact forces (stress fractures). The end result is inflammation of the involved structure with complaints of pain, tenderness, swelling, and disability.

Bursae, tendons, muscles, ligaments, joints, and bones are all subject to overuse. Some of the common overuse syndromes are briefly outlined in Table 39-4. Plantar fasciitis is very common in athletes, and Osgood-Schlatter disease is seen in children who do a lot of jumping.

Stress Fractures

With intensity and duration of training many young athletes suffer stress fractures, especially after a recent increase in training regimens. They occur as a result of repeated mus-

Table 39-4 Selected overuse injuries

DISORDER	CAUSE	MANIFESTATIONS
Plantar fasciitis	Repetitive stretching of the plantar fascia (calcaneus to metatarsal heads)	Pain in arch or heel
Achilles tendinitis	Repeated forcible traction on short tendon	Pain on palpation; pain with plantar flexion against resistance
Severs disease	Epiphysitis of the calcaneus	Pain over insertion of Achilles tendon into tip of calcaneus
Anterior leg pain ("shin splints")	Irritation of posterior tibial muscle in unconditioned athlete or one not conditioned to a new sport	Pain in leg along anterior or medial edge of midshaft or distal third of tibia
Osgood-Schlatter disease	Traction apophysitis of tibial tubercle	Pain and tenderness; overprominence of involved tubercle
Sinding-Larsen syndrome ("jumper's knee")	A variant of Osgood-Schlatter disease; traction apophysitis on inferior pole of patella	Same as above; pain slightly lower than Osgood-Schlatter
Patellofemoral syndromes	Malalignment of extensors, increased patellar compression, and increased training intensity	Chronic knee pain, especially following forced leg extension from flexion or after running
"Tennis elbow"	Lateral epicondylitis from repetitive strain on elbow	Pain in elbow, aggravated by use
"Little League elbow"	Osteochondritis of the capitellum; tendinitis of flexor-origin medial epicondyle from repetitive valgus strain to elbow from throwing	Pain in elbow that increases with activity
"Little League shoulder"	Microfracture of proximal humeral growth plate from repetitive throwing	Pain and characteristic contracture; loss of internal rotation and increased external rotation
"Swimmer's shoulder"	Supraspinatus tendinitis from repetitive shoulder movement	Pain in shoulder that increases with activity

cle contraction and are seen most often in repetitive weight-bearing sports such as running, gymnastics, and basketball. They occur less often in swimmers (upper extremity). The sites in order of frequency are the tibia (50%), metatarsals (18%), fibula (12%), femur (6%), and other (less than 1%) (Orava, 1980).

The most common symptoms of stress fracture are a sharp, persistent, progressive pain or a deep, persistent dull ache located over the bone. Sometimes there is pain on impact (heel strike), but the most important clinical sign is pain over the involved bony surface. Diagnosis is established on the basis of clinical observation. Occasionally a bone scan may be needed.

Therapeutic Management

Development of inflammation is common to all overuse syndromes; therefore the management is directed toward rest or alteration of activities, physical therapies, and medication. Rest is the primary therapy, usually interpreted as reduced activity and use of alternative exercise—*not* bed rest or immobilization with casting. The primary purpose is to alleviate the repetitive stress that initiated the symptoms. It is important to keep the youngster mobile, and training can be continued. Alternative exercise is selected that maintains conditioning without aggravating the injury. For example, pool running (treading water in the deep end of a pool) can use the same movements as running but without the weight bearing; bicycling, swimming, and rowing are viable alternatives.

Other modalities include cryotherapy and cold whirlpools, and sometimes taping, bracing, splinting, and other orthotics are employed, very specific to the injury. Medications, such as nonsteroidal antiinflammatory drugs (see Table 26-4), are sometimes prescribed to reduce inflammation and pain. Topical medications are of questionable value.

HEAT INJURY

Infants, children, and adolescents are at high risk for heat-related illness. Several characteristics of infants and children render them more vulnerable to heat injury. The greater ratio of surface area to body mass in infants and young children leads to increased transfer of heat between the body and the environment. Children produce more metabolic heat for body mass during exercise and have a reduced capacity to convey heat from body core to the skin.

Also, children do not have the sweating capacity of adults and take longer to become acclimated to hot conditions (Rosenstein, 1989).

Heat cramps are caused by sodium depletion, which in turn potentiates the effects of calcium on skeletal muscle. It most often occurs as a result of strenuous exercise in a hot environment. Cramps most often involve the leg muscles. Vital signs are usually normal, but the core temperature may be elevated. The child sweats profusely, but mentation is normal. Treatment is rest and replacement of lost sodium (Robinson and Seward, 1987).

Heat exhaustion, or heat collapse, is a common condition that usually occurs during vigorous exercise in a hot environment. It results from excessive loss of fluids, especially in poorly acclimated and dehydrated children. The onset may be gradual with initial complaints that include thirst, headache, fatigue, dizziness, anxiety, or nausea and vomiting. The child usually has a clear sensorium but may be somewhat disoriented. The temperature can be normal or mildly elevated; sweating is profuse. Tachycardia, hypotension (usually postural), and syncope may be observed secondary to intravascular volume depletion. Treatment is to move the child to a cool environment, provide rest, and replace fluid volume. The child with a clear sensorium can be given cool water; otherwise water and salt are replaced intravenously. External cooling methods are not necessary.

Heatstroke represents a failure of normal thermoregulatory mechanisms. Heatstroke usually occurs during or immediately following physical activity, especially in the unacclimatized adolescent who is exercising vigorously. The onset is rapid with initial symptoms of headache, weakness, and disorientation. Central nervous system manifestations may be agitation, confusion, and lethargy; loss of consciousness may occur without warning and may be accompanied by nuchal rigidity, posturing, and convulsions. Sweating may not be present. The temperature is elevated typically greater than 40° C (104° F), and there is severe volume depletion. Immediate care is relocation to a cool environment, removal of clothing, application of cool water (wet towels or immersion), and use of fans. The child is transported to the hospital for intensive care.

Hospital care includes rapid cooling, careful monitoring of temperature and other vital signs, supportive care (fluid and electrolyte replacement, supplemental oxygen), and treatment of any complications. Antipyretics are of no value.

Nonexertional, or classic, heatstroke has a slow onset with insidious development of anorexia, nausea, vomiting, headache, development of mental manifestations, and loss of intravascular volume. Classic heatstroke occurs primarily in children with abnormal thermoregulation (e.g., children with cystic fibrosis) and infants subjected to prolonged neglect in a hot environment (Robinson and Seward, 1987).

UNDERWATER SPORTS–RELATED INJURIES

Children who venture into water at least waist deep generally start to play underwater. It is not unusual for children to be able to swim underwater before they are able to swim on the surface. The injuries that are sustained from diving or swimming underwater are serious and deserve brief mention. Near drowning is primarily a respiratory and neurologic problem and is discussed in Chapters 32 and 37; the major injury from diving or surfing is damage to the cervical spine (see Spinal Cord Injuries, Chapter 40).

Male teenagers are typical victims of shallow-water blackout when they attempt to swim long distances (several lengths of the pool) underwater. Before entering the water, the youngster hyperventilates, reducing carbon dioxide to very low levels and thus decreasing the need to breathe. However, this action reduces respiratory stimulation from carbon dioxide accumulation and stretch receptors in the lung. The physical activity of swimming consumes the existing oxygen supply before the P_{CO_2} level rises sufficiently high to stimulate breathing. Consequently the P_{O_2} reaches a dangerous level before the respiratory center is stimulated, resulting in hypoxia and unconsciousness. Unfortunately, hyperventilation does not significantly increase the body's stores of oxygen—mainly stored in arterial hemoglobin and already saturated in normal individuals (Strauss, 1982).

In addition, breath-holding with hyperinflated lungs (Valsalva maneuver) causes further decrease in oxygen to the brain. The cerebral hypoxia causes the youngster to lose consciousness before there is the desire to surface for air. Often these youngsters are found dead at the bottom of a lake or pool. The result is drowning unless the youngster is rescued quickly. Similarly, persons who engage in breath-holding while diving in deep water suffer hypoxia as a result of decreasing P_{O_2} as they ascend from the depths. These are usually older (and experienced) divers who are unaware of this danger.

Other underwater sports injuries include ear squeeze, which occurs when middle ear pressures are not equalized during diving; decompression sickness (the bends) and air emboli from too rapid decompression after deep dives; and nitrogen narcosis.

Sports and Accidental Drowning

Death by drowning contributes significantly to the mortality among the relatively healthy teenage age-group. Each year 1200 adolescents between ages 10 and 19 years die by drowning. At highest risk are males between ages 15 and 19 years, with concurrent alcohol use present in 40% of drowning incidents. Alcohol not only impairs judgment but also increases the likelihood of water aspiration. Preventive measures to decrease the number of deaths have been unsuccessful. Suggested methods of intervention have been to (1) reduce the amount of alcohol consumed by adolescents, (2) increase the proportion of the population who are able to swim, and (3) encourage routine use of protective devices, such as life vests, when boating or fishing. Since most drownings are witnessed but resuscitation methods are not quickly or appropriately initiated, public education programs have been suggested as a potential remedy for this problem (Runyan and Gerken, 1989).

HEALTH CONCERNS ASSOCIATED WITH SPORTS

A number of health concerns that are related to sports activities may affect athletic performance and/or the physical well-being of the participant.

Nutrition

Most athletes are motivated to enhance their performance by any and all means available. They are eager to learn about nutrition, and many become subject to misconceptions, fads, and superstitions regarding certain foods. Physical perfomance is affected by energy and body composition. The young athlete must maintain a diet that provides sufficient nutrients and energy to meet metabolic needs for optimum functioning. Physical training increases the need for energy as well as for more nutrients that convert food energy into chemical energy for physical performance.

There is no evidence to indicate that food supplements, extra vitamins, or high-protein diets are needed to meet the demands of heavy physical exercise or improve physical performance. However, young athletes need considerably more calories than the recommended daily allowance. When the basic requirements for growth and activity are met by a balanced diet of protein, grains and cereals, fruits and vegetables, and dairy products, the additional calories needed for the extra exertion can be selected as desired. These extra caloric needs can be supplied by eating additional helpings from any of the basic four food groups, but many of the additional calories are provided by complex carbohydrates found in such foods as vegetables, pastas, and bread. A summary of nutrition pointers for young athletes is presented in Box 39-13.

Water and electrolytes. Considerable water is lost from the body through perspiration, urination, and evaporation from the respiratory tract. Water losses, especially from the skin, increase with the duration and intensity of exercise and in higher environmental temperatures. Although the thirst mechanism is experienced early in dehydration, it is unreliable as an indicator of fluid deficit. Athletes participating in multiple daily exercise sessions in warm environments are at risk for dehydration and should receive all the water they desire (Primos and Landry, 1989).

Very little water is exchanged in the stomach and must reach the intestines for absorption. The best fluids for rapid gastric emptying are those that are cold, of low osmolality (Costill, 1984), and of a large volume. Those containing simple sugars or glucose polymers with little or no electrolytes are better than plain water (Murray, 1987). Gatorade and other types of "sports" drinks contain excess carbohydrate and should be diluted with one or two parts of water to one part drink (Primos and Landry, 1989).

Small amounts of electrolytes are lost during exercise, especially sodium and chloride. Because sweat is quite dilute relative to plasma concentrations, excessive perspiration can result in excessive loss of water and an increase in plasma concentrations of sodium chloride. Therefore, it is more important to replace water than sodium and chloride. Salt tablets are unnecessary and may actually be harmful. Athletes derive sufficient salt replacement from their diet (Primos and Landry, 1989).

Box 39-13 FIFTEEN STEPS TO GOOD SPORTS NUTRITION

1. A well-balanced diet consists of elements from the four basic food groups. The recommended percentages of major nutrients are 55% to 75% carbohydrates, 25% to 30% fat, and 15% to 20% protein.
2. Athletes should take water at regular intervals during exercise.
3. For each pound of fluid lost through exercise, the athlete should consume 16 ounces of water.
4. Any athlete who loses more than 3% of body weight in an exercise session should not return to activity until the fluid is restored. Monitoring body weight can prevent chronic dehydration.
5. Beverages with small amounts of simple sugars or glucose polymers with little or no electrolytes may be better sources of hydration than plain water.
6. Salt tablets are rarely needed and may actually do harm by increasing dehydration.
7. Glycogen loading is of value only for endurance exercises that take more than 1 hour, such as marathons and cross-country ski races. It is not recommended for children.
8. Protein and amino acid supplementation are potentially harmful and should be discouraged.
9. Vitamin supplements are usually unnecessary and a waste of money; excessive doses may be harmful. One daily multivitamin is not harmful for youngsters who do not consume well-balanced meals.
10. Mineral supplements are usually not needed, except for young athletes who develop a specific deficiency such as iron.
11. Any weight loss program should be designed to lose body fat primarily and not lean body tissue or water. The goal should be to achieve a certain percentage of body weight as fat.
12. Athletes should not lose more than 1 to 2 pounds per week. They should not reduce daily caloric intake to less than 1200 calories for girls and 1500 calories for boys.
13. Athletes who wish to gain weight can do so by combining increased caloric intake with muscle work (i.e., weight training). Nutritional supplements are not usually needed.
14. Athletes should gain weight no more rapidly than 1 to 2 pounds per week. They should be monitored for percentage of body fat.
15. The pregame meal should be eaten at least 2½ hours before competition. It should consist primarily of carbohydrates and not foods that are slowly digested (fats, desserts) or have excessive concentrated sugars.

From Primos, W.A., and Landry, G.L.: Fighting the fads in sports nutrition, Contemp. Pediatr. 6(9):14-50, 1989.

Minerals. The basic diet will not satisfy the iron requirement of 10% to 15% of female athletes. The largest group are those teenage girls who may become iron depleted after menarche. Young boys who are experiencing rapid adolescent growth and who have irregular and inadequate diets also are at risk of iron depletion. These youngsters will need medicinal iron supplements (Smith, 1984).

Adequate calcium intake during puberty is essential to promote mineralization of the growing skeleton. In addition, calcium plays a vital role in nerve transmission, muscle contraction, and blood coagulation. Female athletes who engage in intensive training and subsequently develop amenorrhea may require additional calcium intake to prevent osteoporosis (Squire, 1987). The best sources of calcium for athletes are nonfat dairy products (Loosli, 1990).

Glycogen. Energy is derived primarily from glycogen previously stored in muscles and the liver. Energy for prolonged exercise is derived from high-carbohydrate food (e.g., bread, cereals, pancakes, potatoes, rice, spaghetti) consumed 24 to 48 hours before the activity, not from a meal eaten just before the activity. The meal before a physical contest should be eaten at least 2½ hours before the exertion and consist mainly of carbohydrates. Carbohydrate (glycogen) loading is a technique reserved for competition in prolonged aerobic endurance events and requires dietary changes a week before the competitive event. For more information regarding carbohydrate loading and other techniques for improving athletic performance, the readers are directed to excellent texts on sports medicine and sports training.

Weight. Control of body weight by restriction of water intake, food restriction, or encouragement of sweat loss is dangerous, and these are highly undesirable means for meeting a minimum weight classification. Young athletes need to learn something about nutrition to dispel the allure of prevalent fads and fallacies about diet and performance (Narins, Belkengren, and Sapala, 1983). The optimum diet for an athlete is one that contains the essential food groups and that is adjusted to the energy requirements of the sport in which the youngster is engaged. Such a diet plan should provide adequate nutrition for top physical efficiency and performance, maintenance of physical fitness and desirable body weight, and optimum function of all organ systems.

Exercise-Related Menstrual Dysfunction

Considerable interest has been generated regarding delayed or secondary amenorrhea associated with the physical stress of ballet dancing and some types of athletics, for example, running and gymnastics. The phenomenon has been attributed to a complex interplay of physical, genetic, hormonal, nutritional, psychologic, and environmental factors that include the stress of competition, decreased protein consumption, and altered lean-to-fat ratio.

Delayed menarche has been reported for girls who engage in strenuous exercise. Except for swimmers, menarche is attained later in athletes than in nonathletes. Gymnasts, figure skaters, and ballet dancers have the latest mean ages of menarche; track athletes have less of a delayed maturity than gymnasts and ballet dancers, who also tend to be smaller, lighter, and leaner than other female athletes. Swimmers, who tend to be larger, have a mean age of menarche that approximates that for nonathletes. Also, there appears to be an association between delayed menarche and more advanced competitive levels; that is, athletes at the more advanced levels have a greater delay than those at lower competitive levels (Malina, Meleski, and Shoup, 1982).

It is not clear whether exercise delays menarche or menarcheal delay promotes athletic success. Some observers believe strenuous prepubertal activity delays menarche (Frische and others, 1981; Warren, 1980). It is also postulated that the delayed puberty promotes athletic success, which in turn encourages perseverance (Shangold and Mirkin, 1985). Also, the selection process for various sports may favor certain body types, for example, the smaller, more slender gymnasts (Malina, Meleski, and Shoup, 1982).

Some observers (Diddle, 1983) attribute delayed menarche and maintenance of regular ovulation to lack of development of body fat with the subsequent effect on feedback mechanisms as the critical factor. These observations established that girls do not begin menses until at least 17% body fat content has been attained. This has been challenged by others who found no level of body fat that can be termed "critical" (Garn, LaVelle, and Pilkington, 1983).

Alterations in established menstrual bleeding patterns are often observed in girls who engage in strenuous exercise. The incidence varies with the type of exercise and the intensity of the exercise program. Circulating gonadotropins are decreased with exercise, but the association between strenuous exercise and menstrual irregularity is still puzzling (Ziporyn, 1984). Increased serum androgen levels have also been reported with intense exercise (Jurkowski and others, 1978). Other factors, including diet and stress, prevent the identification of any typical profile. Not all girls are affected, but the activities that appear to be associated with delayed or altered menstruation are ballet dancing, running, gymnastics, and competitive swimming.

There is consensus regarding a correlation between strenuous exercise and menstruation, although the exact roles played by the various factors have not been defined satisfactorily. Few detrimental effects have been detected, and normal patterns are established spontaneously or with cessation of exercise. A lower incidence of dysmenorrhea has been reported in girls who engage in vigorous exercise (Hale, 1983).

It has also been found that women competing in ballet dancing and gymnastics are subject to decreased bone density, stress fractures, and symptoms of anorexia nervosa (Braisted and others, 1985; Loucks and Horvath, 1985; Warren and others, 1986). The peak of bone density is reached in late adolescence and is related to circulating estrogen levels. Girls with diminished estrogen secretion in delayed menarche will reach late adolescence with low bone density and will be subject to osteoporosis. Hypoestrogenic bone loss greatly increases the risk of injury (Warren, 1989). Teenage girls need to be counseled to increase calcium intake to four to six servings per day, which may not be well accepted because most adolescents think of fat in association with dairy products.

An additional area for counseling the female athlete with delayed menarche regards pregnancy. Sexually active teenagers, regardless of menstruation, need to be reminded to take precautions. Most erroneously believe that because they do not menstruate, they cannot become pregnant.

Drug Misuse by Athletes

Young athletes have used various substances in the attempt to augment their athletic performance. These substances, known as *ergogenic aids,* are believed by athletes to increase strength and endurance, delay onset of fatigue, increase the ability to concentrate, and decrease sensitivity to pain. Although use of these substances is prohibited in international Olympic competition, there are no means at present to enforce a prohibition on their use in other sports participation.

The principal drugs misused by athletes are the psychomotor stimulants (e.g., amphetamines) and the anabolic steroids. Amphetamines and related drugs, such as methylphenidate (Ritalin) and phenmetrazine (Preludin), are taken to provide a sense of increased alertness and relief of fatigue; however, obscuring fatigue may permit participants to exceed their limits and precipitate a sudden collapse (Dyment, 1982). These drugs can also make the users more aggressive, which can contribute to injuries to themselves and others. Although use of amphetamines is declining, ingestion of caffeine and caffeine-related substances, readily available as cola drinks, tea, and coffee, has increased (American Academy of Pediatrics, Committee on Sports Medicine, 1983).

Anabolic steroids, such as nandrolone phenpropionate (Durabolin) and methandrostenolone (Dianabol), are a source of concern to health professionals. The majority of these drugs are no longer manufactured in the United States by legitimate companies. Black market supplies of anabolic steroids are of poor quality and potency. In the attempt to enhance muscle strength, these drugs are administered to athletes by coaches, managers, athletic trainers, and even physicians. The user develops larger-appearing muscles and increased body weight and body water, but reports on the effectiveness in improving performance have been conflicting. Although the psychologic effect may be beneficial, many valid studies have failed to demonstrate any improvement in performance (American Academy of Pediatrics, Committee on Sports Medicine, 1983).

The precise incidence of use by adolescent athletes remains debatable. Self-report surveys have documented use patterns ranging from 5% to 11% of high-school athletes (Johnson and others, 1989). Coaches and health professionals who work with youth report a trend toward increased use of these agents. Teenagers rely on poor sources of information about the potential hazards of steroids (friends, television, muscle magazines) and are generally poorly informed of their potential negative side effects (Johnson and others, 1989; Nelson, 1989). Health professionals need to be aware of the clinical manifestations of steroid use. Clinical signs such as severe acne, sudden increase in strength and muscle, sudden decrease in body fat, male pattern of baldness, and water retention are common. In females, male pattern of hair growth and deepening voice are significant observations.

The dangers of continued use are well known and include hypertension; virilization in females; oligospermia, testicular atrophy, infertility, and gynecomastia in males; and premature closure of the epiphyses, acne, increased blood cholesterol, and hepatocellular carcinoma in both sexes. Mood changes have been observed, including aggressiveness, changes in libido, and mood swings. Health hazards outweigh any potential gain that might be induced, and the American Academy of Pediatrics, Committee on Sports Medicine (1989) and the American College of Sports Medicine both condemn the use of anabolic steroids.

Other drugs that are often misused include nutritional aids, local anesthetic agents, beta blockers (to reduce circulating catecholamines and thus reduce anxiety related to somatic-type stress), and antiinflammatory drugs, such as dimethylsulfoxide (DSMO) (which is not approved for use and is available only as a veterinary or an industrial preparation) and corticosteroids. The possibility of their use by the adolescent athlete should be considered when performing a health assessment.

Sudden Death

A death associated with sports produces renewed anxiety in both parents and health professionals. The term *sudden,* or *instantaneous, death* is applied to death that occurs within minutes of the onset of the cause of death, within an hour or within 24 hours of the episode. Sudden death occurs in three areas: (1) in those sports with a high inherent risk for sport-related sudden death; (2) in children with recognized or unknown underlying medical problems; and (3) in the sport environment (i.e., the rules, equipment, practice fields or areas of sports participation, and the ambient temperature of the geographic area), which may be a contributing or causal factor (Luckstead, 1982).

Sports. Sports that create the greatest risk are those involving collision and frequent body contact. Examples of collision sports include football, ice hockey, rugby, and boxing. There is a high potential for serious injury or fatality in sports such as mountain or rock climbing and hang gliding. Sports that involve high-velocity objects, such as baseball and ice hockey, may cause death as a result of serious head or chest injuries. Riding vehicles such as mopeds, minibikes, and motorcycles can be considered as sports.

Medical conditions. The most frequent medical causes of sudden death during sports activity are cardiac abnormalities, especially idiopathic hypertrophic subaortic stenosis (hypertrophic cardiomyopathy). Manifestations suggestive of hypertrophic cardiomyopathy include a typical triad of severe chest pain with dizziness, prominent pulses, and a murmur at the left lower sternal border. A history of sudden death of a relative, or relatives, in the second and third decade often offers a clue to recognition.

Well-trained athletes often display evidence of hypertrophic cardiomyopathy, the so-called athlete's heart, but the condition is not pathologic. Congenital heart problems are infrequent causes of sudden death in sports involving children and adolescents. Children with systemic hypertension, some types of cardiac arrhythmias, and some forms of heart block will require restrictions in the type and amount of exercise they can tolerate safely.

Environmental causes. Environmental factors that are potential causes of death include playing conditions, clothing, equipment, rules used by officials governing a sport, and outdoor temperature. Heat stroke and hypothermia are probably the most serious uncontrollable environmental causes of death in athletes.

NURSE'S ROLE IN CHILDREN'S SPORTS

Nurses may become involved in sports activities in the areas of preparation and evaluation for activities, prevention of injury, treatment of injuries, and rehabilitation after injury. Selecting an appropriate sport for both recreation and competition is a joint effort of youngster, parents, and health professionals. Children are introduced to sports as part of family activities, neighborhood games, and school physical education programs, and both parents and children are influenced by media exposure to a variety of sports. Children are highly influenced by the popularity and exposure afforded athletics in the school setting, especially in high school.

The American Academy of Pediatrics has established guidelines for programs in elementary school (American Academy of Pediatrics, Committee on Pediatric Aspects of Physical Fitness, Recreation, and Sports, 1981) and for sports for children of all ages (American Academy of Pediatrics, Committee on Sports Medicine, 1983). Nurses who work with children involved in sports activities should be aware of the recommendations regarding children's athletics and understand some of the motivating factors, developmental characteristics of children, and pressures for participation.

The best approach to counseling children and parents regarding sports participation is to encourage activities that are most likely to provide pleasure and physical benefits throughout childhood into adulthood. Exposure to a variety of sports activities is probably better for young children than limiting them to only one sport. Parents should be cautioned against overprogramming children in order that the children have ample time for other activities and associations.

Nurses are sometimes members of a sports medicine team, although the training and rehabilitation are usually managed by certified sports trainers and other specialists in sports medicine. Nurses should be able to provide emergency treatment for any type of injury and know when to refer the injured child for evaluation and care. Sports injuries can occur in free play as well as in organized athletic programs, and a school nurse is often the first person who attends an injured child.

When children sustain athletic injuries, nurses are often responsible for instructing the children and their parents regarding care. Instructions, such as schedule for appointments, application of ice, and any restrictions in activity, should be made clear, preferably accompanied by written directions. The importance of taking medications as prescribed is emphasized, since they may be needed for an extended period of time and compliance may be difficult. For children continuing with activities, drug administration an hour before practice or competition is advantageous.

Prevention of sports injuries is probably the most important aspect of any athletic program. The children should be suited to the activity, the environment and equipment made safe for physical activity, and the children adequately prepared for the sports, especially those requiring strenuous and or continuous physical exertion. Nurses collaborate with coaches and athletic trainers to ensure that safety measures are carried out. Stretching exercises, warming up and cooling down activities, and an appropriate training program are only some of the requisites for safe participation. Protective measures, such as pads, taping, wrapping, or other devices, are employed for areas at risk (Fig. 39-29). Nurses are also on the alert for environmental safety risks.

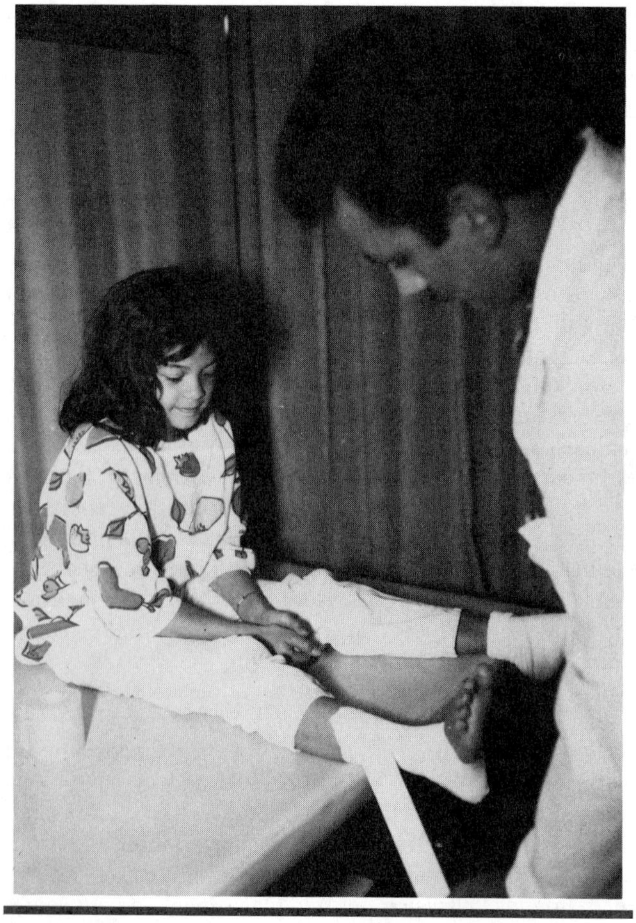

Fig. 39-29. Competent care is essential to prevention of sports injury.

Participation of youth in sports programs has grown significantly in the past several decades. The number of females in sports programs has grown 600% since 1970 (Squire, 1987). This trend toward greater participation by both genders has been encouraged because of its demonstrated effect on reducing obesity and lowering blood pressure, and its beneficial impact on lowering cholesterol and lipid levels.

Nurses can provide education to coaching staff, parents, and players on the detrimental effects of steroid use on athletes. Teenagers who participate in sports programs need to know that the use of steroids constitutes cheating and can result in dismissal from play. In addition to education about the potential side effects, nurses should be alert to physical signs and counsel those youths appropriately.

Parental Pressure

There is a lot of peer and parental pressure to participate in sports, and the stress on the adolescent to perform in competitive situations is poorly understood. There is much fear of failure related to the pressure to be like friends or parents. When children need medical attention because of repeated injuries, disinterest should be suspected and investigated. It is best to obtain separate histories from the youth and the parents in an attempt to illuminate possible psychologic complications as a cause of injury (Pillemer and Micheli, 1988). Alternative sports or other means for gaining self-esteem and regard from parents and peers can be explored and encouraged for children not interested in or suited for athletic competition.

Attrition and exercise aversion are sometimes the aftermath of declining interest in sports after participation during the school years and adolescence. Motivation can be altered or permanently destroyed by failure to appreciate youngsters' needs related to sports activities. Ridicule or derogation during acquisition of motor skills can shatter a youngster's self-esteem, producing anxiety and self-doubt that may result in a lifelong aversion to sports. Every child should have the opportunity to develop a strong sense of personal worth through the process of motor learning and acquisition of skills (Ogilvie, 1982). They need positive encouragement. *All* participants should have the opportunity to participate and be rewarded for their contribution, no matter how small; all participants should be rewarded for what they do right.

Both coaches and parents are guilty of exploiting youngsters for their own purposes. Although the positive aspects are important and inherent in sports activities, nurses should be alert to some parental behaviors and motivations that interfere with a youngster's enjoyment of the activities. However, many parents are notoriously resistant to the idea of altering their behavior.

First, there are parents who are unwilling to allow the activity to remain child-oriented and who often place unrealistic demands on the child. Both the youngster's physical and emotional age must be considered. Second, there are parents who are unable to maintain the appropriate emotional distance from the activity and make the youngsters' involvement in sports an extension of their own ego. These youngsters may recognize that they are being exploited and exhibit extreme forms of rebellion. Third, parents' manipulative behaviors can have a profound negative effect on their youngsters. Guilt-producing verbal manipulation (e.g., pointing out what they and others have sacrificed for the child) is a powerful weapon that creates a form of emotional bondage. Fourth, there are parents who lose sight of the meaning of the sport because they become entrapped in dreams and fantasies that their youngsters' athletic ability can become a passport to status and economic freedom (Ogilvie, 1982).

The pressures that some parents impose on their children negate most of the psychologic values, such as fun, emotional release, and learning to relate effectively with peers. Winning becomes more important than playing. Overemphasis on sports has the potential for interfering with the emotional and social growth of a child, especially when ego integration is tied to recognition and reward through such a narrow range of personal characteristics. Ego vulnerability is great in youngsters whose identity, self-esteem, and feelings of self-worth depend entirely on the psychologic and social rewards of athletic achievement.

■ MUSCULOSKELETAL DYSFUNCTION

The disorders affecting the skeletal structures and associated musculature are primarily congenital, traumatic, secondary to metabolic dysfunction, or idiopathic in origin. Some appear at any age, such as fractures, whereas others have a predilection for a different stage of the childhood span of growth and development. There are those detected at birth or shortly after, such as congenital foot and hip deformities (see Chapter 11); Legg-Calvé-Perthes disease affects children in middle childhood; and slipped femoral capital epiphysis and scoliosis are more characteristic of late childhood and adolescence.

TORTICOLLIS

Torticollis (wry neck) is a congenital or acquired condition of limited neck motion in which the neck is flexed and turned to the affected side as a result of shortening of the sternocleidomastoid muscle. In early infancy a firm, nontender mass may be felt in the midportion of the muscle. The mass regresses and is replaced by fibrous tissue. If the condition remains untreated, there is permanent limitation of neck movement and the head and face become asymmetric, probably related to impaired blood supply to the depressed side of the head.

Treatment consists of gentle stretching exercises. The face is turned toward the affected muscle while the head is tilted in the opposite direction with the neck extended. The position is held for a count of 5 and repeated 10 times, twice daily (Watts, 1987). The exercises are best performed by two persons—one to control the torso and one to manipulate the head. If stretching exercises are unsuccessful, surgical release of the sternocleidomastoid muscle may be needed.

Nursing Considerations

Nurses are alert to the possibility of torticollis in infants with limited head movement. After diagnosis it is frequently a nursing responsibility to teach and supervise the family in performing the exercises. The exercise requires very explicit instructions to the family, and compliance is mandatory. The nurse also suggests that the child be placed in the crib or playpen in a way that encourages turning the head away from the deformity in order to observe activities and interesting items. Feeding and play with the child can be used to encourage turning the head in the direction desired for correction.

LEGG-CALVÉ-PERTHES DISEASE

Legg-Calvé-Perthes disease (LCPD), sometimes called *coxa plana* or *osteochondritis deformans juvenilis,* is a self-limited disorder in which there is aseptic necrosis of the femoral head. The disease affects children 3 to 12 years, but most cases occur in males between 4 and 8 years as an isolated event. In approximately 10% to 15% of cases the involvement is bilateral; most of the affected children have a skeletal age significantly below their chronologic age. The male/female ratio is 4:1 or 5:1; white children are affected 10 times more frequently than black children.

Pathophysiology

The cause of the disease is unknown, but there is a disturbance of circulation to the femoral capital epiphysis that produces an ischemic aseptic necrosis of the femoral head. During middle childhood circulation to the femoral epiphysis is more tenuous than at other ages, being supplied almost entirely by lateral retinacular vessels. These can become obstructed by trauma, inflammation, coagulation defects, and a variety of other causes (Staheli, 1986). This circulatory impairment appears to extend to the epiphysis and acetabulum as well. The pathologic events seem to take place in four stages (Box 39-14). The entire process may encompass as little as 18 months or continue for several years. The reformed femoral head may be severely altered or appear entirely normal.

BOX 39-14 STAGES OF LEGG-CALVÉ-PERTHES DISEASE

Stage I: Aseptic necrosis or infarction of the femoral capital epiphysis with degenerative changes producing flattening of the upper surface of the femoral head—the *avascular stage.*

Stage II: Capital bone absorption and revascularization with fragmentation (vascular resorption of the epiphysis) that gives a mottled appearance on radiographs—the *fragmentation,* or *revascularization, stage.*

Stage III: New bone formation, which is represented on radiographs as calcification and ossification or increased density in the areas of radiolucency; this filling-in process appears to take place from the periphery of the head centrally—the *reparative stage.*

Stage IV: Gradual reformation of the head of the femur without radiolucency and, it is hoped, to a spherical form—the *regenerative stage.*

Clinical Manifestations

The onset is insidious and the history may reveal only intermittent appearance of a limp on the affected side or a symptom complex including hip soreness, ache, or stiffness that can be constant or intermittent. The pain may be experienced in the hip, along the entire thigh, or in the vicinity of the knee joint. The pain and limp are usually most evident on arising and at the end of a long day of activities. The pain is usually accompanied by joint dysfunction and limited range of motion. There may be a vague history of trauma. The diagnosis is established by radiographic examination.

Therapeutic Management

Since deformity occurs early in the disease process, the aim of treatment is to keep the head of the femur "contained" in the acetabulum, which serves as a mold to preserve the spherical shape of the head and to maintain a full range of motion. Activity causes microfractures of the soft, ischemic epiphysis, which tend to induce synovitis, stiffness, and adductor contracture (Staheli, 1986). The initial therapy is rest, and non–weight bearing, which helps reduce inflammation and restore motion. Later active motion is encouraged. In some cases traction is applied to stretch tight adductor muscles.

Containment can be accomplished by non-weight-bearing devices, such as an abduction brace, leg casts, or a leather harness sling, that prevent weight bearing on the affected limb; by various weight-bearing appliances such as abduction-ambulation braces or casts after a period of bed rest and traction; and by surgical reconstruction and containment procedures. Conservative therapy must be continued for 2 to 4 years, although braces constructed from lightweight materials allow the child to maintain a nearly normal activity level. Surgical correction, although a relatively recent advance and subject to additional risks (e.g., from anesthesia, infection, blood transfusion), returns the child to normal activities in 3 to 4 months.

The disease is self-limited, but the ultimate outcome of therapy depends on early and efficient treatment and the age of onset of the disorder. Younger children, whose epiphyses are more cartilaginous, have the best prognosis for complete recovery. The later the diagnosis is made, the more femoral damage has occurred before treatment is implemented. In most cases, with good patient compliance, the prognosis is excellent.

Nursing Considerations

Nurses are often the first health professionals to identify affected children and to refer them for medical evaluation.

They are also persons on whom the child and family can rely to help them understand and adjust to the therapeutic measures. Since most care of these children is conducted on an outpatient basis, the major emphasis of nursing care is teaching the family the care and management of the corrective appliance selected for therapy. The family needs to learn the purpose, function, application, and care of the corrective device and the importance of compliance in order to achieve the desired outcome.

One of the most difficult aspects associated with the disorder is coping with normally active children who feel well but must remain relatively inactive. It is important to emphasize that children continue to attend school and engage in former activities that can be adapted to the therapeutic appliance. School adaptation may need to be arranged with school personnel.

Suitable activities must be devised to meet the needs of the child in the process of developing a sense of initiative or industry. Activities that meet the creative urges are well received. This is also an opportune time to encourage the child to begin a hobby such as collections, model building, or crafts.*

SLIPPED FEMORAL CAPITAL EPIPHYSIS

Slipped femoral capital epiphysis (SFCE), or *coxa vara,* refers to the spontaneous displacement of the proximal femoral epiphysis in a posterior and inferior direction. It develops most frequently shortly before or during accelerated growth and the onset of puberty (children between the ages of 10 and 16 years—median age, 13 for boys, 11 for girls) and is most frequently observed in obese children. Bilateral involvement has been reported variously as 16% to 40%.

Pathophysiology

The cause of SFCE is unknown, but it occurs most often in "overlarge" youngsters or very tall, thin, rapidly growing children. There has been some evidence to implicate hormonal factors; for example, resistance of the growth plate to shear stress is decreased by growth hormone and increased by sex hormone, suggesting that the disorder may be related to excess growth hormone in the tall child and decreased sex hormone in the obese child. It has also been associated with endocrine abnormalities, renal osteodystrophy, and growth hormone therapy. SFCE has been reported to precede the diagnosis of hypothyroidism in an impressive number of cases (Puri and others, 1985).

The pathologic processes as seen in radiographs involve first a rarefaction of bone on the lower femoral side of the epiphysis with widening of the growth plate. After trauma or slight injury the femoral portion of the epiphysis slides upward but remains attached by the thick, continuous periosteum. As slipping increases, the epiphyseal displacement becomes posterior and inferior. The slipping produces deformity of the femoral head and stretches the blood vessels to the epiphysis.

Clinical Manifestations

The following different varieties of clinical behavior have been observed: (1) an episode of trauma in which the epiphysis is acutely displaced in a previously functional joint; (2) gradual displacement without definite injury with progressively increased hip disability; (3) intermittent bouts of displacement alternating with periods of well-being with gradual appearance of symptoms associated with ambulation (e.g., external rotation); and (4) a combined gradual and traumatic displacement, in which there is gradual slippage with further displacement caused by injury.

Slipped femoral epiphysis is suspected when an adolescent or preadolescent youngster, especially one who is obese or tall and lanky, begins to limp and complains of pain in the hip continuously or intermittently. The pain is frequently referred to the groin, anteromedial aspect of the thigh, or knee. Physical examination reveals early restriction of internal rotation on adduction and external rotation deformity with loss of abduction and internal rotation as the severity increases. The diagnosis is confirmed by radiographic examination.

Therapeutic Management

The treatment varies with the degree of displacement but involves surgical stabilization and correction of deformity. In mild cases simple pin fixation is sufficient. More extensive displacement requires skeletal traction followed by pin fixation or osteotomy. The prognosis depends on the degree of deformity and the occurrence of complications, such as avascular necrosis and cartilaginous necrosis. As in other disorders, early diagnosis and implementation of therapy increase the likelihood of a satisfactory cure.

Nursing Considerations

Nursing care is the same as that for a child in a cast or a child in traction, discussed earlier in this chapter.

KYPHOSIS AND LORDOSIS

The spine, consisting of numerous segments, can acquire deformation curves of three types: kyphosis, lordosis, and scoliosis (Fig. 39-30).

Kyphosis

Kyphosis is an abnormally increased convex angulation in the curvature of the thoracic spine (Fig. 39-30, *B*). It can occur secondary to disease processes such as tuberculosis, chronic arthritis, osteodystrophy, or compression fractures of the thoracic spine. The most common form of kyphosis is "postural." Children, especially during the time when skeletal growth outpaces growth of muscle, are prone to exaggeration of a tendency toward kyphosis. They assume bizarre sitting and standing positions. This is particularly common in self-conscious adolescent girls who assume a

*See Nursing Care Plan: The Child with Legg-Calvé-Perthes Disease in Wong, D.L., and Whaley, L.F.: Clinical manual of pediatric nursing, ed. 3, St. Louis, 1990, Mosby–Year Book, Inc.

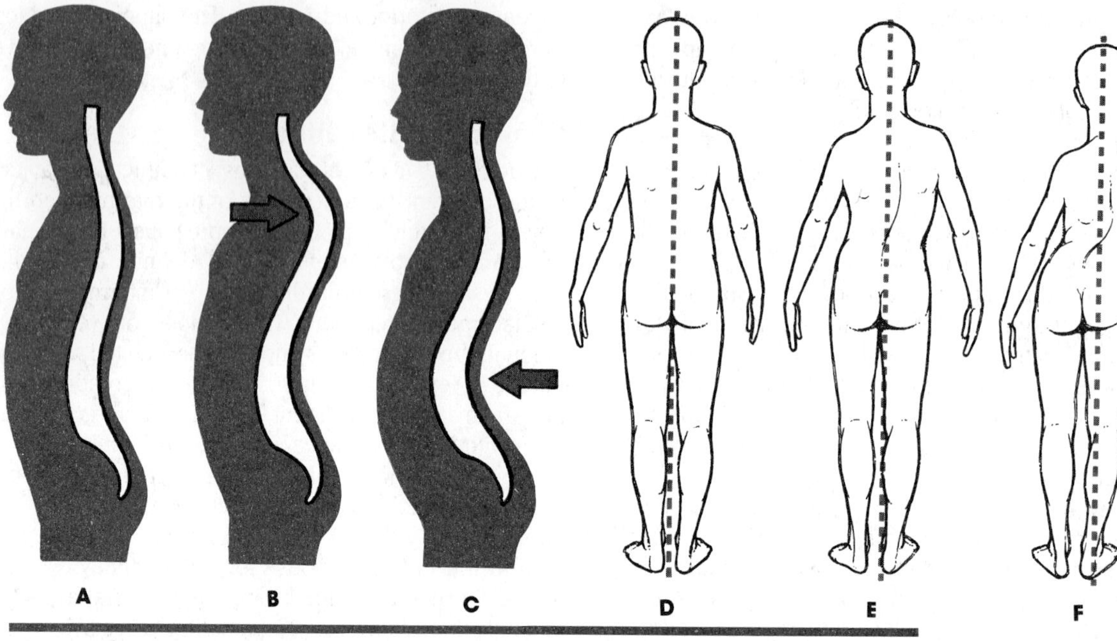

Fig. 39-30. Defects of spinal column. **A,** Normal spine. **B,** Kyphosis. **C,** Lordosis. **D,** Normal spine in balance. **E,** Mild scoliosis in balance. **F,** Severe scoliosis not in balance. **G,** Rib hump and flank asymmetry seen in flexion caused by rotary component.
Redrawn from Hilt, N.E., and Schmitt, E.W.: Pediatric orthopedic nursing, St. Louis, 1975, Mosby–Year Book, Inc.

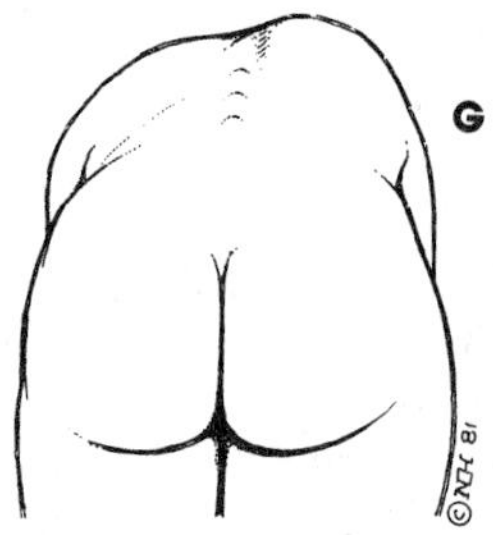

round-shouldered slouching posture in the attempt to hide their developing breasts and increasing height.

Postural kyphosis is almost always accompanied by a compensatory postural lordosis, an abnormally exaggerated concave lumbar curvature. Treatment consists of postural exercises to strengthen shoulder and abdominal muscles and bracing for more marked deformity. Unfortunately treatment is difficult because of the nature of the adolescent personality. The normal rebellious tendencies of the adolescent together with continual parental nagging to "stand up straight" often interfere with compliance to a therapeutic regimen. The best approach is to emphasize the cosmetic value of corrective therapy and to place the responsibility on the adolescent for carrying out an exercise program at home with regular visits to and assessments by a therapist.

Most adolescents respond well to selected sports as a supplement to regular exercise. Boys prefer weight lifting (preferably performed from a prone or supine position on a bench) and track sports. Girls respond well to dancing classes (ballet or modern dancing). Swimming is excellent and has the added advantages of exercising all muscles, eliminating gravity, and teaching breath control.

Lordosis

Lordosis is an accentuation of the lumbar curvature beyond physiologic limits (Fig. 39-30, *C*). It may be a secondary complication of a disease process, the result of trauma, or idiopathic. Lordosis is a normal observation in toddlers and, in older children, is often seen in association with flexion contractures of the hip, obesity, congenital dislocated hip, and slipped femoral capital epiphysis. During the pubertal growth spurt lordosis of varying degrees is observed in teenagers, especially girls. In obese children the weight of the abdominal fat alters the center of gravity, causing a compensatory lordosis. Unlike kyphosis, severe lordosis is usually accompanied by pain.

Treatment involves management of the predisposing cause when possible, such as weight loss and correction of deformities. Postural exercises and/or support garments are helpful in relieving symptoms in some cases; however, these do not usually effect a permanent cure.

SCOLIOSIS

Scoliosis, the most common spinal deformity, is a lateral curvature of the spine usually associated with a rotary deformity (produced by rotation of affected vertebrae) that eventually causes cosmetic and physiologic alterations in the spine, chest, and pelvis. It can appear at any age but is more frequent in adolescent girls during their growth spurt.

Etiology

Scoliosis can be caused by a number of etiologic agents and may occur spontaneously or in association with other diseases or deformities. Scoliosis can be *structural* or *functional.* Functional, postural, or nonstructural scoliosis is caused by some other deformity, such as unequal leg length. The curve is flexible and corrects by bending. The curve may be postural with a slight curve that disappears when the child lies down or tries to compensate for a leg-length discrepancy. A transient scoliosis may be produced by pressure on a nerve root or inflammation. Functional scoliosis can be corrected by treating the underlying problem.

Structural scoliosis is characterized by changes in the spine and its supporting structures that cause loss of flexibility and noncorrectable deformity. The spine fails to straighten on side bending, and a truly structural deformity displays a rotational deformity not observed in functional curvatures. Structural scoliosis may be congenital or a secondary defect associated with other disorders, especially neuromuscular disease or paralysis. In 70% of cases it is "idiopathic" without apparent cause; however, evidence indicates that it is probably genetic and transmitted as an autosomal-dominant trait with incomplete penetrance or is multifactorial. The various causes of structural scoliosis are outlined in Box 39-15.

Recent evidence has implicated neurologic deficits in the etiology of idiopathic scoliosis, although the site of damage is not apparent (Barrack and others, 1984). The primary deficit appears to be somehow related to proprioception, which could involve neural pathways of visual, vestibular, and proprioceptive afferent nerves that have connections with numerous neural pathways involving the brain and spinal cord.

Clinical Manifestations

Idiopathic scoliosis is seldom apparent before 10 years of age and is most noticeable at the beginning of the preadolescent growth spurt. Parents will often bring a child for evaluation because of "ill-fitting" clothes such as uneven pant lengths or uneven skirt hems. There are rarely discomfort and few outward signs until the deformity is well established. Early detection and treatment are essential to successful management (see also Back and Extremities, Chapter 7).

Diagnostic Evaluation

Diagnosis is made by observation and radiographic examination. The undressed child viewed from the posterior side will often reveal primary curvature and a compensatory curvature that places the head in alignment with the gluteal fold (Fig. 39-30, *E*). In uncompensated scoliosis the head and hips are not in alignment (Fig. 39-30, *F*). In advanced cases with rotary deformity, rib hump and flank asymmetry are observed when the child bends from the waist unsup-

Box 39-15 CAUSES OF STRUCTURAL SCOLIOSIS

Idiopathic (Genetic) Scoliosis
Infantile
- Age of onset—birth to 3 years of age
- More common in males
- Usually left thoracic curve
- Poor prognosis

Juvenile
- Age of onset—4 to 10 years of age
- More equal distribution between sexes
- Usually right thoracic curve
- Severity increases with growth

Adolescent
- Age of onset—10 years of age to skeletal maturity
- Predominant in females, about 7:1
- Right thoracic and thoracolumbar curves more common

Congenital Scoliosis
Associated with meningomyelocele or other dysrhaphism
Hemivertebrae

Neuromuscular (Paralytic) Scoliosis
Caused by muscular imbalance
Neurogenic
- Lower motor neuron disease such as poliomyelitis, spinal muscular atrophy
- Upper motor neuron disease such as cerebral palsy

Myogenic
- Progressive disease such as muscular dystrophy
- Static disease such as amyotonia congenita

Mixed—weakness and overpull by stronger trunk muscles, such as in Friedreich ataxia

Neurofibromatosis
Short sharp thoracic curve often associated with kyphosis

Traumatic
Thoracogenic—result of thoracotomy and thoracoplasty with rib resection
Spinal trauma
- Irradiation such as tumor therapy
- Fractures

Spinal Irritation
Spinal cord tumor
Nerve root irritation

Miscellaneous
Secondary to irritation
- Tumor
- Inflammation

Nutritional—rickets
Metabolic—renal osteodystrophy

Mesenchymal Disease
Congenital disorders
- Dwarfism
- Disease of connective tissue such as arachnodactyly, arthrogryposis multiplex congenita
- Disease of bone such as osteogenesis imperfecta

Acquired disorders—rheumatoid arthritis

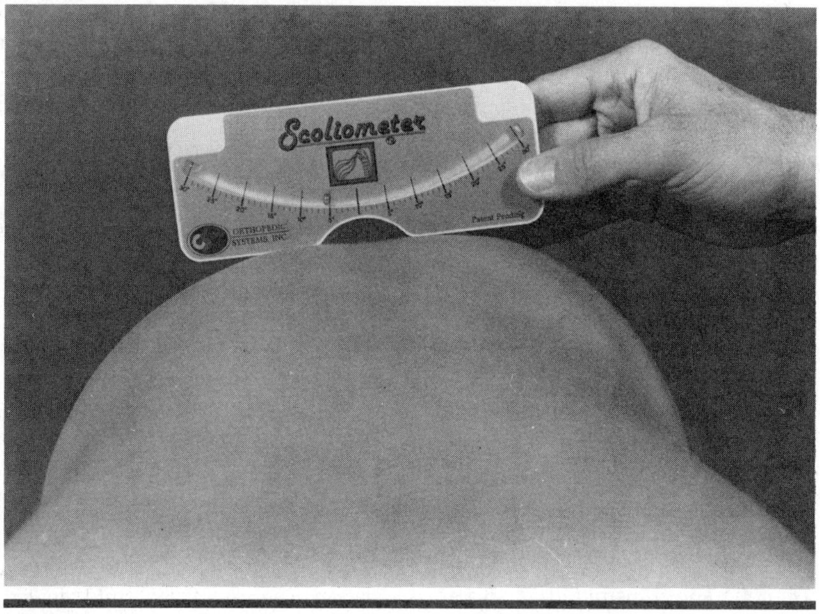

Fig. 39-31. Scoliometer used to document clinical deformity seen in patients with scoliosis.

From Bunnell, W.P.: Nonoperative treatment of spinal deformity: the case for observation. In AAOS: Instructional course lectures, vol. 36, St. Louis, 1985, Mosby–Year Book, Inc.

QUESTIONS AND CONTROVERSIES

Is mass scoliosis screening necessary?

Until recently scoliosis was considered to be dangerous and, if untreated, would progress until pulmonary function was compromised. Presently it is believed that only persons with severe thoracic curves are at risk for pulmonary complications and that the major damages inflicted are discomfort and cosmetic problems (Ziporyn, 1985).

Screening is relatively simple to accomplish and is designed to detect the deformity early to arrest its progress before it becomes severe. Proponents of screening state that early detection permits use of bracing rather than surgery for correction and identifies mild cases that would otherwise become so severe that they require surgery. Advocates cite population studies that indicate back surgery has decreased as screening programs spread (Allen and Ferguson, 1985; Berwick, 1985). Screening is also endorsed by the American Academy of Orthopedic Surgeons (Allen and Ferguson, 1985).

Opponents argue that the incidence of scoliosis requiring treatment is not high enough to justify mass testing (Wynne, 1984) and is not cost-effective (Morais and others, 1985). Small curvatures rarely require treatment, and only 0.14% of children screened need bracing or surgery (Cross, 1985). Moreover, the number of false-positive results causes unneeded anxiety and stress (Berwick, 1985). Many children are being subjected to excessive radiography (Ziporyn, 1985), and those who will not progress often undergo bracing unnecessarily (Berwick, 1985; Wynne, 1984). Many cases would be detected by parents or practitioners without screening (Berwick, 1985).

ported with the arms (Fig. 39-30, *G*). A clinical deformity can be documented by placing a scoliometer, a modified inclinometer, across the back at the point of maximum deformity while the child is in the forward-bent position (Bunnell, 1984) (Fig. 39-31). Radiographs taken in the standing position establish the degree of spinal curvature.

Screening for scoliosis by school nurses is now routine in most schools and mandated by law in many states. Although asymmetry suggests scoliosis, it is not diagnostic and screening has both supporters and detractors (see Questions and Controversies). Until the debate is resolved, screening continues to be a widespread practice.

Therapeutic Management: Nonoperative

A thorough examination, history, and assessment of the child are carried out in order to evaluate the status of the deformity, factors contributing to the defect, and factors that may influence the outcome of therapy. Treatment is best undertaken in a center in which a team is available that specializes in management of scoliosis. Current management involves straightening and realignment of the vertebrae by either external (bracing) or internal (surgical) fixation techniques. Although there is some question regarding whether or not bracing is effective in preventing progression of curvatures (Miller, Nachemson, and Schultz, 1984), it still remains the primary mode of therapy for minor curvatures. Bracing is not curative but may slow the progression of the deformity until the spine has reached the more adult size.

Bracing and exercise. Exercises can often help postural scoliosis but are rarely of value with structural defects. Nonoperative treatment by application of a properly constructed and well-fitted external bracing device and close

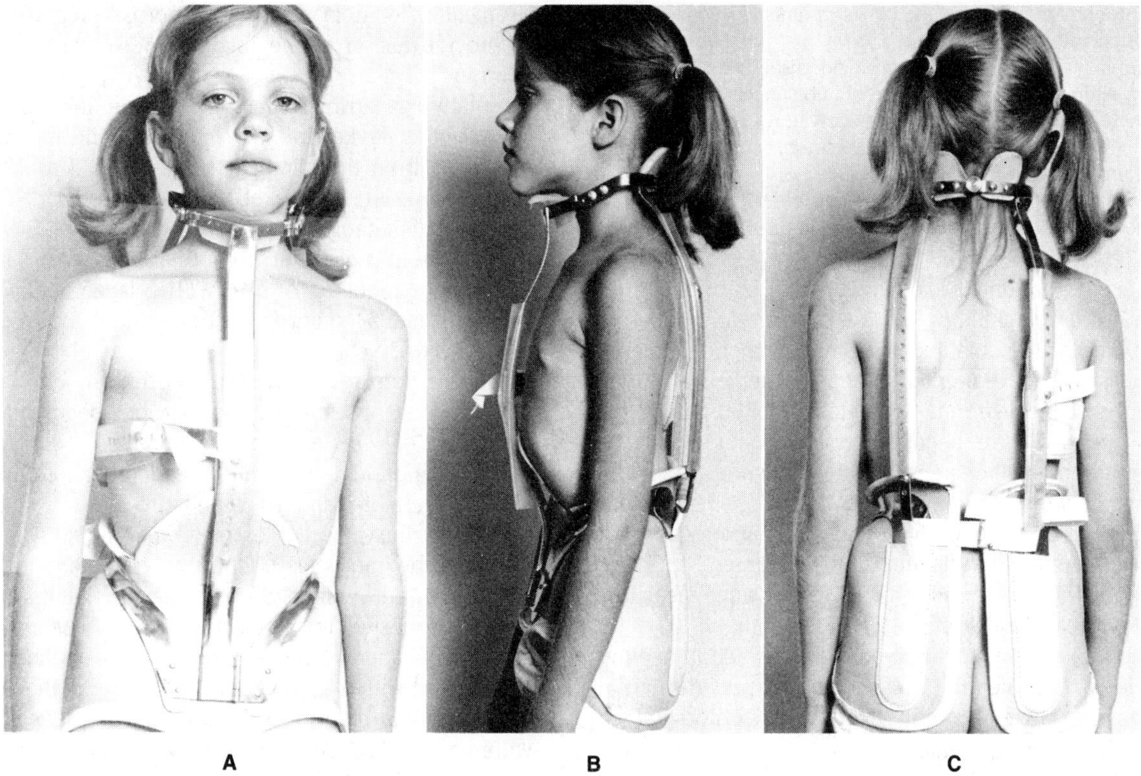

Fig. 39-32. Milwaukee brace. **A,** Front view. **B,** Side view. **C,** Rear view.
From Blount, W.P. and Mueller, K.H.: Praxis 8:139-149, June 1972.

supervision are successful in halting the progression of most curvatures. There are basically two types of braces in use: (1) the Milwaukee brace, an individually adapted steel and leather brace that extends from a chin cup and neck pads to the pelvis, where lumbar pads rest on the hips (Fig. 39-32), and (2) an underarm brace, of which there are numerous varieties, used primarily for lumbar curvatures. The Milwaukee brace is suitable for virtually all curves and is the benchmark of current orthotic treatment (Renshaw, 1985). The brace is used for minimum curvatures and is worn 23 hours a day but offers little interference with normal activity.

Supplemental exercises are employed daily both in and out of the brace to prevent atrophy of spinal and abdominal muscles. The brace is adjusted at regular trimonthly intervals and, when radiographic examinations reveal bone maturity, the child is gradually weaned from the brace over a 1- to 2-year period. The brace is then worn only at night until the spine is absolutely mature. An underarm modification of the Milwaukee brace has been designed that is receiving greater patient acceptance. An orthoplast jacket is molded with specific built-in corrective forces for each patient. However, its use is limited to patients with low curvatures.

Electrical stimulation. Many young patients with mild to moderate curvatures have an alternative to bracing in the form of electrical stimulation. An electrical stimulator generates an electrical pulse that is transmitted to muscles on the convex side of the curvature. The electrical stimulation causes the muscles to contract at regular and frequent intervals, straightening the spine. Stimulators currently available involve either electrodes taped to the skin surface over standard electrode gel and attached to a battery-operated mechanism or surgically implanted receiver and leads coupled to an external transmitter by an external antenna. The devices are worn at night, allowing unrestricted activity during waking hours.

The stimulation, although not painful, may be associated with an uncomfortable sensation, and transient sleep problems are usual during the first month of treatment. Surface stimulators are poorly tolerated by children under 10 years of age. The cost of surface stimulation compares favorably with the cost of bracing, but the implanted option is considerably higher and involves hospitalization for the implant procedure.

Reports indicate that stimulation prevents progression of scoliosis in the majority of patients. There are advantages and disadvantages to the treatment, however. Skin irritation is a common complication of surface stimulation, and the implant stimulators require two surgical procedures—one for placement and one for removal (McCollough, 1985).

Therapeutic Management: Operative

Surgical intervention may be required for correction. The indications for surgery are:

Physiologic—pulmonary function is diminished considerably, approximately 50%.

Functional—children with neurologic disabilities have difficulty sitting or walking because of imbalance.

Cosmetic—some children whose curvature is amenable to bracing are unable to use that therapy because of a self-image problem.

Pain—although rare in children, some older youngsters may have chronic discomfort from sitting on one buttock continually; pressure sores become a problem.

With few exceptions the techniques consist of spinal realignment and straightening by way of external or internal fixation and instrumentation combined with bony fusion (arthrodesis) of the realigned spine. The degree of curvature and the cause determine the decision for surgery. Bracing and exercise have been universally disappointing in curves greater than 40 degrees, and paralytic and congenital curves, which will eventually progress, are best treated with early surgical stabilization. Age of the child and location of the curvature influence the decision for surgery, and any curve that does not respond to more conservative measures requires surgical correction.

For the most severe scoliotic curvatures, traction is often needed for a time before spinal fusion to provide partial correction and more flexibility. Methods incorporating either continuous or intermittent traction are employed. One type consists of a leather head halter and pelvic girdle attached to a system of ropes and pulleys that can be manipulated by the patient. More rigid deformities are best managed by skeletal traction techniques.

The traction is applied to the spine by way of a metal ring, or halo, attached to the skull and pins inserted into either the distal femur or the iliac wings of the pelvis. With halo-femoral traction the child is placed on a special Stryker frame, and progressive traction is applied by weight in twice-daily increments. Halo-pelvic traction is applied by means of turnbuckles, and the child can remain ambulatory. Another alternative is halo-wheelchair traction, applied by means of a pulley system and weights suspended from behind the chair, using the weight of the child's upright body for countertraction. The halo is used both preoperatively and postoperatively. Casting is used by some orthopedists, but success with these techniques is variable.

Harrington instrumentation. The most frequently performed operative techniques for correction of the deformity involve the implantation of a rigid metal appliance. The *Harrington distraction* system consists of a metal rod applied to the *concave* side of the scoliotic curve, with cannulated hooks attached to the vertebra at each end of the curve. The spine is straightened by progressive distraction between the hooks in a manner similar to the mechanism of an automobile jack. The *Harrington compression* system employs compression to the *convex* curve of the spine posteriorly by means of hooks attached to either end of the curve and a semirigid, threaded rod. Progressive compression is applied to the convexity by advancing small nuts along the threaded rod from opposite directions, shortening the distance between the hooks. The two techniques are frequently used in combination. Chips and strips of bone (from ilium or tibia) are placed across prepared vertebrae to provide fusion to the involved portion of the vertebral column.

Following Harrington instrumentation, the child is immobilized on a Stryker frame. When the child has sufficiently recovered from the surgery, usually after 8 to 12 days, an immobilizing plaster jacket is applied from occiput to pelvis, which is changed at 3 months and maintained for a total of 6 months. Further immobilization with a removable cast may be required for sites with delayed healing. Regular follow-up management is continued at 3- to 6-month intervals for 3 to 5 years.

Luque segmental instrumentation. The Luque segmental spinal instrumentation provides segmental stabiiity by the use of wires and flexible L-shaped rods. By way of a posterior approach, wires are threaded beneath the laminae of each vertebra and tightened around the rods resting along the transverse processes so that the spinal column is stabilized by transverse traction on each vertebra. After the rods are wired in place, the anesthesia is lightened and the patient requested to wiggle the toes to ensure no spinal cord involvement. The patient is reanesthetized and the spine fused with a bone graft taken from the iliac crest. The advantages to this procedure are that the patient can walk within a few days and that no postoperative immobilization is required. The disadvantage is a possibility of spinal nerve damage.

Dwyer instrumentation. The Dwyer instrumentation and fusion technique involves transfixing cannulated screws to each vertebra in the curvature, then threading a titanium cable through the cannulae of the screw heads. When satisfactory correction is achieved, the screw heads are crimped to the cable, and bone chips (obtained from the iliac bone) are placed between adjacent vertebral bodies to facilitate fusion. Tension is then applied to the cable to maintain alignment. This procedure requires an anterior approach, but because the cable does not provide rigid fixation, a supplemental fusion via a posterior approach is needed. The Dwyer procedure is performed less frequently in children with idiopathic scoliosis but is well suited to treatment of spina bifida. Children with Dwyer instrumentation are cared for in bed.

Other. Other surgical procedures have been tried and proved successful in selected cases. Many of the current procedures combine the features of the methods previously described. Various modifications of the Harrington procedure are used. One that is used infrequently combines the Harrington and Dwyer (Zielke) procedures. A newer approach uses the distraction force of the Harrington rods plus the strength of Luque segmentation (Cotrel-Dubousset procedure) (Fig. 39-33).

Nursing Considerations

Treatment for scoliosis extends over a significant portion of the affected child's period of growth. In adolescents this period is the one in which their identity, physical and psychologic, is formed. For some youngsters much of this time is spent in the hospital setting immobilized in complex, unat-

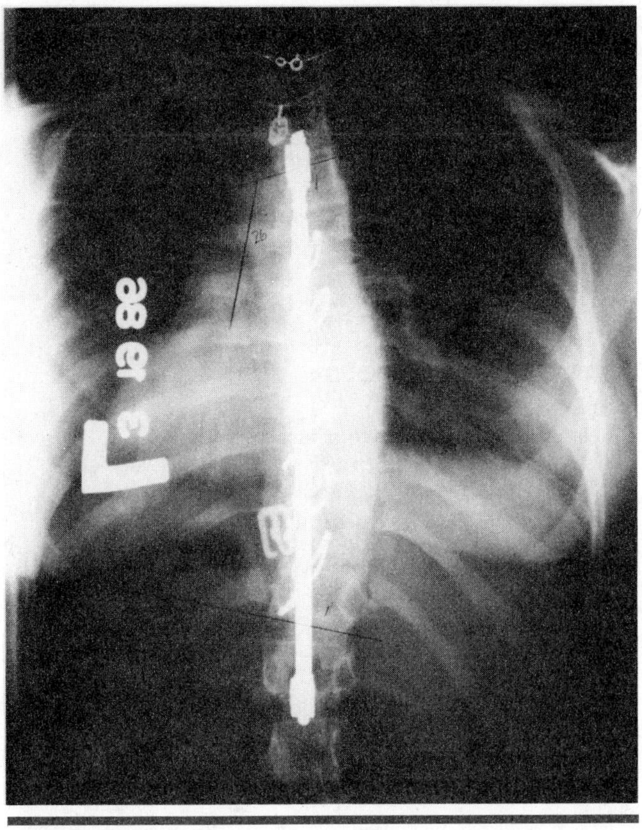

Fig. 39-33. Harrington rod with Luque wires (Cotrel-Dubousset).

tractive appliances. For those treated on an outpatient basis it means a modified life-style and being "different" from their peers, even though they are usually able to engage in many activities enjoyed by other youngsters.

Assessment

One of the major functions of nurses is to learn to detect the presence of scoliosis. School nurses routinely evaluate children in their care, and most are a part of scoliosis screening programs. The methods of assessment are those described in Chapter 7 and in relation to Diagnostic Evaluation, p. 1887.

Screening procedures are simple and require only a 30-second observation. Unfortunately, studies have indicated that current screening procedures are less than ideal (Morais and others, 1985; Viviani and others, 1984), and too many children are exposed to radiographs in the attempt to rule out scoliosis in normal children. Methods of improving the effectiveness of screening and the application to all school children should be a goal of nursing.

Nursing Diagnoses

Based on a thorough assessment, several nursing diagnoses are identified. The more common diagnoses for the child with scoliosis are included in the Nursing Care Plan on pp. 1892-1893. Others may apply in specific situations.

Planning

Nursing objectives for the child with scoliosis include the following:

1. Help the child adjust to the method of therapeutic management.
2. Prevent complications.
3. Provide support and encouragement to the child and family.

Implementation

When the child first faces the prospect of a prolonged period in a brace, cast, or other device, the therapy program and the nature of the device must be explained thoroughly to the child and parents so that they will have an understanding of the anticipated results, how the appliance corrects the defect, the freedoms and constraints imposed by the device, and what they can do to help achieve the desired goal. The management involves the skills and services of a team of specialists, including the orthopedist, physical therapist, orthotist (a specialist in fitting orthopedic braces), nurse, social worker, and sometimes a pulmonary specialist.

It is difficult for a child to be restricted at any phase of development, but the teenager needs continual positive reinforcement, encouragement, and as much independence as can be safely assumed during this time. Although adolescents cope well for the first year or two after casting, problems may arise as the time extends. Nurses need to be aware of this and be prepared to provide support and encouragement if problems arise (Davis and Lewis, 1984). Guidance and assistance regarding anticipated problems, such as selection of clothing and participation in social activities, are appreciated by adolescents. Socialization with peers should be encouraged and every effort expended to help the adolescent feel attractive and worthwhile.

Since many persons view any disability as deviant, the child will need help in learning how to deal with reactions of others to the appliance. Preparation for such responses places the child at an advantage. The best approach is usually to initiate the interaction by mentioning the device and its purpose. This alleviates the ambiguity surrounding the appliance and its purpose and reduces the anxiety on the part of the child and the other person. Most importantly the child should be helped to view the condition and appliance in a positive way and avoid seeing them as a stigma. There are youngsters who have the education and peer counseling and support who find positive aspects to wearing a brace in addition to improved posture and relief of symptoms. They enjoy the increased attention from peers and the experience of "being different" (Gratz and Papalia-Finlay, 1984).

Preoperative care. The child hospitalized for surgical management requires preparation for the procedures involved, which are puzzling and often frightening to the very young patient. They need to know what is going to happen,

NURSING CARE PLAN
The Child with Structural Scoliosis

NURSING DIAGNOSIS: Potential for injury related to unaccustomed brace

GOAL 1
Prevent injury

INTERVENTIONS

Assess environment for hazards
Teach safety precautions such as using handrail on stairways and avoiding slippery surfaces
Help develop safe methods of mobilization

EXPECTED OUTCOME

Child remains free of injury related to wearing brace

GOAL 2
Help child adjust to restricted movement

INTERVENTIONS

Demonstrate alternative modes of accomplishing tasks such as getting in and out of bed, dressing
Help devise alternatives for restricted activities and coping with awkwardness

EXPECTED OUTCOME

Child demonstrates appropriate adaptation to corrective device (specify)

NURSING DIAGNOSIS: Potential impaired skin integrity related to corrective device

GOAL 1
Prevent skin irritation and breakdown

INTERVENTIONS

Examine skin surfaces in contact with brace for signs of irritation
Implement corrective action to treat or prevent skin breakdown
Suggest nonirritating fabrics and clothing such as cotton T-shirts

EXPECTED OUTCOME

Skin remains clean with no evidence of irritation

NURSING DIAGNOSIS: Body image disturbance related to perception of defect in body structure

GOAL 1
Assist in physical adjustment to appliance

INTERVENTIONS

Plan *with* the child
Attempt to determine source of any discomfort
Refer to orthotist for needed adjustment and service
Assist with plan for personal hygiene
Help in selection of appropriate apparel to wear over brace and footwear to maintain proper balance
Reinforce teaching regarding removal and reapplication of appliance
Investigate any complaints of discomfort

EXPECTED OUTCOMES

Brace fits well and produces no discomfort
Child complies with directions for wear and care of brace
Child is well groomed and wears attractive attire

GOAL 2
Promote positive body image

INTERVENTIONS

Encourage child to discuss feelings about wearing brace
Emphasize positive aspects and eventual outcome

EXPECTED OUTCOMES

Child verbalizes feelings and concerns
Child plans in terms of long-range goals as well as short-range ones

See also Nursing Care Plan: The Child with a Chronic Illness or Disability, Chapter 22

Operative care

See Nursing Care Plan: The Child Undergoing Surgery, Chapter 27

Postoperative care

NURSING DIAGNOSIS: Potential for injury related to surgery

GOAL 1
Promote active movement

INTERVENTIONS

Encourage child to exercise by contracting and relaxing thigh and calf muscles periodically

EXPECTED OUTCOME

Child maintains optimum movement of lower extremities

NURSING CARE PLAN
The Child with Structural Scoliosis—cont'd

GOAL 2

Prevent injury to surgical repair

INTERVENTIONS

Place on Stryker frame for care (Harrington instrumentation)
Maintain proper body alignment; avoid twisting movements
Logroll with care when moving child
Keep flat for 12 hours before logrolling (Luque procedure)
Beginning activity—have child roll from side-lying to sitting position
Walk slowly with aid of safety belt and walker; unassisted ambulation allowed by sixth day
Assist with physical therapy and range of motion exercises
Perform regular tests of neurologic integrity

EXPECTED OUTCOME

Child attains ambulation without injury

GOAL 3

Prevent abdominal distention (from paralytic ileus)

INTERVENTIONS

*Insert and maintain nasogastric suction
Assess for returning bowel function (e.g., bowel sounds)

EXPECTED OUTCOME

Child exhibits no evidence of bowel distention

NURSING DIAGNOSIS: Pain related to surgical procedure

GOAL 1

Relieve pain
See Nursing Care Plan: The Child in Pain, Chapter 26

INTERVENTIONS

*Administer opioids around the clock until pain can be controlled with nonopioids
Consider patient-controlled analgesia for child able to follow instructions

EXPECTED OUTCOME

Child exhibits evidence of only minimum discomfort

NURSING DIAGNOSIS: Altered patterns of urinary elimination related to surgical procedure, loss of blood, renal hypoperfusion

GOAL 1

Facilitate urinary elimination

INTERVENTIONS

*Insert indwelling catheter

EXPECTED OUTCOME

Urinary bladder remains empty

GOAL 2

Promote urinary output

INTERVENTIONS

Maintain intravenous infusion
Encourage oral fluids when allowed

EXPECTED OUTCOME

Child has a sufficient urinary output

NURSING DIAGNOSIS: Impaired physical mobility related to spinal surgery and instrumentation

See Nursing Care Plan: The Child Who Is Immobilized, p. 1845

NURSING DIAGNOSIS: Altered family processes related to a child with a physical disability

GOAL 1

Support family

INTERVENTIONS

See Nursing Care Plan: The Family of the Ill or Hospitalized Child, Chapter 26

EXPECTED OUTCOME

Family members avail themselves of services

See also Nursing Care Plan: The Child in the Hospital, Chapter 26

*Dependent nursing action.

especially during the traction procedures, and a full explanation of why the procedure is necessary (one child thought that the traction was applied to "break" the bones) and of the potential outcome of the surgery.

During the progressive traction application the patient needs to be observed carefully for signs of neurologic impairment. Assessments of neurologic function are performed regularly and include assessment of the nerves both distal and proximal to the curvature. Particular attention should be paid to the cranial nerves and deep tendon reflexes in the extremities. (See The Child in Traction, p. 1862, for specific management and care.)

✦ **NURSING ALERT:** Loss of lateral gaze and the inability to follow a moving object is an early sign of excessive neurologic traction. Other early signs include hyperreflexia of the lower extremities and dysesthesia in a glove and stocking distribution (Micheli, Magin, and Rouvales, 1979).

Postoperative care. Postoperatively patients are monitored in an intensive care unit. They are placed on an Egg-crate mattress to prevent pressure areas, and the child with Harrington instrumentation will be placed on a Stryker frame, which facilitates care and lessens the possibility of damage to the fusion and indwelling instruments from twisting the spine and the possibility of "popping out" the rods. Nurses who work with these appliances should become familiar with their mechanism before assuming responsibility for patient care. The child who is not on a Stryker frame must be carefully logrolled when turned.

In addition to the usual postoperative assessments—of wound, circulation, and vital signs—the neurologic status of the patient requires special attention, especially that of the extremities. Prompt recognition of any neurologic impairment is imperative because delayed paralysis may develop that requires removal of the instrumentation. The patient is encouraged to exercise by contracting and relaxing the thigh and calf muscles periodically.

There is usually some degree of paralytic ileus following the procedure; therefore nursing includes care of the nasogastric intubation and assessment for returning bowel function. Urinary retention is common and often requires insertion of an indwelling catheter. Because of the extensive blood loss during the surgical procedure and renal hypoperfusion, observation of urinary output is especially important.

The child usually has considerable pain for the first few days following surgery and requires frequent administration of pain medication (see Pain Management, Chapter 26). Because of the anterior approach, patients with Dwyer instrumentation also require thoracotomy care in addition to the care related to the fusion and realignment procedures.

Children with a Luque procedure are kept flat for 12 hours before logrolling is begun. The head of the bed can be elevated on the second day and range of motion exercises begun. Activity is begun by instructing the patient to roll from a side-lying position to a sitting position. Next, walking slowly with the aid of a safety belt and walker is allowed, and finally unassisted ambulation, which is usually achieved by the sixth day.

All patients are started on physiotherapy as soon as they are able, beginning with range of motion exercises and many of the activities of daily living. Self-care such as washing and eating is always encouraged. Some simple physical therapy may be begun during this acute stage. Throughout the hospitalization diversionary activities and contact with family and friends are an important part of nursing care and planning.

The family is encouraged to become involved with the patient's care to facilitate the transition from hospital to home management. Family members learn to apply and care for the brace or learn cast care, with special attention to jagged edges on the cast, padding of the appliance, and daily skin checks for reddened areas, especially in areas such as under the arms or over the hips. They may need assistance in modifying the environment for limited ambulation and acquiring needed home care items such as an Egg-crate mattress, straight-backed chair, and a raised toilet seat. The child and family need to learn efficient ways to move and carry out various activities of daily living. The diet may require modification. Overeating and constipation can be problems related to limited activity.

Several organizations provide education and services to both families and professionals. The **National Scoliosis Foundation, Inc.*** is devoted to awareness and action for early detection and prevention of spinal deformity. They offer educational support materials for parents, schools, and health care providers. A list of books, pamphlets, and other materials is available on request. The **Scoliosis Association, Inc.†** a national self-help group, has a number of chapters throughout the United States, and the **Scoliosis Research Society,‡** an organization of physicians and scientists, has published an excellent book, *Scoliosis: A Handbook for Patients.*

5 Evaluation

The effectiveness of nursing interventions is determined by continual reassessment and evaluation of care based on the following observational guidelines and expected outcomes:

1. Observe and interview the child relative to problems and solutions experienced.
2. Observe child for evidence of proper usage of the method of management and signs of complications (e.g., skin irritation).
3. Observe and interview the child and family regarding their feelings and concerns.

Expected outcomes:
See Nursing care plan, pp. 1892-1893.

---

*P.O. Box 547, Belmont, MA 02178; (617) 489-0880.

†P.O. Box 51353, Raleigh, NC 27609; (919) 846-2639.

‡P.O. Box 2001, Park Ridge, IL 60068; (708) 698-1627. The book can be purchased by sending $1.00 to the organization.

■ ORTHOPEDIC INFECTIONS

Infections of bones and joints are not uncommon and often pose a problem with diagnosis because of their similarity of symptoms. The most frequently observed infection is osteomyelitis, and in populations where tuberculosis is endemic, this disease is encountered increasingly in nursing practice.

OSTEOMYELITIS

Osteomyelitis, an infectious process of bone, can occur at any age but occurs most frequently between ages 5 and 14 years. It is twice as common in boys as in girls.

Etiology

Any organism can cause osteomyelitis, and there is some relationship between the age of the child and the type of organism responsible. In older children staphylococci are the most common organisms, approximately 80% of which are *Staphylococcus aureus;* in younger children other organisms predominate, especially *Haemophilus influenzae.* One report describes *Pseudomonas aeruginosa* osteomyelitis acquired from puncture wounds. The organism was present in the soles of the sneakers the children were wearing (Fisher, Goldsmith, and Gilligan, 1985). In children with sickle cell anemia *Salmonella* organisms are frequently responsible for osteomyelitis.

Osteomyelitis can be acquired from *exogenous* or *hematogenous* sources. Exogenous osteomyelitis is acquired by invasion of the bone by direct extension from the outside as a result of a penetrating wound, open fracture, contamination during surgery, or secondary extension from an overlying abscess or burn.

Hematogenous spread of organisms from a preexisting focus is the most common source of infection. Common sources of foci include furuncles, skin abrasions, impetigo, upper respiratory tract infection, acute otitis media, tonsillitis, abscessed teeth, pyelonephritis, or infected burns. Other factors that predispose to development of osteomyelitis are poor physical condition, poor nutrition, and surroundings that are not hygienic.

Pathophysiology

Infective emboli from the focus of infection travel to the small end arteries in the bone metaphysis, where they set up an infectious process. The infection does not spread to the epiphysis, since it has a blood supply separate from the metaphysis. The infectious process leads to local bone destruction and abscess formation. The abscess with its collected necrotic debris exerts pressure within the rigid, unyielding bone and ruptures into the subperiosteal space, where the pressure lifts and strips the periosteum. The infection spreads beneath the periosteum, causing thrombosis of vessels and adding further to the bony necrosis.

In infants and very young children the elevated periosteum attempts to wall off the infection by forming new bone—*involucrum.* Underneath, the cortex, deprived of blood supply, dies, and the necrotic bone that cannot be absorbed continues to produce more intraosseous tension and necrosis. Granulation forms around the dead bone, or *sequestrum.* Sinuses may form between the sequestra and the skin surface or into a joint to create a suppurative arthritis. Small areas of sequestrum may be absorbed, but larger areas surrounded by dense bone become honeycombed with sinuses that retain infective material and cause exacerbations for years (the chronic stage of osteomyelitis).

Clinical Manifestations

Signs and symptoms of *acute* hematogenous osteomyelitis begin abruptly and build up to a maximum intensity during the first few days of the disease, usually less than 1 week. There is frequently a history of trauma to the affected bone.

Children with acute osteomyelitis appear very ill. They are irritable and restless with elevated temperature, rapid pulse, and dehydration. There is usually localized tenderness, increased warmth, and diffuse swelling over the involved bone. The extremity is painful, especially on movement. The child holds it in semiflexion, and the surrounding muscles are tense and resist passive movement. Most cases involve the femur or tibia and to a lesser extent the humerus and hip. In infants the diagnosis is more difficult because of lack of systemic symptoms. The disorder may involve multiple bones or joints because of the difficulty in confining an infectious process in children in this age-group.

In *subacute* hematogenous osteomyelitis symptoms have been present for a longer period and the child sometimes has been treated with antibiotics, often for another infection, which modify the clinical symptoms. In some instances the infection may produce a walled-off abscess rather than a spreading infection.

Diagnostic Evaluation

In acute osteomyelitis there is marked leukocytosis and an elevated erythrocyte sedimentation rate. Blood culture is usually positive during the early stage, but radiographic findings are often negative or show only soft tissue swelling for 10 to 14 days. After this time the radiographic findings reveal new bone formation. Computed tomography may reveal bone changes at an early stage, and scintigraphy reveals a greater uptake of radionucleotides in osteomyelitic bone than in normal bone.

Similar symptoms are observed in rheumatic fever, rheumatoid arthritis, leukemia and other malignant lesions, cellulitis, erysipelas, and scurvy. Sometimes the osteomyelitis may be unrecognized if it occurs as a complication of a severe toxic and debilitating illness.

Therapeutic Management

As soon as blood cultures have been drawn, prompt and vigorous intravenous antibiotic therapy is initiated. The choice is influenced by age, and the dosage determined is sufficient to ensure high blood and tissue levels. Since most cases of osteomyelitis are caused by staphylococci, large doses of penicillin G are administered and supplemented by methicillin or oxacillin. In children younger than 3 years of age, the infectious agents are more apt to be penicillin-resistant staphylococci or gram-negative organisms; therefore the agents of choice are usually methicillin, nafcillin, or clindamycin in conjunction with ampicillin. Neonates in whom coliform organisms are likely to be involved are given kanamycin or gentamicin, either intramuscularly or *slowly* intravenously in addition to intravenously administered ampicillin. In selected cases antibiotics may be administered orally following a short, intensive intravenous course.

When the infective agent is identified, the appropriate antibiotic is usually continued for at least 3 to 4 weeks, but the length of therapy is determined by the duration of symptoms, the initial response to treatment, and the sensitivity of the organism in the specific case. Because of prolonged high-dose therapy, it is important to monitor hematologic, renal, hepatic, and other organ systems that might be adversely affected by the drugs (e.g., ototoxic).

Antibiotic therapy is accompanied by local treatment. The child is placed on complete bed rest, and immobilization of the affected extremity, which may require a splint or bivalved cast, is continued throughout therapy to limit the spread of infection and, when it is a complication of a fracture, to maintain alignment of bone fragments. Weight bearing on the nonfractured leg is prohibited to avoid the possibility of pathologic fracture.

Opinions differ regarding surgical intervention, but many advocate sequestrectomy and surgical drainage to decompress the metaphyseal space before pus erupts and spreads to the subperiosteal space to form abscesses that strip the periosteum from bone or form draining sinuses. When these complications occur, a chronic infection usually persists. When surgical drainage is carried out, polyethylene tubes are placed in the wound—one tube instills an antibiotic solution directly into the infected area by gravity, and the other, connected to a suction apparatus, provides drainage.

Nursing Considerations

During the acute phase of illness any movement of the affected limb will cause discomfort to the child; therefore the child is positioned comfortably with the affected limb supported. Moving and turning are carried out carefully and gently to minimize discomfort. The child may require pain medication or sedation. Vital signs are taken and recorded frequently, and measures are implemented to reduce a significant temperature elevation.

Antibiotic therapy requires careful observation and monitoring of the intravenous equipment and site. Since more than one antibiotic is usually administered, the compatibility of the drugs must be determined and care taken to avoid mixing noncompatible drugs. A double, or piggyback, setup is safest so that there is less opportunity for the two drugs to come in contact with each other. The stability of the drugs and their toxic nature are also considered when determining the rate of administration. The needle must be well situated in the vein to ensure that the drug does not infiltrate into surrounding tissues, where it may produce tissue damage. For this type of long-term antibiotic therapy, the heparin lock is the preferred method of intravenous administration.

Children with an open wound are placed on body substance precautions, depending on the policies of the institution. The wound is managed according to the directions of the practitioner. Antibiotic solution administered directly into the wound is most efficiently accomplished with a regular intravenous infusion setup that is prepared and regulated as any intravenous infusion. The drainage tubes are connected to low Gomco or wall suction for continuous removal. Intake and output are measured and recorded, and the character of the wound drainage is noted. The amount and character of drainage on the wound dressing are also noted.

Casts are sometimes employed for immobilization, and, if so, routine cast care is carried out. The extremity is examined for sensation, circulation, and pain, and the area over the inflammation is usually left open for observation. The affected area, casted or uncasted, is assessed for color, swelling, heat, movement, and tenderness.

The child usually has a poor appetite and may be subject to vomiting. Nourishment in the form of high-calorie liquids such as fruit juices, gelatin, and juice bars should be encouraged until the child begins to feel better. The appetite returns as the acute symptoms subside. During convalescence adequate nutrition must be maintained to aid healing and reconstitution of new bone.

When the acute stage subsides, children begin to feel better, the appetite improves, and they become interested in their surroundings and relationships. They wish to move about in bed and are allowed to do so. However, weight bearing on the affected limb is not permitted until healing is well under way in order to avoid pathologic fractures. Diversional and constructive activities become important nursing interventions. Children are usually confined to bed for some time after the acute phase but may be allowed to move about the unit on a gurney or in a wheelchair when isolation and bed rest are no longer necessary. At this stage the continuous intravenous infusion may be replaced by a heparin lock to allow greater freedom.

As the infection subsides, physical therapy is instituted to ensure restoration of optimum function. The child is usually discharged with oral antibiotics, and progress is followed closely for some time.*

SEPTIC (SUPPURATIVE, PYOGENIC, PURULENT) ARTHRITIS

Infection of the joints, like infection of bone, usually develops through hematogenous dissemination from another focus; occasionally it may result from direct extension of a soft tissue infection. Joint infections occur predominantly in males, especially in the adolescent age-group. In infancy, however, the incidence in boys and girls is more nearly

*See Nursing Care Plan: The Child with Osteomyelitis in Wong, D.L., and Whaley, L.F.: Clinical manual of pediatric nursing, ed. 3, St. Louis, 1990, Mosby–Year Book, Inc.

equal. Any joint may be involved, but the hip, knee, shoulder, and other large joints are more commonly affected. Usually only one joint is involved.

The signs and symptoms of suppurative arthritis, unlike osteomyelitis, are usually characteristic. The presence of a warm and tender joint, painful on even gentle pressure, is sufficient to differentiate it from osteomyelitis, in which gentle passive motion is tolerated. When superficial joints are involved, they are exquisitely painful and swollen; deep-seated joints show little superficial evidence. In most instances there is history of a traumatic injury to the affected joint. Fever, leukocytosis, and increased erythrocyte sedimentation rate are present but may not be demonstrated in affected infants.

The most common pathogens are *Staphylococcus aureus,* group A streptococci, and *Haemophilus influenzae.* Diagnosis is made from blood culture, joint fluid aspirate, and radiographs.

Therapeutic Management and Nursing Considerations

Treatment consists of open surgical drainage of hip and shoulder joint disease and repeated needle aspirations of the joint space in other joints. The goals are (1) to cleanse the joint to avoid destruction of articular cartilage, (2) to decompress the joint to avoid interference with the blood supply to the epiphysis, (3) to eradicate the infection with adequate antibiotic therapy, and (4) to prevent secondary bone infection and hematogenous spread. Therapy is similar to that for osteomyelitis: intravenous antibiotic therapy, relief of pain, immobilization of the joint, and prohibition of weight bearing until healing is complete. Nursing care is the same as that for osteomyelitis.

TUBERCULOSIS

Tubercular infection of the bones is acquired by hematogenous dissemination from a primary tubercular focus. The most common sites in infants and small children are the carpals and phalanges and corresponding bones of the feet. One or several bones may be involved, with spindle-shaped swelling and tenderness as soft tissues are affected. The process, relatively painless, persists with intermittent symptoms for several months and may leave a permanent deformity. Affected areas are immobilized with a splint or cast.

Tuberculosis of Spine (Tuberculous Spondylitis)

In older children the infection attacks the body of one or more vertebrae, destroying the bone, and spreads to all the articular tissues, producing a kyphotic deformity. The lower thoracic spine is most frequently affected. Symptoms are insidious. The child will be irritable and complain of persistent or intermittent pain over the areas innervated by spinal nerves that arise adjacent to the affected vertebrae. There is muscle splinting and pain when increased pressure is placed on the child's head. The child assumes a position that best eases the weight on the diseased vertebrae, such as avoiding bending and walking stiffly on the toes, and prefers to rest on the abdomen or across a chair or a lap.

Treatment is immobilization with extension or plaster body cast until there is no evidence of active infection followed by spinal fusion. Antimicrobial therapy and drainage of tubercular abscess are standard therapies. The reparative process is slow, but in most instances recovery takes place with little or no deformity. Nursing care is similar to care of the child with scoliosis.

Tuberculosis of Hip

The hip is the joint most commonly affected by tuberculosis, but the process usually begins in the epiphysis of the femoral head and then erupts into the joint capsule. The initial manifestation is a limp that occurs intermittently, most often on arising in the morning or after exercise. There is progressive destruction of the femoral head with symptoms of pain, and the thigh gradually becomes fixed and adducted with internal rotation. There may be swelling around the hip and abscess formation.

Treatment involves bed rest, traction to reduce muscle spasm, and appropriate drug therapy. Hip fusion may be necessary in severe cases.

■ SKELETAL AND ARTICULAR DYSFUNCTION

There are a variety of disorders involving bones. Fractures of bones are relatively common in childhood (see p. 1851). Rickets is less common but is still a preventable disease in most instances, and uncommon disorders of bone and connective tissue such as arachnodactyly (Marfan syndrome) and achondroplasia do not cause immobilization. Bone tumors (see Chapter 36) are dreaded diseases, and bone infections are responsible for significant morbidity. There are other rare disorders, but only one—osteogenesis imperfecta—is elaborated further.

The most prominent articular disorder in children is rheumatoid arthritis. Although usually classified as a collagen disease, lupus erythematosus is also considered in this section because a frequent symptom is joint discomfort.

OSTEOGENESIS IMPERFECTA

Osteogenesis imperfecta (OI) is a group of heterogenous inherited disorders of connective tissue characterized by connective tissue and bone defects, including one or more of the following: varying degrees of bone fragility leading to fractures, blue sclerae, progressive bone deformities, presenile hearing loss, and dentinogenesis imperfecta, hypoplastic teeth with an opalescent blue or brown discoloration (Cohen, 1984). The inheritance pattern is autosomal dominant in the majority of cases, although the most severe form demonstrates autosomal-recessive inheritance.

Persons with OI have normal calcium and phosphorus levels but appear to have abnormal precollagen type I that prevents the formation of collagen, the major component of

Table 39-5 Classification of osteogenesis imperfecta

TYPE		CHARACTERISTICS
I*	A	Mild bone fragility, blue sclerae, normal teeth, presenile deafness (age 20-30 years); autosomal-dominant inheritance
	B	Same as A except dentinogenesis imperfecta instead of normal teeth
	C	Same as B; no bone fragility
II		Lethal; stillborn or die in early infancy; severe bone fragility, multiple fractures at birth; 10% of OI cases; autosomal-recessive inheritance
III		Severe bone fragility leads to severe progressive deformities; normal sclerae; marked growth failure; most autosomal-recessive; few autosomal-dominant
IV	A	Mild to moderate bone fragility; normal sclerae; short stature; variable deformity; autosomal dominant
	B	Same as A except dentinogenesis imperfecta instead of normal teeth; approximately 6% of OI cases

*Two thirds of cases are type I.

connective tissue. The precollagen remains relatively inert and unable to undergo final transformation into collagen. Consequently, bone of these patients consists of large areas of osseous tissues devoid of an organized trabecular pattern and increased numbers of large osteoblasts. Lamellae, when present, are very thin. The more severe the degree of OI, the greater is the number of osteocytes and the greater the disruption of the normal architectural patterns of the bone.

At present OI is believed to consist of four different variations, as outlined in Table 39-5. Type II, the most severe form of OI, is characterized by multiple intrauterine or perinatal fractures and severe deformity and, often, early death. The brittle nature of the bones renders them easily fractured by the slightest trauma.

The diseases of later onset run a milder course. The tendency to fracture appears later (at variable ages) and disappears after puberty. During childhood the shafts of long bones are slender with reduced cortical thickness resulting from defective periosteal bone formation. In addition to the features already described, the child with OI has thin skin, hyperextensibility of ligaments, a tendency to recurrent epistaxis, excess diaphoresis, tendency to bruise easily, and mild hyperpyrexia. The disease shows variable expressivity; that is, the number and extent of pathologic features appear in any individual range, from severe to minimum involvement. The incidence of fractures decreases at puberty, when the body's production of hormones helps strengthen bones.

Therapeutic Management

The treatment of OI is primarily supportive. The goals of a rehabilitation approach to management are directed to preventing (1) positional contractures and deformities, (2) muscle weakness and osteoporosis, and (3) malalignment of lower extremity joints prohibiting weight bearing.

Several drugs have been tried but appear to be of limited benefit. Lightweight braces and splints help support limbs, prevent fractures, and aid in ambulation. Physical therapy helps prevent disuse osteoporosis and strengthens muscles, which in turn improves bone density. Exercises are usually simple ones against light resistance or water exercises with swimming. Patients with milder disease are encouraged to participate in sports. Exercise also gives children a sense of well-being and confidence in their bodies (Root, 1984).

Surgery is sometimes used to help treat the manifestations of the disease. Surgical techniques are used to correct deformities that interfere with bracing, standing, or walking. For the child with recurrent fractures, inserting an intermedullary rod provides stability to bones. Unfortunately the rods must be replaced as the child grows; otherwise fractures may occur through the unprotected portion of the bone.

Nursing Considerations

Infants and children with this disorder require careful handling to prevent fractures. They must be supported when they are turned, positioned, moved, and fondled. Even changing a diaper may cause a fracture in severely affected infants. These children should never be held by the ankles when being diapered but should be gently lifted by the buttocks.

One of the most distressing features of OI is its frequent confusion with child abuse. Numerous fractures and easy bruising characteristic of OI are signs usually observed in child abuse; parents must often deal with accusations of abuse until a correct diagnosis is made. This is very traumatic for parents; therefore they need considerable nonjudgmental support during this time.

Both parents and the affected child need education regarding the child's limitations and guidelines in planning suitable activities that promote optimum development as well as protect the child from harm. Realistic occupational planning and genetic counseling are part of the long-term goals of care. Educational materials and information can be obtained from the **Osteogenesis Imperfecta Foundation, Inc.*** This organization also has a network that can put a family in contact with other families with a similar problem.

JUVENILE ARTHRITIS

Clinically and pathologically, juvenile arthritis (JA), juvenile rheumatoid arthritis (JRA), or juvenile chronic polyarthritis (CJA) is an inflammatory disease with an unknown inciting agent and a slight tendency to occur in families. Both infectious and autoimmune theories have been presented, but there is no convincing evidence to establish either one as an etiologic agent. There are two peak ages of onset: between 2 and 5 and between 9 and 12 years of age. Females

*P.O. Box 14807, Tampa, FL 34629-4807; (813) 855-7077.

are affected somewhat more frequently than males. In many instances the disease remains undiagnosed for years.

JA is, in many ways, similar to the adult disease, but there are many features that are quite distinct. A distinguishing feature is its tendency to occur in the prepubertal child. Characteristics of JA include negative results in the latex fixation test in 90% of cases; classic symptoms of spiking fever, skin rash, or pericarditis in 5% to 10% of cases; tendency to be very mild in 70% of cases, with few joints involved; development of iridocyclitis as a complication in 8% to 20% of milder forms; and "burning itself out" over 2 to 3 years in milder forms and over 8 to 10 years in most other forms.

Pathophysiology

The rheumatic process is characterized by a chronic inflammation of the synovium with joint effusion and eventual erosion, destruction, and fibrosis of the articular cartilage. Adhesions between joint surfaces and ankylosis of joints occur if the process persists long enough.

Clinical Manifestations

Whether a single joint or multiple joints are involved, stiffness, swelling, and loss of motion develop in the affected joints. They are swollen and warm to the touch but seldom red. The swelling results from edema, joint effusion, and synovial thickening. The affected joints may be tender and painful to the touch or relatively painless. The limited motion early in the disease is the result of muscle spasm and joint inflammation; later it is caused by ankylosis or soft tissue contracture. Morning stiffness or "gelling" of the joint(s) is characteristic and present on arising in the morning or after inactivity. Infections, injuries, or surgical procedures often precipitate a flare-up of the arthritis; therefore prompt recognition and treatment of infections are necessary.

Growth may be retarded during periods of active disease, usually with growth spurts during remissions. In severe long-standing cases growth is significantly retarded. Corticosteroid therapy is also a contributing factor. There may be growth disturbances, either overgrowth or undergrowth, adjacent to the inflamed joints—for example, altered leg length after knee involvement and micrognathia (receding chin) from temporomandibular arthritis.

JA is a variable disease and is now recognized to pursue three major disease courses: *systemic onset, monoarticular* or *pauciarticular* (involving few joints, usually less than five), and *polyarticular* (simultaneous involvement of four or more joints). These groups, including subgroups, and the manifestations associated with each are outlined in Table 39-6.

Course. The outcome and sources of morbidity are variable and unpredictable in any individual patient. The disease, even in severe forms, is rarely life-threatening. Chronic joint pain is characteristic of polyarticular and systemic disease; the major morbidity in type I patients is chronic iridocyclitis (inflammation of the iris and ciliary body) and spondyloarthropathy in type II disease. There may be exacerbations and remissions or the symptoms may continue for years. The symptoms may cause little disability or (less commonly) are severe with joint destruction and permanent deformity. Although the disease usually remits at puberty, some patients continue to have active arthritis into adulthood.

The overall prognosis for children with JA is good. At least 75% eventually enter long remissions without significant residual deformity or impaired function. The poorest prognosis is associated with rheumatoid factor–positive polyarthritis and systemic-onset disease. The most debilitating complications are severe hip disease and loss of vision from iridocyclitis.

Diagnostic Evaluation

The diagnosis of JA is one of exclusion, that is, differentiation from a variety of disorders with similar manifestations at the onset of the disease. Radiographic findings are variable, but the earliest manifestations are widening joint spaces followed by gradual evidence of fusion and articular destruction. There may be evidence of soft tissue swelling, osteoporosis, and periostitis around affected joints.

There are no specific diagnostic tests for JA. The erythrocyte sedimentation rate may or may not be elevated, depending on the degree of inflammation present. Leukocytosis is generally present in the early stages of classic systemic disease. The latex fixation test, the most common test used to detect the presence of rheumatoid factor in adults, is negative in 90% of juvenile cases. Rheumatoid factors are found in some children, usually those with disease of later onset. Antinuclear antibodies are found in three fourths of rheumatoid factor–positive and one fourth of rheumatoid factor–negative children and in pauciarticular type I diseases, but not in children with systemic onset or pauciarticular type II disease. There is a strong relationship between the presence of antinuclear antibodies and chronic iridocyclitis but no relationship to the severity of the disease.

Therapeutic Management

There is no specific cure for JA. The major goals of therapy are to (1) preserve joint function, (2) prevent physical deformities, and (3) relieve symptoms without iatrogenic harm. This involves both initial and long-term planning, parent and patient education and counseling, physical and occupational therapy, good health and nutritional education and management, specific drug therapy, orthopedic consultation, and periodic eye examination (Brewer and Arroyo, 1986).

Whenever possible, children are treated at home under the supervision of the health team, and intermittent treatment by qualified professionals is administered. Hospitalization may be needed during severe exacerbations or when intercurrent illness warrants. Iridocyclitis, which is unique to JA, can occur and requires the attention of an ophthalmologist.

Drugs. A variety of antirheumatic drugs is available, and most are effective in suppressing the inflammatory process and relieving pain. The drugs may be given alone or in combination.

Table 39-6 Characteristics of juvenile arthritis related to mode of onset

	SYSTEMIC ONSET	PAUCIARTICULAR (TWO OR THREE SUBTYPES)	POLYARTICULAR (TWO SUBTYPES)
Percentage of patients	30%	45%	25%
Age at onset	Bimodal distribution 1-3 years of age 8-10 years of age	Type I: Less than 10 years Type II: over 10 years	Throughout childhood and adolescence
Sex ratio (female/male)	1.5:1	Type I: almost all female Type II: 1:9	Mostly female
Joints involved	Any Only 20% have joint involvement at time of diagnosis	Usually confined to lower extremities—knee, ankle, and eventually sacroiliac; sometimes elbow	Any joints: usually symmetric involvement of small joints Hip involvement in 50% Spine involved in 50%
Extraarticular manifestations	Fever, malaise, myalgia, rash, pleuritis or pericarditis, adenomegaly, splenomegaly, hepatomegaly	Type I: chronic iridocyclitis; mucocutaneous lesions Type II: acute iridocyclitis; sacroiliitis common; eventual ankylosing spondylitis in many Type III: arthritis only	Systemic signs minimal Possible low-grade fever, malaise, weight loss, rheumatoid nodules, and/or vasculitis
Laboratory tests*	Elevated ESR; RF negative; ANA rarely positive; anemia; leukocytosis	Elevated ESR; ANA positive Type I: HLA-DRW5 positive Type II: HLA-B27 positive Type III: HLA-TMo positive	Elevated ESR Type I: RF positive Type II: RF negative
Long-term prognosis	Mortality—1%-2% of all JA patients Joint destruction in 40%	Continuous disease; eventual remission in 60% Type I: ocular damage; functional blindness in 10% Type II: ankylosing spondylitis Type III: best outlook for recovery	Longer duration; more crippling; remission in 25% Type I: high incidence of disabling arthritis Type II: outlook good

*Abbreviations: ESR, erythrocyte sedimentation rate; RF, rheumatoid factor; ANA, antinuclear antibody; HLA, human leukocyte antigen.

NSAIDs. The primary group of drugs prescribed for JA are the nonsteroidal antiinflammatory drugs (NSAIDs). These include aspirin, tolmetin sodium, ibuprofen, and naproxen (see Table 26-4). All these drugs act in a similar manner, and none is superior to the others in producing the desired effects—analgesic, antipyretic, and antiinflammatory. Reduction in fever takes place in hours, relief of pain occurs in a matter of hours or days (more often in weeks, however), but the antiinflammatory effect (reductions in swelling, pain on motion, tenderness, and limitation of motion of involved joints) does not occur for 30 to 37 days (Brewer and Arroyo, 1986). Consequently, these drugs should not be discontinued without an adequate trial period. Sometimes several drugs are tried before one or two are found that are effective and safe for any given child.

Since there is a narrow margin between effective and toxic doses, the levels are monitored regularly until the dosage is sufficient to maintain the optimum level and a satisfactory clinical response. The total daily dose is divided into four doses to be administered with each meal and at bedtime. Some find better compliance when the drug is given only twice daily.

SAARDs. The second group of drugs used to treat JA are the slower-acting antirheumatic drugs (SAARDs). These include gold, D-penicillamine, and hydroxychloroquine. SAARDs may be added to the regimen when one or two NSAIDs have been ineffective. Injectable gold is the initial SAARD used. The weekly injections can be a problem with young children, but cooperation is important. An oral gold preparation is available but not yet approved for use in children. Hydroxychloroquine, an antimalarial drug that requires a longer period of time to effect a response, is seldom used in the United States.

Other drugs. Cytotoxic drugs such as cyclophosphamide, azathioprine, chlorambucil, and methotrexate are reserved for patients with severe debilitating disease and who have responded poorly to NSAIDs and SAARDs.

Corticosteroids are the most potent antiinflammatory agents available. However, they do not cure the disease or prevent joint damage, and their chronic side effects are undesirable. They are administered in the lowest effective dose, given on alternate days rather than daily, and used for the shortest period possible. Indications for daily corticosteroid (prednisone) therapy are life-threatening disease (e.g., pericarditis), incapacitating systemic disease unresponsive to other antiinflammatory therapy, and iridocyclitis.

Physical management. Programs of physical management are individualized for each child and designed to reach the ultimate goal—preserving function and/or preventing deformity. Physical therapy is directed toward specific joints, focusing on strengthening muscles, mobilizing restricted joint motion, and preventing or correcting deformities; occupational therapy assumes responsibility for generalized mobility and performance of activities of daily living.

General treatment or maintenance programs vary; physiotherapists may be involved several times weekly to monthly in management of a home program (ideally in association with the child's school), or their visits may be limited to infrequent review of the home program for compliance, effectiveness, and need. Strength is frequently lost around the involved joints, and inactivity leads to generalized weakness. However, normal activities of daily living and the child's natural tendency to be active are usually sufficient to maintain muscle strength and joint mobility.

Exercising in a pool is excellent, since it allows freedom of movement with support and minimum gravitational pull. When joints are inflamed, heavy resistance aggravates the pain; at such times, simple isometric or tensing exercises that do not involve joint movement are generally tolerated and should be encouraged. Range of motion exercises are an important aspect of therapy and are continued after evidence of disease has disappeared in order to detect any signs of recurrence.

Most physicians recommend splinting and positioning during rest to help minimize pain and prevent or reduce flexion deformity. Joints most frequently splinted are knees, wrists, and hands. Positioning during rest is also important. The child rests on a firm mattress with no pillow or a very low one and has no support under the knee. Loss of extension in the knee, hip, and wrist causes special problems; vigilance is required to detect the earliest signs of involvement, and vigorous attention must be given to specialized passive stretching, positioning, and resting splints to prevent deformity.

Surgery. The benefits of synovectomy, an established preventive and therapeutic procedure in adults, are questionable in the child with rheumatoid arthritis. It is used primarily in pauciarticular disease. Joint replacement is proving successful in older children but is reserved until the child is fully grown. The cooperation of the child is imperative. Joint fusion is sometimes used.

Nursing Considerations

Children with JA present a challenge to themselves and their family and to the professionals who help them cope with this prototype of chronic illness.

Assessment

Nursing children with JA involves assessment of their general health, the status of involved joints, and children's emotional response to all ramifications of the disease—pain, physical restrictions, therapies, and self-concept.

Nursing Diagnoses

Based on a thorough assessment, several nursing diagnoses are identified. The more common diagnoses for the child with JA are included in the Nursing Care Plan on p. 1902. Others may apply in specific situations.

Planning

Nursing objectives for the child with JA include the following:

1. Relieve pain.
2. Promote general health.
3. Prevent physical deformity and preserve joint function.
4. Promote self-care.
5. Support child and family.

Implementation

The effects of the disease are manifest in every aspect of a the child's life—in physical activities, social experiences, and personality development. Much of the children's adjustment to the stresses and demands of the disease and the level of functioning they achieve are directly related to the reaction and support they receive from their family and the health professionals concerned with their care and management.

Relieve pain. The pain of JA is related to several aspects of the disease—disease severity, functional status, individual pain threshold, family variables, and psychologic adjustment. Although complete pain relief would be highly desirable, it is probably unrealistic. The aim is to provide as much relief as possible with antiinflammatory medication and other therapies to help children tolerate the pain and cope as effectively as possible (Lovell and Walco, 1989). At present, narcotic administration is not a routine therapy for chronic pain of JA. Nonpharmacologic modalities have proved effective in modifying pain perception (see Pain Management, Chapter 26) and activities that aggravate pain.

Promote general health. The general health of children and their siblings must be considered and is frequently overlooked as parents and health personnel con-

NURSING CARE PLAN
The Child with Juvenile Rheumatoid Arthritis

NURSING DIAGNOSIS: Pain related to joint inflammation

GOAL 1

Reduce inflammation

INTERVENTIONS

*Administer antiinflammatory drugs

EXPECTED OUTCOMES

Child exhibits no evidence of discomfort
Joints indicate no evidence of inflammation

GOAL 2

Relieve pain

INTERVENTIONS

Provide heat to painful joints by way of
- Tub baths, including whirlpool
- Paraffin baths
- Warm moist pads
- Soaks

Maintain preventive schedule of drug administration
Avoid overexercising painful, swollen joints
See Nursing Care Plan: The Child in Pain, Chapter 26

EXPECTED OUTCOME

Child is able to move with minimum discomfort

NURSING DIAGNOSIS: Impaired physical mobility related to discomfort

GOAL 1

Preserve joint function

INTERVENTIONS

Carry out or supervise physical therapy regimen
- Muscle-strengthening exercises
- Joint mobilization exercises

Apply splints, sandbags, if needed, to maintain position and reduce flexion deformity
Lie flat in bed with joints extended
Use prone position frequently with no pillow, or a very thin one
Incorporate therapeutic exercises in play activities
- Swimming
- Throwing a ball
- Hanging from monkey bar
- Riding tricycle or bicycle

Supervise and encourage activities of daily living
Encourage child's natural tendency to be active

EXPECTED OUTCOMES

Joint flexibility improves in relation to baseline findings
Child develops no contractures
Child engages in activities suitable to interests, capabilities, and developmental level

NURSING DIAGNOSIS: Bathing/hygiene, dressing/grooming, feeding, toileting self-care deficits related to discomfort, immobility

GOAL 1

Perform activities of daily living

INTERVENTIONS

Encourage maximum independence
Provide and/or help devise methods to facilitate independent functioning
- Select clothes for convenience in putting on and fastening
- Modify utensils (spoons, toothbrush, comb, and so on) for easier grasp
- Elevate toilet seat, if needed
- Install handrails for convenience and safety (hallways, bathroom)

Teach application of splints (when able) and encourage responsibility for their use

EXPECTED OUTCOME

Child is involved in self-help to maximum capabilities

GOAL 2

Conserve energy

INTERVENTIONS

Schedule regular periods for sleep and rest, especially during acute flare-ups

EXPECTED OUTCOME

Child engages in appropriate activities without undue fatigue

NURSING DIAGNOSIS: Altered family processes related to a child with a chronic illness

GOAL 1

Support family

INTERVENTIONS AND EXPECTED OUTCOMES

Refer family to special support group(s) and agencies

See also Nursing Care Plan: The Child with a Chronic Illness or Disability, Chapter 22

*Dependent nursing action.

centrate on the disease. A well-balanced diet and assessment of nutritional status are integral parts of health supervision. The discomfort and increased need for rest may create problems of weight control. Excess weight causes additional strain on inflamed joints, especially those of the lower extremities. Excessive fatigue and overexertion should be avoided by regular periods of rest, especially during acute flare-ups of arthritis. Symptoms may exacerbate during a viral illness.

Posture and body mechanics are important for children with JA, both when they are at rest and when they are active. They must have a firm mattress to maintain good alignment of spine, hips, and knees and no pillow or a very thin one. Children who are confined to bed either at home or in the hospital may require supports or splints to maintain positioning. Waterbeds or an electric blanket (or electric sheet) placed under the bottom sheet provides comforting warmth. Lying in the prone position is encouraged to straighten hips and knees, which they can do during rest periods or while watching television. The family is instructed in the principles and purposes of splints so that they can use them judiciously.

School-age children are encouraged to attend school, even on days when there may be some pain or discomfort. The aid of the school nurse is enlisted so that a child is permitted to take the prescribed medication at school and to arrange for rest in the nurse's office during the day. Split days or half days may help a child remain involved in school. Permitting the child to come to school late allows time to gain joint movement and reduces the time at school to avoid exhaustion. It is important that the child attend school to learn skills and engage in social interaction, especially if the JA continues to limit physical skills. Arranging for two sets of textbooks eliminates the need to carry heavy or numerous books to and from school, thus reducing discomfort and difficulty ambulating.

Facilitate compliance. The child and family are involved in the therapeutic plan. They need to know the purpose and correct use of any splints and appliances and the medication regimen. The family is instructed regarding administration of medications as well as the value of a regular schedule of administration to maintain a satisfactory drug level in the body. They need to know that aspirin should not be given on an empty stomach and to be alert for signs of aspirin toxicity, which include hyperventilation as a sign of acidosis, bleeding from decreased clotting capacity, tinnitus (ringing in the ears) as a sign of cranial nerve VIII involvement, and undue drowsiness that may indicate central nervous system depression. If evidence of drug toxicity is noted, the family is instructed to stop the medication and notify the health professional.

Encourage heat and exercise. Heat has been shown to be beneficial to children with arthritis. Moist heat is best for relieving pain and stiffness, and the most efficient and practical method is in the bathtub. The temperature and duration of the bath are specified by the therapist but usually do not exceed 10 minutes at 37.8° C (100° F). Sometimes a daily whirlpool bath, paraffin bath, or hot packs may be used as needed for temporary relief of acute swelling and pain. Hot packs are easily applied at home using a Turkish towel wrung out after being immersed in hot water or heated in a microwave oven, applied to the area, and covered with plastic for 20 minutes. Painful hands or feet can be immersed in a pan of water for 10 minutes two or three times daily in addition to tub baths.

Pool therapy is the easiest method for exercising a large number of joints. Swimming activities strengthen muscles and maintain mobility in larger joints. Children in urban areas have access to a therapy pool, although transportation may be a problem for some families. Very small children who are frightened of the water can carry out their exercises in the bathtub. Small children love to splash, kick, and throw things in the water.

Activities of daily living provide satisfactory exercise for older children to maintain maximum mobility with minimum pain. These children should be encouraged in their efforts and patiently allowed to dress and groom themselves, to assume daily tasks, and to care for their belongings. It is often difficult for stiff fingers to manipulate buttons, comb or brush hair, and turn faucets, but parents and other caregivers should not offer assistance to them. In addition, children should learn and understand why others do not help them. Many helpful devices, such as self-adhering fasteners, tongs for manipulating difficult items, and grab bars installed in bathrooms for safety, can be employed to facilitate tasks. A raised toilet seat often makes the difference between dependent and independent toileting, since weak quadriceps muscles and sore knees inhibit the ability to raise the body from a low sitting position.

A child's natural affinity for play offers many opportunities for incorporating therapeutic exercises. Throwing or kicking a ball, hanging from monkey bars, and riding a tricycle (with seat raised to achieve maximum leg extension) are excellent moving and stretching exercises for a very young child whose daily living activities are physically limited.

An effective approach to beginning the day's activities is to awaken children early to give them the medication and then to allow them to sleep for an hour. On arising, children take a hot bath (or shower) and perform a simple ritual of limbering-up exercises, after which they commence the activities of the day, such as going to school. Exercise, heat, and rest are spaced throughout the remainder of the day according to individual needs and schedules. Parents are instructed in exercises that fit the needs of the child.

The **Arthritis Foundation*** and the **American Juvenile Arthritis Foundation*** provide services for both parents and professionals, and nurses should refer families to these agencies as an added resource.

The child. JA affects every aspect of the child's daily life. The physical pain and limitations interfere with performance of normal tasks and provision of self-care. Even sim-

*1314 Spring St., N.W., Atlanta, GA 30309; (404) 872-7100. In Canada, the **Arthritis Society,** 250 Bloor St. East, Suite 401, Toronto, Ontario, Canada M4W 2P2.

ple tasks, such as dressing, hair combing, use of the bathroom, cutting food, climbing stairs, manipulating doors and faucets, and using public transportation, are difficult or impossible. There may be school difficulties related to transportation to and from school, stairs, and loss of time as a result of exacerbations and hospitalization. Physical limitations interfere with participation in many activities, both curricular and extracurricular, which limits peer contacts and interaction and increases social isolation. These problems are especially critical for adolescents, for whom peer acceptance and relationships are so vital to personality development. These children increasingly turn to solitary activities and to the family at a time when they are expected to move into greater independence and relationships with peers.

Changes in personality usually accompany JA, as with any chronic illness. These changes may be temporary, such as demanding, irritable behavior, or may be manifest in a more permanent way, such as passive hostility, uncommunicativeness, and manipulativeness. Efforts should be made to break through the child's defenses and to identify anxieties, concerns, and conflicts in order to intervene early to prevent the development of permanent personality problems. (See Chapter 22 for problems of the child with chronic illness.)

Families. The beginning of the disease is often sudden and frightening, and its variable course with cycles of remissions and exacerbations is discouraging. Many parents become susceptible to unorthodox cures advanced by well-meaning friends and advertisers. These should be carefully evaluated. Obviously harmless measures such as wearing a copper bracelet need not be discouraged, but parents must be dissuaded from questionable or conspicuously harmful practices such as active exercising of swollen, feverish joints. Parents' understanding of the disease and their attitude toward the child are the key to the success or failure of a treatment program, and major foci of nursing intervention are parental education and support.

Nurses are alert to cues that signal undue anxiety and guilt that may lead to an unhealthy degree of overprotection, such as preoccupation with causative factors, constant analysis of effects of various therapies, experimenting with diets, and continually searching for a magical cure. The dangers of parental overprotection and overindulgence can be especially detrimental to the progress of the child with JA. Sometimes parents are hesitant to give prescribed medications, keep the child home from school unnecessarily, restrict interaction with age-mates, exhibit reluctance to discipline the child, and assume self-care activities that are best performed by the child.

Most of the reactions, problems, and concerns of families of a child with JA are those of any parents of a child with a chronic illness or diability. The impact of the diagnosis is felt most acutely by the parents, who demonstrate anxiety, guilt, and all the manifestations of the grief process. The problems and needs of these families are discussed extensively in Chapter 22, and the reader is directed to this chapter for additional guidance in planning care.

Evaluation

The effectiveness of nursing interventions is determined by continual reassessment and evaluation of care based on the following observational guidelines and expected outcomes:

1. Observe child's behavior and employ pain assessment techniques.
2. Conduct routine assessment of child's general health.
3. Observe the child during planned and unplanned activities, assess mobility of joints, and observe the use of prescribed appliances.
4. Observe child's ability to perform activities of daily living.
5. Observe and interview child and family regarding feelings and concerns.

Expected outcomes:
See the Nursing Care Plan, p. 1902.

LUPUS ERYTHEMATOSUS

Lupus erythematosus (LE), which literally means "red wolf" because of the characteristic butterfly rash on the face of some affected individuals, is a chronic inflammatory disease of the collagen or supporting tissues of the body. It characteristically follows a course of remissions and exacerbations. Because connective tissue is found practically everywhere, almost any organ or structure can be affected.

LE in childhood consists of two basic types: a transient neonatal disease apparently related to maternal pathology and a group of chronic diseases usually having their onset after infancy that correspond to systemic LE (SLE), discoid LE, disseminated LE, subacute cutaneous LE, or lupus panniculitis seen in adults. The major portion of this discussion is limited to SLE.

Etiology

The cause of SLE is not known. It is believed that an autoimmune response to some inciting event such as stress, infection, extreme fatigue, or exposure to various chemicals, drugs, or excessive sunburn triggers a reaction that alters the body's immune response to its own tissues. Supporting evidence for this finding is that (1) many individuals report such events before onset of symptoms and (2) such events enhance an exacerbation of known lupus disease.

Technically SLE is not an inherited disease, although it demonstrates a tendency to occur within families. In addition, family members without actual disease may have findings suggestive of lupus, such as SLE cells, abnormal sensitivity to sun, a history of arthritis or allergies, or unusual drug reactions. It is well documented that some individuals develop a lupuslike reaction to drugs such as isoniazid, penicillin, tetracycline, sulfa preparations, phenothiazines, and phenytoin (Dilantin).

Clinical Manifestations

Because SLE can affect almost any tissue, the clinical manifestations are variable. The onset is usually insidious, with vague signs such as low-grade fever, arthritis or arthralgia, generalized aching, and rash. However, rapid involvement of vital organs, primarily the kidneys, can herald an acceler-

Box 39-16 MANIFESTATIONS OF SYSTEMIC LUPUS ERYTHEMATOSUS RELATED TO TISSUES INVOLVED

Cutaneous lesions—erythematous blush or scaly erythematous patches over bridge of nose and extending to each cheek symmetrically ("butterfly rash"); may extend to scalp, neck, chest, and extremities; sometimes pruritic; resemble severe sunburn or hives or may become bullous
Musculoskeletal system—generalized weakness, usually accompanied by arthritis, myalgia, joint swelling, and stiffness; usually not severe enough to cause deformity; pain may cause temporary disability
Central nervous system—varies from forgetfulness, excitability, and headache to seizures and frank psychosis; seizures may be early sign; any cranial nerves can be affected; paralysis (spinal cord involvement)
Heart and lungs—serous linings may be inflamed; pleurisy (lungs), pericarditis (heart); usually reversible with rest
Kidneys—glomerulus usual site of destruction; proteinuria; kidney failure
Blood—anemia from decreased erythrocytes common; amenorrhea secondary to anemia; platelets and plasma proteins may be affected
Lymphoid system—spleen and cervical, axillary, and inguinal lymph nodes enlarged (sometimes); LE hepatitis may develop
Gastrointestinal tract—nausea, vomiting, diarrhea, and abdominal pain possible

ated course with minimum or absent involvement of other sites. Box 39-16 describes manifestations related to various tissues involved.

The majority of children (approximately 90%) with SLE have cutaneous involvement at some time during their illness, and about one third of children have skin disease as the chief complaint. Some patients experience sensitivity to cold (Raynaud phenomenon), especially in the hands and feet. Cyanosis may be present, and ulcers often develop in dry, cracked skin. Patchy areas of alopecia may occur, although during remission the hair usually regrows.

Renal involvement is a serious complication of SLE. Presumably antigen-antibody complexes deposited primarily in the glomerular basement membrane initiate an inflammatory response that results in tissue damage and consequent kidney failure. Although supportive approaches, such as hemodialysis and kidney transplant, have improved the outlook for these patients, tissue damage in other vital organs, especially the heart and lungs, may foreshorten the benefits derived from life-supporting techniques.

Diagnostic Evaluation

SLE has been called the "great imitator," since its clinical manifestations may point to a variety of unrelated conditions. The diagnosis of SLE is established by the demonstration of any four of eleven diagnostic criteria (Box 39-17).

A neurologic examination should be done to provide baseline data for evaluating subtle changes in behavior and function. Sometimes a psychiatric evaluation may also be warranted, since personality alterations caused by steroids and renal damage are difficult to distinguish from those resulting from central nervous system involvement.

Box 39-17 CRITERIA FOR DIAGNOSIS OF SYSTEMIC LUPUS ERYTHEMATOSUS

1. Butterfly rash
2. Discoid rash
3. Photosensitivity
4. Oral ulcers
5. Arthritis
6. Serositis
7. Renal disorder
8. Neurologic disorder(s) (psychosis, coma, seizures, paresis)
9. Hematologic disorder(s) (anemia, thrombocytopenia, leukopenia)
10. Immunologic disorder(s) (anti-DNA, LE prep, anti-SM, STS)
11. Antinuclear antibody

Therapeutic Management

The objectives of medical treatment are (1) to reverse the autoimmune and inflammatory processes and (2) to prevent exacerbations and complications. Therapy involves the use of specific and supportive medications and regulation of activity and diet.

Drugs. The principal drugs used to control inflammation are the corticosteroids, administered in doses sufficient to suppress symptoms, then tapered to the lowest suppressive dose. One alternative is the "pulse" method, the administration of a large dose of steroids intravenously over a 20- to 30-minute period on 3 consecutive days. Large doses may be needed to treat seizures and other central nervous system manifestations. Sometimes the immunosuppressive agent azathioprine (Imuran) helps reduce the amount of steroids needed.

Another group of drugs effective in relieving the dermatologic, arthritic, and renal symptoms of the disease are antimalarial preparations, such as hydroxychloroquine (Plaquenil) and chloroquine (Aralen). Although the exact action of these drugs on SLE is not known, often they permit a continued remission with a lowered dose of steroids.

NSAIDs, such as aspirin, relieve muscle and joint pains and reduce tissue inflammation. Drugs used to control various complications include anticonvulsants, antihypertensives, and antibiotics. The selection of appropriate medication in each of these categories is essential, since many of them greatly aggravate the disease process and affect renal function.

Regulation of activity and diet. The goal of restricted activity is to prevent a recurrence of the disease. Although the exact relationship is unclear, fatigue, stress, or sudden exertion brings about a relapse of symptoms. An effective schedule must provide for gradual resumption of pre-SLE activity and maximum rest periods, usually 8 to 10 hours of sleep a night and one or two rest times during the day.

Diet may be restricted depending on weight gain and/or fluid retention from steroids and renal damage. The most frequently prescribed diet modification is moderate or low salt. Low-protein diets may be necessary to prevent elevated nitrogen levels. Weight reduction may help preserve maximum joint function and conserve energy.

Nursing Considerations

The principal nursing goals are to (1) help the child and family adjust to the limitations and treatments of the disease and (2) prevent exacerbations and complications. Since older female adolescents are the most likely group to be affected, the nurse must have an awareness of their special needs, such as body image changes, present and future vocational activities, social relationships, and emerging sexuality. Although this is a potentially fatal disorder, nurses are encouraged to apply those principles of adjusting to a chronic illness that are discussed in Chapter 22.

Assist family in adjusting to disease and its treatment. SLE is a complex disease. Although much is known about its effect on connective tissues and appropriate types of treatment, few concrete facts are available. However, family members need an understanding of the disease process to gain an appreciation of the necessity of regular, uninterrupted drug administration, moderate activity, and dietary modifications. Usually diagnostic tests are performed during hospitalization, which allows the nurse an opportunity to help the family learn about the disease.

Several organizations have been formed to help children and families learn about and adjust to the disease. These include the **American Lupus Society*** and the **Lupus Foundation of America.†** The nurse should be aware of what information the family is receiving, because learning about joint deformity, sudden bouts of pain and disability, a disfiguring rash, and the possibility of renal failure can be overwhelming. Nurses should also be aware of advertised nonmedical approaches to treatment, since quackery abounds when no known cure exists.

The nurse has the responsibility of helping the adolescent adjust to drug therapy. The side effects of steroids and immunosuppressant drugs are discussed under Modes of Therapy, Chapter 36, and outlined in Table 36-3. Most of the antimalarial drugs have few side effects. However, hydroxychloroquine and chloroquine can cause irreversible retinal damage; therefore frequent ophthalmic examinations are necessary. In addition, after exposure to the sun, the skin may tan less and become more erythematous and the hair may lighten.

Body image changes from both the disease and the drugs are a major concern. Each of these should be approached in a positive manner by discussing the use of cosmetics and wigs. Sometimes health professionals fail to assess adequately the child's adjustment reactions and regard the depression and withdrawal as effects of the disease rather than a response to body image changes.

Lifelong restricted activity imposes many hardships for these children, although they may be able to continue to participate in moderation. The child and family need to weigh the consequences of activity against the pleasures. For example, a day of skiing, with proper sun precautions, may be worth the achiness for the following day or even week. This provides the youngster with some sense of control over events. The severity of the disease is also a factor if the risk of irreversible damage is great.

Prevent exacerbations and complications. The list of "don'ts" for these individuals is long; therefore compliance may be a serious problem. The need for adherence to the medication schedule is paramount. Some adolescents, in an attempt to lessen the side effects of steroids, may elect to skip a few doses. Adherence is important to maintain a remission but must be taken daily (or as prescribed) to prevent sudden withdrawal from the drug, which may precipitate a serious physiologic crisis. The dosage may need to be altered at times of stress. Affected persons should carry an identification card or Medic Alert tag emphasizing their dependence on steroids.

Skin care is important. In those individuals who are sensitive to the sun, exposure must be avoided. It is important to stress that reflected sun through clouds, on snow, on water, or on white cement can cause a severe reaction. Although clothes can protect most areas of the body, special sunscreening agents are necessary for the face (see Chapter 18). A large-brimmed hat helps to shade the face.

Sometimes patients are requested to check their urine routinely for protein. The youngster with kidney involvement is subject to long-term management that may entail hemodialysis and/or kidney transplant. Nursing considerations for each procedure are discussed in Chapter 30.

KEY POINTS

- Trauma is the leading cause of death in children and is caused by accidental injury, child abuse injury, and birth injuries.
- Immobility has a profound effect on all elements of growth and development.
- The major consequences of immobilization are loss of muscle strength, endurance, and muscle mass; bone demineralization leading to osteoporosis; loss of joint mobility; and contractures.
- In the care of the immobilized child, nurses are concerned with position changes, adequate dietary intake, adequate hydration, promotion of activity, and involvement of child in self-care.

*23751 Madison St., Torrence, CA 90505; (213) 373-1335.

†1717 Massachusetts Ave, N.W., Suite 203, Washington, DC 20036; (202) 328-4550.

- Features of children's fractures not observed in the adult include presence of growth plate, thicker and stronger periosteum, porosity of bone, more rapid healing, and less stiffness.
- Types of fractures seen in children are bends, buckle, greenstick, and complete.
- Goals of fracture management in children are to regain alignment and length of the bony fragments, retain alignment and length, and restore function to injured parts.
- The method of fracture reduction is determined by the age of the child, degree of displacement, amount of overriding, amount of edema, condition of skin and soft tissues, sensation, and circulation distal to fracture.
- The primary purposes of traction are to fatigue involved muscle and reduce muscle spasm, to position bone ends in desired realignment, and to immobilize fracture site until realignment has been achieved to permit casting or splinting.
- Complications of fractures are circulatory impairment, nerve compression syndromes, compartment syndromes, epiphyseal damage, nonunion, malunion, infection, kidney stones, and pulmonary emboli.
- Participation in sports predisposes adolescents to acute injuries, such as contusions, dislocations, sprains, and strains, and overuse syndromes, such as stress fractures.
- Health concerns associated with sports are related menstrual dysfunction, drug misuse, and sudden death.
- Musculoskeletal dysfunctions in childhood include torticollis, Legg-Calvé-Perthes disease, slipped femoral capital epiphyses, kyphosis and lordosis, and scoliosis.
- Nonoperative management of scoliosis includes bracing, exercise, and electrical stimulation.
- Nursing care of the child with osteomyelitis is directed at positioning, careful monitoring of vital signs, drugs, intravenous equipment and site, and nutrition.
- Osteomyelitis is acquired by direct or secondary invasion or hematogenous spread of infectious organisms.
- Goals of therapy for juvenile arthritis are to preserve joint function, prevent physical deformities, and relieve symptoms without iatrogenic harm.
- Nursing care of juvenile arthritis involves promoting general health, facilitating compliance, and encouraging exercise.
- Objectives of therapy for lupus erythematosus are to reverse autoimmune and inflammatory processes and to prevent exacerbations and complications.

REFERENCES

Allen, B.L., Jr., and Ferguson, R.L.: Management of the child with school referral for scoliosis, Pediatr. Clin. North Am. 32:1333-1345, 1985.

American Academy of Pediatrics, Committee on Aspects of Physical Fitness, Recreation, and Sports, Pediatrics 67:927-928, 1981.

American Academy of Pediatrics, Committee on Sports Medicine: Sports medicine: health care for young athletes, Evanston, IL, 1983, American Academy of Pediatrics.

American Academy of Pediatrics, Committee on Sports Medicine: Participation in boxing among children and young adults, Pediatrics 74:311-312, 1984.

American Academy of Pediatrics, Committee on Sports Medicine: Recommendations for participation in competitive sports, Pediatrics 81:737-739, 1988.

American Academy of Pediatrics, Committee on Sports Medicine: Anabolic steroids and the adolescent athlete, Pediatrics 83:127-128, 1989.

Barrack, R.L., and others: Proprioception in idiopathic scoliosis, Spine 9:681-685, 1984.

Berwick, D.M.: Scoliosis screening: a pause in the chase, Am. J. Public Health 75:1371-1374, 1985.

Braisted, J.R., and others: The adolescent ballet dancer: nutritional practices and characteristics associated with anorexia nervosa, J. Adolesc. Health Care 6:365-371, 1985.

Brewer, E.J., and Arroyo, M.: Use of nonsteroidal anti-inflammatory drugs in children, Pediatr. Ann. 15:575-581, 1986.

Bunnell, W.P.: An objective criterion for scoliosis screening, J. Bone Joint Surg. 66-A:1381-1385, 1984.

Cohen, F.L.: Clinical genetics in nursing practice, Philadelphia, 1984, J.B. Lippincott Co.

Cook, D.E., and Gustafson, P.R.G.: Sports health care for children and adolescents, Pediatr. Nurs. Update 1(15):1-8, 1986.

Costill, D.L.: Water and electrolyte requirements during exercise, Clin. Sports Med. 3:639-644, 1984.

Cross, A.W.: Health screening in schools, part III, J. Pediatr. 107:653-661, 1985,

Davis, S.E., and Lewis, S.A.: Managing scoliosis: fashions for the body and mind, MCN 9:186-187, 1984.

Diddle, A.W.: Athletic activity and menstruation, South. Med. J. 76:619-624, 1983.

Dyment, P.G.: Initial management of minor acute soft-tissue injuries, Pediatr. Ann. 17:99-106, 1988.

Fisher, M.C., Goldsmith, J.F., and Gilligan, P.H.: Sneakers as a source of *Pseudomonas aeruginosa* in children with osteomyelitis following puncture wounds, J. Pediatr. 106:607-609, 1985.

Frishe, R.E., and McArthur, J.W.: Menstrual cycles: fatness as a determinant of minimum weight for height necessary for their maintenance and onset, Science 186:4543-467, 1974.

Garn, S.M., LaVelle, M., and Pilkington, J.J.: Comparison of fatness in premenarcheal and postmenarcheal girls of the same age, J. Pediatr. 103:328-331, 1983.

Gratz, R.R., and Papalia-Finlay, D.: Psychosocial adaptation to wearing the Milwaukee brace for scoliosis: a pilot study of adolescent females and their mothers, J. Adolesc. Health Care 5:237-242, 1984.

Hale, R.W.: Exercise, sports, and menstrual dysfunction, Clin. Obstet. Gynecol. 26:728-735, 1983.

Johnson, M.D., and others: Anabolic steroid use by male adolescents, Pediatrics 83:921-924, 1989.

Jurkowski, J.E., and others: Ovarian hormonal responses to exercise, J. Appl. Physiol. 44:109-114, 1978.

Loosli, A.R.: Athletes, food and nutrition, Food Nutr. News 62(3):15-20, 1990.

Loucks, A.B., and Horvath, S.M.: Athletic amenorrhea: a review, Med. Sci. Sports Exerc. 17:56-72, 1985.

Lovell, D.J., and Walco, G.A.: Pain associated with juvenile rheumatoid arthritis, Pediatr. Clin. North Am. 36:1015-1027, 1989.

Luckstead, E.F.: Sudden death in sports, Pediatr. Clin. North Am. 29:1355-1362, 1982.

Malina, R.M., Meleski, B.W., and Shoup, R.F.: Anthropometric, body composition, and maturity characteristics of selected school-age athletes, Pediatr. Clin. North Am. 29:1305-1323, 1982.

McCullough, F.L., and Evans, L.M.: Assessment of neurovascular status in children, Orthop. Nurs. 4(4):19-25, 1985.

McCollough, N.C., III: Electrical stimulation in management of idiopathic scoliosis. In Stauffer, E.S., editor: Instructional course lectures, vol. 36, St. Louis, 1985, Mosby–Year Book, Inc.

Micheli, L.J., Magin, M.A., and Rouvales, R.: The patient with scoliosis: surgical management and nursing care, Am. J. Nurs. 79:1599-1607, 1979.

Miller, J.A.A., Nachemson, A.L., and Schultz, A.B.: Effectiveness of braces in mild idiopathic scoliosis, Spine 9:632-635, 1984.

Morais, T., and others: Age- and sex-specific prevalence of scoliosis and the value of school screening programs, Am. J. Public Health 75:1377-1380, 1985.

Murray, R.: The effects of consuming carbohydrate-electrolyte beverages on gastric emptying and fluid absorption during and following exercise, Sports Med. 4:322-328, 1987.

Narins, D.M., Belkengren, R.P., and Sapala, S.: Nutrition and the growing athlete, Pediatr. Nurs. 9:163-168, 1983.

Nelson, M.A.: Androgenic-anabolic steroid use in adolescents, J. Pediatr. Health Care 3:175-180, 1989.

Nichols, H.H.: Nursemaid's elbow: reducing it to simple terms, Contemp. Pediatr. 5(5):50-57, 1988.

Northrup, C.E., and Kelly, M.E.: Legal issues in nursing, St. Louis, 1987, Mosby–Year Book, Inc.

Ogilvie, B.C.: The orthopedist's role in childen's sports, Orthop. Clin. North Am. 14:361-372, 1982.

Orava, S.: Stress fractures, Br. J. Sports Med. 14:40-44, 1980.

Pillemer and Micheli; Psychological considerations in youth sports, Clin. Sports Med. 7:679-689, 1988.

Primos, W.A., and Landry, G.L.: Fighting the fads in sports nutrition, Contemp. Pediatr. 6(9):14-50, 1989.

Puri, R., and others: Slipped upper femoral epiphysis and primary juvenile hypothyroidism, J. Bone Joint Surg. 67-B:14-20, 1985.

Ramenofsky, M.L., and Morse, T.S.: Standards of care for the critically injured pediatric patient, J. Trauma 22:921-933, 1983.

Renshaw, T.S.: Orthotic treatment of idiopathic scoliosis and kyphosis. In Stauffer, E.S., editor: Instructional course lectures, vol. 36, St. Louis, 1985, Mosby–Year Book, Inc.

Rivara, F.P., Parish, R.A., and Mueller, B.A.: Extremity injuries in children: predictive value of clinical findings, Pediatrics 78:803-807, 1986.

Robinson, M.D., and Seward, P.N.: Heat injury in children, Pediatr. Emerg. Care 3:114-117, 1987.

Root, L.: The treatment of osteogenesis imperfecta, Orthop. Clin. North Am. 15:775-790, 1984.

Rosenstein, B.J.: Summer tips: heat exhaustion and heatstroke, Contemp. Pediatr. 6(5):92-93, 1989.

Runyan, C.W., and Gerken, E.A.: Epidemiology and prevention of adolescent injury: a review and research agenda, JAMA 262:2273-2279, 1989.

Shangold, M.M., and Mirkin, G.: The adolescent athlete. In Lavery, J.P., and Sanfilippo, J.S., editors: Pediatric and adolescent obstetrics and gynecology, New York, 1985, Springer-Verlag New York, Inc.

Sibinga, M.S., and Freedman, C.J.: Restraint and speech, Pediatrics 48:116-122, 1971.

Smith, N.J.: Nutrition in children's sports. In Micheli, L.J., editor: Pediatric and adolescent sports medicine, Boston, 1984, Little, Brown & Co., Inc.

Squire, D.L.: Female athletes, Pediatr. Rev. 9:183-187, 1987.

Staheli, L.T.: The hip. In Gellis, S.S., and Kagan, B.M.: Current pediatric therapy 12, Philadelphia, 1986, W.B. Saunders Co.

Strauss, R.H.: Medical concerns in underwater sports, Pediatr. Clin. North Am. 29:1431-1440, 1982.

Van Allen, M.W.: The deadly degrading sport (editorial), JAMA 249:249-250, 1983.

Viviani, G.R., and others: Assessment of accuracy of the scoliosis school screening examination, Am. J. Public Health 74:497-498, 1984.

Warren, M.P.: The effects of exercise on pubertal progression and reproductive function in girls, J. Clin. Endocrinol. Metab. 51:1150-1155, 1980.

Warren, M.P.: Amenorrheic athletes may heed MD's warning of injury risk, Obstet. Gyencol. News 24:12, 1989.

Warren, M.P., and others: Scoliosis and fractures in young ballet dancers: relation to delayed menarche and secondary amenorrhea, N. Engl. J. Med. 309:1348-1353, 1986.

Watts, H.G.: Orthopedic problems. In Behrman, R.E., and Vaughan, V.C., III: Textbook of pediatrics, ed. 13, Philadelphia, 1987, W.B. Saunders Co.

Wynne, E.J.: Scoliosis screening: to screen or not to screen, Can. J. Public Health 75:1377-1380, 1985.

Ziporyn, T.: Latest clue to exercise-induced amenorrhea, JAMA 252:1259-1263, 1984.

Ziporyn, T.: Scoliosis management now subject of numerous questions, JAMA 254:3009-3019, 1985.

BIBLIOGRAPHY

General

Blatzheim, L.L., Edberg, A., and Lacy, L.: Operationalizing primary nursing in the pediatric rehabilitation setting, J. Pediatr. Nurs. 2:434-437, 1987.

Brady, M., and Grey, M.: Growing pains: a myth or a reality, J. Pediatr. Health Care 3:219-220, 1989.

Dudek, G.: Nursing update: hypophosphatemic rickets, Pediatr. Nurs. 15:45-50, 1989.

Mason, K.J.: Pediatric orthopaedics: developmental norms, Orthop. Nurs. 8(4):45-50, 1989.

Peterson, H.: Growing pains, Pediatr. Clin. North Am. 33:1365-1372, 1986.

Quan, L., and Marcuse, E.K.: The epidemiology and treatment of radial head subluxation, Am. J. Dis. Child. 139:1194-1197, 1985.

Sigmon, H.D.: Helping your long-term trauma patient travel the road to recovery, Nursing '84 14(1):58-63, 1984.

Sills, E.M.: What's causing the back pain? Contemp. Pediatr. 5(11):85-96, 1988.

Szer, I.S.: Are those limb pains "growing" pains? Contemp. Pediatr. 6(3):143-148, 1989.

Trauma

Alexander, R., and others: Serial abuse in children who are shaken, Am. J. Dis. Child. 144:58-60, 1990.

Campbell, P.M.: Transportation of the critically ill and injured child, Crit. Care Q. 8(1):1-12, 1985.

Crawford, A.H., and Cionni, A.S.: Management of pediatric orthopedic injuries by the emergency medicine specialist. In Pierog, J.E., and Pierog, L.J., editors: Pediatric critical illness and injury, Rockville, MD, 1984, Aspen Systems Corp.

Haller, J.A., and others: Organization and function of a regional pediatric trauma center: does a system of management improve outcome? J. Trauma 23:691-696, 1983.

Harris, B.H.: Management of multiple trauma, Pediatr. Clin. North Am. 32:175-181, 1985.

Harris, B.H., and others: The crucial hour, Pediatr. Ann. 16:301-304, 1987.

Jamison, D.W.: When emergency care is up to you, RN 50(4):26-31, 1987.

King, D.R.: Trauma in infancy and childhood: initial evaluation and management, Pediatr. Clin. North Am. 32:1299-1310, 1985.

King, R.C.: Dealing with abrasions and lacerations, RN 47(6):53-56, 1984.

Leyendecker, M., and others: Rescuing a multiple trauma victim, Nursing '89 19(10):54-61, 1989.

Morse, T.S.: The child with multiple injuries, Emerg. Med. Clin. North Am. 1:175-185, 1983.

Phelps, E.D.: Trauma assessment of the pediatric patient, Point of View 24(3):8, 1987.

Ragiel, C.A.: The impact of critical injury on patient, family, and clinical systems, Crit. Care Q. 7(3):73-78, 1984.
Rich, J.: Principles of trauma care, Point of View 24(3):4-5, 1987.
Stevens, W.S., Rodgers, B.M., and Newman, B.M.: Pediatric trauma associated with all-terrain vehicles, J. Pediatr. 109:25-29, 1986.
Thomas, D.O.: The ABCs of pediatric emergencies, RN 47(3):34-41, 1984.
Veise-Berry, S.W.: Nursing considerations during radiologic examination of the massively injured trauma patient, Crit. Care Q. 6(1):55-63, 1983.
Wong, D.L.: Childhood trauma: its developmental aspects and nursing interventions, Crit. Care Q. 5(2):47-59, 1982.

Immobilization

Baird, S.E.: Development of a nursing assessment tool to diagnose altered body image in immobilized patients, Orthop. Nurs. 4(1):47-54, 1985.
Cuzzell, J.Z.: Readers' remedies for pressure sores, Am. J. Nurs. 86:923-924, 1986.
Karn, M.A., and Ragiel, C.A.: The psychologic effects of immobilization on the pediatric patient, Orthop. Nurs. 5(6):12-16, 1986.
Olson, E.V.: The hazards of immobility, Am. J. Nurs. 90:43-52, 1990.
Rubin, M.: The physiology of bed rest, Am. J. Nurs. 88:50-58, 1988.
Willey, T.: High-tech beds and mattress overlays, Am. J. Nurs. 89:1142-1145, 1989.

Fractures

Benz, J.: The adolescent in a spica cast, Orthop. Nurs. 5(3):22-23, 1986.
Cochran, S.: Open fracture, Nursing '87 17(5):33, 1987.
Conrad, E.U., and Rang, M.C.: Fractures and sprains, Pediatr. Clin. North Am. 33:1523-1540, 1986.
Cuddy, C.M.: Caring for a child in a spica cast: a parent's perspective, Orthop. Nurs. 5(3):17-20, 1986.
Evers, J.A., and Werpachowski, D.: Dealing with fractures, RN 47(11):53-57, 1984.
Feller, N.G., Stroup, K., and Christian, L.: Helping staff nurses become mini-specialists, Am. J. Nurs. 89:991-992, 1989.
Gamron, R.: Taking the pressure out of compartment syndrome, Am. J. Nurs. 88:1076-1080, 1988.
Hamdan, J.A., Taleb, Y.A., and Ahmed, M.S.: Traction induced hypertension in children, Clin. Orthop. 185:87-89, 1984.
Hansell, M.J.: Fractures and the healing process, Orthop. Nurs. 7(1):43-49, 1988.
Ibrahim, K.: An overview of childhood fractures, Pediatr. Nurs. 10:57-65, 1984.
Lane, P.L., and Lee, M.M.: Synthetic materials have changed casts and cast care, Nursing '83 13(7):50-51, 1983.
Lavin, R.J.: The high-pressure demands of compartment syndrome, RN 52(2):22-25, 1989.
Mather, M.L.S.: The secret to life in a spica, Am. J. Nurs. 87:56-58, 1987.
McCullough, F.L.: Skeletal trauma in children, Orthop. Nurs. 8(2):41-50, 1989.
Morris, L., and others: Special care for skeletal traction, RN 51(2):24-29, 1988.
Morris, L., and others: Nursing the patient in traction, RN 51(1):26-31, 1988.
Rang, M., and Wright, J.: Pitfalls in fractures, Pediatr. Ann. 18:53-68, 1989.
Redheffer, G.M., and Bailely, M.: Assessing and splinting fractures, Nursing '89 19(6):51-59, 1989.
Robinson, J.E., and Marx, L.O.: A nail-safe method, Am. J. Nurs. 85:158-161, 1985.
Rockwood, C.A., Jr., Wilkins, K.E., and King, R.E., editors: Fractures in children, vol. 3, Philadelphia, 1984, J.B. Lippincott Co.
Swingle, M.: Children's cast care, Child. Nurse 6(5):1-3, 1988.
Wise, L.B.: A comparison of orthopedic casts: breaking the mold, MCN 11:174-176, 1986.

Amputation

Barker-Stotts, K.A.: Traumatic amputation, Nursing '88 18(5):51, 1988.
Cmiel, P.A., and Cavanaugh, C.E.: Digital replantation in children, Am. J. Nurs. 89:1158-1161, 1989.
Miller, R.A., and Evans, W.E.: Immediate postop prosthesis, Am. J. Nurs. 87:310-311, 1987.
Varni, J.W., and others: Family functioning, temperament, and psychologic adaptation in children with congenital or acquired limb deficiencies, Pediatrics 84:323-330, 1989.

Disorders Related to Sports

American Academy of Pediatrics, Committee on Drugs and Committee on Sports Medicine: Dimethyl sulfoxide (DMSO), Pediatrics 71:76, 1983.
American Academy of Pediatrics, Committee on Sports Medicine: Amenorrhea in adolescent athletes, Pediatrics 84:394-395, 1989.
American Academy of Pediatrics, Committee on Sports Medicine: Knee brace use by athletes, Pediatrics 85:228, 1990.
Backous, D.D., and others: Soccer injuries and their relation to physical maturity, Am. J. Dis. Child. 142:839-842, 1988.
Bar-Or, O.: Exercise in prepubertal girls: what are the limits? Contemp. Pediatr. 4(1):124-129, 1987.
Council on Scientific Affairs: Drug abuse in athletes, JAMA 259:1703-1705, 1988.
Dickson, T.B., and Kichline, P.D.: Functional management of stress fractures in female athletes using a pneumatic leg brace, Am. J. Sports Med. 15:86-89, 1987.
Garrett, W.E., Jr.: Strains and sprains in athletes, Postgrad. Med. 73(3):200-209, 1983.
Garrick, J.G.: Sports medicine, Pediatr. Clin. North Am. 33:1541-1550, 1986.
Goldberg, B., and others: Injuries in youth football, Pediatrics 81:255-261, 1988.
Kris-Etherton, P.M.: Nutrition and athletic performance, Contemp. Nutr. 14(8), 1989.
Krowchuk, D.P., and others: High school athletes and the use of ergogenic aids, Am. J. Dis. Child. 143:486-489, 1989.
Latinis, B.: Frequent sports injuries of children: etiology, treatment, and prevention, Issues Compr. Pediatr. Nurs. 6:167-178, 1983.
McLain, L.G., and Reynolds, S.: Sports injuries in a high school, Pediatrics 84:446-450, 1989.
Micheli, L.J.: Overuse injuries in children's sports: the growth factor, Orthop. Clin. North Am. 14:337-360, 1983.
Nickerson, H.J., and others: Causes of iron deficiency in adolescent athletes, J. Pediatr. 114:657-663, 1989.
Ouellette, M.D., MacVicar, M.G., and Harlan, J.: Relationship between percent body fat and menstrual patterns in athletes and nonathletes, Nurs. Res. 35:330-333, 1986.
Pope, H.G., and Katz, D.L.: Affective and psychotic symptoms associated with anabolic steroid use, Am. J. Psychiatry 145:487-491, 1988.
Pratt, M.: Strength, flexibility, and maturity in adolescent athletes, Am. J. Dis. Child. 143:560-563, 1989.
Puhl, J.: Iron and exercise interactions, Contemp. Nutr. 12(2), 1987.
Rowland, T.W., and Kelleher, J.F.: Iron deficiency in athletes, Am. J. Dis. Child. 143:197-200, 1989.
Stover, C.N., and DeBald, M.: Guide to lateral ankle sprain management, Orthop. Nurs. 5(3):34-39, 1986.
Strong, W.B., and Wilmore, J.H.: Unfit kids: an office-based approach to physical fitness, Contemp. Pediatr. 5(4):33-48, 1988.
Sullivan, J.A.: Recurring pain in the pediatric athlete, Pediatr. Clin. North Am. 31:1097-1112, 1984.
Terney, R., and McLain, L.G.: The use of anabolic steroids in high school students, Am. J. Dis. Child. 144:99-103, 1990.
Tsimoyianis, G.V., and others: Reduction in pulmonary function and increased frequency of cough associated with passive smoking in teenage athletes, Pediatrics 80:32-36, 1987.

Williams, M.H.: Nutritional ergogenic aids and athletic performance, Nutr. Today, pp. 7-14, Jan./Feb. 1989.
Wilson, M.C., and Fischer, R.G.: Drug use in sports, Pediatr. Nurs. 12:452, 1986.
Yelverton, G.A.: Anabolic steroids, Pediatr. Nurs. 15:63, 1989.

Musculoskeletal Disorders

Benchot, R.J.: The adolescent with slipped capital femoral epiphysis, Point of View 19:6-9, 1982.
Bunnell, W.P.: Back pain in children, Orthop. Clin. North Am. 13:587-603, 1982.
Colter, J.M.: Office management in Legg-Calvé-Perthes syndrome, Orthop. Clin. North Am. 13:619-627, 1982.
Malkiewicz, J.: A pragmatic approach to musculoskeletal assessment, RN 45(11):57-62, 1982.

Scoliosis

Allard, J.L., and Dibble, S.L.: Scoliosis surgery: a look at Luque rods, Am. J. Nurs. 84:609-611, 1984.
Axelgaard, J., and Brown, J.C.: Lateral electrical surface stimulation for the treatment of progressive idiopathic scoliosis, Spine 8:242-260, 1983.
Bridwell, K.H.: Cotrel-Dubousset instrumentation, Orthop. Nurs. 7(1):11-16, 1988.
Bunnell, W.P.: Spinal deformity, Pediatr. Clin. North Am. 33:1475-1487, 1986.
DiRaimondo, C.V., and Green, N.E.: Brace-wear compliance in patients with adolescent idiopathic scoliosis, J. Pediatr. Orthop. 8:143-146, 1988.
Eckerson, L.F., and Axelgaard, J.: Lateral electrical surface stimulation as an alternative to bracing the treatment of idiopathic scoliosis: treatment protocol and patient acceptance, Phys. Ther. 64:483-490, 1984.
Fitz, C.R.: Diagnostic imaging in children with spinal disorders, Pediatr. Clin. North Am. 32:1537-1558, 1985.
Francis, E.E.: Lateral electrical surface stimulation treatment for scoliosis, Pediatr. Nurs. 13:157-160, 1987.
Hall, J.E.: Preoperative assessment of the patient with a spinal deformity. In Stauffer, E.S., editor: Instructional course lectures, vol. 36, St. Louis, 1985, Mosby–Year Book, Inc.
Jacobs-Zacny, J.M., and Horn, M.J.: Nursing care of adolescents having posterior spinal fusion with Cotrel-Dubousset instrumentation, Orthop. Nurs. 7(1):17-21, 1988.
Johnson, J.B., and Killman-Young, J.: Adolescence, anxiety, and adaptation: preparing for posterior spine fusion with instrumentation, J. Pediatr. Nurs. 3:348-349, 1988.
Jones, M.C.: Clinical approach to the child with scoliosis, Pediatr. Rev. 6:219-222, 1985.
Kahanovitz, N., and Weiser, S.: Lateral electrical surface stimulation (LESS) compliance in adolescent female scoliosis patients, Spine 7:753-755, 1987.
Luque, E.R.: Segmental spinal instrumentation for correction scoliosis, Clin. Orthop. 163:192-198, 1982.
Rauen, K.K., and Ho, M.: Children's use of patient-controlled analgesia after spine surgery, Pediatr. Nurs. 15:589-593, 1989.
Thomas, P.: Nursing care of patients undergoing posterior spinal fusion with segmental (Luque) spinal instrumentation, Orthop. Nurs. 2(3):13-20, 1983.
Voznak, L.: My life with scoliosis, Orthop. Nurs. 7(1):22-26, 1988.

Orthopedic Infections

Aronoff, S.C., and Scoles, P.V.: Treatment of childhood skeletal infections, Pediatr. Clin. North Am. 30:271-280, 1983.
Barton, L.L., Dunkle, L.M., and Habib, F.H.: Septic arthritis in childhood, Am. J. Dis. Child. 141:898-900, 1987.
Kilcoyne, R.F., and Plumly, T.F.: Infections of bones and joints, Nurs. Pract. 8(3):12, 63, 66, 1983.
Morrissy, R.T., and Shore, S.L.: Bone and joint sepsis, Pediatr. Clin. North Am. 33:1551-1564, 1986.
Volberg, F.M., and others: Unreliability of radiographic diagnosis of septic hip in children, Pediatrics 73:118-120, 1984.

Osteogenesis Imperfecta

Binder, H., and others: Osteogenesis imperfecta: rehabilitation approach with infants and young children, Arch. Phys. Med. Rehabil. 65:537-541, 1984.
Guerrein, A.T.: Osteogenesis imperfecta: a disorder that breaks more than our hearts, MCN 7:315-318, 1982.
Sillence, D.: Osteogenesis imperfecta: an expanding panorama of variants, Clin. Orthop. 159:11, 1981.
Varni, M.A., and Jaffe, M.: Osteogenesis imperfecta: the basics, Pediatr. Nurs. 10:29-33, 1984.
Wynne-Davies, R., and Gormley, J.: Clinical and genetic patterns in osteogenesis imperfecta, Clin. Orthop. 159:26, 1981.

Juvenile Arthritis

Baum, J.: Treatment of juvenile arthritis, Am. Fam. Physician 27:133-139, 1983.
Giannini, E.H., Brewer, E.J., and Person, D.A.: Auranofin in the treatment of juvenile rheumatoid arthritis, J. Pediatr. 102:138-141, 1983.
Gorman, T.K., and Marsh, M.E.: Arthritis at an early age, Am. J. Nurs. 84:1472-1477, 1984.
Manners, P.J., and Ansell, B.M.: Slow-acting antirheumatic drug use in systemic onset juvenile chronic arthritis, Pediatrics 77:99-103, 1986.
Mortensen, M.E., and Rennebohm, R.M.: Clinical pharmacology and use of nonsteroid anti-inflammatory drugs, Pediatr. Clin. North Am. 36:1113-1139, 1989.
Haugen, M.S., and Lynch, P.A.: Diagnostic tests in pediatric rheumatology: application for nurses, Pediatr. Nurs. 13:389-393, 1987.
Ignatavicius, D.D.: Meeting the psychosocial needs of patients with rheumatoid arthritis, Orthop. Nurs. 6(3):16-20, 1987.
Rennebohm, R., and Correll, J.K.: Comprehensive management of juvenile rheumatoid arthritis, Nurs. Clin. North Am. 19:647-662, 1984.
Rosenberg, A.M.: Advanced drug therapy for juvenile rheumatoid arthritis, J. Pediatr. 114:171-178, 1989.
Southwood, T.R., and others: Unconventional remedies used for patients with juvenile arthritis, Pediatrics 85:150-154, 1990.
Winkel, M.F.: Juvenile rheumatoid arthritis—parent support group: do parents perceive a need? Pediatr. Nurs. 14:131-132, 1988.
Witter, D.C.: When children have arthritis, Arthritis Today 1(2):10-13, 1987.

Systemic Lupus Erythematosus (SLE)

Emery, H.: Clinical aspects of systemic lupus erythematosus in childhood, Pediatr. Clin. North Am. 33:1177-1190, 1986.
Feutren, G., and others: Effects of cyclosporine in severe systemic lupus erythematosus, J. Pediatr. 111:1063-1068, 1987.
Lee, L.A., and Weston, W.L.: Lupus erythematosus in childhood, Dermatol. Clin. 4:151-160, 1986.
Lehman, T.J.A., and others: Systemic lupus erythematosus in the first year of life, Pediatrics 83:235-239, 1989.
Miller, M.L., Magilavy, D.B., and Warren, R.W.: The immunologic basis of lupus, Pediatr. Clin. North Am. 33:1191-1202, 1986.
Nass, T.: Helping the patient who has lupus, RN 50(10):69-74, 1987.
Olson, N.Y., and Lindsley, C.B.: Neonatal lupus syndrome, Am. J. Dis. Child. 141:908-910, 1987.
Phadke, K., and others: Acute renal failure as the initial manifestation of systemic lupus erythematosus in children, J. Pediatr. 105:38-41, 1984.
Szer, I.S.: The diagnosis and management of systemic lupus erythematosus in childhood, Pediatr. Ann. 15:596-604, 1986.

CHAPTER 40

The Child with Neuromuscular Dysfunction

RELATED TOPICS

The child with cerebral dysfunction, Ch. 37
Genetic counseling, Ch. 5
The immobilized child, Ch. 39
Myelomeningocele (meningomyelocele), Ch. 11
Neurologic assessment, Chs. 7 and 8

GLOSSARY

ADL Activities of daily living
CP Cerebral palsy
DMD Duchenne muscular dystrophy
EMG Electromyogram
GBS Guillain-Barré syndrome
hypertonia Increased muscle tension
hypotonia Decreased muscle tension
MD Muscular dystrophy
MG Myasthenia gravis
MVA Motor vehicle accident
paraplegia Paralysis of lower extremities
quadriplegia Paralysis of all four extremities; usually greater involvement of legs than arms
spasticity Hyperactivitly of muscle stretch reflex, which gets worse with rapid passive motion
TIG Tetanus immune globulin
TAT Tetanus antitoxin

Disorders of muscle or muscle innervation interfere with physical movement and are, in most instances, more difficult to manage than those involving traumatic injury as discussed in the early segments of Chapter 39. This chapter is primarily concerned with impairment of innervation to muscles and to a lesser extent with muscle pathology.

NEUROMUSCULAR DYSFUNCTION

Weakness or abnormal performance of skeletal muscle may represent a defect in the muscle itself or reflect a pathologic disorder at some point along the neural pathway from the cortex of the brain to the neuromuscular junction. The identification of the source of muscle dysfunction includes not only the testing of muscle function but also the systematic elimination of possible disorders of neural structures on which muscle function depends for its stimulus. In a few disorders muscle disease may be accompanied by a neural disorder.

Some clinical features are shared by muscle disease, *(myopathy)*, which differs in many ways from muscle dysfunction resulting from disorders of neuronal structures—brain, cranial nerve nuclei, long nerve tracts, anterior horn cells of the spinal cord, and peripheral nerves. Motor function is accomplished by means of the simple reflex arcs or by way of impulses transmitted from the cerebral cortex and other centers in the brain through the various nerve pathways of the central nervous system. The upper motor neurons consist of cells that lie in the cerebral cortex and fibers that traverse the brainstem and spinal cord to terminate at their synapses with the anterior horn cells. The anterior horn cells, axons, and peripheral nerve branches constitute the lower motor neurons. The motor unit consists of the lower motor neuron, the neuromuscular junction, and the muscle fibers it supplies (Fig. 40-1). The upper motor neuronal pathways from the cerebrum to the lower motor neuron are described as (1) pyramidal—those whose fibers extend from the cortex, come together in the medulla, cross from one side to the other, then extend down the cord to synapse with anterior horn motor neurons; and (2) extrapyramidal—a complex network of motor neurons that comprise relays between motor areas of the cortex, basal ganglia, thalamus, cerebellum, and brainstem.

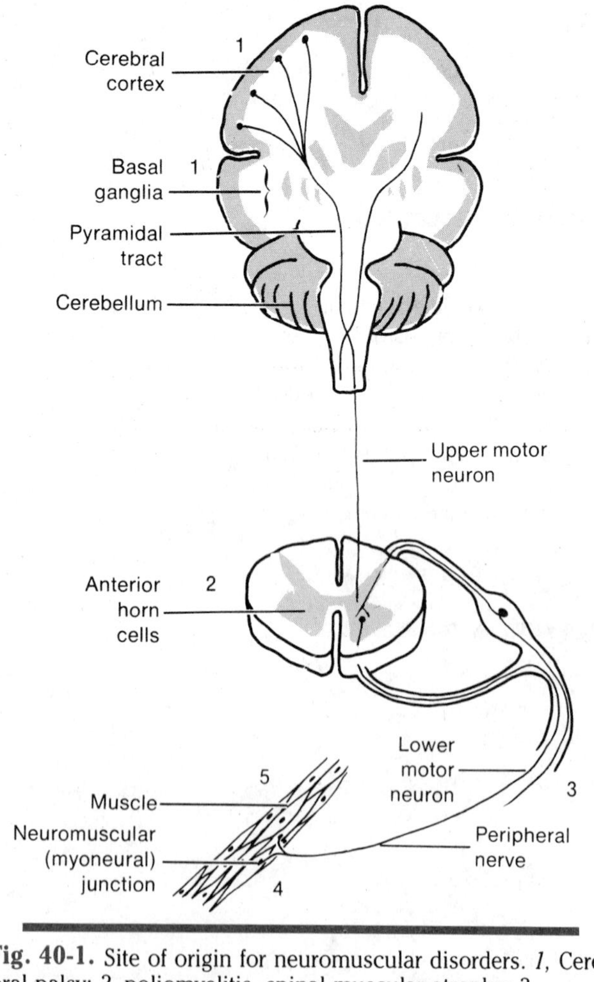

Fig. 40-1. Site of origin for neuromuscular disorders. *1,* Cerebral palsy; *2,* poliomyelitis, spinal muscular atrophy; *3,* mononeuropathies, polyneuropathies; *4,* myasthenia gravis, neurotoxic disorders; *5,* muscular dystrophies.

CLASSIFICATION AND DIAGNOSIS

The site of pathologic disturbance determines the type of muscular dysfunction. In general, *upper motor neuron* lesions produce weakness associated with spasticity, increased deep tendon reflexes, and abnormal superficial reflexes. The primary disorder of upper motor neuron dysfunction is cerebral palsy. Lesions of *lower motor neurons* interrupt the reflex arc, causing weakness and atrophy of the skeletal muscles involved with associated hypotonia or flaccidity, which eventually progress to atrophy with varying degrees of contracture deformity. A disorder of the *extrapyramidal pathway* and the cerebellum rarely produces muscle weakness.

Lower motor neuron involvement is usually symmetric (except that of poliomyelitis and single peripheral nerve disease), whereas disorders of the pyramidal tract are more often asymmetric. Muscle wasting is characteristic of lower motor neuron lesions and more marked than in diseases of muscles. Deep tendon reflexes are briskly active in upper motor neuron disease, are diminished or absent in lower motor neuron disease, and depend on the progress of muscle degeneration in the myopathies.

These disorders can also be categorized according to onset: those in which there is acute onset of flaccid paralysis and those with more gradual onset and progressive degeneration. In most instances the sudden appearance of flaccid paralysis in a previously healthy child can be attributed to an infectious process. Neurotoxins (e.g., botulism, tick paralysis, or heavy metal poisoning), pressure on the spinal cord from tumors or abscesses, and spinal cord injury are less likely causes. Hereditary factors and metabolic disease are more often responsible for muscular weakness and atrophy of gradual onset.

Classification

The most useful classification of neuromuscular disorders is one that defines the site of origin of the pathologic lesion: the anterior horn cells of the spinal cord, the peripheral nerves, the myoneural junction, and the muscles.

Diseases of anterior horn cells. Diseases and disorders that affect the anterior horn cells are the result of destruction or atrophy of the anterior horn of the spinal column with the inability to transfer impulses from sensory neurons to motor neurons. Enteroviruses, which have a worldwide distribution, are prominent etiologic agents that selectively affect anterior horn cells. These include the polioviruses, of which there are three types: coxsackieviruses, groups A and B, and the ECHO viruses. Degeneration of the anterior horn cells is caused by inherited disorders, primarily the spinal muscular atrophies.

Neuropathies. Disorders affecting peripheral nerves may be *mononeuropathies,* involving a single nerve and the muscles it innervates, or *polyneuropathies,* which involve multiple nerves and the muscles they supply. Neuropathies are caused by a number of hereditary diseases, traumatic injury, infections, poisons, and (secondarily) some metabolic diseases. Polyneuropathy can be restricted to specific areas (as in diabetes mellitus); some hereditary diseases involve skeletal muscles extensively. Usually distal limbs (feet and hands) are affected first, with gait disturbance and footdrop as early manifestations. The involvement gradually progresses medially as the disorder becomes more severe.

In some polyneuropathies there is segmented or patchy loss of the myelin sheath of nerve fibers; in others the primary process appears to be progressive degeneration of nerve fibers. Examples of acute and chronic polyneuropathies are infectious polyneuritis and peroneal atrophy, respectively.

Neuromuscular junction disease. Disorders involving a neurohormonal deficiency interfere with transmission of nerve impulses to muscles at the neuromuscular junction. Normally, nerve impulses are transmitted to skeletal muscles across the neuromuscular junction by acetylcholine. This is accomplished in three steps: (1) acetylcholine is released from vesicles in the terminal nerve endings; (2) it then diffuses across the junction and contacts receptor sites in the muscle membrane, stimulating the muscle to contract; and (3) it is removed by the action of cholinesterase. Interference at any of these three steps will block transmission of nerve impulses and prevent muscular contraction.

Several toxic substances act at the myoneural junction to inhibit nerve impulses to the skeletal muscles. Examples of toxins that prevent release of acetylcholine are those that produce the paralysis of botulism and tick paralysis. Action at receptor sites is blocked by the drug curare. Paralysis resulting from inhibition of cholinesterase release is caused by poisoning with organic phosphate insecticides.

Diseases of muscles. Disorders that affect the muscles directly may be a result of inflammatory, degenerative, or metabolic causes. Chief among these are the muscular dystrophies.

Diagnostic Tools

To aid in differentiating between diseases with similar manifestations, several general diagnostic tools are used. In addition, a number of more definitive tests are used to establish a specific diagnosis. The neurologic examination is a basic test that helps to assess the extent of motor and sensory function.

The *electromyogram* (EMG) measures the electric potentials generated in individual muscles. A small metal disk is placed on the skin overlying the muscle to be tested, or a sterile needle electrode is inserted directly into the muscle. The electric activity generated in the skeletal muscles is measured at rest, with slight voluntary contraction, and with maximal contraction. The electric activity is amplified and displayed on a cathode ray oscilloscope. Needle electrodes are sensitive enough to pick up the activity of a single muscle fiber; thus this is usually the method of choice.

Nerve conduction velocity, the velocity of electric impulse conduction along motor or sensory nerves, is frequently measured in conjunction with electromyography. Certain diseases affect the peripheral nerves, prolonging the conduction time from the point of stimulation of the nerve to the muscle and increasing the duration of the evoked potential of the muscle.

Muscle biopsy is the most useful laboratory examination to confirm and classify muscle disorders. *Serum enzyme measurements* are helpful in diagnosis and monitoring the course of muscular disease. These are outlined in Box 40-1.

HYPOTONIA

Decreased muscle tone in an infant is not an unusual observation in the newborn nursery and is one of the most common presenting symptoms in neuromuscular disorders. It may also indicate a variety of systemic conditions. Frequent causes are cerebral trauma or hypoxia at birth, but most neuromuscular disorders with hypotonia as the presenting symptom are genetically determined, especially Down syndrome and infantile spinal muscular atrophy.

Clinical Manifestations

Hypotonia, sometimes called the *floppy infant syndrome,* is marked by diminished muscle tone and weakness in both

Box 40-1 SERUM ENZYME MEASUREMENTS

Creatine phosphokinase (CPK)—found in skeletal muscle and a few other organs and elevated in skeletal muscle disease; the most specific test

Aldolase—present in skeletal and heart muscle and significantly elevated in muscle damage

Serum glutamic-oxaloacetic transaminase (SGOT)—elevated in muscle disease but has wider distribution in organs

Lactic dehydrogenase (LDH)—elevated in muscle disease but has wider distribution

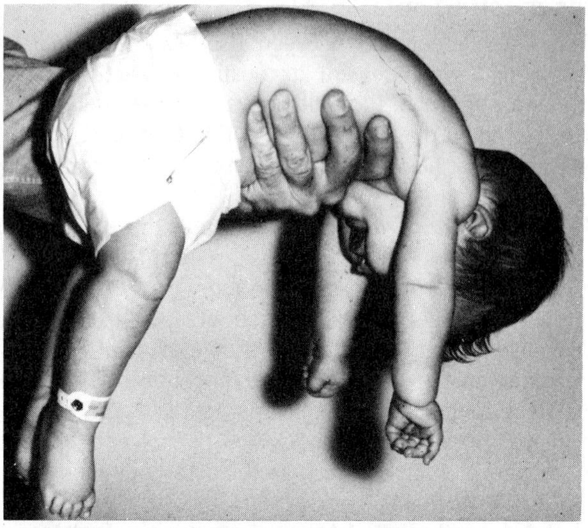

Fig. 40-2. Hypotonicity demonstrated by horizontal suspension in an infant with Werdnig-Hoffmann disease.
From Swaiman, K.F., and Wright, F.S.: The practice of pediatric neurology, ed. 2, St. Louis, 1982, Mosby–Year Book, Inc.

spontaneous and passive motion and reflex testing. The infant, when placed in a supine position, assumes a characteristic "frog posture" or lies in some other unusual position at rest. Normally, the young infant who is held in horizontal suspension (i.e., with the examiner's hand supporting the infant under the chest) will respond by slightly raising the head with the back relatively straight, arms flexed and slightly abducted, and knees partly flexed. The hypotonic infant droops over the supporting hand with head and extremities hanging loosely, resembling an inverted U (Fig. 40-2). The muscles feel flabby when palpated, and there is marked head lag when the infant is pulled to a sitting position. Poor sucking may be noted.

Therapeutic Management and Nursing Considerations

The management of these infants is determined by the cause of the hypotonia. It is a nursing responsibility to record and report findings that suggest hypotonia in an infant so that further evaluation can be carried out and therapeutic measures implemented if indicated.

CEREBRAL PALSY

Cerebral palsy (CP) is a nonspecific term applied to disorders characterized by impaired movement and posture and early onset. It is nonprogressive and may be accompanied by intellectual and language deficits. The etiology, clinical features, and course are variable, characterized by abnormal muscle tone and coordination as the primary disturbances. It is the most common permanent physical disability of childhood, and, although the incidence is not known, various studies suggest that it varies from 1.2 to 2 in every 1000 live births (Healy and Smith, 1988; Nelson, 1989).

Box 40-2 APPROXIMATE DISTRIBUTION OF CAUSES IN CEREBRAL PALSY

Low birth weight, preterm birth	35% to 40%
Perinatal asphyxia in term infants	25% to 30%
Congenital and perinatal infections (CMV, rubella, toxoplasma, neonatal meningitis)	5% to 10%
Intrauterine ischemic events	5% to 10%
Congenital brain anomalies not evident on clinical examination	5% to 10%
Perinatal metabolic conditions other than asphyxia (hyperbilirubinemia, hypoglycemia, hyperosmolarity, amino acid disorders)	5%
Genetic origin	2% to 5%

From Paneth, N.: Etiologic factors in cerebral palsy, Pediatr. Ann. 15:191, 194-201, 1986.

Etiology

A variety of prenatal, perinatal, and postnatal factors contribute to the etiology of CP, singly or multifactorially (Box 40-2). The dominant mechanism of damage is ischemia and/or asphyxia, to which the preterm/low-birth-weight infant is particularly vulnerable. Next in frequency are those infants who experience severe perinatal asphyxia. Congenital infections, metabolic conditions, and intrauterine ischemic events are implicated less often, and genetic factors as such rarely cause CP (Paneth, 1986). The multifactorial implication is exemplified by the preterm infant of low birth weight who suffers perinatal asphyxia, infection, or a metabolic condition.

Pathophysiology

It is difficult to establish a precise location of neurologic lesions based on etiology or clinical signs because there is no characteristic pathologic picture. In some cases there are gross malformations of the brain. In others there may be evidence of vascular occlusion, atrophy, loss of neurons, and laminar degeneration that produce narrower gyri, wider sulci, and low brain weight. Anoxia plays the most significant role in the pathologic state of brain damage, which is frequently secondary to other causative mechanisms.

There are a few exceptions. In some cases the manifestations or etiology can be related to anatomic areas. For example, CP associated with prematurity is usually spastic diplegia caused by hypoxic infarction or hemorrhage in the area adjacent to the lateral ventricles. In the athetoid type of CP caused by kernicterus and hemolytic disease of the newborn, there are pigment deposits in the basal ganglia and some cranial nerve nuclei. Hemiparetic CP is frequently associated with mechanical trauma to the cortex or cerebrovascular accident of the middle cerebral artery. Cerebral hypoplasia and sometimes neonatal hypoglycemia are related to ataxic CP. Generalized cortical and cerebral atrophy have been shown to cause severe quadriparesis with mental retardation and microcephaly.

Clinical Manifestations

The alert observer may suspect CP when a child demonstrates some of the following groups of manifestations.

Delayed gross motor development. This is a universal manifestation of CP. The child shows a delay in all motor accomplishments, and the discrepancy between motor ability and expected achievement tends to increase with successive developmental milestones as growth advances. It is especially significant if other developmental behavior, such as language and personal-social achievement, is normal.

Abnormal motor performance. Neuromotor dysfunction is particularly evident in motor performance. An early sign is preferential unilateral hand use that may be apparent at about 6 months of age. Hand dominance does not normally develop until the preschool years. Abnormal crawling with propulsion by hand movements only and with lower extremities and hips hiked along, much like a "bunny hop," is seen in diplegia. Children with hemiplegia have an asymmetric crawl, using the unaffected arm and leg to propel themselves on either the buttocks or the abdomen. Spasticity may cause the child to stand or walk on the toes. Uncoordinated or involuntary movements are characteristic of dyskinetic CP, and facial grimacing and writhing movements of the tongue, fingers, and toes are signs of athetosis. Other significant signs of motor dysfunction are poor sucking and feeding difficulties, with persistent tongue thrust. Head staggering, tremor on reaching, and truncal ataxia may be observed as well.

Alterations of muscle tone. Increased or decreased resistance to passive movements is a sign of abnormal muscle tone. The child may exhibit opisthotonic postures (exaggerated arching of the back) and may feel stiff on handling or dressing. Also, there is difficulty in diapering because of spasticity of hip adductor muscles and lower extremities. When pulled to a sitting position, the child may extend the entire body, rigid and unbending at the hip and knee joints. This is an early sign of spasticity.

Abnormal postures. Children with spastic CP assume abnormal postures at rest or when their position is changed. From an early age a child lying in a prone position will maintain the hips higher than the trunk with the legs and arms flexed or drawn under the body. In the supine position spasticity is evident by scissoring (legs in crossed position, knees, hips, and ankles stiff) and extension of legs and with the feet plantar flexed. This posture is exaggerated when the child is suspended vertically or when others try to make him bear weight. Spasticity may be mild or severe, depending on the degree of impairment. A persistent infantile resting and sleeping posture (i.e., arms abducted at shoulders, elbows flexed, and hands fisted) is a sign of spasticity when it remains constant after 4 to 5 months of age. The hemiparetic child may rest with the affected arm adducted and held against the torso with the elbow pronated and slightly flexed and the hand closed.

Reflex abnormalities. Persistence of primitive infantile reflexes is one of the earliest clues to CP—for example, obligatory tonic neck reflex at any age or nonobligatory persistence beyond 6 months of age and the persistence or even hyperactivity of the Moro, plantar, and palmar grasp reflexes. Hyperreflexia, ankle clonus, and stretch reflexes can be elicited from many muscle groups on fast passive movements—for example, resistance to passive abduction when hips are suddenly separated (adductor catch).

Associated disabilities. Some of the disabilities associated with CP are subnormal learning and reasoning capacity (mental retardation), impaired behavioral and interpersonal relationships (attention deficit–hyperactivity disorder), seizures, and impairment of special senses.

Mental retardation. The most serious disability is mental retardation. One third of the children with CP have normal intelligence (fewer have high normal or superior intelligence compared with the normal population); one third are mildly retarded; and one third are moderately retarded or below (low-grade deficiency is more common in persons with CP than in the general population). As a group, children with athetosis and ataxia are intellectually superior to those with other types of CP. Incidence of severe or profound retardation is highest in rigid, atonic, and quadriparetic CP.

Seizures. Seizures are more apt to accompany postnatally acquired hemiplegia. They are an unusual finding in athetosis and diplegia. The most common type is generalized tonic-clonic seizures, and the peak incidence of commencement is between 2 and 6 years of age.

Attention deficit—hyperactivity disorder. The manifestations of attention deficit–hyperactivity disorder may occur in children with CP. The primary presenting symptoms are poor attention span, marked distractibility, hyperactive behavior, and defects of integration (see Chapter 18).

Sensory impairment. Abnormalities of vision occur more often in CP, and hearing loss is frequently an associated disability. Strabismus is much higher in spastic children, and hearing loss is often seen in athetosis.

Clinical Classification

CP has been classified in several ways, but the most useful classification is based on the nature and distribution of neuromuscular dysfunction.

Spastic cerebral palsy. The most common clinical type, spastic CP, represents an upper motor neuron type of muscular weakness. The reflex arc is intact, and the characteristic physical signs are increased stretch reflexes, increased muscle tone, and (often) weakness. Early neurologic manifestations are usually generalized hypotonia or decreased tone that lasts for a few weeks or may extend for months or even as long as a year. The clinical features of spastic CP are outlined in Box 40-3.

Dyskinetic cerebral palsy. Dyskinesis implies abnormal involuntary movements. These movements originate in the basal ganglia, especially the globus pallidus, and the nuclei of cranial nerve VIII and of other cranial nerves. Movements disappear in sleep and are aggravated by stress. The major manifestation is athetosis, characterized by slow, wormlike, writhing movements that usually involve all extremities, the trunk, neck, facial muscles, and tongue. Dys-

Box 40-3 TYPES OF SPASTIC CEREBRAL PALSY

Hemiparesis—one side of body affected
- Most common form of spastic cerebral palsy
- Motor deficit usually greater in upper extremity; most children able to walk; underdevelopment of affected limbs
- Pattern of spasticity
  - Leg—increased tone of calf, hamstring, and hip adductor muscles
  - Gait—walk with foot inverted and plantar flexed, knee flexed, and leg adducted
  - Arm—increased tone in shoulder adductor and internal rotator muscles, elbow flexor and pronator muscles, and wrist and finger flexor muscles
- Parietal lobe syndrome—impairment of cortical sensory function (absence or inability to recognize size, shape, or texture of objects held in affected hand); impaired two-point discrimination and position sense

Quadriparesis or **tetraparesis**—all four extremities involved
- Highest incidence of severe disability
- Upper and lower limbs equally affected
- Same physical manifestations as hemiparesis bilaterally except lower extremities more involved than in hemiparesis, which causes considerable tightness of hip adductor muscles; difficulty in separating legs or even crossing them over one another ("scissors" gait)
- One fourth only mildly affected with minimum functional limitations on ambulation, self-care, and other activities; one half moderately impaired and impeded in self-care and independence in a sheltered situation; and one fourth severely damaged and require almost total care
- Delay in attaining developmental milestones proportionate to degree of motor deficit
- Speech dysarthric; swallowing may be impaired; tongue protrusion incomplete
- Emotions more labile with inappropriate laughing or crying

Diplegia—similar parts on both sides of the body involved, such as both arms
- Spasticity in legs greater than in arms
- Late attainment of gross motor milestones, sitting, standing, and walking; development of hand skills generally appropriate for age

Monoplegia*—involving only one extremity
Triplegia*—involving three extremities
Paraplegia*—pure cerebral paraplegia of lower extremities

*Rare occurrences.

kinetic movements of tongue and other pharyngeal, laryngeal, and oral muscles cause drooling and dysarthria (imperfect speech articulation), which makes it difficult to understand what the child is saying. There is often high-frequency hearing loss or deafness and conjugate upward gaze palsy, in which the eyes are converged toward the midline and displaced upward.

Involuntary movements may take on choreiform (involuntary, irregular, jerking movements) and dystonic (disordered muscle tone) manifestations that increase in intensity under emotional stress and during adolescence. In rare instances deformities develop as a result of continuous uncontrollable movements that maintain joint mobility.

Ataxic cerebral palsy. The least common type of CP, ataxia, is caused by a defect in the cerebellum or its pathways and is characterized by nonprogressive failure of muscle coordination and irregular muscle action. Affected children have a wide-based gait and perform rapid, repetitive movements poorly. There is disintegration of movements of the upper extremities when the child reaches for objects. Cerebellar coordination tends to improve as the child grows, but there is very slow development in the first 3 to 5 years of life.

Mixed-type cerebral palsy. A combination of spasticity and athetosis is described as mixed-type CP. Many affected children are severely disabled. This combination is sometimes observed after traumatic postnatal head injury.

Rigid, tremor, and atonic types. These types are uncommon. Both rigid and atonic types have a poor prognosis, with deformities and lack of active movement. Tremors as a leading manifestation in CP are rare. The tremor is seen at rest and on movement, but motor accomplishments are favorable and musculoskeletal complications do not occur.

Diagnostic Evaluation

Infants at risk based on known etiologic factors associated with CP warrant careful assessment during early infancy to identify signs of muscular dysfunction as early as possible. Careful assessment of the low-birth-weight or preterm infant, the infant with a low Apgar score at 5 minutes, and the infant who demonstrated other perinatal or neonatal abnormalities such as seizures, intracranial hemorrhage, or metabolic disturbances should be carried out. Early recognition is made more difficult by lack of reliable neonatal neurologic signs. Cortical control of movement does not occur until later in infancy; therefore motor impairment associated with voluntary control is usually not apparent until after 2 to 4 months of age at the earliest. More often the likelihood of a diagnosis cannot be confirmed until the second half of the first year. Motor dysfunction in some mildly affected infants may be overlooked until they exhibit delay or abnormality of some advanced motor skills such as standing or walking.

Persistence of primitive reflexes may be of value, and two offer assistance in diagnosis: the asymmetric tonic neck reflex, persistent Moro reflex (beyond 4 months of age), and the crossed extensor reflex. The tonic neck reflex normally disappears between 4 and 6 months of age. An "obligatory" response is considered abnormal. This is elicited by turning the infant's head to one side, holding it there for 20 seconds. When a crying infant is unable to move from the asymmetric posturing of the tonic neck reflex when crying, it is considered to be "obligatory" and an abnormal response. The crossed extensor reflex, which normally disappears by 4 months, is elicited by applying a noxious stimulus to the sole of one extremity with the knee extended. Normally the contralateral foot will respond with extensor, abduction, and then adduction movements. Finding these reflexes after the age when they should have disappeared suggests the possibility of CP (Taft, 1984).

The neurologic examination and history are the primary modalities for diagnosis. A thorough knowledge of normal variations of motor development is required for detecting abnormal progress, and a careful history is elicited to detect possible etiologic factors. The child's spontaneous movements and behavior are observed, including posture, attitude, and muscle size, function, and tone.

Supplemental diagnostic tests may be used, such as electroencephalography, tomography, screening for metabolic defects, and serum electrolyte values. The possibility of slowly progressive degenerative disease and early onset, slow-growing brain tumors must be ruled out.

Therapeutic Management: General Concepts

The goals of therapy for children with CP are early recognition and promotion of an optimum developmental course to enable affected children to attain their potential within the limits of their brain dysfunction. The disorder is permanent, and therapy is chiefly symptomatic and preventive. To be effective it requires the services of an organized team of health professionals that considers (1) the nature of the physical disability, (2) defects associated with the disorder, and (3) the interpersonal and social influences encountered by the affected child.

The beneficial influences of a habilitation program on both child and family are based on recognition of the disability as early as possible and implementation of treatment. Parents are essential to a treatment program, and their cooperation and confidence are considered in all aspects of management. With early diagnosis parents can begin to provide sensorimotor experiences that are essential for cognitive development, since central nervous system structures depend on stimulation and use to attain and maintain their functional integrity.

The broad aims of therapy are (1) to establish locomotion, communication, and self-help; (2) to gain optimum appearance and integration of motor functions; (3) to correct associated defects as effectively as possible; and (4) to provide educational opportunities adapted to the needs and capabilities of the individual child. Each child is evaluated and managed on an individual basis. The plan of therapy may involve a variety of settings, facilities, and specially trained persons, including the parents. The scope of the child's needs may require, in addition to the pediatrician and nurse, such professionals as a psychologist and/or psychiatrist, orthopedist, physical therapist, teacher, social worker, speech pathologist and/or therapist, neurologist, orthotist, audiologist, and occupational therapist.

Mobilizing devices. Braces and other devices are often used to help prevent or reduce deformity. Braces can increase the energy efficiency of gait, control joint alignment, or both. Most bracing is poorly tolerated by young children, and children with functioning upper extremities often remove a lower extremity brace.

Some of the more commonly used mobility devices include wheeled scooter boards that allow children to propel themselves while the abdomen or total body is supported and legs positioned with wedges to prevent scissoring.

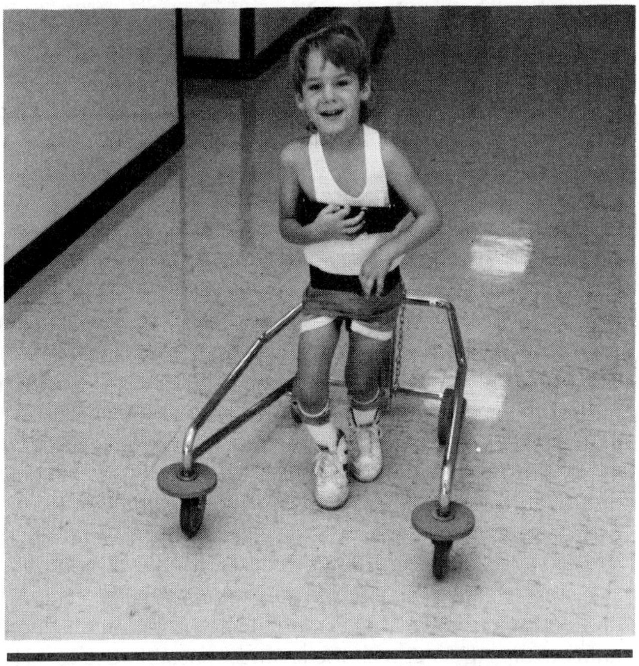

Fig. 40-3. Child in ambulation device that allows arm freedom.

Wheeled go-carts provide good sitting balance and serve as an early "wheelchair" experience for young children (see Fig. 39-6). Strollers can be equipped with custom seats for dependent mobilization. Special devices for independent mobilization that allow the upper extremities to remain free are particularly valuable for children with lower extremity involvement (Fig. 40-3). A number of wheelchairs can be customized to meet the needs and preferences of older children (see Mobilization Devices, Chapter 39).

The use of infant walkers is discouraged. They have been found to pose a risk of injury to normal children and are especially hazardous for children with CP. It has been observed that infant walkers bring out and exaggerate abnormal motor patterns, prevent integration of primitive reflexes, and delay development of normal balance and protective responses in children with CP (Holm, Harthun-Smith, and Tada, 1983).

Surgery. Orthopedic surgery may be required to decrease or abolish spastic muscle imbalance. This includes tendon lengthening procedures (especially heel-cord lengthening), release of spastic wrist flexor muscles, and correction of hip and adductor muscle spasticity or contracture to improve locomotion. Selective dorsal rhizotomy has provided marked improvement in some children with CP. However, achieving the benefits from the surgery requires intensive physical therapy and family commitment (Brucker, 1990).

Surgical intervention is usually reserved for the child who does not respond to the more conservative measures, but it is also indicated for the child whose spasticity causes progressive deformities. Surgery is primarily used to improve function rather than for cosmetic purposes and is followed by physical therapy. Neurosurgical procedures are used only in selected cases.

Medication. Drugs to decrease spasticity have little usefulness in improving function in CP. Antianxiety agents have been used to some extent to relieve excessive motion and tension, particularly in the athetoid child. Skeletal muscle relaxants, such as dantrolene (Dantrium), baclofen, and methocarbamol (Robaxin), may be used on a short-term basis for older children and adolescents. Diazepam (Valium) is used frequently but should be restricted to older children and adolescents (Sternfeld, 1986). The drugs have been successful in relieving stiffness and thus facilitating ease of motion. Local nerve block to motor points of a muscle with a neurolytic agent such as phenol solution reduces spasticity temporarily.

Anticonvulsant medications are used routinely for children who have seizures. Generally phenobarbital and phenytoin are most widely prescribed and appear to be effective in most instances. Other anticonvulsants or combinations are needed in special situations. Regular periodic monitoring of blood levels is required to obtain the desired anticonvulsant effect with the smallest possible dosage. Hyperactive, dyskinetic children perform better when given dextroamphetamine or other drugs used for the child with attention deficit–hyperactivity disorder.

Technical aids. A wide variety of technical aids are available to improve the functioning of children with CP. For example, specially designed electromechanical toys that employ the concept of biofeedback operate from a head unit. The toy is manipulated only when the head and trunk are in correct alignment. Eye-hand coordination can also be enhanced by appropriately designed toys and games.

The most numerous devices are those that facilitate nonvocal communication. Microcomputers combined with voice synthesizers aid children with speech difficulties to "speak." These and others print messages onto screen monitors and paper. These devices have made it apparent that some children have been erroneously considered to be mentally retarded (Sternfeld, 1986).

Many other electronic devices allow independent functioning. Sensors can be activated and deactivated by using a head-stick, tongue, or other voluntary muscle movement over which the child has control. The application of this technology makes it possible for persons with CP to eventually function in their own apartments and can be extended into the workplace.

Other considerations. Care of visual and auditory deficits requires the attention of appropriate specialists, and speech therapy involves the services of a speech therapist (see Chapter 25). Dental care is especially important for children with CP and is all too frequently overlooked. Regular visits to the dentist and dental prophylaxis, including brushing, fluoride, and flossing (after several teeth are present), should be instituted as soon as the teeth erupt. This is especially important for children on phenytoin, who often develop gum hyperplasia.

Therapeutic Management: Physiotherapy

Physical therapy is one of the most frequently used conservative treatment modalities. It requires the specialized skills of a qualified therapist with an extensive repertoire of exercise methods who can design a program to stimulate each child to achieve functional goals. In general, physical therapy is directed toward good skeletal alignment for the spastic child; training in purposeful acts, even in the face of involuntary motion, for the athetoid child; and maximum development of proprioceptive sense in ataxia.

An active therapy program involves the family, the physical therapist, and often other members of the health team, especially the nurse. The major approach employs traditional types of therapeutic exercises that consist of stretching, passive, active, and resisted movements applied to specific muscle groups or joints to maintain or increase range of motion, strength, or endurance. Another approach is one of "patterning," which attempts to alter abnormal tone and posture and elicit desired movements through positional manipulation or other means of modifying or augmenting sensory output. These programs require intensive daily manipulation and a legion of volunteers to carry out the program. The American Academy of Pediatrics (1982) has issued a strong statement against this form of treatment for neurologically disabled children. Therefore this option will not be discussed further.

No therapeutic approach is able to achieve spectacular changes in the ultimate outcome of motor disability. Therefore the most practical approach is to select a mode of intervention that is most appropriate for the specific problem and that best suits the need of the individual child at any given time. Early efforts are focused on alleviating abnormal postures by positioning and range of motion exercises. For example, rather than being pulled to a sitting position by the arms, which stimulates hypertonic extensor muscles of the back, the spastic infant is slowly pushed forward by hands placed posteriorly on the trunk. Extensor spasticity and scissoring of legs can be avoided if the infant straddles a thigh or hip when carried in the sitting position.

Passive range of motion exercises, stretching, and elongation exercises are valuable at any age, even at early ages when the child is unable to cooperate. They are of particular value for postural abnormalities around various joints. For example, stretching of the gastrocnemius muscle and its tendon helps to prevent tightness and spasticity, which lead to toe walking and equinus position of the ankle. When the child is old enough to cooperate, some active extension can be performed, with passive motion applied to complete joint extension. Prevention of contracture deformity is a prime function of physical therapy.

Functional and adaptive training (occupational therapy). Training in manual skills and activities of daily living (ADL) proceeds along developmental lines and according to the child's functional level. Sitting, balance, crawling, and walking are encouraged at appropriate ages, accompanied by stimulation of protective extension and equilibrium reactions. When standing is attempted, therapy may be needed to strengthen and improve balance, which is sometimes facilitated by the use of braces, especially to control plantar flexion and less often to prevent knee flexion caused by hamstring muscle spasticity and inadequate control of hip and knee extensor muscles. Walking, using reciprocal leg motion, should be attempted at the appropriate age, even if the child requires considerable assistance from braces and other persons, and the child should be encouraged to progress to parallel bars or other ambulatory aids as soon as possible.

Hand activities are begun early to improve motor function and provide the child with sensory experiences and information about his environment. Use of extremities requires some stability of the trunk; therefore a gross motor position in which the child has some active control is selected. Objects and toys are chosen to provide needed sensory input, using a variety of shapes, forms, and textures. The child will electively use the less affected or unaffected hand as the dominant one, and there are differing opinions about whether or not the child should be therapeutically encouraged to use the deficient extremity. Undue insistence often provokes an adverse emotional reaction. Play that encourages the use of hands for unimanual and bimanual activities is initiated early. Large balls, a doll carriage to push, or other toys that require some manner of manipulation are accepted without resistance and promote assistive use of both hands. Play is a valuable tool in a therapeutic program and is selected to combine therapy with the child's ability and interest. This often requires a great deal of ingenuity and inventiveness on the part of those involved in the child's care.

The child may need considerable help (and patience) in learning to feed, dress, and care for personal hygiene needs, the most important and earliest tasks on which to concentrate. Children should be fed in the normal eating position. When they have difficulty with sucking and swallowing, it is a temptation to hold them in a semireclining posture to make use of gravity flow. This method does not promote active swallowing, however, and the neck hyperextension may even interfere with swallowing. A more flexed sitting position with arms brought forward to decrease the tendency toward back and neck extension is more natural during bottle- or spoon-feeding and encourages active swallowing.

Because jaw control is compromised, more normal control can be achieved if the feeder provides stability of the oral mechanism from the side or front of the face. When directed from the front, the middle finger of the nonfeeding hand is placed posterior to the body portion of the chin, the thumb below the bottom lip, and the index finger parallel to the child's mandible (Fig. 40-4). Manual jaw control from the side assists with poor head control, neck and trunk hyperextension, and jaw stabilization. The middle finger of the nonfeeding hand is placed posterior to the bony portion of the chin, the index finger on the chin below the lower lip, and the thumb placed obliquely across the cheek to provide lateral jaw stability (Fig. 40-5) (Logigian and Ward, 1989).

Speech training under the supervision of a speech therapist is begun early, before the child learns poor habits of communication. Parents and others can help by following the directions of the speech therapist and by talking to the child slowly and using pictures or handling objects about which the adult is speaking. Feeding techniques, such as

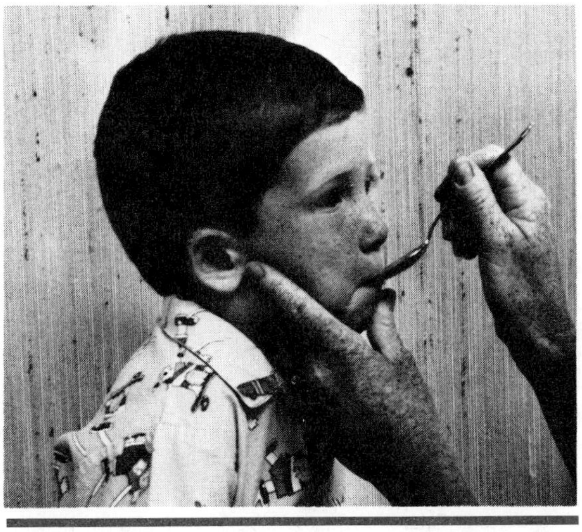

Fig. 40-4. Manual jaw control provided anteriorly.

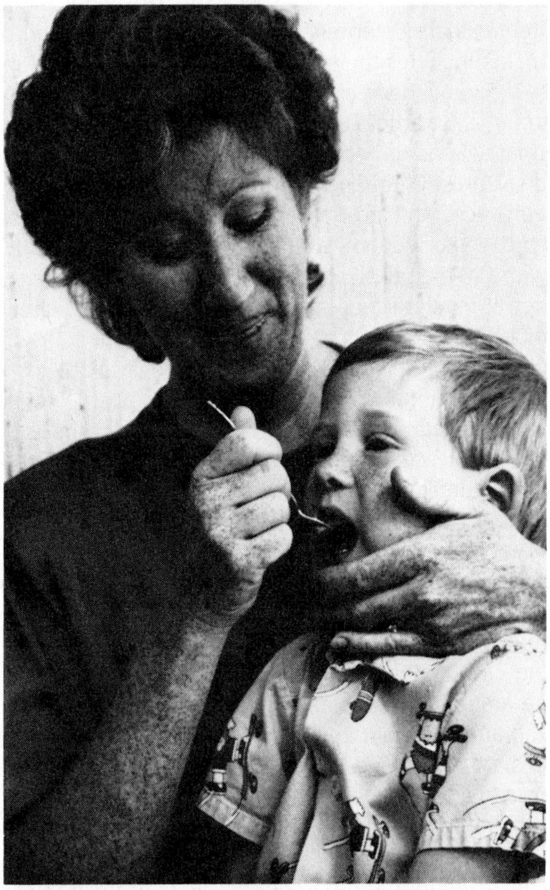

Fig. 40-5. Manual jaw control provided from the posterior.

forcing the child to use the lips and tongue in eating, help to facilitate speech—for example, placing food at the side of the tongue, first one side then the other; making the child use the lips to take food from a spoon rather than placing it directly on the tongue; and avoiding using the teeth to remove the food from the utensil. If severe dysarthria prevents articulate speech and the child has reasonable intelligence, nonverbal communication is taught.

As the child progresses from simple feeding and self-care activities, training is extended to include other tasks that are within the child's developmental and functional capabilities, such as cooking or typing. It should be remembered that children should not be expected to learn a task until they are at the developmental stage at which it would normally be accomplished. In all ADL it is important to capitalize on the child's assets and compensate for liabilities. For example, a child with visual-motor dysfunction would be helped by substituting an electric typewriter for the laborious task of handwriting. Learning one-handed tying of shoelaces would be needed by a hemiparetic child. The level of expected independence is related to both gross and fine motor manipulation, and even when complete independence in a specific activity is not realistic, the child should learn any masterable part of the task. However, motor function is not the sole purpose of learning as much independence as possible. Any accomplishment promotes self-reliance and self-esteem for healthier personality development.

Education. As in all aspects of care, educational requirements are determined by the child's needs and potential. This includes the severity of the child's disease and the presence and degree of associated conditions that affect learning and participation, such as learning impairment, abnormal actions or behavior, impaired vision and/or hearing, and seizures. Children with mild physical disability, normal intelligence, and no associated learning disability should attend regular school, although this is sometimes difficult because of the physical structure of the school. When attendance at regular school is not appropriate for the child, special classes or school facilities designed to meet the special needs of children with disabilities are available in most larger communities. For those who are unable to benefit from formal education, a training program may be appropriate. At adolescence prevocational and vocational counseling and guidance are arranged. At any phase or in any setting, education is geared toward the child's assets.

Recreation. Recreational activities are also a necessary part of growing up. Recreational outlets and after-school activities should be considered for the child who is unable to participate in regular athletic and other peer activities. Some can compete in athletic and artistic endeavors, and there are many games and pastimes that are suited to their capabilities. Sports, physical fitness, and recreation programs are encouraged for children with CP, and young children should be exposed to all physical activities available to children without disabilities.

There are numerous developmental centers that have facilities for indoor and outdoor activities designed to appeal to children of all ages. If these are not available, they should be instigated. Such programs require adequate supervision to avoid any harmful effects, however. Recreational activities serve to stimulate children's interest and curiosity, help them adjust to their disability, improve their functional abilities, and build self-esteem. Competitive sports are also becoming increasingly available to these children and offer an added dimension to physical activities. Information on training programs and competition on local, state, regional, and national levels can be obtained from the **National Association of Sports for Cerebral Palsy.***

Nursing Considerations

Nurses in a community setting, especially those in public health, in physicians' offices and clinics, and in schools, are more likely to become involved with a family in which there is a child with CP. Both the child and the family need the help, support, and encouragement that nurses are prepared to offer, and nurses can be involved in all aspects of the child's management. Nurses who know the family and their special needs and problems are in the best position to provide guidance and support.

Assessment

Early recognition of CP is often a result of alert observation by the nurse. Detection begins at birth, and the nurse should be especially observant for signs in an infant who has a history that includes any of the prenatal and perinatal conditions that predispose to brain damage. Unusual manifestations in a newborn can be signs of a variety of conditions, but an infant who displays poor feeding, rigidity, tenseness, or hypotonia merits closer scrutiny. A history of these unexplained signs is cause for repeated assessment. The disorder is not readily identifiable in the early months of life; often evidence is not apparent until the child begins to walk. Delayed attainment of developmental milestones is one of the most valuable clues to recognizing CP; therefore slow development in a child offers one of the earliest indications of neurologic impairment.

Nursing Diagnoses

Based on a thorough assessment, several nursing diagnoses are identified. The more common diagnoses for the child with CP are included in the Nursing Care Plan on pp. 1922-1923. Others may apply in specific situations.

Planning

Nursing objectives for the child with CP include the following:

1. Establish locomotion and communication.
2. Encourage self-help.

*United Cerebral Palsy Association, Inc., 66 East 34th St., New York, NY 10016; (800) USA-1UCP or (212) 481-6300.

3. Facilitate acquisition of educational opportunities adapted to the needs and capabilities of the child.
4. Promote a positive self-image in the child.
5. Support the family in its efforts to meet the needs of the child.
6. Care for the child during hospitalization.

Implementation

Nurses working with children need to be well acquainted with normal child growth and development and the tools of assessment. The earlier any deviation from normal is detected, the better the outlook for optimum developmental attainment. It is also important that the child receive appropriate therapy from persons or agencies qualified to provide such services. Parents are sometimes tempted to follow advice from unreliable sources. Nurses who are acquainted with services and facilities can refer the family to qualified practitioners.

Nurses who work directly with the child in the home or in the therapeutic setting are members of the health team who plan and carry out a program of therapy. Since children are being treated at an earlier age, parents are participating earlier in treatment programs for their child. They are taught the proper handling and home care of young children with CP. Parents need carefully programmed steps so that their change of role from parent to therapist can be melded into the already established relationship. The nurse or therapist needs to have documented data about the parent-child relationship before teaching the parent how to facilitate the child's posture or inhibit certain reflex patterns.

Parents learn how to posture children, how to introduce and carry out appropriate exercises, and how to place children in appropriate positions for play, dressing, eating, bathing, toileting, and other daily activities. Nurses are acquainted with the special needs of the child and the physical therapy objectives and modalities; thus they are able to reinforce the plan and assist the family in devising and modifying equipment and activities to follow through and reinforce the therapy program in the home, for example, modifying eating utensils by building up spoon handles for easier grasp and modifying clothes to facilitate self-help (see also Chapter 24).

Because children with CP expend so much energy in their efforts to accomplish activities of daily living, more frequent rest periods should be arranged to avoid fatigue that may aggravate their limited capabilities. The diet should include extra calories to help meet these extra energy demands. Safety precautions are implemented, such as children wearing bicycle helmets if they are subject to falls or there is a chance of injuring their heads on hard objects. Furniture should be upholstered, or sharp edges padded to protect a child from injury. Because their respiratory muscles are less efficient, these children are more susceptible to common upper respiratory infections and should avoid contact with infected persons. Dental problems are more frequent in children with CP, which creates a need for meticulous attention to all aspects of dental care.

Parents are sometimes very preoccupied with their ability to perform activities such as positioning their child; as a result, a child's personal comfort and satisfaction may be overlooked. They often perceive their children's inability to perform or behave to be a direct result of their own inadequacy in working with their children. The parents are so intent on achieving a desired goal, such as flexing a child's knees, that they repeatedly remind their children of their errors but fail to acknowledge or support their less-than-successful efforts to comply, even though the children are willing. Nurses can help parents integrate therapy into play activities in more natural and less frustrating ways.

Some children have difficulty in keeping their heads upright. Because of this, they cannot explore much of their environment and process the information. Parents need to be complimented on their efforts to provide a stimulating environment for these children. These infants are "at risk" for delayed development in holding up their heads, righting their shoulders and trunks for stable posture, sitting, pulling, standing, and crawling. Most parents of children with impaired movements benefit from support and practical suggestions for feeding, moving, holding, and encouraging the infant to explore hands and feet and begin to play.

Although practical advice is important, the nurse or physical therapist should offer suggestions at a pace that can be absorbed by the parents to avoid making them feel inadequate in their parenting abilities. The parents are encouraged to define their concern, and nurses should acknowledge the concern as genuine and ask the parents how long they have tried a certain approach. In this way the nurse is able to find out what works, what does not work, and *what the parents* would like to try next. The parents are given positive feedback for their observations of the infant, the progress *they* note, and how *they* differentiate the child's needs.

Sometimes parents need support simply because the demands made on them are very fatiguing. It is probably better for parents of young children with CP to reduce the *quantity* of involvement with their children, rather than reduce the *quality* of the interactions. As normal preschool children acquire autonomous skills, language, and mobility, they spend less time with their parents and are less dependent.

Probably the nursing interventions most valuable to the family are support and help in coping with the emotional aspects of the disorder, many of which are discussed in relation to the child with a disability (Chapter 22). Initially the parents need supportive counseling directed toward understanding the implications of the diagnosis and all the feelings that it engenders. Later they need clarification regarding what they can expect from the child and from health professionals. Having a child with CP implies numerous problems of daily management and changes in family life.

There are constant demands with few rewards, and the day-by-day changelessness of these demands is trying to parents. Many find that their child with CP gives them little pleasure. The nurse needs to support the parents in their frustration, their problem solving, their concerns, their ap-

NURSING CARE PLAN
The Child with Cerebral Palsy

NURSING DIAGNOSIS: Impaired physical mobility related to neuromuscular impairment

GOAL 1
Establish locomotion

INTERVENTIONS
Encourage sitting, crawling, and walking at appropriate ages
Carry out therapies that strengthen and improve control
Assist child in using reciprocal leg motion when learning to walk
Provide incentives to locomote
Ensure adequate rest before attempting locomotion activities
Incorporate play that encourages desired behavior
Employ aids that facilitate locomotion such as parallel bars, crutches
Prepare child and family for surgical procedures if indicated

EXPECTED OUTCOME
Child acquires locomotion within capabilities (specify)

GOAL 2
Prevent deformity

INTERVENTIONS
Apply and correctly use braces
Carry out and teach family to perform stretching exercises
Employ appropriate range of motion exercises
Perform preoperative and postoperative care for child who requires corrective surgery

EXPECTED OUTCOME
Child benefits from appropriate preventive measures (specify measures and child's expected response)

NURSING DIAGNOSIS: Bathing/hygiene, dressing/grooming, feeding, toileting self-care deficits related to physical disability

GOAL 1
Promote self-help

INTERVENTIONS
Encourage child to assist with care as age and capabilities permit
Select toys and activities that allow maximum participation by child and that improve motor function and sensory input
Avoid undue persistence to accomplish a goal
Encourage activities that require both unimanual and bimanual activities
Adapt utensils, foods, and clothing to facilitate self-help, e.g., large-bowled spoon with padded handle, finger foods and foods that adhere to, rather than slip from, utensil, and clothing that opens from front with self-adhering closings rather than buttons
Assist parents in toilet training the child

EXPECTED OUTCOME
Child engages in self-help activities commensurate with capabilities

NURSING DIAGNOSIS: Potential for injury related to physical disability, neuromuscular impairment, perceptual and cognitive impairment

GOAL 1
Prevent physical injury

INTERVENTIONS
Provide safe physical environment
- Padded furniture
- Siderails on bed
- Sturdy furniture that does not slip
- Avoid scatter rugs and polished floors

Select toys appropriate to age and physical limitations
Encourage sufficient rest
Use restraints when child is in chair or vehicle
Provide child who is prone to falls with protective helmet and enforce its use
Institute seizure precautions for susceptible child
*Administer anticonvulsant drugs as prescribed

EXPECTED OUTCOMES
Family provides a safe environment for the child (specify)
Child is free of injury

NURSING DIAGNOSIS: Impaired verbal communication

GOAL 1
Facilitate communication

INTERVENTIONS
Enlist the services of a speech therapist early
Talk to child slowly
Use articles and pictures to reinforce speech
Employ feeding techniques that help facilitate speech such as using lips, teeth, and various tongue movements
Teach and use nonverbal communication methods to dysarthric child who would benefit, e.g., Blissymbols
Help family acquire electronic equipment to facilitate nonverbal communication (e.g., typewriter, microcomputer with voice synthesizer)

*Dependent nursing action.

NURSING CARE PLAN
The Child with Cerebral Palsy—cont'd

EXPECTED OUTCOME

Child is able to communicate needs to caregivers (specify desired communication and means of accomplishment)

NURSING DIAGNOSIS: Fatigue related to increased energy expenditure

GOAL 1

Ensure balanced diet

INTERVENTIONS

Provide extra calories to meet energy demands of increased muscle activity
Monitor weight gain
Provide vitamin, mineral, and/or protein supplements if eating habits are poor
Devise aids and techniques to facilitate feeding

EXPECTED OUTCOMES

Child eats a balanced diet
Weight remains within acceptable limits (specify)

GOAL 2

Promote relaxation

INTERVENTIONS

Maintain a well-regulated schedule that allows for adequate rest and sleep periods
Be alert for evidence of fatigue, which tends to aggravate symptoms

EXPECTED OUTCOMES

Child is sufficiently rested

GOAL 3

Promote general health

INTERVENTIONS

Ensure regular routine health maintenance
- Physical assessment
- Dental care
- Immunizations

EXPECTED OUTCOMES

Child receives regular health assessments (specify schedule)
Child receives appropriate immunizations (specify) and dental care (specify)

NURSING DIAGNOSIS: Body image disturbance related to perception of disability

GOAL 1

Promote a positive body image

INTERVENTIONS

Capitalize on child's assets and provide compensation for liabilities
Praise child for accomplishments and "near" accomplishments such as partial completion of a task
Plan activities and goals *with* the child
See Nursing diagnosis: Body image disturbance in Nursing Care Plan: The Child with a Chronic Illness or Disability, Chapter 22

EXPECTED OUTCOME

Child exhibits behaviors that indicate positive body image (specify)

NURSING DIAGNOSIS: Altered family processes related to a child with a lifelong disability

GOAL 1

Support family

INTERVENTIONS

See Nursing diagnosis: Altered family processes in Nursing Care Plan: The Child with a Chronic Illness or Disability, Chapter 22
Refer to special support group(s) and agencies

EXPECTED OUTCOMES

Family contacts special support group

See also:
Nursing Care Plan: The Child with a Chronic Illness or Disability, Chapter 22
Nursing Care Plan: The Child with Mental Retardation, Chapter 24
Nursing Care Plan: The Child with Vision Impairment, Chapter 25
Nursing Care Plan: The Child with Hearing Impairment, Chapter 25

proaches to helping the child, and their lack of gratification, as well as the positive approaches they use. All of these aspects must be explored and discussed. Parents, as well as other members of the family, require a great deal of support and counseling. Siblings of a child with a disability are affected and may respond to the presence of the child with overt or less evident behavioral problems. The family needs a relationship with nurses who can provide continued contact, support, and encouragement through the long process of habilitation.

Parents can also find help and solace from parent groups with whom they can share problems and concerns and from whom they can derive comfort and practical information. The national organization, **United Cerebral Palsy Associations,*** has branches in most communities. The address of the nearest branch can be obtained from a local telephone directory, local agency directory, or a local health department or by writing to the national headquarters. The association provides a variety of services for children and families. There are also a number of excellent books available to serve as guides for parents and nurses who work with the child with CP.

Hospitalized child. CP is not a disorder that requires hospitalization; therefore, when children with CP are hospitalized, they are usually admitted for another reason or for corrective surgery. Consequently, many nurses are not accustomed to handling these children. Nurses who have never been associated with a child with cerebral palsy may react in a variety of ways, including with fear, revulsion, or overwhelming pity. The basic concept to keep in mind when caring for these children is that they are, first of all, children who happen to be afflicted with a disorder that limits their capacities in performing some activities of daily living and, for some, communicating with others. They should be approached and treated the same as any child in the hospital. The nurse's actions should convey acceptance, affection, and friendliness and promote a feeling of trust and dependability in the child. This is especially true with older children who have normal intelligence but who may have communication problems. These children often appear to be mentally retarded because of speech impairment. Frequently nurses tend to "talk down" to them and do things for them that they are perfectly capable, although not as adeptly as children without a disability, of doing for themselves. This is especially humiliating to a teenager who values independence and self-esteem.

To facilitate the care and management of these children, the therapy program should be continued, insofar as their condition allows, during the time they are hospitalized. This should be incorporated into the nursing care plan, and every effort expended to make certain that the ground that has been so laboriously gained is not lost. Encouraging the parents to room-in and actively participate in care facilitates a continuation of the home therapy routine and helps children adjust to an unfamiliar environment.

Children with CP frequently display behavioral problems. In some of these children the emotional disturbance is probably a reflection of the brain lesion. However, in most cases the behavioral problem is the result of conscious or unconscious rejection by others, particularly the parents. This is not surprising, since this condition is often frightening and unpleasant to others. These children may be viewed by some as being socially unacceptable, which may cause a parent to reject the child. When parents are helped to accept the child, the behavioral problems are significantly reduced.

Evaluation

The effectiveness of nursing interventions is determined by continual reassessment and evaluation of care based on the following observational guidelines and expected outcomes:

1. Observe the child's movements and speech.
2. Observe the child's activities, especially those related to self-care.
3. Interview the family regarding the child's activities and school attendance.
4. Observe the child's interactions with others and the choice of activities; interview the child regarding feelings and concerns.
5. Interview the family regarding their feelings and concerns and observe the members' interaction with the child.
6. Observe the child's behavior and responses during hospitalization.

Expected outcomes:
See Nursing Care Plan, pp. 1922-1923.

PROGRESSIVE INFANTILE SPINAL MUSCULAR ATROPHY (WERDNIG-HOFFMANN DISEASE)

Progressive infantile spinal muscular atrophy (Werdnig-Hoffmann disease) is a disorder characterized by progressive weakness and wasting of skeletal muscles caused by degeneration of anterior horn cells. It is inherited as an autosomal-recessive trait and is the most common paralytic form of the "floppy infant syndrome." The site of the pathologic condition is the anterior horn cells of the spinal cord and the motor nuclei of the brainstem, but the primary effect is atrophy of skeletal muscles.

Clinical Manifestations

The age of onset is variable, but, the earlier the onset, the more fulminating the course and the more disseminated and severe the motor weakness. The disorder may be manifest early, often at birth, frequently in utero, and almost always before 2 years of age. The manifestations and prognosis are categorized according to age of onset.

Group 1. This group comprises the infants who acquire the disease in utero or during the first 2 months of life. Inactivity is the most prominent feature. The infant lies in the

*66 E. 34th St., New York, NY 10016; (800) USA-1UCP or (212) 481-6300. In Canada: **Canadian Cerebral Palsy Association,** 40 Dundas Street West, Suite 222, P.O. Box 110, Toronto, Ont. M5G 2C2, Canada; (416) 979-7923.

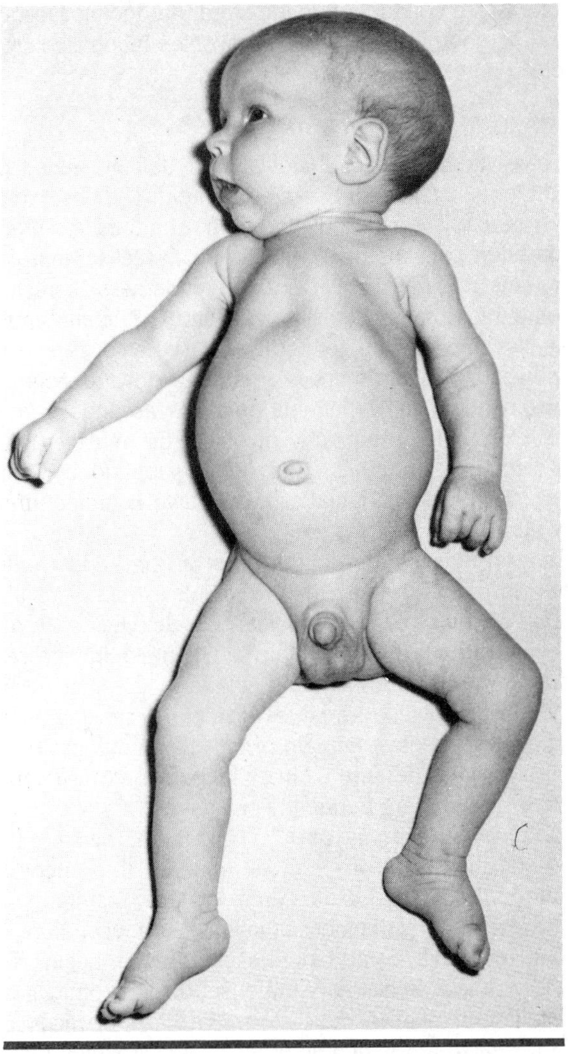

Fig. 40-6. Patient with group 1 Werdnig-Hoffmann disease lying in typical posture of abduction of legs at hips and flexion of knees. Arms are flexed slightly with little movement at shoulders. Movements of fingers and toes are present. Pectus excavatum deformity of chest is common and is result of unopposed diaphragmatic breathing.

From Swaiman, K.F., and Wright, F.S.: The practice of pediatric neurology, ed. 2, St. Louis, 1982, Mosby–Year Book, Inc.

frog position with legs externally rotated, abducted, and flexed at the hips (Fig. 40-6). There is weakness and limited movements of the shoulder and arm muscles, but active movement is usually limited to fingers and toes. Breathing is diaphragmatic, with sternal retractions caused by intercostal muscle paralysis. The cry and cough are weak, and secretions tend to pool in the pharynx. The facies are alert, and sensation and intellect are normal. These infants do not progress to roll over, sit alone, or walk. Early death (usually by 3 years of age) from respiratory failure or infection is usual. The most common complication is pneumonia.

Group 2. The infants in this group manifest the disease between 2 and 12 months of age. The symptoms are less devastating than in group 1. The weakness is confined to the arms and legs at first but later becomes generalized. The legs are usually involved to a greater extent than the arms. Pectus excavatum is prominent and is the result of unopposed diaphragmatic breathing. Movements are absent during complete relaxation or sleep. Some of these infants are able to sit if placed in position and in rare instances can stand holding onto furniture. The life span varies from 7 to 84 months.

Group 3. Children in this group experience onset of symptoms in the second year of life. They have normal head control and sit unassisted by 6 to 8 months of age. Thigh and hip muscles are weak; those who manage to walk have lumbar lordosis, waddling gait, genu recurvatum, and protuberant abdomen. Ambulation becomes increasingly difficult; children are confined to a wheelchair by the second decade. Deep tendon reflexes may be present early but disappear. It is often difficult to distinguish these children from those with juvenile spinal muscular atrophy.

Therapeutic Management

The diagnosis is established from electromyography demonstrating a denervation pattern and is confirmed by muscle biopsy. Treatment is symptomatic and preventive, primarily prevention of infection and treating orthopedic problems, the most serious of which is scoliosis. Many children benefit from powered chairs, lifts, special mattresses, and accessible environmental controls. Vigorous antibiotic therapy and pulmonary physical therapy are implemented during upper respiratory infections.

Nursing Considerations

The infant or small child with extensive paralysis requires frequent change of position to prevent physical injury and complications, especially pneumonia. The pharynx requires frequent suctioning to remove secretions, and feeding must be carried out slowly and carefully to prevent aspiration. Since these children are intellectually normal, verbal, tactile, and auditory stimulation are important aspects of care. Supporting them so that they can see the activities around them and transporting them in a buggy for a change of environment provide stimulation and a broader scope of contacts.

Children who are able to sit require proper support and attention to alignment to prevent deformities and other complications. Children with group 2 or group 3 disease will need attention to education needs and opportunities for social interaction with other children. Parents of a child with a chronic or potentially fatal illness require a great deal of support and encouragement (see Chapters 22 and 23). The parents of children with a genetically transmitted disorder also need to be encouraged to seek genetic counseling.

JUVENILE SPINAL MUSCULAR ATROPHY (KUGELBERG-WELANDER DISEASE)

Juvenile spinal muscular atrophy (Kugelberg-Welander disease, juvenile proximal hereditary muscular atrophy) is also the result of anterior horn cell and motor nerve degeneration. The disease is characterized by a pattern of muscular weakness similar to that of infantile spinal muscular atrophy. Several modes of inheritance have been reported for the disease—autosomal-recessive, autosomal-dominant, and X-linked recessive.

The onset occurs between 2 and 17 years of age, with symptoms resembling group 3 infantile spinal muscular atrophy, although proximal muscle weakness (especially of the pelvic girdle) appears later, in early childhood or adolescence, and the progression is slower. Muscles of the lower arms and legs are involved relatively late, and muscles of the trunk and those supplied by the cranial nerves are usually unaffected. The disease runs a slowly progressive course. Some children lose the ability to walk 8 to 9 years after onset of symptoms, but many can still walk after 20 years or more. Many affected persons have a normal life expectancy.

Therapeutic Management and Nursing Considerations

The management is primarily symptomatic and supportive and related to maintaining mobility as long as possible, preventing complications, and providing child and family support.

INFECTIOUS POLYNEURITIS (GUILLAIN-BARRÉ SYNDROME)

Infectious polyneuritis, also known as infectious neuronitis, Guillain-Barré syndrome (GBS), and Landry's paralysis, is probably the most common form of polyneuritis and may occur at any age. It is an acute polyneuropathy in which motor dysfunction predominates over sensory disturbance; there is bilateral facial paresis or paralysis and occasionally weakness of the bulbar and respiratory musculature. Although children are less often affected than adults, the incidence in the pediatric age-group appears to be increasing, with higher susceptibility in children between ages 4 and 10 years. Both sexes are affected with equal frequency.

The precise etiologic agent is unknown. Since the disease has been associated with a number of viral infections or the administration of vaccines, it has been suggested that it may be a toxic sequela of an original infection, an activated latent virus, or a manifestation of an acute infection. Among illnesses that have been associated with the disease are infectious mononucleosis, measles, mumps, and a glandular feverlike syndrome. It may also be associated with *Mycoplasma* and *Pneumocystis* infections or gram-negative organisms. There has been an association with a vaccination process (the swine flu immunization of 1976). Some believe that it may represent a cell-mediated immunologic response directed at the peripheral nerves.

Pathophysiology

Pathologic changes in spinal and cranial nerves consist of inflammation and edema with rapid, segmented demyelination and compression of nerve roots within the dural sheath. Nerve conduction is impaired, producing ascending partial or complete paralysis of muscles innervated by the involved nerves.

Clinical Manifestations

The paralytic manifestations of GBS are usually preceded by a mild influenza-like illness or sore throat. The onset can be rapid, reaching peak activity within 24 hours, or gradual progression of symptoms over days or weeks. Neurologic symptoms initially involve muscle tenderness, sometimes accompanied by paresthesia and cramps. Proximal muscle weakness progressing to paralysis usually occurs before distal weakness, and there is a tendency toward symmetric involvement. In most patients paralysis ascends from the lower extremities, frequently involving the muscles of the trunk, upper extremities, and those supplied by cranial nerves. The seventh (facial) cranial nerve is almost universally affected.

Tendon reflexes are depressed or absent, and paralysis is flaccid. Paralysis may involve facial, extraocular, labial, lingual, pharyngeal, and laryngeal muscles. Evidence of intercostal and phrenic nerve involvement includes breathlessness in vocalizations and shallow, irregular respirations. There may be variable degrees of sensory impairment. Most patients complain of muscle tenderness or sensitivity to slight pressure. Urinary incontinence or retention and constipation are frequently present.

Course and prognosis. The general health of the child and the extent of paralysis influence the outcome of the illness. Almost all deaths are caused by respiratory failure; therefore early diagnosis and access to respiratory support are especially important. Muscle function begins to return 2 days to 2 weeks after the onset of symptoms, and recovery is complete in most cases. The rate of recovery is usually related to the degree of involvement, which may extend from a few weeks to months. The greater the degree of paralysis, the longer the recovery phase.

Diagnostic Evaluation

Criteria for diagnosis of GBS are listed in Box 40-4.

Box 40-4 CRITERIA FOR DIAGNOSIS OF GUILLAIN-BARRÉ SYNDROME

1. The paralysis may follow a nonspecific infection, but an illness known to be associated with polyradiculoneuropathy, such as herpes zoster or diphtheria, should not be present.
2. Findings should include multiple or diffuse lower motor unit paralysis that is rapid or gradual in onset, symmetric involvement, progressive weakness, and areflexia.
3. Sensory involvement may be present but generally is less severe than the motor weakness.
4. Cerebrospinal fluid examination should contain fewer than 10 white cells/mm^3.
5. Cerebrospinal fluid protein concentration should equal or exceed 60 mg/dl.

Therapeutic Management

Treatment of Guillain-Barré syndrome is symptomatic. Corticosteroid therapy has been of benefit in the early stages. Respiratory and pharyngeal involvement requires assisted ventilation, frequently with tracheostomy. Recent studies indicate that plasma exchange (plasmapheresis) may be beneficial both in shortening the length of illness and lessening the long-term disability (Briscoe and others, 1987).

Nursing Considerations

Nursing care is essentially supportive and is the same as that required for quadriplegia from any cause. Since the care of the quadriplegic child is discussed in relation to spinal cord injury later in the chapter, it will not be considered at length here. The emphasis of care is on close observation to assess the extent of paralysis and prevention of complications.

During the acute phase of the disease the child's condition should be carefully observed for possible difficulty in swallowing and respiratory involvement. There should be a respirator on standby, with a cardiac monitor attached, and suction apparatus, tracheostomy tray, and vasoconstrictor drugs available at the bedside. Vital signs and level of consciousness are monitored frequently. For the child who develops respiratory dysfunction, the care is the same as that of any child with respiratory distress requiring mechanical ventilation (see Chapter 31 and care of the child with tetanus who is given muscle relaxant drugs).

Throughout the recovery phase special emphasis is placed on prevention of complications, including good postural alignment, frequent change of position, and passive range of motion exercises. Children with oral and pharyngeal involvement are usually fed via a nasogastric tube to ensure adequate feeding. Bowel and bladder care is needed to avoid constipation and urine retention. Sensory impairment makes the child susceptible to burns and trophic ulcers.

Physical therapy is limited to passive range of motion exercises during the evolving phase of the disease. Later, as the disease stabilizes and recovery begins, an active physical therapy program is implemented to prevent contracture deformities and facilitate muscle recovery. This may include active exercise, gait training, and bracing.

Throughout the course of the illness child and parent support is paramount. The usual rapidity of the paralysis and the long period of recovery tax the emotional reserves of all family members greatly. The parents and child benefit from repeated reassurance that recovery is occurring and from realistic information regarding the possibility of permanent disability. In the event of a residual disability, the family needs assistance in accepting and adjusting to the loss of function (see Chapter 22). The **Guillain-Barré Syndrome Support Group*** is a nonprofit organization devoted to support, education, and research. It provides support to families from recovered persons, publishes informational literature and a newsletter, and maintains a list of practitioners experienced with the disease.

*P.O. Box 262, Wynnewood PA 19096, (215) 642-6855.

TETANUS

Tetanus, or lockjaw, is an acute, preventable, and often fatal disease caused by an exotoxin produced by the anaerobic spore-forming, gram-positive bacillus *Clostridium tetani.* It is characterized by painful muscular rigidity primarily involving the masseter and neck muscles. There are four requirements for the development of tetanus: (1) presence of tetanus spores or vegetative forms of the bacillus, (2) injury to the tissues, (3) wound conditions that encourage multiplication of the organism, and (4) a susceptible host.

Tetanus spores are found in soil, dust, and the intestinal tracts of humans and animals, especially herbivorous animals. The organisms are more prevalent in rural areas but are readily carried to urban areas by the wind. They are not invasive but enter the body by way of wounds, particularly a puncture wound, burn, or crushed area. They may enter through a very minor, unnoticed break in the skin such as a thorn or needle prick, bee sting, or scratch. In the newborn infection may occur through the umbilical cord, usually in situations in which infants are delivered in contaminated surroundings. The disease has the greatest incidence in months when persons are more involved in outdoor activities. Drug addicts are especially susceptible because of poor injection technique and the use of street heroin, which is often mixed with quinine, a protoplasmic poison that favors the growth of the organism.

Pathophysiology

When conditions are favorable, the organisms proliferate and form two exotoxins: (1) tetanospasmin, a potent toxin that affects the central nervous system to produce the clinical manifestations of the disease, and (2) tetanolysin, which appears to have no significance. The ideal conditions for growth of the organisms are devitalized tissues without access to air, such as puncture wounds, wounds that have not been washed or kept clean, and those that have crusted over, trapping pus beneath. The exotoxin appears to reach the central nervous system by way of either the neuron axons or the vascular system. The toxin becomes fixed on nerve cells of the anterior horn of the spinal cord and the brainstem. The toxin acts at the myoneural junction to produce the muscular stiffness and lower the threshold for reflex excitability.

The incubation period for tetanus varies from 3 days to 3 weeks but average is 8 days. The more extensive the injury, the shorter the incubation period and the more severe the symptoms, although this is debatable.

Clinical Manifestations

There are several forms of the disease. *Local tetanus* is a less severe form characterized by persistent rigidity of muscles near the inoculation site, which may persist for weeks or months, but some cases resolve without sequelae. *Otogenous tetanus* is generalized or local tetanus that follows chronic otitis media, whereas *C. tetani* is a secondary invader, surviving in purulent discharge. *Cephalic tetanus,* a rare form, follows infection of the head or face and can occur as a complication of acne or otitis media. This form is often limited to cranial nerves III, IV, VII, IX, X, and XII but may progress to generalized tetanus.

Generalized tetanus is the most common and dangerous form of the disease. The manner of onset varies, but the initial symptoms are usually a progressive stiffness and tenderness of the muscles in the neck and jaw. The characteristic difficulty in opening the mouth (trismus), caused by sustained contraction of the jaw-closing muscles, is evident early and gives the disease its common name, lockjaw. Spasm of facial muscles produces the so-called sardonic smile *(risus sardonicus).* Progressive involvement of the trunk muscles causes opisthotonos and a boardlike rigidity of abdominal and limb muscles. There is difficulty in swallowing, and the patient is highly sensitive to external stimuli. The slightest noise, a gentle touch, or bright light will trigger convulsive muscular contractions that last seconds to minutes. The paroxysmal contractions recur with increased frequency until they become almost continuous.

Mentation is unaffected; the patient remains alert, and pain and distress are reflected in rapid pulse, sweating, and an anxious expression. Laryngospasm and tetany of respiratory muscles and accumulated secretions predispose to respiratory arrest, atelectasis, and pneumonia. Fever is usually absent or only mild; presence of fever generally indicates a poor prognosis. As the child recovers from the disease, the paroxysms become less and less frequent and gradually subside. Survival beyond 4 days usually indicates recovery, but complete recovery may require weeks.

The mortality rate is about 30%, but the disease is almost invariably fatal in the newborn. The first symptom is difficulty sucking, which progresses to total inability to suck, excessive crying, irritability, and nuchal rigidity.

Therapeutic Management: Prevention

Preventive measures are based on the immune status of the affected child and the nature of the injury. Specific prophylactic therapy after trauma is administration of either tetanus toxoid or tetanus antitoxin. For clean, minor wounds in children who have completed the immunization series (see Chapter 12) or received a booster within the previous 10 years, a dose of tetanus toxoid is not necessary. Protective levels of antibody are maintained for at least 10 years; therefore antitoxin is not indicated for the fully immunized child. (See also Table 12-10.) Children with more serious wounds (e.g., contaminated, puncture, crush, or burn wounds) are given a tetanus toxoid booster prophylactically as soon as possible after injury.

The unprotected or inadequately immunized child who sustains a "tetanus-prone" wound (e.g., contaminated soil, crush injury, burn, compound fracture, retained foreign body, or a wound unattended for 24 hours) should receive tetanus immune globulin (TIG), human TIG. TIG is preferred to tetanus antitoxin (TAT) because of its absence of sensitivity reactions and longer half-life. Once the toxin has bound to central nervous system tissue, antitoxin has no effect, but if the binding has taken place only peripherally, administration of human tetanus immune globulin or bovine or horse tetanus antitoxin will prevent binding in the central areas. Concurrent administration of both TIG and toxoid at separate sites is recommended both to provide protection and to initiate the active immune process. Completion of active immunization is carried out according to the usual pattern.

Proper surgical cleansing and debridement of contaminated wounds reduce the chance of infection.

Therapeutic Management: Treatment

The affected child is best treated in an intensive care facility where close and constant observation and equipment for monitoring and respiratory support are readily available. A quiet environment is preferred to reduce external stimuli. Neonates are placed in an open unit or incubator in which a constant environmental temperature can be maintained and oxygen supplied.

General supportive care, including maintenance of adequate fluid and electrolyte balance and caloric intake, is indicated. Indwelling oral or nasogastric feedings are used whenever possible, but severe laryngospasm may necessitate intravenous alimentation or gastrostomy feeding. Recurrent laryngospasm or excessive accumulation of secretions may require endotracheal intubation.

Antitoxin therapy to neutralize toxins not yet bound to nervous tissue is the most specific therapy for tetanus. TIG is preferred, but, if unavailable, TAT is given. Antibiotics are administered to control the proliferation of the vegetative forms of the organism at the site of infection. The American Academy of Pediatrics (1988) recommends therapy for 10 to 14 days. When the child recovers, active immunization should take place, since the disease does not confer a permanent immunity.

Local care of the wound by surgical debridement and cleansing helps reduce the numbers of proliferating organisms at the site of injury. An antibacterial agent such as pHisoHex or povidone-iodine (Betadine) followed by a dilute solution of hydrogen peroxide has proved effective. The cleansing should be repeated several times during the first 48 hours, and deep, infected lacerations are usually exposed and debrided.

Sedatives or muscle relaxants are administered to help reduce muscle spasm and prevent convulsions. Patients with severe tetanus and those who do not respond to other sedatives may require the administration of a neuromuscular blocking agent, usually pancuronium bromide (Pavulon) or *d*-tubocurarine. Because of their paralytic effect on respiratory muscles, use of these drugs requires mechanical ventilation and constant attendance by trained personnel until muscle spasms are controlled.

Endotracheal tube or tracheostomy is often indicated and should be performed before severe respiratory distress develops. Administration of corticosteroids has met with success in some instances.

Nursing Considerations

In caring for the child with tetanus, every effort should be made to control or eliminate stimulation from sound, light, and touch. Although a darkened room is ideal, sufficient light is essential in order that the child can be carefully observed; light appears to be less irritating than vibratory or auditory stimuli. The infant or child is handled as little as possible, and extra effort is expended to avoid any sudden and/or loud noise.

Medications are administered as prescribed, and vital signs are observed and recorded at frequent intervals. The location and extent of muscle spasms and assessment of their severity are important nursing observations. Respiratory status is carefully evaluated for any signs of embarrassment, and appropriate emergency equipment is kept available at all times. Muscle relaxants and sedatives that may be prescribed can also cause respiratory depression; therefore the child must be assessed for excessive central nervous system depression. Blood gases are obtained frequently to evaluate the respiratory status. Attention to hydration and nutrition may involve monitoring an intravenous infusion, monitoring nasogastric or gastrostomy feedings, and suctioning oropharyngeal secretions when indicated.

If a potent muscle relaxant such as pancuronium bromide (Pavulon) is used, the total paralysis makes oral communication impossible. Therefore all the child's needs must be anticipated, and procedures carefully explained beforehand. As the dose of medication is decreased, the child regains movement of the eyelids and facial muscles, which gives the child some opportunity to express emotions and indicate choices through a signal system, for example, blinking the lids to indicate "yes" or "no."

Although most affected children are neonates and receive the nursing care and assessment of any high-risk infant (Chapter 10), older children may acquire a tetanus infection. Since their mental status is clear, they are aware of what is happening to them and are often in a state of terror. They should not be left alone, and all efforts should be made to reduce anxiety, which can contribute to muscular spasms. A calm and reassuring manner and sympathetic understanding can help immeasurably in getting a child through this crisis situation. Parents are encouraged to stay with the child to offer security and support.

BOTULISM

Botulism is a serious food poisoning that results from ingestion of the preformed toxin produced by the anaerobic bacillus *Clostridium botulinum.* Botulism toxin exerts its effect by inhibiting the release of acetylcholine at the myoneural junction, thereby impairing motor activity of muscles innervated by affected nerves. There is wide variation in severity of the disease, from constipation to progressive sequential loss of neurologic function and respiratory failure.

Types of Botulism

Three forms of the disease are recognized: infantile botulism, classic botulism, and wound botulism.

Classic botulism. The classic form of the disease is usually seen in adults but may occur in children and adolescents. The most common source of the toxin is improperly sterilized home-canned foods. Central nervous system symptoms appear abruptly about 12 to 36 hours after ingestion of contaminated food and may or may not have been preceded by acute digestive disturbance. Early symptoms include blurred vision, diplopia, weakness, dizziness, difficulty talking and speaking, vomiting, and dysphagia. These are followed by descending paralysis and dyspnea. Progressive respiratory paralysis is life-threatening.

Infant botulism. Infant botulism, unlike the disease in older persons, is caused by ingestion of spores or vegetative cells of *C. botulinum* and the subsequent release of the toxin from organisms colonizing the gastrointestinal tract. There appears to be no common food or drug source of the organisms; however, the *C. botulinum* organisms have been found in honey fed to affected infants, and light as well as dark corn syrup has been reported to contain spores (American Academy of Pediatrics, 1988).

One study (Spika and others, 1989) identified risk factors for infant botulism in the United States. They appear to be decreased frequency of bowel movements (less than one per day for at least 2 months) in infants 2 months of age or older, and ingestion of corn syrup and living in a rural area or on a farm for infants less than 2 months of age. Thus preexisting host factors may be the most important risk factors for developing the disease.

The affected infant is usually well before the onset of symptoms. Constipation is a common presenting symptom, and almost all infants exhibit generalized weakness and a decrease in spontaneous movements. Deep tendon reflexes are usually diminished or absent; cranial nerve deficits are common (especially CN VII, IX, X, and XI), as evidenced by loss of head control, difficulty in feeding, weak cry, and reduced gag reflex. The most frequently recognized form of the disease is consistent with the "floppy infant syndrome."

Wound botulism. Wounds contaminated with *C. botulinum* and subsequent elaboration of the toxin produces classic symptoms in about 4 to 14 days after tissue trauma. The disease has been described in a small number of adolescents and adults, and most wounds are sustained in open fields or on farms.

Therapeutic Management

Diagnosis is made on the basis of history, physical examination, and laboratory detection of toxin or the organism in the patient or the implicated food. Treatment consists of aggressive supportive measures, primarily respiratory and nutritional. Botulinal antitoxin is sometimes used in adults and older children but is not administered to infants. Evidence indicates that the infants recover without it and that its therapeutic efficacy is lacking. Furthermore, since the antitoxin is made from horse serum, it may cause serum sickness or anaphylaxis and may induce a lifelong hypersensitivity (Arnon, 1986). Toxins vary in protein-binding capacity. Some have a relatively short half-life and do not bind to tissues firmly; therefore therapy is continued until paralysis abates. Other toxins appear to bind irreversibly to nerve endings and are therefore not amenable to neutralization. Respiratory support is often needed and should be available at the bedside ready for use if indicated.

The prognosis is generally good if the patient is adequately supported, although recovery may be very slow, requiring weeks to months following severe illness.

Nursing Considerations

Nursing responsibilities include observing for and reporting signs of muscle impairment and providing intensive nursing care when the infant is hospitalized (see Nursing Care of High-Risk Infants, Chapter 10). Parental support and reassurance are important. Most infants recover when the disorder is recognized and therapy implemented. Parents should be aware that during recovery patients fatigue easily when muscular action is sustained. This has important implications for timing the resumption of feedings because of the risk of aspiration. They should also be advised that normal bowel action may not return for several weeks; therefore a stool softener can be beneficial. Cathartics and enemas are not advised.

Home supervision of the outpatient and education regarding possible modes of infection (such as use of honey as formula sweetener) are nursing responsibilities. Since the prime sources of botulism toxin are inadequately cooked or improperly canned food, families are advised about the danger of home-canned foods, especially vegetables, fruits, fish, and condiments. Boiling is not always adequate, particularly in high altitudes where water boils at a lower temperature, which does not destroy the organisms (Parke, 1990).

MYASTHENIA GRAVIS

Myasthenia gravis (MG) is relatively uncommon in childhood. Juvenile MG appears to be identical to that seen in adults and usually has its onset after age 10 years, but it may appear as early as age 2 years. Girls are affected six times as often as boys. Juvenile and adult forms of the disease are autoimmune disorders associated with attack of circulating antibodies on the acetylcholine receptors on the muscle end plate, blocking their function.

Clinical Manifestations

The most common symptoms are general paralysis of the optic muscles with ptosis and diplopia. Difficulty in swallowing, chewing, and speaking is also prominent, accompanied by weakness and paralysis of all skeletal muscles. The signs and symptoms are more pronounced in the late afternoon and evening. They are relieved by rest and made worse by exercise and stress.

Diagnostic Evaluation

The diagnosis is made on the basis of the characteristic distribution of muscle weakness and the progressive weakness on repeated or sustained muscular contraction. The diagnosis is established by observation of the response to the anticholinesterase drugs. Intravenous administration of a small test dose of edrophonium (Tensilon) produces a beneficial effect in 1 minute but lasts for less than 5 minutes. Electrophysiologic studies are helpful in diagnosis and help document transmission failure at the myoneural junction. Antibodies to human muscle acetylcholine are detected in serum of almost all affected persons.

Therapeutic Management

Treatment consists of the oral administration of anticholinesterase drugs, the least toxic of which is pyridostigmine (Mestinon). The initial dose is 30 mg every 4 hours in the older child and 5 mg every 4 hours in the infant. The dosage is gradually increased until a satisfactory result is obtained. The child must be observed for signs of parasympathetic stimulation from overmedication. These include lacrimation, salivation, abdominal cramps, sweating, diarrhea, vomiting, bradycardia, and weakness of respiratory muscles.

Other therapies directed at the immunologic mechanism include thymectomy, corticosteroid therapy, and immunosuppression. All have disadvantages. Plasmapheresis has been used for short-term intensive intervention.

The prognosis of juvenile MG is relatively good. However, the course of the disease is marked by fluctuating remissions and exacerbations.

Nursing Considerations

These children need continuous medical and nursing supervision. The parents are taught the importance of accurate administration of medications, with special emphasis on recognizing side effects with the dangers of choking, aspiration, and respiratory distress.

Parents are counseled regarding promoting a life-style that minimizes stress and maximizes relaxation. Strenuous activity is discouraged. They are also warned of the possibility of a sudden exacerbation of symptoms during times of physical or emotional stress (myasthenia crisis) that requires immediate medical attention. They should receive instruction in providing respiratory assistance until help arrives or the child can be transported to medical aid.

Neonatal Myasthenia Gravis

A *transient* form of MG occurs in approximately 15% of infants born to mothers with myasthenia gravis who may not be aware that they have the disease. The muscular weakness results from transplacentally acquired maternal acetylcholine receptor antibodies. These infants display generalized weakness and hypotonia at birth with a depressed Moro reflex, ptosis, ineffective sucking and swallowing reflexes, and weak cry. There is no evidence of neurologic damage. In this form the symptoms usually disappear within 2 to 4 weeks.

Persistent neonatal MG is a familial abnormality of neuromuscular transmission that is not immunologically mediated. It appears indistinguishable from the transient form, but the mother usually does not have the disease. The disease persists throughout life, and more than one sibling may be affected, which suggests a genetic etiology. Sex distribution is equal. The disorder is relatively resistant to drug therapy, and the eyelid and extraocular muscles seem to be the muscles most severely affected.

The prognosis in persistent neonatal MG is usually good. Although there is gradual worsening of symptoms with age, the life span is not affected significantly.

SPINAL CORD INJURIES

Spinal cord injuries with major neurologic involvement are not a common cause of physical disability in childhood. However, a sufficient number of children with these injuries are admitted to major medical centers, and because of the increased survival as the result of improved management, nurses are more likely to become involved with such children. In addition, the catastrophic nature of spinal cord injury with its serious sequelae and the importance of preventive and functional rehabilitation justify a discussion of the topic. The principles of management and nursing care apply to all spinal cord lesions, regardless of etiology, particularly myelomeningocele, the most common cause of paraplegia in the pediatric age-group.

In addition to care related to the immobilized child as discussed in Chapter 39, children with damage to the spinal cord present additional problems, specifically complications related to the neuropathology of the central and autonomic nervous systems. A high level of paraplegia may create major problems in the ability to sit upright without support, whereas children with paraplegia with lower level injuries can walk with minimum assistance. The extent of paralysis is determined by both neurologic and clinical assessment. Although the majority of children with spinal cord injuries are paraplegic, many are quadriplegic. Some children with quadriplegia are able to move only their face and neck muscles, whereas others are able to lift and bend their arms but are unable to perform fine hand movements. Almost every physiologic system is disrupted in a child with high-level quadriplegia. Not only are the central and peripheral nerves impaired, but there is also autonomic nervous system dysfunction. Vital structures such as blood vessels, lungs, bladder, and bowel are affected. Therefore an understanding of neuromuscular physiology is essential to effectively care for the child with damage or injury to the spinal cord.

Review of Essential Neuromuscular Physiology

The spinal cord extends from the medulla oblongata to the lower border of the first lumbar vertebra and contains millions of nerve fibers (Fig. 40-7). However, because of its protected location, a considerable amount of direct trauma is required to cause injury. Posteriorly the cord is protected by the spinous processes, which are stabilized by related ligaments and muscles. It is further protected by the spinal fluid, which surrounds it and absorbs some of the shock.

Spinal nerves. The 31 nerves of the spinal cord are divided into five segments. The eight *cervical* cord segments lie within the first seven vertebrae. The remaining cord segments— *thoracic* (12), *lumbar* (five), *sacral* (five), and *coccygeal* (one)— extend from the first thoracic vertebra to the lower level of the first lumbar vertebra. Therefore the cord constituents do not anatomically match by number the 30 associated vertebrae. However, nerves that arise from the spinal cord exit from the spinal column at the numerically

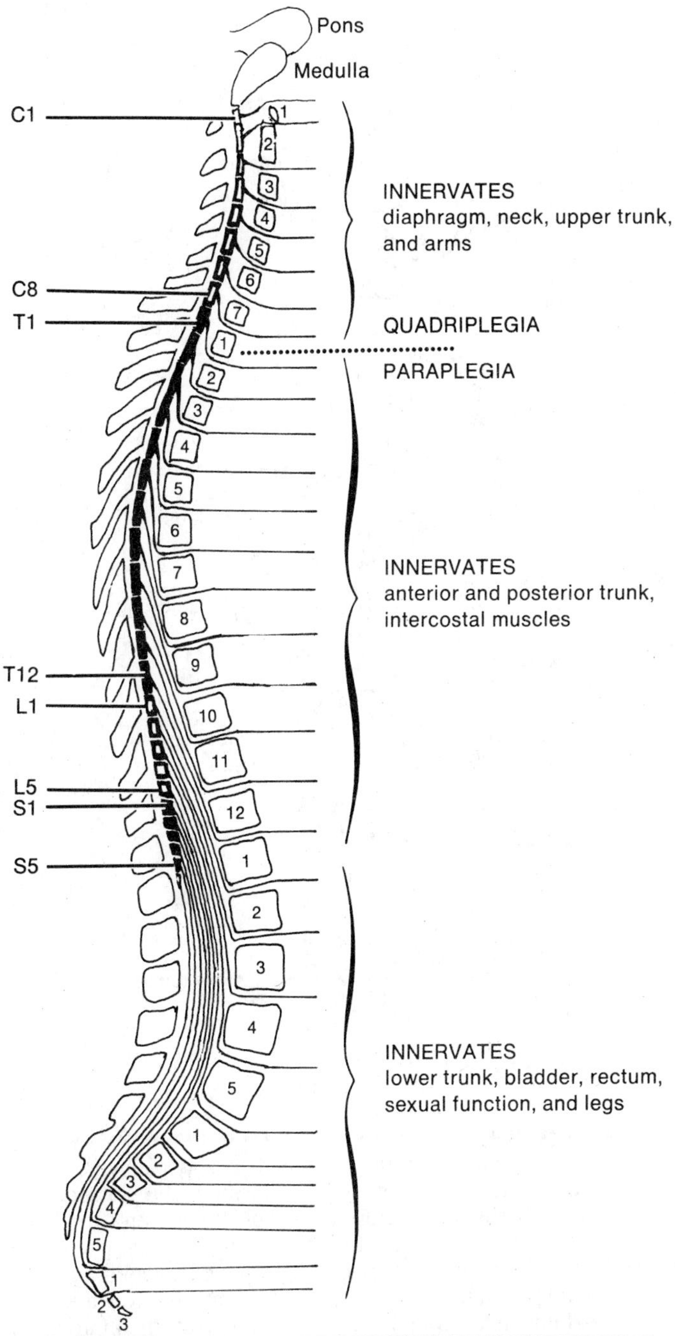

Fig. 40-7. Relationships of spinal cord segments and spinal nerves to vertebral bodies. Cervical nerves exit through intervertebral foramina above their respective vertebral bodies (seven cervical vertebrae and eight cervical nerves). Spinal cord ends at L1 and L2 vertebral level.

corresponding vertebrae. In describing injuries to the spinal cord, the highest point at which there is normal function is referred to in relation to the vertebra, for example, an intact cord at the sixth cervical vertebra is designated as a C6 injury.

Certain areas of the curved vertebral column are less stable and more prone to damage from severe flexion and twisting. These sites are the cervical area and the junction of the thoracic and lumbar regions. The cervical vertebrae are fractured most frequently, and this high level of injury causes extensive paralysis and many associated neurologic problems (see Table 40-1). Also, traumatic tearing or embolic occlusion of arteries supplying these areas can markedly jeopardize the cord tissue. Impaired blood supply frequently produces severe neurologic deficit, which can extend to complete loss of cord function at the level of injury.

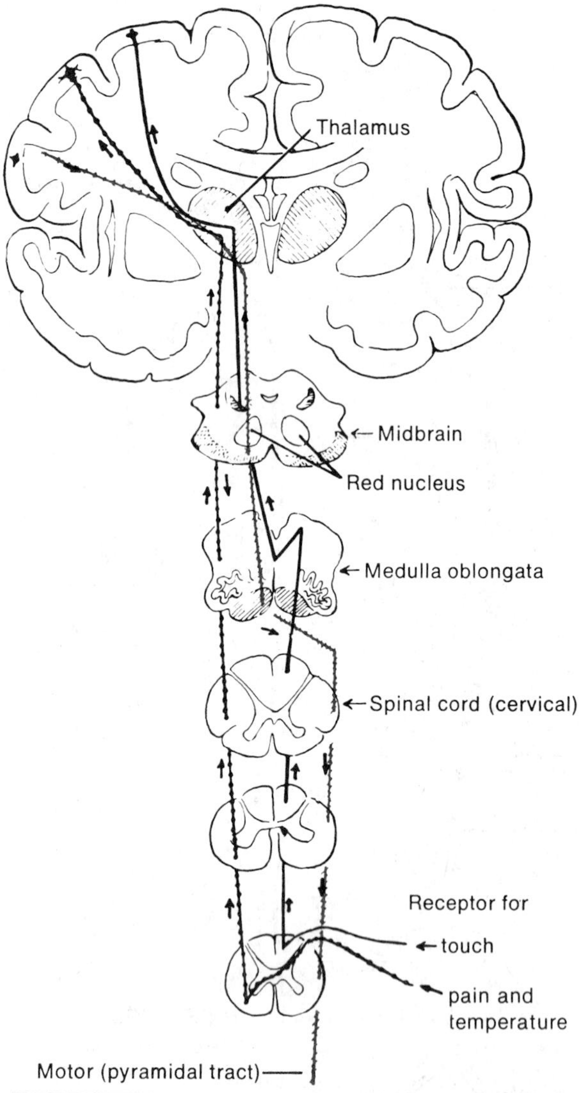

Fig. 40-8. Diagram of main motor and sensory pathways. Perception of touch, passive motion, position, and vibration is transmitted through posterior tract in spinal cord through medial lemniscus in brainstem to thalamus and through internal capsule to cortex (this pathway is represented by solid line). Pain and temperature sensations are transmitted through anterolateral tract and lateral lemniscus to thalamus, then through internal capsule to cortex *(irregular line)*. Motor impulses are transmitted by pyramidal tract, descending from cerebral cortex, crossing in medulla to opposite side, and continuing to anterior horns of spinal cord *(red line)*.

From Conway, B.L.: Carini and Owens' neurological and neurosurgical nursing, ed. 7, St. Louis, 1978, Mosby–Year Book, Inc.

Cell bodies of interneurons and motor neurons within the spinal cord are identified as H-shaped gray matter surrounded by columns of white myelinated nerve fibers, each column serving as a route for a specific type of impulse, such as touch, vibration, pain, and temperature (Fig. 40-8). Nerve pathways in the spinal cord transmit sensory and motor impulses between peripheral receptors and the brain, conduct impulses through the reflex arc, and convey sympathetic and parasympathetic nerve impulses from the brain to peripheral structures.

Sensory transmission begins when peripheral receptors pick up a wide variety of stimuli and transfer the impulses, by means of peripheral nerves, to the spinal nerves, where they make ganglionic connections and enter the cord posteriorly. At this point the impulses travel in two directions: (1) across the intraneuron connection and then to the motor neurons (reflex arc), or (2) up the spinal cord to predetermined areas of the brain. *Motor* impulses are transmitted from the cerebral cortex to the medulla (where nerve tracts cross) and then proceed down descending motor pathways to the desired level within the spinal cord. Here they connect with the anterior horn cells and are transmitted to the muscle fibers by means of the lower motor neurons to complete a meaningful movement.

A network of nerves that serves the major muscle groups constitutes a *plexus*. Total involvement of any one of these plexuses seriously impairs function to the areas it innervates. The three major plexuses are described in Box 40-5.

Upper vs lower motor neurons. *Upper motor neurons* extend from cerebral centers to cells in the spinal column; *lower motor neurons* consist of anterior horn cells and spinal and peripheral nerves. Motor fibers of the reflex arc are lower motor neurons, an important point for relative dominance of the higher central nervous system (CNS) over reflex arcs suppresses some reflex responses. In spinal cord injury when the higher centers no longer exert an influence, spastic responses are observed in muscles innervated by the intact lower motor neurons. Most spinal cord injuries involve upper motor neurons; children born with spinal

Box 40-5 THE THREE MAJOR PLEXUSES

Cervical plexus (C1 through C4), which innervates the neck and diaphragm
Brachial plexus (C4 through T1), which supplies the shoulders, chest, and arms
Lumbosacral plexus (L1 through S4), which transmits impulses to the lower trunk and legs

Box 40-6 DIFFERENCES IN CLINICAL MANIFESTATIONS BETWEEN UPPER AND LOWER MOTOR NEURON SYNDROMES

Upper Motor Neuron Syndrome	Lower Motor Neuron Syndrome
Spastic paralysis in muscle groups below lesion (reflex arcs below lesion are intact)	Flaccid paralysis caused by muscle atonia (reflex arcs are permanently damaged)
Hyperreflexia with tendon reflexes exaggerated, Babinski reflex present	Reflex with associated muscle response absent
No wasting of muscle mass because of increased muscle tone	Marked atrophy of atonic muscle
Flexion contractures and spasms of muscle groups below lesion level common	Fasciculations (local twitching of muscle groups) common No flexor spasms
No skin or tissue changes	Loss of hair Skin and tissue changes Cornified nails

cord defects have primarily lower motor neuron deficits. (See also Fig. 40-1.) Manifestations of upper and lower motor neuron syndromes are outlined in Box 40-6.

Effect on sensory and motor tracts. Voluntary muscle control is lost following complete transection of the cord. In partial transection function is altered to varying degrees, depending on the areas innervated by involved nerves. Crossing of motor tracts at various levels makes it possible for an injured person to have motor paralysis in one leg but retain pain and temperature sensation to that leg while losing these sensations in the opposite leg, which retains its motor function.

Although a transected cord injury leads to sensory loss, it is not uncommon for the injured person to have pain experiences. For example, smooth or skeletal muscle spasms, destruction of the myelin sheath (impulses cross to adjacent nerves), and scar formation or irritation of nerve endings may cause pain. Pain suffered by a person with quadriplegia or paraplegia is often intensified because of loss of sensation in other parts. Severe and prolonged pain should be medically evaluated for treatable pathology.

Effect on autonomic system. Sympathetic and parasympathetic systems receive both excitatory and inhibitory stimuli from autonomic centers in the cerebral cortex, limbic system, and hypothalamus. The stimuli are transmitted by means of a feedback mechanism within the ascending fibers of the cord that normally controls descending input. Axons of the many CNS neurons synapse with autonomic preganglionic fibers and thus are able to alter their patterned responses. The most significant effects of autonomic disruption are described in Box 40-7.

Box 40-7 SIGNIFICANT EFFECTS OF AUTONOMIC DISRUPTION

Decreased muscle tone and impairment of vasoconstrictive effects of sympathetic innervation cause venous pooling, diminished venous return to the heart, decreased cardiac output, and hypotension, especially orthostatic hypotension

Thermoregulatory disruption in the hypothalamus and skin receptors causes blood vessels to remain dilated during the initial stage, inability to sweat in response to increased environmental temperature, and possible rapid elevation in body temperature

Voluntary bowel and bladder function is lost because of damage to nerve fibers that innervate these organs

Altered sexual function (lack of erection, ejaculation, and orgasm) resulting from interference with numerous autonomic nerve fibers and plexuses

Etiology

The most common cause of serious spinal cord damage in children is congenital defects of the spinal cord (e.g., myelomeningocele). Postnatal causes are primarily accidental injury, especially motor vehicle accidents (MVAs) (including automobile-bicycle and all-terrain vehicle accidents), sports injuries (especially from diving, trampoline activities, and football), and birth trauma. The large majority of diving injuries (60% to 100%) occur outside organized sports programs (Bruce, Schut, and Sutton, 1984).

Transverse myelitis (inflammation of the spinal cord) has also been reported to develop from inadvertent intraarterial administration of long-acting penicillin when injected into the buttocks. Damage can be extensive enough to result in paraplegia or even lower limb amputation (Schanzer and Jacobson, 1985; Stoller and Losey, 1985).

Mechanisms of injury. In MVAs most spinal cord injuries in children are the result of indirect trauma caused by sudden hyperflexion or hyperextension of the neck, often combined with a rotational force. Trauma to the spinal cord without evidence of vertebral fracture or dislocation is particularly apt to occur in MVAs when proper restraints are not used. An unrestrained child becomes a projectile during sudden deceleration and is subject to injury from contact with a variety of objects inside and outside the automobile. Few persons receive spinal injuries when secured with properly fitting seat belts, that is, cross-chest restraints. Stretch injuries and internal injuries are sustained from use of only a lap restraint. High cervical spine injuries have been reported in children less than 2 years of age restrained in forward-facing car seats (Fuchs and others, 1989).

Falling from heights occurs less often in children than in adults, but vertebral compression of the spine from blows to the head or buttocks occurs in water sports (diving and surfing) or falls from horses or other athletic injuries. Birth injuries may occur in breech delivery from traction force on the cord during delivery of the head and shoulders. A number of teenagers receive cord injuries when they are accidentally shot or stabbed in the back. Infants sustain cervical cord damage (as well as brain and eye damage, mental retardation, and death) when they are shaken. Infants have very weak neck muscles, and during vigorous shaking their heavy heads wobble rapidly back and forth.

Fracture dislocation is the most frequent immediate cause of spinal cord injury, particularly in the lower cervical region, because of the marked mobility of the neck. Spinal cord injury without fracture, although unusual in adults, is not uncommon in the child whose spine is suppler, weaker, and more mobile than that of the adult, so the force is more easily dissipated over a larger number of segments. In children the vertebral column, composed of cartilaginous rings, is capable of considerable elongation, whereas the cord itself, its meninges, and its vascular supply are unable to withstand the same degree of traction.

Pathophysiology

The severity of the force, the mechanisms of the injury, and the degree of the individual's muscular relaxation at the time of the injury greatly influence the extensiveness of the trauma. Compression, contusion, laceration, and anatomic transection are the basic types of cord injuries and usually involve four interrelated pathologic changes: (1) cellular damage to cord tissue, (2) hemorrhage and vascular damage, (3) structural changes of white and gray matter related to vascular disruption, inflammation, and edema, and (4) local biochemical response to trauma. Changes in one of these can lead to another. For example, an acute injury produces a decreased blood supply to the cord tissue, with resulting ischemia that can lead to cellular necrosis. Acid metabolites accumulate during the hypoxic state and can contribute to further cellular damage. A concurrent inflammatory process produces cord edema above and below the traumatized segment, which further decreases the blood supply. Research on spinal cord trauma indicates that the neurotransmitters norepinephrine and dopamine can be markedly altered in the first few hours after injury, which causes further development of hemorrhagic necrosis in the central gray matter.

Clinical Manifestations

As a result of these pathologic responses to the initial trauma, spinal cord injury causes three stages of response; therefore the extent and severity of damage cannot be determined at first. Immediate loss of function is caused by both anatomic and impaired physiologic function, and improved function may not be evident for weeks or even months.

First stage. Manifestation of the initial response to acute injury is flaccid paralysis below the level of the damage. This stage is known as diaschisis or *spinal shock syndrome* and is caused by the sudden disruption of central and autonomic pathways. Local effects of cord edema and ischemia produce a physiologic transection with or without an anatomic severance. Most children with a spinal cord injury experience some spinal shock. Manifestations include absence of reflexes at or below the cord lesion with flaccidity or limpness of the involved muscles, loss of sensation and motor function, and autonomic dysfunction (symptoms of hypotension, low or high body temperatures, loss of bladder and bowel control, and autonomic dysreflexia) (see p. 1939).

These symptoms occur soon after the injury and last 1 to 6 weeks with much autonomic reflex cord function returning in about 3 weeks. The length of this stage indicates to some degree the extent of later recovery. In general, the shorter the duration of spinal shock, the more neurologic return can be anticipated. Problems related to this first stage are the serious consequences of prolonged immobility: atrophy of both paralyzed and noninvolved muscles, negative nitrogen balance, calcium loss from bone, atonic bladder and urinary retention, risk of skin breakdown, reduced cardiac output and plasma volume, and respiratory compromise (especially with high involvement).

Autonomic paralysis also affects thermoregulatory functions. Afferent impulses from temperature receptors in the skin are not integrated; therefore the patient is subject to temperature increase or decrease in response to alterations in environmental temperature. Hyperthermia can result from excessive ambient temperature, such as too many covers.

Second stage. Except in the situations previously mentioned, flaccid paralysis is replaced by spinal reflex activity and increasing spasticity or, in partial lesions, greater or lesser degree of neurologic recovery. Diagnosis may be confused in infants since spinal reflexes in paralyzed limbs may be misinterpreted as the normal movements in the infant. Even minor stimuli, such as rubbing the mattress, are sufficient to elicit spinal reflexes. Concurrent crying may also lead to the erroneous impression that sensation is intact. Absence of spontaneous leg movement of the extremities when the infant is held vertically suspended under the axilla suggests paralysis. Reflex withdrawal or extension of the limb after tactile or pinprick stimulus confirms a diagnosis.

Problems related to spasticity include contractures (especially of the hip adductor, hip and knee flexor muscles, and heel cords). Contraction of spastic muscles reduces bone demineralization and nitrogen loss somewhat. The atonic bladder becomes hypertonic, and, instead of continuous dribbling, urine is expelled involuntarily at intervals by reflex action.

The paralytic nature of autonomic function is replaced by *autonomic dysreflexia,* especially when the lesions are above the midthoracic level. This autonomic phenomenon is caused by visceral distention or irritation, particularly bowel or bladder. This triggers sensory impulses, which travel to the cord lesion, where they are blocked, causing activation of sympathetic reflex action with disturbed central inhibitory control. Excessive sympathetic activity is manifested by flushing of the face, sweating of the forehead, pupillary constriction, marked hypertension, headache, and bradycardia. The precipitating stimulus may be merely a full bladder or rectum or other internal or external sensory input. It can be a catastrophic event unless the irritation is relieved (see p. 1939).

Third stage. In the final stage neurologic signs are stabilized in terms of loss and recovery of function. The major emphasis is on rehabilitation. A problem unique to injury in childhood is progressive spinal deformity usually not seen in adults or in adolescents near the end of the growth period. Scoliosis develops in the major percentage of children with high thoracic and cervical lesions and is almost certain to occur in children with quadriplegia whose injury occurred in infancy or early childhood. Consequently affected infants and children are placed in carefully constructed trunk supports. Kyphosis usually appears locally at the site of the initial injury, especially when it results from hyperflexion-type injuries. Proper immobilization during vertebral healing helps to prevent progressive deformity. Increasing lordosis occurs with the development of hip contracture caused by spasticity or by prolonged sitting in nonambulatory children.

Diagnostic Evaluation

A history of the nature of the injury provides valuable clues regarding the possible type of damage incurred and direction for further assessment without the risk of additional damage. A complete neurologic examination is performed to determine if damage was incurred and, if so, the level and extent of any nerve impairment. A neurologic unit of the CNS is considered normal if reflex arcs are functioning, sensory tracts are intact when each dermatome is examined separately, and voluntary motor response demonstrates ability to move a body part against gravity on command.

Testing a reflex arc is accomplished by stimulating peripheral receptors at a specific site, such as eliciting the patellar reflex. Symmetric testing is performed to determine unilateral or bilateral neurologic deficit. A sufficient number of reflexes are examined to test motor function thoroughly. The blunt end of a safety pin is used to assess pressure sensitivity, and the sharp point to elicit pain. Hot and cold water, a tuning fork, and cotton may also be used to determine specific sensory loss, for example, temperature, vibration, and light touch.

Body surface zones, or dermatomes, accurately correspond to the spinal cord segment receiving the sensory input from the peripheral nerves in that zone. Systematically pinpricking the body surface in each zone determines intactness of sensory pathways. The zones and the spinal cord segments they represent are illustrated in Fig. 40-9. The examiner tests for each specific sensory fiber in the dermatome areas in which there is a suspected neurologic deficit. Proprioception, or knowing where one's extremities are, is a very vital sense for ambulating safely.

Matching cord level to vertebra is more difficult in infants and young children than it is in older children and adults because the sacral and several lower lumbar cord segments lie at a lower position, especially during the first 2 years of life (see Fig. 4-8). The spinal anatomy approaches adult configuration by the time the child reaches 7 or 8 years; by late adolescence the conus medullaris has usually reached the level of L1.

Motor system evaluation includes observation of gait if the child is able to walk, noting balance maintenance with eyes open and closed, and ability to lift, flex, and extend arms and legs. Testing muscle strength with and without resistance and against gravity will give clues to the specific nature and degree of motor dysfunction. The number of muscles in any muscle group that remain completely intact in the upper extremities makes a marked difference in the individual's ability to provide self-care, especially at high injury levels. The presence of abdominal muscles is valuable in bladder and bowel training and in maintaining an upright sitting position. Hip movement is necessary for ambulation with braces and crutches.

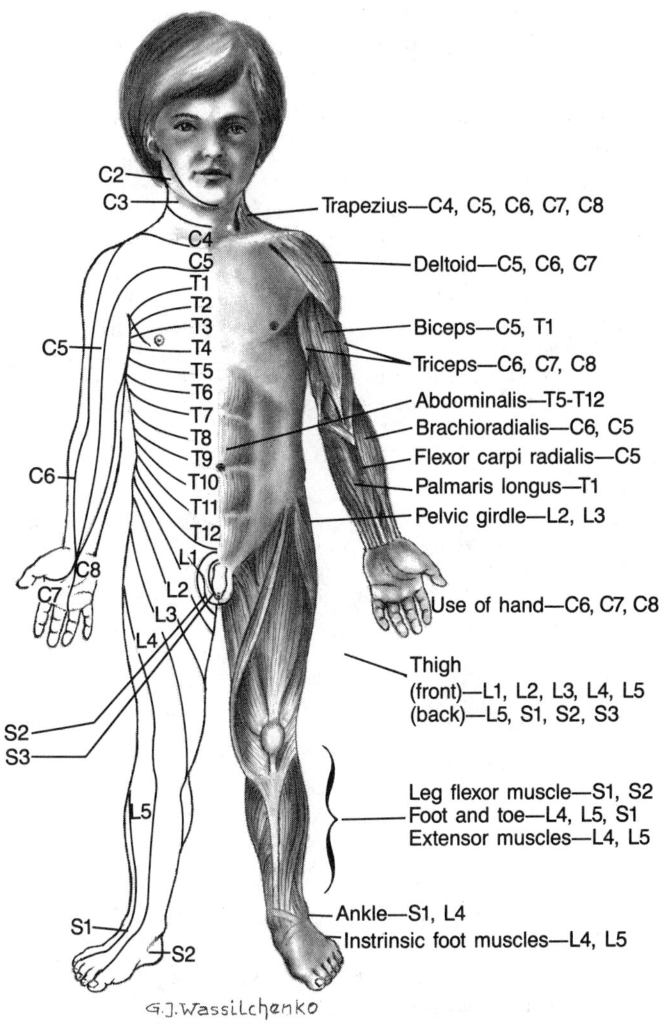

Fig. 40-9. Dermatomes and innervation of major muscles needed for performing activities of daily living.

The degree to which supportive aids are needed for ambulation is determined by the strength, stability, and movement of the pelvis, trunk, hip flexor muscles, and quadriceps muscles. A general guideline for determining the capacity for self-help is that a person with paraplegia who has function down to and including the quadriceps muscle or muscle function below the L3 level will have little difficulty

Table 40-1 Functional significance of spinal cord lesions

HIGHEST INTACT CORD SEGMENT	FUNCTIONAL CAPACITY	FUNCTIONAL GOALS
C1-3 Muscle innervation: None below chin, including phrenic nerve to diaphragm	No voluntary control below chin Respiratory paralysis complete May cause bradycardia or tachycardia, vomiting	Artificial ventilation; can be taught glossopharyngeal breathing to be used for short periods Electric wheelchair Adaptive equipment for special tasks in bed or wheelchair using mouth stick
C4 (high quadriplegia) Muscle innervation: Intact sternocleidomastoid, trapezius, upper cervical paraspinous muscles	No voluntary function of upper extremities, trunk, or lower extremities All neck movements Respirator dependent	Electric wheelchair Externally powered devices and adaptive equipment for special tasks in bed or wheelchair with mouth stick, such as turning pages, using electic typewriter Totally dependent for activities of daily living
C5 Muscle innervation: Partial deltoid, biceps, major muscles of rotator cuffs at shoulders Diaphragm	Abduction, flexion, and extension of arm Flexion and extension of forearm Unable to roll over or attain sitting position Abdominal respiration Poor respiratory reserve	Electric wheelchair Requires attendant to assist in moving and transfer to wheelchair Adaptive devices for self-feeding, grooming, using electric typewriter Vocational potential with adaptive devices
C6 Muscle innervation: Pectoralis major, serratus anterior, latissimus dorsi muscles Complete deltoid and brachioradialis muscles Partial triceps muscle	Significant increase in function over that with lesion at C5 level Adduction and medial rotation of arm Wrist extension Good elbow flexion	Cuff strapped to hand permits use of implements for self-care and other activities Able to assist in dressing and transfer Hand rim extension permits independence in wheelchair
C7 Muscle innervation: Triceps and finger flexor and extensor muscle Shoulder depressor muscles Still nerve disruption to intercostal muscles	With elbow stabilized in extension and intact shoulder depressor muscles able to lift body weight Grasp and release still weak; dexterity lacking	Almost complete independence within limitations of wheelchair Requires some assistance in transfer and lower extremity dressing Hand splints helpful Can roll over in bed, sit up in bed, and eat independently Homebound employment possible Outside work usually not feasible
T1-10 (high paraplegia) Muscle innervation: Full innervation of upper extremity muscles	Full use of upper extremities, including intrinsic muscles of hand Trunk balance poor May have difficulty in lifting sufficiently to put on lower extremity clothing Considerable energy expenditure to put on long leg braces with extensive attachments	Completely wheelchair dependent Trunk balance benefits from training Able to drive automobile with hand controls May be braced for standing May hold job away from home Cannot manage public transportation
T10-L2 Muscle innervation: Full abdominal and upper back muscle control	Good trunk balance Good respiratory reserve Can accomplish moderate hiphiking using external oblique and latissimus dorsi muscles	Ambulation with bilateral long braces using four-point or swing-through crutch gait Usually able to negotiate curbs Some able to use public transportation Few vocational limitations as long as does not require much walking or standing
L3 or below Muscle innervation: Quadriceps muscle Partial gluteus and hamstring muscles	May be lumbar lordosis Floppy ankles	Ambulates well, often with short leg braces with or without cane Difficulty in getting out of wheelchair May never require wheelchair

in learning to walk with or without braces and crutches. It is especially vital that children with lumbar levels of injury be taught to walk functionally so that they are weight bearing at least part of the time to minimize the risk of osteoporosis and hypercalcemia. The functional significance of spinal cord lesion level is summarized in Table 40-1.

If CNS pathology is detected, a body system assessment is performed to determine the degree of autonomic impairment. Because the cord and CNS directly influence the function of the autonomic nerves, the specific sympathetically related organ systems are examined for skeletal muscle and vascular tone and body temperature regulation. For example, bladder and gastrointestinal function have sympathetic and parasympathetic innervation and local reflexes.

Radiographic examination is important for localizing the lesion, but the nature of the spine in childhood frequently creates difficulty in interpretation. Radiograms must be taken carefully and with sufficient help to prevent further damage to the spine. Several persons may be needed to log roll the patient and to support the head during turning or transfer.

Therapeutic Management

The management of the child with spinal cord injury is complex and controversial. Initial care begins at the scene of the accident; therefore education and training of rescue personnel in stabilization and transfer techniques to prevent or reduce the severity of injury are of utmost importance. In any situation in which spinal cord injury is suspected or a possibility, the child should be calmed, reassured, and advised not to move; no one should be allowed to move the child unless they are able to do so carefully. The child should be lifted gently and without undue haste (preferably by a coordinated team) to avoid twisting or bending the spine. If conscious, the child is placed supine on a rigid surface to prevent sagging. Infants and small children are removed in their car seats; no attempt should be made to take them out of the seat. Because of the complexity and relative infrequency of these injuries, it is usually recommended that these persons be transferred to a spinal injury center for care by specially trained personnel.

Management during the first stage is primarily supportive, with efforts directed toward preventing further neuronal damage, avoiding complications, and maintaining vital functions. Children with cervical lesions often have compromised respiratory function and may require ventilatory assistance. Cervical lesions may require skeletal traction or other device to maintain position, and corticosteroids are administered in an attempt to prevent destructive edema. Operative intervention may be necessary to remove bone fragments and debris, but routine surgical exploration is not usually recommended.

The focus of the second phase is primarily rehabilitative and is aimed at returning the patient to the home and community. The focus is on maximizing the potential for self-help, education, and, for the older child, vocational counseling.

Prognosis. The ultimate outlook for spinal cord function after injury depends on the completeness of the cord transection, the site of injury, and the complicating damage to the neuronal tissue. Healing of the injury and return of neurologic function are related to two factors:

1. Although individual nerve fibers do regenerate, they do not necessarily reconnect or make synaptic connections with the distal portion of the severed fibers; the chance of numerous fibers reconnecting is highly unlikely.
2. The damage resulting from cord ischemia produces necrosis in the gray and white matter of the cord tissue, which does not regenerate if the axon cylinder is not intact.

In general, recovery in thoracic lesions is usually hopeless for motor function, and victims are relegated to life in a wheelchair. Cervical injuries are variable in extent of damage. Incomplete lesions produce hemiplegia, and complete transection implies some involvement of all extremities from partial use of upper extremities to complete paralysis, including the need for artificial maintenance of respiration. Lumbar injury may involve partial or complete loss of function in lower extremities and bladder.

Nursing Considerations

The nursing care of the paralyzed child is complex and challenging. As a member of acute care and rehabilitation teams, the nurse is involved in all aspects of care. Ideally, initial care takes place in a special intensive care unit with personnel trained to handle spinal cord injuries, and nursing management is concerned primarily with prevention of complications and maintenance of functions.

Once the acute period is over, the lesion is usually static and nonprogressive, regardless of whether the paralysis is secondary to trauma, congenital defects, infection, treated tumor, or surgery. The nurse is a member of a team of specialists, including physicians from a number of specialty areas, physical and occupational therapists, psychologists, social workers, teachers, and vocational counselors. Each team member has a unique contribution to make, and mutual agreement for specific areas of responsibility and evaluation of progress are determined during regularly scheduled team conferences.

Although care of the child with a spinal cord injury is, in most aspects, the same as that of any immobilized child, there are some important differences (see The Immobilized Child, Chapter 39).

Respiratory care. The child with a high-level injury (quadriplegia) will require continuous ventilatory assistance. In most instances a tracheostomy is the method of choice for greater ease in clearing secretions and for less trauma to tissues for long-term respirator dependence. Respiratory therapy personnel are responsible for establishing and maintaining the equipment, but the nurse must understand how it works and recognize deviations from the prescribed rate and volume and mechanical malfunction. In case of malfunction the nurse must be prepared to maintain respirations manually with a ventilation bag. In some youngsters breathing pacemaker devices (phrenic nerve stimulators) are implanted to stimulate the phrenic nerve and produce diaphragmatic contractions and lung expansion without a ventilator. If the child has a pacemaker, part of the nursing function is understanding its function and operation.

Children with lesions below the C4 level are seldom ventilator dependent, but their vital capacity is significantly reduced. They should be positioned for optimum chest expansion, and a variety of breathing exercises and assistive devices are used to stimulate deep breathing. Intermittent positive-pressure breathing by machine may be needed, and vital capacity and blood gases are monitored periodically. Chest physiotherapy is performed several times daily, and nebulized oxygen may be needed occasionally. Regular routine monitoring of breath sounds to assess for adequate ventilation in all lobes is part of routine care.

The cough reflex is markedly diminished and, together with weak intercostal muscles, the youngster may have difficulty with secretions. Increasing the elastic qualities of the lung by exercise will help to achieve a productive cough.

Temperature regulation. Temperature regulation usually creates few problems, although environmental conditions can influence body temperature. During the spinal shock stage the dilated capillaries conducting body heat to the subcutaneous tissues cause heat loss to the environment. In hot weather, without the capacity to sweat, the body retains heat. Consequently, clothing and blankets are added or removed according to the body temperature. An elevated temperature that cannot be corrected by environmental measures should be evaluated for urinary tract or upper respiratory infection. However, excessive perspiration observed in sentient areas usually indicates an elevated ambient temperature. Since the skin is a less reliable indicator in these children, the oral or rectal route is usually the preferred method of temperature measurement.

Skin care. In cases in which spinal cord injury is associated with vertebral fracture, cervical traction is maintained for several weeks until there is sufficient evidence of bone healing (see The Child in Traction, Chapter 39). Initially the child is turned every 2 hours around the clock by specially trained personnel. An alternating pressure mattress, Eggcrate mattress, or sheepskin is kept underneath the child, and the skin is thoroughly inspected at least once a day for signs of pressure, especially over bony prominences. Prevention of decubiti is much easier than treatment. A number of factors contribute to the risk of skin breakdown in these children: decreased sensation, poor nutrition from negative nitrogen balance, low hemoglobin level, spasticity, and improper positioning.

The areas most apt to be affected are the sacrum, scapulae, heels, and occiput when the child is in a supine position; the trochanters and the lateral aspect of the ankles, heels, and knees when in a side-lying position; and the ischial tuberosities when in a sitting position. The common type of pressure lesion begins in deeper tissues and is only visible on the surface at a later stage; therefore areas that feel firm, irregular, or warm or appear to be only slightly reddened require careful evaluation. Keeping the skin clean and dry is particularly important in these children, especially those who are incontinent. Treatment of pressure areas or decubiti is instituted early, according to the protocol of the institution.

Physiotherapy. Maintaining good body alignment, preventing pressure from bed linen, providing proper support, and applying splints as ordered and padded booties to hold the feet in correct position are important in daily care. Range of motion, passive, and active exercises are carried out under the guidance of a physical therapist. In children with upper motor neuron involvement, the spasticity that develops may require administration of an antispasmodic, usually diazepam. Decreasing stimuli to the muscles also helps reduce spasticity. For example, tight clothing and bed linen are avoided, and extremities are handled at the joints rather than by the belly of the muscle. Anticipating the possibility of spasms when the child is moved and providing the necessary safety precautions prevent possible injury during transport.

During the period of immobilization, unless there are contraindications, exercises are aimed at maintaining and increasing strength of the child's intact musculature. Upper extremity strengthening is especially important to the paraplegic child who must rely on these muscle groups for turning, transferring, dressing, crutch walking, and other activities. Children are usually eager to use their muscles and respond to interesting and innovative activities.

Neuropathic bladder. When the bladder is denervated, as in the acute stage of spinal shock syndrome or after lower motor neuron damage, the bladder wall is flaccid. Lack of muscle tone inhibits the bladder's ability to respond to changes in passive pressure causing overextension. Therefore it is important to prevent overdistention by periodic emptying, even though there may be dribbling between emptying.

In contrast, an upper motor neuron lesion causes increased bladder tone and contractions that often include the urinary sphincter. Thus although the bladder empties periodically by reflex action, complete emptying is prevented, resulting in urinary retention and ureteral reflux. Administration of antispasmodics such as dicyclomine (Bentyl) relaxes bladder musculature and promotes increased bladder capacity and more adequate emptying. Intervals of urination depend on many factors, including patterns of fluid intake and perspiration. Most children require some type of external collecting device. This is relatively simple in males, but no satisfactory device is available for females, who usually must rely on diapers and incontinent pants. From the beginning attempts are made to keep the child relatively dry by regulating fluid intake and output and periodically emptying the bladder by intermittent catheterization. Older children can be taught to perform self-catheterization.* Bladder-training programs usually begin with intermittent bladder emptying at regular intervals, which are gradually increased. Periodic urine cultures and, in manual emptying, periodic catheterization for residual volume are performed until the child achieves regular, complete empty-

*Home care instructions are available in Wong, D.L., and Whaley, L.F.: Clinical manual of pediatric nursing, ed. 3, St. Louis, 1990, Mosby–Year Book, Inc.

ing. Surgical implantation of a Scott sphincter may help continence in some children.

The urine is kept acidic to decrease the likelihood of stone formation and to inhibit bacterial growth. Ascorbic acid, 1 to 4 g daily, is most effective. The traditional cranberry juice may also be advised. Oral antimicrobials are frequently administered prophylactically. Maintenance of bladder dynamics and control of urinary tract infections are of utmost importance. Pyelonephritis and renal failure are the most significant causes of death in long-standing paraplegia.

Bowel training. Successful bowel training is easier to institute than bladder management. The aim is to control defecation until an appropriate time and place are found. A diet with sufficient roughage for adequate stool bulk and insertion of a glycerin or bisacodyl (Dulcolax) suppository at a convenient time, either morning or evening, are often all that are necessary to induce a bowel movement within a short time. The probability of an accident between times is diminished once the bowel is completely evacuated. Stool softeners, such as dioctyl sodium sulfonsuccinate (Colace), are usually prescribed, and manual anal stimulation may help initiate evacuation, especially in spastic paraplegia. Sometimes an oral laxative such as bisacodyl may be necessary. Once an appropriate regimen is established, little modification is required.

Autonomic dysreflexia. Children with high-level lesions are very susceptible to the development of autonomic dysreflexia, which requires prompt action to prevent encephalopathy and shock. As soon as a quick assessment has ruled out other causes, such as orthostatic hypertension, someone should take the blood pressure while the bladder is checked for distention (the usual precipitating cause). The bladder is drained slowly, and if this does not relieve symptoms, any tight clothing is loosened, and the bowel is checked for the pressure of impacted feces. If removal of the causative agent is unsuccessful in controlling the syndrome, intravenous administration of an antihypertensive drug is indicated followed by oral maintenance doses. Antispasmodics may also be administered.

Remobilization. As soon as the condition warrants, the child is moved from a reclining to an erect position. Cardiovascular deconditioning and impaired autonomic responses below the level of injury will cause pooling of blood in the extremities because of peripheral vasodilation, a drop in blood pressure, and a feeling of light-headedness, dizziness, or fainting on sudden assumption of an upright posture. Therefore an upright position must be accomplished gradually by first placing the child (secured by passive restraint) on a tilt table. The table is then slowly elevated from a horizontal to a 30-degree semireclining position (Fig. 40-10). This is performed twice daily for 20 to 30 minutes, gradually increasing the angle until the vertical angle is reached.

During the procedure vital signs are monitored, and behavior is observed for subjective symptoms of syncope. Elastic hose or wrapping the lower extremities with elastic bandage from instep to groin and applying an abdominal binder reduce the pooling of blood. The process of achieving upright posture may require several weeks. After tolerance is achieved, the child will be ready to begin to use a wheelchair. Getting the child up should be accomplished slowly by gradually elevating the bed over 20 to 30 minutes before placing the child in the wheelchair, then gradually lowering the legs after being in the chair a short time.

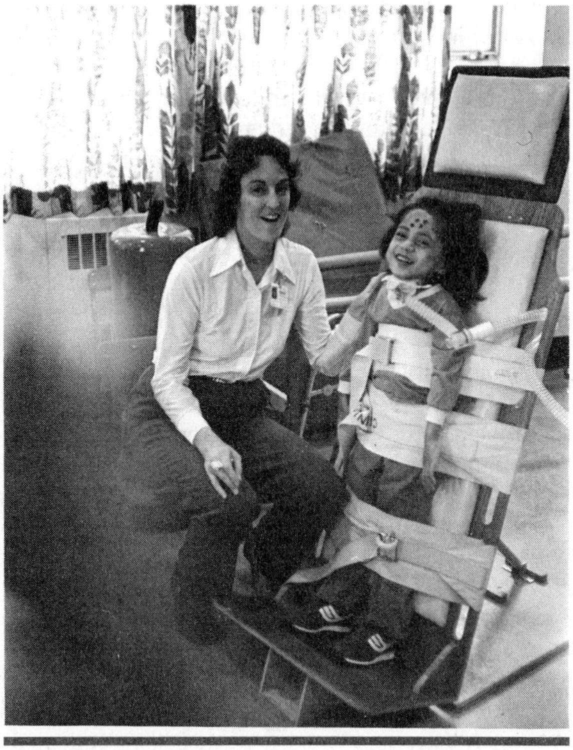

Fig. 40-10. Child on tilt table with physical therapist.

All adaptive devices help children increase their mobility, function, and endurance. The child with some lower extremity function progresses to parallel bars and then to a walker; the child with quadriplegia learns to use a wheelchair—among the most valuable aids available to the child with a spinal cord injury. Selection of a wheelchair should be made carefully in relation to where it will be used, architectural barriers, and the functional capacity of the child. For lower extremity paralysis the wheelchair described earlier is applicable. For children with severe upper extremity paralysis, a variety of motorized wheelchairs are used, but the more complex they are, the greater their cost, weight, and tendency to break down (see Fig. 39-5). Wheelchair tolerance is gained over a period of time accompanied by measures to prevent orthostatic hypotension and pressure sores.

A variety of braces and other appliances can be adapted for use by many children. The primary purpose of lower extremity bracing in the child with a spinal cord injury is for ambulation, although correction of deformities may be attempted. However, the efficacy is limited because of the tendency to develop pressure lesions over insensate areas.

The higher the lesion, the more support required, with the accompanying difficulties of getting into the brace and the greater energy expended in using the appliance. The energy required in ambulating with crutches and braces is two to four times greater than that required for normal walking.

Children, with their natural and overwhelming propensity for mobility, usually attain or may even surpass the maximum expectation in ambulation. However, as they approach adulthood, the increasing weight and energy cost usually cause them to resort to predominant use of the wheelchair for mobility and the pursuit of more intellectual and vocational interests. Wheelchair mobility has the advantages of requiring no more energy than normal walking and allowing the person with paraplegia to maintain the speed of other pedestrians on level ground.

Physical rehabilitation. The major aims of physical rehabilitation are to prepare the child and family to resume life at home and in the community. Members of the complex rehabilitation team work collaboratively to identify the child's problems and to plan realistic interventions. Integration of activities is coordinated by one team member, most often a specialist in physical medicine and rehabilitation. Through mutual trust, good communication, professional respect, and sincere interest in the child and the family, members of the team attempt to achieve their collaborative goals. Training in the rehabilitation center involves maximum achievement commensurate with each child's physical capacities. Instruction for home routine is stressed and includes all the precautions and management implemented in the hospital, such as skin care, nutrition, bladder and bowel training, and an exercise program. The overall goals of rehabilitation are listed in Box 40-8.

Physical rehabilitation of children with quadriplegia takes approximately 6 months; children with paraplegia can achieve these goals in 1 to 3 months, but they require constant vigilance to avoid complications. Emotional adjustments take longer, especially in older children and adolescents. In most children the outlook is favorable unless life-threatening consequences of urinary pathology are severe or emotional adjustment is poor.

Psychosocial rehabilitation. Early acquired or congenital disability is usually more readily accepted by children than paralysis that appears later in childhood. Rehabilitation includes not only the child's emotional responses but also those of the persons who maintain the closest contacts with the child. It involves intensive education so that members of the family understand the nature of the disability, the therapeutic regimen, and complications so that they are able to provide the physical and emotional support needed by the children. As with any disability, children should be treated as normally as possible and encouraged in developmental tasks at the age at which they would normally be expected to acquire abilities and perform activities. However, goals must be realistic, and children should not be forced beyond their capabilities.

Severe depression can be emotionally and intellectually immobilizing, but it indicates that the child is no longer hiding behind denial. In rehabilitation it is desirable for the child to begin to express negative feelings toward the situation, since these feelings, redirected by efforts of the rehabilitation team, are the ones that will motivate the child toward learning a new way of life.

The responses to loss have been discussed in Chapter 23, and the multiple problems related to altered self-image, especially in older children and adolescents, have been discussed in relation to children with disabilities in Chapter 22. Children with severe disabilities need to alter some concepts about self and social roles. If they describe adults as persons with complete control over their body and the ability to do what they want when they want to, they will need to develop a more realistic definition of interdependent adult living. The needs of youngsters who are permanently disabled must be reevaluated periodically by the total rehabilitation team, including the youngsters and their families. As young adults, these teenagers may not be financially independent, which alters the choice of occupation or profession. Vocational rehabilitation involves not only helping teenagers with permanent disabilities find meaningful work activities but also assisting them in enrolling in formal educational programs.

The outlook for children with spinal cord injury is favorable for integration into society. Increased awareness of the needs of persons with disabilities has removed many structural and occupational barriers. The success of a rehabilitation program is not judged by how well children manage within the rehabilitation setting but by how well they function on the outside. In addition to agencies that offer assistance to children with disabilities in general, some agencies provide specific assistance to paralyzed persons, including children.* The **Spinal Injury Hotline** supplies victims and their families with information, hope, and peer support.†

Sexuality. The problems of self-concept are particularly marked when children with a spinal cord injury reach puberty and are likely to be even more intense if the disability occurs during adolescence. Sexual development and aware-

Box 40-8 GOALS OF REHABILITATION FOR THE CHILD WITH A SPINAL CORD INJURY

Maximizing function and minimizing the disabling effects of the pathology

Assisting the child and family in setting realistic goals for the child, learning to be good problem solvers, and using the assets the child has

Helping the child to cope with the stigma of being different and to build a valued self-concept

*A complete listing of organizations and resources can be obtained by contacting **Spinal Network,** P.O. Box 4162, Boulder, CO 80306; (800) 338-5412. Other sources of information and assistance are listed in Appendix E.

†(800) 526-3456. In Maryland, (800) 638-1733.

ness and changing perceptions of body image are prominent aspects of adolescence, and a loss in these areas is a severe blow to these youngsters. Development of secondary sex characteristics does not seem to be altered by spinal cord injury, and it is now believed that with comprehensive rehabilitation, well-motivated young people can look forward to successful participation in marital and family activities.

In females, if the injury occurs after the onset of menstruation, there is usually a temporary cessation and irregularity in menstrual flow, but in the majority menstruation usually resumes. Ovulation and conception are possible, but females will not experience vulval or clitoral orgasms, although they can learn to use other erogenous zones for a sexual experience. This is important to emphasize in sex education, because many females have the misconception that because they lack sensation, they are unable to conceive. Also, the pregnant paraplegic or quadriplegic may be unaware that she is in labor, and those with a high-level injury are subject to autonomic hyperreflexia during labor.

As soon as adolescent males become aware of their functional loss, they will be concerned about sexual capacities, regardless of the type of sexual activities experienced before the spinal cord injury. The practitioner will provide them with information about what can be expected regarding erection, ejaculation, and other sexual experiences. The health professional should take the initiative in discussing sexuality with youngsters and their families. Parents of younger children will want to know about their children's sexual and reproductive potential. As their interest and understanding increase, children need to know the specifics of physiology, prognosis, and sexual techniques related to their particular problems.

A knowledgeable rehabilitation team will be valuable to children as they experience loss as a sexual being. This is especially true of paraplegia or quadriplegia. Most sexual counseling for adolescents with spinal cord injury focuses on developing the idea that sex means different things to individuals, and youngsters are encouraged to discuss their ideas. Most rehabilitation teams have an active program in sexual counseling to help youngsters learn intimacy and how to function sexually within their limitations. Through individual and group counseling they gain new attitudes concerning sexuality, experiences exclusive or inclusive of intercourse.

MUSCULAR DYSFUNCTION

As skeletal development is responsible for linear growth, muscle growth accounts for a significant portion of the increase in body weight. The number of muscle fibers is established by the fourth or fifth month of fetal life and remains constant throughout life. Differences in muscle size between individuals and differences in one person at various times during a lifetime are a result of the ability of the separate muscle fibers to increase in size. The increase in muscle fiber length that accompanies growth is also associated with an increase in the number of nuclei in the fibers. This increase is most apparent during the adolescent growth spurt. At this time the increase in secretion of growth hormone and adrenal androgens stimulates the growth of muscle fibers in both sexes, but the growth in boys is further stimulated by the secretion of testosterone.

At about 6 months of prenatal life, muscle mass constitutes approximately one sixth of the body weight; at birth, about one fourth; and at adolescence, one third. The variability in size and strength of muscle is influenced by genetic constitution, nutrition, and exercise. At all ages muscles increase in size with use and shrink with inactivity. Consequently, maintaining muscle tone to minimize the amount of atrophy in skeletal muscle through active or passive range of motion exercises is an important protective nursing function.

Skeletal muscles are subject to a large number of disorders that cause degeneration of muscle fibers with subsequent loss of function. In most instances there is fibrous connective tissue replacement of muscle fibers, proximal muscles are affected more severely than distal ones, and the lower extremities are affected to a greater extent than the upper extremities. Children with muscle disease characteristically develop a waddling gait and have difficulty in running, climbing, and rising from a sitting position. Innervation is not affected.

Diseases of skeletal muscles can be inflammatory (such as polymyositis), the result of endocrine dysfunction (such as hypothyroidism and hyperthyroidism), or caused by congenital defects (such as absence of muscle, periodic paralysis, and the various muscular dystrophies and myotonias). Inflammation occurs in a number of infectious illnesses such as trichinosis, toxoplasmosis, and those caused by coxsackievirus.

In addition to the electromyogram, measurement of serum enzyme activity, especially creatine phosphokinase, is often helpful in differential diagnosis of muscle disease. The intracellular enzyme creatine phosphokinase is present in muscle tissues and very few other organs and is released in large amounts in some diseases of muscles such as muscular dystrophy. Creatine phosphokinase is not elevated in neurogenic disease. Although the treatment in a large number of muscle disorders is palliative and symptomatic rather than curative, an accurate diagnosis is essential for purposes of rehabilitation, counseling, and treatment in those amenable to specific therapy.

JUVENILE DERMATOMYOSITIS

Dermatomyositis is a multisystem inflammatory disorder of unknown etiology and often difficult to distinguish from muscular dystrophy. There is proximal limb and trunk muscle weakness and loss of reflexes. Neck muscles are frequently affected, and the child may have difficulty in lifting the head or supporting it in an upright position. Muscles tend to be stiff and sore. Masseter involvement with atrophy may occur, making it difficult to chew food during the active stage of disease. Soft palate dysfunction may make

Table 40-2 Characteristics of the major muscular dystrophies

PRIMARY MYOPATHY/ INHERITANCE PATTERN	AGE OF ONSET	INITIAL MANIFESTATIONS	PROGRESSION	THERAPY
Pseudohypertrophic (Duchenne) X-linked recessive; sporadic	Early childhood; age 1-3 years	Lordosis Waddling gait Difficulty in rising from floor and climbing stairs Fat deposits replace wasted gastrocnemius muscles	Rapid Ultimately involves all voluntary muscles Death usually occurs between ages 15 and 25 years	Supportive Physical therapy to prevent disuse atrophy of unaffected muscles
Limb-girdle Autosomal recessive (usually)	Late childhood or during adolescence; over age 8 years	Weakness of proximal muscles of both pelvic and shoulder girdles	Variable but usually slow Most become incapacitated within 20 years of onset, in some, disability may remain slight	Supportive Physical therapy to prevent disuse atrophy of unaffected muscles
Facioscapulohumeral (Landouzy-Déjerine) Autosomal dominant	Early adolescence; over age 8 years	Lack of facial mobility Difficulty in raising arms over head Forward slope of shoulders	Very slow May be intervals with no progression Considerable disability in time but life span unaffected	Supportive

speech difficult and interfere with breathing. Distal muscle strength and reflex response remain unaffected. Dermatomyositis, frequently classified as a collagen disease, is characterized by red, indurated skin lesions over the malar areas and nose and a violet discoloration of the eyelids. The skin over extensor muscle surfaces may be erythematous, scaly, and atopic.

Dermatomyositis responds to corticosteroid therapy, and with early and vigorous treatment most affected children recover. Physical therapy is essential to prevent contracture deformity and to rebuild muscle strength. Bracing or splinting may be needed.

MUSCULAR DYSTROPHIES

The muscular dystrophies (MDs) constitute the largest and most important single group of muscle diseases of childhood. They all have a genetic origin in which there is gradual degeneration of muscle fibers and are characterized by progressive weakness and wasting of symmetric groups of skeletal muscles with increasing disability and deformity. In all forms of muscular dystrophy there is insidious loss of strength, but each differs in regard to muscle groups affected, age of onset, rate of progression, and inheritance patterns.

The basic defect in muscular dystrophy is unknown, although it appears to be caused by a metabolic disturbance unrelated to the nervous system. Serum creatine phosphokinase is consistently increased in affected individuals, which assists in diagnosis and affords a means for early detection of the disorder in asymptomatic children in families at risk. Electromyography (EMG) and muscle biopsy are important diagnostic procedures.

Treatment of the muscular dystrophies consists mainly of providing supportive measures, including physical therapy, orthopedic procedures to minimize deformity, and assisting the affected child in meeting the demands of daily living.

The major forms of muscular dystrophy are summarized in Table 40-2, and the initial sites of muscle involvement are illustrated in Fig. 40-11.

PSEUDOHYPERTROPHIC (DUCHENNE) MUSCULAR DYSTROPHY

The most severe and the most common muscular dystrophy of childhood is pseudohypertrophic MD (DMD). An X-linked inheritance pattern is identified in 50% of cases; the remainder appear as sporadic cases and probably represent fresh mutations. As in all X-linked disorders, males are affected almost exclusively. The incidence is approximately 1:3500 male births (Thomas and Dubowitz, 1989). Box 40-9 describes the characteristics of DMD.

Recent studies indicate that dystrophin, a protein product in skeletal muscle, is absent from the muscle of children with DMS, although it is present but in reduced amounts or abnormal in character in children with Becker MD, a milder variant (Hoffman, Brown, and Kunkel, 1987).

Clinical Manifestations

Evidence of muscle weakness usually appears during the third year, although there may have been a history of delay in motor development, particularly walking. Difficulties in running, riding a bicycle, and climbing stairs are usually the first symptoms noted. Later abnormal gait on a level surface becomes apparent. In the early years rapid developmental gains may mask the progression of the disease. Questioning

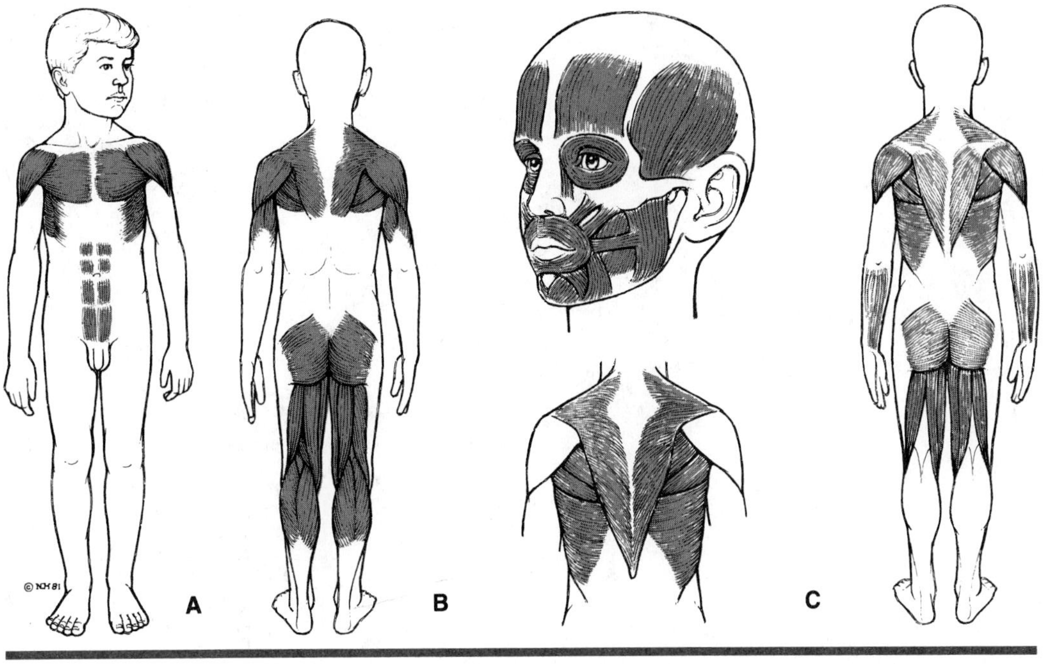

Fig. 40-11. Initial muscle groups involved in muscular dystrophies. **A,** Pseudohypertrophic. **B,** Facioscapulohumeral. **C,** Limb-girdle.

of parents may reveal that the child has difficulty in rising from a sitting or supine position. Occasionally enlarged calves may be noticed by parents.

Typically affected males have a waddling gait and lordosis, fall frequently, and develop a characteristic manner of rising from a squatting or sitting position on the floor (Gower sign) (Fig. 40-12). Muscles, especially of calves, thighs, and upper arms, become enlarged from fatty infiltration and feel unusually firm or woody on palpation. The name *pseudohypertrophy* is derived from this muscular enlargement. Profound muscular atrophy occurs in later stages, and as the disease progresses, contractures and deformities involving large and small joints are common complications. Ambulation usually becomes impossible by 12 years of age. Facial, oropharyngeal, and respiratory muscles are spared until the terminal stages of the disease. Ultimately the disease process involves the diaphragm and auxiliary muscles of respiration, and cardiomegaly is common. The cause of death is usually respiratory tract infection or cardiac failure.

Mild mental retardation is commonly associated with muscular dystrophy. The mean intelligence quotient is about 20 points below the normal, and frank mental deficit is present in 25% of these children.

Complications. The major complications of muscular dystrophy include contractures, disuse atrophy, infections, obesity, and cardiopulmonary problems.

Contracture deformities of hips, knees, and ankles occur from early selective muscle involvement and often exaggerate the weakness. Passive range of motion exercises, stretching, and active exercises under the supervision of a physical therapist are effective in treating reducible contractures. Nonreducible contractures require wedge casting or surgical reduction. Scoliosis caused by muscle imbalance is common and tends to progress even when the child becomes dependent on a wheelchair. Bracing with a rigid corset may be needed for support, although it may interfere with mobility, and children with DMD do not tolerate rigid spinal bracing. Frequent rest periods in the recumbent position are often beneficial. For correction of deformities it is essential to select a procedure that immobilizes the child for as short a period as possible to minimize the chances of developing disease atrophy.

Atrophy of disuse from prolonged inactivity occurs readily when children are immobilized or confined to bed with illness, injury, or surgery. To minimize this complication, physical therapy should be implemented if bed rest extends beyond a few days. A daily goal for well children

recumbent: lying down or leaning backward.

Box 40-9 CHARACTERISTICS OF DUCHENNE MUSCULAR DYSTROPHY

- Early onset, usually between 3 and 5 years of age
- Progressive muscular weakness, wasting, and contractures
- Calf muscle hypertrophy in most cases
- Loss of independent ambulation by 9 to 11 years of age
- Slowly progressive generalized weakness during teenage years
- Relentless progression until death from respiratory or cardiac failure

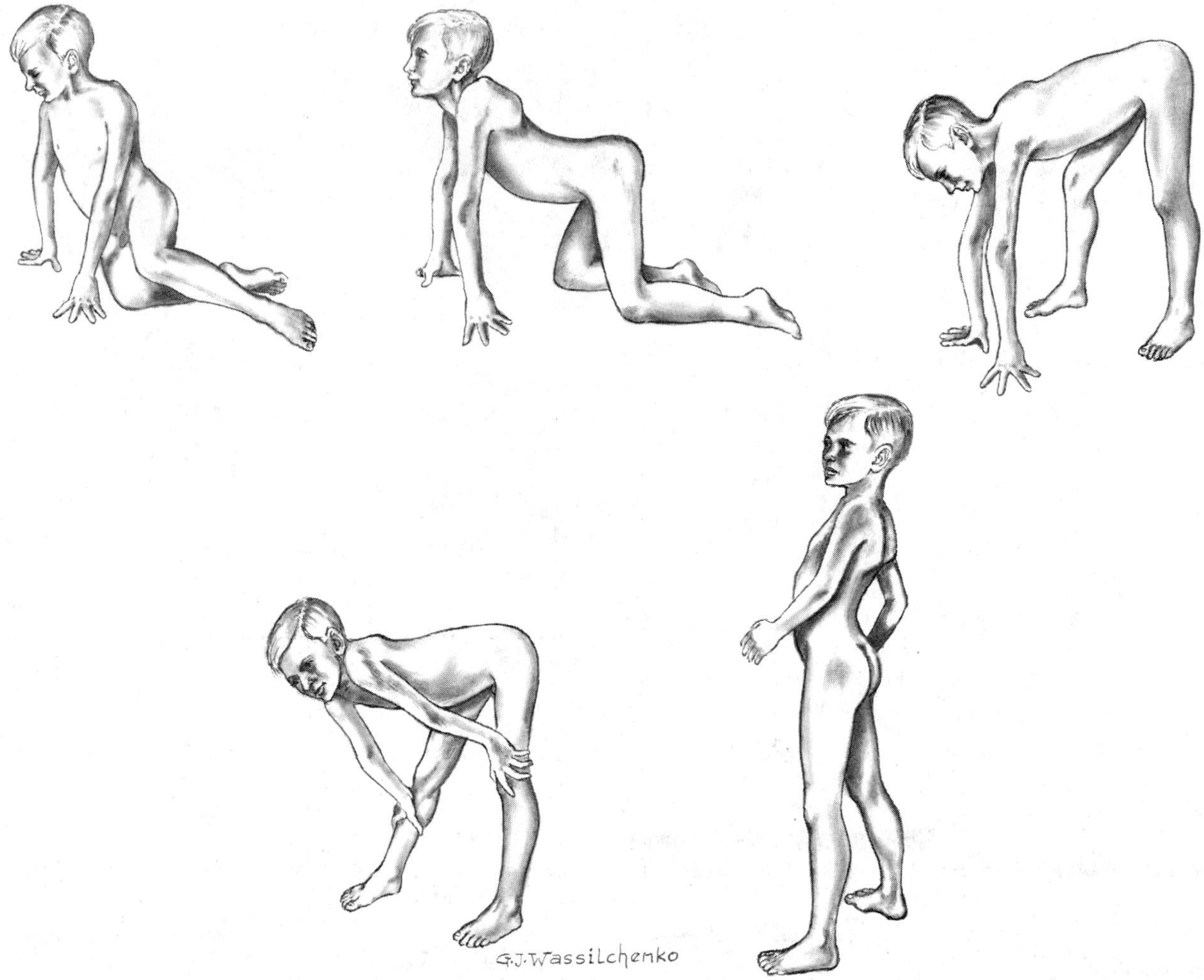

Fig. 40-12. Child with Duchenne muscular dystrophy attains standing posture by assuming a kneeling position, then gradually pushing his torso upright (with knees straight) by "walking" his hands up his legs (Gower sign). Note marked lordosis in upright position.

should be at least 3 hours of ambulation when disability is moderate to maintain muscle strength.

Infections become increasingly frequent as the dystrophic process produces a progressive decrease in vital capacity resulting from weakness of primary, secondary, and associated muscles of respiration. Consequently, even minor upper respiratory infections may become serious problems in these children. Prompt and vigorous antibiotic therapy supplemented by postural drainage and intermittent respiratory therapy is effective. Because these children are unable to cough, secretions collect easily.

Obesity is a frequent complication that contributes to premature loss of ambulation. Children with restricted opportunity for physical activity and who suffer from boredom easily consume calories in excess of their needs. This is compounded by overfeeding by well-meaning family and friends. Proper dietary intake and a diversified recreational program help reduce the likelihood of obesity and enable children to maintain ambulation and functional independence for a longer time.

Cardiac manifestations are usually late events but may occur in ambulatory children. Most significant of these, cardiac failure, is difficult to correct in advanced cases, but treatment with digoxin and diuretics is often beneficial in the early stages of the disease.

Diagnostic Evaluation

The disease is confirmed by serum enzyme measurement, muscle biopsy, and EMG. The serum creatine phosphokinase, aldolase, and serum glutamic-oxaloacetic transaminase levels are extremely high in the first 2 years of life before onset of clinical weakness. They diminish with muscle deterioration but do not reach normal levels until severe muscle wasting and incapacitation have occurred. Muscle biopsy reveals degeneration of muscle fibers with fibrosis and fatty tissue replacement. EMG readings show a decrease in amplitude and duration of motor unit potentials. Diagnosis poses few problems in children 2 to 7 years of age, but in older children the similarity of symptoms to those of limb-girdle muscular dystrophy and some other myopathies confuses the diagnosis.

Some success has been reported in prenatal diagnosis of DMD but is subject to uncertainties (Darras, Harper, and Francke, 1987).

Therapeutic Management

There is no effective treatment for childhood muscular dystrophy. Increased muscle bulk and muscle power has been reported following a course of corticosteroid (Mendell and others, 1989; Brooke and others, 1987). However, the beneficial effects from administration of corticosteroids will need further evaluation before it becomes routine therapy.

Maintaining function in unaffected muscles for as long as possible is the primary goal. It has been found that children who remain as active as possible are able to avoid wheelchair confinement for a longer period. Early recourse to a wheelchair accelerates deconditioning and promotes the development of lower extremity contractures. Maintenance of function often includes range of motion exercises, surgery to release contracture deformities, bracing, and performance of activities of ADL. Some surgical techniques allow early sitting and ambulation if children are still ambulating without bracing or casting and improve the quality of their remaining years. Genetic counseling is recommended for parents, female siblings, and maternal aunts and their female offspring (see Chapter 5).

Nursing Considerations

The care and management of a child with muscular dystrophy involve the combined efforts of a comprehensive health team. Nurses can help clarify the roles of these health professionals to family and others. The major emphasis of nursing care is to assist the child and family to cope with the progressive, incapacitating, and fatal nature of the disease, to help design a program that will afford a greater degree of independence and reduce the predictable and preventable disabilities associated with the disorder, and to assist them to deal constructively with the limitations the disease imposes on their daily lives.

Working closely with other team members, nurses help the family in developing the child's self-help skills to give the child the satisfaction of being as independent as possible for as long as possible. It is tempting for parents to overprotect their affected children. Children derive pleasure and build self-esteem from performing actions that produce visible pleasure in their parents. Even the physical weakness that prevents the child from physical competition with other children has little effect on the child as long as it does not affect the parents' attitude toward the child as an individual. Therefore parents must be helped to develop a balance between limiting the child's activity because of muscular weakness and allowing the child to accomplish things alone. This requires continual evaluation of the child's capabilities, which are often difficult to assess. It is not always possible to know when the child seeks parental assistance to get a little extra attention or because of overtired muscles. Fortunately most children with muscular dystrophy instinctively recognize this need to be as independent as possible and strive to do so.

Practical difficulties faced by families are physical limitations of housing and mobility. Families often live in houses or apartments that are unsuited to wheelchairs—no street-level entrance, upstairs bedrooms and bathrooms, no tub. Many of these families have no independent means of transportation. Assisting with these problems involves team problem solving. Parents also need help in buying and modifying clothing for their child. It is difficult to find clothing and footwear to wear comfortably in a wheelchair, to fit over contracted limbs, or to fit an obese child. Diet, nutritional needs, and nutrition modification are discussed according to the needs of the individual child and family.

Parents' social activities are also restricted, and the family's activities must be continually modified to the needs of the affected child (see Chapter 22). The child cannot be left with an ordinary teenage baby-sitter but requires a specially trained person, such as a student nurse. Consequently, parents, too, tend to lead more isolated lives. When the child becomes increasingly helpless, the family may consider a skilled nursing facility to provide the care needed. Nurses can assist with decision making and support the family in the decision.

Each child's therapy program is tailored to individual needs and capabilities, and families should be active participants. Parents need assistance with the physical therapy program and education regarding a home regimen of exercises and activity. Many parents erroneously believe that by exerting sufficient effort, the child can overcome the weakness and prevent progression of the disease process. They should also be advised to notify the nurse or other designated person when the child becomes even temporarily bedridden so that the exercise program can be continued, although modified, during this time.

Children with muscular dystrophy are typically passive, frequently withdrawn, and emotionally immature. As their physical condition deteriorates to the point where they can no longer keep up with friends and classmates, they tend to become socially isolated. Their physical capabilities diminish, and their dependency increases at the ages when most children are expanding their range of interests and relationships. To gain associations, they often learn behaviors that bring them the rewards of other children's company. These friends are often children who have been rejected by more able-bodied classmates.

No matter how successful the program and how well the family adapts to the disorder, superimposed on the physical and emotional problems associated with a child with a long-term disability is the constant presence of the ultimate outcome of the disease. All the manifestations seen in the child with a fatal illness are encountered in these families (see Chapter 23). The guilt feelings of the mother may be particularly pronounced in this disorder because of the mother-to-son transmission of the defective gene.

Nurses are especially valuable health professionals as they come to know the family and the family's problems. Nurses can be alert to problems and needs of the families and make necessary referrals when supplementary services are indicated. The **Muscular Dystrophy Association of America, Inc.*** has branches in most communities to provide assistance to families in which there is a member with muscular dystrophy.

*810 Seventh Ave., New York, NY, 10019; (212) 586-0808.

KEY POINTS

- Upper motor neuron lesions produce weakness associated with spasticity, increased deep tendon reflexes, and abnormal superficial reflexes; lower motor neuron lesions interrupt the reflex arc, causing weakness and atrophy of the skeletal muscles.
- The most useful classification of neuromuscular disorders defines the source of the lesion: cerebral cortex, anterior horn cells of the spinal cord, peripheral nerves, myoneural junction, and muscles.
- Clinical manifestations of cerebral palsy include delayed gross motor development, abnormal motor performance, alterations of muscle tone, abnormal postures, reflex abnormalities, and associated disabilities such as mental retardation, seizures, attention deficit disorder, and sensory impairment.
- Therapy for cerebral palsy takes into account the nature of the physical disability, defects associated with the disorder, and interpersonal and social influences encountered by the affected child.
- Werdnig-Hoffmann disease is characterized by progressive weakness and wasting of skeletal muscles caused by degeneration of anterior horn cells.
- Nursing care of the child with Guillain-Barré syndrome consists of monitoring vital signs, ensuring alignment and positioning, physical therapy, and support of the family.
- Tetanus occurs when tetanus spores or vegetative bacilli enter a wound and multiply in a susceptible host.
- Infant botulism results from toxins produced by *C. botulinum;* toxin is ingested from poorly preserved food or released in the gastrointestinal tract by ingested spores.
- Primary management of myasthenia gravis is oral administration of anticholinesterase drugs.
- Spinal cord injuries usually involve the following four interrelated pathologic changes: cellular damage to cord tissue, hemorrhage and vascular damage, structural changes of white and gray matter related to vascular disruption, inflammation and edema, and local biochemical response to trauma.
- Therapeutic management of spinal cord injury is directed toward preventing further neuronal damage, avoiding complications, and maintaining vital functions.
- Goals of rehabilitation in spinal cord injury are to maximize function, assist the child and family in realistic goal setting, and help the child cope with stigma and build self-concept.
- Muscular dystrophies are the largest and most important group of muscular dysfunctions in childhood.
- Major complications of Duchenne muscular dystrophy include contractures, disuse atrophy, infections, obesity, and cardiopulmonary problems.

REFERENCES

American Academy of Pediatrics: Report of the Committee on Infectious Diseases, Elk Grove, IL, 1988, American Academy of Pediatrics.

American Academy of Pediatrics Policy Statement: The Doman-Delacato treatment of neurologically handicapped children, Pediatrics 70:810-812, 1982.

Arnon, S.S.: Infant botulism. In Gellis, S.S., and Kagan, B.M.: Current pediatric therapy 12, Philadelphia, 1986, W.B. Saunders Co.

Briscoe, D.M., McMenamin, J.B., and O'Donohoe, N.V.: Prognosis in Guillain-Barré syndrome, Arch. Dis. Child. 62:733-735, 1987.

Brooke, M.H., and others: Clincial investigation of Duchenne muscular dystrophy: interesting results in a trial of prednisone, Arch. Neurol. 44:82-817, 1987.

Bruce, D.A., Schut, L., and Sutton, L.N.: Brain and cervical spine injuries occurring during organized sports activities in children and adolescents, Primary Care 11:175-194, 1984.

Brucker, J.M.: Selective dorsal rhizotomy: neurosurgical treatment of cerebral palsy, J. Pediatr. Nurs. 5:105-114, 1990.

Darras, B.T., Harper, J.F., and Francke, U.: Prenatal diagnosis and detection of carriers with DNA probes in Duchenne's muscular dystrophy, N. Engl. J. Med. 316:985-992, 1987.

Fuchs, S., and others: Cervical spine fractures sustained by young children in forward-facing car seats, Pediatrics 84:348-354, 1989.

Healy, A., and Smith, B.: Cerebral palsy: setting the stage for the future, Contemp. Pediatr. 5(2):44-64, 1988.

Hoffman, E.P., Brown, R.H., Jr., and Kunkel, L.M.: Dystrophin: the protein product of the Duchenne muscular dystrophy locus, Cell 51:919-928, 1987.

Holm, V.A., Harthun-Smith, L., and Tada, W.L.: Infant walkers and cerebral palsy, Am. J. Dis. Child. 137:1189-1190, 1983.

Logigian, M.K., and Ward, J.D.: Pediatric rehabilitation, Boston, 1989, Little, Brown & Co., Inc.

Mendell, J.R., and others: Randomized, double-blind six-month trial of prednisone in Duchenne's muscular dystrophy, N. Engl. J. Med. 320:1592-1597, 1989.

Nelson, K.B.: Cerebral palsy. In Swaiman, K.F.: Pediatric neurology, St. Louis, 1989, Mosby–Year Book, Inc.

Paneth, N.: Etiologic factors in cerebral palsy, Pediatr. Ann. 15:191, 194-201, 1986.

Parke, J.T.: Diseases of the neuromuscular junction. In Oski, F.A., and others, editors: Principles and practice of pediatrics, Philadelphia, 1990, J.B. Lippincott Co.

Schanzer, H., and Jacobson, J.H.: Tissue damage caused by the intramuscular injection of long-acting penicillin, Pediatrics 75:741-744, 1985.

Spika, J.A., and others: Risk factors for infant botulism in the United States, Am. J. Dis. Child. 143:828-832, 1989.

Sternfield, L.: Cerebral palsy. In Gellis, S.S., and Kagan, B.M.: Current pediatric therapy 12, Philadelphia, 1986, W.B. Saunders Co.

Stoller, K.P., and Losey, R.: Inadvertent intra-arterial injection of penicillin: an unseen danger, Pediatrics 75:785-786, 1985.

Taft, L.T.: Cerebral palsy, Pediatr. Rev. 6:35-44, 1984.

Thomas, N.H., and Dubowitz, V.: Muscular dystrophy and other muscle disorders, Curr. Opin. Pediatr. 1:296-300, 1989.

BIBLIOGRAPHY

General

Downey, J.A., and Low, N.L., editors: The child with disabling illness, ed. 2, Philadelphia, 1984, W.B. Saunders Co.

Eng, G.D., and Binder, H.: Rehabilitation of infants and children with neuromuscular disorders, Pediatr. Ann. 17:745-754, 1988.

Greenberg, F., and others: X-linked infantile spinal muscular atrophy, Am. J. Dis. Child. 12:217-219, 1988.

Lenox, A.C.: When motor nerves die, Am. J. Nurs. 83:540-546, 1983.

Martinson, I.M., and Widmer, A.: Home health care nursing, Philadelphia, 1989, W.B. Saunders Co.

Silver, B.: How could I have thought James couldn't be helped? RN 51(1):23-24, 1988.

Swaiman, K.F.: Pediatric neurology, St. Louis, 1989, Mosby–Year Book, Inc.

Cerebral Palsy

Accardo, P., and Whitman, B.: Toe walking: a marker for language disorders—in the developmentally disabled, Clin. Pediatr. 28:347-350, 1989.

Barabas, G., and Taft, L.T.: The early signs and differential diagnosis of cerebral palsy, Pediatr. Ann. 15:203-214, 1986.

Coffman, S.P.: Parents' perceptions of needs for themselves and their children in a cerebral palsy clinic, Issues Compr. Pediatr. Nurs. 6:67-77, 1983.

Diamond, M.: Rehabilitation strategies for the child with cerebral palsy, Pediatr. Ann. 15:230-236, 1986.

Fee, M.A., Charney, E.B., and Robertson, W.W.: Nutritional assessment of the young child with cerebral palsy, Inf. Young Child. 1:33-40, 1988.

Harris, S.R.: Early diagnosis of spastic diplegia, spastic hemiplegia, and quadriplegia, Am. J. Dis. Child. 143:1356-1360, 1989.

Logigian, M.K.: Cerebral palsy. In Logigian, M.K., and Ward, J.D, editors: Pediatric rehabilitation: a team approach for therapists, Boston, 1989, Little, Brown & Co., Inc.

Magill, J., and others: The self-esteem of adolescents with cerebral palsy, Am. J. Occup. Ther. 40:402-407, 1986.

Matthews, D.J.: Controversial therapies in the management of cerebral palsy, Pediatr. Ann. 17:762-764, 1988.

Naelye, R.L., and others: Origins of cerebral palsy, Am. J. Dis. Child. 143:1154-1161, 1989.

Nelson, K.B., and Ellenberg, J.H.: The asymptomatic newborn and risk of cerebral palsy, Am. J. Dis. Child. 141:1333-1335, 1987.

Niswander, K.R.: Does substandard care cause cerebral palsy? Contemp. Pediatr. 5(1):56-76, 1988.

Pilon, B.H., and Smith, K.A.: A parent group for the Hispanic parents of children with severe cerebral palsy, Child. Health Care 14:96-102, 1985.

Staudt, L.A., Peacock, W.J., and Oppenheim, W.: The role of selective posterior rhizotomy in the management of cerebral palsy, Inf. Young Child. 2(3):48-58, 1990.

Steele, S.: Young children with cerebral palsy: practical guidelines for care, Pediatr. Nurs. 11:259-267, 1985.

Stern, F.M., and Gorga, D.: Neurodevelopmental treatment (NDT): therapeutic intervention and its efficacy, Inf. Young Child. 1(1):22-32, 1988.

Task Force on Joint Assessment of Prenatal and Perinatal Factors Associated with Brain Disorders: National Institutes of Health report on causes of mental retardation and cerebral palsy, Pediatrics 76:457-458, 1985.

Torfs, C.P., and others: Prenatal and perinatal factors in the etiology of cerebral palsy, J. Pediatr. 116:615-619, 1990.

Wolraich, M.L.: Counseling families of children with cerebral palsy, Pediatr. Ann. 15:239-244, 1986.

Neuromuscular Dysfunction

Dezfulian, M., Yolken, R., and Bartlett, J.: Rapid diagnosis of a case of infant botulism by enzyme immunoassay, Pediatr. Infect. Dis. 4:399-401, 1985.

Engel, A.G.: Myasthenia gravis and myasthenic syndromes, Ann. Neurol. 16:519-523, 1984.

Jemison-Smith, P., and Hubbell, H.: Guillain-Barré syndrome, Crit. Care Update 10(6):12-16, 1983.

Kess, R.: Suddenly in crisis: unpredictable myasthenia, Am. J. Nurs. 84:994-998, 1984.

Lancaster, M.J.: Botulism: north to Alaska, Am. J. Nurs. 90:60-62, 1990.

Lefvert, A.K., and Osterman, P.O.: Newborn infants to myasthenic mothers: a clinical study and an investigation of acetylcholine receptor antibodies in 17 children, Neurology 33:133-138, 1983.

Miller, D.K.: The challenge of infant botulism, MCN 7:180-183, 1982.

Roach, E.S., and others: Early-onset myasthenia gravis, J. Pediatr. 108:193-197, 1986.

Sebilia, A.J.: "When was your last tetanus shot?" RN 47(8):18-24, 1985.

Turick-Gibson, T.: Infant botulism, Pediatr. Nurs. 14:280-283, 1988.

Wilkinson, W.J., and Clore, E.R.: Infant botulism: a dilemma for nursing, J. Pediatr. Nurs. 3:164-168, 1988.

Spinal Cord Injury

Agee, B.L., and Herman, C.: Cervical logrolling on a standard hospital bed, Am. J. Nurs. 84:315-318, 1984.

Barker, E., and Higgins, R.: Managing a suspected spinal cord injury, Nursing '89 19(4):52-59, 1989.

Bauer, S.B.: Neurogenic bladder dysfunction, Pediatr. Clin. North Am. 34:1121-1132, 1987.

Birdsall, C.: How do you teach female self-catheterization? Am. J. Nurs. 85:1226-1227, 1985.

Chadwick, A.T., and Oesting, H.H.: Caring for patients with spinal cord injuries, Nursing '89 19(11):53-56, 1989.

Nurse's hotline helps the spinal cord-injured, Am. J. Nurs. 87:720-721, 1987.

Peterson, T.: Autonomic dysreflexia, Nursing '87 17(8):33, 1987.

Romeo, J.H.: The critical minutes after spinal cord injury, RN 51(4):61-67, 1988.

Romeo, J.H.: Spinal cord injury: nursing the patient toward a new life, RN 51(5):31-35, 1988.

Soloway, M., and Smith, R.: Cranberry juice as a urine acidifier, JAMA 260:1465, 1988.

Sullivan-Bolyai, S., Swanson, M., and Shurtleff, D.B.: Toilet training the child with neurogenic impairment of bowel and bladder function, Issues Compr. Pediatr. Nurs. 7:33-43, 1984.

Muscular Dysfunction

Carroll, J.E.: Diagnosis and management of Duchenne muscular dystrophy, Pediatr. Rev. 6:195-200, 1985.

Firth, M., and others: Interview with parents of boys suffering from Duchenne muscular dystrophy, Dev. Med. Child Neurol. 25:466-471, 1983.

Pachman, L.M.: Juvenile dermatomyositis, Pediatr. Clin. North Am. 33:1097-1117, 1986.

Spencer, C.H., and others: Course of treated juvenile dermatomyositis, J. Pediatr. 105:399-408, 1984.

Vaughan, S.M., and Whittle, E.: Caring for the child with dermatomyositis, Issues Compr. Pediatr. Nurs. 7:255-267, 1984.

APPENDIX A

Family Assessment

Family APGAR questionnaire

PART I

The following questions have been designed to help us better understand you and your family. You should feel free to ask questions about any item in the questionnaire.

The space for comments should be used when you wish to give additional information or if you wish to discuss the way the question is applied to your family. Please try to answer all questions.

Family is defined as the individual(s) with whom you usually live. If you live alone, your "family" consists of persons with whom you now have the strongest emotional ties.*

For each question, check only one box

	Almost always	**Some of the time**	**Hardly ever**
I am satisfied that I can turn to my family for help when something is troubling me. Comments: ______	☐	☐	☐
I am satisfied with the way my family talks over things with me and shares problems with me. Comments: ______	☐	☐	☐
I am satisfied that my family accepts and supports my wishes to take on new activities or directions. Comments: ______	☐	☐	☐
I am satisfied with the way my family expresses affection and responds to my emotions, such as anger, sorrow, and love. Comments: ______	☐	☐	☐
I am satisfied with the way my family and I share time together. Comments: ______	☐	☐	☐

*According to which member of the family is being interviewed the interviewer may substitute for the word 'family' either spouse, significant other, parents, or children.

A

Fig. A-1. Family APGAR questionnaire. **A,** Part I.

Modified from Smilkstein, G.: The Family APGAR: a proposal for a family function test and its use by physicians, J. Fam. Pract. 6(6):1231-1239, 1978. May be photocopied for clinical use.

Family APGAR questionnaire

PART II

Who lives in your home?* List by relationship (eg, spouse, significant other,** child, or friend).

Please check below the column that best describes how you now get along with each member of the family listed.

Relationship	Age	Sex	Well	Fairly	Poorly
______	__	__	☐	☐	☐
______	__	__	☐	☐	☐
______	__	__	☐	☐	☐
______	__	__	☐	☐	☐
______	__	__	☐	☐	☐
______	__	__	☐	☐	☐

If you don't live with your own family, please list below the individuals to whom you turn for help most frequently. List by relationship, (eg, family member, friend, associate at work, or neighbor).

Please check below the column that best describes how you now get along with each person listed.

Relationship	Age	Sex	Well	Fairly	Poorly
______	__	__	☐	☐	☐
______	__	__	☐	☐	☐
______	__	__	☐	☐	☐
______	__	__	☐	☐	☐
______	__	__	☐	☐	☐
______	__	__	☐	☐	☐

*If you have established your own family, consider home to be the place where you live with your spouse, children, or significant other; otherwise, consider home as your place of origin, eg, the place where your parents or those who raise you live.

***"Significant other" is the partner you live with in a physically and emotionally nurturing relationship, but to whom you are not married.

B

Fig. A-1, cont'd. B, Part II.

Infant/Toddler HOME Inventory

Bettye M. Caldwell and Robert H. Bradley

Family Name ______________________ Visitor ______________ Date ________

Address __________________________________ Phone ______________

Child's Name ______________________ Birthdate __________ Age _____ Sex _____

Parent Present ______________________ If other than parent, relationship to child ______________

Family Composition ____
(persons living in household, including sex and age of children)

Family Ethnicity ______________ Language Spoken ________ Maternal Education ________ Paternal Education ________

Is Mother Employed? ________ Type of work when employed ______ Is Father Employed? ________ Type of work when employed ______

Current child care arrangements ______________________________

Summarize past year's arrangement ______________________________

Other persons present during visit ______________________________

Comments: ____

____

SUMMARY

	Subscale	Score Fourth	Lowest Half	Middle Fourth	Upper
I.	RESPONSIVITY		0 - 6	7 - 9	10 - 11
II.	ACCEPTANCE		0 - 4	5 - 6	7 - 8
III.	ORGANIZATION		0 - 3	4 - 5	6
IV.	LEARNING MATERIALS		0 - 4	5 - 7	8 - 9
V.	INVOLVEMENT		0 - 2	3 - 4	5 - 6
VI.	VARIETY		0 - 1	2 - 3	4 - 5
	TOTAL SCORE		0 - 25	26 - 36	37 - 45

Fig. A-2. Home Inventory questionnaires. AUTHOR'S NOTE: HOME inventories for families and preschoolers (3 to 6 years) and elementary age children (6 to 10 years) are available from Center for Research on Teaching and Learning, Education Building, Room 205, University of Arkansas at Little Rock, 2801 S. University Ave., Little Rock, AR 72204; (501) 569-3422.

From Caldwell, B., and Bradley, R.: Manual of Home Observation for Measurement of the Environment, rev. ed., Little Rock, 1984, University of Arkansas at Little Rock.

Infant/Toddler HOME Inventory

Place a plus (+) or minus (-) in the box alongside each item if the behavior is observed during the visit or if the parent reports that the conditions or events are characteristic of the home environment. Enter the subtotal and the total on the front side of the Record Sheet.

I. RESPONSITIVITY		24. Child has a special place for toys and treasures.	
1. Parent spontaneously vocalizes to child at least twice.		25. Child's play environment is safe.	
2. Parent responds verbally to child's vocalizations or verbalizations.		**IV. LEARNING MATERIALS**	
3. Parent tells child name of object or person during visit.		26. Muscle activity toys or equipment.	
4. Parent's speech is distinct, clear and audible.		27. Push or pull toy.	
5. Parent initiates verbal interchanges with Visitor.		28. Stroller or walker, kiddie car, scooter, or tricycle.	
6. Parent converses freely and easily.		29. Parent provides toys for child to play with during visit.	
7. Parent permits child to engage in "messy" play.		30. Cuddly toy or role-playing toys.	
8. Parent spontaneously praises child at least twice.		31. Learning facilitators—mobile, table and chair, high chair, play pen.	
9. Parent's voice conveys positive feelings toward child.		32. Simple eye-hand coordination toys.	
10. Parent caresses or kisses child at least once.		33. Complex eye-hand coordination toys.	
11. Parent responds positively to praise of child offered by Visitor.		34. Toys for literature and music.	
II. ACCEPTANCE		**V. INVOLVEMENT**	
12. Parent does not shout at child.		35. Parent keeps child in visual range, looks at often.	
13. Parent does not express overt annoyance with or hostility to child.		36. Parent talks to child while doing household work.	
14. Parent neither slaps nor spanks child during visit.		37. Parent conciously encourages developmental advance.	
15. No more than 1 instance of physical punishment during past week.		38. Parent invests maturing toys with value via personal attention.	
16. Parent does not scold or criticize child during visit.		39. Parent structures child's play periods.	
17. Parent does not interfere with or restrict child 3 times during visit.		40. Parent provides toys that challenge child to develop new skills.	
18. At least 10 books are present and visible.		**VI. VARIETY**	
19. Family has a pet.		41. Father provides some care daily.	
III. ORGANIZATION		42. Parent reads stories to child at least 3 times weekly.	
20. Child care, if used, is provided by one of three regular substitutes.		43. Child eats at least one meal a day with mother and father.	
21. Child is taken to grocery store at least once a week.		44. Family visits relatives or receives visits once month or so.	
22. Child gets out of house at least 4 times a week.		45. Child has 3 or more books of his/her own.	
23. Child is taken regularly to doctor's office or clinic.			

	I	II	III	IV	V	VI	TOTAL
TOTALS							

Fig. A-2, cont'd.

Developmental/Sensory Assessment

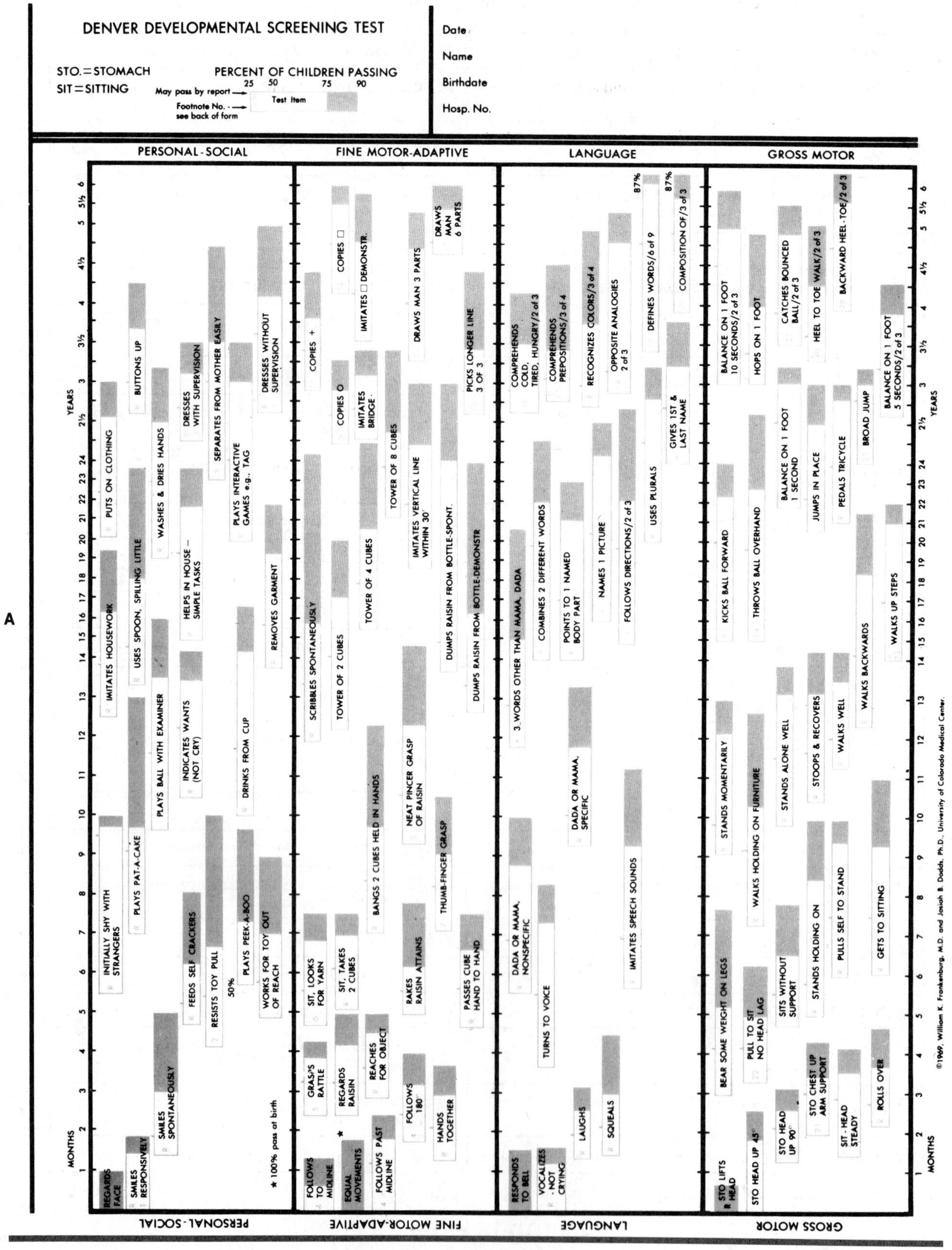

Fig. B-1. A, Denver Developmental Screening Test.
A from W.K. Frankenburg and J.B. Dodds, University of Colorado Medical Center, 1969.

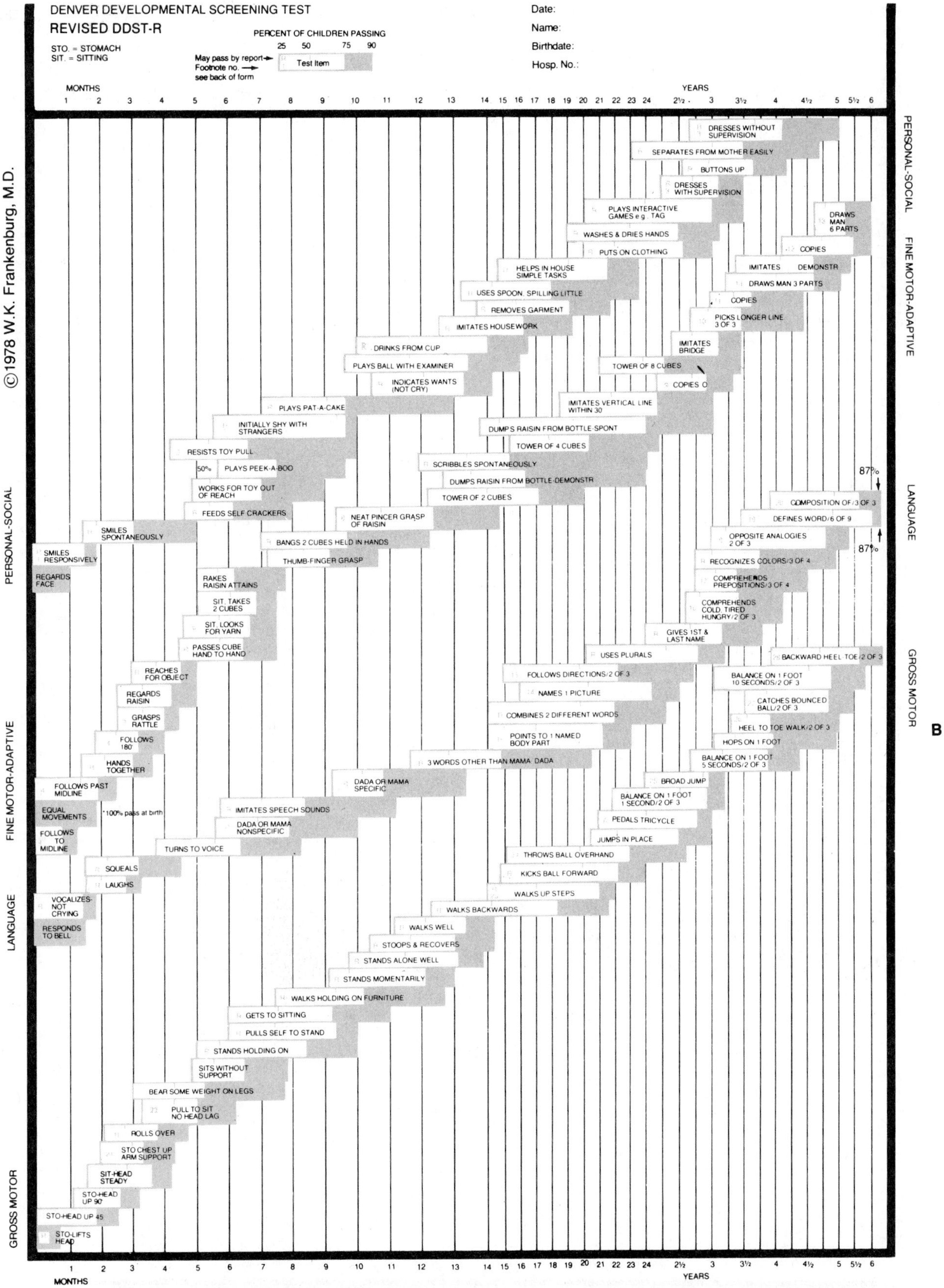

Fig. B-1, cont'd. B, DDST revised (DDST-R). Resembling a growth curve, this form places items at lowest age level starting at bottom left and progresses upward to right with increasing age.

B from Frankenburg, W.K., Sciarillo, W., and Burgess, D.: The newly abbreviated and revised Denver Developmental Screening Test, J. Pediatr. 99(6):995-999, 1981.

DIRECTIONS

DATE:
NAME:
BIRTHDATE:
HOSP. NO.:

1. Try to get child to smile by smiling, talking or waving to him. Do not touch him.
2. When child is playing with toy, pull it away from him. Pass if he resists.
3. Child does not have to be able to tie shoes or button in the back.
4. Move yarn slowly in an arc from one side to the other, about 6" above child's face. Pass if eyes follow 90° to midline. (Past midline; 180°)
5. Pass if child grasps rattle when it is touched to the backs or tips of fingers.
6. Pass if child continues to look where yarn disappeared or tries to see where it went. Yarn should be dropped quickly from sight from tester's hand without arm movement.
7. Pass if child picks up raisin with any part of thumb and a finger.
8. Pass if child picks up raisin with the ends of thumb and index finger using an over hand approach.

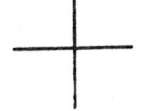

9. Pass any enclosed form. Fail continuous round motions.
10. Which line is longer? (Not bigger.) Turn paper upside down and repeat. (3/3 or 5/6)
11. Pass any crossing lines.
12. Have child copy first. If failed, demonstrate

When giving items 9, 11 and 12, do not name the forms. Do not demonstrate 9 and 11.

13. When scoring, each pair (2 arms, 2 legs, etc.) counts as one part.
14. Point to picture and have child name it. (No credit is given for sounds only.)

C

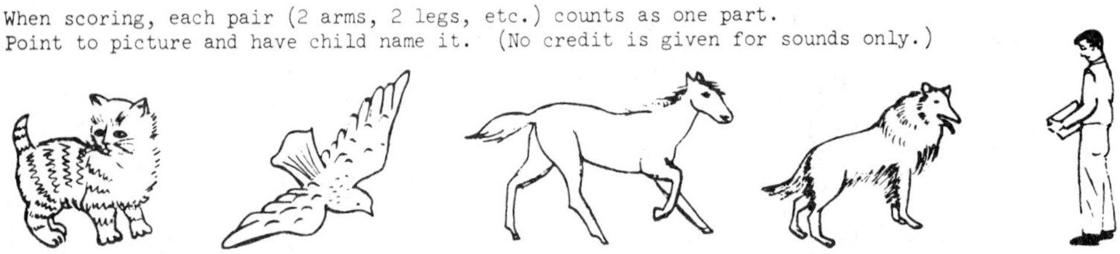

15. Tell child to: Give block to Mommie; put block on table; put block on floor. Pass 2 of 3. (Do not help child by pointing, moving head or eyes.)
16. Ask child: What do you do when you are cold? ..hungry? ..tired? Pass 2 of 3.
17. Tell child to: Put block <u>on</u> table; <u>under</u> table; <u>in front</u> of chair, <u>behind</u> chair. Pass 3 of 4. (Do not help child by pointing, moving head or eyes.)
18. Ask child: If fire is hot, ice is ?; Mother is a woman, Dad is a ?; a horse is big, a mouse is ?. Pass 2 of 3.
19. Ask child: What is a ball? ..lake? ..desk? ..house? ..banana? ..curtain? ..ceiling? ..hedge? ..pavement? Pass if defined in terms of use, shape, what it is made of or general category (such as banana is fruit, not just yellow). Pass 6 of 9.
20. Ask child: What is a spoon made of? ..a shoe made of? ..a door made of? (No other objects may be substituted.) Pass 3 of 3.
21. When placed on stomach, child lifts chest off table with support of forearms and/or hands.
22. When child is on back, grasp his hands and pull him to sitting. Pass if head does not hang back.
23. Child may use wall or rail only, not person. May not crawl.
24. Child must throw ball overhand 3 feet to within arm's reach of tester.
25. Child must perform standing broad jump over width of test sheet. (8-1/2 inches)
26. Tell child to walk forward, heel within 1 inch of toe. Tester may demonstrate. Child must walk 4 consecutive steps, 2 out of 3 trials.
27. Bounce ball to child who should stand 3 feet away from tester. Child must catch ball with hands, not arms, 2 out of 3 trials.
28. Tell child to walk backward, toe within 1 inch of heel. Tester may demonstrate. Child must walk 4 consecutive steps, 2 out of 3 trials.

<u>DATE AND BEHAVIORAL OBSERVATIONS</u> (how child feels at time of test, relation to tester, attention span, verbal behavior, self-confidence, etc,):

Fig. B-1, cont'd. C, Directions for numbered items on testing forms for DDST and DDST-R.

C from W.K. Frankenburg and J.B. Dobbs, University of Colorado Medical Center, 1969.

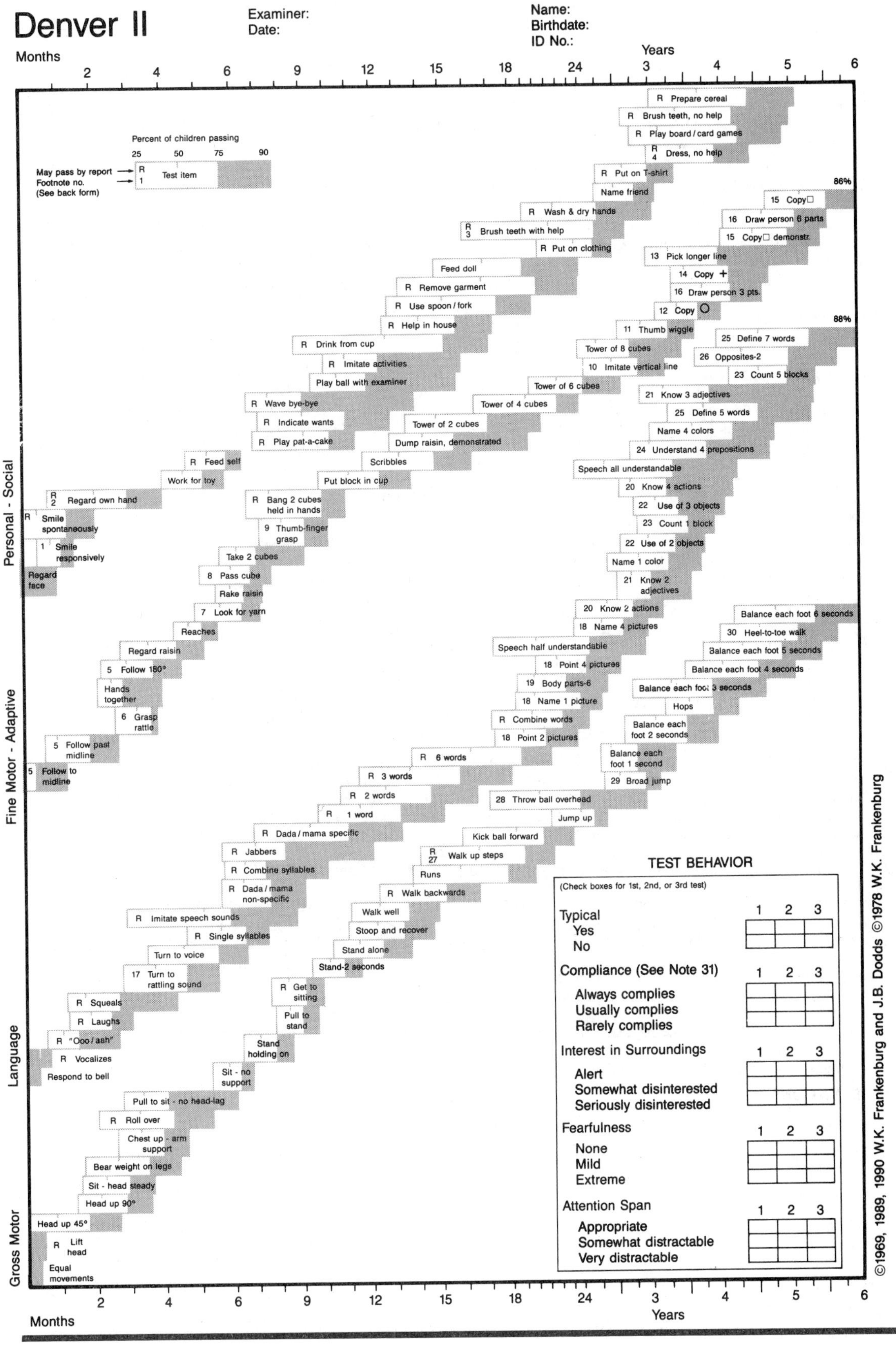

A

Fig. B-2. A, Denver II.
From W.K. Frankenburg and J.B. Dodds, 1990.

DIRECTIONS FOR ADMINISTRATION

1. Try to get child to smile by smiling, talking or waving. Do not touch him/her.
2. Child must stare at hand several seconds.
3. Parent may help guide toothbrush and put toothpaste on brush.
4. Child does not have to be able to tie shoes or button/zip in the back.
5. Move yarn slowly in an arc from one side to the other, about 8" above child's face.
6. Pass if child grasps rattle when it is touched to the backs or tips of fingers.
7. Pass if child tries to see where yarn went. Yarn should be dropped quickly from sight from tester's hand without arm movement.
8. Child must transfer cube from hand to hand without help of body, mouth, or table.
9. Pass if child picks up raisin with any part of thumb and finger.
10. Line can vary only 30 degrees or less from tester's line.
11. Make a fist with thumb pointing upward and wiggle only the thumb. Pass if child imitates and does not move any fingers other than the thumb.

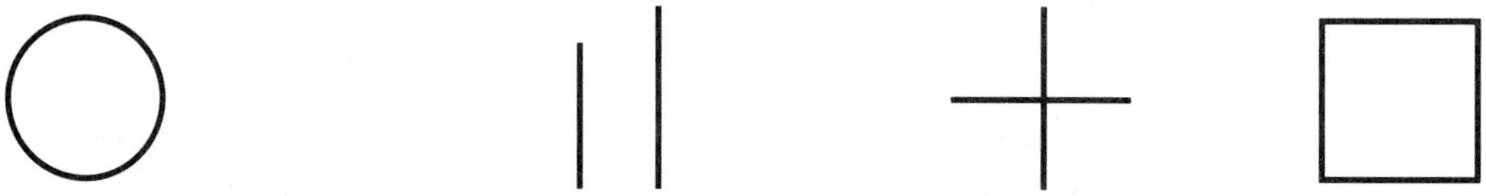

12. Pass any enclosed form. Fail continuous round motions.
13. Which line is longer? (Not bigger.) Turn paper upside down and repeat. (pass 3 of 3 or 5 of 6)
14. Pass any lines crossing near midpoint.
15. Have child copy first. If failed, demonstrate.

When giving items 12, 14, and 15, do not name the forms. Do not demonstrate 12 and 14.

16. When scoring, each pair (2 arms, 2 legs, etc.) counts as one part.
17. Place one cube in cup and shake gently near child's ear, but out of sight. Repeat for other ear.

B

18. Point to picture and have child name it. (No credit is given for sounds only.) If less than 4 pictures are named correctly, have child point to picture as each is named by tester.

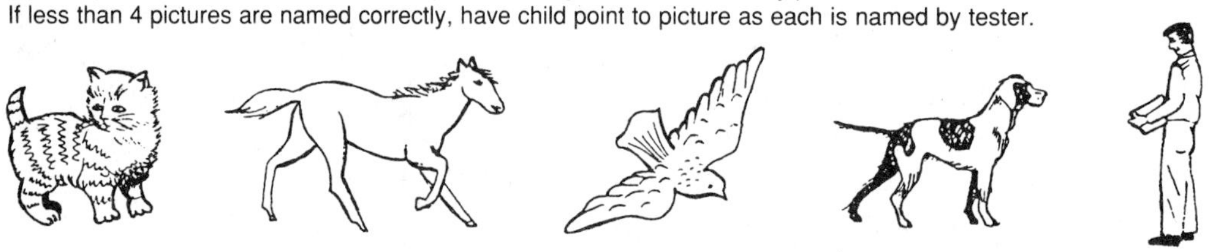

19. Using doll, tell child: Show me the nose, eyes, ears, mouth, hands, feet, tummy, hair. Pass 6 of 8.
20. Using pictures, ask child: Which one flies?... says meow?... talks?... barks?... gallops? Pass 2 of 5, 4 of 5.
21. Ask child: What do you do when you are cold?... tired?... hungry? Pass 2 of 3, 3 of 3.
22. Ask child: What do you do with a cup? What is a chair used for? What is a pencil used for? Action words must be included in answers.
23. Pass if child correctly places and says how many blocks are on paper. (1, 5).
24. Tell child: Put block **on** table; **under** table; **in front of** me, **behind** me. Pass 4 of 4. (Do not help child by pointing, moving head or eyes.)
25. Ask child: What is a ball?... lake?... desk?... house?... banana?... curtain?... fence?... ceiling? Pass if defined in terms of use, shape, what it is made of, or general category (such as banana is fruit, not just yellow). Pass 5 of 8, 7 of 8.
26. Ask child: If a horse is big, a mouse is __? If fire is hot, ice is __? If the sun shines during the day, the moon shines during the __? Pass 2 of 3.
27. Child may use wall or rail only, not person. May not crawl.
28. Child must throw ball overhand 3 feet to within arm's reach of tester.
29. Child must perform standing broad jump over width of test sheet (8 1/2 inches).
30. Tell child to walk forward, → heel within 1 inch of toe. Tester may demonstrate. Child must walk 4 consecutive steps.
31. In the second year, half of normal children are non-compliant.

OBSERVATIONS:

Fig. B-2. B, Directions for administration of numbered items on Denver II.
From W.K. Frankenburg and J.B. Dodds, 1990.

0-9 MONTHS (R-PDQ)

REVISED DENVER PRESCREENING DEVELOPMENTAL QUESTIONNAIRE

Child's Name ______

Person Completing R-PDQ: ______

Relation to Child: ______

For Office Use

Today's Date: ____ yr ____ mo ____ day

Child's Birthdate: ____ yr ____ mo ____ day

Subtract to get Child's Exact Age: ____ yr ____ mo ____ day

R-PDQ Age: (____ yr ____ mo ____ completed wks)

CONTINUE ANSWERING UNTIL 3 **"NOs"** ARE CIRCLED

		For Office Use
1. Equal Movements When your baby is lying on his/her back, can (s)he move each of his/her arms as easily as the other and each of the legs as easily as the other? Answer **No** if your child makes jerky or uncoordinated movements with one or both of his/her arms or legs.	**Yes** **No**	(0) FMA
2. Stomach Lifts Head When your baby is on his/her stomach on a flat surface, can (s)he lift his/her head off the surface?	**Yes** **No**	(0-3) GM

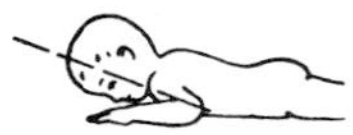

		For Office Use
3. Regards Face When your baby is lying on his/her back, can (s)he look at you and watch your face?	**Yes** **No**	(1) PS
4. Follows To Midline When your child is on his/her back, can (s)he follow your movement by turning his/her head from one side to facing directly forward?	**Yes** **No**	(1-1) FMA

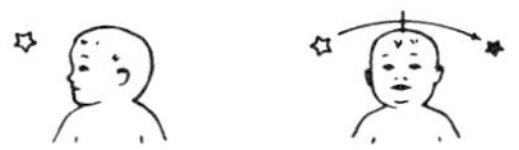

		For Office Use
5. Responds To Bell Does your child respond with eye movements, change in breathing or other change in activity to a bell or rattle sounded outside his/her line of vision?	**Yes** **No**	(1-2) L
6. Vocalizes Not Crying Does your child make sounds other than crying, such as gurgling, cooing, or babbling?	**Yes** **No**	(1-3) L
7. Smiles Responsively When you smile and talk to your baby, does (s)he smile back at you?	**Yes** **No**	(1-3) PS
8. Follows Past Midline When your child is on his/her back, does (s)he follow your movement by turning his/her head from one side ***almost all the way to the other side?***	**Yes** **No**	(2-2) FMA

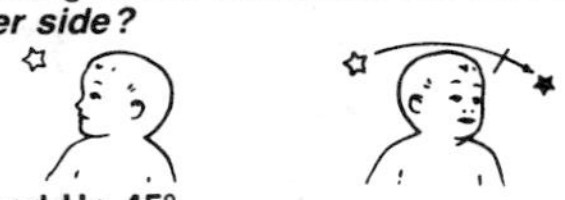

		For Office Use
9. Stomach, Head Up 45° When your baby is on his/her stomach on a flat surface, can (s)he lift his/her head 45°?	**Yes** **No**	(2-2) GM

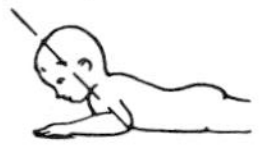

		For Office Use
10. Stomacn, Head Up 90° When your baby is on his/her stomach on a flat surface, can (s)he lift his/her head 90°?	**Yes** **No**	(3) GM

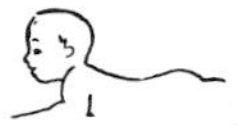

		For Office Use
11. Laughs Does your baby laugh out loud without being tickled or touched?	**Yes** **No**	(3-1) L
12. Hands Together Does your baby play with his/her hands by touching them together?	**Yes** **No**	(3-3) FMA
13. Follows 180° When your child is on his/her back, does (s)he follow your movement from one side ***all the way*** to the other side?	**Yes** **No**	(4) FMA

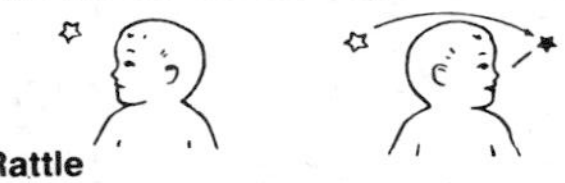

		For Office Use
14. Grasps Rattle ***It is important that you follow instructions carefully.*** Do ***not*** place the pencil in the palm of your child's hand. When you touch the pencil to the back or tips of your baby's fingers, does your baby grasp the pencil for a few seconds?	**Yes** **No**	(4) FMA

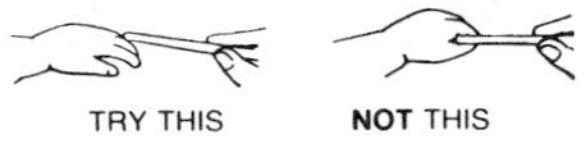

(Please turn page)

Fig. B-3. Revised Prescreening Developmental Questionnaire. (Sample of first page only.)
The *first* page is reprinted with permission of William K. Frankenburg. Copyright 1975, 1986, W.K. Frankenburg.

DENVER ARTICULATION SCREENING EXAM
for children 2½ to 6 years of age

Instructions: Have child repeat each word after you. Circle the underlined sounds that he pronounces correctly. Total correct sounds is the Raw Score. Use charts on reverse side to score results.

Name:

Hosp. No.:

Address:______________________
____

Date: __________ Child's age: __________ Examiner: __________ Raw score: ____
Percentile: ______ Intelligibility: __________ Result: __________

1. table	6. zipper	11. sock	16. wagon	21. leaf
2. shirt	7. grapes	12. vacuum	17. gum	22. carrot
3. door	8. flag	13. yarn	18. house	
4. trunk	9. thumb	14. mother	19. pencil	
5. jumping	10. toothbrush	15. twinkle	20. fish	

Intelligibility: (circle one)
1. Easy to understand
2. Understandable ½ the time
3. Not understandable
4. Can't evaluate

Comments:

A

Date: __________ Child's age: __________ Examiner: __________ Raw score: ____
Percentile: ______ Intelligibility: __________ Result: __________

1. table	6. zipper	11. sock	16. wagon	21. leaf
2. shirt	7. grapes	12. vacuum	17. gum	22. carrot
3. door	8. flag	13. yarn	18. house	
4. trunk	9. thumb	14. mother	19. pencil	
5. jumping	10. toothbrush	15. twinkle	20. fish	

Intelligibility: (circle one)
1. Easy to understand
2. Understandable ½ the time
3. Not understandable
4. Can't evaluate

Comments:

Date: __________ Child's age: __________ Examiner: __________ Raw score ____
Percentile: ______ Intelligibility: __________ Result: __________

1. table	6. zipper	11. sock	16. wagon	21. leaf
2. shirt	7. grapes	12. vacuum	17. gum	22. carrot
3. door	8. flag	13. yarn	18. house	
4. trunk	9. thumb	14. mother	19. pencil	
5. jumping	10. toothbrush	15. twinkle	20. fish	

Intelligibility: (circle one)
1. Easy to understand
2. Understandable ½ the time
3. Not understandable
4. Can't evaluate

Fig. B-4. A, Denver Articulation Screening Examination for children 2½ to 6 years of age.
From A.F. Drumwright, University of Colorado Medical Center, 1971.

To score DASE words: Note raw score for child's performance. Match raw score line (extreme left of chart) with column representing child's age (to the closest previous age group). Where raw score line and age column meet number in that square denotes percentile rank of child's performance when compared to other children that age. Percentiles above heavy line are ABNORMAL percentiles, below heavy line are NORMAL.

PERCENTILE RANK

Raw Score	2.5 yr.	3.0	3.5	4.0	4.5	5.0	5.5	6 years
2	1							
3	2							
4	5							
5	9							
6	16							
7	23							
8	31	2						
9	37	4	1					
10	42	6	2					
11	48	7	4					
12	54	9	6	1	1			
13	58	12	9	2	3	1	1	
14	62	17	11	5	4	2	2	
15	68	23	15	9	5	3	2	
16	75	31	19	12	5	4	3	
17	79	38	25	15	6	6	4	
18	83	46	31	19	8	7	4	
19	86	51	38	24	10	9	5	1
20	89	58	45	30	12	11	7	3
21	92	65	52	36	15	15	9	4
22	94	72	58	43	18	19	12	5
23	96	77	63	50	22	24	15	7
24	97	82	70	58	29	29	20	15
25	99	87	78	66	36	34	26	17
26	99	91	84	75	46	43	34	24
27		94	89	82	57	54	44	34
28		96	94	88	70	68	59	47
29		98	98	94	84	84	77	68
30		100	100	100	100	100	100	100

B

To score intelligibility:

	NORMAL	ABNORMAL
2½ years	Understandable ½ the time, or, "easy"	Not understandable
3 years and older	Easy to understand	Understandable ½ time Not understandable

Test result: 1. NORMAL on Dase and Intelligibility = NORMAL

2. ABNORMAL on Dase and/or Intelligibility = ABNORMAL

*If abnormal on initial screening rescreen within 2 weeks.
If abnormal again child should be referred for complete speech evaluation.

Fig. B-4, cont'd. B, Percentile rank.

Lit. 217

DENVER EYE SCREENING TEST

Name:
Hospital No.:
Ward:
Address:

Vision Tests	1ST SCREENING: DATE: Right Eye Normal	1ST SCREENING: Right Eye Abnormal	1ST SCREENING: Right Eye Untestable	1ST SCREENING: Left Eye Normal	1ST SCREENING: Left Eye Abnormal	1ST SCREENING: Left Eye Untestable	RESCREENING: DATE: Right Eye Normal	RESCREENING: Right Eye Abnormal	RESCREENING: Right Eye Untestable	RESCREENING: Left Eye Normal	RESCREENING: Left Eye Abnormal	RESCREENING: Left Eye Untestable
1. "E" (3 years and above—3 to 5 trials)	3P	3F	U	3P	3F	U	3P	3F	U	3P	3F	U
2. Picture card (2 1/2 - 2 11/12 yrs.—3 to 5 trials)	3P	3F	U	3P	3F	U	3P	3F	U	3P	3F	U
3. Fixation (6 months - 2 5/12 years)	P	F	U	P	F	U	P	F	U	P	F	U
4. Squinting		yes			yes			yes			yes	

Tests for Non-Straight Eyes	1ST SCREENING: Normal	1ST SCREENING: Abnormal	1ST SCREENING: Untestable	RESCREENING: Normal	RESCREENING: Abnormal	RESCREENING: Untestable
1. Do your child's eyes turn in or out, or are they ever not straight?	NO	YES	U	NO	YES	U
2. Cover Test	P	F	U	P	F	U
3. Pupillary Light Reflex	P	F	U	P	F	U

Total Test Rating (Both Eyes)	1ST SCREENING	RESCREENING
Normal (passed vision test plus no squint, plus passed 2/3 tests for non-straight eyes)	Normal	Normal
Abnormal (abnormal on any vision test, squinting or 2 of 3 procedures for non-straight eyes)	Abnormal	Abnormal
Untestable (untestable on any vision test or untestable on 2/3 tests for non-straight eyes)	Untestable	Untestable
Future Rescreening Appointment for Total Test Rating (Abnormal or Untestable)	Date:	Date:

Fig. B-5. Denver Eye Screening Test.
From W.K. Frankenburg and J.B. Dobbs, University of Colorado Medical Center, 1969.

SNELLEN SCREENING*

Preparation

1. Hang the Snellen chart on a light-colored wall so that the 20- to 30-foot lines are at eye level when children 6 to 12 years old are tested in the standing position.
2. Secure the chart to the wall with double-stick tape on the back side of all four corners. If the chart must be reversed for use of the letter or E chart, secure it at the top and bottom with tacks. Make sure that the chart does not swing when in place.
3. The illumination intensity on the chart should be 10 to 30 foot-candles, without any glare from windows or light fixtures. The illumination should be checked with a light meter.
4. Mark an exact 20-foot distance from the chart. Mark the floor with a piece of tape or "footprints" positioned so that the heels touch the 20-foot line.

Procedure

1. Place the child at the 20-foot mark, with the heel edging the line if the child is standing or with the back of the chair placed at the marker if the child is seated.
2. If the E chart is used, accustom the child to identifying which direction the "legs of the E" are pointing. Use a demonstration E card for this purpose.
3. Teach the child to use the occluder to cover one eye. Instruct child to keep both eyes open during the test. Provide a clean cover card for each child and then discard after use.
4. If the child wears glasses, test only with glasses on.
5. Test both eyes together, then right eye, then left eye.
6. Begin with the 40- or 30-foot line and proceed with test to include the 20-foot line.
7. With the child suspected of low vision, begin with the 200-foot line and proceed until the child can no longer correctly read three out of four or four our of six symbols on a line.
8. Use covers on the Snellen chart to expose only one symbol or one line at a time. When screening kindergarten or older children, expose one line but may use a pointer to point to one symbol at a time.

Recording and Referral

1. Record the last line the child read correctly (three out of four or four out of six symbols).
2. Record visual acuity as a fraction. The numerator represents the distance from the chart, and the denominator represents the last line read correctly. For example, 20/30 means that the child read the 30-foot line at a 20-foot distance.
3. Observe the child's eyes during testing and record any evidence of squinting, head tilting, thrusting the head forward, excessive blinking, tearing, or redness.
4. Only make referrals after a second screening has been made on children who are potential candidates for referral.
5. The following children should be referred for a complete eye examination:
   a. Three-year-old children with vision in either eye of 20/50 or less (inability to correctly identify one more than half the symbols on the 40-foot line) *or* a two-line difference in visual acuity between the eyes in the passing range; for example, 20/20 in one eye and 20/40 in the other
   b. All other ages and grades with vision in either eye of 20/40 or less (inability to correctly identify one more than half the symbols on the 30-foot line)
   c. All children who consistently show any of the signs of possible visual disturbances, regardless of visual acuity

*Modified from recommendations of the National Society to Prevent Blindness: Guide to testing distance visual acuity, Schaumburg, IL, 1988, The Society.

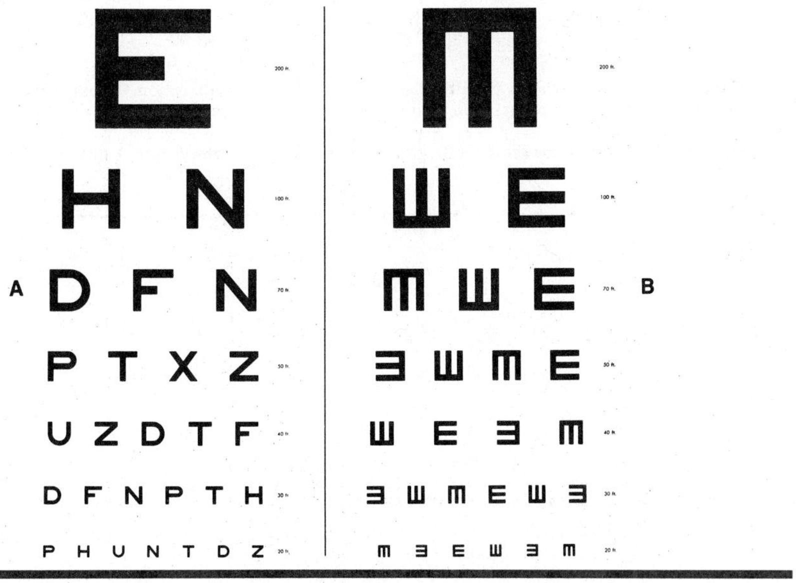

Fig. B-6. Snellen chart. **A,** Letter (alphabet) chart. **B,** Symbol E chart.
From National Society to Prevent Blindness, Inc., Schaumburg, IL.

APPENDIX C

Growth Measurements

HEIGHT AND WEIGHT MEASUREMENTS FOR BOYS

	HEIGHT BY PERCENTILES						WEIGHT BY PERCENTILES					
	5		50		95		5		50		95	
AGE*	CM	INCHES	CM	INCHES	CM	INCHES	KG	LB	KG	LB	KG	LB
Birth	46.4	18¼	50.5	20	54.4	21½	2.54	5½	3.27	7¼	4.15	9¼
3 months	56.7	22¼	61.1	24	65.4	25¾	4.43	9¾	5.98	13¼	7.37	16¼
6 months	63.4	25	67.8	26¾	72.3	28½	6.20	13¾	7.85	17¼	9.46	20¾
9 months	68.0	26¾	72.3	28½	77.1	30¼	7.52	16½	9.18	20¼	10.93	24
1	71.7	28¼	76.1	30	81.2	32	8.43	18½	10.15	22½	11.99	26½
1½	77.5	30½	82.4	32½	88.1	34¾	9.59	21¼	11.47	25¼	13.44	29½
2†	82.5	32½	86.8	34¼	94.4	37¼	10.49	23¼	12.34	27¼	15.50	34¼
2½†	85.4	33½	90.4	35½	97.8	38½	11.27	24¾	13.52	29¾	16.61	36½
3	89.0	35	94.9	37¼	102.0	40¼	12.05	26½	14.62	32¼	17.77	39¼
3½	92.5	36½	99.1	39	106.1	41¾	12.84	28¼	15.68	34½	18.98	41¾
4	95.8	37¾	102.9	40½	109.9	43¼	13.64	30	16.69	36¾	20.27	44¾
4½	98.9	39	106.6	42	113.5	44¾	14.45	31¾	17.69	39	21.63	47¾
5	102.0	40¼	109.9	43¼	117.0	46	15.27	33¾	18.67	41¼	23.09	51
6	107.7	42½	116.1	45¾	123.5	48½	16.93	37¼	20.69	45½	26.34	58
7	113.0	44½	121.7	48	129.7	51	18.64	41	22.85	50¼	30.12	66½
8	118.1	46½	127.0	50	135.7	53½	20.40	45	25.30	55¾	34.51	76
9	122.9	48½	132.2	52	141.8	55¾	22.25	49	28.13	62	39.58	87¼
10	127.7	50¼	137.5	54¼	148.1	58¼	24.33	53¾	31.44	69¼	45.27	99¾
11	132.6	52¼	143.3	56½	154.9	61	26.80	59	35.30	77¾	51.47	113½
12	137.6	54¼	149.7	59	162.3	64	29.85	65¾	39.78	87¾	58.09	128
13	142.9	56¼	156.5	61½	169.8	66¾	33.64	74¼	44.95	99	65.02	143¼
14	148.8	58½	163.1	64¼	176.7	69½	38.22	84¼	50.77	112	72.13	159
15	155.2	61	169.0	66½	181.9	71½	43.11	95	56.71	125	79.12	174½
16	161.1	63½	173.5	68¼	185.4	73	47.74	105¼	62.10	137	85.62	188¾
17	164.9	65	176.2	69¼	187.3	73¾	51.50	113½	66.31	146¼	91.31	201¼
18	165.7	65¼	176.8	69½	187.6	73¾	53.97	119	68.88	151¾	95.76	211

Adapted from National Center for Health Statistics (NCHS), Health Resources Administration, Department of Health, Education and Welfare, Hyattsville, MD. Conversion of metric data to approximate inches and pounds by Ross Laboratories.
*Years unless otherwise indicated.
†Height data include some recumbent length measurements, which make values slightly higher than if all measurements had been of stature (standing height).

HEIGHT AND WEIGHT MEASUREMENTS FOR GIRLS

	HEIGHT BY PERCENTILES						WEIGHT BY PERCENTILES					
	5		50		95		5		50		95	
AGE*	CM	INCHES	CM	INCHES	CM	INCHES	KG	LB	KG	LB	KG	LB
Birth	45.4	17¾	49.9	19¾	52.9	20¾	2.36	5¼	3.23	7	3.81	8½
3 months	55.4	21¾	59.5	23½	63.4	25	4.18	9¼	5.4	12	6.74	14¾
6 months	61.8	24¼	65.9	26	70.2	27¾	5.79	12¾	7.21	16	8.73	19¼
9 months	66.1	26	70.4	27¾	75.0	29½	7.0	15½	8.56	18¾	10.17	22½
1	69.8	27½	74.3	29¼	79.1	31¼	7.84	17¼	9.53	21	11.24	24¾
1½	76.0	30	80.9	31¾	86.1	34	8.92	19¾	10.82	23¾	12.76	28¼
2†	81.6	32¼	86.8	34¼	93.6	36¾	9.95	22	11.8	26	14.15	31¼
2½†	84.6	33¼	90.0	35½	96.6	38	10.8	23¾	13.03	28¾	15.76	34¾
3	88.3	34¾	94.1	37	100.6	39½	11.61	25½	14.1	31	17.22	38
3½	91.7	36	97.9	38½	104.5	41¼	12.37	27¼	15.07	33¼	18.59	41
4	95.0	37½	101.6	40	108.3	42¾	13.11	29	15.96	35¼	19.91	44
4½	98.1	38½	105.0	41¼	112.0	44	13.83	30½	16.81	37	21.24	46¾
5	101.1	39¾	108.4	42¾	115.6	45½	14.55	32	17.66	39	22.62	49¾
6	106.6	42	114.6	45	122.7	48¼	16.05	35½	19.52	43	25.75	56¾
7	111.8	44	120.6	47½	129.5	51	17.71	39	21.84	48¼	29.68	65½
8	116.9	46	126.4	49¾	136.2	53½	19.62	43¼	24.84	54¾	34.71	76½
9	122.1	48	132.2	52	142.9	56¼	21.82	48	28.46	62¾	40.64	89½
10	127.5	50¼	138.3	54½	149.5	58¾	24.36	53¾	32.55	71¾	47.17	104
11	133.5	52½	144.8	57	156.2	61½	27.24	60	36.95	81½	54.0	119
12	139.8	55	151.5	59¾	162.7	64	30.52	67¼	41.53	91½	60.81	134
13	145.2	57¼	157.1	61¾	168.1	66¼	34.14	75¼	46.1	101¾	67.3	148¼
14	148.7	58½	160.4	63¼	171.3	67½	37.76	83¼	50.28	110¾	73.08	161
15	150.5	59¼	161.8	63¾	172.8	68	40.99	90¼	53.68	118¼	77.78	171½
16	151.6	59¾	162.4	64	173.3	68¼	43.41	95¾	55.89	123¼	80.99	178½
17	152.7	60	163.1	64¼	173.5	68¼	44.74	98¾	56.69	125	82.46	181¾
18	153.6	60½	163.7	64½	173.6	68¼	45.26	99¾	56.62	124¾	82.47	181¾

Adapted from National Center for Health Statistics, Health Resources Administration, Department of Health, Education and Welfare, Hyattsville, MD. Conversion of metric data to approximate inches and pounds by Ross Laboratories.
*Years unless otherwise indicated.
†Height data include some recumbent length measurements, which make values slightly higher than if all measurements had been of stature.

GROWTH STANDARDS OF HEALTHY CHINESE CHILDREN AND ADOLESCENTS (URBAN)*

AGE (MONTHS OR YEARS)	BOYS				GIRLS			
	WEIGHT (KG)	HEIGHT (CM)	HEAD CIRCUMFERENCE (CM)	CHEST CIRCUMFERENCE (CM)	WEIGHT (KG)	HEIGHT (CM)	HEAD CIRCUMFERENCE (CM)	CHEST CIRCUMFERENCE (CM)
Birth	3.27	50.6	34.3	32.8	3.17	50.0	33.7	32.6
1 mo	4.97	56.5	38.1	37.9	4.64	55.5	37.3	36.9
2 mo	5.95	59.6	39.7	40.0	5.49	58.4	38.7	38.9
3 mo	6.73	62.3	41.0	41.3	6.23	60.9	40.0	40.3
4 mo	7.32	64.4	42.0	42.3	6.69	62.9	41.0	41.1
5 mo	7.70	65.9	42.9	42.9	7.19	64.5	41.9	41.9
6 mo	8.22	68.1	43.9	43.8	7.62	66.7	42.8	42.7
8 mo	8.71	70.6	44.9	44.7	8.14	69.0	43.7	43.4
10 mo	9.14	72.9	45.7	45.4	8.57	71.4	44.5	44.2
12 mo	9.66	75.6	46.3	46.1	9.04	74.1	45.2	45.0
15 mo	10.15	78.3	46.8	46.8	9.54	76.9	45.6	45.8
18 mo	10.67	80.7	47.3	47.6	10.08	79.4	46.2	46.6
21 mo	11.18	83.0	47.8	48.3	10.56	81.7	46.7	47.3
24 mo	11.95	86.5	48.2	49.2	11.37	85.3	47.1	48.2
2½ yr	12.84	90.4	48.8	50.2	12.28	89.3	47.7	49.0
3 yr	13.63	93.8	49.1	50.8	13.1	92.8	48.1	49.8
3½ yr	14.45	97.2	49.4	51.5	14.0	96.3	48.5	50.5
4 yr	15.26	100.8	49.7	52.2	14.89	100.1	48.9	51.2
4½ yr	16.07	103.9	50.0	53.0	15.63	103.1	49.1	51.8
5 yr	16.88	107.2	50.2	53.6	16.46	106.5	49.4	52.5
5½ yr	17.65	110.1	50.5	54.4	17.18	109.2	49.6	53.0
6 yr	19.25	114.7	50.8	55.6	18.67	113.9	50.0	54.2
7 yr	21.01	120.6	51.1	57.1	20.35	119.3	50.2	55.5
8 yr	23.08	125.3	51.4	58.8	22.43	124.6	50.6	57.1
9 yr	25.33	130.6	51.7	60.8	24.57	129.5	50.9	58.6
10 yr	27.15	134.4	51.9	62.0	27.05	134.8	51.3	60.7
11 yr	30.13	139.2	52.3	64.3	30.51	140.6	51.7	63.5
12 yr	33.05	144.2	52.7	66.5	34.82	146.6	52.3	67.2
13 yr	36.90	149.3	53.0	68.9	38.52	150.7	52.8	70.3
14 yr	42.03	156.5	53.5	72.4	42.26	153.7	53.1	73.3
15 yr	46.91	162.0	54.3	76.0	45.37	155.5	53.4	75.6
16 yr	50.90	165.6	54.9	78.8	47.43	156.8	53.8	76.6
17 yr	53.11	167.7	55.2	80.8	48.57	157.4	53.9	77.9

Adapted from Practical Pediatrics; edited by Peking Children's Hospital, 1979.
*Measurements of rural Chinese children are slightly lower.
NOTE: A comparison of the average growth of American and Chinese children demonstrates that on the standard NCHS growth charts the mean height and weight for Chinese children fall in the 10th percentile, as compared with the mean growth measurements for American children, which comprise the 50th percentile.

HEAD CIRCUMFERENCE CHARTS

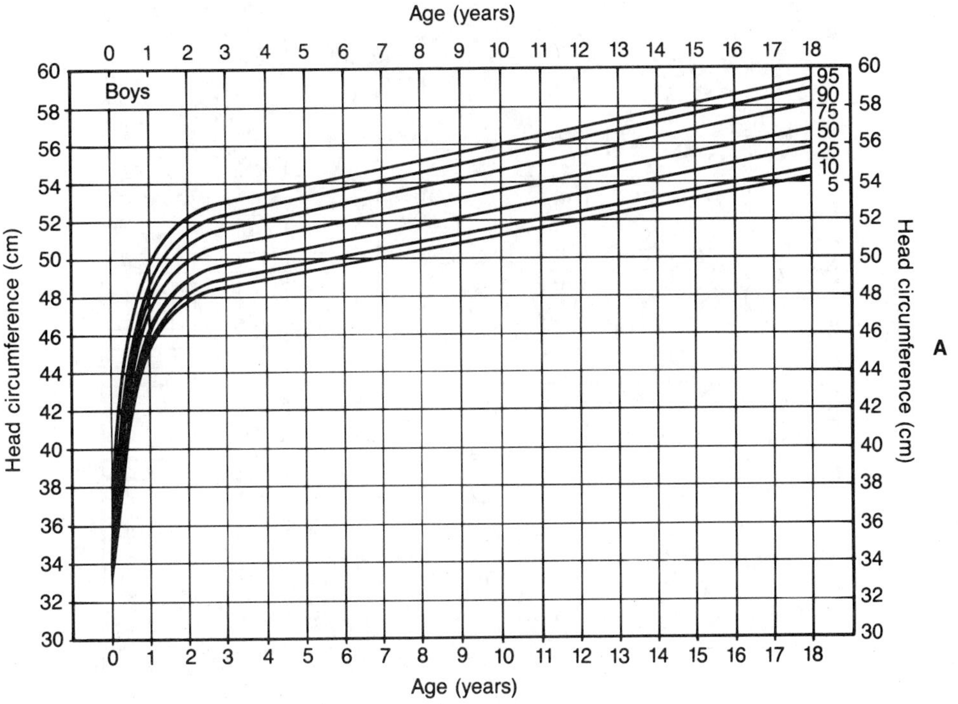

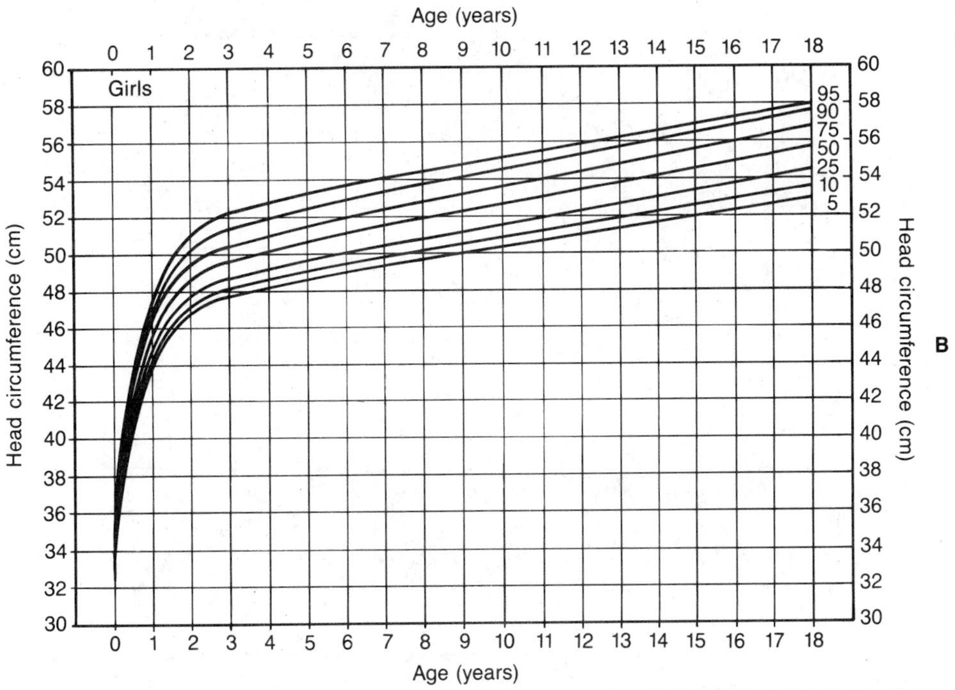

Fig. C-1. Selected percentiles for smoothed head circumference values of children from birth to 18 years. **A,** Boys. **B,** Girls.

From Roche, A.F., and others: Head circumference reference data: birth to 18 years, Pediatrics 79(5):706-712, 1987.

MEASUREMENT OF TRICEPS SKINFOLD THICKNESS

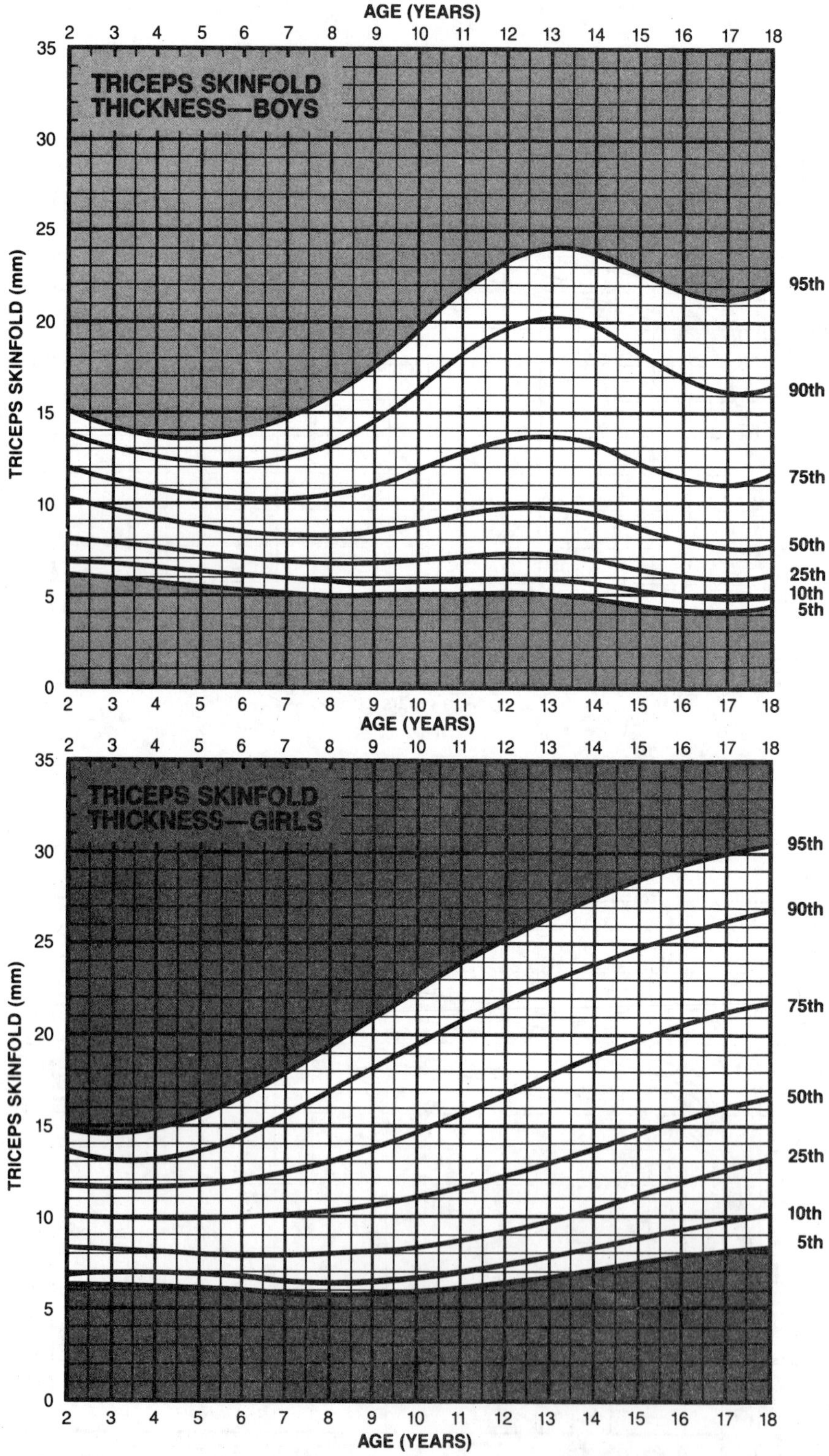

Fig. C-2. Triceps skinfold.

Modified from Johnson, C.L., and others: Basic data on anthropometric measurements and angular measurements of the hip and knee joints for selected age-groups, 1-74 years of age, United States, 1972-1975, Vital and Health Statistics Series 11, No. 219. DHHS Publication No. (PHS) 81-1669, 1981. Provided as a service of Ross Laboratories, Copyright 1983, Columbus, Ohio, 43216. May be copied for individual patient use.

MEASUREMENT OF MIDARM CIRCUMFERENCE

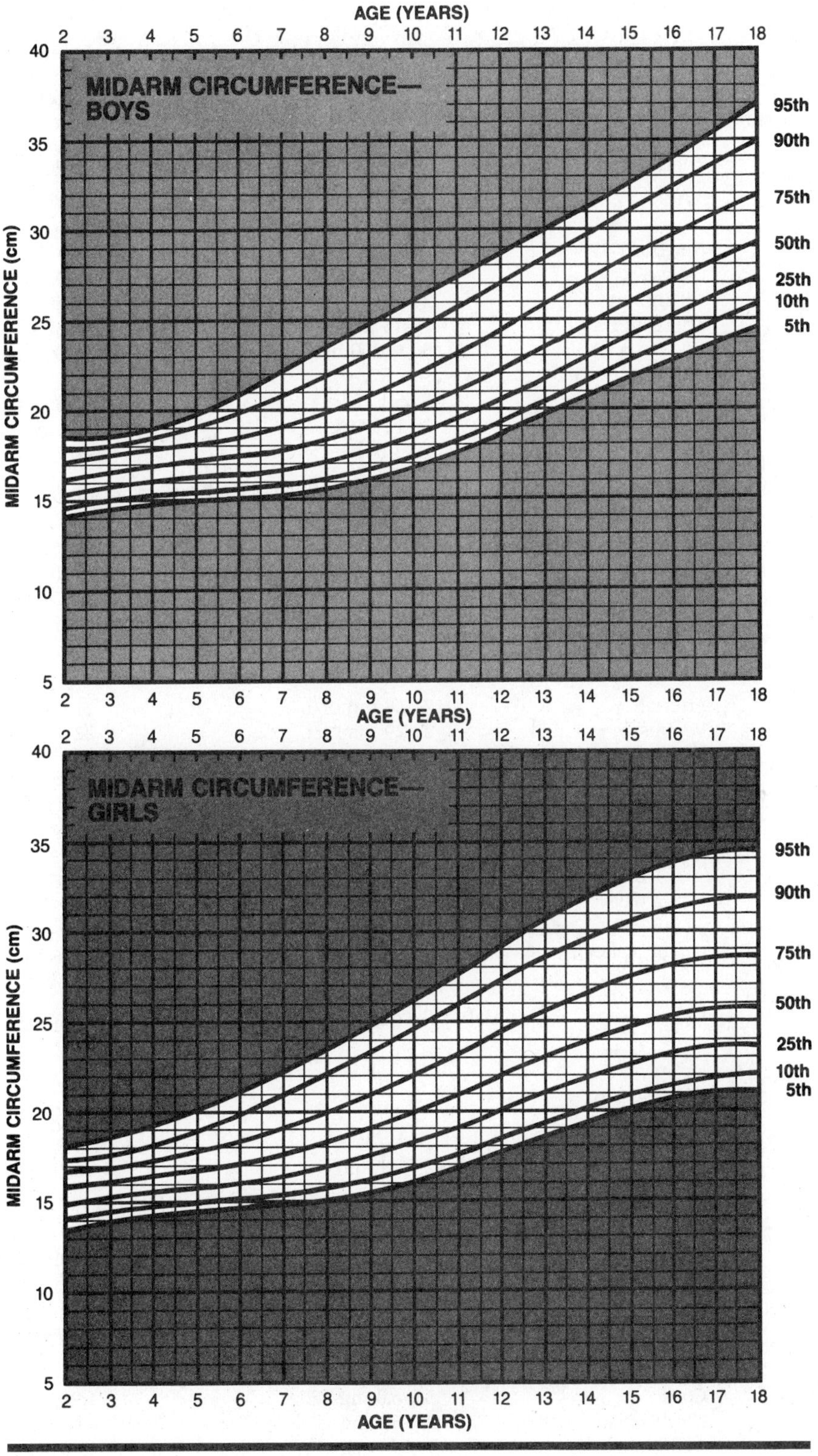

Fig. C-3. Midarm circumference.

Modified from Johnson, C.L., and others: Basic data on anthropometric measurements and angular measurements of the hip and knee joints for selected age-groups, 1-74 years of age, United States, 1971-1975, Vital Health Statistics Series 11, No. 219. DHHS Publication No. [PHS] 81-1669, 1981. Provided as a service of Ross Laboratories, Copyright 1983, Columbus, Ohio, 43216. May be copied for individual patient use.

APPENDIX D

Common Laboratory Tests

Test/specimen	Age/sex/reference	Conventional units	International units
		Normal ranges	
Acetaminophen			
Serum, plasma	Therap. conc.	10-30 μg/ml	66-200 μmol/L
	Toxic conc.	>200 μg/ml	>1300 μmol/L
Ammonia nitrogen			
Plasma or serum	Newborn	90-150 μg/dL	64-107 μmol/L
	0-2 weeks	79-129 μg/dL	56-92 μmol/L
	>1 month	29-70 μg/dL	21-50 μmol/L
	Thereafter	15-45 μ/dL	11-32 μmol/L
Urine, 24 hr		500-1200 mg/d	36-86 mmol/d
Amylase	Newborn	5-65 U/L	5-65 U/L
Serum	>1 yr	25-125 U/L	25-125 U/L
Urine, timed specimen		1-17 U/hr	1-17 U/hr
Antistreptolysin O titer (ASO)		<166 Todd units	
Serum	School-age children	170-330 Todd units	
Base excess			
Whole blood	Newborn	(−10)-(−2) mmol/L	(−10)-(−2) mmol/L
	Infant	(−7)-(−1) mmol/L	(−7)-(−1) mmol/L
	Child	(−4)-(+2) mmol/L	(−4)-(+2) mmol/L
	Thereafter	(−3)-(+3) mmol/L	(−3)-(+3) mmol/L
Bicarbonate (HCO_3)			
Serum	Arterial	21-28 mmol/L	21-28 mmol/L
	Venous	22-29 mmol/L	22-29 mmol/L

Test/specimen	Age/sex/reference	Premature (mg/dL)	Full-term (mg/dL)	Premature (μmolL)	Full-term (μmolL)
Bilirubin, total					
Serum	Cord	<2.0	<2.0	<34	<34
	0-1 day	8.0	<6.0	<137	<103
	1-2 days	12.0	<8.0	<205	<137
	2-5 days	16.0	<12.0	<274	<205
	Thereafter	2.0	0.2-1.0	<34	3.4-17.1

Test/specimen	Age/sex/reference	Conventional units	International units
Bilirubin, direct (conjugated)			
Serum		0.0-0.2 mg/dL	0-3.4 μmol/L
Bleeding time			
Blood from skin puncture			
Ivy	Normal:	2-7 min	2-7 min
	Borderline:	7-11 min	7-11 min
Simplate (G-D)		2.75-8 min	2.75-8 min
Blood volume			
Whole blood	Male	52-83 mL/kg	0.052-0.083 L/kg
	Female	50-75 mL/kg	0.050-0.075 L/kg
C-reactive protein (CRP)			
Serum	Cord	10-350 ng/mL	10-350 μg/L
	Adult	68-8200 ng/mL	68-8200 μg/L
Calcium, ionized			
Serum, plasma, or whole blood	Cord	5.0-6.0 mg/dL	1.25-1.50 mmol/L
	Newborn	4.3-5.1 mg/dL	1.07-1.27 mmol/L
	24-48 hr	4.0-4.7 mg/dL	1.00-1.17 mmol/L
	Thereafter	4.48-4.92 mg/dL or 2.24-2.46 mEq/L	1.12-1.23 mmol/L

Modified from Behrman, R.E., and Vaughan, V.C., III, editors: Nelson textbook of pediatrics, ed. 13, Philadelphia. 1987, W.B. Saunders Co.

Test/specimen	Age/sex/reference	Conventional units	International units
		Normal ranges	
Calcium, total			
Serum	Cord	9.0-11.5 mg/dL	2.25-2.88 mmol/L
	Newborn, 3-24 hr	9.0-10.6 mg/dL	2.3-2.68 mmol/L
	24-48 hr	7.0-12.0 mg/dL	1.75-3.0 mmol/L
	4-7 d	9.0-10.9 mg/dL	2.25-2.73 mmol/L
	Child	8.8-10.8 mg/dL	2.2-2.70 mmol/L
	Thereafter	8.4-10.2 mg/dL	2.1-2.55 mmol/L
Urine (24 hr)	Ca free diet:	5-40 mg/d	0.13-1.0 mmol/d
	Low to average Ca in diet:	50-150 mg/d	1.25-3.8 mmol/d
	Average Ca in diet:	100-300 mg/d	2.5-7.5 mmol/d
CSF		4.2-5.4 mg/dL or 2.1-2.7 mEq/L	1.05-1.35 mmol/L
Feces	Average	0.64 g/d	16 mmol/d
Carbon dioxide, partial pressure (Pco_2)			
Whole blood, arterial	Newborn	27-40 mm Hg	3.6-5.3 kPa
	Infant	27-41 mm Hg	3.6-5.3 kPa
	Thereafter: Male	35-48 mm Hg	4.7-6.4 kPa
	Female	32-45 mm Hg	4.3-6.0 kPa
Carbon dioxide, total (tCO_2)			
Serum or plasma	Cord	14-22 mmol/L	14-22 mmol/L
	Premature (1 week)	14-27 mmol/L	14-27 mmol/L
	Newborn	13-22 mmol/L	13-22 mmol/L
	Infant	20-28 mmol/L	20-28 mmol/L
	Child	20-28 mmol/L	20-28 mmol/L
	Thereafter	23-30 mmol/L	23-30 mmol/L
Cerebrospinal fluid pressure			
CSF		70-180 mm water	70-180 mm water
Cerebrospinal fluid volume			
CSF	Child	60-100 mL	0.006-0.10 L
	Adult	100-160 mL	0.1-0.16 L
Chloride			
Serum or plasma	Cord	96-104 mmol/L	96-104 mmol/L
	Newborn	97-110 mmol/L	97-110 mmol/L
	Thereafter	98-106 mmol/L	98-106 mmol/L
CSF		118-132 mmol/L	118-132 mmol/L
Urine, 24 hr	Infant	2-10 mmol/d (diet-dependent)	2-10 mmol/d
	Child	15-40 mmol/d	15-40 mmol/d
	Thereafter	110-250 mmol/d (varies with Cl intake)	110-250 mmol/d
Sweat	Normal (homozygote)	0-35 mmol/L	0-35 mmol/L
	Marginal (e.g., asthma, Addison disease, malnutrition)	30-60 mmol/L	30-60 mmol/L
	Cystic fibrosis	60-200 mmol/L	60-200 mmol/L
*Cholesterol, total			
Serum or plasma	Cord	45-100 mg/dL	1.17-2.59 mmol/L
	Newborn	53-135 mg/dL	1.37-3.50 mmol/L
	Infant	70-175 mg/dL	1.81-4.53 mmol/L
	Child	120-200 mg/dL	3.11-5.18 mmol/L
	Adolescent	120-210 mg/dL	3.11-5.44 mmol/L

*Normal cholesterol values for children are not universally defined. The mean cholesterol levels for children ages 1 to 19 are reported as 160.9 mg/dl to 166.4 mg/dl (as cited in Resnicow, Morley-Kotchen, and Wynder, 1989). Cutoff values for determining risk for future coronary heart disease in children are inconsistent. The American Academy of Pediatrics (1989) recommends a cutoff value of 176 mg/dl (75th percentile) for children 0 to 19 years of age (See also p. 1591.)

Continued.

Common Laboratory Tests—cont'd

Test/specimen	Age/sex/reference	Conventional units	International units
		Normal ranges	
Clotting time (Lee-White)			
Whole blood		5-8 minutes (glass tubes)	5-8 min
		5-15 minutes (room temp)	5-15 min
		30 minutes (silicone tube)	30 min
Copper			
Serum	Birth-6 mo	20-70 μg/dL	3.14-10.99 μmol/L
	6 yr	90-190 μg/dL	14.13-29.83 μmol/L
	12 yr	80-160 μg/dL	12.56-25.12 μmol/L
	Adult: Male	70-140 μg/dL	10.99-21.98 μmol/L
	Female	80-155 μg/dL	12.56-24.34 μmol/L
Creatine kinase (CK, CPK)			
Serum	Newborn	68-580 U/L	68-580 U/L
	Adult: Male	12-70 U/L	12-70 U/L
	Female	10-55 U/L	10-55 U/L
	Ambulatory: Male	25-90 U/L	25-90 U/L
	Female	10-70 U/L	10-70 U/L
		Higher after exercise	Higher after exercise
Creatinine			
Serum	Cord	0.6-1.2 mg/dL	53-106 μmol/L
	Newborn	0.3-1.0 mg/dL	27-88 μmol/L
	Infant	0.2-0.4 mg/dL	18-35 μmol/L
	Child	0.3-0.7 mg/dL	27-62 μmol/L
	Adolescent	0.5-1.0 mg/dL	44-88 μmol/L
	Adult: Male	0.6-1.2 mg/dL	53-106 μmol/L
	Female	0.5-1.1 mg/dL	44-97 μmol/L
Urine, 24 hr	Infant	8-20 mg/kg/d	71-180 μmol/kg/d
	Child	8-22 mg/kg/d	71-195 μmol/kg/d
	Adolescent	8-30 mg/kg/d	71-265 μmol/kg/d
	Adult	14-26 mg/kg/d	124-230 μmol/kg/d
Creatinine clearance (endogenous)			
Serum or plasma and urine	Newborn	40-65 ml/min/1.73 m^2	
	<40 yr: Male	97-137 ml/min/1.73 m^2	
	Female	88-128 ml/min/1.73 m^2	
Digoxin			
Serum, plasma; collect at least 12 hr after dose	Therap. conc.		
	CHF	0.8-1.5 ng/ml	1.0-1.9 nmol/L
	Arrhythmias:	1.5-2.0 ng/ml	1.9-2.6 nmol/L
	Toxic conc.		
	Child	>2.5 ng/mL	>3.2 nmol/L
	Adult	>3.0 ng/mL	>3.8 nmol/L
Eosinophil count			
Whole blood, capillary blood		50-350 cells/mm^3 (μL)	50-350 $\times 10^6$ cells/L
Erythrocyte (RBC) count			
Whole blood	cord	3.9-5.5 million/mm^3	3.9-5.5 $\times 10^{12}$ cells/L
	1-3 d	4.0-6.6 million/mm^3	4.0-6.6 $\times 10^{12}$ cells/L
	1 wk	3.9-6.3 million/mm^3	3.9-6.3 $\times 10^{12}$ cells/L
	2 wk	3.6-6.2 million/mm^3	3.6-6.2 $\times 10^{12}$ cells/L
	1 mo	3.0-5.4 million/mm^3	3.0-5.4 $\times 10^{12}$ cells/L
	2 mo	2.7-4.9 million/mm^3	2.7-4.5 $\times 10^{12}$ cells/L
	3-6 mo	3.1-4.5 million/mm^3	3.1-4.5 $\times 10^{12}$ cells/L
	0.5-2 yr	3.7-5.3 million/mm^3	3.7-5.3 $\times 10^{12}$ cells/L
	2-6 yr	3.9-5.3 million/mm^3	3.9-5.3 $\times 10^{12}$ cells/L
	6-12 yr	4.0-5.2 million/mm^3	4.0-5.2 $\times 10^{12}$ cells/L
	12-18 yr: Male	4.5-5.3 million/mm^3	4.5-5.3 $\times 10^{12}$ cells/L
	Female	4.1-5.1 million/mm^3	4.1-5.1 $\times 10^{12}$ cells/L

Test/specimen	Age/sex/reference	Conventional units		International units	
		Normal ranges			
Erythrocyte sedimentation rate (ESR)					
Whole blood					
Westergren (modified)	Child	0-10 mm/hr		0-10 mm/hr	
	<50 yr: Male	0-15 mm/hr		0-15 mm/hr	
	Female	0-20 mm/hr		0-20 mm/hr	
Wintrobe	Child	0-13 mm/hr		0-13 mm/hr	
	Adult: Male	0-9 mm/hr		0-9 mm/hr	
	Female	0-20 mm/hr		0-20 mm/hr	
ZETA		41-54%		41-54 AU	
Fat, fecal					
Feces (72 hr)	Infant, breast-fed	<1 g/d		<1 g/d	
	0-6 yr	<2 g/d		<2 g/d	
	Adult	<7 g/d		<7 g/d	
Fatty acids, free					
Serum or plasma	Adults	8-25 mg/dL		0.30-0.90 mmol/L	
	Children and obese adults	<31 mg/dL		<1.10 mmol/L	
Fibrinogen					
Plasma	Newborn	125-300 mg/dL		1.25-3.00 g/L	
	Thereafter	200-400 mg/dL		2.00-4.00 g/L	
Galactose					
Serum	Newborn	0-20 mg/dL		0-1.11 mmol/L	
	Thereafter	<5 mg/dL		<0.28 mmol/L	
Urine	Newborn	≤60 mg/dL		≤3.33 mmol/L	
	Thereafter	<14 mg/dL		<0.08 mmol/L	
Glucose					
Serum	Cord	45-96 mg/dL		2.5-5.3 mmol/L	
	Premature	20-60 mg/dL		1.1-3.3 mmol/L	
	Neonate	30-60 mg/dL		1.7-3.3 mmol/L	
	Newborn, 1 d	40-60 mg/dL		2.2-3.3 mmol/L	
	Newborn, >1 d	50-90 mg/dL		2.8-5.0 mmol/L	
	Child	60-100 mg/dL		3.3-5.5 mmol/L	
	Thereafter	70-105 mg/dL		3.9-5.8 mmol/L	
Whole blood	Adult	65-95 mg/dL		3.6-5.3 mmol/L	
CSF	Adult	40-70 mg/dL		2.2-3.9 mmol/L	
Urine (quantitative)		<0.5 g/d		<2.8 mmol/d	
(Qualitative)		Negative		Negative	
Glucose tolerance test (GTT), oral					
Serum					
Dosages		**Normal**	**Diabetic**	**Normal**	**Diabetic**
Adult: 75 g	Fasting	70-105 mg/dL	>115 mg/dL	3.9-5.8 mmol/L	>6.4 mmol/L
Child: 1.75 g/kg of ideal weight up to maximum of 75 g	60 min	120-170 mg/dL	≥200 mg/dL	6.7-9.4 mmol/L	≥11 mmol/L
	90 min	100-140 mg/dL	≥200 mg/dL	5.6-7.8 mmol/L	≥11 mmol/L
	120 min	70-120 mg/dL	≥140 mg/dL	3.9-6.7 mmol/L	≥7.8 mmol/L
Growth hormone (hGH, Somatotropin)					
Plasma	Cord	10-50 ng/mL		10-50 μg/L	
Fasting, at rest	Newborn	10-40 ng/mL		10-40 μg/L	
	Child	<5 ng/mL		<5 μg/L	
	Adult: Male	<5 ng/mL		<5 μg/L	
	Female	<8 ng/mL		<8 μg/L	

Continued.

Common Laboratory Tests—cont'd

Test/specimen	Age/sex/reference	Conventional units	International units
		Normal ranges	
Hematocrit (HCT, Hct)			
Whole blood	1 d (cap)	48-69%	0.48-0.69 vol. fraction
	2 d	48-75%	0.48-0.75 vol. fraction
	3 d	44-72%	0.44-0.72 vol. fraction
	2 mo	28-42%	0.28-0.42 vol. fraction
	6-12 yr	35-45%	0.35-0.45 vol. fraction
	12-18 yr: Male	37-49%	0.37-0.49 vol. fraction
	Female	36-46%	0.36-0.46 vol. fraction
Hemoglobin (Hb)			
Whole blood	1-3 d (cap)	14.5-22.5 g/dL	2.25-3.49 mmol/L
	2 mo	9.0-14.0 g/dL	1.40-2.17 mmol/L
	6-12 yr	11.5-15.5 g/dL	1.78-2.40 mmol/L
	12-18 yr: Male	13.0-16.0 g/dL	2.02-2.48 mmol/L
	Female	12.0-16.0 g/dL	1.86-2.48 mmol/L
Hemoglobin A			
Whole blood		>95% of total	0.95 fraction of Hb
Hemoglobin F			
Whole blood	1 d	63-92% HbF	0.62-0.92 mass fraction HbF
	5 d	65-88% HbF	0.65-0.88 mass fraction HbF
	3 wk	55-85% HbF	0.55-0.85 mass fraction HbF
	6-9 wk	31-75% HbF	0.31-0.75 mass fraction HbF
	3-4 mo	<2-59% HbF	<0.02-0.59 mass fraction HbF
	6 mo	<2-9% HbF	<0.02-0.09 mass fraction HbF
	Adult	<2.0% HbF	<0.02 mass fraction HbF
Immunoglobulin A (IgA)			
Serum	Cord	0-5 mg/dL	0-50 mg/L
	Newborn	0-2.2 mg/dL	0-22 mg/L
	½-6 mo	3-82 mg/dL	30-820 mg/L
	6 mo-2 yr	14-108 mg/dL	140-1080 mg/L
	2-6 yr	23-190 mg/dL	230-1900 mg/L
	6-12 yr	29-270 mg/dL	290-2700 mg/L
	12-16 yr	81-232 mg/dL	810-2320 mg/L
	Thereafter	60-380 mg/dL	600-3800 mg/L
Immunoglobulin D (IgD)			
Serum	Newborn	None detected	None detected
	Thereafter	0-8 mg/dL	0-0.44 μmol/L
Immunoglobulin E (IgE)			
Serum	Male	0-230 IU/mL	0-230 k/U/L
	Female	0-170 IU/mL	0-170 k/U/L
Immunoglobulin G (IgG)			
Serum	Cord	760-1700 mg/dL	7.6-17 g/L
	Newborn	700-1480 mg/dL	7-14.8 g/L
	½-6 mo	300-1000 mg/dL	3-10 g/L
	6 mo-2 yr	500-1200 mg/dL	5-12 g/L
	2-6 yr	500-1300 mg/dL	5-13 g/L
	6-12 yr	700-1650 mg/dL	7-16.5 g/L
	12-16 yr	700-1550 mg/dL	7-15.5 g/L
	Adults	600-1600 mg/dL (higher in blacks)	6-16 g/L
Immunoglobulin M (IgM)			
Serum	Cord	4-24 mg/dL	40-240 mg/L
	Newborn	5-30 mg/dL	50-300 mg/L
	½-6 mo	15-109 mg/dL	150-1090 mg/L
	6 mo-2 yr	43-239 mg/dL	430-2390 mg/L
	2-6 yr	50-199 mg/dL	500-1990 mg/L
	6-12 yr	50-260 mg/dL	500-2600 mg/L
	12-16 yr	45-240 mg/dL	450-2400 mg/L
	Thereafter	40-345 mg/dL	400-3450 mg/L

Test/specimen	Age/sex/reference	Conventional units	International units
		Normal ranges	
Iron			
Serum	Newborn	100-250 μg/dL	17.90-44.75 μmol/L
	Infant	40-100 μg/dL	7.16-17.90 μmol/L
	Child	50-120 μg/dL	8.95-21.48 μmol/L
	Thereafter, Male	50-160 μg/dL	8.95-28.64 μmol/L
	Female	40-150 μg/dL	7.16-26.85 μmol/L
	Intoxicated child	280-2550 μg/dL	50.12-456.5 μmol/L
	Fatally poisoned child	>1800 μg/dL	>322.2 μmol/L
Iron-binding capacity, total (TIBC)			
Serum	Infant	100-400 μg/dL	17.90-71.60 μmol/L
	Thereafter	250-400 μg/dL	44.75-71.60 μmol/L
Lead			
Whole blood	Child	<25 μg/dL	<1.21 μmol/L
	Adult	<40 μg/dL	<1.93 μmol/L
	Acceptable for industrial exposure	<60 μg/dL	<2.90 μmol/L
	Toxic	≥100 μg/dL	≤4.83 μmol/L
Urine, 24 hr		<80 μg/L	<0.39 μmol/L
Leukocyte count (WBC count)		**×1000 cells/mm³ (μL)**	**×10⁹ cells/L**
Whole blood	Birth	9.0-30.0	9.0-30.0
	24 hr	9.4-34.0	9.4-34.0
	1 mo	5.0-19.5	5.0-19.5
	1-3 yr	6.0-17.5	6.0-17.5
	4-7 yr	5.5-15.5	5.5-15.5
	8-13 yr	4.5-13.5	4.5-13.5
	Adult	4.5-11.0	4.5-11.0
		×1000 cells/mm³ (μL)	**×10⁶ cells/L**
CSF	Premature	0-25 mononuclear	0-25
		0-100 polymorphonuclear	0-100
		0-1000 RBC	0-1000
	Newborn	0-20 mononuclear	0-20
		0-70 polymorphonuclear	0-70
		0-800 RBC	0-800
	Neonate	0-5 mononuclear	0-5
		0-25 polymorphonuclear	0-25
		0-50 RBC	0-50
	Thereafter	0-5 mononuclear	0-5

Test/specimen	Age/sex/reference	Conventional units (%)	Conventional units (cells)	International units
Leukocyte differential count				
Whole blood	Myelocytes	0%	0 Cells/mm³ (μL)	number fraction 0
	Neutrophils—"bands"	3-5%	150-400 Cells/mm³ (μL)	number fraction 0.03-0.05
	Neutrophils—"segs"	54-62%	3000-5800 Cells/mm³ (μL)	number fraction 0.54-0.62
	Lymphocytes	25-33%	1500-3000 Cells/mm³ (μL)	number fraction 0.25-0.33
	Monocytes	3-7%	285-500 Cells/mm³ (μL)	number fraction 0.03-0.07
	Eosinophils	1-3%	50-250 Cells/mm³ (μL)	number fraction 0.01-0.03
	Basophils	0-0.75%	15-50 Cells/mm³ (μL)	number fraction 0-0.0075

Continued.

Common Laboratory Tests—cont'd

Test/specimen	Age/sex/reference	Conventional units (Normal ranges)	International units (Normal ranges)
Mean corpuscular hemoglobin (MCH)			
Whole blood	Birth	31-37 pg/cell	0.48-0.57 fmol/L
	1-3 d (cap)	31-37 pg/cell	0.48-0.57 fmol/L
	1 wk-1 mo	28-40 pg/cell	0.43-0.62 fmol/L
	2 mo	26-34 pg/cell	0.40-0.53 fmol/L
	3-6 mo	25-35 pg/cell	0.39-0.54 fmol/L
	0.5-2 yr	23-31 pg/cell	0.36-0.48 fmol/L
	2-6 yr	24-30 pg/cell	0.37-0.47 fmol/L
	6-12 yr	25-33 pg/cell	0.39-0.51 fmol/L
	12-18 yr	25-35 pg/cell	0.39-0.54 fmol/L
	18-49 yr	26-34 pg/cell	0.40-0.53 fmol/L
Mean corpuscular hemoglobin concentration (MCHC)			
Whole blood	Birth	30-36% Hb/cell or g Hb/dL RBC	4.65-5.58 mmol or Hb/L RBC
	1-3 d (cap)	29-37% Hb/cell or g Hb/dL RBC	4.50-5.74 mmol or Hb/L RBC
	1-2 wk	28-38% Hb/cell or g Hb/dL RBC	4.34-5.89 mmol or Hb/L RBC
	1-2 mo	29-37% Hb/cell or g Hb/dL RBC	4.50-5.74 mmol or Hb/L RBC
	3 mo-2 yr	30-36% Hb/cell or g Hb/dL RBC	4.65-5.58 mmol or Hb/L RBC
	2-18 yr	31-37% Hb/cell or g Hb/dL RBC	4.81-5.74 mmol or Hb/L RBC
	>18 yr	31-37% Hb/cell or g Hb/dL RBC	4.81-5.74 mmol or Hb/L RBC
Mean corpuscular volume (MCV)			
Whole blood	1-3 d (cap)	95-121 μm^3	95-121 fL
	0.5-2 yr	70-86 μm^3	70-86 fL
	6-12 yr	77-95 μm^3	77-95 fL
	12-18 yr: Male	78-98 μm^3	78-98 fL
	Female	78-102 μm^3	78-102 fL
Osmolality			
Serum	Child, adult:	275-295 mOsmol/kg H_2O	
Urine, random		50-1400 mOsmol/kg H_2O, depending on fluid intake. After 12 hr fluid restriction: >850 mOsmol/kg H_2O	
Urine, 24 hr		≃300-900 mOsmol/kg H_2O	
Oxygen, partial pressure (pO_2)			
Whole blood, arterial	Birth	8-24 mm Hg	1.1-3.2 kPa
	5-10 min	33-75 mm Hg	4.4-10.0 kPa
	30 min	31-85 mm Hg	4.1-11.3 kPa
	>1 hr	55-80 mm Hg	7.3-10.6 kPa
	1 d	54-95 mm Hg	7.2-12.6 kPa
	Thereafter (decreased with age)	83-108 mm Hg	11-14.4 kPa
Oxygen saturation			
Whole blood, arterial	Newborn	40-90%	Fraction saturated 0.40-0.90
	Thereafter	95-99%	Fraction saturated 0.95-0.99
Partial thromboplastin time (PTT)			
Whole blood (Na citrate)			
Nonactivated		60-85 s (Platelin)	60-85 s
Activated		25-35 s (differs with method)	25-35 s

Test/specimen	Age/sex/reference	Conventional units	International units
		Normal ranges	
pH			H^+ concentration:
Whole blood, arterial	Premature (48 hr)	7.35-7.50	31-40 nmol/L
	Birth, full term	7.11-7.36	43-77 nmol/L
	5-10 min	7.09-7.30	50-81 nmol/L
	30 min	7.21-7.38	41-61 nmol/L
	>1 hr	7.26-7.49	32-54 nmol/L
	1 d	7.29-7.45	35-51 nmol/L
	Thereafter	7.35-7.45	35-44 nmol/L
	Must be corrected for body temperature		
Urine, random	Newborn/neonate	5-7	0.1-10 μmol/L
	Thereafter	4.5-8	0.01-32 μmol/L
	(average ≃6)		(average ≃1.0 μmol/L)
Stool		7.0-7.5	31-100 nmol/L
Phenylalanine			
Serum	Premature	2.0-7.5 mg/dL	0.12-0.45 mmol/L
	Newborn	1.2-3.4 mg/dL	0.07-0.21 mmol/L
	Thereafter	0.8-1.8 mg/dL	0.05-0.11 mmol/L
Urine, 24 hr	10 d-2 wk	1-2 mg/d	6-12 μmol/d
	3-12 yr	4-18 mg/d	24-110 μmol/d
	Thereafter	trace-17 mg/d	trace-103 μmol/d
Plasma volume			
Plasma	Male	25-43 mL/kg	0.025-0.043 L/kg
	Female	28-45 mL/kg	0.028-0.045 L/kg
Platelet count (thrombocyte count)			
Whole blood (EDTA)	Newborn	84-478 × 10^3/mm^3 (μL)	84-478 × 10^9/L
	(After 1 wk, same as adult)		
	Adult	150-400 × 10^3/mm^3 (μL)	150-400 × 10^9/L
Potassium			
Serum	Newborn	3.9-5.9 mmol/L	3.9-5.9 mmol/L
	Infant	4.1-5.3 mmol/L	4.1-5.3 mmol/L
	Child	3.4-4.7 mmol/L	3.4-4.7 mmol/L
	Thereafter	3.5-5.1 mmol/L	3.5-5.1 mmol/L
Plasma (heparin)		3.4-4.5 mmol/L	
Urine, 24 hr		2.5-125 mmol/d varies with diet	
Protein			
Serum Total			
	Premature	4.3-7.6 g/dL	43.0-76.0 g/L
	Newborn	4.6-7.4 g/dL	46.0-74.0 g/L
	Child	6.2-8.0 g/dL	62.0-80.0 g/L
Electrophoresis			
Albumin	Premature	3.0-4.2 g/dL	30-42 g/L
	Newborn	3.6-5.4 g/dL	36-54 g/L
	Infant	4.0-5.0 g/dL	40-50 g/L
	Thereafter	3.5-5.0 g/dL	35-50 g/L
α_1-Globulin	Premature	0.1-0.5 g/dL	1-5 g/L
	Newborn	0.1-0.3 g/dL	1-3 g/L
	Infant	0.2-0.4 g/dL	2-4 g/L
	Thereafter	0.2-0.3 g/dL	2-3 g/L
α_2-Globulin	Premature	0.3-0.7 g/dL	3-7 g/L
	Newborn	0.3-0.5 g/dL	3-5 g/L
	Infant	0.5-0.8 g/dL	5-8 g/L
	Thereafter	0.4-1.0 g/dL	4-10 g/L

Continued.

Common Laboratory Tests—cont'd

Test/specimen	Age/sex/reference	Conventional units	International units
		Normal ranges	
β-Globulin	Premature	0.3-1.2 g/dL	3-12 g/L
	Newborn	0.2-0.6 g/dL	2-6 g/L
	Infant	0.5-0.8 g/dL	5-8 g/L
	Thereafter	0.5-1.1 g/dL	5-11 g/L
γ-Globulin	Premature	0.3-1.4 g/dL	3-14 g/L
	Newborn	0.2-1.0 g/dL	2-10 g/L
	Infant	0.3-1.2 g/dL	3-12 g/L
	Thereafter	0.7-1.2 g/dL	7-12 g/L
		Higher in blacks	Higher in blacks
Total			
Urine, 24 hr		1-14 mg/dL	10-140 mg/L
		50-80 mg/d (at rest)	50-80 mg/L
		<250 mg/d after intense exercise	<250 mg/L after exercise
Total			
CSF		Lumbar: 8-32 mg/dL	80-320 mg/L
Prothrombin time (PT)			
One-stage (Quick)			
Whole blood (Na citrate)	In general	11-15 s (varies with type of thromboplastin)	11-15 s
	Newborn	Prolonged by 2-3 sec	Prolonged by 2-3 sec
Two-stage modified (Ware and Seegers)			
Whole blood (Na citrate)		18-22 sec	18-22 sec
RBC count, see erythrocyte count			
Red cell volume			
Whole blood	Male	20-36 mL/kg	0.020-0.036 L/kg
	Female	19-31 mL/kg	0.019-0.031 L/kg
Reticulocyte count			
Whole blood	Adults	0.5-1.5% of erythrocytes or 25,000-75,000/mm^3 (μL)	0.005-0.015 (number fraction) 25,000-75,000 × 10^6/L
Capillary	1 d	0.4-6.0%	0.004-0.060 (number fraction)
	7 d	<0.1-1.3%	<0.001-0.013 (number fraction)
	1-4 wk	<0.1-1.2%	<0.001-0.012 (number fraction)
	5-6 wk	<0.1-2.4	<0.001-0.024 (number fraction)
	7-8 wk	0.1-2.9%	0.001-0.029 (number fraction)
	9-10 wk	<0.1-2.6%	<0.001-0.026 (number fraction)
	11-12 wk	0.1-1.3%	0.001-0.013 (number fraction)
Salicylates			
Serum, plasma	Therap. conc.:	15-30 mg/dL	1.1-2.2 mmol/L
	Toxic conc.:	>30 mg/dL	>2.2 mmol/L
Sedimentation rate, see erythrocyte sedimentation rate			
Sodium			
Serum or plasma	Newborn	136-146 mmol/L	134-146 mmol/L
	Infant	139-146 mmol/L	139-146 mmol/L
	Child	138-145 mmol/L	138-145 mmol/L
	Thereafter	136-146 mmol/L	136-146 mmol/L
Urine, 24 hr		40-220 mmol/L (diet dependent)	40-220 mmol/L
Sweat		10-40 mmol/L	10-40 mmol/L
	Cystic fibrosis	>70 mmol/L	>70 mmol/L

Test/specimen	Age/sex/reference	Conventional units	International units
		Normal ranges	
Specific gravity			
Urine, random	Adult	1.002-1.030 >1.025	1.002-1.030 >1.025
Urine, 24 h	After 12 hr fluid restriction	1.015-1.025	
Theophylline			
Serum, plasma	Therap. conc.		
	Bronchodilator	8-20 μg/mL	44-110 μmol/L
	Prem. apnea	6-13 μg/mL	33-72 μmol/L
	Toxic conc.	>20	>110 μmol/L
Thrombin time			
Whole blood (Na citrate)		Control time ± 2 sec when control is 9-13 sec	Control time ± 2 sec when control is 9-13 sec
Thyroxine, total (T_4)			
Serum	Cord	8-13 μg/dL	103-168 nmol/L
	Newborn	11.5-24 (lower in low birth weight infants)	148-310 nmol/L
	Neonate	9-18 μg/dL	116-232 nmol/L
	Infant	7-15 μg/dL	90-194 nmol/L
	1-5 yr	7.3-15 μg/dL	94-194 nmol/L
	5-10 yr	6.4-13.3 μg/dL	83-172 nmol/L
	Thereafter	5-12 μg/dL	65-155 nmol/L
	Newborn screen (filter paper)	6.2-22 μg/dL	80-284 nmol/L
Tourniquet test (capillary fragility)		<5-10 petechiae in 2.5 cm circle on forearm (halfway between systolic and diastolic pressure for 5 min); 0-8 petechiae in 6 cm circle (50 torr for 15 min); 10-20 petechiae in 5 cm circle (80 mm Hg)	<5-10 petechiae in 2.5 cm circle on forearm (halfway between systolic and diastolic pressure for 5 min); 0-8 petechiae in 6 cm circle (50 torr for 15 min); 10-20 petechiae in 5 cm circle (80 mm Hg)

Test/specimen	Age/sex/reference	mg/dL M	mg/dL F	g/L M	g/L F
Triglycerides (TG)					
Serum, after ≥12 hr fast					
	Cord blood	10-98	10-98	0.10-0.98	0.10-0.98
	0-5 yr	30-86	32-99	0.30-0.86	0.32-0.99
	6-11 yr	31-108	35-114	0.31-1.08	0.35-1.14
	12-15 yr	36-138	41-138	0.36-1.38	0.41-1.38
	16-19 yr	40-163	40-128	0.40-1.63	0.40-1.28

Test/specimen	Age/sex/reference	Conventional units	International units
Triiodothyronine, free			
Serum	Cord	20-240 pg/dL	0.3-3.7 pmol/L
	1-3 d	200-610 pg/dL	3.1-9.4 pmol/L
	6 wk	240-560 pg/dL	3.7-8.6 pmol/L
	Adults (20-50 yr)	230-660 pg/dL	3.5-10.0 pmol/L
Triiodothyronine, total (T_3-RIA)			
Serum	Cord	30-70 ng/dL	0.46-1.08 nmol/L
	Newborn	72-260 ng/dL	1.16-4.00 nmol/L
	1-5 yr	100-260 ng/dL	1.54-4.00 nmol/L
	5-10 yr	90-240 ng/dL	1.39-3.70 nmol/L
	10-15 yr	80-210 ng/dL	1.23-3.23 nmol/L
	Thereafter	115-190 ng/dL	1.77-2.93 nmol/L

Continued.

Common Laboratory Tests—cont'd

Test/specimen	Age/sex/reference	Conventional units	International units
		Normal ranges	
Urea nitrogen			
Serum or plasma	Cord	21-40 mg/dL	7.5-14.3 mmol urea/L
	Premature (1 wk)	3-25 mg/dL	1.1-9 mmol urea/L
	Newborn	3-12 mg/dL	1.1-4.3 mmol urea/L
	Infant/Child	5-18 mg/dL	1.8-6.4 mmol urea/L
	Thereafter	7-18 mg/dL	2.5-6.4 mmol urea/L
Uric acid (serum)	Newborn	2.0-6.2 mg/dL	119-369 µmol/L
Phosphotungstate	Adult: Male	4.5-8.2 mg/dL	268-488 µmol/L
	Female	3.0-6.5 mg/dL	178-387 µmol/L
Uricase	Child	2.0-5.5 mg/dL	119-327 µmol/L
	Adult: Male	3.5-7.2 mg/dL	208-428 µmol/L
	Female	2.6-6.0 mg/dL	155-357 µmol/L
Urine volume			
Urine, 24 hr	Newborn	50-300 mL/d	0.050-0.300 L/d
	Infant	350-550 mL/d	0.350-0.500 L/d
	Child	500-1000 mL/d	0.500-1.000 L/d
	Adolescent	700-1400 mL/d	0.700-1.400 L/d
	Thereafter: Male	800-1800 mL/d	0.800-1.800 L/d
	Female	600-1600 mL/d (varies with intake and other factors)	0.600-1.600 L/d
WBC, see Leukocyte			

REFERENCES

American Academy of Pediatrics, Committee on Nutrition: Indications for cholesterol testing in children, Pediatrics 83(1):141-142, 1989.

Resnicow, K., Morley-Kotchen, J., and Wynder, E.: Plasma cholesterol levels of 6585 children in the United States: results of the Know Your Body screening in five states, Pediatrics 84(6):969-976, 1989.

APPENDIX E

Resources for Families and Health Care Professionals

GENERAL RESOURCES: CHILD HEALTH AND SPECIAL SERVICES*

American Academy of Pediatrics
Publications Department
P.O. Box 927
141 Northwest Point Blvd.
Elk Grove Village, IL 60007
(708) 228-5005
(800) 433-9016
(800) 421-0589

American Dietetic Association
216 W. Jackson Blvd., Suite 800
Chicago, IL 60606
(312) 899-0040

American Hospital Association
840 N. Lake Shore Drive
Chicago, IL 60611
(312) 280-6000

Association of Birth Defects in Children
3526 Emerywood Lane
Orlando, FL 32812
(407) 859-2821

Association for the Care of Children's Health
7910 Woodmont Ave., Suite 300
Bethesda, MD 20814
(301) 654-6549

Association for Neuro-Metabolic Disorders
5223 Brookfield Lane
Sylvania, OH 43560
(419) 885-1497

Boys Town
Communications and Public Service Division
Father Flanagan's Boys' Home
Boys Town, NE 68010
(402) 498-1111
(800) 448-3000 (hotline)

Canadian Institute of Child Health
17 York St., Suite 105
Ottawa, Ontario K1N 557
(613) 238-8425

Cancer Information Services
National Cancer Institute
Office of Cancer Communications
Building 31, Room 10A-24
9000 Rockville Pike
Bethesda, MD 20892
(301) 496-5583
(800) 4-CANCER (hotline)

Centering Corporation
P.O. Box 3367
Omaha, NE 68103-0367
(402) 553-1200

Children's Defense Fund
122 'C' St., N.W., Suite 400
Washington, DC 20001
(202) 628-8787

Child and Youth Services Administration
1120 19th St., N.W., Suite 700
Washington, DC 20036
(202) 673-7783

Child Welfare League of America
440 First St., N.W., Suite 310
Washington, DC 20001
(202) 638-2952

Federation for Children with Special Needs, Inc.
95 Berkeley St., Suite 104
Boston, MA 02116
(617) 482-2915

Government Printing Office
Superintendent of Documents
Washington, DC 20402-9325
(202) 275-3050

Human Resource Center
201 I.U. Willets Rd.
Albertson, NY 11507
(516) 747-5400

March of Dimes Birth Defects Foundation
1275 Mamaroneck Ave.
White Plains, NY 10605
(914) 428-7100

Mead Johnson
Nutritional Division
2400 W. Lloyd Expressway
Evansville, IN 47721
(812) 429-5000

Medic-Alert Foundation International
P.O. Box 1009
Turlock, CA 95381
(209) 668-3333
(800) 344-3226

National Center for Education in Maternal and Child Health
38th and 'R' Streets, N.W.
Washington, DC 20057
(202) 625-8400

*Organizations serving the needs of children and families with specific disorders are listed as appropriate throughout text.

National Center for Health Statistics
Department of Health and Human Services
Public Health Services
3700 East-West Highway, Room 157
Hyattsville, MD 20782
(301) 436-8500

National Dairy Council
6300 N. River Rd.
Rosemont, IL 60018-4233
(708) 696-1020

National Easter Seal Society for Crippled Children
70 E. Lake St.
Chicago, IL 60612
(312) 726-6200
(312) 726-4258 (TDD)
(800) 221-6827

National Foundation for Jewish Genetic Diseases, Inc.
250 Park Ave., Suite 1000
New York, NY 10177
(212) 371-1030

National Heart, Lung and Blood Institute
National Institutes of Health
9000 Rockville Pike
Building 31, Room 4A21
Bethesda, MD 20892
(301) 496-4236

National Information Center for Children and Youth with Handicaps (NICHCY)
P.O. Box 1492
Washington, DC 20013
(703) 893-6061 (Virginia telephone number)
(800) 999-5599

National Information System for Health Related Services
University of South Carolina
Benson Building
Columbia, SC 29208
(800) 922-9234

National Institutes of Child Health and Human Development
Building 31, Room 2A-32
9000 Rockville Pike
Bethesda, MD 20892
(301) 496-5133

National Institute of Marriage and Family Relations
6116 Rolling Rd., Suite 306
Springfield, VA 22152
(703) 569-2400

National Mental Health Association
1021 Prince St.
Alexandria, VA 22314
(703) 684-7722

National Rehabilitation Association
633 S. Washington St.
Alexandria, VA 22314
(703) 836-0850

National Safety Council
444 N. Michigan Ave.
Chicago, IL 60611
(312) 527-4800
(800) 621-7615

Pediatric Projects
P.O. Box 571555
Tarzana, CA 91357
(818) 705-3660

"Plain Talk" and "Caring About Kids" Series
U.S. Department of Health and Human Services
Public Health Service
Alcohol, Drug Abuse, and Mental Health Association
5600 Fishers Lane
Rockville, MD 20857
(301) 443-3875

Public Affairs Information Services
521 W. 43rd St., 5th Floor
New York, NY 10036
(212) 736-6629

Ross Laboratories
Division Abbott Laboratories
Creative Services and Information
625 Cleveland Ave.
Columbus, OH 43215
(614) 227-3333

Sarah K. Davidson Family–Patient Health Education Library
Strong Children's Medical Center
University of Rochester Medical Center
P.O. Box 777
601 Elmwood Ave.
Rochester, NY 14642
(716) 275-7129

SKIP (Sick Kids Need Involved People) of New York
990 2nd Ave.
New York, NY 10022
(212) 421-9161

Sudden Infant Death Syndrome National Headquarters
10500 Little Patuxen Parkway
Columbia, MD 21044
(301) 964-8000
(800) 221-SIDS

U.S. Consumer Product Safety Commission
5401 Westbard Ave.
Washington, DC 20207
(301) 492-5500
(800) 492-8104 (Maryland only)
(800) 638-CPSC (Outside Maryland)
(800) 638-8270 (TDD)

U.S. Department of Agriculture
Office of Public Information
Food and Nutrition Service
3101 Park Center Dr.
Alexandria, VA 22302
(703) 756-3276

Wyeth Laboratories
P.O. Box 8299
145 King of Prussia
Radnor, PA 19087
(215) 383-0600

NATIONAL CLEARINGHOUSES

Clearinghouse on Child Abuse and Neglect
P.O. Box 1182
Washington, DC 20013
(703) 821-2086 (Virginia telephone number)

Consumer Information Catalog
P.O. Box 100
Pueblo, CO 81009
(719) 948-3334

Food and Drug Administration
Office of Consumer Affairs
5600 Fishers Lane
Rockville, MD 20857
(301) 443-1544

High Blood Pressure Information Center
120/80 National Institutes of Health
Bethesda, MD 20892
(301) 496-2411

Human Nutrition Information Service
Department of Agriculture
6505 Belcrest Rd., Room 360
Hyattsville, MD 20782
(301) 436-7725

National Digestive Diseases Information Clearinghouse
Box NDDIC
Bethesda, MD 20892
(301) 468-6344

National Health Information Clearinghouse "Healthfinder"
ONHIC
P.O. Box 1133
Washington, DC 20013-1133
(301) 565-4167 (Maryland telephone number)
(800) 336-4797

National Highway Traffic Safety Administration
NES-11 HL
U.S. Department of Transportation
400 7th St., S.W.
Washington, DC 20590
(202) 366-9550

National Information System and Clearinghouse
University of South Carolina
Benson Building
Columbia, SC 29208
(800) 922-9234

National Institute of Mental Health
Public Inquiries Branch
Parklawn Building, Room 15C-05
5600 Fishers Lane
Rockville, MD 20857
(301) 443-4513

National Library Service for the Blind and Physically Handicapped
Library of Congress
1291 Taylor St., N.W.
Washington, DC 20542
(202) 707-5100

National Maternal and Child Health Clearinghouse
38th and 'R' Streets, N.W.
Washington, DC 20057
(202) 625-8400

National Rehabilitation Information Center
8455 Colesville Rd., Suite 935
Silver Spring, MD 20910-3319
(301) 588-9284
(800) 346-2742

National Self-Help Clearinghouse
33 W. 42nd St., Room 620N
New York, NY 10036
(212) 642-2944

National Technical Information Service
Agency of the Department of Commerce
5285 Port Royal Rd.
Springfield, VA 22161
(703) 487-4650

Self-Help Center
1600 Dodge Ave., Suite S-122
Evanston, IL 60201
(708) 328-0470

Sudden Infant Death Syndrome Clearinghouse
8201 Greensboro Dr., Suite 600
McLean, VA 22102
(703) 821-8955

APPENDIX F

NANDA-Approved Nursing Diagnoses

Activity intolerance
Activity intolerance, potential
Adjustment, impaired
Airway clearance, ineffective
Anxiety
Aspiration, potential for
Body image disturbance
Body temperature, altered, potential
Bowel incontinence
Breastfeeding, effective
Breastfeeding, ineffective
Breathing pattern, ineffective
Cardiac output, decreased
Communication, impaired verbal
Constipation
Constipation, colonic
Constipation, perceived
Coping, defensive
Coping, family: potential for growth
Coping, ineffective family: compromised
Coping, ineffective family: disabling
Coping, ineffective individual
Decisional conflict (specify)
Denial, ineffective
Diarrhea
Disuse syndrome, potential for
Diversional activity deficit
Dysreflexia
Family processes, altered
Fatigue
Fear
Fluid volume deficit (1)
Fluid volume deficit (2)
Fluid volume deficit, potential
Fluid volume excess
Gas exchange, impaired
Grieving, anticipatory
Grieving, dysfunctional
Growth and development, altered
Health maintenance, altered
Health-seeking behaviors (specify)
Home maintenance management, impaired
Hopelessness
Hyperthermia
Hypothermia
Incontinence, functional
Incontinence, reflex
Incontinence, stress
Incontinence, total
Incontinence, urge
Infection, potential for
Injury, potential for
Knowledge deficit (specify)
Mobility, impaired physical
Noncompliance (specify)
Nutrition, altered: less than body requirements
Nutrition, altered: more than body requirements
Nutrition, altered: potential for more than body requirements
Oral mucous membrane, altered
Pain
Pain, chronic
Parental role conflict
Parenting, altered
Parenting, altered, potential
Personal identity disturbance
Poisoning, potential for
Post-trauma response
Powerlessness
Protection, altered
Rape-trauma syndrome
Rape-trauma syndrome: compound reaction
Rape-trauma syndrome: silent reaction
Role performance, altered
Self-care deficit, bathing/hygiene
Self-care deficit, dressing/grooming
Self-care deficit, feeding
Self-care deficit, toileting
Self-esteem disturbance
Self-esteem, chronic low
Self-esteem, situational low
Sensory/perceptual alterations (specify) (visual, auditory, kinesthetic, gustatory, tactile, olfactory)
Sexual dysfunction
Sexuality patterns, altered
Skin integrity, impaired
Skin integrity, impaired, potential
Sleep pattern disturbance
Social interaction, impaired
Social isolation
Spiritual distress (distress of the human spirit)
Suffocation, potential for
Swallowing, impaired
Thermoregulation, ineffective
Thought processes, altered
Tissue integrity, impaired
Tissue perfusion, altered (specify type) (renal, cerebral, cardiopulmonary, gastrointestinal, peripheral)
Trauma, potential for
Unilateral neglect
Urinary elimination, altered patterns
Urinary retention
Violence, potential for: self-directed or directed at others

APPENDIX G

Recommendations for *Haemophilus Influenzae* Type B Conjugate Vaccines

On October 4, 1990, The U.S. Food and Drug Administration (FDA) approved one of the *Haemophilus influenzae* type b (Hib) conjugate vaccines, commonly referred to as HbOC, for use in infants beginning at 2 months of age. Because this announcement occurred near the time of publication for *Nursing Care of Infants and Children,* the section on Hib vaccines in Chapter 12 could not be changed to include these recommendations. Therefore, the statement that Hib should be administered at 15 months of age should be disregarded and replaced with the following recommendations. Additional developments in relation to Hib vaccines are expected, especially the possibility of other Hib conjugate vaccines (PRP-D and PRP-OMP) receiving FDA approval for use in infants. The reader is urged to be alert for such changes.

RECOMMENDATIONS*

1. All children should be immunized with an *H. influenzae* type b conjugate vaccine at 2 months of age or as soon as possible thereafter rather than at 15 months of age as previously recommended. Currently, only HbOC has been approved by the FDA for administration to children younger than 15 months of age.
2. For routine immunization beginning at 2 to 3 months of age, HbOC should be administered in a three-dose series with the doses given at approximately 2-month intervals. *H. influenzae* type b immunization may be given at the same time as DTP and OPV immunizations. HbOC should be given intramuscularly in a separate syringe and at a separate site from other immunizations.
3. Administration of a booster (fourth) dose is recommended at 15 months of age or as soon as possible thereafter. For this dose, any licensed conjugate vaccine, PRP-OMP, PRP-D, or HbOC, is acceptable. The *H. influenzae* type b conjugate vaccine and MMR can be administered simultaneously but should be given at separate sites with separate syringes. Because several injections are required to complete the routine childhood immunizations recommended at this age, some may choose to give these injections in more than one patient visit. In this situation, for patients who have not previously been immunized against measles, priority should be given to administration of MMR.
4. Immunization of children older than 2 months of age at the time of the first dose should be performed as follows:
   a. Unimmunized children between 3 and 6 months of age should receive a four-dose regimen. Optimally, the first three doses of HbOC should be given at 2-month intervals with a minimum of 1 month between doses. A fourth dose of any licensed conjugate vaccine should be given at 15 months of age or as soon as possible thereafter.
   b. Unimmunized infants 7 to 11 months of age should receive a three-dose regimen. Optimally, the first two doses of HbOC should be given at 2-month intervals with a minimum of 1 month between doses. A third dose of any licensed conjugate vaccine should be given at 15 months of age or as soon as possible thereafter.
   c. Unimmunized children 12 to 14 months of age should receive a two-dose regimen at an optimal interval of 2 months with a minimum of 1 month between doses. No additional doses are indicated for these children. In this situation, HbOC is given for the first dose. Any licensed conjugate vaccine is appropriate for the second dose.
   d. Unimmunized children 15 months of age or older who have not yet reached their fifth birthday (i.e., until 59 months of age) should receive one dose of any licensed conjugate vaccine.

Table G-1 Summary of Recommendations

AGE AT INITIATION OF IMMUNIZATION (MONTHS)	NUMBER OF DOSES TO BE ADMINISTERED	CURRENTLY RECOMMENDED *H. INFLUENZAE* TYPE B VACCINE REGIMEN
2-6	4	HbOC for initial three doses; HbOC, PRP-OMP, or PRP-D for fourth dose*
7-11	3	HbOC for initial two doses; HbOC, PRP-OMP, or PRP-D for third dose*
12-14	2	HbOC for first dose; HbOC, PRP-OMP, or PRP-D for second dose*
15-59	1	HbOC, PRP-OMP, or PRP-D*
60	1†	HbOC, PRP-OMP, or PRP-D*

*Safety and efficacy are likely to be equivalent for PRP-OMP (PedvaxHIB), PRP-D (ProHIBit), and HbOC (HibTITER) administered to children 15 months of age and older.
†Only indicated for children with chronic illness known to be associated with an increased risk for *H. influenzae* type b disease (see recommendation No. 5 on p. 1984).

*Reprinted with permission from *AAP News,* November 1990; 6(11). Copyright © 1990, American Academy of Pediatrics.
See Table G-1 for summary.

5. Unimmunized children 5 years of age or older with a chronic illness known to be associated with increased risk of *H. influenzae* type b disease should be given a single dose of any licensed conjugate vaccine. Examples include children with anatomic or functional asplenia or sickle cell anemia, or those who have undergone a splenectomy. Until further data are available, patients with Hodgkin disease should be immunized 10 to 14 days or more prior to the initiation of chemotherapy or, if this cannot be accomplished, 3 months or more after the cessation of chemotherapy. No known contraindications exist to simultaneous administration for *H. influenzae* type b vaccine with pneumococcal or meningococcal vaccine when they are given in separate syringes at different sites.
6. Unimmunized children who experience invasive *H. influenzae* type b disease when younger than 24 months of age should be subsequently immunized according to the age-appropriate recommendations. Children whose disease occurred at 24 months of age or older do not need immunization because the disease most likely induced immunity.

INDEX

C

D

E

I

J

K

N

O

P

Q

R

W

CONVERSION OF POUNDS TO KILOGRAMS FOR PEDIATRIC WEIGHTS*

POUNDS → ↓	0	1	2	3	4	5	6	7	8	9
0	0.00	0.45	0.90	1.36	1.81	2.26	2.72	3.17	3.62	4.08
10	4.53	4.98	5.44	5.89	6.35	6.80	7.35	7.71	8.16	8.61
20	9.07	9.52	9.97	10.43	10.88	11.34	11.79	12.24	12.70	13.15
30	13.60	14.06	14.51	14.96	15.42	15.87	16.32	16.78	17.23	17.69
40	18.14	18.59	19.05	19.50	19.95	20.41	20.86	21.31	21.77	22.22
50	22.68	23.13	23.58	24.04	24.49	24.94	25.40	25.85	26.30	26.76
60	27.21	27.66	28.22	28.57	29.03	29.48	29.93	30.39	30.84	31.29
70	31.75	32.20	32.65	33.11	33.56	34.02	34.47	34.92	35.38	35.83
80	36.28	36.74	37.19	37.64	38.10	38.55	39.00	39.46	39.93	40.37
90	40.82	41.27	41.73	42.18	42.63	43.09	43.54	43.99	44.45	44.90
100	45.36	45.81	46.26	46.72	47.17	47.62	48.08	48.53	48.98	49.44
110	49.89	50.34	50.80	51.25	51.71	52.16	52.61	53.07	53.52	53.97
120	54.43	54.88	55.33	55.79	56.24	56.70	57.15	57.60	58.06	58.51
130	58.96	59.42	59.87	60.32	60.78	61.23	61.68	62.14	62.59	63.05
140	63.50	63.95	64.41	64.86	65.31	65.77	66.22	66.67	67.13	67.58
150	68.04	68.49	68.94	69.40	69.85	70.30	70.76	71.21	71.66	72.12
160	72.57	73.02	73.48	73.93	74.39	74.84	75.29	75.75	76.20	76.65
170	77.11	77.56	78.01	78.47	78.92	79.38	79.83	80.28	80.74	81.19
180	81.64	82.10	82.55	83.00	83.46	83.91	84.36	84.82	85.27	85.73
190	86.18	86.68	87.09	87.54	87.99	88.45	88.90	89.35	89.81	90.26
200	90.72	91.17	91.62	92.08	92.53	92.98	93.44	93.89	94.34	94.80

*To obtain kilogram equivalent of 15 pounds, read 10 pounds on side scale, then 5 pounds on top scale. The kilogram equivalent is 6.80.

CONVERSION OF POUNDS AND OUNCES TO KILOGRAMS FOR PEDIATRIC WEIGHTS

POUNDS	KILOGRAMS	POUNDS	KILOGRAMS	OUNCES	KILOGRAMS	OUNCES	KILOGRAMS
1	0.454	9	4.082	1	0.028	9	0.255
2	0.907	10	4.536	2	0.057	10	0.283
3	1.361	11	4.990	3	0.085	11	0.312
4	1.814	12	5.443	4	0.113	12	0.340
5	2.268	13	5.897	5	0.142	13	0.369
6	2.722			6	0.170	14	0.397
7	3.175			7	0.198	15	0.425
8	3.629			8	0.227		

CONVERSION FACTORS FOR TEMPERATURE*

CELSIUS	FAHRENHEIT	CELSIUS	FAHRENHEIT	CELSIUS	FAHRENHEIT	CELSIUS	FAHRENHEIT
34.0	93.2	36.4	97.5	38.6	101.5	41.0	105.9
34.2	93.6	36.6	97.9	38.8	101.8	41.2	106.1
34.4	93.9	36.8	98.2	39.0	102.2	41.4	106.5
34.6	94.3	37.0	98.6	39.2	102.6	41.6	106.8
34.8	94.6	37.2	99.0	39.4	102.9	41.8	107.2
35.0	95.0	37.4	99.3	39.6	103.3	42.0	107.6
35.2	95.4	37.6	99.7	39.8	103.6	42.2	108.0
35.4	95.7	37.8	100.0	40.0	104.0	42.4	108.3
35.6	96.1	38.0	100.4	40.2	104.4	42.6	108.7
35.8	96.4	38.2	100.8	40.4	104.7	42.8	109.0
36.0	96.8	38.4	101.1	40.6	105.2	43.0	109.4
36.2	97.2			40.8	105.4		

*(°C × 9/5) + 32 = °F
(°F − 32) × 5/9 = °C

°C = Temperature in Celsius (centigrade) degrees
°F = Temperature in Fahrenheit degrees